DISEASES/CONDITIONS AND ICD-9-CM CODES

Abruptio placentae	641.2**
Acne vulgaris	706.1
Acromegaly	253.0
Actinic keratosis	702.0
Acute bronchitis	466.0
Acute and chronic viral hepatitis	070.9
Acute diarrhea (NOS)	787.91
Acute leukemia (plain leukemia)	208.0**
Acute myocardial infarction	410.9**
Acute otitis media	382.9
Acute pancreatitis	577.0
Acute peripheral facial paralysis (Bell's palsy)	351.0
Acute renal failure	584.9
Acute respiratory failure	518.81
Acute stress disorder	308.9
Adrenocortical insufficiency	255.4
Adverse reactions to blood transfusions	999
Alcoholism	303.9**
Allergic reactions to drugs	995.2
Allergic reactions to insect stings	989.5
Allergic rhinitis	477.8
Alopecia areata	704.01
Alzheimer's disease	331.0
Amebiasis	006.9
Amenorrhea	626.0
Anal fissure .	565.0
Anaphylaxis, NOS	995.0
Angina pectoris	413.9
Angioedema	995.1
Ankle fracture	824.8
Ankylosing spondylitis	720.0
Anorectal abscess	566.
Anorexia nervosa	307.1
Aortic aneurysm and dissection	441.00
Aplastic anemia	284.9
Asthma	493.9**
Atelectasis	518.0
Atopic dermatitis	691.8
Atopic fibrillation	427.31
Attention deficit/hyperactivity disorder	314.01
Autoimmune hemolytic anemia	283.0
Bacterial meningitis	320
Bacterial pneumonia	482.9
Bacterial vaginitis	616.1
Benign prostatic hyperplasia	600
Blastomycosis	116.0
Bleeding esophageal varices	456.0
Brain abscess	324.
Brain tumors	239.6
Breast cancer	174
Brucellosis	023
Bulimia nervosa	307.51
Bullous diseases	694
Burns	940-949
Bursitis	726-727
Cancer of the endometrium	182.0
Cancer of the skin	172-173
Cancer of the uterine cervix	180
Cardiac arrest, sudden cardiac death	427.5
Care after myocardial infarction	414.8
Cellulitis	682.
Chancroid	099.3
Chlamydia trachomatis infection	079.88
Cholelithiasis and cholecystitis	574.1-574.9
Cholera	001
Chronic fatigue syndrome	780.71
Chronic leukemia	208.1**
Chronic obstructive pulmonary disease	491.2**
Chronic pancreatitis	577.1
Chronic renal failure	585
Chronic serous otitis media	381.1**
Coccidioidomycosis	114*
Colorectal cancer	153
Concussion	850
Congenital heart disease	745-747
Congenital rubella	771.0
Congestive heart failure	428.0
Conjunctivitis, acute	372.0**
Connective tissue disease	710*
Constipation	564.0
Contact dermatitis	692
Cough	786.2
Cushing's syndrome	255.0
Delirium	780.0
Dementia, multi-infarct, uncomplicated	294.8
Depression psychosis	298.0
Depression with anxiety	300.4
Diabetes insipidus	253.5
Diabetes mellitus, I	250.01
Diabetes mellitus, II	250.02
Diabetic ketoacidosis	276.2**
Diphtheria	032*
Diseases of the mouth	528*
Disseminated intravascular coagulation	286.6
Diverticulitis	562.11
Drug abuse (nondependent)	305.9**
Dysfunctional uterine bleeding	626.6
Dysmenorrhea	635.5
Dysphagia and esophageal obstruction	530.3
Ectopic pregnancy	633*
Elbow dislocation	832.0**
Encephalitis	323*
Endometriosis	617*
Enuresis	786.30
Epididymitis	604**
Episodic vertigo	386.11
Erythema multiforme	695.1
Fetal lung immaturity	770.4
Fever	780.6
Fibrocystic diseases of the breast	610.1
Fibromyositis	729.1
Fifth disease	057.0
Finger dislocation, closed	834.0**
Finger fracture	816.0**
Fistula (anal)	565.1
Fitting of diaphragm	V25.02
Folliculitis	704.8
Food allergy	693.1
Food poisoning	005*
Foot fracture	825.2**
Frostbite	991*
Gangrene	785.4
Gastritis	535**
Gastroesophageal reflux disease (GERD)	530.81
Generalized anxiety disorder	300.02
Generalized epilepsy	345.1**
Genital warts (condylomata acuminata)	078.11
Giant cell arteritis	446.5
Giardiasis	7.1
Gilles de la Tourette syndrome	307.23
Glaucoma	365**
Gonorrhea	098.0
Gout	274.9
Granuloma inguinale (donovanosis)	099.2
Guillain-Barré syndrome	357.0
Headache	784.0
Heart block	426.1**
Heat exhaustion	992.3
Heat stroke	992.0
Hemochromatosis	285.0
Hemolytic disease of the fetus and newborn	773.2
Hemophilia and related conditions	286.0
Hemorrhoids	455.6
Herpes gestationis	646.8**
Herpes simplex	054*
Herpes zoster	053*
Hiccups	786.8
High-altitude sickness	993.2
Histoplasmosis	115**
HIV-associated infections	042.0
HIV infection, asymptomatic	V08
HIV infection, early symptomatic	042
HIV infection, late symptomatic	042
Hyperlipoproteinemias	272*
Hyperparathyroidism	252.0
Hyperprolactinemia	253.1
Hypersensitivity pneumonitis	495
Hypertension (essential)	401*
Hyperthyroidism	242**
Hypertrophic cardiomyopathy	425.4
Hypoparathyroidism	252.1
Hypothyroidism	244*
Immunization practices	V03, V04, V05, V06**
Impetigo	684
Impotence	302.72
Indigestion	536.8
Infectious diarrhea	009.2
Infectious mononucleosis	075
Infective endocarditis	424.9**
Influenza	487.2
Ingrowing nail	703.0
Insect and spider bite	989.5
Insertion of intrauterine device	V25.1
Insomnia (NOS)	780.52
Intracerebral hemorrhage	431
Iron deficiency anemia	280.0-280.9
Irritable bowel syndrome	564.1
Jellyfish sting	989.5

*4th digit needed
**5th (or 4th and 5th) digit needed

Juvenile rheumatoid arthritis	714.3**
Keloids	701.4
Laryngitis	464.00
Lead poisoning	984*
Legionnaires' disease	482.84
Leishmaniasis	085*
Leprosy	030*
Lichen planus	697.0
Low back pain	724.2
Lyme disease	088.81
Lymphogranuloma venereum	099.1
Malabsorption	579*
Malaria	084.6
Measles (rubeola)	055.9
Meconium aspiration	770.1
Melanoma, malignant	172*
Méniére's disease	386.0**
Meningitis	320-322
Menopausal	627.2
Migraine headache	346**
Mitral valve prolapse	424.0
Monilial vulvovaginitis	121.1
Multiple myeloma	203.0**
Multiple sclerosis	340
Mumps	072.9
Myasthenia gravis	358.0**
Mycoplasmal pneumonias	483.0
Mycosis fungoides	202.1**
Nausea and vomiting	787.01
Neoplasm of the vulva	239.5
Neutropenia	288.0
Nevi	216*
Newborn physiologic jaundice	774.6
Nongonococcal urethritis	099.4**
Non-Hodgkin's lymphomas	202.8**
Non-autoimmune hemolytic anemia	283.1**
Normal delivery	650
Obesity	278.0**
Obsessive-compulsive disorders	300.3
Onychomycosis	110.1
Optic neuritis	377.3**
Osteoarthritis	715**
Osteomyelitis	730**
Osteoporosis	733.00
Otitis externa	380.10
Paget's disease of bone	731.0
Panic disorder	300.01
Pap smear	V72.3
Parkinsonism	332.0
Paronychia	681.0**
Partial epilepsy	345.4**
Patent ductus arteriosus	747.0
Pediculosis	132*
Pelvic inflammatory disease	614*
Peptic ulcer disease	533*
Pericarditis	432.9
Peripheral arterial disease	443.9
Peripheral neuropathies	356*
Pernicious anemia	281.0
Personality disorder	301**
Pheochromocytoma	227.0
Phobia	300.2**
Pigmentary disorders—vitiligo	709.01
Pinworms	127.4
Pityriasis rosea	696.3
Placenta previa	641**
Plague	020*
Platelet-mediated bleeding disorders	287.1
Pleural effusion	511.9
Polycythemia vera	238.4
Polymyalgia rheumatica	725
Porphyria	277.1
Postpartum hemorrhage	666.1**
Post-traumatic stress disorder	309.81
Pregnancy	V22.2
Pregnancy-induced hypertension	642**
Premature beats	427.6**
Premenstrual tension syndrome (PMS)	625.4
Prescribed oral contraceptive	V25.01
Pressure ulcers	707.0
Preterm labor	644.2**
Primary glomerular disease	581-583
Primary lung abscess	513.0
Primary lung cancer	162.9
Prostate cancer	185
Prostatitis	601*
Pruritus	698.9
Pruritus ani	698.0
Pruritus vulvae	698.1
Psittacosis (ornithosis)	073*
Psoriasis	696.1
Pulmonary embolism	415.1
Pyelonephritis	590**
Q fever	083.0
Rabies	071
Rat-bite fever	026*
Relapsing fever	087*
Renal calculi	592
Reye syndrome	331.81
Rheumatic fever	390
Rheumatoid arthritis	714.0
Rib fracture	807.0**
Rocky Mountain spotted fever	082.0
Rosacea	695.3
Roseola	057.8
Rubella	056*
Salmonellosis	003.0
Sarcoidosis	135
Scabies	133.0
Schizophrenia	295**
Seborrheic dermatitis	690.1**
Septicemia	038*
Sezary's syndrome	202.2**
Shoulder dislocation	831.0**
Sickle cell anemia	282.6**
Silicosis	502
Sinusitis, chronic	473*
Skull fracture	800, 801, 803
Sleep apnea	780.57
Sleep disorders	780.50
Snakebite	989.5
Stasis ulcers	454.0
Status epilepticus	345.3
Stomach cancer	151*
Streptococcal pharyngitis	034.0
Stroke	436
Strongyloides infection	127.2
Subdural or subarachnoid hemorrhage	852**
Sunburn	692.71
Syphilis	090-097
Tachycardias	785.0
Tapeworm infections	123*
Telogen effluvium	704.02
Temporomandibular joint syndrome	524.6**
Tendonitis	726.90
Tetanus	037
Thalassemia	282.4**
Therapeutic use of blood components	V59.0**
Thrombotic thrombocytopenic purpura	446.6
Thyroid cancer	193
Thyroiditis	245*
Tinea capitis	110.0
Tinnitus	388.3**
Toe fracture	826.0
Toxic shock syndrome	040.82
Toxoplasmosis	130*
Transient cerebral ischemia	435*
Trauma to the genitourinary tract	958, 959
Trichinellosis	124
Trichomonal vaginitis	131.01
Trigeminal neuralgia	350.1
Tuberculosis, pulmonary	011**
Tularemia	021*
Typhoid fever	002.0
Typhus fevers	080, 081
Ulcerative colitis	556*
Urethral stricture	598*
Urinary incontinence	788.30
Urticaria	708*
Uterine inertia	661.0**
Uterine leiomyoma	218*
Varicella	052*
Venous thrombosis	453.8
Viral pneumonia	480.9
Viral respiratory infections	465.9
Vitamin deficiency	264-269
Vitamin K deficiency	269.0
Warts (verrucae)	078.10
Wegener's granulomatosis	446.4
Whooping cough (pertussis)	033*
Wrist fracture	814.0**

*4th digit needed
**5th (or 4th and 5th) digit needed

CONN'S
Current Therapy 2011

CONN'S
Current
Therapy
2011

Edward T. Bope, MD
Chief of Medicine, Columbus VA
Clinical Professor, Department of Family Medicine
The Ohio State University College of Medicine
Columbus, Ohio

Rick Kellerman, MD
Professor and Chair, Department of Family and
 Community Medicine
University of Kansas School of Medicine–Wichita
Wichita, Kansas

Robert E. Rakel, MD
Professor, Department of Family and
 Community Medicine
Baylor College of Medicine
Houston, Texas

LATEST APPROVED METHODS
OF TREATMENT FOR THE
PRACTICING PHYSICIAN

ELSEVIER
SAUNDERS

ELSEVIER
SAUNDERS

1600 John F. Kennedy Blvd.
Ste 1800
Philadelphia, PA 19103–2899

Acquisitions Editor: Kate Dimock
Developmental Editor: Joan Ryan
Publishing Services Manager: Anne Altepeter
Senior Project Manager: Cheryl A. Abbott
Design Direction: Steven Stave

Printed in the United States of America

Last digit is the print number: 9 8 7 6 5 4 3 2 1

Contributors

Charles S. Abrams, MD
Associate Chief, Division of Hematology-Oncology, University of
Pennsylvania School of Medicine; Staff Physician, Division of
Hematology-Oncology, University of Pennsylvania Medical Center,
Philadelphia, Pennsylvania
Platelet-Mediated Bleeding Disorders

Mark J. Abzug, MD
Professor of Pediatrics (Infectious Diseases), University of Colorado–
Denver School of Medicine; Medical Director, The Children's
Hospital Clinical Trials Organization, The Children's Hospital,
Aurora, Colorado
Viral Meningitis and Encephalitis

Horacio E. Adrogué, MD
Medical Director, Pancreas Transplant Program; Medical Director,
Methodist Transplant Network, The Methodist Hospital Transplant
Center, Houston, Texas
Hypertension

Tod C. Aeby, MD
Residency Program Director, Department of Obstetrics, Gynecology,
and Women's Health, University of Hawaii John A. Burns School of
Medicine, Honolulu, Hawaii
Uterine Leiomyomas

Lee Akst, MD
Assistant Professor, Department of Otolaryngology, Loyola
University Chicago Stritch School of Medicine, Maywood, Illinois
Hoarseness and Laryngitis

Mahboob Alam, MD
Section of Cardiology, Baylor College of Medicine, Houston, Texas
Hypertrophic Cardiomyopathy

Brian K. Albertson, MD
University Physicians Group, Harrisburg, Pennsylvania
Osteomyelitis

Madson Q. Almeida, MD
Section on Endocrinology and Genetics, Program on Developmental
Endocrinology and Genetics, *Eunice Kennedy Shriver* National
Institute of Child Health and Human Development (NICHD),
National Institutes of Health (NIH), Bethesda, Maryland
Cushing's Syndrome

Girish Anand, MD
Fellow in Gastroenterology, Albert Einstein Medical Center,
Philadelphia, Pennsylvania
Dysphagia and Esophageal Obstruction

Deverick J. Anderson, MD
Clinical Associate, Duke University Medical Center, Durham,
North Carolina
*Rickettsial and Ehrlichial Infections (Rocky Mountain Spotted Fever
and Typhus)*

Kelley P. Anderson, MD
Clinical Associate Professor of Medicine, University of Wisconsin
School of Medicine and Public Health–Marschfield Clinic Campus,
Marshfield, Wisconsin
Heart Block

Emmanuel Andrès, MD, PhD
Service de Médecine Interne, Diabète et Maladies Métaboliques,
Clinique Médicale B, Hôpital Civil–Hôpitaux Universitaires de
Strasbourg, Strasbourg, France
Pernicious Anemia and Other Megaloblastic Anemias

Gregory M. Anstead, MD
Associate Professor of Medicine, University of Texas Health Science
Center at San Antonio School of Medicine; Director,
Immunosuppression and Infectious Diseases Clinics, South Texas
Veterans Healthcare System, San Antonio, Texas
Coccidioidomycosis

Aydin Arici, MD
Professor, Department of Obstetrics, Gynecology, and Reproductive
Sciences, Yale University School of Medicine, New Haven,
Connecticut
Abnormal Uterine Bleeding

Ann M. Aring, MD
Assistant Clinical Professor, Department of Family Medicine, The
Ohio State University College of Medicine; Assistant Program
Director, Family Medicine Residency, Riverside Methodist Hospital,
Columbus, Ohio
Fever

Isao Arita, MD
Chairman, Agency for Cooperation in International Health–
Kumamoto, Kumamoto City, Japan
Smallpox

Cecilio Azar, MD
Professor of Medicine, Division of Gastroenterology, Department of
Internal Medicine, American University of Beirut Medical Center,
Beirut, Lebanon
Bleeding Esophageal Varices

Masoud Azodi, MD
Associate Professor, Division of Gynecology Oncology, Yale
University School of Medicine, New Haven, Connecticut
Cancer of the Endometrium

Adrianne Williams Bagley, MD
Pediatrician, Lincoln Community Health Center, Inc., Durham,
North Carolina
Pelvic Inflammatory Disease

Federico Balagué, MD
Privat Docent, Rheumatology, Medical School, Geneva
University, Geneva, Switzerland; Adjunct Associated Professor,
Orthopedics, New York University, New York, New York; Médecin
Chef Adj Service de Rhumatologie, HFR-Hôpital, Cantonal Fribourg,
Switzerland
Spine Pain

Ashok Balasubramanyam, MD
Professor of Medicine, Division of Diabetes, Endocrinology and
Metabolism, Baylor College of Medicine, Houston, Texas
Diabetes Insipidus

Arna Banerjee, MD
Assistant Professor of Anesthesiology and Surgery, Department
of Anesthesiology and Critical Care and Department of
Surgery, Vanderbilt University Medical Center, Nashville,
Tennessee
Delirium

Nurcan Baykam, MD
Associate Professor of Infectious Diseases, University of Ankara
Faculty of Medicine; Staff, Infectious Diseases and Clinical
Microbiology Clinic, Ankara Numune Education and Research
Hospital, Ankara, Turkey
Brucellosis

Sheryl Beard, MD
Assistant Clinical Professor, Department of Family and Community
Medicine, University of Kansas School of Medicine; Associate
Director, Via Christi Regional Medical Center, Wichita, Kansas
Otitis Externa

Meg Begany, RD, CSP, LDN
Neonatal Nutritionist; Nutrition Support Service Coordinator,
Newborn/Infant Intensive Care Unit, The Children's Hospital of
Philadelphia, Philadelphia, Pennsylvania
Normal Infant Feeding

David I. Bernstein, MD
Professor of Medicine and Environmental Health, University of
Cincinnati College of Medicine, Cincinnati, Ohio
Hypersensitivity Pneumonitis

John P. Bilezikian, MD
Professor, Department of Medicine, Columbia University College of
Physicians and Surgeons; Attending Physician, New York-
Presbyterian Hospital, New York, New York
Primary Hyperparathyroidism and Hypoparathyroidism

Federico Bilotta, MD, PhD
University of Rome La Sapienza, Rome, Italy
Hiccups

Natalie C. Blevins, PhD
Assistant Professor of Clinical Psychology in Clinical Psychiatry,
Department of Psychiatry, Indiana University School of Medicine,
Indianapolis, Indiana
Anxiety Disorders

Roberta C. Bogaev, MD
Texas Heart Institute, Houston, Texas
Hypertrophic Cardiomyopathy

Diana Bolotin, MD, PhD
Section of Dermatology, The University of Chicago, Chicago,
Illinois
Cancer of the Skin

Mary Ann Bonilla, MD
Assistant Clinical Professor, Columbia University College of
Physicians and Surgeons, New York, New York; Attending Physician,
St. Joseph's Regional Medical Center, Paterson, New Jersey
Neutropenia

Zuleika L. Bonilla-Martinez, MD
Wound Healing Fellow, Department of Dermatology and Cutaneous
Surgery, University of Miami Miller School of Medicine, Miami, Florida
Venous Ulcers

David Borenstein, MD
Clinical Professor of Medicine, The George Washington University
Medical Center, Washington, DC
Spine Pain

Patrick Borgen, MD
Chief, Breast Service, Department of Surgery, Memorial Sloan-
Kettering Cancer Center, New York, New York
Diseases of the Breast

Krystene I. Boyle, MD
Clinical Instructor, Department of Obstetrics and Gynecology,
University of Cincinnati College of Medicine; Clinical Fellow,
Department of Obstetrics/Gynecology, Division of Reproductive
Endocrinology, University of Cincinnati Medical Center, Cincinnati,
Ohio
Menopause

Mark E. Brecher, MD
Adjunct Professor, Department of Pathology and Laboratory
Medicine, University of North Carolina at Chapel Hill School of
Medicine, Chapel Hill, North Carolina; Chief Medical Officer/Senior
Vice President, Laboratory Corporation of America, Burlington,
North Carolina
Therapeutic Use of Blood Components

Sylvia L. Brice, MD
Associate Professor of Dermatology, University of Colorado, Denver,
Colorado
Viral Diseases of the Skin

Patricia D. Brown, MD
Associate Professor of Medicine, Division of Infectious Diseases,
Wayne State University School of Medicine; Chief of Medicine,
Detroit Receiving Hospital, Detroit, Michigan
Pyelonephritis

Patrick Brown, MD
Assistant Professor of Oncology and Pediatrics, The Johns Hopkins
University School of Medicine; Director, Pediatric Leukemia
Program, Sidney Kimmel Comprehensive Cancer Center at Johns
Hopkins, Baltimore, Maryland
Acute Leukemia in Children

Richard B. Brown, MD
Professor of Medicine, Tufts University School of Medicine,
Boston; Senior Clinician, Baystate Medical Center, Springfield,
Massachusetts
Toxic Shock Syndrome

Peter Buckley, MD
Interim Dean, School of Medicine, Medical College of Georgia, Augusta,
Georgia
Schizophrenia

Irina Burd, MD, PhD
Instructor, Department of Obstetrics and Gynecology, University of Pennsylvania School of Medicine; Staff, Hospital of the University of Pennsylvania, Philadelphia, Pennsylvania
Menopause

Diego Cadavid, MD
Consultant in Immunology and Inflammatory Diseases, Massachusetts General Hospital, Charlestown, Massachusetts
Relapsing Fever

Grant R. Caddy, MD
Consultant Physician and Gastroenterologist, Ulster Hospital, Belfast, Northern Ireland
Cholelithiasis and Cholecystitis

Thomas R. Caraccio, PharmD
Associate Professor of Emergency Medicine, Stony Brook University Medical Center School of Medicine, Stony Brook, New York; Assistant Professor of Pharmacology and Toxicology, New York College of Osteopathic Medicine, Old Westbury, New York
Medical Toxicology: Ingestions, Inhalations, and Dermal and Ocular Absorptions

Enrique V. Carbajal, MD
Associate Clinical Professor of Medicine, University of California–San Francisco School of Medicine, San Francisco, California; Department of Medicine, Veterans Affairs Central California Health Care System, Fresno, California
Premature Beats

Steve Carpenter, MD
Associate Professor, Baylor College of Medicine, St. Luke's Episcopal Hospital, Houston, Texas
Hodgkin's Disease: Radiation Therapy

Petros E. Carvounis, MD, FRCSC
Assistant Professor, Cullen Eye Institute, Baylor College of Medicine; Chief of Ophthalmology (interim), Ben Taub General Hospital, Harris County Hospital District, Houston, Texas
Uveitis

Donald O. Castell, MD
Professor of Medicine, Division of Gastroenterology and Hepatology, Medical University of South Carolina, Charleston, South Carolina
Gastroesophageal Reflux Disease

Alvaro Cervera, MD
University of Barcelona, Barcelona, Spain; National Stroke Research Institute, Heidelberg Heights, Victoria, Australia
Ischemic Cerebrovascular Disease

Lawrence Chan, MD
Professor of Medicine, Rutherford Chair, and Division Chief, Diabetes, Endocrinology, and Metabolism, Baylor College of Medicine; Chief, Diabetes, Endocrinology, and Metabolism, St. Luke's Episcopal Hospital, Houston, Texas
Dyslipoproteinemias; Primary Aldosteronism

Miriam M. Chan, BSc Pharm, PharmD
Director of Pharmacy Education, Riverside Methodist Hospital Family Medicine Residency; Clinical Assistant Professor of Family Medicine and Pharmacy, The Ohio State University, Columbus, Ohio; Adjunct Professor of Pharmacy, Ohio Northern University, Lima, Ohio
New Drugs in 2009 and Agents Pending FDA Approval; Popular Herbs and Nutritional Supplements

Emery Chen, MD
Endocrine Surgeon, Woodland Clinic, Woodland, California
Thyroid Cancer

Venkata Sri Cherukumilli, BS
Medical Student, University of California–San Diego, School of Medicine, La Jolla, California
Rheumatoid Arthritis

Meera Chitlur, MD
Assistant Professor of Pediatrics, Wayne State University School of Medicine; Staff Physician, Carman and Ann Adams Department of Pediatrics, Division of Hematology/Oncology, Children's Hospital of Michigan, Detroit, Michigan
Hemophilia and Related Bleeding Disorders

Saima Chohan, MD
Assistant Professor of Medicine, Section of Rheumatology, University of Chicago, Chicago, Illinois
Hyperuricemia and Gout

Peter E. Clark, MD
Associate Professor of Urologic Surgery, Vanderbilt University School of Medicine, Nashville, Tennessee
Malignant Tumors of the Urogenital Tract

Claus-Frenz Claussen, MD
Julius-Maximilians-Universitat Wurzburg, Wurzburg; Head, 4-G Research Institute, Neurootologisches Forschungsinstitut, Bad Kissingen, Germany
Tinnitus

Keith K. Colburn, MD
Professor of Medicine and Chief of Rheumatology, Loma Linda University, Loma Linda, California
Bursitis, Tendinitis, Myofascial Pain, and Fibromyalgia

Gary C. Coleman, DDS, MS
Associate Professor, Department of Diagnostic Sciences, Baylor College of Dentistry, Dallas, Texas
Diseases of the Mouth

Patricia A. Cornett, MD
Associate Chair for Education, Medicine, University of California–San Francisco; Chief, Hematology/Oncology, Veterans Affairs Medical Center–San Francisco, San Francisco, California
Nonimmune Hemolytic Anemia

Fiona Costello, MD
Clinical Associate Professor, Departments of Clinical Neurosciences and Surgery, University of Calgary Faculty of Medicine, Calgary, Alberta, Canada
Optic Neuritis

John F. Coyle II, MD
Clinical Professor, Department of Medicine, University of Oklahoma College of Medicine–Tulsa, Tulsa, Oklahoma
Disturbances Caused by Heat

Lester M. Crawford, PhD
Formerly Research Professor, Georgetown University School of Medicine, Washington, DC, and Head, Department of Physiology, University of Georgia College of Medicine, Athens, Georgia
Foodborne Illness

Burke A. Cunha, MD
Professor of Medicine, Stony Brook University Medical Center School of Medicine, Stony Brook; Chief, Infectious Disease Division, Winthrop-University Hospital, Mineola, New York
Urinary Tract Infections in Women; Viral and Mycoplasmal Pneumonias

Contributors

vii

F. William Danby, MD, FRCPC
Assistant Professor of Surgery (Dermatology), Dartmouth Medical School, Hanover, New Hampshire; Associate Staff, Elliot Hospital Consulting Staff, Catholic Medical Center, Manchester, New Hampshire
Anogenital Pruritus

Ralph C. Daniel, MD
Department of Dermatology, St. Dominic-Jackson Memorial Hospital, Jackson, Mississippi
Diseases of the Nails

Athena Daniolos, MD
Associate Professor, Department of Dermatology, University of Wisconsin School of Medicine and Public Health; Attending Physician, University Health Services, University of Wisconsin, Madison, Wisconsin
Condyloma Accuminata (Genital Warts)

Stella Dantas, MD
Physician, Department of Obstetrics and Gynecology, Beaverton Medical Office, Northwest Permanente PC Physicians and Surgeons, Beaverton, Oregon
Uterine Leiomyomas

Andre Dascal, MD, FRCPC
Associate Professor, Departments of Medicine, Microbiology, and Immunology, McGill University Faculty of Medicine; Senior Infectious Disease Physician, Sir Mortimer B. Davis-Jewish General Hospital, Montreal, Quebec, Canada
Acute Infectious Diarrhea

Susan Davids, MD, MPH
Associate Professor of Medicine, Medical College of Wisconsin; Associate Program Director, Internal Medicine Residency, Clement J. Zablocki Veterans Affairs Medical Center, Milwaukee, Wisconsin
Acute Bronchitis

Susan A. Davidson, MD
Associate Professor, University of Colorado–Denver School of Medicine; Chief, Gynecologic Oncology, University of Colorado Hospital, Aurora, Colorado
Neoplasms of the Vulva

Melinda V. Davis-Malesevich, MD
Resident, Bobby R. Alford Department of Otolaryngology – Head & Neck Surgery, Baylor College of Medicine, Houston, Texas
Obstructive Sleep Apnea

Francisco J.A. de Paula, MD, PhD
Assistant Professor, Department of Internal Medicine, School of Medicine of Ribeirao Preto, USP, Ribeirao Preto, Brazil
Osteoporosis

Prakash C. Deedwania, MD
Professor of Medicine, University of California–San Francisco School of Medicine, San Francisco, California; Chief, Cardiology Section, Veterans Affairs Central California Health Care System, Fresno, California
Premature Beats

Phyllis A. Dennery, MD
Professor of Pediatrics, University of Pennsylvania School of Medicine; Werner and Gertrude Henle Chair and Chief, Division of Neonatology, Children's Hospital of Philadelphia, Philadelphia, Pennsylvania
Hemolytic Disease of the Fetus and Newborn

Stephen R. Deputy, MD
Assistant Professor of Neurology, Louisiana State University School of Medicine; Staff Neurologist, Children's Hospital, New Orleans, Louisiana
Traumatic Brain Injury in Children

Daniel Derksen, MD
Professor and Vice Chair of Service, Department of Family and Community Medicine, University of New Mexico School of Medicine, Albuquerque, New Mexico
Nausea and Vomiting

Richard D. deShazo, MD
Professor of Medicine and Pediatrics and Billy S. Guyton Distinguished Professor, University of Mississippi College of Medicine; Chair, Department of Medicine, University of Mississippi Medical Center, Jackson, Mississippi
Pneumoconiosis

Clio Dessinioti, MD, MSc
Attending Dermatologist, Andreas Sygros Hospital, Athens, Greece
Parasitic Diseases of the Skin

Douglas DiOrio, MD
Adjunct Clinical Professor, The Ohio State University College of Medicine; Fellowship Director, Riverside Sports Medicine, Riverside Methodist Hospital, Columbus, Ohio
Common Sports Injuries

Sunil Dogra, MD, DNB, MNAMS
Assistant Professor, Department of Dermatology, Venereology, and Leprology, Post Graduate Institute of Medical Education and Research, Chandigarh, India
Leprosy

Basak Dokuzoguz, MD
Chief, Infectious Diseases and Clinical Microbiology Clinic, Ankara Numune Education and Research Hospital, Ankara, Turkey
Brucellosis

Joseph Domachowske, MD
Professor of Pediatrics, Microbiology, and Immunology, State University of New York Upstate Medical University, Syracuse, New York
Infectious Mononucleosis

Geoffrey A. Donnan, MD
Department of Neurology, University of Melbourne Faculty of Medicine, Dentistry, and Health Sciences; Florey Neuroscience Institutes, Carlton South, Victoria, Australia
Ischemic Cerebrovascular Disease

Craig L. Donnelly, MD
Dartmouth Medical School, Hanover, New Hampshire; Chief, Child and Adolescent Psychiatry, Dartmouth-Hitchcock Medical Center, Lebanon, New Hampshire
Attention-Deficit-Hyperactivity Disorder

John Dorsch, MD
Associate Professor, Family and Community Medicine, University of Kansas School of Medicine – Wichita, Wichita, Kansas
The Red Eye

Douglas A. Drevets, MD, DTM&H
Professor and Interim Chief, Section of Infectious Diseases, University of Oklahoma Health Sciences Center School of Medicine; Staff Physician, Veterans Affairs Medical Center, Oklahoma City, Oklahoma
Plague

Jean Dudler, MD
Associate Professor of Medicine, Division of Rheumatology, Centre Hospitalier Universitaire Vaudois and University of Lausanne, Lausanne, Switzerland
Rat-Bite Fever

Peter R. Duggan, MD
Assistant Clinical Professor, University of Calgary, Calgary, Alberta, Canada
Polycythemia Vera

Kim Eagle, MD
Albion Walter Hewlett Professor of Internal Medicine, Chief of Clinical Cardiology, and Director, Cardiovascular Center, University of Michigan Health System, Ann Arbor, Michigan
Angina Pectoris

Genevieve L. Egnatios, MD
Department of Dermatology, Mayo Clinic Scottsdale, Scottsdale, Arizona
Contact Dermatitis

Julian Elliott, MB, BS, FACP
Conjoint Senior Lecturer, National Centre in HIV Epidemiology and Clinical Research, University of New South Wales, Sydney; Infectious Diseases Physician, Alfred Hospital, Melbourne; HIV Clinical Advisor, International Health Research Group, Macfarlane Burnet Institute for Medical Research and Public Health, Melbourne, New South Wales, Australia
Psittacosis

Sean P. Elliott, MD
Assistant Professor, University of Minnesota Medical School, Minneapolis, Minnesota
Trauma to the Genitourinary Tract

Dirk M. Elston, MD
Director, Department of Dermatology, Geisinger Medical Center, Danville, Pennsylvania
Diseases of the Hair

John Embil, MD
Associate Professor of Internal Medicine, University of Manitoba, Winnipeg, Manitoba, Canada
Blastomycosis

Tobias Engel, MD
Pediatric and Reproductive Endocrinology Branch, National Institute of Child Health and Human Development, National Institutes of Health, Bethesda, Maryland
Pheochromocytoma

Scott K. Epstein, MD
Dean for Educational Affairs and Professor of Medicine, Tufts University School of Medicine, Boston, Massachusetts
Acute Respiratory Failure

Andrew M. Evens, DO, MSc
Associate Professor of Medicine and Director, Translational Therapeutics, Division of Hematology/Oncology, Northwestern University Feinberg School of Medicine/The Robert H. Lurie Comprehensive Cancer Center of Northwestern University, Chicago, Illinois
Non-Hodgkin's Lymphoma

Walid A. Farhat, MD
Associate Professor, Department of Surgery, Pediatric Urologist, The Hospital for Sick Children, Toronto, Ontario, Canada
Childhood Incontinence

Dorianne Feldman, MD, MSPT
Instructor of Physical Medicine and Rehabilitation, The Johns Hopkins University School of Medicine, Baltimore, Maryland
Rehabilitation of the Stroke Patient

Gregory Feldman, MD
Surgical Resident, Stanford Hospitals and Clinics, Stanford, California
Peripheral Arterial Disease

Steven R. Feldman, MD, PhD
Professor of Dermatology, Wake Forest University School of Medicine, Winston-Salem, North Carolina
Acne Vulgaris and Rosacea

Barri J. Fessler, MD, MSPH
Associate Professor of Medicine, Division of Clinical Immunology and Rheumatology, University of Alabama at Birmingham, Birmingham, Alabama
Polymyalgia Rheumatica and Giant Cell Arteritis

Terry D. Fife, MD
Associate Professor of Clinical Neurology, University of Arizona; Director, Arizona Balance Center, Barrow Neurological Institute, Phoenix, Arizona
Ménière's Disease

David Finley, MD
Surgeon, Thoracic Service, Memorial Sloan-Kettering, New York, New York
Pleural Effusions and Empyema Thoracis

Robert S. Fisher, MD
Lorber Professor of Medicine and Chief, Gastroenterology Section and Digestive Disease Center, Temple University School of Medicine, Philadelphia, Pennsylvania
Irritable Bowel Syndrome

William E. Fisher, MD
Professor of Surgery, Baylor College of Medicine, Houston, Texas
Acute and Chronic Pancreatitis

Alan B. Fleischer, Jr., MD
Professor and Chair, Department of Dermatology, Wake Forest University School of Medicine, Winston-Salem, North Carolina
Acne Vulgaris and Rosacea

Raja Flores, MD
Surgeon, Thoracic Service, Memorial Sloan-Kettering, New York, New York
Pleural Effusions and Empyema Thoracis

Brian J. Flynn, MD
Associate Professor of Urology, University of Colorado–Denver School of Medicine, Aurora, Colorado
Urethral Strictures

Nathan B. Fountain, MD
Professor of Neurology and Director, Dreifuss Comprehensive Epilepsy Program, University of Virginia
Seizures and Epilepsy in Adolescents and Adults

Jennifer Frank, MD
Department of Family Medicine; University of Wisconsin, Appleton, Wisconsin
Syphilis

Ellen W. Freeman, PhD
Research Professor, Departments of Obstetrics/Gynecology and Department of Psychiatry, University of Pennsylvania School of Medicine, Philadelphia, Pennsylvania
Premenstrual Syndrome

Theodore M. Freeman, MD
San Antonio Asthma and Allergy Clinic, San Antonio, Texas
Allergic Reaction to Stinging Insects

Aaron Friedman, MD
Ruben Bentson Professor and Chair, Pediatrics, University of Minnesota, Minneapolis, Minnesota
Parenteral Fluid Therapy in Children

R. Michael Gallagher, DO
Director, Headache Center of Central Florida, Melbourne, Florida
Headache

John Garber, MD
Instructor in Medicine, Harvard Medical School; Fellow in Gastroenterology, Massachusetts General Hospital, Boston, Massachusetts
Acute and Chronic Viral Hepatitis

Khalil G. Ghanem, MD, PhD
Assistant Professor of Medicine, The Johns Hopkins University School of Medicine, Baltimore, Maryland
Gonorrhea

Donald L. Gilbert, MD, MS
Professor of Medicine, University of Cincinnati College of Medicine; Associate Professor, Cincinnati Children's Hospital Medical Center, Cincinnati, Ohio
Gilles de la Tourette Syndrome

Robert Giusti, MD
Assistant Professor of Pediatrics, Division of Pediatric Pulmonology, New York University School of Medicine; New York University Langone Medical Center, New York, New York
Cystic Fibrosis

Mark T. Gladwin, MD
Professor of Medicine, University of Pittsburgh School of Medicine; Chief; Division of Pulmonary, Allergy and Critical Care Medicine, University of Pittsburgh, Pittsburgh, Pennsylvania
Sickle Cell Disease

Andrew W. Goddard, MD
Professor of Psychiatry, Indiana University Hospital, Indianapolis, Indiana
Anxiety Disorders

Mark S. Gold, MD
Distinguished Professor and Chairman, Psychiatry, Neuroscience, Anesthesiology and Community Health and Family Medicine, University of Florida College of Medicine, Gainesville, Florida
Drug Abuse

Robert Goldstein, MD
Director of Cardiac Device Clinic, Assistant Professor of Medicine, Division of Cardiology, Case Medical Center, Cleveland, Ohio
Tachycardias

Robert C. Goldstein, MD
Fellow, Infectious Diseases, Beth Israel Medical Center, New York, New York
Toxoplasmosis

Marlís González-Fernández, MD, PhD
Assistant Professor of Physical Medicine and Rehabilitation, The Johns Hopkins University School of Medicine; Medical Director, Outpatient Physical Medicine and Rehabilitation Clinics, The Johns Hopkins Hospital, Baltimore, Maryland
Rehabilitation of the Stroke Patient

E. Ann Gormley, MD
Professor of Surgery (Urology), Dartmouth Medical School, Hanover, New Hampshire; Staff Urologist, Dartmouth-Hitchcock Medical Center, Lebanon, New Hampshire
Urinary Incontinence

Eduardo Gotuzzo, MD
Principal Professor of Medicine, Universidad, Peruana Cayetano Heredia; Chief, Department of Infectious, Tropical, and Dermatologic Diseases, Hospital National Cayetano Heredia, Lima, Peru
Cholera

Luigi Gradoni, PhD
Research Director, Vector-Borne Diseases and International Health, Istituto Superiore di Sanità, Rome, Italy
Leishmaniasis

Jane M. Grant-Kels, MD
Professor and Chair, Department of Dermatology; Dermatology Residency Director; and Assistant Dean of Clinical Affairs, University of Connecticut School of Medicine; Director of Dermatopathology and Director, Cutaneous Oncology and Melanoma Center, University of Connecticut Health Center, Farmington, Connecticut
Melanocytic Nevi

William Greene, MD
Assistant Professor, Psychiatry, University of Florida, Gainesville, Florida
Drug Abuse

Joseph Greensher, MD
Professor of Pediatrics, Stony Brook University Medical Center School of Medicine, Stony Brook, New York; Medical Director and Associate Chair, Department of Pediatrics, Long Island Regional Poison and Drug Information Center, Winthrop-University Hospital, Mineola, New York
Medical Toxicology: Ingestions, Inhalations, and Dermal and Ocular Absorptions

David Gregory, MD
Assistant Clinical Professor of Family Medicine, University of Virginia School of Medicine, Charlottesville, Virginia; Assistant Clinical Professor of Family Medicine, Virginia Commonwealth University School of Medicine, Richmond, Virginia; Director of Didactic Curriculum, Lynchburg Family Medicine Residency; Staff Physician in Family Medicine and Obstetrics, Lynchburg General Hospital and Virginia Baptist Hospital, Lynchburg, Virginia
Resuscitation of the Newborn

Priya Grewal, MD
Assistant Professor, Division of Liver Diseases, Mount Sinai School of Medicine, New York, New York
Cirrhosis

Charles Grose, MD
Professor of Pediatrics, University of Iowa Carver College of Medicine; Director of Infectious Diseases Division, Children's Hospital of Iowa, Iowa City, Iowa
Varicella (Chickenpox)

Robert Grossberg, MD
Assistant Professor of Medicine, Infectious Diseases, Albert Einstein College of Medicine, Bronx, New York
Fungal Diseases of the Skin

Michael Groves, MD
Resident, Bobby R. Alford Department of Otolaryngology–Head & Neck Surgery, Baylor College of Medicine, Houston, Texas
Nonallergic Perennial Rhinitis

Eva C. Guinan, MD
Associate Professor of Pediatrics and Director, Linkages Program, Harvard Catalyst, Harvard Medical School, Boston, Massachusetts
Aplastic Anemia

Tawanda Gumbo, MD
Associate Professor of Medicine, University of Texas Southwestern Medical School; Attending Physician, Parkland Memorial Hospital and University Hospital-St. Paul, Dallas, Texas
Tuberculosis and Other Mycobacterial Diseases

Juliet Gunkel, MD
Assistant Professor, University of Wisconsin School of Medicine and Public Health; Staff Physician, University of Wisconsin Hospitals and Clinics and Meritor Hospital, Madison, Wisconsin
Premalignant Cutaneous and Mucosal Lesions

Amita Gupta, MD, MHS
Assistant Professor, Division of Infectious Diseases, The Johns Hopkins University School of Medicine, Baltimore, Maryland
The Patient with HIV Disease

David Hadley, MD
Urology Resident, University of Utah Health Sciences Center, Salt Lake City, Utah
Urethral Strictures

Rebat M. Halder, MD
Professor of Medicine, Department of Dermatology, Howard University College of Medicine, Washington, DC
Pigmentary Disorders

Ronald Hall II, PharmD
Associate Professor, Texas Tech University Health Sciences Center School of Pharmacy, Dallas, Texas
Tuberculosis and Other Mycobacterial Diseases

Nicola A. Hanania, MD, MS
Associate Professor of Medicine, Section of Pulmonary, Critical Care and Sleep Medicine; Director, Asthma Clinical Research Center, Baylor College of Medicine, Houston, Texas
Chronic Obstructive Pulmonary Disease

Rashidul Haque, MB, PhD
International Centre for Diarrhoeal Disease Research, Dhaka, Bangladesh
Amebiasis

David R. Harnisch, Sr., MD
Associate Professor, Department of Family Medicine, University of Nebraska Medical Center, Omaha, Nebraska
Dysmenorrhea

George D. Harris, MD, MS
Professor and Dean, Year 1 and 2 Medicine, University of Missouri–Kansas City School of Medicine; Faculty, Family Medicine Residency Program at Truman Medical Center–Lakewood, Kansas City, Missouri
Osteomyelitis

J. Owen Hendley, MD
Professor, Division of Pediatric Infectious Diseases, University of Virginia Health System, Charlottesville, Virginia
Otitis Media

Emily J. Herndon, MD
Assistant Professor, Department of Family and Preventive Medicine, Emory University School of Medicine; Staff Physician, Department of Community Medicine, Grady Health System, Atlanta, Georgia
Contraception

David G. Hill, MD
Yale University School of Medicine, New Haven, Connecticut; Waterbury Pulmonary Associates, Waterbury, Connecticut
Cough

L. David Hillis, MD
Chair, Department of Medicine, University of Texas Health Science Center, San Antonio, Texas
Congenital Heart Disease

Christopher D. Hillyer, MD
President and CEO, New York Blood Center; Professor, Division of Hematology, Department of Medicine, Weill Cornell Medical College, New York, New York
Adverse Effects of Blood Transfusion

Stacey Hinderliter, MD
Clinical Assistant Professor of Family Medicine, University of Virginia School of Medicine, Charlottesville, Virginia; Clinical Assistant Professor of Family Medicine, Virginia Commonwealth University School of Medicine, Richmond, Virginia; Pediatric Faculty, Lynchburg Family Medicine Residency; Staff Physician, Lynchburg General Hospital, Lynchburg, Virginia
Resuscitation of the Newborn

Molly Hinshaw, MD
Assistant Professor of Dermatology, University of Wisconsin School of Medicine and Public Health, Madison, Wisconsin; Dermatopathologist, Dermpath Diagnostics, Brookfield, Wisconsin
Autoimmune Connective Tissue Disease; Cutaneous Vasculitis

Bryan Ho, MD
Assistant Professor of Neurology, Tufts Medical Center, Boston, Massachusetts
Myasthenia Gravis

David C. Hodgson, MD, MPH
Associate Professor, Department of Radiation Oncology, University of Toronto Faculty of Medicine; Radiation Oncologist, Princess Margaret Hospital, Toronto, Ontario, Canada
Hodgkin's Lymphoma

Raymond J. Hohl, MD, PhD
Professor of Internal Medicine and Pharmacology, University of Iowa Carver College of Medicine, Iowa City, Iowa
Thalassemia

Sarah A. Holstein, MD, PhD
Assistant Professor, Department of Internal Medicine, University of Iowa Carver College of Medicine, Iowa City, Iowa
Thalassemia

Marisa Holubar, MD
Clinical Teaching Fellow, Warren Alpert Medical School of Brown University, Providence, Rhode Island
Severe Sepsis and Septic Shock

M. Ekramul Hoque, MBBS, MPH (Hons), PhD
Lecturer in Community Health, School of Medicine, Deakin
University, Geelong, Victoria, Australia
Giardiasis

Ahmad Reza Hossani-Madani, MD
Department of Dermatology, Howard University College of
Medicine, Washington, DC
Pigmentary Disorders

Christine Hsieh, MD
Department of Family Medicine, Thomas Jefferson University,
Philadelphia, Pennsylvania
Constipation

Judith M. Hübschen, PhD
Scientist, Institute of Immunology, Laboratoire National de Santé/
Centre de Recherche Public–Santé, Luxembourg
Rubella and Congenital Rubella

Christine Hudak, MD
Summa Health System, Akron, Ohio
Vulvovaginitis

William J. Hueston, MD
Professor and Chair, Department of Family Medicine, Medical
University of South Carolina, Charleston, South Carolina
Hyperthyroidism; Hypothyroidism

Joseph M. Hughes, MD
Associate Professor of Clinical Medicine, Columbia University
College of Physicians and Surgeons, New York, New York; Attending
Physician, Department of Medicine, Division of Endocrinology,
Bassett Healthcare, Cooperstown, New York
Adrenocortical Insufficiency

Scott A. Hundahl, MD
Professor of Surgery, University of California–Davis School of
Medicine, Sacramento, California; Chief of Surgery, Veterans Affairs
Northern California Health Care System, Mather, California
Tumors of the Stomach

Stephen P. Hunger, MD
Professor of Pediatrics, University of Colorado–Denver School of
Medicine; Section Chief, Center for Cancer and Blood Disorders and
Ergen Family Chair in Pediatric Cancer, The Children's Hospital,
Aurora, Colorado
Acute Leukemia in Children

Gerald A. Isenberg, MD
Associate Professor of Surgery and Director of Surgical
Undergraduate Education, Jefferson Medical College of Thomas
Jefferson University; Program Director, Colorectal Residency,
Thomas Jefferson University Hospital, Philadelphia, Pennsylvania
Tumors of the Colon and Rectum

Alan C. Jackson, MD, FRCPC
Professor of Medicine (Neurology) and Medical Microbiology,
University of Manitoba Faculty of Medicine; Head, Section of
Neurology, Winnipeg Regional Health Authority, Winnipeg,
Manitoba, Canada
Rabies

Danny O. Jacobs, MD, MPH
David C. Sabiston, Jr., Professor and Chair, Department of Surgery,
Duke University School of Medicine, Durham, North Carolina
Diverticula of the Alimentary Tract

Kurt J. Jacobson, MD
Cardiovascular Medicine Fellow, University of Wisconsin Hospitals
and Clinics, Madison, Wisconsin
Mitral Valve Prolapse

Robert M. Jacobson, MD
Professor of Pediatrics, College of Medicine, Mayo Clinic; Chair,
Department of Pediatric and Adolescent Medicine, Mayo Clinic,
Rochester, Minnesota
Immunization Practices

James J. James, MD, DrPH, MHA
Director, Center for Public Health Preparedness and Disaster
Response; Editor-in-Chief, Journal of Disaster Medicine and Public
Health Preparedness, American Medical Association, Chicago,
Illinois
*Biologic Agents Reference Chart: Symptoms, Tests, and Treatment;
Toxic Chemical Agents Reference Chart: Symptoms and Treatment*

Katarzyna Jamieson, MD
Associate Professor of Medicine, University of Iowa, Iowa City,
Iowa
Chronic Leukemias

James N. Jarvis, MD
CMRI/Arthritis Foundation Oklahoma Chapter Endowed Chair,
Professor of Pediatrics and Section Chief, Pediatric Rheumatology,
University of Oklahoma College of Medicine, Oklahoma City,
Oklahoma
Juvenile Idiopathic Arthritis

Nathaniel Jellinek, MD
Department of Dermatology, Warren Alpert Medical School of
Brown University, Providence, Rhode Island
Diseases of the Nails

Roy M. John, MD, PhD
Clinical Assistant Professor, Harvard Medical School; Associate
Director, Cardiac Electrophysiology Laboratory, Brigham and
Women's Hospital, Boston, Massachusetts
Cardiac Arrest: Sudden Cardiac Death

James F. Jones, MD
Research Medical Officer, Chronic Viral Diseases Branch, National
Center for Zoonotic, Vector-Borne, and Enteric Diseases, Centers for
Disease Control and Prevention, Atlanta, Georgia
Chronic Fatigue Syndrome

Marc A. Judson, MD
Professor of Medicine, Medical University of South Carolina,
Charleston, South Carolina
Sarcoidosis

Tamilarasu Kadhiravan, MD
Assistant Professor of Medicine, Department of Medicine, Jawaharlal
Institute of Postgraduate Medical Education and Research–
Puducherry, Puducherry, India
Typhoid Fever

Harmit Kalia, DO
Division of Gastroenterology, University of Medicine and Dentistry–
New Jersey Medical School, Newark, New Jersey
Cirrhosis

Walter Kao, MD
Associate Professor of Medicine, University of Wisconsin School of Medicine and Public Health; Attending Cardiologist, Heart Failure and Transplant Program, University of Wisconsin Hospitals and Clinics, Madison, Wisconsin
Heart Failure

Dilip R. Karnad, MD
Department of Medicine, King Edward Memorial Hospital, Mumbai, India
Tetanus

Andreas Katsambas, MD, PhD
Professor of Dermatology, Department of Dermatology, University of Athens School of Medicine; Andreas Sygzos Hospital, Athens, Greece
Parasitic Diseases of the Skin

Philip O. Katz, MD
Clinical Professor of Medicine, Jefferson Medical College of Thomas Jefferson University; Chairman, Division of Gastroenterology, Albert Einstein Medical Center, Philadelphia, Pennsylvania
Dysphagia and Esophageal Obstruction

Arthur Kavanaugh, MD
Professor of Medicine, University of California–San Diego, School of Medicine, La Jolla, California
Rheumatoid Arthritis

Clive Kearon, MRCPI, FRCPC, PhD
Professor of Medicine, McMaster University Faculty of Health Sciences; Attending Physician, Henderson General Hospital, Hamilton, Ontario, Canada
Venous Thromboembolism

B. Mark Keegan, MD, FRCPC
Assistant Professor and Consultant of Neurology; Section Chair, Multiple Sclerosis and Autoimmune Neurology, Mayo Clinic, Rochester, Minnesota
Multiple Sclerosis

Paul R. Kelley, MD
Assistant Professor, Psychiatry, Quillen College of Medicine, East Tennessee State University, Johnson City, Tennessee
Mood Disorders

Stephen F. Kemp, MD
Professor of Medicine and Associate Professor of Pediatrics, University of Mississippi College of Medicine; Director, Allergy and Immunology Fellowship Program, Departments of Medicine and Pediatrics, University of Mississippi Medical Center, Jackson, Mississippi
Anaphylaxis and Serum Sickness

Kevin A. Kerber, MD
Assistant Professor, Department of Neurology, University of Michigan Health System, Ann Arbor, Michigan
Episodic Vertigo

Haejin Kim, MD
University of Cincinnati Medical Center, Cincinnati, Ohio
Hypersensitivity Pneumonitis

Paul S. Kingma, MD, PhD
Assistant Professor, The Perinatal Institute, Cincinnati Children's Hospital Medical Center, Cincinnati, Ohio
Care of the High-Risk Neonate

Robert S. Kirsner, MD, PhD
Professor, Vice Chairman and Stiefel Laboratories Chair, Department of Dermatology and Cutaneous Surgery and Chief of Dermatology, University of Miami Miller School of Medicine, Miami, Florida
Venous Ulcers

Joseph E. Kiss, MD
Associate Professor of Medicine, Division of Hematology-Oncology, University of Pittsburgh School of Medicine; Medical Director, Hemapheresis and Blood Services, The Institute for Transfusion Medicine, Pittsburgh, Pennsylvania
Thrombotic Thrombocytopenic Purpura

Joel D. Klein, MD, FAAP
Professor of Pediatrics, Jefferson Medical College of Thomas Jefferson University, Philadelphia, Pennsylvania; Division of Pediatric Infectious Diseases, Alfred I. duPont Hospital for Children, Wilmington, Delaware
Mumps

Luciano Kolodny, MD
Merck & Co., Inc., North Wales, Pennsylvania
Erectile Dysfunction

Gerald B. Kolski, MD, PhD
Clinical Professor of Pediatrics, Temple University School of Medicine; Adjunct Clinical Professor of Pediatrics, Drexel University College of Medicine, Philadelphia, Pennsylvania; Attending Physician, Crozer Chester Medical Center, Upland, Pennsylvania
Asthma in Children

Frederick K. Korley, MD
Robert E. Meyerhoff Assistant Professor of Emergency Medicine, Johns Hopkins University School of Medicine; Staff, The Johns Hopkins Medicine Institutions, Baltimore, Maryland
Disturbances Caused by Cold

Kristin Kozakowski, MD
Pediatric Urology Senior Fellow, The Hospital for Sick Children, Toronto, Ontario, Canada
Childhood Incontinence

Robert A. Kratzke, MD
John Skoglund Chair of Lung Cancer Research, University of Minnesota Medical School; Associate Professor, University of Minnesota Medical Center, Minneapolis, Minnesota
Primary Lung Cancer

Jeffrey A. Kraut, MD
Professor of Medicine, David Geffen School of Medicine at UCLA; Chief of Dialysis, Veterans Affairs Greater Los Angeles Healthcare System, Los Angeles, California
Chronic Renal Failure

Jacques Kremer, PhD
Postdoctoral Program, Institute of Immunology, National Laboratory of Health, Luxembourg
Measles (Rubeola)

John N. Krieger, MD
Professor of Urology, University of Washington School of Medicine; Chief of Urology, Veterans Affairs Puget Sound Health Care System, Seattle, Washington
Bacterial Infections of the Male Urinary Tract; Nongonococcal Urethritis

Leonard R. Krilov, MD
Chief, Pediatric Infectious Diseases and International Adoption, Winthrop University Hospital, Pediatric Specialty Center, Mineola, New York
Travel Medicine

Lakshmanan Krishnamurti, MD
Department of Medicine, Vascular Medicine Institute, University of Pittsburgh School of Medicine, Pittsburgh, Pennsylvania
Sickle Cell Disease

Roshni Kulkarni, MD
Professor, Department of Pediatrics and Human Development, Michigan State University College of Medicine, East Lansing, Michigan
Hemophilia and Related Bleeding Disorders

Bhushan Kumar, MD, MNAMS
Former Professor and Head, Department of Dermatology, Postgraduate Institute of Medical Education and Research, Chandigarh, India
Leprosy

Seema Kumar, MD
Assistant Professor of Pediatrics, Mayo Clinic College of Medicine; Consultant, Division of Pediatrics, Endocrinology, and Metabolism, Department of Pediatrics, Mayo Clinic, Rochester, Minnesota
Obesity

Louis Kuritzky, MD
Assistant Professor, Family Medicine Residency Program, University of Florida, Gainesville, Florida
Prostatitis

Robert A. Kyle, MD
Professor of Medicine, Laboratory Medicine and Pathology, Mayo Clinic College of Medicine, Rochester, Minnesota
Multiple Myeloma

Lori M.B. Laffel, MD, MPH
Associate Professor of Pediatrics, Harvard Medical School; Chief, Pediatric, Adolescent, and Young Adult Section and Investigator, Section on Genetics and Epidemiology, Joslin Diabetes Center, Boston, Massachusetts
Diabetes Mellitus in Children and Adolescents

Richard A. Lange, MD
Executive Vice Chairman, Department of Medicine, University of Texas Health Science Center, San Antonio, Texas
Congenital Heart Disease

Julius Larioza, MD
Attending Physician, Bay State Medical Center, Springfield, Massachusetts
Toxic Shock Syndrome

Jerome Larkin, MD
Assistant Professor of Medicine, Warren Alpert Medical School at Brown University; Attending Physician, Rhode Island Hospital, Providence, Rhode Island
Severe Sepsis and Septic Shock

Andrew B. Lassman, MD
Department of Neurology and Brain Tumor Center, Memorial Sloan-Kettering Cancer Center, New York, New York
Brain Tumors

Barbara A. Latenser, MD
Clara L. Smith Professor of Burn Treatment, Department of Surgery, University of Iowa Carver College of Medicine; Medical Director, Burn Treatment Center, University of Iowa Hospitals and Clinics, Iowa City, Iowa
Burn Treatment Guidelines

Christine L. Lau, MD
Assistant Professor of Surgery, Division of Thoracic and Cardiovascular Surgery, University of Virginia School of Medicine, Charlottesville, Virginia
Atelectasis

Susan Lawrence-Hylland, MD
Clinical Assistant Professor, Rheumatology Section, University of Wisconsin Hospital and Clinics, Madison, Wisconsin
Autoimmune Connective Tissue Disease; Cutaneous Vasculitis

Miguel A. Leal, MD
Clinical Instructor and Cardiovascular Medicine Fellow, University of Wisconsin Hospital and Clinics, Madison, Wisconsin
Pericarditis and Pericardial Effusions

Paul J. Lee, MD
Winthrop University Hospital, Pediatric Specialty Center, Mineola, New York
Travel Medicine

Jerrold B. Leikin, MD
Professor of Emergency Medicine, Northwestern University Feinberg School of Medicine, Chicago, Illinois; Professor of Medicine, Rush Medical College, Chicago, Illinois; Director of Medical Toxicology, Evanston Northwestern Healthcare-Omega, Glenbrook Hospital, Glenview, Illinois
Disturbances Caused by Cold

Albert P. Lin, MD
Assistant Professor, Ophthalmology, Baylor College of Medicine; Staff Physician, Eye Care Line, Michael E. DeBakey VA Medical Center, Houston, Texas
Glaucoma

Morten Lindbaek, MD
Professor of General Practice, University of Oslo, Oslo, Norway
Sinusitis

Jeffrey A. Linder, MD, MPH, FACP
Assistant Professor of Medicine, Harvard Medical School; Associate Physician, Division of General Medicine and Primary Care, Brigham and Women's Hospital, Boston, Massachusetts
Influenza

Gary H. Lipscomb, MD
Professor and Director, Division of General Obstetrics and Gynecology, Department of Obstetrics and Gynecology, Northwestern University Feinberg School of Medicine, Chicago, Illinois
Ectopic Pregnancy

James A. Litch, MD, DTMH
Clinical Assistant Professor, University of Washington School of Medicine and School of Public Health and Community Medicine, Seattle, Washington
High-Altitude Illness

James Lock, MD
Professor of Child Psychiatry and Pediatrics, Stanford University School of Medicine and School of Public Health and Community Medicine, Seattle, Washington
Bulimia Nervosa

Robert C. Lowe, MD
Associate Professor of Medicine, Boston University School of Medicine, Boston, Massachusetts
Gastritis and Peptic Ulcer Disease

Benjamin J. Luft, MD
Edmund D. Pellegrino Professor of Medicine, Stony Brook University Medical Center School of Medicine, Stony Brook, New York
Toxoplasmosis

Michael F. Lynch, MD
Medical Epidemiologist, Malaria Branch, Centers for Disease Control and Prevention, Atlanta, Georgia
Malaria

Kelly E. Lyons, PhD
Research Associate Professor, Department of Neurology, University of Kansas School of Medicine, Kansas City, Kansas
Parkinsonism

James M. Lyznicki, MS, MPH
Associate Director, Center for Public Health Preparedness and Disaster Response, American Medical Association, Chicago, Illinois
Biologic Agents Reference Chart: Symptoms, Tests, and Treatment; Toxic Chemical Agents Reference Chart: Symptoms and Treatment

Kimberly E. Mace, PhD
Malaria Branch, Centers for Disease Control and Prevention, Atlanta, Georgia
Malaria

Judith Mackall, MD
Associate Professor of Medicine, Division of Cardiology, University Hospitals of Cleveland, Cleveland, Ohio
Tachycardias

Bahaa S. Malaeb, MD
Resident Urologist, University of Minnesota Medical School, Minneapolis, Minnesota
Trauma to the Genitourinary Tract

Christopher R. Mantyh, MD
Associate Professor, Faculty of Biology, Chemistry, and Pharmacy, Free University of Berlin; Head of Laboratory, Division of Viral Infection, Robert Koch Institute, Berlin, Germany
Diverticula of the Alimentary Tract

Woraphong Manuskiatti, MD
Professor of Dermatology, Department of Dermatology, Faculty of Medicine, Siriraj Hospital, Mahidol University, Bangkok, Thailand
Keloids

Lynne Margesson, MD, FRCPC
Assistant Professor of Surgery (Dermatology) and Obstetrics and Gynecology, Dartmouth Medical School, Lebanon, New Hampshire; Associate Staff, Elliot Hospital; Consulting Staff, Catholic Medical Center, Manchester, New Hampshire
Anogenital Pruritus

Paul Martin, MD
Chief, Division of Hepatology, Schiff Liver Institute/Center for Liver Diseases, University of Miami Miller School of Medicine, Miami, Florida
Cirrhosis

Vickie Martin, MD
Resident, Department of Obstetrics and Gynecology, Kingston General Hospital, Kingston, Ontario, Canada
Amenorrhea

Maria Mascarenhas, MBBS
Associate Professor of Pediatrics, University of Pennsylvania School of Medicine; Section Chief, Nutrition Division of Gastroenterology and Nutrition and Director, Nutrition Support Service, The Children's Hospital of Philadelphia, Philadelphia, Pennsylvania
Normal Infant Feeding

Pinckney J. Maxwell IV, MD
Assistant Professor of Surgery, Division of Colon and Rectal Surgery, Jefferson Medical College of Thomas Jefferson University, Philadelphia, Pennsylvania
Tumors of the Colon and Rectum

Ali Mazloom, MD
Graduate Student, University of Texas School of Public Health, Houston, Texas
Hodgkin's Disease: Radiation Therapy

Anthony L. McCall, MD, PhD
James M. Moss Professor of Diabetes, University of Virginia School of Medicine; Endocrinologist, University of Virginia Health Care System, Charlottesville, Virginia
Diabetes Mellitus in Adults

Jill D. McCarley, MD
Assistant Professor of Psychiatry, Quillen College of Medicine, East Tennessee State University, Johnson City, Tennessee
Mood Disorders

Laura J. McCloskey, PhD
Assistant Professor of Pathology, Anatomy, and Cell Biology, Jefferson Medical College of Thomas Jefferson University; Associate Director, Clinical Laboratories, Thomas Jefferson University Hospitals, Philadelphia, Pennsylvania
Reference Intervals for the Interpretation of Laboratory Tests

Michael McGuigan, MD
Medical Director, Long Island Regional Poison and Drug Information Center, Winthrop-University Hospital, Mineola, New York
Medical Toxicology: Ingestions, Inhalations, and Dermal and Ocular Absorptions

Donald McNeil, MD
Associate Professor of Clinical Medicine, Department of Immunology, The Ohio State University College of Medicine and Public Health, Columbus, Ohio
Allergic Reactions to Drugs

Genevieve B. Melton, MD, MA
Assistant Professor of Surgery, University of Minnesota, Minneapolis, Minnesota
Hemorrhoids, Anal Fissure, and Anorectal Abscess and Fistula

Mario F. Mendez, MD, PhD
Professor, Department of Neurology and Department of Psychiatric and Biobehavioral Sciences, David Geffen School of Medicine at UCLA; Attending Physician, Neurobehavior Unit, Veterans Affairs Greater Los Angeles Healthcare System, Los Angeles, California
Alzheimer's Disease

Moises Mercado, MD
Professor of Medicine, Faculty of Medicine, Universidad Nacional Autonoma de Mexico; Head, Endocrine Service, and Experimental Endocrinology Unit, Hospital de Especialidades, Centro Medico Nacional Siglo XXI, Institute Mexicano del Segero Social, Mexico City, Mexico
Acromegaly

Ralph M. Meyer, MD
Edith Eisenhauer Chair in Clinical Oncology and Professor, Departments of Oncology, Medicine, and Community Health and Epidemiology, Queen's University Faculty of Medicine; Director, Institute of Canada Clinical Trials Group at Queen's University, Kingston, Ontario, Canada
Hodgkin's Lymphoma

Jeffrey Wm. Milks, MD
Director, Geriatric Fellowship, Riverside Methodist Hospital; Medical Director, Senior Independence Hospice-Ohio, Ohio Presbyterian Retirement Services, Columbus, Ohio
Pain

Brian Miller, MD, MPH
Assistant Professor of Psychiatry, Medical College of Georgia, Augusta, Georgia
Schizophrenia

Peter A. Millward, MD
Medical Director, Transfusion Medicine, William Beaumont Hospital, Royal Oak, Michigan
Therapeutic Use of Blood Components

Howard C. Mofenson, MD
Professor of Pediatrics and Emergency Medicine, Stony Brook University Medical Center School of Medicine, Stony Brook, New York; Professor of Pharmacology and Toxicology, New York College of Osteopathic Medicine, Old Westbury, New York
Medical Toxicology: Ingestions, Inhalations, and Dermal and Ocular Absorptions

Enrique Morales, MD
Attending Nephrologist, Hospital 12 de Octubre, Madrid, Spain
Primary Glomerular Diseases

Jaime Morales-Arias, MD
Assistant Professor of Pediatrics; Pediatric Hematology/Oncology, Louisiana State University Health Sciences Center; New Orleans, Louisiana
Disseminated Intravascular Coagulation

Timothy I. Morgenthaler, MD
Associate Professor of Medicine, Pulmonary and Critical Care Medicine, Center for Sleep Medicine, Mayo Clinic and Foundation, Rochester, Minnesota
Sleep Disorders

Warwick L. Morison, MD
Professor of Dermatology, The Johns Hopkins University School of Medicine, Baltimore, Maryland
Sunburn

Scott Moses, MD
Medical Staff, Fairview Lakes Regional Medical Center, Wyoming, Minnesota
Pruritus

Ladan Mostaghimi, MD
Clinical Assistant Professor, University of Wisconsin School of Medicine and Public Health; Clinical Assistant Professor, University of Wisconsin Hospital and Clinics, Madison, Wisconsin
Psychocutaneous Medicine

Judd W. Moul, MD
Professor and Chief, Division of Urology; Director, Duke Prostate Center, Department of Surgery, Duke University Medical Center, Durham, North Carolina
Benign Prostatic Hyperplasia

Claude P. Muller, MD
Scientist, Institute of Immunology, Laboratoire National de Santé/Centre de Recherche Public–Santé, Luxembourg
Measles (Rubeola); Rubella and Congenital Rubella

Michael Murphy, MD
Associate Professor, Department of Dermatology, University of Connecticut School of Medicine; Attending Physician, John Dempsey Hospital-University of Connecticut Health Center, Farmington, Connecticut
Melanocytic Nevi

Diya F. Mutasim, MD
Chairman, Department of Dermatology and Professor of Dermatology and Pathology, University of Cincinnati College of Medicine, Cincinnati, Ohio
Bullous Diseases

Nicole Nader, MD
Instructor, Mayo Clinic College of Medicine; Fellow, Division of Pediatric Endocrinology and Metabolism, Department of Pediatrics, Mayo Clinic, Rochester, Minnesota
Obesity

Alykhan S. Nagji, MD
Resident, Department of Surgery, University of Virginia School of Medicine, Charlottesville, Virginia
Atelectasis

David G. Neschis, MD
Associate Professor of Surgery, Division of Vascular Surgery, University of Maryland School of Medicine, Baltimore, Maryland
Acquired Diseases of the Aorta

David H. Neustadt, MD
Clinical Professor of Medicine, University of Louisville School of Medicine; Senior Attending, University Hospital, Jewish Hospital, Louisville, Kentucky
Osteoarthritis

Douglas E. Ney, MD
Assistant Professor, University of Colorado–Denver School of Medicine; Attending Physician, University of Colorado Hospital, Aurora, Colorado
Brain Tumors

Lucybeth Nieves-Arriba, MD
Case Western Reserve University School of Medicine; Gynecologic Oncology, Women's Health Institute, Cleveland Clinic, Cleveland, Ohio
Cervical Cancer

Enrico M. Novelli, MD
Department of Medicine, Vascular Medicine Institute, University of Pittsburgh School of Medicine, Pittsburgh, Pennsylvania
Sickle Cell Disease

Jeffrey P. Okeson, DMD
Professor and Chair, Oral Health Science; Director, Orofacial Pain Program, College of Dentistry, University of Kentucky, Lexington, Kentucky
Temporomandibular Disorders

David L. Olive, MD
Professor of Obstetrics and Gynecology, University of Wisconsin School of Medicine and Public Health, Madison, Wisconsin
Endometriosis

Peck Y. Ong, MD
Assistant Professor of Clinical Pediatrics, Keck School of Medicine of the University of Southern California; Attending Physician, Children's Hospital Los Angeles, Los Angeles, California
Atopic Dermatitis

Silvia Orengo-Nania, MD
Professor of Ophthalmology, Baylor College of Medicine, Houston, Texas
Glaucoma

Bernhard Ortel, MD
Associate Professor of Dermatology, University of Chicago, Chicago, Illinois
Cancer of the Skin

Matthew T. Oughton, MD, FRCPC
Assistant Professor, Department of Medicine, McGill University Faculty of Medicine; Infectious Disease Physician, Sir Mortimer B. Davis-Jewish General Hospital, Montreal, Quebec, Canada
Acute Infectious Diarrhea

Gary D. Overturf, MD
Professor Emeritus of Pediatrics and Pathology, University of New Mexico School of Medicine; Medical Director, Infectious Diseases, TriCore Reference Laboratories, Albuquerque, New Mexico
Bacterial Meningitis

Scott Owings, MD
Clinical Assistant Professor, Department of Family and Community Medicine, University of Kansas School of Medicine, Wichita, Kansas; Associate Director, Smoky Hill Family Medicine Residency, Salina, Kansas
Gaseousness and Dyspepsia

Kerem Ozer, MD
Clinical and Research Fellow and Instructor, Departments of Medicine and Endocrinology, Baylor College of Medicine, Houston, Texas
Diabetes Insipidus; Dyslipoproteinemias

Karel Pacak, MD, PhD, DSc
Professor of Medicine and Chief of the Section on Medical Neuroendocrinology, National Institute of Child Health and Human Development, National Institutes of Health, Bethesda, Maryland
Pheochromocytoma

Richard L. Page, MD
Professor and Head, Division of Cardiology, Department of Medicine; Robert A. Bruce Endowed Chair in Cardiovascular Research, University of Washington School of Medicine, Seattle, Washington
Atrial Fibrillation

Rajesh Pahwa, MD
Professor of Neurology, University of Kansas School of Medicine, Kansas City, Kansas
Parkinsonism

Pratik Pandharipande, MD, MSCI
Anesthesiology Service, Veterans Administration Tennessee Valley Healthcare Systems; Associate Professor of Anesthesiology/Critical Care, Vanderbilt University Medical Center, Nashville, Tennessee
Delirium

Diane E. Pappas, MD, JD
Professor of Pediatrics, University of Virginia, Charlottesville, Virginia
Otitis Media

Sangtae Park, MD, MPH
Clinical Assistant Professor of Urology, University of Chicago Pritzker School of Medicine, Chicago, Illinois
Renal Calculi

Jotam Pasipanodya, MD
Research Scientist, University of Texas Southwestern Medical Center at Dallas, Dallas, Texas
Tuberculosis and Other Mycobacterial Diseases

Manish R. Patel, DO
Assistant Professor, University of Minnesota Medical Center, Minneapolis, Minnesota
Primary Lung Cancer

Paul Paulman, MD
Assistant Dean for Clinical Skills and Quality, Family Medicine, University of Nebraska College of Medicine, Omaha, Nebraska
Iron Deficiency

Alexander Perez, MD
Assistant Professor of Surgery, Duke University School of Medicine, Durham, North Carolina
Diverticula of the Alimentary Tract

Allen Perkins, MD, MPH
Professor and Chairman, Department of Family Medicine, University of South Alabama College of Medicine, Mobile, Alabama
Marine Poisonings, Envenomations, and Trauma

William A. Petri, Jr., MD, PhD
Chief, Division of Infectious Disease and International Health, University of Virginia Medical Center, Charlottesville, Virginia
Amebiasis

Vesna Petronic-Rosic, MD, MSc
Associate Professor and Clinic Director, University of Chicago Section of Dermatology, Chicago, Illinois
Melanoma

Michael E. Pichichero, MD
Director of Research, Department of Immunology and Center for Infectious Disease, Rochester General Hospital Research Institute, Rochester, New York
Whooping Cough (Pertussis)

Claus A. Pierach, MD
Professor of Medicine, University of Minnesota Medical School, Abbott Northwestern Hospital, Minneapolis, Minnesota
Porphyrias

Antonello Pietrangelo, MD, PhD
Professor of Internal Medicine, Department of Internal Medicine, University of Modena and Reggio Emilia, Modena, Italy
Hemochromatosis

Daniel K. Podolsky, MD
Professor of Internal Medicine, University of Texas Southwestern Medical School; Philip O'Bryan Montgomery Jr., MD, Distinguished Presidential Chair in Academic Administration and Doris and Bryan Wildenthal Distinguished Chair in Medical Science, University of Texas Southwestern Medical Center, Dallas, Texas
Inflammatory Bowel Disease: Crohn's Disease and Ulcerative Colitis

Michael A. Posencheg, MD
Medical Director, Newborn Nursery; Associate Medical Director, Intensive Care Nursery; Assistant Professor of Clinical Pediatrics, Division of Neonatology and Newborn Services, Hospital of the University of Pennsylvania, Philadelphia, Pennsylvania
Hemolytic Disease of the Fetus and Newborn

Manuel Praga, MD
Associate Professor of Medicine, Universidad Complutense; Head, Nephrology Department, Hospital 12 de Octubre, Madrid, Spain
Primary Glomerular Diseases

Abhiram Prasad, MD
Associate Professor of Medicine, Mayo Clinic College of Medicine, Rochester, Minnesota
Acute Myocardial Infarction

Daniel Pratt, MD
Assistant Professor of Medicine, Harvard Medical School; Director, Liver-Biliary-Pancreas Center, Massachusetts General Hospital, Boston, Massachusetts
Acute and Chronic Viral Hepatitis

Richard A. Prinz, MD
Helen Shedd Keith Professor and Chairman, Department of General Surgery, Rush Medical College; Chairman, Department of General Surgery, Rush University Medical Center, Chicago, Illinois
Thyroid Cancer

David Puchalsky, MD
Associate Professor of Dermatology, University of Wisconsin School of Medicine and Public Health, Madison, Wisconsin
Papulosquamous Eruptions—Psoriasis

David M. Quillen, MD
Associate Professor, Department of Community Health and Family Medicine, University of Florida College of Medicine, Gainesville, Florida
Allergic Rhinitis Caused by Inhalant Factors; Epididymitis

Beth W. Rackow, MD
Assistant Professor, Department of Obstetrics, Gynecology, and Reproductive Sciences, Yale University School of Medicine, New Haven, Connecticut
Abnormal Uterine Bleeding

Peter S. Rahko, MD
Professor of Medicine, University of Wisconsin School of Medicine and Public Health; Director of Echocardiography, University of Wisconsin Hospitals and Clinics, Madison, Wisconsin
Mitral Valve Prolapse

S. Vincent Rajkumar, MD
Professor of Medicine and Chair, Myeloma Amyloidosis Dysproteinemia Group, Division of Hematology, Mayo Clinic, Rochester, Minnesota
Multiple Myeloma

Kirk D. Ramin, MD
Associate Professor and Director, Maternal-Fetal Medicine Fellowship Program, Department of Obstetrics and Gynecology, University of Minnesota Medical School, Minneapolis, Minnesota
Antepartum Care

Julio A. Ramirez, MD
Professor of Medicine, University of Louisville School of Medicine; Chief, Division of Infectious Diseases, Department of Veterans Affairs Medical Center, Louisville, Kentucky
Legionellosis

Didier Raoult, PhD
Professor, Faculté de Médecine, Université de la Méditerranée, Marseille, France
Q Fever

Lakshmi Ravindran, MD
Assistant Professor, University of Toronto Faculty of Medicine; Staff Psychiatrist, Mood and Anxiety Program, Centre for Addiction and Mental Health, Toronto, Ontario, Canada
Panic Disorder

Elizabeth Reddy, MD
Fellow, Department of Medicine, Division of Infectious Disease, Duke University, Durham, North Carolina
Intestinal Parasites

Guy S. Reeder, MD
Professor of Medicine, Mayo Clinic College of Medicine, Rochester, Minnesota
Acute Myocardial Infarction

Ian R. Reid, MD
Professor of Medicine and Endocrinology, University of Auckland Faculty of Medical and Health Sciences School of Medicine, Auckland, New Zealand
Paget's Disease of Bone

Robert L. Reid, MD
Professor, Department of Obstetrics and Gynecology, Queen's University Faculty of Medicine; Chair, Division of Reproductive Endocrinology and Infertility, Kingston General Hospital, Kingston, Ontario, Canada
Amenorrhea

John D. Reveille, MD
Professor of Internal Medicine and Director, Rheumatology and Clinical Immunogenetics, The University of Texas Medical School, Houston, Texas
Ankylosing Spondylitis

Robert W. Rho, MD
Associate Professor of Medicine, Division of Cardiology, University of Washington Medical Center, Seattle, Washington
Atrial Fibrillation

Jason R. Roberts, MD
Gastrointestinal Fellow, Medical University of South Carolina, Charleston, South Carolina
Gastroesophageal Reflux Disease

Malcolm K. Robinson, MD
Assistant Professor of Surgery, Harvard Medical School; Metabolic Support Service, Department of Surgery, Brigham and Women's Hospital, Boston, Massachusetts
Parenteral Nutrition in Adults

Nidra Rodriguez, MD
Assistant Professor of Pediatric Hematology, University of Texas Medical School at Houston and University of Texas M. D. Anderson Cancer Center, Houston Texas
Autoimmune Hemolytic Anemia

Giovanni Rosa, MD
University of Roma La Sapienza, Rome, Italy
Hiccups

Jonathan Rosand, MD, MSc
Director, Division of Neurocritical Care and Emergency Neurology, Massachusetts General Hospital; Independent Faculty, Center for Human Genetic Research, Massachusetts General Hospital, Boston, Massachusetts
Intracerebral Hemorrhage

Peter G. Rose, MD
Case Western Reserve University School of Medicine; Section Head, Gynecologic Oncology, Women's Health Institute, Cleveland Clinic, Cleveland, Ohio
Cervical Cancer; Ovarian Cancer

Clifford J. Rosen, MD
Professor of Medicine, Tufts University School of Medicine, Boston, Massachusetts; Senior Scientist, Maine Medical Center Research Institute, Maine Medical Center, Portland, Maine
Osteoporosis

Richard N. Rosenthal, MD
Professor of Clinical Psychiatry, Columbia University College of Physicians and Surgeons; Chairman, Department of Psychiatry, St. Luke's-Roosevelt Hospital Center, New York, New York
Alcoholism

Anne E. Rosin, MD
Associate Professor of Dermatology, University of Wisconsin School of Medicine and Public Health; Attending Physician, University of Wisconsin Hospital and Clinics, Madison, Wisconsin
Warts (Verruca)

Anne-Michelle Ruha, MD
Clinical Assistant Professor, Department of Emergency Medicine, University of Arizona College of Medicine, Tucson, Arizona; Director, Medical Toxicology Fellowship, Department of Medical Toxicology, Banner Good Samaritan Medical Center, Phoenix, Arizona
Spider Bites and Scorpion Stings

Susan L. Samson, MD, PhD
Assistant Professor, Department of Medicine, Baylor College of Medicine; Attending Physician, Ben Taub General Hospital, Houston, Texas
Hyponatremia

J. Terry Saunders, PhD
Assistant Professor of Medical Education in Internal Medicine, University of Virginia School of Medicine, Charlottesville, Virginia
Diabetes Mellitus in Adults

Barry M. Schaitkin, MD
Professor of Otolaryngology, University of Pittsburgh School of Medicine; Residency Program Director, University of Pittsburgh Medical Center, Pittsburgh, Pennsylvania
Acute Peripheral Facial Paralysis (Bell's Palsy)

Ralph M. Schapira, MD
Professor and Vice Chair, Department of Medicine, Medical College of Wisconsin; Staff Physician, Milwaukee Veterans Affairs Medical Center, Milwaukee, Wisconsin
Acute Bronchitis

Michael Schatz, MD, MS
Clinical Professor, Department of Medicine, University of California–San Diego, School of Medicine, La Jolla, California; Chief, Department of Allergy, Kaiser Permanente, San Diego, California
Asthma in Adolescents and Adults

Stacey A. Scheib, MD
Resident Physician, Department of Obstetrics and Gynecology, Thomas Jefferson University Hospital, Philadelphia, Pennsylvania
Menopause

Lawrence R. Schiller, MD
Clinical Professor of Internal Medicine, University of Texas Southwestern Medical School; Attending Physician, Digestive Health Associates of Texas; Program Director, Gastroenterology Fellowship, Baylor University Medical Center, Dallas, Texas
Malabsorption

Janet A. Schlechte, MD
Professor, Department of Internal Medicine, University of Iowa Hospital, Iowa City, Iowa
Hyperprolactinemia

Kerrie Schoffer, MD, FRCPC
Assistant Professor in Neurology, Dalhousie University Faculty of Medicine; Neurologist, QEII Health Sciences Centre, Halifax, Nova Scotia, Canada
Peripheral Neuropathies

Kevin Schroeder, MD
Program Director, Transitional Year, and Medical Director of Acute Dialysis, Riverside Methodist Hospital, Columbus, Ohio
Acute Renal Failure

Daniel Schuller, MD
Professor of Medicine and Chief, Pulmonary-Critical Care and Sleep Medicine Division, Creighton University, Omaha, Nebraska
Primary Lung Abscess

Carlos Seas, MD
Associate Professor of Medicine, Universidad Peruana Cayetano Jeredia; Chief, Inservice Department, Hospital National Cayetano Heredia, Lima, Peru
Cholera

Steven A. Seifert, MD, FAACT, FACMT
Professor, University of New Mexico School of Medicine; Medical Director, New Mexico Poison Center, Albuquerque, New Mexico
Venomous Snakebite

Edward Septimus, MD
Affiliated Professor, George Mason University School of Public Policy, Fairfax, Virginia; Medical Director, Infection Prevention, HCA Healthcare System, Nashville, Tennessee
Bacterial Pneumonia

Daniel J. Sexton, MD
Professor of Medicine, Duke University School of Medicine, Durham, North Carolina
Rickettsial and Ehrlichial Infections (Rocky Mountain Spotted Fever and Typhus)

Beejal Shah, MD
Assistant Professor, Department of Medicine, Baylor College of Medicine; Attending Physician, Ben Taub General Hospital, Houston, Texas
Hyponatremia; Primary Aldosteronism

Jamile M. Shammo, MD
Associate Professor of Medicine and Pathology, Division of Hematology/Oncology, Rush University Medical Center, Chicago, Illinois
Myelodysplastic Syndromes

Amir Sharafkhaneh, MD, PhD
Associate Professor of Medicine, Section of Pulmonary, Critical Care and Sleep Medicine; Director, Sleep Fellowship Program, Baylor College of Medicine, Houston, Texas
Chronic Obstructive Pulmonary Disease

Ala I. Sharara, MD
Professor of Medicine and Head, Division of Gastroenterology, American University of Beirut Medical Center; Consulting Professor, Duke University Medical Center, Durham, North Carolina
Bleeding Esophageal Varices

Chelsea A. Sheppard, MD
Principal, Gold Standard Laboratory Consulting Group, LLC, Springfield, Missouri
Adverse Effects of Blood Transfusion

Julie Shott, MD
Sports Medicine Fellow, Riverside Methodist Hospital, Columbus, Ohio
Common Sports Injuries

Dan-Arin Silasi, MD
Assistant Professor, Gynecologic Oncology, Yale University School of Medicine, New Haven, Connecticut
Cancer of the Endometrium

Michael J. Smith, MD, MSCE
Assistant Professor, Department of Pediatrics, University of Louisville School of Medicine; Attending Physician, Division of Pediatric Infectious Diseases, Kosair Children's Hospital, Louisville, Kentucky
Cat-Scratch Disease

Suman L. Sood, MD
Assistant Professor of Medicine, Division of Hematology/Oncology, University of Michigan, Ann Arbor, Michigan
Platelet-Mediated Bleeding Disorders

Erik K. St. Louis, MD
Senior Associate Consultant, Neurology, Mayo Clinic and Foundation, Rochester, Minnesota
Sleep Disorders

Murray B. Stein, MD
Professor of Psychiatry and Family and Preventive Medicine, University of California–San Diego School of Medicine, La Jolla, California; Adjunct Professor of Psychology, San Diego State University, San Diego, California
Panic Disorder

Todd Stephens, MD
Clinical Instructor, Family and Community Medicine, University of Kansas School of Medicine–Wichita; Associate Director, Family Medicine Residency, Via Christi Family Medicine Residency Program, Wichita, Kansas
Genital Ulcer Disease: Chancroid, Granuloma Inguinale, and Lymphogranuloma

Dennis L. Stevens, MD, PhD
Professor of Medicine, University of Washington School of Medicine, Seattle, Washington; Chief, Infectious Diseases, Veterans Affairs Medical Center, Boise, Idaho
Bacterial Diseases of the Skin

Catherine Stevens-Simon, MD
Formerly Associate Professor of Pediatrics, Division of Adolescent Medicine, University of Colorado–Denver School of Medicine; Staff Physician, The Children's Hospital, Aurora, Colorado
Chlamydia trachomatis

Brenda Stokes, MD
Assistant Clinical Professor of Family Medicine, Instructional Faculty, University of Virginia School of Medicine, Charlottesville, Virginia; Assistant Clinical Professor, Department of Family Medicine, Virginia Commonwealth University School of Medicine, Richmond, Virginia; Medical Staff, Central Health-Lynchburg General and Virginia Baptist Hospitals, Lynchburg, Virginia
Hypertensive Disorders of Pregnancy; Postpartum Care

Constantine A. Stratakis, MD, PhD
Program Head, Program on Developmental Endocrinology and Genetics and Director, Pediatric Endocrinology Training Program, National Institutes of Health, Bethesda, Maryland
Cushing's Syndrome

Harris Strokoff, MD
Child and Adolescent Psychiatrist, Northwestern Counseling and Support Services, Saint Albans, Vermont
Attention-Deficit-Hyperactivity Disorder

Paniti Sukumvanich, MD
Fellow, Breast Service, Department of Surgery, Memorial Sloan-Kettering Cancer Center, New York, New York
Diseases of the Breast

Prabhakar P. Swaroop, MD
Assistant Professor of Internal Medicine, University of Texas Southwestern Medical Center at Dallas, Dallas, Texas
Inflammatory Bowel Disease: Crohn's Disease and Ulcerative Colitis

Jessica P. Swartout, MD
Fellow in Maternal-Fetal Medicine, Department of Obstetrics and Gynecology, University of Minnesota Medical School, Minneapolis, Minnesota
Antepartum Care

Masayoshi Takashima, MD
Director, The Sinus Center, and Director, Sleep Medicine Fellowship–OTO Section, Bobby R. Alford Department of Otolaryngology–Head and Neck Surgery, Baylor College of Medicine, Houston, Texas
Nonallergic Perennial Rhinitis; Obstructive Sleep Apnea

Matthew D. Taylor, MD
Resident, Department of Surgery, University of Virginia Medical Center, Charlottesville, Virginia
Atelectasis

Edmond Teng, MD, PhD
Assistant Professor, Department of Neurology, David Geffen School of Medicine at UCLA; Neurobehavioral Unit and Geriatric Research Education and Clinical Center, Veterans Affairs Greater Los Angeles Healthcare System, Los Angeles, California
Alzheimer's Disease

Joyce M.C. Teng, MD, PhD
Assistant Professor of Dermatology and Pediatrics, University of Wisconsin School of Medicine and Public Health; Attending Physician, University of Wisconsin Hospital and Clinics, Madison, Wisconsin
Urticaria and Angioedema

Nathan Thielman, MD, MPH
Duke Global Health Institute, Duke University, Durham, North Carolina
Intestinal Parasites

David R. Thomas, MD
Professor of Medicine, Division of Geriatric Medicine, Saint Louis University School of Medicine; Attending Physician, Saint Louis University Hospital, St. Louis, Missouri
Pressure Ulcers

Kenneth Tobin, DO
Clinical Assistant Professor and Director, Chest Pain Center, University of Michigan Medical Center, Department of Internal Medicine, Division of Cardiovascular Disease
Angina Pectoris

David E. Trachtenbarg, MD
Medical Director, Methodist Diabetes Care Center; Clinical Professor, Family and Community Medicine, University of Illinois College of Medicine, Peoria, Illinois
Diabetic Ketoacidosis

Maria Trent, MD, MPH
Assistant Professor of Pediatrics, The Johns Hopkins University School of Medicine; Active Staff, The Johns Hopkins Hospital Children's Center, Baltimore, Maryland
Pelvic Inflammatory Disease

Debra Tristram, MD
Clinical Professor, Department of Pediatrics, Brody School of Medicine, Greenville, North Carolina
Necrotizing Skin and Soft Tissue Infections

Elaine B. Trujillo, MS, RD
Nutritionist, National Cancer Institute, National Institutes of Health, Bethesda, Maryland
Parenteral Nutrition in Adults

Arvid E. Underman, MD, FACP, DTMH
Clinical Professor of Medicine and Microbiology, Keck School of Medicine of the University of Southern California, Los Angeles, California; Director of Graduate Medical Education, Huntington Hospital, Pasadena, California
Salmonellosis

Utku Uysal, MD
Epilepsy and EEG Fellow, University of Virginia, Charlottesville, Virginia
Seizures and Epilepsy in Adolescents and Adults

David van Duin, MD, PhD
Assistant Professor, Medicine, Cleveland Clinic Lerner College of Medicine; Staff Physician, Infectious Diseases, Cleveland Clinic Foundation, Cleveland, Ohio
Histoplasmosis

Mary Lee Vance, MD
Professor of Internal Medicine and Neurosurgery and Associate Director, General Clinical Research Center, Department of Medicine, Division of Endocrinology and Metabolism, University of Virginia Health System
Hypopituitarism

Erin Vanness, MD
Clinical Assistant Professor, University of Wisconsin School of Medicine and Public Health, Madison, Wisconsin
Erythema Multiforme, Stevens-Johnson Syndrome, and Toxic Epidermal Necrolysis

Vahan Vartanian, BS
Department of Urology, University of Chicago Pritzker School of Medicine, Chicago, Illinois
Renal Calculi

Brenda R. Velasco, MD
Gastroenterology Fellow, Temple University Hospital, Philadelphia, Pennsylvania
Irritable Bowel Syndrome

Donald C. Vinh, MD, FRCPC
Division of Infectious Diseases, Department of Medicine, and Department of Medical Microbiology, McGill University Health Center, Montreal General Hospital, Montreal, Quebec, Canada
Blastomycosis

Todd W. Vitaz, MD
Assistant Professor, Department of Neurological Surgery, University of Louisville School of Medicine; Director of Neurosurgical Oncology and Co-Director, Neurosciences ICU, Norton Hospital, Louisville, Kentucky
Management of Head Injuries

Thomas W. Wakefield, MD
S. Martin Lindenauer Professor of Surgery, Section of Vascular Surgery, Department of Surgery, University of Michigan, Ann Arbor, Michigan
Venous Thrombosis

Ellen R. Wald, MD
Professor and Chair, Department of Pediatrics, University of Wisconsin School of Medicine and Public Health; Pediatrician-in-Chief, American Family Children's Hospital, Madison, Wisconsin
Urinary Tract Infections in Infants and Children

Andrew Wang, MD
Associate Professor of Medicine/Cardiology, Duke University Medical Center, Durham, North Carolina
Infective Endocarditis

Bryan K. Ward, MD
Resident Physician, The Johns Hopkins University School of Medicine, Baltimore, Maryland
Acute Peripheral Facial Paralysis (Bell's Palsy)

Ruth Weber, MD, MSEd
Clinical Assistant Professor, Family and Community Medicine, University of Kansas School of Medicine–Wichita; Associate Program Director, Wesley Family Medicine Residency, Wichita, Kansas
Pharyngitis

Anthony P. Weetman, MD, DSc
Professor of Medicine, The Medical School, University of Sheffield; Honorary Consultant Endocrinologist, Sheffield Teaching Hospitals, Sheffield, United Kingdom
Thyroiditis

Arthur Weinstein, MD, FACP, FACR
Professor of Medicine, Georgetown University School of Medicine; Associate Chairman, Department of Medicine, and Director, Section of Rheumatology, Washington Hospital Center, Washington, DC
Lyme Disease

David N. Weissman, MD
Adjunct Professor of Medicine and Microbiology (Immunology), West Virginia University School of Medicine; Director, Division of Respiratory Disease Studies, National Institute for Occupational Safety and Health, Morgantown, West Virginia
Pneumoconiosis

Robert C. Welliver, Sr., MD
Professor, State University of New York at Buffalo School of Medicine; Co-Director, Division of Infectious Diseases, Women and Children's Hospital of Buffalo, Buffalo, New York
Viral Respiratory Infections

Ryan Westergaard, MD
Postdoctoral Fellow, Division of Infectious Diseases, The Johns Hopkins University School of Medicine, Baltimore, Maryland
The Patient with HIV Disease

Meir Wetzler, MD, FACP
Professor of Medicine and Chief, Leukemia Section, Roswell Park Cancer Institute, Buffalo, New York
Acute Leukemia in Adults

Steven R. Williams, MD
Clinical Assistant Professor, Department of Obstetrics and Gynecology, The Ohio State University College of Medicine and Public Health, Columbus, Ohio
Infertility

Elaine Winkel, MD
Associate Professor of Medicine, University of Wisconsin School of Medicine and Public Health; Attending Cardiologist, Heart Failure and Transplant Program, University of Wisconsin Hospital and Clinics, Madison, Wisconsin
Heart Failure

Jennifer Wipperman, MD
Instructor, Department of Family and Community Medicine, University of Kansas School of Medicine–Wichita, Wichita, Kansas
Otitis Externa

Michael Wolfe, MD
The Charles H. Rammelkamp Jr. Professor of Medicine, Case Western Reserve University; Chair, Department of Medicine, MetroHealth Medical Center, Cleveland, Ohio
Gastritis and Peptic Ulcer Disease

Gary S. Wood, MD
Professor and Chairman, Department of Dermatology, University of Wisconsin School of Medicine and Public Health; Attending Physician, Veterans Affairs Medical Center, Madison, Wisconsin
Cutaneous T-Cell Lymphomas, Including Mycosis Fungoides and Sézary Syndrome

Jamie R.S. Wood, MD
Instructor in Pediatrics, Harvard Medical School; Research Associate, Sections on Genetics and Epidemiology and Vascular Cell Biology; and Staff Physician, Pediatric, Adolescent, and Young Adult Section, Joslin Diabetes Center, Boston, Massachusetts
Diabetes Mellitus in Children and Adolescents

Jon B. Woods, MD
Associate Professor of Pediatrics, Uniformed Services University of the Health Sciences, F. Edward Hebert School of Medicine, Bethesda, Maryland; Pediatric Infectious Diseases, Wilford Hall Medical Center, Lackland Air Force Base, San Antonio, Texas
Anthrax

Steve W. Wu, MD
Assistant Professor, University of Cincinnati College of Medicine; Assistant Professor, Cincinnati Children's Hospital Medical Center, Cincinnati, Ohio
Gilles de la Tourette Syndrome

Elizabeth Yeu, MD
Assistant Professor of Ophthalmology, Baylor College of Medicine, Houston, Texas
Vision Correction Procedures

James A. Yiannias, MD
Associate Professor and Chair, Department of Dermatology, Mayo Clinic Scottsdale, Scottsdale, Arizona
Contact Dermatitis

Ronald F. Young, MD
Medical Director, Swedish Radiosurgical Center, Swedish Medical Center and Swedish Neuroscience Institute, Seattle, Washington
Trigeminal Neuralgia

Jami Star Zeltzer, MD
Associate Professor, Department of Obstetrics and Gynecology, Division of Maternal-Fetal Medicine, University of Massachusetts Medical School, Worcester, Massachusetts
Vaginal Bleeding in Late Pregnancy

Wei Zhou, MD
Associate Professor of Surgery, Stanford University School of Medicine, Stanford, California
Peripheral Arterial Disease

Mary Zupanc, MD
Heidi Marie Bauman Chair of Epilepsy and Professor, Departments of Neurology and Pediatrics; Chief, Division of Pediatric Neurology, Medical College of Wisconsin; Director, Pediatric Comprehensive Epilepsy Program; and Director, Pediatric Neurology, Children's Hospital of Wisconsin, Milwaukee, Wisconsin
Epilepsy in Infants and Children

Preface

Conn's Current Therapy in 2011 brings the same excellent source of information to the desktop of the physician that it did in 1949 when Dr. Conn put together the first edition to provide in one source the most recent advances in therapy for conditions encountered in practice. Experts were asked to give their "method" of treatment in a format that allowed quick reference for the busy doctor. Some less common diseases have always been included in Conn's Current Therapy because, although they may present less often, they can have serious consequences if not recognized. Furthermore, because they are rarer, the need is even greater for guidance. Robert E. Rakel, MD, well-known scholar, became the editor in 1994 after Dr. Conn's rather sudden death and has continued the traditions of Conn's Current Therapy. Edward T. Bope, MD, teacher and clinician, joined Dr. Rakel in 2001 and serves today as the chief editor. In 2010, Rick Kellerman, MD, joined Drs. Rakel and Bope in continuing the tradition.

Each year, new experts are asked to write their method for every topic. They are chosen based on recommendations from other experts and authors or because of their scholarly activity and research. Changing authors each year keeps the book crisp and up to date. Having experts explain their methods adds a personal and practical tone to the book. Such practical wisdom is of immense value to today's physician, who typically is inundated with sometimes-conflicting information from multiple sources. The authors provide references for their chapters in case the reader needs additional information or wants to see the evidence firsthand. Each year the topics are reviewed and new ones are added to keep the book current.

New features, such as electronic access to previous editions, are also added. The reader can thereby compare articles from year to year and find favorite topics and authors. It is possible to note variation in the way a disease is managed, providing options that fit the physician's practice style and population needs.

This year you will find more tables and boxes of information, features that will save you time in getting to the critical information. An effort is made to include evidence where it exists. New applications for this classic book appear from time to time and recently physicians studying for maintenance of certification Board exams have appeared as fans. Conn's Current Therapy is possible to read in a year and is comprehensive enough to be worth the effort.

Conn's Current Therapy is indeed an international book. Contributing authors from around the world offer advice about the diagnosis and management of conditions not common in the United States but increasingly seen here because we have a mobile society. The contribution of these international experts adds greatly to the comprehensive nature of the book, making it one of the only sources for treatment of diseases of the world.

Each chapter includes Current Diagnosis and Current Therapy lists. These allow quick reference on a busy day or a review of material previously read. As always, tables, graphs, and figures are used in the chapters when possible to present in-depth data in a convenient format. Careful attention is given to ensuring that all the information is correct and current. All of the material is reviewed by our pharmacist, Miriam Chan, PharmD, and by Drs. Bope, Rakel, and Kellerman for accuracy and readability. It is our habit to use trade names as well as generic drug names to help the clinician identify the treatment by whatever name is most familiar. The treatment recommendations are those that the author has found to work best. When a drug is not approved by the FDA for the use indicated, a footnote is added with this information. Such a notation may merely reflect a case in which approval for the indication being discussed was never requested. Dosages outside the usual FDA-approved range are also noted.

We greatly appreciate the assistance of the very capable editorial staff at Elsevier and are always humbled by and grateful for the knowledge and experience of our pharmacist reviewer, Miriam Chan.

Edward T. Bope, MD

Rick Kellerman, MD

Robert E. Rakel, MD

Contents

SECTION 3
Diseases of the Head and Neck

SECTION 4
The Respiratory System

SECTION 5
The Cardiovascular System

SECTION 6
The Blood and Spleen

SECTION 7
The Digestive System

SECTION 8
Metabolic Disorders

SECTION 13
Diseases of the Skin

SECTION 14
The Nervous System

Contents

xxx

SECTION 15
The Locomotor System

SECTION 16
Obstetrics and Gynecology

SECTION **17**
Psychiatric Disorders

SECTION **18**
Physical and Chemical Injuries

SECTION **19**
Appendixes

Symptomatic Care Pending Diagnosis

Pain

Method of
Jeffrey Wm. Milks, MD

The concept of pain is almost universally understood; however, an exact definition would be extremely complex if not impossible to create. Most disease states involve some element of pain, and it is the most common reason people visit health care providers. Pain is often referred to as the fifth vital sign. The manifestation of pain is a product of the physical, psychological, social, and spiritual experiences of that person. Pain is not only a reflex reaction to a noxious stimulus but also a cognitive reaction modified by a person's global response to the discomfort. This chapter deals primarily with the management of acute pain.

A numerical scale, usually 0 to 10, is used to describe the intensity of pain. Pain scales are a common and reproducible method of quantifying pain in adults as well as children. Zero is the absence of any pain and 10 represents the worst pain imaginable (Fig. 1). The pain scale can be used over time to assess the effectiveness of treatment. It is important for the practitioner to avoid underestimating pain. How the pain interferes with function needs to be understood. Different people have a marked variability as to how functional or incapacitated they may be with their pain.

Classification

Pain can be classified using several different parameters. Pain can be acute, meaning that it had an abrupt onset and has been present for less than 6 weeks. Depending on the severity this may or may not require treatment for the pain syndrome. Acute pain usually resolves. Chronic pain generally is more gradual in onset and is, by definition, more persistent. This pain usually requires long-term tools to manage the discomfort that improves when treated adequately.

Pain is also commonly described as nociceptive or neuropathic. The differentiation of pain into these categories often allows the practitioner to initiate a more effective treatment plan.

Nociceptive pain results from irritated tissue (such as a finger stick). Nociceptive pain has origin from either musculoskeletal tissue (somatic) or organ tissue (visceral). The cause is usually apparent or can be discovered with testing. Nociceptive pain usually responds to analgesics including acetaminophen, nonsteroidal antiinflammatory drugs (NSAIDs), and low-potency narcotics. Medications including

CURRENT DIAGNOSIS

- Pain is often referred to as the fifth vital sign.
- The pain scale can be used over time to assess the effectiveness of treatment.
- Nociceptive pain results from irritated tissue (such as a finger stick). The etiology of this pain is usually apparent and the duration is usually limited to shorter periods.
- Neuropathic pain results from irritation of the nerve tissue. The etiology of this pain is more difficult to elucidate and is almost always associated with chronic pain.
- Management of pain requires incorporating modalities that are effective and are acceptable to the patient.
- Several diseases respond best to disease-specific medications:
  - Restless legs syndrome: dopamine antagonists
  - Migraine headache: tryptans
  - Gout: colchicine
  - Temporal arteritis: corticosteroids
  - Cauda equina syndrome: surgical decompression
  - Acute glaucoma: acetazolamide, topical β-blocker, and a topical steroid

cyclooxygenase 2 (COX-2) selective inhibitors and corticosteroids may also be used. Swelling responds best to physical modalities: Rest, ice (cold therapy), compression, and elevation, often referred to by the acronym RICE.

Neuropathic pain results from irritation of the nerve tissue. The cause may be difficult to elucidate, and treatment is usually for extended periods of time with multiple modalities. Chronic pain almost always has a neuropathic component. Neuropathic pain responds better to nonnarcotic medications. Anticonvulsants such as carbamazepine (Tegretol),[1] gabapentin (Neurontin),[1] and lamotrigine (Lamictal)[1] may be beneficial as well as antidepressant medications such as tricyclic antidepressants, venlafaxine ER (Effexor XR),[1] or duloxetine (Cymbalta). Antidepressant medications may be helpful even if depression is not present. When opioid medications are required, long-acting forms are preferred. The centrally

---

[1]Not FDA approved for this indication.

PAIN RATING SCALE

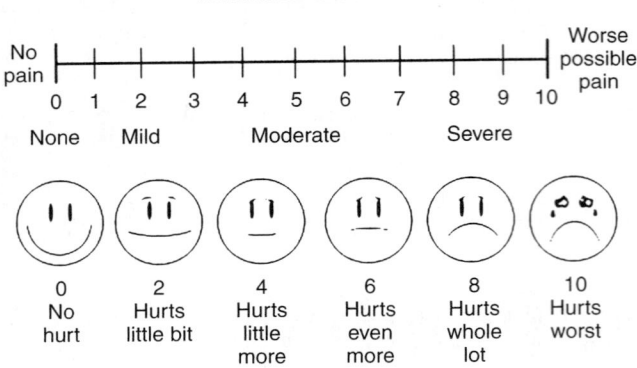

FIGURE 1. Pain scale: 0 = no pain; 1-3 = mild pain (nagging, annoying, interfering little with activities of daily living [ADLs]); 4–6 = moderate pain (interferes significantly with ADLs); 7-10 = severe pain (disabling; unable to perform ADLs). (Adapted from McCaffery M, Pasero C: Pain: Clinical Manual. St. Louis, Mosby, 1999. Faces pain rating scale modified from Wong DL: Whaley & Wong's Essentials of Pediatric Nursing, 5th ed. St. Louis: Mosby, 1997.)

acting synthetic opioid analgesic, tramadol (Ultram) is often used with significant benefit. The short-acting forms of narcotic medications should be used only for occasional breakthrough pain.

Treatment

Numerous modalities are available for treatment of pain. It is important to determine which treatments are acceptable to the patient. The use of multiple modalities can prove more beneficial with fewer side effects than the use of any single approach. Culture, gender, previous personal experiences, and comorbidities including depression and fear are variables that can affect the choice of treatment. Alleviating pain totally is not usually a realistic goal, and therefore the goals of pain management should be established. This is especially true in chronic pain management.

NONPHARMACOLOGIC TREATMENT (ALPHABETIC LISTING)

Acupuncture

Acupuncture and electroacupuncture therapy have been used to treat a broad spectrum of illnesses and injuries and are particularly effective at treating anatomically localized neuromusculoskeletal injuries caused by repetitive stress or trauma. The anatomic neuromusculoskeletal injuries that are most typically treated by acupuncture and electroacupuncture result from trauma, sports injuries, auto accidents, and work-related repetitive stress injuries of the tendon, ligament, and bursa, and injuries in and around joint areas and the soft tissues (e.g., muscles, ligaments) surrounding the spine. Acupuncture and electroacupuncture are also commonly used to treat chronic or postoperative pain, headaches, nausea, menstrual-related pain, and other conditions that may be anatomically, neurologically, or physiologically based.

Bracing (Immobilization)

Bracing includes splints, casting, and external hardware. Bracing effectively limits motion and thus prevents stimulation of nociceptive pain receptors. This is a very effective tool for managing pain from trauma. Effective immobilization often eliminates the need for systemic analgesics.

Chiropractic Manipulation

Collectively, systematic reviews of research in chiropractic have not demonstrated that spinal manipulation is more effective for pain management than allopathic medicine treatments, with the possible

 CURRENT THERAPY

- Effective pain management may include pharmacologic or nonpharmacologic treatment.
  - Nonpharmacologic treatment: Acupuncture, bracing, chiropractic manipulation, electrical nerve stimulation, hypnotherapy, iontophoresis and/or phonophoresis, massage therapy, physical therapy, yoga
  - Pharmacologic treatment: Acetaminophen, corticosteroids, NSAIDs, opioid-based analgesics, topical analgesics
- Acute pain should be treated with short-acting medications when pain medication is deemed necessary.
- Long-acting opioid preparations are generally only appropriate for chronic pain.
- Using multiple modalities may prove more beneficial with fewer side effects than the use of any single approach.
- Nociceptive pain usually responds to analgesics including acetaminophen, NSAIDs, and low potency narcotics.
- Neuropathic pain responds better to non-narcotic medications.
- No NSAID has ever been proved more effective for pain relief than any other NSAID.
- There is significant variation in the potency and side effects of opioid medications as well as the patient's response to the medication.
- The placebo effect with all treatments is substantial and should not be discredited if the treatment is safe (causing no harm) and is perceived as effective by the patient.

NSAID, nonsteroidal antiinflammatory drug.

exception of treatment of back pain, where there is significant literature substantiating chiropractic benefit. Chiropractic care usually incorporates multiple different modalities.

Electrical Nerve Stimulation

Electrical nerve stimulation (ENS) is most commonly used for chronic pain and postoperative pain. Despite the widespread use of transcutaneous electrical nerve stimulation (TENS) units, the analgesic effectiveness of TENS remains controversial in many pain conditions including fibromyalgia. Studies have shown that the use of TENS units for neck pain and chronic low back pain are no more effective than sham treatments. On the other hand, a well-performed meta-analysis demonstrated statistical benefit for the treatment of musculoskeletal pain, osteoarthritis pain, and postoperative pain. Implanted ENS units are complex and expensive medical devices that are appropriate and effective for a variety of chronic refractory pain conditions, including pain associated with cancer, failed back syndromes, arachnoiditis, visceral pain, drug-refractory chronic cluster headaches, and chronic reflex sympathetic dystrophy. Studies have confirmed benefit in these situations.

Hypnosis

Hypnotherapy is used for acute and chronic pain. Many studies show benefit, but skeptics suggest a strong placebo effect as the main contributing factor. As with many other nonpharmacologic modalities, the danger or risk is minimal.

Physical Therapy

Physical therapy is often used for acute injuries. Physical therapy has been accepted as effective by the medical community for a long time, but recent critical reviews have questioned the benefit. Modalities used can include hot packs, cold packs, infrared heat, paraffin bath, hydrotherapy, short-wave or microwave diathermy, ultrasound, and traction. There is more risk and cost associated with this therapy than the other nonpharmacologic treatments, but the treatment is generally covered by insurers.

Ionophoresis and Phonophoresis

Ionophoresis and phonophoresis involve the use of topically applied medications in which the delivery is reportedly enhanced by the use of electrical current in the case of ionophoresis or ultrasound in the case of phonophoresis. No studies have been able to show conclusive evidence of benefit of either of these modalities.

Massage Therapy

Massage may relieve pain, reduce swelling, and help loosen tight (contracted) tissue. Few would challenge the benefit. It is at least as effective as other more expensive nonpharmacologic and some pharmacologic treatments for acute and chronic pain. Massage therapy should not be used when there is active infection or if there is any increased risk of deep vein thrombosis.

Meditation

Several well-performed studies have been able to document improved pain control with the use of meditation. However, meditation is used infrequently for pain management in the United States.

Nutraceuticals

The use of vitamins, food supplements, and herbs has grown tremendously in the past 20 years. Deficiency of nutrients is associated with many disease states, including rickets, scurvy, pernicious anemia, and others. Supplementation with nutraceuticals in persons without deficiency does not improve health. There are no controlled studies showing benefit and numerous reports of harm. Use of these agents is generally discouraged. A prescribing practitioner must be knowledgeable of the treatment, potential side effects, and drug interactions.

Yoga

Yoga involves integration of stretching and strengthening of musculoskeletal tissue with control of breathing, meditation, and often spirituality. Some controlled studies have shown benefit and other reports have shown lack of benefit for pain management. There are some reports of musculoskeletal injury from the practice of yoga techniques.

PHARMACOLOGIC TREATMENT

Acute pain should be treated with short-acting medications when pain medication is deemed necessary. These medicines can be used on an as-needed basis. There is usually good patient acceptance of these medications. To be effective, short-acting medicines need to have a rapid onset of action. These medicines tend to be inexpensive, and many are available over the counter, including acetaminophen, aspirin, ibuprofen (Advil), naproxen (Aleve). Toxicity is generally less of a problem when treating acute pain than the use of the same medicines for chronic pain because of the short duration of use.

Long-acting preparations are generally only appropriate for chronic pain. The long half-life helps smooth the blood concentration peak and trough effect and thus provides better pain control. Short-acting medications can be used for breakthrough pain. Patients and sometimes their family members often are concerned about the possibility of becoming "addicted" to pain medications, especially opioid-based pain relievers. Reassurance usually alleviates that concern.

Some general rules for pain management are listed in Box 1. Box 2 lists the advantages of various routes of administration. Box 3 lists types of pain medication.

BOX 1 General Rules for Pain Management

Choose the best medication that fits the pain
Start low and titrate up
Reevaluate at appropriate intervals
Begin one medicine at a time
Short-acting agents are most appropriate for acute pain, long-acting agents for chronic pain
Choose the most appropriate route of administration

BOX 2 Routes of Pain Medication Administration

Oral: Liquid or Pill
Preferred by most
Least expensive

Intranasal
Rapid delivery
Avoids breakdown by gastrointestinal mechanisms

Injectable (Intravenous, Subcutaneous, Intramuscular)
Most rapid onset of action
Most predictable method of delivery

Transdermal
Slow, but more uniform delivery over time
Requires the least dosing frequency

Epidural, Intrathecal
Minimizes systemic side effects

Rectal
Use if the oral route is not desirable
Readily absorbed
Usually more rapid onset of action than oral by the oral route

Transmucosal
Rapid onset of action
Does not require swallowing medication

BOX 3 Pain Medications

- Acetaminophen
- Nonsteroidal antiinflammatory drugs
  - Salicylates
  - Nonselective cyclooxygenase inhibitors
  - Selective cyclooxygenase 2 inhibitors
- Capsaicin
- Lidocaine
- Diclofenac topical
- Corticosteroids
- Tramadol
- Opioids

Acetaminophen

Acetaminophen is a well-known and accepted analgesic. Acetaminophen has antipyretic as well as analgesic properties. This inexpensive pain medication is available in multiple forms including, pills, liquids, extended release, and suppositories. Acetaminophen is pregnancy category B.

The usual dose for a normal adult without liver disease is 625 mg up to every 4 hours. In 2009, the FDA Advisory Board recommended that the total daily dose of acetaminophen not exceed 4 g per day for adults and that no more than 650 mg per dose be given except by prescription. Use of combination prescription medications is discouraged owing to the common use of over-the-counter analgesics. When used together, combination prescription medicines (particularly those with acetaminophen) combined with self-administered over-the-counter preparations (which often contain acetaminophen) have resulted in numerous cases of accidental overdosing. Acetaminophen overdose is the most common overdose reported to poison control centers. Liver toxicity secondary to acetaminophen overdose is by far the most common cause of acute liver failure in the United States.

Nonsteroidal Antiinflammatory Drugs

NSAIDs are well known and accepted analgesics (Table 1). They are a heterogeneous group of medications with similar actions but different pharmacokinetics. The half-life varies from 3 hours to 60 hours depending on the NSAID. All NSAIDs create an increased risk for cardiovascular events as well as the potential for renal toxicity and at least some degree of gastrointestinal toxicity. Gastrointestinal toxicity is where there is the greatest variability among NSAIDs' side effects.

There are two groups of NSAIDs: nonselective cyclooxygenase (COX) inhibitors and COX-2 inhibitors. Nonselective COX inhibitors block the synthesis of proinflammatory prostaglandins by inhibiting both COX-1 and COX-2 enzymes. Selective COX-2 inhibitors preferentially inhibit the COX-2 enzymes, thereby circumventing many of the side effects typically caused by COX-1 inhibition. A COX-3 inhibitor and several other selective COX-2 inhibitors are available outside the United States. Examples of nonselective COX inhibitors include ibuprofen (Motrin), naproxen (Naprosyn), diclofenac (Voltaren), and numerous prescription medications. Examples of COX-2 selective drugs include celecoxib (Celebrex), meloxicam (Mobic), and nabumetone (Relafen), although meloxicam and nabumetone possess more COX-1 activity then celecoxib. Only celecoxib (Celebrex) is considered to be highly selective for COX-2 enzymes. Highly selective COX-2 medications have a lower risk for gastrointestinal bleeding.

No NSAID has ever been proved more effective for pain relief than any other NSAID.

Capsaicin

Capsaicin is an extract from the jalapeno pepper. It is used topically for management of pain including postherpetic neuralgia, diabetic peripheral neuropathy,[1] and musculoskeletal pain. Capsaicin is available over the counter as a cream (0.025%, 0.035%, 0.075%, 0.1%, and 0.25%), lotion (0.025%, 0.075%), roll-on (0.075%), gel (0.025%, 0.05%), and patch (0.025%). It should be applied 4 times a day. Its mode of action is believed to occur by depletion of substance P, one of the body's neurotransmitters for pain and heat. Treatment usually takes several weeks to achieve maximum benefit, limiting its use in acute pain. Capsaicin can burn mucus membranes if applied incorrectly.

---

[1]Not FDA approved for this indication.

TABLE 1 Examples of Nonsteroidal Antiinflammatory Drugs

Generic Name (Brand Name)	Dosages Available	Dosing Schedule	Maximum Daily Dosing
Short Acting			
Aspirin	Tabs: 81, 162, 325, 500, 650, mg Supps: 120, 200, 300, 600 mg	q4h	4 g
Ibuprofen (Motrin, Advil)	OTC: Tabs: 100, 200-mg Susp: 100 mg/5 mL, 200 mg/5 mL Rx: Tabs: 400, 600, 800 mg	qid	2.4-3.2 g
Indomethacin (Indocin)	Caps: 25, 50 mg ER caps: 75 mg Syrup: 25 mg/5 mL Supps: 50 mg	tid	200 mg
Diclofenac (Voltaren)	Caps: 25 mg Tabs: 50 mg DR tabs: 75 mg ER tabs: 100 mg Supps[2]: 50 mg	bid-tid	150-200 mg
Mefenamic acid (Ponstel)	Caps: 250 mg	2 tabs initially, then 1 tab qid Max course: 7 d	1.25 g
Intermediate Acting			
Naproxen (OTC: Aleve; Rx: Naprosyn)	OTC: Tabs and liquid pills: 200 mg Rx: Susp: 125 mg/5 mL Tabs: 250, 375, 500 mg CR tabs: 375, 500, 750 mg	q12h	1-1.5 g
Sulindac (Clinoril)	Tabs: 150, 200 mg	q12h	400 mg
Celecoxib (Celebrex)	Caps: 100, 200 mg	q12h	800 mg[3]
Long Acting			
Piroxicam (Feldene)	Caps: 10, 20 mg Supps[2]: 20 mg	Once daily	20 mg
Oxaprozin (Daypro)	Caplets: 600 mg	Once daily	1800 mg
Meloxicam (Mobic)	Tabs: 7.5, 15 mg	Once daily	15 mg

[2]Not available in the United States.
[3]Exceeds dosage recommended by the manufacturer.
cap, capsule; CR, controlled release; DR, delayed release; ER, extended release; max, maximum; OTC, over the counter; Rx, prescription; supp, suppository; susp, suspension; tab, tablet.

Lidocaine

Lidocaine is a local anesthetic used topically for analgesia. Lidocaine works by inhibiting the sodium ion channels, thus stabilizing neuronal cell membranes and inhibiting nerve impulse initiation and conduction. The medication is pregnancy category B.

Lidocaine patches (Lidoderm) are available as a 5% patch which can be applied for up to 12 hours per day and up to 3 patches at a time. Lidoderm is indicated for pain associated with postherpetic neuralgia. Lidocaine patches are usually used as an adjunct for pain control. According to the package insert, only 3% of the dose applied is expected to be absorbed systemically. Toxicity is possible if there is excessive dosing, inappropriate application, or renal compromise. Topical lidocaine solution (Xylocaine Viscous 2%) can be used for sore throat, painful mucous membrane lesions such as herpetic ulcerations, and pharyngeal and esophageal pain. For sore throat it is usually recommended that the medication be swished in the back of the throat and expectorated; 10 to15 mL can be used every 3 to 4 hours, with a maximum of 6 doses per day. When used for esophageal or pharyngeal pain, the medication may be swallowed. The total daily dosage of topical lidocaine solution should not exceed 60 mL or 1200 mg of lidocaine. Lidocaine gel (Xylocaine Jelly 2%) is indicated as an anesthetic lubricant for gastrointestinal and genitourinary procedures. Owing to increased absorption by the respiratory tree, dosing should be limited to 400 mg per day when used for this indication. Lidocaine gel can also be used on painful mucous membranes such as herpetic ulcerations.[1] Topical lidocaine may need to be applied every 3 hours.

Diclofenac

Diclofenac is an NSAID with a relatively short half-life of 1.9 hours. It is indicated for treating pain associated with osteoarthritis and other musculoskeletal pain. The mechanism of action is uncertain, but it is believed to exert its benefit through COX and lipoxygenase inhibition, which results in reduced prostaglandin synthesis. It is available as a 1.3% patch (Flector Patch), usually applied twice daily, and a 1% gel (Voltaren Gel) that can be applied to painful joints four times per day. Two grams of the gel is the recommended dose to the upper extremities and 4 g to the lower extremities. The maximum recommended dose is 32 g per day. It comes in 100-g tubes. Occlusion should be avoided.

Corticosteroids

Corticosteroids have been available to help control pain and inflammation since the mid 20th century. Numerous formulations are available including pills, oral suspension, suppositories, enemas, topical creams and ointments, and injection for intraarticular, intramuscular, or intravenous use (Table 2). Some common systemic forms include prednisone, dexamethasone (Decadron), and methylprednisolone (Medrol). High-dose corticosteroids (prednisone equivalents of 40-80 mg) are typically used for acute inflammation for short periods (less than 2 weeks). Long-term use of corticosteroids is associated with osteoporosis, avascular necrosis, and adrenal suppression. When used for longer than 2 weeks, it is recommended that the medication be tapered. Patients on prolonged corticosteroid therapy are at significantly increased risk for addisonian crisis during periods of acute illness or if there is rapid withdrawal.

Corticosteroids increase the risk for gastrointestinal bleeding, elevate blood glucose levels in people with glucose intolerance, stimulate appetite, raise blood pressure, and often produce mild euphoria. Corticosteroids have been known to cause steroid psychosis. Dexamethasone is less likely to cause edema owing to its decreased mineralocorticoid effect. Corticosteroids are particularly effective for rheumatologic disorders such as rheumatoid arthritis, polymyalgia rheumatica, and temporal arteritis. Corticosteroids have also been reported as particularly effective for bone pain secondary to metastatic disease. Intraarticular or local injection helps decrease some of the systemic effects that result from the prolonged use of higher doses necessary to achieve the same analgesic results as injection therapy.

[1]Not FDA approved for this indication.

TABLE 2 Examples of Corticosteroids

Glucocorticoid	Approximate Equivalent Dose	Biological Half-Life (hours)
Short-Acting		
Cortisone	25 mg	8-12
Hydrocortisone (Cortef)	20 mg	8-12
Intermediate-Acting		
Methylprednisolone (Medrol)	4 mg	18-36
Prednisolone	5 mg	18-36
Prednisone	5 mg	18-36
Triamcinolone (Kenalog)	4 mg	18-36
Long-Acting		
Betamethasone (Celestone)	0.6-0.75 mg	36-54
Dexamethasone (Decadron)	0.75 mg	36-54

Dixon JS: Second-line Agents in the Treatment of Rheumatic Diseases. London, Informa Health Care, 1991; Meikle AW, Tyler FH: Potency and duration of action of glucocorticoids. Effects of hydrocortisone, prednisone and dexamethasone on human pituitary-adrenal function. Am J Med 1977;63;200–207; Webb R, Singer M: Oxford Handbook of Critical Care. Oxford: Oxford University Press, 2005.

Opioid-Type Analgesics

Opioid-based analgesia (Table 3) has been around for several thousand years. These medications are effective analgesics with common although manageable side effects. There are long-acting forms and short-acting forms of these powerful pain relievers. The short-acting forms are most commonly used for acute pain of relatively short duration, and the longer-acting preparations are appropriate for chronic pain. There is significant variation in the potency and side effects of each of the medications as well an individual patient's response to the medication. Starting at lower doses is necessary to avoid the most dangerous side effects, which are sedation and decreased respiratory drive. The amount of analgesic can be increased at specified intervals to achieve effective analgesia without oversedation.

Common side effects of all opioid medications include constipation, nausea with or without vomiting, and pruritus. It is important to prevent constipation, and it is customary to begin a bowel regimen at the same time that any narcotic is initiated. Use of docusate sodium (Colace) 100 mg twice a day and senna (Senokot) 8.6 mg twice a day along with increased fluid intake is an appropriate first step. Glycerin suppositories, milk of magnesia, sorbitol 70%, lactulose (Cephulac), or polyethylene glycol (MiraLax) may be added if necessary. Enemas and rectal suppositories may be used when oral laxatives are ineffective or undesirable. Side effects of opiates include central nervous system symptoms such as sedation, cognitive impairment, hallucinations, and depression.

The method of delivery affects the time to the onset of action. Intravenous formulations have a more-rapid onset of action (5 to 10 min). Intramuscular, subcutaneous, transmucosal, or rectal methods of administration have an onset of action of about 10 to 20 minutes. Oral medications typically have an onset of action of 15 to 30 minutes. Transdermal preparations have the slowest onset of action (up to 12 hours).

There is no identified maximum dose for many narcotic medications. Exceptions include codeine, meperidine (Demerol), nalbuphine (Nubain), pentazocine (Darvon), propoxyphene (Darvon-N), and tramadol (Ultram). Side effects are usually the limiting factor. Current pain-management therapy recommends the use of single-entity formulations, especially for treating chronic pain. Care must be used when using combination medications, which often add acetaminophen or a NSAID to the opioid, because the additional ingredient can become toxic when higher doses are used. Toxicity has commonly been reported in patients taking multiple different analgesic medications containing similar adjuncts such as acetaminophen.

TABLE 3 Opioid-Based Analgesic Used for Acute Pain

Medication/form	Half-life	Usual Beginning Dose	Duration	Usual Dosing	Maximum Daily Dose	Comments
Butorphanol (Stadol)	4.7 h	1 mg SC,[1] IV 2 mg IM	3-4 h	0.5-2 mg IV q3-4h prn 1-4 mg IM q3-4h prn	No benefit in exceeding 4 mg per dose IM	Agonist and antagonist properties
Butorphanol (Stadol NS)	4.7 h	1 mg (1 spray) per nostril May repeat in 60-90 min if required	3-4 h	1-2 sprays q3-4h	Not to exceed 2 sprays q3-4h	Agonist and antagonist properties
Codeine phosphate	2.5-3.5 h	15-60 mg SC, IV	4-6 h	15-60 mg q4-6h	360 mg	7% of population unable to metabolize to the active ingredient
Codeine sulfate	2.5-3.5 h	15-60 mg PO	3-4 h	15-60 mg bid-qid[3]	360 mg	More constipation than other opioid medications
Codeine + acetaminophen	15, 30, 60 mg/ 300 mg	30 mg/300 mg	3-4 h	1-2 tabs q4-6h	12 tabs/day	Use caution with other acetaminophen products
Fentanyl (Sublimaze)[1]	3.7 h	50-100 µg IV	1-2 h	50-100 µg		Usually used as adjunct to anesthesia
Fentanyl buccal tablets (Fentora)	2.6-11.7 h	100 µg × 1, may repeat in 30 min Multiple strengths are available	3-4 h[3]	Complex titration schedule	Adjust long-acting meds to achieve no more than 4 doses/d	Oral formulations are not for acute pain Use primarily in opioid-tolerant patients
Fentanyl transmucosal (Atiq)	7 h	200 µg PO, may repeat in 30 min if needed	3-4 h[3]	Complex titration schedule	Adjust long-acting meds to achieve no more than 4 doses/day	Oral formulations are not for acute pain Use primarily in opioid-tolerant patients
Fentanyl transdermal (Duragesic Patch)	17 h	25 µg/h q72h	72 h	25 µg/h Titrate every 3-6 days		Not for acute pain management Caution as the drug is stored in the skin and can take several days to lose its effect after patch removal
Hydrocodone plus acetaminophen (oral) (Vicodin, Lortab)	*	5, 7.5, 10 mg hydrocodone, variable doses of acetaminophen	4-6 h	1-2 tabs q4h	Less than 4 g acetaminophen per day	Watch acetaminophen dose/day
Hydrocodone plus ibuprofen (oral) (Vicoprofen)	*	2.5, 5, 7.5, 10 mg hydrocodone 200 mg ibuprofen	4-6 h	1 tab up to q4-6h	5 tabs/day	
Hydromorphone (parenteral) (Dilaudid)	2.6 h	0.2-0.6 mg IV 0.8-1.0 mg SC, IM	2-3 h 4-6 h	0.2-0.6 mg IV 0.8-1.0 mg SC, IM		
Hydromorphone (oral) (Dilaudid)	2.6 h	2 mg	3-4 h	2 mg-8 mg PO q3-4h		
Hydromorphone (rectal) (Dilaudid)	2.6 h	3 mg PR	6-8 h	3 mg q6-8h		
Meperidine (Demerol)	2.5-4 h	50 mg PO 50 mg IM 50 mg SC 50 mg IV (must be diluted)	3-4 h	50-150 mg IM, PO, SC q3-4h	600 mg	Active metabolites Avoid use for >48 h due to seizure risk
Methadone (Dolophine)	Average 23 h Long and variable half-life	Tab: 5 mg, 10 mg, 40 mg Soln: 5 mg/5 mL, 10 mg/5 mL SC, IM, and IV preparations available	8-12 h	5 mg PO q4h[3] prn Titrate and monitor closely		Not for acute pain management Complex dosing regimen, multiple drug interactions, most commonly used for chronic pain
Morphine parenteral	2-4 h	2.5 mg SC, IV, IM	2-6 h	2-10 mg IV, SC, IM q2-6h prn		IV should be diluted
Morphine (oral)	2-4 h	10 mg PO	3-4 h	10-30 mg PO q3-4h		
Morphine (rectal)	2-4 h	10 mg PR	4 h	10-20 mg PR q4h prn		
Nalbuphine (Nubain)	5 h	10 mg IV, IM, SC	3-6 h	10 mg IV, SC, IM q3-6h	20 mg/dose 160 mg/day	Agonist and antagonist properties

Drug						Comments
Pentazocine lactate (parenteral) (Talwin)	2-3 h	30 mg IM, IV, SC	3-4 h	30 mg IM, IV, SC q3-4h	60 mg max IM, SC dose; 30 mg max IV dose	Agonist and antagonist properties
Pentazocine/naloxone 50 mg/0.5 mg (Talwin NX)	2-3 h	50 mg PO	3-4 h	1-2 tabs q3-4h	360 max daily dose; 12 tabs/day	
Propoxyphene HCl (Darvon)	6-12 h	65 mg	4 h	65 mg q4h prn	390 mg	
Propoxyphene napsylate (Darvon-N)	6-12 h	100 mg	4 h	100 mg PO q4h prn	600 mg	
Oxycodone	3.2 h	5 mg	4 h	5-30 mg q4h prn		Reports less nausea
Tapentadol (Nucynta)	4 h	50 mg	4-6 h	50-100 mg PO q4-6h	600 mg/day	Increased risk for serotonin syndrome; Works on both ascending and descending neurologic pain pathways
Tramadol (Ultram)	6.3 hr metabolite 7.4 h	50 mg; IR: 25 mg PO, then increase 25 mg/day to 25 mg qid, then increase every 3 days to 50 mg qid	IR: 4-6 h	IR: 50-100 mg q4-6h	IR: 400 mg	Increased risk for serotonin syndrome
(Ultram ER)		ER: 100 mg qd, titrate every 5 days	ER: Daily due to extended-release formation	ER: 100-300 mg qd	ER: 300 mg; Elderly: 300 mg	

[1]Not FDA approved for this indication.
[3]Exceeds dosage recommended by the manufacturer.
ER, extended release; IR, instant release; max, maximum; med, medication; soln, solution; tab, tablet.

The treatment of chronic pain often requires multiple medicines to achieve satisfactory pain control.

Pseudo-addiction and pseudo-allergy to opioids are two problems that occur often enough to warrant special discussion. Pseudo-addiction occurs when the patient demonstrates drug-seeking behavior due to ineffective pain control. Concern about addiction is the most commonly cited reason for undertreatment of pain. Proper pain management requires monitoring and adjusting medications to achieve an optimal balance between pain control and side effects. Pseudo-allergy occurs when the patient reports pruritus, which is a side effect of the opiate, which causes histamine release. Codeine, morphine, and meperidine are the most common causative agents of pseudo-allergy. When the only symptom of allergy is pruritus, it would be reasonable to use an alternative narcotic before labeling the patient "allergic to narcotics."

Disease-Specific Analgesics

Restless Legs Syndrome

Restless legs syndrome (RLS) is a condition with leg pain that can only be relieved with walking or movement. The disorder can be quite distressing and be difficult to treat. Restless legs syndrome responds better to dopamine agonists such as ropinirole (Requip), pramipexole (Mirapex), or carbidopa/levodopa (Sinemet),[1,2] than to typical analgesics.

Migraine Headaches

The medication group known as the triptans are available as numerous formulations. The prototype drug was sumatriptan (Imitrex), which is available as a subcutaneous injection of 6 mg, a nasal spray of 5-20 mg, or oral tablets of 25-100 mg. The sumatriptan dose may be repeated after 2 hours to a maximum daily oral dose of 200 mg. This relatively new class of medications is more effective and has fewer side effects and more rapid onset of action than other analgesics for treating migraine headaches. Numerous medications can be used preventatively.

Gout

Gout is a severe inflammatory condition of joints. The great toe is the most common site involved. Colchicine (Colcrys) can have a dramatic effect in a relatively short period of time. The dosing has changed recently to: 0.6 mg tablet, 2 tablets initially then 1 tablet 1 hour later if necessary. The maximum dose is 1.8 mg per treatment dose per attack. Allopurinol (Zyloprim) may be used to prevent recurrences.

Glaucoma

Closed-angle glaucoma can appear suddenly and is usually painful. Visual loss can progress quickly, but the discomfort often leads patients to seek medical attention before permanent damage occurs. The treatment of acute angle-closure glaucoma consists of urgent reduction of intraocular pressure (IOP), suppression of inflammation, and the reversal of angle closure. Once glaucoma is diagnosed, the initial intervention includes acetazolamide (Diamox), a topical β-blocker, and a topical steroid. Acetazolamide should be given as a stat dose of 500 mg IV followed by 500 mg PO. Ophthalmologic topical β-blockers including carteolol (Ocupress) and timolol (Timoptic) also aid in lowering intraocular pressure. Studies have not conclusively demonstrated superior protectiveness of one β-blocker over another. Both β-blockers and acetazolamide are thought to decrease production of aqueous humor and to enhance opening of the angle. An α-agonist can be added for a further decrease in intraocular pressure.

Cauda Equina Syndrome

Cauda equina syndrome is an acute emergency. It is a serious neurologic condition in which there is acute loss of function of the neurologic elements (nerve roots) of the spinal canal below the

termination (conus) of the spinal cord. Symptoms include paraplegia, urinary and rectal sphincter weaknesses, sexual dysfunction, saddle anesthesia, bilateral leg pain, and bilateral absence of ankle reflexes. Pain may be wholly absent. The patient might complain only of lack of bladder control and of perineal anesthesia. Surgical decompression usually by laminectomy in less than 48 hours is critical.

Temporal Arteritis

This somewhat common condition manifests with a headache, fever, jaw claudication, and tenderness over the temporal artery. The disease did has a smoldering course; however, it usually manifests with these symptoms. Blindness is a well-known complication and is more likely to occur if the disease is not treated promptly with corticosteroids. The erythrocyte sedimentation rate is typically greater than 60 mm/hour. The disease is confirmed by biopsy of the temporal artery; however, treatment should begin at the time the disease is suspected. Prednisone[1] 20 mg twice daily for 2 weeks and then tapered to maintain a normal sedimentation rate for up to 2 years is one effective approach to management.

Summary

Pain is the most common reason patients seek medical attention. Practitioners need to be competent in the diagnosis of pain syndromes and effective pain treatments. People react differently to pain. Management of discomfort requires incorporation of modalities that are effective as well as acceptable to the patient. Elimination of the pain completely is not a reasonable goal. Effectiveness of therapy must be reevaluated at regular intervals, and multiple modalities are often more effective than single-entity treatments. Even though there is considerable controversy regarding numerous pharmacologic and nonpharmacologic interventions, the practitioner needs to be aware of different possible therapies. When one treatment is less than optimally effective, additional interventions need to be prescribed. The placebo effect with all treatments is substantial and should not be discredited if the treatment is safe (causing no harm) and is perceived as effective by the patient.

---

[1]Not FDA approved for this indication.

REFERENCES

British Pain Society. Spinal cord stimulation for the management of chronic pain: Recommendations for best clinical practice. PDF available at www.britishpainsociety.org/SCS_2005.pdf; [accessed 5.06.10].

Council of Acupuncture and Oriental Medicine Associates (CAOMA). Foundation for Acupuncture Research: Acupuncture and electroacupuncture. Evidence-based treatment guidelines. Calistoga, CA: Council of Acupuncture and Oriental Medicine Associates; 2004.

Ernst E. Chiropractic: a critical evaluation. J Pain Symptom Manage 2008; 35(5):544–62.

Hartrick C, Van Hove I, Stegmann J-U, Oh C, Upmalis D. Efficacy and tolerability of tapentadol immediate release and oxycodone HCl immediate release in patients awaiting primary joint replacement surgery for end-stage joint disease: A 10-day, phase III, randomized, double-blind, active- and placebo-controlled study. Clin Ther 2009;31(2):1–12.

Johnson M, Martinson M. Efficacy of electrical nerve stimulation for chronic musculoskeletal pain: A meta-analysis of randomized controlled trials. Pain 2006;130(1):157–65.

Kaye AD, Kaye AM, Hegazi A, et al. Nutraceuticals: potential roles and potential risks for pain management. Pain Pract 2002;2(2):122–8.

Larson AM, Polson J, Fontana RJ, et al. Acute Liver Failure Study Group: Acetaminophen-induced acute liver failure: results of a United States multicenter, prospective study. Hepatology 2005;42:1364–72.

Morone NE, Greco CM, Weiner DK. Mindfulness meditation for the treatment of chronic low back pain in older adults: A randomized controlled pilot study. Pain 2008;134(3):310–9.

Nnoaham KE, Kumbang J. Transcutaneous electrical nerve stimulation (TENS) for chronic pain. Cochrane Database Syst Rev 2008;(3): CD003222.

Ohio Hospice and Palliative Care Organization. Palliative Care Pocket Consultant. 3rd ed. Dubuque, IA: Kendall/Hunt; 2008.

---

[1]Not FDA approved for this indication.
[2]Not available in the United States.

Nausea and Vomiting

Method of
Daniel Derksen, MD

Nausea and vomiting are common symptoms with a broad differential diagnosis. Nausea—a vague, subjective feeling that vomiting is imminent—is most often the first symptom. It may be followed by vomiting (emesis), which is the forceful expulsion of gastric contents. Retching differs in that gastric contents are not expelled, most often after prolonged bouts of vomiting. Reflux is characterized by the return of gastric content to the lower esophagus and even up into the mouth, accompanied by a sour taste or burning (heartburn) sensation. Recent advances in the treatment of nausea and vomiting related to cancer chemotherapy and postoperative care have identified the neurotransmitters involved in the pathophysiology of nausea and vomiting and have expanded treatment options. An organized approach to the assessment of these symptoms requires an understanding of the underlying pathophysiology as well as a methodical approach to taking the history, conducting a thorough physical examination, ordering appropriate laboratory and imaging studies, and treating causes and the symptoms of nausea and vomiting.

Epidemiology

Nausea and vomiting (ICD-9 code 787.01) is one of the top reasons patients see a primary care provider. Infectious diseases causing nausea and vomiting, gastroenteritis, diarrhea, and dehydration are leading causes of death in developing countries and the leading causes of sick days and reduction of employee productivity in the United States. Nausea and vomiting postoperatively and during cancer chemotherapy add significant costs, pain, and discomfort to hospital and ambulatory treatment.

Risk Factors

Previous gastrointestinal (GI) surgery, certain medications and chemotherapeutic regimens, substance abuse, pregnancy, infectious diseases, medical conditions, and central nervous system disorders increase the risk of nausea and vomiting symptoms.

Pathophysiology

Multiple afferent and efferent pathways regulate nausea and vomiting. The components of the complex pathways include a chemoreceptor trigger zone in the floor of the fourth ventricle, the nucleus tractus solitarius in the medulla, motor nuclei that control the vomiting reflex, vagal afferent nerves from the GI tract, and sympathetic afferent neurons that synapse in the spinal cord and ascend to brain stem nuclei and the hypothalamus. The sympathetic and parasympathetic nervous systems are also involved in conjunction with the smooth muscle cells and the enteric brain within the wall of the stomach and intestine. Neurotransmitters include acetylcholine, dopamine, histamine, and serotonin and form the basis of treatment modalities to suppress nausea and vomiting.

Prevention

Once the diagnosis has been established, appropriate treatment of the underlying cause of the symptoms can be instituted. When the cause of nausea and vomiting is related to medication, the dose can be adjusted or the medication switched as appropriate.

Clinical Manifestations

Nausea and vomiting are often associated with or preceded by other autonomic symptoms such as sweating and flushing. When dehydration results from prolonged vomiting or decreased oral fluid intake, clinical manifestations include dry mucous membranes, delayed capillary refill, a depressed fontanel in infants, decreased lacrimation and urination, and tachycardia. Later and more ominously with severe dehydration, hypotension and altered mental status are manifest. Especially in the very young, those with underlying chronic medical conditions, and in the elderly, hydration status must be assessed and quickly addressed. In most cases, dietary changes, antiemetics, and oral rehydration are sufficient. Intravenous hydration, hospitalization, and inpatient monitoring may be necessary for those with more serious clinical manifestations of dehydration (altered mental status, cardiovascular compromise, hypotension).

Diagnosis

HISTORY

The first step in the assessment of patients with nausea and vomiting is to obtain a thorough history, including comprehensive review of over-the-counter, recreational, and prescribed medications, substances, herbs, and other remedies. The wide range of possible etiologies of nausea and vomiting require a methodic approach to the history: past medical history including surgeries, habits, sexual activity, review of systems, physical examination, and diagnostic work-up. The duration of symptoms, the frequency of episodes, recent travel, association of symptoms with certain foods or beverages, what the patient has done to alleviate the symptoms, and whether others in the household are ill can help narrow down the possible causes.

CURRENT DIAGNOSIS

- Obtain a thorough history, including review of over-the-counter, recreational, and prescribed medications.
- The wide range of possible etiologies of nausea and vomiting requires a methodic approach to the history, physical examination, and diagnostic work-up of diarrhea.
- In women of childbearing age, obtain a urine pregnancy test.
- For chronic, severe, or recurrent symptoms, start with a complete blood count and differential, serum chemistries, liver function tests, thyroid-stimulating hormone, amylase or lipase, and other blood work, tests, and imaging as guided by the history and examination.

PHYSICAL EXAMINATION

A targeted examination based on the history includes numerous elements. Vital signs are checked: temperature, heart rate, and blood pressure. The eye is examined for evidence of exophthalmos (hyperthyroidism). The retina and optic disk are examined for papilledema (loss of venous pulsation or blurring of the optic disk margin occur early in patients with increased intracranial pressure) or retinopathy (in diabetics and hypertensives). The external ear canal and tympanic membranes are examined for evidence of otitis media or fluid behind the eardrum. The thyroid gland is palpated for enlargement, nodules, or tenderness. Mucous membranes are examined for evidence of dehydration. Teeth are checked for enamel abnormalities (bulimia). An abdominal examination is performed for distension (obstruction, gastroparesis), bowel sounds (absence suggests perforation or ileus), masses, liver enlargement or tenderness, rebound or guarding (suggesting acute appendicitis or cholecystitis). The pelvic examination in female patients looks for torsion of the ovary, cervicitis, urethritis, or pelvic inflammatory disease; male patients have a genital, testicular, and rectal examination for evidence of urethritis, epididymitis, torsion, and prostatitis. A rectal examination also looks for impaction or occult blood in the stool. The skin is examined for delayed capillary refill and poor turgor (dehydration), evidence of jaundice, or scars from past surgeries.

LABORATORY AND IMAGING STUDIES

In women of childbearing age, obtain a urine pregnancy test. For chronic, severe, or recurrent symptoms, start with a complete blood count and differential, serum chemistries, renal function, liver function tests, serum protein and albumin, thyroid stimulating hormone, amylase or lipase, and other blood work, tests, and imaging as guided by the history and examination. Further work-up might include collection of stool samples (*Camphylobacter, Shigella, Salmonella*) and studies to assess for *Giardia lamblia* or antibiotic-associated diarrhea (*Clostridium difficile*). Drug screening may be ordered if substance abuse is suspected. Imaging include radiographs with the patient lying flat and sitting or standing upright to check for free air under the diaphragm when suspecting perforation, dilated loops of bowel, or air-fluid levels in obstruction. Computed tomography (CT), magnetic resonance imaging (MRI), and esophagogastroduodenoscopy (EGD) are guided by availability of testing and the history, examination, and laboratory findings.

Differential Diagnosis

Box 1 summarizes the wide differential diagnosis of nausea and vomiting.

Treatment

Antiemetics, hydration, and dietary changes are the first-line treatments for acute episodes of nausea and vomiting. Controlling the symptoms may be all that is necessary in acute, self-limited bouts of nausea and vomiting symptoms. Oral rehydration with cool water can be accomplished by encouraging the patient to take small amounts (6 ounces or less) on a frequent basis. Beverages with high fructose or sugar content can exacerbate symptoms and cause an osmotic diarrhea. Once clear liquids are tolerated, simple foods such as rice, toast, and other items are added.

CURRENT THERAPY

- Antiemetics, dietary changes, and hydration are the first-line treatments for acute episodes of nausea and vomiting.
- Controlling the symptoms may be all that is necessary in acute, self-limited bouts of nausea and vomiting symptoms, including rehydration.
- Severity and duration of symptoms guide use of additional medications given by oral, intravenous, intramuscular, or rectal routes.

About 75% of pregnant women suffer from nausea and or vomiting; most have mild symptoms (morning sickness) that peak in the first trimester, but 2% develop the most severe form, hyperemesis gravidarum. Most pregnant women with morning sickness can be treated with dietary changes (small, more-frequent high-carbohydrate, low-fat meals), lifestyle modifications (shortening work days, short

---

BOX 1   Differential Diagnosis of Nausea and Vomiting

Central Nervous System
- Demyelinating disorders
  - Multiple sclerosis
- Increased intracranial pressure
  - Tumor
  - Intracranial bleed
  - Infarction
  - Abscess
  - Meningitis
  - Trauma
- Labyrinthitis
  - Meniere's disease
  - Vestibular neuritis
  - Motion sickness
- Migraine headaches
- Seizure disorders

Endocrine System
- Addison's disease
- Diabetes (ketoacidosis, gastroparesis)
- Hyperthryoidism
- Hypothyroidism
- Hyperparathyroidism
- Hypoparathryoidism
- Porphyria

Gastrointestinal System
- Appendicitis
- Gastric bypass procedures
- Gastroparesis (e.g., in chronic diabetes)
- Hepatobiliary disease

- Cholecystitis
- Hepatitis
- Neoplasia
- Ileus
  - After surgery, infection, or radiation
  - Related to medications
- Inflammatory bowel disease
  - Crohn's disease
  - Ulcerative colitis
- Irritable bowel disease
- Ischemia
  - Mesenteric
  - Small bowel
- Obstruction
  - Scarring or adhesions from previous surgeries
  - Small bowel obstruction
  - Esophageal spasm
- Pancreatitis
  - Obstructing stone or tumor
  - Alcohol related
- Peptic ulcer disease
  - Esophagitis
  - Gastritis
  - Gastroesophageal reflux
- Peritonitis

Genitourinary System
- Nephritis
- Nephrolithiasis
- Torsion (ovary, testicle)
- Uremia

Continued

BOX 1 Differential Diagnosis of Nausea and Vomiting—Cont'd

Infection
- Bacterial
  - *Camphylobacter*
  - *Salmonella*
  - *Shigella*
  - Enterogenic *Escherichia coli*
- Viral
  - Rotavirus
  - Influenza
- Otitis media, bacterial or viral
- Sexually transmitted infection
  - Cervicitis
  - Epdidymitis
  - Pelvic inflammatory disease
  - Prostatitis
  - Urethritis
  - Numerous organisms including gonorrhea and chlamydia
- Urinary tract infection
  - Lower (cystitis)
  - Upper (pyelonephritis)

Medication and Other Drugs
- Acetaminophen (Tylenol)
- Acyclovir (Zovirax)
- Alcohol abuse
- Antibiotics
  - Azithromycin (Zithromax)
  - Sulfasalazine (Azulfidine)
  - Erythromycin
  - Metronidazole (Flagyl)
  - Sulfonamides (e.g., trimethoprim-sulfamethoxazole [Bactrim])
  - Tetracycline
- Antidepressants
  - Selective serotonin reuptake inhibitors
- Antihypertensives
  - β-blockers (atenolol [Tenormin], metoprolol [Lopressor])
  - Calcium channel blockers
  - Diuretics (hydrochlorothiazide)
- Chemotherapeutic agents
  - Cisplatinum (Cisplatin [Platinol])
  - Cyclophosphamide (Cytoxan)
  - Nitrogen mustard (Mustargen)
  - Dacarbazine (DTIC-Dome)
  - Methotrexate (Trexall)
  - Vinblastine (Velban)

- Diabetes treatment
  - Metformin (Glucophage), sulfonylureas
- Digoxin (Lanoxin)
- Ergotamines
  - Dihydroergotamine (Migranal)
  - Methysergide (Sansert)[2]
- Ferrous gluconate, ferrous sulfate
- Gout treatment
  - Allopurinol (Zylprim)
- Hormones
  - Estrogen
  - Progesterone
  - Oral and injected contraceptives
- Levodopa (L-dopa), carbidopa (Lodosyn)
- Nicotine
  - Patch, gum
  - Smokeless tobacco
  - Cigarette, pipe, or cigar tobacco
- Nonsteroidal antiinflammatory drugs
  - Aspirin
  - Ibuprofen (Motrin)
  - Naproxen (Naprosyn)
- Opioids
  - Codeine
  - Heroin
  - Hydrocodone
  - Oxycodone
  - Morphine
  - Burprenorphine/naloxone (Suboxone)
- Prednisone
- Seizure medications
  - Phenobarbital
  - Phenytoin (Dilantin)
- Theophylline (Uniphyl)

Pregnancy
- Morning sickness
- Hyperemesis gravidarum
- Intrauterine and tubal pregnancies.

Psychiatric Disorders
- Anorexia
- Anxiety
Bulimia
Depression

[2]Not available in the United States.

naps or rest periods) and oral fluids and do not require hospitalization. Pregnant women and those contemplating pregnancy should take a daily prenatal multivitamin. Ginger[7] 250 mg by mouth four times per day (1 g/day) with pyridoxine[1] 10 mg and doxylamine (Aldex AN)[1] 10 mg combination can be used to treat more-persistent nausea and vomiting that does not respond to dietary and lifestyle changes. From there, an antihistamine such as diphenhydramine (Benadryl)[1] 25 to 50 mg PO or IV every 6 hours can be added. Promethazine (Phenergan) 12.5 to 25 mg (PO, IM, IV, PR) is the next line of treatment. For persistent symptoms, dehydration, and hyperemesis gravidarum, hospitalization, intravenous fluids, and additional antiemetics may be necessary.

Severity and duration of symptoms guide use of additional medications given by oral, intravenous, intramuscular, or rectal routes. Side effects include sleepiness, decreased energy, and, in some cases, extrapyramidal effects such as tardive dyskinesia with centrally acting antiemetics used in higher doses. Table 1 lists the common agents, dosages, and side effects of medications used to treat nausea and vomiting.

Monitoring

For patients who have complications related to nausea and vomiting, following serum electrolytes, renal function, nutritional status, and other parameters may be necessary until hydration is restored, electrolytes are replaced, and laboratory results and clinical status return to normal.

[1]Not FDA approved for this indication.
[7]Available as dietary supplement.

TABLE 1 Medications for Nausea and Vomiting

Drug Class	Class Side Effects	Drug (Trade Name)	Adult Dosing	Comments
Antibiotics		Erythromycin[1]	3 mg/kg IV q8h in acute gastroparesis, then 250 mg q8h PO × 5-7 d	Nausea, abdominal pain, *Clostridium difficile* diarrhea
Anticholinergics	Sedation, dry mouth, dizziness, hallucinations, confusion, exacerbate narrow angle glaucoma, blurred vision	Scopolamine (Transderm Scop)	1 patch q3d	Act as primary antimuscarinic agents
Antihistamines	Sedation, dry mouth, confusion, urinary retention, blurred vision	Diphenhydramine (Benadryl)[1]	50 mg PO, IM, IV q6h	
		Doxylamine (Aldex AN)[1]	5-10 mg PO qd	For nausea and vomiting related to pregnancy
		Hydroxyzine (Vistaril)[1]	25-100 mg PO, IM q6h	
		Meclizine (Antivert)	25-50 mg POq6h[3]	
		Promethazine (Phenergan)	12.5-25 mg PO, IM, IV, PR q4-6h	
Benzamides	Sedation, hypotension, extrapyramidal effects, diarrhea, neuroleptic syndrome, supraventricular tachycardia, CNS depression	Metoclopramide (Reglan)[1]	10 mg PO, IM, IV q6h	Prokinetic agents
Butyrophenones	Sedation, hypotension, extrapyramidal effects, tachycardia, dizziness, QT prolongation and torsades de pointes, neuroleptic malignant syndrome	Droperidol (Inapsine)	0.625-1.25 mg IM, IV q4h	Dopamine antagonists
		Haloperidol (Haldol)[1]	0.5-5 mg PO, IM, IV q8h	
Cannabinoids				Medical marijuana (access limited by federal and state laws)
Glucocorticoids	GI upset, anxiety, euphoria, flushing, insomnia	Dexamethasone (Decadron)[1]	4-10 mg PO, IM, IV q6-12h	
		Methylprednisolone (Medrol)[1]	40-100 mg PO, IM, IV qd	
Ginger		Ginger[7]	250 mg PO q6h or 1 g PO qd	Can help relieve the nausea and vomiting due to pregnancy (morning sickness)
Phenothiazines	Sedation, hypotension, extrapyramidal effects, neuroleptic malignant syndrome, cholestatic jaundice	Chlorpromazine (Thorazine)	10-25 mg PO, IM, PR q6h	Dopamine antagonist
		Prochlorperazine (Compazine)	10 mg PO, IM, IV or 25 mg PR q6h	
Pyridoxine (Vitamin B6)[1]		Pyridoxine (Vitamin B6)[1]	10 mg PO q6h	Can reduce mild to moderate nausea, and useful in treatment of morning sickness in pregnancy
Serotonin (5HT3) antagonists	Fever, constipation, diarrhea, dizziness, sedation, nervousness, altered liver function tests, headache, fatigue	Dolasetron (Anzemet)	100 mg PO, IV q24h	
		Granisetron (Kytril)	2 mg PO, IV q24h	
		Ondansetron (Zofran)	4-8 mg PO, IV q8-12h	

[1]Not FDA approved for this indication.
[3]Exceeds dosage recommended by the manufacturer.
[7]Available as a dietary supplement.
CNS, central nervous system; GI, gastrointestinal.

Complications

The complications of prolonged nausea and vomiting are dehydration, electrolyte disturbances (hypokalemia, hypophosphatemia, and hypomagnesemia), depletion of vitamin and trace elements, metabolic alkalosis, and malnutrition. Usually these can be corrected with oral or intravenous hydration, correction of electrolyte deficiencies, and treating the underlying cause. In patients whose nausea and vomiting are accompanied by gastroenteritis, symptoms and clinical status might not return to baseline unless all electrolytes (potassium, magnesium, phosphorous) and trace elements (such as zinc) are replaced.

REFERENCES

American College of Obstetrics and Gynecology. Nausea and vomiting in pregnancy. ACOG Practice Bulletin No. 52. Obstet Gynecol 2004;103 (4):803–14.

Braun C. Nausea and vomiting. In: Rakel RE, Bope ET, editors. Conn's Current Therapy, 2007. Philadelphia, WB: Saunders; 2006. pp. 5–9.

Flake ZA, Scalley RD, Bailey AG. Practical selection of antiemetics. Am Fam Physician 2004;69:1169–74.

Hasler WL, Chey WD. Nausea and vomiting. Gastroenterology 2003; 125:1860–7.

Kraft R. Nausea and vomiting. In: Rakel RE, Bope ET, editors. Conn's Current Therapy 2010. Philadelphia, WB: Saunders; 2009. pp. 5–9.

Gaseousness and Dyspepsia

Method of
Scott Owings, MD

Gaseousness

Gaseousness includes three disorders: belching, flatulence, and bloating. Because patients may interpret symptoms of abdominal pain, early satiety, nausea, and constipation as excess gas, it is important for the physician to elicit a careful description of the patient's complaint. Often, an exact etiology is not found, making treatment difficult. Although the symptoms are usually benign and secondary to diet and eating habits, one must consider etiologies such as gastrointestinal infection, obstruction, malabsorptive processes, dysmotility syndromes, irritable bowel syndrome (IBS), and psychiatric illness.

NORMAL PHYSIOLOGY

The normal volume of gas in the gastrointestinal tract is less than 200 mL, and normal expulsion during a 24-hour period averages 600 to 700 mL. Up to 25 episodes of flatus daily is considered normal, with the average being 14. Ninety-nine percent of intestinal gas consists of nitrogen (N_2), oxygen (O_2), carbon dioxide (CO_2), hydrogen (H_2), and methane (CH_4). The concentration and quantity of gas are determined primarily by three mechanisms: air swallowing, intraluminal production, and diffusion from blood. Air swallowing is responsible for the majority of N_2 and O_2. Intraluminal gas production is responsible for the majority of CO_2, H_2, and CH_4, which are products of bacterial metabolism. Some CO_2 can be produced by the interaction of acid and bicarbonate. The majority of gas in flatus is a product of colonic bacterial metabolism.

PATHOGENESIS

Gaseousness, in particular symptoms of bloating and increased flatus, are most commonly the result of excess gas production, abnormal gas transit, or increased visceral sensitivity to normal amounts of gas. Increased intestinal gas production is commonly caused by carbohydrate maldigestion, such as that seen in patients with lactose intolerance or a diet high in fructose, sorbitol, and starches, which are poorly absorbed. High-fiber diets, celiac disease, and small intestine bacterial overgrowth can increase gas production. Dysmotility is seen with gastroparesis and chronic intestinal pseudo-obstruction, both of which are associated with diabetes mellitus, scleroderma, amyloidosis, and endocrine disease. Patients with previous Nissen fundoplication, fat intolerance, and various familial conditions may have dysmotility. Increased visceral sensitivity is thought to be the pathophysiology in patients with functional bowel disorders such as IBS and functional dyspepsia.

EVALUATION

Typically, a thorough history and physical examination are all that are needed in the evaluation of gaseousness, unless underlying organic disease is suggested. Symptoms such as weight loss, rectal bleeding, fever, vomiting, steatorrhea, nocturnal abdominal pain, and diarrhea indicate structural disease and warrant further evaluation. The dietary history may reveal a close association with specific foods such as certain vegetables and fruits, legumes, or foods containing lactose or fructose. The history may also elicit underlying anxiety or psychiatric illness. The physical examination should include a detailed abdominal inspection and a search for signs of endocrine or neurologic processes as well as nutritional deficiency. Laboratory testing should be aimed at excluding organic disease and may include a complete blood count (CBC), complete metabolic profile (CMP), amylase, erythrocyte sedimentation rate, thyroid-stimulating hormone, and stool studies. Serum testing for anti-endomysium (EMA) and tissue transglutaminase (TTG) antibodies is helpful in screening for celiac sprue. Imaging techniques such as plain films, barium studies, ultrasonography, and computed tomography may be helpful, particularly if ileus or obstruction is suspected. Endoscopy may be warranted when biopsies are necessary. Hydrogen breath testing is indicated in the work-up of carbohydrate maldigestion or of small intestinal bacterial overgrowth. Gastric emptying scanning and gastrointestinal manometry are helpful in the evaluation of dysmotility syndromes and chronic intestinal pseudo-obstruction.

Belching

Belching, or eructation, is the retrograde expulsion of esophageal or gastric gas from the mouth. It may result from increased air swallowing with eating meals; drinking carbonated beverages; chewing gum; smoking; anxiety; or aerophagia, which is a functional disorder caused by habitual air swallowing. Patients with gastroesophageal reflux disease (GERD) often increase air swallowing in an attempt to decrease heartburn. It may also be caused by relaxation of the lower esophageal sphincter, which is associated with certain foods such as mints and chocolate. Treatment should be aimed at decreasing air swallowing by eating and drinking slowly, avoiding causative agents, stopping smoking, and treating heartburn.

Flatulence

As mentioned earlier, up to 25 episodes of flatus daily is considered normal. Most patients complaining of increased flatus are not exceeding this level. Because gas volume is difficult to determine, counting episodes of flatus over a 24-hour period is the most reliable measure. Because increased flatus is a common early symptom in patients with maldigestive diseases, the diagnosis should be considered in patients found to have excessive flatus production. A thorough history and physical examination may be all that are necessary for the evaluation of flatulence. If no organic etiology is suspected, treatment should be aimed at dietary modifications. Undergarments and cushions made to reduce malodorous flatus are available.

Bloating

Bloating is perceived by patients to be the sensation of excess abdominal gas. However, studies have failed to confirm a difference in volume or composition of gas between patients complaining of bloating and asymptomatic controls. Although more studies are needed, the symptom of bloating that accompanies functional bowel disorders, such as IBS, is thought to be caused by delayed transit times and visceral hypersensitivity. Functional bloating is a diagnosis of exclusion, and causes such as dysmotility syndromes, malabsorptive processes, infection, and intestinal obstruction should be considered.

TREATMENT

If a cause of gaseousness is not found, treatment may be difficult. Mainstays of management include dietary modification and prescription of nonmedicinal and medicinal therapies. Avoiding foods that are contributory, such as those containing lactose, fructose, sorbitol, high fiber, and starches, may be all that is necessary. Various cooking methods have been proposed, as well as a low-gas diet that includes decreased amounts of complex carbohydrates. Hypnotherapy may be helpful in reducing bloating and flatulence in IBS patients and in patients with intractable eructation.

Many medications are available to treat gaseousness and bloating, but there are limited data to support their use. Enzyme preparations such as B-galactosidase (lactase) and encapsulated pancreatic enzymes may be helpful if a deficiency is suspected. Bacterial α-galactosidase (Beano)[7] may be helpful in legume-rich diets. Simethicone (Mylicon) has not been proven to be helpful. Activated charcoal[1] and bismuth compounds such as Pepto-Bismol[1] have some supporting evidence in decreasing the amount of flatus and its odor. Antibiotics are helpful when small intestinal bacterial overgrowth is suspected. Prokinetics such as metoclopramide (Reglan) are helpful in dysmotility syndromes such as diabetic gastroparesis but are not beneficial in the treatment of postoperative ileus. Cisapride (Propulsid) and tegaserod (Zelnorm), both prokinetics pulled from the U.S. market, were beneficial in specific populations. At this point, there are insufficient data to support the use of probiotics such as *Lactobacillus* and *Acidophilus*. In general, narcotics and anticholinergics should be avoided.

---

[1]Not FDA approved for this indication.
[7]Available as dietary supplement.

CURRENT DIAGNOSIS

Gaseousness

- Perform a thorough history and physical examination.
- Identify associated triggers such as smoking, medication, diet, and psychosocial factors.
- Identify warning symptoms, such as weight loss, rectal bleeding, fever, vomiting, steatorrhea, and diarrhea, that warrant further work-up.
- Laboratory and imaging studies should be reserved for ruling out organic disease.
- Hydrogen breath testing is done for maldigestion, malabsorption, and bacterial overgrowth.
- Gastric emptying scanning and manometry are done for dysmotility syndromes and pseudo-obstruction.

Dyspepsia

- Rule out common diagnoses (gastroesophageal reflux disease, use of nonsteroidal antiinflammatory drugs, peptic ulcer disease, irritable bowel syndrome).
- If patient is <55 years of age and no alarm features are present, test for *Helicobacter pylori*.
- *H. pylori* testing is done by serology, urea breath test, stool antigen, or biopsy.
- If patient is >55 years of age or alarm features are present, consider esophagogastroduodenoscopy.
- Alarm features include family history of upper gastrointestinal cancer, weight loss, gastrointestinal bleeding, persistent vomiting, dysphagia, and anemia.
- In 60% of cases, the diagnostic evaluation does not identify a cause; this is termed functional dyspepsia.

Dyspepsia

Dyspepsia has recently been redefined by the so-called Rome III committee, replacing the previous definition of a persistent or recurrent pain or discomfort centered in the upper abdomen. The new definition requires one or more symptoms of postprandial fullness, early satiation, or epigastric pain or burning. Dyspepsia need not be associated with meals, as the term "indigestion" would suggest. Classic heartburn and regurgitation are not included in the definition and are typically more indicative of GERD. The diagnosis is often difficult clinically, because there is significant overlap between symptoms and the pathophysiology is poorly understood.

DIFFERENTIAL DIAGNOSIS

The differential diagnosis can be divided into the categories of functional (nonulcer) dyspepsia and dyspepsia caused by structural or biochemical disease. Functional dyspepsia is defined as symptoms of persistent or recurrent dyspepsia experienced for at least 12 weeks during the preceding 12 months with no evidence of organic disease. Functional dyspepsia accounts for up to 60% of patients with dyspepsia. The pathogenesis is unclear, but current investigation involves the study of gastric motor function, visceral sensitivity, *Helicobacter pylori* infection, and psychosocial factors.

The three most common causes of structural disease are peptic ulcer disease (15%-25%), reflux esophagitis (5%-15%), and gastric or gastroesophageal cancer (1%-2%). Other causes of structural disease include biliary tract disease, gastroparesis, pancreatitis, ischemic bowel disease, and chronic abdominal wall pain. Causes of biochemical disease include drug-induced dyspepsia, carbohydrate malabsorption, and metabolic disturbances.

DIAGNOSIS AND MANAGEMENT

Because functional dyspepsia is a diagnosis of exclusion, a thorough workup is necessary. The medical history may be helpful to identify other common diagnoses, such as GERD, use of nonsteroidal antiinflammatory drugs or cyclooxygenase 2 inhibitors, peptic ulcer disease, and IBS. The physical examination is usually normal in isolated dyspepsia. Signs of anemia or other disease processes should be investigated. Stool should be checked for occult blood. Laboratory studies should include a CBC to check for anemia. Other testing may include pancreatic enzyme levels, liver function tests, and electrolytes if other etiologies are suggested.

The American Gastroenterological Association suggests that patients 55 years of age or younger who have none of the so-called alarm symptoms should be tested for *H. pylori*, using the urea breath test or a stool antigen test, and treated if positive. If *H. pylori* tests are negative or symptoms persist despite eradication, then it is reasonable to try a proton pump inhibitor (PPI) for 4 to 6 weeks. If symptoms continue, the physician should consider doubling the dose of the PPI or assessing the patient with esophagogastroduodenoscopy. Patients older than 55 years of age and younger patients with alarm features should be directly evaluated with endoscopy and *H. pylori* testing. If the work-up is negative and a trial of a PPI has failed, then reevaluation is indicated. If no other source is found and IBS, gastroparesis, and pancreatic, colon, biliary tract, and psychological disorders can be reasonably excluded, then the condition should be treated as for functional dyspepsia.

THERAPY

If a cause of dyspepsia is diagnosed, treatment should be aimed at the underlying diagnosis. The remainder of this section focuses solely on the treatment of functional dyspepsia. It is important to validate the

CURRENT THERAPY

Gaseousness

- Etiology indentified; treat appropriately
- Decrease air swallowing (stop smoking, carbonated beverages, and chewing gum; eat and drink more slowly, treat heartburn)
- Avoid causative agents (lactose, fructose, sorbitol, high fiber, starches, caffeine, mint, chocolate)
- Simethicone (Mylicon) has not proved to be helpful.
- Enzyme preparations such as lactase and pancreatic enzymes if deficiency is suspected
- Bacterial α-galactosidase (Beano)[7] in legume-rich diets
- Antibiotics for small intestinal bacterial overgrowth
- Prokinetics such as metoclopramide (Reglan) for dysmotility syndromes
- Avoid narcotics and anticholinergics.
- Cisapride (Propulsid) and tegaserod (Zelnorm) have been pulled from the U.S. market.

Dyspepsia

- Etiology indentified; treat appropriately
- *Helicobacter pylori* eradication
- Functional dyspepsia
  - Validate diagnosis; provide education and reassurance.
  - Address associated psychosocial factors.
  - Smoking cessation
  - Avoidance of triggers
  - Antidepressants, prokinetics, and H_2 receptor antagonist therapy are beneficial in some groups.
  - Empiric proton pump inhibitor therapy has established efficacy.

---

[7]Available as dietary supplement.

diagnosis, provide education, and reassure the patient of the benign nature of the diagnosis. The physician should set realistic treatment goals while limiting invasive testing and targeting pharmacotherapy toward predominant symptoms. Patients should be advised to quit smoking, discontinue ulcerogenic medications if feasible, and avoid foods or other contributory triggers. Addressing associated psychosocial factors may help alleviate symptoms.

Multiple trials have been performed to evaluate the effectiveness of a wide range of pharmacologic treatments, primarily by comparing them to placebo response (which is 30%-60%). Groups of medications with insufficient evidence of effectiveness or lack of a statistically significant response include H_2 receptor antagonists, prokinetics, misoprostol (Cytotec),[1] sucralfate (Carafate),[1] anticholinergics and antimuscarinics, antidepressants, psychological therapies, herbal therapies, and antacids, although some treatment trials do support the use of antidepressants, prokinetics, and H_2 receptor antagonist therapy in selected groups. PPI therapy has established efficacy in the treatment of functional dyspepsia. If *H. pylori* is present, eradication may improve symptoms.

---

[1]Not FDA approved for this indication.

REFERENCES

Bazaldua OV, Schneider FD. Evaluation and management of dyspepsia. Am Fam Physician 1999;60(6):1773–84, 1787–8.

Hasler WL. Approach to the patient with gas and bloating. In: Yamada T, editor. Textbook of Gastroenterology. Philadelphia: Lippincott Williams & Wilkins; 2003. p. 802–10.

Longstreth GF. Functional dyspepsia, UpToDate; June 2008. Available at http://www.uptodate.com (accessed May 26, 2009).

Suzuki H, Nishizawa T, Hibi T. Therapeutic strategies for functional dyspepsia and the introduction of the Rome III classification. J Gastroenterol 2006;41(6):513–23.

Talley NJ. American Gastroenterological Association medical position statement: Evaluation of dyspepsia. Gastroenterology 2005;129(5):1753–5.

Talley NJ, Holtmann G. Approach to the patient with dyspepsia and related functional gastrointestinal complaints. In: Yamada T, editor. Textbook of Gastroenterology. Philadelphia: Lippincott Williams & Wilkins; 2003. p. 655–71.

Talley NJ, Vakil NB, Moayyedi P. American Gastroenterological Association technical review on the evaluation of dyspepsia. Gastroenterology 2005;129:1756–80.

Hiccups

Method of
Federico Bilotta, MD, PhD, and
Giovanni Rosa, MD

Epidemiology

Hiccups—brief bursts of intense inspiratory activity involving the diaphragm and inspiratory intercostal muscles, with reciprocal inhibition of the expiratory intercostal muscles—might result from structural or functional disturbances of the medulla or afferent-efferent nerves of the respiratory muscles. Hiccups are common, benign, and usually transient; it affects almost everyone in a lifespan. Some conditions, including gastric distention, excessive alcohol intake, anesthesia, and neck, thoracic, or abdominal surgery facilitate hiccups. Rarely, it becomes persistent or intractable and can lead to significant adverse effects including malnutrition, weight loss, fatigue, dehydration, insomnia, and wound dehiscence. Intractable hiccups can also reflect serious underlying disease. Hiccups, have no known physiologic function, and can be defined according to the duration of the episodes distinguishing hiccup attack or bout (<48 hours), persistent hiccup (>48 hours), chronic hiccup (hiccup lasting >2 months). Hiccups that are resistant to nonpharmacologic and pharmacologic therapies described in the literature should be defined as refractory.

Pathophysiology

Hiccups result from stimulation of one or more components of the "hiccup reflex arc" that comprises nerve and muscle structures between the base of the fourth cerebral ventricle, the vagus and phrenic nerves (from their origin at C3-C5 and along their course), the anterior scalene, intercostals, and diaphragmatic muscles. The hiccup reflex arc also has connections with the truncus and the mesencephali, the respiratory center, the medullary reticular formation, the hypothalamus, and the phrenic nerve nuclei.

CURRENT DIAGNOSIS

- Hiccup is a spasm of the diaphragm resulting in a rapid, involuntary inhalation stopped by the sudden closure of the glottis.
- When hiccups persist (i.e., last >48 hours), the suggested diagnostic work-up includes esophagogastroduodenoscopy, complete blood count, and chest X-ray. If these investigations yield negative findings, noninvasive brain imaging should be performed.

Benign, self-limited bouts of hiccups often arise after gastric distention from excessive food or alcohol intake, aerophagy, gastric insufflations, or strong thermic excursions. Persistent and refractory hiccups have different origins: organic, psychogenic, or idiopathic. Organic triggering mechanisms belong to three subgroups: central, peripheral, toxic, and metabolic or pharmacologic. Central causes include infectious organic lesions of the brain such as meningitis, encephalitis, and syphilis; cerebral or spinal tumor; vascular causes, such as ischemic episodes and hemorrhagic stroke (especially subarachnoid hemorrhage); head trauma; and cerebral arteriovenous malformations (i.e., dolichoectasia). Peripheral causes include any irritation of the vagus and phrenic nerves, stimulation of the meningeal afferents by meningitis, and stimulation of the pharyngeal or laryngeal nerve by pharyngitis, peritonsillar abscess, goiter, cysts, or tumor of the neck. Stimulation of the thoracic branches can result from chest trauma, bronchial or mediastinal tumor, pulmonary edema, pleuritis, mediastinitis, esophagitis, dissection of the thoracic aorta, pneumonia, bronchitis, empyema, and direct surgical manipulation. Hiccups related to indirect nerve stimulation arise from stimulation of the afferent vagus nerve branches, for example by peptic ulcer, gastritis, intestinal obstructions, intestinal inflammatory diseases, disorders of the genitourinary apparatus, hepatitis, or surgical manipulation of the abdominal organs. Other possible causes include hiatal hernia and diaphragmatic inflammation secondary to a perihepatic or subphrenic abscess. Hiccups developing during or after general anesthesia are variably attributed to central nervous system suppression, hyperextension of the neck, glottal stimulation due to intubation, or gastric distention secondary to mask ventilation. Several toxic and pathologic metabolic states such as uremia, sepsis, and alcohol intoxication can cause hiccups. Psychogenic causes, accounting for up to 50% of the cases of persistent refractory hiccups, include stress, excitement, suicidal ingestion of toxic substances, and anorexia nervosa.

Complications

The major complications are dehydration and weight loss resulting from inability to tolerate fluids and food. Hiccups can occasionally lead to cardiac arrhythmias due to low blood potassium levels. Ingesting large amounts of fluids to stop hiccups can result in low blood sodium levels, a condition that itself stimulates neurogenic hiccup.

Therapy

Treatment modalities for hiccups can be roughly categorized as nonpharmacologic or pharmacologic. Nonpharmacologic management consists of reversing possible underlying causes, including relieving esophageal obstruction or gastric distention. Raising carbon dioxide pressure reduces hiccup frequency; this therapeutic approach provides the physiologic basis for the common and often effective "breathe-into-a-paper-bag" technique. Several methods of vagal stimulation, including tongue, larynx, and external auditory canal stimulation, have been used in attempts to terminate hiccup episodes. In selected cases phrenic nerve or diaphragmatic pacing stimulation or surgical interruption of the phrenic nerve have been used.

CURRENT THERAPY

- Nonpharmacologic therapies include various forms of vagal stimulation, hypercapnia, and phrenic nerve or diaphragmatic pacing stimulation or surgical interruption.
- Pharmacologic therapies include long-lasting local anesthetics for phrenic nerve blockade (bupivacaine)[1] and several systemic drugs (baclofen,[1] carbamazepine,[1] chlorpromazine, haloperidol,[1] ketamine,[1] lidocaine,[1] metoclopramide,[1] nefopam,[2] nifedipine,[1] nimodipine,[1] and phenytoin[1]).

[1]Not FDA approved for this indication.
[2]Not available in the United States.

Among the pharmacologic therapies, the selective infiltration of phrenic nerve with long-lasting local anesthetics (bupivacaine [Marcaine][1]) has been described. Systemic pharmacologic therapies include administration of baclofen (Lioresal),[1] carbamazepine (Tegretol),[1] chlorpromazine (Thorazine), haloperidol (Haldol),[1] ketamine (Ketalar),[1] lidocaine (Xylocaine),[1] metoclopramide (Reglan),[1] nefopam (Acupan),[2] nifedipin (Adalat),[1] nimodipine (Nimotop),[1] and phenytoin (Dilantin).[1] Baclofen (Lioresal), a drug active on the smooth muscles with antispasticity properties, is often effective when given at 5 mg orally up to 3 times a day. Chlorpromazine and haloperidol, antipsychotic drugs, are among the most widely used systemic therapies for in-hospital hiccups treatment. Carbamazepine and phenytoin, anticonvulsant drugs, often effective in patients having hiccups of central origin. Metoclopramide, an antiemetic drug with central antidopaminergic effects, is effective in patients with hiccups of central or gastric origin; it should be given orally or IV at the dose of 10 mg up to 4 times daily. Nifedipine and nimodipine, calcium antagonist drugs, are often effective probably owing to antispasticity effects on smooth muscles. In some cases of hiccups resistant to several of these therapies, the nonopioid analgesic drug nefopam, injected at a dose of 10 mg IV over 10 seconds, was effective in treating hiccups of central and peripheral origin.

---

[1]Not FDA approved for this indication.
[2]Not available in the United States.

Conclusions

Hiccup is a rare clinical condition that can occur as isolated symptom of an underlying disease; when persistent or chronic can lead to devastating consequences. A standard therapeutic approach does not exist. Noninvasive and nonpharmacologic therapies should be considered as first-line treatment. A dedicated diagnostic work-up for patients with persisting hiccups (lasting >48 hours) and chronic intractable hiccups might be helpful in ruling out underlying diseases that could be treated causally. A diagnostic work-up for persistent and chronic intractable hiccups includes the following: esophagogastroduodenoscopy, complete blood count, and chest x-ray and, if these investigations yield negative findings, noninvasive brain imaging.

REFERENCES

Bilotta F, Doronzio A, Martini S. Bulbar compression due to vertebrobasilar artery dolichoectasia causing persistent hiccups in a patient successfully treated with diuretics and corticosteroids. J Clin Chin Med 2008; 3:706–8.

Bilotta F, Pietropaoli P, Rosa G. Nefopam for refractory postoperative hiccups. Anesth Analg 2001;93:1358–60.

Bilotta F, Rosa G. Nefopam for severe hiccups. N Engl J Med 2000; 343:1973–2204.

Dunst MN, Margolin K, Horak D. Lidocaine for severe hiccups. N Engl J Med 1993;329:890–1.

Hernandez JL, Fernandez-Miera MF, Sampedro E, et al. Nimodipine treatment for intractable hiccups. Am J Med 1999;106:600.

Howard SR. Persistent hiccups. Br Med J 1992;305:1237–8.

Kolodzik PW, Eilers MA. Hiccups (singultus): review and approach to management. Ann Emerg Med 1991;20:565–73.

Newsom Davis J. An experimental study of hiccup. Brain 1970;93:851–72.

Souadjian J, Cain J. Intractable hiccups: etiological factors in 220 cases. Postgrad Med 1968;43:72–7.

Wagner M, Stapezynski J. Persistent hiccups. Ann Emerg Med 1982;11:24–6.

Acute Infectious Diarrhea

Method of
Matthew T. Oughton, MD, FRCPC, and Andre Dascal, MD, FRCPC

Diarrhea is defined as production of at least 200 g of stool per day. However, accurate measurement of stool mass is impractical and is most often used only in clinical trials. A more functional definition of diarrhea is an increase in stool frequency and liquidity compared to the patient's usual bowel habit. Diarrhea is generally classified as acute if it lasts no more than 14 days, persistent if longer than 14 days, and chronic if longer than 30 days.

Clinically, there are two major types of diarrhea. Secretory diarrhea is watery, usually produced in large volumes, and contains little or no blood or leukocytes. Inflammatory diarrhea is bloody, usually has leukocytes, and is produced in smaller volumes. Recognizing the class of diarrhea can be useful in suggesting etiologies and in managing the diarrhea.

The precise cause of a case of diarrhea is usually difficult to ascertain, because diarrhea is a nonspecific reaction by the intestine to numerous insults, including infections, toxins, and autoimmune disorders. Acute infectious diarrhea, by definition, is caused by a microbial pathogen. Although infections are the leading cause of diarrhea, many different pathogens cause acute infectious diarrhea, and the likelihood of any particular agent depends on the patient's age, symptoms, and epidemiologic risk factors.

In immunocompetent adults in the developed world, acute infectious diarrhea is most often a minor and self-resolving ailment. Recent data for the United States estimate an annual burden of between 211 million and 375 million cases, with more than 900,000 hospitalizations and 6000 deaths. However, acute infectious diarrhea can cause severe illness in infants, immunocompromised patients, and malnourished patients; it remains a major cause of global morbidity and mortality. The World Health Organization (WHO) estimates that more than 4 billion cases of acute infectious diarrhea occur each year worldwide and attributes 2 million deaths (5% of all deaths) to diarrheal diseases annually. Most of these deaths are in children who are younger than 5 years and live in developing countries.

Thorough investigation of a patient with acute diarrhea should include a detailed history, physical examination, and laboratory tests (Boxes 1 and 2). In general, clinical investigation of an individual case of acute infectious diarrhea is more useful in identifying sequelae of diarrhea, such as dehydration, than it is in revealing the exact etiologic agent. However, identification of the causative organism can sometimes reveal the existence of a common-source outbreak. One well-known example occurred in 1994, when the state public health laboratory in Minnesota noted an increase in *Salmonella* serotype enteritidis detected in submitted samples; this ultimately led to the recognition of a multistate *Salmonella* outbreak related to improperly cleaned ice cream trucks.

BOX 2   Physical Examination for Acute Infectious Diarrhea

- Vital signs
  - Blood pressure (look for postural changes)
  - Heart rate (look for postural changes)
  - Respiratory rate
  - Temperature
  - Weight (particularly useful to assess effects of rehydration)
- Cardiovascular examination
  - Volume status (jugular venous pressure)
- Respiratory examination
- Rule out hyperventilation (compensatory respiratory alkalosis for metabolic acidosis due to dehydration and loss of bicarbonate)
- Abdominal examination
  - Focal tenderness
  - Guarding
  - Hepatosplenomegaly
  - Consider rectal examination (look for bloody stool)
- Integument examination
  - Lymphadenopathy
  - Rashes (rose spots)

Etiology

It is uncommon to identify the exact etiologic agent in a case of acute infectious diarrhea. However, in some clinical situations, exact identification is important for determining optimal management or possible sequelae. The treatment of inflammatory diarrhea varies depending on the causative organism, and some diseases require alterations in therapy (e.g., suspected *Campylobacter* resistance to fluoroquinolones) or even avoidance of antibiotic therapy (e.g., enterohemorrhagic *Escherichia coli*, in which antibiotic therapy has been associated with more frequent adverse outcomes) (Boxes 3 and 4).

BACTERIA

Escherichia coli

E. coli is a versatile pathogen that causes a wide spectrum of disease affecting numerous organ systems. This is illustrated by the wide variety of diarrheagenic *E. coli*, including enterotoxigenic (ETEC),

---

BOX 1   Clinical History for Acute Infectious Diarrhea

- Description of diarrhea
  - Duration
  - Frequency
  - Presence of blood, pus, "grease" in stool
  - Symptoms of fever, tenesmus, dehydration
  - Weight loss
- Other GI symptoms
  - Anorexia
  - Cramping
  - Emesis
  - Nausea
- Previous episodes with similar symptoms
- Ill contacts with similar symptoms
- Recent antibiotic exposure
- Other medication exposure
  - Anticholinergics
  - Antimotility agents
  - Aspirin (ASA)
  - Proton pump inhibitors (PPIs)
- Recent dietary history
  - Shellfish
  - Undercooked meat (chicken)
  - Unsanitary water
- Animal contacts
  - Turtles
  - Other reptiles
- Travel history
  - Travel to endemic or epidemic areas
- Sexual history
- Vaccination history
- Contact with institutions, e.g., hospitals, nursing homes, daycare facilities
- Employment history
- Immune status
  - Presence of HIV
  - Presence of other congenital or acquired immunodeficiencies

---

BOX 3   Etiologic Agents of Predominantly Secretory Diarrhea

Bacterial
- Enteroaggregative *Escherichia coli* (EAEC)
- Enterotoxigenic *E. coli* (ETEC)
- Vibrio cholerae

Viral
- Adenovirus (types 40 and 41)
- Astrovirus
- Caliciviruses (Norwalk, Sapporo)
- Rotavirus

Protozoal
- *Cryptosporidium*
- *Cyclospora*
- *Dientamoeba fragilis*
- *Giardia lamblia*
- *Isospora belli*
- Microspora species (especially *Enterocytozoon bieneusi*)

BOX 4   Etiologic Agents of Predominantly Inflammatory Diarrhea

Bacterial
- *Aeromonas* sp.
- *Bacteroides fragilis* (enterotoxigenic strains)
- *Campylobacter* sp. (particularly FQ-resistant strains)
- *Clostridium difficile* (toxigenic strains)
- *Escherichia coli* (enterohemorrhagic, enteroinvasive)
- *Pleisomonas* sp.
- *Shigella* sp.
- *Salmonella enterica* serotypes *typhi* and *paratyphi*
- Nontyphoid *Salmonella* species
- Noncholera *Vibrio* species
- *Yersinia*

Protozoal
- *Entamoeba histolytica*

enteroaggregative (EAEC), enterohemorrhagic (EHEC), enteropathogenic (EPEC), and enteroinvasive (EIEC) strains. In general, people are exposed to diarrheagenic *E. coli* by consuming contaminated food and water.

ETEC is a major cause of infantile diarrhea and traveler's diarrhea. Infantile diarrhea affects infants usually in developing countries, particularly during warm and wet conditions, and traveler's diarrhea affects the immunologically naive tourist under similar conditions. In both cases, a large inoculum is required to cause disease. Major virulence factors of ETEC strains include species-specific fimbriae for enterocyte adherence, as well as heat-stable and heat-labile plasmid-encoded enterotoxins. After a relatively brief incubation period of 1 to 2 days, the infected patient develops a secretory diarrhea that lasts up to 5 days. The cornerstones of management are prevention (through dietary hygiene) and adequate rehydration. Antibiotics use is controversial and usually reserved for moderate to severe disease.

EAEC is recognized as a major cause of children's and traveler's diarrhea. Since the initial identification of EAEC in 1985, studies have identified numerous putative virulence factors, including specific aggregative adherence fimbriae. However, no one factor has been identified in all EAEC strains. This suggests that apart from their aggregative adherence to enterocytes, EAEC strains are probably a heterogeneous collection. However, the clinical disease caused by EAEC is relatively consistent and includes persistent secretory diarrhea with low-grade fever. Management of disease from EAEC requires adequate rehydration; the role of antibiotics remains controversial.

The notorious virulence of EHEC (also known as Shiga-like toxin–producing *E. coli*) has led to frequent media reports of "hamburger disease." *E. coli* O157:H7 is the most common strain of EHEC, although several others have been documented. Unlike most other categories of diarrheagenic *E. coli*, EHEC can cause disease with an infectious dose as low as 10 to 100 organisms. Sequelae of EHEC infection include hemorrhagic diarrhea, hemolytic-uremic syndrome, and thrombotic thrombocytopenic purpura. The primary virulence factor is Shiga-like toxin, which damages ribosomes. The gene for Shiga-like toxin is transmitted between EHEC strains by a bacteriophage vector. A separate virulence plasmid has been identified in certain strains of EHEC, but its significance is uncertain. Management of EHEC disease is supportive, because some evidence suggests that antibiotics can enhance the release of Shiga-like toxin and increase the risk of developing hemolytic-uremic syndrome.

EPEC has been associated most strongly with pediatric diarrhea in both epidemic and sporadic forms. EPEC adheres to enterocytes, causing the pathognomic attaching and effacing lesion seen on pathologic section. It then secretes proteins that initiate signal transduction within the enterocyte, ultimately resulting in secretory diarrhea. Because EPEC causes persistent diarrhea that can lead to significant dehydration, rehydration and antibiotic therapy are usually indicated.

As its name implies, EIEC invades enterocytes, where it then replicates and spreads to adjacent cells. The resulting diarrhea may be secretory or inflammatory and lasts up to 7 days. EIEC is closely related to *Shigella* genetically and in the clinical disease that they both cause. As with *Shigella*, antibiotic treatment reduces duration of symptomatic illness.

Shigella Species

The genus *Shigella* consists of four serovars pathogenic to humans: *Shigella sonnei* (Group A), *Shigella flexneri* (Group B), *Shigella boydii* (Group C), and *Shigella dysenteriae* (Group D). *S. sonnei*, the most commonly isolated species, typically causes secretory diarrhea, and the remaining *Shigella* species cause bacillary dysentery with fever, bloody diarrhea, cramping, and tenesmus. As with the typhoid group of *Salmonella*, humans are the sole host for *Shigella* species; however, the low infectious dose required by *Shigella* species to cause disease is more similar to the nontyphoid *Salmonella* species.

Salmonella Species

For clinical purposes, the genus *Salmonella* can be divided into two broad groups: typhoid and nontyphoid.

The typhoid group, consisting of *Salmonella enterica* serotypes *typhi* and *paratyphi*, causes typhoid (enteric) fever. These organisms exclusively infect human hosts and are transmitted via contaminated food or water. A large inoculum of typhoid group bacteria is required to experimentally produce infection. Some infected persons become chronic carriers who can transmit infection to others, such as the infamous Typhoid Mary. Typhoid fever is endemic in the developing world. The classic presentation of typhoid fever evolves over 3 weeks: a stepwise fever with temperature-pulse dissociation in the first week, abdominal pain and rose spots on the trunk in the second week, and hepatosplenomegaly with intestinal bleeding in the third week. Because these species are only transmitted between human hosts, identification of one case of typhoid fever becomes a public health issue that mandates contact tracing. Possible complications include bacteremia, gastrointestinal bleeding or perforation, cholangitis, pneumonia, and osteomyelitis.

The nontyphoid group consists of all *Salmonella* species except *S. enterica* serotypes *typhi* and *paratyphi*. These species generally incubate in animals and are transmitted to humans through consumption of contaminated food or water; direct human-to-human transmission is exceedingly rare. In contrast to the typhoid group, nontyphoid *Salmonella* species can cause disease with inocula as low as 10 to 100 organisms. The disease that results is most often a gastroenteritis with fever, emesis, and diarrhea that can be secretory or inflammatory, lasting up to 7 days. Possible complications include bacteremia, endovascular infection from seeding of atherosclerotic plaques or prosthetic grafts, and Reiter's syndrome.

Campylobacter Species

Campylobacter species are common bacterial causes of acute infectious diarrhea; *Campylobacter jejuni* is the major species that causes human disease. Infection is contracted through consumption of contaminated poultry, milk, or water. After an incubation period of 2 to 7 days, the patient develops bloody diarrhea. *Campylobacter* diarrhea is also notable for its manifold extraintestinal complications, including autoimmune phenomena such as reactive arthritis and Guillain-Barré syndrome. Antibiotic therapy is usually reserved for severe disease or immunocompromised patients, in whom recurrent disease is more frequent.

Vibrio cholerae

Vibrio cholerae is the prototype of an enterotoxic bacterium that causes secretory diarrhea. It is almost exclusively a disease of developing countries with poor sanitation. There have been several pandemics in the last century, with the most recent affecting South America and Central America as well the more typical regions in Africa and Asia. The only two serotypes to cause human disease are O1 and O139; serotype O1 is divided into biotypes *cholerae* and *eltor*.

Cholera toxin affects enterocytes to produce a secretory diarrhea described as *rice-water stools*. Disease severity ranges from mild to severe with profound dehydration. Rehydration is the cornerstone of treatment, via oral or intravenous routes as dictated by clinical severity.

Clostridium difficile

Clostridium difficile has been recognized as one cause of antibiotic-associated diarrhea and the leading cause of pseudomembranous colitis since the late 1970s. *C. difficile*–associated diarrhea was conventionally thought to only be a health issue for institutionalized patients who have had recent exposure to antibiotics or chemotherapy. In the last 5 years, however, significant expansions in *C. difficile*–associated diarrhea disease severity and host range have been described by researchers in North America and Europe. Disease severity ranges from asymptomatic colonization to mild diarrhea to fulminant pseudomembranous colitis resulting in colectomy, need for intensive care, and high attributable mortality rate.

Other Bacteria

Several other bacteria are less-common causes of acute infectious diarrhea. They merit some discussion because of their specific clinical presentations or potential for causing severe disease.

Vibrio parahemolyticus

Vibrio parahemolyticus causes gastrointestinal illness associated with consumption of raw or undercooked oysters and other seafood. The spectrum of illness varies widely. Immunocompetent patients usually develop self-limited secretory diarrhea or gastroenteritis with fever lasting from 1 to 3 days, and immunocompromised patients present with severe diarrhea, septicemia, and a profound hemolytic anemia.

Staphylococcus aureus

Staphylococcus aureus causes a variety of gastrointestinal illnesses. It is a common cause of enterotoxin-mediated foodborne illness, manifesting with emesis, watery diarrhea, and cramping after a brief incubation period of 1 to 6 hours. *S. aureus*, particularly methicillin-resistant *S. aureus* (MRSA), is also an uncommon but recognized cause of pseudomembranous colitis.

Bacteroides fragilis

Although *Bacteroides fragilis* is recognized as part of the normal flora of the large intestine, certain strains produce a metalloprotease that has been associated with diarrhea in several studies of human and animal populations. Some studies have suggested that these enterotoxigenic *B. fragilis* strains may be more likely than nontoxigenic strains to cause blood infections.

Clostridium perfringens

Clostridium perfringens is a ubiquitous pathogen that is a common cause of enterotoxin-mediated secretory diarrhea. Its specific enterotoxin (CPE) has been found in all five toxinotypes of *C. perfringens*. Gastrointestinal disease can result from ingestion of preformed toxin, with a short incubation period before clinical disease, or ingestion of a large bacterial inoculum, requiring a longer incubation before disease. Treatment is usually supportive.

PROTOZOA

Giardia lamblia

Giardia lamblia is a protozoan pathogen that causes diarrhea that can be chronic and refractory to treatment. The infectious cyst form is ingested in contaminated food or water, and the trophozoite then attaches to the intestinal wall. *Giardia* has expanded its environmental niche in recent years from the beaver fever endemic to isolated rivers and lakes, becoming a global pathogen.

Entamoeba histolytica

Entamoeba histolytica can cause amoebic dysentery, which can manifest as acute, subacute, or chronic diarrhea. Diagnosis of *E. histolytica* is complicated by the highly similar but nonpathogenic *Entamoeba dispar*. Other than the rare situation where microscopy of stool detects ingested erythrocytes (pathognomic of *E. histolytica*), the two species are morphologically identical and can only be distinguished by methodologies such as serology, antigen detection, or nucleic acid testing.

VIRUSES

Rotavirus

Rotavirus primarily affects infants and children from 3 to 36 months of age, resulting in a spectrum of disease from asymptomatic shedding to severe gastroenteritis with dehydration. Globally, it is the leading viral cause of severe gastroenteritis. Other groups affected include travelers, the immunocompromised, and patients in hospitals or other institutions.

Calicivirus

Norwalk virus is the most well-known member of the calicivirus family. Outbreaks of Norwalk often occur in long-term care facilities, cruise ships, and hospitals. It is highly contagious, with attack rates often greater than 10%. The clinical syndrome of Norwalk infection usually features rapid onset of severe nausea and emesis along with varying degrees of diarrhea.

Differential Diagnosis

OTHER INFECTIONS

Infections that cause diarrhea are not necessarily primarily gastrointestinal (Box 5). Systemic infections that result in diarrhea are probably underrecognized as a distinct etiology; however, the astute clinician should usually be able to recognize a systemic infection after a proper history, physical examination, and appropriate laboratory tests. Bacterial infections such as Group A streptococcosis, legionellosis, leptospirosis, and some tick-borne infections (including borreliosis, ehrlichosis, tularemia, and Rocky Mountain spotted fever) can

---

BOX 5   Diseases That Can Mimic Acute Infectious Diarrhea

Infectious Etiologies
- Dengue fever
- *Francisella* sp.
- Hantavirus
- *Legionella* sp.
- Leptospirosis
- Lyme borreliosis
- Malaria
- SARS

Noninfectious Etiologies
- Antibiotic-associated diarrhea
- Bacterial overgrowth
- Brainerd diarrhea (infectious etiology suspected but unproved)
- Endocrinopathies (e.g., VIPoma)
- Inflammatory bowel disease
- Irritable bowel syndrome
- Other medications

Abbreviations: SARS = severe acute respiratory syndrome; VIP = vasoactive intestinal peptide.

manifest with diarrhea as an initial symptom. Septicemia, caused by a variety of pathogens such as gram-negative enteric organisms, can also cause diarrhea and other gastrointestinal symptoms. Viremia is another cause of diarrhea; the most common cause is probably influenza, but other viruses including severe acute respiratory syndrome–associated coronavirus (SARS-CoV), hantaviruses, dengue virus (*Flavivirus* sp.), and hemorrhagic fever viruses should be considered in the presence of correlating exposures. *Plasmodium falciparum* malaria can result in diarrhea severe enough to mimic bacillary dysentery, particularly in children, and severe diarrhea has been associated with poor outcome.

OTHER NONINFECTIOUS ETIOLOGIES

A variety of noninfectious causes can result in acute diarrhea (see Box 5). For instance, diarrhea is a common adverse effect of antimicrobial agents and other medications. The mechanism varies by antibiotic, but common reasons include direct stimulation of gut motility, increased gut osmolality, and disruption of the normal gut flora.

Although not strictly an infection, diarrhea is one of the most common symptoms of bacterial overgrowth. This disease occurs after disruption of host mechanisms that normally regulate bacterial intestinal colonization, such as pancreatitis or intestinal dysmotility. Definitive treatment should address the underlying condition, but broad-spectrum antibiotics can result in a long-lasting cure.

Brainerd diarrhea was initially described after an outbreak in Brainerd, Minnesota, in 1983. It manifests as an acute secretory diarrhea that can last for several months. Its etiology remains unknown, but several outbreaks have demonstrated epidemiologic links to consumption of unpasteurized milk and undertreated water.

Some endocrinopathies, such as VIPoma, can cause profuse diarrhea. Inflammatory bowel diseases (e.g., Crohn's disease, ulcerative colitis) can manifest with an inflammatory diarrhea and constitutional symptoms. Irritable bowel syndrome can result in periods of diarrhea; however, there are alternating periods of constipation and a lack of constitutional symptoms.

Special Cases

TRAVELER'S DIARRHEA

According to the Centers for Disease Control and Prevention (CDC), 20% to 50% of international travelers develop diarrhea related to their travels. The etiologic agents vary by exposure, geographic region, and local outbreaks. Bacteria are the most commonly implicated pathogens, with ETEC being the most commonly identified cause. Other etiologic agents include the other common bacterial, viral, and protozoal enteric pathogens described earlier. Diarrhea is usually mild to moderate and self-limited; 90% of patients report resolution of symptoms after 1 week, and 98% after 4 weeks. Although it is usually a nuisance rather than a severe threat to health, diarrhea can significantly limit the traveler's activities.

Because traveler's diarrhea is self-limited, investigations of the cause are usually reserved for diarrhea that is prolonged or manifests with higher-risk features such as fever or bloody stool. Stool should be examined for ova and parasites (O&P) if the travel history is supportive.

The focus for management should be supportive care. People seen for travel medicine advice should be counseled to avoid consuming water or food not known to be safe. The safest diet for travelers consists of freshly prepared foods served thoroughly heated, fruits and vegetables that are peeled or are washed with safe water, and beverages that are bottled or boiled before consumption. Ice and tap water should be considered contaminated. Patients for whom diarrhea could be catastrophic should be advised to avoid traveling unless it is strictly necessary.

After the traveler has developed diarrhea, a variety of medications are available for treatment (Box 7). One review determined that antibiotics shorten the duration of traveler's diarrhea but had higher rates of adverse effects compared with placebo.

IMMUNOCOMPROMISED STATES

Gastrointestinal illness is a common problem in immunocompromised patients. Apart from the infectious etiologies of diarrhea described earlier, other causes found in immunocompromised patients include the agent causing the immunocompromised state (such as HIV or chemotherapeutic agents), opportunistic organisms, adverse effects of medications, dysfunction of intestinal absorption, and idiopathic enteropathies.

Opportunistic organisms that can cause diarrhea include parasites (e.g., *Cryptosporidium parvum, Cyclospora cayetanensis, Isospora belli,* microsporidia), fungi (e.g., disseminated fungal infections from *Histoplasma capsulatum* and *Cryptococcus neoformans*), bacteria (e.g., *Mycobacterium avium-intracellulare* complex), and viruses (e.g., cytomegalovirus, herpes simplex virus). In general, treatment requires prolonged courses of antimicrobial agents and can be complicated by concomitant medications or diseases; consultation with an appropriate specialist is suggested.

Prevention

Methods of prevention are listed in Box 6.

AVOIDANCE

An effective method for preventing acute infectious diarrhea is to eliminate exposures that put one at risk. This applies particularly to patients who would be at high risk for contracting acute infectious diarrhea or having adverse outcomes, for example, patients who are immunocompromised or physically debilitated. Exposure avoidance is usually situational and patient-specific, such as suggesting that travel be postponed to a region currently undergoing a cholera epidemic or cautioning against consumption of raw seafood.

HYGIENE

Proper handwashing by health care workers caring for patients with acute diarrhea is essential to prevent institutional transmission, and its importance cannot be overstated. Barrier precautions are also commonly implemented, particularly if the patient is incontinent of stool. Other precautions, such as tailoring environmental cleaning practices to specific pathogens during outbreaks, are also proven effective.

PROPHYLACTIC ANTIBIOTICS

There is a limited role for antibiotics in preventing acute infectious diarrhea, particularly traveler's diarrhea. The normally mild severity and self-limited nature of the disease, along with the risk of adverse effects from antibiotics, means that prophylactic antibiotics are most often reserved for brief durations in patients at high risk for contracting acute infectious diarrhea or for experiencing adverse outcomes.

BOX 6   Prevention of Acute Infectious Diarrhea

- Avoidance
- Hygiene
- Prophylactic antibiotics
- Probiotics
- Vaccines
  - Cholera/ETEC (Dukoral)[2]
  - Rotavirus (RotaTeq)
  - *Salmonella typhi* (Vivotif Berna, Typhim Vi)

---

[2]Not available in the United States.
Abbreviation: ETEC = enterotoxigenic *Escherichia coli*.

PROBIOTICS

There has been a surge of publications concerning the role of probiotics in preventing diarrhea of varying etiologies. Although individual studies have produced varied results for diarrhea caused by *C. difficile*–associated diarrhea and traveler's diarrhea, one meta-analysis of 34 studies supported a role for probiotics in preventing diarrhea, with an overall risk reduction of at least 21%. Stratification by type of diarrhea found a much larger reduction in antibiotic-associated (52%) than traveler's (8%) diarrhea. However, these findings were challenged due to the variety of organisms and treatment regimens between different studies, and the low proportion of adult patients in those studies reporting reductions in antibiotic-associated diarrhea.

VACCINES

Rotavirus

A live human-bovine reassortant rotavirus oral vaccine (RotaTeq) has been licensed since February 2006 in the United States for infants 6 to 32 weeks of age. The vaccine appears efficacious in preventing rotaviral gastroenteritis, and consequently it reduces the need for outpatient and inpatient assessment. A large phase III trial demonstrated no increased risk over placebo of intussusception, an adverse effect that led to the withdrawal of a previous rotavirus vaccine. An attenuated human rotavirus vaccine (RotaRix) is licensed in countries throughout Europe, Asia, and Africa, but not North America.

Vibrio cholerae and ETEC

An oral inactivated cholera vaccine (Dukoral), available in Canada but not in the United States, has demonstrated some efficacy in preventing traveler's diarrhea. The B subunit of *V. cholerae* toxin used in this vaccine has sufficient structural homology with ETEC heat-labile toxin to provide moderate short-term protection against this common cause of traveler's diarrhea, lasting up to 3 months.

CURRENT DIAGNOSIS

History

- Duration and frequency of diarrhea
- Other gastrointestinal symptoms (emesis, tenesmus, abdominal pain)
- Presence of bloody stool, fever
- Medication use, including recent antibiotic use
- Recent contact with ill persons, travel, and animal contact
- Consumption of raw or undercooked poultry or seafood
- Immunocompromised state (rule out)

Physical Examination

- Hydration status
- Gastrointestinal examination
- Other systems as indicated by symptoms

Laboratory Tests

- For limited secretory diarrhea: usually none
- For bloody diarrhea: complete blood count (CBC), stool for culture (rule out O157:H7); consider ova and parasites test (O&P)
- For chronic diarrhea: consider *C. difficile* assay, O&P
- For traveler's diarrhea: CBC, stool for culture, and O&P
- For immunocompromised patients: CBC, stool for culture, and O&P

Salmonella typhi

Enteral and parenteral vaccines are available to prevent typhoid. The enteral form (Vivotif Berna) is a live attenuated strain of *S. typhi*, which is taken as four capsules over 7 days and confers immunity for approximately 5 years. The parenteral form (Typhim Vi) is purified capsular polysaccharide that is given as a single intramuscular injection. This is the preferred route for patients with contraindications to live attenuated vaccines, such as immunocompromised status. Neither vaccine is completely protective, and neither provides protection against *S. paratyphi*.

Treatment

Management of acute infectious diarrhea is listed in Box 7.

REHYDRATION

Maintaining adequate hydration is usually the cornerstone of management for acute diarrhea. The route of administration depends on the patient's hydration status and disease severity; enteral hydration is preferred to parenteral, if possible.

In 2003 the WHO reformulated their well-known oral rehydration solution (ORS). The new lower-osmolarity formula has been found to reduce stool volume, emesis, and the need for switching to intravenous therapy in children with diarrhea. This new formulation has 75 mmol/L sodium, 75 mmol/L glucose, and a total osmolarity 245 mOsm/L, which can be achieved with a recipe of 2.6 g sodium chloride, 13.5 g anhydrous glucose, 1.5 g potassium chloride, 2.5 g sodium bicarbonate and 1.5 g trisodium citrate dihydrate per liter of water.

A homemade solution can be prepared with 40 mL sugar and 5 mL table salt per liter of clean water; however, this preparation lacks potassium. Furthermore, commercially prepared rehydration solutions should be preferred to homemade in order to minimize the chance of errors in preparing the solution. Most sports drinks are not equivalent to actual rehydration solutions, because sports drinks often have higher carbohydrate and lower electrolyte loads.

Parenteral rehydration is usually intravenous, although intraosseous administration can be used for infants in whom intravenous access cannot be obtained and enteroclysis can be used in adult patients with difficult vascular access who do not require large volumes of replacement fluid. Sufficient volumes of fluid should be given to replace preexisting fluid deficits as well as ongoing losses and maintenance requirements.

BOX 7 Management of Acute Infectious Diarrhea

Rehydration
- Enteral
  - World Health Organization formulation
  - Commercially available rehydration solutions
  - Home remedies
- Parenteral
  - Intravenous
  - Intraosseous
  - Enteroclysis

Medications
- Antidiarrheals
  - Bismuth subsalicylate
  - Morphine derivatives
- Antibiotics
- Probiotics

CURRENT THERAPY

- Supportive care
- Rehydration (always replace previous losses and provide maintenance)
  - Enteral
  - Parenteral (intravenous, intraosseous, enteroclytic)
- Antidiarrheal medications (only if patient is afebrile and stools are not bloody)
  - Morphine derivatives
  - Bismuth subsalicylate (Pepto-Bismol)
- Antibiotics (only if necessary as indicated by symptoms, severity, and risk factors)
  - Empiric therapy
    - Adults
      - Ciprofloxacin (Cipro) 500 mg PO bid for 3-5 d
      - Levofloxacin (Levaquin)[1] 500 mg PO qd for 3-5 d
    - Children
      - Azithromycin (Zithromax)[1] 5-10 mg/kg PO qd for 3-5 d
      - Trimethoprim-sulfamethoxazole (Septra) 5-25 mg/kg/d PO in two equally divided doses for 3-5 d *plus*
      - Erythromycin 10 mg/kg/d PO qid for 5 d
  - Specific therapy as directed by pathogen identification and susceptibilities
- Probiotics

[1]Not FDA approved for this indication.

ANTIDIARRHEAL MEDICATIONS

Some medications reduce intestinal motility by affecting the myenteric motor plexus to inhibit peristalsis. Opioid derivatives, such as loperamide (Imodium), are the class of medications most commonly used for this purpose. Although licensed for use with acute, chronic, and traveler's diarrhea, loperamide is contraindicated in the presence of fever or bloody stool or in situations where inhibition of peristalsis is otherwise undesirable or potentially harmful.

Other medications are classified as antidiarrheal but have different mechanisms of action. Bismuth subsalicylate (Pepto-Bismol) appears to function by multiple mechanisms including intestinal secretion reduction, intestinal reabsorption of fluids and electrolytes, toxin binding, and direct antimicrobial effects. It has proven efficacy in the management of traveler's diarrhea, although its dosing frequency may be difficult for some patients. Racecadotril (or acetorphan)[2] is a new synthetic enkephalinase inhibitor that acts by the same mechanism as the opioid derivatives and has been studied for its antidiarrheal effect in pediatric patients.

ANTIBIOTICS

Antibiotics should be used cautiously in the treatment of acute infectious diarrhea. Most clinical cases adequately resolve without antibiotic therapy. Furthermore, their use may lead to further diarrhea (including antibiotic-associated diarrhea), contribute to selective pressures favoring development of antibiotic-resistant organisms, and prolong the carriage of certain pathogens. Recommendations in the empiric and pathogen-specific treatment of acute infectious diarrhea are given in Tables 1 and 2.

[2]Not available in the United States.

TABLE 1 Empiric Therapy of Diarrheal Disease

Clinical Syndrome	Adult Patients	Pediatric Patients
Febrile dysenteric diarrhea in industrialized regions, or moderate to severe traveler's diarrhea	Ciprofloxacin (Cipro) 500 mg PO bid *or* levofloxacin (Levaquin)[1] 500 mg PO qd for 3-5 d	Azithromycin (Zithromax)[1] 5-10 mg/kg PO qd for 3-5 d *or* trimethoprim-sulfamethoxazole (Septra) 5-25 mg/kg/d PO in two divided doses for 3-5 d *plus* erythromycin[1] 10 mg/kg PO qid for 5 d
Persistent diarrhea (≥14 d in duration) in industrialized countries	Consider anti-*Giardia* therapy: metronidazole (Flagyl)[1] 250 mg PO tid for 7 d	Consider anti-*Giardia* therapy: metronidazole (Flagyl)[1] 20 mg/kg/d PO in three divided doses for 7 d

[1]Not FDA approved for this indication.
Adapted from Montes M, DuPont HL: Enteritis, enterocolitis and infectious diarrhea syndromes. In Cohen J, Powderly WD: Infectious Diseases, 2nd ed. St Louis: Mosby, 2004, pp 477-489.

TABLE 2 Pathogen-Specific Therapy of Diarrheal Disease

Pathogen	Adult Patients	Pediatric Patients
Campylobacter jejuni	Azithromycin (Zithromax)[1] 500 mg PO qd for 3 d	Erythromycin stearate[1] 40 mg/kg/d in four divided doses for 5 d *or* azithromycin[1] 10 mg/kg/d
Clostridium difficile	Initial disease: metronidazole (Flagyl) 250 mg PO qid for 10-14 d or vancomycin (Vancocin) 125-500 mg PO qid for 10-14 d	Initial disease: metronidazole 20 mg/kg/d in three divided doses for 10-14 d or vancomycin 125-500 mg PO qid for 10-14 d
EAEC, EIEC, EPEC, ETEC	Same as empiric therapy for febrile dysentery and traveler's diarrhea (see Table 1)	Azithromycin[1] 10 mg/kg/d. If resistance is suspected, use ceftriaxone (Rocephin),[1] cefixime (Suprax),[1] or cefotaxime (Claforan)[1]
EHEC*	No antimicrobial therapy (increased risk of increasing toxin release and hemolytic-uremic syndrome)	No antimicrobial therapy (increased risk of increasing toxin release and hemolytic-uremic syndrome)
Entamoeba histolytica	Metronidazole 500 mg PO tid for 10 d or tinidazole (Tindamax) 1 g PO bid for 3 d Follow with paromomycin (Humatin) 500 mg PO tid for 7 d	Metronidazole 50 mg/kg/d IV in three divided doses plus diiodohydroxyquin (Yodoxin) 40 mg/kg/d in three divided doses for 20 d

Continued

TABLE 2 Pathogen-Specific Therapy of Diarrheal Disease—Cont'd

Pathogen	Adult Patients	Pediatric Patients
Giardia lamblia	Metronidazole[1] 250 mg PO tid for 7 d *or* albendazole (Albenza)[1] 400 mg PO qd for 5 d *or* tinidazole 2 g PO in one dose	Metronidazole[1] 20 mg/kg/d in three divided doses for 7 d *or* furazolidone (Furoxone) 6 mg/kg/d divided in four doses for 7 d
Shigella sp.	Ciprofloxacin (Cipro) 500 mg PO bid for 3-5 d *or* levofloxacin (Levaquin)[1] 500 mg PO qd for 3-5 d	Azithromycin[1] 10 mg/kg/d. If resistance is suspected, use ceftriaxone,[1] cefixime,[1] or cefotaxime[1]
Salmonella sp.		
non-typhoid group	Asymptomatic or mild: no antimicrobial therapy At risk for complications: ciprofloxacin[1] 500 mg PO bid or levofloxacin[1] 500 mg PO qd for 5-7 d Alternatives: azithromycin[1] or erythromycin stearate (Erythrocin stearate)[1] 500 mg PO bid for 5 d	≤6 mo old: ceftriaxone[1] 50 mg/kg IV qd >6 mo old and healthy, and asymptomatic or with mild illness: no antimicrobial therapy At risk for complications: ceftriaxone[1] 50 mg/kg IV qd (not to exceed 2 g/d)
typhoid group	Ciprofloxacin (Cipro) 500 mg PO bid for 7-10 d or levofloxacin (Levaquin)[1] 500 mg PO OD for 7-10 d or ceftriaxone 2 g IV q 24h for 14 d	Ceftriaxone 75-100 mg/kg IVq 24h for 14 d (not to exceed 4 g/d) or azithromycin 20 mg/kg PO OD for 5-7 d (not to exceed 1 g/d)
Vibrio cholerae	Doxycycline 300 mg PO for one dose or ciprofloxacin[1] 1 g PO for one dose Recurrent disease can require prolonged courses of antibiotics or adjunctive therapy (e.g., IVIG,[1] resins[1])	TMP-SMX (Septra)[1] 1 DS tab PO bid for 3 d or azithromycin[1] 20 mg/kg PO for one dose (not to exceed 1 g)

[1]Not FDA approved for this indication.
*Shiga toxin and Shiga-like toxin–producing *E. coli*.
Abbreviations: DS = double strength; EAEC = enteroaggregative *E. coli*; EHEC = enterohemorrhagic *E. coli*; EIEC = enteroinvasive *E. coli*; EPEC = enteropathogenic *E. coli*; ETEC = enterotoxigenic *E. coli*; IVIG = intravenous immunoglobulin; TMP-SMX = trimethoprim-sulfamethoxazole.
Adapted from Montes M, DuPont HL: Enteritis, enterocolitis and infectious diarrhea syndromes. In Cohen J, Powderly WD: Infectious Diseases, 2nd ed. St Louis: Mosby, 2004, pp 477-489.

PROBIOTICS

As with the prevention of diarrhea, a growing body of evidence has yet to provide definite conclusions on the use of probiotics for treating acute infectious diarrhea. One of the major limitations to using probiotics is the variation in species and doses used in different clinical trials. However, there may be a class effect that is most likely a combination of competition for intestinal binding sites or nutritional resources, elaboration of antibacterial compounds, and immune stimulation. Another recognized limitation is the rare but serious case of blood infection from the probiotic organism; documented cases have occurred not only in recipients but also in other patients being cared for in close proximity to the recipient.

REFERENCES

Aranda-Michel J, Giannella RA. Acute diarrhea: A practical review. Am J Med 1999;106:670–6.
DuPont HL. What's new in enteric infectious diseases at home and abroad. Curr Opin Infect Dis 2005;18:407–12.
Dupont HL, the Practice Parameters Committee of the American College of Gastroenterology. Guidelines on acute infectious diarrhea in adults. Am J Gastroenterol 1997;92(11):1962–75.
Guerrant RL, Van Gilder T, Stiner TS, et al. Practice guidelines for the management of infectious diarrhea. Clin Infect Dis 2001;32:331–50.
Hahn S, Kim Y, Garner P. Reduced osmolarity oral rehydration solution for treating dehydration due to diarrhea in children: Systematic review. Br Med J 2001;323:81–5.
Helton T, Rolson DD. Which adults with acute diarrhea should be evaluated? What is the best diagnostic approach? Cleve Clin J Med 2004;71(10):778–85.
Musher DM, Musher BL. Contagious acute gastrointestinal infections. N Engl J Med 2004;351(23):2417–27.
Reisinger EC, Fritzsche C, Krause R, Krejs GJ. Diarrhea caused by primarily non-gastrointestinal infections. Nat Clin Practice Gastroenterol Hepatol 2005;2(5):216–22.
Sazawal S, Hiremath G, Dhingra U, et al. Efficacy of probiotics in prevention of acute diarrhoea: A meta-analysis of masked, randomised, placebo-controlled trials. Lancet Infect Dis 2006;6:374–82.
Thielman NM, Guerrant RL. Acute infectious diarrhea. N Engl J Med 2004;350:38–47.
World Health Organization. Oral rehydration salts: Production of the new ORS. PDF available at http://www.who.int/child-adolescent-health/New_Publications/CHILD_HEALTH/WHO_FCH_CAH_06.1.pdf (accessed April 5, 2007).

Constipation

Method of
Christine Hsieh, MD

Constipation is a common complaint and accounts for about 2.5 million physician visits annually. The estimates of the prevalence of constipation vary widely from 2% to 28%, with increasing prevalence in older adults, women, and persons from lower socioeconomic levels.

Definition

Physicians generally define constipation as having fewer than three bowel movements per week; however, patients might also consider hard stools, excessive straining, or a sense of incomplete evacuation to be constipation. An international working group of experts has revised a consensus definition of constipation, known as the Rome III criteria (Box 1).

Pathophysiology

Constipation can be divided into primary or secondary disorder. A thorough medical history and physical examination are needed to exclude constipation secondary to an underlying medical condition (Box 2) or medication (Box 3). Primary causes of constipation can be classified into three groups: normal-transit constipation, slow-transit constipation, and pelvic floor dysfunction. Normal transit constipation, also known as functional constipation, occurs most commonly. In functional constipation, stool passes through the colon at a normal rate. Slow-transit constipation, colonic inertia, is a colonic motor disorder characterized by prolonged delay in the passage of stool through the colon. Pelvic floor dysfunction is the inefficient coordination of the pelvic musculature in the emptying of stool from the rectum. The cause for pelvic floor dysfunction is unclear, but is likely multifactorial.

Clinical Features and Diagnosis

Secondary medical conditions may be excluded with a thorough history and physical examination, as well as specific laboratory tests such as metabolic panel and thyroid function test. A barium enema or colonoscopy may be indicated to exclude structural diseases such as colon cancer, especially in patients age 50 years and older. Alarm symptoms such as weight loss, gastrointestinal bleeding, and anemia also necessitate a thorough evaluation with radiography or endoscopy. A comprehensive review of the patient's medication lists, including prescription and over-the-counter medications, is important. Medications are a common secondary cause of constipation, especially those that affect the central nervous system, nerve conduction, and smooth muscle function.

 CURRENT DIAGNOSIS

- A thorough history and physical examination are needed to exclude secondary medical causes of constipation.
- Review the patient's medication lists to evaluate for medications that can cause constipation.
- Patients with alarm symptoms such as weight loss, gastrointestinal bleeding, and anemia and patients 50 years and older need a thorough evaluation with radiography or endoscopy.
- Patients who fail conservative medical management should be referred to a specialist for further diagnostic evaluation including colonic motility, anorectal manometry, defacography, and balloon expulsion test to assess colonic transit and anorectal function.

Patients with normal or slow-transit constipation might complain of abdominal bloating and infrequent bowel movements. A colonic transit marker study is useful once secondary causes are excluded to differentiate normal transit, slow transit, or pelvic floor dysfunction. Slow transit is characterized by markedly delayed colonic transit time. Pelvic floor dysfunction is characterized by normal transit time but stagnant markers in the rectum. Patients with pelvic floor dysfunction are more likely to complain of a feeling of incomplete evacuation, a sense of obstruction, and a need for digital manipulation. Additional studies to diagnose pelvic floor dysfunction are anal manometry demonstrating inappropriate contraction of the anal sphincter during straining, impaired expulsion of barium in defecography, and impaired balloon expulsion from the rectum.

Treatment

GENERAL MEASURES FOR TREATING CONSTIPATION

If a secondary cause of constipation is identified, treating the underlying medical condition or eliminating certain medications might relieve the constipation. Otherwise, initial management should begin with nonpharmacologic methods to improve bowel regularity but may proceed to the use of laxatives to relieve constipation. Patients who fail conservative medical management should be referred to a specialist for further diagnostic evaluation.

NONPHARMACOLOGIC TREATMENTS

Counseling on normal bowel habits and simple lifestyle changes might improve bowel regularity. Having a bowel movement may be partly a conditioned reflex, and patients should be educated on

CURRENT THERAPY

- If a secondary cause of constipation is identified, eliminating the offending medication or treating the underlying medical condition can relieve the constipation.
- Counseling on normal bowel habits and simple lifestyle changes such as increasing dietary fiber can improve bowel regularity.
- Empiric treatment with fiber and laxatives can increase bowel movement frequency and improve symptoms of constipation.
- Biofeedback therapy is the treatment of choice for pelvic floor dysfunction.
- Surgery is reserved for patients proved to have slow colonic transit constipation without small bowel motility delay or pelvic floor dysfunction.

recognizing and responding to the urge to defecate. Patients should be encouraged to attempt to stimulate defecation first thing in the morning when the bowel is 2 to 3 times more active and 30 minutes after meals to take advantage of the gastrocolic reflex.

In Western society, inadequate fiber intake is a common reason for constipation. The daily recommended fiber intake is 20-35 g per day. If fiber intake is substantially less, patients should be encouraged to increase their intake of fiber-rich foods such as bran, fruits, vegetables, and nuts. The recommendation is to increase fiber by 5 g per day until reaching the daily recommended intake. Adding fiber to the diet too quickly can cause excessive gas and bloating.

Adequate hydration and physical activity is considered important in maintaining bowel motility, but there has been inconsistent evidence that hydration and regular exercise relieves constipation.

PHARMACOLOGIC TREATMENT

There are few studies comparing specific treatment approaches for constipation. There are limited data about the superiority among the various treatments and the long-term benefits and harms of laxatives and fiber preparations. There are no evidence-based guidelines for the order of use of the various types of laxatives (Table 1).

Bulk laxatives can contain soluble (psyllium [Metamucil], wheat dextrin [Benefiber], pectin,[7] or guar[7]) or insoluble (cellulose [Citrucel]) products. Both types absorb water from the intestinal lumen and increase stool mass and soften the stool consistency. Patients with normal-transit constipation have the most benefit, but slow-transit constipation or functional outlet problems might not be relieved with bulking agents. Similar to increasing fiber-rich foods, bloating and excessive gas production may be a complication of bulk laxatives.

Emollient laxatives or stool softeners such as docusates (Colace, Surfak) act by lowering surface tension, allowing water to penetrate and soften the stool. They are generally well tolerated but are not as effective in the treatment of constipation. Stool softeners may be more useful for patients with anal fissures or hemorrhoids that cause painful defecation. Mineral oil is not recommended due to the potential risk of aspiration.

Saline or osmotic laxatives, such as magnesium salts, cause secretion of water into the intestinal lumen by osmotic activity. In general, these agents are thought to be relatively safe because they work within the colonic lumen and do not have a systemic effect. However, they should be used cautiously in patients with congestive heart failure and chronic renal insufficiency because they can precipitate electrolyte imbalance and volume overload.

Alternative hyperosmotic laxatives are sorbitol, lactulose (Cephulac), and polyethylene glycol (PEG) 3350 (MiraLax). Sorbitol and lactulose are indigestible agents that are metabolized by bacteria to hydrogen and organic acids. Poor bacterial absorption of these agents

---
[7]Available as dietary supplement.

TABLE 1 Medication Treatment for Chronic Constipation

Medication	Dosage
Bulk Laxatives	
Psyllium (Metamucil)	1 tbsp, qd-tid
Methylcellulose (Citrucel)	1 tbsp, qd-tid
Polycarbophil (Fibercon, Konsyl)	2-4 tabs/day
Wheat dextrin (Benefiber)	1-2 tsp, qd-tid
Guar gum[7]	
Stool Softner	
Docusate sodium (Colace)	100 mg bid
Docusate calcium (Surfak)	240 mg daily
Osmotic Laxatives	
Magnesium hydroxide (Milk of Magnesia)	30-60 mL daily
Magnesium citrate	296 mL (0.5 to 1 bottle) daily
Sorbitol 70%	15-30 mL qd-bid
Lactulose (Cephulac)	15-30 mL qd-bid
Polyethylene glycol 3350 (MiraLax)[3]	17 g qd-bid
Stimulant Laxatives	
Bisacodyl (Ducolax, Correctol)	5-15 mg qd
Senna (Senokot)	8.6 mg tab, 2-4 tabs/day
Prokinetic Agents	
Tegaserod (Zelnorm)*	
New Agent	
Lubiprostone (Amitiza)	24 µg bid

[3]Exceeds dosage recommended by the manufacturer.
[7]Available as a dietary supplement.
*Suspended from marketing in March 2007.
tab, tablet.

can lead to flatulence and abdominal distention. PEG is not degraded by bacteria and is associated with less abdominal discomfort.

The stimulant laxatives include products containing senna (Senokot) and bisacodyl (Dulcolax). These laxatives increase intestinal motility and stimulate fluid secretion into the bowel. They generally produce bowel movements within hours, but they can cause abdominal cramping due to the increased peristalsis. Chronic use of stimulant laxatives containing anthraquinones (cascara [Black Draught], senna) can cause a brown-black pigmentation of the colonic mucosa, known as melanosis coli. This condition is benign and might resolve as the stimulant laxative is discontinued.

A number of prokinetic agents have been studied for the treatment of slow-transit constipation. Colchicine[1] and misoprostol (Cytotec)[1] have been found to accelerate colonic transit time and increase stool frequency in constipated patients, but neither has received FDA approval for this indication.

In women with irritable bowel syndrome characterized by constipation, Tegaserod (Zelnorm)[2] is a colonic prokinetic agent that improves stool consistency and frequency. However, Tegaserod was removed from the market in March 2007 due to increased cardiovascular events.

Lubiprostone (Amitiza) is an intestinal chloride channel activator that promotes intestinal fluid secretion of chloride, enhancing intestinal motility. A common side effect is nausea, which is dose dependent, occurring in about 30% of patients. The long-term safety of this medication has not been established.

BIOFEEDBACK

Biofeedback or pelvic floor retraining is beneficial for patients with pelvic floor dysfunction. Biofeedback is used to emphasize normal coordination and function of the anal-sphincter and pelvic-floor muscles. A systematic review of biofeedback studies revealed an overall success rate of 67%.

---
[1]Not FDA approved for this indication.
[2]Not available in the United States.

SURGERY

Surgery is considered only in patients proved to have slow colonic transit constipation without small bowel motility delay or pelvic floor dysfunction. A subtotal colectomy with ileorectostomy is the procedure of choice for patients with slow-transit constipation that is persistent and intractable.

REFERENCES

Diamant NE, Kamm MA, Wald A, Whitehead WE. AGA technical review on constipation. American Gastroenterological Association. Gastroenterology 1999;116:735–60.
Enck P. Biofeedback training in disordered defecation: A critical review. Dig Dis Sci 1993;38:1953–60.
Johanson JF, Ueno R. Lubiprostone, a locally acting chloride channel activator, in adult patients with chronic constipation: A double-blind, placebo-controlled, dose-ranging study to evaluate efficacy and safety. Aliment Pharm Ther 2007;25:1351–61.
Koch A, Voderholzer WA, Klauser AG, Muller-Lissner SA. Symptoms in chronic constipation. Dis Colon Rectum 1997;40:902–6.
Lembo A, Camilleri M. Chronic constipation. NEJM 2003;349:1360–8.
Longstreth GF, Thompson WG, Chey WD, et al. Functional bowel disorders. Gastroenterology 2006;130:1480–91.
Muller-Lissner SA, Fumagalli I, Bardhan KD, et al. Tegaserod, a 5-HT$_4$ receptor partial agonist, relieves symptoms in irritable bowel syndrome patients with abdominal pain, bloating and constipation. Aliment Pharmacol Ther 2001;15:1655–66.
Prather CM, Ortiz-Camacho CP. Evaluation and treatment of constipation and fecal impaction in adults. Mayo Clin Proc 1998;73:881–996.
Rao SSC. Constipation: Evaluation and treatment. Gastroenterol Clin North Am 2003;32:659–83.
Schiller LR. Constipation and fecal incontinence in the elderly. Gastroenterol Clin North Am 2001;30:497–515.
Stocchi L, Pemberton JH. Surgical management of constipation. In: Cameron JL, editor. Current Surgical Therapy. St. Louis: Mosby; 2001. p. 260–4.
Tramonte SM, Brand MB, Mulrow CD, et al. The treatment of chronic constipation in adults: A systematic review. J Gen Intern Med 1997;12:15–24.
Voderholzer WA, Schtke W, Mihldorfer BE, et al. Clinical response to dietary fiber treatment of chronic constipation. Am J Gastroenterol 1997;92:95–8.

Fever

Method of
Ann M. Aring, MD

Patients often come to the physician's office with a fever. Fever can be present in a wide variety of clinical presentations ranging from self-limited viral illnesses to serious bacterial infections. Most febrile conditions can be easily diagnosed with other presenting symptoms and a problem-focused physical examination. However, fever produces anxiety for patients, parents, and health care providers, which can lead to overtreatment. Typically, fever is transient and only requires treatment to provide patient comfort.

Definitions

The definition of fever is arbitrary, because temperature varies daily within individual persons. The hypothalamic thermostat maintains core body temperature at about 37°C (98.6°F). Normal body temperature varies in a regular pattern each day. This circadian temperature rhythm, or diurnal variation, results in lower body temperatures in the early morning and temperatures approximately 1°C higher in the late afternoon or early evening.

CURRENT DIAGNOSIS

- The definition of fever is arbitrary, because temperature varies within individual persons daily. Oral temperatures of 37.5°C (99.5°F) or rectal temperatures of 100.4°F (38°C) are consistent with fever.
- Temperature accuracy depends on the measurement technique. Oral temperatures are preferred in patients older than 5 years. Rectal temperatures are preferred in infants.
- Fever in infants younger than 3 months or in neutropenic patients is considered a medical emergency that warrants immediate further evaluation.
- Fever is beneficial but is associated with increased cardiac demand and increased metabolic needs. Benign febrile seizures can occur in young children with a fever.
- Fever of unknown origin (FUO) in children merits a thorough evaluation based on the age of the child. FUO in adults is defined as a temperature higher than 101°F that is of at least 3 weeks' duration and whose cause remains undiagnosed after 3 days in the hospital or after three outpatient visits.
- Hyperthermia is characterized by a temperature above the upper limit of the hypothalamic set point of 41.1°C (106°F).

The word *fever* is derived from the Latin *fovere* (to warm). In adults and children older than 12 years, fever is generally accepted as a rectal temperature higher than 38°C (100.4°F), an oral temperature higher than 37.5°C (99.5°F), or an axillary temperature higher than 37°C (98.6°F).

The methods of determining body temperature are oral, rectal, and axillary. The oral route of determining temperature is preferred in children older than 5 years and in adults. Typically, rectal temperatures are obtained in infants by placing a lubricated thermometer in the rectum. In general, axillary temperatures are inaccurate and should not be used. Liquid crystal strips applied to the forehead and temperature-sensitive pacifiers are popular with parents but are inaccurate and miss fevers in many children.

The temperature considered to be the physiologic limit to febrile illness is 41.1°C (106°F). Hyperthermia is characterized by a temperature higher than this hypothalamic set point. Hyperthermia is due to an interference within the normal mechanisms that balance heat production and dissipation or an insult to the hypothalamus.

When the cause of a fever is unknown, two terms may be used: fever of unknown origin (FUO) and fever of unknown source. The definition of FUO in adults includes a temperature higher than 101°F that is of at least 3 weeks' duration and whose source remains undiagnosed after 3 days in the hospital or after three outpatient visits. FUO is also used to define a fever that occurs at different periods over weeks or months. Fever of unknown source is defined as a fever in the first week of an illness.

Pathogenesis and Physiology

Fever is a physiologic mechanism that occurs when an inciting stimulus causes an inflammatory response. Fever may be caused by infections, vaccines, tissue injury, malignancy, drugs, collagen vascular diseases, granulomatous disease, inflammatory bowel disease, endocrine disorders such as thyrotoxicosis and pheochromocytoma, and central nervous system abnormalities. Dehydration, increased physical activity, and heat exposure can all cause an elevation in temperature. Infections cause most fevers in all age groups.

Monocytes or tissue macrophages are activated by the microbial or nonmicrobial stimuli to produce various cytokines with pyrogenic activity. The list of currently recognized pyrogenic cytokines includes interleukin-1 (IL-1), tumor necrosis factor α (TNF-α), IL-6, interferon-β (IFN-β), and interferon-γ (IFN-γ). These cytokines activate the arachadonic acid cascade and increase production of prostaglandin E_2 (PGE_2). PGE_2 then resets the thermoregulatory set point in the hypothalamus at a higher level.

Thermoregulatory responses include redirecting blood to or from cutaneous vascular beds, increased or decreased sweating, and behavioral responses such as seeking warmer or cooler environmental temperatures. The body dissipates heat via evaporation of water from the body surface and lungs through radiation (60%), convection (12%), and conduction (3%).

Risks and Benefits of Fever

Fever is beneficial and not usually harmful to the host, with a few exceptions. Fever is associated with increased cardiac demand and increased metabolic needs. In pregnancy, fever is associated with harmful clinical effects. Many animal studies have shown that fever enhances the immunologic response to infectious agents. Use of antipyretic medications to lower fever increases both morbidity and mortality in infected laboratory animals and prolongs varicella infections in humans.

Febrile seizures are usually benign but can cause considerable parental anxiety. Febrile seizures are divided into two types: simple (generalized, last <15 minutes, and do not recur within 24 hours) and complex (prolonged, recur more than once in 24 hours, or are focal). Recent studies have shown that in previously normal children, most simple febrile seizures are not associated with recurrent seizures or brain damage.

Fever of Unknown Origin

ADULTS

The evaluation of FUO remains among the most challenging problems facing the clinician. There are four categories. Classic FUO is commonly caused by infections, drug fever, malignancy, and inflammatory diseases. Neutropenic FUO (neutrophils <500/mm³) is seen in periodontal and perianal infections; candidemia and aspergillosis are major causes. Nosocomial FUO is commonly caused by septic thrombophlebitis, drug fever, and *Clostridium difficile* colitis. In HIV-associated FUO, *Mycobacterium avium* complex infections, tuberculosis, non-Hodgkin's lymphoma, cytomegalovirus, and drug fever are important etiologies.

CHILDREN

Febrile illness in infants and young children is common. A complete history and physical examination, including vital signs, skin color and exanthems, behavior state, and hydration status, do not reveal a source of infection in 20% of febrile children. The child's age determines the need for further investigation. Febrile infants younger than 28 days should have a complete blood count (CBC) with differential; electrolytes; serum glucose; cerebrospinal fluid (CSF) Gram stain and cell count; cultures from blood, CSF, and urine; group B streptococcal antigen from urine and CSF; and a chest x-ray. Management requires hospitalization and empiric parenteral antibiotics.

For children 28 to 90 days old, obtain a CBC with differential and urinalysis with culture. A low-risk child is defined as a previously healthy term infant who has no focal bacterial infection on examination. If the white blood cell count (WBC) is greater than 15,000/mm³, blood cultures should be obtained, as well as CSF Gram stain, culture, cell count, glucose, and protein. For a positive CSF Gram stain or abnormal CSF count, the patient should be admitted and parenteral antibiotics should be given. For negative CSF Gram stain, normal CSF cell count, and negative urinalysis, the child should be

given ceftriaxone (Rocephin) 50 mg/kg (maximum dose, 1 g) and reevaluated in 24 hours. For a positive urinalysis or urine culture, the patient may be given oral antibiotics as an outpatient and reexamined in 24 hours. If the child cannot take oral antibiotics, he or she must be admitted for parenteral antibiotics. For a WBC less than 15,000 mm³ with a negative urinalysis and CSF Gram stain, the child may be followed closely as an outpatient. The child should be reevaluated in 24 hours. High-risk infants are toxic appearing with lethargy, signs of poor perfusion, hypoventilation, hyperventilation, or cyanosis. High-risk infants need to be admitted to the hospital with parental antibiotics.

For children 3 to 36 months old who have a fever without a source, no diagnostic tests or antibiotics are needed if the child appears well and the fever is less than 39°C (102.2°F) (low risk). Acetaminophen (Tylenol) 10 mg/kg may be given with instructions to give every 6 hours as needed. The child's caregiver should also be instructed to return to the clinician if the fever persists longer than 48 hours or if the patient's condition worsens. If the temperature is greater than 39°C, obtain a CBC with differential. In addition, a boy younger than 6 months or a girl younger than 2 years should have a urine culture. Blood cultures are indicated if the WBC is greater than 15,000/mm³ and the fever is higher than 39°C. CSF cultures are indicated when the diagnosis of sepsis or meningitis is suspected based on history, observation, and physical examination. Empiric antibiotic therapy with ceftriaxone 50 mg/kg (maximum dose, 1 g) should be given if the temperature is higher than 39°C and the WBC is greater than 15,000/mm³. The child needs to be followed up in 24 to 48 hours. High-risk children in this age group should be admitted to the hospital for broad-spectrum parenteral antibiotics.

Treatment

Antipyretic medications are commonly used for the symptomatic relief of fever. Acetaminophen, ibuprofen (Advil, Motrin), and aspirin are inhibitors of hypothalamic cyclooxygenase, thus inhibiting PGE_2 synthesis. These drugs are all equally effective antipyretic agents. Ibuprofen and aspirin are also antiinflammatory agents; acetaminophen does not have any antiinflammatory properties.

Acetaminophen is available in a wide variety of dosage forms including drops, elixir, syrup, capsule, tablet, chewable tablet, and suppository. Dosing is generally 10 to 15 mg/kg every 4 to 6 hours in children older than 3 months. For adults, acetaminophen dosing is 650 to 1000 mg every 6 hours. Maximum daily dose of acetaminophen is 75 mg/kg (or 720 mg) in children and 4000 mg in adolescents and adults.

Ibuprofen is a nonsteroidal antiinflammatory (NSAID) drug that may be given to febrile children 6 months or older. Ibuprofen is quickly absorbed and produces a more rapid temperature fall and longer duration of action than acetaminophen. This advantage might not be maintained after the first dose is given. Dosing in children is 10 mg/kg every 6 to 8 hours. Adults and adolescents may take doses of 200 to 400 mg every 6 hours. Ibuprofen is also available in a wide variety of dosage forms including drops, elixir, syrup, capsule, tablet, and chewable tablet.

Aspirin (salicylic acid) remains an effective treatment for fever in adults. Because aspirin is associated with Reye's syndrome in children, aspirin is not recommended for treating fever in children. Adult dosing is 325 to 650 mg every 4 to 6 hours as needed.

Combining two antipyretics for fever, such as ibuprofen and acetaminophen, is common clinical practice. Combinations have not been proved to produce quicker or longer-lasting responses. The American Academy of Pediatrics (AAP) cautions against using multiple antipyretics because of an increase in the likelihood of dosing errors. Combining drugs is more expensive and could also delay proper diagnosis or therapy.

Nonpharmacologic treatment can also provide relief from the discomfort of fever. Extra oral fluids should be encouraged to prevent dehydration. Sponge bathing with tepid water may be used. Alcohol or ice water should not be used for sponge bathing. Alcohol is absorbed through the skin and can cause hypoglycemia or dehydration. Both alcohol and ice water increase shivering and can cause more discomfort.

REFERENCES

Aronoff DM, Neilson EG. Antipyretics: Mechanisms of action and clinical use in fever suppression. Am J Med 2001;111(4):304–15.

Baraff LJ. Management of fever without source in infants and children. Ann Emerg Med 2000;36:602–14.

Crocetti M, Moghbeli N, Serwint J. Fever phobia revisited: Have parental misconceptions about fever changed in 20 years? Pediatrics 2001;107 (6):1241–6.

Finkelstein JA. Fever in pediatric primary care: Occurrence, management, and outcomes. Pediatrics 2000;105:260–6.

Greisman LA, Mackowiak PA. Fever: Beneficial and detrimental effects of antipyretics. Curr Opin Infect Dis 2002;15(3):241–5.

Kourtis AP, Sullivan DT, Sathian U. Practice guidelines for the management of febrile infants less than 90 days of age at the ambulatory network of a large pediatric health care system in the United States: Summary of new evidence. Clin Pediatr 2004;43(1):11–6.

Knockaert DC, Vanderschueren S, Blockmans D. Fever of unknown origin in adults: 40 years on. J Intern Med 2003;253:263–75.

Mackowiak PA. Temperature regulation and the pathogenesis of fever. In: Mandell GL, Bennett JE, Donlin R, editors. Principles and Practices of Infection Diseases, Vol 1. Philadelphia: Churchill Livingstone; 2000. p. 604–22.

McCarthy PL. Fever without apparent source on clinical examination. Curr Opin Pediatr 2004;16(1):94–106.

Mourad O, Palda V, Detsky A. A comprehensive evidence-based approach to fever of unknown origin. Arch Intern Med 2003;163:545–51.

Roth AR, Basello GM. Approach to the adult patient with fever of unknown origin. Am Fam Phys 2003;68(11):2223–8.

Cough

Method of
David G. Hill, MD

Cough is among the most common presenting complaints of outpatients in the United States. It serves as a protective reflex against foreign material and as a method to clear secretions from the airway. The cough center is located in the medulla, and the cough reflex is mediated by way of multiple nervous system pathways including the trigeminal, glossopharyngeal, vagus, and phrenic nerves. Cough is mediated by separate neural pathways from bronchoconstriction.

When cough occurs there is a synchronized activation of muscles, the glottis opens, and the lungs expand. At the peak of inspiration the glottis closes and expiratory muscles contract. This results in increased intrathoracic pressure; when the glottis opens airflow can reach 500 miles per hour. The cough reflex varies in different patient populations. Women have a more sensitive cough reflex than men. Smokers' cough reflexes are depressed despite the increased frequency of cough in this population. Patients who have a decreased cough sensitivity following cerebral vascular accidents have an increased incidence of pneumonia. Angiotensin-converting enzyme (ACE) inhibitors increase cough reflex sensitivity and have been shown to decrease the risk of pneumonia in patients with cerebrovascular accidents. The evaluation of cough as a patient complaint may best be pursued by examining the duration of the symptoms. Cough can be subcategorized into acute and chronic cough. Cough that occurs following an acute respiratory infection may narrow the differential diagnosis and is addressed separately.

Acute Cough

Acute cough may be defined as cough that has been present for less than 8 weeks. Because all causes of chronic coughs initially cause acute symptoms, patients with acute cough may actually have cough caused by one of the etiologies discussed later in this section; however, acute cough more commonly is the result of a less indolent process (Box 1). Infectious etiologies are a frequent cause of acute cough. Most acute cough is the result of viral infections, specifically the common cold. Most cough resulting from the common cold is self-limited and lasts less than 3 weeks. Most episodes of sinusitis are of viral etiology; however, bacterial sinusitis can also result in acute cough. The presence of a significant smoking history raises the possibility of an acute exacerbation of chronic obstructive pulmonary disease (COPD) as the cause of acute cough, especially in patients with previously documented COPD. *Bordetella pertussis* infection may also be the etiology of an acute episode of cough. Noninfectious processes that lead to acute cough include allergic rhinitis, congestive heart failure, asthma, and aspiration. The clinical history, physical examination, and diagnostic testing are of particular importance in differentiating these disease states and often point to the diagnosis.

Postinfectious Cough

Postinfectious cough begins with an acute upper respiratory tract infection but persists following the resolution of the other acute symptoms (Box 2). Postnasal drip syndrome may present following

---

BOX 1   Causes of Acute Cough

- Viral upper respiratory infections (the common cold)
- Acute sinusitis (usually viral, occasionally bacterial)
- Exacerbation of chronic obstructive pulmonary disease
- Allergic rhinitis
- *Bordetella pertussis* infection

BOX 2   Causes of Postinfectious Cough

- Postnasal drip syndrome
- Bronchospasm
- *Bordetella pertussis* infection
- Bacterial sinusitis
- *Mycoplasma pneumoniae/Chlamydia pneumoniae* infection

the common cold or sinusitis. Bronchospasm may lead to post-infectious cough either as a result of a single episode of postinfectious wheezing or an exacerbation of underlying asthma. Postinfectious cough may be the initial presentation of asthma. Recurrent episodes of airflow obstruction are required to confirm the diagnosis of this chronic illness. Because *B. pertussis* can present with an indolent course, this infection can be confused with a post-infectious cough. Similarly, bacterial sinusitis can be confused with postinfectious cough. Both of these etiologies of cough are the result of ongoing infection rather than true postinfectious cough. *Mycoplasma pneumoniae* and *Chlamydia pneumoniae* infections may also result in postinfectious cough likely because of persistent airway inflammation and increases in cough reflex sensitivity.

Chronic Cough

Chronic cough presents the most difficult diagnostic dilemma for the health care practitioner. Cough of greater than 8 weeks' duration can be considered chronic. Lesser duration of symptoms may still be indicative of one of the etiologies discussed in this section, but such cough is more likely the result of one of the infectious or postinfectious etiologies described previously. In patients who have never smoked, chronic cough is most likely the result of asthma, postnasal drip syndrome, or gastroesophageal reflux. These three etiologies are the most common cause of chronic cough regardless of patient age. In nonsmokers with a normal chest radiograph who are not taking an ACE inhibitor, these three etiologies alone or in combination are the cause of more than 85% of chronic cough (Box 3). Postnasal drip syndrome is the most common of these etiologies. Cough may be the sole presenting symptom of any of these conditions; they are not mutually exclusive and may coexist, particularly in the patient with troublesome, persistent symptoms. Most patients with problematic, persistent cough have multiple etiologies contributing to their symptoms. COPD must be considered in current smokers and in those patients with a significant smoking history. Smokers can have a cough of any etiology, however, and it should not be assumed that their cough is the result of smoking or COPD. Although smokers frequently admit to cough when a history is taken, they infrequently seek medical attention for this symptom. Cough resulting from the use of ACE inhibitors must be considered in all patients being treated with these medications. Less common, yet frequent causes of cough include chronic bronchitis from irritants other than tobacco smoke and eosinophilic bronchitis. Occasionally, chronic cough may be the result of:

- Bronchogenic carcinoma
- Metastatic carcinoma
- Bronchiectasis
- Sarcoidosis
- Pulmonary fibrosis
- Pneumoconiosis
- Hypersensitivity pneumonitis
- Congestive heart failure
- Chronic infection, such as tuberculosis or *Mycobacterium avium* complex
- Recurrent aspiration because of pharyngeal or esophageal abnormalities

---

BOX 3   Causes of Chronic Cough

- Postnasal drip syndrome
- Asthma
- Gastroesophageal reflux disease (GERD)
- Eosinophilic bronchitis
- Angiotensin-converting enzyme inhibitors

CURRENT DIAGNOSIS

All Patients Presenting With Cough

- Perform thorough history and physical examination.
- Review timing and nature of cough along with exacerbating or mitigating factors.
- Review prior history of cough, allergies, asthma, or gastroesophageal reflux.
- Take medication history, particularly use of ACE inhibitors.
- Focus physical examination on head, neck, and thorax.

Patients With Postinfectious or Chronic Cough

- Obtain chest radiograph, particularly in patients with an abnormal respiratory examination.
- Evaluate airflow obstruction with spirometry.
- Stop ACE inhibitors and assess for improvement.
- Administer empiric therapy for postnasal drip, asthma, or gastroesophageal reflux.
- Consider methacholine challenge testing to evaluate for airway hyperreactivity.
- Induce sputum for eosinophils or empiric trial of corticosteroids for eosinophilic bronchitis.
- If cough persists, consider esophagoscopy, 24-hour pH probe monitoring, high-resolution chest CT, or bronchoscopy.

Abbreviations: ACE = angiotensin-converting enzyme; CT = computed tomography.

Key Diagnostic Points

The evaluation of acute cough should focus on the history and physical examination. Most acute cough will be the result of self-limited viral upper respiratory infections. More thorough evaluation is necessary in the workup of cough of longer duration particularly if the cough has been present for more than 2 months. The history of onset of the cough and whether it was associated with an acute infectious episode should be elicited. Exposure to sick contacts particularly to a known case of *B. pertussis* are important historic considerations. The timing and nature of the cough and any associated sputum must be described. Factors that mitigate or worsen the cough should be examined, and prior history of episodic cough, allergies, wheezing, asthma, and gastroesophageal reflux should be questioned. A thorough medication history particularly regarding use of ACE inhibitors must be obtained. Environmental factors both at home and in the work place should be reviewed. Although smoking history is important, it is again noted that smoking-related cough is an infrequent reason for a patient to seek medical attention. The physical examination should focus most on the head, neck, and thorax with a thorough examination of the upper respiratory tract including the auditory canal, nose, and oropharynx. The cardiopulmonary examination should also be thorough to elicit signs of less common illnesses.

Acute cough associated with an acute respiratory illness and prominent upper airway symptoms can be assumed to be secondary to the common cold. Diagnostic testing is not indicated in such patients; a chest radiograph would be normal and is thus not recommended. Patients who have abnormal sinus transillumination, purulent nasal secretions, sinus pain or tenderness, or maxillary toothache could possibly have bacterial sinusitis. Again, a viral etiology of sinusitis is more likely than bacterial sinusitis, and antibiotic therapy should be initiated only in patients with persistent symptoms despite symptomatic therapy. Patients with documented COPD who present with acute cough, purulent sputum, dyspnea, and wheezing have an exacerbation of their underlying COPD and should be treated appropriately. Allergic rhinitis usually presents with a clear clinical history of episodic nasal and other allergy symptoms, and allergen avoidance can be initiated. It is important to note that allergic rhinitis can present with perennial symptoms.

Postinfectious cough should be evaluated with thorough history and physical examinations followed by limited diagnostic evaluation and empiric therapies. Patients should be treated for postnasal drip syndrome, particularly in the setting of described rhinitis, postnasal drip, or frequent throat clearing. The presence of nasal inflammation and congestion, cobblestoning of the pharyngeal mucosa, or mucus in the oropharynx should also lead to empiric therapy for postnasal drip syndrome. If cough persists in the patients with suspected postnasal drip syndrome, evaluation of the sinuses with imaging and treatment of those patients with evidence of bacterial sinusitis should be pursued. Computed tomography (CT) imaging of the sinuses is the gold standard for diagnosing bacterial sinusitis. Patients with postinfectious cough and an abnormal respiratory examination should have a chest radiograph. Patients with a normal radiograph and evidence of bronchospasm can be empirically treated for airway hyperreactivity. Again, the diagnosis of asthma requires recurrent airflow obstruction and cannot be made on the basis of a single episode of postinfectious wheezing or airway hyperreactivity. In subjects with cough and vomiting, known exposure to a case of B. pertussis, or in the presence of a B. pertussis epidemic in the community, empiric therapy for this illness should be pursued.

Before the vaccine era, B. pertussis was an endemic disease, which occurred in cyclic epidemics. It has been documented that B. pertussis continues to circulate in the adult population despite control of the disease in the pediatric population by vaccination. Immunity to B. pertussis, whether as a result of primary infection or immunization, is shortlived. The longer the elapsed interval since prior infection or immunization and repeat infection, the more likely repeat infection will be symptomatic. Perhaps repeat adolescent and adult booster immunization programs should be implemented to effectively control or eliminate this infection.

History and physical examinations remain paramount in the patient presenting with chronic cough. The majority of patients should have a chest radiograph obtained as part of their evaluation. If the history and physical examination suggest that postnasal drip, asthma, or gastroesophageal reflux is the etiology of a patient's symptoms, empiric therapy for these conditions should be initiated. Cough triggered by environmental factors or changes may be secondary to rhinitis and postnasal drip or airway hyperreactivity and asthma. Substernal burning or a sour taste in the mouth, particularly when triggered by supine positioning or bending, should increase the suspicion of gastroesophageal reflux.

If asthma is suspected, spirometry should be performed to document whether airflow obstruction is present. Response to inhaled bronchodilator with normal spirometry is indicative of airway hyperreactivity. Improvement in symptoms and spirometry with empiric asthma therapy even in the setting of normal baseline flow rates also confirms an asthmatic etiology. A methacholine challenge can be performed to confirm airway hyperreactivity. If cough in the setting of a positive methacholine challenge shows absolutely no response to empiric asthma therapy with inhaled corticosteroids and bronchodilators, consider a trial of systemic steroids. If the cough does not respond to aggressive asthma therapy, the methacholine challenge test results were probably false positive; asthma therapy can be discontinued and diagnostic efforts focused elsewhere.

Cough patients being treated with ACE inhibitors should cease these medications. Up to 30% of patients treated with ACE inhibitors will develop a persistent cough, more commonly in women, nonsmokers, and patients of Chinese ancestry. It may take 4 weeks or more for cough caused by ACE inhibitors to resolve following cessation of these medications. In the presence of ACE inhibitor use, further evaluation of dry cough should not be pursued until the patient has been withdrawn from these medications for 1 month.

An abnormal chest radiograph can direct further diagnostic studies and therapies, whereas a normal chest radiograph makes less common etiologies of chronic cough such as carcinoma, congestive heart failure, sarcoidosis, or interstitial lung disease unlikely. Evidence of basilar infiltrates or fibrosis may suggest interstitial lung disease or chronic aspiration. Severe gastroesophageal reflux must be considered in those patients with radiographic evidence of chronic aspiration.

Chronic cough without a definitive etiology can be troubling to both patient and health care provider. A systematic approach can simplify both diagnosis and treatment (Figure 1). It is again stressed that such a cough may be the result of multiple etiologic factors. In the absence of specific factors that help to point to an etiology of chronic cough, empiric treatment for postnasal drip syndrome should be pursued. Methacholine challenge testing will rule out asthma if it is negative and should also be performed early in the evaluation of chronic cough. Cough may be the sole manifestation of asthma in nearly 60% of patients presenting with chronic cough. A positive methacholine challenge does not have 100% predictive value but should lead to empiric asthma therapy.

Empiric therapy for silent gastroesophageal reflux should be initiated in those who do not respond to treatment for postnasal drip syndrome and do not have evidence of or respond to treatment for asthma. Cough may be the only manifestation of gastroesophageal reflux up to 30% of the time. Definitive diagnosis of gastroesophageal reflux requires invasive testing and may require more than one testing modality. Therefore it is recommended that empiric therapy for reflux be pursued before diagnostic testing. Reflux therapy should include conservative approaches such as dietary and lifestyle changes, bed positioning, and pharmacologic treatment. Gastroesophageal reflux–related cough can be particularly troublesome and persistent and may take weeks or months to respond to appropriate and intensive antireflux therapy. This may include higher-than-normal doses of proton pump inhibitors and

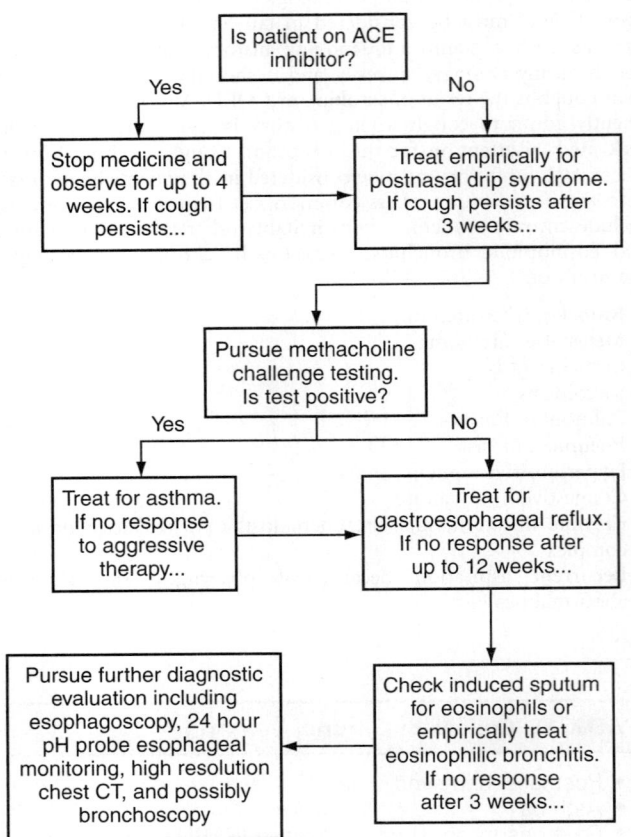

FIGURE 1. Approach to chronic cough of uncertain origin. ACE = angiotensin-converting enzyme; CT = computed tomography

promotility agents. Surgical treatment of reflux may be necessary to effectively treat reflux related cough in some patients. In patients with persistent cough, the common etiologies of cough often coexist and exacerbate one another. Therapy should often be additive, for instance treating both asthma and reflux, rather than mutually exclusive. Persistent cough should result in further diagnostic evaluation including sputum studies, esophagoscopy, 24-hour pH probe esophageal monitoring, high-resolution chest CT, and possibly bronchoscopy. In the presence of normal chest imaging, bronchoscopy is unlikely to yield beneficial diagnostic information in the patient with chronic cough.

Eosinophilic bronchitis in the absence of asthma is also a frequent cause (up to 13% of cases) of chronic cough. Patients with eosinophilic bronchitis will have normal spirometry and a negative methacholine challenge. The disease may be diagnosed by appropriate induced sputum analysis showing at least 3% eosinophils. Alternatively it can be empirically treated with a course of inhaled corticosteroids. Most patients appear to respond to inhaled corticosteroids within 3 weeks. Systemic corticosteroids may be required to improve the symptoms in some cases. There may be an association of gastroesophageal reflux with eosinophilic bronchitis. Patients with gastroesophageal reflux have been found to have increased sputum eosinophilia.

 CURRENT THERAPY

Treatment of Acute Cough

- Common cold: Supportive care with dexbrompheniramine, 6 mg, and pseudoephedrine, 120 mg (Drixoral Cold and Allergy Tablets); or ipratropium nasal spray (Atrovent, 0.06%), two 42-mcg sprays in each nostril 3 times daily for 4 to 7 d depending on duration of symptoms.
- Acute sinusitis: Treat as a common cold. Add oxymetazoline (Afrin), two sprays twice daily for three days. If symptoms persist, consider antibiotic therapy directed against *Haemophilus influenzae* and *Streptococcus pneumoniae* such as azithromycin (Zithromax), 500 mg daily for 3 d.
- Exacerbation of chronic obstructive pulmonary disease: Antibiotics directed against *H. influenzae* and *S. pneumoniae* for 3 to 7 d such as clarithromycin (Biaxin), 500 mg twice daily for 7 d; systemic corticosteroids such as prednisone (Deltasone), 40 mg tapered over 10 d; inhaled anticholinergics such as tiotropium (Spiriva), one inhalation daily; and short-acting β-agonists such as albuterol (Proventil), two inhalations every 4 h as needed; smoking cessation.
- Allergic rhinitis: Nasal corticosteroids such as mometasone (Nasonex), two sprays in each nostril daily; nonsedating antihistamines such as fexofenadine (Allegra), 180 mg daily; allergen avoidance if possible.
- *Bordetella pertussis*: Erythromycin 500 mg four times daily for 14 d or trimethoprim 160 mg/sulfamethoxazole (Bactrim DS),[1] 800 mg twice daily for 14 d. Other macrolide antibiotics such as azithromycin (Zithromax)[1] or clarithromycin (Biaxin)[1] are likely effective and may be better tolerated.

Treatment of Postinfectious Cough

- Postnasal drip syndrome: Dexbrompheniramine, 6 mg, and pseudoephedrine (Drixoral Cold and Allergy Tablets), 120 mg for up to 3 wk; ipratropium (Atrovent), 0.06% nasal spray for up to 3 wk; azelastine (Astelin) nasal spray (137 mcg), two sprays each nostril twice daily for up to 3 wk.
- Bronchospasm: Inhaled corticosteroid such as budesonide (Pulmicort),[1] two inhalations daily with or without inhaled long-acting β-agonist such as formoterol (Foradil), two inhalations twice daily; short-acting β-agonist such as albuterol (Ventolin), two puffs every 4 h as needed. Oral steroids such as prednisone (Deltasone), 40 mg tapered over 10 d.
- *Bordetella pertussis*: Erythromycin, 500 mg four times daily for 14 d, or trimethoprim 160 mg/sulfamethoxazole, 800 mg (Bactrim DS)[1] twice daily for 14 d. Other macrolide antibiotics such as azithromycin (Zithromax)[1] or clarithromycin (Biaxin)[1] are likely effective and may be better tolerated.
- Bacterial sinusitis: Dexbrompheniramine, 6 mg, and pseudoephedrine (Drixoral Cold and Allergy Tablets), 120 mg for up to 3 wk; oxymetazoline (Afrin), two sprays twice daily for 3 d; azithromycin (Zithromax), 500 mg daily for 3 d.
- Chlamydia/mycoplasma: Clarithromycin (Biaxin), 500 mg twice daily for 14 d.

Treatment of Chronic Cough

- Postnasal drip syndrome
  Nonallergic: Dexbrompheniramine, 6 mg, and pseudoephedrine (Drixoral Cold and Allergy Tablets), 120 mg for up to 3 wk; ipratropium (Atrovent), 0.06% nasal spray for up to 3 wk; azelastine (Astelin) nasal spray (137 mcg), two sprays each nostril twice daily for up to 3 wk.
  Allergic: Fluticasone (Flonase) (50 mcg), two sprays each nostril daily; fexofenadine (Allegra), 180 mg daily; allergen avoidance.
- Asthma: Albuterol (Proventil), two puffs every 4 hours as needed; inhaled corticosteroid such as budesonide (Pulmicort), two inhalations daily with or without inhaled long-acting β-agonist such as formoterol (Foradil), two inhalations twice daily; combination of long-acting β-agonist and inhaled steroid such as fluticasone/salmeterol (Advair) (100/50 mcg), inhaled twice daily; montelukast (Singulair), 10 mg daily; prednisone (Deltasone), 40 mg daily with tapering dose over 10 d.
- Gastroesophageal reflux: Dietary and lifestyle modifications, lansoprazole (Prevacid), 30 mg daily for up to 3 mo; metoclopramide (Reglan), 10 mg before meals and sleep.
- Eosinophilic bronchitis: Fluticasone (Flovent)[1] (110 mcg), two inhalations twice daily; prednisone (Deltasone), 30 mg daily for 3 wk.
- ACE inhibitor: Discontinue medication.

---
[1]Not FDA approved for this indication.

Bronchiectasis may infrequently result in chronic cough. Bronchiectasis is characterized by the abnormal dilatation of one or more branches of the bronchial tree. It can effectively be diagnosed by high resolution CT scan of the thorax. Bronchiectasis may occur following a severe infection, distal to an area of airway obstruction, congenitally, from chronic inflammatory processes, and as a result of chronic parenchymal scarring and traction. Patients with bronchiectasis may present with productive or nonproductive coughs. They may have recurrent episodes of infection resulting from persistent colonization of the abnormal bronchial segment. Infectious agents may include routine bacterial organisms and typical or atypical mycobacterium. Bronchiectasis may be seen in a variety of chronic illnesses. The presence of bronchiectasis in a patient without a known predisposing cause should prompt the clinician to look for appropriate clinical states such as:

- Primary or acquired immunodeficiencies
- Abnormalities of ciliary function, such as ciliary dyskinesia or cystic fibrosis
- Postinfectious inflammatory processes, such as allergic bronchopulmonary aspergillosis
- Collagen vascular diseases
- Inflammatory bowel disease
- Sarcoidosis
- Yellow nail syndrome

The presence of localized bronchiectasis may be an indication to pursue flexible fiberoptic bronchoscopy to rule out an obstructing lesion and to obtain appropriate culture specimens. Treatment of bronchiectasis is aimed at the underlying disease state if one can be identified. Infections should be treated with appropriate antibiotics. Clearance of bronchial secretions can be aided with mucolytics and chest physiotherapy including use of percussive devices. In some cases surgical therapy to remove the bronchiectatic segment can be considered.

Treatment

The key treatments for cough are best described based on the suspected etiology. Acute cough therapy should focus on supportive treatment of the underlying suspected etiology, which will likely be a viral upper respiratory infection. Therapy for exacerbation of chronic obstructive pulmonary disease, allergic rhinitis, bacterial sinusitis, or *B. pertussis* infection is more specific. Postinfectious cough should focus on therapy for postnasal drip syndrome or airways reactivity if suspected. In chronic cough of uncertain etiology (see Figure 1), cough therapy should begin with empiric treatment of postnasal drip syndrome, evaluation and treatment of asthma, empiric treatment of gastroesophageal reflux syndrome, and finally evaluation or empiric therapy for eosinophilic bronchitis.

Cough is a frequent and troublesome symptom for both patient and health care provider. Acute cough although at times troubling is usually self-limiting. Postinfectious cough and chronic cough are more problematic, but can effectively be evaluated and treated by performing a thorough history and physical examination and pursuing a systematic approach to diagnostic evaluation and both empiric and guided therapies. The resolution of chronic troubling cough is a therapeutic relief for the patient and a gratifying experience for the caregiver.

REFERENCES

Barnes TW, Afessa B, Swanson KL, Lim KG. The clinical utility of flexible bronchoscopy in the evaluation of chronic cough. Chest 2004;126:268–72.
Breitling CE, Ward R, Goh KL. Eosinophilic bronchitis is an important cause of chronic cough. Am J Respir Crit Care Med 1999;160:406–10.
Cherry JD. Epidemiological, clinical, and laboratory aspects of pertussis in adults. Clin Infect Dis 1999;28(Suppl2):S112–7.
Cohen M, Sahn SA. Bronchiectasis in systemic diseases. Chest 1999;116:1063–74.
Irwin RS, Madison JM. Symptom research on chronic cough: A historical perspective. Ann Intern Med 2001;134:809–14.
Irwin RS, Madison JM. The diagnosis and treatment of cough. N Engl J Med 2000;343:1715–21.
Irwin RS, Madison JM. The persistently troublesome cough. Am J Respir Crit Care Med 2002;165:1469–74.
Kiljander TO. The role of proton pump inhibitors in the management of gastroesophageal reflux disease-related asthma and chronic cough. Am J Med 2003;115(3A):S65–71.

Pruritus

Method of
Scott Moses, MD

Because pruritus is the most common symptom in dermatology, clinicians are often asked to reduce its distressing effect on comfort and sleep. Left untreated, itch and its associated persistent scratching increases risk of chronic skin changes and secondary infection. Although pruritus is most often caused by a dermatologic condition, it can also be a symptom of underlying systemic disease.

The sensation of itch starts in the skin's free nerve endings, travels via unmyelinated C-fibers to the spine, and finally travels via the spinothalamic tract to the brain. Histamine, commonly associated with allergic rhinitis and urticaria, is only one of several chemical mediators of pruritus. Serotonin is integral to the pruritus of uremia, cholestasis, polycythemia vera, lymphoma, and morphine-associated pruritus. In atopic dermatitis, proinflammatory mediators (e.g., cytokines) are released in an immune-mediated response. Pruritus has been attributed to neuropathy in a wide variety of conditions including herpes zoster, brachioradial pruritus, notalgia paresthetica, spinal tumors, and multiple sclerosis.

Diagnosis

History is the key to identifying the cause of pruritus. Most causes are evident from the associated dermatitis (Box 1), distribution (Figure 1), or exogenous exposure history (Box 2). Clinicians should focus on the timing of pruritus and associated rash development, food and medication exposures, possible allergen and irritant exposures, pet exposure, and travel history.

In children, pruritus rarely has a systemic cause. However, clinicians should be alert for children who demonstrate red flag symptoms such as growth failure, anorexia, fatigue, associated bowel or bladder changes, and nighttime awakenings due to pruritus.

Underlying systemic disease is responsible for up to 50% of pruritus in older adults and should be considered in refractory cases and where skin findings are absent. Reassuring findings that suggest a non-systemic cause include recent onset, localized itch, pruritus limited to exposed skin, household members also with pruritus, and recent travel history.

CURRENT DIAGNOSIS

- Reassuring findings that suggest a nonorganic cause include recent onset, localized itch, pruritus limited to exposed skin, household members also with pruritus, and recent travel history.
- Underlying systemic disease is responsible for up to 50% of pruritus in older adults and is uncommon in children.
- Laboratory testing to consider in atypical cases includes a complete blood count, ferritin, thyroid-stimulating hormone, serum bilirubin, alkaline phosphatase, serum creatinine, blood urea nitrogen, HIV test, and skin scrapings, biopsy, and culture.

BOX 1 Dermatitis-Associated Causes of Pruritus

Allergic Contact Dermatitis
- Sharply demarcated erythematous lesion with overlying vesicles
- Reaction within 2-7 d of exposure (see Box 4)

Atopic Dermatitis
- Atopic patients (allergic rhinitis, asthma) with the itch that rashes
- Affects flexor wrists and ankles, antecubital and popliteal fossa

Bullous Pemphigoid
- Initially pruritic urticarial lesions, often in intertriginous areas
- Tense blisters form after urticaria

Cutaneous T-Cell Lymphoma (Mycosis Fungoides)
- Oval eczematous patch on non–sun-exposed skin (e.g., buttocks)
- Can also manifest as erythroderma (exfoliative dermatitis)
- Can also manifest as a new eczematous disorder in older adults

Dermatitis Herpetiformis
- Rare vesicular dermatitis affects lumbosacral spine, elbows, knees

Folliculitis
- Pruritus out of proportion to appearance of dermatitis
- Papules and pustules at follicular sites on chest, back, or thighs

Lichen Planus
- Lesions often on the flexor wrists
- 6 Ps: pruritus, polygonal, planar, purple papules, and plaques

Lichen Simplex Chronicus
- Complication of chronic scratching (e.g., atopic dermatitis)
- Thickened plaques over lower legs, posterior neck, and groin

Parasitic Skin Infections
Insects
- Chigger bites (harvest mite): Southeastern United States
- Cutaneous myiasis (bot fly): Central and South America, Africa
- Leishmaniasis (sand fly): Central and South America, Africa, Asia

Pediculosis (lice)
- Occiput of school-aged child
- Genitalia affected in adults (STD)

Scabies
- Burrows at hand web spaces, axillae, and genitalia
- Hyperkeratotic plaques, pruritic papules or scale present
- Face and scalp affected in children but not adults

Prurigo nodularis
- Complication of chronic scratching (variant of lichen simplex)
- 1-2 cm nodules on extensor arms and legs

Psoriasis
- Plaques on extensor extremities, low back, palms, soles, and scalp

Sunburn
- Consider photosensitizing causes (e.g., NSAIDs, cosmetics)

Xerotic Eczema
- Intense itching during winter in northern climates
- Involves back, flanks, abdomen, waist, and distal extremities

Abbreviations: NSAIDs = nonsteroidal antiinflammatory drugs; STD = sexually transmitted disease.

Dermatitis distribution and appearance often indicate the cause. The examination can also reveal the chronicity of pruritus.

Excoriations and impetigo are seen acutely, and postinflammatory pigment changes and lichenification are seen with chronic scratching. Clinicians should be alert for findings consistent with thyroid disease, renal disease, liver disease, anemia, and hematologic malignancy. Examination should include careful palpation of the lymph nodes, liver, and spleen. Systemic causes of pruritus are listed in Box 3. Pruritic conditions specific to pregnancy are summarized in Box 4.

CURRENT THERAPY

- Pruritus is usually self-limited and responds well to nonspecific measures such as liberal use of skin lubricants and avoidance of provocative factors.
- Antihistamines are not uniformly effective in reducing itch.
- Left untreated, itch and its associated persistent scratching increases risk of impetigo and cellulitis in the short term and lichen simplex chronicus and prurigo nodularis in chronic cases.

In cases refractory to 2 weeks of symptomatic therapy or in which an underlying systemic cause is considered, a limited laboratory evaluation is indicated and is summarized in Table 1. When itch persists or is refractory to general measures, remember that up to one half of older adults have pruritus caused by an underlying systemic problem.

Treatment

Pruritus is usually self-limited and responds well to nonspecific measures such as liberal use of skin lubricants and avoidance of provocative factors (Box 5). Oral antihistamines are not uniformly effective in all causes of pruritus. Specific management of dermatitis, as with atopic dermatitis, scabies, and contact dermatitis, can relieve symptoms.

In the atypical case, where these measures fail, a systemic condition may be uncovered. In these patients, the itch should be alleviated by treating the underlying condition, as with thyroid replacement in hypothyroidism or iron supplementation in iron deficiency anemia. Uremia and cholestasis-related pruritus have established effective therapies beyond treating the causative chronic renal or hepatic insufficiency (Box 6).

CAUSES OF PRURITUS

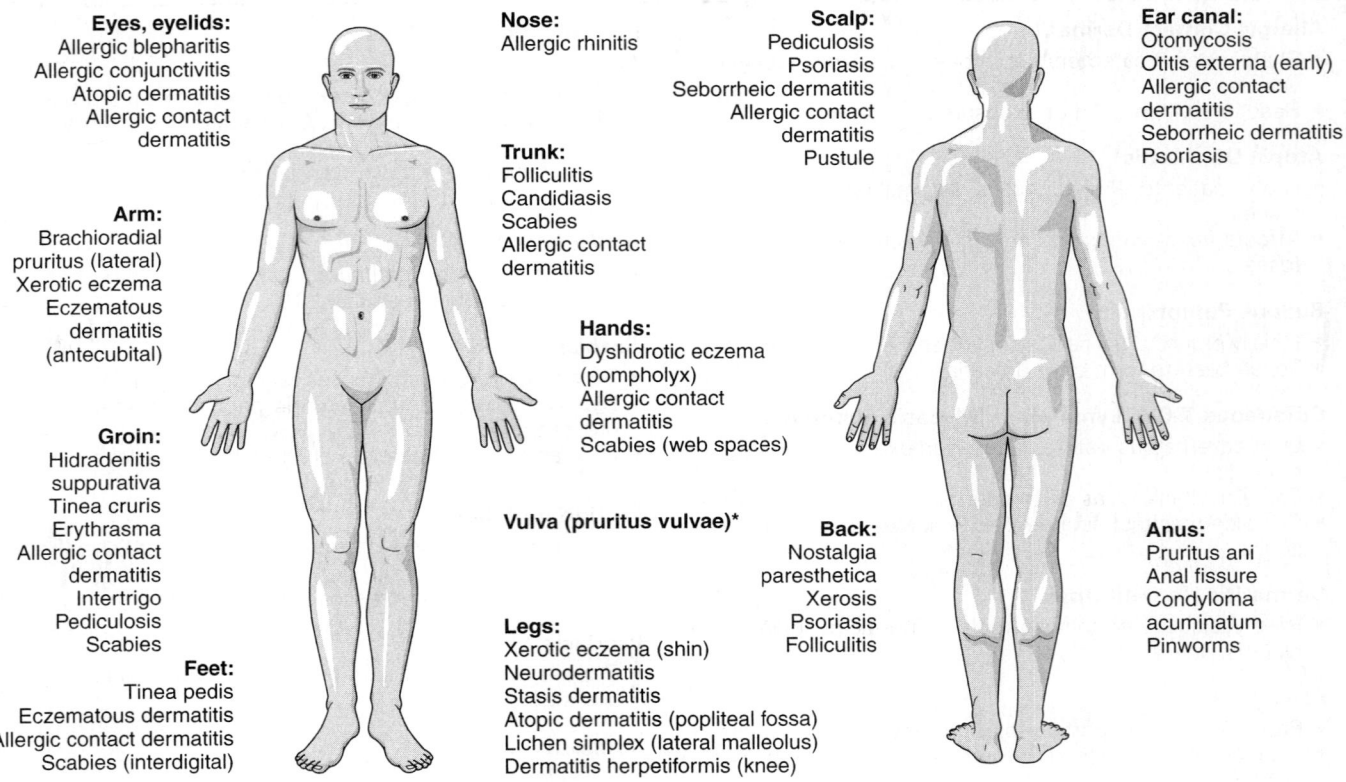

Eyes, eyelids:
Allergic blepharitis
Allergic conjunctivitis
Atopic dermatitis
Allergic contact
dermatitis

Arm:
Brachioradial
pruritus (lateral)
Xerotic eczema
Eczematous
dermatitis
(antecubital)

Groin:
Hidradenitis
suppurativa
Tinea cruris
Erythrasma
Allergic contact
dermatitis
Intertrigo
Pediculosis
Scabies

Feet:
Tinea pedis
Eczematous dermatitis
Allergic contact dermatitis
Scabies (interdigital)

Nose:
Allergic rhinitis

Trunk:
Folliculitis
Candidiasis
Scabies
Allergic contact
dermatitis

Hands:
Dyshidrotic eczema
(pompholyx)
Allergic contact
dermatitis
Scabies (web spaces)

Vulva (pruritus vulvae)*

Legs:
Xerotic eczema (shin)
Neurodermatitis
Stasis dermatitis
Atopic dermatitis (popliteal fossa)
Lichen simplex (lateral malleolus)
Dermatitis herpetiformis (knee)

Scalp:
Pediculosis
Psoriasis
Seborrheic dermatitis
Allergic contact
dermatitis
Pustule

Back:
Nostalgia
paresthetica
Xerosis
Psoriasis
Folliculitis

Ear canal:
Otomycosis
Otitis externa (early)
Allergic contact
dermatitis
Seborrheic dermatitis
Psoriasis

Anus:
Pruritus ani
Anal fissure
Condyloma
acuminatum
Pinworms

*Causes of pruritus vulvae: prepubertal girls—poor hygiene, streptococcal infection, *Escherichia coli* infection, pinworms, scabies, allergic contact dermatitis; young women—vaginitis, allergic contact dermatitis, hidradenitis suppurativa, lichen simplex chronicus; postmenopausal women—atrophic vaginitus, lichen sclerosus, vulvar cancer, Paget's disease; females with diabetes mellitus—candidiasis, other dermatophyte infections.

FIGURE 1. Causes of pruritus (by distribution). (Adapted from Moses S: Pruritus. Am Fam Physician 2003;68:1135-1146.)

BOX 2 Exposure-Related Pruritus

Allergic Contact Dermatitis
- Topical medications: Neomycin, benzocaine (Americaine)
- Nickel, latex, cosmetics, black hair dye
- Laundry detergents or fabric softeners
- Paint-on tattoos (paraphenylenediamine)
- Tattoo dye: cadmium yellow, mercuric sulfide (red)
- Ointments highly concentrated in inert oil

Heat Exposure
- Miliaria rubra (prickly heat)
- Cholinergic urticaria (response to hot bath, fever, exercise)

Occupational Exposure
- Dyes (e.g., glyceryl monothioglycolate)
- Potassium dichromate in cements and dyes
- Rosins or epoxy resins in adhesives
- Rubber, methyl methacrylate, fiberglass

Systemic Medications
- Drug hypersensitivity (rifampin [Rifadin], vancomycin [Vancocin])
- Itraconazole (Sporanox), fluconazole, ketoconazole (Nizoral)
- Niacinamide (niacin), B vitamins, aspirin, quinidine (Quinidex)
- Nitrates (food preservatives)
- Spinal narcotics (pruritus affects face, neck, and upper chest)

Water Exposure
- Aquagenic pruritus (associated with polycythemia vera)
- Cholinergic urticaria (response to warm water)
- Itching within 15 min of any water contact
- Polycythemia vera
- Swimmer's itch (7-d eruption after freshwater swimming)

BOX 3 Systemic Causes of Pruritus

Cholestasis
- Intense itching, worse at night
- Affects hands, feet, and pressure sites
- Reactive hyperpigmentation spares midback (butterfly appearance)

Chronic Renal Failure
- Severe paroxysms of generalized itching
- Worse in summer

Delusions of parasitosis
- Focal erosions on exposed areas of arms and legs

Human Immunodeficiency Virus
- Pruritus is a common presenting symptom due to secondary causes
- Causes: Eczema, drug reaction, eosinophilic folliculitis, seborrhea

Hodgkin's Lymphoma
- Prolonged generalized pruritus often precedes diagnosis

Hyperthyroidism
- Skin is warm and moist
- Pretibial edema may be present
- Onycholysis, hyperpigmentation, and vitiligo have been associated

Iron-Deficiency Anemia
- Other dermatologic signs include glossitis and angular cheilitis

Malignant Carcinoid
- Intermittent head and neck flushing
- Explosive diarrhea

Multiple Myeloma
- Affects elderly with bone pain, headache, cachexia, anemia, and renal failure

Neurodermatitis or Neurotic Excoriations
- Bouts of intense itching that can awaken the patient from a sound sleep

- Affects scalp, neck, wrist, extensor elbow, outer leg, ankle, perineum

Parasitic Infection (usually in returning travelers or immigrants)
- Filariasis: Tropical parasite responsible for lymphedema
- Onchocerciasis: Transmitted by black fly in Africa, Latin America
- Schistosomiasis: Fresh water exposure in Africa, Mediterranean, South America
- Trichinosis: Undercooked pork, bear, wild boar, or walrus meat

Parvovirus B19
- Slapped cheek appearance in children
- Arthritis in some adults

Peripheral Neuropathy
- Brachioradial pruritus: Affects lateral arms of white patients in the tropics
- Notalgia paresthetica: Midback pruritus with hyperpigmented patch
- Herpes zoster: Accompanies painful prodrome 2 d before rash

Polycythemia Rubra Vera
- Pricking-type itch persists for hours after hot shower or bath

Scleroderma
- Nonpitting extremity edema, erythema, and intense pruritus
- Edema phase with pruritus precedes fibrosis of the skin

Urticaria
- Response to allergen, cold, heat, exercise, sunlight, or direct pressure

Weight Loss (Rapid) in Eating Disorders
- Other signs include hair loss or fine lanugo hair on back and cheeks
- Also yellow skin discoloration and petechiae

BOX 4 Causes of Pruritus in Pregnancy

Pruritic Urticarial Papules and Plaques of Pregnancy
- Common in the third trimester
- Intense pruritus involves abdomen
- Spreads to thighs, buttocks, breasts, and arms

Prurigo of Pregnancy
- Common in second half of pregnancy
- Extensor arms and abdomen with excoriated papules and nodules
- Associated with atopic dermatitis

Herpes Gestationis or Pemphigoid Gestationis
- Uncommon
- Autoimmune condition associated with Graves' disease
- Vesicles and bullae on abdomen and extremities in second half of pregnancy
- Responds to prednisone[1] 0.5 mg/kg (Level A)

Intrahepatic Cholestasis of Pregnancy
- Uncommon
- Trunk and extremity itching without rash in late pregnancy
- Jaundice not present in the mild form (prurigo gravidarum)
- Responds to cholestyramine (Questran) and Vitamin K$_1$ (Aquamephyton)[1](Level B)

Pruritic Folliculitis of Pregnancy
- Uncommon, occurs in second half of pregnancy
- Erythematous follicular papules over trunk, with spread to extremities
- May be a variant of prurigo of pregnancy

Other Common Pruritic Conditions Exacerbated in Pregnancy
- Atopic dermatitis
- Contact dermatitis

[1]Not FDA approved for this indication.
Levels of evidence: Level A: Evidence from high-quality randomized controlled clinical trials or meta-analyses; Level B: Evidence from nonrandomized clinical studies or nonquantitative systematic reviews.

TABLE 1 Diagnostic Evaluation of Pruritus for Atypical, Persistent, or Refractory Cases

Tests	Findings
Complete blood count,* serum ferritin*	Iron deficiency anemia, polycythemia rubra vera, Hodgkin's lymphoma, multiple myeloma, parasitic infection
Serum bilirubin, alkaline phosphatase*	Cholestasis (e.g., cirrhosis)
Serum creatinine, blood urea nitrogen*	Uremia (e.g., chronic renal failure)
Thyroid stimulating hormone*	Hyperthyroidism
Microscopy of skin scrapings, skin culture, skin biopsy	Dermatophytes, scabies; skin bacterial, fungal or viral infection; mastocytosis, mycosis fungoides, bullous pemphigoid
HIV test	HIV infection
Chest radiograph	Hodgkin's lymphoma, multiple myeloma
Stool tests	Parasites, *Helicobacter pylori*
	Children: pinworms, perianal streptococcus

*Denotes a first-line test. Unmarked tests are performed if history indicates.

BOX 5 Nonspecific Management of Pruritus

- Use skin lubricants liberally
  - Petrolatum or skin lubricant cream at bedtime
  - Apply alcohol-free, hypoallergenic lotions frequently during day
- Avoid excessive bathing
  - Briefly pat dry after bath and immediately apply skin lubricants
  - Decrease bathing frequency
  - Limit bathing to brief exposure to tepid water
- Limit soap use
  - Use mild, unscented, hypoallergenic soap 2 or 3 times per wk
  - Daily use of soap only in groin and axillae; spare legs, arms, and torso
- Minimize dryness
  - Humidify dry indoor environment (especially in winter)
- Choose clothing that does not irritate the skin
  - Doubly rinsed cotton clothes and silk are best
  - Add bath oil (e.g., Alpha Keri) to rinse cycle when washing sheets
  - Avoid heat-retaining fabrics (synthetics)
  - Avoid wool and smooth-textured cotton clothes
- Avoid vasodilators
  - Avoid caffeine, alcohol, spices, hot water, and excessive sweating
- Avoid provocative topical medications
  - Avoid prolonged topical corticosteroids (risk of skin atrophy)

- Avoid topical anesthetics and antihistamines
- May sensitize exposed skin and risk contact dermatitis
- Standard antipruritic topical agents
  - Menthol and camphor (e.g., Sarna Lotion)
  - Oatmeal baths (e.g., Aveeno)
  - Pramoxine[1] (e.g., PrameGel [pramoxine + menthol], Pramosone [pramoxine + hydrocortisone])
  - Calamine lotion (Use on weeping lesions only, not on dry skin)
- Antipruritic topical agents for refractory cases (used in severe atopic dermatitis)
  - Doxepin 5% cream (Zonalon)
  - Burow's solution (wet dressings with aluminum acetate 5% in water)
  - Unna's boot[1] (zinc oxide paste bandages)
  - Coal tar emulsion[1] (Zetar)
- Systemic antipruritic agents (used in allergic and urticarial disease)
  - Doxepin (Sinequan)[1] 1 mg/kg up to 25 mg at bedtime (Level A)
  - Hydroxyzine (Atarax) 0.5 mg/kg up to 25-50 mg at bedtime
  - Nonsedating antihistamines (e.g., Fexofenadine [Allegra], Level A)
- Prevent complications of scratching
  - Keep fingernails short and clean
  - Rub skin with palms if urge to scratch is irresistible

[1]Not FDA approved for this indication.
Level A: Evidence from high-quality randomized controlled clinical trials or meta-analyses.

Complications

Itch and the scratch it induces are not benign. When scratching is left unchecked, fingernails introduce bacteria into abraded skin, and impetigo or cellulitis can ensue. Lichen simplex chronicus and prurigo nodularis are chronic skin changes seen with long-term scratching and in particular with atopic dermatitis.

Medications to treat pruritus are also not without adverse effects. Antihistamines can affect alertness and learning if used during the day, and with chronic use, the associated dry mouth can predispose to tooth decay.

Follow-Up

General measures to treat pruritus should be reviewed at each visit. Consistent practice of these simple home strategies can prevent sleepless nights, frequent evaluations, unnecessary medications, and the complications of scratching.

BOX 6 Specific Management of Pruritic Conditions

Cholestasis

- Cholestyramine (Questran) (Level B)
  - Adult: 4 g 30 min before meals
  - Child: 240 mg/kg/d divided tid (up to 6 g/d)
- Ursodiol (Actigall)[1] 15 mg/kg/d divided before meals
- Ondansetron (Zofran)[1] 4-8 mg IV, then 4 mg PO q8h (Level B)
- Opioid receptor antagonist (Level A)
  - Naloxone (Narcan)[1] 0.002 mcg/kg/h IV, titrate to max 0.25 mcg/kg/h
  - Naltrexone (Revia)[1] 12.5 mg PO qd (advance to 50 mg PO qd)
- Rifampin (Rifadin)[1] 10 mg/kg/d divided bid (max: 300 mg bid) (Level B)
- Bile duct stenting from extrahepatic cholestasis (Level A)
- Lidocaine (Xylocaine)[1] IV has been used
- Bright light therapy (Level B)
- Plasmapheresis

Neurotic Excoriation

- Pimozide (Orap)[1] for delusions of parasitosis
- Selective serotonin reuptake inhibitor (SSRI)

Notalgia Paresthetica

- Topical capsaicin (Zostrix)[1] applied 4-6 times per d for several wk (Level B)

Polycythemia Vera

- Aspirin[1] 500 mg PO q8-24h (Level B)
- Paroxetine (Paxil)[1] 10-20 mg PO qd (Level B)
- Interferon-α (Intron A)[1] 3-35 million IU/wk (Level B)

Spinal Opioid–Induced Pruritus

- Ondansetron (Zofran)[1] 8 mg IV concurrent with opioid (Level A)
- Nalbuphine (Nubain)[1] 5 mg IV concurrent with opioid (Level B)

Uremia

- UV B phototherapy twice weekly for 1 mo (Level A)
- Activated charcoal[1] 6 g/d (Level A)
- Topical capsaicin[1] 0.025% cream to localized areas (Level A)
- Ondansetron and naltrexone are not efficacious in uremia (Level A)

---

[1]Not FDA approved for this indication.
Level A: Evidence from high-quality randomized controlled clinical trials or meta-analyses; Level B: Evidence from nonrandomized clinical studies or nonquantitative systematic reviews.

REFERENCES

Belsito DV. The diagnostic evaluation, treatment and prevention of allergic contact dermatitis in the new millennium. J Allergy Clin Immunol 2000;105:409–20.

Bender BG. Sedation and performance impairment of diphenhydramine and second-generation antihistamines: A meta-analysis. J Allergy Clin Immunol 2003;111:770–6.

Bergasa NV. An approach to the management of the pruritus of cholestasis. Clin Liver Dis 2004;8:55–66.

Berger R, Gilchrest BA. Skin disorders. In: Duthie EH, Katz PR, editors. Practice of Geriatrics. 3rd ed. Philadelphia: WB Saunders; 1998. p. 467–72.

Boiko S, Zeiger R. Diagnosis and treatment of atopic dermatitis, urticaria, and angioedema during pregnancy. Immunol Allergy Clin North Am 2000;20:839.

Callen JP, Bernardi DM, Clark RAF, Weber DA. Adult-onset recalcitrant eczema: A marker of noncutaneous lymphoma or leukemia. J Am Acad Dermatol 2000;43:207–10.

Correale CE, Walker C, Lydia M, Craig TJ. Atopic dermatitis: A review of diagnosis and treatment. Am Fam Physician 1999;60:1191–210.

Cyr PR, Dreher GK. Neurotic excoriations. Am Fam Physician 2001;64:1981–4.

Diehn F, Tefferi A. Pruritus in polychaemia vera: Prevalence. Laboratory Correlates and Management 2001;115:619–21.

Fagan EA. Intrahepatic cholestasis of pregnancy. Clin Liver Dis 1999;3:603–32.

Finn AF, Kaplan AP, Fretwell R, et al. A double-blind, placebo-controlled trial of fexofenadine HCl in the treatment of chronic idiopathic urticaria. J Allergy Clin Immunol 1999;103:1071–8.

Fisher AA. Aquagenic pruritus. Cutis 1993;51:146–7.

Gelfand JM, Rudikoff D. Evaluation and treatment of itching in HIV-infected patients. Mt Sinai J Med 2001;68:298–308.

Ghent CN. The pruritus of cholestasis. Hepatology 1999;29:1003–6.

Gupta MA, Gupta AK, Voorhees JJ. Starvation-associated pruritus: A clinical feature of eating disorders. J Am Acad Dermatol 1992;27:118–20.

Habif TP. Clinical Dermatology. 3rd ed. Chicago: Mosby–Year Book; 1996.

Harrigan E, Rabinowitz LG. Atopic dermatitis. Immunol Allergy Clin North Am 1999;19:383–96.

Heymann WR. Chronic urticaria and angioedema associated with thyroid autoimmunity: Review and therapeutic implications. J Am Acad Dermatol 1999;40:229–32.

Koblenzer CS. Itching and atopic skin. J Allergy Clin Immunol 1999;104: S109–3.

Krajnik M, Zylicz Z. Understanding pruritus in systemic disease. J Pain Symptom Manage 2001;21:151–68.

Kroumpouzos G, Cohen LM. Dermatoses of pregnancy. J Am Acad Dermatol 2001;45:1–19.

Leung AKC. Pruritus in children. J Roy Soc Health 1998;118:280–6.

Lidofsky S, Scharschmidt BF. Jaundice. In: Feldman M, Scharschmidt BF, Sleisenger MH, Fordtran JS, editors. Sleisenger and Fordtran's Gastrointestinal and Liver Disease. 6th ed. Philadelphia: WB Saunders; 1998. p. 230–1.

Moses S. Pruritus. Am Fam Physician 2003;68:1135–46.

Parker F. Structure and function of skin. In: Goldman L, Bennett JC, editors. Cecil Textbook of Medicine. 21st ed. Philadelphia: WB Saunders; 2000. p. 2266.

Paus R, Schmeiz M, Biró T, Steinhoff M. Frontiers in pruritus research: Scratching the brain for more effective itch therapy. J Clin Invest 2006;116:1174–85.

Robinson-Bostom L, DiGiovanna JJ. Cutaneous manifestations of end-stage renal disease. J Am Acad Dermatol 2000;43:975–86.

Shellow WVR. Evaluation of pruritus. In: Goroll AH, Mulley AG, editors. Primary Care Medicine. 4th ed. Philadelphia: Lippincott Williams & Wilkins; 2000. p. 1001–4.

Stambuk R, Colvin R. Dermatologic disorders. In: Gabbe SG, Niebyl JR, Simpson JL, editors. Obstetrics: Normal and Problem Pregnancies. 4th ed. New York: Churchill Livingstone; 2002. p. 1283–90.

Tennyson H. Neurotropic and psychotropic drugs in dermatology. Dermatol Clin 2001;19:179–97.

Tormey WP, Chambers JPM. Pruritus as the presenting symptom in hyperthyroidism. Br J Clin Pract 1994;48:224.

Valsecchi R, Cainelli T. Generalized pruritus: A manifestation of iron deficiency. Arch Dermatol 1983;119:630.

Veien NK, Hattel T, Laurberg G, Spaun E. Brachioradial pruritus. J Am Acad Dermatol 2001;44:704–5.

Villamil AG, Bandi JC, Galdame OA, et al. Efficacy of lidocaine in the treatment of pruritus in patients with chronic cholestatic liver disease. Am J Med 2005;118:1160–3.

Waxler B, Dadabhoy Z, Stojiljkovic L, Rabito SF. Primer of postoperative pruritus for anesthesiologists. Anesthesiology 2005;103:168–78.

Zirwas MJ, Seraly MP. Pruritus of unknown origin: A retrospective study. J Am Acad Dermatol 2001;45:892–6.

Tinnitus

Method of
Claus-Frenz Claussen, MD

Tinnitus is noise(s) in the ear, which is usually subjective and can be extremely disturbing and frustrating to those affected. According to studies of the American Tinnitus Association, approximately 36 million Americans older than 40 years suffer from tinnitus.

Tinnitus has been regarded as a disease entity for many centuries. During the second half of the 20th century, physicians were able to discriminate among several different kinds of tinnitus including bruits, maskable tinnitus, and nonmaskable tinnitus. Under the influence of Shulman and his team, the term *tinnitology* was coined.

The present interest of researchers in the field of tinnitology is split into two fields of action: suggestions for improvement of objective and quantitative differential diagnostics in tinnitus and research and development to improve various types of treatment for different kinds of tinnitus.

General Phenomena of Tinnitus

A noise without any human information function, a tinnitus, can be a normal as well as a pathologic function of human hearing. On the one hand, tinnitus can be regarded as a problem of acoustic resolution of the inner ear microphone, that is, the cochlear noise-to-signal ratio. In a well-dampened soundproof chamber, most normal-hearing persons experience a sizzling sound in their ears because of their perception of molecular vibrations from inner ear fluids (as known from thermodynamics). Yet this underlying percept is masked in everyday life by normal environmental noise.

On the other hand, tinnitus patients regularly tell their physicians about subjective ear noises that they describe, for example, as pulsating, humming, roaring, whistling, hissing, fullness of the ear, and pressure and/or pain in the ear.

Table 1 presents the subjective sensational qualities of tinnitus in 823 tinnitus patients (77.52% male and 22.48% female with a mean age of 50.87 years ± 8.68 years) from Bad Kissingen, Germany, who underwent clinical inpatient rehabilitation therapy for several weeks for severe disabling tinnitus.

CURRENT DIAGNOSIS

Irritating subjective or objective perception of irritating acoustic noise or sound in the ear, head, or body that may be described, for example, as:

- Pulsating
- Humming
- Roaring
- Whistling
- Hissing

TABLE 1 Subjective Classification of Ear Noises in 823 (=100%) Tinnitus Patients

Complaints	Right Ear (%)	Left Ear (%)
Pulsating	1.94	1.94
Humming	7.41	6.93
Roaring	14.10	14.22
Whistling	50.67	51.76
Hissing	9.96	10.81
Pressure in the ear	6.32	5.83
Pain in the ear	14.10	14.22

TABLE 2 Subjective Classification of Different Time/Intensity Patterns of Tinnitus in 823 (=100%) Patients

Time/Intensity Patterns	%
Permanent	59.17
Intermittent	19.97
Swelling up and going down	43.26

In these same patients, we looked for descriptions of different time/intensity patterns of their tinnitus (Table 2), and the subjective background of discomfort was investigated as shown in Table 3. Additionally, the patients named the most irritating factors related to their tinnitus (Table 4).

Sleep disturbance is a common and frequent complaint. Scientific studies report decreased tolerance and increased discomfort when insomnia and depression are associated with tinnitus.

In 1991, a sample of 338 New Zealanders regularly experiencing tinnitus completed and returned questionnaires to associations for people with tinnitus or hearing impairment. Nearly half the sample was sometimes depressed because of tinnitus. Those reporting depression and those reporting more severe problems as a consequence of the tinnitus saw more health care professionals and used more coping strategies. Most respondents did not remember exactly when they first noticed the tinnitus.

A questionnaire investigation comprising 1091 patients from Bispebjerg Hospital, Copenhagen (1993), concerning "tinnitus-incidence and handicap," was conducted at a hearing center. A majority of patients, 59%, claimed that they were troubled by tinnitus. Neither a greater degree of hearing loss nor a longer duration of tinnitus was associated with more severe tinnitus. Among patients with both subjective hearing loss and tinnitus, 23% stated that tinnitus was the greater problem, and 38% said that tinnitus and hearing loss were equally troublesome. The corresponding figures for patients with hearing impairment of such a degree that a hearing aid was

TABLE 3 Subjective Classification of Subjective Background of Discomfort in 823 (=100%) Patients

Subjective Complaints About Factors of Discomfort	%
Headache	69.02
Migraine	4.13
Exhaustion	59.99
Lacking in drive	42.16
Feeling of weakness	55.29
Forgetfulness	68.41
Disorientation	0.49
Daze	44.84
Tiredness	63.91
Insomnia	69.50

TABLE 4 Subjective Classification of Most Irritating Factors Related to Their Tinnitus in 823 (=100%) Patients

Most Irritating Factors Related to Tinnitus	%
All patients with specific additional statements	25.76
Difficulties in going to sleep	10.69
Difficulties in sleeping through the night	11.06
Depression	0.24
Abnormal sounds (also hallucinations)	2.67
Acute hearing loss	8.38

deemed necessary were 9% and 41%, respectively. Stress symptoms such as headache, tension of facial muscles, and sleep disturbances were correlated to tinnitus. Of patients with tinnitus, 83% were interested in obtaining treatment for it.

The so-called Copenhagen Male Study reported on the results from a 10-year follow-up examination concerning hearing and factors known to cause hearing problems. The original sample comprised 5050 subjects, and at the present examination, 3387 (67%) men at a median of 63 years of age (range, 53 to 75 years) participated. An increasing prevalence of 30% to 40% of hearing problems was demonstrated with increasing age. A prevalence of 17% of tinnitus of more than 5 minutes' duration was found; 3% indicated that tinnitus was so annoying that it interfered with sleep, reading, and/or concentration. The prevalence of tinnitus increased up to 70 years of age and seemed to remain constant thereafter.

In Norway, 15% of the adult population has experienced shorter or longer periods of tinnitus. Three percent of these, in total approximately 7000 to 10,000 persons, suffer from continuous tinnitus followed by symptoms that represent a handicap or occupational disability. Similar observations were reported from many other countries.

Clinical Types

Tinnitus is no longer considered to be a syndrome or a single disease. Because of improvements in neuro-otometry, several different types of tinnitus can be differentiated.

By means of modern audiometry, the framework for normal hearing can be described objectively and quantitatively. Therefore, in any tinnitus case, a thorough analysis of the hearing function and pathways needs to be performed including threshold audiometry, audiometric tinnitus masking (if possible), acoustic dynamics between the measurable thresholds of hearing and acoustic discomfort, speech audiometry, otoacoustic emissions, acoustic brainstem-evoked potentials, and acoustic late-evoked potentials. Thereby signs of pathology within the hearing pathways between the ear and the human brain cortex can be measured.

Thus, we know from thorough neuro-otologic studies that approximately 24% of cases of disabling tinnitus have their source within the otoacoustic periphery (i.e., inner ear and the eighth cranial nerve). Approximately 35% originate from the acoustic pathways within the brainstem. Approximately 41% have their cause within supratentorial structures and/or functions. These pathologies also should serve as basic information for planning systematic pharmacotherapy directed to the central nervous system (CNS) focus of dysfunction.

At least four different kinds of tinnitus (Figure 1) can be discriminated, which can be determined by the physician using a simple question-and-answer procedure as follows.

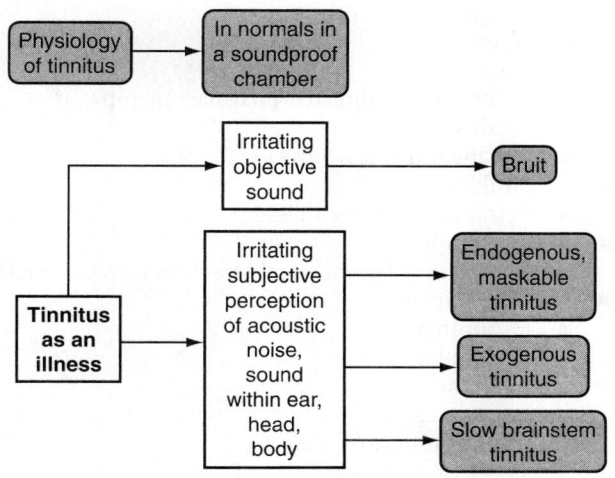

FIGURE 1. Categories of physiologic and clinical types of tinnitus.

BRUITS

Q: Has someone informed you that he or she could hear a noise coming from your head?
A: Yes. Their description of what they heard listening from outside my head is similar to what I perceive.

By means of auscultation through a stethoscope or a microphone, a real sound can be objectively heard emanating from the patient's skull. Patients frequently report, for example, a bubbling, hissing, or pulsating sound.

The cause can be vascular in origin, that is, abnormal curling of blood caused by atheromas, vascular dissections, scars, compressions, or high blood pressure amplitudes, for example.

Bruits also can originate from the middle ear and its connections toward the epipharynx: middle ear inflammations with bubbling sounds of gas from within the effusions, whizzing middle ear muscles, or an open eustachian tube.

Cracking sounds, which are misinterpreted as tinnitus, are reported from arthritic and other mandibular joint disorders. Also, sounds can be transferred from the cervical spine and its joints as well as its vessels into the cranial structures so that they become misinterpreted as tinnitus.

ENDOGENOUS TINNITUS

Q: Where is your feeling of well-being better, in a busy and noisy environment or in cavelike silence?
A: I much prefer a busy and noisy environment.

The patient with a maskable or endogenous tinnitus prefers covering it with external sounds. When using masking procedures, easily three zones of tinnitus can be discriminated within the hearing field:

1. Low-tone tinnitus (at and below 750 Hz)
2. Middle-frequency tinnitus (1 to 2 kHz)
3. High-frequency tinnitus (above 2 kHz until 10 kHz or even 12 kHz)

Low-tone tinnitus is more frequently found in Ménière's disease and some other cochlear-apical disorders, and middle-tone tinnitus is more frequently found in diseases such as otosclerosis. Most frequently tinnitus is matched in the high-tone range and is related, for example, to noise trauma, whiplash, head and skull trauma, cardiovascular failure, stress, acoustic neuromas, and toxic events including those associated with pharmaceutical, nicotine, or drug abuse. Also, several masking points may exist simultaneously.

Dysfunctions of the inner ear contribute to the development of tinnitus. But tinnitus by itself depends on a cortical process of the human brain. A sleeping patient does not suffer from any kind of tinnitus.

Since approximately 1985, the Würzburg neuro-otology group of Claussen et al. has been able to detect by means of vestibular evoked potentials (VestEP) and brain electrical activity mapping (BEAM) groups of patients suffering from a maskable or endogenous tinnitus that respond cortically in a typical, reproducible, and measurable manner:

1. Location of the site of the potentials around the upper gyrus of the temporal lobe (Brodmann's area 41)
2. Typical shortening of the latencies of evoked quantitative electro-encephalograms (QEEGs) (i.e., VestEP waves I, II, III)
3. Enlarged DC shift of the evoked QEEGs (i.e., difference between VestEP waves III and IV)
4. Typical cortical electrical burst expansion in three phases on the brain surface

Since approximately 1990, the New York group of Shulman, Strashun, and Goldstein has followed a neuroradiologic path for deciphering the cortical modalities in tinnitus patients by using single-photon emission computer tomography (SPECT). They discovered remarkably elevated metabolic processes in the temporal lobes of patients suffering from a maskable tinnitus.

Thereafter we were able to prove in therapeutic trials with pharmacotherapy (e.g., extractum ginkgo biloba [EGB 761]*), as well as with physiotherapy (competitive kinesthetic interaction therapy [KKIT]), that the subjective reduction or abolition of tinnitus goes together with an electrophysiologic measurable normalization of the VestEP with BEAM or QEEG. So the endogenous tinnitus could be proven to be a CNS network phenomenon.

EXOGENOUS TINNITUS

Q: Where is your feeling of well-being better, in a busy and noisy environment or in cavelike silence?
A: I much prefer a cavelike silence because noise and/or a group of people speaking at the same time are most confusing. It provokes ringing and shrieking sounds within my ears.

Unlike endogenous tinnitus, patients suffering from exogenous tinnitus cannot benefit from masking noises from their surroundings. Some physicians wrongly call this condition *hyperacusis,* but these patients do not hear better as this term suggests. Seemingly better is the named syndrome of the hypersensitive ear.

In exogenous tinnitus, pure-tone audiometry may be normal or exhibit regular deficits of the hearing threshold, but there is no maskable tinnitus. However, when measuring the acoustic dynamics by adding the audiometrically recorded discomfort threshold, the discomfort level, which is usually between 1 and 8 kHz below 95 dB, rises below this level to values of 90 to 60 dB or even 50 dB. The person being exposed to sound exceeding the level of his low discomfort threshold experiences a loss of understanding together with subjective pain and noise in the ears accompanied by possible vegetative reactions.

Hearing aids can adjust the incoming sounds by filtering, peak clipping, and cleaning of the sound signals so they fit optimally into the remaining acoustic dynamics of the individually existing hearing field. Thus, hearing aids are the first choice for treating exogenous tinnitus. Some other methods for treating this type of tinnitus are physiotherapy, psychotherapy, stress reduction, and supportive pharmacotherapy.

TINNITUS IN SLOW BRAINSTEM SYNDROME (CLAUSSEN)

Q: How would you best describe your tinnitus?
A: I am becoming increasingly more in a daze and more disoriented and hear ringing and other sounds, which I cannot really localize in my ears or my head. The noise disturbs me as much as my mental instability.

We regularly see older patients who complain about a hazy tinnitus in combination with vertigo, giddiness, and dizziness and also report a reduced state of alertness. These patients have a connected statoacoustic problem. Objectively, affected patients exhibit an increase in the latencies of the experimentally provoked vestibular nystagmus as well as of the acoustically evoked brainstem potentials.

Especially in this group, we have noted by evaluating our therapeutic responses that a combination of cocculus† (picrotoxin), conium† (coneine), amber and petrol oil (Vertigoheel†) has a so-called tuning-up effect on the brainstem. Then the typical symptoms also disappear.

COMBINED ENDOGENOUS AND EXOGENOUS TINNITUS

A combination of both types of subjective tinnitus, endogenous and exogenous, is also found in tinnitus patients. Affected patients report that the noise they hear is present during both the day and night; however, the noise fluctuates. Especially the intensity of the noise can be very increased, for example when the patient is in a noisy environment or busy place or in a conversation with several participants.

Even though patients with combined endogenous and exogenous tinnitus have maskable tinnitus, they report that therapeutic acoustic maskers do not reduce their symptoms. They need a thorough audiometric and neuro-otologic workup.

Contemporary and Practical Treatment

Modern therapy of tinnitus appears to be complex and sometimes incomprehensible. But when talking about therapy of disabling tinnitus, we emphasize a main therapeutic approach in the sense that we have to break and inhibit the psychosomatic cycle of deterioration from tinnitus to stress, to insomnia, to panic. Some aspects of this reactional behavior are similar to pain.

The steps for individual tinnitus therapy must be chosen according to the kind of tinnitus diagnosed. Tinnitus is frequently associated with conditions such as stress, hearing loss, noise trauma, otorhinolaryngologic disorders (e.g., Ménière's disease, otosclerosis, perilymphatic fistula, acoustic neuroma), high blood pressure, metabolic disorders, allergy, intoxications, whiplash and other head and neck traumas, functional disorders of the neck, burnout syndrome, mandibular joint problems, and extracranial and intracranial vascular problems.

The Current Therapy box lists different therapeutic approaches to tinnitus. These therapies must be individually interrelated with the different types of tinnitus (see Figure 1). Besides the severe disabling types of tinnitus, minor forms of tinnitus also occasionally occur that may be event related or may be time limited.

CURRENT THERAPY

- Avoidance of noise, ototoxic drugs, allergens
- Treatment of bruits by medical or surgical measures
- Instrumental therapy
- Tinnitus maskers
- Hearing aids
- Electrostimulation
- Specific pharmacotherapy
    - Lidocaine (Xylocaine)[1]
    - Carbamazepine (Tegretol)[1]
- Calming pharmacotherapy
    - Diazepam (Valium)[1]
    - Amitriptyline (Elavil)[1]
- Nontropic pharmacotherapy
    - Gingko*
    - Flunarizine[2]
- Neurotransmitter-directed pharmacotherapy
    - Betahistine*
    - Gabapentin (Neurontin)
- Psychotherapy
    - Retraining therapy (TRT)
- Physiotherapy
    - Competitive kinesthetic interaction therapy (KKIT)
- Other therapies
    - Hypnotherapy
    - Counseling
    - Acupuncture

[1]Not FDA approved for this indication.
[2]Not available in the United States.
*Available as dietary supplement.

---

*Available as dietary supplement.
†Available as homeopathic remedy.

NOISE AVOIDANCE AND BASICS OF THERAPY

Avoidance can help in noise-related tinnitus by the prevention of noise exposure or at least by wearing ear protection. The use of ototoxic drugs must be controlled and limited. Inflammatory ear disease needs specific treatment of the external and the middle ear with antibiotics and anti-inflammatory drugs. Control and maintenance of a satisfactory degree of aeration of the middle ear is necessary. Acoustic neuroma calls for surgical removal of the tumor. Surgery is also necessary in otosclerosis and perilymphatic fistula. Specific gnathologic therapy by a dentist is recommended in a temporomandibular joint syndrome.

INSTRUMENTATIONS FOR THERAPY

Instrumentations currently available and frequently used according to the type and the chronicity of tinnitus are as follows:

1. Tinnitus maskers/tinnitus instruments, tapes/CDs for masking and relaxation
2. Acoustic ultra-high-frequency stimulation
3. Hearing aids
4. External electrical stimulations
5. External magnetic stimulation

PHARMACOTHERAPY

Pharmacotherapy, that is, treatment with pharmaceutical agents, is important in the management of tinnitus. It may be the main therapy or may play only a supportive, palliative, or intermittent role. The four lines of therapeutic agents used in the treatment of tinnitus may overlap and may be combined.

First-Line Agents

First-line therapeutic agents can relieve tinnitus either slowly or quickly. Lidocaine (Xylocaine),[1] a local anesthetic drug, only has a temporary effect in suppressing tinnitus. It is an aminoethylamide, which is well soluble in water.

A daily intravenous dose of lidocaine of 1 mg per kg of body weight can temporarily alleviate the phenomenon of endogenous tinnitus. The duration, however, depends on the blood level. As soon as the level of lidocaine in the blood is lowered below a threshold, tinnitus returns.

In tinnitus, lidocaine is best applied by iontophoresis through an electrical field with an active electrode in the external ear and a passive electrode at an arm, after instillation of a solution of lidocaine (1:100,000) into the external meatus.

This therapy temporarily relieves the disturbing tinnitus, so that the patients at least get some hours of rest and sleep. However, the untoward side effects of lidocaine also have to be taken into consideration.

Some forms of tinnitus also have an acoustic hallucinatory component, as in epilepsia. Therefore, carbamazepine (Tegretol),[1] which is an important antiepileptic agent used for bipolar affective disorders, is also used in tinnitus with a supratentorial focus. We have seen beneficial effects in very specific cases of endogenous tinnitus. Chemically, carbamazepine belongs to the tricyclic antidepressants. In adults, we give a daily dose of 200 mg. However, renal, hepatic, and hematologic parameters have to be monitored thoroughly.

Second-Line Agents

This group of drugs is especially used to treat the emotional effects seen in endogenous tinnitus, exogenous tinnitus, and combined endogenous and exogenous tinnitus, which can lead via sleeplessness to anxiety and panic. Here we see an indication for alprazolam (Xanax)[1] and similar substances. Alprazolam is administered to tinnitus patients in a daily dosage of 0.75 to 1.5 mg. Also chlordiazepoxide (Librium)[1] can alternatively be applied in a daily dosage of 15 to 30 mg. Even diazepam (Valium)[1] is used in a daily dosage of 4 to 30 mg.

The mood changes associated with tinnitus can lead to psychosis and insomnia. Here a tricyclic antidepressant such as amitriptyline (Elavil)[1] in a daily dosage of 75 to 150 mg can be helpful.

Additionally, this agent has a desired sedative component. Other sedatives and psychotropic drugs are also used to treat the psychologic effects associated with tinnitus, but they must be applied very carefully.

Third-Line Agents

Third-line therapeutic agents comprise the so-called nootropic drugs. These are pharmacologic agents that activate brain function through improved metabolism, leading to a better adaptation and interconnection. They were originally developed to treat senile dementia. Within this group, in Germany, we use piracetam (Nootrop, Normabraïn) in a daily dosage of 800 to 1200 mg.

We have seen very beneficial effects from extract of ginkgo biloba (EGB 761*) (Tebonin, Rökan), which is administered in a daily dosage of 120 mg.

We also use calcium channel antagonists, among which flunarizine (Sibelium),[2] in a daily dosage of 15 to 30 mg, is effective in tinnitus with irritative foci, especially in mesencephalic and diencephalic areas. Cinnarizin[2] was the predecessor. This holds especially for the endogenous tinnitus group.

Fourth-Line Agents

The fourth line of therapy involves neurotransmitter-directed pharmacotherapy. According to the chemical structures of the neurotransmitters, we mainly use one system of the amines (i.e., the histamine mechanism) and one system of amino acids (i.e., γ-aminobutyric acid [GABA]).

Because it is known that inner ear functions are regulated at the neurotransmission level of the histaminergic H_1, H_2, and H_3 receptors, betahistine (Serc)[2] plays an important role in inner ear receptor-targeted therapy. The daily dosage that we administer in peripheral cochlear tinnitus is 16 to 48 mg.

The inhibitory neurotransmitter GABA is extremely potent in its ability to alter neuronal discharges because of failures in the supratentorial CNS neurotransmission. According to recent findings, endogenous tinnitus with a supratentorial dysregulation can be influenced by gabapentin (Neurontin).[1] It is used in dosages starting with 300 mg daily and can be increased to 900 mg daily. Originally gabapentin was used as an additional therapy in partial epilepsia without secondary generalized seizures. Like with other antiepileptic drugs, the parameters from kidney, liver, and blood have to be supervised.

ADAPTED PSYCHOTHERAPY

Nowadays so-called tinnitus retraining therapy (TRT) is widely applied. It includes a therapeutic wide-band low-level noise generator. It is based on habituation, which is defined as a reduced response to a stimulus after repeated exposure. It is a state in which the tinnitus signal no longer elicits any response. Resetting or reprogramming neuronal networks involved in subcortical signal detection brings about habituation.

Also, in cases with a known interrelation of stress and tinnitus, a stress–diathesis model for tinnitus was proposed by Shulman et al. Stress management techniques require a counselor and the close cooperation of the patient, physician, biofeedback therapist, and psychologist.

A cognitive therapy that provides significant support to the patient with severe disabling tinnitus, particularly for control of the effect, is strongly recommended and encouraged.

ADAPTED PHYSIOTHERAPY

A specific program of physiotherapy successfully applied in endogenous tinnitus is KKIT. This therapy uses expressive movements of body language. In a special rehabilitation program, different groups

---

[1]Not FDA approved for this indication.

*Available as dietary supplement.
[1]Not FDA approved for this indication.
[2]Not available in the United States.

of muscles in the hand, arm, leg, foot, and body, rising from the feet up to the face, are activated, which guides the tinnitus patient into a situation of peaceful resting, reduction of tension, and finally into relaxation. This scheme was adapted from a program of treating pain. KKIT points toward mechanisms of interference of expressive gestural movements with facilitating tinnitus from around the basal ganglia of the brain.

OTHER METHODS OF THERAPY

During the recent years, the external magnetotherapy in tinnitus cases of the type of endogenous tinnitus has been developed. Several authors have proved that pulsating electromagnetic fields applied over the temporal lobe of the brain can reduce the tinnitus complaints or even abolish the complaints during the application. The effect can also be longer lasting after the application. The basis of assessment for the magnetic intensities of the pulsating fields should extend from 2 to 100 mT. The frequency rate should lie between 3 and 12 Hz.

Worldwide, many innovations now take place in this field of a broadened scope of modern tinnitus therapy in special cases. Other methods of tinnitus therapy recommended in the literature include acupuncture, counseling, group therapy, and hypnotherapy.

ACKNOWLEDGMENT

Sponsored by grant Projekt D. 1417, durch die LVA Baden-Württemberg, Stuttgart, Germany.

REFERENCES

Alster J, Shemesh Z, Ornan M, Attias J. Sleep disturbance associated with chronic tinnitus. Biol Psychiatry 1993;34:84–90.

Arnesen AR, Engdahl B. Tinnitus—etiology, diagnosis and treatment. Tidsskr Nor Laegeforen 1996;116:2009–12.

Bergmann JM, Bertora GO. Cortical and brainstem topodiagnostic testing in tinnitus patients—a preliminary report. Int Tinnitus J 1996;2:151–8.

Bertora GO, Bergmann JM. Tinnitus: Supratentorial areas study through brain electric tomography (LORETA), ASN 2004;2:2. ISSN 1612–3352. Available at http://www.neurootology.org.

Claussen CF. Treatment of the slow brainstem syndrome with Vertigoheel. Biol Med 1985;3:447–70, 4:510–4.

Claussen CF. Medical classification of tinnitus between bruits: exogenous and endogenous tinnitus and other types of tinnitus, ASN 2004;2 (ISSN):1612–3352. Available at http://www.neurootology.org.

Claussen CF, Kolchev C, Schneider D, Hahn A. Neurootological brain electrical activity mapping in tinnitus patients. Proceedings of the 4th International Tinnitus Seminar. Bordeaux 1991;1092:351–5.

Claussen CF, Schneider D, Koltchev C. On the functional state of central vestibular structures in monaural symptomatic tinnitus patients. Int Tinnitus J 1995;1:5–12.

George RN, Kemp S. A survey of New Zealanders with tinnitus. Br J Audiol 1991;25:331–6.

Jastreboff PJ, Hazell JWP. A neurophysiological approach to tinnitus: clinical implications. Br J Audiol 1993;27:1–11.

Kersebaum M. Clinical therapy of tinnitus by means of exogenous magnetic stimulation. 19th IFOS-Congress. Sao Paulo: Brasil; 2009.

Kleinjung T, Eichhammer P, Langguth B, et al. Long-term effects of repetitive transcranial magnetic stimulation (rTMS) in patients with chronic tinnitus. Otolaryngol Head Neck Surg 2005;132:566–9.

Parving A, Hein HO, Suadicani P, et al. Epidemiology of hearing disorders. Some factors affecting hearing. The Copenhagen Male Study. Scand Audiol 1993;22:101–7.

Plewnia C, Bartels M, Gerloff C. Transient suppression of tinnitus by transcranial magnetic stimulation. Ann Neurol 2003;53:263–6.

Quaranta A, Assennato G, Sallustio V. Epidemiology of hearing problems among adults in Italy. Scand Audiol Suppl 1996;42:9–13.

Shulman A. A final common pathway for tinnitus—the medial temporal lobe system. Tinnitus J 1996;2:115–26.

Shulman A, Aran JM, Feldmann H, et al. Tinnitus diagnosis/treatment. Philadelphia: Lea & Febiger; 1991.

Shulman A, Strashun AM, Afriyie M, et al. SPECT imaging of brain and tinnitus—neurotologic/neurologic implications. Int Tinnitus J 1995; 1:13–29.

Spine Pain

Method of
David Borenstein, MD, and
Federico Balagué, MD

Spine pain is a common symptom that is diagnosed and treated by a wide variety of health care professionals. The interest in this medical problem is not limited to its incidence as a patient problem but also the likelihood of spine pain being experienced by the treating physician as well. The good news about spine pain is that the vast majority of patients (about 90%) improve over 2 months with minimal intervention. The bad news is that the smaller number of patients who develop chronic spine pain utilize more than the majority of health resources expended on this expensive medical problem. The goal of therapy is to relieve spine pain while it is acute so that chronic pain does not develop.

The axial skeleton may be divided into cervical, thoracic, lumbar, sacral, and coccygeal locations. The lumbar and cervical areas are the most mobile and at greatest risk for damage. These two areas will be the primary subjects of this article.

Epidemiology

Spine pain is the most common musculoskeletal complaint worldwide and produces direct and indirect costs of hundreds of billions of dollars each year in the United States. More than 80% of the world's population at some time during their lives will have an episode of low back pain. An estimated 20% of the U.S. population has back pain every year. Neck pain occurs at a variable rate ranging from 0.055/1000 person-years (disk herniation with radiculopathy) to 213/1000 person-years (self-reported neck pain). Thoracic spine pain is relatively rare compared to the incidence of pain in the other two locations in the axial skeleton.

Persons of all ages develop spine pain. Younger people are at risk for developmental problems (idiopathic scoliosis, spondylolysis, spondylolisthesis), and older patients develop disorders associated with degeneration of spinal structures (osteoarthritis, spinal stenosis).

Risk Factors

Psychosocial factors are stronger predictors of incident low back pain than mechanical factors in adolescent populations. In adults, psychosocial difficulties are risk factors for chronicity more strongly related to outcome than any clinical or mechanical variables. Previous episodes of spine pain are strong predictors of future ones.

Studies of cohorts of twins have shown that nonspecific low back pain is more than 60% genetically determined, and work and leisure-time physical activities play a minor role. Other environmental factors, such as smoking and obesity, have not been shown to be a predictor of the development of spine pain on a consistent basis.

Pathophysiology

Most of the structures of the axial skeleton receive sensory input. The presence of anatomic alterations in these structures is not sufficient to predict the presence of pain. In general, spine pain is referred to as nonspecific because no definite pain generator can be identified. The nociceptive inputs generated by musculoskeletal structures is referred to as somatic pain.

In the first few decades of life, muscular sprains and strains of the paraspinous muscles in the lumbar and cervical regions are the most likely source of spinal pain. These muscular injuries occur when lifting in a position that places stress on paraspinous structures. Often the spine is in an awkward position and is mechanically disadvantaged. The subsequent muscle injury results in reflexive muscular contraction that can recruit muscles in the same myotome. Tonic contraction approximates the damaged components of the muscle but results in relative anoxia that causes the production of anaerobic metabolites that stimulate nociceptors. The number of recruited muscles may be extensive, manifested by severe spinal stiffness and limitation of motion. Most of these soft tissue injuries to the muscle heal spontaneously without any long-term structural alterations.

Simultaneously, as people age, intervertebral disks become flatter as the nucleus pulposus loses its absorbency and the annulus fibrosus fissures and degenerates. The process results in the loss of disk integrity. Degeneration of normal biomechanical and biochemical disk properties results. Biomechanical insufficiency inevitably results in a transfer of stresses posterior to the facet joints and ligaments that are ill suited to assume compressive, tensile, and shear loads. Osteophytes form in response to these abnormal pressures, compromising the space for the neural elements. Disk degeneration itself might not be a painful process until alterations in facet joint alignment result in the onset of articular pain.

Spondylolysis is a developmental abnormality associated with a stress fracture in the growth plate of the pars interarticularis. This abnormality may be discovered as a radiographic abnormality in an asymptomatic patient. An increased risk of low back pain occurs with spondylolisthesis, the abnormality associated with instability of spinal elements in the setting of spondylolysis.

Pain generation in the axial skeleton may be somatic or neuropathic in origin. The joints, ligaments, muscles, fascia, blood vessels, and disks can be the source of localized somatic spine pain. Somatic pain, when it does radiate, tends to be less focused in distribution and exacerbated by specific positions of the spine.

Neuropathic or radicular pain is the sensation generated by damage of neural elements. Intervertebral disk herniation with compression of spinal nerve roots causes neural inflammation resulting in neuropathic and radicular pain. Radicular pain follows the path of the corresponding spinal nerve root. In addition to pain, sensory deficits and muscle weakness can occur, depending on the intensity of the nerve compression.

Prevention

Since the turn of the century, adolescents report nonspecific spine pain at an incidence similar to that in adult populations. This finding suggests that primary prevention must be given at a very early age to have any chance of efficacy.

Among papers reporting on primary prevention, only exercise has shown effectiveness, with effect sizes ranging from 0.39 to 0.69. Other techniques, such as stress management, shoe inserts, back supports, education, and reduced lifting, were found ineffective.

Clinical Manifestations

The most common symptoms of spinal disorders are regional pain and decreased range of motion associated in a minority of patients with radiating pain. For the majority of patients, pain has mechanical characteristics: Its intensity increases with physical activity, movements, or some postures and decreases with rest. However, it has been demonstrated that nocturnal pain is not uncommon in the absence of serious specific spinal disorders. The precise topography of pain is often difficult for the patient to describe, and its interpretation is difficult owing to the overlap of the cutaneous projections between adjacent spinal levels and the similarities between dermatomes, myotomes, and sclerotomes.

Diagnosis

The diagnosis of spine pain is based upon the patient's history and physical examination. The history and physical examination should include description of pain as detailed as possible (e.g., past episodes, precise

CURRENT DIAGNOSIS

- Most spine pain is mechanical in origin in 95% or more of patients
- Symptoms of mechanical acute spine pain resolve in most patients in 1 to 8 weeks
- Most patients with spine pain do not require laboratory tests or radiographs to achieve resolution of their symptom of spine pain

location, beginning of symptoms, factors increasing or decreasing pain intensity, radiating pain, neurologic symptoms, systemic symptoms), patient's medical history (e.g., past spinal surgery, neoplasia, corticosteroid treatments), and a limited physical examination focused on the posture of the spine, range of motion, muscle contraction, pain on palpation or percussion, and a brief neurologic examination.

Besides the high rate of false positives and financial costs, imaging studies have a negative effect on a patient's quality of life. Therefore, unless there is a clear-cut surgical indication or a suspicion of an underlying life-threatening disorder, no imaging studies should be ordered on the first encounter for a patient with acute nonspecific low back or neck pain. Similarly, laboratory testing is not required unless a patient presents with clinical symptoms that suggest a systemic illness (e.g., fever, weight loss).

Differential Diagnosis

A number of guidelines are available in the literature to help a clinician in the diagnosis and treatment of patients with spine pain. The purpose of these approaches is to differentiate the vast majority of patients with mechanical disorders who will improve with noninvasive therapy without the need for radiographic or laboratory investigation from the small minority with a specific cause of spinal pain.

Traditionally, red flags have been used to identify patients with a systemic disorder causing spine pain. The red flags have included questions regarding prior history of cancer, weight loss, prolonged morning stiffness, bladder dysfunction, and bowel dysfunction. The presence of these findings suggests a diagnosis of malignancy, infection, spondyloarthropathy, or cauda equina syndrome, respectively. A study has reported that red flag disorders occur so infrequently and have false positive findings as not to be helpful in the primary care setting at the initial visit. The one exception was spine pain associated with osteoporotic vertebral compression fractures.

Despite the findings of this one report, clinicians need to be mindful of patients who would be harmed to a significant degree by delayed therapy. The three disorders that require expeditious evaluation and treatment are intraabdominal vascular disorders with tearing pain and hemodynamic instability (expanding aortic aneurysm); cauda equina syndrome with bilateral sciatica; saddle anesthesia; bladder or bowel incontinence (lumbar space-occupying compressive lesions); and cervical myelopathy with balance difficulties, autonomic dysfunction, and hyperreflexia with spasticity and Babinski's sign (cervical space-occupying compressive lesions). These disorders require expeditious vessel repair or decompression surgery.

The differential diagnosis of mechanical low back pain (Table 1) and mechanical neck pain (Table 2) includes disorders ranging from muscle strain and herniated disk to scoliosis and whiplash injuries. The age of patients, pain pattern with exacerbating and mitigating factors, tension signs, and findings of plain radiographs can help differentiate among these common causes of spine pain.

Nonspecific is a term used commonly to describe the pain associated with mechanical disorders. On occasion, physicians have confused the use of "nonspecific" as an absence of pathology causing pain associated with mechanical disorders. The "nonspecific" designation refers to the inability to identify the specific pain-generating anatomic structure, not the absence of somatic pain.

TABLE 1 Mechanical Low Back Pain

Feature	Muscle Strain	Herniated Nucleus Pulposus	Osteoarthritis	Spinal Stenosis	Spondylolisthesis	Scoliosis
Age (yr)	20-40	30-50	>50	>60	20	30
Pain Pattern						
Location	Back (unilateral)	Back/leg (unilateral)	Back (unilateral)	Leg (bilateral)	Back	Back
Onset	Acute	Acute (previous episodes)	Insidious	Insidious	Insidious	Insidious
Standing	↑	↓	↑	↑	↑	↑
Sitting	↓	↑	↓	↓	↓	↓
Bending	↑	↑	↓	↓	↑	↑
Straight leg	−	+	−	+ (stress)	−	−
Plain radiograph*	−	−	+	+	+	+

*Possibility of seeing the abnormality, not a recommendation to get radiographs.
↑, increased; ↓, decreased; +, present; −, absent
Reprinted with permission from Mechanical low back pain. In Borenstein DG, Wiesel SW, Boden SD (eds): Low back and neck pain, 3rd ed. Philadelphia, WB Saunders, 2004.

TABLE 2 Mechanical Neck Pain

Feature	Neck Strain	Herniated Nucleus Pulposus	Osteoarthritis	Myelopathy	Whiplash
Age (yr)	20-40	30-50	>50	>60	30-40
Pain Pattern					
Location	Neck	Neck/arm	Neck	Arm/leg	Neck
Onset	Acute	Acute	Insidious	Insidious	Acute
Flexion	+	+	−	−	+
Extension	−	+/−	+	+	+
Plain radiograph*	−	−	+	+	−

*Possibility of seeing the abnormality, not a recommendation to get radiographs.
+, present; −, absent.
(Reprinted with permission from Mechanical neck pain. In Borenstein DG, Wiesel SW, Boden SD (eds): Low back and neck pain, 3rd ed. Philadelphia, WB Saunders, 2004.)

Therapy

Many mechanical disorders of the spine are self-limited in duration, with a vast majority of patients improving gradually over time (Box 1). This progression to "natural healing" makes placebo look efficacious in many clinical trials investigating therapies for spine pain. This situation results in evidence-based reviews of spine pain therapies revealing very few categories that have a clinically significant impact on improvement. Nonetheless, physicians need to make therapeutic choices for their patients despite this relative paucity of

---

BOX 1 Management of Low Back Pain

Acute (<6 weeks)
First consultation: gather information on core outcome domains
Rule out pain of nonspinal origin
Rule out specific causes (red flags)
No routine imaging
Inform and reassure the patient. Advise to stay active and continue daily activities, if possible, including work
Prescribe analgesia, if necessary. First choice: acetaminophen; second choice: NSAIDs
Consider adding muscle relaxants (short course) or referring for spinal manipulation
Avoid overmedicalizing, especially in patients with favorable outcome
Be aware of yellow flags: inappropriate attitudes and beliefs about back pain, inappropriate pain behavior, emotional problems

Subacute (6-12 weeks)
Reassessment

Bear in mind minimum clinically important difference of core outcome tools
Consider patients' expectations
Consider yellow flags if outcome is not favorable
Reassess regularly by valid outcome tools to evaluate response to treatment
Focus on function
Give priority to active treatments
Consider multidisciplinary program in occupational setting for workers with subacute low back pain and sick leave (>4-8 weeks)

Chronic (> 12 weeks)
Repeat thorough clinical examination
In cases of low impairment and disability, simple evidence-based therapies (e.g., exercises, medication, brief interventions might be sufficient)
In cases of more-severe disability or chronicity, give priority to multidisciplinary approaches (biopsychosocial)

NSAID, nonsteroidal antiinflammatory drug.
From Balagué F, Mannion AF, Pellisé F, Cedraschi C. Clinical update: low back pain. Lancet 2007;369(9563):726-728.

- Localized neck or low back pain
  - Encouragement to remain active out of bed
  - Patient education about the natural history to improvement
  - Reassurance about the incidence of resolution
  - Effective oral drug therapy: NSAIDs, analgesics, muscle relaxants
  - Physical therapy with exercise program
- Radicular pain
  - Encouragement to remain active out of bed
  - Patient education about the potential for improvement
  - Efficacy of oral drug therapy: NSAIDs, analgesics, muscle relaxants, corticosteroids, antiseizure medication, epidural corticosteroid injections
  - Physical therapy: Mackenzie exercises for disk herniation
  - Surgical decompression for cauda equina, motor weakness, or intractable pain

NSAID, nonsteroidal antiinflammatory drug.

evidence. Therapy for spine pain includes controlled physical activity, nonsteroidal antiinflammatory drugs (NSAIDs), skeletal muscle relaxants, local and epidural corticosteroid injections, and long-term pain therapy. Surgical intervention is reserved for patients who have surgically correctable abnormalities and who have cauda equina syndrome, increasing motor weakness, spasticity, or intractable pain.

The treatment of an individual patient has to be tailored based on the patient's expectations and preferences. Goals of the treatment should be clearly defined and the patient informed about the expected benefits and side effects of the treatment at the first encounter. A short trial limited to a few days may be a good start.

Self-management with education of the patient about maintaining physical activities as tolerated has been encouraged for neck and low back pain. Information on nonpharmacologic pain-management strategies and daily life activities may be provided by health care providers, but patients adhere more to the former than to the latter.

Exercises are slightly effective for pain and function in patients with chronic low back pain. No specific form of exercise is clearly better than others.

The use of manipulative physical techniques in the care of spine pain patients remains controversial. The absence of clear-cut distinctions between manipulative techniques with or without thrust adds to the confusion when one analyzes the efficacy of manual therapy treatments. Overall there is some clinical trial evidence in favor of spinal manipulation for acute low back pain.

NSAIDs have short-term efficacy for both acute and chronic low back pain; however, the effect sizes are not very large. The efficacy of these drugs for patients with radicular pain has not been evaluated well enough to make general recommendations. No single class of NSAIDs has superiority to another. Cyclooxygenase 2 (COX-2) inhibitors have a better gastrointestinal (GI) safety profile but no greater efficacy. A patient's response cannot be predicted, and a trial and error approach is often necessary.

Opiates have not demonstrated any favorable influence in the outcome of low back pain patients. Side effects are quite common and the risk of addiction is real. When these kinds of drugs are effective, the improvement is more important in pain intensity than in terms of function. Muscle relaxants do have some efficacy for acute and chronic low back pain, but the effect size is limited.

Antidepressants are not generally prescribed owing to an inconsistent improvement of patients. For patients with chronic low back pain and depression, an optimized antidepressant treatment shows a better effect on depression than pain and functional capacity.

Evidence is lacking to support the prescription of systemic corticosteroids. However, corticosteroids have the advantage of not being toxic to the kidneys. Oral corticosteroids may be considered in patients with radicular pain from a herniated disk or spinal stenosis where epidural injections are relatively contraindicated (chronic warfarin therapy).

Some patients will have persistent neuropathic pain despite surgical decompression or as a result of postsurgical fibrosis. Opioid therapy is ineffective in many patients with chronic neuropathic pain. Antiseizure medicines, such as gabapentin (Neurontin)[1] and pregabalin (Lyrica) have efficacy in peripheral neuropathic pain. These same medicines are prescribed in patients with chronic neuropathic radicular pain[1] with the hope that the mechanisms that work with peripheral neuropathy will also work for spine pain patients. Other medicines including antidepressants (duloxetine [Cymbalta],[1] tricyclic antidepressants) have been tried when other drugs have been ineffective.

Epidural, selective nerve root, or facet joint injections have not shown adequate efficacy to be recommended on a regular basis. However, a limited number (2 or 3) of spinal injections may be attempted for patients with radicular pain who do not improve with oral medication.

Spinal surgery is indicated for disk herniation with radicular compromise, cervical or lumbar spinal stenosis with myelopathy or neurogenic claudication, and unstable spondylolisthesis. Controversy remains however, concerning the relative benefit of surgical versus medical therapy for radiculopathy. Diskectomy significantly shortens (by about 8 weeks) the acute phase of pain associated with radiculopathy. However, studies with longer follow-up periods have never shown a clear difference between conservative and surgical therapies. Some studies have shown that intensive multidisciplinary conservative programs can be compared with surgical fusion procedures for patients with spinal instability.

For the most chronically disabled spine pain patients only, intensive multidisciplinary programs including, among others, physical reconditioning and cognitive-behavioral methods, have shown effectiveness.

Monitoring

From the standpoint of monitoring of the efficacy of the treatment, five main dimensions have been recommended to evaluate the outcome of patients with spine pain. The intensity of pain is relevant, but also the perceived functional capacity, generic health status, work disability, and satisfaction with treatment. Many tools are available for the evaluation of each specific dimension. The clinician who decides to start using any specific tool needs to know, among other information, the minimal clinically meaningful changes for each tool because differences that may be statistically significant when comparing two groups of patients may be irrelevant at the individual patient level. For example, in terms of intensity of pain, the threshold is usually accepted is 3.5 to 4.7 and 2.5 to 4.5 for patients with acute and chronic pain, respectively.

Precisely evaluating several domains with specific tools is rather time consuming. However, for busy clinicians, there are brief instruments (core set of measures) with roughly 7 or 8 questions that include all the previously mentioned dimensions and that have been properly validated.

Complications

The clinician should inform the patient about the possible side effects of therapies as they are initiated. At subsequent visits, specific questions regarding the potential side effects are asked. For example, the presence of hypertension, peripheral edema, and hepatic and renal dysfunction need to be evaluated in patients who are taking chronic NSAID therapy.

[1]Not FDA approved for this indication.

In addition, a majority of NSAIDs have potential GI toxicity including mild mucosal irritation, ulcers, and perforations. Hematologic and neurologic toxicity are quite variable depending on the prescribed drug. Cardiovascular toxicity may clearly be an issue, particularly for long-term treatments. The benefit of persistent use of NSAIDs for patients with chronic spine pain needs to be weighed against the increased risk of toxicities.

The use of opiates induces constipation and urinary retention that may be a serious problem for some patients. These drugs can also produce drowsiness, headache, nausea, or vomiting.

Antidepressants also produce drowsiness and anticholinergic symptoms during the first couple of weeks of use. These drugs have specific side effects including tachycardia, weight gain, or sexual problems.

REFERENCES

Balagué F, Mannion AF, Pellisé F, Cedraschi C. Clinical update: Low back pain. Lancet 2007;369(9563):726–8.

Bigos SJ, Holland J, Holland C, et al. High-quality controlled trials on preventing episodes of back problems: Systematic literature review in working-age adults. Spine J 2009;9(2):147–68.

Borenstein DG. Chronic neck pain: How to approach treatment. Curr Pain Headache Rep 2007;11(6):436–9.

Briggs AM, Smith AJ, Straker LM, Bragge P. Thoracic spine pain in the general population: Prevalence, incidence and associated factors in children, adolescents and adults. A systematic review. BMC Musculoskelet Disord 2009;10:77.

Chou R, Qaseem A, Snow V, et al. Diagnosis and treatment of low back pain: A joint clinical practice guideline from the American College of Physicians and the American Pain Society. Ann Intern Med 2007;147:478–91.

Chou R, Huffman LH. Medications for acute and chronic low back pain: A review of the evidence for an American Pain Society/American College of Physicians clinical practice guideline. Ann Intern Med 2007;147:505–614.

Chou R, Fu R, Carrino JA, Deyo RA. Imaging strategies for low-back pain: systematic review and meta-analysis. Lancet 2009;373(9662):463–72.

Chou R, Atlas SJ, Stanos SP, Rosenquist RW. Nonsurgical interventional therapies for low back pain: A review of the evidence for an American Pain Society clinical practice guideline. Spine 2009;34(10):1078–93.

Chou R, Baisden J, Carragee EJ, et al. Surgery for low back pain: A review of the evidence for an American Pain Society Clinical Practice Guideline. Spine 2009;34(10):1094–109.

Costa Lda C, Maher CG, et al. Prognosis for patients with chronic low back pain: Inception cohort study. BMJ 2009;339:b3829.

Deyo RA, Mirza SK, Turner JA, Martin BI. Overtreating chronic back pain: Time to back off? J Am Board Fam Med 2009;22(1):62–8.

Henschke N, Maher CG, Refshauge KM, et al. Prevalence of and screening for serious spinal pathology in patients presenting to primary care settings with acute low back pain. Arthritis Rheum 2009;60(10):3072–80.

The Infectious Diseases

The Patient with HIV Disease

Method of

*Ryan Westergaard, MD, and
Amita Gupta, MD, MHS*

Since its first description in the early 1980s, the acquired immunodeficiency syndrome (AIDS) has become one of the most devastating epidemics in human history. Millions of new infections occur every year, predominantly in resource-poor settings where access to diagnosis and treatment of human immunodeficiency virus (HIV) infection remains inadequate. The natural history of HIV infection remains one of progressive immune system dysfunction with inevitable acute and chronic infectious complications. With few exceptions, the inexorable decline in T-lymphocyte function eventually leads to the death of untreated patients. Remarkable advances in therapeutics, leading to the development of highly active antiretroviral therapy (HAART), have transformed HIV infection from an almost universally fatal illness to a chronic disease that can be managed over decades with an enlarging repertoire of treatment options. This chapter provides an overview of the current understanding of HIV pathogenesis and epidemiology and reviews guidelines for the initial evaluation and long-term management of HIV infection in adult patients.

Epidemiology

According to the Joint United Nations Programme on HIV/AIDS, an estimated 33 million people were living with HIV at the end of 2007; roughly half of them were women, and more than 2 million were children. Of the estimated 7400 new infections that occur daily, 96% occur in low- and middle-income countries, and approximately 1000 of those infected are children younger than 15 years of age. The prevalence of HIV infection in populations varies widely across the world, with the highest documented rates occurring in southern Africa, where prevalence rates derived from surveillance of asymptomatic pregnant women have exceeded 30% in some settings. AIDS is now the leading cause of death worldwide for persons aged 15 to 59 years, and this trend is associated with particularly dire social and economic consequences in sub-Saharan Africa, where more than half of global AIDS deaths occur. In some sub-Saharan countries such as Swaziland, Botswana, and Lesotho, life expectancy has been reduced by more than 20 years. However, with a rapid and significant increase in funding and commitment from the U.S. government (President's Emergency Plan for AIDS Relief [PEPFAR]) and many multilateral agencies such as the Global Fund, a dramatic increase in prevention, care, and treatment services is now underway. A stabilization and initial trend illustrating a global decrease in AIDS deaths is being observed.

North America has experienced a striking decline in AIDS deaths since the advent of HAART, although a sizeable reduction in the annual number of new HIV infections has not yet been achieved. In the United States, an estimated 1.1 million people are living with HIV. The Centers for Disease Control and Prevention (CDC) estimates that 21% of these individuals are unaware of their HIV status. The CDC estimates that approximately 56,300 people were newly infected with HIV in 2006. Ethnic minorities, particularly African Americans, are disproportionately represented among those with new infections. As is the case worldwide, sexual contact accounts for the majority of HIV transmission for both men and women. In the United States, male-to-male sexual contact represents the mode of acquisition for the majority (61%) of new cases among men, whereas most women are infected via heterosexual contact. Injection drug use accounts for roughly 20% of new HIV infections in both men and women.

The risk of HIV transmission per exposure has been estimated from studies of discordant couples and cohort studies. The average risk of HIV transmission per coital act in serodiscordant heterosexual couples is approximately 0.1%. The presence of other sexually transmitted infections and higher viral load (VL) increase the risk of transmission; condom use and male circumcision considerably reduce the risk. Female-to-male transmission is less effective than male-to-female transmission. Receptive anal intercourse is associated with a higher risk of transmission compared with vaginal intercourse. Even though the risk of transmission by oral sex is very low, it should not be considered completely safe.

Mother-to-child transmission can occur in utero, in the peripartum period, and during breast-feeding. The probability of transmission is most influenced by maternal plasma VL. Other risk factors include maternal CD4+ T-cell count (discussed later), hepatitis C infection, premature rupture of membranes, preterm birth, and duration of breast-feeding. In United States, mother-to-child transmission has been markedly reduced (from 20%-25% to <1%) through routine HIV testing and effective interventions. These interventions include HAART, elective cesarean delivery if the VL is greater than 1000 copies per milliliter at week 38, and recommendation to avoid breast-feeding. The risk of HIV transmission with breast-feeding is 10% to 16% in the absence of intervention and is thought to be highest during the first 2 to 4 months. Factors that increase transmission include inflammatory or ulcerative conditions of the breast, mastitis, and breast abscess. Infants with thrush are more likely to acquire HIV from an infected mother via breast-feeding. In many low-income countries where breast-feeding is critical for infant nutrition and survival, the issue is complex and is the subject of ongoing investigation.

Pathophysiology

HIV is an enveloped, single-stranded RNA virus belonging to the family Retroviridae. It was recognized as the causative agent of AIDS within 3 years after the initial description of the syndrome in 1981, and ongoing characterization of its molecular biology has provided the identification of multiple targets for drug development. Two human immunodeficiency viruses exist: HIV-1 and HIV-2. HIV-1 has worldwide distribution, accounts for most infections outside western Africa, and is the focus of this chapter.

HIV-2 infection causes a similar clinical syndrome but is less efficiently transmitted and results in lower levels of viremia and slower progression to AIDS. A key difference in terms of management between HIV-1 and HIV-2 is that HIV-2 is naturally resistant to non-nucleoside reverse transcriptase inhibitors (see later discussion). For this reason, it is important to assess for HIV-2 by Western blot in persons who are from regions of the world where HIV-2 is present or coexists with HIV-1.

Genetic heterogeneity of HIV-1 is reflected in categorization of the virus into three groups (M, O, and N) and several clades (e.g., B, C, D, AE, CRF01_AE), some of which have overlapping geographic distribution around the world. Subtype C is prevalent in southern and eastern Africa, China, India, South Asia, and Brazil and accounts for 50% of HIV subtypes, whereas subtype B, the most common subtype in the United States, accounts for 12%.

The HIV viral genome is encoded in single-stranded RNA, packaged in core protein structures, and surrounded by a lipid bilayer envelope that is derived from the cell membrane of the host cell as the virus buds from the cell surface after replication. This outer viral membrane contains HIV-specific glycoproteins, including gp120 and gp41, which facilitate attachment and entry into host cells through interaction with the cell surface receptor, CD4, and coreceptors CCR5 and CXCR4. $CD4^+$ helper T lymphocytes are the predominant host cell affected by HIV; this molecular tropism explains the immune system destruction manifested in chronic HIV infection and provides the rationale for clinical staging of HIV infection using $CD4^+$ T-cell counts. The interaction of HIV with the coreceptor CCR5 has been an area of research interest leading to the recent development of coreceptor antagonist drugs.

After host cell entry, the key enzyme responsible for viral replication is reverse transcriptase, an RNA-dependent DNA polymerase that is packaged within the virion core. This enzyme facilitates conversion of the HIV genome into a double-stranded DNA intermediate molecule. The second key enzymatic step is integration of this intermediate nucleic acid product into the host genome, which is facilitated by the viral protein integrase. Protein synthesis with packaging of new viral particles ensues, utilizing an HIV-specific protease. The integrase inhibitor class of drugs acts by blocking this step of integration.

Natural History

The natural history of HIV infection reflects the progressive depletion of circulating $CD4^+$ cells, in addition to diverse effects on other immune cells and tissues that are incompletely understood. Within 1 to 4 weeks after the initial HIV infection, seroconversion may be accompanied by a nonspecific, self-limited illness, often referred to as the acute retroviral syndrome. This illness has variable manifestations but may include fever, malaise, myalgias, arthralgias, generalized lymphadenopathy, pharyngitis, and rash. The associated rash has been described as maculopapular, urticarial, or roseola-like. An illness resembling acute infectious mononucleosis syndrome, similar to that caused by Epstein-Barr virus or cytomegalovirus (CMV), and aseptic meningitis have been described. Very rarely has an acute opportunistic infection (OI) been reported in the setting of acute seroconversion. The proportion of patients experiencing such an illness is not precisely known, because many do not present to medical facilities, and for those who do, HIV infection is commonly not considered. Diagnosis of acute HIV infection requires a high index of suspicion, which does not commonly occur unless the patient reports a recent history of a high-risk exposure.

During the acute phase of infection, high levels of viremia are present (often exceeding 10 million copies per milliliter) as HIV becomes widely disseminated throughout the body and the host defenses are just beginning to counteract circulating virus through cell-mediated and humoral (antibody-mediated) immune mechanisms. Antibodies against HIV usually become detectable between 2 and 4 months after infection. The initial, high-level viremia becomes attenuated as neutralizing antibodies are established and equilibrium is reached whereby ongoing replication is partially controlled by the immune response, resulting in a steady-state level of viremia. This so-called virologic set point differs from patient to patient and is one of the determinants of the rate of disease progression. A small number of HIV-infected persons are able to control viral replication to levels below the limit of detection, and they tend to have a more benign course of disease. In these patients, designated elite suppressors by researchers, HIV replication continues to occur, and HIV RNA can be isolated from latently infected cells by means of specialized laboratory techniques.

After the establishment of HIV infection and seroconversion, a period of asymptomatic infection ensues, during which patients are free of evidence of immune suppression and OIs are uncommon. This phase of clinical latency lasts a median of 8 to 10 years, based on observational studies in the West from the pre-HAART era. Ongoing viral replication leads to gradual decline in the CD4 count.

The symptomatic stage of HIV infection can begin at any time after infection, but clinical manifestations become more likely as the CD4 count falls farther below the normal range of 800 to 1200 cells/mm^3. Both the absolute CD4 count and the percentage of $CD4^+$ T cells correlate with the risk of developing OIs and should be monitored longitudinally to assess patients' candidacy for prophylactic interventions and initiation of HAART. For example, *Pneumocystis jirovecii* (formerly *Pneumocystis carinii*) pneumonia (PCP) usually occurs in patients with a CD4 count of less than 200 cells/mm^3 or a percentage of less than 10%. CMV retinitis occurs almost exclusively in patients with a CD4 count of less than 50 cells/mm^3 or a percentage of less than 5%. Mucocutaneous candidiasis (oral thrush), herpes zoster, HIV-associated nephropathy, peripheral neuropathy, tuberculosis, and community-acquired bacterial pneumonia occur with increased frequency at earlier stages of infection and are less reliably predicted by $CD4^+$ cell measurement.

Diagnosis

Diagnosis of HIV infection during the acute retroviral syndrome requires detection of circulating HIV RNA because of the absence of HIV-specific antibodies at this stage. Other laboratory findings that can raise the suspicion for acute HIV infection include a decreased total lymphocyte count; the T-cell count characteristically decreases during the first several weeks after infection and later often returns to preinfection levels, after the initial spike in viremia is brought under control by immune defenses. The erythrocyte sedimentation rate and hepatic transaminases may also be elevated. Cerebrospinal fluid pleocytosis has been documented in patients undergoing lumbar puncture in the setting of acute HIV infection.

HIV RNA can be detected by reverse transcriptase polymerase chain reaction (RT-PCR) or branched-chain DNA testing. In the acute retroviral syndrome, the VL is usually very high, and ultrasensitive RT-PCR is not generally needed. Although commercially available PCR and branched DNA tests are licensed for disease monitoring and not for diagnosis of HIV infection, their specificity is sufficiently high that finding high levels of HIV RNA in a patient with suspected acute HIV infection provides convincing evidence for infection. In all such cases, close follow-up with repeat HIV antibody testing to confirm seroconversion within 2 to 4 months is essential.

Diagnosis of HIV at all other stages of disease relies on commercially available assays for detecting HIV-specific antibodies. A standard protocol involves screening with the highly sensitive enzyme immunoassay (EIA) that detects antigens of both HIV-1 and HIV-2. Negative EIA is sufficient to rule out HIV infection, except in cases where acute HIV infection is suspected, as just described.

Positive EIA tests require further confirmation with the more specific Western blot test. The CDC has established criteria for Western blot positivity, which include the presence of at least two of the HIV-specific bands p24, gp41, and gp160/120. The Western blot is considered negative if no bands are present and indeterminate if an HIV band is present but the criteria for positivity are not met. Indeterminate Western blot results usually include a single p24 band and can occur during early infection, while seroconversion is in progress, or in advanced AIDS when antibody production is impaired. Causes of indeterminate Western blot results that are unrelated to HIV include pregnancy, autoimmune disease, and cross-reacting antibodies resulting from blood transfusion or organ transplantation.

Other HIV antibody kits have been developed for ease of administration or achievement of rapid results, and they have utility in settings such as community-based screening programs, emergency departments, and even patient-initiated home testing. OraSure, an office-based test that employs a special swab for collecting oral fluid specimens rather than blood, was licensed in 1996. Specimens are collected at the point of care and sent to a central laboratory, where antibodies are detected; the sensitivity and specificity are similar to those of traditional blood-based methods. OraQuick Advance, a rapid HIV test that can utilize whole blood, plasma, or oral fluid, was approved in 2004 and can provide results comparable in accuracy to EIA within about 20 minutes. An advantage of this technique is the ability to provide reliable negative results at the point of care. Positive results still need to be confirmed with standard EIA and Western blot serologic testing.

Screening

The traditional paradigm for screening of asymptomatic patients for HIV has included targeting patients with behavioral risk factors for HIV transmission and patients seeking care for sexually transmitted diseases. Documentation of separate, written consent and administration of formal pretest and posttest counseling has been recommended and is still required by statute in many U.S. states.

In response to the consistent observations that many people are not diagnosed with HIV until late in the course of disease and that transmission rates for infected persons who are unaware of their serostatus are several times higher than for persons who are aware that they are infected, the CDC issued new guidelines for routine HIV testing in September 2006 to make HIV testing a routine part of medical care. Voluntary (opt-out) screening is now recommended in health care settings for all persons aged 13 to 64 years, regardless of risk. Screening should be repeated annually for persons with behavioral risk factors for HIV and should be repeated each time a person seeks treatment for symptoms related to sexually transmitted disease. The CDC advocates that requirements for separate, written consent for HIV testing are no longer needed; instead, general consent to receive medical care can be considered sufficient.

CURRENT DIAGNOSIS

- Revised national guidelines recommend universal screening for HIV infection for patients aged 13 to 64 years in all settings after notification that testing will be done, unless the patient specifically declines (opt-out testing). Patients with behavioral risk factors, sexually transmitted diseases, or tuberculosis should be screened annually.
- Acute HIV infection is recognized as a variable syndrome including fever, pharyngitis, rash, and arthralgias.
- As antiretroviral therapy has prolonged survival for patients living with HIV, non–HIV-related outcomes such as cardiovascular and renal disease have gained importance as preventable causes of morbidity and mortality.

Approach to the Patient with HIV Infection

HIV care is a continuously evolving field, and new drugs and classes of drugs have been introduced in recent years. Professional guidelines for antiretroviral therapy (ART) are updated frequently as data from clinical trials are published and accumulating clinical evidence influences beliefs about best practices in HIV care. For these reasons, the receipt of appropriate care by HIV$^+$ patients is determined in large part by the experience of the care provider. The volume of HIV$^+$ patients seen in one's practice is known to correlate with measures of quality care. A U.S. Department of Health and Human Services panel recommends that HIV patients receive care from a health care provider who routinely cares for at least 20 and preferably 50 HIV-infected patients. Referral to a specialist is warranted in cases of treatment failure due to drug resistance or for management of complications of HIV or antiretroviral drugs. Because of the multifaceted nature of the longitudinal care of HIV-infected patients, an interdisciplinary approach, integrated and coordinated by an experienced primary care provider, is optimal.

The initial history and physical examination of HIV-infected patients should be systematic and comprehensive, owing to the multiorgan system nature of diagnoses associated with HIV infection. A thorough review of current and recent symptoms should assess for presence of OIs and malignant or premalignant conditions. Symptoms such as unexplained weight loss, fever, chronic diarrhea, recurrent oral or genital ulcers, dysphagia, dyspnea, or gastrointestinal bleeding should prompt further investigation for the presence of undiagnosed manifestations of HIV-related complications. Because patients with HIV infection have a higher incidence of cognitive impairment, mental illness, and substance abuse than the general population, symptoms of neurocognitive impairment (e.g., impaired memory), depression, suicidality, and unhealthy alcohol and drug use should also be carefully assessed.

The past medical and surgical history should focus on conditions that may follow a more malignant course in the setting of HIV infection, such as chronic viral hepatitis, and conditions that can be exacerbated by HIV or by ART, such as cardiovascular or renal disease and metabolic abnormalities such as dyslipidemia or impaired glucose tolerance. The circumstances surrounding the patient's HIV acquisition should be formally assessed. The provider should understand previous and current patterns of risk behaviors for the purpose of counseling regarding transmission prevention (positive prevention) and to assess the patient's risk of acquisition of drug-resistant virus and current risk for concomitant sexually transmitted infections.

A complete physical examination should be performed at the time of initial evaluation and at subsequent visits. Signs such as temporal wasting, lymphadenopathy, and hepatomegaly or splenomegaly can provide clues to the stage of disease and alert the provider to the presence of OIs or AIDS-related malignancies. The oral cavity should be examined for the presence of thrush, oral hairy leukoplakia, and mucosal lesions of Kaposi sarcoma. A complete skin examination is important on initial evaluation and longitudinally, because many OIs and medication toxicities have cutaneous manifestations. A funduscopic examination should be done, and, in those patients with a CD4 count of less than 50 to 100 cells/mm^3, referral to an ophthalmologist is necessary to screen for evidence of CMV retinitis. Close examination of the anogenital area may identify treatable sexually transmitted infections and premalignant lesions associated with human papillomavirus infection. Recommended laboratory evaluations are presented in Table 1.

Antiretroviral Therapy

Antiretroviral drugs that are currently approved for the treatment of HIV fall into six classes: nucleoside reverse transcriptase inhibitors (NRTIs), non-nucleoside reverse transcriptase inhibitors (NNRTIs), protease inhibitors (PIs), fusion inhibitors, integrase inhibitors, and chemokine (CC) receptor 5 (CCR5) antagonists (Table 2). The goals of therapy are to increase disease-free survival, achieve maximal and sustained suppression of viral replication to undetectable levels (<50 copies/mL), preserve immunologic function, and improve quality of life.

(Text continued on p. 53)

TABLE 1 Initial Laboratory Evaluation

Test	Frequency	Comments
HIV antibody testing	At initial visit	If prior documentation is not reliable or if HIV RNA is undetectable
CD4+ T-cell count	At initial visit, then every 3–6 mo	Levels may be falsely elevated in splenectomized patients and with concurrent HTLV-1 infection.
Plasma HIV RNA (viral load)	At initial visit, before ART initiation, every 3 mo while on ART	Ultrasensitive viral load assay detects levels as low as 50 copies/mL and should be used to monitor response while on treatment.
Resistance testing	At initial visit, and with treatment failure before change in ART regimen	Genotype and phenotype tests are available; genotypes are more commonly used.
HLA-B*5701 testing	Before treatment initiation if considering abacavir (Ziagen)	—
Coreceptor tropism assay	Before treatment initiation if considering CCR5 antagonist (maraviroc [Selzentry])	—
Complete blood count	At initial visit, then every 3–6 mo	AZT can cause bone marrow suppression and macrocytosis.
Serum chemistry panel	At initial visit	Up to 75% of HIV-infected patients have elevated hepatic transaminases at diagnosis.
Fasting lipid profile and blood glucose level	At initial visit	Every 3–6 mo
Hepatitis screen (anti-HCV, anti-HAV, anti-HBsAg, anti-HBcAg)	At initial visit	HAV, HBV vaccinations are indicated for nonimmune patients.
Syphilis serology	At initial visit and annually in sexually active patients	Confirm with FTA-ABS test if positive; up to 6% of HIV-infected patients have biologic false-positive RPR result.
Urine NAAT for gonorrhea and *Chlamydia*	Consider at initial visit and annually in sexually active patients	Testing every 3–6 mo is recommended for very-high-risk patients.
Toxoplasma gondii serology	At initial visit and if CD4+ count is <100 cells/mm³	Most cases of toxoplasmosis represent reactivation of latent infection.
Tuberculin skin test (PPD)	At initial visit, then annually in high-risk persons (e.g., homeless, injection drug users) if initial test is negative	Cutoff of >5 mm of induration is indication for treatment of LTBI.
PAP smear	At initial visit	Annually
G6PD screen	At initial visit	Identifies patients at risk for hemolysis induced by dapsone or primaquine
Chest radiograph	If patient has pulmonary symptoms or a positive PPD result	Not recommended routinely

Abbreviations: ART = antiretroviral therapy; AZT = azidothymidine (zidovudine); FTA-ABS = fluorescent treponemal antibody, absorbed; G6PD = glucose-6-phosphate dehydrogenase; HAV = hepatitis A virus; HBcAg = hepatitis B core antigen; HBsAg = hepatitis B surface antigen; HCV = hepatitis C virus; HLA = human leukocyte antigen; HTLV-1 = human T-lymphotropic virus 1; LTBI = latent tuberculosis infection; NAAT = nucleic acid amplification test; PAP smear = Papanicolaou test; PPD = purified protein derivative; RPR = rapid plasma reagin test.

TABLE 2 Approved Antiretroviral Medications

Generic Name (Trade Name)	Abbreviation	Formulations and Coformulations	Recommended Adult Dosing	Important Points
Nucleoside Analogue Reverse Transcriptase Inhibitors (NRTIs)				
Abacavir (Ziagen)	ABC	300 mg tablets; 20 mg/mL oral solution *Coformulations:* Trizivir (ABC 300 mg + ZDV 300 mg + 3TC 150 mg) Epzicom (ABC 600 mg + 3TC 300 mg)	300 mg bid or 600 mg qd Trizivir 1 tablet bid Epzicom 1 tablet qd	Hypersensitivity reaction (FDA black box warning); screen patients for the HLA-B*5701 haplotype Possible increase in acute MI No food restrictions
Didanosine (Videx)	ddI	125, 200, 250, 400 mg capsules; 2, 4 g powder for oral solution	Body weight ≥60 kg: 400 mg (with TDF 250 mg) qd Body weight <60 kg: 250 mg (with TDF 200 mg) qd	Pancreatitis, peripheral neuropathy, nausea, lactic acidosis; concurrent use of TDF causes increased ddI levels and higher rate of toxicity Take on an empty stomach Must be swallowed whole
Emtricitabine (Emtriva)	FTC	200 mg capsule; 10 mg/mL oral solution *Coformulations:* Atripla (EFV 600 mg + FTC 200 mg + TDF 300 mg) Truvada (FTC 200 mg + TDF 300 mg)	200 mg capsule qd or 240 mg (24 mL) oral solution qd Atripla 1 tablet qd Truvada 1 tablet qd	Skin discoloration, rare nausea and vomiting No food restrictions

Continued

TABLE 2 Approved Antiretroviral Medications—Cont'd

Generic Name (Trade Name)	Abbreviation	Formulations and Coformulations	Recommended Adult Dosing	Important Points
Lamivudine (Epivir)	3TC	150, 300 mg tablets; 10 mg/mL oral solution *Coformulations:* Combivir (3TC 150 mg + ZDV 300 mg) Epzicom (see ABC) Trizivir (see ABC)	150 mg bid or 300 mg qd Combivir 1 tablet bid	Minimal toxicity Requires dosage adjustment in renal insufficiency. No food restrictions
Stavudine (Zerit)	d4T	15, 20, 30, 40 mg capsules; 1 mg/mL oral solution	30 mg bid (weight-based dosing is no longer recommended)	Peripheral neuropathy, lipodystrophy, pancreatitis, lactic acidosis, dyslipidemia No food restrictions
Tenofovir (Viread)	TDF	300 mg tablet *Coformulations:* Atripla (see FTC) Truvada (see FTC)	1 tablet qd	Renal insufficiency, Fanconi's syndrome, headache, nausea, vomiting, diarrhea No food restrictions
Zidovudine (Retrovir)	AZT, ZDV	100 mg capsules; 300 mg tablets; 10 mg/mL IV solution; 10 mg/mL oral solution *Coformulations:* Combivir (see 3TC) Trizivir (see ABC)	300 mg bid or 200 mg tid	Bone marrow suppression (macrocytic anemia, neutropenia), GI disturbance, lactic acidosis with hepatic steatosis (rare) No food restrictions

Non-nucleoside Analogue Reverse Transcriptase Inhibitors (NNRTIs)

Generic Name (Trade Name)	Abbreviation	Formulations and Coformulations	Recommended Adult Dosing	Important Points
Delavirdine (Rescriptor)	DLV	100, 200 mg tablets	400 mg tid (four 100-mg tablets may be dispersed in >3 oz water to produce a slurry; 200-mg tablets should be taken as intact tablets)	Rash, elevated hepatic transaminases, headache No food restrictions
Efavirenz (Sustiva)	EFV	50, 200 mg capsules; 600 mg tablets *Coformulation:* Atripla (see FTC)	600 mg qd on an empty stomach at or before bedtime	Rash, CNS symptoms (vivid dreams, impaired concentration, dizziness), hyperlipidemia, false-positive cannabinoid test Take on an empty stomach, preferably at bedtime
Etravirine (Intelence)	ETR	100 mg tablets	200 mg bid after a meal	Rash, nausea Take after a meal Tablets may be dispersed in water
Nevirapine (Viramune)	NVP	200 mg tablets; 50 mg/5 mL oral suspension	200 mg qd for 14 d, then 200 mg PO bid	Hepatotoxicity, rash, lipodystrophy No food restrictions

Protease Inhibitors (PIs)

Generic Name (Trade Name)	Abbreviation	Formulations and Coformulations	Recommended Adult Dosing	Important Points
Atazanavir (Reyataz)	ATV	100, 150, 200, 300 mg capsules	PI-naive patients only: ATV 400 mg qd PI-experienced patients: 300 mg (with RTV 100 mg) qd (when given with TDF, EFV, NVP)	Indirect hyperbilirubinemia, first-degree atrioventricular block, hyperglycemia, fat maldistribution, nephrolithiasis. Avoid taking simultaneously with antacids. Take with food.
Darunavir (Prezista)	DRV	75, 300, 400, 600 mg tablets	PI-naive patients only: 800 mg (with RTV 100 mg) qd PI-experienced patients: 600 mg (with RTV 100 mg) bid	Rash (contains sulfa moiety), hepatotoxicity, diarrhea, nausea, headache, hyperlipidemia, hyperglycemia, fat maldistribution Take with food.
Fosamprenavir (Lexiva)	FPV	700 mg tablet or 50 mg/mL oral suspension	PI-naive patients only: 1400 mg bid *OR* 1400 mg (with RTV 100-200 mg) qd *OR* 700 mg (with RTV 100 mg) bid PI-experienced patients: 700 mg (with RTV 100 mg) bid (once-daily dosing not recommended)	Rash, GI intolerance, headache, hyperlipidemia, hepatotoxicity, fat maldistribution No food restrictions

Continued

TABLE 2 Approved Antiretroviral Medications—Cont'd

Generic Name (Trade Name)	Abbreviation	Formulations and Coformulations	Recommended Adult Dosing	Important Points
Indinavir (Crixivan)	IDV	100, 200, 333, 400 mg capsules	800 mg q8h *OR* 800 mg (with RTV 100–200 mg) bid	Nephrolithiasis, GI intolerance, indirect hyperbilirubinemia, hyperlipidemia, headache, blurred vision, alopecia Should be administered without food but with water 1 h before or 2 h after a meal for optimal absorption
Lopinavir/ritonavir (Kaletra)	LPV/r	100 mg (+RTV 25 mg), 200 mg (+RTV 50 mg) tablets; 400 mg (+RTV 100 mg)/5 mL oral solution	PI-naive patients only: 4 × 200/50 mg tablets or 10 mL qd PI-experienced patients: 2 × 200/50 mg tablets or 5 mL bid	GI intolerance, diarrhea, hyperlipidemia, elevated hepatic transaminases, hyperlipidemia, fat maldistribution No food restrictions
Nelfinavir (Viracept)	NFV	250, 625 mg tablets; 50 mg/g oral powder	1250 mg bid *OR* 750 mg tid	Diarrhea, hyperlipidemia, hyperglycemia, fat maldistribution, elevated hepatic transaminases Take with food May be dispersed in water
Ritonavir (Norvir)	RTV	100 mg capsules; 80 mg/mL oral solution	Refer to other PIs for dosing recommendations	GI intolerance, headache, hyperlipidemia, hyperglycemia, dysgeusia, paresthesias Take with food
Saquinavir (Invirase)	SQV	200 mg hard gel capsules; 500 mg tablets	1000 mg (with RTV 100 mg) PO bid	GI intolerance, headache, elevated hepatic transaminaes, hyperlipidemia, hyperglycemia, fat maldistribution Take within 2 h after a meal
Tipranavir (Aptivus)	TPV	250 mg capsules	500 mg (with RTV 200 mg) PO bid	Hepatotoxicity, rash (contains sulfa moiety), rare cases of intracranial hemorrhage have been reported Take with food
Fusion Inhibitor Enfuvirtide (Fuzeon)	T20	90 mg/1 mL powder for injection	90 mg SQ bid	Injection site reactions (erythema, pain, induration), increased risk of bacterial pneumonia, hypersensitivity reaction
Coreceptor (CCR5) Antagonist Maraviroc (Selzentry)	MVC	150, 300 mg tablets	150 mg bid when given with strong CYP3A inhibitors (± CYP3A inducers) including PIs (except TPV/RTV) *OR* 300 mg bid when given with NRTIs, T20, TPV/RTV, NVP, and other drugs that are not strong CYP3A inhibitors *OR* 600 mg bid when given with CYP3A inducers (e.g., EFV, ETR, rifampin) without a CYP3A inhibitor	Abdominal pain, cough, dizziness, musculoskeletal symptoms, pyrexia, rash, upper respiratory tract infections, hepatotoxicity, orthostatic hypotension. No food restrictions
Integrase Inhibitor Raltegravir (Isentress)	RAL	400 mg tablets	400 mg bid	Nausea, headache, diarrhea, fever, CPK elevation No food restrictions

Abbreviations: ART = antiretroviral therapy; CNS = central nervous system; CPK = creatine phosphokinase; CYP3A = cytochrome P-450 isoenzyme 3A; GI = gastrointestinal; HLA = human leukocyte antigen; MI = myocardial infarction.

WHEN TO INITIATE ANTIRETROVIRAL THERAPY

In the mid-1990s, when combination HAART became available, the treatment paradigm was to "hit early and hit hard," because it was believed that the virus could be eradicated with treatment and rapid immune restoration could be achieved. However, as more data accumulated, there was recognition that the virus establishes itself within hours after infection and cannot be eradicated with HAART. In addition, during this early HAART era, it was observed that several of the regimens used were complicated, were associated with several toxicities and reduced quality of life, and, importantly, were not associated with marked clinical benefits. Therefore, between 1996 and 2006, the recommended CD4 count threshold for starting therapy steadily declined, with 2006 recommendations of the U.S. Department of Health and Human Services (DHHS), the International AIDS Society–USA, and the British HIV Society all generally indicating a threshold of 200 cells/mm³ for initiation of treatment in asymptomatic patients.

More recently, however, accumulating evidence of the beneficial effects of earlier versus later treatment has resulted in a shift toward earlier initiation of HAART. There are now several classes of drugs, and many of the newer ART regimens are more potent, better tolerated, and less complex than before (i.e., low pill burden and once-daily dosing). The newer regimens, such as PIs boosted with ritonavir (Norvir) and NNRTIs used in triple-drug combinations, are more effective at achieving and sustaining virologic suppression (HIV-1 RNA <50 copies/mL) than the older regimens that used unboosted PIs and NRTIs. Most cases of virologic failure now occur when patients are lost to follow-up, are nonadherent, or discontinue their treatment. Furthermore, there is mounting evidence from several cohorts with long-term follow-up of HIV-infected patients that demonstrates a benefit of starting ART earlier. Consistently, persons starting treatment at a CD4 count threshold below 200 cells/mm³ have a two to four times greater risk of AIDS or death than patients who start when their CD4 count is between 201 and 350 cells/mm³.

There is also increasing recognition of the importance of non–AIDS-defining illnesses, such as cardiovascular, renal, and liver disease, at higher CD4 counts (>350 cells/mm³). Cohort data (e.g., North American AIDS Cohort Collaboration on Research and Design [NA-ACCORD], ART-Collaborative) and one large trial (Strategies for Management of Anti-Retroviral Therapy [SMART]) reported significant benefits in reducing these complications when ART was initiated at higher CD4 thresholds (>350 or >500 cells/mm³). Earlier initiation of HAART also appears to be associated with reduced risk of transmission, greater preservation of the R5-tropic virus, improved immune restoration (including CD4 counts); it also may be cost-effective.

CURRENT RECOMMENDATIONS FOR ANTIRETROVIRAL THERAPY

Current guidelines for HIV treatment in the United States are shown in Tables 3 and 4. Current U.S. guidelines advocate treating all patients with a CD4 count of less than 500 cells/mm³ and any patient

---

TABLE 3 US DHHS Guidelines for HIV Treatment, 2009

Clinical Condition or CD4 Count (cells/mm³)	Recommendation	Strength of Recommendation and Quality of Evidence*
History of AIDS-defining illness		AI
CD4 count <350		AI
Pregnant women		AI
Patients with HIV-associated nephropathy	ART should be initiated	AII
CD4 count 350–500		A/B-II†
Patients with HBV infection, when treatment for HBV is indicated		AIII
CD4 count >500	Initiation of ART should be considered	B/C-III‡

From US DHHS Guidelines, 2009. Available at http://www.aidsinfo.nih.gov/Guidelines/ (accessed July 28, 2010).
*Strength of Recommendations: A = strong evidence to support the recommendation; B = moderate evidence to support the recommendation.
Quality of Evidence: I = randomized trials with either clinical or validated laboratory outcomes (e.g., viral load); II = nonrandomized trials or well-designed observational cohort studies with long term-clinical outcomes; III = recommendation based on expert opinion.
†45% of expert panel voted for strong recommendation (A) and 55% voted for moderate recommendation (B).
‡50% of expert panel members favor starting ART (B); the other 50% of members view treatment as optional (C) in this setting.

TABLE 4 International AIDS Society (IAS)–USA Guidelines, 2010

Measure	Recommendation	Strength of Recommendation and Quality of Evidence*
Specific Conditions		
Symptomatic HIV disease		AI
Pregnant Women		AI
HIV-1 RNA >100 000 copies/mL		AII
Active hepatitis B or C virus coinfection		BII, AII
Active or high risk for cardiovascular disease	ART should be initiated regardless of CD4 count	BII
HIV-associated nephropathy		BII
Symptomatic primary HIV infection		BII
Risk for secondary HIV transmission is high (e.g., serodiscordant couples)		BII
Asymptomatic, CD4 cell count ≤500 cells/mm³		
CD4 count <350	ART should be initiated	AI
CD4 count 350–500	ART should be initiated	AII
CD4 count >500	ART should be considered unless patient is an elite controller (HIV-1 RNA <50 copies/mL) or has stable CD4 cell count and low-level viremia in the absence of ART	CIII

From Thompson MA, Aberg JA; Cahn P, et al: Antiretroviral treatment of adult HIV infection: 2010 Recommendations of the International AIDS Society–USA Panel. JAMA. 2010;304(3):321–333
*Strength of Recommendations: A = strong evidence to support the recommendation; B = moderate evidence to support the recommendation.
Quality of Evidence: I = randomized trials with either clinical or validated laboratory outcomes (e.g., viral load); II = nonrandomized trials or well-designed observational cohort studies with long term-clinical outcomes; III = recommendation based on expert opinion.

with an AIDS-defining illness. For patients whose CD4 count is greater than 500 cells/mm^3, current guidelines recommend considering individualized treatment for specific scenarios such as active hepatitis B co-infection or pregnancy. Critical to all these recommendations, however, is ensuring that the patient is ready to start therapy and understands the regimen, the importance of adherence to it, and the need to continue therapy for life.

SELECTION OF AN ANTIRETROVIRAL REGIMEN

Table 5 presents the regimens recommended for ART initiation in treatment-naive HIV-1–infected adults residing in the United States and other high-income countries. Current ART strategies that represent the standard of care are based on combining at least three potent antiretroviral agents. Therapy is individualized in high-income settings and takes into account several factors such as comorbidities, concomitant medications, possible drug interactions, pill burden, dosing schedule, adherence issues, risk for side effects, and pregnancy. Triple-NRTI regimens are inferior to PI- and NNRTI-containing regimens and therefore are not recommended.

Efavirenz (Sustiva) is the preferred NNRTI because it has the best long-term treatment response to date, based on clinical trial data. It is available with tenofovir (Viread) and emtricitabine (Emtriva) in a coformulation, called Atripla (efavirenz 600 mg + tenofovir 300 mg + emtricitabine 200 mg), that can be taken once a day. Nevirapine (Viramune) is an alternative NNRTI; it should not be used in women with a CD4 count of less than 250 cells/mm^3 or in men with less than 400 cells/mm^3, because it is associated with increased risk of severe hepatotoxicity in such patients. Efavirenz-based regimens are equivalent to boosted-PI regimens in terms of efficacy and durability but have the advantages of low pill burden and limited long-term toxicity. The main drawback to NNRTI-containing regimens is their low barrier to resistance; for this reason, NNRTIs are less favored in patients for whom adherence is likely to be a problem.

The preferred PIs are the newer ones: atazanavir (Reyataz) boosted with ritonavir, lopinavir coformulated with ritonavir (Kaletra), and darunavir (Prezista) boosted with ritonavir. They are potent, have a high genetic barrier to resistance, and can be dosed once daily in many treatment-naive patients. The main drawbacks with PIs as a class are their interactions with other drugs, gastrointestinal intolerance, and metabolic complications (for most members of the class). The relative advantages and disadvantages of initial ART regimens are shown in Table 6.

TABLE 5 Starting Regimens for Antiretroviral Naïve Patients*

	Column A	Column B		
	Dual NRTI backbone	NNRTI	PI	INSTI
Preferred	TDF/FTC	EFV	ATV/r DRV/r	RAL
Alternative	ABC/(3TC or FTC) ZDV/(3TC or FTC)†	AND NVP	OR LPV/r† FPV/r SQV/r	OR

From US DHHS guidelines, 2008. Available at http://www.aidsinfo.nih.gov/ Guidelines/ (accessed July 28, 2010).
*Select one component from column A (dual NRTI combination) and one from column B (NNRTI, PI or INSTI).
†3TC/ZDV plus LPV/r is the preferred regimen for pregnant women.
Abbreviations: 3TC = lamivudine (Epivir®); ABC = abacavir (Ziagen®); ABC/3TC = abacavir/lamivudine (Epzicom®); ATV = atazanavir (Reyataz®); DRV = darunavir (Prezista®); EFV = efavirenz (Sustiva®); FPV = fosamprenavir (Lexiva®); FTC = emtricitabine (Emtriva®); INSTI = integrase strand transfer inhibitor; LPV/r = lopinavir/ritonavir (Kaletra®); NNRTI = non-nucleoside reverse transcriptase inhibitor; NRTI = nucleoside reverse transcriptase inhibitor; NVP = nevirapine (Viramune®); PI = protease inhibitor; r = ritonavir (Norvir®); RAL = raltegravir (Isentress®); SQV = saquinavir (Invirase®); TDF = tenofovir (Viread®); TDF/FTC = tenofovir/ emtricitabine (Truvada®); ZDV = zidovudine (Retrovir®).

TABLE 6 Advantages and Disadvantages of Initial Antiretroviral Regimens

Drugs	Advantages	Disadvantages
Non-Nucleoside Reverse Transcriptase Inhibitors		
Class	• Extensive experience • Saves PI option • Fewer drug interactions than PIs	• Low genetic barrier to resistance • Class resistance with single mutation • Drug interactions, especially with methadone • ADRs: skin rash, especially NVP
EFV	• Potent and never beaten in a clinical trial • Low pill burden (coformulated with TDF and FTC), once-daily dosing	• Teratogenic (avoid use in pregnancy or with potential for pregnancy) • Compared to LPV/r: lower CD4 response, more resistance mutations, and increased lipoatrophy
NVP	• Low pill burden • ART potency comparable to EFV	• ADRs: rash and hepatotoxicity including hepatic necrosis • Contraindicated in women with baseline CD4 >250 cells/mm^3 and men with CD4 >400 cells/mm^3 • Single dose may cause class resistance
Protease Inhibitors		
Class	• Extensive experience • Saves NNRTI option • Higher genetic barrier to resistance	• ADRs: metabolic complications • Multiple drug interactions • GI intolerance
ATV/r	• High genetic barrier to resistance with boosting • Potency • Once-daily dosing • Low pill burden • No hyperlipidemia • Less GI intolerance	• ADRs: jaundice (harmless) and PR interval prolongation (usually inconsequential) • Drug interaction with TDF and ATV (can be overcome by ATV/r 400/100 mg qd with EFV) • Absorption requires food and gastric acid
DRV/r	• Once-daily dosing • High potency	• ADRs: skin rash • Food requirement

Continued

Drugs	Advantages	Disadvantages
LPV/r	• Potency • Coformulated with RTV • No significant food effect • Option for once-daily therapy in treatment-naïve patients • Preferred in pregnancy	• ADRs: GI intolerance • RTV boosting required (coformulated) • Hyperlipidemia
FPV/r	• Potency • No significant food effect • Option for once-daily dosing • RTV boosting not required in treatment-naïve patients (preferred) • Appears equivalent to LPV/r	• ADRs: skin rash (has sulfa moiety) • Cross-resistance with DRV/r
SQV/r	• Potency • Reduced pill burden with Invirase • 500 mg tab • Once-daily option	• ADRs: GI intolerance • Boosting with RTV required
Integrase Inhibitor		
RAL	• Virologic response noninferior to EFV when used with TDF/FTC • Well tolerated • No food effect • Minimal drug interactions	• Twice-daily dosing • Few data comparing RAL with boosted PI in treatment-naïve patients • Lower genetic barrier to resistance than PI-based regimens
Nucleoside Reverse Transcriptase Inhibitor Combinations		
ZDV/3TC/ ABC	• Coformulated • Minimal drug interactions • Low pill burden • ABC may be associated with risk of cardiovascular disease and higher rate of viral failure in patients with baseline VL >100,000 copies/mL	• ADRs: ABC hypersensitivity and AZT marrow suppression, GI intolerance • HBV flare[†] • Requires twice daily dosing
ZDV/3TC	• Extensive experience • Coformulated • No food effect	• ADRs: GI intolerance and marrow suppression (ZDV) • HBV flare[†] • Requires twice-daily dosing (ZDV)
TDF/FTC*	• Well tolerated • Coformulated • Long half-life of each drug may give pharmacologic barrier to resistance. • No thymidine analog mutations • Extensive experience	• HBV flare[†] • Rare cases of nephrotoxicity (ddI/3TC or FTC) • Once-daily dosing • HBV flare[†] • Food effect
ABC/3TC*	• Coformulated • Once-daily dosing • No food effect	• ADRs: ABC hypersensitivity • HBV flare[†] • Risk of cardiovascular disease
Nucleoside Combinations to Avoid		
d4T/ddI	—	ADRs: peripheral neuropathy, lipoatrophy, pancreatitis, lactic acidosis. High rate of virologic failure
ABC/TDF/ 3TC TDF/ ddI/3TC	—	High rate of virologic failure
NNRTI/ddI/ TDF	—	
d4T/AZT	—	Antagonistic effects
TDF/ddI	—	Drug interaction requiring dose adjustment; avoid with NNRTI

*FTC and 3TC are similar except for convenience of coformulations; FTC has longer intracellular half-life and less extensive experience.
[†]In hepatitis B virus (HBV) co-infection (HBV surface antigen positive), hepatitis B flare may be caused by discontinuation of agent or by HBV resistance to NRTI (3TC, FTC, TDF).
Abbreviations: 3TC = lamivudine (Epivir); ABC = abacavir (Ziagen); ATV = atazanavir (Reyataz); ddI = didanosine (Videx); d4t = stavudine (Zerit); DRV = darunavir (Prezista); EFV = efavirenz (Sustiva); FPV = fosamprenavir (Lexiva); FTC = emtricitabine (Emtriva); INSTI = integrase strand transfer inhibitor; LPV/r = lopinavir/ritonavir (Kaletra); NNRTI = non-nucleoside reverse transcriptase inhibitor; NRTI = nucleoside reverse transcriptase inhibitor; NVP = nevirapine (Viramune); PI = protease inhibitor; r = ritonavir (Norvir); RAL = raltegravir; SQV = saquinavir (Invirase); TDF = tenofovir (Viread); ZDV = zidovudine (Retrovir).

MONITORING RESPONSE TO ANTIRETROVIRAL THERAPY

After ART is initiated, the CD4 count usually increases within a few weeks, largely because of redistribution of cells. Subsequently, the CD4 count improves over years of therapy, at an average rate of 100 cells/mm^3 per year, and then reaches a plateau. The starting CD4 count appears to influence the plateau reached (i.e. people starting at a lower count also plateau at a lower count than do those whose baseline count was higher). In approximately 5% to 10% of individuals, the CD4 response is less than this or does not increase from baseline. This is not evidence of treatment failure if the VL is undetectable. The plasma HIV VL rapidly decreases after initiation of HAART, and by 4 weeks most patients have at least a 1 log$_{10}$ drop in VL. In most individuals, it should become undetectable (<50 copies/mL) by 24 weeks.

The CD4 count should be assessed at 3 months after ART initiation and then every 3 to 6 months thereafter. The VL should be measured 2 to 8 weeks after ART initiation, every 1 to 2 months until undetectable, and thereafter every 3 to 4 months. If a patient has been on a long-term stable suppressive regimen, visits can be reduced to every 6 months, with VL and CD4 testing performed at that interval. If a change in ART is motivated by drug toxicity or regimen simplification, it is recommended that VL be measured 2 to 8 weeks afterward, to confirm potency of the new regimen.

Other laboratory tests and their frequency of monitoring are shown in Table 1.

Treatment Failure

Treatment failure can be virologic, immunologic, or clinical. Virologic failure is defined as failure to achieve a VL of less than 400 copies/mL by 24 weeks or less than 50 copies/mL by 48 weeks, or a consistent finding (two consecutive measurements) of more than 50 copies/mL after a fall to less than 50 copies/mL. Most patients should have a decrease of at least 1 $\log_{10}$ in VL within 4 weeks. Immunologic failure is the failure to increase the CD4 count by 25 to 50 cells/mm^3 during the first year. In treatment-naive patients, current regimens are associated with an average increase of 150 cells/mm^3 in the first year. Clinical failure is the occurrence or recurrence of HIV-related events 3 months or longer after HAART initiation; this is not to be confused with immune reconstitution syndromes (discussed later).

Today, with the use of appropriate combinations, newer fixed-dose formulations, and more tolerable regimens, treatment failure in patients on their first-line therapy usually occurs because of inadequate adherence or treatment discontinuation (e.g., loss to follow-up, intolerance) rather than regimen inefficacy. Occasionally, pharmacokinetic issues such as a reduced drug level due to genetic polymorphism or a drug interaction (e.g., omeprazole [Prilosec] with atazanavir [Reyataz]) or transmitted resistance can be causes of treatment failure. In the United States, primary resistance seems to be declining, and in most places it is identified in fewer than 10% of HIV-infected acute seroconverters assessed.

Drug Resistance and Resistance Testing

A patient may be infected with a drug-resistant HIV virus to begin with (primary resistance), or, more commonly, resistance can emerge as a result of treatment (secondary resistance).

Several NNRTI-associated resistance mutations confer resistance to other NNRTIs, including K103N, 106M, and Y181C.

Among NRTIs, the resistance mutation most commonly detected when regimens containing lamivudine (Epivir) or emtricitabine are used is M184V. This mutation also makes the virus hypersusceptible to tenofovir or zidovudine (Retrovir), so in many situations lamivudine or emtricitabine may be kept in the regimen if tenofovir or zidovudine is being used. Other NRTIs can be associated with thymidine analogue mutations, or TAMS (e.g., 41L, 210W, 215Y); accumulation of TAMS or presence of multinucleoside mutations (e.g., Q151M, T69 insertion) confers cross-resistance to other NRTIs.

With PIs, accumulation of mutations generally leads to significant cross-resistance. Ritonavir-boosted PIs, particularly lopinavir (i.e., Kaletra) and darunavir, have high barriers to resistance, so development of resistance does not occur as easily as with the NNRTI class. Indications for resistance testing include the baseline resistance (prior to initial therapy), acute HIV infection, suboptimal viral suppression (VL >1000 copies/mL), and virologic failure with VL greater than 1000 copies/mL. Resistance testing should be performed while the patient is on therapy or within 1 month after discontinuation, because, after that point, the wild-type virus may re-emerge and predominate.

Current standard methods of genotyping do not detect minority variants (resistant virus populations accounting for <10% to 20% of plasma virus). Resistance testing is usually a genotypic test and should be performed early in cases of virologic failure. The phenotypic resistance assay is more expensive and is typically used in patients who have multiple resistance mutations after multiple virologic failures. Interpretation of resistance testing should include adherence assessment, prior history of antiretroviral agents, and prior resistance testing results, because a history of resistance mutations remains relevant even if they are not detected on the current resistance test. Because resistance testing interpretation is complex, special expertise should be sought.

Adverse Drug Reactions and Drug-Drug Interactions

Adverse drug reactions (ADRs) are common with ART and are a reason for patient nonadherence or treatment discontinuation. ADRs can be idiosyncratic, dose related, time related (delayed), or dose and time related (cumulative). A particular ADR may be drug specific (e.g., hypersensitivity to abacavir [Ziagen]) or class related (e.g., hyperlipidemia because of PIs). It is important to inform patients of potential common or serious ADRs associated with their therapy. Often, the challenge in managing ADRs is that the patient is taking several concomitant medications that may have overlapping toxicities and ADR profiles. A symptom-based approach is often most practical (Table 7). Although many of the ADRs can be managed conservatively, some, such as symptomatic lactic acidosis, systemic hypersensitivity reactions, Stevens-Johnson syndrome, acute pancreatitis, and severe hepatotoxicity, are potentially life threatening. Serious ADRs necessitate withdrawal of the offending drug, and rechallenge with the drug should not be attempted in these situations.

Numerous important drug-drug interactions exist among antiretroviral agents and other medications of various classes. Familiarity with common interactions and ready access to reliable HIV pharmacology reference materials or a clinical pharmacologist with expertise in ART is essential for the clinician prescribing ART. Table 8, although not exhaustive, lists important drug-drug interactions, including combinations that are contraindicated and those that require adjustments to prescribe dosages. Tables 9 and 10 show dose adjustments that must be made with coadministration of certain antiretroviral drugs.

 CURRENT THERAPY

- Multiple studies have demonstrated that superior clinical outcomes are achieved in patients who receive care from clinicians with substantial experience in HIV care.
- Accumulating evidence suggests that earlier initiation of antiretroviral therapy (with CD4$^+$ T-cell counts of 350–500 cells/mm^3) improves outcomes.
- New classes of antiretroviral medications, including integrase inhibitors and CCR5 coreceptor antagonists, give treatment-experienced patients additional therapeutic options.
- Revised and updated guidelines for prevention and management of opportunistic infections were released in 2009, with emphasis on the importance of antiretroviral therapy for prevention and treatment of opportunistic infections, especially for those for which specific therapy does not exist.

Adverse Effect	Manifestations	Causative Drugs		Stepwise Action
		Antiretrovirals	Other Drugs	
SJS/TEN[†]	Usually in first few weeks, with rash, mucosal ulcerations (± blistering), fever, hepatic dysfunction	NVP (0.5%-1%); less common with EFV (0.1%), ETR (<1%); rare with FPV, DRV, TPV, LPV/r, ATV, IDV, ABC, ZDV, ddI	Cotrimoxazole (Bactrim), sulfadiazine, dapsone, atovaquone (Mepron), voriconazole (Vfend)	Discontinue all antiretroviral agents and any other possible drug; manage like severe burns; do not rechallenge with offending drug
Hypersensitivity reaction[‡]	In rank order: high fever, diffuse rash, nausea, headache, abdominal pain, diarrhea, arthralgias, pharyngitis, dyspnea. Almost all have two or more systems involved. Always progresses with ABC, 90% present within first 6 wk	ABC (6%-7%); very rare if HLA-B*5701 is negative. Less common in African Americans	Cotrimoxazole, sulfadiazine, dapsone	Discontinue ABC and any other possible drug; rule out other causes; do not rechallenge with ABC. Symptoms resolve 48 h after ABC is stopped
Skin rash	Maculopapular rash ± pruritus	NVP, EFV, FPV > TPV >> ABC, DRV/r[§]	Cotrimoxazole, sulfadiazine, dapsone, atovaquone, voriconazole	Rule out SJS/TEN and hypersensitivity. Antihistamines; continue offending drug; watch for progression of rash (if so, discontinue)
GI intolerance[¶]	Anorexia, nausea, vomiting, epigastric pain; begins with first dose	PIs, ddI, ZDV; common	Isoniazid (Nydrazid), rifamycins, pyrazinamide	Administer with food (not for ddI or unboosted IDV); antiemetics; switch to less emetogenic antiretroviral agent
	Diarrhea; usually begins with first dose.	PIs, especially NFV, LPV/r, and buffered ddI formulations	Clindamycin (Cleocin), atovaquone	Antimotility agents, calcium salts, bulk-forming agents; rehydration (if needed)
Hepatotoxicity[#]	Abrupt onset of GI symptoms, fever, rash, jaundice, eosinophilia, hepatic necrosis; encephalopathy can occur	NVP (usually ≤6 wk but up to 18 wk reported). Increased risk for baseline CD4 >250 (women) or CD4 >400 (men)	Isoniazid, rifamycins, pyrazinamide	Discontinue all antiretroviral agents and any other possible drug; rule out viral hepatitis; supportive management; do not rechallenge with NVP
	Symptomatic or subclinical hepatic enzyme elevations	NNRTIs, especially d4T, ddI, ZDV. PIs, especially TPV, MVC. 3TC, FTC, TDF can cause this with HBV co-infection and NRTI withdrawal or HBV resistance	Isoniazid, rifamycins, pyrazinamide, azithromycin (Zithromax), clarithromycin (Biaxin), all azole antifungals	If symptomatic, discontinue all antiretroviral agents and switch to nonhepatotoxic antiretrovirals after normalization; if asymptomatic, monitor closely. Many discontinue drugs if ALT >5-10 × upper limit of normal
Lactic acidosis, fatty liver**	Nonspecific GI symptoms, wasting, fatigue, tachypnea, tachycardia, hepatomegaly, pancreatitis, hyperlactatemia, respiratory or multiorgan failure	d4T + ddI > d4T > ddI > ZDV (rare or never with other NRTIs); associated with long duration of use, female gender, obesity	Metformin (Glucophage)	Discontinue all antiretroviral agents; hydration; supportive care; roles of intravenous thiamine[1]/riboflavin,[1] steroids, carnitine,[7] plasmapheresis are unclear; switch to ABC/3TC/TDF or NRTI-sparing regimen
Pancreatitis**	Epigastric pain (postprandial), vomiting, fever, elevated amylase, lipase	ddI, d4T, high-dose RTV; concurrent d4T, ddI, and TDF without ddI dose adjustment; ddI + ribavirin contraindicated	Alcohol, cotrimoxazole, pentamidine (Pentam)	Discontinue offending drugs; manage like acute pancreatitis related to any other cause; do not rechallenge

Continued

TABLE 7 Approach to Adverse Drug Reactions in the HIV-Infected Patient*—Cont'd

Adverse Effect	Manifestations	Causative Drugs		Stepwise Action
		Antiretrovirals	**Other Drugs**	
Peripheral neuropathy**	Numbness, paresthesia (often painful after weeks to months); depressed ankle jerks; recovery possibly incomplete	ddl, d4T (10%-30% or higher based on duration)	Isoniazid	Switch to ABC/3TC/TDF; gabapentin (Neurontin), tricyclic antidepressants, narcotic analgesics
Myopathy**	Myalgia, muscle tenderness, proximal weakness, elevated creatine kinase	ZDV (uncommon with current doses)	Statins, fibrates, steroids	Switch to another NRTI; improves in 3–4 wk after discontinuation; roles of coenzyme Q10,[7] L-carnitine[7] are unproven
Nephrolithiasis, crystalluria††	Flank pain, nondescript abdominal pain, dysuria, hematuria, renal dysfunction	IDV	Cotrimoxazole, sulfadiazine, acyclovir (Zovirax)	Discontinue IDV; hydration and analgesics; IDV can be resumed with plenty of oral fluids; if symptoms recur, consider switching
Nephrotoxicity	Renal dysfunction; nephrogenic diabetes insipidus; Fanconi's syndrome	IDV, TDF Occurs primarily in patients with inadequate dose adjustment, baseline renal dysfunction, or concurrent nephrotoxic drugs Risk for Fanconi's with TDF associated with older age, low BMI, low CD4	Acyclovir, amphotericin B (Fungizone), cotrimoxazole, pentamidine	Discontinue offending drug; hydration; generally reversible
Hematologic	Anemia, neutropenia usually after weeks to months‡‡	ZDV	Cotrimoxazole, dapsone, sulfadiazine, pyrimethamine (Daraprim), flucytosine (Ancobon), trimetrexate (Neutrexin), amphotericin B, ganciclovir (Cytovene), valganciclovir (Valcyte), rifabutin (Mycobutin)	Discontinue concomitant marrow suppressant, if any; exclude marrow involvement by opportunistic infections/ malignancy; erythropoietin (Procrit) or filgrastim (Neupogen); switch to another NRTI
	Bleeding tendency in hemophiliacs	PIs	—	Factor VIII infusion (Advate); consider NNRTI-based regimens
	Eosinophilia	Enfuvirtide (Fuzeon)	Cotrimoxazole, dapsone, sulfadiazine	Exclude disseminated strongyloidiasis, malignancy; watch for hypersensitivity
Central nervous system symptoms§§	Drowsiness, insomnia, vivid dreams, nightmares, hallucination, impaired concentration/attention Usually resolves in 2–3 wk Worsening of psychiatric disorders, suicidal ideation	EFV; effects can begin with first dose	Isoniazid, dapsone, steroids	Usually resolves in 2-4 wk; consider discontinuation, if symptoms are persistent or psychiatric illness is exacerbated
Fat atrophy	Loss of subcutaneous fat (face, buttocks, extremities) Associated with long-term use	d4T > ZDV, ddl; less common with EFV	Steroids	Discontinue d4T, ZDV early if possible; either slow reversal or irreversible changes
Fat accumulation	Increase in abdominal girth, breast size, buffalo hump	PIs, EFV	—	Consider change in regimen for cosmetic reasons; restorative surgery
Hyperlipidemia	Increase in total and low-density lipoproteins, triglycerides; begins within weeks	PIs, except ATV (rank: TPV/r > LPV/r, FPV/r > IDV/r > SQV/r), EFV, d4T	—	Follow NCEP guidelines, statins (preferably pravastatin, atorvastatin, rosuvastatin [Crestor] but may need dose adjustment)¶¶

Continued

TABLE 7 Approach to Adverse Drug Reactions in the HIV-Infected Patient*—Cont'd

Adverse Effect	Manifestations	Causative Drugs Antiretrovirals	Other Drugs	Stepwise Action
Insulin resistance	Fasting blood sugar >126 mg/dL, abnormal glucose tolerance test, DM symptoms More likely with family history of DM	PIs, except ATV	—	Diet, exercise, if indicated: metformin, rosiglitazone (Avandia), insulin (no major drug interactions with antiretroviral agents); consider switch to other non-PI regimens

Based on Guidelines for the Use of Antiretroviral Agents in HIV-1-Infected Adults and Adolescents, U.S. Department of Health and Human Services, January 2008.

[1]Not FDA approved for this indication.

[2]Not available in the United States.

[7]Available as dietary supplement.

*Only common and serious side effects are dealt with; side effects such as osteoporosis, avascular osteonecrosis (PIs), unconjugated hyperbilirubinemia, retinoid-like effects (IDV), and cranial malformations (EFV) are also known to occur.

[†]Approximately 0.3%-1% with NVP; a low dose lead-in period for NVP may decrease the risk; less common (0.1%) with EFV; occurs in the initial weeks after initiation; safety of replacing NVP with another NNRTI is unknown.

[‡]Approximately 5% with ABC; once-daily dosing possibly increases the risk; if ABC-related, symptoms resolve within 48 h after discontinuation of ABC.

[§]FPV and TPV are sulfonamide derivatives; potential cross-hypersensitivity with sulfonamides.

[¶]Symptoms begin with first doses; may abate with time.

[#]Low-dose lead-in period for NVP may reduce the risk; onset within the first few weeks with NNRTIs, after weeks to months with PIs, and after months to years with NRTIs; discontinuation of 3TC, FTC, or TDF in HBV co-infected patients may cause acute flare-up of hepatitis; safety of replacing NVP with another NNRTI is unknown.

**Class-specific adverse effect of NRTIs, because of mitochondrial toxicity; do not combine ddI/d4T/ddC; ABC, 3TC, and TDF are less prone; all four syndromes can occur in variable combinations; symptomatic lactic acidosis is rare but is associated with high mortality.

[††]Approximately 10% of patients taking IDV experience at least one episode of colic; occurrence is seen in only 50%, if fluid intake is improved (at least 1.5-2 L of noncaffeinated fluid, preferably water).

[‡‡]Almost all ZDV-treated patients have isolated macrocytosis; anemia and neutropenia occur in approximately 1%-4% and 2%-8%, respectively.

[§§]Occurs during initial weeks of treatment; patients are to be warned to restrict risky activities.

[¶¶]Only atorvastatin (Lipitor) and pravastatin (Pravachol) among statins, and gemfibrozil (Lopid) and fenofibrate (Triglide) among fibrates, can be coadministered with PIs.

Abbreviations: 3TC = lamivudine (Epivir); ABC = abacavir (Ziagen); ALT = alanine aminotransferase; ATV = atazanavir (Reyataz); BMI = body mass index; CD4 = CD4+ T-cell count (in cells/mm[3]); d4T = stavudine (Zerit); ddC = zalcitabine (Hivid)[2]; ddI = didanosine (Videx); DM = diabetes mellitus; DRV = darunavir (Prezista); EFV = efavirenz (Sustiva); ETR = etravirine (Intelence); FPV = fosamprenavir (Lexiva); FTC = emtricitabine (Emtriva); GI = gastrointestinal; HBV = hepatitis B virus; HLA = human leukocyte antigen; IDV = indinavir (Crixivan); LPV/r = lopinavir/ritonavir (Kaletra); MVC = maraviroc (Selzentry); NARTI = nucleoside reverse transcriptase inhibitor; NCEP = National Cholesterol Education Program; NFV = nelfinavir (Viracept); NNRTI = non-nucleoside reverse transcriptase inhibitor; NVP = nevirapine (Viramune); PI = protease inhibitor; r = RTV as a booster; RTV = ritonavir (Norvir); SJS = Stevens-Johnson syndrome; SQV = saquinavir (Invirase); TDF = tenofovir (Viread); TEN = toxic epidermal necrolysis; TPV = tipranavir (Aptivus); ZDV = zidovudine (Retrovir).

TABLE 8 Drug Interactions with Antiretroviral Agents*

Class	Agent	Antiretroviral Agent	Comments
α-Adrenergic blockers	Alfuzosin (Uroxatral)	RTV, All PIs	Consider tamsulosin (Flomax) or doxazosin (Cardura)
Antianginals	Ranolazine (Ranexa)	All PIs	—
Antiarrhythmics	Flecainide (Tambocor), propafenone (Rythmol), amiodarone (Cordarone), quinidine	All PIs	—
Antihistamines	Astemizole (Hismanal),[2] terfenadine (Seldane)[2]	All PIs, EFV	Loratadine (Claritin), fexofenadine (Allegra), cetirizine (Zyrtec), or desloratadine (Clarinex)
Antimycobacterials	Rifampin (Rifadin)	All PIs, NVP	Use rifabutin (Mycobutin) with PIs
	Rifapentine (Priftin)	All PIs, NNRTIs	Rifabutin
Antineoplastics	Irinotecan (Camptosar)	ATV, caution with other PIs	—
Calcium channel blockers	Bepridil (Vascor)	All PIs	—
Ergot alkaloids	Ergotamine (Cafergot)	All PIs, EFV	Sumatriptan (Imitrex)
Gastrointestinal agents	Cisapride (Propulsid)[2]	All PIs, EFV	Metoclopramide (Reglan)
	Proton pump inhibitors	ATV, NFV	
Herbs	St. John's wort[7]	All PIs, NNRTIs	Other antidepressants
Intranasal steroids	Fluticasone (Flonase)	All PIs	Beclomethasone (Beconase AQ)
Lipid-lowering drugs	Simvastatin (Zocor), lovastatin (Mevacor)	All PIs	Pravastatin (Pravachol), fluvastatin (Lescol), possibly atorvastatin (Lipitor), rosuvastatin (Crestor)
Neurotropics	Pimozide (Orap)	All PIs	—
Psychotropics	Midazolam (Versed), triazolam (Halcion)	All PIs	Temazepam (Restoril), lorazepam (Ativan)

Adapted from John G. Bartlett's Pocket Guide to Adult HIV/AIDS Treatment 2008-2009. Fairfax, VA, Johns Hopkins HIV Care Program, 2008.

[2]Not available in the United States.

[7]Available as dietary supplement.

*Delavirdine (Rescriptor) drug interactions are not shown as this drug is no longer used in clinical practice. Detailed information about drug interactions and searchable drug interaction databases are available at http://www.hopkins-aids.edu/, http://www.hiv-druginteractions.org/, http://hivinsite.ucsf.edu.

Abbreviations: ATV = atazanavir (Reyataz); EFV = efavirenz (Sustiva); NFV = nelfinavir (Viracept); NRTI = nucleoside reverse transcriptase inhibitor; NNRTI = non-nucleoside reverse transcriptase inhibitor; NVP = nevirapine (Viramune); PI = protease inhibitor; RTV = ritonavir (Norvir).

TABLE 9 Combinations Requiring Dose Adjustments: NRTIs

Drug	Zidovudine (Retrovir, AZT)	Stavudine (Zerit, d4T)	Didanosine (Videx, ddl)	Tenofovir (Viread, TDF)
Methadone (Dolophine)	AZT AUC increase 40%; no dose change Monitor CBC	d4T decreased 27%; no dose change	ddl EC: no interaction	No change in methadone or TDF levels
Didanosine (Videx, ddl)	—	Increased toxicity: pancreatitis, peripheral neuropathy lactic acidosis Avoid	-	ddl increases 44% >60 kg: 250 mg/d ddl EC <60 kg: 200 mg/d ddl EC
Ribavirin (Rebetol)	Monitor for severe anemia In vitro inhibition of AZT activation; not shown in vivo	No data	Magnifies ddl toxicity; contraindicated	Ribavirin unchanged; no data on TDF level
Atazanavir (Reyataz, ATV)	AZT AUC unchanged but C_{min} decrease 30%; significance unknown	No data	Buffered ddl: take ATV 2 h before or 1 h after ddl or use ddl EC (separate dosing due to food restrictions)	ATV AUC decreases 25%; TDF AUC increases 24% Avoid concomitant use unless ATV is combined with RTV (ATV/r)
Indinavir (Crixivan, IDV)	—	No data	Buffered ddl: take 1 h apart	IDV C_{max} increases 14%; clinical significance unknown
Cidofovir (Vistide), ganciclovir (Cytovene), valganciclovir (Valcyte)	Ganciclovir + AZT increases marrow toxicity Monitor CBC	No data	ddl and oral ganciclovir: ddl AUC increased 111% (PO) and 50%-70% (IV); use with caution or avoid	Combination may increase levels of both drugs; monitor for toxicity
Lopinavir/ritonavir (Kaletra, LPV/r)	No pharmacokinetics data but interaction unlikely due to favorable clinical data	No data	No data	TDF AUC increases 34% Use standard doses and monitor for TDF toxicity
Tipranavir (Aptivus, TPV)	AZT decreased 33%-43%; clinical significance unknown	No interaction	Separate dose of ddl EC by >2 h	TPV AUC decreases 9%-18%; clinical significance unknown

Adapted from John G. Bartlett's Pocket Guide to Adult HIV/AIDS Treatment 2008–2009. Fairfax, VA, Johns Hopkins HIV Care Program, 2008.
Abbreviations: AUC = area under the concentration-versus-time curve; CBC = complete blood count; C_{max} = maximum plasma concentration; C_{min} = minimum plasma concentration; EC = enteric coated; NRTI = nucleoside reverse transcriptase inhibitor.

TABLE 10 Combinations Requiring Dose Adjustments: PIs and NNRTIs

Drug	Efavirenz (Sustiva, EFV)	Nevirapine (Viramune, NVP)	Etravirine (Intelence, ETR)
Atazanavir (Reyataz)/ritonavir (Norvir, RTV) combination (ATV/r)	ATV 400 mg + RTV 100 mg (with food) + EFV SD (avoid coadministration in PI-experienced patients)	Avoid	Avoid
Darunavir (Prezista)/ritonavir combination (DRV/r)	DRV/r SD + EFV SD (dose not established; consider TDM)	DRV/r SD + NVP SD (dose not established; consider TDM)	DRV/r-SD + ETR-SD
Fosamprenavir (Lexiva, FPV)	FPV 1400 mg qd + RTV 300 mg qd + EFV SD FPV 700 mg bid + RTV 100 mg bid + EFV SD	FPV 700 mg + RTV 100 mg bid + NVP SD	Avoid
Indinavir (Crixivan, IDV)	IDV 1000 mg q8h + EFV SD IDV 800 mg q12h + RTV 200 mg bid + EFV SD	IDV 1000 mg q8h + NVP SD IDV 800 mg q12h + RTV 200 mg q12h + NVP SD	Avoid
Lopinavir/ritonavir coformulation (Kaletra, LPV/r)	LPV/r 600/150 mg bid + EFV SD	LPV/r 600/150 mg bid + NVP SD	ETR: SD LPV/r: SD
Nelfinavir (Viracept, NFV)	NFV SD + EFV SD	NVP SD + NFV SD	Avoid
Saquinavir Invirase, SQV)	SQV/r 1000/100 mg bid + EFV SD	SQV 1000 mg bid + RTV 100 mg bid + NVP SD	SQV/r 1000/100 mg bid + ETR SD
Tipranavir (Aptivus)/ritonavir combination (TPV/r)	TPV 500 mg bid + RTV 200 mg bid + EFV SD	Inadequate data; NVP may decrease TPV	Avoid

Adapted from John G. Bartlett's Pocket Guide to Adult HIV/AIDS Treatment 2008-2009. Fairfax, VA, Johns Hopkins HIV Care Program, 2008.
Abbreviations: SD = standard dose; NNRTI = non-nucleoside reverse transcriptase inhibitor; PI = protease inhibitor; TDM = therapeutic drug monitoring.

Complications

DIAGNOSIS AND MANAGEMENT OF OPPORTUNISTIC INFECTIONS

OIs are the most common cause of disability and death in patients who are not receiving ART. Clinical experience from the pre-HAART era demonstrated that the risk of OIs increases proportionately with the severity of immune system dysfunction and can be roughly predicted by the CD4 count in patients receiving and not receiving HAART. Guidelines for initiating and discontinuing antimicrobial prophylaxis against OIs are based on the CD4 count, as summarized in Table 11.

Diagnosis of OIs requires that clinicians recognize that a diverse array of bacterial, fungal, viral, and parasitic pathogens can cause overlapping clinical syndromes. A broad differential diagnosis must be considered when evaluating an HIV-infected patient with specific or generalized symptoms. Aside from infectious complications, symptoms may arise from toxicities inherent to antiretroviral or other medications. Patients infected with HIV have increased rates of cardiovascular, renal, and hematologic abnormalities, which may also cause nonspecific symptoms. A syndromic approach to recognizing complications of HIV infection is described in the following paragraphs. Recommended treatment regimens for the most common OIs are presented in Table 12. Detailed treatment guidelines that are periodically updated are available from the CDC and the HIV Medicine Association of the Infectious Diseases Society of America (http://aidsinfo.nih.gov/contentfiles/Adult_OI.pdf [accessed June 5, 2009]).

Neurologic Complications

Both central nervous system disease and peripheral nerve abnormalities are common in advanced AIDS. Peripheral neuropathy has been associated with some NRTI medications, most commonly stavudine (d4T, Zerit), as a result of the mitochondrial toxicity inherent to these drugs. HIV infection can directly cause distal sensory neuropathy, which may manifest as dysesthesia or hypersensitivity, decreased reflexes, and chronic neuropathic pain. Inflammatory demyelinating polyneuropathy (e.g., Guillain-Barré syndrome), which has known associations with some enteric pathogens, causes ascending motor weakness, typically without sensory involvement. CMV infection may cause polyradiculopathy, transverse myelitis, and encephalitis/ventriculitis in patients with CD4 counts lower than 50 cells/mm^3. CMV end-organ disease, including retinitis (a vision-threatening condition), requires prompt diagnosis and initiation of appropriate anti-CMV therapy.

TABLE 11 Antimicrobial Prophylaxis for Opportunistic Infections

Infection	Indications for Initiating Prophylaxis	Preferred Regimen	Alternative Regimen	Indications for Discontinuing Prophylaxis
Pneumocystis jirovecii pneumonia (PCP)	CD4 <200	TMP-SMX (Bactrim DS) 1 DS tablet PO qd, or TMP-SMX (Bactrim SS) 1 SS tablet PO qd	TMP-SMX (Bactrim DS) 1 DS tablet PO three times weekly[3] Dapsone[1] 100 mg PO qd or 50 mg PO bid Dapsone 50 mg PO qd + pyrimethamine (Daraprim)[1] 50 mg PO weekly + leucovorin[1] 25 mg PO weekly Aerosolized pentamidine (NebuPent) 300 mg via Respirgard II nebulizer monthly Atovaquone (Mepron) 1500 mg/d Atovaquone 1500 mg/d + pyrimethamine 25 mg/d + leucovorin 10 mg/d	CD4 >200 for 3 mo in response to HAART
Toxoplasma gondii encephalitis	CD4 <100 and toxoplasma IgG positive	TMP-SMX[1] 1 DS tablet PO qd	TMP-SMX 1 DS tablet PO three times weekly TMP-SMX 1 SS tablet PO qd Dapsone[1] 50 mg PO qd + pyrimethamine 50 mg PO weekly + leucovorin[1] 25 mg PO weekly Dapsone 200 mg + pyrimethamine 75 mg + leucovorin 25 mg, all PO weekly Atovaquone[1] 1500 mg ± pyrimethamine 25 mg + leucovorin 10 mg, all PO qd	CD4 >200 for 3 mo in response to HAART
Mycobacterium avium-intracellulare (MAI)	CD4 <50	Azithromycin (Zithromax) 1200 mg PO once weekly Clarithromycin (Biaxin) 500 mg PO bid Azithromycin 600 mg PO twice weekly	Rifabutin (Mycobutin) 300 mg PO qd	CD4 >100/mm^3 for 3-6 mo and undetectable viral load in response to HAART
Mycobacterium tuberculosis	Positive diagnostic test for LTBI	Isoniazid (INH) 300 mg PO qd (or 900 mg PO twice weekly for 9 mo) + pyridoxine 50 mg PO qd	Rifampin (Rifadin) 600 mg PO qd × 4 mo	Completion of treatment for LTBI

[1]Not FDA approved for this indication.
Abbreviations: CD4 = CD4$^+$ T-cell count (in cells/mm^3); DS = double-strength; HAART = highly active antiretroviral therapy; IgG = immunoglobulin G; LTBI = latent tuberculosis infection; SS = single-strength; TMP-SMX = trimethoprim-sulfamethoxazole.

TABLE 12 Recommended Treatment for Opportunistic Infections

Infection	Preferred Regimen	Alternative Regimen	Maintenance Therapy	Important Points
Pneumocystis jirovecii pneumonia (PCP)	TMP-SMX (Bactrim) (15–20 mg TMP and 75–100 mg SMX)/kg/day IV divided q6h or q8h May switch to PO after clinical improvement Duration of therapy: 21 d	Pentamidine (Pentam) 4 mg/kg IV q24h infused over ≥60 min, or Primaquine[1] 15–30 mg PO q24h + clindamycin[1] (Cleocin) 600–900 mg IV q6–8h or 300–450 mg PO q6–8h	Drug regimens for secondary prophylaxis same as for primary prophylaxis	Indications for corticosteroids: PaO₂ <70 mm Hg on room air, A-a gradient >35 mm Hg Prednisone[1] doses: 40 mg PO bid on days 1–5, 40 mg PO qd on days 6–10, 20 mg PO qd on days 11–21
Toxoplasma gondii encephalitis	Pyrimethamine (Daraprim) 200 mg PO × 1, then 50 mg (weight <60 kg) or 75 mg (≥60 kg) PO qd + sulfadiazine 1000 mg (<60 kg) or 1500 mg (≥60 kg) PO q6h + leucovorin[1] 10–25 mg PO qd	Pyrimethamine + leucovorin in same doses as for preferred regimen + clindamycin[1] 600 mg IV or PO q6h, or TMP-SMX[1] (5 mg/kg TMP and 25 mg/kg SMX) IV or PO bid	Pyrimethamine 25–50 mg PO qd + sulfadiazine 2000–4000 mg PO qd (in two to four divided doses) + leucovorin 10–25 mg PO qd	Duration of acute therapy: at least 6 wk; longer if clinical or radiographic response is incomplete at 6 wk
Mycobacterium avium-intracellulare (MAI)	At least two drugs as initial therapy with clarithromycin 500 mg PO bid + ethambutol (Myambutol)[1] 15 mg/kg PO qd Optional third drug in severe disease: rifabutin (Mycobutin) 300 mg PO qd (dosage adjustment may be necessary based on drug-drug interactions)	Azithromycin (Zithromax) 500–600 mg + ethambutol 15 mg/kg PO qd Alternative third drugs include fluoroquinolones: levofloxacin (Levaquin),[1] ciprofloxacin (Cipro),[1] moxifloxacin (Avelox),[1] amikacin (Amikin)[1]	Same as initial treatment	Criteria for discontinuing therapy: CD4 is >100 × 6 mo as a result of ART, symptoms have resolved, and at least 12 mo of therapy has been received
Cryptococcus neoformans meningitis	Induction therapy: amphotericin B deoxycholate 0.7 mg/kg IV qd + flucytosine 100 mg/kg PO qd in 4 divided doses for at least 2 wk	Lipid formulation amphotericin B 4–6 mg/kg IV qd + flucytosine 100 mg/kg PO qd in 4 divided doses for at least 2 wk, or Amphotericin B (without flucytosine) at same dose, or Fluconazole 400–800 mg PO once daily for 10–12 weeks	Consolidation therapy: Fluconazole 400 mg PO qd for 8–10 wk after induction therapy Maintenance therapy: Fluconazole 200 mg PO qd lifelong or until CD4 ≥200 for >6 mo as a result of ART	Managing elevated intracranial pressure is key to preventing morbidity and mortality; serial lumbar puncture and lumbar drainage is indicated in some cases
Cytomegalovirus (CMV) retinitis	Sight-threatening lesions: Ganciclovir intraocular implant + valganciclovir 900 mg PO (bid for 14–21 d, then once daily) Small or peripheral lesions: Valganciclovir 900 mg PO bid for 14–21 d, then 900 mg PO qd	Ganciclovir 5 mg/kg IV q12h for 14–21 d, then valganciclovir 900 mg PO qd, or Foscarnet 60 mg/kg IV q8h or 90 mg/kg IV q12h for 14–21 d, then 90–120 mg/kg IV q24h, or Cidofovir 5 mg/kg/wk IV for 2 wk, then 5 mg/kg every other week	Valganciclovir 900 mg PO qd, or ganciclovir implant (may be replaced q6–8mo) + valganciclovir 900 mg PO qd until immune recovery	Maintenance therapy for CMV retinitis can be safely discontinued in patients with inactive disease and sustained CD4 >100 for ≥3–6 mo; consultation with ophthalmologist is advised
CMV esophagitis or colitis	Ganciclovir 5 mg/kg IV q12h for 21–28 d or until symptoms resolve Oral valganciclovir may be used if symptoms are not severe enough to interfere with oral absorption	Foscarnet 60 mg/kg IV q8h or 90 mg/kg IV q12h for 21–28 d	Maintenance therapy is usually not necessary but should be considered after relapses	Patients with CMV gastrointestinal disease should undergo ophthalmologic screening
Esophageal candidiasis	Fluconazole 100 mg (up to 400 mg) PO or IV qd for 14–21 d	Itraconazole oral solution 200 mg PO qd Voriconazole 200 mg PO or IV bid Posaconazole 400 mg PO bid Caspofungin 50 mg IV qd Micafungin 150 mg IV qd Anidulafungin 100 mg IV × 1, then 50 mg IV qd Amphotericin B deoxycholate 0.6 mg/kg IV qd	Not routinely recommended	Patients with fluconazole-refractory oropharyngeal or esophageal candidiasis with response to echinocandin should be started on voriconazole or posaconazole for secondary prophylaxis until ART produces immune reconstitution

[1]Not FDA approved for this indication.
Abbreviations: A-a gradient = alveolar-arterial difference in partial pressure of oxygen (PaO₂ − PaO₂); ART = antiretroviral therapy; CD4 = CD4⁺ T-cell count (in cells/mm³); PaO₂ = arterial partial pressure of oxygen.

Focal central nervous system lesions may be caused by infectious and malignant conditions. Cerebral toxoplasmosis usually occurs in patients with prior exposure to *Toxoplasma gondii* who develop reactivation disease when the CD4 count is lower than 100 cells/mm^3. The main differential diagnosis for one or several enhancing brain lesions includes toxoplasmosis and primary central nervous system lymphoma (PCNSL). PCNSL is almost always associated with Epstein-Barr virus, and detection of nucleic acid for Epstein-Barr virus in cerebrospinal fluid carries a high specificity for this condition in the proper radiographic context. Progressive multifocal leukoencephalopathy, a rare and potentially devastating demyelinating condition, is caused by reactivation of JC virus and can manifest as focal neurologic deficit, seizures, or cognitive dysfunction. *Cryptococcus neoformans* is a common cause of meningitis in AIDS patients and can also manifest with central nervous system mass lesions, pulmonary disease, or gastrointestinal disease. Worldwide, tuberculosis accounts for a large proportion of HIV-associated meningitis; less commonly, it can manifest as single or multiple focal lesions (tuberculomas). Neurosyphilis should be considered in patients with unexplained neurologic disease and sexual risk factors.

Respiratory Complications

Respiratory illnesses are among the most common causes of morbidity in HIV patients. Community-acquired bacterial pneumonia occurs at a significantly higher rate in HIV-infected compared with HIV-noninfected hosts, regardless of CD4 count, and is one of the most common reasons for hospitalization. *Pneumocystis jirovecii* (formerly *Pneumocystis carinii*) pneumonia (PCP) manifests with fever, cough, and dyspnea. Findings on physical examination and chest radiography can be variable, making the diagnosis difficult in the absence of high clinical suspicion. Elevated lactate dehydrogenase and oxygen desaturation with ambulation can be diagnostic clues. More than 90% of cases occur among patients with CD4 counts lower than 200 cells/mm^3. The diagnosis is established by visualization of organisms in induced sputum (sensitivity, 50%-90%) or in bronchoalveolar lavage specimens (sensitivity, 90%-99%), most commonly with the use of immunofluorescent staining. Slight worsening of clinical symptoms after initiation of treatment for PCP is common, particularly when adjunctive corticosteroids are not administered.

The risk of reactivation of latent TB is increased 100-fold in patients with HIV infection. HIV$^+$ persons who are latently infected have a 10% annual risk of developing symptomatic tuberculosis, compared with a 10% lifetime risk among the general population. The risk of reactivation increases with decreasing CD4 count, and patients with counts lower than 350 cells/mm^3 are more likely to have atypical radiographic presentations, including middle- and lower-lobe infiltrates without cavitation. Patients with very low CD4 counts are more likely to have extrapulmonary tuberculosis. Diagnostic approaches to tuberculosis are similar in HIV$^+$ and HIV$^-$ patients. Tuberculin skin testing can still be used to diagnose latent tuberculosis infection, although the recommended cutoff for a positive test is 5 mm of induration. Treatment of co-infection with *Mycobacterium tuberculosis* and HIV requires consultation with experienced clinicians and pharmacists because of extensive drug-drug interactions among antiretroviral drugs and rifamycins.

Gastrointestinal Complications

Diagnosis of OIs affecting the gastrointestinal tract is made difficult by the numerous infections and complications of therapies that can result in nonspecific syndromes such as nausea, vomiting, abdominal pain, and diarrhea. Oropharyngeal candidiasis (thrush) commonly manifests as white plaques on the tongue, palate, or buccal mucosa that are painless and can easily be scraped off. Although thrush is typically uncomplicated and easily treatable with topical preparations such as nystatin (Mycostatin) and clotrimazole (Mycelex troches), in the proper clinical setting it can alert the clinician to the presence of esophageal candidiasis. Esophageal involvement should be suspected in patients with dysphagia and odynophagia; retrosternal chest pain may also be present. Thrush is usually present but is not required for the diagnosis, which is often made on clinical grounds rather than being confirmed with endoscopy. Patients with esophageal candidiasis typically respond after several days of treatment, and 7 to 14 days of antifungal therapy is usually sufficient. For cases not responsive to empiric treatment for candidiasis, referral for endoscopy should be considered. Esophagitis caused by CMV or herpes simplex virus requires a histopathologic diagnosis.

Acute diarrhea, defined as three or more loose or watery stools per day for 3 to 10 days, is common among HIV$^+$ patients, and more than 1000 different enteric pathogens have been described. Data from a large cohort indicate that the most common pathogens isolated are *Clostridium difficile*, *Shigella* spp., *Campylobacter jejuni*, *Salmonella* spp., *Staphylococcus aureus*, and *Mycobacterium avium-intracellulare* (MAI). Culture of the stool can yield a microbiologic diagnosis in many cases, particularly for acute diarrheal illnesses caused by *Campylobacter*, *Yersinia*, *Salmonella*, and *Shigella* species. Infection with *C. difficile*, the most common bacterial enteric pathogen in the United States for both HIV-infected and HIV-uninfected persons, is diagnosed in most settings by detection of cytotoxin in the stool, although the more laborious tissue culture is considered the gold standard. Enteric viruses are present in 15% to 30% of HIV-infected persons with acute diarrhea. Definitive diagnosis is not feasible in most clinical laboratories; viral enteritis should be suspected in the setting of community outbreaks, because of the high transmissibility of viral pathogens. Treatment is supportive with fluid resuscitation and antimotility agents.

Chronic diarrhea (duration >30 days) was a common manifestation of advanced-stage AIDS in the pre-HAART era and is still considered an AIDS-defining condition. Most pathogens that cause acute gastroenteritis can also cause chronic symptoms. Pathogens that should be suspected in cases of chronic watery diarrhea include protozoa such as *Cryptosporidium parvum*, *Isospora belli*, and *Microsporidia* spp. These entities are self-limited in the absence of severe immunosuppression. In advanced HIV, pathogen-specific antimicrobial therapy is infrequently effective, and symptoms commonly do not improve without immune reconstitution in response to ART. *Giardia lamblia* causes watery diarrhea, abdominal bloating, and occasionally malabsorption syndrome and can occur at any CD4 count. CMV infection can affect any segment of the gastrointestinal tract and is a common cause of chronic diarrhea. Diagnosis of gastrointestinal CMV disease is difficult without biopsy. Detection of CMV viremia with PCR does not correlate well with presence of CMV disease in HIV-infected patients, and CMV can be undetectable in serum in patients with extensive gastrointestinal disease.

Other Conditions

Mycobacterium avium and *Mycobacterium intracellulare* are closely related mycobacteria that are ubiquitous in the environment. They are discussed as a single pathologic entity and referred to as MAI or *Mycobacterium avium* complex (MAC). MAI is a common cause of chronic pulmonary disease in patients with structurally abnormal airways. In advanced HIV infection, it can cause a multiorgan system disease characterized by fever, night sweats, diarrhea, and abdominal pain. Infiltration of the bone marrow and liver may occur, leading to hematologic abnormalities and abnormal liver function tests, which can be a clue to the diagnosis. Biopsy of a lymph node or of bone marrow is sometimes necessary to diagnose disseminated MAI, but it is most often diagnosed by means of blood culture using specialized culture media.

IMMUNE RECONSTITUTION INFLAMMATORY SYNDROME

Recovery of cellular and humoral immune system function in response to ART is occasionally associated with severe symptoms resulting from inflammatory responses directed against opportunistic pathogens. Risk factors for this immune reconstitution inflammatory syndrome (IRIS) include a low nadir CD4 count, a high baseline VL, and PI-containing HAART regimens. Most cases of IRIS occur within the first 2 months after initiation of HAART, and onset can occur as early as within the first week. Disseminated MAI accounts for up to one third of the cases of IRIS in the United States. Other important causes of IRIS are tuberculosis, CMV infection, viral hepatitis, and candidal infections. It may be possible to decrease the risk of IRIS by delaying initiation of HAART by several weeks, until therapy for OIs has been instituted, but the risks of other complications of untreated AIDS often outweigh any potential benefit of this strategy. When it occurs, IRIS usually can be managed with nonsteroidal anti-inflammatory drugs or corticosteroids. HAART should not be interrupted except in life-threatening illnesses.

Management of HIV in Pregnant Women

Periodically updated guidelines for the treatment of HIV in pregnancy are available on the U.S. Department of Health and Human Services AIDSinfo website (http://www.aidsinfo.nih.gov [accessed June 5, 2009]). Pregnancy is not known to have an effect on HIV progression. HIV progression has been shown to increase rates of preterm delivery and low birth weight in developing countries, but this link has not been established in resource-rich settings. All pregnant women should be offered HAART to reduce perinatal transmission and improve maternal health, regardless of CD4 count or VL. Guidelines for ART are otherwise similar for pregnant and nonpregnant patients, with the important exception that drugs with unacceptable or inadequately studied safety profiles should be avoided. Efavirenz, tenofovir, didanosine (Videx), and stavudine should be avoided. If possible, preferred regimens should include zidovudine and lamivudine with either lopinavir/ritonavir (Kaletra) or nelfinavir (Viracept). Data suggest that nevirapine (Viramune) should be avoided in women who have CD4 counts higher than 250 cells/mm^3 at the time of initiation of therapy. This recommendation does not pertain to the practice of giving a single dose of nevirapine in the intrapartum period in resource-poor settings to prevent perinatal transmission. Elective cesarean should be offered at 38 weeks, gestation to women who are likely to have VLs greater than 1000 copies/mL at the time of delivery. After delivery, administration of zidovudine to the infant for 6 weeks is also recommended.

Postexposure Prophylaxis of HIV Infection

The scarcity of data describing occupationally acquired HIV infection makes it difficult to quantify the risk of transmission associated with exposure of health care workers to an HIV-infected source. Pooled data from multiple studies demonstrated HIV transmission in 20 health care workers, out of more than 6000 workers who sustained a needlestick injury from an HIV-infected patient, yielding a transmission rate of 0.33%. HIV transmission due to mucosal exposure was even more uncommon (0.09%), and transmission from exposure of intact skin has not been described.

Despite poorly characterized risks and benefits, postexposure prophylaxis with ART is recommended for health care workers sustaining percutaneous, mucus membrane, or nonintact skin exposure to an HIV-infected source. HIV antibody testing of the worker should be done at the time of exposure and repeated at 6 weeks, 12 weeks, and 6 months after exposure. If given, prophylaxis should be administered as soon as possible, preferably within hours after the exposure. Recommended prophylactic regimens typically contain a two-drug combination of NRTIs; coformulations of zidovudine plus lamivudine (Combivir) and emtricitabine plus tenofovir (Truvada) are used extensively and have good tolerability. Three-drug HAART regimens including a PI are recommended for more severe exposures. The duration of postexposure prophylaxes is typically 4 weeks. The recommendations for prophylaxis have been expanded to include nonoccupational exposures such as unanticipated sexual or needle-sharing behavior. Most recently, strategies for preexposure prophylaxis have been discussed as a strategy for HIV prevention in settings where unsafe sexual practices or injection drug use are likely.

REFERENCES

Adult Prevention and Treatment of Opportunistic Infections Guidelines Working Group. Guidelines for prevention and treatment of opportunistic infections in HIV-infected adults and adolescents [draft]. 2008. Available at: http://aidsinfo.nih.gov/contentfiles/Adult_OI.pdf [accessed June 5, 2009].

Branson B. Current HIV epidemiology and revised recommendations for HIV testing in health care settings. J Med Virol 2007;79(Suppl. 1):S6–10.

Hammer SM, Eron JJ Jr, Reiss P, et al. Antiretroviral treatment of adult HIV infection: 2008 recommendations of the International AIDS Society–USA Panel. JAMA 2008;300(5):555–70.

Hirsch MS. Initiating therapy: What to start, what to use. J Infect Dis 2008;197(Suppl. 3):S252–60.

Joint United Nations Programme on HIV/AIDS. 2008 Report on the Global AIDS Epidemic. Available at: http://www.unaids.org/en/KnowledgeCentre/HIVData/GlobalReport/2008/2008_Global_report.asp [accessed June 5, 2009].

Landon BE, Wilson IB, McInnes K, et al. Physician specialization and the quality of care for human immunodeficiency virus infection. Arch Intern Med 2005;165(10):1133–9.

Panel on Antiretroviral Guidelines for Adults and Adolescents. Guidelines for the use of antiretroviral agents in HIV-1-infected adults and adolescents, Department of Health and Human Services; 2008. Available at: http://www.aidsinfo.nih.gov/ContentFiles/AdultandAdolescentGL.pdf [accessed June 5, 2009].

Amebiasis

Method of
Rashidul Haque, MB, PhD, and
William A. Petri, Jr., MD, PhD

Amebiasis, a disease caused by the protozoan parasite *Entamoeba histolytica*, is estimated to be the third leading parasitic cause of deaths worldwide in humans. There are noninvasive species of ameba including *Entamoeba dispar* and *Entamoeba moshkovskii* that are morphologically indistinguishable from *E. histolytica* by traditional light microscopy. Amebiasis is distributed worldwide, but the majority of cases are found in developing countries. The World Health Organization estimates that approximately 50 million people suffer from invasive amebiasis each year, resulting in 40,000 to 100,000 deaths annually. For example, a prospective study of preschool children in an urban slum of Dhaka, Bangladesh, demonstrated a 39% incidence of *E. histolytica* infection during the first year of observation.

Human beings are the only known host of the parasite *E. histolytica*. Individuals become infected with *E. histolytica* when they ingest cysts in fecally contaminated food or water. When these cysts reach the intestine, they swell and release the motile, symptom-inducing form of *E. histolytica*, called the trophozoite. Trophozoites can remain in the intestine and even form new cysts without causing disease symptoms. They colonize the large intestine by adhering to colonic mucins via a galactose and *N*-acetyl-d-galactosamine (Gal/GalNAc)–specific lectin. Reproduction of trophozoites is without a recognized sexual cycle, and the overall population structure of *E. histolytica* appears to be clonal. Aggregation of amebae in the mucin layer likely signals encystation via the Gal/GalNAc lectin. Cysts excreted in stool perpetuate the life cycle by further fecal–oral spread. Invasive disease results when the trophozoite penetrates the intestinal mucus layer, which acts as barrier to invasion by inhibiting amebic adherence to the underlying epithelium and by slowing trophozoite motility. In addition, trophozoites can be carried through the blood to other organs, most commonly the liver, where they form life-threatening abscesses.

Intestinal Amebiasis

There are several clinical classifications of amebiasis based on the invasiveness and site of infection with different treatments. Intestinal amebiasis is a term that encompasses the entire spectrum of clinical intestinal disease, including amebic colitis. Patients with amebic colitis typically present with a several week history of cramping abdominal pain, weight loss, and watery or, less commonly, bloody diarrhea. The insidious onset and variable signs and symptoms make diagnosis difficult, with fever and grossly bloody stool absent in most cases. Differential diagnosis of a diarrheal illness with occult or grossly bloody stools should include *Shigella*, *Salmonella*, *Campylobacter*, and enteroinvasive and enterohemorrhagic *Escherichia coli*. Noninfectious causes include inflammatory bowel disease, ischemic colitis, diverticulitis, and arteriovenous malformation.

Unusual manifestations of amebic colitis include acute necrotizing colitis, toxic megacolon, ameboma, and perianal ulceration with potential fistula formation. Acute necrotizing colitis is rare (<0.5% of cases) and is associated with a greater than 40% mortality. Patients with acute necrotizing colitis are typically very ill-appearing with fever, bloody mucoid diarrhea, abdominal pain with rebound tenderness, and peritoneal signs of irritation. Surgical intervention is indicated if there is bowel perforation or if the patient fails to improve on antiamebic therapy. Toxic megacolon is rare (approximately 0.5% of cases) and typically is associated with corticosteroid use.

Amebic Liver Abscess

Amebic liver abscess is 10 times more common in men than women and is a rare disease in children. Approximately 80% of patients with amebic liver abscess present with symptoms that develop relatively acutely (typically < 2 to 4 weeks in duration) with fever, cough, and a constant, dull, aching abdominal pain in the right upper quadrant or epigastrium. Involvement of the diaphragmatic surface of the liver may lead to right pleural pain or referred shoulder pain. Associated gastrointestinal symptoms occur in up to 10% to 35% of cases and include nausea, vomiting, abdominal cramping, abdominal distention, diarrhea, or constipation. Hepatomegaly with point tenderness over the liver, below the ribs, or in the intercostal spaces is a typical finding. Complications from amebic liver abscess may arise from rupture of the abscess with extension into the peritoneum, pleural cavity, or pericardium. Extrahepatic amebic abscesses have occasionally been described in the lung, brain, and skin, and presumably reach these sites hematogenously.

Diagnosis

Historically, diagnosis of amebiasis was complicated and often unreliable for various reasons. The signs and symptoms of amebiasis can provide means to obtain clinical diagnosis. However, the confirmation of an amebic infection rests with laboratory identification. Over the last 25 years, various molecular diagnostic tests have been developed to diagnose *E. histolytica*. The diagnosis of intestinal amebiasis must be based on tests that distinguish *E. histolytica* from *E. dispar*. *E. histolytica*-specific antigen detection test and polymerase chain reaction (PCR) tests are now available for specific diagnosis of *E. histolytica* (Table 1). Enzyme-linked immunoabsorbent assay–based antigen detection kits are now commercially available. Field studies that directly compared PCR to stool culture or antigen-detection tests for the diagnosis of *E. histolytica* infection suggest that these three different methods perform equally well. An important aid to antigen detection and PCR-based tests is the detection of serum antibodies to amebae, which are present in 70% to 90% of patients with symptomatic *E. histolytica* infection. A drawback of current serologic tests is that patients remain positive for years after infection, making it difficult to distinguish new from past infection in regions of the world where amebiasis is endemic. Colonic mucosal biopsies and

TABLE 1 Sensitivity of Laboratory Tests for the Diagnosis of Amebiasis

Laboratory Tests	Amebic Colitis	Amebic Liver Abscess
Microscopy (stool)*	25%–60%	8%–44%
Microscopy (abscess fluid)	N/A	<20%
Stool antigen detection†	>90%	40%
Serum antigen detection†	<65%	>90% (before therapy)
PCR/real-time PCR (stool)	>90%	>40%
PCR/real-time PCR (abscess fluid)	N/A	90%–100% (before therapy)
Serology		
Acute	50%–70%	70%–90%
Convalescent	>90%	>90%

†TechLab *E. histolytica* II antigen detection test.
Abbreviation: PCR = polymerase chain reaction.
*Does not distinguish *Entamoeba histolytica* from the commensal parasites *Entamoeba dispar* and *Entamoeba moshkovskii*.

exudates can reveal a range in histopathologic appearance and severity of intestinal lesions associated with amebic colitis.

Amebic liver abscess patients may reveal a mild to moderate leukocytosis and anemia. Patients with an acute presentation of amebic liver abscess tend to have a normal alkaline phosphatase and elevated aspartate transaminase with the opposite true for patients with a chronic presentation. Ultrasound, abdominal computed tomography scan, and magnetic resonance imaging of the liver are all excellent imaging modalities for detecting liver lesions (most commonly single and in the right lobe) but are not specific for amebic liver abscess. The differential diagnosis of a liver mass should include pyogenic liver abscess, necrotic hepatoma, and echinococcal cyst (usually an incidental finding that would not be the cause of fever and abdominal pain). Patients with amebic abscess are more likely than patients with pyogenic liver abscesses to be male and younger than age 50 years; have immigrated from or traveled to an endemic country; and lack jaundice, biliary disease, or diabetes mellitus. Fewer than half of patients with amebic liver abscess have parasites detected in their stool by antigen detection. Helpful clues to the diagnosis include the presence of epidemiologic risk factors for amebiasis and the presence of serum antiamebic antibodies (present in 70% to 80% of patients at the time of presentation; see Table 1). Occasionally, aspiration of the abscess is required to rule out a pyogenic abscess. Amebae are visualized in the abscess pus in a minority of patients with amebic liver abscess. Traditional PCR and real-time PCR tests can be used for the detection of *E. histolytica* DNA in the stool and liver abscess pus samples and have been found to be sensitive and specific (see Table 1).

Therapy

Therapy differs for invasive versus noninvasive infections (Table 2). Noninvasive infections can be treated with lumen active agents such as paromomycin (Humatin) to eradicate cysts and lumen-dwelling trophozoites. Nitroimidazoles, particularly metronidazole (Flagyl), are the mainstay of therapy for invasive amebiasis (see Table 2). Nitroimidazoles with longer half-lives (namely tinidazole [Tindamax], secnidazole,[2] and ornidazole[2]) are better tolerated and allow shorter duration of treatment; they are recently available in the United States. Approximately 90% of patients presenting with mild to moderate amebic colitis or dysentery respond to nitroimidazole treatment. In the rare case of fulminant amebic colitis, it is prudent to add broad-spectrum antibiotics to treat intestinal bacteria that may spill into the peritoneum, with patients occasionally requiring surgical

---

[2]Not available in the United States.

TABLE 2 Drug Therapy for the Treatment of Amebiasis*

Type of Infection	Drug	Adult Dosage	Pediatric Dosage
Asymptomatic intestinal colonization	Paromomycin (Humatin) or	25–35 mg/kg/d in 3 doses × 7 d	25–35 mg/kg/d in 3 doses × 7 d
	Diloxanide furoate (Furamide)*	500 mg tid × 10 d	20 mg/kg/d in 3 doses × 10 d
Amebic liver abscess[†]	Metronidazole (Flagyl) or	750 mg tid × 7–10 d in 3 doses × 7–10 d	35–50 mg/kg/d
	Tinidazole (Tindamax) *followed by luminal agent*	800 mg tid × 5 d[3] in 3 doses × 5 d	60 mg/kg/d[3]
	Paromomycin (Humatin)	25–35 mg/kg/d in 3 doses × 7 d	25–35 mg/kg/d in 3 doses × 7 d
	Diloxanide furoate (Furamide)[5] or	500 mg tid × 10 d in 3 doses × 10 d	20 mg/kg/d
Amebic colitis[†]	Metronidazole (Flagyl) *followed by luminal agent (similar to amebic liver abscess)*	500–750 mg tid × 7–10 d in 3 doses × 7–10 d	35–50 mg/kg/d

[3]Exceeds dosage recommended by the manufacturer.
[5]Investigational drug in the United States.
*The information is updated annually by the Medical Letter on Drugs and Therapeutics at http://www.medletter.com/htmlprm.htm#Parasitic.
[†]Treatment of amebic liver abscess and amebic colitis should be followed by a treatment with a luminal agent.

intervention for acute abdomen, gastrointestinal bleeding, or toxic megacolon. Parasites persist in the intestine in as many as 40% to 60% of metronidazole (Flagyl)-treated patients. Therefore, metronidazole (Flagyl) treatment should be followed with paromomycin (Humatin) or the second-line agent diloxanide furoate (Furamide)[2] to cure luminal infection (see Table 2). Do not treat with metronidazole (Flagyl) and paromomycin (Humatin) at the same time because the diarrhea, a common side effect of paromomycin (Humatin), may make it difficult to assess response to therapy.

Therapeutic aspiration of an amebic liver abscess is occasionally required as adjunctive treatment to antiparasitic therapy. Abscess drainage should be considered in patients who fail to clinically respond to drug therapy within 5 to 7 days or those with high risk of abscess rupture as defined by cavity size greater than 5 cm or location in the left lobe. Bacterial coinfection of amebic liver abscess has been occasionally observed (both prior to and as a complication of drainage), and it is reasonable to add antibiotics or drainage, or both, to the treatment regimen if a prompt response to nitroimidazole therapy is not observed. Imaging-guided percutaneous treatment (needle aspiration or catheter drainage) has replaced surgical intervention over more recent years as the procedure of choice for therapeutically reducing abscess size.

---

[2]Not available in the United States.

REFERENCES

Diamond LS, Clark CG. A redescription of *Entamoeba histolytica* Schaudin 1903 (amended Walker 1911) separating it from *Entamoeba dispar* (Brumpt 1925). J Eukaryot Microbiol 1993;40:340–4.

Haque R, Mollah NU, Ali IKM, et al. Diagnosis of amebic liver abscess and intestinal infection with the TechLab *Entamoeba histolytica* II antigen detection and antibody tests. J Clin Microbiol 2000;38:3235–9.

Haque R, Ali IKM, Akther S, Petri Jr WA. Comparison of PCR, isoenzyme analysis, and antigen detection for diagnosis of *Entamoeba histolytica* infection. J Clin Microbio 1998;36:449–52.

Haque R, Ali IKM, Sack RB, et al. Amebiasis and mucosal IgA antibody against the *Entamoeba histolytica* adherence lectin in Bangladeshi children. J Infect Dis 2001;183:1787–93.

Haque R, Huston CD, Hughes M, et al. Current concepts: Amebiasis. N Engl J Med 2003;348:1565–73.

Petri WA Jr, Haque R, Lyerly D, Vine RR. Estimating the impact of amebiasis on health. Parasitol Today 2000;16:320–1.

Petri WA Jr, Singh U. State of the art: Diagnosis and management of amebiasis. Clin Infect Dis 1999;29:1117–25.

Stanley SL Jr. Amoebiasis. Lancet 2003;22(9362):1025–34.

Tanyuksel M, Petri WA Jr. Laboratory diagnosis of amebiasis. Clin Microbiol Rev 2003;16:713–29.

World Health Organization WA. Amoebiasis. Wkly Epidemiol Rec 1997;72:97–100.

Giardiasis

Method of
M. Ekramul Hoque, MBBS, MPH (Hons), PhD

Background

Giardiasis is a parasitic infection of the upper small intestine caused by a flagellated protozoan, *Giardia lamblia* (also called *Giardia intestinalis* and *Giardia duodenalis*). This ubiquitous parasite is a major cause of intestinal infection among adults and children in developing and developed countries. The existence of this parasite was reported in the prehistoric era across the continents. However, pathogenicity of the organism among humans was known only in the latter part of the last century.

Organism

Giardia is a microscopic organism that exists in two life forms. The trophozoite, which is environmentally unstable, causes clinical illness, and the resistant cysts are responsible for the transmission of infection. Trophozoites are binucleated, flagellated, and pear shaped, measuring 12 to 15 µm long and 6 to 8 µm wide. They have a pair of claw-shaped median bodies and a concave ventral disk used for nourishment and attachment on the wall of the small intestine of vertebrate hosts. Cysts are smaller and oval, usually 8 to 12 µm long and 7 to 10 µm wide, and contain four nuclei.

Epidemiology

Giardiasis is one of the most common intestinal infections in the world. More than 200 million people are reported to have symptoms of giardiasis, and some 500,000 new cases are reported annually. Some estimates suggest the worldwide prevalence of giardiasis is 20% to 60%. Others report from 2% to 7% in industrialized countries and 20% to 30% in developing countries. In the United States, giardiasis became nationally notifiable in 2002. In 2008, there were 18,913 giardiasis cases reported from 47 states/jurisdictions, with an incidence rate of 7.4 cases per 100,000 population.

The incidence varied by state from 2.2 to 32.8 cases per 100,000 population; rates were higher in the northern states than the southern states. *Giardia* infection is highly underreported, and therefore the true burden of giardiasis in the United States is probably underestimated. An estimate suggests there are 2 million giardiasis cases in the United States annually, and 5000 people are hospitalized due to severe infection. On average, New Zealand reports nearly 44.1 cases of giardiasis per 100,000 population every year, which is one of the highest among the industrialized countries. *Giardia* infection is reported to be more prevalent both in urban and rural populations.

Humans are the primary reservoir of the parasite. Other possible hosts are farm, wild, and domestic animals. Polymerase chain reaction (PCR) testing of samples of human feces from different geographic locations has so far associated *G. intestinalis* genotypes (assemblages) A and B with human infections. The role of animals in transmitting *G. intestinalis* to humans and the most likely routes of infection remain unclear.

Transmission of the *Giardia* infection is through the fecal-oral route following direct or indirect contact with cysts of *Giardia*. Cysts are infectious immediately after being excreted in feces. An infected person can excrete a maximum of 10^9 cysts per day for several months. Cysts may be killed by simple drying and heat, but they can survive for several weeks in cool and wet environments. Infectious dose is low; ingestion of as few as 10 cysts can cause infection. Commonly, the organism spreads by water or food or directly through person-to-person contact. Outbreaks of waterborne giardiasis have been reported year round, suggesting frequent contamination of water sources and longer survival of cysts in water.

Giardiasis shows a bimodal pattern of age distribution, peaking in children younger than 5 years and in adults 25 to 44 years (Figure 1). Incidence of infection varies by season, peaking in late summer and early autumn and dropping in winter. Persons at increased risk for infection include (among others) children of diaper age, children attending daycare centers, daycare workers, immunocompromised persons, pregnant women, institutionalized persons, travelers to endemic regions, people drinking contaminated water during outdoor activities, sewage and irrigation workers, and men who have sex with men.

It is not clear whether giardiasis causes malnutrition or malnutrition predisposes to *Giardia* infection. However, nutritional insufficiency can contribute to chronicity of the disease. Repeated exposure to the parasite can elicit an immune response, which might explain asymptomatic giardiasis cases. Breast-fed infants of immune mothers might acquire temporary protection against giardiasis, but this is not conclusive.

Pathogenesis

Clinical illness results from the interaction of *Giardia* organisms with the human host and the host's subsequent response to the parasite. *Giardia* isolates can vary in virulence, which might further explain the intensity of the symptoms.

After a person ingests *Giarda* cysts, excystation begins in the duodenum in the presence of gastric acid, pancreatic enzymes, and parasite-derived cysteine protease. Two tropozoites are formed from each cyst by binary fission (miotic division). The motility of parasites and the inflammatory cytokine response to parasitic attachment on the mucosal brush borders results in secretion of fluid and electrolytes, hence diarrhea and malabsorption. Trophozoites frequently slough off villi, which are swept into the fecal stream and replaced by new sets. After 4 to 15 days of colonization, some trophozoites encyst in the jejunum under an alkaline environment of bile secretion. Immotile cysts undergo a single cell division to form four nuclei, which are then passed intermittently in the feces.

Giardia trophozoites remain adherent to the intestinal mucosa but are not invasive. This close association might directly affect the brush border and its enzyme system. Hospital-based investigation observed partial villous atrophy in up to 25% of patients. Malabsorption of vitamin B_{12} occurs in 20% to 40% cases. Parasites are also found in extraintestinal sites such as the gallbladder and the urinary tract.

Clinical Features

Clinical manifestations of giardiasis vary from asymptomatic infection to severe diarrhea. The incubation period for *Giardia* infection varies from 1 week to several weeks. However, a period of 5 to 25 days is average.

Freshly exposed persons in an endemic area can present with acute symptoms that usually begin about 15 days (range, 1–46 days) following exposure. The symptoms include nausea, anorexia, upper abdominal discomfort, malaise, low-grade fever, and chills followed by the sudden onset of explosive, watery, foul-smelling diarrhea associated with foul flatulence and abdominal distention. Generally, the acute stage resolves spontaneously within 2 to 4 weeks. Some patients become asymptomatic passers of cysts for a period. Others have periodic brief recurrences of acute symptoms.

About 30% to 50% of infected patients go on to a subacute or chronic stage. Overseas travelers to *Giardia*-endemic areas often do not recognize or remember the infection during their travel and subsequently present periodically with persistent or recurrent mild to moderate symptoms. Features of subacute to chronic *Giardia* infection include flatulence, mushy foul stools, upper abdominal cramps, abdominal distention, steatorrhea, marked weight loss, and fatigue. Uncommon manifestations are cholecystitis, pancreatitis, immunologic reactions (including arthritis, retinal arteritis, and iridocyclitis), and occasionally rash and urticaria, mostly in adults. In rare cases, symptoms persist for years, but most cases resolve spontaneously after a variable period of weeks or months.

Generally, 10% to 30% of infected people remain symptom free, but the true percentage may be as high as 60%. The prevalence of asymptomatic infection is higher among children than among adults, especially among those in daycare. The duration of the asymptomatic cyst-passing state is not determined.

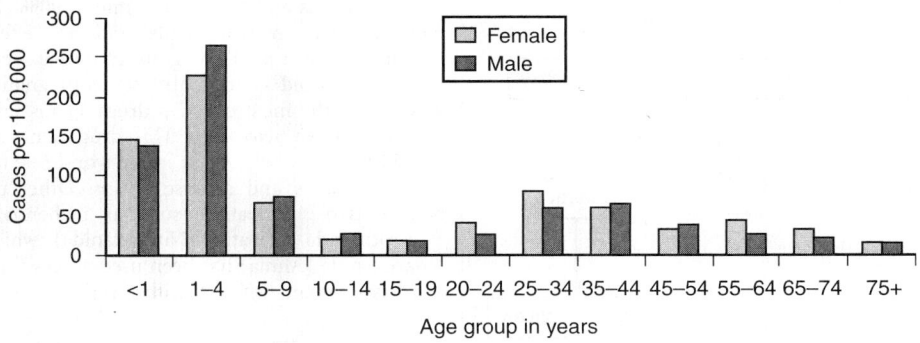

FIGURE 1. Notification rate of giardiasis in New Zealand by age and gender.

Diagnosis

Clinical signs and symptoms along with the history of risk behavior and exposure to *Giardia* risk factors can lead to a preliminary diagnosis of the disease. Laboratory diagnostic procedures are then applied to confirm the infection (Figure 2).

Traditionally, diagnosis is based on microscopic detection of *Giardia* cysts or trophozoites in the fecal specimens. At least three specimens of feces collected on consecutive days may be required to recover the parasite. The sensitivity of parasite detection is 50% to 70% in one specimen and 90% in three specimens.

Immunologic methods for detecting *Giardia* have superior sensitivity and specificity compared with other conventional methods of diagnosis. Widely used methods are enzyme immunoassay (EIA) detecting soluble antigens, direct fluorescent antibody (DFA) detecting intact organisms, and immunochromatographic lateral-flow immunoassays or rapid assay. Sensitivity of immunoassay varies between 94% and 97%, and specificity varies between 99% and 100%. EIA and rapid assay can pick up antigens of recently cured cases; DFA detects *Giardia* cysts. Immunoassay tests are quick and costs are reasonable.

Serologic tests do not have great diagnostic value in clinical practice because immunoglobulin G (IgG) persists even after infection; IgM, however, can indicate active infection. Negative serology does not exclude infection.

Duodenal aspirates or string test and duodenal mucosal biopsy are costly and invasive. They should be reserved for situations when giardiasis is strongly suspected despite persistent negative feces tests. PCR is used mostly in epidemiologic studies.

Treatment

Giardiasis, if diagnosed, should be treated. There are unresolved debates on the significance of treatment of asymptomatic cases. However, asymptomatic cases can remain a potential source of infection and can turn symptomatic at any moment.

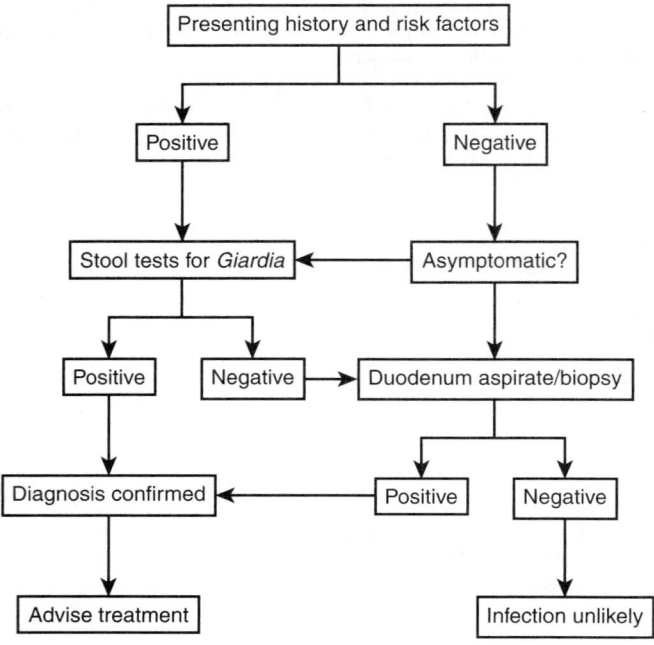

FIGURE 2. Diagnostic algorithm for giardiasis.

CURRENT DIAGNOSIS

- Giardiasis is a common parasitic infection of the small intestine.
- Children, caregivers, travelers, and persons exposed to contaminated water are at greater risk for infection.
- Clinical manifestations vary widely.
- A large fraction of infected persons remain asymptomatic.
- Infective cysts pass intermittently with patients' feces.
- Diagnosis is by detection of *Giardia* parasites in feces by repeated microscopy or by immunologic assays.
- Assays can give false positives in recently cured persons.
- Infection can resolve spontaneously or can go into a chronic stage lasting for months with marked weight loss.

PHARMACOLOGIC THERAPY

A number of effective antigiardial drugs are available (Table 1).

Metronidazole (Flagyl)[1] is preferred and widely used because of its broad-spectrum coverage. It is not approved by the FDA for routine treatment of giardiasis in the United States. Metronidazole is effective and well tolerated and has a cure rate of 80% to 95%. The common side effects are gastrointestinal upset, headache, nausea, leukopenia, and metallic taste in the mouth. It is contraindicated in the first trimester of pregnancy due to its suspected carcinogenic, teratogenic, and mutagenic effects. Although the drug on therapeutic doses has shown no significant increased risk of cancer in humans. Other minor side effects are peripheral neuropathy, seizures, depression, irritability, restlessness, and insomnia. Drug resistance is not yet widespread.

Furazolidone (Furoxone)[2] is the primary drug of choice in the United States. It is available in liquid form and is widely used to treat children. Cure rates are between 80% and 89%. It is not recommended in pregnancy. Side effects include gastrointestinal disturbances, hemolytic anemia, disulfiram-like reactions with alcohol, hypersensitivity reactions, brown discoloration of the urine, orthostatic hypotension, and hypoglycemia.

Albendazole (Albenza)[1] is an anthelminthic whose efficacy is equal to that of metronidazole and with cure rates of 62% to 95%. Absence of anorexia in using this drug is an advantage for treating children. Notable side effects are gastrointestinal upset, abdominal pain, nausea, vomiting, diarrhea, dizziness, vertigo, fever, increased intracranial pressure, alopecia, and (reversible) increase in serum transaminases after prolonged use. Albendazole is contraindicated in pregnancy due to teratogenicity. Paromomycin (Humatin)[1] is a poorly absorbed aminoglycoside that is excreted in the feces without being metabolized. Its efficacy rate is between 60% and 70%. It is recommended for giardial infection in pregnant patients. Common side effects are nausea, increased gastrointestinal motility, abdominal pain, and diarrhea. 5-Nitroimidazole compounds, tinidazole (Tindamax) ornidazole (Tiberal), and secnidazole (Noameba-DS, Secnil)[1,2] are effective as first-line agents and have a cure rate of 90%. They have longer serum half-lives than metronidazole and are effective in single doses. Common side effects are gastrointestinal upset, vertigo, and bitter taste. They need caution to use in pregnant patients. Quinacrine[2] was one of the most effective drugs against giardial infection, with a cure rate of 92% to 95%. This drug is no longer produced in the United States and elsewhere in the world due to a number of pharmacokinetic issues and adverse effects. Other potential drugs include benzimidazole derivatives such as mebendazole (Vermox)[1] and a 5-nitrothiazole derivative (Nitazoxanide), which are not used widely. Nitazoxanide (Alinia) has been used successfully in France in resistant giardiasis patients infected with HIV.

---

[1]Not FDA approved for this indication.
[2]Not available in the United States.

TABLE 1 Therapeutic Doses of Antigiardial Drugs

Drugs	Adult Dose	Pediatric Dose
Metronidazole (Flagyl)[a]	250 mg tid × 5–7 d	5 mg/kg tid × 5–7 d
Tinidazole (Tindamax)[b]	2 g single dose	50 mg/kg single dose (max, 2 g)
Ornidazole (Tiberal)[c]	2 g single dose	40–50 mg/kg single dose (max, 2 g)
Secnidazole (Noameba-DS, Secnil)[b]	2 g single dose	30 mg/kg single dose
Quinacrine (Atabrine)[c]	100 mg tid × 5–7 d[e]	2 mg/kg tid × 5–7 d (max 300 mg/d)[e]
Furazolidone[d]	100 mg qid × 7–10 d	1.5 mg/kg qid × 10 d
Paromomycin[a]	500 mg tid × 10 d[f]	8–10 mg/kg tid × 5–10 d[f]
Albendazole	400 mg qd × 5 d	15 mg/kg/day × 5–7 d (max 400 mg/d)
Nitrazoxanide	500 mg bid × 3 d	7.5 mg/kg bid × 3 d

[a]Not a U.S. FDA approved indication; [b]Not available in the U.S.; [c]No longer produced in the U.S.; [d]Available in liquid formulation; [e]After meal; [f]With meal
qd, once a day; bid, twice a day; tid, three times a day; qid, four times a day

OTHER MEASURES

Diet modification can reduce acute symptoms, improve host defense mechanisms, and inhibit growth and replication of *Giardia* trophozoites in the lumen of the intestine. General advice is to consume a diet of whole foods that is high in fiber, low in simple carbohydrates, and low in fat.

Follow-up

Follow-up stool tests are advised to ensure resolution of infection. Hygiene practices should be enhanced during outbreaks. Symptomatic persons should be kept away from public contact.

Prognosis

Giardiasis is usually a self-limited intestinal infection. Effective antigiardial agents shorten the infection period. If untreated, giardiasis often resolves spontaneously in a few weeks. Prognosis is, therefore, generally excellent.

CURRENT THERAPY

- Metronidazole (Flagyl)[1] is widely used because of its broad-spectrum coverage, but it is contraindicated in the first trimester of pregnancy.
- Furazolidone (Furoxone)[2] is available in liquid form to treat children.
- Absence of anorexia with albendazole (Albenza)[1] is an advantage for treating children.
- Paromomycin (Humatin)[1] is recommended in pregnancy due to its poor absorption rate.
- Tinidazole (Tindamax), ornidazole (Tiberal); and secnidazole (Noameba-DS, Secnil)[2] are effective in single doses.
- Nitazoxanide (Alinia) is used in drug-resistant giardiasis.
- Some diet modifications can reduce acute symptoms, improve host defense, and inhibit trophozoite replications.

[1]Not FDA approved for this indication.
[2]Not available in the United States.

Prevention

Eradication of giardiasis is not possible because the disease is endemic in the human population, animal population, and environment. Prevention and control methods are the way forward. Health departments in all countries, including the Centers for Disease Control and Prevention in the United States, publish recommendations for prevention and control of giardiasis. These include decontamination of water supplies and sanitary and hygiene practices. Potentially contaminated water may be treated by boiling for more than 1 minute or filtering through a pore size of 1 μm or smaller. Chlorination and iodination are unreliable. Laws and regulations to protect provisions of safe water should be enforced and monitored. Regular surveillance and reviews of sanitation can ensure quality.

People involved in recreational water activities and persons traveling overseas must be informed about the possibility of exposure to the parasite. Persons with symptomatic infection should not swim in a pool until 2 weeks after the treatment. Other occupational groups (e.g., daycare workers, medical personnel, irrigation and sewage workers) need to be cautioned. In daycare centers, hand washing with soap after changing diapers and a separate diaper-changing area should be implemented. All symptomatic family members, daycare center teachers, and children in daycare should be treated for giardiasis. Treatment of asymptomatic cases should be considered if the infected person is suspected to be a potential source of transmission of the disease.

REFERENCES

Cacciò SM, Thompson RCA, McLauchlin J, Smith HV. Unravelling *Cryptosporidium* and *Giardia* epidemiology. Trends Parasitol 2005;21(9):430–7.

Centers for Disease Control and Prevention. Parasitic disease information: Giardiasis fact sheet. Available at http://www.cdc.gov/ncidod/dpd/parasites/giardiasis/factsht_giardia.htm [accessed 5.04.07].

Escobedo AA, Cimerman S. Giardiasis: a pharmacotheraphy review. Expert Opin Pharmacother 2007;8(12):1885–902.

Falagas ME, Walker AM, Jick H. Late incidence of cancer after metronidazole use: a matched metronidazole user/nonuser study. Clin Infect Dis 1998;26(2):384–8.

Gardner TB, Hill DR. Treatment of giardiasis. Clin Microbiol Rev 2001;14(1):114–28.

Hanson KL, Cartwright CP. Use of an enzyme immunoassay does not eliminate the need to analyze multiple stool specimens for sensitive detection of *Giardia lamblia*. J Clin Microbiol 2001;39(2):474–7.

Hetsko ML, McCaffery JM, Svard SG, et al. Cellular and transcriptional changes during excystation of *Giardia lamblia* in vitro. Exp Parasitol 1998;88(3):172–83.

Hlavsa MC, Watson JC, Beach MJ. Giardiasis surveillance—United States, 1998–2002. MMWR Surveill Summ 2005;54(SS01):9–16.

Hoque ME, Hope VT, Scragg R. *Giardia* infection in Auckland and New Zealand: Trends and international comparison. The N Z Med J 2002;115(1150):121–3.

Islam A, Stoll BJ, Ljungstrom I, et al. *Giardia lamblia* infections in a cohort of Bangladeshi mothers and infants followed for one year. J Pediatr 1983;103 (6):996–1000.

Kulda J, Nohynkova E. Flagellates of the human intestine and of intestines of other species. In: Kreier JP, editor. Protozoa of Veterinary and Medical Interest, vol. II. New York: Academic Press; 1978. p. 69–104.

Lebwohl B, Deckelbaum RJ, Green PHR. Giardiasis. Gastrointest Endosc 2003;57(7):906–13.

Mineno T, Avery MA. Giardiasis: Recent progress in chemotherapy and drug development. Curr Pharm Des 2003;9:841–55.

New Zealand Ministry of Health. Communicable disease control manual. Wellington: New Zealand Ministry of Health; 1998.

Snel SJ, Baker MG, Venugopal K. The epidemiology of giardiasis in New Zealand, 1997–2006. N Z Med J 2009;122(1290):62–75.

Yoder JS, Beach MJ. Giardiasis surveillance–United States, 2003–2005. MMWR 2007;56(SS07):11–8. Erratum: MMWR 2007;56(43):1141.

Yoder JS, Harral C, Beach MJ. Giardiasis surveillance—United States, 2006–2008. MMWR 2010;59(SS-6):15–25.

Severe Sepsis and Septic Shock

Method of
Jerome Larkin, MD, and Marisa Holubar, MD

Epidemiology

The true prevalence and incidence of sepsis remain unknown. A study by Martin and colleagues in 2003 analyzed data from the National Hospital Discharge Survey from 1979 to 2000. Although some limitations apply, particularly shifts in the understanding of and use of coding, their findings have the advantage of assessing a large sample size over a prolonged period of observation. The most striking finding was a rise in the incidence of sepsis in the United States over this period, from an annual occurrence of 164,000 cases in 1979 to 660,000 cases in 2000. This reflects an average annual increase on average of 8.7% for more than 20 years. Coincident with this increase was a rise in the percentage of patients with a diagnosis of sepsis due to fungal organisms (4.6% in 2000). Gram-positive organisms supplanted gram-negatives as the largest group of pathogens after 1987 (52% versus 37%).

Mortality was highest among African American men and was associated with failure of three or more organs. Men were more likely to become septic than women (relative risk, 1.90). In-hospital mortality fell from 27.8% to 17.9% between 1995 and 2000. Total mortality increased, most likely as a result of the increase in the total burden of disease. This increase, although perhaps in part attributable to greater use of the diagnostic code for sepsis, is thought to have resulted from a combination of aging of the population, greater numbers of immunosuppressed individuals surviving longer, greater use of prosthetic devices, and greater number and more invasive medical interventions. Diabetes, hypertension, chronic obstructive pulmonary disease, congestive heart failure, and HIV infection all increased as a proportion of medical conditions contributing to sepsis, whereas the proportion of patients with cancer and that of pregnant patients declined. The percentage of patients with one or more organs failing (i.e., severe sepsis) increased from 17% to 35% of all patients with a diagnosis of sepsis.

A study by Dombrovskiy and associates described an even greater increase in the proportion of severe sepsis, from 25.6% in 1993 to 43.8% in 2003. They also found an absolute increase in the number of cases of sepsis, as well as an increase in total mortality, again likely due to increased incidence. Case-fatality rates fell from 45.8% to 37.8%, but mortality was substantially higher at both the beginning and the end of their study period than was described by Martin. These findings suggest acceleration in both severity and incidence of severe sepsis and septic shock.

Sepsis is the 10th most common cause of death in the United States. The incidence is highest during the winter, most likely reflecting increased respiratory viral infections that precede the development of community-acquired pneumonia, which is itself a medical condition with increased risk of developing severe sepsis.

A remarkable aspect of sepsis, severe sepsis, and septic shock is the relatively small number of associated pathogens out of the more than 1000 microorganisms known to cause human disease. *Staphylococcus aureus*, streptococci, enterococci, and gram-negative rods are the most commonly isolated species. *Escherichia coli, Klebsiella, Pseudomonas, Serratia, Acinetobacter, Enterobacter, Citrobacter,* and *Neisseria meningitidis* (a gram-negative coccus) constitute the most common gram-negative pathogens. This relative paucity of etiologic bacterial pathogens has implications for empiric antimicrobial therapy. The emergence of resistant organisms, particularly methicillin-resistant *S. aureus* (MRSA) and gram-negative bacteria harboring extended-spectrum β-lactamases, increases the risk of antibiotic failure and attendant mortality. Fungal pathogens, particularly non-candidal species, continue to increase in incidence. This is most likely the result of better empiric management of gram-negative and candidal sepsis in patients with hematologic malignancies.

Although sepsis is most typically a disease of the elderly, the immune suppressed, and those with chronic medical problems, otherwise young and healthy individuals can also be stricken with no clear cause or known risk factor, such as in meningococcemia, toxic shock syndrome, and necrotizing fasciitis.

Definitions

The term sepsis derives from a Greek word that generally implies putrefaction. It also has a colloquial meaning, understood by most lay people to mean a serious, potentially overwhelming infection. Historically, it has been intuitively understood by physicians to mean an infection, once localized, that has now disseminated and is life threatening. Bacteremia is implied if not always proven. Sepsis was usually fatal in the preantibiotic era, and its morbidity and mortality remain substantial.

In 2001, a consensus conference, sponsored by the American College of Chest Physicians and the Society of Critical Care Medicine and involving the European Society of Intensive Care Medicine, the Surgical Infection Society, and the American Thoracic Society, was convened to arrive at a specific definition of sepsis. Achieving such a definition is critically important to ongoing research on interventions aimed at improving mortality. Their deliberations, building on the work of a previous conference and published in 2003, elaborated several key concepts. They defined systemic inflammatory response syndrome (SIRS) as a state of immune activation characterized by the findings of fever with tachycardia, tachypnea, and/or leukocytosis or leukopenia. Although sensitive, this definition is so overly broad as to be rather unhelpful to an experienced clinician who would not need to resort to such terms to understand that a patient is seriously ill. Nonetheless, it provides a useful construct in beginning to arrive at a specific definition of sepsis. Both infectious and noninfectious processes—severe burn and pancreatitis being the most notable examples of the latter—can cause SIRS.

Sepsis is defined as the finding of SIRS in the presence of known or suspected invasion by a microbe into a normally sterile body site. Severe sepsis is sepsis that has become more generalized. The cardinal finding is organ dysfunction that is unrelated to the primary site of infection. Other typical findings include hyperglycemia, thrombocytopenia, hyperbilirubinemia, acidosis, coagulopathy, edema, oliguria, hypotension, ileus, hypoxia, and poor perfusion. Heart, kidney, and respiratory failure are the most common forms of organ dysfunction. Altered sensorium is also common. Septic shock refers to the presence of hypotension with systolic blood pressure lower than 90 mm Hg or mean arterial pressure lower than 60 mm Hg despite adequate fluid resuscitation. These terms (sepsis, severe sepsis, and septic shock) are all part of a continuum, implying a progressively graver degree of illness with associated increasing mortality. No single symptom, physical finding, organ dysfunction, or laboratory abnormality serves to make or exclude the diagnosis, although isolation of a microorganism in the setting of such findings is highly suggestive. Increasing numbers of physical findings and other abnormalities correlates with an increasing likelihood of the diagnosis of sepsis.

The consensus conference put forward a staging system for sepsis based on host predisposition, nature of infection, host response, and organ dysfunction (mnemonic: PIRO). By this, it is understood that a given patient may be predisposed to infection based on medical conditions such as diabetes, vascular disease, sickle cell anemia, or inherited or acquired immunodeficiencies. Additionally, there are likely to be more subtle genetic predispositions to the development of sepsis, as well as age-related factors. The nature of infection in terms of the site, inoculum, and virulence of the infecting organism clearly plays a role in determining the development of sepsis. The host response—ranging from localization and clearing of the infection without deleterious effect on the host to a state of immunologic dissonance whereby the inflammatory response is itself the driver of pathology—is signaled by the development of organ dysfunction. This staging system allows patients to be stratified at different points and serves as a template for evaluating the efficacy of various interventions as the characterization of sepsis and research into novel therapies progresses.

Pathophysiology

Infection of the immunocompetent host by a microorganism typically leads to immune activation. This serves to isolate the site and source of infection. Local tissue is often damaged, but eventually the infection is cleared, and repair and regeneration occur. This process is highly regulated, with a number of different cell types and mediators involved, all in delicate balance between proinflammatory and antiinflammatory effects. The patient may have few or no symptoms, or there may be systemic evidence of infection (i.e., SIRS). Sepsis is the failure of localization such that the process becomes generalized and leads to tissue destruction remote from the site of infection. Why the immune system enters this state of dysregulation remains unknown, although an enormous amount of research over the last 4 decades has elucidated many of the pathways and mediators involved. Tumor necrosis factor, platelet-activating factor, interleukins, eicosanoids, interferons, and nitric oxide are among the biologically active molecules characterized to date. Particular microbes also contribute to this process through the elaboration of toxins (typically by gram-positive organisms) and endotoxins (gram negative–derived lipopolysaccharide). These events lead to tissue destruction as a result of ischemic insult, direct cytotoxicity, and accelerated apoptosis. The characterization of inflammatory mediators has led to attempts to modify the immune response through the use of novel therapies such as monoclonal antibodies directed against tumor necrosis factor. To date such attempts have not met with success, and investigation continues.

Diagnosis

The diagnosis of sepsis ultimately relies on the clinical suspicion of infection in the setting of SIRS. A constellation of other supportive evidence establishes a greater or lesser likelihood of the presence of sepsis (see the Current Diagnosis box). It is rare that specific microbiologic evidence for infection is available in a manner timely enough to determine that sepsis is present or to help guide the initial, typically urgent, therapy. When it is available, it usually is a Gram stain or other type of specialized microbiology stain that confirms the presence of a potential pathogen in a site where none should be (e.g., gram-positive cocci in cerebrospinal fluid). Early therapy therefore relies on aggressive resuscitative measures and the administration of empiric antibiotics.

CURRENT DIAGNOSIS

Systemic inflammatory response syndrome (SIRS)

- Diagnosis is based on the presence of two or more of the following:
  - Temperature >38°C or <36°C
  - Pulse >90 beats/min
  - Respirations >20 breaths/min or arterial partial pressure of carbon dioxide ($Paco_2$) <32 mm Hg
  - White blood cell count >12,000 or <4000 cells/mm³ or >10% bands

Sepsis

- Diagnosis is based on a finding of SIRS plus proven or suspected infection as the cause

Severe Sepsis

- Diagnosis is based on a finding of sepsis plus organ dysfunction of one or more major systems (typically kidney, lung, or heart; less often, central nervous system)

Septic Shock

- Diagnosis is based on a finding of severe sepsis plus persistent hypotension despite aggressive fluid resuscitation (i.e., vasopressors are required to maintain mean arterial pressure >65 mm Hg)

Supportive Laboratory Findings

- Hyperglycemia
- Lactic acidosis
- Hyperbilirubinemia
- Acute renal failure
- Thrombocytopenia
- Coagulopathy
- Leukocytosis or leukopenia
- Elevated erythrocyte sedimentation rate or C-reactive protein

Supportive Physical Findings

- Decreased capillary refill or mottling of skin
- Mental status changes or obtundation
- Tachypnea or respiratory failure
- Tachycardia
- Anuria or oliguria
- Edema

Treatment

EARLY GOAL-DIRECTED RESUSCITATION: THE FIRST SIX HOURS

Initial treatment of sepsis should focus on correction of hemodynamic parameters, early administration of antibiotics, and source control of potential sites of infection. The 2008 guidelines from the Surviving Sepsis Campaign, an international initiative to improve sepsis outcomes, emphasized the importance of aggressive fluid resuscitation. Therapy should be implemented according to a protocol directed at achieving the following specific goals:

- Central venous pressure 8 to 12 mm Hg, or 12 to 15 mm Hg in those who are mechanically ventilated or have decreased left ventricular compliance
- Central venous or mixed venous oxygen saturation 70% or greater
- Mean arterial pressure (MAP) 65 mm Hg or greater
- Urine output 0.5 mL/kg/hour or greater

Administration of fluid boluses of 1000 mL or more of crystalloids or 300 to 500 mL of colloids over 30 minutes should begin as soon as hypoperfusion is recognized. There is no evidence that one type of fluid is superior to the other, although crystalloid is substantially cheaper. In cases of profound intravascular volume depletion, more rapid and more frequent fluid administration may be needed. Hemodynamic improvement (decreased heart rate, increased blood pressure, increased urine output) and the goal central venous pressure should direct the need for continued infusion of fluid while avoiding the development of volume overload and pulmonary edema. Transfusion of packed red blood cells should be considered if anemia is present, with a goal of achieving a hemoglobin level of 7.0 to 9.0 g/dL. If tissue hypoperfusion or hypoxia persists (central mixed venus oxygen saturation <70%) despite achieving a central venous pressure of 12 mm Hg, therapy with dopamine (Intropin) or norepinephrine (Levophed) should be initiated with a goal of achieving a MAP of 65 mm Hg. There is no role for the use of low-dose dopamine for renal protection. An arterial line for more precise and continuous measurement of blood pressure should be inserted as soon as possible after the initiation of vasopressor therapy. Ideally, vasopressors should not be introduced to increase MAP until after the fluid deficit has been corrected. However, in cases of severe shock, vasopressor therapy may be needed early in the resuscitation effort to improve perfusion to the peripheral vascular beds. If there is no response to dopamine and norepinephrine, the patient should be treated with epinephrine (Adrenalin).[1]

Appropriate antibiotics should be administered within 1 hour after diagnosis of severe sepsis or septic shock, because mortality increases in a linear fashion with each hour of delay. All efforts should be made to obtain appropriate cultures, in particular at least two sets of blood cultures. At least one of these should be peripheral, with the second from any long-term (>48 hours) vascular device. Cultures of urine, sputum, wounds, abscesses, and cerebrospinal fluid should also be obtained as appropriate and before the administration of antibiotics, assuming that such specimens can be obtained during the first hour. Specific antibiotic choices are discussed later.

SOURCE CONTROL

A survey for potential sources of infection should be performed, and early resuscitation efforts should occur concomitantly. Elimination of the source of infection is critical to reversing septic shock. Conditions that require emergent intervention, such as necrotizing fasciitis, cholangitis, and intestinal infarction, should be ruled out within the first 6 hours after presentation. Potentially infected indwelling devices should be removed as soon as possible. Necrotic tissue should be débrided and abscesses drained if either condition is detected. Practitioners must consider the risks and benefits of the specific invasive procedures and the timing of such interventions for each patient individually. Every effort should be made to limit the invasiveness of necessary procedures, to avoid further stress in patients with an already hemodynamically fragile state. Imaging studies such as computed tomography of the head, chest, abdomen, and pelvis are necessary to identify or rule out potential sources of infection. An exception to the mandate to drain or débride infected collections is the presence of infected pancreatic necrosis, in which case surgical intervention should be delayed.

OTHER INTERVENTIONS

After hemodynamic parameters have been stabilized with fluid and vasopressors, cultures have been obtained, antibiotics have been administered, and initial source control of infected foci has been achieved, other interventions may be appropriate. Many of these are typical components of good critical care.

CURRENT THERAPY SUMMARY

Initial Six Hours

- Initiate fluid resuscitation with crystalloid or colloid to achieve central venous pressure of 12 mm Hg (or 15 mm Hg if intubated).
- Add dopamine (Intropin) or norepinephrine (Levophed) for persistent hypotension (mean arterial pressure <65 mm Hg).
- Obtain blood, urine, and other appropriate cultures (cerebrospinal fluid, abscess drainage, catheter tip, tissue, sputum).
- Administer empiric antimicrobial therapy.
- Perform appropriate imaging studies with urgent source control as indicated and allowed by clinical status; remove potentially infected foreign bodies.
- All interventions should be undertaken simultaneously and initiated within 1 hour after making a presumptive diagnosis of sepsis.

Subsequent Interventions

- Maintain glycemic control with a target blood glucose level of less than 150 mg/dL.
- Use unfractionated or low-molecular-weight heparin for prophylaxis against deep venous thrombosis.
- Use a histamine 2 (H_2) blocker or proton pump inhibitor for gastric ulcer prophylaxis.
- Initiate therapy with dobutamine (Dobutrex) for low cardiac output in the face of adequate filling pressures.
- Consider therapy with activated protein C (drotrecogin alfa [Xigris]) for patients with an Acute Physiology and Chronic Health Evaluation (APACHE) II score of 25 or greater.
- Consider therapy with hydrocortisone (Solu-Cortef)[1] for patients with continued hypotension despite adequate fluid resuscitation and vasopressors.
- Achieve adequate sedation.

[1]Not FDA approved for this indication.

Cardiac Dysfunction

Patients who have adequate left ventricular filling pressures (as determined by a central venous pressure ≥12 mm Hg) but low cardiac output may benefit from therapy with dobutamine (Dobutrex) to increase cardiac output and improve tissue perfusion.

Corticosteroid Therapy

Activation of the hypothalamic-pituitary axis and the consequent increase in serum cortisol levels are vital aspects of the body's acute stress response to shock. Recent data suggest that critical illness–related corticosteroid insufficiency is more prevalent in septic shock than previously thought, with rates as high as 60%. Therapy with corticosteroids is indicated only for those patients who have continued hypotension in the face of adequate fluid resuscitation and vasopressor support. Hydrocortisone (Solu-Cortef)[1] should be administered intravenously 200–300 mg/day for seven days either divided every 6 hours or as a continuous infusion. Dexamethasone (Decadron)[1] should not be used unless hydrocortisone is not available. Because of the unclear long-term benefits and the known immunosuppressive side effects of corticosteroids, patients should

---

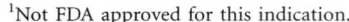

[1]Not FDA approved for this indication.

[1]Not FDA approved for this indication.

be weaned from hydrocortisone as soon as vasopressors are no longer necessary. If another form of corticosteroid other than hydrocortisone is used, then fludrocortisone (Florinef)[1] at a dose of 50 mcg/day should be added for mineralocorticoid effect.

Activated Protein C

Patients who are at increased risk of death with Acute Physiology and Chronic Health Evaluation (APACHE) II scores of 25 or higher and those with multiple organ dysfunction may benefit from infusion of activated protein C (drotrecogin alfa [Xigris]). This drug has numerous contraindications, including current active bleeding, recent (within 3 months) hemorrhagic stroke, recent (within 2 months) severe head trauma or intracranial or intraspinal surgery, trauma with a risk of life-threatening bleeding, presence of an epidural catheter, and intracranial neoplasm or mass lesion or evidence of herniation. It is not recommended for use in children. It is given as a 96-hour continuous infusion.

Glycemic Control

Maintenance of the blood glucose concentration lower than 150 mg/dL is associated with decreased mortality and length of stay in the intensive care unit. Control should be achieved with intravenous insulin, paying close attention to serum glucose levels every 1 to 2 hours until stable, with adjustments made on the basis of a validated protocol. Patients receiving intravenous insulin should simultaneously receive some form of glucose as a calorie source to minimize the risk of hypoglycemia.

Sedation and Paralytics

Sedation and treatment of pain should be aggressively managed according to validated protocols. Daily interruption of sedation allows for more accurate titration of drug and decreases the total time of mechanical ventilation. Paralytics should be avoided or used only briefly if required.

---

[1]Not FDA approved for this indication.

Anticoagulation

Patients should receive prophylaxis for deep venous thrombosis with either low-molecular-weight heparin or unfractionated heparin unless contraindicated by severe thrombocytopenia, recent intracranial bleeding, or coagulopathy. Those patients who cannot receive heparin should receive prophylaxis with graduated compression stockings or intermittent compression devices. Patients who are at especially high risk for deep venous thrombosis (e.g., prior history of clot, orthopedic surgery, trauma) should receive both pharmacologic and mechanical prophylaxis. Low-molecular-weight heparin is preferred to unfractionated heparin in high-risk patients.

Ulcer Prophylaxis

Patients should receive prophylaxis with a proton pump inhibitor or a histamine 2 (H$_2$) blocker to prevent upper gastrointestinal bleeding.

Bicarbonate Therapy

There is no role for the administration of bicarbonate to correct acidosis or improve hemodynamic status.

ANTIBIOTICS

Antibiotic choices should take into account the most likely pathogens for the suspected site or process. In general, initial empiric therapy (Table 1) should be broad, with an intention to narrow therapy once a microorganism has been isolated or a more precise clinical diagnosis has been made. Such a reevaluation should take place approximately 72 hours after the initiation of therapy. Numerous studies have documented the mortality associated with initial therapy that did not include agents active against the pathogen eventually isolated. In general, drugs from the β-lactam and related classes of antibiotics should be preferred for at least a part of most empiric regimens.

Special considerations include patients with neutropenia and fever, who should always be treated with at least one agent active against *Pseudomonas*. Some debate continues regarding the use of

TABLE 1 Empiric Antibiotic Choices for Severe Sepsis*

Source	Antibiotic and Dose	Comments
Community-acquired pneumonia	Ceftriaxone (Rocephin) 2 g q24h *plus* azithromycin (Zithromax) 500 mg q24h	Should include atypical coverage; alternative is moxifloxacin (Avelox)
Health care–associated pneumonia	Piperacillin/tazobactam (Zosyn) 4.5 g q6h *or* meropenem (Merrem)[1] 2 g q8h[3] *plus* vancomycin (Vancocin)[1] 1 g q12h	Should cover for *Pseudomonas* and other resistant gram-negative rods
Neutropenia/fever	Piperacillin/tazobactam[1] 4.5 g q6h *or* meropenem[1] 2 g q8h[3]	Consider empiric fungal coverage for prolonged neutropenia
Abdominal sepsis	Ampicillin/sulbactam (Unasyn) 3 g q6h *or* piperacillin/tazobactam 4.5 g q6h	Consider coverage for yeast, MRSA
Urosepsis	Ampicillin/sulbactam[1] 3 g q6h or piperacillin/tazobactam[1] 4.5 g q6h	Obtain imaging and decompression as appropriate
Foreign body/vascular catheter–related sepsis	Piperacillin/tazobactam[1] 4.5 g q6h *or* meropenem[1] 2 g q8h[3] *plus* vancomycin 1 g q12h	Vascular catheters or other foreign bodies should be removed urgently
Meningitis	Ceftriaxone 2 g q12h *plus* vancomycin[1] 750 mg q8h *plus* rifampin (Rifadin)[1] 600 mg q24h	Consider steroid therapy before or simultaneously with administration of antibiotics
Soft-tissue infection	Cefazolin (Ancef) 2 g q8h *plus* vancomycin 1 g q12h	Image for abscess with débridement as appropriate
Necrotizing fasciitis	Ampicillin/sulbactam 3 g q6h *plus* vancomycin 1 g q12h *plus* clindamycin (Cleocin) 900 mg q8h	Obtain urgent surgical consultation
Unknown	Piperacillin/tazobactam 4.5 g q6h *or* meropenem 2 g q8h[3] *plus* vancomycin 1 g q12h *plus* tobramycin (Tobrex) 7 mg/kg q24h	Obtain appropriate imaging studies, especially of abdomen, pelvis, central nervous system

[1]Not FDA approved for this indication.
[3]Exceeds dosage recommended by the manufacturer.
*In all cases, prior antimicrobial therapy, kidney and liver dysfunction, and the probable source of sepsis should be carefully considered. Always consider coverage for methicillin-resistant *Staphylococcus aureus* (MRSA) in areas where incidence in bloodstream isolates is >10%.

two anti-pseudomonal drugs as part of the initial antibiotic regimen. Given the possibility of resistance on the part of this pathogen, it would seem reasonable to use two drugs initially, until *Pseudomonas* has been isolated (if present) and its susceptibilities are known, allowing coverage to be narrowed. The Surviving Sepsis Campaign guidelines advocate this approach. There is no benefit in treating with two drugs known to be active in an attempt to achieve a supposed synergy.

Patients with hematologic malignancies are at increased risk for sepsis from fungal organisms. Severe sepsis or septic shock in such patients warrants empiric treatment with an echinocandin, a broad-spectrum azole such as voriconazole (Vfend) or posaconazole (Noxafil), or amphotericin (Fungizone).

MRSA continues to increase in incidence nationally and is now common as a community-acquired pathogen. It is also to be suspected as a cause of postinfluenza bacterial pneumonia. Empiric treatment with an antibiotic active against this bacterium, such as vancomycin (Vancocin), linezolid (Zyvox), or daptomycin (Cubicin), should be strongly considered in septic patients in communities where the rate of MRSA in bloodstream infections exceeds 10%. This pathogen should always be considered in a patient with a long-term intravenous catheter, prosthetic device, or other indwelling foreign body. Although vancomycin-resistant *S. aureus* is extremely rare, caution should be taken when using daptomycin and linezolid as empiric therapy, because resistance has been reported.

Prior administration of antibiotics and the attendant risk of infection by a pathogen resistant to the previous therapy should be considered in arriving at a course of empiric therapy. A typical scenario is a patient who presents with a catheter-related bloodstream infection while taking vancomycin. One would expect a gram-negative bacterium, a fungal organism, or, potentially, a vancomycin-resistant enterococcus as the pathogen. Recent hospitalization or residence in a nursing home places patients at risk for colonization and subsequent infection with resistant gram-negative rods.

Prognosis and Limits of Care

Patients who present with severe sepsis or septic shock often have substantial prior medical morbidity, decreasing their chance of survival. The overall mortality rate remains between 20% and 40%. Patients often have expressed wishes regarding limits of care to family members or others close to them before becoming ill. It is always appropriate to discuss goals of therapy, possible and probable outcomes, and plans for further evaluation and treatment with patients (if possible) and their proxies in all instances. Decisions to proceed with or limit care should be made within the context of a patient's expressed or expected wishes and should take into account unfolding clinical data and circumstances. Time spent in this endeavor can substantially decrease the amount of futile care rendered to a patient and lead to care that more truly reflects the patient's wishes regarding life-prolonging measures. The stress and anxiety experienced by family members may also be reduced.

Substantial progress has been made in the last 3 decades in decreasing the mortality associated with severe sepsis and septic shock. Nevertheless, the mortality rate remains unacceptably high, and the overall incidence and severity of disease appear to be increasing, by as much as 1.5% annually by some estimates. The risk of death for an individual patient appears to stabilize approximately 6 months after the original illness. Many patients who do survive remain with the same risk factors (e.g., diabetes, vascular disease, prosthetic devices, immunosuppression) that contributed to their infection and therefore are at risk for recurrence. Moreover, certain organisms, such as MRSA, resistant gram-negative rods, and fungi, remain difficult to treat, and success rates are relatively low despite aggressive, timely, and prolonged therapy.

There is some cause for optimism. The Surviving Sepsis Campaign has now entered phase III. This is a program in which a core set of recommendations, described in the guidelines, are being implemented with opportunities to measure outcomes, assess physician behavior, and provide feedback to improve survival through evidence-based interventions. This effort involves more than 12,000 patients in 239 hospitals in 17 countries and will undoubtedly change the future course of this lethal disease.

REFERENCES

Bone RC. Immunologic dissonance: A continuing evolution in our understanding of the systemic inflammatory response syndrome (SIRS) and the multiple organ dysfunction syndrome (MODS). Ann Intern Med 1996; 125:680–7.

Delinger RP, Levy MM, Carlet JM, et al. Surviving Sepsis Campaign: International guidelines for management of severe sepsis and septic shock—2008. Crit Care Med 2008;36:296–327.

Dombrovskiy VY, Martin AA, Sunderram J, Paz HL. Rapid increase in hospitalization and mortality rates for severe sepsis in the United States: A trend analysis from 1993 to 2003. Crit Care Med 2007;35:1244–50.

Ibrahim EH, Sherman G, Ward S, et al. The influence of inadequate antimicrobial treatment of bloodstream infections on patient outcomes in the ICU setting. Chest 2000;118:146–55.

Jimenez MF, Marshall JC. Source control in the management of sepsis. Intensive Care Med 2001;27(Suppl. 1):S49–62.

Kumar A, Roberts D, Wood KE, et al. Duration of hypotension before initiation of effective antimicrobial therapy is the critical determinant of survival in human septic shock. Crit Care Med 2006;34:1589–96.

Leibovici L, Shraga I, Drucker M, et al. The benefit of appropriate empirical antibiotic treatment in patients with bloodstream infection. J Intern Med 1998;244:379–86.

Levy MM, Fink MP, Marshall JC, et al. 2001 SCCM/ESICM/ACCP/ATS/SIS International Sepsis Definitions Conference. Intensive Care Med 2003;29:530–8.

Martin GS, Mannino DM, Easton S, et al. The epidemiology of sepsis in the United States from 1979 through 2000. N Engl J Med 2003;348:1546–54.

McDonald JR, Friedman ND, Stout JE, et al. Risk factors for ineffective therapy in patients with bloodstream infection. Arch Intern Med 2005;165:308–13.

Miller PJ, Wenzel RP. Etiologic organisms as independent predictors of death and morbidity associated with bloodstream infection. J Infect Dis 1987;156:471–7.

Sasse KC, Nauenberg E, Long A, et al. Long-term survival after intensive care unit admission with sepsis. Crit Care Med 1995;23:1040–7.

Brucellosis

Method of
Basak Dokuzoguz, MD, and Nurcan Baykam, MD

Brucellosis is a common bacterial zoonotic disease. It has become more significant in recent years as a bioterrorism agent. Brucellosis is known as a historic disease, and the sequencing of the *Brucella melitensis* genome was completed in 2002.

Etiology

The disease is caused by bacteria of the genus *Brucella*, which are nonmotile, gram-negative, aerobic, unencapsulated cocci or short rods. *Brucella* species are divided into six subtypes based on the main host animals (Table 1). Of these, *B. abortus*, *B. melitensis*, *B. suis*, and *B. canis* are known human pathogens. Two new species, provisionally called *B. pinnipediae* and *B. cetaceae*, have been shown to cause human diseases.

Epidemiology

Brucellosis is one of the major zoonotic diseases and occurs all over the world. Some countries in Europe and North America have achieved control and prevention of the disease based on vaccination

TABLE 1 Subtypes and Hosts of *Brucella* Species

Species	Host Animal	Human
B. abortus	Cows, camels, yaks, buffalo	+
B. melitensis	Goats, sheep, camels	+
B. suis	Pigs, wild hares, caribou, reindeer, wild rodents	+
B. canis	Canines	+
B. neotomae	Rodents	–
B. ovis	Sheep	–
B. pinnipediae	Minke whales, dolphins	+
B. cetaceae	Seals	+

programs. However, brucellosis remains endemic in other parts of the world, especially in the Mediterranean, the Middle East, Central Asia, Africa, and Latin America. The real incidence of the disease is not known because underreporting of the disease is believed to be common.

The most common causes of human brucellosis are reported as *B. melitensis* followed by *B. abortus*. The biotypes of *Brucella* species vary by geographic region.

The disease is transmitted to humans by direct contact with infected animals, by ingestion of raw or unpasteurized milk and milk products, through cuts and abrasions, or by inhalation of aerosols. It is an occupational disease of farmers, veterinarians, slaughterhouse workers, and health care workers, especially laboratory staff. Some individual cases occur as a result of ingesting contaminated dairy products, handling infected animal tissue or body fluids, or handling aborted animal fetuses and placentas. However, the transmission route for outbreaks is usually inhalation of aerosols. Human-to-human transmission of brucellosis is very rare, but there are a few case reports of humans infected through sexual contact, transplacental transmission, or transplantation.

Pathogenesis

The *Brucella* species are pathogenic for humans and animals. *Brucella* species prefer to survive and multiply within phagocytic cells of the host. Unlike other pathogenic bacteria, they do not have classic virulence factors such as exotoxins, cytolysins, capsules, fimbria, plasmids, and endotoxic lipopolysaccharides. Instead of these factors, the bacteria have molecular determinants that are necessary for cell invasion and survival in the cellular compartment. The major one of these molecular determinants is S lipopolysaccharide (S LPS).

The bacteria are phagocytosed by M cells, macrophages, and neutrophils after invasion of mucosa. Fc receptors, complement, lectin, and fibronectin receptors mediate the bacteria for internalization. Most intracellular *Brucella* species are eliminated in phagolysosomes, but some of them reproduce in the acidic compartment. The intracellular mechanism of the organism is not completely described, but intracellular replication of bacteria does not destroy the cell or the cell's function. Replication of *Brucella* spp. within human osteoblastic cell lines can directly mount a proinflammatory response which may have a role in the chronic inflammation and bone/joint destruction in osteoarticular brucellosis.

After they are taken up by local tissue lymphocytes, the bacteria disseminate into the circulation, and with tropism to the reticuloendothelial system, they become localized within bone marrow, liver, spleen, and lymph nodes. The characteristic feature of the disease is the formation of granulomas in these tissues.

As a host humoral immune response to the disease, the titers of IgM antibodies increase within the first week of infection, and IgG synthesis follows after the second week. Cell-mediated immunity is probably the main mechanism for recovery from the infection.

Clinical Features

Human brucellosis is a multisystem disease that can manifest with a broad spectrum of clinical features. The musculoskeletal, genital, cardiac, respiratory, and nervous systems are involved. The definition and the classification of cases recommended by the World Health Organization (WHO) is presented in Box 1. Some authors classify the disease course as acute, subacute, or chronic, but such a classification has no clinical significance.

The onset of symptoms can be insidious or acute after the incubation period, which is 2 to 8 weeks. A broad spectrum of symptoms such as fever, headache, back pain, weakness, profuse sweating, chills, depression, and joint pain can be observed. These symptoms can also mimic various infectious and noninfectious diseases. Usually an undulant fever pattern is accompanied by so much sweating that the patient needs to change clothes frequently. On the other hand, the physical examination might not reveal any specific finding (Table 2). In children, the range of clinical signs and symptoms may be different than in adults, because children have fewer constitutional symptoms but more hepatic and splenic involvement.

Hepatomegaly, elevated transaminase levels, and granulomatous lesions are the presentations of hepatic involvement in brucellosis. The most common complication of brucellosis is osteoarticular disease, which occurs as peripheral arthritis, sacroiliitis, and spondylitis. This complication is reported in 10% to 80% of cases, and this range may be related to the age and genetic predisposition (HLA-B39) of patients and the infecting *Brucella* species. Genitourinary system involvements exist in 2% to 20% of patients with brucellosis.

BOX 1 Recommended Case Definitions and Classifications by the World Health Organization

Clinical Description

An illness characterized by acute or insidious onset, with continued, intermittent, or irregular fever of variable duration; profuse sweating, particularly at night; fatigue; anorexia; weight loss; headache; arthralgia and generalized aching. Local infection of various organs can occur.

Laboratory Criteria for Diagnosis

- Isolation of *Brucella* spp. from clinical specimen *or*
- Brucella agglutination titer (e.g., standard tube agglutination tests: STA>160) in one or more serum specimens obtained after onset of symptoms *or*
- ELISA (IgA, IgG, IgM), 2-mercaptoethanol test, complement fixation test, Coombs' test, fluorescent antibody test (FAB), radioimmunoassay for detecting antilipopolysaccharide antibodies, counterimmunoelectrophoresis (CIE)

Case Classification

Suspected

A case that is compatible with the clinical description and is epidemiologically linked to suspected or confirmed animal cases or contaminated animal products.

Probable

A suspected case that has a positive rose bengal test.

Confirmed

A suspected or probable case that is laboratory confirmed.

Abbreviations: ELISA = enzyme-linked immunosorbent assay; Ig = immunoglobulin.

TABLE 2 Clinical Presentation and Laboratory Findings of Human Brucellosis

Feature	Percentage
Signs and Symptoms	
Fever	72–91
Constitutive symptoms (e.g., malaise, arthralgias)	26–90
Hepatic involvement	17–31
Splenomegaly	14–16
Osteoarticular involvement	9–22
CNS disorder	3–13
Lymphadenopathy	2–7
Genitourinary involvement	1–5.7
Respiratory disorders	0.2–6
Cardiovascular disorders	0.4–1.8
Skin rashes	0.4–3
Laboratory Findings	
Hematologic	
Relative lymphocytosis	40
Anemia	31
Leukopenia	2–27
Thrombocytopenia	5–15
Pancytopenia	2
Biochemistry	
Elevated transaminase	24–31

Data derived from Aygen B, Doganay M, Sümerkan B, et al: Clinical manifestations, complications and treatment of brucellosis: An evaluation of 480 patients. Med Mal Infect 2002;32:485–493; Dokuzoguz B, Ergonul O, Baykam N, et al: Characteristics of *B. melitensis* versus *B. abortus* bacteremias. J Infect 2005;50(1):1–5; Pappas G, Akritidis N, Bosikovski M, Tsianos E: Brucellosis. N Engl J Med 2005;352:2325–2336.
Abbreviation: CNS = central nervous system.

Prostatitis, epididymo-orchitis, cystitis, pyelonephritis, interstitial nephritis, exudative glomerulonephritis, and renal abscess are the clinical manifestations of this complication. Neurobrucellosis can develop at any stage of disease and can have widely variable manifestations, including encephalitis, meningoencephalitis, radiculitis, myelitis, peripheral and cranial neuropathies, subarachnoid hemorrhage, and psychiatric manifestations. Brucellosis can cause a variety of ocular lesions and different types of skin rash that are nonspecific and reported rarely. Another rare (<2%) but severe complication of brucellosis is endocarditis, which most often involves the aortic valve and requires surgery. Mortality from brucellosis is rare and is usually related to endocarditis.

Diagnosis

The absolute diagnosis of brucellosis is based on identification of bacteria from blood, bone marrow, and materials from affected organs such as cerebrospinal fluid, liver, lymph nodes, synovial fluid, or prostatic fluid by culture. The rate of bacteria isolation from the blood is between 15% and 70%. Lysis centrifugation technique and automated systems improve the range of culture positivity. Lysis centrifugation technique is inexpensive and easier method which can be used in laboratories with limited expertise or equipment if all safety precautions are taken.

Compatible clinical findings with a serum agglutinin titer of at least 1/160 in the standard tube agglutination test (STA) have diagnostic value. In endemic areas, the titer of at least 1/320 is recommended in the diagnosis. False-negative results of STA may be attributed to blocking antibodies; results can be improved by testing with 2-mercaptoethanol or antihuman immunoglobulin. Negative results in the early phase of the disease can be overcome by repeating the test after 2 weeks. Diagnosis of *B. canis* infection is unavailable with routine STA. False-positive results may be related to cross-reactions of some gram-negative bacterial infections.

CURRENT DIAGNOSIS

- The common symptoms of brucellosis, which can also mimic various infectious and noninfectious diseases, are fever, headache, back pain, weakness, profuse sweating, chills, depression, and joint pain.
- The absolute diagnosis of brucellosis is based on identification of bacteria from blood, bone marrow, and materials of affected organs such as cerebrospinal fluid, liver, lymph nodes, synovial fluid, and prostatic fluid by culture.
- Compatible clinical findings with a serum agglutinin titer of ≥ 1/160 in the standard tube agglutination test (STA) have diagnostic value.

CURRENT THERAPY

- The treatment requires combined regimens for their synergistic effect plus agents with good penetration capacity into the macrophages.
- At least 6 weeks of therapy may be extended to 6 months, according to the complications of the disease.
- Rifampin (Rifadin)[1] plus doxycycline (Vibramycin) treatment is a favorable regimen and the most synergistic one.
- Rifampin may be replaced by streptomycin or gentamycin (Garamycin)[1] as the first-line therapy choice.
- Combinations with trimethoprim-sulfamethoxazole (TMP-SMX; Bactrim)[1] is usually recommended in the second-line treatment regimens.
- Quinolones[1] are alternative drugs in cases with side effects due to first-line drugs and relapses.
- Rifampin in a combination with TMP-SMX[1] or an aminoglycoside are the main regimens for children younger than 8 years.
- Rifampin and TMP-SMX[1] combination is preferred in pregnancy
- Although the use of ceftriaxone (Rocephin)[1] is controversial in brucellosis, it could be preferred in the treatment of central nervous system involvement.
- Rifampin[1] (600–900 mg qd) plus doxycycline (100 mg bid) regimen for 2–3 weeks is recommended as postexposure prophylaxis.

[1]Not FDA approved for this indication.

Enzyme-linked immunosorbent assay (ELISA) is another serologic test that has higher specificity and sensitivity compared with STA. Although it is not used in current clinical practice because of standardization problems, polymerase chain reaction (PCR) is a promising diagnostic tool in brucellosis. Duration of diagnosis can be shortened by automated culture systems and PCR techniques. Rose bengal and a new dipstick test are also rapid tests useful for early diagnosis, but positive results should be confirmed by STA.

Treatment

Because the *Brucella* species are intracellular pathogens, treatment requires not only combined regimens for their synergistic effect but also agents with good penetration into the macrophages. For success of the therapy, adequate duration of drug therapy is another

TABLE 3 Drug Combinations Used to Treat Brucellosis

Generic Name (Trade Name)	Adult Dose	Pediatric Dose	Dose Adjustment		Adverse Effects
			Renal Failure	Hepatic Insuffiency	
Ciprofloxacin[1] (Cipro)	500–750 mg PO q12h or 400 mg IV q8–12h	Not suggested	Necessary	No change	Drug fever, rash, seizures, Achilles tendon rupture or tendinitis
Doxycycline (Vibramycin, Vibra-tabs)	100 mg PO q12h	2.2–4.4 mg/kg[3] PO div q12h (≥ 8 y)	No change	No change	Nausea, vomiting, eosinophilia, photosensitivity
Gentamicin[1] (Garamycin)	2 mg/kg IM/IV q8h or 5 mg/kg IM/IV q24h[1] or 240 mg q24h	2.5 mg/kg q8–12h IM/IV	Necessary	No change blockade (rapid infusion)	Ototoxicity, nephrotoxicity, neuromuscular
Ofloxacin[1] (Floxin, Oflox)	400 mg PO bid	Not suggested	Necessary	Moderate: no change Severe: necessary	Drug fever, rash, mild neuroexcitatory symptoms
Rifampin[1] (Rifadin, Rimactane)	600–900 mg PO qd	20 mg/kg PO qd Do not exceed 600 mg qd	No change	Moderate: caution Severe: avoid	Red/orange discoloration of body secretions, flu-like symptoms, elevated AST/ALT, drug fever, rash, thrombocytopenia
Streptomycin	15 mg/kg IM q24h or 1 g IM qd for 2–3 wk	20–40 mg/kg IM qd	Necessary	No change	Ototoxic, nephrotoxic
TMP-SMX[1] (Bactrim, Septra)	1 DS tab PO q12h (160 mg TMP/800 mg SMX)	Do not exceed 1 g qd 8–12 mg/kg TMP PO q12h	Necessary; avoid use	No change	Folate deficiency, hyperkalemia, leukopenia, thrombocytopenia, hemolytic anemia ± G6PD, aplastic anemia, elevated AST/ALT, hypersensitivity reactions (Stevens-Johnson syndrome, erythema multiforme)

[1]Not FDA approved for this indication.
[3]Exceeds dosage recommended by the manufacturer.
Abbreviations: ALT = alanine aminotransferase; AST = aspartate aminotransferase; DS = double strength; G6PD = glucose-6-phosphate dehydrogenase; TMP-SMX = trimethoprim-sulfamethoxazole.

important factor. At least 6 weeks of drug therapy is recommended by the WHO. This duration may be extended to 6 months, depending on such complications of the disease as neurobrucellosis, spondylodiskitis, and abscesses.

The drug combinations listed in Table 3 are widely used in brucellosis. Rifampin (Rifadin)[1] plus doxycycline (Vibramycin) treatment for human brucellosis was recommended by WHO two decades ago; it is still a favorable regimen and was found to be the most synergistic one. Rifampin may be replaced by streptomycin or gentamycin (Garamycin)[1] as first-line therapy choices. According to a recently reported meta-analysis, doxycycline-streptomycin resulted in a significantly higher rate of failure than doxycycline-rifampicin-aminoglycoside regimen. Combinations with trimethoprim-sulfamethoxazole (TMP-SMX, Bactrim)[1] is usually recommended in second-line treatment regimens. Combination rifampin plus a quinolone[1] is not preferred in the initial therapeutic regimen because of the reported decreased activity in pH 5 and lack of synergism between quinolones and other antibiotics that are used in brucellosis. Quinolones are alternative drugs for patients who have relapses or who have side effects from first-line drugs.

Rifampin[1] in combination with TMP-SMX[1] or an aminoglycoside are the main regimens for children younger than 8 years. The rifampin and TMP-SMX combination may be prescribed for pregnant patients.

Although the use of ceftriaxone (Rocephin)[1] is controversial in brucellosis, it may be preferred for treating central nervous system involvement. Because their activity is decreased in an acidic environment, macrolides are not used in brucellosis treatment.

Because there are no significantly important resistance problems for antibiotics targeted to *Brucella* species, susceptibility tests are not recommended routinely except in epidemiologic studies and for some rare recurrent cases. Most of the recurrences are related to noncompliance or to short duration of therapy. In tuberculosis-endemic populations, community-acquired rifampin resistance should be taken into consideration in treating brucellosis.

Supportive therapy might be useful depending on the clinical situation. The cognitive and emotional disturbances in neurobrucellosis can be improved by antibiotics without any antidepressant or antipsychotic therapy.

In the management of *Brucella* endocarditis, medical treatment alone is often effective in patients with early diagnosis and no cardiac failure. However, in most cases, surgery is required in addition to medical treatment.

Prevention

Various vaccines have been applied to humans in some countries in the 20th century, but an acceptable vaccine has not yet been developed for humans. Although investigations of the *B. melitensis* outer membrane protein 25 and cytoplasmic protein BP26 are promising for future vaccine development, prevention of the disease in humans is related to controlling and eliminating animal brucellosis. In this respect, vaccination and slaughter programs of animals, pasteurization of milk and milk products, and education programs about contact precautions for persons at risk must be emphasized.

Because *Brucella* bacteria can be transmitted via the inhalational route, laboratory workers should be warned about the risk, and biosafety level 2 prevention measures should be applied.

[1]Not FDA approved for this indication.

Because of laboratory accidents and biological warfare, rifampin[1] (600–900 mg qd) plus doxycycline (100 mg bid) for 2 to 3 weeks is recommended as postexposure prophylaxis.

REFERENCES

Aygen B, Doganay M, Sümerkan B, et al. Clinical manifestations, complications and treatment of brucellosis: An evaluation of 480 patients. Med Mal Infect 2002;32:485–93.

Baykam N, Esener H, Ergonul O, et al. In vitro antimicrobial susceptibility of *Brucella* species. Int J Antimicrob Agents 2004;23(4):405–7.

Bossi P, Tegnell A, Baka A, et al. Bichat guidelines for the clinical management of brucellosis and bioterrorism-related brucellosis. Euro Surveill 2004;9(12):E15–6.

Dokuzoguz B, Ergonul O, Baykam N, et al. Characteristics of *B. melitensis* versus *B. abortus* bacteremias. J Infect 2005;50(1):1–5.

Delpino MV, Fossati CA, Baldi PC. Proinflammatory response of human osteoblastic cell lines and osteoblast-monocyte interaction upon infection with Brucella spp. Infect Immun. 2009;77(3):984–95.

Eren S, Bayam G, Ergonul O, et al. Cognitive and emotional changes in neurobrucellosis. J Infect 2006;53:184–9.

Ergonul O, Celikbas A, Tezeren D, et al. Analysis of risk factors for laboratory-acquired *Brucella* infections. J Hosp Infect 2004;56:223–7.

Espinosa BJ, Chacaltana J, Mulder M, et al. Comparison of culture techniques at different stages of brucellosis. Am J Trop Med Hyg 2009;80(4):625–7.

Falagas ME, Bliziotis IA. Quinolones for treatment of human brucellosis: Critical review of the evidence from microbiological and clinical studies. Antimicrob Agents Chemother 2006;50(1):22–33.

Giannacopoulos I, Nikolakopoulou NM, Eliopoulou M, et al. Presentation of childhood brucellosis in Western Greece. Jpn J Infect Dis 2006;59:160–3.

Joint Food and Agriculture Organization/World Health Organization, FAO-WHO Expert Committee on Brucellosis (sixth report). In: WHO Technical Report Series No. 740. Geneva: World Health Organization, 1986. p. 56–7.

Pan American Health Organization. Case definition: Brucellosis, Epidemiol Bull 2000;21(3):13. PDF available at http://www.paho.org/english/dd/ais/EB_v21n3.pdf [accessed 27.04.07].

Pappas G, Akritidis N, Bosilkovski M, Tsianos E. Brucellosis. N Engl J Med 2005;352:2325–36.

Skalsky K, Yahav D, Bishara J, et al. Treatment of human brucellosis: systematic review and meta-analysis of randomised controlled trials. BMJ 2008;336(7676):701–4.

Young EJ. *Brucella* species. In: Mandel GL, Bennett JE, Dolin R, editors. Mandell, Douglas and Bennett's Principles and Practice of Infectious Diseases, 7th ed. Philadelphia: Churchill Livingstone; 2010. p. 2921–5.

---

[1]Not FDA approved for this indication.

Varicella (Chickenpox)

Method of
Charles Grose, MD

Chickenpox is caused by varicella zoster virus (VZV). After chickenpox occurs, VZV enters the sensory nerve and establishes latency in the dorsal root ganglia along the spinal cord. When VZV reactivates in late adulthood, the virus causes the disease known as shingles (herpes zoster).

Pathogenesis of Chickenpox

Chickenpox is an airborne infection. The virus first infects the mucosa tissues of the nose and subsequently establishes an infection in the tonsils or lymph nodes around the neck. After 4 to 6 cycles of replication, the primary viremia occurs (Figure 1). The virus then disperses to multiple organs in the body. After a second period of replication, the second viremia occurs. The virus is carried within lymphocytes in the bloodstream. The vesicular lesions occur after the virus exits the capillaries and enters the epidermis.

Epidemiology after Approval of the Vaccine

The varicella vaccine was approved for administration to children in the United States in 1995, and the vast majority of states have approved the administration of varicella vaccine to all young children. Approximately 4 million cases of chickenpox occurred annually in the United States prior to 1995. There were also approximately 100 deaths annually, the vast majority in otherwise healthy children, and more than 14,000 hospitalizations per year.

More than 15 years later, the effect of universal varicella immunization in the United States is dramatic. The number of hospitalizations and deaths was reduced by 75%. Similarly, the total number of cases of chickenpox in the United States has also decreased dramatically. Nevertheless, more than one half million cases of chickenpox will probably continue to occur annually. These cases will include many immunocompromised children who remain unimmunized.

ADMINISTRATION OF VARICELLA VACCINE

Varicella vaccine is a live attenuated virus. Each dose of vaccine (0.5 mL) is administered subcutaneously. The virus must replicate in the infected child for an immune response to occur (Figure 2). The initial virus replication can cause a few vesicles near the site of infection. The replication can also lead to a viremia with a short-lived rash anywhere on the body. The vaccine virus can, in very few cases, replicate to a sufficient extent that the infection transfers to another person who will subsequently develop a mild case of vaccine-related chickenpox. In 1995, a single dose of varicella vaccine was originally recommended. As of 2007, two doses of varicella vaccine are recommended for every child. The first dose is given between 12 and 15 months. The second dose is routinely recommended between 4 and 6 years. Instead of single-dose vials of vaccine (Varivax), the vaccine can also be administered as a component of the 4-in-1 vials of measles-mumps-rubella-varicella vaccine (Pro Quad). This approach reduces the number of injections given to a child. Children 13 years and above, who have never received varicella vaccine, should be given 2 doses of vaccine (Varivax), separated by a 4-week interval.

RISK FACTORS FOR BREAKTHROUGH CHICKENPOX

Breakthrough chickenpox refers to a wild-type chickenpox that is usually a mild illness with less than 50 vesicles that occurs in children given varicella vaccine at least 42 days previously. Thus, breakthrough chickenpox is a form of vaccine failure. Breakthrough chickenpox was believed to be relatively uncommon during the prelicensure clinical studies. However, by 2000 it was apparent that breakthrough chickenpox was not a rare event. Several reports documented large outbreaks of wild-type chickenpox in immunized children who were attending large daycare facilities or grade schools.

A major risk factor is believed to be immunization with one dose of vaccine. The 2-dose regimen of varicella vaccine should eliminate most cases of breakthrough chickenpox.

CURRENT DIAGNOSIS

- Diagnosis of chickenpox is usually made by observation or rash.
- Diagnosis is confirmed by a rapid viral diagnosis kit performed on a vesicle smear.
- Diagnosis of past varicella infection is made by serology.
- Commercial antibody kits may not be sensitive enough to detect serum antibody after varicella vaccination.

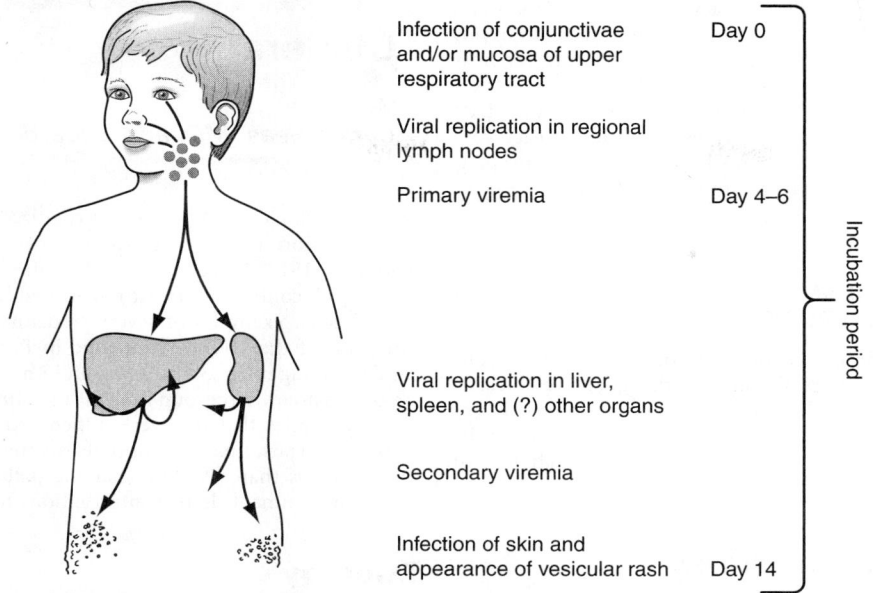

Infection of conjunctivae and/or mucosa of upper respiratory tract — Day 0

Viral replication in regional lymph nodes

Primary viremia — Day 4–6

Viral replication in liver, spleen, and (?) other organs

Secondary viremia

Infection of skin and appearance of vesicular rash — Day 14

Incubation period

FIGURE 1. Diagrammatic representation of the pathogenesis of acute varicella infection. There are two viremias during the 14-day incubation period. The first viremia occurs after local replication at the site of infection. The typical chickenpox rash appears at the end of the second viremia. See Grose (2005) for a more detailed description.

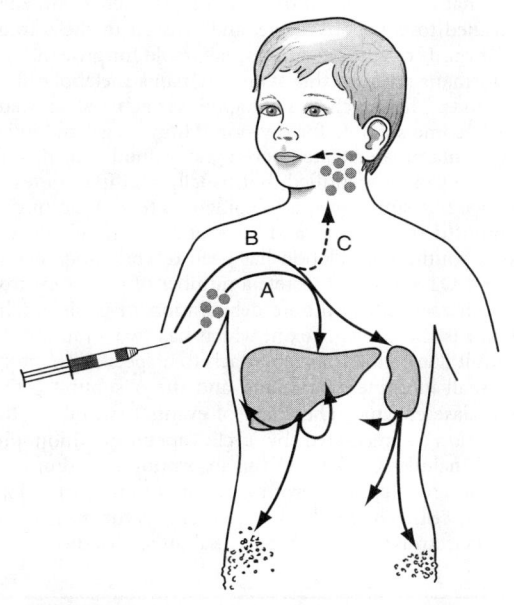

FIGURE 2. Pathways of infection following administration of vari-cella vaccine. Pathway A shows a rash that sometimes appears at the site of injection after local replication of the virus. Pathway B shows a viremia with appearance of a few small papulovesicular lesions on the skin distant from the site of injection. Pathway C shows the virus as it travels to the respiratory tract where infection can be spread on rare occasions to other individuals. See Grose (2005) for a more detailed description.

Treatment

TREATMENT OF SEVERE CHICKENPOX IN HEALTHY CHILDREN

Chickenpox is considered a more severe disease in children younger than 1 year and in postpubertal adolescents. VZV is highly suscepti-ble to acyclovir and two second-generation antiviral agents: famciclo-vir (Famvir) and valacyclovir (Valtrex). Acyclovir is now a generic drug and very economic. Every case of chickenpox in a child younger than 1 year should be treated with acyclovir. The oral dosage is 20 mg/kg four times a day for 5 to 7 days. Chickenpox in children older than 1 year can also be treated with acyclovir to reduce the severity and duration of disease. The maximum dosage is 800 mg four times a day. Acyclovir is available in a liquid suspension and tablets containing 200, 400, or 800 mg. The 800-mg tablet is very large and may be difficult for some children to swallow.

Famciclovir (Famvir) or valacyclovir (Valtrex) are the preferred antiviral agents for adolescents because these are better adsorbed than acyclovir. However, they are much more expensive. The dosage of famciclovir (Famvir) is 500 mg orally three times a day. The dos-age of valacyclovir (Valtrex) is 1 g three times a day. For most adoles-cents, a 5-day regimen should be sufficient treatment.

TREATMENT OF CHICKENPOX IN CHILDREN WITH AN UNDERLYING IMMUNODEFICIENCY

Children with HIV infection who contract chickenpox can usually be managed with oral acyclovir treatment as long as their HIV is under control. The majority of children diagnosed with acute chickenpox who have cancer or have undergone organ transplantation should be considered for admission to the hospital and begin immediate treatment with intravenous (IV) acyclovir. The dosage of IV acyclovir is 10 mg/kg every 8 hours. The dosage can be raised to 15 mg/kg every 8 hours in patients presenting varicella pneumonia or varicella encephalitis. The serum creatinine level should be monitored daily and the acyclovir dosage adjusted downward if the serum creatinine reaches 1 mg/dL.

 CURRENT THERAPY

- Severe chickenpox in infants and immunosuppressed chil-dren is treated with intravenous acyclovir (30 mg/kg/d).
- Severe chickenpox in healthy children is treated with oral acyclovir (80 mg/kg/d).
- Severe chickenpox in adolescents is treated with either famciclovir (Famvir) (500 mg tid) or valacyclovir (Val-trex) (1 g tid).
- Prophylaxis following exposure to chickenpox can be managed with a course of oral acyclovir (40 mg/kg/d).

The efficacy of oral famciclovir or valacyclovir is better than oral acyclovir, allowing older children with chickenpox and an immunosuppressive condition to be discharged more quickly from the hospital. Discharge is generally considered after no new vesicle formation is noted for 24 hours. Antiviral therapy (combined IV and oral) for 10 to 14 days is usually suggested, although each case must be assessed individually. Children who have varicella encephalitis or varicella pneumonia may require more than 2 weeks of antiviral therapy.

TREATMENT OF CHICKENPOX IN CHILDREN RECEIVING CORTICOSTEROIDS

Children receiving high-dose oral corticosteroid treatment for conditions such as acute asthma are also at high risk of severe chickenpox. These children should be treated with antivirals just as aggressively as those with cancer. Children receiving only intermittent inhaled corticosteroids do not appear to be at high risk of severe chickenpox.

TREATMENT OF ZOSTER IN CHILDREN

Zoster in otherwise healthy children is usually a benign illness. The disease is normally improving by the time the diagnosis is made. However, zoster in immunocompromised children may persist for 2 weeks or longer, requiring immediate treatment with one of the oral antiviral drugs recommended. The dosage is the same as for severe chickenpox.

ALTERNATIVES TO VARICELLA-ZOSTER IMMUNE GLOBULIN

Varicella-zoster immune globulin (VZIG) has been given in the past to infants and children with cancer who were exposed to chickenpox. VZIG has been discontinued after 2005. Physicians can consider the administration of IV gammaglobulin as a single infusion of 500 mg/kg for infants who are exposed to varicella shortly after birth. An alternative regimen is oral acyclovir suspension at 40 mg/kg per day divided every 6 hours. Acyclovir should be initiated on the day of exposure and continued for 10 days.

Prophylaxis with oral acyclovir also can be considered for VZV-nonimmune children with cancer after an exposure to chickenpox. The recommended dosage is one half of the therapeutic dosage, meaning oral acyclovir can be given at 40 mg/kg per day. The daily dosage for children who can swallow tablets can be divided three times a day rather than four times a day during the 10-day therapy period. Children who develop chickenpox despite oral acyclovir treatment should be admitted to the hospital for treatment with IV acyclovir at 10 mg/kg every 8 hours. There are extremely few examples of true acyclovir-resistant VZV; most failures are caused by inadequate absorption of the oral formulation.

REFERENCES

Davis MM, Patel MS, Gebremariam A. Decline in varicella-related hospitalizations and expenditures for children and adults after introduction of varicella vaccine in the United States. Pediatrics 2004;114:786–92.

Grose C. Varicella vaccination of children in the United States: Assessment after the first decade, 1995–2005. J Clin Virol 2005;33:89–95.

Grose C, Widerman J. Generic acyclovir vs. famciclovir and valacyclovir. Pediatr Infect Dis J 1997;16:838–41.

Hay M, Kimura H, Oshiro M, et al. Varicella exposure in a neonatal medical center: Successful prophylaxis with oral acyclovir. J Hosp Infect 2003;54:212–5.

Nguyen HQ, Jumaan AO, Seward JF. Decline in mortality due to varicella after implementation of varicella vaccination in the United States. N Engl J Med 2005;352:450–8.

Takahashi M. Effectiveness of live varicella vaccine. Expert Opin Biol Ther 2004;4:199–216.

Cholera

Method of
Carlos Seas, MD, and Eduardo Gotuzzo, MD

Cholera is an ancient scourge recognized since the time of Hippocrates. More accurate descriptions of the disease began approximately in 1817. Since then, cholera has caused seven pandemics, affecting all continents, and it remains endemic in almost all affected areas. Recent examples of severe epidemics are the Latin American extension of the seventh pandemic in Peru in 1991, explosive epidemics among refugees in Africa, and unexpected epidemics of cholera due to a new serogroup in Asia since 1992. We can conclude from these epidemics that it is very difficult to predict when a new epidemic will start, that appropriate treatment reduces the mortality to values less than 1%, and that the pathogen continues to evolve in the environment despite interventions to control its spread.

Etiology

Cholera is caused by a curved gram-negative bacillus that belongs to the family Vibrionaceae. Two serogroups, O1 and O139, are associated with clinical cholera, and both cause the same clinical entity. These serogroups have shown both regional and pandemic potential. *Vibrio cholerae* is a natural inhabitant of certain aquatic environments, where it lives attached to copepods, algae, and crustacean shells in a symbiotic association. If conditions are not favorable for growth, *V. cholerae* adopts a dormant state. In this state it remains metabolically inactive for long periods. The switch to a metabolically active state occurs when conditions become suitable for division. Humans get the infection by consuming contaminated water, beverages, or food. During epidemics, a single source can be identified, but usually multiple routes of transmission play a role simultaneously. Epidemics tend to occur during the warmest months of the year, and association with climate variability and El Niño southern oscillation has been recently documented.

V. cholerae O1 and O139 secrete a number of potent exotoxins that induce the characteristic isotonic dehydration of cholera. The better studied toxin is the cholera toxin, which has two subunits, A and B. The B subunit allows the toxin to attach to a specific receptor present along the small intestine of humans, and the A subunit activates the adenylate cyclase enzyme. The chain of events that follows this enzymatic activation is mediated by cyclic adenosine monophosphate (cAMP) and includes blockage of the absorption of sodium and chloride by the microvillus and promotion of secretion of chloride and water by crypt cells. The result of these events is the massive liberation of water and electrolytes into the intestinal lumen, as shown in Table 1.

CURRENT DIAGNOSIS

- History of travel to an endemic area.
- Acute voluminous watery diarrhea with rice-water appearance, leading to severe dehydration in a matter of hours.
- Muscle cramps, vomiting, and signs of severe dehydration such as loss of skin elasticity (slow skin-pinch retraction), hoarse voice, sunken eyes, and wrinkled hands and feet (washerwoman hands).
- Fever is absent in most patients.
- Milder forms of dehydration cannot be distinguished from other common causes of acute diarrhea.
- Stool culture using proper media is positive for *V. cholerae* O1 or O139. Dark field microscopy of a fresh stool sample can detect the presence of vibrio; specific antisera confirm the serogroup.

TABLE 1 Electrolyte Concentrations (mmol/L)

Substance	Sodium	Chloride	Potassium	Bicarbonate	Osmolality
Cholera Stool					
Adults		130	100	20	44
Children		100	90	33	30
Rehydration Solution					
Ringer's lactate*	130	109	4	28*	271
Normal saline	154	154	0	0	308
Rice-based ORS	75	65	20	10	180
WHO ORS‡	75	65	20	10†	245

*Ringer's lactate contains lactate instead of bicarbonate.
†Bicarbonate is replaced with trisodium citrate, which stays fresh longer than bicarbonate in sachets.
‡Reduced osmolality formula.
Abbreviations: ORS = oral rehydration solution; WHO = World Health Organization.

Treatment

The objectives of therapy are to replace the fluid and electrolyte losses caused by diarrhea and vomiting, to maintain hydration, and to reduce the volume of diarrhea and excretion of vibrios to the environment. The treatment is divided into two phases: the rehydration phase and the maintenance phase.

REHYDRATION PHASE

The objective of the rehydration phase is to replace the losses that occurred before the patient was admitted. This phase begins with a thorough evaluation of the degree of dehydration. Table 2 shows the clinical signs according to the degree of dehydration.

Patients with severe dehydration present with a constellation of signs that reflect a deficit of at least 10% of body weight. The pulse is feeble and very rapid, the blood pressure is not measurable, the skin elasticity is lost, the eyes are sunken, and the voice is inaudible or hoarse. The intravenous route is recommended for rehydrating all patients with severe dehydration. The rate and speed of the infusion is recommended at 50 to 100 mL/kg/hour for the first 2 to 4 hours. After this time, the patient must be fully rehydrated to begin the maintenance phase. The preferred intravenous solution is Ringer's lactate solution. If this solution is not available, normal saline may be used, but the recovery from metabolic acidosis is less efficient. Oral rehydration solutions (ORS) should be started as soon a possible in these patients.

Milder forms of dehydration due to cholera cannot be clinically distinguished from other common causes of acute diarrhea. Symptoms due to some degree of dehydration are seen when water deficit is greater than 5% of body weight. The intravenous route may be used in these patients if the stool output is high (<10–20 mL/kg/hour) or if the patient does not tolerate the oral route. The great majority of patients with milder forms of dehydration can be rehydrated by the oral route.

Laboratory abnormalities in patients with severe cholera reflect hemoconcentration and include a high hematocrit, increase in white blood cell count, azotemia, and elevation of specific gravity and total proteins. These laboratory parameters are good indicators of the degree of dehydration on admission, but they are not useful for following the rehydration status. Metabolic acidosis with a high anion gap is typically seen in patients with severe cholera. Hypokalemia or normal values (due to acidosis) and normal or low serum sodium and chloride are also observed in these patients. Hyperglycemia results from high levels of epinephrine, glucagon, and cortisol stimulated by hypovolemia. Hypoglycemia is rare but carries a poor prognosis, particularly in children.

MAINTENANCE PHASE

The maintenance phase begins when the patient has been fully rehydrated. A good indicator of the recovery of the normal hydration status is not only the absence of clinical signs of dehydration but also the volume of urine output. Urine outputs greater than 0.5 mL/kg/hour are expected in fully hydrated patients. The maintenance phase has the objective of preserving the normal hydration status, and it lasts until the diarrhea abates.

The oral route is advised for the maintenance phase, and the ORS recommended by the World Health Organization (WHO) is the preferred oral solution. Recently, WHO has promoted the use of ORS with lower osmolality (75 mmol/L of sodium and total osmolality of 245 mOsm/L vs. the former solution containing 90 mmol/L of sodium and total osmolality of 311 mOsm/L) to treat all kinds of acute diarrheal diseases. Adults should be observed for hyponatremia when using this reduced-osmolality ORS. ORS uses the principle of common transportation of solutes, electrolytes, and water not affected by cholera in the intestine. ORS containing rice instead of glucose is also preferred, because the purging rate is lower with solutions containing rice than with glucose-based solutions. If ORS in packets is not available, a solution can be made with 2.6 g sodium chloride, 2.9 g sodium citrate, 1.5 g potassium chloride, and 13.5 g glucose or 50 g rice powder to 1 L of boiled water.

The amount of oral fluids should match the ongoing losses to prevent dehydration during this phase. Periodic review of the patient's chart is advised for this purpose. Predesigned forms to register intake and output and vital signs should be available to monitor the hydration status regularly. Cholera cots or cholera chairs facilitate the collection and measurement of stools and urine during treatment.

TABLE 2 Clinical Findings by Degree of Dehydration

	Degree of Dehydration	
Clinical Finding	**Some**	**Severe**
Loss of fluid (% of body weight)	5%–10%	>10%
Mentation	Restless	Drowsy or comatose
Radial pulse rate	Rapid	Very rapid
Radial pulse intensity	Weak	Feeble or impalpable
Respiration	Normal or deep	Deep and rapid
Systolic blood pressure	Low	Very low or undetectable
Skin elasticity	Retracts slowly	Retracts very slowly
Eyes	Sunken	Very sunken
Voice	Hoarse	Not audible
Urine production	Scant	Oliguria

CURRENT THERAPY

- Identify the degree of dehydration on admission.
- Register the intake and output regularly in predesigned charts.
- Rehydrate the patient in two phases. The rehydration phase lasts 2–4 hours. The maintenance phase lasts until diarrhea abates.
- Use the intravenous route for patients who have severe dehydration during the rehydration phase, those who purge more than 10–20 mL/kg/h, and those who do not tolerate the oral route during the maintenance phase. The amount and speed of the intravenous infusion vary between 50 and 100 mL/kg/h.
- The preferred intravenous solution is Ringer's lactate solution. Normal saline may be used, but the acidosis resolves less efficiently.
- Use the oral rehydration solution advised by the World Health Organization during the maintenance phase for severely dehydrated patients and for milder forms of dehydration in the rehydration phase. The amount of oral fluids advised is 500–1000 mL/h.
- Start antibiotics once the patient can tolerate the oral route. Doxycycline (Vibramycin) in a single dose of 300 mg, is the preferred regimen, given with a light meal.
- Start a normal diet as soon as the patient tolerates anything by mouth.
- Discharge patients when all the following criteria are fulfilled: oral tolerance <600–800 mL/h, stool output >400 mL/h, urine output <30–40 mL/h.

Discharging patients from the hospital is a critical issue, particularly when health centers are overloaded with patients with varying degrees of dehydration. Patients can be safely discharged if all the following criteria are met: oral intake between 600 and 800 mL/hour, urine output between 30 and 40 mL/hour, and stool output lower than 400 mL/hour. Case fatality rates in centers with experience in the treatment of cholera are extremely low, about 0.14%.

PHARMACOLOGIC THERAPY

An oral antibiotic is advised to reduce the volume of diarrhea, the requirement for intravenous fluids, and the hospital stay. Antibiotics are not lifesaving and should not be offered if the patient cannot tolerate the oral route. A reduction in almost 50% of the volume and duration of diarrhea and a reduction in the excretion of vibrios to 1 to 2 days have been documented with the use of effective antimicrobials. Single-dose regimens are preferred over multiple-dose regimens. A single dose of doxycycline (Vibramycin) 300 mg, given with a light meal, is the preferred regimen. Alternative regimens are listed in Table 3.

The quinolones are the group of antimicrobials more extensively studied to date, and excellent results in both clinical and bacteriologic parameters have been reported in clinical trials. Quinolones should not be used in children or pregnant women. Resistance to the quinolones has emerged in endemic areas of India and Bangladesh. Oral azithromycin (Zithromax)[1] (1 g in a single dose) is an alternative to treat infections by quinolone-resistant strains in both children and adults. Chemoprophylaxis with antimicrobials to prevent transmission of cholera is not recommended.

Complications and Prognosis

The most severe complication of cholera is acute renal failure. A careful evaluation of the medical charts of these patients disclosed improper replacement of fluids during the rehydration or maintenance phases. The nonoliguric form predominates. All age groups are affected, and the mortality rate is very high.

The presentation of cholera in children is similar to that in adults. Certain features are distinctive in children, however, such as fever, seizures, mental alteration, and hypoglycemia.

Cholera in the elderly carries a bad prognosis. The common presence of comorbidities, the difficulties in properly evaluating the hydration status, and the higher incidences of acute renal failure and pulmonary edema account for the higher mortality observed in this population.

Cholera in pregnant women is associated with more severe illness and with fetal losses.

---

[1]Not FDA approved for this indication.

TABLE 3 Antimicrobial Regimens for the Treatment of Cholera

Drug	Antimicrobial Regimen	
	Adult	**Children**
Preferred Regimen		
Doxycycline (Vibramycin)	300 mg with food	
Alternative Regimens		
Azithromycin (Zithromax)[1]	1 g as a single dose	20 mg/kg as a single dose
Ciprofloxacin (Cipro)[1]	1 g single-dose or 250 mg qd for 3 d or 500 mg bid for 3 d	Not recommended
Cotrimoxazole (Bactrim)[1]	TMP 160 mg and SMX 800 mg bid for 3 d	TMP 8 mg/kg and SMX 40 mg/kg divided in 2 doses for 3 d
Doxycycline (Vibramycin)	300 mg as a single dose	Not evaluated
Erythromycin[1]	250 mg qid for 3 d	12.5 mg/kg q6h for 3 d
Furazolidone (Furoxone)	100 mg qid for 3 d	5 mg/kg qid for 3 d or 7 mg/kg as a single dose
Norfloxacin (Noroxin)[1]	400 mg bid for 3 d	Not recommended
Tetracycline	500 mg qid for 3 d	50 mg/kg body weight qid for 3 d*

[1]Not FDA approved for this indication.
*Only for children older than 8 years.
Abbreviations: SMX = sulfamethoxazole; TMP = trimethoprim.

REFERENCES

Griffith DC, Kelly-Hope LA, Miller MA. Review of reported cholera outbreaks worldwide, 1995–2005. Am J Trop Med Hyg 2006;75:973–7.

Khan WA, Bennish ML, Seas C, et al. Randomized controlled comparison of single-dose ciprofloxacin and doxycycline for cholera caused by *Vibrio cholerae* O1 or O139. Lancet 1996;348:296–300.

Khan WA, Saha D, Rahman A, et al. Comparison of single-dose azithromycin and 12-dose, 3-day erythromycin for childhood cholera: A randomized, double-blind trial. Lancet 2002;360(9347):1722–7.

Nalin DR, Hirschhorn N, Greenough III W, et al. Clinical concerns about reduced-osmolarity oral rehydration solution. JAMA 2004;291:2632–5.

Sack DAW, Sack RB, Nair GB, Siddique AK. Cholera. Lancet 2004;363:223–33.

Saha D, Karim MM, Khan WA, et al. Single-dose azithromycin for the treatment of cholera in adults. N Engl J Med 2006;354:2452–62.

Seas C, Gotuzzo E. Cholera. In: Mandell GL, Bennett JE, Dolin R, editors. Principles and Practice of Infectious Diseases. Philadelphia: Churchill-Livingstone; 2005. p. 2536–44.

Foodborne Illness

Method of
Lester M. Crawford, PhD

History

In the 1920 edition of *Principles and Practice of Medicine*, Sir William Osler devoted three of the 1168 pages to food poisoning. He got virtually everything right, even by today's standards. He just had very little to report on a disease complex that was vitally important in his time. Today, the Centers for Disease Control and Prevention (CDC) estimates approximately 76 million illnesses, 325,000 hospitalizations, and 5000 deaths from foodborne disease each year in the United States. Viruses account for 67% of these infections, bacteria for 30%, and parasites for 2%.

Therapy of foodborne disease has passed through a variety of stages. In Osler's time, treatment primarily consisted of stomach lavage and enemas. After World War II, antibiotics were freely used. By the 1980s, competitive exclusion by antibiotic-resistant bacteria had dictated a more conservative approach that relied on supportive therapy including fluids. In severe cases, selective use of specific targeted antibacterials remained necessary. The remarkable success rate of oral rehydration therapy under primitive conditions in developing countries underscored the critical importance of maintaining fluid balance. Today, fluid therapy has become the cornerstone of the treatment of foodborne disease.

Etiology, Diagnosis, and Treatment

There are 30 principal foodborne diseases. Waterborne diseases are classified as foodborne diseases. Six of the 30 diseases are dealt with in other chapters. These are hepatitis, salmonellosis, typhoid, cholera, giardiasis, and toxoplasmosis. This chapter deals with the remaining major causes of this group of diseases.

AEROMONAS SPECIES

Although the role of *Aeromonas* in foodborne disease was elucidated in the 1890s, it has only recently been appreciated as the ubiquitous pathogenic organism that it is. These are, in fact, aquatic organisms, but *Aeromonas* has been isolated from a variety of plants, animals, and foodstuffs. *Aeromonas* has also been found in stool cultures, skin, and sputum samples from healthy persons. Gastrointestinal infections caused by this organism are characterized by mucoid, bloody stools, watery diarrhea typical of dysentery, and low-grade fever. This syndrome can progress to pneumonia, arthritis, osteomyelitis, endocarditis, and urinary tract infections, particularly in children, the elderly, and immunocompromised patients. *Aeromonas* can affect virtually any organ system and can cause hemolytic uremic syndrome.

The organism is amenable to antibiotic therapy and may be successfully treated with trimethoprim-sulfamethoxazole (Bactrim),[1] aminoglycosides, tetracyclines, cephalosporins, and the quinolones. Antibiotic resistance has now become a problem; it has been demonstrated that *Aeromonas* spp. can produce β-lactamases and transferable tetracycline R-plasmids. Therefore, it may be preferable to initiate therapy with trimethoprim-sulfamethoxazole or one of the fluoroquinolones when *Aeromonas* is isolated.

BACILLUS CEREUS

Bacillus cereus was not recognized as a significant foodborne pathogen until the 1950s, and the first major outbreak was not until 1971 in England. This organism is ubiquitous in the environment but is not pathogenic until conditions favor its growth. Pathogenesis is accomplished through a wide variety of extracellular toxins and enzymes. There is a diarrheagenic toxin and an emetic toxin.

Foods become toxic when the levels of *B. cereus* approach millions of organisms per gram. The usual syndrome involves nausea (but not vomiting), watery diarrhea, rectal straining, and abdominal pain. There is an incubation period of 8 to 19 hours; the duration of illness is usually 12 to 24 hours. In some cases, an emetic syndrome occurs that is more severe and acute than the diarrheal syndrome. The emetic syndrome is characterized by an incubation period of approximately 3 hours and is typified by severe vomiting. Diarrhea is generally not present in the emetic syndrome. The emetic syndrome closely mirrors staphylococcal food poisoning.

The diarrheal syndrome generally requires minimal therapeutic intervention other than monitoring of fluid and food intake. The emetic syndrome, although brief, can require intravenous fluids and medication such as phenobarbital[1] to moderate the frequency of vomiting.

CALICIVIRUSES

Caliciviruses cause the majority of foodborne illness in the United States and, most likely, the rest of the world. Indeed, without the cases caused by norovirus, cases of foodborne disease would be reduced by approximately two thirds according to some estimates, and there would likely be little need for or interest in this chapter.

Norwalk, Ohio, was the site of the first reported outbreak (1968) of this disease complex. The virus was therefore named *Norwalk virus*. The name was later changed to *Norwalk-like virus* (NLV), and the current name is *norovirus*.

There are three genotypes of enteric caliciviruses. In addition to norovirus, the calicivirus family includes Desert Shield virus, Hawaii virus, Mexico virus, Snow Mountain virus, and others.

Etiology

Fecal-oral transmission is the most common route of infection, but vomitus can also transmit infectious doses of the agent. Although swimming pools and uncooked or partially cooked food can transmit the infection, the primary source is drinking water. The recent spate of cruise ship infections has generally been traced to drinking water. Properly chlorinated water is generally safe, but nonchlorinated water is problematic. Inadequately chlorinated or brominated water can transmit norovirus, as can chlorinated water that comes from an overwhelmingly contaminated source. Leakage of sewage into treated water can result in individual cases or outbreaks.

Diagnosis

The disease entity is characterized by epidemic diarrhea. Symptoms include gastroenteritis, vomiting, diarrhea, headache, and 2 to 3 days

---

[1]Not FDA approved for this indication.

of low-grade fever. People of all ages are affected. In the United States, older children and adults are more likely to be infected, and in the Third World, young children are more often involved. Diagnosis may be by isolation of the virus from feces and confirmation by radioimmunoassay (RIA) or enzyme-linked immunosorbent assay (ELISA), or both.

Treatment

There is no specific treatment for norovirus infection. Supportive therapy, especially including fluids, is generally adequate for most patients. For patients in developing countries, oral rehydration therapy is generally the treatment of choice.

A specific vaccine for norovirus is being developed. The virus has been isolated, cloned, and sequenced, and an experimental vaccine is in clinical trials.

CAMPYLOBACTER SPECIES

Campylobacter has gone from not being recognized as a human pathogen to being the leading cause of bacterial diarrhea in just over 25 years. The agent is estimated to cause about 2.5 million illnesses, which is 12% of all foodborne disease in the United States. Moreover, serious sequelae such as Guillain-Barré syndrome (1:1000 cases) and Reiter's syndrome (1:100 cases) infrequently supervene.

Diagnosis

Difficulty in culturing Campylobacter prevented isolation and characterization of the organism until the early 1970s. Campylobacter jejuni is the species most associated with foodborne illness. Campylobacteriosis is characterized by abdominal pain, diarrhea, and fever lasting 2 to 5 days. Longer durations of illness and relapses are not uncommon. Diagnosis is confirmed by direct microscopic examination of the stool or through the use of selective media.

Treatment

Seriously ill patients should be treated with antibiotics, as should infants, older people, and the immunosuppressed. Seriously ill patients are defined as those with persistent high fever or refractory or bloody diarrhea. Clarithromycin (Biaxin)[1] is generally accepted as the antibiotic of choice, and fluoroquinolones such as ciprofloxacin (Cipro)[1] are the first alternative. The tetracyclines are also useful. Campylobacteriosis is resistant to the cephalosporins, vancomycin (Vancocin), and rifampin (Rifadin). Supportive therapy aimed at electrolyte replacement and hydration is also important.

CLOSTRIDIUM BOTULINUM

Clostridium botulinum elaborates one of the most potent substances in nature. One nanogram per kilogram of body weight is sufficient to paralyze an otherwise healthy person. When the toxin is ingested in food in sufficient quantities to cause illness, near total paralysis occurs in humans, often requiring artificial ventilation for extended periods. Mild botulism can consist of nothing more than double vision or a few days of dysphagia.

The mechanism of action of botulism is to block release of acetylcholine at the neuromuscular junction by attaching to specific receptors on the nerve terminal side of the junction. Nerve conduction restores activity at the neuromuscular junction.

Any food can contain botulinum toxin, but the most common vehicles in the United States are fruits and vegetables. Infant botulism is usually associated with consumption of honey.

Diagnosis

Diagnosis is confirmed by isolation of botulinum toxin either from the suspect food or from the patient's blood serum or feces. Resorting to symptomatic diagnosis can lead to confusing botulism with Guillain-Barré syndrome or even stroke.

---

[1]Not FDA approved for this indication.

Treatment

Therapy must center around the management of respiratory impairment. This requires accessibility to an intensive care unit. The Centers for Disease Control and Prevention (CDC) can provide polyvalent vaccines[5,10] that are effective against the six botulism toxins (A, B, C, D, E, F). The toxin can persist in the patient's serum for as much as a month after ingestion, and relapses and exacerbations are possible. The toxicity to the neuromuscular junctions can continue for months and, in rare cases, for as long as a year. Careful management and diagnostic advances have reduced mortality to well under 10%.

CLOSTRIDIUM PERFRINGENS

McClane has written, "Clostridium perfringens is ideally suited for its role as a major foodborne pathogen." He was referring to its ubiquity in soil and in human and animal feces; moreover, the organism has a doubling time of less than 10 minutes once established in foods. Finally, C. perfringens is heat resistant and it elaborates two toxins that can induce specific pathology in the human intestinal tract. Indeed, C. perfringens is the third leading cause of foodborne illness in the United States, after norovirus and B. cereus.

Diagnosis

The two forms of human disease caused by this organism are C. perfringens type A food poisoning and C. perfringens type C food poisoning, better known as necrotic enteritis. The type A syndrome is much more common but type C is a more serious disease.

Abdominal cramps and diarrhea typify the type A disease. These symptoms develop 8 to 16 hours after ingestion of contaminated food and persist for 12 to 24 hours, with a complete recovery in most patients. However, severe illness and even death can supervene in older or debilitated patients.

The necrotic enteritis form of the disease is characterized by vomiting, intense abdominal pain, bloody diarrhea, and severe gastroenteritis. The incubation period is 1 to 5 days after exposure. The more advanced cases can progress to jejunal necrosis and death if not managed well.

Treatment

Treatment for the type A disease is supportive therapy. Necrotic enteritis can require surgical repair of the small intestine, including removal of the affected area. C. perfringens is quite susceptible to penicillin, and some authorities report that the antibiotic may be useful in the management of severe cases of type C.

ENTEROBACTER SAKAZAKII

Enterobacter sakazakii causes meningitis or necrotizing enterocolitis in neonates, which results in a mortality rate of 40% to 80%. Surviving patients sometimes develop hydrocephalus, paralysis, or neurologic deficits. E. sakazakii has been isolated from dry infant formulas. The natural source of the organism is not well known.

Enterobacters are generally resistant to the cephalosporins but are responsive to medium-spectrum penicillins, such as carbenicillin (Geocillin),[1] piperacillin (Pipracil),[1] and ticarcillin (Ticar).[1] The aminoglycosides and the fluoroquinolones are also indicated.

ESCHERICHIA COLI O157:H7

This variant of Escherichia coli burst on the scene in North America in the late 1970s, and now it can be found in practically every country in the world. The reservoir for the disease is believed to be cattle, but wildlife of various kinds can likewise harbor the organism. In cattle, the disease is silent, causing no overt signs.

---

[1]Not FDA approved for this indication.
[5]Investigational drug in the United States.
[10]Available in the United States from the Centers for Disease Control.

In humans, the verocytotoxin, a Shiga-like toxin that has been genetically incorporated into the organism, can cause hemorrhagic colitis and hemolytic-uremic syndrome, which leads, in some cases, to disseminated intravascular coagulation (DIC). DIC can result in a layer of fibrin forming in the glomerular capillary bed and acute renal failure. These sequelae are most likely to occur in children and older persons and in pregnant women. The young patients generally fully recover but sometimes require dialysis.

The number of cases is low and the fatality rate is small, but the severity and permanence of some of the sequelae have given great prominence to the disease. Major outbreaks such as the Jack-in-the-Box event of 1993 and the 2006 spinach outbreak have focused public attention on *E. coli* O157:H7. Control of this organism depends on proper cooking and handling of food, assiduous hand washing, and effective water-treatment programs. There is much interest in a vaccine for cattle or humans for *E. coli* O157:H7.

Diagnosis

Diagnosis is made by serotyping for specific antibodies to *E. coli* O157:H7. Transmission of the organism generally occurs from ingesting contaminated food but can occur from direct contact. The incubation period is 12 to 60 hours.

Treatment

Therapy consists of fluid replacement. Antibiotics are of no use because the lesional insult is caused by a combination of toxins that continue to be pathogenic for a period of time after the elaborating organism is no longer active. In fact, the U.S. Food and Drug Administration (FDA) has issued (January 2007) a warning against the use of antibiotics in enterohemorrhagic *E. coli* cases because such therapy could adversely affect the outcome. Dialysis is indicated in cases that progress to kidney failure. In the more severe cases of intestinal hemorrhage, blood transfusion may be necessary.

LISTERIA MONOCYTOGENES

Although *Listeria monocytogenes* infects a relatively small number of patients, listeriosis results in a 25% to 40% fatality rate, and severe aftereffects are relatively common in affected patients. It is extremely difficult to identify the specific food responsible because of the highly variable incubation period, which ranges from 3 to 70 days.

There are three modes of transmission: contaminated food, direct contact with the organism or with contaminated soil, and inhalation of the organism. Initial symptoms include fever, headache, and vomiting, but these may be followed by endocarditis, meningoencephalitis, and septicemia. These later symptoms can lead to hemorrhagic shock, disorientation, and coma. Listeriosis is a leading cause of stillbirth and miscarriage and must be handled aggressively in pregnant women. Neonatal cases likewise must be managed with care. Almost one half of all listeriosis cases are in neonates.

Confirmation of the diagnosis is accomplished by isolation of the organism from blood or cerebrospinal fluid. Virtually all β-lactam antibiotics are effective against *L. monocytogenes* including potassium penicillin G (Pfizerpen). Erythromycin (Ery-Tab),[1] tobramycin (Nebcin),[1] and other antibiotics in the macrolide and aminoglycoside families also are effective against *L. monocytogenes*.

STAPHYLOCOCCUS AUREUS

Whereas most food borne illnesses have incubation periods of days and even weeks, *Staphylococcus aureus* infections usually trigger symptoms in 2 to 6 hours. The organism elaborates a complex system of toxins in food under certain conditions that results in nausea, vomiting, retching, and abdominal cramping. Severe cases result in muscle cramping, vacillations in blood pressure and heart rate, and severe headaches. The disease usually runs its course in 2 days, but some cases last longer. Death can occur in the young, the elderly, and the debilitated.

Incriminated foods in *Staphylococcal* outbreaks are generally those that require a great deal of human handling such as salads and various

---

[1]Not FDA approved for this indication.

meats, although canned foods have caused clusters of infection. The usual inciting factor is not keeping the prepared foods hot enough or cold enough to prevent the proliferation of organisms and the formation of the causative toxins. Stored foods should be maintained at temperatures of 45°F (7.2°C) or kept warm at 140°F (60°C). Foods should be brought to these temperatures as rapidly as technologically possible.

Supportive therapy is indicated. Antibiotic therapy is not useful because the causative agent, the toxin, is not affected by antibiotics. Persistent vomiting or dehydration can indicate fluid therapy, such as 5% dextrose, together with electrolyte replacement, particularly potassium.

REFERENCES

Allos BM, Blaster MJ. *Campylobacter jejuni* and the expanding spectrum of related infections. Clin Infect Dis 1995;20:1092–101.

Ball JM, Graham DY, Opekum AR, et al. Recombinant Norwalk-like particles given orally to volunteers: Phase I study. Gastroenterology 1999;117:40–8.

Bennett RW. *Bacillus cereus*. In: Labbé RG, García S, editors. Guide to Foodborne Pathogens. New York: John Wiley and Sons; 2001. p. 51–60.

Gill DM. Bacterial toxins: A table of lethal amounts. Microbiol Rev 1982;46:86–94.

Greatorex JS, Thorne GM. Humoral immune response to Shiga-like toxins and *Escherichia coli* O157:H7 lipopolysaccharide in hemolytic-uremic syndrome patients and healthy subjects. J Clin Microbiol 1994;32:1172–8.

Lawrence GW. The pathogenesis of enteritis necroticans. In: Rood JA, McClane, Songer JG, et al (editors), The Clostridia: Molecular Genetics and Pathogenesis. London: Academic Press; 1997. p. 198–207.

Lederberg J, Shope RE, Oaks SC, editors. Emerging Infections: Microbial Threats to Health in the United States. Washington, DC: National Academies Press; 1992.

Miliotis MD, Bier JW, editors. International Handbook of Foodborne Pathogens. New York: Marcel Dekker; 2003.

Olsen SJ, MacKinnon LC, Goulding JS, et al. Surveillance for foodborne-disease outbreaks—United States, 1993–1997. MMWR CDC Surveill Summ 2000;49(1):1–62.

Schlech WF. Foodborne listeriosis. Clin Infec Dis 2000;31:770–5.

Necrotizing Skin and Soft Tissue Infections

Method of
Debra Tristram, MD

Epidemiology

Necrotizing skin and soft tissue infections (nSSTIs) are uncommon; an annual incidence of approximately 1000 cases/year is estimated for the United States. The microorganisms responsible for nSSTIs are numerous (Table 1) and can be mixtures of aerobic and anaerobic organisms acting synergistically to produce infection, or a single, highly virulent pathogen.

Polymicrobial infections with 4 or 5 different organisms present the most common form of the disease (55%-75% of all nSSTIs). These infections involve the trunk and perineal areas and are more common in immunocompromised patients. In contrast, monomicrobial infections occur much more often in young, healthy persons. Involvement of the extremities is common, resulting from seemingly minor trauma in more than 75% of cases. A subgroup of nSSTIs is associated with exposure to contaminated water or fish, especially in warmer waters. *Vibrio vulnificus* is the primary pathogen in this scenario, but nSSTIs have also been increasingly reported secondary to other gram-negative waterborne organisms (see Table 1).

Fungal pathogens are also emerging as important causes of nSSTIs. Usually these are infections are caused by septated molds, but aseptated zygomyces are reported with increasing frequency (see Table 1).

TABLE 1 Most Common Pathogens Involved in Necrotizing Skin and Soft Tissue Infections

Risk Factors	Organisms	Location	Special Types by Anatomic Location
Polymicrobial Immunosuppression Diabetes mellitus Peripheral vascular disease Obesity Chronic renal disease, dialysis HIV Ethanol abuse Bites Blunt or penetrating trauma Surgical incisions Varicella Perforation of the GI tract Malnutrition, cachexia Chronic dermatosis Diabetes mellitus Iron overload and deferoxamine therapy Immunocompromised states (particularly prolonged neutropenia) Soft tissue trauma, especially with soil contamination	Mixture of aerobes, anaerobes, and facultative organisms: *Bacteroides* spp., *Clostridium* spp., *Eikenella corrodens*, *Enterobacter* spp., *Escherichia coli*, *Fusobacter* spp., *Haemophilus influenzae* type B, *Klebsiella* spp., *Peptococcus* spp., *Peptostreptococcus* spp, *Prevotella* spp., *Porphyromonas* spp., *Proteus* spp., *Pseudomonas* spp., *Stapylococcus aureus* (MSSA and MRSA), *Streptococcus* spp. Fungal: *Absidia* spp., *Aspergillus* spp., *Fusarium* spp., *Mucor* spp., *Rhizopus* spp., and others Fungal: *Absidia* spp., *Aspergillus* spp., *Fusarium* spp., *Mucor* spp., *Rhizopus* spp., and others	Perineal area and trunk	Fournier's gangrene: perineal and scrotal necrosis Lemierre's disease: deep neck space infections with dissemination (*Fusobacter necrophorum* and other oral flora) Malignant otitis externa: *Pseudomonas areuginosa*, *Staphylococcus aureus*, invasive fungi, especially *Aspergillus* spp. Meleney's synergistic gangrene (MRSA and anaerobic streptococci) Rhinocerebral infections: Invasive fungal pathogens in persons with diabetes mellitus or in profoundly neutropenic patients
Monomicrobial Otherwise young, healthy persons Occasionally, recent trauma, operation or IV drug use	*S. pyogenes, S. aureus*, and anaerobic streptococci (i.e., *Peptostreptococcus*)	Extremities, occasionally trunk	
Exposure to contaminated water or fish, especially seawater: Skin break due to fish finning, trauma in water or handling seafood	*Vibrio vulnificus* and other *Vibrio* spp.: warm seawater Fresh or brackish water: *Aeromonas hydrophia, Edwardisella tarda, Pseudomonas* spp., and other enterics; *Schewanella putrificiens; Streptococcus iniae*	Extremities	

GI, gastrointestinal; HIV, human immunodeficiency virus; MRSA, methicillin-resistant *Staphylococcus aureus*; MSSA, methicillin-susceptible *Staphylococcus aureus*.

Risk Factors

Risk factors for the development of skin and soft tissue infections are numerous and are outlined in Table 1. Loss of skin integrity through trauma and immunocompromised states are the most common antecedent risk factors.

Pathophysiology

Necrotizing SSTIs are capable of breaking down and crossing anatomic barriers rapidly by direct spread, causing extensive destruction of the subcutaneous, fascial, or muscle layers of the integument, with little surface evidence of infection. Trivial injuries from cuts, abrasions, scratches, or insect bites provide a portal of entry through direct inoculation. Thrombosis of cutaneous vessels, vasculitis, and necrosis follows microbial and leukocytic invasion of the deep dermal tissue and fascial layer. A smaller percentage of patients have no visible portal of entry; systemic spread from an unrecognized focus through the vasculature or lymphatics might play a role in these cases.

Prevention

Maintenance of skin integrity is the cornerstone of prevention. Cleaning of traumatized skin with antibacterial soaps and removal of all foreign material can reduce the risk for infection. Use of proper skin preparation, perioperative antibiotics, and sterile surgical technique can cut the risk of postoperative infections to nearly zero. Education of patients who have risk factors regarding when to seek medical attention can aid in decreasing serious consequences for compromised hosts.

Clinical Manifestations

Necrotizing SSTIs in the earliest stages can appear like a cellulitis or erysipelas. Localized warmth, erythema, induration, and swelling are characteristic of early nSSTIs. As the disease process progresses, violaceous or darker maroon areas can appear within the margins of initial erythema, and bullae can form, initially filled with clear fluid but progressively filled with hemorrhagic fluid (Fig. 1). A peau d'orange appearance to the skin is a late finding. The skin can have a

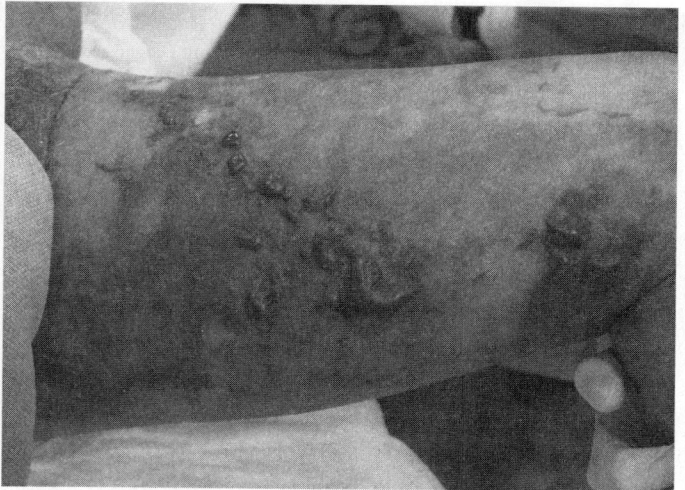

FIGURE 1. Necrotizing skin and soft tissue infection in an otherwise healthy male patient who sustained an abrasion to his shin several days before presentation. Violaceous patches within the initial area of cellulitis and development of hemorrhagic bullae and skin sloughing are demonstrated. Group A streptococci were recovered from surgery.

wooden or hardened feel in contrast to the palpable soft tissue structures underlying simple cellulitis. Crepitus in the tissue (common in *Clostridium* infection) is not seen if the responsible organisms are not gas producing (e.g., group A streptococci). Examination of the affected area can reveal pain out of proportion to the observed clinical appearance due to involvement of the cutaneous nerve roots; anesthesia of the area is a more ominous sign, indicating further spread of the infection and destruction of the nerve tissue. Systemic toxicity with high fever, muscle aches, fatigue, and anorexia can usher in more-severe toxic shock–like features with vascular collapse, altered mental status, and respiratory distress.

Diagnosis

Diagnosis of nSSTIs depends on a strong clinical suspicion and is confirmed only by surgical exploration. Laboratory findings are nonspecific and do not differentiate between cellulitis and deeper tissue infections. Muscle enzymes may be elevated if there is muscle necrosis either from direct infection or by compression from edema causing a compartment syndrome. Imaging with computed tomography (CT) or magnetic resonance imaging (MRI) might reveal underlying edema extending along fascial planes, but the sensitivity and specificity of these procedures is unknown. Absence of gas in the tissues does not eliminate nSSTI; other pathogens that cause nSSTIs might not form gas (e.g., group A streptococci).

CURRENT DIAGNOSIS

- Prompt surgical intervention confirms the diagnosis and can be life and limb saving.
- Empiric antibiotic coverage should target organisms obtained from the details of injury.
- Physical examination of the affected area should focus on the following:
    - Exquisite pain and tenderness out of proportion to the visible physical signs of infection
    - Presence of hemorrhagic bullae, skin sloughing, skin anesthesia
    - Palpable gas in the tissue (uncommon)

Imaging should not delay surgical intervention. At the time of surgery, the underlying tissue is swollen, the fascia is grey, and a brownish exudate may ooze from the area. The exudate is replete with microorganisms and provides an early clue to the pathogen(s) on Gram stain. If nSSTI is suspected but not certain, a small incision can be made by the surgeon in the suspect area for inspection, biopsy, and cultures.

Differential Diagnosis

There are multiple other infectious and noninfectious conditions in the differential diagnosis of nSSTIs; these are outlined in Box 1. Many can be eliminated from the differential by a careful history.

Therapy

Necrotizing infection is a surgical emergency; all patients with suspected nSSTI should be seen by a surgeon immediately. Because most nSSTIs begin as cellulitis, administration of empiric antibiotics should not be withheld while awaiting full evaluation; if treated early enough, some patients might avoid more extensive, disfiguring surgical débridement. Cultures of drainage and of tissue obtained from the surgical procedure should be sent for aerobic, anaerobic, and fungal stains and cultures. Pus or exudate samples sent in sterile cups or syringes in addition to tissue samples are preferable to swab specimens because the recovery of anaerobes is inhibited by exposure to air. Gram stains done at the time of surgery may be helpful to guide therapy in cases where antibiotic pretreatment inhibits bacterial growth. Empiric antibiotics can be tailored to target the specific organisms isolated from cultures when susceptibilities are available.

CURRENT THERAPY

- Necrotizing skin and soft tissue infections are rapidly progressive infections capable of breaking down and crossing anatomic barriers quickly, causing extensive destruction of the subcutaneous, fascial or muscle layers of the integument with little surface evidence of infection.
- Unrecognized or seemingly minor breaks in the skin or mucosa initiate the process in more than 80% of cases.
- A high index of suspicion is needed for prompt, aggressive surgical débridement and treatment with antibiotics to prevent significant morbidity, limb loss, and mortality.

Empiric antibiotic coverage of *all* potential pathogens that cause nSSTIs is difficult to achieve. Consultation with an infectious disease specialist for antibiotic management is strongly recommended. Careful attention to the details surrounding the onset and circumstances of infection can give clues to the potential cause(s), but empiric antibiotics should include coverage for gram-positive organisms (especially methicillin-resistant *Staphylococcus aureus* [MRSA]) and anaerobes as well as gram-negative organisms. Certain clinical scenarios noted in Table 1 can give added guidance to the organisms requiring coverage, but nothing can replace cultures for the exact drug(s) of choice for the given infection. All nSSTIs should be suspected to be polymicrobial until proved otherwise; initial empiric therapy for mixed infections should contain an extended-spectrum β-lactam such as ampicillin-sulbactam (Unasyn) or pipercillin-tazobactam (Zosyn) *and* clindamycin (Cleocin) *and* ciprofloxacin (Cipro) or other fluoroquinolone. In areas with a high incidence of MRSA isolates with inducible clindamycin resistance, vancomycin (Vancocin) or daptomycin (Cubicin) should be used instead of clindamycin until culture results are available.

Adjunctive therapies such as hyperbaric oxygen and intravenous immunoglobulin (IVIg, Gammagard)[1] have been used in some cases. Neither has been evaluated in a controlled fashion and is not considered standard therapy but may be useful for certain cases. Nonrandomized observational studies suggest that IVIg infusions reduce morbidity and mortality, but further studies are warranted.

Monitoring

Patients with nSSTIs can have severe systemic reactions, leading to shock, acute respiratory distress syndrome (ARDS), and multiorgan failure. Such patients are best managed in an intensive care setting. Second-look surgery is often beneficial to further assess the extent of the infection and to reculture and débride as needed.

Complications

Necrotizing infections nearly always cause skin scarring as well as the potential for disfigurement and limb loss. Survivors can require multiple revisions of the débrided area to provide satisfactory coverage with grafting and flaps. Despite great improvements in medical care, mortality associated with nSSTIs remains 25% to 35%; mortality is directly proportional to the interval between time of onset and the time of intervention. Mortality rates can be even higher in patients with underlying conditions.

[1]Not FDA approved for this indication.

REFERENCES

Anaya DA, Dellinger EP. Necrotizing soft-tissue infection: Diagnosis and management. Clin Infect Dis 2007;44:705–10.
Miller LG, Perdreau-Remington F, Rieg G, et al. Necrotizing fasciitis caused by community-associated methicillin-resistant *Staphylococcus aureus* in Los Angeles. N Engl J Med 2005;352:1445–53.
Napolitano LM. Severe soft tissue infections. Infect Dis Clin North Am 2009;3:571–91.
Saranti B, Strong M, Pascual J, Scwab CW. Necrotizing fasciitis: Current concepts and review of the literature. J Am Coll Surg 2009;208:279–88.
Stevens DL, Bisno AL, Chambers HF, et al. Practice guidelines for the diagnosis and management of skin and soft-tissue infections. Clin Infect Dis 2005;41:1373–406.

Toxic Shock Syndrome

Method of
Julius Larioza, MD, and Richard B. Brown, MD

Toxic shock syndrome (TSS) is an acute illness caused by the production of local exotoxins capable of diffusing into the mucosa and exerting an exaggerated immunologic response resulting in the development of multisystem disease. These substances are superantigens belonging to a family of pyrogenic toxins produced by bacteria that include *Staphylococcus aureus* and *Streptococcus pyogenes*. The former produces classic TSS, whereas the latter causes a modified form of TSS known as toxic shock-like syndrome (TSLS). A high burden (colonization or infection) with these organisms in the setting of certain parameters allows for the production of superantigens and the subsequent development of the syndrome.

CURRENT DIAGNOSIS

- Toxic shock syndrome (TSS) and toxic shock-like syndrome (TSLS) are rapid-onset illnesses causing fever, hypotension, rash, vomiting, diarrhea, and the potential for multiorgan failure.
- TSS and TSLS are associated with elaboration of bacterial toxins, which results in a vigorous cytokine cascade, rather than direct bacterial invasion.
- Diagnosis of TSS and TSLS is based on fulfillment of criteria that involve identification of a constellation of clinical and laboratory data.

CURRENT TREATMENT

- Bacteremia is present more commonly in TSLS and may contribute to higher mortality.
- Treatment consists of strategies to decrease bioburden and toxin production, directed antibiotic therapy at maximal parenteral doses, and clinical support with close monitoring of end-organ function.

Epidemiology

TSS was first described in 1978 and is now recognized in both menstrual and nonmenstrual forms. The former, as initially described, was typically noted after several days of menstruation and was commonly related to use of high-absorbency tampons, such as the Rely brand, which have since been taken off the market. Currently, nonmenstrual TSS has become almost as common as menstrual TSS, with most cases reported after surgical procedures (e.g., sinonasal manipulation with packing). It has also been linked with use of contraceptive diaphragms, chronic peritoneal dialysis catheters, viral influenza, sinusitis, intravenous drug use, and burn wounds.

TSLS was first described in 1987. Similar in clinical appearance to TSS, it was associated with *S. pyogenes* and was initially labeled as streptococcal toxic shock syndrome. Most commonly, organisms produce streptococcal pyrogenic exotoxin type A. However, other toxins and other streptococci have been occasionally implicated. Although those at the extremes of life and persons with underlying comorbidities appear to be at risk, most cases of TSLS occur in otherwise healthy persons between the ages of 20 and 50 years. It may be a result of the absence of protective immunity.

Clinical Manifestations

TSS is a rapid-onset illness that causes fever, hypotension, rash, vomiting, diarrhea, and, eventually, multiple organ failure. If not treated promptly, it can be lethal. TSLS displays many of the typical TSS symptoms with the addition of severe soft tissue necrosis. Menstrual and nonmenstrual TSS share similar features. The rash is most commonly a diffuse erythema that may resemble severe sunburn. However, a rash mimicking that of scarlet fever may also be seen. Hyperemia of conjunctiva and mucous membranes and strawberry tongue may also be present. Desquamation of the palms and soles, as noted in many bacterial toxin-mediated disorders, often appears during convalescence. When it occurs after surgery, the classic signs of localized infection, such as erythema, tenderness, and purulence, may be absent, making diagnosis more difficult. Multiple organ involvement may include the gastrointestinal, hepatic, renal, musculoskeletal, hematologic, or central nervous systems.

There are several notable differences between TSS and TSLS. The skin is often the portal of entry in TSLS, with soft tissue infections developing in 80% of patients. Cutaneous signs may include localized erythema and edema, a bullous or hemorrhagic cellulitis, necrotizing fasciitis, myositis, or gangrene. Soft tissue involvement of this nature is uncommonly encountered in TSS. Bacteremia is present in more than 50% of patients with TSLS, compared to 15% of those with TSS. Perhaps as a result of this fact, the mortality rate is as much as five times greater with TSLS, reaching 25%.

Pathogenesis

Production of toxic shock syndrome toxin type 1 (TSST-1) has been associated with the majority of menstrual TSS cases (90%); non-menstrual cases are mediated by TSST-1 or by staphylococcal enterotoxins B and C. The dependence of menstrual TSS on TSST-1 may be related to the ability of this protein, but not other pyrogenic toxins, to cross vaginal mucosa. Toxin production is regulated by the *agr* gene, which is expressed under conditions that include high protein levels, relatively neutral pH, and high partial pressures of CO_2 and O_2. All of these conditions are met when menstruation occurs in the setting of high-absorbency tampon use.

Most TSS-susceptible patients lack specific antibodies capable of blocking the responsible superantigens. Nonmenstrual onset of TSS is most likely related to clinically trivial *S. aureus* infections in the vagina and elsewhere (e.g., sinonasal passages). A major subclass of nonmenstrual TSS is viral influenza–associated *S. aureus,* which can infect nasopharyngeal tissues damaged by influenza infection and cause TSS by secreting TSST-1 or staphylococcal enterotoxins.

S. pyogenes causes TSLS by secreting streptococcal pyrogenic exotoxins of three serotypes: A, B, and C. Infection usually occurs after minor injury or surgery, although a portal of entry may never be identified.

Diagnosis

The diagnosis of TSS or TSLS is based on identification of a constellation of clinical and laboratory data proposed by the Centers for Disease Control and Prevention (Table 1).

Differential diagnosis for patients presenting with components of this syndrome includes sepsis caused by other bacteria, staphylococcal scalded skin syndrome, Rocky Mountain spotted fever, meningococcemia, exanthematous viral syndromes, and leptospirosis. Noninfectious causes include severe hyperthermia, drug reactions, and insect-related allergic reactions.

Additional laboratory data that are helpful in diagnosis include complete blood count (CBC) with differential, serum electrolytes, assessment of muscle enzymes, and renal and liver function studies. Urinalysis, chest radiography, and electrocardiography may also help in identification of end-organ complications. Blood, wound, urine, and respiratory cultures should always be performed before initiation of antibiotic therapy. If menstrual TSS is suspected, vaginal cultures for *S. aureus* should be obtained. Testing for TSST-1 should be undertaken if the test is available.

TABLE 1 Diagnostic Criteria for Toxic Shock Syndrome (Staphylococcal) and Toxic Shock-Like Syndrome (Streptococcal)

TSS*	TSLS
Fever	Isolation of group A streptococci from a sterile site (definite case) or from a nonsterile site (probable case)
Hypotension	
Diffuse macular rash with subsequent desquamation	
Plus involvement of three of the following organ systems:	Hypotension
Liver	Plus two of the following:
Blood	Renal dysfunction
Renal	Liver dysfunction
Mucous membrane	Erythematous macular rash
Gastrointestinal	Coagulopathy
Muscular	Soft tissue necrosis
Central nervous system	Adult respiratory distress syndrome
Negative serologic tests for measles, leptospirosis, Rocky Mountain spotted fever	
Negative cultures from blood or cerebrospinal fluid for organisms other than *Staphylococcus aureus*	

Adapted from McCormick JK, Yarwood JM, Schlievert PM. Toxic Shock syndrome and bacterial superantigens: An update. Annu Rev Microbiol 2001; 55:77–104.
*Proposed revision of diagnostic criteria for TSS secondary to *Staphylococcus aureus* includes isolation of *S. aureus* from a mucosal or normally sterile site, production of TSS-associated superantigen by the isolate, lack of antibody to the implicated toxin at the time of acute illness, and development of antibody to the toxin during convalescence.
TSLS = toxic shock-like syndrome; TSS = toxic shock syndrome.

TABLE 2 Recommended Doses of Selected Antibiotics Useful in the Management of Toxic Shock Syndrome and Toxic Shock-Like Syndrome

Agent	Dose
Vancomycin* (Vancocin)	15 mg/kg q12h
Daptomycin* (Cubicin)	6 mg/kg q24h
Clindamycin (Cleocin)	900 mg q8h

*Adjust for renal dysfunction.

Treatment

Treatment strategies for TSS and TSLS are similar. Initial management should include cleaning of any obvious wounds, removal of foreign bodies (e.g. tampons, nasal packing), and drainage or débridement of affected tissues. Such strategies result in decreased bioburden and toxin production.

Antibiotics active against offending pathogens should be employed parenterally and in the highest dose appropriate for the patient's circumstances. With the emergence of methicillin-resistant *Staphylococcus aureus* (MRSA), vancomycin (Vancocin) and daptomycin (Cubicin) are agents likely to be effective against typical pathogens, even if associated with bacteremia. The former is often monitored by measuring trough levels and maintaining them at 15 to 20 µg/mL. The latter has the additional potential advantage of killing organisms without major cell lysis, which may spare cytokine release and elaboration of sepsis cascades. Clindamycin (Cleocin) should be employed as a second agent, because of its activity against likely pathogens and because it may terminate toxin production at a cellular level. Table 2 depicts usual doses. Because of their potential for affecting renal function, agents such as vancomycin and daptomycin need to be assessed carefully for optimal dosing during the period of illness. Duration of therapy is typically 7 days, although bacteremic patients may be treated for more extended periods.

As appropriate, local wound management may include use of topical agents. In vitro studies of silver sulfadiazine (Silvadene)[1] cream suggest that sublethal concentrations may actually increase toxin production by *S. aureus*. For that reason, mupirocin (Bactroban) or povidine iodine (Betadine) may be a better choice. Management and monitoring of end organs and treatment of shock are mandatory, and severely ill patients are best managed in the critical care unit. Corticosteroids and specialized forms of intravenous gamma globulin[1] have been employed but are not considered standard care.

Prevention

Awareness of these syndromes may help with prevention. Patients who have developed menstrual TSS should be encouraged to avoid tampon use for at least three cycles, and to then employ the lowest-absorbency tampon feasible. Careful cleansing of skin wounds, drainage of abscesses, and judicious use of topical antimicrobials for injuries may help to prevent colonization and subsequent toxin production.

REFERENCES

Davies HD, McGeer A, Schwartz B, et al. Invasive group A streptococcal infections in Ontario, Canada. Ontario Group A Streptococcal Study Group [see comment and author reply]. N Engl J Med 1996;335:547–54.

Edwards-Jones V, Foster HA. The effect of topical antimicrobial agents on the production of toxic shock syndrome toxin-1. J Med Microbiol 1994; 41:408–13.

---

[1]Not FDA approved for this indication.

Jamart S, Denis O, Deplano A, et al. Methicillin-resistant *Staphylococcus aureus* toxic shock syndrome. Emerg Infect Dis 2005;11(4):636–7.

Manders SM. Toxin-mediated streptococcal and staphylococcal disease. J Am Acad Dermatol 1998;39:383–98.

McCormick J, Yarwood JM, Schlievert PM, et al. Toxic shock syndrome and bacterial superantigens: An update. Ann Rev Microbiol 2001;55:77–104.

Parsonnet J, Hansmann MA, Delaney ML, et al. Prevalence of toxic shock syndrome toxin 1-producing *Staphylococcus aureus* and the presence of antibodies to this superantigen in menstruating women. J Clin Microbiol 2005;43(9):4628–34.

Schlievert PM. Staphylococcal toxic shock syndrome: Still a problem. Med J Aust 2005;182(12):651–2.

Stevens DL. The toxic shock syndromes. Infect Dis Clin North Am 1996;10 (4):727–46.

Tierno PM Jr. Reemergence of staphylococcal toxic shock syndrome in the United States since 2000. J Clin Microbiol 2005;43(4):2032; author reply 2032–3.

Wood TF, Potter MA, Jonasson O. Streptococcal toxic shock-like syndrome: The importance of surgical intervention. Ann Surg 1993;217:109–14.

Influenza

Method of
Jeffrey A. Linder, MD, MPH, FACP

Influenza is a highly contagious viral infection that should be considered in any patient with respiratory symptoms between October and May in North America. Influenza infects 5% to 20% of the population of the United States in a typical year and is responsible for up to 226,000 hospitalizations and 36,000 deaths per year. Influenza can range in severity from mild illness to life-threatening disease. Those at highest risk of hospitalization, death, or complications from influenza are children younger than 5 years, adults older than 65 years, adults older than 50 years who have underlying medical conditions, those infected with HIV, and pregnant women.

Information about influenza changes rapidly. To optimally care for patients with influenza-like illness during the influenza season, clinicians need to keep abreast of updated recommendations and the current prevalence of influenza in their community. The influenza vaccine remains the best means of reducing the incidence, severity, and complications from influenza, but antiviral medications and symptomatic treatments have an important role in the prevention and treatment of influenza as well (Box 1).

Microbiology

There are two types of influenza viruses, A and B. Influenza A is separated into subtypes based on two surface antigens: hemagglutinin (H) and neuraminidase (N). The predominant circulating strains of influenza in recent decades have been influenza A (H1N1), influenza A (H3N2), and influenza B. Influenza A (H3N2) subtypes generally cause more severe influenza and are associated with higher mortality than other types. Influenza viruses undergo slight genetic changes from year to year, termed *antigenic drift*. Major changes in surface glycoproteins are termed *antigenic shift* and can result in severe pandemic influenza in a nonimmune population. Because of antigenic drift and because immunity to a given type or subtype of influenza provides limited cross-immunity to other types and subtypes, the influenza vaccine needs to be reformulated and administered each year.

Patients contract influenza by being exposed to large-sized respiratory droplets from an infected person or contact with surfaces harboring influenza virus. Influenza has a latency of 1 to 4 days before the onset of symptoms. Adults are infectious from the day before symptom onset through about day 5 of illness, but immunosuppressed adults and children shed virus for longer periods. Symptoms generally last from 7 to 14 days.

Highly pathogenic influenza A (H5N1), also called *avian influenza*, spreads rapidly among birds and has very high mortality. To date, there have been several hundred cases of influenza A (H5N1) among humans, with about 60% mortality. Influenza A (H5N1), if it acquires the ability to be highly transmissible among humans, is a threat to cause pandemic influenza. To date, there have also been several hundred cause of a novel swine-origin influenza A (H1N1) virus, which also has the potential to cause pandemic influenza.

Prevention

Influenza vaccination is between 30% and 90% effective in preventing influenza or complications of influenza. Influenza vaccination is highly cost-effective and can even be cost-saving in high-risk groups. Influenza vaccination is less effective in younger children, in adults older than 65 years, in adults with comorbid conditions, and if there is a poor match between the influenza vaccine and circulating influenza. The Centers for Disease Control and Prevention's (CDC) Advisory Committee on Immunization Practices puts out annual recommendations and supplementary updates on the prevention and treatment of influenza (www.cdc.gov/flu). At present, there are two types of influenza vaccine: the trivalent inactivated vaccine (TIV) and the live, attenuated influenza vaccine (LAIV).

The TIV (Fluzone, Fluvirin, Fluarix, FluLaval, Afluria) is administered as an intramuscular injection. The main adverse effect of the TIV is soreness at the injection site. Patients often report a mild immune response of fever, malaise, myalgia, and headache that can last for 1 to 2 days, but rates of most of these symptoms are no different from those who receive placebo injection. The TIV should not be administered to patients with egg allergies. Allergic reactions to egg proteins or other vaccine components (e.g., antibiotics and inactivating compounds) include angioedema, hives, asthma, and anaphylaxis. Vaccination should be deferred in patients with acute febrile illness, but patients with more moderate illness can be vaccinated. Guillain–Barré syndrome was associated with the 1976 swine flu vaccine, but there is no consistent evidence that modern influenza vaccines are associated with Guillain–Barré syndrome.

The LAIV (FluMist) is administered as a nasal spray and is approved for patients ages 2 to 49 years. The LAIV is contraindicated in children with recurrent wheezing, in patients with comorbid conditions, in pregnant women, and in family members or close contacts of severely immunosuppressed patients who require a protected environment (e.g., hematopoetic stem cell transplant recipients). The LAIV should not be administered to those with severe nasal congestion. Adverse effects of the LAIV include runny nose, nasal congestion, headache, sore throat, chills, and tiredness, although these are only slightly more common than in patients receiving placebo. Those receiving the LAIV should avoid contact with severely immunosuppressed persons for 7 days.

Patients should begin to be vaccinated in the fall when the seasonal vaccine becomes available, generally starting in October. In the event of vaccine shortages, higher-risk patients should receive priority. Patients should continue to be vaccinated until February and beyond because in the majority of recent influenza seasons, the peak has been February or later. Children 6 months to 8 years of age who have not been previously immunized against influenza should be given two doses separated by at least 4 weeks for both vaccines.

Evaluation

COMMUNITY PREVALENCE OF INFLUENZA

In caring for a patient with suspected influenza, the single most important piece of data is the community prevalence of influenza among patients with influenza-like illness. This ranges from near 0% during summer months to about 30% during a typical influenza seasonal peak. The prevalence may be higher during a particularly severe outbreak. Clinicians can check the local prevalence of influenza among patients with influenza-like illness through the CDC (www.cdc.gov/flu) and their state department of public health.

HISTORY AND PHYSICAL EXAMINATION

Beyond the local prevalence of influenza, the diagnosis of influenza rests on the patient's history. All methods of diagnosing influenza—symptom complexes, clinician judgment, and testing—generally are highly specific but have poor sensitivity. Thus, it is important to consider a diagnosis of influenza in any patient with respiratory symptoms during influenza season. Influenza is classically described as the very sudden onset of fever, headache, sore throat, myalgias, cough, and nasal symptoms. Children can also have otitis media, nausea, and vomiting. In differentiating influenza from nonspecific upper respiratory tract infections, it is most useful to consider the circulating prevalence of influenza, the abruptness of onset, and the severity of symptoms.

Certain symptom complexes have been shown in trials of antiviral treatment to strongly suggest influenza. For example, in an area with circulating influenza, the acute onset of cough and fever can have a positive predictive value as high as 85%. Similarly, several clinical trials found patients likely to have influenza while influenza was circulating if patients had symptoms for 48 hours or less, subjective fevers, or a measured temperature of at least 100.5°F, and any two symptoms of headache, cough, sore throat, or myalgias. Other studies, outside of clinical trials, have shown that clinician judgment performed as well as or better than hard-and-fast symptom complexes or rapid testing.

The physical examination in influenza primarily serves to identify the severity of influenza, complications, and worsening of underlying medical conditions. Clinicians should record vital signs and perform examinations of the ears, nose, sinuses, throat, neck, lungs, and heart for all patients suspected to have influenza.

TESTING

Rapid influenza test kits, some of which can distinguish influenza A from influenza B, can provide a point-of-care result in about 30 minutes and are available as nasopharyngeal swabs, nasal washes, and nasal aspirates. All forms of rapid testing have a sensitivity of about 70% and are more than 90% specific. Testing is likely most useful when there is an intermediate probability of influenza (e.g., a community prevalence of influenza among patients with influenza-like illness of 10%-30%), and patients have an intermediate probability of complications from influenza. If circulating prevalence of influenza is low (e.g., <10%), testing is unlikely to be positive and is not necessary. If the circulating prevalence of influenza is high (e.g., >30%), the relatively low sensitivity of rapid tests makes the risk of a false-negative test unacceptably high. In the event of a high prevalence of influenza or a high risk of complications from influenza, empiric antiviral treatment is indicated. Testing may be particularly helpful for hospitalized patients to rule out a need for antibiotics. Chest radiography, cultures, and blood tests are not routinely indicated, but they should be obtained for patients with suspected pneumonia or to identify other suspected complications.

Complications

Complications of influenza include primary complications, suppurative complications, and worsening of comorbid conditions. Primary complications of influenza include viral pneumonia, which is a feared complication and is likely a main cause of mortality in pandemic influenza. Other, less common primary complications of influenza include myositis and rhabdomyolysis, Reye's syndrome, myocarditis, pericarditis, toxic shock syndrome, and central nervous system disease (e.g., encephalitis, transverse myelitis, and aseptic meningitis). Children can have a severe course with influenza, including signs and symptoms of sepsis along with febrile seizures. Suppurative complications of influenza include bacterial pneumonia, otitis media, and sinusitis. Influenza can cause worsening of comorbid conditions like asthma, chronic obstructive pulmonary disease, congestive heart failure, and chronic kidney disease.

Chemoprophylaxis

Antiviral medications can be used to prevent influenza in patients who did not receive the influenza vaccine, cannot receive the influenza vaccine, received the vaccine in the prior 2 weeks (before reliable immunity develops) or in the event of poor matching between vaccine and circulating influenza strains (Table 1). Chemoprophylaxis should also be considered for close contacts of patients with confirmed influenza or for patients with immune deficiency who are unlikely to respond to the influenza vaccine but who are at high risk for having complications from influenza.

Amantadine (Symmetrel) and rimantadine (Flumadine) are no longer recommended for chemoprophylaxis or treatment because of a high prevalence of resistant influenza A strains. The neuraminidase inhibitors oseltamivir (Tamiflu) and zanamivir (Relenza) had been shown to be about 80% effective in preventing influenza in household contacts of persons with influenza and more than 90% effective in preventing influenza in institutional settings. However, most influenza A (H1N1) strains circulating early in the 2008–2009 influenza season were resistant to oseltamivir. Chemoprophylaxis should be taken for a minimum of 2 weeks or until 1 week after the end of an outbreak. For patients allergic to or unable to respond to the vaccine, chemoprophylaxis should be used for the duration of circulating influenza. The TIV can be given to patients receiving chemoprophylaxis. The LAIV should not be given from 2 days before to 14 days after taking an antiviral medication. Patients who receive the LAIV in this window should be revaccinated at a later date.

CURRENT DIAGNOSIS

- Influenza should be considered in any patient with respiratory symptoms between October and May in North America.
- The single most important piece of information when considering a diagnosis of influenza is the community prevalence of influenza.
- During outbreaks, sudden onset of fever and cough has a positive predictive value of about 85%.
- Rapid testing should be used when the community prevalence of influenza among patients with influenza-like illness is between 10% and 30%.

TABLE 1 Antiviral Agents for the Treatment and Prophylaxis of Influenza

Antiviral Agent	Treatment*		Prophylaxis†		Comments
	Children	Adults	Children	Adults	
Oseltamivir (Tamiflu)	Approved for children ≥1 y Dose for 5 d bid: ≤15 kg: 30 mg 16–23 kg: 45 mg 24–40 kg: 60 mg >40 kg: 75 mg	75 mg bid for 5 d	Approved for children ≥1 y Dose qd: ≤15 kg: 30 mg 16–23 kg: 45 mg 24–40 kg: 60 mg >40 kg: 75 mg	75 mg qd	Oseltamivir should only be used if predominant circulating strains are influenza A (H3N2) or influenza B or testing is positive for influenza B. For patients with creatinine clearance <30 mL/min, oseltamivir dosing should be reduced to qd for treatment and to qod for prophylaxis.
Zanamivir (Relenza)	Approved for children ≥7 y 10 mg (2 inhalations) bid for 5 d	10 mg (2 inhalations) bid for 5 d	Approved for children ≥5 y 10 mg (2 inhalations) qd	10 mg (2 inhalations) qd	

Adapted from Centers for Disease Control and Prevention: Prevention and control of influenza: Recommendations of the Advisory Committee on Immunization Practices (ACIP), 2008. MMWR 2008:57(RR-7); 1–60 and interim recommendations from the Centers for Disease Control and Prevention.
*Treatment must be started within the first 48 hours of symptoms.
†Prophylaxis should be given for at least 2 weeks or until 1 week after the end of an outbreak.

CURRENT THERAPY

- The influenza vaccine is the best means of preventing influenza. The trivalent inactivated influenza vaccine is recommended for health care workers, children aged 6 months to 4 years, all persons 50 years old and older, and patients with chronic conditions.
- The antivirals zanamivir (Relenza; for all influenza types) and oseltamivir (Tamiflu; for influenza A [H3N2] and influenza B) can be used for prophylaxis of influenza in unimmunized patients, in close contacts of infected patients, and during institutional outbreaks of influenza.
- Zanamivir (for all influenza types) and oseltamivir (for influenza A [H3N2] and influenza B) can be used to treat influenza, but they must be started within 48 hours of symptom onset.

Treatment

The influenza vaccine is the best means of reducing influenza-related morbidity and mortality, but its limitations include production problems, low vaccination rates, and the variable effectiveness of the vaccine itself. Given these limitations, there is an important role in management for influenza-specific antiviral medications (see Table 1). Antiviral medications reduce the duration of influenza symptoms by 1 to 2 days, reduce complications requiring antibiotics by 30% to 40%, might decrease hospitalizations and mortality, and are cost-effective.

Again, amantadine and rimantadine are no longer recommended for the treatment of influenza because of a high prevalence of resistant influenza A strains, and oseltamivir should not be used if the influenza strain is likely to be influenza A (H1N1). To date, swine-origin influenza A (H1N1) has been sensitive to both oseltamivir and zanamivir. Zanamivir is taken as an oral inhaled powder and is not recommended for patients with underlying lung or heart disease. Adverse effects of zanamivir include worsening of underlying lung disease and allergic reactions. Oseltamivir is taken as a capsule or oral suspension. The dose of oseltamivir should be reduced in patients with renal disease. Adverse effects of oseltamivir include nausea, vomiting, and, extremely rarely, behavioral changes.

Antibiotics are generally not necessary, but they should be prescribed to treat suppurative complications of influenza. Antitussives such as guaifenesin with codeine (Robitussin AC) help coughing patients sleep at night. β-Agonists, such as albuterol (Proventil),[1] can help patients with cough, especially if there is wheezing on examination. Analgesics and antipyretics like acetaminophen (Tylenol) and ibuprofen (Motrin) reduce fever and generally help patients feel better. Patients should be encouraged to rest and drink plenty of fluids. Patients with suspected influenza should minimize contact with others to avoid spreading the infection.

REFERENCES

Centers for Disease Control and Prevention. Prevention and control of influenza: Recommendations of the Advisory Committee on Immunization Practices (ACIP), 2008. MMWR 2008;57(RR-7):1–60.

Cooper NJ, Sutton AJ, Abrams KR, et al. Effectiveness of neuraminidase inhibitors in treatment and prevention of influenza A and B: Systematic review and meta-analyses of randomised controlled trials. BMJ 2003;326(7401):1235.

Falsey AR, Murata Y, Walsh EE. Impact of rapid diagnosis on management of adults hospitalized with influenza. Arch Intern Med 2007;167(4):354–60.

Rothberg MB, Bellantonio S, Rose DN. Management of influenza in adults older than 65 years of age: Cost-effectiveness of rapid testing and antiviral therapy. Ann Intern Med 2003;139:321–9.

Stein J, Louie J, Flanders S, et al. Performance characteristics of clinical diagnosis, a clinical decision rule, and a rapid influenza test in the detection of influenza infection in a community sample of adults. Ann Emerg Med 2005;46(5):412–9.

[1]Not FDA approved for this indication.

Leishmaniasis

Method of
Luigi Gradoni, PhD

Epidemiology

Leishmaniases are diseases caused by members of the genus *Leishmania*, protozoan parasites infecting numerous mammal species including humans. The flagellated forms (promastigotes) are transmitted by the bite of phlebotomine sand flies and multiply as aflagellated forms (amastigotes) within cells of the mononuclear phagocyte system. The diseases range over the intertropical zones of America and Africa and extend into temperate regions of Latin America, Southern Europe, and Asia. About 20 named *Leishmania* species and subspecies are pathogenic for humans, and 30 sand fly species are proven vectors. Each parasite species circulates in natural foci of infection where susceptible phlebotomines and mammals coexist. The epidemiology and clinical manifestations of the diseases are largely diverse, being usually grouped into two main entities: zoonotic leishmaniases, where domestic or wild animal reservoirs are involved in the transmission cycle and humans play a role of an accidental host, and anthroponotic leishmaniases, where humans are the sole reservoir and source of the vector's infection.

Visceral leishmaniasis (VL) is caused by *Leishmania donovani* in the Indian subcontinent and East Africa (anthroponotic entity) and by *L. infantum* (*L. chagasi*) in the Mediterranan basin, parts of Central Asia, and in Latin America (a zoonotic entity with domestic dogs acting as the main reservoir host). Several species of *Leishmania* cause cutaneous leishmaniasis (CL) or mucocutaneous (MCL) leishmaniasis. The most common are *L. major* (rural zoonotic entity) and *L. tropica* (urban anthroponotic entity) in the Old World and *L. mexicana*, *L. braziliensis*, *L. amazonensis*, *L. panamensis*, *L. guyanensis*, and *L. peruviana* (sylvatic zoonotic entities) in the New World.

Globally, 66 Old World and 22 New World countries are endemic for human leishmaniasis, with an estimated yearly incidence of 1 million to 1.5 million cases of CL forms and 500,000 cases of VL forms. Overall estimated prevalence is 12 million people with a disability-adjusted life years burden of 860,000 for men and 1.2 million for women. The disease affects the poorest people in the poorest countries: 72 are developing countries, of which 13 are among the least developed. The incidence is not uniformly distributed in endemic areas: 90% of CL cases are found in only seven countries (Afghanistan, Algeria, Brazil, Iran, Peru, Saudi Arabia, and Syria), whereas 90% of VL cases occur in rural and suburban areas of five countries (Bangladesh, India, Nepal, Sudan, and Brazil). These figures, however, must be regarded as underestimates; currently, it appears that the global incidence of human leishmaniases is higher than before, owing to environmental and human behavioral factors contributing to the changing landscape of these diseases.

Risk Factors

Risk factors for leishmaniasis are primarily associated with geographically and temporally defined human exposure to phlebotomine vectors. In the Old World, colonization and urbanization of desert areas have been identified as the major risk factor for outbreaks of zoonotic CL. Tourists and military forces are often exposed to *L. major* or *L. tropica* infections in rural or urban endemic settings of North African and Middle East countries. In the New World, the colonization of the primary forest associated with activities of deforestation, road building, mining, and tourism is responsible for the domestication of sylvatic cycles of CL and MCL agents. Increase in density and geographic range of phlebotomine vectors resulting from climate changes, together with the increased mobility of infected pet dogs, have been identified as a cause of northward spreading of zoonotic VL in Europe.

Individual risk factors play a major role in VL disease. Most of the *L. donovani* and *L. infantum* infections are asymptomatic or subclinical in well-nourished immunocompetent persons. Malnourished persons, infants younger than 2 years, and severely immunosuppressed adults are at high risk for acute VL when exposed to infection. Before the era of HAART (highly active antiretroviral therapy), the AIDS epidemics in southern Europe caused more than 2000 HIV and VL co-infection cases among men aged 39 years on average. Other conditions have been reported that influence the clinical outcome of VL, such as immunosuppressive therapies following organ transplantation, corticosteroid and anti–tumor necrosis factor α (TNF-α) treatments for immunologic disorders, hematologic neoplasia, and chronic conditions of hepatic cirrhosis. However, most of acute VL episodes in adults remain unexplained. Other factors associated with impaired immune response to *Leishmania* (e.g., genetic factors) are probably involved.

Pathophysiology

Ingestion of metacyclic promastigotes inoculated by the vector in the skin is mediated by several types of receptors found in resident macrophages, monocytes, neutrophils, and dendritic cells. *Leishmania* lipophosphoglycan, the most abundant surface glycoconjugate, is the main factor of virulence. Once in the cell phagolysosome, amastigotes survive from hydrolase activity through pH acidification while selectively inhibiting production of reactive oxygen species. Multiplication of parasites, infection of new cells, and dissemination to tissues are contrasted by the host's inflammatory and specific immune responses. Even in most susceptible natural mammal hosts, the majority of infections are efficiently controlled, giving rise to asymptomatic latent infections. Leishmaniases have typical immunological polarity: Cure or control are associated with robust cellular immune responses driven by production of interleukin (IL) 12, whereas acute or chronic diseases are characterized by the absence of such responses and the presence of high levels of nonprotective serum antibodies, a condition often associated with high levels of IL-10 production. In spite of this polarity, analysis of cytokine patterns in tissues reveals a less-polar situation, as both T_H1 and T_H2 cytokines were found to be secreted in specimens from tissues infected with CL, MCL, and VL.

Prevention

There are no human vaccines available for the immune protection against leishmaniasis. Promising data on safety and immunogenicity have been provided for the only *Leishmania* candidate vaccine under development, consisting of the recombinant polyprotein antigen LEISH-F1 with MPL-SE as adjuvant. Preventive measures are thus limited to the individual protection from sand fly bites or to community protection through reservoir control. Individual protection is through the use of repellents or insecticide-impregnated nets. Reservoir control measures are largely diverse depending on the epidemiologic entity of leishmaniasis. Examples related to zoonotic entities with synanthropic reservoir hosts are the destruction of rodent populations around human dwellings (e.g., to control zoonotic CL due to *L. major*) and the fight against canine infections through the mass use of topical insecticides or drug treatments (e.g., to control zoonotic VL due to *L. infantum*). Early diagnosis and treatment of human cases is the main control measure against anthroponotic entities of VL (*L. donovani*) and CL (*L. tropica*).

Clinical Manifestations

VISCERAL DISEASE

VL, also known as kala-azar, results from the multiplication of *Leishmania* in the phagocytes of the reticuloendothelial system. In endemic settings, the ratio of incident asymptomatic infections to incident clinical cases varies from 4:1 to 50:1 depending on the epidemiologic type (anthroponotic VL is normally more virulent) and the poverty of the affected country. Classic VL manifests as pallor, fever, and hard splenomegaly; hepatomegaly is less common. Laboratory findings document pancytopenia and hypergammaglobulinemia. The clinical incubation period ranges from 3 weeks (exceptional) to more than 2 years, but 4 to 6 months is average. Patients report a history of fever resistant to antibiotics; on physical examination, the spleen is typically appreciated 5 to 15 cm below the left costal margin. Symptomatic VL is 100% fatal when left untreated.

CUTANEOUS DISEASE

CL results from multiplication of *Leishmania* in the phagocytes of the skin. In the classic course of the disease, lesions appear first as papules, advance slowly to nodules or ulcers, and then spontaneously heal with scarring over months to years. The clinical incubation period ranges from 1 week (exceptional) to several months; lesions caused by *L. major* and *L. mexicana* tend to evolve and resolve quickly, whereas those caused by *L. braziliensis*, *L. tropica*, and dermotropic strains of *L. infantum* can have longer periods of incubation and spontaneous healing.

MUCOSAL DISEASE

MCL results from parasitic metastasis in the nasal mucosal that eventually extends to the oropharynx and larynx. It can develop from CL lesions caused by *L. braziliensis* and *L. panamensis*. Typically, MCL evolves slowly (3 years on average) and does not heal spontaneously.

Diagnosis

The standard diagnosis method for all forms of leishmaniasis is still the microscopy demonstration of *Leishmania* organisms in Giemsa-stained impression smears or cultures from samples of infected tissues. In general, sensitivity increases when both staining and culture are performed. Polymerase chain reaction (PCR) detection of *Leishmania* DNA on samples further increases the diagnostic sensitivity and also might allow species identification by target DNA sequencing or restriction fragment length polymorphism analysis.

Different tissue samplings must be performed depending on the clinical form of leishmaniasis. For VL, aspirate or biopsy specimens are obtained from spleen, bone marrow, the liver, or enlarged lymph nodes. Higher diagnostic yields are obtained with spleen aspirates (more than 98%), although bone marrow aspirates (80% to 98% of yield) are usually preferred. For CL and MCL, material is obtained by scraping tissue juice from a nodular lesion or from the edge of an ulcer or by taking punch biopsies of inflamed tissue. Diagnostic yields of about 80% are obtained with impression smears and cultures during the first half of the natural course of the lesion. After that, standard parasitologic diagnosis becomes more difficult and PCR remains the only reliable method.

Serology is useful when the diagnosis of VL proves difficult with other methods. Commercially available dipstick tests using recombinant antigen K39 can be employed in decisions for or against treatment. Negative serology results are common in CL and MCL, as well as in VL when patients are severely immunosuppressed.

 CURRENT DIAGNOSIS

- Infected tissues must be sampled for microscopy demonstration of *Leishmania* organisms in Giemsa-stained impression smears or cultures. Polymerase chain reaction (PCR) detection of *Leishmania* DNA increases diagnostic sensitivity.
- Different tissue samplings are performed depending on the clinical form of leishmaniasis: For visceral leishmaniasis, aspirate or biopsy specimens are obtained from spleen, bone marrow, the liver, or enlarged lymph nodes. For cutaneous and mucocutaneous leishmaniasis the material is obtained by skin lesion scraping or biopsy.
- Serology is useful when the diagnosis of visceral leishmaniasis proves difficult with other methods.

Differential Diagnosis

VISCERAL DISEASE

The differential diagnosis depends on the local disease pattern associated with endemic areas. In many of them it includes chronic malaria, disseminated histoplasmosis, hepatosplenic schistosomiasis, typhoid fever, brucellosis, tuberculosis, endocarditis, relapsing fever, and African trypanosomiasis. Other cosmopolitan diseases include syphilis, lymphomas, chronic myeloid leukemia, sarcoidosis, malignant histiocytosis, and liver cirrhosis.

CUTANEOUS DISEASE

A typical history of CL—an inflammatory, slowly developing, and painless skin lesion associated with recent exposure to sand fly bites—can strongly support a clinical diagnosis of disease. However, there is an extensive differential diagnosis, which includes acute or chronic forms of CL. For the former, insect bites, furuncular myiasis, and bacterial tropical ulcers are the most common; for the latter, keloid, lupus vulgaris, discoid lupus erythematosus, and sarcoidosis.

Treatment

The therapy of leishmaniasis relies on a limited number of drugs, most of which are old and relatively toxic compounds. Systemic drug administration requires hospitalizing and monitoring the patient.

 CURRENT THERAPY

- The therapy of leishmaniasis relies on a limited number of drugs, most of which are old and relatively toxic. Systemic drug administration requires hospitalization and monitoring of the patient.
- The pentavalent antimony (Sb) drugs sodium stibogluconate (Pentostam)[10] and meglumine antimoniate (Glucantime)[2] are equivalent and used in all clinical forms of leishmaniasis. Dosage is Sb 20 mg/kg/day IM for 21 to 28 days. In cases of uncomplicated cutaneous leishmaniasis, use intralesional administration intermittently over 20 to 30 days.
- Liposomal amphotericin B (Ambisome) is the gold standard for treating visceral leishmaniasis. Dosage: Total dose of 18 to 21 mg/kg IV using one of the following schedules: 3 mg/kg/day on days 1 to 5 and 10; 3 mg/kg on days 1 to 5, day 14, and day 21; 10 mg/kg/day for 2 days.
- Amphotericin B desoxycholate (Fungizone) is used in visceral leishmanaisis[1] and mucocutaneous leishmaniasis. Dosage is 0.5 mg/kg IV every other day for 14 days.
- Other parenteral drugs: Pentamidine isethionate (Pentam 300)[1] is used to treat some forms of New World cutaneous leishmaniasis; dosage is 2 mg/kg IM every other day for 7 days. Paromomycin (aminosidine) sulfate[2] is used for Indian visceral leishmanaisis; dosage is 11 mg/kg/day IM for 21 days.
- Miltefosine (Impavido)[5] is recommended for visceral leishmaniasis therapy in India and Ethiopia and for cutaneous leishmaniasis therapy in Colombia and Bolivia. Dosage is 2.5 mg/kg/day (not exceeding 100 mg/day) PO for 28 days.

---

[1]Not FDA approved for this indication.
[2]Not available in the United States.
[5]Investigational drug in the United States.
[10]Available in the United States from the Centers for Disease Control and Prevention.

PENTAVALENT ANTIMONIALS

Organic salts of pentavalent antimony (Sb) are still the mainstay therapy for all clinical forms of leishmaniasis. Two preparations are available that are equal in efficacy and toxicity when used in equivalent Sb doses: sodium stibogluconate (Pentostam),[10] available in English-speaking countries, and meglumine antimoniate (Glucantime)[2] available in Southern Europe and Latin America. The recommended dosage of Sb is 20 mg/kg/day for 21 to 28 days, given intramuscularly or intravenously. Treatment should be prolonged for 40 to 60 days in areas with documented Sb-resistant VL (e.g., in Bihar State, India). The drugs can be administered intralesionally in cases of uncomplicated CL, intermittently over 20 to 30 days. Systemic toxicity caused by the antimonials relates to the total dose administered and includes anorexia, pancreatitis, and changes on electrocardiography (e.g., prolongation of the Q-T interval), which can precede dangerous arrhythmias.

AMPHOTERICIN B DRUGS

Liposomal amphotericin B (Ambisome) is the current gold standard for VL treatment, being highly effective and nontoxic. However the high cost of the drug precludes its use in developing countries where leishmaniasis is endemic. Liposomal amphotericin B is given intravenously at the total dose of 18 to 21 mg/kg, with various treatment schedules similarly effective: 3 mg/kg/day on days 1 to 5 and 10; 3 mg/kg on days 1 to 5, 14 and 21; or 10 mg/kg/day for 2 days.

Amphotericin B desoxycholate (Fungizone) is a relatively toxic compound used in Sb-resistant VL[1] and MCL, administered intravenously at the low dosage of 0.5 mg/kg every other day for 14 days. Doses in excess of 1 mg/kg/day commonly result in severe infusion-related side effects (fever, chills, and bone pain) and delayed side effects (toxic renal effects).

OTHER PARENTERAL DRUGS

Other parenteral drugs include old second-line drugs whose use is limited. Pentamidine isethionate (Pentam 300)[1] is a toxic compound used to treat some forms of New World CL resistant to Sb therapy and is given intramuscularly at the low dose of 2 mg/kg every other day for 7 days. Treatment in excess of this dosage can result in common side effects such as myalgias, nausea, headache, and hypoglycemia. Paromomycin (aminosidine) sulfate injection[2] (manufactured by Gland Pharma, India, on behalf of Institute of One World Health) is an old aminoglycoside that is being reevaluated as a first-line drug for Indian VL. It is given intramuscularly at the dose of 11 mg base per kg per day for 21 days. Elevation of alanine aminotranferease (ALT) and aspartate aminotransferase (AST) liver enzymes is usually seen during therapy.

MILTEFOSINE, THE FIRST ORAL DRUG FOR LEISHMANIASIS

Miltefosine (Impavido)[5] is a hexadecylphosphocholine originally developed as an anticancer agent. It is the first recognized oral treatment for leishmaniasis and is available in Germany and India. So far, it is recommended for VL therapy in India and Ethiopia and for CL therapy in Colombia and Bolivia. The drug is administered at 2.5 mg/kg/day (not exceeding 100 mg/day) for 28 days. Miltefosine administration does not require the patient to be hospitalized for monitoring. Mild gastrointestinal toxicity may be common. The drug is contraindicated in pregnancy.

---

[1]Not FDA approved for this indication.
[2]Not available in the United States.
[5]Investigational drug in the United States.
[10]Available in the United States from the Centers for Disease Control and Prevention.

Monitoring

In VL patients, fever recedes by day 3 to 5 of treatment, and well-being returns by the first week. Hematologic indices start to improve during the second week. Hemoglobin, serum albumin, and body weight are the most useful indicators of progress. The spleen tends to normalize 1 to 2 months after the end of therapy, although it can take up to 1 year to regress completely. Parasitologic assessment of cure is not normally necessary. Relapses can occur after apparent clinical cure from 2 to 8 months after treatment has been discontinued.

In CL patients, clinical response to drugs is rapid, but complete reepithelialization of lesions is observed in only one third of patients by the end of 3- to 4-week treatment courses.

REFERENCES

Alvar J, Aparicio P, Aseffa A, et al. The relationship between leishmaniasis and AIDS: The second 10 years. Clin Microbiol Rev 2008;21:334–59.

Berman JJ. Treatment of leishmaniasis with miltefosine: 2008 status. Expert Opin Drug Metab Toxicol 2008;4:1209–16.

Bern C, Adler-Moore J, Berenguer J, et al. Liposomal amphotericin B for the treatment of visceral leishmaniasis. Clin Infect Dis 2006;43:917–24.

Bhattacharya SK, Sinha PK, Sundar S, et al. Phase 4 trial of miltefosine for the treatment of Indian visceral leishmaniasis. J Infect Dis 2007;196:591–668.

Chappuis F, Sundar S, Hailu A, et al. Visceral leishmaniasis: what are the needs for diagnosis, treatment and control? Nat Rev Microbiol 2007;5:873–82.

González U, Pinart M, Rengifo-Pardo M, et al. Interventions for cutaneous and mucocutaneous leishmaniasis. Cochrane Database Syst Rev 2009;(2): CD004834 .

Gradoni L, Soteriadou K, Louzir H, et al. Drug regimens for visceral leishmaniasis in Mediterranean countries. Trop Med Int Health 2008;13:1272.

Gramiccia M, Gradoni L. The current status of zoonotic leishmaniases and approaches to disease control. Int J Parasitol 2005;35:1169–80.

Sundar S, Agrawal N, Arora R, et al. Short-course paromomycin treatment of visceral leishmaniasis in India: 14-day vs 21-day treatment. Clin Infect Dis 2009;49:914–8.

Leprosy

Method of
Bhushan Kumar, MD, MNAMS, and Sunil Dogra, MD, DNB, MNAMS

Leprosy is a chronic, very mildly infectious disease of the skin and peripheral nerves caused by *Mycobacterium leprae*. The first historical descriptions of leprosy came from India in about 600 BC when it was called *kushta*. Leprosy is also known as *Hansen's disease* after the demonstration of *M. leprae* by Gerhard Armauer Hansen in 1873. The damage to peripheral nerves results in sensory and motor impairment with the characteristic hideous deformities and disabilities so deeply associated with the disease. Leprosy was once widely distributed in Europe and Asia but now occurs mainly in resource-poor countries in tropical and warm temperate regions. Stigma remains a major obstacle to leprosy control, despite advances in bacteriology, chemotherapy, and epidemiology.

Epidemiology

After the successful implementation of and subsequently very encouraging results reported with multidrug therapy (MDT), a highly effective treatment regimen, in 1991 the World Health Assembly developed the global strategy for eliminating leprosy as a public health problem by 2000. The goal to reduce the prevalence of leprosy to less than one case per 10,000 population at the global level by 2000 was achieved; however, pockets of high endemicity still remain in some areas of Angola, Brazil, the Central African Republic, the Democratic Republic of the Congo, India, Madagascar, Mozambique, Nepal and the United Republic of Tanzania. There were 213,036 registered prevalent cases at the beginning of 2009; 249,007 cases were detected in 2008. The number of new cases detected globally has fallen by 9126 (a 4% decrease) during 2008 compared with 2007.

Major achievements of the leprosy elimination strategy have included achieving elimination in 119 of 122 countries where the disease was considered a public health problem in 1985. (including cure of more than 18 million patients), free supply of MDT drugs, increased coverage of leprosy services, and integration of the leprosy elimination strategy within general health services.

However, reaching a prevalence level of less than one per 10,000 population is not the end of leprosy or leprosy work. The new challenge is to build on the success of the leprosy campaign and deliver sustainable care for leprosy patients who have been treated successfully or who are likely to trickle in because of the long incubation of the disease.

Etiopathogenesis

Modern-day leprosy dates from 1873 following the discovery of *M. leprae* (the first bacillus to be associated with a human disease). *M. leprae* is an acid- and alcohol-fast, gram-positive, obligate intracellular, noncultivable bacterium, which has been successfully inoculated and has multiplied in the nine-banded armadillo and nude mouse.

The principal means of transmission of *M. leprae* is probably through nasal or respiratory mucosa and skin-to-skin transmission in contacts of heavily infected multibacillary (MB) patients. The incubation period varies widely from months to 30 years, and the average time is usually 5 to 7 years. Apart from humans, nine-banded armadillos and, very rarely, sooty mangabey monkeys are the only known reservoir of infection.

More than 95% of adults are resistant to the infection. Subclinical infections occur more commonly in endemic areas, but clinical disease manifests in only a small fraction having specific impairment of cell-mediated immunity (CMI) to *M. leprae*.

The disease presents a broad spectrum of clinical and histopathologic manifestations ranging from bacteriologically scanty tuberculoid to highly bacilliferous lepromatous leprosy. The clinicopathologic bipolarity stems from the immunologic status, which guides the dual response of monocytes and macrophages to *M. leprae*. In cases located at the tuberculoid pole, these cells can destroy and eliminate all the bacilli; in cases near the lepromatous pole, the bacilli proliferate and persist in these cells and can be also partially killed simultaneously.

Clinical Features

The clinical features of leprosy reflect the pathology, which in turn depends on the balance between bacillary multiplication and the host cell–mediated immune response (Table 1). Leprosy affects skin and nerves and produces systemic involvement in lepromatous disease. Patients commonly present with skin lesions, weakness or numbness caused by involvement of a peripheral nerve trunk, deformities, resorption of fingers and toes, or a burn or ulcer in an anesthetic hand or foot. Sometimes patients present with nerve pain, sudden palsy, new skin lesions, painful red eye, or a systemic febrile illness.

Inspection of the whole body in good light is important because otherwise lesions with faint erythema or slight hypopigmentation (more often on covered areas in borderline disease) might be missed. Skin lesions should be examined for hypoesthesia to light touch and temperature and for anhidrosis.

The morbidity and disability associated with leprosy are secondary to nerve damage. About 25% of leprosy patients have some degree of disability, which is greatest in patients with BL and LL disease. Early recognition and treatment are crucial to prevention of deformities.

Systemic Involvement

Features of systemic involvement occur usually in longstanding disease and are mainly seen in patients near the lepromatous pole because of bacillary infiltration and the associated granulomatous infiltration that affects various organs, especially the nasal mucosa, eyes, bones, testes, kidneys, lymph nodes, liver, and spleen. Besides the disease, systemic manifestations in the form of such constitutional symptoms as fever, malaise, joint pains, and acute inflammation of eyes, joints, and the reticuloendothelial system (among others) can occur as a part of a type 2 lepra reaction.

Diagnosis

CLINICAL DIAGNOSIS

The diagnosis and classification of leprosy have been based on clinical features and skin smears when facilities are available. Clinical diagnosis of leprosy is based on patients having one or more of the three cardinal signs. The cardinal signs are hypopigmented or erythematous skin lesion(s), with definite loss of or impairment of sensations; involvement of the peripheral nerves, as demonstrated by definite thickening, with sensory impairment; and skin smear positive for AFB.

LABORATORY DIAGNOSIS

Laboratory diagnostic tests such as slit skin smears, histologic examination of involved tissues, serology, and polymerase chain reaction (PCR) studies have been confined to areas where such facilities are available and in academic and research centers.

Slit Skin Smears

The diagnostic specificity of skin smears is almost 100%; however, the sensitivity is rarely more than 50% because smear-positive patients represent only 10% to 50% of cases. The inherent problems of skin smears are the logistics and the reliability of the technique of taking, staining, and interpreting the smears. Skin smears help identify patients with MB disease and patients who are experiencing clinical relapse.

Skin Biopsies

The biopsy helps to confirm the clinical diagnosis and classification of disease, but it cannot be regarded as the diagnostic gold standard because a number of the histologic features can be nondiagnostic or doubtful. In practice, a clinical and histopathologic correlation may be necessary for resolving a diagnostic difficulty.

Serology and Polymerase Chain Reaction

Serology and PCR are rarely used in endemic countries because of their limited availability and lack of uniform diagnostic values across the disease spectrum. The basis of serologic tests is to determine the presence of anti-phenolic glycolipid-1 (PGL-1) antibodies by the *M. leprae* particle agglutination assay (MLPA) and the enzyme-linked immunosorbent assay (ELISA) techniques. The PGL-1 antibody test is specific and more sensitive in patients with MB disease, but unfortunately it is not very helpful in the diagnosis of paucibacillary (PB) disease, and it has low predictive value for diagnosis of early disease. Antibodies to the 35-kD protein of *M. leprae* have been studied for their role in diagnosis of disease with comparable results. PCR for detection of *M. leprae* DNA encoding specific genes is highly sensitive and specific, because it detects *M. leprae* DNA in 95% of MB and 55% of PB patients. Currently, PCR is not used in routine clinical practice.

Lepromin Test

The lepromin test is not a diagnostic test, but it is helpful for identifying the level of CMI against *M. leprae* in a given patient. It is a nonspecific test of some value in classifying a case of leprosy. It is

CURRENT DIAGNOSIS

A case of leprosy is diagnosed in the presence of one or more of the following cardinal signs and who has yet to complete a full course of treatment:
- Hypopigmented or erythematous skin lesion(s) with definite loss or impairment of sensations
- Involvement of the peripheral nerves, as demonstrated by definite thickening with sensory impairment
- Skin smear positive for acid-fast bacilli

strongly positive in TT; weakly positive in BT; negative in BB, BL, and LL; and unpredictable in indeterminate leprosy. Lepromin (lepromin A, 160 million bacilli/mL) 0.1 mL is injected intradermally, and the reaction is read at 48 hours (Fernandez reaction) and at 3 to 4 weeks (Mitsuda reaction). Neither test is diagnostic, because both may be positive in persons with no evidence of leprosy. However, close contacts of an MB patient who have negative lepromin tests have a greater risk of developing disease.

Classification Of Disease

Ridley and Jopling (1966) defined five groups on the basis of clinical, bacteriologic, histologic, and immunologic features. These groups are tuberculoid, borderline tuberculoid, midborderline (borderline borderline), borderline lepromatous, and lepromatous leprosy. This is a very useful classification for research purposes, but it is often not feasible in field conditions and primary health centers. This classification does not include the indeterminate and pure neuritic type of leprosy. In general, PB disease is equivalent to indeterminate, tuberculoid, and BT leprosy, and MB disease is equated with BB, BL, and LL disease.

In 1998, the WHO Expert Committee on Leprosy declared skin-slit smears as not essential for institution of MDT. This was necessitated by the unavailability or unreliability of technical expertise for the skin smear in many leprosy-control programs and the potential for transmitting HIV and hepatitis by nonsterile techniques.

Recently, for field workers, WHO has classified leprosy based on the number of skin lesions for treatment purposes. PB leprosy is leprosy with one to five skin lesions. MB leprosy includes more than five skin lesions. If facilities are available, any patient with a positive slit-skin smear should be considered to have MB leprosy.

Rare Variants

Lucio Leprosy

Lucio leprosy (LuLp) is a diffuse form of LL. It is common in Mexico and Costa Rica and less common in the Gulf Coast, but it is quite rare in the rest of the world. It manifests as slowly progressive, diffuse, shiny infiltration of skin of the face and most of the body (*lepra bonita*, "beautiful leprosy"). There is loss of eyebrows, hoarseness of voice, and numbness and edema of hands and feet that mimic myxedema. This form of the disease is liable to the most severe of all reactional states, the Lucio phenomenon, in which destructive vasculitis leads to skin necrosis and ulcers.

Pure Neuritic Leprosy

Pure neuritic leprosy is characterized in the absence of any skin patch by an area of sensory loss along the distribution of a thickened nerve trunk with or without motor deficit. This form is seen most often, but not exclusively, in India and Nepal, where it accounts for 5% to 10% of leprosy cases. Histology of a cutaneous nerve might reveal an infiltrate that is characteristic of any type of leprosy.

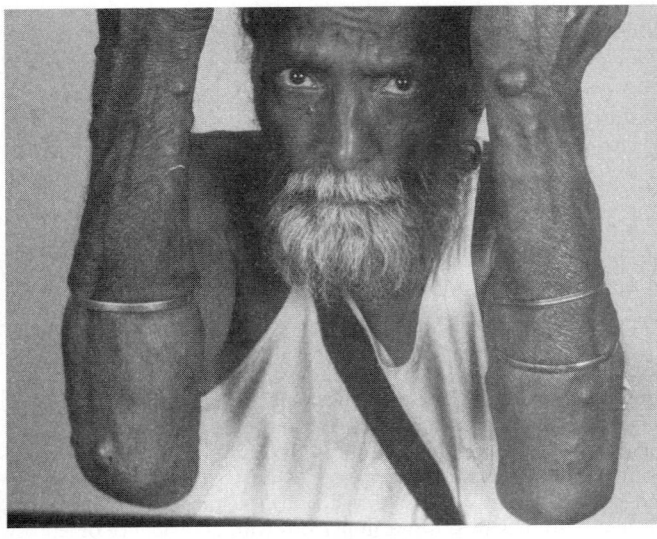

FIGURE 7. Histoid leprosy.

Histoid Leprosy

Histoid leprosy, first described in 1960, is now a well-recognized but rarely reported entity. Controversy still remains whether to consider histoid leprosy as a separate entity. It usually occurs in patients who had received irregular or inadequate treatment or dapsone monotherapy or as a spectrum under lepromatous leprosy. It manifests as superficially or deeply fixed cutaneous nodules, plaques, or pads (Figure 7). In a given patient, the number of lesions can vary from a few to a hundred. Histopathologically, the striking feature is predominance of spindle-shaped cells and unusually large numbers of AFB.

Treatment

The concept of chemotherapy for leprosy has undergone a phenomenal change over the last two decades. The WHO MDT has been successful in eliminating leprosy in many countries. However, the search for new drugs and new drug regimens continues. The goals of advanced therapy include improved patient compliance, alternative agents against clofazimine- and rifampin-resistant bacilli, more efficient killing of persistent bacteria, uniform MDT for all types of leprosy, and supervised short regimens for preventing drug resistance.

WHO MULTIDRUG THERAPY

The MDT introduced in 1982 has proved to be the most effective tool in controlling leprosy. More than 18 million patients have been cured of the disease, with acceptable cumulative relapse rates of 0.77% for MB and 1.07% for PB disease. MDT as recommended by WHO remains the current and most accepted treatment by all countries with endemic leprosy. A single dose of rifampin (Rifadin)[1] 600 mg plus ofloxacin (Floxin)[1] 400 mg and minocycline (Minocin)[1] 100 mg (ROM therapy) is an acceptable and cost-effective alternative regimen for PB leprosy with one skin lesion, although most still favor the conventional WHO MDT PB regimen.

OTHER REGIMENS FOR SPECIAL SITUATIONS

Drug Substitutions

For adult MB patients who cannot take rifampin, the Seventh WHO Expert Committee on Leprosy recommended daily administration of 50 mg of clofazimine (Lamprene), together with two of the following

---

[1]Not FDA approved for this indication.

 CURRENT THERAPY

Multidrug Therapy Regimen for Paucibacillary Leprosy (6 months)

ADULT (50–70 KG)

- Dapsone: 100 mg daily
- Rifampin (Rifadin)[1]: 600 mg once a mo under supervision

CHILD (10–14 Y)

- Dapsone: 50 mg daily
- Rifampin: 450 mg once a mo under supervision

Adjust dose appropriately for a child younger than 10 y. For example, dapsone 25 mg daily and rifampicin 300 mg given once a mo under supervision.

Multidrug Therapy Regimen for Multibacillary Leprosy (12 months)

ADULT (50–70 KG)

- Dapsone: 100 mg daily
- Rifampin:[1] 600 mg once a mo under supervision
- Clofazimine (Lamprene): 50 mg daily and 300 mg once a mo under supervision

CHILD (10–14 Y)

- Dapsone: 50 mg daily
- Rifampin[1]: 450 mg once a mo under supervision
- Clofazimine: 50 mg daily and 150 mg once a mo under supervision

Adjust dose appropriately for a child less than 10 y. For example, dapsone 25 mg daily and rifampin 300 mg given once a mo under supervision, clofazimine 50 mg given twice a wk, and clofazimine 100 mg given once a mo under supervision.

---

[1]Not FDA approved for this indication.

---

three drugs: 400 mg ofloxacin,[1] 100 mg minocycline,[1] or 500 mg clarithromycin (Biaxin)[1] once daily for 6 months, followed by daily administration of 50 mg clofazimine plus 100 mg minocycline or 400 mg ofloxacin for at least an additional 18 months. For MB patients who cannot take clofazimine, it should be replaced with ofloxacin 400 mg daily or minocycline 100 mg daily. Alternatively, the patient may be treated with a monthly administration of a combination consisting of rifampin[1] 600 mg, ofloxacin 400 mg, and minocycline 100 mg (ROM therapy) for 24 months. MB patients who cannot tolerate dapsone should receive only daily clofazimine with no substitution; in PB cases dapsone should be replaced with clofazimine.

Accompanied Multidrug Therapy

Accompanied MDT (A-MDT) recommended by WHO is an essential element of the "flexible and patient friendly MDT delivery system" suitable to migrant populations, patients living in remote areas, and patients living in areas of civil war. In this policy, the patient is provided the entire supply of MDT drugs at the time of diagnosis: 6 months of medication for a PB patient and 12 months for an MB patient, while asking "someone close or important to the patient" to assume the responsibility of helping the patient complete the full course of treatment. However, poor adherence to self-administration of treatment, a common phenomenon in tuberculosis and leprosy patients, and the associated risk of drug resistance and relapses are to be expected.

---

[1]Not FDA approved for this indication.

Pregnancy and Lactation

Leprosy is exacerbated during pregnancy, so it is important that the standard multidrug therapy be continued during pregnancy. The standard MDT regimens are safe, both for the mother and the child, and therefore should be continued unchanged during pregnancy and lactation.

Concomitant Active Tuberculosis

If the patient has both leprosy and active tuberculosis, it is necessary to treat both infections at the same time. Give appropriate antituberculosis therapy in addition to the MDT appropriate to the type of leprosy. Rifampin is common to both regimens, and it must be given in the doses required for tuberculosis.

Concomitant HIV Infection

The management of a leprosy patient infected with HIV is the same as that of any other leprosy patient without infection with HIV.

NEWER DRUGS

A few new drugs are available to complement or replace the currently used MDT (Box 1). The objective of the new drugs is not to induce quick clinical regression but to minimize relapses or to address special situations like drug resistance or drug intolerance. Promising bactericidal activity of ofloxacin,[1] clarithromycin,[1] and minocycline[1] against *M. leprae* has been demonstrated in the mouse foot-pad system and then confirmed in clinical trials. Strong bactericidal effects against *M. leprae* of moxifloxacin (Avelox),[1] rifapentine (Priftin),[1] and other derivatives have been identified in *in vitro* studies. However, no precise recommendation of their use is available yet.

Reactions

During the course of leprosy, immunologically mediated episodes of acute or subacute inflammation known as *reactions* can occur. Most reactions belong to one of the two major types; reversal reaction (RR or type 1) or erythema nodosum leprosum (ENL or type 2). Reversal reactions can occur throughout the spectrum of leprosy but are more

---

[1]Not FDA approved for this indication.

| BOX 1 | Newer Drugs and Alternative Drugs |

Quinolones
- Clinafloxacin[5]
- Moxifloxacin (Avelox)[1]
- Ofloxacin (Floxin)[1]
- Pefloxacin (Pefocin)[2]
- Sparfloxacin (Zagam)[2]
- Temafloxacin (Omniflox)[2]

Macrolides
- Clarithromycin (Biaxin)[1]

Tetracyclines
- Minocycline (Minocin)[1]

Ansamycins
- KRM-1648[5]
- KRM-1657[5]
- KRM-1668[5]
- Rifabutin (Mycobutin)[1]
- Rifapentine (Priftin)[1]

---

[1]Not FDA approved for this indication.
[2]Not available in the United States.
[5]Investigational drug in the United States.

---

common in patients with borderline leprosy. On the other hand, ENL occurs exclusively in patients with MB disease, especially lepromatous and borderline lepromatous leprosy. Reactions can be disastrous; they cause acute nerve damage resulting in deformities. Almost 30% of MB patients develop reactions during the course of their disease. Reactions may be seen at presentation, during treatment, and even after treatment.

The principles of treatment of reactions are to control the acute inflammation in skin and nerves, ease the pain, halt eye damage, and prevent spread of the disease. Standard antileprosy chemotherapy should be started or continued along with antireaction treatment. Clinical evidence of ongoing neuritis (nerve tenderness, new anesthesia, motor loss) should be carefully sought and, if neuritis is present, corticosteroid treatment should be started immediately.

TYPE 1 REACTIONS

The type 1 reaction is a type IV hypersensitivity (delayed-type hypersensitivity) reaction, and it typically occurs in borderline disease. It is characterized by acutely inflamed skin lesions or acute neuritis, or both. Existing skin lesions become erythematous or edematous and can desquamate or, rarely, ulcerate. Often, new small lesions also appear at distant sites (Figure 8). Occasionally, edema of face, hands, or feet is the presenting symptom; however, constitutional symptoms are unusual. Although type 1 reactions can occur spontaneously and at any time during the course of the disease, the usual times are after starting treatment and during the puerperium.

Because of the high risk of permanent damage to peripheral nerve trunks, RR needs to be diagnosed as soon as possible and managed adequately. The drug of choice is prednisolone (Delta-Cortef). The usual course begins with 40 to 60 mg daily (up to a maximum of 1 mg/kg), gradually reducing the dose weekly or biweekly and eventually stopping in about 12 weeks. Early neural impairment (usually up to 6 months' duration) may be helped by systemic corticosteroid therapy tapered over a period of 4 to 6 months. Adverse effects associated with long-term corticosteroid therapy must be kept in mind.

TYPE 2 REACTIONS

The type 2 reaction, a type III hypersensitivity reaction (immune-complex mediated) occurs in patients with LL and BL disease. Attacks are often acute in onset but can become chronic or recur over several years. ENL typically manifests as painful, red evanescent nodules on the face and extensor surfaces of the limbs. Rarely, they appear as bullous, pustular, necrotic forms. ENL is often accompanied by systemic symptoms producing fever and malaise, and in severe form it may be complicated by uveitis, dactylitis, arthritis, neuritis, lymphadenitis, myositis, and orchitis.

Acute or subacute neuritis with or without nerve function impairment is one of the major criteria for distinguishing mild and severe ENL. The treatment of ENL should start with general measures as in type 1 reaction. Mild ENL can be treated with analgesics like

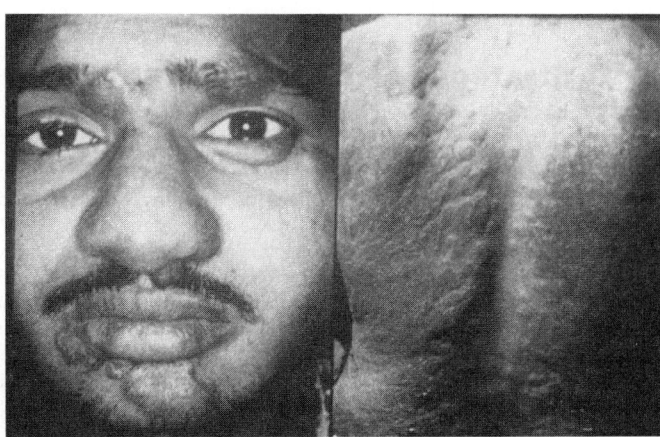

FIGURE 8. Borderline tuberculoid leprosy with type 1 reaction.

aspirin. In moderate and severe ENL, corticosteroids or thalidomide (Thalomid) are more useful and may be life saving. Thalidomide (100 mg q8h) has a dramatic effect in controlling ENL, and it may be useful in preventing recurrent ENL, but its teratogenic effects preclude its use in women of childbearing age. Clofazimine (Lamprene) has a useful anti-inflammatory effect in ENL and can be used at a dose of 300 mg daily in divided doses as an adjuvant to prednisolone and tapered over several months. Injectable antimonials are often used by Indian leprologists.

LUCIO'S PHENOMENON

The Lucio phenomenon occurs only in patients with Lucio leprosy. It results from infarction consequent on deep cutaneous vasculitis, causing the appearance of irregularly shaped erythematous patches. The patches sometimes darken and heal, but sometimes they form bullae that necrose, leaving deep, painful ulcers that are slow to heal. The systemic features are severe and can be fatal. Treatment with glucocorticoids (prednisolone) should be instituted at doses of 60 to 80 mg in two equal daily doses supplemented preferably with an augmented daily dose (200–300 mg) of clofazimine.

Prevention of Disabilities and Rehabilitation

The socioeconomic impact resulting from the physical and psychological disabilities of leprosy continues to be a burden in endemic countries. Approximately 25% of leprosy patients have some degree of disability, which is greatest in patients with long-standing BL and LL disease.

Preventing patients with nerve damage from progressing to disability and deformity is a challenge that will last for the patient's lifetime. Among the important efforts for prevention are periodic measurement of neural impairment, early and adequate management of reactions, and advice for care of eyes, hands, and feet. Special footwear needs to be provided for patients with foot deformities to prevent ulceration. Early detection and treatment of reactions significantly reduce and prevent such complications as nerve damage with its resultant impairment, eye involvement, and loss of vision. Socioeconomic rehabilitation is another important component of caring for patients.

Prevention

Large population-based trials in different countries suggest that bacille Calmette-Guérin (BCG) vaccine[1] gives variable protection against leprosy, ranging from 34% to 80%. Therefore, BCG immunization of children for tuberculosis can contribute to leprosy control.

In a recently published large study from India, vaccine containing cultivable mycobacterium, ICRC,[5] provided a protective efficacy of 65% (heat-killed *M. leprae* + BCG provided 64% protective efficacy). The role of chemoprophylaxis with bactericidal drugs in contacts of leprosy patients is still debated.

WHO Strategy for 2006 Through 2010

The WHO Technical Advisory Group (TAG) recognizes that new cases will continue to appear in most of the currently endemic countries, and therefore, expertise will have to be maintained at the appropriate level even within an integrated system. The main aim of the strategy is to sustain antileprosy services and the gains made so far. It is expected that by 2010 the disease burden will be further reduced to very low levels through services that would ensure enhancing community awareness, quality diagnosis, adequate management of patients including referral facilities, reduction of stigma, prevention of disabilities, rehabilitation, long-term care of the disabled, and effective partnerships among all stake holders.

---

[1]Not FDA approved for this indication.
[5]Investigational drug in the United States.

REFERENCES

Abulafia J, Vignale RIA. Leprosy: Pathogenesis updated. Int J Dermatol 1999;38:321–34.

Bhattacharya SN, Sehgal VN. Reappraisal of the drifting scenario of leprosy multi-drug therapy: New approach proposed for the new millennium. Int J Dermatol 2002;41:321–6.

Britton WJ, Lockwood DN. Leprosy. Lancet 2004;363:1209–19.

Grosset JH. Newer drugs in leprosy. Int J Lepr Other Mycobact Dis 2001;69(2 Suppl.):S14–S18.

Gupte MD. South India immunoprophylaxis trial against leprosy: Relevance of the findings in the context of trends in leprosy. Lepr Rev 2000;71 (Suppl.):S43–S47; discussion S47–9.

Kumar B, Dogra S, Kaur I. Epidemiological characteristics of leprosy reactions: 15 years experience from North India. Int J Lepr Other Mycobact Dis 2004;72:125–33.

Kumar B, Kaur I, Dogra S, Kumaran MS. Pure neuritic leprosy in India: An appraisal. Int J Lepr Other Mycobact Dis 2004;72:284–90.

Lockwood DN, Kumar B. Treatment of leprosy. BMJ 2004;328:1447–8.

Naafs B. Current views on reactions in leprosy. Indian J Lepr 2000;72:97–122.

Noordeen SK. Vision beyond 2005. Indian J Lepr 2004;76:171–2.

Pfaltzgraff RE, Bryceson A. Clinical leprosy. In: Hastings RC, editor. Leprosy. New York: Churchill Livingstone; 1989. p. 134–76.

WHO Expert Committee on Leprosy. Seventh Report. WHO Technical Report Series No. 874. Geneva: World Health Organization; 1998.

World Health Organization. The Weekly Epidemiological Record No. 6, 2010, 85, 37–48. (33):293–300. PDF available for download at http://www.who.int/wer [accessed July 23, 2010].

Malaria

Method of
Kimberly E. Mace, PhD, and Michael F. Lynch, MD*

Malaria is an intraerythrocytic infection caused by protozoa of the genus *Plasmodium*. It is transmitted by the bite of an infective female *Anopheles* mosquito, which serves as the vector and definitive host.

Malaria is one of the most significant parasitic diseases in the world, with an unacceptably high global burden. There were an estimated 243 million clinical cases with 863,000 deaths in 2008, mostly in children younger than 5 years living in sub-Saharan Africa, making malaria one of the world's leading killers. World Malaria Report 2009 describes 108 countries and territories with areas at risk for malaria transmission resulting in nearly half the world's population at risk for malaria infection. Each year, approximately 1400 cases of malaria are reported in the United States. The overwhelming majority of these illnesses occur among travelers to malaria endemic areas, but rare instances of local mosquito-borne transmission in the United States have occurred.

Malaria should always be considered in the differential diagnosis of fever in a traveler returning from a malarious area or in those with fever of unknown origin regardless of travel history. Prompt diagnosis and treatment are imperative because untreated *Plasmodium* infections can progress to coma, kidney failure, pulmonary edema, and death. Appropriate chemoprophylaxis and the use of personal protective measures are important in preventing malaria infection.

Risk Factors for Transmission

Malaria is a vector-borne disease most commonly transmitted through infective mosquitoes. Rarely, it can be transmitted through exposure to infected blood and blood products, organ transplantation, or contaminated needles (induced malaria) or by vertical transmission (congenital malaria). Most cases of malaria among persons from countries

---

*The findings and conclusions in this chapter are those of the authors and do not necessarily represent the views of the Centers for Disease Control and Prevention.

where it is not endemic are acquired while traveling in an endemic area (imported malaria). Imported malaria poses a potential for reintroduction of malaria into a nonendemic country. If a competent mosquito vector exists, a local mosquito could acquire the parasite by biting an infected person and then could transmit that infection to another person. In the United States, 63 outbreaks due to locally acquired mosquito-borne malaria transmission (introduced malaria) were identified from 1957 to 2003.

Etiology and the Parasite's Life Cycle

Infection with protozoa of the genus *Plasmodium* causes malaria. Typically, four species of *Plasmodium* cause clinical disease in humans: *P. falciparum*, *P. vivax*, *P. ovale*, and *P. malariae*; however,

data from Southeast Asia describes an increasing number of human infections caused by *P. knowlesi*, a simian species.

The life cycle of malaria starts with inoculation of sporozoites into the human bloodstream from the bite of a female *Anopheles* mosquito. Sporozoites travel rapidly to the liver, where asexual replication occurs (exo-erythrocytic phase, tissue schizogony). Thousands of merozoites are released from the infected liver cells to invade red blood cells (RBCs), where they multiply every 24 to 72 hours (erythrocytic cycle, blood schizogony), depending on the species. Some parasites differentiate into gametocytes (sexual erythrocytic stage), which can subsequently be ingested by a female *Anopheles* mosquito, develop into sporozoites in the mosquito's midgut, and eventually migrate into the salivary glands, continuing the malaria transmission cycle with the mosquito's next blood meal (Fig. 1).

In *P. vivax* and *P. ovale* infections, some sporozoites do not enter the exo-erythrocytic cycle but instead develop into latent hepatic

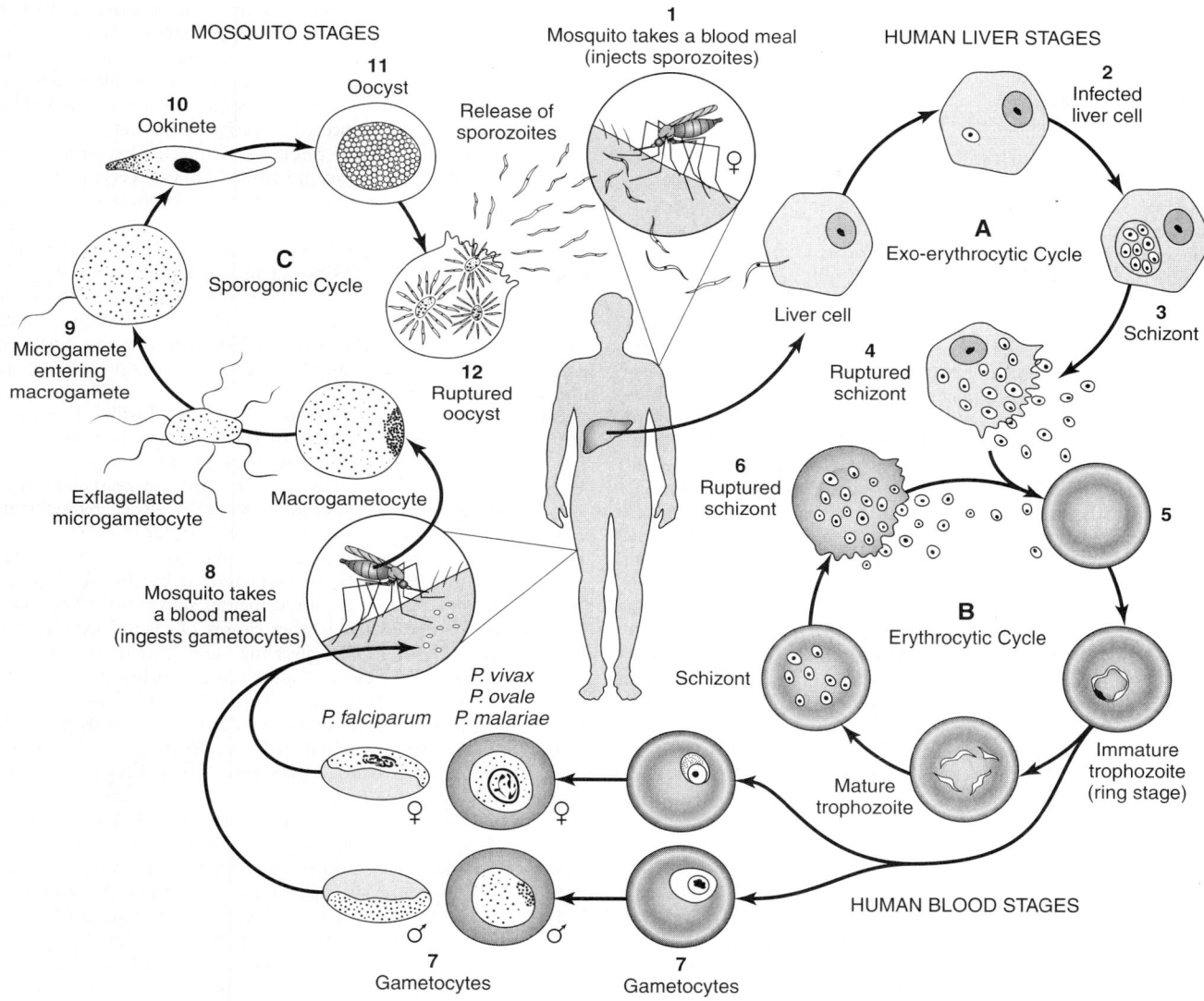

FIGURE 1. The malaria parasite life cycle involves two hosts. During a blood meal, a malaria-infected female *Anopheles* mosquito inoculates sporozoites into the human host **1**. Sporozoites infect liver cells **2** and mature into schizonts **3**, which rupture and release merozoites **4**. (In *Plasmodium vivax* and *Plasmodium ovale*, a dormant stage [hypnozoites] can persist in the liver and cause relapses by invading the bloodstream weeks or even years later.) After this initial replication in the liver (exoerythrocytic cycle or tissue schizogony **A**), the parasites undergo asexual multiplication in the erythrocytes (erythrocytic cycle or blood schizogony **B**). Merozoites infect red blood cells **5**. The ring stage trophozoites mature into schizonts, which rupture, releasing merozoites **6**. Some parasites differentiate into sexual erythrocytic stages (gametocytes) **7**. Blood stage parasites are responsible for the clinical manifestations of the disease. The gametocytes, male (microgametocytes) and female (macrogametocytes), are ingested by an *Anopheles* mosquito during a blood meal **8**. The parasites' multiplication in the mosquito is known as the sporogonic cycle **C**. While in the mosquito's stomach, the microgametes penetrate the macrogametes, generating zygotes **9**. The zygotes in turn become motile and elongated (ookinetes) **10** and invade the midgut wall of the mosquito, where they develop into oocysts **11**. The oocysts grow, rupture, and release sporozoites **12**, which make their way to the mosquito's salivary glands. Inoculation of the sporozoites **1** into a new human host perpetuates the malaria life cycle.

forms, or hypnozoites. These forms can reactivate later and cause acute illness. The resulting infection, a relapse, can occur months to years after the initial infection and can occur repeatedly. If *P. vivax* or *P. ovale* infections are acquired congenitally or through exposure to blood or blood products, there is no liver phase, and therefore relapses cannot occur. Neither *P. falciparum* nor *P. malariae* have latent hepatic forms and therefore do not cause relapse. However, subsequent illness, called *recrudescence*, can occur in all species if the parasite is not cleared after suboptimal therapy. For example, if *P. malariae* infection is not treated, symptomatic recrudescences, often associated with immunosuppression, can occur decades after the primary infection.

The incubation period, or the period from infection to the appearance of symptoms, is species-dependent. The incubation period is usually 9 to 14 days for *P. falciparum*, 12 to 17 days for *P. vivax*, 16 to 18 days for *P. ovale*, and 18 to 40 days (or longer) for *P. malariae*. Persons taking chemoprophylaxis and those who have acquired partial immunity from repeated exposure to malaria infection can experience a prolonged incubation period.

Epidemiology

Malaria is endemic to much of Africa, Asia, and parts of Central Asia, Oceania, Central America, South America, the Caribbean, and the Middle East (Fig. 2). *P. falciparum* is the most common species in the tropics and subtropics. *P. malariae*, although less common, follows a similar geographic distribution. *P. vivax* is prevalent in many temperate zones as well as in the tropics and subtropics and has the widest geographic distribution. *P. ovale* is found mainly in West Africa. *P. knowlesi*, a simian strain, has been reported to infect humans in Southeast Asia. Together, *P. falciparum* and *P. vivax* account for more than 90% of clinical malaria illnesses worldwide.

The development of resistance to antimalarial drugs has complicated malaria prophylaxis and treatment. Chloroquine-resistant *P. falciparum* is widespread with few exceptions, and chloroquine-resistant *P. vivax* is an issue in Papua New Guinea, Indonesia, and East Timor. *P. falciparum* resistance to sulfadoxine-pyrimethamine (Fansidar) is widespread in the Amazon River Basin areas and much of Southeast Asia and Africa, whereas mefloquine resistance is so far limited to Southeast Asia. Perhaps most troubling, there have been reports from Southeast Asia of artemisinin resistance manifesting as failure to clear parasites by day 3 of treatment. Knowledge of species-specific resistance patterns is essential to making appropriate decisions about chemoprophylaxis and treatment. Up-to-date information regarding areas where malaria transmission occurs and local patterns of drug resistance can be found on websites of the Centers for Disease Control and Prevention (CDC): http://www.cdc.gov/malaria/map/ or http://wwwn.cdc.gov/travel/default.aspx.

Clinical Manifestations

The clinical presentation of malaria is nonspecific, though it invariably includes fever. Therefore, clinicians must routinely obtain a travel history from febrile patients and maintain a high index of suspicion for malaria among febrile patients returning from malarious areas. The clinical presentation of malaria can vary substantially, depending on the infecting species, the level of parasitemia, and the immune status of the patient. The initial clinical symptoms usually include a flulike prodrome with headache, malaise, and myalgias that is followed by fever.

Malaria paroxysms of chills, high fevers, and then sweats are produced when infected red blood cells rupture and release merozoites. After a number of cycles of erythrocytic schizogony, the release of merozoites may become synchronized, resulting in classic cyclic fevers. With *P. falciparum*, *P. vivax*, and *P. ovale* infections, the paroxysms can occur in 48-hour cycles (tertian malaria); *P. malariae* infections have 72-hour cycles (quartan malaria) and *P. knowlesi* infections have 24-hour cycles (quotidian malaria). However, many patients,

particularly those with *P. falciparum*, do not develop cyclic paroxysms at all, and so a lack of cyclic fevers should not rule out a diagnosis of malaria. Other symptoms include headache, febrile seizures, rigors, cough, chest pain, diarrhea, nausea, vomiting, myalgias, and abdominal pain. On physical examination, a patient can appear well without physical findings or might have signs of jaundice, tachycardia, hypotension (usually secondary to volume depletion), mild hepatomegaly, and splenomegaly. Laboratory abnormalities in cases of uncomplicated malaria can include anemia, an elevated reticulocyte count, thrombocytopenia, lymphopenia, hyperbilirubinemia, and mildly elevated transaminases. Appropriately treated, uncomplicated malaria has a good prognosis with a case fatality rate around 0.1%.

An uncomplicated malaria infection can progress to severe disease or death within hours. Risk factors for severe malaria include lack of acquired immunity and inadequate, inappropriate, or delayed treatment, a high parasite burden, and age older than 50 years. *P. falciparum*, more than any other species of *Plasmodium*, is responsible for severe disease and death associated with malaria. This severity is attributed to several factors unique to this species. The tissue and blood schizonts release a larger number of merozoites when they rupture, resulting in a rapid rise in parasitemia, and they can also invade red blood cells of all developmental stages, producing more-profound anemia. In addition, the processes of cytoadherence of *P. falciparum*–infected erythrocytes to the vascular endothelium, rosetting of infected erythrocytes with uninfected erythrocytes, and agglutination of infected erythrocytes with other infected erythrocytes contribute to tissue hypoxia and end-organ dysfunction. Even the immune response itself can contribute to many of the cellular and humoral processes that manifest in severe malaria illness. Pro-inflammatory cytokines including TNF-α and IFN-γ likely contribute to endothelial dysfunction, which manifests in cerebral malaria or in acute respiratory distress syndrome (ARDS) secondary to malaria. The complex balance of proinflammatory versus antiinflammatory immune responses might determine if one is protected or predisposed to severe disease.

Severe malaria due to *P. falciparum* is associated with a 15% to 20% mortality rate. Clinical indicators of severe malaria include impaired consciousness, coma, generalized seizures, severe anemia, acute renal failure, ARDS, circulatory collapse, disseminated intravascular coagulation, abnormal bleeding, metabolic (lactic) acidosis, hypoglycemia, hemoglobinuria, jaundice, or a parasitemia greater than 5%.

Cerebral malaria, an ominous complication with an estimated 10% to 40% mortality rate, is characterized by diffuse symmetric encephalopathy. Coma or impaired mental status caused by malaria has to be distinguished from other causes of altered mental status, including hyperpyrexia, hypoglycemia, and concurrent infections such as meningitis. The clinical spectrum of cerebral malaria ranges from odd behavior to delirium, generalized seizures, and coma with extensor posturing (opisthotonos). Children, more commonly than adults, can suffer from cerebral malaria and its residual neurologic sequelae. On the other hand, ARDS, jaundice, and renal impairment occur more often in adults. ARDS can occur as a secondary manifestation of malaria, and it often ensues after initial clinical improvement or clearance of peripheral parasitemia. Severe anemia and hypoglycemia, more common in children and pregnant women, are important features of severe malaria and predict poor prognosis. Acidosis due to an increase in lactate levels and its associated acidotic breathing are also poor prognostic factors.

Non–*P. falciparum* infections are not without risk of severe disease. Severe manifestations of *P. vivax*, in particular, are not uncommon. Notably, *P. vivax* accounted for three of 34 deaths (9%) that occurred in the United States between 2002 and 2008. *P. falciparum* caused 24 deaths (71%) and *P. malariae* infections, mixed *P. falciparum*, and unknown species contribute to the remaining seven deaths (21%). Severe manifestations of *P. vivax*, in adults and children, are often pulmonary. However, jaundice, kidney failure, and acidosis have also been associated with *P. vivax*. Splenic rupture has been described in patients with persistent, untreated *P. vivax* infection who have developed massive splenomegaly. Chronic complications of malarial infections include hyperreactive malarial syndrome (tropical splenomegaly syndrome), nephrotic syndrome (a rare complication of persistent *P. malariae* infection), and possibly Burkitt's lymphoma.

Diagnosis

Malaria should be considered in any febrile patient with a history of travel to an area of malaria transmission even if the patient gives a history of taking appropriate prophylactic therapy. Information on the location and duration of the trip, the date of return, the history of prophylaxis choice and adherence, and the date of symptom onset enables the physician to assess the risk of malaria and, if necessary, choose an appropriate course of treatment.

To provide appropriate therapy, it is essential to identify the infecting malaria species, determine where the infection was acquired, and determine the parasite density. Health care providers evaluating patients for possible malaria must obtain thick and thin blood smears, the most valid diagnostic test, to demonstrate asexual forms of the parasite. Malaria smears should be read immediately without delays; sending specimens to offsite laboratories can delay results. In rare instances, if the patient is extremely ill with symptoms consistent with severe malaria and has a history of malaria exposure, treatment should be started immediately before results are available. Initial blood smears may be negative, particularly in symptomatic semi-immune persons and those taking prophylaxis. Therefore, blood smears should be repeated every 12 to 24 hours for a total of three sets before the diagnosis of malaria can be excluded.

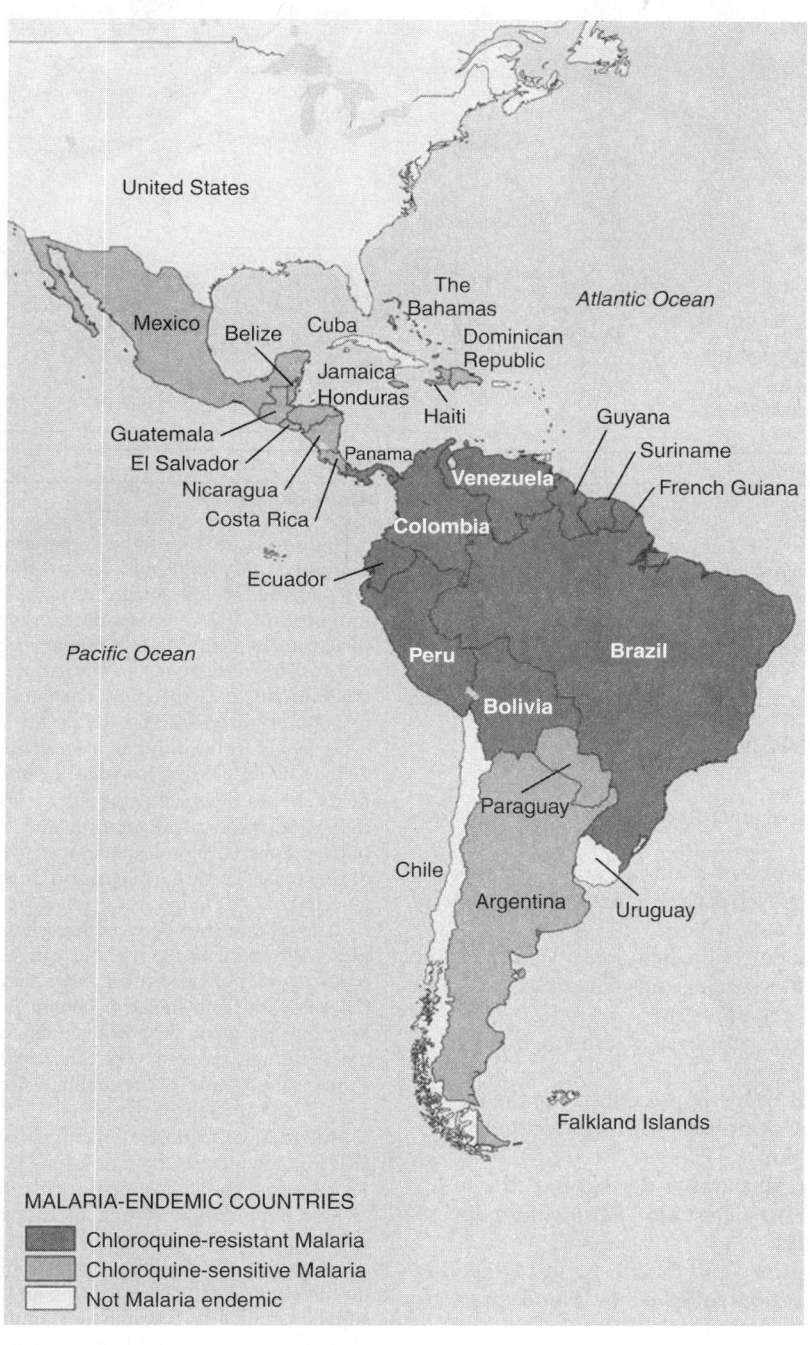

MALARIA-ENDEMIC COUNTRIES

- Chloroquine-resistant Malaria
- Chloroquine-sensitive Malaria
- Not Malaria endemic

A

FIGURE 2. Malaria-endemic countries in the Western and Eastern Hemispheres. Malaria transmission occurs in large areas of Central and South America, parts of the Caribbean, Africa, Asia (including South Asia, Southeast Asia, and the Middle East), Eastern Europe, and the South Pacific. (Reprinted with permission from Brunette G, Kozarsky P, Magill A, Shlim D (eds): CDC Health Information for International Travel 2010. Atlanta: U.S. Department of Health and Human Services, Public Health Service, 2009.)

(Continued)

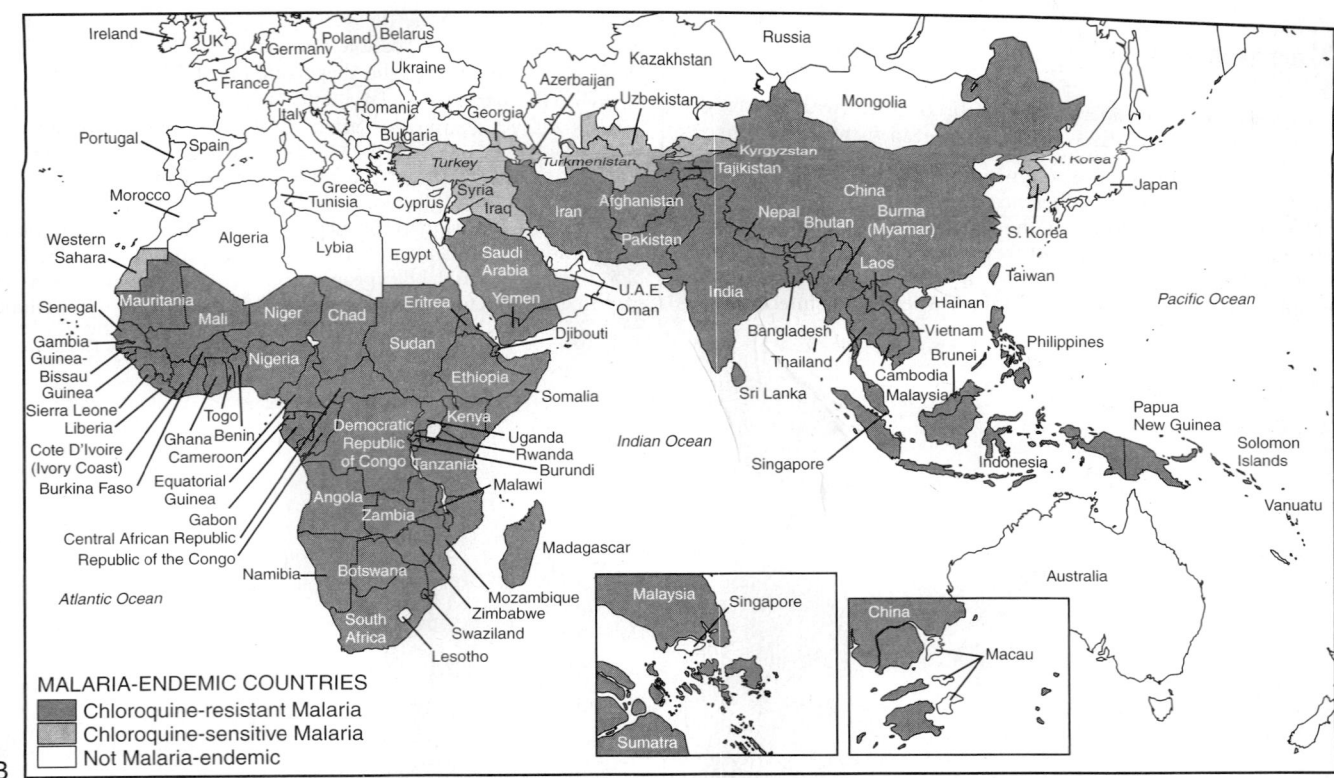

MALARIA-ENDEMIC COUNTRIES
- Chloroquine-resistant Malaria
- Chloroquine-sensitive Malaria
- Not Malaria-endemic

B

FIGURE 2. (Cont'd)

Initial laboratory evaluation of patients with suspected malaria should include a complete blood count, electrolytes, creatinine, urea, glucose, and bilirubin. In patients with severe disease or respiratory symptoms, lactate level, arterial blood gas, and additional coagulation studies should also be obtained.

CURRENT DIAGNOSIS

History
- Does the patient have fever (with or without other flu-like symptoms)?
- Did the patient travel to a malaria-endemic area?
  - When did the travel occur? What was the date of symptom onset?
  - Where was the infection acquired? What are the prevalent parasite species and drug-resistance patterns from this region?
- Did the patient take prophylaxis during travel to a malaria-endemic region?
  - Was prophylaxis properly prescribed for the region?
  - Was the patient compliant with the regimen?

Diagnostic Confirmation
- Thick blood smear for parasite detection
- Thin blood smear to determine *Plasmodium* species and parasite density
- An alternative is to use rapid diagnostic test (RDT) for faster parasite detection followed by blood smear to determine species and parasite density
- Signs of severe malaria: Parasite density >5%; altered consciousness, seizures or coma; severe anemia; hypoglycemia; respiratory distress/acute respiratory distress syndrome (ARDS); hypotension; acute renal failure; acidosis; hyperbilirubinemia

Blood smears should be prepared with Giemsa stain (pH 7.2) and examined under light microscopy. Both thick and thin smears should be scanned at low magnification and then examined under oil immersion (1000× magnification). The thick smear concentrates the parasites, resulting in a higher diagnostic sensitivity than the thin smear. The easiest way to determine the percent parasitemia using the thin smear is to count the parasitized erythrocytes among 500 to 2000 erythrocytes and divide the number of parasitized erythrocytes by the total number of erythrocytes counted and multiply by 100. To avoid missing low-density infections, at least 200 high-power fields should be examined before a slide is considered negative. Further details about preparation and diagnostic assistance on digital photographs of blood smears can be found at the CDC's Division of Parasitic Diseases diagnostic Internet site: http://www.dpd.cdc.gov/dpdx.

The relationship between parasitemia and clinical severity is complex. Although severe malaria can occur even with apparently low parasitemia, persons with greater than 5% parasitemia are at higher risk of death from malaria. Thus it is essential to determine the parasite burden at the time of diagnosis as an indicator of disease severity. Although gametocytes can persist much longer, blood smears should be negative for asexual parasites within 48 to 72 hours following the completion of therapy.

Alternative diagnostic tests for malaria include rapid diagnostic tests (RDTs), polymerase chain reaction (PCR), and serology. RDTs identify *P. falciparum* specific antigens such as histidine-rich protein-2 (HRP-2) or common enzymes such as aldolase and lactate dehydrogenase (pLDH) present in all *Plasmodium* species infecting humans. Determination of parasite density is not possible with RDTs, and therefore they do not eliminate the need for thin and thick blood smears. BinaxNOW supplies an RDT to hospitals and commercial laboratories in the United States that detects two different malaria antigens: HRP-2 and aldolase. Therefore, this test identifies *P. falciparum* infections but does not differentiate *P. vivax*, *P. ovale*, *P. malaria*, or mixed infections. All malaria RDTs must be performed with proper controls.

PCR may be more sensitive for detecting parasites than microscopy. PCR is particularly valuable for identifying the species of a parasite when that cannot be determined by morphology or RDT alone.

Currently, PCR is used mostly as a research tool and is available only in reference laboratories. As access to quality PCR increases, routine species confirmation by PCR might become the standard of care. Malaria serology can detect antibodies to any of the four major species but cannot be used to diagnose acute infections. However, it may be useful for identifying an infective donor in cases of transfusion-related malaria, investigating congenital cases, assessing the validity of clinical malaria diagnoses in empirically treated nonimmune travelers, and diagnosing hyperreactive malarial syndrome.

Antimalarial Drugs

Because of the emergence and spread of drug-resistance, the slow rate of development of new antimalarial drugs, and the infrequency with which newly developed drugs are submitted for U.S. Food and Drug Administration (FDA) approval, relatively few drugs are available for the prophylaxis and treatment of malaria infections in the United States. The choice of antimalarial drugs used for treatment should be guided by several factors: local availability of the drug, the infecting species, where it was likely acquired (according to travel history) and drug resistance patterns in that area, severity of symptoms, and percent parasitemia.

Antimalarial drugs can be categorized by their ability to kill the organism at various stages in its life cycle (see Fig. 1). Drugs that kill malaria parasites infecting liver cells during the exo-erythrocytic cycle are referred to as tissue schizonticides, whereas blood schizonticides kill malaria parasites that have been released into the bloodstream and are asexually replicating in the erythrocytic cycle. Rapidly acting blood schizonticides are the essential components of acute malaria treatment regimens, and tissues schizonticides targeted toward latent forms can prevent relapse in certain species. Certain drugs can also have activity against gametocytes. Gametocidal activity does not affect a patient's clinical response but can decrease the probability that infection is transmitted to another person. Currently no medications are available that have activity against malaria sporozoites.

Chloroquine phosphate (Aralen) and hydroxychloroquine sulfate (Plaquenil) are used to prevent and treat malaria. They are blood schizonticides that are active against the erythrocytic stages of all *Plasmodium* species and have gametocytocidal activity against *P. vivax*, *P. ovale*, and *P. malariae*. Chloroquine is the treatment of choice for susceptible strains of all *Plasmodium* species, although the widespread prevalence of chloroquine-resistant forms of *P. falciparum* and *P. vivax* have limited its use in most malaria endemic areas. Chloroquine can be taken safely by pregnant women and children. Side effects include gastrointestinal disturbance, dizziness, blurred vision, insomnia, headache, and pruritus. Although extremely rare, long-term administration of chloroquine, usually associated with its use in the treatment of rheumatologic conditions, can lead to retinopathy, ototoxicity, and peripheral neuropathy.

Quinine sulfate (Qualaquin) (oral) and its dextro isomer, quinidine gluconate, (parenteral) are commonly used for the treatment of malaria in the United States, and are particularly useful for chloroquine-resistant malaria. They are blood schizonticides that are effective against the erythrocytic stages of all species of plasmodia and are also active against the gametocytes of *P. vivax*, *P. ovale*, and *P. malariae*. Parenteral quinidine is currently the only FDA-approved treatment for severe malaria in the United States, whereas intravenous or intramuscular formulations of quinine are used in other countries. Owing to their potential cardiac toxicity, intravenous quinidine should be administered with telemetry monitoring. Common side effects include cinchonism (a syndrome of tinnitus, hearing loss, headache, nausea, and visual disturbance) and hyperinsulinemic hypoglycemia. As the duration of therapy increases, so does the risk for adverse events. To shorten the course of therapy (from 7 to 3 days), quinine and intravenous quinidine are combined with doxycycline (Vibramycin),[1] tetracycline,[1] or clindamycin (Cleocin)[1] (see

Table 1 for details). Malaria acquired in Southeast Asia exhibits decreased responsiveness to quinine and quinidine; therefore, the treatment regimen for cases acquired there should not be shortened.

Mefloquine (formerly Lariam, now only available in generic) is a long-acting blood schizonticide that is used for both prevention and treatment of malaria. It is effective against the erythrocytic stages of all species. Side effects include nausea, vomiting, diarrhea, abdominal pain, myalgia, a mild skin rash, fatigue, and mild neuropsychiatric complaints (dizziness, headache, somnolence, sleep disorders, fuzzy thinking). Mefloquine has also been associated with rare serious adverse reactions such as seizures and psychoses at prophylactic doses. Although mefloquine can be used to treat chloroquine-resistant *P. falciparum*, adverse reactions are more common at the higher doses used for treatment than at prophylactic doses. Any traveler receiving a prescription for mefloquine must receive a copy of the FDA Medication Guide (http://www.accessdata.fda.gov/drugsatfda_docs/label/2003/19591slr 022_lariam_lbl.pdf).

Because other options that have fewer adverse events are available for treatment, mefloquine normally is not recommended. Mefloquine is contraindicated for use in patients with known hypersensitivity to the drug and persons with a history of psychiatric disease. Mefloquine is also contraindicated in persons with a history of seizures (not including febrile seizures in childhood). It should be avoided in patients with cardiac conduction disorders because it prolongs the QTc interval, and it should be used with caution in persons taking β-blockers. Concomitant administration of mefloquine and quinine or quinidine should be avoided because it can produce arrhythmias and increase the risk of seizures.

Mefloquine prophylaxis in the second and third trimesters is not associated with an adverse fetal or pregnancy outcome. More limited data suggest that though it is rarely used, it is probably safe in the first trimester.

Atovaquone-proguanil (Malarone), a fixed-combination antimalarial drug that is both a blood and tissue schizonticide, can be used for chemoprophylaxis and for treatment of chloroquine-resistant *P. falciparum*. Though it has tissue schizonticidal activity, it does not prevent relapses of *P. vivax* and *P. ovale*. Side effects are rare, but abdominal pain, nausea, vomiting, and headache have been reported. Treatment efficacy, safety, and pharmacokinetic data in children 5 to 11 kg have been extrapolated, allowing prophylaxis doses in these children.[1] Providers should note that this prophylactic dosing for children weighing less than 11 kg constitutes off-label use in the United States. Atovaquone-proguanil is contraindicated in children who weigh less than 5 kg, pregnant women, women who are breast-feeding infants who weigh less than 5 kg, and persons with severe renal impairment.

Tetracyclines are blood schizonticides that are effective against the erythrocytic stages of all species of *Plasmodium*. Because of their relatively slow onset of action, tetracyclines should never be used alone for treatment. Combined with quinine or quinidine, they are effective against chloroquine-resistant *P. falciparum* and *P. vivax*. Doxycycline[1] alone is effective as prophylaxis against chloroquine-resistant and mefloquine-resistant *P. falciparum*. Side effects include gastrointestinal symptoms, *Candida* vaginitis or stomatitis, and idiosyncratic photosensitivity reactions. Tetracyclines should not be used in pregnant women or in children younger than 8 years old.

Clindamycin[1] is active against blood schizonts of all species of *Plasmodium*. Like the tetracyclines, clindamycin should never be used alone to treat malaria. Clindamycin can be used in combination with quinine to treat chloroquine-resistant *P. falciparum* infections in people who are not able to take tetracyclines. Side effects include diarrhea, nausea, and skin rashes.

Derivatives of artemisinin (such as artesunate,[10] artemether,[2] and dihydroartemisinin[2]) are compounds derived from the Chinese medicinal plant quinghaosu (*Artemisia annua*) that are active against

---

[1]Not FDA approved for this indication.

[1]Not FDA approved for this indication.
[2]Not available in the United States.
[10]Available in the United States from the Centers for Disease Control and Prevention.

blood schizonts and gametocytes. Artemisinin and its derivatives are short-acting, highly effective antimalarial drugs for the treatment of uncomplicated multidrug-resistant *P. falciparum* and severe *P. falciparum* infection. These drugs are available in oral, rectal, and intravenous formulations. Although they can be used alone for at least 7 days, combining them with other antimalarial drugs can treat malaria infections effectively, decrease the length of treatment, and safeguard against selecting for drug-resistant parasites.

Common artemisinin-based combination therapies (ACTs) used worldwide include artesunate copackaged with mefloquine (Artequin)[2] and artemether coformulated with lumefantrine (Coartem or Riamet). Coartem (Novartis Pharmaceuticals) has been FDA approved for use in the United States. This lipid-soluble drug should be taken with fatty food or whole milk to improve absorption. Adverse drug reactions are not common but include abdominal pain, headache, anorexia, dizziness, physical weakness, joint pain, and muscle pain. Additionally, parenteral artesunate, an investigational new drug, is available through the CDC for the treatment of severe malaria if quinidine is not available or is not well tolerated. Inquiries regarding artesunate treatment should be directed to the CDC malaria hotline: 770-488-7788 Monday through Friday 9 AM to 5 PM Eastern time or 770-488-7100 after hours, on weekends, and on holidays.

Primaquine phosphate, a tissue schizonticide with gametocytocidal activity, is the only drug available to prevent relapse of *P. vivax* and *P. ovale* infections. Primaquine (up to 30 mg/day)[3] has the following uses: primary prophylaxis for destinations where *P. vivax* is the main species[1]; presumptive antirelapse therapy (PART) to treat the liver stages (hypnozoites) of *P. vivax* and *P. ovale* for persons who have had prolonged exposure in malaria-endemic areas such as missionaries, Peace Corps volunteers, and the military[1]; and radical cure of acute *P. vivax* and *P. ovale* infection to prevent relapses. Primary prophylaxis with primaquine eliminates the need for PART. The duration of therapy for PART and radical cure is 14 days, given after the patient has left the malarious area and in conjunction with a blood schizonticide.

Primaquine can cause hemolysis and methemoglobinemia in glucose-6-phosphate dehydrogenase (G6PD)-deficient persons. Before primaquine is used the first time, G6PD deficiency must be ruled out by appropriate laboratory testing. The most common side effects are abdominal pain and headache. Primaquine is contraindicated in pregnant women because of the unknown G6PD status of the fetus and in breast-feeding women if the G6PD status of the infant is unknown.

Other antimalarials often encountered in malaria endemic countries, such as sulfadoxine-pyrimethamine (Fansidar), amodiaquine (Camoquin),[2] proguanil (Paludrine),[2] or halofantrine (Halfan),[2] are not recommended for use in the United States either because of limited efficacy or the side-effect profile.

Treatment

Ideally, treatment for malaria should not be initiated until the diagnosis has been confirmed by laboratory investigations. However, health care providers should not delay treatment when malaria is strongly suspected and smear results are not available in a timely manner. Once the diagnosis is confirmed, appropriate antimalarial therapy must be initiated immediately. The choice of treatment should be guided by the species of *Plasmodium* found, the level of parasitemia, the clinical status of the patient, and the likely drug susceptibility of the infecting species as determined by where the infection was acquired. All species require treatment with a rapidly acting blood schizonticide; patients with *P. vivax* or *P. ovale* also require treatment with primaquine phosphate to decrease the likelihood of a relapse.

---

[1]Not FDA approved for this indication.
[2]Not available in the United States.
[3]Exceeds dosage recommended by the manufacturer.

CURRENT THERAPY

- Promptly diagnose and initiate treatment to avert severe manifestations or death
- Determine where the patient acquired the infection to assess local drug resistance patterns and develop a treatment strategy
- Distinguish between uncomplicated and severe malaria
  - Severe malaria: Treat with parenteral therapy (quinidine or artesunate[10]) in an intensive care setting
  - Uncomplicated malaria: Distinguish between *P. falciparum* and non-*P. falciparum*
    - *P. falciparum* malaria: Strongly consider admitting to hospital
    - *P. vivax* or *P. ovale*: Assess G6PD status and prevent relapsing infections by prescribing primaquine

---

[10]Available in the United States from the Centers for Disease Control and Prevention.

Species identification is necessary to distinguish *P. falciparum* malaria from non–*P. falciparum* malaria. *P. falciparum* can cause rapid progression of disease and death; therefore, patients with *P. falciparum*, mixed infections with *P. falciparum*, or infections in which the species cannot be identified immediately should he hospitalized and monitored closely to assess for the development of severe malaria and subsequent complications. Although uncommon, *P. knowlesi* infections also have the capacity to rapidly result in high parasitemia and progress to a potentially fatal outcome. If the infecting species or probable origin of infection cannot be determined, patients should be treated for multidrug-resistant *P. falciparum* until another pathogen is identified. Using available clinical and laboratory data, physicians must determine whether a patient has uncomplicated or severe malaria. Patients with uncomplicated malaria typically can be treated with oral therapy but might need parenteral therapy if they are unable to tolerate oral medications. Patients with severe malaria should be immediately started on parenteral malaria therapy and monitored in an intensive care setting.

After initiating treatment, when clinically indicated, patients should have repeat blood smears to assess appropriate response. Due to the release of sequestered *P. falciparum*-parasitized RBCs from vascular capillary beds, it is not uncommon for parasite density to increase within the first 24 hours after treatment. In such instances, if the patient is improving clinically, the treatment regimen should be continued with monitoring, until blood smears are negative. If the patient does not improve or blood smears remain positive after 7 days, then the clinician should consider drug failure and initiate an alternative treatment regimen.

For detailed treatment information, including doses and frequency of therapy, refer to Tables 1 and 2.

CHLOROQUINE-SENSITIVE *P. FALCIPARUM*, *P. VIVAX*, *P. OVALE*, *P. MALARIAE*, AND *P. KNOWLESI*

For *P. malariae*, *P. ovale*, *P. knowlesi*, chloroquine-sensitive *P. vivax*, and chloroquine-sensitive *P. falciparum* infection, prompt treatment with oral chloroquine phosphate (Aralen) is recommended. If chloroquine is not available, then other treatments can be used. In addition, infections with *P. vivax* and *P. ovale* require primaquine to reduce the likelihood of a relapse, if patients have a documented normal level of G6PD activity.

---

[1]Not FDA approved for this indication.

TABLE 1 Recommended Drugs for Treatment of Specific Types of Malaria

Diagnosis	Recommended Drug
Uncomplicated chloroquine-sensitive *P. falciparum*	Chloroquine phosphate (Aralen)
Uncomplicated chloroquine-resistant *P. falciparum*	Quinine sulfate* (Qualaquin) **plus one of the following**:
or	Doxycycline[1,†] *or*
Resistance unknown	Tetracycline[1,†] *or*
or	Clindamycin (Cleocin)[1]
Species unknown	**or**
	Atovaquone/proguanil (Malarone)
	or
	Artemether-lumefantrine (Coartem)
	or
	Mefloquine[‡]
Uncomplicated *P. malariae*	Chloroquine phosphate (Aralen)
Uncomplicated *P. vivax* or *P. ovale* (except chloroquine-resistant *P. vivax*)	Chloroquine phosphate (Aralen) **plus**
	Primaquine phosphate[§]
Uncomplicated chloroquine-resistant *P. vivax*	Quinine sulfate* (Qualaquin) **plus one of the following**:
	Doxycycline[1,†] *or*
	Tetracycline[1,†]
	plus
	Primaquine phosphate[§]
	or
	Atovaquone/proguanil **plus** primaquine phosphate[§]
	or
	Mefloquine[‡] **plus** primaquine phosphate[§]
Chloroquine-sensitive malaria during pregnancy	Chloroquine phosphate (Aralen)
Chloroquine-resistant *P. falciparum* during pregnancy	Quinine sulfate* (Qualaquin) **plus** Clindamycin[1]
Chloroquine-resistant *P. vivax* during pregnancy	Quinine sulfate* (Qualaquin)
Severe malaria	Parenteral quinidine gluconate **plus one of the following**:
	Doxycycline[1,†] *or*
	Tetracycline[1,†] *or*
	Clindamycin[1]
	or
	Parenteral artesunate[¶] followed by another oral treatment

[1]Not FDA approved for this indication.
*Quinidine/quinine course = 7 d if infection was acquired in Southeast Asia; = 3 d if infection was acquired in Africa or South America.
[†]Not indicated for use in children younger than 8 y.
[‡]Because of resistant strains, treatment with mefloquine is not recommended in persons who have acquired infections in parts of Thailand, Burma, Cambodia, Laos, China, and Vietnam.
[§]All persons who take primaquine should have a documented normal glucose 6 phoshate dehydrogenase level before starting the medication.
[¶]Investigational new drug; contact Centers for Disease Control and Prevention for information.

DRUG-RESISTANT *P. FALCIPARUM*

For *P. falciparum* infections acquired in chloroquine-resistant areas, there are four treatment options: quinine sulfate (Qualaquin) plus doxycycline,[1] tetracycline,[1] or clindamycin[1]; atovaquone-proguanil; artemether-lumafantrine; and mefloquine. Because mefloquine has a higher rate of severe neuropsychiatric reactions at treatment doses, it is recommended only when the other options are not available. Mefloquine is also not recommended for the treatment of falciparum malaria in persons who acquired the infection in Southeast Asia, especially Thailand, Cambodia, Burma (Myanmar), Laos, and Vietnam, because of the potential that the infection results from a mefloquine-resistant strain. Because artemisinin-tolerant strains have been limited to patients in Southeast Asia, and artemether-lumafantrine has only recently been released in the United States, the impact of artemisinin-tolerant strains on clinical management of U.S. patients with malaria remains to be seen.

DRUG-RESISTANT *P. VIVAX*

P. vivax infections acquired in areas with chloroquine resistance can be treated with either of three treatment options: quinine sulfate plus doxycycline[1] or tetracycline,[1] atovaquone-proguanil, or mefloquine alone. As noted earlier, its use is limited by the preponderance of severe neuropsychiatric adverse effects when mefloquine is administered at the treatment dosage. In addition to either of those regimens, persons who have a

[1]Not FDA approved for this indication.

normal level of G6PD activity and who are infected with *P. vivax* should be treated with primaquine phosphate to prevent relapse.

SEVERE MALARIA

Patients with severe malaria, regardless of species, and those who are unable to take oral medications should be treated with parenteral antimalarial therapy. Severe malaria is a medical emergency, and treatment with intravenous medication should be initiated immediately (see Tables 1 and 2). In the United States, quinidine gluconate is the only parenteral rapidly acting blood schizonticide approved by the FDA. Under an investigational new drug protocol, artesunate, a parenteral drug for the treatment of severe malaria, is available now through the CDC in the United States. Health care providers caring for patients with severe malaria should contact the CDC to assess the need for artesunate (CDC Malaria Hotline: 770-488-7788, Monday through Friday, 9 AM to 5 PM Eastern time); emergency consultation: 770-488-7100 after hours). In addition to antimalarial therapy, patients should receive the necessary supportive care.

The patient should be admitted to an intensive care unit with continuous cardiac monitoring (to assess the QTc interval) and regular measurements of blood pressure and blood glucose. Fluid status, level of consciousness, and vital signs should be monitored closely. Because these patients are at risk for hypoglycemia, severe anemia, renal failure, and acidosis, regular assessment of blood glucose, hemoglobin and hematocrit, creatinine, urea, electrolytes, and acid-base status also is required. Severe anemia requires blood transfusion with packed red blood cells. Hemodialysis or hemofiltration is usually needed in patients with acute renal failure. Oxygen and other respiratory support

TABLE 2 Treatment Dosages of Antimalarial Drugs

Drug	Adult Dosage	Pediatric Dosage*
Artesunate[†]	2.4 mg/kg IV push at 0, 12, 24, and 48 h	2.4 mg/kg IV push at 0, 12, 24, and 48 h
Atovaquone-proguanil (Malarone)	4 adult tabs (each adult tab contains 250 mg atovaquone and 100 mg proguanil) PO as a single daily dose for 3 consecutive days	Dosage is based on weight Each ped tab contains 62.5 mg atovaquone and 25 mg proguanil Daily dose to be taken for 3 consecutive days: 5–8 kg: 2 ped tabs 9–10 kg: 3 ped tabs 11–20 kg: 1 adult tab 21–30 kg: 2 adult tabs 31–40 kg: 3 adult tabs ≥41 kg: 4 adult tabs
Artemether-lumefantrine (Coartem)	1 tablet = 20 mg artemether and 120 mg lumefantrine A 3-d treatment schedule with a total of 6 oral doses is recommended for both adult and pediatric patients based on weight The patient should receive the initial dose, followed by the second dose 8 h later, then 1 dose PO bid for the following 2 d. Medication should be taken with food or whole milk to improve absorption. 5 to <15 kg: 1 tab per dose 15 to <25 kg: 2 tabs per dose 25 to <35 kg: 3 tabs per dose ≥35 kg: 4 tabs per dose	
Chloroquine phosphate (Aralen)	600 mg base (=1 g salt) PO, then 300 mg base (=500 mg salt) and 6, 24 and 48 h	10 mg base/kg PO, then 5 mg base/kg at 6, 24 and 48 h
Clindamycin, oral (Cleocin)[1]	20 mg base/kg/d PO divided tid × 7 d	20 mg base/kg/d PO divided tid × 7 d
Clindamycin, parenteral[1]	10 mg base/kg IV followed by 5 mg base/kg IV q8h Switch to oral clindamycin as soon as patient is able to complete 7-d course	10 mg base/kg IV followed by 5 mg base/kg IV q8h Switch to oral clindamycin as soon as patient is able to complete 7-d course
Doxycycline (Vibramycin)[1,‡]	100 mg PO or IV bid × 7 d	2.2 mg/kg PO or IV bid × 7 d[‡]
Mefloquine	750 mg salt (=684 mg base) PO followed by 500 mg salt (=456 mg base) PO 6–12 h after the initial dose	15 mg salt/kg (=13.7 mg base/kg) PO followed by 10 mg salt/kg (=9.1 mg base/kg) PO 6–12 h after the initial dose
Primaquine phosphate[¶]	30 mg base PO qd × 14 d[3]	0.5 mg base/kg PO qd × 14 d[3]
Quinidine gluconate	6.25 mg base/kg (=10 mg salt/kg) loading dose[§] IV over 1–2 h, then 0.0125 mg base/kg/min (=0.02 mg salt/kg/min) continuous infusion for at least 24 h Alternative regimen: 15 mg base/kg (=24 mg salt/kg) loading dose IV infused over 4 h, followed by 7.5 mg base/kg (=12 mg salt/kg) infused over 4 h q8h, starting 8 h after the loading dose Once parasite density <1% and patient can take oral medication, complete treatment with oral quinine	6.25 mg base/kg (=10 mg salt/kg) loading dose[§] IV over 1–2 h, then 0.0125 mg base/kg/min (=0.02 mg salt/kg/min) continuous infusion for at least 24 h Alternative regimen: 15 mg base/kg (=24 mg salt/kg) loading dose IV infused over 4 h, followed by 7.5 mg base/kg (=12 mg salt/kg) infused over 4 h q8h, starting 8 h after the loading dose Once parasite density <1% and patient can take oral medication, complete treatment with oral quinine
Quinine sulfate (Qualaquin)	650 mg salt (=542 mg base) PO tid × 3 or 7 d (×7 d if acquired in Southeast Asia)	10 mg salt/kg (=8.3 mg base/kg) PO tid × 3 d (×7 d if acquired in Southeast Asia)
Tetracycline[1,‡]	250 mg PO qid × 7 d	25 mg/kg/d PO divided qid × 7 d[‡]

[1]Not FDA approved for this indication.
[3]Exceeds dosage recommended by the manufacturer.
*Pediatric dose should *never* exceed adult dose.
[†]Available only through the Centers for Disease Control and Prevention in the United States.
[‡]Doxycycline and tetracycline are not indicated for use in children younger than 8 years.
[§]Patients should be given a loading dose of quinidine unless they have received >40 mg/kg of quinine in the preceding 48 h or if they received mefloquine treatment within the preceding 12 h.
[¶]All persons who take primaquine should have a documented normal glucose 6 phosphate dehydrogenase level prior to starting the medication.

may be required in patients with ARDS. Thrombocytopenia is common with malaria and should be managed appropriately, but it is not an indicator of severe malaria. One should consider exchange transfusion if parasitemia is greater than 10% or if the patient has altered mental status, ARDS, or renal complications. Blood smears should be initially repeated every 12 hours to monitor response. Once parasite density is lower than 1% and the patient is able to eat and drink, the treatment course should be completed with oral medications.

Various adjunctive therapies for malaria have been shown to be ineffective and sometimes even harmful. These include corticosteroids[1] for the treatment of cerebral malaria, phenobarbital for seizure prophylaxis,

heparin for coagulation abnormalities, iron chelators[1] to reduce parasite clearance time, pentoxifylline (Trental)[1] to inhibit tumor necrosis system, and dichloroacetate[1] for treatment of metabolic acidosis.

CONGENITAL AND PREGNANCY-ASSOCIATED MALARIA

Malaria in pregnancy affects both the mother and her fetus. Infection with *P. falciparum* during pregnancy can increase the mother's risk of developing severe disease and anemia as well as increasing the risk of stillbirth, prematurity, and low birth weight, especially for women in

[1]Not FDA approved for this indication.

[1]Not FDA approved for this indication.

their first or second pregnancies and those immunocompromised. Babies born to nonimmune mothers with acute malaria are at risk for congenital malaria, but empiric treatment is not recommended. Congenital malaria often manifests as fever, anemia, or failure to thrive at 1 to 2 months of age and can be difficult for an unsuspecting clinician to detect. If the child is asymptomatic at the time of the delivery, blood smears are not recommended. Instead, health care providers should remain alert for the development of signs and symptoms consistent with malaria and initiate a prompt diagnostic evaluation. Treating physicians should judge each case individually, considering such factors as reliability of follow-up and access to medical care. Educating the mother about the risk of congenital malaria and instructing her to seek medical care if the infant develops symptoms of malaria may be appropriate in most cases, while presumptive treatment of the newborn may be warranted in others. Primaquine treatment of infants is unnecessary because there is no liver phase with congenitally acquired infections.

For pregnant women with uncomplicated malaria caused by *P. malariae*, *P. ovale*, chloroquine-sensitive *P. vivax*, and chloroquine-sensitive *P. falciparum*, prompt treatment with chloroquine (Aralen) is recommended. For pregnant women who acquired *P. vivax* in a region of chloroquine-resistance, treatment with quinine (Qualaquin) for 7 days is recommended. After treatment, all pregnant women with *P. vivax* and *P. ovale* should be given chloroquine prophylaxis for the duration of the pregnancy to avoid relapses; women may be treated with primaquine after delivery if they (and infant, if breastfeeding) have a normal G6PD screening test. For pregnant women with uncomplicated chloroquine-resistant *P. falciparum* malaria, prompt treatment with quinine and clindamycin[1] is recommended.

MALARIA IN CHILDREN

For pediatric patients, treatment options are the same as those for adults except that the drug dosage is adjusted by the patient's weight. The pediatric dosage should never exceed the recommended adult dosage. For treatment of chloroquine-resistant *P. falciparum* in children younger than 8 years, doxycycline and tetracycline should not be used. Quinine sulfate (if appropriately dosed) or quinidine may be given in combination with clindamycin[1] to children. Alternatively, children weighing >5 kg can be treated with atovaquone-proguanil or artemether-lumefantrine. Mefloquine can be considered if these options are not available. In rare instances, doxycycline[1] or tetracycline[1] can be used in combination with quinine in children younger than 8 years if other treatment options are not available or are not tolerated and the benefit of adding doxycycline or tetracycline is judged to outweigh the risk.

Prevention

A combination of personal protective measures and chemoprophylaxis can be highly effective in preventing malaria in travelers and those living in malaria-endemic areas. Malaria-endemic countries have focused on delivering person- and household-level protection through insecticide-treated nets and indoor residual spraying with insecticides. Chemoprophylaxis in the form of intermittent preventive treatment of high-risk groups, pregnant women, and infants has been adopted by several malaria-endemic countries.

Other protective measures include mosquito avoidance (indoors and outdoors) during the peak *Anopheles* biting period between dusk and dawn by wearing clothing that minimizes the amount of exposed skin and applying insect repellents that contain DEET (diethylmethyltoluamide). DEET may be used on adults, children, and infants older than 2 months. Higher concentrations of DEET can have a longer repellent effect; however, concentrations over 50% provide no added protection. Alternatively, repellents that contain picaridin (e.g., Cutter Advanced Insect Repellent) and IR3535 (e.g., Skin So Soft Bug Guard Plus) are also recommended by the CDC. Travelers who are not staying in well-screened or air-conditioned rooms should sleep under insecticide-treated bed nets.

For travelers to malaria-endemic areas, chemoprophylaxis with an appropriate antimalarial drug is effective in preventing malaria infection. The choice of prophylactic medication should be made in light of the traveler's destination, length of stay, the presence of resistant strains, age, drug allergies, other medications, and medical history. Often, potential side effects, convenience of the dosing regimen, and cost affect patients' choices of medications. Detailed prophylaxis recommendations are presented in Table 3.

Malaria infection in pregnant women can be more severe than it is in nonpregnant women. Women who are pregnant or likely to become pregnant should be advised to avoid travel to malaria-risk areas. However, pregnant women who choose to travel to these areas should take appropriate antimalarial prophylaxis and use personal protective measures.

Travelers should be advised that they can contract malaria despite the use of prophylaxis and personal protective measures. Travelers should be aware of the signs and symptoms of malaria and should urgently seek medical care if they develop fever or experience flulike symptoms. Because many health care providers do not always ask about a history of recent travel, travelers should be advised to specifically inform providers of their recent travel to a malaria-endemic area so that the appropriate diagnostic evaluation and treatment can be initiated.

A malaria vaccine to protect against the development of illness or to dampen the severity of disease has been elusive despite the development of more than 45 vaccine candidates from 1990 to 2008. The Malaria Vaccine Initiative, partnered with GlaxoSmithKline, have brought a vaccine candidate, RTS,S/AS01, to phase III clinical trials, the first in recent years to progress to such levels. RTS,S is a pre-erythrocytic vaccine designed to promote antibody and T_H1 cell-mediated responses to the circumsporozoite protein expressed on the surface of *P. falciparum* sporozoites. This strategy aims to prevent clinical malaria illness by interfering with parasite progression to blood-stage disease. Studies to date show RTS,S to be of promising efficacy in children and infants living in endemic areas. Though a vaccine is not currently available for travelers or the military, RTS,S is a prospective future tool to decrease malaria burden in endemic areas, and in the most vulnerable populations.

TABLE 3 Malaria Chemoprophylaxis Recommendations

Drug	Use	Adult Dosage	Pediatric Dosage	Comments
Atovaquone/ proguanil (Malarone)	Prophylaxis in all malaria risk areas	Adult tabs contain 250 mg atovaquone and 100 mg proguanil HCl 1 adult tab PO qd	Ped tabs contain 62.5 mg atovaquone and 25 mg proguanil HCl 5–8 kg[1]: 2 ped tabs PO qd 9–10 kg[1]: 3 ped tab PO qd 11–20 kg: 1 adult tab PO qd 21–30 kg: 2 adult tabs PO qd >31–40 kg: 3 adult tabs PO qd >40 kg: 4 adult tabs PO qd	Begin 1-2 d before travel to malarious areas Take daily at the same time each day while in the malarious area and for 7 d after leaving such areas Contraindicated in persons with severe renal impairment (creatinine clearance <30 mL/min) Atovaquone/proguanil should be taken with food

Continued

TABLE 3 Malaria Chemoprophylaxis Recommendations—Cont'd

Drug	Use	Adult Dosage	Pediatric Dosage	Comments
Chloroquine phosphate* (Aralen and generic)	Prophylaxis only in areas with chloroquine-sensitive *P. falciparum*	300 mg base (500 mg salt) PO 1×/wk	5 mg/kg base (8.3 mg/kg salt) PO 1×/wk, up to max adult dose of 300 mg base	Not recommended for prophylaxis for children <5 kg or pregnant women Partial tab dosages may need to be prepared by a pharmacist and dispensed in individual caps Begin 1-2 wk before travel to malarious areas Take weekly on the same day of the week while in the malarious area and for 4 wk after leaving such areas Can exacerbate psoriasis
Doxycycline[†]	Prophylaxis in all malaria risk areas	100 mg PO qd	≥8 yr of age: 2 mg/kg up to adult dose of 100 mg/d*	Begin 1-2 d before travel to malarious areas Take daily at the same time each day while in the malarious area and for 4 wk after leaving such areas Contraindicated in children <8 yr of age and pregnant women
Hydroxychloroquine sulfate (Plaquenil)	An alternative to chloroquine for prophylaxis only in areas with chloroquine-sensitive *P. falciparum*	310 mg base (400 mg salt) PO 1×/wk	5 mg/kg base (6.5 mg/kg salt) PO 1×/wk, up to max adult dose of 310 mg base	Begin 1-2 wk before travel to malarious areas Take weekly on the same day of the week while in the malarious area and for 4 wk after leaving such areas
Mefloquine	Prophylaxis in areas with mefloquine-sensitive *P. falciparum*	228 mg base (250 mg salt) PO 1×/wk	≤9 kg: 4.6 mg/kg base (5 mg/kg salt) PO 1×/wk 10–19 kg: ¼ tab PO 1×/wk 20–30 kg: ½ tab PO 1×/wk 31–45 kg: ¾ tab PO 1×/wk ≥46 kg: 1 tab PO 1×/wk	Begin 1-2 wk before travel to malarious areas Take weekly on the same day of the week while in the malarious area and for 4 wk after leaving such areas Contraindicated in persons allergic to mefloquine or related compounds (e.g., quinine and quinidine) and in persons with active depression, a recent history of depression, generalized anxiety disorder, psychosis, schizophrenia, other major psychiatric disorders, or seizures Use with caution in persons with psychiatric disturbances or a previous history of depression Not recommended for persons with cardiac conduction abnormalities
Primaquine phosphate[1,‡]	Prophylaxis in areas with mainly *P. vivax*	30 mg base (52.6 mg salt) PO qd[3]	0.6 mg/kg base (1.0 mg/kg salt) up to adult dose PO qd[3]	Begin 1-2 d before travel to malarious areas Take daily at the same time each day while in the malarious area and for 7 ds after leaving such areas Contraindicated in persons with G6PD[‡] deficiency Contraindicated during pregnancy and lactation unless the infant being breast-fed has a documented normal G6PD level
Primaquine phosphate[‡]	Used for presumptive antirelapse therapy (terminal prophylaxis) to decrease the risk of relapses of *P. vivax* and *P. ovale*	30 mg base (52.6 mg salt) PO qd × 14 d after departure from the malarious area[3]	0.6 mg/kg base (1.0 mg/kg salt) up to adult dose PO qd × 14 d after departure from the malarious area[3]	Indicated for persons who have had prolonged exposure to *P. vivax* or *P. ovale* or both Contraindicated in persons with G6PD[‡] deficiency Contraindicated during pregnancy and lactation unless the infant being breast-fed has a documented normal G6PD level

cap = capsule; G6PD = glucose 6 phosphate dehydrogenase; max = maximum; ped = pediatric; tab = tablet.
[1]Not FDA approved for this indication.
[3]Exceeds dosage recommended by the manufacturer.
*All pregnant women with *P. vivax* and *P. ovale* should be given chloroquine prophylaxis for the duration of pregnancy to avoid relapses and can be treated with primaquine after delivery.
[†]Doxycycline and tetracycline are not indicated for use in children younger than 8 y.
[‡]All persons who take primaquine should have a documented normal G6PD level before starting the medication.

REFERENCES

Baird JK. Effectiveness of antimalarial drugs. N Engl J Med 2005;352(15): 1565–77.

Centers for Disease Control and Prevention. Guidelines for Treatment of Malaria in the United States. PDF available at: http://www.cdc.gov/malaria/pdf/treatmenttable.pdf; [accessed 18.06.10].

Food and Drug Administration. FDA Approves Coartem Tablets to Treat Malaria. PDF available at: http://www.fda.gov/NewsEvents/Newsroom/PressAnnouncements/2009/ucm149559.htm; [accessed 18.06.10].

Griffith KS, Lewis LS, Mali S, Parise ME, et al. Treatment of malaria in the United States: A systematic review. JAMA 2007;297(20):2264–77.

Lalloo DG, Hill DR. Preventing malaria in travellers. BMJ 2008;336 (7657):1362–6.

Mali S, Steele S, Slutsker L, Arguin PM. Centers for Disease Control and Prevention (CDC): Malaria surveillance—United States. 2006. MMWR Surveill Summ 2008;57(5):24–39.

Newman RD, Parise ME, Barber AM, Steketee RW. Malaria-related deaths among U.S. travelers, 1963–2001. Ann Intern Med 2004;141(7):547–55.

Price RN, Douglas NM, Anstey NM. New developments in *Plasmodium vivax* malaria: Severe disease and the rise of chloroquine resistance. Curr Opin Infect Dis 2009;22(5):430–5.

Rosenthal PJ. Artesunate for the treatment of severe falciparum malaria. N Engl J Med 2008;358(17):1829–36.

Targett GA, Greenwood BM. Malaria vaccines and their potential role in the elimination of malaria. Malar J 2008;7(Suppl. 1):S10.

World Health Organization. Severe falciparum malaria. World Health Organization, Communicable Diseases Cluster. Trans R Soc Trop Med Hyg 2000;94(Suppl. 1):S1–90.

World Health Organization. World Malaria Report 2009. Geneva: World Health Organization; 2009.

Bacterial Meningitis

Method of
Gary D. Overturf, MD

Acute bacterial meningitis occurs in all age groups, but predominantly in children younger than 2 years and the elderly (older than 60 years). With the introduction of effective protein conjugate vaccines for *Haemophilus* and pneumococcal infection, the incidence of bacterial meningitis is rapidly declining in children, and adults are now the major population affected. Bacterial meningitis is a medical emergency requiring rapid and decisive action to prevent death or neurologic sequelae. Since the introduction of chloramphenicol (Chloromycetin) in the early 1950s, the mortality has remained between 5% and 40% depending on the age of the patient and the etiology. Of the survivors, 10% to 30% suffer permanent neurologic deficits. Prognosis is affected by the timeliness of therapy, the age of the patient, and the etiology. Presumptive diagnosis and administration of therapy are critical.

Diagnosis

Acute bacterial meningitis must be considered in the differential diagnosis of persons of any age presenting with fever and headache or signs of meningeal irritation or acute central nervous system dysfunction. Presentations can be subtle at the extremes of age or in patients who have received partially effective antibiotic therapy. The diagnosis of bacterial meningitis requires the examination of the cerebrospinal fluid (CSF), which must be performed as expeditiously as possible. Studies indicate that lumbar puncture may be safely performed on patients who have normal mental status or are without focal neurologic signs or papilledema; clinical impression are predictive of the computed tomography (CT) findings. If there are signs or symptoms suggesting the presence of an intracranial mass

CURRENT DIAGNOSIS

- Patient age and epidemiology:
  - Clinical symptoms: Fever, headache, meningeal signs
  - CSF examination: High opening pressure >300 mm Hg
  - Elevated white blood cell count (>10–>5000)
  - >60% polymorphonuclear cells
- Low CSF glucose (<40 mg/dL or <50% serum glucose)
- High CSF protein (>50–>1.0 g/dL)
- Bacteria present on Gram stain of CSF

Abbreviation: CSF = cerebrospinal fluid.

(e.g., tumor, cerebral hematoma, or brain abscess), blood cultures should be obtained and empirical antibiotics should be administered prior to the performance of a CT scan.

The CSF findings in bacterial meningitis include a cell count of greater than 500 to 5000 white blood cells (WBC) per mm^3 with a predominance of neutrophils, a protein concentration of greater than 150 mg/mL, and a low glucose (e.g., less than 35 to 40 mg/dL). No single value is absolute, and a single value may be normal in up to a third of the cases. The Gram-stained sediment of centrifuged CSF is the critical examination leading to a specific diagnosis. In patients who have not received antibiotics capable of reaching the CSF, the Gram stain is positive in 80% to 90% of culture-confirmed cases. In persons previously treated with antibiotics (e.g., beta-lactam antibiotics, tetracycline, fluoroquinolones), the frequency of positive Gram stains is much reduced (e.g., 60% to 70%), but the cells, cell type, protein, and glucose concentrations are not significantly affected. CSF antigen tests are not reliable, and high false-positive and false-negative rates direct against relying on the use of such tests. Clinical judgment is paramount, and antibiotics should be given in situations of ambiguous results of the CSF examination.

Antibiotic Selection

The outcome of bacterial meningitis is closely related to the timely use of antibiotics. Hypotension, seizures, an altered mental status, and hypoglycorrhachia at the time of initial antibiotic administration are predictive of higher case fatality and neurologic sequelae. Because prompt administration of antibiotics is critical, the choice of antibiotics usually is made before results of the CSF cultures are known. If organisms are seen on Gram stain, therapy may be directed by the probable bacterial etiology (Table 1). In the event the CSF Gram stain fails to reveal a possible pathogen, empirical antibiotic therapy should be begun based on the age of the patient for those persons who have acquired their infection in the community (Table 2). For those persons who are members of special risk groups, empirical therapy should be based on the likely etiology (Table 3). Once the CSF cultures are completed, therapy can be modified according to results of the culture and sensitivity data.

Antibiotics used in bacterial meningitis should be rapidly bactericidal and achieve high concentrations in the CSF. Antibiotics should be given in maximal doses (Table 4). Because the bactericidal activity of antibiotics in CSF is dose dependent, the fractional CSF-to-serum ratio is very small. Finally, the use of combinations of antibiotics should be minimized to avoid antagonizing the bactericidal activity.

Special Considerations for Antibiotic Therapy

During the past two decades, resistance to penicillin and some third-generation cephalosporins (e.g., ceftriaxone [Rocephin], cefotaxime [Claforan]) has steadily increased among strains of *Streptococcus*

TABLE 1 Cerebrospinal Fluid Gram Stain Morphology and Antibiotic Recommendations

Morphology	Possible or Probable Pathogens	Treatment Options	Alternative Therapies
Gram-positive cocci, short chains or pairs	*Streptococcus pneumoniae, Streptococcus agalactiae* (group B streptococci)	Ceftriaxone (Rocephin) or cefotaxime (Claforan) plus vancomycin (Vancocin)	Chloramphenicol (Chloromycetin)
Gram-positive cocci, clusters; or gram-positive bacilli	*Staphylococcus aureus, Listeria monocytogenes*	Vancomycin, ampicillin plus gentamicin (Garamycin)	Nafcillin (Unipen) or Oxacillin, trimethoprim-sulfamethoxazole (Bactrim)
Gram-negative diplococci	*Neisseria meningitidis*	Ceftriaxone or cefotaxime	Ampicillin, Penicillin G, or chloramphenicol
Gram-negative coccobacilli	*Haemophilus influenzae*	Ceftriaxone or cefotaxime	Chloramphenicol
Gram-negative bacilli	*Escherichia coli, Klebsiella* species, *Pseudomonas aeruginosa*	Cefepime (Maxipime) or ceftazidime (Fortaz)	Imipenem (Primaxin) or meropenem (Merrem)

TABLE 2 Antibiotic Recommendations for Bacterial Meningitis Acquired in the Community, by Age Group and Probable Pathogen

Age Group	Probable Pathogens	Empirical Therapy
Neonate < 1 mo	Group B streptococcus; *Escherichia coli*, or other gram-negative enteric rod; occasionally *Listeria monocytogenes*	Ampicillin plus cefotaxime (Claforan)
Infants 1–3 mo	*H. influenzae, N. meningitidis, S. pneumoniae,* Group B streptococci	Ceftriaxone (Rocephin) or cefotaxime (Claforan)
Children 3 mo–7 y and older children and adults 7–50 y	*H. influenzae, S. pneumoniae, N. meningitidis*	Ceftriaxone or cefotaxime plus vancomycin (Vancocin)
Older adults > 50 y	*S. pneumoniae, N. meningitidis, L. monocytogenes*	Ceftriaxone plus ampicillin

TABLE 3 Antibiotic Recommendations for Presumed Bacterial Meningitis in Persons with Special Risks

Condition or Risk Factor	Common Pathogens	Antibiotic Recommendations
Impaired immunity (e.g., HIV, early complement deficiency, agammaglobulinemia)	*Listeria monocytogenes, Streptococcus pneumoniae, Haemophilus influenzae*	Ampicillin plus ceftriaxone (Rocephin) or cefotaxime (Claforan)
Closed head trauma with CSF leak	*S. pneumoniae, H. influenzae*	Ceftriaxone or cefotaxime plus vancomycin (Vancocin)
Asplenia	*S. pneumoniae, H. influenzae*	Ceftriaxone or cefotaxime plus vancomycin
Terminal complement deficiency	*Neisseria meningitidis*	Ceftriaxone or cefotaxime
Neurosurgical procedures	*Staphylococcus aureus*	Vancomycin plus ceftriaxone or cefotaxime
CSF shunt infections	Coagulase-negative staphylococci, gram-negative bacilli	
Elderly patients (> 65 y)	*S. pneumoniae, Listeria monocytogenes*	Ceftriaxone or cefotaxime plus vancomycin
Recurrent bacterial meningitis (see CSF leak)	*Streptococcus pneumoniae*	Ceftriaxone or cefotaxime plus vancomycin
Alcoholic patients	*Streptococcus pneumoniae* and gram-negative bacilli	Ceftriaxone or cefotaxime plus vancomycin

Abbreviation: CSF = cerebrospinal fluid.

pneumoniae. Currently, approximately 30% to 50% of isolates are either intermediately (inhibitory concentration, 0.1 to 1.0 µg/mL) or fully (inhibitory concentration more than 2.0 µg/mL) resistant to *Penicillin* G and ampicillin. Resistance to ceftriaxone (Rocephin) and cefotaxime (Claforan) may occur as well in 10% to 15% of strains. Vancomycin (Vancocin) is recommended in those regimens for meningitis when pneumococci are considered. However, higher maximal doses are required for vancomycin because of its relatively poor penetration into the CSF. In general, lumbar puncture with CSF culture should be repeated in 48 hours in those cases where vancomycin therapy is the primary drug because of demonstrated penicillin or cephalosporin resistance.

Meningitis caused by gram-negative bacilli such as *Pseudomonas aeruginosa, Escherichia coli,* or *Enterobacter cloacae* should be treated with a cephalosporin with an extended spectrum of gram-negative activity, such as ceftazidime (Fortaz) or cefepime (Maxipime). A carbapenem, such as imipenem (Primaxin) or meropenem (Merrem), can also be used for antibiotic-resistant gram-negative enteric and pseudomonas meningitis. Meropenem is associated with less risk of drug-induced seizures and may be a better choice for bacterial meningitis.

TABLE 4 Antibiotic Doses for Adults and Children for Treatment of Bacterial Meningitis

Antibiotic	Daily Adult Dose	Daily Pediatric Dose	Dose Interval
Amikacin (Amikin)	15 mg/kg	15–20 mg/kg	8 h
Ampicillin	12 g	200–400 mg/kg	4–6 h
Cefotaxime (Claforan)	12 g	200–300 mg/kg	4–6 h
Ceftriaxone (Rocephin)	4 g	100 mg/kg	12 h
Ceftazidime (Fortaz)	6 g	150–200 mg/kg	8 h
Cefepime (Maxipime)	6 g	100–150 mg/kg	8 h
Gentamicin (Garamycin)	5 mg/kg	7.5 mg/kg	8 h
Meropenem (Merrem)	6 g	120 mg/kg	8 h
Nafcillin (Unipen)	12 g	200 mg/kg	4–6 h
Penicillin G	24 million U	250,000 units/kg	4 h
Tobramycin (Nebcin)	5 mg/kg	6–7.5 mg/kg	8 h
Trimethoprim-sulfamethoxazole (Bactrim)	10–15 mg/kg	10–20 mg/kg	8 h
Vancomycin (Vancocin)	2 g	60 mg/kg	12 h

Adapted from Bradley JS, Nelson JD: 2002–2003 Nelson's Pocket Book of Pediatric Antimicrobial Therapy, 15th ed. Philadelphia and New York, Lippincott Williams & Wilkins, 2002.
Gilbert DN, Moellering RC, Sande MA. The Sanford Guide to Antimicrobial Therapy 2005. Hyde Park, Antimicrobial Therapy Inc., 2005.

Patients with ventriculoatrial and ventriculoperitoneal shunt–associated meningitis and ventriculitis usually require removal of the shunt for cure, as well as the administration of antibiotics to clear the infection. Certain patients with infections caused by organisms of reduced virulence, such as coagulase-negative staphylococci, or those with exquisitely antibiotic-susceptible infections, can be treated with a trial of antibiotics alone.

Because of the extreme sensitivity of *Neisseria meningitidis* to antibiotics, uncomplicated meningitis may be treated with as little as 5 to 7 days of antibiotics. Pneumococcal meningitis may be treated with 10 to 14 days of antibiotics and haemophilus infections are treated successfully with 7 to 10 days of antibiotics. Gram-negative meningitis was treated in the past with 3 weeks of aminoglycosides, but current experience with newer extended-spectrum cephalosporins (ceftriaxone, cefotaxime, carbapenems) suggests that 2 weeks of therapy is often sufficient in neonates as well as in some elderly patients and postoperative infections.

All patients with bacterial meningitis should be monitored carefully throughout the treatment period. Infectious disease consultation is recommended for most infections of the central nervous system.

CURRENT THERAPY

- Neonates < 2 mo
  - Group B streptococcal infection: cefotaxime (Claforan) or ampicillin
  - Gram-negative rods, other than *Pseudomonas:* cefotaxime
  - *Pseudomonas:* cefepime (Maxipime), ceftazidime (Fortaz), or meropenem (Merrem)
  - *Listeria:* Ampicillin + gentamicin (Garamycin)
- Children > 2 mo
  - Empirical for unknown etiology: cefotaxime or ceftriaxone (Rocephin)
  - *Streptococcus pneumoniae:* cefotaxime or ceftriaxone
  - *Haemophilus influenzae:* cefotaxime or ceftriaxone
  - *Neisseria meningitidis:* ampicillin or cefotaxime
- Older children and adults
  - Empirical for unknown etiology: cefotaxime or ceftriaxone
  - *S. pneumoniae:* cefotaxime or ceftriaxone
  - *N. meningitidis:* ampicillin or cefotaxime
  - Gram negative, postoperative, or *Staphylococcus aureus* (see Tables 1–4)
  - Add vancomycin if at risk for infection with resistant pneumococcus

Repeated lumbar punctures are not routinely recommended for patients with fully susceptible bacterial isolates or in those who show good response to therapy. Repeated sampling of the CSF with lumbar puncture or, when appropriate, shunt or ventricular reservoir puncture should be performed in those with known resistant bacterial isolates, in patients who have an inadequate response, in those patients who deteriorate on therapy, or in those for whom clinical response may correlate poorly with the microbiologic response (shunt infections, neonates, and elderly patients).

Adjunctive Therapy

Corticosteroids reduce the incidence of permanent neurologic sequelae in children with bacterial meningitis, particularly when caused by *Haemophilus influenza* type b. Data in support of steroids in either pneumococcal or meningococcal infections are less robust. Dexamethasone (Decadron[1]), 0.15 mg/kg every 6 hours for the first 2 to 4 days of treatment, was evaluated in children older than 2 months with bacterial meningitis. The first dose of dexamethasone should be given before, at the start, or within no later than 12 hours after beginning antibiotics.

Use of corticosteroids in adults is more controversial. Although doses of dexamethasone are recommended by some experts for adults with bacterial meningitis, its efficacy in adult meningitis has not been evaluated in a well-designed prospective trial. A recent study in adults found that corticosteroids significantly reduced the risk for unfavorable outcomes, particularly in patients with pneumococcal meningitis. There has been concern that the anti-inflammatory properties of dexamethasone may decrease the penetration of antibiotics, especially vancomycin, into the CSF. One study in children did not show this to be the case. Dexamethasone[1] should be administered in adults with proven or suspected pneumococcal meningitis, only if it can be given prior to the first dose of antibiotics in a dose of 10 mg every 6 hours for 4 days. In patients with meningitis caused by *Streptococcus pneumoniae* highly resistant to penicillin (minimum inhibitory concentration [MIC] >2.0 µg/mL) or cephalosporins (MIC >4.0 µg/mL), vancomycin should not be used as a single agent if corticosteroids are used. The addition of rifampin (Rifadin[1]) is often recommended in these situations.

Chemoprophylaxis for Bacterial Meningitis

Prophylactic antibiotics are recommended in case of meningitis caused by *Neisseria meningitidis* and *Haemophilus influenzae* type b. Prophylaxis is provided to eliminate the carriage of organisms among

---

[1]Not FDA approved for this indication.

contacts and prevent spread to hosts susceptible to invasive disease. In cases of meningococcal meningitis, prophylaxis is indicated only for those with household or close intimate contact with the index case. Administration of prophylaxis to large groups (e.g., college students, schoolchildren, or preschool classes) requires a special assessment and a recommendation of local or regional health departments. Chemoprophylaxis is not necessary for casual contacts or medical personnel unless there is a direct exposure to respiratory secretions. The recommended dose of rifampin (Rifadin) is 10 mg/kg (600 maximal, adults) twice a day for 2 days; ciprofloxacin (Cipro[1]), 500 mg as single dose, is also effective for adults. Third-generation cephalosporins used in treatment of the index case of meningitis are sufficient to eliminate carriage of the organism.

Chemoprophylaxis for *H. influenzae* type b is recommended for all household contacts of an index case if one of the contacts is an unvaccinated child younger than 4 years. If the index case is treated with ceftriaxone (Rocephin) or cefotaxime (Claforan), prophylaxis is not required, but if treated with ampicillin or chloramphenicol (Chloromycetin), prophylaxis is recommended to eliminate carriage. The recommended regimen for prophylaxis is rifampin,[1] 20 mg/kg (or 600 mg in adults) once a day for 4 days. With the near elimination of invasive infections caused by *Haemophilus influenzae* type b, with the use of routine immunization of children with conjugate haemophilus vaccines, *Haemophilus influenzae* types A, F, and rarely other serotypes have emerged, and the use of prophylaxis is not recommended in these situations because sufficient data are not available to support its efficacy, nor has spread within contacts been documented.

Vaccines for Bacterial Meningitis

The universal recommendation for the use of protein-polysaccharide conjugate *Haemophilus influenzae* type b (HIB) vaccines in 1987 reduced the incidence of bacterial meningitis by this organism by greater than 97%. Three HIB vaccines (PedvaxHIB, ActHIB, HibTITER), licensed in the United States, are routinely given to children in dosage schedules employing three to four doses by 12 to 18 months of age (see www.cdc.gov).

A pneumococcal protein-polysaccharide conjugate vaccine (Prevnar) licensed in 2000 is routinely recommended for children and has markedly reduced the incidence of invasive infections with seven serotypes of pneumococci in children. This vaccine is also recommended for children at high risk of pneumococcal infections (e.g., HIV infection, asplenia, sickle cell disease, and others). A pneumococcal polysaccharide vaccine (Pneumovax 23) is recommended for adults older than 65 years or for those over 50 years with risk factors (e.g., alcoholism, diabetes or other metabolic or renal disease, chronic pulmonary or cardiac disease). Although clear evidence for prevention of bacterial meningitis is lacking, evidence supports its efficacy against invasive pneumococcal diseases, many of which are the preceding infections leading to bacteremia and meningitis.

Currently two vaccines remain available for prevention of meningococcal disease caused by four serotypes, A, C, Y, and W-135. The meningococcal polysaccharide vaccine (Menomune) was recommended for persons older than 2 years at high risk for severe meningococcal infections including adolescents and college students (particularly those residing in dormitories), military recruits, and those with complement deficiencies and asplenia. A quadrivalent protein-polysaccharide conjugate vaccines (Menactra) was licensed in 2005. This vaccine is now recommended for routine immunization of all children 11 to 12 years of age and adolescents and college students at high risk as well as those more than 2 to 55 years of age with high-risk factors for meningococcal infection, including all those for whom the polysacharide vaccine was previously recommended.

---

[1]Not FDA approved for this indication.

REFERENCES

Anderson EJ, Yogev LR. A rational approach to the management of ventricular shunt infections. Pediatric Infect Dis J 2005;24:557–8.

Andes DR, Craig WA. Pharmacokinetics and pharmacodynamics of antibiotics in meningitis. Infect Dis Clin North Am 1999;13(2):595–618.

De Gans J, van de Beek. Dexamethasone in adults with bacterial meningitis. N Engl J Med 2002;347:1549–64.

Gray LD, Fedorko DP. Laboratory diagnosis of bacterial meningitis. Clin Microbiol Rev 1992;5:130–45.

Hussein AS, Shafran SD. Acute bacterial meningitis in adults: A 12-year review. Medicine (Baltimore) 2000;79:360–8.

Klinger G, Chin C-Y, Beyene J, et al. Predicting the outcome of neonatal bacterial meningitis. Pediatrics 2000;106:477–82.

Klein JO. Bacterial sepsis and meningitis. In: Remington JS, Klein JO, editors. Infectious Diseases of the Fetus and Newborn Infant. 5th ed. New York and Saint Louis: WB Saunders; 2002. p. 943–98.

Odio CM, Faingezicht I, Paris M, et al. The beneficial effects of early dexamethasone administration in infants and children with bacterial meningitis. N Engl J Med 1991;324:1525–31.

Ronan A, Hogg GG, Klug CL. Cerebrospinal fluid shunt infections in children. Pediatr Infect Dis J 1995;14:782–6.

Schuchat A, Robinson K, Wenger JD, et al. Bacterial meningitis in the United States in 1995. N Engl J Med 1997;337:970–6.

Unhanand M, Mustapha MM, McCracken GH, et al. Gram-negative enteric bacillary meningitis: A twenty-one year experience. J Pediatr 1993; 122:15–7.

Van de Beek D, de Gans J, Spanjaard L, et al. Clinical features and prognostic factors in adults with bacterial meningitis. N Engl J Med 2004;351: 1849–58.

Infectious Mononucleosis

Method of
Joseph Domachowske, MD

Infectious mononucleosis (IM) is a clinical syndrome consisting of fever, lymphadenopathy, exudative tonsillopharyngitis, splenomegaly, and atypical lymphocytosis. Because most cases are caused by Epstein-Barr virus (EBV), many clinicians use the term IM synonymously with acute EBV infection. Less common causes of IM include primary cytomegalovirus infection, hepatitis A, hepatitis B, toxoplasmosis, HIV, adenovirus, and rubella.

CURRENT DIAGNOSIS

- Fever
- Lymphadenopathy
- Exudative pharyngitis
- Splenomegaly
- Atypical lymphocytosis

CURRENT THERAPY

- Supportive therapy including hydration and analgesics
- Antiviral medications are not effective.
- Glucocorticoids are reserved for patients with airway obstruction.

Classic Syndrome and Disease Course

Humans are the only known reservoir for EBV. Transmission occurs efficiently, usually through direct contact with oral secretions. The incubation period of EBV in IM is between 30 and 50 days. This is followed by a prodrome characterized by malaise, headache, and fatigue, after which fever, sore throat, and cervical lymphadenopathy occur. The adenopathy is symmetrical and involves the posterior and anterior cervical lymph node chains. More generalized adenopathy is not uncommon. The pharynx is erythematous with an associated white or green-gray exudate. Severe fatigue can be predominant. Less common signs include palatal or pharyngeal petechiae; periorbital, palpebral, or forehead edema; and a maculopapular or morbilliform rash, particularly if the patient takes penicillin or amoxicillin (Amoxil). Gastrointestinal complaints are also relatively common. The nausea and anorexia may be secondary to mild hepatitis, which is present in almost all infected individuals. Splenomegaly is also common, whereas jaundice and hepatomegaly are uncharacteristic.

Although most patients with IM develop pharyngitis, adenopathy predominates in the so-called glandular form of IM, and there are minimal or no pharyngeal symptoms. Patients may also present with a more systemic illness characterized by prolonged fever and fatigue. The vast majority of individuals who develop IM recover uneventfully. Acute symptoms resolve in 1 to 2 weeks, although fatigue often persists for months. The frequency with which clinical signs and symptoms occur in children and in adults are summarized in Table 1.

Complications of Infectious Mononucleosis

SPLENIC RUPTURE

As many as 2 patients per 1000 develop splenic rupture as a direct complication of IM. Approximately half of these events are spontaneous, and, for reasons that are poorly understood, almost all are reported in males. Rupture has occurred between days 4 and 24 of symptomatic infection and was not able to be predicted based on symptom severity, laboratory findings, or even physician-documented palpable splenomegaly. Despite the life-threatening potential of splenic rupture, fatalities are rare. Nonoperative treatment with intensive supportive care is successful for some patients, whereas others require splenectomy. Specific guidelines have not been established regarding the timing of safe return to athletic participation after IM without risk of splenic rupture. Because rupture can occur even in the absence of trauma, precluding strenuous activity, including weight lifting and contact sports, for the first 3 to 4 weeks after the onset of illness is usually recommended. For patients who compete in higher-risk contact sports, radiologic evaluation of spleen size may be reasonable before clearance, although this approach remains a debated issue.

AIRWAY OBSTRUCTION

Obstruction of the upper airway is another known complication of IM. Patients with massive lymphadenopathy, mucosal edema, and severe tonsillopharyngitis need to be carefully evaluated and monitored. The administration of glucocorticoids is advocated for individuals with incipient obstruction. Some patients require endotracheal intubation or tracheostomy placement.

Unusual Manifestations of Infectious Mononucleosis

A full spectrum of illness and laboratory abnormalities have been described for primary EBV- associated IM. Mild hematologic abnormalities (anemia, mild thrombocytopenia, atypical lymphocytosis) are common (Table 2), and more severe changes can also occur. Hemolytic anemia, aplastic anemia, thrombocytopenic purpura, hemolytic uremic syndrome, and disseminated intravascular coagulation are among the most serious hematologic perturbations described. EBV infection is also the most commonly recognized infectious trigger for the development of hemophagocytic lymphohistiocytosis (sometimes called macrophage activation syndrome). Patients with this syndrome develop fever, generalized lymphadenopathy, hepatosplenomegaly with hepatitis, pancytopenia, and coagulopathy. A detailed discussion of the important association of EBV infection with the development of lymphoproliferative disorders (including those seen in transplant patients), Burkitt's lymphoma, T-cell lymphoma, smooth muscle tumors, Hodgkin's disease, and nasopharyngeal carcinoma are beyond the scope of this chapter.

Neurologic manifestations of primary EBV infection may include meningoencephalitis, "Alice in Wonderland" syndrome with associated metamorphopsia (visual-spatial hallucinations), Guillain-Barré syndrome, facial nerve palsy, optic neuritis, and peripheral neuritis. Patients with neurologic manifestations of EBV infection may not have other evidence of IM.

TABLE 1 Clinical Signs and Symptoms of Primary Epstein-Barr Virus Infection in Children and Adults

Sign or Symptom	Frequency (%)	
	Children <16 y	Adults
Lymphadenopathy	94–100	93–100
Malaise/fatigue	85–100	90–100
Fever	92–100	63–100
Tonsillopharyngitis	67–75	70–91
Pharyngeal exudate	45–59	40–74
Splenomegaly	53–82	32–51
Hepatomegaly	30–63	6–24
Cough	15–51	5–31
Rash	17–34	3–15
Nausea, abdominal pain	0–17	2–14
Eyelid or forehead edema	10–14	5–34
Genital ulcers	1–2	Uncommon, perhaps underreported
Meningoencephalitis and other neurologic findings	Uncommon	Uncommon

TABLE 2 Laboratory Abnormalities in Acute Epstein-Barr Virus Infectious Mononucleosis

Findings	% Positive
EBV-specific antibody	100
Lymphocytosis	95–100
Elevated liver transaminases	80–100
Atypical lymphocytosis	90–99
Heterophile antibody	80–90 in adults*
Leukocytosis	60–80
Neutropenia	60–80
Anemia (mild-moderate)	40–60
Thrombocytopenia (usually mild)	25–45
Increased cold agglutinins	10–45
Leukopenia	10–20
Positive direct Coombs' test	Rare
Significant anemia	Rare
Anti-platelet antibodies	Rare
False-positive HIV ELISA	Rare

*Age dependent (see text).
EBV, Epstein-Barr virus; ELISA, enzyme-linked immunosorbent assay.

Lymphoproliferative disorders and malignancies associated with EBV persistence and reactivation are recognized complications in immunocompromised individuals; however, persistent, recurrent, or reactivated EBV infection is extremely rare in immunocompetent individuals. Care must be taken to carefully interpret laboratory results of EBV antibody titers (see later discussion). If IM does recur in an otherwise healthy individual, it is likely that the separate episodes of IM were each caused by a different etiologic agent (e.g., EBV and then cytomegalovirus), rather than true recurrence of the EBV infection.

Diagnosis

The clinical diagnosis of IM is not always straightforward, so confirmatory testing is usually performed. In addition, hematologic and liver enzyme perturbations are common, so complete blood counts with evaluation of the peripheral smear and detection of serum liver transaminases are prudent. By the second week of infection, it is not uncommon to see 20% or more atypical lymphocytes on the peripheral blood smear. These atypical cells, sometimes referred to as Downey cells, have a higher cytoplasm-to-nucleus ratio than normal lymphocytes, and prominent nucleoli are occasionally seen. The cytoplasm is more basophilic and vacuolated than usual, so an untrained eye might suspect the presence of peripheral blasts. These lymphocytes represent activated T lymphocytes that are directed against the EBV-infected B lymphocytes.

Most cases of IM are caused by EBV, so confirming the etiologic agent of IM starts with EBV testing. Primary EBV infection stimulates the production of serum antibodies directed against viral antigens, as well as unrelated antigens found on sheep and horse erythrocytes. The latter antibodies, referred to as heterophile antibodies, are a group of proteins (mostly immunoglobulin M [IgM]) that do not recognize EBV antigens. Although it is not specific for a diagnosis of EBV infection (i.e., other conditions can lead to the production of heterophile antibodies), a positive heterophile antibody test result obtained from an adolescent or adult patient with symptoms consistent with IM is presumptive evidence for EBV infection. Although the heterophile antibody tests have a sensitivity of up to 90% in patients older than 12 years of age, these types of tests are not recommended for use in young children, because children do not reliably generate these nonspecific antibody responses. Approximately 50% of children between 2 and 4 years of age, and fewer than 10% of children younger than 2 years with primary EBV infection are heterophile antibody positive.

A number of rapid spot tests are commercially available for the detection of heterophile antibodies. The assay itself is simple and inexpensive to perform and requires minimal training. The results can be available within minutes, making this an attractive, popular diagnostic tool that is available in many office and urgent care settings.

The specific diagnosis of acute EBV infection is based on the appearance of IgM antibody directed against the EBV viral capsid antigen (anti-EBV-VCA-IgM). This is the first EBV-specific antibody produced, and it is usually detectable by the time the patient is symptomatic. The detection of anti-EBV-VCA-IgM establishes that the patient has a current (or has had a very recent) primary EBV infection and is the single most useful EBV specific antibody titer used to diagnose the etiologic agent of IM. Further on during the course of the illness, the patient also develops additional antibodies directed against the VCA (anti-EBV-VCA-IgG), early antigen (anti-EBV-EA), and nuclear antigen (anti-EBNA). Many clinical laboratories perform these antibody tests as an EBV antibody panel, requiring interpretation of each of the results. Table 3 provides details regarding the appearance and persistence of each of these antibodies. Because IgG titers to VCA and EBNA can persist for life, their presence alone simply confirms a past infection.

The most common cause of EBV-negative IM is cytomegalovirus infection, but toxoplasmosis, hepatitis A, hepatitis B, HIV, adenovirus, and rubella are recognized to cause fever, adenopathy, and fatigue with atypical lymphocytosis. The diagnosis of IM caused by these other agents can be established by standard serologic testing. IgM testing is available to establish toxoplasmosis, hepatitis A, hepatitis B, and rubella. Alternatively, IgG antibody titers can be collected from the patient's serum during the acute phase of infection and compared with titers obtained during convalescence (usually 4–6 weeks apart). A fourfold rise in IgG antibody titer establishes the etiologic agent. HIV testing is performed as a two-step process consisting of a screening enzyme linked immunoassay for anti-HIV IgG antibodies, followed by confirmatory Western blotting. Adenovirus infection can be confirmed by viral culture or nucleic acid–based amplification tests, if available.

Treatment

The mainstay of treatment for individuals with IM is supportive care. Acetaminophen (Tylenol) or nonsteroidal antiinflammatory medications are recommended for the treatment of fever and throat pain. Maintaining adequate hydration in the face of fevers and severe pharyngitis can be challenging. Intravenous hydration is necessary in a minority of cases. No specific treatment has been identified to relieve the prolonged fatigue that many adolescents and young adults experience after the acute infection.

The use of corticosteroids for uncomplicated IM remains controversial. Studies evaluating steroids for use in IM suggest that they do reduce lymphoid and mucosal swelling, and clinicians should consider administering steroids to patients with impending airway obstruction. However, routine use of glucocorticoids is probably best avoided. The clinical manifestations of IM represent the immune response to infection with EBV, a herpes-group virus that establishes lifelong latency and has oncogenic potential. For this reason, therapy with immunomodulatory agents (e.g., glucocorticoids) could alter the immune response, potentially predisposing the patient to a lifelong lymphoproliferative complication.

Specific antiviral therapy of acute EBV infection with oral and intravenous acyclovir (Zovirax)[1] has been tested. Although short-term

---

[1]Not FDA approved for this indication.

TABLE 3 Serologic Testing for Epstein-Barr Virus Infection

Antibody	Time of Appearance from Onset of Symptoms	Patients with Positive Test (%)	Antibody Persistence
Heterophile	End of 1st wk	See text	Up to 1 y
VCA-IgM	1–3 wk	100	2–3 mo
VCA-IgG	<3 wk	100	Lifelong
Early antigen	After the 1st wk	70–80	3–6 mo
EBNA	3–4 wk	100	Lifelong

EBNA, Epstein-Barr nuclear antigen; Ig, immunoglobulin; VCA, viral capsid antigen.

suppression of virus shedding can be demonstrated, measurable clinical benefits are lacking. These results are not unexpected, because there is little evidence that ongoing viral replication contributes to disease pathogenesis. Available data support the hypothesis that the symptoms of IM are secondary to the immunopathology generated in response to EBV-transformed lymphocytes during the acute phase of the disease.

REFERENCES

Barnes CJ, Alió AB, Cunningham BB, et al. Epstein-Barr virus-associated genital ulcers: An under-recognized disorder. Pediatr Dermatol 2007;24:130–4.

Cameron B, Bharadwaj M, Burrows J, et al. Prolonged illness after infectious mononucleosis is associated with altered immunity but not with increased viral load. J Infect Dis 2006;193:664–71.

Candy B, Hotopf M. Steroids for symptom control in infectious mononucleosis. Cochrane Database Syst Rev 2006;(3):CD004402.

Domachowske JB, Cunningham CK, Cummings DL, et al. Acute manifestations and neurologic sequelae of Epstein Barr virus encephalitis in children. Pediatr Infect Dis J 1996;15:871–5.

Gershburg E, Pagano JS. Epstein-Barr virus infections: Prospects for treatment. J Antimicrob Chemother 2005;56:277–81.

Gulley ML, Tang W. Laboratory assays for Epstein-Barr virus-related disease. J Mol Diagn 2008;10:279–92.

Klein E, Kis LL, Klein G. Epstein-Barr virus infection in humans: From harmless to life endangering virus-lymphocyte interactions. Oncogene 2007;26: 1297–305.

Kutok JT, Wang F. Spectrum of Epstein-Barr virus-associated diseases. Annu Rev Pathol 2006;1:375–404.

Stephenson JT, Dubois JJ. Nonoperative management of spontaneous splenic rupture in infectious mononucleosis: A case report and review of the literature. Pediatrics 2007;120:e432–e435.

Thompson SK, Doerr TD, Hengerer AS. Infectious mononucleosis and corticosteroids: Management practices and outcomes. Arch Otolaryngol Head Neck Surg 2005;131:900–4.

Waninger KN, Harcke HT. Determination of safe return to play for athletes recovering from infectious mononucleosis: A review of the literature. Clin J Sport Med 2005;15:410–6.

> ### BOX 1 International Consensus Definition of Chronic Fatigue Syndrome
>
> - Clinically evaluated, unexplained, persistent or relapsing chronic fatigue (lasting more than 6 months) that is of new or definite onset (has not been lifelong); is not the result of ongoing exertion; is not substantially alleviated by rest; and results in substantial reduction in previous levels of occupational, educational, social, or personal activities.
> - Four or more of the following symptoms are concurrently present for more than 6 months:
>   - Impaired memory or concentration
>   - Multijoint pain
>   - Muscle pain
>   - New headaches
>   - Postexertional malaise
>   - Sore throat
>   - Tender cervical or axillary lymph nodes
>   - Unrefreshing sleep
> - Exclusionary clinical diagnoses:
>   - Any active medical condition that could explain the chronic fatigue
>   - Any previously diagnosed medical condition whose resolution has not been documented beyond reasonable clinical doubt and whose continued activity can explain the chronic fatiguing illness
>   - Psychotic major depression, bipolar affective disorder, schizophrenia, delusional disorders, dementias, anorexia nervosa, bulimia nervosa
>   - Alcohol or other substance abuse within 2 years prior to the onset of the chronic fatigue and at any time afterward
>
> Adapted from Fukuda K. Straus SE, Hickie I, et al: The chronic fatigue syndrome: A comprehensive approach to its definition and study. Ann Intern Med 1994;121:953–959.

Chronic Fatigue Syndrome

Method of
James F. Jones, MD

Definition

Chronic fatigue syndrome (CFS) is the name applied to an illness of unknown origin that at face value resembles unresolved infections, depression, endocrinologic and metabolic disorders, sleep disorders, and many other conditions that include fatigue in their diagnostic criteria.

In the modern era, interest in this illness began with the question of a relationship with a chronic active Epstein-Barr virus infection. Subsequent studies did not support Epstein-Barr virus as the only cause of this syndrome, but several recent studies have found 10% of patients with acute infectious mononucleosis and other infectious diseases might have a similar illness or postinfection fatigue syndrome.

The lack of association with a specific infectious agent led to the generation in 1988 of a definition based on the presence of incapacitating fatigue and varying combinations of signs and symptoms. Any preexisting medical or psychiatric condition was exclusionary. Evaluation of this definition at a number of centers in the United States, Great Britain, and Australia led to the current definition published in 1994 (Box 1). The definition was altered so that preexisting medical conditions that were treated satisfactorily were allowed, as well as certain psychiatric and syndromic diagnoses. Additional changes in the definition included a decrease in the number of symptoms and removal of the signs; signs had been shown to be somewhat arbitrary, and patients could be identified in their absence. The greater number of symptoms in the 1988 version did not allow identification of a specific illness, and they increased the possibility that patients who had primary psychiatric illnesses (e.g., somatiform disorders) would be mislabeled with CFS. The 1994 definition still requires more than 6 months of fatigue, but it dropped the 50% level of activity present in the 1988 definition because the requirement was impossible to apply evenly across all patients.

The diagnostic criteria, including exclusion of other illnesses, are described in the Current Diagnosis box. The definition was originally designed as a research tool and included suggestions for unifying the measurement of fatigue and evaluation of the mental status of patients.

Epidemiology

The prevalence of the syndrome using the 1988 definition is approximately 13 per 100,000, whereas the 1994 definition identified approximately 300 per 100,000. Application of an empiric definition (see later) in a population recruited with unwellness, rather than fatigue, identified a higher prevalence of CFS (Reeves et al, 2007). An increase in CFS cases in an unwell population highlights the need to address illness in general and not just fatigue when considering this diagnosis. One demographic variable that has remained stable is the 3:1 ratio of women to men.

BOX 2   Screening Laboratory Tests

- Alanine aminotransferase
- Albumin
- Alkaline phosphatase
- C-reactive protein
- Complete blood count
- Creatinine
- Electrolytes
- Globulin
- Glucose
- Thyroid-stimulating hormone and free T_4
- Total protein
- Urinalysis

Abbreviation: T_4 = thyroxine.

Diagnosis

Diagnosis of CFS begins with exclusion of other illness processes associated with fatigue and unwellness and subsequent suspicion of the syndrome after taking a history and performing a physical examination and screening laboratory tests (Box 2). It should not be assumed that a patient with fatigue as a presenting complaint has CFS. The history shows whether the illness began acutely or more gradually and whether there are preexisting symptoms. History often provides insight into previously identified factors that influence patient perception of illness. Questioning about typical episodes provides information about cyclic events, possible triggers of symptoms, and possible exposures.

The interviewer gives the patients the opportunity to describe the history of the illness. The interviewer simply guides the patient and tries not to ask leading questions. This process not only gathers information but also serves as an ice breaker between the interviewer and the patient. It allows the interviewer to determine the mental status of the patient, the patient's concentration and memory capabilities, and what may be on the patient's agenda. It usually allows the examiner to determine the kind and scope of prior medical and alternative care evaluations the patients has received.

The diagnosis of CFS should not be made on the first visit. Attempts should be made to determine the duration, the mode of onset, the magnitude, and the consequences of each complaint, although these are not included in the working definition. Only with such thorough questioning will an underlying process responsible for the illness be identified or suspected.

A more recent application of the definition uses three validated questionnaires: the Medical Outcomes Survey Short Form-36 (SF-36), the Multidimensional Fatigue Inventory (MFI), and the CDC Symptom Inventory. These questionnaires provide numeric scores that identify persons with CFS and provide a record of their level of impairment. The Symptom Inventory collects information about the presence, frequency, and intensity of 19 fatigue- and illness-related symptoms during the month preceding the interview; these include all eight CFS-defining symptoms (postexertional fatigue, unrefreshing sleep, problems remembering or concentrating, muscle aches and pains, joint pain, sore throat, tender lymph nodes and swollen glands, and headaches). Perceived frequency of each symptom is rated on a four-point scale (1 = a little of the time, 2 = some

of the time, 3 = most of time, 4 = all of the time), and severity or intensity of symptoms is measured on a three-point scale (1 = mild, 2 = moderate, 3 = severe).

The case definition specifies that CFS causes substantial reduction in occupational, educational, social, or recreational activities. *Substantial reduction* is defined as scores lower than the 25th percentile on the SF-36 using the following four factors: physical function ($\leq$70), or role physical ($\leq$50), or social function ($\leq$75), or role emotional ($\leq$66.67) subscales of the SF-36, related to published norms of the U.S. population according to Ware and Sherbourne. We defined severe fatigue using the Multidimensional Fatigue Inventory as a score of 13 or higher on the general fatigue scale or 10 or higher on the reduced activity scales of the MFI (their respective medians). Finally, because the case definition specifies that characteristic symptoms accompany fatigue, subjects reporting at least 4 symptoms and scoring at least 25 on the Symptom Inventory Case Definition Subscale were considered to have substantial accompanying symptoms.

Routine laboratory evaluations are recommended to address contributory illnesses (see Box 2). Routine testing does not include specific antibody testing, tests of immune function per se, or single-photon emission computed tomography (SPECT) or magnetic resonance imaging (MRI) of the brain. Negative screening test results do not automatically exclude an alternative diagnosis. Specific testing, for example, for a sleep disorder or chronic sinusitis may be necessary. A mental status examination, either informally or by using a standard instrument when indicated, is equally important.

A working diagnosis of CFS may then be made if the evaluation fails to identify an underlying illness. This approach is warranted because the patient's underlying disease might declare itself in the future. Continued adherence to a diagnosis of CFS in the face of an evolving or readily identifiable medical or psychiatric illness is the single most detrimental outcome of a premature or prolonged diagnosis of CFS.

Additional laboratory or other diagnostic testing is based on the individual patient's complaints. The interview techniques listed earlier assist in this process. An additional valuable tool that will lead the interviewer to identify a specific illness or symptoms requiring intervention is simply to ask the patient to list the problems described in decreasing order of magnitude. Which problem causes the most difficulty? Or which problems interfere with the ability to carry out daily functions? Patients often use this exercise to list the consequences of their illness.

Therapy

Treatment regimens vary with the needs of the individual patient and how he or she perceives the illness. The goals of treatment depend on the person's specific symptoms and eventually the patient's identified needs within a framework of providing reentry into their premorbid condition. Complete return to normal might not be possible immediately, however, nor is this goal appropriate if it is too lofty. In fact, the desire for total immediate recovery can hamper clinical improvement. The patient's adaptation to this new, albeit temporary, state is often a more realistic short-term goal. Therapeutic modalities include education regarding the boundaries and limitations of the diagnosis, development of coping skills, institution of a graduated exercise program when possible, and use of medications to treat symptoms. If the patient is being seen in a multidisciplinary setting, these approaches may be combined into a specific program. If CFS is an infrequent diagnosis in a practice, identifying the problems that cause loss of function becomes critical.

EDUCATION

All physicians who make the diagnosis must provide information regarding the illness in general and the specific criteria that allowed recognition of the problem. Just as education regarding asthma and diabetes mellitus is a critical component of therapy for those diseases, education regarding the origin, specific components, and outcome of the syndrome is more critical in this situation.

CURRENT DIAGNOSIS

- Identify duration of fatigue and its consequences.
- Identify primary symptoms.
- Exclude other illnesses/diseases.
- Reconsider the diagnosis on an ongoing basis.
- Chronic fatigue syndrome is a working diagnosis.

CURRENT THERAPY

- Education regarding the advantages and disadvantages of CFS as a diagnosis
- Development of coping skills
- Cognitive behavior therapy
- Initiation of a graded exercise program
- Symptomatic medication

The literature supports CFS as a condition that is not life threatening or progressive. Lay representations, which are readily available, are often incorrect in painting a uniformly dismal outcome. Physicians should counsel their patients that all illness symptoms should not be attributed to CFS, and patients should seek medical advice when new problems arise or old problems become more prominent. Patients should also be taught that persistent efforts to find a cure via experiences of their acquaintances or the newest information in magazines or on the Internet are not as productive as their participation in a specifically designed program as outlined here. Paramount in this process is their consideration of acceptance of their current, albeit temporary, status. Wanting their lives back and attempting to regain them with a pill are not effective approaches.

A major part of the education and treatment process is the interview process. Giving the patient the opportunity to describe the illness and its consequences in a nonjudgmental situation is critical to gaining the patient's confidence. A physician who makes the diagnosis of CFS literally establishes a contract for long-term care with the patient, and it must be based on mutual trust.

DEVELOPMENT OF COPING SKILLS

To recommend coping strategies, the provider must know the needs of the patient, another rationale for the patient-generated problem list. If the patient complains of problems with memory and concentration, simple advice regarding using lists and audiotaping activities or needs is logical. If they cannot perform on the job or their behavioral responses to these complaints aggravate the consequences, formal neuropsychological testing or therapy, or both, is required. Assistance with understanding losses is also very important. Depending on the magnitude of the consequences of their illness, patients can lose self-respect and the appreciation of their families, employees, and coworkers. They need to learn that as individuals they are not responsible for these losses but that they are responsible, at least in part, for their recovery. They need to go through a grieving process and then learn how to adapt to their current state. They need to learn to accept and desire incremental levels of progress. Formal psychological therapy may be required to achieve these goals.

The origin of the illness and the character of the fatigue dictate the approach in many cases. If the origin is with an apparent, usually unidentified, flu-like illness that does not resolve, or if the character of the fatigue simulates the malaise of such an illness, the patient needs to know that the symptoms are normal responses. The duration and consequences in the eyes of society and the individual patient are the factors that differentiate a normal resolution of an illness from a prolonged or chronic condition.

The patient also needs to know that resumption of normal activity is not the correct approach. Most patients have symptoms on a daily basis, but they also have days when the symptoms are more or less pronounced (bad and good days). A typical patient performs on the good days as if there were no illness. This action is then followed in 1 or 2 days by an exacerbation of symptoms. Learning to compartmentalize activities and to never exceed their personal limits are critical steps in coping with CFS.

On the other hand, total acceptance of such a program is not appropriate either. Usually, acute-onset patients notice that they can be more active without exacerbation of symptoms regardless of their therapeutic program. This observation usually heralds resolution of the illness. In some instances, the illness is resolving, but the patient perceives the outcome of increased physical activity (e.g., muscle aches and tiredness) as illness symptoms rather than simply the expected consequences of increased activity. The recurrence of the patient's whole syndrome following activity, however, suggests that resolution has not taken place.

EXERCISE

It seems contradictory to follow the discussion about listening to one's body and avoiding excessive activity with a section that recommends regular exercise. The studies on muscle function show that patients are tired after performing repetitive acts and that there appears to be no primary problem in muscle function. There may a problem in fitness or conditioning, however. Whether this result is a consequence of the illness or the inactivity that accompanies the syndrome is not known.

Lessons from the rehabilitation of patients with cardiac and pulmonary diseases teach us that anaerobic exercise to regain strength should precede exercises to improve aerobic fitness and overall conditioning. A program that includes active stretching followed by range-of-motion contractions and extensions that eventually includes resistance is usually an effective start. Five minutes per day is a typical starting point for a patient who has been totally inactive. The endpoint of each session should be preset by the clock or number of repetitions and should be reached before the patient becomes tired. This endpoint is based on the fact that either tiredness is a trigger for the production of biological changes that are a part of the host's attempt to limit activity or the perception that tiredness triggers illness behavior. At this stage in the understanding of the illness, prevention of activation of either of these pathways and an increase in overall fitness are appropriate goals. This section may be summarized by the adage that no exercise is bad, some is good, and too much exercise is not helpful.

The previous sections on education, coping skills, and exercise provide the kinds of therapy that are offered in cognitive behavior therapy programs.

SYMPTOMATIC THERAPY

One usually associates symptomatic therapy with medication. Some interventions require alterations in patient habits or changes in biological processes that do not require medication per se.

Sleep Therapy

The primary example is treatment of sleep problems. A very large percentage of patients presenting for evaluation of fatigue, many of whom carry the diagnosis of CFS, have sleep disorders or disturbances. Some have problems with sleep hygiene. They may read or watch television for prolonged periods (longer than 15 minutes) before trying to go to sleep. This habit can actually allow arousal of the brain within several hours following sleep onset, thus leading to interrupted sleep. Caffeine ingestion after 6 PM and exercise within 4 hours of bedtime can impede getting to sleep.

Patients are often given medication for insomnia that is manifested by going to bed at 11 PM but not being able to get to sleep until 1 or 2 AM, with a waking time of 10 AM. A hypnotic might be prescribed that allows induction of sleep at an earlier time, but the patient might still not experience restorative sleep. One explanation for this series of events is that the patient has a phase-delay syndrome and needs to alter the sleep cycle with prescribed light therapy before improvement is expected. Appropriate use of hypnotics may be important in allowing initial normalization of sleep cycling, but these agents are not sufficient as the sole mode of therapy, nor should they be used for prolonged periods.

Daytime sleepiness is another common problem with multiple origins. Ill-advised symptomatic therapy includes self- or physician-generated use of stimulants. These drugs include caffeine, herbs that contain ephedrine such as Ma huang (*Ephedra sinica*), and antidepressants that actually serve as stimulants (serotonin and norepinephrine reuptake inhibitors [SNRIs]). These substances might allow short-term improvement in daytime function, but they block identification of the underlying nighttime or daytime origin of the sleep problem.

Pharmacologic Therapy

Premature treatment can prevent adequate diagnosis and treatment of readily remediated problems. However, symptomatic medications have a definite place in the therapy of CFS. Many CFS patients do not tolerate standard doses of any of the medications used for symptomatic relief.

Classes of drugs that might have beneficial effects for symptom relief include hypnotics of various types, antidepressants of several types if depression is evident, and non-narcotic analgesics. As used in the treatment of fibromyalgia, tricyclic antidepressants and SNRIs are used for symptomatic therapy in the absence of formal depression. Because these classes of medications are being used as adjuncts to the other modes of therapy, they are not always successful. They might need to be changed during the course of the illness.

Often patients come to the physician using a large number of medications. It might not be possible to determine by the history alone whether the patient's symptoms are not at least in part due to the medication regimen. Often the medications need to be tapered and stopped to sort out their influence on the manifesting complaints.

Popular remedies for CFS are discussed primarily to familiarize the practitioner with them and to support previous warnings regarding lack of efficacy. The primary problem with their use is that proof is lacking that such intervention has been uniformly beneficial. This statement is particularly true in cases of parenteral (injectable) repetitious therapy with any substance.

Alternative Therapies

The effectiveness of diet manipulations and ingestion of herbs, enzymes, amino acids, vitamins, minerals, or hormones, although usually safe, is equally unproven. These agents constitute a large component of the therapeutic armamentarium in use by patients with CFS. Herbs are particularly in vogue. Many of them have medicinal qualities and if taken in excessive amounts may be injurious. Because many of these substances are readily available, they are used by patients who are anxious for improvement in their illness. If the reader has such patients or is such a patient, one must make sure that the remedy in question is safe and that its use is affordable and does not hide illness parameters that require specific identification.

If patients are intent on taking these types of remedies, they should be advised to at least seek the advice of a responsible care provider who is knowledgeable in their use and adverse consequences. Alternative care in many forms is also in vogue and may be helpful if provided in a responsible fashion. Some patients with myalgias and other pain complaints find particular benefit from acupuncture and therapeutic massage.

Therapeutic Plan

Therapy for CFS patients continues to be directed at relieving symptoms and consequences of the syndrome. It is clear, however, that one approach or one medication is not satisfactory for all patients. Identifying the patient's most problematic symptoms and using a variety of modalities that address those problems in the treatment plan are the most effective ways of assisting the patient. Patients should be reminded not to expect total return to their premorbid state to occur immediately.

Because the use of medications remains arbitrary, failure of one regimen may be followed by successful relief using the more effective modes of therapy, such as cognitive behavior therapy and graduated exercise. Eventually the origins of symptom production will be understood and therapy can be directed with some authority. As it stands now, one must always be careful that whatever the treatment, it must not aggravate the illness.

REFERENCES

Bazelmans E, Prins JB, Lulofs R, et al. The Netherlands Fatigue Research Group Nijmegen. Cognitive behaviour group therapy for chronic fatigue syndrome: A non-randomised waiting list controlled study. Psychother Psychosom 2005;74(4):218–24.

Jones JF, Maloney EM, Boneva RS, et al. Complementary and alternative medical therapy utilization by people with chronic fatiguing illnesses in the United States. BMC Complement Altern Med 2007;7:12.

Jones JF, Nisenbaum R, Reeves WC. Medication use by persons with chronic fatigue syndrome: Results of a randomized telephone survey in Wichita, Kansas. Health Qual Life Outcomes 2003;I(1):74.

Moss-Morris R, Sharon C, Tobin R, Baldi JC. A randomized controlled graded exercise trial for chronic fatigue syndrome: Outcomes and mechanisms of change. J Health Psychol 2005;10(2):245–59.

Nater UM, Wagner D, Solomon L, et al. Coping styles in people with chronic fatigue syndrome identified from the general population of Wichita, KS. J Psychosom Res 2006;60(6):567–73.

Reeves WC, Jones JF, Maloney E, et al. Prevalence of chronic fatigue syndrome in metropolitan, urban, and rural Georgia. Popul Health Metr 2007;5:5.

Reeves WC, Wagner D, Nisenbaum R, et al. Chronic fatigue syndrome: A clinically empirical approach to its definition and study. BMC Med 2005; 3(1):19.

Wagner D, Nisenbaum R, Heim C, et al. Psychometric properties of the CDC Symptom Inventory for assessment of chronic fatigue syndrome. BioMed Central Popul Health Metr 2005;3:8.

Ware JE, Sherbourne CD. The MOS 36-item short form health survey (SF-36): Conceptual framework and item selection. Med Care 1992;30: 473–83.

Whiting P, Bagnall AM, Sowden AJ, et al. Interventions for the treatment and management of chronic fatigue syndrome: A systematic review. JAMA 2001;286:1360–8.

Mumps

Method of
Joel D. Klein, MD, FAAP

Mumps is a respiratory viral infection caused by mumps virus, an RNA virus in the family Paramyxoviridae. The virus is spread from human to human through direct contact with airborne droplets.

Epidemiology

Before the introduction of mumps vaccine, there were large yearly epidemics, usually occurring in the winter and early spring. Infection generally occurred among young children (younger than 15 years), with rare cases in young adults. With the introduction of the mumps vaccine in 1967, there was a dramatic decrease in the number of cases. However, in 1986 and 1987, there was a resurgence of mumps among teenagers and young adults, most of whom were born before routine immunization with the mumps vaccine.

Outbreaks were also seen among some children who had received mumps vaccine, because a single dose of the vaccine did not always confer immunity. In 1989, a second dose of mumps vaccine was recommended to address this issue. Mumps vaccine currently is usually administered as part of a combined vaccine such as measles-mumps-rubella (MMR) or most recently measles-mumps-rubella-varicella (MMRV) (Proquad).

Despite these changes, outbreaks of mumps occasionally occur, usually among college-aged persons. Recent examples include an epidemic in the United Kingdom in the winter of 2004 to 2005 and in the United States in 2006.

Clinical Manifestations

The incubation period of mumps is 14 to 25 days and involves nonspecific complaints of malaise, low-grade fever, and anorexia. The single most diagnostic physical finding in mumps is unilateral or bilateral parotitis, which occurs in up to 40% of cases.

CURRENT DIAGNOSIS

- Painful parotid swelling
- Edema of the face in the area of the parotid
- Elevation of serum amylase
- Headache and occasional meningismus
- Viral isolation or serology can confirm diagnosis

Mumps parotitis can occur early in the disease and may be associated with swelling and pain in other salivary glands. There often is erythema of the area and tenderness with palpation of the affected parotid. Patients at times also complain of earache and headache. Swelling over the parotid and related glands can occur rapidly and can result in distortion of the contours of the face, pushing the earlobe upward and outward. Edema can extend to the anterior chest wall as well. Examination of the oral cavity can reveal erythema of the orifice of Stensen's duct without purulent discharge. Parotitis generally resolves within 1 week.

The most commonly reported complications of mumps are aseptic meningitis and encephalitis, which can occur individually or together. Meningitis occurs in 10% to 15% of cases but probably is underreported. There is a typical viral-like pleocytosis in the cerebrospinal fluid (CSF), but the CSF glucose may be low. Encephalitis is rare and is seen in 1 or 2 per 100,000 cases.

Orchitis, either unilateral or bilateral, may be seen in as many as 50% of infected men. This complication can have a rapid onset and can be associated with increased fever, abdominal pain, nausea, and testicular swelling. This complication generally resolves within 1 week and can result in testicular atrophy but rarely infertility. Pancreatitis is sometimes seen, is usually mild, and may be associated with transient hyperglycemia. Table 1 lists the incidence of complications of mumps.

Diagnosis

Diagnosis of mumps is usually made by clinical examination and history. It should be considered in any patient with sudden onset of parotid swelling and fever. Mumps virus isolation may be attempted on fluids obtained by nasopharyngeal swab and urine. Virus may be excreted for 1 week before and 1 week after the onset of parotitis. When available, PCR may also be used to detect mumps virus in secretions.

Serum amylase determinations, although not specific, may be helpful in situations where mumps is suspected. Serology, which is readily available, may be diagnostic as well. Mumps IgM obtained during the acute infection is usually elevated and diagnostic. Acute and convalescent-paired sera can also be used to retrospectively confirm the diagnosis. Other commonly ordered laboratory tests, including complete blood count (CBC) are not particularly helpful. The CBC might show mild leukopenia with lymphocytosis.

Differential diagnosis of mumps parotitis includes many infections that are listed in Box 1.

TABLE 1 Complications of Mumps Infection

Mumps Complications	Incidence of Complications
Central nervous system	40%–50%
Orchitis and epididymitis	15%–30%
Oophoritis	7%
Pancreatitis	2%–5%
Deafness	1 in 20,000 reported cases
Myocarditis	Rare
Arthritis	Rare
Thyroiditis	Rare

BOX 1 Differential Diagnosis of Mumps Parotitis

- Parainfluenza virus infection
- Enterovirus infection
- Epstein-Barr virus
- Cytomegalovirus infection
- HIV
- Suppurative bacterial infection (Staphylococcus aureus, Streptococcus pneumoniae)
- Nontuberculous mycobacterial infection

Treatment

There is no specific therapy for mumps. Adequate analgesia is important, because many patients are quite uncomfortable. Because most patients are febrile, hydration also plays an important role. This is particularly critical because there may be difficulty swallowing and pain with mastication.

Children with mumps should be excluded from school for 9 days from onset of parotid swelling. Droplet precautions are recommended for patients with mumps admitted to the hospital for a period of 9 days from onset of parotid swelling.

Prevention

Mumps vaccine should be administered to children at age 12 to 15 months. A second dose should be given at age 4 to 6 years. Patients with HIV who are not severely immunocompromised may receive a combination mumps vaccine. Adults born in 1957 or later, in whom immunity is not known, should receive one dose of a mumps combination vaccine (MMR). Persons born before 1957 are usually considered immune, but they might benefit from immunization during a mumps community outbreak.

CURRENT THERAPY

- Analgesia for pain
- Warm or cold compresses
- Droplet isolation in the hospital
- Patient may return to school 5 days after the onset of parotid swelling

REFERENCES

American Academy of Pediatrics Committee on Infectious Diseases. Mumps. In: Pickering LK, editor. Red Book: 2006 Report of the Committee on Infectious Diseases. 27th ed. Elk Grove Village, Ill: American Academy of Pediatrics; 2006. p. 464–8.

Cherry JD. Mumps Virus. In: Feigin RD, Cherry JD, Demmler GJ, Kaplan SL, editors. Textbook of Pediatric Infectious Diseases. 5th ed. Philadelphia: WB Saunders; 2004. p. 2305–14.

Gupta RK, Best J, MacMahon E. Mumps and the UK epidemic 2005. BMJ 2005;330:1132–5.

Litman N, Baum SG. Mumps virus. In: Mandell GL, Bennett JE, Dolin R, editors. Principles and Practice of Infectious Diseases. 6th ed. Philadelphia: Churchill Livingstone; 2005. p. 2003–8.

Maldonado Y. Mumps. In: Behrman RE, editor. Nelson Textbook of Pediatrics. 17th ed. Philadelphia: WB Saunders; 2004. p. 1035–6.

McQuone SJ. Acute viral and bacterial infections of the salivary glands. Otolaryngol Clin North Am 1999;32(5):793–811.

Plague

Method of
Douglas A. Drevets, MD, DTM&H

Plague caused by *Yersinia pestis* is an ancient disease, and historical descriptions indicate that it probably caused Justinian's Plague (AD 541) that led into the first plague pandemic. The second plague pandemic, also known as the Black Death, began in Central Asia in 1347 and then spread to Europe, Asia, and Africa. It killed an estimated 50 million persons. The third and current plague pandemic began in China and then disseminated throughout the world by shipping routes in 1899–1900. *Y. pestis* is a gram-negative, nonmotile, facultatively anaerobic, non-spore-forming coccobacillus that is approximately 0.5 to 0.8 µm in diameter and 1 to 3 µm in length. Genomic sequencing shows that *Y. pestis* is a recently emerged clone of *Y. pseudotuberculosis*.

Epidemiology

Plague is a zoonosis that is usually spread between mammalian hosts by the bite of infected fleas. The most important enzootic reservoirs are urban and sylvatic rodents; however, domestic cats and dogs have been linked to human disease. Human plague occurs in North and South America, Asia, and Africa. An average of 2577 (range 876–5419) cases of human plague were reported yearly to the World Health Organization between 1989 and 2003, 80.3% of which were from Africa, with an overall average case fatality rate of 8.14%. In North America, 82% of 295 indigenous cases were from Arizona, Colorado, and New Mexico. Bubonic plague is the most common form in humans, accounting for 84% of U.S. cases reported between 1947 and 1996, with septicemic and pneumonic plague accounting for 13% and 2%, respectively. An outbreak in Algeria in 2003 demonstrated the ability of this organism to reemerge in areas where the disease had been absent for decades.

Modes of Transmission

Most human infections are transmitted from rodent to humans via the bite of an infected flea. Infection also can be acquired by contact with body fluids from infected animals, such as during field dressing of game or by inhalation of respiratory droplets from animals, particularly cats, or humans with pneumonic plague.

Bioterrorism Threat

Plague was used as an agent of biowarfare by the Japanese in World War II and was a focus of intensive research and development in the former Soviet Union during the Cold War. Primary pneumonic plague is the most likely form of exposure because of biowarfare or bioterrorism. Recent increases in terrorism worldwide have increased the focus of public health management groups to develop comprehensive statements regarding plague as a biological weapon.

Pathogenesis and Clinical Syndromes

Transdermal inoculation of bacilli from the bite of an infected flea ultimately leads to infection of the regional lymph nodes in which massive replication of bacteria creates the bubo (derived from the Greek "bubon" or "groin"), a swollen, erythematous, and painful

CURRENT DIAGNOSIS

- Travel to a plague endemic area or contact with a case of animal or human plague.
- Abrupt onset of fever and prostration.
- Bubo in groin, axillae, or cervical areas.
- Gram-negative coccobacilli with bipolar staining identified in aspirate from bubo, on blood smear, or from blood-tinged sputum.

lymph node in the groin, axilla, or cervical region. Bacteremia and septicemia frequently develop and lead to secondary infection of other organs including lungs, spleen, and the central nervous system. Primary pneumonic plague is a rare natural occurrence and results from the inhalation of respiratory droplets containing *Y. pestis* bacilli from another case of pneumonic plague, usually in humans or in cats. Secondary pneumonic plague results from seeding of the lungs by blood-borne bacteria in the setting of either bubonic or septicemic plague. Septicemic plague also begins with a transdermal exposure but manifests as primary bacteremia/septicemia without the bubo. Less common manifestations include meningitis, pharyngitis, and gastroenteritis.

Bubonic plague is an acute febrile lymphadenitis that develops 2 to 8 days after inoculation. Inflamed lymph nodes are usually 1 to 6 cm and painful. Abrupt onset of fever is an almost universal finding and occurs simultaneously with, or up to 24 hours before, the appearance of the bubo. Headache, malaise, and chills are frequent, along with nausea, vomiting, and diarrhea. Most patients are tachycardic, hypotensive, and appear prostrate and lethargic with episodic restlessness. Leukocytosis with a left shift is typical. Complications include pneumonia, shock, disseminated intravascular coagulation, purpuric skin lesions, acral cyanosis, and gangrene. The differential diagnosis of bubonic plague includes tularemia and Group A β-hemolytic streptococcal adenitis with bacteremia.

The symptoms of septicemic plague are not distinct from those caused by other gram-negative bacteria, and they are very similar to those of bubonic plague except that abdominal pain is more common in septicemic plague. Septicemic plague must be differentiated from fulminate septicemia caused by other gram-negative bacteria. Primary pneumonic plague has an abrupt onset of fever and influenza-like symptoms 1 to 5 days after inhalation exposure. Symptoms include shortness of breath, cough, chest pain, and bloody sputum with rapid progression to fulminate pneumonia and respiratory failure. Patients with secondary pneumonic infection show respiratory symptoms in addition to those attributed to the bubo or sepsis. Radiographic findings include patchy bronchopneumonia, multilobar consolidations, cavitations, and alveolar hemorrhage and are not pathognomonic of *Y. pestis*. Plague pneumonia must be differentiated from severe influenza, inhalation anthrax, and overwhelming community-acquired pneumonia.

Diagnosis

Plague is diagnosed by demonstrating *Y. pestis* in blood or body fluids such as a lymph node aspirate, sputum, or cerebrospinal fluid. A tentative diagnosis of bubonic plague can be made rapidly with fluid aspirated from a bubo showing gram-negative coccobacilli with bipolar staining. Serology showing a fourfold rise in antibody titers to F1 antigen or a single titer of more than 1:128 is also diagnostic. Rapid diagnostic tests that use monoclonal antibodies to detect *Y. pestis* F1 antigen in bubo aspirates and sputum have been developed and field tested.

Treatment

The aminoglycosides (gentamicin and streptomycin), the fluoroquinolones ciprofloxacin (Cipro) and levofloxacin (Levaquin), and doxycycline (Vibramycin) are the first-, second-, and third-line

CURRENT THERAPY

- Prompt administration of gentamicin or ciprofloxacin.
- Aggressive supportive care.
- Respiratory isolation of hospitalized cases.
- Postexposure prophylaxis to close contacts.

classes of antibiotics, respectively. Typical minimal inhibitory concentrations for 90% (MIC_{90}) of tested strains for the fluoroquinolones are less than 0.03 to 0.25 µg/mL compared with less than 1.0 µg/mL and less than 1.0 µg/mL to 4.0 µg/mL for gentamicin and streptomycin, respectively, and less than 1.0 µg/mL for doxycycline. Streptomycin (15 mg/kg up to 1 g intermuscularly [IM] every 12 hours) and gentamicin (5 to 7 mg/kg/day intravenously [IV]/IM in one or two doses daily) are the drugs of choice for severe infection. Standard doses for the fluoroquinolones include ciprofloxacin, 400 mg IV/500 mg orally every 12 hours; levofloxacin, 500 mg IV/orally daily; and ofloxacin, 400 mg IV/orally every 12 hours. Doxycycline is administered at 100 mg IV/orally every 12 hours. Chloramphenicol (25 mg/kg IV/orally every 6 hours) can be used in select circumstances. Antibiotic therapy should be continued for a total of 10 days.

Prevention and Control

Standard infection control procedures that should be used when caring for patients with suspected plague include a disposable surgical mask, latex gloves, devices to protect mucous membranes, and good hand washing. Hospitalized patients with known or suspected pneumonic plague should be placed in strict isolation for at least 48 hours after appropriate antibiotics are initiated. Postexposure prophylaxis should be given to individuals with close contact (defined as less than 2 meters) with an infectious case or who have had a potential respiratory exposure. The recommended adult antibiotics for prophylaxis are doxycycline or ciprofloxacin in the same doses used for treatment. Postexposure prophylaxis can be given orally and should be continued for 7 days following exposure. Currently, there is no licensed plague vaccine.

REFERENCES

Butler T. A clinical study of bubonic plague. Observations of the 1970 Vietnam epidemic with emphasis on coagulation studies, skin histology and electrocardiograms. Am J Med 1972;53:268–76.

Boulanger LL, Ettestad P, Fogarty JD, et al. Gentamicin and tetracyclines for the treatment of human plague: Review of 75 cases in New Mexico, 1985–1999. Clin Infect Dis 2004;38:663–9.

Cler DJ, Vernaleo JR, Lombardi LJ, et al. Plague pneumonia disease caused by Yersinia pestis. Semin Respir Infect 1997;12:12–23.

Gage KL, Dennis DT, Orloski KA, et al. Cases of cat-associated human plague in the Western US, 1977–1998. Clin Infect Dis 2000;30:893–900.

Hull HF, Montes JM, Mann JM. Septicemic plague in New Mexico. J Infect Dis 1987;155:113–8.

Inglesby TV, Dennis DT, Henderson DA, et al. Plague as a biological weapon: Medical and public health management. Working Group on Civilian Biodefense. JAMA 2000;283:2281–90.

Perry RD, Fetherston JD. Yersinia pestis—etiologic agent of plague. Clin Microbiol Rev 1997;10:35–66.

Prentice MB, Rahalison L. Plague. Lancet 2007;369:1196–207.

Ratsitorahina M, Chanteau S, Rahalison L, et al. Epidemiological and diagnostic aspects of the outbreak of pneumonic plague in Madagascar. Lancet 2000;355:111–3.

Weekly epidemiological record. World Health Organization. August 13, 2004, 79th year, No. 33, 2004, 79:301–8. http://www.who.int/wer.

Wong JD, Barash JR, Sandfort RF, Janda JM. Susceptibilities of Yersinia pestis strains to 12 antimicrobial agents. Antimicrob Agents Chemother 2000;44:1995–6.

Anthrax

Method of
Jon B. Woods, MD

Anthrax has been a significant disease for both humans and their livestock for millennia. It was the first disease to fulfill Koch's postulates in 1876, as well as the first bacterial disease for which an effective vaccine was developed, for livestock, in 1880. This gram-positive rod-shaped bacillus species differs from the more benign members of its genera in containing two additional plasmids, one encoding for an antiphagocytic poly-D-glutamic acid capsule and the other encoding for two toxins. Three distinct toxin components combine to form two toxins, edema toxin and lethal toxin; the common component, protective antigen (PA), forms a pore through eukaryotic cell walls that allows the other two toxin components, edema factor (EF) and lethal factor (LF), to enter affected host cells. EF is an adenylate cyclase affecting many cell types and is responsible for the edema associated with anthrax infections. LF is a zinc metalloprotease that seems to have its greatest affect on macrophages; within the cells it cleaves mitogen-activated protein kinase and disrupts the cellular response to infection.

Background

Anthrax is an enzootic, and occasionally epizootic, disease of grazing animals worldwide. The incredibly durable spores of this bacillus can persist in soil for decades. These spores, when inadvertently ingested by herbivores while grazing, can germinate and then replicate in a rapid progression to bacteremia and subsequent death of the animal. At the time of death these animals can have as many as 10^8 vegetative bacilli per milliliter of blood. Those bacilli, which are exposed to oxygen upon the animal's death, can sporulate and then reenter the soil to begin the cycle anew.

Human anthrax can take several forms, most commonly cutaneous, but also intestinal, oropharyngeal, and inhalational disease. Naturally occurring human anthrax disease has typically been the result of exposure to infected animals or contaminated animal products such as hair or wool, bone meal, hides, or meat. Less commonly, human cutaneous anthrax has resulted from the bites of flies that have recently fed on infected animals. Gastrointestinal and oropharyngeal anthrax can result from ingestion of the raw or inadequately cooked flesh of an animal infected with anthrax. Endemic inhalational anthrax, or woolsorter's disease, results from inhalation of anthrax spores aerosolized during the manipulation of contaminated animal products, especially hair or wool; this was an exceedingly rare form of disease even prior to the institution of more stringent control measures and closure of most of the U.S. textile mills processing foreign-acquired goat hair by the 1970s. More recently, inhalational anthrax and cutaneous cases have resulted from exposure to spores intentionally processed and disseminated as biologic weapons. The extreme environmental stability of the spores, their ease of production, and their infectivity via the aerosol route are some features that have made *Bacillus anthracis* a top candidate for both nations and terrorists seeking biologic weapons. An apparently accidental aerosol release of dried anthrax spores from a biologic weapons facility in the Soviet city of Sverdlovsk in 1979 resulted in as many as 68 deaths because of inhalational anthrax. More recently, anthrax spores intentionally sent through the U.S. postal system resulted in 11 cases of inhalational anthrax and perhaps as many as 11 cases of cutaneous anthrax.

Clinical Features

Cutaneous anthrax represents approximately 95% of naturally occurring human anthrax cases. It typically occurs 1 to 7 days after exposure to infected livestock or contaminated livestock products, but rarely it is transmitted to humans by the bites of flies that have recently fed on infected animals. The lesion begins as a painless or mildly pruritic papule at the site of spore inoculation, progressing into an expanding round ulcer by the following day. Over the following several days the ulcer dries to a dark, almost black eschar, which resolves over the ensuing 1 to 2 weeks. The lesion can be surrounded by significant local edema and may be accompanied by regional lymphadenopathy. Treated, cutaneous anthrax is rarely fatal, although without antibiotics, progression to bacteremia and ultimately death can occur in up to 10% to 20% of cases.

Both forms of gastrointestinal anthrax are acquired via ingestion of insufficiently cooked meat from infected animals. The infectious dose is unknown. Intestinal anthrax may be initially misdiagnosed as either gastroenteritis or acute abdomen, typically presenting 1 to 6 days following contaminated meat consumption with fever, nausea, vomiting, and focal abdominal pain. Without prompt initiation of antibiotic therapy, disease can progress to hematemesis, hematochezia or melena, massive serosanguineous or hemorrhagic ascites, and sepsis, with mortality rates greater than 50%. Oropharyngeal anthrax typically presents after a 1- to 6-day incubation period with severe pharyngitis and fever, followed by appearance of pharyngeal or tonsillar ulcers. Gray or tan pseudomembranes can form over the ulcers, which are often accompanied by significant cervical lymphadenopathy and unilateral neck edema. Mortality of oropharyngeal anthrax varies from 10% to 50%.

Inhalation of aerosolized anthrax spores into the pulmonary alveoli can result in inhalational anthrax. The lethal dose via inhalation for 50% of humans (LD_{50}) is thought to be between 8000 and 55,000 spores. The alveolar spores are ingested by macrophages and carried to regional lymphatics, where they can germinate and replicate, eventually leading to hemorrhagic mediastinitis. The incubation period is presumably dose dependent, and although typically 1 to 6 days was suspected in at least one human case to be 43 days. Early inhalational anthrax presents suddenly as a nonspecific syndrome consisting of fever, malaise, headache, fatigue, and drenching sweats. Other common symptoms include nausea, vomiting, confusion, a nonproductive cough, and mild chest discomfort. Upper respiratory symptoms are notably absent. Physical findings are nonspecific in the early phase of the disease, but tachycardia is common. Auscultatory lung exam is typically normal at this stage, but dullness to percussion can develop over time in the lower lung fields as hemorrhagic pleural effusions accumulate. These early findings generally persist for 2 to 5 days before progressing fulminantly to tachypnea, cyanosis, shock, and multiorgan system failure. These late findings typically herald impending death within 24 to 36 hours. Gastrointestinal hemorrhage and hemorrhagic meningitis are common at autopsy. Prognosis is poor in the absence of intensive supportive care and early initiation of appropriate antibiotic combinations. Mortality ranges from 45% to more than 85% historically.

Diagnosis

None of the forms of human anthrax disease can be diagnosed on the basis of clinical findings alone (Table 1). For example, diagnosis of cutaneous anthrax requires the presence of a compatible skin lesion accompanied by confirmatory laboratory studies; an exposure history, or a known risk may also be present. Both forms of gastrointestinal anthrax are typically accompanied by a history of ingestion of the meat of anthrax-infected animals. Early intestinal anthrax can be difficult to differentiate clinically from other causes of gastrointestinal illness to include acute gastroenteritis, dysentery, or even peritonitis. Later in the course of intestinal disease, surgical or autopsy findings may include ileal or cecal ulceration, and bowel edema and necrosis is

---

TABLE 1 Empirical Antibiotic Therapy for Anthrax*

Cutaneous Anthrax (without Systemic Symptoms)	Inhalational, Gastrointestinal, or Cutaneous Disease with Systemic Symptoms
Ciprofloxacin (Cipro[1]) • 500 mg PO twice daily (adults) • 15 mg/kg (up to 500 mg/dose) PO twice daily (children) or Doxycycline (Vibramycin) • 100 mg PO twice daily (adults) • 2.2 mg/kg (up to 100 mg/dose) PO bid (children < 45 kg) or (if strain susceptible): Penicillin G procaine (Bicillin C-R) • 1,200,000 U IM q12h (adults) • 25,000 U/kg (maximum 1,200,000 U) q12h (children) or Penicillin V Potassium (Veetids) • 500 mg PO q6h (adults) or Amoxicillin (Amoxil[1]) • 500 mg PO q8h (adults and children > 40 kg) • 15 mg/kg q8h (children <40 kg) According to CDC recommendations, amoxicillin prophylaxis is appropriate only after 14–21 d of fluoroquinolone or doxycycline and only for populations with relative contraindications to the other drugs (children, pregnancy)	Ciprofloxacin (Cipro IV[1]) • 400 mg IV q12h (adult) • 15 mg/kg/dose (up to 400 mg/dose) q12h (children) or Doxycycline (Vibramycin IV) • 200 mg IV, then 100 mg IV q12h (adults) • 2.2 mg/kg (100 mg/dose maximum) q12h (children < 45 kg) or (if strain susceptible): Penicillin G (Pfizerpen) • 4 million U IV q4h (adults) • 50,000 U/kg (up to 4M U) IV q6h (children) plus One or two additional antibiotics with activity against anthrax. Clindamycin (Cleocin[1]) plus rifampin (Rifadin[1]) may be a good empiric choice, pending susceptibilities. Potential additional antibiotics include one or more of the following clindamycin (Cleocin), rifampin (Rifadin), gentamicin[1] (generic), macrolides (erythromycin [generic], vancomycin (Vancocin[1]), imipenem (Pimaxin[1]), and chloramphenicol[1] (generic). Convert from IV to oral therapy when patient is stable, to complete at least 60 d of antibiotics. **Meningitis** Add Rifampin (Rifadin[1]) 20 mg/kg IV once daily or vancomycin (Vancocin[1]) 1 g IV q12h Oral dosing may be necessary for treatment of systemic disease in a mass casualty situation.

Adapted from Woods JB (ed): USAMRIID's Medical Management of Biological Warfare Casualties Handbook, 6th ed. 2005.
[1]Not FDA approved for this indication.
*Should be adjusted for susceptibilities.
Abbreviations: CDC = Centers for Disease Control and Prevention; IV = intravenous; PO = orally.

CURRENT DIAGNOSIS

Cutaneous/Oropharyngeal

- Painless or pruritic lesion beginning 1–7 d after exposure
    - Typical lesion progression from papule to ulcer to dark eschar (see text), often with significant edema

Plus

- Lesion gram stain, culture usually positive if patient has not received antibiotics
    - If negative, punch biopsy of lesion margin for IHC may still be positive
- Blood culture rarely positive in absence of systemic symptoms

Acute and convalescent serology or may give evidence of infection.

Gastrointestinal

- Gastrointestinal symptoms (variable) beginning 1–6 d after ingestion exposure.
    - Focal abdominal pain with hematochezia or melena common.
    - Nonspecific bowel wall edema, air–fluid levels, and ascites on radiographs.

Plus

- Stool culture (variably +).
- Blood culture (variably +).
- Acute and convalescent serology or blood sample for PCR may give evidence of infection.
- Ascites: often hemorrhagic.
    - Gram stain and culture, and IHC or PCR, if available, may be positive.

Surgical findings: hemorrhagic mesenteric adenitis, bowel edema, ileal and/or cecal ulcerations.

Inhalational

- Nonspecific febrile syndrome beginning abruptly 1–6 (but up to 43) d after aerosol exposure (see text).
    - Absence of upper respiratory findings, no pneumonia.
    - Widened mediastinum ± effusions on CXR or chest CT in *all* cases.

Plus

- Blood culture often positive if patient has not received antibiotics.
- Acute and convalescent serology or blood sample for PCR may give evidence of infection.
- Laboratory studies show hemoconcentration, mildly increased WBC with left shift, mildly increased AST and ALT, hypoalbuminemia.
- CSF (if meningitis) and pleural effusions are hemorrhagic.
- Gram stain and culture often positive.

If negative, IHC or PCR may be positive.

Abbreviations: AST = serum aspartate aminotransferase (level); ALT = serum alanine aminotransferase (level); CSF = cerebrospinal fluid; CXR = chest radiograph; CT = computed tomography study; IHC = immunohistochemical staining; PCR = polymerase chain reaction (study); WBC = white blood count.

associated with hemorrhagic mesenteric adenitis and serosanguineous to hemorrhagic ascites. Oropharyngeal anthrax can clinically resemble diphtheria, with pharyngeal lesions and an edematous so-called bull neck. Early inhalational anthrax is a nonspecific febrile syndrome that may be difficult to distinguish clinically from many other infectious diseases. However, the presence of mental status changes, profuse sweating, and absence of upper respiratory symptoms or pneumonia in inhalational anthrax may aid in differentiating it from influenza-like respiratory illnesses.

Gram stain and culture of skin lesions are ideally performed on the fluid of an unopened vesicle and are often positive in the cutaneous anthrax patient who has not received antibiotics. Tissue biopsy can be performed on lesions for immunohistochemical staining in culture-negative patients. Blood culture should be collected in any systemically ill patient suspected of having any form of anthrax disease. *B. anthracis* grows quickly in standard laboratory culture media. Paired acute and convalescent serologic studies may suggest infection in patents that have negative cultures, albeit these studies are not well validated. Stool culture can be positive in intestinal anthrax, although it is only variably so. Peritoneal fluid, pleural effusions, or cerebrospinal fluid (CSF) (when meningitis is present) can potentially demonstrate organisms on Gram stain and culture or may be positive via immunostaining or polymerase chain reaction (PCR) studies.

For patients with inhalation anthrax during the attacks of 2001, the complete blood count (CBC) revealed a mean white blood cell count of 9800/μL, with a predominance of neutrophils and a mildly elevated hematocrit. Mildly elevated serum sodium, aspartate transaminase (AST), and alanine aminotransferase (ALT) were common, as was hypoalbuminemia.

A widened mediastinum caused by adenitis, as well as pleural effusions, may be visible on chest radiograph in patients with inhalational anthrax. Negative chest radiograph in a patient suspected of inhalational anthrax should prompt a chest computerized tomography (CT) scan. In the 2001 attacks, either the chest radiograph or CT was abnormal in all cases of inhalational disease. Abdominal radiographs in intestinal anthrax may demonstrate any number of nonspecific findings, to include ascites, diffuse air–fluid levels, and bowel edema.

Treatment

Patient survival for all forms of severe anthrax disease hinges on prompt initiation of appropriate antibiotics. Initial empirical therapy for patients with inhalational anthrax, gastrointestinal anthrax, or cutaneous anthrax with systemic symptoms should include intravenous (IV) ciprofloxacin (Cipro IV) or doxycycline (Vibramycin IV) combined with one or two additional antibiotics effective against anthrax (Table 2). One suggested combination includes a quinolone (ciprofloxacin [Cipro IV]), clindamycin (Cleocin[1]), and rifampin (Rifadin[1]). Antibiotic choices should be adjusted to reflect the specific susceptibilities of the infecting strain. Rifampin (Rifadin[1]), vancomycin (Vancocin[1]), or chloramphenicol[1] (generic) should be added if meningitis is suspected. IV antibiotics can be switched to oral treatment as the patent's clinical condition improves, to complete at least 60 days of total antibiotic therapy. Specific antidotes for anthrax toxins are in development, including human anthrax immune globulin, which may be available as an investigational therapy for severe anthrax disease through the Centers for Disease Control and Prevention (CDC).

---

[1]Not FDA approved for this indication.

CURRENT THERAPY

Cutaneous Anthrax (without Systemic Symptoms)

- Oral antibiotics (see Table 2 for details)
  - Doxycycline (Vibramycin), or
  - Ciprofloxacin (Cipro[1])
- Consider nonsteroidal anti-inflammatory agents (NSAIDs) or corticosteroids for severe edema
- Infection control:
  - Contact precautions

Do not debride lesions

Inhalational, Gastrointestinal, or Cutaneous Disease with Systemic Symptoms

- Supportive care
  - May need assisted ventilation and/or vasopressors
  - Drain pleural effusions and large peritoneal fluid collections
- Combination IV antibiotics (see Table 2 for details)
  - Doxycycline (Vibramycin IV), or
  - Ciprofloxacin (Cipro IV[1])

Plus

- One or two additional antibiotics
- Consider corticosteroids for severe edema or meningitis
- Consider human anthrax immune globulin (investigational), if available
- Infection control:
  - Contact precautions (not transmitted by droplet or aerosol)

Avoid autopsy or invasive procedures prior to receipt of antibiotics.

[1]Not FDA approved for this indication.

Patients with systemic anthrax disease often require aggressive supportive therapy, including fluid resuscitation, blood products, vasopressor agents, and airway management. Patients may also benefit from drainage of large hemorrhagic pleural or peritoneal fluid accumulations. Although clinical data are lacking, severe edema or meningitis in anthrax disease may benefit from administration of corticosteroids.

Uncomplicated naturally acquired cutaneous anthrax should be treated empirically with 7 to 10 days of either oral ciprofloxacin (Cipro[1]) or doxycycline (Vibramycin). For cutaneous disease thought to have been acquired via exposure to an anthrax aerosol, at least 60 days of antibiotics is recommended.

A licensed anthrax vaccine (BioThrax) has been available in the United States to the armed forces, veterinarians, and textile and laboratory workers since 1970. It is derived from the sterile supernatant of a liquid culture of an attenuated (nonencapsulated) strain of *B. anthracis* and is administered subcutaneously in a six-shot primary series over 18 months followed by annual boosters. The vaccine is licensed only for preexposure prophylaxis of persons 18 to 65 years of age but is available investigationally for postexposure and pediatric use.

Individuals exposed to aerosolized anthrax spores should immediately receive postexposure prophylaxis consisting of both oral antibiotics and anthrax vaccine. Oral doxycycline (Vibramycin) or ciprofloxacin (Cipro) are the preferred empiric antibiotics for postexposure prophylaxis. Antibiotics should be continued for variable lengths of time depending on the patient's anthrax immune status and the suspected inhaled dose of anthrax (Table 2). Exposed individuals should also receive the anthrax vaccine[1] (BioThrax) to counter delayed incubation of residual alveolar anthrax after discontinuation of antibiotics.

[1]Not FDA approved for this indication.

TABLE 2 Anthrax Aerosol Postexposure Prophylaxis*

Immunized[†]	Not Immunized and Vaccine Available	Not Immunized and Vaccine Not Available
Ciprofloxacin (Cipro) • 500 mg PO bid for adults • 10–15 mg/kg PO twice daily (up to 1 g/d) for children *or* Doxycycline (Vibramycin) • 100 mg PO bid for adults or children > 8 y and > 45 kg • 2.2 mg/kg PO bid (up to 200 mg/d) for children < 8 y		
If antibiotic susceptibilities allow, patients who cannot tolerate tetracyclines or quinolone antibiotics can be switched to amoxicillin (Amoxil[1]), 500 mg PO tid for adults and 80 mg/kg divided tid (≥ 1.5 g/d) in children.		
Continue antibiotics for *at least* 30 d	Receive at least 3 doses of anthrax vaccine[1] (BioThrax) at 2-wk intervals, and then continue antibiotics for *at least* 1–2 wk after receipt of 3rd dose of vaccine.	Continue antibiotics for *at least* 60 d.
Patients should be closely observed after discontinuation of antibiotics.		
If suspected clinical signs of anthrax disease occur, then resume empirical antibiotics.		

Adapted from Woods JB (ed): USAMRID's Medical Management of Biological Warfare Casualties Handbook, 6th ed. 2005.
[1]Not FDA approved for this indication.
*Unknown antibiotic susceptibilities.
[†]Immunized = completed 6 doses of anthrax vaccine and up to date on boosters, or minimum of 3 doses within past 6 mo. Those who have already received 3 doses within 6 mo of exposure should continue with their routine vaccine schedule.
Abbreviation: PO = orally.

REFERENCES

Beatty ME, Ashford DA, Griffin PM, et al. Gastrointestinal anthrax, a review of the literature. Arch Intern Med 2003;163:2527–31.

Centers for Disease Control and Prevention. Notice to readers: Use of anthrax vaccine in response to terrorism: Supplemental recommendations of the Advisory Committee on Immunization Practices. MMWR 2002;51(45):1024–6.

Inglesby TV, O'Toole T, Henderson DA, et al. Anthrax as a biological weapon 2002: Updated Recommendations for Management. JAMA 2002;287 (17):2236–52.

Jernigan JA, Stephens DS, Ashford DA, et al. Bioterrorism-related inhalational anthrax: The first 10 cases reported in the United States. Emerg Infect Dis 2001;7:933–44.

Kuehnert MJ, Doyle TJ, Hill HA, et al. Clinical features that discriminate inhalational anthrax from other acute respiratory illnesses. Clin Infect Dis 2003;36:328–36.

Turnbull PCB. Guidelines for the Surveillance and Control of Anthrax in Humans and Animals. 3rd ed. World Health Organization Report WHO/EMC/ZDI/98.6; 1998.

Woods JB editor. USAMRIID's Medical Management of Biological Warfare Casualties Handbook; 2005. 6th ed.

Psittacosis

Method of
Julian Elliott, MB, BS, FACP

Epidemiology

Psittacosis is the disease caused by infection with the bacterium *Chlamydophila psittaci*, formerly known as *Chlamydia psittaci*. It affects men more than women, and the main age group affected is adults older than 40 years. The main reservoir for psittacosis is birds, particularly psittacine birds (parrots, parakeets, budgerigars, and cockatoos), but other bird species and mammals can be infected. The most common form of acquisition is exposure to infected birds, by breathing in an aerosol of dried feces or from nose or eye secretions.

Risk factors for disease include contact with pet birds—especially a new, sick, or dead bird—and occupational exposure, for example work as a veterinarian, as a zoo keeper, or in a poultry-processing plant. Most cases are sporadic, but outbreaks have occurred associated with pet shops, aviaries, and poultry-processing plants and with mowing lawns in areas with large numbers of psittacine birds. Person-to-person transmission is rare. There is no evidence of infection acquired through ingestion of poultry products.

Clinical Features

The incubation period varies from 4 to 14 days or longer. The typical presentation of psittacosis is of an influenza-like illness with sudden onset of fever, chills, and prominent headache, but a more gradual onset is also seen. Rigors may be present. Cough is usually later in onset, dry, and not very marked. There may also be diarrhea, pharyngitis, altered mental state, or shortness of breath. Chest examination is usually abnormal, but the findings are often minimal and less prominent than symptoms or x-ray findings would suggest. Pleural effusions are rare.

Patients might present with a fever of unknown origin without obvious respiratory involvement, or the disease can be misdiagnosed as meningitis due to prominent headache, sometimes with photophobia. The degree of illness varies from asymptomatic to life threatening. Elderly persons and pregnant women are susceptible to more severe illness.

Other, less common findings include hemoptysis, proteinuria, hepatosplenomegaly, and encephalitis. Cardiac manifestations include relative bradycardia and rarely myocarditis, culture-negative endocarditis, and pericarditis. Erythema nodosum and other skin manifestations have also been described. *C. psittaci* has also been demonstrated by PCR to be present in a variable proportion of ocular adnexal MALT lymphomas with up to one half of cases responding to antibiotic treatment.

Diagnosis

Diagnosis depends on eliciting a history of recent bird contact from a patient with a compatible clinical syndrome, most commonly an influenza-like presentation, community-acquired pneumonia (CAP), or fever of unknown origin. The diagnosis should also be considered in a patient with CAP and prominent headache, splenomegaly, or failure to respond to β-lactam antibiotics. If the presentation is of an atypical CAP, the differential diagnosis includes infection with *Legionella* species, *Mycoplasma pneumoniae*, or *Chlamydophila pneumoniae*.

The white cell count is usually normal or slightly elevated, but there is often a left shift or toxic changes. Increases in the C-reactive protein (CRP) and erythrocyte sedimentation rate (ESR) are common. Mildly abnormal liver function tests, hyponatremia, and mild renal impairment are also common. The cerebrospinal fluid sometimes contains a few mononuclear cells but is otherwise normal. The chest x-ray usually shows more than predicted by the examination findings, but is nonspecific. The most common finding is lobar consolidation, but bilateral consolidation or interstitial opacities are also commonly seen.

Culture of *C. psittaci* is difficult and hazardous, so confirmation of diagnosis is more commonly performed using serology. The complement fixation (CF) test is widely used, but it cannot differentiate between *Chlamydophila* species. A fourfold rise in titer, using samples collected at least 14 days apart, or a single titer of 1:128 or higher, is interpreted as a positive result. The antibody rise may be delayed or diminished by antibiotic treatment. A microimmunofluorescent (MIF) test is more specific for each *Chlamydophila* species, with a fourfold rise in titer or an IgM antibody titer of 1:16 interpreted as positive, but this test is not widely available. Polymerase chain reaction (PCR) assays have been developed, but they are not yet available for routine clinical use.

CURRENT DIAGNOSIS

- The key to successful management of psittacosis is considering it as a possible diagnosis and asking about bird contact.
- The commonest clinical scenarios are influenza-like illness, community-acquired pneumonia, or fever of unknown origin. The typical presentation is sudden onset of fever and chills, with prominent headache. The diagnosis should also be considered in a patient with community-acquired pneumonia and failure to respond to β-lactam antibiotics.
- Nonspecific findings on investigation include a normal or slightly elevated white blood cell count with a left shift or toxic changes, increase in C-reactive protein (CRP) or erythrocyte sedimentation rate (ESR), mildly abnormal liver function tests, hyponatremia, mild renal impairment, and a chest x-ray with more abnormalities than predicted by the examination findings.
- Diagnosis can be confirmed with serology using either the complement fixation test, which is widely used but unable to differentiate between *Chlamydia* species, or the microimmunofluorescent test, which is specific for individual *Chlamydia* species. Either a single high titer or a fourfold rise in titer using samples collected at least 14 days apart are interpreted as positive.

CURRENT THERAPY

- Empiric therapy should be commenced when the diagnosis is suspected on clinical presentation and initial investigations.
- Tetracyclines are the drugs of choice; for example, doxycycline (Vibramycin) 100 mg bid for 10 to 14 days.
- Macrolides are usually recommended for pregnant women, children, and people with intolerance of tetracyclines, but they are probably less effective.
- Defervescence and improvement in symptoms usually occur within 24 to 48 hours of initiating a tetracycline; subsequent mortality is less than 1%.
- Notification to health authorities facilitates public health investigation and interventions to reduce transmission and control outbreaks.

Management

When the diagnosis is suspected on clinical presentation and initial investigations, empiric therapy should be commenced. Tetracyclines are the drugs of choice, for example, doxycycline (Vibramycin) 100 mg bid for 10 to 14 days. This class usually leads to defervescence and improvement in symptoms within 24 to 48 hours, and subsequent mortality is less than 1%. Macrolides are usually recommended for pregnant women, children, and patients with intolerance of tetracyclines, but erythromycin (Erythrocin)[1] has been shown to fail in situations where a tetracycline was effective, and there are few clinical data on the efficacy of the other agents in this class. Some data suggest that quinolones may be effective, but further evidence is needed. Tetracycline hydrochloride[2] or doxycycline (4.4 mg/kg/d divided into two infusions) is given intravenously for critically ill patients.

Notification of health authorities is important for initiating public health investigations and interventions to reduce transmission and control of outbreaks.

REFERENCES

Centers for Disease Control and Prevention. Compendium of measures to control Chlamydia psittaci infection in humans (psittacosis) and pet birds (avian chlamydiosis), 2000. MMWR Morb Mortal Wkly Rep 2000;49 (RR08):1–17.
Crosse BA. Psittacosis: A clinical review. J Infect 1990;21:251–9.
Grayston JT, Thom DH. The chlamydial pneumonias. Curr Clin Top Infect Dis 1991;11:1–18.
Gregory DW, Schaffner W. Psittacosis. Semin Resp Infect 1997;12:7–11.
Hughes P, Chidley K, Cowie J. Neurological complications in psittacosis: A case report and literature review. Respir Med 1995;89:637–8.
Husain A, Roberts D, Pro B, et al. Meta-Analyses of the association between Chlamydia psittaci and ocular adnexal lymphoma and the response of ocular adnexal lymphoma and the response of ocular adnexal lymphoma to antibiotics. Cancer 2007;110:809–15.
Richards M. Psittacosis, UpToDate 2006; Available at http://www.uptodate.com/physicians/pulmonology_toclist.asp [accessed August 18, 2007; subscription required].
Williams J, Tallis G, Dalton C, et al. Community outbreak of psittacosis in a rural Australian town. Lancet 1998;351:1697–9.
Yung AP, Grayson ML. Psittacosis: A review of 135 cases. Med J Aust 1988;148:228–33.

---

[1]Not FDA approved for this indication.
[2]Not available in the United States.

Q Fever

Method of
Didier Raoult, PhD

Q fever is widespread zoonosis caused by *Coxiella burnetii*, a small, coccoid, strict intracellular gram-negative bacterium. It lives within the phagolysosome of its eukaryotic host cell at very low pH (4.5-4.8). It had previously been classified in the rickettsial family; however, recent phylogenic data based on study of the 16S rRNA gene sequence have shown that it belongs to *Legionellales* with the *Legionella* species and *Francisella tularensis*.

The bacterium has a sporelike life cycle, which explains its marked resistance to physicochemical agents. In cultures, *C. burnetii* exhibits a phase variation (from virulent phase I to avirulent phase II) caused by a spontaneous chromosome deletion. The avirulent form paradoxically generates high antibody levels in patients, but only patients with chronic infection have high antiphase I immunoglobulin G (IgG) and IgA antibody titers.

C. burnetii is a potent biological weapon. The reservoir of *C. burnetii* is wide, and nearly all tested mammals, birds, and ticks can be infected. Outbreaks have also been reported in association with the birth products of mammals (including ungulates and pets), raw milk, slaughterhouses, and farm work. Laboratory outbreaks have been reported. The disease is prevalent everywhere in the world but in New Zealand, but because its clinical spectrum is wide and nonspecific, the observed incidence is directly related to physician interest in Q fever.

Clinical Features

Q fever is a reportable disease in the United States. In humans, infection is symptomatic in only 50% of patients. Most symptomatic patients experience a flulike syndrome lasting 2 to 7 days and consisting of severe headaches and cough; 5% to 10% of infected patients may be sick enough to be investigated. They initially have high fever and one or several of pneumonia, hepatitis, meningoencephalitis, rash, myocarditis, and pericarditis. Routine laboratory investigation commonly shows mildly elevated transaminase levels and mild thrombocytopenia.

In special hosts such as immunocompromised patients (specifically those with lymphoma or splenectomy), *C. burnetii* can cause chronic infection. In pregnant women it can lead to recurrent miscarriage, low-birth-weight offspring, and prematurity.

In patients with valvular heart disease and those with arterial aneurysms or a vascular prosthesis, it can cause chronic endocarditis or vascular infection in patients in the 2 years following primary infection. The clinical picture is that of a chronic blood culture–negative endocarditis; the modified Duke criteria are of diagnostic value in such cases. It is spontaneously fatal in most cases.

Diagnosis

Because Q fever is pleomorphic, the diagnosis is based mainly on comprehensive serum testing in patients with an unexplained infectious syndrome. Liver biopsy may be of diagnostic value because the typical doughnut granuloma is quasispecific to acute Q fever. Valves obtained at surgery or autopsy can be used for culture, direct immunostaining, and polymerase chain reaction (PCR).

Three serologic techniques are used. Complement fixation lacks sensitivity, and one third of patients with acute Q fever do not exhibit complement-fixing antibodies within 1 month after onset of the disease. However, a fourfold increase in antibodies to phase II antigen indicates acute Q fever, and antibody levels against phase I that are higher than 1:200 indicate chronic Q fever. Indirect immunofluorescence assay is the reference method. A single titer of 1:200 for IgG antiphase II associated with a titer of 1:50 for IgM is diagnostic of acute infection. IgG antibody levels against phase I that are great than 1:800

and IgA antibody levels greater than 1:50 are highly predictive of chronic infection. Enzyme-linked immunosorbent assay (ELISA) is useful for diagnosing acute infection in detecting IgM antiphase II.

PCR has recently been developed to detect *C. burnetii* DNA in the sera of patients with Q fever. Real-time PCR using multicopy gene *IS1111* is the more-sensitive technique. It is positive in the sera of patients with acute Q fever before IgG antibodies to *C. burnetii* become apparent. It is also positive in patients with untreated chronic Q fever. Contamination of PCR can occur, and many unconfirmed results are reported in the literature. Detection of patients at risk for chronic infection may be provided by systematic echocardiography in patients with acute Q fever specifically seeking for aortic bicuspidy and serologic fellow-up at 3 and 6 months after acute infection.

Treatment

To be active against Q fever, an antibiotic compound has to enter the cell, be effective at an acidic pH (where *C. burnetii* multiplies), and have activity against *C. burnetii*. No antibiotic is bactericidal, but bactericidal activity can be achieved by the addition of hydroxychloroquine (Plaquenil)[1] to doxycycline (Vibramycin).

For acute Q fever, the reference treatment is doxycycline 100 mg orally twice daily for 2 to 3 weeks. Other compounds have been reported to be effective, such as trimethoprim-sulfamethoxazole (TMP-SMX) (Bactrim),[1] Rifampin (Rifadin)[1] 300 mg twice daily, and ofloxacin (Floxin)[1] 200 mg twice daily. In the case of Q fever in pregnant women, one double-strength TMP-SMX tablet (trimethoprim 160 mg, sulfamethoxazole 800 mg)[1] twice daily until delivery prevents fetal death (Table 1).

Chronic endocarditis should be treated for 3 years, and antibody levels should be monitored. When IgG antiphase I is less than 800 and IgA is less than 50, treatment may be stopped before 3 years. Two protocols have been evaluated: doxycycline 200 mg daily combined with ofloxacin[1] 400 mg daily for 4 years to lifetime, and doxycycline combined with hydroxychloroquine[1] for 1.5 to 3 years in an amount to achieve a 1 ± 0.20 µg/mL plasma concentration. Doxycycline serum levels greater than 4.5 µg/mL of serum are associated with a more rapidly favorable outcome. This last regimen is apparently more efficacious in terms of relapse. However, regular ophthalmologic surveillance is critical to detect the accumulation of chloroquine in the retina. Both regimens expose the patient to a major risk of photosensitization.

---

[1]Not FDA approved for this indication.

TABLE 1 Treatment

Q fever	Recommended Treatment	Alternative Treatment
Acute	Doxycycline (Vibramicyn) 100 mg PO q12h[2] × 14 d	Ofloxacin (Floxin)[1] 200 mg PO q8h[2] × 14 d Cotrimoxazole (Bactrim)[1] 160/800 mg/PO q12h × 14 d
Chronic	Doxycycline 100 mg PO q12h *plus* hydroxychloroquine (Plaquenil)[1] 200 mg PO q8h[2] × 18-36 mo	Doxycycline 100 mg PO q12h *plus* ofloxacin[1] 200 mg PO q 8h[2] for 3 y to lifetime
Acute in a patient with a valvular lesion	Same as chronic Q fever for 12 mo	
In pregnancy	Cotrimoxazole (Bactrim)[1] 160/800 mg PO q12h until term	

[1]Not FDA approved for this indication.
[2]Exceeds dosage recommended by the manufacturer.

The combination of doxycycline and hydroxychloroquine for 1 year has demonstrated efficacy in preventing endocarditis.

Prevention

Prevention depends on avoiding exposure, particularly by pregnant women and patients with valvulopathy. No vaccine is currently available outside Australia.

REFERENCES

Carcopino X, Raoult D, Bretelle F, et al. Managing Q fever during pregnancy: The benefits of long-term cotrimoxazole therapy. Clin. Infect Dis 2007;45:548–55.
Klee SR, et al. Highly sensitive real-time PCR for specific detection and quantification of Coxiella burnetii. BMC Microbiol 2006;19:2.
Landais C, Fenollar F, Thuny F, Raoult D. From acute Q fever to endocarditis: Serological follow-up strategy. Clin Infect Dis 2007;44:1337–40.
Maurin M, Raoult D. Q fever. Clin Microbiol Rev 1999;12:518–53.
Rolain JM, Maurin M, Raoult D. Bacteriostatic and bactericidal activities of moxifloxacin against Coxiella burnetii. Antimicrob Agents Chemother 2001;45:301–2.

Rabies

Method of
Alan C. Jackson, MD, FRCPC

Rabies is an acute infection of the nervous system caused by rabies virus, which is a member of the family Rhabdoviridae in the genus *Lyssavirus*. Other lyssaviruses have only very rarely caused rabies in Europe, Africa, and Australia.

Pathogenesis

Rabies virus is usually transmitted by bites from rabid animals. Transmission has rarely occurred through an aerosol route (in a laboratory accident or bat cave containing millions of bats) or by transplantation of infected organs and tissues. The virus is in the saliva of the rabid animal and inoculated into subcutaneous tissues or muscles. During most of the long incubation period (lasting 20 to 90 days or longer), the virus is close to the site of inoculation. The virus binds to the nicotinic acetylcholine receptor at the postsynaptic neuromuscular junction and travels toward the central nervous system (CNS) in peripheral nerves by retrograde fast axonal transport. There is rapid dissemination throughout the CNS by fast axonal transport. Under natural conditions, degenerative neuronal changes are not prominent, and it is thought that the rabies virus induces neuronal dysfunction by mechanisms that are not well understood. In rabies vectors, the encephalitis is associated with behavioral changes that lead to transmission by biting. After the CNS infection is established, the virus spreads by autonomic and sensory nerves to multiple organs, including the salivary glands of rabies vectors in which the virus is secreted in high titer.

Clinical Features

In North America, where the bat is the most common rabies vector, a history of an animal bite is usually absent, and there may be no known contact with animals. The incubation period is usually between 20 and 90 days, but it may occasionally last 1 or more years. Prodromal features are nonspecific and include malaise, headache, and fever, and patients may also have anxiety or agitation. Approximately half of patients may experience pain, paresthesias, or pruritus at the site of the wound, which has often healed; this may reflect involvement of local sensory ganglia. Approximately 80% of patients with rabies have encephalitic rabies; approximately 20% have paralytic rabies. In encephalitic rabies, there are characteristic periods of generalized arousal or hyperexcitability separated by lucid periods. Autonomic dysfunction occurs frequently and includes hypersalivation, gooseflesh, cardiac arrhythmias, and priapism. Hydrophobia is the most characteristic feature of rabies and occurs in 50% to 80% of patients; contractions of the diaphragm and other inspiratory muscles occur on swallowing. This may become a conditioned reflex, and even the sight or thought of water can precipitate the muscle contractions. Hydrophobia is thought to be caused by inhibition of inspiratory neurons near the nucleus ambiguus.

In paralytic rabies, prominent muscle weakness usually begins in the bitten extremity and progresses to quadriparesis; typically there is sphincter involvement. Patients have a longer clinical course than in encephalitic rabies. Paralytic rabies is frequently misdiagnosed as the Guillain-Barré syndrome. Coma subsequently develops in both clinical forms. With aggressive medical therapy, a variety of medical complications develop, and multiple organ failure is a frequent occurrence. Survival is very rare and has usually occurred in the context of incomplete postexposure rabies prophylaxis that included administration of some rabies vaccine.

Epidemiology

Worldwide more than 55,000 human deaths per year are attributed to rabies. The impact is particularly significant in terms of years of life lost because children are frequently the victims. Most human rabies cases occur through transmission from dogs in developing countries with endemic dog rabies, particularly in Asia and Africa. In the United States and Canada, the most common human cases are from insect-eating bats, and often, there is no known history of a bat bite or exposure to bats. A bat bite may not be recognized. The rabies virus variant responsible for most human cases is found in silver-haired bats and eastern pipistrelle bats. These are small bats not frequently in contact with humans. There are a variety of other rabies vectors in North American wildlife, including skunks, raccoons, and foxes, but these species are rarely responsible for transmission to humans. This is likely because of effective postexposure rabies prophylaxis.

Diagnosis

Most cases of rabies can be diagnosed clinically or the diagnosis strongly suspected, which is particularly important to initiate appropriate barrier nursing techniques and prevent exposures of many health care workers. Some cases may be candidates for an aggressive therapeutic approach. A serum neutralizing titer can be useful in a previously unimmunized individual, but a positive titer may not develop until the second week of clinical illness, and the result of the

test may not be readily available. Detection of rabies virus antigen on a skin biopsy obtained from the nape of the neck using a fluorescent antibody technique is a useful diagnostic test. Detection of rabies virus ribonucleic acid (RNA) in saliva or in skin biopsies using reverse transcription polymerase chain reaction (RT-PCR) amplification is an important recent advance in rapid rabies diagnosis. Rabies virus antigen can be detected in brain tissue obtained by brain biopsy or postmortem.

Prevention

After recognition of a rabies exposure, rabies can be prevented with initiation of appropriate steps, including wound cleansing and active and passive immunization. After a human is bitten by a dog, cat, or ferret, the animal should be captured, confined, and observed for a period of at least 10 days. The animal should also be examined by a veterinarian prior to its release. If the animal is a stray, unwanted, shows signs, or develops signs of rabies during the observation period, the animal should be killed immediately, and its head should be transported under refrigeration for a laboratory examination. The brain should be examined via an antigen-detection method using the fluorescent antibody technique and viral isolation using cell culture or mouse inoculation.

The incubation period for animals other than dogs, cats, and ferrets is uncertain; these animals should be killed immediately after an exposure, and the head submitted for examination. If the result is negative, one may safely conclude that the animal's saliva did not contain rabies virus and, if immunization has been initiated, it should be discontinued. If an animal escapes after an exposure, it should be considered rabid unless information from public health officials indicates this is unlikely, and rabies prophylaxis should be initiated. The physical presence of a bat may warrant postexposure prophylaxis when a person (such as a small child or sleeping adult) is unable to reliably report contact that could have resulted in a bite.

Local wound care should be given as soon as possible after all exposures, even if immunization is delayed, pending the results of an observation period. All bite wounds and scratches should be washed thoroughly with soap and water. Devitalized tissues should be debrided.

Purified chick embryo cell culture vaccine (RabAvert) and human diploid cell vaccine (Imovax) are licensed rabies vaccines in the United States and Canada. Other vaccines grown in either primary cell lines (hamster or dog kidney) or continuous cell lines (Vero cells) are also satisfactory and available in other countries. A regimen of four 1-mL doses of rabies vaccine should be given intramuscularly (IM) in the deltoid area (anterolateral aspect of the thigh is also acceptable in children). Ideally, the first dose should be given as soon as possible after exposure, but failing that, it should be given regardless of the length of a delay. Four additional doses should be given on days 3, 7, and 14. Pregnancy is not a contraindication for immunization. Live vaccines should not be given for 1 month after rabies immunization. Local and mild systemic reactions are common. Systemic allergic reactions are uncommon, and anaphylactic reactions may be treated with epinephrine and antihistamines. Corticosteroids may interfere with the development of active immunity. Immunosuppressive medications should not be administered during postexposure therapy unless they are essential. The risk of developing rabies should be carefully considered before deciding to

---

CURRENT DIAGNOSIS

- A history of animal bite or exposure is frequently absent in North America.
- Pain, paresthesias, and pruritus are early neurologic symptoms of rabies, probably reflecting infection in local sensory ganglia.
- Autonomic features are common.
- Hydrophobia is a highly specific feature of rabies.
- Paralytic features may be prominent, and the clinical presentation may resemble the Guillain-Barré syndrome.
- Saliva samples for reverse transcription polymerase chain reaction (RT-PCR) and a skin biopsy should be obtained for detection of rabies virus antigen.

CURRENT THERAPY

- Details of an exposure determine whether postexposure rabies prophylaxis should be initiated.
- Wound cleansing is very important after a potential rabies exposure.
- Active immunization with a schedule of 5 doses of rabies vaccine at intervals is recommended.
- Passive immunization (if previously unimmunized) consists of human rabies immune globulin infiltrated into the wound and the remainder of the 20 IU/kg dosage given intramuscularly.

discontinue vaccination because of an adverse reaction. A serum neutralizing antibody determination is necessary only after immunization of immunocompromised patients. Less expensive vaccines, derived from neural tissues, are still used in some developing countries; these vaccines are associated with serious neuroparalytic complications.

Human rabies immune globulin (Imogam or BayRab) should also be administered as passive immunization for protection before the development of immunity from the vaccine. It should be given at the same time as the first dose of vaccine and no later than 7 days after the first dose. Rabies vaccine and human rabies immune globulin should never be administered at the same site or in the same syringe. The recommended dose of human rabies immune globulin is 20 international units (IU)/kg; larger doses should not be given because they may suppress active immunity from the vaccine. After wounds are washed, they should be infiltrated with human rabies immune globulin (if anatomically feasible), and the remainder of the dose should be given IM in the gluteal area. If the exposure involves a mucous membrane, the entire dose should be administered IM. With multiple or large wounds, the human rabies immune globulin may need to be diluted for adequate infiltration of all of the wounds. Adverse effects of human rabies immune globulin include local pain and low-grade fever.

After an exposure, a previously immunized patient should receive two 1-mL doses of rabies vaccine on days 0 and 3, but the patient should not receive human rabies immune globulin.

Management of Human Rabies

Only seven people have survived rabies, and six received rabies vaccine prior to the onset of their disease. The possibilities for an aggressive approach were recently reviewed (see Jackson et al., 2003). There was one survivor in Wisconsin in 2004 who did not receive rabies vaccine. It is now doubtful whether the therapy she received played a significant role in her favorable outcome because a similar approach has failed in many cases (Wilde et al. 2008). Palliation is an alternative approach and may be appropriate for many patients who develop rabies.

REFERENCES

Jackson AC. Human disease. In: Jackson AC, Wunner WH, editors. Rabies. 2nd ed. London: Elsevier, Academic Press; 2007. p. 309–40.
Jackson AC. Rabies. Curr Treat Options Infect Dis 2003;5:35–40.
Jackson AC. Rabies: New insights into pathogenesis and treatment. Curr Opin Neurol 2006;19(3):267–70.
Jackson AC. Update on rabies diagnosis and treatment. Curr Infect Dis Rep 2009;11:196–201.
Jackson AC, Warrell MJ, Rupprecht CE, et al. Management of rabies in humans. Clin Infect Dis 2003;36:60–3.
Jackson AC, Wunner WH. Rabies. 2nd ed. London: Elsevier, Academic Press; 2007.
Manning SE, Rupprecht CE, Fishbein D, et al. Human rabies prevention–United States, 2008: recommendations of the Advisory Committee on Immunization Practices. MMWR Recomm Rep 2008;57(RR-3):1–28.
World Health Organization. WHO expert consultation on rabies. First report (First Report Edition). Geneva: WHO; 2005.

Rat-Bite Fever

Method of
Jean Dudler, MD

Rat-bite fever (RBF) is a systemic febrile disease caused by infection with *Streptobacillus moniliformis*. As its name implies, it is transmitted by rat bite. However, it can also be transmitted by simple contact with infected rats or even through ingestion of food contaminated with rat excreta. Diagnosis can be difficult, and a high degree of awareness is necessary to make a correct diagnosis. Recognition and early treatment are crucial, because case fatality can be higher than 10% in untreated cases.

Epidemiology

S. moniliformis is part of the normal respiratory flora of the rat. From 50% to 100% of healthy wild, laboratory, and pet rats harbor *S. moniliformis* in the nasopharynx. *S. moniliformis* is also excreted in the urine, and *Spirillum minus* has been demonstrated in conjunctival secretions and blood. Thus, rat-bite fever can be transmitted not only from a bite but also through scratches, handling of dead rats, and even handling of litter material.

Although the rat is the natural reservoir and major vector of the disease, *S. moniliformis* has also been found in other rodents such as mice, squirrels, and gerbils, as well as in other mammals such as weasels and in pets that prey on rodents, such as cats and dogs, which can also act as vectors of the disease.

The major risk factor is exposure to rats, either as an occupational hazard for persons such as laboratory workers, veterinarians, or pet shop employees, or for persons who have rats for pets or feed rats to snakes, especially children. Classically, homelessness and lower socioeconomic status were described as major factors, but most cases reported in the last few years have involved pet rats.

No precise data are available on the true incidence of rat-bite fever because it is not a reportable disease. It appears to be unusual in Western countries, a rarity that could reflect failed diagnosis or a spontaneous recovery in most cases, considering the high percentage of *S. moniliformis* carriage, the frequency of contacts between humans and rats in modern society, and the fairly high risk—estimated around 10%—of developing rat-bite fever after being bitten or scratched.

Clinical Presentation

Rat-bite fever is a systemic febrile disease. Classically, following a rat bite and a short incubation of 1 to 3 days (but up to 3 weeks), systemic dissemination of the organism is associated with an abrupt onset with intermittent relapsing fever, rigors, myalgias, arthralgias, headache, sore throat, malaise, and vomiting. These symptoms are followed within the first week by the development of a maculopapular rash in 75% of patients. The rash can be pustular, purpuric, or petechial, and it typically involves the extremities, in particular the palms and soles. The bite site typically heals promptly, with minimal inflammation and absent or minimal regional adenopathy.

Up to 50% of infected patients develop an asymmetric migrating polyarthritis, which appears to be exceedingly painful and affects large and middle-sized joints. Joint effusion appears more common in adults. Infection can occur in any tissues. Anemia, meningitis, bronchitis, pneumonia, endocarditis, myocarditis, pericarditis, brain abscess, and infarcts of the spleen and kidneys have been reported as complications of rat-bite fever.

Although most cases seem to resolve spontaneously within 2 weeks, persistence up to 2 years has been reported. The mortality rate in untreated cases is around 10% to 15%, and it rises to more than 50% in the rare cases with cardiac involvement.

Two closely related variants have been described. In Haverhill fever, the organism is transmitted by ingestion of contaminated food. It tends to occur in epidemics and also causes rashes and arthritis, but upper respiratory tract symptoms and vomiting appear more prominent. Sodoku is a rat-bite fever caused by *Spirillum minus*; it is common in Japan. The course is more subacute, arthritic symptoms are rare, and if the bite initially heals, it then ulcerates and is associated with regional lymphadenopathy and a distinctive rash.

Diagnosis

Diagnosis is difficult, with nonspecific clinical findings, broad differential diagnosis, and difficulties in identifying the responsible organism. Rat-bite fever should not be dismissed in the absence of bite history, because transmission can occur without a bite, and pet lovers or laboratory workers can minimize or forget the bite, especially in the absence of a local reaction.

No reliable serologic test is available, and the definitive diagnosis requires isolation of *S. moniliformis* from the wound, the blood, or the synovial fluid. The microbiology laboratory should be specifically notified of any clinical suspicion because of the hurdles in identification.

S. moniliformis is a highly pleomorphic, nonencapsulated, non-motile gram-negative rod, which may stain positively on Gram stain. It is often dismissed as proteinaceous debris because of its numerous bulbous swellings with occasional clumping (*moniliformis* = "necklace-like"). It grows slowly and requires a microaerophilic environment with 5% to 10% CO_2 or anaerobic conditions and media supplementation with 20% normal rabbit serum. Cultures should be held for more than 5 days and should not be dismissed as contamination. *S. moniliformis* is also inhibited by sodium polyanethol sulfonate, a common adjunct in most commercial blood culture media. Identification using polymerase chain reaction amplification and gene sequencing has been used. It can be performed on samples from the patient or animal in question if available.

Differential Diagnosis

Differential diagnosis is broad and depends on the clinical presentation. Malaria, typhoid fever, and neoplastic disease can cause relapsing fevers, and the presence of a rash and polyarthritis might suggest viral and rickettsial diseases. An asymmetric oligoarthritis points more toward a bacterial etiology, in particular disseminated gonococcal and meningococcal diseases in the context of cutaneous lesions. Lyme disease or secondary syphilis occasionally have such a clinical presentation, but 25% to 50% of patients infected with *S. moniliformis* or *S. minus* have a false-positive VDRL (Venereal Disease Research Laboratory) test. Finally, when classic infectious symptoms such as fever or rash are missing, any causes of polyarthritis, from crystal-related arthropathies to rheumatoid arthritis, can be entertained.

Treatment

All established cases of rat-bite fever should be treated with antibiotics. Despite being potentially lethal, rat-bite fever is easily treatable by a simple course of penicillin. The Centers for Disease Control and Prevention recommends intravenous penicillin G 1.2 million units per day for 5 to 7 days followed by oral penicillin V (Pen Vee K)[1] or ampicillin (Omnipen)[1] 500 mg qid for an additional week. For allergic patients, or if an intravenous line cannot be established, oral tetracycline (Achromycin)[1] 500 mg qid or streptomycin[1] 7.5 mg/kg bid intramuscularly are alternatives. Numerous other antibiotics have been reported to

---

[1]Not FDA approved for this indication.

CURRENT DIAGNOSIS

- The examiner must maintain a high index of suspicion.
- Nonspecific initial symptoms are followed by a maculopapular rash and septic arthritis.
- Exposure to rats is the major risk factor. Transmission can occur with simple contact with infected animals or excreta.
- Notify microbiology laboratory of suspicion (slow growth, 5%–10% CO_2 microaerophilic conditions, 20% normal rabbit serum media supplementation, and avoidance of sodium polyanethol sulfonate).

CURRENT THERAPY

Bite Site

- Clean and disinfect bite site.
- Local treatment does not prevent further dissemination.
- Administer tetanus toxoid (Td), if indicated.
- Do not give antirabies prophylaxis.

Established Cases

- Intravenous penicillin G (Bicillin) 1.2 million U/d for 5 to 7 d, followed by oral penicillin V[1] or ampicillin (Omnipen)[1] 500 mg qid for an additional wk (CDC recommendations).
- Oral tetracycline[1] 500 mg qid or streptomycin[1] 7.5 mg/kg bid IM are alternatives.
- Numerous other antibiotics are reported useful (macrolides, cephalosporins, quinolones).

Prophylaxis

- The role of prophylactic antibiotic is unknown. Some authors recommend oral penicillin V.[1]
- Encourage patients with an occupational risk to use protective gloves to handle animals or cages.

---

[1]Not FDA approved for this indication.

---

be potentially useful, including clarithromycin (Biaxin),[1] cephalosporins, and quinolones, but none has been subjected to any clinical trial.

Typically the bite site heals promptly. It should be cleaned and disinfected, even if local treatment does not appear to prevent further dissemination. Tetanus prophylaxis (Td) administration is indicated as required by the patient's immunization record, but antirabies prophylaxis is usually not required for rodent bite.

The role of prophylactic antibiotics is unknown, but some authors recommend the use of oral penicillin V.[1] Primary prevention by using protective gloves to handle animals or cages should be encouraged for patients with occupational risk.

---

[1]Not FDA approved for this indication.

REFERENCES

Abdulaziz H, Touchie C, Toye B, Karsh J. Haverhill fever with spine involvement. J Rheumatol 2006;33:1409–10.

Albedwawi S, LeBlanc C, Show A, Slinger RW. A teenager with fever, rash and arthritis. CMAJ 2006;175:354.

Berger C, Altwegg M, Meyer A, Nadal D. Broad range polymerase chain reaction for diagnosis of rat-bite fever caused by *Streptobacillus moniliformis*. Pediatr Infect Dis J 2001;20:1181–2.

Centers for Disease Control and Prevention. Fatal rat-bite fever—Florida and Washington, 2003. MMWR Morb Mortal Wkly Rep. 2005;53: 1198–202.

Holroyd KJ, Reiner AP, Dick JD. *Streptobacillus moniliformis* polyarthritis mimicking rheumatoid arthritis: An urban case of rat bite fever. Am J Med 1988;85:711–4.

Rupp ME. *Streptobacillus moniliformis* endocarditis: Case report and review. Clin Infect Dis 1992;14:769–72.

Schachter ME, Wilcox L, Rau N, et al. Rat-bite fever. Canada Emerg Infect Dis 2006;12:1301–2.

Stehle P, Dubuis O, So A, Dudler J. Rat bite fever without fever. Ann Rheum Dis 2003;62:894–6.

van Nood E, Peters SH. Rat-bite fever. Neth J Med 2005;63:319–21.

Washburn RG. *Streptobacillus moniliformis* (rat-bite fever). In: Mandell GL, Bennett JE, Dolin R, editors. Mandell, Douglas, and Bennett's Principles and Practice of Infectious Diseases. 4th ed. Philadelphia: Churchill-Livingstone; 2000. p. 2422–4.

Relapsing Fever

Method of
Diego Cadavid, MD

Relapsing fever is one of several diseases caused by spirochetes. Other human spirochetal diseases are syphilis, Lyme disease, and leptospirosis. Notable features of spirochetes are wavy and helical shapes, length-to-diameter ratios of as much as 100 to 1, and flagella that lie between the inner and outer cell membranes. The spirochetes that cause relapsing fever are in the genus *Borrelia*. Other *Borrelia* species cause Lyme disease, avian spirochetosis, and epidemic bovine abortion. Table 1 shows the main *Borrelia* species of relapsing fever, their vectors, and an estimate of their geographic ranges. In the United States relapsing fever was considered a disease endemic only in the West. However, the recent finding of relapsing fever–like *Borrelia* in ticks and dogs in the eastern United States suggests that the risk of relapsing fever may extend into the East.

Epidemiology

There are two forms of relapsing fever: epidemic transmitted to humans by the body louse *Pediculus humanus* (louse-borne relapsing fever, LBRF) and endemic transmitted to humans by soft-bodied ticks of the genus *Ornithodoros* (tick-borne relapsing fever, TBRF). In LBRF itching caused by skin infestation with lice leads to scratching, which may result in crushing of lice and release of infected hemolymph into areas of skin abrasion. Louse infestation is associated with cold weather and a lack of hygiene. Migrant workers and soldiers at war are particularly susceptible to this infection. Historically, massive outbreaks of LBRF occurred in Eurasia, Africa, and Latin America, but currently the disease is found only in Ethiopia and neighboring countries. However, immigrants can spread LBRF to other parts of the world.

The main risk factor for TBRF is exposure to endemic areas (Table 1). The risk of infection increases with outdoor activities in areas where rodents nest, like entering caves or sleeping in rustic cabins. *Ornithodoros* ticks are soft-bodied and feed for short periods of time (minutes), usually at night. They can live many years between blood meals and may transmit spirochetes to their offspring transovarially. Infection is produced by regurgitation of infected tick saliva into the skin wound during tick feeding. There are several natural vertebrate reservoirs for TBRF, but most common are rodents (deer mice, chipmunks, squirrels, and rats). In contrast, the body louse *Pediculus humanus* is a strict human parasite, living and multiplying in clothing.

Clinical Diagnosis

Relapsing fever should be suspected in any patient presenting with two or more episodes of high fever and constitutional symptoms spaced by periods of relative well-being. The index of suspicion

CURRENT DIAGNOSIS

- There are two forms of relapsing fever: epidemic and endemic.
- Epidemic relapsing fever is transmitted from person to person by the body louse *Pediculus humanus*.
- Endemic relapsing fever is transmitted from rodent reservoirs to humans exposed to endemic areas by soft-bodied ticks of the genus *Ornithodoros*.
- The hallmark of relapsing fever is two or more febrile episodes separated by periods of relative well-being.
- The diagnosis is confirmed by visualization of the etiologic spirochetes in thin peripheral blood smears prepared at times of febrile peaks by phase-contrast or darkfield microscopy or light microscopy after Wright or Giemsa staining.

increases if the patient has been exposed to endemic areas for TBRF or to countries where LBRF still occurs (Table 1). Whereas LBRF is usually associated with a single febrile relapse, TBRF usually has multiple relapses (up to 13). In LBRF the second episode of fever is typically milder than the first; in TBRF the multiple febrile periods are usually of equal severity. The febrile periods last from 1 to 3 days, and the intervals between fevers last from 3 to 10 days. During the febrile periods, numerous spirochetes are circulating in the blood. This is called spirochetemia and is sometimes unexpectedly detected during routine blood smear examinations. Between fevers, spirochetemia is not observed because the numbers are low. The fever pattern and recurrent spirochetemia are the consequences of antigenic variation of abundant outer membrane lipoproteins of relapsing fever *Borrelia* species that are the target for serotype-specific antibodies.

The mean latency between exposure to ticks in the endemic form or to lice in the epidemic form and onset of symptoms is 6 days (range, 3 to 18 days). Because *Ornithodoros* ticks feed briefly and painlessly at night, patients with TBRF may not be able to recall having been bitten by a tick. The clinical manifestations of TBRF and LBRF are similar, although some differences do exist. Table 2 lists the frequency of the most common manifestations of TBRF. The usual initial presentation is sudden onset of chills followed by high fever, tachycardia, severe headache, vomiting, myalgia and arthralgia, and often delirium. In the early stages, a reddish rash may be seen over the trunk, arms, or legs. The fever remains high for 3 to 5 days, and then it clears abruptly. After an asymptomatic period of 7 to 10 days, the fever and other constitutional symptoms can reappear suddenly. The febrile episodes gradually become less severe, and the person eventually recovers completely. As the disease progresses, fever, jaundice, hepatosplenomegaly, cardiac arrhythmias, and cardiac failure may occur, especially with LBRF. Jaundice is more common at times of relapses. Patients with LBRF are more likely to develop petechiae on the trunk, extremities, and mucous membranes; epistaxis; and blood-tinged sputum. Rupture of the spleen may rarely occur. Multiple neurologic complications can occur as a result of

TABLE 1 Relapsing Fever *Borrelia* Species Pathogenic to Humans

Relapsing Fever	*Borrelia* Species	Arthropod Vector	Distribution of Disease
Endemic	B. hermsii	Ornithodoros hermsi	Western North America
	B. turicatae	O. turicata	Southwestern North America and northern Mexico
	B. venezuelensis	O. rudis	Central America and northern South America
	B. hispanica	O. marocanus	Iberian peninsula and northwestern Africa
	B. crocidurae	O. erraticus	North and East Africa, Middle East, southern Europe
	B. duttoni	O. moubata	Sub-Saharan Africa
	B. persica	O. tholozani	Middle East, Greece, Central Asia
	B. uzbekistan	O. pappilipes	Tajikistan, Uzbekistan
Epidemic	B. recurrentis	Pediculus humanus	Worldwide (recently only in East Africa including immigrants to Europe)

TABLE 2 Frequent Clinical Manifestations of Tick-Borne Relapsing Fever

Sign or Symptom	Frequency (%)
Headache	94
Myalgia	92
Chills	88
Nausea	76
Arthralgia	73
Vomiting	71
Abdominal pain	44
Confusion	38
Dry cough	27
Ocular pain	26
Diarrhea	25
Dizziness	25
Photophobia	25
Neck pain	24
Rash	18
Dysuria	13
Jaundice	10
Hepatomegaly	10
Splenomegaly	6

disseminated intravascular coagulation in LBRF and as a result of infection of the meninges and cranial and spinal nerve roots by spirochetes in TBRF. The most common neurologic complications of TBRF are aseptic meningitis and facial palsy. Relapsing fever in pregnant women can cause abortion, premature birth, and neonatal death. Sometimes patients can have nonfebrile relapses, consisting of periods of severe headache, backache, weakness, and other constitutional symptoms without fever that occur at the time of expected relapses. Delirium may persist for weeks after the fever resolves, and rarely symptoms may be protracted.

Relapsing fever may be confused with many diseases that are relapsing or cause high fevers. These include typhoid fever, yellow fever, dengue, African hemorrhagic fevers, African trypanosomiasis, brucellosis, malaria, leptospirosis, rat-bite fever, intermittent cholangitis, cat-scratch disease, echovirus 9 infection, among others. Relapsing fever *Borrelias* have antigens that are cross reactive with Lyme disease *Borrelias* and inasmuch as the endemic areas of relapsing fever and Lyme disease overlap to some extent, confusion between the two infections can be expected.

Laboratory Diagnosis

Although the pattern of recurring fever is the clue to diagnosing relapsing fever, confirmation of the diagnosis requires demonstration of spirochetes in peripheral blood taken during an episode of fever. The comparatively large number of spirochetes in the blood during relapsing fever provides the opportunity for the simplest method for laboratory diagnosis of the infection, light microscopy of Wright or Giemsa stained thin blood smears or darkfield or phase-contrast microscopy of a wet mount of plasma. The blood should be obtained during or just before peaks of body temperature. Between fever peaks, spirochetes often can be demonstrated by inoculation of blood or cerebrospinal fluid (CSF) into special culture medium (BSK-H with 6% rabbit serum available from Sigma) or experimental animals. Enrichment for spirochetes is achieved by using the platelet-rich fraction of plasma or the buffy coat of sedimented blood. In the United States the most common causes of relapsing fever are *Borrelia hermsii* and *Borrelia turicatae*; both grow in BSK-H medium and in young mice or rats. Whereas direct visual detection of organisms in the blood is the most common method for laboratory confirmation of relapsing fever, immunoassays for antibodies are the most common means of laboratory confirmation for Lyme disease. Although serologic assays have been developed for the agents of relapsing fever, these are not widely available and of dubious utility. The antigenic variation displayed by the relapsing fever species means there are

hundreds of different "serotypes." If a different serotype or species is used for preparing the antigen, only antibodies to conserved antigens may be detected. For this reason, a standardized enzyme-linked immunosorbent assay (ELISA) with Lyme disease *Borrelia* as antigen may be the best available serologic assay for relapsing fever. ELISA for *Borrelia burgdorferi* antibodies is routinely done across the United States and Europe. If a positive result for IgM or IgG antibodies is obtained, the Western blot for antibodies to *B. burgdorferi* antigens would be expected to discriminate current or past Lyme disease from relapsing fever, as well as from syphilis, another cause of false-positive Lyme disease ELISA results. Other frequent laboratory abnormalities can occur in relapsing fever but are not diagnostic. These include elevated white blood cell count with increased neutrophils, thrombocytopenia, increased serum bilirubin, proteinuria, microhematuria, prolongation of the prothrombin time (PT) and partial thromboplastin time (PTT), and elevation of fibrin degradation products.

Treatment

Relapsing fever *Borrelias* are very sensitive to several antibiotics, and antimicrobial resistance is rare. Table 3 summarizes the treatment options for adults and children younger than 8 years. Children older than 8 years can be treated with the same antibiotics as adults, but the doses should be adjusted by weight. Before antibiotics are given, the possibility of causing the Jarisch-Herxheimer reaction should be considered (see later). The tetracycline antibiotics are most commonly used for treatment of LBRF and TBRF. The first antibiotic of choice in adults and children older than 8 years is doxycycline (Doryx). In general, shorter treatments are needed for LBRF than for TBRF. Single-dose therapy is usually recommended for LBRF. In contrast, in TBRF even multiple doses of tetracyclines for up to 10 days may fail to prevent relapses, and retreatment can be required.

TABLE 3 Treatment Options for Tick-Borne Relapsing Fever*

Adults
Nonsevere forms

1. Doxycycline (Doryx oral), 100 mg PO bid for 1–2 wk[†]
2. Tetracycline (Sumycin), 500 mg PO qid for 1–2 wk
3. Erythromycin (Erythrocin),[1] 500 mg PO tid for 1–2 wk

Severe forms

1. Ceftriaxone (Rocephin),[1] 2 g IV qd for 1–2 wk
2. Penicillin G parenteral aqueous (Pfizerpen),[1] 4 million U IV q4h for 1–2 wk

Children (≤8 y)
Nonsevere forms

1. Erythromycin suspension oral (EryPed),[1] 30–50 mg/kg/d divided tid for 1–2 wk
2. Azithromycin oral suspension (Zithromax),[1] 20 mg/kg on the first day followed by 10 mg/kg/d for 4 more days
3. Penicillin V (Pen-Vee K),[1] 25–50 mg/kg/d divided qid for 1–2 wk
4. Amoxicillin (Amoxil),[1] 50 mg/kg/d divided tid for 1–2 wk

Severe forms

1. Ceftriaxone (Rocephin),[1] 75–100 mg/kg/d IV for 1–2 wk
2. Penicillin G parenteral aqueous (Pfizerpen),[1] 300,000 U/kg/d given IV in divided doses q4h for 1–2 wk

[1]Not FDA approved for this indication.
*The same oral agents are used for treatment of louse-borne (epidemic) relapsing fever but given as a single dose.
[†]In general, treatment for 1 wk is recommended in early/milder cases and for up to 2 wk for more severe cases.
Abbreviations: IV = intravenous; PO = orally.

CURRENT THERAPY

- The antibiotic of choice for treatment of relapsing fever is doxycycline (Doryx) except in children or pregnant women. In children < 8 y, erythromycin (E-Mycin)[1] or oral penicillin[1] is used instead of tetracycline (Table 3).
- Relapsing fever if severe or complicated with neuroborreliosis requires treatment with the intravenous antibiotics ceftriaxone (Rocephin) or penicillin G (Table 3).
- The louse-borne epidemic form is treated with a single dose, whereas the endemic tick-borne form is treated with multiple doses for at least 1 week (Table 3).
- Antibiotic treatment of relapsing fever results in the Jarisch-Herxheimer reaction in as many as 60% of cases, more often in the epidemic than in the endemic form. It is characterized by the sudden onset of tachycardia, hypotension, chills, rigors, diaphoresis, and high fever. To reduce the risk of the JHR, antibiotics should be started between but not at times of febrile peaks.

[1]Not FDA approved for this indication.

Alternative oral antibiotics to the tetracyclines are erythromycin (E-Mycin),[1] azithromycin (Zithromax),[1] amoxicillin (Amoxil),[1] penicillin,[1] and chloramphenicol (Chloromycetin).[1] However, oral chloramphenicol is no longer available in the United States. Erythromycin, azithromycin, and penicillin do not appear as effective as the tetracyclines; however, they are recommended for children younger than 8 years and for pregnant women. Amoxicillin is another alternative for young children with early Lyme disease; however, it is ineffective for human granulocytic ehrlichiosis, which sometimes occurs as a co-infection with Lyme disease.

Although treatment with antibiotics is usually given orally, they may need to be given intravenously if severe vomiting makes swallowing impractical. If there are symptoms and signs of meningitis or encephalitis without clinical and/or radiologic signs of increased intracranial pressure, the CSF should be examined to rule out central nervous system (CNS) infection. The finding of elevation of CSF cells and protein demands the use of parenteral antibiotics, such as penicillin G or ceftriaxone (Rocephin). Optimally, antibiotic treatment should be started during afebrile periods when the spirochetemia is low. Starting therapy near the peak of a febrile period may induce the Jarisch-Herxheimer reaction, in which high fever and a rise and subsequent fall in blood pressure, sometimes to dangerously low levels, may occur. Dehydration should be treated with fluids given intravenously. Severe headache can be treated with pain relievers such as codeine, and nausea or vomiting can be treated with prochlorperazine.

Jarisch-Herxheimer Reaction

Antibiotic treatment of relapsing fever causes the Jarisch-Herxheimer reaction (JHR) in as many as 60% of cases. The JHR is more common in LBRF than in TBRF. It is characterized by the sudden onset of tachycardia, hypotension, chills, rigors, diaphoresis, and high fever. Patients with the JHR have said that they felt as if they were going to die. The JHR is caused by the rapid killing of circulating spirochetes 1 to 4 hours after the first dose of antibiotic, which results in the release of large amounts of Borrelia lipoproteins in the circulation followed by massive release of tumor necrosis factor and other cytokines. If possible, patients with the JHR should be transferred to an

intensive care unit for close monitoring and treatment. During several hours, the temperature declines and the patient feels better. Large amounts of intravenous fluids (0.9% sodium chloride solution) may be required to treat hypotension. Steroids and nonsteroidal antiinflammatory agents have no effect on the frequency or severity of the JHR. One study found that pretreatment with anti-TNF-alpha monoclonal antibody (Humira)[1] suppressed the JHR after penicillin treatment for LBRF and reduced the associated increases in plasma cytokines. Death can occur as a result of the JHR secondary to cardiovascular collapse in up to 5% of patients with treated LBRF and much less frequently in TBRF.

Outcome

Complete recovery occurs in 95% or more of adequately treated patients. The prognosis for untreated cases or if treatment is delayed varies. Mortality as high as 40% is reported in untreated epidemics of LBRF. Relapsing fever also has a high mortality in neonates. Some neurologic sequelae can occur in patients with TBRF complicated with neuroborreliosis.

Prevention

Prevention of TBRF involves avoidance of rodent- and tick-infested dwellings such as animal burrows, caves, and abandoned cabins. Wearing clothing that protects skin from tick access (e.g., long pants and long-sleeved shirts) is also helpful. Repellents and acaricides provide additional protection. Diethyltoluamide (DEET) repels ticks when applied to clothing or skin, but it must be used with caution. It loses its effectiveness within 1 to several hours when applied to skin and must be reapplied; it is absorbed through the skin and may cause CNS toxicity if used excessively. Picaridin (KBR 3023), which has been used as an insect repellent for years in Europe and Australia, is now available in the United States in 7% solution as Cutter Advanced Repellent (Spectrum Brands). The U.S. Centers for Disease Control and Prevention (CDC) is recommending it as an alternative to DEET. Permethrin Insect Repellent, an acaricide, is more effective than DEET but should not be applied directly to skin. When applied to clothing, it provides good protection for 1 day or more. In LBRF, prevention can be achieved by promoting personal hygiene and by dusting undergarments and the inside of clothing with malathion[1,2] or lindane powder[2] when available. Widespread antibiotic use may be necessary to control epidemics of LBRF, using one or two doses of 100 mg doxycycline given within 1 week of exposure.

REFERENCES

Barbour AG, Hayes SF. Biology of Borrelia species. Microbiol Rev 1986;50:381–400.

Bryceson AD, Parry EH, Perine PL, et al. Louse-borne relapsing fever. Q J Med 1970;39:129–70.

Cadavid D, Barbour AG. Neuroborreliosis during relapsing fever: Review of the clinical manifestations, pathology, and treatment of infections in humans and experimental animals. Clin Infect Dis 1998;26:151–64.

Fekade D, Knox K, Hussein K, et al. Prevention of Jarisch-Herxheimer reactions by treatment with antibodies against tumor necrosis factor alpha. N Engl J Med 1996;335:311–5.

Kazragis RJ, Dever LL, Jorgensen JH, Barbour AG. In vivo activities of ceftriaxone and vancomycin against Borrelia spp. in the mouse brain and other sites. Antimicrob Agents Chemother 1996;40:2632–6.

Melkert PW. Fatal Jarisch-Herxheimer reaction in a case of relapsing fever misdiagnosed as lobar pneumonia. Trop Geogr Med 1987;39:92–3.

Southern P, Sanford J. Relapsing fever. Medicine 1969;48:129–49.

Taft W, Pike J. Relapsing fever. Report of a sporadic outbreak including treatment with penicillin. JAMA 1945;129:1002–5.

[1]Not FDA approved for this indication.

[1]Not FDA approved for this indication.
[2]Not available in the United States.

Lyme Disease

Arthur Weinstein, MD, FACP, FACR

Epidemiology

Lyme disease, or borreliosis, is a tick-transmitted infection caused by *Borrelia burgdorferi*. It is the most common insect-borne illness in the United States with more than 20,000 new cases reported annually. It occurs worldwide with hyperendemicity in temperate regions. In the United States, most cases originate from states in the Northeast, mid-Atlantic, upper Midwest, and Pacific coast regions. The life cycle of the Ixodes tick ensures that most cases of human borrelial infection occur from spring to fall. Three genospecies of *B. burgdorferi* account for human disease: *B. burgdorferi sensu stricto*, *B. garinii*, and *B. afzelii*. Although all three are found in Europe and the latter two in Asia, *B. burgdorferi sensu stricto* is the only cause of Lyme disease in the United States. Lyme disease occurs in all age groups with highest frequencies in young children and adults older than 30 years and is equally common in men and women. It often manifests clinically in stages, with exacerbations and remissions in each stage.

Clinical Features

EARLY LYME DISEASE

Localized skin infection and early disseminated infection occur within days to weeks after the bite of an infected tick. Erythema migrans (EM) rash, the hallmark of early Lyme disease, occurs in up to 70% to 80% of patients at the site of the tick bite. It usually is macular and asymptomatic but may burn or itch, and it is commonly found at the belt line, inguinal area, or in and around the axilla. It expands over days, often to a very large circumference and with central clearing, giving a bull's-eye appearance. Approximately 10% of patients have multiple skin lesions (disseminated EM), a sign of hematogenous spread of the borrelia. At this early stage, patients may have nonspecific flulike complaints, namely fever, fatigue, myalgia, arthralgia, and headache, resembling a viral syndrome. These symptoms occasionally occur without the rash. In untreated patients, EM resolves spontaneously within days to several weeks after onset, but treatment often accelerates its resolution.

Early disseminated disease occurs days to weeks after the tick bite and may occur without preceding localized EM. Certain subtypes of *B. burgdorferi* are associated with higher frequency of spirochetemia and dissemination to other organs. For instance, in Europe, EM is often an indolent, localized infection, whereas in the United States, it is associated with more intense inflammation and signs that suggest dissemination of the spirochete. The clinical manifestations of dissemination can be highly variable and may include disseminated EM rash and neurologic, cardiac, and musculoskeletal features either alone or in combination. Neurologic features (neuroborreliosis) are seen in approximately 10% of patients and include acute lymphocytic meningitis, cranial neuropathy, especially facial paresis, which may be bilateral, and radiculoneuritis. Neuroborreliosis is more common in Europe where neurotropic subspecies of borrelia (*B. garinii*, *B. afzelii*) are found. Meningitis usually resolves spontaneously, whereas treatment of other neurologic features can hasten recovery and prevent progression to the later stages of Lyme disease. Carditis, which includes varying degrees of atrioventricular block or mild myopericarditis, may develop in approximately 8% of untreated patients, but early treatment can prevent its occurrence. In more recent series, the incidence of Lyme carditis was reported as less than 1% in the United States. Rheumatic features at this stage consist of migratory, episodic joint, tendon, or bursal pains with or without objective signs of inflammation. Typically there is acute localized pain that lasts days to weeks, remits spontaneously, and then recurs in another region. Inflammatory polyarthritis is not a feature of early or late Lyme disease.

The diagnosis of early Lyme disease relies to a great degree on the clinical presentation. In an endemic area, with a history of possible tick exposure, the presence of a classical EM lesion is sufficient for the diagnosis. With very early infection and isolated EM, laboratory tests for antibodies to *B. burgdorferi* may be negative. Conversely, with disseminated early Lyme disease, antibody testing is frequently positive.

LATE LYME DISEASE

Late Lyme disease occurs months to years after initial infection (mean, 6 months) and may present de novo without prior features of early Lyme disease. Systemic symptoms are generally minimal or absent. Musculoskeletal complaints, the most common manifestation, are seen in 80% of untreated patients and include intermittent oligoarthritis (50%) and acute or subacute inflammatory arthritis that most often affects one or both knees. This arthritis may begin abruptly with knee pain and a large joint effusion. Synovial fluid is inflammatory with white counts ranging in the thousands or tens of thousands. Radiographs may be normal except for soft-tissue swelling and joint effusion but may also demonstrate osteopenia, bone cysts, and even mild cartilage loss with small erosions. Untreated, these attacks of arthritis generally last many months, recur for several years but eventually may remit. *B. burgdorferi* is not culturable from the synovial fluid of patients with Lyme arthritis, but borrelial DNA can be detected by polymerase chain reaction (PCR) in over 80% of untreated patients. The PCR test is generally negative after appropriate antibiotic therapy.

Neurologic features of late Lyme disease are seen more frequently in Europe because *B. garinii* is the most neurotropic subspecies. There are a wide range of neurologic abnormalities, especially encephalomyelitis and peripheral neuropathy. In the United States, Lyme encephalopathy or polyneuropathy is described with subtle disturbances of memory and concentration, spinal radicular pain, or distal paresthesias. Nerve conduction studies reveal axonal polyneuropathy. Pleocytosis of the cerebrospinal fluid (CSF) is unusual in late neurologic Lyme disease. High CSF protein may be seen, but borrelial organisms by culture or PCR are not commonly found. Important to the diagnosis of neuroborreliosis is the demonstration of increased intrathecal synthesis of borrelia-specific antibodies.

A chronic skin lesion, acrodermatitis chronica atrophicans, caused by *B. afzelii*, is seen most commonly in Europe.

Laboratory Testing in Lyme Disease

Lyme disease should not be diagnosed purely on serologic tests because false-positive tests are common. Instead, serologic tests should be used to confirm the diagnosis in the appropriate clinical setting. Even a true positive test only confirms recent or past exposure to *B. burgdorferi*, but this must be evaluated in the context of the patient's past and current symptoms.

Despite these methodologic and diagnostic issues, measurement of antibodies to *B. burgdorferi* by enzyme-linked immunoassay (ELISA) is a useful screening test for early and late Lyme disease. This so-called Lyme test is positive in most cases of late Lyme disease and virtually always positive in late Lyme arthritis. It may be negative very early after infection or in those individuals who receive early antibiotic therapy. However, the high rate of false positivity has led to a two-test strategy whereby all sera that show positive or equivocal ELISA tests for borrelial antibodies are tested again by more specific Western (immuno) blotting. In patients with CNS disease, demonstration of intrathecal antibodies by ELISA in relatively higher concentration than serum antibodies is suggestive of neuroborreliosis.

Immunoblotting is usually performed for both IgM and IgG antibodies to borrelial proteins. Although this technique is not as automated or quantitative as ELISA, it is more specific because it identifies the borrelial antigens to which the antibodies are directed. There are recommendations for standardized testing and interpretation of Western blot results. IgM antibodies usually appear 2 to 4 weeks after EM, peak at 6 to 8 weeks, and decline thereafter, although IgM reactivity may occasionally persist for many years. An IgM blot

CURRENT DIAGNOSIS

- Erythema migrans is usually asymptomatic and expansile.
- Lyme disease can present with only flulike symptoms: fever, arthralgia, myalgia.
- Antibody testing for borrelial infection is often negative during early infection.
- A two-test strategy (serum ELISA, immunoblot) is recommended for diagnosis.
- IgM antibodies are commonly seen in early infection (4–8 wk) but may persist for many months.
- IgG antibodies are characteristic of late Lyme disease, especially Lyme arthritis.
- Intrathecal antibody synthesis is an important diagnostic marker for neuroborreliosis.
- Clinical symptoms combined with antibody status are of diagnostic importance.
- A positive IgM Western blot result should not be used to diagnose Lyme disease in a patient with chronic and non-specific symptoms.

Abbreviation: ELISA = enzyme-linked immunosorbent assay.

CURRENT THERAPY

- Early antibiotic therapy hastens resolution of symptoms and prevents late complications.
- In adults, oral therapy with doxycycline (Vibramycin)[1] is preferred for most features of Lyme disease.
- Neuroborreliosis is usually treated with IV ceftriaxone.
- Duration of therapy is generally 2–4 wk.
- Lyme disease is cured after antibiotic treatment (one or two courses) in most patients.
- Some patients with Lyme arthritis develop persistent antibiotic-resistant synovitis, which may be autoimmune and is treated with antirheumatic drugs.
- Patients with chronic fatigue, arthralgia, and myalgia that begins, persists, or recurs after antibiotic treatment for Lyme disease generally have a post–Lyme disease syndrome and not ongoing infection.
- There is no scientific support for prolonged courses of oral or IV antibiotics for Lyme disease.

[1]Not FDA approved for this indication.
Abbreviation: IV = intravenous.

is considered to be positive if two of three specified bands (23, 39, 41 kd) are present. The results of an IgM blot are best interpreted in the first weeks after symptom onset when the true positive rate exceeds the false-positive rate. A positive IgM blot found in a patient with long-standing symptoms should be interpreted with caution because it likely represents a false-positive result. IgG antibodies appear after 4 to 6 weeks, peak at 4 to 6 months, and then remain positive for many years, even decades. An IgG immunoblot is considered to be positive if 5 of 10 specified bands (18, 23, 28, 30, 39, 41, 45, 58, 66, 93 kd) are present. IgG seroconversion, with or without IgM seroconversion, can be taken as presumptive evidence of exposure to *B. burgdorferi* and in the proper clinical context supports the diagnosis of Lyme disease. However, a positive IgG immunoblot does not necessarily mean current or ongoing borreliosis. Conversely, a negative IgG immunoblot is presumptive evidence against the diagnosis of late Lyme disease. A major issue in the laboratory diagnosis of Lyme disease using the standard two-test strategy is the misinterpretation of a positive IgM Western blot in a patient with chronic and non-specific symptoms, leading to a misdiagnosis of infection with *B. burgdorferi*. An ELISA assay for antibodies to a borrelial-specific surface protein (C6 peptide of VlsE) was demonstrated to be a sensitive and specific single test for the diagnosis of Lyme disease and is commercially available but as yet has not replaced standard ELISA and Western blot testing for diagnosis.

Culture of *B. burgdorferi* requires special medium and conditions and takes many weeks. Even so, in expert laboratories the organism can be recovered from the EM lesion in a high percentage of patients and from the blood in patients with disseminated early Lyme disease. Risk for spirochetemia starts the day the patient notices the rash and continues for 2 weeks.

B. burgdorferi is cultured only rarely from the CSF of patients with neuroborreliosis.

PCR to detect borrelial DNA is also positive with the same or higher frequency as culture from the skin, blood, and CSF. However, it is most useful in the synovial fluid of patients with suspected and untreated Lyme arthritis where it can be positive in more than 80% of patients despite universally negative cultures. PCR analysis of synovial tissue may be more likely to yield positive results than synovial fluid because *B. burgdorferi* associates with connective tissue. However, because virtually all cases of Lyme arthritis are strongly positive by ELISA and immunoblotting for IgG antibodies to *B. burgdorferi*, the diagnosis can usually be made with reasonable certainty using these tests alone.

Treatment

The goals of treatment of Lyme disease are to resolve the clinical symptoms by eradication of the organism and to prevent late stage disease with early therapy. Although most manifestations resolve spontaneously without treatment, clinical trials demonstrated that treatment with antibiotics hastens resolution and prevents late manifestations of Lyme borreliosis. In most of the trials, treatment of 3 weeks' duration was effective. Revised evidence-based guidelines for treatment have recently been published by the Infectious Diseases Society of America. Generally, early Lyme disease is treated with antimicrobials for 2 to 3 weeks, although studies showed that EM treatment with oral doxycycline for 10 days is as effective as treatment for 20 days. Long-term outcomes are similar for both regimens. Effective oral medications include doxycycline (Vibramycin),[1] tetracycline, second-generation cephalosporins such as cefuroxime axetil (Ceftin), and amoxicillin (Amoxil).[1] Erythromycin (E-Mycin)[1] and azithromycin (Zithromax)[1] are somewhat less effective. Doxycycline and tetracycline should not be used in children younger than 8 years or in pregnant women. Oral therapy is sufficient for certain clinical features: EM, facial palsy without signs of meningitis, and first-degree heart block. Oral therapy with doxycycline (Vibramycin) is associated with fewer side effects and is much less expensive than the also employed intravenous (IV) therapy with ceftriaxone (Rocephin).[1] Although amoxicillin and doxycycline appear to be equally efficacious, doxycycline has the distinct advantage of also being effective in treating *Anaplasma phagocytophila* infection, which causes human granulocytic ehrlichiosis (HGE) and is also transmitted by the Ixodes tick. In general, patients with neurologic manifestations, either early or late, other than isolated facial palsy, are treated de novo with IV ceftriaxone (Rocephin)[1] for 3 to 4 weeks, although aqueous penicillin (Penicillin G)[1] is also effective. Carditis with heart block may resolve spontaneously, but patients with higher grades of heart block and with cardiomyopathy are generally treated with IV antibiotics. If the oral regimen fails, as may occur with 20% of patients, parenteral therapy with ceftriaxone or cefotaxime (Claforan)[1] is warranted. In patients with persistent symptoms, a second parenteral regimen is usually administered. There is no need to change the medication because *B. burgdorferi* does not show resistance to any of the antimicrobials recommended.

[1]Not FDA approved for this indication.

TABLE 1 Suggested Treatment of Lyme Disease

Clinical Features/Indication	Antibiotic regimen	Regimen		Duration of Therapy
		Adults	Children	
Early Infection (Local and Disseminated Disease)	Doxycycline (Vibramycin)[1]	100 mg bid	<8 y: not recommended >8 y: 1–2 mg/kg bid; maximum 100 mg	2–3 wk
	Tetracycline[1]	500 mg qid	Not for pregnant women	2–3 wk
	Amoxicillin[1]	500 mg tid	As above	2–3 wk
	Cefuroxime axetil (Ceftin)	500 mg bid	50 mg/kg/d in 3 divided doses	2–3 wk
	Azithromycin (Zithromax)[1]	500 mg daily	30 mg/kg/d in 2 divided doses	7–10 d
	Erythromycin[1]	500 mg qid	50 mg/kg/d	2–3 wk
Neuroborreliosis Failure to Respond to Oral Therapy	Ceftriaxone (Rocephin)[1] Cefotaxime (Claforan)[1]	2 g IV daily	75–100 mg/kg/d	2–4 wk
	Penicillin G[1]	2 g IV tid 4–5 million U IV q4h	90–180 mg/kg/d in 3–4 divided doses 2–4 million U IV q4 h	2–4 wk 2–4 wk
Carditis	Oral or IV regimen			2–3 wk
Late Lyme Arthritis	Oral or IV regimen			4 wk*
Pregnancy	Amoxicillin or cefuroxime axetil Penicillin G Ceftriaxone Cefotaxime			2–4 wk

*May give another course if poor response.
[1]Not FDA approved for this indication.
Abbreviation: IV = intravenous.

Oral and parenteral therapies are both used with success in treating Lyme arthritis with treatment duration of 3 to 4 weeks. Occasionally a second month of treatment is needed to eradicate the organism from the joint. Even with successful treatment, the arthritis may resolve quite slowly with synovitis persisting over several months (Table 1).

PERSISTENT (TREATMENT-RESISTANT) LYME ARTHRITIS

Approximately 10% of patients with Lyme arthritis in the United States are treatment resistant, with recurrent inflammatory effusions, usually in one knee, for months to several years despite appropriate antibiotic therapy. This antibiotic-resistant Lyme arthritis is thought to be related to an intra-articular autoimmune response in predisposed individuals. There is no evidence for persistent infection because borrelial DNA by PCR in synovial fluid or synovial tissue is not found in these individuals. A genetic predisposition is suggested by the increased frequency of HLA-DR4 and HLA-DRB1*0401, 0101, and related alleles, similar to that seen in rheumatoid arthritis. In this situation, treatment consists of nonsteroidal anti-inflammatory drugs, intraarticular steroid injections, and antirheumatic agents such as hydroxychloroquine (Plaquenil),[1] sulfasalazine (Azulfidine),[1] and even methotrexate (Rheumatrex).[1] In some cases, arthroscopic synovectomy proves effective. This arthritis usually remits after several years.

POST–LYME DISEASE SYNDROME

Although the long-term prognosis of treated Lyme disease is excellent, some patients develop arthralgia, myalgia, and fatigue, during or soon after infection, which persists despite adequate courses of antibiotics. Other features of this symptom complex include memory and concentration difficulties, neuropathic pains, headache, and unrefreshed sleep. This condition is often called post–Lyme disease syndrome, post-treatment chronic Lyme disease, or chronic Lyme disease. The actual frequency of this condition after Lyme disease is unclear but is likely no more than 5%. Some studies suggested that delay in initiating antibiotic treatment for borrelial infection is more likely to result in post–Lyme disease syndrome. In none of these studies did current serologic status correlate with persistent symptoms. Although these patients have significant somatic complaints and functional disability, they lack objective findings of an inflammatory condition. Although

virtually all patients with this syndrome complain of problems with memory and concentration, demonstrable abnormalities on neuro-cognitive testing are not universally present. The pathogenesis of this chronic post-treatment symptomatic state and its relationship to Lyme disease are unclear. Patients may feel better during antibiotic therapy, but the effect is not durable and relapse is common when antibiotics are discontinued. The symptoms wax and wane, but the overall course is chronic. Controversy has raged as to whether chronic, relatively resistant borrelial infection plays a role and hence whether chronic antibiotic therapy is warranted. However, an important study on post–Lyme syndrome patients failed to document the presence of B. burgdorferi in the plasma or spinal fluid of these patients by culture or PCR. In addition, a controlled trial failed to show a response to a 3-month course of antibiotics (1 month of IV ceftriaxone [Rocephin][1] followed by 2 months of oral doxycycline[1]). This suggests that chronic infection is not the cause of post–Lyme disease syndrome, that the condition spontaneously waxes and wanes, and that prolonged antibiotic treatment does not result in long-term symptom remission. A recent review critically examined the concept of "chronic Lyme disease" and the causes of clinical symptoms following Lyme disease treatment.

Prevention

The best currently available method for preventing infection with B. burgdorferi and other tick-transmitted infections is to avoid tick infested areas through the summer. If exposure is unavoidable, use of protective clothing (shirt tucked into pants and pants tucked under socks) may interfere with attachment by ticks. Wearing light-colored clothing makes it easier to identify ticks. Daily inspection of the entire body to locate and remove ticks also decreases the transmission of infection. Attached ticks should promptly be removed with fine-toothed forceps, if possible. Tick and insect repellent applied to the skin and clothing provides additional protection. The most effective repellent is DEET (diethyltoluamide). Permethrin, a pesticide that kills ticks and mites when applied to clothing, decreases the risk of tick bite. Strategies to reduce the number of ticks may be somewhat effective in decreasing tick-borne illnesses, including the application of acaricides and landscaping to provide desiccating barriers. Although vaccination is available for dogs and

[1]Not FDA approved for this indication.

a recombinant outer surface protein A (OspA)-based vaccine (LYMErix) is effective and relatively safe in humans, currently no marketed vaccine is available to prevent Lyme disease in humans.

AFTER TICK BITE

It is not recommended to treat all patients after a tick bite because several prospective studies demonstrated that the risk of drug-associated rash is as great as the risk of developing Lyme disease. Conversely, it may be reasonable to treat persons believed to be at higher risk for the development of borrelial infection prophylactically. Studies showed that transmission of *B. burgdorferi* from tick to host occurs with greater frequency when there has been tick attachment for more than 48 hours resulting in a blood-engorged tick. Because a controlled study demonstrated that a single 200-mg dose of doxycycline[1] effectively prevents Lyme disease when given within 72 hours of a tick bite, the threshold for treating patients after tick bites with this benign regimen is lower than in the past.

---

[1]Not FDA approved for this indication.

REFERENCES

Feder HM Jr, Johnson BJB, O'Connell S, et al. A critical appraisal of "chronic Lyme disease." N Engl J Med 2007;357:1422–30.

Klempner MS, Hu LT, Evans J, et al. Two controlled trials of antibiotic treatment in patients with persistent symptoms and a history of Lyme disease. N Engl J Med 2001;345:85–92.

Nadelman RB, Nowakowski J, Fish D, et al. Prophylaxis with single dose doxycycline for the prevention of Lyme disease after an Ixodes scapularis tick bite. N Engl J Med 2001;345:79–84.

Steere AC. Lyme disease. N Engl J Med 2001;345:115–25.

Steere AC, Dhar A, Hernandez J, et al. Systemic symptoms without erythema migrans as the presenting picture of early Lyme disease. Am J Med 2003;114:58–62.

Treatment of Lyme disease. The Medical Letter 2005;47:41–3.

Tugwell P, Dennis DT, Weinstein A, et al. Clinical guideline 2: Laboratory evaluation in the diagnosis of Lyme disease. Ann Intern Med 1997;127:1109–23.

Weinstein A. Laboratory testing for Lyme disease: time for a change? Clin Infect Dis 2008;47:196–7.

Weinstein A, Britchkov M. Lyme arthritis and post-Lyme disease syndrome. Curr Opin Rheum 2002;14:383–7.

Wormser GP, Dattwyler RJ, Shapiro ED, et al. The clinical assessment, treatment, and prevention of Lyme disease, human granulocytic anaplasmosis, and babesiosis: Clinical practice guidelines by the Infectious Diseases Society of America. Clin Infect Dis 2006;43:1089–134.

Wormser GP, Ramanathan R, Nowakowski J, et al. Duration of antibiotic therapy for early Lyme disease. A randomized, double-blind, placebo-controlled trial. Ann Intern Med 2003;138:697–704.

Rubella and Congenital Rubella

Method of
Judith M. Hübschen, PhD, and Claude P. Muller, MD

Rubella is normally a mild self-limiting rash-fever illness. Infection during pregnancy, however, can result in fetal death or congenital defects known as congenital rubella syndrome (CRS). Rubella virus is a single-stranded RNA virus (family *Togaviridae*) of which only one serotype but several genotypes are known.

Epidemiology

Humans are the only known natural host for rubella virus, and before the first licensed vaccine was introduced in 1969, the virus circulated worldwide, causing epidemics every few years.

Rubella spreads mainly via aerosols, but in contrast to measles, a close and prolonged contact is usually required for transmission. Children with CRS can shed large quantities of virus for many months after birth. In unvaccinated populations, approximately 15% to 20% of women of childbearing age are susceptible to the disease and can become infected during pregnancy.

Effective vaccination programs have already led to the elimination of rubella and CRS in some countries (e.g., the United States and Finland). However, routine rubella vaccination has not yet been introduced in many developing countries in Africa and Asia, and endemic virus continues to circulate in many countries worldwide. Insufficient vaccination rates in industrialized countries and the refusal to be vaccinated for religious and other reasons represent a considerable threat to control and elimination goals of the World Health Organization (WHO).

Reinfections with rubella virus are possible and have been reported more often after vaccination than after natural primary infection. Normally, reinfections are asymptomatic and congenital malformations seem to be very rare.

Clinical Manifestations

Rubella virus normally causes only a mild disease, and it is estimated that depending on the cohort, between 20% and 50% of infections are subclinical. The incubation period lasts about 2 weeks (range, 12-23 days), at the end of which a maculopapular rash can appear, which spreads from the face to the trunk and limbs. Lymphadenopathy can develop before the rash and can persist for up to 2 weeks after rash. Especially in adults, a prodromal phase may be observed with fever, malaise, and other uncharacteristic symptoms. Viremia occurs for about 1 week before onset of rash, and virus can be transmitted from around 1 week before, until up to nearly 2 weeks (and exceptionally longer) after onset of rash.

Complications

Rubella infection acquired after birth is rarely associated with complications other than arthralgia and arthritis in post-pubertal women. Male patients and prepubertal girls only rarely have these symptoms. Joint symptoms normally last a few days, but they sometimes persist for up to 1 month. Encephalopathy and thrombocytopenia are other rare complications associated with rubella.

Infection during pregnancy can lead to miscarriage and, especially if acquired in the first trimester, is likely to result in congenital defects. The range and severity of the damages is related to the developmental stage of the fetus at the time of infection. The most common manifestations of CRS include defects of the eyes (e.g., cataracts, glaucoma, pigmentary retinopathy), ears (e.g., deafness), heart (e.g., patent ductus arteriosus, pulmonary artery stenosis, ventricular septal defect, neonatal myocarditis) and the central nervous system (e.g., microcephaly, meningoencephalitis, mental and motor retardation, speech, behavior and psychiatric disorders). Most of the clinical features are permanent, but some are transient (e.g., intrauterine growth retardation, hepatosplenomegaly, thrombocytopenic purpura, haemolytic anemia, bone lesions). Not all manifestations are apparent at birth; some appear only later in life (e.g., type 1 diabetes mellitus, thyroid dysfunction).

Diagnosis and Differential Diagnosis

A rubella diagnosis based on clinical symptoms alone is unreliable. Laboratory confirmation is necessary to exclude other rash-fever diseases such as infections caused by measles virus, parvovirus B19, human herpesvirus 6, dengue virus, enteroviruses, and group A *Streptococcus*. Rubella-specific immunoglobulin (Ig) M, which normally persists for 2 to 3 months but occasionally much longer, points to a current or recent infection. False-positive IgM results occur more often with indirect serologic assays than with antibody capture assays

CURRENT DIAGNOSIS

- Laboratory confirmation of rubella is necessary to exclude other diseases with similar clinical symptoms.
- Laboratory diagnosis is normally done by serologic testing and increasingly also by molecular diagnostic methods, including reverse-transcriptase polymerase chain reaction.

and are sometimes linked to rheumatoid factor or cross-reacting non-rubella IgM antibodies. During pregnancy, false-positive IgM tests are of particular concern. A significant increase in rubella-specific IgG antibody titer between acute and convalescent phase sera also indicates a recent infection with rubella virus. IgG avidity testing can also differentiate between old and recent infections. The virus can also be detected by reverse transcription polymerase chain reaction (RT-PCR) or virus isolation in cell culture.

Fetal infections are usually diagnosed either by rubella-specific IgM in fetal blood or by rubella virus in amniotic fluid. However, the time point for testing is critical. After birth, laboratory confirmation of CRS is normally done by detecting rubella-specific IgM, which is almost always detectable during the first 3 months of life but only very rarely after the age of 18 months. Detection of rubella-specific IgG antibodies at a time when maternal antibodies have normally disappeared also suggests a congenital infection. In addition, detecting rubella virus by isolation in cell culture or by RT-PCR in respiratory secretions, oral fluid, urine, cerebrospinal fluid, or lens aspirates of infants with CRS may be possible for up to 1 year and sometimes even longer.

Treatment

No specific therapy exists, either for acute cases of rubella or for CRS cases, and emphasis must therefore be on prevention. Rubella infection during pregnancy requires a careful laboratory diagnosis, comprehensive risk assessment, and counseling. Depending on the defects, children with CRS should be referred to specialists as early as possible.

Prevention

The first rubella vaccine was licensed in 1969 in the United States and contained a live-attenuated strain obtained after serial passaging of a wild-type isolate. Since then, several other vaccine strains have been prepared, and strain RA 27/3, which was licensed in 1979, is currently the most widely used worldwide. Rubella vaccine is available in combination with measles and mumps vaccines (MMR) and as a quadrivalent vaccine containing additionally a varicella component (MMRV) (ProQuad). About 95% of all vaccinees develop an immune response; occasional failures may be due to inappropriate storage and handling of the vaccine, coexisting infections, or the presence of passively acquired antibodies. Antibodies induced by

CURRENT THERAPY

- There is no specific therapy for the treatment of acute rubella or congenital rubella syndrome.
- Rubella in pregnant women requires a careful diagnosis and counseling based on thorough risk assessment.
- Patients with congenital rubella syndrome should be referred to specialists depending on their congenital defects.
- Protection against rubella and congenital rubella syndrome relies on vaccination.

vaccination are thought to be long-lasting (> 20 years) and to provide lifelong protection in most vaccinees.

Immunity against rubella infection is usually assumed if a rubella-specific IgG titer of at least 10 IU/mL is present. The immune status of women should be checked before pregnancy, and, if necessary, vaccination should be offered. Health care workers in contact with pregnant women should also be immune.

Vaccination is contraindicated in pregnancy, although inadvertent vaccination is no indication for therapeutic abortion. Although some studies reported cases of congenital infection after vaccination during pregnancy, cases of CRS due to rubella vaccine strains do not seem to occur or must be very rare. Other contraindications include severe immunosuppression and severe allergic reactions to components of the vaccine. Only very few and rare side effects are known following rubella vaccination, but lymphadenopathy, joint symptoms, and rash are sometimes observed.

REFERENCES

Banatvala JE, Brown DW. Rubella. Lancet 2004;363(9415):1127–37.
Best JM. Rubella. Semin Fetal Neonatal Med 2007;12(3):182–92.
Best JM, Castillo-Solorzano C, Spika JS, et al. Reducing the global burden of congenital rubella syndrome: Report of the World Health Organization Steering Committee on research related to measles and rubella vaccines and vaccination, June 2004. J Infect Dis 2005;192(11):1890–7.
Cooper LZ, Alford Jr CA. Rubella. In: Remington, Klei, Wilson Bake, editors. Infectious Diseases of the Fetus and Newborn Infant. 6th ed. Philadelphia: Elsevier Saunders; 2006. p. 893–926.
da Silva e Sá GR, Camacho LA, Siqueira MM, et al. Seroepidemiological profile of pregnant women after inadvertent rubella vaccination in the state of Rio de Janeiro, Brazil, 2001–2002. Rev Panam Salud Publica 2006;19(6):371–8.
Reef SE, Redd SB, Abernathy E, et al. The epidemiological profile of rubella and congenital rubella syndrome in the United States, 1998–2004: The evidence for absence of endemic transmission. Clin Infect Dis 2006;43 (Suppl. 3):S126–S132.

Measles (Rubeola)

Method of
Claude P. Muller, MD, and Jacques Kremer, PhD

Measles is an acute systemic disease associated with a maculopapular rash, fever, and respiratory symptoms caused by a single-stranded RNA virus of the family of Paramyxoviridae and the genus *Morbillivirus*.

Epidemiology

With a basic reproduction number of 15, measles virus is the most infectious pathogen. It is transmitted via aerosol to susceptibles (e.g., in kindergarten classes or doctors' offices), and humans are the only natural host. At least 95% of a population must be immune in order to prevent the virus from circulating.

Before the introduction of vaccination, epidemics occurred at regular intervals, and virtually all children had measles during early childhood. Measles induces high levels of antibodies and lifelong protection against the disease. Although vaccine-induced immunity is probably somewhat less robust than immunity after natural infection because of lower and waning antibodies, measles morbidity and mortality have dramatically declined since the introduction of a live-attenuated vaccine in 1963.

As of 2004, endemic circulation of the virus had been interrupted in the Western Hemisphere, as well as in several countries in Europe and the Western Pacific. The success in measles control has encouraged the World Health Organization (WHO) to introduce a timetable for measles elimination in most regions of the world.

In many developing countries, where 98% of global measles deaths occur, measles continues to be a serious condition. Although the 164,000 deaths estimated in 2008 represent a 78% reduction in global measles mortality compared with 2000, measles vaccines are still underused in many developing countries.

Clinical Features

Eight to 14 days after infection, the patient develops characteristic prodromal symptoms including fever and cough, coryza, or conjunctivitis. A maculopapular rash appears 2 to 4 days later (typically on day 12 after exposure) behind the ears and the hairline, spreading from the head to the trunk and the extremities. One or 2 days before the onset of rash, Koplik's spots, the pathognomonic enanthema, appear on the buccal mucosa and fade again as the skin rash evolves.

Uneventful measles lasts about 7 to 10 days, and cough is usually the last symptom to disappear. Patients are infectious from 4 to 5 days before until 4 days after the onset of rash. The course of disease can be complicated by otitis media (3%–9%), bronchitis or bronchopneumonia (1%–6%), and gastrointestinal and neurologic involvement. Postinfectious encephalitis complicates about 1 in 1000 infections, and subacute sclerosing panencephalitis (SSPE) affects approximately 1 in 1,000,000 cases, usually 7 to 10 years after acute measles. Measles also causes immunosupression, facilitating secondary bacterial infections, which are responsible for most measles deaths, especially in developing countries.

Measles outbreaks have sometimes been observed in highly vaccinated populations. A mild, vaccine-modified form of measles, not necessarily covered by the clinical case definition, can occur in vaccinated persons with low-level immunity. In contrast, patients who contracted measles after vaccination with a formalin-inactivated measles vaccine, licensed in 1961 and withdrawn from the market in 1966, suffered from a severe illness referred to as *atypical measles*.

Diagnosis

The clinical case definition includes any person with fever (>38.3°C), maculopapular rash (≥3 d), and at least one of the symptoms of cough, coryza, or conjunctivitis. Laboratory confirmation is based on measles-specific IgM by enzyme-linked immunosorbent assay (ELISA), detected from onset of rash until weeks later. When IgM and IgG are negative early after onset of rash, repeat testing is warranted. The diagnosis can also be confirmed by an increase in measles-specific IgG between paired sera, detection of viral RNA by reverse-transcriptase polymerase chain reaction (RT-PCR), or virus isolation. Nasopharyngeal swabs, oral fluid, peripheral blood mononuclear cells (PBMCs), and the cellular fraction of urine are appropriate specimens for measles RT-PCR and virus isolation, as well as for genotyping of the virus in specialized laboratories. In most countries, confirmed or even suspected cases must be reported to the national health authorities.

CURRENT DIAGNOSIS

- Fever (>38.3°C) and maculopapular rash (≥3 d) in association with cough, conjunctivitis, or coryza or some combination of these (CDC clinical case definition)
- Pathognomonic Koplik's spots on the buccal mucosa
- Detection of measles-specific IgM or increase in measles-specific IgG in paired sera
- Detection of viral RNA by reverse transcriptase polymerase chain reaction (RT-PCR) in nasopharyngeal swabs, oral fluid, urine, peripheral blood mononuclear cells (PBMCs), (or dried blood spots) with or without virus isolation

Treatment

There is no specific treatment for acute measles. Supportive therapy includes hydration, antipyretics, bedrest, and protection from light for patients with photophobia. Secondary bacterial infections are treated with antibiotics. Vitamin A supplementation[1] has been shown to improve the clinical outcome in malnourished patients and patients with vitamin A deficiency. Ribavirin (Virazole)[1] and isoprinosin,[2] combined with interferon-α (IFN-α), have been used with limited success in experimental treatments of SSPE.

Prevention

Measles virus has only one serotype, and current live-attenuated vaccines are effective against all of the 24 known genotypes. Vaccination induces long-lasting protection against the disease even after a single dose. Transplacentally acquired maternal antibodies and immaturity of the infant immune system interfere with seroconversion rates, which, after the first dose, range between 80% and 95% depending on the age of the vaccinee. Improper handling of the vaccine can be another reason for primary vaccine failures. Therefore, two-dose vaccination programs are necessary to achieve a population immunity greater than 95%, which is necessary to interrupt virus circulation.

Measles vaccination is recommended in virtually all countries, but immunization schedules depend on the specific epidemiologic situation of each country. Many industrialized countries use measles-mumps-rubella (MMR) combined vaccines, with a first dose given at 12 to 15 months of age and a second dose at 3 to 6 years of age to catch up children with primary or secondary vaccine failure after the first dose. In many developing countries with large birth cohorts and a higher measles incidence, monovalent measles vaccines (Attenuvax) are administered at 6 to 9 months of age to offset the higher risk of early exposure to wild-type virus and the earlier loss of maternal antibodies. A second dose should be provided as a routine revaccination during early childhood or in follow-up campaigns including broader age groups. Transient fever and rash are observed in 5% to 10% of patients vaccinated with live attenuated strains. Much publicized links to autism or other chronic diseases have never been confirmed by national or international scientific panels. Because of these treatment options, contact tracing is recommended (e.g., after in-flight exposure).

---

[1]Not FDA approved for this indication.
[2]Not available in the United States.

CURRENT THERAPY

Treatment

- There is no specific therapy for treating acute measles.
- Patient care is limited to supportive therapy.
- Secondary bacterial infections are treated with antibiotics.
- Vitamin A supplementation[1] might improve the clinical outcome.

Supportive Therapy

- Hydration
- Antipyretics
- Rest
- Protection from light
- Vitamin A[1]
- Treatment for secondary bacterial infections

---

[1]Not FDA approved for this indication.

The vaccine is not recommended for children with primary or acquired severe immunodeficiency, except for children with asymptomatic HIV infection. The disease may be prevented in susceptible persons by hypergammaglobulin given within 6 days or by active immunization within 3 days after exposure. Passive immunization is also recommended in persons with some malignant diseases or deficits in cellular immunity.

REFERENCES

Bannister BA, Begg NT, Gillespie SH. Childhood Infections: Measles. Infectious Disease. Oxford: Blackwell Science; 1996. p. 256–60.

Campbell C, Levin S, Humphreys P, et al. Subacute sclerosing panencephalitis: Results of the Canadian Paediatric Surveillance Program and review of the literature. BMC Pediatr 2005;5:47.

Centers for Disease Control and Prevention (CDC) . Global measles mortality, 2000–2008. MMWR Morb Mortal Wkly Rep. 2009 Dec 4;58(47):1321–6. http://www.ncbi.nlm.nih.gov/pubmed/19959985.

Gershon AA. Measles virus. In: Mandell GL, Bennett JE, Dolin R, editors. Principles and Practice of Infectious Diseases. New York: Churchill Livingstone; 1995. p. 1519–25.

Griffin DE. Measles virus. In: Knipe DM, Howley PM, editors. Fields Virology. Philadelphia: Lippincott Williams & Wilkins; 2001. p. 1401–24.

Kremer JR, Bouche FB, Schneider F, Muller CP. Re-exposure to wild-type virus stabilizes measles-specific antibody levels in late convalescent patients. J Clin Virol. 2006;35(1):95–8. Epub 2005 Aug 30. http://www.ncbi.nlm.nih.gov/pubmed/16137922.

Tetanus

Method of
Dilip R. Karnad, MD

Tetanus is a potentially fatal illness caused by the neurotoxin produced by the spore-bearing anaerobic bacterium *Clostridium tetani*. Because the causative organism and its spores are ubiquitous, nonimmune persons in any part of the world can get tetanus unless protected by the highly effective vaccine.

Epidemiology

As a result of effective universal immunization, tetanus is rare in the developed world. An average of 31 cases is reported annually from the United States and 12 to 15 cases per year from the United Kingdom in the last few years. Although progressively declining in the developing world, more than a 1000 cases each were reported in 2008 from Bangladesh, China, India, Ghana, Philippines, and Uganda by the World Health Organization (WHO). Tetanus affects persons of all ages, but a significant number of patients in developed countries are elderly people who have not received primary immunization or adequate booster doses to maintain protective immunity. In developing countries, most patients are neonates (tetanus neonatorum), who are born to nonimmunized mothers and hence lack transplacentally acquired passive immunity. Infection of the umbilical stump due to poor hygiene results in severe tetanus that has mortality in excess of 60%.

The infection is caused by the gram-positive spore-bearing bacterium, *Clostridium tetani*, whose spores exist in the soil, animal feces, and even the human gastrointestinal tract. Spores remain dormant and viable for several months and are destroyed by autoclaving at 1 atmosphere pressure at 120°C for 15 minutes. When inoculated into human or animal tissues, they transform into motile bacilli in an anaerobic environment and produce a potent exotoxin, tetanospasmin, which produces the manifestations of tetanus. Tetanus is not transmitted from humans to humans, and patients do not require isolation.

Risk Factors

Elderly persons are at increased risk because they might not have received adequate immunization or have waning immunity. Other predisposed groups include immigrants from countries with an unreliable immunization program, immunosuppressed patients (HIV infection or those receiving immunosuppressive drugs), and intravenous drug addicts. Local factors include wounds with crushed, devitalized tissue or contaminated with dirt or rust such as open fractures, punctures, and abscesses. However, even scratches, chronic ulcers, and tattooing may cause tetanus. In developing countries, unsafe practices related to termination of pregnancy can cause maternal tetanus, and newborn babies not born in medical facilities are at risk for neonatal tetanus.

Pathophysiology

Tetanospasmin is highly toxic protein released by *C. tetani*. It is absorbed into the circulation and reaches ends of motor axons all over the body, from where it is transported proximally along the axonal cytoplasm to motor nuclei in the brainstem and spinal cord at a rate of 3 to 13 mm/hour. A fragment of the toxin then binds inhibitory interneurons that produce γ-amino butyric acid (GABA) and glycine and inactivates synaptobrevin, a protein that is essential for release of neurotransmitters from presynaptic vesicles.

Loss of normal inhibition at motor and autonomic neurons results in spontaneous discharge of nerve impulses and exaggerated responses to stimuli manifesting as tonic muscle contraction with superadded intermittent muscle spasms. Because tetanospasmin reaches motor nuclei of the shortest motor axons first, muscles innervated by motor cranial nerves are affected first, followed by trunk muscles and finally the extremities. Autonomic overactivity results in severe tachycardia, swings in blood pressure, profuse sweating, and rarely ileus. An exaggerated startle-like response to stimuli with motor and autonomic components is also typical. Generalized spasms can mimic tonic seizures.

Clinical Manifestations

The predisposing wounds, such as cuts, abrasions, burns, puncture wounds, and other skin lesions, should be looked for. Uncommon causes include needle-sticks in intravenous drug abusers, ulcerated malignant tumors, and chronic middle ear infection in children (otogenic tetanus). In up to 30% of patients no site of infection is found. The incubation period is the interval between the injury and onset of symptoms and can range from a few days to a few months (usually 3-21 days). A short incubation period (<7 days) suggests likelihood of developing severe tetanus, but a long incubation period does not necessarily indicate milder disease. The period of onset (interval between the first symptom and first muscle spasm) is a better predictor of severity: Early elective tracheal intubation and mechanical ventilation are usually required if the interval is less than 48 hours.

GENERALIZED TETANUS

Initial symptoms include inability to open the mouth (lockjaw or trismus), difficulty in chewing and swallowing, and stiffness of neck muscles. Contraction of facial muscles produces the characteristic sneering smile (risus sardonicus) (Fig. 1). In severe cases, intermittent spasms are provoked by attempts to speak or swallow. Pooled saliva due to hypersalivation and dysphagia can trigger cough and laryngeal spasms, which, if prolonged, may be fatal. Rigidity of paraspinal muscles follows, and hyperextension of the spine results in opisthotonos (Fig. 2). Proximal muscles of the extremity, too, are affected. Deep tendon reflexes are always exaggerated, and ankle clonus is common. Tonic muscle spasms can affect head and neck muscles and laryngeal muscles or may be generalized. Spasms occur spontaneously or in response to loud noise, bright lights, or

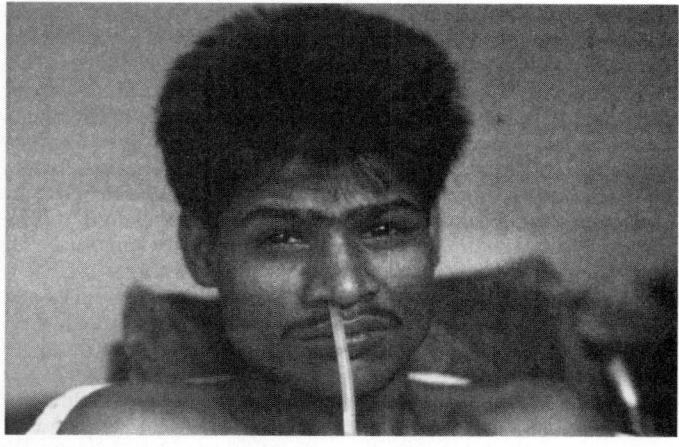

FIGURE 1. Typical facial expression with the sneering smile (risus sardonicus), wrinkled forehead, narrow palpebral fissures and crow's feet at the lateral palpebral margins due to tonic contraction of muscles of facial expression in moderate tetanus.

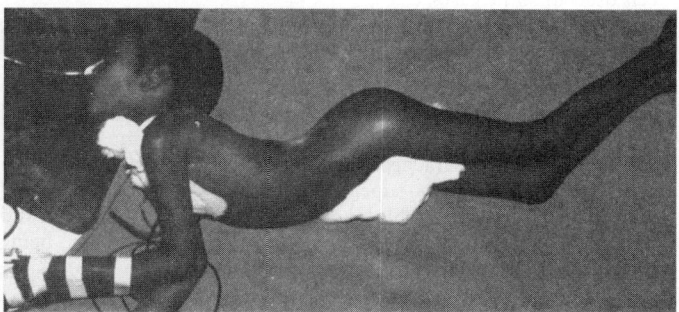

FIGURE 2. Spasm of paraspinal muscles producing the hyperextended opisthotonic posture in severe tetanus.

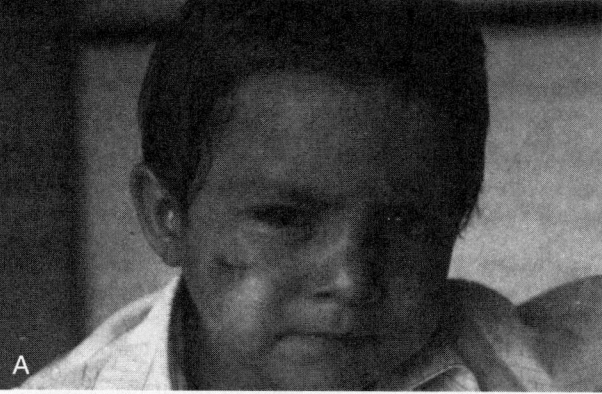

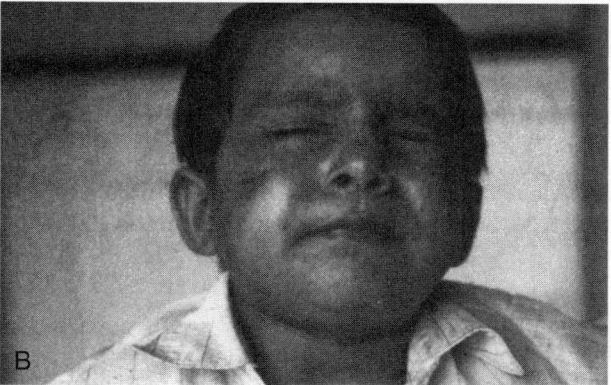

FIGURE 3. Cephalic tetanus: This 6-year-old child developed mild tetanus following a wound on his right cheek 3 weeks after it was sutured. He had cephalic tetanus characterized by partial paralysis of the right facial nerve along with overactivity of the unaffected nerve fibers. **A,** Note the overactivity of the facial muscles with a narrow palpebral and prominent nasolabial fold on the same side as the injury. **B,** On asking him to shut his eyes tight, the weakness of the orbicularis oculi and other facial muscles on the right side become manifest.

attempts to speak or swallow. Prolonged spasms can compromise breathing.

The Ablett classification is commonly used to grade severity of tetanus. Grade I (mild) tetanus is characterized by moderate trismus and general spasticity without spasms, dysphagia, or respiratory distress. Grade II (moderate) tetanus has severe trismus, intermittent short spasms, mild tachypnea, and dysphagia. Grade III (severe) tetanus is associated with severe rigidity, prolonged spasms, severe dysphagia, tachypnea, apneic spells, and tachycardia. Presence of additional violent autonomic disturbances with persistent or intermittent episodes of severe hypertension and tachycardia alternating with hypotension and bradycardia is classified as grade IV (very severe) tetanus. Cardiac arrhythmias, peripheral vasoconstriction, and sudden asystole can also occur in very severe tetanus.

Despite use of antitetanus immune globulin (Baytet) to neutralize circulating tetanus toxin, the disease can progress for up to 2 weeks as more intra-axonal toxin continues to reach the central nervous system. Manifestations persist for another 2 to 3 weeks before gradually subsiding. During this period, an apparently stable patient is at risk for developing sudden asphyxia due to severe generalized or laryngeal spasms. Patients can develop fever and hyperthermia due to excessive muscular activity.

CEPHALIC TETANUS

Following injuries on the head or face, in some patients the toxin reaches the local motor nuclei earlier and produces a combination of partial paralysis and overactivity. More severely affected motor neurons stop functioning, and the remaining fibers are overactive and cause muscle spasm (Fig. 3).

LOCALIZED TETANUS

In localized tetanus, a rare form, manifestations are restricted to muscles in the region of the wound. These patients have a good prognosis.

Diagnosis

C. tetani can be isolated from the wound in less than 30% of cases, and microbiological and other laboratory tests do not help in confirming the diagnosis. The diagnosis is entirely clinical. In a patient with a predisposing injury, presence of trismus; rigidity of neck, abdominal, and paraspinal muscles; and severe hyperreflexia are suggestive. The spatula test is a useful bedside test: A spatula (tongue depressor) is inserted into the mouth to touch the posterior pharyngeal wall. Normally, a gag reflex is activated in an attempt to expel the spatula. In tetanus, severe spasms of the masseters results in the patient biting on the spatula, making it difficult to withdraw it, a positive test. In one study, the spatula test was positive in 94% of patients with tetanus and in none without tetanus. The electromyogram shows continuous discharge of motor units in moderate tetanus and absence of the normal silent period.

Differential Diagnosis

Although the diagnosis of tetanus is easy in severe tetanus, in initial stages it may be mistaken for other conditions (Table 1). The spatula test is negative in other conditions causing trismus. Abdominal

TABLE 1 Conditions that Mimic Clinical Manifestations of Tetanus

Clinical Feature	Differential Diagnosis
Trismus	Acute tonsillar abscess, temporomandibular joint disease, extrapyramidal reaction to drugs, dental pathology
Neck stiffness	Cervical spine disease, extrapyramidal reaction to drugs like antipsychotics, antiemetics or metoclopramide (Reglan), meningitis, subarachnoid hemorrhage
Abdominal rigidity	Acute abdomen
Dysphagia	Myasthenia gravis, acute bulbar paralysis, rabies
Muscle spasms	Seizures, spasticity due to spinal cord disease, stiff man syndrome

muscles usually relax after adequate sedation. As in spasticity due to cord compression, deep reflexes are exaggerated, but the plantar response, which is extensor in spinal cord disorders, is always flexor in tetanus. Unlike seizures or other intracranial disease, the patient is always fully alert and awake in tetanus.

Treatment

In patients with life-threatening spasms, prompt adequate sedation is the first step in management. Patients must be observed in an intensive care unit (ICU) because the disease can rapidly worsen. They should be nursed in a quiet, dimly lit room to keep external stimuli to a minimum, which is difficult in modern intensive care units.

NEUTRALIZATION OF TOXIN

Although unsupported by randomized studies, human tetanus immune globulin (Baytet) (3000 to 6000 units) is administered intramuscularly to neutralize circulating toxin. This does not bind to toxin that has already entered neurons. There is insufficient evidence favoring intrathecal administration[1] of tetanus immune globulin over the usual intramuscular route. Equine antiserum[2] (10,000 units) may be administered after skin testing for hypersensitivity. Though rarely used nowadays due to risk of anaphylaxis or serum sickness, it has the advantage of being administered intravenously.

CONTROL OF CLOSTRIDIAL INFECTION

Benzylpenicillin (penicillin G) in a dose of 10 million to 12 million units per day is given intravenously for 10 days. In one study, metronidazole (Flagyl) (500 mg every 6 h for 10 days) was superior to procaine penicillin (Wycillin),[1] presumably because procaine and penicillin are GABA antagonists and can worsen manifestations of tetanus. However, a more-recent study showed that a single intramuscular injection of 1.2 million units of benzathine penicillin (Bicillin LA)[1] was as effective as benzylpenicillin or metronidazole. Débridement of the infected wound and abscess drainage should be performed after adequate control of spasms.

CONTROL OF MUSCLE SPASMS

Benzodiazepines (diazepam [Valium] or lorazepam [Ativan][1]) are the preferred drugs and act by enhancing the effect of GABA on its receptor on the postsynaptic membrane, thus potentially antagonizing the effect of tetanospasmin. However, because very little GABA is

released in tetanus, large doses (up to 1000 mg/day)[3] of diazepam may be required to achieve adequate sedation and muscle relaxation. Diazepam may be administered intravenously (10 to 30 mg in 5-mg boluses every 5 min[3]) or through a nasogastric tube (10 to 40 mg every 1 to 2 hours).[3] Barbiturates and chlorpromazine (Thorazine) are alternative agents. Other sedative hypnotic agents, such as midazolam (Versed)[1] and propofol (Diprivan),[1] have also been used with good effect.

In mild to moderate tetanus, drug doses can be titrated to achieve moderate sedation and control rigidity and spasms without causing respiratory depression. In severe cases, however, spasms might not be controlled despite large doses, increasing risk of severe CNS depression. In these patients, heavy sedation combined with neuromuscular blockade and mechanical ventilation is required. In about 10% of cases, benzodiazepines produce paradoxical excitation instead of sedation; increasing doses make the patient more wakeful, agitated, and delirious, with increased spasms. Discontinuation of diazepam and use of barbiturates and chlorpromazine can prevent paralysis and the need for mechanical ventilation. Pancuronium (Pavulon),[1] vecuronium (Norcuron),[1] and rocuronium (Zemuron)[1] are often used for neuromuscular blockade. Atracurium (Tracrium)[1] could also be used but can have unfavorable cardiovascular effects. Intravenous and intrathecal baclofen (Lioresal Intrathecal)[1] have been used in some cases.

AIRWAY MANAGEMENT

Tracheostomy or endotracheal intubation is required in moderate and severe tetanus to prevent respiratory failure due to laryngeal spasm and aspiration of oropharyngeal secretions. In most developing countries, elective tracheostomy is performed early in severe tetanus. In countries with superior intensive care facilities, heavy sedation, neuromuscular blockade, endotracheal intubation, and mechanical ventilation are preferred, with tracheostomy being reserved for those needing prolonged ventilation.

CONTROL OF AUTONOMIC DISTURBANCES

With good intensive care, mortality due to respiratory failure has drastically reduced, and autonomic dysfunction is now the major challenge in patients with severe tetanus. Various measures to control autonomic fluctuations include intravenous fluid loading, oral and parenteral β-blockers, α-blockers, centrally acting sympatholytics like clonidine (Catapres),[1] and epidural or spinal bupivacaine (Marcaine).[1] Many patients develop sudden asystole, possibly due to sudden parasympathetic discharge, catecholamine-induced myocardial damage, or sudden loss of sympathetic drive. Consequently, long-acting antiadrenergic drugs should not be used. Increasing the level of sedation itself is also effective to a significant extent.

The agent most commonly used for autonomic dysfunction is intravenous magnesium sulfate.[1] A randomized, controlled trial in Vietnamese patients showed that magnesium sulfate did not decrease mortality, length of stay in the intensive care unit, or need for mechanical ventilation but reduced the dose of sedatives and neuromuscular blocking drugs required. This study used a loading dose of 40 mg/kg over 30 min, followed by intravenous infusion of 2 g/hour in patients weighing more than 45 kg and 1.5 g/hour in patients weighing 45 kg or less. Infusion was titrated to maintain serum magnesium levels between 2 and 4 mmol/L.

OTHER MEASURES

Continuous muscle hyperactivity and spasms greatly increase caloric requirements. Most patients require nasogastric tube feeding because of trismus and dysphagia. A catabolic state similar to sepsis can develop in very severe tetanus. Consequently, patients to lose up to 15% of body weight during the illness. Good nursing care is essential to prevent pressure sores and aspiration pneumonia. Urinary catheterization is required in most patients because urinary retention is

---

[1]Not FDA approved for this indication.
[2]Not available in the United States.
[3]Exceeds dosage recommended by the manufacturer.

---

[1]Not FDA approved for this indication.
[3]Exceeds dosage recommended by the manufacturer.

common and distention of the urinary bladder can provoke spasms and autonomic overactivity. All patients should be started on a primary immunization schedule against tetanus.

Complications

Respiratory failure can occur owing to laryngeal obstruction, prolonged spasm of respiratory muscles, aspiration pneumonia, or sedative drugs. Severe spasms can result in tongue-bite, compression fractures of mid-thoracic vertebrae, rhabdomyolysis, myoglobinuria, and kidney failure. Rarely, patients develop acute respiratory distress syndrome (ARDS) either due to tetanus itself or as a result of secondary bacterial sepsis. Cardiac arrhythmias and sudden asystole are common in patients with autonomic dysfunction. Acute myocardial infarction can occur in elderly patients with underlying coronary artery disease. Deep vein thrombosis and pressure sores are preventable complications. The overall mortality ranges from 40 to 60% in countries with inadequate health care facilities. With good intensive care, mortality as low as 10% is reported in some series. Mortality is higher in neonates, elderly patients, and patients with short incubation period and period of onset.

Prevention

Adsorbed tetanus toxoid (Tt), derived from formaldehyde-treated tetanus toxin, is extremely effective in inducing active immunity. It is available as a single-antigen preparation or in combination with diphtheria toxoid as pediatric diphtheria-tetanus toxoid (DT) or adult tetanus-diphtheria (Td), and with both diphtheria toxoid and acellular pertussis vaccine as DTaP (Infanrix, Tripedia) or Tdap (Adacel, Boostrix). Pediatric vaccines (DT and DTaP) contain amounts of tetanus toxoid identical to those in adult vaccines, but three to four times as much diphtheria toxoid. The usual schedule for primary immunization in children younger than 7 years consists of four doses of DTaP or DT at age 2, 4, 6, and 15 to18 months. A booster dose is recommended at 4 to 6 years of age. In persons 7 years or older, three doses of the adult formulation (Td) are administered; the second dose is given 4 to 8 weeks after the first and the third dose after another 4 to 6 months. Further booster doses are needed every 10 years to maintain antibody titers above the protective level of 0.1 IU/mL.

After administration of Tt to patients with wounds, protective titers of antibody are achieved after at least 2 weeks, and passive immunization with 250 units of human tetanus immune globulin (Baytet) or 1500 units of equine anti-tetanus serum[2] administered intramuscularly is needed to confer protection in these initial few weeks. This is especially required in patients with tetanus-prone wounds who have not received at least three doses of tetanus toxoid in the past.

Previously unimmunized patients with clean, minor wounds that are not tetanus prone do not need any passive immunization, but they should receive active immunization. Passive immunization is not necessary in those who have received three or more doses of the toxoid. These patients should receive a dose of Tt (or Td) if more than 10 years has elapsed since the last booster dose and the wound is not tetanus prone or if more than 5 years has elapsed after the booster dose and they have a tetanus-prone wound. In countries where neonatal tetanus is common, primary immunization of women during pregnancy has been advocated as a public health program to prevent neonatal tetanus.

REFERENCES

Apte NM, Karnad DR. The spatula test: A simple bedside test to diagnose tetanus. Am J Trop Med Hyg 1995;53:386–447.
Attygalle D, Rodrigo N. New trends in the management of tetanus. Expert Rev Anti Infect Ther 2004;2:73–84.
Centers for Disease Control and Prevention. Tetanus. In: Atkinson W, Wolfe S, Hamborsky J, McIntyre L, editors. Epidemiology and Prevention of Vaccine-Preventable Diseases. 11th ed. Washington DC: Public Health Foundation; 2009. p. 273–82.
Farrar JJ, Yen LM, Cook T, et al. Tetanus. J Neurol Neurosurg Psychiatry 2000;69:292–301.
Gibson K, Uwineza JB, Kiviri W, Parlow J. Tetanus in developing countries: A case series and review. Can J Anesth 2009;56:307–15.
Rhee P, Nunley MK, Demeriades D, et al. Tetanus and trauma: A review and recommendations. J Trauma 2005;58:1082–8.
Roper MH, Vandelaer JH, Gasse FL. Maternal and neonatal tetanus. Lancet 2007;370:1947–59.
Thwaites CL, Yen LM, Loan HT, et al. Magnesium sulphate for treatment of severe tetanus: A randomized controlled trial. Lancet 2006;368:1436–43.
Trujillo MH, Castillo A, Espana J, et al. Impact of intensive care management on the prognosis of tetanus. Analysis of 641 cases. Chest 1987;92:63–5.

Whooping Cough (Pertussis)

Method of
Michael E. Pichichero, MD

Pertussis, or whooping cough, is a highly contagious acute respiratory tract infection caused by *Bordetella pertussis*. It causes prolonged cough illness, without associated fever, characterized by paroxysms of coughing, inspiratory "whoops," and post-tussive vomiting in severe cases and persistent intermittent staccato cough episodes in teenagers and adults. The incidence of pertussis is rising in the United States despite record-high vaccination coverage. In 2004, more cases occurred in adolescents and in adults than children.

Microbiology and Pathophysiology

B. pertussis is a gram-negative coccobacillus that is difficult to grow with standard media. *B. pertussis* does not invade the human host; bacteremia does not occur. The systemic effects of illness are produced by the organism's toxins, especially pertussis toxin. *B. pertussis* attaches to the nasopharynx and tracheobronchial tree with adhesins such as fimbriae, filamentous hemagglutinin, and pertactin where it produces toxins such as pertussis toxin, adenylate cyclase toxin, and tracheal cytotoxin that paralyze the respiratory cilia, resulting in inflammation of the respiratory tract.

Epidemiology

B. pertussis is a human pathogen transmitted from person to person via aerosolized droplets. Pertussis is highly contagious, similar to varicella, infecting 80% to 90% of susceptible contacts. Persons with pertussis are most contagious in the 2 weeks before cough onset and during the first 2 weeks of cough, typically a time frame before medical care is sought or clinicians consider the possibility of the diagnosis.

In 2004, approximately 20,000 cases of pertussis were reported to the Centers for Disease Control and Prevention (CDC); because substantial underreporting is a recognized problem, current estimates of true pertussis incidence per year in the United States probably is in the range of 1 to 3 million cases. A new development is the recognition that pertussis is a disease of adolescents and adults as well as children. Several studies showed that among teenagers and adults who seek care for cough illness of more than 1 week duration, approximately 20% have pertussis.

Immunity

It has been known for decades that immunity to tetanus wanes over time and boosters are needed approximately every 10 years to sustain protective antibody levels. The phenomenon of waning immunity to pertussis is a newer observation and one of the explanations of the rising incidence of pertussis in the United States. Apparently boosters of pertussis vaccines are also needed, perhaps, like tetanus, approximately every 10 years. Two new adolescent/adult pertussis vaccine formulations that are combined with tetanus and diphtheria vaccines (Boostrix, Adacel) were licensed and recommended for universal use in 2005 to address this problem.

Clinical Symptoms

Classic pertussis is a 30- to 90-day illness that presents in three stages: catarrhal, paroxysmal, and convalescent. The stages may be shorter in immunized children, adolescents, and adults. Pertussis is most severe when it occurs during the first 6 months of life.

In the catarrhal stage, nonspecific symptoms similar to the common cold predominate. The paroxysmal stage is characterized by a persistent cough, sometimes with bursts of numerous rapid coughs. A long inspiratory effort sometimes causes a high-pitched whoop. Typically, the patient is afebrile and, between coughing attacks, usually appears normal. The paroxysmal stage usually lasts 6 weeks. The cough gradually lessens over 2 to 3 weeks during the convalescent period. Milder paroxysms may recur with subsequent respiratory infections for many months following a pertussis infection. Infants may appear very ill and distressed during the paroxysmal stage and require close observation and supportive care. Older children, adolescents, and adults have a prolonged cough with paroxysms but no whoop.

Complications

Complications occur most commonly among young infants with pertussis. The most common complication is secondary bacterial pneumonia. Hypoxia or effects of pertussis toxin may contribute to neurologic complications including seizures and encephalopathy. In the United States, 90% of deaths occur in children younger than 6 months. Complications from pertussis in adolescents and adults are not uncommon (Table 1).

TABLE 1 Complications From Pertussis in Adolescents and Adults

Symptoms/Signs	Minnesota	Massachusetts Adolescents	Adults
Paroxysmal cough	100%	85%	87%
Whooping	26%	30%	35%
Post-tussive emesis	56%	45%	41%
Apnea	–	19%	37%
Cyanosis	–	6%	9%
Hospitalization	0%	1.4%	3.5%

Diagnosis

A clinical diagnosis of pertussis is typically made based on the characteristic cough, although patients are often seen several times before the correct diagnosis is considered absolute lymphocytosis (>10,000 lymphcytes/mm^3) may be seen during the late catarrhal and paroxysmal stages but is less common among adults and immunized children. Chest radiographs may show peribronchial consolidation, interstitial edema, or variable atelectasis. The presence of fever and consolidation with pertussis suggests a secondary bacterial pneumonia.

Isolation of *B. pertussis* from a culture of nasal secretions remains the gold standard for laboratory diagnosis. A nasopharyngeal specimen is obtained by inserting a small flexible Dacron or calcium alginate swab through the nose to the posterior nasopharynx (attempting to touch the adenoids) where it is held for a few seconds, perhaps inducing a cough. The specimen is transferred to *Bordetella*-specific transport media and subsequently plated on Regan-Lowe charcoal agar or Stainer-Scholte agar. Cultures are usually positive if obtained in the catarrhal or early paroxysmal stage of disease. Success in isolating *B. pertussis* diminishes if patients have received pertussis vaccine or recent antimicrobials or if specimens are obtained beyond the first 2 weeks of cough.

Polymerase chain reaction (PCR) is more sensitive among persons with mild or atypical symptoms and those who have received prior antimicrobial therapy. The CDC recommends using PCR as a presumptive assay in conjunction with culture. Direct fluorescent antibody (DFA) testing has a low sensitivity and variable specificity, requiring experienced laboratory personnel for consistent results. DFA testing should only be performed as a adjunct to culture or PCR. Serologic testing methods have recently emerged as a very valuable diagnostic tool. Single samples of 100 µL of blood can be used to measure pertussis antibodies that are compared to age-specific standards to confirm a clinical diagnosis. These methods are not widely available in hospitals or private laboratories, but state laboratories often can provide this testing.

Treatment

Infants and children with severe cough paroxysms associated with cyanosis or apnea require hospitalization and intensive care. Infants younger than 3 months should be admitted routinely for observation of their paroxysmal episodes, their need for supportive interventions, and their ability to feed appropriately. Continuous monitoring of heart rate, respiratory rate, and oxygen saturation is indicated.

All patients should receive antibiotics. Macrolides are the treatment of choice: erythromycin, clarithromycin (Biaxin),[1] azithromycin (Zithromax),[1] or telithromycin (Ketek).[1] Fluoroquinolones are also effective therapy for pertussis. Trimethoprim-sulfamethoxazole (Bactrim)[1] is an alternative choice although less effective.

---

[1]Not FDA approved for this indication.

TABLE 2 Licensed Vaccines for the Prevention of Pertussis in Infants, Children, Adolescents, and Adults

Indicated Age Group	Sanofi Pasteur Tripedia infants/children[†]	GlaxoSmithKline Infanrix* Infants/children[†]	Sanofi Pasteur Daptacel infants/children[†]	GlaxoSmithKline Boostrix adults/adolescents	Sanofi Pasteur Adacel adults/adolescents
Antigens					
PT (μg)	23.4	25	10	8	2.5
FHA (μg)	23.4	25	5	8	5
PRN (μg)	–	8	3	2.5	3
FIM 2 + 3 (μg)	–	–	5	–	5
D (Lf)	6.7	25	15	2.5	2
T (Lf)	5	10	5	5	5

*PEDIARIX also contains these DTaP components
[†]6 wk to < 7 y
Abbreviations: D = diphtheria toxoid; FHA = filamentous hemagglutinin; FIM 2 + 3 = fimbrial agglutinogen 2 and 3; PRN = pertactin; PT = pertussis toxoid; T = tetanus toxoid.

Prevention

Pertussis is a preventable disease by vaccination. Vaccines are available and recommended for universal use in infants, children, adolescents, and selected adult populations (health care workers, adults caring for infants younger than 6 months, and those with chronic respiratory conditions, e.g., chronic obstructive pulmonary disease). Table 2 lists the vaccines licensed in the United States.

REFERENCES

Farizo KM, Cochi SL, Zell ER, et al. Epidemiological features of pertussis in the United States, 1980–1989. Clin Infect Dis 1992;14(3):708–19.

Lee LH, Pichichero ME. Costs of illness due to *Bordetella pertussis* in families. Arch Fam Med 2000;9(10):989–96.

Pichichero ME, Rennels MB, Edwards KM, et al. Combined tetanus, diphtheria, and 5-component pertussis vaccine for use in adolescents and adults. JAMA 2005;293(24):3003–11.

Purdy KW, Hay JW, Botteman MF, et al. Evaluation of strategies for use of acellular pertussis vaccine in adolescents and adults: A cost-benefit analysis. Clin Infect Dis 2004;39:20–8.

Skowronski DM, De Serres G, MacDonald D, et al. The changing age and seasonal profile of pertussis in Canada. J Infect Dis 2002;185(10):1448–53 [Epub 2002 Apr 22].

Strebel P, Nordin J, Edwards K, et al. Population-based incidence of pertussis among adolescents and adults, Minnesota, 1995–1996. J Infect Dis 2001;183(9):1353–9 [Epub 2001 Mar 30].

Yih WK, Lett SM, des Vignes FN, et al. The increasing incidence of pertussis in Massachusetts adolescents and adults, 1989–1998. J Infect Dis 2000;182(5):1409–16 [Epub 2000 Oct 09].

Immunization Practices

Method of
Robert M. Jacobson, MD

Routine immunizations represent the cutting edge for consensus-driven, evidence-based practice guidelines in the care of children and adults. Perhaps no other office-based task is as universally accepted and evidenced as immunizations. We should model the rest of our practices on the success that we have enjoyed with immunizations.

That is not to say that we are providing immunizations as well as we should; the practice of immunization is difficult, complex, and evolving. Other chapters deal with the specific diseases to which we direct our vaccines, but office practitioners must consider a variety of aspects that go beyond the understanding of the individual vaccine-preventable diseases. These include the adoption of a comprehensive immunization schedule, using a number of immunization-specific practices, and the understanding of common problems associated with immunization in the office.

The Adoption of a Comprehensive Immunization Schedule

In recent years, we have benefited from efforts made at the national level to harmonize and systematically update recommended schedules for routine immunizations. The Advisory Committee on Immunization Practices (ACIP), sponsored by the Centers for Disease Control and Prevention (CDC), works closely with the American Academy of Pediatrics (AAP) and the American Academy of Family Physicians (AAFP) to publish a single set of recommendations for routine immunizations for infants, children, and adolescents up to 18 years of age (Tables 1 and 2). The Adult Immunization Schedule is similarly approved by the ACIP, the American College of Obstetricians and Gynecologists, the AAFP, and the American College of Physicians (Table 3). These are published widely in a number of journals as well as on the Internet. The harmonized schedules address the use of both individual vaccine components as well as all licensed combination vaccines. The vaccine schedules give ranges of target age ranges for immunization rather than prescribe individual ages. For example, the measles-mumps-rubella combination is to be given from 12 to 15 months of life rather than either 12 months or 15 months. Furthermore, the pediatric schedule includes catch-up schedules for children who did not receive immunizations at the recommended ages. The adult schedule includes common conditions with vaccine-specific recommendations (such as for pregnancy).

Each of the 50 states in the United States has specific immunization requirements for day care, school, and even college attendance. These vary state by state and in some states affect not only initial enrollment but also continued participation in schools. The Immunization Action Coalition collates and publishes online (www.immunize.org/laws/) an up-to-date listing of the state-specific state mandates on immunization and vaccine-preventable diseases as well as links to the individual state health departments.

(*Text continued on p. 154*)

TABLE 1 Recommended Childhood and Adolescent Immunization Schedule

Recommended Immunization Schedule for Persons Aged 0 Through 6 Years—United States • 2010

For those who fall behind or start late, see the catch-up schedule

Vaccine ▼ Age ►	Birth	1 month	2 months	4 months	6 months	12 months	15 months	18 months	19–23 months	2–3 years	4–6 years
Hepatitis B[1]	HepB	HepB			HepB						
Rotavirus[2]			RV	RV	*RV*[2]						
Diphtheria, Tetanus, Pertussis[3]			DTaP	DTaP	DTaP	*see footnote[3]*	DTaP				DTaP
Haemophilus influenzae type b[4]			Hib	Hib	*Hib*[4]	Hib					
Pneumococcal[5]			PCV	PCV	PCV	PCV				PPSV	
Inactivated Poliovirus[6]			IPV	IPV		IPV					IPV
Influenza[7]					Influenza (Yearly)						
Measles, Mumps, Rubella[8]						MMR		*see footnote[8]*			MMR
Varicella[9]						Varicella		*see footnote[9]*			Varicella
Hepatitis A[10]						HepA (2 doses)				HepA Series	
Meningococcal[11]										MCV	

Range of recommended ages for all children except certain high-risk groups

Range of recommended ages for certain high-risk groups

This schedule includes recommendations in effect as of December 15, 2009. Any dose not administered at the recommended age should be administered at a subsequent visit, when indicated and feasible. The use of a combination vaccine generally is preferred over separate injections of its equivalent component vaccines. Considerations should include provider assessment, patient preference, and the potential for adverse events. Providers should consult the relevant Advisory Committee on Immunization Practices statement for detailed recommendations: **http://www.cdc.gov/vaccines/pubs/acip-list.htm**. Clinically significant adverse events that follow immunization should be reported to the Vaccine Adverse Event Reporting System (VAERS) at **http://www.vaers.hhs.gov** or by telephone, **800-822-7967**.

1. **Hepatitis B vaccine (HepB).** (Minimum age: birth)
   At birth:
   - Administer monovalent HepB to all newborns before hospital discharge.
   - If mother is hepatitis B surface antigen (HBsAg)-positive, administer HepB and 0.5 mL of hepatitis B immune globulin (HBIG) within 12 hours of birth.
   - If mother's HBsAg status is unknown, administer HepB within 12 hours of birth. Determine mother's HBsAg status as soon as possible and, if HBsAg-positive, administer HBIG (no later than age 1 week).
   After the birth dose:
   - The HepB series should be completed with either monovalent HepB or a combination vaccine containing HepB. The second dose should be administered at age 1 or 2 months. Monovalent HepB vaccine should be used for doses administered before age 6 weeks. The final dose should be administered no earlier than age 24 weeks.
   - Infants born to HBsAg-positive mothers should be tested for HBsAg and antibody to HBsAg 1 to 2 months after completion of at least 3 doses of the HepB series, at age 9 through 18 months (generally at the next well-child visit).
   - Administration of 4 doses of HepB to infants is permissible when a combination vaccine containing HepB is administered after the birth dose. The fourth dose should be administered no earlier than age 24 weeks.
2. **Rotavirus vaccine (RV).** (Minimum age: 6 weeks)
   - Administer the first dose at age 6 through 14 weeks (maximum age: 14 weeks 6 days). Vaccination should not be initiated for infants aged 15 weeks 0 days or older.
   - The maximum age for the final dose in the series is 8 months 0 days
   - If Rotarix is administered at ages 2 and 4 months, a dose at 6 months is not indicated.
3. **Diphtheria and tetanus toxoids and acellular pertussis vaccine (DTaP).** (Minimum age: 6 weeks)
   - The fourth dose may be administered as early as age 12 months, provided at least 6 months have elapsed since the third dose.
   - Administer the final dose in the series at age 4 through 6 years.
4. *Haemophilus influenzae* **type b conjugate vaccine (Hib).** (Minimum age: 6 weeks)
   - If PRP-OMP (PedvaxHIB or Comvax [HepB-Hib]) is administered at ages 2 and 4 months, a dose at age 6 months is not indicated.
   - TriHiBit (DTaP/Hib) and Hiberix (PRP-T) should not be used for doses at ages 2, 4, or 6 months for the primary series but can be used as the final dose in children aged 12 months through 4 years.
5. **Pneumococcal vaccine.** (Minimum age: 6 weeks for pneumococcal conjugate vaccine [PCV]; 2 years for pneumococcal polysaccharide vaccine [PPSV])
   - PCV is recommended for all children aged younger than 5 years. Administer 1 dose of PCV to all healthy children aged 24 through 59 months who are not completely vaccinated for their age.
   - Administer PPSV 2 or more months after last dose of PCV to children aged 2 years or older with certain underlying medical conditions, including a cochlear implant. See *MMWR* 1997;46(No. RR-8).

6. **Inactivated poliovirus vaccine (IPV)** (Minimum age: 6 weeks)
   - The final dose in the series should be administered on or after the fourth birthday and at least 6 months following the previous dose.
   - If 4 doses are administered prior to age 4 years a fifth dose should be administered at age 4 through 6 years. See *MMWR* 2009;58(30):829–30.
7. **Influenza vaccine (seasonal).** (Minimum age: 6 months for trivalent inactivated influenza vaccine [TIV]; 2 years for live, attenuated influenza vaccine [LAIV])
   - Administer annually to children aged 6 months through 18 years.
   - For healthy children aged 2 through 6 years (i.e., those who do not have underlying medical conditions that predispose them to influenza complications), either LAIV or TIV may be used, except LAIV should not be given to children aged 2 through 4 years who have had wheezing in the past 12 months.
   - Children receiving TIV should receive 0.25 mL if aged 6 through 35 months or 0.5 mL if aged 3 years or older.
   - Administer 2 doses (separated by at least 4 weeks) to children aged younger than 9 years who are receiving influenza vaccine for the first time or who were vaccinated for the first time during the previous influenza season but only received 1 dose.
   - For recommendations for use of influenza A (H1N1) 2009 monovalent vaccine see *MMWR* 2009;58(No. RR-10).
8. **Measles, mumps, and rubella vaccine (MMR).** (Minimum age: 12 months)
   - Administer the second dose routinely at age 4 through 6 years. However, the second dose may be administered before age 4, provided at least 28 days have elapsed since the first dose.
9. **Varicella vaccine.** (Minimum age: 12 months)
   - Administer the second dose routinely at age 4 through 6 years. However, the second dose may be administered before age 4, provided at least 3 months have elapsed since the first dose.
   - For children aged 12 months through 12 years the minimum interval between doses is 3 months. However, if the second dose was administered at least 28 days after the first dose, it can be accepted as valid.
10. **Hepatitis A vaccine (HepA).** (Minimum age: 12 months)
    - Administer to all children aged 1 year (i.e., aged 12 through 23 months). Administer 2 doses at least 6 months apart.
    - Children not fully vaccinated by age 2 years can be vaccinated at subsequent visits
    - HepA also is recommended for older children who live in areas where vaccination programs target older children, who are at increased risk for infection, or for whom immunity against hepatitis A is desired.
11. **Meningococcal vaccine.** (Minimum age: 2 years for meningococcal conjugate vaccine [MCV4] and for meningococcal polysaccharide vaccine [MPSV4])
    - Administer MCV4 to children aged 2 through 10 years with persistent complement component deficiency, anatomic or functional asplenia, and certain other conditions placing tham at high risk.
    - Administer MCV4 to children previously vaccinated with MCV4 or MPSV4 after 3 years if first dose administered at age 2 through 6 years. See *MMWR* 2009; 58:1042–3.

The Recommended Immunization Schedules for Persons Aged 0 through 18 Years are approved by the Advisory Committee on Immunization Practices (**http://www.cdc.gov/vaccines/recs/acip**), the American Academy of Pediatrics (**http://www.aap.org**), and the American Academy of Family Physicians (**http://www.aafp.org**). Department of Health and Human Services • Centers for Disease Control and Prevention

Recommended Immunization Schedule for Persons Aged 7 Through 18 Years—United States • 2010
For those who fall behind or start late, see the schedule below and the catch-up schedule

Vaccine ▼ Age ►	7–10 years	11–12 years	13–18 years
Tetanus, Diphtheria, Pertussis[1]		Tdap	Tdap
Human Papillomavirus[2]	see footnote[2]	HPV (3 doses)	HPV Series
Meningococcal[3]	MCV	MCV	MCV
Influenza[4]	Influenza (Yearly)		
Pneumococcal[5]	PPSV		
Hepatitis A[6]	HepA Series		
Hepatitis B[7]	HepB Series		
Inactivated Poliovirus[8]	IPV Series		
Measles, Mumps, Rubella[9]	MMR Series		
Varicella[10]	Varicella Series		

Legend:
- Range of recommended ages for all children except certain high-risk groups
- Range of recommended ages for catch-up immunization
- Range of recommended ages for certain high-risk groups

This schedule includes recommendations in effect as of December 15, 2009. Any dose not administered at the recommended age should be administered at a subsequent visit, when indicated and feasible. The use of a combination vaccine generally is preferred over separate injections of its equivalent component vaccines. Considerations should include provider assessment, patient preference, and the potential for adverse events. Providers should consult the relevant Advisory Committee on Immunization Practices statement for detailed recommendations: **http://www.cdc.gov/vaccines/pubs/acip-list.htm**. Clinically significant adverse events that follow immunization should be reported to the Vaccine Adverse Event Reporting System (VAERS) at **http://www.vaers.hhs.gov** or by telephone, **800-822-7967**.

1. **Tetanus and diphtheria toxoids and acellular pertussis vaccine (Tdap).** (Minimum age: 10 years for Boostrix and 11 years for Adacel)
   - Administer at age 11 or 12 years for those who have completed the recommended childhood DTP/DTaP vaccination series and have not received a tetanus and diphtheria toxoid (Td) booster dose.
   - Persons aged 13 through 18 years who have not received Tdap should receive a dose.
   - A 5-year interval from the last Td dose is encouraged when Tdap is used as a booster dose; however, a shorter interval may be used if pertussis immunity is needed.
2. **Human papillomavirus vaccine (HPV).** (Minimum age: 9 years)
   - Two HPV vaccines are licensed: a quadrivalent vaccine (HPV4) for the prevention of cervical, vaginal and vulvar cancers (in females) and genital warts (in females and males), and a bivalent vaccine (HPV2) for the prevention of cervical cancers in females.
   - HPV vaccines are most effective for both males and females when given before exposure to HPV through sexual contact.
   - HPV4 or HPV2 is recommended for the prevention of cervical precancers and cancers in females.
   - HPV4 is recommended for the prevention of cervical, vaginal and vulvar precancers and cancers and genital warts in females.
   - Administer the first dose to females at age 11 or 12 years.
   - Administer the second dose 1 to 2 months after the first dose and the third dose 6 months after the first dose (at least 24 weeks after the first dose).
   - Administer the series to females at age 13 through 18 years if not previously vaccinated.
   - HPV4 may be administered in a 3-dose series to males aged 9 through 18 years to reduce their likelihood of acquiring genital warts.
3. **Meningococcal conjugate vaccine (MCV4).**
   - Administer at age 11 or 12 years, or at age 13 through 18 years if not previously vaccinated.
   - Administer to previously unvaccinated college freshmen living in a dormitory.
   - Administer MCV4 to children aged 2 through 10 years with persistent complement component deficiency, anatomic or functional asplenia, or certain other conditions placing them at high risk.
   - Administer to children previously vaccinated with MCV4 or MPSV4 who remain at increased risk after 3 years (if first dose administered at age 2 through 6 years) or after 5 years (if first dose administered at age 7 years or older). Persons whose only risk factor is living in on-campus housing are not recommended to receive an additional dose. See *MMWR* 2009;58:1042–3.

4. **Influenza vaccine (seasonal).**
   - Administer annually to children aged 6 months through 18 years.
   - For healthy nonpregnant persons aged 7 through 18 years (i.e., those who do not have underlying medical conditions that predispose them to influenza complications), either LAIV or TIV may be used.
   - Administer 2 doses (separated by at least 4 weeks) to children aged younger than 9 years who are receiving influenza vaccine for the first time or who were vaccinated for the first time during the previous influenza season but only received 1 dose.
   - For recommendations for use of influenza A (H1N1) 2009 monovalent vaccine. See *MMWR* 2009;58(No. RR-10).
5. **Pneumococcal polysaccharide vaccine (PPSV).**
   - Administer to children with certain underlying medical conditions, including a cochlear implant. A single revaccination should be administered after 5 years to children with functional or anatomic asplenia or an immunocompromising condition. See *MMWR* 1997;46(No. RR-8).
6. **Hepatitis A vaccine (HepA).**
   - Administer 2 doses at least 6 months apart.
   - HepA is recommended for children aged older than 23 months who live in areas where vaccination programs target older children, who are at increased risk for infection, or for whom immunity against hepatitis A is desired.
7. **Hepatitis B vaccine (HepB).**
   - Administer the 3-dose series to those not previously vaccinated.
   - A 2-dose series (separated by at least 4 months) of adult formulation Recombivax HB is licensed for children aged 11 through 15 years.
8. **Inactivated poliovirus vaccine (IPV).**
   - The final dose in the series should be administered on or after the fourth birthday and at least 6 months following the previous dose.
   - If both OPV and IPV were administered as part of a series, a total of 4 doses should be administered, regardless of the child's current age.
9. **Measles, mumps, and rubella vaccine (MMR).**
   - If not previously vaccinated, administer 2 doses or the second dose for those who have received only 1 dose, with at least 28 days between doses.
10. **Varicella vaccine.**
    - For persons aged 7 through 18 years without evidence of immunity (see *MMWR* 2007;56[No. RR-4]), administer 2 doses if not previously vaccinated or the second dose if only 1 dose has been administered.
    - For persons aged 7 through 12 years, the minimum interval between doses is 3 months. However, if the second dose was administered at least 28 days after the first dose, it can be accepted as valid.
    - For persons aged 13 years and older, the minimum interval between doses is 28 days.

The Recommended Immunization Schedules for Persons Aged 0 Through 18 Years are approved by the Advisory Committee on Immunization Practices (**http://www.cdc.gov/vaccines/recs/acip**), the American Academy of Pediatrics (**http://www.aap.org**), and the American Academy of Family Physicians (**http://www.aafp.org**). Department of Health and Human Services • Centers for Disease Control and Prevention

TABLE 2 Recommended Catch-Up Immunization Schedule

Catch-up Immunization Schedule for Persons Aged 4 Months Through 18 Years Who Start Late or Who Are More Than 1 Month Behind—United States • 2010

The table below provides catch-up schedules and minimum intervals between doses for children whose vaccinations have been delayed. A vaccine series does not need to be restarted, regardless of the time that has elapsed between doses. Use the section appropriate for the child's age.

PERSONS AGED 4 MONTHS THROUGH 6 YEARS

Vaccine	Minimum Age for Dose 1	Minimum Interval Between Doses			
		Dose 1 to Dose 2	Dose 2 to Dose 3	Dose 3 to Dose 4	Dose 4 to Dose 5
Hepatitis B[1]	Birth	4 weeks	8 weeks (and at least 16 weeks after first dose)		
Rotavirus[2]	6 wks	4 weeks	4 weeks[2]		
Diphtheria, Tetanus, Pertussis[3]	6 wks	4 weeks	4 weeks	6 months	6 months[3]
Haemophilus influenzae type b[4]	6 wks	4 weeks if first dose administered at younger than age 12 months / 8 weeks (as final dose) if first dose administered at age 12–14 months / No further doses needed if first dose administered at age 15 months or older	4 weeks[4] if current age is younger than 12 months / 8 weeks (as final dose)[4] if current age is 12 months or older and first dose administered at younger than age 12 months and second dose administered at younger than 15 months / No further doses needed if previous dose administered at age 15 months or older	8 weeks (as final dose) This dose only necessary for children aged 12 months through 59 months who received 3 doses before age 12 months	
Pneumococcal[5]	6 wks	4 weeks if first dose administered at younger than age 12 months / 8 weeks (as final dose for healthy children) if first dose administered at age 12 months or older or current age 24 through 59 months / No further doses needed for healthy children if first dose administered at age 24 months or older	4 weeks if current age is younger than 12 months / 8 weeks (as final dose for healthy children) if current age is 12 months or older / No further doses needed for healthy children if previous dose administered at age 24 months or older	8 weeks (as final dose) This dose only necessary for children aged 12 months through 59 months who received 3 doses before age 12 months or for high-risk children who received 3 doses at any age	
Inactivated Poliovirus[6]	6 wks	4 weeks	4 weeks	6 months	
Measles, Mumps, Rubella[7]	12 mos	4 weeks			
Varicella[8]	12 mos	3 months			
Hepatitis A[9]	12 mos	6 months			

PERSONS AGED 7 THROUGH 18 YEARS

Vaccine	Minimum Age for Dose 1	Dose 1 to Dose 2	Dose 2 to Dose 3	Dose 3 to Dose 4	
Tetanus, Diphtheria/ Tetanus, Diphtheria, Pertussis[10]	7 yrs[10]	4 weeks	4 weeks if first dose administered at younger than age 12 months / 6 months if first dose administered at age 12 months or older	6 months if first dose administered at younger than age 12 months	
Human Papillomavirus[11]	9 yrs	Routine dosing intervals are recommended[11]			
Hepatitis A[9]	12 mos	6 months			
Hepatitis B[1]	Birth	4 weeks	8 weeks (and at least 16 weeks after first dose)		
Inactivated Poliovirus[6]	6 wks	4 weeks	4 weeks	4 weeks[6]	
Measles, Mumps, Rubella[7]	12 mos	4 weeks			
Varicella[8]	12 mos	3 months if the person is younger than age 13 years / 4 weeks if the person is aged 13 years or older			

1. Hepatitis B vaccine (HepB).
- Administer the 3-dose series to those not previously vaccinated.
- A 2-dose series (separated by at least 4 months) of adult formulation Recombivax HB® is licensed for children aged 11 through 15 years.

2. Rotavirus vaccine (RV).
- The maximum age for the first dose is 14 weeks 6 days. Vaccination should not be initiated for infants aged 15 weeks 0 days or older.
- The maximum age for the final dose in the series is 8 months 0 days.
- If Rotarix was administered for the first and second doses, a third dose is not indicated.

3. Diphtheria and tetanus toxoids and acellular pertussis vaccine (DTaP).
- The fifth dose is not necessary if the fourth dose was administered at age 4 years or older.

4. Haemophilus influenzae type b conjugate vaccine (Hib).
- Hib vaccine is not generally recommended for persons aged 5 years or older. No efficacy data are available on which to base a recommendation concerning use of Hib vaccine for older children and adults. However, studies suggest good immunogenicity in persons who have sickle cell disease, leukemia, or HIV infection, or who have had a splenectomy; administering 1 dose of Hib vaccine to these persons who have not previously received Hib vaccine is not contraindicated.
- If the first 2 doses were PRP-OMP (PedvaxHIB or Comvax), and administered at age 11 months or younger, the third (and final) dose should be administered at age 12 through 15 months and at least 8 weeks after the second dose.
- If the first dose was administered at age 7 through 11 months, administer the second dose at least 4 weeks later and a final dose at age 12 through 15 months.

5. Pneumococcal vaccine.
- Administer 1 dose of pneumococcal conjugate vaccine (PCV) to all healthy children aged 24 through 59 months who have not received at least 1 dose of PCV on or after age 12 months.
- For children aged 24 through 59 months with underlying medical conditions, administer 1 dose of PCV if 3 doses were received previously or administer 2 doses of PCV at least 8 weeks apart if fewer than 3 doses were received previously.
- Administer pneumococcal polysaccharide vaccine (PPSV) to children aged 2 years or older with certain underlying medical conditions, including a cochlear implant, at least 8 weeks after the last dose of PCV. See MMWR 1997;46(No. RR-8).

6. Inactivated poliovirus vaccine (IPV).
- The final dose in the series should be administered on or after the fourth birthday and at least 6 months following the previous dose.

- A fourth dose is not necessary if the third dose was administered at age 4 years or older and at least 6 months following the previous dose.
- In the first 6 months of life, minimum age and minimum intervals are only recommended if the person is at risk for imminent exposure to circulating poliovirus (i.e., travel to a polio-endemic region or during an outbreak).

7. Measles, mumps, and rubella vaccine (MMR).
- Administer the second dose routinely at age 4 through 6 years. However, the second dose may be administered before age 4, provided at least 28 days have elapsed since the first dose.
- If not previously vaccinated, administer 2 doses with at least 28 days between doses.

8. Varicella vaccine.
- Administer the second dose routinely at age 4 through 6 years. However, the second dose may be administered before age 4, provided at least 3 months have elapsed since the first dose.
- For persons aged 12 months through 12 years, the minimum interval between doses is 3 months. However, if the second dose was administered at least 28 days after the first dose, it can be accepted as valid.
- For persons aged 13 years and older, the minimum interval between doses is 28 days.

9. Hepatitis A vaccine (HepA).
- HepA is recommended for children aged older than 23 months who live in areas where vaccination programs target older children, who are at increased risk for infection, or for whom immunity against hepatitis A is desired.

10. Tetanus and diphtheria toxoids vaccine (Td) and tetanus and diphtheria toxoids and acellular pertussis vaccine (Tdap).
- Doses of DTaP are counted as part of the Td/Tdap series
- Tdap should be substituted for a single dose of Td in the catch-up series or as a booster for children aged 10 through 18 years; use Td for other doses.

11. Human papillomavirus vaccine (HPV).
- Administer the series to females at age 13 through 18 years if not previously vaccinated.
- Use recommended routine dosing intervals for series catch-up (i.e., the second and third doses should be administered at 1 to 2 and 6 months after the first dose). The minimum interval between the first and second doses is 4 weeks. The minimum interval between the second and third doses is 12 weeks, and the third dose should be administered at least 24 weeks after the first dose.

Information about reporting reactions after immunization is available online at http://www.vaers.hhs.gov or by telephone, 800–822–7967. Suspected cases of vaccine-preventable diseases should be reported to the state or local health department. Additional information, including precautions and contraindications for immunization, is available from the National Center for Immunization and Respiratory Diseases at http://www.cdc.gov/vaccines or telephone, 800-CDC-INFO (800-232-4636).

Department of Health and Human Services • Centers for Disease Control and Prevention

TABLE 3 Recommended Adult Immunization Schedule

Recommended Adult Immunization Schedule
UNITED STATES • 2010
Note: These recommendations *must* be read with the footnotes that follow
containing number of doses, intervals between doses, and other important information.

Figure 1. Recommended adult immunization schedule, by vaccine and age group

VACCINE ▼ AGE GROUP ►	19–26 years	27–49 years	50–59 years	60–64 years	≥65 years
Tetanus, diphtheria, pertussis (Td/Tdap)[1,*]	Substitute 1-time dose of Tdap for Td booster; then boost with Td every 10 yrs				Td booster every 10 yrs
Human papillomavirus (HPV)[2,*]	3 doses (females)				
Varicella[3,*]	2 doses				
Zoster[4]				1 dose	
Measles, mumps, rubella (MMR)[5,*]	1 or 2 doses		1 dose		
Influenza[6,*]	1 dose annually				
Pneumococcal (polysaccharide)[7,8]	1 or 2 doses				1 dose
Hepatitis A[9,*]	2 doses				
Hepatitis B[10,*]	3 doses				
Meningococcal[11,*]	1 or more doses				

*Covered by the Vaccine Injury Compensation Program.

For all persons in this category who meet the age requirements and who lack evidence of immunity (e.g., lack documentation of vaccination or have no evidence of prior infection)	Recommended if some other risk factor is present (e.g., on the basis of medical, occupational, lifestyle, or other indications)	No recommendation

Report all clinically significant postvaccination reactions to the Vaccine Adverse Event Reporting System (VAERS). Reporting forms and instructions on filing a VAERS report are available at www.vaers.hhs.gov or by telephone, 800-822-7967.

Information on how to file a Vaccine Injury Compensation Program claim is available at www.hrsa.gov/vaccinecompensation or by telephone, 800-338-2382. To file a claim for vaccine injury, contact the U.S. Court of Federal Claims, 717 Madison Place, N.W., Washington, D.C. 20005; telephone, 202-357-6400.

Additional information about the vaccines in this schedule, extent of available data, and contraindications for vaccination is also available at www.cdc.gov/vaccines or from the CDC-INFO Contact Center at 800-CDC-INFO (800-232-4636) in English and Spanish, 24 hours a day, 7 days a week.

Use of trade names and commercial sources is for identification only and does not imply endorsement by the U.S. Department of Health and Human Services.

Figure 2. Vaccines that might be indicated for adults based on medical and other indications

INDICATION ► VACCINE ▼	Pregnancy	Immuno-compromising conditions (excluding human immunodeficiency virus [HIV])[3–5,13]	HIV infection[3–5,12,13] CD4+ T lymphocyte count <200 cells/μL	HIV infection[3–5,12,13] CD4+ T lymphocyte count ≥200 cells/μL	Diabetes, heart disease, chronic lung disease, chronic alcoholism	Asplenia[12] (including elective splenectomy and persistent complement component deficiencies)	Chronic liver disease	Kidney failure, end-stage renal disease, receipt of hemodialysis	Health-care personnel
Tetanus, diphtheria, pertussis (Td/Tdap)[1,*]	Td	Substitute 1-time dose of Tdap for Td booster; then boost with Td every 10 yrs							
Human papillomavirus (HPV)[2,*]		3 doses for females through age 26 yrs							
Varicella[3,*]	Contraindicated			2 doses					
Zoster[4]	Contraindicated			1 dose					
Measles, mumps, rubella (MMR)[5,*]	Contraindicated			1 or 2 doses					
Influenza[6,*]	1 dose TIV annually								1 dose TIV or LAIV annually
Pneumococcal (polysaccharide)[7,8]	1 or 2 doses								
Hepatitis A[9,*]	2 doses								
Hepatitis B[10,*]	3 doses								
Meningococcal[11,*]	1 or more doses								

*Covered by the Vaccine Injury Compensation Program.

For all persons in this category who meet the age requirements and who lack evidence of immunity (e.g., lack documentation of vaccination or have no evidence of prior infection)	Recommended if some other risk factor is present (e.g., on the basis of medical, occupational, lifestyle, or other indications)	No recommendation

These schedules indicate the recommended age groups and medical indications for which administration of currently licensed vaccines is commonly indicated for adults ages 19 years and older, as of January 1, 2010. Licensed combination vaccines may be used whenever any components of the combination are indicated and when the vaccine's other components are not contraindicated. For detailed recommendations on all vaccines, including those used primarily for travelers or that are issued during the year, consult the manufacturers' package inserts and the complete statements from the Advisory Committee on Immunization Practices (www.cdc.gov/vaccines/pubs/acip-list.htm).

The recommendations in this schedule were approved by the Centers for Disease Control and Prevention's (CDC) Advisory Committee on Immunization Practices (ACIP), the American Academy of Family Physicians (AAFP), the American College of Obstetricians and Gynecologists (ACOG), and the American College of Physicians (ACP).

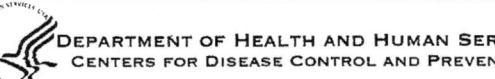

DEPARTMENT OF HEALTH AND HUMAN SERVICES
CENTERS FOR DISEASE CONTROL AND PREVENTION

Immunization Practices

153

Recommended Adult Immunization Schedule—UNITED STATES • 2010

For complete statements by the Advisory Committee on Immunization Practices (ACIP), visit www.cdc.gov/vaccines/pubs/ACIP-list.htm.

1. Tetanus, diphtheria, and acellular pertussis (Td/Tdap) vaccination

Tdap should replace a single dose of Td for adults aged 19 through 64 years who have not received a dose of Tdap previously.

Adults with uncertain or incomplete history of primary vaccination series with tetanus and diphtheria toxoid-containing vaccines should begin or complete a primary vaccination series. A primary series for adults is 3 doses of tetanus and diphtheria toxoid-containing vaccines; administer the first 2 doses at least 4 weeks apart and the third dose 6–12 months after the second. However, Tdap can substitute for any one of the doses of Td in the 3-dose primary series. The booster dose of tetanus and diphtheria toxoid-containing vaccine should be administered to adults who have completed a primary series and if the last vaccination was received 10 or more years previously. Tdap or Td vaccine may be used, as indicated.

If a woman is pregnant and received the last Td vaccination ≥10 years previously, administer Td during the second or third trimester. If the woman received the last Td vaccination < 10 years previously, administer Tdap during the immediate postpartum period. A dose of Tdap is recommended for postpartum women, close contacts of infants aged < 12 months, and all health-care personnel with direct patient contact if they have not previously received Tdap. An interval as short as 2 years from the last Td is suggested; shorter intervals can be used. Td may be deferred during pregnancy and Tdap substituted in the immediate postpartum period, or Tdap may be administered instead of Td to a pregnant woman.

Consult the ACIP statement for recommendations for giving Td as prophylaxis in wound management.

2. Human papillomavirus (HPV) vaccination

HPV vaccination is recommended at age 11 or 12 years with catch-up vaccination at ages 13 through 26 years.

Ideally, vaccine should be administered before potential exposure to HPV through sexual activity; however, females who are sexually active should still be vaccinated consistent with age-based recommendations. Sexually active females who have not been infected with any of the four HPV vaccine types (types 6, 11, 16, 18 all of which HPV4 prevents) or any of the two HPV vaccine types (types 16 and 18 both of which HPV2 prevents) receive the full benefit of the vaccination. Vaccination is less beneficial for females who have already been infected with one or more of the HPV vaccine types. HPV4 or HPV2 can be administered to persons with a history of genital warts, abnormal Papanicolaou test, or positive HPV DNA test, because these conditions are not evidence of prior infection with all vaccine HPV types.

HPV4 may be administered to males aged 9 through 26 years to reduce their likelihood of acquiring genital warts. HPV4 would be most effective when administered before exposure to HPV through sexual contact.

A complete series for either HPV4 or HPV2 consists of 3 doses. The second dose should be administered 1–2 months after the first dose; the third dose should be administered 6 months after the first dose.

Although HPV vaccination is not specifically recommended for persons with the medical indications described in Figure 2, "Vaccines that might be indicated for adults based on medical and other indications," it may be administered to these persons because the HPV vaccine is not a live-virus vaccine. However, the immune response and vaccine efficacy might be less for persons with the medical indications described in Figure 2 than in persons who do not have the medical indications described or who are immunocompetent. Health-care personnel are not at increased risk because of occupational exposure, and should be vaccinated consistent with age-based recommendations.

3. Varicella vaccination

All adults without evidence of immunity to varicella should receive 2 doses of single-antigen varicella vaccine if not previously vaccinated or the second dose if they have received only 1 dose, unless they have a medical contraindication. Special consideration should be given to those who 1) have close contact with persons at high risk for severe disease (e.g., health-care personnel and family contacts of persons with immunocompromising conditions) or 2) are at high risk for exposure or transmission (e.g., teachers; child-care employees; residents and staff members of institutional settings, including correctional institutions; college students; military personnel; adolescents and adults living in households with children; nonpregnant women of childbearing age; and international travelers).

Evidence of immunity to varicella in adults includes any of the following: 1) documentation of 2 doses of varicella vaccine at least 4 weeks apart; 2) U.S.-born before 1980 (although for health-care personnel and pregnant women, birth before 1980 should not be considered evidence of immunity); 3) history of varicella based on diagnosis or verification of varicella by a health-care provider (for a patient reporting a history of or presenting with an atypical case, a mild case, or both, health-care providers should seek either an epidemiologic link with a typical varicella case or to a laboratory-confirmed case or evidence of laboratory confirmation, if it was performed at the time of acute disease); 4) history of herpes zoster based on diagnosis or verification of herpes zoster by a health-care provider; or 5) laboratory evidence of immunity or laboratory confirmation of disease.

Pregnant women should be assessed for evidence of varicella immunity. Women who do not have evidence of immunity should receive the first dose of varicella vaccine upon completion or termination of pregnancy and before discharge from the health-care facility. The second dose should be administered 4–8 weeks after the first dose.

4. Herpes zoster vaccination

A single dose of zoster vaccine is recommended for adults aged 60 years regardless of whether they report a prior episode of herpes zoster. Persons with chronic medical conditions may be vaccinated unless their condition constitutes a contraindication.

5. Measles, mumps, rubella (MMR) vaccination

Adults born before 1957 generally are considered immune to measles and mumps.

Measles component: Adults born during or after 1957 should receive 1 or more doses of MMR vaccine unless they have 1) a medical contraindication; 2) documentation of vaccination with 1 or more doses of MMR vaccine; 3) laboratory evidence of immunity; or 4) documentation of physician-diagnosed measles.

A second dose of MMR vaccine, administered 4 weeks after the first dose, is recommended for adults who 1) have been recently exposed to measles or are in an outbreak setting; 2) have been vaccinated previously with killed measles vaccine; 3) have been vaccinated with an unknown type of measles vaccine during 1963–1967; 4) are students in postsecondary educational institutions; 5) work in a health-care facility; or 6) plan to travel internationally.

Mumps component: Adults born during or after 1957 should receive 1 dose of MMR vaccine unless they have 1) a medical contraindication; 2) documentation of vaccination with 1 or more doses of MMR vaccine; 3) laboratory evidence of immunity; or 4) documentation of physician-diagnosed mumps.

A second dose of MMR vaccine, administered 4 weeks after the first dose, is recommended for adults who 1) live in a community experiencing a mumps outbreak and are in an affected age group; 2) are students in postsecondary educational institutions; 3) work in a health-care facility; or 4) plan to travel internationally.

Rubella component: 1 dose of MMR vaccine is recommended for women who do not have documentation of rubella vaccination, or who lack laboratory evidence of immunity. For women of childbearing age, regardless of birth year, rubella immunity should be determined and women should be counseled regarding congenital rubella syndrome. Women who do not have evidence of immunity should receive MMR vaccine upon completion or termination of pregnancy and before discharge from the health-care facility.

Health-care personnel born before 1957: For unvaccinated health-care personnel born before 1957 who lack laboratory evidence of measles, mumps, and/or rubella immunity or laboratory confirmation of disease, health-care facilities should consider vaccinating personnel with 2 doses of MMR vaccine at the appropriate interval (for measles and mumps) and 1 dose of MMR vaccine (for rubella), respectively.

During outbreaks, health-care facilities should recommend that unvaccinated health-care personnel born before 1957, who lack laboratory evidence of measles, mumps, and/or rubella immunity or laboratory confirmation of disease, receive 2 doses of MMR vaccine during an outbreak of measles or mumps, and 1 dose during an outbreak of rubella.

Complete information about evidence of immunity is available at www.cdc.gov/vaccines/recs/provisional/default.htm.

6. Influenza vaccination

Vaccinate all persons aged 50 years and any younger persons who would like to decrease their risk of getting influenza. Vaccinate persons aged 19 through 49 years with any of the following indications.

Medical: Chronic disorders of the cardiovascular or pulmonary systems, including asthma; chronic metabolic diseases, including diabetes mellitus; renal or hepatic dysfunction, hemoglobinopathies, or immunocompromising conditions (including immunocompromising conditions caused by medications or HIV); cognitive, neurologic or neuromuscular disorders; and pregnancy during the influenza season. No data exist on the risk for severe or complicated influenza disease among persons with asplenia; however, influenza is a risk factor for secondary bacterial infections that can cause severe disease among persons with asplenia.

Occupational: All health-care personnel, including those employed by long-term care and assisted-living facilities, and caregivers of children aged <5 years.

Other: Residents of nursing homes and other long-term care and assisted-living facilities; persons likely to transmit influenza to persons at high risk (e.g., in-home household contacts and caregivers of children aged <5 years, persons aged ≥50 years, and persons of all ages with high-risk conditions).

Healthy, nonpregnant adults aged <50 years without high-risk medical conditions who are not contacts of severely immunocompromised persons in special-care units may receive either intranasally administered live, attenuated influenza vaccine (FluMist) or inactivated vaccine. Other persons should receive the inactivated vaccine.

7. Pneumococcal polysaccharide (PPSV) vaccination

Vaccinate all persons with the following indications.

Medical: Chronic lung disease (including asthma); chronic cardiovascular diseases; diabetes mellitus; chronic liver diseases, cirrhosis; chronic alcoholism; functional or anatomic asplenia (e.g., sickle cell disease or splenectomy [if elective splenectomy is planned, vaccinate at least 2 weeks before surgery]); immunocompromising conditions including chronic renal failure or nephrotic syndrome; and cochlear implants and cerebrospinal fluid leaks. Vaccinate as close to HIV diagnosis as possible.

Other: Residents of nursing homes or long-term care facilities and persons who smoke cigarettes. Routine use of PPSV is not recommended for American Indians/Alaska Natives or persons aged <65 years unless they have underlying medical conditions that are PPSV indications. However, public health authorities may consider recommending PPSV for American Indians/Alaska Natives and persons aged 50 through 64 years who are living in areas where the risk for invasive pneumococcal disease is increased.

8. Revaccination with PPSV

One-time revaccination after 5 years is recommended for persons with chronic renal failure or nephrotic syndrome; functional or anatomic asplenia (e.g., sickle cell disease or splenectomy); and for persons with immunocompromising conditions. For persons aged ≥65 years, one-time revaccination is recommended if they were vaccinated ≥5 years previously and were younger than aged <65 years at the time of primary vaccination.

9. Hepatitis A vaccination

Vaccinate persons with any of the following indications and any person seeking protection from hepatitis A virus (HAV) infection.

Medical: Men who have sex with men and persons who use injection drugs.

Behavioral: Persons working with HAV–infected primates or with HAV in a research laboratory setting.

Occupational: Persons with chronic liver disease and persons who receive clotting factor concentrates.

Other: Persons traveling to or working in countries that have high or intermediate endemicity of hepatitis A (a list of countries is available at wwwn.cdc.gov/travel/contentdiseases.aspx).

Unvaccinated persons who anticipate close personal contact (e.g., household contact or regular babysitting) with an international adoptee from a country of high or intermediate endemicity during the first 60 days after arrival of the adoptee in the United States should consider vaccination. The first dose of the 2-dose hepatitis A vaccine series should be administered as soon as adoption is planned, ideally ≥2 weeks before the arrival of the adoptee.

Single-antigen vaccine formulations should be administered in a 2-dose schedule at either 0 and 6–12 months (Havrix), or 0 and 6–18 months (Vaqta). If the combined hepatitis A and hepatitis B vaccine (Twinrix) is used, administer 3 doses at 0, 1, and 6 months; alternatively, a 4-dose schedule, administered on days 0, 7, and 21–30 followed by a booster dose at month 12 may be used.

10. Hepatitis B vaccination

Vaccinate persons with any of the following indications and any person seeking protection from hepatitis B virus (HBV) infection.

Behavioral: Sexually active persons who are not in a long-term, mutually monogamous relationship (e.g., persons with more than one sex partner during the previous 6 months); persons seeking evaluation or treatment for a sexually transmitted disease (STD); current or recent injection-drug users; and men who have sex with men.

Occupational: Health-care personnel and public-safety workers who are exposed to blood or other potentially infectious body fluids.

Medical: Persons with end-stage renal disease, including patients receiving hemodialysis; persons with HIV infection; and persons with chronic liver disease.

Other: Household contacts and sex partners of persons with chronic HBV infection; clients and staff members of institutions for persons with developmental disabilities; and international travelers to countries with high or intermediate prevalence of chronic HBV infection (a list of countries is available at wwwn.cdc.gov/travel/contentdiseases.aspx).

Hepatitis B vaccination is recommended for all adults in the following settings: STD treatment facilities; HIV testing and treatment facilities; facilities providing drug-abuse treatment and prevention services; health-care settings targeting services to injection-drug users or men who have sex with men; correctional facilities; end-stage renal disease programs and facilities for chronic hemodialysis patients; and institutions and nonresidential daycare facilities for persons with developmental disabilities.

Administer or complete a 3-dose series of HepB to those persons not previously vaccinated. The second dose should be administered 1 month after the first dose; the third dose should be administered at least 2 months after the second dose (and at least 4 months after the first dose). If the combined hepatitis A and hepatitis B vaccine (Twinrix) is used, administer 3 doses at 0, 1, and 6 months; alternatively, a 4-dose schedule, administered on days 0, 7, and 21–30 followed by a booster dose at month 12 may be used.

Adult patients receiving hemodialysis or with other immunocompromising conditions should receive 1 dose of 40 g/mL (Recombivax HB) administered on a 3-dose schedule or 2 doses of 20 g/mL (Engerix-B) administered simultaneously on a 4-dose schedule at 0, 1, 2 and 6 months.

11. Meningococcal vaccination

Meningococcal vaccine should be administered to persons with the following indications.

Medical: Adults with anatomic or functional asplenia, or persistent complement component deficiencies.

Other: First-year college students living in dormitories; microbiologists routinely exposed to isolates of Neisseria meningitidis; military recruits; and persons who travel to or live in countries in which meningococcal disease is hyperendemic or epidemic (e.g., the "meningitis belt" of sub-Saharan Africa during the dry season [December through June]), particularly if their contact with local populations will be prolonged. Vaccination is required by the government of Saudi Arabia for all travelers to Mecca during the annual Hajj.

Meningococcal conjugate vaccine (MCV4) is preferred for adults with any of the preceding indications who are aged ≤55 years; meningococcal polysaccharide vaccine (MPSV4) is preferred for adults aged ≥56 years. Revaccination with MCV4 after 5 years is recommended for adults previously vaccinated with MCV4 or MPSV4 who remain at increased risk for infection (e.g., adults with anatomic or functional asplenia). Persons whose only risk factor is living in on-campus housing are not recommended to receive an additional dose.

12. Selected conditions for which *Haemophilus influenzae* type b (Hib) vaccine may be used

Hib vaccine generally is not recommended for persons aged 5 years. No efficacy data are available on which to base a recommendation concerning use of Hib vaccine for older children and adults. However, studies suggest good immunogenicity in patients who have sickle cell disease, leukemia, or HIV infection or who have had a splenectomy. Administering 1 dose of Hib vaccine to these high-risk persons who have not previously received Hib vaccine is not contraindicated.

13. Immunocompromising conditions

Inactivated vaccines generally are acceptable (e.g., pneumococcal, meningococcal, influenza [inactivated influenza vaccine]) and live vaccines generally are avoided in persons with immune deficiencies or immunocompromising conditions. Information on specific conditions is available at www.cdc.gov/vaccines/pubs/acip-list.htm.

For your office practice, you are encouraged to adopt a more specific schedule. For example, where the harmonized schedule might give you some latitude with what age to give the dose for the measles-mumps-rubella vaccine, it would be more appropriate for you and your colleagues to pick either 12 or 15 months. When all practitioners sharing an office adopt a uniform practice, they reduce parental and staff confusion and misunderstanding as well as mistakes in vaccine administration and patient scheduling.

Adoption of Immunization-Specific Practices

EDUCATION OF SELF AND STAFF

Immunization practices certainly have evolved over the last century, and much of the development has accelerated since the enactment of the National Childhood Vaccine Injury Act of 1986 (PL 99-660), which established the national Vaccine Injury Compensation Program (VICP), a no-fault alternative to the tort system for resolving vaccine injury claims. This legislation protects vaccine providers and manufacturers from frivolous lawsuits directed against routine childhood immunization.

Although in the 1980s it was routine for a child in the first year of life to receive three injections and three oral doses of polio, now the typical infant by 12 months of age may receive 24 separate injections against vaccine-preventable disease. Almost each year the routine childhood vaccine schedule is altered in a substantive way. Most recently, the newest routine vaccination schedule includes annual influenza vaccinations for children and adolescents through 18 years of age. Such changes require a practitioner's continuing education and practice advancement.

A number of electronic web sites provide announcements and updates of vaccines in form delivered for health care practitioners; the CDC provides a web site (www.cdc.gov/vaccines) with information resources for both parents and health care practitioners including sections on updates. In addition, the Immunization Action Coalition, a not-for-profit group dedicated to the dissemination of scientifically correct immunization information, also has a very useful web site (www.immunize.org). The latter invites practitioners to sign up for routine mailings of updates on immunization practices. Similarly, providers can access the CDC's Morbidity and Mortality Weekly Report (MMWR) online. These provide updates and statements from ACIP. Furthermore, the AAP publishes on its web site (www.aap.org) its policy statements and recommendation online for members and nonmembers alike.

Paper-based resources are more difficult to keep up to date, but important ones include the paper-based publication *MMWR* published by the CDC and the *Red Book* published by the AAP. The *Red Book* not only does an outstanding job with vaccine-related issues but also includes a host of information for a general practitioner on pediatric and adolescent infectious diseases. The CDC publishes the "Pink Book" both in paper and online too. It is formally entitled *Epidemiology and Prevention of Vaccine Preventable Diseases*.

The CDC and the Medical University of South Carolina have sponsored the development of an electronic-based educational program called Teaching Immunization Delivery and Evaluation (TIDE). Its web site is http://www2.edserv.musc.edu/tide, and the program is endorsed by the Academic Pediatric Association and the Society of Adolescent Medicine. It is a flexible tool to teach immunization delivery, and it uses clinical scenarios that inspire problem solving. Self-contained modules are available that provide continued education credit.

ASSESSMENT OF INDIVIDUAL NEEDS

Each patient is unique, but the success of the routine immunization schedule depends on its universality. Precautions and contraindications exist, and the children and adults who most frequently attend health care providers' offices have relatively higher rates of chronic conditions than the general population. These conditions raise questions of contraindications and precautions. Therefore, individuals must be assessed for their individual needs. Even misperceptions of contraindications can lead to delays and require catch-up. Practitioners should be familiar with the routine schedules (Tables 1, 2, and 3) as well as the general precautions of contraindications associated with each vaccine.

One of the most important resources available for the busy practitioner is a chart developed by the CDC organized by condition that specifies which vaccines are contraindicated by that condition. This chart is on the CDC web site under the tab of Healthcare Professionals. It is entitled "Guide to Contraindications" (www.cdc.gov/vaccines/recs/vac-admin/contraindications.htm).

The CDC has developed survey tools that are available freely to download from its web site (www.cdc.gov/vaccines). The practitioner can use this with the individual patient to assess vaccine needs. Assessment tools are available online for both adults and children.

PATIENT EDUCATION

Patient and parent education is incredibly important in applying immunizations. After all, we are giving a form of a biologic with known rates and associations with adverse events to large numbers of persons who are often well and without a medical need or condition. We should inform the patient, and, in the case of a child or adolescent not yet at the age of majority, the parent as best we can about the immunizations, the diseases for which we are vaccinating, the nature of the benefits from the vaccines, as well as the common adverse reactions and possible severe adverse reactions that might occur. The patients and parents should learn who should receive the vaccines and who should not and what they should do in case of an adverse event. This information is complex in depth and breadth, but the National Childhood Vaccine Injury Act of 1986 that created protection for vaccine providers and manufacturers at the same time created regulations with a uniform system of vaccine information statements to be provided. The National Immunization Program publishes brief vaccine-specific statements for all of the routine vaccines given to children and adults. These Vaccine Information Statements (VISs) are published in a highly readable format (www.cdc.gov/vaccines/pubs/vis) and are required by U.S. law to be provided to the parent and recipient before each dose of certain vaccines including those on a routine childhood vaccine schedule. VISs also exist for some of the more exotic vaccines, such as the Japanese encephalitis vaccine, the smallpox vaccine, the typhoid vaccines, the yellow fever vaccine, as well as for the rabies vaccines. The Immunization Action Coalition (www.immunize.org) has partnered with the CDC and has translated the VISs for each vaccine into more than 20 different languages. More detailed information for the vaccines can be obtained from the statements from the ACIP (www.cdc.gov/vaccines/recs/acip), the Food and Drug Administration-approved package inserts, and the AAP's *Red Book*.

PREVACCINATION PREPARATION

Not only should the parent and recipient of the vaccine be provided the VIS, but efforts should be taken to minimize the discomfort of the recipient. Information plays a large role. A study done at the Mayo Clinic demonstrated that informing the child prior to the visit actually decreased the amount of distress observed at the time of the visit. Furthermore, efforts at the time of the visit including distraction or relaxation techniques can prevent or reduce distress associated with the vaccine. Office staff should learn methods of successful communication, distraction, and relaxation techniques to facilitate routine immunizations.

 CURRENT DIAGNOSIS

- At each patient contact, practitioners should review the patient's immunization record for vaccines due and overdue.

For some of the vaccines, antipyretics such as acetaminophen (e.g., Tylenol or FeverAll) or ibuprofen (e.g., Advil or Motrin) might be administered at the time of immunization and then at regular intervals specific to that drug for the following 24 hours to reduce the occurrence and the severity of fever as well as the local injection pain that might occur with immunization.

The *Red Book* Committee, the Committee on Infectious Diseases of the AAP, recommends that practitioners consider a variety of efforts to minimize the discomfort of immunization including specific injection techniques, the use of multiple vaccinators to immunize simultaneously rather than serially, as well as possibly local anesthetics and nonpharmacologic agents.

VACCINE DELIVERY

Some vaccines are given intramuscularly (IM) or subcutaneously (SC); still others, via the mouth or nose. IM vaccines should be given deep into a muscle mass. Practitioners should use the anterolateral thigh muscle injections for children younger than 18 months and then move to the deltoid muscle in children older than 18 months when the muscle mass of the deltoid is large enough. SC injections should be given in subcutaneous fat of the anterolateral thigh or triceps with a shorter needle inserted at an angle.

PREVENTION OF NEEDLE INJURY

For the safety of the patient, parent, and provider, efforts should be made to minimize the exposure to an accidental needle stick. Although the risk of accidental inoculation with the patient's blood is minimal in immunization, as with the use of sharps in any office, employees should examine the safety needles available and choose a safety needle appropriate for minimizing accidental needle sticks. The office should provide a child-proof sharps container that allows for rapid disposal of the needle with a minimal amount of effort. The container should be checked regularly for function and emptied frequently to avoid overfilling during the workday.

DOCUMENTATION AND RECORDS

All offices should adopt a standard of documentation of immunizations. The physician's or nurse's order for a vaccine should not be used in place of documentation that the vaccine was given. Documentation of the vaccine administered should include the species and the brand name given as well as the lot number. The patient record should also include the location, date, and time. Such a record would be made more useful if all the vaccine-antigens could be viewed at once with regard to series and dates. To best manage combinations currently available as well as future possibilities, the record should be organized by vaccine-antigen and not common vaccine combinations. This requires that a combination vaccine then appear in several antigen categories. Furthermore, the record would be enhanced by clarification when vaccines were not given because of precaution or contraindication as the basis. We have an ongoing problem with the adoption of chickenpox vaccine (Varivax). Those children who previously acquired chickenpox do not need the chickenpox vaccine, but we need to document the occurrence of that disease and its date to prevent overvaccination.

CURRENT THERAPY

- Providing routine immunizations requires an office to organize its educational activities, practice standards, communication methods, and documentation strategies.

RECORD SHARING AND REGISTRIES

Vaccine registries at the community level or regional level dramatically reduce the miscommunication and the need for occurrence of both overimmunization as well as empowering physicians and nurses to feel better about taking advantage of missed opportunities in vaccinating children. Most parents whose children are undervaccinated report that their children are "up to date." Records that accurately reflect the child's full vaccine record would better equip the practitioner in best managing those patients.

VACCINE STORAGE

Storage requirements are much more complex than traditionally practiced. Offices must provide proper refrigeration as well as freezers for vaccines. Certain vaccines require refrigeration, other vaccines require freezing, and some vaccines are more heat labile or cold labile than others. Proper care and maintenance of refrigerator includes the purchase of appropriate dedicated equipment, the monitoring of the temperatures, the purchase of proper containers to be used on the shelves, and adequate space to allow for prevention of errors with storage. Furthermore, the staff must be trained and scheduled to provide oversight in the case of a power or equipment failure.

ASSESSMENT OF THE OVERALL PROCESS AND ITS OUTCOMES

Assessing an individual's immunization needs, providing the vaccines, and recording them properly in the individual's record is no longer adequate for the assessment of the overall process. Each office should make efforts to assess its overall practice. Each office must monitor the rates of on-time immunizations as well as up-to-date immunization and look for opportunities to improve these metrics. The effort of collecting this information has led to improvements in rates of on-time vaccination. Immunization practices are evolving and the maintenance of quality as well as the rapid adoption and improvement of practices require regular office meetings of staff. Physicians, nurses, and receptionists must be aware of new changes. Receptionists' misunderstanding of the vaccine needs frequently leads to missed opportunities to vaccinate. Misunderstanding between physicians and other clinicians can also lead to failed attempts. Regular office meetings should occur throughout the year to evaluate the vaccine schedule, the success of vaccinating the panel of patients, and considerations for practice improvements.

STANDING ORDERS

One of the most successful approaches in the office to make real efforts to improve immunization rates above and beyond that driven by the well child care schedule is to create standing orders that permit nursing staff to provide vaccines to patients without a doctor visit. This is particularly helpful with flu season and for acute care contacts with the patient. Such standing orders need to be written in such a way that they meet state law, facilitate nurse assessment of the patient's vaccine needs, as well as rule out any precautions or contraindications for the child's immunization. Materials exist online at the Immunization Action Coalition (www.immunize.org) that can help in writing such standing orders.

RECALL REMINDERS AND TRACKING

A second method for improving office vaccination rates are recall reminders and tracking. Providers should develop proactive approaches toward their patient panels to ensure compliance with the routine childhood schedule. Offices should contact patients when vaccines are due. Additional efforts should be made for those subjects who are behind in immunizations. Finally, offices should have systems to identify those children in families for whom the flu vaccine is indicated and make efforts every autumn to contact the families proactively and schedule immunization visits. The broadening of the flu vaccine indications has made this a major issue for office practices who care for either children or adults or both.

REPORTING ADVERSE EVENTS

The same laws that created the vaccine information statements and the protection for vaccine providers from frivolous lawsuits have also created the Vaccine Adverse Events Reporting System (VAERS). This system, set up by the federal government, collects information on adverse events believed to be related to immunization. These include certain ones required by regulation as well as those temporally associated with the immunizations that strike the provider or family as potentially significant. Vaccine manufacturers and providers are in fact required to report certain adverse events occurring after immunization whether or not they were caused by the immunization.

VAERS has actually led to the discontinuation of certain office-based immunization practices including the use of the tetravalent oral rhesus rotavirus vaccine (RotaShield). It has also helped to protect vaccines from unwarranted claims of harm. Although it has its weaknesses, statistical approaches have made it a powerful tool. Participation for providers of vaccines is required. All office staff, including receptionists, must understand the legal requirements of reporting.

VACCINES FOR CHILDREN

The U.S. government set up a program entitled Vaccines for Children (VFC) that enables providers to receive free-of-charge vaccines that can be given to patients with certain conditions including those who are younger than 18 years and are Medicaid eligible, uninsured, American Indian or Alaska Native, or whose health insurance benefit plan does not include vaccinations. Some recipients may be charged a vaccine provider fee, which is a limited amount. The federal government purchases vaccine for the VFC program and then distributes it to the state's health departments, which redistributes to the qualified providers. To learn how an office can participate, the VFC program can be contacted at the CDC through its web pages.

Common Problems

Offices that provide vaccines to their patients struggle with common problems in immunization practice. These include missed or delayed vaccinations, vaccine shortages, catch-up, change-ups, decisions not to vaccinate, true and false contraindications, multiple providers, and incomplete records. One cannot make these problems disappear, but one can prepare for them, prevent them from happening in many cases, and minimize the harm when they do occur.

MISSED OR DELAYED VACCINATIONS

Although daycare and school-based requirements have resulted in very high vaccine rates by school entry, on-time immunization is tragically low. Many children do not get their vaccines when due and are left at risk. Although this occurs more frequently among those with multiple providers and those who do not have health insurance, practitioners can change their office practices to reduce the problems in delayed immunizations. First of all, do not relegate routine immunization to the well child visit. Second, be assertive in obtaining the complete vaccine records from your patient's previous providers of health care. Third, create standing order policies to facilitate your office staff providing vaccines without a physician visit.

Furthermore, the practitioner should have charts available in the office explaining how to proceed with a child who has not received vaccines on time. Practitioners cannot be expected to memorize this information. It is complex, age dependent, and vaccine specific. The information must be available for ready reference. With the American Academies of Pediatrics and Family Practitioners, the ACIP has created catch-up schedules (www.cdc.gov/vaccines/recs/schedules).

There are two catch-up schedules: one for children 4 months to 6 years of age and one for 7 to 18 years of age (Table 2).

LOCUS OF RESPONSIBILITY

Providers cannot expect their patients or their patients' parents to take responsibility for timely vaccination. Patient-held immunization records have failed to improve vaccination rates. Office practitioners must also consider that even in a specialty practice their patients may be expecting them to monitor their immunization needs along with providing them the vaccines that they need. Providers, whether of specialty or primary care, must assess their individual patients and determine who is monitoring the patients' vaccination status and needs. Specialists must never assume that the patient is cognizant of the need or that a primary care provider is actively playing that role. All too often, patients relinquish their relationships with primary care providers once they begin an ongoing relationship with a specialist.

VACCINE SHORTAGES

Ongoing shortages do occur with vaccine supplies. Most famously are the shortages with the influenza vaccine, but we also have shortages with vaccines when there have been changes in use or recommendations such as the adoption of the adolescent diphtheria/tetanus (Td) at 11 years of age and the rapid acceptance of the pneumococcal conjugate vaccine (Prevnar). Manufacturers struggle to produce adequate supplies knowing the expense of creating inadequate supplies actually leads to distrust and anger directed toward the manufacturer as well as difficulties in completing on-time immunizations. Manufacturing too much vaccine can lead to unusable stockpiles of expired vaccine product. Therefore manufacturers seek to reach a balance. Shortages are communicated best to office practices in the United States through the CDC's web site (http://www.cdc.gov/vaccines/vac-gen/shortages/), where information is provided for the basis of shortages as well as explanations for what the practitioners should do during this time. In most situations the vaccine providers are expected to record those people who have not received the vaccine on time because of the shortage and are to be called back in a timely manner when vaccine supplies are available.

CATCH-UP

Catching children up on missed or delayed vaccinations is a major problem. This activity results not just because of shortages but because of parents' delays in immunization. The third and fourth children in a family often suffer delays in immunizations because of parents' issues with the organization and scheduling of appropriate on-time well child visits. Offices that rely on the well child visit schedules as the only basis for immunization have higher rates of vaccine delays and more problems with catch-up than those who use every opportunity of every visit to assess vaccine status of the child and to vaccinate on time. To make matters worse, the current schedule when on time can call for five injections at once. Imagine the child who has accumulated significant delays and now needs to be caught up. One of the major difficulties of catch-up is the problem of information. I previously mentioned the chart that all vaccine providers should have available to facilitate catching up immunizations (see Table 2).

CHANGE-UPS

Change-ups are also difficult because the new adoption of a vaccine can lead to some confusion for those who previously received an older moiety. For example, most recipients of the meningococcal polysaccharide vaccine (Menomune) do not need the newer meningococcal conjugate vaccine (Menacta, Menveo), but those who previously received the adolescent tetanus-diphtheria (Td) vaccine may certainly benefit from the new adolescent tetanus-diphtheria-reduced-dose-acellular pertussis vaccine (Adacel, Boostrix).

DECISIONS NOT TO VACCINATE

There are many reasons why patients may fail to be vaccinated. Common reasons include misunderstandings by the practitioner or parent of contraindications regarding vaccines. These are vaccine specific and complex in language in application. Many more people fail to get vaccines because of contraindications than those who truly have them. Other common reasons include parents' failure to attend to the well-visit schedule and the practitioners' failures to use other visits as the basis for immunization.

Some parents, however, actually consider immunization and choose to refuse. They are suspicious that the vaccines do not work, are not necessary or at least no longer necessary, are not safe, weaken the immune system, provide a poorer immunity than the actual diseases they target, that children receive too many vaccines, and that some vaccine lots are contaminated. Practitioners should be familiar with these concerns and their rebuttals. Two good sources for information on these include CDC (www.cdc.gov/vaccines) and the Immunization Action Coalition (www.immunize.org). The latter organization has actually collected stories of parents who chose not to vaccinate their children and then suffered the consequences of vaccine-preventable disease.

TRUE AND FALSE CONTRAINDICATIONS

Perhaps one of the most common problems with immunization delivery in the United States with regard to the failure of the provider stems from common misconceptions regarding the presence or absence of contraindication to immunization. Although some contraindications are vaccine specific, certain principles apply. First, family histories of adverse events are never contraindications to immunization. Second, household pregnancy or breast-feeding is never a contraindication to immunization. Third, the presence of an illness or injury by itself is not a contraindication. If the illness is moderate or severe, with or without a fever, then a vaccine's administration may be contraindicated. Although local and systemic adverse reactions do occur with vaccines, these are in general not contraindications to further doses.

It would be impossible for a practitioner to memorize contraindications. The CDC (www.cdc.gov/vaccines) has prepared a user-friendly online table that is indexed by disease and condition to guide the practitioner. This table should be available for ready use throughout the day.

MULTIPLE PROVIDERS AND INCOMPLETE RECORDS

Both under- and overimmunization occur much more frequently among patients who use more than one provider. Regional registries that allow practitioners to share their vaccine records greatly reduce both missed opportunities to vaccinate as well as the inadvertent administration of unnecessary doses. Practitioners should work with their local and state health departments to develop regional vaccine registries.

For all of the problems we face, for all of the intricacies of practices we must adopt, there is perhaps no one practice more important to the health of the community than the delivery of routine immunizations. Although it is worth the effort, it requires an ongoing commitment to continuing education, practice assessment, and evidence-based improvement of the office practice.

REFERENCES

American Academy of Family Physicians. Immunization, http://www.aafp.org/online/en/home/clinical/immunizationres.html; 2010 [Accessed August 9, 2010]. This web site provides links to specific AAFP recommendations for immunizations.

American Academy of Pediatrics. AAP Policy. http://aappolicy.aappublications.org/ [Accessed August 9, 2010]. This web site provides links to the AAP policies including its online Red Book with its recommendations regarding vaccines and immunization.

American Academy of Pediatrics. Pickering LK, Baker CJ, Kimberlin DW, Long SS, eds. Red Book: 2009 Report of the Committee on Infectious Diseases. 28th ed. Elk Grove Village, IL: American Academy of Pediatrics, 2009.

Centers for Disease Control and Prevention. ACIP Recommendations, http://www.cdc.gov/vaccines/pubs/ACIP-list.htm. This page last modified on July 27, 2010 [Accessed August 9, 2010]. This web site provides links to the ACIP recommendations, which are updated annually as new data dictate. All of the documents listed on this page are current, regardless of their publication dates.

Centers for Disease Control and Prevention. 2010 Child & Adolescent Immunization Schedules, http://www.cdc.gov/vaccines/recs/schedules/child-schedule.htm. This page last modified on June 15, 2010 [Accessed August 9, 2010]. This web site provides the harmonized schedule for children and adolescents with informative footnotes and additional charts for catch-up for children between the ages of 4 months and 18 years.

Centers for Disease Control and Prevention. Adult Immunization Schedule. http://www.cdc.gov/vaccines/recs/schedules/adult-schedule.htm. This page last modified on June 15, 2010 [Accessed August 9, 2010]. This web site provides a harmonized schedule for anyone over 18 years old with informative footnotes.

Centers for Disease Control and Prevention. Vaccine Information Statements. http://www.cdc.gov/vaccines/pubs/vis/default.htm. This page last modified on August 3, 2010 [Accessed August 9, 2010]. This web page lists links to all of the federally mandated Vaccine Information Statements that vaccine providers must use when informing parents of the recommended vaccines to be given to children.

Centers for Disease Control and Prevention. Vaccine Management: Recommendations for Storage and Handling Selected Biologicals. April, 2009. http://www.cdc.gov/vaccines/pubs/vac-mgt-book.htm; 2007. This page last modified on March 16, 2010 [Accessed August 9, 2010]. This document provides vaccine-specific instructions on storage of vaccines.

Immunization Action Coalition. State Information. http://www.immunize.org/laws/. Last updated April 22, 2010 [Accessed August 9, 2010]. This web site provides specific state-by-state rules for school and day-care attendance.

Shefer A, Briss P, Rodewald L, et al. Improving immunization coverage rates: an evidence-based review of the literature. Epidemiologic Rev 1999;21(1):96–142. A systematic review of the published studies of interventions to improve vaccine uptake.

Travel Medicine

Method of
Leonard R. Krilov, MD, and Paul J. Lee, MD

More than 50 million Americans travel internationally every year, with increasing numbers choosing exotic destinations in underdeveloped countries. About half of American international travelers are immigrants going for a VFR (visiting friends and relatives) trip. The ease of global travel potentially increases exposure to health risks and conditions not typically encountered in the United States. Travel medicine has developed as an interdisciplinary specialty to keep travelers healthy by providing appropriate immunizations and by educating the traveler, identifying and assessing potential health risks based on the planned trip, discussing preventive measures and contingency planning, and providing treatment should illness occur.

The critical cornerstone of travel medicine is a pretravel consultation. Patients should schedule an appointment witir travel medicine provider well in advance of the trip: at least 2 weeks, but preferably 4 to 6 weeks. A questionnaire (Box 1), especially if completed before the consultation, allows the health care provider to quickly and completely identify intrinsic (traveler) and extrinsic (travel-related) risks. Both providers and travelers can learn about the destination(s) and associated accommodations, food, water, medical services, infectious risks, and so on from reputable, up-to-date sources such as Centers for Disease Control and Prevention (CDC) Traveler's Health website and the World Health Organization (WHO) International Travel and Health website.

BOX 1 **Sample Health Questionnaire to Prepare for International Travel**

When are you traveling, and how long will you be at each location?

Where are you traveling: country(s), region(s), town/city(s), urban vs. rural?

What kinds of accommodations exist where you will be staying? (e.g., hotel with air conditioning, outdoor camping)

What is the purpose of the trip: business, vacation, both:

How will you be traveling: airplane, ship, train, motor vehicle?

Have you traveled internationally in the past? Where did you go and when?

How old are you?

What is your current health status?

Do you have any significant medical history? (e.g., past major illnesses, surgery, chronic health problems, immune disorder, underling medical conditions)

Do you have any food or environmental allergies? To what? (e.g., eggs, latex, yeast)

What medications (prescription, nonprescription) are you currently taking, or have taken in the past 3 months?

What vaccinations have you had previously, how many doses did you receive, and when (as precisely as possible) were the doses given?

Did you have any reaction to any previous vaccinations? Which vaccines and what happened?

If you are female, are you pregnant now? Are you trying to become pregnant, or planning on becoming pregnant in the next 3 months? Are you breast-feeding?

BOX 2 **Sample Traveler's Emergency Medical Kit**

Prescription medications: Check with airlines about having needles, liquids, and medications (e.g., insulin) in carry-on bags

A list of included medications and the traveler's medical conditions; list allergies in red

Over the counter medicines and supplies

Analgesics and antipyretics for pain and fever (acetaminophen, ibuprofen)

Antihistamine (for allergic reactions)

Topical antibiotic and antifungal preparations, topical hydrocortisone

Bismuth subsalicylate (Pepto-Bismol, available as tablets, caplets, liquid), antacid

Bandages, gauze, tape, Ace wraps

Insect repellant, sunscreen, lip balm

Tweezers, scissors, thermometer

Obtain a directory of English-speaking physicians at your destination(s); the International Association for Medical Assistance to Travelers (IAMAT) (http://www.iamat.org) is a good starting point

If traveling with infants or children, schedule an appointment with the pediatrician and/or travel medicine clinic, and complete all steps above

---

Travelers should prepare an emergency medical kit, which should include the items listed in Box 2. Travelers should be aware of how to obtain medical care while traveling. A helpful starting point is the International Association for Medical Assistance to Travelers (IAMAT) website, listed in the references. Standard health insurance gives little to no coverage for medical expenses incurred outside the United States, including air evacuation, so travelers should review their policies carefully and consider purchasing additional coverage for their trip.

Prevention of Environmental Illnesses

An absolute contraindication to air travel is having a pneumothorax and/or pneumomediastinum (because of the pressurized cabin) and having an highly contagious disease such as active tuberculosis, measles, or varicella. Relative contraindications include significant cardiovascular, pulmonary, and neuropsychiatric illnesses, which could potentially become acute or unstable during the flight. Flying is relatively contraindicated for women in late pregnancy and for newborns younger than 2 weeks. The pressurized cabin can cause barotrauma in those with upper respiratory infections or with recent middle ear surgery. Jet lag, motion sickness, and deep vein thrombosis are also potential complications of travel.

Because many travelers head for warmer destinations, adequate sun protection is important because sunburn is the most common skin problem in travelers. Those preferring winter sports or a more adventurous trip may be susceptible to altitude sickness. Altitude sickness can occur in travelers who will be at 6000 feet or higher and can manifest as acute mountain sickness (AMS), high-altitude cerebral edema (HACE) or high-altitude pulmonary edema (HAPE). Symptoms typically develop 1 to 2 days after arriving at the high altitude and always include headache along with gastrointestinal upset (anorexia, nausea, vomiting), dizziness or lightheadedness, fatigue, weakness, or unusual difficulty sleeping. HAPE and HACE can become life threatening, and HAPE is the most common altitude-related cause of death.

Prevention of altitude sickness involves descent or "climbing high, sleeping low" when possible, keeping well hydrated, and avoiding alcohol, sedatives, and overexertion. Travelers should not go higher until symptoms decrease, and they should descend if symptoms worsen.

Travelers should also have a complete medical examination if not done recently, or if a trip longer than 1 month is planned, travelers should obtain a letter from the health care provider regarding their health history, medications, allergies, and immunization records. It is important that travelers and providers realize almost half of deaths in travelers are caused by cardiovascular events, even in those younger than 60 years. Extra prescriptions for any medications and a letter from the health care provider should be obtained. The letter should explain the medical indication for the prescription, because some countries have strict laws regarding narcotics. Travelers should discuss how medications will be taken while crossing time zones and know the generic names of their medications because pharmaceutical companies overseas might use different brand names.

Basic Travel Precautions and Recommendations

The second leading cause (about a quarter) of deaths in travelers is from accidental injury, primarily caused by motor vehicle and swimming accidents. Travelers on vacation might take risks they might otherwise not at home, and unfamiliarity with local traffic laws, customs, and patterns can result in injury or death. Motor vehicle accidents, including motorbikes and motorcycles, are the leading cause of death in young travelers, and travelers may be at higher risk than the indigenous population to become involved in an accident. Motor vehicle travel is significantly more dangerous in developing countries, where the majority of fatalities involve passengers, pedestrians, and cyclists, so even the nondriving traveler remains at risk. Basic water safety should be reviewed, and use of alcohol avoided when driving, swimming, or even traveling at night. Travelers should be reminded about personal safety because homicides still account for more travel-related deaths than do infectious diseases.

Travelers should be aware of altitude illness symptoms and not dismiss them or attribute them to other causes. Acute mountain sickness usually self resolves within 2 to 4 days. Acetazolamide (Diamox 125 mg twice daily beginning 1 to 2 days before ascent and continuing until descent or the 3rd day at maximum altitude) while commonly used, should be limited to those whose initial destination is at 10,000 feet or higher, who must rapidly ascend more than a 1000 feet a day, or who have a history of recurrent acute mountain sickness.

Prevention of Infectious Diseases

Most U.S. citizens who travel to developing countries are less likely to contract a serious infectious disease than the local populace because of a strong immune system, previous immunizations, good health and nutrition, and a relatively short exposure time to pathogens. However, widespread prevalence of novel pathogens being presented to a naive immune system and high infectivity rates can result in illness.

Although there are many different diseases that international travelers can contract, they can be grouped into three general categories: foodborne and waterborne diseases, vectorborne diseases, and airborne diseases. The most common infectious diseases travelers experience are travelers' diarrhea (TD) and common upper respiratory infections.

Prevention of Foodborne and Waterborne Disease

Traveler's diarrhea ("turista") affects 30% to 70%, or 40,000 to 50,000 cases daily, depending on the location and its associated risks. High-risk areas include developing countries in Central and tropical South America, Africa, the Middle East, and Asia. TD is caused by a broad spectrum of pathogens, primarily enterotoxigenic *Escherichia coli*, *Salmonella* spp., and *Shigella* spp., and it can be best defined as an acute change from a normal stool pattern, with increased frequency (three or more episodes per day) and change to an unformed consistency. Associated symptoms include nausea, vomiting, abdominal cramping and pain, bloating, urgency, fever, and malaise. Most cases resolve within 48 hours, and 90% resolve within 1 week. However, long-lasting immunity does not seem to develop after each episode, and more than one episode can occur during a single trip.

Prevention of TD and other foodborne and waterborne diseases is best achieved by adhering closely to dietary precautions. The phrase "Boil it, cook it, peel it, or forget it," summarizes this approach. Foods should be well cooked, and liquids should be bottled, carbonated, or boiled. Raw fruits, vegetables, and meat, as well as under-cooked meat, foods washed in water, and food from street vendors are high risk and should be avoided. If a fresh fruit or vegetable is chosen, it should be fully peelable by the traveler, because most of the pathogens are microscopic and do not penetrate through the peel.

CURRENT DIAGNOSIS

- Most morbidity and mortality related to international travel is caused by common preventable health concerns, not by unusual diseases.
- For every 100,000 travelers who go to an underdeveloped country for 1 month, 50,000 develop a health issue and 8000 will see a physician. However, only 300 will be admitted to a hospital, and only 1 dies.
- Traveler's diarrhea is by far the most common illness of international travelers, affecting 30% to 70% depending on the location and duration of travel. It is rarely life threatening.

Infants and children are at higher risk of becoming dehydrated from the fluid losses of TD because of their higher proportion of water per body mass and higher daily turnover of total body water. Their hydration status and fluid intake should be monitored closely. Probiotics have been studied as prophylaxis for TD, but studies have shown no clear benefit. Where possible, infants should continue being breast-fed to benefit from maternal antibodies as well as to avoid exposure to potentially contaminated fluids. Formula-fed infants should be given full-strength bottled or canned formula. Patients who are on antacids, H₂ blockers, and proton pump inhibitors are at increased risk of developing TD because these drugs decrease gastric acidity, which can allow pathogens to pass into the small and large bowel.

Antimotility agents and antibiotic prophylaxis are still not recommended by most experts and the CDC except in rare cases. Prophylactic antibiotics will be ineffective against viruses, parasites, and the increasing number of bacteria that have developed resistance to commonly used antibiotics. More seriously, they lull users into a false sense of security, causing them to forget or ignore the aforementioned food and water precautions that are critical for preventing TD. Bismuth subsalicylate (Pepto Bismol, two 262 mg tablets or 60 mL 4 times a day for up to 3 weeks) has been shown to significantly reduce TD through its antimicrobial and antisecretory effects. Patients should be aware that bismuth subsalicylate contains aspirin, with its concomitant risks, and that this compound can decrease absorption of medications like doxycycline and can turn the tongue and stool black. Because of potential adverse side effects, use longer than 3 weeks is not recommended.

Treatment is usually supportive, with oral fluid rehydration, and should not require hospitalization or prescription medications. If infection becomes severe, with signs of infectious colitis (fever, abdominal pain, hematochezia), it can be treated with a single dose of ciprofloxacin (Cipro)[1] 500 mg. If there is no response, treatment can be extended for up to 3 days. Azithromycin (Zithromax)[1] can be used for children (10 mg/kg/day) or for areas with fluoroquinolone-resistant *Campylobacter* (500 mg daily for adults). Rifaximin (Xifaxan) 200 mg three times a day for 3 days is an alternative for travelers older than 12 years who have *E. coli* TD, but it is not effective against *Campylobacter* and *Shigella*.

Other infections that can be transmitted through water and food contaminated with fecal pathogens include viruses such as hepatitis A and B and rotavirus (15%-20% of TD) and parasites such as *Giardia intestinalis* and *Cryptosporidia* spp. (~10%). Travelers should also remember that infections such as schistosomiasis and leptospirosis can occur through exposure to water in lakes and rivers, so wading and swimming in freshwater bodies should be avoided.

Prevention of Vectorborne Diseases

Vector-borne diseases are a second category of infections that travelers are at risk of contracting. These are viruses and parasites that are transmitted by mosquito and other insect bites, such as dengue fever, chikungunya fever, yellow fever, Japanese encephalitis, and West Nile virus, and can result in incapacitating symptoms, severe sequelae, or even death. Personal protective measures, such as use of insect repellant, are the primary means of preventing these diseases, because there is typically no treatment, other than supportive care, once the traveler becomes ill.

Permethrin (e.g., Sawyer Permethrin Clothing Spray) is an insecticide that can be applied to clothing and bedding, giving protection for about 2 weeks, even when these items are laundered. It can be sprayed in bedrooms and indoor areas, but travelers should not enter the room for 30 minutes after spraying. Permethrin should not be directly applied to skin.

---

[1]Not FDA approved for this indication.

- Treatment for traveler's should be supportive. Prophylactic antibiotics are not recommended except in rare cases. Bismuth subsalicylate (Pepto Bismol, 262 mg tablets or 60 mL 4 times/day for up to 3 weeks) has been shown to significantly reduce traveler's diarrhea through its antimicrobial and antisecretory effects. Rifaximin (Xifaxan) 200 mg three times daily for 3 days is an alternative for *E. coli* traveler's diarrhea.
- Infectious colitis (fever, abdominal pain, hematochezia) can be treated with a single dose of ciprofloxacin (Cipro)[1] 500 mg or azithromycin (Zithromax)[1] 10 mg/kg daily for children, 500 mg daily for adults.
- Malaria prophylaxis depends on age, travel location and duration.
- Vaccinations should be up to date and include required and recommended ones.

---

[1]Not FDA approved for this indication.

Diethyltoluamide (DEET) is the best-studied insect repellant available, with an excellent safety profile for more than 40 years. In high concentrations (35%) it can provide 6 to 8 hours of protection against mosquito bites. High concentrations of other repellants like picaridin (KBR 3023) (e.g., Skin So Soft Bug Guard) and oil of lemon eucalyptus seem to be equivalent to low concentrations of DEET, and they must be applied more frequently to maintain protection. DEET should not be applied to cuts or irritated skin. Use of DEET concentrations up to 30% is safe for children and infants older than 2 months, but areas around the eyes, mouth, and hands of young children should be avoided to prevent unintentional ingestion and absorption.

Other personal protective measures include covering exposed skin with light-colored tightly woven fabrics and avoiding perfumes and colognes. Sleeping with insect netting is only necessary if sleeping outdoors or if there are no doors or windows indoors. Avoiding outdoor activities from dusk to dawn can help prevent many mosquito bites, but species like *Aedes aegypti*, which transmit dengue and yellow fever, are daytime feeders and found in urban and rural areas.

Malaria is the first vector-borne illness travelers think about, which is not surprising, given that up to a half billion people contract malaria annually, and 1 million die. Every year, 125 million people travel to more than 100 countries where malaria remains endemic, and malaria is diagnosed in more than 10,000 after their return home. Malaria prevention is summarized by ABCD: **A**wareness of the level of risk, timing, and symptoms of malaria; **B**ite prevention through personal protective measures; **C**ompliance with Chemoprophylaxis; and **D**octor evaluation for prompt **D**iagnosis and treatment. Malaria is caused one of five *Plasmodium* protozoa, and chemoprophylactic medicines are available. The medications, indications, dosing, and contraindications and adverse reactions are listed in Table 1. The choice of chemoprophylactic drug should be based on the travel destination, tolerability to the patient, adverse effects, and cost. Because personal protective measures and chemoprophylaxis cannot guarantee 100% protection against malaria, travelers should be advised that they could still contract malaria and should seek medical attention immediately if fever occurs 1 week or more after exposure. Malaria can develop up to a year after travel. Malaria and antimalarial medications can cause adverse effects in pregnant women and the fetus, so travel should be discouraged until after delivery or at least the second trimester.

Prevention of Airborne Disease and Sexually Transmitted Diseases

Although diseases such as measles and varicella are extremely contagious, spreading rapidly through the air, appropriate vaccinations (see later) remain the only effective means of protecting travelers against these highly transmissible and serious infections. Travelers who develop a respiratory infection usually acquire it the same way, through direct, inadvertent contact with infectious droplets rather than inhalation. Tuberculosis, which is one of the most common global infections, is not common in travelers, because infection usually requires close repeated exposure to an infectious patient for prolonged periods. Studies have shown there is very little risk of transmission on modern aircraft because the cabin air is completely changed every 2 to 3 minutes, with any recirculated air passing through HEPA (high-efficiency particulate air) filters, trapping pathogens.

Sexually transmitted diseases (STDs) remain one of the most common global infections with more than 1/3 billion infections annually. In one survey, nearly a quarter of international travelers had sexual contact with someone encountered during their trip, ranging from a casual relationship to using a commercial sex worker. Some tourists travel to a destination solely for commercial sex services (sex tourism). Diseases that can be transmitted sexually include hepatitis A, B, and C and the usual sexually transmitted diseases: HIV, syphilis, gonorrhea, and chlamydia. Because abstinence-only recommendations can be ineffective or are ignored by sexually active travelers, safe-sex practices, including correct and consistent use of male latex condoms, to prevent pregnancy and spread of STDs, should be reinforced.

Prevention of Infection: Travel Vaccines

All travelers should be up to date on all recommended vaccines as outlined by the Centers for Disease Control and Prevention (CDC). See http://www.cdc.gov/vaccines/recs/schedules/adult-schedule.htm and http://www.cdc.gov/vaccines/recs/schedules/child-schedule.htm for the current adult and child/adolescent immunization schedule, respectively. For those not previously vaccinated, hepatitis A, hepatitis B, typhoid, influenza, polio, and Japanese encephalitis virus vaccines may be recommended, depending on the destination and duration of travel. Yellow fever vaccine (YFV, YF-VAX) is the only mandatory travel vaccine, and only for travel at any time of year to rural and urban areas in certain sub-Saharan Africa and Central and South America countries. The most up-to-date YFV travel requirements are available on the CDC website at http://wwwnc.cdc.gov/travel/yellowbook/2010/chapter-2/yellow-fever-vaccine-requirements-and-recommendations.aspx.

Rare complications such as viscerotropic and neurotropic disease have been reported, with a three to four times higher risk in patients with thymic dysfunction or other immunodeficiency, and in travelers older than 60 years. YFV should not be given to children younger than 4 months, and it should only be given to children younger than 9 months in consultation with a travel medicine expert or the CDC Vector-Borne Diseases Branch (970-221-6400). Children too young for immunization and immunosuppressed patients should be given a medical waiver letter.

YFV must be given by a certified provider. A relatively comprehensive listing of sites providing YFV and the International Certificate of Vaccination or Prophylaxis (ICVP), which is the only accepted documentation of YF vaccination, is available from the CDC website at http://wwwnc.cdc.gov/travel/yellow-fever-vaccination-clinics-search.aspx. Travelers who arrive to or from an endemic country without a complete or valid ICVP may be denied entry or quarantined, unless the traveler has a valid medical waiver letter or agrees to onsite vaccination. Meningococcal vaccine (Menactra, Menomune) is required for travel to Saudi Arabia during the Hajj. Table 2 lists information about vaccine licensed in the United States specifically for travelers, including age restrictions, dosing, and adverse effects.

TABLE 1 Malaria Prophylactic Agents

Drug (Trade)	Prophylactic Indication	Formulations	Dosage (Patient's Weight)	Schedule	Contraindications and Adverse Reactions
Mefloquine (Lariam and generic)	Areas with chloroquine-resistant *Plasmodium falciparum* (most malaria-endemic areas except Caribbean and Middle East)	250 mg tab	≤9 kg: 5 mg/kg PO q wk; 10-19 kg: ¼ tab PO q wk; 20-30 kg: ½ tab PO qk; 31-45 kg: ¾ tab PO q wk; ≥46 kg: 1 tab PO q wk	Begin 1-2 wk before travel to malaria area, same day each week during stay, and for 4 wk after leaving the malaria area	Contraindicated in patients with active depression, recent history of depression, generalized anxiety disorder, psychosis, schizophrenia, other major psychiatric disorders, or seizures. Contraindicated if allergic to mefloquine or other quinine-containing compounds. Use with caution in patients with psychiatric disturbances or a previous history of depression. Not recommended for patients with cardiac conduction abnormalities. Psychiatric disturbances (sensory and motor neuropathies: paresthesias, tremor, ataxia, agitations, restlessness, mood changes, panic attacks, forgetfulness, confusion, hallucinations, aggression, paranoia, and encephalopathy) and seizures are *rare* with prophylactic use. Other reported side effects with prophylactic use: GI disturbance, headache, insomnia, abnormal dreams, visual disturbances, depression, anxiety, and dizziness
Atovaquone/proguanil (Malarone)	Areas with chloroquine-resistant *P. falciparum* (most malaria-endemic areas except Caribbean and Middle East)	250/100 mg tab; 62.5/25 mg ped tab	5-8 kg[1]: 2 ped tabs PO qd; 9-10 kg[1]: 3 ped tab PO qd; 11-20 kg: 1 adult tab PO qd; 21-30 kg: 2 adult tabs PO qd; >31-40 kg: 3 adult tabs PO qd; >40 kg: 4 adult tabs PO qd	Begin 1-2 days before travel to malaria area, same time each day during stay, and for 7 d after leaving the malaria area	Contraindicated for patients with severe renal impairment (creatinine clearance <30 mL/min). Not recommended for children <5 kg, pregnant women, or women breast-feeding infants <5 kg
Doxycycline (Adoxa, Doryx, Vibramycin, and generic)	Areas with chloroquine resistant or mefloquine resistant *P. falciparum* (most or some malaria-endemic areas)	50, 100 mg cap; 75, 100 mg delayed-release caps; 75, 100 mg tab; 25 mg/5 mL susp; 50 mg/5 mL syrup	2 mg/kg PO qd up to adult max of 100 mg PO qd	Begin 1-2 d before travel to malaria area, same time each day during stay, and for 4 wk after leaving the malaria area	Contraindicated if ≤8 yr old or if pregnant, secondary to potential effects on bone, enamel, and the fetus. Delay oral typhoid vaccine >24 h after taking doxycycline, because of its antibacterial effect on the live attenuated vaccine. Adverse reactions: photosensitivity reaction, increased frequency of *Candida vaginitis*, GI side effects (nausea, vomiting, esophagitis)
Chloroquine phosphate (Aralen and generic)	Areas with chloroquine sensitive *P. falciparum* (only Caribbean, Middle East)	500 mg tab (contains 300 mg chloroquine base)	8.3 mg/kg (5 mg/kg base) PO q wk	Begin 1-2 wk before travel to malaria area, same day each wk during stay, and for 4 wk after leaving the malaria area	Adverse reactions: GI disturbance, headache, dizziness, blurred vision, pruritus. Can exacerbate psoriasis. If unable to tolerate chloroquine, drugs for chloroquine-resistant *P. falciparum* may be used
Hydroxychloroquine sulfate (Plaquenil)	Areas with chloroquine sensitive *P. falciparum* (only Caribbean, Middle East)	200 mg tab (contains 155 mg of hydroxychloroquine base)	6.5 mg kg (5 mg/kg base) PO q wk	Begin 1-2 wk before travel to malaria area, same day each week during stay, and for 4 wk after leaving the malaria area	Less evidence for hydroxychloroquine being effective as an antimalarial drug. Same adverse reactions and comments as chloroquine

[1]Not FDA approved for this indication.

cap = capsule; GI = gastrointestinal; max = maximum; ped = pediatric; susp = suspension; tab = tablet

TABLE 2 U.S. Licensed Travel-Specific Vaccines

Infection and Pathogen	Vaccine (Manufacturer)	Type	Minimum Age	Administration	Booster (as Needed)	Adverse Effects
Yellow fever (yellow fever virus)	YF-VAX (Sanofi Pasteur)	Live attenuated YF 17D-204 strain	4[1]-9 mo	0.5 mL SC × 1, at least 10 d before entry to YF region	10 y (see text)	25% local reaction at vaccine site, fever, myalgias Rare hypersensitivity, neurotropic, and viscerotropic complications
Typhoid fever (*Salmonella typhi*)	ViCPS (Typhim Vi) (Sanofi pasteur)	*S. typhi* Ty2 purified capsule polysaccharide	2 y	0.5 mL IM × 1, at least 2 wk before travel	2 y	<7%, fever headache, local pain at vaccine site
	Ty21a (Vivotif Berna) (Berna Biotech Ltd.)	Live attenuated *S. typhi* Ty21a strain	6 y	1 cap PO qod × 4, complete 1 wk before travel	5 y	<5%, fever, headache, abdominal discomfort, nausea, vomiting, rash
Japanese encephalitis (Japanese encephalitis virus)	JE-VAX (Sanofi Pasteur) (discontinued 2006; existing supplies will be used until gone)	Inactivated Japanese encephalitis virus	12 mo	1.0 mL SC given days 0, 7, 30 for age >3 y, 0.5 mL dose for age 1-3 y Complete 10 d before travel Abbreviated schedule option (given days 0, 7, 14) for imminent travel	1 SC dose, 2 y	20% local reaction at vaccine site, 10% fever, chills, headache, myalgias, abdominal pain, nausea, vomiting, rash, dizziness 0.5% immediate and delayed hypersensitivity reactions 1/50,000 seizures
	IXIARO (Novartis)	Inactivated Japanese encephalitis virus	18 y	0.5 mL IM × 2, given 28 d apart, complete 1 week before travel	No data at present	≥10% headache, myalgias, pain/tenderness at vaccine site

[1]Not FDA approved for this indication.

REFERENCES

Centers for Disease Control and Prevention. Travellers Health. Available at: http://wwwnc.cdc.gov/travel; [accessed 19.06.10].

Centers for Disease Control and Prevention. Travelers Health–Yellow Book. Health Information for International Travel 2010. Available at: http://wwwnc.cdc.gov/travel/content/yellowbook/home-2010.aspx; [accessed 19.06.10].

Department of State. Travel Information: Travel Warnings; Travel Alerts. http://travel.state.gov; [accessed 19.06.10].

Dietz TE. High Altitude Medicine Guide. Available at http://www.high-altitude-medicine.com; [accessed 19.06.10].

International Association for Medical Assistance to Travelers (IAMAT). Home page. Available at http://www.iamat.org; [accessed 19.06.10].

International Society of Travel Medicine. Home page. Available at http://www.istm.org; [accessed 19.06.10].

World Health Organization. International Travel and Health. Available at http://www.who.int/ith/en/index.html; [accessed 19.06.10].

Toxoplasmosis

Method of

Robert C. Goldstein, MD, and
Benjamin J. Luft, MD

Toxoplasmosis is the disease caused by the ubiquitous, obligate intracellular protozoan *Toxoplasma gondii*. Samuel T. Darling first described toxoplasmosis in the adult human in 1908. Nicolle and Manceaux named the organism in 1909. In the immunocompetent host, toxoplasmosis is usually self-limited and may cause asymptomatic lymphadenopathy or, rarely, acute chorioretinitis. If *Toxoplasma* is acquired within 3 months of conception or during the first or second trimester of pregnancy, potentially grave congenital infection may result. If it is acquired during the third trimester, transmission occurs with greater frequency but the infant tends to be asymptomatic at birth, only to have manifestations of the disease later in life. The immunocompromised host is especially at risk for newly acquired infection (e.g., through solid organ transplantation) and for reactivation of latent organisms (e.g., AIDS, bone marrow transplantation, severe immunosuppression secondary to chemotherapy) with infection involving all tissues but manifesting most prominently within the central nervous system.

Pathophysiology and Epidemiology

The protozoan exists in three main forms: sporozoite, tachyzoite, and bradyzoite. Although *T. gondii* may infect humans, other mammals, and birds (intermediate hosts), its definitive host is the cat family, Felidae. It is only in the cat that the organism can undergo its entire life cycle. Asexual and then sexual replication of the organism occurs in the epithelium of cat small intestine, producing environmentally hardy oocysts. Oocysts are shed in cat feces for 3 to 14 days after the primary infection. In favorable environmental conditions (i.e., soil of high humidity and moderate temperatures [4°C-37°C]), sporulation occurs in 2 to 5 days, creating a sporozoite within the oocyst. This infectious state may remain for up to a year, or possibly longer.

The sporozoites are ingested by hosts in contaminated meat, water, and soil to initiate the tachyzoite form. In the intermediate host, this is produced by an extraintestinal asexual cycle. In this rapidly multiplying stage, tachyzoites disseminate in the bloodstream and infect many tissues, including central nervous system, heart muscle, skeletal muscle, liver, spleen, and placenta. Clinical manifestations are caused by the inflammatory response to tachyzoite infestation. This includes helper T-cell (Th1) production and production of cytokines interleukin-12, tumor necrosis factor-α, and interferon-γ. In turn, this response leads to the formation of bradyzoites within cysts, which can persist in tissues, causing latent infection.

Transmission to humans occurs by oral ingestion of infected undercooked meat containing cysts, eating of undercooked food that has come into contact with infected meat, ingestion of contaminated water or soil containing sporulated oocysts, organ transplantation from an infected donor, blood transfusion, laboratory accidents, and vertically by congenital transmission.

Seroprevalence of infection increases with age; is roughly equal in males and females; is lower in regions that are cold, hot, arid, or of high elevation (possibly because *T. gondii* oocysts do not survive well in the soil of these areas); and varies according to health and hygiene practices. Prevalence is higher in Western Europe (e.g., 65%-85% in France) than in the United States (20%-40%). This may be related to higher consumption of raw or undercooked meat in Europe. This also holds true for tropical parts of South America and sub-Saharan Africa, where the humid climate favors survival of oocysts and there is an abundance of cats.

CURRENT DIAGNOSIS

- *Toxoplasma*-specific immunoglobulin G can be used as an initial screening test for all patients.
- *Toxoplasma*-specific immunoglobulin M can be used to help differentiate between acutely acquired and latent infection, but results may not be fully reliable, and samples should be sent to a *Toxoplasma* reference laboratory for confirmation.
- Treat all immunocompromised patients who have multiple ring-enhancing brain lesions for presumed toxoplasmosis and monitor for response.

Each year in the United States, there are between 400 and 4000 congenital infections, 1.26 million cases of ocular infection, and many cases of systemic or neurologic infection among immunocompromised persons. Approximately 23% of U.S. adolescents and adults have been exposed to *T. gondii*. There are approximately 750 deaths per year, with 50% to 60% of these infections probably acquired through food. Overall, *Toxoplasma* complications account for 21% of food-related deaths, third after *Salmonella* and *Listeria*.

In a recent study conducted by the Centers for Disease Control and Prevention (CDC), the overall age-adjusted seroprevalence of persons aged 6 to 49 years in the United States was 10.8%. Seroprevalence is lower among U.S.-born individuals than among immigrants. For example, the seroprevalence was 7.7% among U.S-born women and 28.1% among foreign-born women. There was also a higher prevalence among people living below the poverty index level. When looking at ethnic groups of U.S.-born persons between 1999 and 2004, the immunoglobulin G (IgG) seroprevalence was highest in non-Hispanic blacks and lowest in Mexican Americans, with non-Hispanic whites being in between. Among U.S. and foreign-born members of different ethnic groups between 6 and 49 years of age, Mexican Americans had the highest prevalence (13.7%) and non-Hispanic whites the lowest (8.7%). Overall, there was a significant drop in seroprevalence among U.S.-born persons between 12 and 49 years of age between 1988–1994 (14.1%) and 1999–2004 (9.0%). This may be due to improved food, livestock, and pet hygiene.

Diagnosis and Testing

Detection is available via indirect methods (serology) and directly (polymerase chain reaction [PCR] of DNA, hybridization, culture, and pathology). Serology is often used for diagnosis in immunocompetent patients (Fig. 1). Immunocompromised patients often require direct evidence to definitively establish the diagnosis; biopsy with evidence of tachyzoites is diagnostic of acute infection.

IgG is used as a screening test in all categories of patients, including immunocompromised patients, pregnant patients, newborns, and those with eye infection. The Sabin-Feldman dye test, the IgG avidity

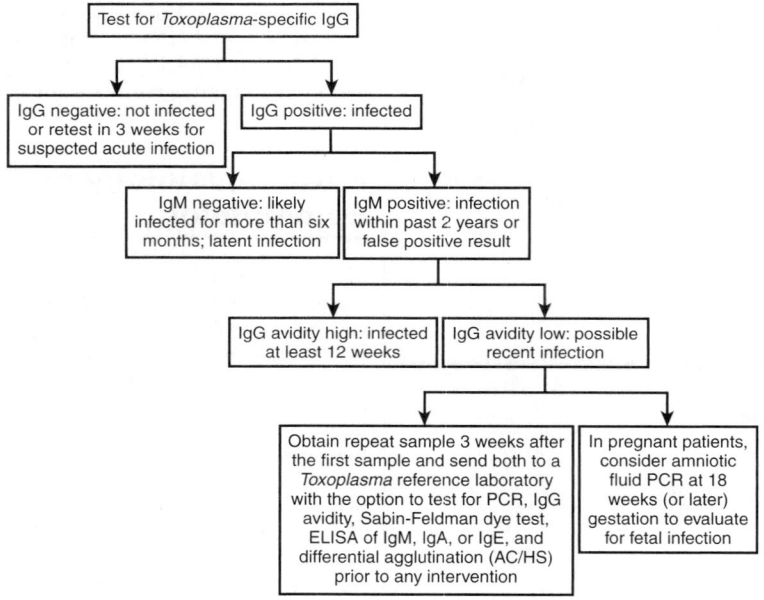

FIGURE 1. Suggested algorithm for serologic testing of *Toxoplasma gondii* in people older than 1 year of age. Equivocal results should be repeated and sent for confirmatory testing at a reference laboratory. *Abbreviations:* AC/HS = agglutination and differential agglutination test; ELISA = enzyme-linked immunosorbent assay; Ig = immunoglobulin; PCR = polymerase chain reaction. (Adapted with permission from Wilson M, Jones JL, McAuley JB: Toxoplasma. In Murray PR, Baron EJ, Landry ML, et al [eds]: Manual of Clinical Microbiology, 9th ed. Washington, DC, ASM Press, 2007, pp 2070–2081.)

test, the immunofluorescent antibody test, the enzyme-linked immunosorbent assay (ELISA), or the agglutination and differential agglutination (AC/HS) test can be used for IgG detection. Antibody develops within 1 to 8 weeks after infection and persists for life. In newborns, maternal IgG may persist for up to 1 year, so differentiation is needed by a Western blot or enzyme-linked immune filtration assay (ELIFA).

A positive IgG high avidity test, which measures the strength with which IgG binds to *Toxoplasma*, can be used to rule out infection within the past 3 to 5 months in pregnant patients and in those with ocular infection. High-avidity antibodies develop 12 to 16 weeks after infection, depending on the testing kit used. A positive result in a pregnant woman during the first 3 months of pregnancy indicates that the woman most likely was infected before she became pregnant, so the fetus is not at high risk for having acquired *Toxoplasma*. The absence of IgG antibodies in early pregnancy identifies mothers who are at risk for acquiring acute infection.

IgM, detectable within 2 weeks, is generally used to rule out recently acquired infection. A negative IgM test during the first two trimesters of pregnancy rules out acute infection. In early pregnancy, more power can be attained by testing for both IgM and IgG. Negative IgM results with ocular disease may indicate reactivation of congenital infection, whereas high titers may signify an acutely acquired infection. IgM can also be used for neonatal screening of toxoplasmosis. The particularly sensitive and specific IgM immunosorbent agglutination assay (ISAGA) can be used for this purpose. IgM has low sensitivity in immunocompromised patients. Confirmation of positive results should be attained from a *Toxoplasma* reference laboratory, because many commercially available IgM testing kits have had problems with specificity (ranging from 77.5% to 99.1%), leading to high rates of false-positive results. In a recent examination of 100 consecutive serum samples of IgM-positive results received for confirmatory testing by the Palo Alto Medical Foundation Toxoplasma Serology Laboratory, 62% were found to be negative. Therefore, the greatest benefit of a positive IgM antibody test is that it demonstrates the possibility of a recently acquired infection, making it necessary to send the sample for confirmatory testing at a reference laboratory.

IgA, peaking in 2 months, can persist for prolonged periods (usually 1 to 5 years) and can be used in newborn testing. Combining IgA and IgM tests greatly increases sensitivity in neonates. Up to 75% of affected infants can be identified.

IgE is highly specific in pregnant patients but has low sensitivity. It can be used in combination with other serologic tests.

In addition to tissue diagnosis by immunohistochemistry, cell culture, and mouse inoculation, PCR amplification of specific genes can be used for direct detection. Amniotic fluid, blood, urine, vitreous or aqueous fluid, cerebrospinal fluid, peritoneal fluid, pleural fluid, bone marrow aspirate, and organ tissue can all be tested using PCR. With appropriate precautions to minimize contamination, PCR specificity and positive predictive value approach 100%. Mixed results are obtained with sensitivity and negative predictive value when dealing with amniotic fluid, although PCR is useful in prenatal testing for *T. gondii* by allowing for early diagnosis. PCR testing of amniotic fluid after 18 weeks of gestation caries a sensitivity of approximately 60% and a specificity of 100%. Amniotic fluid PCR should be considered in pregnant women with serology results suggestive of recently acquired infection, in those with ultrasound findings of possible toxoplasmosis, and in patients who are immunocompromised. Caution is advised, however, for pregnant women with HIV infection who may be coinfected with *T. gondii*, because of the risk of infecting the fetus with HIV during the amniocentesis. PCR is of great utility in immunocompromised patients, but it may not distinguish between acute (e.g., tachyzoites) and chronic (e.g., tissue cysts) infection. In immunocompromised patients, PCR amplification can be combined with parasite isolation from body fluids to demonstrate tachyzoites and tissue histologic findings.

Histologic findings in lymph nodes infected with *T. gondii* include reactive follicular hyperplasia, irregular clusters of epithelial-like histiocytes encroaching on germinal centers, and monocyte-like cells causing distention of sinuses. Neural tissue findings consist of multiple foci of necrosis and microglia nodules. Presence of tissue cysts

indicates past infection but does not, on its own, indicate active infection. Wright-Giemsa stain may be used to visualize the cysts, but immunoperoxidase staining is more sensitive.

Neuroimaging should be done for any focal or nonfocal clinical neurologic findings in immunocompromised patients. In cases of *Toxoplasma* encephalitis, they may guide therapy and aid in diagnosis. Clinical and radiologic response to therapy, usually seen within 10 to 14 days, supports a diagnosis of toxoplasmosis without the need of invasive brain biopsy. Computed tomography or magnetic resonance imaging (MRI) may be used, although the latter is more sensitive. A noncontrast computed tomogram of the brain may show hypodense lesions with surrounding vasogenic edema in acute or subacute cases. Chronic lesions, especially after treatment, may appear calcified. MRI, preferably with gadolinium contrast, may show multiple ring-enhancing lesions that can occupy the basal ganglia, lobar gray-white junction, periventricular white matter, cerebral cortex, or posterior fossa. Surrounding edema is often disproportionately large compared with the lesion size. It is difficult to differentiate between toxoplasmosis brain lesions and lymphoma (an important differential in immunosuppressed patients). Positron emission tomography and single-photon emission tomography may have a role in making this distinction in the near future.

Infection in Immunocompetent Patients

Infection in immunocompetent hosts, including pregnant women, is usually asymptomatic. Between 10% and 20% of patients develop a nonspecific flu-like or mononucleosis-like illness with low-grade fever, malaise, or predominantly isolated cervical or occipital lymphadenopathy that is nontender. Nodes may stay enlarged for up to 6 weeks, but a fluctuating, chronic form has also been described. Myocarditis, polymyositis, encephalitis, pneumonitis, and hepatitis are possible but rare. In general, if signs and symptoms develop, they are self-limited and resolve within weeks to months.

Important and more common differential diagnoses that can cause similar symptoms are cytomegalovirus and Epstein-Barr virus infection. The differential diagnosis also includes cat scratch disease, lymphoma, tuberculosis, sarcoidosis, and metastatic cancer. To help establish a diagnosis, serology and lymph node biopsy should be performed.

Infection in Immunocompromised and AIDS Patients

Infection in immunocompromised patients usually occurs as a result of reactivation of chronic infection and may be life threatening. Multiorgan involvement is possible, including *Toxoplasma* pneumonia and septic shock, but the most typical findings involve the central nervous system. Meningeal signs rarely occur, but there may be altered mental status, seizures, cerebellar signs, focal neurologic deficits (i.e., speech abnormalities and hemiparesis), and neuropsychiatric findings.

The finding of multiple brain abscesses in an immunocompromised patient is highly suggestive of *Toxoplasma* encephalitis. There is usually bilateral hemisphere involvement, especially in the basal ganglia. Pulmonary toxoplasmosis is another possibility; it may manifest as a pneumonia, pneumonitis, or effusion.

Ocular Toxoplasmosis

Ocular infection may produce acute chorioretinitis, which can lead to necrotizing retinitis. The vitreous humor may become exudative, with tachyzoites and cysts possibly visible within the retina. The typical finding is areas of white focal lesions with a surrounding vitreal inflammatory reaction, the classic "headlight in the fog."

CURRENT THERAPY

- Pyrimethamine (Daraprim) plus sulfadiazine[1] plus folinic acid (Leucovorin)[1] is the mainstay of therapy for toxoplasmosis.
- Spiramycin (Rovamycine)[2] should be used for therapy in pregnancy if treatment is needed before 18 weeks of gestation, because of the possible teratogenic effects of pyrimethamine.
- Prophylactic treatment should be initiated for immunocompromised patients who have a CD4[+] count of less than 100 cells/mm[3] and should be continued for the life of the patient or until immunosuppression has ended.

[1]Not FDA approved for this indication.
[2]Not available in the United States.

Ocular disease may result from congenital or acutely acquired infection. Acute infection is thought to be more common. Patients with congenitally acquired infection typically have bilateral eye disease, whereas those with acutely acquired infection usually have unilateral signs.

Congenital Toxoplasmosis and Toxoplasmosis in Pregnancy

In the United States, approximately 85% of women of child-bearing age are at risk for acquiring *T. gondii*. Mother-to-fetus vertical transmission can occur through an infected placenta. If a mother obtains a primary infection more than 3 months before conception (i.e., only positive IgG is present), there is little risk to the fetus. There is a small but discernible increased risk if the infection is obtained within 3 months of conception, and this risk progressively increases throughout gestation. The frequency of transmission is inversely related to the severity of disease. Although the rate of toxoplasmosis transmission between mother and fetus is low (10%-20%), maternal infection in the first two trimesters can result in severe congenital toxoplasmosis and possibly fetal death. Maternal third-trimester infection leads most often to fetal toxoplasmosis (80%-90%) but also often results in subclinical infection in newborns. If this is left untreated, chorioretinitis and growth retardation may develop in the second or third decade of life. Immunocompromised patients with chronic infection can rarely transmit infection via the placenta.

There are no specific diagnostic ultrasound findings of fetal toxoplasmosis. Findings include increased placental thickness, intracranial calcifications, ventricular dilatation, liver enlargement, and ascites. Hydrocephalus demonstrated by ultrasonography has been used as an indication to terminate pregnancy.

In infected infants, pathologic examination of brain tissue typically reveals periaqueductal and periventricular vasculitis and necrosis. Calcification of necrotic areas may be revealed on imaging. Hydrocephalus can develop secondary to obstruction. However, the classic triad of hydrocephalus, chorioretinitis, and cerebral calcifications is a rare occurrence. Instead, several nonspecific signs are microcephaly, blindness, strabismus, epilepsy, mental retardation, anemia, thrombocytopenia, hepatosplenomegaly, jaundice, and rash. These signs are included in the TORCH (toxoplasmosis, other infections, rubella, cytomegalovirus, and herpes simplex) syndrome.

Treatment

Suggested toxoplasmosis treatment regimens are summarized in Table 1.

IMMUNOCOMPETENT HOSTS

Lymphadenitis usually is not treated unless symptoms persist or are severe. Combination therapy with pyrimethamine (Daraprim), sulfadiazine,[1] and folinic acid (leucovorin)[1] for 2 to 6 weeks is the typical regimen. Infection acquired through blood products or laboratory accidents is usually more serious and requires treatment.

PREGNANCY

Although not universally utilized, spiramycin (Rovamycine),[2] available through the CDC, is recommended for suspected or confirmed acute maternal infection acquired during gestation in the first and early second trimester or pyrimethamine plus sulfadiazine[1] in the late second and third trimesters. Definitive diagnosis of acute infection requires conversion of a negative titer to a positive one or a significant rise in titers. In addition, infection of the mother does not necessarily indicate infection of the fetus. Therefore, it is necessary to have prenatal diagnostic testing by amniotic fluid PCR (sensitivity ranges from 68% to 98.8%).

If the PCR result is negative, spiramycin prophylaxis should be given until at least the 17th week of pregnancy. In Austria and Germany, this is followed by 4 weeks of pyrimethamine plus sulfadiazine[1] plus leucovorin.[1] In the United States and France, spiramycin[2] is continued throughout pregnancy, in addition to monthly ultrasound examinations.

If the PCR result is positive and the possibility of fetal infection is high (e.g., by ultrasound findings) or the infection was acquired after 18 weeks of gestation, it is recommended to use the pyrimethamine and sulfadiazine regimen after 18 weeks of gestation (although in some countries this may start as early as 16 weeks). In some countries, this regimen is alternated with spiramycin, but it does not reliably cross the placenta to treat fetal infection. Treatment is continued throughout pregnancy, along with monthly ultrasound examinations and folinic acid to reduce bone marrow toxicity. Pyrimethamine is potentially teratogenic and should not be given during the first 16 to 18 weeks of pregnancy. In most countries, treatment is continued for the newborn through the first year of life.

Treatment of acute infection during pregnancy has been associated with a reduction in the rate of fetal infection by about 50%. The European Research Network on Congenital Toxoplasmosis sponsored studies of the effects of treatment in pregnant mothers. One of the studies confirmed prenatal infection with amniocentesis or cordocentesis. These women were treated with pyrimethamine plus sulfadiazine or pyrimethamine plus sulfadoxine (Fansidar).[1] The congenital transmission rate was 39% in women who received therapy and 72% in those who did not; this difference was not statistically significant when time of gestation was taken into account. The percentage of infants born with severe congenital signs of toxoplasmosis in mothers who received prenatal treatment was 3.5%, compared with 20% in those who did not receive treatment. The earlier antibiotics were given, the greater their efficacy in preventing severe infection. Additionally, The National Collaborative Chicago-Based Congenital Toxoplasmosis Study prospectively studied 120 infected infants who were treated between 1981 and 2004 with pyrimethamine, sulfadiazine, and leucovorin for 1 year; there were significantly fewer occurrences of cognitive, motor, vision, and hearing abnormalities. Patients with congenital toxoplasmosis who are not treated or are treated for only 1 month have been shown to have poor outcomes.

Caution must be taken in the use of antibiotics to treat congenital infection. Sulfonamides given late in pregnancy have been associated with kernicterus in the newborn. Pyrimethamine is a folic acid antagonist (dihydrofolate reductase inhibitor) that can cause neural tube defects, because folic acid serves as a coenzyme in the formation of DNA, RNA, myelin, and lipids. Folinic acid (leucovorin)[1] should be given with pyrimethamine to compensate for the reduction of folic acid. Pyrimethamine has also been associated with kidney and heart malformations in newborns and with increased risk of central nervous

[1]Not FDA approved for this indication.
[2]Not available in the United States.

TABLE 1 Suggested Toxoplasmosis Treatment Regimens

Population	Drug	Dosage	Duration
Acute infection in an immunocompetent patient or in a pregnant patient infected ≥6 mo before conception	Treatment not recommended or, if acutely ill, Pyrimethamine (Daraprim) plus	200 mg PO loading dose, then 50–75 mg PO daily	4–6 wk, or 1–2 wk after symptoms resolve
	Sulfadiazine[1] plus Leucovorin (folinic acid)[1]	1–1.5 g PO q6h 5–20 mg PO TIW	During and 1 week after pyrimethamine use
Acute infection in a pregnant patient acquired <18 wk gestation ≥18 wk gestation	Spiramycin (Rovamycine)[2] See fetal infection (or, if amniotic PCR test is negative, consider switch to spiramycin)	1g PO q8h without food	Throughout pregnancy or until fetal infection is documented
Fetal infection (after 16–18 wk gestation)	Pyrimethamine plus Sulfadiazine[1] plus	Loading dose 50 mg PO q12h × 2 d, then 50 mg PO daily Loading dose 75 mg/kg PO, then 50 mg/kg q12h (maximum, 4 g daily)	Throughout pregnancy Throughout pregnancy
	Leucovorin	10–20 mg PO daily	During and for 1 wk after pyrimethamine use
Congenital infection in the infant	Pyrimethamine plus	Loading dose 2 mg/kg PO daily × 2 d, then 1 mg/kg PO daily × 2–6 mo, then 1 mg/kg TIW	1 y
	Sulfadiazine plus Leucovorin and possibly	50 mg/kg PO q12h 10 mg PO TIW	1 y During and for 1 wk after pyrimethamine use
	Prednisone (if CSF protein is ≥1 g/dL and if chorioretinitis threatens vision)	1 mg/kg daily in two divided doses	Until signs resolve
Adult chorioretinitis	Pyrimethamine[1] plus Sulfadiazine plus Leucovorin and possibly	200 mg PO loading dose, then 50–75 mg PO daily 1–1.5 g PO q6h 5–20 mg PO TIW	1–2 wk after symptoms resolve 1–2 wk after symptoms resolve During and 1 wk after pyrimethamine use
	Prednisone	1 mg/kg daily in two divided doses	Until signs and symptoms resolve
Immunocompromised patients and patients with encephalitis*	Pyrimethamine plus Leucovorin plus either Sulfadiazine or Clindamycin (Cleocin)[1]	Loading dose 200 mg PO, then 50–75 mg PO daily 10–20 mg PO or IV or IM daily (maximum, 50 mg daily) 1–1.5 g PO q6h 600 mg PO or IV q6h (maximum, 1200 mg q6h)	At least 4–6 wk after signs and symptoms resolve During and for 1 wk after pyrimethamine use At least 4–6 wk after signs and symptoms resolve
	Alternatives: Trimethoprim-sulfamethoxazole (Bactrim)[1] alone, or Pyrimethamine plus leucovorin plus one of the following: Clarithromycin (Biaxin)[1] Atovaquone (Mepron)[1] Azithromycin (Zithromax)[1] Dapsone[1]	5 mg/kg trimethoprim PO or IV q12h (maximum, 15–20 mg/kg/day) Same as above pyrimethamine/ leucovorin doses 500 mg PO q12hr 750 mg PO q6h 1200–1500 mg PO daily 100 mg PO daily	Same as above Same as above
Primary prophylaxis for immunocompromised patients (i.e., CD4+ count ≤100 cells/mm³ and Toxoplasma IgG+)	Trimethoprim-sulfamethoxazole (Bactrim DS)[1] Alternatives: Pyrimethamine[1] plus dapsone[1] plus leucovorin	1 double-strength tablet (160/800 mg) PO daily 50–75 mg/wk pyrimethamine plus 50 mg/day dapsone plus 25 mg/wk leucovorin	For life or until immunosuppression has abated (see text) Same as above
	Pyrimethamine-sulfadoxine (Fansidar)[1] plus leucovorin Atovaquone (Mepron)	1 tablet twice weekly Fansidar plus 25 mg/wk leucovorin 1500 mg PO daily	

Adapted with permission from Montoya JG, Liesenfeld O: Toxoplasmosis. Lancet 2004;363(9425):1965–1976.
[1]Not FDA approved for this indication.
[2]Not available in the United States.
*After the initial phase of therapy, maintenance therapy must be continued as long as the patient remains immunocompromised. See text for details.
Abbreviations: CSF = cerebrospinal fluid; IM = intramuscular; PCR = polymerase chain reaction; PO = orally; TID = three times daily; TIW = three times per week.

system cancers in children. There is also danger of bone marrow suppression in mother and fetus from treatment with pyrimethamine and sulfadiazine (a dihydrofolate synthetase inhibitor), requiring weekly blood count monitoring. Risks and benefits must be weighed before treatment for toxoplasmosis is implemented in the pregnant patient.

CHORIORETINITIS

Treatment is recommended for severe inflammatory reaction and for close proximity of retinal lesions to the fovea or optic disk. Small peripheral retinal lesions in immunocompetent patients may not need treatment, because the disease may be self-limited. If treatment is warranted, a common regimen consists of pyrimethamine (with leucovorin), sulfadiazine, and prednisone continued for at least 1 week after the resolution of symptoms. Alternatively, clindamycin (Cleocin)[1] and trimethoprim-sulfamethoxazole (TMP/SMX [Bactrim])[1] may be used. In cases of recurrent chorioretinitis, a long-term intermittent regimen of TMP-SMX may be of benefit. A short course of steroids may be given to patients with ocular or neural toxoplasmosis if there is suspicion of a significant inflammatory component of pathology.

IMMUNOCOMPROMISED HOSTS

In patients who have undergone organ transplantation, particularly those who are donor positive and recipient negative for *T. gondii*, prophylactic treatment with TMP-SMX[1] is recommended.

Immunocompromised patients are particularly susceptible to toxoplasma encephalitis. Neuroimaging by computed tomography or MRI should be done for any suspicion of neurologic infection. It is standard practice to initiate anti-*Toxoplasma* therapy in the setting of multiple ring-enhancing lesions found on imaging with positive IgG titers in an immunocompromised patient. The most common regimen consists of pyrimethamine (with leucovorin) plus sulfadiazine[1] (or clindamycin[1] in sulfa-allergic patients) continued for at least 4 to 6 weeks after resolution of signs and symptoms. TMP-SMX[1] may be an acceptable alternative to pyrimethamine plus sulfadiazine, especially in developing countries where there is a limited supply of medications. Other alternatives, in combination with pyrimethamine and leucovorin, include atovaquone (Mepron)[1] (750 mg PO every 6 hours), dapsone[1] (100 mg PO daily), clarithromycin (Biaxin)[1] (500 mg PO every 12 hours),* azithromycin (Zithromax)[1] (1200–1500 mg PO daily), and clindamycin[1] (600–1200 mg IV or PO every 6 hours).

After the initial phase of therapy has ended, maintenance therapy should be continued. This usually consists of the same regimen of medications, but at half the doses, for the life of the patient or until immunosuppression has concluded. In AIDS patients whose symptoms of toxoplasmosis have resolved, this usually coincides with a CD4[+] count greater than 200 cells/mm[3] that has been sustained for at least 6 months and an HIV viral load that has been controlled for at least 6 months. An example regimen may be pyrimethamine 25 mg daily plus sulfadiazine 500 mg four times daily plus folinic acid 10–20 mg daily. Alternative regimens may consists of atovaquone 750 mg two to four times daily alone, or clindamycin 600 mg three times daily plus pyrimethamine 25 mg daily plus folinic acid.

Prevention

The best treatment is prevention. HIV-positive patients and pregnant women should avoid extensive contact with cats whenever possible. If cats are present, they should not be fed undercooked meat, and they should be kept indoors to avoid contact with potentially infected soil. Litter boxes should be cleaned daily (and gloves should be worn) and disinfected with near-boiling water for 5 minutes before refilling. Petting of cats probably poses little risk of transmission of *Toxoplasma*. This may be due to generally frequent self-grooming by housecats and the fact that not much, if any, fecal material adheres to cat fur. Serologic testing of cats has not been shown to be of clinical utility.

Cats may not develop antibodies during the oocyst-shedding period; they may test positive after already having shed the oocysts; and they may shed oocysts more than once. In addition, cats shed oocysts for only 1 to 2 weeks, making stool testing unhelpful.

Gloves should be worn when handling soil or gardening. It is also important to thoroughly wash hands after contact with animals, soil, and raw meat and to appropriately cook meat. Beef, lamb, and veal roasts and steaks should be cooked to at least 145°F. Pork, ground meat, and wild game should be cooked to at least 160°F. Poultry should be cooked to 180°F in the thigh. Fruits and vegetables need to be thoroughly washed or peeled before eating. Freezing food to −12°C can kill tissue cysts, and appropriate levels of irradiation may kill oocysts. Microwave ovens are not reliable because of uneven heating. Cooking utensils and appliances should be cleaned if they are contacted by undercooked or raw foods. To prevent contamination of food and water, felines should be kept away from farms and water sources.

Although there is no currently available human vaccine, prophylactic treatment should be offered to immunocompromised patients who are IgG positive. AIDS patients who have a CD4[+] count of less than 100 cells/mm[3] and are seropositive for *T. gondii* can receive primary prophylaxis with one double-strength tablet of TMP-SMX (160/800 mg [Bactrim DS])[1] daily. Alternative regimens although less effective, include pyrimethamine 50 to 75 mg/week plus dapsone[1] 50 mg/day or, as another option, pyrimethamine/sulfadoxine (Fansidar)[1] one tablet twice weekly or atovaquone 1500 mg once daily. It has been suggested that primary prophylaxis should be discontinued in those patients who have responded to an effective HIV regimen and maintain a CD4 count >200 cells/mm[3] for more than 3 months.

Other options in preventing the spread of toxoplasmosis include health care provider and patient education about treatment and the interpretation of tests. Universal prenatal screening is used in some European nations (e.g., Austria, France). Cost-benefit analysis is still underway to determine whether the United States may adopt these methods, but there is the overlying risk of equivocal and false-positive results that may lead to further testing, stress, and unnecessary treatment.

---

[1]Not FDA approved for this indication.

REFERENCES

Bakshi R. Neuroimaging of HIV and AIDS related illnesses: A review. Front Biosci 2004;9:632–46.

Chirgwin K, Hafner R, Leport C, et al. Randomized phase II trial of atovaquone with pyrimethamine or sulfadiazine for treatment of toxoplasmic encephalitis in patients with acquired immunodeficiency syndrome: ACTG 237/ANRS 039 Study. Clin Infect Dis 2002;34:1243–50.

Dubey JP. The history of *Toxoplasma gondii*—the first 100 years. J Eukaryot Microbiol 2008;55(6):467–75.

Fisher MA, Levy J, Helfrich M, et al. Detection of *Toxoplasma gondii* in the spinal fluid of a bone marrow transplant recipient. Pediatr Infect Dis 1987;6:81–3.

Foulon W, Villena I, Stray-Pedersen B, et al. Treatment of toxoplasmosis during pregnancy: A multicenter study of impact on fetal transmission and children's sequelae at age 1 year. Am J Obstet Gynecol 1999;180:410–5.

Gilber DN, Moellering RC, Eliopoulos GM, et al. [eds.]. The Sanford Guide to Antimicrobiol Therapy, 40th ed. Sperryville, VA: Antimicrobial Therapy, Inc.; 2010.

Hughes JM, Colley DG, Lopez A, et al. Preventing congenital toxoplasmosis. Morb Mortal Wkly Rep MMWR 2000;49(RR02):57–75.

Jones JL, Kruszon-Moran D, Sanders-Lewis K, et al. *Toxoplasma gondii* infection in the United States, 1999–2004: Decline from the prior decade. Am J Trop Med Hyg 2007;77(3):405–10.

Jones JL, Lopez A, Wilson M. Congenital toxoplasmosis. Am Fam Physician 2003;67(10):2131–8.

Jones JL, Lopez A, Wilson M, et al. Congenital toxoplasmosis: A review. Obstet Gynecol Surv 2001;56(5):296–305.

Kaplan JE, Benson C, Holmes KH, et al. Guidelines for prevention and treatment of opportunistic infections in HIV-infected adults and adolescents: Recommendations from CDC, the National Institutes of Health, and the HIV Medicine Association of the Infectious Diseases Society of America. MMWR Recomm Rep 2009;58:1–207.

Luft BJ, Conley F, Remington JS, et al. Outbreak of central-nervous system toxoplasmosis in Western Europe and North America. Lancet 1983;1:781–3.

Luft BJ, Hafner R, Korzun AH, et al. Toxoplasmic encephalitis in patients with acquired immunodeficiency syndrome: Development of objective criteria for early diagnosis and treatment. N Engl J Med 1993;329(14):995–1000.

---

[1]Not FDA approved for this indication.

*In a recent CDC report, doses of clarithromycin above 500 mg twice daily may be associated with increased mortality in patients treated for disseminated *Mycobacterium avian* complex.

Luft BJ, Remington JS. Acquired toxoplasmic encephalitis. In: Remington JS, Swartz MW, editors. Current Clinical Topics in Infectious Diseases, vol. 6. New York: McGraw-Hill; 1985.

McAuley JB. Toxoplasmosis in children. Pediatr Infect Dis J 2008;27:161–2.

McLeod R, Boyer K, Karrison T, et al. Outcome of treatment for congenital toxoplasmosis, 1981–2004: The National Collaborative Chicago-Based, Congenital Toxoplasmosis Study. Clin Infect Dis 2006;42(10):1383–94.

Montoya JG, Boothroyd JC, Kovacs JA. *Toxoplasma gondii*. In: Mandell GL, Bennett JE, Dolin R, [eds.]: Mandell, Douglas, and Bennett's Principles and Practice of Infectious Diseases, 7th ed. Philadelphia, PA: Churchill Livingstone-Elsevier; 2010. pp. 3495–526.

Montoya JG, Liesenfeld O. Toxoplasmosis. Lancet 2004;363:1965–76.

Montoya JG, Remington JS. Management of *Toxoplasma gondii* infection during pregnancy. Clin Infect Dis 2008;47(4):554–66.

Remington JS. Toxoplasmosis in the adult. Bull N Y Acad Med 1974;50(2):211–26.

Wilson M, Jones JL, McAuley JB. Toxoplasma. In: Murray PR, Baron EJ, Landry ML, et al., Manual of Clinical Microbiology. 9th ed. Washington, DC: ASM Press; 2007. p. 2070–81.

Cat-Scratch Disease

Method of
Michael J. Smith, MD, MSCE

Cat-scratch disease (CSD), regional lymphadenopathy following a cat scratch or bite, has been described since the 1950s. *Bartonella henselae*, a pleomorphic, facultative intracellular gram-negative bacillus, was not identified as the etiologic agent until 40 years later. As the laboratory detection of *B. henselae* has improved, it has become associated with an increasing number of clinical entities. These have traditionally been divided into typical CSD, the classic finding of unilateral regional lymphadenopathy following a cat scratch or bite, and atypical CSD, which includes all other presentations.

Epidemiology

As CSD is not a reportable disease, the true incidence remains unknown. However, there are an estimated 24,000 cases in the United States each year. Predominantly a disease of childhood and adolescence, CSD has the highest age-specific incidence rate occurring in children younger than 10 years of age. Although less frequent, CSD does occur in older individuals as well. A recent study found that 6% of patients with confirmed CSD were older than the age of 60 years.

Nearly 90% of patients with CSD have exposure to cats and approximately half recall a definitive scratch or bite. Early epidemiologic evidence suggested an increased risk of CSD in patients with kittens as compared to patients with adult cats. It was subsequently shown that kittens have a higher rate of *B. henselae* bacteremia than adult cats. In contrast, adult cats are more likely to have antibodies indicative of past infection. Most bacteremic cats are asymptomatic, so even a healthy-appearing animal can transmit disease.

The cat flea, *Ctenocephalides felis*, has been implicated in the transmission between cats. Consequently, CSD is more prevalent in warm and humid environments that support the growth of fleas with infection occurring primarily in the fall and winter months. To date, no evidence exists for human to human transmission.

Clinical Manifestations

Typical CSD is the most common form of CSD in immunocompetent patients. Initially, papules develop at the site of inoculation within the first week after a cat scratch or bite. This is followed by the gradual onset of unilateral regional lymphadenopathy over the next several weeks. Occasionally these lymph nodes may suppurate. The location of lymphadenopathy depends on the site of inoculation but most

commonly occurs in the axillary, inguinal or cervical chains. In contrast to bacterial lymphadenitis, the lymph nodes are not inflamed. Patients are usually well-appearing and afebrile. Lymphadenopathy gradually resolves over several months without specific therapy.

The most common form of atypical CSD is Parinaud's oculoglandular syndrome (POGS), which occurs when bacteria are inoculated directly into the eye or eyelid. Small papules develop, almost always in the palpebral conjunctiva, in association with ipsilateral preauricular lymphadenopathy. There is also a painless, nonpurulent conjunctivitis. Similar to typical CSD, these symptoms resolve without antimicrobial therapy over several weeks.

Typical CSD and POGS share a similar pathophysiology; direct inoculation followed by a local immune response. In contrast, the other types of atypical CSD are due to systemic infection with *B. henselae*. These include hepatosplenic CSD, osteomyelitis, endocarditis, encephalitis, and neuroretinitis. *Bartonella* has also been implicated in the etiology of fever of unknown origin (FUO). One recent study revealed that 5% of all children with FUO of infectious etiology had antibodies against *B. henselae* indicative of current or recent infection.

In immunocompromised individuals, *B. henselae* can cause life-threatening invasive disease. Bacillary angiomatosis (BA), which is also caused by other *Bartonella* species, is caused by the angioproli-ferative effects of *Bartonella* and results in multiple vascular tumors in the skin and subcutaneous tissues. Bacillary peliosis (BP) is another form of vasoproliferative disease that leads to the development of blood-filled cysts in the reticuloendothelial element of the liver, spleen, and bone marrow of severely immunocompromised patients.

Diagnosis

A detailed history and physical examination are essential for the diagnosis of CSD. Any contact with cats or kittens, especially if bites or scratches occurred, should raise suspicion for CSD, regardless of the patient's age and clinical presentation.

Bartonella is a fastidious organism that takes several weeks to grow, making culture impractical. Therefore, serologic testing has become the mainstay of diagnosis. Indirect fluorescent antibody testing for IgM and IgG against *B. henselae* is performed by most commercial laboratories as well as the Centers for Disease Control. A single elevated titer or a fourfold or greater increase between acute and convalescent titers is diagnostic of CSD.

The combination of history, physical examination, and serologic testing may obviate the need for biopsy in cases of typical CSD. If a node is removed, the characteristic histopathologic finding is the formation of granulomas with microabscesses and central necrosis. Rarely, gram-negative bacilli may be identified using the Warthin-Starry silver stain. These are both nonspecific findings, and any patient undergoing biopsy should have samples sent for cytology as well as fungal, mycobacterial, and standard bacterial culture and sensitivity to rule out other etiologies of lymphadenopathy. Polymerase chain reaction (PCR) testing of tissue is emerging as a highly specific diagnostic tool. Sensitivity of PCR testing varies with the specific DNA target used but is usually quite high. It is becoming increasingly available in commercial laboratories.

 CURRENT DIAGNOSIS

- Suspect CSD in any patient with lymphadenopathy and a history of cat exposure, regardless of age.
- Serologic testing can confirm the diagnosis.
- If biopsy is performed, specimens should be sent for pathology as well as fungal, mycobacterial, and routine bacterial cultures.
- Granulomas with central necrosis are characteristic of CSD but are not specific. When available, PCR is highly specific for CSD.

Abbreviations: CSD = cat-scratch disease; PCR = polymerase chain reaction.

CURRENT THERAPY

Immunocompetent Patients

- Typical CSD only requires supportive treatment.
- No antibiotics are indicated.
- For atypical CSD there are no definitive treatment recommendations.
- Endocarditis requires surgery and antibiotic therapy, which should include at least 14 days of an aminoglycoside.

Immunocompromised Patients

- BA or BP treatment for at least 3 months with either
  - Erythromycin (E.E.S.)[1] 500 mg PO qid or
  - Doxycycline (Vibramycin) 100 mg PO bid.

---

[1]Not FDA approved for this indication.
Abbreviations: BA = bacillary angiomatosis; BP = bacillary peliosis; CSD = cat-scratch disease.

Treatment

Treatment of typical CSD is supportive and mainly consists of needle aspiration of suppurative lymph nodes when required. There is no evidence to suggest that treatment with antibiotics significantly alters the course of disease. In the only prospective, randomized, double blinded study of typical CSD, a 5-day course of azithromycin (Zithromax) or placebo was given to 29 patients with clinical CSD. Although the subjects who received azithromycin had a more rapid reduction in lymphadenopathy as measured by ultrasound at 30 days, the long-term outcomes were identical for both groups.

Evidence for the treatment of atypical CSD in immunocompetent patients is limited to case reports and retrospective reviews. Success has been reported using a range of oral antibiotics including trimethoprim-sulfamethoxazole (Bactrim, Septra),[1] rifampin (Rifadin),[1] azithromycin (Zithromax),[1] doxycycline (Vibramycin), and ciprofloxacin (Cipro),[1] as well as intravenous gentamicin (Garamycin).[1] Nevertheless, most cases of atypical CSD are thought to resolve without antibiotic therapy. A notable exception is endocarditis, which requires surgical replacement of the damaged valve in addition to antibiotic therapy. One retrospective review found that treatment of endocarditis with a regimen that included an aminoglycoside for at least 14 days was significantly associated with a higher rate of survival.

Immunocompromised patients with BA or BP warrant antimicrobial treatment. There have been no controlled studies to determine optimal therapy, but either erythromycin (E.E.S.)[1] or doxycycline (Vibramycin) is effective. Most experts recommend a treatment course of at least 3 months to prevent relapse.

Prevention

Cat owners should avoid activities that may result in a cat scratch or bite, and should promptly wash any cat-inflicted wounds. Appropriate flea control will also reduce the likelihood of CSD. Because of the risk for invasive disease caused by *B. henselae*, immunocompromised individuals should be specifically warned of the risks of cat exposure. If possible, they should avoid purchasing or adopting kittens.

REFERENCES

American Academy of Pediatrics. Cat-scratch disease. In: Pickering LK, editor. Red Book: 2003 Report of the Committee on Infectious Diseases. 26th ed. Elk Grove Village, IL: American Academy of Pediatrics; 2006. p. 232–4.

---

[1]Not FDA approved for this indication.

Bass JW, Freitas BC, Freitas AD, et al. Prospective randomized double blind placebo-controlled evaluation of azithromycin for treatment of cat-scratch disease. Pediatr Infect Dis J 1998;17:447–52.

Batts S, Demers DM. Spectrum and treatment of cat-scratch disease. Pediatr Infect Dis J 2004;23:1161–2.

Ben-Ami R, Ephros M, Avidor B, et al. Cat-scratch disease in elderly patients. Clin Infect Dis 2005;41:969–74.

Hansmann Y, DeMartino S, Piemont Y, et al. Diagnosis of cat scratch disease with detection of *Bartonella henselae* PCR: A study of patients with lymph node enlargement. J Clin Microbiol 2005;43:3800–6.

Jacobs RF, Schutze GE. *Bartonella henselae* as a cause of prolonged fever and fever of unknown origin in children. Clin Infect Dis 1998;26:80–4.

Massei F, Gori L, Machhia P, Maggiore G, et al. The extended spectrum of bartonellosis in children. Infect Dis Clin North Am 2005;19:691–711.

Raoult D, Fournier PE, Vandenesch F, et al. Outcome and treatment of *Bartonella* endocarditis. Arch of Int Med 2003;163:226–30.

Rolain JM, Brouqui P, Koehler JE, et al. Recommendations for treatment of human infection caused by *Bartonella* species. Antimicrob Agents Chemother 2004;48:1921–33.

Zangwill KM, Hamilton DH, Perkins BA, et al. Cat scratch disease in Connecticut: Epidemiology, risk factors, and evaluation of a new diagnostic test. N Engl J Med 1993;329:8–13.

Salmonellosis

Method of
Arvid E. Underman, MD, FACP, DTMH

Salmonellosis refers to a group of infections caused by members of the genus *Salmonella*. This genus is named after Salmon, a pathologist who first isolated the organism, later designated as *Salmonella choleraesuis*, from the intestine of pigs with diarrhea. *Salmonellae* are widely distributed throughout nature and are adapted to a myriad of warm and cold-blooded hosts. In humans there are four main clinical presentations:

1. Acute gastroenteritis
2. Bacteremia
3. Focal extraintestinal infection
4. Chronic carriage (Table 1)

Microbiology

Salmonellae are motile, Gram-stain negative, nonspore-forming bacilli that are differentiated from other *Enterobacteriaceae* by inability to ferment lactose and sucrose while producing acid, hydrogen sulfide, and gas (except *Salmonella typhi*). Members of the genus were more accurately classified into serotypes using the Kauffman-White schema that differentiated and grouped them serologically dependent on their lipopolysaccharide somatic (O) and flagellar (H) antigens.

More recently, DNA analysis has divided the genus into two species. Initially the first of the two species was named *Salmonella choleraesuis* and was divided into six subspecies, each of which was then divided into more than 2400 serotypes (serovars) by Kauffman-White methodology. The second species, *Salmonella Bongori*, is inconsequential. Serotypes were named historically from the host or the geographic locale of the first isolate, such as *Salmonella typhimurium* or *Salmonella dublin*. However, under the new DNA division, *choleraesuis* was both a species and a serotype. To avoid confusion the name *Salmonella enterica* has been widely adopted. The first of the six subspecies (Group I) is also named *enterica*. It contains the more than 1400 serotypes that occur in warm-blooded animals. Using nomenclature employed by the United States Centers for Disease Control and the World Health Organization (WHO), the species and subspecies name is understood; and the serotype is capitalized.

TABLE 1 Clinical Presentations of Salmonellosis

Acute gastroenteritis (90%–95% of cases)
Bacteremia (< 5% of cases)
- Transient during acute gastroenteritis
- Enteric fever (nontyphoid)
- Persistent or recurrent (especially HIV)
Focal complications following bacteremia
- Bronchopneumonia, empyema, chest wall abscess
- Aortitis with mycotic aneurysm
- Prosthetic graft or valve infection
- Endocarditis, endarteritis
- Osteomyelitis (especially with sickle cell anemia)
- Septic arthritis
- Soft tissue abscess
- Hepatic or splenic abscess
- Meningitis or brain abscess
- Suppurative urogenital disease
Carriage (asymptomatic)
- Convalescent excretors (<2 mo)
- Convalescent carriers (2–12 mo)
- Chronic carriers (> 12 mo)

Thus, the formal *S. enterica* subspecies *enterica* serotype *typhimurium* becomes simply *S. Typhimurium*, which except for the capital T is where we started!

Epidemiology

In the last 25 years, the incidence of nontyphoid salmonellosis has increased two- to threefold with approximately 1.5 million cases occurring annually in the United States. This is an underestimate because most cases are sporadic (endemic) and go unreported. Children younger than 5 years of age have the highest incidence of gastroenteritis and constitute the greatest number of cases.

Animals are the source of nontyphoid salmonella infection in humans. Infection occurs from food of animal origin such as meat, poultry, eggs, and dairy products. Contamination may occur during the production, slaughter, processing, or distribution of these products. Outbreaks have been associated with eggs, ice cream, and processed meats. Increasingly there have been outbreaks associated with raw vegetables (e.g., scallions) that are crosscontaminated during growth and distribution. Restaurant or home outbreaks occur in the context of improper preparation, cooking, and refrigeration. Most of the outbreaks can be attributed to centralized mass production and preparation of food along with globalization of the food trade. Novel sources of human salmonella include pet turtles, lizards, iguanas, African hedgehogs, rattlesnakes, and even marijuana contaminated by manure.

Emergence of antibiotic resistant species is a formidable problem. It is believed that resistance is driven worldwide by improper antibiotics use. However, in developed countries it is attributable to widespread use in animal feeds. Large numbers of transferable resistance plasmids have been described. Resistance rates of more than 50% to ampicillin, chloramphenicol (Chloromycetin), and trimethoprim-sulfamethoxazole (TMP-SMZ) (Bactrim) occur in parts of Asia, Africa, and Latin America. One strain of *S. Typhimurium* (DT104) is resistant to five antimicrobials; the three mentioned previously plus tetracycline and streptomycin. This organism has spread widely in livestock throughout the United States, Canada, United Kingdom, Europe, and the Middle East. Likewise, resistance to third-generation cephalosporins is increasing and is mediated by plasmids producing both regular and extended-spectrum beta-lactamases (ESBLs). Even more disturbing is fluoroquinolone resistance caused by mutated DNA gyrase, topoisomerase IV, or efflux pumps. The latter literally expel the quinolone from the bacterium before it can act on its target. Fluoroquinolone resistance is most pronounced in Southeast Asia, Europe, and the Middle East.

Pathogenesis

Human infection usually requires 10^6 organisms. Fewer organisms may cause disease in patients who have hypochlorhydria or achlorhydria, have impaired cellular immunity, are at the extremes of age, or are taking certain drugs (Table 2). *Salmonellae* predominately infect the terminal ileum and proximal colon through attachment. Initially host response is by neutrophils followed by lymphocytes and macrophages. Strains vary genetically in their virulence and invasiveness. The organisms can survive intracellularly, thus avoiding antibiotic agents that lack intracellular penetration. Bacteria that are not contained regionally in the gut or lymph nodes may enter the blood. There are many predisposing factors associated with this and subsequent focal complications (see Table 2).

Clinical Presentation

GASTOENTERITIS

Acute gastroenteritis is by far the most common clinical presentation of salmonellosis. It should be emphasized that there is considerable overlap in its presentation with other infectious intestinal pathogens such as *Campylobacter* species. Given this, the incubation ranges from 6 to 96 hours but most commonly occurs between 12 and 48 hours. Initial symptoms include nausea and vomiting, followed by headaches, myalgias, malaise, chills, low-grade fever, abdominal cramps, and diarrhea. High temperatures (40°C [104°F]) should alert the clinician to invasive disease. Stools may be merely loose or profuse and watery. On direct examination, they may or may not contain polymorphonuclear leukocytes or occult blood. The presence of mucus or gross blood in the absence of hemorrhoids or fissures should alert the clinician to organisms causing dysentery such as *Shigella* species. The white count is most often normal or slightly elevated, with a left shift containing 10 to 15 bands. Low white counts with greater numbers of bands should alert the clinician to possible bacteremia or enteric fever. The diagnosis can be confirmed only by stool or blood culture. Serum serology examinations are not helpful. Most healthy adults have a self-limited, uncomplicated course, with resolution of symptoms without treatment within 48 to 72 hours.

TABLE 2 Predisposing Factors for Salmonellosis

Gastrointestinal
- Achlorhydria
- Gastric surgery
- Inflammatory bowel disease
Immune or structural compromise
- Age (<6 mo, >60 y)
- Lymphoma
- Splenectomy
- Cirrhosis with portal hypertension
- Diabetes mellitus
- Chronic uremia
- Hemolytic anemia (iron overload)
- Sickle cell (bone infarct, autosplenectomy)
- Systemic lupus
- Atheromata, aortic aneurysm
Infections
- HIV/AIDS (decreased T-cells)
- Malaria
- Bartonellosis
- Schistosomiasis
Drugs
- H_2-blockers, $H+^+$ proton pump inhibitors
- Antibiotic administration
- Antimotility agents
- Chemotherapy
- Corticosteroids
- Transplant antirejection agents

CURRENT DIAGNOSIS

- More than 95% of nontyphoid Salmonellosis presents as uncomplicated acute gastroenteritis.
- The clinical presentation of different causes of gastro-enteritis and diarrhea overlaps significantly.
- The physician should be familiar with groups of patients at risk for complicated Salmonellosis.
- Specific diagnosis requires culture of the stool or blood.
- Focal complications are always suspect in high-risk patients who are blood culture positive for nontyphoid *Salmonellae* (e.g., aortitis or mycotic aneurysm in patients older than age 60 years with atherosclerosis).

Treatment

FLUID AND ELECTROLYTE REPLACEMENT

The sine qua non in the treatment of diarrhea is fluid and electrolyte replacement. In most cases increased oral intake of bland juices coupled with clear broth and temporary elimination of lactose-containing foods will suffice. Commercial electrolyte solutions (Pedialyte) may be useful. Although not readily available in the United States, rehydration salts are widely employed in many developing countries. WHO distributes packets containing its recommended formula of 90 mmol of sodium, 20 of potassium, 80 of chloride, 30 of bicarbonate, along with 111 mmol of glucose to dissolve in 1 L of sterile or boiled water. This mixture should be consumed at a rate sufficient to compensate for diarrheal losses while maintaining an adequate output of dilute appearing urine. Within 24 to 48 hours, the diet can be supplemented with bland, soft foods given in small, frequent feedings. If the patient has profuse vomiting or severe dehydration as determined by orthostatic changes in blood pressure, parenteral rehydration should be used. Frequently, this can be accomplished as an outpatient in an infusion room or with a home agency rather than through admission to hospital. When there is persistent emesis, profuse diarrhea, systemic toxicity, or abnormalities in serum electrolytes, parenteral rehydration in hospital is prudent.

ANTIMOTILITY AND ANTINAUSEA AGENTS

The use of agents such as atropine-diphenoxylate (Lomotil) or loperamide (Imodium) should be discouraged. Although they may result in symptomatic improvement in cramps and diarrhea, they can increase complications and even predispose to bacteremia. In general, if the patient has a fever and the diarrhea contains blood or mucus, their use should be eschewed. Most pediatricians feel they should never be used in children younger than 5 years of age. An alternative is bismuth subsalicylate (Pepto-Bismol). The adult dose is 1 ounce (2 tablespoons) or 2 tablets (262.5 mg) every 30 minutes for 8 hours. The pediatric dose is 1.1 mL/kg at 4-hour intervals for up to 5 days. Although nausea and vomiting are occasional presenting symptoms with enterocolitis, they rarely persist. Prochlorperazine (Compazine) or trimethobenzamide (Tigan) may be helpful. Both are available in oral, suppository, or parenteral form, even though injectable prochlorperazine (Compazine) has been in short supply. Suppositories usually stimulate further diarrhea. Vomiting may preclude oral administration. A singular muscular injection of prochlorperazine (Compazine) 5 to 10 mg, is often all that is needed. This may be repeated every 4 to 6 hours as needed. Promethazine hydrochloride (Phenergan) is more frequently used in children and may be used orally (0.5 mg/pound or 1 mg/kg every 6 hours) or intramuscularly in the same doses. A 5-HT$_3$ receptor antagonist such as ondansetron (Zofran)[1] is expensive and inefficacious.

 CURRENT THERAPY

- Fluid and electrolyte replacement is of paramount importance.
- The physician should avoid routine empiric antibiotic in acute uncomplicated patients.
- The physician should avoid antimotility agents for diarrhea presenting with fever or with mucus and blood present.
- More than 95% of patients with nontyphoid salmonellosis *will get better* on their own.
- Fluoroquinolone antibiotics should be reserved for when they are truly indicated clinically.
- Increasing resistance mandates sensitivity testing (including tests for ESBL) to guide therapy of bacteremia and its complications.
- Do not prescribe *prophylactic* antibiotics to prevent diarrhea in travelers.
- Stress personal hygiene and prudent food choice with proper preparation.

Abbreviation: ESBL = extended spectrum beta lactamases.

ANTIBIOTICS

The routine empiric use of antibiotics, especially fluoroquinolones, for any and all cases of diarrhea is not only unjustifiable but should be decried. Certainly antibiotics are not needed in the treatment of uncomplicated *Salmonella* gastroenteritis in otherwise healthy children or adults. Studies have shown that they neither shorten the course nor improve symptoms. No doubt some of this usage is patient driven. However, overuse is contributing to the emergence of resistance, and may increase risk of symptomatic and bacteriologic relapse. Indeed antibiotic use may actually prolong the convalescent excretion or contribute to chronic carriage of the organism. Postponing antibiotic therapy until the return of a stool culture often provides the physician with a way to avert the frequent demand for antibiotic therapy. Often patients are better by the time results become available. Nevertheless, high-risk patients, as previously identified (see Table 2), should receive treatment to prevent potential complications from bacteremia. Additionally, if patients are sick enough to require hospitalization, antibiotic therapy should be considered.

Appropriate antibiotic therapy should be guided by susceptibility testing. Initially, TMP-SMZ (cotrimoxazole, Bactrim, or Septra)[1] may be administered to the nonsulfonamide-sensitive patient. The dose is 5 to 8 mg/kg trimethoprim every 12 hours for children or 1 double-strength tablet (160 mg trimethoprim/800 mg sulfamethoxazole) every 12 hours for adults. Although widely used, trimethoprim-sulfamethoxazole has not yet received FDA approval. If the organism is susceptible, ampicillin, 50 mg/kg orally to 100 mg/kg/day intravenously, each in four divided doses for children, or 2 to 4 g/day in four divided doses for adults, may be administered. Amoxicillin (Amoxil)[1] in equivalent oral dosage may be substituted. The duration of therapy is generally 5 days.

Newer fluoroquinolone antibiotics, such as ciprofloxacin,[1] ofloxacin,[1] and norfloxacin,[1] are among the most effective agents with excellent oral bioavailability and intracellular concentration. They are contraindicated in prepubertal children and pregnant women. Adult doses are ciprofloxacin (Cipro), 500 mg twice daily; ofloxacin (Floxin), 400 mg twice daily; or norfloxacin (Noroxin), 400 mg twice daily. It must be emphasized that the trend in the United States to use these agents empirically for all suspected bacterial diarrhea should be vigorously resisted by the thoughtful clinician.

[1]Not FDA approved for this indication.

[1]Not FDA approved for this indication.

Bacteremia and Focal Infection

Bacteremia in acute uncomplicated *Salmonella* gastroenteritis is infrequent. Therefore, blood cultures are not routinely necessary except for patients who are in high-risk categories. Shaking chills or high fever (40°C [104°F]) should alert the clinician to possible bacteremia. Focal suppurative infection following bacteremia is also infrequent but may occur at any site. Thus, *Salmonella* has been associated with bronchopneumonia, soft tissue infection, aortic mycotic aneurysms, endocarditis, septic arthritis, splenic or hepatic abscesses, meningitis, and osteomyelitis. The clinician should suspect an endovascular mycotic aneurysm in all blood culture positive patients older than 50 years of age. *Salmonella* should always be suspected in individuals with sickle cell disease in whom bone and joint infection is the most frequent cause of extraintestinal infection. Meningitis occurs primarily in infants younger than 5 months of age. The diagnosis of a *Salmonella* bacteremia in HIV patients will almost always be accompanied by recurrent episodes.

Treatment

ANTIBIOTICS

Bacteremia and localized suppurative infection require antibiotic therapy. The choice of effective treatment is less predictable with the emergence of resistance. Therapy must be altered according to the results of susceptibility testing. Therefore the recovery of the organism is extremely important, and adequate cultures of blood or infected material must be obtained before initiation of therapy.

Parenteral ampicillin, 100 to 200 mg/kg/day divided into four doses, or TMP/SMZ,[1] 8 to 10 mg/kg of trimethoprim per day in three divided doses, may be used. In the case of resistance or allergy to the foregoing, third-generation cephalosporins such as cefotaxime (Claforan) or ceftriaxone (Rocephin) have reasonable activity, but intracellular concentrations are not optimal. Cefotaxime, 1 to 2 grams every 6 to 8 hours for adults, or 100 to 200 mg/kg/day in three or four divided doses for children, has been found effective in bacteremia, osteomyelitis, septic arthritis, and a variety of other focal *Salmonella* infections. The use of chloramphenicol (Chloromycetin) is not recommended but a preparation of it in oil (Typhomycine)[2] is in use in developing countries. Ciprofloxacin (Cipro)[1] 7.5 mg/kg intravenously twice daily is becoming a favored agent; not only is it effective but oral bioequivalence facilitates the change to 500 to 750 mg by mouth twice daily. If fluoroquinolone resistance is encountered, imipenem (Primaxin)[1] may be tried. Efficacy data for it or other agents such as azithromycin (Zithromax)[1] are scant.

SURGERY

Focal infection often requires surgery. Often this is as simple as the drainage of localized suppuration or lavage of a septic joint. However, in the case of infected aortic aneurysms, extensive resection and vascular reconstruction are required. Infected prosthetic grafts must be removed in nearly all cases with courses of antibiotics before and after surgery.

The duration of therapy for simple bacteremia is 10 to 14 days. Septic arthritis is usually treated 4 weeks whereas osteomyelitis and endovascular infections require 6 weeks. Oral fluoroquinolones such as ciprofloxacin (Cipro), 500 mg twice daily, may be helpful in treating osteomyelitis. TMP-SMZ (Bactrim)[1] can also be used in this manner. Both have adequate blood levels after oral administration. I have had to use continuous prophylaxis of either TMP-SMZ or ciprofloxacin in several HIV patients to prevent recurrent bacteremia. Because prophylactic TMP-SMZ is used chronically for *Pneumocystis*, it may be preferred.

---

[1]Not FDA approved for this indication.
[2]Not available in the United States.

Enteric Fever

The clinical picture of nontyphoid *Salmonella* enteric fever is indistinguishable from that of typhoid fever, which is discussed elsewhere in this publication. However, the following discussion also applies to enteric fever caused by nontyphoid *Salmonellae*.

TREATMENT

The adjunct and antibiotic therapy of nontyphoid enteric fever parallels that of the treatment of typhoid. Antibiotics should be adjusted and altered once the results of susceptibility testing are available. Acceptable regimens include ampicillin, amoxicillin,[1] and TMP-SMZ (Bactrim),[1] along with third-generation cephalosporins and fluoroquinolone antibiotics. My preference was cefotaxime (Claforan)[1] in the same doses as for bacteremic salmonellosis. The duration is 10 to 14 days. Relapse rates are low and is seen within 2 to 6 weeks. Relapse requires an equivalent course of therapy in both dose and duration. Currently, I prefer ciprofloxacin (Cipro)[1] intravenously 7.5 mg/kg every 12 hours continued until the patient is afebrile and clinically able to start it orally. Comparative studies are ongoing using both third-generation cephalosporins, such as ceftriaxone (Rocephin)[1] or cefixime (Suprax),[1] and oral fluoroquinolones in short-course therapy of typhoid as well as nontyphoid enteric fever. Although these show some promise, they are currently not the standard of practice in the United States. Nevertheless, a strong case can be made for oral fluoroquinolones use, with obvious cost saving. Otherwise healthy young adults may be treated orally as outpatients. This advantage, if for no other reason, should *prevent* the physician from prescribing quinolones for uncomplicated gastroenteritis or other self-limited diarrheas of bacterial origin.

Adjunctive measures are of importance, including attention to fluid and electrolyte balance and nutrition. As in typhoid the routine use of corticosteroids is controversial. Use in patients who are steroid dependent or believed to be hypoadrenal is indicated. In those who are delirious, obtunded, comatose, or in shock it may be warranted; but there are little supportive data. It has been my overall impression that nontyphoid enteric fever is somewhat milder than typhoid itself, and complications such as gastrointestinal bleeding or ileal perforation are exceedingly rare.

Carrier State

Asymptomatic excretion of organisms invariably occurs following clinical *Salmonella* gastroenteritis. It exceeds 8 weeks in 5% to 10% of patients. Chronic carriage, either in the stool or urine, is defined as excretion of the organism for more than 1 year. Its incidence is stated to be 1% in adults and 5% in children younger than 5 years of age. This is somewhat less than that seen with *S. typhi*. Convalescent excreters need only maintain strict personal hygiene to prevent transmission of the organism. Those involved in food preparation or in child and health care should be kept off work until three successive cultures are negative at intervals required by the public health department. It goes without saying that all positive cases of salmonellosis are reportable by law to local public health authorities.

Recently, oral quinolones have been used (ciprofloxacin [Cipro],[1] 500 to 750 mg twice daily for 5 to 14 days), to curtail institutional outbreaks, as in nursing homes or psychiatric facilities. Although this may be expeditious, eliminating or preventing the source of the outbreak in a prospective fashion is preferable. In the case of food handlers and health or child care workers, some feel that quinolone therapy eliminates the problem of convalescent excretion, hence individuals may return to work without delay. The data are debatable and the successive negative stool requirement will not be obviated.

---

[1]Not FDA approved for this indication.

The management of the chronic carriage of nontyphoidal salmonellosis is the same as that of *S. typhi*, which is discussed in detail elsewhere. A 4- to 6-week course of oral antibiotics may be tried when no evidence of gallbladder disease exists. However, if chronic cholecystitis and/or cholelithiasis are present, cholecystectomy is almost always necessary. Despite cholecystectomy, a certain number of individuals will continue to excrete organisms thought to be of hepatobiliary origin. Chronic carriage is seen, albeit rarely, in the United States with either *Schistosoma mansoni* or *Schistosoma haematobium*. When these parasites are treated, subsequent therapy of the *Salmonella* results in termination of the stool or urinary carrier state.

Prevention

Prevention of salmonellosis has both personal and public health dimensions. Food and leftovers should be rapidly refrigerated. I recommend separate plastic (not wood) cutting boards for meats and vegetables that are washed after each use. Spillage of raw animal juices should be immediately cleaned. All preparation surfaces should be washed and dried after each meal. Detergent rather than antibacterial cleaners should be used; bleach is beautiful.

Public health surveillance is essential with regular inspection of restaurants, food retailers, and industrial food processors. National efforts to coordinate and computerize surveillance systems such as FoodNet should be expanded and fully funded so as to guarantee our food supply. Preservation technologies including irradiation need study.

Finally, the practicing physician should take the time to reiterate to patients with HIV or malignancies or other immune compromised patients (see Table 2) how they can avoid food-borne pathogens.

REFERENCES

Brenner FW, Villar RG, Angulo FJ, et al. Salmonella nomenclature. J Clin Microbiol 2000;38:2465.

Fierer J, Swancutt M. Non-typhoid *Salmonella*: A review. In: Remington JS, Swartz MN, editors. Current Clinical Topics in Infectious Diseases 20. Boston: Blackwell Science; 2000. p. 134–57.

Herikstad H, Hayes P, Mokhtar M, et al. Emerging quinolone-resistant Salmonella in the United States. Emerg Infect Dis 1997;3:371–2.

Molbak K. Human health consequences of antimicrobial drug resistant *Salmonella* and other foodborne pathogens. Clin Infect Dis 2005;41:1613–20.

Sirinivan S, Garner P. Antibiotics for treating Salmonella gut infections. Cochrane Database Sys Rev 2000;93:CD001167.

Su LH, Chiu CH, Chu CS, et al. Antimicrobial resistance in nontyphoid *Salmonella*: A global challenge. Clin Infect Dis 2004;39:546–51.

Voetsch AC, Van Gilder TJ, Angulo FJ, et al. FoodNet estimate of the burden of illness caused by nontyphoidal Salmonella infections in the United States. Clin Infect Dis 2004;38(Suppl. 3):S127–S134.

Typhoid Fever

Method of
Tamilarasu Kadhiravan, MD

Typhoid fever is a bacteremic infection caused by the gram-negative bacillus *Salmonella enterica* serotype Typhi. *S. Paratyphi* also causes an illness clinically indistinguishable from typhoid fever. Humans are the only known host of *S.* Typhi, and it is transmitted by ingestion of contaminated food or water. Improvement in sanitation and hygiene led to the elimination of typhoid fever from the developed world long before the advent of antibiotics. On the other hand, in parts of the world lacking sanitation, it continues to be an important cause of febrile illness despite the availability of effective antibiotics.

Epidemiology

Typhoid fever is endemic in the developing world, especially the South and South East Asian countries of India, Nepal, Pakistan, Bangladesh, Vietnam, and Indonesia. Annual incidence in endemic settings is typically more than 100 cases per 100,000 population, and it predominantly affects children and young adults. Apart from sick persons with typhoid fever, convalescent carriers and asymptomatically infected food handlers (long-term carriers) are the sources of infection. Potential vehicles of infection include food or water consumed from roadside eateries, ice cubes and ice cream made from contaminated water, and raw vegetables and fruits. In contrast, most cases of typhoid fever in developed countries are imported by travel, especially to the Indian subcontinent.

Pathogenesis and Clinical Features

Following ingestion, the bacilli invade and multiply in the small intestinal lymphoid tissue before entering the bloodstream. This primary bacteremia leads to widespread seeding of the reticuloendothelial system and intestinal lymphoid tissue, where the infection is amplified and spills over into the circulation. Onset of symptoms usually coincides with this secondary bacteremia. Interestingly, unlike other Gram-negative bacteremic infections, septic shock develops relatively late in the course of illness, and the infection can be eminently cured by oral antibiotic therapy. Nonetheless, it should be emphasized that any delay in initiating antibiotic therapy increases the risk of complications (Box 1).

During the first week, temperature gradually increases in a stepladder fashion. Localizing symptoms are usually minimal. Anorexia, lassitude, and malaise are often marked. Headache and vomiting are common; however, a supple neck helps rule out meningitis. Abdominal symptoms such as constipation, loose stools, and abdominal pain are not infrequent, but they are nonspecific and often overlooked. Soft, tender enlargement of liver or spleen is seen in about half the patients. Rose spots and relative bradycardia, though classic, are rare. When the infection goes untreated, hypertrophied lymphoid tissue of the Peyer's patches can ulcerate toward the end of the second week, resulting in torrential gastrointestinal bleeding, small intestinal perforation, and secondary bacterial peritonitis. Patients with severe illness can present with a muttering delirium described as *coma vigil*.

BOX 1   Complications of typhoid fever

Abdominal
Paralytic ileus
Intestinal hemorrhage
Intestinal perforation
Secondary peritonitis
Symptomatic liver dysfunction
Acalculous cholecystitis

Long-term
Gallbladder cancer

Extra-abdominal
Encephalopathy
Cerebellar dysfunction
Myocarditis
Osteomyelitis and soft tissue abscesses
Multiorgan dysfunction syndrome
Hemophagocytic syndrome
Hemolysis
Glomerulonephritis

Untreated typhoid fever often resolves spontaneously in about 4 to 6 weeks. However, the risk of death is high (>10%), and relapses are frequent. Many patients excrete *S.* Typhi in feces and urine during convalescence (convalescent carriers), and some of them continue to excrete beyond 1 year (long-term carriers).

Current Pattern of Antimicrobial Susceptibility

Since 1990, a sea change has occurred in the antimicrobial susceptibility of *S.* Typhi in endemic countries and elsewhere. Unregulated use of fluoroquinolones has resulted in emergence of *S.* Typhi strains with decreased susceptibility. These strains have a subthreshold increase in minimal inhibitory concentration that is not detected by conventional disk-diffusion testing. Resistance to nalidixic acid (NegGram) (a quinolone) is a surrogate marker for such strains. In fact, most infections in the community are now caused by nalidixic acid–resistant *S.* Typhi (NARST). Not surprisingly, this change is reflected in far-away geographic locales such as the United States and the United Kingdom.

Diagnosis

Clinical features are nonspecific, and laboratory testing is essential to confirm a diagnosis of typhoid fever. A soft splenomegaly, absence of leukocytosis, mild leukopenia, and modest elevation of transaminases are subtle pointers to a diagnosis of typhoid fever. Blood culture drawn early in the illness before initiation of antibiotics is often fruitful and is the gold standard for the diagnosis of typhoid fever. The time-honored Widal test, which detects agglutinating antibodies to somatic and flagellar antigens of *S.* Typhi, adds little to decision making. Initial enthusiasm about rapid serologic tests such as Typhidot and Tubex TF has not been confirmed in community-based studies. None of these tests are sensitive enough to rule out typhoid. In a patient who has nonlocalizing acute febrile illness lasting more than 5 to 7 days in a suggestive epidemiologic setting (residence in or travel to endemic area; outbreaks), it is prudent to treat presumptively for typhoid fever, after reasonably ruling out competing diagnoses such as malaria, dengue, leptospirosis, and rickettsial infection.

CURRENT DIAGNOSIS

- Typhoid fever typically manifests as an undifferentiated acute febrile illness.
  Soft splenomegaly, normal or low white cell count, and elevated liver enzymes are subtle diagnostic pointers.
- Blood culture, drawn before antibiotic administration, is the most useful investigation.
- Consider presumptive treatment in appropriate epidemiologic settings.

Treatment

Fluoroquinolones (ciprofloxacin [Cipro] or ofloxacin [Floxin][1] 7.5 mg/kg twice a day for 5 to 7 days) are unparalleled in efficacy for treating fully susceptible *S.* Typhi strains. However, their use is associated with frequent treatment failures, prolonged defervescence, and higher rates of complications in NARST infections. Given the widespread emergence of NARST, fluoroquinolones are no longer to be considered the drug of choice. Several alternatives have been evaluated in randomized, controlled trials for treating uncomplicated typhoid fever caused by NARST (Table 1). Ease of oral administration, proven efficacy, and safety make azithromycin (Zithromax)[1] a reasonable first choice for uncomplicated typhoid fever. In hospitalized seriously ill patients and treatment failures, parenteral ceftriaxone (Rocephin)[1] is preferred. Usually, it takes about 4 to 7 days for defervescence after the initiation of antibiotics. Antipyretics should be used for symptom relief; ibuprofen (Motrin; 10 mg/kg every 6 hours) is superior to acetaminophen (Tylenol; 12 mg/kg every 6 hours). However, ibuprofen should be avoided when dengue fever is a possibility. A soft, low-residue diet is traditionally advised to prevent intestinal perforation. Such a practice, however, is not founded on scientific evidence. Treatment of *S.* Paratyphi infection is identical to that of *S.* Typhi infection.

[1]Not FDA approved for this indication.

TABLE 1 Outcomes of Alternative Treatments for Nalidixic Acid–Resistant *S.* Typhi (NARST) Infection Evaluated in Randomized, Controlled Trials

Drug	Dosage	Fever Clearance Time (Median or Mean)	Rate of Treatment Failure	Relapse Rate	Comments
High-dose ofloxacin (Floxin)[1]	10 mg/kg[3] bid × 7 d	8.2 d	36%	< 1%; insufficient data	Not recommended
Gatifloxacin (Tequin)[2]	10 mg/kg qd × 7 d	4.4 d	9%	3%	Serious concerns about dysglycemia
Azithromycin (Zithromax)[1]	10-20[3] mg/kg qd × 7 d	4.4 d	9%	< 1%; insufficient data	Unproven in complicated typhoid fever
Cefixime (Suprax)[1]	10 mg/kg[3] bid × 7 d	5.8 d	27%	9%	High cost; not recommended
Ceftriaxone* (Rocephin)[1]	60-75 mg/kg qd × 10-14 d	6.1 d	9%	5%	High relapse rate (14%) with 7-day regimen

Data from Dolecek C, Tran TP, Nguyen NR, et al: A multi-center randomised controlled trial of gatifloxacin versus azithromycin for the treatment of uncomplicated typhoid fever in children and adults in Vietnam. PLoS One 2008;3:e2188; Pandit A, Arjyal A, Day JN, et al: An open randomized comparison of gatifloxacin versus cefixime for the treatment of uncomplicated enteric fever. PLoS One 2007;2:e542; and Parry CM, Ho VA, Phuong le T, et al: Randomized controlled comparison of ofloxacin, azithromycin, and an ofloxacin-azithromycin combination for treatment of multidrug-resistant and nalidixic acid-resistant typhoid fever. Antimicrob Agents Chemother 2007;51:819.
[1]Not FDA approved for this indication.
[2]Not available in the United States.
[3]Exceeds dosage recommended by the manufacturer.
*No trials on treatment of NARST infection; extrapolated data from Parry CM, Hien TT, Dougan G, White NJ, Farrar JJ: Typhoid fever. N Engl J Med 2002;347 (22):1770-1782.

CURRENT THERAPY

- Decreased susceptibility to fluoroquinolones is widespread among *Salmonella enterica* serotype Typhi.
- High-dose fluoroquinolones are suboptimal for treating such infections.
- Azithromycin (Zithromax)[1] is the preferred drug for uncomplicated typhoid fever.
- Ceftriaxone (Rocephin)[1] is preferred for treating hospitalized and seriously ill patients.

[1]Not FDA approved for this indication.

Prevention

Sustained improvement in sanitation and access to safe drinking water are essential to control typhoid fever in endemic areas. Avoiding potentially contaminated food and beverages and pretravel vaccination decrease the risk of typhoid fever among travelers (see the article on travel medicine). Recently, mass administration of the Vi polysaccharide vaccine (Typhim Vi, Typherix [outside United States]) has been found to confer herd immunity and is a potential tool for the control of typhoid fever in endemic settings.

REFERENCES

Bhutta ZA. Current concepts in the diagnosis and treatment of typhoid fever. BMJ 2006;333:78.

Dolecek C, Tran TP, Nguyen NR, et al. A multi-center randomised controlled trial of gatifloxacin versus azithromycin for the treatment of uncomplicated typhoid fever in children and adults in Vietnam. PLoS ONE 2008;3:e2188.

Dutta S, Sur D, Manna B, et al. Evaluation of new-generation serologic tests for the diagnosis of typhoid fever: data from a community-based surveillance in Calcutta, India. Diagn Microbiol Infect Dis 2006;56:359.

Effa EE, Bukirwa H. Azithromycin for treating uncomplicated typhoid and paratyphoid fever (enteric fever). Cochrane Database Syst Rev 2008;(4): CD006083.

Lynch MF, Blanton EM, Bulens S, et al. Typhoid fever in the United States, 1999–2006. JAMA 2009;302:859.

Ochiai RL, Acosta CJ, Danovaro-Holliday MC, et al. A study of typhoid fever in five Asian countries: Disease burden and implications for controls. Bull World Health Organ 2008;86:260.

Pandit A, Arjyal A, Day JN, et al. An open randomized comparison of gatifloxacin versus cefixime for the treatment of uncomplicated enteric fever. PLoS ONE 2007;2:e542.

Parry CM, Ho VA, Phuong le T, et al. Randomized controlled comparison of ofloxacin, azithromycin, and an ofloxacin-azithromycin combination for treatment of multidrug-resistant and nalidixic acid-resistant typhoid fever. Antimicrob Agents Chemother 2007;51:819.

Vinh H, Parry CM, Hanh VT, et al. Double blind comparison of ibuprofen and paracetamol for adjunctive treatment of uncomplicated typhoid fever. Pediatr Infect Dis J 2004;23:226.

Rickettsial and Ehrlichial Infections (Rocky Mountain Spotted Fever and Typhus)

Method of
Deverick J. Anderson, MD, and
Daniel J. Sexton, MD

Rickettsial Infections

ROCKY MOUNTAIN SPOTTED FEVER

Rocky Mountain spotted fever (RMSF) is the most lethal of several tickborne illnesses that occur in the United States. Between 20% and 25% of infections are fatal if not treated appropriately. *Rickettsia rickettsii*, the obligate intracellular bacterium that causes RMSF, circulates in nature in a complex cycle between ticks and small rodents. Humans are only occasional and accidental hosts for this organism.

Epidemiology

RMSF is a highly seasonal disease that predominantly occurs in the spring and early summer months; cases occasionally occur in the autumn and even the winter in warmer climates. RMSF occurs with varying frequency in western Canada, much of the continental United States, Mexico, Central America, Brazil, and Colombia. The incidence of RMSF varies by geographic area and, although reporting of cases of RMSF is primarily through passive surveillance, the average reported annual incidence of RMSF is approximately 2.2 cases per 1 million persons.

Pathogenesis

In the United States, *R. rickettsii* is primarily transmitted by *Dermacentor variabilis* (the American dog tick) in the eastern United States and *Dermacentor andersoni* (the wood tick) in the western United States. Recently, *Rhipicephalus sanguineus* (the common brown dog tick) was recognized as the vector for RMSF in an outbreak in eastern Arizona; this finding is not surprising because this vector also transmits RMSF in Mexico and Central America. Although most infections occur after a tick bite, transmission rarely occurs from crushing or removing infected ticks from humans or animals. Indeed, infection can be experimentally induced with aerosols of infected tick tissues or by mucosal contact. Tick bites are painless and often go unnoticed. Thus, many patients with RMSF have no knowledge of a tick bite prior to the onset of their illness.

Clinical Features and Diagnosis

After inoculation from a tick bite, *R. rickettsii* proliferates and spreads throughout the body via the bloodstream and lymphatics, as well as by contiguous spread from cell to cell. *R. rickettsii* has a specific tropism for endothelial cells, resulting in widespread vasculitis, increased vascular permeability, edema, and activation of the humoral inflammatory and coagulation mechanisms. Organ dysfunction, hypovolemia, and shock can result from microvascular thrombosis and hemorrhage. Risk factors associated with increased severity and fatal outcomes include increasing age, male gender, diabetes mellitus, glucose-6-phosphate dehydrogenase (G6PD) deficiency, alcohol use, and delay in effective therapy for longer than 6 days after onset of symptoms.

The incubation period for RMSF ranges from 2 to 14 days. Most patients with RMSF develop a rash between the third and fifth days of illness. The typical rash of RMSF begins on the ankles and wrists and spreads both centrally and to the palms and soles. The skin rash often begins as a macular or maculopapular eruption and then usually becomes petechial. As many as 10% of patients do not, however, develop a rash (*spotless RMSF*). Additionally, the rash can be difficult to recognize in patients with dark skin.

Other symptoms of RMSF are nonspecific and include fever, headache, myalgias, malaise, and anorexia. As the disease progresses and becomes more severe, symptoms such as cough, bleeding, nausea, vomiting, abdominal pain, edema (especially in children), delirium, and focal neurologic symptoms (including seizures) can occur. In the absence of the classic triad of tick bite, fever, and rash, patients with RMSF may be erroneously believed to have an array of other infections such as ehrlichiosis, infectious mononucleosis, viral hepatitis, viral meningitis, measles, influenza, toxic shock syndrome, meningococcemia, leptospirosis, or typhoid fever. Because of shared residence and shared risks for tick exposure, family clusters of infection occasionally occur. When such clusters do occur, assumed person-to-person transmission of a viral or bacterial pathogen may lead to misdiagnosis and delay in treatment. If ineffective antibiotics are prescribed empirically before a typical rash appears, patients with RMSF may be erroneously assumed to have a drug eruption. Such cases can end tragically if the rash is presumed to occur because of (ineffective) drug therapy rather than in spite of it.

Most patients with RMSF have normal white blood cell (WBC) counts. As the severity of illness progresses, thrombocytopenia almost always develops, and WBC counts can become quite low. Although fibrinogen concentrations may be low and fibrin split products can become elevated in patients with RMSF, disseminated intravascular coagulation is uncommon. Other common laboratory abnormalities in patients with RMSF include hyponatremia, elevated serum transaminases, hyperbilirubinemia, and elevated creatinine.

There is no timely diagnostic test for RMSF in the early phase of illness. Thus, it is imperative that therapy be based on individual clinical features and the epidemiologic setting. Patients who have symptoms suggesting RMSF and who present in the spring or summer in an endemic area usually require empiric therapy.

Treatment

The preferred therapy is doxycycline (Vibramycin) 100 mg orally or intravenously every 12 hours for adults and children who weigh more than 45 kg. For children younger than 8 years or for children older than 8 years but weighing less than 45 kg, the dose is 2.2 mg/kg divided into two doses (maximum dose 200 mg/day).[1] In severe cases, adjunctive therapy such as mechanical ventilation, oxygen therapy, or hemodialysis may be necessary and useful.

The optimal duration of therapy is unknown. Doxycycline can usually be discontinued 2 or 3 days after the patient becomes afebrile. Most clinicians treat patients with RMSF for 7 to 10 days, but this is probably longer than is necessary for cure in all but the most severe cases. Therapy can and should be discontinued within 4 or 5 days in children with RMSF who respond promptly to treatment because the risk of dental staining is minimal when short courses of doxycycline are given. In general, doxycycline use should be avoided in pregnant women. Instead, pregnant women should be given chloramphenicol (Chloromycetin) 500 mg intravenously or orally every 6 hours. Doxycycline may, however, be the preferred agent for treatment of RMSF in pregnant women at the end of pregnancy because chloramphenicol use in such situations can result in the gray baby syndrome, a potentially fatal drug reaction due to chloramphenicol's effect on bilirubin conjugation in term infants.

CURRENT DIAGNOSIS

- There are no widely available tests to rapidly and accurately diagnose Rocky Mountain spotted fever (RMSF) in its early phases.
- If morulae are not found in patients with HME or HGA, the diagnosis cannot be established with certainty in the acute phases of these illnesses.

Although the diagnosis of RMSF can rarely be made in its acute phase by immunohistochemical staining of skin biopsy samples or by polymerase chain reaction, these diagnostic techniques are available only in a few large referral centers. In routine practice, the diagnosis of RMSF is usually proved long after symptoms and treatment have ceased. The mainstay of diagnosis is indirect fluorescent antibody testing, which is available through all state health laboratories. Antibodies typically appear 10 to 12 days after the onset of illness. The optimal time to obtain a convalescent antibody titer is 14 to 21 days after the onset of symptoms. The minimum diagnostic titer in most laboratories is 1:64.

Prevention

Prevention of many cases of RMSF is impossible because ticks are ubiquitous and many patients with RMSF are unaware of having had a tick bite. Persons with frequent exposure to tick-infested environments should frequently inspect their bodies and clothes for ticks. Early detection and removal of attached ticks can prevent disease transmission. Several hours of feeding are usually required for an infected tick to transmit *R. rickettsii*; thus, RMSF might not occur if infected ticks are removed during this preactivation period. Embedded ticks should be carefully removed by tweezers or by fingers shielded by a cloth, tissues, paper towels, or gloves. Prophylactic antimicrobial therapy is *not* recommended following tick exposure, because only a minuscule percentage of ticks in endemic areas are infected with *R. rickettsii*.

OTHER RICKETTSIAL INFECTIONS

Rickettsiae other than *R. rickettsii* can also cause human infection. For example, a single case of *Rickettsia parkeri* infection was reported in an otherwise healthy 40-year-old man from coastal Virginia in 2002. *R. parkeri* was first isolated from Gulf Coast ticks in the southern United States more than 60 years ago, but until this Virginia case was recognized, *R. parkeri* was not known to cause infections in humans. The patient presented with symptoms similar to those of RMSF and multiple eschars on his lower extremities. Erythematous papules, which then developed into eschars, preceded the other symptoms by 4 days. The patient failed to respond to other antibiotics but improved with doxycycline therapy. Subsequently, the authors of a serologic study of 15 patients with presumed RMSF reported that four of these 15 patients had higher titers for *R. parkeri* than for *R. rickettsii*, suggesting that infection with *R. parkeri* may be more common than previously realized and that some patients with presumed RMSF actually have *R. parkeri* infection.

Ehrlichial Infections

Ehrlichia and *Anaplasma* are obligate intracellular bacteria that grow within membrane-bound vacuoles in human and animal leukocytes. As yet, there is no clear understanding of the mechanism by which *Ehrlichia* produces disease in humans. Humans infected with *Ehrlichia* do not show tissue necrosis, abscess formation, or a severe inflammatory response. Ehrlichial and anaplasmal infections do not lead to vasculitis, thrombosis, or acute endothelial injury as seen in rickettsial infections. *Ehrlichia* replicates within phagosomes in infected leukocytes and produces intracellular colonies called *morulae*.

Ehrlichiosis typically leads to one of two types of illness in humans: human monocytotropic ehrlichiosis (HME) caused by *Ehrlichia chafeensis* or human granulocytic anaplasmosis (HGA) caused by *Anaplasma phagocytophilum*.

EPIDEMIOLOGY

Like other tickborne diseases, the actual incidence of ehrlichiosis is difficult to ascertain because reporting is based on a passive surveillance system that undoubtedly fails to detect or report many cases.

The best available evidence suggests that HME has an annual incidence of approximately 0.7 cases per 1 million persons and primarily occurs in the southeastern, south-central, and mid-Atlantic regions of the United States. *E. chafeensis* was first isolated from a soldier in Fort Chaffee, Arkansas, in 1990. Since then, cases of HME have been recognized in New England and the Pacific Northwest as well. First described in 1994, HGA has an annual incidence of approximately 1.6 cases per 1 million persons and has been described in the upper Midwest, California, and almost the entire Atlantic seaboard.

PATHOGENESIS

The principal vector of *E. chafeensis* is *Amblyomma americanum* (the Lone Star tick); the principal vector of *A. phagocytophilum* is *Ixodes scapularis* (the black-legged tick) in the eastern United States and *I. pacificus* (the western black-legged tick) in the western United States. As opposed to rickettsia, survival of ehrlichia requires horizontal transmission by ticks to and persistent infection in a wild vertebrate host (typically the white-tailed deer or white-footed mouse).

At least two other ehrlichial genogroups cause human disease. Infection of the neutrophils by *E. ewingii* causes mild disease that has mainly been diagnosed in immunocompromised patients in the Midwest. The ehrlichial-like *Neorickettsia sennetsu* group causes a mild mononucleosis-like illness that has never been reported outside East and Southeast Asia.

CLINICAL FEATURES AND DIAGNOSIS

Both HGE and HMA typically occur from May to September and have similar symptoms. After an incubation period of 7 to 14 days, patients most often present with fever, malaise, myalgias, headaches, and chills. An important minority of patients have nausea, vomiting, arthralgias, cough, or neurologic symptoms including altered mental status or stiff neck. Rash is uncommon in ehrlichiosis, though a faint rash occurs more commonly in patients with HGE than in those with HMA. When a rash is present as a prominent sign, coinfection with another rickettsial or other tickborne pathogen should be suspected. Rarely, patients with severe illness develop meningoencephalitis, septic shock, respiratory insufficiency, congestive heart failure, and acute renal failure.

Mortality rates of 3% for patients with HGE and 1% for patients with HMA have been reported, but these numbers may be inaccurate because many mild cases or cases that are empirically treated with doxycycline escape detection or definitive diagnosis. Immunocompromised patients may have severe illnesses and higher mortality rates.

The most common laboratory abnormalities seen in patients with ehrlichiosis are leukopenia and thrombocytopenia, but elevated serum transaminases, lactate dehydrogenase, and alkaline phosphatase levels also occur commonly. Cerebrospinal fluid abnormalities including pleocytosis are common and can mimic the changes seen in patients with viral or other forms of aseptic meningitis.

Distinguishing between RMSF and ehrlichiosis on the basis of clinical features may be impossible, although the presence of leukopenia and the absence of rash are more typical of ehrlichiosis. There are five methods to diagnose ehrlichiosis:

- Examination of peripheral blood or buffy coat for the presence of characteristic morulae in leukocytes
- Indirect fluorescent antibody (IFA) testing
- Polymerase chain reaction testing of tissues
- Immunochemical staining of erhlichial or anaplasmal antigens in tissue
- Synthesis of the history, clinical, laboratory, and epidemiologic features of individual cases

Culture of *Ehrlichia* is extremely difficult, and laboratories able to perform such cultures are few and often inaccessible to clinicians in daily practice. Although only a minority of patients with ehrlichiosis have morulae detectable in blood smears, a blood film should be examined in all patients with suspected infection; morulae are more commonly seen in patients with HGA than in those with HME.

Convalescent serologic antibody testing should be performed 2 to 3 weeks after onset of symptoms. The minimum diagnostic IFA titer is 1:64, and a fourfold-antibody rise is considered confirmatory of recent infection.

CURRENT THERAPY

- In most patients with Rocky Mountain spotted fever (RMSF), human monocytotropic ehrlichiosis (HME), or human granulocytic anaplasmosis (HGA), the cornerstone of management is empiric therapy based on clinical judgment and the epidemiologic setting.
- Doxycycline 100 mg PO or IV bid is the treatment of choice for patients with RMSF, HME, and HGA.
- For children who weigh <45 kg or who are younger than 8 y, the recommended dose of doxycycline is 2.2 mg/kg/d in two divided doses.[1]
- Most clinicians treat patients with RMSF for 7 to 10 d; treatment can usually be discontinued 2 to 3 d after the patient becomes afebrile.
- Treat ehrlichiosis for approximately 7 d or for 3 d after defervescence.
- Chloramphenicol (Chloromycetin) 500 mg IV every 6 h should be used to treat pregnant patients with RMSF and patients with adverse reactions to tetracyclines.
- Alternative therapies for HGE and HMA include chloramphenicol and rifampin (Rifadin),[1] although these should only be used to treat HGE or HMA in pregnant patients or in patients with adverse reaction to doxycycline. Doxycycline, however, may be necessary when life-threatening illness occurs in a pregnant patient.

[1]Not FDA approved for this indication.

TREATMENT

As with rickettsial infection, doxycycline[1] is the treatment of choice for ehrlichiosis. Doxycycline can be administered either orally or intravenously at a dose of 100 mg twice per day. For children who weigh less than 45 kg or are younger than 8 years old, the recommended dose is 2.2 mg/kg each day in two divided doses.[1]

There have been no randomized trials of optimal therapy for either HME or HGA, but the consensus of most experienced clinicians is that therapy should be continued for approximately 7 days or for 3 days after defervescence. Defervescence typically occurs within 48 hours of initiation of therapy.

All tetracyclines can cause dental staining, but this risk remains low if a short course is administered. Chloramphenicol[1] has also been used effectively, but, given the higher risk of hematologic toxicity, this medication should be reserved for pregnant patients or patients with adverse reaction to doxycycline. Additionally, some ehrlichia have been shown to be resistant to chloramphenicol in vitro. Thus, doxycycline may be necessary when life-threatening illness occurs in a pregnant patient. Rifampin (Rifadin)[1] has been used to successfully treat a few pregnant patients with HGA, but at present the efficacy of such therapy can only be considered an anecdotal observation; rifampin does not have an FDA approval for this indication.

[1]Not FDA approved for this indication.

REFERENCES

Bakken JS, Dumler JS. Human granulocytic ehrlichiosis. Clin Infect Dis 2000;31:554–60.

Chapman AS, Bakken JS, Folk SM, et al. Diagnosis and management of tickborne rickettsial diseases: Rocky Mountain spotted fever, ehrlichioses, and anaplasmosis—United States: A practical guide for physicians and other health-care and public health professionals. MMWR Recomm Rep 2006;55(RR-4):1–27.

Holman RC, Paddock CD, Curns AT, et al. Analysis of risk factors for fatal Rocky Mountain spotted fever: Evidence for superiority of tetracyclines for therapy. J Infect Dis. 2001;184:1437–44.

Kaplan JE, Schonberger LB. The sensitivity of various serologic tests in the diagnosis of Rocky Mountain spotted fever. Am J Trop Med Hyg 1986;35:840–4.

Kirk JL, Sexton DJ, Fine DP, Muchmore HG. Rocky Mountain spotted fever: A clinical review based on 48 confirmed cases. Medicine (Baltimore) 1990;69:35–45.

Paddock CD, Holman RC, Krebs JW, Childs JE. Assessing the magnitude of fatal Rocky Mountain spotted fever in the United States: Comparison of two national data sources. Am J Trop Med Hyg 2002;67:349–54.

Parola P, Raoult D. Ticks and tickborne bacterial diseases in humans: An emerging infectious threat. Clin Infect Dis 2001;32:897–928.

Pretzman C, Daugherty N, Poetter K, Ralph D. The distribution and dynamics of *Rickettsia* in the tick population of Ohio. Ann N Y Acad Sci 1990;590:227–36.

Stone JH, Dierberg K, Aram G, Dumler JS. Human monocytic ehrlichiosis. JAMA 2004;292:2263–70.

Smallpox

Method of
Isao Arita, MD

This chapter discusses the diagnosis and treatment of smallpox. However, in the unlikely event that a patient appears to have smallpox, it is essential to contact your local public health service office to obtain any updates, including vaccination, other methods of preventing further transmission, and protection for yourself and your personnel from the infection.

In 1980, the World Health Organization (WHO) declared that smallpox was eradiated throughout the world and would not return to the human community, and they recommended that smallpox vaccination be discontinued based on their assessment that risk of return of the disease is unlikely. Thus, all the nations in the world discontinued smallpox vaccination, and smallpox virus stocks in laboratories were destroyed except for those in two WHO collaborating centers in the United States and the Soviet Union. These stocks have been maintained to complete necessary research under strict biocontainment measures.

Since then, there has been no smallpox despite continuing global surveillance of the disease. Although the world has been apparently enjoying the benefit of successful smallpox eradication, the terrorist suicide attacks in New York City and Washington, D.C., on September 11, 2001, completely altered the situation: Subsequent deliberate delivery of *Bacillus anthracis* from an unknown source alerted the U.S. and global community to the potential threat of bioterrorism, including smallpox as the bioweapon.

These circumstances urgently revived the necessity to remember the experience in smallpox eradication, which was once thought to be the technology of the past and which did not progress much in terms of prevention and treatment. Fortunately, such experience was described in detail and comprehensively by the experts who actually worked in the eradication program in WHO's 1988 publication "Smallpox and Its Eradication." In this section, special efforts are made to describe salient features of such experiences and knowledge for medical professionals at medical facilities, who may employ them in their emergency work for minimizing possible hazard, if smallpox infection occurs.

As in the past, there is no specific treatment for smallpox. In fact, this was one of the reasons international efforts were made to eradicate smallpox. Smallpox was greatly feared because of its 30% case-fatality rate and its ability to spread in any country and in any season. The second reason was that vaccination had been a very effective tool for prevention, but the complications, such as postvaccinal encephalitis, eczema vaccinatum, and progressive vaccinia, were relatively frequent and severe. For example, 10 to 50 persons per 1 million primary vaccinees suffered adverse effects in the United States. These complications prompted a strong consensus that the only way to eliminate such vaccine complications was to eradicate the disease, thereby making vaccination unnecessary.

Clinical Features

The clinical pictures of smallpox is distinct for diagnosis and surveillance. There is no subclinical infection of epidemiologic significance. If the national security office warns of a possible return of smallpox, the disease ought to be, without much difficulty, suspected by medical personnel, who are concerned about the risk.

Surveillance of deliberate release of smallpox virus will be done by the appropriate national security offices, which require full cooperation by medical professionals. In fact, such cooperation is indispensable. Experience has shown that medical facilities are a common contact point, where persons infected with such severe disease as smallpox will visit, seeking consultation and medical treatment.

Clinical Course

After the incubation period (usually 10–14 days, ranging rarely 7–19 days), prodromal symptoms begin with fever and malaise. The exanthem develops in a very regular stepwise fashion of macules, papules, vesicles, and pustules (Figure 1). The exanthem is quite characteristic, with uniform features at each step and typical distribution on the body. The lesions are distributed more on the face and extremities, the extensor side is more affected than the flexor side, and there are fewer lesions on the trunk. The appearance is so classic that medical personnel can suspect smallpox once they have seen the good pictures of smallpox exanthems.

Within one week, the skin lesions become pustules, which, in a few days, become confluent and reach maximum size. By the end of the second week, scabbing starts. The scabs fall from the skin, leaving depigmented spots in the affected skin (see Figure 1H). The scabs can persist for as long as 1 month. Within a few months, the depigmented areas become blackish pigmented spots. These are signs with which surveillance identified the presence of transmission retrospectively in the affected community in the recent past, if the surveillance missed the actual presence of smallpox. Finally, the pustules on the face become pockmark scars.

As for the severity of the disease, *Variola major* is the severest type, with a fatality rate of 30%. For smallpox terrorism, V. major is the likely strain. V. minor causes mild disease, with a fatality rate of a few percent. Intermediate-type disease has been found in some areas, including Africa. The clinical pictures of mild and intermediate smallpox are similar to those caused by V. major. Hence, V. minor disease should be treated just as V. major disease is in practice, when surveillance and control measures are to take place. Only laboratory study can verify the type of V. virus. Pregnancy appears to augment the severity of the disease.

History of smallpox vaccination modifies the course of the disease. Vaccinated patients who have smallpox have an accelerated clinical course and fewer skin lesions. This applies to persons vaccinated either before immunization programs ended, when smallpox had not yet been eradicated, or during special containment vaccination programs against the risk of infection. However, the percentage of unvaccinated persons among the global population is rapidly increasing. For clinical diagnosis, it is important to refer to the clinical characteristics, as described earlier.

Meanwhile, in emergency or unexpected circumstances, where the public health service has not yet been ready to organize personnel, persons who were vaccinated in the past may be requested (subject to their agreement to help), after a fresh vaccination, to participate in some emergency activities for surveillance or related activities.

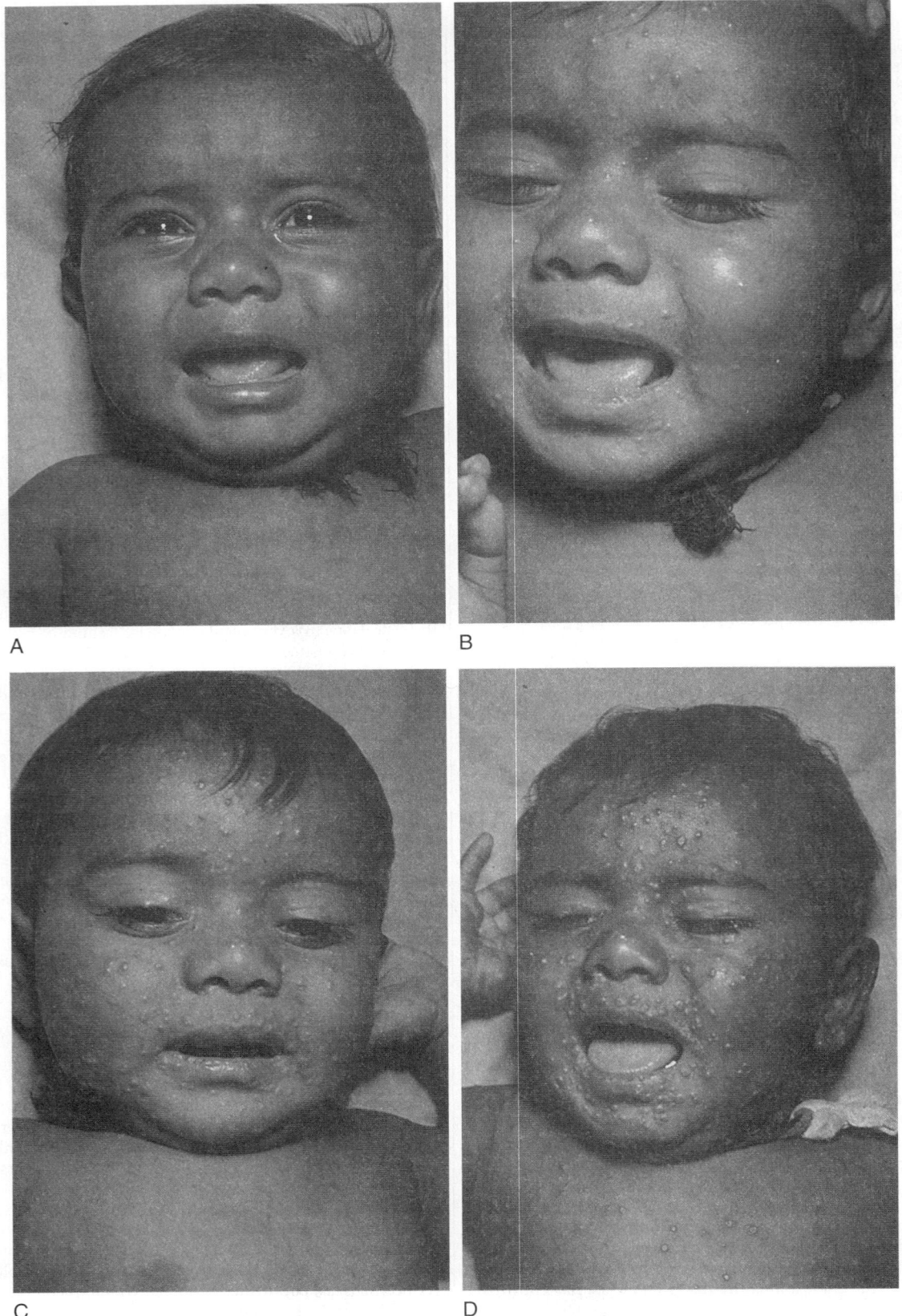

FIGURE 1. Lesions of smallpox. **A,** Day 1: The rash appears 1 day after the onset of fever. A few small papules are visible on the face and upper arms. An enanthem is usually present in the oropharynx at this time, but it cannot be seen in this photograph. **B,** Day 3: Additional lesions continue to appear, and some of the papules are becoming obviously vesicular. **C,** Day 4: All lesions have usually appeared by this time. Those that appeared earliest on the face and upper extremities are somewhat more mature than those that appeared later on other parts of the body, but on any specific area of the body all lesions are at approximately the same stage of development. Lesions are present on the palms. **D,** Day 5: Almost all the papules have now become vesicular or pustular, the true vesicular stage usually being very brief. Some of the lesions on the upper arms show early umbilication.

(Continued)

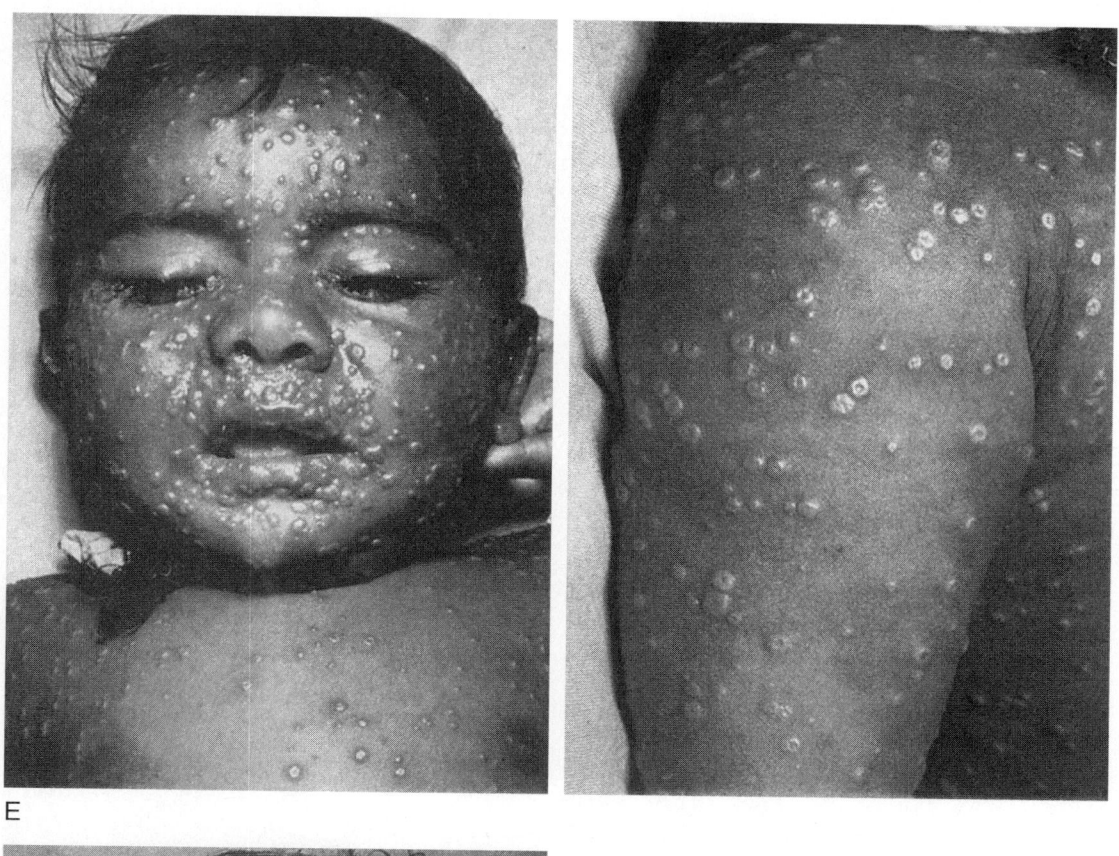

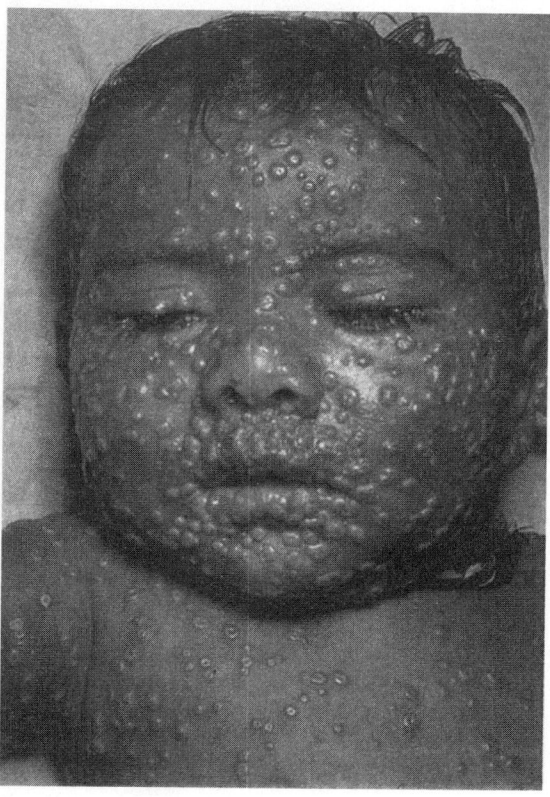

FIGURE 1. (Cont'd) E, Day 6: All the vesicles have now become pustules, which feel round and hard to the touch ("shotty"), like a foreign body. **F,** Day 7: Many of the pustules are now umbilicated and all lesions now appear to be at the same stage of development.

(Continued)

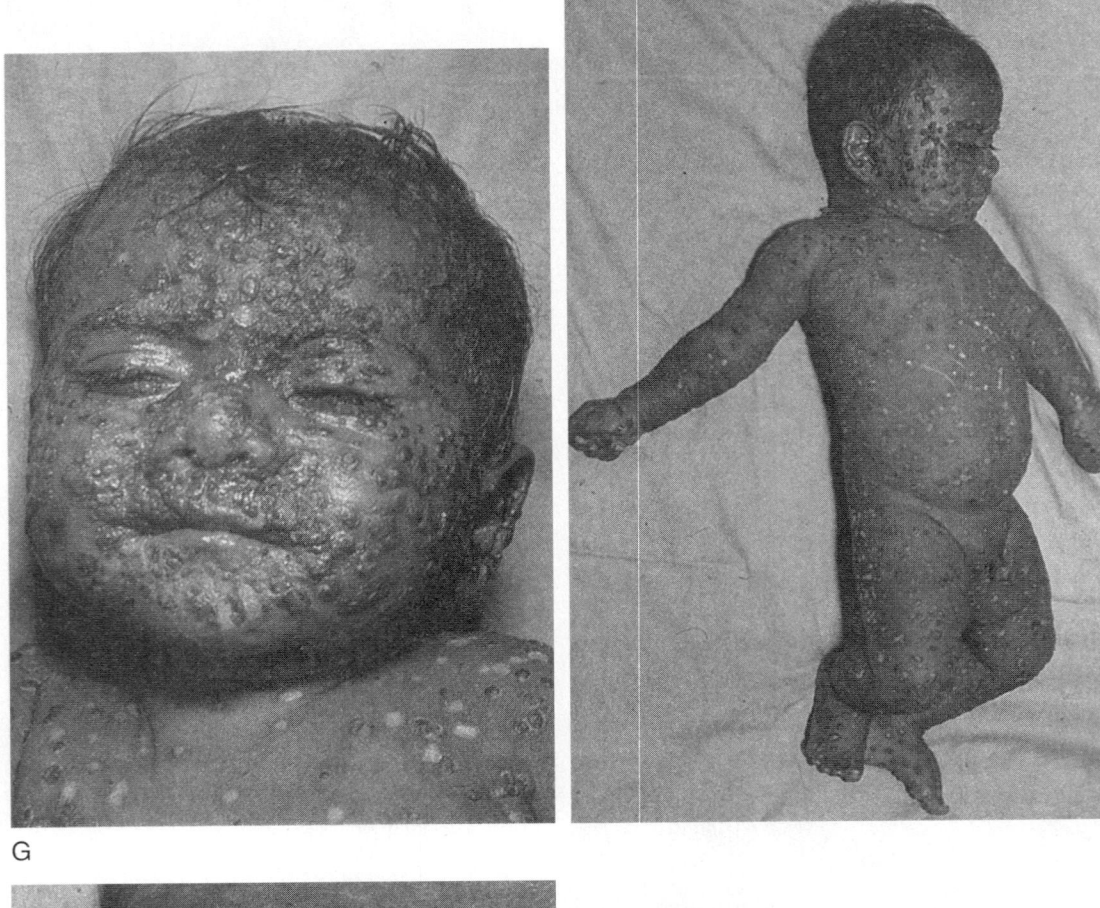

G

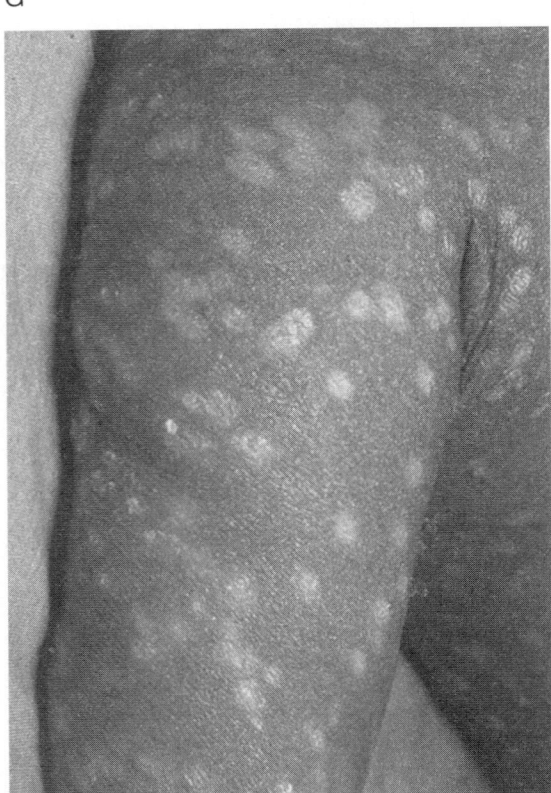

H

FIGURE 1. (Cont'd) G, Day 13: The lesions are now scabbing, but the eyelids are more swollen than at earlier times. There is no evidence of secondary bacterial infection of the skin lesions. **H,** Day 20: The scabs have separated except on the palms and the soles, leaving depigmented areas.

Differential Diagnosis and Laboratory Studies

During the program of smallpox eradication (1967–1980), surveillance was based on the clinical diagnosis in endemic nations, and only during the last 3 years of the program was laboratory diagnosis practiced by WHO reference laboratories in the United States and the Soviet Union. However, in today's world, it is important to pay special attention to the differential diagnosis, both clinical and laboratory, because a diagnosis of smallpox will necessarily result in a national health emergency including control of traffic, social events, and economic affairs and psychological calamity.

 CURRENT DIAGNOSIS

- Smallpox was declared eradicated in 1980.
- Smallpox is one of the priority diseases requiring biodefense preparedness.
- Preliminary diagnosis of smallpox should be regarded as a national emergency.
- Smallpox has a characteristic progression of exanthems after prodromal symptoms: macules, papules, vesicles, and pustules. The entire rash is uniform at each stage. The rash lasts about 1 wk after the onset of fever. Check the type of rash on the patient against photos of the exanthems.
- If you suspect smallpox, report it to the local public health service office immediately to get instructions for further emergency action.
- Be prepared to collect specimens from the rash, based on established procedures, and to dispatch them to the designated laboratory.

The clinical differential diagnosis includes varicella and other diseases of rash and fever (Table 1). In varicella, the features of the exanthem are different from those of smallpox. The varicella exanthem is a mixture of different types of rash, and the lesions are more abundant on the trunk (Figure 2). For clinicians, it may be difficult to suspect smallpox for the first 2 to 3 days of smallpox rash, because the rash may be mistaken for varicella or some other skin eruption. However, by day 3 to 4, it should be apparent that the rash is smallpox. Human monkeypox is another possible diagnosis, because the type of rash and distribution on the skin are very similar to those of smallpox, but the lymphadenopathy (maxillar, inguinal, etc.) is distinctive in monkeypox (Figure 3).

In the differential diagnosis of smallpox, it is important to pay attention to the case history of the patient regarding whether the patient has had contact with a smallpox-like disease. In the case of a smallpox attack, there are two possible scenarios. In the first one, a case of deliberate release of smallpox virus through aerosol or contaminated materials, the case history does not arouse suspicion. The second scenario is a patient with secondary transmission from a primary smallpox patient. In this situation, the case history might show the contact with a smallpox-like disease within 17 days before the onset of rash.

The methods of laboratory diagnosis include electron microscopic test, rapid DNA test, virus isolation, and genetic sequence study. These should be operative services of a laboratory network of either a national reference laboratory or a contracted reference laboratory from another country. WHO should be in a position to assist in these laboratory networks.

The electron microscopic or rapid DNA test can be completed within a day, and virus isolation and genetic sequence tests can be completed in a few days in a designated laboratory in the network. Collection and dispatch of specimens (usually from skin lesions) should be according to the accepted protocol, namely, specimen placed in a leak-proof double container and packed according to the rules of the International Association of Transportation Regulators (IATR) (Figure 4).

TABLE 1 Alternative Diagnoses in Suspected but Unconfirmed Cases of Smallpox

Final Diagnosis	England and Wales, 1946–1948* (Variola major)	India, 1976† (Variola major)	Somalia, 1977–1979‡ (Variola minor)
Chickenpox	41	53	20
Erythema multiforme	7	1	0
Allergic dermatitis	7	1	1
Drug rash	6	2	1
Syphilis	3	4	4
Impetigo	3	2	0
Scabies	1	1	0
Psoriasis	1	1	0
Vaccinia	5	0	1
Herpes	2	0	0
Measles	2	0	0
Rubella	1	0	0
Molluscum contagiosum	0	0	1
Septicemia	4	0	0
Skin diseases (various)	14	5	0
Other (including no diagnosis made)	0	30	1
Total	97	100	29

Source: World Health Organization.
*Data from Conybeare ET: Cases in which smallpox was suspected but unconfirmed. Mon Bull Min Health Public Health Lab Serv 1950:9:56–61.
†During posteradication surveillance in India. Data from Basu RN, Jezek Z, Ward NA: The eradication of smallpox from India. New Delhi: World Health Organization, 1979.
‡During posteradication surveillance in Somalia. Data from Jezek Z, Kriz B, Masar I, et al: [Liquidation of the last foci of variola in the world—Somalia (author's transl)] Cesk Epidemiol Mikrobiol Imunol 1981;30(12):113–124, Czech.

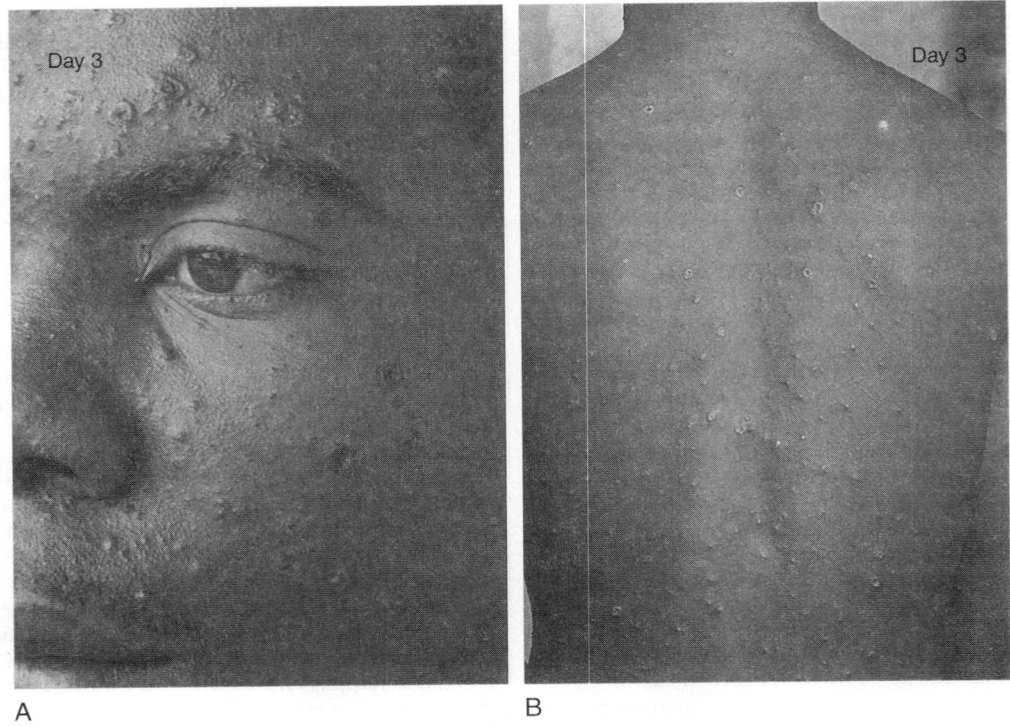

FIGURE 2. Chickenpox. **A** and **B**, On the third day of rash, pocks are at different stages of development (papules and vesicles). There are many lesions on the trunk (**B**) and few on the limbs. (Photographs from the World Health Organization.)

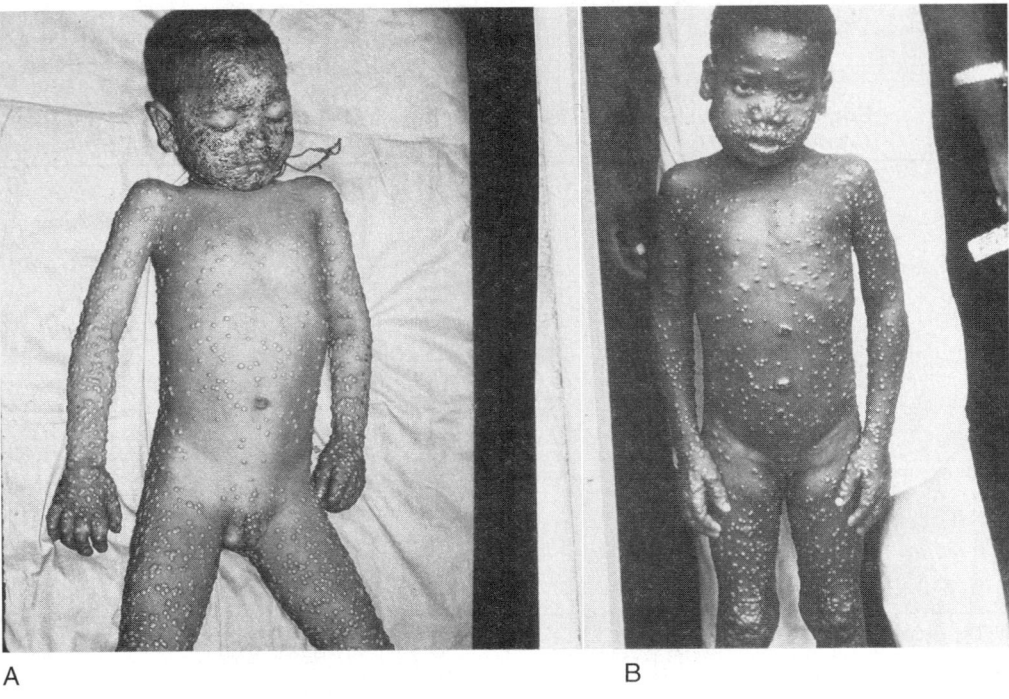

FIGURE 3. Similar exanthem in patients infected with smallpox virus (**A**) and monkeypox virus (**B**) on day 7 of exanthem. (Photographs from the World Health Organization.)

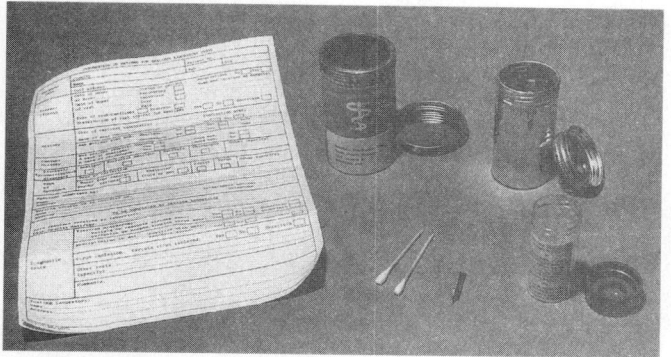

FIGURE 4. Container for smallpox specimen collection. Transportation of dangerous pathogens or specimens requires a special double container to ensure safety. (Photograph from the World Health Organization.)

The preparedness of the laboratory network is the first priority in any nation that wishes to handle smallpox bioterrorism surveillance properly.

Treatment

The patient with diagnosed smallpox must be safely transported and admitted to an isolated station or ward for treatment by trained hospital personnel. Patients with suspected smallpox should be also isolated and vaccinated. Patients with suspected smallpox *must not* be treated in the same isolation facilities with smallpox patients.

Currently, there is no effective therapeutic substance licensed for treating smallpox in humans. Before and after the smallpox eradication period (1967–1980), strenuous efforts were made to develop treatment for smallpox, but they have failed. As recently experienced in the United States, immunization of the population as preparedness for biodefense has also failed due to vaccine complications. Most nations, to date, are not in favor of conducting mass vaccination campaigns as preemptive measures. Thus, the research to produce a safer vaccine and the research on an antiviral drug are warranted and continued.

If smallpox reemerges, all patients should receive supportive care. Supportive care can include infection control, such as antibiotics to prevent secondary infection, and intensive rehydration therapy. Ventilator assistance may be needed. In special cases, such as the severe type of hemorrhagic smallpox, patients must also be treated for shock. Attention should be paid to likely renal failure and malnutrition. These medical practices are complicated by the precautions for protection and disinfection that are necessary to prevent smallpox virus contamination of the environment and population.

CURRENT THERAPY

- We have no specific antiviral drug or treatment of smallpox.
- Provide supportive care as symptoms suggest.
- Consult the local health service office for all the necessary pubic health measures, such as protection for yourself and your staff from infection, disinfection, isolation, vaccination, transport, and other relevant containment methods as required.

Experience has shown that smallpox vaccination during the incubation period, within 4 to 5 days after the exposure to the infection, can prevent the infection. However, in practice, any person in contact with a smallpox patient or suspected smallpox patient should be vaccinated as soon as possible. Vaccinia immune globulin intravenous (VIGIV) can reduce some complications of vaccination, but there has been no evidence that it is effective for treating smallpox.

Smallpox was once eradicated by the unified efforts of humankind. The strategy was through immunization as a preventive measure, not through curative treatment, which is not available even today, when bioterrorism by smallpox is threatening us. Research is needed to develop a further attenuated vaccine and antiviral drug as well, but use of the vaccine should still play a greater role, as was done in the eradication efforts a quarter century ago.

This article was written in 2006, and because the technical progress will be very rapid, readers are requested to seek updated information that will be available from the World Health Organization (http://www.who.int/csr/disease/smallpox/en/) and the U.S. Centers for Disease Control and Prevention (http://www.bt.cdc.gov/agent/smallpox/index.asp) in 2008.

Acknowledgments

I am grateful to Dr. D. A. Henderson of Johns Hopkins University, who advised on the preparation of this article and to Ms. M. Nakane of the Agency for Cooperation in International Health (in Japan), who sorted out all important references during the preparation of this article.

REFERENCES

Arita I. Smallpox vaccine and its stockpile in 2005. Lancet Infect Dis 2005;5(10):647–52.

Breman JG, Henderson DA. Diagnosis and management of smallpox, N Engl J Med 2002;346(17):1300–8. Available from http://content.nejm.org/cgi/content/full/346/17/1300 [accessed May 30, 2007].

Centers for Disease Control and Prevention. Smallpox response plan and guidelines: Annex 1: Overview of smallpox, clinical presentations, and medical care of smallpox patients, Available from http://www.bt.cdc.gov/agent/smallpox/response-plan/files/annex-1-part1of3.pdf [accessed May 30, 2007].

Centers for Disease Control and Prevention. Smallpox response plan and guidelines: Annex 2: General Guidelines for Smallpox Vaccination Clinics. Available from http://www.bt.cdc.gov/agent/smallpox/response-plan/files/annex-2.pdf [accessed May 30, 2007].

Centers for Disease Control and Prevention. Smallpox response plan and guidelines: Annex 3: Guidelines for Large Scale Smallpox Vaccination Clinics: Logistical Considerations and Guidance for State and Local Planning for Emergency, Large-Scale, Voluntary Administration of Smallpox Vaccine in Response to a Smallpox Outbreak. Available from http://www.bt.cdc.gov/agent/smallpox/response-plan/files/annex-3.pdf [accessed May 30, 2007].

Centers for Disease Control and Prevention. Slides and notes: Smallpox disease and its clinical management. Available from http://www.bt.cdc.gov/agent/smallpox/training/overview/pdf/diseasemgmt.pdf [accessed May 30, 2007].

Centers for Disease Control and Prevention. Smallpox fact sheet: Reaction after smallpox vaccination. Available from http://www.bt.cdc.gov/agent/small-pox/vaccination/pdf/reactions-vacc-public.pdf [accessed May 30, 2007].

Fenner F, Henderson DA, Arita I, Jezek Z, Ladnyi ID. Smallpox and Its Eradication, Geneva, Switzerland: World Health Organization, 1988. PDF available at http://whqlibdoc.who.int/smallpox/9241561106.pdf [accessed May 15, 2007].

Institute of Medicine. Assessment of Future Scientific Needs for Live Variola Virus. Washington, DC: National Academies Press; 1999.

University of Pittsburgh Medical Center Center for Biosecurity. Smallpox FAQ, 2005. [on the Internet, cited October 2, 2006]. Available from http://www.upmc-biosecurity.org/website/bioagents/smallpox/smallpox_faq_2005.html.

Diseases of the Head and Neck

Vision Correction Procedures

Method of
Elizabeth Yeu, MD

The term *refractive error* describes any condition where light is poorly focused within the eye, resulting in blurred vision. This is the most common eye problem encountered in the United States and includes such conditions as nearsightedness (myopia), farsightedness (hyperopia), astigmatism, and age-related loss of near vision (presbyopia). A person who is able to see without the aid of spectacles or contact lenses has minimal to no refractive error. A wide variety of techniques are available for correcting refractive errors and restoring visual function. The most common methods employ corrective eyewear, such as eyeglasses and contact lenses. In addition to these noninvasive modalities, several surgical procedures can also be used to treat these conditions. These surgical techniques range from minimally invasive procedures, such as laser vision correction (LVC), to more invasive methods such as refractive lens exchange (RLE) or phakic intraocular lens implantation.

Whichever method is selected, the primary goal of every vision-correcting procedure should be to choose the technique that is most appropriate for each patient. The chosen method should not only correct the patient's visual deficit but also satisfy the patient's goals for visual function. This chapter focuses on the various surgical options that are available for vision correction. To set the groundwork for this discussion, I begin with some background information on ocular anatomy, refractive errors, and the clinical assessment of visual function.

Pathophysiology

BACKGROUND

Although the human eye is a complex structure, from a conceptual standpoint, it can be thought to function much like a simple camera. In general, light enters the eye and needs to be focused on the center of the retina, or the fovea, to generate images. Light first enters through the cornea, a convex transparent window that performs approximately 66% to 75% of the focusing for the eye. After passing through the cornea, the light encounters the iris and pupil. The pupil is an aperture centered within the iris, a muscular diaphragm that controls the diameter of the pupil and thus the amount of light that continues into the eye.

The crystalline lens sits behind the pupil and provides the remaining 25% to 34% of the eye's focusing ability (Figure 1). The lens is suspended by a network of hundreds of supporting cables called zonular fibers. These zonules insert into the ciliary body, a muscular ring that is a peripheral extension of the iris. The refractive power of the lens is somewhat adjustable and can be increased to move the focal point of the eye from distance to near, a process known as *accommodation* (Figure 2). Accommodation results from contraction of the ciliary muscle, which results in a decreased diameter of the ciliary ring, similar to a lens aperture of a camera. This loosens the zonules, which simultaneously reduces zonular tension on the lens, thereby causing the thickness and anterior curvature to increase, along with its amplified refractive power.

After being focused by the lens, light passes through the transparent vitreous humor until it reaches the retina, which lines the inside of the back of the eye. The retina functions like the film in a camera, converting the focused image into an electrical signal that is transmitted to the brain via the optic nerve.

REFRACTIVE ERRORS

Emmetropia is the condition where the eye has essentially no refractive error and requires no correction for distance vision. Refractive errors result when the cornea and lens inadequately focus incoming light, resulting in blurred images projected onto the retina. The unit of measure for refractive error is the diopter (D), which for a thin lens (in air) is defined as the reciprocal of the lens focal length. Most refractive errors refer to the patient's visual status when viewing objects in the distance. For example, a lens that focuses light over a distance of 0.5 m has a refractive power of +2.0 D.

In myopia, or nearsightedness, the focusing powers of the cornea are too strong or the axial length of the eye is too long, or both. The resulting image comes into focus anterior to the retina and is out of focus by the time it reaches the back of the eye. As a result, myopic eyes can see better at near, rather than distance. To correct a myopic eye, its refractive power must be decreased by using a lens with negative refractive power, which weakens the focusing of light and redirects it toward the retina.

Hyperopes, or farsighted persons, are the opposite of myopes. The cornea is flatter and focuses too weakly or the axial length is too short (or both) in the hyperopic eye. The images from objects viewed at a distance are not yet in focus by the time they reach the retina. To see clearly, a hyperopic eye must accommodate to increase its lenticular power to bring distant objects into sharp focus. Because this requires contraction of the ciliary muscle, the farsighted eye is never at rest and must work even harder to see near objects clearly. Because of this, hyperopic refractive corrections must add positive focusing power to the eye (Figure 3).

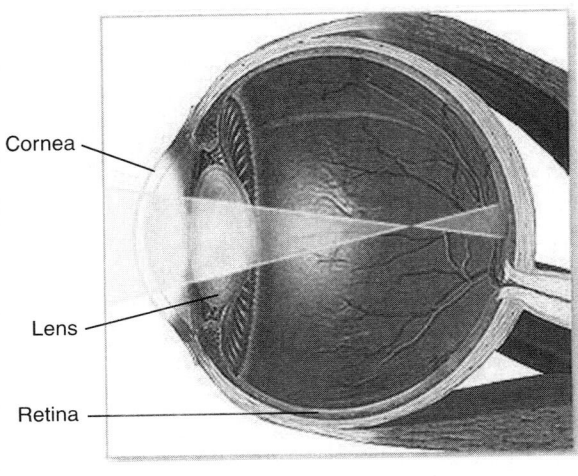

FIGURE 1. The refraction, or bending, of light in the eye occurs through the cornea and the crystalline lens. Refractive errors result when the light is not perfectly focused onto the retina. (Illustration courtesy of A.D.A.M, Inc.)

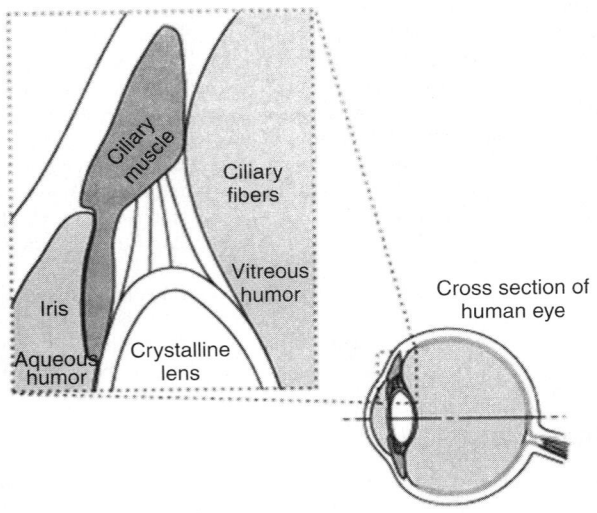

FIGURE 2. The lens is suspended in place by the zonular fibers. These zonules insert into the ciliary body. Accommodation, or the ability to focus at near, occurs as the result of the contraction of the zonules and a change in shape to the crystalline lens.

In astigmatism, the eye has different refractive powers along different meridians; light entering in the vertical direction gets focused differently than light in the horizontal direction. Conceptually, it is easier to think of the astigmatic cornea or lens as shaped like a football rather than a basketball, with the meridian of steeper curvature having greater refractive power. The astigmatic eye produces a blurred image because essentially two focal points of images are being produced. This requires different corrections along each of these meridians to produce a single focused image on the retina (Figure 4).

Presbyopia describes the normal age-related loss of near vision. To see near objects clearly, young distance-corrected eyes must accommodate to increase their refractive power. However, this ability progressively declines with age, usually reaching clinical significance in the 5th decade. Several factors have been implicated in this process, including loss of lens elasticity, decreased zonular tension, and altered ciliary muscle function. Although there is currently no way to reverse this natural consequence of aging, several vision-correction options are available to improve near vision in presbyopic persons.

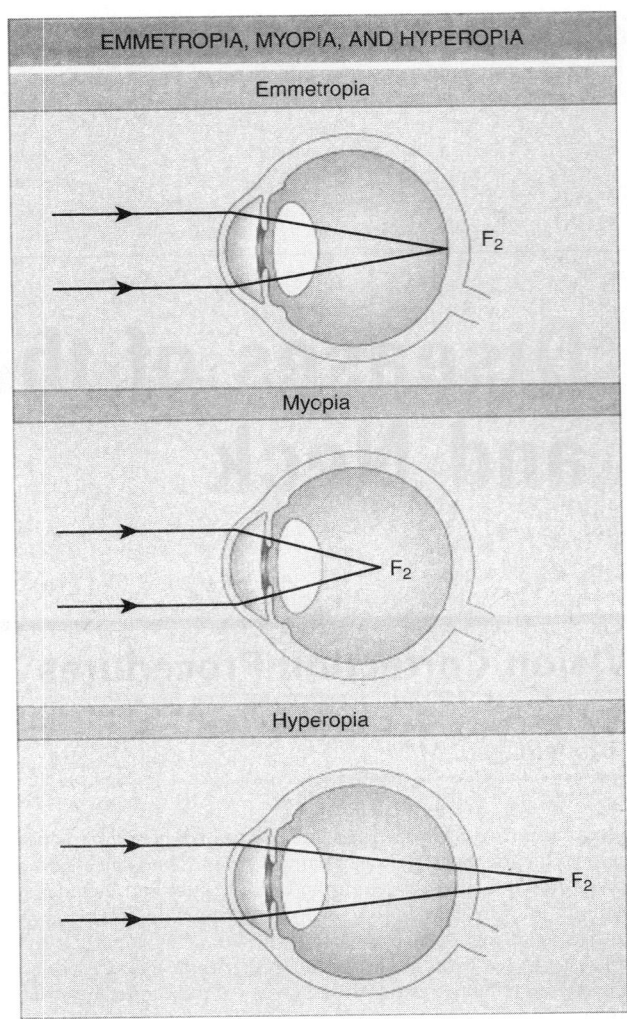

FIGURE 3. Emmetropia, myopia, and hyperopia. In emmetropia, the secondary focal point (F_2) is at the retina. In myopia, the secondary focal point (F_2) is in the vitreous. In hyperopia, the secondary focal point (F_2) is behind the eye. (Reprinted with permission from Mimura T, Azar DT: Part 3: Refractive Surgery. In Yanoff M, Duker JS: Ophthalmology, 3rd ed. St. Louis, Mosby, 2008.)

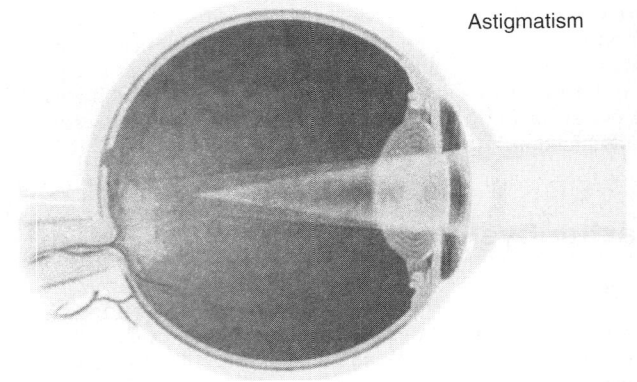

FIGURE 4. Astigmatism occurs when the refractive power of the eye is not symmetrical. The focusing poser of one axis is stronger than the other axis. This effectively leads to multiple focal points of light, which results in blurred images. (Reprinted with permission from Haw WW, Manche EE: Vision correction procedures. In Bope ET, Rakel RE, Kellerman R (eds): Conn's Current Therapy 2010. Philadelphia, Saunders, 2010, pp 193–197.)

Epidemiology

Population-based studies indicate that approximately 25% to 40% of people in their forties have myopia, and 10% to 20% have hyperopia. Myopia is the most common refractive error and affects about 35% of whites and 13% to 30% of African Americans. Approximately three quarters of the American population older than 40 years have refractive errors greater than 0.5 D. Astigmatism of more than 0.5 D is common in adults, and the prevalence increases to approximately 28% in persons in their forties. In general, a higher prevalence of hyperopia and less myopia is observed with increasing age from about 45 to 65 years. This levels off with older age and is eventually followed by an increase in myopia at older ages, which is thought to largely be from cataract formation. Regarding the correction of refractive errors, about 150 million Americans currently use some form of eyewear to correct refractive errors at a cost of approximately 150 billion dollars annually, including 36 million who use contact lenses.

Diagnosis (Assessment of Vision)

There are many aspects of vision, including visual acuity, contrast sensitivity, color perception, and peripheral vision. The most common assessment of visual function is to test the central vision through visual acuity. Visual acuity testing determines a patient's ability to read high-contrast symbols (usually black letters on a white background) of varying sizes at a standard testing distance. This reference distance approximates optical infinity and is typically 20 feet in the United States and 6 meters in Europe. A 20/20 letter on the standard eye chart devised by Snellen is approximately ⅜ inch tall at a distance of 20 feet (subtending a visual angle of 5 minutes of arc). Twenty-twenty vision is considered normal visual acuity.

Visual acuities less than 20/20 are represented by ratios whose denominator is greater than 20. For example, a visual acuity of 20/60 means that the smallest letter the eye can read is three times larger than a 20/20-size letter.

Refractive errors can result in *uncorrected* visual acuities that fall below 20/20. However, in the absence of other disease, the conditions of myopia, hyperopia, astigmatism, and presbyopia can be corrected with restoration of normal visual function. This can be achieved with spectacles, contact lenses, or the various surgical procedures discussed next.

CURRENT DIAGNOSIS

- Refractive errors are an extremely common cause for blurred vision.
- Refractive errors include myopia (nearsightedness), hyperopia (farsightedness), astigmatism, and presbyopia, which is the age-related loss of near vision.
- Medical management includes the use of spectacles, contact lenses, or both.
- Both corneal and intraocular surgical options exist to successfully and permanently correct refractive errors.
- Corneal refractive surgery options include excimer laser, such as laser in situ keratomileusis (LASIK) and photorefractive keratectomy (PRK), to and corneal relaxing incisions for the management of astigmatism.
- In eyes that are not candidates for corneal refractive surgery, intraocular surgery with phakic intraocular lens implants or refractive lens exchange can be considered.
- Increasing advancements now offer, and continue to expand, the various surgical options available to correct myopia, hyperopia, astigmatism, and presbyopia.

Treatment (Surgical Correction of Refractive Errors)

LASER VISION CORRECTION

Laser in situ keratomileusis (LASIK) and photorefractive keratectomy (PRK) use an excimer laser to reshape the anterior surface of the cornea and permanently correct the eye's refractive error. The excimer laser was developed in the 1970s and emits ultraviolet light at a wavelength of 193 nm. This particular wavelength has been found to accurately and efficiently ablate corneal tissue without causing thermal damage to the surrounding collagen. In myopia, the excimer laser treatment flattens the central cornea to decrease its focusing power. Conversely, for hyperopia, laser pulses are applied to the periphery, indirectly steepening the central cornea and thereby increasing its refractive power. Astigmatism is corrected by combining central and peripheral treatments to differentially steepen the flattest corneal meridian and flatten the steepest meridian. Since the first excimer treatment in the late 1980s, LASIK and PRK have been used to treat refractive errors in millions of patients.

LASER IN SITU KERATOMILEUSIS

In LASIK, a lamellar or partial-thickness corneal flap is first created in the cornea. The flap thickness typically varies from about 100 to 180 μm, as compared with a total corneal thickness that usually ranges from 500 to 600 μm. The LASIK flap is reflected at its hinge and the excimer laser ablation is applied directly to the corneal stroma. Once the ablation is complete, the flap is returned to its original position (Figure 5).

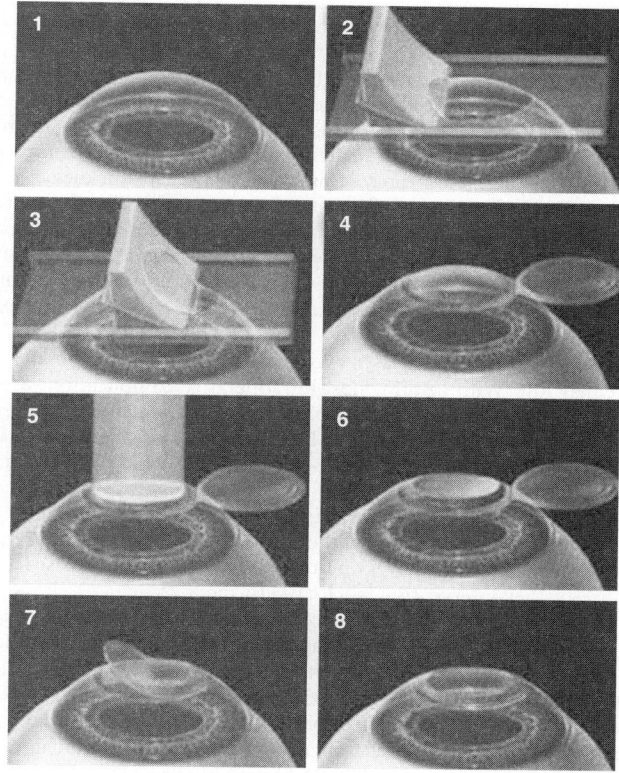

FIGURE 5. LASIK procedure. **1,** The normal cornea. **2** and **3,** A microkeratome (or laser) is used to create a partial-thickness corneal flap attached at a hinge. **4,** The corneal flap is lifted. **5,** The excimer laser ablates the corneal stroma. **6,** The corneal stroma is reshaped. **7** and **8,** The corneal flap is repositioned. (Reprinted with permission from Haw WW, Manche EE: Vision correction procedures. In Bope ET, Rakel RE, Kellerman R (eds): Conn's Current Therapy 2010. Philadelphia, Saunders, 2010, pp 193–197.)

- Laser in situ keratomileusis (LASIK) and photorefractive keratectomy (PRK) use an excimer laser to reshape the anterior surface of the cornea and permanently correct the eye's refractive error. LASIK and PRK can correct myopia, hyperopia, astigmatism and help reduce presbyopia.

- In LASIK, a corneal flap is created and lifted before the excimer laser is applied to correct the refractive error. In contrast, the PRK procedure requires no lamellar flap. In PRK, the laser treatment is applied directly to the anterior stromal surface after the surface epithelium is removed.

- Radial keratotomy (RK) was the first modern form of corneal refractive surgery to correct myopia. In RK, spokelike corneal incisions were created to flatten the central cornea and reduce myopia. Although RK surgery is effective, the results were often unpredictable and unstable and led to overcorrection, with progressive hyperopia.

- Astigmatic keratotomy (AK) incisions are a modification of RK surgery and are used to reduce corneal astigmatism. The two forms of corneal relaxing incisions, astigmatic keratotomy (AK) and limbal relaxing incisions (LRI)—or, more accurately, peripheral corneal relaxing incisions (PCRIs)—are differentiated by their location on the cornea.

- A refractive lens exchange (RLE) is a surgical option that can correct refractive errors by removing and replacing the crystalline lens. In essence, RLE is cataract surgery performed before a visually significant cataract forms; a visually significant cataract is the clouding or opacification of the natural lens. RLE is a viable option for high myopes and hyperopes, where laser vision correction is not an option, and to correct presbyopia.

- Presbyopia correction is a very dynamic field in refractive surgery. Surgical correction options include surgical monovision, which is popularly used with presbyopic contact lens wearers, where one eye is corrected for distance vision and the other eye for near. Monovision can be produced through excimer laser, RLE, or cataract surgery. Also, various intraocular lenses (IOLs) can correct presbyopia.

- Surgically implanted lenses, or phakic intraocular lens implants, can be used to treat myopia only in the United States. Phakic IOLs are an alternative to laser vision correction and can successfully correct myopia in patients for whom keratorefractive surgery is not an option.

- No surgery is without its potential for complications. The more devastating complications of corneal refractive surgery include flap-related complications in LASIK, corneal weakening and ectasias, and vision-limiting haze in PRK. Endophthalmitis is a sight-threatening infection that can occur with any intraocular surgery such as RLE, phakic intraocular lenses, and cataract surgery.

The LASIK flap is created by either a microkeratome, a device containing a motorized oscillating blade connected to a suction ring, or via a femtosecond laser. The femtosecond laser uses ultrashort microscopic pulses of infrared light to define the lamellar flap. The femtosecond laser has allowed greater accuracy with the flap thickness. Also, there are significantly less flap-related complications, such as free (without flap hinge), partial, or buttonhole (doughnut-shaped) flaps.

Recovery of vision usually takes a few days; some patients note gradual improvement over a few weeks. Postoperative medications usually include topical antibiotic and steroid eye drops for approximately 5 to 7 days.

Complications with laser vision correction in general are extremely low. With LASIK, most intraoperative complications associated with LASIK involve the flap. If during the surgery the patient moves the eye (fixation loss), the laser can focus on the wrong part of the eye (decentration of the laser treatment), which can degrade the postoperative vision.

LASIK carries the postoperative risks of flap displacement or induction of flap striae. Most of these cases require a lifting and repositioning the flap. However, more severe or refractory cases can require further intervention, such as suturing.

On rare occasions, epithelial cells from the corneal surface can migrate underneath the LASIK flap and proliferate in the interface. Usually, the peripheral nests of epithelial cells are small and insignificant visually, thus requiring no intervention. Larger collections of cells can compromise vision or cause corneal necrosis and scarring, so they need to be removed. Epithelial ingrowth requires lifting the flap and manually débriding the cells. This treatment might need to be supplemented with alcohol or suturing, or both, to prevent recurrence.

Corneal weakening and subsequent distortion are other potential sequelae of laser vision correction. Certain preoperative corneal shapes suggest a predisposition toward weakening, especially those with steeper curvature in the inferior region as compared with the superior region. Preoperative corneal thicknesses less than 500 μm or post-LASIK residual stromal bed thicknesses less than 250 μm can also be associated with corneal weakening.

As with any surgery, LASIK and PRK are also associated with a risk of infection. The incidence varies, but published rates have been about 0.03%. Staphylococcal and streptococcal species are most common, but atypical organisms such as mycobacteria and fungi have also been reported. Sterile inflammation can also occur in the flap interface and is known as *diffuse lamellar keratitis*. Diffuse lamellar keratitis has been associated with bacterial endotoxin, cleaning solutions, corneal abrasions, and excessive femtosecond laser energy levels. Treatment primarily relies on topical steroid eyedrops, but it may also include oral steroids and irrigation of the flap interface.

PHOTOREFRACTIVE KERATECTOMY

PRK also uses the excimer laser to reshape the cornea, but this procedure requires no lamellar flap. In this method, the laser treatment is applied directly to the anterior stromal surface after the surface epithelium is removed. Several techniques are available to remove the corneal epithelium. Mechanical débridement with a spatula or rotating brush is very common. *Advanced surface ablation* has replaced other techniques used to manipulate the surface epithelium, including a devitalizing 20% alcohol solution, followed by gentle débridement with a blunt spatula or an epikeratome (similar to a LASIK microkeratome) to separate a flap of epithelium at the level of the basement membrane.

Laser-assisted subepithelial keratomileusis (LASEK) is another modification of PRK. An epithelial flap is created with alcohol débridement or with an epikeratome. The epithelial flap is reflected and the laser treatment is performed, similar to LASIK. After the corneal ablation is completed, the epithelial flap is replaced and a contact lens is applied. Some surgeons believe that retention of the epithelium improves postoperative comfort, speeds epithelial healing, and decreases the risk of subepithelial haze following the procedure. Each of these methods has certain advantages and disadvantages, but all do an effective job of preparing the corneal surface for laser ablation.

Once the laser treatment is complete, a soft contact lens is placed on the cornea. The corneal epithelium typically heals in 4 to 7 days, after which the contact lens is removed. Once the contact lens is removed, recovery of vision can take a few more weeks, although some patients experience improvement in vision that continues over several months. Antibiotic eye drops are used until the contact lens is removed, and steroid eye drops may be tapered over several months.

Regarding complications, PRK has fewer intraoperative risks than LASIK because no lamellar flap is being created. Postoperatively, there is a higher risk of subepithelial haze. Fibroblastic transformation of keratinocytes can cause the deposition of disorganized collagen that decreases the smoothness and clarity of the post-PRK cornea. This development is usually associated with higher myopic corrections and may be reversed by increased application of topical steroid eye-drops. Short-duration intraoperative use of low-concentration topical mitomycin-C (Mutamycin) (0.02%) appears to decrease the risk of haze formation. As discussed with LASIK, postoperative infectious or sterile inflammation is a rare but potential risk with PRK as well.

Both PRK and LASIK damage corneal nerves, which appears to have a secondary effect on the ocular hydration status. Postoperative dry eye is greater in LASIK than PRK owing to its greater depth of penetration into the cornea. The increased dryness appears to be temporary, and most patients return to baseline by 6 to 9 months, but a subset of patients experience chronic dry eyes following the procedure. A careful preoperative assessment of dry eye risk factors is recommended, and those at risk may be steered toward PRK or toward no surgery at all.

RADIAL KERATOTOMY

Modern keratorefractive surgery can attribute some of its origins to a flurry of research produced by Sato of Japan in the 1940s that led to radial keratotomy (RK) and astigmatic keratotomy (AK) surgeries. Russian ophthalmologist Fyodorov is credited with advancing keratorefractive surgery in the 1970s through RK surgery. He created up to 16 spoke-like cuts radiating from the central cornea at 90% to 95% corneal depth to balloon the peripheral cornea. This would, in turn, flatten the central cornea and reduce myopia. The combination of RK and AK surgeries were very popular procedures that effectively reduced myopia and astigmatism throughout the 1970s and 1980s. Although RK surgery was effective, the results were often unpredictable and unstable and lad to overcorrection, with progressive hyperopia. RK surgery was quickly replaced by laser vision correction with the introduction of PRK in the late 1980s (Figure 6).

ASTIGMATIC KERATOTOMY

Astigmatic keratotomy incisions are a modification of RK surgery and are used to reduce corneal astigmatism. The two forms of corneal relaxing incisions, astigmatic keratotomy (AK) and limbal relaxing

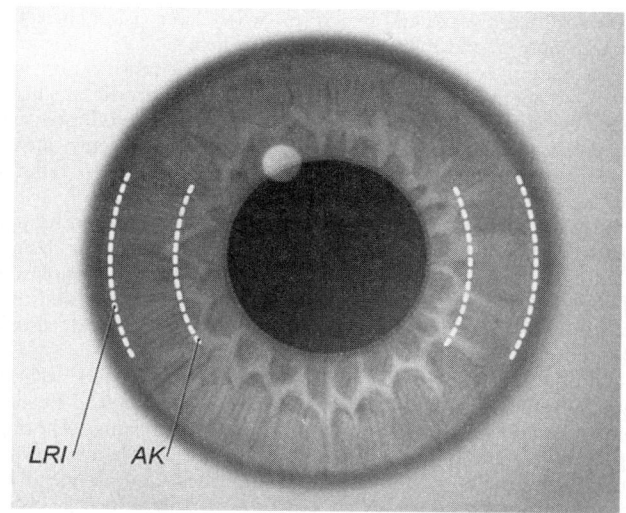

FIGURE 7. Incisions can be placed on the cornea to reduce astigmatism. The more central astigmatic keratotomy (AK) incisions have a greater effect than their peripheral limbal relaxing incision (LRI) counterparts. (Reprinted with permission from Yeu E, Rubenstein JB: Management of astigmatism during lens-based surgery. In American Academy of Ophthalmologists: Focal Points, Clinical Modules for Ophthalmologists, February, 2008.)

incisions (LRI), or more accurately peripheral corneal relaxing incisions (PCRI), are differentiated by their location on the cornea (Figure 7).

Several nomograms exist for AK and PCRIs that consider the age of the patient and the amount and meridian of the steep axis of astigmatism in order to calculate the length of the incisions. In both procedures, incisions are made to a 90% to 95% depth in the cornea to flatten the steep meridian. The basic principles of astigmatism correction hold true for both types of keratotomy surgeries: A greater effect is achieved with longer incisions, with smaller optical zones, with deeper incisions, and in older patients. Hence, the more central AK incisions have a greater effect and can correct upwards of 6 to 7 diopters of astigmatism.

PCRIs have a weaker effect because of their more peripheral location and generally can correct 2 to 3 diopters of astigmatism. Because the incisions are made closer to the limbus, they heal faster, and thus the refractive effect stabilizes more quickly. Given their peripheral location, the ratio of flattening in meridian of incision-to-steepening ratio in the opposite meridian, or *coupling ratio*, is usually 1:1. Patients experience less irregular astigmatism, flare, and foreign body sensation as compared to their more central counterparts. Technically, PCRIs are easier to perform and more forgiving as well.

Corneal relaxing incisions are most commonly performed intraoperatively, at the time of cataract surgery, but are also performed as a separate procedure to treat corneal astigmatism. The procedure is fairly quick to perform and the patient experiences little discomfort. Postoperatively, a topical antibiotic is used for 4 to 7 days, and a topical analgesic is used as needed.

Regarding complications of corneal relaxing incisions, patients commonly experience a foreign body sensation during the first few days. Less-common complications include glare, undercorrection or overcorrection, irregular astigmatism from the incisions, wound gape or perforation, decreased corneal sensation, and dry eye syndrome.

REFRACTIVE LENS EXCHANGE

Unlike the corneal procedures that have been discussed, refractive lens exchange (RLE) is a surgical option that can correct refractive errors by removing and replacing the crystalline lens. In essence, RLE is cataract surgery without a visually significant cataract, which is the clouding or opacification of the natural lens. RLE is a viable

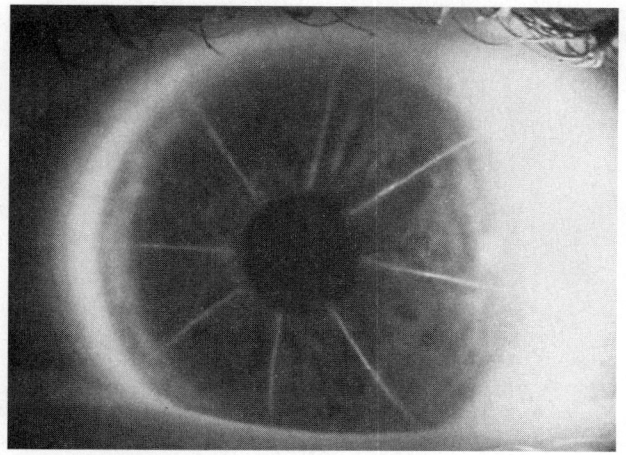

FIGURE 6. Radial keratotomy was the first modern form of refractive surery for the correction of myopia. Up to 16 spokelike cuts radiating from the central cornea at 90% to 95% of corneal depth can be created to flatten the central cornea and balloon the peripheral cornea to correct myopia.

option for high myopes and hyperopes, where laser vision correction is not an option, and for correcting presbyopia.

The natural crystalline lens is removed via emulsification with ultrasound energy. This lens is then replaced by an acrylic or silicone intraocular lens (IOL) implant that can effectively and accurately correct refractive errors. Preoperative biometric measurements, including the corneal curvature and axial length, are used in different formulas to calculate the proper intraocular lens power.

Since the turn of the century, a variety of IOLs has been brought forth to address presbyopia correction. There are different designs, including multifocal designs and accommodating IOLs. Monovision, popularly used with presbyopic contact lens wearers (one eye is corrected for distance vision and the other eye for near), can also be reproduced permanently with RLE and cataract surgery.

Although currently available presbyopia-correcting IOL technology is effective in providing a greater range of vision and freedom from spectacle use, the IOLs are not without their faults. Although improved, the multifocal IOL can cause glare and halos from its inherent concentric ring design, and diminished contrast sensitivity can result from the light's being "split" for distance and near vision. The only currently FDA-approved accommodating IOL has neither of these disadvantages of the multifocal IOLs, but it does not provide UV light protection and also provides less predictable near vision (Figure 8).

Because RLE is intraocular, it is much more invasive than the previous extraocular corneal procedures. Hence, although both eyes can undergo corneal procedures simultaneously, elective intraocular procedures should always be performed as two separate staged surgeries. Being intraocular, RLE procedures likely have a similar risk of endophthalmitis (severe postoperative intraocular infection) as modern cataract surgeries do, which is between 0.05% to 0.10%. Other postoperative complications of RLE include retinal detachment in high myopes (1.85%-8%) and a likely need for a laser capsulotomy procedure to treat capsular haze that commonly occurs behind the IOL after surgery.

In addition to the postoperative risks of RLE, other common obstacles can be encountered intraoperatively because operating on soft lenses, very long eyes (high myopes) and very short eyes (high hyperopes) has its own set of potential complications. Preoperative surgical planning and strategy are key to a successful RLE.

PHAKIC INTRAOCULAR LENS IMPLANT

Surgically implanted lenses, or phakic intraocular lens implants, may be used only to treat myopia in the United States. Phakic IOLs are an alternative to laser vision correction and can successfully correct myopia in patients for whom keratorefractive surgery is not an option. As compared to laser vision correction for myopia, some studies suggest that the quality of vision with a phakic IOL is superior. Phakic IOLs function very similarly to contact lenses that are permanently implanted inside the eye. Regarding the two FDA-approved phakic IOLs available today, a phakic IOL can be implanted to sit in front of and attached to the iris (see Figure 8) or just behind the iris. As in RLE, the implantation of a phakic IOL is intraocular, and surgery should be performed on only one eye at a time to respect the risks involved in the more-invasive procedure. Unlike RLE, all structures inside the eye, including the crystalline lens, are left untouched when a phakic IOL is implanted.

As do all surgical procedures, phakic IOLs are subject to various complications, of which cataract formation is a more common one (up to 9%). Other surgical complications include infection, retinal detachment, acute glaucoma, and loss of corneal endothelial cells, which are the nonregenerating cells on the back surface of the cornea that are responsible for maintaining corneal clarity.

Future Outlook

Refractive surgery technology continues to evolve. Regarding corneal refractive surgery, there are several options on the horizon for the correction of presbyopia. These include the excimer laser creation of a multifocal cornea (PresbyLASIK) to provide both distance and near vision, and different corneal implants that can be placed on top (onlays) or within (inlays).

For intraocular refractive surgery options, phakic IOL technology, which is currently only approved in the United States for the correction of myopia, may be available for hyperopic correction, as it is in Europe. Also, potentially safer phakic IOLs will be continue to be released. Lastly, new IOL options to correct presbyopia are an expanding focus in cataract surgery and refractive lens exchange surgeries.

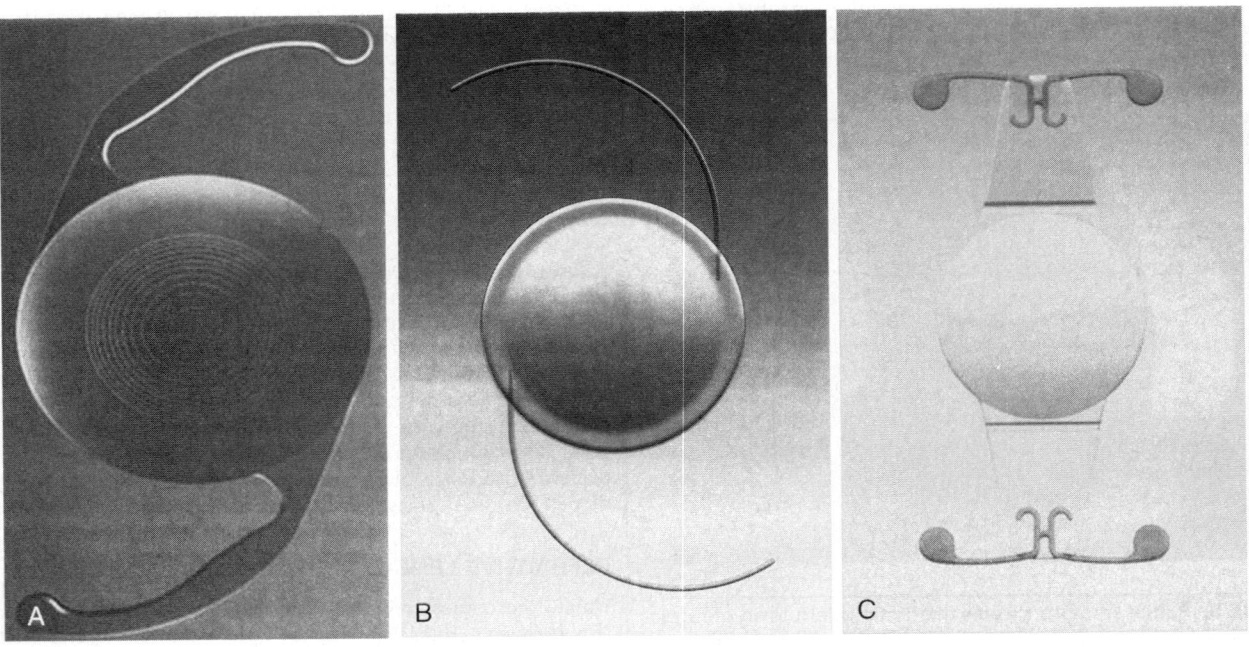

FIGURE 8. Examples of currently FDA-approved intraocular lens implants. **A** and **B**, Multifocal. **C**, Accommodating. (**A**, From Alcon Labs, Fort Worth, TX. **B**, From Abbott, Abbott Park, IL. **C**, From Bausch and Lomb, Rochester, NY.)

REFERENCES

Buratto L. Phakic IOLs: Which approaches are likely to be effective and safe? Program and abstracts of the 2006 Joint Meeting of the American Academy of Ophthalmology and Asia Pacific Academy of Ophthalmology, Las Vegas, Nevada. Refractive Surgery Subspecialty Day. November 2006.

Cowden JW, Bores LD. A clinical investigation of the surgical correction of myopia by the method of Fyodorov. Ophthalmology 1981;88(8):737–41.

Donders RC, Moore WD. On the anomalies of accommodation and refraction of the eye. London: New Sydenham Society; 1864.

Packard R. Refractive lens exchange for myopia: A new perspective? Curr Opin Ophthalmol 2005;16(1):53–6.

Price FW, Grene RB, Marks RG, Gonzales JS. Astigmatism reduction clinical trial: A multicenter prospective evaluation of the predictability of arcuate keratotomy. Evaluation of surgical nomogram predictability. ARC-T Study Group. Arch Ophthalmol 1995;113(3):277–82.

Stulting RD, Carr JD, Thompson KP, et al. Complications of laser in situ keratomileusis for the correction of myopia. Ophthalmology 1999;106(1):13–20.

Vitale S, Ellwein L, Cotch MF, et al. Prevalence of refractive error in the United States, 1999–2004. Arch Ophthalmol 2008;126(8):1111–9.

The Red Eye

Method of
John Dorsch, MD

In the primary care office, the most common causes of red eye are conjunctivitis, subconjunctival hemorrhage, and foreign body causing corneal abrasions. Other common causes of red eye include blepharitis and hordeolum. Less common but serious causes of red eye include viral keratitis, uveitis, scleritis, and angle-closure glaucoma. Other usually less serious causes of red eye include episcleritis, pingueculum, and pterygium. All primary care physicians should have expertise in recognizing and treating the common causes of red eye, and recognize and refer patients with higher-stakes diagnoses (Boxes 1 and 2).

Physical Examination

Always check visual acuity in any patient with an eye complaint. Fluorescein strips (Flu-Glo, Fluorets), topical anesthetic drops, and cobalt blue light are used to examine the cornea for abrasions, keratitis, and ulceration. Cotton-tipped applicators are used to evert the upper eyelid and look for a foreign body.

Pupillary reaction is often affected by angle closure glaucoma and uveitis, but it is rarely affected by conjunctivitis, blepharitis, and corneal disorders. The pupil may be irregular in the patient with uveitis.

 CURRENT DIAGNOSIS

■ Patients with traumatic injury to the eye, loss of vision, extreme pain not explained by pathology, keratitis, suspected uveitis or glaucoma, chemical injury, or nonhealing corneal abrasion should be referred to an ophthalmologist.

■ Bacterial, viral, and allergic conjunctivitis can often be distinguished by the type of ocular discharge present.

■ Subconjunctival hemorrhage can occur from trauma, from increased intrathoracic pressure, from anticoagulants, or idiopathically.

Patients with uveitis often have pain in the closed affected eye when light is shined in the normal eye with a bright light or with convergence of the eyes. This is due to consensual reflex of the pupils to light and accommodation.

The diagnosis of conjunctivitis is made by pulling the lower eyelid down with the examiner's finger. If the bulbar or palpebral conjunctivae are inflamed (i.e., hyperemic, edematous, discharge), conjunctivitis is present. Palpable preauricular nodes may be present with viral conjunctivitis and chlamydial conjunctivitis.

BOX 1   Approach to the Patient with Red Eye

The following questions are often helpful in making the diagnosis in patients with red eyes.

- *Is one eye or are both eyes involved?* Infections, allergy, and systemic illness are more likely to cause bilateral eye involvement.
- *Does the patient have intense eye pain?* If yes, likely diagnoses include acute angle closure glaucoma, uveitis, scleritis, keratitis, foreign body, or corneal abrasion.
- *Does the patient have a foreign body sensation?* If so, consider corneal abrasion, trauma, dry eye, keratitis, and other corneal disorders.
- *Is there a discharge?* If it is *very* copious and purulent, consider gonococcal conjunctivitis. If it is discolored and purulent, consider bacterial conjunctivitis. Copious watery discharge is typical of viral conjunctivitis. Stringy, mucoid discharge is typical of allergic or chlamydial conjunctivitis.
- *Do the eyes itch?* If so, consider blepharitis or allergy in the differential.
- *Are the eyelids swollen?* Consider allergy or infection.
- *Do the eyelids have lumps?* Hordeolum and chalazion should be considered.
- *Do the eyes burn?* Consider blepharitis or dry eye.
- *Is the eye redness recurrent?* Consider herpes keratitis, uveitis, and allergic conjunctivitis.
- *Does the patient have photophobia?* Corneal problems (abrasions, keratitis) and uveitis should be considered.
- *Is there loss of vision?* Consider corneal ulcer, uveitis, and angle-closure glaucoma.
- *Is the patient using ocular medications?* Prolonged use of neomycin and sulfa ophthalmic medications can cause sensitization and redness of the eyes.

BOX 2   Red Eye

Common Causes
- Conjunctivitis: bacterial, viral, allergic
- Subconjunctival hemorrhage
- Corneal abrasion
- Blepharitis

Less Common Causes
Less serious
- Episcleritis
- Pingueculum
- Pterygium

More serious
- Viral keratitis
- Uveitis
- Scleritis
- Angle closure glaucoma

Conjunctivitis

Conjunctivitis is the most common cause of red eye encountered by primary care providers. Among the etiologies of conjunctivitis, viral conjunctivitis is the most common. Although patients with conjunctivitis might have some minor irritation of the eyes, they usually do not complain of pain in the eye or loss of vision. Ocular discharge is generally considered to be an important diagnostic feature of conjunctivitis (Table 1). Although much has been written about characterizing conjunctivitis by the nature of the discharge, one meta-analysis failed to find evidence of the diagnostic usefulness of clinical signs and/or symptoms in distinguishing bacterial conjunctivitis from viral conjunctivitis.

VIRAL CONJUNCTIVITIS

Viral conjunctivitis is often seen in epidemics and is most commonly caused by species of the genus *Adenovirus*. Typically, viral conjunctivitis starts in one eye and spreads to the other eye a few days later. The conjunctivae appear red and swollen, with copious watery discharge (Figure 1). The natural course of viral conjunctivitis self-limiting, lasting 10 to 14 days. Management should be directed at scrupulous hygiene. Patients must be informed that their infection is highly contagious. They should avoid close contact with other persons (e.g., towels, direct contact, swimming pools) for 2 weeks and wash hands frequently to prevent the spread of their infection. Topical antibiotics have been prescribed to try to prevent bacterial superinfection, but there is no good evidence that they have any significant impact. Symptomatic treatment with cold compresses and topical vasoconstrictors may be helpful.

BACTERIAL CONJUNCTIVITIS

Bacterial conjunctivitis typically starts abruptly in one eye and spreads to the other eye in 1 to 2 days. Usually a purulent discharge is present that persists throughout the day. A variety of gram-positive and gram-negative organisms cause bacterial conjunctivitis, but the most common etiologies are *Staphylococcus aureus*, *Streptococcus pneumoniae*, *and Haemophilus pneumoniae*. Treatment of bacterial conjunctivitis is usually empiric, but conjunctival scraping for smears and cultures should be done in infants, immunocompromised patients, and patients with hyperacute conjunctivitis in which *Neisseria gonorrhoeae* or *Chlamydia trachomatis* infection is suspected. Treatment of bacterial conjunctivitis (excluding gonococcal or chlamydial conjunctivitis) usually consists of a topical antibiotic used four times a day (Table 2). Topical antibiotics are usually prescribed for 5 to 7 days, and resolution of conjunctivitis is expected within that time.

Hyperacute bacterial conjunctivitis has an abrupt onset, copious purulent discharge, and rapid progression, and it is usually associated with gonococcal infection in a sexually active patient. Chemosis (edema of the conjunctivae) may be present.

Chlamydial conjunctivitis is acquired through exposure to infected secretions from the genital tract, either direct or indirect. The infection is usually unilateral (at least initially), and often there is involvement of the preauricular node on the ipsilateral side. Gonococcal and chlamydial infections are treated systemically (Box 3).

TABLE 1 Conjunctivitis

Type	Course	Characteristics	Discharge
Bacterial	Starts in one eye, often spreads to other eye		Purulent
Allergic	Accompanies allergic rhinitis	Itchy eyes	Mucus
Viral	Usually bilateral	Very red eyes	Watery

TABLE 2 Topical Antibiotics Used to Treat Bacterial Conjunctivitis

Drug	Dosage
Bacitracin (Ak-Tracin, Bacticin) ointment	Apply 0.5 inch in eye q3-4h
Ciprofloxacin (Ciloxan) 0.3% ophthalmic solution	1-2 gtt in eye q15min × 6 h, then q30min × 18 h, then q1h × 1 d, then q4h × 12 d[3]
Gatifloxacin (Zymar) 0.3% ophthalmic solution	1 gt in eye q2h up to 8 ×/day × 2 days, then 1 gt qid × 5 days
Gentamicin (Gentak, Gentasol) 0.3% ophthalmic solution or ointment	Ointment: 0.5 inch applied to eye 2-3 × per day Solution: 1-2 gtt in eye q4h
Levofloxacin (Quixin) 0.5% ophthalmic solution	1-2 gtt in eye q2h × 2 days while awake, then q4h while awake × 5 days
Moxifloxacin (Vigamox) 0.5% ophthalmic solution	1 gt in eye tid × 7 d
Neomycin/polymyxin B/ gramicidin (Neosporin) ophthalmic solution	1-2 gtt in eye q4h × 7-10 d
Ofloxacin (Ocuflox) 0.3% ophthalmic solution	1-2 gtt in eye q2-4h × 2 d, then 1-2 gtt in eye qid × 5 d
Polymyxin B and trimethoprim (Polytrim) ophthalmic solution	1 gt in eye q3h × 7-10 d
Sulfacetamide (Isopto Cetamide, Ocusulf-10, Sodium Sulamyd, Sulf-10, AK-Sulf) 10% ophthalmic solution, ointment	Ointment: 0.5-inch ribbon in eye q3-4h and qhs × 7 d Solution: 1-2 gtt in eye q2-3h × 7-10 d
Tobramycin (AK-Tob, Tobrex) 0.3% ophthalmic solution	1-2 gtt in eye q4h

[3]Exceeds dosage recommended by the manufacturer.

BOX 3 Treatment of Chlamydial and Gonococcal Conjunctivitis

Chlamydial Conjunctivitis
- Erythromycin (Ery-Tab)[1] 250 mg PO qid × 14 d
or
- Doxycycline (Vibramycin) 100 mg PO bid × 14 d
- Treat partners

Gonococcal Conjunctivitis
- Ceftriaxone (Recephin 1 g IM)

[1]Not FDA approved for this indication.

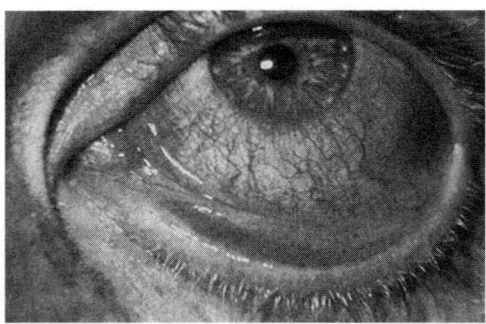

FIGURE 1. Viral conjunctivitis. (Reproduced with permission from the University of Michigan Kellogg Eye Center, http://www.kellogg.umich.edu.)

CONJUNCTIVITIS OF THE NEWBORN

Chlamydial conjunctivitis is the most common cause of infectious conjunctivitis of the newborn in the United States. Onset of conjunctivitis is 3 to 10 days after birth, but it has been reported as late as 2 months after birth. *Chlamydia trachomatis* infection can also cause pneumonia, otitis media, proctitis, and vulvovaginitis in infants. Treatment consists of erythromycin (EryPed Drops) orally 50 mg/kg/day in four divided doses for 14 days. Erythromycin ointment (Ilotycin 0.5%) or tetracycline ointment[2] given shortly after delivery is effective in preventing chlamydial conjunctivitis but not systemic chlamydial infections.

Gonococcal conjunctivitis of the newborn is a hyperacute infection that occurs 2 to 4 days after birth. It can cause corneal ulceration and loss of vision. Gonococcal conjunctivitis can be prevented with silver nitrate drops[2] or erythromycin (Ilotycin) or tetracycline ointment[2] administered shortly after delivery. Silver nitrate commonly causes a self-limited chemical conjunctivitis, which can delay visual bonding of the infant to the parents in the first few hours of life. Therapy of gonococcal conjunctivitis of the newborn consists of IV penicillin G[1] given four times a day for 7 days or ceftriaxone (Rocephin) IV or IM once a day for 7 days or gentamicin (Garamycin)[1] IM given twice a day for 7 days.

CONJUNCTIVITIS–OTITIS MEDIA SYNDROME

Conjunctivitis-otitis media syndrome is a common condition in which children with otitis media also have purulent bilateral ocular discharge. It responds to treatment of otitis media; no topical treatment of conjunctivitis is required.

 CURRENT THERAPY

- Do not use eye patches in patients with corneal abrasions.
- Do not use topical anesthetics for the eye outside a clinic or hospital setting, because corneal toxicity can occur.
- Patients with corneal abrasions should be reexamined the following day.
- Patients with corneal abrasions from extended-wear contact lenses often become colonized with *Pseudomonas aeruginosa* and should be treated with appropriate antibiotics (quinolones).

---

[1]Not FDA approved for this indication.
[2]Not available in the United States.

METHICILLIN-RESISTANT *STAPHYLOCOCCUS AUREUS* CONJUNCTIVITIS

Increasing numbers of cases of bacterial conjunctivitis are caused by methicillin-resistant *S. aureus* (MRSA). MRSA conjunctivitis manifests as bacterial conjunctivitis resistant to conventional therapy and is treated with the same drugs used to treat MRSA in other parts of the body (Doxycycline [Vibramycin],[1] vancomycin [Vancocin], sulfamethoxazole-trimethoprim [Bactrim][1]). Cultures should be obtained when MRSA is suspected.

ALLERGIC CONJUNCTIVITIS

Allergic conjunctivitis is an immunoglobulin E (IgE)-mediated condition characterized by bilateral eye involvement, itchy eyes, and mucoid discharge. *Seasonal* conjunctivitis is caused by exposure to common allergens (e.g., pollens, dander) and usually accompanies allergic rhinitis. *Perennial* allergic conjunctivitis is similar to seasonal allergic conjunctivitis, but the symptoms are usually less severe. Patients are usually treated with a systemic antihistamine. Ophthalmic (topical) medications include antihistamine or decongestants, mast cell inhibitors, nonsteroidal antiinflammatory drugs (NSAIDs), H_1-antagonists, and various combinations of these (Table 3). Milder cases can be treated with a decongestant-antihistamine combination for about 2 weeks. Moderate to more severe cases can require longer use of these medications or the addition of systemic antihistamines or mast cell inhibitors. Some patients require topical corticosteroids or cyclosporine (Restasis)[1] for severe allergic conjunctivitis, but these should be evaluated by an ophthalmologist because of potential complications of therapy.

Subconjunctival Hemorrhage

In subconjunctival hemorrhage, the redness of the eye is localized and sharply circumscribed, and the underlying sclera is not visible (Figure 2). Conjunctivitis is not present, and there is no discharge. There is typically no pain or visual change. Subconjunctival hemorrhage may be spontaneous, but it can also result from trauma, hypertension, bleeding disorders, or increased intrathoracic pressure (e.g., straining, coughing, retching). No treatment is necessary, but investigation may be warranted if the etiology is in question or the hemorrhage is recurrent. Referral to an ophthalmologist should be considered if the subconjunctival hemorrhage is from trauma or has not resolved within 2 to 3 weeks.

---

[1]Not FDA approved for this indication.

TABLE 3 Topical Medications for Allergic Conjunctivitis

Generic Name	Brand Name(s)	Dosing	Mode of Action
Azelastine 0.05% solution	Optivar	1 gt in eye(s) bid	H_1-antagonist, mast cell inhibitor
Cromolyn 4% solution	Crolom, generic	1-2 gtt in eye(s) 4-6 times per day	Mast cell inhibitor
Emedastine 0.05% solution	Emadine	1 gt in eye(s) qid	H_1-antagonist
Epinastine 0.05% solution	Elestat	1 gt in eye(s) bid	H_1- and H_2-antagonist, mast cell inhibitor
Ketorolac 0.5% solution	Acular	1 gt in eye(s) qid up to 1 wk	NSAID
Diclofenac 0.1% solution[1]	Voltaren ophthalmic	1 gt in eye(s) qid × 2 wk	NSAID
Lodoxamide 0.1% solution	Alomide	1-2 gtt in eye(s) qid up to 3 mo	Mast cell inhibitor
Loteprednol 0.2% susp.	Alrex	1 gt in eye(s) qd	Corticosteroid
Naphazoline/pheniramine (solution)	Naphcon-A (OTC) Opcon-A (OTC) Visine-A (OTC)	1-2 gtt in eye(s) qd-qid prn	Antihistamine, decongestant
Nedrocomil 2% solution	Alocril	1-2 gtt in eye(s) bid	H_1-antagonist, mast cell inhibitor
Olopatadine 0.1% solution	Patanol	1 gt in eye(s) bid	H_1-antagonist, mast cell inhibitor
Olopatadine 0.2% solution	Pataday	1 gt in eye(s) qd	Mast cell inhibitor

[1]Not FDA approved for this indication.
Abbreviation: NSAID = nonsteroidal antiinflammatory drug.

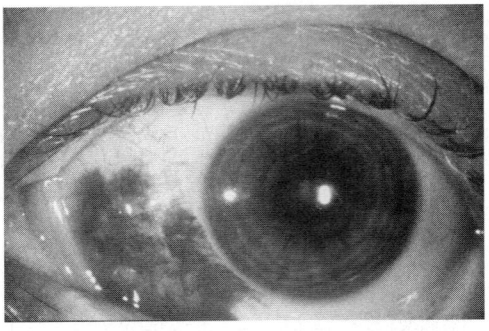

FIGURE 2. Subconjunctival hemorrhage. (Reprinted with permission from American Academy of Ophthalmology: Managing the Red Eye. Eye Care Skills for the Primary Care Physician Series. San Francisco: American Academy of Ophthalmology, 2001.)

Corneal Abrasion

Corneal abrasions typically result from scratching of the corneal epithelium due to trauma, but they can also occur from extended-wear contact lenses. Patients with corneal abrasions present with pain, excessive tearing from the involved eye, photophobia, a foreign-body sensation (like having sand in the eye), and blurry vision.

Corneal abrasions are identified by staining the cornea with fluorescein and examining under cobalt blue light (Figure 3). The eye should also be examined carefully to check for foreign bodies. Topical anesthetic is administered to make the patient comfortable during the examination, but continued use can cause corneal damage.

Management of corneal abrasions consists of pain relief and prevention of infection. Pain can be relieved with topical NSAIDs such as ketorolac (Acular)[1] and Diclofenac (Voltaren),[1] oral over-the-

---

[1]Not FDA approved for this indication.

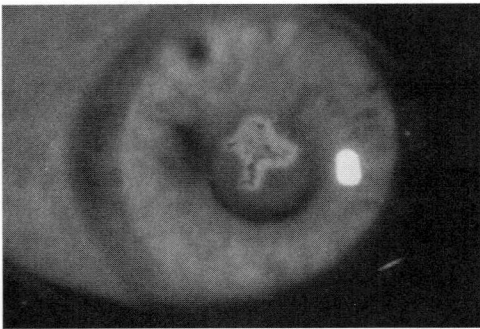

FIGURE 3. Corneal abrasion with fluorescein stain with cobalt blue light. (Reprinted with permission from American Academy of Ophthalmology: Managing the Red Eye. Eye Care Skills for the Primary Care Physician Series. San Francisco: American Academy of Ophthalmology, 2001.)

counter analgesics, and occasionally oral narcotics. Topical antibiotics are usually prescribed to prevent infection. Antibiotic ointments are lubricating and soothing to the eye, making them a good option for traumatic corneal abrasions. Topical ophthalmic antibiotic ointments commonly used are bacitracin (Bacticin), erythromycin (Ilotycin), and gentamicin (Gentak).

In patients who have corneal abrasions from contact lens overwear, eyes are commonly colonized with *Pseudomonas aeruginosa*. These patients should be treated with topical antibiotics such as ciprofloxacin (Ciloxan) or ofloxacin (Ocuflux) solutions.

Patching of the eye, though a common practice of the past, has not shown evidence of benefit in recent studies. It was found that eye patching can actually cause harm, so this practice is no longer recommended.

Infrequently, patients have traumatic uveitis accompanying corneal abrasion. Traumatic uveitis usually causes significantly more pain than a corneal abrasion, and, if uveitis is suspected, the patient should be evaluated by an ophthalmologist.

Patients with corneal abrasions should be reexamined in 24 hours. Corneal abrasions typically should be healed or greatly improved in 24 hours. If the abrasion is not completely healed after 24 hours, the patient should be examined again in 2 or 3 days. Referral should be considered if any worsening occurs or if the abrasion does not heal within 5 days. Corneal abrasions can be prevented by using protective eyewear.

Other Causes of Red Eye

Other causes of red eye are somewhat less common.

BLEPHARITIS

Blepharitides are inflammatory conditions of the eyelid caused by infection or obstruction of eyelid glands (Table 4). Blepharitis may be accompanied by conjunctivitis. *Staphylococcal* blepharitis arises from the accessory glands to the eyelashes and causes discharge from the eyelid, often associated with erythema, induration, loss of eyelashes, and crusting of the eyelid (Figure 4). This is treated with hot, moist packs to the eyes, baby shampoo scrubs, and erythromycin ointment (Ilotycin) at bedtime. *Seborrheic* blepharitis, a more chronic form of blepharitis, arises from the meibomian glands and causes **scaling** of the eyelids (Figure 5). Seborrheic blepharitis is often associated with skin disorders such as rosacea, eczema, and seborrheic dermatitis. This is treated with hot, moist packs and baby shampoo scrubs. Resistant cases are treated with oral tetracycline (Sumycin) (or one of its derivatives).

HORDEOLUM (STYE)

A hordeolum is an acute, painful mass of the eyelid that is caused by inflammation of the glands (Figure 6). It does not usually cause the eye to become red as well. Warm compresses to the eyelid four times a day for 3 to 5 minutes typically causes resolution within 1 week. Because they arise from the same glands, hordeola and blepharitis commonly occur together.

TABLE 4 Blepharitis			
Type	**Site of Origin**	**Clinical Characteristics**	**Treatment**
Staphylococcal	Accessory glands of eyelids	Erythema and induration of eyelid; crusting; discharge; loss of eyelashes	Warm compresses Baby shampoo scrubs Erythromycin ointment (Ilotycin)
Seborrheic	Meibomian glands	More chronic, scaling	Warm compresses Baby shampoo scrubs Oral tetracycline for resistant cases

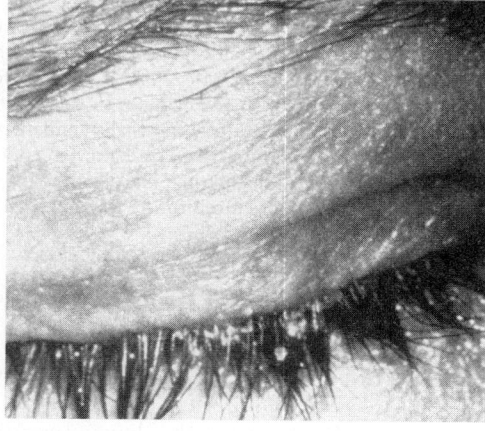

FIGURE 4. Staphylococcal blepharitis. (Reprinted with permission from American Academy of Ophthalmology: Managing the Red Eye. Eye Care Skills for the Primary Care Physician Series. San Francisco: American Academy of Ophthalmology, 2001.)

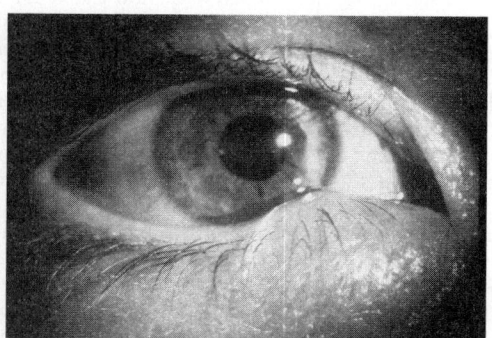

FIGURE 5. Seborrheic blepharitis. (Reprinted with permission from American Academy of Ophthalmology: Managing the Red Eye. Eye Care Skills for the Primary Care Physician Series. San Francisco: American Academy of Ophthalmology, 2001.)

FIGURE 6. Hordeolum. (Reprinted with permission from American Academy of Ophthalmology: Managing the Red Eye. Eye Care Skills for the Primary Care Physician Series. San Francisco: American Academy of Ophthalmology, 2001.)

EPISCLERITIS

Episcleritis is a self-limited inflammation of the episcleral vessels and is believed to be autoimmune. It has a rapid onset and usually minimal discomfort. Redness is most often confined to a sector of the eye. Episcleritis usually resolves in 7 to 10 days. Recurrence is not uncommon. Oral NSAID drugs may be prescribed, but treatment is usually not necessary.

SCLERITIS

Scleritis is, fortunately, much less common than episcleritis. Patients with scleritis experience intense inflammation and deep eye pain. Scleritis is commonly associated with rheumatoid arthritis and inflammatory bowel disease. The patient should be promptly referred to an ophthalmologist if scleritis is suspected.

ACUTE ANGLE CLOSURE GLAUCOMA

Acute angle closure glaucoma is characterized by acute ocular pain and is often accompanied by vomiting, blurred vision, acute photophobia, pupils unreactive to light, and circumcorneal redness (ciliary flush). Treatment of glaucoma with pilocarpine (Isopto Carpine), topical timolol (Timoptic), and acetazolamide (Diamox) should be started, and the patient should be given an urgent referral to an ophthalmologist.

ANTERIOR UVEITIS

Uveitis is the inflammation of the iris and ciliary muscle, often associated with autoimmune disease. Trauma can also cause uveitis. Signs of uveitis include ocular pain, ciliary flush, and occasionally irregularity of the pupil. Prompt referral should be arranged for a patient in whom uveitis is suspected.

In general, referral to an ophthalmologist should strongly be considered for:

- Traumatic injury to the eye
- Loss of vision
- Extreme eye pain not explained by pathology
- Keratitis
- Suspected uveitis or glaucoma
- Chemical injury (especially alkali)
- Corneal abrasion not healing

REFERENCES

American Optometric Association. Optometric clinical practice guideline: Care of the patient with anterior uveitis. Revised March 1999. PDF available at www.aoa.org/documents/CPG-7.pdf; June 23, 1994 [accessed 20.06.10].

Arbour JD, Brunette I, Boisjoly HM, et al. Should we patch corneal abrasions? Arch Ophthalmol 1997;115(3):313–7.

Au YK, Henkind P. Pain elicited by consensual pupillary reflex: a diagnostic test for acute iritis. Lancet 1981;2:1254–5.

Avdic E, Cosgrove SE. Management and control strategies for community-associated methicillin-resistant *Staphylococcus aureus*. Expert Opin Pharmacother 2008;9(9):1463–79.

Boder F, Marchant C, et al. Bacterial etiology of conjunctivitis-otitis media syndrome. Pediatrics 1985;76:26–8.

Bradford CA. Basic Ophthalmology. 8th ed. San Francisco: American Academy of Ophthalmology; 2004.

De Toledo AR, Chandler JW. Conjunctivitis of the newborn. Infect Dis Clin North Am 1992;6(4):807–13.

Frith P, Gray R, MacLennan S, et al. The Eye in Clinical Practice. Oxford: Blackwell Scientific; 1994.

Jackson WB. Blepharitis: Current strategies for diagnosis and treatment. Can J Ophthalmol 2008;43(2):170–9.

Liebowitz HM. The red eye. N Engl J Med 2000;343(5):345–51.

Patterson J, Fetzer D, Krall J, et al. Eye patch treatment for the pain of corneal abrasion. South Med J 1996;89(2):227–9.

Prochazka AV. Diagnosis and treatment of red eye. Primary Care Case Reviews 2001;4:23–31.

Rietveld RP, van Weert H, Riet G, Bindels P. Diagnostic impact of signs and symptoms in acute infectious conjunctivitis: Systematic literature search. BMJ 2003;327(4):789.

Tarabishy A, Jeng B. Bacterial conjunctivitis: A review for internists. Cleve Clin J Med 2008;75(7):507–12.

Talbot EM. A simple test to diagnose iritis. BMJ 1987;295:812–3.

Trobe JD. The Physician's Guide to Eye Care. 2nd ed. San Francisco: Foundation of the American Academy of Ophthalmology; 2001.

Wilson SA, Last A. Management of corneal abrasion. Am Fam Physician 2004;70:123–30.

Wong AH, Barg SS, Leung AK. Seasonal and perennial allergic conjunctivitis. Recent Pat Inflamm Allergy Drug Disc 2009;3(2):118–27.

Optic Neuritis

Method of
Fiona Costello, MD

Idiopathic optic neuritis (ON) is an acquired, inflammatory, demyelinating optic nerve injury that commonly affects young adults. ON can occur as a clinically isolated syndrome (CIS) or in association with multiple sclerosis (MS). In 20% of cases, patients present with ON as their first manifestation of MS; and a significant proportion of MS patients develop ON during the course of their disease.

Clinical Presentation

Patients with ON often describe acute to subacute onset of vision loss, with associated pain on eye movement. Women make up the majority of cases, and approximately one third of patients experience positive visual phenomena, such as sparkles, flashes of light, or other photopsias. Loss of color vision, or dyschromatopsia, is also common. A variety of visual field loss patterns occur, including cecocentral, arcuate, and altitudinal defects. Patients with unilateral ON have a relative afferent pupil defect in the affected eye, but this clinical finding may be absent in cases of bilateral ocular involvement. The fundus examination is normal in most adult patients at presentation, but mild hyperemia of the optic disc occurs in approximately one third of cases. Visual recovery typically occurs 4 to 6 weeks after symptom onset, at which time optic disc pallor often becomes evident in the affected eye.

Atypical clinical features such as hemorrhages and exudates should serve as "red flags" and prompt the clinician to consider possible ON mimics. Failure of clinical improvement, for example, may indicate an underlying compressive lesion, such as an optic nerve sheath tumor or a suprasellar mass. Bilateral simultaneous vision loss may lead to a diagnosis of Leber's hereditary optic neuropathy. Abundant vitreous cells or florid optic disc edema at the time of presentation suggests the diagnosis of neuroretinitis, and careful clinical follow-up of these patients often reveals the development of a "macular star." Patients with vascular risk factors may present with abrupt-onset vision loss and optic disc swelling due to anterior ischemic optic neuropathy. In such cases, the patients have a specific morphologic appearance of the optic disc, with a small or absent physiologic cup to suggest the diagnosis. Posterior ischemic optic neuropathy may be more challenging to distinguish from ON, because optic disc swelling is not apparent at initial presentation. Again, a compatible clinical history and clinical course should suggest this diagnosis, which is considered one of exclusion. Systemic clinical manifestations including fever, rash, joint pain, alopecia, and lymphadenopathy are not typical for ON, and patients with these signs and symptoms should be investigated for underlying disorders including lymphoma, sarcoidosis, or systemic lupus erythematosus.

CURRENT DIAGNOSIS

- Age greater than 45 years
- Optic disc pallor at "acute" presentation
- Bilateral simultaneous vision loss
- Absence of pain, or pain that progresses over weeks
- Atypical fundus features (abundant vitreous cells, florid optic disc edema, hemorrhages, and exudates)
- Poor or no visual recovery
- History of myelitis with poor clinical recovery
- Associated systemic signs and symptoms (rash, joint swelling, fever, or lymphadenopathy)

Neuromyelitis optica is a severe inflammatory process of the optic nerves and spinal cord that is associated with poor clinical recovery. In addition to optic nerve involvement, patients with neuromyelitis optica typically develop clinical and magnetic resonance imaging (MRI) evidence of myelitis, with absent lesions on brain imaging. The recently described neuromyelitis optica immunoglobulin G autoantibody can be used to expedite diagnosis and treatment of this distinct clinical syndrome.

Investigations

ON remains a clinical diagnosis, yet its association with MS serves as an impetus for additional investigations, including cranial MRI. Many ON patients demonstrate clinically silent lesions on their baseline MRI study (50%-70%) and harbor abnormal cerebrospinal fluid constituents (60%-70%), increasing their future risk of MS. The Optic Neuritis Treatment Trial (ONTT) experience has shown that the presence or absence of white matter lesions on the baseline cranial MRI scan can predict the future risk of clinically definite MS (CDMS) after ON. Twenty-five percent of ON patients with no brain lesions on their baseline cranial MRI scan developed CDMS after 15 years of follow-up, compared with 72% of patients with one or more lesions. Furthermore, among ON patients with no MRI lesions, male gender, optic disc swelling, and atypical clinical features (e.g., no light perception vision, lack of pain, severe optic disc edema, peripapillary hemorrhages, retinal exudates) were associated with a reduced future risk of CDMS.

Current Approach to Therapy: Acute and Long-term Management

Much of our understanding regarding the clinical presentation and acute management of ON has come from the ONTT, which was designed to compare the speed and level of visual recovery after treatment with oral prednisone, intravenous methylprednisolone (IVMP; Solu-Medrol), or placebo. Patients were randomized into three groups within 8 days after symptom onset. Those treated with oral prednisone (1 mg/kg/day for 14 days) demonstrated an increased incidence of recurrent ON, compared to those treated with IVMP (250 mg every 6 hours for 3 days in hospital, followed by oral prednisone for 11 days), or those given oral placebo (for 14 days). IVMP therapy decreased the likelihood of developing CDMS after 2 years, although this effect was not sustained after 3 years. According to the American Academy of Neurology practice parameter for the role of corticosteroids in the management of acute monosymptomatic ON, oral prednisone in doses of 1 mg/kg/day has not demonstrated efficacy in promoting visual recovery and therefore has no proven value in treating ON. Higher-dose oral corticosteroids or IVMP may hasten the speed of visual recovery, but there is no evidence of long-term benefit for visual function. Hence, the decision to use these medications should be made with the intention to increase the speed of recovery but not to improve eventual visual outcome.

In light of the future risk of MS after ON, efforts have become more proactive to initiate disease-modifying drug therapies as early as the first demyelinating event so as to delay or possibly prevent this diagnosis. Three studies have addressed the role of interferon therapy in patients with ON and other CIS. The first of these was the Controlled High-Risk Subjects Avonex Multiple Sclerosis Prevention Study (CHAMPS), which included 383 CIS patients who were enrolled into a randomized, placebo-controlled trial if they had two or more clinically silent lesions on their baseline cranial MRI scan. Fifty percent (192 patients) of the CIS patients included in this study had ON. After initial treatment with high-dose IVMP, half of the patients received weekly interferon beta-1a (Avonex)[1] 30 µg once weekly,

---

[1]Not FDA approved for this indication.

CURRENT THERAPY

- Investigate for clinical mimics in patients with atypical signs or symptoms.
- Request cranial magnetic resonance imaging to predict future risk of multiple sclerosis.
- Avoid standard dose of oral prednisone (1 mg/kg/day).
- Consider treatment with high-dose corticosteroids (equivalent to intravenous methylprednisolone 1000 mg/day) to enhance the rate of visual recovery in appropriate patients.
- Consider initiating a disease-modifying therapy in optic neuritis patients deemed to be at high risk for multiple sclerosis in the future.

and half received placebo. There was a significantly lower rate (44%) of MS and a relative reduction of new MRI lesions in patients treated with interferon versus placebo. A second study, the Early Treatment of Multiple Sclerosis (ETOMS) study, enrolled 308 CIS patients with four asymptomatic white matter lesions (or three lesions if one of them enhanced with gadolinium) on the baseline cranial MRI scan. Half of the patients received subcutaneous interferon beta-1a (Rebif)[1] 22 µg once weekly, and half received placebo. After 2 years, fewer patients developed clinically significant MS in the interferon-treated group (34%) as compared to the placebo group (45%). The Betaferon in Newly Emerging Multiple Sclerosis for Initial Treatment (BENEFIT) trial included CIS patients with at least two brain MRI lesions, who were randomized to receive interferon beta-1b (Betaseron)[1] 250 µg subcutaneously on alternate days or placebo until the diagnosis of CDMS or a 24-month follow-up point was reached. Treatment with interferon beta-1b delayed the time to diagnosis of MS. In the recent PreCiSe study, 481 patients presenting with a CIS were randomly assigned to receive either subcutaneous glatiramer acetate 20 mg per day ($n = 243$) or placebo ($n = 238$) for up to 36 months, unless they converted to clinically definite multiple sclerosis. Glatiramer acetate reduced the risk of developing clinically definite multiple sclerosis by 45% compared with placebo (hazard ratio 0.55; 95% CI 0.40-0.77; $p = 0.0005$).

Prognosis and Future Considerations

Most patients with ON have an excellent visual prognosis and achieve visual acuity of 20/40 or better after 12 months of follow-up. Nevertheless, many patients report subtle and persistent visual problems after ON, including loss of stereovision, loss of depth perception, and altered motion perception. Patients with prior ON may also describe Uhthoff's phenomenon, which refers to recurrent symptoms of visual disturbance induced by exercise or increased body temperature.

The prognosis for ON patients depends in large part on their risk of recurrent MS-related relapses, and long-term management must be tailored to meet the needs of the individual. Patients with MRI abnormalities who are deemed to be at future risk of MS can benefit from early treatment, and initiation of disease-modifying drug therapy should be considered in these individuals.

---

[1]Not FDA approved for this indication.

REFERENCES

Beck RW, Cleary PA, Anderson MM. A randomized controlled trial of corticosteroids in the treatment of acute optic neuritis. N Engl J Med 1992;326:581–8.
Comi G, Filippi M, Barkof F. Effect of early interferon treatment on conversion to definite multiple sclerosis: A randomized study. Lancet 2001;357:1576–82.
Comi G, Martinelli V, Rodegher M, et al. PreCISe study group. Effect of glatiramer acetate on conversion to clinically definite multiple sclerosis in patients with clinically isolated syndrome (PreCISe study): a randomised, double-blind, placebo-controlled trial. Lancet 2009;374(9700):1503–11. Epub 2009 Oct 6.
Hickman SJ, Dalton CM, Miller DH. Management of acute optic neuritis. Lancet 2002;360:1953–62.
Jacobs LD, Beck RW, Simon JH. Intramuscular interferon beta-1a therapy initiated during a first demyelinating event in multiple sclerosis. N Engl J Med 2000;343:898–904.
Kappos L, Polman CH, Freedman MS, et al. Treatment with interferon beta-1b delays conversion to clinically definite and McDonald MS in patients with clinically isolated syndromes. Neurology 2006;67:1242–9.
Kaufman DI, Trobe JD, Eggenberger ER, et al. Practice parameter: The role of corticosteroids in the management of acute mononysymptomatic optic neuritis. Neurology 2000;54:2039–44.
Lennon VA, Wingerchuk DM, Kryzer TJ, et al. A serum autoantibody marker of neuromyelitis optica: Distinction from multiple sclerosis. Lancet 2004;354:2106–12.
Miller D, Barkhof F, Montalban X, et al. Clinically isolated syndromes suggestive of multiple sclerosis. Part 1: Natural history, pathogenesis, diagnosis and prognosis. Lancet Neurol 2005;4:281–8.
Optic Neuritis Study Group. The clinical profile of optic neuritis: Experience of the Optic Neuritis Treatment Trial. Arch Ophthalmol 1991;109:1673–8.
Optic Neuritis Study Group. High and low risk profiles for the development of mutiple sclerosis within 10 years after optic neuritis. Arch Ophthalmol 2003;121:944–9.
Optic Neuritis Study Group. Multiple sclerosis risk after optic neuritis: Final optic neuritis treatment trial follow-up. Arch Neurol 2008;65:727–32.
Soderstrom M, Ya-Ping J, Hillert J. Optic neuritis prognosis for multiple sclerosis from MRI, CSF, and HLA findings. Neurology 1998;50:708–14.

Uveitis

Method of
Petros E. Carvounis, MD, FRCSC

Uveitis refers to intraocular inflammation: it comprises multiple disease entities, some of which are caused by infectious agents and some of which are immune mediated. Uveitis can be classified by the predominant anatomic location of the inflammation: if it is in the anterior chamber, it is an anterior uveitis (previously known as iritis or iridocyclitis); if it is in the vitreous, it is an intermediate uveitis; and if it is in the retina or choroid, it is a posterior uveitis. In panuveitis, inflammation involves all of these sites. Uveitis is said to be limited if it lasts less than 3 months or persistent if it lasts longer than 3 months.

Clinical Features and Diagnosis

ANTERIOR UVEITIS

Anterior uveitis is the most commonly encountered type. It typically manifests with sudden-onset severe photosensitivity, pain, blurred vision, and red eye. Clinical examination documents decreased vision, limbal injection, keratic precipitates (cells and protein on the corneal endothelium), and an anterior chamber reaction (white cells and flare-increased light scatter in the anterior chamber caused by the increased protein concentration resulting from inflammation-induced vascular permeability). The anterior uveitis associated with juvenile idiopathic arthritis in children may be asymptomatic.

Anterior uveitis is commonly idiopathic but may be associated with human leukocyte antigen (HLA) B27; other HLA-B27 conditions, such as ankylosing spondylitis, Achilles' tendonitis, plantar fasciitis, and dactylitis, should be sought. It may also be associated with psoriatic arthropathy, Reiter's syndrome (although conjunctivitis is its most common feature), inflammatory bowel disease (which is also associated with intermediate uveitis), or sarcoidosis. Rheumatoid arthritis does not cause uveitis, although it may cause scleritis. In a patient with prior intraocular surgery or recent trauma, postoperative infectious endophthalmitis is a possibility. Infectious causes such as tuberculosis, syphilis, and Lyme disease need to be excluded, because they are curable. Viral infections (e.g., herpes simplex virus, varicella-zoster virus) can lead to an anterior uveitis, but they more frequently cause keratitis. Other rare associations are possible.

A good history, including a very thorough systems review combined with a good clinical examination including dilated funduscopy (to rule out retina or choroid involvement) by an ophthalmologist with expertise and interest in uveitis is mandatory for appropriate diagnosis and management.

A first occurrence of anterior uveitis that readily responds to topical corticosteroids (see later discussion) does not require further investigation unless there is strong suggestion of an associated systemic disorder based on the history and general physical examination. Investigation for anterior uveitis that is recurrent or is unresponsive to topical corticosteroids should be tailored based on the clinical examination findings but should not neglect to rule out syphilis, tuberculosis, Lyme disease, and HIV.

INTERMEDIATE UVEITIS

Intermediate uveitis typically manifests in a young or middle-aged adult with pain, photosensitivity, blurred vision, and floaters. The most important finding on clinical examination is a vitreitis (white cells in the vitreous and vitreous haze).

Intermediate uveitis is commonly idiopathic (pars planitis) or may be associated with tuberculosis, sarcoidosis, Lyme disease, syphilis, inflammatory bowel disease, or, rarely, multiple sclerosis. Intraocular lymphoma should be considered in patients older than 50 years of age who have vitreitis. Investigation of intermediate uveitis is mandatory, because it is usually unresponsive to topical corticosteroid drops.

POSTERIOR UVEITIS

Posterior uveitis is commonly infectious. Patients complain of visual loss and floaters. Clinical signs include decreased visual acuity, vitreous cells and haze, and some of the following: retinal infiltrates, serous retinal detachment, retinal hemorrhage, chorioretinal scars, choroidal granulomas, venular sheathing, or arteriolar sheathing.

The most common cause of posterior uveitis is *Toxoplasma* retinochoroiditis. Viral infections such as varicella-zoster or herpes simplex can uncommonly cause acute retinal necrosis, and cytomegalovirus retinitis can be devastating in immunocompromised individuals. Tuberculosis, Lyme disease, and syphilis are bacterial causes of posterior uveitis. *Pneumocystis jiroveci* (formerly called *Pneumocystis carinii*) and *Cryptococcus* can cause a choroiditis in the immunocompromised individual. Sarcoidosis can also cause posterior uveitis. There is a plethora of well-defined posterior uveitides without associated systemic findings (e.g., serpiginous chorioretinitis). Intraocular lymphoma can masquerade as posterior uveitis and needs be considered in older patients.

CURRENT DIAGNOSIS

- The most common form of uveitis is anterior uveitis.
- Anterior uveitis is commonly idiopathic.
- Posterior uveitis is most likely infectious.
- In any form of uveitis, syphilis, tuberculosis, and Lyme disease need to be ruled out.
- In immunosuppressed individuals, the uveitis is most likely infectious: the patient's HIV status needs to be determined, because a positive status completely changes the diagnostic approach.
- The key to correct diagnosis is a good history, including a thorough review of systems and a careful ophthalmologic examination as well as dilated funduscopy; laboratory and radiographic investigations, sometimes including aqueous or vitreous polymerase chain reaction or cytologic studies, are frequently necessary.
- Involvement of an ophthalmologist with expertise in the diagnosis and treatment of uveitis is mandatory.

Unless a clinical diagnosis is possible (e.g., in *Toxoplasma* chorioretinitis), further investigations are required. If a rapid plasma reagin test is negative, a diagnostic vitrectomy should be considered in all patients and is mandatory in immunocompromised patients; otherwise, tailored laboratory and radiographic investigations need be performed.

PANUVEITIS

Panuveitis combines the signs and symptoms of anterior and posterior uveitis, although early in the course one location may predominate. Bacterial or fungal endophthalmitis needs be considered. Vogt-Koyanagi-Harada syndrome is a common cause in the Far East and in patients of Native American ancestry. Adamantiades-Behçet syndrome, sympathetic ophthalmia, tuberculosis, syphilis, and, rarely, Lyme disease need be considered, among others.

Sequelae and Complications of Uveitis

Uncontrolled uveitis can be a blinding condition. Visual loss results commonly from cystoid macular edema or from cataracts, glaucoma, band keratopathy, hypotony maculopathy, macular scar, macular necrosis, or retinal detachment.

Current Treatment

Almost all of the medications employed in the treatment of uveitis are used off-label (FDA approved for an indication other than the treatment of uveitis).

CURRENT THERAPY

- Uveitis resulting from a systemic infection (e.g., syphilis, Lyme disease, tuberculosis) needs to be treated as a central nervous system infection.
- Idiopathic anterior uveitis or anterior uveitis related to an autoimmune disease responds to topical corticosteroids (e.g., prednisolone acetate [Pred Forte] 1% 1 drop every 2 hours while awake[3]) and cycloplegia (e.g., homatropine [Isopto Homatropine][1] 2% 1 drop three times daily).
- Periocular steroids (posterior or anterior sub-Tenon's steroid injection) is useful in the management of severe anterior uveitis and in intermediate uveitis.
- Intraocular triamcinolone acetonide injection (Kenalog)[1] or implantation of a sustained-release fluocinolone implant (Retisert) is reserved for cases of severe uveitis.
- Oral steroids (prednisone 1–2 mg/kg PO) can be effective in cases of severe uveitis that is unresponsive to topical, periocular, and intraocular steroids.
- Systemic immunosuppressants can control uveitis unresponsive to steroids or be used as steroid-sparing agents. Some specific uveitides mandate systemic immunosuppression as first-line treatment.
- Commonly used immunosuppressants are azathioprine (Imuran),[1] methotrexate (Trexall),[1] cyclosporine (Neoral),[1] and mycophenolate mofetil (CellCept).[1]
- Anti-tumor necrosis factor-α agents are promising immunomodulators.

---

[1]Not FDA approved for this indication.
[3]Exceeds dosage recommended by the manufacturer.

ANTERIOR UVEITIS

If photosensitivity is a prominent complaint, topical cycloplegia affords considerable relief. Homatropine (Isopto Homatropine) 2% or 5%, scopolamine (Isopto Hyoscine) 0.25%, or tropicamide (Mydriacyl) 1% may be used. Cyclopentolate (Cyclogyl) should be avoided, because it has chemoattractant properties in vitro. Topical cycloplegia is also necessary with severe anterior uveitis to prevent posterior synechiae.

Topical corticosteroid drops are the first line of treatment for anterior uveitis (e.g., prednisolone acetate [Pred Forte] 1% 1 drop every 2 hours while awake).[3] Patient education to ensure compliance is of paramount importance. Rimexolone (Vexol) 1% is considered an alternative by some authorities.

After 1 to 2 weeks, a slow taper of the drops is commenced (administer four times daily for 7–10 days, then taper by 1 drop every 7–10 days), provided that the anterior chamber cells have resolved. If there is an increase in activity during the taper, an increase in the dosing frequency to re-achieve a complete response, followed by a slower taper, is performed. Occasionally, patients have to be maintained for the long term on topical prednisolone; this is acceptable, provided that no adverse side effects occur.

If there is incomplete response prednisolone acetate 1% given every 2 hours or if the drops cannot be tapered without recurrence and investigations are negative, the next step to be considered could be a sub-Tenon's (under the conjunctiva) injection of 0.5 to 1.0 mL triamcinolone acetonide 40 mg/mL (Kenalog),[1,6,*] which forms a depot providing continuous steroid release for up to 6 months; alternatively, oral corticosteroids (usually prednisone) may be used in patients with especially severe bilateral uveitis, although this is uncommon. For the rare severe anterior uveitis that is unresponsive to these treatments or to decreases in the steroid dose, immunosuppressant medications such as methotrexate,[1] cyclosporine,[1] or mycophenolate mofetil[1] or an anti-tumor necrosis factor-α (anti-TNF-α) agent such as infliximab)[1] may be given (see later discussion for recommended doses).

It cannot be overemphasized that a severe "anterior uveitis," especially with a hypopyon, occurring after recent intraocular surgery or trauma should alert the physician to the possibility of endophthalmitis. Emergent anterior chamber and vitreous cultures need be obtained, and intravitreous nonpreserved vancomycin (Vancocin) 1.0 mg/0.1 mL[6] and ceftazidime (Fortaz) 2.25 mg/0.1 mL[6] must be injected.

The main side effects of topical steroid use are cataract formation and ocular hypertension, which can lead to glaucoma. Untreated uveitis can cause the same side effects; therefore, inflammation needs be controlled promptly, and then the corticosteroids need to be tapered off as soon as possible without precipitating a recurrence. Topical steroid use also predisposes to cornea infection, including reactivation of herpes simplex or varicella-zoster keratitis.

INTERMEDIATE UVEITIS, POSTERIOR UVEITIS, AND PANUVEITIS

Uveitis associated with systemic infection (e.g. syphilis, Lyme disease) is treated in consultation with an infectious disease specialist, because intraocular involvement is considered central nervous system involvement. Adjuvant topical corticosteroids and mydriatics can afford relief without jeopardizing cure in most cases (as for anterior uveitis).

Ocular toxoplasmosis, the most common posterior uveitis, is self-limited. Treatment is required in cases in which the optic nerve or macula is threatened or the vitreitis is particularly severe. Treatment consists of pyrimethamine (Daraprim) (loading dose 50 mg, then 25 mg twice daily), sulfadiazine (1 g four times daily), and folinic acid (Leucovorin)[1] 5 mg three times weekly. More recently, clindamycin (Cleocin)[1] 150 to 300 mg PO four times daily or trimethoprim-sulfamethoxazole[1] (Bactrim DS 800 mg sulfamethoxazole/160 mg trimethoprim twice daily) have been found to be equally efficacious

---

[1]Not FDA approved for this indication.
[3]Exceeds dosage recommended by the manufacturer.
[6]May be compounded by pharmacists.
[*]Kenalog is commercially available as 40 mg/mL. Special compounding is needed for the concentration of 4 mg/mL.

---

and are more widely used. Prednisone 40 mg/day is added 24 to 48 hours later. Treatment duration is usually 30 to 40 days, with a prednisone taper guided by the clinical response.

For intermediate uveitis, posterior uveitis, or panuveitis not associated with systemic infection, treatment options are to be considered in the following order:

1. Periocular steroids (posterior sub-Tenon's injection of triamcinolone acetonide)[1] are commonly efficacious for intermediate uveitis.
2. Oral corticosteroids are very efficacious but have ocular as well as systemic side effects. If the uveitis cannot be controlled with less than prednisone 10 mg after 6 months of treatment, one of the other options needs to be considered.
3. In very severe cases of intermediate uveitis and in cases of severe posterior uveitis or panuveitis, intravitreous triamcinolone acetonide (Kenalog 4 mg[1,*] or a fluocinolone implant (Retisert) inserted with a pars plana vitrectomy can be used; whether the latter is superior to systemic immunosuppression is the subject of an ongoing clinical trial (the Multicenter Uveitis Steroid Treatment [MUST] trial).
4. Systemic immunosuppression with azathioprine (Imuran)[1] up to 2.5 to 4 mg/kg/day, cyclosporine (Neoral)[1] 2.5 to 5.0 mg/kg/day in 2 divided doses, tacrolimus (Prograf)[1] 0.15 to 0.30 mg/kg/day, mycophenolate mofetil (CellCept)[1] 500 to 1000 mg twice daily, methotrexate (Trexall)[1] (12.5 to 25 mg weekly, or an anti-TNF-α agent (e.g., infliximab [Remicade])[1] have all been used with success as steroid-sparing agents or to control uveitis poorly responsive to corticosteroids alone.

There are specific uveitis entities that mandate the use of immunosuppression as first-line treatment (together with steroids initially). These include Wegener's retinal vasculitis, Adamantiades-Behçet's syndrome, sympathetic ophthalmia, and possibly birdshot choroidopathy, uveitis related to Vogt-Koyanagi-Harada syndrome, and serpiginous chorioretinitis.

---

[1]Not FDA approved for this indication.
[*]Kenalog is commercially available as 40 mg/mL. Special compounding is needed for the concentration of 4 mg/mL.

REFERENCES

Harper SL, Chorich LJ, Foster CS. Diagnosis of uveitis. In: Foster CS, Vitale A, editors. Diagnosis and Treatment of Uveitis. Philadelphia: WB Saunders; 2002. p. 79–97.

Jabs DA, Rosenbaum JT, Foster CS, et al. Guidelines for the use of immunosuppressive drugs in patients with ocular inflammatory disorders: Recommendations of an expert panel. Am J Ophthalmol 2000;130:492–513.

Nussenblatt RB. Philosophy, goals and approaches to medical therapy. In: Nussenblatt SM, Whitcup SM, editors. Uveitis, Fundamentals and Clinical Practice. 3rd ed. Philadelphia: Mosby; 2004. p. 95–136.

The Standardization of Uveitis Nomenclature (SUN) working group. Standardization of uveitis nomenclature for reporting clinical data: Results of the first international workshop. Am J Ophthalmol 2005;140:509–16.

Glaucoma

Method of
Albert P. Lin, MD, and Silvia Orengo-Nania, MD

Glaucoma is an optic neuropathy with characteristic optic nerve head appearance: narrowing of the neuroretinal rim. The optic nerve is a collection of more than 1 million axons from the retinal ganglion cells. The anterior 1-mm portion of the optic nerve within the globe is referred to as the *optic disk* or simply the disk. When the disk is examined with direct or indirect ophthalmoscopy, a cup, or a physiologic empty space, is observed centrally. The remainder of the disk,

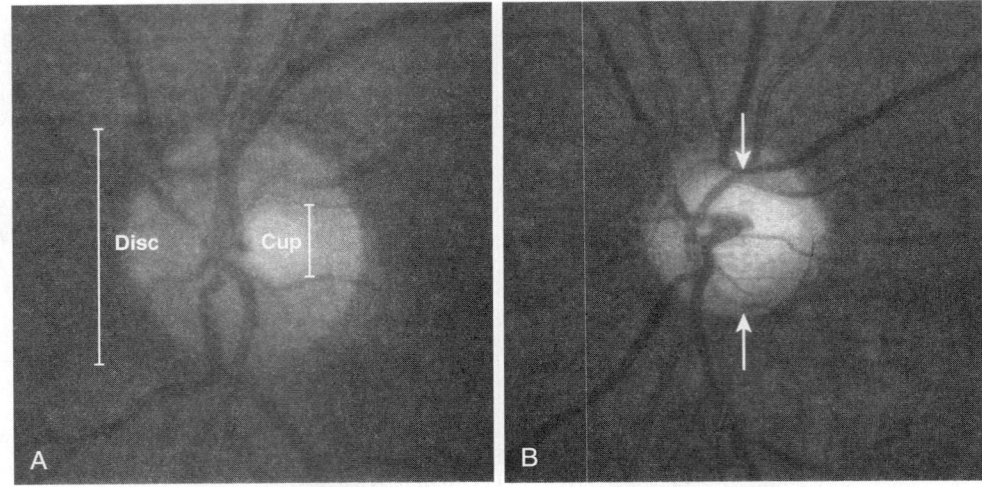

FIGURE 1. Disk appearance. **A,** Normal disk. Cup-to-disk ratio is less than 0.4. **B,** Glaucoma. Increased cup-to-disk ratio and narrow neuroretinal rim superiorly and inferiorly *(arrows)*.

which has a yellow-orange appearance, contains the axons and is referred to as the *neuroretinal rim*. The area of the cup compared to the entire disk is the cup-to-disk ratio, which is normally less than 0.4 (Figure 1A). When patients develop glaucoma, axons are lost from the neuroretinal rim and the size of the cup increases in relation to the disk. Narrowing of the neuroretinal rim and increased cup-to-disk ratio are the hallmarks of glaucomatous optic neuropathy (Figure 1B).

Glaucoma can result in significant and irreversible loss of vision and is one of the leading causes of blindness in the United States. Early in the disease state, glaucoma is asymptomatic. As the disease progresses, the patient develops decreased peripheral vision and eventually loss of the central vision.

Glaucoma is typically associated with increased intraocular pressure (IOP), but it is possible to have normal-tension or low-tension glaucoma. Glaucoma treatment is focused on the reduction of IOP to prevent or slow optic nerve damage and preserve visual function.

Glaucoma is classified in many ways, and it is most useful to approach it clinically based on the status of the angle, the area between the cornea and iris where aqueous exits the globe. We further discuss primary open angle glaucoma, the most common form of glaucoma in the United States, and the management of acute angle closure, one of the true ophthalmic emergencies.

Primary Open Angle Glaucoma

Glaucoma is one of the leading causes of blindness in older adults, especially in patients of African-American descent. Vision loss from glaucoma is irreversible, and the treatment goal is to reduce IOP, slow disease progression, and preserve visual function during the patient's lifetime. Glaucoma is a slowly progressive disease, and progression to blindness often takes more than 10 years, even in untreated patients. Given its slow progression and the fact that central vision loss occurs in late disease, most patients do well with early diagnosis and treatment. Treatment is more difficult in late disease because the rate of disease progression and visual deterioration is accelerated, sometimes despite good control of IOP.

Due to the early asymptomatic nature of the disease, the patient's adherence and persistence with treatment is often less than optimal. Studies have shown patients who obtain glaucoma information from physicians other than their ophthalmologists have a higher rate of medication adherence. Ophthalmologists have the options to use treatment modalities such as laser and surgery to obtain pressure control and decrease or eliminate the need for medication use.

 CURRENT DIAGNOSIS

Primary Open Angle Glaucoma

- Primary open angle glaucoma is an irreversible optic neuropathy typically associated with elevated intraocular pressure.
- Primary open angle glaucoma is the most common form of glaucoma and is projected to affect more than 3 million Americans in 2020. It is more common in African-Americans (6%-7%), Asians (2%-3%), and Hispanics (2%) and less common in whites (1%). It is more common in older adults: 1%-2% in 50-year-olds compared to 6%-12% in 80-year-olds.
- Primary open angle glaucoma is diagnosed by a complete ophthalmic examination, including dilated stereoscopic optic nerve exam and formal visual field.
- Untreated primary open angle glaucoma can lead to slow irreversible loss of vision and blindness. Other common causes of slow and progressive vision loss in older adults include cataracts, macular degeneration, and diabetic retinopathy.

Acute Angle Glaucoma

- Pupillary block in susceptible patients leads to block of aqueous drainage and sudden and extreme rise of intraocular pressure. Acute angle closure can damage the optic nerve, resulting in acute angle closure glaucoma.
- About 0.5%-1.0% of U.S. adults is at risk for acute angle closure. It is more common in Inuits and Asians and rare in blacks. The risk of acute angle closure increases with age. It is also more common in hyperopes.
- Patients can present with blurry vision, red eye, pain, headache, nausea, or vomiting. Acute angle closure is sometimes misdiagnosed as migraines or gastrointestinal illnesses. Patients with conjunctivitis, keratitis, uveitis, and corneal abrasion can also present with the same symptoms.
- Peripheral iridotomy prevents acute angle closure in susceptible patients. High intraocular pressure can result in irreversible damage of the optic nerve within hours, making acute angle closure one of the true ophthalmic emergencies.

The American Academy of Ophthalmology recommends asymptomatic patients older than 40 years be referred for ophthalmic evaluation once every several years for early detection of glaucoma and other chronic eye diseases. However, the US Preventive Services Task Force found insufficient evidence to recommend for or against screening for glaucoma in adults. Risks, benefits, and cost effectiveness of screening are beyond the scope of this chapter, but symptomatic patients or patients at high risk for glaucoma (African-American ethnicity and family history) might benefit from ophthalmology consultation. It is possible to diagnose glaucoma by direct ophthalmoscopy, but it is not a substitute for binocular assessment of the disk through dilated pupils and formal visual field testing. If glaucoma is suspected or diagnosed, primary care visits should include inquiries regarding glaucoma medication use, medication side effects, and the time of last eye examination. Primary care physicians can improve glaucoma outcome by promoting adherence to medication and follow-up. Glaucoma patients need to follow up with their ophthalmologists at least annually, and in severe cases every 3 months, for intraocular pressure checks.

TREATMENT

TOPICAL GLAUCOMA MEDICATIONS

Topical glaucoma medications are administered once or twice daily. Patients should look up, pull down their lower eye lid, drop the medication on the inferior conjunctival cul-de-sac, and keep their eyes closed for 5 minutes. Applying gentle pressure next to the bridge of the nose to occlude the puncta can improve absorption of the medication. Medication bottle caps are color-coded by their class, and patients can usually identify their eye drops by color. Glaucoma medications are not subject to first-pass effect through the liver and can sometimes have significant systemic side effects, especially the β-blockers. Topical glaucoma medications are described later and summarized in Table 1.

Prostaglandin Analogues

Latanoprost (Xalatan), travoprost (Travatan), and bimatoprost (Lumigan) are prostaglandin analogues and are color-coded by teal caps. They are administered once at bedtime but may be administered once at any time during the day to promote adherence. They decrease IOP by increasing aqueous outflow. Side effects are primarily local and include increased conjunctival hyperemia, increased lash growth, and possible irreversible increase in periocular and iris pigmentation.

β-Blockers

Timolol (Betimol, Istalol, Timoptic), levobunolol (Betagan), and betaxolol (Betoptic) are color-coded by yellow caps. They are administered once or twice daily and decrease IOP by decreasing aqueous production. Side effects include bradycardia, exacerbation of chronic obstructive pulmonary disease (COPD) and asthma, impotence, and decreased serum high-density lipoprotein (HDL) cholesterol. Physicians need to be aware that a topical β-blocker is a potential cause of acute changes in cardiovascular or pulmonary status. There are several reported incidents of death following the use of topical β-blockers mostly due to exacerbation of asthma.

 CURRENT THERAPY

Primary Open Angle Glaucoma

- Topical eye drops, including β-blockers, selective α_2 agonists, carbonic anhydrase inhibitors, and prostaglandin analogues can be used to reduce intraocular pressure.
- Oral carbonic anhydrase inhibitors are typically used in recalcitrant cases until surgery can be performed.
- Laser trabeculoplasty may be used as first-line or adjunct therapy.
- Glaucoma surgery, including trabeculectomy, tube shunt, and cyclodestruction, may be performed if goal intraocular pressure cannot be reached with medical therapy or in nonadherent patients.

Acute Angle Glaucoma

- All glaucoma eye drops except prostaglandin analogues are used to reduce intraocular pressure.
- Oral and intravenous medications are added sequentially to reduce intraocular pressure as needed.
- Laser iridotomy can be performed as prophylactic treatment or acutely to break the pupillary block if the patient is unresponsive to medical intervention.
- Emergent trabeculectomy is performed if the patient is unresponsive to all other treatments.

Selective α_2 Agonists

Brimonidine (Alphagan) and apraclonidine (Iopidine) belong to the class of Selective α_2 receptor agonists, and brimonidine is more commonly prescribed; it is color-coded by purple caps. It is administered twice daily and decreases IOP by decreasing aqueous production. Allergic conjunctivitis has been reported in up to 25% of patients. Rarely, it causes dry mouth and chronic fatigue and drowsiness in the elderly.

Carbonic Anhydrase Inhibitors

Dorzolamide (Trusopt) and brinzolamide (Azopt) are color-coded by orange caps and are sulfa-based medications. They are administered twice daily and decrease IOP by decreasing aqueous production. This class of medication has minimal systemic side effects. However, some patients complain about transient stinging and a bitter taste in the mouth after administration. These side effects, if tolerable, are not indications for discontinuing therapy.

Combined Topical Medications

Timolol and dorzolamide (Cosopt) and timolol and brimonidine (Combigan) are color-coded by blue caps. Combined medications decrease exposure to preservatives and can decrease irritation and problem with dry eyes. Adherence might also be improved.

TABLE 1 Topical Glaucoma Medications: Carbonic Anhydrase Inhibitors

Class	β-Blocker	Selective α_2 Agonist	Carbonic Anhydrase Inhibitor	Prostaglandin Analogue	Combination
Medication	Timolol (Timoptic) Betaxolol (Betoptic) Levobunolol (Betagan)	Brimonidine (Alphagan)	Dorzolamide (Trusopt) Brinzolamide (Azopt)	Latanoprost (Xalatan) Travoprost (Travatan) Bimatoprost (Lumigan)	Timolol/Dorzolamide (Cosopt) Timolol/Brimonidine (Combigan)
Dosing	bid	bid	bid	qhs	bid
Cap color	Yellow	Purple	Orange	Teal	Blue
Side effects	Bradycardia COPD and asthma exacerbation	Allergic conjunctivitis, dry mouth, fatigue in elderly	Stinging, bitter taste	Hyperemia, lash growth, increased pigmentation	See individual components

COPD = chronic obstructive pulmonary disease.

ORAL CARBONIC ANHYDRASE INHIBITORS

Oral carbonic anhydrase inhibitors include acetazolamide (Diamox), 250 mg or 500 mg given twice daily, and methazolamide (Neptazane), 25 mg or 50 mg given twice daily. They are sulfa-based medications and decrease IOP by decreasing aqueous production. Oral carbonic anhydrase inhibitors are not commonly used today because effective topical medications are available. They are typically used on a short-term basis to achieve IOP control in acute or refractory cases. Side effects can include aplastic anemia, kidney stones, bitter taste, indigestion, paresthesia of the extremities, tinnitus, and polyuria. Clinicians need to consider the possibility of hypokalemia when patients take other diuretics to control blood pressure (Table 2). Acetazolamide may also be given intravenously.

LASER TRABECULOPLASTY

Argon or selective laser trabeculoplasty can be used to increase aqueous outflow. Laser trabeculoplasty is noninvasive and safe, and it can be performed in the office in less than 10 minutes. Compared to surgery, IOP reduction is limited, up to 25% as primary treatment, but less as an adjunct modality. It is ineffective or less effective in some patients with light trabecular meshwork pigmentation. The effect of laser decreases over time but may be repeated in the case of selective laser trabeculoplasty.

SURGERY

The most commonly performed glaucoma surgeries are trabeculectomy, tube shunt, and cyclodestruction. Trabeculectomy and tube shunt are procedures that create an opening in the sclera to increase aqueous outflow. Cyclodestruction destroys the ciliary body and decreases aqueous production. The procedure can be trans-scleral or endoscopic; the endoscopic method is typically done at the time of cataract surgery. Alternative surgical methods, such as deep sclerectomy, Trabectome, canaloplasty, and iStent, are being developed and performed to minimize the invasiveness and potential complications associated with traditional glaucoma surgery.

Visual Impairment and Blindness

Patients who are visually impaired (Snellen vision of less than 20/40) or legally blind (Snellen vision of less than 20/200 or visual field of less than 20 degrees) may have significantly decreased mobility and ability to function. Continued glaucoma treatment is still important in these patients because even maintenance of count-finger vision can allow the patients some degree of independence. Low vision devices and services, including high-contrast video magnifiers, audiobooks, eccentric viewers, and mobility training, can allow patients maximal use of their residual vision and improve their confidence and quality of life.

Acute Angle Closure Glaucoma

Pupillary block in susceptible patients blocks aqueous drainage and leads to sudden and extreme rise of intraocular pressure. Acute angle closure can damage the optic nerve, resulting in acute angle closure glaucoma.

About 0.5% to 1.0% of U.S. adults is at risk for acute angle closure. It is more common in Inuits and Asians and rare in African Americans. The risk of acute angle closure increases with age. It is also more common in hyperopes.

MECHANISM OF ACUTE ANGLE CLOSURE: PUPILLARY BLOCK

After aqueous is produced in the ciliary body in the posterior chamber, it travels through the pupil and exits the anterior chamber through the trabecular meshwork located between the iris and the cornea. Pupillary block occurs when the iris comes in contact with the lens and obstructs the flow of aqueous through the pupil. Increased posterior chamber pressure displaces the iris anteriorly against the trabecular meshwork and stops aqueous outflow.

Patients at risk for acute angle closure have narrow occludable angles. These patients have smaller eyes, allowing the lens to contact the iris to initiate papillary block. The distance between the iris and the lens is the shortest when the pupil is mid-dilated. Therefore, patients who present with acute angle closure might have a history of dim light exposure (movies) or use of medications with anticholinergic properties (antihistamines, decongestants, antispasmodics). High IOP causes iris and corneal endothelial cell dysfunction, resulting in nonreactive pupil and hazy cornea, respectively. High IOP also results in inflammation and red eye as well as severe pain, nausea, and vomiting (Figure 2). Elevated IOP can damage the optic nerve within hours, and acute angle closure needs to be treated emergently to prevent permanent loss of vision.

DIAGNOSIS

Patients with acute angle closure can present with blurry vision, red eye, pain, headache, nausea, or vomiting. History can include hyperopia, onset after exposure to a dim environment, or taking anticholinergic medications. Examination findings include decreased vision, conjunctival hyperemia, mid-dilated, nonreactive pupil with or without an afferent papillary defect, and increased IOP (by palpation or tonometry). Acute angle closure is sometimes misdiagnosed as migraines or gastrointestinal illness. Patients with conjunctivitis, keratitis, uveitis, and corneal abrasion can also present with the same symptoms.

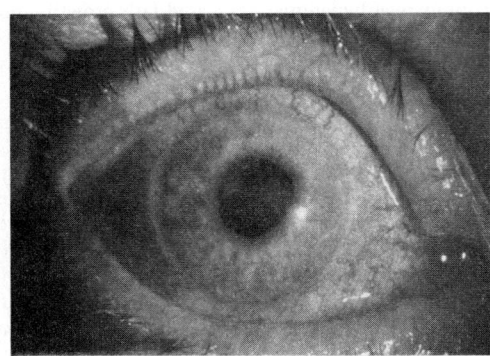

FIGURE 2. Acute angle closure patient with red eye and mid-dilated and nonreactive pupil.

TABLE 2 Oral and Intravenous Glaucoma Medications

Medication	Acetazolamide (Diamox)	Methazolamide (Neptazane)	Mannitol (Osmitrol)	Glycerin 50% (Osmoglyn)
Class	CAI	CAI	Hyperosomtic	Hyperosmotic
Dosage	250 or 500 mg bid	25 mg or 50 mg bid	1 g/kg in 30 min	1 g/kg once
Route	PO or IV	PO	IV	PO
Side Effects	Bitter taste, indigestion, paresthesia, tinnitus, polyuria, kidney stones, hypokalemia, aplastic anemia, sulfa allergy.		Polyuria, dehydration Exacerbate CHF and diabetes (glycerin).	

Abbreviations: CAI = carbonic anhydrase inhibitor; CHF = congestive heart failure.

TREATMENT

If acute angle closure is suspected, an emergent referral to ophthalmology is indicated. If an ophthalmologist is not immediately available, the goal will be to medically control the IOP as soon as possible. One drop of topical aqueous suppressant—β-blocker, selective α_2 agonist, or carbonic anhydrase inhibitor—should be administered (timolol, brimonidine, dorzolamide) (see Table 1). The maximum dose of oral or intravenous carbonic anhydrase inhibitor is given: acetazolamide 500 mg or methazolamide 50 mg (see Table 2). The patient is placed in the supine position to allow the lens and iris to fall posteriorly. The patient is reassessed in 30 minutes, and if the condition is not improved, topical drops are repeated. If there is no improvement after another 30 minutes, a hyperosmotic, oral glycerin (Osmoglyn) 1 g/kg or intravenous mannitol (Osmitrol) 1 g/kg over 30 minutes, is administered. Hyperosmotics may be contraindicated in patients with congestive heart failure, and glycerin can cause severe hyperglycemia in diabetic patients.

An ophthalmologist can break the papillary block by medically lowering the IOP or by performing anterior chamber paracentesis, compression gonioscopy, laser peripheral iridotomy, and, in recalcitrant cases, emergent trabeculectomy. Once the pressure is controlled, it is important to perform an iridotomy in both eyes to prevent future episodes. Patients with patent iridotomies may safety take anticholinergic medications.

REFERENCES

Allingham RR, Damji KF, Freedman S, et al., editors, Shield's Textbook of Glaucoma. 5th ed. Philadelphia: Lippincott Williams & Wilkins; 2005. p. 155–90.

American Academy of Ophthalmology. Practice guidelines. Preferred practice patterns. Primary angle closure. Available at: http://www.aao.org/CE/Practice Guidelines/PPP_Content.aspx?cid=a6a3402d-3fc6-44a4-9a52-46b74d37b830; September 2005 [accessed 20.06.10].

American Academy of Ophthalmology. Practice guidelines. Preferred practice patterns. Primary open-angle glaucoma. Available at: http://one.aao.org/CE/PracticeGuidelines/PPP_Content.aspx?cid=a5a59e02-450b-4d50-8091-b2dd21ef1ff2; September 2005 [accessed 20.06.10].

Congdon N, O'Colmain B, Klaver CC, et al. Eye Diseases Prevalence Research Group; Causes and prevalence of visual impairment among adults in the United States. Arch Ophthalmol 2004;122:477–85.

Friedman DS, Wolfs RC, O'Colmain BJ, et al. Eye Diseases Prevalence Research Group: Prevalence of open-angle glaucoma among adults in the United States. Arch Ophthalmol 2004;122(4):532–8.

Lin AP, Orengo-Nania S, Braun UK. PCP's role in chronic open-angle glaucoma. Geriatrics 2009;64:20–8.

Nordstrom BL, Friedman DS, Mozaffari E, et al. Persistence and adherence with topical glaucoma therapy. Am J Ophthalmol 2005;140:598–606.

Schwartz GF, Quigley HA. Adherence and persistence with glaucoma therapy. Surv Ophthalmol 2008;54:S57–S68.

US Preventive Services Task Force. Screening for glaucoma. Available at: http://www.ahrq.gov/CLINIC/uspstf/uspsglau.htm#summary; March, 2005 [accessed 20.06.10].

Otitis Externa

Method of
*Sheryl Beard, MD, and
Jennifer Wipperman, MD*

Acute otitis externa (AOE) is an inflammatory condition of the external auditory canal, which can also include the tympanic membrane or pinna. Every year, 1 to 2.5 in 100 people are affected. More often, otitis externa occurs during the summer.

Risk Factors

Conditions that disrupt cerumen or the skin barrier of the ear canal predispose to infection. Chronic trauma (cotton swabs, hearing aids, ear plugs), prolonged water exposure, dermatologic disorders, or obstructions (sebaceous cyst, canal stenosis) can alter cerumen and cause skin edema, leading to infection.

Pathophysiology

The external auditory canal is approximately 35 mm long and curves in an S-shape toward the tympanic membrane. The inner two thirds of the canal is osseous. The outer third is cartilaginous, and the overlying epithelium contains hair follicles and cerumen-producing glands. Cerumen acts as a moisture barrier, and its slightly acidic pH and lysozymes inhibit bacterial growth. Removal of cerumen exposes the epithelium, allowing bacterial infection and inflammation.

Prevention

Removing obstructing cerumen prevents moisture buildup. Using a hair dryer or acidifying ear drops after water exposure is beneficial. Swimmers may use ear plugs. Patients should also avoid aggressive cleaning with cotton swabs.

Clinical Manifestations

Patients present with itching and progressive pain that is worse with traction on the pinna. Initially, the ear canal is erythematous with minimal discharge. Later, the canal becomes narrowed from edema, drainage, and debris. Otorrhea, aural fullness and hearing loss are common. Tenderness is often disproportionate to physical examination findings. Some patients exhibit surrounding cellulitis or lymphadenitis.

Diagnosis

Diagnostic criteria for AOE include rapid onset of symptoms and signs of ear canal inflammation for less than 3 weeks. Pneumatic otoscopy and tympanometry are useful to differentiate AOE from AOM and also can demonstrate an intact tympanic membrane. Cultures of the ear canal are beneficial in refractory or recurrent cases. Imaging studies may be useful if malignant otitis externa is suspected.

Differential Diagnosis

AOM can occur separately or in conjunction with AOE. If purulent secretions from middle ear disease enter the ear canal, an inflammatory reaction known as *infectious eczematous dermatitis* can occur. *Contact dermatitis* causes pain and itching, with associated maculopapular lesions on the conchal bowl and a thickened ear canal. A common cause is neomycin otic preparations. Chronic dermatosis such as *psoriasis* or *allergic contact dermatitis* can cause ear canal itching, hyperkeratosis, and lichenification. *Otomycosis*, a fungal infection of the ear canal, is more common in patients with diabetes, immunocompromised states, or prolonged topical antibiotic treatment. The ear canal can have white debris sprouting hyphae *(Candida)* or a moist white plug dotted by black debris *(Aspergillus)*. Itching and thick otorrhea of various colors are common. Concomitant bacterial infection can occur, and fungal culture should be obtained in cases of refractory AOE. Finally, *furunculosis* is an infected hair follicle that is manifested by a tender, erythematous papule or pustule.

TABLE 1 Common topical otic preparations for treating Acute Otitis Externa

Active Drug	Trade Name	Dose (mL)	Cost (US$) Trade	Generic
Anti-infective				
Acetic acid, aluminum acetate	Otic Domeboro	60	31	22
Acetic acid, hydrocortisone	VoSol HC	10	110	24
Antibiotic				
Ciprofloxacin, hydrocortisone	Cipro HC	10	108	—
Ciprofloxacin, dexamethasone	Ciprodex	7.5	110	—
Neomycin, polymixin B, hydrocortisone	Cortisporin Otic	10	80	22
Ofloxacin	Floxin Otic	5	80	60
Antifungal				
Clotrimazole 1%[1]	Clotrimazole 1%	10	—	18

Modified from Rosenfeld FM, Brown L, Cannon CR, et al: Clinical practice guideline: Acute otitis externa. Otolaryngal Head Neck Surg 2006;134(Suppl. 4):S4–S23.
[1]Not FDA approved for this indication.

Treatment

Treatment of otitis externa generally consists of topical antimicrobial agents and pain control (Table 1). In most cases, NSAIDs or acetaminophen provides pain relief. Benzocaine otic solution (Oticaine 20% otic drops) should be used with caution because it can mask the progression of underlying disease. If benzocaine is used, the patient should be reexamined within 48 hours. Topical steroids also hasten pain relief by a median of 1 day compared to topical antibiotics alone.

Topical antibiotic otic preparations are the mainstay of therapy. *Pseudomonas* species are the most common causative bacteria, followed by *Staphylococcus*. Aminoglycoside and fluoroquinolone antibiotics have a 70-90% clinical response rate. Fluoroquinolones have a shorter and less-frequent dosing schedule, but they are more costly. Aminoglycoside and acidic solutions should be avoided in patients with tympanic membrane perforation or tympanostomy tubes. Neomycin should be avoided if contact dermatitis is suspected. Systemic antibiotics should be used if patients are immunocompromised or have surrounding cellulitis or if topical antibiotics cannot be delivered effectively.

Patients should avoid water exposure and ear trauma during treatment. Removal of obstructing debris ensures drug delivery. If the canal is extremely edematous, a Merocel wick may be inserted to allow better drug absorption. Anti-infective ribbon (glycerin and ichthammol[1] ribbon gauze) has also used with efficacy similar to that of topical antibiotics.

Monitoring

Significant improvement usually occurs within 48 to 72 hours. Most patients are symptom free in 4 to 7 days. If symptoms do not improve, the patient should be reevaluated. Clinical failure may be due to inadequate drug delivery, noncompliance, obstruction, or misdiagnosis.

Complications

Malignant otitis externa, a life-threatening complication, is mainly seen in diabetic or immunocompromised patients. Progressive infection invades the temporal bone, causing osteomylitis, and further spread can lead to cranial neuropathies (most often facial paralysis), dural sinus thrombosis, meningitis, or cerebral abscess. Clinical signs include severe pain, ottorhea, and granulation tissue at the bone–cartilaginous junction of the canal. Diagnosis may be confirmed by computed tomography scan, and cultures. Intravenous antibiotics are usually required, and in severe cases surgical débridement may be necessary.

Other complications include surrounding cellulitis or chondritis and perforation of the tympanic membrane. Chronic otitis externa can cause fibrous scarring, leading to obstruction of the medial canal, which requires surgical treatment.

REFERENCES

Carfrae MJ, Kesser BW. Malignant otitis externa. Otolaryngol Clin North Am 2008;41(3):537–49 viii–ix.
Hornigold R, Gillet D, Kiverniti E, et al. The management of otitis externa: A randomised controlled trial of a glycerol and icthammol ribbon gauze versus topical antibiotic and steroid drops. Eur Arch Otorhinolaryngol 2008;265(10):1199–203.
Manolidis S, Friedman R, Hannley M, et al. Comparative efficacy of aminoglycoside versus fluoroquinolone topical antibiotic drops. Otolaryngol Head Neck Surg 2004;130(Suppl. 3):S83–8.
Rosenfeld RM, Brown L, Cannon CR, et al. Clinical practice guideline: Acute otitis externa. Otolaryngol Head Neck Surg 2006;134(Suppl. 4):S4–S23.
Rosenfeld RM, Singer M, Wasserman JM, et al. Systematic review of topical antimicrobial therapy for acute otitis externa. Otolaryngol Head Neck Surg 2006;134(Suppl. 4):S24–S48.
Ruckenstein MJ. Infections of the external ear. In: Cummings CW, editor. Otolaryngology: Head and Neck Surgery. 4th ed. Philadelphia: Mosby; 2005.

Otitis Media

Method of
*Diane E. Pappas, MD, JD, and
J. Owen Hendley, MD*

Otitis media is a common pediatric diagnosis, accounting for an average of 12.8 million visits per year in children age 12 years and younger. Although most ear infections in the United States are still treated with antibiotics, increasing concern over antibiotic resistance coupled with increased understanding of inflammation of the tympanic membrane require an ongoing reassessment of the proper diagnosis and treatment of otitis media.

Epidemiology

Otitis media is most common during early childhood, and at least one such illness is diagnosed in more than 70% of children by the age of 5 years. Approximately one third of these children have recurrent otitis media, and about 5% to 10% develop chronic middle ear disease.

[1]Not FDA approved for this indication.

Peak incidence occurs during the last half of the first year of life; in infants 6 to 12 months of age, at least one episode of acute otitis media is diagnosed in 62%, and three or more episodes of acute otitis media are diagnosed in 17%. The majority of these infections (70%) are associated with viral respiratory infections, and they are most common during the fall and winter months as the respiratory viruses spread in successive waves through the community.

The most common bacterial pathogens are *Streptococcus pneumoniae* (25%-50%), *Haemophilus influenzae* (about 15%-30%), and *Moraxella catarrhalis* (about 3%-20%), all of which are common flora in the nasopharynx. Bacterial resistance is common, and approximately 100% of *M. catarrhalis*, 50% of *H. influenzae*, and 30% of *S. pneumoniae* are resistant. Resistance in *H. influenzae* and *M. catarrhalis* is due to the production of β-lactamase, enzymes that destroy the antibacterial effectiveness of penicillins. Resistance in *S. pneumoniae* operates via a different mechanism; the penicillin-binding protein of the bacteria is altered such that antibiotics cannot bind and exert their antibacterial effects on the bacterial cell wall. The resistant *S. pneumoniae* can be further classified based on the degree of resistance, with about half having intermediate resistance (minimum inhibitory concentration between 0.1 and 1 μg/mL) and about half classified as highly resistant (minimum inhibitory concentration >2 μg/mL).

Viral pathogens can also be present. Viral pathogens alone have been found by tympanocentesis in as many as 5% to 22% of episodes of acute otitis media, including respiratory syncytial virus, rhinovirus, coronavirus, parainfluenza, and adenovirus.

Risk Factors

The development of acute otitis media is the result of the interplay of multiple factors, including genetics, environment, and infectious factors (Box 1). Acute otitis media is more common in certain ethnic groups; it is more common in American Indians and Eskimos than in white children, and it is more common in white children than in black children. Craniofacial abnormalities (cleft lip or palate, cleft uvula, submucosal cleft) and some genetic syndromes (Down syndrome) are also associated with an increased risk of acute otitis media. Environmental factors, including time of year, daycare attendance, and parental smoking are also significant. The most important risk factor seems to be the presence of a preceding viral respiratory infection; the majority of children with acute otitis media have viral respiratory symptoms.

BOX 1   Risk Factors for Development of Acute Otitis Media

Genetic Factors
Ethnicity
- Eskimo
- American Indian
- White

Sex
- Male

Environmental Factors
- Seasonal (follows respiratory viruses)
- Parental smoking
- Sibling(s) in the home
- Out-of-home child care
- Family history of recurrent otitis media
- Anatomic abnormalities
- Down syndrome

Infectious Factors
- Preceding respiratory viral infection
- Carriage of bacterial pathogens in the nasoparynx

Pathophysiology

Bacterial acute otitis media typically develops 3 to 7 days after the onset of a viral respiratory infection. The middle ear is normally sterile, but bacteria and secretions from the nasopharynx can reach the middle ear during swallowing and yawning. Eustachian tube dysfunction caused by the viral respiratory infection can interfere with the normal clearance of the nasopharyngeal secretions from the middle ear by the mucociliary lining of the tube. Eustachian tube dysfunction evidenced by abnormal middle ear pressures is common during the usual course of a cold, affecting almost half of children with colds. Bacteria that are a normal part of the flora of the nasopharynx, including *S. pneumoniae*, *H. influenzae*, and *M. catarrhalis*, may be trapped and replicate in the middle ear, producing the purulent bulging tympanic membrane typical of bacterial acute otitis media. Symptomatic viral infection appears to be a necessary prerequisite for eustachian tube dysfunction, because neither the presence of bacteria nor the presence of viral replication without symptomatic illness are sufficient to induce eustachian tube dysfunction. It is hypothesized that the host response in symptomatic respiratory infection is responsible for the eustachian tube dysfunction.

Prevention

Many of the predisposing factors for development of acute otitis media, such as genetic makeup and time of year, are not alterable, but there are some strategies that one can employ to decrease the risk of developing acute otitis media. Breast-feeding for at least the first 6 months of life seems to be protective. Routine vaccination with seasonal flu vaccine (Fluzone)[1] has also been shown to be an effective method for reducing the incidence of acute otitis media. The use of pneumococcal conjugate vaccine (Prevnar) can reduce the incidence of pneumococcal otitis media caused by vaccine serotypes, but it resulted in a minimal reduction in diagnosed acute otitis media. Decreased attendance at daycare might also reduce the incidence of acute otitis media. Exposure to tobacco smoke should be avoided.

Clinical Manifestations

Bacterial acute otitis media typically manifests as a nonspecific respiratory illness. Most children have had a cold for 3 or 4 days with cough and runny nose when they present to the physician with other complaints, which might include otalgia or otalgia equivalents (excessive crying, decreased sleep, ear pulling, fever, decreased appetite, diarrhea, vomiting). Unfortunately, none of these symptoms is specific for bacterial acute otitis media. The acute onset of purulent otorrhea secondary to perforation of the tympanic membrane is a specific sign of bacterial acute otitis media.

Diagnosis

The normal tympanic membrane, translucent gray with sharp light reflex and visible handle of the malleus (Figure 1A), is easily identified. The abnormal findings diagnostic of acute otitis media have not been so clearly defined. In 2004, the American Academy of Pediatrics and the American Academy of Family Physicians published a clinical guideline to clarify the diagnosis and treatment of acute otitis media (AAP/AAFP criteria, Box 2). Under these guidelines, evidence of middle ear effusion, signs of tympanic membrane inflammation, and acute onset of symptoms are diagnostic of acute otitis media. These criteria are effective for diagnosing inflammation of the middle ear, but they do not distinguish between a viral and bacterial etiology; as many as 22% of middle ear effusions have viral pathogens alone, without bacterial pathogens.

---

[1]Not FDA approved for this indication.

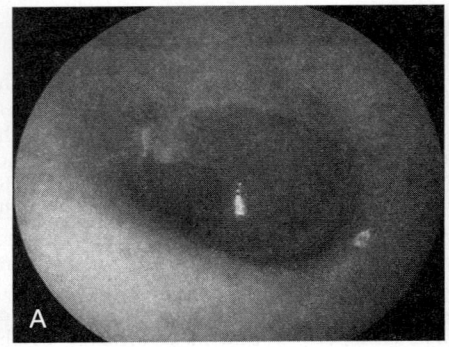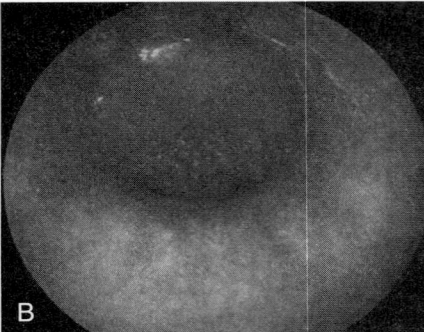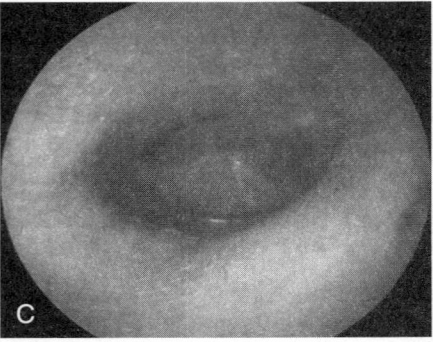

FIGURE 1. Appearance of the tympanic membrane. **A,** Normal tympanic membrane, with translucent gray color, sharp light reflex, and visible malleus. **B,** Bacterial acute otitis media is characterized by a completely bulging tympanic membrane, with injection and the appearance of a doughnut or bagel suggested by the attachment of the tympanic membrane to the umbo, commonly referred to as a "pus" drum. **C,** Viral acute otitis media is characterized by an inflamed tympanic membrane with injection and some fluid layered inferiorly, but the malleus is still visible and the tympanic membrane is not bulging. (Photos courtesy of Dr. Carlos Armengol, Pediatric Associates of Charlottesville, Va.)

BOX 2   Diagnosis of Acute Otitis Media

Bacterial
- "Pus" drum (complete bulging of tympanic membrane with purulent fluid)
or
- Otorrhea

Viral
- Middle ear effusion
- Limited tympanic membrane mobility
- Air-fluid level behind tympanic membrane
and
- Signs of tympanic membrane inflammation
  - Erythema of tympanic membrane
  - Distinct otalgia that interferes with sleep or activities
and
- Acute onset

 CURRENT DIAGNOSIS

- Inflammation of the middle ear is common during the course of an otherwise uncomplicated viral respiratory infection and resolves spontaneously.
- There are no specific signs and symptoms of bacterial acute otitis media, except in the case of otorrhea.
- American Academy of Pediatrics/American Academy of Family Physicians criteria for diagnosis of acute otitis media are effective for diagnosis of inflammation of the middle ear, but they do not distinguish between a viral and bacterial etiology.
- Complete bulging of the tympanic membrane with purulent fluid (pus drum) or otorrhea is bacterial acute otitis media.
- Middle ear effusion (limited tympanic membrane mobility or air-fluid level behind the tympanic membrane), coupled with signs of tympanic membrane inflammation (erythematous tympanic membrane, distinct otalgia) and acute onset signify viral acute otitis media and will resolve spontaneously.

Inflammation of the middle ear can result from bacterial acute otitis media, but it is also commonly found during the course of otherwise uncomplicated viral respiratory infections and resolves spontaneously. In a recently completed (as yet unpublished) study presented at the 2009 Pediatric Academic Societies Conference, it was found that the AAP criteria for acute otitis media were met in 35% of colds in children, most commonly during the first week of cold symptoms. The majority of these resolved spontaneously without medical intervention.

Because most episodes of acute otitis media resolve spontaneously, the diagnosis of *bacterial acute otitis media* should be reserved for the tympanic membrane that is completely bulging, commonly referred to as a *pus drum*, or for cases in which there is acute onset of otorrhea (see Figure 1B). The likelihood of recovering a bacterial pathogen from the middle ear fluid is significantly increased in the presence of a completely bulging tympanic membrane; in one study of 96 patients, 91% of the cultures recovered from completely bulging tympanic membranes were positive for bacterial pathogens, compared with only 10% of the cultures recovered from tympanic membranes with erythema or minimal bulging (or both). The current AAP/AAFP criteria are quite useful for identifying tympanic membrane inflammation, and, in the absence of complete bulging or acute onset of otorrhea, condition should be termed *viral acute otitis media* (see Figure 1C).

Differential Diagnosis

The most critical differentiation is between viral acute otitis media and bacterial acute otitis media. The presence of a completely bulging tympanic membrane or otorrhea should distinguish clearly between the two. In the case of otorrhea, other conditions to consider include foreign body in the ear canal and external otitis media. Careful examination of the ear canal should distinguish between these etiologies. Otorrhea from a ruptured tympanic membrane is purulent, yellow-green, and wet. Otitis externa is characterized by yellow-green, often clumped-appearing debris in the canal and extreme tenderness when the external ear is manipulated; the tympanic membrane is usually not visualized.

Treatment

Appropriate treatment of bacterial acute otitis media is complicated by concerns for complications and the increasing incidence of bacterial resistance. Available studies evaluating treatment for acute otitis media, which include both viral and bacterial acute otitis media, have shown that a majority (77%) of episodes of acute otitis media in children will resolve spontaneously without treatment. There are no studies evaluating antibiotic versus placebo for bacterial acute otitis media (pus drum). In some European countries, a strategy of watchful waiting is employed, and antibiotic treatment of acute otitis media is not common. Most children in the United States (83%) with a diagnosis of acute otitis media are treated with antibiotics. Slightly more than half were treated with amoxicillin (Amoxil), and the rest were treated with broader spectrum antibiotics.

Given the incidence of resistance of *S. pneumoniae*, the most appropriate initial treatment of bacterial acute otitis media (Table 1) is high-dose amoxicillin at 80 to 90 mg/kg/day[3]; at this level, concentrations are adequate to eradicate sensitive and most moderately resistant *S. pneumoniae*. As for *H. influenzae* and *M. catarrhalis*, resistance is commonplace owing to β-lactamase production, but these infections generally resolve with treatment with β-lactam antibiotics like amoxicillin. If there is no improvement after a course of high-dose amoxicillin, then second-line therapy may include amoxicillin-clavulanate (Augmentin) or a second- or third-generation cephalosporin. The optimal duration of oral therapy for treatment of bacterial acute otitis media is unknown, but 5 to 10 days is common. If the pus drum persists, then third-line therapy with an intramuscular injection of ceftriaxone (Rocephin) at 50 mg/kg/day for a course of 1 to 3 days should be initiated. This option is also useful as first- or second-line therapy in cases of children who are vomiting and unable to take oral medications. Failure to respond to these measures should prompt referral to an otolaryngologist for further evaluation. In published studies, myringotomy provided no benefit over antibiotic alone in treatment of acute otitis media.

---

[3]Exceeds dosage recommended by the manufacturer.

TABLE 1 Treatment of Bacterial Acute Otitis Media

Drug	Dosage
First-Line Therapy	
Amoxicillin (Amoxil, etc.)	90 mg/kg/day[3] divided bid
Alternatives for amoxicillin allergy with hives	
Azithromycin (Zithromax)	10 mg/kg/d on day 1, then 5 mg/kg/d × 4 days, as a single daily dose
Clindamycin (Cleocin)[1]	30-40 mg /kg/d[3] divided tid
Second-Line Therapy	
Amoxicillin-clavulanate (Augmentin)	45 mg/kg/day divided bid
Second- or third-generation oral cephalosporins	
Cefdinir (Omnicef)	14 mg/kg/d as a single daily dose
Cefpodoxime (Vantin)	10 mg/kg/d as a single daily dose[3]
Cefuroxime (Ceftin)	30 mg/kg/d divided bid
Third-Line Therapy	
Ceftriaxone (Rocephin)	50 mg/kg IM in a single dose for 1 or 3 days

[1]Not FDA approved for this indication.
[3]Exceeds dosage recommended by the manufacturer.

CURRENT THERAPY

- For bacterial acute otitis media (complete pus drum or otorrhea), first-line therapy is as follows:
  - High-dose amoxicillin: 90 mg/kg/day[3] divided twice daily
  - Alternatives for amoxicillin allergy with hives include:
    - Azithromycin: 10 mg/kg/d on day 1, then 5 mg/kg/day as a single daily dose for 4 days
    - Clindamycin[1]: 30-40 mg/kg/day[3] divided three times a day
- For viral acute otitis media, antibiotic therapy is not indicated. However, pain control is important and may include the following:
  - Acetaminophen: 15 mg/kg every 4 to 6 hours as needed
  - Ibuprofen: 10 mg/kg every 6 to 8 hours as needed for fever or pain; do not use in children younger than 6 months.
  - Antipyrine-benzocaine otic drops (Auralgan): 2 to 4 drops to affected ear every 2 hours as needed for pain; do not use in children younger than 6 months or in patients with acute perforation or tympanostomy tubes

---

[1]Not FDA approved for this indication.
[3]Exceeds dosage recommended by the manufacturer.

Viral acute otitis media (Table 2) should be treated symptomatically and is likely to resolve spontaneously without further intervention. Pain control is very important and may include acetaminophen (Tylenol), ibuprofen (Motrin, Advil), and antipyrine-benzocaine otic drops (Auralgan). If no improvement is noted in 48 to 72 hours, then treatment with high-dose amoxicillin may be considered. Parents may be given a prescription and instructed to fill it only if symptoms, especially otalgia and fever, are not improving within 48 to 72 hours. In a study comparing this delayed-prescribing strategy to immediate prescription of antibiotics for diagnosed acute otitis media, immediate treatment did not significantly reduce pain or distress but did result in about 1 day less of illness, less crying, and less nighttime disturbance. These effects were not noted until after 24 hours, when symptoms would be expected to improve anyway. Parents were comfortable with the delayed-prescribing strategy, and the final result was a 70% reduction in the use of antibiotics.

Monitoring

Routine ear rechecks are unnecessary, because routine monitoring is not needed for bacterial acute otitis media treated with appropriate antibiotic with resolution of symptoms. If symptoms persist despite

TABLE 2 Treatment of Viral Acute Otitis Media

Drug	Dosage	Indications	Contraindications
First-Line Therapy			
Acetaminphen (Tylenol)	15 mg/kg q4-6h prn	Fever or pain	Do not use in children younger than 6 mo
Ibuprofen (Motrin, Advil)	10 mg/kg q6-8h prn	Fever or pain	Do not use in cases of perforation or PE tubes
Antipyrine-benzocaine otic drops (Auralgan)	2-4 drops to affected ear q2h prn	Pain	Do not use in children younger than 6 mo
Second-Line Therapy			
Amoxicillin (Amoxil)	90 mg/kg/day[3] divided bid	If no improvement after 48-72 h	

therapy, reassessment by the primary care physician is recommended. Persistent pus drum suggests chronic suppurative otitis media and requires referral to otolaryngology, where further management, including myringotomy and culture, is available.

Complications

Complications of acute otitis media can include mastoiditis, intracranial abscess, chronic otitis media with effusion, and perforation of the tympanic membrane. Mastoiditis classically occurs following diagnosis of acute otitis media with systemic symptoms, postauricular inflammation, and anterior displacement of the pinna. Patients with mastoiditis tend to be school-aged and present with a history of prolonged symptoms. Treatment of the acute otitis media with antibiotics has little effect on the incidence of mastoiditis. Mastoiditis is uncommon and is not increased in patients managed with initial observation in whom continued observation and initiation of antibiotic treatment for persistent symptoms is provided.

REFERENCES

Armengol CE, Hendley JO, Winther B. The natural history of acute otitis media during colds in young children. Presented at the 2009 Pediatric Academic Societies Conference, May 4, 2009, Baltimore, MD.

American Academy of Pediatrics and American Academy of Family Physicians. Clinical practice guideline: Diagnosis and management of acute otitis media. Pediatrics 2004;113:1451–65.

Halsted C, Lepow ML, Balassanian N, et al. Otitis media: Clinical observations, microbiology, and evaluation of therapy. Am J Dis Child 1968;115:542–51.

Ho D, Rotenberg BW, Berkowitz RG. The relationship between acute mastoiditis and antibiotic use for acute otitis media in children. Arch Otolaryngol Head Neck Surg 2007;134:45–8.

Little P, Gould C, Williamson I, et al. Pragmatic randomized controlled trial of two prescribing strategies for childhood acute otitis media. BMJ 2001; 322:336–42.

Niemela M, Uhari M, Jounio-Ervasti K, et al. Lack of specific symptomatology in children with acute otitis media. Pediatr Infect Dis J 1994;13:765–8.

Rosenfield RW, Vertrees JE, Carr J, et al. Clinical efficacy of antimicrobials for acute otitis media: Meta-analysis of 5,400 children from 33 randomized trials. J Pediatr 1994;124:355–67.

Ruuskanen O, Arola M, Heikkinen T, et al. Viruses in acute otitis media: Increasing evidence for clinical significance. Pediatr Infect Dis J 1991;10:425–7.

Thorne MC, Chawaproug L, Elden LM. Suppurative complications of acute otitis media: Changes in frequency over time. Arch Otolaryngol Head Neck Surg 2009;135:638–64.

Winther B, Gwaltney Jr JM, Phillips CD, et al. Radioopaque contrast dye in nasopharynx reaches the middle ear during swallowing and/or yawning. Acta Otolaryngol 2005;125:625–8.

Winther B, Hayden FG, Hendley JO. Middle ear pressure in preschool age children: Influence of respiratory illness, season, and picornavirus or bacteria in the nasopharynx. Acta Otolaryngol 2007;127:796–800.

Winther B, Alper CM, Mandel EM, et al. Temporal relationships between colds, upper respiratory viruses detected by polymerase chain reaction and otitis media in young children followed through a typical cold season. Pediatrics 2007;119:1069–75.

Episodic Vertigo

Method of
Kevin A. Kerber, MD

Vertigo is a type of dizziness symptom. Dizziness is a nonspecific term that refers to any sensation of spatial disorientation; vertigo means an illusion of movement—typically, true visualized spinning of the environment. Vertigo can also mean a sense of linear displacement or tilt, although it is best to report these symptoms using the patient's own words. Other common types of dizziness include lightheadedness, presyncope, and unsteadiness while walking. True vertigo is highly suggestive of vestibular system involvement, although by itself it cannot differentiate a peripheral localization (i.e., inner ear or vestibular nerve) from a central localization (i.e., brainstem or cerebellum). Because vertigo does not discriminate peripheral from central pathology, localization of the lesion and subsequent diagnosis depend on the features of the vertigo and the presence or absence of other signs or symptoms.

To effectively evaluate patients who present with vertigo, an understanding of the key aspects of the vestibular system is of central importance, because the dilemma is often discriminating a benign peripheral vestibular disorder from a small focal brain lesion. Many clinicians make a diagnosis of peripheral disease if other neurologic features (e.g., motor, sensory, or language deficits) are not present, but this approach is flawed. A more effective approach is to aim to diagnose one of the specific peripheral vestibular disorders. If a specific peripheral vestibular disorder does not fit, then a work-up for a central nervous system lesion may be warranted. The three common peripheral vestibular disorders all have highly characteristic history and examination features.

The Vestibular System

The peripheral vestibular system maintains a balanced tonic input to the brain. The input represents the circuitry linking the inner ear to brain structures that control eye movements. This circuitry is called the vestibulo-ocular reflex. A normal functioning vestibulo-ocular reflex is important for balance and for maintaining clear vision when moving. When an imbalance is caused by a lesion or aberrant stimulation, then vertigo ensues. A hallmark sign of vestibular system imbalance is nystagmus.

Nystagmus is a term used to describe rhythmic slow and fast movements of the eyes in opposite directions. The slow phase is caused by the imbalance in the vestibular system, whereas the fast phase represents the brain's attempt to correct for the slow drift. The pattern of nystagmus is determined by the location of pathology and whether the pathology is inhibitory or stimulatory. Pathology at the level of the semicircular canal causes nystagmus in the plane of the affected canal. In other words, vertical canals (i.e., posterior and anterior canals) lead to vertical and torsional nystagmus, whereas the horizontal canal leads to nystagmus in the horizontal plane. At the vestibular nerve level (i.e., cranial nerve 8), a mixed horizontal-torsional pattern of nystagmus is generated, because inputs from all of the semicircular canals converge at this level, and the signals from the vertical canals mostly cancel each other out. Patterns of nystagmus become less predictable with central lesions, although some general rules apply. Patterns of central dysfunction include the following: pure vertical (downbeat or upbeat) spontaneous nystagmus, bidirectional gaze-evoked nystagmus (look left, beats left; look right, beats right), gaze-evoked down-beating nystagmus, and persistent downbeating positional nystagmus.

Another hallmark sign of vestibular disturbance is a positive head-thrust test. A subject with an intact vestibulo-ocular reflex will maintain gaze on a stationary, straight-ahead target after a brief, small amplitude, high acceleration movement of the head to one side. A subject with vestibular impairment on one side loses this reflex on the ipsilateral side and therefore, after the quick head movement, needs to make a refixation voluntary eye movement (i.e., a "saccade") back to the target because the eyes moved with the head. This so-called catch-up or corrective saccade is easily appreciated at the bedside and indicates vestibular de-afferentiation.

THREE COMMON PERIPHERAL VESTIBULAR DISORDERS

The three common peripheral vestibular disorders are vestibular neuritis, Meniere's disease, and benign paroxysmal positional vertigo (BPPV). Each has characteristic bedside features.

A patient with vestibular neuritis presents with the abrupt onset of severe vertigo, nausea, and imbalance. No other neurologic symptoms are present. The disorder is presumed to be caused by a viral disturbance of the vestibular nerve, although no viral tests are reliable for confirming this cause in individual patients. This situation is analogous to that of Bell's palsy. On examination, the acute peripheral vestibular pattern of nystagmus is seen. This pattern consists of unidirectional spontaneous nystagmus with a horizontal greater than torsional component. "Uni-directional" means that the nystagmus beats toward only one side. Looking in the direction of the fast phase increases the velocity of the nystagmus, whereas looking in the opposite direction decreases the velocity—but the direction of the fast phase never changes. If the nystagmus does change direction, then the pathology localizes to the brain. The affected ear is on the side opposite the fast phase of nystagmus. The other characteristic finding is a corrective saccade after the head-thrust test toward the affected side. Treatment with a short course of an oral corticosteroid within 3 days of symptom onset may result in a more complete recovery of vestibular function than if this therapy is not used. In addition, a program of vestibular rehabilitation can improve the outcome. It is important to note that small strokes of the cerebellum or brainstem can closely mimic vestibular neuritis.

Meniere's disease is characterized by recurrent episodes of vertigo, nausea, and imbalance typically lasting hours. Unilateral auditory features (i.e., hearing loss, roaring tinnitus, or fullness) must be present and prominent to make the diagnosis. Early in the course, auditory symptoms fluctuate along with vertigo attacks, but later the auditory symptoms become fixed and progressive. Some patients develop bilateral Meniere's disease. The initial treatment of Meniere's disease is a low-salt diet (<1500–2000 mg/day) or a diuretic. However, neither of these treatments is of established efficacy. Ablative surgical procedures are appropriate in cases of refractory vertigo. Transient ischemic attacks should be considered in the differential diagnosis whenever the vertigo attacks are brief (minutes) and new in onset. The dizziness of migraine can also closely mimic Meniere's disease.

CURRENT DIAGNOSIS

Vestibular Neuritis

- A single, severe and prolonged (days) episode of vertigo, nausea, and imbalance
- Nystagmus: spontaneous, unidirectional, horizontal more than torsional; fast phase beats away from affected side
- Head-thrust test: positive toward affected side (e.g., opposite to the direction of fast phase of nystagmus)
- Red flags for stroke: any other pattern of nystagmus, negative head-thrust test, and stroke risk factors

Meniere's Disease

- Recurrent episodes of vertigo (typically lasting hours) with unilateral and prominent auditory features (hearing loss, roaring tinnitus, or fullness)
- Unilateral hearing loss eventually becomes permanent and progressive
- Red flags for transient ischemic attacks: new onset, brief episodes (i.e., minutes), stroke risk factors

Benign Paroxysmal Positional Vertigo (BPPV)

- Recurrent, brief (<1 minute), positionally triggered vertigo attacks
- A burst of upbeat-torsional nystagmus triggered by the Dix-Hallpike test occurs with the most common variant, posterior canal BPPV
- Resolution of positional nystagmus with the Epley maneuver
- Red flags for central structural pathology: persistent down-beating nystagmus, other neurologic signs or symptoms

Patients with BPPV report very brief episodes (<1 minute) of vertigo triggered by certain head movements. The most common positional triggers are tilting the head back to look up, getting in or out of bed, or rolling over in bed. It is important to note that dizziness of any cause may worsen after certain movements, but the dizziness of BPPV is *triggered* by certain movements. The most common form of BPPV occurs when particles that stem from the otolith organ break free and enter the posterior canal. Posterior canal BPPV is identified at the bedside with the use of the Dix-Hallpike test (Figure 1). In response to the Dix-Hallpike test, the particles move in the canal and, by doing so, trigger a burst of upbeat-torsional nystagmus lasting 20 to 30 seconds. This disorder is cured in minutes by the particle repositioning maneuver described by Epley and others. BPPV is less commonly caused by particles in the horizontal canal or, very rarely, in the anterior canal. If the particles are in one of these other canals, both the pattern of nystagmus and repositioning maneuvers are different. Positional vertigo and nystagmus are common in patients with migraine. If a persistent down-beating nystagmus is seen during the Dix-Hallpike test, a central nervous system cause (e.g., Chiari malformation, cerebellar tumor, cerebellar degeneration) should be considered.

OTHER PERIPHERAL VESTIBULAR DISORDERS

Many other disorders can involve the peripheral vestibular system, but an understanding of the three most common peripheral vestibular disorders allows one to recognize features of pathology that stems from the peripheral structures. Many physicians order magnetic resonance imaging to exclude an acoustic neuroma in patients with vertigo; however, recurrent vertigo is an atypical presentation of this very rare disorder. Although case reports suggest that acoustic neuroma can manifest with isolated recurrent dizziness, epidemiologic research shows that up to one third of the general population report a history of bothersome dizziness, including vertigo. The more typical presentation of acoustic neuroma is gradually progressive unilateral hearing loss.

Vestibular paroxysmia is a label for very brief (seconds) spontaneous recurrent vertigo attacks, often preceded by auditory symptoms. The mechanism causing vestibular paroxysmia is believed to be analogous to that of trigeminal neuralgia and hemifacial spasm: aberrant stimulation within the system leads to transient symptoms.

Superior canal dehiscence syndrome is characterized by brief vertigo (seconds) triggered by sound or pressure changes.

CENTRAL VESTIBULAR DISORDERS

The central vestibular system involves many pathways within the brainstem and the cerebellum. Any pathology that affects the central vestibular pathways can cause an imbalance within the system. Acute or recurrent transient pathology causes vertigo; gradually progressive pathology causes abnormal eye movements and unsteadiness.

Stroke should be on the differential diagnosis of any acute vertigo presentation. Although the true probability of stroke as a cause of acute-onset severe vertigo is unknown, the best estimates suggest that between 3% and 20% of patients with acute vertigo harbor a stroke etiology. This probability drops substantially if there are no other neurologic features, the peripheral vestibular pattern of nystagmus is identified, and a corresponding head-thrust test is positive.

Other central structural lesions can cause acute vertigo, but again the likelihood of these causes is extremely low in the absence of central neurologic signs and symptoms. The characteristic finding in a Chiari malformation is down-beating nystagmus triggered by positional testing. Episodic vertigo is a common feature in some types of the genetic disorder known as episodic ataxia.

Approach to the Patient

If the symptom is true vertigo (i.e., visualized spinning of the environment), then the vestibular system is involved. A mild internal spinning sensation is probably less specific for a vestibular system localization. The next step is to define the characteristics of the symptom. Is this a new symptom or recurrent? If it is recurrent, what is the duration and

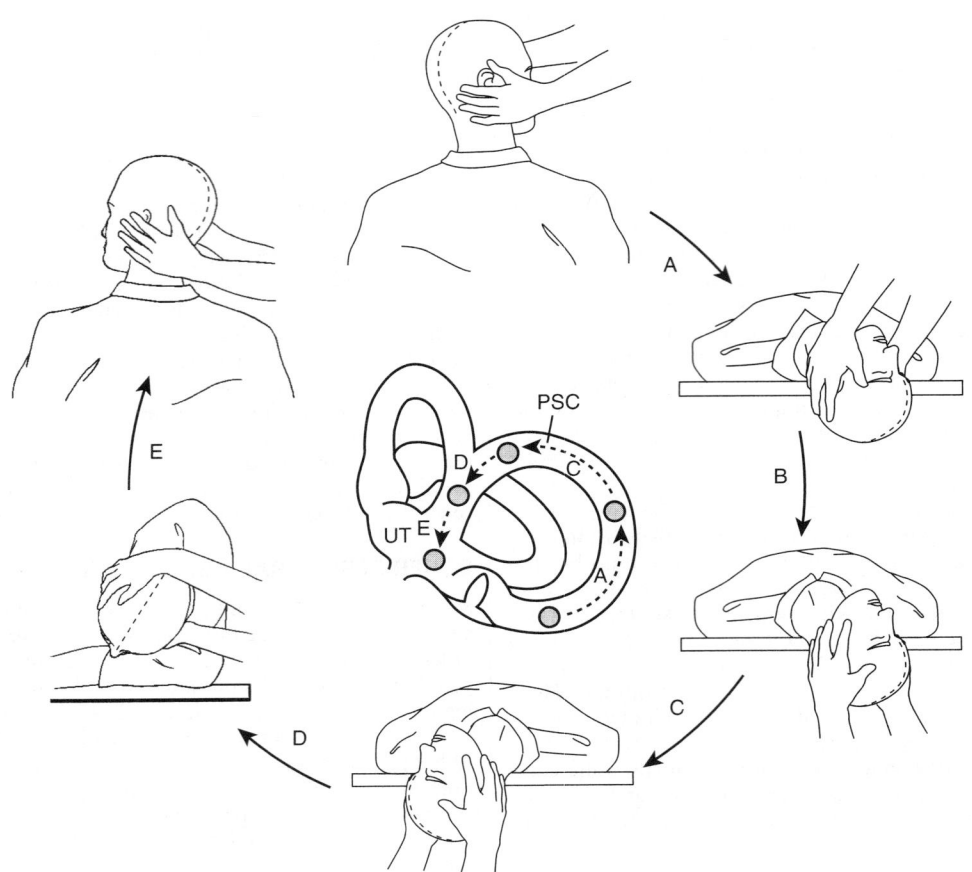

FIGURE 1. Treatment maneuver for benign paroxysmal positional vertigo affecting the right ear. To treat the left ear, the procedure is reversed. The drawing of the labyrinth in the center shows the position of the particle as it moves around the posterior semicircular canal (PSC) and into the utricle (UT). The patient is seated upright, with head facing the examiner, who is standing on the right. **A,** The patient is rapidly moved to head-hanging right position (Dix-Hallpike test). This position is maintained until the nystagmus ceases. **B,** The examiner moves to the head of the table, repositioning hands as shown. **C,** The head is rotated quickly to the left with right ear upward. This position is maintained for 30 seconds. **D,** The patient rolls onto the left side while the examiner rapidly rotates the head leftward until the nose is directed toward the floor. This position is then held for 30 seconds. **E,** The patient is rapidly lifted into the sitting position, now facing left. The entire sequence should be repeated until no nystagmus can be elicited. After the maneuver, the patient is instructed to avoid head-hanging positions to prevent the particles from reentering the posterior canal. (Reprinted with permission from Rakel RE: Conn's Current Therapy 1995. Philadelphia, WB Saunders, 1995, p 839.)

frequency of the episodes, and are there any triggers? Next, ask about aggravating or alleviating factors and about accompanying symptoms. The patient's past medical history may predict a risk for certain disorders. The family history may reveal a familial pattern of similar symptoms (e.g., benign recurrent vertigo often has a familial pattern).

 CURRENT THERAPY

- Vestibular neuritis: Both oral corticosteroids and vestibular rehabilitation have a high level of evidence supporting efficacy. Consider a burst and taper of oral corticosteroids if the diagnosis is made within 3 days after onset. Consider referral for vestibular rehabilitation.
- Meniere's disease: Consider a trial of a low-salt diet or a diuretic as initial therapy, although both lack evidence to support efficacy. Consider an ablative surgical procedure in refractory cases.
- Benign paroxysmal positional vertigo (BPPV): The Epley maneuver has a high level of evidence supporting efficacy in the treatment of posterior canal BPPV.

The examination is critical for localizing the lesion. Whenever possible, it is always preferable to examine the patient while symptoms are active. Hearing should be tested one ear at a time with tuning forks or finger rub. If the general medical and general neurologic examinations are unrevealing, then the focus should shift to the ocular motor examination to search for signs of vestibular or brain dysfunction. Does the patient have nystagmus? If so, what type and pattern? Is the head-thrust test positive? Instruct the patient to follow your finger back and forth and assess whether the eyes move smoothly. This is a test of the smooth pursuit system, and pathologically impaired smooth pursuit is a central nervous system sign. If the patient reports that symptoms are triggered by head or body turns, then positional testing should be performed. Start with the Dix-Hallpike test. If this test does not trigger nystagmus, then have the patient lie supine and turn the head to each side; this can trigger the nystagmus of horizontal canal BPPV.

If the patient's features do not fit with a common peripheral vestibular disorder, central nervous system causes should be considered. There are two main questions to ask when trying to decide whether the vertigo localizes to the brain: Are there other symptoms that must stem from the brainstem or cerebellum? and Are there examination findings (e.g., central pattern of eye movements) that localize to the brainstem or cerebellum rather than the peripheral vestibular system?

If the symptom has been present for longer than several months, the features do not fit with a peripheral vestibular disorder, and the neurologic examination is normal, then chronic dizziness or benign recurrent vertigo is the appropriate label. This diagnosis is inclusive of migraine-related dizziness, dizziness with panic disorder, and psychophysiologic dizziness. These causes may represent focal chemical or signaling changes within the brain or a hypersensitivity disorder. Although much remains to be known about the underlying mechanisms of chronic dizziness symptoms, genetics does seem to play a role.

Management

First, attempt to identify a specific disorder and focus on the treatment of that disorder. Patients with prolonged symptoms usually require symptomatic treatment with standard doses of an antihistamine, an antiemetic, or a benzodiazepine. However, these symptomatic medications are not appropriate as long-term therapy. Patients with chronic dizziness may benefit from lifestyle modifications, such as cardiovascular exercise, optimizing sleep and stress management, and eliminating any food triggers. Migraine prophylactic agents are reasonable to try, but their effectiveness for dizziness has not been established.

REFERENCES

Baloh RW, Honrubia V. Clinical Neurophysiology of the Vestibular System. 3rd ed. New York: Oxford University Press; 2001.
Epley JM. The canalith repositioning procedure: For treatment of benign paroxysmal positional vertigo. Oto Head Neck Surg 1992;107:199.
Hillier SL, Hollohan V. Vestibular rehabilitation for unilateral peripheral vestibular dysfunction. Cochrane Database Syst Rev 2007;(4):CD005397.
Hilton M, Pinder D. The Epley (canalith repositioning) manoeuvre for benign paroxysmal positional vertigo. Cochrane Database Syst Rev 2004;(2):CD003162.
James AL, Thorp M. Meniere's disease. BMJ Clin Evid 2006;15:797–803.
Kerber KA, Brown DL, Lisabeth LD, et al. Stroke among patients with dizziness, vertigo, and imbalance in the emergency department: A population-based study. Stroke 2006;37:2484–7.
Lee H, Sohn SI, Cho YW, et al. Cerebellar infarction presenting isolated vertigo: Frequency and vascular topographical patterns. Neurology 2006;67:1178–83.
Lewis RF, Carey JP. Images in clinical medicine: Abnormal eye movements associated with unilateral loss of vestibular function. N Engl J Med 2006;355:e26.
Neuhauser HK, von Brevern M, Radtke A, et al. Epidemiology of vestibular vertigo: A neurotologic survey of the general population. Neurology 2005;65:898–904.
Newman-Toker DE, Kattah JC, Alvernia JE, Wang DZ. Normal head impulse test differentiates acute cerebellar strokes from vestibular neuritis. Neurology 2008;70:2378–85.
Strupp M, Zingler VC, Arbusow V, et al. Methylprednisolone, valacyclovir, or the combination for vestibular neuritis. N Engl J Med 2004;351:354–61.
Thirlwall AS, Kundu S. Diuretics for Meniere's disease or syndrome. Cochrane Database Syst Rev 2006;(3):CD003599.

Ménière's Disease

Method of
Terry D. Fife, MD

Ménière's disease is a disorder of the inner ear that results in recurrent spontaneous episodes of vertigo, hearing loss, ear fullness and tinnitus affecting the same ear. The hearing loss often fluctuates early in Ménière's disease, but fluctuating hearing is not always present. Eventually permanent hearing loss occurs, affecting the low frequencies initially but ultimately affecting all frequencies.

Epidemiology

The reported prevalence of Ménière's disease varies from about 50 to 200 per 100,000. Both sexes are equally affected.

Risk Factors

Possible risk factors for later development of Ménière's syndrome include syphilitic otitis and viral infection of the inner ear, head trauma, and a family history of Ménière's disease.

Pathophysiology

The underlying mechanism is generally believed to be due to endolymphatic hydrops, a type of swelling of the endolymphatic compartment that ultimately leads to permanent damage of the inner ear structures. Possible reasons for this periodic swelling of the endolymph compartment include mechanical obstruction of endolymph flow or at least dysregulation of the electrochemical membrane potential between endolymph and perilymph compartments.

Endolymphatic hydrops appears to be the mechanism for a number of conditions that can lead to Ménière's syndrome. When no primary cause is identified, the idiopathic form of the syndrome is called Ménière's disease. When an underlying cause is found, it is referred to as Ménière's syndrome or secondary Ménière's or secondary endolymphatic hydrops. Secondary Ménière's syndrome can result from delayed endolymphatic hydrops in which symptoms come on years after a prior disorder or viral injury of the labyrinth, syphilitic otitis, autoimmune inner ear disease, and trauma.

Prevention

There is no known way of preventing the development of Ménière's disease because it occurs in many people with no risk factors.

Clinical Manifestations

Ménière's can manifest with periodic unilateral (or, less commonly, bilateral) hearing loss or isolated attacks of vertigo. Not uncommonly, Ménière's has both elements present at its onset, but the vertigo is usually the symptom that gets the most attention. Vertigo usually lasts 1 to 6 hours but can last as little at 30 minutes or as long as all day. Patients prone to motion sickness often report that their dizziness lasts longer because the after-effect of vertigo lingers longer in those who are motion sensitive. Vertigo attacks in Ménière's disease are often quite severe and generally render patients unable to move around owing to the vertigo, nausea, and recurrent vomiting.

The hearing loss is usually unilateral, and patients might notice fluctuation in hearing accompanied by ear fullness and a low-pitched roaring tinnitus either before or coincident with the vertigo. If audiometry can be performed during this time, low-frequency (250-1000 Hz) hearing loss may be documented and might improve after the attack ceases. This signature fluctuating low-frequency sensorineural hearing loss is very helpful (Figure 1) when found, but getting patients with vertigo attacks in for testing while they are in the acute stage of vertigo is usually not feasible.

Occasionally, patients with Ménière's have sudden random drop attacks in which they abruptly fall without loss of consciousness. These spells, referred to as otolithic crises of Tumarkin, can lead to serious injury and should prompt aggressive treatment. The mechanism is presumed to be related to sudden mechanical deformation or sudden neural discharges related to the otolith structures of the inner ear. Because there is no specific treatment for Tumarkin crises, treatment entails the standard treatments for Ménière's disease in general.

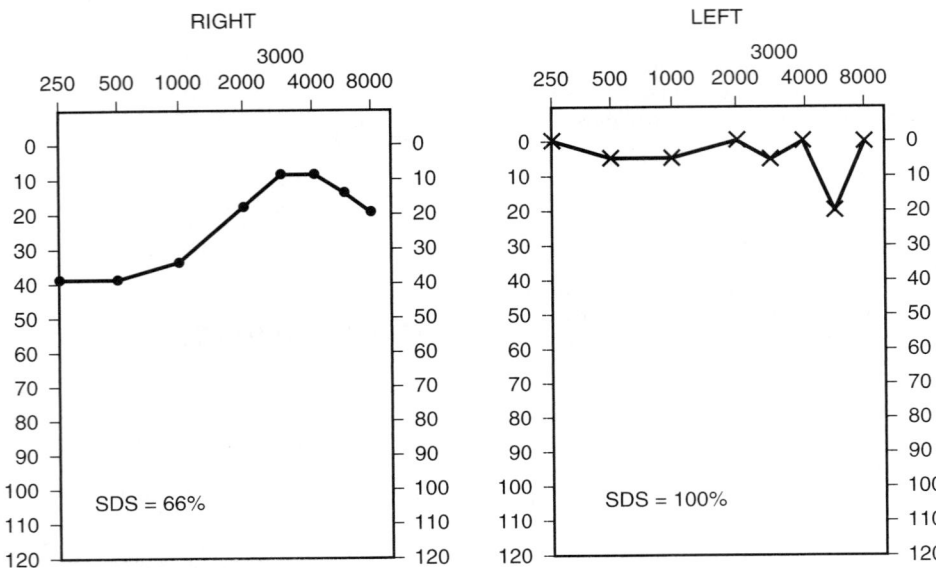

FIGURE 1. Audiogram showing typical low-frequency hearing trough of Ménière's disease affecting the right ear.

As Ménière's disease progresses, usually over months to years, permanent low-frequency hearing loss develops that gives way to hearing loss at all frequencies. Eventually, it the patient can lose all or most hearing on that side. Meanwhile, with each vertigo attack, some vestibular function is lost, and so as vertigo attacks continue, vestibular loss ensues, often paralleling the hearing loss. Ménière's occasionally burns out, meaning that enough vestibular function has been lost that acute hydrops no longer produces vertigo. Patients might report less severe dizziness or just a vague feeling of unsteadiness. This usually indicates advanced Ménière's, and unilateral hearing and vestibular loss should be expected.

Bilateral Ménière's has treatment implications because treating one side alone will be unlikely to stop the vertigo attacks because they could be emanating from the untreated side. Surgical treatment of both sides is also problematic because it could leave the patient with bilateral hearing loss, vestibular loss, or both.

Diagnosis

The diagnosis of Ménière's disease is a made clinically based on the unilateral hearing loss, tinnitus, ear fullness, and episodic vertigo typically lasting 1 to 6 hours. The criteria for definite, probable, and possible Ménière's are listed in Box 1.

 CURRENT DIAGNOSIS

- Ménière's disease is characterized by recurrent attacks of severe vertigo, nausea, and vomiting typically lasting 1 to 6 hours.
- Ménière's disease causes tinnitus on the side of the affected ear; the tinnitus can change in pitch and loudness during attacks of vertigo.
- Attacks of vertigo are associated with reduced or muffled hearing on the side of the affected ear.
- Fluctuating unilateral hearing loss and low-frequency hearing loss on the side of the affected ear is characteristic.

BOX 1   Diagnostic Criteria for Ménière's Disease

Possible Ménière's Disease
- Episodic vertigo of the Ménière's type without documented hearing loss or sensorineural hearing loss, fluctuating or fixed, with dysequilibrium but without definitive episodes
- Other causes excluded

Probable Ménière's Disease
- One definitive episode of vertigo
- Audiometrically documented hearing loss on at least one occasion
- Tinnitus or aural fullness in the treated ear
- Other causes excluded

Definite Ménière's Disease
- Two or more definitive spontaneous episodes of vertigo lasting 20 minutes or longer
- Audiometrically documented hearing loss on at least one occasion
- Tinnitus or aural fullness in the treated ear
- Other causes excluded.

Criteria from Committee on Hearing and Equilibrium: Committee on Hearing and Equilibrium guidelines for the diagnosis and evaluation of therapy in Ménière's disease. Otolaryngol Head Neck Surg 1995;113:181-185.

Differential Diagnosis

Vestibular neuritis causes a single attack of vertigo, sometimes with acute hearing loss (labyrinthitis), but it can usually be distinguished from Ménière's because vestibular neuritis has a lifetime recurrence rate of only 2%, whereas Ménière's vertigo attacks recur multiple times and cause fluctuating and gradual decline in hearing.

When a patient reports episodic vertigo attacks in the absence of unilateral tinnitus, ear fullness, and hearing loss, one must be cautious in diagnosing Ménière's disease because migrainous vertigo (basilar-type migraine) can produce a similar pattern. The longer a patient has recurrent spells of vertigo without demonstrable unilateral hearing loss, the more it favors a diagnosis of migrainous vertigo.

Benign paroxysmal positional vertigo causes brief recurrent spells of spinning without hearing loss, so it is rarely confused with Ménière's disease.

Vertebrobasilar insufficiency can cause isolated vertigo, but the duration is usually only several minutes and without hearing loss, whereas Ménière's attacks last hours and are associated with unilateral auditory symptoms.

Acoustic neuroma (vestibular schwannoma) typically leads to slowly progressive unilateral sensorineural hearing loss, but vertigo is infrequently a prominent feature because patients compensate gradually as their vestibular function wanes due to compressive effects of the tumor.

Fluctuating unilateral hearing loss, ear fullness, and tinnitus can occur without vertigo and is referred to as cochlear hydrops. Such symptoms can precede the development of vertigo but may be treated as Ménière's nonetheless. Lermoyez's syndrome refers to transiently improved hearing and tinnitus during attacks of vertigo. More commonly, however, hearing declines around and during vertigo spells.

Treatment

MEDICAL MANAGEMENT

Treatment of Ménière's disease is mainly aimed at preventing the vertigo attacks, but no treatments are known that reliably restore or arrest hearing loss or tinnitus. It is presumed that if attacks of vertigo, ear fullness, fluctuating hearing, and tinnitus are all stopped, hearing should stabilize, but this is still a supposition. The management of Ménière's is hierarchical, starting with a low-sodium diet and a diuretic and proceeding to more-invasive or destructive surgical procedures only when initial medical treatment fails. When a patient has very frequent vertigo attacks and is disabled, more-aggressive treatment may be considered sooner.

CURRENT THERAPY

- Initial therapy includes a sodium-restricted diet (preferably <1500 mg of sodium daily) and a diuretic agent (e.g., thiazide diuretics).
- Betahistine,[1] a medication widely used in Europe that may be obtained at compounding pharmacies in the United States, may be helpful in selected patients at a dosage of 8-16 mg three times daily.
- Transtympatic infusion of gentamicin[1] or corticosteroids and endolymphatic sac surgery may be considered as minimally invasive options in patients with serviceable hearing because these procedures have a reasonably low risk of inducing hearing loss.
- Vestibular nerve sectioning is highly effective in stopping vertigo attacks with reasonable low risk of causing further hearing loss but is a more invasive procedure.
- Labyrinthectomy is highly effective in stopping vertigo attacks but causes complete hearing loss, so it is only an option for patients who have already lost all useful hearing.

Patients who have undergone procedures that cause acute loss of vestibular function often have vertigo for a while after the surgery; the vertigo improves more quickly with vestibular rehabilitative therapy.

---

[1]Not FDA approved for this indication.

Dietary sodium should be restricted to 1000 to 1500 mg daily. The average person consumes about 4000 mg daily, and the maximum recommended daily intake of sodium is 2300 mg. Because more than 70% of the daily sodium comes from processed foods, this dietary restriction generally requires more than simply stopping the use of table salt, which generally accounts for only about 10% of daily sodium intake for most people.

A diuretic is usually added to the sodium restriction. The most commonly prescribed diuretic is hydrochlorothiazide 25 mg combined with triamterene 37.5 mg (Dyazide)[1] because this combination usually obviates the need for potassium supplementation. Acetazolamide (Diamox)[1] 125 to 250 mg bid or furosemide (Lasix)[1] 10 to 20 mg daily are also options. Patients with severe sulfa allergy can use low-dose ethacrynic acid (Edecrin)[1] 12.5-25 mg daily.

An acute attack of vertigo from Ménière's disease can be managed with vestibular suppressants such as dimenhydrinate (Dramamine)[1] 50 mg, meclizine (Antivert) 25 to 50 mg, diazepam (Valium)[1] 2 to 5 mg, or promethazine (Phenergen)[1] 12.5 to 50 mg. Scopolamine in patch form (Transderm-Scop)[1] is too slow to be useful because it takes hours to be absorbed transdermally; oral scopolamine tablets (Scopace)[1] 0.4 mg may be effective. Nausea can additionally be managed with prochlorperazine (Compazine) 10 mg orally or 25 mg by suppository, with oral or sublingual ondansetron (Zofran)[1] 4 to 8 mg, or with other antiemetics. Generally the vertigo attacks subside in several hours even without treatment.

Betahistine (Serc)[1,2] may also be helpful in Ménière's, though it is not commonly used in the United States. The role of betahistine is not firmly established although it is widely prescribed for vertigo throughout the world. Betahistine may be helpful when successful medical management with diet and diuretic has helped but is inadequate to stop attacks. Betahistine is a vasodilator, a modest H_1 histamine agonist and a powerful H_3 histamine receptor antagonist. Its method of action in Ménière's is unknown, though it increases blood flow and might also influence endolymphatic fluid regulation and receptors in the endolymphatic sac. Doses of betahistine may start at 8 mg PO three times daily and may be increased to 16 mg three times daily. It is available outside the United States in the form of Serc (Solvay Pharmaceuticals, Belgium). Betahistine may also be made within the United States at compounding pharmacies with a physician prescription and may also be imported from outside the United States for individual use. Side effects are few, though occasionally patients report some headache. Betahistine is not histamine, and we have not found it to cause or aggravate urticaria.

Oral corticosteroids are often used but rarely seem effective except in cases of bilateral Ménière's resulting from autoimmune inner ear disease (AIED). Oral corticosteroids rarely seem to be effective in typical Ménière's disease.

Ménière's attacks have been said to be triggered by caffeine, chocolate, stress, visual stimuli, and dropping barometric pressure. Such triggers should be avoided when possible, but strong associations with these triggers can also occur in migrainous vertigo. Vestibular rehabilitative therapy is not generally helpful in Ménière's because most vertigo attacks remit and the patients have few vestibular symptoms between attacks.

BILATERAL MÉNIÈRE'S DISEASE

The estimated incidence of bilateral Ménière's varies in the literature but is estimated to occur in about 15% of cases and tends to become bilateral within the first few years of onset in most cases. The possibility of bilateral involvement weighs on the decision making for any procedures that sacrifice hearing or vestibular function because it leaves the patient with only one functioning labyrinth.

SERVICEABILITY OF HEARING

Serviceable hearing is residual hearing that can be useful to the patient by wearing hearing aids. In general, because hearing loss is permanent, one should avoid sacrificing any serviceable hearing.

---

[1]Not FDA approved for this indication.
[2]Not available in the United States.

INJECTIONS AND SURGICAL TREATMENTS

Patients who continue to have disabling vertigo despite a low-salt diet, diuretics, and possibly betahistine are considered to have failed conservative medical therapy. The next step in treatment depends on the age, health status, and residual hearing and vestibular function of the patient and also on the surgeon's opinion and experience with the various options. If spells are infrequent, symptomatic management of vertigo attacks may be the best option. Table 1 outlines some of the additional interventional options.

TRANSTYMPANIC GENTAMICIN

Transtympanic gentamicin (Garamycin)[1] administration has become increasingly used as an effective treatment of Ménière's. This is partly due to its ease of administration of gentamicin and its relative safety. Gentamicin is a commonly used aminoglycoside antimicrobial agent with activity against gram-negative bacteria that also happens to be ototoxic. It damages hair cells of the labyrinth and preferentially affects hair cells of the vestibular neuroepithelium over that of the cochlea. Even so, transtympanic administration still has some risk of causing hearing loss. Gentamicin is performed by injecting a small amount (usually about 0.5 mL) of gentamicin sulfate (80 mg/2 mL) solution through the tympanic membrane into the middle ear space. To avoid rapid drainage through the eustachian tube, the injection is done with the patient supine and kept in that position for an hour or so to allow the gentamicin to absorb through the round window into the inner ear. There are many protocols, but commonly an injection is given once, and additional injections can be considered every 3 to 4 weeks until improvement in vertigo attacks is realized.

ENDOLYMPHATIC SAC SURGERY

Another option for patients with residual functional hearing is endolymphatic sac shunt or decompression. This procedure eliminates vertigo in 50% to 75% of those treated. Nevertheless, its effectiveness compared to placebo has remained a point of contention based on a number of studies. It has been suggested that the procedure's effectiveness depends on the operative technique and experience of the surgeon.

---

[1]Not FDA approved for this indication.

INTRATYMPANIC STEROIDS

Sometimes, a trial of intratympanic corticosteroids may be tried, though its effectiveness in controlled trials is still not compelling. Even so, a trial of corticosteroids administered in this manner poses little risk.

VESTIBULAR NEURECTOMY

The most definitive procedure for stopping vertigo attacks in Ménière's when the goal is to preserve hearing is vestibular neurectomy. This procedure involves craniotomy and severing the vestibular nerve while preserving the cochlear nerve. This procedure requires overnight hospitalization and general anesthesia, and it does pose some risk for facial nerve function and hearing on the affected side.

LABYRINTHECTOMY

For patients who have unilateral Ménière's and no serviceable hearing, labyrinthectomy is a commonly used procedure. This procedure entails the removal of the membranous labyrinth and is highly effective in stopping recurrent vertigo attacks from that ear. In elderly patients or those that are poor surgical candidates, a more limited transtympanic cochleosacculotomy may be performed.

MENIETT TREATMENT

The Meniett device is a portable low-frequency pressure-wave delivery system that administers a wave of pressure of about 12 cm H_2O to the middle ear via a tympanostomy tube for about 0.6 seconds pulsed at 6 Hz for 5 minutes about three to five times daily. Quality randomized trials demonstrating the effectiveness of this treatment are very limited, however. This method has few risks and only requires myringotomy and a pressure equalization tube. A practical limitation is the cost of the device, which is not often paid for by many health insurance companies.

Monitoring

Following patients with Ménière's disease should include monitoring of the frequency and severity of vertigo spells and the fluctuation in hearing, ear fullness, and tinnitus. Periodic audiometry is probably the most sensitive measure of stabilization of the condition. Vestibular testing may be considered when changes might alter the treatment strategy. Brain imaging is only helpful in excluding other disorders, but it has no role in the management of Ménière's disease.

TABLE 1 Procedures Used in the Management of Ménière's Disease

Method	Technique	Advantage	Disadvantage
Procedures Intended to Spare Serviceable Hearing			
Meniett device	Applies repetitive low-pressure pulses of air with the aim of enhancing endolymph drainage	Minimally invasive; no significant side effects and no risk of hearing loss	Requires tympanostomy tube placement; usually not covered by insurance; rate of effectiveness still unclear
Intratympatic corticosteroids	Injection of steroid through the tympanic membrane to the middle ear to be absorbed in the inner ear	Minimally invasive, few side effects	Effectiveness unclear when compared to placebo
Transtympanic gentamicin (Garamycin)[1]	Injection of gentamicin through the tympanic membrane to the middle ear to be absorbed in the inner ear	Simple office-based procedure, low risk profile	Number of injections is unpredictable; some risk of hearing loss
Endolymphatic mastoid shunt	Placing a shunt from the endolymphatic sac to the mastoid air cells	Effective in 50%-75%; low risk of hearing loss; day procedure	Vertigo can recur; effectiveness depends on surgical experience and technique
Vestibular neurectomy	Surgical sectioning of the vestibular part of cranial nerve VIII, sparing the auditory part of the nerve	Highly effective in eliminating vertigo attacks	Requires general anesthesia; risk of facial weakness, hearing loss
Procedures Expected to Eliminate Residual Hearing			
Labyrinthectomy or cochleosacculotomy	Several methods of removing all or part of the labyrinth	Highly effective in stopping vertigo attacks	Inevitable complete hearing loss

[1]Not FDA approved for this indication.

Complications

Known complications include the progression of unilateral and occasionally bilateral hearing and vestibular function. There may also be complications associated with some of the treatments as described earlier. Owing to the unpredictability of the vertigo attacks, many patients avoid certain activities and might even develop agoraphobic features because the attacks are so severe and disruptive. In most cases, these avoidance behaviors improve if Ménière's can be controlled.

Conclusion

The management of Ménière's disease is still part art and part science. Treatment options are many, but patients should be reassured that in most cases, something can be offered to help improve the vertigo and quality of life.

REFERENCES

Committee on Hearing and Equilibrium. Committee on Hearing and Equilibrium guidelines for the diagnosis and evaluation of therapy in Ménière's disease. Otolaryngol Head Neck Surg 1995;113:181–5.

DeBeer L, Stokroos R, Kingma H. Intratympanic gentamicin therapy for intractable Ménière's disease. Acta Otolaryngol 2007;127:605–12.

Garduño-Anaya M, De Toledo H, Hinojosa-González R, et al. Dexamethasone inner ear perfusion by intratympanic injection in unilateral Ménière's disease: A two-year prospective, placebo-controlled, double-blind, randomized trial. Otolaryngol Head Neck Surg 2005;133:285–94.

Kaylie DM, Jackson CG, Gardner EK. Surgical management of Ménière's disease in the era of gentamicin. Otolaryngol Head Neck Surg 2005;132 (3):443–50.

Rosenberg SI. Vestibular surgery for Ménière's disease in the elderly: A review of techniques and indications. Ear Nose Throat J 1999;78(6):443–6.

Sinusitis

Method of
Morten Lindbaek, MD

Epidemiology of Acute Sinusitis

The incidence of sinusitis-like illness severe enough to prompt a visit to the doctor is between 1.6 and 3.5 episodes per 100 adults per year in Western developed countries. There is seasonal variation, with the highest frequency in the winter and lowest in the summer and autumn.

Acute sinusitis is diagnosed more often in women than in men; two thirds of patients with sinusitis are women. The higher incidence in women may be due to differences in health care–seeking behavior, greater exposure to upper respiratory infections from child care duties, and increased mucosal thickening due to estrogen exposure leading to a greater likelihood of ostial obstruction and subsequent sinus infection.

Pathogenesis, Etiology and Definitions

Sinusitis means inflammation of the mucosa of the paranasal sinuses irrespective of the cause. By definition, acute sinusitis lasts less than 30 days, subacute sinusitis lasts from 1 to 3 months, and chronic sinusitis lasts longer than 3 months. Most cases of sinusitis involve more than one of the paranasal sinuses, most commonly the maxillary and ethmoid sinuses.

PREDISPOSING FACTORS

Viral upper respiratory infections and allergic rhinitis can lead to mucosa edema, ostial narrowing, increased secretion, and decreased mucociliary activity. A dysfunctional mucociliary system, anatomic malformations, polyps, septal deviation, foreign bodies, and tumors can cause ostial obstruction, leading to sinusitis. In some cases, sinusitis is caused by upper tooth infections that spread directly to the maxillary sinus.

VIRAL (SEROUS) SINUSITIS

Viral infections cause mucosal thickening that can narrow or close the ostium, causing decreased oxygen concentration, increased carbon dioxide concentration, and formation of a serous secretion in the sinus. This condition is called *serous sinusitis* and can cause modest symptoms of facial pressure. Most of these cases resolve spontaneously.

BACTERIAL (PURULENT) SINUSITIS

Acute bacterial sinusitis is usually a secondary infection resulting from sinus ostia obstruction or impaired mucus clearance mechanisms caused by an acute viral upper respiratory tract infection. When bacteria enter via the ostium and serous secretions and good growth conditions are present, bacteria grow rapidly. The body responds with an inflammatory reaction, and polymorphonuclear leukocytes are mobilized, resulting in pus formation, or *acute mucopurulent sinusitis*. Occasionally the inflammatory system of the body does not limit bacterial growth. The infection progresses and the pus becomes thinner, homogeneous, and foul smelling. When this occurs, there is greater risk of irreversible damage to the sinus mucosa and complications.

The most common bacterial pathogens are *Streptococcus pneumoniae, Haemophilus influenzae, Moraxella catarrhalis,* and group A β-hemolytic streptococci.

Diagnosis of Acute Bacterial Sinusitis

Four studies from primary care provide useful information on symptoms, signs, and blood tests that help discriminate bacterial sinusitis from viral sinusitis and viral upper respiratory infections (Table 1). Purulent rhinorrhea as a symptom and the finding of purulent secretions in the nasal cavity were associated with bacterial sinusitis in three of the four studies. Tooth pain was associated with bacterial infection in two. Other findings are less-consistent predictors of bacterial sinusitis. A biphasic history with worsening following initial improvement and lack of effect of decongestants were associated with bacterial infection in one study each and were not investigated in the others. The value of palpation as a diagnostic tool has not been proved in any diagnostic study. An erythrocyte sedimentation rate (ESR) greater than 10 for men and greater than 20 for women was associated in the two studies where it was investigated, and C-reactive protein (CRP) greater than 10 mg/L was associated in one, but not in the other where it was investigated. Because acute bacterial sinusitis usually develops as a complication of viral upper respiratory tract infections, experts have proposed that duration of illness of less than 7 days be used as a negative diagnostic criterion.

The value of plain sinus x-rays in the diagnosis of bacterial sinusitis is limited. When using fluid level or opacity as the criterion for bacterial sinusitis, the sensitivity and specificity of x-ray is 76% and 79%, respectively. The test characteristics of ultrasonography are unstable and unsatisfactory. The average specificity is low, 69%, giving a high proportion of false positive cases. However, a normal plain x-ray or ultrasound is good evidence against bacterial infection. Sinus CT has a high specificity of about 90%, when using presence of a fluid level or total opacification as the diagnostic criteria for acute bacterial sinusitis.

TABLE 1 Symptoms, Signs, and Blood Tests Independently Associated with a Confirmed Diagnosis of Acute Sinusitis

	Study				
Feature	Hansen	Lindbaek	Williams	van Duijn	Total
Reference standard	Puncture	CT sinus	X-ray	Ultrasound	
Number of patients	$n = 174$	$n = 201$	$n = 247$	$n = 441$	
Association	LR (frequency)	LR (frequency)	LR (frequency)	LR (frequency)	
Symptoms*					
Purulent rhinorrhea	—	1.5 (78)	1.5 (59)	1.9 (47)	3+ 1−
Pain in teeth	—	—	2.5 (11)	2.1 (26)	2+ 2−
Beginning with common cold	—	—	—	1.4 (78)	1+ 3−
Unilateral maxillary pain	—	—	—	1.8 (27)	1+ 3−
Two phases in history	0	2.1 (59)	0	0	1+
Lack of response to nasal decongestants	0	0	2.1 (28)	0	1+
Signs*					
Purulent secretion in nasal cavity	—	5.5 (42)	2.1 (34)	—	2+ 2−
Pain in bending forward	—	—	—	1.6 (52)	1+ 3−
Transillumination of sinus	—	—	1.6 (56)	0	1+
Blood Tests*					
ESR>10®/20	2.9 (39)	1.7 (61)	0	0	2+
CPR>10	1.8 (57)	—	0	0	1+ 1−
Predictive Values					
Positive (numbers of factors)	0.68 (2 of 2)	0.86 (3 of 4)	0.80 (4 of 5)	—	Not stated
Negative (numbers of factors)	—	0.74 (2 of 2)	0.53 (3 of 4)	0.66 (4 of 5)	Not stated

*Association given by likelihood ratio (frequency of trial in percentage)
— = no association; 0 = not investigated.
Hansen JG, Schmidt H, Rosborg J, Lund E: Predicting acute maxillary sinusitis in a general practice population. BMJ 1995;311(6999):233-236.
Lindbaek M, Hjortdahl P, Johnsen UL: Use of symptoms, signs, and blood tests to diagnose acute sinus infections in primary care: Comparison with computed tomography. Fam Med 1996;28(3):183-188.
van Duijn NP, Brouwer HJ, Lamberts H: Use of symptoms and signs to diagnose maxillary sinusitis in general practice: comparison with ultrasonography. BMJ 1992;305(6855):684-687.
Williams JW Jr, Simel DL, Roberts L, Samsa GP: Clinical evaluation for sinusitis. Making the diagnosis by history and physical examination. Ann Int Med 1992;117(9): 705-710.
Reprinted with permission from Lindbaek M, Hjortdahl P: The clinical diagnosis of acute purulent sinusitis in general practice—a review. Br J Gen Pract 2002;52:491-495. ©British Journal of General Practice, 2002.

 CURRENT DIAGNOSIS

- By definition, acute sinusitis lasts less than 30 days, subacute sinusitis lasts from 1 to 3 months, and chronic sinusitis lasts longer than 3 months.
- Most cases of sinusitis involve more than one of the paranasal sinuses, most commonly the maxillary and ethmoid sinuses.
- The following symptoms and signs are associated with acute bacterial sinusitis: purulent rhinorrhea, purulent secretions in the nasal cavity, tooth pain, biphasic history with worsening following initial improvement, elevated erythrocyte sedimentation rate or C-reactive protein (or both), and history of more than 7 days' duration.
- Duration of illness of less than 7 days may be used as a negative diagnostic criterion.
- The value of plain sinus x-rays in the diagnosis of bacterial sinusitis is limited, though a normal plain sinus x-ray is good evidence against bacterial infection.
- A fluid level or opacification of a sinus on computed tomography is 90% specific for acute bacterial sinusitis.
- Patients with recurrent sinusitis constitute 7% to 9% of all patients with acute sinusitis.

Differential Diagnosis

A serious common cold is the condition most often confused with acute bacterial sinusitis. A number of recurring pain conditions such as atypical migraine, tension headache, trigeminal neuralgia, and dysfunction of the temporomandibular joint must be considered because these conditions can mimic bacterial sinusitis.

Treatment of Acute Bacterial Sinusitis

SYMPTOMATIC TREATMENT

Topically or orally administered α-adrenergic agents (decongestants), proteolytic enzymes, nasal irrigation with salt water, mucolytic agents, and antihistamines have been used for symptom relief in acute sinusitis. Use of topical corticosteroids has given conflicting evidence. However, in patients with recurrent sinusitis, a combination of steroids and antibiotics gave signficant higher cure rate than antibiotics alone.

ANTIBIOTIC TREATMENT

Patients presenting with less than 7 days of mild to moderate symptoms consistent with acute sinusitis should be given symptomatic treatment only. Antibiotic treatment should be reserved for patients with moderately severe symptoms of bacterial sinusitis of greater than 7 days' duration and for those with severe sinusitis symptoms (severe pain or fever >39°C) regardless of duration of illness. More than half of the patients with acute bacterial sinusitis are cured without any antibiotic treatment.

CURRENT THERAPY

- In patients with a clinically diagnosed acute sinusitis, no significant difference has been demonstrated between antibiotics and placebo.
- In patients with confirmed sinusitis, a significant difference between antibiotics and placebo has been demonstrated, with a number needed to treat (NNT) of 7 to 15.
- In most countries, amoxicillin is the drug of choice; more broad-spectrum antibiotics have not shown a higher cure rate.
- For patients presenting with less than 7 days of mild to moderate symptoms consistent with acute sinusitis, give symptomatic treatment only.
- Antibiotic treatment should be reserved for patients with moderately severe symptoms of bacterial sinusitis of greater than 7 days' duration and for those with severe symptoms (severe pain or fever >39°C) regardless of duration of illness.
- More than half of the patients with acute bacterial sinusitis are cured without any antibiotic treatment.

In patients with clinically diagnosed acute sinusitis, no significant difference has been demonstrated between antibiotics and placebo. In patients with a confirmed sinusitis (CT scan, x-ray, or bacteriology) various meta-analyses have found a significant difference between antibiotics and placebo with a pooled difference of 7% to 15%, giving a number needed to treat (NNT) of 7 to 15. Three meta-analyses have concluded that newer and broad-spectrum antibiotics are not significantly more effective than narrow-spectrum agents. Initial treatment should be with the narrowest-spectrum agent that is active against the likely pathogens, *S. pneumoniae* and *H. influenzae*. Knowledge of local antibiotic resistance patterns should guide antibiotic selection, though amoxicillin (Amoxil) is considered the drug of choice in most countries and erythromycin (Ery-Tab) or trimethoprim-sulfamethoxazole (Bactrim, Septra) for patients allergic to penicillin.

A meta-analysis of individual patient data found no clinical feature that could predict a significant effect of antibiotic treatment.

SINUS PUNCTURE

The indication for puncture and irrigation of the sinuses is sinus empyema when antibiotic treatment has produced no improvement. In these cases, antibiotics have low penetration and the mucosal concentration does not reach bactericidal levels, even with high dosages. However, the need for puncture in the treatment of acute bacterial sinusitis seems to be rare, only 1% to 2% of the patients.

Complications

Serious complications of sinusitis include brain abscess, orbital cellulitis, subdural empyema, and meningitis. There is no mention of such complications among more than 2700 patients in 27 clinical trials of sinusitis treatment. Another important complication is the development of chronic sinusitis from inadequately treated acute sinusitis, found in 1% to 2 % of patients with acute sinusitis.

Recurrent Sinusitis

Patients with recurrent sinusitis constitute 7% to 9% of all patients with acute sinusitis. They can have an underlying physiologic or anatomic abnormality such as allergic rhinitis, immune compromise, or an underlying anatomic abnormality. Nasal polyps or abnormalities in the ostiomeatal complex can cause reduced drainage of the sinuses.

REFERENCES

Ahovuo-Saloranta A, Borisenko OV, Kovanen N, et al. Antibiotics for acute maxillary sinusitis. Cochrane Database Syst Rev 2008;(2):CD000243.

Ah-See K. Sinusitis (acute). Clin Evid (Online) 2008;pii:0511.

de Ferranti SD, Ioannidis JP, Lau J, et al. Are amoxycillin and folate inhibitors as effective as other antibiotics for acute sinusitis? A meta-analysis. BMJ 1998;317(7159):632–7.

Hickner JM, Bartlett JG, Besser RE, et al. Centers for Disease Control and Prevention: Principles of appropriate antibiotic use for acute rhinosinusitis in adults: Background. Emerg Med 2001;37(6):703–10.

Lindbaek M. Acute sinusitis: guide to selection of antibacterial therapy. Drugs 2004;64(8):805–19.

Lindbaek M, Hjortdahl P. The clinical diagnosis of acute purulent sinusitis in general practice—a review. Br J Gen Pract 2002;52:491–5.

van Buchem FL, Knottnerus JA, Schrijnemaekers VJ, Peeters MF. Primary-care–based randomised placebo-controlled trial of antibiotic treatment in acute maxillary sinusitis. Lancet 1997;349(9053):683–7.

Williamson IG, Rumsby K, Benge S, et al. Antibiotics and topical nasal steroid for treatment of acute maxillary sinusitis: A randomized controlled trial. JAMA 2007;298(21):2487–96.

Young J, De Sutter A, Merenstein D, et al. Antibiotics for adults with clinically diagnosed acute rhinosinusitis: A meta-analysis of individual patient data. Lancet 2008;371(9616):908–14.

Nonallergic Perennial Rhinitis

Method of
Michael Groves, MD, and Masayoshi Takashima, MD

Although rhinitis, defined strictly, means "inflammation of the nasal mucosa," it can be generally defined as a disorder of the nasal mucosa characterized by one or more of the common symptoms of sneezing, rhinorrhea, nasal congestion, and nasal pruritus. It is thought to affect as many as 30% of the world population, and it is a significant detriment to quality of life. Rhinitis therefore represents an important disease entity worthy of specific attention by physicians in primary care clinics. For allergic rhinitis alone, the direct costs of medical care and the indirect costs, including loss of productivity and missed days of school or work, are estimated to be greater than $11 billion annually in the United States. It may be assumed that this dollar amount would be much higher if all forms of rhinitis were included. A better understanding of the pathophysiology, diagnosis, and treatment of the various forms of rhinitis can decrease these costs through the employment of more effective therapeutic strategies.

Classification

Rhinitis is a family of disorders with multiple causes (Figure 1). It can be divided into two categories by making the distinction between infectious (bacterial or viral) and noninfectious etiologies. The noninfectious group can be further divided into allergic and nonallergic forms. Allergic rhinitis is characterized by mucosal inflammation produced by immunoglobulin E–mediated responses to a variety of aeroallergens. Nonallergic rhinitis can produce periodic or perennial nasal symptoms that are not the result of these IgE-dependent mechanisms. Perennial nonallergic rhinitis is loosely defined as the presence of two or more symptoms—such as hypersecretion, sneezing, nasal congestion, and postnasal drip—for more than 3 months per year. It is estimated that up to 25% of rhinitis patients fit into this purely nonallergic category; however, other studies have found that between 44% and 87% of rhinitis patients have mixed disease. As discussed later in this chapter, diagnosis is made on the basis of exclusion of an identifiable allergy, structural abnormality, sinus disease, or cerebrospinal fluid rhinorrhea.

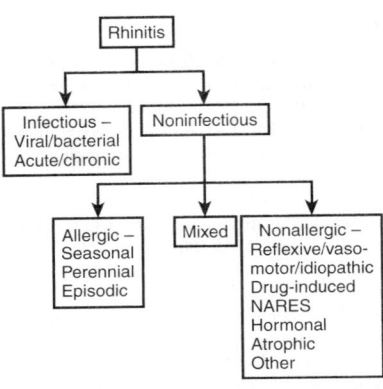

FIGURE 1. Classification of rhinitis. NARES = nonallergic rhinitis with eosinophilia syndrome.

Nasal Physiology

The nose is the gatekeeper between the outside environment and the more fragile lower airways. It performs critical functions, including warming and humidifying inhaled air and filtering out harmful airborne particles before they reach the lungs.

The nasal vasculature consists of an intricate network of resistance vessels (small arteries, arterioles, and arteriovenous anastomoses) and capacitance vessels (valveless veins and venous sinusoids). The sinusoids are particularly numerous in the lamina propria (erectile tissue) of the nasal turbinates. They are fed by inflow from the resistance vessels, which are primarily under sympathetic control. Increased sympathetic stimulation results in α-adrenergically mediated vasoconstriction. This leads to a decrease in blood pooling in the venous sinusoids, turbinate shrinkage, and increased nasal airflow.

Sensory nerve endings are distributed throughout the nasal mucosa from the ophthalmic and maxillary branches of the trigeminal nerve. They are able to detect touch, temperature, pain, itch, and airflow. The small, unmyelinated, nociceptive C-fibers are responsible for the detection of pain and noxious chemical stimuli. Excitation of these fibers induces reflexive parasympathetic responses. The parasympathetic nervous system's primary postganglionic neurotransmitter, acetylcholine, acts on muscarinic (M) receptors concentrated in the glands, blood vessels, and epithelium of the nasal mucosa, leading to an increase in glandular secretion and vasodilation.

Pathophysiology

REFLEXIVE AND IDIOPATHIC (VASOMOTOR) RHINITIDES

Many noninfectious, nonallergic rhinitis syndromes are caused by the reflexive parasympathetic production of nasal congestion or increased nasal secretions in response to C-fiber activation by a known stimulus. Included in this group is gustatory rhinitis, in which patients develop rhinitis after the ingestion of food, especially spicy foods that contain capsaicin. This compound directly activates C-fibers. Cold/dry air and environmental or occupational irritants such as tobacco smoke, perfume, or chemical fumes may also initiate rhinitis symptoms. On the other hand, many patients have no identifiable cause for their rhinitis. The terminology for this condition is in constant flux in the medical literature, but the most commonly used names are idiopathic rhinitis or vasomotor rhinitis.

Although many of these nonallergy stimuli are able to produce mild symptoms in normal subjects, they tend to create far more persistent and intense nasal pathology in rhinitic patients. Some have proposed that the central nervous system is incorrectly interpreting signals from the sensory fibers of the nasal mucosa—a so-called central hyperresponsiveness. Another theory posits that nasal hyperresponsiveness is caused by an imbalance between parasympathetic and sympathetic effects on the nasal mucosa as it reacts to stimuli. Finally, some believe that the underlying mechanism is a phenomenon called neurogenic edema. Nociceptive C-fibers are known to release multiple inflammatory neuropeptides. These neurons can be antidromically stimulated, meaning that their dendrites can be triggered to release neuropeptides by action potentials generated at axon terminals on the same nerve (the so-called axon reflex). Repeated stimuli may lead to high neuropeptide levels in the mucosa. The neuropeptides, in turn, cause increased vascular permeability, vasodilation, and a cascade of inflammatory cell responses leading to edema, nasal congestion, and rhinorrhea.

DRUG-INDUCED RHINITIS

Aspirin-sensitive patients often develop rhinitis symptoms in addition to nasal polyposis and intrinsic asthma. In sensitive patients, aspirin's effects on arachidonic acid metabolism may lead to abnormally high levels of leukotrienes and subsequent inflammation of the nasal mucosa. There may also be some inhibition of eosinophil apoptosis related to the increased levels of leukotrienes.

Rhinitis medicamentosa is a separate type of drug-induced rhinitis caused by excessive use of topical α-adrenergic agonists. These drugs produce vasoconstriction of nasal blood vessels. With long-term use, the α-adrenergic receptors are downregulated, and the patient is forced to use higher and higher doses to achieve adequate symptom relief. Sudden discontinuation of the product leads to an intense rebound nasal congestion. Many other drugs, including angiotensin-converting enzyme inhibitors, β-blockers, chlorpromazine (Thorazine), methyldopa (Aldomet), nonsteroidal antiinflammatory drugs, immunosuppressive drugs, and oral contraceptives, can also cause nasal congestion.

NONALLERGIC RHINITIS WITH EOSINOPHILIA SYNDROME (NARES)

Patients with nonallergic rhinitis with eosinophilia syndrome (NARES) have perennial rhinitis symptoms with paroxysmal exacerbations of sneezing, profuse watery rhinorrhea, nasal pruritus, and, occasionally, loss of the sense of smell. They have greatly increased levels (5%-20%) of eosinophils in their nasal secretions. NARES may be an early stage of aspirin sensitivity or nasal polyposis. Nasal biopsies from patients with NARES show mast cells with bound IgE despite no evidence of allergy on skin testing. This may point to a local allergic reaction as the main culprit in symptom production. These patients respond well to nasal corticosteroids.

HORMONAL RHINITIS

Rhinitis symptoms are common during pregnancy but can also occur in conjunction with the menstrual cycle. It is presumed that increased levels of estrogen lead to vascular smooth muscle relaxation, pooling of blood in the venous sinusoids, and increased plasma leakage. Not all pregnant women with rhinitic symptoms have hormonally induced rhinitis, because allergic rhinitis, infectious rhinosinusitis, and rhinitis medicamentosa are also very common in this patient group. A previous history of rhinitis or asthma is not a risk factor for pregnancy-induced rhinitis. Hypothyroidism is believed to cause rhinitis in up to 2% of patients, but a strong link has never been established.

ATROPHIC RHINITIS

Primary atrophic rhinitis is a progressive, chronic nasal disease characterized by atrophy of the nasal mucosa and glands with subsequent resorption of the bone of the nasal turbinates. There is extensive nasal crusting, dryness, and a fetid odor in addition to the sensation of nasal congestion despite widely patent nasal cavities. Infection with the bacteria *Klebsiella ozaenae* is the most commonly implicated cause of primary atrophic rhinitis, although hereditary and vascular anomalies may also play a role.

Secondary atrophic rhinitis can be caused by overly aggressive turbinate surgery, chronic sinus infections, granulomatous disease, trauma, or irradiation.

OTHER CAUSES

Emotional stress (e.g., crying) and sexual arousal can also produce nasal congestion and rhinitic symptoms, presumably through autonomic mechanisms. Gastroesophageal reflux also has been linked to nasal inflammation and subsequent rhinitis. Lastly, a growing body of evidence supports the idea of a "local allergic rhinitis" characterized by allergen-specific, IgE-mediated nasal inflammation without associated atopy on intradermal skin testing.

Diagnosis

As with any medical condition, the proper diagnosis of perennial nonallergic rhinitis begins with a careful history and differential diagnosis (Box 1). Important elements include the age at symptom onset, time course, perennial versus seasonal symptoms, possible inciting factors, detailed questions about occupational exposures, the character of the mucus, pertinent related symptoms such as itching eyes, past medical history, family history, and previous medical evaluation or therapy for the problem. Features of the patient's story that would suggest a nonallergic cause include onset after age 20 years and isolated postnasal drainage. Features that might suggest an allergic cause include seasonal exacerbations, concomitant eye symptoms, and frequent sneezing or nasal pruritus. Rhinitis syndromes with specific inciting factors, such as gustatory rhinitis, cold/dry air rhinitis, or rhinitis medicamentosa, can often be diagnosed from the history alone.

Another important element of the history is an assessment of how the symptoms affect the patient's quality of life. This is important in establishing a baseline against which symptomatic improvement can be compared.

Next, a thorough head and neck examination is necessary. The careful physician will examine the ears for effusions or other middle ear pathology, palpate the neck for evidence of lymphadenopathy suggestive of an infectious etiology, and inspect the face for classic allergic signs such as periorbital venous congestion (allergic shiners) and the so-called allergic salute—a transverse nasal crease created by frequent wiping of a chronically dripping nose with the back of the hand. The latter two signs are more often found in patients with allergic disease but can be identified in patients with nonallergic rhinitis as well.

A comprehensive nasal examination requires proper lighting with a headlight or indirect light reflected from a head mirror (the use of which has unfortunately been lost in most primary care clinics despite its ubiquity in images of physicians from decades past). A nasal speculum is used to examine the nasal cavity. Septal perforations can cause crusting, nasal irritation, and epistaxis due to the increased air turbulence in the nasal vault caused by air criss-crossing across the hole. Deviations of the nasal septum should be noted, as well as any turbinate hypertrophy, because obstruction can block the flow of nasal secretions and lead to rhinorrhea, postnasal drip, and nasal congestion. The turbinate and nasal mucosa may have a pale appearance or a bluish hue in both allergic and nonallergic rhinitis. It tends to be hyperemic in patients with infections and in those with rhinitis medicamentosa. Quantity and quality of secretions should be noted, with profuse, watery rhinorrhea possible in both allergic and vasomotor rhinitis.

BOX 1 Differential Diagnosis

- Allergic rhinitis
- Nasal/valve collapse
- Nasal tumors
- Foreign body
- Choanal stenosis
- Septal deviation
- Enlarged turbinates/Concha bullosa
- Adenoid hypertrophy
- Nasal polyps
- Acute/chronic infectious rhinosinusitis
- Ciliary defects
- Cerebrospinal fluid rhinorrhea

 CURRENT DIAGNOSIS

- Check for possible stimuli and severity and duration of disease.
- Check drug use, exposure at the workplace, hormonal status, and history of asthma.
- Exclude other nasal diseases with an endoscopy.
- Exclude allergy.
- Exclude chronic rhinosinusitis with a computed tomographic scan.
- Exclude cerebrospinal fluid rhinorrhea (if suggested by the history) with a β_2-transferrin test of the nasal fluid.

Physicians with expertise in the use of rigid or flexible nasopharyngoscopes may choose to use these instruments when assessing the posterior septum, choanae, nasopharynx, and middle meatus. Adenoidal hypertrophy is a common cause of nasal obstruction and mouth breathing, especially in children. Unilateral choanal atresia is occasionally diagnosed in adults. Patients with unilateral nasal obstruction, discharge, and possibly pain should be assessed for a nasal neoplasm or foreign body. Purulent secretions emanating from the middle meatus may indicate infectious rhinosinusitis. Finally, a scope examination can easily identify nasal polyps, which are distinguished from mucosal hypertrophy because they are freely mobile and insensate and fail to shrink with application of α-adrenergic vasoconstrictors.

In daily clinical practice, the diagnosis of nonallergic rhinitis and its subgroups is based primarily on a thorough history and physical examination. If this evaluation suggests clinically relevant noninfectious rhinitis, other possible diagnoses are excluded in a stepwise fashion (see Current Diagnosis box). Perform nasal cytology (looking for eosinophilia); if the result is positive, consider an oral aspirin challenge.

Although a detailed history and physical examination are often sufficient to establish a diagnosis of allergic versus nonallergic rhinitis and initiate treatment, it is often helpful to obtain further testing to clearly delineate the two. The preferred method for doing so is intradermal skin testing. This method is fast, sensitive, and easily performed in the office setting. Serum immunoassays for specific IgE are also available but are, on average, not as sensitive as skin testing.

Treatment

There are many modalities in the clinician's armamentarium against perennial nonallergic rhinitis. An evaluation of the severity of the disease should be performed to confirm the need for therapy.

 CURRENT THERAPY

- Make the correct diagnosis of nonallergic perennial rhinitis (diagnosis of exclusion).
- Classify it correctly as to the type of nonallergic perennial rhinitis; effective therapy depends on correct classification of the disorder.
- Evaluate the severity of the disease to confirm need for therapy.
- Lifestyle changes may be sufficient for therapy.
- If medical therapy fails, a vidian neurectomy is an option for treatment.

INTRANASAL CORTICOSTEROIDS

Intranasal corticosteroids have been shown to effectively relieve symptoms in a number of nonallergic rhinitides, especially NARES and idiopathic rhinitis. Because their therapeutic action is predominantly through their antiinflammatory effects, they are much less likely to be effective in noninflammatory conditions such as hormonally induced rhinitis. There are a large number of drugs available in this category, with varying dosage amounts and schedules (Table 1).

No single corticosteroid has been proven to be more effective than any of the others. Local side effects can include a burning or stinging sensation and minor epistaxis, typically manifested as blood-streaked mucus. Septal perforation is rare but can occur if the patient consistently directs the spray at the septum. Proper instruction on delivering the spray in a slightly lateral direction helps avoid this complication. Systemic side effects are rare when these compounds are used at recommended doses.

ORAL ANTIHISTAMINES

Oral antihistamines have been shown to be generally ineffective in relieving symptoms of nonallergic rhinitis. In addition, the first-generation antihistamines, such as diphenhydramine (Benadryl) and hydroxyzine (Vistaril),[1] commonly induce drowsiness and impairment.

INTRANASAL ANTIHISTAMINES

Two intranasal antihistamines are available in the United States, azelastine (Astelin) and olopatadine (Patanase).[1] Both have been shown to be effective compared with placebo for control of rhinorrhea, postnasal drip, sneezing, and reducing nasal congestion. Intranasal azelastine has been shown to be effective in reducing symptoms caused specifically by nonallergic rhinitis. Azelastine comes in a 0.1% aqueous solution, whereas olopatadine is available as a 0.6% aqueous solution. Both are delivered by means of a metered-dose spray device, placing 2 sprays in each nostril twice daily. This should be considered as primary therapy for patients with allergic or nonallergic rhinitis. Systemic absorption does exist and can cause some sedation; patients should be warned of this side effect before initiation of therapy.

TOPICAL DECONGESTANTS

The topical decongestants, all α-adrenergic agonists, include phenylephrine (Neo-Synephrine) and oxymetazoline (Afrin). Both are effective in reducing nasal congestion by decreasing blood flow to the nasal mucosa, but they have no effect on the other symptoms of rhinitis. In addition, both carry the risk of inducing rhinitis

[1]Not FDA approved for this indication.

TABLE 1 Intranasal Corticosteroids Used to Treat Nonallergic Rhinitis

Generic Drug Name	Trade Name	Adult Dosage (sprays per nostril)
Beclomethasone dipropionate monohydrate	Beconase AQ	1–2 bid
Budesonide	Rhinocort Aqua[1]	1–4 qd
Ciclesonide	Omnaris[1]	2 qd
Flunisolide	Nasarel[1]	2 bid-qd
Fluticasone furoate	Veramyst[1]	2 qd
Fluticasone propionate	Flonase	2 qd
Mometasone	Nasonex[1]	2 qd
Triamcinolone	Nasacort AQ[1]	1–2 qd

[1]Not FDA approved for this indication.

medicamentosa, as discussed earlier. Therefore, they are recommended only as short-term therapies (i.e., <4–5 days) for acute exacerbations of rhinitis syndromes.

If rhinitis medicamentosa develops, therapy consists of discontinuation of the offending topical decongestant and initiation of an intranasal corticosteroid to help mitigate rebound nasal congestion. In some cases, surgical reduction of the size of the inferior turbinates may be required.

ORAL DECONGESTANTS

In nonallergic rhinitis patients with nasal congestion, an oral decongestant, such as pseudoephedrine (Sudafed), may be of some benefit. They should be used with caution in patients with medical comorbidities. There is a risk of adverse outcomes in patients with hypertension, vascular disease, hyperthyroidism, closed-angle glaucoma, or bladder obstruction. Even in healthy individuals, these agents can cause unpleasant side effects such as insomnia, palpitations, irritability, and loss of appetite.

INTRANASAL ANTICHOLINERGICS

Because the reflexive production of increased nasal secretions is mediated by the parasympathetic nervous system, application of an anticholinergic to the nasal mucosa might be expected to decrease this response. Intranasal ipratropium bromide (Atrovent) has been shown to be effective at decreasing rhinorrhea in nonallergic rhinitis without impairment of normal nasal functions such as olfaction or mucociliary clearance. It comes in 0.3% and 0.6%[1] preparations, with the lower concentration being more commonly used for rhinorrhea associated with perennial nonallergic rhinitis. Ipratropium can also be used safely and effectively in conjunction with an antihistamine or an intranasal corticosteroid. In addition, patients with reflexive rhinitis caused by specific stimuli (e.g., gustatory rhinitis, cold/dry air rhinitis) may benefit from the application of an intranasal anticholinergic agent shortly before exposure to the stimulus.

OTHER PHARMACEUTICAL AGENTS

Several other medications used for the treatment of allergic rhinitis have unclear utility in patients with nonallergic rhinitis. Cromolyn sodium (Nasalcrom)[1] inhibits the degranulation of sensitized mast cells, but the importance of histamine release in the pathogenesis of nonallergic rhinitis is uncertain. Therefore, only a modest benefit may be expected with use of this medication, and studies thus far have shown mixed results.

Despite the possible role of leukotrienes in the development of drug-induced rhinitis, there are no studies that demonstrate a place for leukotriene receptor antagonists, such as montelukast (Singulair),[1] in the treatment of this syndrome.

SALINE RINSES

A favorite of otolaryngologists, saline rinses in either isotonic or hypertonic concentrations may have modest benefits in reducing nasal congestion and sneezing. This is perhaps a result of improved mucociliary clearance, removal of mucosal irritants, and reduction of nasal bacteria and secretions. Delivery method and preparation are not standardized and depend mostly on patient and physician preference. Common delivery methods include squeeze bottles, neti pots, and water picks with irrigating adaptors.

BEHAVIOR MODIFICATION AND AVOIDANCE MEASURES

Patients with known triggers of hyperreactive rhinitis symptoms should be encouraged to avoid them if possible. Also, some rhinitides may respond to simple behavioral modifications. For example, rhinitis of pregnancy may improve with elevation of the head of the bed, gentle exercise, use of nasal valve dilators, and saline rinses. Cautious use of topical decongestants and intranasal corticosteroids may be of benefit if these measures fail.

[1]Not FDA approved for this indication.

INTRANASAL CAPSAICIN

A short course of topical applications of capsaicin[1,6] to the nasal mucosal has been shown to control symptoms of nonallergic rhinitis for up to 1 year. Capsaicin therapy is thought to work by repeatedly stimulating nociceptive C-fibers, causing depletion of their inflammatory neuropeptides and eventual nerve degeneration. Capsaicin is not available in any standardized form in the United States, and this therapeutic strategy remains in its experimental phase.

SURGERY

Surgical intervention can often help decrease the sensation of nasal congestion, drainage, and decreased airflow through correction of anatomic abnormalities. Septoplasty, inferior turbinate reduction, endoscopic nasal polypectomy, adenoidectomy, and nasal valve reconstruction all seek to relieve obstructions to nasal airflow. Multiple methods exist for the performance of each of these procedures, and the particular strategy used depends on the surgeon's expertise and the patient's specific anatomy.

Since the 1960s, when Golding-Wood first described the procedure, vidian neurectomy has been used to treat idiopathic or vasomotor rhinitis that is recalcitrant to medical therapy. The procedure is aimed at eliminating the proposed autonomic imbalance caused by a dominant parasympathetic system. Postganglionic sympathetic neurons from the deep petrosal nerve and preganglionic parasympathetic neurons from the greater superficial petrosal nerve combine to form the vidian nerve as it courses through the vidian canal. Destruction of the vidian nerve as it exits the canal interrupts the parasympathetic input, but most of the sympathetic tone remains, because fibers traveling in the carotid plexus continue to reach the nasal mucosa. Many surgeons have shied away from this procedure over the last several decades because of the difficulties associated with accessing the vidian nerve. Long-term relief of symptoms was rarely achieved, but this may have been related to incorrect identification of the vidian nerve. Newer endoscopic techniques, which allow for direct visualization of the nerve, have led to renewed interest by increasing the safety and effectiveness of the procedure.

Conclusion

The perennial nonallergic, noninfectious rhinitides make up a diverse group of disease entities producing derangements in nasal physiology and aggravating nasal symptoms such as congestion and rhinorrhea. A careful history and physical examination are crucial to proper diagnosis, and treatment options are as varied as the disease entities themselves. It is incumbent on primary care providers to understand the syndromes of rhinitis in order to reduce the burden of rhinitis symptoms in their patients.

[1]Not FDA approved for this indication.
[6]May be compounded by pharmacists.

REFERENCES

Bachert C, van Cauwenberge P, Khaltaev N, et al. Allergic rhinitis and its impact on asthma. In collaboration with the World Health Organization. Executive summary of the workshop report. Geneva, Switzerland, December 7–10, 1999. Allergy 2002;57(9):841–55.

Dykewicz MS, Fineman S, Skoner DP, et al. Diagnosis and management of rhinitis: Complete guidelines of the Joint Task Force on Practice Parameters in Allergy, Asthma and Immunology. Ann Allergy Asthma Immunol 1998;81(2):478–518.

Greiner AN, Meltzer EO. Pharmacologic rationale for treating allergic and nonallergic rhinitis. J Allergy Clin Immunol 2006;118(5):985–96.

Jaradeh SS, Smith TL, Torrico L, et al. Autonomic nervous system evaluation of patients with vasomotor rhinitis. Laryngoscope 2000;110:1828–31.

Robinson SR, Wormald PJ. Endoscopic vidian neurectomy. Am J Rhinology 2006;20(2):197–202.

Sapci T, Yazici S, Evcimik MF, et al. Investigation of the effects of intranasal botulinum toxin type a and ipratropium bromide nasal spray on nasal hypersecretion in idiopathic rhinitis with eosinophilia. Rhinology 2008;46:45–51.

Sarin S, Undem B, Sanico A, et al. The role of the nervous system in rhinitis. J Allergy Clin Immunol 2006;118(5):999–1014.

van Rijswijk JB, Boeke EL, Keizer JM, et al. Intranasal capsaicin reduces nasal hyperreactivity in idiopathic rhinitis: A double blind randomized application regimen study. Allergy 2003;58:754–61.

Wallace DV, Dykewicz MS, Bernstein DI, et al. The diagnosis and management of rhinitis: An updated practice parameter. J Allergy Clin Immunol 2008;122(2 Suppl):S1–S84.

Hoarseness and Laryngitis

Method of
Lee Akst, MD

Voice is an essential component of communication. Vocal difficulty is very distressing to patients and can have a negative impact on physical, social, and emotional qualities of life. To understand the pathophysiology, evaluation, and treatment of voice complaints, it is important to understand the anatomy and physiology of normal voice production. Looking first at how good voice quality is achieved makes it readily apparent how alterations in vocal fold vibration, symmetry, or closure can lead to various vocal difficulties.

To aid discussion of voice complaints, clarification of terminology is necessary. Although "hoarseness" is a term that most patients use to describe any type of voice complaint and "laryngitis" is the presumptive explanation that many patients provide for their symptoms, each of these terms has a more precise meaning. Dysphonia is the general term for vocal difficulty. Hoarseness implies a rough or raspy change in voice quality and is one type of dysphonia. Other categories include limited vocal projection, strained vocal effort, and change in pitch—each of which may occur with or without vocal roughness. The term laryngitis specifically describes inflammation of the larynx. This inflammation may be acute or chronic, and again it describes some but certainly not all cases of dysphonia. This distinction will be made clear as the evaluation and management of dysphonia are described.

Normal Laryngeal Function

The larynx plays a central role in voice production by serving as a vibrating instrument that turns airflow from the lungs into sound. The sound is shaped into intelligible speech through the resonating and articulating functions of the pharynx and oral cavity. The ability of the larynx to create vibration and serve as a sound source is a function of its complex layered microanatomy. The deeper layers of the vocal fold include the thyroarytenoid muscle and the vocal ligament, which position the more superficial layers of the superficial lamina propria and epithelium during phonation. Compared with the fibrous nature of the vocal ligament, the superficial lamina propria is a loose gelatinous layer whose pliability allows for voice production.

During inspiration (Figure 1A), the vocal folds are abducted so that air can move past the larynx without resistance. During phonation (see Figure 1B), the vocal folds are held in an adducted position while the lungs drive air toward the larynx. Air pressure builds in the subglottis, beneath the vocal folds, until it overcomes the forces of vocal fold closure, pushes past the vocal folds, and generates negative pressure in its wake as it moves past the larynx. A combination of the vocal folds' intrinsic viscoelasticity and the negative pressure created through Bernoulli's effect draws the vocal fold edges back together, allowing subglottic pressure to rebuild and the cycle to repeat. Repeated cycles of opening and closing at the level of the vocal fold edges generate a so-called mucosal wave, which travels from the inferior edge of each vocal fold up across the medial and superior edges

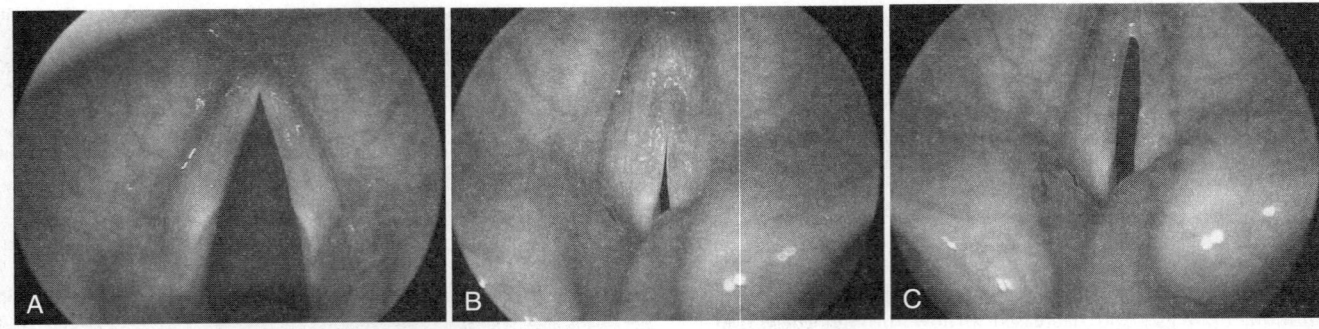

FIGURE 1. A, Normal vocal folds in abducted position for inspiration. **B**, Normal vocal folds in adducted position for phonation. **C**, Displacement of the vocal fold medial edges creates mucosal wave propagation during phonation and produces voice.

(see Figure 1C). These waves may repeat hundreds of times each second, depending on pitch. This cycled opening and closing of the vocal folds during phonation imparts pressure waves to the air column that moves the vocal folds, generating sound. The ability of vocal folds to vibrate easily and symmetrically in this very rapid fashion allows for clear, smooth voicing.

Evaluation of Dysphonia

Central to the evaluation of dysphonia is the understanding that any disruption of vocal fold closure, symmetry, or vibration impairs the ability of the vocal folds to generate a clear sound source. Most voice complaints arise from anatomic or functional limitations in glottal closure or mucosal wave formation, although other parts of the respiratory tree are also responsible for components of the voice. General points concerning evaluation of dysphonia are discussed in this section, with specific causes discussed afterward.

HISTORY

A careful history can provide many clues that point toward the proper diagnosis in patients with dysphonia. Although many patients offer the complaint of "hoarseness" as a general term, a careful historian distinguishes between complaints related to voice quality, vocal projection, vocal effort or strain, vocal fatigue, and so on. Two questions that can help a patient organize his or her own thoughts related to poor voice are, "What abnormal things does your voice do now that it did not do before?" and "What normal things did your voice do before that it now no longer can do?" The acuteness of onset, duration, severity, and progression of any complaint should be determined.

The history should also determine what other factors or events might have caused or exacerbated the dysphonia. Recent sources of laryngeal inflammation might include intubation, excessive voice use, or upper respiratory tract infection. Baseline conditions that foster chronic laryngeal inflammation include environmental allergies, rhinitis, and laryngopharyngeal reflux. Laryngopharyngeal reflux can exist in the absence of heartburn, with reflux-associated inflammation of the larynx and pharynx providing symptoms of globus pharyngeus, throat clearing, nonproductive cough, effortful swallowing, and even mild dysphagia in association with dysphonia.

Concerning the possibility of laryngeal malignancy, any patient with dysphonia should be asked about smoking and alcohol use, because these are risk factors for squamous cell carcinoma. Another important question in distinguishing inflammatory dysphonia from a mass lesion of the vocal fold concerns whether there are any periods of normal voice or the dysphonia is constant—inflammation may wax and wane, but dysphonia associated with mass lesions is usually progressive and unremitting. Finally, the history should elicit other possible head and neck complaints, including dyspnea, stridor, dysphagia, odynophagia, otalgia, sore throat, and pain with speaking (odynophonia). If hoarseness is associated with some of these symptoms for longer than 2 weeks, the suspicion of malignancy is increased.

PHYSICAL EXAMINATION

The physical examination for patients with dysphonia includes a complete head and neck evaluation with focus on the larynx and laryngeal function. Although much of the head and neck examination can be performed in a general setting, some portions of the laryngeal examination require specialized equipment found only in some otolaryngology offices that specialize in voice care. Routine head and neck evaluation should include systematic examination of the ears, nose, oral cavity, oropharynx, and neck.

Complaint of otalgia in the setting of an unremarkable ear examination suggests a possibility of referred pain from a lesion of the larynx or pharynx, and is concerning for possible malignancy. Edematous and erythematous nasal mucosa suggests rhinitis, with the possibility of postnasal drip contributing to laryngeal inflammation. Tremor of the tongue or palate might suggest neurologic disorder, whereas pharyngeal erythema and exudate suggest possible acute infection. Pachydermia (cobblestoning) of the posterior pharyngeal wall suggests the possibility of laryngopharyngeal reflux. Tenderness with manipulation of the hyoid bone suggests tension of the strap muscles and correlates closely with complaint of odynophonia and the possibility of muscle tension dysphonia. A neck mass might represent either metastatic lymphadenopathy from a laryngeal malignancy or a primary lesion which itself compresses the recurrent laryngeal nerve and causes paralytic dysphonia. Surgical scarring along the neck suggests the possibility that prior thyroid surgery, carotid endarterectomy, or anterior approach to the cervical spine might have led to vocal fold paralysis.

LARYNGEAL EXAMINATION

Beyond a general examination of the head and neck, there should be directed evaluation of the larynx and laryngeal function. The examiner should listen to the voice carefully, because vocal characteristics such as roughness, breathiness, strain, vocal breaks, and diplophonia (pitch instability, with two different pitches present simultaneously) can help guide the differential diagnosis of dysphonia. Visual examination of the larynx has many forms, ranging from mirror examination to flexible fiberoptic laryngoscopy to videostrobolaryngoscopy.

Mirror examination offers an adequate view of the vocal folds in many patients but may be limited by patient tolerance, physician inexperience, and inherent limitations of this technique to brightly illuminate the larynx or record the examination for later review. Flexible laryngoscopy is routinely available in almost all otolaryngology offices, is well tolerated by patients, and offers good views of the larynx that can be recorded with appropriate equipment. Mirror examination and flexible laryngoscopy are limited to observation of vocal fold motion and anatomy but cannot observe laryngeal function because they do not visualize vibration of the vocal folds. To examine vocal fold vibration, videostroboscopy uses a strobe light to create the impression of slow motion analysis of mucosal waves. Stroboscopy is typically available only in selected otolaryngology practices in which laryngologists specialize in the treatment of voice disorders.

CURRENT DIAGNOSIS

- The general term to describe vocal difficulty is dysphonia. Hoarseness is a specific term for rough voice quality, which is one type of dysphonia. Laryngitis signifies laryngeal inflammation, which is one possible cause of dysphonia.
- An accurate history and physical examination guide the diagnosis of voice complaints. Although many portions of the examination for dysphonia can be done in a general setting, videostroboscopy is often necessary for diagnosis and may be available only in specialized laryngology offices.
- The most common cause of acute hoarseness is viral laryngitis. Symptoms are self-limited and usually resolve within 2 weeks.
- Dysphonia persisting for longer than 2 weeks suggests the possibility of another diagnosis, such as vocal cord paralysis, neoplasm, phonotraumatic lesion, or chronic laryngitis.
- Indications for referral of a patient with voice complaints to an otolaryngologist include dysphonia that persists for longer than 2 weeks, that is of acute onset during voicing, or that is accompanied by other symptoms such as otalgia, dysphagia, or difficulty breathing.

OTHER TESTING

Videostroboscopic evaluation, combined with a thorough history and routine physical examination, can establish the diagnosis for almost all patients with voice complaints, but further testing is sometimes indicated. For instance, electromyography is used by some laryngologists for further evaluation of vocal fold paralysis or paresis. More commonly, radiographic studies are used for further evaluation of some voice complaints. Computed tomography (CT) scans are ordered most often in the evaluation of suspected laryngeal neoplasms and for patients with vocal fold paralysis.

In the case of neoplasm, CT scanning is useful to assess the extent of the primary lesion and to evaluate possible metastatic cervical lymphadenopathy. In patients with laryngeal malignancy, chest radiography is also important to assess for pulmonary metastases. For patients with vocal fold paralysis who do not have a clear history of surgical injury of the recurrent laryngeal nerve, a CT scan from skull base to thoracic inlet identifies possible lesions along the course of the recurrent laryngeal nerve. Central problems are less likely, but if they are suspected as a cause of vocal fold paralysis, then magnetic resonance imaging of the brain may be indicated as well.

Types of Dysphonia

Although not comprehensive, the conditions discussed here account for the vast majority of voice complaints. Some patients with voice complaints have more than one condition, and not every patient will fit neatly into a single category. Nevertheless, understanding how each of these conditions creates dysphonia, and knowing which particular history and physical examination findings might be associated with each cause, can help a physician to appropriately diagnose and manage voice complaints.

ACUTE LARYNGITIS

Acute laryngitis is the most common cause of hoarseness and dysphonia. It is most often viral in nature, and onset of laryngeal symptoms may be associated with other symptoms of upper respiratory tract infection, including fever, myalgia, sore throat, and rhinorrhea.

Viral inflammation of the vocal folds leads to diminished and more effortful vocal fold vibration, yielding a voice characterized by increased effort and a harsh, strained quality with decreased projection. Characteristic findings on laryngoscopy include vocal fold edema and erythema with decreased amplitude of the mucosal wave. Treatment of acute viral laryngitis is supportive, with counseling for hydration, humidification, and mucolytics. Symptoms generally are self-limited and resolve within 2 weeks. During this time, patients should be instructed to use the voice in a comfortable fashion, rather than straining or pushing to get loudness, because pushing behaviors may lead to the development of persistent muscle tension dysphonia.

Bacterial or fungal infections also cause acute laryngitis in rare cases. With appropriate physical findings and in the right clinical setting, antibiotic or antifungal therapy may be used to treat these conditions. Amoxicillin-clavulanate (Augmentin) is often the antibiotic of choice, and fluconazole (Diflucan) is a commonly used antifungal agent.

CHRONIC LARYNGITIS

Chronic laryngitis is the nonspecific condition of prolonged laryngeal inflammation; the term itself does not indicate an etiology for the inflammation. Among the many possible sources for this inflammation are mechanical irritation from traumatic coughing or prolonged speaking, chemical irritation from environmental irritants (e.g., smoking, inhaled medications), and irritation from postnasal drip or laryngopharyngeal reflux. More than one cause may exist simultaneously. Issues related to cigarette use, excessive voice use, medication effect, and rhinitis can identified with careful history taking. Laryngopharyngeal reflux is a very common source of chronic laryngitis. It may manifest with several nonspecific symptoms, such as throat irritation, globus pharyngeus, frequent throat clearing, and nonproductive cough, with or with accompanying heartburn. Because vocal fold inflammation increases with continued mechanical trauma, the hoarseness of chronic laryngitis typically gets worse with prolonged voice use and improves with voice rest. Examination findings in chronic laryngitis include generalized laryngeal edema and erythema, and careful inspection may also reveal interarytenoid hyperplasia, subglottic edema, laryngeal ventricular obliteration, and an increase in thick glottic secretions.

Treatment of chronic laryngitis is tailored to the cause of the inflammation. Vocal hygiene with moderate voice use and instructions to reduce throat clearing and coughing may diminish mechanical irritation, and smoking cessation is recommended to any smoker with laryngeal complaints. Several studies have suggested that an appropriate trial of proton pump inhibitors for treatment of laryngopharyngeal reflux includes twice-daily therapy for at least 2 months, in contrast to the once-daily dosing often used for typical heartburn complaints. Lifestyle counseling to limit consumption of caffeine, carbonation, alcohol, and acidic foods can improve reflux, and attention to hydration and humidification decreases the viscosity of glottic secretions. For patients who are troubled by vocal difficulties associated with chronic laryngitis, referral to a speech language pathologist for voice therapy can improve compliance with suggested lifestyle changes and help foster vocal improvement.

VOCAL FOLD PARALYSIS

The dysphonia in cases of vocal fold paralysis usually relates to poor vocal fold closure (Figure 2). The result is a breathy voice with limited projection and increased vocal effort. The farther from midline the immobile vocal fold, the more air leaks through the incompetent glottal valve without being turned into sound. Patients whose immobile vocal fold sits in a lateral position may have severely weak and breathy voices, whereas patients whose immobile vocal fold sits near midline may have a perceptually near-normal conversational voice and complain only of mild increase in effort, vocal fatigue, or problems with loud projection. Because of their glottal insufficiency, patients may complain of "running out of air" with prolonged speech. Impaired glottal closure may also decrease airway protection during swallowing, so patients with vocal fold paralysis need to be questioned about aspiration as well. Whereas rehabilitation of poor voice may be elective, patients with increased aspiration risk need prompt therapy.

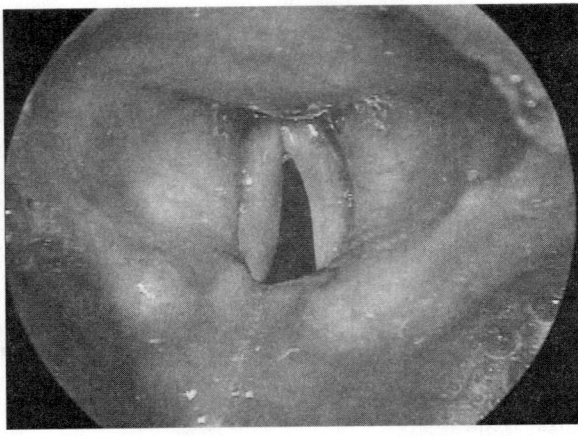

FIGURE 2. Vocal fold paralysis prevents the right vocal fold from closing to midline and creates dysphonia.

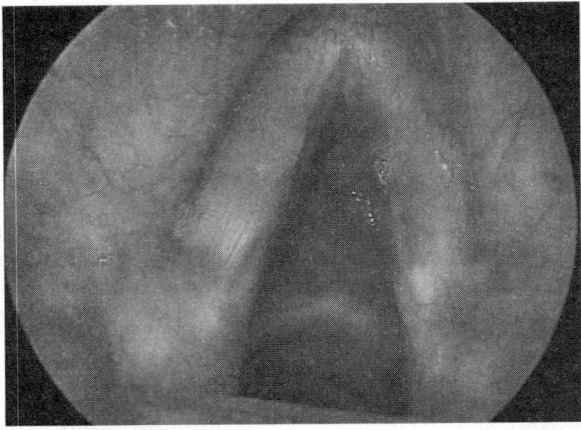

FIGURE 3. A large right hemorrhagic polyp, which can impair vocal fold vibration.

Evaluation of vocal fold paralysis includes identification of the cause of paralysis. Surgical injury to the recurrent laryngeal nerve accounts for almost half of all cases of unilateral vocal fold paralysis, and cervical or thoracic neoplasm and idiopathic paralysis account for most of the remaining cases. In a patient without a clear surgical history explaining the paralysis, CT scanning from skull base to mediastinum can identify any possible lesions along the course of the recurrent laryngeal nerve. In those patients whose histories suggest other possible causes (e.g., central neurologic injury, Lyme disease), further investigations, such as magnetic resonance imaging of the brain or blood work may be indicated as well. Some physicians perform laryngeal electromyography to help with the prognosis of paralysis or to differentiate neurologic injury from cricoarytenoid joint fixation; however, this study is neither standardized nor routine in many practices. Although flexible laryngoscopy alone may be satisfactory to document vocal fold immobility, stroboscopy can be added to investigate the impact of glottal insufficiency on vocal cord vibration and possible vocal fold flutter.

Treatment of vocal fold paralysis might include any combination of voice therapy, injection laryngoplasty, transcervical medialization laryngoplasty, and laryngeal reinnervation. Depending on the cause of the paralysis, some patients experience gradual recovery with synkinetic reinnervation or recovery of purposeful vocal fold motion over a period of several months. Based on the degree of voice and swallowing handicap, treatment of patients with vocal fold paralysis may be optional rather than necessary. Voice therapy can help teach patients to produce a stronger voice despite the paralysis, but by itself will not help a paralyzed vocal cord to recover motion. Various medialization techniques have been developed to help reposition an immobile vocal fold in the midline, where the contralateral mobile vocal fold can provide for complete glottal closure and lead to improved voice and swallowing. Injection medialization can be performed in the office or in the operating room, with temporary or permanent materials; if recovery of vocal fold motion is thought possible, then temporary injection is preferred. Transcervical medialization is a permanent but reversible surgical technique performed by otolaryngologists that repositions an immobile vocal fold in the midline. Laryngeal reinnervation offers the possibility of midline positioning of the immobile vocal fold with restored tone and bulk of the vocal fold musculature; however, because results may not mature for several months, this technique is less commonly performed than either injection or transcervical medialization.

PHONOTRAUMATIC LESIONS: NODULES, POLYPS, AND CYSTS

During vibration, vocal folds are subject to the shearing stresses of vibration. Although vocal fold structure is designed to accommodate these stresses in most circumstances, patients with vocal abuse or excessive voice use are at risk for development of lesions as the result of cumulative phonotrauma. Depending on the location and nature of these lesions, they are categorized as nodules, polyps, or cysts.

Vocal fold nodules are areas of fibrovascular scarring that are located just beneath the epithelium, at the level of basement membrane and superficial lamina propria. They are typically bilateral and symmetrical, sitting at the junction of the anterior one third and the posterior two thirds of each vocal fold. Polyps are typically unilateral lesions that may be edematous or fibrous in nature and may contain hemorrhage (Figure 3). They usually are exophytic and extend outward from the vocal fold epithelium, although the fibrous base of a polyp may extend into the superficial lamina propria of a vocal fold. In contrast to an epithelial-based lesion such as a polyp, a vocal fold cyst is a subepithelial encapsulated lesion that sits entirely within the vocal fold; its size may exert a mass effect that deforms the medial edge of the involved vocal fold. These cysts are occasionally noted as congenital lesions in children, but in adults they are more often caused by traumatic occlusion of the ducts of the seromucinous glands within the larynx.

Nodules, polyps, and cysts cause dysphonia by disturbing vocal fold vibration, leading to rough voice quality. These lesions get larger as traumatic voice use accumulates, and vocal roughness usually becomes more severe and more constant as the lesions progress. Because vibration is more easily disturbed at high pitch, performers with these lesions may notice that high pitch is affected first. Effort of phonation often increases, but projection remains intact. Lesions large enough to limit vocal fold closure may also cause a slightly breathy voice quality. Because patients with excessive voice use are at risk for these lesions, a history of social and occupational voice demands is valuable in cases of suspected phonotrauma.

Treatment for these lesions always begins with voice therapy designed to modify the patient's voice use so as to diminish trauma. Voice therapy may be all that is necessary to allow resolution of some early traumatic changes, particularly in the case of edematous nodules. If dysphonia persists despite voice therapy and other conservative measures, surgery may be considered. Surgery with the goal of voice preservation and restoration (phonosurgery) is typically performed by otolaryngologists who specialize in the care of persons with vocal difficulties. The goal of phonosurgery for these lesions is to remove the lesion that impairs vibration while preserving as much of the remaining, pliable superficial lamina propria as possible, so that vocal fold vibration can be restored.

REINKE'S EDEMA

Reinke's edema, also known as polypoid corditis, is a benign swelling of the vocal folds that is most commonly seen in patients with a long-term smoking history. The edema, a reaction to long-term irritation, accumulates within the superficial lamina propria. The edema is most often bilateral and occurs diffusely along the entire length of the vocal fold, rather than being limited to a more discrete area, as

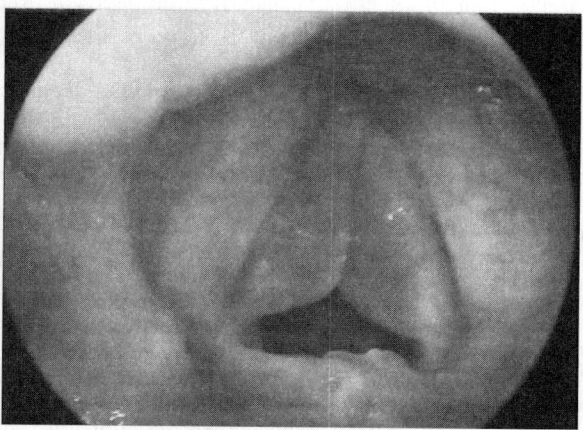

FIGURE 4. Symmetrical polypoid degeneration of the bilateral vocal folds, characteristic of Reinke's edema.

is seen with phonotraumatic polyps (Figure 4). As vocal fold mass increases with disease progression, the pitch of the voice decreases, and this is the change in voice most associated with Reinke's edema. A classic presentation of this condition is a female in her fifth or sixth decade of life who provides a long history of smoking and progressive deepening of her voice. In rare circumstances, the vocal folds gradually accumulate enough edema to compromise the airway, so breathing complaints should be evaluated as well.

Because a significant smoking history is also a risk factor for vocal fold leukoplakia and malignancy, good visualization of the vocal folds is necessary to evaluate for other lesions in these patients. If benign edema of the vocal folds is truly the only lesion noted, management depends on the degree to which voice quality is disturbing to the patient or the degree to which the airway is narrowed. Smoking cessation can lead to stabilization of pitch at its current level, and phonosurgery to remove excess vocal fold mass can help lead to normalization of pitch and improve the airway. Phonosurgery may be performed with cold instruments or with the pulsed photoangiolytic lasers, an emerging therapy; in either case, there is a risk of creating a vocal fold scar that might limit vocal fold vibration even as vocal fold contours are improved.

RECURRENT RESPIRATORY PAPILLOMATOSIS

Recurrent respiratory papillomatosis (Figure 5) is a benign laryngeal neoplasm that is caused by the human papilloma virus. It is the most common source of hoarseness in children, although adults also may

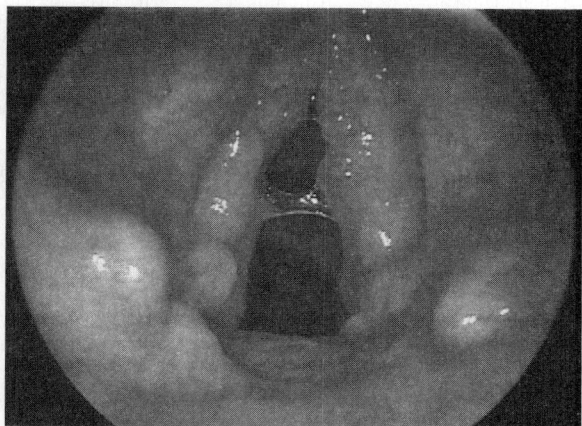

FIGURE 5. Recurrent respiratory papillomatosis, whose presence along each vocal fold medial edge disrupts sound production.

be affected. As the lesions grow on the laryngeal epithelium, they create hoarseness and sometimes effortful voice by disrupting vocal fold vibration, particularly if the lesions are located along the medial edge of either vocal fold. Large and bulky lesions may lead to airway compromise, and advanced disease may spread throughout the mucosa of the upper aerodigestive tract rather than being limited to the larynx. Although accurate diagnosis depends on histopathologic analysis, a diagnosis of benign papilloma can be suspected from the characteristic appearance of the vascular fronds, which can be seen under magnified visualization in the office or in the operating room.

Treatment of recurrent respiratory papillomatosis is surgery, which is performed with a carbon dioxide laser, microdebrider, cold instruments, or the emerging technology of pulsed potassium titanyl phosphate (KTP) laser. As its name implies, the condition is recurrent: Even though surgery may reduce or remove the papilloma temporarily, the tissue continues to harbor the papilloma virus, and the disease usually grows back. Because repeated surgeries are expected, the goal of any single procedure is to remove as much disease as possible while limiting surgical scarring of the vocal folds. Scarring created as a result of surgery is cumulative, and over time patients develop persistent dysphonia caused as much from repeated surgeries as from recurrence of the disease. An ability to treat epithelial lesions while limiting scarring at the level of the superficial lamina propria is one main advantage of pulsed laser photoangiolysis; that these pulsed laser procedures can be performed in the office as well as the operating room is another. To help limit the need for repeated surgical procedures, adjunct medical therapies such as interferon and cidofovir are sometimes used for treatment of advanced disease.

VOCAL CORD CANCER

In 2008, an estimated 12,250 new cases of laryngeal cancer and 3,670 deaths attributable to laryngeal cancer occurred in the United States. The annual incidence of laryngeal cancer is 6.4 cases per 100,000 for men and 1.3 cases per 100,000 for women. Smoking is the single largest risk factor for laryngeal cancer, and excessive alcohol use has a synergistic effect as a risk factor as well. Survival rates for laryngeal cancer depend on the stage of the tumor at the time of diagnosis, which is a function of tumor size and possible tumor spread to the cervical lymph nodes or distant metastatic sites. Cancers that occur on the medial edge of the vocal fold produce dysphonia while still small, and many laryngeal cancers are diagnosed early.

The dysphonia associated with laryngeal cancer is constant, progressive, and unremitting, without the intermittent vocal improvement that may occur in inflammatory conditions. The presence of dysphagia, odynophagia, otalgia, hemoptysis, or unexplained weight loss further increases the index of suspicion for malignancy. Cervical lymphadenopathy is associated with advanced tumors. Diagnosis may be suspected on the basis of laryngeal examination and is confirmed with biopsy. The presence or absence of mucosal waves on the involved vocal fold on videostroboscopic examination can help predict the depth of the lesion. Both a CT scan of the neck and chest radiographs are indicated to assess for tumor size and spread. Early cancers are treated with surgery or radiation therapy, with similar cure rates. Emerging technologies such as pulsed photoangiolytic lasers may allow for surgical treatment of early disease with better preservation of surrounding normal tissue. More advanced tumors are usually treated with a combination of radiation therapy and surgery or chemotherapy.

Leukoplakia, or a raised white plaque on the epithelial surface, is a visual marker for the likely presence of dysplasia or carcinoma in situ. As a very early lesion, vocal fold leukoplakia may manifest with mild dysphonia or may be found incidentally on head and neck examination performed for other reasons. This early disease may take many years before progressing to invasive carcinoma, and recognition of leukoplakia presents an opportunity for early treatment to prevent progression of disease. Pulsed laser photoangiolysis has emerged as a state-of-the-art therapy for treatment of this epithelial lesion with preservation of the underlying vocal fold pliability.

Neurologic Disorders and the Voice

Neurologic conditions that affect the voice usually do so by causing poor coordination of vocal fold motion. Spasmodic dysphonia, for instance, leads to involuntary spasms that either bring the vocal folds tightly together (adductor spasmodic dysphonia) or apart (abductor spasmodic dysphonia) during phonation. These spasms lead to vocal breaks that are strained or breathy, respectively. Although the cause of spasmodic dysphonia is thought to lie within the central nervous system, the gold standard treatment of botulinum toxin is targeted at the end organ. Injection of botulinum toxin (Botox)[1] into appropriate laryngeal muscles can weaken these muscles and diminish the spasm.

Vocal fold tremor is a neurologic disorder that is distinct from spasmodic dysphonia. Its hallmark is tremulous voice quality caused by tremor of the larynx, which may occur both during phonation and at rest. Vocal fold tremor may exist alone or as part of systemic tremor. Botulinum toxin[1] can decrease the amplitude of the tremor but may exacerbate the loss of projection that many tremor patients also have as a complaint. Medications such as anxiolytics or β-blockers that are used to treat systemic tremor may also improve the voice in patients with vocal fold tremor without worsening hypophonia.

Functional Voice Disorders

Functional dysphonia may exist by itself or in combination with an anatomic or neurologic source of dysphonia. The most common form of functional voice disorder is muscle tension dysphonia, which describes inappropriate hyperfunction of the supraglottic muscles. This hyperfunction often occurs in response to another source of hoarseness, as the patient tries to force out a strained voice with improved projection rather than accept the limited voice quality that may accompany the other disorder. The hyperfunction may then become an entrenched habit separate from the original pathology. In this sense, a classic scenario for muscle tension dysphonia is a patient who strains to speak more loudly during an acute laryngitis and whose strained, squeezed voice pattern persists even after the acute laryngitis has resolved. Patients with muscle tension dysphonia may complain of odynophonia as tension in the involved supraglottic muscles leads to muscular pain with prolonged speaking. Once other lesions have been evaluated, the treatment of muscle tension dysphonia is expert voice therapy with an emphasis on decreased hyperfunction.

Presbylaryngis

Presbylaryngis is the term that is used to describe the aging voice. It typically manifests in the seventh or eighth decade but can develop earlier. Acoustically, presbylaryngis results in a characteristic thinned voice, often with decreased projection and increased vocal strain. The condition occurs as cumulative voice use leads to traumatic thinning of the superficial lamina propria, particularly at the mid-cord level. This loss of superficial lamina propria leads to deficiency at the medial edge of each vocal fold, and a spindle-shaped defect in glottal closure may be noticed with close evaluation. Many patients with a complaint of presbylaryngis find that appropriate voice therapy to address breath support and vocal projection leads to satisfactory improvement in the voice without altering the vocal fold anatomy. For those patients who remain unsatisfied with their voice after therapy, vocal fold medialization procedures can restore straight vocal cord edges and may lead to improved projection; however, currently available injectables and implants that address contour defects cannot restore pliability.

CURRENT THERAPY

- Appropriate treatment of voice complaints depends on accurate diagnosis.
- Supportive therapy is all that is necessary for most cases of acute laryngitis associated with viral upper respiratory tract infections.
- Laryngopharyngeal reflux is a common cause of chronic laryngitis, and appropriate therapy often requires twice-daily administration of proton pump inhibitors for at least 2 months.
- Microlaryngeal phonosurgery may be indicated for some patients with benign phonotraumatic lesions.
- Vocal cord medialization can rehabilitate the voice in a patient with unilateral vocal cord paralysis.
- Many patients with dysphonia benefit from voice therapy, alone or in combination with other treatment strategies.

Conclusion

Understanding the anatomy and physiology of normal voice production provides a framework through which dysphonia can be evaluated. Application of this knowledge during the history and physical examination guides the diagnosis of hoarseness and allows clinicians to distinguish among conditions as varied as acute laryngitis, benign phonotraumatic lesions, vocal fold paralysis, and laryngeal cancer as part of a differential diagnosis. Videostrobolaryngoscopy allows evaluation of vocal fold function as well as structure and can confirm diagnosis. As with any condition, accurate diagnosis directs appropriate therapy. Because no further evaluation or management is necessary for acute viral laryngitis, many patients with hoarseness require no more than a careful history and physical examination. However, if dysphonia persists for longer than 2 weeks or is accompanied by other laryngopharyngeal symptoms that are not thought to be related to an upper respiratory tract infection, referral should be made to an otolaryngologist for further evaluation.

REFERENCES

Koufman JA, Aviv JE, Casiano RR, et al. Laryngopharyngeal reflux: Position statement of the committee on speech, voice, and swallowing disorders of the American Academy of Otolaryngology-Head and Neck Surgery. Otolaryngol Head Neck Surg 2002;127:32–5.

Merati AL, Heman-Ackah YD, Abaza M, et al. Common movement disorders affecting the larynx: A report from the neurolaryngology committee of the AAO-HNS. Otolaryngol Head Neck Surg 2005;133:654–65.

Swibel Rosenthal LH, Benninger MS, Deeb RH. Vocal fold immobility: A longitudinal analysis of etiology over 20 years. Laryngoscope 2007;117:1864–70.

Wilson JA, Deary IJ, Millar A, et al. The quality of life impact of dysphonia. Clin Otolaryngol 2002;27:179–82.

Zeitels SM, Casiano RR, Gardner GM, et al. Management of common voice problems: Committee report. Otolaryngol Head Neck Surg 2002;126:333–48.

Zeitels SM, Healy GB. Laryngology and phonosurgery. N Engl J Med 2003;349:882–92.

---

[1]Not FDA approved for this indication.

Pharyngitis

Method of
Ruth Weber, MD, MSEd

Epidemiology

Pharyngitis is common and has substantial medical and societal costs. "Sore throat" accounts for over 7 million outpatient visits by children annually. The estimated total cost of pharyngitis in children is $540 million dollars per year.

An estimated 30% of childhood pharyngitis is caused by group A β-hemolytic streptococcus (GABHS). In temperate climates, pharyngitis occurs in outbreaks during winter and early spring, predominantly involving children age 5 to 15 years of age. GABHS is uncommon in preschool-aged children and in adults. Group C β-hemolytic streptococcus pharyngitis occurs mainly in college students and young adults.

Of other causes of pharyngitis (Table 1), gonococcal pharyngitis is most common in older adolescents and young adults. Transmission is by oral-genital contact. If gonococcal pharyngitis is diagnosed in a prepubertal child, sexual abuse must be considered.

Risk Factors

The major risk factors for GABHS pharyngitis are age and exposure such as in crowded schools or through household contacts. Oral sexual activity is implicated in gonococcal pharyngitis. Swimming pools have been implicated in transmission of Group C and D β streptococcal pharyngitis.

Pathophysiology

Pathogenic strains of *Streptococcus pyogenes* can be differentiated by Lancefield antigens and by hemolysis on blood agar. The strain containing group A antigen and displaying β hemolysis causes pharyngitis (GABHS). The M protein is responsible for virulence. The M protein cross-reacts with cardiac myosin and laminin, potentially causing rheumatic heart disease. More than 100 M-protein serotypes have been identified. Some streptococcus strains produce erythrogenic toxins,

TABLE 1 Pharyngitis: Distribution of Causative Organisms (All Age Groups)

Pathogen	Percentage of Population
Group A β-hemolytic streptococcus	15-30
Rhinovirus	20
Adenovirus	2-5
Coronavirus	2-5
Coxsackievirus	2-5
Group C β-hemolytic streptococcus	2-5
Herpes simplex virus	2-5
Influenza virus	2-5
Chlamydia trachomatis	<1
Corynebacterium diphtheriae	<1
Epstein-Barr virus	<1
Human immunodeficiency virus	<1
Arcanobacterium haemolyticum	<1
Mycoplasma spp.	<1
Neisseria gonorrhoeae	<1

causing the rash of scarlet fever. Patients develop lifelong immunity to one serotype after infection, but reinfection with a different serotype is possible.

Prevention

GABHS is transmitted by droplet spread. No evidence supports other forms of transmission. Patients and household/close contacts should be educated on minimizing droplet spread to reduce the transmission of GABHS.

Phase I trials have been completed on a multivalent vaccine targeting streptococcus M proteins that cause pharyngitis, invasive disease, and rheumatic fever.

Clinical Manifestations

The type of pharyngitis cannot be identified by history and clinical findings. Microbiologic confirmation is necessary to diagnose GABHS pharyngitis.

GROUP A STREPTOCOCCAL PHARYNGITIS

In patients age 3 years to adult, sudden onset of sore throat, pain on swallowing, and fever (101-104°F) suggest GABHS pharyngitis. Nausea and vomiting can also occur in school-aged children. Clinical signs can include tonsillar erythema with or without exudate, anterior cervical lymphadenitis, soft palate petechiae, red swollen uvula, and scarletiniform rash. Infants rarely present with exudative pharyngitis but have coryza with excoriation and crusting of the nares. Posttonsillectomy patients with GABHS can have milder symptoms and clinical signs.

Patients with suppurative complications of GABHS have unusually severe symptoms, with neck swelling, drooling, and "hot potato" voice. The clinician must look for peritonsillar abscess and infections in the parapharyngeal and submandibular spaces (Ludwig's angina).

SCARLET FEVER

Some strains of GABHS produce a pyogenic exotoxin that causes scarlet fever in susceptible patients. The clinical signs and symptoms are identical to GABHS pharyngitis plus development of the characteristic rash within 24 to 48 hours of symptom onset. The fine, papular, bright red rash blanches with pressure, begins on the neck, and spreads to the extremities and trunk. It is more pronounced in creases, and feels rough, with a goose-pimple appearance. The punctate rash spares the face but patients have flushed cheeks and forehead, with pallor around the mouth. The rash fades in 3 to 4 days and is followed by desquamation. After desquamation of an initial white coating, the tongue has a classical strawberry appearance caused by edematous papillae.

POST-STREPTOCOCCAL GLOMERULONEPHRITIS

Renal symptoms of hypertension, edema, and hematuria can occur 1-3 weeks after GABHS pharyngitis. Glomerulonephritis is an autoimmune response to M proteins. It is not preventable by antibiotics.

VIRAL PHARYNGITIS

Coryza, hoarseness, cough, diarrhea, viral exanthem, anterior stomatitis, and conjunctivitis can indicate a viral etiology for pharyngitis. Adenovirus infections can cause fever for 7 days, and conjunctivitis can persist for 14 days. Adenoviral outbreaks are often associated with swimming pools.

Enterovirus pharyngitis (Coxsackievirus, echovirus, enterovirus) occurs in summer and fall. Fever, cervical adenopathy, and erythema of the tonsils are common, but exudates are rare. Herpangina (Coxsackie virus A/B) manifests with fever and painful papulovesicular lesions in the posterior oropharynx that resolve in 7 days. Hand, foot, and mouth disease (Coxsackie virus A-16) manifests with painful vesicles and ulcers in the mouth plus painful vesicles on the palms, soles, and occasionally trunk. Lesions resolve in 7 days.

Primary oral herpes simplex infection occurs in young children. It manifests as acute gingivostomatitis, with ulcerating vesicles on the anterior mouth and lips but not on the posterior pharynx. High fever with intense pain is common, and dehydration can occur. Symptoms last for 14 days.

Diagnosis

The necessity of obtaining microbiologic confirmation of infection before treating for presumed GABHS pharyngitis remains controversial. If the clinical symptoms suggest GABHS pharyngitis, throat culture or rapid antigen detection test (RADT) are indicated. If the clinical symptoms suggest viral pharyngitis, the pretest probability of GABHS infection is low, and a diagnostic test should not be performed.

Several methods for determining the probability of GABHS infection have been proposed. The Centor Criteria (for adults) are widely accepted. A score of 1 is given for each of the following characteristics: tonsillar exudate, tender anterior cervical adenopathy, history of fever, absence of cough. A score of 3 or more indicates a positive predictive value for GABHS of 40% to 60%. A score of 0 to 1 indicates a positive predictive value for GABHS of 1% to 5%

Throat culture is the gold standard for diagnosing GABHS infection. The tonsils and the posterior pharynx should be aggressively swabbed. Other areas of the mouth should not be touched when obtaining the culture. Culture should be obtained before beginning antibiotic therapy, because even a single dose of antibiotics can cause the culture to be negative. The swab is plated on a sheep's blood agar plate and incubated. The plate must be read at both 24 and 48 hours of incubation. When done correctly, throat culture has 90% to 95% sensitivity. Although throat culture is considered the gold standard for diagnosing GABHS infection, it does not differentiate a carrier state from clinical infection.

RADT has high specificity but low sensitivity. The many tests available have different performance characteristics. In children, a throat culture should be performed if the RADT test is negative in order to identify patients who have a false negative RADT result. In adults, throat culture is not necessary after a negative RADT because of the low incidence of GABHS and extremely low risk of acute rheumatic fever. The use of RADT has allowed clinicians to begin antibiotic therapy early in those with a positive test. This decreases the risk of spread of GABHS, allows earlier return to school or work, and modestly improves clinical signs and symptoms.

Streptococcal antibody testing has no value in the acute diagnosis of GABHS pharyngitis. Testing has some value in confirming prior GABHS infection in patients in whom acute rheumatic fever or acute post-streptococcal glomerulonephritis is suspected. The two antibodies that can be identified are antistreptolysin O (ASO) and anti-deoxyribonuclease B (ARB). Positive, elevated, or increasing titers are confirmation of recent GABHS infection. ASO titers rise within a week of infection and peak 3 to 6 weeks after infection. ARB titers rise within 1 to 2 weeks of infection and peak at 6 to 8 weeks. Titers are higher in school-aged children than in adults.

CURRENT DIAGNOSIS

- Patients prioritize symptom relief over microbiological cure.
- Most pharyngitis is viral; microbiological confirmation is required for group A β-hemolytic streptococcus pharyngitis.
- In adults, throat culture is not necessary if rapid antigen detection test is negative.
- Stop presumptive antibiotic therapy if throat culture results are negative for group A β-hemolytic streptococcus.

Differential Diagnosis

INFECTIOUS MONONUCLEOSIS

Classically a triad of severe sore throat, lymphadenopathy, and fever (up to 104°F) in 15- to 25-year-olds, mononucleosis begins with a prodrome of chills, sweats, fever, and malaise. Clinical signs include enlarged tonsils; posterior and anterior cervical, axilliary and inguinal adenopathy; and hepatosplenomegally. Approximately 15% of patients present with jaundice and 5% with rash. Patients with mononucleosis who are treated with amoxicillin (Amoxil)[1] often develop a pruritic maculopapular rash. Complete blood count (CBC) shows an absolute lymphocytosis with greater than 10% atypical lymphocytes. Within 2 to 3 weeks the heterophile antibody test (Mono Spot) becomes positive. The antibody test has a higher false-negative rate in children than adults. If a false-negative test is suspected, an IgM antibody to viral capsid antigen is indicated to confirm the diagnosis.

ACUTE RETROVIRAL SYNDROME

Primary infection with HIV can manifest as a syndrome of fever, nonexudative pharyngitis, arthralgia, myalgia, and lymphadenopathy. Some 40% to 80% of patients develop a rash. HIV antibodies are negative. Assay for HIV type 1 RNA or p24 antigen is positive.

NEISSERIA GONORRHEA

N. gonorrhea pharyngitis is usually asymptomatic and associated with oral sexual practices. The diagnosis is confirmed by isolating the organism on Thayer-Martin medium. All patients should be screened and treated for co-infection with *Chlamydia*.

LEMIERRE'S SYNDROME

Lemierre's syndrome is a rare etiology of severe pharyngitis is caused by *Fusobacterium necrophorum*. Infection spreads from the pharynx to include the surrounding tissues, with subsequent thrombophlebitis of the internal jugular vein.

Treatment

A major therapeutic decision is to determine if the patient needs an antibiotic in addition to symptomatic treatment.

The goal of treatment of viral pharyngitis is control of symptoms, especially relief of pain. Acetaminophen (Tylenol) alone is as effective as formulations of acetaminophen plus a decongestant or antihistamine. No evidence supports Chinese herbs for symptom relief. Oral steroids can relieve pain but the risks of use outweigh the benefit. Many patients mistakenly believe that antibiotic therapy relieves pain. Ancillary treatment options include rest, adequate fluid intake, and antipyretic medications.

The goals of antibiotic treatment of GABHS pharyngitis are to decrease infectivity and prevent supperative and other complications, especially acute rheumatic fever. Symptoms generally improve within 3 to 4 days without treatment. Delay of treatment of GABHS pharyngitis for up to 9 days after symptoms begin does not appear to increase the risk of acute rheumatic fever and a delay of 24 to 48 hours while awaiting culture results does not increase the risk of acute rheumatic fever. Early treatment of GABHS pharyngitis does reduce infectivity, lessens morbidity, and promotes early return to normal activities. Nevertheless, criteria for initiating antibiotics remain controversial.

The choice of antibiotic is determined by the bacteriology of GABHS, clinical efficacy, patient adherence to treatment regimen, adverse effects, and cost. If antibiotics are initiated while awaiting throat culture result, the antibiotic must be discontinued if the culture is negative.

Penicillin remains the antibiotic of choice for GABHS pharyngitis. GABHS has never shown resistance to penicillin or cephalosporins. Amoxicillin can replace penicillin for treatment. (Liquid amoxicillin has a better taste than liquid penicillin.) In the penicillin-allergic patient, a first-generation cephalosporin or macrolide may be substituted. In some areas of the United States up to 5% of GABHS is resistant to macrolides and less than 1% is resistant to clindamycin (Cleocin). Antibiotics should be given for 10 days to eradicate GABHS from the pharynx. At this time, short-course (≤5 days) treatment cannot be recommended, except with azithromycin (Zithromax).

No clear evidence supports antibiotic treatment for group C or group G streptococcal pharyngitis. Treatment might shorten the course of infection. Treatment options are identical to those for GABHS pharyngitis.

TREATMENT REGIMENS

- Oral penicillin: PenicillinVK (Veetids): 40 mg/kg/day (up to adult dose of 1000 mg /day) in divided doses two or three times daily for 10 days.
- Amoxicillin: 50 mg/kg/day (up to adult dose of 1000 mg/day) twice daily for 10 days; FDA has approved Moxatag for patients older than 12 years at 775 mg once a day.
- Penicillin G benzathine (Bicillin-LA): Patients weighing less than 27 kg, 600,000 units IM; patients weighing 27 kg or more, 1.2 million units IM once. Penicillin G is used for patients who are unlikely to complete a full 10-day course of oral medication and for those with a personal or family history of rheumatic fever.
- First-generation oral cephalosporin: Cephalexin (Keflex) 25 to 50 mg/kg/day (up to adult dose of 1000 mg/day) twice daily for 10 days. This regimen should be used if the patient is allergic to penicillin; shorter courses are not FDA approved.
- Macrolides should be used if the patient is allergic to penicillin: Erythromycin 20 to 40 mg/kg/day (up to adult dose of 1000 mg/kg/day) in three or four doses for 10 days. Azithromycin (patients older than 6 months): Day 1: 10mg/kg once (up to adult dose of 500 mg); days 2 to 5: 5 mg/kg once daily (up to adult dose of 250 mg/day). The dose of azithromycin is not established in infants younger than 6 months.

Tetracycline, sulfonamides and older fluroquinalones are not recommended because of high rates of resistance. All patients should be considered infectious until they have completed 24 hours of antibiotic therapy.

Monitoring

In general, follow-up throat cultures or RADT for patients successfully treated for GABHS pharyngitis (i.e., test for cure) are not necessary. An additional throat culture is required if symptoms do not abate, symptoms recur, or the patient had previous rheumatic fever.

Patients who have repeated symptomatic episodes of GABHS have either recurrent new infections or are carriers of GABHS, with repeated superimposed viral infections.

GABHS carriers have positive cultures for GABHS without clinical symptoms. Approximately 20% of school-aged children are carriers. GABHS carrier status is suspected if the clinical picture is of viral pharyngitis but the patient has positive RADT or cultures both when symptomatic and when asymptomatic. Carriers do not respond to antibiotics and have no serologic response to ASO and anti-DNA B. These patients do not need to be identified or treated. These patients do not develop rheumatic fever and are not important in the spread of GABHS to others.

Patients with repeated GABHS pharyngitis have a clinical picture of recurrent bacterial pharyngitis. They respond to antibiotics and have negative RADT and culture when they are asymptomatic. They have a serologic response to ASO and anti-DNA B. Prophylactic antibiotics are not recommended for these patients. Tonsillectomy may be considered when infection attack rates do not decrease over time and no other explanation of recurrent infection can be found. Meta-analyses have found inconclusive evidence of benefit from tonsillectomy compared to nonsurgical treatment.

CURRENT THERAPY

- Penicillin is the drug of choice for group A β-hemolytic streptococcus pharyngitis. A macrolide is indicated if the patient is allergic to penicillin.
- Treatment is necessary for 10 days to eradicate group A β-hemolytic streptococcus from the pharynx.
- Amoxicillin can be substituted for penicillin. Patients older than 12 years may be treated with once-daily amoxicillin (Moxatag).
- Patients are not infectious after 24 hours of appropriate antibiotic treatment.

Patients with GABHS pharyngitis who remain symptomatic and continue to have positive cultures should receive a second course of antibiotics, with either the same antimicrobial agent or intramuscular penicillin. If a patient experiences repeated infections and there is concern that the GABHS infection is being spread among close contacts, all close and family contacts should be cultured and only those who are positive should be treated. Family pets are not reservoirs and do not spread disease.

Mass screening for GABHS should be considered in outbreaks of GABHS in a closed or semiclosed community or in outbreaks of acute rheumatic fever or post-streptococcal glomerulonephritis.

Non-GABHS pharyngitis (i.e., group C or G β-hemolytic streptococcus) is not associated with rheumatic fever and no evidence supports treatment or follow-up culture.

Complications

The complications of GABHS pharyngitis can be classified as suppurative and nonsuppurative.

Suppurative complications occur when the infection spreads to cause conditions such as lateral pharyngeal abscess, cervical lymphadenitis, sinusitis, otitis media, retropharyngeal abscess, Lemierre's syndrome, and mastoiditis. Appropriate treatment of GABHS with antibiotics decreases these complications.

Nonsuppurative complications include acute rheumatic fever, acute post-streptococcal glomerulonephritis, and post-streptococcal reactive arthritis. Acute rheumatic fever occurs 2 to 3 weeks after GABHS pharyngitis. It is not seen after GABHS skin infections. Starting antibiotics within 9 days of symptoms can prevent acute rheumatic fever. Acute post-streptococcal glomerulonephritis can occur 10 days after pharyngeal infection and 21 days after skin infection. Antibiotics do not alter the attack rate. Post-streptococcal reactive arthritis is similar to other reactive arthritis, and the attack rate is not altered by antibiotics.

Potential complications from treatment of GABHS pharyngitis include anaphylactic reaction to antibiotics and antibiotic resistance.

REFERENCES

Choby BA. Diagnosis and treatment of streptococcal pharyngitis. Am Fam Physician 2009;79(5):383–90.

Gerber MA. Diagnosis and treatment of pharyngitis in children. Pediatr Clin North Am 2005;52:729–47.

Gerber MA, Baltimore RS, Eaton CB, et al. Prevention of rheumatic fever and diagnosis and treatment of acute streptococcal pharyngitis: A scientific statement from the American Heart Association Rheumatic Fever, Endocarditis, and Kawasaki Disease Committee of the Council on Cardiovascular Disease in the Young, the Interdisciplinary Council on Functional Genomics and Translational Biology, and the Interdisciplinary Council on Quality of Care and Outcomes Research: Endorsed by the American Academy of Pediatrics. Circulation 2009;119(11):1541–51.

Halsey ES. Pharyngitis, bacterial. Available at:http://emedicine.medscape.com/article/225243-overview; [accessed 10.06.10].

The Respiratory System

Acute Respiratory Failure

Method of
Scott K. Epstein, MD

The respiratory system serves many complex physiologic functions, the most important of which is gas exchange. Using the interface between the alveolar space and capillaries, O_2 is taken up and CO_2 is eliminated. Acute respiratory failure, a life-threatening entity, is present when this system fails, over the course of minutes to hours, resulting in hypoxemia (type I) or hypercapnia (type II), or both. Most patients with acute respiratory failure present with dyspnea, although the correlation with disease severity is poor. Indeed, dyspnea might seem mild in those with baseline chronic respiratory failure, and it might be absent in those with an underlying neurologic process (e.g., drug overdose). Other symptoms and signs such as cough, chest pain, orthopnea, fever, tachypnea, rales, and wheezing are insensitive and nonspecific.

This chapter outlines the general pathophysiology and therapeutic approach to acute respiratory failure by using the examples of three common entities: acute lung injury (ALI), cardiogenic pulmonary edema (congestive heart failure [CHF]), and acute exacerbation of chronic obstructive pulmonary disease (COPD).

Definitions and Pathophysiology

ACUTE HYPOXIC RESPIRATORY FAILURE

Hypoxic respiratory failure is conventionally defined as an arterial oxygen tension (Pao_2) of less than 60 mm Hg. Because this definition ignores the inspired fraction of oxygen (Fio_2), some favor a Pao_2/Fio_2 ratio of less than 300. To account for the arterial CO_2 tension ($Paco_2$), others favor an alveolar–arterial (A–a) O_2 gradient greater than 250 mm Hg, using the equation

$$A - a \; O_2 \text{ gradient} = PAo_2 - Pao_2$$
$$= (713 \times Fio_2) - (PAo_2 + Paco_2/0.8)$$

where 713 is the barometric pressure (760) minus the water vapor pressure. A normal A–a O_2 is less than 10 mm Hg, but this threshold value increases with age. The determination of Pao_2 requires an invasive test, an arterial blood gas. Oxygenation can be continuously monitored noninvasively by pulse oximetry, which provides an estimate of arterial oxygen saturation (Sao_2). In general, an Sao_2 of 0.90 corresponds to a Pao_2 of 60 mm Hg, but the relation depends on temperature, pH, $Paco_2$, and 2,3-diphosphoglycerate (2,3-DPG).

Accuracy is adversely affected by low perfusion states, dark skin pigmentation, nail polish, dyshemoglobins (e.g., carboxyhemoglobin, methemoglobin), intravascular dyes, motion, and ambient light.

Clinicians tend to focus on Pao_2 and Sao_2, but the real parameter of interest is O_2 delivery (Do_2) to organs and tissues. Do_2 depends on cardiac output and O_2 carrying capacity of arterialized blood (Cao_2):

$$Do_2 = CO \times Cao_2$$

where

$$Cao_2 = k(Hb \times Sao_2) + 0.003 \, Pao_2$$

where k is a constant. Do_2 decreases when cardiac output or hemoglobin is reduced despite a normal Pao_2 and Sao_2. The peripheral response to reduced Do_2 is an increased O_2 extraction ratio (O_2ER), allowing oxygen uptake ($\dot{V}o_2$), an indicator of metabolic demand, to remain constant. Cellular and organ dysfunction occurs when Do_2 and O_2ER are outstripped by metabolic demand. The balance between Do_2 and demand can be estimated by examining the mixed venous O_2 saturation ($\overline{Mvo_2}$) using the rearranged Fick equation:

$$Mvo_2 = Sao_2 - (\dot{V}o_2/CO \times Hb)$$

When Mvo_2 falls below 65% to 75%, imbalance is present.

When cellular injury is present, extraction capabilities are limited and cellular hypoxia occurs despite "adequate" Do_2. Under these circumstances, the Mvo_2 can be paradoxically normal. These parameters can be determined using a pulmonary artery catheter. The data obtained may be useful in individual patients, but randomized, controlled trials show no benefit when the pulmonary artery catheter is used routinely to guide therapy.

The pathophysiologic mechanisms of type I respiratory failure are listed in Table 1. The most common mechanism is ventilation–perfusion ($\dot{V}/\dot{Q}$) mismatch, characterized by a widened A–a O_2 gradient, a dramatic increase in Pao_2 in response to supplemental O_2, and a variable $Paco_2$. When areas of low $\dot{V}/\dot{Q}$ predominate (e.g., reduced ventilation with normal perfusion), the $Paco_2$ may be low as the patient hyperventilates in an effort (only partially effective) to increase the Pao_2. When areas of high $\dot{V}/\dot{Q}$ predominate, much ventilation is wasted, and hypercapnia is also present. Areas of lung that are perfused but not ventilated characterize shunt. The resulting fall in Pao_2 depends on the percentage of cardiac output circulating through the shunt and the O_2 content of that blood. Supplemental O_2 has minimal or small effect on Pao_2 because the shunted blood is not exposed to the increased Fio_2. Therefore, treatment is aimed at decreasing shunt by improving ventilation to the affected area or reducing perfusion to that area. When shunt results from a unilateral process (e.g., pneumonia, atelectasis), placing the good lung down decreases shunt perfusion, and oxygenation improves.

TABLE 1 Pathophysiologic Mechanisms of Acute Hypoxic Respiratory Failure

Mechanism	A–ao$_2$ Gradient	Paco$_2$	Response to 100% O$_2$	Cause
Diffusion abnormality	↑	↑ normal	↑↑	Severe interstitial lung disease
Hypoventilation	Normal	↑	↑↑↑	Narcotic overdose, obesity hypoventilation syndrome, respiratory muscle weakness
↓ Fio$_2$	Normal	Usually ↓	↑↑↑	High altitude, smoke inhalation
↓ Mvo$_2$	↑	Usually ↓	↑	ALI, shock, CHF, PE
Shunt	↑	Usually ↓	None or ↑	ALI, CHF, atelectasis, PE
V̇/Q̇ mismatch	↑	↑, normal, ↓	↑↑↑	Acute exacerbation of COPD, asthma, PE

↑ = increased; ↓ = decreased; A–ao$_2$ = alveolar–arterial O$_2$; ALI = acute lung injury; CHF = cardiogenic pulmonary edema; COPD = chronic obstructive pulmonary disease; Fio$_2$ = fraction of inspired oxygen; Mvo$_2$ = mixed venous oxygen saturation; Paco$_2$ = partial pressure of arterial CO$_2$; PE = pulmonary embolism: V̇/Q̇ = ventilation–perfusion ratio.

ACUTE HYPERCAPNEIC RESPIRATORY FAILURE

Hypercapneic respiratory failure is defined as a Paco$_2$ greater than 45 mm Hg. The equation used to determine Paco$_2$ provides insight into the three basic mechanisms underlying hypercapnia:

$$Paco_2 = k(\dot{V}Co_2)/V_E(1 - V_D/V_T)$$

where k is a constant, V_E is total minute ventilation (respiratory rate times tidal volume) and V_D/V_T is the dead space. Therefore, hypercapnia can result from increased CO$_2$ production ($\dot{V}Co_2$), increased physiologic dead space (V_D/V_T), and decreased minute ventilation (Box 1). Increased $\dot{V}Co_2$ alone is usually insufficient to cause hypercapnia because the respiratory system responds by increasing minute ventilation to keep Paco$_2$ normal (37–43 mm Hg). Conversely, with abnormalities of respiratory muscle function or respiratory drive or with increased dead space (and diminished reserve), the respiratory response to increased $\dot{V}Co_2$ may be insufficient, and hypercapnia results.

Treatment

Treatment of acute hypoxemic and hypercapneic respiratory failure combines nonspecific (e.g., supplemental O$_2$, mechanical ventilation) and specific therapy (Boxes 2 and 3).

OXYGEN THERAPY

In the hospital, 100% O$_2$ is supplied from a wall source with a regulator determining flow rate in liters per minute. The final delivered oxygen concentration (Fio$_2$) depends on this flow rate and the amount of room air breathed by the patient. The O$_2$ flow rate is almost never sufficient to meet all of the patient's ventilatory demands, so varying amounts of room air are entrained to meet these needs. The final inspired oxygen concentration depends on

---

BOX 1 Pathophysiologic Mechanisms of Hypercapnia

Increased Carbon Dioxide Production ($\dot{V}Co_2$)
Fever
Overfeeding
Seizure
Sepsis
Thyrotoxicosis

Decreased Ventilation (V_E)
Depressed respiratory drive
Phrenic nerve injury
Respiratory muscle weakness

Increased Dead Space (V_D/V_T)
Acute exacerbation of chronic obstructive pulmonary disease
Interstitial lung disease
Pulmonary vascular disease

BOX 2 Causes of and Treatments for Acute Hypoxemic Respiratory Failure

Acute Exacerbation of Chronic Obstructive Pulmonary Disease
Antibiotics
Bronchodilators
Systemic steroids

Acute Lung Injury or Acute Respiratory Distress Syndomre
Efforts to decrease lung water
Lung-protective mechanical ventilation

Congestive Heart Failure
Afterload reduction
Diuretics
Inotropes

Lobar Collapse or Atelectasis
Bronchoscopy
Pulmonary toilet (airway suctioning to improve clearance of secretions)

Pneumonia
Antibiotics
Chest physiotherapy

Pneumothorax
Tube thoracostomy to drain pleural air and facilitate lung re-expansion

Pulmonary Embolism
Anticoagulation
Thrombolytic therapy

Status Asthmaticus
Bronchodilators
Systemic steroids

BOX 3 Causes of and Treatments for Acute Hypercapneic Respiratory Failure

Acute Exacerbation of Chronic Obstructive Pulmonary Disease
Antibiotics
Bronchodilators
Systemic steroids

Acute Respiratory Muscle Weakness (e.g., myasthenic crisis)
Acetylcholinesterase therapy

Drug Overdose
Flumazenil (Romazicon)
Naloxone (Narcan)
Other antidotes

Guillain-Barré Syndrome
Immunoglobulin
Plasmapheresis

Spinal Cord Injury
Intravenous methylprednisolone

Status Asthmaticus
Bronchodilators
Systemic steroids

Toxin (e.g., botulinum toxin)
Antitoxin

binding of CO_2, and minute ventilation inadequate for the amount of CO_2 produced. Therefore, the goal in these patients is to achieve a Pao_2 of 55 to 60 mm Hg (Sao_2 88%–90%) with low-flow oxygen (~24%–28% O_2). If this (often delicate) balance between maintaining tissue oxygenation and avoiding significant respiratory acidosis cannot be achieved, short-term mechanical ventilation may be required. In most nonhypercapneic patients, high flow of oxygen (50%–100%) can be administered safely for 24 hours with a goal Pao_2 of between 65 and 80 mm Hg.

MECHANICAL VENTILATION

Mechanical ventilation can be delivered noninvasively through a tight-fitting face mask or invasively via an endotracheal tube. The goals of mechanical ventilation are to correct severe arterial blood gas abnormalities, provide respiratory support while specific therapy is used, and unload and rest the respiratory muscles. The ventilator should be set to optimize patient–ventilator interaction and avoid dynamic hyperinflation and intrinsic positive end-expiratory pressure (PEEPi). PEEPi can worsen gas exchange, predispose to barotrauma, and cause hypotension.

Noninvasive Ventilation

Noninvasive ventilation is most commonly applied as continuous positive airway pressure (CPAP), when airway pressure is kept constant throughout the respiratory cycle, or by bilevel positive airway pressure (BiPAP), when inspiratory pressure support actively assists each inspiration. Noninvasive ventilation offers numerous advantages over invasive ventilation, including increased comfort; maintenance of normal swallowing, speech, and cough; less need for sedation; and avoiding the trauma of intubation.

The effective application of noninvasive ventilation starts with carefully explaining the procedure to the patient, followed by selection of a proper-fitting face mask. The mask is placed close to the face to acclimate the patient to high inspiratory flow. The mask is then secured using straps (but not too tightly), and ventilator settings are adjusted to minimize leak and ensure comfort. The patient is reassessed frequently. Failure to improve within 2 to 4 hours (e.g., reduction in dyspnea, respiratory rate, accessory muscle use, and hypercapnia) signals noninvasive ventilation failure and need for intubation.

Noninvasive ventilation improves outcome (avoids intubation, decreases length of stay, improves survival) in a number of conditions (Table 3). Although randomized, controlled trials show dramatic benefit in AECOPD, other studies show no or uncertain benefit in

the relative fraction of each gas, total minute ventilation, and the pattern of breathing (including the inspiratory to expiratory ratio). O_2 may be administered using nasal prongs, a facial mask, or high-flow devices designed to deliver higher Fio_2 (Table 2).

In hypercapneic patients (e.g., with acute exacerbation of COPD), high-flow O_2 can lead to worsening hypercapnia and acute respiratory acidosis. The mechanisms are multifactorial: worsening $\dot{V}/\dot{Q}$ matching (increased dead space), decreased intracellular

TABLE 2 Short-Term Oxygen Delivery Systems

Delivery System	O₂ Flow Rate (L/min)	Fio₂ Range	Comments
Basic Systems			
Nasal cannula (prongs)	1–6	0.22–0.40	Comfortable Facilitates communication and oral intake Humidification required at high flow rates
Simple masks	5–6	0.30–0.50	Mask acts as reservoir to increase Fio₂ High flow combats CO₂ rebreathing Less comfortable Must be removed to facilitate communication and oral intake Easily displaced with movement
Reservoir Masks			
Nonrebreathing	4–10	0.60–1.00	One-way valve between the mask and the reservoir bag Inspired O₂ from wall source and reservoir bag
Partial rebreathing	5–10	0.35–0.90	Lacks one-way valve
Venturi masks	4–10	0.24–0.40	Uses Bernoulli principle (fixed amount of entrained room air added to O₂) Maximum delivered Fio₂ can be controlled Often used in COPD to avoid excessive Fio₂ and risk for hypercapnia

COPD = chronic obstructive pulmonary disease; Fio₂ = fraction of inspired oxygen.

TABLE 3 Efficacy of Noninvasive Ventilation in Various Conditions

Condition	Quality of Evidence	Comment
AECOPD	Strong	↓ Need for intubation ↑ Survival
Acute cardiogenic pulmonary edema	Strong	↓ Need for intubation ↑ Survival
Hypoxemic respiratory in ICH with diffuse pulmonary infiltrates	Strong	↓ Need for intubation ↑ Survival
Facilitating weaning in select patients	Strong	↓ Duration of intubation Most effective in AECOPD
High risk for extubation failure	Strong	↓ Need for reintubation
Extubation failure in heterogeneous patient population	Moderate	Not effective, two RCTs
Routinely after extubation	Moderate	Not effective, single RCT
Extubation failure in acute exacerbation of COPD	Moderate	Single case-control study
Type I RF, diffuse infiltrates, not ICH	Moderate	↓ Need for intubation
Asthma	No RCTs	Probably effective in ↓ need for intubation
Obesity hypoventilation	No RCTs	Probably effective in ↓ need for intubation
Postoperative respiratory failure	Small RCTs	Probably effective in ↓ need for reintubation
Do not intubate patients	Observational studies	Most effective with CHF, COPD
Pulmonary fibrosis	Observational studies	Not effective

AECOPD = acute exacerbation of chronic obstructive pulmonary disease; CHF = cardiogenic pulmonary edema; COPD = chronic obstructive pulmonary disease; Fio_2 = fraction of inspired oxygen; ICH = immunocompromised host; RCT = randomized, controlled trial; RF = respiratory failure.

BOX 4 Screening Criteria to Assess Readiness to Undergo a Trial of Spontaneous Breathing

Required Criteria

$Pao_2/Fio_2 \geq 150$ or $Sao_2 \geq 90\%$ or $Fio_2 \leq 40\%$ and (PEEP) ≤ 5 cm H_2O
Absence of hypotension

Additional Criteria (optional criteria)

Weaning parameters*

- Negative inspiratory force < -20 to -25 cm H_2O
- Respiratory rate (f) ≤ 35 breaths/min
- Spontaneous tidal volume (V_T) >5 mL/kg
- $f/V_T < 105$ breaths/L/min

Absence of significant anemia (e.g., Hb $\geq 8–10$ mg/dL)
Absence of fever (e.g., core temperature $\leq 38.5°C$)
Adequate mental status: patient awake and alert or easily aroused

---

*Recent studies indicate that these parameters are often unnecessary in deciding whether to initiate trials of spontaneous breathing.
Hb = hemoglobin; PEEP = positive end-expiratory pressure

---

dysfunction can result. Most patients require sedation, but excessive sedation levels are associated with worse outcomes. Therefore, strategies to minimize continuous intravenous sedation using a sedation protocol or once-daily interruption of sedation are recommended.

Invasive mechanical ventilation, especially when prolonged, is associated with numerous complications including ventilator-associated pneumonia, sinusitis, airway injury, thromboembolism, and gastrointestinal bleeding. Therefore, once significant clinical improvement occurs efforts should focus on rapidly removing the patient from the ventilator. This is achieved by daily screening for readiness (Box 4) followed by a 30- to 120-minute spontaneous breathing trial on minimal or no ventilator support. Patients tolerating the spontaneous breathing trial are extubated if they have a good cough, manageable respiratory secretions, and an adequate mental status to protect the airway. Approximately 25% of patients do not tolerate the spontaneous breathing trial; they should be returned to full ventilator support for 24 hours and undergo careful evaluation for reversible causes. The clinician should consider a more gradual approach to weaning these patients.

Specific Causes of Acute Respiratory Failure

ACUTE EXACERBATION OF CHRONIC OBSTRUCTIVE PULMONARY DISEASE

Patients with COPD can experience two or three exacerbations per year, especially if they are actively smoking, resulting in 500,000 hospitalizations every year in the United States. Hospital mortality ranges from 2% to 11%, rising to 25% for those requiring critical care.

Acute exacerbation of COPD is defined by increased sputum volume, purulence, and dyspnea. Physical examination is notable for tachypnea, use of accessory respiratory muscles, diminished breath sounds, prolonged expiratory phase with wheezing, thoraco-abdominal paradox (inward inspiratory abdominal motion), and Hoover's sign (inward inspiratory motion of the lower rib cage). The latter two physical signs indicate the presence of dynamic hyperinflation and diaphragmatic dysfunction. Acute exacerbation of COPD is further characterized by hypoxemia (resulting from $\dot{V}/\dot{Q}$ mismatch) and hypercapnia. Patients with more severe underlying disease might demonstrate evidence of acute and chronic respiratory acidosis.

---

community acquired pneumonia, acute respiratory distress syndrome (ARDS), pulmonary fibrosis, and routinely after planned extubation. One mechanism for improved outcome is the reduction in infection (pneumonia, sepsis) seen with noninvasive ventilation compared with intubated patients. Noninvasive ventilation should not be used in the presence of respiratory arrest, shock, excessive secretions, inability to protect the airway, an agitated or uncooperative patient, and facial abnormalities that preclude proper application of the mask.

Invasive Ventilation

Invasive mechanical ventilation is delivered via an endotracheal tube. The set parameters include Fio_2 and positive end-expiratory pressure (PEEP). For volume-assist control, the clinician chooses respiratory rate and tidal volume. For pressure support, the clinician chooses the inspiratory pressure level above PEEP, and the patient determines respiratory rate. The resulting tidal volume depends on inspiratory pressure level and patient factors including respiratory muscle strength and respiratory system mechanics. Initially the ventilator is set to meet most of the patient's minute ventilation, allowing respiratory muscle rest. Such full support should not be prolonged because diaphragmatic

CURRENT DIAGNOSIS

- History and physical examination can give insight into the etiology of hypoxic and hypercapneic respiratory failure but may be insufficient to make a definitive diagnosis and guide therapy.
- An arterial blood gas is mandatory to define severity and whether hypoxic or hypercapneic (or both) respiratory failure is present.
- Additional diagnostic modalities, including chest radiograph, electrocardiogram, cardiac laboratory tests (troponin, brain natriuretic peptide), echocardiography, and selected use of a pulmonary artery catheter, can help identify a specific etiology.

Etiology and Diagnosis

Approximately 50% of acute exacerbations of COPD result from bacterial infection (e.g., *Pneumococcus* species, *Haemophilus influenzae*, *Moraxella catarrhalis*, and *Pseudomonas* species). The remainder result from viral infection and air pollution. In many cases a cause cannot be identified, although there is increasing appreciation that acute myocardial infarction and pulmonary embolism may be present in up to 25%. Pulmonary embolism may be suggested by a $Paco_2$ lower than baseline and the need for a higher than expected Fio_2 to maintain the Sao_2 at greater than 90%. Computed tomographic pulmonary arteriogram is recommended to make the diagnosis, because $\dot{V}/\dot{Q}$ scanning is nondiagnostic in nearly one half of COPD patients, and false-positive high-probability scans occur.

Treatment

Treatment for acute exacerbation of COPD is based on high-quality evidence consisting of numerous randomized, controlled trials and well-performed meta-analyses. Bronchodilator therapy is essential. Nebulized combination therapy (albuterol and ipratropium [DuoNeb]) is effective, but it is not demonstrably superior to single-agent therapy delivered via a metered-dose inhaler. Theophylline should generally be avoided because toxicity outweighs benefits.

Antibiotics improve outcome, especially in the presence of fever and increased sputum purulence and volume. Older agents, such as amoxicillin and tetracycline, appear to be less effective than newer macrolides and fluoroquinalones.

Corticosteroids enhance β-agonist activity and counteract the inflammatory state seen in acute exacerbations of COPD. Oral prednisone at a dose of 30 to 40 mg is recommended. Intravenous therapy (methylprednisolone [SoluMedrol] 125 mg every 6 hours for 72 hours followed by oral prednisone) should be used in the critically ill patient or when response to oral therapy is suboptimal.

There is no role for mucolytic agents or chest physiotherapy.

Admission to the intensive care unit (ICU) is indicated for patients with hemodynamic instability, confusion, lethargy and coma, severe dyspnea unresponsive to emergency management, or severely abnormal gas exchange despite initial therapy (Pao_2 <40 mm Hg, $Paco_2$ >60 mm Hg, pH <7.25).

Randomized, controlled trials demonstrate that noninvasive ventilation decreases the risk for intubation and improves survival in acute exacerbations of COPD when there are severe dyspnea, hypoxemia, tachypnea, and significant respiratory acidosis ($Paco_2$ >45 mm Hg and pH <7.35). Patients who fail noninvasive ventilation or who are not candidates require intubation and mechanical ventilation.

A major risk is the development of dynamic hyperinflation (PEEPi), which can worsen gas exchange, predispose to barotrauma (e.g., pneumothorax), and cause hypotension. PEEPi is minimized by keeping delivered minute ventilation at 5 L/min or less; this is achieved by lowering tidal volume (e.g., 6 mL/kg ideal body weight) or respiratory rate (8–10 breaths/min), or by increasing inspiratory flow rate, allowing more time for expiration. PEEPi is suggested by an elevated plateau pressure or persistent expiratory flow at the time

CURRENT THERAPY

- Treatment of acute respiratory failure often begins with nonspecific approaches such as oxygen and mechanical ventilation (noninvasive or invasive).
- The goal of mechanical ventilation is to improve gas exchange and rest the respiratory muscles while waiting for the beneficial effects of specific therapy aimed at the underlying cause (e.g., bronchodilators, antibiotics, and corticosteroids in acute exacerbations of chronic obstructive pulmonary disease [COPD]).
- Noninvasive ventilation avoids many complications associated with invasive ventilation and improves outcomes for patients with acute cardiogenic pulmonary edema and acute exacerbations of COPD.
- Invasive mechanical ventilation can be lifesaving but can cause clinical deterioration if not properly administered.
- Using low tidal volumes (6 mL/kg ideal body weight) can help avoid dangerous dynamic hyperinflation in acute exacerbations of COPD and further lung injury in acute lung injury (e.g., volutrauma, barotrauma).
- Once signs of improvement are evident, focus rapidly shifts to liberating the patient from the ventilator using spontaneous breathing trials to assess the need for ventilatory support followed by airway assessment to determine readiness for extubation.

of the next ventilator breath. PEEPi can also increase work of breathing by increasing the patient's inspiratory effort to trigger the ventilator. When extrinsic PEEP is at or just below the PEEPi level, the patient triggers more easily and work of breathing is reduced.

The approach to weaning and extubation in acute exacerbations of COPD is similar to that for other conditions, although the risk of failing a spontaneous breathing trial is increased.

ACUTE LUNG INJURY AND ACUTE RESPIRATORY DISTRESS SYNDROME

ALI is the result of an acute process and is characterized by hypoxemia (Pao_2/Fio_2 <300), bilateral diffuse alveolar infiltrates, and no evidence of cardiac etiology. When the Pao_2/Fio_2 is less than 200, the patient is said to have ARDS. ALI results from pulmonary and extrapulmonary etiologies. Pulmonary causes include pneumonia, gastric aspiration, near drowning, toxic gas inhalation, and lung contusion. Extrapulmonary causes include sepsis, pancreatitis, fat embolism, drug overdose, nonthoracic trauma, and massive transfusion. Conditions that can mimic the clinical findings of ALI include CHF, diffuse alveolar hemorrhage (DAH), acute cryptogenic organizing pneumonia (COP), and acute eosinophilic pneumonia (AEP). These latter three entities can be diagnosed by bronchoscopy (DAH, AEP) or by open lung biopsy (COP), all are treated with high doses of corticosteroids. Studies indicate that corticosteroids do not improve the outcome of ALI/ARDS.

Differentiating cardiogenic pulmonary edema from ALI can be challenging, especially because these conditions can coexist. Physical findings of jugular venous distention and a positive third heart sound, abnormal electrocardiogram (ECG), elevated brain natruretic peptide (BNP), and positive cardiac enzymes (troponin) point to a cardiac etiology. A chest radiograph showing cardiomegaly, vascular redistribution, widened vascular pedicle, perihilar alveolar infiltrates and pleural effusions also suggest a cardiac cause. Bedside echocardiography can demonstrate reduced left ventricular function. A pulmonary artery catheter provides definitive evidence of an elevated pulmonary capillary wedge pressure and reduced cardiac output. That said, recent randomized, controlled trials demonstrate no improvement in survival with routine use of the pulmonary artery catheter in ALI.

ALI causes heterogeneous effects in the lung, resulting in poorly ventilated, atelectatic, dependent regions of lung. Traditional tidal volumes of 10 to 15 mL/kg can cause lung injury by creating significant shear stress by repeatedly opening these atelectatic areas (atelectrauma) and overdistending less affected areas (volutrauma, barotrauma). Indeed, experimental and clinical studies demonstrate that a lung-protective strategy, using a tidal volume of 6 mL/kg ideal body weight, improves survival in ALI. Using small tidal volumes often results in significant hypercapnia, which can have an independent protective effect (permissive hypercapnia). The application of PEEP recruits and opens atelectatic lung, thereby reducing harmful shear forces. The optimal level of PEEP remains uncertain: Recent multicenter studies found no difference in mortality in patients randomized to high ($\sim$14 cm H_2O) or low ($\sim$8 cm H_2O) PEEP when all patients received a tidal volume of 6 mL/kg ideal body weight.

CARDIOGENIC PULMONARY EDEMA

CHF occurs in patients with cardiomyopathy or acutely when ischemia is present. Diagnosis is suggested by jugular venous distension, a third heart sound, diffuse rales, abnormal ECG, and a chest radiograph showing cardiomegaly, diffuse alveolar infiltrates, and bilateral pleural effusion. A markedly elevated BNP or pro-BNP further suggests a cardiac etiology.

Therapy consists of oxygen, nitrates, diuretics, afterload reduction, and anti-ischemic therapy if the history or ECG is suggestive. Mechanical ventilation produces positive intrathoracic pressure, which improves cardiac function by decreasing both left ventricular preload and afterload, reversing hypoxemia, and decreasing work of breathing. In hemodynamically stable patients without active ischemia, CPAP at levels of 8 to 12 cm H_2O should be used. A meta-analysis of 15 randomized, controlled trials showed that noninvasive ventilation decreased the need for intubation and improved survival. CPAP and BiPAP appear to be equivalent, although many prefer BiPAP when hypercapnia is present.

Because cardiogenic pulmonary edema is rapidly reversible, intubated patients can often be extubated within 24 hours. That said, the transition from positive pressure ventilation to negative ventilation (e.g., T-piece or extubation) can precipitate pulmonary edema.

REFERENCES

Acute Respiratory Distress Syndrome Network. Ventilation with lower tidal volumes as compared with traditional tidal volumes for acute lung injury and the acute respiratory distress syndrome. N Engl J Med 2000;342:1301–8.

Bach PB, Brown C, Gelfand SE, et al. Management of acute exacerbations of chronic obstructive pulmonary disease: A summary and appraisal of published evidence. Ann Intern Med 2001;134:600–20.

Brower RG, Lanken PN, MacIntyre N, et al. Higher versus lower positive end-expiratory pressures in patients with the acute respiratory distress syndrome. N Engl J Med 2004;51:327–36.

Ely EW, Baker AM, Dunagan DP, et al. Effect on the duration of mechanical ventilation of identifying patients capable of breathing spontaneously. N Engl J Med 1996;335:1864–9.

Epstein SK. Complications in ventilator supported patients. In: Tobin M, editor. Principles and Practice of Mechanical Ventilation. New York: McGraw Hill; 2006. p. 877–902.

Kress JP, Pohlman AS, O'Connor MF, et al. Daily interruption of sedative infusions in critically ill patients undergoing mechanical ventilation. N Engl J Med 2000;342:1471–7.

MacIntyre NR, Cook DJ, Ely EW Jr, et al. Evidence-based guidelines for weaning and discontinuing ventilatory support: A collective task force facilitated by the American College of Chest Physicians, the American Association for Respiratory Care, and the American College of Critical Care Medicine. Chest 2001;120:375S–95S.

Majid A, Hill NS. Noninvasive ventilation for acute respiratory failure. Curr Opin Crit Care 2005;11:77–81.

Masip J, Orque M, Sanchez B, et al. Noninvasive ventilation in acute cardiogenic pulmonary edema: Systematic review and meta-analysis. JAMA 2005;294:3124–30.

Schumaker G, Epstein SK. Management of acute respiratory failure in acute exacerbations of COPD. Resp Care 2004;49:766–82.

Atelectasis

Method of
Christine L. Lau, MD; Alykhan S. Nagji, MD; and Matthew D. Taylor, MD

Atelectasis refers to the collapse of alveoli that affects segmental or lobar regions of the lung or the entire lung and results in hypoventilation. However, recent studies have suggested that the alveoli are not collapsed but are filled with fluid and foam. These hypotheses are not mutually exclusive; collapsed alveoli and fluid- and foam-filled alveoli may be present concurrently in an atelectatic lung. Although atelectasis is considered a benign condition, early treatment, reversal, and prevention are essential to an overall improved outcome.

Etiology

COMPRESSION ATELECTASIS

Compression atelectasis occurs when the transmural pressure distending the alveolus is reduced to a level that allows the alveolus to collapse. To best illustrate this mechanism, consider the patient who has undergone induction of anesthesia. The diaphragm is relaxed and is displaced cephalad. In the supine position, the pleural pressures increase to the greatest extent in the dependent lung regions and can compress the adjacent lung tissue.

SURFACTANT IMPAIRMENT

Surfactant serves to reduce the alveolar surface tension, thereby stabilizing the alveoli and preventing collapse. Reduction in surfactant occurs with certain types of anesthesia. Studies have shown that hyperinflation by means of increased tidal volume, sequential air inflations to the total lung capacity, or even a single cycle of increased tidal volume can increase the release of surfactant, aiding in recruitment and stabilization of alveoli.

GAS RESORPTION

One mechanism by which gas resorption results in atelectasis involves the patent airway. In regions of the lung with increased ventilation compared to perfusion, which produces a ventilation/perfusion ($\dot{V}/\dot{Q}$) mismatch, there is low alveolar oxygen tension. Increasing the fraction of inspired oxygen (F_{IO_2}) initiates a cascade of events that increases alveolar oxygen tension (P_{AO_2}) and decreases alveolar nitrogen tension (P_{AN_2}), which results in loss of alveolar volume secondary to increased absorption of oxygen.

Another mechanism by which gas resorption leads to atelectasis occurs after complete airway occlusion. In such cases, gas is trapped distal to the obstruction. Gas uptake by the proximal blood flow continues without additional gas inflow. This causes the alveoli to collapse.

Pathophysiology

The trapping of air and hyperinflation of the alveoli are produced from the aforementioned mechanisms. The gases that are trapped are absorbed by the blood perfusing through that region of the lung, which eventually causes collapse of the alveoli. The atelectasis produces alveolar hypoxia and pulmonary vasoconstriction to prevent $\dot{V}/\dot{Q}$ mismatching and to minimize arterial hypoxia. This vascular response is effective only if a large part of the lung is not collapsed; otherwise, intrapulmonary shunting occurs.

CURRENT DIAGNOSIS

- Hypoxia
- Tachypnea
- Diminished breath sounds
- Wheezing
- Radiologic signs of atelectasis

Clinical Presentation

The signs and symptoms of atelectasis are often nonspecific. The natural course of atelectasis may lead to fever, cough, tachypnea, wheezing, rhonchi, and chest pain. On physical examination, atelectasis may manifest as an area of localized reduced breath sounds with constant wheeze or reduced chest wall expansion or both.

Diagnosis

Chest radiographs aid in the diagnosis of atelectasis. They provide both direct and indirect signs that may indicate an atelectatic etiology for the patient's symptoms.

Direct signs include:

- Displaced pulmonary vessels
- Air bronchograms
- Displacement of intralobar fissures (most reliable sign)

Indirect signs include:

- Pulmonary opacification
- Diaphragmatic elevation
- Hyperexpansion of unaffected lung
- Tracheal, heart, and mediastinal shift toward atelectatic side
- Shift of the hilum toward the collapsed lobe
- Segmental ipsilateral rib approximation

Treatment

Treatment of atelectasis is geared toward the underlying cause. It is important to recognize respiratory distress and to intubate the patient if appropriate.

If the etiology is that of an obstructive atelectasis, chest percussion or vibration and nasotracheal or bronchoscopic suctioning may help in the clearing of secretions. With regard to lung re-expansion, incentive spirometry, continuous or intermittent positive-pressure ventilation, and early ambulation may be used.

Those patients who have a nonobstructive atelectasis caused by a pneumothorax or pleural effusion benefit from tube thoracostomy or thoracentesis. Additionally, appropriate pain management in the postoperative setting allows for proper ventilation.

CURRENT THERAPY

- Chest percussion or vibration
- Nasotracheal or bronchoscopic suctioning
- Incentive spirometry
- Positive-pressure ventilation
- Ambulation
- Postoperative pain control

REFERENCES

Duggan M, Kavanagh BP. Pulmonary atelectasis: A pathogenic perioperative entity. Anesthesiology 2005;102:838–54.
Duggan M, Kavanagh BP. Atelectasis in the perioperative patient. Curr Opin Anaesthesiol 2007;20:37–42.

Hubmayr RD. Perspective on lung injury and recruitment: A skeptical look at the opening and collapse story. Am J Respir Crit Care Med 2002;165:1647–53.
Peroni DG, Boner AL. Atelectasis: Mechanisms, diagnosis and management. Paediatr Respir Rev 2000;1:274–8.
Wagner PD, Laravuso RB, Uhl RR, West JB. Continuous distributions of ventilation-perfusion ratios in normal subjects breathing air and 100 per cent O2. J Clin Invest 1974;54:54–68.

Chronic Obstructive Pulmonary Disease

Method of
*Nicola A. Hanania, MD, MS, and
Amir Sharafkhaneh, MD, PhD*

Epidemiology

Chronic obstructive pulmonary disease (COPD) is the sixth most prevalent chronic medical condition in the United States, affecting more than 5% of the population. It is estimated that COPD is not diagnosed in 50% of patients suffering from it, probably because symptoms early in the disease are very subtle, causing delay in seeking medical attention, and because spirometry testing is underutilized. For many years, COPD was thought to be a disease of "old men"; however, its incidence has dramatically increased in women, and middle-aged (45-65 years) persons are also at risk. COPD causes more than 700,000 hospitalizations every year. COPD is the fourth leading cause of death in the United States, leading to more than 120,000 deaths every year. COPD-related mortality in women has now surpassed that of men in the United States. The annual cost of COPD in the United States exceeds $42 billion, with the majority of costs being secondary to issues related to COPD exacerbations.

Risk Factors

Cigarette smoking is the most common cause of COPD, and most patients report a smoking history of more than 20 pack-years upon diagnosis. Genetic susceptibility is important in this disease because only 20% to 30% of smokers develop the disease. α_1-Antripsyn deficiency is currently the only known genetic risk factor, but it is a rare cause of the disease and several other genes remain to be identified. In addition to cigarette smoke, other environmental exposures can lead to COPD; these include environmental tobacco smoke, occupational exposures, and exposures to air pollution. The role of recurrent respiratory infections in causing COPD is still debatable.

Pathophysiology

COPD is a multicomponent disease caused by exposure to noxious agents including cigarette smoke. The increased exposure to oxidative stress is believed to be the most important trigger for this disease in susceptible persons. COPD manifests with impaired lung function (including expiratory airflow limitation, hyperinflation, and abnormalities of gas exchange), which leads to respiratory symptoms including dyspnea, exercise limitation, and deconditioning. Airflow limitation in this disease is caused by airway inflammation, mucociliary dysfunction, and structural changes in the lung parenchyma (destruction and loss of elastic recoil), small airways (airway remodeling), and pulmonary vasculature (pulmonary hypertension).

Large airways show hypertrophy of mucous glands and infiltration of the airway walls with inflammatory cells.

Clinically, chronic bronchitis with cough and sputum production occurring in the majority of patients is a manifestation of large airways involvement; however, physiologically, this large airways involvement does not contribute markedly to the airflow limitation. Small airways involvement includes airway inflammation which occurs in all stages of severity and is characterized by infiltration with neutrophils, macrophages, and T-lymphocytes (particularly CD8$^+$), luminal obstruction with inflammatory mucus, airway wall thickening, and hypertrophy of airway smooth muscles.

Lung parenchymal involvement in COPD manifests with destruction of alveolar walls and enlargement of alveolar spaces beyond terminal bronchioles (emphysema). With disease advancement, the airspace enlargement creates large empty spaces called *bullae*. Loss of lung tissue results in reduced alveolar-capillary membrane that is needed for gas exchange and reduced lung elastic recoil. These changes cause impaired gas exchange, increased lung volume and hyperinflation, airflow limitation, and exercise impairment. Involvement of vasculature includes thickening of the vessel wall and endothelial dysfunction. Loss of capillaries due to emphysema and associated hypoxemia in advanced COPD results in pulmonary hypertension.

Prevention

COPD is a preventable disease. Because more than 90% of patients with the disease are smokers, smoking cessation is an important intervention to prevent this disease. In patients with the disease, smoking cessation was shown to slow the decline in lung function and mortality. Other preventive measures should include avoiding exposure to respiratory irritants such as environmental tobacco smoke (secondhand smoke) and respiratory infections (by receiving vaccinations). None of the pharmacologic interventions available for treating COPD can diminish the deterioration in lung function that occurs with this disease.

Clinical Manifestations

COPD is a slowly progressive disease that ultimately causes severe limitation of physical activity, deterioration of quality of life, and ultimately premature death. COPD commonly occurs in patients who are 40 years of age and older. In most instances, the smoking history is very prominent (>20 pack-years). Cough and sputum production (chronic bronchitis) are present in the majority of patients. Early in the disease, symptoms may be subtle, and many patients relate them to the aging process. Fatigue and activity limitation are very common. Dyspnea on exertion is common, although many patients limit their activity and might not report dyspnea until late in the disease. Dyspnea is usually progressive and leads to exercise intolerance.

The course of COPD is often complicated with repeated exacerbations, which are the first presenting symptoms in some cases. Several extrapulmonary morbidities can complicate its course, including cardiac disease, depression, osteoporosis, and muscle wasting. Several clinical phenotypes for COPD that can have therapeutic implications have been described, although these need to be further explored.

Diagnosis

The diagnosis of COPD should be considered in any smoker who is 40 years of age or older who presents with respiratory symptoms such as smoker's cough, sputum production, dyspnea, or activity limitation. Many patients with COPD do not perceive symptoms, and therefore thorough questioning by clinicians is of paramount importance.

CURRENT DIAGNOSIS

- COPD is a preventable disease most commonly caused by cigarette smoke exposure.
- COPD is not diagnosed in approximately 50% of patients suffering from it.
- COPD should be ruled out in any smoker 40 years or older presenting with respiratory symptoms (cough, dyspnea, sputum production or activity limitation).
- The diagnosis of COPD is confirmed by spirometry.
- A post-bronchodilator FEV$_1$/FVC less than 70% is diagnostic of COPD.
- Staging of severity of this disease is based on percentage of predicted FEV$_1$: mild is greater than 80%, moderate is 50% to 80%, severe is between 30% and 50%, and very severe less than 30% (or less than 50% in the presence of signs of chronic respiratory failure).
- The course of COPD may be complicated by multiple extrapulmonary comorbidities such as cardiac disease, depression, osteoporosis, and muscle wasting.

Abbreviations: COPD = chronic obstructive pulmonary disease; FEV$_1$ = forced expiratory volume in 1 second; FVC = forced vital capacity.

Physical examination of the COPD patient may be normal, and the classic "blue bloater" and "pink puffer" phenotypes are rarely seen early in the disease process. Patients with advanced emphysema may have evidence of hyperinflation on chest examination (barrel-shaped chest and hyperresonance), use of accessory muscles, and muscle wasting (cachexia). Spirometry should be performed on patients who report symptoms. The diagnosis of COPD is made based on the demonstration airway obstruction following bronchodilator administration: forced expiratory volume in 1 second per forced vital capacity (FEV$_1$/FVC) less than 70%. The severity of the disease is based on the percentage of predicted FEV$_1$ and is classified into four stages (Table 1).

Lung volume measurements as well as measurement of the diffusion capacity (D$_{LCO}$) of the lung can aid in assessing the presence of hyperinflation (increased lung volume) and lung destruction (low D$_{LCO}$). A 6-minute walk test can help in assessing exercise tolerance and to rule out exercise-induced hypoxemia, although it not routinely needed in patients with mild disease. Although the role of the chest radiograph in diagnosing COPD is limited, it is usually needed during the initial evaluation to rule out other pathologies such as lung cancer. Screening for α$_1$-antitrypsin deficiency is also

TABLE 1 Stepwise Approach to the Pharmacologic Management of COPD

Severity	Spirometric Findings	Intervention
Stage I: mild	FEV$_1$/FVC < 70% FEV$_1$ ≥ 80%	Add a *short-acting bronchodilator* to be used when needed; anticholinergic or β$_2$-adrenoceptor agonist
Stage II: moderate	FEV$_1$/FVC < 70% 50% ≤ FEV$_1$ < 80%	Add *one or more long-acting bronchodilators* on a scheduled basis Consider pulmonary rehabilitation.
Stage III: severe	FEV$_1$/FVC < 70% 30% ≤ FEV$_1$ < 50%	Add inhaled steroids if repeated exacerbations
Stage IV: very severe	FEV$_1$/FVC < 70% FEV$_1$ < 30%	Evaluate for adding oxygen Consider surgical options

Abbreviations: FEV$_1$ = forced expiratory volume in 1 sec; FVC = forced vital capacity.

recommended in all patients with COPD. Routine use of computed tomography (CT) has no utility in the routine diagnosis of COPD, although it may be helpful in detecting early emphysema.

Differential Diagnosis

Several diseases can manifest with symptoms and signs of COPD. Asthma and COPD have similar symptoms and signs. Asthma usually has an early onset as opposed to COPD, which rarely occurs before the fourth decade. The presence of allergy history, family history, and the absence of smoking history favors the diagnosis of asthma. Spirometry can show complete reversibility in asthma, and partial reversibility is usually observed in COPD. Another lung disease that can mimic COPD is bronchiectasis. Dyspnea may be a presenting symptom in diseases other than COPD in the elderly population; these include congestive heart failure and coronary insufficiency.

Treatment

GOALS OF THERAPY

The main goals of therapy of COPD are focused on relieving symptoms, improving health status, preserving lung function from decline, improving exercise performance, preventing exacerbations, and decreasing mortality. These goals should be reached with minimal side effects from treatment. Traditional COPD therapies have focused on controlling symptoms and aim to alleviate the problems of reduced airflow and declining lung function. However, with our improved knowledge about the multicomponent nature of the disease, therapeutic approaches aim to target both the symptoms and the inflammation that underlies and drives COPD.

 CURRENT THERAPY

- COPD is a treatable disease.
- The goals for treatment of COPD are to reduce symptoms, exacerbations, complications, progression of the disease, and mortality and improve lung function, exercise tolerance, and health status (quality of life).
- Several pharmacologic and nonpharmacologic interventions are available.
- Smoking cessation is the most important intervention in the management of COPD.
- Nonpharmacologic interventions include influenza vaccination, exercise, and pulmonary rehabilitation.
- All symptomatic patients with COPD should be treated with medications.
- Pharmacologic agents available include bronchodilators (short-acting and long-acting) and inhaled corticosteroids in combination with long-acting β$_2$-agonists.
- Short-acting bronchodilators should be considered for rescue of symptoms, and long-acting bronchodilators (β$_2$-agonists and anticholinergics) should be considered for maintenance therapy in all stages of severity.
- Inhaled corticosteroids should be considered in patients with recurrent exacerbations and those with severe disease (FEV$_1$ <50% predicted).
- Oxygen therapy should be considered in stable patients who on optimal therapy have documented hypoxemia on room air (Po$_2$ <55 mm Hg).
- Surgical interventions in COPD are limited to some patients with severe emphysema.

Abbreviations: COPD = chronic obstructive pulmonary disease; FEV$_1$ = forced expiratory volume in 1 second; FVC = forced vital capacity.

NONPHARMACOLOGIC INTERVENTIONS

Vaccination

Reducing further damage to lung tissue is a main goal of therapy in any chronic lung disease. With that in mind, yearly influenza vaccination (killed [Fluzone, Fluarix] or live inactive [FluMist] viruses) can reduce more-severe forms of influenza and acute exacerbations of COPD (by 60%). Pneumococcal vaccination (Pneumovax 23) reduces invasive pneumococcal disease and is recommended in COPD patients with more-severe lung disease (FEV$_1$ < 40%) and elderly patients.

Smoking Cessation

Smoking cessation is the single most effective and cost-effective intervention to reduce the progression of COPD and should be attempted in all patients. Unfortunately, even with the best intervention strategies, less than a third of smokers become sustained quitters. Once patients develop demonstrable airflow obstruction, their symptoms and airway inflammation can persist even after smoking cessation. Several effective therapies for tobacco dependence are available and should be considered in patients interested in quitting smoking. These include behavioral techniques, support groups, and pharmacotherapy (Table 2) including nicotine supplements, bupropion (Zyban), and nicotine-receptor partial agonists like varenicline (Chantix).

Exercise and Pulmonary Rehabilitation

Pulmonary rehabilitation is currently recommended to be considered in the management of patients with moderate or worse COPD. Pulmonary rehabilitation is an individualized multidisciplinary program that aims to optimize patients' performance and self-control. The program includes upper and lower body and breathing exercises; nutritional, psychological, and behavioral interventions; and education. Pulmonary rehabilitation produces significant improvement in respiratory symptoms, exercise capacity, quality of life, and health care utilization

Surgical Therapies

Lung volume reduction surgery (LVERS) includes resection of severely emphysematous areas of the lungs. The procedure can be performed through thoracoscopy or median sternotomy. In the National Emphysema Treatment Trial (NETT), LVRS improved spirometry, lung

TABLE 2 Pharmacologic Therapies for Smoking Cessation

Drug	Dose	Frequency
Oral		
Nicotine polacrilex (Nicotine gum, Nicorette)	2 mg, 4 mg	10-20 mg/day, q1-2h
Nicotine lozenges/ tablets (Commit)	2 mg, 4 mg	10-20 mg/day 1 piece every h
Bupropion sustained-release (Zyban)	150 mg	150 mg × 3 d, then 300 mg qd
Varenicline (Chantix)	1 mg	Initial 1-week dose titration, then 1 mg bid × 12 wk
Patch		
Nicotine Transdermal System Step 1, 2, 3	21, 14, 7 mg	Over 24 h
Nicoderm CQ Step 1, 2, 3	15, 10, 5 mg	Over 16 h
Nicotrol Step 1, 2, 3 Prostep	22, 11 mg	Over 24 h
Inhaled		
Nicotine nasal spray (Nicotrol NS)	0.5 mg/ inhalation	10-40 mg/day in hourly or prn dosing
Nicotine inhaler (Nicotrol Inhaler)	10 mg/ ampule	6-10 ampules/day

volumes, exercise tolerance, dyspnea, and quality of life. Subjects with upper lobe disease and low baseline exercise capacity had improved longevity when compared to optimal medical therapy. In contrast, NETT showed that patients with very advanced COPD including FEV_1 of 20% or less, diffusing capacity of 20% or less, or diffuse emphysema had shorter longevity with LVRS. LVRS can help COPD patients with severe lung disease as long as it is performed in centers with experience in this type of surgery.

COPD patients with giant bulla (>1/3 hemithorax) might benefit from bullectomy with improvement in symptoms (dyspnea), lung function, oxygenation and ventilation, exercise capacity, and quality of life.

In selected patients with advanced COPD, lung transplant can improve pulmonary function, exercise capacity, and quality of life.

PHARMACOLOGIC INTERVENTIONS

Evidence-based guidelines for COPD emphasize the comprehensive and stepwise approach to the management of COPD and stipulate that all patients who are symptomatic merit a trial of pharmacologic intervention (see Table 1). Short-acting bronchodilators given when needed are recommended for patients with intermittent symptoms such as cough, wheeze, or exertional dyspnea. However, maintenance therapy should be initiated in patients who have persistent symptoms such as dyspnea or nighttime awakenings, despite use of as-needed short-acting agents. In this setting, maintenance treatment should be initiated with a long-acting bronchodilator or, alternatively, a short-acting agent given four times per day. Rescue therapy with albuterol (Proventil, Ventolin) should be continued as needed. If the benefit of treatment is limited, then a bronchodilator from another drug class or a combination of two drug classes (e.g., long-acting bronchodilator plus inhaled corticosteroids [ICS]) should be attempted. The addition of regular ICS therapy should be considered in patients with FEV_1 less than 50% of predicted who had disease exacerbations requiring a course of oral steroids or antibiotic at least once in the preceding year.

Bronchodilators

Bronchodilators work through their direct relaxation effect on airway smooth muscle cells, although many have non-bronchodilator activities that might contribute to their beneficial effects in COPD. Three classes of bronchodilators—β_2-agonists, anticholinergics, and theophylline—are currently available and can be used individually or in combination (Box 1).

Several issues need to be considered when assessing the response to bronchodilator therapy. First, the lack of acute response to one class of bronchodilator does not necessarily imply nonresponsiveness to another. One further consideration is that a patient's FEV_1 response to acute bronchodilator therapy does not predict long-term response to bronchodilator therapy and can vary from day to day. The clinical efficacy of bronchodilators has traditionally been assessed by the degree of improvement in FEV_1. However, other physiologic measures such as the change in inspiratory capacity (IC) correlate better with change in symptoms, such as dyspnea and exercise tolerance. This suggests that assessment of bronchodilator treatment using indices of hyperinflation or air trapping might provide a better indicator of efficacy. Although changes in lung volumes are independent of changes in FEV_1, several studies have demonstrated that the more-sustained airway patency offered by long-acting bronchodilators reduces air trapping.

Several other outcome measures are now used to assess response to bronchodilator therapy. COPD exacerbation is an important but occasionally overlooked parameter. The use of long-acting β_2-adrenoceptor agonists and long-acting anticholinergic agents reduce the frequency of exacerbation and severity of individual exacerbations. The effects of long-acting bronchodilators on health status have been well documented in several clinical trials. The long-term effects of tiotropium (Spiriva) on the decline in postbronchodilator FEV_1 over 4 years was investigated in the Understanding of Potential Long-term Impact on Function with Tiotropium trial (UPLIFT). Although tiotropium failed to slow the decline in lung function over

---

BOX 1 Commonly Used Pharmacologic Agents for COPD

Short-Acting Agents
β_2-Adrenoceptor Agonists
Albuterol (Ventolin, Proventil, ProAir, AccuNeb) (MDI, NS)
Levalbuterol (Xopenex) (MDI, NS)
Pirbuterol (Maxair) (MDI)

Anticholinergic
Ipratropium bromide (Atrovent) (MDI, NS)

Fixed Combination
Albuterol-ipratropium (Combivent, DuoNeb) (MDI, NS)

Long-Acting Agents
β_2-Adrenoceptor Agonists
Salmeterol (Serevent Diskus) (DPI)
Formoterol (Foradil, Perforomist) (DPI, NS)
Arformoterol (Brovana) (NS)

Anticholinergic
Tiotropium bromide (Spiriva) (DPI)

Fixed Combination
Salmeterol-fluticasone (Advair Diskus, Advair HFA)* (DPI, MDI)
Formoterol/Budesonide (Symbicort)† (MDI)

Methylxanthines
Theophylline (Uniphyl, Theo-24) (PO)

---

*Only one dose formulation (250/50) is approved for COPD in the United States.
†Only one dose formulation (160/4.5) approved for COPD in the United States.
Abbreviations: COPD = chronic obstructive pulmonary disease; DPI = dry powder inhaler; MDI = metered dose inhaler; NS = nebulized solution; PO = oral preparation.

---

the 4 years of the study, it had a significant effect on improving health status and reducing exacerbations.

To achieve maximal benefit, a bronchodilator must be correctly delivered to the airway using a proper technique. Inhaled bronchodilators have traditionally been delivered to the lung using a metered dose inhaler (MDI). However, a significant number of patients with COPD cannot effectively coordinate their breathing using an MDI. This problem may be remedied by the use of a dry-powder device (DPI), an MDI with a spacer device, or a nebulizer.

Inhaled Corticosteroids

Given the prominence of airway inflammation in COPD, highly potent but nonspecific antiinflammatory agents such as corticosteroids could be expected to have some effects on lung function and health outcomes of COPD patients. Although these agents appear to have minimal significant effects on key inflammatory chemoattractants, there are data to suggest an association with reduced neutrophil chemotaxis. Current guidelines recommend the use of regular treatment with ICS for symptomatic patients who suffer frequent exacerbations and whose FEV_1 is less than 50% of predicted. Several, large 3-year randomized trials have failed to show a significant effect of ICS on the rate of decline of FEV_1, compared with placebo.

Although both ICS and long-acting β_2-agonists (LABAs) are effective by themselves in improving lung function and reducing exacerbations, their beneficial effects are amplified when they are given together. There is a large and growing body of experimental and clinical evidence supporting the use of combination therapy with inhaled corticosteroids and LABAs for the long-term treatment of

COPD patients with moderate to severe disease. The use of ICS and LABA combination products has been shown to improve lung function, symptoms, and health status and reduce exacerbations in patients with moderate to severe COPD. More recently, a large ($N = 6112$) 3-year study, TORCH, demonstrated a significant effect of therapy with salmeterol-fluticasone combination (SFC) (Advair) over 3 years on several COPD outcomes. SFC had a 2.6% absolute risk reduction in all-cause mortality compared to placebo ($P = 0.052$) and was significantly superior to placebo and both component drugs in reducing moderate-to-severe exacerbations and improving health status ($P < 0.001$). Over the 3-year treatment period, patients taking SFC experienced a 25% reduction in the annual rate of moderate-to-severe exacerbations compared with placebo ($P < 0.001$).

Oropharyngeal candidiasis was reported as the most common adverse event for the use of LABA-ICS combination relative to placebo over a period of 24 to 52 weeks, with headache, upper respiratory tract infection, and musculoskeletal pain reported less frequently. Data from TORCH showed that neither SFC, salmeterol alone (Serevent) or fluticasone alone (Flovent) led to increased cardiac disorders, ophthalmic adverse events, or increased probability of bone fractures over the 3-year treatment period. However, an unexpected safety finding was an increased incidence of pneumonia reported in patients taking fluticasone and SFC.

Oxygen

Supplemental long term oxygen therapy (LTOT) has been associated with a variety of beneficial effects in patients with severe COPD who are hypoxemic in room air. These include prolonged survival, reduced secondary polycythemia, improved cardiac function during rest and exercise, reduction in the oxygen cost of ventilation, and improved exercise tolerance. Patients with Pao_2 less than 55 mm Hg (Sao_2 <88%) whose disease is stable despite receiving otherwise comprehensive medical treatment are candidates to receive LTOT. Patients whose Pao_2 is 55 to 59 mm Hg (Sao_2 89%) are eligible to receive LTOT if they show signs of pulmonary hypertension, cor pulmonale, erythrocytosis, edema from right heart failure, or impaired mental state. If oxygen desaturation only occurs during exercise or sleep, then oxygen therapy should be considered specifically under those conditions.

Mucolytics

Mucus impaction contributes to worsening of symptoms of patients with COPD. A number of studies investigating the role of mucolytics such as potassium iodide (SSKI, Pima)[1] and guaifenesin (Mucinex)[1] failed to demonstrate significant clinical efficacy of these agents in the management of patients with COPD, although some have shown some decrease in COPD exacerbations. A variety of new agents addressing mucociliary clearance and mucus production are under investigation.

Antibiotics

Although empiric treatment with antibiotics has been shown to be of benefit in COPD exacerbations (see later), their role in chronic management is not well defined and is currently not recommended. The role of chronic macrolide therapy in COPD is under investigation.

Augmentation Therapy for α_1-Antitrypsin Deficiency

Replacement therapy with α_1-proteinase inhibitor (Prolastin) has been approved for patients with emphysema due to the α_1-antiprotease deficiency. Given in weekly infusions to patients with ZZ or null AAT phenotypes, therapy can increase serum levels above the target threshold of 11 μM and can provide protective levels within the epithelial lining of the lung. Although AAT augmentation therapy has a sound theoretical basis, proof of its efficacy has been difficult to document. However, available evidence supports the use of this therapy in patients with AAT serum levels less than 11 μM and FEV_1 between 30% and 65% predicted, but it might not be useful in other subsets of patients with COPD.

---

[1]Not FDA approved for this indication.

Complications

COPD EXACERBATIONS

Acute exacerbation of COPD (AECOPD) is defined as worsening of respiratory symptoms including dyspnea, cough, and sputum production beyond daily variations that warrant change in therapy. AECOPD is associated with worsening quality of life and faster decline of lung function. AECOPD has a 10% in-hospital mortality rate and up to 25% mortality in patients admitted to ICU. Although AECOPD is usually caused by bacterial or viral infections, environmental pollution, and lack of compliance with medications, in many cases the cause is not clear. Differential diagnosis of AECOPD includes pneumonia, myocardial ischemia, congestive heart failure, pneumothorax, pleural effusion, pulmonary embolism, cardiac arrhythmias, and noncompliance with medications.

For treatment purposes, AECOPD severity is divided to level I (ambulatory), level II (requiring hospitalization), and level III (acute respiratory failure). The evaluation of patients during AECOPD should include the severity of COPD, comorbid medical conditions, history of prior AECOPD, and its outcomes including hospitalization and intubation. Effect of AECOPD on respiratory and hemodynamic function should be evaluated and considered for severity classifications. Initial diagnostic procedures, depending on the severity of AECOPD, include saturation of oxygen, chest radiography, electrocardiogram (ECG), and routine blood tests including complete blood count (CBC) and basic metabolic panel. Other diagnostic tests may be indicated to rule out other diagnoses.

Early treatment of AECOPD is associated with faster recovery. Main pharmacotherapy includes increased short-acting bronchodilators, antibiotics, and systemic steroid. Short-acting β-agonists (albuterol [Proventil, Ventolin]) and anticholinergics (ipratropium [Atrovent]) offer similar benefits. Several studies showed reduction in treatment failure and mortality (especially for in-patient treatment) with the use of antibiotics for AECOPD. Systemic corticosteroids reduce treatment failure and length of hospital stay and improve FEV_1 but are associated with increased side effects, particularly hyperglycemia. Nonpharmacotherapeutic interventions include supplemental oxygen and ventilatory support.

Outpatient therapy of AECOPD includes educating the patient and reviewing how to use various inhalational agents. Optimization of short-acting bronchodilator use with a spacer or in the form of nebulized therapy is the mainstay of therapy in mild AECOPD. Systemic steroids at a dose of 40 to 60 mg daily for 10 to 14 days, and oral antibiotics (in patients with altered sputum characteristics) may be indicated. First-line antibiotic therapy includes macrolides, doxycycline, and cephalosporins. In case of treatment failure, respiratory fluoroquinolones or amoxicillin-clavulanate (Augmentin) are recommended.

For patients with level II AECOPD or hospitalized patients, in addition to optimization of short-acting bronchodilator therapy and systemic steroids, antibiotics should be started in patients with changed sputum characteristics. Antibiotic should be chosen on the basis of the local bacterial resistant patterns. In level III AECOPD, special attention should be given to more-resistant bacteria, such as *Pseudomonas* spp. In such cases, combination antibiotics should be considered.

Patients with more-severe AECOPD (levels II and III) need supplemental oxygen if oxygen saturation is less than 90%. In case of respiratory failure, noninvasive or invasive ventilator support may be needed. Noninvasive ventilatory support reduces the risk of intubation, in-hospital mortality, and the length of hospitalization.

REFERENCES

Agusti AG. COPD, a multicomponent disease: implications for management. Respir Med 2005;99:670–82.
American Thoracic Society/European Respiratory Society. Statement: Standards for the diagnosis and management of individuals with alpha-1 antitrypsin deficiency. Am J Respir Crit Care Med 2003;168:818–900.
Calverley PM, Anderson JA, Celli B, et al. Salmeterol and fluticasone propionate and survival in chronic obstructive pulmonary disease. N Engl J Med 2007;356:775–89.

Carlin BW. Pulmonary rehabilitation: A focus on COPD in primary care. Postgrad Med 2009;121(6):140–7.

Cazzola M, Hanania NA, Jones PW, et al. It's about time—directing our attention toward modifying the course of COPD. Respir Med 2008;102(Suppl. 1):S37–48.

Celli BR, Barnes PJ. Exacerbations of chronic obstructive pulmonary disease. Eur Respir J 2007;29:1224–38.

Celli BR, Macnee W. Standards for the diagnosis and treatment of patients with COPD: A summary of the ATS/ERS position paper. Eur Respir J 2004;23:932–46.

Edwards MA, Hazelrigg S, Naunheim KS. The National Emphysema Treatment Trial: Summary and update. Thorac Surg Clin 2009;19(2):169–85.

Fiore MC. US public health service clinical practice guideline: treating tobacco use and dependence. Respir Care 2000;45:1200–62.

Hanania NA. Optimizing maintenance therapy for chronic obstructive pulmonary disease: Strategies for improving patient-centered outcomes. Clin Ther 2007;29(10):2121–33.

Hanania NA, Donohue JF. Pharmacologic interventions in chronic obstructive pulmonary disease: Bronchodilators. Proc Am Thorac Soc 2007;4(7):526–34.

Hanania NA, Sharafkhaneh A. Update on the pharmacologic therapy for chronic obstructive pulmonary disease. Clin Chest Med 2007;28(3):589–607.

Mundey K. An appraisal of smoking cessation aids. Curr Opin Pulm Med 2009;15(2):105–12.

Nocturnal Oxygen Therapy Trial Group. Continuous or nocturnal oxygen therapy in hypoxemic chronic obstructive lung disease: A clinical trial. Ann Intern Med 1980;93:391–8.

Quon BS, Gan WQ, Sin DD. Contemporary management of acute exacerbations of COPD: a systematic review and metaanalysis. Chest 2008;133(3):756–66.

Rabe KF, Hurd S, Anzueto A, et al. Global strategy for the diagnosis, management, and prevention of COPD—2006 update. Am J Respir Crit Care Med 2007;176(6):532–55.

Tashkin DP, Celli B, Senn S, et al. UPLIFT Study Investigators. A 4-year trial of tiotropium in chronic obstructive pulmonary disease. N Engl J Med 2008;359(15):1543–54.

Varkey JB, Varkey AB, Varkey B. Prophylactic vaccinations in chronic obstructive pulmonary disease: Current status. Curr Opin Pulm Med 2009;15(2):90–9.

Cystic Fibrosis

Method of
Robert Giusti, MD

Cystic fibrosis (CF), an autosomal recessive disease, is the most common lethal inherited disease in the white population. In this population the carrier rate is approximately 1 in 30, with an incidence of 1 in 3200 births. CF also occurs in African Americans (1 in 15,000), Hispanic Americans (1 in 8000) and Asian Americans (1 in 31,000), but diagnosis may be delayed because of a low index of suspicion in these ethnic groups. Lung disease is the primary cause of morbidity and mortality in CF. Progressive fibrosis and destruction of lung tissue from chronic cycles of infection and inflammation lead to respiratory failure. The median survival for CF patients is 37.4 years.

Pathophysiology

The defect that results in CF is an abnormal gene located on the long arm of chromosome 7 that codes for a protein known as the cystic fibrosis transmembrane regulator (CFTR). This protein becomes incorporated into the lipid bilayer of the epithelial surface of the cell and functions as a chloride channel. Defective cyclic adenosine monophosphate (cAMP)-regulated chloride secretion through a mutated CFTR protein results in dehydrated airway surface fluid, which impedes the normal ciliary function, resulting in chronic infection and atelectasis. In addition, CFTR also down-regulates an epithelial sodium channel (ENaC). When CFTR is defective, this down-regulation is diminished, resulting in increased sodium reabsorption and a further reduction in airway surface fluid. The CFTR gene is expressed in the biliary ducts, vas deferens, pancreatic ducts, sweat glands, and the mucous glands of the lung.

More than 1500 specific mutations have been discovered in the CF gene, and the functional consequences of these mutations at the cellular level have been classified into five types. Clinical features correlate with the amount of CFTR activity at the epithelial surface. As the amount of residual CFTR declines, more organ systems are involved. Classes I, II, and III mutations result from abnormal protein production, trafficking through the cell, and regulation at the apical cell surface. These mutations result in 1% CFTR activity and are associated with more severe disease, worse pulmonary function, and pancreatic insufficient (PI) phenotype. The ΔF508 mutation, the most common mutation affecting 70% of CF mutations in the U.S. population, results from the deletion of a phenylalanine at amino acid position 508. In the presence of two copies of this mutation, a patient manifests a PI phenotype.

In Classes IV and V mutations, CFTR is present on the apical surface but chloride channel conduction is defective, resulting in 5% residual CFTR activity and the pancreatic sufficient (PS) phenotype. In the PS phenotype, respiratory symptoms might not present until adulthood, and sufficient pancreatic function is maintained to prevent malabsorption. Because PS patients have residual pancreatic function, there is adequate pancreatic tissue to become inflamed, and these patients might present with recurrent pancreatitis. Residual CFTR function is also manifested in the sweat gland, with sweat tests in the borderline range (40–60 mEq/L). The presence of a class IV or V mutation with a Δ508 mutation results in a PS phenotype.

At the end of intron 8, a noncoding region of the CFTR gene, a stretch of 5, 7, or 9 thymidine residues is found, designated the 5T, 7T, or 9T allele. A lower number of thymidines results in less efficient splicing of CFTR transcripts and therefore a lower amount of functional CFTR protein. The 5T allele has been classified as a mutation causing mild disease with partial penetrance. The 5T polymorphism is found on about 21% of the CFTR genes derived from patients with congenital bilateral absence of the vas deferens (CBAVD). In CBAVD there is 10% CFTR activity, which is sufficient to have obstructive azoospermia as the only clinical manifestation (Box 1).

BOX 1 Differentiating Between Criteria of CFTR Genotypes

Pancreatic Insufficient

Class I, II, or III mutation
1% CFTR activity
Absent or minimal chloride channel function
Elevated sweat chloride >60 mmol/L
Classic early presentation (50% diagnosed by 6 months of age)
Median survival is 37.4 years
Patients require pancreatic enzymes
Fecal pancreatic elastase-1 <100 µg/g
Atrophic scarred pancreas
Risk of diabetes mellitus increases with age

Pancreatic Sufficient

Class IV or V mutation
5% CFTR activity
Some chloride channel function
Borderline or mildly elevated sweat chloride (40–60 mmol/L)
Atypical late presentation (sometimes in adulthood)
Survival to 50 years is not uncommon
No pancreatic enzyme supplement required
Fecal pancreatic elastase-1 >250 µg/g
Adequate functional pancreatic tissue to develop recurrent pancreatitis
Lower risk of diabetes mellitus

CFTR=cystic fibrosis transmembrane regulator (protein).

Clinical Presentation

GASTROINTESTINAL

About 15% of infants present with meconium ileus, obstruction of the distal ileum with thickened viscid meconium. Prenatal ultrasound might detect echogenic bowel, which suggests CF. Infants present shortly after birth with feeding intolerance and a distended abdomen that requires surgical intervention. Colostomies are placed to permit irrigation to dilate the underdeveloped microcolon, and resection of the terminal ileum is sometimes required. In utero perforation of the bowel can occur, manifesting with calcifications on abdominal x-ray.

The distal intestinal obstruction syndrome (DIOS) is an intestinal obstruction seen in older CF patients. It manifests with abdominal pain, constipation, and a palpable mass in the right lower quadrant consisting of viscous mucus and undigested fecal material that causes obstruction at the ileocecal valve. This can predispose to intussusception. The obstruction is treated by oral or nasogastric administration of polyethylene glycol and electrolytes (GoLYTELY),[1] an osmotic agent, which causes water to be retained in the intestine, inducing diarrhea. Rectal prolapse and the meconium plug syndrome, in which there is delayed passage of meconium in the newborn period, are additional reasons for referring a child for a sweat test.

Infants might also present with prolonged obstructive jaundice, which can progress to hepatic steatosis, complete biliary obstruction, and acholic stools. In the biliary tree, sludging of bile due to inadequate chloride and fluid transfer into the bile canaliculus can result in focal biliary cirrhosis and cholethiasis. Approximately 2% of patients progress to multilobular cirrhosis with portal hypertension, hypersplenism, and esophageal varices. Progression to liver failure and the need for transplantation is a possibility. Ursodeoxycholic acid (Actigall),[1] a cholorectic bile acid that increases the flow of bile, has been shown to lower hepatic enzymes and delay the progression of liver disease.

Chloride channel dysfunction in the pancreas results in thickened secretions within the pancreatic ducts and obstruction to the flow of pancreatic chyle. Approximately 85% of patients with CF develop exocrine pancreatic insufficiency. The inadequate production of pancreatic lipase and amylase results in fat and protein malabsorption, steatorrhea, failure to thrive, hypoalbuminemia, and edema. The buffering capacity of pancreatic chyle is diminished, resulting in decreased effectiveness of pancreatic enzyme replacement therapy, which is optimally effective at a neutral pH.

The 72-hour recording of dietary intake and stool collection for quantitative determination of fecal fat content is inconvenient and prone to collection errors in the nonresearch setting. The pancreatic enzyme elastase-1 is stable during intestinal transit and is not affected by porcine pancreatic replacement therapy. The measurement of fecal elastase-1 in stool has been found to be a less cumbersome and a sensitive assay to assess pancreatic function. This can be performed on a small specimen and does not require a timed collection.

Treatment with pancreatic enzyme replacement (pancrelipase [Creon, Pancrease]) improves linear growth and weight gain. The recommended dose per meal is 1000 to 2500 U/kg/dose. A high-fat diet is recommended to increase caloric intake to 150 kcal/kg of body weight, which is necessary to ensure optimal growth. The report of the Cystic Fibrosis Foundation Patient Registry indicates that 14% of CF patients are below the 5th percentile for height and 22% are below the 10th percentile for weight. Because nutritional failure as measured by body mass index (BMI) has been shown to be a predictor of progressive pulmonary deterioration, aggressive use of nutritional supplementation and nighttime gastrostomy feeds are advocated to improve the quality of life and lung function. Supplementation of fat-soluble vitamins is necessary to prevent nutritional deficiency.

Because CF patients are living longer, progressive fibrosis of the pancreas results in an increased incidence of diabetes, which is seen in 15% of CF patients. Annual glucose tolerance testing has become the standard of care in adolescents and adults to diagnose glucose intolerance before the onset of diabetes, which has been found to result in deterioration of lung function. Respiratory infection and steroid therapy can result in hyperglycemia, leading to a need for insulin before the patient develops frank diabetes. Because there are reductions of both insulin and glucagon, ketoacidosis is rare.

Infants with CF lose a great deal of salt in their sweat and can develop hyponatremic dehydration, heat prostration, and hypochloremic alkalosis. Salt supplementation is the norm, especially during warm summer months.

PULMONARY

The lungs in CF are normal at birth. In young CF patients *Staphylococcus aureus* and *Haemophilus influenzae* are common early colonizers, but as patients age, *Pseudomonas aeruginosa* becomes the predominant organism and is present in the sputum of 80% of adults. *P. aeruginosa* undergoes a mucoid transformation, which interferes with the effectiveness of antibiotic therapy. Because the acquisition of *P. aeruginosa* has been correlated with a more rapid deterioration of lung function and decreased survival, aggressive antibiotic therapy is initiated when this organism is isolated to prevent chronic colonization of the airway.

Burkholderia cepacia, an organism that is intrinsically resistant to a broad range of antibiotics, has been associated with poorer lung function. Nine genetically distinct species, known as genomovars, make up the *B. cepacia* complex. *Burkholderia cenocepacia* and *Burkholderia multivorans* are most commonly isolated from CF patients. The transmission of these organisms and other multiply resistant gram-negative bacteria from person to person in CF clinics and summer camps has resulted in strict infection-control guidelines.

A chronic cough, recurrent chest infections, purulent sputum, digital clubbing, chronic sinusitis, and nasal polyps are common presenting symptoms in CF. The incidence of recurrent pneumothorax is increased in CF, and chemical pleurodesis or pleurectomy are often required. Massive hemoptysis and recurrent episodes of hemoptysis are often a result of collateral bronchial arteries that can require embolization. CF patients often have opacification of the sinuses and nasal polyposis (Box 2).

BOX 2 Clinical Presentation of Cystic Fibrosis

Gastrointesinal

Failure to thrive
Malabsorption
Meconium ileus
Meconium plug syndrome
Rectal prolapse
Recurrent pancreatitis
Steatorrhea

Pulmonary

Bronchiectasis
Chronic cough
Chronic sinusitis
Digital clubbing
Nasal polyps
Purulent bronchitis
Recurrent and persistent pneumonia

Other

Growth failure
Hyponatremia and dehydration
Male infertility

---

[1]Not FDA approved for this indication.

Diagnosis

Sweat testing remains the standard for making the diagnosis of CF. The elevation of the chloride results from CFTR chloride channel dysfunction in the sweat ducts, where reabsorption of chloride occurs. Pilocarpine is iontophoresized into the skin to stimulate sweating. A chloride level greater than 60 mEq/L is consistent with the diagnosis of CF, but the result must be interpreted in the context of the clinical picture. The borderline range for sweat chloride is 40 to 60 mEq/L. Additional testing is necessary to confirm the diagnosis when the sweat test is in the borderline range. False-positive sweat test results can occur with malnutrition, Addison's disease, and ectodermal dysplasia, so it is essential to confirm the diagnosis with a confirmatory sweat test or a genetic analysis, or both. Sweat tests can be performed after 2 weeks of age, at which time a sufficient quantity of sweat can be collected to ensure a proper analysis.

Genetic analysis for mutations known to cause CF symptoms is an alternative diagnostic approach. The presence of two abnormal CFTR mutations known to cause CF disease predicts with a high degree of certainty that a patient has CF. Prenatal screening is recommended by the American College of Obstetrics and Gynecology for pregnant white women. When both parents are found to be carriers, amniocentesis and chorionic villous sampling can be used to assess the 25% chance of having an infant affected by CF.

The active transport of ions generates a transepithelial electrical potential difference (PD). Abnormalities of chloride ion transport in patients with CF are associated with a different pattern of PD compared with normal epithelium. This assay thus provides a direct view of the physiology at the ion channel level. Nasal PD measurements help to resolve diagnostic dilemmas in atypical patients and a change of PD measurement toward normal is an outcome measure of therapeutic interventions that correct the chloride channel dysfunction.

Three features distinguish the nasal PD in a patient with CF. A high basal PD reflects enhanced sodium transport across a relatively chloride impermeable membrane. A larger inhibition of PD after nasal perfusion with the sodium channel inhibitor amilorlide reflects inhibition of accelerated sodium transport. Little or no change in PD in response to perfusion of the nasal epithelial surface with a chloride-free solution in conjunction with isoproterenol reflects an absence of CFTR-mediated chloride secretion.

Newborn screening for CF has been shown to improve nutritional and neurodevelopmental outcomes. Trypsinogen, a precursor of trypsin, is commonly elevated in the serum of newborns with CF. Infants with CF have elevated immunoreactive trypsinogen (IRT) levels for 2 to 3 weeks after birth. When the IRT is elevated in a blood specimen collected shortly after birth, then an analysis for the presence of CF mutations on the same blood specimen or a persistent elevation of IRT at 2 to 3 weeks of age in a repeat blood specimen are two different methods to determine which infants should be referred for sweat testing. Mutation analysis performed during newborn screening detects carriers of CF mutations, and genetic counseling for these families is warranted to permit informed decisions concerning future pregnancies.

Treatment

Therapeutic interventions are shown in Figure 1.

GENE THERAPY

The goal of gene therapy is to correct the basic defect by inserting a normal functioning gene into the ciliated cells in the submucous glands that express abnormal CFTR function. Initial attempts using the adenovirus as the vehicle for transporting the gene into the cells lining the airway appeared promising; however, the host immune response to the virus has limited the effectiveness of this approach. The ideal vector would efficiently deliver the gene to the appropriate target cell without causing toxicity or an inflammatory response.

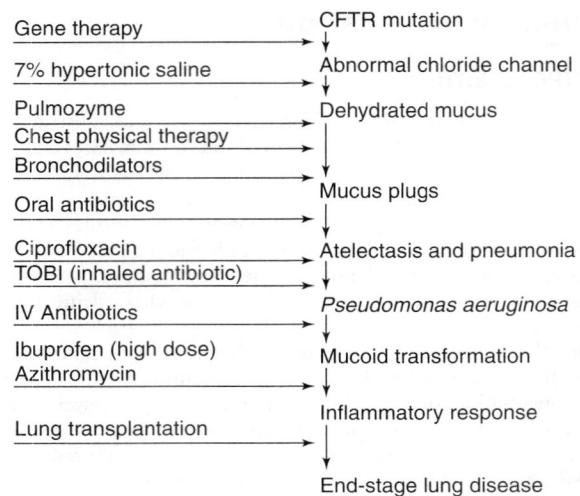

FIGURE 1. Therapeutic interventions for cystic fibrosis lung disease.

Although gene therapy offers the potential to correct the basic defect of CF, many technical barriers to effective gene therapy need to be addressed to permit this form of therapy to become an effective treatment. Liposomes are being evaluated as an alternate delivery system for administering the normal gene into epithelial cells.

HYDRATION OF AIRWAY SURFACE FLUID

Hypertonic saline (Hyper-sal), at a 7% concentration,[6] has been shown to increase the hydration of the airway surface fluid and reduce the frequency of pulmonary exacerbations. This recent addition to the therapeutic treatment regimen has been shown to facilitate the clearance of airway mucus, resulting in improved pulmonary function, and to decrease the frequency of pulmonary exacerbations. Hypertonic saline induces coughing and bronchospasm and is administered following bronchodilator therapy.

PHYSICAL THERAPY

Airway clearance can be performed using various techniques, including conventional percussion therapy, pneumatically inflated chest vest percussion device, oscillating positive pressure devices such as the Flutter or Acapella, autogenic drainage, and exercise. These techniques are recommended on a daily basis to help mobilize secretions and prevent the complications related to persistent accumulation of airway mucus.

BRONCHODILATORS

Airway hyperreactivity is present in 50% to 60% of CF patients. β-Agonists keep airways open and facilitate airway clearance by increasing ciliary beat frequency and smooth muscle relaxation. The spirometric response to β-agonists should be monitored because with worsening bronchiectasis and the development of floppy airways, airflow may be impaired. Because anticholinergics alter viscosity of mucus and can have an adverse effect on gastrointestinal motility, this class of bronchodilator has not been recommended for routine use in CF by a consensus conference of the Cystic Fibrosis Foundation.

ANTIBIOTICS

Aggressive use of antibiotics for the chronic bacterial colonization of the airways in CF has resulted in improving longevity and quality of life. Prophylactic inhaled antibiotics have been effective in CF

---

[6]May be compounded by pharmacists.

patients to decrease the bacterial burden in the CF airway. Alternate-month therapy with a 300-mg aerosol preparation of tobramycin (TOBI) improves lung function, delays the time to the onset of pulmonary exacerbation, and decreases the need for hospitalization. A preparation of aztreonam (Cayston) for inhalation,[1] which is administered by a very efficient portable nebulizer (Altera nebulizer system), has recently been approved by the FDA.

Pulmonary exacerbations are characterized by an increased cough, copious purulent sputum, decreased appetite, weight loss, and decreased exercise tolerance. Quinolone antibiotics are effective for treating *P. aeruginosa* in an oral preparation, but the development of resistance to this class of drug is a limiting factor. Ciprofloxacin (Cipro) is not approved by the FDA for use in children, but there is considerable experience with this drug in children with CF. When oral and inhaled antibiotics are not effective, hospitalization for aggressive airway clearance and a 10- to 14-day course of IV antibiotics is indicated. A combination of two drugs (usually an aminoglycoside and a β-lactam semisynthetic penicillin or a cephalosporin) is selected based on susceptibility of the organism recovered by culture of sputum or a deep throat swab. In young children who are not able to produce sputum, bronchoscopy may be performed to obtain a specimen for culture and sensitivity and to assess the amount of airway inflammation.

MUCOLYTIC THERAPY

DNase (Pulmozyme) is a nebulized mucolytic agent that cleaves neutrophil-derived DNA that contributes to the thick airway secretions that clog the CF airways. Daily inhalation therapy (2.5 mg) reduces sputum viscosity, facilitating airway clearance and resulting in a 5% improvement in lung function. This therapy has largely replaced treatment with *N*-acetylcysteine (Mucomyst),[1] which causes bronchial irritation.

ANTIINFLAMMATORY THERAPY

There has been growing awareness of the role of the host inflammatory responses in the progression of CF lung disease. Chronic endobronchial colonization with bacteria results in the release of proinflammatory mediators interleukin (IL)-8 and nuclear factor (NF)-κB. These mediators recruit neutrophils into the airway; the neutrophils release elastase, protease, superoxide ions, and hydroxyl radicals, which damage lung tissue and contribute to the development of bronchiectasis.

Corticosteroids

Alternate-day systemic steroids were studied in a multicenter placebo-controlled study as a therapeutic intervention to decrease the inflammatory response in the CF airway. Significant risks of growth impairment, diabetes, and cataracts were found. Although inhaled steroids are commonly prescribed for CF patients, there is no double-blind study to demonstrate benefit of long-term therapy in CF patients who do not have a component of asthma.

Nonsteroidal Antiinflammatory Drugs

Oral administration of twice-daily high-dose ibuprofen[1] (20–30 mg/kg)[3] to achieve peak plasma concentration of 50 to 100 μg/mL interferes with neutrophil migration and inhibits the activation of NF-κB. Konstan studied 85 CF patients and found that ibuprofen therapy results in less decline in lung function, fewer hospitalizations, and improved weight gain. This effect is most pronounced in patients who are younger than 13 years and have minimal lung disease. Although prolonged use of this therapy has been shown to have ongoing benefit, the risk of GI side effects has limited the implementation of this therapy by most CF patients.

Macrolide antibiotics (azithromycin [Zithromax])[1] are not considered effective in the treatment of infection with *P. aeruginosa*, but a number of clinical trials have demonstrated a modest improvement in lung function and a decrease in the frequency of infectious exacerbations and need for antibiotic therapy in CF patients chronically colonized with *P. aeruginosa*. The mechanisms of action are not well understood but are believed to be related to a number of antiinflammatory and immunomodulatory effects of this class of antibiotic. The expression of *P. aeruginosa* pathogenicity factors and neutrophil recruitment appear to be altered by chronic macrolide therapy.

Oxygen therapy to correct alveolar hypoxia is effective to prevent pulmonary hypertension in CF patients with severe lung disease. Pulmonary hypertension results from pulmonary vascular remodeling, which results in increased pulmonary vascular resistance. Cor pulmonale contributes to the morbidity of CF with right heart failure, progressive exercise intolerance, and risk of syncope.

LUNG TRANSPLANTATION

Approximately 150 patients receive bilateral cadaveric lung transplants per year. Evaluation at a lung transplant center is considered when progressive deterioration in lung function results in a forced expiratory volume in one second (FEV_1) less than 30% predicted. Survival rates in CF lung-transplant recipients are comparable with other groups of patients. The availability of donor organs continues to be a limiting factor, and the disparity between donor availability and a growing recipient pool has progressively lengthened the waiting time for organs and has increased the mortality for patients awaiting lung transplantation. Living-donor lobar transplantation, which involves removal of both diseased lungs from the recipient and the implantation of two lower lobes donated by two donors, is an alternative for CF patients awaiting lung transplantation.

REFERENCES

http://www.genet.sickkids.or.ca/cftr/app

Cystic Fibrosis Foundation. Cystic Fibrosis Foundation Patient Registry, 2005 Annual Data Report to the Center Directors. Bethesda Md: Cystic Fibrosis Foundation; 2006.

Solomon MP, Wilson DC, Corey M, et al. Glucose intolerance in children with cystic fibrosis. J Pediatr 2003;142:128–32.

Konstan MW, Byard PJ, Hoppel CL, Davis PB. Effect of high-dose ibuprofen in patients with cystic fibrosis. N Engl J Med 1995;332(13):848–54.

Obstructive Sleep Apnea

Method of
Melinda V. Davis-Malesevich, MD, and
Masayoshi Takashima, MD

Sleep-disordered breathing encompasses the spectrum from upper airway resistance syndrome to obstructive sleep apnea (OSA). OSA is characterized by episodes of partial or complete upper airway collapse leading to cessation or reduction of airflow. Such events lead to oxygen desaturation and sleep fragmentation, causing excessive daytime sleepiness, morning headaches, depression, memory loss, impaired alertness, decreased libido, and reduced cognitive function. Nighttime symptoms are often more telling, and obtaining a sleep history from a bed partner is exceptionally helpful. The most common symptoms include loud snoring, restless sleep, choking or gasping episodes, and awakenings during sleep. Nocturnal perspiration, nocturia, and symptoms of nocturnal gastroesophageal reflux are also commonly associated with severe OSA.

As the severity of OSA typically increases with age, nightly hypoventilation and activation of the sympathetic nervous system lead to pathophysiologic derangements, such as hypertension, ischemic heart disease, myocardial infarction, stroke, arrhythmia, and premature death.

---

[1]Not FDA approved for this indication.
[3]Exceeds dosage recommended by the manufacturer.

Apnea–hypopnea index (AHI): Sum of apneas and hypopneas per hour of sleep.
Obstructive apnea: Cessation of airflow for ≥10 seconds associated with ongoing ventilatory effort.
Obstructive hypopnea: Decreased airflow of ≥50% for ≥10 seconds despite ongoing effort, resulting in oxyhemoglobin desaturation of ≥4%.
Obstructive sleep apnea (OSA): AHI >5 events per hour of sleep, often associated with oxygen desaturation <90%. Mild OSA is defined by an AHI of 5 to 15. Moderate OSA is an AHI 15 to 30, and severe OSA is an AHI >30.
Obstructive sleep apnea syndrome: OSA in association with daytime symptoms of excessive sleepiness or other neurobehavioral symptoms.
Primary snoring: Snoring with an AHI <5 and no complaints of excessive daytime sleepiness.
Respiratory effort–related arousals: Sleep fragmentation that is caused by arousals from increasing respiratory effort but that does not meet criteria for an apnea or hypopnea. The event lasts longer than 10 seconds.
Respiratory disturbance index: Sum of apneas, hypopneas, and respiratory effort–related arousals per hour of sleep.
Upper airway resistance syndrome (UARS): Snoring in association with AHI <5, frequent arousals, and abnormally negative midesophageal pressure (less than −10 cm H_2O) or increased diaphragmatic electromyogram activity.

An apnea–hypopnea index (AHI) of greater than 5 has been shown to be associated with increased risk of cerebrovascular accident, AHI greater than 20 is associated with increased mortality, and patients with oxygen desaturation below 90% have an elevated incidence of cardiac arrhythmias. These potentially severe consequences, along with a patient's decreased quality of life, substantiate the need for early recognition and treatment.

Definitions of terms related to sleep apnea are listed in Box 1.

Epidemiology

Based on available population-based studies, the prevalence of OSA among adults between 30 and 60 years of age is estimated to be 9% for women and 24% for men, and approximately 9% of men and 4% of women have at least moderate disease (AHI 15 to 30). OSA remains undiagnosed in 70% to 80% of patients because their symptoms are often vague, and OSA must be diagnosed with polysomnography.

Risk Factors

Elderly persons 65 years and older have a higher prevalence of obstructive sleep apnea secondary to decreased muscle tone.

Obesity (body mass index [BMI] greater than 30 kg/m^2) is a risk factor for OSA. A 10% increase in weight is associated with a sixfold increase in risk for development of OSA, and a 10% weight loss is associated with 26% decrease in AHI. There is evidence of a potential link between OSA and insulin resistance.

Approximately 30% of hypertensive persons have OSA. Patients with moderate to severe OSA have a 2.9 odds ratio of developing hypertension. Up to 50% of patients with cardiovascular disease have OSA, even after adjusting for hypertension and other comorbid conditions.

Male patients are nearly twice as likely to have OSA as female patients. Estrogen and progesterone might have a protective role because population-based studies have demonstrated that postmenopausal women have a two- to threefold increased risk of OSA compared to premenopausal women.

African Americans and Asians are at greater risk for OSA than whites. Being African American is an independent risk factor for severe sleep-disordered breathing, with an odds ratio of 2.55 compared with whites. Asians have a narrower cranial base, a higher Mallampati score, smaller thyromental distance, and steeper thyromental plane than whites, which might account for their increased risk.

Pathophysiology

Airway obstruction leading to OSA can occur anywhere along the pathway from the nostrils, soft palate, hypopharynx, base of tongue, and the epiglottis. The airway lacks skeletal structure and is vulnerable to influences such as muscle tone, fat deposition, and tissue redundancy.

Prevention

Lifestyle modification can prevent OSA. Patients should adopt a healthy and athletic lifestyle to develop good muscle tone and weight loss, avoid sedatives and alcohol at bedtime, establish regular sleeping patterns, avoid the supine sleeping position, and elevate the head when sleeping.

Diagnosis

Definitive diagnosis of OSA is made by polysomnography. Mild OSA is defined as an AHI of 5 to 15 per hour, moderate OSA is an AHI of 15 to 30 per hour, and severe OSA is an AHI greater than 30 per hour. Patients spend the night in a sleep laboratory during which multiple physiologic variables are continuously monitored. These include electroencephalogram (EEG), electrooculogram (EOG), electromyogram (EMG), oronasal airflow, chest wall effort, body position, snore volume, electrocardiogram (ECG), and oxyhemoglobin saturation. Laboratory testing also includes a complete accounting of sleep variables, monitoring of cardiac rhythm, and assessment of possible restless legs syndrome (RLS) or periodic limb movements (PLMs) during sleep. This information enables the clinician to determine the severity of the condition and identifies potentially relevant comorbidities.

 CURRENT DIAGNOSIS

Symptoms

- Excessive daytime fatigue and somnolence
- Morning headaches
- Loud snoring and gasping for air
- Witnessed apneic episodes following loud snoring
- Frequent nocturia with no other underlying etiology
- Hypertension

Clinical Signs and Risk Factors

- Central obesity with body mass index (BMI) >30 kg/m^2
- Large neck circumference (>17 inches in men, >16 inches in women)
- Being male or a postmenopausal woman
- Use of sedatives or alcohol before going to bed
- Family history of sleep apnea
- Craniofacial abnormalities: retrognathia, micrognathia, congenital malformations

A thorough diagnostic study requires at least 6 hours of sleep, allowing assessment of variability related to sleep stages. If there are sufficient apneas or hypopneas during the first half of the study (ideally 4 hours of diagnostic testing, with a minimum of 2 hours if an AHI >40 is confirmed), a split-night study may be performed, in which the second half of the night (minimum of 3 hours of sleep) is devoted to titration of continuous positive airway pressure (CPAP) therapy. If the criteria for a split-night sleep study are not achieved during the night, a second night for titration study is ordered. The split-night protocol is a cost-effective use of laboratory resources that is particularly well suited for patients with severe OSA.

According to the Institute for Clinical Systems Improvement (ICSI), polysomnography should be performed in patients with symptoms of OSA and one or more of the following: cardiovascular disease, hypertension, coronary artery disease, obesity, sleep complaint, type 2 diabetes mellitus, recurrent atrial fibrillation, and large neck circumference.

Treatment

Initially, patients should be counseled to avoid practices that can potentially worsen the severity of OSA. Relaxation caused by the use of CNS depressants before sleep (alcohol, sleep medications, pain medications) can worsen upper airway collapse during sleep and should be discouraged. In some patients with positional OSA, avoiding the supine position during sleep might suffice in helping normalize ventilation during sleep. Sewing a tennis ball onto the backs of pajamas or wearing a knapsack filled with polystyrene foam (Styrofoam) has been useful in promoting non-supine sleep. If significant upper airway pathology is identified (nasal septum deviation, enlarged tonsils, craniofacial abnormalities), surgical consultation should be pursued. Weight loss and maintenance should always play a role in the treatment of these patients.

CONTINUOUS POSITIVE AIRWAY PRESSURE THERAPY

CPAP remains the therapeutic mainstay for primary treatment of OSA. It serves as a pneumatic stent for the upper airway and is effective in reducing the physiologic abnormalities measured on polysomnography. Additionally, CPAP is believed to augment lung volumes and elicit a reflex that increases tone in the upper airway musculature. Overall, it has been shown to reduce AHI, improve quality of life, and reduce cardiovascular risk.

There are many manufacturers of CPAP devices and many interfaces that help maximize comfort with treatment. Expiratory pressure release (EPR) is available through a couple of CPAP manufacturers. EPR does not seem to compromise the effectiveness of CPAP therapy and improves the patient's sense of comfort with therapy, but it does not seem to systematically improve the level of adherence.

CURRENT THERAPY

- Gold standard for treatment is positive airway pressure
- Weight loss, smoking cessation, avoidance of sedatives
- Improvement of sleep hygiene and sleep schedule
- Minimally invasive procedures (oral appliances, palatal stents, radiofrequency turbinate reductions) may be beneficial for a select patient population
- Surgical therapy is usually reserved for patients not tolerating or unable to use CPAP or BiPAP
- Initial procedures are focused on decreasing upper airway resistance to improve compliance with CPAP or BiPAP
- Identification of anatomic sites of obstruction is critical to successful surgical outcomes

Abbreviations: BiPAP = bilevel positive airway pressure; CPAP = continuous positive airway pressure.

Bi-level respiratory-assist devices deliver alternating levels of positive airway pressure and might be considered an alternative therapeutic option when standard CPAP is not tolerated or when oxygen saturation is not raised sufficiently with standard CPAP. In some cases of severe OSA (in particular among patients with underlying pulmonary conditions), supplemental oxygen can be used in conjunction with CPAP therapy.

The main disadvantage with positive airway pressure treatment is poor compliance. Short-term adherence data reveal compliance with CPAP therapy is variable, with 29% to 83% of patients using CPAP for less than 4 hours per night. Treatment is effective as long as the patient uses the device for the entire night, every night. The use of integrated heated humidifiers has minimized issues of upper airway dryness and has helped improve adherence to therapy.

ORAL APPLIANCES

Prostheses worn in the mouth during sleep can help maintain a patent airway, especially in patients who sleep on their back and experience airway collapse secondary to the tongue. In general, there are two types of appliances, mandibular-advancement appliances and tongue-retaining devices. The mandibular-advancement appliances are currently used more often and have been more widely studied. They require viable dentition for retention. They are fitted to the maxillary and mandibular dentition to enable the protrusion of the mandible and therefore increase oropharyngeal patency. The most common side effect is drooling. Temporomandibular joint pain might limit the viability of this therapy. Chronic use of the appliance can result in a change of the dental occlusion. A dentist with expertise in sleep medicine should ideally implement and monitor this type of treatment.

SURGICAL PROCEDURES

Patients with an identifiable anatomic upper airway (soft tissue) obstruction or craniofacial abnormality might benefit from surgery. A variety of soft-tissue procedures help stabilize the retropalatal region, and others are intended to stabilize the retrolingual airway (Box 2). Office-based procedures are available, such as radiofrequency ablation of the soft palate and soft palate stents, which are intended to stiffen the soft palate and thereby decrease snoring and respiratory events. A substantially more invasive procedure, the maxillomandibular advancement, has been shown very effective in a number of case series. Of course, a tracheostomy completely bypasses the upper airway, curing sleep apnea, but it is not without its comorbidities, such as wound care issues.

BOX 2   Treatments for Obstructive Sleep Apnea

Nasal Obstruction
Septoplasty
Rhinoplasty or nasal valve surgery
Turbinate reduction

Retropalatal Obstruction
Uvulopalatopharyngoplasty
Z-palatoplasty
Lateral pharyngoplasty
Palatal stents
Radiofrequency soft palate surgery

Retrolingual Obstruction
Radiofrequency reduction of the base of the tongue
Lingual tonsillectomy
Genioglossus advancement
Hyoid suspension
Partial glossectomy
Tongue base suspension
Maxillomandibular advancement

It is hard to predict which patients are likely to have a successful surgical outcome. Part of the reason is the difficulty associated with accurately identifying the site(s) of obstruction. Sleep endoscopy, a relatively new technique, helps define this better. Patients are examined in a drug-induced sleep-resembling relaxed state. As the patient snores and obstructs while sleeping, a flexible fiberoptic scope is passed through the nose to evaluate the upper airway to reveal the site of obstruction. The data on the validity of this procedure are scant yet promising.

Monitoring

The patient's response to therapy needs to be monitored. In the case of CPAP therapy, monitoring of CPAP adherence is critical, because subjective reports are inaccurate. Resolution of excessive sleepiness is the desired outcome for patients who are symptomatic at baseline. If excessive sleepiness remains problematic despite documentation of desirable CPAP adherence, treatment with modafinil (Provigil) 100 to 400 mg in the morning might be considered. Other potential conditions affecting sleep need to be monitored and, if necessary, treated. Often, other conditions such as poor sleep hygiene, restless legs syndrome, periodic limb movements, or psychophysiologic insomnia interfere with adequate response to therapy.

For patients who undergo surgery, retesting is indicated. The interval at which retesting should be done depends on the type of surgery that was performed. Retesting 3 months following the surgical intervention is adequate in most cases.

REFERENCES

Al Lawati NM, Patel SR, Ayas NT. Epidemiology, risk factors, and consequences of obstructive sleep apnea and short sleep duration. Prog Cardiovasc Dis 2009;51:285–93.
Ancoli-Israel S, Klauber MR, Stepnowsky C, et al. Sleep-disordered breathing in African-American elderly. Am J Respir Crit Care Med 1995;52:1946–9.
Fujita S, Conway W, Zorick F, Roth T. Surgical correction of anatomic abnormalities in obstructive sleep apnea syndrome; Uvulopalatopharyngoplasty. Otolaryngol Head Neck Surg 1981;89(6):923–34.
Institute for Clinical Systems Improvement (ICSI) . Diagnosis and Treatment of Obstructive Sleep Apnea in Adults. Bloomington, MN: Institute for Clinical Systems Improvement; 2008.
Li KK, Powell NB, Kushida C, et al. A comparison of Asian and white patients with obstructive sleep apnea syndrome. Laryngoscope 1999;109:1937–40.
Peppard PE, Young T, Palta M, et al. Prospective study of the association between sleep-disordered breathing and hypertension. N Engl J Med 2000;342:1378–84.
Peppard PE, Young T, Palta M, et al. Longitudinal study of moderate weight change and sleep-disordered breathing. JAMA 2000;284:3015–21.
Punjabi NM. The epidemiology of adult obstructive sleep apnea. Proc Am Thorac Soc 2008;5:136–43.
Quan SF, Howard BV, Iber C, et al. The Sleep Heart Health Study: Design, rationale, and methods. Sleep 1997;20:1077–85.
Sher AE, Schechtman KB, Piccirillo JF. The efficacy of surgical modifications of the upper airway in adults with obstructive sleep apnea syndrome. Sleep 1996;19(2):156–77.

Primary Lung Cancer

Method of
Robert A. Kratzke, MD, and Manish R. Patel, DO

Lung cancer is the leading cause of cancer-related death in North America for both men and women. It is not the most common cancer, but most patients with lung cancer are diagnosed at a late stage, accounting for the excess mortality. In the United States, lung cancer accounts for only 13% of new cancer cases but almost one third of cancer-related deaths. Although approximately one third of patients are diagnosed at an early stage, the 5-year survival rate for all patients with lung cancer is less than 20%.

Lung cancer is broadly divided into two groups, small cell lung cancer (SCLC) and non–small cell lung cancer (NSCLC). Approximately 80% of lung cancers are NSCLC, and most of those are squamous carcinomas, adenocarcinomas, or bronchoalveolar carcinomas. Carcinoid tumors and other neuroendocrine tumors are less common, and adenoid cystic carcinomas are rare. Although there is increasing awareness of the importance of histologic subtype in determining responses to newer therapies, the concept of histology-targeted therapy is still evolving, and the standard treatments for NSCLC are generally the same regardless of the histologic subtype.

Epidemiology

Lung cancer occurs most commonly in middle-aged and elderly people. The peak incidence occurs in those aged 65 to 85 years. It is extremely rare in people younger than 30 years of age, and the incidence decreases after 85 years. Before the 1960s, lung cancer was rare among women. However, in North America, the current incidence of lung cancer is almost equal between men and women.

The incidence is decreasing among men and has leveled off in women over the past decade. Lung cancer occurs at a higher frequency in African Americans. This most likely reflects socioeconomic status more than genetic risk, because cigarette smoking remains more common among African Americans. However, there is some evidence that African Americans are more vulnerable to the effects of tobacco-related carcinogens.

Etiology

Cigarette smoking is the established cause of the lung cancer in general. In particular, there is a positive smoking history in 95% of all cases of SCLC. Eighty percent of newly diagnosed lung cancers are in patients who are current or former smokers. Current smokers with a greater than 20-pack-year smoking history have a 2000-fold greater risk of developing lung cancer compared with nonsmokers. Smoking cessation decreases the risk but does not eliminate it. The risk of developing lung cancer in former smokers remains increased by 2- to 10-fold over that in nonsmokers even decades after smoking cessation. There is also clearly a dose-response relationship in tobacco smoke–induced lung cancer in that the risk is highest among those with the greatest prior cigarette exposure. Pipe and cigar smoke also increase the risk of lung cancer. Among nonsmokers, there is a twofold increased risk of developing lung cancer that is clearly associated with inhalation of second-hand smoke.

 CURRENT DIAGNOSIS

- A history of cigarette smoking is the greatest risk factor.
- Cough, dyspnea, and chest pain are the most common presenting symptoms.
- Diagnosis is made by needle biopsy or pleural fluid cytology.
- The initial staging evaluation should include
  - Positron-emission tomography/computed tomography to evaluate for distant metastasis
  - Magnetic resonance imaging of the brain for small cell lung cancer
- Patients with resectable cancers should have an additional evaluation of mediastinum before resection (i.e., mediastinoscopy or endoscopic ultrasonography)

Other environmental factors have been associated with the development of lung cancer. Up to 20% of lung cancer cases occur among nonsmokers, and this population of patients appears to be rising. Certainly, some of this increase is a result of second-hand exposure to cigarette smoke, but this is difficult to quantify. Asbestos exposure has been associated with the development of lung cancer, and the risk is particularly accentuated by combination with cigarette smoke. Radon exposure has also been associated with the development of lung cancer, particularly in uranium mine workers, in whom the risk approaches 10 times that of the general population. Several other environmental exposures, including chromium, arsenic, and polyvinyl chloride, have been implicated in the development of lung cancers; however, a clear causal link is less well established. Although a patient with a family history of lung cancer has an approximately twofold higher risk, the genetic basis of this finding is not well understood.

Clinical Presentation

The location of tumors and the appearance of paraneoplastic syndromes often determine the clinical presentation of patients with lung cancer (Table 1). Many patients with early-stage disease are asymptomatic and have a mass discovered incidentally on chest radiography or computed tomography (CT) scanning done for some other reason. Centrally located tumors often cause symptoms associated with local effects of the tumor, such as cough, hemoptysis, wheezing, or stridor. Obstruction of the bronchi can lead to postobstructive pneumonia (i.e., pneumonia distal to the obstruction) as the presenting sign, and obstruction of the superior vena cava can lead to the superior vena cava syndrome, with facial edema, bluish discoloration of the upper chest, and shortness of breath. Mediastinal lymph node involvement can cause disruption of the recurrent laryngeal nerve, leading to hoarseness. Tumors arising in the superior sulcus (Pancoast tumors) can lead to a lower brachial plexopathy and Horner's syndrome. Peripheral tumors tend to manifest later as pain when they involve the chest wall or pleura. Pleural effusion may also be the presenting sign for lung cancer.

Lung cancer frequently metastasizes early, and symptoms caused by metastatic lesions may be the first sign of malignancy. Brain metastases are a common presentation, particularly in patients with SCLC, but also in NSCLC. Symptoms such as seizures, nausea and vomiting, headache, and focal neurologic signs may be the initial presentation in such patients. Bony metastases are common in all types of lung cancer and can manifest with pain, pathologic fracture, or spinal cord compression. Liver metastases can cause biliary obstruction and jaundice, but this is not particularly common.

Lung cancers are notable for ectopic production of hormones leading to several paraneoplastic syndromes. These are most commonly described in SCLC but also occur in NSCLC. Probably the most common paraneoplastic syndromes in NSCLC are tumor cachexia and hypercalcemia. Although the causes of tumor cachexia are not well characterized, hyperkalemia is mediated by the production of parathyroid hormone–related peptide. This leads to release of calcium from bones and elevation of calcium in the blood. This syndrome is effectively treated with bisphosphonate therapy. Hypertrophic pulmonary arthropathy can occur with NSCLC or SCLC and is characterized by digital clubbing and periostitis of the long bones demonstrable on plain radiographs. SCLC frequently manifests with paraneoplastic syndromes, the most common being the Lambert-Eaton myasthenic syndrome. Approximately 50% of patients who present with this syndrome have an underlying malignancy, and 95% of those are SCLCs. Other paraneoplastic syndromes related to SCLC are the syndrome of inappropriate antidiuretic hormone, Cushing's syndrome caused by ectopic production of corticotropin, and cerebellar degeneration associated with the elaboration of anti-Yo autoantibodies.

Diagnosis and Evaluation

Once lung cancer is suspected, tissue biopsy is required to make a definitive diagnosis. Several methods can be used to obtain tissue, depending on the location of the tumor. Mediastinal involvement can be assessed by mediastinoscopy; endoscopic ultrasonography is also being increasingly used. Transbronchial biopsy can be performed for centrally located tumors, and the yield may be increased by using endobronchial ultrasonography techniques. For peripheral lesions, CT-guided needle biopsy is usually recommended. If equivocal results are obtained, open procedures using video-assisted thoracoscopic surgery (VATS) are occasionally required. For patients presenting with pleural effusion, cytologic examination of pleural fluid can establish the diagnosis.

Once the diagnosis is confirmed, accurate staging of disease is important to determine the prognosis and appropriate therapy. The first step is to rule out metastatic disease. For NSCLC, fusion positron-emission tomography (PET)-CT scanning is often the best test. Although SCLC tumors are PET-avid tumors, the added benefit of PET-CT over the CT scan is not clear for this disease. For NSCLC, additional imaging of the brain or the bones is not necessary unless symptoms warrant additional evaluation. In SCLC, the frequency of metastasis to these sites warrants a baseline evaluation with bone scanning and magnetic resonance imaging of the brain at the time of diagnosis.

In patients that are potentially resectable, accurate staging of the mediastinum becomes paramount. Abnormal lymphadenopathy on CT is not adequate to determine lymph node involvement for NSCLC. PET-CT scans have higher sensitivity and specificity, but these tests do not replace direct sampling of the lymph nodes by mediastinoscopy. Endoscopic and endobronchial ultrasonography techniques are less invasive, can be combined with lymph node sampling, and are emerging as an appropriate method of staging the mediastinum in experienced hands.

All patients should be evaluated with baseline blood work including a complete blood count, liver function tests, and assessment of renal function. Assessment of the patient's performance status has important prognostic and therapeutic implications and should be

TABLE 1 Clinical Manifestations of Lung Cancer

Tumor Local Effects	Distant Metastases	Paraneoplastic Syndromes
Cough	Bone pain	Hypercalcemia
Dyspnea	Neurologic symptoms	SIADH
Hemoptysis	Headache	Lambert-Eaton syndrome
Chest pain	Nausea and vomiting	Cerebellar ataxia
Hoarseness	Weight loss	Encephalitis
Horner's syndrome	Fatigue	Cachexia/anorexia
SVC syndrome	Abdominal pain	Cushing's syndrome
Postobstructive pneumonia	Spinal cord compression	
Pericardial effusion	Pathologic fracture	

Abbreviations: SIADH = syndrome of inappropriate antidiuretic hormone; SVC = superior vena cava.

CURRENT THERAPY

Non–small cell lung cancer

- Stage I: Surgical resection
- Stage II: Surgery + adjuvant chemotherapy
- Stage IIIA: Induction chemotherapy
  - Responders: Surgery with or without XRT
  - Nonresponders: Concurrent chemotherapy + XRT
- Stage IIIB: Concurrent chemotherapy and XRT
- Stage IV: Chemotherapy and drugs targeting the epidermal growth factor receptor
  - 1st line: Platinum doublet chemotherapy with bevacizumab (Avastin) or cetuximab (Erbitux)
  - 2nd line: Pemetrexed (Alimta), docetaxel (Taxotere), or erlotinib (Tarceva) as a single agent

Small cell lung cancer

- Limited stage: Concurrent chemotherapy + XRT; PCI for responders
- Extensive stage:
  - 1st line: Carboplatin (Paraplatin)/etoposide (VePesid) or cisplatinum (Platinol)/irinotecan (Camptosar) for four cycles; PCI for responders; supportive care
  - 2nd line: Topotecan (Hycamtin)

Abbreviations: PCI = prophylactic cranial irradiation; XRT = radiation therapy.

documented for all patients. Furthermore, for patients who are considered surgically resectable, it is important to assess the tolerability of lobectomy or pneumonectomy. A forced expiratory volume in 1 second (FEV_1) greater than 2 L generally predicts the ability to tolerate pneumonectomy, whereas an FEV_1 of less than 1 L predicts worse outcome with lobectomy. The diffusion capacity of carbon monoxide (DL_{CO}) can also be a useful measurement in borderline cases.

Treatment

NON-SMALL CELL LUNG CANCER

For NSCLC, the stage at diagnosis is the best predictor of overall survival and the most appropriate therapy (Tables 2 and 3).

Stage I

In the tumor-node-metastasis (TNM) staging system, stage I comprises T1 (stage IA) and T2 (stage IB) tumors that do not have any nodal involvement (N0) and no evidence of distant metastasis (M0). The primary mode of therapy for these patients is surgical resection, which results in 5-year survival rates of approximately 70%. Whenever possible, lobectomy with complete mediastinal lymph node dissection is recommended for accurate pathologic staging. Occasionally, pneumonectomy is required based on the location of the primary tumor; however, the morbidity and mortality of this procedure are much higher than with lobectomy. Video-assisted thoracoscopy approaches, if possible, are often desirable and may result in lower surgical morbidity. Surgical resection may not be feasible for all patients, particularly those with poor pulmonary function or poor performance status. For such patients, primary radiotherapy may be considered. Traditional external-beam radiation

TABLE 3 Staging Groups*

Stage	T	N	M
IA	T1	N0	M0
IB	T2	N0	M0
IIA	T1–2a	N0	M0
	T2b	N0	M0
IIB	T2b	N1	M0
	T3	N0	M0
IIIA	T1–2	N2	M0
	T3	N1	M0
	T4	N0–1	M0
IIIB	T4	N2	M0
	Tx	N3	M0
IV	Tx	NX	M1

*For staging of tumors (T), nodes (N), and metastases (M), see Table 2.

TABLE 2 Tumor-Node-Metastasis (TNM) Staging*

Primary Tumor (T)	
T0	No demonstrable tumor
T_{is}	Carcinoma in situ
T1	Tumor <3 cm
T1a	Tumor <2 cm
T1b	Tumor >2 cm and <3 cm
T2	Tumor >3 cm but <7 cm
T2a	Tumor >3 cm but <5 cm
T2b	Tumor >5 cm but <7 cm
T3	Tumor >7 cm or any of the following: • Directly invades the chest wall, diaphragm, phrenic nerve, mediastinal pleura, pericardium, or main bronchus <2 cm from carina • Atelectasis or obstructive pneumonitis of the entire lung • Separate tumor nodules within the same lobe
T4	Tumor of any size that invades the mediastinum, heart, great vessels, esophagus, trachea, recurrent laryngeal nerve, vertebral body, or carina or separate tumor nodule in a different ipsilateral lobe

Regional Lymph Nodes (N)	
N0	No regional lymph node disease
N1	Ipsilateral involvement of hilar, peribronchial, or interlobar nodes including by direct extension of the primary tumor
N2	Involvement of ipsilateral mediastinal nodes
N3	Involvement of contralateral mediastinal or hilar nodes or involvement of ipsilateral or contralateral scalene or supraclavicular nodes

Distant Metastasis (M)	
M0	No metastasis identified
M1	Distant metastasis
M1a	Separate tumor nodule in contralateral lobe, tumor with pleural nodules, or malignant pleural or pericardial effusion
M1b	Distant metastasis

*For staging groups, see Table 3.

therapy results in much poorer outcomes than surgery, although newer techniques are emerging; for example, stereotactic radiosurgery is becoming an effective method of providing local control for stage I tumors.

Several studies have evaluated the role of adjuvant chemotherapy in this group of patients, but no clear survival benefit has emerged. The Cancer and Leukemia Group B (CALGB) 9633 study randomized 344 patients with stage IB tumors to receive either surgery alone or surgery followed by carboplatin (Paraplatin)[1] and paclitaxel (Taxol). A survival benefit was demonstrated only for patients with tumors larger than 4 cm. The JBR.10 study, conducted by the National Cancer Institute of Canada, showed a survival benefit for carboplatin and vinorelbine (Navelbine) adjuvant therapy; however, this study included patients with stage IB, II, and III disease. Additional studies from Europe and Asia have also demonstrated advantages to adjuvant chemotherapy in resected NSCLC, but typically not in tumors smaller than 4 cm. The LACE (Lung Adjuvant Cisplatin Evaluation) meta-analysis incorporated data from five large, randomized trials and also found no significant benefit for adjuvant chemotherapy in stage I patients. In light of these findings, adjuvant therapy in NSCLC is not routinely recommended for small stage I tumors (<4 cm) except as part of a clinical trial. Larger stage I tumors may benefit from adjuvant chemotherapy, and this decision is largely left to the practicing oncologist and patient.

There does not appear to be any added benefit for the use of radiation therapy after surgical resection of stage I tumors. If the surgical margins are positive, adjuvant radiation therapy is routinely recommended, but this occurs infrequently. As discussed later, some patients with a clinical stage I NSCLC are upstaged by the finding of malignant disease in the mediastinum, and in this group postoperative radiation therapy improves local control and, potentially, survival when combined with adjuvant chemotherapy.

Stage II

The approach to treating stage II NSCLC is largely the same as for stage I, with surgical resection as the primary modality of treatment. Again, lobectomy using a minimally invasive video-assisted thoracoscopic approach is preferred whenever possible. Adjuvant chemotherapy offers a more clear survival advantage in patients with stage II disease. All of the aforementioned studies and the meta-analysis showed a benefit for adjuvant chemotherapy in stage II patients.

Stage III

Stage III NSCLC denotes metastasis to mediastinal lymph nodes. The hallmark of treatment in stage III patients is a multimodal approach in which surgery, radiation, and chemotherapy all may play a significant role. The division of this stage into IIIA and IIIB denotes ipsilateral and contralateral nodal involvement, respectively. Whereas the overall prognosis in this group of patients is poor, treatment with curative intent results in long-term survival in 10% to 30% of cases. This also represents the stage with the most heterogeneity, so the approach should be individualized, taking into consideration the patient's performance status, resectability, and extent of disease.

Whether patients with stage III disease should undergo resection of the tumor is still open to some debate. The Intergroup 0139 trial randomized stage IIIA and selected stage IIIB patients to receive concurrent chemoradiation with cisplatin (Platinol)[1] and etoposide (VePesid)[1] plus 45 Gy of radiation followed by surgical resection, or the same chemoradiation with 61 Gy of radiation therapy. Patients in the surgical arm who experienced progression while receiving the chemotherapy were given additional radiation therapy to 61 Gy. There was no difference in overall survival between the two groups (23.6 versus 22.2 months for trimodality and chemoradiation therapy, respectively). Recurrence rates and progression-free

survival were much more favorable for the surgery arm. Much of the excess mortality in the surgery arm occurred among those patients who required a pneumonectomy for complete resection. Forty-six percent of patients were downstaged by induction chemotherapy to N0 disease at the time of resection. Among those patients, the 5-year survival rate was 40%, suggesting that good response to induction chemoradiotherapy may predict a benefit for surgical resection. Therefore, for patients with stage IIIA, two cycles of induction chemotherapy with or without irradiation should be offered, followed by restaging. Those with a good response to chemotherapy could be considered for complete resection followed by consolidation chemotherapy. Radiation therapy to the mediastinum should be offered to patients who have residual mediastinal disease at the time of resection. Pneumonectomy for complete resection should be undertaken only in patients who have an excellent performance status and after careful discussion of the risks of this procedure.

In general, stage IIIB disease is inoperable. Patients who have satellite tumors within the same lobe may be considered for resection provided that they do not have disease in the mediastinum and that resection can be accomplished with no more than a lobectomy. For patients with inoperable stage III disease, chemotherapy with irradiation is clearly superior to irradiation alone and can lead to long-term survival, with a 3-year survival rate as high as 30%. The optimal strategy is not known, but a commonly used regimen is the combination of cisplatin[1] and etoposide[1] given concurrently with radiation therapy to 66 Gy for 6 weeks. The use of induction chemotherapy followed by chemoradiation has been evaluated, as has the use of consolidation chemotherapy, but neither regimen has clearly been proven to be superior. For patients with poor performance status, a sequential chemotherapy followed by irradiation might be preferred; for those deemed unfit for chemotherapy, palliative irradiation might be the most appropriate therapy.

Stage IV

For patients with metastatic NSCLC, the treatment is mainly palliative; however, prolongation of survival is a reasonable goal. Despite best therapy, however, median survival time remains less than a year. Several platinum combinations have efficacy in NSCLC. Schiller and colleagues randomized 1207 patients to receive either cisplatin[1] in combination with paclitaxel, docetaxel (Taxotere), or gemcitabine (Gemzar), or a combination of carboplatin[1] and paclitaxel, with survival as the primary endpoint. Response rates were highest with the cisplatin/gemcitabine combination; however, overall survival was not significantly different for any of the groups. Based on tolerability, carboplatin-containing regimens have largely replaced cisplatin doublets for patients with metastatic disease. Carboplatin can be combined with one of the previously mentioned drugs or with newer agents such as pemetrexed (Alimta) and irinotecan (Camptosar).[1] All have demonstrated efficacy, but no single regimen has emerged with clear superiority. Recently, the addition of bevacizumab (Avastin), a monoclonal antibody against vascular endothelial growth factor, to carboplatin and paclitaxel was shown to prolong median survival to 12.3 months, compared with 10.3 months for chemotherapy alone. This study excluded patients with squamous histology and brain metastasis because of the risk of bleeding complications in those subgroups. Therefore, in patients with nonsquamous NSCLC, this regimen is standard of care. It remains to be seen whether the addition of bevacizumab to other platinum doublets results in similar improvements in survival. In one trial, the combination of cisplatin, gemcitabine, and bevacizumab did not provide any additional benefit to cisplatin and gemcitabine alone.

There has also been interest in the use of drugs targeting the epidermal growth factor receptor (EGFR). Data presented at the 2008 American Society of Clinical Oncology annual meeting demonstrated a modest benefit for the addition of cetuximab (Erbitux),[1] a monoclonal antibody against EGFR, to a regimen of cisplatin[1] and

---

[1]Not FDA approved for this indication.

[1]Not FDA approved for this indication.

vinorelbine, compared with the chemotherapy regimen alone, in patients whose tumors expressed EGFR. Targeting of EGFR in combination with chemotherapy has not extended to the oral EGFR tyrosine kinase inhibitors, erlotinib (Tarceva) and gefitinib (Iressa). Four phase III randomized trials, two with gefitinib and two with erlotinib, failed to show a survival benefit for EGFR tyrosine kinase inhibitors in combination with platinum doublet chemotherapy in unselected NSCLC patients, although subgroup analysis did demonstrate a benefit for never-smokers, patients with bronchioalveolar histology, and patients with somatic mutations in EGFR. Therefore, cetuximab with cisplatin and vinorelbine can be considered for first-line therapy, but this should be limited to patients with squamous histology and those who have brain metastases, because such patients are not eligible for bevacizumab therapy.

Patients are commonly evaluated for response after two cycles of treatment and continued for four cycles if they have responsive or stable disease. There has been controversy as to whether additional chemotherapy after four cycles of treatment offers any benefit, and the general trend among North American oncologists is to limit the first-line chemotherapy to four cycles. Thus far, no clear benefit to maintenance chemotherapy or extended chemotherapy beyond six cycles has been demonstrated. It should be noted that in the bevacizumab trial and the cetuximab trial, these agents were maintained after completion of four cycles of chemotherapy, until progression or unacceptable toxicity developed. Maintenance pemetrexed resulted in an improvement in progression-free survival, without a clear improvement in overall survival; but it was not clear whether this strategy was better than simply using second-line pemetrexed at the time of progression.

When relapse occurs, there continues to be a survival and quality-of-life benefit associated with salvage therapy. Single-agent regimens should be used to avoid excess toxicity in this poor-prognosis population. Approved second-line treatments include docetaxel and erlotinib, based on improved survival compared with best supportive care. Pemetrexed has also been approved based on non-inferiority to docetaxel in the second-line setting and is better tolerated than docetaxel. If these therapies fail, salvage therapy can be attempted with several active chemotherapy agents, although none of these has demonstrated a clear survival benefit in this population. Chemotherapy should be considered only for patients who have good performance status, and careful emphasis should be placed on palliation of symptoms.

Supportive care is an important adjunct to chemotherapy in the treatment of stage IV lung cancer. Palliative irradiation can be applied to tumors that are causing significant pain or symptoms. Palliative response is seen in more than 50% of patients. Patients with superior vena cava syndrome benefit from the addition of palliative irradiation, as do patients with obstructive pneumonia. One or a few metastases to the brain should be treated with surgical resection followed by whole-brain radiotherapy whenever possible. Stereotactic radiosurgery is an alternative if surgery is not feasible.

SMALL CELL LUNG CANCER

SCLC is hallmarked by aggressive growth and early metastasis. If it is left untreated, median survival time is only 2 to 4 months. However, these tumors are highly sensitive to chemotherapy, and response rates of 60% to 80% are expected. These tumors are also highly radiosensitive, but radiation therapy is limited by the extent of metastatic disease. Although the TNM staging system for NSCLC is applicable, in practical terms SCLC is usually referred to as being of limited stage (if the disease is limited to one radiation field) or extensive stage (if not so limited). Surgery is not usually a viable treatment option except in those with very small tumors and no evidence of metastasis to the mediastinum or distant sites.

Patients with limited-stage disease should be treated with four cycles of cisplatin[1] and etoposide with concurrent radiotherapy to the involved field. With this approach approximately 20% of patients are disease free at 3 years. Extensive-stage SCLC is incurable, and median survival is in the range of 8 to 12 months. Chemotherapy can result in dramatic improvements in performance status, and this is one of the few situations in which chemotherapy should be offered even to very moribund patients. The standard of care is carboplatin[1] plus etoposide. Despite numerous trials of multiagent chemotherapy and novel targeted agents, no other regimen has surpassed the results of the standard of care. The combination of carboplatin and irinotecan[1] was shown to be superior to the standard of care in a large, randomized, phase III trial in Japan, but an American trial showed no benefit for this approach. Therefore, cisplatin and irinotecan could be considered an acceptable alternative to the standard of care. The toxicity profile is similar, with the irinotecan regimen causing significant gastrointestinal toxicity and the etoposide regimen having mainly hematologic toxicity. If first-line therapy fails, topotecan (Hycamtin) has been shown to improve quality of life and overall survival when used as second-line therapy. There are no other second- or third-line agents with proven survival or palliative benefit, and, given the dismal prognosis, patients should be considered for a clinical trial whenever possible.

For both limited- and extensive-stage disease, relapse in the brain is a significant cause of morbidity and mortality and has prompted the use of prophylactic cranial irradiation. This approach has consistently proved to be of benefit for patients who have a good response to primary therapy. The benefit has been seen to prevent symptomatic brain metastasis and also to improve overall survival. Cognitive dysfunction after prophylactic cranial irradiation can occur, particularly if it is given concurrently with chemotherapy. Therefore, whenever possible, it should be given only after chemotherapy is completed.

REFERENCES

Arriagada R, Bergman B, Dunant A, et al. Cisplatin-based adjuvant chemotherapy in patients with completely resected non-small-cell lung cancer. N Engl J Med 2004;350:351–60.

DeVita VT, Hellman S, Rosenberg SA. Cancer: Principles and practice of oncology. 4th ed. Philadelphia: Lippincott; 1993.

Noda K, Nishiwaki Y, Kawahara M, et al. Irinotecan plus cisplatin compared with etoposide plus cisplatin for extensive small-cell lung cancer. N Engl J Med 2002;346:85–91.

Pignon JP, Tribodet H, Scagliotti GV, et al. Lung adjuvant cisplatin evaluation: A pooled analysis by the LACE Collaborative Group. J Clin Oncol 2008;26:3552–9.

Sandler A, Gray R, Perry MC, et al. Paclitaxel-carboplatin alone or with bevacizumab for non-small-cell lung cancer. N Engl J Med 2006;355: 2542–50.

Schiller JH, Harrington D, Belani CP, et al. Comparison of four chemotherapy regimens for advanced non-small-cell lung cancer. N Engl J Med 2002;346:92–8.

Shepherd FA, Rodrigues Pereira J, Ciuleanu T, et al. Erlotinib in previously treated non-small-cell lung cancer. N Engl J Med 2005;353:123–32.

Slotman B, Faivre-Finn C, Kramer G, et al. Prophylactic cranial irradiation in extensive small-cell lung cancer. N Engl J Med 2007;357:664–72.

Strauss GM, Herndon JE 2nd, Maddaus MA, et al. Adjuvant paclitaxel plus carboplatin compared with observation in stage IB non-small-cell lung cancer: CALGB 9633 with the Cancer and Leukemia Group B, Radiation Therapy Oncology Group, and North Central Cancer Treatment Group Study Groups. J Clin Oncol 2008;26:5043–51.

van Meerbeeck JP, Kramer GW, Van Schil PE, et al. Randomized controlled trial of resection versus radiotherapy after induction chemotherapy in stage IIIA-N2 non-small-cell lung cancer. J Natl Cancer Inst 2007;99: 442–50.

Winton T, Livingston R, Johnson D, et al. Vinorelbine plus cisplatin vs. observation in resected non-small-cell lung cancer. N Engl J Med 2005;352: 2589–97.

---

[1]Not FDA approved for this indication.

---

[1]Not FDA approved for this indication.

Coccidioidomycosis

Method of
Gregory M. Anstead, MD

Coccidioidomycosis is caused by soil fungi of the genus *Coccidioides*, divided genetically into *Coccidioides immitis* (California isolates) and *Coccidioides posadasii* (isolates outside California). There are no distinct clinical differences between the two species. *Coccidioides* occurs only in the Western hemisphere, primarily in the southwestern United States (Arizona and parts of California, New Mexico, Utah, Nevada, and Texas) and in northern Mexico, areas characterized by arid to semiarid climates, hot summers, low altitude, alkaline soil, and sparse vegetation. Hyperendemic areas include the San Joaquin Valley of California and Pima, Pinal, and Maricopa Counties in Arizona. *Coccidioides* is also found in parts of Latin America (Guatemala, Honduras, Nicaragua, Argentina, Paraguay, Venezuela, and Colombia). Cases may be observed in nonendemic areas because of travel or reactivation of prior infection. In the United States, an estimated 150,000 cases of coccidioidomycosis occur annually, with the clinical presentation ranging from a self-limited respiratory infection to devastating disseminated disease. Persons with occupations involving exposure to soil are at risk for coccidioidomycosis. Immunocompromised persons are also at high risk, including patients with AIDS, transplant recipients (especially those who received *Coccidioides*-infected organs), patients receiving tumor necrosis factor-α antagonists, pregnant women, and cancer patients. Filipinos, African Americans, and persons with blood group B are also at increased risk for disseminated disease. Outbreaks may occur after dust storms, earthquakes, droughts, and activities causing soil disruption, such as construction and archeological digs.

Coccidioides is dimorphic; in the soil, the organism exists in its mycelial form, which produces barrel-shaped arthroconidia. The usual means of infection is the inhalation of arthroconidia; uncommon routes include direct cutaneous inoculation and organ transplantation. Arthroconidia germinate to produce spherules filled with endospores, the characteristic tissue phase. Spherules rupture to release endospores, which form additional spherules. The spherules become surrounded by neutrophils and macrophages, which leads to granuloma formation. Both B and T lymphocytes are essential for host defense against this pathogen.

Clinical Manifestations

Coccidioidomycosis is asymptomatic in 60% of infected individuals. In the remaining 40% a self-limited, flu-like illness, with dry cough, pleuritic chest pain, myalgias, arthralgia, fever, sweats, anorexia, and weakness, develops 1 to 3 weeks after exposure. Primary infection may be accompanied by immune complex–mediated complications, including an erythematous macular rash, erythema multiforme, and erythema nodosum. Acute infection usually resolves without therapy, although symptoms may persist for weeks. In 5% of these patients, asymptomatic pulmonary residua persist, including pulmonary nodules and cavitation. Immunocompromised patients may develop chronic progressive pulmonary infection, with the evolution of thin-walled cavities that may rupture, leading to bronchopleural fistula and empyema formation.

Extrapulmonary disease develops in 1 of every 200 patients and can involve the skin, soft tissues, bones, joints, and meninges. The most common cutaneous lesions are verrucous papules, ulcers, or plaques. The spine is the most frequent site of osseous dissemination, although the typical lytic lesions may also occur in the skull, hands, feet, and tibia. Joint involvement is usually monoarticular and most commonly involves the ankle and knee. Fungemia may occur in immunocompromised patients and carries a poor prognosis.

In coccidioidal meningitis, the basilar meninges are usually affected. Cerebrospinal fluid findings include lymphocytic pleocytosis (often with eosinophilia), hypoglycorrhachia, and elevated protein levels. The mortality rate is greater than 90% at 1 year without therapy, and chronic infection is the rule. Hydrocephalus or hydrocephalus coexisting with brain infarction is associated with a higher mortality rate.

Coccidioidomycosis is a great imitator and has many diverse clinical presentations, including immune thrombocytopenia, ocular involvement, massive cervical lymphadenopathy, laryngeal and retropharyngeal abscesses, endocarditis, pericarditis, peritonitis, hepatitis, and lesions of the male and female genitals and urogenital tracts.

Diagnosis

Coccidioidomycosis may be diagnosed by direct observation of spherules in tissues or in wet mounts of sputa or exudates. The growth of *Coccidioides* in culture usually occurs in 3 to 5 days, with sporulation after 5 to 10 days. Definitive identification is made by DNA probe or exoantigen testing. Laboratory personnel should exercise extreme caution when handling cultures of *Coccidioides*.

Serologic methods are quite useful in establishing the diagnosis and for monitoring the course of the infection. Immunoglobulin M (IgM) antibodies are present soon after infection or relapse but then wane; quantification does not correlate with disease severity. The IgG antibody appears later and remains positive for months. Rising titers of IgG are associated with progressive disease, and declining titers are associated with resolution. The IgG antibodies are able to fix complement when combined with coccidioidal antigen, and can be detected by immunodiffusion for complement fixation (IDCF); titers of 1:16 or greater suggest disseminated disease. In the cerebrospinal fluid, a positive IDCF of any titer is considered diagnostic of meningitis and is much more sensitive than culture in making the diagnosis. An enzyme immunoassay is also available, but it is less specific. Recently, a specific urinary antigen test became available for the diagnosis of coccidioidomycosis; this assay has a sensitivity of 71% in moderate-to-severe disease, compared with 84% for culture, 29% for histopathologic examination, and 75% for serologic testing.

Treatment

In most patients, primary pulmonary infection resolves spontaneously without treatment. However, all patients require observation for at least 2 years to document resolution of infection and to identify any complications as soon as possible. For patients who have risk factors for disseminated disease (listed earlier), treatment is necessary. Other indications for treatment are severe disease (infiltrates involving both lungs or more than half of one lung; significant hilar or mediastinal lymphadenopathy; complement fixation titers >1:16) and highly symptomatic disease (weight loss >10%; night sweats present for >3 weeks; symptoms present for >2 months).

For diffuse or severe pneumonia, therapy with amphotericin B deoxycholate (Fungizone) 0.5 to 1.5 mg/kg/day, or a lipid formulation of amphotericin B (Abelcet or AmBisome)[1] 2 to 5 mg/kg/day should be given for several weeks, followed by an oral azole, such as itraconazole (Sporanox)[1] 200 mg twice daily or fluconazole (Diflucan)[1] 400 to 800 mg/day). The total duration of therapy should be at least 1 year; for immunosuppressed patients, oral azole therapy should be maintained as secondary prophylaxis. In HIV patients with CD4-positive T-cell counts greater than 250 cells/mm[3] who had focal pneumonias that responded to azoles, antifungals may be discontinued. Azole therapy may be used initially for less severe disease. During pregnancy, amphotericin B is the preferred drug, because of the teratogenicity of azoles.

An asymptomatic patient with a solitary nodule or pulmonary cavitation due to *C. immitis* does not require specific antifungal therapy or resection. However, the development of complications from the cavitation, such as hemoptysis or bacterial or fungal superinfection, necessitates initiation of azole therapy. Resection of the cavities is an alternative to antifungal therapy. Rupture of a cavity into the pleural space requires surgical intervention with closure by lobectomy with decortication, in addition to antifungal therapy. For chronic pneumonia, the initial treatment should be an oral azole for at least 1 year. If the disease persists, one may switch to another oral azole, increase the dose if fluconazole was initially selected, or switch to amphotericin B. Resection should be performed for patients with refractory focal lesions or severe hemoptysis.

The treatment of disseminated infection without central nervous system involvement is based on oral azole therapy, such as itraconazole or fluconazole (400 mg/day, or higher in case of fluconazole). If there is little or no improvement or if there is vertebral involvement, treatment with amphotericin B is recommended (dosage as for diffuse pneumonia). Concomitant surgical débridement or stabilization is also recommended. In patients with refractory coccidioidomycosis that has failed to respond to fluconazole, itraconazole, and amphotericin B and its lipid formulations, treatment with posaconazole (Noxafil)[1] 200 mg four times daily has been successful.

---

[1]Not FDA approved for this indication.

For coccidioidal meningitis, lifetime treatment with azoles is indicated. Fluconazole, at doses of 800 mg/day or higher,[3] is recommended. There have been a few reports of successful treatment of coccidioidal meningitis with voriconazole (Vfend)[1] 200 mg orally twice daily after a loading dose. Itraconazole is not recommended because of its irregular oral absorption. Obstructive hydrocephalus requires shunting. Intrathecal amphotericin B[1] was previously used for meningeal coccidioidomycosis, but it is now strictly reserved for infections that are refractory to high-dose azoles.

REFERENCES

Anstead GM, Graybill JR. Coccidioidomycosis. Infect Dis Clin North Am 2006;20:621–43.

Blair JE. State-of-the art treatment of coccidioidomycosis skeletal infections. Ann N Y Acad Sci 2007;1111:422–33.

Blair JE. State-of-the-art treatment of coccidiodomycosis skin and soft tissue infections. Ann N Y Acad Sci 2007;1111:411–21.

Crum NF, Lederman ER, Stafford CM, et al. Coccidioidomycosis: A descriptive survey of a reemerging disease—Clinical characteristics and emerging controversies. Medicine (Baltimore) 2004;83:149–75.

Crum-Cianflone NF, Truett AA, Teneza-Mora N, et al. Unusual presentations of coccidioidomycosis: A case series and review of the literature. Medicine (Baltimore) 2006;85:263–77.

Galgiani J, Ampel N, Blair J, et al. Coccidioidomycosis. Clin Infect Dis 2005;41:1217–23.

Parish JM, Blair JE. Coccidioidomycosis. Mayo Clin Proc 2008;83:343–8; quiz 348–349.

Saubolle MA, McKellar PP, Sussland D. Epidemiologic, clinical, and diagnostic aspects of coccidioidomycosis. J Clin Microbiol 2007;45:26–30.

Williams PL. Coccidioidal meningitis. Ann N Y Acad Sci 2007;1111:377–84.

---

[1]Not FDA approved for this indication.
[3]Exceeds dosage recommended by the manufacturer.

Histoplasmosis

Method of
David van Duin, MD, PhD

Mycology and Pathogenesis

Histoplasma capsulatum var. *capsulatum* and *H. capsulatum* var. *duboisii* are the two varieties of *H. capsulatum* that cause human histoplasmosis. *H. capsulatum* var. *duboisii* is the causative agent of African histoplasmosis, which is characterized by skin, bone, lymph node, and subcutaneous tissue involvement. This chapter focuses solely on the manifestations and treatment of *H. capsulatum* var. *capsulatum*, hereafter referred to as *H. capsulatum*.

H. capsulatum is a thermally dimorphic fungal pathogen, which grows as a mold in the environment, and converts to a yeast at 37°C during infection. During mold growth, *H. capsulatum* forms macroconidia, which are 8 to 15 µm and have thick walls and protuberances, as well as microconidia, which are 2 to 4 µm and have a smooth surface.

Disruption of soil containing *H. capsulatum*, such as during a construction project, results in the aerosolization of microconidia, which are the infectious particles. Inhaled microconidia are phagocytized but are able to survive and convert to yeast phase inside pulmonary macrophages. The resulting dissemination through the reticuloendothelial system is usually quickly contained in immunocompetent hosts, but it can lead to severe disease in the absence of normal immunity. Microconidia can be carried for several miles by air currents. Therefore, persons who are not in the direct vicinity of the disrupted soil are also at risk for developing histoplasmosis.

In tissues, *H. capsulatum* is recognized as 2- to 4-μm oval yeast forms with narrow-based budding. *H. capsulatum* does not have a capsule; the name is derived from the erroneous interpretation by Samuel Darling of an apparent clearing surrounding these yeasts in tissues as a capsule.

Epidemiology

Histoplasmosis is most common in North and Central America, but cases occur worldwide, some in microfoci of infection. Areas of high prevalence include the Mississippi and Ohio River valleys in the United States and Rio de Janeiro State in Brazil. *H. capsulatum* thrives in soil that is enriched with bird or bat guano, and it can be found in high quantities near bird roosts, chicken coops, abandoned old buildings, and bat-infested caves. Because *H. capsulatum* can enter a state of latency and reactivate years later, cases have been described in patients who have a remote history of living in or visiting endemic areas. A complete geographic history and a high index of suspicion are required for the correct diagnosis of such cases in nonendemic areas.

Clinical Manifestations

Most *H. capsulatum* infections are asymptomatic; it is estimated that less than 5% of infections lead to clinical symptoms. The occurrence and severity of a clinical syndrome are thought to be related to the immune status of the host, as well as the size of the infectious inoculum. The most common clinical scenario is acute pulmonary histoplasmosis, but a variety of other symptomatic histoplasmosis syndromes have been described. Also, a substantial number of cases come to clinical attention years after the initial infection during the course of a pulmonary nodule work-up, when malignancy is suspected. Although they are asymptomatic, these cases can lead to anxiety, as well as the morbidity and health care costs associated with radiographic exposures and biopsy procedures.

ACUTE PULMONARY HISTOPLASMOSIS

Most commonly, acute pulmonary histoplasmosis is a self-limited flu-like illness. Symptoms are generally nonspecific and include fevers, chills, malaise, a nonproductive cough, and chest pain. Chest radiographs can show diffuse infiltrates in one or more lobes, often with hilar lymphadenopathy. The differential diagnosis includes more common infections such as bacterial and viral pneumonias. Symptoms usually resolve without treatment in 2 to 3 weeks. However, more-severe cases do occur, even in seemingly immunocompetent hosts. In these cases, severe respiratory distress, prolonged symptoms, and even death can occur in the absence of adequate treatment. This highlights the importance of timely diagnosis and treatment when indicated.

CHRONIC PULMONARY HISTOPLASMOSIS

Some patients with acute pulmonary histoplasmosis fail to clear their infection and go on to develop a chronic pulmonary infection. A subset of these patients has chronic cavitary disease.

Chronic pulmonary histoplasmosis may be arbitrarily defined when the duration of symptoms from pulmonary histoplasmosis exceeds 6 weeks. The classic patient is a white middle-aged to elderly man with chronic obstructive pulmonary disease (COPD). Although these are clearly risk factors for the development of chronic disease, case series have illustrated that even never-smokers without preexisting lung disease are at risk for developing this complication.

A combination of systemic and pulmonary signs and symptoms is usually found in chronic pulmonary histoplasmosis. Fevers, night sweats, weight loss, lack of appetite, subjective loss of energy, and malaise are common systemic symptoms, and pulmonary symptoms include cough, sometimes with minimal hemoptysis, dyspnea, and sputum production. In patients with preexisting lung disease it may be difficult to distinguish these symptoms from baseline

symptomatology. Radiology studies classically show cavitary disease without hilar lymphadenopathy. However, nodules, infiltrates, and lymphadenopathy are also seen, especially in nonsmoking women.

Untreated, this form of histoplasmosis can lead to death secondary to respiratory failure. With treatment, prognosis depends on coexisting pulmonary disease, and is generally favorable with regard to microbiological cure. However, relapses occur in up to 20% of cases even after prolonged treatment.

DISSEMINATED HISTOPLASMOSIS

Most, if not all, episodes of histoplasmosis have a period of dissemination, during which infected macrophages spread throughout the body via the reticuloendothelial system. In the majority of cases this is a self-limited event, which is quickly contained upon activation of the immune system. However, about 1 in 2000 infections results in progressive disseminated disease. Almost invariably, these cases occur in immunocompromised hosts. Patients at risk for progressive disseminated disease include those with advanced HIV infection, solid organ transplant recipients, patients with hematologic malignancies, and those treated with immunomodulating agents, most notably corticosteroids or tumor necrosis factor α (TNF-α) inhibitors. Infants are also at risk.

Recognition of disseminated histoplasmosis can be challenging. Symptoms include fevers, malaise, anorexia, respiratory symptoms, and weight loss. Laboratory investigations often reveal elevated acute phase reactants, abnormal liver function tests, and pancytopenia. Hepatosplenomegaly and lymphadenopathy occur in about half of cases. Severe cases can be clinically indistinguishable from bacterial sepsis, and patients present with hypotension and multiorgan failure. A potential diagnostic clue to the diagnosis is the presence of mucosal ulcerations, which are generally painful and can occur anywhere in the oral, pharyngeal, or laryngeal mucosa. Various morphologies may be seen, ranging from superficial to verrucous. Adrenal involvement resulting in adrenal insufficiency can occur. These patients present with enlarged adrenals on imaging and clinical symptoms of Addison's disease.

Although survival without antifungal therapy has been described, disseminated histoplasmosis is generally fatal if left untreated.

MEDIASTINAL MANIFESTATIONS OF HISTOPLASMOSIS

Mediastinal disease can manifest itself as mediastinal fibrosis or granulomatous mediastinitis. Mediastinal fibrosis or fibrosing mediastinitis is an uncommon complication of pulmonary disease, in which extensive fibrotic tissue develops in the mediastinum in response to infection. Men between ages of 20 and 40 years are at the highest risk for this complication. The fibrosis consists of mature collagen, rather than granulomatous tissue, which encases the structures of the mediastinum and can have a progressive course eventually leading to death. The prognosis depends on the extent of involvement of mediastinal structures. Bilateral disease in which the pulmonary veins are involved is especially associated with poor outcomes. No satisfactory treatment is available.

In contrast, granulomatous mediastinitis, also known as mediastinal granuloma, is characterized by a caseous inflammatory mass of mediastinal lymph nodes. Most patients remain asymptomatic, and cases are often recognized only as an incidental imaging finding. However, a subset of patients develops symptoms related to compromise of mediastinal structures. The prognosis is more benign; usually the process resolves and the involved lymph nodes calcify. The role of treatment in this entity remains unclear.

CENTRAL NERVOUS SYSTEM HISTOPLASMOSIS

Central nervous system (CNS) involvement during *H. capsulatum* infection occurs infrequently. Like other extrapulmonary disease, CNS disease may be seen as a part of progressive disseminated histoplasmosis in about 5% to 10% of disseminated histoplasmosis cases. Additionally, isolated cases in which no other signs of dissemination are found have been reported. CNS histoplasmosis typically results in chronic lymphocytic meningitis, but parenchymal lesions can also be found. Symptoms are similar to those of other chronic infectious meningitides. The typical presentation is a combination of systemic symptoms including fevers, weight loss, and night sweats and localizing symptoms of headache, focal neurologic deficits, or behavioral changes. Treatment failures and relapses are common. Prognosis in the context of adequate treatment is dependent on the degree and the reversibility of immunosuppression.

OTHER MANIFESTATIONS OF HISTOPLASMOSIS

Involvement of all organ systems with *H. capsulatum* has been reported, either in the setting of clinical disseminated histoplasmosis or as an isolated extrapulmonary site of infection.

H. capsulatum as a cause of endovascular and cardiac infections is well established. In endocarditis cases, native and prosthetic valves may be involved. Pericarditis is found in around 5% of patients with pulmonary histoplasmosis, and it appears to represent an immunologic reaction. Consistent with this, symptoms usually resolve with nonsteroidal antiinflammatory drugs (NSAIDs) or corticosteroids. Bone, joint, and skin infections can also occur and can present diagnostic difficulty.

Urogenital involvement is often documented in autopsy series, but it infrequently results in clinical symptoms. Few cases of *H. capsulatum* causing symptomatic prostatitis, nephritis, epididymitis, vaginal and penile ulcers, and ovarian involvement have been reported. Similarly, although autopsy series report gastrointestinal involvement in disseminated histoplasmosis in up to 70% to 90% of cases, specific symptoms attributable to the gastrointestinal tract are much less common. Diarrhea, gastrointestinal bleeding, bowel perforation, or bowel obstruction can result from gastrointestinal histoplasmosis.

Diagnosis

Diagnosing histoplasmosis can be complicated, and the available specific diagnostic tests each have their limitations. If the diagnosis is suspected, using available modalities in combination is generally the right approach. Turn-around time can vary depending on circumstances, and in severe or disseminated cases, empiric therapy may be warranted. Obtaining tissue, when it is feasible to do so, is essential for a pathologic diagnosis.

HISTOPATHOLOGY

One of the most useful modalities in reaching a diagnosis is histopathology. Necrotizing or non-necrotizing granulomas are often seen. An experienced pathologist can recognize the specific pattern of yeast forms, mostly inside but also outside of macrophages. The yeast forms are best visualized by a methamine silver stain, such as the Gomori-Grocott methenamine silver stain (GMS). Alternatively, periodic acid–Schiff (PAS) staining may be used. Confusion with other pathogens or, more commonly, staining artifacts can occur, and expert consultation is required in such cases. Obtaining tissue for histopathology is usually the real challenge, and a careful evaluation of the risk-to-benefit ratio for each individual patient needs to be made.

CURRENT DIAGNOSIS

- The most common symptomatic manifestation of histoplasmosis is acute pulmonary histoplasmosis, which is generally characterized by nonspecific symptoms including fevers, chills, malaise, a nonproductive cough, and chest pain.
- Other presentations of histoplasmosis include chronic pulmonary histoplasmosis, disseminated histoplasmosis in immunocompromised hosts, and extrapulmonary disease such as mediastinal histoplasmosis.
- A multimodality approach to diagnosis, which may include serology, histopathology, antigen testing, and culture, should be considered in the appropriate setting.

CULTURES

Culture confirmation of histoplasmosis is desirable, but often the yield of cultures is limited. In addition, cultures may be subject to a substantial time delay of several weeks. In disseminated histoplasmosis, cultures are often positive from several sites, including blood and bone marrow. In acute pulmonary histoplasmosis, the yield of respiratory cultures is estimated to be between 9% and 40%, depending on the degree of lung involvement. In mild to moderate cases, cultures are rarely positive. In chronic cavitary lung disease, the yield of culture improves, probably as a reflection of the increased fungal burden in these patients, and cultures can grow *H. capsulatum* in as many as 85% of cases. A positive fungal culture, with microscopic characteristics suggesting *H. capsulatum,* should be confirmed by specific testing. This is usually accomplished by DNA probing.

SEROLOGY

Antibody testing can be helpful when used in conjunction with the clinical scenario and other specific testing. The presence of antibodies to *H. capsulatum* may be determined by complement fixation (CF) or immunodiffusion (ID). Immunodiffusion methods evaluate the presence of M and H precipitin bands. Mild acute infections may be characterized by presence of an M band in isolation. Presence of an H band generally indicates more severe or chronic infection and is usually found in combination with an M band. Complement fixation determines the level of antibodies directed against mycelial and yeast antigens separately. For diagnosis, a fourfold rise in either mycelial or yeast CF antibody titer is required.

The incidence of detectable antibodies in persons in endemic areas is much lower than the incidence of positive skin testing, which suggests that detectable antibodies probably wane after exposure to undetectable levels. Therefore, although an isolated antibody titer of 1:32 or greater is not diagnostic, it is very suggestive of histoplasmosis in a patient with a consistent clinical presentation. In addition, any positive titer should lead to additional work-up because a substantial number of patients with confirmed histoplasmosis have antibody titers that are in the low positive range. Antibodies take 2 to 6 weeks to appear, which limits their use in acute cases. Immunosuppressed states clearly diminish the sensitivity of serology, but positive serologies are found in around 50% of disseminated histoplasmosis in immunocompromised patients. Antibody testing may be particularly helpful in CNS histoplasmosis, where cerebrospinal fluid (CSF) cultures are often negative. The finding of detectable anti–*H. capsulatum* antibodies in the CSF is diagnostic in the right clinical setting.

ANTIGEN DETECTION

A commercial assay is available to determine the presence of polysaccharide antigens shed by *H. capsulatum* in urine or serum. Previously, urine assays appeared to outperform serum assays, but the most recent generation of antigen assays seems to be equivalent in urine and serum. Measuring antigen shedding in bronchoalveolar lavage (BAL) fluid is a new and promising development. Preliminary data indicate that yields from BAL may be increased in pulmonary disease. In general, antigen detection assays are a valuable adjunct to diagnosis and should be obtained in any case in which histoplasmosis is suspected. Because direct shedding is measured, the yield of this test is not diminished in immunocompromised hosts. In limited disease with a minimal fungal burden, antigens are unlikely to be detected.

Treatment

In 2007, the Infectious Diseases Society of America (IDSA) published updated management guidelines for the treatment of histoplasmosis (Table 1). The IDSA emphasizes that all of its guidelines "cannot always account for individual variation among patients. They are not intended to supplant physician judgment with respect to particular patients or special clinical situations." Regarding acute pulmonary histoplasmosis, no evidence from clinical trials is available to guide treatment decisions, and the IDSA guidelines are relatively conservative,

TABLE 1 2007 IDSA Guidelines for Treating Histoplasmosis

Clinical Manifestation	Induction	Duration	Maintenance	Total Duration
Acute Pulmonary				
Mild to moderate <4 weeks	None			
Mild to moderate >4 weeks	None		Itra*	6-12 wk
Moderately severe to severe	AmB[†]	1-2 wk	Itra*	12 wk
Chronic Pulmonary				
	Itra*	3 day	Itra*	1-2 yr
Disseminated				
Mild to moderate	Itra*	3 day	Itra*	1 yr
Moderately severe to severe	AmB[†]	1-2 wk	Itra*	1 yr
Granulomatous mediastinitis	Itra*	3 day	Itra*	6-12 wk
CNS	AmB[†]	4-6 wk	Itra*	1 yr

[1]Not FDA approved for this indication.

*Itraconazole (Sporanox) dosing for mild to moderate disease is 200 mg qd or bid; for all other indications a loading dose of 200 mg tid × 3 d is recommended followed by 200 mg qd or bid, guided by blood levels.

[†]Amphotericin B, in general liposomal (AmBisome)[1] or lipid formulations (Abelcet)[1] are preferred, but deoxycholate formulation of amphotericin B (Fungizone) may be used as an alternative in the treatment of acute pulmonary histoplasmosis. In CNS histoplasmosis, liposomal amphotericin B[1] is preferred.

Abbreviations: AmB = amphotericin B; CNS = central nervous system; ISDA = Infectious Diseases Society of America; Itra = itraconazole.

reserving treatment only for "moderately severe to severe" cases. No explicit definition of severity is provided. Also, when mild to moderate symptoms persist, treatment is not recommended until the patient has been symptomatic for more than 4 weeks. Here, careful clinical judgment is warranted. Although poor long term outcomes are uncommon in these patients, symptom resolution upon antifungal treatment is the rule. Therefore, some experts treat even mild to moderate acute pulmonary disease with a symptom duration of less than 4 weeks, in contrast to IDSA guideline recommendations.

Recommended induction treatment for the first 1 to 2 weeks in moderately severe to severe acute pulmonary histoplasmosis is a lipid formulation of amphotericin B (AmBisome, Abelcet)[1] 3-5 mg/kg IV daily. During induction therapy, methylprednisolone (Solu-Medrol) may be used as needed for respiratory complications. After that, oral itraconazole (Sporanox) can be used (200 mg three times daily for 3 days and then 200 mg twice daily) for a total duration of treatment of 12 weeks. Oral itraconazole for 6 to 12 weeks is the treatment of choice when the decision is made to treat mild to moderate acute pulmonary histoplasmosis.

When itraconazole is used, careful instructions should be given to ensure optimal oral absorption. Using the solution results generally in higher blood levels, but the unpleasant taste can be an issue for patients. To optimize absorption of the capsules, encourage patients to take them with a cola beverage. Because of substantial interpersonal variability in itraconazole metabolism, blood levels remain unpredictable. As a result, levels should be monitored on all patients whose treatment exceeds 2 weeks. In general, blood levels between 1.0 and 10.0 µg/mL are recommended, even though strong evidence for these cutoffs is lacking.

[1]Not FDA approved for this indication.

CURRENT THERAPY

- Oral itraconazole is the treatment of choice for most forms of histoplasmosis.
- Serum levels of itraconazole are unpredictable and should be monitored during treatment.
- Depending on localization and severity of disease, induction with amphotericin B formulations may be required.
- Careful monitoring of patients during and after treatment is recommended, because relapses are observed in a subset of patients.

Chronic pulmonary histoplasmosis requires oral itraconazole therapy for 1 to 2 years. As noted earlier, relapses can occur even with prolonged therapy, and some patients require lifelong suppressive therapy. When an asymptomatic pulmonary nodule is found to be a histoplasmoma in the course of a malignancy work-up, no treatment is generally indicated.

In disseminated histoplasmosis with moderately severe to severe symptoms, induction treatment with liposomal amphotericin B[1] (3 mg/kg IV daily) is recommended for the first 1 to 2 weeks. This is followed by oral itraconazole for a total of at least 1 year. When symptoms of disseminated histoplasmosis are mild to moderate, the induction phase can be omitted, and treatment with oral itraconazole for 1 year should suffice. The role of treatment in mediastinal complications of histoplasmosis depends on the etiology. If symptomatic and inflammatory findings predominate, as in granulomatous mediastinitis, treatment with oral itraconazole is warranted. In mediastinal fibrosis, antifungal treatment generally does not improve the prognosis. CNS histoplasmosis should be aggressively treated with liposomal amphotericin B (5 mg/kg daily intravenously) for 4 to 6 weeks, followed by oral itraconazole for at least 1 year.

[1]Not FDA approved for this indication.

REFERENCES

Ashbee HR, Evans EG, Viviani MA, et al. Histoplasmosis in Europe: Report on an epidemiological survey from the European Confederation of Medical Mycology Working Group. Med Mycol 2008;46(1):57–65.

Assi MA, Sandid MS, Baddour LM, et al. Systemic histoplasmosis: A 15-year retrospective institutional review of 111 patients. Medicine (Baltimore) 2007;86(3):162–9.

Cuellar-Rodriguez J, Avery RK, Lard M, et al. Histoplasmosis in solid organ transplant recipients: 10 years of experience at a large transplant center in an endemic area. Clin Infect Dis 2009;49(5):710–6.

Deepe Jr GS. Immune response to early and late *Histoplasma capsulatum* infections. Curr Opin Microbiol 2000;3(4):359–62.

Gugnani HC. Histoplasmosis in Africa: A review. Indian J Chest Dis Allied Sci 2000;42(4):271–7.

Hage CA, Bowyer S, Tarvin SE, et al. Recognition, diagnosis, and treatment of histoplasmosis complicating tumor necrosis factor blocker therapy. Clin Infect Dis 2010;50(1):85–92.

Hage CA, Davis TE, Fuller D, et al. Diagnosis of histoplasmosis by antigen detection in bronchoalveolar fluid. Chest 2010;137(3):623–8.

Hage CA, Wheat LJ, Loyd J, et al. Pulmonary histoplasmosis. Semin Respir Crit Care Med 2008;29(2):151–65.

Kahi CJ, Wheat LJ, Allen SD, Sarosi GA. Gastrointestinal histoplasmosis. Am J Gastroenterol 2005;100(1):220–31.

Kauffman CA. Histoplasmosis: A clinical and laboratory update. Clin Microbiol Rev 2007;20(1):115–32.

Kauffman CA. Diagnosis of histoplasmosis in immunosuppressed patients. Curr Opin Infect Dis 2008;21(4):421–5.

Kauffman CA. Histoplasmosis. Clin Chest Med 2009;30(2):217–25, v.

Kennedy CC, Limper AH. Redefining the clinical spectrum of chronic pulmonary histoplasmosis: A retrospective case series of 46 patients. Medicine (Baltimore) 2007;86(4):252–8.

Mata-Essayag S, Colella MT, Rosello A, et al. Histoplasmosis: A study of 158 cases in Venezuela, 2000-2005. Medicine (Baltimore) 2008;87(4):193–202.

Nosanchuk JD, Gacser A. *Histoplasma capsulatum* at the host–pathogen interface. Microbes Infect 2008;10(9):973–7.

Pasqualotto AC, Oliveira FM, Severo LC. *Histoplasma capsulatum* recovery from the urine and a short review of genitourinary histoplasmosis. Mycopathologia 2009;167(6):315–23.

Thompson 3rd GR, Cadena J, Patterson TF. Overview of antifungal agents. Clin Chest Med 2009;30(2):203–15, v.

Wheat LJ. Approach to the diagnosis of the endemic mycoses. Clin Chest Med 2009;30(2):379–89, viii.

Wheat LJ, Freifeld AG, Kleiman MB, et al. Clinical practice guidelines for the management of patients with histoplasmosis: 2007 update by the Infectious Diseases Society of America. Clin Infect Dis 2007;45(7):807–25.

Wheat LJ, Kauffman CA. Histoplasmosis. Infect Dis Clin North Am 2003;17(1):1–19, vii.

Wheat LJ, Musial CE, Jenny-Avital E. Diagnosis and management of central nervous system histoplasmosis. Clin Infect Dis 2005;40(6):844–52.

Blastomycosis

Method of

John M. Embil, MD, and Donald C. Vinh, MD, FRCPC

Blastomyces dermatitidis is the thermally dimorphic fungus that causes blastomycosis. The mycelial form of *B. dermatitidis* exists in the environment but grows as a yeast at body temperature. Although *B. dermatitidis* is endemic to certain specific regions within North America, numerous cases have been reported from areas where it is not considered endemic. It is presumed that those patients acquired infection in the endemic areas and subsequently presented outside of these geographic locations. The clinical manifestations of blastomycosis can be diverse, and therefore this infection should be suspected within the appropriate clinical context in persons with a history of residence or travel to such endemic areas.

Epidemiology

Our knowledge of the exact geographic distribution of *B. dermatitidis* is limited by the fact that the fungus cannot be readily recovered from nature; thus, identification of the endemic area has been largely derived from outbreak investigations and small case series. Most epidemiologic studies have depended upon recovery of *B. dermatitidis* in culture from clinical specimens or histologic visualization to establish the diagnosis. In addition, the incidence and prevalence of blastomycosis has been difficult to establish because suitable serologic or skin-prick assays (demonstrating acceptable sensitivity and/or specificity) to confirm infection are lacking. The geographic niche of *B. dermatitidis* may therefore be greater than is currently believed.

The currently known areas of endemicity for *B. dermatitidis* are the south central and upper midwestern United States, including areas surrounding the Great Lakes. *B. dermatitidis* is also endemic in Wisconsin (1.3 cases per 100,000 population) and Mississippi (1.4 cases per 100,000 population), as well as parts of Missouri, Kentucky, Tennessee, Arkansas, and Alabama. In Canada, the major areas of endemicity include the province of Manitoba (0.62 cases per 100,000 population) and the Kenora region of the province of Ontario (7.11 cases per 100,000 population). Although most cases of blastomycosis are concentrated in these regions, it should be remembered that persons can acquire infection with *B. dermatitidis* in these areas but present at a later time to health care providers in locations where blastomycosis is not usually observed. Inquiring about residence or travel to these areas is important to help establish the diagnosis.

Risk factors for acquiring blastomycosis have been defined by case reports, case series, and a small number of case-control studies and have not been conclusively established. Exposure while in endemic regions to soil, decaying wood, or to dust clouds generated by soil disruption is important; however, specific outdoor occupations or activities have not been confirmed. The fungus may also be associated with exposure to river waterways.

Race may be a contributing factor to disease. In one study from Mississippi, African-American race and prior history of pneumonia were independent risk factors for blastomycosis; however, neither environmental nor socioeconomic risk factors were detected. These findings were in contrast to previously noted studies where race and gender were not identified as specific risk factors for acquisition of blastomycosis. One study in Canada noted an increased incidence among the aboriginal population of Manitoba. Thus, it remains unclear if certain ethnic groups are at increased risk for disease or simply reflect differences in exposure.

Immunosuppression may also be an important risk factor, particularly for the tendency to develop severe disease. Blastomycosis has been reported in pregnant women, persons with diabetes mellitus, organ transplant recipients, and persons infected with HIV.

Dogs and humans are the species most commonly affected by *B. dermatitidis*. Anecdotally, dogs can serve as a sentinel marker for human disease (i.e., dogs present with systemic infection before their owners), leading to early suspicion of human infections by astute veterinarians. In such cases, it is speculated that humans and their pet dogs have a simultaneous exposure to the same source of fungus and therefore develop synchronous infection. This hypothesis, however, remains to be confirmed, and in a more recent study, canine blastomycosis was not deemed to predict human disease among the human owners. Additional studies are required to establish the relationship between blastomycosis in humans and disease in their pet dogs.

The most common mode of transmission is presumed to be by inhalation of aerosolized conidia from the environment. There are, however, reports of cutaneous blastomycosis occuring after accidental cutaneous inoculation, for example in the laboratory setting during autopsy or after dog bites. The median incubation period, established by reviewing the results of point-source outbreaks, ranges from 30 to 45 days.

Pathophysiology

Following inhalation of conidia into the lungs, the fungus is phagocytosed by alveolar macrophages. The human body temperature allows the fungus to transform to the yeast phase. It is speculated that a process similar to infection with *Mycobacterium tuberculosis* then occurs. The fungus might spread to other organs via the bloodstream and lymphatics. The primary defense against *B. dermatitidis* is through a suppurative response initially with neutrophils, followed by influx of monocytes with establishment of cell mediated immunity, resulting in noncaseating granuloma. The patient with intact immunologic responses can contain the process without progression to clinical disease. Alternatively, the patient can develop a symptomatic pneumonia and then mount a suitable immunologic response and recover. Impaired immunity favors the development of progressive pulmonary disease with or without extrapulmonary manifestations. It has also been suggested that reactivation of disease can occur at pulmonary or extrapulmonary sites. A vaccine that protects humans against infection with *B. dermatitidis* is unavailable.

Clinical Manifestations

After inhalation of the conidia, an initial infection can occur. Most primary infections (at least 50%) are asymptomatic or mild and usually go unrecognized, resolving spontaneously. In others, a symptomatic pneumonia can develop; recovery can occur either spontaneously or with therapy, without further progression. Some persons develop progressive pneumonia or extrapulmonary manifestations. The type of clinical manifestations (localized, extrapulmonary or disseminated disease) can have a seasonal variation: Persons with manifestations occurring early after exposure (1 to 6 months) developed localized pneumonia, whereas those who presented later after exposure (4 to 9 months) tended to have isolated extrapulmonary or disseminated disease. Blastomycosis has been termed "the great mimic," because its clinical manifestations are nonspecific and can be similar to those of many different clinical entities. The most common organ systems involved in blastomycosis, in descending order of frequency, include lung, skin, bone, genitourinary, and central nervous systems (CNS). Box 1 summarizes the key clinical manifestations of blastomycosis.

Blastomycosis in Special Populations

Children account for a small percentage of the cases of blastomycosis, ranging from 2% to 11%. Children demonstrate a similar spectrum of manifestations as in adults (excluding prostatic disease). The most common symptoms include cough, headache, chest pain, weight loss, fever, abdominal pain, and night sweats. It is postulated that children experience disseminated infection more frequently than adults.

Although there are few published reports of blastomycosis in pregnancy, disease has been observed in pregnant women, with presumed subsequent intrauterine and perinatal transmission.

Blastomycosis has been reported in persons with advanced HIV and among those who have undergone solid organ transplants. In immunocompromised hosts, it appears that a significant percentage developed rapidly progressive pulmonary disease, leading to respiratory failure and death. For those who are immunocompromised, the reported mortality rates range is 30% to 40%, with death occurring within the first few weeks of disease onset.

Diagnosis

The most reliable technique for confirming the diagnosis of blastomycosis is recovery of the fungus in culture. Alternatively, direct observation of the pathogen by light microscopy or with calcofluor white stain or in histopathologic examination of tissue establishes a presumptive diagnosis. *B. dermatitidis* is characteristically observed as a thick-walled, broad-based budding yeast. Because colonization does not occur, identification of *B. dermatitidis* should never be considered a contaminant. Serologic assays are extremely variable in their

---

BOX 1   Clinical Manifestations of Blastomycosis

Lung

Acute Pneumonia

Acute pneumonia is clinically indistinguishable from bacterial pneumonia.

Patients may present with fevers, chills, dyspnea, and cough, which initially might not be productive but, with time, may be accompanied by sputum production.

Radiographic findings can also be difficult to discern from those due to a bacterial pneumonia.

The radiographic pattern of pulmonary blastomycosis includes the following:

- Lobar infiltrates that mimic bacterial pneumonias
- Cavitary lung lesions and miliary patterns, which can mimic tuberculosis
- Mass lesions that may be mistaken for neoplasms
- Cystic lesions that resemble abscesses

There is no definitive plain radiograph or computed tomographic scan findings characteristic of pulmonary blastomycosis.

The spectrum of clinical pulmonary disease ranges from spontaneous resolution to pneumonia, with or without the acute respiratory distress syndrome, which is accompanied by high (50%-89%) mortality rates.

Chronic Pneumonia

A nonresolving pneumonia is one of the hallmarks of pulmonary blastomycosis.

Chronic pneumonia may be associated with fever, chills, weight loss, sputum-producing cough, and hemoptysis.

There is no characteristic radiographic appearance to help establish the diagnosis.

Skin

Cutaneous lesions are the most common extrapulmonary manifestations of blastomycosis. Lesions usually result from dissemination of a primary pulmonary lesion or rarely from direct inoculation.

Lesions can have a number of different appearances, with verrucae (wartlike lesions) and ulcers being the most common manifestations. The verrucous lesions have a heaped-up appearance with a raw excoriated center. These lesions can mimic squamous cell carcinomas. Cutaneous abscesses may be associated with these lesions.

Ulcerative lesions initially manifest as pustules that eventually erode, producing a bed of granulation tissue that is friable and bleeds when traumatized. Other skin lesions include subcutaneous nodules and isolated abscesses.

Bone and Joint

The most common manifestation of extrapulmonary blastomycosis, after cutaneous disease, is involvement of bones and joints.

Any bone may be involved, although the long bones and axial skeleton are the most commonly affected.

The radiographic findings are indistinguishable from bacterial osteomyelitis and arthritis.

Genitourinary Tract

In the genitourinary tract, the prostate has been reported to be commonly affected by blastomycosis.

Symptoms can mimic prostatitis, and patients can present with obstructive uropathy.

Central Nervous System

The CNS is infrequently affected by *B. dermatitidis*. However, in persons infected with advanced HIV, CNS blastomycosis appears to occur more commonly than in immunocompetent hosts.

Clinical manifestations depend on the area of involvement and range from focal neurologic findings (e.g., due to mass lesions in the brain parenchyma) to symptoms of meningitis due to involvement of the meninges.

Radiographically, the findings may be indistinguishable from bacterial processes. Other sites of involvement have been described but are infrequent compared to those summarized above.

BOX 2 Establishing the Diagnosis of Blastomycosis

Direct Examination

A wet preparation of respiratory secretions or a touch preparation of tissues examined under high magnification by light microscopy can reveal the characteristic thick-walled, broad-based budding yeast form. However, this method has a low diagnostic yield: 36% for a single specimen and 46% for multiple specimens.

Calcofluor white stains can help in identifying the pathogen but require fluorescence microscopy.

Histopathologic Examination

The fungus may be difficult to identify with hematoxylin and eosin stain.

If there is a high index of suspicion, the Gomori methenamine-silver stain should be used to optimize detection of thick-walled, broad-based budding yeast forms compatible with *B. dermatitidis*.

Culture

Diagnostic yield ranges from approximately 86% from sputum to 92% from specimens obtained by bronchoscopy.

Culture is the gold standard for diagnosis. However, the fungus can take several weeks to be isolated in culture.

Confirmation of identity traditionally requires demonstration of thermal-dimorphism (mycelial-to-yeast conversion), which can further delay diagnosis.

Isolation of *B. dermatitidis* should not be considered a contaminant.

Serology

Current serologic assays are neither sensitive nor specific, and they should not be used to establish or refute a diagnosis or in therapeutic decision making.

Nucleic Acid Detection

This method permits genetic-based identification of *B. dermatitidis* from culture of clinical specimens, rather than relying on thermal-dimorphism to confirm identity of the fungus, thus reducing the time required for its identification.

Antigen Detection

The only currently available antigen detection assay has its greatest sensitivity in urine, although antigens can be detected in serum and other body fluids.

Cross reaction with antigens from other fungi (e.g., *Histoplasma* spp.) can occur.

The greatest benefit of the antigen detection assay may be to follow efficacy of treatment in patients with established disease (antigen levels decrease with successful treatment or rise with recurrence).

Skin Testing

A commercially available standardized reagent for skin testing is not available.

Modified from Chapman SW, Bradsher RW, Campbell GD, et al: Practice guidelines for the management of patients with blastomycosis. Cin Infect Dis 2000;30:679-83; and Martynowicz MA, Prakash UBS: Pulmonary blastomycosis: An appraisal of diagnostic techniques. Chest 2002;121:768-773.

---

sensitivity and specificity and do not play a role in confirming or excluding the diagnosis, thus limiting their value in therapeutic decision making. A reliable skin test is unavailable, but a urinary antigen detection assay exists that may be of benefit to follow the efficacy of treatment in established infections. Box 2 summarizes techniques for establishing the diagnosis of blastomycosis.

 CURRENT DIAGNOSIS

- Blastomycosis is caused by the thermally dimorphic fungus *Blastomyces dermatitidis*.
- *B. dermatitidis* is endemic to the United States (southeastern and south central states bordering Mississippi and Ohio rivers; upper Midwestern states bordering the Great Lakes) and to Canada (Manitoba and Ontario bordering the Great Lakes; Quebec adjacent to St. Lawrence River).
- Blastomycosis should be suspected in the appropriate clinical context in patients who have resided or traveled to an endemic area.
- Blastomycosis has a broad range of manifestations, mimicking other infectious (e.g., bacteria, mycobacteria) and neoplastic processes.
- Blastomycosis may be asymptomatic, or it can manifest with disease involving the lung, bones and joints, skin, or central nervous system.
- Diagnosis requires culture or microscopic examination of clinical specimens. Serology has no diagnostic value.

Treatment

The treatment recommendations for blastomycosis from the Infectious Diseases Society of America (IDSA) are summarized in Table 1. Amphotericin B deoxycholate (Fungizone) is the agent with which there is the greatest experience, particularly for the treatment of patients with severe blastomycosis or for those who have CNS involvement. Lipid preparations of amphotericin B (Abelect, Amphotec, AmBisome)[1] have been shown to be effective in animal models, although clinical trial data are unavailable for these agents in humans. Clinical experience suggests that the lipid formulations are as effective but less toxic than the deoxycholate preparation.

It is generally accepted that in patients with severe disease or CNS involvement, amphotericin B should be used to initiate therapy until the patient is stable, followed by step-down to an azole, specifically itraconazole (Sporanox), to complete the total duration of therapy. Ketoconazole (Nizoral), although once recommended as the agent of choice, is less effective and more toxic than itraconazole. Experience with fluconazole (Diflucan)[1] for the treatment of blastomycosis is limited, although *in vitro* studies have demonstrated that fluconazole is effective against *B. dermatitidis*. Fluconazole does, however, have excellent penetration into the CNS; therefore, fluconazole may be

---

[1]Not FDA approved for this indication.

 CURRENT THERAPY

- Treatment varies with the severity of disease.
- Long-term suppressive therapy may be required for those who are immunosuppressed.

TABLE 1 Treatment Suggestions for Infections Caused by *Blastomycosis dermatitidis*

Manifestation	Treatment Recommendations		Comments
	Primary Recommendation	*Alternative Recommendation*	
Pulmonary Infection			
Mild to moderate	Itraconazole (Sporanox) 200 mg PO od or bid × 6-12 mo	Fluconazole (Diflucan)[1] 400-800[3] mg/day or ketoconazole (Nizoral) 400-800 mg/kg × 6-12 mo	
Moderate to severe	Amphotericin B deoxycholate (Fungizone) 0.7-1 mg/kg/d × 1-2 wk until stable followed by itraconazole 200 mg PO bid × 6-12 mo	Lipid preparations of amphotericin B (Abelect, Amphotec, AmBisome)[1] 3-5 mg/kg/d for 1-2 wk until stable followed by itraconazole 200 mg PO bid × 6-12 mo	An alternative approach is to use amphotericin B deoxycholate for a total dose of 1.5-2.5 g Amphotericin B toxicity can be attenuated by minimizing the duration of therapy and switching to oral therapy when the patient is stable
Disseminated Infection Not Involving the Central Nervous System			
Mild to moderate	Itraconazole 200 mg PO od or bid × 6-12 mo		
Moderate to severe	Amphotericin B deoxycholate 0.7-1 mg/kg/d × 1-2 wk followed by itraconazole 200 mg PO bid to complete 12 mo of therapy	Lipid preparations of amphotericin B[1] 3-5 mg/kg/d for 1-2 wk followed by itraconazole 200 mg PO bid to complete 12 mo of therapy	An entire treatment course can be completed with amphotericin B deoxycholate to achieve a total dose of 2 g To minimize toxicity, switching to oral therapy once the patient is stable should be considered Bone and joint infections are usually treated for 12 mo with itraconazole
Central Nervous System Involvement (with or without other manifestations)			
	Lipid preparations of amphotericin B[1] 5 mg/kg/d × 4-6 wk followed by an oral azole for ≥12 mo		It has been suggested that liposomal amphotericin B achieves higher CNS levels than other lipid formulations When switching to oral azole, options include fluconazole[1] 800 mg PO qd,[3] itraconazole 200 mg PO bid or tid,[3] or voriconazole (Vfend)[1] 200-400[3] mg PO bid Longer durations of therapy may be necessary in the immunocompromised host
Special Populations			
Immunocompromised	Amphotericin B deoxycholate 0.7-1 mg/kg/d × 1-2 wk followed by itraconazole 200 mg PO bid to complete 12 mo of therapy	Lipid preparations of amphotericin B[1] 3-5 mg/kg/d × 1-2 wk followed by itraconazole 200 mg PO bid to complete 12 mo of therapy	Lifelong suppression with itraconazole 200 mg PO qd may be required for those in whom immunosuppression cannot be reversed
Pregnant patients	Amphotericin B deoxycholate 0.7-1 mg/kg/d × 1-2 wk followed by itraconazole 200 mg PO bid to complete 12 mo of therapy	Lipid preparations of amphotericin B[1] 3-5 mg/kg/d × 1-2 wk followed by itraconazole 200 mg PO bid to complete 12 mo of therapy	During pregnancy, azoles should be avoided because of potential teratogenicity If the newborn demonstrates evidence of infection, give amphotericin B deoxycholate 1.0 mg/kg/d
Children: mild to moderate	Itraconazole[1] 10 mg/kg/d for 6-12 mo		Maximum dose of itraconazole should be 400 mg/d
Children: moderate to severe	Amphotericin B deoxycholate 0.7-1 mg/kg/d × 1-2 wk followed by itraconazole 10 mg/kg/d × 12 mo	Lipid preparation of amphotericin B[1] 3-5 mg/kg/d × 1-2 wk followed by itraconazole 10 mg/kg/d × 12 mo	

[1]Not FDA approved for this indication.
[3]Exceeds dosage recommended by the manufacturer.
Modified from Chapman SW, Bradsher RW, Campbell GD, et al: Practice guidelines for the management of patients with blastomycosis. Clin Infect Dis 2000;30:679; and Chapman SW, Dismukes WE, Proia LA, et al: Clinical practice guidelines for the management of blastomycosis: 2008 update by the Infectious Diseases Society of America. Clin Infect Dis 2008;46:1801-1812.

considered as an alternative treatment of CNS blastomycosis. There are also a number of reports of voriconazole (Vfend)[1] being used for the successful treatment of CNS blastomycosis, as well as in persons with refractory blastomycosis. A case series of patients with CNS blastomycosis suggested that voriconazole may be the most desirable azole for the management of CNS disease. The echinocandins (caspofungin [Cancidas][1], micafungin [Mycamine][1] and anidulafungin [Eraxis][1]) have limited activity against *B. dermatitidis* and are not considered appropriate choices.

Box 2 summarizes the therapeutic options for treatment of various types of blastomycosis. Amphotericin B is usually the treatment option of choice in persons who have severe disease. Whenever the patient is clinically stable, it is desirable to switch from the potentially toxic amphotericin B to a less-toxic agent (usually an azole). It is important to note that amphotericin B in cumulative doses of 1.5 to 2.5 grams for persons with disseminated blastomycosis, with life-threatening disease, or in those who are immunocompromised or pregnant, can lead to cure without relapses.

In patients with overwhelming pulmonary disease, amphotericin B is the therapeutic agent of choice. Although acute respiratory distress syndrome (ARDS) can complicate the management of these patients, data on the role of corticosteroids in the management of patients with overwhelming pulmonary disease or ARDS is unavailable. For patients with less-severe pulmonary disease, an alternative to amphotericin B is a 6- to 12-month course of oral itraconazole. A similarly prolonged course of oral itraconazole is also appropriate for persons with bone and joint disease. The precise duration of therapy, however, is unknown and should be individualized. The same is true for cutaneous blastomycosis. For persons with CNS blastomycosis, an initial treatment course of 4 to 6 weeks with intravenous amphotericin B should be followed with an oral azole to complete at least 12 months of therapy. For those who are immunocompromised, prolonged therapy is also necessary. Patients who are immunosuppressed and in whom the immunosuppression cannot be reversed can require lifelong suppressive itraconazole therapy at 200 mg per day. Additional details for the management of the various stages of blastomycosis should be sought from the most current version of the IDSA guidelines.

---

[1]Not FDA approved for this indication.

REFERENCES

Bariola JR, Perry P, Pappas PG, et al. Blastomycosis of the central nervous system: a multicenter review of diagnosis and treatment in the modern era. Clin Infect Dis 2010;50:797–804.

Chapman SW, Sullivan DC. Blastomyces dermatitidis. In: Mandell GL, Bennett JE, Dolin R, editors. Mandell, Douglas, and Bennett's Principles and Practice of Infectious Diseases, 7th ed. Philadelphia: Elsevier; 2010. pp. 3319–32.

Chapman SW, Lin AC, Hendricks KA, et al. Endemic blastomycosis in Mississippi: Epidemiological and clinical studies. Semin Respir Infect 1997;12:219–28.

Chapman SW, Bradsher RW, Campbell GD, et al. Practice guidelines for the management of patients with blastomycosis. Cin Infect Dis 2000;30: 679–83.

Chapman SW, Dismukes WE, Proia LA, et al. Clinical practice guidelines for the management of blastomycosis: 2008 update by the Infectious Diseases Society of America. Clin Infect Dis 2008;46:1801–12.

Choptiany M, Wiebe L, Limerick B, et al. Risk factors for acquisition of endemic blastomycosis. Can J Infect Dis Med Microbiol 2009;20:117–21.

Crampton TL, Light RB, Berg GM, et al. Epidemiology and clinical spectrum of blastomycosis diagnosed at Manitoba hospitals. Clin Infect Dis 2002;34:1310–6.

Martynowicz MA, Prakash UBS. Pulmonary blastomycosis: An appraisal of diagnostic techniques. Chest 2002;121:768–73.

Meyer KC, McManus EJ, Maki DG. Overwhelming pulmonary blastomycosis associated with the adult respiratory distress syndrome. N Engl J Med 1993;329:1231–6.

Oppenheimer M, Cheang M, Trepman E, et al. Orthopedic manifestations of blastomycosis. South Med J 2007;100:570–8.

Pappas PG. Blastomycosis in the immunocompromised patient. Semin Respir Infect 1997;12:243–51.

Ward BA, Parent AD, Raila F. Indications for the surgical management of central nervous system blastomycosis. Surg Neurol 1995;43:379–88.

Pleural Effusions and Empyema Thoracis

Method of
David Finley, MD, and Raja Flores, MD

Pleural effusions have multiple etiologies, making the diagnosis and management a common clinical issue. Though the amount of fluid produced varies significantly, an average 0.1 to 0.2 mL/kg is maintained within the pleural space. Production of fluid is matched with removal during normal physiologic states, but aberrations of this homeostasis with local or systemic diseases lead to the formation of an effusion. Symptoms are related to the volume of fluid and the etiology of the fluid accumulation, including both benign and malignant processes. Secondary infection of a pleural effusion, known as an empyema, is a significant complication necessitating aggressive treatment of both the underlying cause and the empyema itself.

Symptoms are variable and include dyspnea, shortness of breath, cough, and chest discomfort, though patients can be asymptomatic, even with very large effusions. Dullness to percussion and decreased breath sounds are often hallmarks of effusions, but these signs are also seen with lung masses and consolidative pneumonias. A clinical history, physical examination, and imaging studies are often needed in combination to diagnose an effusion.

Etiology

Many local and systemic illnesses are associated with the formation of a pleural effusion. Systemic symptoms can indicate the most common cause of the effusion, but diagnostic procedures are often necessary to delineate the etiology. Determination of an exudative or transudative effusion can point out possible disease that may be the cause (Box 1).

Fluid that is low in total protein is a transudative effusion, which is most commonly caused by decreased oncotic pressure or increased capillary hydrostatic pressure. Transudative effusions can also be caused by fluid traversing the diaphragm, as seen in patients with ascites.

BOX 1 Etiologies of Transudative and Exudative Effusions

Transudative
Congestive heart failure
Cirrhosis
Pulmonary emboli
Peritoneal dialysis
Renal disorders
Myxedema
Sarcoidosis

Exudative
Malignancy
Infection
Drugs (e.g., nitrofurantoin [Marcodantin, Macrobid], methotrexate [Trexall])
Chylothorax
Pulmonary emboli
Gastrointestinal diseases (e.g., pancreatitis)
Collagen vascular disease (e.g., rheumatoid arthritis)
Asbestos exposure
Trauma (e.g., hemothorax, chest surgery)
Postpericardiectomy or postmyocardial infarction syndrome
Pleuropericarditis

Exudative effusions are high in total protein (pleural fluid-to-serum ratio >0.5) and often have an elevated cell count. Increased capillary permeability and decreased lymphatic clearance, usually due to a local or systemic inflammatory illness, produce exudative effusions. The causes are varied, but the most common causes are malignancy, infection, and pulmonary emboli.

Diagnosis

IMAGING

Approximately 200 to 500 mL of pleural fluid is necessary before it can be visualized on a posteroanterior upright chest x-ray, usually as blunting of the costophrenic angle. A lateral chest x-ray is more sensitive, often discerning fluid with as little as 100 mL present; layering of the fluid confirms that it is free flowing. Loculations can be seen on x-ray but may be mistaken for lung or pleural masses. Large effusion can completely opacify the hemithorax where the effusion is located. Ultrasound is useful in defining the location and extent of an effusion and can also identify loculated effusions, pleural thickening, and masses. When used to help guide thoracentesis, it can increase diagnostic accuracy and yield and decrease complications.

Chest computed tomography (CT) has distinct advantages over x-ray and ultrasound, though its utility is significantly decreased when there is a large effusion. Imaging with CT after initial drainage of a large effusion is recommended to obtain the most information regarding the possible etiologies of the effusion and aid in operative planning for treatment of an empyema. It also delineates pleural masses and helps differentiate pleural disease from lung pathology (e.g., loculated effusion vs. lung abscess).

THORACENTESIS

Often it is difficult to discern the cause of an effusion solely based on the patient's clinical presentation and image studies. Also, when concerned about a malignant process or an infected effusion, these studies do not give enough information to make a definitive diagnosis. Thoracentesis is the diagnostic procedure of choice, allowing drainage of the fluid to relieve symptoms for the patient and provide a specimen for evaluation. Ultrasound should be employed to help guide thoracentesis, especially if the effusion is small or loculated. Care must be taken when draining a large amount of fluid in one setting due to the risk of reexpansion pulmonary edema. If a patient becomes symptomatic during the procedure (persistent cough, significant pleuritic pain, or shortness of breath) no more fluid should be remove at that time. Coagulopathy is a contraindication to thoracentesis due to the risk of intrathoracic bleeding.

PLEURAL FLUID

The initial evaluation of pleural fluid is done at the bedside by determining the nature of the fluid: clear, cloudy, bloody, or milky. One should also evaluate the fluid for odor and cellularity. These simple steps can point the clinician toward the correct diagnosis. In addition to bedside evaluation, the fluid should be sent for the following laboratory studies: pH, glucose, lactate dehydrogenase (LDH), protein, cytology, Gram stain, and culture (including fungal and viral). Serum pH, protein, LDH and glucose should be sent at the same time.

Light's criteria are helpful in differentiating between an exudative and transudative effusion (Box 2). The sensitivity and specificity of Light's criteria is 82% to 90%.

BOX 2   Light's Criteria for an Exudative Effusion

Pleural fluid-to-serum ratio of protein >0.5
Pleural fluid-to-serum ration of LDH >0.6
Absolute pleural fluid LDH >2/3 of upper limit of normal
    serum levels

Abbreviation: LDH = lactate dehydrogenase.

Transudative effusions rarely need any further intervention, and the goal of treatment is directed at the underlying condition (see Box 1). For exudative effusions, the cause of the effusion dictates the treatment. Incorporating the clinical picture and radiographs with the pleural fluid chemistry studies, cytology, and cultures, the diagnosis is often obtained. Malignant effusions can have positive cytology, but they are more likely to have a pleural fluid glucose level less than 60 mg/dL and to be bloody. An elevated amylase level is seen in esophageal perforation, pancreatitis, and malignant effusions. Chylothorax can be definitively diagnosed if the triglyceride level is more than 110 mg/dL within the pleural fluid. Finally, pH, glucose, and cultures are useful in the treatment of patients with a presumed infected pleural effusion (empyema).

Up to 25% of patients will not have a definitive diagnosis based on the clinical scenario and pleural fluid evaluation. These patients can require further diagnostic testing, including repeat thoracentesis or evaluation of the chest cavity via video-assisted thoracoscopic surgery (VATS) with pleural biopsies.

Treatment

After initial evacuation of the effusion, treatment is directed at controlling the underlying disease that caused the effusion. Malignant effusions are best managed with pleurodesis, usually employing talc (Sterile Talc), if lung re-expansion can be obtained. This is best performed via VATS, which allows biopsies to be performed, confirming the diagnosis and visually confirming lung re-expansion. Though it can be done via tube thoracostomy at the bedside, VATS pleurodesis has been shown to reduce hospital stay and the risk of recurrence. If the lung cannot expand fully, then the fluid is often best managed with an indwelling long-term silicone-elastic catheter for palliation. In patients with benign disease, pleurodesis is rarely done because of the high complication and failure rates.

Infected Pleural Space and Empyema

A parapneumonic effusion (exudative effusion in the setting of pulmonary infection) is seen in 20% to 40% of patients admitted for pneumonia, of whom 10% to 20% will develop a complicated parapneumonic effusion or empyema (pus in the pleural space). Progression to empyema is most often due to delay in treatment and leads to longer hospital stays and increased morbidity and mortality. Other causes of infected effusions are trauma, thoracic surgical procedures, perforated esophagus, systemic infection, and transdiaphragmatic spread.

Parapneumonic effusions can be separated into three stages: exudative (stage I), fibropurulent (stage II), and organizational (stage III). Though thoracentesis is indicated in each stage, it is usually sufficient for stage I effusions when coupled with appropriate antibiotics. These effusions are free flowing, have negative cultures, and often do not reaccumulate.

Complicated parapneumonic, or stage II, effusions require drainage beyond the initial thoracentesis. The fluid is more viscous and has positive bacterial cultures, a low glucose level, and low pH. Progression to frank pus, or empyema, occurs in this stage, with the formation of loculations as fibrin deposition increases. Complete evacuation of the effusion is required, and initial tube thoracostomy is indicated. If the patient does not improve over the next 24 hours or the space is not completely drained (residual loculations), then surgery is recommended. Randomized, placebo-controlled trials showed no improved outcomes with the use of fibrinolytics as compared to standard tube thoracostomy drainage. The introduction of DNase (Pulmozyme)[1] may be of benefit, but data are insufficient to recommend this treatment. We strongly recommend early intervention with VATS, which has been shown to reduce hospital stay and offers definitive treatment as compared to tube thoracostomy with fibrinolytic therapy.

---

[1]Not FDA approved for this indication.

Delayed or inadequate treatment causes the patient to progress to the organizational stage. This is characterized by heavy fibrin deposit with the formation of a thick peel throughout the pleura with loculations, trapping, and retarding lung re-expansion. Classic CT findings include thickened pleura with multiple loculations and inability of the lung to expand after tube thoracostomy. Decortication, either via VATS or thoracotomy, is required to completely remove the peel off the parietal and visceral pleura. Without obliteration of the empyema space it is very unlikely that the infection can be cleared. In these situations an open thoracostomy, or Eloesser flap, may be required to eradicate the infection.

REFERENCES

Cameron R, Davies HR. Intra-pleural fibrinolytic therapy versus conservative management in the treatment of adult parapneumonic effusions and empyema. Cochrane Database Syst Rev 2008;(2):CD002312.

de Campos JR, Vargas FS, de Campos Werebe E, et al. Thoracoscopy talc poudrage: A 15-year experience. Chest 2001;119:801–6.

Light R. Clinical practice. Pleural effusion. N Engl J Med 2002;346:1971–7.

Light RW. Parapneumonic effusions and empyema. Proc Am Thorac Soc 2006;3:75–80.

Luh SP, Chen CY, Tzao CY. Malignant pleural effusion treatment outcomes: Pleurodesis via video-assisted thoracic surgery (VATS) versus tube thoracostomy. Thorac Cardiovasc Surg 2006;54:332–6.

Luh SP, Hsu GJ, Cheng-Ren C. Complicated parapneumonic effusion and empyema: Pleural decortication and video-assisted thoracic surgery. Curr Infect Dis Rep 2008;10:236–40.

Rahman NM, Chapman SJ, Davies RJ. Diagnosis and management of infectious pleural effusion. Treat Respir Med 2006;5:295–304.

Tokuda Y, Matsushima D, Stein GH, et al. Intrapleural fibrinolytic agents for empyema and complicated parapneumonic effusions: A meta-analysis. Chest 2006;129:783–90.

Primary Lung Abscess

Method of
Daniel Schuller, MD

Definition and Classification

Lung abscess is defined as a focal area of necrosis of the lung parenchyma resulting from microbial infection and usually measuring more than 2 cm in diameter. Smaller or multiple areas of necrosis in contiguous areas are referred to as *necrotizing pneumonia*. Primary lung abscess (80%) is due to direct infection or aspiration. Secondary lung abscess (20%) is secondary to bronchial obstruction, immunodeficiency, pulmonary infarction, trauma, or complications from surgery. Lung abscesses can also be classified according to pathogen (e.g., mixed anaerobic, *Pseudomonas,* mycobacterial, fungal) or duration of symptoms (e.g., chronic with symptoms for more than a month before presentation).

Epidemiology and Risk Factors

Most lung abscesses result from aspiration of oral secretions in patients who harbor high bacterial concentrations in the gingival crevices. Periodontal disease, especially gingivitis, is a major predisposing condition, particularly in hosts impaired by altered sensorium due to alcoholism, anesthesia, coma, drug overdose, seizures, or stroke. Because edentulous persons rarely develop lung abscesses, other causes such as malignancy should be carefully sought. Patients with dysphagia, esophageal disease, poor airway protection, or weak cough and respiratory clearance mechanisms are also at risk for developing lung abscess.

Patients whose immune systems are compromised by malignancy, HIV infection, malnutrition, diabetes, chronic use of corticosteroids, or previous organ transplantation are more likely to be infected with aerobic bacteria, mycobacterial or fungal pathogens. These patients are more likely to have multiple abscesses, less response to treatment, and a worse prognosis.

In children, consider secondary causes including foreign body aspiration, congenital cystic adenomatoid malformation, pulmonary sequestration, cystic fibrosis, bronchiectasis, bronchogenic cyst, congenital immunodeficiency, or severe underlying neurologic abnormality.

Lemierre's disease or jugular vein suppurative thrombophlebitis, usually caused by *Fusobacterium necrophorum,* is a rare infection that begins in the pharynx as a tonsillar or peritonsillar abscess and spreads to involve the internal jugular vein, with septic emboli to the lung with secondary cavitations.

Pathophysiology

The development of a lung abscess usually starts when an insult (e.g., inoculum of highly contaminated oral secretions) overcomes the pulmonary mechanisms of defense and begins a process of pneumonitis in the dependent areas affected by aspiration. Depending on the microbiology and the intensity of the inflammatory response, the acute pneumonitis evolves to tissue necrosis after 7 to 14 days and subsequent cavitation. At first, the enclosing wall is poorly defined, but with time and progressive fibrosis it becomes more discrete. When a communication with the airway exists, the suppurative debris from the abscess can partially drain, leaving an air-containing cavity with a radiographic air-fluid level. Occasionally, abscesses rupture into the pleural cavity yielding an empyema or a bronchopleural fistula (Figure 1). Primary abscesses due to aspiration are much more common on the right side than the left and are most often single. The most common locations include the superior segments of the lower lobes and the posterior segment of the right upper lobe.

Clinical Manifestations

Most patients present with insidious symptoms that evolve over a period of weeks to months. Cough productive of copious amounts of putrid, foul-smelling sputum that occurs in paroxysms after changing position are characteristic. Fevers, chills, night sweats, chest pain, dyspnea, general malaise, and fatigue are common. Hemoptysis can vary from blood-streaked sputum to life-threatening hemorrhage. Physical findings can include fever, tachycardia, periodontal disease, halitosis, signs of lung consolidation or pleural effusion, amphoric breath sounds, and occasionally clubbing of the fingers and toes can appear within a few weeks after the onset of an abscess.

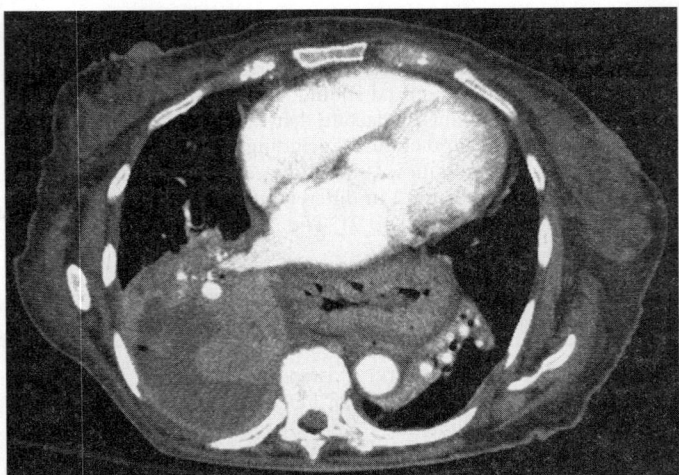

FIGURE 1. Primary lung abscess in the right lower lobe with rupture into the pleural space causing an empyema.

Diagnosis

Lung abscess is easily diagnosed when there is a classic clinical presentation with indolent symptoms lasting more than 2 weeks in a host with predisposing risk factors and a chest radiograph revealing a cavitary infiltrate or an air-fluid level. However, numerous pathogens are associated with this syndrome, and attempts to establish microbiological diagnosis and exclude other conditions are warranted.

Computed tomography (CT) scans can be useful for better anatomic definition, to evaluate possible associated conditions such as malignancy, and to rule out pleural involvement. Distinguishing between a lung abscess and an empyema with an associated bronchopleural fistula leading to an air-fluid level can sometimes be challenging, but it is crucial because the management of these conditions is very different. Features that suggest empyema include a lenticular shape or a larger diameter of the air-fluid level on the lateral view of the chest film, an obtuse angle of the cavity with the chest wall, and a split pleural sign with contrast enhancement of the pleura.

Most lung abscesses are caused by anaerobic or mixed aerobic and anaerobic infections. Anaerobic bacteria include *Peptostreptococcus*, *Prevotella*, *Bacteroides* spp., and *Fusobacterium* spp. and are difficult to isolate owing to technical issues and contamination by upper airway flora. Other pathogens, including *Staphylococcus aureus*, *Klebsiella pneumonia*, *Pseudomonas*, *Burkholderia pseudomallei*, *Nocardia*, *Actinomyces*, and mycobacterial or fungal organisms, are more likely to occur in secondary lung abscesses.

Sputum Gram stains and culture should be performed in all patients but interpreted with caution because prior antimicrobial therapy can inhibit growth, and contaminant strains can be misleading. Even when there is abundant growth of a species of aerobic bacteria, treatment should still be directed at covering anaerobes.

In the absence of positive blood or pleural fluid cultures, microbiological confirmation of a lung abscess requires other invasive methods such as a transthoracic needle aspirates (TTNA) or bronchoscopy with bronchoalveolar lavage (BAL) or protected specimen brush (PSB). The best timing for bronchoscopy is controversial because early intervention has the highest diagnostic yield but at the risk of provoking spillage of a relatively contained abscess into additional lobes or the contralateral lung. In patients who are edentulous or in whom there is a high suspicion for malignancy, the indication for bronchoscopic evaluation is almost universal but should be scheduled when the risk for clinical deterioration (e.g., spillage with resultant respiratory failure) has been minimized.

Differential Diagnosis

In addition to the multiple necrotizing infections or an empyema with a bronchopleural fistula (see earlier), there are many noninfectious diseases that can cause cavitary lung lesions and mimic a lung abscess. The differential diagnosis includes neoplasm (primary or metastatic), bullae or cyst with air-fluid level, bronchiectasis, necrotizing vasculitis, or pulmonary infarction. In patients with multiple cavitary lesions, consider septic emboli.

CURRENT DIAGNOSIS

- Lung abscess is usually a complication of aspiration in patients with gingivitis or periodontal disease.
- Mixed aerobic-anaerobic copathogens are common, but sputum cultures are not reliable.
- Lung abscesses are rare in edentulous patients and should prompt evaluation for bronchial obstruction.
- CT scan of the chest is very useful in the diagnostic evaluation.

Treatment

Lung abscess is best treated with a prolonged course of adequate antimicrobials and postural drainage. Percutaneous or bronchoscopic drainage and surgery are considered only for selected patients whose disease is refractory to standard care.

Initial empiric antibiotic treatment for a typical community-acquired lung abscess should consist of intravenous clindamycin (Cleocin) 600 to 900 mg every 6 to 8 hours, which has been shown to be superior to penicillin. For patients with a nosocomial or health care–associated lung abscess, additional coverage for enteric gram-negative pathogens including *Pseudomonas aeruginosa* and *Staphylococcus aureus* is appropriate.

Alternative antimicrobial options include ampicillin–sulbactam (Unasyn)[1] 1.5 to 3.0 g IV every 6 hours, piperacillin–tazobactam (Zosyn)[1] 3.35 g IV every 6 hours, cefoxitin (Mefoxin) 2 to 3 g every 6 to 8 hours, or a combination of moxifloxacin (Avelox)[1] 400 mg IV daily and metronidazole (Flagyl) 500 mg IV every 6 to 8 hours. The use of metronidazole as single agent has been associated with a high therapeutic failure rate.

After defervescence and radiographic improvement, parenteral antibiotics can be switched to oral bioequivalent therapy for 6 to 8 weeks or longer depending on the course. Shorter antimicrobial courses are associated with a high rate of relapse. Most experts suggest continuing therapy until there is radiographic resolution or a small stable lesion.

Indications for percutaneous or bronchoscopic drainage include persistent sepsis after 5 to 7 days of antimicrobial therapy, abscesses larger than 4 cm that are under tension or enlarging, and need for mechanical ventilator support. Percutaneous drainage should only be considered when there is a reasonable abscess–pleura symphysis and no associated coagulopathy.

Postural drainage and chest physiotherapy facilitate removal of pus, relieving symptoms and improving gas exchange. Surgical resection is required in less than 10% of patients whose disease is refractory to medical management.

Finally, evaluation and management of the predisposing conditions leading to aspiration should take place after the patient is stabilized. This can include swallowing assessment, dental work, or oral surgery.

Prognosis

Primary lung abscesses in nonimmunocompromised hosts have cure rates of 90% to 95% with antimicrobial therapy and postural drainage alone. However, in immunocompromised patients and those with bronchial obstruction due to cancer, the mortality has been reported between 20% and 75%.

---

[1]Not FDA approved for this indication.

CURRENT THERAPY

- Prolonged antimicrobial therapy (6-8 weeks) and postural drainage are the cornerstone of therapy.
- Clindamycin (Cleocin) or alternative anaerobic coverage is required even if sputum cultures grow only aerobic bacteria (colonizers or copathogens).
- Percutaneous or bronchoscopic drainage is reserved for selected cases refractory to medical management or at a high risk for complications.
- Surgical resection is seldom needed because of the success of medical therapy.
- Evaluation and management of underlying predisposing conditions should not be neglected.

REFERENCES

Bartlett JG. Anaerobic bacterial pleuropulmonary infections. Semin Respir Med 1992;13:159–64.

Bartlett JG. The role of anaerobic bacteria in lung abscess. Clin Infect Dis 2005;40:923–5.

Gudiol F, Manresa F, Pallares R, et al. Clindamycin vs. penicillin for anaerobic lung infections. Arch Intern Med 1990;150:2525–9.

Hammer DL, Aranda CP, Galati V, Adams FV. Massive intrabronchial aspiration of contents of pulmonary abscess after fiberoptic bronchoscopy. Chest 1978;7:306–7.

Herth F, Ernst A, Becker HD. Endoscopic drainage of lung abscesses. Technique and outcome. Chest 2005;127:1378–81.

Levinson ME, Mangura CT, Lorber B, et al. Clindamycin compared with penicillin for the treatment of anaerobic lung abscess. Ann Intern Med 1983;98:466–71.

Mandell LA, Wunderink RG, Anzueto A, et al. Infectious Diseases Society of America/American Thoracic Society consensus guidelines on the management of community-acquired pneumonia in adults. Clin Infect Dis 2007;44:S27–72.

Mueller PR, Berlin L. Complications of lung abscess aspiration and drainage. AJR Am J Roentgenol 2002;178:1083–6.

Acute Bronchitis

Method of
Susan Davids, MD, MPH, and
Ralph M. Schapira, MD

Acute bronchitis is one of the most common diagnoses made by primary care physicians in the United States and accounts for nearly 10 million office visits per year. Acute bronchitis is a transient, self-limited inflammatory process of the upper respiratory tract, specifically the trachea and bronchi. Antibiotics are overprescribed to patients with acute bronchitis; this practice has raised significant concern related to the worldwide rise of antibiotic resistance, which is viewed as one of the world's most pressing public health problems.

Acute bronchitis manifests as an acute respiratory illness of less than 3 weeks' duration, with or without sputum production. Acute bronchitis is a clinical diagnosis and must be distinguished from other respiratory diseases, such as pneumonia, acute exacerbation of chronic bronchitis (episode of worsening of symptoms and expiratory airflow obstruction in patients with chronic obstructive pulmonary disease), and the onset of asthma. Most cases of acute bronchitis occur in the fall and winter. The etiology of acute bronchitis is infectious, and viruses appear to be the cause of most cases. Influenzas A and B are the most common viruses isolated, although a wide variety of infectious agents have been identified, such as adenovirus, coronavirus, parainfluenza virus, respiratory syncytial virus, coxsackievirus, *Mycoplasma pneumoniae*, *Bordetella pertussis*, and *Chlamydia pneumoniae*.

Diagnosis of acute bronchitis is based on findings of a prominent cough that may be accompanied by wheezing and sputum production. Most patients are otherwise healthy and without preexisting respiratory disease. Nonspecific constitutional symptoms may also be part of acute bronchitis. Appropriate management of acute bronchitis is essential because it is one of the most common illnesses that present to physicians in the outpatient setting. Antibiotics are often prescribed unnecessarily for acute bronchitis and other respiratory tract illnesses; these prescriptions may potentially lead to adverse events (i.e., allergic reactions and gastrointestinal side effects) and bacterial resistance. Other medications, such as inhaled bronchodilators and antitussives, are often prescribed for acute bronchitis despite questionable evidence to support their routine use.

CURRENT DIAGNOSIS

- Normal healthy adult with cough
- Predominance of cough
- Lasts 1 to 3 weeks
- With or without sputum
- Can be accompanied by other respiratory and constitutional symptoms
- Absence of abnormal vital signs and physical exam suggesting pneumonia, particularly
  - Heart rate >100 beats per minute
  - Respiratory rate >24 breaths per minute
  - Temperature >100.4°F (38°C)
  - Lung findings suggest a consolidation process

Pathophysiology of acute bronchitis involves an acute inflammatory response involving the mucosa of the trachea and bronchi, resulting in injury to the respiratory tract epithelium. Sputum production is increased and bronchoconstriction (potentially resulting in airflow obstruction and wheezing) can occur. Positron emission tomography (PET) of a patient with acute bronchitis confirms that the primary inflammatory changes occur in the trachea and bronchi and not the remainder of the lower respiratory track.

Diagnosis

Cough, phlegm (which may be purulent as both bacteria and viruses can cause purulent sputum), and wheezing help differentiate acute bronchitis from upper respiratory infections such as pharyngitis and sinusitis. Acute bronchitis must be differentiated from acute bacterial pneumonia. The absence of abnormalities in vital signs (heart rate >100 bpm, respiratory rate >24 breath/min, oral temperature >100.4°F [38°C] and physical examination of the chest) supports the diagnosis of acute bronchitis and makes the need for chest radiography unnecessary in most cases. The treatment and outcome of acute bronchitis and pneumonia are very different; a chest radiograph should always be obtained if there is uncertainty about the diagnosis. Chest radiography will demonstrate no lung infiltrates in a patient with acute bronchitis. In contrast, lung infiltrates are present in pneumonia. Pertussis or whooping cough should be considered in adults with cough in the setting of what appears to be an upper respiratory infection, even in those previously immunized. Typically, the cough of pertussis, unlike acute bronchitis, lasts for longer than 3 weeks. Other respiratory diseases, such as previously undiagnosed asthma, can also mimic acute bronchitis, although several features differentiate asthma from acute bronchitis (see Section 12). Rapid testing to diagnose influenza viruses A and B (the most common causes of acute bronchitis) as a cause of acute bronchitis should be considered given the availability of effective treatment if initiated in the first 48 hours.

Treatment

ANTIBIOTICS, INHALED BRONCHODILATORS, AND ANTITUSSIVES

Existing evidence does not support the routine use of antibiotics for uncomplicated cases of acute bronchitis. Although most cases of acute bronchitis are caused by viral infections, upwards of 60% of patients are prescribed antibiotic therapy, which is contributing to the rise of bacterial resistance to commonly used antibiotics. Meta-analyses examining the effectiveness of antibiotic therapy in patients without underlying lung disease suggest no consistent effect of

CURRENT THERAPY

- Antibiotics not routinely recommended
- If influenza is highly probable and patient is presenting within the first 48 hours, consider treatment with
  - Oseltamivir (Tamiflu) 75 mg PO bid with food for 5 days (influenza A/B)
  - Zanamivir (Relenza) 10 mg bid by inhalation for 5 days (influenza A/B)
  - *Amantadine (Symmetrel) 100 mg bid or 200 mg once daily for 5 days (influenza A)
  - *Rimantadine (Flumadine) 100 mg bid for 5 days (influenza A)
- In patients with evidence of bronchial hyperresponsiveness, consider treatment with
  - β_2-agonists for 1 to 2 weeks
  - Antitussives in those with cough for 2 to 3 weeks
  - Antipyretics and analgesics as needed
  - Smoking cessation
- Education: cough likely to last 3 weeks or more.

*Due to antiviral medication resistance, the choice of agent to treat influenza should be based on recommendations from the CDC and local health departments.

antibiotics on the severity or duration of acute bronchitis. A recent study evaluated children and patients with colored sputum and found that they also did not benefit from antibiotics. This study also found that compared to other populations, the elderly were less likely to benefit from antibiotics. Smokers with acute bronchitis are even more likely to be prescribed antibiotics. Their response to antibiotics was either equal to or worse than that of nonsmokers.

One possible reason for overuse of antibiotics is the concern by physicians about patient satisfaction. Studies show that patients presenting to the doctor expecting antibiotics were more likely to be prescribed antibiotics; studies also suggest that satisfaction is more related to appropriate patient education than to receiving antibiotics. Patient education should include information regarding the duration of symptoms associated with acute bronchitis. It was found that patients presented on average after 9 days of cough and that the cough persisted for an additional 12 days after the physician visit. This information can impart a realistic expectation of illness duration to the patient.

If influenza is highly suspected and the patient presents within 48 hours of the onset of symptoms, rapid diagnostic testing and treatment should be considered. Both amantadine (Symmetrel) and rimantadine (Flumadine) are effective for influenza A, and neuraminidase inhibitors, inhaled zanamivir (Relenza), and oral oseltamivir (Tamiflu) are effective for influenzas A and B. If these medications are initiated within the first 48 hours of symptoms (and ideally within 30 hours), the duration of illness can be shortened.

The evidence supporting the use of inhaled bronchodilators for the treatment of the symptoms has been variable. Two small trials reported a shorter duration of cough with the use of inhaled β-agonists; another study reported benefit in those with evidence of bronchial hyperresponsiveness. Current recommendations support the use of β-agonists only in patients with evidence of bronchial hyperresponsiveness (wheezing or spirometry demonstrating a forced expiration volume in 1 second [FEV_1] <80% of predicted).

Antitussive agents have not been shown to improve the acute or early cough but did show some improvements in cough lasting longer than 3 weeks. The current recommendations are to use antitussives, namely dextromethorphan (Benylin) or codeine, in patients with cough of 2 to 3 weeks' duration.

Acute uncomplicated bronchitis is most often a viral illness in which antibiotics are not routinely indicated. Patients presenting with an acute respiratory illness, who are younger than 65 years old without existing pulmonary disease or other significant comorbid illness, should have a thorough physical examination, including vital signs. If the vital signs are normal and physical examination of the chest is clear, pneumonia can most likely be ruled out. In patients who present within 48 hours of onset of symptoms, influenza should be considered as effective therapy is available for acute bronchitis caused by influenzas A or B. Otherwise, the evidence for treatment with antibiotics does not support their routine use. Bronchodilators should be considered in those with evidence of bronchial hyperresponsiveness; cough suppressants should be considered in those with 2 to 3 weeks of cough. Patient education is an integral part of the treatment, and patients should receive information that provides realistic expectations regarding the duration of cough.

REFERENCES

Aagaard E, Gonzales R. Management of acute bronchitis in healthy adults. Infect Dis Clin North Am 2004;18:919–37.
Ebell MH. Antibiotic prescribing for cough and symptoms of respiratory tract infection. JAMA 2005;294(3):3062–4.
Fahey T, Smucny J, Becker L, Glazier R. Antibiotics for acute bronchitis. Cochrane Database Syst Rev 2004;(4) CD000245.
Gonzales R, Sande M. Uncomplicated acute bronchitis. Ann Intern Med 2000;133:981–91.
Kicska G, Zhuang H, Alavi A. Acute bronchitis imaged with F-18 FDG positron emission tomography. Clin Nucl Med 2003;28(6):511–2.
Little R, Rumsby K, Kelly J, et al. Information leaflet and antibiotic prescribing strategies for acute lower respiratory tract infection. JAMA 2005;293 (24):3029–35.
Linder JA, Sim I. Antibiotic treatment of acute bronchitis in smokers. J Gen Intern Med 2002;17:230–4.
Martinez FJ. Acute bronchitis: State of the art diagnosis and therapy. Compr Ther 2004;30(1):55–9.
Smucny J, Flynn C, Becker L, Glazier R. Beta$_2$-agonists for acute bronchitis. Cochrane Database Syst Rev 2004;(1) CD001726.

Bacterial Pneumonia

Method of
Edward Septimus, MD

Pneumonia occurs in about 3 to 4 million patients per year in the United States with approximately 1 million patients requiring hospitalization. The symptoms of pneumonia include cough, shortness of breath, sputum production, and chest pain. Physical examination includes fever in most, with crackles and bronchial breath sounds on auscultation in about 80% of cases. Pneumonia is classified by where it was acquired: community-acquired pneumonia (CAP) and health care–acquired pneumonia (HAP, sometimes called *hospital-acquired pneumonia*). This chapter focuses on adult patients with CAP or HAP.

Community-Acquired Pneumonia

CAP remains a leading cause of death in the United States. One study estimated that more than 900,000 cases of CAP occur in persons older than 65 years each year. The emergence of drug-resistant

Streptococcus pneumoniae (DRSP) and less common pathogens including methicillin-resistant *Staphylococcus aureus* (MRSA) is well documented. Pneumonia in long-term care institutions usually resembles HAP and is discussed later.

DIAGNOSTIC TESTING

Symptoms plus an infiltrate by chest radiograph or other imaging studies are required for the diagnosis. Clinical features and physical findings may be absent in the elderly. All patients should be screened by pulse oximetry. Arterial blood gases should be reserved for patients with suspected CO_2 retention. Routine diagnostic studies to determine the etiology for outpatients with CAP are optional. For patients requiring admission, diagnostic studies to determine the etiology of CAP should be attempted. Increased mortality is more common with inappropriate initial empiric therapy. De-escalation of antimicrobial therapy based on pathogen-specific treatment has been shown to decrease adverse drug effects and selection of antimicrobial resistance.

Blood cultures and sputum for Gram stain and culture (in patients with a productive cough) should be obtained in most patients who are admitted to the hospital. Pretreatment blood cultures have a 5% to 14% yield in patients hospitalized with CAP. The most common positive blood culture to be considered a pathogen is *S. pneumoniae*. In some series, false-positive blood cultures (contaminants) exceed positive blood culture with true pathogens. A false-positive blood culture can lead to extra days in the hospital and unnecessary use of antibiotics, especially vancomycin (Vancocin). The highest yield has been demonstrated with severe CAP (Box 1). Pretreatment Gram stain and culture should be performed only if a good quality specimen can be obtained. A Gram stain can direct initial empiric therapy, especially with less common pathogens such as *S. aureus* or gram-negative bacteria.

Patients with pleural effusions greater than 5 cm on a lateral upright chest radiograph or greater than 1 cm on a lateral decubitus film should undergo a thoracentesis for Gram stain and culture. Urinary antigen tests are available for *S. pneumoniae* and *Legionella pneumophila*. These tests are rapid and specific in adults. For pneumococcal pneumonia, studies in adults show a sensitivity of 50% to 80% and a specificity of greater than 90%. False-positives are seen in children colonized with *S. pneumoniae*; therefore, this test is not recommended in children. For *L. pneumophila*, the urinary antigen can only detect *L. pneumophila* serogroup 1, which accounts for 80% to 90% of legionnaires' disease cases in the United States. The urinary antigen has a sensitivity of 70% to 90% and a specificity of greater than 95%. A new polymerase chain reaction (PCR) test can detect all serotypes of *L. pneumophila* in sputum; however, clinical experience is currently limited.

The diagnosis of atypical pneumonia such as *Chlamydophila pneumoniae*, *Mycoplasma pneumoniae*, and *Legionella* species other than *L. pneumophila* rely on acute and convalescent serologies. In general, management on a single acute serology is unreliable; therefore, serologies are often retrospective and usually do not affect initial antimicrobial therapy.

ADMISSION CRITERIA

The initial decision of the treatment of CAP often revolves around severity of illness and if the patient requires hospitalization. Two severity-of-illness scores are commonly used, CURB-65 and the pneumonia severity index (PSI). CURB-65 stands for confusion, uremia (blood urea nitrogen >20 mg/dL), respiratory rate greater than 30 breaths/minute, systolic *blood* pressure less than 90 mm Hg, and age older than 64 years. The PSI score is based primarily on history of underlying diseases and age that increase the risk of mortality, whereas CURB-65 does not rely on underlying diseases.

With CURB-65, mortality was higher when three (14.5%), four (40%), or five (57%) factors were present. Patients with a score of 0 or 1 can be treated on an outpatient basis, patients with a score of 2 can be admitted to the floor, and patients with scores higher than 3 often require admission to the intensive care unit (ICU). PSI uses 20 different variables and places patients into five risk groups (Table 1). Risk classes I and II patients can be treated as

---

BOX 1 Criteria for Severe Community-Acquired Pneumonia

Minor Criteria

Confusion or disorientation
Hypotension requiring fluid resuscitation
Hypothermia (<36°C)
Leukopenia (WBC <4000 cell/mm^3)
Multilobar infiltrates
Pao$_2$/Fio$_2$ ≤250
Respiratory rate ≥30
Thrombocytopenia (platelet count <100,000 cells/mm^3)
Uremia (BUN ≥20 mg/dL)

Major Criteria

Invasive mechanical ventilation
Septic shock requiring vasopressors

Adapted from Mandell LA, Wunderink RG, Anzueto A, et al: Infectious Diseases Society of America/American Thoracic Society Consensus Guidelines on the Management of Community-Acquired Pneumonia in Adults. Clin Infect Dis 2007;44:S27–S72.
BUN = blood urea nitrogen; Fio$_2$ = fraction of inspired oxygen; Pao$_2$ = partial pressure of arterial oxygen; WBC = white blood cell count.

TABLE 1 Pneumonia Severity Index

Risk Factors	Points
Demographic factors	
Age for men	Age (yr)
Age for women	Age (yr) −10
Nursing home resident	+10
Coexisting illnesses	
Active neoplastic disease	+30
Chronic liver disease	+20
CHF	+10
Cerebrovascular disease	+10
Chronic renal disease	+10
Physical examination	
Altered mental status	+20
Respiratory rate >30	+20
Blood pressure <90 mm Hg	+20
Temperature <35°C or ≥40°C	+15
Pulse ≥125	+10
Laboratory and radiographic findings	
Arterial pH <7.35	+30
BUN ≥30 mg/dL	+20
Sodium <130 mmo/L	+20
Glucose ≥250 mg/dL	+10
Hematocrit <30%	+10
Pao$_2$ <60 mm Hg	+10
Pleural effusion	+10

Adapted from Fine MJ, Auble TE, Yealy DM, et al. A predictive rule to identify low-risk patients with community-acquired pneumonia. N Engl J Med 1997;336:243–250.
Risk classes: I = 0; II < 70 (low risk); III = 71–90 (low risk); IV = 91–130 (moderate risk); V = >130 (high risk).
BUN = blood urea nitrogen; CHF = congestive heart failure; Pao$_2$ = partial pressure of arterial oxygen.

outpatients, risk class III patients can be treated on a short hospitalization or observational unit, and risk classes IV and V patients should be treated as inpatients.

ETIOLOGY

CAP may be caused by a number of pathogens, but only a few account for the majority of cases. Box 2 lists the more common pathogens divided by site of care and severity. According to most studies, an etiology is established in only about 40% of patients with CAP. In confirmed cases, *S. pneumoniae* is the most common bacterial pathogen identified. Atypical pathogens are the most common in mild to moderate CAP; *S. aureus*, gram-negative bacilli, and *L. pneumophila* are more common in severe CAP. Nontypable *Haemophilus influenzae* can be seen in patients with underlying chronic lung disease. *S. aureus* is often associated with preceding influenza. Gram-negative bacilli, including *Pseudomonas aeruginosa*, can be seen in patients who are taking steroids or chemotherapy, who have previously used antibiotics, are alcoholics, or who have underlying pulmonary disease.

TREATMENT

Antimicrobial therapy remains the mainstay of treatment. Until better diagnostic tests are available, initial treatment remains largely empiric. Box 3 reviews the most recent recommended empiric antibiotics. Anaerobic coverage should be considered with a history of loss of consciousness in patients with gingival or esophageal disease. Antibiotics should be modified based on local epidemiology and susceptibilities.

Current levels of penicillin and cephalosporin resistance to *S. pneumoniae* do not usually result in failure when appropriate doses are administered. However, recent studies indicate that resistance to macrolides and older fluoroquinolones (levofloxacin [Levaquin] and ciprofloxacin [Cipro]) have resulted in clinical failures in

---

BOX 2   Community-Acquired Pneumonia Pathogens by Site

Outpatient Setting

Chlamydophlia pneumoniae
Haemophilus influenzae
Mycoplasma pneumoniae
Respiratory viruses: adenovirus, influenza, parainfluenza, respiratory syncytial virus
Streptococcus pneumoniae

Inpatient outside Intensive Care Unit

Aspiration
Chlamydophlia pneumoniae
Haemophilus influenzae
Legionella species
Mycoplasma pneumoniae
Respiratory viruses
Streptococcus pneumoniae

Inpatient in Intensive Care Unit

Gram-negative bacilli
Haemophilus influenzae
Legionella species
Staphylococcus aureus
Streptococcus pneumoniae

Adapted from File TM: Community-acquired pneumonia. Lancet 2003;362:1991–2001.

BOX 3   Empiric Antimicrobial Choice for Community-Acquired Pneumonia

Outpatient Treatment

Healthy patient, no prior antibiotics within the previous 3 months
- Macrolide (azithromycin [Zithromax], clarithromycin [Biaxin], or erythromycin) *or*
- Doxycycline (Vibramycin) (weak recommendation)

Patient with comorbidity (e.g., chronic heart, lung, liver, or renal disease; malignancies; alcoholism; asplenia; diabetes mellitus; immunosuppression) or use of antibiotics in previous 3 months
- Respiratory fluoroquinolone (moxifloxacin [Avelox], gemifloxacin [Factive], or levofloxacin [Levaquin] (750 mg) *or*
- β-Lactam (high-dose amoxicillin or amoxicillin-clavulanate [Augmentin]); alternatives are ceftriaxone (Rocephin), cefpodoxime (Vantin), or cefuroxime (Ceftin) plus a macrolide

In regions with a high rate (>25%) of infection with high-level (MIC ≥16 µg/mL) macrolide-resistant *Streptococcus pneumoniae*
- Use a fluoroquinolone or a β-lactam plus either a macrolide or doxycycline

Inpatients Not in Intensive Care

- Fluroquinolone alone *or*
- β-Lactam (e.g., ceftriaxone, cefotaxime [Claforan], ampicillin, ertapenem [Invanz]) plus a macrolide

Intensive Care Unit Patients

- β-Lactam (e.g., ceftriaxone, cefotaxime, or ampicillin-sulbactam [Unasyn] *plus* either azithromycin or a fluoroquinolone

For *Pseudomonas* infection
- Antipneumococcal, antipseudomonal β-lactam (piperacillin-tazobactam [Zosyn], cefepime [Maxipime], imipenem [Primaxin], or meropenem [Merrem]) plus either ciprofloxacin (Cipro) or levofloxacin (750 mg) *or*
- Antipneumococcal, antipseudomonal β-lactam *plus* an aminoglycoside and azithromycin

Community-Acquired MRSA

- Add vancomycin (Vancocin) or linezolid (Zyvox)

Adapted from Mandell LA, Wunderink RG, Anzueto A, et al: Infectious Diseases Society of America/American Thoracic Society Consensus Guidelines on the Management of Community-Acquired Pneumonia in Adults. Clin Infect Dis 2007;44:S27–S72.
MIC = minimum inhibitory concentration;
MRSA = methicillin-resistant *Streptococcus aureus*.

---

patients with CAP caused by *S. pneumoniae*. Pneumonia caused by community-acquired MRSA may be increasing, especially associated with influenza. Many of these cases are genotypically and phenotypically different from hospital-acquired MRSA. Community-acquired MRSA isolates are less antibiotic resistant and often contain the gene for Panton-Valentine leukocidin (PVL), a toxin associated with necrotizing pneumonia. Anecdotal and in vitro studies suggest clindamycin (Cleocin) (if susceptible) or linezolid (Zyvox) can affect toxin production and improve outcome. More studies are needed to determine the most effective treatment for CAP caused by community-acquired MRSA. Several studies have reported that combination therapy with the combination of a macrolide and a β-lactam for bacteremic pneumococcal pneumonia is associated with lower mortality compared with a single effective drug. A possible explanation might relate to the fact that macrolides have immunomodulatory effects, including cytokine production.

Time to first antibiotic dose for CAP has been studied in two retrospective studies in Medicare patients. These studies demonstrated lower mortality in patients who received timely antimicrobial treatment. The first study showed that if the first dose was given within 8 hours of arrival, mortality was reduced. The second study demonstrated that a 4-hour interval was associated with better outcomes. Treatment should be given for a minimum of 5 days; the patient should be afebrile for 48 to 72 hours and clinically stable. Longer treatment may be needed for CAP caused by *S. aureus*, *L. pneumophila*, or *P. aeruginosa* and in patients with evidence of associated endocarditis, septic arthritis, or meningitis.

PREVENTION

Patients older than 50 years, others at risk for influenza complications, household contacts of high-risk patients, and health care workers with direct patient contact should receive a yearly influenza vaccine. Several reviews have demonstrated that influenza vaccination not only prevents pneumonia but also decreases hospitalizations, decreases cerebrovascular events, and decreases deaths from all causes.

Pneumococcal polysaccharide vaccine (Pneumovax 23) is recommended for all persons older than 65 years and persons with certain underlying illnesses (e.g., functional and anatomic asplenia, cardiopulmonary disease, diabetes). Studies have documented moderate effectiveness for preventing invasive pneumococcal disease (bacteremia and meningitis). The overall efficacy in patients older than 65 years is reported to be between 44% and 75%.

Vaccination status should be determined in all patients admitted to the hospital. Vaccination should be offered year-round for pneumococcal vaccine and during the fall and winter months for influenza vaccine.

Health Care–Acquired Pneumonia

HAP is defined as a pneumonia that occurred more than 48 hours after admission and that was not incubating at the time of admission. Ventilator-associated pneumonia (VAP) is defined as pneumonia that develops 48 to 72 hours after intubation. Health care–associated pneumonia (HCAP) is a new category; HCAP occurs in a patient who attended a hospital or hemodialysis clinic, who was hospitalized in an acute-care hospital for more than 2 days within the prior 90 days, or who resided in a long-term care facility or nursing home. The remaining comments are directed at HAP and VAP.

HAP is the second or third most common health care–associated infection in the United States and is associated with significant morbidity and mortality, resulting in increased length of stay and costs. HAP accounts for about 25% of all ICU infections. VAP occurs in 9% to 27% of intubated patients, and the mortality is double that of similar patients without VAP. The risk of VAP is highest in the first 1 to 2 weeks. Some investigators consider time of onset an important factor in terms of outcomes and pathogens. Early-onset HAP and VAP are pneumonia occurring within 4 to 7 days of hospitalization. Early-onset HAP and VAP usually carry a better prognosis and are more likely to be caused by more sensitive pathogens. Late-onset HAP and VAP are more likely to be caused by multidrug-resistant organisms (MDRO) with a higher mortality.

Aspiration of oropharyngeal secretions or leakage of bacteria around the endotracheal tube is the primary source of bacteria causing HAP or VAP. The stomach and sinuses, blood, and contaminated aerosols are much less common sources. Contaminated biofilm in the endotracheal tube, with subsequent embolization into the lower airway, may be an important factor in the pathogenesis of VAP.

DIAGNOSIS

Unfortunately, there is no universally accepted gold standard for the diagnosis of HAP or VAP. The diagnosis is suspected if a patient has a new or progressive infiltrate along with new-onset fever, purulent sputum (>25 neutrophils per low-power field), leukocytosis, and decreased oxygenation.

Unfortunately, the clinical parameters are overly sensitive; therefore, other diagnostic tests are desirable. For a start, blood and lower respiratory secretions should be collected for culture in all patients with suspected HAP or VAP. A thoracentesis should be performed if a large pleural effusion is present. The microbiological approach favors quantitation or semiquantitation of lower respiratory secretions. The diagnostic threshold used to differentiate colonization versus true infection varies by specimen collection. The proposed diagnostic threshold for endotracheal aspirate is greater than 10^5 colony-forming units (CFU)/mL; for bronchoalveolar lavage, greater than 10^4 CFU/mL; and for protected-specimen brush, greater than 10^3 CFU/mL. A major reservation to this approach is the possibility of false-negative results, which can result if a patient has been started on an antimicrobial agent before the specimens are collected.

TREATMENT

For patients with suspected HAP or VAP, appropriate broad-spectrum antimicrobial therapy should be ordered to cover anticipated pathogens. Consider a Gram stain to guide initial therapy. Whenever possible, select antimicrobial therapy based on local microbiology and epidemiology. Use combination therapy in patients whenever an MDRO is suspected until culture results are available. Risk factors include prolonged hospitalization (>5–7 days), admission from another health care facility, and recent antibiotic therapy. Table 2 summarizes suggested empiric therapy. De-escalation of therapy is strongly recommended when culture results become available. Discontinue antimicrobial therapy if results of cultures and other clinical parameters do not confirm pneumonia. Based on recent studies, a shorter duration of therapy (7–8 days) is now recommended in patients with uncomplicated HAP or VAP who received initial appropriate therapy and have had a good clinical response. *P. aeruginosa*, *Acinetobacter* species, and MRSA can require longer durations of therapy.

PREVENTION

The incidence of HAP and VAP can be reduced by following certain proved measures. An effective infection control program, which includes education, hand-washing compliance, surveillance of ICU infections, and isolation of patients with MDRO to reduce cross-infection should be followed. Noninvasive ventilation should be used whenever possible. If intubation is required, the orotracheal route is preferred to reduce health care–associated infections due to sinusitis and VAP. Consider continuous aspiration of subglottic secretions, if available. Follow a protocol for using sedation with daily interruptions. Perform daily assessment for extubation. For patients on a ventilator, keep the head of the bed at 30 to 45 degrees to prevent aspiration (except when contraindicated). Use agents such as oral chlorhexidine (Peridex) to reduce oropharyngeal colonization. Glucose control to maintain level between 140–180 mg/dL results in lower mortality without increasing the risk of severe hypoglycemia.

TABLE 2 Initial Empiric Therapy for Suspected Health Care–Acquired Pneumonia or Ventilator-Associated Pneumonia

Suspected Pathogen	Recommended Therapy
Patients with No Known Risk Factors for MDRO and Early Onset	
Streptococcus pneumoniae Haemophilus influenzae Methicillin-sensitive Streptococcus aureus Antibiotic-sensitive enteric gram-negative Escherichia coli Klebsiella pneumoniae Enterobacter species Proteus species Serratia marcescens	One of the following: Ceftriaxone (Rocephin) or Fluoroquinolone (levofloxacin [Levaquin], moxifloxacin [Avelox], or ciprofloxacin [Cipro]) or Ertapenem (Invanz) or Piperacillin-tazobactam (Zosyn)
Patients with Risk Factors for MDRO or Late Onset	
Pathogens listed above and MDRO Pseudomonas aeruginosa K. pneumoniae (ESBL)* Acinetobacter species MRSA Legionella species†	Antipseudomonal cephalosporin (e.g., cefepime [Maxipime] or ceftazidime [Fortaz]) or Antipseudomonal carbepenem (e.g., imipenem [Primaxin] or meropenem [Merrem]) or Piperacillin-tazobactam (Zosyn) **plus** Aminoglycoside or Antipseudomonal fluoroquinolone (e.g., ciprofloxacin [Cipro] or levofloxacin [Levaquin]) **plus** Vancomycin (Vancocin) or linezolid (Zyvox)

Modified from American Thoracic Society; Infectious Diseases Society of America: Guidelines for the management of adults with hospital-acquired, ventilator-associated, and healthcare-associated pneumonia, Am J Respir Crit Care Med 171:388–416, 2005.

*If an ESBL strain, a carbepenem is preferred.

†If Legionella suspected, the combination regimen should include either a macrolide (e.g., azithromycin) or a fluoroquinolone.

ESBL = extended-spectrum β-lactamase; MDRO = multidrug-resistant organisms; MRSA = methicillin-resistant Staphylococcus aureus.

REFERENCES

American Thoracic Society; Infectious Diseases Society of America. Guidelines for the management of adults with hospital-acquired, ventilator-associated, and healthcare-associated pneumonia. Am J Respir Crit Care Med 2005;171:388–416.

Chastre J, Wolff M, Fagon JY, et al. Comparison of 8 vs 15 days of antibiotic therapy for ventilator-associated pneumonia in adults: A randomized trial. JAMA 2003;290:2588–98.

Fagon JY, Chastre J, Wolff M, et al. Invasive and noninvasive strategies for management of suspected ventilator-associated pneumonia: A randomized trial. Ann Intern Med 2000;132:621–30.

File TM. Community-acquired pneumonia. Lancet 2003;362:1991–2001.

Fine MJ, Auble TE, Yealy DM, et al. A predictive rule to identify low-risk patients with community-acquired pneumonia. N Engl J Med 1997; 336:243–50.

Houck PM, Bratzler DW, Nsa W, et al. Timing of antibiotic administration and outcomes for Medicare patients hospitalized with community-acquired pneumonia. Arch Intern Med 2004;164:637–44.

Lim WS, van der Eerden MM, Laing R, et al. Defining community acquired pneumonia severity on presentation to hospital: An international derivation and validation study. Thorax 2003;58:377–82.

Mandell LA, Wunderink RG, Anzueto A, et al. Infectious Diseases Society of America/American Thoracic Society Consensus Guidelines on the Management of Community-Acquired Pneumonia in Adults. Clin Infect Dis 2007;44:S27–72.

Metersky ML, Ma A, Houck PM, Bratzler DW. Antibiotics for bacteremic pneumonia: Improved outcomes with macrolides but not fluoroquinolones. Chest 2007;131:466–73.

NICE-SUGAR Study Investigators. Intensive versus conventional glucose control in critically ill patients. N Engl J Med 2009;360:1283–97.

Richards MJ, Edwards JR, Culver DH, Gaynes RP. Nosocomial infections in medical ICUs in the United States: National Nosocomial Infections Surveillance System. Crit Care Med 1999;27:887–92.

van den Berghe G, Wilmer A, Hermans G, et al. Intensive insulin therapy in the medical ICU. N Engl J Med 2006;354:449–61.

Viral Respiratory Infections

Method of
Robert C. Welliver, Sr., MD

Viral infections of the respiratory tract are among the most common infections in humans, and they account for significant morbidity at all ages. Infants and young children can sustain six to eight such infections annually, and adults have an average of nearly two such infections per year.

Rhinoviruses are the most commonly identified etiologic agents and cause illness year-round. Other common causative agents during winter months include influenza viruses and respiratory syncytial virus, and enteroviruses predominate in summer months. The parainfluenza viruses also commonly cause respiratory infection, particularly in autumn (type 1) and late spring or summer (type 3). Coronaviruses, metapneumoviruses, adenoviruses, and other agents are identified less often.

Although each of these agents can cause a common cold, some viral infections are associated with characteristic patterns of respiratory disease. Most of these viruses can also exacerbate asthma, cystic fibrosis, and chronic obstructive pulmonary disease (COPD).

Common Colds

Colds are the most common of the viral respiratory illnesses. Pharyngitis is usually the earliest sign of a cold, beginning a few days after infection has taken place. Nasal congestion and clear or slightly cloudy rhinorrhea usually follow within 24 to 48 hours. Cough occurs in approximately 30% to 40% of those infected, and fluid can accumulate in middle ear or sinus cavities that have become blocked as a result of mucosal swelling. Ear and sinus cavity infections occur when this fluid is trapped for a week or more. Treatment with antibiotics is ineffective before this time, and they are ineffective especially in the absence of other clinical signs of ear and sinus infections.

Colds are a frequent cause of missed school and work, and even of mild morbidity, but they are rarely serious in otherwise healthy persons. The most appropriate approach to treatment therefore entails rest, with adequate nutrition and hydration. Agents that inhibit the activity of cyclooxygenase probably represent the most effective form of pharmacologic intervention. These compounds include acetaminophen (Tylenol) and the nonsteroidal anti-inflammatory agents (NSAIDs) such as ibuprofen (Motrin). They are effective in reducing fever and, perhaps more importantly in most colds, reducing malaise, headache, and pharyngitis.

Nasal congestion and some rhinorrhea during colds are related to dilation of blood vessels in the nose and sinuses. Vasoconstrictors have therefore been used extensively to attempt to reverse these symptoms. Oral decongestants such as pseudoephedrine (Sudafed) have minimal effect on nasal congestion, and can result in systemic hypertension, anxiety, and difficulty sleeping. The propensity for these compounds to cause cardiac arrhythmias in the very young child has led to recommendations against their use in the first year or two of life. Nasal sprays containing vasoconstricting agents such as oxymetazoline (Afrin) can result in mild temporary relief of nasal obstruction. However, the use of these compounds for more than 3 or 4 days can result in rebound vasodilation and paradoxically increased rhinorrhea.

Numerous investigations have evaluated the role of antihistamines in colds. The release of histamine itself is not associated with fever, cough, or malaise, so effects on these symptoms would not be expected. Furthermore, nasal congestion and discharge may be more related to the release of kinins, and not histamine. Indeed, the administration of antihistamines in adults and, particularly, in children has not demonstrated strikingly positive results. As many as 40% of subjects treated with placebo report beneficial effects. Side effects of histamine use, primarily sedation and dry mouth, are commonly encountered.

Cough can be one of the most irritating symptoms during colds. Cough during colds is principally caused by secretions entering the airway (postnasal drip) and not by inflammation of the airway itself. Therefore, it is not surprising that cough suppressants, especially codeine, have little effect on cough induced by colds. Antihistamines have also been found to be ineffective in relief of cough during colds.

Influenza-Like Illness

The influenza syndrome is defined as the abrupt onset of fever, headache, and striking degrees of malaise and prostration, often with intense myalgia. Respiratory symptoms can occur concurrently, but they might not be prominent features. The principal cause is, of course, influenza virus, although infection with many other viruses can cause similar (although not as intense) symptoms. The illness is generally self-limited, and most symptoms resolve over 4 or 5 days. Lassitude can persist for up to 2 weeks.

Influenza virus infection and influenza-like illness are best treated symptomatically, relying on rest, adequate intake of fluids and calories, and appropriate analgesic therapy. Compounds referred to as *M2 inhibitors* such as amantadine (Symmetrel) and rimantadine (Flumadine) have been approved for therapy. Positive outcomes from therapy with these agents are observed only when therapy is instituted within 48 hours after the onset of symptoms, and benefits are not striking. In recent years, resistance to M2 inhibitors has been commonly observed among circulating epidemic strains of influenza virus.

More recently, inhibitors of the activity of influenza viral neuraminidase have been used in treatment and prevention of influenza virus infection in adults and children. The first such compound released, zanamivir (Relenza), was administered by inhalation but was unpopular because of its irritating effects on the airway. An oral compound, oseltamivir (TamiFlu), has been used to prevent and to treat influenza virus infection. As with M2 inhibitors, it is believed that treatment should be started within the first 48 hours of symptoms and that prophylaxis should be instituted within 48 hours of exposure.

Treatment with oseltamivir shortens the duration of subsequent illness by only about 24 hours. Treatment can prevent some of the complications of influenza infection, including pneumonia. The drug may be more effective as a therapeutic agent, because it may be up to 90% effective in preventing culture-positive symptomatic influenza illness. The recommended dose for adults is 75 mg orally every 12 hours for 5 days. In children, the appropriate dose based on body weight is 30 mg twice daily for children weighing less than 15 kg, 45 mg twice daily for children weighing 15 to 23 kg, 60 mg twice daily for children weighing 23 to 40 kg, and 75 mg twice daily for children weighing more than 40 kg. The principal side effect is nausea, which can be reduced by taking the drug with food.

In 2009, a novel H1N1 strain of influenza caused a worldwide pandemic. At the time of this writing, both this epidemic H1N1 strain as well as the seasonal influenza A/H3N2 and type B strains continue to circulate in the world. The considerable majority of these epidemic and seasonal strains continue to show sensitivity to oseltamivir, while most are resistant to M2 inhibitors. All strains continue to show sensitvity to zanamivir.

Croup

Croup is defined by the occurrence of hoarseness or laryngitis, a deep, brassy or barking cough, and inspiratory stridor. Airway obstruction in croup is caused by constriction in the subglottic area, often noted on radiographs by a steeple-shaped narrowing of the air column in this region. Affected children are usually afebrile and nontoxic in appearance.

Parainfluenza virus type 1 is the primary cause of croup, although infection with many different viruses can produce this illness, and influenza virus can cause a particularly severe form of croup. Bacterial secondary infection occurs uncommonly, but it can result in fever and severe obstruction of the airway. Administration of dexamethasone (Decadron)[1] at 0.6 mg/kg either orally or intramuscularly markedly reduces the rate of hospitalization, admission to the intensive care unit, and intubation for croup.

Bronchiolitis

Bronchiolitis represents the most common cause for hospitalization of infants in developed countries. Infants present with a history of several days of upper respiratory symptoms, followed by the rapid onset of wheezing and labored breathing. Respiratory syncytial virus (RSV) is the most common cause and is the agent found in the most severe cases that result in respiratory failure. Contrasting with asthma, obstruction of the airway in bronchiolitis is a result of plugging of bronchioles with detached epithelium and inflammatory cells. Mucus plugging and constriction of smooth muscle are not prominent. Also in contrast with asthma is the absence of a sustained response to bronchodilators and corticosteroids among infants with bronchiolitis.

Therapy of bronchiolitis primarily consists of administration of supplemental oxygen and replacement of fluid deficits as needed. Ribavirin (Virazole)[1] is a compound with antiviral activity against RSV, but controlled studies have not demonstrated meaningful differences

---

[1]Not FDA approved for this indication.

CURRENT DIAGNOSIS

- Rapid diagnostic kits are available for many common respiratory viruses. These tests are used increasingly to establish that antibiotic therapy is not necessary in many patients with febrile respiratory illnesses or with lower respiratory tract infections.
- The presence of wheezing on physical examination virtually excludes bacterial infection from consideration in subjects with lower respiratory disease.

CURRENT THERAPY

- The management of most viral respiratory infections consists of rest, adequate caloric and fluid intake, and management of fever and malaise.
- Corticosteroids are essential in the management of croup.
- Specific antiviral therapy is available only for influenza virus infection, and beneficial effects have been more readily achieved in prevention rather than treatment.

in outcomes between treated and untreated subjects. The compound is quite expensive and must be delivered via a special aerosol generator.

Palivizumab (Synagis), a preparation consisting of a monoclonal antibody against the fusion protein of RSV, has proved to be effective in reducing the rate of hospitalization for RSV infection by approximately 50% when given to high-risk infants. Infants who may be considered candidates for therapy include those with chronic lung disease, those born prematurely, and those with hemodynamically significant congenital heart disease. Doses of palivizumab (15 mg/kg) are given on a monthly basis throughout the local RSV season, usually November through March.

REFERENCES

Akerlund A, Klint T, Olen L, Runderantz H. Nasal decongestant effect of oxymetazoline in the common cold: An objective dose-response study in 106 patients. J Laryngol Otol 1989;103:743–6.

Buckingham SC, Jafri HS, Bush AN, et al. A randomized, double-blind, placebo-controlled trial of dexamethasone in severe respiratory syncytial virus (RSV) infection: Effects on RSV quantity and clinical outcome. J Infect Dis 2002;185:1222–8.

Curley FJ, Irwin RS, Pratter MR, et al. Cough and the common cold. Am J Respir Crit Care Med 1988;138:305–11.

Flores G, Horwitz RI. Efficacy of β_2-agonists in bronchiolitis: A reappraisal and meta-analysis. Pediatrics 1997;100:233–9.

Johnson DW, Jacobson S, Edney PC, et al. A comparison of nebulized budesonide, intramuscular dexamethasone, and placebo for moderately severe croup. N Engl J Med 1998;339:498–503.

Muether PS, Gwaltney JM Jr. Variant effect of first- and second-generation antihistamines as clues to their mechanism of action on the sneeze reflex in the common cold. Clin Infect Dis 2001;33:1483–8.

Randolph AG, Wang EL. Ribavirin for respiratory syncytial virus lower respiratory tract infection. Arch Pediatr Adolesc Med 1996;150:942–7.

Tavorner D, Danz C, Economos D. The effects of oral pseudoephedrine on nasal patency in the common cold: A double-blind single-dose placebo-controlled trial. Clin Otolaryngol 1999;24:47–51.

Treanor JJ, Hayden FG, Vrooman PS, et al. Efficacy and safety of the oral neuraminidase inhibitor oseltamivir in treating acute influenza: A randomized controlled trial. US Oral Neuraminnidase Study Group. JAMA 2000;283:1016–24.

Van Voris LP, Betts RF, Hayden FG, et al. Successful treatment of naturally occurring influenza A/USSR/77 H1N1. JAMA 1981;245:1128–31.

Viral and Mycoplasmal Pneumonias

Method of
Burke A. Cunha, MD

Influenza pneumonia is the most important cause of viral pneumonia in adults. Influenza A is the predominant type of influenza found in adults, and influenza B is more common in children. Influenza A has the potential for severe disease, occurs seasonally, and is the predominant type involved in influenza pandemics. *Mycoplasma pneumoniae* community-acquired pneumonia (CAP) was first recognized decades ago as distinctive from bacterial and viral pneumonias. It was originally described by Eaton as "Eaton agent" pneumonia caused by a pleuropneumonia-like organism (PPLO), later shown to be caused by *M. pneumoniae*. *M. pneumoniae* is a common cause of pneumonia in all age groups, but the peak incidence of *M. pneumoniae* CAP is in young adults. *M. pneumoniae* CAP is a common cause of ambulatory CAP.

The term *atypical pneumonia* was first applied to viral pneumonias because the clinical laboratory and radiologic findings were different from those caused by typical bacterial pulmonary pathogens. In influenza pneumonia, the clinical findings are confined to the trachea, bronchi, lung parenchyma, and central nervous system.

M. pneumoniae CAP is a systemic infection with a pulmonary component. Over the years, atypical pneumonia has come to refer to pneumonia caused by systemic nonviral/nonbacterial pathogen agents that have a pulmonary component. Viral pneumonias are no longer considered atypical pneumonias. Atypical pneumonias may be divided into nonzoonotic and zoonotic atypical CAPs. Nonzoonotic CAPs are most commonly caused by *M. pneumoniae*, *Chlamydia pneumoniae*, or *Legionella* species; whereas the three most common zoonotic atypical pneumonias are caused by *Chlamydia psittaci* (psittacosis), *Francisella tularensis* (tularemia), or *Coxiella burnetii* (Q fever). All of the atypical pneumonias are distinct clinical entities that may be differentiated on the basis of their characteristic pattern of extrapulmonary organ involvement. Although some viruses may occasionally have extrapulmonary manifestations (i.e., influenza, adenovirus with viral pneumonias), the primary clinical features are confined to the lungs. *M. pneumoniae* is a critical cause of nonzoonotic atypical CAP, particularly in the ambulatory setting. *M. pneumoniae* CAP may be severe in patients with impaired host defenses or those with severe, preexisting cardiopulmonary disease.

Influenza (Human, Avian, and Swine)

Viral influenza pneumonia affects children and adults. Influenza B is the primary type causing mild influenza in children and adults. Influenza A is primarily an infection of adults that may be mild to severe. Influenza A has the potential for pandemic spread (e.g., swine influenza [H_1N_1]).

Influenza occurs during the winter months, usually peaking in February. Influenza is spread by aerosolized droplet infection from person to person and via fomites. Influenza A is classified into subtypes based on hemagglutinin (H) and neuraminidase (N) surface proteins. An important characteristic of influenza A virus is antigenic drift, which refers to minor changes in surface protein shift in the neuramidase or hemagglutinin receptors. With influenza A, these surface receptor proteins are important in cellular adherence of the influenza virus and spread of influenza from respiratory epithelial cells. The vaccine for the flu season most often includes the influenza hemagglutinin and neuramidase types seen at the end of the preceding year's season. Prevention of attachment and spread of the virus is helpful to controlling the spread of influenza; vaccine protection conferred by specific antibody response to influenza A is highly protective (approximately 80% in noncompromised hosts).

During the years when influenza B has been prevalent, vaccines for the subsequent year contain an influenza B component.

Clinical manifestations of influenza A in adults varies considerably from mild to fatal infection. Mild infection is usually manifested as an acute febrile illness characterized by headache and myalgias with dry unproductive cough and rhinorrhea. Mild influenza may be due to influenza A or B and usually resolves in a few days without complications in normal hosts who have good cardiopulmonary function.

Severe influenza A (human, avian, swine) occurs in normal healthy adults and may be fatal. The onset of severe influenza A (human, avian, swine) is sudden, and the patient often recalls the exact hour of onset. The patient is febrile with early/extreme prostration rendering the patient bedridden. Fever rapidly rises and may be accompanied by chills. Neck soreness, severe headache, and myalgias are typical. Sore throat, eye pain, conjunctival injection, and hemoptysis are frequently present. Chest pain worsened by deep inspiration is not truly pleuritic but rather reflects influenza A myositis of the intracostal muscles. Shortness of breath is related to the degree of hypoxemia. Severe influenza A causes an oxygen diffusion defect as manifested by an increased A-a gradient (>35). Profound hypoxemia may be accompanied by cyanosis. Hypotension caused by hypoxemia and vascular collapse may follow. The course of fulminant viral influenza A is of short duration.

Physical findings are few in viral influenza (i.e., conjunctival suffusion). Auscultation reveals absolutely quiet lungs because the infectious process is interstitial and not alveolar. Routine blood tests are usually unremarkable except for leukopenia, relative lymphopenia, and thrombocytopenia. Atypical lymphocytes are not present, but low titers of cold agglutinins may be present. Cold agglutinins (if present) have low titers less than or equal to 1:18. In fatal cases, a pale bluelike hue of the skin may be noted, and there may be bleeding from multiple orifices preterminally. The chest radiograph in uncomplicated influenza A is unremarkable or may have minimal perihilar bilateral increased prominence of interstitial markings. In severe influenza A pneumonia, the chest radiograph shows bilateral symmetrical perihilar infiltrates without pleural effusions in <48 hours.

Patients may die from severe influenza A without superimposed bacterial pneumonia. Most deaths during the 1918–1919 pandemic were young military recruits who died early of influenza A pneumonia without bacterial pneumonia. Influenza may be complicated by bacterial pneumonia. Bacterial pneumonias complicating influenza may occur concurrently at presentation or may occur 1 to 2 weeks after an interval of improvement after the presentation of influenza. Influenza A presenting concurrently with bacterial pneumonia is caused by Staphylococcus aureus. In contrast to influenza alone, MSSA/CA-MRSA is manifested by an increase in fever, shaking chills, leukocytosis, purulent sputum, localized rales on auscultation, bacteremia, and focal/segmental infiltrates on chest radiograph that rapidly cavitate in less than 72 hours. Alternately, patients with influenza A may develop a secondary bacterial infection 1 to 2 weeks later. Secondary bacterial pneumonia is less severe and is usually caused by Streptococcus pneumoniae or Haemophilus influenzae.

ANTI-INFLUENZA THERAPY

Therapy of viral influenza is directed at inhibiting viral replication and preventing further infection of respiratory epithelial cells. The neuramidase inhibitors zanamivir (Relenza) and oseltamivir (Tamiflu) have anti-influenza A and B activity. Neuramidase inhibitors decrease the severity and duration of influenza symptoms by 1 to 2 days. Current flu strains are resistant to amantadine and rimantadine, but these drugs may still be useful to increase peripheral airway dilatation and oxygenation, which may be of critical importance in severe influenza A with severe hypoxemia. Mild influenza A/B may be treated with neuramidase inhibitors. Mild cases of influenza A should be treated at the onset of the illness. For severe influenza A, neuramidase inhibitors provide optimal anti-influenza therapy (Table 1). For human and avian influenza (H_5N_1), these antiviral drugs may be ineffective, but are effective against swine influenza.

Mycoplasma pneumoniae Pneumonia

M. pneumoniae is a common cause of ambulatory CAP. It affects all age groups, and in normal hosts with intact cardiopulmonary function, Mycoplasma CAP is usually a mild, self-limiting infection.

TABLE 1 Adult Anti-Influenza Antivirals

Antiviral	Treatment Dose	Prophylactic Dose
Mild Influenza A/B		
Zanamivir (Relenza)†	2 inhalations (5 mg per inhalation) q12h × 5d	2 inhalations (5 mg per inhalation) q24h × 5d
Influenza A		
Oseltamivir (Tamiflu)†	75 mg (PO) q12h × 5d*	75 mg (PO) q24h × 7d

*For avian (H5N1) influenza, 150 mg (PO) q12h may be effective.
†Currently most human and avian influenza strains are resistant.

However, M. pneumoniae derives its importance from difficulty in diagnosis, the necessity for non–β-lactam therapy, and because of its effect on peripheral airways.

Mycoplasma CAP is one of the nonzoonotic causes of CAP (the others being Legionella and Chlamydia pneumoniae). M. pneumoniae is an atypical pneumonia that is a systemic infectious disease with a pulmonary component. It may be distinguished from other atypical pneumonias by its characteristic pattern of extrapulmonary organ involvement. M. pneumoniae CAP most closely resembles C. pneumoniae CAP clinically, but is very different from Legionnaires' disease in terms of its epidemiology, age distribution, pattern of extrapulmonary organ involvement, and severity.

Clinically, M. pneumoniae presents as a subacute febrile illness. Temperatures rarely exceed 102°F (38.9°C). Rigors are not a feature of M. pneumoniae CAP, but patients may complain of chilly sensations. Mild headache and/or myalgias are not uncommon. The most common presenting symptom in Mycoplasma CAP is the prolonged, nonproductive dry cough. Patients with Mycoplasma CAP often complain of or have mild nonexudative pharyngitis. Rhinorrhea and conjunctivitis are not features of M. pneumoniae CAP. Watery diarrhea is commonly present in Mycoplasma CAP, but abdominal pain is not a clinical finding. Other extrapulmonary manifestations are uncommon or rare (e.g., meningoencephalitis, pericarditis, hemolytic anemia, glomerular nephritis, Guillain-Barré syndrome, erythema multiforme). M. pneumoniae has a distinctive pattern of extrapulmonary organ involvement that does not include cardiac involvement (relative bradycardia) or hepatic involvement, including normal serum glutamate-oxaloacetate transaminase (SGOT) or serum glutamate-pyruvate transaminase (SGPT). The distinguishing laboratory feature of M. pneumoniae CAP is elevated cold agglutinin titers. Although a variety of infectious and noninfectious diseases are associated with cold agglutinin elevations, they are usually of low titer (i.e., <1:16). There are no pulmonary infections presenting as CAP that are associated with high elevations of cold agglutinin titers (i.e., ≥1:64). Although elevated cold agglutinins occur early in up to 75% of patients with M. pneumoniae CAP, they are still diagnostically important when present. In a patient with CAP and a cold agglutinin titer greater than or equal to 1:64, the diagnosis of M. pneumoniae CAP is very likely.

M. pneumoniae may be differentiated from the typical bacterial pneumonias because of the presence of extrapulmonary findings, including nonexudative pharyngitis, loose stools or watery diarrhea, erythema multiforme, and high cold agglutinin. Patients with typical bacterial CAP usually have a more acute onset of presentation, a productive cough, and temperatures that may exceed 102°F (38.9°C), often accompanied by chills. Patients with typical pneumonia often have pleuritic chest pain, which is not a feature of M. pneumoniae CAP. Among the atypical pneumonias, the zoonotic pneumonias (i.e., tularemia, psittacosis, Q fever) may be eliminated from consideration if there is a recent zoonotic contact history with the appropriate vector.

C. pneumoniae resembles closely M. pneumoniae CAP. C. pneumoniae may be distinguished by the absence of cold agglutinins and the presence of hoarseness, which is a feature of C. pneumoniae but not M. pneumoniae CAP. Loose stools or watery diarrhea are not usual features of C. pneumoniae CAP. The most common clinical problem is differentiating Legionella from Mycoplasma CAP; this may be done by appreciating the differences in the pattern of extrapulmonary organ involvement with each of these pathogens. Legionella may be clinically differentiated from Mycoplasma by acuteness of onset or severity, the presence of relative bradycardia, temperatures greater than 102°F (38.9°C), and the presence of abdominal pain. From a laboratory standpoint, highly elevated cold agglutinin titers argue strongly against the diagnosis of Legionella and point to M. pneumoniae. Nonspecific laboratory tests in a patient with CAP that suggest Legionella and argue against M. pneumoniae include otherwise unexplained hypophosphatemia, hyponatremia, microscopic hematuria, and increased creatinine. Legionella does not affect the upper respiratory tract as does Mycoplasma (e.g., nonexudative pharyngitis). Ear findings are not a feature of Legionnaires' disease but are common in M. pneumoniae CAP. The finding most likely to cause confusion between M. pneumoniae and Legionella pneumophila is the presence of loose stools or watery diarrhea, which is found in both.

CURRENT DIAGNOSIS

Influenza (human, avian, swine)

- Mild influenza A or B presents acutely with headache, fever, sore throat, plus/minus rhinorrhea.
- Severe influenza A presents with an acute onset (patients often able to name the hour the influenza began) and rapidly become bed bound.
- Headache, myalgias, and prostration are severe.
- With swine influenza, gastrointestinal symptoms (e.g., nausea/vomiting or diarrhea) may be prominent.
- Auscultation of the lungs is quiet, disproportionate to the degree of respiratory distress. Influenza is an interstitial process and not alveolar, which explains the absence of rales.
- With severe influenza, patients rapidly become hypoxemic. Hypoxemia is accompanied by an A-a gradient >35, which indicates a interstitial oxygen diffusing defect.
- Severe tracheobronchitis is common and manifested by hemoptysis.
- Relative lymphopenia occurs early followed by thrombocytopenia and later leukopenia. Low titer elevations of cold agglutinins are not infrequent (≥1:18).
- Patients may have chest pain exacerbated by breathing mimicking pleuritic chest pain. This is the result of direct intracostal muscle involvement with the influenza virus, which results in myositis and pain on inspiration.
- The chest radiograph in early influenza, in mild to moderate cases, is normal or near normal, with minimal, if any, increase in perihilar interstitial markings. The chest radiograph in fulminant cases shows symmetrical bilateral patchy infiltrates without pleural effusion in 48 hours.
- Severe influenza A is accompanied by severe hypoxemia cyanosis, and may be followed by an early fatal outcome.
- Influenza pneumonia most often presents alone without bacterial superinfection, but bacterial infection may accompany (MSSA/CA-MRSA) or follow influenza (S. pneumoniae or H. influenzae).

- Purulent sputum with influenza indicates concurrent bacterial pneumonia usually caused by S. aureus (MSSA/MRSA). Bacterial pneumonia following influenza (after 1 to 2 weeks), is suggested by leukocytosis, focal or segmental pulmonary infiltrates, and purulent sputum; the pathogens are not S. aureus, but most commonly are S. pneumoniae or H. influenzae.
- A laboratory diagnosis may be made by DFA staining of respiratory secretions or viral cultures.

Mycoplasma pneumoniae

- In a patient with CAP and a dry nonproductive cough, without severe headache or myalgias, the most likely diagnosis is M. pneumoniae. M. pneumoniae CAP is commonly accompanied by nonexudative pharyngitis and/or loose stools or watery diarrhea.
- The temperature is usually less than 102°F (38.9°C) and is not accompanied by frank rigors or pleuritic chest pain.
- Relative bradycardia and elevations in the serum transaminases are not features of M. pneumoniae CAP.
- Respiratory viruses are often associated with mild elevations of cold agglutinins (≤1:16) but M. pneumoniae is the only pathogen causing CAP associated with highly elevated cold agglutinin titers (≥1:64). Elevated cold agglutinin titers occur in up to 75% of patients with M. pneumoniae, and occur early and transiently.
- In a patient with CAP, elevated cold agglutinin titers (>1:8) effectively rule out the typical pathogens, as well as Legionella species and C. pneumoniae.
- Elevated M. pneumoniae ELISA IgG titers indicate past exposure/infection and not current infection or co-infection with another pathogen.
- In the absence of an antecedent respiratory tract infection (e.g., nonexudative pharyngitis, otitis, etc., in the preceding 3 months), the presence of an increased M. pneumoniae ELISA IgM titer is diagnostic of acute infection.

CURRENT THERAPY

Viral Influenza

- The aim of therapy is to inhibit the influenza virus and prevent its attachment/spread to uninfected respiratory epithelial cells.
- The neuramidase inhibitors shorten the course of influenza by 1 to 2 days and have antiviral activity. These agents are active against both influenza A and B.
- Most strains of human and avian, but not swine flu strains, are resistant to amantadine (Symmetrel) or rimantadine (Flumadine).
- Amantadine and rimantadine may have an important therapeutic effect in severe influenza A by increasing distal airway dilation and increasing oxygen action.

Mycoplasma pneumoniae

- The agents active against M. pneumoniae are macrolides, tetracyclines, quinolones, and ketolides. β-Lactam

antibiotics are not active against M. pneumoniae because the organisms do not contain a bacterial cell wall.

- Goals of therapy of M. pneumoniae CAP are to eradicate the infection, decrease the shedding of Mycoplasma in respiratory secretions posttherapy, and to prevent posttreatment asthma.
- Therapy is equally efficacious with macrolides, doxycycline (Vibramycin), or a respiratory quinolone intravenously, orally, or in combination for 1 to 2 weeks.
- The mode of administration is determined by the severity of the CAP and the setting. Outpatients are usually treated orally. Patients hospitalized with severe CAP are initially treated intravenously and then changed to an oral agent.
- Resistance to M. pneumoniae with antimicrobials has not been described and is not a clinical consideration.

M. pneumoniae may be cultured from the throat in viral culture media, but the diagnosis is usually made serologically. An elevated enzyme-linked immunosorbent assay (ELISA) or enzyme immunoassay (EIA) IgM titer suggests acute or recent infection, but an elevated IgG titer indicates past exposure but not acute infection. Elevated IgG titers regardless of degree of elevation are not diagnostic of current infection with *M. pneumoniae* and only indicate previous antigenic exposure. *M. pneumoniae* ELISA IgM levels may take up to 3 months to decrease. Therefore, clinicians should take into account recent antecedent respiratory illness in order to properly interpret elevated IgM titers, including patients with nonexudative pharyngitis within 3 months prior to the presentation of CAP. The combination of an increased *M. pneumoniae* IgM titer and highly elevated cold agglutinin titers is virtually diagnostic of acute infection. Cold agglutinin titers are elevated transiently early and rapidly fall; the simultaneously elevated cold agglutinins and IgM titers of *M. pneumoniae* indicate active or current infection. In patients with CAP caused by another organism (e.g., *S. pneumoniae*), the presence of elevated *Mycoplasma* IgG titers does not indicate co-infection but only preexisting serologic exposure to *M. pneumoniae*.

THERAPY

M. pneumoniae has a predilection for the respiratory epithelial cells and resides literally on their surface. Mycoplasmas have no definite cell wall like the typical pathogens causing CAP. Their position on the surface of the respiratory epithelium and their absence of a cell wall necessitates the therapeutic approach, which includes non–β-lactam antibiotics with the capacity to penetrate into the *Mycoplasma* organisms. Traditionally, macrolides and tetracyclines have been used successfully to treat *M. pneumoniae*. Both CAP tetracyclines and macrolides are effective against *Mycoplasma* because they interfere with intracellular protein synthesis at the ribosomal level. Tetracyclines penetrate intracellularly better than macrolides, with the exception of penetration into the alveolar macrophage, which is relevant in *Legionella*, but not *M. pneumoniae*, infections. Macrolides and tetracyclines are both active against *Mycoplasma*; the relative lack of penetration by macrolides into respiratory epithelial cells accounts for differences in therapeutic response. Patients treated with macrolides or tetracyclines defervesce rapidly over 24 to 48 hours. Clinical defervescence manifests by an increased feeling of well-being and a decrease in fever. The dry cough persists during and after therapy regardless of the anti-*Mycoplasma* antimicrobial used.

There are important differences in the shedding rates of *Mycoplasma* from respiratory epithelial cells posttherapy when using tetracyclines instead of macrolides. Tetracycline therapy is associated with a more rapid decrease in shedding. Tetracyclines with better ability to penetrate intracellularly, such as doxycycline (Vibramycin), are the most rapid at decreasing *Mycoplasma* shedding, which is an important public health consideration. Mycoplasmas are transmitted by aerosolized droplet infection. Because patients with *Mycoplasma* have a prolonged cough, organisms not eliminated from respiratory epithelial cells may be aerosolized during coughing for weeks following the acute infection, spreading the infection to susceptible individuals via aerosolized droplets. The aim of therapy is to rapidly treat the patient's pneumonia and extrapulmonary sites of involvement. The secondary goal is to rapidly decrease shedding and aerosolization to prevent the spread of *Mycoplasma* to other individuals. An additional therapeutic goal is to decrease the incidence of post-*Mycoplasma* asthma seen in some patients. *M. pneumoniae* CAP may exacerbate preexisting asthma, but may also cause permanent post-CAP asthma in some individuals.

Until recently, doxycycline was the most active antimicrobial to use against *M. pneumoniae*. Currently, the "respiratory quinolones," levofloxacin (Levaquin) and moxifloxacin (Avelox), are highly active anti-*M. pneumoniae* antimicrobials. The respiratory quinolones and doxycycline penetrate cells efficiently and interfere with intracellular enzymes or protein synthesis of intracellular organisms. Respiratory quinolones and doxycycline are highly effective anti-*Mycoplasma* agents and rapidly decrease shedding of *M. pneumoniae* in respiratory secretions.

Therapy for *M. pneumoniae* is ordinarily 1 to 2 weeks. Patients who have impaired cardiopulmonary disease or compromised host

TABLE 2 Antibiotics Effective Against *M. pneumoniae*

Antibiotic	Dose (Adult)
Mild/Moderate CAP	
Doxycycline	100 mg (IV/PO) q12h
Erythromycin	500 mg (base, estolate, stearate) (PO) q6h
Erythromycin lactobionate	1 g (IV) q6h
Clarithromycin (Biaxin)	500 mg (PO) q12h
Azithromycin (Zithromax)	500 mg (IV) q24h × 2 doses, followed by 500 mg (PO) q24h
Severe CAP	
Levofloxacin (Levaquin)	500 mg (IV/PO) q24h, or 750 mg IV/PO q24h (may allow for shorter duration of therapy)
Moxifloxacin (Avelox)	400 mg (IV/PO) q24h

may require 2 full weeks of therapy. In patients with borderline cardiopulmonary function, *M. pneumoniae* as with other relatively low virulence pathogens may present as severe CAP. Antimicrobial therapy for typical or atypical CAP should be directed against the presumed pathogen and not based on co-morbidities. Normal healthy hosts are treated with the same antimicrobial as patients hospitalized with severe CAP. Patients hospitalized with compromised cardiopulmonary function severe *Mycoplasma* CAP are most often initially treated intravenously with doxycycline (Vibramycin), a macrolide, or a respiratory quinolone. Most patients with *M. pneumoniae* CAP present in the ambulatory setting, which permits therapy with oral doxycycline, macrolide, or a respiratory quinolone (Table 2).

REFERENCES

Ali NJ, Sillis M, Andrews BE, et al. The clinical spectrum and diagnosis of *Mycoplasma pneumoniae* infection. Q J Med 1986;58:241–51.

Cunha BA. Hepatic involvement in *Mycoplasma pneumoniae* community-acquired pneumonia. J Clin Microbiol 2003;3:385–6.

Cunha BA. Influenza: Historical aspects of epidemics and pandemics. Infect Dis Clin North Am 2004;18:141–55.

Cunha BA. The atypical pneumonia: Clinical diagnosis and importance. Clin Microbiol Infect 2006;12:12–24.

Cunha BA. Pneumonia Essentials. 3rd ed. Sudbury, MA, Jones & Bartlett, 2010.

Cunha BA. Urosepsis in the Critical Care Unit. In: Cunha BA, editor. Infectious Diseases in Critical Care Medicine. 3rd ed. New York, NY: Informa Healthcare USA, Inc.; 2009.

Cunha BA. Antibiotic Essentials. 8th ed. Jones and Bartlett: Sudbury, MA; 2009.

Debré R, Couvreur J. Influenza: Clinical features. In: Debré R, Celers J, editors. Clinical Virology: The Evaluation and Management of Human Viral Infections. Philadelphia: WB Saunders; 1970. p. 507–15.

File TM, Tan JS: *Mycoplasma pneumoniae* pneumonia. In: Marrié TJ, editor. Community-Acquired Pneumonia. New York: Kluwer Academic/Plenum Publishers; 2001. p. 487–500.

Hammerschlag MR. *Mycoplasma pneumoniae* infections. Curr Opin Infect Dis 2001;14:181–6.

Hurt AC, Selleck P, Komadina N, et al. Susceptibility of highly pathogenic A(H5N1) avian influenza viruses to the neuraminidase inhibitors and adamantanes. Antiviral Res 2007;73:228–31.

Louria DB, Blumenfield HL, Ellis JT. Studies on influenza in the pandemic of 1957–1958. II. Pulmonary complications of influenza. J Clin Invest 1959;38:213–65.

Marrie TJ. Empiric treatment of ambulatory community-acquired pneumonia: Always include treatment for atypical agents. Infect Dis Clin North Am 2004;18:829–41.

Murray HW, Masur H, Senterfit LS, Roberts RB. The protean manifestations of *Mycoplasma pneumoniae* infection in adults. Am J Med 1975;58:229–42.

Nisar N, Guleria R, Kumar S, et al. Mycoplasma pneumoniae and its role in asthma. Postgrad Med J 2007;83:100–4.

Schmidt AC. Antiviral therapy for influenza: A clinical and economic comparative review. Drugs 2004;6:2031–46.

Waites KB, Talkington DF. *Mycoplasma pneumoniae* and its role as a human pathogen. Clin Microbiol Rev 2004;17:697–728.

Legionellosis

Method of
Julio A. Ramirez, MD

In the summer of 1976, an outbreak of approximately 182 cases of pneumonia occurred in persons attending the American Legion convention in Philadelphia. One year later, Dr. McDade reported the identification of *Legionella pneumophila*, the bacterium responsible for the infection. Today, the family of Legionellaceae is composed of more than 40 species, with some species having different serogroups. *L pneumophila* causes approximately 85% of all *Legionella* infections. *L. pneumophila* serogroup 1 is the single most common member of the family causing clinical infections.

Epidemiology

Legionella is an intracellular organism that lives in natural water. In the aquatic environment, the bacteria live and multiply within freshwater amebae. The number of *Legionella* organisms in the water can increase significantly with appropriate local conditions such as warm temperature, lack of biocides, stagnant water, and presence of amebae and other nutrients. These special conditions can be present in artificial water systems such as cooling towers, whirlpools, decorative fountains, and respiratory therapy devices.

The susceptible host acquires the bacteria from water containing the organism. Infection can be acquired by inhaling aerosols containing *Legionella* organisms or by microaspiration of water contaminated with *Legionella*. The hospitalized patient with *Legionella* pneumonia does not require respiratory isolation because legionellosis is not transmitted from person to person.

Clinical Features

Once *Legionella* organisms reach the respiratory tract, based on the interactions of the organism with the host immune system, the patient can have four possible clinical outcomes: asymptomatic infection, Pontiac fever, legionnaires' disease, or extrapulmonary disease involving the liver, heart brain, or other organs. Pontiac fever is a nonpneumonic form of disease characterized by fever, headaches, myalgias, and malaise. The patient has an influenza-like illness, with resolution of disease in a few days without specific antimicrobial therapy. Patients with legionnaires' disease present with community-acquired pneumonia associated with high fever, gastrointestinal complaints such as diarrhea and central nervous system complaints such as headaches or mental status changes. Hospital-acquired pneumonia can occur if *Legionella* is present in the hospital water supply.

Diagnosis

The currently available laboratory tests for diagnosis of *Legionella* infections include the direct fluorescent antibody stain (DFA), culture, antigen detection in the urine, antibody detection in serum by indirect fluorescent antibody testing (IFA), and DNA amplification using the polymerase chain reaction (PCR). The DFA stain can detect all *L. pneumophila* serogroups, but a large number of bacteria need to be present in sputum for a positive result. *Legionella* can be cultured from respiratory specimens on selective media composed of buffered charcoal–yeast extract agar. The urinary antigen detection has a specificity greater than 95%; the disadvantage is that the test detects only the antigen of *L. pneumophila* serogroup 1. Clinical specimens that have been used to detect *Legionella* by PCR include throat swabs, sputum, tracheal suction, bronchoalveolar lavage fluid, pleural fluid, and lung tissue.

Treatment

In the pulmonary parenchyma, *Legionella* can infect and multiply inside alveolar macrophages, alveolar epithelial cells, and capillary endothelial cells. The poor clinical outcome with β-lactam antibiotics is due to their lack of penetration into cells. Antibiotics with good intracellular penetration that can be used as monotherapy for *Legionella* infections include macrolides, ketolides, tetracyclines, and quinolones (Table 1). Rifampin (Rifadin)[1] is not used as monotherapy because resistance can rapidly emerge when it is used alone.

Therapy of the patient with severe disease is initiated with intravenous antibiotics. Once the patient reaches clinical stability, the intravenous therapy can be switched to oral therapy. Doses for the most common antibiotics for intravenous and oral therapy are depicted in Table 1. In the nonimmunocompromised patient, the recommended duration of therapy is 7 to 10 days. In immunocompromised patients, because they are at risk for relapsing infection, the recommended duration of therapy is 14 to 21 days.

Several antibiotics have demonstrated clinical efficacy in legionnaires' disease. Data with several in vitro and animal studies comparing different anti-*Legionella* antibiotics indicate that erythromycin (Ery-Tab) is a weak anti-*Legionella* agent. If erythromycin is selected for therapy, it is important to add rifampin to the regimen to increase intracellular killing. From the family of macrolides, azithromycin (Zithromax)[1] is the most active. The best bactericidal activity in the laboratory is achieved with quinolones. Retrospective observational studies indicate that patients treated with levofloxacin (Levaquin) have a shorter time to reach clinical stability and shorter duration of hospital stay. These antibiotics are considered primary anti-*Legionella* agents.

In clinical practice, I treat immunocompromised patients who have severe legionnaires' disease with a combination of an intravenous quinolone plus an intravenous macrolide (e.g., levofloxacin plus azithromycin). This regimen is based only on the theoretical consideration that synergistic killing may be obtained using a quinolone to alter DNA synthesis and a macrolide to alter protein synthesis.

---

[1]Not FDA approved for this indication.

TABLE 1 Antibiotic Therapy for *Legionella* Infections

Antibiotic	Oral Dose	Intravenous Dose
Ketolides		
Telithromycin (Ketek)[1]	800 mg qd	—
Macrolides		
Azithromycin (Zithromax)[1]	500 mg qd	500 mg qd
Clarithromycin (Biaxin)[1]	500 mg bid	—
Erythromycin (Ery-Tab)	500 mg q6h	1 g q6h
Quinolones		
Ciprofloxacin (Cipro)[1]	750 mg bid	400 mg bid
Levofloxacin (Levaquin)	750 mg qd	750 mg qd
Moxifloxacin (Avelox)[1]	400 mg qd	400 mg qd
Rifamycins		
Rifampin (Rifadin)[1]	300 mg bid	300 mg bid
Tetracyclines		
Doxycycline (Vibramycin)[1]	100 mg bid	100 mg bid

[1]Not FDA approved for this indication.

Venous Thromboembolism

Method of
Clive Kearon, MRCPI, FRCPC, PhD

Venous thromboembolism (VTE), which includes deep venous thrombosis (DVT) and pulmonary embolism (PE), is the third most common cause of vascular death (after myocardial infarction and stroke) and the leading cause of preventable death among hospitalized patients. Thrombosis starts in the deep veins, and PE occurs when such thrombi break free and lodge in the pulmonary arteries, where they obstruct blood flow and can cause lung damage (i.e., pulmonary infarction). About 90% of the instances of DVT involve the legs, about 5% involve the upper extremities (axillary, subclavian, or jugular veins), and the remaining 5% involve other veins of the body (e.g., internal iliac, renal, ovarian). DVT that is confined to the deep veins of the calf, without involvement of the popliteal vein, is termed isolated distal DVT, whereas that involving the popliteal or a more proximal vein is termed proximal DVT (most proximal DVT also involves the distal veins). Thrombosis of the subcutaneous veins is referred to as superficial vein thrombosis or superficial thrombophlebitis. Superficial vein thrombosis mostly occurs in the legs (e.g., long or short saphenous veins, often in association with varicosities), and its main importance is that it causes pain and swelling and may extend to cause DVT. This chapter focuses on DVT of the legs and PE.

Pathogenesis and Risk Factors

Virchow is credited with identifying stasis, vessel wall injury, and hypercoagulability as the pathogenic triad responsible for thrombosis. This classification of risk factors for VTE remains valuable. Most patients who develop VTE have more than one, and often multiple, risk factors.

VENOUS STASIS

The importance of venous stasis as a risk factor for VTE is demonstrated by the fact that most DVT associated with stroke affects the paralyzed leg, and most DVT associated with pregnancy affects the left leg, due to extrinsic compression of the left common iliac vein by the pregnant uterus and the right common iliac artery. General immobilization, such as in hospitalized patients and in patients with leg injuries or other chronic illness, is also an important risk factor. Venous stasis is thought to predispose to thrombosis by causing local hypoxia (e.g., in venous valve cusps), which attracts inflammatory cells and causes endothelial dysfunction, leading to an increase in the local concentration of clotting factors and tissue factor and an increase in interactions between circulating cells and the venous endothelium.

VESSEL DAMAGE

Venous endothelial damage, usually as a consequence of accidental injury, manipulation during surgery, or iatrogenic injury, is an important risk factor for VTE. Three quarters of proximal DVT that complicates hip surgery occurs in the operated leg, and thrombosis is common with indwelling venous catheters. Venous injury is thought to predispose to thrombosis by exposing blood to subendothelial tissue factor and to collagen, which binds von Willebrand's factor.

HYPERCOAGULABILITY

A complex balance between naturally occurring coagulation and fibrinolytic factors and their inhibitors serves to maintain blood fluidity and hemostasis. Inherited or acquired changes in this balance can predispose to thrombosis. The most important inherited biochemical disorders associated with VTE are defects of the naturally occurring inhibitors of coagulation (i.e., deficiencies of antithrombin,

protein C, or protein S and resistance to activated protein C caused by factor V Leiden) and the G20210A prothrombin gene mutation, which is associated with elevated levels of prothrombin. The first three coagulation deficiencies listed are rare in the normal population (combined prevalence, <1%), have a combined prevalence of approximately 5% in patients with a first episode of VTE, and are associated with a 10- to 40-fold increase in the risk of VTE. The factor V Leiden mutation is common, occurring in approximately 5% of Caucasians and 20% of patients with a first episode of VTE (i.e., a fourfold increase in VTE risk). The G20210A prothrombin gene occurs in approximately 2% of Caucasians and 5% of patients with a first episode of VTE (i.e., a 2.5-fold increase in VTE risk).

Elevated levels of a number of coagulation factors (I, II, VIII, IX, XI) are also associated with thrombosis in a dose-dependent manner. It is probable that such elevations are often inherited, and there is strong evidence for this supposition for factor VIII and factor II; for example, the G20210A prothrombin gene is associated with an increase of approximately 25% in factor II (prothrombin). Abnormalities of the fibrinolytic system have a questionable association with VTE.

Acquired hypercoagulable states include estrogen therapy (threefold increase in VTE, highest during the first 6 months), antiphospholipid antibodies (anticardiolipin antibodies or lupus anticoagulants or both), systemic lupus erythematosus, malignancy, chemotherapy for cancer, and surgery. Patients who develop immunologically related heparin-induced thrombocytopenia also have a very high risk for arterial and venous thromboembolism. Unlike the congenital abnormalities, acquired risk factors are often transient, and this fact has important implications for the duration of anticoagulant prophylaxis and treatment.

COMBINATIONS OF RISK FACTORS AND RISK STRATIFICATION

The risk of developing VTE depends on the prevalence and severity of risk factors (Box 1). By assessment of these factors, hospitalized patients can be categorized as having a low, moderate, or high risk

---

BOX 1 Risk Factors for Venous Thromboembolism (VTE)*

Patient Factors
- Previous VTE[†]
- Age older than 40 years, and particularly older than 70 years[†]
- Pregnancy, puerperium
- Marked obesity
- Inherited hypercoagulable state

Underlying Condition and Acquired Factors
- Malignancy[†]
- Estrogen therapy
- Cancer chemotherapy
- Paralysis[†]
- Prolonged immobility
- Major trauma[†]
- Lower limb injuries[†]
- Heparin-induced thrombocytopenia
- Antiphospholipid antibodies

Type of Surgery
- Lower limb orthopedic surgery[†]
- General anesthesia >30 min

---

*Combinations of factors have an at least an additive effect on the risk of VTE.
[†]Common major risk factors for VTE.

TABLE 1 Risk Stratification for VTE in Hospitalized and Postoperative Patients, Frequency of VTE without Prophylaxis, and Recommended Methods of Prophylaxis*

Risk Factor	Venographic DVT[†] (%)		Pulmonary Embolism (%)		Recommended Prophylaxis
	Calf	Proximal	Symptomatic	Fatal	
Low Risk: Minor (usually same-day) surgery in a mobile patient Medical patients, fully mobile No additional risk factors	2	0.4	0.2	<0.01	Early mobilization
Moderate Risk: Most general surgery patients Most medical patients	20	5	2	0.5	Low-dose UFH (5000 U SQ preoperatively and bid or tid postoperatively) LMWH (~3000 U/d SQ with a preoperative start)[‡] Fondaparinux (Arixtra)[1] GC stockings, alone or with pharmacologic methods
High Risk: Most general surgery patients with previous VTE Major knee or hip surgery Major trauma, spinal cord injury (Heparin-induced thrombocytopenia)	50	15	5	2	LMWH (>3000 U/d) Fondaparinux Warfarin (Coumadin)[§] IPC devices, alone or with GC stockings or pharmacologic methods or both (Specific nonheparin therapy)

[1]Not FDA approved for this indication.
*New anticoagulants (e.g., oral direct thrombin, anti-factor Xa inhibitors) are becoming available for moderate- and high-risk patients.
[†]Asymptomatic DVT detected by screening bilateral venography.
[‡]Higher doses are used in high-risk patients (e.g., ~ 4,000 U once daily with a preoperative start in Europe; ~3,000 U twice daily with a postoperative start in North America).
[§]Usually started postoperatively and adjusted to achieve an international normalized ratio of 2.0–3.0.
Abbreviations: DVT = deep venous thrombosis; GC = graduated compression; IPC = intermittent pneumatic compression; LMWH = low-molecular-weight heparin; UFH = unfractionated heparin; VTE = venous thromboembolism.

of VTE (Table 1). Patients with active cancer are among those with the highest risk of thrombosis, because they often have a large number of major risk factors, such as the hypercoagulable state associated with cancer, recent surgery, chemotherapy, generalized immobility from weakness, localized stasis associated with venous obstruction by tumor, and the presence of indwelling venous catheters.

Epidemiology and Natural History of Venous Thromboembolism

The overall incidence of VTE is about 1.5 per 1000 persons per year in adults, with about two thirds of these episodes being symptomatic DVT and about one third being symptomatic PE (with or without symptoms of DVT). However, the incidence of VTE is highly influenced by age. Before the age of 16 years, most likely because the immature coagulation system is resistant to thrombosis, VTE is very rare and is largely confined to children with major provoking factors such as indwelling venous lines. The risk of VTE increases exponentially with advancing age, with an almost twofold increase every decade, from an annual incidence of 0.3 per 1000 at 40 years to 1 per 1000 at 60 years and 4 per 1000 at 80 years of age.

VTE occurs slightly more frequently in men than in women, although this pattern is reversed before 40 years of age because the association of VTE with estrogen-containing contraceptives and pregnancy. The relative frequency of PE to DVT is somewhat higher in the elderly.

About 50% of the cases of VTE are associated with hospitalization (about half before and half after discharge), which emphasizes the importance of using appropriate prophylaxis to prevent VTE in high-risk patients. Among hospital-associated VTE cases, about half occur in surgical and half in medical patients. About one quarter of VTE cases are associated with cancer; one quarter are associated with minor illnesses, injuries, or estrogen therapy; and one quarter are not associated with any apparent clinical risk factor (referred to as unprovoked or idiopathic VTE). There is overlap among these categories; for example, there is a particularly high risk of VTE among patients with cancer who are hospitalized.

Of all episodes of VTE, about three quarters are first episodes and one quarter are recurrent episodes. Clinically important components of the natural history of VTE are summarized in Box 2.

Diagnosis of Deep Venous Thrombosis

CLINICAL FEATURES

The clinical features of DVT, such as localized swelling, redness, tenderness, and distal edema, are nonspecific, and the diagnosis should always be confirmed by objective tests. About 85% of ambulatory patients with clinically suspected DVT have another cause for their symptoms. The conditions that are most likely to simulate DVT are a ruptured Baker's cyst, cellulitis, muscle tears, muscle cramp, muscle hematoma, external venous compression, superficial thrombophlebitis, and the postthrombotic syndrome. Of patients with symptomatic DVT, about 75% have proximal vein thrombosis; in the rest, thrombosis is confined to the calf. Although clinical features cannot unequivocally confirm or exclude a diagnosis of DVT, clinical assessment can stratify the probability of DVT as high (prevalence of

BOX 2 Natural History of Venous Thromboembolism: Key Points

- Clinical factors can identify high-risk patients.
- VTE starts in the calf veins in >75% of patients.
- Three quarters of asymptomatic DVT detected postoperatively by screening venography are confined to the distal (calf) veins.
- About 20% of symptomatic isolated calf DVT subsequently extends to the proximal veins, usually within 1 week after presentation.
- More than 90% of asymptomatic postoperative DVT resolves without causing symptoms.
- More than 80% of symptomatic DVT involves the popliteal or more proximal veins.
- Symptomatic PE usually arises from proximal DVT.
- Most (70%) patients with symptomatic proximal DVT have asymptomatic PE (high-probability lung scans in 40%), and most patients with symptomatic PE (80%) have DVT.
- Only one quarter of patients with symptomatic PE have symptoms or signs of DVT.
- About 50% of untreated symptomatic proximal DVT is expected to cause symptomatic PE.
- About 10% of symptomatic PE is rapidly fatal.
- Most fatal PE is not diagnosed.
- About 30% of patients with untreated symptomatic nonfatal PE have a fatal recurrence.
- The risk of recurrent VTE after stopping anticoagulant therapy is much lower if VTE was provoked by a reversible risk factor (particularly recent surgery) than if it was unprovoked or provoked by a persistent risk factor.

Abbreviations: DVT = deep venous thrombosis; PE = pulmonary embolism; VTE = venous thromboembolism.

thrombosis, ~60%), intermediate (~25%), or low (~5%) based on: the presence or absence of risk factors (e.g., recent immobilization, hospitalization within the past month, malignancy); whether the clinical manifestations at presentation are typical or atypical and their severity; and whether there is an alternative explanation for the symptoms that is at least as likely as DVT (Table 2).

TABLE 2 Wells Model for Determining Clinical Suspicion of Deep Venous Thrombosis (DVT)*

Variable	Points
Active cancer (treatment ongoing or within previous 6 mo or palliative)	1
Paralysis, paresis, or recent plaster immobilization of the lower extremities	1
Recently bedridden >3 d or major surgery within 4 wk	1
Localized tenderness along the distribution of the deep venous system	1
Entire leg swollen	1
Calf swelling 3 cm greater than on asymptomatic side (measured 10 cm below tibial tuberosity)	1
Pitting edema confined to the symptomatic leg	1
Dilated superficial veins (non-varicose)	1
Alternative diagnosis as likely or greater than that of DVT	−2

*Pretest probability of DVT is calculated from the total points: >2 points, high; 1 or 2, moderate; <1, low.

VENOGRAPHY

Venography, which involves the injection of a radiocontrast agent into a distal vein, is the reference standard for the diagnosis of DVT. Venography detects both proximal and isolated distal DVT. However, it is expensive and technically difficult to perform, can be painful, and requires injection of radiographic contrast, which can cause allergic reactions or renal impairment. For these reasons, venography is now rarely performed.

VENOUS ULTRASONOGRAPHY

Venous ultrasonography is the noninvasive imaging method of choice for diagnosing DVT. It is not painful and is easy to perform. The common femoral vein, the femoral vein (previously called the superficial femoral vein), the popliteal vein, and the calf vein trifurcation (i.e., proximal junction of deep calf veins) are imaged in real time and compressed with the transducer probe (compression ultrasound). Inability to fully compress (i.e., obliterate) the vein lumen with pressure from the ultrasound probe is diagnostic for DVT. Duplex ultrasonography, which combines compression ultrasound with pulsed Doppler or color-coded Doppler technology, facilitates identification of the deep veins (particularly in the calf; see later discussion) and may enable thrombus to be detected if it is not feasible to assess vein compressibility (e.g., iliac or subclavian veins).

Venous ultrasonography is highly accurate for diagnosis of proximal vein thrombosis, with a sensitivity and specificity approaching 95%. The sensitivity for symptomatic calf vein thrombosis is considerably lower and appears to be highly operator dependent. For this reason, many centers do not examine the deep veins of the calf with ultrasonography. Instead, if examination of the proximal veins excludes proximal DVT in a patient with a moderate or high clinical assessment for DVT, the test is repeated in 7 days to detect the small number of calf vein thrombi (~3%) that subsequently extend into the proximal veins. If the test remains negative after 7 days, the risk that thrombus is present and will extend to the proximal veins is negligible, and it is safe to withhold treatment (Box 3).

If the clinical assessment for DVT is low and the result of an initial proximal venous ultrasound scan is normal, it is not necessary to repeat ultrasonography after 7 days, because the prevalence of DVT is only about 2% (mostly distal). If the calf veins below the level of the calf vein trifurcation are also examined and there is no isolated distal DVT as well as no proximal DVT, then DVT is excluded without the need for repeat ultrasonography after 7 days. However, examination of the calf veins has the disadvantage of resulting in diagnosis and treatment of DVT in substantially more patients than does serial examination of the proximal veins, without further reducing the risk of VTE during follow-up (approximately 1% over 3 months in both groups) in those who are not initially diagnosed with DVT.

Ultrasonography is less accurate when its results are discordant with clinical assessment. Therefore, if the clinical suspicion for DVT is low and the ultrasound study shows a localized abnormality (i.e., less convincing findings), or if clinical suspicion is high and the ultrasound is normal, further diagnostic testing (e.g., venography) should be considered.

D-DIMER BLOOD TESTING

D-dimer is formed when cross-linked fibrin in thrombi is broken down by plasmin. Because it is usually increased in patients with acute VTE, low levels of D-dimer can be used to exclude DVT and PE. A variety of D-dimer assays are available, and they vary markedly in their accuracy as diagnostic tests for VTE. All D-dimer assays have a low specificity for DVT; consequently, an abnormal result is associated with a low positive predictive value and cannot be used to diagnose DVT.

D-dimer assays that are used for diagnosis of VTE can be divided into two groups based on their sensitivity and specificity. Very highly sensitive D-dimer assays (e.g., sensitivity >98%; specificity ~40%) have a sufficiently high negative predictive value (>98%) that a normal result can be used to exclude VTE without the need to perform additional diagnostic testing. With moderate to highly sensitive D-dimer assays (sensitivity 85%-97%; specificity 50%–70%), a negative result needs

BOX 3 Test Results That Confirm or Exclude Deep Venous Thrombosis (DVT)

Diagnostic for First DVT

Venography: Intraluminal filling defect in proximal or distal deep veins
Venous ultrasound: Noncompressible popliteal or common femoral vein

Excludes First DVT

Venography: All deep veins seen, and no intraluminal filling defects
D-dimer:

- Normal result on a D-dimer test with a very high sensitivity (i.e., ≥98%) and at least a moderate specificity (i.e., ≥40%)
- Normal result on a D-dimer test with a moderately high sensitivity (i.e., ≥85%) and specificity (i.e., ≥70%), plus low clinical suspicion for DVT at presentation

Venous ultrasound: Fully compressible proximal veins and one or more of the following:

- Low clinical suspicion for DVT
- Normal result on a D-dimer test with a moderately high sensitivity (i.e., ≥85%) and specificity (i.e., ≥70%) at presentation
- Fully compressible distal deep veins (whole leg ultrasound)
- Normal repeat ultrasound of the proximal veins after 7 days

Diagnostic for Recurrent DVT

Venography: Intraluminal filling defect
Venous ultrasound:

- A new, noncompressible common femoral or popliteal vein segment
- A 4.0-mm increase in diameter of the common femoral or popliteal vein compared with a previous test

Excludes Recurrent DVT

Venogram: All deep veins seen, and no intraluminal filling defects
Venous ultrasound: Normal, or ≤1 mm increase in diameter of the common femoral or popliteal veins compared with a previous test, which remains unchanged on repeat testing after 2 and 7 days
D-dimer:

- Normal result on a D-dimer test with a very high sensitivity (i.e., ≥98%) and at least a moderate specificity (i.e., ≥40%)
- Normal result on a D-dimer test with a moderately high sensitivity (i.e., ≥85%) and specificity (i.e., ≥70%), plus low clinical suspicion for DVT

to be combined with another assessment that identifies patients as having a lower prevalence of VTE in order to exclude DVT. Management studies have shown that it is safe to consider DVT excluded in patients who have a normal result on a moderately sensitive D-dimer test in combination with either a low clinical suspicion for DVT or no proximal DVT on venous ultrasonography (see Box 3).

D-dimer testing is much less specific (i.e., fewer negative tests among those without venous thrombosis), and therefore has less clinical utility in postoperative and hospitalized patients and in the elderly (>75 years). Also, D-dimer testing has less clinical utility in patients with a high clinical suspicion of VTE because negative results are rarely obtained, and if a negative test is obtained, its predictive value is lower because of the high prevalence of disease.

COMPUTED TOMOGRAPHIC AND MAGNETIC RESONANCE IMAGING VENOGRAPHY

Computed tomography (CT) and magnetic resonance imaging (MRI) have been reported to have high accuracy (sensitivity and specificity >90%) for the diagnosis of DVT but are rarely used for this purpose, because CT requires the use of radiographic contrast and is associated with high radiation exposure, and both CT and MRI are costly. CT and MRI are expected to be more accurate than ultrasound for DVT that does not involve the limbs, such as that confined to the pelvic veins or the inferior vena cava. Diagnosis of DVT on CT (or, less commonly, on MRI) is most commonly an incidental finding in patients who undergo CT to stage a known malignancy. In this situation, because the clinical suspicion for DVT is low and the examination will not have been designed to diagnose DVT, patients need to be carefully reviewed, often including further testing, before a diagnosis of DVT is accepted.

Diagnosis of Recurrent Deep Venous Thrombosis

The diagnosis of recurrent DVT can be difficult. A negative D-dimer test can exclude recurrent DVT, although the safety of this approach has been less well evaluated than for first episodes of DVT. If D-dimer testing is positive or has not been done, venous ultrasonography is

performed. If the result is normal (i.e., full compressibility of the veins), treatment is withheld, and the test should be repeated twice over the next 7 to 10 days. If the result is positive in the popliteal or common femoral vein segments and the result of a previous test was negative at the same site, a recurrence is diagnosed. Recurrence can also be diagnosed if venous ultrasonography shows other convincing evidence of more extensive thrombosis than was seen on a previous examination (e.g., an increase in compressed thrombus diameter of >4 mm in the common femoral or the popliteal segments; unequivocal extension within the femoral vein of the thigh).

If a comparison between current and previous venous ultrasound findings is equivocal, or if no previous ultrasound is available for comparison, venography should be performed; however, many hospitals no longer perform venography. If the venogram shows an intraluminal filling defect, which is seen with acute rather than remote thrombosis, recurrent DVT is diagnosed. If the venogram outlines all of the deep veins and does not show an intraluminal filling defect, recurrent DVT is excluded. If the venogram is nondiagnostic (i.e., nonfilling of segments of the deep veins) or if venography is not performed in a patient with equivocal findings on ultrasound, the patient can be observed with repeat venous ultrasonography to detect extending DVT or, less satisfactorily, recurrent DVT can be diagnosed based on the results of all assessments, including clinical features. Clinical assessment of the probability of recurrent DVT is less well standardized than for a first episode of DVT; however, many of the factors that are predictive of a first episode are also expected to be predictive of recurrent DVT (Box 3).

Diagnosis of Pulmonary Embolism

CLINICAL FEATURES

Dyspnea is the most common symptom of PE. Chest pain is also common and is usually pleuritic but can be substernal and compressive. Hemoptysis is less frequently present. Tachycardia and tachypnea are common signs. Evidence of right heart failure is less common but of prognostic importance, and a pleural rub may be heard in association

TABLE 3 Wells Model for Determining Clinical Suspicion of Pulmonary Embolism*

Variable	Points
Clinical signs and symptoms of DVT (minimum leg swelling and pain with palpation of the deep veins)	3.0
An alternative diagnosis is less likely than PE	3.0
Heart rate >100 beats/min	1.5
Immobilization or surgery in the previous 4 wk	1.5
Previous DVT/PE	1.5
Hemoptysis	1.0
Malignancy (treatment ongoing or within previous 6 months or palliative)	1.0

*Pretest probability of PE is calculated from the total points: >6 points, high; 4 to 6, moderate; <4, low.
Abbreviations: DVT = deep venous thrombosis; PE = pulmonary embolism.

BOX 4 Test Results That Confirm or Exclude Pulmonary Embolism (PE)

Diagnostic for PE

Pulmonary angiography: Intraluminal filling defect
Computed tomographic pulmonary angiography (CTPA):
- Intraluminal filling defect in a lobar or main pulmonary artery
- Intraluminal filling defect in a segmental pulmonary artery, plus moderate or high clinical suspicion

Ventilation/perfusion scan: High-probability scan, plus moderate to high clinical suspicion
Diagnostic test for deep venous thrombosis: With a nondiagnostic ventilation/perfusion scan or CTPA

Excludes PE

Pulmonary angiogram: Normal
Perfusion scan: Normal
D-dimer:
- Normal result on a D-dimer test with a very high sensitivity (i.e., ≥98%) and at least a moderate specificity (i.e., ≥ 40%)
- Normal result on a D-dimer test with a moderately high sensitivity (i.e., ≥85%) and specificity (i.e., ≥70%), plus low clinical suspicion for PE

Nondiagnostic ventilation/perfusion scan or suboptimal CTPA, plus normal venous ultrasound of the proximal veins and one or more of the following:
- Low clinical suspicion for PE
- Normal result on a D-dimer test with at least a moderately high sensitivity (i.e., ≥85%) and specificity (i.e., ≥ 70%)
- Normal repeat venous ultrasound of the proximal veins after 7 and 14 days

with pulmonary infarction. Although most patients with PE also have DVT, fewer than 25% have symptoms or signs. The clinical features of PE, like those of DVT, are nonspecific, and PE is diagnosed in only about 20% of those in whom it is suspected.

Two groups have published explicit criteria for determining the clinical probability of PE. The model by Wells and colleagues incorporates an assessment of symptoms and signs, the presence of an alternative diagnosis that could account for the patient's condition, and the presence of risk factors for VTE. With this model, a patient's clinical probability of PE can be categorized as low or unlikely (prevalence of PE <10%), moderate (~25%), or high (~ 60%) (Table 3).

CHEST RADIOGRAPHY AND ELECTROCARDIOGRAPHY

In patients with PE, chest radiographs show either normal or nonspecific findings. However, a chest radiograph is useful for exclusion of pneumothorax and other conditions that can simulate PE (e.g., left ventricular failure). The electrocardiogram also frequently shows normal or nonspecific findings but is valuable for excluding acute myocardial infarction. In the appropriate clinical setting, right ventricular strain can suggest PE and a poorer short-term outcome among those with PE.

VENTILATION/PERFUSION LUNG SCANNING

Ventilation/perfusion lung scanning was the most important test for diagnosing PE in the past. Computed tomographic pulmonary angiography (CTPA) has now supplanted lung scanning, although the latter is still used, particularly if CTPA is contraindicated because of renal failure or associated radiation exposure to the chest (e.g., in young women). A normal perfusion scan excludes PE but is obtained in only about 25% of patients; a higher proportion of normal scans is obtained in patients who are young, who do not have chronic lung disease, or who have a normal chest radiograph. An abnormal perfusion scan is nonspecific. Ventilation imaging improves the specificity of perfusion scanning. If the ventilation scan is normal at the site of two or more large (>75% of a segment) perfusion defects, the lung scan is associated with a greater than 85% prevalence of PE and is termed a high-probability scan. About half of patients with PE have a high-probability lung scan. Therefore, among consecutive patients who are investigated for PE, about 25% have a normal perfusion scan and can have the diagnosis excluded; about 15% have a high-probability scan and can have PE diagnosed (provided that the clinical probability is moderate or high) (Box 4); and about 60% have a nondiagnostic lung scan that requires further diagnostic testing.

COMPUTED TOMOGRAPHIC PULMONARY ANGIOGRAPHY

CTPA, performed using helical CT (also known as spiral or continuous-volume CT), is able to directly visualize the pulmonary arteries. CTPA has rapidly advanced from use of single detector scanners to use of progressively larger numbers of detectors (multidetector CT) that enable more rapid and detailed examination of the pulmonary arteries.

Results of the Prospective Investigation of Pulmonary Embolism Diagnosis (PIOPED II) study suggested that CTPA is nondiagnostic in 6% of patients and that, among adequate examinations, sensitivity for PE is 83%, specificity is 96%, positive predictive value is 86% and negative predictive value is 95%. Accuracy varies according to the size of the largest pulmonary artery involved: the positive predictive value was 97% for defects in the main or lobar artery, 68% in segmental arteries, and 25% in subsegmental arteries (4% of PE in this study). Predictive values were also influenced by the clinical assessment of PE probability: the positive predictive value of CTPA was 96% in combination with high, 92% with intermediate, and 58% with low clinical probability (8% of patients); likewise, the negative predictive value was 96% with low, 89% with intermediate, and 60% with high clinical probability (3% of patients). Management studies, in which anticoagulant therapy was withheld in patients with a negative CTPA result suggested that fewer than 2% of patients with a negative CTPA for PE will return with symptomatic VTE during 3 months of follow-up. Taken together, these observations suggest the following conclusions (see Box 4).

- An intraluminal filling defect in a segmental or larger pulmonary artery is generally diagnostic for PE. However, if the clinical probability is low and if there are additional findings that undermine a diagnosis of PE (e.g., technically suboptimal study, negative D-dimer test), further diagnostic testing should be considered (e.g., venous ultrasonography, ventilation/perfusion scanning, repeat CTPA), particularly if the most proximal pulmonary artery involved is at the segmental level.

- A good-quality negative CTPA finding excludes PE. If the CTPA does not show PE but is suboptimal, ultrasonography of the proximal deep veins of the legs should be performed to supplement the findings of the CTPA and exclude DVT.
- Abnormalities suggestive of intraluminal defects that are confined to subsegmental pulmonary arteries are generally nondiagnostic and require further investigation.

MRI is less well evaluated than CTPA for the diagnosis of PE and appears to be less accurate. Both CTPA and MRI have the advantage of identifying alternative pulmonary diagnoses. MRI does not expose the patient to radiation or radiographic contrast media.

D-DIMER BLOOD TESTING

D-dimer testing is a valuable test for the exclusion of PE, either alone (very sensitive D-dimer assay) or in combination with other assessments that are associated with a reduced prevalence of PE (see Box 4 and earlier discussion of D-dimer testing for suspected DVT).

COMPRESSION ULTRASONOGRAPHY

Compression ultrasonography, usually evaluating the proximal deep veins of the legs, can aid in the diagnosis of PE. Demonstration of DVT, which occurs in about 5% of patients with nondiagnostic ventilation/perfusion lung scans, serves as indirect evidence of PE. Exclusion of proximal DVT does not rule out PE in a patient with a nondiagnostic ventilation/perfusion scan, although it does reduce that probability somewhat. However, if there is no proximal DVT on the day of presentation and proximal DVT is not detected on two subsequent examinations performed 1 and 2 weeks later (DVT is diagnosed during serial testing in approximately 2% of patients), anticoagulant therapy can be withheld with a very low risk that the patient will return with VTE (<2% during 3 months of follow-up).

As previously noted for patients with a nondiagnostic ventilation/perfusion lung scan, withholding of anticoagulant therapy and performance of serial ultrasonography is a reasonable approach to management in patients who have a CTPA result that is nondiagnostic, including patients with isolated subsegmental abnormalities.

PULMONARY ANGIOGRAPHY

Although pulmonary angiography was considered to be the reference standard for PE in the past, it is now very rarely performed, because it is invasive and can usually be replaced by CTPA. Combinations of test results that confirm and exclude PE are shown in Box 4.

Prevention of Venous Thromboembolism

The most effective way to reduce mortality from PE and morbidity from the postthrombotic syndrome is to use primary prophylaxis in patients at risk for VTE, particularly during hospitalization. On the basis of well-defined clinical criteria, patients can be classified as being at low, moderate, or high risk for VTE, and use of prophylaxis can then be tailored to the patient's risk (see Table 1). By reducing the need to diagnose and treat VTE, prophylaxis is cost-saving in many situations, rather than just being cost-effective.

Prophylaxis is achieved by reducing blood coagulability or by preventing venous stasis. Anticoagulants, including subcutaneous heparin, low-molecular-weight-heparin (LMWH), and fondaparinux (Arixtra), as well as oral vitamin K antagonists, oral direct thrombin, and factor Xa inhibitors, reduce coagulability. Mechanical methods, including graduated compression stockings and intermittent pneumatic compression (IPC) devices, prevent venous stasis. Antiplatelet agents, such as aspirin,[1] also prevent VTE, but less effectively than the previously stated methods, and they are not usually recommended for this purpose.

Heparin is given subcutaneously at a dose of 5000 U 2 hours before surgery and 5000 U every 8 or 12 hours after surgery. In patients undergoing major orthopedic surgical procedures, low-dose heparin is less effective than LMWH, vitamin K antagonist therapy, or fondaparinux and is not recommended.

LMWH is also given subcutaneously, once or twice a day. It is effective in high-risk patients undergoing elective hip surgery, major general surgery, or major knee surgery and in patients with hip fracture, spinal injury, or acute medical illness. LMWH is more effective than vitamin K antagonist therapy at preventing VTE after major orthopedic surgery while patients are in hospital, but it is also associated with more frequent early postoperative bleeding; both of these differences may be related to the more rapid onset of anticoagulation with LMWH than with vitamin K antagonist therapy.

Graduated compression stockings reduce the risk of venous thrombosis without increasing the risk of bleeding. On their own or in conjunction with IPC, they are indicated in patients who are at high risk for bleeding and in those who are unable to tolerate any bleeding (e.g., neurosurgical patients). In surgical patients, the combined use of graduated compression stockings and pharmacological agents (e.g., low-dose heparin) is more effective than use of either alone. In the absence of a contraindication, pharmacologic prophylaxis is preferred to graduated compression stockings alone, because the evidence of efficacy at preventing PE is greater with the former.

IPC of the legs enhances blood flow in the deep veins and may increase blood fibrinolytic activity. IPC is more effective than graduated stockings alone, particularly after major orthopedic surgery and especially after knee replacement.

Vitamin K antagonist therapy (international normalized ratio [INR], 2.0 to 3.0) is effective for preventing postoperative VTE, including after major orthopedic surgery, but it is difficult to use because of the need for laboratory monitoring.

Fondaparinux, the synthetic pentasaccharide that corresponds to the active component of heparin that binds antithrombin and inhibits factor Xa, has been shown to reduce the frequency of venographically detected DVT by 50%, compared with LMWH, but is associated with an additional risk of bleeding.

GENERAL SURGERY AND MEDICINE

Low-dose heparin or LMWH prophylaxis is the method of choice for moderate-risk general surgical and medical patients. It reduces the risk of VTE by 50% to 70% and is simple, inexpensive, convenient, and safe. If anticoagulants are contraindicated because of an unusually high risk of bleeding, graduated compression stockings, IPC of the legs, or both, should be used. Fondaparinux[1] has also been shown to be effective in these patients.

MAJOR ORTHOPEDIC SURGERY

LMWH, fondaparinux, or vitamin K antagonists provide effective prophylaxis after major orthopedic surgery. If pharmacologic agents are contraindicated because of the risk of bleeding, IPC (with or without graduated compression stockings) is recommended until it becomes safe to use an anticoagulant therapy. Aspirin[1] has also been shown to reduce the frequency of symptomatic VTE and fatal PE after hip fracture; however, because aspirin is expected to be much less effective than anticoagulant therapies, aspirin is not recommended as the sole agent for postoperative prophylaxis. A number of new antithrombotic agents, including oral direct antithrombins (e.g., dabigatran [Pradaxa][2]) and factor Xa inhibitors (e.g., rivaroxaban [Xarelto],[2] apixaban[5]), have been shown to provide effective prophylaxis after major orthopaedic surgery and are being introduced into clinical practice.

A minimum of 10 days of prophylaxis is recommended after major orthopedic surgery, which usually includes treatment after discharge from hospital. In addition, extended prophylaxis for another 10 to 30 days is generally recommended, particularly in patients who have had hip surgery or have other risk factors for thrombosis, such as previous VTE or active cancer.

ENDOSCOPIC GENITOURINARY SURGERY, NEUROSURGERY, AND OCULAR SURGERY

Anticoagulant therapies are avoided in patients undergoing endoscopic genitourinary surgery, neurosurgery, or ocular surgery because of the associated risk of bleeding, particularly close to the time of surgery. Graduated stockings may be used, or IPC in patients with additional risk factors for VTE. If hospitalization is prolonged and the risk of bleeding recedes, patients can subsequently be started on an anticoagulant.

Treatment of Venous Thromboembolism

Anticoagulation is the mainstay of therapy for acute DVT of the leg and PE. The main objectives of anticoagulant therapy are to prevent extension of DVT, early PE, and later recurrences of VTE.

ACUTE ANTICOAGULANT THERAPY

In 1960, it was first established in a randomized trial that heparin (1.5 days) and oral anticoagulants (2 weeks) reduced the risk of recurrent PE and associated death. Based on expert opinion, a regimen of 10 to 14 days of heparin therapy and 3 months of oral anticoagulation became widely adopted in clinical practice. Subsequently, it was shown that 4 or 5 days of intravenous heparin is as effective as 10 days of therapy for the initial treatment of VTE.

In the past 20 years, many trials have established that weight-adjusted LMWH (without laboratory monitoring), given once or twice daily by subcutaneous injection (daily dose of 150–200 IU/kg), is as least as safe and effective as adjusted-dose intravenous unfractionated heparin for the treatment of acute DVT and PE. This enabled treatment of DVT on an outpatient basis, which is now recommended in the absence of very severe symptoms and signs (e.g., impending venous gangrene), severe comorbidity, or marked renal failure that precludes the use of LMWH (which is predominantly renally excreted). Selected patients with PE—those who are without severe symptoms or cardiorespiratory compromise and have good social supports—can also be treated as outpatients, although this approach to treatment has not been evaluated in a randomized trial. In addition to acute anticoagulant therapy, patients with PE should be assessed for possible treatment with thrombolytic therapy (see later discussion).

More recently, once-daily fixed-dose subcutaneous fondaparinux (7.5 mg for body weight 50–100 kg; 5 mg for <50 kg; 10 mg for >100 kg) and twice-daily subcutaneous unfractionated heparin (with or without laboratory monitoring) have also been shown to be as safe and as effective as treatment with LMWH. In the one study that evaluated unmonitored subcutaneous unfractionated heparin, heparin was administered at an initial dose of 333 units/kg followed by 250 units/kg every 12 hours. Danaparoid (Orgaran),[2] argatroban, or lepirudin (Refludan) should be used to treat heparin-induced thrombocytopenia with or without associated thrombosis.

Vitamin K antagonist therapy is usually started on the same day as parenteral anticoagulant therapy. If warfarin (e.g., Coumadin) is used, the initial dose is usually 2.5 to 10 mg, with a lower dose being appropriate in older patients, women, and those with impaired nutrition, and a higher dose being appropriate in younger (<60 years) otherwise healthy outpatients. Subsequent doses should be adjusted to maintain the INR at a target of 2.5 (range, 2.0–3.0). Parenteral anticoagulant therapy is continued until it has been given for 5 days and until the INR is at least 2.0 on two consecutive days.

---

[2]Not available in the United States.

LONG-TERM ANTICOAGULANT THERAPY

The initial demonstration that 3 months of warfarin markedly reduced the frequency of recurrent DVT, compared with 3 months of low-dose subcutaneous heparin, established the need for a prolonged phase of treatment for VTE after initial treatment with intravenous heparin. Subsequently, high-dose subcutaneous heparin and LMWH (50%–75% of the acute treatment dose) was shown to be as effective as warfarin for long-term treatment. Early studies did not monitor patients after anticoagulant therapy was withdrawn to determine whether the risk of recurrent VTE remained acceptable, and they did not compare the risk of recurrence after completion of various durations of therapy to identify the optimal duration. However, during the last 2 decades, a series of well-designed studies have helped to define the optimal duration of anticoagulation for VTE. The findings of these studies can be summarized as follows:

- Shortening the duration of anticoagulation from 3 or 6 months to 4 or 6 weeks results in a doubling of the frequency of recurrent VTE during 1 to 2 years of follow-up.
- Patients with VTE provoked by a transient risk factor have a lower (about one third) risk of recurrence, compared to those with an unprovoked VTE or a persistent risk factor. The greater the provoking transient risk factor (e.g., recent major surgery), the lower the expected risk of recurrence after stopping anticoagulant therapy.
- Three months of anticoagulation is adequate treatment for VTE provoked by a transient risk factor; in the first year after stopping therapy, the risk of recurrence is about 2% if VTE was provoked by a major transient risk factor (e.g., recent surgery) and about 5% if there was a minor risk factor.
- The risk of recurrent VTE is similar if anticoagulant therapy is stopped after 3 months of treatment compared to after 6 or 12 months of treatment; this suggests that 3 months of treatment is sufficient to treat the acute episode of VTE.
- The risk of recurrence is about 10% in the first year, 30% in the first 5 years, and 50% in the first 10 years after stopping anticoagulant therapy in patients with a first unprovoked episode of proximal DVT or PE.
- After 3 months of initial treatment of unprovoked VTE with oral anticoagulants targeted at an INR of 2.5 (range, 2.0–3.0):
  - Oral anticoagulation targeted at an INR of approximately 2.5 reduces the risk of recurrent VTE by more than 90%.
  - Oral anticoagulation targeted at an INR of approximately 1.75 reduces the risk of recurrent VTE by about 75%.
  - Oral anticoagulation with a target INR of approximately 2.5 is more effective than with a target of 1.75, without further increasing the risk of bleeding.
- A second episode of VTE suggests a higher risk of recurrence (increased by about 50%). If both episodes of VTE were provoked by a transient risk factor, 3 months of anticoagulant therapy is expected to be adequate, with subsequent aggressive prophylaxis during transient periods of high risk. A second episode of unprovoked proximal DVT or PE is a strong argument for indefinite anticoagulant therapy.
- The risk of recurrence is lower (about one half) after an isolated calf (distal) DVT than after proximal DVT or PE. This argues against treating unprovoked isolated calf DVT for longer than 3 months.
- The risk of recurrence is similar after an episode of proximal DVT or PE. However, recurrent VTE is about three times as likely to be a PE after an initial PE (about 60% of episodes) than after an initial DVT (about 20% of episodes). This effect is expected to increase mortality from recurrent VTE about twofold after a PE compared with a DVT.
- The risk of recurrence is about threefold higher in patients with active cancer. The risk is higher in patients with metastatic rather than localized disease, and it is expected to be lower if VTE occurred while the patient was receiving chemotherapy and the chemotherapy was subsequently stopped.
- Long-term treatment with LMWH, particularly for the first 3 or 6 months, is more effective than warfarin in patients with VTE associated with cancer and is the preferred treatment for such patients.

- Estrogen therapy is a risk factor for first and recurrent episodes of VTE; consequently, the risk of recurrent VTE after stopping anticoagulants is expected to be lower in women who had VTE while on estrogen therapy, provided that they have stopped taking estrogens, and estrogen therapy should be avoided in patients with a previous VTE who are not on anticoagulant therapy.
- The presence of a hereditary predisposition to VTE does not appear to be a clinically important risk factor for recurrence during or after anticoagulant therapy. Consequently, testing for hereditary thrombophilias is not required in selecting the duration of therapy.
- The presence of an antiphospholipid antibody has uncertain significance as a predictor of recurrence independently of clinical presentation (e.g., provoked versus unprovoked). Absence of an antiphospholipid antibody on routine testing is not a good reason to stop anticoagulant therapy at 3 months in a patient with unprovoked proximal DVT or PE, and presence of an antiphospholipid antibody is not a good reason to treat patients with VTE provoked by a transient risk factor for longer than 3 months.
- Elevated D-dimer levels, measured 1 month after stopping anticoagulant therapy, predict a higher risk of recurrence in patients with a first episode of unprovoked VTE. However, further studies are needed to determine whether negative D-dimer results justify stopping anticoagulant therapy at 3 months in all or selected subgroups of patients with unprovoked proximal DVT or PE.
- Women appear to have a lower risk of recurrence than men. However, further studies are needed to determine whether this risk is low enough to justify stopping anticoagulant therapy in women with unprovoked proximal DVT or PE who have completed 3 months of treatment.
- The presence of residual DVT on ultrasound may be a marker of a heightened risk of recurrence in patients with unprovoked VTE. However, the strength of this relationship is uncertain, and further studies are needed to determine whether absence of residual DVT on ultrasound justifies stopping anticoagulant therapy in patients who have had an unprovoked proximal DVT.
- The presence of an inferior vena caval filter increases the long-term risk of DVT, decreases the risk of PE, and has no net effect on the risk of recurrent VTE. Consequently, the presence of an inferior vena caval filter need not influence the duration of anticoagulant therapy.
- The risk of anticoagulant-induced bleeding is highest during the first 3 months of treatment and stabilizes after the first year.
- The risk of bleeding differs markedly among patients depending on the prevalence of risk factors such as advanced age (particularly >75 years), previous bleeding or stroke, renal failure, anemia, antiplatelet therapy, malignancy, and poor anticoagulant control.
- The risk of major bleeding in younger patients (<60 years) without risk factors for bleeding who have good anticoagulant control (target INR, 2.0–3.0) is about 1% per year, and in those aged 60 to 75 years it is about 2% per year.

Whether anticoagulant therapy (INR, 2.0 to 3.0) is recommended for 3 months or for an indefinite period (with annual review) depends primarily on the presence of a provoking risk factor for VTE (i.e., major or minor transient risk factor, no risk factor, or cancer), risk factors for bleeding, and patient preference (i.e., burden associated with treatment) (Table 4).

THROMBOLYTIC THERAPY

Systemic thrombolytic therapy (e.g., with tissue plasminogen activator) accelerates the rate of resolution of DVT and PE at the cost of an approximately fourfold increase in frequency of major bleeding, and a 10-fold increase in intracranial bleeding. Such therapy can be lifesaving for those who have PE with hemodynamic compromise, and regimens that are administered over 2 hours or less are recommended in this situation. Systemic thrombolytics may reduce the risk of prothrombotic syndrome after DVT, but this does not appear to justify its associated risks.

Catheter-directed therapy, which uses lower doses of thrombolytic agents and is often combined with mechanical disruption of thrombus and stent insertion if there is residual thrombosis, is expected to

TABLE 4 Duration of Anticoagulant Therapy for Venous Thromboembolism

Categories of VTE	Durations of Treatment (Target INR 2.5, Range 2.0–3.0)
Provoked by a transient risk factor*	3 mo
Unprovoked VTE[†]	Minimum 3 mo, then reassess
First unprovoked proximal DVT or PE; no risk factors for bleeding; good anticoagulant control is achievable; and anticoagulation is not a major burden for the patient	Indefinite therapy with annual review
Isolated distal DVT as a first event	3 mo
Second unprovoked VTE	Indefinite therapy with annual review
Cancer-associated VTE	Indefinite treatment[‡]

*Transient risk factors include surgery, hospitalization, or plaster cast immobilization within 3 mo; estrogen therapy; pregnancy; prolonged travel (>8 hr); and lesser leg injuries or immobilizations occurring more recently (≤6 wk). The greater the provoking reversible risk factor (e.g., recent major surgery), the lower the expected risk of recurrence after stopping anticoagulant therapy.
[†]Absence of a transient risk factor or active cancer.
[‡]Initial treatment with LMWH for at least 3 mo is recommended, followed by long-term treatment with either LMWH or warfarin while cancer is active.
Abbreviations: DVT = deep venous thrombosis; INR = international normalized ratio; LMWH = low-molecular-weight heparin; VTE = venous thromboembolism.

be associated with a lower risk of bleeding but requires further evaluation before it can be widely recommended in patients with extensive proximal DVT.

INFERIOR VENA CAVAL FILTERS

Inferior vena caval filters reduce the risk of PE at the expense of increasing the risk of DVT. Their use is usually confined to patients with acute DVT or PE, or both, who cannot be anticoagulated because of a high risk of bleeding. Removable filters can be used for patients with acute VTE who have a temporary contraindication to anticoagulation. Patients who have an inferior vena caval filter inserted should receive anticoagulant therapy if it becomes safe to do so.

GRADUATED COMPRESSION STOCKINGS

Routine early use of graduated compression stockings for 2 years has been shown to reduce the incidence of the postthrombotic syndrome by about 50% after DVT. The efficacy of routinely wearing graduated stockings compared with selectively using stockings in patients who have persistent leg symptoms or new symptoms during follow-up has not been assessed.

Acknowledgment

Dr. Kearon is supported by the Heart and Stroke Foundation of Ontario and a Canadian Institutes of Health Research Team Grant in Venous Thromboembolism (FRN 7846).

REFERENCES

Anderson FA Jr, Spencer FA. Risk factors for venous thromboembolism. Circulation 2003;107:I-9–I-16.

Bernardi E, Camporese G, Buller HR, et al. Serial 2-point ultrasonography plus D-dimer vs whole-leg color-coded Doppler ultrasonography for diagnosing suspected symptomatic deep vein thrombosis: A randomized controlled trial. JAMA 2008;300:1653–9.

Garcia D, Libby E, Crowther MA. The new oral anticoagulants. Blood 2010;115:15–20.

Geerts WH, Bergqvist D, Pineo GF, et al. Prevention of venous thromboembolism: American College of Chest Physicians evidence-based clinical practice guidelines (8th edition). Chest 2008;133:381S–453S.

Kearon C. Natural history of venous thromboembolism. Circulation 2003;107: I-22–I-30.

Kearon C, Kahn SR, Agnelli G, et al. Antithrombotic thereapy for venous thromboembolic disease: ACCP evidence-based clinical practice guidelines (8th edition). Chest 2008;133:454S–545S.

Stein PD, Fowler SE, Goodman LR, et al. Multidetector computed tomography for acute pulmonary embolism. N Engl J Med 2006;354:2317–27.

Torbicki A, Perrier A, Konstantinides S, et al. Guidelines on the diagnosis and management of acute pulmonary embolism: The Task Force for the Diagnosis and Management of Acute Pulmonary Embolism of the European Society of Cardiology (ESC). Eur Heart J 2008;29:2276–315.

Wells PS, Owen C, Doucette S, et al. Does this patient have deep vein thrombosis? JAMA 2006;295:199–207.

Sarcoidosis

Method of
Marc A. Judson, MD

Sarcoidosis is a multisystem granulomatous disease of unknown cause. The lung is most commonly affected, but any organ may be involved. The clinical presentation of sarcoidosis is variable for two main reasons. First, the manifestations of pulmonary sarcoidosis are variable and can range from an asymptomatic state to significant pulmonary dysfunction. Second, extrapulmonary manifestations of sarcoidosis are common and can cause the prominent symptoms of the disease. This variability in disease presentation often makes the diagnosis of sarcoidosis problematic.

Epidemiology

Sarcoidosis occurs worldwide and affects all races and ages. Although the disease shows a predilection for the third decade of life, a smaller second peak in diagnosis occurs in women older than 50 years. There is a slightly higher disease rate in women at younger ages as well. The highest prevalence of sarcoidosis is found in whites in Scandinavia and in persons of African descent in the United States. In the United States, the lifetime risk of sarcoidosis is 0.85% in whites and 2.4% in African Americans, with an age-adjusted incidence rate of 10.9 per 100,000 persons for the white population and 35.5 per 100,000 persons for African Americans. The relative risk for having sarcoidosis increases significantly if a family member has it as well. In the United States, nearly 20% of African Americans with sarcoidosis have an affected first-degree relative, compared with 5% in whites.

The clinical presentation and severity of sarcoidosis vary among racial and ethnic groups. The disease tends to be more severe in African Americans, whereas whites are more likely to be asymptomatic at presentation. Extrathoracic manifestations are more common in certain populations, such as ocular and cardiac sarcoidosis in Japanese populations, chronic uveitis in African Americans, and erythema nodosum in Europeans. There is increasing evidence that genetic polymorphisms affect the risks and manifestations of the disease. This is consistent with the current theory that sarcoidosis does not have a single cause but is the result of an abnormal host (granulomatous) response to one of many potential antigens in a genetically susceptible person.

Immunopathogenesis

The exact immunopathogenesis of sarcoidosis is unknown, but it is thought to be similar to that of other granulomatous diseases. That is, antigen-presenting cells (APCs), usually either macrophages or dendritic cells, process and present an antigen via a human leukocyte antibody (HLA) class II molecule to T lymphocytes and their receptors. These T lymphocytes are usually of the CD4 T-helper 1 (T_H1) class. The antigen involved in this reaction is unknown, and there may be many antigens that are each associated with a specific HLA class II molecule and T-cell receptor. This could explain the inability to determine one specific cause of sarcoidosis and the varied phenotypic expressions of the disease.

The interaction of APCs and T lymphocytes activates the APCs to produce tumor necrosis factor α (TNF-α), and other cytokines. A proliferation of CD4 T_H1 lymphocytes also ensues that results in the secretion of interferon-γ (IFN-γ), interleukin (IL)-2, IL-12, and other cytokines. These cytokines activate and recruit monocytes and macrophages and transform them into giant cells, which are important building blocks of the granuloma.

The typical sarcoidosis lesion is a noncaseating (non-necrotic) granuloma. The sarcoid granuloma consists of a compact core of macrophage-derived epithelioid and multinucleated giant cells surrounded by a perimeter of monocytes, lymphocytes, and fibroblasts. Granulomas can resolve spontaneously or with therapy; however, they can also persist and lead to peripheral hyalinization and fibrosis. The development of such fibrosis can cause permanent organ damage and in large part determines the prognosis.

Clinical Features and Clinical Course

PULMONARY SARCOIDOSIS

Between 30% and 60% of patients with pulmonary sarcoidosis are asymptomatic, and the disease is detected incidentally on chest x-ray. Some patients present with nonspecific pulmonary symptoms, such as dyspnea, cough, wheezing, and chest pain. Respiratory failure from sarcoidosis is extremely rare at presentation. Unlike in many other interstitial lung diseases, crackles are rarely heard on chest auscultation. Abnormalities on the chest radiograph occur in more than 90% of patients with pulmonary sarcoidosis. Bilateral hilar adenopathy occurs in 50% to 85% at disease presentation, and 25% to 50% have parenchymal infiltrates. Sarcoid granulomas have a predilection for the bronchovascular bundles, subpleural locations, intralobular septa, and the airways.

A radiographic staging system was developed several decades ago (Table 1). Groups of patients with higher radiographic stages have more-severe pulmonary dysfunction, lower remission rates, and greater mortality. However, there is significant overlap among these groups, and predictions concerning individual patients based on stage are highly inaccurate.

Advanced pulmonary stage IV sarcoidosis displays destruction of the lung architecture, with upward traction of the hila, lung distortion, upper-lobe volume loss, fibrocystic disease, honeycombed cysts, and decreased lung volumes. Aspergillomas can develop in these large cystic lesions and may be associated with life-threatening hemoptysis. Bronchiectasis from airway distortion also can occur and is an additional potential cause of hemoptysis.

TABLE 1 Chest Radiograph Stages of Sarcoidosis

Lymph Node Stage	Enlargement	Parenchymal Disease
I	Yes	No
II	Yes	Nonfibrotic
III	No	Nonfibrotic
IV	No or yes	Fibrotic

Adapted from Judson MA, Baughman RP: Sarcoidosis. In Baughman RP, du Bois RM, Lynch JP, Wells AU (eds): Diffuse Lung Disease: A Practical Approach. London, Arnold, 2004, pp 109-129.

The majority of patients with pulmonary sarcoidosis have a vital capacity of greater than 70% of predicted at diagnosis. Pulmonary function and the chest radiographic findings are often discordant. In pulmonary sarcoidosis patients with a normal lung parenchyma (stage I), the vital capacity, diffusing capacity, partial pressure of arterial oxygen (Pao_2) at rest, Pao_2 with exercise, and lung compliance are abnormal in 20% to 40% of cases. Patients with abnormal lung parenchyma have abnormal pulmonary function tests 50% to 70% of the time. Patients with stage IV fibrocystic sarcoidosis tend to have the most severe pulmonary dysfunction.

Sarcoidosis is an interstitial lung disease with a restrictive ventilatory defect often found on spirometry. It is underappreciated, however, that endobronchial involvement is common in sarcoidosis, and therefore airflow obstruction may be the major abnormality found on pulmonary function testing. Wheezing may be the prominent presenting symptom of sarcoidosis, and many cases of sarcoidosis are misdiagnosed as asthma in many patients. Airflow obstruction is also common in chronic pulmonary sarcoidosis, where it is caused by airway distortion from fibrosis. The cause of dyspnea in pulmonary sarcoidosis is multifactorial. It may be the result of abnormalities of gas exchange or lung mechanics, weakness of the respiratory muscles, obesity from corticosteroid therapy, pulmonary hypertension, or sarcoidosis involvement of the heart.

Only 3% to 5% of patients die of sarcoidosis. In the United States, 75% of these deaths are the result of pulmonary involvement. Death from pulmonary involvement is rarely acute but normally is an insidious process that develops over 5 to 25 years with the development of progressive pulmonary fibrosis. Several studies have suggested that pulmonary hypertension is a major risk factor for death from pulmonary sarcoidosis. Patients with aspergillomas and stage IV fibrocystic sarcoidosis are also at risk for death from episodes of life-threatening hemoptysis. Other organs that result in fatalities from sarcoidosis are the heart and the central nervous system. In Japan, death from sarcoidosis is more commonly caused by cardiac than pulmonary involvement.

EXTRAPULMONARY SARCOIDOSIS

Sarcoidosis is a multisystem disease that can affect any organ in the body. The extrapulmonary manifestations of sarcoidosis can predominate in many patients. Extrapulmonary disease can affect the prognosis and treatment options for sarcoidosis.

The eyes and skin are the most common extrapulmonary organs involved with sarcoidosis. Ocular manifestations occur in 25% to 50% of patients; anterior uveitis is the most common manifestation. Symptoms of anterior uveitis include red eyes, painful eyes, and photophobia. However, in one third of patients with anterior uveitis from sarcoidosis, the eye is quiet and without symptoms. In addition, an intermediate or posterior uveitis can cause vision problems or can be asymptomatic. For this reason, all patients with sarcoidosis should undergo an eye examination by an ophthalmologist. Other ocular manifestations of sarcoidosis include conjunctivitis, keratoconjunctivitis sicca (dry eyes), scleritis, and optic neuritis.

Skin lesions in sarcoidosis can be classified into two categories: specific lesions that demonstrate noncaseating granulomas on biopsy and nonspecific lesions that do not. The specific skin lesions are often papular and have a predilection for areas of previous scars and tattoos. Lupus pernio is a type of specific skin lesion causing disfiguring lesions on the face, often with erythema and significant induration. These lesions have a predilection for the nose, cheeks, medial and lateral sides of the eyes, and lateral sides of the mouth. Lupus pernio lesions are relatively recalcitrant to therapy and often respond only partially to corticosteroids. The most common nonspecific skin lesion is erythema nodosum, which is often seen with an acute sarcoidosis presentation of fever, arthritis (especially in the ankles), pulmonary symptoms, and bilateral hilar adenopathy on chest radiograph. This syndrome is known as *Löfgren's syndrome* and tends to have a good long-term prognosis.

Cardiac and neurologic sarcoidosis can be life threatening and are therefore important to recognize. Cardiac involvement is detected clinically in 5% of sarcoidosis patients during life but in 25% at autopsy. Cardiac sarcoidosis can cause left ventricular dysfunction and cardiac arrhythmias, possibly resulting in sudden death. All patients with sarcoidosis are recommended to have a 12-lead electrocardiogram; an abnormal result should prompt further evaluation. The diagnosis of cardiac sarcoidosis is problematic, because the disease is patchy and diagnosed less than 25% of the time by endomyocardial biopsy because of sampling error. Often the diagnosis is made noninvasively, if a typical clinical presentation is coupled with detection of abnormalities on echocardiography, gallium scanning, thallium scanning, cardiac magnetic resonance imaging (MRI), or positron emission tomography (PET).

Clinically apparent neurosarcoidosis occurs in less than 10% of sarcoidosis patients. Palsy of the seventh cranial nerve is the most common manifestation of neurosarcoidosis, and it often predates the diagnosis of the disease. Sarcoidosis can affect any part of the peripheral nervous system and central nervous system and can cause a cranial nerve palsy, mononeuropathy or polyneuropathy, aseptic meningitis, seizures, mass lesions in the brain and spinal cord, and encephalopathy.

Sarcoidosis causes clinically apparent peripheral lymphadenopathy in more than 10% of patients. The spleen may be involved in up to 50% of patients, but it is usually asymptomatic and rarely causes hypersplenism.

Bone involvement is occasional, usually occurring as small cysts or cortical defects found in the small bones of the hands and feet. An acute sarcoid arthritis often is present at disease onset and has a good prognosis. This is commonly found in the ankles of patients who present with Löfgren's syndrome. Chronic sarcoid arthritis is rare. It is usually a nondestructive arthropathy of the shoulders, wrists, knees, ankles, and small joints of the hands and feet.

Sarcoidosis of the sinuses is underappreciated. It can occur in the nasopharynx, hypopharynx, larynx, or any of the sinuses and is known as *sarcoidosis of the upper respiratory tract*. Sarcoidosis of the upper respiratory tract is often relatively recalcitrant to therapy.

Histologic evidence of hepatic sarcoidosis is present in 50% to 80% of sarcoidosis patients, although most of these patients are asymptomatic and have normal liver function tests. Hepatomegaly, abdominal pain, and pruritus are the most common symptoms associated with hepatic sarcoidosis but are present only in 15% to 25% of patients with hepatic involvement. Elevation of the serum alkaline phosphatase is the most common liver function test abnormality.

Hypercalcemia or hypercalciuria leading to nephrolithiasis and renal dysfunction can occur with sarcoidosis. These phenomena are the result of the enzyme 1α-hydroxylase in activated macrophages that convert 25-hydroxyvitamin D to 1,25-dihydroxyvitamin D, the active form of the vitamin. This results in increased gut absorption and increased renal excretion of calcium that can cause nephrolithiasis.

Sarcoidosis rarely involves the thyroid, renal parenchyma, and GI tract.

Patients can have constitutional symptoms such as fever, night sweats, weight loss, malaise, and fatigue at presentation. These symptoms occasionally are associated with hepatic sarcoid involvement but together may be a sign of the systemic nature of the disease, presumably from cytokine release, rather than specific organ involvement. Patients who present with Löfgren's syndrome or with asymptomatic bilateral hilar adenopathy on chest radiograph have a good prognosis. African Americans tend to have a worse prognosis than whites, with lower forced vital capacity and more new organ involvement within 2 years of diagnosis. Box 1 lists risk factors associated with a poor prognosis.

Diagnosis and Initial Work-up

The diagnosis of sarcoidosis requires a compatible clinical picture, histologic demonstration of noncaseating granulomas, and exclusion of other diseases capable of producing a similar histologic and clinical picture. Mycobacterial and fungal diseases always must be considered as alternative diagnoses. Therefore, stains and cultures of tissue specimens for mycobacteria and fungi always should be obtained when the diagnosis of sarcoidosis is considered. Because sarcoidosis is a diagnosis of exclusion (granulomatous inflammation of unknown cause), bear a healthy degree of skepticism in the diagnosis and follow the patient closely for additional clues supporting an alternative diagnosis.

Sarcoidosis is a systemic disease, so the signs or symptoms of extrathoracic disease such as uveitis, skin lesions, or an elevated serum alkaline phosphatase should be sought. The diagnosis in a patient who has granulomas on lung biopsy and interstitial infiltrates without adenopathy on radiographic studies is suspect. In this situation, granulomatous infections and bioaerosol exposure causing hypersensitivity pneumonitis should be strongly considered. Because of the varied clinical presentation of sarcoidosis, there is no single diagnostic algorithm.

It is prudent to select a biopsy site associated with less morbidity, such as the skin if a lesion is present. Transbronchial lung biopsy has a diagnostic yield of 40% to more than 90% in pulmonary sarcoidosis. It is recommended that at least four lung biopsy specimens be collected to maximize the diagnostic yield. Endobronchial biopsy has a 40% to 60% sensitivity and adds to the yield of transbronchial biopsy.

Bronchoalveolar lavage (BAL) with examination of lymphocyte populations has been used in the evaluation of possible pulmonary sarcoidosis. In sarcoidosis, there is an increased number of BAL lymphocytes, and these are predominantly CD4$^+$. It has been proposed that an increase in BAL lymphocytes and a BAL CD4/CD8 ratio greater than 3.5 make the diagnosis of sarcoidosis highly likely.

Although serum angiotensin-converting enzyme (ACE) often is elevated in active sarcoidosis, the specificity and sensitivity of this test are inadequate for it to be used diagnostically. Serum ACE may be used as supportive evidence for the diagnosis, and it also may be used in some instances to follow disease activity.

Gallium-67 (^{67}Ga) scanning is cumbersome because it takes several days to complete and is infrequently used as a diagnostic test. However, bilateral hilar uptake and right paratracheal uptake (lambda sign) coupled with lacrimal and parotid uptake (panda sign) with ^{67}Ga strongly suggest a diagnosis of sarcoidosis.

Gadolinium enhancement on MRI and fluorodeoxyglucose PET scanning may replace ^{67}Ga scanning for detecting sarcoidosis activity because evidence suggests that they may be more sensitive in detecting sarcoidosis activity and they can be performed in one sitting.

Ideally, the diagnosis of sarcoidosis requires demonstration of non-caseating granulomas in at least one organ. However, certain clinical presentations are so specific for the diagnosis of sarcoidosis that the diagnosis may be accepted without tissue biopsy. Extreme caution must be used in these situations to ensure that there is no clinical information that would suggest an alternative diagnosis that should prompt a tissue biopsy. Clinical or laboratory findings that strongly support the diagnosis of sarcoidosis without a tissue biopsy are listed in Box 2.

Treatment

Therapy is not mandated for sarcoidosis because the disease can remit spontaneously. Therapy is indicated for potentially dangerous disease that includes neurosarcoidosis, cardiac sarcoidosis, hypercalcemia that does not respond to dietary measures, ocular sarcoidosis that does not respond to topical (eyedrop) therapy, and other life- or organ-threatening disease. Therapy also should be considered when the disease is progressive. Relative indications for therapy include arthritis that fails to respond to nonsteroidal anti-inflammatory drugs (NSAIDs); a systemic inflammatory response syndrome of fever, night sweats, fatigue, and arthralgias; and symptomatic hepatic disease. In general, treatment is discouraged for asymptomatic elevations of serum liver function tests, specific levels of ACE, or asymptomatic uptake on ^{67}Ga scan (with the possible exceptions of the heart or brain).

The decision to treat sarcoidosis can be problematic, because the disease has a variable prognosis that must be weighed against the potential side effects of therapy. It is often most prudent to monitor patients without therapy if they are asymptomatic or have only mild organ dysfunction. For pulmonary sarcoidosis, asymptomatic patients and those with mild disease that might spontaneously remit usually are not treated. For patients with clinical findings that predict spontaneous remission (e.g., erythema nodosum), the benefits of treatment often are offset by the toxicity of therapy. Often these patients can be managed with palliative therapy such as NSAIDs for arthralgias and fever and bronchodilators and inhaled corticosteroids for wheezing and cough.

It is recommended that patients with mild to moderate pulmonary sarcoidosis be observed for 2 to 6 months, if possible. Patients who improve will have avoided the toxicity of corticosteroids, and patients who deteriorate over this period should be considered for treatment. Patients with pulmonary dysfunction who neither improve nor deteriorate during the observation period may be given a corticosteroid trial, or they may be observed further. Patients with severe pulmonary dysfunction or pulmonary symptoms causing significant impairment should be treated.

CURRENT DIAGNOSIS

- The diagnosis of sarcoidosis is one of exclusion.
- Tissue biopsy, confirming noncaseating granulomatous inflammation, is required in most cases.
- Efforts should be made to search for the least-invasive biopsy site.

CURRENT THERAPY

- Many cases of sarcoidosis do not require treatment.
- All patients should be evaluated for possible pulmonary, eye, and cardiac disease.
- When therapy is indicated, corticosteroids are most commonly used.
- Topical corticosteroids should be given whenever possible.

Corticosteroids often are used to treat sarcoidosis, but the dose, duration of therapy, and method by which one can assess effectiveness have not been standardized. Topical corticosteroid therapy should be used whenever possible in an attempt to minimize systemic complications. This includes corticosteroid eye drops for anterior sarcoid uveitis and corticosteroid creams and injections for localized skin lesions. Pulmonary sarcoidosis usually is treated initially with 20 to 40 mg/day of prednisone or its equivalent. Higher doses may be required for neurosarcoidosis and cardiac sarcoidosis. The patient usually is evaluated within 2 to 12 weeks for a response. Patients failing to respond to therapy within 3 months are unlikely to respond to a more protracted course of therapy or a higher dose. Among the responders, the corticosteroid dose is tapered to 5 to 10 mg/day of a prednisone equivalent or an every-other-day regimen. Treatment is usually continued for 12 months.

The relapse rate after corticosteroid therapy is withdrawn may be as high as 70%, and therefore patients need to be followed closely as the corticosteroid dose is tapered and discontinued. In some patients, there may be recurrent relapses requiring long-term low-dose therapy. On occasion, the chronic prednisone dose needed to prevent relapse is less than 5 mg/day. Patients who relapse after corticosteroids have been withdrawn should be re-treated with corticosteroids. Alternative agents, such as corticosteroid-sparing agents, to control the disease in a patient on a chronic low dose of prednisone should be considered. On occasion, alternative agents may completely replace corticosteroid therapy. In general, corticosteroid-sparing agents should not be considered unless the patient requires more than 7.5 mg/day of prednisone to control the disease.

Methotrexate (Rheumatrex)[1] and hydroxychloroquine (Plaquenil)[1] are the most-studied alternative sarcoidosis medications. They are usually used as corticosteroid-sparing agents but at times can be used as replacement therapy. Methotrexate is most useful for pulmonary, skin, joint, and eye sarcoidosis. Hydroxychloroquine is often used for sarcoidosis of the skin, joints, and nerves and for hypercalcemia from sarcoidosis. Azathioprine (Imuran)[1] may be useful for sarcoid uveitis, but usually it is added to corticosteroid plus methotrexate in this instance. Monocycline (Minocin)[1] and doxycycline (Vibramycin)[1] may be useful for skin sarcoidosis. Cyclophosphamide (Cytoxan)[1] is used occasionally and seems to have a potential role in neurosarcoidosis. Recently anti–TNF-α therapies have shown promise in the treatment of sarcoidosis. Such agents include pentoxifylline (Trental),[1] thalidomide (Thalomid),[1] and monoclonal antibodies against TNF-α, such as infliximab (Remicade)[1] and adalimumab (Humira).[1]

---

[1]Not FDA approved for this indication.

REFERENCES

Baughman RP, Teirstein AS, Judson MA, et al. Clinical characteristics of patients in a case control study of sarcoidosis. Am J Respir Crit Care Med 2001;164:1885–9.

Gibson GJ, Prescott RJ, Muers MF, et al. British Thoracic Society Sarcoidosis study: Effects of long term corticosteroid treatment. Thorax 1996;51:238–47.

Hunninghake GW, Costabel U, Ando M, et al. ATS/ERS/WASOG statement on sarcoidosis. Am J Respir Crit Care Med 1999;160:736–55.

Iannuzzi MC, Rybicki BA, Teirstein AS. Sarcoidosis. N Engl J Med 2007;357:2153–65.

Judson MA. An approach to the treatment of pulmonary sarcoidosis with corticosteroids. Chest 1999;111:623–31.

Judson MA. The diagnosis of sarcoidosis. Clinics Chest Med 2008;29:415–27.

Judson MA, Baughman RP. Sarcoidosis. In: Baughman RP, du Bois RM, Lynch JP, Wells AU, editors. Diffuse Lung Disease: A Practical Approach. London: Arnold; 2004, pp. 109–29.

Judson MA, Baughman RP, Teirstein AS, et al. Defining organ involvement in sarcoidosis: The ACCESS proposed instrument. Sarcoidosis Vasc Diffuse Lung Dis 1999;16:75–86.

Lower EE, Baughman RP. Prolonged use of methotrexate in refractory sarcoidosis. Arch Intern Med 1995;155:846–51.

Lynch JP, Kazerooni EA, Gay SE. Pulmonary sarcoidosis. Clin Chest Med 1997;755–85.

Pneumoconiosis

Method of
Richard D. deShazo, MD, and
David N. Weissman, MD

Pneumoconiosis

The pneumoconioses are a group of interstitial fibrotic lung diseases predominantly associated with occupational exposures. They are caused by inhalation of particulate matter in the respirable size range (0.3–5 μm mean aerodynamic diameter), especially mineral or metallic dusts (Table 1). These agents interact with pulmonary target cells, including alveolar macrophages and alveolar epithelial cells, to activate a cascade of inflammatory mediators including growth factors. Although exposure to these dusts can induce other types of respiratory disease as well, the final common pathway leading to pneumoconiosis is alveolar epithelial cell damage and interstitial fibrosis. This chapter focuses on silicosis and asbestosis, two common forms of pneumoconiosis.

Asbestosis

Asbestos is composed of strong, heat-resistant fibers of hydrated magnesium silicate classified morphologically as serpentine (chrysotile) or amphibole (crocidolite [riebeckite asbestos]), amosite [cummingtonite-grunerite asbestos], anthophyllite asbestos, actinolite asbestos, and tremolite asbestos. In addition, certain asbestiform fibers (winchite, richterite, erionite) can cause adverse health effects identical to those of asbestos. Fiber dimensions and persistence in tissues are key determinants of toxicity. There is a dose–response effect between the quantity of asbestos inhaled and the severity of fibrotic lung disease. Asbestos is also a carcinogen, and increasing exposure is associated with increased risk, particularly for lung cancer and mesothelioma.

Although asbestos is no longer mined in the United States, importation of asbestos-containing products continues. Exposures also continue to occur, especially in construction and renovation (due to reservoirs of asbestos that are still present in many older buildings), the heating trades (where asbestos is often encountered), and with exposure to older or imported asbestos-containing automotive friction products such as brake linings and clutch facings. Workers exposed to asbestos can carry it home on their clothing, resulting in exposure of family members. Living near natural amphibole deposits in California has been implicated as a risk factor for mesothelioma.

The Occupational Safety and Health Administration (OSHA) permissible exposure limit (PEL) for asbestos is 0.1 fiber per cc air. This limit was affected in part by the limits of the analytical methodology used in exposure assessment. Exposure to the PEL every day over a 45-year working lifetime has been estimated to be associated with an increased risk of cancer (lung, mesothelioma, and gastrointestinal) of 336 cases per 100,000 exposed persons and an increased risk of asbestosis of 250 cases per 100,000 exposed persons.

Asbestosis causes symptoms of dyspnea and cough. Latency between initial exposure and disease onset is related to exposure intensity. In the United States, this period is generally about two decades. The disease can lead to chronic respiratory failure. Effects of smoking add to the severity of the disease and can cause obstructive findings in addition to the expected decreased lung volume and diffusion capacity associated with fibrotic lung diseases. Bibasilar rubs and inspiratory crackles on auscultation, finger clubbing, and diffuse, bilateral, small, irregular parenchymal opacities and linear streaking at the lung bases on chest x-ray are characteristic.

The International Labour Organization (ILO) has established a system for classification (grading) of radiographs for the presence

TABLE 1 Representative Pneumoconioses

Source	Clinical Features	Occupation	Dust
Crystalline silica	Silicosis, increased susceptibility to TB, airways obstruction, lung cancer	Mining, stone cutting, pottery, foundry work	Free crystalline silica (SiO_2)
Asbestiform fibers	Asbestosis, bronchogenic carcinoma, mesothelioma, various forms of benign pleural disease	Insulation, shipbuilding, construction, some mining (e.g., vermiculite mining in Libby, Mont)	Various asbestiform fibers
Coal	Coal workers' pneumoconiosis, COPD	Coal mining	Coal mine dust
Hard metal	Hard metal lung disease (cobalt lung), asthma	Machinists, metal workers	Hard metal, composed primarily of tungsten carbide and cobalt

COPD = chronic obstructive pulmonary disease; TB = tuberculosis.

of radiographic abnormalities in lung parenchyma and pleura that are associated with pneumoconiosis, as well as their severity. The ILO classification system is widely used in epidemiology, surveillance, administrative, and legal settings. The small opacity profusion grades of 0/1 and 1/0 are often considered as defining the boundary between normal and abnormal lung parenchyma.

High-resolution computed tomography (CT) is the most sensitive imaging method for suspected asbestosis. It detects a range of parenchymal abnormalities related to the fibrotic process, such as ground glass and honeycombing, and pleural abnormalities, such as pleural plaques and diffuse pleural thickening. The presence of pleural plaques on radiography (particularly bilateral calcified pleural plaques); uncoated asbestos fibers or fibers coated with an iron-rich proteinaceous material (asbestos bodies) in sputum, bronchoalveolar lavage, or lung biopsy; and the slower progression of symptoms help differentiate asbestosis from idiopathic pulmonary fibrosis.

CRITERIA FOR DIAGNOSIS

Diagnosis is supported by radiographic chest imaging or lung biopsy findings of interstitial lung disease compatible with asbestosis; documentation of exposure to asbestos by history, the presence of pleural plaques (bilateral pleural plaques are essentially pathognomonic for asbestos exposure), or the presence of asbestos bodies or an excessive burden of uncoated asbestos fibers in lung biopsy tissue or possibly via bronchoalveolar lavage or sputum; and no other likely explanation for the diffuse fibrotic lung disease.

ASBESTOS-RELATED BENIGN PLEURAL DISEASE

Pleural plaques are characteristic forms of localized parietal pleural thickening that are usually bilateral and asymmetrical, involve the lower lung fields or the diaphragm, and spare the costophrenic angles and apices. Pleural plaques are a marker for exposure to asbestos and are often associated with other asbestos-related conditions. Pleural plaques result in minimal reductions in forced vital capacity and do not degenerate into malignant lesions.

In contrast, *diffuse visceral pleural thickening* can result in adhesions between the visceral and parietal pleura with major decreases in forced vital capacity, respiratory insufficiency, and the requirement for decortication.

CURRENT DIAGNOSIS

- History of inhalation of mineral or metal dust
- Respiratory symptoms such as cough and dyspnea
- Spirometry and lung volumes show restriction in advanced disease
- Interstitial lung disease can usually be demonstrated by chest imaging. Biopsy is usually unnecessary
- No other likely cause of interstitial lung disease is present

Benign pleural effusions can occur in the first decade after asbestos exposure and contain erythrocytes and a mixed inflammatory cell infiltrate of lymphocytes, neutrophils, and eosinophils. The thickened visceral pleura and adjacent atelectatic lung tissue can result in a pleural-based area of *rounded atelectasis,* simulating a lung mass on chest radiography. CT can reveal the comet sign, a pleural band connecting the apparent mass to an area of thickened pleura.

LUNG CANCER AND MALIGNANT MESOTHELIOMA

Exposure to all forms of asbestos increases the risk of lung cancer. The peak risk occurs at about 30 to 35 years after the onset of exposure. Tobacco smoking increases this risk in a multiplicative fashion, increasing the sixfold risk associated with asbestos exposure alone to a relative risk of about 60-fold. In contrast, smoking does not further increase the asbestos-associated risk for *malignant mesothelioma.* Asbestos-associated malignant mesothelioma can also affect the peritoneum (and sometimes the pericardium), but when it affects the pleura, this disease manifests with dyspnea, chest pain, and bloody pleural effusion (most often unilateral). A latency period of 30 years or longer after initial exposure is common. Special immunochemical stains and electron microscopy of pleural fluid or pleural biopsies may be necessary to differentiate mesothelioma from adenocarcinoma. There is no evidence of benefit from surveillance for lung cancer in asbestos-exposed populations.

TREATMENT

Treatment of asbestosis is symptomatic and similar to that for other patients with chronic lung disease (Box 1). Lung transplantation should be considered in the setting of end-stage lung disease. Treatment of benign pleural disease is also symptomatic; as already noted, decortication is sometimes required for managing diffuse visceral pleural thickening. Depending on extent of disease, mesothelioma may be treated with surgery, radiation, chemotherapy, or some combination of these. In general, prognosis is poor. Mesothelioma-associated malignant pleural effusion can require palliation through procedures such as pleurodesis, pleurectomy, and decortication. Asbestos-associated lung cancer is managed in the same fashion as lung cancer occurring without a history of exposure to asbestos.

Silicosis

Silicosis is a fibrosing interstitial lung disease resulting from the inhalation of crystalline silicon dioxide (silica) in dust of respirable size. The commonest form of crystalline silica is quartz, which is the main component of sand and is present in most rocks. Noncrystalline (amorphous) silica, like that in diatomaceous earth or glass, does not cause silicosis. However, heating amorphous silica, as occurs in foundries when molten metal is poured into clay castings, can convert amorphous silica into cristobalite, a hazardous form of crystalline silica. Mining, stone cutting, sandblasting, and foundry work are all examples of trades associated with exposure to respirable dust containing crystalline silica. The International Agency for Research on Cancer (IARC) has designated crystalline silica from occupational sources as a Group 1 human lung carcinogen.

The current OSHA PEL for respirable dusts containing crystalline silica is defined according to specified formulas, including one that is most commonly used:

$$(10 \text{ mg/m}^3)/(\% \text{ SiO}_2 \text{ content} + 2)$$

According to this formula, if a respirable dust contains 100% crystalline silica, the PEL for that dust approximates 0.1 mg/m^3.

A number of studies have suggested that this PEL is not fully protective for exposures over an entire working lifetime. The National Institute for Occupational Safety and Health (NIOSH) recommended exposure limit (REL) for respirable crystalline silica is lower than the PEL, at 0.05 mg/m^3. Reporting of silicosis cases to public health authorities is required in some states.

RADIOGRAPHIC PATTERNS OF SILICOSIS

Three main radiographic patterns of silicosis have been described. Two are nodular interstitial patterns and one is an alveolar-filling pattern. The *simple* pattern is associated with nodules that are smaller than 10 mm and that are predominantly rounded and in the upper lung zones. *Progressive massive fibrosis* (PMF) is found in more advanced interstitial disease. It is associated with multiple coalescent larger nodules, upper lobe fibrosis, upward retraction of the hila, and compensatory hyperinflation of the lower lobes. The large upper-zone opacities can cavitate, sometimes in the setting of superimposed mycobacterial infection. Hilar adenopathy can occur, sometimes with an egg-shell pattern of hilar node calcification. A third radiographic pattern is an alveolar-filling process. Overwhelming silica exposure over a short period can cause a pathologic response called

silicoproteinosis, in which alveoli become flooded with proteinaceous fluid. The condition resembles idiopathic pulmonary alveolar proteinosis. The radiographic alveolar filling pattern favors the lower lung zones and is not associated with the changes of simple silicosis or PMF.

SILICOSIS SYNDROMES

Three syndromes of silicosis can be defined based on clinical course and radiographic pattern. *Chronic silicosis* develops slowly, usually 10 to 30 years after first exposure. It most often has the simple radiographic pattern, but it can be associated with PMF.

Accelerated silicosis develops more rapidly, within 10 years after first exposure. It is associated with higher intensity exposures and can be associated with either the simple or PMF radiographic patterns. Accelerated silicosis is differentiated from chronic silicosis by its more rapid course. Patients with accelerated courses are at greater risk for developing PMF. The clinical presentations of chronic and accelerated silicosis are variable but include cough, dyspnea, and a variety of chest findings ranging from a normal chest examination to crackles, rhonchi, or wheezing. PMF is associated with more severe symptoms and respiratory impairment. Findings compatible with both restrictive and obstructive lung disease (decreased forced vital capacity [FVC], forced expiratory volume at 1 sec [FEV$_1$], FEV$_1$/FVC, diffusion capacity) can occur, potentially leading to cor pulmonale and respiratory failure.

Acute silicosis is associated with very intense exposures to silica, leading to symptoms within a few weeks to a few years after exposure. Intense exposure results in lung injury caused by flooding of alveoli with proteinaceous material, or silicoproteinosis. As already noted, the radiographic appearance is that of an alveolar-filling pattern favoring the lower lung zones. Patients present weeks to a few years after exposure with cough, weight loss, fatigue, and occasional pleuritic chest pain, crackles on auscultation, and progression to respiratory failure often complicated by mycobacterial infection.

CRITERIA FOR DIAGNOSIS

The diagnosis of silicosis is predicated on a history of exposure to respirable crystalline silica, typical chest x-ray findings, and the lack of a more likely diagnosis. There is no consensus on the use of high-resolution CT, and lung biopsy is seldom required for diagnosis.

TREATMENT

Treatment is symptomatic and similar to that for other patients with chronic lung disease (see Box 1). Experimental therapies such as oral corticosteroid therapy and whole-lung lavage have been reported, but clinical benefit is unclear. Lung transplantation should be considered for patients with end-stage lung disease.

All forms of silicosis, as well as substantial exposure to crystalline silica in the absence of silicosis, are associated with an increased risk of pulmonary tuberculosis and fungal infections. Patients should be evaluated for latent tuberculosis infection by tuberculin skin testing with interferon gamma release assay. A positive tuberculin skin test in a patient with a history of substantial silica exposure of at least 10 mm of induration should be considered evidence of tuberculosis infection, regardless of previous immunization with bacille Calmette-Guérin. If testing for latent tuberculosis infection is positive, an evaluation for active tuberculosis should be performed and active disease treated. If active tuberculosis is not present, treat for latent infection. For adults, isoniazid (Nydrazid) 5 mg/kg (300 mg maximum) daily or 15 mg/kg (900 mg maximum) twice weekly for 9 months; or rifampin (Rifadin) 10 mg/kg (600 mg maximum) daily for 4 months are effective regimens. Pediatric doses are isoniazid (Nydrazid) 10–20 mg/kg (300 mg maximum) daily or 20–40 mg/kg (900 mg maximum) twice weekly for 9 months; or rifampin (Rifadin) 10–20 mg/kg (600 mg maximum) daily for 4 months. Directly observed therapy must be used with twice-weekly dosing. Pneumococcal vaccine polyvalent (Pneumovax 23, 0.5 mL intramuscularly every 10 years[3]) and yearly influenza immunization should be provided.

---

[3]Exceeds dosage recommended by the manufacturer.

Disclaimer

REFERENCES

American Thoracic Society. Targeted tuberculin testing and treatment of latent tuberculosis infection. MMWR Recomm Rep 2000;49(RR-6):1–54.

Department of Labor. Mine Safety and Health Administration: 30 CFR Parts 56, 57, and 71. Asbestos exposure limit; proposed rule. Fed Reg 2005;70:43950–89.

Miller A. Radiographic readings for asbestosis: Misuse of science—validation of the ILO classification. Am J Ind Med 2007;50:63–7.

Rimal B, Greenberg AK, Rom WN. Basic pathogenic mechanisms of silicosis: Current understanding. Curr Opin Pulm Med 2005;11:169–73.

Ross MH, Murray J. Occupational respiratory disease in mining. Occup Med 2004;54:304–10.

Weissman DN, Banks DE. Silicosis. In: King TE, Schwarz MI, editors. Interstitial Lung Disease. 4th ed. Hamilton, Ontario: B.C. Decker; 2003. p. 387–402.

World Health Organization. Concise international chemical assessment document 24. Crystalline silica quartz. Stuttgart: Wissenschaftliche Verlags GmbH; 2000.

Hypersensitivity Pneumonitis

Method of
David I. Bernstein, MD, and Haejin Kim, MD

Hypersensitivity pneumonitis, also known as extrinsic allergic alveolitis, is an inflammatory disorder of the lungs that is mediated by immunologic hypersensitivity to a specific antigen, usually organic in nature. Table 1 lists causative agents in hypersensitivity pneumonitis.

Pathophysiology

Hypersensitivity pneumonitis is thought to involve primarily type IV (cell-mediated) hypersensitivity. Bronchoalveolar fluid obtained from patients with hypersensitivity pneumonitis shows a predominant $CD8^+$ lymphocytosis supporting T cell–mediated disease. Viruses are thought to play a role in the development of hypersensitivity pneumonitis through upregulation of costimulatory molecules on alveolar macrophages and dendritic cells, leading to increased activation of type 1 helper T cells. Adoptive transfer models in animals have shown that $CD4^+$ T cells and cytotoxic T cells are the most important effector cells in experimental hypersensitivity pneumonitis, rather than cytokines, antibodies, or complement alone.

CURRENT DIAGNOSIS

- Objective evidence of interstitial lung disease by physical exam, spirometry, and radiography associated with exposure to a causative agent
- Improvement in symptoms, lung function, and radiographic abnormalities with avoidance of the causative agent

TABLE 1 Hypersensitivity Pneumonitis: Representative Sources and Causative Agents

Condition or Persons at Risk	Source	Causative Antigens
Dairy farmers	Hay, grains, silage	Thermophilic actinomycetes
Bird fancier's or pigeon breeder's disease	Avian droppings or feathers	Avian proteins
Humidifier lung	Contaminated water	*Aureobasidium pullulans* or other microorganisms
Chemical workers	Polyurethane foam, varnishes, lacquers	Isocyanates
Machine workers	Metalworking fluid	*Pseudomonas fluorescens, Aspergillus niger, Staphylococcus capitis, Rhodococcus* spp., *Bacillus pumilus*
Familial hypersensitivity pneumonitis	Contaminated wood dust in walls	*Bacillus subtilis*
Hot tub lung	Mold on ceiling	*Cladosporium* spp.

From Richerson HB, Bernstein IL, Fink JN, et al: Guidelines for the clinical evaluation of hypersensitivity pneumonitis: Report of the subcommittee on hypersensitivity pneumonitis. J Allergy Clin Immunol 1989;84:839–844; and Hanak V, Golbin JM, Hartman TE, et al: High-resolution CT findings of parenchymal fibrosis correlate with prognosis in hypersensitivity pneumonitis, Chest 2008;134:133–138.

Clinical Presentation and Diagnosis

The main clinical features for hypersensitivity pneumonitis are listed in Table 2. Hypersensitivity pneumonitis is most likely to be diagnosed if the history, physical findings, and pulmonary function tests indicate interstitial lung disease; the chest film is consistent; exposure is documented to a recognized or new causative agent; and there is significant improvement in symptoms, lung function, and radiographic findings with avoidance of the offending cause. Antibody to the offending antigen may be demonstrated but is not required for diagnosis. These are the most widely accepted criteria, but evidence-based diagnostic guidelines have not been established. A careful home, environmental, and occupational history is essential to identify one or more causative antigens.

Treatment

The primary treatment is cessation of exposure to the sources of offending antigens at home or in the workplace. Effective environmental control measures may include modification of work habits, improvement in ventilation, or change in manufacturing procedures. Systemic corticosteroids are often required and aid in recovery during the acute or subacute phases, but there are no long-term studies of their impact on disease progression or survival rates. Referral to a specialist in occupational lung diseases is recommended for proper diagnosis and identification of the sources of causative antigens.

CURRENT THERAPY

- Avoidance of contact with the offending antigen is essential and is often curative if performed early in the course of the disease.
- Systemic corticosteroids are often required during the acute phase of hypersensitivity pneumonitis.

TABLE 2 Clinical Features of Hypersensitivity Pneumonitis

Feature	Acute	Subacute	Chronic
Exposure to antigen	Hours to days	Days to weeks	Months
Symptoms	Influenza-like illness ± cough/dyspnea	Cough and dyspnea with severe cyanosis	Increasing cough and exertional dyspnea; fatigue, weight loss
Physical findings	Fever; lungs normal or bibasilar crackles	Cyanosis; lungs normal or bibasilar crackles	Cyanosis; right-sided heart failure; lungs normal or bibasilar crackles
High-resolution computed tomography	Diffuse ground-glass infiltrates	Reticulation; small centrilobular nodules; air trapping on expiration	Honeycombing, traction bronchiectasis
Pulmonary function testing	↓ FEV$_1$ and FVC (restrictive pattern); ↓ TLC; ↓ PaO$_2$ on exercise challenge; ↓ D$_{LCO}$		
Other findings supportive of a diagnosis of HP	• Positive natural challenge or increase in signs and symptoms on reexposure • Positive precipitating antibodies to HP antigens or antigens cultured directly from the causative environment • Improvement with avoidance • Surgical lung biopsy: interstitial lymphocytic or plasma cell infiltrates and/or noncaseating granulomas; pulmonary fibrosis in advanced cases • BAL lymphocytosis with reduced CD4/CD8 ratio		

From Richerson HB, Bernstein IL, Fink JN, et al: Guidelines for the clinical evaluation of hypersensitivity pneumonitis: Report of the subcommittee on hypersensitivity pneumonitis. J Allergy Clin Immunol 1989;84:839–844; and Bernstein D, Lummus Z, Santilli G, et al: Machine operator's lung: A hypersensitivity pneumonitis disorder associated with exposure to metalworking fluid aerosols. Chest 2006;108:636–641.

Abbreviations: BAL = bronchoalveolar lavage; D$_{LCO}$ = carbon monoxide diffusion in the lungs; FEV$_1$ = forced expiratory volume in 1 second; FVC = forced vital capacity; HP = hypersensitivity pneumonitis; PaO$_2$ = arterial partial pressure of oxygen; TLC = total lung capacity.

REFERENCES

Bernstein D, Lummus Z, Santilli G, et al. Machine operator's lung: A hypersensitivity pneumonitis disorder associated with exposure to metalworking fluid aerosols. Chest 2006;108:636–41.

Girard M, Lacasse Y, Cormier Y. Hypersensitivity pneumonitis. Allergy 2009;65:322–34.

Hanak V, Golbin JM, Hartman TE, et al. High-resolution CT findings of parenchymal fibrosis correlate with prognosis in hypersensitivity pneumonitis. Chest 2008;134:133–8.

Jacobs RL, Andrews CP, Coalson JJ. Hypersensitivity pneumonitis: Beyond classic occupation disease: Changing concepts of diagnosis and management. Ann Allergy Asthma Immunol 2005;95:115–28.

Lacasse Y, Assayag E, Cormier Y. Myths and controversies in hypersensitivity pneumonitis. Semin Respir Crit Care Med 2008;29:631–42.

Richerson HB, Bernstein IL, Fink JN, et al. Guidelines for the clinical evaluation of hypersensitivity pneumonitis: Report of the subcommittee on hypersensitivity pneumonitis. J Allergy Clin Immunol 1989;84:839–44.

Schuyler M, Gott K, French V. The role of MIP-1alpha in experimental hypersensitivity pneumonitis. Lung 2004;182:135–49.

Tuberculosis and Other Mycobacterial Diseases

Method of
Jotam Pasipanodya, MD; Ronald Hall II, PharmD; and Tawanda Gumbo, MD

Mycobacterial diseases are some of the oldest documented infectious diseases in humans, and they still cause significant morbidity and mortality. *Mycobacterium tuberculosis* complex, *Mycobacterium avium* complex (MAC), and *Mycobacterium leprae* are slow-growing, acid-fast bacilli that belong to the family Mycobacteriaceae of the order Actinomycetales. This chapter deals with management of diseases caused by *M. tuberculosis*, MAC, and *M. leprae*. A summary of diseases caused by other, less common mycobacteria is presented in Table 1.

Recent evidence suggests that the mycobacteria causing tuberculosis (TB) might have co-evolved with humans. Clues attesting to the success of mycobacteria as human pathogens include the prolonged period of latency and the ability to cause extensive disease in only a narrow host range. DNA evidence suggests that the *M. tuberculosis* strains causing the current waves of TB epidemics most likely evolved from a common ancestor. *Mycobacterium canetti* and the other strains that form the *M. tuberculosis* complex (i.e., *Mycobacterium africanum*, *Mycobacterium microti*, and *Mycobacterium bovis* strains) also evolved from the ancestral strain through successive loss of DNA. This is contrary to the belief that the *M. tuberculosis* complex evolved from *M. bovis*.

Tuberculosis

EPIDEMIOLOGY

TB remains a global pandemic, with 9.3 million new cases and 1.4 million deaths reported worldwide in 2007. Approximately 1 of every 7 patients who has TB is co-infected with the human immunodeficiency virus (HIV). Whereas global TB incidence trends are stabilizing after reaching a peak in 2004, rates in countries with a low TB burden have been declining gradually. An explanation could be the similar plateau and declines in HIV prevalence observed in the year 2000. On the other hand, this could merely reflect the natural ebbs and increases inherent to epidemic cycles.

Global estimates show that one third of humankind has been infected with *M. tuberculosis*, the TB disease-causing bacillus. About 80% of global TB is accounted for by the 22 high-burden countries. The top five countries in rank order are India, China, Indonesia, Nigeria, and South Africa. TB program priorities and approaches to combating the disease differ among and within countries. These differences are based on the availability of resources and the prevalence of HIV within communities. For example, program goals in areas of low TB incidence, such as the United States, are aimed at TB elimination. Therefore, in the United States, treatment of latent TB is a priority. Reducing TB transmission through increased diagnosis of patients with active TB disease is the primary goal in high-incidence areas.

In 2007, a total of 13,299 TB cases (case rate, 4.4 per 100,000 population) were reported to the Centers for Disease Control and Prevention (CDC) from the 50 U.S. states and the District of

TABLE 1 Species of Mycobacteria

Microbe	Reservoir	Clinical Manifestation
Always Pathogenic in Humans		
M. tuberculosis	Humans	Pulmonary and disseminated tuberculosis
M. bovis	Cattle, humans	TB-like disease
M. africanum	Humans, monkeys	Rarely, TB-like pulmonary disease
M. leprae	Humans	Leprosy
M. canetti	Humans, possibly others	Rarely, TB-like pulmonary disease
Potentially Pathogenic in Humans		
M. avium complex	Soil, water, birds, swine, cattle, environment	Disseminated and pulmonary TB-like disease
M. microti	Rodents, llamas, cats, ferrets, and possibly humans	Rarely, TB-like pulmonary disease
M. kansasii	Water, cattle	TB-like disease
Uncommon or Rarely Pathogenic in Humans		
M. flavescens	Humans, environment	TB-like disease
M. genavense	Humans, birds	Blood-borne disease with AIDS
M. haemophilum	Unknown	Skin, joint, bone, and pulmonary infections in immunocompromised individuals; lymphadenitis in children
M. malmoense	Environment, possibly others	TB-like pulmonary disease in adults; lymphadenitis in children
M. marinum	Fish, water	Skin infections
M. scrofulaceum	Soil, water	Cervical lymphadenitis
M. simiae	Monkeys, water	TB-like pulmonary disease and disseminated disease with AIDS
M. szulgai	Water, environment	TB-like pulmonary disease
M. ulcerans	Humans, environment	Skin infections (Buruli ulcer)
M. xenopi	Water, birds	TB-like pulmonary disease

Adapted from Coberly JS, Chaisson RE: Tuberculosis. In Nelson KE, Williams CM (eds): Infectious Disease Epidemiology: Theory and Practice, 2nd ed. Boston, Jones and Bartlett, 2007.
Abbreviations: M. = genus Mycobacterium; TB = tuberculosis.

Columbia. Foreign-born persons accounted for 58% of the national case total. This means that a high degree of suspicion is needed for the diagnosis of TB when recent immigrants are seen in the clinic. The top five countries of origin for foreign-born persons with TB in the United States were Mexico, the Philippines, India, Vietnam, and China. Since the 1992 TB resurgence peak, the number of cases reported annually in the United States has decreased by 50%.

NATURAL HISTORY

Susceptibility to *M. tuberculosis* infection and the subsequent progression of that infection to active TB disease is influenced by the complex interaction of host, pathogen, and environmental factors. Between 20% and 30% of people exposed to a person with active TB become infected. Animal models, twin studies, segregation studies, and candidate gene analysis studies provide insight into the role of host genetic factors in susceptibility to TB.

The immune system contains the infection in more than 90% to 95% of persons infected. Protective immunity mediated by subsets of T lymphocytes produces soluble lymphokines that enable macrophages to kill intracellular bacilli. The bacilli are often not completely eradicated and remain dormant in macrophages or other cells, with the potential to reactivate to active disease when the immune system wanes. This is termed latent TB infection (LTBI). The lifetime risk of reactivation to active TB disease is 5% to 10%. This risk of reactivation increases with several factors, including development of the acquired immunodeficiency syndrome (AIDS), renal failure, immunomodulatory therapy, and poorly controlled diabetes mellitus.

In a small subgroup of patients, *M. tuberculosis* infection is not brought under control during primary infection and quickly progresses to disseminated disease. TB that follows such a course is called progressive primary TB. Primary TB is associated with a higher mortality rate, and death typically occurs within 2 years after infection. The risk of developing TB disease after being infected is higher in males from infancy to 6 years of age. Males older than 45 years of age are also at an increased risk compared to females of the same age.

Diagnosis of Active Tuberculosis

In immunocompetent persons, pulmonary involvement is the most common presentation, followed by isolated extrapulmonary disease. Involvement of only extrapulmonary sites is rare, and most immunocompromised patients present with both pulmonary and extrapulmonary involvement. The presenting signs and symptoms of active TB disease are site specific. However, constitutional symptoms such as fever, night sweats, and fatigue are common and gradually evolve over many weeks. Patients should be specifically asked about constitutional symptoms, because these symptoms raise the index of suspicion. Atypical presentations are common in patients who are immunosuppressed and can delay diagnosis.

Definitive diagnosis is made on the basis of a positive culture. Therefore, all patients with suspected TB must have the appropriate specimens collected for microscopic and, if appropriate, histologic examination. Mycobacterial culture and sensitivity testing should also be performed, if available. Acid-fast bacillus (AFB) staining and microscopy is limited by poor sensitivity (45%-80% with culture-confirmed TB cases) and poor positive predictive value (50%-80%) for TB in settings where nontuberculous mycobacteria are commonly isolated. TB culture results are available only after 2 to 6 weeks. Nucleic acid amplification (NAA) testing can also be used to confirm a TB diagnosis in 24 to 48 hours, even when the specimen sample is limited. NAA tests can detect the presence of *M. tuberculosis* in 50% to 80% of AFB-negative and culture-positive specimens. The CDC now recommends that evaluation of at least the first diagnostic specimen include NAA testing.

Serial radiologic images can be used to exclude active TB and assess clinical improvement.

Principles of Treatment

The goal of anti-TB therapy is cure. A secondary objective is minimizing the transmission of *M. tuberculosis* to others by curing the patient. Treatment outcomes are best when patient-centered treatments and care are offered, regardless of whether the treatment facility is private or public. Patient management and supervision plans should be tailored to the patient's clinical and social circumstances. Directly observed therapy (DOT) is recommended by regulatory bodies to help ensure adherence to treatment and is regarded as central to current case management. However, the efficacy of DOT compared with self-administration has been questioned in recent studies. There are three types of anti-TB therapy: prophylaxis, definitive TB therapy for drug-susceptible infection, and therapy for drug-resistant TB.

CHEMOPROPHYLAXIS

The confusing terms preventive therapy and chemoprophylaxis are sometimes used to describe treatment of LTBI. Preventive therapy, in this context, does not actually prevent infection; rather, it prevents development of active TB in those already infected. Therefore, the better descriptive term, treatment of LTBI, is preferred. Treatment of minimal or latent TB infection prevents subsequent evolution to active disease. A series of double-blind, placebo-controlled clinical trials done in the 1950s and 1960s provided evidence demonstrating the effectiveness of treatment of LTBI. Priority is usually given to those patients with the highest risk for reactivation.

Treatment of LTBI, particularly when it is targeted toward persons with higher risks of reactivation, is one of the major strategies for elimination of TB in the United States. Targets include people who have been recently infected and those who were remotely infected but have concurrent disease that puts them at higher risk for developing reactivation disease. There are more than 11 million people with LTBI in the United States, each with a 5% to 10% lifetime risk of developing TB disease.

The Mantoux method of tuberculin skin testing is commonly used to diagnosis LTBI as well as active disease. Use of tuberculin skin testing is hampered by low sensitivity in immunocompromised patients, low specificity in persons who have received the bacille Calmette-Guérin (BCG) vaccine, and the requirement to return to a trained person to have the test read after 48 to 72 hours. Results are interpreted based on the patient scenario (Box 1).

Recently, various blood-testing methods that are based on detection of the interferon-γ (IFN-γ) released by T lymphocytes in response to *M. tuberculosis*–specific antigens have become available as an alternative to skin testing. These tests may be more specific than the tuberculin skin test in BCG-vaccinated and immunocompromised populations. However, IFN-γ release assays do not differentiate LTBI from active TB disease. Currently available IFN-γ release assays are QuantiFERON, QuantiFERON-Gold, and ELISPOT. The CDC recommends these tests for LTBI screening of health care workers, recent immigrants, injection drug users, prison and jail inmates and workers, and contacts of TB cases within schools, workplaces, and the military. Prohibitive costs limit the use of these assays in resource-limited places.

Table 2 summarizes the regimens currently recommended by the American Thoracic Society (ATS), CDC, and Infectious Diseases Society of America (IDSA) for treatment of LTBI. Because of high rates of hospitalization and death from liver injury, the ATS and the CDC no longer recommend the 2-month regimen of daily or twice-weekly rifampin (Rifadin) plus pyrazinamide for LTBI. Rifampin or rifabutin (Mycobutin)[1] may be used to treat LTBI in HIV-infected persons exposed to TB that is resistant to isoniazid (INH; Nydrazid) and susceptible to rifampin, with dose adjustments and diligence taken to prevent cytochrome P-450–derived drug interactions with antiretroviral agents.

DEFINITIVE THERAPY

The decision to initiate therapy is made based on local epidemiologic information; the patient's clinical, pathologic, and radiologic data; and the results of microscopic and culture examination. Therapy may be started immediately if the index of suspicion is high or if the patient is gravely ill. However, in general, clinicians should still collect initial specimens for microscopic evaluation and culture before starting treatment. HIV testing and baseline liver function testing, serum creatinine levels, and platelet counts should be conducted as part of standard medical care for patients with suspected or documented TB disease.

---

[1]Not FDA approved for this indication.

BOX 1 Interpretation of a Tuberculin Skin Test

Reaction ≥5 mm of Induration

HIV-positive persons
Recent contacts of TB case patients
Fibrotic changes on chest radiography consistent with prior TB
Organ transplant recipients and other immunosuppressed patients (receiving the equivalent of ≥15 mg/d of prednisone for 1 mo or longer)*

Reaction ≥10 mm of Induration

Recent immigrants (i.e., ≤5 y) from high-prevalence countries
Injection drug users
Residents and employees[†] of the following high-risk congregate settings:
- Prisons and jails
- Nursing homes and other long-term facilities for the elderly
- Hospitals and other health care facilities
- Residential facilities for patients with AIDS
- Homeless shelters
- Mycobacteriology laboratory personnel

Persons with the following clinical conditions that place them at high risk:
- Silicosis
- Diabetes mellitus
- Chronic renal failure
- Certain hematologic disorders (e.g., leukemias, lymphomas)
- Other specific malignancies (e.g., carcinoma of the head, neck, or lung)
- Weight loss (>10% of ideal body weight)
- Gastrectomy and jejunoileal bypass

Children <4 yr of age; infants, children, and adolescents exposed to adults at high risk

Reaction >15 mm of Induration

Persons with no risk factors for TB

Adapted from Centers for Disease Control and Prevention: Screening for tuberculosis and tuberculosis infection in high-risk populations: Recommendations of the Advisory Council for the Elimination of Tuberculosis. Morb Mortal Wkly Rep MMWR 1995;44(No. RR-11):19–34.
*Risk of TB in patients treated with corticosteroids increases with higher dose and longer duration.
†For persons who are otherwise at low risk and are tested at the start of employment, a reaction of >15 mm induration is considered positive.
Abbreviations: AIDS = acquired immunodeficiency syndrome; HIV = human immunodeficiency syndrome; TB = tuberculosis.

Achieving microbiologic cure by killing all bacilli and preventing emergence of clinically significant drug-resistant mutants are the primary goals of definitive TB therapy. Therapy is prolonged despite sputum conversion and resolution of symptoms, because some organisms persist in some tissues. DOT is generally recommended to ensure compliance with prescribed medications.

The four ATS/CDC/IDSA-recommended regimens used for treating TB caused by drug-susceptible organisms are shown in Table 3. Each regimen has an initial phase of 2 months followed by

TABLE 2 CDC-Recommended Treatment for Latent Tuberculosis Infection

Drug	Interval*	Oral Dose (mg/kg) Children	Oral Dose (mg/kg) Adults	Monitoring
Isoniazid (INH, Nydrazid)	Daily	10–20[3]	5	Monthly, LFTs[†] at baseline, repeat in selected patients if initial results are abnormal; hepatitis risk increases with age and alcohol consumption; pyridoxine[1] 10–25 mg/d may prevent peripheral neuropathy and CNS effects
	Twice weekly	20–40[3]	15	
Rifampin (Rifadin)	Daily	10–20	10	Weeks 2, 4, and 8 with pyrazinamide; contraindicated in patients receiving antiretroviral drugs; baseline LFTs[†] and CBC and platelets
	Twice weekly	—	10	
Rifabutin (Mycobutin)[1]	Daily	—	5	Weeks 2, 4, and 8; baseline LFTs[†] and CBC and platelets; use adjusted daily doses of rifabutin and monitor for decreased antiretroviral activity and rifabutin toxicity if PIs or NNRTIs are taken concurrently; contraindicated with saquinavir (Invirase) or delavirdine (Rescriptor)
	Twice weekly	—	5	
Pyrazinamide[‡]	Daily	—	15–20	Weeks 2, 4, and 8; LFTs[†] at baseline; avoid in first trimester of pregnancy
	Twice weekly	—	50	

Adapted from American Thoracic Society: Treatment of tuberculosis. Am J Respir Crit Care Med 2003;167:603–662.
[1]Not FDA approved for this indication.
[3]Exceeds dosage recommended by the manufacturer.
*All intermittent dosing should be given by directly observed therapy (DOT).
[†]LFTs include aspartate aminotransferase (AST), alanine aminotransferase (ALT), and serum albumin.
[‡]Used with either rifampin or rifabutin in combination therapy for 2–4 mo.
Abbreviations: CBC = complete blood count; CDC = Centers for Disease Control and Prevention; CNS = central nervous system; LFT = liver function test; NNRTI = non-nucleoside reverse transcriptase inhibitor; PI protease inhibitor.

a choice of several options for the continuation phase of 4 or 7 months. Treatment of previously untreated TB consists of 2 months of an initial phase of four drugs: isoniazid, rifampin, pyrazinamide, and ethambutol (Myambutol) or streptomycin (generally not used in the United States). The newer rifamycins are also first-line drugs used under certain circumstances. Rifabutin[1] is used if rifampin is contraindicated, as in patients taking certain antiretroviral drugs; rifapentine (Priftin) is used in the once-weekly continuation phase with isoniazid in selected patients (see Table 3). If the organisms are later demonstrated to be susceptible to isoniazid and rifampin, ethambutol is discontinued. The continuation phase is usually 4 months of daily or intermittent isoniazid and rifampin or rifapentine. The 7-month continuation phase is recommended only for those patients with cavitary TB caused by susceptible organisms that remains sputum positive after 2 months of DOT, patients whose initial treatment phase did not include pyrazinamide, and patients on weekly isoniazid and rifapentine whose sputum smear was still positive at the end of the intensive phase. There is evidence from many clinical trials done worldwide that demonstrates the efficacy of supervised intermittent therapy is similar to daily dosing in terms of various clinical outcomes. Routine follow-up to monitor adverse events and adherence to the treatment regimen should occur at least monthly.

Approximately 80% of patients who take the four-drug therapy for susceptible organisms are expected to convert from culture positive to negative after 2 months, and 90% to 95% after 3 months. Failure of treatment is defined by positive culture or, at times, positive smears after 4 months of supervised therapy. Relapse is defined by recurrent TB at any time after completion of treatment or apparent cure. Relapses most commonly occur during the first 6 to 12 months after the end of therapy. Treatment of initially susceptible disease can fail for many reasons, including extensive cavitary disease, drug resistance, malabsorption of drugs, laboratory error, and biologic variation in response. In any case, positive smears or cultures after 2 months of supervised therapy should be carefully evaluated to determine the cause. In addition, a full course of therapy is determined by the number of doses completed. Hence, a 6-month daily regimen (including both initiation and continuation phases) consists of at least 182 doses of isoniazid and rifampin and 56 doses of pyrazinamide (see Table 3). All missed doses should be taken. Patients interrupting therapy by more than 14 days during the initial phase or more than 3 months during continuation phase should be restarted on therapy from the beginning.

TREATMENT OF TUBERCULOSIS IN RESOURCE-POOR SETTINGS

Direct observation of patients taking therapy is just one of five elements of DOTS recommended by the World Health Organization and the International Union Against Tuberculosis and Lung Disease for TB treatment programs in resource-poor settings. The five elements of DOTS are:

- Government commitment to sustained TB control activities
- Case detection by sputum microscopy in symptomatic patients self-reporting to health centers
- Standardized treatment regimen of 6 to 9 months for at least all confirmed sputum smear-positive cases, with DOT for at least the intensive phase
- Regular, uninterrupted supply of essential anti-TB drugs
- Standardized recording and reporting system that allows for patient and program assessments

Smear microscopy for AFB is emphasized because of cost concerns and because access to culture facilities is limited in most countries. Three AFB stains that include early-morning sputum smears are recommended for a diagnosis. However, some recent data refute the need for three sputum samples by suggesting that no significant benefit is derived from the third smear when performed in high-burden countries.

Susceptibility testing is strongly recommended for patients who fail to convert to smear-negative status after 2 months of treatment. The prevalence of drug resistance in areas of high TB burden is unknown because of limited laboratory capacity.

Individualized TB care in resource-limited areas is difficult to implement because most decisions are made based solely on clinical judgment or limited radiologic findings. These challenges result in the use of standardized treatments that emphasize cost-effectiveness for utilitarian returns. This "one size fits all" approach is likely to worsen the financial and clinical outcomes of some patients.

---

[1]Not FDA approved for this indication.

TABLE 3 Drug Regimen for Culture-Positive Pulmonary Tuberculosis Caused by Drug-Susceptible Organisms

Regimen	Drugs	Interval and Minimum Duration*	Dose (Maximum Dose in 24 h or Maximum Duration)	
			Children	Adults
Initial Phase				
1	Isoniazid (INH, Nydrazid)	Once daily on 7 d/wk for 56 doses (8 wk), or	10–20 mg/kg/d[3] (300 mg)	5 mg/kg/d (300 mg)
	Rifampin (Rifadin)	Once daily on 5 d/wk for 40 doses (8 wk)	10–20 mg/kg/d (600 mg)	10 mg/kg/d (600 mg)
	Pyrazinamide		15–30 mg/kg/d (2000 mg)	15–30 mg/kg/d (2000 mg)
	Ethambutol (Myambutol)		15–25 mg/kg/d	15–25 mg/kg/d
2	Isoniazid	Once daily on 7 d/wk for 14 doses (2 wk), then twice weekly for 12 doses (6 wk), or	20–40 mg/kg/d (900 mg)	15 mg/kg/d (900 mg)
	Rifampin		10–20 mg/kg/d (600 mg)	10 mg/kg/d (900 mg)[3]
	Pyrazinamide	Once daily on 5 d/wk for 10 doses (2 wk), then twice weekly for 12 doses (6 wk)	50–70 mg/kg/d (4000 mg)	50–70 mg/kg/d (4000 mg)
	Ethambutol		50 mg/kg/d[3]	50 mg/kg/d[3]
3	Isoniazid	Three times weekly for 24 doses (8 wk)	20–40 mg/kg/d (900 mg)	15 mg/kg/d (900 mg)
	Rifampin		10–20 mg/kg/d (600 mg)	10 mg/kg/d (900 mg)[3]
	Pyrazinamide		50–70 mg/kg/d (3000 mg)	50–70 mg/kg/d (3000 mg)
	Ethambutol		50 mg/kg/d[3]	50 mg/kg/d[3]
4	Isoniazid	Once daily on 7 d/wk for 56 doses (8 wk), or		
	Rifampin	Once daily on 5 d/wk for 40 doses (8 wk)		
	Ethambutol			
Continuation Phase[†]				
1a	Isoniazid	Once daily on 7 d/wk for 126 doses (18 wk), or	182–130 doses (max. 26 wk)	
	Rifampin	Once daily on 5 d/wk for 90 doses (18 wk)		
1b[‡]	Isoniazid	Twice weekly for 36 doses (18 wk)	92–76 doses (max. 26 wk)	
	Rifampin			
1c[§]	Isoniazid	Once weekly for 18 doses (18 wk)	74–58 doses (max. 26 wk)	
	Rifapentine			
2a[‡]	Isoniazid	Twice weekly for 36 doses (18 wk)	62–58 doses (max. 26 wk)	
	Rifampin			
2b[§]	Isoniazid	Once weekly for 18 doses (18 wk)	44–40 doses (max. 26 wk)	
	Rifapentine (Priftin)			
3a	Isoniazid	Three times weekly for 54 doses (18 wk)	78 doses (max. 26 wk)	
	Rifampin			
4a	Isoniazid	Once daily on 7 d/wk for 217 doses (31 wk), or	273–195 doses (max. 39 wk)	
	Rifampin	Once daily on 5 d/wk for 155 doses (31 wk)		
4b	Isoniazid	Twice weekly for 62 doses (31 wk)	118–102 doses (max. 39 wk)	
	Rifampin			

Adapted from the American Thoracic Society: Treatment of tuberculosis. Am J Respir Crit Care Med 2003;167:603–662.
[3]Exceeds dosage recommended by the manufacturer.
*When directly observed therapy (DOT) is used, drugs may be given on 5 d/wk, with the necessary number of doses adjusted accordingly; therapy administered on 5 d/wk should always be given by DOT.
[†]Patients with cavitation on initial chest radiography and positive cultures at 2 mo should receive a 7-mo (31-wk) regimen of either 217 (daily) or 62 (twice weekly) doses in the continuation phase.
[‡]Not recommended for HIV-infected patients with CD4[+] T-cell count <100 cells/mm[3].
[§]Use only in HIV-negative patients who have negative smears at 2 mo and no cavitation on chest radiography.

TREATMENT OF TUBERCULOSIS IN SPECIAL CIRCUMSTANCES

Multidrug-Resistant Tuberculosis

In resource-poor settings, where susceptibility testing facilities usually are not available, the surrogate terms "retreatment" and "chronic" are used to define various forms of drug-resistant strains. In the United States, about 1.1% of TB cases reported in 2007 had primary multidrug resistance, which is defined as resistance to at least isoniazid and rifampin in a patient with no previous history of TB treatment. Combination therapy including first- and second-line drugs is used to treat multidrug-resistant TB, and at least one of the drugs must be an injectable agent. Some of the second-line TB drugs are levofloxacin (Levaquin),[1] cycloserine (Seromycin), ethionamide (Trecator), p-aminosalicylic-acid (Paser), capreomycin (Capastat), kanamycin (Kantrex),[1] and amikacin (Amikin).[1]

Therapy takes several years to complete. Treatment failure, costs, and drug-related side-effects are higher with the second-line drugs. Patients with suspected treatment failure should be managed at specialized facilities with necessary expertise where the full range of drug susceptibilities can be performed. As a general rule, single drugs should never be added to failing regimens because this leads to acquired resistance to each new drug. Drug resistance in

---

[1]Not FDA approved for this indication.

mycobacteria occurs through random genetic mutations, with minimal lateral transfer of genetic material. Chances of detecting primary resistance are greater when the bacillary load is high, for example in patients with multiple cavitary disease. In addition, selective pressure can induce the emergence of drug-resistant mutants.

Extrapulmonary and Sputum-Negative Tuberculosis

TB can involve any organ or tissue in the body. Therefore, histologic examination or smear microscopy with AFB staining of specimens from appropriate sites is necessary to confirm extrapulmonary TB. The specimens may include cerebrospinal, pleural, pericardial, or ascitic fluids and lymph node tissue, bone, bone marrow, or brain biopsy specimens. The yield of bacilli in staining or culture from body fluids is usually very low (<50% for pericardial fluid). A diagnosis of extrapulmonary TB can also be made based on clinical and radiologic improvement on empiric therapy if it is not possible to obtain a specimen.

The same four drugs and dosing regimens used to treat pulmonary TB are also used for extrapulmonary disease. Use of adjunct corticosteroids in patients with pericardial or meningeal TB was associated with lower mortality in some prospective and retrospective studies. Bone and joint TB is treated for 6 to 9 months, and central nervous system TB (including meningitis) for 9 to 12 months. Duration of treatment for TB in all other sites is 6 months if pyrazinamide is given during the first 2 months; otherwise, the continuation phase is prolonged to 7 months. The ATS/CDC/IDSA guidelines also recommend intermittent therapy. Once-weekly administration of isoniazid and rifapentine should be avoided in the continuation phase, because data to support the efficacy of this regimen in patients with extrapulmonary TB is lacking. However, recent data report poor long-term outcomes despite adequate therapy in patients successfully treated for pericardial and meningeal TB. These and other studies question the wisdom of using the same drug exposures to target organisms in different physiologic spaces, given that drug penetration, and therefore drug concentrations, in these spaces differs.

A diagnosis of sputum-negative TB is made in patients for whom the clinical and radiologic findings strongly suggest TB but the culture and AFB smears are negative. In addition, there is clinical and/or radiologic improvements at the end of 2 months of therapy. A 2-month continuation phase of isoniazid and rifampin is used for these patients, rather than the 4 months used for sputum-positive patients.

Mycobacterium avium Complex Infection

In patients with advanced AIDS and other causes of severe cell-mediated immune deficiency, MAC cause disseminated infections. In others with ill-defined immunologic disorders, and in those who are immunocompetent, MAC causes chronic pulmonary disease. Therapy for these patients is long and complicated, with many adverse effects. The same regimens are used for all patients regardless of their HIV/AIDS status. Drug resistance is frequent.

Culture from blood or other sites (e.g., lymph node, bone marrow) is required to demonstrate invasive or disseminated disease. Bacteriologic diagnosis should be based on positive cultures or smears (or both) from sputum or bronchial wash specimens. If sputum specimens are used to diagnose pulmonary disease, at least three positive sputum smears are needed for diagnosis. Clinical and radiologic findings must also be consistent with MAC.

Combination therapy is used to prevent selection of drug-resistant mutants and to capitalize on the additive and synergistic effects of antimycobacterial drugs. Clarithromycin (Biaxin) or azithromycin (Zithromax) together with ethambutol is now the cornerstone of MAC therapy. Three- or four-drug combinations that included ethambutol, a rifamycin (rifampin[1] or rifabutin), clofazimine (Lamprene),[1] isoniazid,[1] or ciprofloxacin (Cipro)[1] were shown to clear bacteremia better in some AIDS patients, especially those with a bacillary burden of greater than 2 $\log_{10}$ colony-forming units per milliliter. However, adherence to therapy was poor because of toxicity. Two-way interactions between antiretroviral medications (e.g. protease inhibitors, non-nucleoside reverse transcriptase inhibitors) and the rifamycins as well as clarithromycin and rifabutin can make patient management complicated. AIDS patients with CD4-positive T-cell counts lower than 50 cells/mm³ should be offered prophylactic therapy to protect against disseminated MAC. Azithromycin has greater efficacy, has fewer drug interactions, and can be given once weekly. Resistance has been observed in 16% of patients treated with azithromycin and in 29% to 58% of those treated with clarithromycin. Resistance of MAC to rifamycin is rare.

Mycobacterium leprae

Leprosy is a legendary disease that has been stigmatized throughout many societies and eras of human history. The causative organism is M. leprae. The global incidence of this disease has been on the decline. Fewer than 200 cases are diagnosed each year in the United States, almost exclusively in immigrants. Most practitioners in the United States will not encounter patients with this disease.

The important clinical features of leprosy are skin lesions, nerve involvement, disfigurement of the face, and reversal reactions. Skin lesions are hypopigmented anesthetic macules and papules. Peripheral nerve enlargement can also occur, as can disfigurement of parts of the face (e.g., leonine faces). Leprosy has a spectrum of manifestations. Some patients have multibacillary leprosy associated with poor cell-mediated immunity. Others have paucibacillary leprosy resulting in a few skin patches with a robust cell-mediated immunity. Skin reactions encountered in paucibacillary leprosy due to delayed hypersensitivity to M. leprae antigens are called reversal reactions. These may also occur when massive numbers of bacilli are killed by chemotherapy.

Diagnosis is established on the basis of a compatible clinical picture and demonstration of M. leprae in smears or on histologic analysis of skin and nerve biopsy specimens. The lepromin skin test is nonreactive in multibacillary disease but reactive in paucibacillary disease. Unlike other mycobacteria, M. leprae has stringent growth requirements; it can only grow when injected into foot pads of some animals and does not grow on artificial laboratory media.

The aim of leprosy treatment is total cure. As with other slow-growing mycobacteria, multidrug therapy is administered. Therapy consists of rifampin,[1] clofazimine (Lamprene), and dapsone. Recently, fluoroquinolones have been investigated for a role in the treatment of leprosy. In the United States, the therapy for paucibacillary leprosy is oral rifampin 600 mg/day and dapsone 100 mg/day for 6 months, followed by dapsone monotherapy for at least 3 years. The treatment of multibacillary leprosy is similar to that of paucibacillary leprosy, with dual therapy being continued for 3 years. Clofazimine is added for reverse reactions and if there is dapsone resistance. After 3 years of dual or even triple therapy, dapsone monotherapy is continued for 10 years. These regimens differ from those recommended by the World Health Organization, which are utilized elsewhere.

Mycobacteria Other Than Tuberculosis

Mycobacteria other than tuberculosis (MOTT) are mycobacterial species that may cause human disease but do not cause TB (see Table 1). The incidence of infection is reported to be about 2 in 100,000, but this may be an underestimate. The common mycobacteria identified in the United States are M. avium, Mycobacterium gordonae, Mycobacterium fortuitum, Mycobacterium kansasii, and Mycobacterium chelonae. MOTT infections are not contagious, but some produce signs and symptoms similar to those of TB, whereas others cause suppurative-like disease. MOTT primarily affect the lungs, and disease progression is slow. MOTT cause reportable disease.

---

[1]Not FDA approved for this indication.

[1]Not FDA approved for this indication.

Diagnosis is based on clinical presentation, radiologic findings, examination of histologic specimens, culture, and smear staining for microscopy of sputa or bronchial washings. The diagnostic criteria for MOTT in AIDS and non-AIDS patients are

- Chest radiographs showing infiltrates or nodular or cavitary disease or computed tomographic scans consistent with bronchiectasis or small nodules
- Three positive cultures with negative AFB smears or two positive cultures and one positive AFB smear from three sputum or bronchial washing specimens obtained within the previous 12 months
- Positive culture from bronchial wash with AFB smear or growth on solid media greater than 2+
- Transbronchial or lung biopsy consistent with mycobacterium histologic features and sputum or bronchial washings that are non-diagnostic of another disease.
- For mycobacteria other than tuberculosis such as *M. abscessus/chelonae* therapy is more with standard antibiotics like ceftriaxone. However, all these patients should be reported to specialist centers.

REFERENCES

Agins BD, Berman DS, Spicehandler D, et al. Effect of combined therapy with ansamycin, clofazimine, ethambutol, and isoniazid for *Mycobacterium avium* infection in patients with AIDS. J Infect Dis 1989;159:784–7.

American Thoracic Society, Centers for Disease Control and Prevention, Council of the Infectious Diseases Society of America. Diagnostic standards and classification of tuberculosis in adults and children. Am J Respir Crit Care Med 2000;161:1376–95.

Bach MC. Treating disseminated *Mycobacterium avium-intracellulare* infection. Ann Intern Med 1989;110:169–70.

Bellamy R, Beyers N, McAdam KP, et al. Genetic susceptibility to tuberculosis in Africans: A genome-wide scan. Proc Natl Acad Sci U S A 2000; 97:8005–9.

Blumberg HM, Burman WJ, Chaisson RE, et al. American Thoracic Society/Centers for Disease Control and Prevention/Infectious Diseases Society of America: Treatment of tuberculosis. Am J Respir Crit Care Med 2003;167:603–62.

Brosch R, Gordon SV, Marmiesse M, et al. A new evolutionary scenario for the *Mycobacterium tuberculosis* complex. Proc Natl Acad Sci U S A 2002; 99:3684–9.

Cegielski JP, Devlin BH, Morris AJ, et al. Comparison of PCR, culture, and histopathology for diagnosis of tuberculous pericarditis. J Clin Microbiol 1997;35:3254–7.

Centers for Disease Control and Prevention. Reported Tuberculosis in the United States, 2007. Atlanta: U.S. Department of Health and Human Services, CDC; 2007.

Comstock GW. Frost revisited: The modern epidemiology of tuberculosis. Am J Epidemiol 1975;101:363–82.

Comstock GW. Tuberculosis in twins: A re-analysis of the Prophit survey. Am Rev Respir Dis 1978;117:621–4.

Comstock GW, Livesay VT, Woolpert SF. Evaluation of BCG vaccination among Puerto Rican children. Am J Public Health 1974;64:283–91.

Dannenberg AM Jr. Delayed-type hypersensitivity and cell-mediated immunity in the pathogenesis of tuberculosis. Immunol Today 1991;12:228–33.

Engel ME, Matchaba PT, Volmink J. Corticosteroids for tuberculous pleurisy. Cochrane Database Syst Rev 2007;(4) CD001876.

Guerra RL, Hooper NM, Baker JF, et al. Use of the amplified *Mycobacterium tuberculosis* direct test in a public health laboratory: Test performance and impact on clinical care. Chest 2007;132:946–51.

Guerra RL, Hooper NM, Baker JF, et al. Cost-effectiveness of different strategies for amplified *Mycobacterium tuberculosis* direct testing for cases of pulmonary tuberculosis. J Clin Microbiol 2008;46:3811–2.

Gumbo T, Louie A, Deziel MR, et al. Concentration-dependent *Mycobacterium tuberculosis* killing and prevention of resistance by rifampin. Antimicrob Agents Chemother 2007;51:3781–8.

Gumbo T, Louie A, Liu W, et al. Isoniazid bactericidal activity and resistance emergence: Integrating pharmacodynamics and pharmacogenomics to predict efficacy in different ethnic populations. Antimicrob Agents Chemother 2007;51:2329–36.

Haas CJ, Zink A, Palfi G, et al. Detection of leprosy in ancient human skeletal remains by molecular identification of *Mycobacterium leprae*. Am J Clin Pathol 2000;114:428–36.

Iseman MD. A Clinician's Guide to Tuberculosis. Philadelphia: Lippincott Williams & Wilkins; 2000.

Kallmann FJ, Reisner D. Twin studies on the significance of genetic factors in tuberculosis. Am Rev Tuberculosis 1943;47:549–74.

Kramnik I, Demant P, Bloom BB. Susceptibility to tuberculosis as a complex genetic trait: Analysis using recombinant congenic strains of mice. Novartis Found Symp 1998;217:120–31.

Kramnik I, Dietrich WF, Demant P, Bloom BR. Genetic control of resistance to experimental infection with virulent *Mycobacterium tuberculosis*. Proc Natl Acad Sci U S A 2000;97:8560–5.

Mabaera B, Lauritsen JM, Katamba A, et al. Sputum smear-positive tuberculosis: Empiric evidence challenges the need for confirmatory smears. Int J Tuberc Lung Dis 2007;11:959–64.

Mabaera B, Lauritsen JM, Katamba A, et al. Making pragmatic sense of data in the tuberculosis laboratory register. Int J Tuberc Lung Dis 2008; 12:294–300.

Mayosi BM, Wiysonge CS, Ntsekhe M, et al. Clinical characteristics and initial management of patients with tuberculous pericarditis in the HIV era: The Investigation of the Management of Pericarditis in Africa (IMPI Africa) registry. BMC Infect Dis 2006;6:2.

Mayosi BM, Wiysonge CS, Ntsekhe M, et al. Mortality in patients treated for tuberculous pericarditis in sub-Saharan Africa. S Afr Med J 2008;98:36–40.

Moonan PK, Weis SE. Assessing the impact of targeted tuberculosis interventions. Am J Respir Crit Care Med 2008;177:557–8.

Moore DF, Guzman JA, Mikhail LT. Reduction in turnaround time for laboratory diagnosis of pulmonary tuberculosis by routine use of a nucleic acid amplification test. Diagn Microbiol Infect Dis 2005;52:247–54.

Nerlich AG, Haas CJ, Zink A, et al. Molecular evidence for tuberculosis in an ancient Egyptian mummy. Lancet 1997;350:1404.

Nuermberger E, Grosset J. Pharmacokinetic and pharmacodynamic issues in the treatment of mycobacterial infections. Eur J Clin Microbiol Infect Dis 2004;23:243–55.

Prasad K, Singh MB. Corticosteroids for managing tuberculous meningitis. Cochrane Database Syst Rev 2000;(1) CD002244.

Stein CM, Nshuti L, Chiunda AB, et al. Evidence for a major gene influence on tumor necrosis factor-alpha expression in tuberculosis: Path and segregation analysis. Hum Hered 2005;60:109–18.

Stein CM, Zalwango S, Malone LL, et al. Genome scan of *M. tuberculosis* infection and disease in Ugandans. PLoS ONE 2008;3:e4094.

Volmink J, Garner P. Directly observed therapy for treating tuberculosis. Cochrane Database Syst Rev 2007;(4) CD003343.

Weis SE, Miller TL, Hilsenrath PE, Moonan PK. Comprehensive cost description of tuberculosis care. Int J Tuberc Lung Dis 2005;9:467–8.

World Health Organisation. Global leprosy situation. Wkly Epidemiol Rec 2005;80:289–95.

World Health Organization. Global Tuberculosis Control: Epidemiology, Strategy, Financing: WHO Report 2009. Geneva: WHO; 2009.

Zink A, Haas CJ, Reischl U, et al. Molecular analysis of skeletal tuberculosis in an ancient Egyptian population. J Med Microbiol 2001;50:355–66.

The Cardiovascular System

Acquired Diseases of the Aorta

Method of
David G. Neschis, MD

Abdominal Aortic Aneurysms

EPIDEMIOLOGY

A ruptured abdominal aortic aneurysm is a devastating event leading to approximately 15,000 deaths per year, and it is the 13th leading cause of death in the United States. It is the 10th leading cause of death in men. Once rupture occurs, there is an 85% chance of death overall and approximately 50% mortality in the patients who make it to the hospital alive. Clearly, the goal is to identify this life-threatening lesion and repair prior to rupture. Abdominal aortic aneurysms are approximately four times more prevalent in men than women. The overall incidence in persons older than 60 years is approximately 3% to 4%, with incidence as high as 10% to 12% in an elderly hypertensive population.

RISK FACTORS

Men are approximately 4 times more likely than women to develop an abdominal aortic aneurysm. Clearly, older persons, particularly those older than 60 years, are higher risk. Tobacco use is probably the strongest preventable risk factor, with tobacco users being approximately eight times more likely to be affected than nonsmokers. Hypertension is present in approximately 40% of patients with abdominal aortic aneurysms. Family history also plays a significant role. In fact, men who have first-degree female relatives who had aneurysms are approximately 18 times more likely than the general population to develop an abdominal aortic aneurysm. There is also a strong correlation between abdominal aortic aneurysms and other peripheral artery aneurysms. Patients with bilateral popliteal artery aneurysms have an approximately 50% to 60% risk of having an abdominal aortic aneurysm.

PATHOPHYSIOLOGY

An aneurysm is a dilatation of a blood vessel that could occur in any blood vessel in the body, even in the veins. Most commonly it is defined as a dilatation of approximately 1.5 to 2 times at that diameter of the adjacent normal vessel.

The definition of a pseudoaneurysm is often misunderstood. The attempt to describe a pseudoaneurysm in terms of the number of layers of the artery wall involved does nothing to help resolve this confusion. A pseudoaneurysm is a walled-off defect in the artery wall. A circular shell of adventitial and surrounding connective tissue contains the blood, preventing free hemorrhage. However, there remains continued flow out and back into the artery lumen, resulting in a classic to-and-fro pattern on duplex ultrasound. The most common cause of a pseudoaneurysm is iatrogenic: from needle puncture, but also can be caused by trauma or focal rupture of the artery at the site of an atherosclerotic ulcer.

The etiology of true aneurysms is not clear, although in the past these have been attributed to atherosclerosis. However, it is well known that the majority of patients with abdominal aortic aneurysms do not have associated significant occlusive disease. Biochemical studies have demonstrated decreased quantities of elastin and collagen in the walls of aneurysmal aortas. It is believed that a family of enzymes known as matrix metalloproteinase (MMP), particularly those that have collagenase and elastase activity, are likely involved in development of arterial aneurysms. The propensity for growth and rupture is based on Laplace's law, $T = PR$, where T represents wall tension (or in other words the propensity to rupture), P is the transmitted pressure, and R is the radius. This explains why patients with hypertension and those with larger aneurysms are at higher risk for aortic rupture.

PREVENTION

Currently the most effective means to prevent aneurysm rupture is early detection and elective repair. Avoidance of smoking and aggressive control of blood pressure would likely be helpful in preventing aneurysmal development and growth. Patients with known abdominal aortic aneurysms that are relatively small and at low risk for rupture are generally serially followed with imaging studies over time. These patients are advised to avoid straining (e.g., heavy lifting), avoid smoking, and keep their blood pressure well controlled.

Investigation is ongoing in efforts to develop a medication that may be helpful in slowing the growth of abdominal aortic aneurysms. It has been known since 1985 that tetracycline antibiotics have activity against MMPs. There had been several animal studies and at least one small human study suggesting that doxycycline (Vibramycin)[1] may be effective at slowing the growth of abdominal aortic aneurysms. Currently, larger human studies are ongoing. At this point, there are no formal recommendations regarding the use of doxycycline for the purpose of slowing aneurysmal growth.

CLINICAL MANIFESTATIONS

Approximately 75% of abdominal aortic aneurysms are asymptomatic and discovered incidentally. Unfortunately, physical examination is an unreliable method for detecting aneurysms or determining

---

[1]Not FDA approved for this indication.

aneurysm size. In heavier patients it may be simply impossible to adequately palpate the aorta. The majority of aneurysms are incidental findings identified on imaging studies performed for other reasons. Occasionally, an aneurysm is first detected upon operation for another condition.

Unfortunately, when an aneurysm becomes symptomatic, this is usually a sign of impending rupture. Symptoms related to abdominal aortic aneurysms can include abdominal or back pain. The classic triad of findings in the setting of abdominal aortic aneurysm rupture includes abdominal pain, hypotension, and a pulsatile abdominal mass. This triad, however, occurs in only approximately 20% of the patients. Often a high index of suspicion needs to be maintained.

The episode of hypotension associated with aneurysm rupture may be manifested as an episode of syncope or near-syncope before the patient arrives at the hospital. It is quite possible for the patient to have a contained rupture of the abdominal aorta and appear quite stable with a normal blood pressure in the emergency department. Although uncommon, a primary fistula between the aneurysm and gastrointestinal tract can occur and manifest as gastrointestinal bleeding.

DIAGNOSIS

Several imaging modalities are available that can accurately diagnose and measure abdominal aortic aneurysms. Real-time B-mode ultrasound has the advantage of being almost universally available, relatively inexpensive, and essentially risk free. The major disadvantage, however, is that it is technician dependent. Computed tomography (CT) scans can provide a very accurate representation of the aorta in a very short study time (Figs. 1 and 2). The use of iodinated contrast is not necessary to obtain a gross size measurement of the aorta. The contrast, however, helps delineate the flow lumen more clearly, and it is quite valuable in planning repair. Disadvantages include the use of ionizing radiation and the use of iodinated contrast material. MRI is also accurate in determining the size of the aneurysm; however, study times are longer, equipment is less widely available, and the expense is considerable. Angiography, while excellent for evaluating the status of important aortic branches and for evaluating occlusive disease, is not an accurate study for the purpose of determining maximal diameter of the aneurysm. Often aneurysms are filled with laminated thrombus, and the flow lumen, which was seen on aortography, is not representative of the true aneurysm size.

 CURRENT DIAGNOSIS

- Because the majority of patients with abdominal aortic aneurysms are asymptomatic, the majority of abdominal aortic aneurysms are detected on imaging studies performed for other indications.
- Patients older than 50 years who present with abdominal or back pain of unclear etiology should be considered for evaluation of possible abdominal aortic aneurysm.
- Asymptomatic men older than 65 years who have ever smoked are eligible for abdominal aortic aneurysms screening.
- All patients older than 60 years who have a strong family history of abdominal aortic aneurysms should be considered for screening.
- Patients presenting with sudden onset of chest or back pain without clear etiology should be evaluated for dissection.
- Dissection can mimic numerous other conditions.

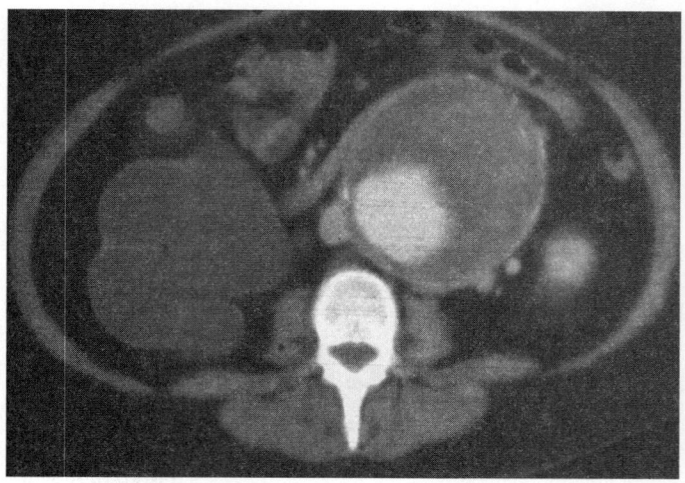

FIGURE 1. Large abdominal aortic aneurysm. Notice how the majority of this aneurysm is filled with laminated thrombus. The flow lumen is only mildly dilated, and this aneurysm could be missed on angiography alone.

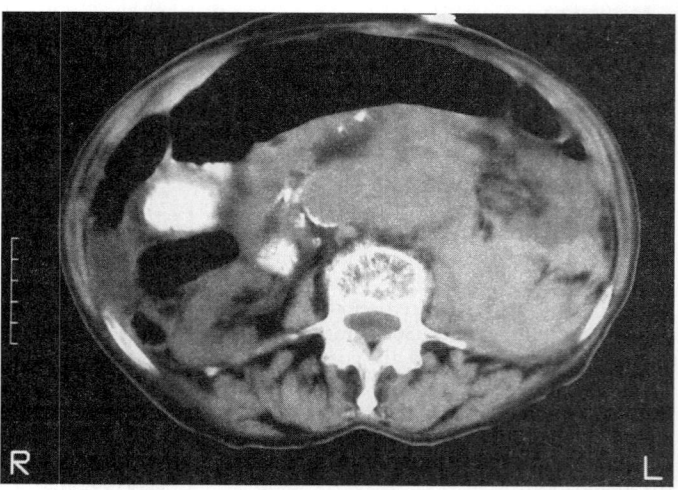

FIGURE 2. Classic image of a ruptured abdominal aortic aneurysm, which in this case can be seen even without the use of intravascular contrast. Note the lack of symmetry and obliteration of tissue planes in the retroperitoneum on the left.

TREATMENT

The decision on when to intervene in an abdominal aortic aneurysm is based on a careful analysis of the patient's risk for rupture verses the risk of operative repair. Historically open repair can be performed with less than 5% in-hospital mortality. Based on historical studies it was estimated that the risk of rupture for an approximately 5-cm aneurysm was about 1% per year, which increased dramatically to 6.6% for aneurysms between 6 cm and 7 cm. It has been fairly well established for years that aneurysms larger than 5.5 cm are generally recommended for repair and those less than 4 cm are generally observed over time. There remained a gray area for moderate aneurysms in the 4 to 5.5 cm category.

Two large prospective randomized trials were developed to answer this question. These include the United Kingdom Small Aneurysm Trial and the Department of Veterans Affairs Aneurysm Detection and Management (ADAM) trial. Both these studies randomized patients with moderately sized aneurysms to observation versus open repair. Results of both trials were fairly similar. The rupture rate for

CURRENT THERAPY

Indications for Repair of Aneurysm

- Fusiform abdominal aortic aneurysms greater than 5.5 cm in maximum diameter
- Most saccular aneurysms and pseudoaneurysms
- Thoracic and thoracoabdominal aortic aneurysms of greater than 6 cm in maximal diameter
- Aneurysms that are symptomatic or are rapidly enlarging.

Indications for Repair of Aortic Dissection

- Dissections involving the ascending aorta
- Dissections involving only the descending aorta are usually managed medically unless complicated by the following: unrelenting pain, end organ ischemia, or significant aneurysmal degeneration to greater than 6 cm in maximal diameter.

aneurysms under observation was 0.5% to 1% per year, and neither trial showed a difference in long-term survival. Both studies concluded that it was relatively safe to observe patients with aneurysms less than 5.5 cm to 6 cm in diameter, particularly in men who would be compliant with the follow-up regimen. The diameter of the aneurysm, however, should not be the only data point used for a decision on whether to repair.

Women seem to have a higher rupture rate for a particular aneurysm diameter than men, perhaps because they are starting with smaller aortas to begin with. Patients with COPD may be at higher risk for rupture as well. Saccular or eccentric-shaped aneurysms may also have a higher propensity to rupture and should not be subject to diameter recommendations for fusiform aneurysms (Figs. 3 and 4). Additionally, rapidly growing aneurysms—growing at a rate faster than approximately 0.5 cm per year—should be considered for repair.

Once it was determined that repair is indicated, a number of options are available. Traditional open repair involves a relatively large abdominal incision, cross clamping of the aorta, and replacement of the aneurysmal segment with a graft of polyethylene terephthalate (Dacron) or polytetrafluoroethylene (PTFE; Teflon). Often the iliac arteries are involved, and in these cases a bifurcated graft is placed. Open repair is quite durable and very effective at preventing aneurysm-related deaths. Long-term complications are rare, and patients following open repair generally enjoy 95% freedom from issues related to the repair over the course of their lifetime. Disadvantages, however, include the large incision and an approximate 1-week hospital stay. Recovery to a relatively normal level of function occasionally takes months. In the past, many patients were deemed too old or frail to be expected to undergo open surgery.

Endograft repair has revolutionized the practice of vascular surgery. Using small incisions placed at the groins and performing the procedure under fluoroscopy guidance, devices can now be advanced into the aorta from the femoral artery. Using angiography as a guide, the graft is deployed typically below the renal arteries and effectively excludes the aneurysm from the circulation. Advantages include small incisions and very short hospital stays. Patients are typically discharged on the first or second day following aneurysm repair. Recovery to normal activity is also quite rapid, taking approximately 1 to 2 weeks. Use of this modality has allowed treatment of older and frailer patients who previously denied treatment due to concerns of operative risk.

Endograft repair, however, is clearly not without its disadvantages. Currently, the durability of endograft repair is unknown, and these patients are subject to frequent serial imaging. Also there is a higher incidence of graft-related complications, which can occur in up to

305

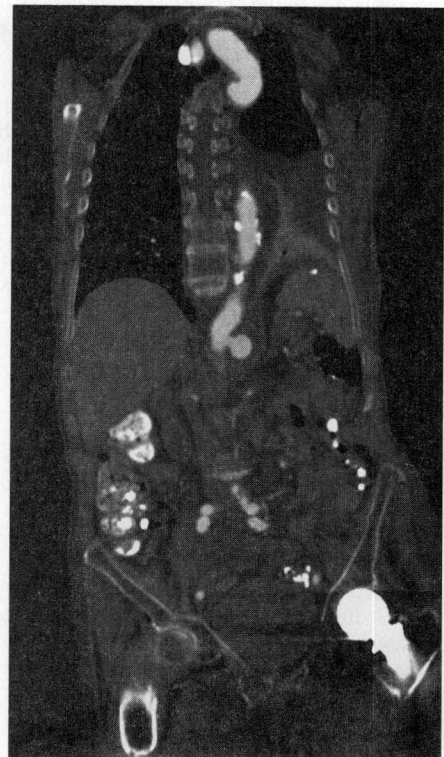

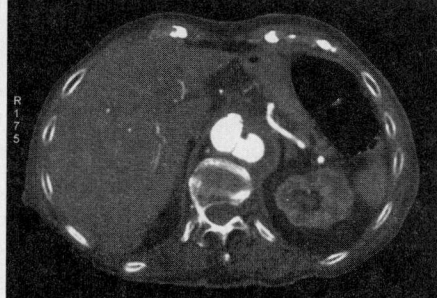

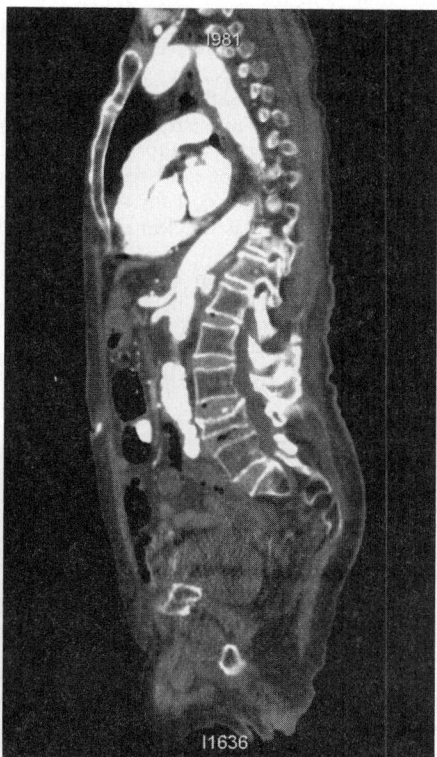

FIGURE 3. Axial CT slice and reconstructed images of a saccular abdominal aortic aneurysm. This lesion could also be described as a pseudoaneurysm. For these, treatment is recommended because it is believed the risk of rupture is higher than for a similarly sized fusiform abdominal aortic aneurysm. I would not recommend following this type of lesion, waiting for it to reach >5 cm in diameter.

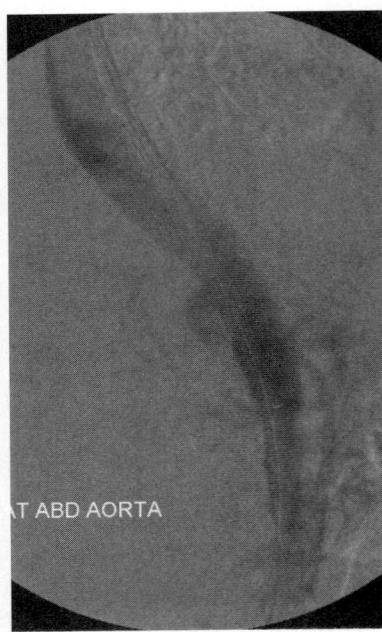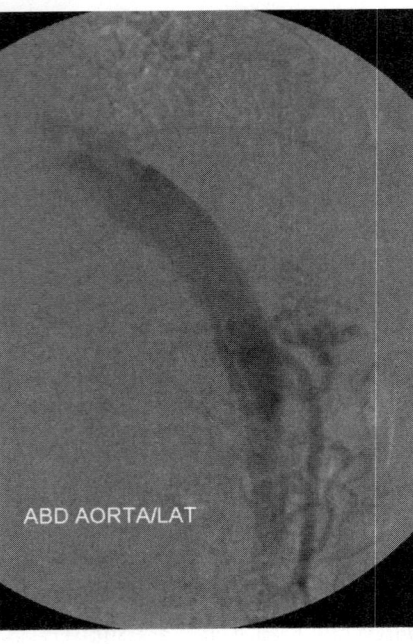

LAT ABD AORTA

ABD AORTA/LAT

FIGURE 4. Angiogram of patient in Figure 3, demonstrating aneurysm before and after deployment of an endograft, which successfully excluded the lesion from the circulation.

35% of the patients. These include the development of leaks of blood into the aneurysm sac outside the graft device, issues related to graft failure and migration, and graft limb thrombosis. These grafts are also quite expensive.

Two major prospective randomized trials studying traditional open versus endograft repair are often cited. These include the United Kingdom–based EVAR-1 trial (first Endovascular Aneurysm Repair trail) and the Dutch-based DREAM trial (Diabetes REduction Assessment with ramipril and rosiglitazone Medication trial). Both these studies randomized patients who were believed to be good risk for open repair to endograft versus traditional open repair. The results of both of these studies were relatively similar in that both studies demonstrated a clear early survival benefit for patients in the endograft group. However, this came at a cost of an increased incidence of graft-related complications in the endograft group and a higher cost for the endograft group. Additionally, at 2 to 4 years, there was no clear difference in long-term survival in either group.

Ultimately, the decision on whether to proceed with open or endograft repair is decision between surgeon and patient based on the patient's aortic anatomy, overall health, and the patient's and physician's preference. It would appear, however, that older and frail patients with good anatomy should be strongly considered for endograft repair.

MONITORING

Patients with abdominal aortic aneurysms should be evaluated for the presence of femoral and popliteal aneurysms (particularly in men) and for thoracic aortic aneurysms. Following open repair, a follow-up CT scan with contrast should be considered in approximately 5 years out to evaluate for the integrity of the graft and for the absence of pseudoaneurysms. Patients who have undergone endograft repair require more-intensive monitoring. Typical regimens include a contrast-enhanced CT scan approximately 2 weeks following repair, then 6 months after repair, and then based on the perceived stability of the graft approximately yearly thereafter. Some centers have used duplex ultrasonography for evaluating patients following endograft repair in efforts to reduce the amount of ionizing radiation the patients receive. However, it should be remembered that duplex ultrasound is highly technician dependent, and follow-up of patients with endograft repairs using only duplex ultrasound should be performed in experienced centers.

Thoracic Aortic Aneurysms

Thoracic aortic aneurysms are limited to the chest cavity. Although they are less common than infrarenal abdominal aortic aneurysms, they share similar risk factors. The male-to-female ratio incidence of the TAA is approximately 1:1.

In the past, the threshold for repair was at a diameter greater than 6 cm. This threshold was chosen due to the higher operative risks associated with repair of the thoracic aorta. Now with the availability of endograft, patients with good anatomy are generally recommended for repair at a diameter similar to those for the infrarenal aorta.

Open repair involves performing a thoracotomy and cross clamping the aorta. Repair in this location is often performed with the addition of extracorporeal bypass to maintain perfusion to the viscera and spinal cord drain performance of the repair. Although the risk of paraplegia in the treatment of infrarenal aortic is exceedingly low, the risk of paraplegia and a repair of an isolated thoracic aortic aneurysm is approximately 6%. Endograft devices for repair of thoracic aortic aneurysm are now widely available and have reduced the incidence of paraplegia to approximately 3%.

Thoracoabdominal Aortic Aneurysms

By definition, thoracoabdominal aortic aneurysms require entrance to both the thoracic and abdominal cavity to perform repair. These lesions are usually true aneurysms of the aorta and should not be confused with dissection. Repair of thoracoabdominal aortic aneurysms is quite complex and carry risks of death and paraplegia as high as 20% in some settings. These procedures are generally performed at larger institutions with considerable experience with this condition. Unfortunately, endograft devices for the repair of thoracoabdominal aortic aneurysms are limited to a handful of centers in the United States.

Thoracic Aortic Dissection

Thoracic aortic dissection is the most common aortic emergency, even more common than ruptured abdominal aortic aneurysm. This potentially fatal condition is rare in patients younger than 50 years and is approximately two times more common in men than women. Patients at risk include patients with a history of connective tissue disorders and patients with severe poorly controlled hypertension.

An aortic dissection occurs when there is loss of integrity of the intima and blood dissects into the media. Once in the media, there is a natural plane through which dissection is quite easy.

Although there are various classification systems for aortic dissection, the Stanford classification is perhaps the most widely used and the most useful. In this classification, any dissection that involves the ascending aorta, whether it involves the ascending aorta alone or both the ascending and descending thoracoabdominal aorta, are classified as type A. Dissections that do not involve the ascending aorta are classified as type B. This classification is useful because type A dissections require urgent surgery. Type B dissections are typically managed medically unless they are associated with complications such as unremitting pain, aneurysmal expansion, and end-organ ischemia. By convention, aortic dissections that are evaluated within 14 days after the onset of symptoms are considered acute and those evaluated beyond 14 days are considered chronic.

Helical CAT scanners with the use of contrast are excellent at defining the location and extent of aortic dissection. However, being alert to the potential for this diagnosis requires a high index of suspicion. Aortic dissection can mimic a variety of common conditions based on the extent of the dissection and the aortic branches involved (Table 1). Uncomplicated type B dissections are typically managed medically. This is usually performed in an intensive care setting with the use of intravenous medications to control contractility and, if necessary, hypertension.

In the past, due to the friability of dissected aortic tissue, the results of operative repair for type B dissections have been particularly poor. Currently, endograft repair with the purpose of excluding the entry point of dissection and reestablishing flow to the true lumen is gaining popularity in the treatment of complex dissection. This at times may be supplemented by stenting of affected aortic side branches and fenestration to establish a connection between the true and false lumen in order to restore perfusion to certain organs. Once the acute phase has passed and medically treated patients are under good hypertensive control, these patients are then converted to an oral medication regimen and transferred out of the intensive care setting. Patients need to be followed with serial CT imaging following discharge to evaluate for aneurysmal degeneration of the false lumen. This evaluation should occur every 6 months until the patient is stable, and then yearly thereafter.

In cases where the total aortic diameter grows to greater than 6 cm, repair for the purpose of preventing rupture is indicated, although this is often technically more complicated than treating a fusiform aneurysm in the absence of a previous dissection. Patients should strictly adhere to their blood pressure medication regimen for life.

TABLE 1 Dissection: The Great Mimicker

Territory Involved or Affected by Dissection	Mimics
Rupture into pericardial sac	Cardiac tamponade
Dissection through aortic valve	Acute aortic insufficiency
Dissection occluding coronary arteries	Myocardial infarction
Involvement of cerebral vessels	Stroke
Involvement of subclavians arteries	Upper extremity ischemia (cold arm)
Dissection running down descending thoracic aorta	Severe back pain and paralysis
Mesenteric artery obstruction	Mesenteric ischemia
Renal artery obstruction	Oliguria and acute renal failure
Iliac artery occlusion	Lower extremity ischemia (cold leg)

REFERENCES

Blankensteijn JD, de Jong SE, Prinssen M, et al. Two-year outcomes after conventional or endovascular repair of abdominal aortic aneurysms. N Engl J Med 2005;352(23):2398–405.

Crawford ES, Crawford JL, Safi HJ, et al. Thoracoabdominal aortic aneurysms: Preoperative and intraoperative factors determining immediate and long-term results of operations in 605 patients. J Vasc Surg 1986;3(3):389–404.

Daily PO, Trueblood HW, Stinson EB, et al. Management of acute aortic dissections. Ann Thorac Surg 1970;10(3):237–47.

EVAR Trial Participants. Endovascular aneurysm repair versus open repair in patients with abdominal aortic aneurysm (EVAR trial 1): Randomised controlled trial. Lancet 2005;365(9478):2179–86.

EVAR Trial Participants. Endovascular aneurysm repair and outcome in patients unfit for open repair of abdominal aortic aneurysm (EVAR trial 2): Randomised controlled trial. Lancet 2005;365(9478):2187–92.

Lederle FA, Wilson SE, Johnson GR, et al. Immediate repair compared with surveillance of small abdominal aortic aneurysms. N Engl J Med 2002;346(19):1437–44.

Lee ES, Pickett E, Hedayati N, et al. Implementation of an aortic screening program in clinical practice: Implications for the Screen For Abdominal Aortic Aneurysms Very Efficiently (SAAAVE) Act. J Vasc Surg 2009;49(5):1107–11.

Nevitt MP, Ballard DJ, Hallett Jr JW. Prognosis of abdominal aortic aneurysms. A population-based study. N Engl J Med 1989;321(15):1009–14.

Nienaber CA, Rousseau H, Eggebrecht H, et al. Randomized comparison of strategies for type B aortic dissection: The INvestigation of STEnt Grafts in Aortic Dissection (INSTEAD) trial. Circulation 2009;120(25):2519–28.

Rentschler M, Baxter BT. Pharmacological approaches to prevent abdominal aortic aneurysm enlargement and rupture. Ann N Y Acad Sci 2006;1085:39–46.

Angina Pectoris

Method of
Kenneth Tobin, DO, and Kim Eagle, MD

Angina pectoris is defined as cardiac-induced pain that is a direct result of a mismatch between myocardial oxygen supply and demand. The initial presentation of ischemic heart disease is chronic stable angina in approximately 50% of patients, and it is estimated that 16.5 million Americans have this diagnosis. Ischemic heart disease is the leading cause of death in the United States.

Stable angina refers to predictable chest discomfort during various levels of exertional activity that is predictably resolved with rest or administration of sublingual nitroglycerin (Nitrostat). Unstable angina is an acute ischemic event; this diagnosis includes patients with new-onset cardiac chest pain, angina at rest, postmyocardial infarction angina, or an accelerating pattern of previously stable angina. The terms unstable angina and non–Q wave myocardial infarction are often used interchangeably and should be further defined on the basis of myocardial necrosis as measured by serum biomarkers.

The clinical sensation of angina pectoris is caused by stimulation of chemosensitive and mechanosensitive receptors of unmyelinated nerve cells found within cardiac muscle fibers and around the coronary vessels. This stimulation cascade is thought to occur when lactate, serotonin, bradykinin, histamine, reactive oxygen species, and adenosine are released into the coronary circulation during periods of lactic acidosis. Nerve stimulation via the sympathetic ganglia occurs most commonly between the seventh cervical and fourth thoracic portions of the spinal cord. This explains from an anatomic standpoint why the most commonly recognized pain patterns for angina pectoris involve discomfort in the chest, neck, jaw, and left arm.

The most common cause of angina pectoris is coronary atherosclerosis. As plaque is initially deposited within a coronary vessel, there may be no significant internal luminal compromise during the early positive remodeling phase. However, at the point at which this compensatory mechanism fails, internal luminal compromise ensues. As long as the coronary artery segment distal to the stenosis retains the ability to vasodilate in response to increasing blood flow demands, coronary homeostasis is maintained. Once the critical threshold is passed, the blood supply cannot accommodate this demand, and angina may occur. The four major factors that determine myocardial oxygen demand are heart rate, systolic blood pressure, myocardial wall tension, and myocardial contractility.

Clinical Features

For patients with documented coronary artery disease (CAD) who have predictable episodes of classic symptoms, the diagnosis of angina pectoris is straightforward. Most patients are aware of the levels of exertion that typically induce angina symptoms. Most describe a pain or heaviness across their middle chest that may or may not radiate to the jaw or left arm. Some patients deny chest pain symptoms altogether and instead complain of exertional dyspnea or diaphoresis. Environmental situations such as cold exposure, emotional stress, or heavy meals can induce angina. The Canadian Cardiovascular Society and the New York Heart Association classification systems are used to define angina severity. Both systems use a I through IV scale, with mild angina (class I) referring to episodes that occur with extreme exertion and severe angina (class IV) to episodes that occur with minimal or no exertion. These classification systems are useful for risk stratification and for assessing medical therapy efficacy.

There are clear gender differences in the clinical presentations of angina. Pleuritic, musculoskeletal-type pain, nonexertional pain, and nocturnal pains have been reported as anginal equivalents in women. Fatigue is one of the most common presenting symptoms for CAD in women. The key to the diagnosis in men and women lies in a thorough history, which should always include the quality, location, provoking activities, and duration of pain and factors that relieve the pain. Based on a detailed clinical history, the many diagnoses that can masquerade as angina may be eliminated (Table 1).

Diagnostic Testing

A baseline electrocardiogram (ECG) is often one of the initial tests obtained in a patient with the complaint of chest pain. A normal tracing does not exclude the diagnosis of ischemic heart disease.

More than 50% of patients with diagnosed angina have a normal ECG at rest. The baseline ECG may, however, show evidence of pathologic Q waves or left ventricular hypertrophy, either of which increases the statistical probability of significant CAD. Baseline laboratory data should include a fasting lipid panel to help define the patient's risk factor profile.

Stress testing is an appropriate screening tool for the initial diagnosis of CAD, risk stratification after acute ischemic syndrome, and assessment of treatment efficacy. Whenever feasible, it is more advantageous to obtain an exercise stress test rather than a pharmacologically based study. The additional prognostic data obtained through exercise include blood pressure response, heart rate response, heart rate recovery, metabolic equivalent level attained, and ECG assessment of the ST segment. There are several validated exercise protocols that add additional risk stratification measures to the test results.

The predictive value of exercise treadmill stress testing ranges from 40% for single-vessel disease to 90% for three-vessel disease. A baseline left bundle branch block, paced rhythm, poorly controlled atrial arrhythmia, or left ventricular hypertrophy with secondary ischemic changes often renders the test inconclusive when assessing for ischemic changes. However, if stress testing is being performed for attainment of hemodynamic responses and achievable metabolic equivalent levels, these baseline ECG abnormalities may be overlooked.

Stress test accuracy is markedly improved by the addition of an imaging modality such as echocardiography or nuclear perfusion scanning. The sensitivity and specificity of stress echocardiography and stress nuclear imaging are 85% to 90%. Stress echocardiography is believed to be somewhat more specific, and stress nuclear imaging is thought to be more sensitive. A stress echocardiogram also allows assessment of left ventricular systolic function and valvular function and prediction of right ventricular pressure. In deciding on which stress test to perform, one should rely on the expertise of the testing facility and the individual patient's circumstance.

CURRENT DIAGNOSIS

- The clinical diagnosis of angina depends largely on accurate assessment of a patient's risk factor profile for coronary artery disease and the typicality of the symptom complex.
- The most common symptom of angina pectoris is left-sided chest pain or pressure, with or without associated radiation of pain or pressure to the jaw or left arm, occurring with exertion and relieved with rest or sublingual nitroglycerin.
- Women may present with atypical symptoms such as sharp, nonexertional chest pain; generalized fatigue; or right-sided chest pain.
- Basic screening tests (e.g., 12-lead electrocardiogram, laboratory data, chest radiograph) are normal in most cases.
- For an initial diagnosis, appropriate noninvasive testing or coronary angiography, or both, is important to define the amount of ischemic myocardium and an overall treatment plan.
- Even when invasive procedures are clinically indicated, aggressive medical therapy with high-dose statins, attainment of appropriate blood pressure levels, smoking cessation, and use of antiplatelet therapy is of paramount importance.
- Patients who have clinical evidence of unstable angina and laboratory evidence of myocardial ischemia most often benefit from early invasive treatment strategies.

TABLE 1 Differential Diagnosis of Chest Pain

Cardiac ischemia
Angina
Myocardial infarction
Vasospastic angina
Pericarditis
Aortic dissection (new-onset chest pain and new aortic insufficiency noted on auscultation is an aortic dissection until proven otherwise)
Pulmonary embolism
Esophageal spasm
Gastroesophageal reflux disease
Musculoskeletal pain
Biliary colic
Acute pneumonia

Risk Factor Management

HYPERTENSION

Hypertension is a commonly occurring, well-established, major cardiovascular risk factor. Although the current guidelines (from the seventh report of Joint National Committee on Prevention, Detection, Evaluation and Treatment of High Blood Pressure, known as JNC 7) define hypertension as pressures greater than 140/90 mm Hg, it has been shown that cardiovascular risk progressively increases at blood pressures greater than 115/75 mm Hg.

A meta-analysis of 61 prospective observational trials of hypertension involving 1 million adults with no known vascular disease at baseline revealed several interesting findings. Patient outcomes were related per decade of age to the usual blood pressure at the start of that decade. For example, from ages 40 to 69, for each increase in 20 mm Hg systolic blood pressure, a twofold increase in cardiovascular death rate occurred. These findings were much more pronounced in patients who were between 80 to 89 years old than in the youngest cohort, 40 to 49 years old. Although the relative risk was much higher in the younger group, the absolute risk was greatest among the octogenarians. These increased cardiovascular risks were not confined to subjects with blood pressures greater than 140/90 mm Hg; rather, there was a threshold of risk shown all the way down to 115/75 mm Hg. Even small reductions in blood pressure can have a significant positive impact on cardiovascular disease. Blood pressure reductions of 4 mm Hg systolic and 3 mm Hg diastolic were shown to reduce cardiovascular events by 15% in a cohort of 20,888 patients.

The Heart Outcomes Prevention Evaluation (HOPE) study asked the question whether all patients with atherosclerosis, regardless of blood pressure, should be treated with an angiotensin-converting enzyme inhibitor. Although many subsequent editorials implied that all patients with CAD could benefit from this therapy, a closer look at the data suggests a different interpretation. The mean blood pressure was 139/79 mm Hg, suggesting that a significant portion of the 9297 participants had a baseline blood pressure higher than this value. Compared with placebo, the treatment group had a 22% reduction in the primary outcome composite of myocardial infarction, stroke, or cardiovascular death. A small substudy using 24-hour ambulatory blood pressure monitoring showed blood pressure differences of 11 mm Hg systolic and 4 mm Hg diastolic in the treatment group compared with the placebo group, which may explain the cardiovascular event reductions reported.

HYPERLIPIDEMIA

Dyslipidemia is an important risk factor for atherosclerotic cardiovascular disease. Increased levels of low-density lipoproteins (LDL) and reduced levels of high-density lipoproteins are the main therapeutic targets. Lowering of LDL-cholesterol has been shown to intimately correlate with reductions in cardiovascular disease event rates.

The medical approach to patients with angina should always include aggressive lipid management. Recent guidelines recommend that LDL levels in patients with known CAD should be less than 70 mg/dL. In most patients, it is difficult to achieve these levels without pharmacologic intervention. It has been shown that, regardless of how cholesterol is lowered, there is a concomitant reduction in atherosclerotic cardiovascular disease. However, statins are the first choice for lowering LDL-cholesterol levels among the available pharmacologic agents because of their tolerability profile, positive nonlipid pleiotropic effects, and ability to dramatically lower LDL levels.

The Cholesterol Treatment Trialists' meta-analysis including 90,056 subjects from 14 trials showed a 12% reduction in all-cause mortality per 38.6 mg/dL (1 mmol/L) reduction in LDL-cholesterol, with a 19% reduction in coronary mortality, a 24% reduction in need for revascularization, a 17% reduction in stroke incidence, and a 21% reduction in any major vascular event during a mean follow-up period of 5 years. These benefits were observed in different age groups, across genders, at different baseline cholesterol levels, and equally among those with and without prior CAD and cardiovascular risk factors.

The Heart Protection Study showed that, in patients with established CAD, other atherosclerotic vascular disease, or diabetes, statin therapy reduced cardiovascular events regardless of the baseline LDL-cholesterol level. The trial, which enrolled 20,536 patients aged 40 to 80 years, showed a 24% reduction in major cardiovascular events, a 25% reduction in stroke, and a 13% reduction in overall mortality with statin therapy.

Patients with a recent acute ischemic syndrome were enrolled in the Pravastatin or Atorvastatin Evaluation and Infection Therapy (PROVE IT) trial, known as Thrombolysis in Myocardial Infarction (TIMI) 22, which compared 80 mg atorvastatin (Lipitor) with 40 mg of pravastatin (Pravachol). The atorvastatin group achieved a median LDL level of 62 mg/dL, compared with 96 mg/dL in the pravastatin group. The relative risk reduction for this reduced LDL level was 16%. A substudy looking at the LDL-cholesterol levels achieved with atorvastatin showed that those subjects achieving a level of 40 to 60 mg/dL had a 22% reduction in events, compared with those achieving a level of 80 to 100 mg/dL. Therefore, it appears that high-dose statin therapy and aggressive LDL lowering in this patient population leads to reduced cardiovascular events.

The Treating to New Targets (TNT) trial was the first to compare a more intensely treated group with a less intensely treated group using the same agent. The design of this 10,000-patient study eliminated concerns that outcome differences were induced from dissimilar statin preparations. The mean LDL level achieved was 101 mg/dL with 10 mg atorvastatin (Lipitor), and 77 mg/dL with the 80 mg dose. This LDL reduction was associated with a relative risk reduction of 27% for the primary endpoint of first major cardiovascular event.

It is apparent from both primary and secondary prevention lipid trials that achieving a lower LDL reduces cardiovascular event rates. Following evidence-based data, patients with established CAD benefit from achieving an LDL-cholesterol level of less than 70 mg/dL.

METABOLIC SYNDROME

The combined presence of insulin resistance, hypertension, dyslipidemia, and abdominal obesity define the metabolic syndrome. There is debate about whether this is a true syndrome or simply a clustering of cardiovascular risk factors in a particular individual. The key concept is that the concomitant presence of these particular cardiovascular risk factors markedly increases a patient's chances of developing diabetes mellitus and coronary atherosclerosis. The approach to treatment for this syndrome is no different from that for the individual components. Recognition of the components is key to the treatment of this disorder.

SMOKING

Cigarette smoking is probably the most important of the identified modifiable cardiovascular risk factors. The incidence of CAD is two to four times higher in smokers than in nonsmokers. The pathophysiologic process that leads to atherosclerosis from smoking stems from induced platelet dysfunction, endothelial dysfunction, smooth muscle cell proliferation, and attenuated high-density lipoprotein–cholesterol levels. Smoking cessation must be sought for every CAD patient.

OTHER LIFESTYLE CHANGES

Exercise should be encouraged in patients with stable angina once all appropriate invasive and noninvasive tests have been completed and a stable medical regimen has been established.

Increasing a patient's aerobic capacity can lower the body's oxygen requirement for a given workload, which can lead to increased exercise tolerance and reduced anginal symptoms. Aerobic exercise can improve endothelial function and positively affect baroreflex sensitivity and heart rate variability in patients with CAD.

Endorphins released during exercise are thought to be mood-enhancers as well as effective muscle relaxants. Exercise itself improves sleep patterns. Cortisol levels are reduced with regular exercise, which may attenuate the body's sensation of stress and anxiety. For these reasons, appropriate exercise programs for patients with stable angina have far-reaching positive benefits. Exercise guidelines for CAD patients have been published and should be reviewed before patients begin aggressive secondary prevention efforts.

CURRENT THERAPY

Stable Angina Pectoris

- Treatment with β-blockers, nitrates, calcium channel blockers for symptom control
- Consider addition of ranolazine (Ranexa) if symptoms not adequately controlled
- Aggressive cholesterol treatment based on the National Cholesterol Education Program (NCEP-III) updated guidelines
- Blood pressure management
- Antiplatelet therapy
- Lifestyle modifications:
  - Smoking cessation
  - Exercise prescription
  - Dietary guidelines
- Depression assessment

Unstable Angina

- Positive biomarkers for myocardial ischemia: consider coronary angiography
- Negative biomarkers for myocardial ischemia:
  - Consider noninvasive assessment once symptoms are controlled
  - Substantial ischemic burden identified: consider coronary angiography
  - No or minimal ischemia identified: consider increasing medical therapy
- Persistent symptoms: consider other treatment modalities

TABLE 2 Medications Used for the Treatment of Angina Pectoris

Name	Dosage
β-Blockers	
Atenolol (Tenormin)	25–200 mg PO qd
Metoprolol tartrate (Lopressor)	25–200 mg bid
Metoprolol succinate (Toprol XL)	25–200 mg qd
Carvedilol (Coreg)[1]	6.25–25 mg PO bid
Carvedilol phosphate (Coreg CR)[1]	20–80 mg PO qd
Propranolol (Inderal)	80–320 mg/day, divided bid or tid
Propranolol (Inderal LA)	80–160 mg PO qd
Labetalol (Trandate, Normodyne)[1]	200–800 mg bid
Nitrates	
Isosorbide dinitrate (Isordil)	10–40 mg PO bid or tid
Isosorbide mononitrate (Imdur)	30–240 mg PO qd
Nitroglycerin (Nitrostat)	0.4 mg SL q5min
Nitroglycerin transdermal (Nitro-Dur)	0.2–0.8 mg/h 12–14 h patch
Calcium Channel Blockers	
Dihydropyridines	
Amlodipine (Norvasc)	2.5–10 mg PO qd
Felodipine (Plendil)[1]	2.5–10 mg PO qd
Nifedipine (Procardia XL)	30–90 mg PO qd
Nondihydropyridines	
Verapamil (Calan)	80–120 mg PO tid
Verapamil (Calan SR)	120–480 mg PO qd
Diltiazem (Cardizem)	360 mg/day PO, divided tid or qid
Diltiazem (Cardizem LA)	180–360 mg PO qd

[1]Not FDA approved for this indication.

Major depression affects approximately 25% of people recovering from a myocardial infarction, and another 40% suffer from mild depression. In any given year, one of every three long-term acute ischemic syndrome survivors will develop depression. The Heart and Soul Study examined 1017 patients with stable CAD over a period of 4.8 years. Patients identified with depression were twice as likely to experience recurrent cardiovascular events. Physical inactivity was associated with a 44% greater rate of cardiovascular events. Patients with symptoms of depression were less likely to follow dietary, exercise, and medication recommendations.

Approach to Treatment

MEDICAL THERAPY

Medications used to treat angina pectoris and typical dosages are listed in Table 2.

Nitrates

Nitrates provide an exogenous source of nitric oxide which serves to relax smooth muscle and inhibit platelet aggregation. Nitrates exert their antianginal effect by reducing myocardial oxygen demand through coronary and systemic vasodilatation. Nitrates are strong venodilators, and in higher doses they can also induce arterial dilatation. Reducing the preload through venodilitation reduces myocardial oxygen demand. Coronary artery dilatation of stenotic vessels and intracoronary collaterals directly increases myocardial oxygen delivery. Through these mechanisms, nitrates have been shown to prevent recurrent episodes of angina and to increase exercise tolerance.

There are several nitrate preparations, which differ mainly in route of administration, onset of action, and effective half-life. Nitrate tolerance can occur with long-term use of any nitrate preparation and can be avoided by providing a 10- to 12-hour nitrate-free interval.

β-Blockers

β-Blockers are considered first-line therapy for patients with chronic stable angina pectoris. They competitively inhibit catecholamines from binding to β-receptors. Over time, β-blocker therapy leads to an increase in β-receptor density. Because of receptor upregulation, acute β-blocker withdrawal may lead to a transient supersensitivity to catecholamines and subsequent angina or even myocardial infarction. There are three classes of β-receptors. Some β-blockers are receptor specific, and some exert an effect over all three receptors. However, at higher doses, even β-selective agents have cross-reactivity for all β-receptors. β-Blockers reduce myocardial oxygen demand through a negative inotropic effect, a chronotropic effect, and a reduction in left ventricular wall stress.

Several cardioselective β-blockers, including atenolol (Tenormin) and metoprolol (Lopressor), have been shown to be effective antianginals that are fairly well tolerated in patients with underlying bronchospastic disease. Dosing is important for β-blocker efficacy. A study comparing atenolol with placebo showed that all doses from 25 through 200 mg/day were effective in reducing angina, but only the two highest doses led to an increase in exercise tolerance. Certain β-blockers have intrinsic sympathomimetic activity, including pindolol (Visken)[1] and acebutolol (Sectral).[1] Although they may be effective in reducing angina, they should be used with caution in patients with a prior history of myocardial infarction and in those with left ventricular dysfunction, because they may not reduce heart rate or blood pressure at rest.

When β-blockers are used to treat angina, a goal resting heart rate should be between 55 and 60 beats/min. Caution should be used in patients with resting bradycardia and in those with known reactive airway disease. Atenolol is renally excreted and should be used with caution in the elderly and in those with known renal dysfunction.

[1]Not FDA approved for this indication.

Calcium Channel Blockers

Calcium channel blockers are classified as either dihydropyridines or nondihydropyridines. The former group includes amlodipine (Norvasc), felodipine (Plendil),[1] nifedipine (Procardia), and nicardipine (Cardene); the latter includes diltiazem (Cardizem) and verapamil (Calan). There are differences among the two subclasses in regard to chronotropic, dromotropic, and inotropic effects.

Calcium channel blockers positively alter myocardial oxygen supply and demand, mainly through direct arterial vasodilatation. The nondihydropyridines also exhibit negative chronotropic and inotropic effects, thus further lowering myocardial oxygen demands.

One of the early quick-release preparations of a dihydropyridine calcium channel blocker, nifedipine, was reported to potentially induce myocardial infarction when used to treat angina. This was most likely due to a rapid drop in afterload leading to reflex adrenergic activation. Sustained-release preparations of nifedipine (Procardia XL), as well as the other dihyropyridines, have been proven safe and effective in patients with cardiovascular disease. Although amlodipine and felodipine are tolerated in patients with left ventricular systolic dysfunction, other calcium channel blockers should be avoided in this patient subset.

Ranolazine (Ranexa)

Ranolazine (Ranexa) is a new and unique antianginal drug approved for the treatment of stable angina. It is a sustained-release preparation that has been approved for patients who remain symptomatic while on standard angina pharmacotherapy. Its mechanism of action may be through reduction of fatty acid oxidation or effects on sodium shifts and intracellular calcium levels. QT prolongation has been reported, but a significant increase in arrhythmias has not been seen. Side effects include dizziness, constipation, and nausea. Dosing is 500 or 1000 mg twice daily, and the major route of metabolism is the cytochrome P-450 system. Ranolazine should be used cautiously in patients who are taking other pharmacologic agents that have the potential to prolong the QT interval.

Medication Combinations

Many patients with chronic stable angina require more than one antianginal medication to control their symptoms. There are no published data available to guide firm treatment recommendations. However, it is important to recognize medication side effects when deciding which agents to combine. β-Blockers block the atrioventricular (AV) node and exert a portion of their effectiveness through this mechanism. The nondihydropyridine calcium channel blockers also have AV-nodal blocking properties, and therefore should be used cautiously with β-blockers, especially in patients with preexisting conduction system disease. The dihydropyridine agents do not have AV-nodal blocking effects and may be a safer choice when used in combination with β-blockers. Nitrates do not have a side effect profile that raises concerns when they are used with β-blockers or with calcium channel blockers.

Antiplatelet Therapy

The common etiology leading to an acute ischemic syndrome is a platelet-rich clot occurring at the site of a significant coronary artery stenosis, often after a plaque rupture. Antiplatelet medications have been shown to consistently decrease morbidity and mortality in a wide array of cardiovascular disease patients. A meta-analysis suggested that, for patients with stable cardiovascular disease, low-dose aspirin therapy (50–100 mg daily) is as effective as higher doses (>300 mg). In this patient population, aspirin therapy resulted in a 26% reduction in myocardial infarction; the number of patients needed to treat to prevent a myocardial infarction was 83.

The Antiplatelet Trialists' Collaboration study demonstrated a reduction in myocardial infarction, stroke, and death in high-risk cardiovascular patients treated with antiplatelet therapy. Consensus guidelines recommend indefinite oral aspirin for the secondary prevention of cardiovascular events in all angina patients.

Clopidogrel (Plavix) is an effective alternative to aspirin for the treatment of stable cardiovascular disease in those patients with a true aspirin allergy. However, there are no data to indicate that clopidogrel is superior to aspirin in this particular patient population. In patients with unstable angina, dual antiplatelet therapy with aspirin and clopidogrel is recommended.

INVASIVE ASSESSMENT

The decision to pursue an invasive treatment approach differs significantly in patients with chronic stable angina and in those with acute coronary syndromes. Within both groups, accurate risk stratification is the key consideration in choosing who will benefit from coronary angiography and subsequent percutaneous coronary intervention. An invasive strategy in unstable angina patients has been shown to reduce recurrent acute coronary syndrome events consistently in many trials. A routine invasive strategy is recommended for patients with non-ST segment acute ischemic syndromes who have refractory ischemia, elevated cardiac biomarkers suggesting myocardial necrosis, or new ST-segment depression on ECG monitoring.

In patients with unstable angina, there are significant gender differences in outcomes related to the use of invasive therapy. Both men and women with elevated biomarkers from myocardial necrosis have comparable reductions in rates of death, myocardial infarction, and rehospitalization with invasive treatment strategies. However, in the absence of positive biomarkers, women appear to have potentially negative outcomes with an invasive approach. The current American College of Cardiology and American Heart Association guidelines recommend a conservative approach in such women.

Patients diagnosed with stable angina comprise a vast array of clinical presentations. The two most fueled debates in this arena concern the initial choice of medical therapy versus an invasive approach, and when to cross over from a medical treatment plan to an invasive one. The Atorvastatin Versus Revascularization Treatment (AVERT) trial studied the effects of intensive lipid-lowering therapy on ischemic events in a relatively low-risk population of patients with single- or two-vessel disease compared with percutaneous transluminal coronary angioplasty. AVERT randomized 341 patients to medical therapy plus atorvastatin (Lipitor) 80 mg or to angioplasty followed by usual medical care (which included the option of statin therapy at the choice of the treating physician). The medical treatment group experienced a 36% reduction in the composite endpoint of ischemic events compared with the angioplasty group. This difference was due primarily to repeated angioplasty, coronary artery bypass grafting, or hospitalization for worsening angina. The primary outcome of this trial from a practical standpoint was that high-dose statin therapy was safe in this patient population and did not increase cardiovascular events, compared with an angioplasty-based treatment plan.

One of the keys in interpreting the available data is recognizing that, by the time many of these trials are published, the percutaneous treatment choices are often outdated. Early trials used mainly balloon angioplasty, and later trials used early-generation bare metal stents. Equally as important is to determine what the background medical treatment plans were for any particular trial on this subject. Often, lipid therapy was not aggressive, hypertension management was not confirmed to be adequate, and intravenous glycoprotein IIb/IIIa antagonists were either not available or not used as a standard protocol when indicated.

The Clinical Outcomes Utilizing Revascularization and Aggressive Drug Evaluation (COURAGE) trial was designed to address the potential advantages of current medical therapy over a percutaneous approach in patients with demonstrable ischemia but stable CAD. Of the 35,000 patients screened, only 2287 met the study inclusion criteria. All participants of the COURAGE trial underwent a coronary angiography, and patients with high-risk anatomic findings such as severe left main coronary artery stenosis were excluded. The biggest difference in this trial compared with previous studies was that strict guideline-based medical therapy was followed in both groups. In the

---

[1]Not FDA approved for this indication.

entire cohort, 85% of subjects were taking a β-blocker, 93% were taking a statin, and 85% were taking aspirin. The final interpretation of the COURAGE trial results was not that medical therapy is superior for all patients with CAD but that, in selected cohorts, aggressive medical therapy is an appropriate first step in the treatment of ischemic heart disease.

NOVEL THERAPIES

Transmyocardial Laser Revascularization

Transmyocardial laser revascularization is an invasive treatment that can be performed as an open heart procedure or percutaneously. The mechanism was originally thought to be the creation of myocardial channels leading to collateral circulation to ischemic zones, but this concept has been called into question. Current theories suggest cardiac denervation, laser-induced angiogenesis, or placebo effect. Likely selection bias within trials has also limited published outcomes data. In a randomized trial involving patients with class III or IV angina and percutaneously untreatable CAD, there was no reduction in angina, no improvement in exercise tolerance, and no decrease in adverse cardiac events after percutaneous transmyocardial laser revascularization, compared with maximal medical therapy. In this trial, the placebo effect was dramatically reduced through extensive blinding protocols for patients and treating physicians.

Angiogenesis leading to the induction of newly formed coronary vessels has been an active area of research for many years. Three main angiogenic growth factors that have been studied: fibroblastic growth factors, vascular endothelial growth factor, and platelet-derived growth factor. Major research limitations for these agents are that they do not act independently, and their biologic properties are poorly understood. Potential complications such as aberrant vascular proliferation, tumor development or proliferation, and proatherogenic effects have made patient enrollment difficult. Although there are some trial results suggesting that the ischemic burden shown on perfusion imaging may be reduced, no firm positive outcome data have yet been published.

External Counterpulsation

External counterpulsation is a noninvasive method of increasing coronary blood flow through diastolic augmentation. Large blood pressure cuffs are placed on both legs and thighs and are inflated to a pressure of 300 mm Hg in early diastole (triggered by the patient's ECG), promoting venous return to the heart. The mechanism is unclear but may be related to enhanced endothelial function, improved myocardial perfusion, and possibly placebo effect. Several small studies have suggested a clinical reduction in angina episodes, but no positive mortality benefit has yet been published. Contraindications to this treatment include certain aortic valvular diseases, aortic aneurysm, and peripheral vascular disease.

Spinal Cord Stimulation

For patients whose angina is refractory to medical therapy and who are not candidates for revascularization, spinal cord stimulation may be considered. Few intermediate or long-term data are available, but many short-term studies suggest reduced angina episodes. Placement of the device and subsequent stimulation at the C7-T1 level suggests that the mechanism of action is reduced pain sensation.

Other Causes of Angina

SYNDROME X

The cardiac syndrome X refers to patients who have normal or near-normal epicardial coronary arteries and episodic chest pain. This disorder is much more common in women and is often seen in patients younger than 50 years of age. The chest pain episodes may last longer than 30 minutes and may have a variable response to sublingual nitrates. Patients with syndrome X often describe typical stress-induced angina. Risk factors include hypertension, diabetes, and

hyperlipidemia. Female patients are typically postmenopausal and frequently have stress-induced symptoms and ischemia on stress imaging. They often respond to standard angina medications and typically have a better prognosis than patients with significant epicardial plaque.

VASOSPASTIC OR PRINZMETAL'S ANGINA

The classic definition of Prinzmetal's angina is chest pain with documented ST-segment elevation during symptoms or during exercise in the face of angiographically normal or near-normal coronary arteries. Over the years, the definition has expanded to include patients who have classic angina symptoms commonly relieved with nitrates or calcium channel blockers and minimal or no CAD. It has been shown that patients with nonobstructive CAD may be prone to focal artery spasm at the stenosis site; therefore, the previous requirement of normal coronary arteries is not an absolute necessity. Other disease states (e.g., Raynaud's phenomenon) can increase a patient's development of coronary artery spasm, as can illicit drug usage (e.g., cocaine). Vasospasm is more common in active smokers. β-Blockers should be used cautiously in these patients, because they may exacerbate coronary spasm. Patients with angiographically documented intramyocardial bridging may be prone to focal coronary spasm and subsequent angina pectoris.

Newer Imaging Techniques

CALCIUM SCORING

Coronary artery calcium scoring is a well-studied imaging modality used to assess a patient's pretest probability of CAD. With respect to evaluation for angina, one must remember that electron-beam computed tomographic (CT) scanning does not offer physiologic data and therefore does not allow determination of myocardial ischemia. This study is most useful in the work-up of a low-risk patient with an atypical chest pain syndrome. If such a patient has an elevated calcium score, other studies may be reasonable.

COMPUTED TOMOGRAPHIC CORONARY ANGIOGRAPHY

CT coronary angiography is a noninvasive way to image the coronary arteries. Like electron-beam CT, it does not provide physiologic data regarding coronary artery perfusion, but it does provide anatomic information such as the presence and percentage of coronary artery stenosis. Although selected patients with stable or unstable angina may be considered candidates for CT angiography, its main utility is in patients being evaluated for chest pain who are otherwise at low risk and have a low pretest probability. Because of the volume of intravenous contrast required by CT angiography, the risk of contrast nephropathy must be considered when contemplating this study.

Summary

The approach to the patient with angina should be based on a global assessment and intensive treatment of all identified cardiovascular risk factors. Noninvasive testing is helpful for an initial diagnosis and to guide the decision for a more invasive approach. Familiarity and adherence to current treatment guidelines is of paramount importance. There are important gender differences that should not be overlooked in the clinical presentation of angina and in the approach to optimal therapy.

REFERENCES

Anderson JL, Adams CD, Antman EM, et al. ACC/AHA 2007 guidelines for the management of patients with unstable angina/non-ST-elevation myocardial infarction: A report of the American College of Cardiology/American Heart Association Task Force on Practice Guidelines. J Am Coll Cardiol 2007;5067:e1–157.
Antithrombotic Trialists C. Collaborative meta-analysis of randomized trials of antiplatelet therapy for prevention of death, myocardial infarction, and stroke in high risk patients. BMJ 2002;423:71–86.

Berger J, Brown D, Becker R, et al. Low-dose aspirin in patients with stable cardiovascular disease: A meta-analysis. Am J Med 2008;121(1):43–9.

Blood Pressure Lowering Treatment Trialists Collaboration. Effects of different blood pressure lowering regimens on major cardiovascular events: Results of prospectively-designed overviews of randomized trials. Lancet 2003;362:1527–45.

Boden WE, O'Rourke RA, Teo KK, et al. Optimal medical therapy with or without PCI for stable coronary disease. N Engl J Med 2007;35:1503–16.

Cholesterol Treatment Trialists' Collaborators. Efficacy and safety of cholesterol-lowering treatment: Prospective meta-analysis of data from 90056 participants in 14 trials of statins. Lancet 2005;366:1267–78.

Gibbons RJ, Abrams J, Chatterjee K, et al. ACC/AHA 2002 guideline update for the management of patients with chronic stable angina: A report of the American College of Cardiology/American Heart Association Task Force on Practice Guidelines (Committee to Update the 1999 Guidelines for the Management of Patients with Chronic Stable Angina), Available at www.acc.org/qualityandscience/clinical/guidelines/stable/stable_clean.pdf (accessed October 2009).

Grundy SM, Cleeman JI, Merz NB, et al. Implications of recent clinical trials for the National Cholesterol Education Program Adult Treatment Panel III guidelines. Circulation 2004;110:227–39.

Heart Outcomes Prevention Evaluation Study Investigators. Effects of an angiotensin-converting-enzyme inhibitor, ramipril, on cardiovascular events in high-risk patients. N Engl J Med 2000;342:145–53.

Mehta SR, Cannon CP, Fox KA, et al. Routine vs selective invasive strategies in patients with acute coronary syndromes: A collaborative meta-analysis of randomized trials. JAMA 2005;293(23):2908–17.

Ray K, Cannon C. Optimal goal for statin therapy use in coronary artery disease. Curr Opin Cardiol 2005;20:525–9.

Stone G, Teirstein P, Rubenstein R, et al. A prospective, multicenter, randomized trial of percutaneous transmyocardial laser revascularization in patients with nonrecanalizable chronic total occlusions. J Am Coll Cardiol 2002;39:1581–7.

Wenger NK. Cardiac rehabilitation: A guide to practice in the 21st century. New York: Marcel Dekker; 1999.

Whooley MA, Jonge P, Vittinghoff E, et al. Depressive symptoms, health behaviors, and risk of cardiovascular events in patients with coronary heart disease. JAMA 2008;300:2379–88.

Cardiac Arrest: Sudden Cardiac Death

Method of
Roy M. John, MD, PhD

Cardiac arrest, or sudden cardiac death, accounts for 60% of deaths from cardiac disease. It may be the initial manifestation or a complication of preexisting heart disease. Most cases are the result of potentially correctable arrhythmias, but the rate of successful resuscitation from an out-of-hospital cardiac arrest to neurologically intact survival remains dismally low. Recognition of patients who are at high risk for sudden cardiac arrhythmic death is critical for prevention. The ability to recognize those at risk for sudden death has increased appreciably, such that prophylactic measures can be implemented in a number of cardiac conditions to minimize risk.

Whereas specific antiarrhythmic drugs have proved disappointing in the prevention of sudden death, drugs that block the effects of β-adrenergic stimulation, angiotensin, and aldosterone have consistently led to reduced mortality among patients with cardiac disease and left ventricular (LV) dysfunction, partly through their salutary effects on sudden death. The implantable cardioverter-defibrillator (ICD) has emerged as a dominant therapeutic strategy based on clinical trials of its efficacy. This review addresses the clinical conditions associated with a high risk for sudden death and the current therapeutic options.

Definition and Causes

Sudden cardiac death is defined as abrupt, unexpected natural death occurring within a short time period (generally <1 hour) after onset of acute symptoms. Primary cardiac arrhythmia is responsible for most of the cases, but acute severe myocardial dysfunction, intracardiac obstruction, and acute aortic dissection are other important causes (Table 1). Structural abnormalities of the myocardium resulting from hypertrophy, scarring, and fibrosis serve as substrates for malignant arrhythmias. The majority of patients who die suddenly have atherosclerotic coronary artery disease (CAD). However, only about 20% of those who survive a cardiac arrest demonstrate evidence of an acute myocardial infarction. Instead, a large number have evidence of prior myocardial infarction and LV dysfunction. It is now recognized that chronic LV dysfunction is the most important predictor of sudden death in ischemic and nonischemic cardiomyopathy.

A significant number (10%) of sudden deaths occur in the absence of obvious structural heart disease. Young, active, and otherwise healthy individuals are often the victims. Inherited or spontaneous mutations in genes coding for ion channels are responsible for most of these cases. A number of specific syndromes have been recognized, allowing for screening of relatives.

TABLE 1 Causes of Sudden Cardiac Death

Electrophysiologic abnormalities
- Conduction system disease involving the His-Purkinje conduction system
- Primary ventricular arrhythmia associated with cardiac conditions listed here

Abnormalities of the QT interval
- Brugada syndrome
- Wolff-Parkinson-White syndrome
- Catecholaminergic ventricular tachycardia
- Idiopathic ventricular fibrillation
- Malignant ventricular arrhythmia resulting from metabolic abnormalities
- Commotio cordis

Coronary artery disease
- Atherosclerotic disease
- Congenital anomalies
- Spasm
- Arteritis
- Dissection
- Embolism

Primary cardiomyopathies
- Nonischemic dilated cardiomyopathy
- Hypertrophic cardiomyopathy

Myocarditis

Valvular heart disease

Arrhythmogenic right ventricular dysplasia

Pulmonary hypertension

Hypertensive heart disease

Congenital heart disease

Noncompaction of the left ventricle

Inflammatory and infiltrative diseases of the myocardium
- Sarcoidosis
- Chagas' disease
- Hemochromatosis
- Amyloidosis
- Hydatid cyst

Neuromuscular diseases
- Muscular dystrophy
- Myotonic dystrophy
- Kearns-Sayre syndrome
- Friedreich's ataxia

Intracardiac obstruction
- Primary cardiac tumors (e.g., myxoma)
- Intracardiac thrombus
- Massive pulmonary embolism

Acute aortic dissection

Tests to Identify Risk for Sudden Death

Electrocardiography (ECG) and echocardiography can provide several clues. Assessment of ventricular function provides the most information in determining the risk for sudden death.

Several noninvasive tests, including detection of microvolt T-wave alternans, signal-averaged ECG, and heart rate variability, have been developed to predict the future risk of sudden death. These tests have poor generalized applicability because of their low positive predictive value. In addition, most have not been coupled with a therapeutic intervention to show that therapy based on them can reduce the risk of dying.

Intracardiac electrophysiologic testing has retained some value, especially in patients with CAD. Inducibility of a sustained arrhythmia can be a marker for arrhythmic events, and therapy based on results of electrophysiologic testing has been shown to reduce mortality.

Treatment

This article summarizes the treatment modalities that have been shown to be effective in the various conditions leading to sudden cardiac death. Data based on randomized clinical trials are limited to common conditions such as CAD and the cardiomyopathies. The rarer diseases lack large clinical experience, and recommendations are based on the current consensus.

ACUTE MANAGEMENT OF SURVIVORS OF CARDIAC ARREST

Once stabilized with the use of standard advanced cardiac life support guidelines, patients should undergo cardiac evaluation by echocardiography and cardiac catheterization. Electrolyte abnormalities should be sought and corrected. Mild hypokalemia (3.0–3.5 mmol/L) is common after a cardiac arrest and resuscitation and is related to hypotension and transient acidosis. Hence, it is often the result and not the cause of the cardiac arrest. Similarly, in the acute phase after resuscitation, it is not uncommon to find global LV hypokinesis, but this should not be taken as a marker for preexisting heart disease. LV function tends to improve over the next 24 to 48 hours and should then be reassessed.

Ventricular fibrillation that occurs during the acute phase of a myocardial infarction (within the first 24–48 hours) is presumed to be secondary to electrical instability resulting from myocardial ischemia and reperfusion. If treated promptly by defibrillation, this arrhythmia has little prognostic value so long as overall myocardial function is preserved.

If acute ischemia or infarction is the documented cause of a cardiac arrest, revascularization by percutaneous angioplasty or coronary bypass surgery is the best treatment. The risk of recurrence is determined by the residual LV ejection fraction. In the Antiarrhythmic Versus Implantable Defibrillator (AVID) trial and Canadian trial of Implantable Defibrillators (CIDS), ICDs did not offer any survival benefit for patients with preserved LV function (>35%). Therefore, postrevascularization electrophysiologic evaluation is recommended only for patients with impaired ejection fraction or significant LV scarring.

Survivors of a malignant arrhythmia other than that due to a reversible cause such as severe metabolic disturbance, toxic drug effect, or acute myocardial infarction are best treated with an ICD. In the largest prospective, randomized trial of drugs versus an ICD (the AVID trial), the ICD reduced mortality by 39% at 1 year and by 31% at 3 years, compared with amiodarone (Cordarone) or sotalol (Betapace). In the absence of specific contraindication, ICD therapy is currently the standard of care for secondary prevention of life-threatening arrhythmic events.

Primary Prevention of Ventricular Arrhythmias and Sudden Cardiac Death

CORONARY ARTERY DISEASE

There are considerable data to guide efforts at primary prevention of sudden death in patients with CAD. β-Adrenergic blockers and angiotensin-converting enzyme inhibitors reduce mortality after myocardial infarction and should be routinely prescribed in the absence of major contraindications (Table 2). Part of the benefit on mortality offered by these drugs is achieved through reduction of the incidence of sudden death. There is no role for the use of antiarrhythmic drugs in primary prevention. Amiodarone, sotalol, and dofetilide (Tikosyn) have largely neutral effects, but class 1 antiarrhythmic drugs such flecainide (Tambocor) and propafenone (Rythmol) are clearly harmful and increase mortality in patients with ventricular dysfunction.

Ventricular arrhythmias occurring late (>24 hours) after a myocardial infarction usually indicate a persisting propensity for recurrent arrhythmia and risk of death. Commonly, these patients have impaired LV function and benefit from treatment with an ICD; an intracardiac electrophysiologic study is helpful in determining the risk of recurrence. Inducibility of ventricular tachycardia (VT) on electrophysiologic study is considered a predictor of sudden death, and treatment of such patients with an ICD lowers mortality.

For the stable patient with CAD, depressed ejection fraction and nonsustained VT are recognized risk factors for sudden death. If severe LV dysfunction is present (ejection fraction <30%), implantation of an ICD will significantly reduce sudden death mortality. In the presence of moderate LV dysfunction (ejection fraction 30%-40%), a defibrillator is indicated if patients have New York Heart Association class II or III heart failure symptoms. Nonsustained VT occurring in the context of moderate LV dysfunction warrants an intracardiac electrophysiologic study. In 40% and 60% of patients, sustained ventricular arrhythmia is inducible; these patients will benefit from ICD therapy (Table 3).

IDIOPATHIC DILATED CARDIOMYOPATHY

Unlike CAD, nonischemic dilated cardiomyopathy is more variable in its course. This is partly because the etiology is often unclear; the disease process may be progressive in some and self-limited with spontaneous improvement in others. Consequently, benefit from ICD therapy is not as convincing as in patients with CAD. Nonsustained VT, syncope, and heart failure symptoms are predictors of high risk of sudden death in this population. In the Defibrillators in Nonischemic Cardiomyopathy Treatment Evaluation trial (DEFINITE), implantation of an ICD based on the presence of LV dysfunction, symptomatic heart failure, and nonsustained VT resulted in a reduction in arrhythmic mortality. The Sudden Death in Heart Failure trial (SCD Heft) showed that ICDs reduce mortality in the presence of heart failure symptoms and an LV ejection fraction of 35% or less.

Syncope in the presence of cardiomyopathy can be a harbinger of sudden death and merits the use of ICD therapy if another cause of syncope cannot be identified.

TABLE 2 Drugs That Have Been Shown to Reduce Sudden Cardiac Death

β-Adrenergic blockers: metoprolol (Lopressor), carvedilol (Coreg)
Angiotensin-converting enzyme inhibitors
Angiotensin receptor blockers
Aldosterone antagonists
Antiplatelet drugs
Lipid-lowering agents
Fish oil[1]

[1]Not FDA approved for this indication.

TABLE 3 Indication for ICD Therapy Based on the ACC/AHA 2008 Guidelines

Class I Indication*
1. Cardiac arrest due to VF or VT not due to a transient or reversible cause
2. Spontaneous sustained VT in association with heart disease
3. Recurrent syncope of undetermined origin in the presence of ventricular dysfunction and inducible ventricular arrhythmias on electrophysiologic study
4. NYHA class II or III heart failure and persistent systolic left ventricular dysfunction with LVEF ≤35%
5. Coronary artery disease and systolic left ventricular dysfunction (LVEF ≤30%) persisting >40 days after myocardial infarction or revascularization
6. Nonsustained VT with coronary disease, prior myocardial infarction, left ventricular dysfunction, and inducible VF or sustained VT on electrophysiologic study

Class II Indication[†]
1. Familial or inherited conditions with a high risk for life-threatening ventricular tachyarrhythmia
2. Unexplained syncope in the presence of left ventricular dysfunction and nonischemic cardiomyopathy
3. Patients with cardiac sarcoid, Chagas' disease, or giant cell myocarditis
4. Adult congenital heart disease with high risk for sudden cardiac death

---

*There is good clinical evidence and general agreement that ICD is beneficial.
[†]There is inadequate data or some divergence of opinion regarding ICD benefit.
ACC/AHA, American College of Cardiology/American Heart Association Task Force; ICD, implantable cardioverter-defibrillator; LVEF, left ventricular ejection fraction; NYHA, New York Heart Association; VF, ventricular fibrillation; VT, ventricular tachycardia.

HYPERTROPHIC CARDIOMYOPATHY

Hypertrophic cardiomyopathy is a genetically heterogenous disease with an autosomal dominant mode of inheritance caused by mutations in genes coding for sarcomeric proteins. Unrecognized hypertrophic cardiomyopathy is a frequent cause of sudden death in young athletes.

Sudden death in hypertrophic cardiomyopathy is caused by ventricular arrhythmias and can be prevented by implantation of an ICD. A number of risk factors for sudden death have been identified in retrospective studies and are outlined in Table 4. The presence of any one of the major risk factors is an indication for ICD implantation. Electrophysiologic testing has no major value in risk stratification.

There are some families with mutations in the cardiac troponin T gene in whom the phenotypic features may not be diagnostic of hypertrophic cardiomyopathy but who nevertheless have a higher risk of sudden death. Currently, however, the value of genetic screening for risk stratification is unknown and is not considered standard of care.

TABLE 4 Clinical Risk Factors for Sudden Death in Hypertrophic Cardiomyopathy

Major Risk Factors
Cardiac arrest
Spontaneous sustained or nonsustained ventricular tachycardia
History of sudden cardiac death in first-degree relatives
Syncope
Left ventricular thickness ≥30 mm
Abnormal blood pressure response to exercise

Possible Risk Factors
Atrial fibrillation
Myocardial ischemia
Left ventricular outflow obstruction
High-risk mutations
Intense (competitive) physical exertion

ARRHYTHMOGENIC RIGHT VENTRICULAR DYSPLASIA

Arrhythmogenic right ventricular dysplasia is characterized by progressive replacement of myocytes with fibrofatty tissue due to an inherited autosomal dominant abnormality in the genes coding for cell-to-cell junction proteins. Typically, the right ventricle is involved, but progressive involvement of the LV has been described. Right bundle branch blockade with late potentials (epsilon wave) and T-wave inversion in the precordial lead may be present on ECG. Ventricular arrhythmia and sudden death are common modes of presentation between the ages of 20 and 40 years, although occasionally heart failure is the presenting symptom.

Patients presenting with stable VT may respond to radiofrequency ablation and antiarrhythmic therapy, but the recurrence rates are high. Consequently, most patients will require ICD therapy. ICD is the first line of treatment for patients with prior cardiac arrest, inducible ventricular arrhythmias on electrophysiologic study, and unexplained syncope.

Sudden Death Associated with Abnormalities of the QT Interval

Congenital long QT (LQT) syndrome is caused by inherited abnormalities of the potassium channel (LQT1 and LQT2) or of the sodium channel (LQT3) that result in abnormal cardiac repolarization. These patients carry a risk of developing torsades de pointes VT. Torsades de pointes can lead to syncope but is frequently self-limited. However, the arrhythmia can degenerate to ventricular fibrillation, and sudden death may be the initial manifestation.

The mortality rate is high in untreated patients (approximately 1% per year). Once syncopal episodes begin, the risk of death increases; in one study, 20% of patients had died within 1 year after a syncopal spell. However, ideal management of the congenital LQT syndrome remains controversial. β-Adrenergic blockers and left stellate ganglionectomy, at times in conjunction with cardiac pacing, have been shown to reduce symptoms and mortality. However, β-blockers provide incomplete protection for patients with LQT2 or LQT3. Because most patients are children or teenagers at the time of diagnosis, there is concern about long-term therapy with implantable devices because of the need for generator changes, potential lead malfunction, and risk of infection. ICD therapy is currently reserved for high-risk patients identified by prior cardiac arrest, recurrent syncope, or VT while on β-blockers, QTc exceeding 500 msec, siblings with sudden death, and symptoms in the patient with LQT3 and possibly LQT2.

One of the major precipitants of torsades in the asymptomatic patient is iatrogenic effects. Numerous drugs have the potential to prolong the QT interval (Table 5). In addition, hypokalemia and hypomagnesemia can induce QT prolongation and torsades de pointes.

TABLE 5 Drugs Known to Cause QT Prolongation and Torsades de Pointes

Common
Quinidine
Sotalol (Betapace)
Dofetilide (Tikosyn)
Ibutilide (Corvert)
Disopyramide (Norpace)
Procainamide (Pronestyl)

Less Common
Amiodarone (Cordarone)
Antibiotics: clarithromycin (Biaxin), erythromycin, pentamidine (Pentam), sparfloxacin (Zagam)[2]
Antiemetic agents: domperidone (Motilium),[2] droperidol (Inapsine)
Antipsychotic agents: chlorpromazine (Thorazine), haloperidol (Haldol), mesoridazine (Serentil),[2] thioridazine (Mellaril)

---

[2]Not available in the United States.

In patients without a recognized QT abnormality, drug-induced torsades is treated by discontinuation and avoidance of the offending drug. A number of risk factors have been recognized for drug-induced torsades. They include female gender, hypokalemia and hypomagnesemia, bradycardia, congestive heart failure, baseline QT prolongation, and high drug concentrations (with the exception of quinidine). Conversion of atrial fibrillation with rapid heart rates to sinus rhythm in the presence of a QT-prolonging drug is a known risk for torsades because of the relative bradycardia interacting with QT prolongation. Administration of class III antiarrhythmic drugs such as sotalol, ibutilide (Corvert), and dofetilide used for conversion and prevention of atrial fibrillation should be commenced under telemetric monitoring. The potential for accumulation of antiarrhythmic drugs in the face of renal dysfunction (e.g., sotalol, dofetilide) should be recognized and dosing adjusted.

A familial form of the short QT syndrome associated with sudden death has been described. A family history of sudden death appears to confer a high risk of sudden arrhythmic death in these patients, warranting ICD therapy.

BRUGADA SYNDROME

Brugada syndrome is characterized by ECG features of incomplete right bundle branch block, J-point elevation with ST-segment elevation in the right precordial leads, normal QT interval, and risk of ventricular fibrillation. The condition has been shown to be caused by an inherited abnormality of the sodium channel involving the same gene (SCN5A) that is responsible for LQT3. The clinical features share similarities with those of LQT3: relative inefficacy of β-blockade, high mortality in symptomatic patients, and sudden death occurring during rest or sleep. Diagnostic criteria are equivocal. ST-segment abnormalities may be transient and dynamic and tend to be augmented by administration of sodium channel blockers.

The general consensus is that symptomatic patients should be treated with an ICD. Asymptomatic patients with a malignant family history should also be considered for ICD therapy. As with the LQT syndromes, drugs have a potential for provoking arrhythmias; sodium channel blockers, including tricyclic antidepressants, have the potential for inducing ventricular arrhythmias and are best avoided in these patients.

CATECHOLAMINERGIC VENTRICULAR TACHYCARDIA

Inherited defects in genes coding for handling of calcium by the sarcoplasmic reticulum result in ventricular arrhythmia triggered by exercise or emotional stress. The resting ECG is normal. Children are usually affected, but late onset of this condition has been recognized. An autosomal dominant form is caused by mutations in the gene coding for the cardiac ryanodine receptor. The autosomal recessive form is caused by mutation in the gene encoding for calsequestrin, a calcium-buffering protein in the sarcoplasmic reticulum. β-Blockers are the primary form of treatment. However, those patients who have had ventricular fibrillation or continue to have VT or syncope despite β-blocker therapy are considered to be at high risk and should receive ICD therapy.

WOLFF-PARKINSON-WHITE SYNDROME

In the Wolff-Parkinson-White (WPW) syndrome, atrial fibrillation can be conducted rapidly via an accessory pathway with a short refractory period, resulting in ventricular fibrillation and death. The risk of sudden death in patients with WPW syndrome is estimated to be less than 1 in every 1000 patient-years of follow-up. Although the risk is reportedly very low among asymptomatic patients, a potentially lethal arrhythmia can be the initial manifestation in a small number of patients (up to 10%).

The treatment of choice for WPW syndrome is catheter ablation of the accessory pathway; this is successful in 95% of patients. If ablation is ineffective or preferentially avoided because of a high risk of heart block, use of antiarrhythmic drugs such as flecainide or propafenone is an alternative. Rarely, amiodarone may be required to suppress arrhythmias including atrial fibrillation.

Management in the asymptomatic individual who exhibits the WPW pattern on ECG is controversial. Until recently, the consensus was that asymptomatic patients did not require invasive evaluation. Patients with intermittent ventricular preexcitation and those in whom the refractory period of the accessory pathway can be determined to be long are at low risk for sudden death. If a benign nature of the accessory pathway cannot be confirmed by noninvasive evaluation, intracardiac electrophysiologic testing should be considered, with radiofrequency ablation if appropriate. A recent study showed that prophylactic ablation in asymptomatic patients younger than 35 years of age significantly reduced subsequent arrhythmias. Prophylactic ablation should also be considered for individuals in situations in which there is minimal tolerance of a potential for arrhythmias, such as in airline pilots.

Idiopathic Ventricular Fibrillation

A small number of patients who are resuscitated from sudden death episodes have no identifiable structural, electrical, or genetic abnormalities. The term idiopathic ventricular fibrillation is applied to these patients. Clinically silent focal myocarditis, cardiomyopathy, or unrecognized ionic channel abnormalities may be responsible and may become apparent during subsequent follow-up. The current consensus is that drug therapy is ineffective, and ICD therapy is the safest and most effective secondary prevention strategy.

Adult Congenital Heart Disease

A number of congenital heart diseases can be corrected or palliated by surgery, and survival into adulthood is common. However, sudden arrhythmic cardiac death is a leading cause for late mortality. Unexplained syncope in such patients warrants evaluation by electrophysiologic testing. Intracardiac repair of tetralogy of Fallot has been accomplished since the mid-1950s, with favorable long-term outcome. Risk of late arrhythmic death increases with wide QRS duration, right ventricular dilatation from pulmonary regurgitation, and LV dysfunction. Ventricular arrhythmias or complete heart block may lead to sudden death. Syncope in such patients is an ominous symptom and should be investigated by electrophysiologic evaluation. Pulmonary valve replacement is known to reduce subsequent arrhythmia risk. Inducible VT and evidence for spontaneous ventricular arrhythmias should prompt the consideration of ICD therapy.

A rare condition called noncompaction, caused by an arrest in development of the LV, is known to be associated with sudden death. Prophylactic ICD implantation is recommended.

Neuromuscular Diseases

Some neuromuscular diseases are associated with conduction system disease and ventricular arrhythmias leading to sudden death. Myotonic dystrophy and Kearns-Sayre syndrome are situations in which prophylactic cardiac pacing at the first sign of conduction system disease can be life-saving. If evidence of cardiac disease precedes the onset of respiratory muscle disease, the risk of cardiac arrhythmia is high, and ICD implantation is often necessary.

Bradyarrhythmia

Bradyarrhythmias resulting from atrioventricular blockade below the atrioventricular node is a cause for sudden death. Most cases of Mobitz type II block or complete heart block below the His bundle are caused by sclerodegenerative changes in the specialized conduction system. Occasionally, cardiac sarcoid or other infiltrative diseases may be responsible. Chagas' disease is a common cause in endemic areas in South America. A familial form of progressive heart block caused by a defect in the *SCN5A* gene has been identified in some families.

Symptomatic bradyarrhythmias and heart block due to disease in the His-Purkinje system are indications for permanent cardiac pacing. In the absence of the other structural heart disease, permanent cardiac pacing can restore longevity to match that of age-matched controls.

REFERENCES

Antiarrhythmics Versus Implantable Defibrillators (AVID) Investigators. A comparison of antiarrhythmic drug therapy with implantable defibrillators in patients resuscitated from near fatal ventricular arrhythmias. N Engl J Med 1997;337:1576–83.

Ezekowitz JA, Armstrong PW, McAlister FA. Implantable cardioverter defibrillators in primary and secondary prevention: A systematic review of randomized, controlled trials [see comments]. Ann Intern Med 2003;138:445–52.

Goldberg I, Moss AJ, Peterson DR, et al. Risk factors for aborted cardiac arrest and sudden cardiac death in children with the congenital long QT syndrome. Circulation 2008;117:2184–91.

Pappone C, Santinelli V, Manguso F, et al. A randomized study of prophylactic catheter ablation in asymptomatic patients with the Wolff-Parkinson-White syndrome. N Engl J Med 2003;349:1803–11.

Priori SG, Schwartz PJ, Napolitano C, et al. Risk stratification in the long-QT syndrome. N Engl J Med 2003;348:1866–74.

Santinelli V, Radinovic A, Manguso F, et al. The natural history of asymptomatic ventricular pre-excitation: A long-term prospective follow-up study of 184 asymptomatic children. J Am Coll Cardiol 2009;53:275–80.

Zipes DP, Camm AJ, Borggrefe M, et al. ACC/AHA/ESC 2006 Guidelines for management of patients with ventricular arrhythmias and the prevention of sudden cardiac death. Circulation 2006;114(10):e385–484.

Atrial Fibrillation

Method of
Robert W. Rho, MD, and Richard L. Page, MD

Atrial fibrillation (AF) is the most common arrhythmia requiring treatment. Patients with AF can suffer from significant symptoms or can have no symptoms at all. Regardless of whether a patient has symptoms or not, all patients with AF are at increased risk for stroke and heart failure, which may be the first clinical event drawing attention to the arrhythmia. The clinical impact of AF is far ranging and includes sinus node dysfunction, iatrogenic complications from the treatment of AF, and a significant decrease in quality of life. As a consequence, AF exerts a tremendous impact on health care resources and expenditures. Significant advancements in our understanding of the pathophysiology, diagnosis, and treatment of AF have led to the ability to approach each patient who has AF with an evidence-based strategy for care.

Epidemiology

It is estimated that more than 2 million persons suffer from AF in the United States. Every year more than 70,000 patients in the United States die from stroke or heart failure that occurs as a consequence of AF. The incidence of AF increases with age and with the presence of structural heart disease. The prevalence of AF is 2% to 3% in patients older than 40 years, 6% in patients older than 65 years, and 9% in patients older than 80 years. With the aging of the population in the United States and the improvement in survival among patients with structural heart disease, the prevalence of AF is increasing at an alarming pace. It is estimated that by 2050, more than 5 million Americans will suffer from AF.

Definitions

Paroxysmal AF is AF that starts and terminates spontaneously without any intervention. *Persistent AF* is AF that continues for more than 7 days or requires pharmacologic or electrical cardioversion to sinus rhythm. *Permanent AF* is AF that has been present for more than 1 year and in which attempts at cardioversion either have not been attempted during this time interval or have failed. *Lone AF* is found in patients younger than 65 years who have AF but who have no clinical evidence of cardiovascular disease and are at low risk for thromboembolism.

Risk Factors

Risk factors for AF include advanced age, hypertension, congestive heart failure, ischemic cardiomyopathy, valvular heart disease, systolic left ventricular (LV) dysfunction, diastolic dysfunction, obstructive sleep apnea, and hyperthyroidism. Acute clinical situations during which patients are at high risk for developing AF include cardiac surgery, acute pulmonary embolism, acute pericarditis, and alcohol binges. In many cases of AF, there is no identifiable cause.

Pathophysiology

AF results from triggers that initiate multiple wavelets of reentry within the left atrium. Triggers responsible for initiation of AF are usually atrial premature depolarizations (APDs) that originate from the pulmonary veins, but other supraventricular tachycardias, including atrial flutter, can also serve as triggers that initiate AF. Largely owing to the coupling interval of the triggering APD and the heterogeneity of conduction properties and repolarization times at that instant in time surrounding the site of origin of the APD, this electrical event can initiate wavelets of reentry that can spin randomly around islands of functionally refractory tissue and around fixed anatomic obstacles. These functional wavelets of reentry are facilitated by the following left atrial characteristics: short refractory periods, regional heterogeneity of atrial refractory periods, regions of slow conduction velocities, and increased left atrial size.

These electrophysiologic properties (excluding left atrial size) can vary as a function of the degree of prematurity of the triggering APD. In addition, exposure of the atria to AF or other rapid atrial arrhythmias can lead to electrophysiologic and structural changes (electrophysiologic remodeling) that result in a more favorable environment for the perpetuation of AF. As a consequence, AF begets more AF. Structural and electrophysiologic changes can occur from the hemodynamic consequences of structural heart abnormalities (i.e., LV dysfunction and mitral regurgitation), resulting in left atrial enlargement and fibrosis. The frequency of triggers and the electrophysiologic characteristics of the atrium determine the clinical burden (frequency and duration) of AF. Because continued exposure to AF itself causes electrophysiologic and structural remodeling, the natural history of paroxysmal AF is to become persistent and then permanent.

Prevention

Prevention of AF should focus on identification and optimal treatment of known risk factors of AF such as hypertension, congestive heart failure, valvular heart disease (valve surgery if appropriate), obstructive sleep apnea, hyperthyroidism, excessive alcohol intake, and ischemia from coronary artery disease. Unfortunately, in many instances, AF occurs in the absence of any known predisposing condition or despite optimal treatment of known risk factors. In such cases, future bouts of AF may be prevented by the addition of an antiarrhythmic agent (secondary prevention).

Among patients who undergo cardiac surgery, the risk of AF may be as high as 30% to 50%. Most of the time AF occurs on postoperative day 2 or 3. Postoperative AF following cardiac surgery can contribute significantly to morbidity, mortality, prolonged hospital stays, and increase cost. Significant attention has been directed at interventions to prevent postoperative AF following cardiac surgery. Some perioperative interventions that have been demonstrated to decrease the risk of postoperative AF include preoperative initiation of β-adrenergic blocking agents, amiodarone, and sotalol.

Clinical Manifestations

SYMPTOMS

Although most patients who seek medical attention experience symptoms from AF, many patients are asymptomatic. These asymptomatic patients might discover that they have AF coincidently during a routine physical examination or after suffering a stroke or presenting with symptoms of congestive heart failure. Symptoms are generally caused by a combination of irregularity of the heart rhythm, rapid ventricular rate, and loss of atrial contribution to ventricular filling. Symptomatic patients might complain of palpitations, shortness of breath, lightheadedness, chest pressure, weakness, and fatigue.

Symptoms of AF are not a reliable indicator of the clinical burden of AF. In one study of patients with symptomatic paroxysmal AF, asymptomatic episodes occurred 12 times more frequently than symptomatic recurrences. In another study of patients with AF who had an implantable atrial recording device, 60% of patients were found to have asymptomatic AF. These studies highlight how unreliable symptoms may be in assessing the duration of an episode and the efficacy of treatments aimed at rhythm control. Absence of symptoms does not mean absence of AF (or absence of risk of stroke).

QUALITY OF LIFE

Patients with AF have a significantly impaired quality of life. In a study of patients referred for electrophysiologic procedures, patients with supraventricular arrhythmias had lower SF-36 scores (a measure of quality of life) compared to those with heart failure or a history of myocardial infarction. In general, patients with symptomatic AF demonstrate an improvement in quality of life measures with successful rhythm control. This has not been demonstrated among patients with asymptomatic AF. A quality of life substudy of the Canadian Trial of Atrial Fibrillation, a study that prospectively evaluated the efficacy of three antiarrhythmic agents among patients with symptomatic AF, demonstrated an improvement in quality of life measures among patients who were successfully treated compared to patients who remained in AF. A similar improvement in quality of life has not been demonstrated in the RACE (Rate Control versus Electrical Cardioversion) study. RACE was a study that evaluated the strategy of rate versus rhythm control and therefore, most patients enrolled in this study were relatively asymptomatic in order to agree to randomization into a rate-control arm.

STROKE

Patients with AF have a significantly higher risk of stroke than patients in sinus rhythm. The annual risk of stroke in patients with AF is 3% to 5% (or even higher in certain groups). The risk of stroke increases with age, history of hypertension, history of congestive heart failure, a prior history of stroke, and diabetes (Box 1). In the Stroke Prevention in Atrial Fibrillation (SPAF) study, prior thromboembolism, a systolic blood pressure of greater than 160 mm Hg, female sex, age greater than 75 years, recent stroke, and LV fractional shortening of less than 25% were independent risk factors for stroke. Patients with paroxysmal AF have the same risk as patients with chronic AF. In a subanalysis of the SPAF study, no significant difference in stroke rate was observed between patients with paroxysmal AF versus permanent AF (3.2% versus 3.3%; $P = NS$).

BOX 1   Risk Factors for Stroke (Nonvalvular Atrial Fibrillation)
Age >75 years
History of hypertension
History of congestive heart failure or left ventricular dysfunction
Prior history of transient ischemic attack, stroke, or systemic embolus
Diabetes

Stroke may be the first presentation of patients suffering from AF. In a study of patients with cryptogenic stroke, 24% of the subjects were found subsequently to have asymptomatic bouts of AF. In contrast, patients with lone AF (i.e., without any risk factors for stroke, including no prior history of hypertension and age <65 years) had a low annual stroke risk.

CONGESTIVE HEART FAILURE

Atrial fibrillation and heart failure often coexist. The incidence of AF in patients with heart failure ranges from 10% to 50%, with the highest incidence in patients with the most severe heart failure symptoms. In patients with heart failure, AF may be either the consequence of or the cause of decompensated heart failure. Patients with AF and poor ventricular rate control can suffer acute hemodynamic decompensation due to abbreviated filling times and loss of atrial contribution to ventricular filling. Prolonged exposure to rapid rates can contribute to a chronic deterioration in LV function. This phenomenon, called *tachycardia-mediated cardiomyopathy*, is a common cause of reversible LV dysfunction. In general, patients who have an average heart rate of greater than 110 beats/min are at risk for developing a tachycardia-mediated cardiomyopathy. This may be the primary etiology of newly diagnosed LV dysfunction, or it might contribute to the worsening of a preexisting cardiomyopathy. The development of heart failure in patients with AF is associated with a higher mortality.

SICK SINUS SYNDROME

A strong association exists between sinus node dysfunction and AF. Patients with sinus node dysfunction may be completely asymptomatic or could have significant postconversion pauses resulting in presyncope, syncope, or, rarely, cardiac arrest. Sinus node dysfunction can result directly from the same myopathic process affecting the atrium, predisposing it to AF. Additionally, sinus node dysfunction can result from electrical remodeling from the chronic bombardment of electrical activity during repetitive bouts of AF. The contribution of the latter etiology may be reversible. An electrophysiologic study of sinus node function assessed before and after AF ablation revealed significant improvement in sinus node function 6 months after successful ablation of AF.

Significant sinus node dysfunction should be suspected in all patients with advanced age and in patients with AF conducting with a slow ventricular rate who are not on atrioventricular (AV) node blocking agents. Caution should be taken in these patients because they are more likely to experience significant postcardioversion pauses. Antiarrhythmic agents can further exacerbate sinus node dysfunction after cardioversion and suppress any atrial, junctional, or ventricular escape mechanisms. Sinus node dysfunction must be considered when performing electrical or pharmacologic cardioversion or when antiarrhythmic agents are employed for maintaining sinus rhythm. Elective cardioversion and antiarrhythmic agents should be used cautiously in patients with a history of sinus node dysfunction, advanced age, slow ventricular response without AV nodal agents, or history of presyncope or syncope. Rarely, temporary pacing may be necessary in such patients following elective cardioversion. In some patients, permanent pacing may be necessary to allow rate control medications to be titrated up and to prevent symptomatic pauses following spontaneous conversion to sinus rhythm.

Diagnosis

Patients with AF may be completely asymptomatic or can complain of fatigue, lack of energy, dyspnea on exertion, palpitations, chest pressure, lightheadedness, and lower extremity edema. Findings on physical examination include absence of the A wave on the jugular venous pulse, irregularly irregular ventricular rate, slight variations in the intensity of the first heart sound, and a weak, rapid, and irregularly irregular pulse. The radial pulse might not reflect the true apical pulse, and therefore auscultation of the apical pulse provides a more accurate assessment of the ventricular rate (pulse deficit). In patients with evidence of heart failure, an S_3 gallop may be auscultated, but an S_4 gallop is absent during AF.

The 12-lead electrocardiogram (ECG) shows absence of P-waves and irregular R-to-R intervals. Occasionally a wide QRS complex may be observed following a long-short R-to-R interval sequence, which is the manifestation of aberrancy, usually in the right bundle, and is known as *Ashman's phenomenon*. At times, AF might appear regular in lead V1 and can be mistaken for atrial flutter. An irregular R-to-R interval and absence of flutter waves in the inferior leads are a clue that the rhythm is AF and not atrial flutter (Fig. 1).

Asymptomatic AF can escape diagnosis for years. In some patients, asymptomatic AF may be discovered incidentally on routine examination or after the patient presents with congestive heart failure or stroke. AF should be suspected in all patients presenting with cryptogenic stroke or in patients who present with new-onset heart failure or acute decompensation of previously controlled heart failure. In such patients, continuous telemetry monitoring during their hospitalization followed by an ambulatory ECG monitor might lead to the diagnosis of AF. Patients with existing pacemakers or implantable defibrillators should have programmed diagnostic features optimized to capture episodes of asymptomatic AF.

In all patients with new-onset AF, causes of secondary AF should be sought (Box 2). Clinical evidence of thyrotoxicosis should be ruled out. Patients who have a pulmonary embolism can present with new-onset AF as their only clinical sign. In such cases, a careful history and high index of suspicion lead to the appropriate diagnosis. After a careful history and physical examination, additional tests for new-onset AF should include pulse oximetry and laboratory assessment with a complete blood count, electrolytes, and thyroid function test. An echocardiogram should be performed to assess LV function, valvular morphology and function, and left atrial size. In patients with pacemakers or implantable defibrillators (especially with atrial leads present), diagnostic information may be stored in the device and can be analyzed with an interrogator. It is important to recognize that undersensing AF in the atrial lead and double counting in the atrial lead can to misrepresentation of the true clinical burden of atrial high rate episodes or mode switching episodes, which are device parameters that are often used as surrogate markers of how much AF a patient is having. This potential pitfall should be taken under consideration in interpreting the diagnostic data available in the pacemaker or defibrillator.

CURRENT DIAGNOSIS

- The diagnosis of ongoing atrial fibrillation (AF) can be made by a 12-lead electrocardiogram.
- Paroxysmal AF can require longer-term monitoring with an appropriate ambulatory electrocardiogram.
- Asymptomatic AF can escape diagnosis. It may be discovered coincidently or not until the patient presents with a stroke or heart failure.
- Patients who present with a cryptogenic stroke should be evaluated for the possibility of paroxysmal AF. AF may be responsible for up to 24% cases of cryptogenic stroke.
- AF should be ruled out among patients who present with new-onset congestive heart failure or an acute exacerbation of preexisting heart failure.

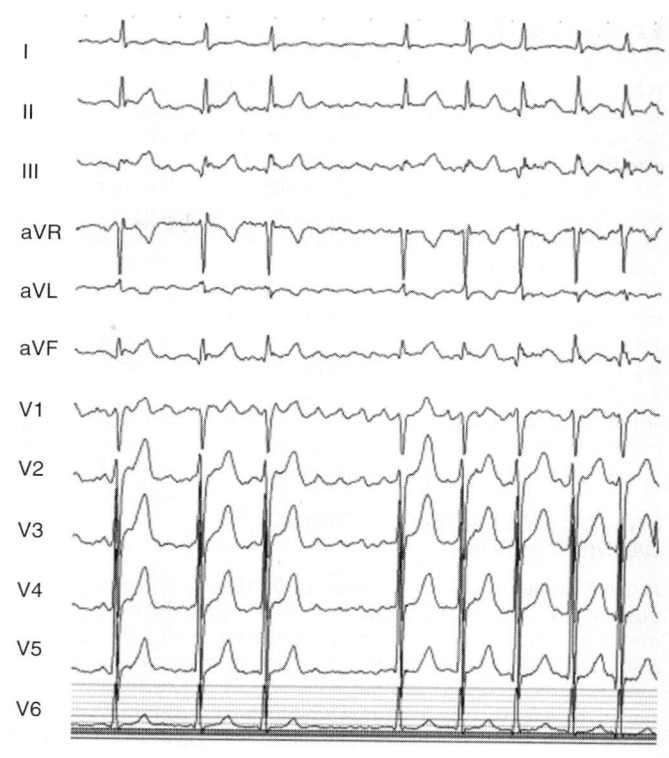

FIGURE 1. Atrial fibrillation mimicking atrial flutter. Atrial fibrillation can look regular in lead V1; however, the irregularly irregular R-to-R intervals and absence of flutter waves in the inferior leads are clues that this is atrial fibrillation and not atrial flutter.

BOX 2	Secondary Causes of Atrial Fibrillation

Cardiac

Ischemia
Hypertension
Mitral valve disease
Heart failure
Pericarditis
Endocarditis
Myocarditis
Wolff-Parkinson-White syndrome
Cardiac tumor
Congenital heart disease
Cardiac surgery

Noncardiac

Thyrotoxicosis
Electrolyte abnormalities
Drugs (sympathomimetics)
Ethyl alcohol
Hypothermia
Pneumonia
Pulmonary embolism
Trauma
Pheochromocytoma
Noncardiac surgery
Lung cancer

Treatment

When approaching a patient with AF, four general questions should be asked: Should the patient undergo acute cardioversion? What is the patient's stroke risk, and is aspirin or warfarin indicated to mitigate the risk? Is the patient's rate adequately controlled while in AF? Is a rate-control or rhythm-control strategy more appropriate? Once each question has been answered, treatment options for patients with AF (shown in Box 3) include cardioversion with direct current electrical cardioversion or pharmacologic cardioversion; stroke prevention with heparin (short term), warfarin, or aspirin; rate control with pharmacologic AV node blocking agents or by radiofrequency ablation of the AV junction and implantation of a pacemaker; and rhythm control with antiarrhythmic drugs, percutaneous catheter-based AF ablation, or surgical maze procedure. Selection of the appropriate treatment options for patients with AF depends on age, presence and degree of symptoms, assessment of stroke risk, comorbid conditions, and hemodynamic effects of AF.

SHOULD THE PATIENT UNDERGO CARDIOVERSION?

Patients should undergo immediate cardioversion if they are clinically unstable, as with hypotension, worsening heart failure, or ongoing ischemia. In all other situations, cardioversion is elective, and careful consideration of stroke risk must accompany all decisions to perform cardioversion. Patients who have been in AF for less than 48 hours can safely undergo cardioversion without anticoagulation. Patients who have been in AF for an unknown period or who have been in AF longer than 48 hours have two options: transesophageal echocardiogram-guided cardioversion while anticoagulated with heparin or warfarin (Coumadin), or treatment with warfarin for at least 3 to 4 weeks before cardioversion. With the second option, we recommend at least weekly laboratory studies targeting an INR greater than 2, with a goal of 2 to 3. In patients who have been in AF for longer than 48 hours, cardioversion is associated with a 5% to 7% risk of stroke without anticoagulation and a 1% risk of stroke with anticoagulation. This risk is irrespective of the method of cardioversion (electrical or pharmacologic). Patients should continue anticoagulation therapy for a minimum

CURRENT THERAPY

- Treatment is directed at four aspects of atrial fibrillation:
  - Does the patient need cardioversion?
  - What is the patient's stroke risk and can the risk be mitigated by aspirin or warfarin?
  - Is rate control adequate in this patient?
  - Is a rate or rhythm control strategy appropriate for the patient?
- Stroke prevention is addressed by evaluating the patient's clinical risk for stroke and choosing the appropriate stroke prevention intervention for the patient. Depending on the patient's risk profile, either aspirin alone or warfarin is recommended.
- Rate control is usually achieved with drugs that slow conduction in the atrioventricular node (digoxin, non-dihydropyridine calcium channel blocker, and β-adrenergic blocking agents).
- Rhythm control requires a careful assessment of whether a rhythm-control strategy is appropriate. If it is appropriate, antiarrhythmic agents and catheter ablation are possible options.

of 4 weeks after cardioversion because mechanical activity might not resume immediately after sinus rhythm has been reestablished. This period of 4 weeks is the absolute minimum, and we recommend long-term anticoagulation in patients who have two or more risk factors for stroke associated with AF.

Patients with symptomatic AF who have not converted spontaneously within 24 to 36 hours may be candidates for cardioversion. We typically perform cardioversion once before initiating an antiarrhythmic agent. Cardioversion should be discouraged in patients with frequent paroxysms of AF without the aid of an antiarrhythmic agent because the risk of recurrence after cardioversion is high. Patients

---

BOX 3   Treatment Options

Cardioversion
Electrical Cardioversion
External (biphasic or monophasic waveforms)
Internal

Pharmacologic Cardioversion
Ibutilide (Corvert) 1 mg IV
Propafenone (Rythmol) 450-600 mg PO
Flecainide (Tambocor) 300 mg PO

Rate Control
Pharmacologic Rate Control
β-Blockers

- Atenolol[1] (Tenormin) PO
- Metoprolol[1] (Lopressor) PO or IV
- Esmolol (Brevibloc) IV (IV drip available)

Calcium channel blockers

- Diltiazem (Cardizem) PO[1] or IV (IV drip available)
- Verapamil (Calan) IR tablet or IV

Digoxin (Lanoxin)

Nonpharmacologic Rate Control
Atrioventricular node ablation and pacemaker

Rhythm Control
Antiarrhythmic Drugs (Vaughan-Williams classification)
Amiodarone (Cordarone)[1] (I, II, III) 100-400 mg/d
Propafenone (Rythmol) (IC) 450-900 mg/d divided tid
Flecainide (Tambocor) (IC) 100-300 mg/d divided bid
Sotalol (Betapace) (III,II) 160-320 mg/d divided bid
Dofetilide (Tikosyn) (III) 500-1000 µg/d divided bid
Dronedarone (Multaq) (I, II, III) 400 mg bid
Procainamide (Pronestyl)[1] (IA) 1000-4000 mg/d divided qid
Quinidine (IA) 600-1500 mg/d divided tid
Disopyramide (Norpace)[1] (IA) 400-750 mg/d divided qid

Nonpharmacologic Rhythm Control
Atrial fibrillation ablation
Surgical maze procedure

Stroke Prevention
Aspirin 325 mg/day
Warfarin (Coumadin) dosed for target INR 2-3

Abbreviations: INR = international normalized ratio; IR = intermediate release.
[1]Not FDA approved for this indication.

TABLE 1 Guidelines for Choosing Antiarrhythmic Drugs

Underlying Disorder	First Line	Second Line
No structural heart disease	Flecainide (Tambocor)* Propafenone (Rythmol)* Sotalol (Betapace)†	Amiodarone (Cordarone)[1] Dofetilide (Tikosyn)
LV dysfunction	Amiodarone‡ Dofetilide§	
Coronary artery disease	Dofetilide Sotalol	Amiodarone
Hypertension with LV hypertrophy <1.4 cm	Flecainide Propafenone	Amiodarone Dofetilide Sotalol
Hypertension with LV hypertophy >1.4 cm	Amiodarone	

*Avoid in patients with coronary artery disease.
†Prolongs QT. Avoid in kidney dysfunction.
‡Associated with pulmonary fibrosis, hepatotoxicity, photosensitivity, and thyrotoxicosis. Patients on amiodarone should be screened for toxicity.
§Prolongs QT. Multiple drug interactions. Special dosing in renal impairment.
Abbreviation: LV = left ventricular.

with structural heart disease and AF of longer duration are less likely to remain in sinus rhythm after cardioversion, whereas patients who have structurally normal hearts and AF duration of less than 7 days are more likely to remain in sinus rhythm after cardioversion. In patients with AF for longer than 3 months, prior failed cardioversion, structural heart disease, or increased left atrial size, an appropriate antiarrhythmic agent (Table 1) may be necessary to maintain sinus rhythm successfully after cardioversion.

Electrical Cardioversion

Although some studies have demonstrated a failure rate in more than 20% of patients, with meticulous technique, success rates of 95% can be achieved. Studies of biphasic shock waveforms have demonstrated higher success rates with less energy and less evidence of skin burns in comparison to conventional monophasic waveforms. Electrical cardioversion requires anesthesia and should be performed with an initial synchronized shock energy of 300 J when performed with monophasic shock and 150 J when performed with a biphasic shock. For best results, the shock electrodes should be placed in an anterior-to-posterior configuration.

Pharmacologic Cardioversion

Advantages of antiarrhythmic agents for cardioversion are convenience and not requiring anesthesia. Disadvantages include modest efficacy and the risk of proarrhythmia. Antiarrhythmic agents demonstrating efficacy in cardioversion include ibutilide (intravenous) (Corvert), amiodarone (intravenous or oral) (Cordarone),[1] flecainide (oral) (Tambocor), and propafenone (oral) (Rythmol). Intravenous ibutilide, flecainide, and propafenone should not be used in patients with structurally abnormal hearts or coronary artery disease. Intravenous ibutilide is associated with a risk of torsades de pointes, and therefore careful monitoring in an intensive care unit is warranted for 4 hours after administration. The risk of torsades de pointes is low in patients with no structural heart abnormalities, no coronary disease, and normal baseline QT interval.

WHAT IS THE PATIENT'S STROKE RISK AND SHOULD WARFARIN OR ASPIRIN BE INITIATED?

Patients with AF and rheumatic mitral valve disease have an 18-fold risk of stroke and therefore should be anticoagulated with warfarin. Risk factors for stroke have been identified in patients with

[1]Not FDA approved for this indication.

nonvalvular AF and include age older than 65 years, prior history of stroke, history of hypertension (even if currently well treated), history of heart failure or LV dysfunction, and diabetes. Pooled data from studies comparing warfarin and aspirin to placebo have demonstrated a 62% and 22% reduction in the risk of stroke with warfarin and aspirin, respectively. Patients who have strokes while being treated with warfarin have smaller strokes and suffer less morbidity from their strokes.

Despite the abundance of data on the beneficial effects of warfarin in stroke prevention, warfarin is underused in clinical practice. Studies of patients with AF reveal that only half of patients eligible for anticoagulation are prescribed warfarin. This is especially true in the elderly population, who are at greatest risk for stroke and who would benefit the most from anticoagulation.

Numerous studies have been performed to identify risk factors for stroke among patients with AF. Risk factors that are strongly and consistently associated with stroke in AF include a prior history of stroke, transient ischemic attack (TIA), or embolism and mitral stenosis. Moderate risk factors include age older than 75 years, hypertension, diabetes, a history of heart failure, and LV ejection fraction of less than 35%. Less-validated risk factors include age 65 to 74 years, female sex, coronary artery disease, and thyrotoxicosis.

Several criteria have been used to segregate patients into risk groups based on clinical risk factors. One such method of risk stratification on which to base treatment recommendations for stroke preventions is the CHADS2 risk score. CHADS2 is an acronym for congestive heart failure, hypertension, age greater than 75 years, diabetes, and stroke (or TIA). For stroke or TIA, a score of 2 is given because prior stroke or TIA is a strong predictor of recurrent stroke. The other risk factors are given a score of 1. The predictive value of the CHADS 2 scoring system was evaluated in a series of 1733 Medicare patients with AF who were discharged without anticoagulation. Patients with a CHADS2 score of 1, 2, 3, and 4 had an annual odds ratio of stroke of 1.9, 2.8, 4.0, and 5.9 respectively. This was an elderly population of patients (aged 65-94 years). The 2006 American College of Cardiology/American Heart Association/European Society of Cardiology (ACC/AHA/ESC) Guidelines for the Management of Atrial Fibrillation recommends aspirin 81 to 325 mg/day for patients with a CHADS2 score of 0, aspirin or warfarin (INR 2-3) for patients with CHADS2 score of 1, and warfarin anticoagulation (INR 2-3) for patients with a CHADS2 score of 2 or greater (Fig. 2).

IS THE RATE CONTROL ADEQUATE?

Goals of rate control are to manage symptoms and to prevent tachycardia-mediated cardiomyopathy. It is important to control rate not only at rest but also with exercise. Current guidelines recommend a goal of 60 to 80 beats/min at rest and 90 to 115 beats/min with moderate exercise. Assessment of adequate rate control should include a baseline assessment of rate at rest and with exercise. A 6-minute walk test, exercise stress testing, and a 24-hour ambulatory ECG monitor may be useful tools to assess adequate rate control with exercise.

Adequate rate control may be difficult to achieve in some patients despite treatment with multiple rate-control agents. It is important that secondary causes of rapid rates such as anemia, hypoxia, anxiety, pain, and heart failure are addressed in addition to prescribing rate-control agents. In a subset of patients, an ablate-and-pace strategy may be a good solution to this problem (discussed later). Another obstacle to adequate rate control is the presence of sinus node dysfunction and tachy-brady syndrome. In such patients, implantation of a pacemaker may be necessary in order to treat rapid rates appropriately with AV nodal agents.

Pharmacologic Rate-Control Strategies

Several pharmacologic agents are effective in achieving ventricular rate control. These drugs include β-blockers, calcium channel blockers (nondihydropyridine), and digoxin (Lanoxin). Digoxin should not be used alone for rate control because its efficacy is poor during periods of exercise or emotional excitement. However, digoxin has been shown to be effective in combination with a β-blocker or a calcium channel blocker. The two calcium channel blockers used for

ANTICOAGULATION FOR ATRIAL FIBRILLATION

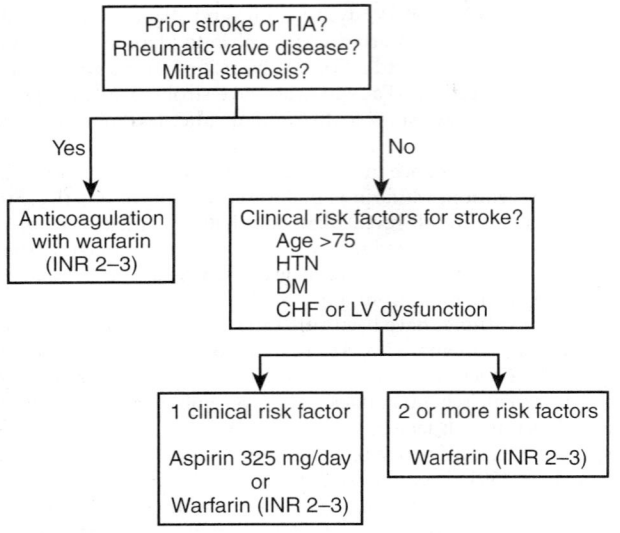

FIGURE 2. A suggested algorithm for stroke prevention with the use of aspirin or warfarin. All patients with rheumatic heart disease (especially with rheumatic mitral valve disease) should receive anticoagulation. In patients with one or more risk factors, warfarin (Coumadin) is the most effective treatment to prevent stroke. A prior history of stroke or transient ischemic attack is given a CHADS2 score of 2. All other risk factors are given a CHADS2 score of 1. See text. *Abbreviation:* CHADS2 = *c*ongestive heart failure, *h*ypertension, *a*ge greater than 75 years, *d*iabetes, and *s*troke (or TIA).

ventricular rate control are intravenous diltiazem (Cardizem) and intravenous and immediate-release verapamil (Calan). Diltiazem has the added benefit of being available as a continuous infusion for patients hospitalized with hemodynamic compromise due to excessive ventricular rates. β-Blockers, as a class, are also effective agents for rate control in patients with AF and may be the first choice in patients with coronary artery disease.

Nonpharmacologic Rate-Control Strategies

Rate control might not be achievable in some patients despite maximal doses of AV nodal agents. Furthermore, it may be difficult to treat patients who are hypotensive or those who have paroxysmal AF with rapid ventricular response but significant sinus bradycardia (tachy-brady syndrome). Percutaneous radiofrequency ablation of the AV node is an effective means to achieve rate control in patients with drug-refractory rate control. This procedure causes complete heart block, and therefore a permanent pacemaker is required and depended upon. Patients remain in AF after the procedure, and therefore life-long anticoagulation is required after the procedure. Several observational clinical studies have demonstrated improvement in symptoms and quality of life after the procedure. We reserve this procedure for elderly patients after all other means of rate control have been exhausted. In patients with tachy-brady syndrome, implantation of a pacemaker can allow treatment with AV nodal agents that could not be used previously owing to bradycardia.

IS A RATE-CONTROL OR RHYTHM-CONTROL STRATEGY MORE APPROPRIATE?

Randomized trials comparing the strategy of rate control versus rhythm control in patients with AF have shown no difference in mortality or stroke risk. AFFIRM (Atrial Fibrillation Follow-Up Investigation of Rhythm Management) was the largest of the studies and randomized 4060 patients with one or more risk factors for stroke to a strategy of rate control or rhythm control. Physicians were given the option of discontinuing anticoagulation in the rhythm control group. Over a 5-year follow-up period, 63% of patients in the rhythm control group were in sinus rhythm, and more than 80% of patients in the rate-control group had adequate rate control. Although no significant difference in cumulative mortality was observed between groups, there was a trend toward reduced survival in the rhythm control group. An important finding in AFFIRM was that ischemic stroke was observed in 5.5% of the rate control and 7.1% of the rhythm control arm. Most of these strokes occurred in patients who did not receive anticoagulation or whose INRs were subtherapeutic on warfarin.

Important conclusions from AFFIRM are that a rhythm-control strategy does not protect patients from stroke, and that a rate-control strategy is a reasonable treatment strategy for patients with AF. Important limitations in the ability to generalize this study into clinical practice is that the average age of patients in AFFIRM was approximately 70 years and that the majority of patients were asymptomatic. Furthermore, antiarrhythmic agents were employed for rhythm control, and it is not known whether similar conclusions can be drawn about nonpharmacologic rhythm control treatments (e.g., AF ablation, surgical maze). Therefore, it is difficult to apply these results to young symptomatic patients with paroxysmal AF in whom rhythm control may be more appropriate.

Based on the data available, the preferred treatment strategy for elderly asymptomatic patients is rate control and chronic anticoagulation. Patients who have symptoms despite adequate rate control are not likely to tolerate a rate-control strategy and may be treated with antiarrhythmic agents and cardioversion if necessary. If antiarrhythmic drugs are ineffective, AF ablation may be considered in selected patients. In patients with one or more risk factors for stroke, continued anticoagulation is recommended even if the patient has no symptomatic evidence of recurrent AF.

Rhythm-Control Strategies

A list of antiarrhythmic agents is provided in Table 1. Most antiarrhythmic drugs carry a risk of serious adverse effects. These toxicities relate to the underlying cardiac condition, and therefore selection of antiarrhythmic drug therapy should be made after evaluation for structural heart disease and coronary disease. The physician must carefully consider comorbidities (especially kidney and liver function), current medications, and the patient's compliance history.

The long-term efficacy for maintaining sinus rhythm with antiarrhythmic agents is modest. The 1-year efficacy for maintaining sinus rhythm (based on symptomatic recurrence) with antiarrhythmic drugs is approximately 40% to 60%, and 30% to 40% of patients stop medications because of side effects and adverse effects.

Amiodarone (Cordarone)[1] is the most effective in maintaining sinus rhythm, but it is associated with a number of serious side effects, including pulmonary fibrosis, hepatotoxicity, and thyroid abnormalities. Toxicity from amiodarone is proportional to cumulative doses, and therefore it is a good option at the low doses used to treat AF (typically 200 mg/day) in patients older than 65 years. Amiodarone should not be used for lifelong therapy in patients younger than 60 years.

The current algorithm for antiarrhythmic drug choices published in the ACC/AHA/HRS guidelines is included in Table 1. Dronedarone (Multaq) was approved since this algorithm was published, and it will fit in a newer algorithm as first- or second-line therapy for many patients. This agent has demonstrated benefit in moderate-risk patients with AF by reducing the combined endpoint of mortality and cardiovascular hospitalization. It is contraindicated in patients with class IV heart failure or class II or III heart failure with a recent decompensation requiring hospitalization or referral to a specialized heart failure clinic.

[1]Not FDA approved for this indication.

Nonpharmacologic Strategies for Rhythm Control

Radiofrequency Ablation

Since the turn of the century, percutaneous catheter-based radiofrequency ablation has emerged as a viable option for patients with paroxysmal AF. Ideal candidates for AF ablation are young patients with symptomatic paroxysmal AF and structurally normal hearts. In most cases, the expected success rate for patients with AF who undergo one procedure is approximately 70% to 80%. The benefits associated with AF ablation include an improvement in symptoms and improvement in LV function among patients with tachycardia induced cardiomyopathy. To date there has been no evidence that AF ablation improves survival or eliminates the need for warfarin anticoagulation among patients at high risk for stroke. Complications of catheter ablation include pulmonary vein stenosis, cardiac perforation and tamponade, atrial-esophageal fistula, and stroke. Comorbidities, severity of symptoms associated with AF, and the operator's experience are important factors to consider in recommending this procedure for patients.

Surgical Maze Procedure

In the surgical maze procedure lines of conduction block are strategically created in atrial tissue to create a pathway for conduction from the sinus node to the AV node. As a result, the atria are compartmentalized and propagation of multiple wavelets of reentry is prevented. The original maze procedure was performed by cutting and sewing to create these lines of conduction block. Other surgical methods to create these conduction barriers are now used, such as radiofrequency, microwave, and cryoablation. This procedure should be reserved for patients with AF with other indications for cardiac surgery, but a number of minimally invasive techniques for AF surgery are under investigation.

Monitoring

Monitoring is performed to initially diagnose AF, evaluate the clinical burden of AF (frequency and duration), and to assess the ventricular rate in AF. Additional information that is important in monitoring AF includes the presence of sinus node dysfunction, evidence of proarrhythmia from antiarrhythmic agents used to treat AF, significant postconversion pauses, and the coexistence of other arrhythmias that may be triggering AF (atrial flutter, supraventricular tachycardia). In many cases, the identification of a specific triggering arrhythmia is very important because the triggering arrhythmias can be treated successfully, resulting in a significant reduction and even elimination of AF.

Monitoring tools used to diagnose and characterize the frequency and duration of AF include the 12-lead ECG and ambulatory ECG monitors. Ambulatory ECG monitors that are used most often are classified as continuous short-term monitors or event recorders.

CONTINUOUS SHORT TERM MONITORS

The Holter monitor is the prototype for continuous ambulatory ECG monitors. Modern continuous monitors provide high-quality ECGs from 3 to up to 12 electrodes, with full disclosure for usually 24 to 48 hours. This type of monitor is ideal for patients who have symptoms that occur frequently (at least once per day), but it has limited application in situations where symptoms are infrequent.

EVENT RECORDERS

Event recorders are ambulatory ECG monitors that are designed to be worn for up to 30 days. There are two types of event recorders. Loop recorders (before symptom onset) constantly store and dump 30 seconds to 4 minutes (depending on the manufacturer) of ECG data. When activated by the patient, the last 30 seconds to 4 minutes of ECGs are stored for analysis. This type of monitor requires that the patient wear electrodes and leads constantly. Nonloop recorders (after symptom onset) are event recorders that do not require that the patient wear electrodes continuously. These are small devices that are kept by the patient nearby (in a pocket or purse), and when the patient has symptoms, he or she places the electrodes on the chest and the ECG is then recorded.

Event recorders are ideal monitors for identifying a correlation between symptoms and rhythm for intermittent symptoms. Limitations of event recorders are that patient-triggered monitors cannot detect asymptomatic arrhythmias; devices with automatic triggers can allow detection of very slow or very rapid arrhythmias but can miss AF that is slower than the detection rate of the device. The primary limitation to looping event recorders are discomfort, poor compliance, and premature termination of monitoring (patients often complain of wearing the electrodes and leads for extended periods). The limitation specifically to the nonlooping event recorder is the inability to detect short-lived arrhythmias and poor electrogram quality in some cases.

Selection of the appropriate monitoring tool depends on the clinical information that the ordering physician wishes to gain. The most common uses of ambulatory monitoring are for the initial diagnosis of AF and to evaluate the adequacy of rate control among patients with AF. The initial diagnosis of a patient with paroxysmal AF may be very difficult. Short-lived bouts of AF can evade diligent attempts to capture the event on a recording device. The diagnostic yield of a 24-hour Holter monitor in patients with paroxysmal AF that occurs relatively infrequently is poor. In such cases, a looping event recorder may be more useful to capture an episode. Among patients with a diagnosis of AF in whom the physician wishes to assess adequate rate control, a 24 hour Holter monitor can be helpful in obtaining a minimum, maximum, and average heart rate through a range of the patient's activity during the 24 hour monitoring period. These data may be helpful in deciding whether adequate rate control has been achieved.

Conclusion

Atrial fibrillation is a common arrhythmia associated with significant comorbidities. Effective treatment strategies for stroke prevention, rate control, and rhythm control are available to physicians caring for patients with AF. With a thorough understanding of the mechanisms, clinical issues, and treatment options, along with careful consideration of the patient's individual clinical presentation, physicians may now make evidence-based decisions for the management of patients with AF.

REFERENCES

Atrial Fibrillation Follow-up Investigation of Rhythm Management (AFFIRM) Investigators. A comparison of rate control and rhythm control in patients with atrial fibrillation. N Engl J Med 2002;347:1825–33.

Dorian P, Jung W, Newman D, et al. The impairment of health-related quality of life in patients with intermittent atrial fibrillation: Implications for the assessment of investigational therapy. J Am Coll Cardiol 2000;36:1303–9.

Fuster V, Ryden LE, Cannom DE, et al. American College of Cardiology/ American Heart Association/European Society of Cardiology 2006 Guidelines for the Management of Patients with Atrial Fibrillation. J Am Coll Cardiol 2006;48:854–906.

Go AS, Hylek EM, Phillips KA, et al. Prevalence of diagnosed atrial fibrillation in adults: National implications for rhythm management and stroke prevention: The Anticoagulation and Risk Factors in Atrial Fibrillation (ATRIA) study. JAMA 2001;285:2370–5.

Hocini M, Sanders P, Jais P, et al. Techniques for curative therapy of atrial fibrillation. J Cardiovasc Electrophys 2004;15:1467–71.

Hylek EM, Go AS, Chang Y, et al. Effect of intensity of oral anticoagulation on stroke severity and mortality in atrial fibrillation. N Engl J Med 2003;349:1019–26.

Israel CW, Gronefeld G, Ehrlich JR. Long-term risk of recurrent atrial fibrillation as documented by an implantable monitoring device: Implications for optimal patient care. J Am Coll Cardiol 2004;43:47–52.

Klein AL, Grimm RA, Murray RD, et al. Assessment of cardioversion using transesophageal echocardiography. Use of transesophageal echocardiography to guide cardioversion in patients with atrial fibrillation. N Engl J Med 2001;344:1411–20.

Page RL, Wilkinson WE, Clair WK, et al. Asymptomatic arrhythmias in patients with symptomatic paroxysmal atrial fibrillation and paroxysmal supraventricular tachycardia. Circulation 1994;89:224–7.

Rho RW. Management of atrial fibrillation after cardiac surgery. Heart 2009; 95(5):422–9.

Rho RW, Page RL. Long term ambulatory monitors. In: Saksena S, Camm AJ, editors. Electrophysiological Disorders of the Heart. 2nd ed. Philadelphia, WB: Saunders; 2005.

Van Gelder IC, Hagens Ve, Bosker HA, et al. A comparison of rate control and rhythm control in patients with recurrent persistent atrial fibrillation. N Engl J Med 2002;347:1834–40.

Wang TJ, Larson MG, Levy D. Temporal relations of atrial fibrillation and congestive heart failure and their joint influence on mortality. The Framingham Heart Study. Circulation 2003;107:2920–5.

Premature Beats

Method of

Prakash C. Deedwania, MD, and
Enrique V. Carbajal, MD

Premature beats are the most common form of cardiac arrhythmia encountered in clinical practice. Premature beats are one of the most common causes of irregular pulse and palpitations. In many instances, premature beats are not associated with any symptoms. They result from electrical depolarization of myocardium that occurs earlier than the sinus impulse. Premature beats have been referred to by a variety of names, including premature contractions, premature complexes, ectopic beats, and early depolarizations. Although no single term is ideal, most electrophysiologists refer to them as premature complexes because although the term *ectopic beat* denotes the abnormal site of origin of the depolarization, it does not necessarily require the beat to be premature, and, in some cases, ectopic rhythm indeed occurs as an escape phenomenon.

Although premature beats generally occur in patients with organic heart disease, they frequently can be seen in the absence of any structural heart disease, especially in elderly patients. Premature beats can be triggered by, or increase in frequency with, myocardial ischemia and heart failure. Premature beats can be provoked by, or occur in association with, a variety of systemic abnormalities, including electrolyte disturbances, acid-base imbalance, toxins from recreational drug and/or alcohol abuse, metabolic perturbations, systemic illnesses such as thyroid disorders, pulmonary disease, infections, and febrile illnesses, and any condition associated with increased catecholamine levels.

Most premature beats occur as a result of enhanced automaticity, but other electrophysiologic mechanisms, including reentry and triggered activity, might play a role. Based on the corresponding site of origin, premature electrical depolarizations are called *premature atrial complexes* (PACs), *premature junctional complexes* (PJCs), and *premature ventricular complexes* (PVCs). Morphologic features and timing of the premature beat on electrocardiographic (ECG) recording(s) help determine the site of origin and the nature of premature complexes. Premature beats can occur in a repetitive fashion as *bigeminy* (after every other normal beat), *trigeminy* (after each sequence of two normal beats), or *quadrigeminy* (after each sequence of three normal beats). They also can occur as two or three successive premature beats, defined as *couplets* and *triplets*, respectively. In this article, the primary focus is on single premature beats.

Premature Atrial Complexes

PACs are the most common form of atrial arrhythmias that can originate at any site in the atria. The exact morphology of the atrial activation (P wave) varies depending on the site of origin of the PAC. Careful and systematic examination of the ECG features of PACs usually can distinguish them from PVCs.

ELECTROCARDIOGRAPHIC FEATURES

The cardinal features of PACs include their prematurity with reference to sinus beats, abnormal P wave morphology, and, in most cases, QRS morphology that is similar to that of sinus beats. The P wave morphology of the PAC generally differs from the sinus P wave unless the premature complex originates in the high right atrial area adjacent to the sinus node, in which case distinguishing PACs from sinus arrhythmia may be difficult. Although sinus arrhythmias are generally phasic in nature, being influenced by the respiratory cycle, this feature would be helpful in differentiating from high right atrial PACs only when the PACs are frequent and repetitive. When the PAC occurs quite early in the diastolic phase, the P wave may not be obvious on surface ECG because it is often hidden in the preceding T wave and would be evident only by watching carefully for the notched or peaked T wave.

If the PAC is too premature, it might fail to conduct to the ventricles if the atrioventricular (AV) node is refractory owing to conduction of the preceding sinus impulse. Such nonconducted PACs are called *blocked PACs*, and they are important because they can be confused with instances of AV block. Such erroneous interpretation can be avoided by simply remembering a common rule of thumb that requires normal successive P-P intervals for all sinus beats, including the interval for a blocked P wave, before considering the diagnosis of AV block. Although most PACs have a normal or prolonged PR interval, the relationship of the PAC to the subsequent QRS complex depends on the site of origin of the PAC and the prematurity index. For example, a PAC originating in the lower atrial area near the AV node generally has a shorter PR interval, whereas a PAC that is quite premature and originates in the upper left atrial area might have a longer than usual PR interval. In general, the PR interval of a PAC is inversely related to its prematurity.

Because most PACs are able to depolarize the sinus node, they usually can reset the sinus automaticity; therefore, the subsequent pause following most PACs is generally less than compensatory because the sinus node fires earlier than expected. In this case, measurement of the P-P interval between the sinus P wave preceding the PAC and the P wave following the PAC is generally less than twice the basic sinus cycle length. This is in contrast to the full compensatory pause often observed in conjunction with PVCs. In some cases, the PAC collides with the sinus impulse in the perinodal tissue and thus fails to reset the sinus node, thereby resulting in a full compensatory pause.

In general, electrical depolarization below the AV node is normal with PAC and results in an unchanged (baseline) QRS complex. Aberrant conduction, however, may be encountered when the PAC reaches the infranodal tissue during the period when it is still partially refractory. Most frequently, the aberrant conduction usually occurs when a short coupled PAC follows a long pause in patients with sinus bradycardia (long-short cycle). This usually results in a right bundle-branch block pattern and is commonly referred to as the *Ashman phenomenon*.

CURRENT DIAGNOSIS

- Premature beats are identified by their occurrence at times considerably shorter than the regular sinus rhythm cycles.
- The origin of the premature beats is determined by the presence or absence of P waves, morphology of the P wave (when present), QRS configuration, and the presence or absence of a compensatory period.
- The presence of frequent PVCs (≥10 per hour) during the postdischarge evaluation of survivors of acute MI predicts increased risk of arrhythmic death and overall cardiac mortality.

CLINICAL FEATURES

Although PACs can occur in normal individuals of all ages, they are quite infrequent except in the elderly. Their frequency increases with age; as many as 50% to 70% of the elderly may have occasional PACs. Some elderly individuals without organic heart disease have frequent PACs and occasionally atrial bigeminy or two to three PACs in a row. Whether the increased frequency of PACs in these individuals is secondary to senile amyloidosis, myocardial fibrosis, or diastolic dysfunction secondary to aging-related changes in the heart is not known. PACs are extremely common in patients with heart disease and in patients with acute as well as chronic respiratory failure. The frequency of PACs can increase markedly during periods of acute febrile illness, shock states, and metabolic disorders, especially in patients with hyperthyroidism and conditions associated with increased catecholamine levels. Use of excessive caffeine, alcohol, tobacco, and recreational drugs can increase the frequency of PACs. In patients with acute myocardial infarction (MI), frequent PACs usually are precursors of atrial fibrillation and occur in association with ventricular failure. In general, the presence of frequent PACs in the setting of acute MI is an indicator of poor prognosis.

In general, PACs are benign except when they are a marker of an underlying cardiopulmonary disorder(s). The major clinical importance of PACs is related to the increased risk of atrial tachyarrhythmias in patients with an established history of such arrhythmias as well as in the elderly who are generally at high risk for atrial fibrillation. As indicated earlier, in rare instances the blocked PACs may be confused with episodes of AV nodal block; however, careful examination of the ECG features described previously easily establishes the correct diagnosis and avoids unnecessary pacemaker implantation.

TREATMENT

The correction of an underlying structural cardiopulmonary disorder and other precipitating factors (e.g., electrolyte or metabolic abnormalities) usually is all the treatment that is needed. No specific treatment is generally required in most patients because PACs usually are benign except in patients with a history of recurrent atrial tachyarrhythmias, for example, atrial flutter/fibrillation. In such patients, specific treatment may be indicated and could include a β-blocker or a heart rate-modulating calcium channel blocking agent such as verapamil (Calan) or diltiazem (Cardizem). Recent studies have shown that verapamil is quite effective in patients with frequent PACs and multifocal atrial tachycardia in the setting of acute or chronic ventilatory insufficiency. In patients who are at risk for recurrent atrial fibrillation, treatment with a specific antiarrhythmic agent, such as propafenone (Rythmol) or flecainide (Tambocor), may be beneficial; however, these drugs should be used only when the patient has a history of recurrent atrial flutter/fibrillation because of the increased risk of proarrhythmia, especially in the presence of organic heart disease such as recurrent ischemia or heart failure.

CURRENT THERAPY

- In general, premature beats in patients without evidence of organic heart disease do not require any specific antiarrhythmic therapy because generally there is no significant increased risk of life-threatening arrhythmia.
- Correction of any underlying structural cardiopulmonary disorder and other precipitating factors (e.g., electrolyte or metabolic abnormalities).
- Suppression of PVCs using currently available antiarrhythmic drugs (except for amiodarone) is not advisable for most patients primarily because of the increased risk of proarrhythmic effects of these drugs.
- In the occasional patient who is disabled by annoying symptoms due to PVCs, a trial of β-blocker therapy should be considered and often is effective in many patients.

Premature Junctional Complexes

PJCs are rarely seen in normal individuals and are infrequently encountered even in patients with organic heart disease. When present, PJCs can occur due to abnormal automaticity or reentry phenomenon. Although digitalis toxicity is cited as a common etiologic factor, PJCs also can occur in the setting of MI, myocarditis, and electrolyte/metabolic disturbances.

ELECTROCARDIOGRAPHIC FEATURES

The ECG characteristics of PJCs are distinct from those of PACs in that the P wave usually is inverted in the inferior leads (II, III, and aVF) because of retrograde conduction to the atria from the ectopic foci in the junctional area. The second feature of PJCs is that the PR interval almost always is shorter than the normal PR interval because of the proximity of ectopic foci to the AV node and bundle of His. In most cases, the P wave might not even be visible on surface ECGs because it lies hidden within the QRS complex. Rarely, the P wave precedes the QRS complex when the ectopic impulse traverses to the atria before traveling down to depolarize the ventricle. In general, the infranodal conduction of PJCs is normal, and thus the QRS morphology of the conducted PJCs is similar to that noted during sinus rhythm. When the PJC is closely coupled to the preceding sinus beat, aberrant conduction might occur if the impulse traverses down the bundle branch during the relative refractory period (most frequently manifesting as a right bundle-branch block pattern). Because in many instances no obvious P wave accompanies a PJC, aberrantly conducted PJCs may be hard to differentiate from PVCs.

In some instances when PJCs occur during the period when the AV node as well as the infranodal conduction systems both are refractory, the PJC may encounter both retrograde and antegrade blocks for impulse propagation. In such situations, no P wave or QRS complex is related to the PJC. Although the ectopic impulse would be invisible on a surface ECG, it would penetrate a portion of the conduction system and thus make it partially or completely refractory to conduction of the subsequent sinus impulse. This would be manifested as a sudden prolongation of subsequent PR interval in case of partial refractoriness or as an episode of "pseudo AV nodal block" due to the blocked sinus beat if the infranodal tissue were unable to conduct the sinus impulse. Thus, even though some PJCs might not have any surface ECG complexes, their presence can be suspected based on their influence on the conduction of the following sinus beat owing to the electrophysiologic phenomenon described as "concealed conduction."

CLINICAL FEATURES

PJCs usually are not seen in normal persons and are rarely encountered in cardiac patients except in the setting of digitalis intoxication and infrequently in the setting of MI or myocarditis. In patients with digitalis toxicity, PJCs may lead to junctional tachycardia, occasionally resulting in palpitation, but are rarely associated with hemodynamic compromise. Because in some cases concealed conduction of PJCs might result in periods of varying degrees of pseudo AV blocks, it is clinically important to recognize their presence in order to prevent undue concern and avoid inappropriate pacemaker implantation.

Premature Ventricular Complexes

PVCs are the most common form of arrhythmia and can be encountered frequently in both healthy individuals as well as in patients with a variety of cardiac disorders. PVCs are often triggered by electrolyte abnormalities, acid-base imbalance, metabolic perturbations, hypoxia, and ischemia.

ELECTROCARDIOGRAPHIC FEATURES

PVCs occur as a result of premature depolarization of the ventricles due to ectopic foci in the ventricular myocardium or Purkinje fibers. In general, PVCs result in wide QRS complexes with the T wave axis usually opposite to that of the QRS. In the vast majority of cases, PVCs do not conduct retrogradely and thus do not result in a distinct P wave. The sinus beats may, however, continue uninterrupted and thus manifest as an instance of AV dissociation in conjunction with PVCs. For the same reason, because PVCs usually do not conduct retrogradely and depolarize the atrium and the sinus node, there usually is a full compensatory pause in contrast to the partial compensatory pause generally seen with PACs. In patients with slow sinus rates, however, interpolated PVCs might occur. If the ectopic foci for PVCs are located high in the His-Purkinje system, the resulting premature complexes may have a narrow QRS morphology quite similar to that seen during sinus rhythm. Additionally, if the PVCs occur rather late, in close proximity to the sinus impulse, there may also be a narrow complex QRS because of fusion between the normal depolarization due to sinus impulse and the abnormal activation sequence from the ectopic foci. In the instance of fusion beats, a normal P wave precedes the QRS. The PR interval is shorter, and the QRS morphology may be only partially altered. In some cases, this might give the appearance of an intermittent bundle-branch block or preexcitation (Wolff-Parkinson-White syndrome) pattern.

Based on the morphologic features of PVCs, they have been classified as *uniform* or *multiform;* they also have been referred to as *unifocal* or *multifocal.* Also recommended is classification of PVCs based on their coupling interval with the preceding sinus beat. PVCs with a short coupling interval near or on the previous T wave have been described as showing R-on-T phenomenon; alternatively PVCs may have long coupling intervals. Based on the underlying electrophysiologic mechanism responsible for PVCs, the coupling interval may be *fixed,* as in reentrant beats, or *variable,* as seen with ventricular parasystole. PVCs may have a repetitive pattern, for example, bigeminy or trigeminy, or they may occur in pairs. It is now believed that repetitive PVCs, such as couplets and triplets, are prognostically more important than just the frequency of isolated PVCs.

CLINICAL FEATURES

PVCs can be recorded frequently in normal individuals, and, similar to PACs, their frequency increases with age. In patients without organic heart disease or without prior evidence of sustained ventricular tachyarrhythmias, the mere presence of frequent PVCs is not considered prognostically important. However, individual exceptions do exist, and the clinician is advised to evaluate each given patient accordingly. In patients with organic heart disease, PVCs are the most common form of arrhythmia and carry significant prognostic importance, especially in survivors of acute MI and patients with recurrent ischemia and advanced heart failure. It has been well established during the past 2 decades that frequent PVCs occurring during the acute phase of MI are associated with an increased risk of sustained ventricular arrhythmias in the initial 48 hours, but they do not predict long-term outcome or risk of arrhythmic events. More recently, it has been shown in patients receiving thrombolytic therapy that PVCs, particularly episodes of nonsustained ventricular tachycardia, increase in frequency but are generally short-lived and represent a sign of myocardial reperfusion. However, the presence of frequent PVCs during the postdischarge evaluation of survivors of MI is indicative of a poor prognosis.

Although as many as 80% to 90% of patients with chronic heart failure have frequent PVCs, the results of several recent studies have shown that only the presence of nonsustained ventricular tachycardia (defined as three or more PVCs in a row) at a rate greater than 100 bpm is strongly predictive of an increased risk of sudden cardiac death in these patients. This is in clear contrast to the findings of several large clinical trials, which showed that more than 10 PVCs per hour in post-MI patients are predictive of a poor prognosis and an increased risk of arrhythmic death.

Overall, the association between PVCs and an increased risk of ventricular tachyarrhythmias and sudden cardiac death appears to be related not only to the frequency and complexity of PVCs but also to the severity of underlying structural heart disease. For example, a patient with mitral valve prolapse and frequent PVCs would be at

relatively lower risk for arrhythmic events compared to a patient with advanced heart failure who has repetitive PVCs and episodes of nonsustained ventricular tachycardia. Proper evaluation of the risk of PVCs has become more crucial than ever because most currently available antiarrhythmic drugs have the potential for causing serious adverse reactions, including proarrhythmias, in patients with advanced cardiac disorders.

TREATMENT

In general, PVCs in patients without evidence of organic heart disease do not require any specific antiarrhythmic therapy because generally there is no significantly increased risk of life-threatening arrhythmia. However, when PVCs are associated with disabling palpitations, reassurance and treatment with β-blockers (atenolol [Tenormin], metoprolol [Toprol-XL]) may help in relieving symptoms. In patients with systemic illness or other provoking factors (e.g., electrolyte abnormalities or acid-base imbalance), immediate correction of the underlying abnormality usually is associated with beneficial effects.

Because of the associated poor prognosis with PVCs in the setting of acute MI, common practice in the past consisted of routine administration of intravenous lidocaine (Xylocaine) in an effort to suppress PVCs during the initial phase of acute MI. However, because recent data suggest that the routine use of lidocaine is not necessary and often can be harmful, lidocaine should be avoided because of the risk of serious adverse reactions, especially central nervous system side effects such as seizures in the elderly. With the ready availability of cardiac monitoring, it now is possible to accurately identify a harbinger of ventricular tachyarrhythmias early in the coronary care unit, so prophylactic use of lidocaine is generally not recommended. Furthermore, results from several studies and their meta-analyses have demonstrated that routine use of prophylactic lidocaine during the acute or healing phase of MI does not alter the overall mortality in patients with acute MI.

In contrast, it is well established that the presence of frequent PVCs ($\geq$10 per hour) during the postdischarge evaluation of survivors of acute MI predicts an increased risk of arrhythmic death and overall cardiac mortality. Numerous trials have been conducted with a variety of different antiarrhythmic drugs. Many of the studies demonstrated that suppression of PVCs with most currently available antiarrhythmic drugs is not beneficial in reducing the increased risk associated with PVCs. The Cardiac Arrhythmia Suppression Trials (CAST I and II) clearly demonstrated that, compared to placebo, treatment with class Ic antiarrhythmic drugs (which primarily work by slowing conduction) was associated with an increased risk of arrhythmic death despite adequate suppression of PVCs. The findings from CAST I and II, as well as several other clinical trials, indicate that although frequent PVCs may be a marker for an adverse event, suppression of PVCs with type I antiarrhythmic agents does not favorably influence the associated increased risk of death. Results from the Canadian Amiodarone Myocardial Infarction Arrhythmia Trial (CAMIAT) and the European Myocardial Infarct Amiodarone Trial (EMIAT) suggest that in patients with frequent PVCs in the post-MI setting, use of amiodarone (Cordarone), a complex drug with predominantly class III antiarrhythmic properties, in combination with β-blockers is associated with improved outcome. However, because of the associated drug toxicity with long-term amiodarone use, it is generally considered suitable only for the high-risk cohort (although many patients with low left ventricular ejection fraction now undergo implantation of an automatic internal cardiac defibrillator).

In general, suppression of PVCs using currently available antiarrhythmic drugs (except for amiodarone) is not advisable for most patients, primarily because of the increased risk of proarrhythmic effects of these drugs. In the occasional patient who is disabled by annoying symptoms due to PVCs, an initial trial of β-blocker therapy should be considered and is effective in many patients. Correction of the provoking factors and appropriate management of any underlying heart disease often are beneficial in managing patients with frequent PVCs.

REFERENCES

Barrett PA, Peter CT, Swan HJ, et al. The frequency and prognostic significance of electrocardiographic abnormalities in clinically normal individuals. Prog Cardiovasc Dis 1981;23:299.

Boutitie F, Boissel J-P, Connolly SJ, et al. EMIAT and CAMIAT Investigators: Amiodarone interaction with β-blockers: Analysis of the merged EMIAT (European Myocardial Infarct Amiodarone Trial) and CAMIAT (Canadian Amiodarone Myocardial Infarction Trial) databases. Circulation 1999;99:2268.

Brodsky M, Wu D, Denes P, et al. Arrhythmias documented by 24 hour continuous electrocardiographic monitoring in 50 male medical students without apparent heart disease. Am J Cardiol 1977;39:390.

Cairns JA, Connolly SJ, Roberts R, et al. Randomised trial of outcome after myocardial infarction in patients with frequent or repetitive ventricular premature depolarisations: CAMIAT. Lancet 1997;349:675.

Echt DS, Liebson PR, Mitchell B, et al. Mortality and morbidity in patients receiving encainide, flecainide, or placebo. N Engl J Med 1991;324:781.

Fleg J, Kennedy H. Cardiac arrhythmias in a healthy elderly population. Chest 1982;81:302.

Julian DG, Camm AJ, Frangin G, et al. Randomised trial of effect of amiodarone on mortality in patients with left-ventricular dysfunction after recent myocardial infarction: EMIAT. Lancet 1997;349:667.

Morganroth J. Premature ventricular complexes. Diagnosis and indications for therapy. JAMA 1984;252:673.

Romhilt D, Chaffin C, Choi S, et al. Arrhythmias on ambulatory electrocardiographic monitoring in women without apparent heart disease. Am J Cardiol 1984;54:582.

Rosen KM, Rahimtoola SH, Gunnar RM. Pseudo A-V block secondary to premature nonpropagated His bundle depolarizations: Documentation by His bundle electrocardiography. Circulation 1970;42:367.

Ruskin JN. Ventricular extrasystoles in healthy subjects. N Engl J Med 1985;312:238.

Simpson Jr RJ, Cascio WE, Schreiner PJ, et al. Prevalence of premature ventricular contractions in a population of African American and white men and women: The Atherosclerosis Risk in Communities (ARIC) study. Am Heart J 2002;143:535.

Heart Block

Method of
Kelley P. Anderson, MD

Heart block is at once a syndrome, a set of electrocardiographic (ECG) patterns, and a mechanism of serious signs and symptoms including sudden death and syncope. Interest has accelerated since conventional pacemaker therapy, once considered to be a straightforward, definitive treatment, has been associated with serious consequences in many patients. The development of new forms of pacing has magnified the complexity of pacemaker therapy selection and many aspects remain controversial. This has underscored the importance of recognizing preventable and reversible causes of heart block to reduce the need for permanent pacing and to eliminate unnecessary implantation.

The details of risk stratification of heart block, assessment of the benefits and risks of the therapeutic options, and patient education and guidance are largely in the domain of heart rhythm specialists. However, heart block may be encountered unexpectedly in any patient during any clinical encounter. Furthermore, some patients can require evaluation in the absence of known cardiac disease because of increased risk of conduction disorders in themselves, family members, or future children. A basic understanding of heart block may be useful in order to initiate emergency treatment when necessary and to recognize patients who might benefit from further evaluation or specialist referral.

Mechanisms

The function of the cardiac conduction system is to initiate and coordinate cardiac contractions in order to circulate blood according to physiologic needs. Electrical activation is initiated by pacemaker cells of the sinus node regulated by the autonomic nervous system. Unlike conduction in common electrical circuits in which electrons flow along a conductor according to the voltage gradient, electrical activity in cardiac cells propagates from segment to segment of the cell membrane in cardiac myocytes (myocardial cells) and in specialized cardiac conduction cells. Energy-requiring ion pumps maintain an electrochemical gradient across the insulating cell membrane. Electrical activity opens voltage-sensitive ion channels, causing regenerative electrical activity as ions shift along their electrochemical gradient.

Electrical activity in a single cell excites several adjacent cells via gap junctions. This cascade effect makes it possible for a single cell impulse to spread rapidly throughout the myocardium so that myocytes are excited in the shortest possible time to enhance contraction synchrony, and it provides a vital safety mechanism in that each myocardial cell can be activated by many electrical paths. In addition, specialized conduction cells exhibit automaticity. Although normally latent, because normal activation inhibits spontaneous discharge, when the normal impulse is blocked, discharges from these subsidiary pacemakers provide vital heart rate support.

Block of electrical activation can occur due to failure of any step in the process, such as lack of energy, electrolyte imbalance, inflammatory disruption of the membrane, block of ion channels by drugs, or loss of gap junctions with infiltration of fibrous tissue (Box 1).

BOX 1   Some Mechanisms of Conduction Disturbances

Calcium channel blockade
- Diltiazem
- Verapamil

Cell death
- Ablation
- Apoptosis
- Inflammatory necrosis
- Ischemic necrosis
- Surgical trauma

Cell dysfunction
- Barotrauma
- Inflammation
- Thermal injury

Congenital structural defects
- Endocardial cushion defects

Energy depletion
- Cyanide
- Ischemia

Gap junction disturbances
- Edema
- Fibrosis
- Genetic defects
- Inflammation

Genetic defects
- *NKX2.5* mutation
- *SCN5A* mutation

Prolonged refractory period
- Drugs
- Ischemia
- Vagal activity

Sarcolemmal ion gradient disturbances
- Hyperkalemia
- Hypokalemia

Sodium channel dysfunction
- *SCN5A* mutations
- Sodium channel blocking drugs such as lidocaine, procainamide, flecainide, amiodarone, and imipramine

---

Because of the extensive redundancy and interconnectedness of system elements and because of the capacity to compensate for injury by electrical and anatomic remodeling, extensive damage can occur before signs or symptoms of heart block. Regions of the heart where there are fewer alternative paths for electrical activation, such as proximal portions of the His–Purkinje system, where all conducting fibers are confined to a relatively small area, are more vulnerable to complete block. Subclinical preexisting injury might explain why subsidiary pacemakers often fail to provide adequate rate support when heart block occurs.

If the patient survives the initial insult, there is a possibility for recovery due to remodeling. However, remodeling can be maladaptive and result in an adverse long-term outcome by further conduction system damage, by left ventricular dysfunction, and perhaps by increasing the propensity for bradycardia-induced ventricular tachyarrhythmias (VTAs). The mechanisms of bradycardia-induced VTA are not known, but bradyarrhythmias precipitate torsades de pointes, a specific form of VTA, in the presence of drugs that block potassium channels, electrolyte disturbances, certain genetic abnormalities of ion channel function, heart failure, and myocardial hypertrophy. A comprehensive list of drugs that can account for bradyarrhythmia-related ventricular arrhythmias is available at www.torsades.org.

Etiology

Although there are many potential causes of heart block, the pathophysiology is not known for the vast majority of cases because there are no tests that allow detailed structural or functional examination in patients. By the time of death, morphologic examination can reveal only nonspecific changes such as fibrosis. Instead, most etiologies are inferred by history of recent or past exposures (e.g., trauma or radiation), concomitant disorders (e.g., muscular dystrophy, amyloidosis), abnormal test results (Lyme disease), or family history (Lenègre's disease) (Box 2). Because most etiologies cannot be verified, the clinician must remain open to alternative explanations and accept the likelihood of multiple contributors.

Some patients, usually young, otherwise healthy persons, present with prolonged asystole due to heart block but have no other detectable abnormalities and have excellent outcomes in the absence of intervention beyond counseling. This suggests that autonomic influences alone can cause severe heart block and suppression of subsidiary pacemakers. It is not known if such responses result from an abnormality or an exaggerated normal reflex. However, the identification of such patients is important because most can be managed without pacemakers.

Other patients who should be identified are those with conditions that place them, their relatives, or their unborn children at risk for heart block. This includes patients and family members with genetic disorders associated with heart block. It also includes women with anti-Ro/SSA and/or anti-La/SSB antibodies whose children are at increased risk for congenital heart block, a rare, but devastating disorder. Members of this group can benefit from counseling and anticipatory evaluation and treatment of offspring.

Signs and Symptoms

Most of the symptoms experienced by patients with heart block are common and nonspecific, such as syncope, lightheadedness, fatigue, and dyspnea. Because other arrhythmias and other cardiac and noncardiac disturbances may be responsible for the same symptoms, it is important to document the cause. Proof, which requires documentation of rhythm and the abnormal hemodynamics responsible for the symptoms, is almost never accomplished. Sometimes a cardiac rhythm disturbance can be related to a clinical event, such as several seconds of asystole due to atrioventricular (AV) block and syncope. More commonly, a patient complaining of fatigue or

---

BOX 2   Etiologies of Heart Block

Often Permanent or Progressive
Alcohol septal ablation (acute, delayed)
Cardiomyopathies (hypertrophic, idiopathic, mitochondrial)
Catheter ablation (atrioventricular nodal reentry, accessory atrioventricular connections)
Congenital heart block (neonatal lupus)
Congenital heart disease (endocardial cushion defects)
Genetic disorders (sodium channel mutations, Lenègre's disease)
Hypertension
Idiopathic fibrosis and calcification (previously Lev's disease, Lenègre's disease)
Infectious disorders (destructive, e.g., endocarditis)
Infiltrative disorders (amyloidosis)
Myocardial infarction
Neuromyopathic disorders (myotonic dystrophy, Erb's dystrophy, peroneal muscular atrophy)
Noninfectious inflammatory disorders (HLA-B27–associated disorder, sarcoidosis)
Tumors (mesothelioma)
Valvular heart disease

Often Transient or Reversible
Blunt trauma (baseball)
Cardiac surgery (valve replacement)
Cardiac transplant rejection
Central nervous system
Drugs (antiarrhythmics, digoxin, edrophonium [Tensilon])
Electrolyte disturbances (hyperkalemia)
Increased vagal activity
Infectious disorders—nondestructive (Lyme disease)
Metabolic disturbances (hypothermia, hypothyroidism)
Myocardial ischemia
Myocarditis (Chagas' disease, giant cell myocarditis)
Rheumatic fever

---

lightheadedness is bradycardic due to high-grade AV block. Asymptomatic complete AV block is also not uncommon. A favorable response to pacemaker implantation is inconclusive due to a powerful placebo effect. Rarely, first-degree AV block results in significant symptoms (e.g., fatigue, palpitations, chest fullness) due to atrial contraction against a partially closed mitral valve. In such cases it is often possible to identify a recent change in PR interval.

ELECTROCARDIOGRAPHIC PATTERNS

Cardiac conduction disturbances are classified by the pattern of ECG complexes. A normal 12-lead ECG lessens the probability of significant fixed conduction disturbances, but it does not eliminate the possibility of transient third-degree block due to reversible functional effects such as intense vagal activity or ischemia. A normal ECG rhythm during symptoms is very helpful for excluding heart block as the mechanism.

PR prolongation and intraatrial delay rarely require immediate action but can have adverse hemodynamic consequences and occasionally cause symptoms due to suboptimal coordination between atrial and ventricular contraction. Significant disease of the His bundle may be electrocardiographically silent, but more often, concomitant distal disease is evident in the form of fascicular or bundle branch block or a nonspecific intraventricular conduction delay. In a patient with syncope, the presence of bifascicular block raises the possibility of transient third-degree block as the mechanism and of progression to permanent complete block.

Most patients with conduction disorders are not symptomatic and do not progress to complete block. However, the combination of right bundle branch block (RBBB) and left posterior fascicle block has a greater tendency to progress to complete block than the more common RBBB and left anterior fascicle block. Nevertheless, conduction disturbances of the His-Purkinje system should not be assumed to be responsible for syncope or cardiac arrest because they are relatively common in patients with cardiovascular disorders that cause syncope or cardiac arrest due to other mechanisms. Conduction disturbances can cause dyssynchronous contraction and result in adverse remodeling. In addition, they can mask or mimic the ECG signs of myocardial infarction.

Alternating bundle branch block is a changing ECG pattern in which both RBBB and left bundle branch block are observed or when the bifascicular block pattern switches between the anterior and posterior fascicle involvement. This pattern is considered a harbinger of complete block with or without symptoms and warrants continuous monitoring and evaluation for permanent pacemaker implantation.

The challenge in second-degree and transient third-degree AV block is distinguishing between block in the AV node, which is rarely permanent, and infranodal block, which often progresses to permanent third-degree block. ECG clues that block is in the AV node include normal QRS duration (<100 ms), type I (Wenckebach) pattern, PR prolongation before blocked impulses and PR shortening after pauses, occurrence during enhanced vagal activity (e.g., sleep), narrow QRS escape complexes, and no factors favoring infranodal block. ECG clues for infranodal block include prolonged QRS duration ($\geq$120 ms), type II pattern, and escape QRS complexes broader than intrinsic complexes. Whereas type II second-degree AV block is almost always due to block in the His-Purkinje system, other second-degree AV block ECG patterns have poor sensitivity and specificity for the site of the block.

Unsustained polymorphic ventricular tachycardia is an ominous sign in any context and can result from a variety of cardiac, metabolic, and autonomic abnormalities. However, in the presence of heart block it suggests that heart rate support may be necessary to prevent sustained VTA. QT prolongation and post-pause U-wave accentuation should be sought as other harbingers of bradycardia-related VTA.

The importance and value of ECG documentation of heart block to the patient's management and well-being cannot be overemphasized. ECGs are subject to artifact and may be misleading when standards for acquisition and analysis are not followed. Multiple tracings of suspicious events should be obtained in multiple leads when possible. A 12-lead simultaneous rhythm recording mode is available on most modern ECG machines and should be used when continuous recordings are obtained to document arrhythmias.

METHODS USED IN THE ASSESSMENT OF HEART BLOCK

Clinicians encounter heart block in three general contexts. For the patient with documented heart block, the clinician selects therapy based, in part, on whether or not the arrhythmia is permanent or likely to recur. There are no tests that provide information about the pathologic state of the AV conduction system; therefore, these outcomes must be inferred from the ECG and past experience. Additional testing including invasive tests such as electrophysiologic studies, coronary angiography, and myocardial biopsy, as well as a large number of specific laboratory tests are occasionally helpful but usually do not provide information about the choice of therapy for heart block.

Another common context is the patient with symptoms for whom the objective is to verify or exclude heart block as the mechanism by correlating the cardiac rhythm with symptoms. Real-time monitoring, such as inpatient telemetry, is used for patients who might require immediate access to drugs or pacing devices to prevent or terminate asystole or bradycardia-dependent VTA. Holter monitoring is useful for patients who have more than one event in a 24-hour window and for capturing asymptomatic rhythm events. External loop recorders are carried for a month or longer and are very helpful to associate rhythm abnormalities with symptoms and to rule out a rhythm disorder as the cause of symptoms. Patients with infrequent events may be candidates for implantable loop recorders that monitor for longer than 1 year.

 CURRENT DIAGNOSIS

- Assess risk for heart block in the absence of symptoms or evidence of asystole
- Review ECG pattern, family history, maternal antibodies, cardiac interventions, and surgery
- Evaluate documented heart block with asystole or bradycardia
- Classify bradyarrhythmia: Transient, recurrent, progressive, permanent
- Grade signs and symptoms: none, mild, severe
- Evaluate signs or symptoms of possible transient heart block with no documentation
- Establish temporal pattern: Single, recurrent, rare, often, recent onset, long-standing
- Grade signs and symptoms: none, mild, severe
- Document rhythm during symptoms: Telemetry monitoring, Holter monitor, external loop recorder, implantable recorder

Electrophysiologic studies allow precise measurements of AV node and His-Purkinje system function and can provide definitive information regarding the site of block if the conduction disturbance occurs during the study. Additional tests have been developed that stress the AV conduction system, including rapid atrial and ventricular pacing, administration of antiarrhythmic drugs such as procainamide and disopyramide, combinations of drugs, and pacing maneuvers. The provocation of heart block is assumed to indicate a propensity for spontaneous AV block. Unfortunately, the sensitivity is low and a negative test does not imply a low risk of future episodes. Electrophysiologic studies have the additional advantage of providing immediate test results, as well as providing the results of programmed stimulation for provocation of supraventricular and ventricular tachyarrhythmias.

The third important context for clinicians is patients who might be at high risk for adverse consequences of heart block but are asymptomatic. Addressing this is a challenge for the future because few methods are currently available. Possible applications include screening for mutations and polymorphisms that predispose to heart block, measurements of mechanical dyssynchrony to identify patients prone to develop adverse cardiac remodeling due to conduction disorders or right ventricular pacing, and methods capable of assessing electrophysiologic and metabolic function of conducting tissue in vivo.

Treatment

Selecting the correct therapeutic approach balances the risks and benefits of therapy against the risks of heart block for both immediate and long-term management. Pharmacologic agents are useful for emergency, temporary, and standby heart support in select circumstances. The standby mode is accomplished by a prepared infusion at the bedside. To avoid excessive doses at the time of sudden heart block, the optimal dose can be established in advance by test doses starting at low infusion rates.

PHARMACOLOGIC TREATMENT

Atropine 0.5 to 3.0 mg[3] or 0.04 mg/kg IV is useful for treatment or pretreatment of patients who develop heart block at the level of the AV node in the context of elevated vagal tone, such as in association with nausea or endotracheal tube suction. Atropine should be avoided in patients with infranodal AV block because prolonged asystole sometimes occurs due to more frequent His-Purkinje system depolarization from increased sinus rate. Vagal activity inhibits sympathetic activity,

---

[3]Exceeds dosage recommended by the manufacturer.

Methods of Heart Rate Support

- Immediate: Intravenous catecholamines, transcutaneous pacing
- Short-term: Transvenous temporary pacing
- Long-term: Permanent pacemakers

Pacemaker Configuration

- Number of leads: 1,2,3,4
- Lead locations: Right atrial appendage, Bachmann's bundle, right ventricular apex, outflow tract, left ventricle, coronary sinus
- Programming to minimize ventricular pacing (manufacturer dependent)

and therefore reduction of vagal tone by atropine disinhibits sympathetic activity and can account for the unpredictable effects of atropine on heart rate. Elevations in heart rate after atropine can persist for hours and cannot be readily reversed.

Aminophylline 2.5 to 6.3 mg/kg IV is reported to reverse heart block resistant to atropine and epinephrine by antagonizing adenosine. Stimulation of β-adrenergic receptors increases sinus and subsidiary pacemaker rates, AV node and His-Purkinje system conduction velocities, and myocardial contractility. The effective refractory period shortens in most tissue, but this effect varies with dose and specific tissue type.

Dobutamine 2.5 to 40 μg/kg/minute is a useful β-receptor agonist because it increases cardiac output and lowers filling pressures without excessive rise or fall of blood pressure.

Isoproterenol (Isuprel) in a 0.02 to 0.06 mg IV bolus or 0.5 to 10.0 μg/min IV infusion, stimulates β$_1$- and β$_2$-adrenergic receptors and enhances vasodilation more than the other catecholamines. This can result in unwanted hypotension in some circumstances, but it is also less likely to cause a reflex increase in vagal tone than other drugs.

Epinephrine in 1 mg IV boluses for cardiac arrest, 0.2 to 1 mg subcutaneously, or 0.5 to 5 μg/min IV stimulates both α- and β-adrenergic receptors. It is recommended for asystolic cardiac arrest in part because it increases myocardial and cerebral flow. However, the increase of systemic vascular resistance may be detrimental by augmenting metabolic acidosis and decreasing cardiac performance in patients with poor left ventricular function. The suggested dose ranges are broad because the response, such as improved AV conduction, to β-adrenergic stimulants varies widely and may be affected by β-adrenergic receptor down-regulation in patients with chronic elevations in sympathetic activity, such as patients with long-standing heart failure.

Any of these agents can precipitate tachyarrhythmias by direct electrophysiologic effects mediated by adrenergic receptors and indirect effects such as myocardial ischemia, and they can worsen hemodynamic status. The adverse effects of catecholamines are time dependent and cumulative. Ischemia and receptor-mediated electrophysiologic effects occur immediately after administration, and changes in gene expression of ion channels begin as early as several hours. Long-term changes such as myocardial hypertrophy, apoptosis, and fibrosis usually begin to occur within 24 hours but can progress over much longer periods. This suggests that the duration and dose of catecholamine infusions should be minimized.

PACING

Temporary pacing includes transcutaneous, transvenous, transthoracic, transesophageal, and transgastric approaches. Transcutaneous pacing provides noninvasive heart rate support as well as immediate access to countershock, but it is often painful, so most patients require sedation, and capture is not achieved in some patients. For these reasons, its principal uses are for short-term pacing during

cardiopulmonary resuscitation and for standby pacing in patients at risk for bradyarrhythmias. If the risk of bradycardia is high, ventricular capture should be verified in advance. Capture is often difficult to ascertain because transcutaneous stimuli cause large deflections on the ECG, and pectoral muscle stimulation can be confused with a pulse. Capture should be verified by careful ECG analysis at sub- and suprathreshold stimulus amplitudes and confirmed by appropriately timed femoral artery pulses, Korotkoff sounds, or arterial pressure waveforms.

Transvenous insertion of an electrode catheter is the method of choice for most patients who require temporary pacing. This approach is reliable and safe when performed by competent staff with strict aseptic technique, fluoroscopic guidance, and appropriate catheters. Complications include inadequate pacing or sensing thresholds, vascular complications, pneumothorax, myocardial perforation, infection, and dislodgment. Small studies suggest that long-term (>5 days) temporary pacing can be accomplished with active-fixation permanent pacemaker leads attached to an external pulse generator.[1] Tunneling the lead can enhance stability and reduce the risk of infection.

Permanent pacemakers are highly effective, safe, and cost-effective and have few contraindications. Although the complications are rarely life threatening, they should be carefully considered and acknowledged. Septicemia or endocarditis has been reported in 0.5% of patients. In patients with pacemaker-related endocarditis, the in-hospital mortality rate is reported to be greater than 7%, with a 20-month mortality greater than 25%. The rate of significant complications has been reported to be 3.5%. About 10% of pacemakers become infected or develop some other type of failure that can require extraction. In one series, the rate of major complications associated with extraction was 1.4%. There is a long-term continuous risk of infection, thrombosis, and erosion. Conventional pacing, that is, from the right ventricular apex, is now known to be detrimental and can cause adverse ventricular remodeling, atrial fibrillation, heart failure, and premature death.

In young persons there is a periodic need to replace generators and leads, which limits venous access sites, and unused leads accumulate or must be extracted. Perhaps of greater consequence is the constant inconvenience of lifelong follow-up, electromagnetic interference, and false alarms from electronic surveillance devices as well as exclusion from important procedures, such as magnetic resonance imaging of the thorax.

Although it has been shown that patients with reduced left ventricular function are at greater risk for adverse effects, it is not known how to identify other patients at risk. Many strategies for reducing the adverse effects of conventional pacing have been proposed and many have been studied, but there is no consensus about which method should be used in the many settings that are encountered. Therefore, the decision for pacemaker implantation also includes selection of lead configuration, lead locations, and pacing mode. Because some configurations change the short- and long-term risks of implantation, patient guidance and education are more complex as well.

Approach to the Patient

The object of the evaluation and management for heart block is to prevent adverse effects by heart rate support in patients with poorly tolerated bradycardia; monitoring and standby heart rate support in stable patients at high risk for asystole or severe bradycardia; identifying and treating reversible causes of heart block; identifying patients at high risk for sudden death, syncope, or recurrent symptoms; and selecting and implanting the appropriate rate support device as soon as safety permits.

Advanced cardiac life-support guidelines apply to the patient who is unresponsive or severely compromised by heart block. However, heart block is rarely the primary problem. Therefore, evaluation

---

[1]Not FDA approved for this indication.

and treatment of other disorders should continue while efforts to increase heart rate are under way.

The initial evaluation should include a thorough history and physical examination, review of current and previous ECGs and rhythm strips, and laboratory tests to determine if heart block is present or if there is a significant risk of heart block occurring in the future and, if so, a differential diagnosis of possible etiologies. The patient should then be stratified for the appropriate level of care: the unstable patient who requires ongoing evaluation and treatment in an intensive care setting, the stable patient at high risk for asystole or complications who needs temporary transvenous pacing or other invasive procedures, the patient at moderate risk who requires continuous monitoring and standby noninvasive heart rate support measures, the patient at low risk who requires rapid but not immediate access to heart rate support measures that hospital monitoring provides, and the patient at low risk who can be evaluated and managed as an outpatient.

Patients who present after resuscitated cardiac arrest or syncope or with ECG abnormalities that indicate conduction system abnormalities usually belong in one of the first four categories. The fifth category usually includes patients with mild symptoms and no suggestive ECG abnormalities and patients whose risk is estimated to be low after inpatient monitoring or previous evaluation. The most common presentation is the patient who has symptoms that could be due to heart block as well as other arrhythmic or nonarrhythmic causes. In such patients, ECG confirmation of the relationship between heart block and symptoms should be obtained.

Determining the need for long-term heart rate support, as well as other issues that can affect selection of implantable devices (e.g., risk for VTAs), should be accomplished as soon as possible because the risks of complications and anxiety associated with temporary heart rate support measures increase over time. Medical societies have developed guidelines for implantable rhythm management devices (http://content.onlinejacc.org/cgi/content/full/51/21/e1). The reasons for the selected therapy, including the rationale for any deviation from established guidelines, should be documented and provided to the patient. This will reduce future confusion or misunderstanding about the original rationale for implantation that can affect management of patients with device complications and those with a compelling need for device upgrade or explanation.

Patients with acute coronary syndromes require special consideration. The incidence of heart block in patients with myocardial infarction based on creatine phosphokinase as the marker of necrosis is approximately 10%. Although the incidence is probably lower using more sensitive markers such as troponin, heart block is still likely to be associated with increased in-hospital mortality due to larger infarct size. Bradycardia reduces myocardial oxygen consumption. Therefore, overcorrection of heart rate must be avoided, and ischemia should be relieved by increasing perfusion as soon as possible.

Studies in the prethrombolytic era did not demonstrate a benefit in mortality with prophylactic temporary transvenous pacing, and complications were common. The risks of transvenous insertion may be higher in patients requiring administration of thrombolytics and other anticoagulants. Catheter-based revascularization methods should be given strong consideration because of established effectiveness, because thrombolytic drugs might be avoided, and because transvenous temporary pacing, if needed, is readily and safely accomplished during the procedure. Suggestions for standby temporary pacing (Box 3) should take into consideration the risks of transvenous pacing based on local circumstances (e.g., experience, fluoroscopic guidance, insertion site, use of anticoagulants).

Most conduction disturbances associated with myocardial ischemia or infarction resolve quickly but can persist for days or weeks. The need for permanent pacemaker implantation as a consequence of myocardial infarction is rare, and prophylactic pacemaker implantation in high-risk subsets has not been shown to reduce mortality. Guidelines for temporary and permanent pacing in acute myocardial infarction have been published (http://www.escardio.org/guidelines-surveys/esc-guidelines//Pages/cardiac-pacing-and-cardiac-resynchronisation-therapy.aspx).

BOX 3 Suggestions for Temporary Pacing in Acute Myocardial Infarction

Transvenous Pacing

Asystole or poorly tolerated bradycardia unresponsive to atropine or aminophylline

Persistent third-degree AV block

Alternating RBBB and LBBB, or RBBB and alternating LAFB and LPFB

Bifascicular block (new)

Second-degree AV block (any type) and QRS $\geq$110 ms

Any indication listed for standby transcutaneous pacing at time of cardiac catheterization if performed

Standby Transcutaneous Pacing

Any indication listed for transvenous pacing until the transvenous pacing system is inserted

Transient asystole or poorly tolerated bradycardia

Bifascicular block (uncertain time of onset or old)

Second-degree AV block (any type) and QRS <110 ms

New first-degree AV block

AV = atrioventricular; LAFB = left anterior fascicle block; LPFB = left posterior fascicle block; LBBB = left bundle branch block; RBBB = right bundle branch block.

Conclusions

Heart block remains a challenge because the cellular mechanisms responsible are poorly understood, prediction of symptomatic heart block (who and when) is unreliable, treatments that restore normal conduction do not exist for most conditions, and pacemaker therapy can have significant long-term adverse consequences. Fortunately, ongoing clinical trials will provide guidance in pacemaker configurations and programming that will minimize adverse effects. Recent achievements in molecular biology suggest we are on the threshold of advances that will elucidate mechanisms and produce treatments that will relegate artificial pacemakers to museum pieces.

Acknowledgments

The author thanks the Marshfield Clinic Research Foundation for its support through the assistance of Linda Weis and Alice Stargardt in the preparation of this chapter.

REFERENCES

Barold SS, Hayes DL. Second-degree atrioventricular block: A reappraisal. Mayo Clin Proc 2001;76:44–57.

Carlson MD, Wilkoff BL, Maisel WH, et al. Recommendations from the Heart Rhythm Society Task Force on Device Performance Policies and Guidelines Endorsed by the American College of Cardiology Foundation (ACCF) and the American Heart Association (AHA) and the International Coalition of Pacing and Electrophysiology Organizations (COPE). Heart Rhythm 2006;3:1250–73.

Elizari MV, Acunzo RS, Ferreiro M. Hemiblocks revisited. Circulation 2007;115:1154–63.

Pierpont ME, Basson CT, Benson DW Jr, et al. Genetic basis for congenital heart defects: Current knowledge: A scientific statement from the American Heart Association Congenital Cardiac Defects Committee, Council on Cardiovascular Disease in the Young: Endorsed by the American Academy of Pediatrics. Circulation 2007;115:3015–38.

Zipes DP, Camm AJ, Borggrefe M, et al. ACC/AHA/ESC 2006 guidelines for management of patients with ventricular arrhythmias and the prevention of sudden cardiac death: A report of the American College of Cardiology/American Heart Association Task Force and the European Society of Cardiology Committee for Practice Guidelines (writing committee to develop Guidelines for Management of Patients with Ventricular Arrhythmias and the Prevention of Sudden Cardiac Death): Developed in collaboration with the European Heart Rhythm Association and the Heart Rhythm Society. Circulation 2006;114:e385–484.

Tachycardias

Method of
Robert Goldstein, MD, and Judith Mackall, MD

Tachycardia refers to a cardiac rhythm with a rate faster than 100 beats/min. Patients presenting with tachycardia typically present with symptoms of palpitation, lightheadedness or near syncope, dyspnea, and chest pain or pressure. Less often they are hypotensive, in congestive heart failure, or unresponsive. The tachycardia can be supraventricular or ventricular in origin and manifest on the surface electrocardiogram (ECG) as a narrow complex tachycardia (NCT), defined as QRS 120 msec or less, or a wide complex tachycardia, defined as a QRS greater than 120 msec.

Mechanisms of Tachycardia

Abnormal heart rhythms result from an abnormality in propagation or formation of impulses. Most tachycardias are caused by reentrant excitation, an abnormality of impulse propagation. Reentry is the mechanism for atrial flutter, atrioventricular (AV) node reentry tachycardia (AVNRT), some atrial tachycardias, AV reciprocating tachycardia (AVRT), some ventricular tachycardias (VTs), and ventricular fibrillation (VF). The three elements necessary for reentry are two pathways, unidirectional block, and an area of slow conduction. The two pathways can be anatomic, such as in dual AV node (AVN) pathways, or functional, such as occurs in some intra-atrial tachycardias. For reentry to initiate, the impulse finds one pathway refractory, resulting in unidirectional block. The impulse then propagates via the second, conducting, pathway. The propagating impulse must have traveled far enough or slowly enough that when it returns to the area previously refractory it now conducts and re-enters the pathway (Fig. 1A).

Arrhythmias due to abnormal impulse formation can be classified into automatic and triggered rhythms. Cells that depolarize generate an action potential or impulse that results in a depolarizing wavefront that propagates through the heart, resulting in a beat. The cardiac action potential results from significant ion shifts through specialized ion channels and other transport mechanisms. The cardiac action potential is divided into phases 0 through 4 (Fig. 1B). During each phase, different ion channel currents are active, depending on their kinetic properties. Cardiac muscle cells normally have a constant resting membrane potential during phase 4.

Cardiac cells in the sinus node, AVN, and His-Purkinje system exhibit *automaticity*. Automaticity is due to phase 4 depolarization caused by a net depolarizing (inward) current. As membrane potential reaches the threshold voltage for sodium current, an action potential is generated. The slope of phase 4 determines the rate at which the cell will reach threshold. Cells in the sinus node typically have the steepest phase 4 and result in heart rates of 60 to 80 beats/min at rest. Cells in the Purkinje system reach threshold at 40 beats/min. Myocardial cells that exhibit increased or enhanced automaticity have a steeper phase 4 slope and fire more rapidly than the sinus node cells. This can occur in the setting of acute ischemia or high catecholamine states. The tachycardia tends to warm up and decelerate slowly, in contrast to reentrant and triggered rhythms, which have sudden onset and offset.

Triggered arrhythmias are different from automatic arrhythmias because they require a triggering beat. Triggered activity due to early after depolarizations (EADs) or delayed after depolarizations (DADs) occurs in atrial and ventricular tissue and is a mechanism of torsades de pointes, atrial tachycardia seen in the setting of digitalis toxicity, and some atrial and VTs that occur in structurally normal hearts. Triggered arrhythmias result from EADs occurring in phase 2 or 3 or DADs occurring in phase 4. EADs are primarily due to the inward depolarizing calcium current that reactivates when phase 2 of the action potential is significantly prolonged. If large enough, an EAD can reach the threshold potential for sodium current and initiate an action potential (Fig. 1C). DADs occur during phase 4 and are caused by a transient inward current. This transient inward current is generated when intracellular calcium overload occurs and spills out from internal stores, activating calcium-sensitive currents. If the DAD is large enough in amplitude, it can reach threshold and initiate an impulse (Fig. 1D).

Narrow Complex Tachycardias

NCTs are diagnosed by the ECG criteria of a QRS duration of 120 msec or less. This implies that the ventricle is being activated by the His-Purkinje system. Entry into the His-Purkinje system occurs via the AVN. All narrow complex tachycardias therefore arise at the level of the AVN or above (from the atrium) and are designated supraventricular tachycardia. Although all NCTs are supraventricular, not all supraventricular tachycardias are NCTs. Some supraventricular tachycardias occur as wide complex tachycardia, which is discussed in the next section.

Initial evaluation of the patient with NCT includes a hemodynamic assessment and a 12-lead ECG. If the patient is hypotensive or unresponsive, or both, synchronized DC (direct current) cardioversion should be performed immediately, using anesthesia if the patient is conscious. If the patient is stable, there is time to assess the regularity of the ventricular rate on the ECG and observe the response of the tachycardia to vagal maneuvers or adenosine (Adenocard).

Irregularly Irregular Ventricular Rhythms

The differential diagnosis of an irregularly irregular rhythm includes atrial fibrillation (AF), atrial flutter (AFl) with variable conduction, and multifocal atrial tachycardia. These arrhythmias are often associated with underlying structural heart disease and conditions of hypertension, pulmonary disease, or valvular heart disease, but AF and AFl can occur in patients without underlying heart disease.

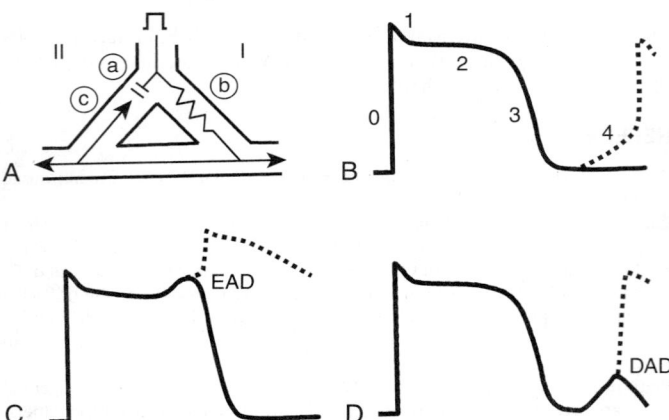

FIGURE 1. A, Diagram of reentry. The impulse is initiated at Π. I and II represent two distinct pathways. *a* represents unidirectional block, *b* represents slow conduction, and *c* shows the propagation of the wavefront reentering the circuit. **B,** A cardiac action potential. The different phases of the action potential are 0-4. Phase 4 demonstrates automaticity, which, when it reaches threshold, will initiate the next cardiac action potential. **C,** A cardiac action potential demonstrating early after depolarization (EAD) at the end of phase 2. **D,** A cardiac action potential demonstrating a delayed after depolarization (DAD) during phase 4.

- A hemodynamic assessment and a 12-lead electrocardiogram should be obtained on every patient presenting with tachycardia.
- A narrow complex tachycardia, defined as a QRS duration of less than 120 msec, can be converted to normal sinus rhythm with the administration of IV adenosine.
- If the rhythm does not convert with adenosine, it is most likely atrial fibrillation or flutter, and the rate can be controlled by administration of an atrioventricular node blocking agent.
- A wide complex tachycardia, defined as a QRS duration of greater than 120 msec, should be considered ventricular in origin if the patient has a history of prior myocardial infarction.
- Ventricular tachycardia can occur in patients with structurally normal hearts; an underlying ion channelopathy or right ventricular dysplasia should be excluded because long-term management differs.
- Radiofrequency ablation is often successful in curing supraventricular tachycardias and some ventricular tachycardias.

ATRIAL FIBRILLATION

AF is the most common arrhythmia. The diagnosis can be made from the surface ECG demonstrating p waves that are chaotic and low amplitude. Originally thought to represent multiple reentrant wave fronts, it is now evident that most result from foci located in the myocardial sleeves of the pulmonary veins. The foci act as drivers that cause fibrillatory conduction resulting in disorganized atrial activation. Because of the disorganized atrial activation, the atria do not contract and the risk of thromboembolism is increased. Refer to the article on AF for treatment options.

ATRIAL FLUTTER

In typical AFl, a macroreentrant wavefront in the right atrium travels counterclockwise around the tricuspid valve. The atrial activation resembles a sawtooth pattern in leads 2, 3, and aVF (Fig. 2). Because

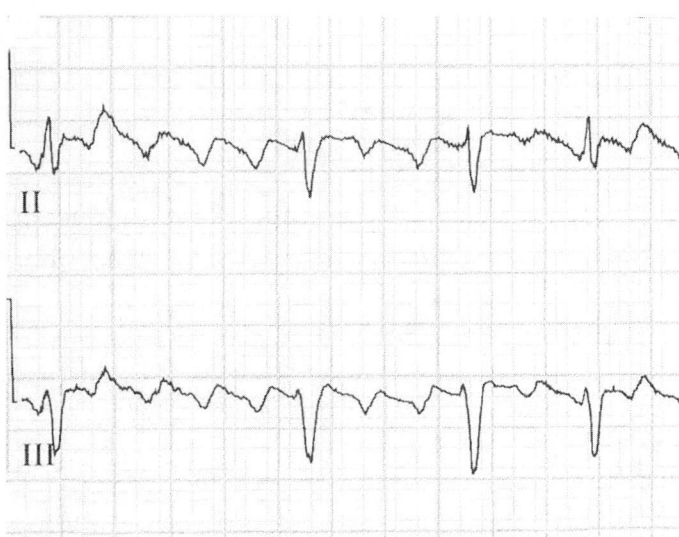

FIGURE 2. Electrocardiogram of leads II and III depicting typical atrial flutter. Note the sawtooth atrial activity.

AFl is not AVN dependent, adenosine[1] will not terminate the arrhythmia. Transient block in the AVN will unmask the atrial activity on the ECG to allow the atrial activity to be evaluated. Acute management focuses on ventricular rate control using AVN blocking agents such as β-blockers or calcium channel blockers. Digoxin (Lanoxin)[1] does not work quickly but may be added for long term additional rate control.

The treatment of AFl is similar to that for AF with regard to anticoagulation. If the duration of the arrhythmia is less than 48 hours, cardioversion can be performed with low risk of thromboembolism. However, if the onset of the AFl is unknown, then anticoagulation with warfarin (Coumadin) should be initiated. The dose should be adjusted to an international normalized ratio (INR) of 2.0 to 3.0. Elective cardioversion can be safely performed after 3 weeks of therapeutic INR.

If the patient is symptomatic or the ventricular rate is difficult to control, a transesophageal echocardiogram can be performed to exclude atrial thrombus, and cardioversion can be undertaken to expedite restoration of normal sinus rhythm. Long-term suppression of AFl requires the use of antiarrhythmic drugs of either class IC (if there is no underlying heart disease) or class III. Because class IC agents slow atrial conduction, recurrent AFl can have a slower atrial rate, resulting in 1:1 AV conduction; therefore, an AVN blocking agent is usually administered with the class 1C drug.

Cure of AFl can be achieved with radiofrequency ablation (RFA) in more than 98% of patients. The macroreentrant circuit in AFl uses the atrial tissue between the tricuspid valve annulus and the inferior vena cava, and radiofrequency energy delivered across the cavotricuspid isthmus prevents AFl from recurring. RFA is the treatment of choice for patients with recurrent AFl.

MULTIFOCAL ATRIAL TACHYCARDIA

The diagnosis of multifocal atrial tachycardia is made from the ECG. In addition to a heart rate greater than 100 beats/min, there are at least three distinct p wave morphologies. The mechanism is either triggered or automatic. It is often seen in patients with hypoxia, respiratory distress, and acidosis. Both β-blockers and verapamil (Calan)[1] have been used, although β-blockers may be contraindicated in the setting of respiratory insufficiency. RFA is not an effective treatment.

Regular Ventricular Rhythms

ATRIOVENTRICULAR NODE REENTRY TACHYCARDIA

The most common regular NCT is AVNRT, and it usually occurs in the setting of a normal structural heart. The ECG demonstrates a regular NCT with no obvious p waves (Fig. 3).

The mechanism of the tachycardia is reentry. In AVNRT, there are dual AVN pathways. The normal or fast pathway lies anteriorly and conducts rapidly with slower recovery time (longer refractory period). The slow pathway lies more inferiorly and conducts slower but has rapid recovery (shorter refractory period). A single premature beat, either premature atrial contraction or premature ventricular contraction, can initiate AVNRT (Fig. 4). In the typical form, a wave of

---

[1]Not FDA approved for this indication.

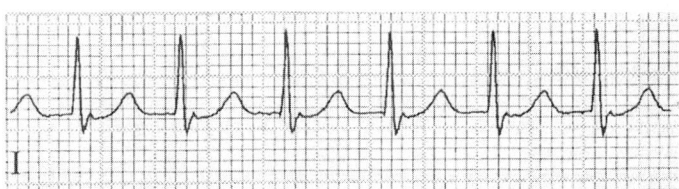

FIGURE 3. A 12-lead electrocardiogram depicting typical atrioventricular node reentry tachycardia. Note the absence of obvious atrial activity or p wave.

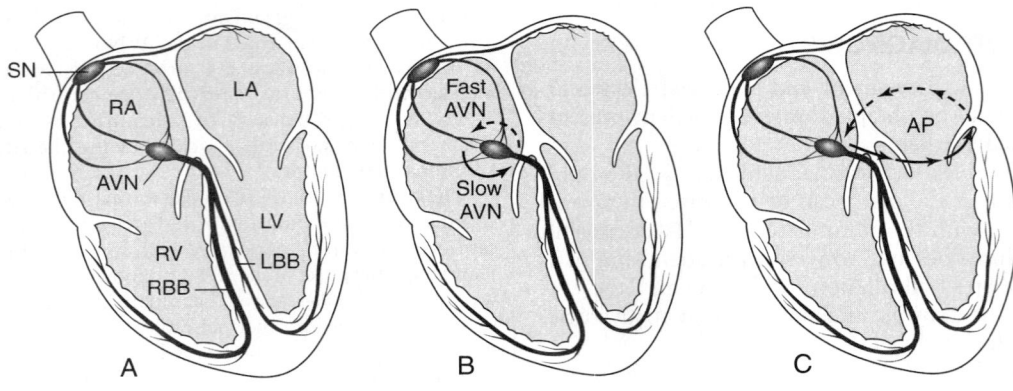

FIGURE 4. A, Normal conduction system. AVN, atrioventricular node; LA = left atrium; LBB, left bundle branch; LV = left ventricle; RA, right atrium; RBB, right bundle branch; RV = right ventricle; SN, sinus node. **B,** Diagram of heart depicting typical atrioventricular node reentry tachycardia (AVNRT) with antegrade conduction via the slow AVN and retrograde conduction via the fast AVN. **C,** Diagram of the heart depicting orthodromic atrioventricular reciprocating tachycardia (o-AVRT) with antegrade conduction via the AVN and retrograde conduction via the accessory pathway (AP).

depolarization from the premature beat finds the fast AVN pathway refractory, and the impulse travels via the slow AVN. Once across the AVN, the impulse continues down the His-Purkinje system to activate the ventricles. At the same time it approaches the His bundle it finds the fast AVN pathway recovered, and the impulse quickly travels retrograde. The retrograde atrial activation and the ventricular activation occur almost simultaneously, which is why the p wave is obscured by the QRS complex on the ECG. Once the impulse reaches the atrium, the slow AVN pathway has recovered and reentry occurs.

In *atypical* AVNRT, the circuit is reversed. The antegrade limb is the fast AVN pathway and the retrograde limb is the slow pathway. Because the retrograde conduction via the slow AVN pathway takes longer, the retrograde p wave occurs well after the QRS complex, and the morphology of the p wave is usually negative in leads 2, 3, and AVF.

Acute management includes administration of adenosine 6 mg IV push, which can be repeated at higher doses if initially unsuccessful. Because adenosine is metabolized by red blood cells, it should be given rapidly via a proximal vein, which will result in a higher dose of adenosine reaching the receptors in the heart. Adenosine, having a half-life of only 9 seconds, causes transient block in AVN conduction. Most often the block occurs in the slow pathway, but it can occur in the fast AVN pathway as well. Because AVNRT is an AVN-dependent rhythm, block in the AVN terminates the tachycardia (Fig. 5). Long-term therapy with a β-blocker or calcium channel blocker can prevent recurrence. RFA of the slow pathway is curative, and because of the high success rate and low risk of complication it is the treatment of choice for recurrent AVNRT.

ATRIOVENTRICULAR RECIPROCATING TACHYCARDIA

Approximately 30% of regular NCT occurs in the presence of an accessory pathway and a single AVN pathway. The accessory pathway is a muscle-like strand connecting the atrium to the ventricle, present since birth, which demonstrates electrophysiologic properties different from the AVN. Many accessory pathways are only able to conduct

retrogradely: the concealed accessory pathway. In patients with an antegradely conducting accessory pathway, activation of the ventricles may be evident in normal sinus rhythm. The ventricles begin to be activated via the accessory pathway, which, because it does not connect to the His-Purkinje system, results in cell-to-cell activation. This inscribes a delta wave at the onset of the QRS. The PR is markedly shortened (<120 msec) because of the ventricular preexcitation via the accessory pathway (Fig. 6).

AVRT can initiate with a premature beat as in AVNRT. When the reentry circuit travels antegrade via the AVN and retrograde via the accessory pathway it is known as *orthodromic* AVRT (see Fig. 4). Because the ventricles activate via the His-Purkinje system, the QRS is narrow. The atria and ventricles do not get activated simultaneously (Fig. 7).

Patients with evidence of accessory pathway conduction on the ECG and symptomatic palpitation are said to have Wolff-Parkinson-White (WPW) syndrome. The incidence of ventricular preexcitation is about 1:1000. Patients often give a history of palpitations since childhood.

Ebstein's anomaly is associated with the presence of posteroseptal and right free wall accessory pathways. Approximately 10% of Ebstein's patients have one or more accessory pathways. Accessory pathways are located throughout the atrioventricular annulus, although they are most commonly at the left lateral mitral valve annulus. Rarely, the accessory pathway has an epicardial course, which can have ramifications regarding therapy.

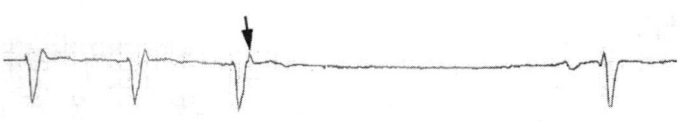

FIGURE 5. Electrocardiogram lead V1 recorded during administration of adenosine. Termination of atrioventricular node reentry tachycardia occurs in the antegrade slow pathway. The *arrow* points to retrograde atrial activity at the terminal portion of the QRS that is sometimes apparent during tachycardia.

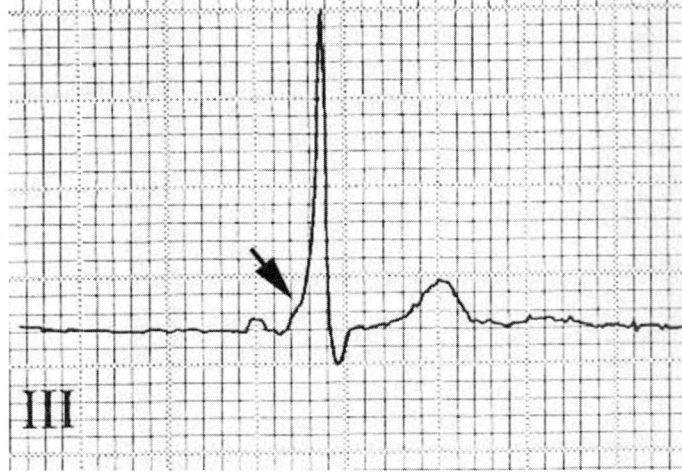

FIGURE 6. Electrocardiogram lead III recording of a QRS demonstrating ventricular preexcitation *(arrow),* also called Wolff-Parkinson-White pattern.

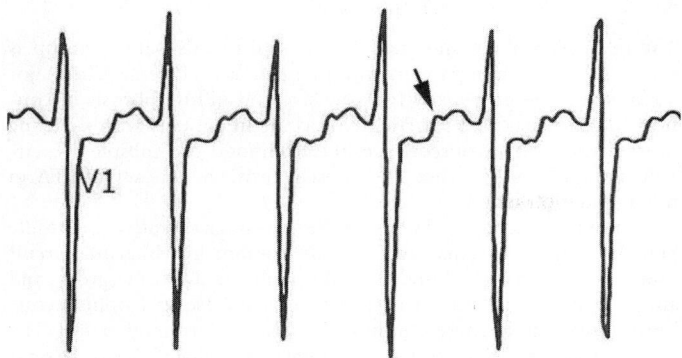

FIGURE 7. A 12-lead electrocardiogram depicting orthodromic atrioventricular reciprocating tachycardia. The *arrow* highlights the atrial activity, which is occurring well after the QRS complex.

Orthodromic AVRT is an AVN-dependent rhythm, and therefore administration of adenosine will terminate the tachycardia. Caution should be used if administering longer-acting AVN-blocking agents because blocking AVN conduction can allow more impulses to travel antegradely via the accessory pathway. Some accessory pathways have short refractory periods, and rapid conduction to the ventricles can occur in AF, with resultant degeneration into VF. This is the mechanism of sudden death in WPW syndrome. Additionally, administration of adenosine can precipitate atrial fibrillation in 10% to 15% of patients. Therefore, if it is unknown whether or not the patient has an antegradely conducting accessory pathway, it is good practice to have a defibrillator present at the bedside during administration of adenosine. For patients with known WPW syndrome (or delta wave on baseline ECG), procainamide (Pronestyl)[1] or ibutilide (Corvert)[1] (drugs that slow conduction over the accessory pathway) can be administered.

ATRIAL TACHYCARDIA

Atrial tachycardia (AT) can be reentrant, automatic, or triggered. They represent 10% of all regular NCT. Because ATs are not AVN-dependent rhythms, administration of adenosine *usually* does not terminate the arrhythmia. In 12% of patients, adenosine does terminate the AT, indicating a triggered mechanism. In automatic atrial tachycardias it can transiently slow the rate. AVN-blocking agents such as β-blockers or calcium channel blockers can be given to control ventricular rate. Treatment can include cardioversion, administration of antiarrhythmic drugs (class IC or class III), calcium channel blockers for triggered AT, or RFA.

SINUS TACHYCARDIA

Sinus tachycardia occurs in the setting of underlying pathologic conditions such as fever, hypoxia, hypovolemia, anemia, postural orthostatic tachycardia syndrome (POTS), or hyperadrenergic states. The treatment should be directed at the underlying condition and not directed at the sinus tachycardia. Sinus tachycardia does not usually exhibit AV block. Uncommonly, isolated sinus tachycardia—sometimes called inappropriate sinus tachycardia—can occur. The pathophysiology of this syndrome is not well established. β-Blockers, calcium channel blockers, and RFA have been used.

Wide Complex Tachycardias

Wide complex tachycardia is defined on the ECG by a QRS duration longer than 120 msec. The differential diagnosis is listed in Box 1. Patients with a wide complex tachycardia in the setting of hemodynamic compromise should undergo electrical cardioversion for

[1]Not FDA approved for this indication.

BOX 1 Differential Diagnosis of a Wide Complex Tachycardia

Supraventricular Origin

Wolff-Parkinson-White (WPW) disease with atrioventricular reciprocating tachycardia or atrial fibrillation
Any supraventricular tachycardia with aberrant conduction or ventricular pacing

Ventricular Origin

Ventricular tachycardia
Arrhythmogenic right ventricular dysplasia
Right ventricular outflow tract ventricular tachycardia
Left ventricular outflow tract ventricular tachycardia
Genetic ion abnormalities: long QT syndrome, Brugada syndrome, catecholaminergic polymorphic ventricular tachycardia

---

prompt restoration of normal sinus rhythm, and only thereafter should the differential diagnosis be considered. If the patient has a history of prior myocardial infarction, the diagnosis is likely VT. Conversely, a wide complex tachycardia in a younger healthy patient with vigorous LV function is likely supraventricular in origin.

If there is ECG evidence of prior myocardial infarction, or the wide QRS complex is a different morphology compared to normal sinus rhythm, the diagnosis is likely VT. When the QRS morphology is identical to the baseline ECG, the arrhythmia is more likely to be supraventricular in etiology.

Several ECG criteria have been published as an aid to help distinguish VT from supraventricular tachycardia (Box 2). Although these are general guidelines, the ECG distinction between VT and supraventricular tachycardia might not be easily discernible. In such situations one should err on the side of assuming VT as the diagnosis, because this is statistically more likely.

Two clinically important wide complex tachycardias occur in patients with WPW syndrome, antidromic AVRT, and AF with rapid, preexcited ventricular conduction. The more common presentation of AVRT is orthodromic AVRT, in which the antegrade limb of the reentrant circuit uses the AV node and the retrograde limb uses the accessory pathway (see Fig. 4C). In antidromic AVRT, seen in patients with WPW syndrome, the accessory pathway is used for antegrade conduction and the AVN is used for retrograde conduction. A single premature atrial contraction or premature ventricular contraction can both initiate and terminate AVRT.

Acute treatment of a patient presenting with wide complex tachycardia should focus on the restoration of normal sinus rhythm. Because antidromic AVRT is an AVN-dependent rhythm, adenosine terminates the tachycardia. Because of the risk of AF in this setting,

---

BOX 2 Electrocardiographic Criteria to Diagnose Ventricular Tachycardia

Atrioventricular dissociation
Right superior QRS axis
QRS duration >140 msec in right bundle branch block morphology
QRS duration >160 msec in left bundle branch block morphology
Precordial lead concordance (QRS complex all positive or all negative)
Absence of an R-S transition in the precordial leads

a defibrillator should be at the bedside. If one suspects AF with WPW, it is critical to avoid AV nodal blocking agents because they can exacerbate the rhythm disturbance by inhibiting AV nodal conduction, thereby preferentially causing rapid conduction to the ventricles via the accessory pathway. In these clinical scenarios, administration of procainamide[1] or ibutilide, which slow conduction in the accessory pathway, is recommended. Curative treatment of antidromic AVRT can generally be achieved safely and effectively with RFA. In most cases, ablation of the accessory pathway also prevents recurrence of AF.

An important area of clinical ambiguity involves the therapeutic dilemma in patients with an asymptomatic WPW ECG pattern. It is generally agreed that patients in high-risk professions (e.g., pilots) should undergo an electrophysiology study and RFA. Some clinicians recommend RFA as first-line therapy even for asymptomatic patients in order to avoid the complications that can arise with this disorder.

Ventricular Tachycardia in Structural Heart Disease

The mechanism of VT in patients with structural heart disease (SHD) is reentry related to the replacement of normal myocardial tissue with fibrotic scar or infiltrative substances, coupled with regions of partial viability resulting in areas of slow conduction and unidirectional block. The three diseases discussed in this section represent the most common causes for VT in SHD.

ISCHEMIC HEART DISEASE

In the United States, the most common clinical presentation of VT is in patients with ischemic heart disease with an incidence of about 5%. Left ventricular function in these patients may be severely compromised with large segments of infarcted tissue. The mainstay of treatment for scar-related VT in patients with ischemic heart disease is the implantation of an implantable cardioverter-defibrillator (ICD) to prevent sudden death from VT or VF.

Despite ICD therapy, additional treatment might be necessary in patients with frequent episodes of VT resulting in ICD discharges. The administration of a class III antiarrhythmic drug or β-blocker, or both, can aid in reducing episodes of VT. Likewise, catheter-based therapy with RFA (targeting reentrant circuits) can improve morbidity from repeated ICD shocks. In patients with depressed ejection fraction (<35%) and ischemic heart disease, ICD implantation is indicated for primary prevention of sudden cardiac death due to VT or VF. Studies suggest that RFA of inducible VTs at the time of ICD implantation can reduce ICD discharges in these patients. Cure of VT related to ischemic heart disease is difficult to achieve owing to the potential for multiple reentrant VT circuits. The goal for treatment following ICD therapy should focus on preventing ICD discharges in this group.

---

[1]Not FDA approved for this indication.

CURRENT THERAPY

- The majority of narrow QRS complex tachycardias are amenable to curative therapy using radiofrequency ablation.
- Wide QRS complex tachycardias are commonly secondary to ventricular tachycardia in the setting of structural heart disease, and effective therapy is accomplished with cardioverter-defibrillator implantation.
- Adjunctive therapy for ventricular tachycardia in structural heart disease includes radiofrequency ablation and antiarrhythmic drug treatment.
- Outflow tract ventricular tachycardia in the structurally normal heart can be effectively treated with radiofrequency ablation.

NONISCHEMIC HEART DISEASE

The pathophysiology and treatment of VT in this patient group is very similar to that of patients with ischemic heart disease. The major difference is the propensity for extensive and diffuse fibrosis in contrast to more localized scarring that occurs in patients with ischemic heart disease. As a consequence, the likelihood of multiple VT circuits is significantly higher, and subsequently, the efficacy of RFA in this population is limited.

A notable exception in which RFA is often curative is bundle branch reentry VT. This is a reentrant rhythm in which the circuit uses the left and right bundles as the limbs of the tachycardia, and although it can be seen in ischemic heart disease and nonischemic heart disease it is most common in dilated cardiomyopathy. The diagnosis should be suspected in patients with dilated cardiomyopathy and a baseline ECG with first-degree AV block and bundle branch block. The clinical VT often has the identical QRS morphology and axis to the patient's baseline bundle branch block. Cure is achieved by RFA of the right bundle branch.

ARRHYTHMOGENIC RIGHT VENTRICULAR DYSPLASIA

Arrhythmogenic right ventricular dysplasia is less common than the aforementioned causes for VT in the SHD population, yet it remains an important cause for VT that should be recognized. It is characterized by fibrofatty infiltration of predominantly the right ventricle (RV), although it rarely involves both ventricles. This is a genetic disorder that has been linked to specific chromosomal defects resulting in mutations in a desmosomal protein gene.

The clinical presentation can vary over a wide spectrum, from asymptomatic patients to those with sudden cardiac death. The ECG VT morphology generally consists of a left bundle branch block with a negative QRS in the inferior limb leads, which suggests origin in the RV free wall. The diagnosis should be suspected in any VT with a left bundle branch block in a younger patient population.

There is currently no single diagnostic test for arrhythmogenic right ventricular dysplasia. A constellation of tests taken together can aid in the diagnosis. An echocardiogram is often nondiagnostic, although on occasion it demonstrates RV dysfunction. Other tests should include an exercise treadmill test, signal-averaged ECG, cardiac MRI, RV angiogram, and RV biopsy. A recent study showed that RV biopsy can identify desmosomal abnormalities, even in grossly normal RV locations.

The mainstay of therapy for VT related to arrhythmogenic right ventricular dysplasia is ICD implantation. There is a minor role for RFA that is predominantly palliative in situations of frequent ICD discharges, and it often requires an epicardial approach.

Ventricular Tachycardia in the Structurally Normal Heart

Ventricular arrhythmias in the structurally normal heart are pathophysiologically distinct from the VT seen in patients with SHD. The mechanism of VT is usually enhanced automaticity or triggered activity rather than reentry. The majority of these patients do not require ICD implantation.

VENTRICULAR OUTFLOW TRACT TACHYCARDIA

RVOT VT is the most common cause for VT in the patient with a structurally normal heart. There is a wide spectrum of clinical presentations varying from occasional premature ventricular contractions to sustained VT. The ECG QRS morphology and axis is distinct, with a left bundle branch block and positive QRS in the inferior limb leads. The mechanism of the VT is triggered activity, and consequently it is often responsive to pharmacologic treatment with adenosine[1] and calcium channel blockers. Additional therapy with

---

[1]Not FDA approved for this indication.

RFA generally has excellent results, with cure achievable in most instances. ICD implantation is contraindicated.

LVOT VT comprises the minority of outflow tract VT (20%), and is pathophysiologically similar to its RVOT counterpart. The ECG usually demonstrates a right bundle branch block morphology with positive QRS in the inferior limb leads.

ION CHANNELOPATHIES

Uncommon causes of VT and VF result from diseases related to cardiac ion channel mutations. These ion channelopathies can cause abnormal repolarization of the ventricles that create a milieu favoring VT and VF. The three most common disorders are long QT syndrome, Brugada's syndrome, and catecholaminergic polymorphic VT. Although the specific mechanism underlying each of these genetic abnormalities differs, the therapy in patients presenting with ventricular arrhythmias is ICD implantation. Primary preventive therapy is unique to each disorder and is a topic of current debate that is beyond the scope of this work.

PACEMAKER-RELATED TACHYCARDIAS

In the majority of pacemaker patients with implanted pacemakers, the paced QRS complex is greater than 120 msec. This is secondary to the cell-to-cell conduction that results from RV pacing bypassing the normal His-Purkinje system. Thus, any tachycardia of atrial origin can give rise to a wide complex tachycardia in pacemaker patients with ventricular tracking of atrial events.

Pacemaker-mediated tachycardia is a second mechanism of pacemaker-related tachycardia. The simplest way of understanding this tachycardia is to compare it to orthodromic AVRT (see Fig. 4). However, rather than the accessory pathway's acting as the antegrade connection, the pacemaker lead acts as the additional pathway. Retrograde conduction is similar to antidromic AVRT using the AVN. A minor pacemaker programming adjustment corrects this abnormality. Placing a magnet over the pacemaker interrupts the tachycardia.

REFERENCES

Blomström-Lundqvist C, Scheinman MM, et al. European Society of Cardiology Committee, NASPE-Heart Rhythm Society. ACC/AHA/ESC guidelines for the management of patients with supraventricular arrhythmias—executive summary. A report of the American College of Cardiology/American Heart Association Task Force on Practice Guidelines and the European Society of Cardiology Committee for Practice Guidelines (Writing Committee to Develop Guidelines for the Management of Patients with Supraventricular Arrhythmias) developed in collaboration with NASPE-Heart Rhythm Society. J Am Coll Cardiol 2003;42(8):1493–531.

Delacretaz E. Supraventricular tachycardia. N Eng J Med 2006;354:1039–51.

Epstein AE, Dimarco JP, Ellenbogen KA, et al. American College of Cardiology/American Heart Association Task Force on Practice; American Association for Thoracic Surgery; Society of Thoracic Surgeons: ACC/AHA/HRS 2008 guidelines for Device-Based Therapy of Cardiac Rhythm Abnormalities: executive summary. Heart Rhythm 2008;5(6):934–55.

Haqqani HM, Morton JB, Kalman J. Using the 12-lead ECG to localize the orgin of atrial and ventricular tachycardias. Part 2: Ventricular tachycardia. J Cardiovasc Electrophysiology 2009;20:825–32.

Monteforte N, Priori S. The long QT syndrome and catecholaminergic polymorphic ventricular tachycardia. Pacing Clin Electrophysiol 2009;32:S52–7.

Pappone C, Santinelli V, Manguso F, et al. A randomized study of prophylactic catheter ablation in asymptomatic patients with the Wolff-Parkinson-White syndrome. N Eng J Med 2003;349:1803–11.

Teh AW, Kistler PM, Kalman JM. Using the 12-lead ECG to localize the orgin of ventricular and atrial tachycardias. Part I: Focal atrial tachycardia. J Cardiovasc Electrophysiol 2009;20:706–9.

Vereckei A, Duray G, Szénási G, et al. Application of a new algorithm in the differential diagnosis of a wide QRS complex tachycardia. Eur Heart J 2007;28:589–600.

Wellens HJ, Bär FW, Lie KI. The value of the electrocardiogram in the differential diagnosis of a tachycardia with a widened QRS complex. Am J Med 1978;64:27–33.

Zipes DP, Camm AJ, Borggrefe M, et al. European Heart Rhythm Association; Heart Rhythm Society, American College of Cardiology; American Heart Association Task Force; European Society of Cardiology Committee for Practice Guidelines. ACC/AHA/ESC 2006 guidelines for management of patients with ventricular arrhythmias and the prevention of sudden cardiac death: A report of the American College of Cardiology/American Heart Association Task Force and the European Society of Cardiology Committee for Practice Guidelines (Writing Committee to Develop Guidelines for Management of Patients With Ventricular Arrhythmias and the Prevention of Sudden Cardiac Death). J Am Coll Cardiol 2006;48(5):e247–e346.

Congenital Heart Disease

Method of
Richard A. Lange, MD, and L. David Hillis, MD

Congenital heart disease affects 0.4% to 0.9% of live births. Nowadays, most survive to adulthood because of improved diagnosis and treatment. Congenital cardiac defects can be categorized according to the presence or absence of cyanosis (due to right-to-left shunting) and the amount of pulmonary blood flow (Box 1).

Acyanotic Conditions

ATRIAL SEPTAL DEFECT

Atrial septal defect (ASD) occurs in female patients two to three times as often as in male patients. Although most result from spontaneous genetic mutations, some are inherited.

The physiologic consequences of ASD result from the shunting of blood from one atrium to the other; the direction and magnitude of shunting are determined by the size of the defect and the relative compliances of the ventricles. A small defect (<0.5 cm in diameter) is associated with a small shunt and no hemodynamic sequelae, whereas a sizable defect (>2 cm in diameter) usually is associated with a large shunt, with substantial hemodynamic consequences. In most patients with ASD, the right ventricle is more compliant than the left; as a result, left atrial blood is shunted to the right atrium, causing increased pulmonary blood flow and dilatation of the atria, right ventricle, and pulmonary arteries (Fig. 1). Eventually, if the right ventricle fails or its compliance declines, the magnitude of left-to-right shunting diminishes.

BOX 1   Categorization of Congenital Heart Disease

Acyanotic Cardiac Defects
Increased pulmonary blood flow
- Atrial septal defect
- Ventricular septal defect
- Atrioventricular canal defect
- Patent ductus arteriosus
Normal pulmonary blood flow
- Aortic stenosis
- Pulmonic stenosis
- Aortic coarctation

Cyanotic Cardiac Defects
Normal pulmonary blood flow
- Ebstein's anomaly
Decreased pulmonary blood flow
- Tetralogy of Fallot
- Eisenmenger's syndrome

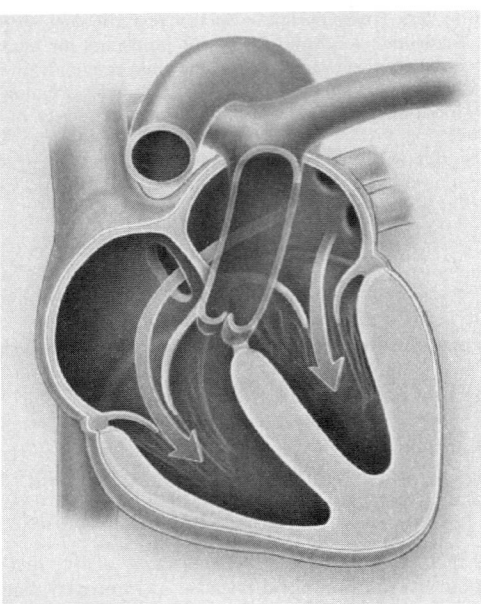

FIGURE 1. Atrial septal defect. Blood from the pulmonary veins enters the left atrium, after which some of it crosses the atrial septal defect into the right atrium and ventricle *(longer arrow)*. Thus, left-to-right shunting occurs. (Reprinted with permission from Brickner ME, Hillis LD, Lange RA: Congenital heart disease in adults. First of two parts. N Engl J Med 2000;342:256-263.)

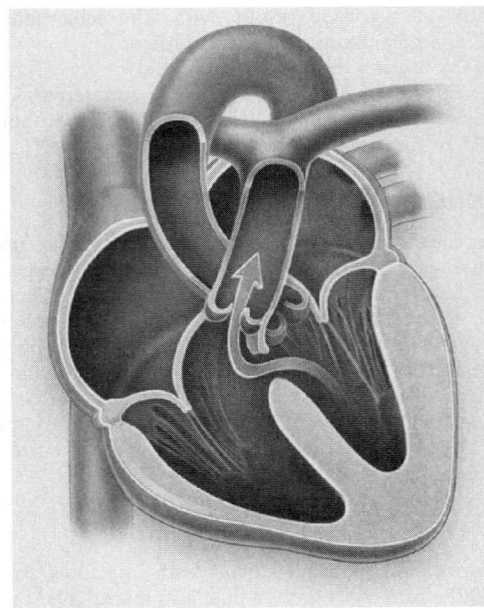

FIGURE 2. Ventricular septal defect. When the left ventricle contracts, it ejects some blood into the aorta and some across the ventricular septal defect into the right ventricle and pulmonary artery *(arrow)*, resulting in left-to-right shunting. (Reprinted with permission from Brickner ME, Hillis LD, Lange RA: Congenital heart disease in adults. First of two parts. N Engl J Med 2000;342:256-263.)

In a patient with a large ASD, a right ventricular or pulmonary arterial impulse may be palpable, and wide, fixed splitting of the second heart sound is present. A systolic ejection murmur, audible in the second left intercostal space, is caused by increased blood flow across the pulmonic valve; flow across the ASD itself does not produce a murmur.

Because ASDs initially produce no symptoms or striking physical examination findings, they are often undetected for years. Small defects with minimal left-to-right shunting cause no symptoms or hemodynamic abnormalities, so they do not require closure. Even patients with moderate or large ASDs (characterized by a ratio of pulmonary to systemic blood flow of 1.5 or more) often have no symptoms until the third or fourth decades of life. Over the years, the increased blood volume flowing through the right heart chambers usually causes right ventricular dilatation and failure. Obstructive pulmonary vascular disease (Eisenmenger's syndrome) occurs uncommonly in adults with ASD.

The symptomatic patient with an ASD typically reports fatigue or dyspnea on exertion. Alternatively, the development of supraventricular tachyarrhythmias, right heart failure, paradoxical embolism, or recurrent pulmonary infections might prompt the patient to seek medical attention. Although an occasional patient with an unrepaired ASD survives to an advanced age, those with sizable shunts often die of right ventricular failure or arrhythmias in their 30s or 40s.

Echocardiography can reveal atrial and right ventricular dilatation and identify the ASD's location. The sensitivity of echocardiography may be enhanced by injecting microbubbles in solution into a peripheral vein, after which the movement of some of them across the defect into the left atrium can be visualized.

An ASD with a pulmonary to systemic flow ratio of 1.5 or more should be closed (surgically or percutaneously) to prevent worsening right ventricular dysfunction. Prophylaxis against infective endocarditis is not recommended for patients with ASD (repaired or unrepaired) unless a concomitant valvular abnormality is present.

VENTRICULAR SEPTAL DEFECT

Ventricular septal defect (VSD) is the most common congenital cardiac abnormality, with similar incidence in boys and girls. Approximately 25% to 40% of them close spontaneously by 2 years of age.

The physiologic consequences of a VSD are determined by the size of the defect and the relative resistances in the systemic and pulmonary vascular beds. A small defect causes little or no functional disturbance, because pulmonary blood flow is only minimally increased. In contrast, a large defect causes substantial left-to-right shunting, because systemic vascular resistance exceeds pulmonary vascular resistance (Fig. 2). Over time, however, the pulmonary vascular resistance usually increases, and the magnitude of left-to-right shunting declines. Eventually, the pulmonary vascular resistance equals or exceeds the systemic resistance; the shunting of blood from left to right ceases; and right-to-left shunting begins (e.g., Eisenmenger's physiology).

A small, muscular VSD can produce a high-frequency systolic ejection murmur that terminates before the end of systole (when the defect is occluded by contracting heart muscle). With a moderate or large VSD and substantial left-to-right shunting, a holosystolic murmur, loudest at the left sternal border, is audible and is usually accompanied by a palpable thrill. If pulmonary hypertension develops, the holosystolic murmur and thrill diminish in magnitude and eventually disappear as flow through the defect decreases.

Echocardiography is usually performed to confirm the presence and location of the VSD and to delineate the magnitude and direction of shunting. With catheterization, one can determine the magnitude of shunting and the pulmonary vascular resistance.

The natural history of VSD depends on the size of the defect and the pulmonary vascular resistance. Adults with small defects and normal pulmonary arterial pressure are generally asymptomatic, and pulmonary vascular disease is unlikely to develop. In contrast, patients with large defects who survive to adulthood usually have left ventricular failure or pulmonary hypertension (or both) with associated right ventricular failure.

Surgical closure of VSDs is recommended if the pulmonary vascular obstructive disease is not severe. Prophylaxis against infective endocarditis is recommended for patients with unrepaired VSD and those with a residual shunt despite surgical correction.

ATRIOVENTRICULAR CANAL DEFECT

The endocardial cushions normally fuse to form the tricuspid and mitral valves as well as the atrial and ventricular septa. Atrioventricular (AV) canal defects are caused by incomplete fusion of the endocardial cushions during embryonic development. They are the most common congenital cardiac abnormality in patients with Down syndrome.

Such cushion defects include a spectrum of abnormalities, ranging from ASD with a cleft anterior mitral valve leaflet to a common AV canal defect in which a single AV valve in association with a large ASD and VSD is present.

A common AV canal defect permits substantial left-to-right shunting at both the atrial and ventricular levels, which leads to excessive pulmonary blood flow and resultant pulmonary congestion within months of birth. Eventually, the excessive pulmonary blood flow leads to irreversible pulmonary vascular obstruction (e.g., Eisenmenger's physiology).

In the patient with an AV canal defect and left-to-right intracardiac shunting, the physical examination reveals a loud holosystolic murmur audible throughout the precordium. As pulmonary vascular resistance increases, the holosystolic murmur diminishes in intensity and duration, eventually disappearing as flow through the defect decreases.

AV canal defects require surgical repair if the magnitude of pulmonary vascular obstructive disease is not prohibitive. Although such patients might initially benefit from medical treatment with diuretics and afterload reduction, the onset of heart failure symptoms is generally the point at which surgery is considered. Prophylaxis against infective endocarditis is recommended for patients with repaired and unrepaired AV canal defects.

PATENT DUCTUS ARTERIOSUS

The ductus arteriosus connects the descending aorta (just distal to the left subclavian artery) and the left pulmonary artery. In the fetus, it permits pulmonary arterial blood to bypass the unexpanded lungs and to enter the descending aorta for oxygenation in the placenta. Although it normally closes spontaneously soon after birth, it fails to do so in some infants, so that continuous flow from the aorta to the pulmonary artery (i.e., left-to-right shunting) occurs (Fig. 3). The incidence of patent ductus arteriosus (PDA) is increased in pregnancies complicated by persistent perinatal hypoxemia or maternal rubella infection as well as among infants born prematurely or at high altitude.

A patient with PDA and a moderate or large shunt has bounding peripheral arterial pulses and a widened pulse pressure. A continuous "machinery" murmur, audible in the second left intercostal space, begins shortly after the first heart sound, peaks in intensity at or immediately after the second heart sound (thereby obscuring it), and diminishes in intensity during diastole. If pulmonary vascular obstruction and hypertension develop, the murmur decreases in duration and intensity and eventually disappears.

With echocardiography, the PDA can usually be visualized, and Doppler studies demonstrate continuous flow in the pulmonary trunk. Catheterization and angiography allow one to quantify the magnitude of shunting and the pulmonary vascular resistance and to visualize the PDA.

The subject with a small PDA has no symptoms attributable to it and a normal life expectancy. However, it is associated with an elevated risk of infective endarteritis. A PDA of moderate size might cause no symptoms during infancy; during childhood or adulthood, fatigue, dyspnea, or palpitations can appear. Additionally, the PDA can become aneurysmal and calcified, with subsequent rupture. Larger shunts can precipitate left ventricular failure. Eventually, pulmonary vascular obstruction can develop; when the pulmonary vascular resistance equals or exceeds the systemic vascular resistance, the direction of shunting reverses.

One third of patients with an unrepaired moderate or large PDA die of heart failure, pulmonary hypertension, or endarteritis by 40 years of age, and two thirds die by 60 years of age. Surgical ligation, generally accomplished without cardiopulmonary bypass, carries a mortality of less than 0.5%. Because of the risk of endarteritis associated with unrepaired PDA (about 0.45% annually after the second decade of life) and the safety of ligation, even a small PDA should be ligated surgically or occluded percutaneously. Once severe pulmonary vascular obstructive disease develops, ligation or closure is contraindicated.

AORTIC STENOSIS

A bicuspid aortic valve is found in 2% to 3% of the population and is four times more common in male than female patients. The bicuspid valve has a single fused commissure and an eccentrically oriented orifice. Although the deformed valve is not stenotic at birth, it is subjected to abnormal hemodynamic stress, which can lead to leaflet thickening and calcification. In many patients, an abnormality of the ascending aortic media is present, predisposing the patient to aortic root dilatation. Twenty percent of patients with bicuspid aortic valve have an associated cardiovascular abnormality, such as PDA or aortic coarctation.

In patients with severe aortic stenosis (AS), the carotid upstroke is usually delayed and diminished. The aortic component of the second heart sound is diminished or absent. A systolic crescendo–decrescendo murmur is audible over the aortic area and often radiates to the neck. As the magnitude of AS worsens, the murmur peaks progressively later in systole.

In most patients, echocardiography with Doppler flow permits an assessment of the severity of AS and of left ventricular systolic function. Cardiac catheterization is performed to assess the severity of AS and to determine if concomitant coronary artery disease is present.

The symptoms of AS are angina pectoris, syncope or near syncope, and those of heart failure (dyspnea). Asymptomatic adults with AS have a normal life expectancy. Once symptoms appear, survival is limited: The median survival is 5 years once angina develops, 3 years once syncope occurs, and 2 years once symptoms of heart failure appear. Therefore, patients with symptomatic AS should undergo valve replacement.

PULMONIC STENOSIS

Pulmonic stenosis (PS) is the second most common congenital cardiac malformation (after VSD). Although typically an isolated abnormality, it can occur in association with VSD.

The patient with PS is usually asymptomatic, and the condition is identified by auscultation of a loud systolic murmur. When it is severe, dyspnea on exertion or fatigue can occur; less often, patients have retrosternal chest pain or syncope with exertion. Eventually, right ventricular failure can develop, with resultant peripheral edema and abdominal swelling.

In patients with moderate or severe PS, the second heart sound is widely split, with its pulmonic component soft and delayed. A crescendo-decrescendo systolic murmur that increases in intensity with inspiration is audible along the left sternal border. If the valve

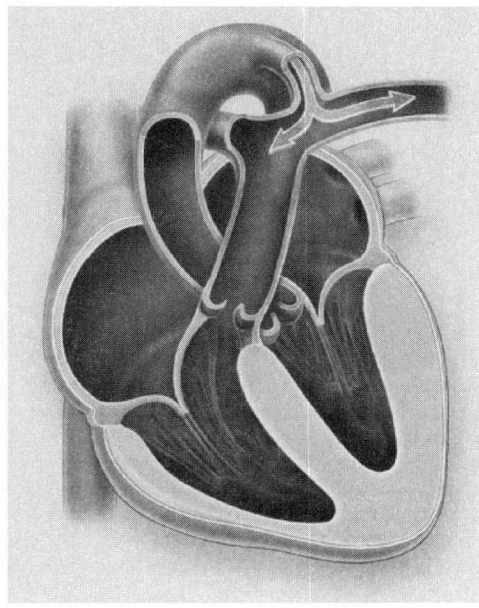

FIGURE 3. Patent ductus arteriosus. Some of the blood from the aorta crosses the ductus arteriosus into the pulmonary artery *(arrows)*, with resultant left-to-right shunting. (Reprinted with permission from Brickner ME, Hillis LD, Lange RA: Congenital heart disease in adults. First of two parts. N Engl J Med 2000;342:256-263.)

is pliable, an ejection click often precedes the murmur. On echocardiography, right ventricular hypertrophy is evident; the severity of PS can usually be assessed with measurement of Doppler flow.

Adults with mild PS are usually asymptomatic and do not require a corrective procedure. In contrast, patients with moderate or severe PS should undergo percutaneous balloon dilatation.

AORTIC COARCTATION

Aortic coarctation typically consists of a diaphragm-like ridge extending into the aortic lumen just distal to the left subclavian artery (Fig. 4), resulting in an elevated arterial pressure in both arms. Less commonly, the coarctation is located immediately proximal to the left subclavian artery, in which case a difference in arterial pressure is noted between the arms. Extensive collateral arterial circulation to the lower body through the internal thoracic, intercostal, subclavian, and scapular arteries often develops in patients with aortic coarctation. The condition, which is two to five times as common in male as in female patients, can occur in conjunction with gonadal dysgenesis (e.g., Turner's syndrome), bicuspid aortic valve, VSD, or PDA.

On physical examination, the arterial pressure is higher in the arms than in the legs, and the femoral arterial pulses are weak and delayed. A harsh systolic ejection murmur may be audible along the left sternal border and in the back, particularly over the coarctation. A systolic murmur, caused by flow through collateral vessels, may be heard in the back.

On chest radiography, increased collateral flow through the intercostal arteries causes notching of the posterior third through eighth ribs. The coarctation may be visible as an indentation of the aorta, and one may see prestenotic and poststenotic aortic dilatation, producing the "reversed E" or "3" sign. Computed tomography, magnetic resonance imaging, and contrast aortography provide precise anatomic delineation of the coarctation's location and length.

Most adults with aortic coarctation are asymptomatic. When symptoms are present, they are usually those of hypertension: headache, epistaxis, dizziness, and palpitations. Complications of aortic coarctation include hypertension, left ventricular failure, aortic dissection, premature coronary artery disease, infective endocarditis, and cerebrovascular accidents (due to rupture of an intracerebral aneurysm). Two thirds of patients older than 40 years who have uncorrected aortic coarctation have symptoms of heart failure. Three fourths die by the age of 50 years and 90% by the age of 60 years.

Surgical repair or intraluminal stenting should be considered for patients with a transcoarctation pressure gradient greater than 30 mm Hg, with the choice of procedure influenced by the age of the patient, anatomic considerations of the coarctation, and the presence of concomitant cardiac abnormalities. Persistent hypertension is common despite surgical or percutaneous intervention.

Cyanotic Conditions

EBSTEIN'S ANOMALY

With Ebstein's anomaly, the tricuspid valve's septal leaflet and often its posterior leaflet are displaced into the right ventricle, and the anterior leaflet is usually malformed and abnormally attached or adherent to the right ventricular free wall. As a result, a portion of the right ventricle is atrialized, in that it is located on the atrial side of the tricuspid valve, and the remaining functional right ventricle is small (Fig. 5). The tricuspid valve is usually regurgitant, but it may be stenotic. Eighty percent of patients with Ebstein's anomaly have an interatrial communication (atrial septal defect or patent foramen ovale), through which right-to-left shunting of blood can occur.

The severity of the hemodynamic derangements in patients with Ebstein's anomaly depends on the magnitude of displacement and the functional status of the tricuspid valve leaflets. On the one extreme, patients with mild apical displacement of the tricuspid valve leaflets have normal valvular function; on the other extreme, those with severe leaflet displacement or abnormal anterior leaflet attachment, with resultant valvular dysfunction, have an elevated right atrial pressure and right-to-left interatrial shunting.

The clinical presentation of subjects with Ebstein's anomaly ranges from severe right heart failure in the neonate to the absence of symptoms in the adult in whom it is discovered incidentally. Older

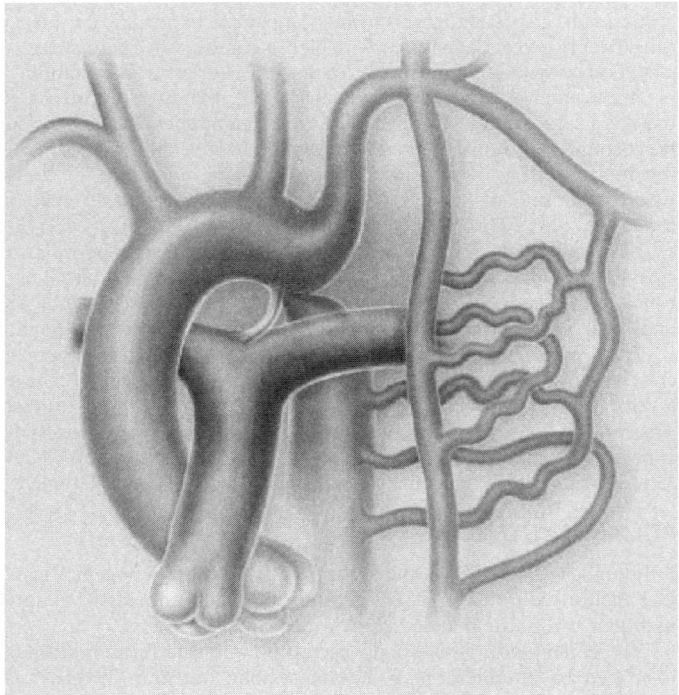

FIGURE 4. Coarctation of the aorta. Coarctation causes obstruction to blood flow in the descending thoracic aorta; the lower body is perfused by collateral vessels from the axillary and internal thoracic arteries through the intercostal arteries. (Reprinted with permission from Brickner ME, Hillis LD, Lange RA: Congenital heart disease in adults. First of two parts. N Engl J Med 2000; 342:256-263.)

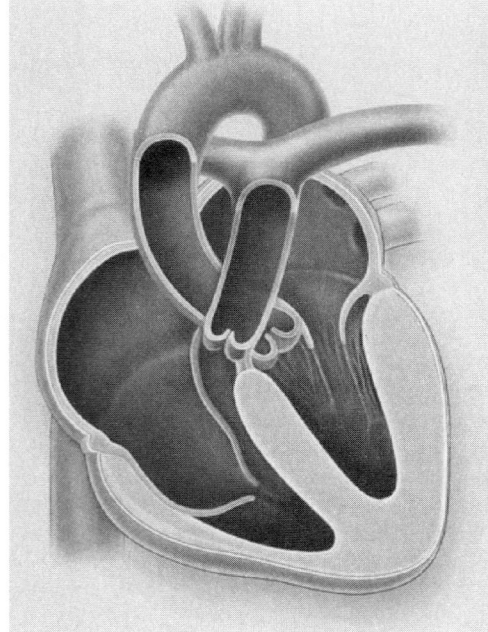

FIGURE 5. Ebstein's anomaly. With Ebstein's anomaly, the tricuspid valve is displaced apically, a portion of the right ventricle is atrialized (i.e., located on the atrial side of the tricuspid valve), and the functional right ventricle is small. (Reprinted with permission from Brickner ME, Hillis LD, Lange RA: Congenital heart disease in adults. Second of two parts. N Engl J Med 2000;342:334-342.)

children with Ebstein's anomaly often come to medical attention because of an incidental murmur, whereas adolescents and adults may be identified because of a supraventricular arrhythmia.

On physical examination, the severity of cyanosis depends on the magnitude of right-to-left shunting. The first and second heart sounds are widely split, and a third or fourth heart sound is often present, resulting in triple or even quadruple heart sounds. A systolic murmur caused by tricuspid regurgitation is usually present at the left lower sternal border.

Echocardiography is used to assess the presence and magnitude of right atrial dilatation, anatomic displacement and distortion of the tricuspid valve leaflets, and the severity of tricuspid regurgitation or stenosis.

Prophylaxis against infective endocarditis is recommended. Patients with symptomatic right heart failure should receive diuretics. Tricuspid valve repair or replacement in conjunction with closure of the interatrial communication is recommended for older patients with severe symptoms despite medical therapy and those with less severe symptoms who have cardiac enlargement.

TETRALOGY OF FALLOT

Tetralogy of Fallot is characterized by a large VSD, an aorta that overrides both ventricles, obstruction to right ventricular outflow (subvalvular, valvular, supravalvular, or in the pulmonary arterial branches), and right ventricular hypertrophy (Fig. 6).

Most patients with tetralogy of Fallot have substantial right-to-left shunting through the large VSD because of increased resistance to flow in the right ventricular outflow tract; the magnitude of right ventricular outflow tract obstruction determines the magnitude of shunting. Because the resistance to flow across the right ventricular outflow tract is relatively fixed, changes in systemic vascular resistance affect the magnitude of right-to-left shunting: A decrease in systemic vascular resistance increases right-to-left shunting, whereas an increase in systemic resistance decreases it.

Patients with tetralogy of Fallot typically have cyanosis from birth or beginning in the first year of life. In childhood, they might have

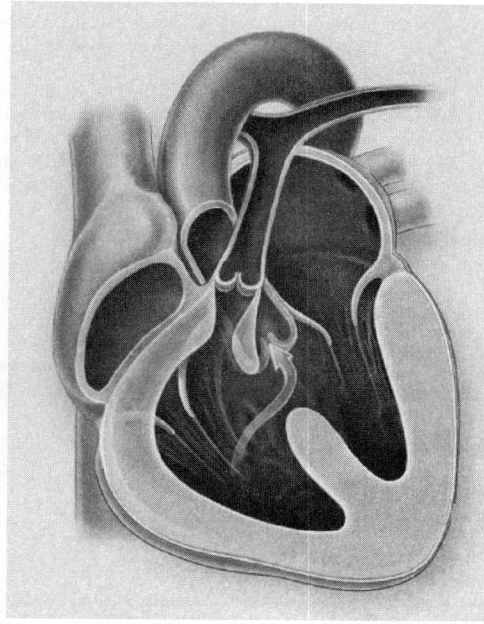

FIGURE 6. Tetralogy of Fallot. Tetralogy of Fallot is characterized by a large ventricular septal defect, obstruction of the right ventricular outflow tract, right ventricular hypertrophy, and an aorta that overrides the left and right ventricles. With right ventricular outflow tract obstruction, blood is shunted through the ventricular septal defect from right to left *(arrow)*. (Reprinted with permission from Brickner ME, Hillis LD, Lange RA: Congenital heart disease in adults. Second of two parts. N Engl J Med 2000;342:334-342.)

sudden hypoxic spells, characterized by tachypnea and hyperpnea, followed by worsening cyanosis and, in some cases, loss of consciousness, seizures, cerebrovascular accidents, and even death. Such spells do not occur in adolescents or adults. Without surgical intervention, most patients die in childhood.

On physical examination, patients with tetralogy of Fallot have cyanosis and digital clubbing. A right ventricular lift or tap is palpable. The second heart sound is single, because its pulmonic component is inaudible. A systolic ejection murmur, audible along the left sternal border, is caused by the obstruction to right ventricular outflow. The intensity and duration of the murmur are inversely related to the severity of right ventricular outflow obstruction; a soft, short murmur suggests that severe obstruction is present.

Laboratory examination reveals arterial oxygen desaturation and compensatory erythrocytosis. Echocardiography can be used to establish the diagnosis and to assess the location and severity of right ventricular outflow tract obstruction.

Complete surgical repair (closure of the VSD and relief of right ventricular outflow tract obstruction) is recommended to relieve symptoms and to improve survival; it should be performed when patients are very young. Those with tetralogy of Fallot (repaired or unrepaired) are at risk for endocarditis and therefore should receive antibiotic prophylaxis before dental or elective surgical procedures.

Patients with repaired tetralogy of Fallot require careful follow-up, because they can subsequently develop atrial or ventricular arrhythmias, pulmonic regurgitation, right ventricular dysfunction, or recurrent obstruction of the right ventricular outflow tract.

EISENMENGER'S SYNDROME

With substantial left-to-right shunting, the pulmonary vasculature is exposed to increased blood flow under increased pressure, often resulting in pulmonary vascular obstructive disease. As the pulmonary vascular resistance approaches or exceeds systemic resistance, the shunt is reversed (right-to-left shunting develops), and cyanosis appears (Fig. 7).

Most patients with Eisenmenger's syndrome have impaired exercise tolerance and exertional dyspnea. Palpitations are common and most often result from atrial fibrillation or flutter. As erythrocytosis (due to arterial desaturation) develops, symptoms of hyperviscosity (visual disturbances, fatigue, headache, dizziness, and paresthesias) can appear. Patients with Eisenmenger's syndrome can experience hemoptysis, bleeding complications, cerebrovascular accidents, brain abscess, syncope, and sudden death.

Eisenmenger's syndrome patients typically have digital clubbing and cyanosis, a right parasternal heave (due to right ventricular hypertrophy), and a prominent pulmonic component of the second heart sound. The murmur caused by a VSD, PDA, or ASD disappears when Eisenmenger's syndrome develops.

The chest x-ray reveals normal heart size, prominent central pulmonary arteries, and diminished vascular markings (pruning) of the peripheral vessels. On transthoracic echocardiography, evidence of right ventricular pressure overload and pulmonary hypertension is present. The underlying cardiac defect can usually be visualized, although shunting across the defect may be difficult to demonstrate by Doppler because of the low jet velocity.

 CURRENT DIAGNOSIS

- Examine blood pressures in arms and legs, pulse oximetry, mucous membranes and nail beds, respiratory rate, and peripheral pulses.
- In addition to listening over the precordium for heart sounds and murmurs, palpate for thrills and evidence of right or left chamber enlargement.
- Ancillary testing should include chest radiography, electrocardiography, and echocardiography.
- Consult a cardiologist if the physical examination or ancillary tests suggest congenital heart disease.

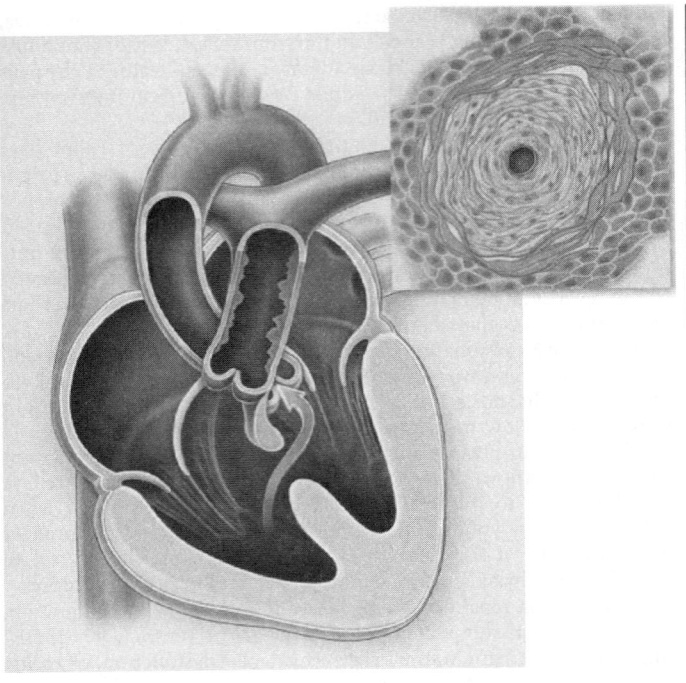

FIGURE 7. Eisenmenger's syndrome. In response to substantial left-to-right shunting, morphologic alterations occur in the small pulmonary arteries and arterioles *(inset),* leading to pulmonary hypertension and the resultant reversal of the intracardiac shunt *(arrow).* In the small pulmonary arteries and arterioles, medial hypertrophy, intimal cellular proliferation, and fibrosis lead to narrowing or closure of the vessel lumina. With sustained pulmonary hypertension, extensive atherosclerosis and calcification often develop in the large pulmonary arteries. (Reprinted with permission from Brickner ME, Hillis LD, Lange RA: Congenital heart disease in adults. Second of two parts. N Engl J Med 2000;342:334-342.)

 ## CURRENT THERAPY

- All congenital heart disease patients should have long-term follow-up for possible complications.
- Endocarditis prophylaxis is recommended for subjects with:
    - Unrepaired cyanotic congenital heart disease
    - Recently repaired congenital heart disease (<6 months after surgical or percutaneous repair)
    - Repaired congenital heart disease with residual defects
- Closure of defects with large left-to-right shunts (i.e., atrial septal defect, ventricular septal defect, atrioventricular canal, or patent ductus arteriosus) is recommended unless pulmonary vascular obstructive disease is far advanced.
- Patients with bicuspid aortic valves should be monitored for aortic root dilatation.
- Pregnancy should be avoided in women with cyanotic congenital heart disease because of high maternal and fetal morbidity and mortality.

Even though patients with Eisenmenger's syndrome have severe pulmonary hypertension, they have a favorable long-term survival: 80% at 10 years after diagnosis, 77% at 15 years, and 42% at 25 years. Death is usually sudden, presumably caused by arrhythmias, but some patients die of heart failure, hemoptysis, brain abscess, or stroke.

Phlebotomy with isovolumic replacement should be performed in patients with moderate or severe symptoms of hyperviscosity; it should not be performed in asymptomatic or mildly symptomatic patients regardless of the hematocrit. Repeated phlebotomy can result in iron deficiency, which can worsen the symptoms of hyperviscosity, because iron-deficient erythrocytes are less deformable than iron-replete ones. Anticoagulants and antiplatelet agents should be avoided, because they exacerbate the hemorrhagic diathesis.

Patients with Eisenmenger's syndrome should avoid intravascular volume depletion, high altitude, and the use of systemic vasodilators. Because of high maternal and fetal morbidity and mortality, pregnancy should be avoided. Patients with Eisenmenger's syndrome who are undergoing noncardiac surgery require meticulous management of anesthesia, with attention to maintenance of systemic vascular resistance, minimization of blood loss and intravascular volume depletion, and prevention of iatrogenic paradoxical embolization. In preparation for noncardiac surgery, prophylactic phlebotomy (usually of 1 to 2 units of blood, with isovolumic replacement) is recommended for patients with a hematocrit greater than 65% to reduce the likelihood of perioperative hemorrhagic and thrombotic complications.

Lung transplantation with repair of the cardiac defect or combined heart–lung transplantation are options for patients with Eisenmenger's syndrome who are deemed to have a poor prognosis (as reflected by the presence of syncope, refractory right heart failure, a high New York Heart Association (NYHA) functional class, or severe hypoxemia). Because of the somewhat limited success of transplantation and the reasonably good survival among patients treated medically, careful selection of patients for transplantation is imperative. Although pulmonary vasodilators improve exercise capacity, they have not been proved to improve survival.

REFERENCES

Brickner ME, Hillis LD, Lange RA. Congenital heart disease in adults. First of two parts. N Engl J Med 2000;342:256–63.
Brickner ME, Hillis LD, Lange RA. Congenital heart disease in adults. Second of two parts. N Engl J Med 2000;342:334–42.
Deanfield J, Thaulow E, Warnes C, et al. Management of grown up congenital heart disease. Eur Heart J 2003;24:1035–84.
Lange RA, Hillis LD, Vongpatanasin WP, Brickner ME. The Eisenmenger syndrome in adults. Ann Int Med 1998;128:745–55.
Marelli AJ, Mackie AS, Ionescu-Ittu R, et al. Congenital heart disease in the general population: Changing prevalence and age distribution. Circulation 2007;115:163–72.
Warnes CS, Williams RG, Bashore TM, et al. ACC/AHA 2008 Guidelines for the management of adults with congenital heart disease: Executive summary. A report of the American College of Cardiology/American Heart Association Task Force on Practice Guidelines (Writing Committee to Develop Guidelines for the Management of Adults With Congenital Heart Disease). Circulation 2008;118:2395–451.

Hypertrophic Cardiomyopathy

Method of
Mahboob Alam, MD, and
Roberta C. Bogaev, MD

Definition

Hypertrophic cardiomyopathy (HCM) is defined as left ventricular (LV) hypertrophy that is not associated with LV dilation and that occurs in the absence of another systemic or cardiac disease capable of producing wall thickening (e.g., systemic hypertension, aortic valve stenosis).

Epidemiology

Hypertrophic cardiomyopathy (HCM) is a common but complex genetic disorder of the heart. It is equally prevalent in men and women and affects people of many races and nationalities. Echocardiographic studies show that approximately 1 in 500 adults in the general population has the HCM phenotype.

HCM is the most common cause of sudden cardiac death (SCD) in young people in the United States. In community-based patient populations uncontaminated by tertiary center referral bias (and whose HCM is, therefore, more representative of the true disease state), overall HCM-related annual mortality rates have been estimated at 1% in adults and 2% in children.

Although HCM occurs with equal frequency in men and women, it is usually diagnosed in women at older ages and with more pronounced symptoms of heart failure. Most elite athletes who die of SCD, irrespective of its cause, are African-Americans, a group in whom HCM is clinically underrecognized. Yamaguchi syndrome (apical hypertrophy) is most common in Japanese patients.

Pathophysiology

Left ventricular outflow tract (LVOT) obstruction in patients with HCM occurs in mid-systole, is dynamic, and results from the narrowing of the LVOT. This narrowing results in an increased ejection velocity, which produces a Venturi effect that leads to systolic anterior motion of the anterior mitral valve leaflet, thereby further limiting the ejection of blood from the left ventricle. As discussed later in this chapter, risk of sudden death in patients with HCM is multifactorial.

Molecular Genetics

HCM is inherited in an autosomal dominant mendelian pattern and has a diverse genetic etiology; to date, more than 400 mutations affecting at least 11 contractile proteins of the cardiac sarcomere have been associated with HCM. The most commonly involved genes include the genes for β-myosin heavy chain and myosin-binding protein C. Others include the genes for troponin T and I, regulatory and essential myosin light chains, titin, α-tropomyosin, α-actin, β-myosin heavy chain, and muscle LIM protein. The characteristic diversity of the HCM phenotype is attributable to the diversity of causal mutations and, probably, to the influence of modifier genes and environmental factors.

Clinical Manifestations

The clinical presentation of HCM largely depends on the degree of hypertrophy (which manifests as reduced diastolic function) it causes and whether there is also dynamic LVOT obstruction (which can cause syncope, arrhythmias, or both). Sudden cardiac death is often the initial presentation of HCM in young athletes. Usually, HCM patients present with dyspnea on exertion, chest pain, dizziness, and syncope. Chest pain is believed to result from a supply-and-demand mismatch between the hypertrophic LV myocardium and the reduced luminal diameter of the intramural coronary arteries. Dyspnea and reduced exercise capacity result from the stiffness and elevated filling pressure of the LV; in cases of the obstructive form of HCM, mitral regurgitation also contributes to these symptoms. Syncope and SCD are related to dynamic LVOT obstruction and ventricular arrhythmia in disarrayed myocardium, respectively.

Physical Examination Findings

Classic physical examination findings in a patient with dynamic LVOT obstruction include pulsus bisferiens (spike and dome), double or triple apical impulse (triple if a wave is felt), and a fourth heart sound. Patients also typically have pansystolic apical (mitral regurgitation–related) and right upper sternal border mid-systolic ejection murmurs that vary with exercise, Valsalva maneuver, and the degree of dynamic LVOT obstruction. Likewise, it is the particular characteristics (bifid or triple apical impulses), and not the force, of the apical impulse that indicate HCM.

Sudden Cardiac Death

MARKERS OF SUDDEN CARDIAC DEATH

Several markers are used to assess a patient's risk of SCD, including family history of sudden, premature death (especially one or more HCM-related deaths); extreme LV hypertrophy (>30 mm), especially in young patients; a personal history of cardiac arrest or sustained ventricular tachycardia; multiple, repetitive (or prolonged), nonsustained ventricular tachycardia on serial ambulatory Holter electrocardiographic recording; unexplained (non-neural) syncope, particularly exertion-related syncope in young patients; and hypotensive or attenuated blood pressure response during upright exercise. Patients with multiple risk factors have an increased risk of SCD and often require an implantable cardiac defibrillator (ICD). However, a single risk factor, such as family history of multiple sudden deaths, massive LV hypertrophy in a young patient, or frequent or prolonged runs of nonsustained ventricular tachycardia on Holter electrocardiography, can also justify prophylactic ICD implantation. Severe LV hypertrophy was reported to be one of the most important predictors of SCD by Elliott and colleagues, although in their cohort, only 12% of patients had severe LV hypertrophy, and the majority of SCDs occurred in patients with mild to moderate LV hypertrophy.

RISK STRATIFICATION FOR SUDDEN CARDIAC DEATH

Hypertrophic cardiomyopathy is the most common cause of SCD in young persons, including elite athletes. In contrast, elderly patients are not usually targeted for risk stratification because HCM-related SCD is uncommon in this age group and because survival to an advanced age (without overt disease manifestations) itself generally indicates lower risk.

Implanting an ICD remains the only effective therapy for primary and secondary prevention of SCD in patients with HCM. Patients with a history of SCD have a much higher risk of a recurrent event (about 11%) than patients without prior SCD (4%). Antiarrhythmic therapy (with amiodarone (Cordarone),[1] β-blockers, or calcium-channel blockers) has no significant value in preventing SCD.

Diagnosis

Electrocardiography mostly reveals voltage criteria for LV hypertrophy, left atrial enlargement, septal Q waves, and ST-T wave changes in lateral leads. Figure 1 shows a diagram of the clinical decision-making process used when a patient's initial clinical evaluation results suggest HCM.

IMAGING MODALITIES

The usual initial imaging modality is two-dimensional echocardiography, which reveals evidence of LV hypertrophy. About two thirds of patients have asymmetric septal hypertrophy—that is, a ratio of septal thickness to posterior wall thickness greater than 1.3. Other echocardiographic findings include systolic anterior motion of the anterior mitral leaflet contributing to a mid-systolic dynamic LV outflow gradient and some degree of mitral regurgitation; left atrial enlargement; elevated LV filling pressure; and impaired LV relaxation.

Cardiac magnetic resonance imaging (MRI) has increasingly been used to assess LV remodeling, especially after surgical and nonsurgical septal reduction. In patients who have undergone alcohol septal ablation, cardiac MRI can also provide valuable information on the size of induced infarcts, LV diastolic function, and changes in the degree of dynamic obstruction.

---

[1]Not FDA approved for this indication.

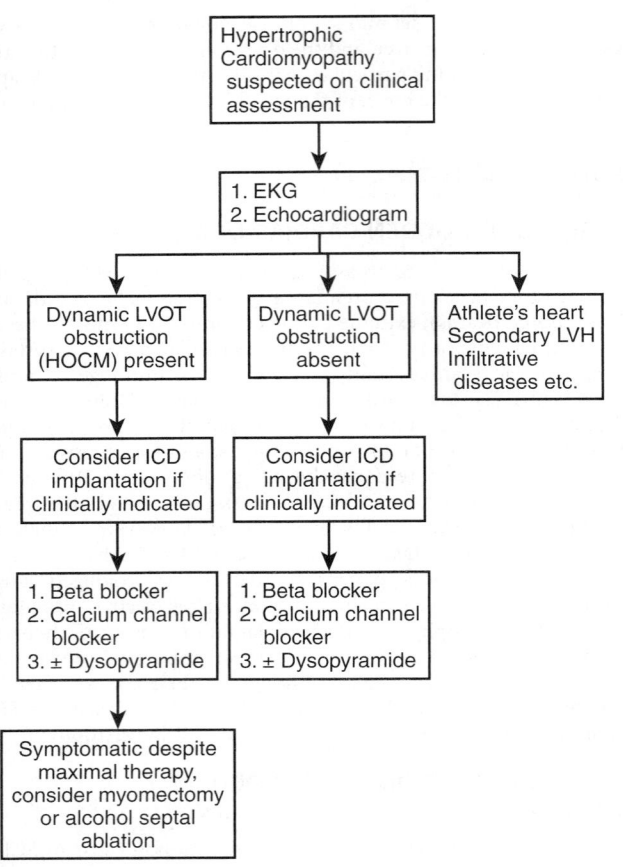

FIGURE 1. Clinical decision-making pathway used when hypertrophic cardiomyopathy is suspected.

Differential Diagnosis

ATHLETE'S HEART

Intensive physical training in endurance sports can lead to a physiologic increase in LV wall thickness, as well as LV mass and cavity size. In some athletes, the LV wall thickness may be comparable to that of patients with HCM. Because HCM is responsible for about one third of SCDs in trained athletes, it is crucial to understand the features that distinguish the physiologic athlete's heart from the HCM patient's heart (Table 1). In a study of 720 trained athletes, Sharma and colleagues found that only 5% had an LV wall thickness that exceeded normal physiologic limits, and only 0.4% had an LV wall thickness greater than 12.0 mm. All of the trained athletes had an enlarged LV cavity (54.4 ± 2.1 mm; range, 52-60 mm). Sharma's group also found lower peak oxygen consumption and anaerobic threshold in patients with HCM than in trained athletes.

SECONDARY LEFT VENTRICULAR HYPERTROPHY (HYPERTENSION OR AORTIC STENOSIS)

A personal or family history of hypertension might advocate secondary LV hypertrophy rather than HCM. Carnitine is an essential substance for β-oxidation of long-chain fatty acids. Patients with HCM have been found to have impaired myocardial fatty acid metabolism and thus higher serum carnitine levels than patients with hypertensive heart disease have. Carotid artery intima-media thickness is a surrogate marker for atherosclerosis associated with hypertension and other risk factors. Carotid intima-media thickness is usually normal in patients with HCM. Differences in serum carnitine levels and measurement of the intima-media thickness of the carotid artery can therefore assist in distinguishing between hypertensive heart disease and HCM.

Aortic stenosis can be distinguished from HCM on the basis of physical examination findings, echocardiography, or hemodynamics measurements made in the catheterization laboratory. Aortic stenosis, in contrast to HCM, is characterized by a delayed and slow rise

---

<table>
<tr><td></td><td></td></tr>
</table>

CURRENT DIAGNOSIS

- Symptoms of dyspnea on exertion, chest pain, syncope, or presyncope.
- Physical examination consistent with pulsus bisferiens, murmurs of mitral regurgitation, and left ventricular outflow tract obstruction.
- Electrocardiographic evidence of left ventricular hypertrophy, left atrial enlargement, and unusual repolarization abnormalities.
- Echocardiogram can reveal hypertrophy, which can be apical or asymmetrical septal; systolic anterior motion of anterior mitral valve leaflet; and mid-systolic left ventricular outflow tract obstruction with resting or provoked gradient.
- Left heart catheterization reveals elevated resting or provoked left ventricular outflow tract gradient with Brockenbrough-Braunwald-Morrow sign.

Hemodynamic evaluation can be performed echocardiographically by using a measured velocity to calculate an estimated pressure gradient. However, left heart catheterization allows a more accurate assessment with simultaneous direct measurement of the LV pressure and the aortic pressure. In patients with the obstructive form of HCM, a gradient can exist at rest or after induction of a premature ventricular contraction. The Brockenbrough-Braunwald-Morrow sign is defined as either a reduction or no change in pulse pressure (LV pressure minus aortic pressure) after a premature ventricular contraction or an extrasystolic beat.

TABLE 1 Characteristics of Patients with Physiologic Athlete's Heart versus Patients with Hypertrophic Cardiomyopathy

Parameter	Athlete's Heart	HCM
Family history of HCM	Negative	May be positive
Family history of SCD	Negative	May be positive
Genetic test for sarcomeric mutation	Negative	May be positive
Echocardiographic Criteria		
LV wall thickness	Usually <10 mm	Usually >12 mm
Asymmetric septal hypertrophy	Absent	May be present
LV mass	Increased	Increased
LV cavity dimensions	Dilated (>55 mm)	Not dilated (may be small)
LV diastolic function	Normal	Impaired
LV filling pressure	Normal	May be elevated
Regression of LV hypertrophy	After deconditioning	Absent
Metabolic Oxygen Consumption		
Anaerobic threshold	Normal to increased	Reduced
Peak oxygen consumption	Normal to increased	Reduced

Abbreviations: HCM = hypertrophic cardiomyopathy; LV = left ventricle; SCD = sudden cardiac death.

of the carotid arterial pulse (pulsus parvus et tardus), systolic ejection murmur, concentric and symmetric LV hypertrophy, abnormalities of the aortic valve structure (e.g., calcification and bicuspid aortic valve), the absence of dynamic LVOT obstruction, systolic anterior motion of the anterior mitral valve leaflet, and the Brockenbrough-Braunwald-Morrow sign. In patients with severe LV dysfunction, dobutamine echocardiography can assist with the diagnosis of severe aortic stenosis.

INFILTRATIVE DISEASES

Infiltrative diseases classically produce a restrictive cardiomyopathy that phenotypically manifests with marked biatrial enlargement and normal-sized ventricles. Patients can have evidence of right ventricular hypertrophy in addition to LV hypertrophy. Serum iron studies demonstrating iron overload and genetic testing for the *HFE* gene are pathognomonic of hemachromatosis.

Other forms of infiltrative disease can be confirmed with endomyocardial biopsy. Sarcoidosis causes caseating granulomas, but these may be too patchy to be evident on limited biopsies, leading to a high false-negative rate. Historically, the gold standard method of confirming cardiac amyloid is the appearance of apple-green birefringence under polarized light after Congo red staining of endomyocardium. Additionally, amyloidosis, sarcoidosis, and HCM each have specific cardiac MRI features that can be used to differentiate among them.

Glycogen-storage diseases, such as Fabry's disease and Pompe's disease, are often diagnosed from their noncardiac clinical manifestations. Mass spectroscopy has increased our ability to diagnose these diseases in newborns. The initial diagnosis of glycogen storage diseases is infrequently made in adult patients.

INFANTILE AND PEDIATRIC CARDIOMYOPATHIES

Infiltrative disorders, including Pompe's disease, Fabry's disease, Kearns-Sayre syndrome, and Danon's disease, can manifest with features of HCM. These disorders cause metabolic or myocardial dysfunction. Genetic defects, coexisting physical examination characteristics, or both can distinguish heritable cardiomyopathies from HCM.

Left ventricular noncompaction is a rare disorder that has been increasingly recognized in adults. The spongy myocardium that develops in these patients is believed to be secondary to an arrest in the final stages of myocardial development, resulting in prominent ventricular trabeculae interspersed with deep recesses. Two forms of LV noncompaction occur: isolated noncompaction, and noncompaction associated with other congenital heart defects. Isolated LV noncompaction in adults has been diagnosed from echocardiographic findings that show the trabeculae associated with the disease.

Treatment

MEDICAL MANAGEMENT

Medical management of HCM aims at treating symptoms of heart failure (mostly diastolic, rarely systolic). The most commonly used agents are β-blockers, calcium-channel blockers, and disopyramide (Norpace).[1] Traditionally, β-blockers, especially long-acting ones, such as metoprolol (Lopressor,[1] Toprol XL), atenolol (Tenormin), propranolol (Inderal),[1] and nadolol (Corgard),[1] are used as first-line agents. β-Blockers slow heart rate and reduce LV myocardial contractility, thus augmenting ventricular filling and relaxation, which decreases myocardial oxygen demand. Additionally, the sympatholytic action of β-blockers can blunt the LVOT gradient during exercise.

CURRENT THERAPY

- Medical therapy, including β-blockers, calcium channel blockers, and disopyramide.
- Surgical myectomy is the preferred therapy for patients with obstruction who remain symptomatic despite maximal medical therapy.
- Alcohol septal ablation is a minimally invasive alternative to surgical myectomy for carefully selected patients who have obstruction and who remain symptomatic despite medical therapy.
- Dual-chamber atrioventricular pacing has been used in the past with little success.

Other agents that have been used include calcium channel blockers (e.g., verapamil [Calan SR, Verelan, Isoptin SR][1]) and disopyramide.[1] Verapamil relieves symptoms and improves exercise capacity, mainly in patients without markedly obstructed LV outflow, because of its beneficial effect on ventricular relaxation and filling. Diltiazem (Cardizem)[1] has been used in HCM patients, but its effects have not been studied. Amlodipine (Norvasc),[1] felodipine (Plendil),[1] and nicardipine (Cardene, Cardene SR)[1] should be avoided because they have vasodilative effects but do not slow the heart rate. Calcium-channel blockers pose a risk of hypotension, particularly in patients with LVOT obstruction. Disopyramide, a negative inotrope and antiarrhythmic, is typically considered the third option and is usually used in combination with β-blockers. If patients remain symptomatic (New York Heart Association [NYHA] class III or IV) on maximally tolerated medications, invasive therapies are considered.

DUAL-CHAMBER PACING

Dual-chamber pacing, once promoted as an alternative to surgical septal reduction, has gradually fallen out of favor. In several randomized studies, dual-chamber pacing did not improve objective measures of elevated LVOT gradient, such as exercise time and maximal oxygen consumption.

Subjective improvement in symptoms has been reported but is widely believed to be a placebo effect. Several small nonrandomized studies of dual-chamber pacing have reported subjective improvement in the absence of significant objective improvement in patients with HCM. For example, Ommen and colleagues showed that when compared to surgical myomectomy, dual-chamber pacing produced subjective, but not objective, improvements in exercise tolerance. Patients with HCM and nonreversed septal curvature (i.e., preservation of the elliptical shape of the LV cavity, which is common in elderly HCM patients) were found to have a better response to dual-chamber pacing than patients with reversed septal curvature (i.e., a crescent-shaped LV cavity, which is common in young HCM patients).

ALCOHOL SEPTAL ABLATION

Introduced in 1995 by Dr. Ulrich Sigwart, alcohol septal ablation has been one of the most commonly performed procedures for relieving LVOT obstruction in patients with HCM. Patients selected for this procedure are NYHA class III ot IV despite maximal medical therapy and have a resting LVOT gradient of at least 30 mm Hg or an induced gradient of at least 50 mm Hg. This procedure involves injecting 1 to 3 mL of absolute ethanol into one of the septal perforator branches of the left anterior descending coronary artery. Care is taken to ensure that there are no septal-apical collaterals (which are rare but important to exclude, because they can induce an anterior infarction) by injecting an echo-contrast agent into the first septal perforator and identifying the septal area that will be affected by the injection.

This procedure has been modified since its introduction to include standard echo-contrast, smaller amounts of intravenous alcohol, and use of a temporary transvenous pacemaker. Significant complications of this procedure include complete heart block requiring a permanent pacemaker (which occurs in about 10% of patients). Procedure-related cardiovascular mortality is comparable to that associated with surgical myomectomy (about 1%). Alcohol septal ablation has been shown to effectively reduce the LVOT gradient at immediate, early, and mid-term follow-up.

Although the 2003 American College of Cardiology and European Society of Cardiology (ACC/ESC) guidelines for the treatment of HCM maintain myomectomy as the gold standard, alcohol septal ablation is an emerging and less-invasive therapeutic strategy that is useful as long as it is performed in carefully selected patients at centers with clinical expertise in treating HCM. Longer-term follow-up data are lacking, and there are theoretical concerns about the risk of aggravating ventricular arrhythmia by creating a myocardial scar in the basal septum, although the clinical significance of this risk remains unclear.

MYECTOMY

Surgical septal reduction has been performed successfully for the past 4 decades, producing excellent outcomes. Surgical septal myectomy is the primary treatment option for patients with severe drug-refractory heart failure symptoms (NYHA class III and IV) associated with obstructed LV outflow under basal conditions or with physiologic exercise (gradient $\geq$50 mm Hg). The most commonly used technique (Morrow's myectomy) involves removing 4 to 12 g of basal septal myocardial tissue to abolish the dynamic LVOT obstruction. Follow-up studies have found survival rates of 98% at 1 year, 96% at 5 years, and 83% at 10 years. When performed in centers of excellence, surgical myectomy has a very low operative mortality (<1%).

Athletes with Hypertrophic Cardiomyopathy

All athletes with the HCM phenotype are identified as being at high risk for SCD during competitive sports and should therefore not be allowed to participate in such sports for several reasons. Risks include the possibility of ventricular arrhythmias (under stressful conditions), hemodynamic and autonomic changes, electrolyte abnormalities, and other, as yet poorly understood mechanisms. These athletes are usually allowed to participate in low-static- and low-dynamic-intensity sports, such as golf and bowling.

Conclusion

Although the clinical presentation of HCM is variable and the disease can be caused by diverse genetic mutations, the greatest threat to patients remains the risk of SCD. Appropriate risk stratification and early referral for ICD implantation are the most important measures for decreasing mortality risk in HCM patients. The current risk-stratification algorithm is probably incomplete; some patients who do not meet the current criteria for ICD implantation remain at risk for sudden cardiac death. Other therapeutic strategies (medical therapy, dual-chamber pacing, alcohol septal ablation, and surgical myectomy) attempt to alleviate LVOT obstruction, thereby increasing exercise capacity and diminishing dyspnea.

REFERENCES

Elliott PM, Poloniecki J, Dickie S, et al. Sudden death in hypertrophic cardiomyopathy: identification of high risk patients. J Am Coll Cardiol 2000;36:2212–8.

Kitaoka H, Doi Y, Casey SA, et al. Comparison of prevalence of apical hypertrophic cardiomyopathy in Japan and the United States. Am J Cardiol 2003;92:1183–6.

Maron BJ. Hypertrophic cardiomyopathy: A systematic review. JAMA 2002;287:1308–20.

Maron BJ, McKenna WJ, Danielson GK, et al. American College of Cardiology/European Society of Cardiology clinical expert consensus document on hypertrophic cardiomyopathy. A report of the American College of Cardiology Foundation Task Force on Clinical Expert Consensus Documents and the European Society of Cardiology Committee for Practice Guidelines. J Am Coll Cardiol 2003;42:1687–713.

Maron BJ, Towbin JA, Thiene G, et al. Contemporary definitions and classification of the cardiomyopathies: An American Heart Association Scientific Statement from the Council on Clinical Cardiology, Heart Failure and Transplantation Committee; Quality of Care and Outcomes Research and Functional Genomics and Translational Biology Interdisciplinary Working Groups; and Council on Epidemiology and Prevention. Circulation 2006;113:1807–16.

Olivotto I, Maron MS, Adabag AS, et al. Gender-related differences in the clinical presentation and outcome of hypertrophic cardiomyopathy. J Am Coll Cardiol 2006;46:480–7.

Ommen SR, Nishimura RA, Squires RW, et al. Comparison of dual-chamber pacing versus septal myectomy for the treatment of patients with hypertrophic obstructive cardiomyopathy: A comparison of objective hemodynamic and exercise end points. J Am Coll Cardiol 1999;34:191–6.

Seidman JG, Seidman C. The genetic basis for cardiomyopathy: From mutation identification to mechanistic paradigms. Cell 2001;104:557–67.

Sharma S, Elliott PM, Whyte G, et al. Utility of metabolic exercise testing in distinguishing hypertrophic cardiomyopathy from physiologic left ventricular hypertrophy in athletes. J Am Coll Cardiol 2000;36:864–70.

Sharma S, Maron BJ, Whyte G, Firoozi S, Elliott PM, McKenna WJ. Physiologic limits of left ventricular hypertrophy in elite junior athletes: Relevance to differential diagnosis of athlete's heart and hypertrophic cardiomyopathy. J Am Coll Cardiol 2002;40:1431–6.

Sigwart U. Non-surgical myocardial ablation for hypertrophic obstructive cardiomyopathy. Cardiologia 1998;43:157–61.

Towbin JA. Hypertrophic cardiomyopathy. Pacing Clin Electrophysiol 2009;32 (Suppl. 2):S23–31.

Mitral Valve Prolapse

Method of
Kurt M. Jacobson, MD, and Peter S. Rahko, MD

Mitral valve prolapse (MVP) has been known by many names, including floppy valve syndrome, Barlow's syndrome, click/murmur syndrome, myxomatous mitral valve disease, and billowing mitral cusp syndrome. MVP is a common cardiac valvular abnormality characterized by redundant, floppy mitral valve leaflets; it is often detected initially by characteristic nonejection clicks or a middle- to late-peaking crescendo systolic murmur on physical examination.

Prevalence

MVP is the most common congenital cause of mitral regurgitation (MR) in adults and the most common indication for mitral valve surgery in the United States today. Previously, it was one of the most overdiagnosed conditions within cardiology, with suggested prevalence rates ranging from 5% to 15%. With the use of current diagnostic standards, rates are much lower; the overestimation was a consequence of diverse and nonuniformly accepted two-dimensional echocardiographic diagnostic criteria. Freed and colleagues, using the Framingham study population and applying consistent and more stringent echocardiographic diagnostic criteria, demonstrated a much lower prevalence of MVP (approximately 2.4%). The incidence appeared to be similar among men and women. Gender differences do exist, however. Women tend to have a more benign course, whereas men tend to have more advanced myxomatous disease resulting in a greater chance of more severe MR.

Classification

Primary MVP is characterized by idiopathic myxomatous change of the mitral valve leaflets or the chordal structures or both. Secondary MVP is present when underlying conditions such as Marfan's syndrome, Ehlers-Danlos syndrome, osteogenesis imperfecta, or other collagen vascular disorders are evident. Certain congenital cardiac abnormalities, including Ebstein anomaly, aortic coarctation, hypertrophic cardiomyopathy, and ostium secundum atrial septal defects, are also associated with MVP. Familial variants with an autosomal dominant pattern of inheritance have been identified, and work to identify the genes involved is underway. The reported prevalence of MVP in first-degree relatives is between 30% and 50%.

Pathology

Macroscopic and microscopic changes can involve both the anterior and posterior leaflets as well as the chordal structures of the leaflet apparatus. Macroscopically, the surface area of the leaflet is increased, providing the accentuated, billowing appearance of the valve leaflets. Additional notable changes are thickening of the individual leaflets, increased leaflet length, thinning and stretching of the chordae, and increased circumference of the mitral valve annulus. At the microscopic level (Fig. 1), normal mitral valves have three well-defined layers, each containing cells and a characteristic composition and configuration of the extracellular matrix: the fibrosa, composed predominantly of collagen fibers densely packed and arranged parallel to the free edge of the leaflet; the centrally located spongiosa, composed of loosely arranged collagen and proteoglycans; and the atrialis, composed of elastic fibers. In myxomatous mitral valves, the spongiosa layer is expanded by loose, amorphous extracellular matrix that has more proteoglycans but less collagen and more fragmented elastic fibers. What collagen is present appears to be disorganized and fragmented, giving the appearance of a haphazard layering of the spongiosa. It is this thickening that produces the classic macroscopic appearance of the myxomatous valve on two-dimensional echocardiography.

Clinical Presentation

Most patients with MVP are asymptomatic and will remain so, testifying to the often benign nature of this disease. Previously, various nonspecific symptoms, including fatigue, dyspnea, palpitations, postural orthostasis, anxiety, and panic attacks, were described as an MVP syndrome when present in association with the characteristic nonejection systolic click or middle- to late-peaking crescendo systolic murmur. Other symptoms, including chest discomfort, near-syncope, and syncope, have also been described by patients with MVP. However, in a community-based study, the prevalence of various clinical complaints including chest pain, dyspnea, and syncope was no higher in patients with MVP than in those without evidence of MVP, making such findings nonspecific. In a controlled study that compared symptomatic MVP patients with first-degree relatives with and without echocardiographic evidence of MVP, there also was no association of MVP with atypical chest pain, dyspnea, panic attacks, or anxiety. There was, however, a significant association of MVP with physical findings of systolic clicks, systolic murmurs, thoracic bony abnormalities, low body weight, and low blood pressure. Congestive heart failure, atrial fibrillation,

CURRENT DIAGNOSIS

- A midsystolic click with or without a middle- to late-peaking crescendo systolic murmur is the classic auscultatory finding of mitral valve prolapse (MVP).
- Key examination maneuvers can help differentiate MVP from other valvular heart diseases.
- Diagnostic echocardiographic findings of MVP are systolic billowing of the mitral valve leaflets 2 mm above the annulus into the left atrium.
- The presence of significant myxomatous thickening of the valve leaflets (>5 mm) is significant for prognosis.

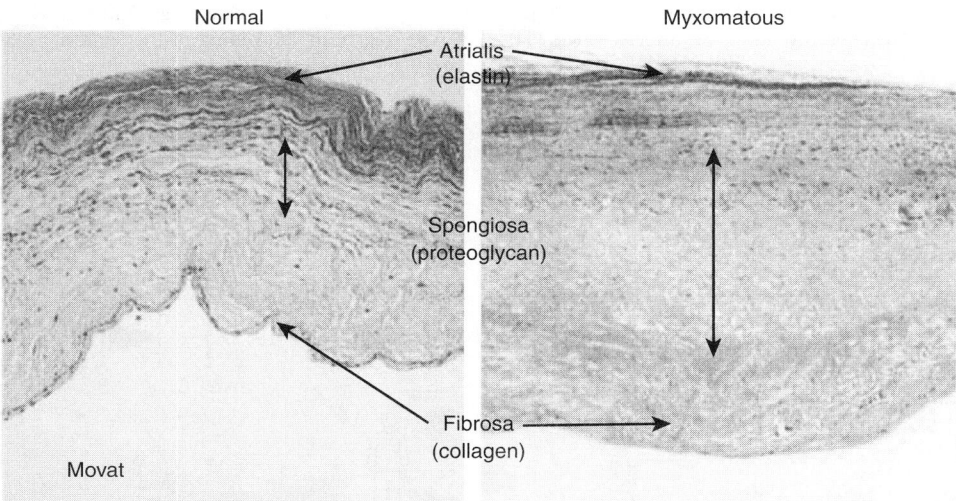

FIGURE 1. Morphologic features of normal mitral valves *(left)* and valves with myxomatous degeneration *(right)*. Myxomatous valves have an abnormal layered architecture: loose collagen in fibrosa, expanded spongiosa strongly positive for proteoglycans, and disrupted elastin in atrialis *(top)*. Movat pentachrome stain (collagen stains yellow, proteoglycans blue-green, and elastin black). (Modified from Rabkin E, Aikawa M, Stone JR, et al: Activated interstitial myofibroblasts express catabolic enzymes and mediate matrix remodeling in myxomatous heart valves. Circulation 2001;104:2525.)

stroke or transient ischemic attack, hypertension, diabetes, and hypercholesterolemia are no more likely in patients with MVP than in those without MVP. However, previous retrospective studies suggested a higher incidence of cerebral embolic events, infectious endocarditis, severe MR, and need for mitral valve replacement in patients with classic (complicated) versus nonclassic MVP. Symptoms of poor cardiac reserve, such as reduced exercise tolerance, dyspnea on exertion, and fatigue, may reflect the presence of significant MR and warrant clinical concern.

Diagnosis

Symptoms are not predictive of the presence or absence of MVP. Certain physical and auscultatory characteristics on examination do support the diagnosis of MVP. Patients with MVP more often have a lower body mass index, have a lower waist-to-hip ratio, and are taller. Findings of scoliosis, pectus excavatum, and hyperextensibility are also prevalent among patients with MVP. The classic auscultatory findings include a midsystolic click and a middle- to late-peaking crescendo systolic murmur heard best at the apex. The auscultatory findings are best elicited with the diaphragm of the stethoscope, and they change in relation to the first and second heart sounds (S_1 and S_2) in response to changes in left ventricular (LV) volume. Therefore, the patient should be examined in several positions: supine (including lateral decubitus), sitting, standing, and, if possible, squatting. Changes in LV filling and volume affect the degree of prolapse.

The most important and most specific finding on auscultation is the presence of a nonejection midsystolic click or clicks caused by snapping of the valve apparatus as parts of the valve leaflets billow into the atrium during systole. Although these clicks can be heard over the entire precordium, they are best heard at the apex. The click can be misinterpreted as a split S_1, a true S_1 with an S_4, or a true S_1 with an early ejection click from a bicuspid valve. It can be differentiated from an ejection click heard in bicuspid aortic valves by its timing relative to the beginning of the carotid upstroke. Ejection clicks occur as the aortic valve opens and therefore precede the carotid upstroke, whereas the nonejection clicks of MVP occur afterward. Clicks from atrial septal aneurysms are uncommon but can be difficult to distinguish from those of MVP. Ejection clicks and clicks from atrial septal aneurysms are not altered by changes in loading characteristics, allowing them to be differentiated from clicks of MVP. Often, but not always, a middle- to late-peaking crescendo systolic murmur can be appreciated by itself or after a click. The

murmur terminates with closure of the aortic valve (A2). This represents MR, and, in general, the duration of the murmur correlates with the severity of the MR. The earlier in systole the murmur is detected, the more severe the MR. Eventually, with more severe MR, the murmur becomes holosystolic. MVP manifestations on examination vary, and they may not always be reproducible, even in the same patient.

Certain maneuvers can aid in more accurately diagnosing MVP on examination (Fig. 2). MVP is very sensitive to LV filling, and subtle changes in auscultatory findings elicited by careful examination maneuvers can be instrumental in separating MVP from other valvular abnormalities. Generally, measures that decrease LV volume or increase contractility produce earlier and more prominent systolic prolapse of the mitral leaflets, causing the systolic click and murmur to move closer to S_1. For example, in the transition from squatting to standing, LV volume is reduced, and the onset of the click and murmur is moved closer to S_1. Conversely, anything that increases LV volume, such as leg-raising, squatting, or slowing the heart rate (increased diastolic filling), delays the onset of the click or murmur and usually diminishes its duration and intensity.

Use of Echocardiography

Two-dimensional echocardiography has proved to be the most accurate noninvasive tool for the diagnosis, assessment, and follow-up of clinically suspected MVP. In fact, physical signs of MVP in an asymptomatic patient are an American College of Cardiology/American Heart Association (ACC/AHA) class I indication for use of echocardiography to make the diagnosis of MVP and assess the severity of MR, leaflet morphology, and ventricular size and function. Once the diagnosis is made, follow-up is determined by the severity of MVP. Routine echocardiographic follow-up of asymptomatic patients with MVP is not recommended unless there are significant findings of MR or LV structural changes. Frequency of follow-up in patients with prolapse and MR is determined by the severity of MR and should be at least annual in patients with severe MR.

Diagnostic criteria for MVP on two-dimensional echocardiography are

- Billowing of one or both mitral valve leaflets or their prolapse superiorly across the mitral annular plane in the parasternal long-axis view by greater than 2 mm during systole
- The degree of thickening of the leaflets

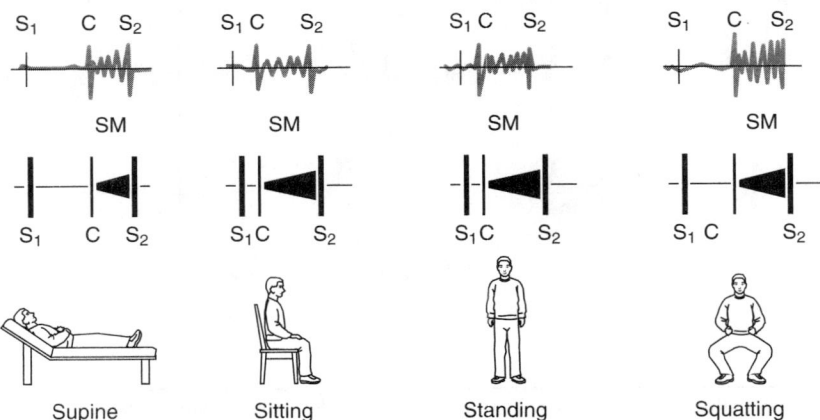

FIGURE 2. Auscultative findings with changes in position in patients with mitral valve prolapse (MVP). *Abbreviations*: C, click of MVP; S_1, mitral valve closure; S_2, aortic valve closure. (Modified from Devereux RB, Perloff JK, Reichek N, et al: Mitral valve prolapse. Circulation 1976;54[1]:3–14.)

CURRENT THERAPY

- Patients with physical findings of mitral valve prolapse (MVP) should have an echocardiogram to confirm the diagnosis, determine the severity of prolapse, determine the amount of myxomatous thickening, document the severity (if present) of mitral regurgitation, and determine left ventricular size and function.
- Uncomplicated MVP without significant mitral regurgitation can be evaluated clinically every 3 to 5 years.
- Complicated MVP (associated with significant mitral regurgitation, left ventricular structural changes, pulmonary hypertension, atrial fibrillation, or stroke) should be observed closely with serial clinical evaluation and echocardiography.
- Surgery may be required for complicated MVP associated with severe mitral regurgitation. Repair rather than replacement is the procedure of choice and should be performed at surgical centers experienced with mitral valve repair.
- Recommendations for surgery are the same for MVP as for other forms of chronic severe mitral regurgitation.

Combined leaflet prolapse of greater than 2 mm and leaflet thickness greater than 5 mm are supportive of classic MVP, whereas prolapse in the absence of increased thickness is considered nonclassic MVP. In addition to more often being associated with the auscultative findings of the click and murmur, the classic form is more commonly associated with increased risk of endocarditis, stroke, progressive MR, and need for mitral valve repair or replacement.

Because the mitral apparatus is saddle-shaped, certain echocardiographic views are more specific than others for determining leaflet prolapse. Most practitioners agree that the parasternal long-axis and apical two-chamber or apical long-axis views are the most accurate for determining prolapse. A finding of prolapse as determined on other views, particularly the apical four-chamber view, is much less specific and frequently leads to a false-positive diagnosis.

Medical Management

Most patients with MVP remain asymptomatic and require no additional management aside from careful observation over time. It is appropriate to provide reassurance that uncomplicated (nonclassic) MVP is a non–life-threatening condition and is unlikely to affect longevity. Periodic clinical evaluation every 3 to 5 years is reasonable. Patients who develop palpitations, lightheadedness, dizziness, or syncope should undergo Holter or event monitoring for detection of arrhythmias. Palpitations are frequently controlled with β-blockers or calcium channel blockers, although the presence of specific arrhythmias may mandate additional therapy. Endocarditis prophylaxis is no longer recommended for patients with MVP unless they have a history of endocarditis or valve replacement. Prophylaxis is recommended for patients who have undergone repair if prosthetic material was used (e.g., in ring repairs). Aspirin or warfarin (Coumadin) therapy may be recommended for certain symptomatic patients with neurologic events who have atrial fibrillation, significant MR, hypertension, or heart failure (Table 1).

Patients with classic (complicated) MVP deserve regular clinical follow-up, particularly if MR is present. These patients are more likely to develop moderate or severe MR over time. Patients with mild to moderate MR and normal LV function should be clinically evaluated at least annually and should undergo echocardiography every second or third year if stable. Patients with severe MR should have an annual echocardiogram and closer clinical follow-up. Those who have severe MR and develop symptoms or impaired LV systolic

TABLE 1 ACC/AHA Recommendations for Oral Anticoagulation in Patients with Mitral Valve Prolapse

Class	Recommendation
I	ASA therapy (75–325 mg/d) for cerebral TIAs
	Warfarin (Coumadin) therapy for patients ≥65 years in atrial fibrillation with hypertension, MR, or history of congestive heart failure
	ASA therapy (75–325 mg/d) for patients <65 years in atrial fibrillation with no history of MR, hypertension, or congestive heart failure
	Warfarin therapy after stroke for patients with MR, atrial fibrillation, or left atrial thrombus
IIa	ASA therapy is reasonable in patients after stroke who do not have MR, atrial fibrillation, left atrial thrombus, or echocardiographic evidence of thickening >5 mm or redundancy of leaflets
	Warfarin therapy is reasonable after stroke for patients without MR, atrial fibrillation, or left atrial thrombus who have echocardiographic evidence of thickening >5 mm or redundancy of leaflets
	Warfarin therapy is reasonable for TIAs that occur despite ASA therapy
	ASA therapy (75–325 mg/d) can be beneficial for patients with a history of stroke who have contraindications to anticoagulants
IIb	ASA therapy (75–325 mg/d) may be considered for patients in sinus rhythm with echocardiographic evidence of complicated mitral valve prolapse

Adapted from Bonow RO, Carabello BA, Chatterjee K, et al: ACC/AHA 2006 guidelines for the management of patients with valvular heart disease. J Am Coll Cardiol 2006;48(3):e1–e148. [Erratum in J Am Coll Cardiol 2007;49(9):1014.]

Abbreviations: ACC/AHA = American College of Cardiology/American Heart Association; ASA = aspirin; MR = mitral regurgitation; TIA = transient ischemic attack.

function require cardiac catheterization and evaluation for mitral valve surgery. Often the valve can be repaired rather than replaced, with a low operative mortality rate and excellent short- and long-term results when performed at experienced centers. Preservation of the native valve allows for lower risks of thrombosis and endocarditis than does prosthetic valve replacement.

Surgical Management

MVP is the most common cause of adult MR requiring mitral valve surgery. Symptoms of heart failure, severity of MR, presence or absence of atrial fibrillation, LV systolic function, LV end-diastolic and end-systolic volumes, and pulmonary artery pressure (at rest and with exercise) influence the decision to recommend mitral valve surgery. Indications for surgery in patients with MVP and MR mirror those with other forms of nonischemic severe MR. Patient outcomes after mitral valve repair are typically very good, and the surgical risk is lower than for many other forms of cardiac surgery, including mitral valve replacement.

Based on a Cleveland Clinic review of 1072 patients who underwent primary isolated mitral valve repair for MR due to myxomatous disease, the in-hospital mortality rate was 0.3%. The Mayo Clinic reviewed 1173 patients who underwent mitral valve repair for MVP from 1980 to 1999, observing mortality rates of 0.7%, 11.3%, and 29.4% at 30 days, 5 years, and 10 years, respectively.

Because of the remarkably low mortality rates associated with MVP repair, some experts advocate earlier rather than later repair of MVP in asymptomatic patients with severe MR and no evidence of LV dysfunction, pulmonary hypertension, or atrial fibrillation. Class I ACC/AHA recommendations for surgery are shown in Table 2.

TABLE 2 ACC/AHA Recommendations for Mitral Valve Surgery in Patients with Chronic Severe Mitral Regurgitation

Class	Recommendation
I	MV surgery is beneficial for patients in NYHA functional class II, III, or IV symptoms in the absence of severe LV dysfunction.*
	MV surgery is beneficial for asymptomatic patients with mild to moderate LV dysfunction.*
	MV repair is recommended over MV replacement in most patients who require surgery, and patients should be referred to experienced surgical centers.
IIa	MV repair is reasonable in experienced surgical centers for asymptomatic patients with normal LV function* if the likelihood of successful repair without residual mitral regurgitation is >90%.
	MV surgery is reasonable for asymptomatic patients with preserved LV function and new onset of atrial fibrillation.
	MV surgery is reasonable for asymptomatic patients with preserved LV function and pulmonary hypertension.†
	MV surgery is reasonable for patients who have a primary abnormality of the mitral apparatus and NYHA class III-IV symptoms and severe LV dysfunction* in whom MV repair is highly likely.
III	MV surgery is not indicated for asymptomatic patients with mitral regurgitation and preserved LV function* if repair seems unlikely.
	Isolated MV surgery is not indicated for patients with mild or moderate mitral regurgitation.

Adapted from Bonow RO, Carabello BA, Chatterjee K, et al: ACC/AHA 2006 guidelines for the management of patients with valvular heart disease. [Erratum in J Am Coll Cardiol 2007;49(9):1014.] J Am Coll Cardiol 2006;48(3):e1-e148.

*Normal (or preserved) LV function is defined as EF >60% and ESD <40 mm; mild to moderate LV dysfunction is defined as EF 30%-60% and/or ESD between 40 and 55 mm; severe LV dysfunction is defined as EF <30% and/or ESD >55 mm.

†Pulmonary hypertension is defined as a pulmonary artery systolic pressure >50 mm Hg at rest or >60 mm Hg with exercise.

Abbreviations: ACC/AHA = American College of Cardiology/American Heart Association; EF = ejection fraction; ESD, end-systolic dimension; LV = left ventricular; MV = mitral valve; NYHA, New York Heart Association.

REFERENCES

Bonow RO, Carabello BA, Chatterjee K, et al. ACC/AHA 2006 guidelines for the management of patients with valvular heart disease: A report of the American College of Cardiology/American Heart Association Task Force on Practice Guidelines (Writing Committee to Revise the 1998 guidelines for the management of patients with valvular heart disease) developed in collaboration with the Society of Cardiovascular Anesthesiologists endorsed by the Society for Cardiovascular Angiography and Interventions and the Society of Thoracic Surgeons. J Am Coll Cardiol 2006;48(3): e1-148 [Erratium in J Am Coll Cardiol 2007;49(9):1014].

Devereux RB, Kramer-Fox R, Brown WT, et al. Relation between clinical features of the mitral prolapse syndrome and echocardiographically documented mitral valve prolapse. J Am Coll Cardiol 1986;8:763-72.

Flack JM, Kvasnicka JH, Gardin JM, et al. Anthropometric and physiologic correlates of mitral valve prolapse in a biethnic cohort of young adults: The CARDIA study. Am Heart J 1999;138:486.

Freed LA, Benjamin EJ, Levy D, et al. Mitral valve prolapse in the general population: The benign nature of echocardiographic features in the Framingham Heart Study. J Am Coll Cardiol 2002;40:1298-304.

Freed LA, Levy D, Levine RA, et al. Prevalence and clinical outcome of mitral-valve prolapse. N Engl J Med 1999;341:1-7.

Gillinov AM, Cosgrove DM, Blackstone EH, et al. Durability of mitral valve repair for degenerative disease. J Thorac Cardiovasc Surg 1998;116(5):734-43.

Levy D, Savage D. Prevalence and clinical features of mitral valve prolapse. Am Heart J 1987;113:1281-90.

Marks AR, Choong CY, Sanfilippo AJ, et al. Identification of high-risk and low-risk subgroups of patients with mitral-valve prolapse. N Engl J Med 1989;320:1031-6.

Rabkin E, Aikawa M, Stone JR, et al. Activated interstitial myofibroblasts express catabolic enzymes and mediate matrix remodeling in myxomatous heart valves. Circulation 2001;104:2525-32.

Savage DD, Devereux RB, Garrison RJ, et al. Mitral valve prolapse in the general population: 2. Clinical features: The Framingham Study. Am Heart J 1983;106:577-81.

Savage DD, Garrison RJ, Devereux RB, et al. Mitral valve prolapse in the general population: 1. Epidemiologic features: The Framingham Study. Am Heart J 1983;106:571-6.

Suri RM, Schaff HV, Dearani JA, et al. Survival advantage and improved durability of mitral repair for leaflet prolapse subsets in the current era. Ann Thorac Surg 2006;82(3):819-26.

Heart Failure

Method of
Elaine Winkel, MD, and Walter Kao, MD

Despite the decrease in the incidence of other circulatory conditions, or perhaps rather because of improvements in the management of related circulatory conditions, heart failure represents the major clinical challenge facing all clinicians who manage patients with cardiac disease today. It continues to be the most common cause of hospitalization for patients older than 65 years of age and results in the expenditure of almost 40 billion dollars annually in the United States. Heart failure is a chronic degenerative disease; if left untreated, it will result in progressively deteriorating functional capacity and premature death. For optimal patient outcome, it must be managed aggressively and proactively.

This discussion focuses exclusively on heart failure resulting from systolic dysfunction, the management of which has been most extensively studied. However, it is now recognized that diastolic dysfunction, particularly of the left ventricle (LV), is an increasingly common condition, particularly in the elderly, and can result in similar symptoms. The optimal management of this vexing condition has yet to be determined with certainty, although there are ongoing efforts to establish evidence-based approaches to this disease as well.

Definition

Although heart failure is defined traditionally as a condition in which the heart is unable to pump enough blood to satisfy the metabolic demands of the body, this expression has little direct clinical relevance. On a practical level, heart failure is perhaps better thought of as a condition involving abnormality of cardiac emptying or filling associated with increased intracardiac filling pressures or decreased cardiac output, exercise intolerance, frequent arrhythmias, and early death. The abnormalities in cardiac structure and function typically precede, often by many years, the onset of symptoms. Therefore, to most effectively treat this disease, it is critically important to affirmatively seek out and diagnose cardiac dysfunction before overt symptoms develop.

History and Physical Examination

In the United States, the most common cause of cardiac dysfunction is coronary artery disease due to atherosclerotic cardiovascular disease (ASCVD). Because ASCVD is typically a systemic rather than a localized phenomenon, any suggestion of atherosclerotic disease in any vascular bed should prompt a thorough cardiac evaluation as well.

Exercise intolerance due to dyspnea or fatigue is the most common presenting symptom in patients with heart failure, although other symptoms may also be present, such as orthopnea, paroxysmal nocturnal dyspnea, dependent edema, or palpitations. Many of these symptoms are nonspecific, and a high index of suspicion is necessary to diagnose underlying heart failure. Other historical findings that should heighten the suspicion for underlying heart failure include the presence of predisposing conditions such as hypertension, diabetes mellitus or metabolic syndrome, obesity, prior exposure to known cardiotoxic agents, ASCVD, and a family history of premature ASCVD, documented cardiomyopathy, or unexplained premature death. When such characteristics are present, particularly in concert with other suggestive findings from the history or physical examination, they should prompt a more directed evaluation, including strong consideration of imaging studies to measure cardiac function.

Physical examination findings are often subtle, especially if the underlying disease has been progressing insidiously for an extended period before presentation, as is often the case. The vital signs may be normal, although the heart rate is frequently elevated due to the compensatory hyperadrenergic state associated with untreated cardiac dysfunction. Tachycardia, especially sinus tachycardia, should always be considered a symptom of underlying systemic disease and should spur further investigation. Chronic arterial hypertension is a frequent cause of heart failure, particularly in non-Caucasian populations; it often persists despite substantial degrees of cardiac dysfunction and should prompt additional cardiac evaluation. Increased central venous pressure may manifest as an elevation in measured jugular venous pressure or as systemic edema; however, the latter symptom is frequently nonspecific, being often seen in older individuals with venous insufficiency, obesity, or sedentary lifestyles. In contrast, visceral edema, when detected, is more specifically associated with increased central venous pressure. The carotid impulse is typically normal, although in patients with severe degrees of LV systolic dysfunction the impulse may be less dynamic than normal. Asymmetrical arterial pulses or bruits suggest systemic atherosclerotic disease, including likely coronary artery disease.

The presence of pulmonary rales, although classically described in patients with cardiogenic or noncardiogenic intraalveolar pulmonary edema, is typically seen only with new and rapid onset of cardiac dysfunction, the prototype of which is acute myocardial infarction with associated LV dysfunction. The compensatory potential of pulmonary venous and lymphatic drainage is such that more insidious, slowly developing cardiac dysfunction is most often not associated with intraalveolar fluid; for this reason, the lung fields may be clear on auscultation or even on radiographic examination. In patients with disease of longer standing, in whom one or both ventricular chambers has had a chance to dilate, the apical (LV) impulse may be laterally displaced; in more severe degrees of LV dysfunction, it may not be palpable at all.

The heart sounds are often subtly decreased in intensity due to decreased LV contractile power, but they remain physiologic in the absence of conduction disease. With an acute onset, gallops may be present, particularly an early diastolic sound (S_3); however, a slowly dilating dysfunctional heart may retain a substantial degree of compliance, lessening the chance of an audible filling sound even if LV filling pressures are elevated. In more advanced stages of disease, evidence of impaired peripheral or end-organ perfusion may be present, such as jaundice, cool extremities, delayed capillary refill, or decreased intensity of peripheral pulses. These symptoms are typically accompanied by unequivocal symptoms or other suggestive cardiopulmonary signs of cardiac disease.

Laboratory and Diagnostic Procedures

The chest radiography and 12-lead electrocardiography are simple, rapid, and low-risk procedures that can frequently add to the initial diagnostic impression. Depending on the degree of cardiac chamber dilation, the radiographic cardiac silhouette may be variably affected.

The LV silhouette is most often enlarged in patients with slowly progressive disease, because the LV chamber has had a opportunity to dilate significantly, whereas in instances of acute onset (e.g., acute myocardial infarction without antecedent disease), the LV may appear normal sized. Patients with chronic valvular or coronary atherosclerotic disease may also demonstrate calcification that can be detected on plain chest films. The presence of intraalveolar pulmonary edema typically is easily detected on standard chest radiographs, although pulmonary interstitial edema can be much more subtle and difficult to detect. More commonly, in patients with chronic LV dysfunction and resultant secondary postcapillary pulmonary hypertension, the central pulmonary arteries are dilated and more prominent than normal.

Many electrocardiographic abnormalities associated with heart failure are nonspecific. Because the most common cause of heart failure is coronary artery disease, any indication of ongoing myocardial ischemia or pattern of prior infarction or injury should prompt further intensive evaluation. The presence of arrhythmias, especially those of ventricular origin, also suggests underlying organic cardiac disease.

Standard laboratory results are typically nonspecific but in more advanced cases can yield findings of impaired end-organ perfusion, such as elevations in serum urea nitrogen, creatinine, or liver transaminases. Patients with chronic heart failure may also be anemic and may manifest other chemical evidence of malnutrition or chronic disease. However, patients who have progressed to this degree of impairment typically have a host of other symptoms and signs that point unequivocally to a severe heart failure syndrome. More recently, the presence of elevated levels of plasma brain natriuretic peptide has been associated with cardiac disease in patients with dyspnea. This test has gained increasing popularity as an initial diagnostic tool, although its utility in the diagnosis of nondecompensated heart failure remains to be fully elucidated.

Transthoracic echocardiography has emerged as the most common method of definitively diagnosing LV systolic dysfunction. It is typically available at short notice in most clinical settings and can provide a wealth of structural and functional data in a noninvasive fashion. After the history, physical examination, and standard laboratory studies discussed earlier, echocardiography should be the next diagnostic study performed if cardiac dysfunction is suspected. Although a complete review of the echocardiographic findings typically seen in heart failure is beyond the scope of this discussion, standard studies can establish the diagnosis, provide clues to the underlying etiology, and help guide initial therapy. Moreover, an echocardiographic study obtained at initial diagnosis establishes an important baseline data set to which subsequent studies can be compared to gauge the efficacy of therapy and assist in determining prognosis.

Once the diagnosis of LV systolic dysfunction has been established, an effort should be made to determine the underlying etiology, because it may dictate therapy. Cardiac catheterization, including coronary angiography and right heart catheterization for hemodynamic assessment, should be strongly considered in all patients with newly diagnosed LV systolic dysfunction, because noncontracting or poorly contracting myocardium, if ischemic or hibernating (viable but hypoperfused), may regain contractile strength after proper revascularization. In addition, hemodynamic data obtained during catheterization can assist in guiding medical and surgical therapy for heart failure; moreover, like other initial imaging studies, it can provide valuable baseline information for future comparison. The use of supplemental catheter-based procedures such as endomyocardial biopsy remains controversial, predominantly because of the risk associated with these procedures and the variable sensitivity of routine endomyocardial biopsy in the diagnosis of infiltrative myocardial processes such as myocarditis. In specific cases in which the index of suspicion for certain infiltrative diseases is particularly high, biopsy may be used to confirm the diagnosis. If this procedure is employed, it is important that a sufficient volume and distribution of specimens be collected, to optimize diagnostic yield, and that the procedure be performed by an experienced operator, to minimize the risk of complications.

Provocative testing (e.g., treadmill exercise testing), with or without supplemental imaging modalities such as radionuclide perfusion imaging, is less useful in patients with already established cardiac dysfunction, although the response to exercise testing in a patient with previously undiagnosed heart failure can be revealing. In addition to the likely finding of decreased exercise performance, the blood pressure and heart rate response to increasing exercise demand may be impaired. Further scrutiny (e.g., cardiac catheterization) should follow the demonstration of inducible or fixed myocardial perfusion defects with exercise or of a decreased left ventricular ejection fraction (LVEF). Resting radionuclide ventriculography can also be employed to determine global LV systolic function (LVEF) in patients in whom effective imaging cannot be achieved with echocardiography. Exercise testing with expired gas analysis may be used to determined peak exercise oxygen consumption and has been demonstrated to correlate with prognosis in patients with chronic heart failure. However, its value when measured before optimization of therapy in patients with newly diagnosed heart failure is uncertain.

Classification

Patients with heart failure are classified according to their self-described degree of functional impairment and assigned a New York Heart Association (NYHA) functional class (Table 1). Although it is subjective on the part of both the patient and the interviewer, this classification has long been used for gross estimation of functional status. The NYHA class has been reported to correlate with mortality risk, but its ability to discriminate among patients and its relevance in an individual patient over time remains questionable.

Heart failure can also be classified by evolutionary stage (Table 2), based predominantly on management strategy (pharmacologic, nonpharmacologic, or surgical).

Management of Heart Failure

NONPHARMACOLOGIC THERAPY

Nonpharmacologic heart failure therapy reduces symptoms and improves functional capacity and quality of life. It is vital to provide ongoing patient and family education about dietary restrictions, avoidance of unhealthy behaviors, stress reduction, and energy conservation. Participation in an exercise program to combat deconditioning and promote weight loss improves functional capacity. Close outpatient monitoring, including a heart failure disease management program, improves compliance and reduces hospitalization. Identification and treatment of sleep-disordered breathing, present in as many as 40% of patients with heart failure, can dramatically improve symptoms.

PHARMACOLOGIC THERAPY

Angiotensin-converting enzyme (ACE) inhibitors and selected β-blockers have been shown in randomized clinical trials to improve symptoms and survival in patients with LV systolic dysfunction and are the cornerstones of medical therapy for heart failure. Angiotensin receptor blocking agents, or the combination of hydralazine (Apresoline)[1] and a nitrate, provide similar (but not superior) benefit in patients with contraindications to use of ACE inhibitors. Digoxin (Lanoxin) provides no survival benefit but improves symptoms in patients with atrial fibrillation and in those patients who remain symptomatic on optimal doses of vasodilators. Diuretics provide symptomatic relief if volume overload is present. Antialdosterone agents should be prescribed for all patients with LV dysfunction after acute myocardial infarction and for all other heart failure patients who remain symptomatic despite optimal doses of vasodilator and β-blocker therapy. Antiarrhythmics should be used only for symptomatic atrial or ventricular arrhythmias, because they may be proarrhythmic. Table 3 describes the use of various medications in patients with heart failure.

---

[1]Not FDA approved for this indication.

CURRENT DIAGNOSIS

- Identify the presence of characteristics associated with left ventricular systolic dysfunction.
- Document the degree of left ventricular dysfunction by imaging.
- Ascertain clinical volume and perfusion status.
- Determine the cause of cardiac dysfunction, if possible, with special attention to coronary artery disease.

TABLE 1 New York Heart Association Functional Classification of Chronic Heart Failure

Class*	Symptoms
I	No perceived limitation of physical activity
II A/B	Symptoms with moderate physical exertion
III A/B	Symptoms with low levels of physical exertion (i.e., activities of daily living)
IV	Resting symptoms

*A = early stage; B = late stage.

TABLE 2 Stages of Heart Failure

Stage	Description	Examples
A	High risk for development of HF due to presence of conditions strongly associated with HF development No identified structural or functional abnormalities of the pericardium, myocardium, or cardiac valves No history of signs or symptoms of HF	Systemic hypertension Coronary artery disease Diabetes mellitus Prior cardiac drug therapy Prior alcohol abuse Family history of cardiomyopathy
B	Presence of structural heart disease strongly associated with HF development No history of signs or symptoms of HF	LV hypertrophy or fibrosis LV dilation or dysfunction Asymptomatic valvular heart disease Previous myocardial infarction
C	Current or prior symptoms of HF with underlying structural heart disease	Dyspnea or fatigue from LV systolic dysfunction Asymptomatic patient undergoing treatment for prior symptoms of HF
D	Advanced structural heart disease and marked symptoms of HF at rest despite maximal medical therapy Requirement for specialized interventions	Frequent HF hospitalizations and cannot be discharged In hospital awaiting heart transplantation Home continuous inotropic or mechanical support In hospice setting for HF management

HF, heart failure; LV, left ventricular.

TABLE 3 Heart Failure Medications

Drug Class	Name/Dose	Comments
ACEIs (in enalapril [Vasotec] equivalents)	10–20 mg bid	Likely a class effect, so agent choice depends on duration of action and tolerability. Higher doses decrease hospitalization rates. Hyperkalemia limits use. Reduced doses may be necessary to allow adequate β-blocker dose titration.
Angiotensin receptor blockers	Valsartan (Diovan) 40–160 mg bid Candesartan (Atacand) 4–32 mg/d	The only two agents in this class to show benefit in randomized clinical trials. Good for patients intolerant of ACEIs. Noninferior but not superior to ACEIs, so use second line. Hyperkalemia limits use.
Hydralazine and nitrates	Hydralazine (Apresoline)[1] 25–100 mg qid with isosorbide dinitrate (Isordil Titradose)[1] 20–40 mg qid	Agents of choice in patients with significant renal insufficiency or other contraindications to ACEIs or aldosterone receptor antagonists.
β-Blockers	Metoprolol succinate (Toprol XL) 100–200 mg/d Carvedilol (Coreg) 25–50 mg bid Bisoprolol (Zebeta)[1] 2.5–10 mg/d	The only three agents in this class to show benefit in randomized clinical trials. Dose is based on body size. Some clinical and survival improvement with lower doses, but target dose is recommended.
Loop diuretics (expressed as furosemide [Lasix] equivalents)	40–100 mg qd or bid	Dietary compliance, fluid restriction, and titration of other heart failure drugs affect dose required.
Aldosterone receptor antagonists	Spironolactone (Aldactone) 12.5–25 mg/d	For patients who remain NYHA functional class III despite adequate doses of vasodilators and β-blockers. Hyperkalemia limits use.
	Eplerenone (Inspra) 25–50 mg/d	For patients with left ventricular dysfunction after acute myocardial infarction. Fewer side effects than spironolactone. Hyperkalemia limits use.
Digoxin (Lanoxin)	0.125–0.25 mg/d	Adjust for renal insufficiency. Women need lower doses. Serum level measurement not routinely necessary; only to confirm toxicity.

[1]Not FDA approved for this indication.
Abbreviations: ACEI = angiotensin-converting enzyme inhibitor; NYHA, New York Heart Association.

353

Parenteral agents for heart failure, including dobutamine (Dobu-trex), milrinone (Primacor), and nesiritide (Natrecor), are used primarily in the inpatient setting to treat acutely decompensated heart failure and are beyond the scope of this discussion. However, it should be noted that intravenous inotropic agents (dobutamine, milrinone) have been shown in uncontrolled trials to improve symptoms and quality of life but to increase mortality. Therefore, they should be used only for short periods, at the lowest possible doses, and in a monitored setting. Short-term inpatient use of nesiritide also improves symptoms.

DEVICE THERAPY

Implantable cardioverter-defibrillators (ICDs) have been shown in randomized clinical trials to improve survival in heart failure patients with ischemic or nonischemic cardiomyopathy. Indications for implantation are an LVEF of less than 30% and mild-to-moderate symptoms of heart failure in a patient whose anticipated survival exceeds 1 year or ischemic cardiomyopathy and an LVEF of less than 35% regardless of symptoms.

Cardiac resynchronization therapy, with or without implantation of a cardioverter-defibrillator, has been shown in randomized clinical trials to improve symptoms and survival in selected heart failure patients when added to optimal medical heart failure therapy. One third of heart failure patients with low LVEF and moderate to severe symptoms have ventricular dyssynchronous contraction, which is associated with increased mortality. Indications for cardiac resynchronization therapy include an LVEF lower than 35%, NYHA functional class III-IV symptoms, and a QRS duration of greater than 120 msec, which is a marker for ventricular dyssynchrony.

THERAPY FOR ADVANCED HEART FAILURE

Patients with heart failure that has become refractory to medical and resynchronization therapy should be referred to an advanced heart failure center experienced in the surgical treatment of heart failure. Surgical therapies improve symptoms and survival and are now considered the standard of care for heart failure patients in whom standard medical therapy has failed.

Heart transplantation is the only definitive surgical therapy for advanced heart failure, but alternative surgical approaches include coronary revascularization, valve surgery, LV reconstruction, and the use of ventricular assist devices. In patients with ischemic cardiomyopathy and hibernating myocardium, coronary revascularization improves LV function, functional capacity, and survival, compared with medical therapy. Mitral valve repair or replacement can improve symptoms in selected patients. Ventricular reconstruction may benefit patients with LV aneurysms or recurrent ventricular arrhythmias.

Left ventricular assist devices are implantable pumps that work in parallel with the native heart to provide short-term mechanical circulatory support in patients who are expected to recover heart function (e.g., patients with myocarditis, after acute myocardial infarction, after coronary artery bypass grafting) and in patients awaiting heart transplantation. In addition, these devices are approved as a permanent alternative to transplantation (destination therapy) in patients for whom heart transplantation is not an option. Early identification and referral of patients who might benefit from these therapies is essential for the best surgical outcomes.

Common Management Errors

Heart failure management errors result in increased hospitalizations and mortality. ACE inhibitors remain underused, despite evidence from clinical trials in more than 10,000 patients. Although Losartan (Cozaar)[1] is commonly used for the patient who cannot tolerate ACE inhibitors, only two members of the angiotensin receptor blocker class, valsartan (Diovan) and candesartan (Atacand), have been shown in clinical trials to provide benefit. The combination of hydralazine (Apresoline)[1] and isosorbide dinitrate (Isordil Titradose)[1] is also underused, despite evidence that these drugs improve exercise tolerance and survival.

[1]Not FDA approved for this indication.

CURRENT THERAPY

- Angiotensin-converting enzyme (ACE) inhibitors, angiotensin receptor blocking agents, β-blockers, and aldosterone receptor antagonists improve survival and are integral to the treatment plan.
- Use nonpharmacologic therapy along with medical therapy. Sodium and fluid restriction, smoking and alcohol cessation, stress reduction and treatment of depression, and exercise and weight loss, all improve symptoms and reduce hospitalization.
- Treat comorbidities that exacerbate the heart failure state (e.g., hypertension, arrhythmias, sleep-disordered breathing).
- Consider interventions to treat concomitant structural heart disease, such as coronary revascularization, mitral valve surgery, arrhythmia treatment, and cardiac resynchronization therapy.
- Refer patients with refractory disease early to an advanced heart failure center for implantation of a ventricular assist device or cardiac transplantation.
- Provide palliative care for patients who are not candidates for advanced heart failure therapy.

Only three β-blockers, metoprolol succinate (Toprol XL), carvedilol (Coreg), and bisoprolol (Zebeta),[1] have been shown in trials to improve symptoms and survival in heart failure patients. Metoprolol tartrate (Lopressor)[1] and atenolol (Tenormin)[1] are commonly used as substitutes, even though there are no data supporting their use. β-Blockers are commonly started too early in the course of heart failure, when the patient is experiencing decompensation and fluid overload, and leads to further decompensation.

Patients may receive drugs that worsen the heart failure state, such as first-generation calcium channel blockers, nonsteroidal antiinflammatory drugs, cyclooxygenase 2 inhibitors, and antiarrhythmic drugs. Intravenous inotropic therapy or nesiritide (Natrecor) may be used when the patient would be better served by optimization of his or her oral heart failure regimen. Patients are commonly overdiuresed, which results in symptomatic hypotension and makes initiation and titration of vasodilators and β-blockers difficult.

Many physicians fail to utilize nonpharmacologic therapies as an adjunct to drug therapy. In addition, lack of education and close follow-up can undermine the best medical regimen. Physicians also commonly fail to refer patients who need advanced heart failure therapy, or refer them too late, when end-organ damage is irreversible.

---

[1]Not FDA approved for this indication.

REFERENCES

Bardy GH, Lee KL, Mark DB, et al. Amiodarone or an implantable cardioverter defibrillator for congestive heart failure. N Engl J Med 2005;352:225–37.

Cleland JG, Daubert JC, Erdmann E, et al. The effect of cardiac resynchronization on morbidity and mortality in heart failure. N Engl J Med 2005;352:1539–49.

Cohn JN, Archibald DG, Ziesche S, et al. Effect of vasodilator therapy on mortality in chronic congestive heart failure: Results of a Veterans Administration Cooperative Study. N Engl J Med 1986;314:1547–52.

Cohn JN, Johnson G, Ziesche S, et al. A comparison of enalapril with hydralazine-isosorbide dinitrate in the treatment of chronic congestive heart failure. N Engl J Med 1991;325:303–10.

The Digitalis Investigation Group. Effect of digoxin on mortality and morbidity in patients with heart failure. N Engl J Med 1997;336:525–33.

Hunt SA, Abraham WT, Chin MH, et al. ACC/AHA 2005 Guideline Update for the Diagnosis and Management of Chronic Heart Failure in the Adult: A report of the American College of Cardiology/American Heart Association

Task Force on Practice Guidelines (Writing Committee to Update the 2001 Guidelines for the Evaluation and Management of Heart Failure). Developed in collaboration with the American College of Chest Physicians and the International Society for Heart and Lung Transplantation; endorsed by the Heart Rhythm Society. Circulation 2005;112:e154–235.

International Registry for Heart and Lung Transplantation (ISHLT Registry). Available at: http://www.ishlt.org/registries/heartLungRegistry.asp; May 29, 2009 (accessed).

Metoprolol CR/XL Randomized Intervention Trial in Congestive Heart Failure (MERIT-HF). Effect of metoprolol CR/XL in chronic heart failure. Lancet 1999;353:2001–7.

Packer M, Bristow MR, Cohn JN, et al. The effect of carvedilol on morbidity and mortality in patients with chronic heart failure. U.S. Carvedilol Heart Failure Study Group. N Engl J Med 1996;334:1349–55.

Pitt B, Zannad F, Remme WJ, et al. The effect of spironolactone on morbidity and mortality in patients with severe heart failure. Randomized Aldactone Evaluation Study Investigators. N Engl J Med 1999;341:709–17.

Rose EA, Gelijns AC, Moskowitz AJ, et al. Long-term mechanical left ventricular assistance for end-stage heart failure. N Engl J Med 2001;345:1435–43.

The SOLVD Investigators. Effect of enalapril on mortality and the development of heart failure in asymptomatic patients with reduced left ventricular ejection fractions. N Engl J Med 1992;327:685–91.

Infective Endocarditis

Method of
Andrew Wang, MD

Definition

Infective endocarditis (IE) is a microbial infection of the valves or endocardium of the heart.

Epidemiology, and Risk Factors

The incidence of IE varies regionally from 2.6 per 100,000 population reported in France to 11.6 per 100,000 population in urban United States. This range of incidence has been attributed to differences in predisposing cardiac conditions or risk factors, such as use of injection drugs. The incidence of IE is also affected by age and sex. The incidence of native valve IE increases with age and exceeds 30 per 100,000 after 30 years of age. The average age of the patient with IE has increased over time, likely related to the decreased prevalence of rheumatic heart disease and increased prevalence of degenerative valvular disease in the aging population. IE more commonly is diagnosed in men, with studies showing male-to-female ratios as high as 9:1.

In earlier eras, streptococcal species were the predominant cause of native valve IE. However, changes in the delivery of health care, with increasing exposure to invasive procedures and devices, and the changing demographics of patients and their risk factors for IE have led to major changes in the microbiologic causes of endocarditis. There is an increasing incidence of health care–associated IE, including nosocomial infection and infection related to ambulatory care, which accounts for approximately 25% of IE cases. For example, in one large multinational study, the International Collaboration on Endocarditis (ICE) registry ($N = 2781$ patients with definite native or prosthetic endocarditis), 31% of cases were attributable to *Staphylococcus aureus*, 17% to viridans streptococci, 11% to enterococci, 10% to coagulase-negative staphylococci, 12% to other streptococcal species, 2% to the HACEK (*Haemophilus* spp., *Aggregatibacter* spp., *Cardiobacterium hominis*, *Eikenella corrodens*, *Kingella* spp.) group, 2% to non-HACEK gram-negative bacteria, and 2% to fungi. Among those with *S. aureus* endocarditis, health care–associated infection accounted for 39% of cases.

Predisposing cardiac conditions to the development of IE include degenerative valve disease (in approximately 40% of cases of mitral and 25% of aortic valve IE), presence of prosthetic valve, injection drug use, and rheumatic heart disease.

Pathophysiology

A preexisting valvular or endocardial condition, such as mitral valve prolapse with regurgitation, degenerative aortic valve disease (including bicuspid aortic valve), or congenital heart disease, is a major host factor related to development of IE. Endothelial damage and denudation of the endothelium exposes the underlying basement membrane and fosters platelet and fibrin deposition, a process that occurs spontaneously in persons with valvular heart disease. These deposits are called *nonbacterial thrombotic endocarditis* and form the nidus for vegetation to begin in the setting of bacteremia. The classic lesion of IE, the vegetation, is made up of fibrin, platelets, inflammatory cells, and microorganisms adherent to the endothelium of the heart.

The degree of mechanical stress exerted on the valve might contribute to endothelial denudation and the location of vegetation formation, with left-sided IE more common than right-sided IE. Endocarditis involving the nonvalvular endocardium of the heart similarly occurs at sites of endothelial damage due to mechanical stress, such as the left ventricular outflow tract in patients with hypertrophic obstructive cardiomyopathy and congenital heart defects (ventricular septal defects and patent ductus arteriosus).

The adhesion of bacteria to the denuded endothelium might depend on specific properties of the bacteria. Cell surface characteristics of the organism promote its adherence. For example, the adherence of *S. aureus* to a traumatized animal heart valve has been found to be reduced in the setting of impaired fibronectin binding. Similarly, the ability of bacteria to form biofilm may be associated with their ability to form localized clusters of infections that can make these clusters more resistant to killing by the host immune system and antimicrobial therapy.

With the progressive development of a vegetation, function of the specific heart valve is impaired. Regurgitation or insufficiency of the affected valve most commonly results, leading to predominantly volume overload of the ventricular chamber. In the setting of acute or rapid development of regurgitation, there may be no ventricular adaptation to this volume overload; as a result, acute, severe pulmonary edema and cardiogenic shock may quickly ensue. Less commonly, a large vegetation can result in stenosis of the valve orifice and pressure overload of the proximal or upstream cardiac chamber. As infection extends, destruction of other cardiac tissue, including myocardium and fibrous structures, can occur and result in intracardiac abscess or fistula formation between cardiac chambers.

Prevention

The efficacy of antimicrobial prophylaxis in preventing IE continues to be debated. Current recommendations are generally based on the likelihood of bacteremia occurring as a result of the procedure, the potential for adverse outcome as related to the predisposing cardiac condition, and the level of evidence for antibiotic prophylaxis as effective for the prevention of IE. The American Heart Association has published updated guidelines for IE prophylaxis with a continued trend toward fewer indications for prophylaxis.

Based on an extensive review of published literature and expert consensus, these guidelines have concluded that IE is more likely to result from bacteremia associated with daily activities than with a dental procedure. Antibiotic prophylaxis, even if 100% effective, is estimated to prevent only an extremely small number of cases of IE. These recommendations concluded that antibiotic prophylaxis should not be prescribed solely on the basis of an increased lifetime risk of IE but on the basis of cardiac conditions associated with highest risk of an adverse outcome from IE.

BOX 1 Prophylaxis Against Infective Endocarditis

Procedures Warranting Prophylaxis
Dental procedures that involve manipulating gingival tissue or the periapical region of teeth
Dental procedures that involve perforating the oral mucosa

Cardiac Conditions with High Risk of Adverse Outcome
Prosthetic heart valve or prosthetic material used for valve repair
Previous infective endocarditis
Congenital heart disease including unrepaired cyanotic lesions, palliative shunts or conduits, previous repair with residual defect at site of prosthetic patch or device, and recent repair (<6 months) involving prosthetic device or material
Cardiac transplant with valve regurgitation due to structurally abnormal valve

---

Conditions that warrant IE prophylaxis before dental procedures and procedures on respiratory tract, skin, and musculoskeletal structures are listed in Box 1 and Table 1. The American Heart Association no longer recommends prophylaxis before gastrointestinal or genitourinary procedures solely for the prevention of IE.

Clinical Manifestations and Diagnosis

The diagnosis of IE depends on findings of bacteremia with an organism associated with IE and evidence of endocardial involvement. Because these objective findings may not be sought unless the possibility of IE is considered, careful attention to the patient's history and physical examination is critical to the eventual diagnosis. The clinical presentation of IE is highly variable and can range from chronic fatigue with low-grade fever to acute heart failure due to new, severe valvular regurgitation. Although the virulence of the organism can influence acuity of presentation, the onset of infection is generally followed by the onset of symptoms within 2 weeks of bacteremia. Four processes contribute to the clinical presentation of IE: infection on the valve, including the local intracardiac complications; septic or aseptic embolization to distant organs; continuous bacteremia, often with metastatic foci of infection; and circulating immune complexes and other immunopathologic factors.

 CURRENT DIAGNOSIS

- Infective endocarditis should be considered as a diagnosis in the setting of fever and heart murmur.
- Health care–associated interventions and resulting infections are an increasingly noted cause of IE, changing the epidemiology of this disease.
- Blood cultures show growth in approximately 90% of cases, and multiple sets should be obtained before initiating antibiotics to improve diagnostic yield.
- Echocardiography, particularly transesophageal echocardiography, improves diagnostic sensitivity for infective endocarditis as well as its complications (e.g., intracardiac abscess, fistula).
- The diagnosis of complications, including heart failure, embolic events, and abscess, requires close surveillance, particularly during the first week of therapy, and has adverse prognostic implications.

TABLE 1 Regimens for Dental Procedure

Regimen	Antibiotic Agent	Adult	Children
Oral	Amoxicillin	2 g	50 mg/kg
Penicillin allergy	Cephalexin	2 g	50 mg/kg
	or clindamycin	600 mg	20 mg/kg
	or azithromycin or clarithromycin	500 mg	15 mg/kg
Unable to take oral medication	Ampicillin	2 g IM or IV	50 mg/kg IM or IV
Unable to take oral medication plus penicillin allergy	Cefazolin or ceftriaxone	1 g IM or IV	50 mg/kg IM or IV
	or clindamycin	600 mg IM or IV	20 mg/kg IM or IV

Adapted from Bonow RO, Carabello BA, Kanu C, et al: ACC/AHA 2006 guidelines for the management of patients with valvular heart disease: A report of the American College of Cardiology/American Heart Association Task Force on Practice Guidelines (writing committee to revise the 1998 Guidelines for the Management of Patients With Valvular Heart Disease): Developed in collaboration with the Society of Cardiovascular Anesthesiologists: Endorsed by the Society for Cardiovascular Angiography and Interventions and the Society of Thoracic Surgeons. *Circulation* 2006;114(5):e84-e231.
Note: The antibiotic agent is administered as single dose 30-60 minutes before the procedure.

Approximately 85% of patients present with fever, although this finding might not be present in immunosuppressed states and in patients who have previously been on antibiotic therapy. Nonspecific signs and symptoms such as chills, sweats, anorexia, weight loss, malaise, dyspnea, and cough are common but generally occur in less than half of patients with IE. In addition, predisposing conditions or risk factors for the development of IE, including a history of structural heart disease, injection drug use, or recent invasive procedure, should be sought in the patient's history.

Evidence of a *new or changing* regurgitant murmur in the presence of fever of undetermined origin should prompt additional, timely evaluation for possible IE. Because of the lack of ventricular adaptation to acute volume overload and the resulting hemodynamic changes (tachycardia, hypotension), the murmur in acute aortic insufficiency may be poorly audible. Embolic phenomena, a common extracardiac complication of IE, can manifest with localizing symptoms such as focal neurologic deficit due to stroke or left upper abdominal pain due to splenic infarction. The patient should be carefully examined for any peripheral stigmata of IE such as petechiae, splinter hemorrhages, Janeway lesions, Osler nodes and Roth spots. Many of these findings are immune-mediated, yet infrequently present. Although Janeway lesions, Osler nodes, and Roth spots are more specific abnormalities for IE, they can occur in other conditions and their low incidence in cases of proven IE limits their diagnostic utility.

BLOOD CULTURES

Blood cultures are the definitive microbiologic procedure for the diagnosis of IE. Continuous and low-grade bacteremia makes it unnecessary to await fever spikes or chills to obtain blood cultures, and the first two blood cultures yield an etiologic agent in 90% cases. In patients who have not received antibiotics recently, it is recommended that at least three blood culture sets from separate venipunctures should be obtained over the first 24 hours, which will increase the yield to more than 95% in cases of untreated IE with continuous bacteremia. Each culture media bottle should be inoculated with at least 10 mL of blood to increase the number of colony-forming units per culture. The results of blood cultures should be interpreted based on the specific microorganisms identified as well as the recognized, constant nature of bacteremia in IE.

Other laboratory data may provide clues to the diagnosis yet lack specificity for IE. Hematologic parameters are often abnormal. A normocytic, normochromic anemia (70%-90%), thrombocytopenia (5%-15%), and leukocytosis (30%) are common findings. The erythrocyte sedimentation rate (ESR) and C-reactive protein concentrations are usually elevated. Similarly, the C-reactive protein concentration is also elevated in IE but is a nonspecific finding. Rheumatoid factor assay is positive in up to half of the cases, especially if the illness is protracted. Urinalysis might demonstrate microscopic hematuria and mild proteinuria. Red blood cell casts and heavy proteinuria can be seen in patients with immune complex glomerulonephritis.

ELECTROCARDIOGRAPHY

Although the electrocardiogram (ECG) lacks sufficient sensitivity and specificity for the diagnosis of IE, ECG abnormalities commonly occur in patients with IE and are associated with invasive infection and increased in-hospital mortality. The presence of atrioventricular heart block in a patient with IE is diagnostic of the presence of a ring abscess, typically of the aortic valve, with invasion posteriorly toward the atrioventricular conduction system. One single-center study found that 53% of patients with invasive infection had ECG changes and about a third of the patients with ECG conduction abnormalities died during hospitalization in their cohort of 137 patients with definite IE.

ECHOCARDIOGRAPHY AND DIAGNOSTIC CRITERIA

The diagnosis of IE is based upon clinical suspicion derived from signs and symptoms and, most importantly, the demonstration of associated bacteremia. Given the nonspecific nature of findings from history, physical examination, and even blood cultures, the inclusion of echocardiographic findings has improved the sensitivity of diagnostic criteria for this condition (see modified Duke criteria, Box 2).

ECG findings provide specific evidence of IE that include vegetations, evidence of periannular tissue destruction (abscess), aneurysm, fistula, leaflet perforation, and valvular dehiscence. Box 3 outlines specific definitions of these characteristic findings.

The diagnostic utility of transthoracic echocardiogram (TTE) for suspected IE is highest in patients with intermediate to high likelihood of this disease (e.g., a patient with a new or changed heart murmur and bacteremia). Hence, TTE should be performed in all patients with suspected IE. However, the diagnostic sensitivity of TTE for the visualization of an intracardiac vegetation or abscess is limited, ranging from 40% to 80%, and thus the diagnosis of IE cannot be ruled out on the basis of a negative study. The absence of five clinical criteria has been associated with zero probability of a TTE showing evidence of IE: positive blood cultures, presence of central venous access, recent history of injection drug use, presence of prosthetic valve, and vasculitic or embolic phenomena.

Transesophageal echocardiography (TEE) has greater spatial resolution compared to TTE and so is more sensitive than TTE for detecting intracardiac vegetations (sensitivity, 87%; specificity, 95%). As a result, TEE should be performed in patients with a high likelihood of IE and a negative TTE. Although TTE and TEE have been found to have concordant results in approximately half of patients with suspected IE, TEE provides additional diagnostic information in a high percentage of patients, particularly those with prosthetic valves. Specific subsets of patients in whom TEE should be performed, even as the primary imaging modality (without TTE) include patients with prosthetic heart valves and suspected IE and patients with persistent staphylococcal bacteremia without known source or nosocomial infection. In addition, TEE should be performed in patients with IE when paravalvular abscess is suspected.

BOX 2   The Modified Duke Criteria and Case Definitions of Infective Endocarditis

Modified Duke Criteria

Major Criteria

Positive blood cultures
- Typical microbes consistent with IE from two separate blood cultures: viridans streptococci, *Streptococcus bovis*, HACEK group, *Staphylococcus aureus*; community-acquired enterococci in absence of another focus

or

- Microrganisms consistent with IE from persistently positive blood cultures defined as follows: at least 2 blood cultures drawn more than 12 hours apart or all of three or a majority of more than four separate blood cultures
- Single positive blood culture for *Coxiella burnetti* or antiphase IgG antibody titer >1:800

Evidence of endocardial involvement
  Echo findings of IE, defined as:
- Oscillating intracardiac mass on valve or supporting structure
- Abscess
- New partial dehiscence of prosthetic valve
- New valvular regurgitation

Minor Criteria

Predisposition: predisposing heart condition or injection drug use

Fever, temperature >38°C

Vascular phenomena, major arterial emboli, septic pulmonary infarcts, mycotic aneurysm, intracranial hemorrhage, conjunctival hemorrhage, and Janeway lesions

Immunologic phenomena: glomerulonephritis, Osler's nodes, Roth's spots, rheumatoid factor

Microbiologic evidence: positive blood cultures but does not meet a major criterion as noted above, or serologic evidence of active infection with organism consistent with causing IE

Case Definitions

Definite Infective Endocarditis

Presence of any pathologic criteria:
- Microorganisms demonstrated by culture or histologic examination of a vegetation, a vegetation that has embolized, or an intracardiac abscess specimen

or

- Pathologic lesions; vegetation or intracardiac abscess confirmed by histologic examination showing active endocarditis

If there are no pathologic criteria, then clinical diagnosis of definite IE:
- Two major criteria

or

- One major and three minor criteria

or

- Five minor criteria

Possible Infective Endocarditis

One major criterion and one minor criterion

or

Three minor criteria

Rejected

Firm alternative diagnosis explaining evidence of IE

or

Resolution of IE syndrome with antibiotic therapy for ≤4 days

or

No pathologic evidence of IE at surgery or autopsy, with antibiotic therapy for <4 days

or

Does not meet criteria for possible IE, as above.

Adapted from Li JS, Sexton DJ, Nettles R, et al. Proposed modifications to the Duke criteria for the diagnosis of infective endocarditis. Clin Infect Dis 2003;30(4):633–8.

Abbreviations: HACEK = Haemophilus spp., Aggregatibacter spp., Cardiobacterium hominis, Eikenella corrodens, Kingella spp.; IE = infective endocarditis; Ig = immunoglobulin.

BOX 3   Echocardiographic Findings in Infective Endocarditis

Vegetation

Irregularly shaped, discrete echogenic mass

Adherent to but distinct from endocardial surface or intracardiac device

Oscillation of mass (supportive, not mandatory)

Abscess

Thickened area or mass within the myocardium or valve annulus

Evidence of flow into region (supportive, not mandatory)

Aneurysm

Echolucent space with thin surrounding tissue

Fistula

Blood flow between two distinct cardiac blood spaces or chambers through an abnormal path or channel

Leaflet perforation

Defect in body of valve leaflet with flow through defect

Valve dehiscence

Prosthetic valve with abnormal rocking motion/excursion >15 degrees in at least one direction

Adapted from Sachdev M, Peterson GE, Jollis JG: Imaging techniques for diagnosis of infective endocarditis. Cardiol Clin 2003;21:185-195.

OTHER CARDIAC IMAGING MODALITIES

Cardiac magnetic resonance imaging with contrast appears promising for detecting paravalvular abscesses, thrombus associated with vegetations, valvular complications, and aortocameral fistulas, although temporal resolution might limit its use for detecting vegetation. Cardiac computed tomography has also been used to detect aortic root abscess. However, clinical experience with these techniques in IE patients is limited and their sensitivities and specificities in comparison to echocardiography are not well defined.

Routine coronary angiography is recommended in patients older than 55 years and in those at high risk for coronary artery disease before surgery for IE.

Differential Diagnosis

Given the protean manifestations of IE, the differential diagnosis includes a number of systemic conditions: systemic lupus erythematosus, acute rheumatic fever, atrial myxoma, vasculitis, and renal cell carcinoma.

Treatment, Complications, and Outcome

Antibiotic therapy has improved survival in IE by 70% to 80% and has been shown to reduce the incidence of complications of IE. Detailed descriptions of antibiotic regimens for specific causative organisms are found in guidelines by the American Heart Association (updated in 2008) and the European Society of Cardiology (new in 2009). Recommended antimicrobial regimens against typical organisms causing IE are outlined in Table 2. Although the choice of antimicrobial therapy is mainly guided by the infecting organism and its antibiotic susceptibilities, there are three basic principles of antibiotic treatment for the eradication of native valve infection.

 CURRENT THERAPY

- Because of changes in the epidemiology of infective endocarditis (IE), empiric antibiotic therapy for *Staphylococcus aureus* should be considered before results of blood cultures are available.
- Prompt initiation of antibiotic therapy is important, because the rate of complications such as embolization decreases rapidly within several days.
- Multidisciplinary care for the patient with IE should include evaluation by specialists in infectious diseases, cardiology, and cardiothoracic surgery, especially in cases of complicated IE.
- Surgery for IE has not been studied in randomized, controlled trials compared to medical therapy alone. Surgery should be considered for IE complicated by heart failure, embolism, intracardiac abscess, or persistent bacteremia.
- Although stroke due to embolism is not uncommon in IE, data do not suggest a benefit in delaying cardiac surgery after cerebral infarction if surgery is otherwise indicated.

TABLE 2 Antimicrobial Regimens against Typical Infective Endocarditis Organisms

Organism	Susceptibility	Regimen	Dosage	Duration (wk)
Native Valve				
Streptococcus viridans, Streptococcus bovis	Penicillin	Penicillin	12-18 MU IV q24h	4
	or	Ceftriaxone	2 g IV or IM q24h	4
	or	Vancomycin	30 mg/kg IV q24h in 2 divided doses Max: 2 g/24 h	4
	Penicillin-relative resistance	Penicillin	24 MU IV per 24 h	4
	or	Ceftriaxone	2 g IV/IM per 24 h	4
	plus	Gentamicin	3 mg/kg IV/IM per 24 h in 1 dose	2
	or	Vancomycin	30 mg/kg IV per 24 h in 2 divided doses (limit 2 g/24 h)	4
Enterococcus spp.	Penicillin	Ampicillin	12 g IV per 24 h in 6 divided doses	4-6
	or	Penicillin	18-30 MU IV per 24 h	4-6
	plus	Gentamicin	3 mg/kg IV or IM per 24 h in 3 divided doses	4-6
	or	Vancomycin	30 mg/kg IV per 24 h in 2 divided doses (limit 2 g/24 h)	6
	plus	Gentamicin	3 mg/kg IV or IM per 24 h in 3 divided doses	6
Staphylococcus spp.	Oxacillin	Nafcillin or oxacillin	12 g IV per 24 h in 4-6 divided doses	6
	plus	Gentamicin	3 mg/kg IV/IM per 24 h in 3 divided doses	3-5 days
	or	Cefazolin	6 g IV per 24 h in 3 divided doses	6
	plus	Gentamicin	3 mg/kg IV or IM per 24 h in 3 divided doses	3-5 days
Oxacillin-resistant Staphylococcus spp.		Vancomycin	30 mg/kg IV per 24 h in 2 divided doses Goal: 1-h peak concentration 30-45 µg/mL and trough 10-15 µg/mL	6
Prosthetic Valve				
Staphylococcus spp.	Oxacillin	Nafcillin or oxacillin	12 g IV per 24 h in 4-6 divided doses	6
	plus	Gentamicin	3 mg/kg IV or IM per 24 h in 3 divided doses	
	plus	Rifampin	900 mg IV or PO per 24 h in 3 divided doses	6
	Oxacillin-resistant	Vancomycin	30 mg/kg IV per 24 h in 2 divided doses Goal: 1-h peak concentration 30-45 µg/mL and trough 10-15 µg/mL	6
	plus	Gentamicin	3 mg/kg IV or IM per 24 h in 3 divided doses	
	plus	Rifampin	900 mg IV or PO per 24 h in 3 divided doses	6

Abbreviation: max = maximum.

First, a prolonged course of antibiotic treatment (4 to 6 weeks) is necessary to eradicate infection because bacterial concentration within vegetations is high and organisms deep within vegetations are inaccessible to phagocytic cells. Repeat sets of blood cultures after antibiotic initiation should be obtained every 24 to 48 hours until the resolution of bacteremia is confirmed. If surgery for IE is performed, completion of the 4- to 6-week course of antibiotic therapy is generally favored to reduce the risk of recurrent IE.

Second, parenteral administration of antibiotic therapy is necessary to achieve adequate drug levels required to eradicate infection. Parenteral therapy is typically initiated in the hospital setting, and the patient may receive outpatient parenteral treatment for the remaining duration after an initial period of observation to assess for clinical response to therapy (e.g., clearance of bacteremia and absence of complications).

Third, because of the need for prolonged therapy and rising antimicrobial resistance among organisms, combination therapy typically involving a β-lactam and aminoglycoside antibiotic is recommended. Combination therapy has been shown to reduce the duration of bacteremia in *S. aureus* endocarditis, although this more-rapid resolution of bacteremia was not associated with an improved clinical response or outcome. Both antibiotics should be given temporally close together so that maximum synergistic microcidal effect is obtained. In addition, the dosage and kidney function should be monitored carefully, because combination therapy has been associated with a higher rate of kidney dysfunction.

IE can progress to the development of various intracardiac and extracardiac complications before or despite effective treatment. Heart failure or pulmonary edema is a common complication, occurring in about one third to one half of patients with IE, and it is the most common indication for urgent surgery. Valvular destruction and ensuing insufficiency can result in volume overload and heart failure; in rare cases of large vegetations, heart failure may be a result of valvular stenosis. Heart failure complicates aortic valve IE more often than mitral or tricuspid IE and can result in the setting of moderate, rather than severe, regurgitation, because the left ventricle is unable to compensate for the acute increase in preload and afterload in this condition.

Medical therapy alone is generally insufficient in managing IE complicated by heart failure, particularly in the setting of severe or progressive valvular regurgitation. Surgery should be prompt and unnecessary delays should be avoided.

Para-valvular abscess complicates 30% to 40% cases of IE and is a result of invasive infection that spreads generally along contiguous tissue planes, particularly with aortic valve infection. In the International Collaboration on Endocarditis (ICE) cohort, 22% cases of definite aortic valve IE were complicated by a periannular abscess. These patients were more likely to have prosthetic valves and coagulase-negative staphylococcal infection. TEE is the diagnostic test of choice when an abscess is suspected clinically. An abscess is diagnosed by TEE as the visualization of a periannular area of thickening or mass with a heterogeneous echogenic or echolucent appearance. Rarely, antibiotic therapy alone may be used to treat an intracardiac abscess, though this treatment alone is generally reserved for patients who are poor surgical candidates. The vast majority of patients with an intracardiac abscess require cardiac surgery for débridement. In addition, surgery represents the gold standard for the diagnosis of abscess.

Embolic phenomena often complicate the clinical course in IE. Although clinical signs of embolization occur in approximately one third of patients with IE, at least another third of patients have silent embolism. In the majority of cases, embolic events occur before antibiotic therapy is initiated, whereas less than 10% of events occur after treatment has begun. The most frequent sites of embolic events were central nervous system (approximately 40% of embolic events), lungs (approximately 20%), spleen (20%), peripheral artery (approximately 15%), and kidney (10%).

Factors including vegetation size, mobility, and location as well as the causative organism have been associated with the likelihood of embolic event. Vegetations larger than 10 mm in greatest diameter are associated with an increased risk of embolization. Causative organisms such as *S. aureus* and *Streptococcus bovis* confer an independent risk of embolization. Embolism also occurs with greater frequency in IE caused by enterococci, fastidious gram-negative organisms (HACEK), and fungi as compared to streptococcal IE. In addition to causing infarction of distal vascular beds, embolic events can result in metastatic sites of infection.

Cerebral embolization occurs in 10% to 35% and is at times complicated by meningitis, brain abscess, or intracerebral hemorrhage. The risk of stroke dramatically decreases with initiation of antibiotic therapy. Findings from the ICE merged database suggested a 65% reduction in stroke incidence by week 2 of initiating antimicrobial therapy. Given the low incidence of embolic event after initiation of antibiotic therapy, routine screening for emboli in patients with IE is not recommended. However, patients with persistent fever or bacteremia or localizing symptoms of possible infarction should undergo computed tomographic imaging with radiographic contrast for the diagnosis of embolic complications.

Embolic events have been found to be an independent predictor of in-hospital death in IE. In patients who experience recurrent embolic events, particularly if they occur after initiation of antibiotic therapy, surgical treatment is indicated. For the prevention of embolic events, surgery may be considered for patients with IE who have residual large (>10 mm), mobile vegetations involving mitral or aortic valve.

Surgical intervention for IE may be performed either in the acute or active phase of infection or after the eradication of infection. The optimal timing of surgery in the setting of active IE has not been well evaluated. In patients with serious, life-threatening complications of IE, surgery should be performed emergently. A number of case series have shown that surgery in the active phase of IE can be performed with acceptable risk and without an obvious risk of infecting a prosthetic valve. Surgery during the active phase is generally considered for patients in whom the likelihood of cure of infection with antibiotic therapy alone is low or in whom severe complications have or will likely occur. In contemporary series, surgery is performed in 40% to 50% of patients with IE during the index hospitalization. Surgery after eradication of infection is predominantly performed for adverse hemodynamic effects of valvular regurgitation that results from valve damage.

Indications for surgery in IE are shown in Box 4. Heart failure is a primary indication for urgent surgical intervention, yet even without overt heart failure symptoms, hemodynamic evidence of severe regurgitation (such as premature closure of the mitral valve in severe aortic regurgitation or pulmonary hypertension in severe mitral regurgitation) should also prompt surgical intervention because valvular regurgitation—or rarely, stenosis—is a mechanical complication of IE that will not improve with antimicrobial therapy alone. For mitral valve regurgitation, surgical repair of the native valve without replacing the valve with a prosthesis has been reported in a number of case series However, the role of repair versus replacement has not been evaluated in controlled studies, and its feasibility will be limited by the extent of infection and valvular damage as well as the experience of the surgeon.

Because embolic complications often involve the central nervous system and can worsen neurologic function after cardiopulmonary bypass, the timing of surgery after a cerebral embolic infarct is controversial. One study found that neurologic deterioration did not occur among patients with IE who experienced transient ischemic attacks or asymptomatic emboli, even if surgery was performed acutely.

Regarding persistent bacteremia as an indication for surgery, it is important to recognize that certain microorganisms, particularly *S. aureus*, may be associated with prolonged bacteremia (up to 10 days) after initiation of antibiotic therapy. Because of possible difficulty in eradicating infection from prosthetic materials, all cases of prosthetic valve IE should receive surgical consultation. With valve conservation and improved surgical techniques, the surgical mortality rates have declined over time, with recent reported rates in the range of 7% to 14%. In comparison to medical therapy alone, surgery appears to confer a survival benefit for those patients with major complications of IE, such as heart failure or intracardiac abscess.

Despite the high rate of surgical intervention in IE, the in-hospital mortality rate for native valve IE in the contemporary era remains

BOX 4 Indications for Surgical Intervention in Infective Endocarditis

Class I Indications

Heart failure

Aortic regurgitation or mitral regurgitation with evidence of elevated left ventricular end-diastolic or left atrial pressure

Fungal endocarditis

Highly resistant organism, including persistently positive blood cultures despite ≥1 week of appropriate antibiotic therapy

Echocardiographic evidence of valve perforation, rupture, fistula, or large paravalvular abscess

Prosthetic valve infection with evidence of heart failure, worsening valvular stenosis or regurgitation, valve dehiscence, or abscess formation

Class IIa Indications

Recurrent embolic events with persistent vegetations despite appropriate antibiotic treatment

Class IIb Indications

Mobile, large (>10 mm) vegetation with or without emboli

Adapted from Bonow RO, Carabello BA, Kanu C, et al: ACC/AHA 2006 guidelines for the management of patients with valvular heart disease: A report of the American College of Cardiology/American Heart Association Task Force on Practice Guidelines (writing committee to revise the 1998 Guidelines for the Management of Patients With Valvular Heart Disease): Developed in collaboration with the Society of Cardiovascular Anesthesiologists: Endorsed by the Society for Cardiovascular Angiography and Interventions and the Society of Thoracic Surgeons. *Circulation* 2006;114(5):e84-e231.
Definitions: Class I = benefit >>> risk, surgery should be performed; class IIa = benefit >> risk, reasonable to perform surgery; class IIb: benefit ≥ risk, surgery may be considered, additional studies needed.

high at approximately 15% to 20%, and nearly 25% for prosthetic valve IE. Among host factors, older age, female sex, diabetes mellitus, acute physiology (APACHE II) score, elevated white blood cell count, serum creatinine level greater than 2 mg/dL, and lower serum albumin have been associated with worse outcome. Congestive heart failure, paravalvular complication (e.g., abscess formation), infection with virulent organisms (particularly *S. aureus*), prosthetic valve infection, and absence of surgical intervention are also factors related to higher mortality in IE.

REFERENCES

Bonow RO, Carabello BA, Kanu C, et al. ACC/AHA 2006 guidelines for the management of patients with valvular heart disease: A report of the American College of Cardiology/American Heart Association Task Force on Practice Guidelines (writing committee to revise the 1998 Guidelines for the Management of Patients With Valvular Heart Disease): Developed in collaboration with the Society of Cardiovascular Anesthesiologists: Endorsed by the Society for Cardiovascular Angiography and Interventions and the Society of Thoracic Surgeons. Circulation 2006;114(5):e84–231.

Chu VH, Cabell CH, Benjamin Jr DK, et al. Early predictors of in-hospital death in infective endocarditis. Circulation 2004;109(14):1745–9.

Fowler Jr VG, Miro JM, Hoen B, et al. *Staphylococcus aureus* endocarditis: A consequence of medical progress. JAMA 2005;293(24):3012–21.

Hasbun R, Vikram HR, Barakat LA, et al. Complicated left-sided native valve endocarditis in adults: Risk classification for mortality. JAMA 2003;289 (15):1933–40.

Hoen B, Alla F, Selton-Suty C, et al. Changing profile of infective endocarditis: Results of a 1-year survey in France. JAMA 2002;288(1):75–81.

Li JS, Sexton DJ, Nettles R, et al. Proposed modifications to the Duke criteria for the diagnosis of infective endocarditis. Clin Infect Dis 2000;30(4):633–8.

Moreillon P, Que YA. Infective endocarditis. Lancet 2004;363(9403):139–49.

Nishimura RA, Carabello BA, Faxon DP, et al. ACC/AHA 2008 guideline update on valvular heart disease: Focused update on infective endocarditis: A report of the American College of Cardiology/American Heart Association Task Force on Practice Guidelines endorsed by the Society of Cardiovascular Anesthesiologists, Society for Cardiovascular Angiography and Interventions, and Society of Thoracic Surgeons. Catheter Cardiovasc Interv 2008;72(3):E1–E12.

Task Force on the Prevention, Diagnosis, and Treatment of Infective Endocarditis of the European Society of Cardiology; European Society of Clinical Microbiology and Infectious Diseases; International Society of Chemotherapy for Infection and Cancer; ESC Committee for Practice Guidelines. Guidelines on the prevention, diagnosis, and treatment of infective endocarditis (new version 2009): the Task Force on the Prevention, Diagnosis, and Treatment of Infective Endocarditis of the European Society of Cardiology (ESC). Eur Heart J 2009;30(19):2369–413.

Vikram HR, Buenconsejo J, Hasbun R, et al. Impact of valve surgery on 6-month mortality in adults with complicated, left-sided native valve endocarditis: A propensity analysis. JAMA 2003;290(24):3207–14.

Wang A, Athan E, Pappas PA, et al. Contemporary clinical profile and outcome of prosthetic valve endocarditis. JAMA 2007;297(12):1354–61.

Hypertension

Method of
Horacio E. Adrogué, MD

In 2009, the world was introduced to the pandemic of the H1N1 influenza virus. During the same time period, more people died worldwide of cardiovascular disease than from any other cause. Hypertension is one of the most prevalent and controllable risk factors contributing to cardiovascular disease and kidney disease. It should be considered one of the most far-reaching pandemics of recent history.

It has been more than 33 years since the National Heart, Lung, and Blood Institute published the first Report of the Joint National Committee on Prevention, Detection, Evaluation, and Treatment of High Blood Pressure (JNC 1). The most recent report (JNC 7) was published in 2003, and JNC 8 is due in 2011. This helps to underscore the growing importance of hypertension in the United States and the world. JNC 8 should add a great deal to our approach to the treatment of hypertension in the next decade.

Epidemiology

The current world population is approximately 6.8 billion people, and about one out of every four adults has hypertension. As the world gravitates towards a Western diet and lifestyle, the pandemic of obesity will only worsen, adding to the increasing incidence of hypertension worldwide. In the United States, it is estimated that in the period from 1999 through 2004, 65 million people have hypertension, a tremendous increase from the 50 million people with hypertension estimated from 1988 through 1994. The current population of the Unites States is 308 million, so about 20% of our citizens have hypertension.

Systolic blood pressure (BP) progressively rises as we exceed the age of 40 years. Between 27% and 40% of men and 20% and 45% of women between 40 and 59 years old in the United States have hypertension. The total number of affected people increases to nearly 60% to 75% of adults older than 60 years.

Non-Hispanic whites and Mexican Americans have a similar prevalence of hypertension; non-Hispanic blacks have much higher blood pressure values than the other two groups. In fact, non-Hispanic black men have a 15% to 20% higher prevalence than that of the other two groups, and non-Hispanic black women have up to 25%

higher prevalence. The combination of a higher prevalence and more difficulty in controlling hypertension in the non-Hispanic black population greatly contributes to the disproportionately high representation of this group of Americans on dialysis.

Risk Factors

MODERN WESTERN DIET AND LIFESTYLE

The modern Western diet and lifestyle is one of the most important and potentially modifiable risk factors that most patients and many doctors ignore. It is much easier for both patients and physicians alike to accept a new medication than adopt and implement a healthier life style. Although it takes a lot of work to change our lifestyle, the potential rewards are great. Because most large trials show positive effects of a 2- to 4-mm Hg reduction in systolic BP with the use of antihypertensive medications, it is very important to be aware of similar or better results with lifestyle modification.

As shown in Table 1, improvement in cardiovascular disease (CVD) risk can be attained with modest changes in lifestyle when compared to people who do not make these modifications. Regular aerobic exercise (30 minutes at least three times per week), dietary potassium increase and sodium restriction, moderate alcohol consumption, and low-fat diet have all been shown to improve systolic BP in several studies (Table 2).

AGE

Wish as we might, age is a nonmodifiable risk factor. Between the ages of 18 and 39 years, 10% of American women and 15% of men have hypertension. There is a large increase in the prevalence between ages 40 and 59 years, affecting up to 40% of men and 50% of women. Almost 60% of those older than 60 years, 70% of those older than 70 years, and 80% of those older than 80 years have hypertension, with

TABLE 1 Effect of Diet Modification on Risk of Cardiovascular Disease

Food	Amount	Reduction in CVD (%)
Fish	114 g 4× per week	14
Fruit and vegetables	400 g/d	21
Wine	150 mL/d (5 oz/d)	32
Garlic	2.7 g/d	25
Dark chocolate	100 g/d	21
Almonds	68 g/d	12

Abbreviation: CVD = cardiovascular disease.

TABLE 2 Effect of Lifestyle and Diet Modification on Systolic Blood Pressure

Modification	Amount	Reduction in SBP (mm Hg)
Dietary sodium restriction	<30-50 mmol/d	2-8
Moderation of daily alcohol intake	150-200 mL	2-4
Increased physical activity	30 min 3× per week	4-9
Reduction in body weight	10 kg or 22 lb	5-10
Adoption of DASH eating plan (high potassium)		8-14

Abbreviations: DASH = Dietary Approaches to Stop Hypertension; SBP = systolic blood pressure.

older non-Hispanic blacks having the highest prevalence. This is the trend in the United States, but it might turn out to be somewhat modifiable if we reverse our "expected" weight gain and sedentary lifestyle as we age.

SEX

In general, men have a higher prevalence of hypertension until the age of 45 years. After that, men and women have the same rates. The Prospective Studies Collaboration found that ischemic heart disease mortality associated with hypertension in women was higher than in men. It does not appear that the female sex is a protective state, as we once thought.

ETHNICITY

Non-Hispanic blacks have a higher incidence and prevalence of hypertension in the United States. In addition, the rate of death from CVD among black patients has been shown to be 25% higher than among whites. However, this trend is not present worldwide. Paradoxically, among Hispanics of Mexican origin, there is less hypertension and cardiovascular disease than in whites and blacks even though there is more obesity and diabetes.

BODY WEIGHT

In general, as the population gains weight, their blood pressure rises. In those with hypertension and excess caloric intake, the simple act of decreasing caloric intake can drop blood pressure even before significant weight loss actually occurs. This phenomenon is not completely understood, but insulin might play a role by promoting mild vascular pressor effect and salt retention.

DIET

It has now become very clear that the combination of a high sodium chloride diet exceeding 50 to 100 mmol per day and a low potassium intake of less than 30 to 50 mmol is critical in the pathogenesis of hypertension. Daily consumption of more than approximately 400 mL (13 oz) of alcohol has been shown to contribute to essential hypertension. One study found that excess alcohol consumption correlated even better than sodium chloride intake.

FAMILY HISTORY

Similar to type 2 diabetes mellitus, essential hypertension clearly runs in families. This accounts for one third to one half of the cause of essential hypertension, with the rest due to environmental causes. Monogenic hypertension has been identified in a few select families. This is hypertension caused by mutations in genes that increase the reabsorption of sodium chloride in the renal tubule.

OTHER FACTORS

Smoking, physical inactivity, higher altitudes, and colder weather have all been linked to acute elevations of blood pressure and chronic hypertension. Recent data point to a link between essential hypertension and hyperuricemia (uric acid levels ≥6 mg/dL) in adolescents.

Pathophysiology

The role of excess sodium chloride and inadequate potassium intake is central to the pathogenesis of essential hypertension (Fig. 1). The human kidney was designed to conserve sodium and get rid of potassium because our prehistoric diet was high in potassium and low in sodium. Unfortunately for those of us who partake of the typical Western diet, the end result can be hypertension. The deficit of total body potassium (most being intracellular) contributes to vascular smooth-muscle cell contraction, increased peripheral vascular resistance, and hypertension.

Simultaneously, the excess quantity of sodium expands the extracellular fluid volume, releasing digitalis-like factor, which stimulates the

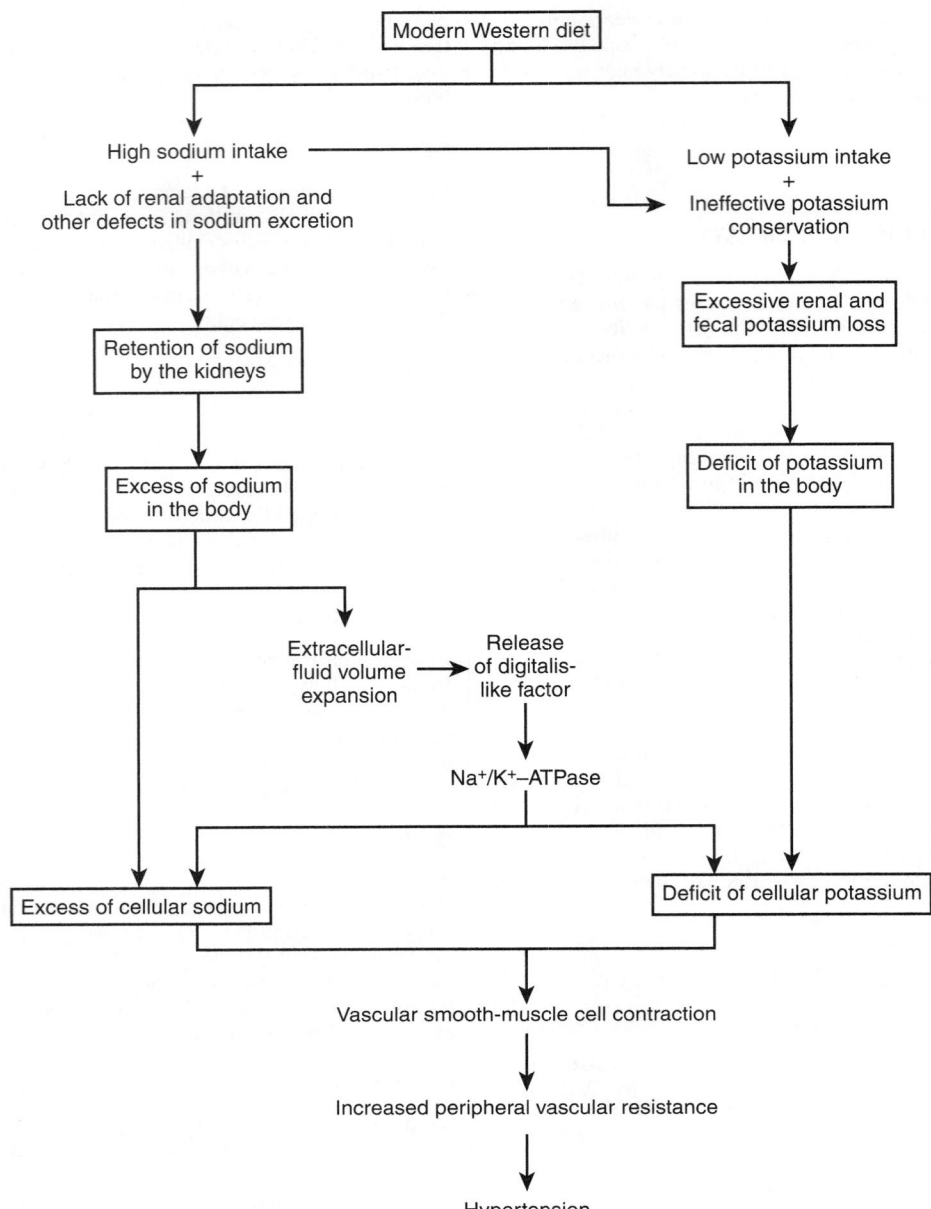

FIGURE 1. Interaction of the modern Western diet and the kidneys in the pathogenesis of primary hypertension. The modern Western diet interacts with the kidneys to generate excess sodium and cause a deficit of potassium in the body; these changes increase peripheral vascular resistance and establish hypertension. An initial increase in the volume of extracellular fluid is countered by pressure natriuresis. (Reprinted with permission from Adrogué HJ, Madias NE: Sodium and potassium in the pathogenesis of hypertension. N Engl J Med 2007;356(19):1966-1978.)

Na^+,K^+-ATPase to conserve sodium and waste potassium. This excess cellular sodium increases vascular smooth-muscle cell contraction, increasing peripheral vascular resistance, leading to hypertension.

Uricase, an enzyme that degrades uric acid to allantoin, is not expressed by humans, which contributes to higher levels of uric acid in humans than in most other mammals. The role of hyperuricemia (uric acid level $\geq$6 mg/dL) in the pathogenesis of hypertension has been the subject of much debate. JNC 7 does not consider it a true risk factor for hypertension. However, more recent data in children might lead to a change of opinion on the role of hyperuricemia and hypertension.

A randomized, double-blind, placebo-controlled, crossover trial of allopurinol (Zyloprim)[1] use was performed in children 11 to 17 years old who had newly diagnosed essential hypertension. Their hypothesis was that the treatment of hyperuricemia ($\geq$6 mg/dL) with allopurinol would lead to a lowering of blood pressure. Thirty adolescents with stage 1 hypertension and obesity (70%) were enrolled and randomized to allopurinol 200 mg twice per day ($n = 15$) or placebo ($n = 15$) for 4 weeks, had a 2-week washout, and then crossed over to the opposite group for an additional 4 weeks. Twenty-two of the 30 allopurinol-treated patients achieved a uric acid level of less than 5 mg/dL by the end of the study. Casual systolic BP decreased by 6.9 mm Hg in the allopurinol group but only 2 mm Hg in the placebo group ($P = 0.009$). Diastolic BP decreased by 5.1 mm Hg in the allopurinol group but only 2.4 mm Hg in the placebo group ($P = 0.05$). An even larger difference was noted in the 24-hour ambulatory blood pressure readings. In addition, plasma levels of renin were noted to decrease in the allopurinol treatment phase, as did the systemic vascular resistance. Although the authors do not conclude that

[1]Not FDA approved for this indication.

this is a new therapy for hypertension, this study does shed light on the role of uric acid in the pathophysiology of essential hypertension. A larger study, done in adults with longer follow-up, could prove critical in finding a new manner of treating hypertension.

Prevention

As previously discussed, being born into a family without hypertension helps prevent hypertension if you also take care of yourself. A low-sodium, high-potassium diet along with physical activity and avoidance of smoking and excess alcohol also help in prevention.

Clinical Manifestations

Essential hypertension is usually asymptomatic unless the blood pressure reaches very high levels. A mean arterial BP of 150 mm Hg causes lesions to appear in arterial walls and can start the syndrome of accelerated malignant hypertension (AMH). AMH is manifested by diastolic BP more than 140 mm Hg, funduscopic changes (bleeding, papilledema, exudates), neurologic changes (vision loss, confusion, headache, seizures, coma), acute kidney injury (oliguria), and gastrointestinal problems such as nausea and vomiting. An extensive description of clinical manifestations of all types of secondary hypertension is beyond the scope of this chapter, but I will discuss clues to these diseases.

Cushing's syndrome is associated with an approximately fourfold higher mortality than essential hypertension. Because obesity is a growing problem, it important to be alert for the sign of truncal obesity (50%-90% incidence) in Cushing's. Other important clues include facial plethora (80%), hirsutism (80%), menstrual disorders or impotence (75%), purple striae (50%-70%), easy bruising (50%), weakness from myopathy (30%-90%), glucose intolerance (75%), and kidney stones and hypokalemia (20%).

Primary hyperaldosteronism can account for up to 10% of those with hypertension and 20% of those with resistant hypertension. This new incidence can reach up to 40% of highly selected groups and is very different from the 1% rate that was commonly quoted in recent years. It is very important to detect this disease early because 75% of cases are due to an adenoma, 20% are due to hyperplasia, and 5% are due to carcinoma. Detection and treatment of this disease can be lifesaving.

Renovascular hypertension is another secondary cause of hypertension that can account for up to 7% of those with elevated blood pressure and suggestive clinical signs and symptoms (Box 1). Once properly diagnosed, it can respond to treatment very well.

Diagnosis

CLASSIFICATIONS

Joint National Committee Classification

According to JNC 7, *normal* BP is defined as systolic BP less than 120 mm Hg and diastolic BP less than 80 mm Hg. *Prehypertension* is systolic BP 120 to 139 mm Hg or diastolic BP 80 to 89 mm Hg (whichever is higher). *Stage 1* hypertension is systolic BP 140 to 159 mm Hg or diastolic BP 90 to 99 mm Hg, and *stage 2* hypertension is systolic BP 160 mm Hg or higher or diastolic BP 100 mm Hg or higher.

International Classification

The World Health Organization, International Society of Hypertension, European Society of Hypertension, and the European Society of Cardiology have also published a classification of hypertension. They define *optimal* blood pressure as a systolic BP less than 120 mm Hg and diastolic BP less than 80 mm Hg. *Normal* is systolic BP 120 to 129 mm Hg and diastolic BP 80 to 84 mm Hg; *high-normal* is systolic BP 130 to 139 mm Hg or diastolic BP 85 to 89 mm Hg. *Stage 1* hypertension is systolic BP 140 to 159 mm Hg or diastolic BP 90 to 99 mm Hg, and *Stage 2* hypertension is systolic BP 160 to 179 mm Hg or diastolic BP 100 to 109 mm Hg. The designation of *stage 3* hypertension is reserved for those with systolic BP 180 mm Hg or higher or diastolic BP 110 mm Hg or higher.

CURRENT DIAGNOSIS

- Blood pressure should be taken in a seated position, with the right arm supported, the patient at rest for 5 minutes, and without recent smoking or caffeine intake.
- Blood pressure should be repeated at least twice on two separate clinic visits before the label of hypertension is given unless stage 2 hypertension is diagnosed on the first visit.
- Every effort should be made to use standard nomenclature when documenting stages of hypertension
- In those whose hypertension does not manifest or behave like essential hypertension, it is imperative to rule out any secondary, treatable, or reversible causes of hypertension.

BOX 1   Clinical Manifestations of Renovascular Hypertension (Renal Artery Stenosis and Fibromuscular Dysplasia)

History

Flash pulmonary edema (recurrent)
Significant (≥30%) elevation in baseline creatinine with the initiation of ACEI or ARB
Past or current smoker
Severe or resistant hypertension (>3 medications)
Sudden onset or sudden worsening of hypertension
Onset of hypertension in a woman younger than 30 years with no family history (suspect fibromuscular dysplasia)

Laboratory Findings

Elevated creatinine for age
Size difference in kidneys by ultrasound of >1.5 cm (the right kidney is normally 0.3-0.5 cm smaller than the left)

Proteinuria (moderate, approximately 1-2 g/d, but is variable)
Evidence of secondary hyperaldosteronism
Low serum sodium
Low serum potassium
High plasma renin

Physical Examination Findings

Advanced hypertensive retinopathy
Abdominal aortic bruits
Femoral arterial bruits

Abbreviations: ACEI = angiotensin-converting enzyme inhibitor; ARB = angiotensin receptor blocker.

American Heart Association Classification

The American Heart Association (AHA) further classifies hypertension into several specific categories.

Isolated systolic hypertension is systolic BP 140 mm Hg or higher and diastolic BP less than 90 mm Hg. *Isolated diastolic* hypertension is systolic BP less than 140 mm Hg and diastolic BP 90 mm Hg or higher. *White coat hypertension* is becoming a more recognized diagnosis and is diagnosed when the clinic BP is more than 140/90 mm Hg while the ambulatory BP averages less than 135/85 mm Hg.

Isolated ambulatory hypertension is a clinic BP of less than 135/85 mm Hg and an average ambulatory BP of more than 140/90 mm Hg. The use of 24-hour ambulatory blood pressure monitors have become much more common in the practice of medicine. People who have a personal history of prehypertension or a family history of hypertension and wish to donate a kidney are evaluated via this method to evaluate their candidacy to donate. Patients with blood pressure that is difficult to control or evaluate benefit greatly from this method. Ambulatory hypertension is a 24-hour average of more than 135/85. In addition, current data show that patients without a normal drop in nighttime blood pressure have an increased cardiovascular morbidity. For this reason, *ambulatory nighttime* hypertension is defined as an average nighttime BP of >125/75 mm Hg and *ambulatory daytime* hypertension is average values of more than 140/90 mm Hg.

The last category is *accelerated or malignant hypertension*, which should be treated as a medical emergency. Diastolic BP is higher than 120 mm Hg and evidence of grade III retinopathy (arteriolar nicking and narrowing, flame-shaped hemorrhages and exudates) or grade IV retinopathy (papilledema) is an indication for hospital admission for careful and monitored treatment of hypertension.

PSEUDOHYPERTENSION

Pseudohypertension is defined as the overestimation of blood pressure when taken by a standard manual sphygmomanometer in certain patients. Hypertension should not be diagnosed in these patients unless the measurements can be verified by the Osler maneuver. It should be suspected in elderly patients and in diabetic patients with known or suspected sclerosis or calcification of radial and brachial arteries. The presence of pseudohypertension can be confirmed in the outpatient setting by the use of the Osler maneuver. The cuff is inflated 30 mm Hg above the auscultated systolic blood pressure and the brachial or radial artery distal to the cuff is palpated and rolled under the examiner's finger. If a pulse is no longer felt but the artery remains palpable like a stiff tube (likely calcified), then the Osler maneuver is positive and pseudohypertension is present.

Other noninvasive clues to the diagnosis include the absence of end-organ damage (left ventricular hypertrophy, retinopathy) and excessive postural hypotension with the use of low doses of antihypertensive agents. An automatic oscillometric recorder or finger BP can also help to detect the patient's true blood pressure. In cases where doubt still remains, intra-arterial pressure measurements should be considered and those values compared to the cuff BP to ensure correct classification of the patient's BP. The importance of proper diagnosis cannot be overstated because these patients will suffer from postural hypotension and risk of injury from antihypertensive medications that they do not need.

Treatment

When all the recent data are viewed in aggregate, the most important message becomes that the degree of blood pressure reduction is the key to reducing the risk of cardiovascular disease regardless of the specific medications that we use. The stage of hypertension dictates when to start medications in addition to lifestyle changes. Patients who present with stage 2 hypertension (JNC 7) need medications initiated at the first visit (Tables 3 and 4).

TABLE 3 Some Common Oral Antihypertensive Drugs

Drug (Trade Name)	Initial Dose	Max Dose	How Supplied	Major Side Effects/Comments
Angiotensin-Converting Enzyme Inhibitors				
Benazepril (Lotensin, generic)*	10 mg qd	80 mg/d†	Tab: 5, 10, 20, 40 mg	Cough, hypotension, renal failure, hyperkalemia, loss of taste, rash, leukopenia, angioedema (rare).
Captopril (Capoten generic)	25 mg bid-tid	450 mg/d	Tab: 12.5, 25, 50, 100 mg	
Enalapril (Vasotec generic)	5 mg qd	40 mg/d†	Tab: 2.5, 5, 10, 20 mg	
Fosinopril (Monopril, generic)	10 mg qd	80 mg/d†	Tab: 10, 20, 40 mg	
Lisinopril (Prinivil, Zestril, generic)	10 mg qd	80 mg/d	Tab: 2.5, 5, 10, 20, 40 mg	
Moexipril (Univasc, generic)	7.5 mg qd	30 mg/d†	Tab: 7.5, 15 mg	
Perindopril (Aceon)	4 mg qd	16 mg/d	Tab: 2, 4, 8 mg	
Quinapril (Accupril, generic)	10-20 mg qd	80 mg/d†	Tab: 5, 10, 20, 40 mg	
Ramipril (Altace, generic)	2.5 mg qd	20 mg/d†	Cap: 1.25, 2.5, 5, 10 mg	
Trandolapril (Mavik)	1-2 mg qd	8 mg/d†	Tab: 1, 2, 4 mg	
Angiotensin Receptor Blockers				
Candesartan (Atacand)	16 mg/d	32 mg/d†	Tab: 4, 8, 16, 32 mg	Similar to ACEIs, but not significantly associated with cough and have lower incidence of angioedema than ACEIs
Eprosartan (Teveten)	600 mg qd	800 mg/d	Tab: 400, 600 mg	
Irbesartan (Avapro)	150 mg qd	300 mg/d	Tab: 75, 150, 300 mg	
Losartan (Cozaar)	50 mg qd	100 mg/d†	Tab: 25, 50, 100 mg	
Olmesartan (Benicar)	20 mg qd	40 mg/d	Tab: 5, 10, 20 mg	
Telmisartan (Micardis)	40 mg qd	80 mg/d	Tab: 20, 40, 80 mg	
Valsartan (Diovan)	80-160 mg qd	320 mg/d	Tab: 40, 80, 160, 320 mg	
Direct Renin Inhibitors				
Aliskiren (Tekturna)	150 mg qd	300 mg qd	Tab: 150, 300 mg	Same as ARBs, but can have more GI side effects such as diarrhea
β-Adrenergic Blockers				
Cardioselective β-Blockers				
Atenolol (Tenormin, generic)	50 mg qd	100 mg qd	Tab: 25, 50, 100 mg	Bradycardia, heart failure, impaired peripheral circulation, fatigue, decreased exercise tolerance, insomnia; bronchospasm at higher doses; can mask hypoglycemia
Betaxolol (Kerlone, generic)	10 mg qd	20 mg qd	Tab: 10, 20 mg	
Bisoprolol (Zebeta, generic)	5 mg qd	20 mg qd	Tab: 5, 10 mg	
Metoprolol (Lopressor, generic), extended-release (Toprol XL)	50 mg bid or 100 mg XL qd	400 mg/d	Tab: 50, 100 mg XL tab: 25, 50, 100, 200 mg	

Continued

TABLE 3 Some Common Oral Antihypertensive Drugs—Cont'd

Drug (Trade Name)	Initial Dose	Max Dose	How Supplied	Major Side Effects/Comments
Noncardioselective β-Blockers				
Nadolol (Corgard, generic)	40 mg qd	320 mg qd	Tab: 20, 40, 80, 120, 160 mg	Bronchospasm, bradycardia, heart failure, impaired peripheral circulation, insomnia, fatigue, decreased exercise tolerance; can mask hypoglycemia
Propranolol (Inderal, generic), long-acting (Inderal LA)	20-40 mg bid or 60-80 mg SR qd	480 mg/d	Tab: 10, 20, 40, 60, 80 mg LA tab: 60, 80, 120, 160 mg	
Timolol (Blocadren, generic)	10 mg bid	60 mg/d	Tab: 5, 10, 20 mg	
Intrinsic Sympathomimetic Agents				
Acebutolol (Sectral, generic)	200 mg bid	600 mg bid	Cap: 200, 400 mg	Same as other β-blockers, except less bradycardia
Carteolol (Cartrol)	2.5 mg qd	10 mg qd	Tab: 2.5, 5 mg	
Penbutolol (Levatol)	20 mg qd	20 mg/d	Tab: 20 mg	
Pindolol (Visken, generic)	5 mg bid	60 mg /d	Tab: 5, 10 mg	
β-Blockers with α-Blocking Activity				
Carvedilol (Coreg, generic)	6.25 mg bid	25 mg bid	Tab: 3.125, 6.25, 12.5, 25 mg	Same as noncardioselective β-blockers
Labetolol (Normodyne, generic)	100 mg bid	600 mg bid	Tab: 100, 200, 300 mg	Same as noncardioselective β-blockers; hepatic toxicity
β-Blockers with Nitric Oxide Activity				
Nebivolol (Bystolic)	5 mg qd	40 mg qd	Tab: 2.5, 5, 10, 20 mg	Similar to other β-blockers; might have lower incidence of side effects
Calcium-Channel Blockers				
Dihydropyridines				
Amlodipine (Norvasc, generic)	2.5-5 mg qd	10 mg qd	Tab: 2.5, 5, 10 mg	Ankle edema, flushing, headache, dizziness, palpitations, gingival hypertrophy
Felodipine (Plendil, generic)	2.5-5 mg qd	10 mg qd	Tab: 2.5, 5, 10 mg	
Isradipine (generic, DynaCirc CR)	5 mg qd	20 mg qd	Tab: 5, 10 mg	
Nicardipine, sustained-release (Cardene SR, generic)	30 mg bid	60 mg bid	Cap: 30, 45, 60 mg	
Nicardipine extended-release (Adalat CC, generic)	30-60 mg qd	120 mg/d	Tab: 30, 60, 90 mg	
Nisoldipine, extended-release (Sular, generic)	20 mg qd	60 mg qd	Tab: 10, 20, 30, 40 mg	
Nondihydropyridines				
Diltiazem, extended-release (Cardizem SR, Cardizem CD, Dilacor XR, Tiazac, generic)	120-180 mg qd	360-480 mg/d	Once daily tab: 60, 90, 120 mg Twice-daily tab: 180, 240, 300, 360, 420 mg	AV block, bradycardia, heart failure, constipation (especially with verapamil), rash (with diltiazem), dizziness, headache, gingival hyperplasia
Verapamil, extended-release (Calan SR, Covera-HS, Isoptin SR, Verelan, generic)	120 mg qd	480 mg qd	Tab: 120, 180, 240 mg Cap: 120, 180, 240 mg Verelan PM: 100, 200, 300 mg	
Diuretics				
Thiazides				
Chlorothiazide (Diuril, generic)	125-250 mg qd-bid	1 g/d	Tab: 250, 500 mg Susp: 250 mg/5 mL	Hypokalemia, hypomagnesemia, hyperuricemia, hypercalcemia, hyperlipidemia, hyperglycemia, hyponatremia, impotence, rashes, photosensitivity, pancreatitis
Hydrochlorothiazide (Esidrix, Oretic, generic)	12.5-25 mg qd	50 mg qd	Tab: 25, 50, 100 mg Soln: 50 mg/5 mL	
Thiazide Congeners				
Chlorthalidone (Hygroton, generic)	12.5-25 mg qd	50 mg/d	Tab: 25, 50, 100 mg	Same as thiazides
Indapamide (Lozol, generic)	1.25 mg qd	5 mg qd	Tab: 1.25, 2.5 mg	Same as thiazides, may have fewer metabolic effects
Metolazone (Zaroxolyn, others)	2.5 mg qd	5 mg qd	Tab: 2.5, 5, 10 mg	Same as thiazides
Loop Diuretics				
Bumetamide (Bumex, generic)	0.5 mg bid	4 mg/d	Tab: 0.5, 1, 2 mg	Same as thiazides, no hypercalcemia
Ethacrynic acid (Edecrin)	12.5 mg bid	50 mg bid	Tab: 25, 50 mg	Same as thiazides, ototoxicity
Furosemide (Lasix, generic)	10-20 mg qd	240 mg/d (bid-tid)	Tab: 20, 40, 80 mg Soln: 10 mg/mL, 40 mg/mL	Same as thiazides, more pancreatitis and allergic reactions
Torsemide (Demadex, generic)	5 mg qd	10 mg qd	Tab: 5, 10, 20, 100 mg	Same as thiazides, more potent
Potassium-Sparing Agents				
Amiloride (Midamor, generic)	5 mg qd	10 mg/d	Tab: 5 mg	More hyperkalemia, nausea, flatulence, skin rash
Triamterene (Dyrenium)	25 mg qd-bid	100 mg/d	Tab: 50, 100 mg	Hyperkalemia; nephrolithiasis; folic acid antagonist; contraindicated in pregnancy

Continued

TABLE 3 Some Common Oral Antihypertensive Drugs—Cont'd

Drug (Trade Name)	Initial Dose	Max Dose	How Supplied	Major Side Effects/Comments
Aldosterone Receptor Antagonists				
Eplerenone (Inspra)	50 mg qd	50 mg bid	Tab: 25, 50, 100 mg	Hyperkalemia, hyponatremia, hypertriglyceridemia, dizziness, cough, fatigue, diarrhea, abdominal pain, mastodynia, gynecomastia
Spironolactone (Aldactone, generic)	12.5 mg qd-bid	50 mg bid	Tab: 25, 50, 100 mg	Hyperkalemia, impotence, gynecomastia in men, breast tenderness in women
α_1-Adrenergic Blockers				
Doxazosin (Cardura, generic)	1 mg qd	16 mg/d	Tab: 1, 2, 4, 8 mg	First-dose hypotension (more with prazosin), dizziness, palpitations, GI disturbances
Prazosin (Minipress, generic)	1 mg bid-tid	20 mg/d	Cap: 1, 2, 5 mg	
Terazosin (Hytrin generic)	1 mg qhs	20 mg/d	Tab or cap: 1, 2, 5, 10 mg	
Central α-Adrenergic Agonists				
Clonidine (Catapres, generic)	0.1 mg bid	1.2 mg/d	Tab: 0.1, 0.2, 0.3 mg	Sedation, drowsiness, depression, dry mouth, impotence, withdrawal hypertension (more with clonidine, less with guanfacine)
Catapres TTS (patch)	TTS-1 q wk	2 TTS-3 patches per wk	Patch: TTS-1, TTS-2, TTS-3	
Guanabenz (Wytensin, generic)	4 mg bid	32 mg bid	Tab: 4, 8 mg	
Guanfacine (Tenex, generic)	1 mg qhs	3 mg qhs	Tab: 1, 2 mg	
Methyldopa (Aldomet, generic)	250 mg bid	3000 mg/d	Tab: 125, 250, 500 mg Susp: 250 mg/5 mL	Same as other central agonists, plus hepatic and hemolytic anemia
Direct Vasodilators				
Hydralazine (Apresoline, generic)	10 mg qid-25 mg bid	200 mg/d	Tab: 10, 25, 50, 100 mg	Headaches, flushing, tachycardia, fluid retention, lupus-like reaction
Minoxidil (Loniten, generic)	5 mg qd	40 mg/d	Tab: 2.5, 10 mg	ECG changes, tachycardia, edema, pericardial effusion, hirsutism
Peripheral Adrenergic Antagonists				
Reserpine (generic)	0.05 mg qd	0.25 mg/d	Tab: 0.1, 0.25 mg	Depression, nasal stuffiness, activation of peptic ulcer

*Reduce diuretic dose before starting ACEI to prevent hypotension; reduce ACEI dosage in renal impairment (except moexipril). Contraindicated in bilateral renal artery stenosis. Pregnancy category C in the first trimester and category D in the second and third trimesters. Nonsteroidal antiinflammatory drugs reduce effect of ACEIs.
†Might require twice-daily dosing for 24-hour control of blood pressure.
Abbreviations: ACEI, angiotensin-converting enzyme inhibitor; cap = capsule; ECG = electrocardiogram; GI = gastrointestinal; soln = solution; susp = suspension; tab = tablet.
Table compiled by Miriam Chan, PharmD.

CURRENT THERAPY

- Lifestyle modification should be the first line of treatment for all patients with hypertension, especially when medications are started on the first clinic visit.
- Secondary causes of hypertension should be treated along with appropriate specialist consultation to ensure the best outcomes for the patient.
- Hypertension should be considered a modifiable risk factor for heart disease, stroke, and chronic kidney disease.
- Cardiovascular risk should be calculated using a published formula to help patients understand how they can affect their own health.
- Every effort should be made to match the drug class used with compelling indications present in each patient.
- Control of hypertension is more important than what medication is used, with the exception of compelling indications.

DIURETICS

Agents targeting the distal convoluted tubule (thiazide-type diuretics) are the preferred agents for the treatment of hypertension. Hydrochlorothiazide (HydroDiuril) (12.5-25 mg/day) is the most commonly used, and chlorthalidone (Hygroton) (12.5-100 mg/day) has been used in all the National Institutes of Health (NIH) trials. Chlorthalidone is a stronger and longer-acting agent than hydrocholothiazide.

It is important to allow up to 4 weeks for full effect of diuretic agents. Creatinine, magnesium, uric acid and electrolyte levels should be measured every 1 to 2 weeks when diuretics are being instituted. When the dosage is stable, laboratory values can be checked every 4 to 6 weeks. In patients whose glomerular filtration rate (GFR) is less than 40 mL/min/1.73 m^2, thiazide-type agents might not work, and loop diuretics will be a better choice.

Furosemide (Lasix) is best dosed every 6 to 8 hours with doses of 20 to 40 mg. Doses up to 400 mg have been used in severe edema, but such high doses require close monitoring of electrolytes. In patients with heart failure and severe proteinuria (>4 g/day), a better choice may be bumetanide (Bumex)[1] 1 to 10 mg/day, which is up to 40 times more potent and twice as orally bioavailable. If hypokalemia

[1]Not FDA approved for this indication.

TABLE 4 Common Combination Products for Hypertension

Drug Combination	Brand Name	Dosage Forms (mg/mg)
Angiotensin-Converting Enzyme Inhibitors and Calcium-Channel Blockers		
Amlodipine/benazepril	Lotrel, generic	2.5/10, 5/10, 5/20, 5/40, 10/20
Amlodipine/valsartan	Exforge	5/160, 5/320, 10/160, 10/320
Enalapril/felodipine	Lexxel	5/5
Trandolapril/verapamil	Tarka	1/240, 2/180, 2/240, 4/240
Angiotensin-Converting Enzyme Inhibitors and Diuretics		
Benazepril/HCTZ	Lotensin HCT, generic	5/6.25, 10/12.5, 20/12.5, 20/25
Captopril/HCTZ	Capozide, generic	25/15, 25/25, 50/15, 50/25
Enalapril/HCTZ	Vaseretic, generic	5/12.5, 10/25
Fosinopril/HCTZ	Monopril HCT, generic	10/12.5, 20/12.5
Lisinopril/HCTZ	Prinzide, Zestoretic, generic	10/12.5, 20/12.5, 20/25
Moexipril/HCTZ	Uniretic, generic	7.5/12.5, 15/12.5, 15/25
Quinapril/HCTZ	Accuretic, generic	10/12.5, 20/12.5, 20/25
Angiotensin Receptor Blocker and Calcium-Channel Blocker		
Telmisartan/amlodipine	Twynsta	40/5, 40/10, 80/5, 80/10
Angiotensin Receptor Blockers and Diuretics		
Candesartan/HCTZ	Atacand HCT	16/12.5, 32/12.5, 32/25
Eprosartan/HCTZ	Teveten-HCT	600/12.5, 600/25
Irbesartan/HCTZ	Avalide	150/12.5, 300/12.5, 300/25
Losartan/HCTZ	Hyzaar, generic	50/12.5, 100/12.5, 100/25
Olmesartan/HCTZ	Benicar HCT	20/12.5, 40/12.5, 40/25
Telmisartan/HCTZ	Micardis HCT	40/12.5, 80/12.5, 80/25
Valsartan/HCTZ	Diovan HCT	80/12.5, 160/12.5, 160/25, 320/12.5, 320/25
β-Blockers and Diuretics		
Atenolol/chlorthalidone	Tenoretic, generic	50/25, 100/25
Bisoprolol/HCTZ	Ziac, generic	2.5/6.25, 5/6.25, 10/6.25
Metoprolol/HCTZ	Lorpressor HCT, generic	50/25, 100/25, 100/50
Nadolol/bendroflumethiazide	Corzide	40/5, 80/5
Propranolol/HCTZ	Inderide LA, generic	40/25, 80/25
Calcium-Channel Blocker, Angiotensin-Converting Enzyme Inhibitor, and Diuretic		
Amlodipine/valsartan/HCTZ	Exforge HCT	5/160/12.5, 5/160/25, 10/160/12.5, 10/160/25, 10/320/25
Centrally Acting Drug and Diuretic		
Methyldopa/HCTZ	Aldoril, generic	250/15, 250/25, 500/30, 500/50
Clonidine/chlorthalidone	Clorpres	0.1/15, 0.2/15, 0.3/15
Direct Vasodilator and Diuretic		
Hydralazine/HCTZ	HydraZide, generic	25/25, 50/50
Diuretic and Diuretic		
Amiloride/HCTZ	Moduretic, generic	5/50
Spironolactone/HCTZ	Aldactazide, generic	25/25, 50/50
Triamterene/HCTZ	Dyazide, Maxzide, generic	37.5/25, 50/25, 75/50
Renin Inhibitor and Angiotensin Receptor Blocker		
Aliskiren/valsartan	Valturna	150/160, 300/320

Abbreviation: HCTZ: hydrochlorothiazide.
Table compiled by Miriam Chan, PharmD.

becomes a problem, the use of a potassium-sparing diuretic such as amiloride (Midamor) 5 to 10 mg/day may be indicated. Care must be taken to avoid hyperkalemia, especially in those with a GFR less than 50 mL/min/1.73 m^2.

The aldosterone blocker spironolactone (Aldactone) has been shown to decrease mortality in patients with congestive heart failure (25 mg/day). It has also been found to help control refractory hypertension at much higher doses (1 mg/kg/day) when used in combination with angiotensin-converting enzyme inhibitors (ACEIs) or angiotensin receptor blockers (ARBs). Great care should be taken to watch for life-threatening hyperkalemia that can develop with this combination of medications.

ADRENERGIC-INHIBITING DRUGS

Central α-agonists such as clonidine (Catapres) are often added to diuretics and act centrally on both imidazoline receptors and α$_2$-receptors. Clonidine can be given 0.1 to 1.4 mg twice per day.

Sedation and dry mouth can be dose-limiting side effects, and rebound hypertension will occur with a sudden cessation of clonidine.

β-Adrenergic receptor blockers can cause worsening bradycardia when used in combination with clonidine. Carvedilol (Coreg) has been tested against metoprolol (Toprol XL) and found to provide survival benefit in heart failure. When used for hypertension, carvedilol is best dosed twice a day starting with 6.25 mg bid to a maximum of 25 mg bid. It is superior to metoprolol because it does not worsen insulin sensitivity and has a limited effect on lipids.

The most notable comparative drug trials for hypertension are ANBP2 (Second Australian National Blood Pressure Study: ACEI superior to thiazide in men only); LIFE (Losartan Intervention For Endpoint reduction: ARB superior to β-blocker) and ACCOMPLISH (Avoiding Cardiovascular Events in Combination Therapy in Patients Living with Systolic Hypertension: ACEI plus calcium-channel blocker superior to ACEI plus thiazide) and the AASK trial (African American Study of Kidney Disease and Hypertension).

The AASK study enrolled 1094 African Americans with hypertensive kidney disease (GFR 20-65 mL/min/1.73 m^2) and studied two blood pressure goals using three different agents. The normal blood pressure control group (mean arterial pressure [MAP], 102-107 mm Hg; $n = 554$) was compared to the tight control group (MAP $\leq$92 mm Hg; $n = 540$). The groups of patients were divided into groups treated with the β-blocker metoprolol (Lopressor) ($n = 441$) or the ACEI ramipril (Altace) ($n = 436$) or the dihydropyridine calcium channel blocker amlodipine (Norvasc) ($n = 217$). Other open-label agents were also allowed. The low-BP group reached an average of 128/78 mm Hg and the normal group reached 141/85 mm Hg.

The conclusion in this study was that ramipril appears to be more effective in slowing progression of chronic kidney disease (CKD) than metoprolol and amlodipine when followed over 3 to 6 years. Only subjects with more than 1 g of proteinuria showed a trend toward slower progression of CKD in the lower BP group. One last very important point was that the amlodipine group showed a significant *increase* in proteinuria (58%) when compared to the *reduction* in the ramipril group (20%) and the metoprolol group (14%).

One very useful algorithm has been proposed and is depicted in Figure 2. Doses should be titrated every 1 to 2 weeks, and great care should be taken to ensure that the physician looks for compelling indications and matches them with appropriate drug therapy.

Blood pressure should be monitored every 2 to 4 weeks while medications are increased or added. Laboratory testing should be individualized to the patient's needs, comorbid conditions, and the medications being used to treat the patient's hypertension. If large doses of diuretics, ACEIs, or ARBs are used, weekly laboratory studies may be indicated.

Complications

The most common complications from long-standing hypertension include stroke, heart disease, and CKD. One of the most important points to remember about hypertension is that it is one factor that must be taken into account in the patient's overall risk for heart disease. There are several great cardiovascular risk calculators. One such calculator can be found at www.qintervention.org. This calculator

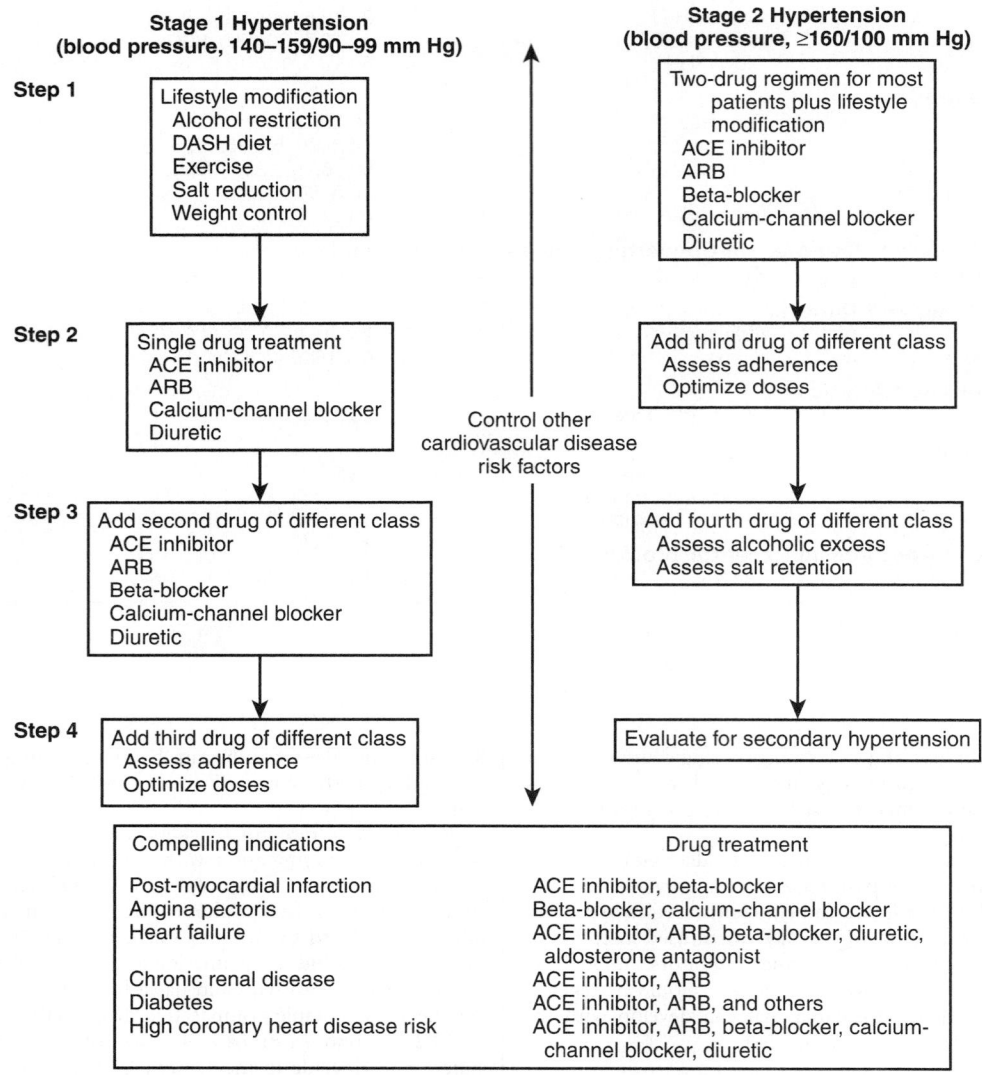

FIGURE 2. Algorithm for management of hypertension. ACE = angiotensin-converting enzyme; ARB = angiotensin receptor blocker; DASH = Dietary Approaches to Stop Hypertension. (Reprinted with permission from Chobanian AV: Shattuck Lecture. The hypertension paradox—more uncontrolled disease despite improved therapy. N Engl J Med 2009;361(9):878-87.)

estimates the 10-year risk for TIA or stroke and heart disease, as well as the 10-year risk of developing type 2 diabetes mellitus. The Framingham score is still considered the gold standard for risk calculation and can be found at http://hp2010.nhlbihin.net/atpiii/calculator.asp?usertype=prof#moreinfo.

CKD is not only a consequence of hypertension but also a newly recognized risk factor for heart disease. CKD is defined as kidney damage for more than 3 months, irrespective of the underlying cause. CKD stage 1 patients have a normal or increased glomerular filtration rate (GFR) (>90 mL/min/1.73 m^2) and evidence of kidney damage (hematuria, proteinuria, abnormal kidney ultrasound). Stage 2 CKD is defined by a GFR of 60 to 89 mL/min/1.73 m^2, and stage 3 CKD is defined by a GFR of 30 to 59 mL/min/1.73 m^2. The most concerning stages of CKD are stage 4 (GFR 15-29 mL/min/1.73 m^2) and stage 5 (GFR <15 mL/min/1.73 m^2). Most patients who have stage 5 CKD are on dialysis. Recipients of a kidney transplant are CKD-staged based on their GFR with the addition of a "T" for transplant following the stage. For example, a kidney transplant recipient with a GFR of 65 mL/min/1.73 m^2 is staged CKD 2T.

According to NHANES III, an estimated 19 million people in the United States have some form of CKD. Almost 400,000 people are on dialysis currently, and about 150,000 have a functioning kidney transplant. The most recent estimate is that by 2020 there will be 530,000 people on dialysis in the United Stages and 250,000 people with a functioning kidney transplant. Hypertension continues to affect almost all dialysis patients and 70% of transplant recipients. It is for this reason that hypertension should be managed as one critical piece of the puzzle in an effort to help our patients live long, productive lives.

Future Therapy

Many new approaches for the treatment of hypertension are on the way. An Australian group has shown that radiofrequency ablation of the renal nerves might hold promise for a selected group of hypertensive patients. Stimulation of carotid baroreceptors has also been looked at to reduce sympathetic outflow and reduce hypertension. Hypertension vaccines are currently in phase II trials and might help treat hypertension by inducing anti-angiotensin II antibodies. These and many trials and medications are in store for those of us who care for patients with hypertension. The next decade is sure to bring as much or more to our endless search for the next best treatment of hypertension.

REFERENCES

Adrogué HJ, Madias NE. Sodium and potassium in the pathogenesis of hypertension. N Engl J Med 2007;356(19):1966–78.

Chobanian AV. Shattuck Lecture. The hypertension paradox—more uncontrolled disease despite improved therapy. N Engl J Med 2009;361(9):878–87. Erratum in: N Engl J Med 2009;361(15):1561.

Collins AJ, Foley RN, Gilbertson DT, Chen SC. The state of chronic kidney disease, ESRD, and morbidity and mortality in the first year of dialysis. Clin J Am Soc Nephrol 2009;4(Suppl. 1):S5–S11.

Cooney MT, Dudina AL, Graham IM. Value and limitations of existing scores for the assessment of cardiovascular risk: A review for clinicians. J Am Coll Cardiol 2009;54(14):1209–27.

Feig DI, Soletsky B, Johnson RJ. Effect of allopurinol on blood pressure of adolescents with newly diagnosed essential hypertension: A randomized trial. JAMA 2008;300(8):924–32.

Kaplan NM. Kaplan's Clinical Hypertension. 9th ed. Philadelphia: Lippincott Williams and Wilkins; 2006.

Katakam R, Brukamp K, Townsend RR. What is the proper workup of a patient with hypertension? Cleve Clin J Med 2008;75(9):663–72.

Molony DA, Craig JC. Evidence-Based Nephrology. Oxford: Blackwell; 2009.

Townsend RR, Textor SC. Hypertension; 2010 Nephrology Self-Assessment Program 9; 2, March 2010.

Acute Myocardial Infarction

Method of
Guy S. Reeder, MD, and Abhiram Prasad, MD

The diagnosis of myocardial infarction (MI) is confirmed by a typical rise and fall in biochemical markers of myocardial necrosis with at least one of the following: ischemic symptoms, changes on the electrocardiogram (ECG) of ischemia (ST elevation or depression), development of pathologic Q waves, or percutaneous coronary intervention (PCI).

Incidence

More than 1 million patients suffer an MI every year in the United States. Despite a 50% decline in cardiovascular death due to advances in diagnosis and management related to MI since the 1970s, MI remains a fatal event in one out of three patients.

Pathophysiology

MI results from reduction in myocardial perfusion sufficient to cause cell necrosis. Atherosclerotic plaque rupture or erosion allows the thrombogenic lipid core to be exposed with complete or partial thrombotic occlusion. Epicardial occlusion may also be accompanied by downstream microvascular constriction. Coronary spasm is an uncommon cause of MI, and spontaneous coronary artery dissection, coronary embolus, and hypercoagulable states are among the rare causes.

Clinical Presentation

Patients with MI usually present with central pressure-like chest discomfort that can radiate to the arms, neck, or back. This is often associated with nausea, diaphoresis, and dyspnea. At least 20% of MIs are clinically unrecognized due to atypical presentation without chest pain, especially in elderly, diabetic, or postoperative patients. Symptoms include back pain, epigastric pain, syncope, dyspnea, or confusion. The differential diagnosis of acute MI includes aortic dissection, acute pulmonary embolism, perimyocarditis, musculoskeletal pain, esophagitis, peptic ulcer disease, cholecystitis, biliary colic, and pancreatitis.

Physical examination is often normal. Some patients have signs of left ventricular (LV) dysfunction including tachycardia, pulmonary rales, and third heart sound. Infarction or ischemia leading to papillary muscle dysfunction or rupture can lead to a murmur of mitral regurgitation. Patients with right ventricular (RV) infarction might have an elevated jugular venous pressure and a positive Kussmaul sign, and those with severe LV dysfunction present with cardiogenic shock. An estimation of prognosis at presentation is possible using the Killip classification or the TIMI (Thombolysis in Myocardial Infarction [trial] risk scores (Tables 1 and 2).

TABLE 1 Killip Class and Hospital Mortality

Killip Class	Clinical Classification	Mortality (%)
I	No heart failure	6
II	Mild heart failure, rales, S$_3$, congestion on chest radiograph	17
III	Pulmonary edema	38
IV	Cardiogenic shock	81

Data from Killip T 3rd, Kimball JT: Treatment of myocardial infarction in a coronary care unit. A two year experience with 250 patients. Am J Cardiol 1967;20(4):457–464.

TABLE 2 TIMI Risk Score for ST-Elevation Myocardial Infarction

Risk Factor	Points	Risk Score	30-Day Mortality (%)
Age ≥ 75 y	3	0	0.8
Age 65–74 y	2	1	1.6
Diabetes or hypertension	1	2	2.2
Systolic BP <100 mm Hg	3	3	4.4
Heart rate >100/min	2	4	7.3
Killip class II-IV	2	5	12.4
Anterior MI or LBBB	1	6	16.1
Weight <67 kg	1	7	23.4
Time to treatment >4 h	1	8	26.8
		>8	35.9

Data from Morrow DA, Antman EM, Charlesworth A, et al: TIMI risk score for ST-elevation myocardial infarction: A convenient, bedside, clinical score for risk assessment at presentation: An intravenous nPA for treatment of infarcting myocardium early II trial substudy. Circulation 2000;102:2031–2037.
BP = blood pressure; TIMI = Thombolysis in Myocardial Infarction (trial).

Evaluation of Suspected Acute Myocardial Infarction

The initial evaluation of a patient with suspected MI should include a focused history, physical examination, ECG, blood sample for cardiac biomarkers, and chest radiograph. The patient's rhythm should be continuously monitored and intravenous access should be established.

ELECTROCARDIOGRAM

A 12-lead ECG should be performed within 10 minutes of arrival into an emergency department. In addition, posterior leads (V7-V9) and leads V3R and V4R should be used in patients with suspected posterior and RV infarctions, respectively. The ECG findings differentiate patients with ST elevation MI (STEMI) and ST depression MI (NSTEMI) (Fig. 1). Patients with STEMI require immediate reperfusion therapy, but those with NSTEMI do not unless there is ongoing ischemic pain or hemodynamic instability.

The ECG diagnosis of MI is difficult in the presence of left bundle branch block (LBBB). However, the presence of ST segment elevation

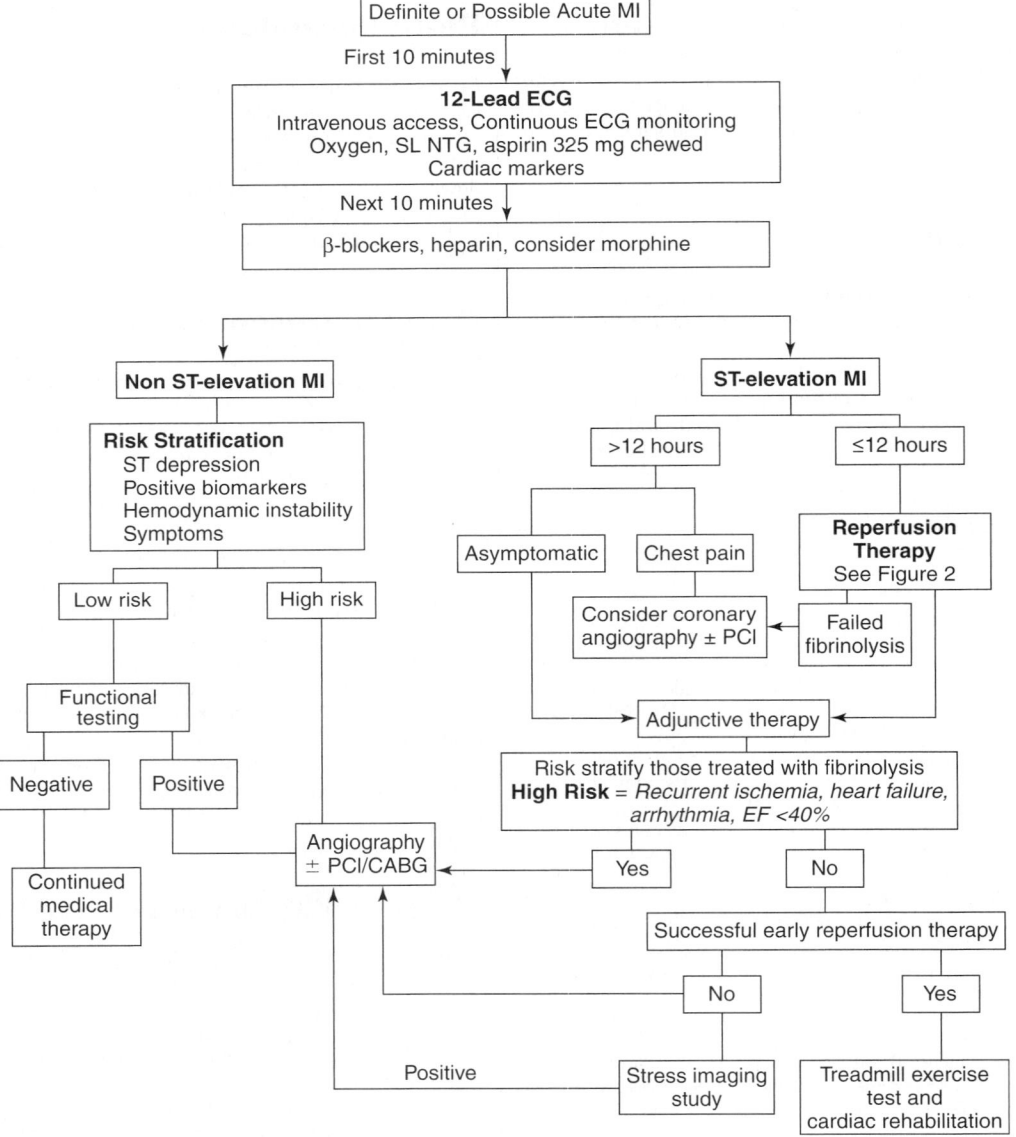

FIGURE 1. Definite or possible acute myocardial infarction (MI). CABG = coronary artery bypass graft; ECG = electrocardiogram; EF = ejection fraction; PCI = percutaneous coronary intervention; SL NTG = sublingual nitroglycerin.

of greater than 1 mm concordant with a QRS complex, ST segment depression greater than 1 mm in leads V1 to V3, or ST segment elevation greater than 5 mm discordant with a QRS complex supports the diagnosis.

SERUM MARKERS

Serum biomarkers of myocardial necrosis include troponins, MB isoforms of creatine kinase (CK-MB), creatine kinase (CK), and myoglobin. Measurement of troponin has replaced other biomarkers due to higher sensitivity, specificity, and prognostic value. Measurements of troponin I or T should be performed at presentation and 6 to 9 hours after the onset of symptoms. If troponin levels are elevated, confirmation with CK-MB may be performed to determine acuteness, because troponin can remain elevated for 10 to 15 days after MI. Likewise, CK-MB is useful for detecting reinfarction during a period of persistent troponin elevations from the initial event. Troponin and CK-MB may be elevated following cardiac surgery, myopericarditis, PCI, tachyarrhythmias, and cardioversion. Troponins may be elevated following pulmonary embolus and decompensated congestive heart failure. All cardiac markers may be initially negative early in acute MI; treatment must never be withheld based on negative initial biomarkers.

Treatment

ST ELEVATION MYOCARDIAL INFARCTION

Initial Approach

These goals should be achieved expeditiously and simultaneously (see Fig. 1): relief of pain, initiation of reperfusion and ancillary therapy, and assessment and treatment of hemodynamic abnormalities. Pain relief is best achieved with oxygen (2 L nasal cannula), nitroglycerin, and morphine sulfate. Patients with ST segment elevation or new LBBB with symptoms for 12 hours or less are candidates for reperfusion therapy.

Reperfusion Therapy

The diagnosis of STEMI mandates immediate reperfusion. PCI is preferred, but it is not promptly available in many areas. Fibrinolytic therapy is widely available, but it is slightly less effective in randomized trials and carries a higher risk of hemorrhagic stroke. The decision regarding which therapy to employ should be made on the basis of a written institution-specific protocol that considers symptom duration, availability of PCI locally, time to transfer to a PCI facility, and fibrinolytic contraindications (Fig. 2). In general, patients presenting within 3 hours of symptom onset derive a large benefit from fibrinolytics; if transfer time to a PCI facility results in a door-to-balloon time of longer than 90 minutes, fibrinolysis is preferred. Guidelines for door-to-needle (30 min) and door-to-balloon (90 min) times recommended by the American College of Cardiology and American Heart Association (ACC/AHA) are one of a number of quality indicators for acute MI care.

Fibrinolytic Therapy

Fibrinolytic therapy should be administered within 30 minutes of arrival to the emergency department. The greatest benefit is seen when this is performed within the first 4 hours of onset of pain resulting in an absolute 3% reduction in mortality, but it is associated with a small (0.4%) increase in stroke rate. There is a 2% absolute reduction in mortality rate for every hour saved in administration of therapy, and no benefit is seen after 12 hours of symptom duration. A benefit is observed in all age groups, including those with prior MI and diabetes, as well as in patients presenting with hypotension and tachycardia. Age older than 75 years, Killip class higher than II, resting tachycardia, hypotension, anterior MI location, and time to reperfusion longer than 4 hours are useful predictors of early mortality, ranging from 0.8% with none of these factors to more than

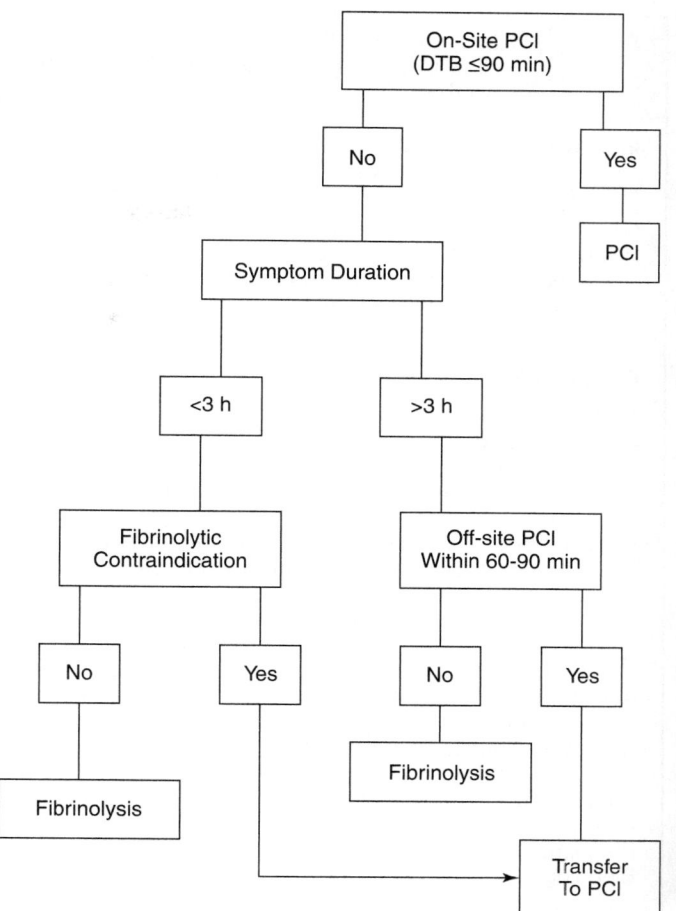

FIGURE 2. Selection of reperfusion therapy. DTB = door-to-balloon time; PCI = percutaneous coronary intervention.

36% for all (see Table 2). Box 1 lists indications and contraindications for fibrinolysis.

Table 3 lists the currently available fibrinolytic agents. These differ primarily with respect to plasma half-life; the longest-acting agent, tenecteplase, requires a single bolus injection. Intravenous heparin must be administered concurrently to reduce the risk of late reocclusion of infarct-related artery.

Primary Percutaneous Coronary Intervention

Although fibrinolytic therapy is easy to administer and widely available, it provides early reperfusion in only 80% of patients and is often not administered due to perceived or actual contraindications in a significant number of patients. In contrast, primary PCI has only rare contraindications and leads to higher reperfusion (approximately 90%). Randomized trials performed in high-volume academic centers comparing fibrinolytic therapy with PCI for acute MI have demonstrated approximately 30% reduction in mortality and reinfarction rates and a significant reduction in cerebrovascular accidents with PCI. Stent deployment during acute MI leads to similar early outcome compared with balloon angioplasty, but it reduces restenosis rates and target vessel revascularization.

Primary PCI should be performed within 60 to 90 minutes of arrival to the hospital by an interventional cardiologist who performs at least 75 procedures a year in a center that has a volume of at least 200 procedures a year and has cardiac surgery capabilities. PCI should also be considered in specific patient populations listed in Box 2. Transfer from one hospital to another for primary PCI should only be considered if it can be achieved within 60 to 90 minutes (total door-to-balloon time); otherwise, fibrinolytic therapy should be administered without delay.

BOX 1 Indications and Contraindications for Fibrinolytic Therapy in Acute Myocardial Infarction

Indications

ST segment elevation ≥ 1 mV in ≥ 2 contiguous limb leads or ≥ 2 mV in contiguous precordial leads

New left bundle branch block

Posterior MI: ST segment depression >2 mV in leads V1 and V2 with either imaging evidence of posterior LV wall motion abnormality or ST segment elevation of 1 mV in the posterior leads V7-V9

Contraindications

Absolute

Active bleeding

Prior intracranial hemorrhage; other strokes or neurologic events within 1 year; intracranial neoplasm

Recent major surgery (<6 wk) or major trauma (<2 wk)

Recent vascular puncture in a noncompressible site (<2 wk)

Suspected aortic dissection

Relative

Active peptic ulcer disease or recent gastrointestinal bleeding (<4 wk)

Severe uncontrolled hypertension on presentation (BP $> 180/110$ mm Hg) or chronic severe hypertension

Cardiopulmonary resuscitation >10 min

Prior nonhemorrhagic stroke

Pregnancy

Bleeding diathesis or INR >2

BP = blood pressure; INR = international normalized ratio.

BOX 2 Indications for Percutaneous Coronary Intervention in Acute Myocardial Infarction

Failed fibrinolysis (rescue PCI)

Contraindication to fibrinolytics

Shock or markers of increased mortality such as TIMI risk score ≥ 5 or Killips classes III-IV

Nondiagnostic ECG changes with ongoing pain or hemodynamic instability

As a preferred strategy when available promptly

ECG = electrocardiogram; PCI = percutaneous coronary intervention; TIMI = Thrombolysis in Myocardial Infarction (trial).

Adjunct Therapy for STEMI

Agents proved to reduce mortality in patients with STEMI include aspirin, β-blockers, statins, and angiotensin-converting enzyme (ACE) inhibitors (Table 4).

Aspirin

Unless there is history of allergic reaction, aspirin 325 mg should be administered immediately on the patient's arrival to the emergency room and continued indefinitely at a dose of at least 81 mg/day. Chewed aspirin has the most rapid onset of action due to absorption from the buccal mucosa, with inhibition of platelets within minutes. Clopidogrel (Plavix) may be administered to patients with an aspirin allergy.

Clopidogrel

is a thienopyridine that blocks the platelet ADP receptor, resulting in reduced platelet aggregation. A loading dose of 300 to 600[3] mg is typically administered at the time of PCI. Some data suggest a benefit of 75 to 300 mg administered with thrombolytic therapy; the lower dose might reduce the bleeding risk in patients older than 75 years. Maintenance dose is 75 mg/day; duration of therapy in PCI with stenting is defined by type of stent. Duration of therapy when administered with fibrinolytics is not well established.

Unfractionated Heparin

Unfractionated heparin has been shown to decrease reocclusion following fibrinolytic therapy, and it should be administered at the time of fibrinolytic infusion. A bolus of 60 U/kg (maximum 4000 units) of unfractionated heparin followed by an infusion of 7–12 U/kg/h may be used to initiate therapy. The activated partial thromboplastin time (aPTT) should be checked at 4 to 6 hours after initiation of heparin and then every 6 to 8 hours. The aPTT should be maintained between 50 and 70 seconds, and therapy should be continued for approximately 48 hours. Heparin may be continued for a longer duration in patients with atrial fibrillation or large anterior MI who are at risk for embolic events. Long-term anticoagulation with warfarin may be indicated in patients with LV thrombus, atrial fibrillation, or an ejection fraction (EF) less than 30% following MI with a target international normalized ratio (INR) of 2 to 3.

Low-Molecular-Weight Heparin

Low-molecular-weight heparins (LMWHs) are produced by fragmentation of unfractionated heparin. These agents have advantages over unfractionated heparin, including a more predictable dose response, greater bioavailability, no need for laboratory monitoring, and a lower rate of thrombocytopenia. LMWHs possess greater

[3]Exceeds dosage recommended by the manufacturer.

TABLE 3 Comparison of Fibrinolytics

Characteristic	Alteplase (Activase) (tPA)	Reteplase (Retavase) (rPA)	Tenecteplase (TNKase)
Dose	15-mg bolus, then 0.75 mg/kg over 30 min (max 50 mg), then 0.5 mg/kg over 60 min (max 35 mg)	10 + 10 MU double bolus 30 min apart	0.5 mg/kg single bolus (max 50 mg)
Plasma half-life	4–6 min	18 min	20 min
Fibrin specificity	++	+	+++
Plasminogen activation	Direct	Direct	Direct
Antigenicity	No	No	No

max = maximum; MU = megaunit; rPA = recombinant plasminogen activator; tPA = tissue plasminogen activator.

TABLE 4 Adjunctive Therapies That Reduce Mortality in Patients with Myocardial Infarction

Drug	Indication	Suggested Drugs and Initial Dose	NNT
Aspirin	All	160–325 mg/day	42 patients for 1 mo
β-Blocker	All except patients with moderate or severe asthma, cardiogenic shock, pulmonary edema or ≥second-degree AV block	Metoprolol (Lopressor) 5 mg IV × 3 (at 5-min intervals), and then 50 mg PO bid *or* Esmolol (Brevibloc) bolus 500 µg/kg and infuse at 50 µg/kg/min	38 patients for 2 y
HMG CoA reductase inhibitors	All	Simvastatin (Zocor) or atorvastatin (Lipitor) 40–80 mg/day	30 patients for 5 y
ACE Inhibitors	Anterior MI, EF <40%, diabetes May consider using in all CAD patients	Captopril (Capoten) 6.25 mg PO tid, increasing at 6h-8h intervals to a maximum of 50 mg tid *or* Lisinopril (Prinivil, Zestril) 2.5-10 mg PO qd Maintain systolic BP >90 mm Hg	20 patients for 3.5 y

ACE, angiotensin-converting enzyme; AV = atrioventricular; BP = blood pressure; CAD = coronary artery disease; EF = ejection fraction; HMG CoA = 3-hydroxy-3-methyl-glutaryl coenzyme A; MI = myocardial infarction; NNT = number needed to treat to save one life.

anti-Xa activity relative to anti-IIa (antithrombin) activity. This may be of potential benefit, because factor Xa generation occurs several steps earlier in the coagulation cascade.

Enoxaparin (Lovenox) is the most widely studied LMWH in STEMI and acute coronary syndromes. Trials of enoxaparin in conjunction with fibrinolysis have shown benefit in terms of preventing reinfarction, no significant mortality advantage, and somewhat increased risk of bleeding. LMWH should be avoided in men with creatinine higher than 2.5 or women with creatinine higher than 2.0.

Glycoprotein IIb/IIIa Antagonists

Platelet glycoprotein IIb/IIIa receptor inhibitors block the final common pathway in platelet aggregation. Currently available drugs include the chimeric monoclonal antibody abciximab (Reopro) and the nonantibody agents tirofiban (Aggrastat) and eptifibatide (Integrilin). Several studies have investigated the role of glycoprotein IIb/IIIa antagonists in STEMI and demonstrated a reduction in the composite endpoints of death, MI, and target vessel revascularization in patients treated with primary PCI. This benefit is due to higher TIMI-3 flow rate in the infarct-related artery, both before and after the coronary intervention procedure. Initial studies investigating the use of glycoprotein IIb/IIIa receptor antagonists with fibrinolytic agents suggested higher TIMI-3 flow rates, but phase III trials have failed to show a superiority of combined therapy over fibrinolytic therapy alone. Thus, intravenous glycoprotein IIb/IIIa inhibitors are indicated in patients being reperfused with PCI, but no indication exists for their combination with fibrinolytic therapy.

β-Adrenergic Antagonist Drugs

Early intravenous β-blocker therapy—metoprolol (Lopressor) 5 mg IV × 3 q5 min, followed by oral administration—is indicated in all patients without contraindications. In patients with borderline LV function, a test dose of intravenous esmolol can be given to assess tolerance to β-blockade. Patients with relative contraindications, such as chronic obstructive pulmonary disease or insulin-dependent diabetes, appear to derive benefit from treatment. Major contraindications to β-blockade include moderate to severe asthma, second- or third-degree atrioventricular block, severe bradycardia, hypotension, and pulmonary edema. β-Blockade should be withheld in these settings.

Angiotensin-Converting Enzyme Inhibitors

ACE activity is markedly increased at the edge of the infarct, and clinical trials have confirmed that ACE inhibitors reduce deleterious LV remodeling. The optimal selection of patients for ACE-inhibitor therapy remains controversial, but the most cost-effective approach is to selectively treat high-risk patients (those with impaired LV function or an anterior MI). However, demonstration of asymptomatic LV dysfunction requires bedside imaging studies, and selection of patients by infarct location alone might not result in early identification of all patients with significant LV dysfunction. Thus, unless the infarct is known to be small, it may be most reasonable to consider initial administration of ACE inhibitors in a nonselective fashion (i.e., in all patients with an acute MI) and then withdraw therapy later based on the absence of high-risk features. Exclusion criteria include allergy to ACE inhibitors, hypotension (systolic blood pressure [BP] <90 mm Hg), shock, history of bilateral renal artery stenosis, and prior worsening of renal function with ACE inhibitors.

ACE inhibitors have a class effect and should be administered orally, initially at low doses, with careful monitoring of the BP. Treatment should be continued indefinitely in patients with symptomatic heart failure or asymptomatic LV dysfunction (LVEF <45%), hemodynamically significant mitral regurgitation, or hypertension. Angiotensin receptor blockers (ARBs) may be used in patients intolerant of ACE inhibitors.

HMG CoA Reductase Inhibitors

Low-density lipoprotein (LDL) cholesterol plays a critical role in the pathogenesis of atherosclerosis. Lipid lowering with HMG CoA (3-hydroxy-3-methyl-glutaryl coenzyme A) reductase inhibitors (statins) are effective in secondary prevention by reducing mortality, recurrent infarction, ischemia, and heart failure. Preliminary studies indicate that treatment with statins can also lead to modest reductions in recurrent ischemia and infarction during acute coronary syndromes. Thus, a lipid profile should be assessed within 24 hours of the MI (before the inflammatory response from the MI leads to a temporary reduction in lipids) or 6 to 8 weeks later. Either way, improved outcomes have been demonstrated by early intensive statin therapy started in the hospital, with a target LDL cholesterol of 60 to 85 mg/dL.

Nitrates

Potential benefits of nitrate therapy include increased perfusion of ischemic zones, decrease in oxygen consumption, improved diastolic function, and enhanced collateral flow. The infusion of intravenous nitroglycerin should be initiated at 5 to 10 µg/min and gradually increased. The goal should be a 10% reduction in systolic BP in normotensive patients and approximately a 30% reduction in systolic pressure in hypertensive patients. Nitrates should be used with caution in patients with RV infarction or dehydration (who are preload dependent) to avoid excessive hypotension. Long-acting oral nitrates may be indicated with significant residual ischemia or heart failure. A nitrate-free interval of 8 to 12 hours must be provided to prevent nitrate tolerance.

Calcium Channel Blockers

Calcium channel blockers have vasodilative, antianginal, and antihypertensive actions. Calcium channel blockers do not reduce mortality in patients with MI and are not recommended for routine therapy or secondary prevention. In patients in whom β-adrenergic antagonists are contraindicated, verapamil or diltiazem may be appropriate as an alternative.

Antiarrhythmic Therapy

Potentially fatal ventricular arrhythmia occurs most commonly in the first 48 hours after an MI, and numerous trials have investigated the effects of antiarrhythmic agents on mortality and the incidence of ventricular fibrillation. Prophylactic therapy with antiarrhythmic drugs has been shown to be ineffective. Lidocaine may be used for 24 to 48 hours to treat ventricular tachycardia and following resuscitation for ventricular fibrillation. Amiodarone (Cordarone) is safe to use in the setting of MI and is the drug of choice for treating symptomatic ventricular arrhythmia.

Implantable Cardioverter-Defibrillator

ICD implantation reduces the occurrence of sudden death in certain high-risk patients such as those with late (>24 hours after the onset of symptoms) sustained ventricular tachycardia and ventricular fibrillation and in patients with EF persistently less than 30% to 35%. An ICD may also be beneficial in patients with late nonsustained ventricular tachycardia who have an EF of less than 40% and ventricular tachycardia induced during an electrophysiology study. ICD implantation should be considered if the patient is judged to be at continuous high risk for ventricular arrhythmia after revascularization for significant spontaneous or inducible ischemia.

NON–ST-ELEVATION MYOCARDIAL INFARCTION

Incompletely occluding coronary thrombus, or extensive collateral arterial supply (or both) is the underlying pathology of NSTEMI. More common than STEMI, especially in the elderly, the presentation is identical except for the absence of ST elevation.

Initial Therapy

Management differs from STEMI in that urgent reperfusion therapy is not indicated; the administration of fibrinolytics may be harmful. Instead, the focus of initial therapy is intensive medical stabilization with antiplatelet and antithrombotic agents to prevent clot propagation, nitrates and β-blockers for anti-ischemic effects, statins for cholesterol lowering, and other agents to control pain and hemodynamic compromise. For patients with continued pain or hemodynamic deterioration, immediate angiography and PCI are indicated. All other patients should undergo risk stratification (see Fig. 1). The TIMI risk score for unstable angina and NSTEMI (Table 5) allows separation of low risk from intermediate and high risks. Low-risk patients are suitable for functional testing, whereas all others undergo elective catheterization plus PCI in 4 to 48 hours.

Adjunct Therapy

In addition to aspirin, clopidogrel is beneficial in NSTEMI. The benefit must be weighed against the bleeding risk if coronary bypass surgery is performed within 5 days of drug administration. We elect to not administer clopidogrel until establishment of coronary anatomy and decision regarding need for bypass surgery. Once started, the drug has shown benefit for 9 to 12 months.

Several large studies have investigated the role of glycoprotein IIb/IIIa antagonists in patients with unstable angina or NSTEMI. Overall, the studies using tirofiban and eptifibatide have demonstrated a small but significant risk reduction in composite endpoints, with the greatest benefit in patients with diabetes, patients with troponin elevations, and patients undergoing PCI. In contrast, the GUSTO-IV ACS (Global Utilization of Strategies To open Occluded coronary arteries trial IV in Acute Coronary Syndromes) trial did not demonstrate any benefit of abciximab in the treatment of NSTEMI. Thus, these studies lead us to recommend that glycoprotein IIb/IIIa receptor antagonists should not be routinely used in all patients with NSTEMI, but they should be considered for high-risk patients requiring PCI, especially those with diabetes, resting ST depression, or elevated troponin.

Enoxaparin has shown modest outcome benefits over unfractionated heparin in patients with NSTEMI. This benefit may be counterbalanced by the inability to measure drug effect if PCI is performed. In our center, where PCI is readily available, we prefer unfractionated heparin.

Bivalirudin (Angiomax) is a direct thrombin inhibitor that compares favorably with unfractionated heparin plus glycoprotein IIb/IIIa inhibition in patients with acute coronary syndromes undergoing PCI. It is also commonly used in the catheterization laboratory for patients with a history of heparin-induced thrombocytopenia. We reserve its use for the latter case.

Fondaparinux (Arixtra) is a synthetic pentasaccharide that binds to antithrombin and compares favorably with enoxaparin in patients with NSTEMI.

The use of β-blockers and statins is similar to that in STEMI. The role of ACE inhibitors is less well defined for all patients, but they are selectively useful for treatment of hypertension and in those with LVEF less than 45%.

Meta-analyses of trials of early elective catheterization and PCI versus initial medical therapy have shown lower rates of mortality, recurrent MI, and rehospitalization for recurrent unstable angina after an early invasive approach. Benefits are predominantly limited to higher-risk patients, especially those older than 65 years and those who have resting ST depression or elevated biomarkers.

SPECIAL SITUATIONS

Cardiogenic Shock

Cardiogenic shock occurs in approximately 7% of patients with MI and has a mortality rate of approximately 80%. It is characterized by systemic hypotension (systolic BP <80 mm Hg), reduced cardiac index (<2.2 L/min/m^2), and elevated pulmonary artery wedge pressure (>16 mm Hg). Initial stabilization should be attempted with inotropes such as dopamine, dobutamine, or epinephrine together with intraaortic balloon counterpulsation. Intraaortic balloon counterpulsation reduces cardiac afterload, improves coronary artery perfusion, and increases systolic BP. However, these interventions do not reduce mortality. Early angiography and revascularization with either PCI or surgery have a significant effect in reducing mortality and should be considered in patients with cardiogenic shock.

Right Ventricular Infarction

RV infarction occurs in approximately 40% of patients with acute inferior MI; however, hemodynamically significant RV dysfunction is less common. Patients usually present with an elevated jugular venous pressure without hemodynamic compromise. Some patients present with hypotension, particularly after the administration of vasodilators such as nitrates. On physical examination, patients might have an elevated jugular venous pressure, Kussmaul sign, clear lungs, and a right-sided gallop. The diagnosis is strengthened by demonstrating the presence of at least 1 mm of ST segment elevation in leads V1, V3R, or V4R or RV dysfunction by echocardiography. The treatment is supportive, with intravenous fluids and inotropic support with dopamine or dobutamine if needed. These interventions may be tailored using guidance from hemodynamic data obtained from a pulmonary artery catheter. Patients with RV infarction are more likely to have

---

TABLE 5 TIMI Risk Score for Unstable Angina and Non–ST-Elevation Myocardial Infarction

Risk Factor	Points	Risk Score	14-Day D, MI, Revascularization
Age ≥65	1	1	4.7
Three risk factors	1	2	8.3
Stenosis ≥50%	1	3	13.2
ST deviation	1	4	19.9
Angina × 2/24 h	1	5	26.2
ASA use	1	6	
Elevated biomarkers	1	7	40.9

ASA = aspirin; MI = myocardial infarction.

complications with bradycardia or atrioventricular block that can require temporary atrial and ventricular pacing. Most patients improve spontaneously after 48 to 72 hours. Patients with shock might benefit from early revascularization with PCI to the right coronary artery.

Mechanical Complications of Acute Myocardial Infarction

Successful reperfusion therapy leads to lower complication rates. Table 6 lists the major ischemic, mechanical, and electrical complications of acute MI and their management.

Cardiac Rehabilitation and Secondary Prevention

Cardiac rehabilitation should be initiated before discharge from the hospital, with the goals of improving quality of life, facilitating return to normal activities, encouraging regular exercise, and promoting secondary prevention. Secondary prevention is aimed at smoking cessation and at aggressive dietary and pharmacologic treatment for hyperlipidemia, hypertension, and diabetes mellitus. Patients with uncomplicated MI may drive a car after 1 to 2 weeks and return to work at 2 to 4 weeks, whereas those with complicated MI require longer cardiac rehabilitation.

Summary

Early recognition and prompt treatment are essential for management of MI. Atypical and painless presentation must always be considered. Urgent reperfusion with fibrinolytic or primary PCI is lifesaving in STEMI, and in-hospital revascularization is beneficial in high-risk NSTEMI and unstable coronary syndromes. Agents that reduce mortality, including aspirin, β-blockers, ACE inhibitors, and lipid-lowering drugs, should always be employed in the absence of contraindications. Most patients benefit from lifestyle changes and risk factor modification in a continuing outpatient setting.

TABLE 6 Complications Associated with Acute Myocardial Infarction

Complications	Clinical Features	Treatment
Ischemic		
Postinfarction angina	Recurrent chest pain after resolution of symptoms	Medical therapy or revascularization
Infarct extension	Recurrent chest pain and biomarker elevation	Urgent angiography and revascularization
Mitral regurgitation	Murmur, heart failure	Treat ischemia, ACE inhibitors
		Consider revascularization with or without mitral valve repair
Mechanical		
LV dysfunction (see Killip classification)	Dyspnea, hypoxia, elevated jugular venous pressure, third heart sound, rales	Diuretics, vasodilators
		Consider revascularization
		Treat associated mechanical complications
Cardiogenic shock	See text	Inotropes and IABP
		Urgent revascularization
Papillary muscle rupture	New mitral regurgitation, pulmonary edema, or shock 2–7 days after MI	IABP
		Emergency mitral valve replacement or repair
Myocardial rupture (lateral wall most often involved)	More common in women, elderly, non-reperfused patients, and inferior MI	Emergency surgery
	3–5 days post MI	
	Recurrent chest pain, pericarditis, vomiting, agitation, bradycardia	
Ventricular septal defect	Equally prevalent with anterior or inferior MI	IABP
	New pansystolic mumur, heart failure, shock	Urgent surgery
Electrical		
Second-degree AV block	Asymptomatic, syncope	Observe
Mobitz type I	More common after inferior MI	Avoid AV node–blocking drugs
Second-degree AV block	Asymptomatic presyncope/syncope	Observe if asymptomatic and temporary pacing with symptoms after inferior MI
Mobitz type II	Presyncope/syncope	
Third-degree AV block		Temporary ± permanent pacing after anterior MI
Atrial fibrillation/flutter	Asymptomatic, palpitations, heart failure	IV heparin for thromboembolic risk
		DC cardioversion for ischemia or hemodynamic compromise
		β-Blockers and digoxin for rate control in asymptomatic patients
		Sotalol or amiodarone for recurrent episodes
Ventricular premature complexes	Asymptomatic, palpitations	No antiarrhythmics indicated
		β-Blockers
		Correct electrolytes
Ventricular tachycardia	Hemodynamic collapse, syncope, palpitations, sudden cardiac death	CPR and DC cardioversion for hemodynamic collapse; otherwise, IV lidocaine or amiodarone
Ventricular fibrillation	Sudden cardiac death	Treat associated ischemia and heart failure
		Correct electrolytes
		Consider revascularization
		If >24 hours after MI, consider EPS and ICD
Torsades de pointes	Hemodynamic collapse, sudden cardiac death	CPR and DC cardioversion
		Correct hypokalemia or hypomagnesemia
		Consider temporary pacing for bradycardia or IV phenytoin

ACE = angiotensin-converting enzyme; AV = strioventricular; CPR = cardiopulmonary resuscitation; DC = direct current; EPS = electrophysiologic study; IABP = intraaortic balloon counterpulsation; ICD = implantable cardioverter-defibrillator; LV = left ventricular; MI = myocardial infarction.

REFERENCES

Alpert JS, Thygesen K, Antman E, et al. Myocardial infarction redefined—a consensus document of the Joint European Society of Cardiology/American College of Cardiology Committee for the redefinition of myocardial infarction. J Am Coll Cardiol 2000;36:959–69.

Anderson JL, Adams CD, Antman EM, et al. ACC/AHA 2007 guidelines for the management of patients with unstable angina/non-ST-elevation myocardial infarction. I Am Coll Cardiol 2007;50:e1–157.

Antman EM, Anbe DT, Armstrong PW, et al. ACC/AHA guidelines for the management of patients with ST-elevation myocardial infarction: A report of the American College of Cardiology/American Heart Association Task Force on Practice Guidelines (Committee to Revise the 1999 Guidelines for the Management of Patients With Acute Myocardial Infarction). J Am Coll Cardiol. 2004;44(3):E1–211.

Antman EM, Cohen M, Bernink PJ, et al. The TIMI risk score for unstable angina/non-ST elevation MI: A method for prognostication and therapeutic decision making. JAMA 2000;284:835–42.

Cannon CP, Hand MH, Bahr R, et al. Critical pathways for management of patients with acute coronary syndromes: An assessment by the National Heart Attack Alert Program. Am Heart J 2002;143:777–89.

Krumholz HM, Anderson JL, Brooks NH, et al. ACC/AHA clinical performance measures for adults with ST-elevation and non—ST-elevation myocardial infarction: A report of the ACC/AHA task force on performance measures (ST-Elevation and Non-ST-Elevation Myocardial Infarction Performance Measures Writing Committee). J Am Coll Cardiol 2006;47:236–65.

Mehta SR, Cannon CP, Fox KA, et al. Routine vs selective invasive strategies in patients with acute coronary syndromes: A collaborative meta-analysis of randomized trials. JAMA 2005;293:2908–17.

Smith Jr SC, Allen J, Blair SN, et al. AHA/ACC guidelines for secondary prevention for patients with coronary and other atherosclerotic vascular disease: 2006 update endorsed by the National Heart, Lung, and Blood Institute. J Am Coll Cardiol 2006;47:2130–9.

Smith Jr SC, Feldman TE, Hirshfeld Jr JW, et al. ACC/AHA/SCA1 2005 guideline update for percutaneous coronary intervention: A report of the American College of Cardiology/American Heart Association Task Force on Practice Guidelines (ACC/AHA/SCAI Writing Committee to Update the 2001 Guidelines for Percutaneous Coronary Intervention). Circulation 2006;113(7):e166–286.

Weaver WD, Cerqueira M, Hallstrom AP, et al. Prehospital-initiated vs hospital-initiated thrombolytic therapy. The Myocardial Infarction Triage and Intervention Trial. JAMA 1993;270:1211–6.

Pericarditis and Pericardial Effusions

Method of
Miguel A. Leal, MD

Embryologic Origin of the Pericardium

During the fifth week of embryonic development, lateral structures called the pleuropericardial folds begin to grow toward the midline. As the folds move medially, they bring along the phrenic nerves, and the root of each fold migrates ventrally. At the end of the fifth week, the pleuropericardial folds fuse, partitioning the thoracic cavity into a pericardial cavity and two partially formed pleural cavities.

The pericardium comprises two juxtaposed layers of connective tissue, which form the parietal and the visceral pericardium. The virtual space between the two layers is called the pericardial space. It normally contains a very small amount of transudative fluid (approximately 5 mL). Its function is not well established, but it could conceptually minimize friction and trauma to the epicardium during the cardiac cycle.

Pathologic Processes Involving the Pericardium

The pericardium can be secondarily involved in a large number of systemic disorders, and it can be primarily affected in an isolated disease process. Clinically, most disease processes involving the pericardium manifest with varying degrees of inflammation, constituting the clinical syndrome of pericarditis. In addition, the amount of pericardial fluid may be increased and may result in a pericardial effusion, which can be transudative or exudative and is sometimes hemodynamically significant.

Although pericarditis and pericardial effusions are distinct phenomena, both manifestations are present in a large group of patients. In some cases, the clinical presentation of acute pericardial inflammation predominates, and the presence of excess pericardial fluid has no clinical significance. In other cases, the effusion and its clinical consequences, such as hemodynamic instability, are the main pathologic mechanism.

Classification

Classically, pericardial disease has been categorized as inflammatory, neoplastic, degenerative, vascular, or idiopathic. Some of the major causes of inflammatory disease are infections (viral infections, including HIV, Coxsackie A and B viruses, echoviruses, influenza and adenoviruses; purulent pericarditis; tuberculosis), myocardial infarction (Dressler's syndrome), and collagen vascular diseases. Neoplastic disease may be related to breast, lung, esophagus, lymphoma, melanoma, or renal cell carcinoma. Degenerative disease is related to mediastinal radiation, whether recent or remote.

Miscellaneous causes of pericardial disease include cardiac surgery, aortic dissection, cardiac contusion (with recent or remote sharp or blunt chest trauma), iatrogenic causes (usually after cardiac diagnostic or interventional procedures, such as coronary angiography or placement of a pacemaker or defibrillator), metabolic causes (uremia, myxedematous state), and idiopathic causes.

Most of these causes of pericardial disease can produce both dry pericarditis (i.e., pericarditis with minimal or no effusion) and pericardial effusive disease. Some causes (e.g., HIV infection, hypothyroidism) are primarily associated with effusion without a significant amount of pericardial inflammation.

The frequencies reported for specific causes of pericardial disease vary significantly in the medical literature, depending on the epidemiology, the population at risk, and how the diagnosis was established. The diagnostic yield of pericardiocentesis or pericardial biopsy is typically higher in patients who are found to have a pericardial effusion than in those who present with apparent acute pericarditis without concomitant effusion.

Clinical Manifestations

ACUTE PERICARDITIS

The typical clinical manifestations of acute pericarditis are chest pain, which is usually pleuritic in nature (i.e., associated with inspiration and positional changes); a pericardial friction rub; and widespread ST-segment elevation on the 12-lead surface electrocardiogram (ECG). Usually, at least two of these features, with or without an accompanying pericardial effusion, should be present for the clinical diagnosis.

The yield of a full diagnostic evaluation is much lower in patients who present with acute pericarditis than in those presenting with pericardial effusion. In two series with a total of 331 patients, a specific diagnosis was established in only 54 (16%). The most common causes of pericarditis were neoplasia (20 patients), tuberculosis (13 patients), nontuberculous infection (7 patients), and collagen vascular disease (7 patients).

In patients with acute pericarditis for which no cause is identified (idiopathic pericarditis), the etiology is frequently presumed to be viral, but evidence for this is often not pursued, given the expense involved and the time required for the results of viral titers to become available. It is likely that some cases for which an identifiable cause exists are labeled idiopathic as the result of an insufficient diagnostic evaluation. However, complex and exhaustive testing strategies are typically not justified by the limited implications for clinical management. An exception to this recommendation is the absence of a prompt and adequate response to standard treatment.

PERICARDIAL EFFUSION

Pericardial effusions are typically diagnosed by chest radiography (Fig. 1) or transthoracic echocardiography (Fig. 2). The latter may reveal a layer of echo-free space between the epicardium and the pericardial sac, sometimes associated with fibrin strands, hematoma, or amorphous material deposited around the heart. The distribution of causes varies with demographics and diagnostic strategies.

In a review of 322 patients with a moderate to large pericardial effusion on echocardiography, the most common causes were idiopathic (20%), iatrogenic (16%), malignancy (13%), chronic idiopathic effusion (9%), acute myocardial infarction (8%), uremia or end-stage renal disease (6%), and collagen vascular disease (5%).

In a different series, including 75 patients presenting to a tertiary care medical center in the United States with a new, unexplained, large pericardial effusion, a diagnosis was made in 53 patients. The most common causes were malignancy (23%), infection (27%), irradiation (14%), collagen vascular disease (12%), uremia or dialysis (12%), and idiopathic (7%). Examination of pericardial fluid yielded a diagnosis in 26%, mostly of malignancy, whereas examination of pericardial tissue was useful for diagnosis in 23%, mostly with infection.

A higher rate of idiopathic disease was found in a review of 204 patients from France; a specific cause was identified in 107 patients (52%). The following distribution was noted: idiopathic (48%), infection (16%), malignancy (15%), collagen vascular disease (10%), hypothyroidism (10%), and renal failure (2%).

Diagnostic Work-up

A careful history and physical examination may reveal a pericardial friction rub, which is usually triphasic (with early diastolic, late diastolic, and systolic components), and the presence of pulsus paradoxus (a drop of 10–12 mm Hg in the systolic blood pressure with inspiration, reflecting enhanced interventricular dependence in the setting of limited pericardial compliance). In addition, laboratory and imaging studies may contribute to establishing the diagnosis.

CURRENT DIAGNOSIS

- Pericarditis usually manifests as a pleuritic-type chest pain syndrome, frequently preceded by a nonspecific prodrome (e.g., malaise, fatigue, recent viral infection).
- The physical examination may reveal a pericardial friction rub, pulsus paradoxus, and signs of elevated filling pressures (e.g., jugular venous distention, congestive hepatomegaly, and edema of the extremities).
- Electrocardiography, chest radiography, and transthoracic echocardiography are diagnostic tests that may contribute to establishing the diagnosis and the need for possible intervention, in the case of an associated hemodynamically significant pericardial effusion.
- Laboratory studies may also be helpful, including cultures, erythrocyte sedimentation rate, C-reactive protein, thyroid-stimulating hormone, creatinine, and markers of autoimmune disease.
- Prognosis is usually favorable, except in specific causes such as malignancy, trauma, or aortic dissection.

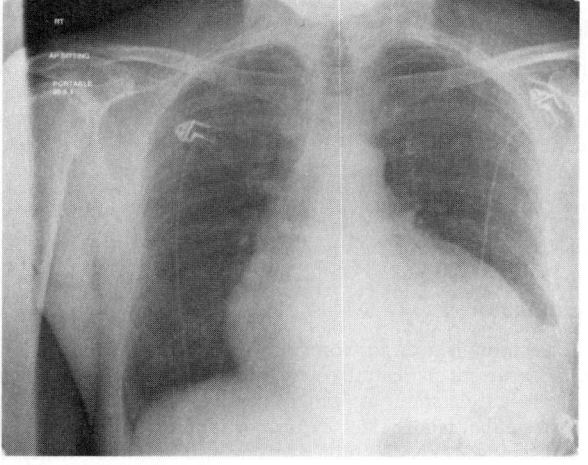

FIGURE 1. Cardiomegaly is demonstrated on a chest radiograph; the double-shadow pattern suggests a large pericardial effusion.

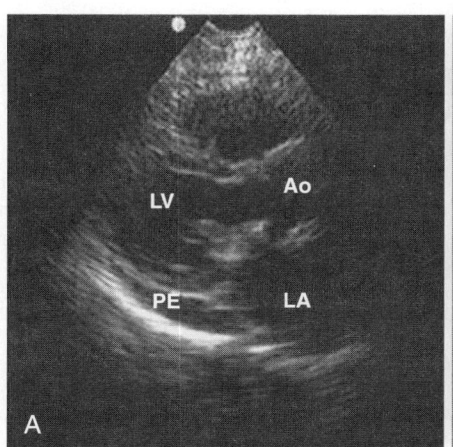
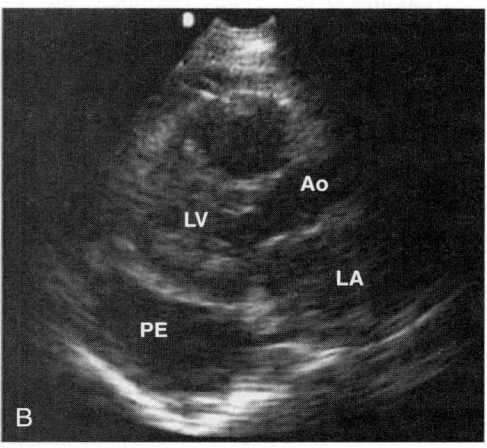

FIGURE 2. Parasternal long-axis views on transthoracic echocardiography demonstrate a large pericardial effusion (PE), lying predominantly posterior to the heart. *Abbreviations:* Ao = aorta; LA = left atrium; LV = left ventricle.

LABORATORY STUDIES

A complete blood count with differential may show leukocytosis. The erythrocyte sedimentation rate and C-reactive protein level are usually elevated, especially if active inflammation is present. Blood urea nitrogen and creatinine levels should also be checked if uremia is suspected.

Cardiac biomarkers are part of the diagnostic work-up and are abnormal in cases of associated myocarditis or myocardial infarction. In a recent study, an elevated troponin I level was found in 32% of patients with viral or idiopathic pericarditis. This was related to the extent of myocardial inflammation but was not a negative prognostic marker.

Further laboratory work may include blood or viral cultures, tuberculin testing with sputum for acid-fast bacilli, rheumatoid factor, antinuclear antibody, and thyroid function tests.

OTHER STUDIES AND PROCEDURES

Chest Radiography

Chest radiography may demonstrate an enlarged cardiac silhouette, which is sometimes the first indication of a large pericardial effusion.

Electrocardiography

Acute pericarditis classically evolves through stages. Initial ECG changes include diffuse, concave upward ST-segment elevation, except in leads aVR and V_1 (where it is usually depressed). T waves are upright in the leads with ST elevation, and the PR segment deviates opposite to P-wave polarity. Several days later, the ST segments return to baseline, followed by flattening of the T waves. The T waves then become inverted, and the ECG eventually returns to baseline weeks to months after the acute episode. The T-wave inversion may persist indefinitely in the chronic inflammation observed with tuberculosis, uremia, or neoplastic processes.

Electrical alternans, the beat-to-beat variability in QRS voltage caused by excessive cardiac mobility, may be seen with a large-size pericardial effusion.

Echocardiography

Universally recommended, echocardiography should be performed urgently if cardiac tamponade is suspected. Cardiac tamponade occurs when the extracardiac pressure from a large effusion causes collapse of the cardiac chambers during diastole. The collapse occurs in a progressive fashion, with right atrial collapse initially, followed by right ventricular collapse and eventual decrement in the cardiac output once the left-sided chambers are affected.

Echocardiograms are particularly helpful if pericardial effusion is suspected on clinical or radiographic grounds, if the illness lasts longer than 1 week, or if myocarditis or purulent pericarditis is suspected. Other causes of pericardial echo-free spaces that must be considered include pleural effusion, pericardial masses, and epicardial fat. Echocardiography can also be used to evaluate for chamber size, tamponade, and ventricular dysfunction.

Computed Tomography

Effusions are easily detected on computed tomography by virtue of the different X-ray coefficients of fluid and pericardium. The nature of the effusion also may be anticipated, given the different attenuation coefficients for blood, exudates, lipid-rich fluids, and serous fluids. Hemopericardium can be difficult to assess without intravenous contrast, because blood has the same radiodensity as myocardium.

Magnetic Resonance Imaging

Magnetic resonance imaging is a sensitive technique for detecting pericardial effusion and loculated pericardial effusion and thickening.

Cardiac Catheterization

Cardiac catheterization can assist in the differentiation between constrictive and restrictive cardiomyopathy.

Pericardiocentesis

Pericardiocentesis is relatively safe when it is guided by angiography or echocardiography, especially with a large, free anterior effusion. One study reported only 3 minor complications in 117 procedures with ultrasound guidance. Heterogeneous exudates may indicate a potentially difficult pericardiocentesis, especially if the fluid is loculated in pockets—a common finding in autoimmune pericarditis, postsurgical cases, and recurrent disease.

In a large study, diagnostic pericardiocentesis led to a diagnosis in only 6% of cases, compared with 29% diagnosed by therapeutic pericardiocentesis. As such, pericardiocentesis should not be performed unless tamponade or suspected purulent pericarditis is present.

If a pericardiocentesis is performed for drainage, an indwelling catheter should be placed in the pericardial space for continued drainage over several days. If the catheter continues to drain a large amount, a more definitive procedure should be performed.

The pericardial fluid should be analyzed for red cells, total protein level, lactic acid dehydrogenase level, adenosine deaminase activity, and cultures. Cytologic studies are also indicated if malignancy is suspected.

Pericardial Window

In the pericardial window procedure, a small area of the pericardium is resected (usually ≤ 10 cm^2). In critically ill patients, a balloon catheter may be used to create a pericardial window. In some studies almost 25% of patients who underwent the procedure required repeat operation within 2 years. Constrictive pericarditis may be a long-term complication if pathologic healing affects the pericardium and leads to thickening of the pericardial sac, usually beyond 1.5 cm.

Pericardiectomy

Pericardiectomy is used for constrictive pericarditis, effusive pericarditis, or recurrent pericarditis with multiple attacks; steroid dependence; or intolerance to other medical management. Studies demonstrate that failure rates are proportional to the amount of pericardium removed (i.e., the more pericardium removed, the less likely it is that the procedure will fail). In effusive pericarditis, the higher failure rate associated with a pericardial window or partial pericardiectomy is probably secondary to continued fluid production from the remaining pericardium, with sealing of the remaining pericardium to the heart.

CURRENT THERAPY

- Nonsteroidal antiinflammatory drugs such as ibuprofen (Advil), indomethacin (Indocin),[1] and ketorolac (Toradol) are the usual treatment modality of choice.
- Colchicine[1] may also be used for prevention of disease recurrence.
- Pericardiocentesis and surgical pericardial windows are needed if there is hemodynamic instability (cardiac tamponade).
- Steroids may be used in refractory cases or if autoimmune causes are involved.

---

[1]Not FDA approved for this indication.

The operative mortality rate was 14% in one series, with a range of 1% for New York Heart Association class I-II, 10% for class III, and 46% for class IV. The 5-year survival rate was 80% for class III-IV and approximately 95% for class I-II.

Treatment

All patients admitted with suspected or established pericarditis, with or without an effusion, should be monitored by telemetry. Other life-threatening causes of chest pain (e.g., myocardial infarction, aortic dissection) should be considered in the differential diagnosis.

In selected cases (young patients with no hemodynamic instability and minor clinical symptoms), pericarditis may be managed on an outpatient basis. In a recent study, fever greater than 38°C, subacute onset, immunosuppression, trauma, oral anticoagulation therapy, failure of therapy with aspirin or nonsteroidal antiinflammatory drugs (NSAIDs), myopericarditis, severe pericardial effusion, and cardiac tamponade were poor prognostic predictors. Patients without these factors were treated on an outpatient basis, without serious complications after a mean follow-up of 38 months.

In another study, the presence of cardiac tamponade and an unfavorable clinical outcome, with persistence of fever, significant pericardial effusion, or general illness lasting longer than 1 week, were highly associated with finding a specific etiology.

If significant clinical activity persists for 3 weeks after admission without an etiologic diagnosis, some authors recommend pericardial biopsy. Complicated cases, such as tuberculous, purulent, or uremic causes, require multidisciplinary involvement, including consultations with a cardiologist, cardiac surgeon, and medical subspecialists (e.g., infectious diseases specialist, nephrologist).

Treatment for specific causes of pericarditis is directed according to the underlying cause. For patients with idiopathic or viral pericarditis, therapy is directed at symptom relief. NSAIDs such as indomethacin[1] (Indocin, 50 mg PO every 8 hours), ibuprofen (Motrin or Advil, 400–800 mg PO every 6–8 hours), or ketorolac (Toradol, 30–90 mg IV/IM every 4 hours[3]) are the mainstay of therapy. These agents have similar efficacies, with relief of chest pain in 85% to 90% of patients within days of treatment. Ibuprofen has the advantage of fewer adverse effects and fewer negative effects on coronary flow. Indomethacin has a poor adverse effect profile and has been shown to reduce coronary flow. Ketorolac is used if the oral route of treatment is not an option. The duration of treatment depends on the clinical course, but common therapeutic courses rarely extend beyond 7 to 10 days.

Aspirin (325 mg PO daily) is recommended for treatment of pericarditis after an ST-elevation myocardial infarction, as part of a secondary prevention regimen against recurrent coronary events. Colchicine[1] (1 mg PO daily), in combination with an NSAID, can be considered in the initial treatment to prevent recurrent pericarditis. Colchicine, alone or in combination with an NSAID, can be considered for patients with recurrent or continued symptoms beyond 14 days.

Corticosteroids (prednisone tapering regimens, starting usually at 40–60 mg PO daily and tapered over the course of 10–14 days) should not be used for initial treatment of pericarditis unless indicated for the underlying disease. Corticosteroids also may be used if the patient has had no response to NSAIDs or colchicine, or if these drugs are contraindicated.

Prognosis

The prognosis depends on the etiology. Pericarditis from idiopathic and viral causes usually has a self-limited course. Purulent, tuberculous, hemorrhagic (Fig. 3) and neoplastic causes of pericarditis and pericardial effusions result in more complicated courses with worse outcomes.

---

[1]Not FDA approved for this indication.
[3]Exceeds dosage recommended by the manufacturer.

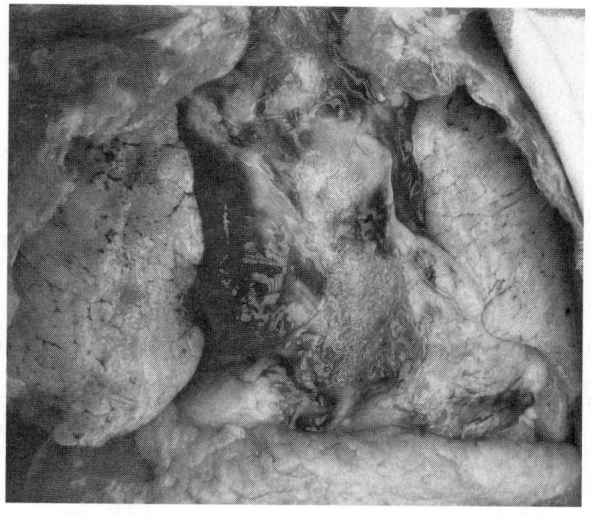

FIGURE 3. Autopsy findings of a large hemorrhagic pericardial effusion.

REFERENCES

Atar S, Chiu J, Forrester JS, Siegel RJ. Bloody pericardial effusion in patients with cardiac tamponade: Is the cause cancerous, tuberculous, or iatrogenic? Chest 1999;116:1564–9.

Corey GR, Campbell PT, van Trigt P, et al. Etiology of large pericardial effusions. Am J Med 1993;95:209–13.

Galve E, Garcia-del-Castillo H, Evangelista A, et al. Pericardial effusion in the course of myocardial infarction: Incidence, natural history, and clinical relevance. Circulation 1986;73:294–9.

Permanyer-Miralda G, Sagrista-Sauleda J, Soler-Soler J. Primary acute pericardial disease: A prospective series of 231 consecutive patients. Am J Cardiol 1985;56:623–30.

Sagrista-Sauleda J, Merce J, Permanyer-Miralda G, Soler-Soler J. Clinical clues to the causes of large pericardial effusions. Am J Med 2000;109:95–101.

Spodick DH. Pericardial disease. In: Braunwald E, Zipes DP, Libby P, editors. Heart Disease: A Textbook of Cardiovascular Medicine. New York: WB Saunders; 2001. p. 183–202.

Troughton RW, Asher CR, Klein AL. Pericarditis. Lancet 2004;363:717–27.

Zayas R, Anguita M, Torres F, et al. Incidence of specific etiology and role of methods for specific etiologic diagnosis of primary acute pericarditis. Am J Cardiol 1995;75:378–82.

Peripheral Arterial Disease

Method of
Gregory Feldman, MD, and Wei Zhou, MD

Peripheral vascular disease comprises a diverse group of conditions that result in significant morbidity and mortality and offers an opportunity for the astute clinician to recognize common but underdiagnosed problems for which effective interventions exist. Peripheral vascular disease is defined as pathology of the blood vessels outside the brain and heart, and peripheral arterial disease (PAD) involves that subset that affects arteries. Most manifestations of PAD follow logically from the consequences of reduced perfusion of end organs and tissues downstream from sites of flow obstruction. Common forms of PAD include extracranial carotid stenosis, aortoiliac disease, and lower extremity occlusive disease (LEOD). This chapter focuses on extracranial carotid and lower extremity diseases; venous conditions are described in the next chapter.

CURRENT DIAGNOSIS

Carotid Artery Diseases

- Presentation: transient ischemic attack and stroke
- Physical examination: bruit and lateralized neurologic deficit
- Diagnostic modalities: carotid ultrasonography, magnetic resonance angiography (MRA), computed tomographic angiography (CTA), and carotid angiography

Lower Extremity Occlusive Diseases

- Presentation: claudication, rest pain, tissue loss, and numbness
- Physical examination: diminished pulse, hair loss, pallor, cool extremities, tissue wasting, ulcerations, and delayed capillary refill (>3 sec).
- Imaging modalities: ankle-brachial index, segmental pressures with waveforms, CTA, MRA, and lower extremity angiography

Epidemiologic data suggest that the prevalence of PAD is 12.2% for American adults older than 60 years of age, increasing to 23.2% for those older than 80 years. Risk factors include increased age, diabetes, past or current tobacco use, renal insufficiency, hypertension, dyslipidemia, and African American or Hispanic ethnicity. More than 95% of patients with PAD have one or more risk factors for cardiovascular disease, and the diagnosis of either condition should raise suspicion for the other. The 10-year risk of death after a diagnosis of PAD is 40%. Alarmingly, an estimated 68% of patients with PAD are undiagnosed by their primary care physicians, although as a group these patients have mainly less advanced cases of atherosclerosis.

The history and physical examination are of paramount importance in detecting peripheral vascular disease and prompting further evaluation. Risk factors for peripheral vascular disease should merit elicitation of common presenting symptoms, including claudication, limb pain at rest, and nonhealing extremity ulcers for LEOD; and amaurosis fugax, transient ischemic attack (TIA), and stroke for carotid occlusive diseases. An appropriate physical examination includes palpation of radial, aortic, femoral, popliteal, and pedal pulses; careful examination of distal extremities for stigmata of arterial insufficiency; cervical and abdominal auscultation for carotid and renal bruits; and a thorough neurologic evaluation.

Carotid Artery Disease

Stroke is the most common cause of permanent disability in the United States, and it remains the third leading cause of death in industrialized countries. Atherosclerotic disease involving the extracranial carotid artery is one of the major causes of all strokes and TIAs. Management of stroke consumes $45 billion annually and is responsible for more than 1 million hospital admissions each year in this country. Neurologic sequelae related to cerebrovascular accidents severely limit a patient's ability to carry out activities of daily living and invariably create an enormous burden on health care costs. As a result, the prevention of cerebrovascular accidents through safe treatment of extracranial carotid occlusive disease remains an important health care goal.

PATHOPHYSIOLOGY

The underlying pathophysiology of atherosclerotic plaque formation continues to be an area of active investigation, with explanatory models incorporating elements of flow dynamics, endothelial damage, lipid deposition, and inflammatory mediators. Plaque deposition frequently occurs at sites of bifurcation, and the carotid bifurcation is a common location for plaque formation. The neurologic sequelae

from carotid disease mostly result from movement of microemboli or macroemboli of disrupted plaque into the cerebral circulation, with symptoms determined by the vascular territory disrupted and the availability of collateral circulation. Rarely, symptoms can also result from critical flow limitation secondary to severe carotid stenosis, although typically the collateral circulation through the vertebral arteries and the contralateral carotid is adequate to compensate. It is not uncommon to find complete occlusion of a single carotid artery without any perceptible neurologic dysfunction.

Carotid stenosis is categorized as symptomatic or asymptomatic, with divergent therapeutic strategies based on this determination. Most patients are asymptomatic. Symptomatic patients can present with TIA or stroke. Although the classification for neurologic insults is constantly evolving, TIA is defined as a focal neurologic deficit that resolves completely within 24 hours. Symptoms of TIA can include generalized confusion, loss of strength or sensation at contralateral upper or lower extremities, and difficulty with speech, vision, or memory. One example of a TIA is amaurosis fugax, in which painless monocular loss of vision results from temporary occlusion of a retinal or ophthalmic artery. Patients often describe this as having the appearance of a curtain being drawn down over the eye. Stroke, in contrast, is defined as a neurologic deficit with acute onset that resolves incompletely or not at all after a thromboembolic or hemorrhagic event.

EVALUATION

Asymptomatic carotid stenosis is detected on auscultation of a cervical bruit (although most stenoses are not accompanied by bruits) or on imaging, which includes screening duplex ultrasonography based on risk factors or, increasingly, incidental findings on computed tomography or magnetic resonance scans performed for other indications. The physical examination for a patient with suspected or confirmed carotid stenosis includes a comprehensive neurologic evaluation, auscultation for cervical bruits, and the palpation of peripheral pulses. Vigorous palpation of carotid pulses is discouraged. Important components of the neurologic examination include a thorough evaluation of cranial nerves, strength, sensation, gait, memory, speech, and comprehension. One needs to pay particular attention to lateralized symptoms.

Imaging modalities are important in diagnosing carotid artery stenosis. The most useful screening imaging modality is a carotid duplex examination, which provides information regarding the estimated degree of stenosis, plaque location and characteristics, and flow dynamics (Fig. 1). Confirmatory imaging includes computed tomographic or magnetic resonance angiography, which can also be used to evaluate intracerebral circulation and to confirm or detect acute or chronic stroke. Of note, magnetic resonance angiography often overestimates the degree of carotid stenosis, particularly for calcified lesions, and should be interpreted in conjunction with

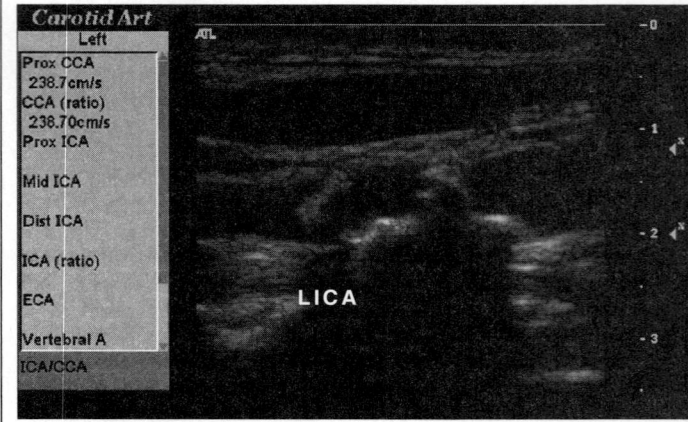

FIGURE 1. Ultrasound scan of left internal carotid artery (LICA) shows severe carotid stenosis and echogenic calcification at the carotid bulb.

duplex results. Carotid and cerebral angiography, historically considered the gold standard, is increasingly being supplanted by these noninvasive imaging modalities. Carotid angiography is now generally reserved for patients who had conflicting findings on two noninvasive diagnostic tests and patients for whom percutaneous interventions are contemplated.

MANAGEMENT

Management options for carotid stenosis include medical optimization, carotid endarterectomy (CEA), and carotid angioplasty and stenting (CAS) (Fig. 2). Medical optimization involves strategies for diet and lifestyle modification, blood pressure control, lipid-lowering agents, and antiplatelet therapy.

Surgical intervention most commonly involves CEA, in which the carotid artery is exposed, controlled, and opened, and atherosclerotic plaque is removed. A patch angioplasty is performed during closure of the artery to avoid luminal narrowing. An estimated 98,000 CEAs were performed in the United States in 2004. Potential perioperative complications include stroke, cranial nerve injury, hematoma, myocardial infarction, and death. Recommendations for surgical intervention are based on balancing the demonstrated benefits of stroke reduction with the incidence of periprocedural complications; such decisions have been shaped by the results of four large, multicenter trials of carotid endarterectomy published during the 1990s. The North American Symptomatic Carotid Endarterectomy Trial (NASCET) randomly assigned 651 patients with severe (70%–99%) symptomatic carotid stenosis to receive either medical therapy alone or CEA in addition to medical therapy. At 2 years, the rate of ipsilateral stroke was 26% in the medical therapy group and 9% in the CEA group, demonstrating a relative risk reduction of 65%. The European Carotid Surgery Trial (ECST) randomized 3024 patients with symptomatic carotid stenosis to CEA versus initial nonoperative management. Rates of stroke, death, and other adverse events were monitored for 3 years and stratified by degree of stenosis. For patients with stenosis equal to or greater than 80%, the risk of major stroke or death at 3 years was 26.5% in the nonoperative group, compared with 14.9% in the CEA group, for a relative risk reduction of 44%. A large Veterans Affairs trial for symptomatic patients with greater than 70% stenosis demonstrated similar results.

The Asymptomatic Carotid Atherosclerosis Study (ACAS) evaluated the utility of CEA in patients with asymptomatic carotid stenosis. A total of 1662 patients with asymptomatic stenosis of 60% or greater were randomized to CEA or medical treatment. The aggregate risk of ipsilateral stroke and perioperative stroke or death at 5 years was 11.0% for patients treated medically and 5.1% for those treated surgically, with an aggregate risk reduction of 53%. Because this represents an absolute risk reduction of only about 1% per year, considerable controversy still exists as to the degree of asymptomatic stenosis that should prompt surgical intervention.

Endovascular techniques represent a recent addition to the arsenal of available treatments for carotid stenosis. CAS, typically with deployment of a distal protection device to minimize the risk of embolization, has emerged as a promising therapeutic option, and the FDA has approved several devices for this purpose. Long-term data are not yet available, but several recent studies suggest that CAS may be comparable in outcome to CEA in selected populations. Indications for the appropriate use of CAS are still being developed, but it is generally agreed that CAS should be considered for symptomatic patients with significant medical comorbidities or high surgical risks, such as recurrent stenosis after CEA, prior neck irradiation or dissection, and inaccessible lesions above the C2 level. After CAS, a second antiplatelet agent, such as clopidogrel (Plavix),[1] is recommended for at least 6 weeks in addition to lifelong aspirin.

Postprocedure restenosis is an uncommon but well-recognized long-term complication after CEA or CAS. A severe restenosis can lead to neurologic symptoms and warrants reintervention. For this reason, routine ultrasound surveillance of the carotid arteries is necessary after CEA or CAS. Higher rates of restenosis have been reported after CAS, compared with CEA, particularly for patients with prior surgeries.

---

[1]Not FDA approved for this indication.

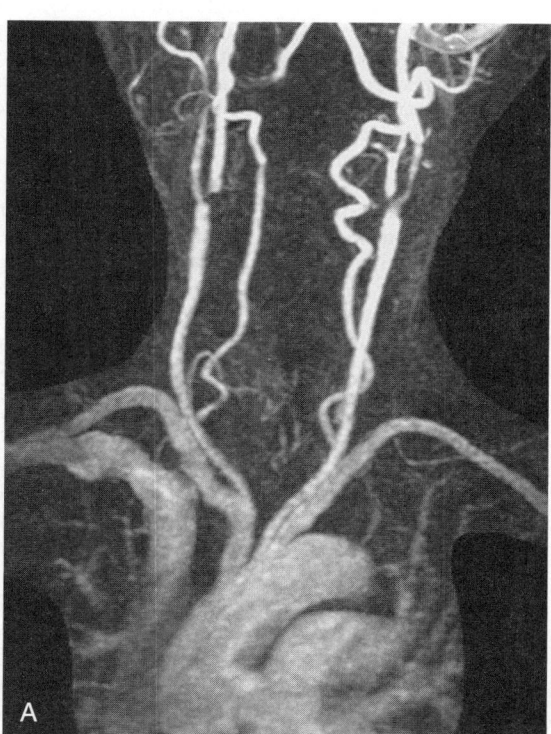
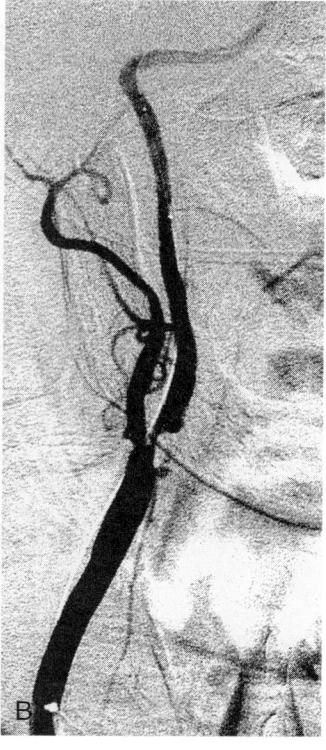

FIGURE 2. A, Time-of-flight magnetic resonance angiogram of the aortic arch and carotid artery demonstrates a severe right carotid artery stenosis. B, Carotid angiography confirms a severe stenosis before carotid stenting procedure. A distal protection device is positioned at middle of the internal carotid artery.

CURRENT THERAPY

Carotid Artery Diseases

- Medical therapy: lifestyle modification and risk factor reduction, lipid-lowering agents, and antiplatelet agents
- Percutaneous carotid stenting procedures
- Carotid artery endarterectomy

Lower Extremity Occlusive Diseases

- Medical management: lifestyle and risk factor modification, pentoxifylline (Trental), and cilostazol (Pletal)
- Exercise regimen
- Percutaneous interventions: angioplasty, stent, and atherectomy
- Surgery: bypass and endarterectomy

A recent consensus statement from the Society for Vascular Surgery issued the following recommendations for the management of carotid stenosis:

- Symptomatic patients with <50% stenosis: optimal medical therapy
- Symptomatic patients with >50% stenosis: CEA. However, most vascular surgeons accept the intervention threshold of >70% stenosis.
- Asymptomatic patients with <60% stenosis: optimal medical therapy
- Asymptomatic patients with >60% stenosis and low perioperative risk: CEA. With improved medical therapy, most vascular surgeons accept >80% stenosis as an indication for CEA in asymptomatic patients.
- Carotid stenting was described as a potential alternative in symptomatic patients with >50% stenosis and high operative risk.

Lower Extremity Occlusive Disease

LEOD is a common form of peripheral vascular disease in which arterial obstruction or stenosis results in inadequate blood flow to meet peripheral tissue demands. Areas of partial or complete occlusion can occur anywhere from the aorta to the pedal vessels, frequently in the iliofemoral, femoropopliteal, or tibial arterial systems. LEOD can best be understood as the peripheral analog to the imbalance between oxygen supply and demand found in coronary artery disease, and it similarly represents a spectrum from mild disease symptomatic only at exertion to severe disease manifesting at rest. The distribution and intensity of symptoms depend on the location and severity of occlusion, the acuteness of onset, and the efficiency of tissue oxygen extraction and utilization. Mild disease can manifest with symptoms of claudication, defined as limb discomfort in specific muscle groups at a reproducible level of exertion. Severe disease can manifest with pain at rest in the affected extremity, tissue loss, or chronic nonhealing wounds.

A distinction should be made between acute and chronic LEOD. Acute LEOD may result from a thrombotic or embolic event and is characterized by an abrupt onset of symptoms. Chronic LEOD is typically less dramatic in presentation and slowly progressive in nature. However, many patients present with acute LEOD. Acute LEOD is a surgical emergency and merits urgent evaluation by a vascular surgeon or specialist.

EVALUATION

The presenting symptoms of PAD are myriad and include cramping or pain in the legs or hips, cool extremities, and diminished extremity sensation. Approximately 50% of patients have atypical symptoms, and the classic symptom of claudication has been observed in only 10% of affected patients in some series. It is worth noting that the term intermittent claudication is frequently misapplied; this term correctly refers to the reproducible nature of the symptoms after a given level of exertion, not to a sporadic manifestation of discomfort. Several

TABLE 1 Rutherford Classification for Peripheral Arterial Occlusive Disease

Symptoms	Grade	Category
Asymptomatic	0	0
Claudication		
Mild	I	1
Moderate	I	2
Severe	I	3
Ischemic rest pain	II	4
Tissue loss		
Minor	III	5
Major	III	6

classification systems have been established to create uniform standards for evaluation and reporting of PAD. Among them, the Rutherford classification is one of the most commonly used (Table 1).

After careful elicitation of presenting symptoms, a focused physical examination is critical in the diagnosis of LEOD. Physical findings of PAD include reduced or absent pulses, hair loss, pallor, cool extremities, tissue wasting, ulcerations, and delayed capillary refill (>3 seconds).

A useful and inexpensive test for diagnosing and monitoring LOED is the ankle-brachial index (ABI), which can be readily performed in a clinic. Doppler ultrasonography is used to measure systolic blood pressures in bilateral dorsalis pedis, posterior tibial, and brachial arteries. The highest pedal systolic value in each leg is then divided by the highest arm pressure to calculate the ABI. An ABI of greater than 0.9 is considered normal. Claudicants typically have ABIs between 0.5 and 0.9. A value lower than 0.5 is concern for critical limb ischemia, and a value lower than 0.3 is often associated with tissue loss. Diabetic patients and patients with noncompressible tibial vessels secondary to calcification often have falsely elevated ABIs that are not dependable predictors of arterial disease. The numeric value of an ABI might not correlate precisely with symptoms or with vascular imaging findings, but it can be used to monitor progression of disease and should be interpreted in the clinical context.

A more sophisticated diagnostic screening test includes segmental pressures with evaluation of arterial waveforms. This test is routinely performed in noninvasive vascular laboratories and can provide both anatomic and functional information regarding blood flow without exposing the patient to radiation or nephrotoxic contrast agents. In segmental pressure measurement, systolic blood pressures are recorded at multiple levels, including the upper thigh, lower thigh, upper calf, ankle, and toes. A decrease of 20 mm Hg pressure between segments indicates significant arterial disease within that segment. For example, a pressure difference of 30 mm Hg between the upper and lower thigh suggests severe superficial femoral artery occlusive disease.

After a careful history and physical examination and noninvasive ultrasound evaluations have been performed, other diagnostic modalities may be required to further delineate anatomy, particularly if interventions are intended. Computed tomographic angiography produces a more detailed anatomic description and is useful for both diagnosis and preoperative planning but requires the use of radiation and intravenous contrast. Magnetic resonance angiography is emerging as a complementary modality, but is typically more expensive than computed tomographic angiography and has limited availability outside academic centers. Traditional angiography is performed if noninvasive modalities are unobtainable. Angiography affords the additional advantage of enabling endovascular intervention at the time of evaluation (Fig. 3).

TREATMENT

Treatment options for PAD include medical optimization, exercise training, and surgical or percutaneous interventions. Patients with mild claudication can benefit from risk factor modification, including smoking cessation and medical optimization for hypertension, diabetes, and dyslipidemia. The role of antiplatelet therapy in mild claudication is controversial, with mixed results from studies on the FDA-approved agents pentoxifylline (Trental) and cilostazol (Pletal).

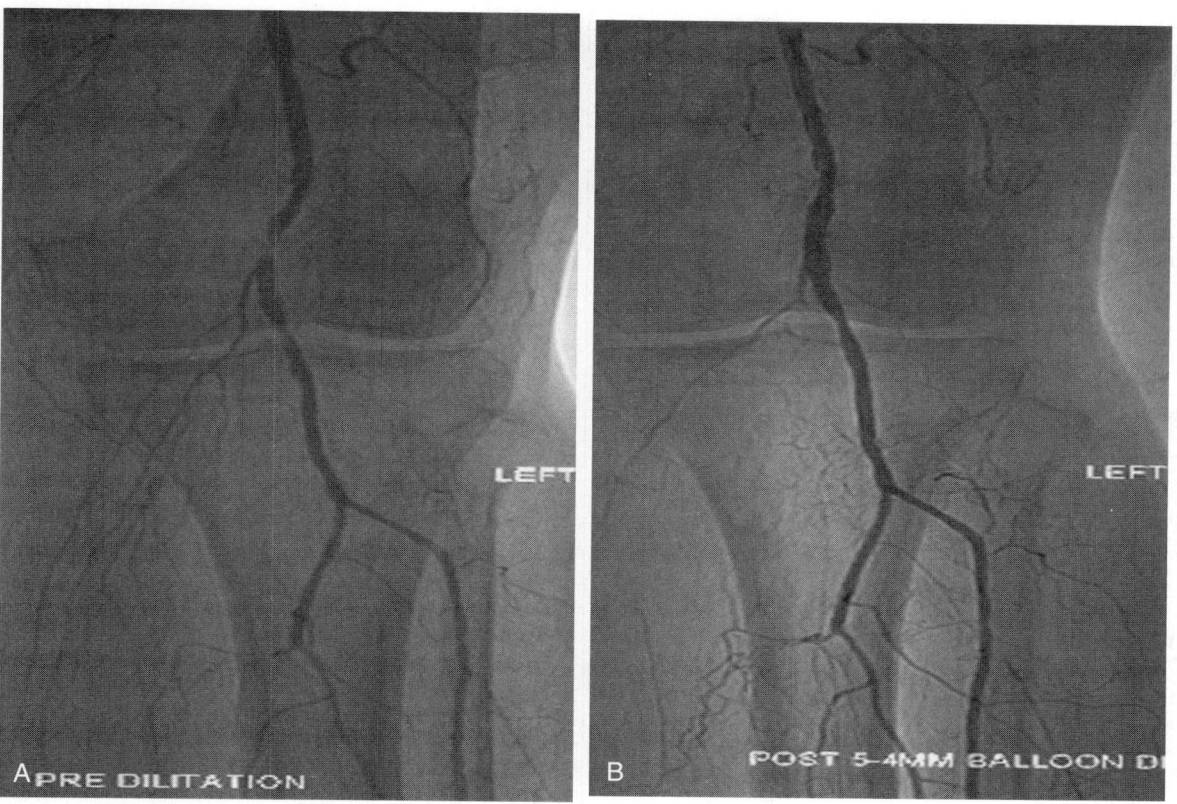

FIGURE 3. **A,** Lower extremity angiogram shows a focal occlusive lesion of the popliteal artery. **B,** Postprocedure angiogram shows complete resolution of the stenosis after balloon angioplasty.

Most claudicants should be prescribed aspirin (ASA) on the basis of cardiovascular risk factors. Medical management alone can lead to improvement in symptoms in a significant proportion of claudicants (as high as 75% in some series), and there is evidence that multimodality therapy is more effective than any single intervention. It is reasonable to perform a trial of medical optimization before more invasive therapeutic modalities are considered, particularly in patients with mild and moderate symptoms.

Supervised exercise regimens have also demonstrated efficacy for some patients with mild and moderate symptoms and should be considered before surgical or percutaneous interventions.

For patients who have not responded to medical optimization, multiple revascularization options exist. As with any surgical intervention, the risks and benefits of the proposed procedure must be carefully weighed against potential improvements in quality of life. Indications for revascularization include critical limb ischemia with rest pain, tissue loss, or nonhealing lesions. Lifestyle-limiting claudication is a relative indication for revascularization. Surgical revascularization options include bypassing the occluded arterial segment with a venous or synthetic graft and removing plaque from an arterial segment (endarterectomy) with local reconstruction. In the acute setting, removal of thromboembolus can be performed by direct exposure, balloon thrombectomy, or purely endovascular techniques. Commonly performed bypass operations that have achieved durable long-term results include aortofemoral bypass for aortoiliac occlusive disease and femoropopliteal and femorotibial bypass for more distal disease. Perioperative morbidity is not insignificant (2%–6%). In this patient population with substantial comorbidity, complications can include myocardial infarction, wound infection, graft infection, graft thrombosis, limb loss, and death. Long-term surveillance of bypass grafts with regular duplex ultrasonographic evaluations is necessary.

Driven by developments in technology and efforts to decrease periprocedural morbidity and mortality, endovascular interventions are increasingly being performed for the treatment of LEOD. Endovascular options include angioplasty alone, angioplasty with stenting, and atherectomy (a percutaneous analog of endarterectomy). In general, endovascular treatment is effective and durable for treatment of focal lesions with good distal run-off vessels. Patients with distal three-vessel run-off have better long-term outcome than those with one-vessel run-off or no run-off vessel. Lesion characteristics are also important. Long segments of occlusion, diffuse lesions, and calcified lesions are associated with poor long-term outcomes. The decreased invasiveness and shorter convalescence achieved with percutaneous approaches are appealing, but fewer long-term data are available than for traditional surgical approaches, and complications can be equally devastating. Endovascular technology is an area of active research and development, and improvements may expand the use of endovascular approaches to LEOD in the future. As with open approaches, routine postintervention surveillance is essential to identify severe restenoses that require secondary intervention. Given that percutaneous interventions can limit options for future reconstruction, patients with LEOD are best managed by vascular specialists familiar with the full range of therapeutic techniques as well as the natural history of disease progression.

REFERENCES

Arain F, Cooper L. Peripheral arterial disease: Diagnosis and management. Mayo Clin Proc 2008;83(8):944–50.

Donnan G, Fisher M, Macleod M, Davis SM. Stroke. Lancet 2008;371:1612–23.

European Carotid Surgery Trialists Collaborative Group. Randomised trial of endarterectomy for recently symptomatic carotid stenosis: Final results of the MRC European Carotid Surgery Trial (ECST). Lancet 1998;351:1379–87.

Ferguson G, Eliasziw M, Barr HW, et al. The North American Symptomatic Carotid Endarterectomy Trial: Surgical results in 1415 patients. Stroke 1999;30:1751–8.

Hobson RW 2nd, Mackey WC, Ascher E, et al. Management of atherosclerotic carotid artery disease: Clinical practice guidelines of the Society for Vascular Surgery. J Vasc Surg 2008;48:480–6.

Ostchega Y, Paulose-Ram R, Dillon CF, et al. Prevalence of peripheral arterial disease and risk factors in persons aged 60 and older: Data from the

National Health and Nutrition Examination Survey 1999–2004. J Am Geriatr Soc 2007;55(4):583–9.

Rosamond W, Flegal K, Friday G, et al. Heart Disease and Stroke Statistics—2007 Update: A Report from the American Heart Association Statistics Committee and Stroke Statistics Subcommittee. Circulation 2007;115:e69–171.

Selvin E, Erlinger T. Prevalence of and risk factors for peripheral arterial disease in the United States: Results from the National Health and Nutrition Examination Survey, 1999–2000. Circulation 2004;110:738–43.

TASC Working Group. Management of peripheral arterial disease. J Vasc Surg 2000;31(1):S1–296.

White C. Intermittent claudication. N Engl J Med 2007;356:1241–50.

Venous Thrombosis

Method of
Thomas W. Wakefield, MD

Epidemiology

Venous thromboembolism (VTE) includes deep venous thrombosis (DVT) and pulmonary embolism (PE). VTE affects up to 900,000 patients per year, and results in 300,000 deaths per year. The incidence has remained constant since the 1980s and increases with age.

Risk Factors

Risk factors for VTE include acquired and genetic factors. Acquired factors include increasing age, malignancy, surgery, immobilization, trauma, oral contraceptives and hormone replacement therapy, pregnancy and the puerperium, neurologic disease, cardiac disease, obesity, and antiphospholipid antibodies. Genetic factors include antithrombin deficiency, protein C deficiency and protein S deficiency, factor V Leiden, prothrombin 20210A, blood group non-O, abnormalities in fibrinogen and plasminogen, elevated levels of clotting factors (e.g., factors XI, IX, VII, VIII, X, and II), and elevation in plasminogen activator inhibitor-1 (PAI-1). When a patient presents with an idiopathic VTE, family history of thrombosis, recurrent thrombosis, or thrombosis in unusual locations, a work-up for hypercoagulability, including testing for the conditions noted in the previous sentence, is indicated. Hematologic diseases associated with VTE include heparin-induced thrombocytopenia and thrombosis syndrome (HITTS), disseminated intravascular coagulation (DIC), antiphospholipid antibody syndrome, myeloproliferative disorders, thrombotic thrombocytopenic purpura (TTP), and hemolytic uremic syndrome (HUS).

Pathophysiology

Although Virchow's triad of stasis, vein injury, and hypercoagulability has defined the events that predispose to DVT formation since the mid-19th century, the understanding today of events that occur at the level of the vein wall including the inflammatory response on thrombogenesis is increasingly becoming appreciated.

Diagnosis

DEEP VENOUS THROMBOSIS

The diagnosis of DVT must be made with duplex ultrasound imaging and laboratory testing, because history and physical examination is inaccurate in up to half the cases. Patients often complain of a dull

CURRENT DIAGNOSIS

- The diagnosis of deep venous thrombosis (DVT) is made with duplex ultrasound imaging and laboratory testing, because history and physical examination are inaccurate in up to half the cases.
- Duplex ultrasound imaging has become the gold standard for the diagnosis of DVT.
- Spiral computed tomographic (CT) scanning is preferred as the initial imaging test to establish the diagnosis of pulmonary embolus, replacing ventilation/perfusion scanning ($\dot{V}/\dot{Q}$).
- Although clinical assessment and D-dimer levels are useful to rule out thrombosis, there is no combination of clinical findings and biomarker testing at this time that can rule in the diagnosis.

ache or pain in the calf or leg. Wells has classified patients into a scoring system that emphasizes physical presentation, and the most common physical finding is edema. Characteristics that score points in the Wells system include active cancer, paralysis or paresis, recent plaster immobilization of the lower extremity, being recently bedridden for 3 days or more, localized tenderness along the distribution of the deep venous system, swelling of the entire leg, calf swelling that is at least 3 cm larger on the involved side than on the noninvolved side, pitting edema in the symptomatic leg, collateral superficial veins (nonvaricose), and a history of previous DVT. With extensive proximal iliofemoral DVT there may be significant swelling, cyanosis, and dilated superficial collateral veins.

Massive iliofemoral DVT can result in phlegmasia alba dolens (white swollen leg) or phlegmasia cerulean dolens (blue swollen leg). If phlegmasia is not aggressively treated, it can lead to venous gangrene when the arterial inflow becomes obstructed owing to venous hypertension. Alternatively, arterial emboli or spasm can occur and contribute to the pathophysiology. Venous gangrene is often associated with underlying malignancy and is always preceded by phlegmasia cerulea dolens. Venous gangrene is associated with significant rates of amputation and pulmonary embolism and with mortality.

Duplex ultrasound imaging has become the gold standard for the diagnosis of DVT. Duplex imaging includes both a B-mode image and Doppler flow pattern. Duplex imaging demonstrates sensitivity and specificity rates greater than 95%. According to the Grade criteria for the strength of medical evidence, duplex ultrasound is given a 2C level of evidence. Even at the level of the calf, duplex is an acceptable technique in symptomatic patients. Duplex imaging is painless, requires no contrast, can be repeated, and is safe during pregnancy. Duplex imaging also identifies other causes of a patient's symptoms. Other tests available for making the diagnosis include magnetic resonance imaging (MRI) (especially good for assessing central pelvic vein and inferior vena cava [IVC] thrombosis), and spiral computed tomographic (CT) scanning (especially with chest imaging during examination for PE).

A single complete negative duplex scan is accurate enough to withhold anticoagulation with minimal long-term adverse thromboembolic complications. This requires that all venous segments of the leg have been imaged and evaluated. If the duplex scan is indeterminate owing to technical issues or to edema, treatment may be based on factors such as biomarkers, with the duplex repeated in 24 to 72 hours. Combining clinical characteristics with a D-dimer assay can decrease the number of duplex scans performed. Although clinical characteristics and D-dimer levels are useful to rule out thrombosis, the converse is not true and there is no combination of biomarkers and clinical presentation that can rule in the diagnosis. Work is ongoing to establish new biomarkers based on the inflammatory response to DVT.

Conditions that may be confused with DVT include lymphedema, muscle strain, muscle contusion, and systemic problems such as cardiac, renal, or hepatic abnormalities. These systemic problems usually lead to bilateral edema.

PULMONARY EMBOLISM

The diagnosis of PE historically has involved ventilation-perfusion ($\dot{V}/\dot{Q}$) scanning and pulmonary angiography. However, the most current techniques include spiral CT scanning and MRI. CT scanning demonstrates excellent specificity and sensitivity. Emboli at the subsegmental level can be identified. The sensitivity for isolated chest CT imaging is increased when clinical analysis is added and when adding lower extremity imaging to the chest scan. Results from the PIOPED II study demonstrate that if the clinical presentation and spiral CT scan results are concordant, therapies can be safely recommended. However, if clinical presentation and spiral CT scanning are discordant, other confirmatory tests are necessary. For the diagnosis of PE, spiral CT imaging is given a 1A level of evidence. MRI is currently being investigated and its usefulness has not yet been definitely defined.

AXILLARY AND SUBCLAVIAN VEIN THROMBOSIS

Thrombosis of the axillary and subclavian veins accounts for less than 5% of all cases of DVT. However, it may be associated with PE in up to 10% to 15% of cases and can be the source of significant disability. Primary axillary and subclavian vein thrombosis results from obstruction of the axillary vein in the thoracic outlet from compression by the subclavius muscle and the costoclavicular space, the Paget-Schrötter syndrome, noted especially in muscular athletes. Secondary axillary and subclavian vein thrombosis results from mediastinal tumors, congestive heart failure, and nephrotic syndrome. Patients with axillary and subclavian vein thrombosis present with arm pain, edema, and cyanosis. Superficial venous distention may be apparent over the arm, forearm, shoulder, and anterior chest wall.

Upper extremity venous duplex ultrasound is used to make the diagnosis of axillary and subclavian vein thrombosis. Thrombolysis and phlebography are considered as next interventions. If phlebography is performed, it is important that the patient undergo positional phlebography with arm abducted to 120 degrees to confirm extrinsic subclavian vein compression at the thoracic outlet once the vein has been cleared of thrombus. Because a cervical rib may be the cause of such obstruction, chest x-ray should be obtained to exclude its presence (although its incidence is quite low).

Treatment

STANDARD THERAPY FOR VENOUS THROMBOEMBOLISM

The traditional treatment of VTE is systemic anticoagulation, which reduces the risk of PE, extension of thrombosis, and thrombus recurrence. Because the recurrence rate for VTE is higher if anticoagulation is not therapeutic in the first 24 hours, immediate anticoagulation should be undertaken. For PE, this usually means anticoagulation and then testing. For DVT, since duplex imaging is rapidly obtained, usually testing precedes anticoagulation. Recurrent DVT can still occur in up to one third of patients over an 8-year period, even with appropriate anticoagulant therapy.

Heparin

Unfractionated heparin or low-molecular-weight heparin (LMWH) is given for 5 days, during which time oral anticoagulation with vitamin K antagonists (usually warfarin) is begun as soon as anticoagulation is therapeutic. It is recommended that the international normalized ratio (INR) be therapeutic for 2 consecutive days before stopping heparin or LMWH.

CURRENT THERAPY

- Initial therapy includes low-molecular-weight heparin (LMWH), compression garments, and ambulation once anticoagulation is therapeutic.
- LMWH should be administered for at least 5 days, during which time an oral anticoagulant (usually warfarin) is begun. Warfarin should be started after heparinization is therapeutic to prevent warfarin-induced skin necrosis. Therapeutic heparinization with LMWH means an appropriate weight-based dose is administered and allowed to circulate. The international normalized ratio (INR) should be therapeutic for 2 consecutive days before stopping LMWH.
- The goal for warfarin dosing is an INR between 2.0 and 3.0.
- The duration of anticoagulation depends on a number of factors, including the presence of risk factors for thrombosis, the type of thrombosis (idiopathic or provoked), the number of times thrombosis has occurred, venous patency, and the level of D-dimer measured approximately 1 month after stopping warfarin.
- Significant iliofemoral deep venous thrombosis should be treated with aggressive pharmocomechanical thrombolysis, and pulmonary embolism causing hemodynamic deterioration or right heart strain should be treated with thrombolysis.

LMWH, derived from the lower molecular weight range of standard heparin, has become the standard for treatment. LMWH is preferred because it is administered subcutaneously, it requires no monitoring (except in certain circumstances such as renal insufficiency or morbid obesity), and it is associated with a lower bleeding potential. Additionally, LMWH demonstrates less direct thrombin inhibition and more factor Xa inhibition. Compared to standard unfractionated heparin, LMWH has significantly improved bioavailability, less endothelial cell binding and protein binding, and an improved pharmacokinetic profile. The half-life of LMWH is dose independent. LMWH is administered in a weight-based fashion.

Use of LMWH in outpatient settings usually requires a coordinated effort of multiple health care providers. Certain LMWHs decrease indices of chronic venous insufficiency compared to standard therapy when used over an extended period. In a study of 480 patients, the LMWH tinzaparin (Innohep) for 12 weeks was superior to warfarin regarding treatment satisfaction, signs and symptoms of post-thrombotic syndrome, and the incidence of leg ulcers. This suggests that there are pleotropic effects of the LMWH or that more consistent anticoagulation is accomplished.

Based on all of the available evidence, LMWH is now preferred over standard unfractionated heparin for the initial treatment of VTE with a level of evidence given 1A.

Warfarin

Warfarin (Coumadin) should be started after heparinization is therapeutic to prevent warfarin-induced skin necrosis. For standard unfractionated heparin, this requires a therapeutic activated partial thromboplastin time (aPTT); for LMWH, warfarin is administered after an appropriate weight-based dose of LMWH is administered and allowed to circulate. Warfarin causes inhibition of protein C and S before factors II, IX and X, leading to paradoxical hypercoagulability at the initiation of therapy. The goal for warfarin dosing is an INR between 2.0 and 3.0. The duration of anticoagulation depends on a number of factors, including the presence of continuing risk factors for thrombosis, the type of thrombosis (idiopathic or provoked), the number of times thrombosis has occurred, the status of the veins when stopping anticoagulation, and the level of D-dimer measured approximately 1 month after stopping warfarin. One study demonstrated a statistically significant advantage to resuming warfarin if the D-dimer assay is elevated over an average 1.4-year follow-up (odds ratio [OR], 4.26; $P = 0.02$), and a meta-analysis has confirmed this relationship.

Duration of Treatment

The recommended duration of anticoagulation after a first episode of VTE is 3 to 6 months, but calf thrombi may be treated with a shorter course of warfarin, usually 6 weeks to 3 months. After a second episode of VTE, the usual recommendation is prolonged warfarin unless the patient is very young at the time of presentation or there are other mitigating factors. VTE recurrence is increased with homozygous factor V Leiden and prothrombin 20210A mutation, protein C or protein S deficiency, antithrombin deficiency, antiphospholipid antibodies, and cancer until resolved. Long-term warfarin is usually recommended in these situations. However, heterozygous factor V Leiden and prothrombin 20210A do not carry the same risk as their homozygous counterparts, and the length of oral anticoagulation is shortened for these conditions.

Regarding idiopathic DVT, most believe this diagnosis requires longer than 6 months of anticoagulation, but the actual length is unknown. One multicenter trial suggested that low-dose warfarin (INR 1.5-2.0) is superior to placebo, with a 64% risk reduction for recurrent DVT after the completion of an initial 6 months of standard therapy. A second study then suggested that full-dose warfarin (INR 2-3) is superior to low-dose warfarin in these patients without a difference in bleeding. Taken together, criteria for discontinuing anticoagulation, including thrombosis risk, residual thrombus burden, and coagulation system activation, are given a level of evidence of 1A.

Complications

Bleeding is the most common complication of anticoagulation. With standard heparin, bleeding occurs over the first 5 days in approximately 10% of patients.

Another complication is heparin-induced thrombocytopenia (HIT), which occurs in 0.6% to 30% of patients. Although historically morbidity and mortality has been high, it has been found that early diagnosis and appropriate treatment have decreased these rates. HIT usually begins 3 to 14 days after heparin is begun, although it can occur earlier if the patient has been exposed to heparin in the past. A heparin-dependent antibody binds to platelets, activates them with the release of procoagulant microparticles leading to an increase in thrombocytopenia, and results in both arterial and venous thrombosis.

Both bovine and porcine unfractionated heparin and LMWH have been associated with HIT, although the incidence and severity of the thrombosis is less with LMWH. Even small exposures to heparin, such as heparin coating on indwelling catheters, can cause the syndrome. The diagnosis should be suspected with a 50% or greater drop in platelet count, when the platelet count falls below 100,000/μL, or when thrombosis occurs during heparin or LMWH therapy.

The enzyme-linked immunosorbent assay (ELISA) detects the antiheparin antibody in the plasma. This test is highly sensitive but poorly specific. The serotonin release assay is another test that can be used, and this test is more specific but less sensitive than the ELISA test.

When the diagnosis is made, heparin must be stopped. Warfarin should not be given until an adequate alternative anticoagulant has been established and until the platelet count has normalized. Because LMWHs demonstrate high cross-reactivity with standard heparin antibodies, they cannot be substituted for standard heparin in patients with HIT. Agents that have been FDA approved as alternatives include the direct thrombin inhibitors hirudin (lepirudin [Refludan]) and argatroban. Fondaparinux (Arixtra)[1] has also been found effective for treatment of HIT in most cases, but it is not FDA approved for this indication. The use of these alternative agents is given either a 2C and 1C level of evidence.

ALTERNATIVE AND FUTURE MEDICAL TREATMENTS FOR DEEP VENOUS THROMBOSIS AND PULMONARY EMBOLISM

New agents for venous thrombosis treatment include factor Xa inhibitors and direct thrombin inhibitors.

Fondaparinux (Arixtra) a synthetic pentasaccharide that has an antithrombin sequence identical to heparin, targets factor Xa. Fondaparinux has been approved for the treatment of DVT and PE; for thrombosis prophylaxis in patient with total hip replacement, total knee replacement, and hip fracture; in extended prophylaxis in patients with hip fracture; and in patients undergoing abdominal surgery. It is administered subcutaneously and has a 17-hour half-life. Dosage is based on body weight. It exhibits no endothelial or protein binding and does not produce thrombocytopenia. However, no antidote is readily available.

In a meta-analysis involving more than 7000 patients, there was more than a 50% risk reduction using fondaparinux begun 6 hours after surgery compared to LMWH begun 12 to 24 hours after surgery. Major bleeding was increased, but critical bleeding was not. Fondaparinux has also been found effective in prophylaxis of other groups of patients including general medical patients.[1] For the treatment of VTE, fondaparinux was found equal to LMWH for DVT, and for PE, it was found equal to standard heparin.

Dabigatran etexilate (Pradaxa)[2] is an oral direct thrombin inhibitor. It is a double prodrug that is converted by esterases into dabigatran. Dabagatran etexilate has been approved for prophylaxis in total hip replacement and total knee replacement in western Europe and Canada. It demonstrates a low risk for bleeding, offers fixed oral dosing without coagulation monitors, and does not show an increase in liver enzymes. It has a predictable anticoagulant effect, uses fixed dosing with no need for monitoring, and directly binds to thrombin with high affinity and specificity. When tested against LMWH given twice daily, it failed to meet the non-inferiority target that was achieved with LMWH once daily. Phase 3 studies are in progress in VTE treatment, atrial fibrillation, and acute coronary syndrome. Dabigatran was recently found to be as effective as warfarin for the treatment of DVT.

Other antithrombotic agents being evaluated include oral heparins, oral anti–factor Xa agents (apixaban[5] and rivaroxaban [Xarelto][5]), difibrinating agents, antiinflammatory agents such as P-selectin inhibitors, factor VIIa inhibitors, tissue factor pathway inhibitor, and activated protein C. P-selectin inhibitors use an antiinflammatory approach to limit thrombus amplification without causing anticoagulation and bleeding.

NONPHARMACOLOGIC TREATMENTS

The rate and severity of postthrombotic syndrome after proximal DVT can be decreased by approximately 50% by the use of compression stockings. This measure is often forgotten by clinicians. Discussion with the patient on its importance is also critical to ensure good compliance. Additionally, walking with good compression does not increase the risk of PE, whereas it significantly decreases the incidence and severity of the postthrombotic syndrome. The use of strong compression and early ambulation after DVT treatment can significantly reduce the pain and swelling resulting from the DVT and carries a 1A level of evidence.

Aggressive Therapies for Venous Thromboembolism

For DVT treatment, the goals are to prevent extension or recurrence of DVT, prevent pulmonary embolism, and minimize the late squeal of thrombosis, namely chronic venous insufficiency. Standard anticoagulants accomplish the first two goals, but not the third goal.

---

[1]Not FDA approved for this indication.

---

[1]Not FDA approved for this indication.
[2]Not available in the United States.
[5]Investigational drug in the United States.

The postthrombotic syndrome (venous insufficiency related to venous thrombosis) occurs in up to 30% of patients after DVT. The following evidence suggests more-aggressive therapies for extensive thrombosis are indicated.

Experimentally, prolonged contact of the thrombus with the vein wall increases damage. The thrombus initiates an inflammatory response in the vein wall that can lead to vein wall fibrosis and valvular dysfunction. Thus, removing the thrombus should be an excellent solution to prevent this interaction. For example, the longer a thrombus is in contact with a vein valve, the more chance that valve will no longer function.

Venous thrombectomy has proved superior to anticoagulation over 6 months to 10 years as measured by venous patency and prevention of venous reflux. Catheter-directed thrombolysis has been employed in many nonrandomized studies and in one small, randomized trial was more effective than standard therapy. Quality of life was improved with thrombus removal, and results appear to be optimized further by combining catheter-directed thrombolysis with mechanical devices. These devices include the Trellis balloon occlusion catheter, the Angiojet rheolytic catheter, and the EKOS ultrasound accelerated catheter. With these devices, thrombolysis is hastened, the amount of thrombolytic agent is decreased, and bleeding is thus decreased. The ACCP has graded aggressive therapy as 2B/C evidence.

Additionally, the use of venous stents for iliac venous obstruction has been shown to decease the incidence of postthrombotic syndrome and chronic venous insufficiency. To more fully elucidate the role of aggressive therapy in proximal iliofemoral venous thrombosis, a study has been approved by the National Institutes of Health (NIH) to compare catheter-directed pharmacomechanical thrombolysis to standard anticoagulation for significant iliofemoral venous thrombosis. This study, the Attract Trial, will evaluate anatomic, physiologic, and quality-of-life endpoints.

For pulmonary embolism, evidence exists that thrombolysis is indicated when there is hemodynamic compromise from the embolism. It is controversial if thrombolysis should be used in situations in which there is no hemodynamic compromise but there is evidence of right heart dysfunction or there are positive biomarkers. Future studies will address thess situations.

Inferior Vena Cava Filters

Traditional indications for the use of IVC filters include failure of anticoagulation, a contraindication to anticoagulation, or a complication of anticoagulation. Protection from pulmonary embolism is greater than 95% using cone-shaped wire-based permanent filters in the IVC. With the success of these filters, indications have expanded to the presence of free-floating thrombus tails, prophylactic use when the risk for anticoagulation is excessive and when the risk of pulmonary embolism is thought to be high, and to allow the use of perioperative epidural anesthesia.

IVC filters can be either permanent or optional (retrievable). If a retrievable filter is left, then it becomes a permanent filter; the long-term fate of these filters has yet to be defined adequately in the literature. Most filters are placed in the infrarenal location in the IVC. However, they may be placed in the suprarenal position or in the superior vena cava.

Indications for suprarenal placement include high-lying thrombi, pregnancy or childbearing age, or previous device failure filled with thrombus. Although some have suggested that sepsis is a contraindication to the use of filters, sepsis has not been found to be a contraindication because the trapped material can be sterilized with intravenous antibiotics.

Filters may be inserted under x-ray guidance or using ultrasound techniques, either external ultrasound and intravascular ultrasound. Other than one randomized prospective study on the use of IVC filters as treatment of DVT (which is not how filters are traditionally used), evidence for the use of filters is rated at a 2C grade of evidence.

REFERENCES

Bruinstroop E, Klok FA, Van De Ree MA, et al. Elevated D-dimer levels predict recurrence in patients with idiopathic venous thromboembolism: A meta-analysis. J Thromb Haemost 2009;7:611.

Comerota AJ, Throm RC, Mathias SD, et al. Catheter-directed thrombolysis for iliofemoral deep venous thrombosis improves health-related quality of life. J Vasc Surg 2000;32(1):130.

Elsharawy M, Elzayat E. Early results of thrombolysis vs. anticoagulation in iliofemoral venous thrombosis. A randomised clinical trial. Eur J Vasc Endovasc Surg 2002;24(3):209.

Fowl RJ, Strothman GB, Blebea J, et al. Inappropriate use of venous duplex scans: An analysis of indications and results. J Vasc Surg 1996;23(5):881.

Gross PL, Weitz JI. New anticoagulants for treatment of venous thromboembolism. Arterioscler Thromb Vasc Biol 2008;28:380.

Hull RD, Pineo GF, Brant R, et al. Home therapy of venous thrombosis with long-term LMWH versus usual care: Patient satisfaction and post-thrombotic syndrome. Am J Med 2009;122:762.

Kearon C, Kahn SR, Agnelli G, et al. Antithrombotic therapy for venous thromboembolic disease: ACCP evidence-based clinical practice guidelines (8th ed). Chest 2008;133:454S.

Merli G, Spyropoulos AC, Caprini JA. Use of emerging oral anticoagulants in clinical practice: Translating results from clinical trials to orthopedic and general surgical patient populations. Ann Surg 2009;250:219.

Neglen P, Hollis KC, Olivier J, et al. Stenting of the venous outflow in chronic venous disease: Long-term stent-related outcome, clinical, and hemodynamic result. J Vasc Surg 2007;46(5):979.

Palareti G, Cosmi B, Legnani C, et al. D-dimer testing to determine the duration of anticoagulation therapy. N Eng J Med 2006;355:1780.

Schulman S, Kearon C, Kakkar AK, et al. Dabigatran versus warfarin in the treatment of acute venous thromboembolism. N Engl J Med 2009;361 (24):2342.

Stein PD, Fowler SE, Goodman LR, et al. Multidetector computed tomography for acute pulmonary embolism. N Engl J Med 2006;354(22):2317.

Turpie AG, Bauer KA, Eriksson BI, et al. Fondaparinux vs. enoxaparin for the prevention of venous thromboembolism in major orthopedic surgery: A meta-analysis of 4 randomized double-blind studies. Arch Intern Med 2002;162(16):1833.

Wakefield TW, Caprini J, Comerota AJ. Thromboembolic diseases. Curr Probl Surg 2008;45(12):844.

Wells PS, Anderson DR, Rodger M, et al. Evaluation of D-dimer in the diagnosis of suspected deep-vein thrombosis. N Engl J Med 2003;349(13):1227.

The Blood and Spleen

Aplastic Anemia

Method of
Eva C. Guinan, MD

The survival of patients with aplastic anemia has improved dramatically in the past several decades. Improved testing for underlying acquired and congenital genetic defects has served to better segregate patients with idiopathic aplastic anemia from those with the very different prognoses associated with an inherited bone marrow failure syndrome (IBMFS) and myelodysplasia (MDS). For patients in the idiopathic (or acquired) aplastic anemia group, advances in transfusion medicine and other supportive care have also certainly contributed. Refinements in both major arms of treatment, immunosuppressive therapy (IST), and allogeneic hematopoietic stem cell transplantation (HSCT), have also contributed to current outcomes (Fig. 1). Although IST survival curves have been stable in the last decade, survival after HSCT regardless of donor source has continued to improve. Greater understanding of pathophysiology and long-term treatment outcomes are having the largest impact on triage of therapy and standards of practice.

Definition

There is no pathognomonic diagnostic test for aplastic anemia. Accordingly, aplastic anemia continues to be diagnosed by a combination of inclusion and exclusion criteria. The definition established by the International Agranulocytosis and Aplastic Anaemia Study states that patients must have bone marrow hypocellularity with two or more of the following: hemoglobin of less than 10 g/dL, platelet count of less than 50×10^9/L, and neutrophil count of less than 1.5×10^9/L. Most commonly, patients said to have aplastic anemia in fact have severe aplastic anemia, which is defined by the absolute neutrophil count (ANC) as shown in Box 1. Severity grading has become part of the diagnostic algorithm and is increasingly used as a predictor of outcome.

Differential Diagnosis

Because many conditions can fulfill these inclusion criteria, care must be taken to consider infectious, metabolic, and toxic exposures that could result in transient pancytopenia. Specific considerations are listed in many current reviews. These diagnoses are wide ranging and include hypoplastic presentations of lymphoma, leukemia, and MDS; anorexia; and transient severe bone marrow suppression due to drug exposure or, albeit rarely, a spectrum of acute viral illnesses.

Patients should be carefully evaluated for other conditions that can require an alternative management approach. A small fraction of pancytopenic and hypocellular patients have clonal cytogenetic abnormalities despite well-reviewed histology that appears to be free of any evidence of dysplasia or infiltrative disease. Accordingly, best practice should include both fluorescent in situ hybridization (FISH) and routine cytogenetics, because the yield for the latter analysis may be inadequate given the hypocellularity of the bone marrow compartment.

Although the prognostic relevance of clonal cytogenetics remains somewhat debatable, evidence of clonality at diagnosis should certainly provoke consideration of MDS as an alternative diagnosis and mandate an aggressive plan of follow-up and determination of HSCT donor status. Clonality also potentially alters immediate treatment depending on the clinical setting and most current literature. Among infectious problems, perhaps the most important consideration from a diagnostic and management perspective is HIV. However, viruses rarely cause a true aplastic picture, and their diagnosis, at present, does not have much therapeutic importance. Aplastic anemia can occur or recur during pregnancy and can resolve with either delivery or termination.

The most important alternative diagnoses are the IBMFSs (Table 1), which should be considered in virtually all patients and certainly in all pediatric patients. Such a diagnosis has important implications for medical management of the extended family, for genetic counseling, for the choice of therapy, for prognosis of the patient, and, in the setting of HSCT, for donor evaluation. A meticulous patient and family history and physical examination should be performed, although uninformative results do not eliminate the possibility of an IBMFS. Genetic testing is now widely available for some IBMFSs; however, it is clear that these syndromes are polygenic, and the relevant genetic defects have not all been defined. Therefore, testing might not be diagnostic. As additional mutations are described and as the natural history and phenotype of various mutations and polymorphisms become better elucidated, this information should be of increasing value.

In addition to IBMFS, an evaluation for paroxysmal nocturnal hemoglobinuria (PNH) should be undertaken. A small clonal population of cells deficient in glycosylphosphatidylinositol (GPI)-linked proteins that characterize PNH can be found in 20% to 50% of adults with aplastic anemia without a concurrent history of clotting or hemolysis. A similar percentage of children has been found to have such cells in their bone marrow. The presence of such cells does not imply a diagnosis of classic PNH, although some patients with apparent aplastic anemia do develop classic PNH. Ongoing clinical investigation into the relation of aplastic anemia and PNH might yield further information that will assist in therapeutic decision making.

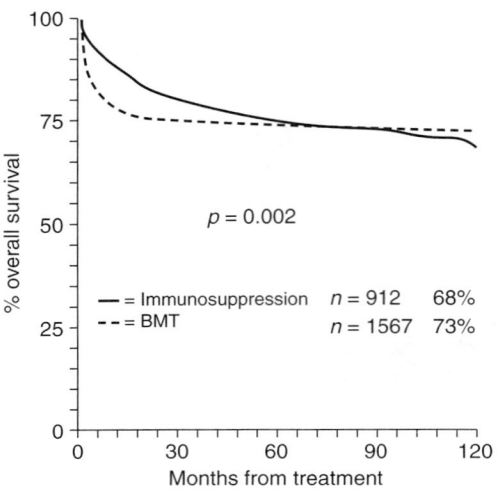

FIGURE 1. The actuarial survival of 2479 patients with acquired severe aplastic anemia. Group A received immunosuppressive therapy (IST) *(solid line)* as first-line therapy and Group B underwent hematopoietic stem cell transplant (BMT) *(dashed line)*. Ten-year survival was 73% with BMT and 68% with IST ($P < 0.002$). Data from Locasciulli A, Oneto R, Bacigalupo A, et al: Outcome of patients with acquired aplastic anemia given first-line bone marrow transplantation or immunosuppressive treatment in the last decade: A report from the European Group for Blood and Marrow Transplantation (EBMT). Haematologica 2007;92:11–18.

Supportive Care

The goals of supportive care in aplastic anemia are alleviating symptoms of anemia and addressing the risks of hemorrhage and infection that result from pancytopenia. Appropriate precautions for minimizing alloimmunization should be taken, such as use of leukodepletion techniques and conservative transfusion goals.

Preemptive counseling can play as important a role as symptom management. There are few evidence-based guidelines for activities of daily living, such as the quality of diet, extent of exercise, and travel restrictions. The best standard is frequent, open communication between physician and patient. Some practical issues, however, are common. For example, the menstrual status of female patients should be ascertained immediately on diagnosis. Because severe menorrhagia

BOX 1   Severity Classification of Aplastic Anemia
Severe Bone marrow cellularity <25% *and* Two peripheral blood findings: • Absolute neutrophil count <0.5 × 10⁹/L • Platelet count <20 × 10⁹/L • Reticulocyte count <20 × 10⁹/L **Very Severe** Same criteria as for severe *and* Peripheral blood absolute neutrophil count <0.2 × 10⁹/L **Nonsevere (Moderate)** Hypocellullar bone marrow *and* Peripheral blood cytopenias not meeting criteria for severe aplastic anemia

- Patient must all meet hematologic criteria.
- Assess severity.
- Adequate cytogenetic analysis is essential.
- Consider diagnoses with treatment implications:
  - Causes of transient pancytopenia.
  - Evaluate for inherited bone marrow failure syndromes, paroxysmal nocturnal hemoglobinuria, myelodysplasia syndrome.
  - Evaluate for malignancy (leukemia, lymphoma), HIV.

can occur in the setting of protracted thrombocytopenia, use of hormonal therapy to suppress menstruation should be addressed with patients and with families of younger patients. Particular regard should be paid to anticipation of menarche in pubertal girls.

With regard to infectious risks, standards widely vary by practitioner and institution. Although the largest single cause of death in patients undergoing either HSCT or IST is infection, there is no current standard for infection prophylaxis in aplastic anemia. Clinical trials to define the best possible approaches to this issue, including the role of novel broad-spectrum anti-infectives and their schedule of use, would be very important. At the least, a detailed history taken in the context of exposure and lifestyle issues should be used to develop a plan for fever and infection prophylaxis with which the patient can be compliant.

Benefit from the use of hematopoietic growth factors to support the ANC, or indeed any lineage, has been unclear in patients with idiopathic aplastic anemia. Some concern has been raised about the association of long-term use of granulocyte colony-stimulating factor (G-CSF) (Neupogen)[1] by patients, particularly children, with aplastic anemia and subsequent development of MDS and acute myelogenous leukemia (AML), although this remains uncertain.

Monitoring of iron status should be routine for patients with ongoing red cell transfusion needs. Chelation should be initiated according to accepted guidelines to minimize complications of iron overload.

Treatment

Observation is not a successful treatment option for patients with severe aplastic anemia; older, retrospective data demonstrate a 1-year mortality with supportive care alone of more than 80%, although clearly more effective current transfusion and support strategies would improve on this outcome. Nonetheless, a recent large report from the European Group for Blood and Marrow Transplantation demonstrates that decreased time from diagnosis to treatment, whether IST or HSCT, is a highly significant predictor of survival. A triage of therapy is shown in Figure 2.

IMMUNOSUPPRESSIVE THERAPY

It is generally held that a significant percentage of aplastic anemia has an immune pathogenesis. A variety of data on immune effector cell function and repertoire, cell surface phenotype, and cytokine production support this belief. In practice, this hypothesis is also supported by the observation that IST with cyclosporine (Neoral)[1] (CSA), antithymocyte globulin (Atgam) (ATG), and corticosteroids results in response in roughly 75% of patients.

Age and response are related, and younger patients generally have a higher likelihood of response. It has also been reported that children with IST and very severe aplastic anemia do better than their age peers with severe aplastic anemia and that children (<16 years)

---

[1]Not FDA approved for this indication.

TABLE 1 Inherited Bone Marrow Failure Syndromes Commonly Associated with Pancytopenia*

Syndrome	Common Hematologic Findings	Diagnostic Tests Available†
Amegakaryocytic thrombocytopenia	Thrombocytopenia with absent or hypolobulated megakaryocytes Macrocytosis Progressive pancytopenia with marrow hypoplasia	Gene mutation analysis
Dyskeratosis congenita	Macrocytosis Thrombocytopenia Progressive pancytopenia with marrow hypoplasia	Gene mutation analysis Telomere length (may be shortened)
Fanconi's anemia	Macrocytosis Single, bilineage, or trilineage cytopenia Progressive pancytopenia with marrow hypoplasia	Abnormal chromosomal breakage or sister-chromatid exchange in the presence of DNA cross-linkers Cell cycle progression in the presence of DNA cross-linkers Gene mutation analysis
Shwachman-Diamond syndrome	Neutropenia Progressive pancytopenia with marrow hypoplasia	Radiologic bony abnormalities Serum trypsinogen and isoamylase levels (may be decreased) Gene mutation analysis

*Diamond-Blackfan anemia, as well as less common disorders such as Pearson's, Seckel's, and Noonan's syndromes; cartilage–hair hypoplasia; and reticular dysgenesis, can progress to marrow failure meeting the definition of aplastic anemia.
†Clinically approved mutation testing is becoming increasingly available, but not all genetic defects have been defined for any of these disorders.

with very severe aplastic anemia have better survival rates than similarly affected adults. Age does not affect the relative survival rate of patients with less severe aplastic anemia.

Randomized studies have demonstrated better response when IST agents are used in combination. Meta-analysis has also shown decreased all-cause mortality. In addition to their general immunomodulatory capacity, the immunologic effects of IST may be specific, because direct lympholytic and bone marrow stimulatory activities have been described. The addition of further immunosuppressive medications, such as mycophenolate, to this regimen has thus far not improved outcomes.

IST responses can be of varying degree and duration and can take 3 to 6 months to become evident. Often, responding patients continue to manifest some evidence of bone marrow failure, with mild degrees of cytopenia or residual macrocytosis commonly observed. Slow taper of CSA in IST responders is advisable, generally over longer than 6 months, and a significant fraction of patients demonstrate prolonged dependence on CSA for persistent hematologic improvement. A second course of IST in patients who failed a first course can produce response in 35% to 50% of patients. Complete or partial loss of response occurs in an appreciable number of patients,

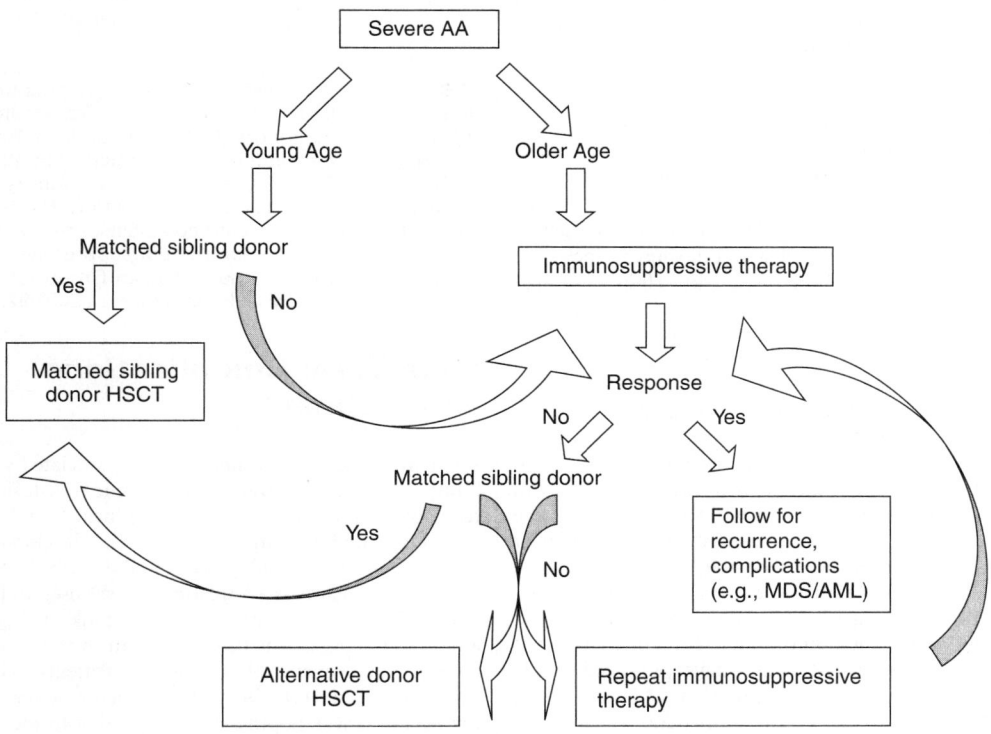

FIGURE 2. Triage of aplastic anemia (AA) therapies. The age limit suggested by young/old is variable from report to report, but generally sits in the 30- to 40-year-old range. AML = acute myelogenous leukemia; HSCT = hematopoietic stem cell transplant; MDS = myelodysplasia.

CURRENT THERAPY

- Minimize interval between diagnosis and initiation of treatment.
- Determine if an MSD is available.
- If the patient is young and has an MSD, proceed to HSCT with non-TBI regimen.
- If has no MSD or is older, proceed to IST with CSA/ATG/steroid.
- For treatment failure, reconsider IST versus HSCT options.

ATG = antithymocyte globulin; CSA = cyclosporine; HSCT = hematopoietic stem cell transplantation; IST = immunosuppressive therapy; MSD = matched sibling donor; TBI = total body irradiation.

approximately one third, and can become manifest years after cessation of IST or immediately on CSA taper. Re-treatment with the same or a similar regimen is often successful.

HEMATOPOIETIC STEM CELL TRANSPLANTATION

HSCT is the only truly curative therapy for aplastic anemia and produces stable survival rates in the range of 60% to 80%, depending on donor type and other HSCT variables (Fig. 3). In young patients with matched sibling donors (MSDs), a short interval from diagnosis to HSCT, and little prior therapy, survival rates up to 97% have been recently reported. Conversely, prior IST or excessive transfusion (or both) are associated with worse outcome. Thus, the general recommendation is for young patients with MSDs to proceed to HSCT as soon as the diagnosis is confirmed. The age cutoff for this decision varies somewhat, but the recommendation certainly holds for patients younger than 30 years and is often implemented for those younger than 40 years.

HSCT for aplastic anemia from MSD can be successfully achieved with radiation-free preparative regimens, of which the most standard and widely used is cyclophosphamide (Cytoxan)[1] (CY) and ATG conditioning. CSA and short-course methotrexate (Trexall)[1] (MTX) provide highly effective graft-versus-host disease (GVHD) prophylaxis in this setting. In a group of adults and children undergoing MSD allogeneic HSCT, this classic CY/ATG/CSA/MTX regimen produced a 96% rate of sustained engraftment, 3% rate of severe acute GVHD, 26% rate of chronic GVHD, and overall survival of 88% at median follow-up of 9 years. A recent study suggests that ATG may not be as essential to this outcome as previously thought. All stem cell sources, including sibling umbilical cord blood, have been used successfully, although use of peripheral blood stem cells appears to result in an unacceptably high rate of chronic GHVD and is not currently advised.

The dearth of alternative therapies for those who fail to respond to IST, coupled with the success of MSD HSCT, have encouraged the use of alternative-donor HSCT for aplastic anemia. Originally, the use of somewhat more aggressive regimens than those necessary with MSD engendered more regimen-related toxicity, and patients coming to alternative-donor HSCT were often late in their clinical course with significant aplastic anemia–associated morbidity. Outcomes were somewhat disappointing. Results have improved significantly over the past decade, and even more so over the past 5 years (see Fig. 3B). Moving HSCT treatment earlier in therapeutic triage, coupled with improvements in histocompatibility typing, better supportive care, and the successful implementation of reduced-intensity regimens and alternative immunosuppressive strategies have produced highly encouraging results, with an overall survival in excess of 70% in some reports. However, the best results are seen when patients are younger, and outcomes in those older than 40 years remain less satisfactory.

[1]Not FDA approved for this indication.

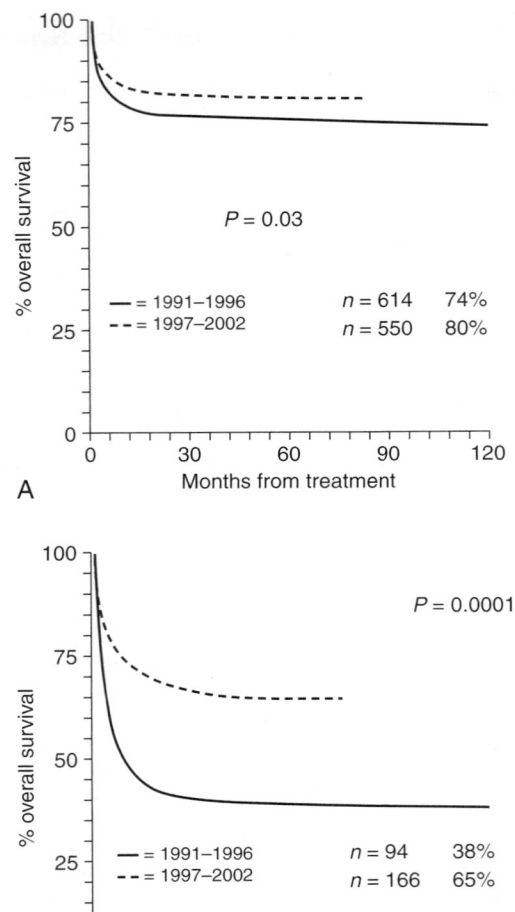

FIGURE 3. The actuarial survival of patients undergoing hematopoietic stem cell transplantation (HSCT) from matched sibling donors (**A**) or alternative donors (**B**) by time periods. Results improved for both donor groups in the later time period (matched sibling donors 74% vs 80%, $P = 0.03$) and alternative donors (38% vs 65%, $P = 0.0001$). Data from Locasciulli A, Oneto R, Bacigalupo A, et al: Outcome of patients with acquired aplastic anemia given first line bone marrow transplantation or immunosuppressive treatment in the last decade: A report from the European Group for Blood and Marrow Transplantation (EBMT). Haematologica 2007;92:11–18.

Long-Term Complications of Treatment

All aplastic anemia treatments can be associated with significant morbidity, be it the iron-overload of chronic transfusion or the more protean problems of IST or HSCT. These include, in both cases, significant regimen-related end-organ toxicity. The development of clonal cytogenetic abnormalities after IST is well described and occurs in patients of all ages, regardless of treatment response, and over a broad time frame. The rate of progression to frank AML is not predictable, although progression is most common in those with monosomy 7 or complex cytogenetic abnormalities. Patients with aplastic anemia who undergo HSCT generally experience fewer toxicities than does the overall HSCT population, in part due to the reduced intensity of aplastic anemia regimens. Growth and fertility may be well preserved, but persistent infectious complications, pulmonary insufficiency, dermatologic pathology, avascular necrosis, and other bone and joint issues, as well as hypothyroidism or other endocrine disturbances, can occur, as can secondary malignancies. Some of these conditions reflect the sequelae of chronic GVHD itself, and others reflect the toxicity of drugs used to manage GVHD. The toll of GVHD is real; decreased quality of life and overall survival are observed in the nearly one half of aplastic anemia patients experiencing chronic GVHD.

Conclusions

Improvements in diagnosis, supportive care, IST, and HSCT have led to significant improvements in survival for patients with severe aplastic anemia. However, there are still controversies over the optimal choice of therapy for individual patients, and any given choice can lead to a number of serious regimen-related toxicities. Further insights into the pathophysiology of bone marrow failure, increased diagnostic accuracy for IBMFS, greater appreciation of the risk and epidemiology of late complications, and steady progress in therapeutics will hopefully combine to yield increasingly well-targeted and more-successful treatment.

Acknowledgments

Eva C. Guinan is a prior recipient of a Specified Established Researcher Award from the Aplastic Anemia & MDS International Foundation and the Distinguished Service Award of the Fanconi Anemia Research Foundation.

REFERENCES

Ades L, Mary JY, Robin M, et al. Long-term outcome after bone marrow transplantation for severe aplastic anemia. Blood 2004;103:2490–7.

Alter BP. Bone marrow failure: A child is not just a small adult (but an adult can have a childhood disease). Hematology (Am Soc Hematol Educ Program) 2005;96–103.

Frickhofen N, Heimpel H, Kaltwasser JP, Schrezenmeier H. Antithymocyte globulin with or without cyclosporin A: 11-year follow-up of a randomized trial comparing treatments of aplastic anemia. Blood 2003;101:1236–42.

Fuhrer M, Burdach S, Ebell W, et al. Relapse and clonal disease in children with aplastic anemia (AA) after immunosuppressive therapy (IST): The SAA 94 experience. German/Austrian Pediatric Aplastic Anemia Working Group. Klin Padiatr 1998;210:173–9.

Gafter-Gvilli A, Ram R, Gurion R, et al. ATG plus cyclosporine reduces all-cause mortality in patients with severe aplastic anemia—systematic review and meta-analysis. Acta Haematol 2008;120:237–40.

Kojima S, Horibe K, Inaba J, et al. Long-term outcome of acquired aplastic anaemia in children: Comparison between immunosuppressive therapy and bone marrow transplantation. Br J Haematol 2000;111:321–8.

Kurre P, Johnson FL, Deeg HJ. Diagnosis and treatment of children with aplastic anemia. Pediatr Blood Cancer 2005;45:770–80.

Locasciulli A, Oneto R, Bacigalupo A, et al. Outcome of patients with acquired aplastic anemia given first line bone marrow transplantation or immunosuppressive treatment in the last decade: A report from the European Group for Blood and Marrow Transplantation (EBMT). Haematologica 2007;92:11–8.

Maciejewski JP, Risitano A, Sloand EM, et al. Distinct clinical outcomes for cytogenetic abnormalities evolving from aplastic anemia. Blood 2002;99: 3129–35.

Marsh JCW, Ball SE, Cavenaugh J, et al. Guidelines for the diagnosis and management of acquired aplastic anaemia. Br J Haematol 2009;147:43–70.

Parker C, Omine M, Richards S, et al. Diagnosis and management of paroxysmal nocturnal hemoglobinuria. Blood 2005;106:3699–709.

Schrezenmeier H, Passweg JR, Marsh JC, et al. Worse outcome and more chronic GVHD with peripheral blood progenitor cells than bone marrow in HLA-matched sibling donor transplants for young patients with severe acquired aplastic anemia: A report from the European Group for Blood and Marrow Transplantation and the Center for International Blood and Marrow Transplant Research. Blood 2007;110(4):1397–400.

Socie G, Gluckman E. Cure from severe aplastic anemia in vivo and late effects. Acta Haematol 2000;103:49–54.

Socie G, Mary JY, Schrezenmeier H, et al. Granulocyte-stimulating factor and severe aplastic anemia: a survey from the European Group for Blood and Marrow Transplantation (EBMT). Blood 2007;109:2794–6.

Young NS. Paroxysmal nocturnal hemoglobinuria: Current issues in pathophysiology and treatment. Curr Hematol Rep 2005;4:103–9.

Young NS, Calado RT, Scheinberg P. Current concepts in the pathophysiology and treatment of aplastic anemia. Blood 2006;108:2509–19.

Iron Deficiency

Method of
Paul Paulman, MD

Epidemiology

Iron is necessary for production of erythrocytes and the normal functioning of several iron-containing cellular enzymes. Iron deficiency is defined as the decrease of total iron stores in the body. Iron deficiency anemia results when iron deficiency is severe enough to decrease erythropoiesis. The most common cause of iron deficiency in the U.S. adult population is blood loss. The most common sources of blood loss are menstrual and gastrointestinal. Other causes of iron deficiency include inadequate intake during high-demand states such as pregnancy, early childhood, or erythropoietin therapy. A diet low in iron-rich foods (vegetarian or vegan) can lead to iron deficiency.

Gastrointestinal diseases including Crohn's disease, sprue, and postgastrectomy states can decrease iron absorption from the gastrointestinal tract, resulting in iron deficiency. Chronic inflammatory states can lead to decreased use of available iron stores, leading to symptoms of iron deficiency.

Iron deficiency is the most common micronutrient deficiency in the world. Iron deficiency affects approximately 2% to 5% of children and adolescents in the United States and 4% of the US adult population, including 20% of women of childbearing age, 50% of pregnant women, and 2% of men.

Risk Factors

Risk factors for iron deficiency include age, socioeconomic status, sex, diet, disease, and medical treatment. Infants, children, and adolescents are at risk, especially during periods of rapid growth. Low socioeconomic status, including minority population group and low income, increase the risk for iron deficiency. Risk is increased in women during the childbearing years and during pregnancy and breastfeeding. Diets low in iron-rich foods, including vegan and vegetarian diets, increase the risk.

Any illness or therapy that leads to decreased absorption of iron or loss of blood also increases the risk. Gastrointestinal diseases causing blood loss or decreased iron absorption can lead to iron deficiency. Antacids cause decreased iron absorption and nonsteroidal antiinflammatory drugs (NSAIDs) cause gastrointestinal blood loss. Erythropoietin therapy depletes iron stores because of increased hematopoiesis. Frequent phlebotomy, including repetitive blood donation or treatment for polycythemia or hemochromatosis, decreases iron stores.

Pathophysiology

Total body iron stores for men are approximately 3.5 g and for women are about 2.5 g. More than 70% of body iron is found in hemoglobin, and the remainder is contained in myoglobin, tissue enzymes, and storage or transport proteins. Iron absorption takes place almost exclusively in the duodenum and upper jejunum. In a non-iron deficient state, only about 6% to 10% of iron from food is absorbed (1 mg of 15 mg/day of dietary iron). Factors that increase iron absorption from the gut include ingestion of heme (meat) iron, iron-deficient states, and coadministration of vitamin C (ascorbic acid). Factors that decrease iron absorption include ingestion of certain foods including vegetable fiber phytates, tea tannates, bran, and medications including tetracyclines and antacids.

Iron deficiency develops in stages. During the early stage, iron needs exceed iron intake and body iron stores are depleted, causing an increase in absorption of dietary iron. As this process continues, erythropoiesis is impaired, leading to iron deficiency anemia, and dysfunction of iron-containing cellular enzymes can occur. This enzyme dysfunction can contribute to the fatigue and loss of stamina seen in patients with iron deficiency anemia. Iron deficiency during childhood can result in deficiencies in growth and cognitive function.

Prevention

Prevention of iron deficiency is focused on providing supplemental dietary iron to populations at risk for iron deficiency. Current recommendations include elemental iron supplementation (1 mg/kg/d) for breast-fed infants after 6 months of age and iron supplementation of infant formula (12 mg/L elemental iron) for formula-fed infants. Iron-enriched cereals should be among the first solid foods offered to infants. Whole cow's milk should be avoided during the first year of life to decrease the possibility of occult gastrointestinal bleeding. Supplemental iron should be taken during pregnancy and breast-feeding.

Clinical Manifestations

Patients with iron deficiency may be asymptomatic. The presence of symptoms and signs of iron deficiency depend on the degree of deficiency, the time course of the development of iron deficiency, and the overall physiologic state of the patient. Common symptoms of iron deficiency include fatigue, weakness, irritability, poor concentration, exercise intolerance, dry mouth, and headache. Severe iron deficiency can cause pica, a craving to eat substances such as ice, dirt, clay, or paint. Signs of iron deficiency include pallor and a systolic heart murmur if anemia is present, alopecia, atrophy of lingual papillae, koilonychias, and chlorosis.

Diagnosis

The gold standard for diagnosis of iron deficiency is the demonstration of decreased iron available for erythropoiesis on a bone marrow aspiration sample. The wide availability of reliable serum iron markers makes bone marrow sampling for diagnosis of iron deficiency unnecessary in most cases. A low serum iron is characteristic of both iron deficiency and anemia of chronic disease. Serum total iron binding capacity is decreased in iron deficiency and elevated in anemia of chronic disease. Serum iron and total iron binding capacity are often ordered together. Many authorities think serum ferritin determination is the most useful laboratory test for iron deficiency. Ferritin levels reflect the quantity of iron stored in the reticuloendothelial system. A low serum ferritin level is diagnostic of iron deficiency. Serum ferritin levels can be falsely elevated in the presence of inflammation.

The diagnosis of iron deficiency anemia requires a decline in serum hemoglobin to less than 13 g/dL in men or 12 g/dL in women along with a decreased mean corpuscular volume and mean corpuscular hemoglobin and the presence of iron deficiency. Other findings in iron deficiency anemia include variation in erythrocyte shape and size (poikilocytosis and anisocytosis) and elevation in the coefficient of red blood cell distribution width (RDW).

Because gastrointestinal blood loss is a common cause of iron deficiency anemia, patients who present with iron deficiency anemia should be considered for appropriate screening for gastrointestinal conditions, including malignancies.

Differential Diagnosis

The differential diagnosis of iron deficiency includes causes of fatigue and exercise intolerance such as hypothyroidism, electrolyte disturbances due to diuretic therapy, left ventricular dysfunction, chronic lung disease, malignancies, or liver disease.

Anemia of chronic disease can mimic iron deficiency anemia. Differentiating characteristics of the two types of anemia can be found in Table 1.

TABLE 1 Difference between Iron Deficiency Anemia and Anemia of Chronic Illness

Test	Iron Deficiency Anemia	Anemia of Chronic Illness
Serum iron	Low	Low
Ferritin	Low	Increased
Red cell morphology	Variable	Normal
C-reactive protein	Normal	Increased

 CURRENT DIAGNOSIS

Symptoms

- Fatigue
- Poor exercise tolerance
- Weakness
- Irritability
- Poor concentration
- Dry mouth
- Headache
- Pica

Signs

- Pallor
- Systolic heart murmur if anemia is present
- Atrophy of lingual papillae
- Koilonychia
- Chlorosis

Laboratory Findings

- Decreased iron seen on bone marrow aspirate (gold standard)
- Low serum ferritin (diagnostic)
- Low serum iron level
- High serum iron-binding capacity
- Low serum hemoglobin
- Low mean corpuscular hemoglobin
- Low mean corpuscular volume
- Variations in size and shape of red blood cells

Treatment

Iron may be replaced via oral or intravenous routes. The most cost-effective oral iron preparation is a non–enteric-coated ferrous sulfate tablet. The most common oral iron replacement regimen consists of one 325 mg ferrous sulfate tablet (Feosol) by mouth three times daily. Each 325 mg ferrous sulfate tablet contains 65 mg of elemental iron.

Other iron salts, ferrous gluconate (Fergon) and ferrous fumarate (Ferro-Sequels) are available for oral replacement. The absorption of oral iron is enhanced by taking the pills on an empty stomach or with an ascorbic acid tablet (500 mg). Because of the gastric distress often caused by oral iron replacement, most practitioners prescribe enteric-coated iron tablets.

Patients who cannot take or cannot tolerate oral iron can be treated with intravenous iron preparations, iron dextran (InFeD), iron sucrose (Venofer),[1] or ferric gluconate (Ferrlecit).[1] Because of the pain associated with the injection and other problems, intramuscular iron is seldom used.

---

[1]Not FDA approved for this indication.

CURRENT THERAPY

Oral Replacement

- Ferrous sulfate (or other equivalent iron preparation) 325 mg three times daily
- Add ascorbic acid tablet 500 mg with each iron tablet to increase iron absorption.
- Consider enteric-coated tablets to decrease gastrointestinal problems associated with oral iron therapy.

Parenteral Replacement

- If oral therapy is not tolerated, parental preparations including iron dextran, iron sucrose, or ferric gluconate may be used.

Unstable Patient

- If the patient is hemodynamically unstable due to anemia, consider blood transfusion.

Treatment Endpoint

- Iron deficiency has been corrected if the serum ferritin is 50 ng/mL or more.

Patients who are severely anemic and hemodynamically unstable may be candidates for blood transfusion. To determine the total dose of iron needed to correct the deficiency, the total iron deficit (depleted stores plus the deficit in red cell hemoglobin iron) should be calculated before beginning therapy. Because the most common cause of iron deficiency is blood loss, the management of iron deficiency should include identification of the source and cause of blood loss.

Monitoring

The earliest marker for successful iron replacement is an increase in the reticulocyte count, which occurs within 5 to 10 days of initiation of iron replacement. A hemoglobin increase of 2 g/dL is considered an appropriate response to oral iron replacement. Complete blood counts should be obtained at 1 month and 2 months after beginning replacement therapy. Iron deficiency should be corrected after 2 months of replacement therapy. Treatment of iron deficiency should continue until the serum ferritin reaches a level of 50 ng/mL. Darkening of stools after 2 or 3 days of starting oral iron replacement is a reliable marker of compliance.

Complications

If properly treated, iron deficiency has few complications in adults. Untreated iron deficiency in infants and small children can lead to cognitive development and growth deficits. Treating iron deficiency without identifying the source and cause of blood loss could result in delay or failure to diagnose gastrointestinal malignancies or other serious clinical problems.

REFERENCES

Anderson GJ, Frazer DM, Mclaren GD. Iron absorption and metabolism. Curr Opin Gastroenterol 2009;25:129–35.

Anemias caused by deficient erythropoiesis. In: Beers MH, Porter RS, Jones TV, et al, editors. Merck Manual of Diagnosis and Therapy. 18th ed. Whitehouse Station, NJ: Merck Research Laboratories; 2006.

Clark SF. Iron deficiency anemia: Diagnosis and management. Curr Opin Gastroenterol 2009;26:122–8.

Clark SF. Iron deficiency anemia. Nutr Clin Pract 2008;23:128–41.

Cook JD. Diagnosis and management of iron deficiency anaemia. Best Pract Res Clin Haematol 2005;18:319–32.

Oski FA. The nonhematologic manifestations of iron deficiency. Am J Dis Child 1979;133:315–22.

Autoimmune Hemolytic Anemia

Method of
Nidra Rodriguez, MD

Hemolysis, the premature destruction of red blood cells (RBCs), leads to hemolytic anemia when the bone marrow cannot compensate for RBC loss. Autoimmune hemolytic anemia (AIHA) occurs as a result of antibody production against self-RBC antigens. Suggested causes for the occurrence of AIHA include alteration in immunoregulatory mechanisms leading to loss of immune tolerance and activation of B cells, T cells, or both. AIHA can be idiopathic, or it can occur secondary to infections, malignancies, or autoimmune disorders. Types of AIHA include warm-antibody AIHA, cold-antibody AIHA, paroxysmal cold hemoglobinuria (PCH), Evans syndrome, and medication-induced AIHA (Box 1).

BOX 1   Classification of Hemolytic Anemia Mediated by Antibodies

I. Warm-autoantibody type
  A. Primary or idiopathic warm-antibody AIHA
  B. Secondary warm-antibody AIHA associated with
    1. Lymphoproliferative disorders (e.g., Hodgkin's disease, lymphoma)
    2. Rheumatic/autoimmune disorders (e.g., SLE, ulcerative colitis)
    3. Certain nonlymphoid neoplasms (e.g., ovarian tumors)
    4. Ingestion of certain drugs (e.g., α-methyldopa [Aldomet])
II. Cold-autoantibody type
  A. Mediated by cold agglutinins
    1. Idiopathic (primary) chronic cold-agglutinin disease (most exhibit evidence of monoclonal B-lymphoproliferation)
    2. Secondary cold-agglutinin hemolytic anemia associated with
      a. Infections (e.g., *Mycoplasma pneumoniae*, infectious mononucleosis)
      b. Clinically evident malignant B-cell lymphoproliferative disorders
  B. Mediated by cold hemolysins
    1. Idiopathic (primary) paroxysmal cold hemoglobinuria
    2. Secondary
      a. Donath-Landsteiner hemolytic anemia, usually associated with an acute viral syndrome in children
      b. Associated with congenital or tertiary syphilis in adults
III. Mixed cold and warm autoantibodies
  A. Primary or idiopathic mixed AIHA
  B. Secondary mixed AIHA
    1. Associated with the rheumatic disorders, especially SLE
IV. Drug-immune hemolytic anemia
  A. Hapten or drug-adsorption mechanism
  B. Ternary (immune) complex mechanism
  C. True autoantibody mechanism

Adapted from Packman CH: Hemolytic anemia due to warm autoantibodies. Blood Rev 2008;22[1]:17–31.
Abbreviations: AIHA = autoimmune hemolytic anemia; SLE = systemic lupus erythematosus.

General Clinical and Laboratory Findings of AIHA

Patients with AIHA typically present with signs and symptoms of anemia, jaundice, and splenomegaly. Anemia may range from mild to severe, and its symptoms may be of acute or insidious onset.

Laboratory findings include anemia, reticulocytosis, increased mean corpuscular volume due to the presence of reticulocytes, indirect hyperbilirubinemia, increased lactate dehydrogenase (LDH), and decreased haptoglobin (Box 2). A positive direct antiglobulin test or Coombs is seen in more than 95% of patients with AIHA. It may be positive for immunoglobulin G (IgG) only, both IgG and complement, or complement alone. The peripheral smear shows polychromasia, spherocytes, and RBC fragments.

Warm-Antibody AIHA

Warm-antibody AIHA is the most common form of AIHA, with an estimated annual incidence of 1 in 80,000. Approximately half of the cases are classified as idiopathic, whereas the remaining cases are often secondary to a predisposing condition. It is mainly identified in the elderly population. However, it is often described in children in association with viral illnesses.

PATHOGENESIS

The antibodies most commonly involved in warm-antibody AIHA are of the IgG type. These IgG antibodies are typically directed against antigens on the Rh system. They bind RBCs at 37°C, allowing their Fc region to remain exposed. This region is recognized by Fc receptors on the macrophages of the spleen, resulting in fragmentation and ingestion of the antibody-coated RBCs. This results in partial or complete phagocytosis. If partial phagocytosis occurs, spherocytes are formed. Splenomegaly results from entrapment of RBCs in the spleen.

BOX 2 Laboratory Values That Suggest Hemolysis

Reticulocytosis >125,000/L of blood
- If automated determination of reticulocyte concentration is unavailable, the value can be derived by multiplying the reticulocyte count (reported as a percentage) by the RBC concentration (RBC/μL) and dividing the total by 100. For example, if the reticulocyte count is 1 and the RBC concentration is 5×10^6/L, the number of reticulocytes per microliter of blood is 50,000.

Indirect bilirubin concentration between 1 and 5 mg/dL
- Patients with Gilbert's disease have an increased indirect bilirubin level in the absence of hemolysis. Unless the patient has underlying liver disease, the direct bilirubin level is rarely elevated in association with hemolysis.

Haptoglobin concentration <50 mg/dL
- Haptoglobin is an acute-phase reactant. When hemolysis occurs in association with inflammatory processes or steroid administration, haptoglobin levels may be within the normal range.

Elevated LDH concentration
- The normal range for LDH depends on the assay and the units of measurement; it therefore varies among laboratories. LDH is mildly to moderately elevated in cases of extravascular hemolysis. Values are much higher in cases of intravascular hemolysis.

Adapted from Rakel RE, Bope ET: Conn's Current Therapy 2008, 60th ed. Philadelphia, Elsevier Saunders, 2008.
Abbreviations: LDH = lactic dehydrogenase; RBC = red blood cells.

CURRENT DIAGNOSIS

- Confirm presence of immune-mediated hemolysis by performing direct antiglobulin test (DAT).
- Determine type of autoimmune hemolytic anemia (AIHA) based on DAT and clinical findings.
- Consider medications in the differential diagnosis of AIHA.
- Consider other tests, such as Donath-Landsteiner antibody testing and cold agglutinin titers, to establish cause of AIHA.

EVALUATION

A positive direct antiglobulin test is seen in more than 95% of patients with warm-antibody AIHA. It may be positive for IgG only or for both IgG and complement C3. Most IgG antibodies are of the IgG1 subtype. Fewer than 5% of patients with warm-antibody AIHA have a negative direct antiglobulin test. In these cases, hemolysis is evident by laboratory results and peripheral smear, but more sensitive assays are needed to confirm the diagnosis. A clinical response to corticosteroids is useful to support the diagnosis.

CLINICAL MANAGEMENT

The goal of treatment is to minimize or eliminate hemolysis. Some mild cases may not require medical intervention. For those patients with moderate to severe AIHA, corticosteroids are the treatment of choice. Approximately 80% of patients have a rapid respond to corticosteroids, typically within 1 week after starting therapy. However, most responses are not sustained. The majority of adult patients receive high-dose oral prednisone (60–100 mg)[3] daily during the initial phase of treatment. Intravenous methylprednisolone (Solu-Medrol) may also be used at daily doses of 100 to 200 mg.[3] In the pediatric population, prednisone is given at doses ranging from 2 to 6 mg/kg/day.[3] These high doses in adults and children are commonly maintained for approximately 2 weeks.

Once the hematocrit has increased and remains stable, the dose may be decreased and subsequently tapered at a slow rate over several months. Patients who require more than 10 to 15 mg of prednisone daily to keep an adequate hematocrit may benefit from splenectomy. More than 50% of splenectomized patients have a partial or complete response. Nevertheless, the rate of relapse is high. Corticosteroids are continued when relapse occurs, but usually at lower doses. Patients who are candidates for splenectomy should receive immunizations against encapsulated organisms at least 2 weeks before the procedure.

Rituximab (Rituxan),[1] a monoclonal antibody directed against CD20 antigen on the surface of B lymphocytes, has produced response in patients with warm-antibody AIHA. In a study published by Zecca and colleagues, 13 of 15 pediatric patients with warm-antibody AIHA were successfully treated with rituximab at a dose of 375 mg/m² weekly for 2 to 4 weeks. Other studies performed in adults have also demonstrated response to this approach. However, the long-term side effects of rituximab are not entirely clear. Therefore, it should be used with caution, and patients should be monitored for side effects. Immunosuppressive drugs such as cyclophosphamide (Cytoxan),[1] azathioprine (Imuran),[1] and cyclosporine (Neoral)[1] have been used primarily in cases refractory to corticosteroids and splenectomy.

The best-described regimen has been cyclophosphamide 50 mg/kg/day for 4 days. Other treatment options that have been used with some success include danazol (Danocrine)[1] and plasmapheresis. High-dose intravenous immune globulin (IVIG, Gammagard)[1] may be effective in some cases, but the response is short lived (1–4 weeks).

---

[1]Not FDA approved for this indication.
[3]Exceeds dosage recommended by the manufacturer.

Supportive care includes RBC transfusions for life-threatening situations and folic acid[1] supplementation to compensate for the increased RBC turnover. If RBC transfusions are needed, the least incompatible unit should be transfused slowly over 3 to 4 hours with careful monitoring for signs of an acute hemolytic reaction. The smallest volume of blood should be transfused to keep the patient hemodynamically stable, to avoid volume overload and an increase in the rate of hemolysis. In cases of secondary warm-antibody AIHA, it is recommended that the underlying condition be treated.

Cold-Antibody AIHA

Primary cold-agglutinin disease is primarily seen in individuals older than 50 years of age, whereas secondary cold-agglutinin disease is most commonly seen in children and young adults. The primary form is idiopathic. The secondary form is caused by infections, auto-immune diseases, or malignancies. Monoclonal autoantibody formation is seen in the primary form, whereas the secondary form is associated with monoclonal or polyclonal autoantibodies.

PATHOGENESIS

Cold agglutinins are typically IgM autoantibodies that cause RBC agglutination at temperatures lower than 37°C, with maximal RBC agglutination at temperatures lower than 4°C. Cold agglutinins may occur in response to infection, as is commonly seen with *Mycoplasma* pneumonia and infectious mononucleosis. The IgM antibody usually reacts with I/i RBC antigen, resulting in complement activation by fixation of antibody to the antigen at low temperatures. Anti-I is characteristic of *Mycoplasma* pneumonia–induced hemolysis, whereas anti-i is characteristic of infectious mononucleosis. However, cold agglutinins have also been reported with other viral or bacterial illnesses, as well as lymphoproliferative disorders.

EVALUATION

Symptoms of anemia are variable and depend on the severity and rapidity of onset. Symptoms, such as acrocyanosis may also occur as a result of RBC agglutination. However, these usually disappear with warming. Other findings include scleral icterus, splenomegaly, and hemoglobinuria. If lymphadenopathy is present, a lymphoproliferative disorder should be suspected.

The Coombs test is typically positive for complement (C3) and negative for IgG. However, if an IgG antibody is present, the Coombs test may also be positive for IgG. Cold agglutinin titers are considered positive if the titer is greater than 1 in 40. These positive titers are variable, typically greater than 1 in 10,000. Signs of hemolysis are usually not evident until the titer is greater than 1 in 1000. Other blood tests that confirm the presence of cold-antibody AIHA include *Mycoplasma* and Epstein-Barr virus titers.

CLINICAL MANAGEMENT

In children, symptoms are usually mild and self-limited. A general approach is to avoid cold exposure. Supportive care to control the underlying disorder is recommended. RBC transfusions warmed to 37°C may be given for life-threatening situations, and the least incompatible unit should be used. For severe anemia, a trial of cyto-toxic drugs such as cyclophosphamide (Cytoxan)[1] or chlorambucil (Leukeran)[1] may be used to decrease the cold agglutinin titer and the rate of hemolysis. Other alternatives that have been used with some success include rituximab[1] and interferon alfa-2b (Intron-A).[1] Plasmapheresis may be used to reduce or eliminate IgM antibodies. However, because its effect is not long-standing, it is used only in the acute setting. Treatment with corticosteroids alone or in combination is generally not effective. In addition, splenectomy is not effective, because the liver is the predominant site of hemolysis.

---

[1]Not FDA approved for this indication.

Paroxysmal Cold Hemoglobinuria

The Donath-Landsteiner autoantibody is responsible for PCH, which is typically characterized by a sudden onset of hemolysis and hemoglobinuria, usually after cold exposure that results in mild to severe anemia. PCH can result from infection, autoimmune disease, syphilis, or it can be idiopathic.

PATHOGENESIS

The Donath-Landsteiner autoantibody is a biphasic, polyclonal IgG that binds RBCs at cooler temperatures (4°C), activates complement, and results in intravascular hemolysis at warmer temperatures (37°C) due to complement fixation. This autoantibody is able to bind several RBC antigens, although its main target is the P antigen.

EVALUATION

The Coombs test is positive for C3 but negative for IgG, because of its dissociation from the RBC surface at warmer temperature. However, the Coombs test may be positive for IgG if it is performed at 4°C. PCH is confirmed by Donath-Landsteiner antibody testing. Plasma is incubated with normal RBCs and cooled to 4°C. If Donath-Landsteiner antibody is present, the cold hemolysin in the plasma binds RBCs. On rewarming to 37°C, the sensitized RBCs are hemolyzed by the complement present in plasma. The presence of hemolysis constitutes a positive antibody test result.

CLINICAL MANAGEMENT

The mainstay of treatment is supportive care and avoidance of cold exposure. Warmed RBCs may be administered in cases of life-threatening hemolysis or symptomatic anemia.

Evans Syndrome

Evans syndrome is the coexistence of Coombs-positive AIHA with immune-mediated thrombocytopenia. The exact pathophysiology is unknown, although defects in immune regulation have been proposed. The typical clinical course is chronic and relapsing, and some patients may also develop neutropenia.

EVALUATION

The Coombs test is positive (often weakly positive) for IgG, C3, or both. Anemia and thrombocytopenia are present with occasional neutropenia or combined cytopenias. Other features of hemolysis are present.

CLINICAL MANAGEMENT

The treatment of choice is corticosteroids, although relapses are frequent during tapering. Other alternatives that have shown some success include intravenous immune globulin (IVIg),[1] immunosuppressive agents, danazol,[1] and splenectomy. Rituximab[1] has been used with varied clinical responses. Supportive care with blood products should be given as needed, although their use should be minimized as possible.

Medication-Induced AIHA

It is well known that medications can cause AIHA. In the past, most cases were secondary to the use of methyldopa (Aldomet) and high-dose penicillin. More recently, the majority of the cases are secondary to the use of cephalosporins.

PATHOGENESIS

Medication-induced AIHA results from three proposed mechanisms based on the interactions among medications, RBC membrane antigens, and antibodies. These mechanisms are induced by drug or hapten adsorption, neoantigen formation, and autoantibody binding (Table 1).

---

[1]Not FDA approved for this indication.

TABLE 1 Major Mechanisms of Drug-Related Hemolytic Anemia and Positive Direct Antiglobulin Tests

	Hapten/Drug Adsorption	Ternary Complex Formation	Autoantibody Binding	Nonimmunologic Protein Adsorption
Prototype drug	Penicillin	Quinidine	α-Methyldopa (Aldomet)	Cephalothin[2]
Role of drug	Binds to RBC membrane	Forms ternary complex with antibody and RBC membrane component	Induces formation of antibody to native RBC antigen	Possibly alters RBC membrane
Drug affinity to cell	Strong	Weak	None demonstrated to intact RBC, but binding to membranes is reported	Strong
Antibody to drug	Present	Present	Absent	Absent
Antibody class predominating	IgG	IgM or IgG	IgG	None
Proteins detected by DAT	IgG, rarely complement	Complement	IgG, rarely complement	Multiple plasma proteins
Dose of drug associated with positive antiglobulin test	High	Low	High	High
Presence of drug required for indirect antiglobulin test	Yes (coating test RBCs)	Yes (added to test medium)	No	Yes (added to test medium)
Mechanism of RBC destruction	Splenic sequestration of IgG-coated RBCs	Direct lysis by complement plus splenic–hepatic clearance of C3b-coated RBCs	Splenic sequestration	None

Adapted from Packman CH: Hemolytic anemia resulting from immune injury. In Lichtman MA, Beutler E, Kipps TJ, et al (eds): Williams Hematology, 7th ed. New York, McGraw-Hill, 2006, Chapter 52.
[2]Not available in the United States.
Abbreviations: DAT = direct antiglobulin test; Ig = immunoglobulin; RBC = red blood cell.

CURRENT THERAPY

Summary

- Corticosteroids are the mainstay of treatment. However, patients unable to be weaned off may require splenectomy.
- Immunosuppressive therapy, primarily cyclophosphamide (Cytoxan),[1] has been used with some success, as has rituximab (Rituxan).[1]
- Red blood cell transfusion may be used for life-threatening situations, and the least incompatible unit should be used.
- Avoid cold exposure if cold-antibody autoimmune hemolytic anemia (AIHA) or paroxysmal cold hemoglobinuria (PCH) is present.
- Discontinue medications if medication-induced AIHA is suspected.

[1]Not FDA approved for this indication.

REFERENCES

Dacie SJ. The immune hemolytic anemias: A century of exciting progress in understanding. Br J Haematol 2001;114:770–85.

D'Arena G, Califano C, Annunziate M, et al. Rituximab for warm-type idiopathic autoimmune hemolytic anemia: A retrospective study of 11 adult patients. Eur J Haematol 2007;79:53–8.

Garratty G. Drug-induced immune hemolytic anemia: The last decade [Review]. Immunohematology 2004;20:138–46.

Glader B. Immune hemolytic anemias. In: Arceci RJ, Hann IM, Smith OP, Hoffbrand AV, editors. Pediatric Hematology. 3rd ed. Hoboken, NJ: Wiley-Blackwell; 2006.

Nydegger UE, Kazatchkine MD, Miescher PA. Immunopathologic and clinical features of hemolytic anemia due to cold agglutinins. Semin Hematol 1991;28:66–77.

Packman CH. Hemolytic anemia resulting from immune injury. In: Lichtman MA, Beutler E, Kipps TJ, et al., Williams Hematology. 7th ed. New York: McGraw-Hill; 2006 [Chapter 52].

Packman CH. Hemolytic anemia due to warm autoantibodies. Blood Rev 2008;22(1):17–31.

Parker CJ. Autoimmune hemolytic anemia. In: Rakel RE, Bope ET, editors. Conn's Current Therapy. 60th ed. Philadelphia: WB Saunders; 2008.

Zecca M, Nobili B, Ramenghi U, et al. Rituximab for the treatment of refractory autoinmune hemolytic anemia in children. Blood 2003;101:3857–61.

Nonimmune Hemolytic Anemia

Method of
Patricia A. Cornett, MD

The nonimmune hemolytic anemias are a heterogeneous group of anemias characterized by the finding of increased red blood cell destruction. A useful classification of these anemias divides the causes into two groups: One group consists of congenital disorders with defects in the red blood cell membrane, enzymes, or hemoglobin, and the other group consists of acquired disorders when, usually, the cause of hemolysis is by extrinsic influences on the red blood cell. Extrinsic factors causing direct injury to the red blood cells include the microangiopathic hemolytic anemias, infections, toxins, and certain systemic illnesses. The one acquired cause of hemolytic anemia where the defect is due to an intrinsic red blood cell abnormality is paroxysmal nocturnal hemoglobinuria.

Pathophysiology

CONGENITAL HEMOLYTIC ANEMIAS

The congenital nonimmune hemolytic anemias are caused by mutations affecting the red blood cell membrane, hemoglobin, or enzymes.

MEMBRANE DISORDERS

The most common red blood cell membrane disorders are hereditary spherocytosis, hereditary elliptocytosis, and hereditary pyropoikilocytosis. Each disorder is caused by a defect in one of the cell wall proteins. The nature of the deformity depends upon the exact structural protein defect. Spherocytes (Fig. 1), and to a lesser extent, elliptocytes (Fig. 5), are not as deformable as the normal biconcave red blood cells and are removed from the circulation by macrophages. This extravascular hemolysis typically occurs predominantly within the spleen. Patients with hereditary pyropoikilocytosis are double heterozygotes, usually inheriting two hereditary elliptocytosis mutations, resulting in the production of tiny, fragmented red blood cells and severe hemolytic anemia.

HEMOGLOBINOPATHIES

Hemoglobin is composed of four subunits held together by noncovalent forces. A number of mutations affect the forces maintaining this structural integrity and can result in degradation and precipitation of the hemoglobin within the cell. These unstable hemoglobins form precipitates, or Heinz bodies, attach to the membrane, and impair the deformability of the red blood cell, ultimately leading to removal of the cells within the spleen. Another hemoglobinopathy, and the most common, sickle cell disease, results from the replacement of valine for glutamic acid in the sixth position of the β-globin subunit. Sickle cell disease has a myriad of downstream physiologic effects that ultimately leads to hemolysis of the sickled red blood cells (Fig. 3).

ENZYME DISORDERS

The red blood cell relies on enzymes functioning in two glycolysis pathways to generate energy. Energy is required to maintain the red blood cell's biconcave shape as well as the integrity of the enzymes, hemoglobin, and membrane through its 120-day life span. The two metabolic pathways are the anaerobic glycolysis (Embden-Meyerhof) pathway and the aerobic glycolysis (hexose monophosphate) pathway. Enzyme defects in the Embden-Meyherhof pathway are generally associated with chronic hemolysis; enzyme defects in the hexose monophosphate pathway are often associated with episodic hemolysis. The most common defect affects the glucose-6-phosphate dehydrogenase (G6PD) enzyme. This enzyme is responsible for diverting glucose from the Embden-Meyerhof pathway to the hexose monophosphate pathway and for restoring intracellular reduced nicotinamide adenine dinucleotide phosphate (NADPH), which functions as an antioxidant. Low levels of G6PD activity result in the inability of the cell to defend itself against oxidant stresses; absent levels result in chronic hemolysis.

ACQUIRED HEMOLYTIC ANEMIAS

For the acquired nonimmune hemolytic anemias, hemolysis results from extrinsic forces affecting the red blood cell. In the microangiopathic hemolytic anemias, red blood cells undergo fragmentation due to high sheer forces generated from abnormal vascular surfaces.

Infections can cause hemolysis due to direct invasion of the organism into the red blood cell (malaria, babesiosis) by release of products that can destabilize the red cell membrane (*Clostridia perfringens*), or by initiating disseminated intravascular coagulation, resulting in microangiopathic hemolysis.

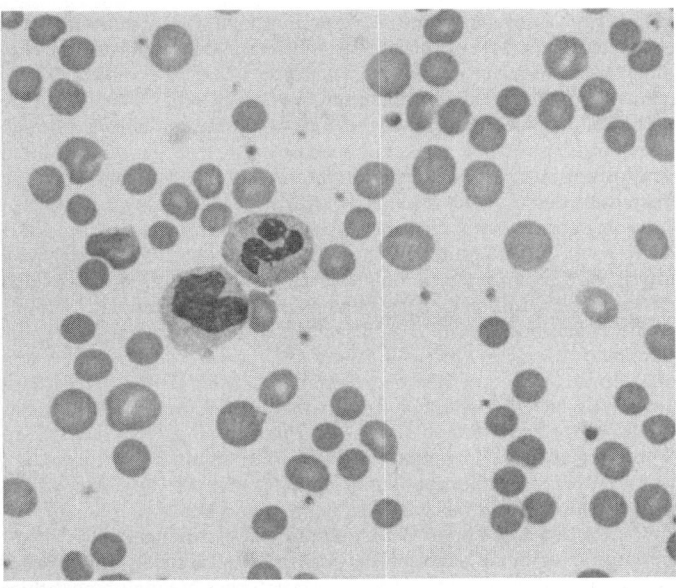

FIGURE 1. Hereditary spherocytosis. Peripheral blood film showing spherocytes.

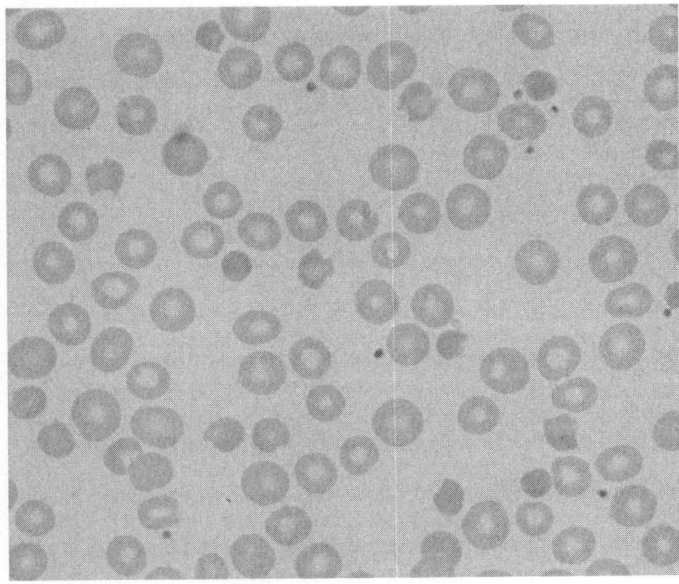

FIGURE 2. Glucose-6-phosphate dehydrogenase deficiency. Peripheral blood film showing bite cells and blister cells.

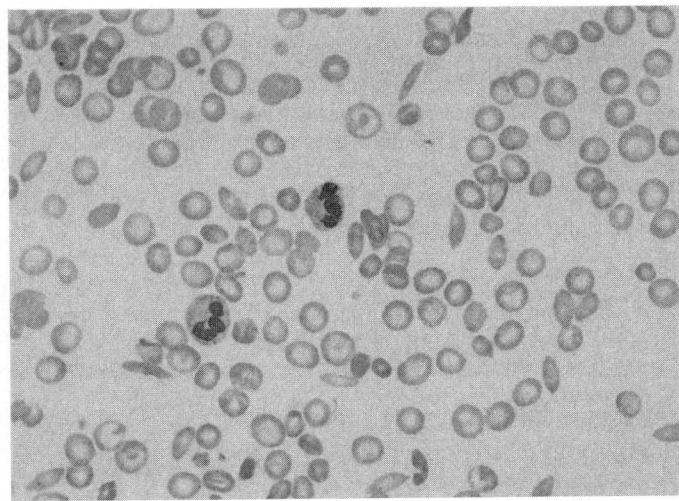

FIGURE 3. Sickle cell anemia. Peripheral blood smear showing sickle cells.

Certain toxic chemicals and physical agents can cause hemolysis through a variety of mechanisms affecting the red blood cell membrane or metabolism. These substances include arsenic, lead, copper, and insect, spider, and snake venoms.

Other systemic disease states causing hemolysis include liver failure and extensive burns. In liver failure, the ratio of cholesterol to phospholipid in the red cell membrane is altered, resulting in membrane instability and hemolysis. Patients with extensive burns can present acutely with a brisk hemolytic anemia; the heat from the burns likely causes mechanical and osmotic damage to red blood cells.

The underlying defect in paroxysmal nocturnal hemoglobinuria is impaired production of a key anchoring cellular membrane protein. Loss of the anchoring protein, glycosylphosphatidylinositol, disrupts a number of cellular proteins including CD59, a protein inhibitor of complement-mediated lysis. Deficiency of CD59 leads to greater sensitivity of red blood cells to hemolysis.

Clinical Manifestations

The clinical manifestations of these disorders, in large part, depend upon the severity of the anemia as well as any associated manifestations related to the underlying cause. General symptoms of anemia include weakness, fatigue, lethargy, and palpitations. Other clinical manifestations of the nonimmune hemolytic anemias, particularly the congenital causes, include jaundice, splenomegaly, formation of pigmented gallstones with the possibility of cholecystitis, and aplastic crisis due to viral infections. Aplastic crisis results from viral suppression of hematopoiesis. Because red blood cell survival at baseline is shortened, abrupt cessation of erythropoiesis results in a rapid fall in the hemoglobin level and relatively acute onset of symptomatic anemia.

Diagnosis

Anemia that is accompanied by reticulocytosis, an indirect hyperbilirubinemia, and an elevated lactate dehydrogenase is usually diagnostic of a hemolytic process. Hemolysis can be immune mediated or due to nonimmune causes. A negative Coombs test should result in an investigation for the causes of nonimmune hemolytic anemia. Further evaluation should then include an examination of the peripheral smear. Other tests used to confirm the presence of hemolysis include serum haptoglobin, plasma and urinary free hemoglobin, and urinary hemosiderin.

CURRENT DIAGNOSIS

- Anemia accompanied by reticulocytosis without evidence of bleeding or recovery from a nutritional anemia should prompt an evaluation for immune and nonimmune causes of hemolytic anemia.
- Key test results that help to confirm the presence of hemolysis include elevated indirect bilirubin and lactate dehydrogenase (LDH) levels, often accompanied by a low haptoglobin level.
- The Coombs test should be done to exclude immune-mediated hemolysis.
- Examination of the peripheral smear often reveals findings that guide further diagnostic testing.
- More-specialized testing may be required to make a definitive diagnosis.
- Both congenital and acquired disorders can lead to nonimmune hemolysis. The most common congenital cause is glucose-6-phosphate dehydrogenase deficiency. The microangiopathic anemias are the most common acquired cause.

Haptoglobin, synthesized by the liver, binds any free hemoglobin in the plasma; the complex is then removed in hepatic parenchymal cells. If the rate of hemolysis exceeds the clearance rate of this complex, the haptoglobin level will be decreased. Intravascular hemolysis can allow detection of free hemoglobin in the plasma if the plasma hemoglobin-binding proteins are saturated and free hemoglobin in the urine if the capacity of renal tubular cells to absorb hemoglobin is exceeded.

Hemoglobin that is filtered in the kidney is stored in the renal tubular cells and excreted in the form of hemosiderin. As these cells slough into the urine, the hemosiderin can be detected by a Prussian blue stain approximately 5 to 7 days following a hemolytic episode. This test is therefore helpful to detect intravascular hemolysis days after the hemolytic event.

For the nonimmune hemolytic anemias, examination of the bone marrow is seldom helpful and generally not necessary in the diagnostic process.

CONGENITAL HEMOLYTIC ANEMIAS

The diagnosis of congenital nonimmune hemolytic anemias is often suspected when the anemia is longstanding. A family history of anemia, splenectomy, or gallstones can also be a clue to a congenital process. Peripheral smear examination is often helpful. The membrane disorders all have findings on the peripheral smear (Table 1), though these findings are not necessarily specific to the disorder. A specialized test, osmotic gradient ektacytometry, can be used to help in diagnosing these disorders.

For patients with certain enzymopathies, most notably G6PD deficiency, bite cells and blister cells may be seen in the peripheral smear during an acute hemolytic event. A supravital stain, such as crystal violet, brilliant cresyl blue, or methylene blue, can demonstrate Heinz bodies. G6PD deficiency is definitely diagnosed by the finding of low G6PD levels in the red cell; however levels can be normal during the acute hemolytic event because red blood cells with low levels have been removed from the circulation. If the diagnosis is still suspected after obtaining a normal result, a repeat test 2 to 3 months after the acute hemolytic episode should be performed.

Most other red blood cell enzymopathies need to be diagnosed by specialized reference laboratories. Hemoglobin electropheresis should be performed to diagnose a suspected hemoglobinopathy. The most common hemoglobinopathy causing hemolysis, sickle cell anemia, is readily diagnosed by this test. However, other hemoglobinopathies causing hemolysis, specifically the unstable hemoglobins, may be electrophoretically silent. If the diagnosis of an unstable hemoglobinopathy is suspected, a supravital stain can demonstrate Heinz bodies and a heat stability test should be obtained for definitive diagnosis.

ACQUIRED NONIMMUNE HEMOLYTIC ANEMIAS

The diagnosis of acquired causes of nonimmune hemolytic anemias is suspected when a hemolytic anemia is new in onset and previous hemoglobin levels have been normal. A notable exception to this general premise is in G6PD-deficient patients presenting with new anemia due to oxidant stresses. Even though the anemia appears to be acquired, the key feature to recognize is the clinical context, which usually includes an infection or a precipitating event of a new drug.

The peripheral smear is usually very helpful in diagnosing the acquired causes of nonimmune hemolytic anemias. Microangiopathic changes found in thrombotic thrombocytopenia purpura (TTP), hemolytic-uremic syndrome (HUS), disseminated intravascular coagulation (DIC), disseminated cancer, and heart valve hemolysis include schistocytes and red blood cell fragments. The ability to recognize these microangiopathic changes can be crucial, particularly in the diagnosis of conditions such as TTP and HUS, both of which require urgent management (Fig. 4). The peripheral smear can also be diagnostic of certain infections (malaria, babesiosis). Other acquired causes are generally diagnosed by the clinical setting.

The diagnosis of paroxysmal nocturnal hemoglobinuria is made by flow cytometry using peripheral blood cells or bone marrow aspirate and the demonstration of deficiency of hematopoietic cell proteins normally linked to the anchoring glycosylphosphatidylinositol protein.

TABLE 1 Classification of Nonimmune Hemolytic Anemias

Diagnosis	Peripheral Smear Findings	Additional Tests
Congenital Disorders		
Membrane disorders		
Hereditary spherocytosis	Spherocytes	Ektacytometry
Hereditary elliptocytosis	Elliptocytes	Ektacytometry
Hereditary pyropoikilocytosis	Microcytes, fragments	Ektacytometry
Hemoglobin disorders		
Sickle cell disease	Sickle cells, targets	Hemoglobin electropheresis
Unstable hemoglobins	Bite cells	Supravital stain, hemoglobin electropheresis, heat stability test
Enzyme disorders		
G6PD deficiency	Bite cells, blister cells	Supravital stain, G6PD level
Others	Variable	Individual enzyme levels
Acquired Disorders		
Microangiopathic hemolytic anemias		
TTP, HUS, DIC, cancer, heart valves	Schistocytes, red blood cell fragments	Targeted to diagnosis
Infections		
Malaria, babesiosis, Clostridium perfringens	Parasite (malaria, babesiosis)	Giemsa stain (babesiosis)
Toxins, Physical Agents		
Arsenic, lead, copper	Basophilic stippling (lead)	Element levels
Insect, spider, snake venoms	Schistocytes, fragments	Targeted to diagnosis
Systemic diseases		
Liver disease	Acanthocytes, target cells	Liver function tests
Burns	Spherocytes, blister cells, fragments	Targeted to diagnosis
Paroxysmal nocturnal hemoglobinuria	Variable	Flow cytometry

Abbreviations: DIC = disseminated intravascular coagulation; G6PD = glucose-6-phosphate dehydrogenase; HUS = hemolytic uremic syndrome; TTP = thrombotic thrombocytopenic purpura.

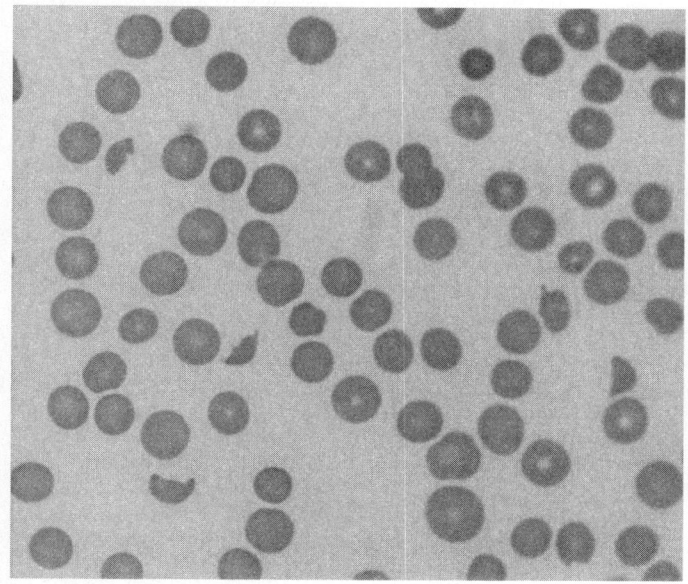

FIGURE 4. Microangiopathic hemolytic anemia. Peripheral blood film showing schistocytes and red blood cell fragments.

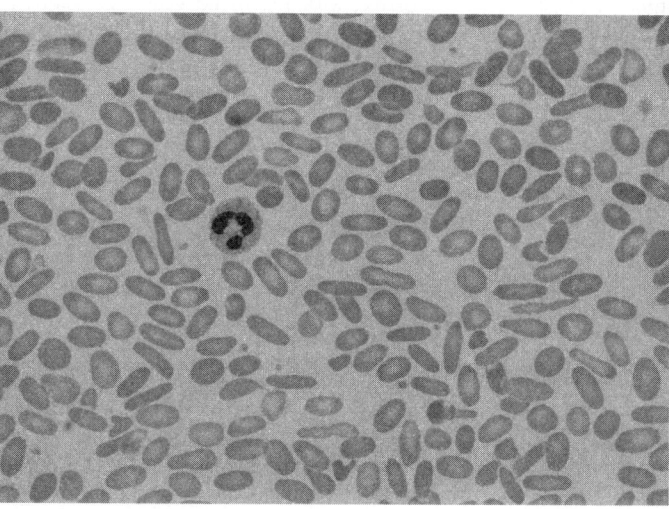

FIGURE 5. Hereditary elliptocytosis. Peripheral blood film showing elliptocytes.

Differential Diagnosis

The differential diagnosis of the nonimmune hemolytic anemias, characterized by reticulocytosis, includes immune hemolytic anemia and the reticulocytosis that can be seen with correction of anemias due to replacement of a deficiency (iron, folate, vitamin B$_{12}$) or recovery from bleeding.

Treatment

CONGENITAL HEMOLYTIC ANEMIAS

For patients who have congenital hemolytic anemias and moderate to severe hemolysis, folate (folic acid) replacement is recommended. Other treatments are more directed at the specific issues that can arise during the patient's lifetime. Because pigmented gallstone formation is common, cholecystectomy may be necessary. Splenectomy, to decrease the rate of hemolysis and improve the lifespan of circulating red blood cells, may be recommended for patients who have

CURRENT THERAPY

- Patients with ongoing moderate to severe hemolysis should be treated with folate (folic acid), 1 mg orally daily.
- Splenectomy can benefit selected patients with congenital hemolytic anemia. Vaccinations for *Streptococcus pneumoniae*, *Haemophilus influenzae* type B, and *Neisseria meningitidis* should be administered before surgery.
- Red blood cell transfusions occasionally are needed to support patients with bone marrow compromise due to infection-induced aplastic crisis.
- Acquired causes of nonimmune hemolytic anemia are generally managed by treating the underlying cause or removing the offending agent.

moderate to severe ongoing hemolysis resulting in symptomatic anemia. Vaccinations for *Streptococcus pneumoniae*, *Haemophilus influenzae* type B, and *Neisseria meningitidis* should be administered before the splenectomy is performed. Patients with G6PD deficiency need to avoid oxidant drugs such as dapsone, primaquine, sulfamethoxazole, and other sulfa based drugs. Parvovirus B19 infection in patients with congenital hemolytic anemias resulting in suppression of bone marrow erythropoiesis can manifest as aplastic crisis characterized by an abrupt fall in the hemoglobin. Red blood cell transfusions may be necessary until bone marrow production recovers and erythropoiesis resumes.

ACQUIRED HEMOLYTIC ANEMIAS

For patients with acquired causes of nonimmune hemolytic anemias, therapy is generally supportive, with red blood cell transfusions as clinically indicated, in addition to therapy directed at the underlying cause of the anemia. For example, infections should be treated appropriately; the underlying cause of DIC or HUS needs to be managed. For TTP and HUS, the initial management consists of emergent plasmapheresis. Exposure to any offending toxins needs to be eliminated; potentially, directed therapy to reduce toxin levels will be required. Specific therapy for paroxysmal nocturnal hemoglobinuria is now available; eculizumab, a humanized monoclonal antibody that inhibits the complement cascade, is used to reduce hemolysis and the need for red blood cell transfusions.

Monitoring

CONGENITAL HEMOLYTIC ANEMIAS

Patients with severe congenital hemolytic anemia require more-frequent monitoring with periodic hemoglobin checks. Patients presenting with worsening anemia should have a reticulocyte count check; a decreased reticulocyte count should prompt an evaluation for reversible causes of anemia (e.g., folate, vitamin B_{12}, or iron deficiency) as well as monitoring for further decline in the hemoglobin. Periodic monitoring for cholelithiasis should also be initiated with abdominal ultrasounds.

ACQUIRED HEMOLYTIC ANEMIAS

For patients with acquired causes of hemolysis, the severity of the hemolysis can be monitored with the hemoglobin and to some extent, the lactate dehydrogenase (LDH) level.

Glucose-6-Phosphate Dehydrogenase Deficiency

G6PD deficiency, reported to affect 400 million people worldwide, is the most common cause of nonimmune hemolytic anemia. G6PD deficiency occurs in geographic areas where malaria is endemic (Africa, Southeast Asia, the Mediterranean, and Middle East), supporting the hypothesis that inheritance of the G6PD mutation has a selective advantage for persons in these malaria-affected areas. The G6PD gene is localized on the X chromosome; thus males are much more commonly affected than females. In some populations, the mutation is found in up to 25% of male natives. Still, female natives may be affected when the gene frequency is sufficiently high to result in homozygous females; additionally, heterozygote females may be symptomatic if by the process of X inactivation or lyonization, sufficient numbers of wild-type X chromosome are inactivated, leaving the abnormal G6PD gene the dominant enzyme expressed.

The G6PD enzyme functions in the aerobic glycolysis hexose monophosphate pathway. An important role of the G6PD enzyme is to reduce NADP to NADPH. NADPH, by virtue of its ability to donate electrons and protons in enzymatic reactions, is able to protect the red blood cell proteins from oxidant stressors.

Many persons are asymptomatic and the deficiency is undiagnosed until a challenging event precipitates an oxidizing stress to the red blood cell. Potential challenging events include exposure to certain classes of drugs, ingestion of fava beans, or an infection. The inability of the red cell to generate sufficient NADPH to maintain reduced glutathione that functions as an antioxidant can result in hemolysis of the cell. Additionally, G6PD deficiency can manifest in newborns as neonatal jaundice, typically within 4 days following birth.

More than 400 mutations in the G6PD gene have been described. The severity of the hemolysis relates to the specific mutation; for instance, the mutation found in male African Americans (type A−) generally is associated with mild, intermittent hemolysis; mutations in Mediterranean and Asian populations tend to cause more severe, and often chronic, ongoing hemolysis.

G6PD deficiency is diagnosed by the finding of a low functional G6PD level in the red cell; however, it is important to recognize that levels can be high during the acute hemolytic event because red blood cells with the least amount of G6PD have been removed from the circulation. If the diagnosis is still suspected after obtaining a normal result, the test should be repeated 2 to 3 months after the acute hemolytic episode. The peripheral smear during the acute hemolytic episode might show bite cells, red cells that have a chunk excised from the edge (see Fig. 2). The bite cells are caused by the spleen's removal of Heinz bodies, which are composed of denatured hemoglobin. Intact Heinz bodies within the red blood cell can be visualized on a peripheral smear stained with supravital stain such as brilliant cresyl blue stain.

Management during an acute hemolytic episode is generally supportive. Patients with mild forms of G6PD deficiency typically have modest reductions of hemoglobin levels; patients with more-severe G6PD deficiency can hemolyze to hemoglobin levels that require transfusion support. Patients who have more-severe G6PD deficiency manifesting with ongoing hemolysis need folate supplements and, rarely, are transfusion dependent. Neonatal jaundice in newborns with G6PD deficiency is managed similarly to other causes of neonatal jaundice with phototherapy and, occasionally, red cell transfusions.

Prevention is the best management strategy for patients with diagnosed G6PD deficiency; drugs that are known to precipitate hemolysis should be avoided. General screening for G6PD deficiency is not routinely done; however, providers might consider screening male patients from ethnic backgrounds having high rates of G6PD deficiency before prescribing known precipitating drugs. For instance, infectious disease clinics often have screening programs for selected patients being considered for prophylactic antibiotics such as trimethoprim-sulfamethoxazole (Bactrim) or dapsone.

Hereditary Spherocytosis

Hereditary spherocytosis is the most common inherited red blood cell membrane defect; its incidence is highest in persons of northern European descent, though it is found in all ethnic groups worldwide. Most cases are inherited in an autosomal dominant fashion.

Hereditary spherocytosis is caused by a defect in one of the proteins that vertically anchor the red blood cell lipid bilayer to the

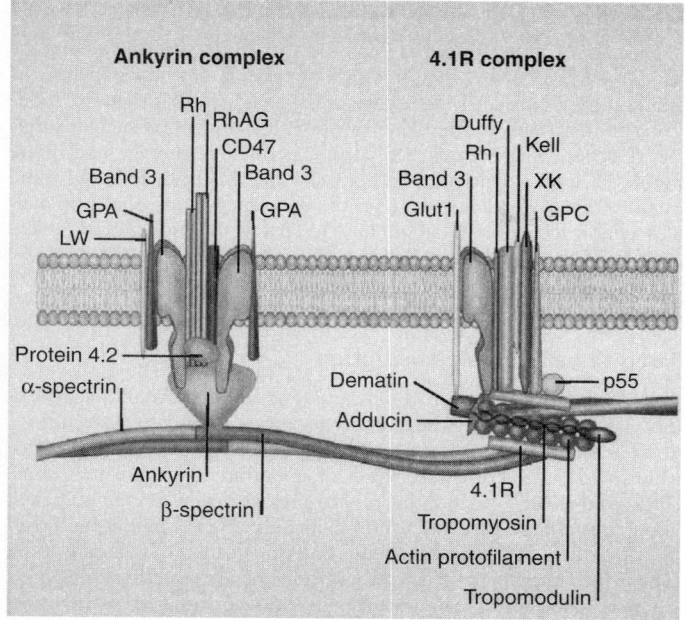

Ankyrin complex   **4.1R complex**

FIGURE 6. Diagram of red blood cell membrane structure. (Reprinted with permission from Mohandas N, Gallagher P: Red cell membrane: Past, present, and future. Blood. 2008;112(10):3939-3948.)

REFERENCES

Bain BJ. Diagnosis from the blood smear. N Engl J Med 2005;353:498–507.

Baker KR, Moake J. Hemolytic anemia resulting from physical injury to red cells. In: Lichtman MA, Beutler E, Kipps TJ, et al, editors. Williams Hematology. 7th ed. New York: McGraw-Hill; 2006. p. 709–16.

Beutler E. Hemolytic anemia resulting from chemical and physical agents. In: Lichtman MA, Beutler E, Kipps TJ, et al, editors. Williams Hematology. 7th ed. New York: McGraw-Hill; 2006. p. 717–21.

Bolton-Maggs P, Stevens R, Dodd N, et al. Guidelines for the diagnosis and management of hereditary spherocytosis. Br J Haematol 2004;126(4):455–74.

Cappellini M, Fiorelli G. Glucose-6-phosphate dehydrogenase deficiency. Lancet 2008;371:64–74.

Crary SE, Buchanan GR. Vascular complications after splenectomy for hematologic disorders. Blood 2009;114:2861–8.

Hill A, Richard SJ, Hillmen P. Recent developments in the understanding and management of paroxysmal nocturnal hemoglobinuria. Br J Haematol 2007;137:181–92.

Mohandas N, Gallagher P. Red cell membrane: Past, present, and future. Blood 2008;112(10):3939–48.

membrane skeleton. Mutations have been described in the trans membranes (band 3, RhAG), anchoring proteins (ankyrin, protein 4.2), and membrane cytoskeleton protein (spectrin) (Fig. 6). Stress forces within the circulation compromise the structural integrity of the flawed hereditary spherocytosis membrane complex, resulting in uncoupling of the cytoskeleton from the lipid bilayer. Microvesicles form within the red blood cell membrane; the separation of the microvesicles from the cell leads to loss of surface area, resulting in the formation of spherocytes. The less-deformable spherocytes are compromised in their ability to navigate through the spleen, leading to splenic sequestration and removal from the circulation.

The clinical manifestations of hereditary spherocytosis are variable and range from mild to severe anemia. As with other hemolytic anemias, patients can have the physical findings of jaundice and splenomegaly and also can be at risk for developing aplastic crisis and gallstones.

The diagnosis is suspected when, in addition to the typical laboratory findings in the hemolytic anemias, the mean cell hemoglobin concentration (MCHC) is elevated and spherocytes are seen on the peripheral smear (see Fig. 1). Classically, an osmotic fragility test has been used to diagnose hereditary spherocytosis. This test, though, can be abnormal in other disorders causing spherocytosis, such as autoimmune hemolytic anemia; additionally, the test was shown to be normal in up to one third of patients with known hereditary spherocytosis. A more reliable, though not widely available, test is osmotic gradient ektacytometry. This test measures red blood cell deformability across an osmolality gradient continuum and can reliably distinguish among the inherited red blood cell membrane disorders.

Management, in addition to the usual supportive measures of daily oral folic acid (1 mg), has also included splenectomy. Removal of the spleen is effective in improving the anemia in hereditary spherocytosis patients. However, concerns over long-term complications from the procedure, including a significant lifetime risk of fatal sepsis and an increased risk of thromboembolic events, have curtailed its routine use. The procedure is now only recommended for those patients who have hereditary spherocytosis with moderate to severe anemia that causes symptoms. Splenectomy should be preceded by vaccination for *S. pneumoniae*, *H. influenzae* type B, and *N. meningitides*.

Pernicious Anemia and Other Megaloblastic Anemias

Method of
Emmanuel Andrès, MD, PhD

Anemia is a common condition, especially in adults, and its prevalence increases with age. It affects quality of life, physical function, and even cognitive function in elderly patients. Anemia is a comorbid condition that affects other diseases (e.g., heart disease, cerebrovascular insufficiency) and is associated with a risk of death. Thus, anemia should not be accepted as a benign condition or a consequence of aging. In adults, many underlying conditions lead to megaloblastic anemia, but the most common ones are nutrient deficiencies, especially folate (folic acid, vitamin B_9) deficiency, vitamin B_{12} (cobalamin) deficiency, and pernicious anemia. Recognition of these conditions is a prerequisite of successful therapy.

Although low hemoglobin levels are often seen with advancing age, anemia should not be assumed to be a normal consequence of aging. Age may be associated with compromised hematopoietic reserve, and the elderly can be more susceptible to anemia in the presence of hematopoietic stress induced by an underlying disorder. Consequently, it is important to identify the underlying disorder. In practice, a hemoglobin (Hb) level less than 10 g/dL is considered a trigger for the investigation of the cause of anemia.

Definition

The World Health Organization (WHO) defines anemia as a hemoglobin concentration less than 12 g/dL for nonpregnant women and less than 13 g/dL for men. Megaloblastic anemia is characterized by many large immature and dysfunctional red blood cells (megaloblasts) in the bone marrow and by hypersegmented or multisegmented neutrophils. Megaloblastic anemia includes nutrient deficiencies related to folate and vitamin B_{12} and pernicious anemia. Megaloblastic anemia is included in the group of macrocytic anemias (mean corpuscular volume [MCV] >100 fL). Macrocytic anemia also includes anemia related to chronic alcohol use (with or without liver disease), thyroid failure, and myelodysplastic syndromes.

Epidemiology

In adults, the prevalence of anemia varies by country, ethnic group, and the health status of the patients. Living conditions can also influence this prevalence. Nevertheless, the prevalence of anemia increases with advancing age, especially after age 60 to 65 years, and rises sharply after the age of 80 years. Results from the third National Health and Nutrition Examination Survey (NHANES III) carried out in the United States indicates that the prevalence of anemia was 11% in community-dwelling men and 10.2% among women 65 years or older. Survey findings also indicate that most anemia among the elderly is mild; only 2.8% of women and 1.6% of men have a hemoglobin less than 11 g/dL.

Results from the Framingham cohort indicate a slightly lower prevalence of anemia among older people living in the United States compared to the NHANES IIII survey. In the Framingham group of 1016 subjects 67 to 96 years of age, the prevalence of anemia in men and women is 6.1% and 10.5%, respectively.

In adults, causes of anemia are divided into three broad groups: nutrient-deficiency anemia, including iron deficiency, folate deficiency, and B_{12} deficiency anemia; anemia of chronic disease, perhaps better termed anemia of chronic inflammation; and unexplained anemia. Table 1 presents the cause of anemia in 300 consecutive patients hospitalized in an internal medicine department.

In the NHANES III study, 34% of all anemia in elderly patients is caused by deficiencies of nutrients including folate, vitamin B_{12}, and iron, alone or in combination. About 60% of nutrient-deficiency anemia is associated with iron deficiency, and most of those cases are the result of chronic blood loss from gastrointestinal lesions. The remaining cases of nutrient-deficiency anemia are usually associated with vitamin B_{12} or folate deficiency (or both) and are easily treated. 12% of anemias were associated with renal insufficiency, 20% were due to chronic diseases, and in 34% the cause remained unexplained.

Etiology

FOLATE DEFICIENCY ANEMIA IN ADULTS

A balanced diet contains 500 to 700 µg of folate. On average, 50% to 60% of dietary folate is absorbed in the duodenum and jejunum. Folate deficiency usually develops as a result of inadequate dietary intake. The body stores very little folate, only enough to last 4 to 6 months. Patients usually have a history of weight loss, poor weight gain, and weakness. In addition, several drugs (methotrexate [Trexall], cotrimoxazole [Bactrim], sulfasalazine [Azulfidine], and anticonvulsants) and alcohol can cause deficiency of folate by inhibiting absorption or by affecting folate metabolism.

TABLE 1 Etiology of Anemia in 300 Consecutive Patients Older than 65 Years Hospitalized in a Department of Internal Medicine in a Tertiary Reference Center

Etiology	Prevalence (%)
Chronic inflammation (chronic disease)	23.0
Iron deficiency	18
Renal failure	9
Liver disease and endocrine disease (chronic disease)	7
Posthemorrhagic	7
Folate deficiency	6*
Myelodysplasia	5
Vitamin B_{12} deficiency	4†
Unexplained causes	21

*10% of these patients have megaloblastic anemia.
†Vitamin B_{12} deficiency is defined as a serum cobalamin level <200 pg/mL (<150 pmol/L) in 2 samples.
Adapted from Andrès E, Federici L, Serraj K, Kaltenbach G: Update of nutrient-deficiency anemia in elderly patients. Eur J Intern Med 2008;19:488-493.

VITAMIN B_{12} DEFICIENCY ANEMIA IN ADULTS

Deficiency of vitamin B_{12} and folate are common, especially among the elderly, each occurring in at least 5% of patients. In these patients, the etiologies of cobalamin deficiency are represented primarily by food-cobalamin malabsorption, other causes of malabsorption such as surgical resection of the stomach or ileum, pernicious anemia, and, more rarely, by intake deficiency. In our work, in which we followed more than 200 elderly patients with a proven deficiency, food-cobalamin malabsorption accounted for about 60% to 70% of the etiologies of cobalamin deficiency, and pernicious anemia accounted for 15% to 25%. Figure 1 presents the principal causes of cobalamin deficiency in 172 patients hospitalized in an internal medicine department.

Food-Cobalamin Malabsorption

Initially described by Carmel in the 1990s, food-cobalamin malabsorption is characterized by the inability to release bound cobalamin from food or intestinal transport proteins, particularly in the setting of hypochlorhydria, where the absorption of unbound cobalamin is normal. This syndrome is defined by cobalamin deficiency despite sufficient food-cobalamin intake and a normal Schilling test. The normal Schilling test rules out pernicious anemia and other causes of malabsorption. The principal characteristics of this syndrome are listed in Box 1.

Food-cobalamin malabsorption is caused primarily by atrophic gastritis. More than 40% of patients older than 80 years have gastric atrophy. Factors that commonly contribute to food-cobalamin malabsorption include *Helicobacter pylori* infection, chronic carriage of *H. pylori*, intestinal microbial proliferation (in which case, cobalamin deficiency can be corrected by antibiotic treatment); long-term ingestion of antacids, H_2-receptor antagonists and proton-pump inhibitors, and biguanides (metformin [Glucophage]); chronic alcoholism; surgery or gastric reconstruction (e.g., bypass surgery for obesity); and complete or partial pancreatic exocrine failure.

Pernicious Anemia

Pernicious anemia, also known as Biermer's anemia or Addison's anemia, is caused by impaired absorption of vitamin B_{12} owing to the neutralization of intrinsic factor action in the setting of immune atrophic gastritis. In elderly patients, this form of megaloblastic anemia is one of the leading causes of cobalamin deficiency. Pernicious anemia has a genetic component. In practice, the diagnosis of pernicious anemia is

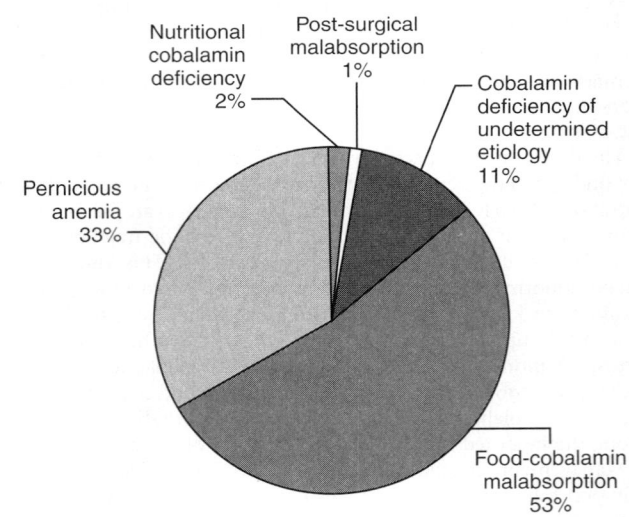

FIGURE 1. Etiologies of cobalamin deficiency in 172 elderly patients hospitalized in the university hospital of Strasbourg, France. (Adapted from Andrès E, Loukili NH, Noel E, et al: Vitamin B_{12} (cobalamin) deficiency in elderly patients. Can Med Assoc J 2004;171: 251-260; and Andrès E, Vidal-Alaball J, Federici L, et al: Clinical aspects of cobalamin deficiency in elderly patients. Epidemiology, causes, clinical manifestations, treatment with special focus on oral cobalamin therapy. Eur J Intern Med 2007;18:456-462.)

BOX 1 Food-Cobalamin Malabsorption Syndrome

Criteria for Food-Cobalamin Malabsorption

Low serum cobalamin (vitamin B_{12}) levels
Normal results of Schilling test using free cyanocobalamin labeled with cobalt-58, or abnormal results of derived Schilling test*
No anti-intrinsic factor antibodies
No dietary cobalamin deficiency

Associated Conditions or Agents

Gastric disease
- Atrophic gastritis
- Type A atrophic gastritis
- Gastric disease associated with *Helicobacter pylori* infection
- Partial gastrectomy
- Gastric bypass
- Vagotomy

Pancreatic insufficiency
- Alcohol abuse
Gastric or intestinal bacterial overgrowth
- Achlorhydria
- Tropical sprue
- Ogylvie's syndrome
- HIV
Drugs
- Antacids (H_2-receptor antagonists and proton-pump inhibitors)
- Biguanides (metformin [Glucophage])
Alcohol abuse
Sjögren's syndrome, systemic sclerosis
Haptocorrin deficiency
Aging or idiopathic

---

*Derived Schilling tests use food-bound cobalamin (e.g., egg yolk, chicken, and fish proteins).
Adapted from Andrès E, Affenberger S, Vinzio S, et al: Food-cobalamin malabsorption in elderly patients: Clinical manifestations and treatment. Am J Med 2005;118:1154-1159.

---

based on the presence of intrinsic factor antibodies in serum (specificity, >98%; sensitivity, around 50%) or biopsy-proven autoimmune atrophic gastritis. The presence of *Helicobacter pylori* infection in gastric biopsies is an exclusion factor. Pernicious anemia is associated with other immunologic diseases such as Sjögren's syndrome, Hashimoto's disease, type 1 diabetes mellitus, and celiac disease.

Other Causes of Cobalamin Deficiency

Cobalamin deficiency caused by dietary deficiency or malabsorption is rare. Dietary causes of deficiency are limited to elderly people who are already malnourished. This mainly concerns elderly patients living in institutions or in psychiatric hospitals. Since the 1980s, the malabsorption of cobalamin has become rare, owing mainly to the decreasing frequency of gastrectomy and surgical resection of the terminal small intestine Other disorders associated with cobalamin malabsorption include deficiency in the exocrine function of the pancreas after chronic pancreatitis (usually alcoholic), lymphomas or tuberculosis of the intestine, Crohn's disease, Whipple's disease, and celiac disease. Uncommon etiology also includes nitrous oxide anesthesia and abuse.

Clinical Features

Box 2 presents features related to vitamin B_{12} deficiency. It should be noted that vitamin B_{12} deficiency may be present in the absence of anemia. The symptoms of folate deficiency are nearly indistinguishable from those of cobalamin deficiency. Box 3 presents the other hematologic manifestations of cobalamin deficiency.

BOX 2 Nonhematologic Manifestations of Vitamin B_{12} Deficiency

Neuropsychiatric

Common

Polyneuritis (especially sensitive ones)
Ataxia
Babinski's phenomenon

Classic

Combined sclerosis of the spinal cord

Rare

Cerebellar syndromes affecting the cranial nerves including optic neuritis, optic atrophy
Urinary incontinence
Fecal incontinence

Under Study

Changes in higher cognitive functions, including dementia
Stroke and atherosclerosis (hyperhomocysteinemia)
Parkinsonian syndromes
Depression
Multiple sclerosis

Digestive

Classic

Hunter's glossitis
Jaundice
Lactate dehydrogenase and bilirubin elevation (intramedullary destruction)

Debatable

Abdominal pain
Dyspepsia
Nausea, vomiting
Diarrhea
Disturbances in intestinal functioning

Rare

Resistant and recurring mucocutaneous ulcers

Other
Under Study

Atrophy of the vaginal mucosa
Chronic vaginal and urinary infections (especially mycosis)
Venous thromboembolic disease
Angina (hyperhomocysteinemia)

Adapted from Andrès E, Loukili NH, Noel E, et al: Vitamin B_{12} (cobalamin) deficiency in elderly patients. Can Med Assoc J 2004;171: 251-260; and Andrès E, Vidal-Alaball J, Federici L, et al: Clinical aspects of cobalamin deficiency in elderly patients. Epidemiology, causes, clinical manifestations, treatment with special focus on oral cobalamin therapy. Eur J Intern Med 2007;18:456-462.

BOX 3   Hematologic Manifestations of Vitamin B$_{12}$ Deficiency

Common
Macrocytosis
Hypersegmentation of neutrophils
Aregenerative macrocytic anemia
Megaloblastic anemia

Rare
Isolated thrombocytopenia and neutropenia
Pancytopenia

Uncommon
Hemolytic anemia
Pseudothrombotic microangiopathy

Adapted from Andrès E, Loukili NH, Noel E, et al: Vitamin B$_{12}$ (cobalamin) deficiency in elderly patients. Can Med Assoc J 2004;171:251-260; and Andrès E, Vidal-Alaball J, Federici L, et al: Clinical aspects of cobalamin deficiency in elderly patients. Epidemiology, causes, clinical manifestations, treatment with special focus on oral cobalamin therapy. Eur J Intern Med 2007;18:456-462.

Diagnosis

Patients with nutrient-deficiency anemia often have mild to moderate anemia with hemoglobin levels between 8 and 10 g/dL. In anemia of exclusive folate and/or vitamin B$_{12}$ deficiency, the erythrocytes are usually macrocytic (MCV >100 fL). Megaloblastic processes are characterized on the peripheral smear by macroovalocytes and hypersegmented neutrophils. Bone marrow aspiration, which is rarely required for diagnosis, demonstrates large immature and dysfunctional red blood cells (megaloblasts) and hypersegmented or multisegmented neutrophils. In cobalamin deficiency (<150 pmol/L), serum vitamin B$_{12}$ level is low (<200 pg/mL), serum methylmalonic acid is increased, and homocysteine levels are increased. In folate deficiency, testing the red cell folate concentration is more reliable than the serum level.

Prevention

Providing food sources of nutrients is best for preventing megaloblastic anemia. Food source supplementation may be is necessary, especially for the very old. The National Academy of Sciences recommends that folate and vitamin B$_{12}$ be supplemented for the elderly in the form of fortified cereal.

CURRENT DIAGNOSIS

- Megaloblastic anemia is a macrocytic anemia characterized by macroovalocytes and hypersegmented neutrophils on the peripheral smear.
- In adults, many underlying conditions lead to megaloblastic anemia, but the most common ones are folate (folic acid, vitamin B$_9$) deficiency, vitamin B$_{12}$ (cobalamin) deficiency, and pernicious anemia.
- In the adult population, folate deficiency usually develops as a result of inadequate dietary intake or as an adverse effect of several drugs (methotrexate [Trexall], cotrimoxazole [Bactrim], sulfasalazine [Azulfidine], anticonvulsants) or alcohol intake.
- In adults and the elderly, vitamin B$_{12}$ deficiency is mainly due to cobalamin malabsorption from food and to pernicious anemia.

Treatment

Treatment of megaloblastic anemia requires particular attention to discerning the cause. In adult patients, vitamin B$_{12}$ deficiency anemia may be treated by vitamin B$_{12}$ supplementation, parenterally or orally. Our working group has developed an effective oral treatment regimen for food-cobalamin malabsorption and pernicious anemia using crystalline cobalamin (cyanocobalamin)[1] (Fig. 2). The effect of oral cobalamin treatment in patients presenting with severe neurologic manifestations has not yet been adequately documented.

For folate deficiency anemia, therapeutic doses of folic acid vary between 1 and 5 mg/day. Usually, these various therapies are continued for at least 3 to 6 months, provided that the underlying causes of the deficiency have been corrected.

If vitamin B$_{12}$ deficiency is present but undiagnosed, folate repletion will correct the megaloblastic anemia, but not the possible neuropathic changes that occur with B$_{12}$ deficiency.

[1]Not FDA approved for this indication.

CURRENT THERAPY

- Recognition of the condition causing megaloblastic anemia is a prerequisite of successful therapy.
- Treatment of nutrient-deficiency megaloblastic anemia is easy with nutrient replacement.
- Vitamin B$_{12}$ deficiency can be treated with both oral and parenteral therapy.
- If vitamin B$_{12}$ deficiency is untreated, folate repletion will correct the megaloblastic anemia but not the associated neuropathic changes that occur with B$_{12}$ deficiency.

Parenteral administration
(Regardless of the etiology of the vitamin deficiency)

Intensification treatment:
Cyanocobalamin: 1000 µg per day for one week, then 1000 µg per week for 1 month

Maintenance treatment:
Cyanocobalamin: 1000 µg per month until the cause is corrected, or for life in the case of pernicious anemia

Oral administration
(for intake deficiency, food-cobalamin malabsorption and pernicious anemia)

Intensification treatment:
Cyanocobalamin: 1000 µg per day for 1 month

Maintenance treatment:
Cyanocobalamin 125 to 500 µg per day for intake deficiency and food-cobalamin malabsorption and
Cyanocobalamin: 1000 µg per day for pernicious anemia

FIGURE 2. Therapeutic schema for vitamin B$_{12}$ deficiency. (Adapted from Andrès E, Affenberger S, Vinzio S, et al: Food-cobalamin malabsorption in elderly patients: Clinical manifestations and treatment. Am J Med 2005;118: 1154-1159; Andrès E, Federici L, Serraj K, Kaltenbach G: Update of nutrient-deficiency anemia in elderly patients. Eur J Intern Med 2008;19:488-493; Andrès E, Loukili NH, Noel E, et al: Vitamin B$_{12}$ (cobalamin) deficiency in elderly patients. Can Med Assoc J 2004;171: 251-260; and Andrès E, Vidal-Alaball J, Federici L, et al: Clinical aspects of cobalamin deficiency in elderly patients. Epidemiology, causes, clinical manifestations, treatment with special focus on oral cobalamin therapy. Eur J Intern Med 2007;18:456-462.

REFERENCES

Andrès E, Affenberger S, Vinzio S, et al. Food-cobalamin malabsorption in elderly patients: Clinical manifestations and treatment. Am J Med 2005;118:1154–9.

Andrès E, Federici L, Serraj K, Kaltenbach G. Update of nutrient-deficiency anemia in elderly patients. Eur J Intern Med 2008;19:488–93.

Andrès E, Loukili NH, Noel E, et al. Vitamin B_{12} (cobalamin) deficiency in elderly patients. Can Med Assoc J 2004;171:251–60.

Andrès E, Vidal-Aball J, Federici L, et al. Clinical aspects of cobalamin deficiency in elderly patients. Epidemiology, causes, clinical manifestations, treatment with special focus on oral cobalamin therapy. Eur J Intern Med 2007;18:456–62.

Carmel R. Malabsorption of food-cobalamin. Baillieres Clin Haematol 1995; 8:639–55.

McDowell MA, Fryar CD, Ogden CL. Anthropometric reference data for children and adults: United States, 1988–1994. Vital Health Stat 2009;11(249):1–68.

Vidal-Aball J, Butler CC, Cannings-John R, et al. Oral vitamin B_{12} versus intramuscular vitamin B_{12} for vitamin B_{12} deficiency. Cochrane Database Syst Rev 2005;(20):CD004655.

Wickramasinghe SN. Diagnosis of megaloblastic anaemias. Blood Rev 2006;20:299–318.

Thalassemia

Method of

Sarah A. Holstein, MD, PhD, and
Raymond J. Hohl, MD, PhD

Globin Gene Arrangements

Thalassemia syndromes encompass a spectrum of hemoglobin disorders that arise from impaired production of globin chains. The genes that encode globins are located in two clusters: the β gene cluster on chromosome 11 and the α gene cluster on chromosome 16 (Fig. 1). The β gene cluster includes the adult globin genes (β and δ) as well as the fetal Aγ and Gγ genes and the embryonic ε gene. The arrangement of the 5′ to 3′ sequence of these genes parallels the order of their developmental expression. Functional hemoglobin is a tetramer that includes two α and two β globin units. The α gene cluster includes two fetal/adult α genes (α1 and α2) and the embryonic ζ genes. In the embryo, three hemoglobins are found ($\zeta_2\varepsilon_2$, $\alpha_2\varepsilon_2$, and $\zeta_2\gamma_2$). Fetal hemoglobin (HbF) is composed of two α chains and two γ chains ($\alpha_2\gamma_2$). In adults, the predominant hemoglobin is hemoglobin A (HbA), consisting of two α chains and two β chains

($\alpha_2\beta_2$) (see Fig. 1). Hemoglobin A2, consisting of two α chains and two δ chains ($\alpha_2\delta_2$), is a normal variant in adults and typically represents less than 3% of the total hemoglobin (see Fig. 1).

In β-thalassemia, there is diminished production of β globin genes, resulting in an excess of α globin chains. Conversely, in α-thalassemia there is impaired production of α globin genes, resulting in an excess of β globin chains. This imbalance of globin production is variable, and the degree of accumulation of unpaired globin chains is directly related to the severity of the disease phenotype. The genetic basis of thalassemia is heterogeneous, and several hundred mutations have been identified. These mutations may affect any level of globin gene expression, including arrangement of the globin gene complex, gene deletion, splicing, transcription, translation, and protein stability. In general, β-thalassemia occurs as a result of mutations, whereas α-thalassemia occurs as a result of gene deletion.

It has been estimated that there are 270 million carriers of thalassemia in the world, including 80 million β-thalassemia carriers. The frequency of β-thalassemia carriers is highest in the malarial tropical and subtropical regions of Asia, the Mediterranean, and the Middle East. The term thalassemia, derived from Greek, refers to the Mediterranean Sea. This distribution is secondary to the selective advantage of heterozygotes against malaria. β-Thalassemia is subdivided into major, intermedia, and minor types (Table 1). α-Thalassemia is classified into four syndromes: α-thalassemia trait 2 (loss of one α globin gene [αα/α−]); α-thalassemia trait 1, also referred to as α-thalassemia minor (loss of two α globin genes [αα/−− or α−/α−]); hemoglobin H (HbH) disease (loss of three alleles [α−/−−]); and hemoglobin Barts hydrops fetalis (loss of all four α globin loci [−−/−−]).

Pathophysiology

The clinical manifestations of thalassemia and their severity are a consequence of the relative excess of unpaired globin chains. In particular, excess α globin chains are unstable and insoluble and therefore precipitate inside the red blood cell (RBC). These inclusions (precipitated hemoglobin) may be visualized as Heinz bodies. The accumulation of α globin chains leads to a variety of insults to the erythrocyte, including changes in membrane deformability and increased fragility. Free β chains are more soluble than free α chains and are able to form a homotetramer (HbH). The hallmark of thalassemia is an anemia that is a consequence of both increased destruction (i.e., hemolysis) and decreased production (i.e., ineffective erythropoiesis). The bone marrow typically displays erythroid hyperplasia.

Oxidant injury is closely linked with the pathology of thalassemia. Under normal conditions, a small amount of methemoglobin (Fe^{3+}) is formed via oxidation and can then be reduced back to hemoglobin (Fe^{2+}). However, isolated globin chains can be oxidized to hemichromes, some forms of which are irreversibly oxidized. The hemichromes can then generate reactive oxygen species, which can oxidize membrane components, leading to cell injury. There is an increase in membrane rigidity in β-thalassemia, and this appears to be secondary to the binding of partially oxidized α globin chains to components of the membrane skeleton. Increased membrane rigidity in turn leads to decreased membrane deformability and increased destruction. In α-thalassemia, HbH has a left-shifted oxygen disassociation curve and therefore does not readily transport oxygen. HbH erythrocytes have increased rigidity, which is thought to be secondary to interactions between excess β globin chains and the membrane. Unlike with β-thalassemia, HbH erythrocytes have increased membrane stability. Inclusion bodies have been identified in HbH cells, and there appears to be a correlation between RBC age and solubility of HbH. As cells age, the amount of soluble HbH decreases, and the level of inclusions increases.

It has also been recognized that there is increased phagocytosis of thalassemia RBCs compared with normal controls. The etiology is not completely understood, but it may be a consequence of reduction in surface levels of sialic acid, increase in surface immunoglobulin G binding, and changes in phosphatidylserine localization.

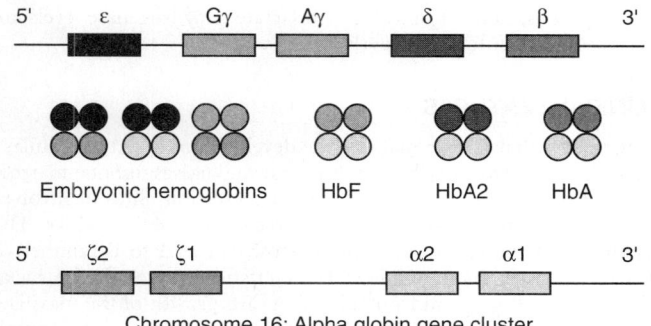

Chromosome 11: Beta globin gene cluster

5′ — ε — Gγ — Aγ — δ — β — 3′

Embryonic hemoglobins   HbF   HbA2   HbA

5′ — ζ2 — ζ1 — α2 — α1 — 3′

Chromosome 16: Alpha globin gene cluster

FIGURE 1. Representation of the β and α globin gene clusters. Also shown are the globin tetramers produced during embryonic development.

TABLE 1   Summary of Hematologic and Clinical Features of the Thalassemias

Type	Hematologic Findings	Hemoglobin Electrophoresis Pattern	Clinical Features
β-Thalassemia major	Severe anemia, microcytosis, hypochromia, target cells, nucleated RBCs	Absence of HbA, markedly elevated HbF, elevated HbA2	Splenomegaly, jaundice, skeletal abnormalities, abnormal facies; transfusion dependent
β-Thalassemia intermedia	Mild to moderate anemia, microcytosis, hypochromia	Elevated HbA2, elevated HbF, decreased HbA	Splenomegaly; variable transfusion dependence
β-Thalassemia minor	Mild anemia, microcytosis, target cells	Elevated HbA2	None
Hemoglobin Barts hydrops fetalis	Severe anemia, anisopoikilocytosis, hypochromia, nucleated RBCs	HbBart; absence of HbA, HbA2, and HbF	Death during gestation; fetus with massive hepatosplenomegaly, generalized edema
Hemoglobin H disease	Moderately severe anemia, anisopoikilocytosis, microcytosis, Heinz bodies	Decreased HbA; HbH and HbBart present	Splenomegaly, jaundice; generally transfusion-dependent
α-Thalassemia trait 1	Mild anemia, hypochromia, microcytosis, target cells	Normal	None
α-Thalassemia trait 2	Normal	Normal	None

Abbreviations: Hb = hemoglobin; RBCs = red blood cells.

CURRENT DIAGNOSIS

- Complete blood count: anemia (very severe in β-thalassemia major, mild in β-thalassemia minor and α-thalassemia trait), low mean corpuscular volume, variable leukocytosis, thrombocytopenia (secondary to splenomegaly) or thrombocythemia (after splenectomy)
- Peripheral blood smear: hypochromia, microcytosis, anisocytosis, poikilocytosis, target cells, Heinz bodies, nucleated red blood cells
- Evidence of hemolytic anemia: indirect hyperbilirubinemia, elevated lactate dehydrogenase, decreased haptoglobin
- Hemoglobin electrophoresis pattern:
  β-Thalassemia minor: elevated HbA2 ($\alpha_2\delta_2$)
  β-Thalassemia intermedia: elevated HbA2, elevated HbF ($\alpha_2\gamma_2$), and decreased HbA ($\alpha_2\beta_2$)
  β-Thalassemia major: absence of HbA, markedly elevated HbF, and elevated HbA2
  α-Thalassemia trait: normal
  Hemoglobin H disease: decreased HbA, presence of HbH (β_4) and HbBart (γ_4)
  Hemoglobin Barts hydrops fetalis: HbBart, absence of HbA, HbA2, and HbF
- Timing of symptomatic disease:
  β-Thalassemia minor: asymptomatic
  β-Thalassemia intermedia: variable
  β-Thalassemia major: within first year of life
  α-Thalassemia trait: asymptomatic
  Hemoglobin H disease: symptomatic at time of birth
  Hemoglobin Barts hydrops fetalis: death during gestation

Despite the pronounced hemolysis and marrow erythroid hyperplasia, patients with thalassemia generally do not display the compensatory reticulocytosis that is indicative of the other basis for anemia, ineffective erythropoiesis. Accumulation of α chain aggregates is thought to lead to death of erythrocyte precursors. Furthermore, abnormal assembly of membrane proteins in erythroid precursors has been demonstrated.

Iron overload is one of the primary causes of morbidity. Even without transfusion, the long-standing anemia, however mild, leads to increased iron absorption in the gut and eventual chronic iron overload. Excessive iron deposition causes devastating damage to multiple organs, particularly affecting the heart, liver, and endocrine organs.

β-Thalassemia Major

Symptoms of β-thalassemia major are not present at birth, because HbF ($\alpha_2\gamma_2$) is present. However, as HbF levels decline over the first year, the signs and symptoms of severe hemolytic anemia begin to manifest. Affected individuals display hepatosplenomegaly from expansion of the reticuloendothelial system as well as extramedullary hematopoiesis, pallor, growth retardation, and abnormal skeletal development. If left untreated, 80% of children with β-thalassemia major will die before the age of 5 years.

LABORATORY FEATURES

Thalassemia major is characterized by a severe microcytic anemia. Hemoglobin levels may be as low as 3 to 4 g/dL. The peripheral blood smear is markedly abnormal and is notable for hypochromia, microcytosis, anisocytosis, poikilocytosis, target cells, and tear drop cells. Routine stains show the presence of precipitated α globin chains as Heinz bodies. The reticulocyte count is often low. The white blood cell count is often high but may be artifactually elevated as a consequence of automated inclusion of high numbers of circulating nucleated RBCs. The platelet count is typically normal, but progressive hypersplenism can result in decreased platelet counts. Patients who have undergone splenectomy often have increased white blood cell and platelet counts. Iron studies reveal elevated serum iron, transferrin saturation, and ferritin. Consistent with hemolysis and ineffective erythropoiesis, indirect bilirubin and lactate dehydrogenase levels are increased and haptoglobin levels are low.

CLINICAL FEATURES

Unique to β-thalassemia major is the development of extramedullary erythropoiesis. This may be so severe that the masses of bone marrow lead to broken bones and spinal cord compression. Sites of involvement include the sinuses and the thoracic and pelvic cavities. The expansion of the erythroid bone marrow can lead to a number of skeletal changes. In particular, characteristic changes in the facial bones and skull result in frontal bossing, overgrowth of the maxillae, and malocclusion. This has sometimes been referred to as chipmunk facies. Other bones are also affected, and premature fusion of the epiphyses results in shortened limbs. Compression fractures of the spine may occur. Even if the disease is managed appropriately with transfusions and iron chelation, patients will still suffer from osteopenia and osteoporosis. Possible mechanisms include changes secondary to hypogonadism or increased bone resorption secondary to vitamin D deficiency.

Hepatomegaly and splenomegaly, secondary to extramedullary erythropoiesis and RBC destruction, are prominent. Injury to Kupffer cells and hepatocytes from chronic overload leads to fibrosis and end-stage liver disease. Hepatic iron overload is probably caused in part by comparatively high levels of transferrin receptors. Iron overload, and perhaps other factors, increase susceptibility to viral hepatitis. Laboratory studies show indirect hyperbilirubinemia, hypergammaglobulinemia, and elevated liver markers. The chronic hemolysis leads to formation of bilirubin gallstones, although cholecystitis or cholangitis is not common. Splenic dysfunction results in immune dysfunction. The shortened erythrocyte survival time leaves patients susceptible to aplastic crisis induced by parvovirus B19 infection. Extramedullary hematopoiesis may also affect the kidneys, and patients often have large kidneys. Rapid cell turnover leads to hyperuricemia, and children may develop gouty nephropathy.

A number of endocrine abnormalities are commonly seen in β-thalassemia major, including hypogonadism, growth failure, diabetes, and hypothyroidism. These abnormalities occur even in chronically transfused patients and may be in part related to iron overload. Endocrine glands, like liver and heart, have high levels of transferrin-receptor and therefore are more susceptible to iron overload. The typical growth pattern for a child with β-thalassemia major is relatively normal until the age of 9 to 10 years. After that time, the growth velocity slows, and the pubertal growth spurt is either absent or reduced. Although secretion of growth hormone does not appear to be altered in thalassemic patients, a reduction in peak amplitude and nocturnal levels of growth hormone has been observed. Amenorrhea is quite common, with 50% of girls presenting with primary amenorrhea. Secondary amenorrhea also develops, particularly in patients who do not receive regular chelation therapy. In males, impotence and azoospermia is common. Primary hypothyroidism typically appears during the second decade of life. The prevalence of diabetes mellitus and impaired glucose intolerance has been estimated at 4% to 20%. Unlike type 1 diabetes mellitus, diabetes associated with thalassemia is rarely complicated by diabetic ketoacidosis. The risk of diabetic retinopathy is lower, but the risk of diabetic nephropathy is higher.

Thalassemic patients suffer from extensive cardiac abnormalities. Chronic anemia causes cardiac dilatation. Although chronic transfusion can help prevent cardiac dilatation, the resulting iron overload leads to cardiac hemosiderosis. Pericarditis, ventricular and supraventricular arrhythmias, and end-stage cardiomyopathy can develop. Ventricular arrhythmia is a common cause of death. Patients may also develop pulmonary hypertension. The degree of iron overload in the heart has traditionally been assessed by cardiac biopsy, but cardiac magnetic resonance imaging (MRI) is increasingly being used.

Vitamin and mineral deficiencies may occur. Folic acid deficiency may develop in patients, presumably as a consequence of increased cell turnover. Although the cause is unknown, patients with β-thalassemia major often have very low serum zinc levels. Serum levels of vitamin E and vitamin C may also be low.

MANAGEMENT OF β-THALASSEMIA MAJOR

Transfusion

The key intervention for the management of β-thalassemia major is chronic transfusion therapy. In particular, during the first decade of life, regular transfusion results in improvements in hepatosplenomegaly, skeletal abnormalities, and cardiac dilatation. Patients typically require 1 to 3 units of packed RBCs every 3 to 5 weeks. The optimal target total hemoglobin level has yet to be determined. Alloimmunization does occur, and some blood centers try to leukodeplete their products, match donors by ethnicity, and limit the donor pool for any particular patient. Although the risk of blood-borne infections is now quite small, regular transfusion of blood products still carries a risk for infections such as HIV and hepatitis C.

CURRENT THERAPY

- Chronic packed red blood cell transfusions for β-thalassemia major (1–3 units of packed leukoreduced erythrocytes every 3–5 weeks) with a target hemoglobin concentration of 9 to 10.5 g/dL; variable transfusion needs for β-thalassemia intermedia and hemoglobin H disease
- Splenectomy with antibiotic prophylaxis and vaccination
- Iron chelation: deferoxamine (Desferal) or deferasirox (Exjade); deferiprone (Ferriprox) does not have FDA approval in the United States
- Osteoporosis management: calcium with vitamin D supplementation; bisphosphonates
- Allogeneic hematopoietic cell transplantation for β-thalassemia major

Splenectomy

The general indication for splenectomy is an increase of more than 50% in the RBC transfusion requirement over the period of 1 year. Splenectomy may initially yield a decrease in the RBC transfusion requirement. It has been noted that thalassemia patients are at higher risk for infection after splenectomy than are those patients splenectomized for other reasons. The bacteria that most frequently cause infections in these patients include *Streptococcus pneumoniae, Haemophilus influenzae, Neisseria meningitidis, Klebsiella, Escherichia coli*, and *Staphylococcus aureus*. The increased susceptibility to infection compared with other splenectomized patients is thought to be a result of greater immune dysfunction secondary to iron overload. In particular, it has been reported that iron-overloaded macrophages lose the ability to kill intracellular pathogens. Antibiotic prophylaxis with penicillin, amoxicillin, or erythromycin is recommended for children up to the age of 16 years. In addition, patients should receive immunizations, including the pneumococcal, influenza, and *Haemophilus influenzae* vaccines.

Iron Chelation Therapy

Because of increased iron absorption and chronic transfusion therapy, iron overload develops. As noted earlier, iron overload causes damage to multiple organs. Because iron is poorly excreted, removal must be accomplished by phlebotomy (not an option in thalassemic patients) or by chelation therapy. Historically, deferoxamine (Desferal) has been the most widely used chelator. This agent may be administered subcutaneously, intramuscularly, or intravenously. The dosing for chronic iron overload is 20 to 40 mg/kg/day SQ or 500 to 1000 mg/day IM + 2 g IV per unit transfused blood. The IV-only route is indicated for patients with cardiovascular collapse. Multiple studies have shown that deferoxamine therapy improves long-term survival. In addition, intensive therapy with deferoxamine has been shown to improve cardiac function in patients with severe iron overload. However, compliance with daily injections has been a particular problem, and, unless regular therapy is given, iron will reaccumulate.

Deferiprone (Ferriprox)[2] was the first orally active chelator to be introduced. It is given three times daily (total of 75 mg/kg/day). Studies have indicated that deferiprone may be as effective as deferoxamine in lowering iron levels. A recent Cochrane Review concluded that deferiprone is indicated in the treatment of iron overload in thalassemia major if deferoxamine therapy is contraindicated or inadequate. Agranulocytosis associated with deferiprone has been reported, and, because of this risk, the drug is currently not available in the United States except through the FDA Treatment Use Program. Deferiprone is available in Europe and Asia. There has also been interest in combined therapy with deferiprone and deferoxamine.

---

[2]Not available in the United States.

Deferasirox (Exjade) is the first orally active agent approved for use in the United States. Its longer half-life in comparison to deferiprone allows this drug to be given once daily (total of 20–40 mg/kg/day). A phase III trial comparing deferasirox to deferoxamine in patients with thalassemia revealed similar decreases in liver iron concentrations. Side effects include gastrointestinal complaints (abdominal pain, nausea, vomiting, diarrhea) and skin rash. There have been postmarketing reports of acute renal failure, hepatic failure, and cytopenias. It is recommended that serum creatinine, ferritin, and alanine aminotransferase be monitored monthly during therapy.

The gold standard for measurement of liver iron concentration has been liver biopsy with iron measurement by atomic absorption spectrometry. More recently, there has been increasing use of MRI technology to measure liver iron levels. In general, iron content determined by MRI methodology correlates with liver iron concentration determined by biopsy. However, the precision of liver MRI measurement appears to be dependent on iron levels, liver fibrosis, and calibration. Hepatic iron concentration has also been measured using a superconducting quantum interference device (SQUID), although reported consistency has varied and widespread use of this technique has been limited by expense and complexity.

Management of Osteoporosis

Even with calcium and vitamin D supplementation, iron chelation, transfusion therapy, and hormonal therapy, bone loss continues to be a significant problem for thalassemia patients. Recently, there has been interest in the use of bisphosphonates. This class of drugs, which includes clodronate (Bonefos),[2] alendronate (Fosamax), pamidronate (Aredia), and zoledronate (Zometa), inhibit osteoclastic bone resorption and have found extensive use in the management of Paget's disease, osteoporosis, and skeletal metastases. Small studies performed in thalassemia patients have failed to show benefit with clodronate 100 mg IM every 10 days or 300 mg IV every 3 weeks. A very small study using alendronate (Fosamax)[1] 10 mg PO daily revealed an increase in bone mineral density only at the femoral level. Conversely, in a study involving pamidronate (Aredia)[1] 30 or 60 mg IV every month, there was an increase in bone density only at the lumbar level. The most promising results have been achieved with the most potent member of the class, zoledronate. Several trials demonstrated that zoledronate (Zometa)[1] 4 mg IV every 3 or 4 months results in significant improvement in femoral and lumbar bone mineral density and reduces bony pain. Larger, long-term trials are necessary before this agent finds widespread use in the management of thalassemia-induced osteoporosis.

Hematopoietic Cell Transplantation

Hematopoietic cell transplantation is the only curative strategy for patients with hemoglobinopathies. Patients are assigned to a risk class (Pesaro class) based on adherence to regular iron chelation therapy, presence or absence of hepatomegaly, and presence or absence of portal fibrosis. Those children with no or little hepatomegaly, no portal fibrosis, and regular iron chelation therapy (class I) have a better than 90% chance of cure, whereas those with both hepatomegaly and portal fibrosis (class III) have long-term survival rates of about 60% in older studies. More recent reports indicate that class III survival has improved to 80%.

The use of human leukocyte antigen (HLA)-identical sibling donors has been preferred, because the use of HLA-mismatched donors has produced inferior results and is associated with increased graft rejection, graft-versus-host disease, and infection. The use of unrelated donors has been explored, and initial studies showed poorer outcomes. However, more recent data suggest that matched unrelated donors might be a viable option if a suitable sibling donor is lacking, thanks to improved donor selection and transplantation techniques.

Another emerging technique is the use of reduced-intensity conditioning regimens, although long-term success has yet to be achieved.

Gene Therapy

Globin gene therapy, achieved through manipulation of autologous stem cells, is an attractive alternative to allogeneic transplantation. There are three major scientific hurdles that must be overcome: design of vectors that yield therapeutic levels of globin gene expression, ability to isolate and transduce autologous stem cells, and development of transplantation conditions that will permit host repopulation. In addition, the safety of viral and nonviral transfection is an issue. At this point, there has been some success in murine models of β-thalassemia. Likewise, although the use of antisense oligonucleotides to manipulate HbA levels has been attempted in cell cultures, no such approach has been used in humans.

Pharmacologic Induction of Fetal Hemoglobin

Induction of HbF expression has been proposed as a therapeutic strategy. For β-thalassemia, induced γ globin gene expression would be predicted to decrease globin chain imbalance by complexing with free α chains. Hydroxyurea (Hydrea)[1] is an antimetabolite thought to interfere with DNA synthesis. It is well established in the management of sickle cell disease, where it has been shown to increase levels of HbF. The use of hydroxyurea in β-thalassemia is much less well established. In the United States, hydroxyurea has been approved for use in sickle cell disease but not for thalassemia. Studies published elsewhere in the world have generally shown improvements in hemoglobin levels in thalassemia intermedia patients, with some patients becoming transfusion independent.

5-Azacytidine (azacitidine [Vidaza]),[1] an inhibitor of DNA methyltransferase, has been shown to induce HbF. However, concerns regarding long-term use have prevented further evaluation in thalassemia. Decitabine (Dacogen),[1] an analogue of 5-azacitidine, has been shown to increase HbF levels in patients with sickle cell disease refractory to hydroxyurea. No data are available for the use of decitabine in thalassemia. Butyrate,[5] an inhibitor of histone deacetylases, is another agent capable of inducing HbF. However, butyrate and its derivatives (arginine butyrate,[5] sodium isobutyramide,[5] and sodium phenylbutyrate [Buphenyl][1]) have failed to show significant clinical benefit in thalassemia patients. Therefore, at this time, no agent has been approved for use in thalassemia patients. A number of hypotheses have been proposed to explain the lack of success of inducers of HbF in thalassemia: there is simply too little γ globin production to significantly affect globin chain balance; these agents decrease expression of partially active β-thalassemia genes; these agents increase expression of α-globin genes; chronic transfusions appear to reduce HbF levels; and these agents suppress erythropoiesis.

Antioxidants

Oxidative damage is believed to be an important cause of tissue damage, and there has been interest in the use of antioxidants in thalassemia patients. A variety of substances have been investigated, including ascorbate,[1] vitamin E,[1] N-acetylcysteine (Mucomyst),[1] flavonoids, and indicaxanthin.[5] A variety of antioxidant effects have been observed in vitro with these agents, but none has been shown to improve anemia in patients with thalassemia.

β-Thalassemia Intermedia

Given the underlying genetic heterogeneity, it is not surprising that the clinical manifestations of β-thalassemia intermedia are also quite varied. Some patients with more mild forms of β-thalassemia intermedia do not require chronic transfusion therapy. There is not a clear consensus as to when chronic transfusion should be initiated.

---

[1]Not FDA approved for this indication.
[2]Not available in the United States.

---

[1]Not FDA approved for this indication.
[5]Investigational drug in the United States.

Factors that are considered for children include growth patterns, spleen size, and bone development. Transfusion may be necessary during infection-induced aplastic crises. In some instances, transfusions are begun in childhood to help with growth and then discontinued after puberty. Some adults gradually become more anemic and eventually require transfusion. Some authors have argued that starting transfusions early in life is advantageous, because the prevalence of alloimmunization appears to increase if transfusion is started after the first few years of life.

Splenomegaly usually develops in all patients, including those who do not require transfusion. With progression of splenomegaly and the accompanying sequestration and hemolysis, there is usually worsening of anemia, to the point at which transfusions may be required. Most patients achieve transfusion independence after splenectomy. Gallstones may develop, and a prophylactic cholecystectomy is sometimes performed at the same time as the splenectomy. As with β-thalassemia major patients, intermedia patients are at increased risk for infection and should be appropriately vaccinated.

For reasons that are not entirely clear, there is an increased risk of thromboembolic complications in intermedia patients compared with thalassemia major patients. An Italian study reported that 10% of thalassemia intermedia and 4% of thalassemia major patients experienced a thromboembolic event. Another study reported that thromboembolism occurred four times more frequently in patients with intermedia versus major disease. This report noted that venous events were more common in the thalassemia intermedia population, whereas arterial events were more common in the thalassemia major population. An even higher rate of venous thrombotic events (29%) was reported in a population of splenectomized patients with thalassemia intermedia. It has been suggested that exposed anionic phospholipids on the surface of damaged RBCs may induce a procoagulant effect. There is no consensus regarding the prophylactic use of antiplatelet agents or anticoagulants in this population.

Patients with thalassemia intermedia may develop iron overload, although it is less severe than in patients with thalassemia major. Even those that are not regularly transfused may develop a degree of iron overload, because there is increased iron absorption. Iron overload may be managed with the iron chelating agents as described earlier. Cardiac toxicity, including congestive heart failure, valvular problems, and pulmonary hypertension (leading to secondary right-sided heart failure), resulting from iron overload is not infrequent in the thalassemia intermedia population.

Bone abnormalities and osteoporosis may develop in thalassemia intermedia patients. In a North American study, the prevalence of fractures in these patients was 12%. Leg ulcers involving the medial malleolus are common and are often difficult to treat. Hypogonadism, hypothyroidism, and diabetes may occur, with frequency related to the severity of anemia and iron overload. Pseudoxanthoma elasticum, a syndrome consisting of skin lesions, angioid streaks in the retina, calcified retinal walls, and aortic valve disease, is more common in thalassemia intermedia than in thalassemia major. Currently, no effective therapy exists, although it has been reported that aluminum hydroxide (Alternagel)[1] reduces skin calcification.

β-Thalassemia Minor

Most patients with β-thalassemia minor are asymptomatic. However, they have an abnormal complete blood count that may sometimes lead to the misdiagnosis of iron deficiency. Although these patients have a microcytic anemia, it is much less severe than in patients with β-thalassemia major. In general, the hematocrit is greater than 30%. The mean corpuscular volume is typically less than 75 fL and the RBC distribution width index is normal, in contrast to iron deficiency, in which the degree of microcytosis is less and the distribution width index is usually increased. The peripheral blood smear shows the presence of target cells. Hemoglobin electrophoresis typically reveals an increase in HbA2. The normal anemia experienced

during pregnancy may sometimes be exacerbated in patients with β-thalassemia minor, necessitating transfusion. Otherwise, no long-term effects of β-thalassemia minor have been described, and no interventions are required.

α-Thalassemia

LABORATORY AND CLINICAL FEATURES

Patients with α-thalassemia trait 2 are asymptomatic and have normal laboratory values, including complete blood count, peripheral smear, and hemoglobin electrophoresis. Individuals with α-thalassemia trait 1 are asymptomatic, and the disease resembles β-thalassemia minor. The peripheral smear shows a hypochromic microcytic anemia with the presence of target cells. Hemoglobin electrophoresis is normal.

HbH disease does produce symptoms. Unlike β-thalassemia major, in which HbF production protects the fetus, individuals with HbH disease develop hemolytic anemia during gestation and are symptomatic at birth. This is because α globin production is required for HbF ($\alpha_2\gamma_2$). As with β-thalassemia major, patients with HbH disease suffer from the consequences of chronic hemolytic anemia, although the severity is somewhat less. The transfusion requirements for HbH patients resemble those for patients with β-thalassemia intermedia, with transfusion support initiated in the second and third decades of life. These patients also develop iron overload, necessitating treatment with chelation therapy.

Hydrops fetalis with hemoglobin Barts is usually fatal in utero. The utter lack of α globin chain production results in absence of HbF. Hemoglobin Barts, a homotetramer consisting of four γ globin genes, is unable to deliver oxygen to tissues. Severe tissue hypoxia develops, leading to widespread tissue ischemia. High cardiac output failure leads to massive edema (hydrops). In most cases, death occurs in the third trimester or late second trimester. There have been reports of live births after intrauterine transfusion, but survival beyond the perinatal period is exceedingly rare. Prenatal diagnosis of hemoglobin Barts hydrops fetalis may be achieved through DNA-based testing using amniocytes from amniocentesis or chorionic villi sampling. Noninvasive testing is under development, including methods that isolate circulating fetal DNA in maternal peripheral blood.

MANAGEMENT

Patients with α-thalassemia 2 and 1 traits do not require treatment. The management of HbH disease is similar to that described for β-thalassemia.

REFERENCES

Angelucci E, Barosi G, Camaschella C, et al. Italian Society of Hematology practice guidelines for the management of iron overload in thalassemia major and related disorders. Haematologica 2008;93:741–52.

Bhatia M, Walters MC. Hematopoietic cell transplantation for thalassemia and sickle cell disease: Past, present, and future. Bone Marrow Transplant 2008;41:109–17.

Borgna-Pignatti C. Modern treatment of thalassemia intermedia. Br J Haematol 2007;138:291–304.

Cohen AR. New advances in iron chelation therapy. Hematology Am Soc Hematol Educ Program 2006;42–7.

Fathallah H, Sutton M, Atweh GF. Pharmacological induction of fetal hemoglobin: Why haven't we been more successful in thalassemia? Ann N Y Acad Sci 2005;1054:228–37.

Gaudio A, Morabito N, Xourafa A, et al. Bisphosphonates in the treatment of thalassemia-associated osteoporosis. J Endocrinol Invest 2008;31:181–4.

Lisowski L, Sadelain M. Current status of globin gene therapy for the treatment of β-thalassemia. Br J Haematol 2008;141:335–45.

Quek L, Thein SL. Molecular therapies in β-thalassemia. Br J Haematol 2006;136:353–65.

Roberts DJ, Brunskill SJ, Doree C, et al. Oral deferiprone for iron chelation in people with thalassaemia. Cochrane Database Syst Rev 2007;(3):CD004839.

Toumba M, Sergis A, Kanaris C, et al. Endocrine complications in patients with thalassaemia major. Pediatr Endocrinol Rev 2007;5:642–8.

---

[1]Not FDA approved for this indication.

Sickle Cell Disease

Method of
*Enrico M. Novelli, MD; Mark T. Gladwin, MD;
and Lakshmanan Krishnamurti, MD*

Epidemiology

Sickle cell disease (SCD) affects 70,000 to 100,000 persons in the United States and millions worldwide. The hemoglobin (Hb) S mutation arose from four geographic areas in Africa and Asia approximately 10,000 years ago and then propagated to vast tropical and subtropical areas due to the selective pressure of malaria infection. It is predominantly found in persons of African, Mediterranean, Arab, or Indian ancestry. In the United States, approximately 1 in 15 African Americans harbors the HbS (sickle hemoglobin) mutation and 1 in 400 is affected by the disease. Most patients with SCD in the United States are homozygous for HbS (SS), with heterozygous HbSC being the second most common abnormality. Conversely, in the Mediterraneum, HbS/β-thalassemia is the most common SCD syndrome, and in the Arab peninsula HbSS in combination with hereditary persistence of fetal hemoglobin (HPFH) is particularly common.

Pathophysiology

SCD consists of a group of inherited hemoglobinopathies characterized by a qualitatively abnormal hemoglobin molecule that affects the structure and integrity of the red blood cells (RBCs). The most common mutation in SCD is a single base substitution in the β-globin gene of the hemoglobin tetramer, leading to an amino acid substitution (valine to glutamic acid, HbS). SCD is an autosomal recessive disease due to homozygosity for HbS or coinheritance of HbS with other abnormal hemoglobins such as hemoglobin C or β-thalassemia.

HbS is less soluble than normal hemoglobin (HbA) in the deoxygenated state and tends to polymerize when sickle RBCs are exposed to hypoxic conditions in the microcirculation. In the classic pathophysiologic explanation of SCD, sickled RBCs containing HbS polymers are less deformable and tend to remain trapped in the microcirculation, causing end-organ ischemia and necrosis. Compounding this mechanism, recent literature has emphasized the role of cellular adhesion, abnormal cytokine levels, and an abnormal endothelial milieu. HbS polymers lead to deformity and fragility of the RBC membrane, with resulting intra- and extravascular hemolysis.

Patients with SCD suffer from severe chronic hemolytic anemia and acute episodes of RBC trapping and destruction in the microvasculature (vaso-occlusive episodes). Vaso-occlusive episodes are the hallmark of SCD and are characterized by more intense episodic vaso-occlusion, often with increasing hemolysis, and are due to exogenous or endogenous factors that acutely alter the rheologic properties of the RBCs. The main determinants of RBC sickling and vaso-occlusion are hypoxemia, RBC dehydration, RBC concentration, high HbS relative to fetal hemoglobin (HbF), and blood viscosity; these can occur in a multitude of clinical settings. Most common clinical inciting events leading to vaso-occlusive episodes are dehydration due to inadequate replacement of fluid losses, thermal changes, surgical stress, exposure to low oxygen tension, infections, and psychological stressors.

Epidemiologic studies indicate that the risk of vaso-occlusive episodes and acute chest syndrome is related to high steady-state hemoglobin levels, leukocytosis, and low HbF levels. These findings are consistent with pathogenic mechanisms of altered red cell rheology, higher viscosity, HbS polymerization, and inflammatory cellular adhesion. Interestingly, the epidemiologic risk factors associated with chronic vascular complications such as pulmonary hypertension, cutaneous leg ulceration, priapism, systemic systolic hypertension, renal failure with proteinuria, and possibly stroke are quite different and include a low steady-state hemoglobin level, increased hemolytic intensity, iron overload, and markers of low nitric oxide bioavailability. One hypothesis is that SCD is driven by two overlapping but different mechanisms of disease, vaso-occlusion, which causes vaso-occlusive episodes and acute chest syndrome, and hemolytic anemia, which leads to endothelial dysfunction and chronic vasculopathy. Both are caused fundamentally by HbS polymerization.

Prevention

BACTERIAL INFECTIONS

Before the antibiotic era, most patients with SCD succumbed to bacterial sepsis, mostly from encapsulated organisms. A landmark multicenter, randomized, double-blind, placebo-controlled clinical trial of prophylaxis with oral penicillin in children with sickle cell anemia published in 1986 showed that bacterial prophylaxis started at birth reduced by about 80% the incidence of infection in the penicillin group, as compared with the group given placebo. This study became the foundation for universal screening of SCD. Results of the Penicillin Prophylaxis in Sickle Cell Study II (PROPS 2) trial show that prophylaxis can be safely discontinued at age 5 years as long as there is no history of prior serious pneumococcal infection or surgical splenectomy and in the setting of appropriate comprehensive care. All children should also receive both the 7-valent pneumococcal conjugate (Prevnar) and 23-valent pneumococcal polysaccharide (Pneumovax) vaccines, and adults should receive Pneumovax every 3 to 5 years.[3] Vaccinations for *H. influenzae* and *N. meningitidis* are also indicated.

NEUROLOGIC EVENTS

Stroke is a devastating complication of SCD and affects predominantly children with HbSS. Abnormal transcranial Doppler results predict future development of stroke in children with SCD. A clinical trial published in 1995 showed that the first stroke can be prevented by placing children on prophylactic monthly transfusion with a target HbS of <30%. A second trial published in 2005 addressed whether transfusional therapy could be safely discontinued after 30 consecutive months of treatment in children who had normalized their transcranial Doppler readings, but this trial unfortunately showed that the transcranial Doppler abnormality recurred in the group in whom transfusion was stopped. An ongoing clinical trial is addressing whether the clinical benefit in reduction of stroke incidence can be maintained when children are switched from chronic transfusion therapy to hydroxyurea (Droxia), in an effort to minimize exposure to blood.

Clinical Manifestations

Multiple genetic and epigenetic factors affect the SCD phenotype. Patients homozygous for HbS (SS) or compound heterozygous for HbS and a nonfunctional β⁰-thalassemia allele tend to display the most severe manifestations. On the other end of the spectrum, hereditary persistence of HbF (HPFH), particularly common in Saudi Arabia, or coinheritance of β-thalassemia tends to mitigate the phenotype. Although the net effect of high HbF levels on the phenotype of SCD is beneficial, coinheritance of one or two α-thalassemia alleles has a more complex effect. α-Thalassemia is present in approximately 30% of patients with SCD and is associated with higher hemoglobin, lower mean corpuscular volume (MCV), and decreased rate of hemolysis. These effects are protective toward cerebrovascular accident (CVA) and leg ulcers, but they can lead to increased rates of vaso-occlusive episodes, osteonecrosis, and acute chest syndrome

---

[3]Exceeds dosage recommended by the manufacturer.

TABLE 1 Severity of the Main Sickle Cell Syndromes

Genotype	Clinical Severity	Hemoglobin (g/dL)
HbSS	Usually marked	6-10
HbS-β⁰-thalassemia	Moderate to marked	6-10
HbS-β⁻-thalassemia	Mild to moderate	9-12
HbSC	Mild to moderate	10-15
HbSS-HPFH	Mild	

HPFH = hereditary persistence of fetal hemoglobin; HbSC = heterozygous phenotype; HbSS = homozygous phenotype.

because of the increased blood viscosity related to the higher hemoglobin level. Patients with HbSC and HbS/β⁺-thalassemia have an intermediate severity phenotype (Table 1). Haplotypes of polymorphic sites in the β-globin gene cluster in chromosome 11, which correspond and are linked to defined geographic regions of origin of the HbS gene, have been associated with different disease severity and rates of complications. Other yet unidentified genetic factors predispose certain patients to develop a particularly severe hemolysis with brisk reticulocytosis and a high rate of specific complications that include leg ulcers, priapism, and pulmonary hypertension.

HEMATOLOGY

This section describes the main clinical manifestations of SCD in each organ system (Fig. 1 and Table 2).

Baseline or Steady-State Hematologic Abnormalities

Chronic intra and extravascular hemolysis causes a chronic anemia of moderate to severe intensity in HbSS and HbS/β⁰-thalassemia, with a hemoglobin range of 6 to 9 g/dL. In HbSC and HbS/β⁺-thalassemia, the anemia may be mild or absent. The anemia of SCD is usually normocytic in HbSS, with anisocytosis and poikilocytosis and a population of small dehydrated dense cells, irreversibly sickled cells, numerous reticulocytes, and schistocytes. Reticulocytosis is common but not compensatory, and nucleated RBCs are seen in acute exacerbations of the anemia such as in splenic or hepatic sequestration. Baseline leukocytosis with neutrophilia is also common and has been associated with acute chest syndrome and CVA in adults and possibly with adverse outcomes such as frequent vaso-occlusive episodes later

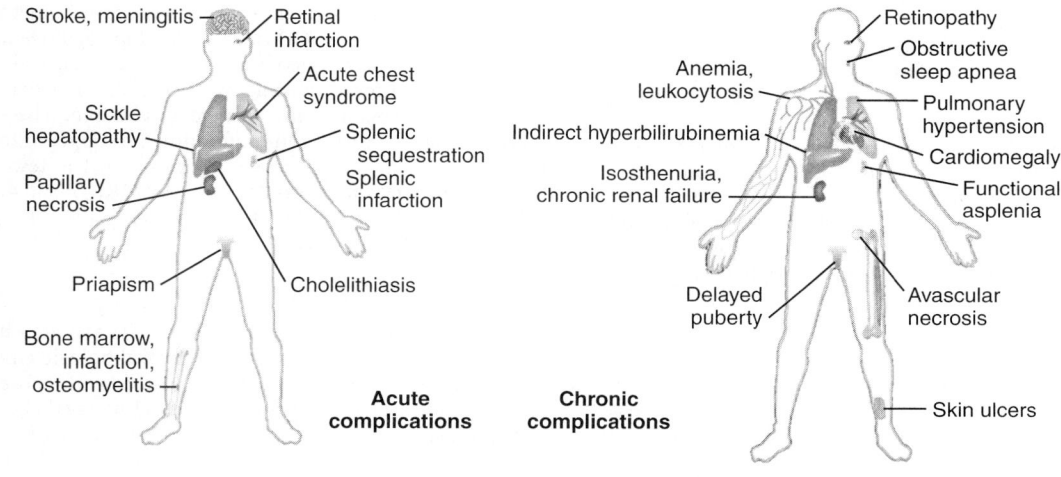

FIGURE 1. Acute and chronic complications of sickle cell disease.

TABLE 2 Landmark Randomized Clinical Trials in Sickle Cell Disease

Year of Publication	Title	Main Findings
1986	Prophylaxis with oral penicillin in children with sickle cell anemia: A randomized trial	84% reduction in incidence of infection and no deaths from pneumococcal septicemia in the penicillin group
1995	Multicenter Study of Hydroxyurea in Sickle Cell Anemia (MSH)	Reduced incidence of painful crises, ACS and transfusion in the hydroxyurea group
		Survival benefit in follow-up study
1995	Preoperative Transfusion in Sickle Cell Disease Study	A conservative transfusion regimen was as effective as an aggressive regimen in preventing perioperative complications in patients with sickle cell anemia
1996	Multicenter investigation of bone marrow transplantation for sickle cell disease	HSCT is safe in SCD with survival and event-free survival at 4 y of 91% and 73% and can lead to cure
1998	Stroke prevention trial in sickle cell anemia (STOP)	Transfusion reduces the risk of a first stroke by 92% in children with sickle cell anemia who have abnormal results on transcranial Doppler ultrasonography
2005	Optimizing primary stroke prevention in sickle cell anemia (STOP 2)	Discontinuation of transfusion for the prevention of stroke in children with sickle cell disease results in a high rate of reversion to abnormal blood-flow velocities on Doppler studies and stroke

Abbreviations: ACS = acute chest syndrome; HSCT = hematopoietic stem cell transplantation; SCD = sickle cell disease; VOE = vaso-occlusive crisis.

in life when present before age 2 years. It is likely that leukocytes are not simply a marker of disease activity and acute phase but also have a direct pathogenic role in cellular adhesion and vaso-occlusion. The platelet count is commonly elevated in SCD, particularly in patients who are autosplenectomized as a result of repeated splenic infarction, and platelet activation is increased. In the subset of patients with HbSC and and HbS/β^+-thalassemia who retain a functional spleen and can have splenomegaly, features of hypersplenism may instead be observed with resulting mild pancytopenia.

Hematologic Indices during Vaso-occlusive Episodes

In acute vaso-occlusive episodes the Hb decreases as a result of hemolysis (by 1.6 g/dL in acute chest syndrome) and sickle cells are observed in the peripheral smear. The lactate dehydrogenase (LDH), reticulocyte count, and other markers of hemolysis such as aspartate transaminase (AST) and indirect bilirubin are elevated in steady state, and in many patients they are further increased during vaso-occlusive episodes. Haptoglobin levels are chronically depressed in SCD and typically not measurable, even in steady state, in patients with HbS homozygosity. In patients with HbSC, vaso-occlusive episodes may be due to increased blood viscosity and RBC sickling, and worsening hemolysis might not be readily appreciated

Splenic sequestration crises occur mostly in childhood and are characterized by anemia disproportionate to the degree of hemolysis, reticulocytosis, and acute enlargement of the spleen. Splenic sequestration and repeated episodes of splenic infarction eventually lead to autosplenectomy, although some patients develop splenomegaly. Splenic infarction usually manifests with acute right upper quadrant pain and occasionally evolves to massive involvement of the spleen (>50% of the splenic tissue).

In severe vaso-occlusive episodes, massive bone marrow infarction can also occur. In these instances, the peripheral blood smear can reveal a leukoerythroblastic picture with immature neutrophilic forms, nucleated RBCs, and teardrop cells. Fat emboli syndrome, a life-threatening complication of vaso-occlusive episodes, can then develop as bone marrow fat embolizes to peripheral capillary beds, leading to multiorgan failure.

Red Blood Cell Alloimmunization

RBC alloimmunization is a common complication of transfusional therapy in SCD and occurs in approximately 30% of patients. It is primarily due to the disparate expression of RBC antigens in African Americans as compared to the donor pool, which is mostly composed of caucasians. Alloimmunization complicates RBC matching and can lead to delayed hemolytic transfusion reactions. Alloantigens can become undetectable by indirect Coombs test 2 months after exposure to mismatched blood, thereby causing future false-negative cross-matching results. A subset of heavily alloimmunized patients with SCD undergo life-threatening hemolytic reactions upon exposure to mismatched RBC units. In these hyperhemolytic crises, there is intense hemolysis of transfused and nontransfused RBCs and acute anemia. Treatment of hyperhemolytic crises includes erythropoietin-stimulating agents (ESA), parenteral steroids, and intravenous immunoglobulins (Gammagard).[1]

Iron Overload

Hemosiderosis is the other major complication of transfusional therapy in SCD and is characterized by iron deposition in the heart, liver, and endocrine glands, leading to organ failure and significant morbidity and mortality. Iron overload is likely in patients who have received more than 10 lifetime transfusions or more than 20 packed RBC units. Liver biopsy is the gold standard for diagnosis but it is an invasive and uncomfortable procedure. Noninvasive imaging methods such as quantitative liver and myocardial MRI and superconducting quantum interference device (SQUID) are not always available, and therefore diagnosis often rests on the finding of an elevated ferritin and transferrin saturation in the appropriate clinical setting.

---

[1]Not FDA approved for this indication.

Hemostatic Activation and Thrombosis

Numerous studies have shown that arterial and venous thrombosis are common in SCD and include pulmonary embolism, in situ pulmonary thrombosis, and stroke. In SCD, alterations at all levels of the hemostatic system have been described: patients with sickle cell disease exhibit increased basal and stimulated platelet activation, increased markers of thrombin generation and fibrinolysis, increased tissue factor activity, and increased von Willebrand factor (vWF) antigen and thrombogenic ultralarge vWF multimers. Interestingly, hemostatic activation is amplified during vaso-occlusive episodes, as shown by increases in multiple markers of thrombosis as compared to steady state, suggesting a link between hemolysis and thrombosis.

NEUROLOGY

Stroke is common in SCD and has a higher prevalence in children as compared to adults with SCD with a ratio of 3 to 1; the highest incidence is between 2 and 5 years of age. Patients can develop overt CVAs from large vessel occlusion (5%-8% of patients with HbSS) or silent infarcts from focal ischemia detectable by MRI without symptoms (20%-35% of patients with HbSS). The pathophysiology of stroke in SCD is unclear, although an unbalance between oxygen demand and supply has been postulated. Patients with repeated strokes may develop anatomic abnormalities and Moyamoya pattern of vascularization, which predisposes to cerebral hemorrhages later in life.

Both overt and silent strokes have a negative impact on the IQ and cause cognitive impairment measurable by psychometric testing. Children and adults with SCD can also develop cognitive impairment and subtle signs of accelerated brain aging and vascular dementia even in the absence of focal ischemia by MRI, with a low hematocrit being a predictor of cognitive impairment in children. These abnormalities are probably due to chronic and diffuse, as opposed to focal, cerebral anoxia and can be unmasked by psychometric testing even in the absence of cerebral lesions detectable by MRI. In patients who do have MRI abnormalities without a history of CVA, the gray matter is predominantly affected.

OPTHALMOLOGY

Retinal abnormalities are common in SCD and are often asymptomatic until the patient presents with opthalmologic emergencies. Retinal disease is due to arteriolar occlusion, with subsequent vascular proliferation, neovascularization, retinal hemorrhage (stage IV) and detachment (stage V). Patients with HbSC are more prone to retinal complications, possibly as a result of increased blood viscosity.

NEPHROLOGY

Renal abnormalities are common in SCD and manifest primarily as hematuria, proteinuria, and renal tubular acidosis, with most patients progressing to overt renal failure in adulthood. Hematuria is usually due to papillary necrosis and is an acute finding that requires supportive care and carries a good prognosis. Rarely, gross hematuria requires urologic consultation. Tubular functional defects include inability to concentrate urine (hyposthenuria) and renal tubular acidosis. Hyposthenuria often manifests with enuresis in childhood, and it is clinically relevant because it predisposes patients to an increased risk of dehydration. Renal tubular acidosis similar to type IV renal tubular acidosis is a common finding in SCD and can lead to hyperkalemia, an important consideration in patients already predisposed to hyperkalemia with intravascular hemolysis and whenever therapy with angiotensin-converting enzyme inhibitors is entertained.

Hyperphosphatemia and hyperuricemia are also often observed in SCD. Microalbuminuria can be detected by early adulthood and tends to progress to nephritic range proteinuria. Focal segmental glomerulosclerosis is the most common glomerular abnormality and it is probably due to glomerular sickling and infarction. There are currently no approved therapies to prevent progression to end-stage renal disease, which occurs in up to 20% of patients with SCD with a median age of 37 years, and renal replacement therapy is often needed in older adults with SCD. Serum creatinine and 24-hour creatinine clearance are not adequate for screening and monitoring of progression of kidney disease, because tubular secretion of creatinine is preserved and glomerular hyperfiltration is common in SCD, leading to relatively low creatinine and high glomerular filtration rate even in patients with underlying kidney impairment. The albumin or protein-to-creatinine ratio and plasma cystatin C levels may instead be used as a screening tool of glomerulopathy in SCD, and they can predict development of chronic kidney disease.

LEG ULCERS

Leg ulcers occur in 10% to 20% of patients with HbSS and have been associated with a chronically high hemolytic rate. They are usually located over the malleolar areas and are exquisitely painful, debilitating, disfiguring, and nonhealing. Vascular and plastic surgery consultation are recommended and aim at excluding local vascular problems that can complicate management of the ulcers and at providing prompt débridement and skin grafting. Although hydroxyurea is associated with development of leg ulcers in patients with myeloproliferative disorders, a review of the literature has failed to show an association with leg ulcers in SCD. Whereas wound healing may be impaired with hydroxyurea use, patients who develop an increase in fetal hemoglobin and have reduced sickling as a result of hydroxyurea therapy might have a net benefit in terms of tissue oxygenation and perfusion. In spite of these theoretical considerations, there is controversy over whether hydroxyurea can be safely used in patients with preexisting or concomitant leg ulcers. Transfusional therapy, including exchange transfusional therapy, and nutritional zinc supplementation, have shown benefit in anecdotal reports, but the evidence is inconclusive.

GASTROENTEROLOGY

Nausea, vomiting, and dyspepsia in SCD are related to delayed gastric emptying and gastrointestinal motility disorders, autonomic neuropathy, or medical therapy. Opiates are often responsible for acute nausea and vomiting, whereas other medications such as hydroxyurea and deferasirox (Exjade) are responsible for chronic symptoms. Gastroparesis may be due to damage of the microvasculature of autonomic nerves (vasa vasorum) from repeated episodes of sickling.

The liver may be episodically affected by hepatic sequestration crises, heralded by direct hyperbilirubinemia, right upper quadrant pain from distention of the hepatic capsule, acute anemia, and reticulocytosis. Elevation of liver injury tests may be drug-induced (hydroxyurea, deferasirox), but also related to hepatic sickling, particularly if it occurs during a vaso-occlusive episode. In older patients, post-transfusion hepatitis C can compound the hepatic manifestations of SCD.

Diarrhea is a common side effect of therapy with deferasirox and is usually self-limited. Lactose-intolerant patients might react to components of deferasirox.

INFECTIOUS DISEASE

Patients homozygous for HbSS develop functional asplenia during childhood. This is due to repeated episodes of splenic infarction leading to fibrosis and autosplenectomy. As a result, children are susceptible to overwhelming bacterial sepsis from encapsulated organisms such as *Staphylococcus pneumoniae*, *H. influenzae*, and *N. meningitidis*. High pediatric mortality from sepsis was therefore common before a landmark study published in 1986 demonstrated the benefit of penicillin prophylaxis instituted at birth. This study was the basis for neonatal screening in the United States. Vaccination for encapsulated organisms is also standard of care in children and adults. In spite of preventive measures, the incidence of life-threatening bacterial infections is increased in SCD, and high fever should be treated empirically as in splenectomized patients, with coverage for penicillin-resistant *S. pneumoniae* pending blood culture results. Patients with indwelling venous catheters are at risk of catheter-related bacteremia.

Viral infections with bone marrow–tropic viruses such as Epstein Barr virus, citomegalovirus, and predominantly parvovirus B19 place the patient at risk for bone marrow suppression, which can further worsen the chronic anemia. In children, infections with parvovirus B19 are responsible for transient red cell aplasia and severe aplastic crises, characterized by acute anemia and reticulocytopenia due to intra marrow destruction of erythroid precursors. Treatment of these episodes includes transfusion and intravenous immunoglobulins,[1] besides supportive measures.

PULMONOLOGY

A subset of patients with vaso-occlusive episodes develop acute chest syndrome, the major pulmonary complication of SCD. Acute chest syndrome is a lung injury syndrome defined by fever, pleuritic chest pain, oxygen desaturation, and multilobar radiographic infiltrates associated with severe vaso-occlusive episodes, infection, and bone marrow fat embolization (Fig. 2). It usually develops a few days after hospitalization for vaso-occlusive episodes and is often misdiagnosed as nosocomial pneumonia or aspiration pneumonia, particularly because it displays a predilection for the lower lobe of the lungs. Although pneumonia often accompanies acute chest syndrome, proper diagnosis is important because acute chest syndrome warrants simple or exchange transfusion in addition to antibiotic therapy and supportive measures. Common infectious pathogens identified in cases of acute chest syndrome include *Chlamidia pneumoniae*, *Mycoplasma pneumoniae*, and *Legionella pneumophyla*, thus dictating inclusion of a macrolide in the antibiotic cocktail. Pulmonary embolism with resulting infarct is also in the differential diagnosis of acute chest syndrome. If not recognized and treated promptly, acute chest syndrome leads to pulmonary failure and carries a high mortality.

Reactive airways disease is common in children with SCD and needs to be actively diagnosed and aggressively treated. Children with chronic respiratory symptoms need to be tested for bronchial hyperresponsiveness.

Chronic complications of SCD include pulmonary fibrosis and pulmonary hypertension. Several adult screening studies have reported that 20% of the population has mild pulmonary hypertension, defined by a pulmonary artery systolic pressure greater than 35 mm Hg (the upper limit of normal pulmonary artery systolic pressure is 32 mm Hg), and that 9% have moderate to severe pulmonary hypertension, defined by a pulmonary artery systolic pressure greater than 45 mm Hg. Despite pulmonary pressure increases that are much lower than those observed in patients with idiopathic or hereditable pulmonary hypertension, the prospective risk of death associated with even mild pulmonary hypertension is extremely high. It is recommended that adult patients with SCD be screened for pulmonary hypertension using transthoracic Doppler echocardiography. In SCD patients, the risk of death associated with high pulmonary artery systolic pressures rises linearly, and even values between 2.5 and 2.9 m/sec are associated with a high risk of death, with an odds ratio for death of 4.4 (95% confidence interval [CI], 1.6-12.2; $P < 0.001$); a test-retest variability of 3 m/sec or more is associated with an odds ratio for death of 10.6 (95% CI, 3.3-33.6; $P < 0.001$).

Right heart catheterization studies of patients with SCD and pulmonary hypertension reveal a hyperdynamic state similar to the hemodynamics characteristic of portopulmonary hypertension. It is increasingly clear that pulmonary pressures rise acutely in vaso-occlusive episodes and even more during acute chest syndrome. This suggests that acute pulmonary hypertension and right heart dysfunction represent a major comorbidity during acute chest syndrome, and right heart failure should be considered in patients presenting with acute chest syndrome.

CARDIOLOGY

Similarly to other conditions with chronic anemia, SCD is associated with a hyperdynamic state, low peripheral vascular resistance, and normal blood pressure or hypotension. In this setting, even mild elevation of the blood pressure can indicate relative hypertension and represent a risk factor for stroke. Because there are no studies on the treatment of hypertension in SCD, general guidelines on antihypertensive therapy are applied.

Coronary artery disease is rarely observed in SCD, although many patients complain of chest pain during vaso-occlusive episodes. In these instances, the usual work-up for acute coronary syndrome is

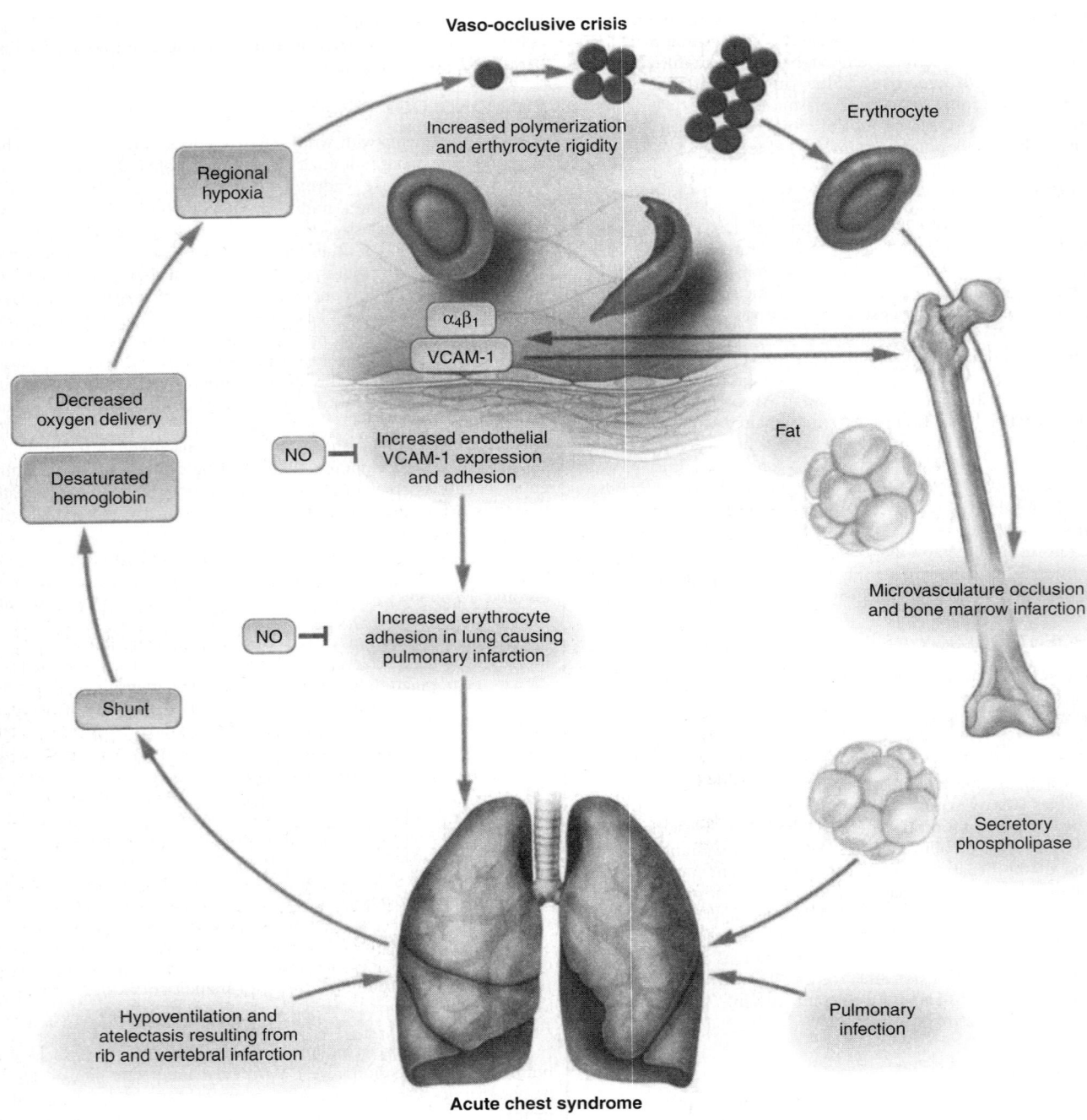

Vaso-occlusive crisis

Regional hypoxia

Increased polymerization and erthyrocyte rigidity

Erythrocyte

Decreased oxygen delivery

Desaturated hemoglobin

$\alpha_4\beta_1$

VCAM-1

NO ⊣ Increased endothelial VCAM-1 expression and adhesion

Fat

NO ⊣ Increased erythrocyte adhesion in lung causing pulmonary infarction

Microvasculature occlusion and bone marrow infarction

Shunt

Secretory phospholipase

Hypoventilation and atelectasis resulting from rib and vertebral infarction

Pulmonary infection

Acute chest syndrome

FIGURE 2. Pathogenesis of the acute chest syndrome. The major triggers associated with the development of acute chest syndrome are infection, bone marrow fat embolization, and direct red cell intravascular sequestration causing lung injury and infarction. Lung injury results in ventilation-perfusion mismatch and hypoxemia, which leads to increased hemoglobin S (HbS) polymerization and erythrocyte vaso-occlusion. This worsens bone marrow infarction and pulmonary vaso-occlusion to promote a vicious cycle. *Abbreviations:* NO = nitric oxide; VCAM-1 = vascular-cell adhesion molecule. (Adapted with permission from Gladwin MT, Vichinsky E: Pulmonary complications of sickle cell disease. N Engl J Med 2008;359:2254-2265.)

recommended. It is possible that myocardial microvascular occlusions are the predominant ischemic event in SCD.

Left-sided heart disease in SCD is primarily due to diastolic dysfunction (present in approximately 13% of patients), although cases of systolic dysfunction and mitral or aortic valvular disease can occur as well; the valves are diseased in approximately 2% of patients. The presence of diastolic dysfunction alone in SCD patients is an independent risk factor for mortality. Patients with both pulmonary vascular disease and echocardiographic evidence of diastolic dysfunction are at a particularly high risk for death (OR, 12.0; 95% CI, 3.8-38.1; $P < 0.001$).

Cardiac dysfunction is a late complication and the major cause of death in patients with iron overload. Heart failure and conduction defects are the most common abnormalities and warrant emergent iron chelation treatment. Both deferoxamine (Desferal) and deferasirox can reduce cardiac iron content and can be used in combination in severe cases.

Methadone (Dolophine) can lead to QTc prolongation, which can place patients at risk for arrhythmia and sudden death, particularly in the setting of pulmonary hypertension and iron overload. Frequent electrocardiographic (ECG) monitoring, as well as reducing the methodone dosage or discontinuing it, are warranted in this group, particularly if the QTc is greater than 500 msec.

ENDOCRINOLOGY

Iron overload is a common cause of endocrinopathy in SCD and thalassemia, with the hypophysis, gonads, and thyroid glands being particularly affected. Patients with iron overload should therefore undergo screening for endocrine dysfunction as it is routinely done in thalassemia.

Patients with SCD are at risk for specific endocrine problems regardless of their iron status. Delayed growth and puberty are relatively common, with delayed age of menarche by 2 to 3 years and small testicular size and hypospermia in boys. A multitude of factors is likely responsible for delayed growth and puberty in SCD, including increased catabolism, chronic hypoxemia, hospitalizations with prolonged immobility, ischemic insults during vaso-occlusive episodes, and chronic use of opiates.

PRIAPISM

Priapism is the most common urogenital manifestation of SCD and manifests predominantly in male patients with HbSS. It is defined as a sustained, painful erection in the absence of sexual stimulation. It is due to occlusion of the penile venous blood return during vaso-occlusive episodes and is defined as stuttering if it lasts from minutes to less than 3 hours and as prolonged if it lasts more than 3 hours. The latter is considered a urologic emergency because it leads to scarring and impotence, and it requires a urologic consultation. Pseudoephedrine (Sudafed)[1] can be used in the nonemergency setting to achieve detumescence, whereas aspiration of the corpus cavernosum is performed under conscious sedation and local anesthesia in the emergency setting. This is usually accompanied by instillation of epinephrine.[1] Other supportive measures such as intravenous fluids and parenteral opiates are usually required. If these measures fail, emergency exchange transfusion can be considered.

A rare neurologic syndrome known as ASPEN syndrome (*ass*ociation of sickle cell disease, *p*riapism, *e*xchange transfusion, and *n*eurologic events) has been described in patients with priapism who have undergone exchange transfusion. It is characterized by headache and seizures occasionally progressing to obtundation requiring mechanical ventilation.

Penile shunts might be required as a last resort to prevent further episodes of priapism by increasing the cavernous blood flow using native vessels or by creating an arteriovenous shunt. Penile shunts invariably result in impotence, which can be ameliorated by implantation of an inflatable penile prosthesis. An ongoing clinical trial is assessing whether sildenafil (Viagra)[1] therapy can prevent priapism by altering vascular smooth muscle tone through inhibition of phosphodiesterase 2 activity.

Diagnosis

The diagnosis of SCD rests on the hemoglobin electrophoresis or high-performance liquid chromatography (HPLC), which allow detection of most hemoglobin variants. In patients with microcytosis in which coinheritance of an α-thalassemia trait is suspected, α globin gene sequencing can be performed.

NEONATAL SCREENING

Children with SCD have an increased susceptibility to bacteremia due to *S. pneumoniae,* which can occur as early as 4 months of age and carries a case fatality rate as high as 30%. Acute splenic sequestration crises also contribute to mortality in infancy. Diagnosis by newborn screening and immediate entry into programs of comprehensive care, including the provision of effective pneumococcal prophylaxis, can reach infants who might otherwise be lost to the health care system and has been demonstrated to decrease morbidity and improve survival in children with SCD. Currently, newborn screening and follow-up of SCD are carried out in all 50 states in the United States as well as in most developed countries.

---

[1]Not FDA approved for this indication.

CURRENT DIAGNOSIS

- Sickle cell disease (SCD) is diagnosed by neonatal screening in the United States
- Persons with congenital hemolytic anemia should be tested for SCD by hemoglobin electrophoresis regardless of their ethnic background.
- Infection with parvovirus B19 should be suspected in children presenting with acute anemia and reticulocytopenia.
- Human leukocyte antigen (HLA) class I and II testing should be performed in all patients with SCD and unaffected siblings to identify donors for bone marrow transplant.
- Acute chest syndrome is diagnosed in patients presenting with fever, hypoxemia, and a radiographic pulmonary infiltrate.
- Screening for iron overload by ferritin, quantitative liver MRI, cardiac MRI, or liver biopsy is indicated in all patients who have received more than 10 lifetime transfusions.
- Pulmonary hypertension screening by transthoracic echocardiogram is indicated in all patients with SCD.

LATE DIAGNOSES AND MISDIAGNOSES

Rarely, patients who were born before universal screening was introduced or who were lost at the time of follow-up of positive neonatal screening only receive the diagnosis late in life. This is particularly the case of patients with HbSC, who might have normal hemoglobin and hematocrit and a mild disease phenotype. Occasionally, the disease is misdiagnosed as iron deficiency in patients with HbS/β$^+$-thalassemia on account of their microcytosis, and they undergo futile and potentially harmful prolonged trials of iron supplementation. Patients who have a low HbS level (<40%) due to recent transfusion or who have only mildly decreased hemoglobin (HbSC or HbS/β$^+$-thalassemia) may have an erroneous diagnosis of sickle cell trait (carrier state).

Treatment

From the original description of SCD in 1910 to the 1970s, there was no efficacious therapy for SCD, and most patients died within the first 2 decades of life, with infectious complications being responsible for the majority of pediatric fatalities. Several preventive and pharmacologic milestones since then, and the realization that care has to occur in a multidisciplinary setting, have profoundly affected the natural history of the disease (Table 3). Median age at death in resource-rich countries was 42 years in male patients and 48 years in female patients with HbSS, according to data from the Cooperative Study of Sickle Cell Disease in the 1980s (a pre-hydroxyurea setting), thereby still lagging approximately 2 to 3 decades behind that of the general African American population. The following sections summarize the therapeutic approach to the most important complications of SCD.

VASO-OCCLUSIVE EPISODES

Acute pain from vaso-occlusive episodes in SCD is extremely intense, affects both children and adults, and is due to ischemia or necrosis of the vascular beds. Most patients report severe pain in the bones and joints of the extremities, as well as lower back, although acute ischemia and pain can affect unusual sites such as the mandibular area. Occasionally, an affected limb displays the typical signs of inflammation, such as edema, warmth, and erythema, but a paucity of signs is the norm. Imaging studies such as MRI and bone scan can reveal signs of acute bone marrow infarction in a painful bony area, but they are not routinely employed in the work-up of a pain episode.

TABLE 3 Manifestations of Sickle Cell Disease with Key Prevention and Treatment Strategies

Manifestation	Prevention	Treatment
Pneumococcal sepsis	Penicillin, Prevnar/Pneumovax vaccination	Antibiotic therapy for penicillin-resistant *Streptococcus pneumoniae*
Splenic or liver sequestration	—	Transfusion
Painful vaso-occlusive episode	Hydroxyurea (Droxia), prevention of exposure to triggers	Intravenous fluids, parenteral opiates, supplemental oxygen
Acute chest syndrome	Incentive spirometry during VOE, hydroxyurea	Transfusion, broad-spectrum antibiotics with atypical coverage
Iron overload	Optimization of transfusion therapy	Iron chelation with deferasirox (Exjade) or deferoxamine (Desferal)
RBC alloimmunization	Transfusion with leukoreduced RBCs	—
CVA	Chronic transfusion in children with high transcranial Doppler velocity	Exchange transfusion and thrombolytics in selected cases
Pulmonary hypertension	Hydroxyurea?, treatment of predisposing conditions such as obstructive sleep apnea, hypoxemia, thromboembolism	Hydroxyurea, chronic transfusion therapy, specific therapy
Kidney disease	Antihypertensive therapy?, hydroxyurea?, ACE inhibitors?	ACE inhibitors?, renal replacement therapy, kidney transplant
Priapism	Chronic transfusion, hydroxyurea?	Pseudoephedrine (Sudafed),[1] aspiration of corpus cavernosum, exchange transfusion, sildenafil (Viagra)[1]?
Leg ulcers	Hydroxyurea?, chronic transfusion?	Surgical débridement, surgical grafting

[1]Not FDA approved for this indication.
ACE = angiotensin-converting enzyme; CVA = cerebrovascular accident; RBC = red blood cells; TCD = transcranial Doppler; VOE = vaso-occlusive crisis.

CURRENT THERAPY

- All children with sickle cell disease (SCD) should receive penicillin prophylaxis.
- High fever should be treated empirically with coverage for *Streptococcus pneumoniae* pending results of blood cultures.
- Children with high transcranial Doppler velocity need to be placed on a chronic transfusion regimen to keep the hemoglobin (Hb) S <30%, indefinitely.
- Painful vaso-occlusive episodes warrant prompt treatment with an individualized intravenous opiate regimen, as well as supportive care with intravenous 5% dextrose in water or half-normal saline and incentive spirometry.
- Preoperative transfusion should aim at a target hemoglobin level of ≤10 g/dL regardless of the HbS percentage and is indicated in all patients with SCD undergoing surgery.
- Therapy with hydroxyurea is indicated in all patients at all ages with HbSS disease, HbSβ-thalassemia, and HbSC with a severe phenotype.

- Erythropoietin-stimulating agents can be used in conjunction with hydroxyurea to prevent or ameliorate reticulocytopenia and in patients with underlying renal insufficiency.
- Iron chelation is indicated in all patients with findings of iron overload.
- Treatment of the acute chest syndrome includes parenteral antibiotics to cover for atypical microorganisms and transfusion, with exchange transfusion reserved for the most severe cases.
- Patients with pulmonary hypertension should receive optimal hematologic care (maximal hydroxyurea and/or chronic transfusion therapy) and specific therapy for pulmonary hypertension in severe cases, with coordination and referral to a pulmonary hypertension specialist.
- Bone marrow transplantation should be offered to all patients who have a matched donor and display a severe phenotype.

High-dose IV opiates, as well as nonsteroidal antiinflammatory drugs (NSAIDs), are the mainstay of treatment of a pain episode. Even in narcotic-naive patients with SCD, opioid dosages often exceed those required for other indications. For instance, doses of intravenous hydromorphone (Dilaudid) of 1 to 2 mg are typical in adult patients. Most patients, however, are on an oral pain regimen at home and have a history of multiple admissions for vaso-occlusive episodes, thereby dictating individualized care based on what has worked in the past and the patient's own perception of the intensity of pain. After an attempt at controlling the pain with three or four closely spaced narcotic boluses is made, patients who are in persistent discomfort or have evidence of underlying complications triggering the vaso-occlusive episode should be admitted and started on patient-controlled analgesia.

Common obstacles to prompt and effective care in SCD are the health professional's fear of overdosing the patient, as well as misconceptions about addiction and pseudoaddiction. In general, health care professionals tend to overestimate the prevalence of opioid abuse and addiction in SCD, and they tend to undertreat patients significantly, leading to patients' frustration and anger when their pain demands are not met (pseudoaddiction).

Nonpharmacological therapies such as biofeedback, relaxation, localized heat, and acupuncture are effective and should be incorporated in the management of pain episodes whenever possible. Care for vaso-occlusive episodes should also include management of possible precipitating factors: dehydration and hypovolemia should be corrected with hypotonic crystalloids, and an infection work-up should be initiated in patients with fever, hypoxemia, or leukocytosis above baseline. Antiemetics and antipruritus therapy is also usually needed.

Prior experiences such as that of the Bronx Comprehensive Sickle Cell Center have shown that a dedicated facility for effective and rapid management of uncomplicated vaso-occlusive episodes reduces hospitalizations and length of stay and facilitates integration of care—psychological, socioeconomic, and nutritional—in a multidisciplinary approach. This experience is at the basis of the concept of day hospital in SCD and relies on the need to provide prompt assessment and treatment of pain, safe dose titration to relief, monitoring of adverse effects, and adequate disposition (emergency department, inpatient admission, home) in a clinical environment familiar with SCD and the individual patient.

CHRONIC PAIN

Chronic pain is common, and recent literature based on pain diaries compiled by patients shows that most patients with SCD experience pain on an almost daily basis. Patients who have successfully transitioned from pediatric to adult care, have a good support system, and are distracted by their work or school schedules tend to cope better and require less pharmacologic support. In most cases, though, short-acting and long-acting opiates are required to empower the patient to manage pain at home and minimize use of the emergency department.

Because analgesic care is life-long, consultation with pain specialists is often valuable, particularly in patients for whom more-sophisticated pain regimens are needed. For instance, the mu-opioid receptor partial agonist buprenorphine (Buprenex), opioid rotation, and methadone used as analgesic can help reduce the total narcotic requirements. Urine toxicology screens are indicated and should be scheduled at regular intervals both to document adherence with the therapy and to screen for use of illicit substances.

TRANSFUSIONAL THERAPY

In SCD, the benefits of transfusion in terms of improved hemodynamics and oxygenation need to be balanced with the risks of iron overload, alloimmunization, transfusion reactions, and viral transmission. Leukoreduced, sickle-negative RBCs with extended phenotypic matching for Rh Cc, Ee, and Kell, which account for 80% of detected antibodies, are required. By employing extended phenotypic matching, the rate of alloimmunization decreased from 3% to 0.5% per unit, and the rate of delayed hemolytic transfusion reactions decreased by 90% in the STOP study. In previously immunized patients, a full RBC match also inclusive of matching for the Duffy, Kidd, and S antigens is recommended. Indications for transfusion include hemoglobin less than 5 g/dL or less than 6 g/dL with symptoms and any severe complication such as stroke, aplastic anemia, splenic or hepatic sequestration, or acute chest syndrome.

Prophylactic transfusions are also standard of care before surgery (with the exclusion of minor procedures such as intravenous port placement). A clinical trial published in 1995 showed that a conservative prophylactic transfusion regimen to achieve a target hemoglobin of 10 g/dL and any HbS value was as effective as an aggressive regimen to achieve a hemoglobin of 10 g/dL and a target HbS value of <30% in preventing postsurgical complications such as acute chest syndrome.

Exchange transfusion (erythrocytapheresis with RBC exchange) is usually reserved for the most severe complications such as acute chest syndrome with impending pulmonary failure, acute stroke and its prevention in children, intractable priapism, multiorgan failure and sepsis. Box 1 summarizes the main indications for simple and exchange transfusion in SCD as well as the areas of uncertainty.

IRON CHELATION

Patients who have received more than 10 transfusions or 20 units of packed RBCs should be screened for iron overload. Liver biopsy is the gold standard for diagnosis of iron overload but is invasive and uncomfortable. Imaging strategies such as liver or cardiac MRI and SQUID are preferred to guide iron chelation but are not always available. Ferritin is therefore often used as a surrogate measurement, although it has poor specificity. Most authorities recommend initiation of iron chelation based on a ferritin level consistently greater than 1000 ng/mL, based on data from the thalassemia literature.

BOX 1   Indications for Transfusion

No Indication
Chronic steady-state anemia
Uncomplicated painful episode
Infections
Minor surgery without general anesthesia
Aseptic necrosis of hip or shoulder
Uncomplicated pregnancy

Unclear Indication
Intractable or frequent painful episodes
Leg ulcers
Before receiving IV contrast dye
Complicated pregnancy
Cerebrovascular accident in adults
Chronic organ failure

Simple Transfusion
Symptomatic anemia
• High output cardiac failure
• Dyspnea
• Angina
• Central nervous system dysfunction
Sudden decrease in hemoglobin
• Aplastic crisis
• Acute spleen or hepatic sequestration
Severe anemia (Hb ~5 g/dL) with fatigue or dyspnea
Preparation for surgery with general anesthesia

Exchange Transfusion
Acute cerebrovascular accident
Multiple organ system failure
Acute chest syndrome
Priapism unresponsive to other treatments
Retinal surgery

In the United States, the oral chelating agent deferasirox and the parenteral deferoxamine are available and should be administered until the ferritin level is less than 500 ng/mL for three consecutive measurements. Patients on iron chelation need to be monitored for hepatic, renal, auditory and visual toxicity, and particular caution has to be exercised in the setting of renal disease, because transient, reversible increases in serum creatinine as well as rare instances of irreversible acute kidney injury have been reported in patients with underlying renal insufficiency. In most patients, however, deferasirox is well tolerated, and dyspepsia and diarrhea are the most common side effects.

ERYTHROPOIETIC STIMULATING AGENTS

Whereas a brisk reticulocytic response is common in SCD, patients who develop renal failure or aplastic crises or who receive therapy with hydroxyurea may experience a relative or absolute reticulocytopenia (<100,000 reticulocytes/mL) and a worsening of their baseline anemia. In these situations, therapy with erythropoietic stimulating agents (ESAs) is indicated. Occasionally, ESAs are used to allow upward titration of hydroxyurea and are used in combination with this medication. A review of the literature and of the experience at the NIH shows that ESAs are safe in patients with SCD, particularly when used in combination with hydroxyurea and when the target hemoglobin is no more than 10 g/dL

Because of bone marrow expansion in patients with HbSS, higher starting doses of erythropoietin (Epogen, Procrit)[1] than in patients

---

[1]Not FDA approved for this indication.

without SCD and on the order of 300 U/kg three times per week (or alternatively as a single dose of 900 U/kg once weekly) may be considered. For darbepoetin (Aranesp),[1] a reasonable starting dose is 100 to 200 μg/weekly or every 2 weeks. ESAs can be titrated by 20% to 25% increases in dose per week in patients who do not respond adequately. Weekly monitoring of hematocrit is essential to avoid overdosage and relative erythrocytosis, which can lead to hyperviscosity and vaso-occlusive episodes.

NUTRITIONAL CONSIDERATIONS

Malnutrition, growth retardation, and stunting with findings of low lean and fat body mass have a high prevalence in children and adolescents with SCD due to their increased caloric demands and a hypermetabolic state. Macronutrient and micronutrient deficiencies are common, and nutritional counseling is therefore warranted. Hypovitaminosis D and low bone mineral density are also prevalent in children and adults. Folic acid[1] is indicated at the dose of 1 mg daily as in other hemolytic diseases. Strategies aimed at decreasing iron intake and absorption should be implemented early. There is also growing interest in antioxidant nutrients, although there are no clear guidelines at present. The small subset of patients who are overweight or obese is at risk for exacerbating or precipitating common orthopedic problems in SCD such as avascular necrosis of the femoral heads and their resulting disability. These patients should also receive targeted nutritional counseling.

HYDROXYUREA

Since the pediatric hematologist Janet Watson suggested in 1948 that the paucity of sickle cells in the peripheral blood of newborns was due to the presence of increased red cell HbF, there has been interest in developing therapies to modulate the hemoglobin switch from fetal to newborn life. Several antineoplastic agents, including 5-azacytidine and hydroxurea, became the focus of attention after they were found to increase HbF levels in nonhuman primates and individuals with SCD.

The landmark Multicenter Study of Hydoxyurea in Sickle Cell Disease (MSH) then showed that the incidence of painful crises was reduced from a median of 4.5 per year to 2.5 per year in hydroxyurea-treated patients with SCD. The rates of acute chest syndrome and blood transfusion were also reduced significantly. A follow-up for up to 9 years of 233 of the original 299 subjects showed a 40% reduction in mortality among those who received hydroxyurea. This study led to the approval of hydroxyurea as the only disease-modifying therapy in SCD. More-recent studies also showed that hydroxyurea is safe and effective in children with SCD.

On a molecular and cellular level, the benefits of hydroxyurea are related to an increased HbF, with levels up to 20% to 25% in some patients. In these patients, increased intracellular levels of HbF prevent the formation of HbS polymers. In addition to this phenomenon, some patients on hydroxyurea who do not adequately increase their HbF levels also display clinical benefits, suggesting that hydroxyurea might have other unknown beneficial rheologic properties.

Although the MSH study only included patients with HbSS, its findings were extrapolated to other sickle cell syndromes such as HbSC and HbS/β-thalassemia. A report from Greece, where S/β-thalassemia is highly prevalent, confirmed that hydroxyurea similarly reduces complications and mortality in patients with HbS/β[0]-thalassemia, with a nonsignificant benefit also observed in HbS/β[+]. Although the NIH guidelines on SCD do recommend hydroxyurea in patients with HbSC disease, there is no direct published evidence of benefit in this population, and some authorities contend it should not be used because the main pathophysiologic alteration in HbSC is increased viscosity, not sickling.

Hydroxyurea should be started in patients with frequent pain episodes, history of acute chest syndrome, other severe vaso-occlusive episodes, or severe symptomatic anemia at a dosage of 15 mg/kg (7.5 mg/kg in patients with renal disease). Endpoints are less pain,

increase in HbF to 15% to 20%, increased hemoglobin level to 7 to 9 g/dL in severely anemic patients, improved well-being, and acceptable myelotoxicity. The dosage can be increased by 500 mg every other day every 8 weeks if no toxicity is encountered to a maximum of 35 mg/kg. Considering the potential myelotoxicity, hepatotoxicity, and nephrotoxicity of this medication, laboratory monitoring needs to be performed every 2 weeks at the time of initiation or escalation and monthly during maintenance therapy. Laboratory studies should include a complete blood cell count (CBC), differential and reticulocyte count, and serum chemistries. Measurements of HbF can be performed every 3 months. An elevated MCV is a marker of adherence to the therapy.

Hydroxyurea should be withheld in patients with an absolute neutrophil count less than 2000/μL, hemoglobin less than 9.0 g/dL with an absolute reticulocyte count less than 80,000/μL, a platelet count of less than 80,000/μL, elevated creatinine, twofold elevation of AST or alanine aminotransferase (ALT). Hydroxyurea should be withheld for 2 months before planned conception and during pregnancy (Fig. 3). Patients need to be counseled on the teratogenic potential as well as the theoretical risk of leukemogenesis, although to date no increase in baseline risk of leukemia in patients with SCD on hydroxyurea has been reported.

Side effects that can affect compliance are weight gain, thinning of the hair, skin and nail hyperpigmentation, nausea and vomiting, and mucosal ulcerations. Because of the toxicity concerns as well as factors intrinsic to long-term preventive therapy, hydroxyurea therapy has had low effectiveness in spite of high efficacy, with poor patient compliance being a major obstacle.

THERAPY OF PULMONARY HYPERTENSION

Because evidence-based guidelines for managing pulmonary hypertension in patients with SCD are not available, recommendations are based upon the pulmonary arterial hypertension literature, case

---

PROTOCOL FOR HYDROXYUREA TREATMENT

Start therapy if one or more of the following conditions are present:
- frequent pain episodes
- history of acute chest syndrome
- other severe VOE
- severe symptomatic anemia

Starting dose: 15 mg/kg or 7.5 mg/kg if the patient has kidney disease

Endpoints:
- less pain
- increase in Hb F to 15–20 percent
- increased hemoglobin level to 7–9 g/dL
- improved well-being
- acceptable myelotoxicity

Dose escalation: increase dose by 500 mg every other day every 8 weeks if no toxicity encountered to a maximum of 35 mg/kg

Lab monitoring:
- At time of initiation or escalation: check CBC/differential/reticulocyte count every 2 weeks; serum chemistries every 2–4 weeks, percent HbF every 6–8 weeks
- During maintenance: check CBC/differential/reticulocyte count. chemistries monthly, percent HbF every 3 months

Criteria to hold:
- ANC <2000
- Hb <9.0 g/dL and retic count <80,000 (alternatively start Epo)
- Platelet count <80,000
- Raising creatinine
- 2-fold elevation of AST or ALT over baseline
- 2 months prior to planned conception/pregnancy

FIGURE 3. Protocol for hydroxyurea treatment.

---

[1]Not FDA approved for this indication.

reports, small open-label studies, and expert opinion. For patients with mild pulmonary hypertension (tricuspid regurgitant velocity [TRV], 2.5-2.9 m/sec), it is important to identify and treat risk factors associated with pulmonary hypertension such as rest, exercise, nocturnal hypoxemia, sleep apnea, pulmonary thromboembolic disease, restrictive lung disease or fibrosis, left ventricular systolic and diastolic dysfunction, severe anemia, and iron overload. In these patients, medical therapy of SCD needs to be maximized, including optimization of hydroxyurea dosage and initiation of a chronic transfusion program in patients who do not tolerate or who respond poorly to hydroxyurea. Consultation with a pulmonologist or cardiologist experienced in pulmonary hypertension is also recommended.

For patients with TRV 3 m/sec or more, we recommend following the guidelines for TRV 2.5 to 2.9 m/sec. In addition, right heart catheterization is necessary to confirm diagnosis and to directly assess left ventricular diastolic and systolic function. We would consider specific therapy with selective pulmonary vasodilator and remodeling drugs if the patient has pulmonary arterial hypertension defined by right heart catheterization and exercise limitation defined by a low 6-minute walk distance.

FDA-approved drugs for primary pulmonary arterial hypertension include the endothelin receptor antagonists (bosentan [Tracleer] and ambrisentan [Letairis]), prostaglandin-based therapy (epoprostenol [Flolan], treprostinil [Remodulin, Tyvaso], and iloprost [Ventavis]), and the phosphodiesterase-5 inhibitors (sildenafil [Revatio]). No published randomized studies in the SCD population exist for any of these agents, although a multicenter placebo-controlled trial of sildenafil for pulmonary hypertension of SCD was stopped early because of an unexpected increase in hospitalizations for vaso-occlusive crisis in the treatment group.

Anticoagulation is indicated in patients who have evidence of pulmonary thromboembolic complications and is supported by evidence of benefit in other populations with pulmonary hypertension.

BONE MARROW TRANSPLANTATION

Despite improvement of supportive care in SCD, life expectancy remains lower than for those not affected. In addition, quality of life for patients with SCD is usually significantly impaired. Although hydroxyurea can decrease acute complications of SCD such as vaso-occlusive episodes and acute chest syndrome, no satisfactory measures exist to prevent the development of irreversible organ damage in adults. Further, therapy with hydroxyurea is lifelong, and only 20% to 30% of eligible patients are prescribed or actually take the drug.

Currently, allogeneic hematopoietic stem cell transplantation (HSCT) remains the only curative treatment. Indications for HSCT have been empirically determined from prognostic factors derived from studies of the natural history of SCD. The most common indications for which patients with SCD have undergone HSCT are a history of stroke, recurrent acute chest syndrome, or frequent vaso-occlusive episodes.

Allogeneic HSCT after myeloablative therapy has been performed in approximately 250 young (<16 years of age) patients with SCD. The backbone of the preparative regimens used have consisted of busulfan (Busulfex)[1] 14 to 16 mg/kg and cyclophosphamide (Cytoxan)[1] 200 mg/kg. Additional immunosuppressive agents used have included antithymocyte globulin (Atgam),[1] rabbit antithymocyte globulin (Thymoglobulin),[1] antilymphocyte globulin, or total lymphoid irradiation (Fig. 4). Cyclosporine A (Neoral),[1] alone or with mercaptopurine (Purinethol)[1] or methotrexate,[1] has been used for post-transplant graft-versus-host disease prophylaxis.

The outcome of HSCT for patients with SCD from matched siblings is excellent, with an overall survival of 93% to 97% and an event-free survival of 85%. Stabilization or reversal of organ damage from SCD has been documented after HSCT. In patients who have stable donor engraftment, complications related to SCD resolve, and there are no further episodes of pain, stroke, or acute chest syndrome. Patients who successfully receive allografts do not experience sickle-related central nervous system complications and have evidence of stabilization of central nervous system disease by cerebral MRI. However, the impact of successful HSCT on reversal of cerebral vasculopathy has been variable. Current research is focused on improving the applicability of HSCT to a greater proportion of patients with SCD by the development of novel conditioning regimens minimizing myeloablation (see Fig. 4) and the use of novel sources of hematopoietic stem cells such as umbilical cord blood.

---

[1]Not FDA approved for this indication.

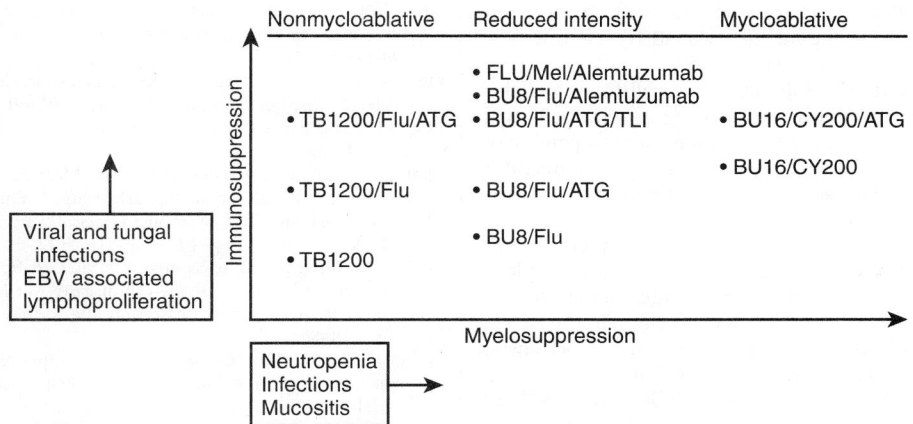

FIGURE 4. Spectrum of immunosuppression and myelosuppression in preparative regimens in hematopoietic stem cell transplantation (HSCT) in sickle cell disease (SCD). Most preparative regimens for HSCT in SCD have employed a backbone of busulfan (BU) (Busulfex)[1] and cyclophosphamide (CY) (Cytoxan).[1] Additional immunosuppressive agents include equine antithymocyte globulin (Atgam) or leporine antithymocyte globulin (Thymoglobulin) (ATG), antilymphocyte globulin, total lymphoid or total body irradiation (TLI or TBI), fludarabine (Flu) (Fludara),[1] and alemtuzumab (Campath).[1] Attempts to reduce the intensity of preparative regimens for patients with SCD have been based on one of two approaches. The first is the use of reduced-intensity conditioning regimens to produce less myeloablation. These require donor marrow infusion for hematopoietic recovery. The second is the use of nonmyeloablative regimens, which do not eradicate host hematopoiesis and allow hematopoietic recovery even without donor stem cell infusion. (Adapted with permission from Krishnamurti L: Hematopoietic cell transplantation: A curative option for sickle cell disease. Pediatr Hematol Oncol 2007;24:569-575.)

EXPERIMENTAL THERAPIES

Modulation of Cellular Dehydration

Cellular dehydration plays a key role in HbS polymerization and sickling and is caused by water loss through the Ca^{2+}-activated K^+ channel (IK1 or Gardos channel) and the K-Cl cotransport (KCC). The Gardos channel inhibitor senicapoc was tested in phase II and phase IIIs clinical trials, where it led to increased hemoglobin and decreased hemolysis but did not result in a reduction in the rate of pain episodes. There is hope that strategies aiming at reducing cellular dehydration may be used in combination with other therapies to prevent vaso-occlusive episodes.

Modulation of Nitric Oxide and Arginine

Nitric oxide (NO) is an active biogas and a free radical species that mediates arterial relaxation, cellular adhesion to endothelium, hemostasis, and blood viscosity. In SCD, NO bioactivity is reduced as a result of decreased production due to endothelial perturbation and NO scavenging by cell-free hemoglobin generated during intravascular hemolysis. Dietary supplementation with arginine,[7] a precursor of NO, and delivery of exogenous NO or NO bioactivity to the microvasculature in SCD, should promote dilatation of the terminal arterioles where obstruction to flow and tissue damage occurs, improvement of lung ventilation and perfusion matching, decrease in pulmonary artery pressures, and inhibition of platelet aggregation and cellular adhesion. Although two recent clinical trials on arginine supplementation and inhaled NO for vaso-occlusive episodes failed to show a clinical benefit, optimization of timing and dosing might lead to valuable NO therapeutics in the future.

SURGICAL ISSUES

Preoperative patient optimization includes prophylactic transfusion, close monitoring of pulse oximetry, adequate analgesia based on the patient's opiate tolerance, and monitoring for sickle cell–related complications.

Avascular necrosis (AVN) of the femoral heads, and more rarely of the humeral heads, is the most common orthopedic problem in SCD. Surgery is usually deferred until the pain and disability from AVN become intolerable and usually involves total hip or shoulder arthroplasty. This is usually a more involved procedure than in the general population on account of the altered bone anatomy in SCD. Patients with bone marrow expansion may experience thinning of the cortical bone and prosthetic instability, and some can suffer from the opposite problem of obliteration of the medullary shaft by sclerotic bone in response to multiple necrotic events.

Patients with SCD tend to develop pigmented gallstones and cholelithiasis. Cholecystectomy is performed in patients with SCD with cholelithiasis, right upper quadrant pain, and a positive hepatobiliary iminodiacetic acid (HIDA) scan. In SCD, the rate of intraoperative complications is higher and so is the rate of reversion from laparoscopic to open cholecystectomy.

Splenectomy is reserved for patients with massive splenic infarction (>50% of the spleen volume); intractable, recurrent splenic pain; and splenic abscess in the setting of splenic infarction. It is important to limit splenectomy to these few specific circumstances, because overwhelming sepsis and acute pulmonary hypertension have been reported in the postsplenectomy period in SCD.

Kidney transplantation has been successfully performed on patients with SCD on chronic renal replacement therapy. Kidney transplantation improves survival in patients with SCD, although survival at 7 years is lower than in African Americans without SCD (67% vs. 83%). This difference is due to vaso-occlusive complications in the transplanted kidney, possibly exacerbated by the higher hematocrit in the postoperative period from resumption of endogenous erythropoietin production and increased blood viscosity. It is therefore critical to closely monitor ESA therapy in the post-transplantation period to prevent overdosing and relative erythrocytosis. A

chronic transfusion program to prevent intrarenal sickling and maximization of hydroxyurea therapy should also be entertained. Combined solid organ and HSCT protocols are being developed to overcome these complications.

REFERENCES

Adams RJ, Brambilla D. Discontinuing prophylactic transfusions used to prevent stroke in sickle cell disease. N Engl J Med 2005;353:2769–78.

Adams RJ, Brambilla DJ, Granger S, et al. Stroke and conversion to high risk in children screened with transcranial Doppler ultrasound during the STOP study. Blood 2004;103:3689–94.

Bunn HF. Pathogenesis and treatment of sickle cell disease. N Engl J Med 1997;337:762–9.

Charache S, Terrin ML, Moore RD, et al. Effect of hydroxyurea on the frequency of painful crises in sickle cell anemia. Investigators of the Multicenter Study of Hydroxyurea in Sickle Cell Anemia. N Engl J Med 1995;332:1317–22.

Falletta JM, Woods GM, Verter JI, et al. Discontinuing penicillin prophylaxis in children with sickle cell anemia. Prophylactic Penicillin Study II. J Pediatr 1995;127:685–90.

Gaston MH, Verter JI, Woods G, et al. Prophylaxis with oral penicillin in children with sickle cell anemia. A randomized trial. N Engl J Med 1986;314:1593–9.

Gladwin MT, Sachdev V, Jison ML, et al. Pulmonary hypertension as a risk factor for death in patients with sickle cell disease. N Engl J Med 2004; 350:886–95.

Gladwin MT, Vichinsky E. Pulmonary complications of sickle cell disease. N Engl J Med 2008;359:2254–65.

Jeong GK, Ruchelsman DE, Jazrawi LM, Jaffe WL. Total hip arthroplasty in sickle cell hemoglobinopathies. J Am Acad Orthop Surg 2005;13:208–17.

Krishnamurti L, Kharbanda S, Biernacki MA, et al. Stable long-term donor engraftment following reduced-intensity hematopoietic cell transplantation for sickle cell disease. Biol Blood Marrow Transplant 2008;14:1270–8.

Lee MT, Piomelli S, Granger S, et al. Stroke Prevention Trial in Sickle Cell Anemia (STOP): Extended follow-up and final results. Blood 2006;108:847–52.

Little JA, McGowan VR, Kato GJ, et al. Combination erythropoietin-hydroxyurea therapy in sickle cell disease: Experience from the National Institutes of Health and a literature review. Haematologica 2006;91:1076–83.

Merkel KH, Ginsberg PL, Parker JC, Post MJ. Cerebrovascular disease in sickle cell anemia: A clinical, pathological and radiological correlation. Stroke 1978;9:45–52.

Morris CR, Kato GJ, Poljakovic M, et al. Dysregulated arginine metabolism, hemolysis-associated pulmonary hypertension, and mortality in sickle cell disease. JAMA 2005;294:81–90.

National Heart, Lung, and Blood Institute . The management of sickle cell disease, 4th ed. NIH Publication N0. 02-2117. PDF available for download at: www.nhlbi.nih.gov/health/prof/blood/sickle/sc_mngt.pdf; 2002 [accessed 10.07.10].

Noguchi CT, Rodgers GP, Serjeant G, Schechter AN. Levels of fetal hemoglobin necessary for treatment of sickle cell disease. N Engl J Med 1988;318:96–9.

Ohene-Frempong K, Weiner SJ, Sleeper LA, et al. Cerebrovascular accidents in sickle cell disease: rates and risk factors. Blood 1998;91:288–94.

Platt OS. The acute chest syndrome of sickle cell disease. N Engl J Med 2000;342:1904–7.

Platt OS, Brambilla DJ, Rosse WF, et al. Mortality in sickle cell disease. Life expectancy and risk factors for early death. N Engl J Med 1994;330:1639–44.

Platt OS, Thorington BD, Brambilla DJ, et al. Pain in sickle cell disease. Rates and risk factors. N Engl J Med 1991;325:11–6.

Reiter CD, Wang X, Tanus-Santos JE, et al. Cell-free hemoglobin limits nitric oxide bioavailability in sickle-cell disease. Nat Med 2002;8:1383–9.

Scheinman JI. Sickle cell disease and the kidney. Nat Clin Pract Nephrol 2009;5:78–88.

Smiley D, Dagogo-Jack S, Umpierrez G. Therapy insight: Metabolic and endocrine disorders in sickle cell disease. Nat Clin Pract Endocrinol Metab 2008;4:102–9.

Steinberg MH. Management of sickle cell disease. N Engl J Med 1999; 340:1021–30.

Steinberg MH, Barton F, Castro O, et al. Effect of hydroxyurea on mortality and morbidity in adult sickle cell anemia: Risks and benefits up to 9 years of treatment. JAMA 2003;289:1645–51.

Vichinsky EP, Neumayr LD, Earles AN, et al. Causes and outcomes of the acute chest syndrome in sickle cell disease. N Engl J Med 2000;342:1855–65.

Walters MC, Patience M, Leisenring W, et al. Bone marrow transplantation for sickle cell disease. N Engl J Med 1996;335:369–76.

Walters MC, Storb R, Patience M, et al. Impact of bone marrow transplantation for symptomatic sickle cell disease: An interim report. Multicenter investigation of bone marrow transplantation for sickle cell disease. Blood 2000;95:1918–24.

---

[7]Available as dietary supplement.

Neutropenia

Method of
Mary Ann Bonilla, MD

Host defense against infection is composed of the humoral and cellular immune systems. B cells provide humoral immunity against extracellular pathogens through antibody production. T cells facilitate antibody production by B cells and also are effectors of antigen-specific cell-mediated immunity that eliminates viruses, mycobacteria, and tumor cells. Phagocytes, such as monocytes and neutrophils, provide protection against invading bacteria and fungi. The neutrophil or polymorphonuclear leukocyte population has two compartments, a marginated pool attached to the vascular endothelium and a circulating pool. In response to an inflammatory stimulus, neutrophils migrate toward the organisms (chemotaxis), ingest them (phagocytosis), and kill them through the process of lysosomal fusion and generation of oxygen radicals.

Neutropenia is defined as an absolute decrease in the number of circulating neutrophils. Normal neutrophil levels are age and race related, with approximately 25% to 50% of persons of African descent and some ethnic groups in the Middle East having lower leukocyte and neutrophil counts without infectious complications (benign ethnic neutropenia). The absolute neutrophil count (ANC) is calculated by multiplying the total white blood cell (WBC) count by the percentage of neutrophils and bands present on the differential: ANC = WBC × (% neutrophils + % bands). An increased susceptibility to infection is proportional to the level of neutropenia. In mild neutropenia (ANC of 1000–1500 cells/mm^3), the patient usually is asymptomatic. In moderate neutropenia (ANC of 500–1000 cells/mm^3), stomatitis or aphthous ulcers, gingivitis, recurrent otitis, or skin infections may be seen. In severe states (ANC <500 cells/mm^3), the risk of pyogenic life-threatening infections increases and includes pneumonias, sinusitis, abscesses, and overwhelming sepsis. Bacteria and fungi that compose the normal oral and enteric flora cause the infections most commonly seen.

The duration of neutropenia influences the risk of infectious complications. Neutropenia may be acute or chronic (lasting >3 months); it may exist as a single cytopenia or as part of a complex disease process; and it may be acquired or congenital. This article provides an approach to the diagnosis, evaluation, and treatment of neutropenia and its complications.

Evaluation of Neutropenia

An accurate and complete clinical history is essential in establishing the onset and possible etiology of the neutropenia. Key points should include the onset, duration, type, frequency, and severity of infections; any exposure to toxins or drugs; and when the neutropenia was first noted by laboratory testing. Obtaining previous complete blood count (CBC) results to document onset can be difficult, because such measurements are not routinely performed in young children, but these data may yield invaluable information.

A detailed physical examination, focusing on adenopathy, splenomegaly, and phenotypic abnormalities including skeletal anomalies, should be performed. Special attention should be given to possible sites of active or chronic infection, especially the oral cavity, gingiva, perirectal area, skin, and sites of chronic infection such as sinuses. Evidence of poor growth suggesting failure to thrive, malabsorption, or nutritional deficiencies must be documented.

Laboratory assays include a CBC with differential and morphologic examination of the peripheral smear for evidence of nutritional deficiency disorders, myelokathexis, Chédiak-Higashi syndrome, or the presence of blasts. Serial blood counts, two to three times weekly, for 4 to 6 weeks are necessary to yield the characteristic 21-day fluctuations in ANC associated with cyclic neutropenia. Viral infections are the most common cause of neutropenia in young children. Titers for hepatitis, Epstein-Barr virus, cytomegalovirus, varicella, influenza, human immunodeficiency virus, and respiratory syncytial virus may be indicated. Assays for T- and B-cell immunophenotyping and function, immunoglobulins, and complement levels may reveal an underlying immunodeficiency.

Positive antineutrophil antibodies detected by agglutination or flow cytometry assays can support the suspected diagnosis of an immune neutropenia. However, a negative result does not exclude this diagnosis, because of the many technical difficulties and reliability of these assays. Gene mutations of ELANE are commonly seen in cyclic, or non-Kostmann's congenital neutropenias. Genetic studies are commercially available for other congenital neutropenias as well (Table 1). Additional studies that may be indicated are antinuclear antibodies and complement to screen for collagen vascular disease; and serum copper, vitamin B$_{12}$, and red blood cell folate levels in adults.

Bone marrow examination is indicated for persistent neutropenia or when more than one lineage abnormality is present, to exclude leukemia, myelodysplasia, metastatic tumor cells, and aplastic anemia. Morphology may reveal a myeloid maturation arrest, or a retention of neutrophils characteristic of a congenital neutropenia. Cytogenetic and fluorescence in situ hybridization (FISH) analysis to detect leukemia or myelodysplastic syndrome–associated abnormalities of chromosomes 5, 7 and 8, should be performed particularly before the initiation of therapy with granulocyte colony-stimulating factor (G-CSF).

Classification

Neutropenia may result from decreased or ineffective marrow production or increased peripheral destruction. A simple classification divides the neutropenias into acquired and congenital forms.

ACQUIRED NEUTROPENIAS

Acquired neutropenias can be caused by infection, drugs, or immune mechanisms, or they may be part of a systemic disorder. The most common cause of acquired neutropenia is infection causing toxic injury or hemophagocytosis. Bacterial infections such as typhoid fever, shigella enteritis, brucellosis, and tularemia are associated with neutropenia. Viral (e.g., hepatitis, Epstein-Barr virus, HIV, cytomegalovirus, herpesvirus-6), rickettsial (e.g., ehrlichiosis) and parasitic (e.g., malaria) infections have been implicated as causative agents.

TABLE 1 Congenital Neutropenia

	Inheritance	Chromosome	Gene Mutation
Severe congenital neutropenia	AD	19p13.3	ELANE
	AD	1p22	2Gfi
Kostmann's neutropenia	AR	1q21.3	HAX
X-linked neutropenia	X-linked	Xp11.232	WAS
Cyclic neutropenia	AD	19p13.36	ELANE
Shwachman-Diamond syndrome	AR?	7q11	SBDS
Barth's syndrome	X-linked	Xq28	TAZ
Chédiak-Higashi syndrome	AR	1q42.1-q42.2	LYST

Reprinted with permission from Pamblad JE, von dem Borne AE: Idiopathic, immune, infectious, and idiosyncratic neutropenias. Semin Hematol 2002;39(2):113.
Abbreviations: AD = autosomal dominant; AR = autosomal recessive.

Some drugs (e.g., chemotherapeutic agents) induce neutropenia because of their cytotoxic effects on the bone marrow and the short half-life of neutrophils. Other medications induce neutropenia by idiosyncratic, immune-mediated, or toxic mechanisms. High-risk categories include antithyroid medications, macrolides, and procainamide (Pronestyl). Other agents include antimicrobials (penicillin, cephalosporin, vancomycin [Vancocin]), analgesics and antiinflammatory agents (indomethacin [Indocin], ibuprofen [Advil]), antipsychotics, antidepressants, anticonvulsants (valproic acid [Depakene], phenytoin [Dilantin]), histamine 2 receptor antagonists (cimetidine [Tagamet], ranitidine [Zantac]), and heavy metals (gold, arsenic, and mercury).

Autoimmune neutropenia of childhood (usually diagnosed before 2 years of age) is considered benign because of the low incidence of serious infections and spontaneous resolution of the neutropenia by 5 years of age. Although patients may respond to intravenous immunoglobulin (GammaGard)[1] and G-CSF (filgrastim [Neupogen]), most require no intervention. Idiopathic neutropenia seen in older children and adults is a diagnosis of exclusion when no other etiology can be elicited. There is a female predominance, serious infections are absent, anemia is occasionally present, splenomegaly is absent, and often there is no spontaneous remission. Other disorders associated with immune-mediated neutropenia include systemic lupus erythematosus, scleroderma, Felty's syndrome, and the inherited autoimmune lymphoproliferative syndrome (ALPS).

CONGENITAL NEUTROPENIA

Although congenital disorders are rare, a family history of neutropenia, severe infection, or sudden death should suggest the diagnosis. Autosomal recessive Kostmann's disease or autosomal dominant non-Kostmann's neutropenia is marked by severe neutropenia (200 cells/mm^3) and a maturational arrest at the promyelocyte level in the bone marrow. Similar features can be seen with a variant of Wiskott-Aldrich syndrome in neutropenic males with monocytopenia, decreased CD4/CD8 ratio, and no eczema. Cardiac or proximal myopathy and hypoglycemia with associated neutropenia (cyclic, chronic, or intermittent) may suggest Barth's syndrome, an X-linked genetic disorder primarily affecting males. Hypoglycemia and neurologic abnormalities manifesting in infancy may reveal metabolic disorders such as glycogen storage disease type 1b. Pancreatic insufficiency resulting in failure to thrive and metaphyseal chondrodysplasia can be signs of Shwachman-Diamond syndrome. Neutropenia in a patient with partial oculocutaneous albinism and giant lysosomes in granulocytes suggest Chédiak-Higashi syndrome. Short stature, thumb abnormalities, or pigment skin anomalies may suggest Fanconi's anemia. The Online Mendelian Inheritance in Man website provides a current comprehensive compendium of human genes and genetic phenotypes of these disorders.

Therapy

TREATMENT OF INFECTION

A diagnosis of neutropenia and fever should be considered a medical emergency. A thorough physical examination, including the ear, nasal, and oral cavities as well as the perirectal areas, is necessary. Imaging of the sinus, mastoids, or lungs may be indicated if symptoms suggest an undocumented infection. A CBC to assess the current ANC and appropriate cultures should be obtained. For patients having an ANC lower than 500 cells/mm^3 and for those who are ill-appearing, broad-spectrum antibiotic therapy should be initiated immediately. Because these patients are at high risk for sepsis from staphylococcal and gram-negative organisms, hospitalization is recommended. Duration of antibiotic therapy is not standardized, but in patients without a focus of infection who subsequently become afebrile and whose cultures are negative, antibiotics may be discontinued after 48 hours of therapy.

TREATMENT OF NEUTROPENIA

In healthy, asymptomatic adults and children, observation alone may be indicated. Offending medications should be withdrawn. The most

[1]Not FDA approved for this indication.

important preventive measure to avoid infection is good hand washing and attention to oral hygiene. Regular dental cleaning, daily flossing, and the use of a mouthwash containing peroxide-based (e.g., Colgate Peroxyl 1.5%) or antibacterial (e.g., Biotene Antibacterial Mouthwash) enzymes may alleviate the gingivitis. Despite this, patients still may be symptomatic, and care to avoid dehydration should be taken if aphthous ulcers are present. So-called magic mouthwash solution, containing viscous lidocaine[6] to provide topical relief from oral ulcers, can be employed. Rectal temperature measurements and rectal suppositories should be avoided.

If the patient has severe neutropenia or develops recurrent or persistent infections, growth factor administration should be considered. G-CSF is now considered the standard of care. In patients with congenital neutropenia (e.g., Kostmann's syndrome, Shwachman-Diamond syndrome, glycogen storage disease type 1b), G-CSF may be started at 5 µg/kg/day. Patients with cyclic neutropenia may respond to a lower dose of 3 µg/kg/day. Those occasional patients with idiopathic or immune neutropenia, who develop significant infections, may respond to a lower dose of 1 µg/kg/day. Dosages should be titrated to achieve an ANC between 1000 and 1500 cells/mm^3 and to maintain the patient infection free. If there is no response to increasing doses of G-CSF (seen more commonly in congenital neutropenia), the dose should be increased every 2 to 4 weeks. Neutropenia that fails to respond to doses greater than 100 µg/kg/day are considered refractory. Patients with refractory disease may be candidates for an HLA-matched related stem cell transplantation.

The development of acute myeloid leukemia and sepsis leading to death has been reported in patients with congenital neutropenia. This may be associated with other abnormalities, such as G-CSF receptor mutations. The current recommendation is to monitor with yearly bone marrow studies in congenital neutropenia patients on chronic G-CSF therapy. The Severe Chronic Neutropenia International Registry maintains long-term data regarding this and other outcomes as well as providing a patient and physician referral database and coordinating research efforts.

[6]May be compounded by pharmacists.

REFERENCES

Hsieh MM, Everhart JE, Byrd-Holt DD, et al. Prevalence of neutropenia in the U.S. population: Age, sex, smoking status, and ethnic differences. Ann Intern Med 2007;146(7):486.

Online Mendelian Inheritance in Man (OMIM) website. Available at: http://www.ncbi.nlm.nih.gov/sites/entrez?db=omim [accessed June 19, 2009].

Pamblad JE, von dem Borne AE. Idiopathic, immune, infectious, and idiosyncratic neutropenias. Semin Hematol 2002;39(2):113.

Rosenberg PS, Alter BP, Bolyard AA, et al. The incidence of leukemia and mortality from sepsis in patients with severe congenital neutropenia receiving long-term G-CSF therapy. Blood 2006;107:4628.

Hemolytic Disease of the Fetus and Newborn

Method of
Michael A. Posencheg, MD, and
Phyllis A. Dennery, MD

Epidemiology

Early-onset hyperbilirubinemia, anemia with or without edema in the fetus or newborn, was previously synonymous with hemolytic disease resulting from Rh-isoimmunization. With the onset of the use of Rh-immunoglobulin (RhIg [RhoGAM]) in pregnant Rh-negative women that is most commonly seen in male infants, but females can also manifest the disease. Interestingly, this disease accounts for a disproportionately large percentage of infants who develop kernicterus. α-Thalassemia is a rare hemoglobinopathy in which all α-globin chain genes are deleted. It is most common in Asian infants and is nearly uniformly fatal, with severe fetal anemia and hydrops fetalis, especially when intrauterine transfusions have not been performed.

in 1968, the landscape of this disorder has changed dramatically. The differential diagnosis of hemolytic disease of the fetus and newborn is broad and can be subdivided into isoimmune and nonimmune categories (Box 1). In this article, we discuss various diseases that result in fetal and neonatal hemolysis, along with recent improvements in diagnosis and management.

Isoimmune hemolytic disease in the fetus and newborn manifests when maternal antibodies cross the placenta and bind to antigens present on the baby's red blood cells. These antigens include Rh factor (D antigen), leading to Rh isoimmunization, the major blood group antigens (e.g., A, B) leading to ABO incompatibility, or minor blood group antigens (e.g., Kell, Kidd, Duffy). The incidence of Rh isoimmunization has now fallen from nearly 14% of pregnancies in the pre-RhIg era to between 1 and 6 per 1000 live births. Incomplete eradication is due to inadvertent failures of RhIg administration, poor prenatal care, or earlier sensitization. Rh-isoimmunization can lead to severe complications, with up to 20% of fetuses having significant anemia and evidence of hydrops in utero.

ABO incompatibility occurs nearly exclusively in fetuses and newborns with type A or B blood born to mothers with type O blood. Although nearly one quarter of pregnancies result in ABO incompatibility, only approximately 1% to 5% of ABO-incompatible infants demonstrate significant hemolytic disease. The incidence of hemolytic disease from minor antigens is more difficult to estimate due to the large number of antigen-antibody reactions that can result in disease. Of the minor antigens, Kell and Duffy antigens are associated with the most severe disease, and Lewis and Lutheran are more likely associated with mild or insignificant hemolysis.

The group of disorders that is nonimmune in nature results in red blood cell destruction in the absence of an antibody-antigen reaction. These include red blood cell membrane defects such as hereditary elliptocytosis or spherocytosis, red blood cell enzyme defects such as glucose-6-phosphate dehydrogenase (G6PD) deficiency and pyruvate kinase deficiency, and hemoglobinopathies such as α-thalassemia. With rates up to 1 in 5000 live births, hereditary spherocytosis is the most common of the RBC membrane defects, occurring most commonly in infants of Northern European descent.

Of the enzyme defects, G6PD is the most common, especially in infants of African or Mediterranean descent. It is an X-linked disorder

Risk Factors

Several elements of the maternal, fetal, and neonatal histories can assist in determining a fetus's or infant's risk of developing one of these hemolytic processes. The results of the maternal blood type and antibody screen are useful to evaluate this risk. Infants born to mothers with type O blood are at risk for ABO incompatibility, whereas infants born to mothers with Rh-negative blood are at risk for Rh isoimmunization. The antibody screen that is performed on maternal blood is specifically searching for antibodies associated with the minor antigen groups that can also be found on red blood cells. Selected minor antigens are listed in Table 1. The presence of a positive direct Coombs' test should raise suspicion of an isoimmune hemolytic process. This test is not always available or warranted.

Assessing the risk of nonimmune disease is based almost entirely on a complete family history. Many of these disorders are associated with certain ethnic or geographic backgrounds. As examples, G6PD deficiency is found more commonly in persons of African or Mediterranean descent, and a family history of persistent anemia requiring splenectomy is often seen in hereditary spherocytosis.

Pathophysiology

The isoimmune forms of fetal and neonatal hemolysis have a similar pathophysiology in that all of them involve the passage of specific maternal IgG antibodies across the placenta, which then interact with their corresponding antigens on the fetal red blood cells. Red cell destruction results when the antibody-coated cells are scavenged by the mononuclear phagocytic system. The production of maternal antibodies is usually the result of previous exposure of the maternal system to fetal red blood cells, which is common during labor or abortion. The initial response of the maternal immune system is to produce IgM antibodies, but repeat exposure elicits an IgG response. This is especially true for Rh isoimmunization, and therefore explains why first-born Rh-positive infants born to Rh-negative mothers are not affected.

In ABO incompatibility, antibodies to A or B antigens already exist, but they are normally IgM antibodies. They do not cross the placenta and therefore do not result in disease. It is only when the antigenicity results in the production of IgG antibodies that passage across the placenta can occur and disease can result. This is exceeding uncommon in blood type A with B incompatibility (mother is type A, baby is type B), but is more common in mothers with blood type O who have a fetus with either blood type A or B. This can occur in first-born infants. As to hemolysis from antibodies to minor antigens, IgG antibody production may be the result of prior exposure to fetal cells such as during a previous pregnancy or via prior blood transfusion.

TABLE 1   Selected Minor Antigens Associated with Fetal or Neonatal Hemolytic Disease

Blood Group	Severe Disease	Rarely Severe Disease	Mild Disease	Usually No Disease
Rh	D, c	C, E, f, Evans, G, Rh29, Rh32, Rh42, Rh46, and others	E,e,f	
Lutheran			Lu^a, Lu^b	
Kell	K	k, Kp^a, Kp^b, Ku, Js^a, Js^b, K11, K22	Ku, Js^a, K11	K23, K24
Lewis				Le^a, Le^b
Duffy		Fy^a	Fy^b, Fy3	
Kidd		Jk^a	Jk^b, Jk3	

Adapted from Eder AF: Update on HDFN: New information on long-standing controversies. Immunohematology 2006;22(4):188-195; and Moise KJ: Fetal anemia due to non–Rhesus-D red-cell alloimmunization. Semin Fetal Neonatal Med 2008;13:207-214.

The pathophysiology of the nonimmune group of hemolytic disease is unique to the specific disease process. Red blood cell membrane defects, such as hereditary spherocytosis, have specific abnormalities of red blood cell membrane proteins that result in abnormal red blood cell shapes. These cells are more prone to destruction from mechanical forces. The enzyme defects such as G6PD and pyruvate kinase deficiency result in an inability of the red blood cell to protect itself from oxidant stress (G6PD) or to produce energy (pyruvate kinase). This makes the cell more prone to hemolysis. Hemoglobinopathies result in anemia from decreased production of stable hemoglobin chains. Specifically, α-thalassemia major involves the lack of production of the α chain of hemoglobin and leads to early fetal anemia, severe hydrops, and death unless intrauterine transfusions are instituted.

Prevention

The administration of Rh-immunoglobulin (RhIg) to mothers who are Rh-negative has dramatically decreased the incidence of hemolytic disease resulting from Rh-isoimmunization. The current recommendation of the American College of Obstetrics and Gynecology (ACOG) is to administer 300 μg of RhIg intramuscularly at 28 weeks' gestation and within 72 hours of delivery of an Rh-positive infant to an Rh-negative mother. RhIg should also be administered to Rh-negative mothers if the mother undergoes amniocentesis, chorionic villus sampling, or cordocentesis, or in the event of maternal bleeding due to placental abruption, placental previa, partial molar pregnancy, spontaneous abortion, or elective termination.

Controversy exists regarding the use of RhIg in the first trimester. As early as 7 weeks of gestation, fetal blood cells can express the D antigen, and women with threatened abortion in the first trimester have been shown to become Rh-sensitized, although this is rare event. Some advocate for administration of RhIg 50 μg (MICRhoGAM) intramuscularly in the first trimester in the setting of spontaneous abortion, elective termination, ectopic pregnancy, or threatened abortion.

The proposed mechanism of action for RhIg involves binding to Rh-positive fetal cells with resultant scavenging by the maternal mononuclear phagocytic system before sensitization and production of maternal antibody against the Rh-D antigen. Sadly, the other forms of hemolytic disease do not have specific preventive strategies.

Clinical Manifestations

The clinical presentation of hemolytic disease in the fetus and newborn varies according to the timing and severity of the disease. Significant and early hemolysis in utero results in fetal anemia, and, as oncotic pressure decreases in the fetal blood vessels, edema forms in the soft tissues and potential spaces. Hydrops fetalis results when there is edema or fluid accumulation in at least two of these spaces: skin, pleura, pericardium, or peritoneum. If this continues unabated, fetal death can result. Of all of the diseases discussed here, Rh-isoimmunization and α-thalassemia are those most commonly associated with fetal anemia and the most severe disease.

Most commonly, hemolytic disease results in early neonatal onset anemia and significant hyperbilirubinemia. Often, infants present with clinical jaundice in the first 24 hours of life and have a significant rate of rise of their serum bilirubin levels or a prolonged course of hyperbilirubinemia. Neonatal anemia with significant hyperbilirubinemia is a common manifestation of ABO incompatibility, hemolysis due to minor antigens, and red blood cell enzyme and membrane defects. The degree of anemia in each, however, is quite variable even within a given diagnosis.

Diagnosis

The assessment of maternal blood type and antibody screen can provide valuable insight into the risk of isoimmune hemolytic anemia. Ultrasound techniques and amniocentesis for the antenatal monitoring of fetal anemia are reviewed later.

CURRENT DIAGNOSIS

- The direct antiglobulin, or Coomb's test (DAT) on neonatal blood is the cornerstone for differentiating isoimmune from non–immune-mediated hemolysis.
- The presence of a positive antibody screen in maternal blood should raise suspicion for hemolytic disease resulting from minor antibody-antigen reactions.
- In utero monitoring for severe fetal anemia includes maternal antibody screen titers, △OD450 measurement, middle cerebral artery peak systolic velocity, and cordocentesis.
- Serial and frequent measurements of bilirubin levels and complete blood counts postnatally can aid the practitioner in determining whether therapy should be escalating.

In the neonate, concern for hemolytic anemia results from a rapidly rising bilirubin level, especially in the first 24 hours of life, a positive direct Coombs' test, hemolysis detected on a blood smear with anemia detected on a complete blood count (CBC), or prolonged hyperbilirubinemia, individually or in combination. In addition to following serial bilirubin levels, in this setting the practitioner should include a neonatal blood type, Coombs' (DAT) test, and complete blood count with reticulocyte count to determine whether hemolysis is occurring. A positive DAT in the appropriate clinical setting suggests isoimmune hemolysis, and a negative DAT nearly rules it out. However, in the setting of ABO incompatibility a significant number of infants can have a positive Coombs' test and not have significant hemolysis.

A G6PD level can be helpful in establishing a diagnosis in infants with the appropriate ethnic background or geographic location. Many states have adopted universal newborn screening for G6PD deficiency. Serum albumin, the primary protein transporter for bilirubin in the blood, can also be measured. Low serum levels of albumin increase the risk of developing neurologic sequelae from the subsequent increased amount of free, unbound bilirubin crossing the blood-brain barrier.

Differential Diagnosis

The differential diagnosis of hemolytic disease starts with determining whether or not the hemolysis is antibody-mediated (see Box 1).

Isoimmune hemolytic disease involves the production of maternal IgG antibodies against antigens on fetal red blood cells, resulting in hemolysis. The major diseases in this group include Rh isoimmunization, ABO incompatibility, and hemolysis resulting from the production of antibodies to minor red blood cell antigens. Examples of these include the broad groups Kell, Duffy, Lutheran, Lewis, and Kidd.

The non–immune mediated hemolytic diseases result from inherent defects in the neonatal red blood cells or hemoglobin productions. Examples of these include the red blood cell membrane defects such as hereditary spherocytosis and hereditary elliptocytosis; red blood cell enzyme defects, including G6PD deficiency and pyruvate kinase deficiency; and hemoglobinopathies, most notably α-thalassemia. Descriptions of these have been included elsewhere in this article.

Treatment

The goals of therapy are different depending on the timing of disease. When significant hemolysis occurs in utero, the fetus becomes progressively anemic. In the fetus, bilirubin is normally processed and excreted through the placenta. Therefore, the primary concern is to treat the anemia and, in doing so, prevent or reverse any signs of edema or hydrops fetalis. In this circumstance, percutaneous umbilical blood sampling (PUBS) and intrauterine blood transfusion can diagnose and treat fetal anemia, respectively.

CURRENT THERAPY

- Intrauterine transfusion may be indicated in the setting of severe fetal anemia with or without edema or hydrops fetalis.
- Phototherapy, the mainstay of postnatal management of hyperbilirubinemia, converts unconjugated bilirubin in a nonenzymatic fashion to a polar, water-soluble form that is more readily excretable.
- Intravenous immunoglobulin (Gammagard)[1] is indicated in infants who have isoimmune hemolytic disease and bilirubin levels approaching the threshold for double-volume exchange transfusion.
- Double-volume exchange transfusion is reserved for infants who fail phototherapy and intravenous immunoglobulin (if indicated). It replaces and removes approximately 86% of the infant's own blood. In the setting of isoimmune hemolytic disease, double-volume exchange transfusion has the added benefit of removing offending maternal antibodies, which contribute to the hemolysis from the infant's circulation.

[1]Not FDA approved for this indication.

In the neonate, the problem is somewhat different. In the absence of placental transfer and maternal clearance of bilirubin, the neonate must now take on this task. However, in the first days of life infants are ill equipped to do so owing to inadequate activity of the glucuronyltransferase enzyme that conjugates bilirubin produced from the high heme load resulting from significant hemolysis. This leads to accumulation of bilirubin because it must be conjugated to be excreted (Fig. 1). Therefore, the more pressing problem faced by the pediatrician is hyperbilirubinemia.

The mainstay of treatment for hyperbilirubinemia is phototherapy. Unconjugated bilirubin absorbs light maximally in the blue portion of the visible spectrum (approximately 450 nm). Phototherapy with a light source that approximates this spectrum results in the photoisomerization of unconjugated bilirubin into a polar, water-soluble, and more readily excretable form. As a result, both configurational and structural isomers are formed; the most common structural isomer is called lumirubin. The efficacy of phototherapy

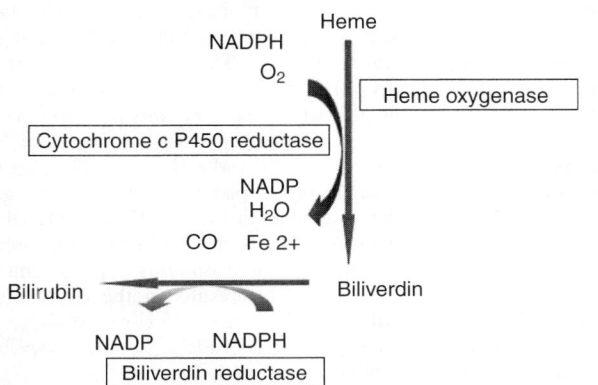

FIGURE 1. Enzymatic pathway leading to the production of bilirubin. Heme is degraded in a rate-limiting, oxygen (O_2) and energy-requiring (NADPH) step by heme oxygenase. This process results in the generation of carbon monoxide (CO) and iron (Fe) and biliverdin. Biliverdin is then converted to bilirubin by biliverdin reductase in another energy-requiring step.

is related to the spectrum of light used, irradiance of light, exposed surface area of the skin, and the distance of the light source from the infant.

In the setting of isoimmune (or antibody-associated) hemolysis, the use of intravenous immune globulin (IVIg [Gammagard])[1] has been shown to decrease the need for exchange transfusion and is a helpful adjunctive therapy. The current recommendation from the American Academy of Pediatrics (AAP) is to administer IVIg 0.5 to 1 g/kg over 2 hours if the total serum bilirubin is rising despite phototherapy or if the total serum bilirubin is within 2 to 3 mg/dL of the exchange transfusion level. This dose may be repeated in 12 hours.

For some infants, the use of phototherapy and IVIg, if indicated, is not sufficient to control the rising bilirubin level. Alternatively, some infants have neurologic manifestations of bilirubin toxicity despite bilirubin levels lower than suggested therapeutic levels. In these instances, a double-volume exchange transfusion is indicated. This procedure involves removing double the infant's blood volume with simultaneous isovolemic replacement of reconstituted whole blood. This process achieves two separate but related goals. First, it removes bilirubin and, second, in the setting of isoimmune hemolytic disease, it removes offending maternal antibodies. Criteria for performing a double-volume exchange transfusion are clearly outlined in the guidelines from the AAP published in 2004, but some experts suggest performing a double-volume exchange transfusion at even lower levels when significant antibody-mediated hemolysis is occurring owing to the added benefit provided by removing maternal antibodies.

Two pharmacologic therapies have been proposed in the treatment of neonatal hyperbilirubinemia. Phenobarbital,[1] when given to mothers just before birth, has been shown to decrease the need for exchange transfusion in their newborn infants. Synthetic metalloporphyrins (e.g., tin-mesoporphyrin, stannsoporfin [Stanate][5]) decrease the production of bilirubin by inhibiting heme oxygenase, the rate-limiting enzyme in the degradation of heme to biliverdin (which is then converted to bilirubin by biliverdin reductase, see Fig. 1). Both of these therapies are still considered experimental because the safety profile of both remains in question.

Monitoring

Monitoring of hemolytic anemia may be performed for the fetus in utero and for the infant after birth. Significant advances have improved our ability to determine the degree of fetal anemia in both invasive and noninvasive manners. Initial concern for the presence of significant antibodies against fetal red blood cells begins with the routine antibody screen performed early in gestation. This is normally an indirect Coombs' test, and most centers consider a titer of 1:16 or 1:32 to be a threshold to suggest significant risk for hemolysis.

Liley first described the relationship between bilirubin level in the amniotic fluid and the degree of fetal anemia in infants greater than 27 weeks gestation. Amniotic fluid is analyzed at a wavelength of 450 nm ($\triangle$OD450) to determine the bilirubin level and the value is plotted on known graphs to assess risk. Interventions including delivery or intrauterine transfusion are suggested if the level, when plotted, falls in the upper 20th percentile of zone II or in zone III. An expanded form of the Liley curve as well as the development of the Queenan curve has provided practitioners with tools to determine the risk of Rh isoimmune fetal anemia as early as 14 weeks' gestation. However, these methods may be less useful when antibodies to the Kell antigens are involved.

The measurement of middle cerebral artery peak systolic velocity (MCA-PSV) by Doppler ultrasonography gives practitioners a noninvasive alternative to amniocentesis for monitoring fetal anemia. Theoretically, as a fetus becomes more anemic, the blood flow velocity increases due to increased cardiac output and vasodilatation,

[1]Not FDA approved for this indication.
[5]Investigational drug in the United States.

resulting in increased MCA-PSV. The measurement is specific for gestational age and can be charted to determine if it is more than 1.5 multiples of the median (MoM), suggesting moderate to severe anemia. The effect of intrauterine transfusions on this measurement is unclear owing to the presence of adult red blood cells, and they can alter the interpretation of MCA-PSV. Large randomized, controlled trials are needed to determine if measurement of MCA-PSV or ΔOD450 are equivalent in assessing the risk of anemia. This would give practitioners a noninvasive way to monitor fetuses at risk for severe anemia.

Cordocentesis is the gold standard for measuring fetal anemia but it comes with severe risk including fetal and perinatal death, cord bleeding, hematomas, further maternal sensitization from fetal-maternal hemorrhage, infection, and placental abruption.

After birth, the neonate at risk for hemolytic anemia must be monitored for degree of anemia and for the development of significant hyperbilirubinemia. In utero, bilirubin is transferred to the maternal circulation via the placenta and processed in the maternal liver, which explains why hyperbilirubinemia is a postnatal event. Early and frequent bilirubin levels and complete blood counts allow the practitioner to evaluate the need for intervention. The availability of hour-specific nomograms that plot the risk of severe hyperbilirubinemia based on the level of bilirubin can be used in term infants to guide therapy and timing of outpatient follow-up. These are published in the AAP position statement from 2004.

Complications

Complications of phototherapy, IVIg,[1] and double-volume exchange transfusions are all possible. Side effects of phototherapy include disruption of mother-baby bonding, increased insensible water loss (less common with modern bilirubin lights), retinal injury from UV light, and, in the setting of an elevated conjugated fraction, a brown discoloration of the skin called "bronze-baby syndrome." The presence of an elevated conjugated fraction or bronzing of the skin is not a contraindication for phototherapy. This is of cosmetic concern only and is usually reversible after removal of the phototherapy.

Complications involving the use of IVIg are rare but include renal dysfunction, increased incidence of thrombotic events, transfusion reactions, and transmission of infections that can occur with transfusion of any blood product, because blood products are derived from pooled plasma.

Many potential complications are associated with double-volume exchange transfusion. These include electrolyte disturbances, arrhythmias, cardiac arrest, thrombotic or embolic sequelae, metabolic acidosis, thrombocytopenia, disseminated intravascular coagulation, infection, necrotizing enterocolitis, temperature instability, and blood transfusion–related complications such as hepatitis, HIV infection, or transfusion reaction.

---

[1]Not FDA approved for this indication.

REFERENCES

American Academy of Pediatrics. Subcommittee on Hyperbilirubinemia: Management of hyperbilirubinemia in the newborn infant 35 or more weeks of gestation. Pediatrics 2004;114(1):297–316.

Dennery PA, Seidman DS, Stevenson DK. Neonatal hyperbilirubinemia. N Engl J Med 2001;344(8):581–90.

Eder AF. Update on HDFN: New information on long-standing controversies. Immunohematology 2006;22(4):188–95.

Harkness UF, Spinnato JA. Prevention and management of RhD isoimmunization. Clin Perinatol 2004;31:721–42.

Moise KJ. Fetal anemia due to non–Rhesus-D red-cell alloimmunization. Semin Fetal Neonatal Med 2008;13:207–14.

Murray NA, Roberts IAG. Haemolytic disease of the newborn. Arch Dis Child Fetal Neonatal Ed 2007;92:F83–88.

Watchko JF. Identification of neonates at risk for hazardous hyperbilirubinemia: Emerging clinical insights. Pediatr Clin North Am 2009;56:671–87.

Hemophilia and Related Bleeding Disorders

Method of
Meera Chitlur, MD, and Roshni Kulkarni, MD

Hemophilia A and Hemophilia B

Hemophilia is an X-linked congenital bleeding disorder caused by a deficiency of factor VIII (hemophilia A) or factor IX (hemophilia B). Hemophilia A is the most common severe bleeding disorder and affects 1 in 5000 males in the United States; hemophilia B occurs in 1 in 30,000 males.

PATHOPHYSIOLOGY

The factor VIII gene is one of the largest genes and spans 186 kb of genomic DNA at Xq28. Inversion mutations account for 40% of severe hemophilia A, and deletions, point mutations, and insertions account for the remainder.

Hepatic and reticuloendothelial cells are presumed sites of factor VIII synthesis. Factor VIII is synthesized as a single chain polypeptide with three A domains (A1, A2, and A3), a large central B domain, and two C domains (Fig. 1). The binding sites for von Willebrand's factor (vWF), thrombin, and factor Xa are on the C2 domain, and factor IXa binding sites are on the A2 and A3 domains. The B domain can be deleted without any consequences. vWF protects factor VIII from proteolytic degradation in the plasma and concentrates it at the site of injury.

The factor IX gene is 34kb long and located at Xq26. It is a vitamin K–dependent serine protease composed of 415 amino acids. It is synthesized in the liver and its plasma concentration is about 50 times that of factor VIII. Gene deletions and point mutations result in hemophilia B.

ROLE OF FACTORS VIII AND IX IN COAGULATION

Factor VIII circulates bound to vWF. It is a cofactor for factor IX and is essential for factor X activation. In the classic coagulation cascade, activation of the intrinsic or extrinsic pathway of coagulation results in sufficient thrombin generation. However, this does not explain bleeding in hemophilia, because the extrinsic pathway is intact. This led to the revised cell-based model of coagulation.

The revised pathway incorporates all coagulation factors into a single pathway initiated by FVII and tissue factor. The contact factors (XI, XII, kallikrein, and high-molecular-weight kininogen) are not essential but serve as a backup. Following injury, encrypted tissue factor is exposed and forms a complex with factor VIIa. The tissue factor–factor VIIa complex activates factor IX to IXa (which moves to the platelet surface) and factor X to Xa. This generates small amounts of thrombin that activates platelets, converts platelet factor V to Va and factor XI to XIa, and releases factor VIII from vWF and activates it. The factor XIa activates plasma factor IX to IXa on the platelet surface, which together with factor VIIIa forms the tenase complex (factor VIIIa/IXa) that converts large amounts of factor X to Xa. Factor Xa forms a prothrombinase complex with FVa and converts large amounts of prothrombin to thrombin, called *thrombin burst*. This results in the conversion of sufficient fibrinogen to fibrin to form a stable clot. (An interactive animation on cell-based coagulation is available at http://www.hemo stasiscme.org/Activities/CellBasedCoagulation/content/).

In hemophilia, lack of factor VIII or IX produces a profound abnormality. Factor Xa generated by FVIIa and tissue factor is insufficient because it is soon inhibited by tissue factor pathway inhibitor (negative feedback), and factors VIII and IX, which are required for amplifying the production of Xa are absent. The primary platelet plug formation and initiation phases of coagulation are normal. Any clot that is formed (from the initiation phase) is friable and porous.

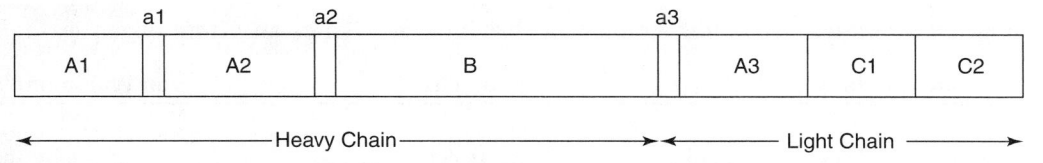

FIGURE 1. Factor VIII protein structure.

CLINICAL FEATURES

The diagnosis of hemophilia is often made following a bleeding episode or because of a family history; 30% of cases, however, have no family history. Based on the plasma levels of factor VIII or IX (normal levels are 50%–150%) that correlate with severity and predict bleeding risk, hemophilia is classified as mild (>5%), moderate (1%-5%) and severe (<1%) (Table 1). Approximately 65% of persons with hemophilia have severe disease, 15% have moderate disease, and 20% have mild disease. Most severe disease manifests by 4 years of age; moderate or mild disease is diagnosed later and often following bleeding secondary to trauma or surgery.

Hemophilia can be diagnosed in the first trimester, using chorionic villus sampling and gene analysis. In the second trimester, fetal blood sampling can be performed. Prenatal diagnosis to determine fetal gender can aid in the management of pregnancy and delivery.

The hallmark of severe hemophilia is hemarthrosis, or bleeding into the joint, that can occur spontaneously or with minimal trauma. Although the immediate effects of a joint bleed are excruciating pain, swelling, warmth, and muscle spasm, the long-term effects of recurrent hemarthrosis include hemophilic arthropathy, which is characterized by synovial thickening, chronic inflammation, and repeated hemorrhages resulting in a target joint. Knees, elbows, ankles, hips, and shoulders are commonly affected. Disuse atrophy of surrounding muscles leads to further joint instability. Limitation of joint range of motion due to hemarthrosis often correlates positively with older age, nonwhite race, and increased body mass index, and it affects quality of life.

Muscle hematomas, another characteristic site of bleeding, can lead to compartment syndrome, with eventual fibrosis and peripheral nerve damage. Iliopsoas bleeds manifest with pain and flexion deformity. Gastrointestinal bleeding and hematuria occur less often.

Central nervous system (CNS) hemorrhage is a rare but serious complication with a 10% recurrence rate and is the leading cause of mortality in hemophiliacs. Although most newborns with severe hemophilia experience an uneventful course following vaginal delivery, vacuum extraction is associated with an increased CNS bleeding risk. The incidence of intracranial hemorrhage in newborns with hemophilia is 1% to 4%.

DIAGNOSIS

Hemophilia A and B are clinically indistinguishable, and specific factor assays are the only way to differentiate and confirm the diagnosis. Both should be differentiated from von Willebrand's disease (vWD).

The prothrombin time (PT), platelet function analyzer (PFA-100), and fibrinogen are normal. (PFA, a platelet-function screening test, is replacing bleeding time, because the bleeding time has low sensitivity and specificity and is operator dependent.) The activated partial thromboplastin time (aPTT) is prolonged when the factor levels are below 30%. Table 2 shows the characteristics and differences between the hemophilias and vWD. Female carriers are usually asymptomatic except for those with extreme lyonization resulting in low factor VIII or IX levels. Factor VIII levels increase throughout pregnancy and drop to prepregnancy levels following delivery, but factor IX levels remain constant throughout pregnancy.

CURRENT DIAGNOSIS

- The hemophilias and von Willebrand's disease (vWD) account for 80% to 85% of inherited bleeding disorders. Hemophilia A and B are X-linked, whereas vWD and rare bleeding disorders (RBDs) are autosomal disorders.
- The diagnosis of hemophilia and other inherited bleeding disorders should be confirmed by specific assays, because screening tests such as prothrombin time (PT) and activated partial thromboplastin time (aPTT) may be normal. Plasma levels of deficient factor determine clinical severity and management.
- Hemarthrosis is the most common and debilitating complication, and central nervous system bleeding is the most common cause of mortality in hemophilia. Mucosal bleeding and menorrhagia are the most common manifestations of vWD. Bleeding manifestations of RBDs are mild, although homozygotes can present with severe disease.
- Newborns have normal levels of factor VIII; therefore, the diagnosis of hemophilia A can be established at birth. Vacuum delivery should be avoided to prevent head bleeds.
- Women and adolescents with menorrhagia and no underlying pathology should be investigated for a bleeding disorder.

TABLE 1 Hemophilia Severity and Clinical Manifestations

Characteristics	Severe (50%–70%)	Moderate (10%)	Mild 30%–40%
Factor VIII or IX activity (normal 50%–150%)	<1%	1%–5%	>5%
Age of diagnosis	At birth to 2 y	Childhood or adolescence	Adolescence or adult
Bleeding patterns	2–4/mo	4–6/y	Rare
Clinical manifestations	Hemarthroses, muscle, central nervous system, gastrointestinal bleeding, hematuria	Bleeding into joints or muscle following minor trauma, surgical procedure, dental bleeding Rarely spontaneous	Surgical procedures (including dental) and major trauma

TABLE 2 Hemophilias and von Willebrand's Disease: Key Characteristics and Differences

Characteristic	Hemophilia A	Hemophilia B	von Willebrand's Disease
Incidence	1:5000	1:30,000	1%–3% of U.S. population
Abnormality	Factor VIII deficiency	Factor IX deficiency	vWF (qualitative and quantitative defect)
Inheritance	X-linked, affects males Gene at the tip of X-chromosome	X-linked, affects males Gene at the tip of X-chromosome	Autosomal dominant (gene: chromosome 12) Some are recessive or compound heterozygotes
Production site	Unknown, liver endothelium	Liver (vitamin K dependent)	Megakaryocytes and endothelial cells
Function	Cofactor; forms tenase complex with factor IX and activates factor X, leading to thrombin burst that results in conversion of large amounts of fibrinogen to fibrin	Serine protease (inactive form: zymogen) Activated by factor XI or VIIa; forms a tenase complex with factor VIII and activates factor X	Platelet adhesion to site of injury or damaged endothelium Protects factor VIII from proteolysis
Classification (normal levels 50%–150%)	Mild (>5%) Moderate (1–5%) Severe (<1%)	Mild (>5%) Moderate (1–5%) Severe (<1%)	Type 1 Type 2 (2A, 2B, 2M, 2N) Type 3
Clinical presentation	Positive family history (30% new mutation) Hemarthroses, hematomas, hematuria, intracranial hemorrhage, gastrointestinal hemorrhage, etc.	Positive family history (30% new mutation) Milder disease, although identical hemorrhage sites as hemophilia A	Positive family history Mucocutaneous bleeding (epistaxis, menorrhagia, postdental bleeding) Type 3 can manifest as hemophilia A.
PFA, bleeding time	Normal	Normal	May be prolonged
PT	Normal	Normal	Normal
aPTT	Prolonged	Prolonged	Prolonged or normal
Factor VIII assay	Decreased or absent	Normal	Decreased or normal (absent type 3)
Factor IX assay	Normal	Decreased or absent	Normal
vWF antigen	Normal	Normal	Decreased or absent (type 3)
vWF:RCo	Normal	Normal	Decreased or abnormal
vWF multimers	Normal	Normal	Abnormal in types 1, 2A, 2B; absent in type 3
Specific treatment	Recombinant factor VIII (preferred) Pathogen-safe plasma-derived concentrates DDAVP for mild cases	Recombinant factor IX Pathogen-safe plasma-derived concentrates DDAVP ineffective	DDAVP (intranasal or intravenous) vWF concentrates (pathogen-safe plasma derived)
Inhibitor patients	Immune tolerance, recombinant factor VIIa, APCC	Immune tolerance, recombinant factor VIIa	Inhibitors are rare
Adjunct therapy	Antifibrinolytics	Antifibrinolytics	Oral contraceptives, antifibrinolytics

APCC = activated prothrombin complex concentrates; aPTT = activated partial thromboplastin time; DDAVP = desmopressin; PFA = platelet function analyzer; PT = prothrombin time; RCo = ristocetin cofactor; vWF = von Willebrand's factor.

TREATMENT

The treatment for hemophilia consists of replacement therapy with intravenous factor VIII or factor IX concentrates produced by purification of donor plasma (plasma derived) or in cell culture bioreactors (recombinant). Careful screening of donors combined with heat treatment and viral inactivation methods have made plasma-derived products safer. Plasma-derived and recombinant products appear to have equivalent clinical efficacy. Recombinant factor concentrates are recommended, but if they are not available, plasma-derived concentrates can be used. Cryoprecipitate is no longer recommended because of concerns regarding pathogen safety.

Treatment administered only during bleeding symptoms is known as *episodic therapy*, and periodic administration of factor concentrates to prevent bleeding is known as *prophylactic therapy*. Response to treatment is more effective when it is administered early. Although prophylaxis prevents the development of joint disease, the high cost of factor replacement coupled with the need for venous access makes it expensive and difficult.

The goal of treatment is to raise factor levels to approximately 30% or more for minor bleeds (hematomas or joint bleeds) and 100% for major bleeds (CNS or surgery). Giving 1 U/kg of factor concentrate raises plasma factor VIII levels by 2% and factor IX levels by 1.5% (except with the recombinant factor IX product, where it increases by 0.8%). The half-life of factor VIII is approximately 8 to 12 hours and that of factor IX is up to 24 hours. Factor concentrates can also be given by continuous infusion (3–4 U/kg/hour). The bolus dose varies from 25 to 50 U/kg depending on the severity, site, and type of bleeding and is dosed to the closest vial because of the cost of the products. Table 3 lists the dosing schedule for various types of bleeds.

For short-term therapy (before dental procedures and minor bleeding episodes) in mild hemophilia A and vWD, the synthetic vasopressin analogue desmopressin acetate (DDAVP [Stimate]) is useful. It increases plasma concentrations of coagulation factor VIII and vWF three- to fivefold by releasing the endothelial stores. A DDAVP trial to determine response is helpful in selecting patients who might benefit from such therapy. For hemostatic purposes, intravenous (0.3 µg/kg in 50 mL of normal saline infused over 15–30 min) or intranasal dose (150 µg) can be used. The intranasal dose is 15 times larger than that recommended for diabetes insipidus. A multidose intranasal spray formulation (Stimate nasal spray) delivers 150 µg per spray. The recommended dosage is one spray for patients who weigh less than 50 kg and two sprays (one in each nostril) for those who weigh more than 50 kg. Desmopressin is ineffective in hemophilia B. Aspirin and aspirin-containing compounds should be avoided in persons with bleeding disorders because they interfere with platelet function and can exacerbate bleeding.

Antifibrinolytics such as ϵ-aminocaproic acid (Amicar) and tranexamic acid (Cyklokapron) are used as adjunct therapies and in mild hemophilia and can obviate the need for factor concentrates. The recommended dosage for = ϵ-aminocaproic acid is 75 to 100 mg/kg/dose IV or orally every 4 to 6 hours (maximum 30 g/24 hours). The recommended dosage for tranexamic acid is 10 mg/kg/dose IV or 25 mg/kg body weight orally, three times daily.

TABLE 3 Treatment of Bleeding Episodes and Desired Plasma Levels in Hemophilias A and B

Type of Bleeding	Desired Factor Level (%)	Factor VIII Dose (U/kg)	Factor IX Dose (U/kg)	Duration of Treatment (Days)	Comments (Dose Factor to the Closest Vial)
Persistent or profuse epistaxis Oral mucosal bleeding (including tongue and mouth lacerations)	20–30	10–15	20–30	1–2	Local pressure, antifibrinolytics, fibrin glue for local control, nosebleed QR for epistaxis Sedation in small children with tongue laceration
Dental procedures	30–50	15–25	30–50	1 h before procedure	Antifibrinolytics for 7–10 d
Acute hemarthrosis, intramuscular hematomas	30–60	15–50	30–60	1–3	Use lower doses if treated early. Non–weight bearing on affected joint.
Physical therapy	30–50	15–25	30–50	Treat before PT	Consider synovectomy (surgical, radioisotope or chemical) for target joints.
Life-threatening bleeding such as intracranial hemorrhage, major surgery, and trauma	80–100	40–50	80–100	10–14 d	Bolus dose followed by continuous infusion (3–4 U/kg/h); may switch to bolus before discharge
Gastrointestinal bleeding	30–50	15–25	30–50	2–3	May use oral antifibrinolytics
Persistent painless gross hematuria	30–50	15–25	30–50	1–2	Increase PO or IV fluids with low-dose antifibrinolytics

PT = physical therapy.

CURRENT THERAPY

- Early and effective treatment and prophylaxis can prevent repeated hemarthrosis and joint destruction in persons with hemophilia. Patients should be tested annually for the presence of inhibitors.
- Wherever available and indicated, recombinant factor concentrates are preferred over plasma-derived products due to potential risk of pathogen transmission. Cryoprecipitate is not recommended. For mild and moderate hemophilia A and von Willebrand's disease, the use of desmopressin coupled with antifibrinolytics can obviate the use of concentrates. Continued vigilance should be implemented for new and emerging bloodborne pathogens.
- All patients with inherited bleeding disorders should be immunized against hepatitis A and B and followed in close collaboration with the local hemophilia treatment center (http://www2a.cdc.gov/ncbddd/htcweb/index.asp). The National Hemophilia Foundation's (www.hemophilia.org) Medical and Scientific Advisory Committee (MASAC) guidelines for updated recommendations and product choice should be followed.

For prophylaxis, factor VIII 25 to 40 U/kg administered every other day or factor IX 25 to 40 U/kg twice weekly (because of the longer half-life of factor IX) is aimed at preventing joint disease. Prophylaxis may begin at 1 to 2 years of age and is continued lifelong. Self-infusion before any planned strenuous activity is recommended. Because of the complications of central venous catheters (infections, thrombosis, and mechanical), use of a peripheral vein is encouraged.

COMPLICATIONS OF TREATMENT

One of the most serious complications of hemophilia treatment is the development of inhibitors or neutralizing antibodies (immunoglobulin [Ig]G) that inhibit the function of substituted factor VIII and factor IX. Approximately 5% to 10% of all hemophiliacs and up to 30%

of patients with severe hemophilia A develop inhibitors. The incidence of inhibitors in hemophilia B is lower (1%–3%). Most factor VIII inhibitors arise after a median exposure of 9 to 12 days in patients with severe hemophilia A. They can be transient or permanent and should be suspected if a patient fails to respond to an appropriate dose of clotting factor concentrate. Inhibitors can exacerbate bleeding episodes and hemophilic arthropathy.

Inhibitor levels, measured using Bethesda units (BU), are classified as high titer (>5 BU) or low titer (<5 BU). In patients with low titer, inhibitors higher than normal doses of factor VIII or IX may be used to treat bleeding. For those with high-titer inhibitors, agents that bypass factor VIII or factor IX are used. These include recombinant activated factor VII and, in the case of hemophilia A, activated prothrombin complex concentrates (APCC) or recombinant porcine factor VIII (currently in prelicensure clinical trials). Immune tolerance induction, a long-term approach designed to eradicate inhibitors, is effective in 70% to 85% of patients with severe hemophilia A; the most important predictor of success of immune tolerance induction is an inhibitor titer of less than 10 BU at the start of immune tolerance induction.

Although inhibitors are rare in hemophilia B, they can result in anaphylaxis with exposure to factor IX–containing products. Immune tolerance regimens are associated with the nephrotic syndrome and are successful in eradicating the inhibitor only in 40% of cases.

Another important complication of treatment is the transmission of bloodborne pathogens such as hepatitis B and C viruses and HIV. In the 1970s, lyophilized plasma factor concentrates of low purity resulted in the transmission of HIV, causing the deaths of many hemophiliacs. Currently, donor screening for pathogens coupled with viral attenuation by heat or solvent detergent technology make these products pathogen safe. However, nonenveloped virus (parvovirus and hepatitis A) and prions can resist inactivation and can be potentially transmitted.

Patients with bleeding disorders should be encouraged to attend the comprehensive hemophilia treatment centers, where they are educated, trained to self-infuse and calculate dosage, maintain treatment logs, and call for serious bleeding episodes. Hemovigilance at the hemophilia treatment centers is maintained through participation in the Centers for Disease Control and Prevention's (CDC) Universal Data Collection project. The mortality rate among patients who receive care at hemophilia treatment centers is lower than among those who do not: 28.1% versus 38.3%, respectively.

Routine vaccination against hepatitis A and B is recommended. Gene therapy offers promise of a cure but has not yet become reality. Two gene-therapy trials for hemophilia B have shown subtherapeutic or transient expression of factor IX.

Von Willebrand's Disease

von Willebrand's disease (vWD) is an inherited (autosomal dominant) bleeding disorder caused by deficiency or dysfunction of von Willebrand Factor (vWF), a plasma protein that mediates platelet adhesion at the site of vascular injury and prevents degradation of factor VIII. A defect in vWF results in bleeding by impairing platelet adhesion or by decreasing factor VIII.

vWF is synthesized in endothelial cells and undergoes dimerization and multimerization, forming low-, intermediate-, and high-molecular-weight (HMW) multimers. The HMW multimers are most effective in promoting platelet aggregation and adhesion. Circulating HMW multimers are cleaved by the protease ADAMTS13, which is deficient in patients with thrombotic thrombocytopenic purpura.

vWD is the most common bleeding disorder, affecting 1% or more of the population. It occurs worldwide and affects all races. vWD is classified into three major categories: partial quantitative deficiency (type 1), qualitative deficiency (type 2), and total deficiency (type 3). There are several different variants of type 2 vWD: 2A, 2B, 2N, and 2M based on the phenotype. About 75% of patients have type 1 vWD.

CLINICAL PRESENTATION

Mucous membrane–type bleeding (e.g., menorrhagia, epistaxis) and excessive bruising are characteristic clinical features in vWD. Bleeding manifestations vary considerably, and in some cases, the diagnosis is not suspected until excessive bleeding occurs with a surgical procedure or trauma. Although excessive menstrual bleeding may be the initial manifestation, it takes 16 years for a diagnosis of bleeding disorder. It is for this reason that the American College of Obstetrics and Gynecology recommended screening for hemostatic disorders in all adolescents and women presenting with menorrhagia and no pathology and before hysterectomy for menorrhagia. In infants or small children with type 3 (severe) vWD, excessive bruising and even joint bleeding (due to very low levels of factor VIII) can mimic hemophilia A.

DIAGNOSIS

Laboratory evaluation for vWD requires several assays to quantitate vWF and characterize its structure and function. Many variables affect vWF assay results, including the patient's ABO blood type. Persons of blood group AB have 60% to 70% higher vWF levels than those of blood group O. Thus, some laboratories interpret vWF levels referenced to specific normal ranges for blood types.

Clinical conditions and disorders with elevated vWF levels include pregnancy (third trimester), collagen vascular disorders, following surgery, in liver disease, and in disseminated intravascular coagulation. Low levels are seen in hypothyroidism and days 1 to 4 of the menstrual cycle.

Symptoms are modified by medications like aspirin or nonsteroidal antiinflammatory drugs (NSAIDs), which can exacerbate the bleeding; oral contraceptives can decrease the bleeding in women with vWD by increasing vWF levels. vWF levels in African American women are 15% higher than in white women. Clinical symptoms and family history are important for establishing the diagnosis of vWD, and a single test is sometimes not sufficient to rule out the diagnosis.

Initial work-up should include a complete blood count, aPTT, PT, fibrinogen level, or thrombin time. These tests do not rule out vWD but help to rule out thrombocytopenia or factor deficiency as the cause for bleeding. The closure times on the PFA-100, which has replaced the bleeding time as a screening test in some centers, may be prolonged. The aPTT in vWD is only abnormal when factor VIII is sufficiently reduced.

Specific tests for vWD include ristocetin cofactor assay, a factor VIII activity, and vWF antigen (vWF Ag) assay. The Ristocetin cofactor activity measures induced binding of vWF to platelet glycoprotein Ib and is the best functional assay of vWF activity. Multimer analysis is done by agarose gel electrophoresis using anti-vWF polyclonal antibody and is available at reference laboratories.

In type I vWD, the vWF is subnormal in amount, with normal multimer structure. Those with types 2A and 2B vWD lack the HMW multimers. In type 2B, the vWF has a heightened affinity for platelets, often resulting in some degree of thrombocytopenia from platelet aggregation. A useful laboratory test for type 2B is the low-dose ristocetin-induced platelet aggregation (RIPA) assay.

In type 3 (severe) vWD, the affected person has inherited a gene for type I vWD from each parent, resulting in very low levels (3%) of vWF (and low factor VIII, because there is no vWF to protect factor VIII from proteolytic degradation). Less commonly, a person with type 3 is doubly heterozygous. Table 4 provides a quick overview of the laboratory findings in the different variants of vWD.

TREATMENT

In type 1 vWD (with subnormal levels of normally functioning vWF), the treatment of choice is DDAVP, which causes a rapid release of vWF from storage sites. It can be given intravenously or by the intranasal route. The recommended dose for IV use is 0.3 μg/kg, given in saline over 10 minutes. Most persons with type 1 vWD have a two- to four-fold increase in plasma levels of vWF within 15 to 30 minutes following infusion. The IV route is often used for surgical coverage or for a severe bleeding episode requiring hospitalization. When necessary, repeat doses may be given at 12- to 24-hour intervals. Tachyphylaxis is less commonly seen in vWD patients than in hemophilia patients. It is important to monitor free water intake following DDAVP administration because it can cause hyponatremia and seizures.

The concentrated form of desmopressin for intranasal use (Stimate nasal spray) may be used. The recommended dosage is one 150-μg spray for patients who weigh less than 50 kg and two sprays (one in each nostril) for those who weigh more than 50 kg. Some young women with menorrhagia have benefited from its use at the onset of

TABLE 4 Clinical Variants of von Willebrand's Disease

Type	Factor VIII	vWF Ag	Ristocetin Cofactor	RIPA	Multimer
1	↓	↓	↓	↓ or normal	Normal
2A	↓ or normal	↓↓	↓	↓↓	Large and intermediate multimers absent
2B	↓ or normal	↓↓	↓ or normal	↓ to low dose	Large multimers absent
2M	Variably ↓	Variably ↓	↓	Variably ↓	Normal
2N	↓↓	Normal	Normal	Normal	Normal
3	↓↓↓↓	↓↓↓↓	↓↓↓↓	None	Absent
Platelet type	↓ or normal	↓ or normal	↓	↓ to low dose	Large multimers absent

Ag = antigen; RIPA = ristocetin-induced platelet aggregation; vWF = von Willebrand's factor.

TABLE 5 Rare Bleeding Disorders: Inheritance, Clinical Features, and Treatment

Factor	Prevalence	Type	Inheritance	Manifestation and Diagnosis	Treatment	Hemostatic Levels	Half-life
Factor I	1:1,000,000	Afibrinogenemia Dysfibrinogenemia Hypofibrinogenemia	AR AD AD	Mild bleeding CNS, umbilical, joint bleeding Recurrent miscarriage PT, aPTT, TT prolonged Low FI levels Paradoxical thrombosis	FFP 15–20 mL/kg Cryoprecipitate 1 bag/5–10 kg Plasma-derived concentrate²* Treatment q3–5d	50 mg–1g/dL	2–5 d
Factor II	1:2,000,000	Type I: hypoprothrombinemia Type II: dysprothrombinemia	AR AR	Hematomas, hemarthroses, menorrhagia CNS, umbilical, postpartum hemorrhage PT abnormal	FFP, PCC 20–30 U/kg for prophylaxis or treatment	20%–30%	3–4 d
Factor V	1:1,000,000	Parahemophilia, labile factor, proaccelerin, Owren's disease	AR	Mucosal bleeding, postpartum hemorrhage, CNS bleeding Platelet factor V deficiency more reflective of bleeding potential Prolonged PT, aPTT Normal TT	FFP Platelet transfusions Antiplatelet antibodies can develop with repeated platelet transfusions	15%–20%	36 h
Factor VII	1: 500,000	Proconvertin or stable factor	AR	Menorrhagia; mucosal, muscle, intracranial bleeds (15%–60%); hemarthrosis Prolonged PT Normal aPTT, TT, FI, liver functions	Recombinant factor VIIa, 15–30 µg/kg q2h for major bleeds FFP, PCC 20–30 U/kg for prophylaxis or treatment Plasma-derived factor VII concentrates²*	15%–20%	4–6 h
Factor X	1:1,000,000		AR	Menorrhagia; umbilical, joint, mucosal, muscle, intracranial bleeding Prolonged PT, aPTT	FFP, PCCs 20–30 U/kg	15%–20%	24–48 h
Factor XI (common in Ashkenazi Jews)	1:1,000,000		AR	Post-traumatic bleeding, menorrhagia Prolonged aPTT Normal PT	Hemoeleven,²* FFP 15–20 mL/ kg Inhibitors can occur	15%–20%	
Factor XIII	1:2,000,000		Ar	Intracranial, joint, umbilical bleeding Delayed wound healing Recurrent miscarriages PT, APTT normal ↓FXIII assay	Fibrogammin P²† 10–20 U/kg FFP 15–20 mL/kg Cryoprecipitate 1 bag/5–10 kg q3–4wk	2%–5%	11–14 d
Combined factor V and VIII	1:2,000,000			Mucosal bleeding Prolonged PT, aPTT (disproportionately)	Factor VIII concentrates and FFP	15%–20%	
Vitamin K-dependent multiple deficiencies	1:2,000,000			Umbilical stump, intracranial, postsurgical bleeding Skeletal abnormalities Hearing loss	Oral vitamin K, FFP, PCC	15%–20%	

²Not available in the United States.
*Available in Europe.
†Compassionate use in the United States.
AD = autosomal dominant; aPTT = activated partial thromboplastin time; AR = autosomal recessive; CNS = central nervous system; FFP = fresh frozen plasma; FI = fibrinogen; PCC = prothrombin complex concentrate; PT = prothrombin time; TT = thrombin time.

menses, with a second dose after 24 hours. Others have used it approximately 45 minutes before invasive dentistry, with good results.

In the type 2 variants (vWF produced is abnormal), desmopressin can cause an increase in abnormal vWF. Although some persons with type 2A might respond, desmopressin is seldom useful in type 2 and might even be contraindicated (as in type 2B, where it can exacerbate the thrombocytopenia).

In type 3 vWD, desmopressin is ineffective because there is no vWF to be released from storage sites. For type 3 patients and in persons with type 1 vWD who do not respond adequately to desmopressin, an intermediate-purity plasma-derived concentrate rich in the hemostatically effective HMW multimers of vWF (such as Humate P) should be used to treat moderately severe or severe bleeding episodes and for before surgery.

As in hemophilia, antifibrinolytics are an effective adjunctive treatment for invasive dental procedures or other bleeding in the oropharyngeal cavity. These may be effective even when used alone in some vWD women with menorrhagia. For epistaxis, Nosebleed QR, a hydrophilic powder, can help.

SPECIAL SITUATIONS

Pregnancy

vWF (and factor VIII) levels increase during the third trimester of pregnancy, and women with type 1 vWD have a decrease in bruising or other bleeding symptoms. However, those with type 2 vWD (abnormal vWF) and type 3 (no vWF) have no change in the bleeding tendency. Even in type 1 vWD, vWF levels fall following delivery, so treatment (with IV desmopressin or Humate P) may be needed.

Acquired von Willebrand's Disease

Acquired vWD occurs in persons who do not have a lifelong bleeding disorder. Conditions associated with acquired vWD include underlying autoimmune disease (lymphoproliferative disorders, myeloproliferative disorders, or plasma cell dyscrasias), valvular and congenital heart disease, Wilms' tumor, chronic renal failure, and hypothyroidism. The mechanism of acquired vWD is unknown. Medications such as valproic acid can also cause vWD. Removal of the underlying condition often corrects the vWF. Desmopressin, Humate P, recombinant factor VIIa, or plasma exchange may be tried, if necessary, to treat bleeding.

Rare Bleeding Disorders

The rare bleeding disorders account for 3% to 5% of inherited coagulation deficiencies, other than factor VIII, factor IX, or vWF deficiencies. They are autosomal recessive and affect both sexes. The prevalence of rare bleeding disorders ranges from 1:500,000 to 1:2,000,000. Bleeding manifestations are restricted to persons who are homozygotes or compound heterozygotes. Rare bleeding disorders are common in countries such as Iran, where consanguineous marriages are customary. Ashkenazi Jews are particularly affected by factor XI deficiency. Deficiency of factor XII is a risk factor for thrombosis, but not for bleeding. Most cases of rare bleeding disorders are identified by abnormal screening tests coupled with specific factor assays.

Factor concentrates (recombinant or plasma derived) are available for some of the deficiencies (mostly in Europe, but not in the United States). Fibrogammin P, a plasma-derived virally purified factor XIII concentrate, is not yet licensed in the United States but is available under an Investigational New Drug (IND) protocol of the Food and Drug Administration through Dr. Diane Nugent, Children's Hospital of Orange County, 500 S. Main St., Orange County, Calif 92868. The advantages of concentrates are pathogen safety and small volume. The use of antifibrinolytics and fibrin glue as adjunct therapy for bleeding manifestations is encouraged. Table 5 lists the inheritance, frequency, manifestations, and treatments of the rare bleeding disorders.

REFERENCES

Arnold WD, Hilgartner MW. Hemophilic arthropathy. Current concepts of pathogenesis and management. J Bone Joint Surg Am 1977;59(3):287–305.

Bolton-Maggs PH, Pasi KJ. Haemophilias A and B. Lancet 2003;361 (9371):1801–9.

Gill JC, Wilson AD, Endres-Brooks J, Montgomery RR. Loss of the largest von Willebrand factor multimers from the plasma of patients with congenital cardiac defects. Blood 1986;67(3):758–61.

Hoffman M, Monroe 3rd DM. A cell-based model of hemostasis. Thromb Haemost 2001;85(6):958–65.

Miller CH, Dilley AB, Drews C, et al. Changes in von Willebrand factor and factor VIII levels during the menstrual cycle. Thromb Haemost 2002;87 (6):1082–3.

Miller CH, Dilley A, Richardson L, et al. Population differences in von Willebrand factor levels affect the diagnosis of von Willebrand disease in African-American women. Am J Hematol 2001;67(2):125–9.

Mulder K, Llinas A. The target joint. Haemophilia 2004;10(Suppl. 4):152–6.

National Hemophilia Foundation Medical and Scientific Advisory Council (MASAC). MASAC recommendations concerning the treatment of hemophilia and other bleeding disorders (Revised October 2006). Available at http://www.hemophilia.org/NHFWeb/MainPgs/MainNHF.aspx?menuid= 57&contentid=693 [accessed May 21, 2008].

Pierce GF, Lillicrap D, Pipe SW, Vandendriessche T. Gene therapy, bioengineered clotting factors and novel technologies for hemophilia treatment. J Thromb Haemost 2007;5(5):901–6.

Soucie JM, Nuss R, Evatt B, et al. Mortality among males with hemophilia; Relations with source of medical care. The Hemophilia Surveillance System Project Investigators. Blood 2000;96(2):437–42.

Veldman A, Hoffman M, Ehrenforth S. New insights into the coagulation system and implications for new therapeutic options with recombinant factor VIIa. Curr Med Chem 2003;10(10):797–811.

Warrier I, Ewenstein BM, Koerper MA, et al. Factor IX inhibitors and anaphylaxis in hemophilia B. J Pediatr Hematol Oncol 1997;19(1):23–7.

Platelet-Mediated Bleeding Disorders

Method of
Suman L. Sood, MD, and Charles S. Abrams, MD

Quantitative and qualitative platelet defects are commonly encountered in clinical practice and can result in bleeding diatheses.

Elements of Platelet Function

The vascular endothelium separates platelets from adhesive substrates in the subendothelial connective tissue. Platelet-mediated hemostasis is initiated by adherence to exposed collagen, fibronectin, and laminin following a breach to the vessel wall. Intracellular signaling cascades lead to secretion of platelet granules, synthesis, and release of thromboxane A_2, and a conformational change in platelet surface glycoprotein IIb/IIIa (GPIIb/IIIa) that enables it to bind soluble fibrinogen or von Willebrand's factor (vWF). Release of thromboxane A_2 and agonists within the secretion granules, such as adenosine diphosphate (ADP) and serotonin, activate neighboring platelets to perpetuate the process.

Fibrinogen binding to GPIIb/IIIa cross-links the platelets into a hemostatic plug, resulting in platelet aggregation and accumulation at the site of injury. Other signaling pathways initiated by agonists such as thrombin, thromboxane A_2, and collagen help promote the process of aggregation. Activated platelet plasma membrane interacts with circulating coagulation factors and provides a surface for assembly and generation of active factor X and thrombin. Secondary hemostasis occurs when the platelet plug is stabilized further by a thrombin-mediated fibrin mesh. The arrest of bleeding in a superficial wound almost exclusively results from the primary hemostatic plug.

Platelet-mediated bleeding disorders are characterized by a prolonged bleeding time, mucocutaneous bleeding, petechiae, and purpura. In contrast, deficiencies in secondary hemostasis result in delayed deep bleeding, such as bleeding into muscles and joints.

Quantitative Bleeding Disorders

Adequate numbers of platelets are required to achieve primary hemostasis. Thrombocytopenia can result from decreased platelet production by bone marrow megakaryocytes, accelerated platelet removal, or platelet sequestration in an enlarged spleen. The clinical context is essential because there is no easy test to differentiate among these possibilities. Most commonly, thrombocytopenia is caused by accelerated platelet removal.

Hemorrhage following trauma or surgery generally does not occur if the platelet count is more than 50,000/μL. In an otherwise hemostatically normal patient, significant spontaneous bleeding usually does not occur with a platelet count greater than 5000 to 10,000/μL. However, there is no absolute threshold for spontaneous bleeding due to thrombocytopenia, and spontaneous bleeding can occur at higher counts when fever, sepsis, severe anemia, and other hemostatic defects are present or when platelet function is impaired by medication. Notably, a prolonged cutaneous bleeding time does not accurately predict clinical bleeding.

THROMBOCYTOPENIA DUE TO DECREASED PLATELET PRODUCTION

Decreased platelet production occurs in primary diseases of the bone marrow such as acute leukemia and aplastic anemia; myelophthisic processes in which marrow is replaced by metastatic carcinoma, fibrosis, or multiple myeloma; following chemotherapy or radiation therapy; with ethanol toxicity; and during infections with viruses such as HIV, cytomegalovirus (CMV), Epstein-Barr virus (EBV), and varicella. Thrombocytopenia also occurs when megakaryocyte proliferation is impaired by myelodysplasia.

Overt bleeding in these disorders, when clearly a result of thrombocytopenia, is treated by platelet transfusion. Prophylactic platelet transfusion, however, is an area of controversy and is complicated by the short life span of platelets (10 days), the 5-day shelf life of stored platelets, and platelet immunogenicity. In patients undergoing treatment for acute leukemia, outcome is unchanged when platelet counts of 5000 to 10,000/μL are used as the threshold for prophylactic transfusion. Single-donor apheresis platelets or platelet donors who are HLA identical to the recipient should be considered to prevent alloimmunization. Preliminary results from the multicenter Platelet Dose trial in patients with malignancy suggest that lower doses of platelets may be safe.

THROMBOCYTOPENIA DUE TO INCREASED PLATELET DESTRUCTION

Nonimmune and immune processes can lead to a shortened platelet life span. Nonimmune causes include sepsis, disseminated intravascular coagulation (DIC), thrombotic thrombocytopenic purpura/hemolytic uremic syndrome (TTP/HUS), preeclampsia and eclampsia, cardiopulmonary bypass, and giant cavernous hemangiomas. The thrombocytopenia resolves with treatment of the underlying disorder, and platelet transfusion is rarely necessary. In TTP/HUS, thrombocytopenia is associated with thrombosis rather than bleeding, and controversial reports exist of clinical deterioration following platelet transfusion.

Immune-mediated platelet destruction can occur due to medication, alloimmune sensitization, or autoimmunity. Medications should always be considered a possible cause of thrombocytopenia. The potential list is long, but drugs with strong evidence of antibody-mediated platelet destruction include quinine (Qualaquin), quinidine, sulfonamides, and gold salts. Besides stopping the offending medication, emergent treatment for severe thrombocytopenia with bleeding includes platelet transfusion, and corticosteroids with or without intravenous immunoglobulin (IVIg).

Heparin-induced thrombocytopenia (HIT) is a special case of drug-induced thrombocytopenia associated with arterial and venous thrombosis rather than bleeding. HIT occurs in 2% to 5% of patients given unfractionated heparin by any route for 5 to 10 days. Antibodies develop to a heparin–platelet factor 4 (PF4) complex. HIT must always be considered when thrombocytopenia is detected in a hospitalized patient. If a patient has HIT, all heparin administration should be stopped, and alternative anticoagulation such as the direct thrombin inhibitors recombinant hirudin and argatroban should be instituted, at least until the platelet count normalizes. Warfarin (Coumadin) should not be used in acute HIT because of its delayed therapeutic effect and association with a syndrome of venous limb gangrene. Platelet transfusions in this disease are controversial, because some reports suggest that they can precipitate thrombotic complications.

Alloimmune thrombocytopenia due to sensitization to alloantigens such as PI^{A1} can result from transfusion (post-transfusion purpura, PTP) or maternal sensitization during pregnancy (neonatal alloimmune thrombocytopenia, NAIT). PTP causes profound thrombocytopenia 7 to 10 days after transfusion and can be treated with IVIg or plasma exchange. NAIT can cause severe thrombocytopenia and bleeding in neonates and is treated with platelet transfusion, corticosteroids, and IVIg.

Autoimmune thrombocytopenia, also known as idiopathic thrombocytopenic purpura (ITP), is caused by circulating antiplatelet autoantibodies. An ITP-like picture can also occur in autoimmune diseases such as systemic lupus erythematosus, in patients with low-grade lymphoproliferative disorders such as chronic lymphocytic leukemia, and in patients with HIV infections. ITP can occur at any age in both sexes and manifests with either mucocutaneous bleeding or unexplained asymptomatic thrombocytopenia. The complete blood count (CBC) is otherwise normal, splenomegaly is absent, and peripheral blood smears are only remarkable for a decreased number of platelets, some of which may be larger than normal. Bone marrow examination is usually not necessary in the absence of other findings suggesting myelodysplasia, but it typically shows normal or increased numbers of megakaryocytes.

Management of ITP is guided by symptoms and platelet count. Asymptomatic patients with platelet counts greater than 30,000/μL can be followed without treatment. With bleeding or a platelet count less than 30,000/μL, treatment with prednisone is initiated. Refractory patients may require splenectomy (60%–75% remission rate), other immunosuppressive medications, or new thrombopoiesis-stimulating agents. Emergent presentation with severe thrombocytopenia (<5000/μL) or internal bleeding should be treated with high doses of pulse corticosteroids or IVIg, or both. Platelet transfusion may be given concurrently with the IVIg for critical bleeding. Anti-D immune globulin may be substituted for IVIg in Rh$^+$ patients who have not undergone splenectomy; however, occasional patients develop severe autoimmune hemolysis.

THROMBOCYTOPENIA DUE TO HYPERSPLENISM

Approximately 30% of the circulating platelet mass is normally present in the spleen. Additional platelets may be sequestered when the spleen enlarges due to portal hypertension or infiltrative diseases. Platelet counts in patients with hypersplenism generally are not lower than 40,000 to 50,000/μL. Consequently, bleeding due to thrombocytopenia from hypersplenism alone is unusual.

Qualitative Platelet Disorders

ACQUIRED QUALITATIVE PLATELET DISORDERS

Acquired disorders of platelet function are relatively common but are usually asymptomatic or mild. Nonetheless, they can be of substantial clinical importance when engrafted on another hemostatic abnormality. They are subclassified as resulting from drugs, hematologic diseases, and systemic disorders. Drugs are the most common cause of dysfunction, most notably aspirin, which irreversibly inactivates the enzyme cyclooxygenase-1 (COX-1), thus inducing a permanent blockade in platelet prostaglandin synthesis and consequently thromboxane A_2 synthesis. Although the antihemostatic effect is minimal in normal persons, it may be quite prominent in a patient with an underlying bleeding disorder. Nonsteroidal anti-inflammatory drugs (NSAIDs) reversibly inhibit platelet prostaglandin synthesis and generally have little effect on hemostasis. Other medications that interfere significantly with platelet function include clopidogrel (Plavix), ticlopidine (Ticlid), and GPIIb/IIIa receptor antagonists. Numerous other drugs have been implicated in platelet dysfunction in case reports, but the evidence for most of these medications is less well established.

Bone marrow processes that can produce intrinsically abnormal platelets include myeloproliferative disorders, leukemias, myelodysplastic syndromes, and dysproteinemias such as multiple myeloma and Waldenström's macroglobulinemia, in which abnormal plasma proteins impair platelet function. In addition, acquired forms of von Willebrand's disease, a rare disorder that can arise secondary to critical aortic stenosis, multiple myeloma, or other clonal lymphoproliferative disorders, can lead to a bleeding diathesis.

Renal failure is the most prominent systemic disorder associated with abnormal platelet function. The hemostatic defect is generally mild and corrects rapidly with the initiation of dialysis. Intravenous desmopressin (DDAVP), a vasopressin analogue that causes release of von Willebrand factor (vWF) from tissue stores, is helpful in uremia, shortening bleeding time in 50% to 75% of patients. Dosing may be repeated, although tachyphylaxis can occur. Maintaining the hemoglobin greater than 10 g/dL can optimize the efficiency of platelets by enhancing the interactions between platelets and the blood vessel wall. DIC can also lead to impaired platelet function. Thrombocytopenia is a consistent feature of cardiopulmonary bypass surgery, typically secondary to hemodilution, platelet membrane activation from interaction with the bypass circuit, and fragmentation from hypothermia. It generally resolves spontaneously within several days after bypass, but platelet transfusions may be helpful if bleeding persists.

CURRENT THERAPY

- In the absence of bleeding, platelet counts of 5000–10,000/μL are used as the threshold for prophylactic transfusion. Single-donor apheresis platelets should be considered to prevent alloimmunization.
- For hemorrhaging patients or for patients scheduled to undergo delicate operations such as neurosurgery, maintaining the platelet count greater than 75,000 to 100,000/μL is recommended.
- When heparin-induced thrombocytopenia is a possibility, all heparin administration must be stopped and alternative anticoagulation instituted, at least until the platelet count returns to normal.
- Because bleeding in patients with ITP is usually minimal to absent until platelet counts decline to <30,000/μL, asymptomatic patients with platelet counts >30,000 can be followed without treatment.
- Treatment for ITP is initiated with prednisone (1 mg/kg); patients who fail to enter clinical remission are candidates for splenectomy or treatment with immunosuppressive agents including rituximab[1] (Rituxan) and azathioprine[1] (Imuran).
- High doses of corticosteroids (methylprednisolone [Solu-Medrol], 1 g/d for 3 d) or IVIg (1 g/kg/d for 2 d) are indicated for emergency treatment of ITP. Platelet transfusion given concurrently with IVIg can be effective for critical bleeding. Anti-D immune globulin (WinRho) may be used instead of IVIg in Rh$^+$ patients, although this treatment can induce clinically significant hemolysis.
- The platelet dysfunction of uremia is usually corrected by dialysis. Maintaining the hemoglobin above 10 g/dL helps minimize bleeding by increasing interactions between platelets and the blood vessel wall. Intravenous desmopressin (DDAVP) given at a dose of 0.3 μg/kg IV over 15 to 30 minutes shortens the bleeding time in most patients with uremia for approximately 4 hours.
- When necessary, treatment of hereditary disorders of platelet adhesion and aggregation usually requires platelet transfusion.

---

[1]Not FDA approved for this indication.
Abbreviations: ITP = idiopathic thrombocytopenic purpura; IVIg = intravenous immunoglobulin.

HEREDITARY QUALITATIVE PLATELET DISORDERS

Bernard-Soulier syndrome (BSS) and Glanzmann's thrombasthenia (GT) are rare autosomal recessive disorders of the platelet membrane glycoproteins GPIb/IX and GPIIb/IIIa, respectively. They manifest with mucocutaneous bleeding in infancy or childhood. Patients with BSS are also thrombocytopenic and have very large platelets that do not agglutinate when exposed to ristocetin. Platelet counts and morphology are normal in GT, but the platelets cannot aggregate in response to ADP or thrombin. Reliable treatment of bleeding in both conditions requires platelet transfusion.

Hereditary disorders of platelet secretion are not uncommon causes of mucocutaneous bleeding and can be due to alpha granule deficiency (gray platelet syndrome), the more common dense granule deficiency (δ storage pool disease [δSPD]), or to aspirin-like defects resulting from abnormalities of the platelet secretory mechanism. δSPD may be associated with albinism (Hermansky-Pudlack and Chédiak-Higashi syndromes) or occur in otherwise normal persons. Patients with δSPD have normal platelet counts with prolonged bleeding times and abnormal platelet aggregation studies with a diagnostic increased adenosine triphosphate-to-adenosine diphosphate (ATP/ADP) ratio due to the absence of platelet dense granule ADP. Although bleeding in patients with secretion disorders can be controlled by platelet transfusion, DDAVP sometimes shortens the bleeding times and improves hemostasis.

REFERENCES

Aster RH, Bougie DW. Drug-induced immune thrombocytopenia. N Engl J Med 2007;357:580–7.

Bolton-Maggs PHB, Chalmers EA, Collins PW, et al. A review of inherited platelet disorders with guidelines for their management on behalf of the UKHCDO. Br J Haematol 2006;135:603–33.

Cines DB, Blanchette VS. Immune thrombocytopenic purpura. N Engl J Med 2002;346:995–1008.

Hedges SJ, Dehoney SB, Hooper JS, et al. Evidence-based treatment recommendations for uremic bleeding. Nat Clin Pract Nephrol 2007;3:138–53.

Lind SE. The bleeding time does not predict surgical bleeding. Blood 1991;77:2547–52.

Mannucci PM. Drug therapy: Treatment of von Willebrand's disease. N Engl J Med 2004;351:683–94.

Nurden AT. Qualitative disorders of platelets and megakaryocytes. J Thromb Hemostasis 2006;3:1773–82.

Nurden AT, Viallard JF, Nurden P. New-generation drugs that stimulate platelet production in chronic immune thrombocytopenic purpura. Lancet 2009;373:1562–9.

Stanworth SJ, Hyde C, Brunskill S, et al. Platelet transfusion prophylaxis for patients with hematological malignancies: Where to now? Br J Haematol 2005;131:588–95.

Warkentin TE. Heparin-induced thrombocytopenia: Pathogenesis and management. Br J Haematol 2003;121:535–55.

Disseminated Intravascular Coagulation

Method of
Jaime Morales-Arias, MD

Disseminated intravascular coagulation (DIC) is an acquired clinicopathologic syndrome that typically occurs as a consequence of a serious underlying condition. It is characterized by systemic activation of the coagulation system. This process initiates a cascade of events that includes the formation of fibrin clots and microthrombi with secondary end-organ ischemia and failure and concomitant consumption of coagulation factors and platelets that can result in hemorrhagic manifestations.

Epidemiology

DIC is a secondary thrombohemorrhagic phenomenon that occurs as a consequence of a multitude of disorders that pathologically activate and dysregulate the intravascular coagulation system. The most common causes are sepsis, cancer, and trauma. DIC is estimated to occur in approximately 1% of hospitalized patients, but it may be present in up to 30% to 50% of those with severe sepsis. DIC carries a high morbidity and mortality risk, usually depending on the severity of the underlying disease and the degree of the hematologic and thrombotic manifestations. Mortality rates have been reported to range from 31% to as high as 86% in some series. Advanced age is associated with a worse outcome.

Risk Factors

The main factor for the occurrence of DIC is the presence of a life-threatening underlying condition that abnormally activates the coagulation process. Severe sepsis (bacterial, viral, fungal) is the major cause. Additionally, serious trauma, especially head trauma, has a high correlation with DIC. Several pregnancy complications have also been implicated in the pathogenesis of DIC. Box 1 summarizes the most common causes.

Pathophysiology

The most common initiating event in DIC is the exposure of blood to tissue factor, which can be secondary to vascular endothelial damage or to activation of tissue factor by circulating monocytes in response to inflammatory cytokines. As a result, this aberrant exposure to tissue factor produces increased amounts of thrombin. In DIC, thrombin generation becomes so excessive that it cannot be counterregulated by the natural antithrombotic pathways, such as tissue factor pathway inhibitor and antithrombin III. Because thrombin activates fibrin, these events create a widespread systemic deposition of fibrin, thus stimulating the formation of microthrombi and end-organ ischemia and damage.

Thrombin promotes the release of tissue plasminogen activator from damaged endothelium. This phenomenon causes a secondary activation of the fibrinolytic pathway, generating fibrin degradation products that in turn interfere with fibrin polymerization and have a deleterious effect on platelet aggregation.

There is generalized consumption of fibrinogen, platelets, and coagulation factors (II, V, VIII), thus promoting bleeding. Coagulation inhibitors such as protein C also get depleted, further impairing the capacity to control the thrombotic manifestations. DIC can also induce a secondary microangiopathic hemolytic anemia, mostly due to intravascular fibrin causing mechanical damage and fragmentation of red blood cells.

Clinical Manifestations

Symptoms may be secondary to either the underlying disease or to DIC. The most common manifestation is that of a bleeding diathesis. A patient might initially have excessive oozing from venipuncture sites or mucosal surfaces, but more severe hemorrhages can also occur. Both venous and arterial thrombosis are seen in DIC and can manifest with secondary organ damage. Other signs include renal, hepatic, and

---

BOX 1   Underlying Conditions in Disseminated Intravascular Coagulation

Sepsis
- Meningococcemia
- Other organisms

Trauma and tissue damage
- Crush injury
- Burns
- Heat stroke

Malignancy
- Acute promyelocytic leukemia
- Solid tumors

Liver disease

Obstetric accidents
- Abruptio placentae
- Amniotic fluid embolism
- Eclampsia

Protein C and S deficiencies (purpura fulminans)

Kasabach-Merritt syndrome

Severe hemolytic transfusion reactions

Toxin exposures (snake and spider bites)

Severe pancreatitis

TABLE 1 Clinical Symptoms in DIC

Sign or Symptom	Incidence (%)
Bleeding	64
Renal impairment	25
Hepatic impairment	19
Pulmonary manifestations	16
Shock	14
Thrombosis	7
Neurologic dysfunction	2

neurologic impairment. Pulmonary hemorrhage and acute respiratory distress syndrome have been reported in severe cases. Table 1 summarizes the most common symptomatology in DIC.

Diagnosis

No single test is diagnostic for DIC, but rather a combination of clinical and laboratory findings can aid in making an accurate diagnosis. Depending on the underlying condition, laboratory abnormalities can vary. However, the most common findings, in decreasing order of frequency, are thrombocytopenia, elevated fibrin degradation products or D-dimers, prolonged prothrombin time (PT), prolonged activated partial thromboplastin time (aPTT), and low fibrinogen. Thrombocytopenia occurs in 98% of patients with DIC, and the platelet count is less than 50,000 per microliter in 50% of them, making this an extremely sensitive, though nonspecific, marker. The PT and aPTT are prolonged in 75% and 60% of patients, respectively, reflecting the degree of consumption of coagulation factors.

Low fibrinogen is another marker for DIC, but its sensitivity has been reported to be as low as 28%. This may be due in part to the fact that fibrinogen is an inflammatory marker and may be falsely elevated in some conditions that cause DIC. Fibrin degradation products and D-dimers are elevated owing to the increased activation of the fibrinolytic pathway. The D-dimer assay has been shown to be more specific for DIC than the measurement of fibrin degradation products. In addition, the thrombin time may be elevated secondary to the increase in fibrin degradation products as well as to the hypofibrinogenemia. Measurement of anticoagulant proteins such as antithrombin III and protein C can demonstrate decreased levels in DIC, but there are limitations owing to the lack of availability of these assays in most centers. In addition, a review of the blood smear can reveal fragmented red blood cells in cases where DIC has caused a microangiopathic hemolytic anemia.

CURRENT DIAGNOSIS

- Disseminated intravascular coagulation (DIC) occurs in the presence of a life-threatening underlying illness and is characterized by systemic pathologic activation of the coagulation system.
- Symptoms may be secondary to either the underlying disease or to DIC, the most common manifestation being a bleeding diathesis.
- A combination of clinical and laboratory findings aid in making an accurate diagnosis.
- Depending on the underlying condition, laboratory abnormalities can vary. The most common laboratory findings are thrombocytopenia, elevated fibrin degradation products, elevated D-dimer assay, prolonged prothrombin time, prolonged activated partial thromboplastin time, low fibrinogen, and microangiopathic hemolytic anemia.
- A validated objective scoring system for the diagnosis of overt DIC based solely on laboratory data is available.

BOX 2 Scoring System for Overt Disseminated Intravascular Coagulation

1. Risk assessment: Does the patient have an underlying disorder known to be associated with overt DIC?
   - Yes: Proceed
   - No: Do not use this algorithm
2. Order global coagulation tests (platelet count, fibrin markers, PT, fibrinogen).
3. Score results.
   - Platelet count: >100 = 0, <100 =1, <50 = 2
   - Elevated fibrin markers such as D-dimers or FDP: No increase = 0, moderate increase = 2, strong increase = 3
   - Prolonged PT: <3 sec = 0, >3 sec but <6 sec = 1, >6 sec = 2
   - Fibrinogen level: >1 g/L = 0, <1 g/L = 1
4. Calculate score:
   - ≥5: compatible with overt DIC. Repeat score daily.
   - <5: Suggestive (not conclusive) for nonovert DIC. Repeat score in next 1 or 2 days.

Abbreviations: DIC = disseminated intravascular coagulation; FDP = fibrin degradation product; PT = prothrombin time.

An objective scoring system for the diagnosis of overt DIC based solely on laboratory data has been established by the Scientific and Standardization Committee of the International Society of Thrombosis and Haemostasis (Box 2). It has been demonstrated to have a sensitivity of 91% and a specificity of 97% and to be an independent prognostic factor for mortality. Following the guidelines of the scoring system, patients with sepsis and DIC have been shown to have a mortality of 43%, as compared to only 27% for those without DIC.

Treatment

To control DIC, the precipitating disease needs to be treated vigorously and promptly. Additionally, aggressive supportive care measures, usually in an intensive care setting, are of utmost importance. In some cases this can indeed be enough. In other instances, a more specific treatment approach, such as replacing platelets or coagulation factor, may be necessary. This should not be based on laboratory parameters alone but rather on the clinical scenario and whether there is active bleeding, thrombosis, or organ dysfunction.

Platelet transfusions in nonbleeding patients are not usually indicated. They should be reserved for patients with a count of <50,000/µL and active bleeding or those who are perceived to be at an increased risk for bleeding, for example, in a preoperative or postoperative setting. A higher platelet count may be desired in specific situations, such as neurotrauma. Platelet support may also be considered in nonbleeding patients if the count is extremely low (<10-20,000/µL).

The same rule applies to factor replacement with fresh frozen plasma. For patients without active bleeding, fresh frozen plasma is rarely indicated. However, in patients with a prolongation of the PT and aPTT and bleeding, or those perceived to be at an increased risk for bleeding or who are undergoing an invasive procedure, fresh frozen plasma should be considered. If the fibrinogen level is significantly low (<1 g/L), cryoprecipitate may be administered.

The use of anticoagulant therapy with heparin in patients with DIC has been controversial. Its use can potentiate the bleeding risks. However, heparin should be considered in cases where thrombosis predominates and is likely to lead to severe tissue injury. For example, heparin or other anticoagulant therapy should be given in the presence of dermal or acral ischemia that might rapidly progress to gangrene, as occurs in purpura fulminans and in some types of bacteremia. Indeed, anticoagulation has been demonstrated to reduce mortality from 90% to 18% in patients with purpura fulminans.

Other instances in which heparin may be of benefit include DIC related to metastatic cancers, aortic aneurysms, retained dead fetus syndrome, and acute promyelocytic leukemias that are unresponsive to initial standard therapy. In addition, heparin therapy may be indicated in the presence of large vessel clots or in cases where intensive replacement of blood products alone has not been effective.

Replacement of anticoagulant factors, including administration of activated protein C (drotrecogin alfa [Xigris] and antithrombin concentrates (Thrombate III, ATryn),[1] is another strategy that has been evaluated. Clinical studies have shown a survival advantage for patients with severe sepsis and DIC using activated protein C, but there was a minor increased risk of bleeding (3.5% versus 2% in placebo), and caution should be exercised in this regard. After several clinical trials studying its potential efficacy in DIC, antithrombin administration has not been demonstrated to decrease mortality.

Antifibrinolytic therapy is usually contraindicated in DIC because of its risk of promoting thrombosis, but it may be considered in patients with severe bleeding whose primary process is a hyperfibrinolytic state. Agents include aminocaproic acid (Amicar) and tranexamic acid (Cyklokapron).[1]

Potential treatment agents undergoing trials include recombinant thrombomodulin, recombinant tissue factor pathway inhibitor, inactivated factor VII (Novoseven), and recombinant nematode anticoagulant protein c2.

---

[1]Not FDA approved for this indication.

REFERENCES

Bernard GR, Vincent JL, Laterre PF, et al. Efficacy and safety of recombinant human activated protein C for severe sepsis. N Engl J Med 2001;344:699–709.

Bick RL. Disseminated intravascular coagulation current concepts of etiology, pathophysiology, diagnosis, and treatment. Hematol Oncol Clin North Am 2003;17:149–76.

Levi M, de Jonge E, van der Poll T. New treatment strategies for disseminated intravascular coagulation based on current understanding of the pathophysiology. Ann Med 2004;36:41–9.

Marder VJ, Feinstein DI, Colman RW, et al. Consumptive thrombohemorrhagic disorders. In: Colman RW, editor. Hemostasis and Thrombosis. 5th ed. Philadelphia: Lippincott Williams and Wilkins; 2006. p. 1571–600.

Seligsohn U, Hoots WK. Disseminated intravascular coagulation. In: Lichtman MA, editor. Williams Hematology. 7th ed. New York: McGraw Hill; 2006. p. 1959–79.

Siegal T, Seligsohn U, Aghai E, et al. Clinical and laboratory aspects of disseminated intravascular coagulation (DIC): A study of 118 cases. Thromb Haemost 1978;39:122–34.

Taylor FB, Toh CH, Hoots WK, et al. Towards definition, clinical and laboratory criteria, and a scoring system for disseminated intravascular coagulation. Thromb Haemost 2001;86:1327–30.

Toh CH, Hoots WK. The scoring system of the Scientific and Standardization Committee on Disseminated Intravascular Coagulation of the International Society on Thrombosis and Haemostasis: A 5-year overview. J Thromb Haemost 2007;5:604–6.

Warren BL, Eid A, Singer P, et al. Caring for the critically ill patient. High-dose antithrombin III in severe sepsis: A randomized controlled trial. JAMA 2001;286:1869–78.

Thrombotic Thrombocytopenic Purpura

Method of
Joseph E. Kiss, MD

Thrombotic thrombocytopenic purpura (TTP) is a life-threatening thrombotic disorder in which unrestrained platelet deposition occurs in the microcirculation of many organs, including the brain, kidneys, heart, and abdominal viscera. Thrombocytopenia develops as platelets are progressively consumed. The term microangiopathic hemolytic anemia refers to the fragmentation of red blood cells (schistocytes) during their passage through partially occluded arterioles and capillaries. Therapeutic plasma exchange, the mainstay of therapy, has markedly improved the mortality rate, from more than 90% in the past to 10% to 20% currently. A high index of suspicion for the diagnosis is necessary, because delays in recognizing the disorder can increase treatment failure and death. Because plasma exchange is very effective, it is appropriate to consider TTP as a provisional diagnosis and to initiate therapy when thrombocytopenia and microangiopathic hemolytic anemia are present without another apparent cause.

Classification

A wide variety of disorders can be associated with TTP or can develop TTP-like manifestations. The primary causes and major secondary forms are outlined in Box 1. This classification is based on clinical and laboratory similarities. There is ongoing controversy as to whether certain secondary causes should be considered in this classification and whether they should be treated with plasma exchange. For example, a TTP-like syndrome can occur in the setting of hematopoietic stem cell transplantation, but the efficacy of plasma exchange has been questioned. Experienced clinical judgment may be necessary to decide on the appropriate diagnosis and the best course of therapy.

Pathogenesis

Remarkable progress has been made over the last few years in understanding the pathogenesis of TTP. Defects in ADAMTS13, a key enzyme that normally clips large, sticky multimers of von Willebrand's factor into smaller subunits, have been found in patients with congenital TTP and in patients with idiopathic TTP. Without the enzyme, long strings of ultra-large von Willebrand's factor remain anchored to the surface of endothelial cells, binding platelets and forming occlusive microthrombi throughout many organs, especially the brain and kidneys. A second hit, presumably endothelial cell injury secondary to the stress of infection, surgery, or pregnancy, triggers an acute episode in the setting of ADAMTS13 deficiency.

Dysfunctional enzyme is found in all cases of congenital TTP. Severe ADAMTS13 deficiency (defined as <10% of normal) caused by an immunoglobulin G autoantibody to ADAMTS13 is reported in 30% to 100% of cases of idiopathic TTP. Typical TTP patients have also been described who do not have ADAMTS13 deficiency, suggesting that alternative, unknown mechanisms can also lead to TTP.

Clinical Presentation

Idiopathic TTP often occurs in young, healthy persons. The peak age group is between 20 and 40 years; women are affected twice as often as men. African Americans are disproportionately affected. The classic

BOX 1   Clinical Classification and Distinguishing Features of TTP and Other Thrombotic Microangiopathies

Primary

Congenital

Caused by mutations in *ADAMTS13* gene
Very rare

Idiopathic

Caused by IgG autoantibody that binds to ADAMTS13
Diagnosed by exclusion of secondary causes
Most common form

Secondary*

Human Immunodeficiency Virus

High response rate reported to plasma infusion and antiretroviral therapy

Collagen Vascular Diseases

Treated in the same way as idiopathic TTP using plasma exchange, immunosuppressants

Drug-Induced Immunologic Disease

Ticlopidine (Ticlid)
Induces antibody to ADAMTS13
Treatment is withdrawing offending drug and performing plasma exchange
Rapid recovery is typical
Related drug, clopidogrel (Plavix), also associated, but the mechanism is uncertain
Quinine also commonly implicated; antiplatelet and antiendothelial antibodies are associated
Must be distinguished from immune thrombocytopenic purpura
ADAMTS13 is not reduced, and efficacy of plasma exchange is questionable

Drug-Induced, Dose-Dependent Toxicity

Associated with cancer chemotherapeutic agents including mitomycin C (Mutamycin) and gemcitabine (Gemzar)
Can develop slowly, sometimes after drug is discontinued
Can also be seen with immunosuppressive agents including cyclosporine (Neoral) and tacrolimus (Prograf)
Treated by stopping drug
Uncertain benefit of plasma exchange

Pregnancy and Postpartum

May be caused by an IgG inhibitor of ADAMTS13
Must be distinguished from HELLP syndrome (HELLP usually occurs during the third trimester of pregnancy or immediately after delivery in association with severe preeclampsia)

Hematopoietic Stem Cell Transplantation–Associated Disease

A TTP-like syndrome that may be caused by infection or graft-versus-host disease
Doubtful benefit of plasma exchange

*If laboratory samples are to be drawn to evaluate a possible secondary cause (e.g., systemic lupus erythematosus), it is important to obtain them before plasma exchange therapy is instituted, to avoid a dilution effect.
Abbreviations: HELLP = hemolysis with elevated liver enzymes and low platelets; IgG = immunoglobulin G; TTP = thrombotic thrombocytic purpura.

---

diagnostic pentad, consisting of thrombocytopenia, microangiopathic anemia, fever, neurologic abnormalities, and renal failure, occurs in only a minority of cases, perhaps because, with increased clinical awareness, the diagnosis is being considered earlier in the course of the disease. Patients might have vague symptoms at first (e.g., malaise, weakness, headache), several days before developing worrisome neurologic complaints including visual disturbances, paresthesias, focal motor weakness, and aphasia (i.e., transient ischemic attacks) or more generalized manifestations such as confusion, seizures, stupor, and coma. The neurologic abnormalities in conjunction with thrombocytopenia and anemia form a common triad that should lead to high diagnostic suspicion. Fever occurs in about 50% of patients at the time of presentation.

Renal injury is associated with rising creatinine and proteinuria and is typically mild in TTP. Cases in which renal failure predominates are termed hemolytic uremic syndrome (HUS). Diarrhea (usually but not always bloody) should prompt consideration of enterotoxin-associated epidemic HUS. Because of frequent clinical overlap with both neurologic and renal manifestations, it may be difficult to distinguish between TTP and HUS in adults.

Gastrointestinal complaints are also common. Abdominal pain, nausea, vomiting, and diarrhea can reflect the presence of visceral ischemia or pancreatitis. These symptoms, along with mental status changes, elevated bilirubin, and thrombocytopenia, may be mistaken for liver disease, further delaying diagnosis. Chest pain and arrhythmias caused by small-vessel myocardial involvement have been reported in up to 18% of patients in some series. These protean clinical manifestations of TTP reflect its multisystemic pathophysiology.

Diagnosis

The hallmark of microangiopathic hemolytic anemia is the presence of fragmented red blood cells on the blood smear. A number of disorders are known to cause microangiopathic hemolysis and thrombocytopenia, which can mimic the clinical and laboratory features of TTP. These include severe hypertension (persisting blood pressure >200/100 mm Hg with or without papilledema), prosthetic cardiac devices (e.g., left ventricular assist devices, intraaortic balloon pump), hemolysis with elevated liver enzymes and low platelets (HELLP) syndrome with severe preeclampsia, and vasculitis. Disseminated intravascular coagulation may be seen in association with sepsis, and a low-grade form is associated with carcinoma. In contrast to disseminated intravascular coagulation, the fibrinogen level in TTP is normal, and fibrin degradation products are also normal or minimally increased. The direct antiglobulin test is used to exclude immune hemolysis, which can occur concomitantly with autoimmune thrombocytopenia (Evan's syndrome).

CURRENT DIAGNOSIS

Recommended Diagnostic Tests for Initial Evaluation

- Complete blood count with differential white blood cell, platelet, and reticulocyte count
- Review of peripheral blood smear
- Coagulation studies including fibrinogen and fibrin degradation products
- Lactate dehydrogenase (LDH)
- Blood urea nitrogen, creatinine, electrolytes
- Liver function tests, including direct and indirect bilirubin
- Haptoglobin
- ADAMTS13 activity and inhibitor level
- Direct antiglobulin test
- Urinalysis

Although measurement of ADAMTS13 is becoming more widely available in clinical laboratories, the usefulness of this test still needs to be validated as a diagnostic and management tool. A number of technical issues affect the analytic sensitivity and specificity of the various assays in use. Therefore, a normal level should not be used to exclude the diagnosis. Severe deficiency of ADAMTS13 has been proposed as a specific test for TTP, but it has also been noted in severe sepsis, disseminated intravascular coagulation, and metastatic malignancy. If these entities can be confidently excluded, a severe deficiency of ADAMTS13 reported by an experienced laboratory strongly supports the diagnosis of TTP.

Treatment

Plasma exchange is the only therapy that has been shown to be effective in a randomized controlled clinical trial. It is believed to work by replacing ADAMTS13 and by removing inhibitory antibodies to the enzyme. It also appears to be effective in patients who are not deficient in ADAMTS13, so other mechanisms may be involved.

If there is a delay in instituting plasma exchange, 15 to 30 mL/kg of plasma should be infused, with attention to avoiding volume overload. Cardiac monitoring in the initial stages of management is advisable in light of the relatively high frequency of cardiac involvement. In the absence of serious bleeding, platelet transfusions are contraindicated because of the potential deposition of platelet microthrombi and the risk of serious clinical sequelae (e.g., transient ischemic attack, myocardial infarction). The role of adjuvant therapy, such as corticosteroids, antiplatelet drugs, and other immunosuppressives, is not firmly established in the routine management of TTP.

Between 1 and 1.5 plasma volumes are exchanged daily, using fresh-frozen plasma or alternative products that have been shown to contain ADAMTS13 (e.g., plasma frozen within 24 hours, cryoprecipitate-reduced plasma, thawed plasma). Plasma exchanges are continued daily while the clinical and laboratory responses are assessed (Fig. 1). The platelet count is the single most useful laboratory parameter to follow. Lactate dehydrogenase (LDH), an indicator of tissue ischemia and hemolysis, typically lags behind changes in platelet levels. The therapeutic goal is to induce remission, consisting of a normal platelet count and near-normal LDH (<1.5 times normal levels).

Plasma exchange is usually continued on a daily schedule for 1 to 2 days after remission is achieved. It is not unusual for the disease activity to quickly reappear, leading some to taper the plasma exchanges over a short period (e.g., every other day × 3, then every 3 days × 2, then stop). A study comparing different institutional tapering practices found no differences in exacerbation rates. A total of 10 to 20 procedures may be needed to achieve a durable response.

Although plasma exchange is considered a safe procedure, serious complications, including catheter-related sepsis, venous thrombosis, and death, have been reported. Patients should be observed closely for 30 days after cessation of plasma exchange. This is a critical time for exacerbation of the disease, which occurs in about 20% of patients. In those who do not respond or who respond slowly, the plasma volume may be increased and immunosuppressive therapy may be considered (e.g., prednisone 1 mg/kg/day). Continuation of the daily plasma-exchange regimen (i.e., patience on the part of the treater) is probably the single most important therapeutic strategy.

Patients who remain refractory or who are plasma exchange dependent after several weeks are considered for additional immunosuppressive therapy. Use of the anti-CD20 monoclonal antibody rituximab (Rituxan)[1] has shown very good results, including disease remission in the majority of patients with refractory disease who were treated with it. Relapses occur in 30% to 40% of patients with idiopathic TTP, months to years later, reflecting the relapsing and remitting autoimmune nature of this disorder.

Prognosis

Because of increased recognition and earlier treatment of TTP, most patients achieve remission and go on to complete recovery. More than half of the deaths occur early, within 48 hours after admission to the hospital. A recent clinical analysis found that age older than 40 years, hemoglobin less than 9 g/dL, and temperature higher than 38.5°C at presentation were associated with increased mortality. Outcome cannot be predicted from the severity of the thrombocytopenia or the LDH level. The ADAMTS13 level appears to have prognostic value: Patients with severe ADAMTS13 deficiency have more autoimmune manifestations, lower platelet counts, less renal insufficiency, and a higher risk of relapse. TTP in association with transplantation and malignancy is often resistant to therapy, and novel approaches are needed.

---

[1]Not FDA approved for this indication.

441

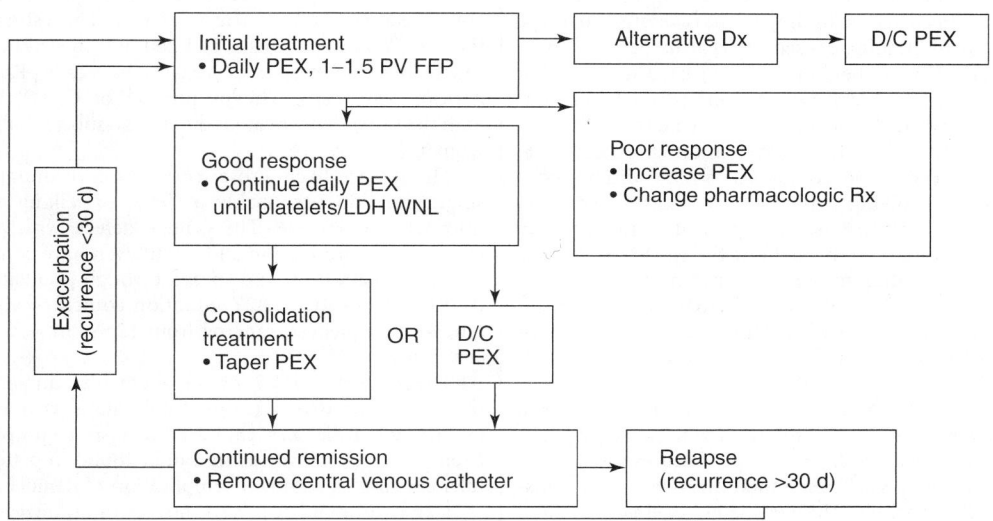

FIGURE 1. Management of thrombotic thrombocytopenic purpura. *Abbreviations:* D/C = discontinue; Dx = diagnosis; FFP = fresh-frozen plasma; LDH = lactate dehydrogenase; PEX = plasma exchange; PV = plasma volume; Rx = prescription; WNL = within normal limits. (Adapted from George JN: How I treat patients with thrombotic thrombocytopenic purpura–hemolytic uremic syndrome. Blood 2000;96:4:1223–29.)

REFERENCES

Allford S, Hunt B, Rose P, et al. Guidelines on the diagnosis and management of the thrombotic microangiopathic haemolytic anemias. Br J Haematol 2003;120:556–73.

Bandarenko N. Members of the United States Thrombotic Thrombocytopenic Purpura Apheresis Study Group (US TTP ASG). Multicenter survey and retrospective analysis of current efficacy of therapeutic plasma exchange. J Clin Apheresis 1998;13:133–41.

Fakhouri F, Vernant JP, Veyradier A, et al. Efficiency of curative and prophylactic treatment with rituximab in ADAMTS13-deficient thrombotic thrombocytopenic purpura: A study of 11 cases. Blood 2005;106:1932–7.

George JN. How I treat patients with thrombotic thrombocytopenic purpura-hemolytic uremic syndrome. Blood 2000;96:41223–9.

Howard MA, Williams LA, Terrell DR. Complications of plasma exchange in patients treated for clinically suspected thrombotic thrombocytopenic purpura-hemolytic uremic syndrome: III. An additional study of 54 consecutive patients. Transfusion 2006;46:154–6.

Kiss JE. Thrombotic thrombocytopenic purpura: recognition and management. Int J Hematol 2010;91:36–45.

Moake JL. Thrombotic microangiopathies. N Engl J Med 2002;347:8589–600.

Qu L, Kiss JE. Thrombotic microangiopathy in transplantation and malignancy. Semin Thromb Hemost 2005;31:691–9.

Vesely SK, George JN, Lammle B, et al. ADAMTS13 activity in thrombotic thrombocytopenic purpura-hemolytic uremic syndrome: Relation to presenting features and clinical outcomes in a prospective cohort of 142 patients. Blood 2003;102(1):60–8.

Hemochromatosis

Method of
Antonello Pietrangelo, MD, PhD

Definition and Classification

Hemochromatosis, or hereditary hemochromatosis, is an iron-loading disorder caused by a genetically determined failure to prevent iron from entering the body when it is not needed. It is characterized by progressive parenchymal iron overload. It has the potential for multiorgan damage and disease, including cirrhosis, diabetes, and cardiomyopathy.

The term *hemochromatosis* was coined in 1889 by von Recklinghausen to describe the necroscopic finding of massive organ damage associated with dark tissue staining caused by what he believed to be a blood-borne pigment. It was Sheldon who suggested in 1935 that the disorder was probably hereditary. Simon demonstrated its hereditary nature and found that the hemochromatosis gene was in linkage with the human leukocyte antigen (HLA) system on chromosome 6. In this genomic region, Feder and colleagues in 1996 discovered a polymorphism (C282Y) involving a novel MHC class I–like gene, named *HFE*. The C282Y polymorphism was present in the majority of patients with hemochromatosis throughout the world.

In addition to C282Y, other minor *HFE* polymorphisms have been reported. The clinical impact of the *HFE* H63D polymorphism appears to be limited. The *HFE* S65C polymorphism can be associated with hemochromatosis when inherited in trans with C282Y on the other parental allele.

As genetic testing for HFE mutations became more widespread, non-*HFE* mutations were found to be associated with hereditary iron overload syndromes in patients with phenotypic features identical to those of classic hemochromatosis. These mutations involve the transferrin receptor 2 *(TfR2)*, hepcidin *(HAMP)*, hemojuvelin *(HJV)*, and ferroportin *(FPN)* genes.

The present definition of hemochromatosis embraces the classic disorder related to *HFE* C282Y homozygosity (the prototype for this syndrome and by far the most common form) and the rare disorders attributed to other genetic mutations (Box 1).

BOX 1   Human Diseases Associated with Iron Overload

Hereditary

Hemochromatosis (from *HFE, TfR2, HIV, HAMP, FPN* genetic mutations)
Ferroportin disease
Aceruloplasminemia
A(hypo)transferrinemia
DMT1 deficiency
H ferritin mutation
Friedreich's ataxia
Porphyria cutanea tarda
Hereditary iron-loading anemias (e.g., thalassemia intermedia)*

Acquired

Dietary
Parenteral
Anemia of inflammation
Transfusion-dependent iron-loading anemia (thalassemia major, hemolytic, sideroblastic)
Long-term hemodialysis
Chronic liver disease (alcoholic, viral, dysmetabolic)
Alloimmune neonatal hemochromatosis[†]
African hemochromatosis (Bantù siderosis)[‡]

---

*Parenchymal iron overload is detectable before transfusion in response to inefficient erythropoiesis and hepcidin downregulation.
[†]This has been historically considered hereditary, but studies suggest an alloimmune pathogenesis.
[‡]Particularly common among Africans in sub-Saharan regions who drink a traditional beer brewed in nongalvanized steel drums. In this disorder, an unidentified iron-loading gene might confer susceptibility to the disease. Ferroportin has been implicated as a possible modifier gene.

Epidemiology

HFE-related hemochromatosis is the most common form of hemochromatosis and the most frequently inherited metabolic disorder found in whites. The reported allelic frequency of C282Y across several screening studies is around 6%. The estimated prevalence of the C282Y polymorphism is 1:200-300 in whites. The prevalence is much lower in Hispanics, Asian Americans, Pacific Islanders, and African Americans. The proportion of C282Y homozygous males with iron-overload-related disease is substantially higher than for women (28% vs. 1%).

The disease likely arose from a chance mutation occurring in a single individual, probably a Celtic or Viking ancestor inhabiting northwestern Europe. The genetic defect, which caused no serious obstacle to reproduction and might even have conferred some advantages, was passed on and spread through population migration. The distribution of the C282Y mutation coincides with its northern origin, with frequencies ranging from 12.5% in Ireland to 0% in southern Europe.

The prevalence of C282Y is higher in certain patient groups, such as those with liver disease (5- to 10-fold higher than in the general population), type 1 diabetes, chondrocalcinosis, or porphyria cutanea tarda. Even higher C282Y incidence can be found in patients with hepatocellular carcinoma, a known complication of hemochromatosis.

Hemochromatosis is associated with homozygosity for the C282Y *HFE* mutation in approximately 80% of clinically characterized patients of European ancestry. Hence, nearly 20% of patients with hemochromatosis have the disease in the absence of C282Y. Other genes associated with clinical hemochromatosis are *TfR2, HJV, HAMP,* and *FPN* (Table 1). None of the related non-*HFE*

TABLE 1 Characteristics of Hemochromatosis

Sex	Ethnicity	Age (y)	When to Suspect — Signs and Symptoms	Fully Expressed Disease	Essential for Diagnosis
Classic *HFE*-related Hemochromatosis					
Male	White	40-50	Fatigue, arthralgia, dark skin, and/or hepatomegaly and elevated ferritin and elevated and serum transferrin saturation	Liver fibrosis or cirrhosis Diabetes Hypogonadism Arthropathy Cardiomyopathy Melanodermia	C282Y *HFE* homozygosity and evidence of iron overload
			Unexplained hyperferritinemia with increased transferrin saturation Parenchymal iron overload at liver biopsy (with decreasing portocentral gradient and iron-spared Kupffer cells) in the absence of end-stage cirrhosis and hematologic disorder		
Non-*HFE* Hemochromatosis: Adult-Onset Forms					
Either	Any	30-40	Symptomatic organ disease (e.g., cirrhosis, diabetes) and elevated serum transferrin saturation and serum ferritin Unexplained hyperferritinemia with increased transferrin saturation in a non-C282Y *HFE* homozygote with signs and symptoms suggesting hemochromatosis Non-C282Y HFE homozygote with signs and symptoms suggesting hemochromatosis, in the absence of end-stage cirrhosis and hematologic disorders with parenchymal iron overload at liver biopsy (with decreasing portocentral gradient and iron-spared Kupffer cells)	Liver fibrosis or cirrhosis Diabetes Hypogonadism Arthropathy Cardiomyopathy Melanodermia	Parenchymal iron overload at liver biopsy (with portocentral gradient and iron-spared Kupffer cells) in a non-C282Y *HFE* homozygote, in the absence of end-stage cirrhosis and hematologic disorders and positive *TfR2* or *FPN* gene mutation analysis
Juvenile Hemochromatosis					
Either	Any	15-30	Impotence or amenorrhea and/or cardiomyopathy and marked elevation of serum iron parameters	Hypogonadotropic hypogonadism Diabetes Cardiomyopathy Liver cirrhosis Arthropathy	Hypogonadism or amenorrhea and/or cardiomyopathy in young patients with marked hyperferritinemia Massive panlobular parenchymal iron overload at liver biopsy in the absence of end-stage cirrhosis or hematologic disorder Positive *HJV* or *HAMP* gene mutation analysis (in rarer cases: combined mutations of *HFE/TfR2* or *HFE/HJV-HAMP*)
			Endocrine disorders and panlobular parenchymal iron overload at liver biopsy in the absence of end-stage cirrhosis or hematologic disorder		
Ferroportin Disease					
Either	Any	10-80	Unexplained hyperferritinemia and normal or inappropriately low transferrin saturation; isolated hyperferritinemia in other family members (including either father or mother)		
			Sinusoidal (Kupffer) cell iron overload at liver biopsy or spleen (and liver), iron accumulation at MRI in patients with unexplained hyperferritinemia and normal or inadequately low transferrin saturation		Heterozygosity for *FPN* mutation and hyperferritinemia with normal or inappropriately low transferrin saturation and sinusoidal (Kupffer) cell iron overload at liver biopsy

hemochromatosis appears to be restricted to Northern Europeans. The frequency of *TfR2* mutations is low and so far has been detected in only a few pedigrees throughout the world, though hemochromatosis associated with the *TfR2* mutation usually occurs earlier in life than *HFE*-related hemochromatosis and has a more-severe phenotype.

Juvenile hemochromatosis is rare, and most cases are due to mutations of *HJV*, particularly the G320V mutation. A small fraction of patients with juvenile hemochromatosis carry mutations in the gene encoding hepcidin (*HAMP*).

A form of hereditary iron overload distinct from hemochromatosis, "the ferroportin disease," is most commonly due to mutations of the *FPN* gene. Unusual *FPN* mutations can cause rare forms of hemochromatosis similar to classic hemochromatosis.

Pathophysiology

The pathogenic basis of all forms of hemochomatosis is hepcidin deficiency. Hepcidin, a defensin-like peptide, is produced by the hepatocytes in response to high serum iron and inflammatory stimuli. It diffuses through the body and results in the degradation of the iron-exporter ferroportin expressed on the surfaces of iron-rich macrophages and intestinal cells. Unneeded iron is not absorbed through the intestine or remains in the macrophages, where it is saved for future needs (Fig. 1). This mechanism ensures the maintenance of circulating iron levels that can meet the body's erythropoietic needs without posing an oxidative threat to the cells.

The most important hepcidin regulators are circulating bone-morphogenetic proteins (BMPs), particularly BMP6, and the BMP coreceptor hemojuvelin (HJV). BMPs appear to respond to serum iron and activate the transcription of hepcidin in the hepatocyte through the HJV/SMAD4 pathway. In mice, loss of BMP6 or SMAD4 leads to severe iron overload, whereas in both mice and humans, loss of HJV causes a dramatic decrease of hepcidin expression and severe hemochromatosis. Therefore, the loss of either causes hepcidin insufficiency, uncontrolled influx of iron into the bloodstream, and hemochromatosis in rodents and humans.

The time of onset and pattern of organ involvement in hemochromatosis varies depending on the rate and magnitude of plasma iron overloading, which depends, in turn, on the underlying genetic mutation and the hepcidin defect. In general, in human hemochromatosis, the more important a given hemochromatosis gene is for hepcidin regulation, the more significant will be the effect of its mutation on iron metabolism and the more severe will be the resulting hemochromatosis phenotype. Milder adult-onset forms of hemochromatosis (mainly *HFE* and rarely *TfR2* or *FPN* related) and more severe juvenile-onset forms (mainly *HJV* and rarely *HAMP* related) are recognized. The main distinguishing features of hemochromatosis are reported in Box 2.

C282Y *HFE* homozygosity results in a genetic predisposition to hemochromatosis, not a disease state. This polymorphism requires the concurrence of host-related or environmental factors to produce disease. Co-inherited mutations in rare hemochromatosis genes, such as *HAMP* and *HJV*, might have a role in disease penetrance of *HFE* hemochromatosis. Debate continues over the roles of fatty liver, high body mass index, and polymorphic changes in oxidative stress–related genes on the expression of hemochromatosis, but there is evidence for a strong association between alcohol consumption and development of hemochromatosis-related cirrhosis. Data from longitudinal studies on hemochromatosis suggest that up to 50% of C282Y homozygotes can develop iron overload, with up to 30% eventually developing hemochromatosis-associated morbidity.

The first biochemical manifestation of hemochromatosis is an increase of transferrin saturation, which reflects an uncontrolled influx of iron into the bloodstream from enterocytes and macrophages. Apart from menstruation, the body has no effective means of significantly reducing plasma iron levels. Iron overload in the plasma compartment leads to the progressive accumulation of iron in the parenchymal cells of key organs, creating a risk for oxidative damage.

Clinical Manifestations

In *HFE*-related hemochromatosis, the clinical presentation, usually in midlife, varies from simple biochemical abnormalities to severe organ damage and disease. Elevated liver enzymes can be found in 30% of C282Y homozygote male patients, liver fibrosis in 18% of male and 5% of female patients, and cirrhosis in 6% and 2%, respectively.

It is important to recall that, variations notwithstanding, all of the genetic mutations causing hemochromatosis result in the same syndrome and the targets of iron toxicity are identical: liver, heart, endocrine glands, and joints. Uncharacteristically severe or early-onset disease in patients with mutations of the adult-onset *HFE* gene might be the result of undetected additional mutations in other hemochromatosis genes. Although additional genotypic abnormalities are rare, the variety of genotypes that can produce a hemochromatosis phenotype highlights the importance of defining and classifying this disease as a unique clinicopathologic entity.

Hemochromatosis should be suspected in a middle-aged men presenting with unexplained cirrhosis of the liver, bronze skin, diabetes and other endocrine failure, or joint inflammation and heart disease. However, this classic syndromic presentation is rare. Today diagnosis is made at earlier stages as an effect of screening and enhanced case detection due to greater awareness and higher index of suspicion among clinicians. The most common presenting symptoms are now fatigue, malaise, and arthralgia, and hepatomegaly is one of the earliest physical signs.

Elevated transferrin saturation, which precedes increased serum ferritin, and moderately increased transaminase levels are common biochemical abnormalities. Increasing serum ferritin levels herald iron accumulation in tissues, and values greater than 1000 micrograms/L can indicate underlying liver fibrosis in *HFE*-related hemochromatosis, even when transaminase levels are normal. The presence of cirrhosis places patients at an increased risk for developing hepatocellular carcinoma.

In patients suffering from juvenile forms of hemochromatosis, the heart and endocrine glands, which are more susceptible to iron toxicity, succumb to its effects earlier, and their failure dominates the clinical picture. These patients usually present with hypogonadism, which is inevitably found in those aged 15 years or older with juvenile-onset hemochromatosis. Cardiomyopathy and endocrine disorders, including diabetes, appear earlier than they do in adult-onset forms. This is probably because the circulatory iron overload develops much more rapidly and reaches much higher levels (reflecting the more-severe hepcidin deficiency associated with mutation of the juvenile-onset genes).

Diagnosis

In patients with signs and symptoms and/or organ disease suggestive of hemochromatosis, the diagnosis is based on the presence of C282Y homozygosity and iron overload. Therefore, C282Y homozygosity is required for the diagnosis of *HFE* hemochromatosis. Any other *HFE* genotype must be interpreted with caution, though *HFE* gene sequencing in suspected cases of hemochromatosis has revealed other *HFE* polymorphisms. Private *HFE* mutations in rare selected pedigrees have also been reported. In C282Y heterozygotes with mildly increased iron stores, compound heterozygosity with other HFE variants including H63D and S65C has been reported. These genotypes as well as homozygosity for the H63D variants can manifest with altered biochemical iron parameters, some degree of hepatic iron deposition, and clinical expression of hemochromatosis (see Table 1).

Before *HFE* was identified, evaluation of the hepatic iron content and distribution by liver biopsy was the method of choice for diagnosing hemochromatosis. Today the demonstration of C282Y homozygosity in a patient with high transferrin saturation and serum ferritin levels is sufficient for diagnosis, even without a liver biopsy. C282Y homozygosity (particularly in those older than 40 years) with serum ferritin greater than 1000 micrograms/L, together with increased transaminases and hepatomegaly, may be an indication

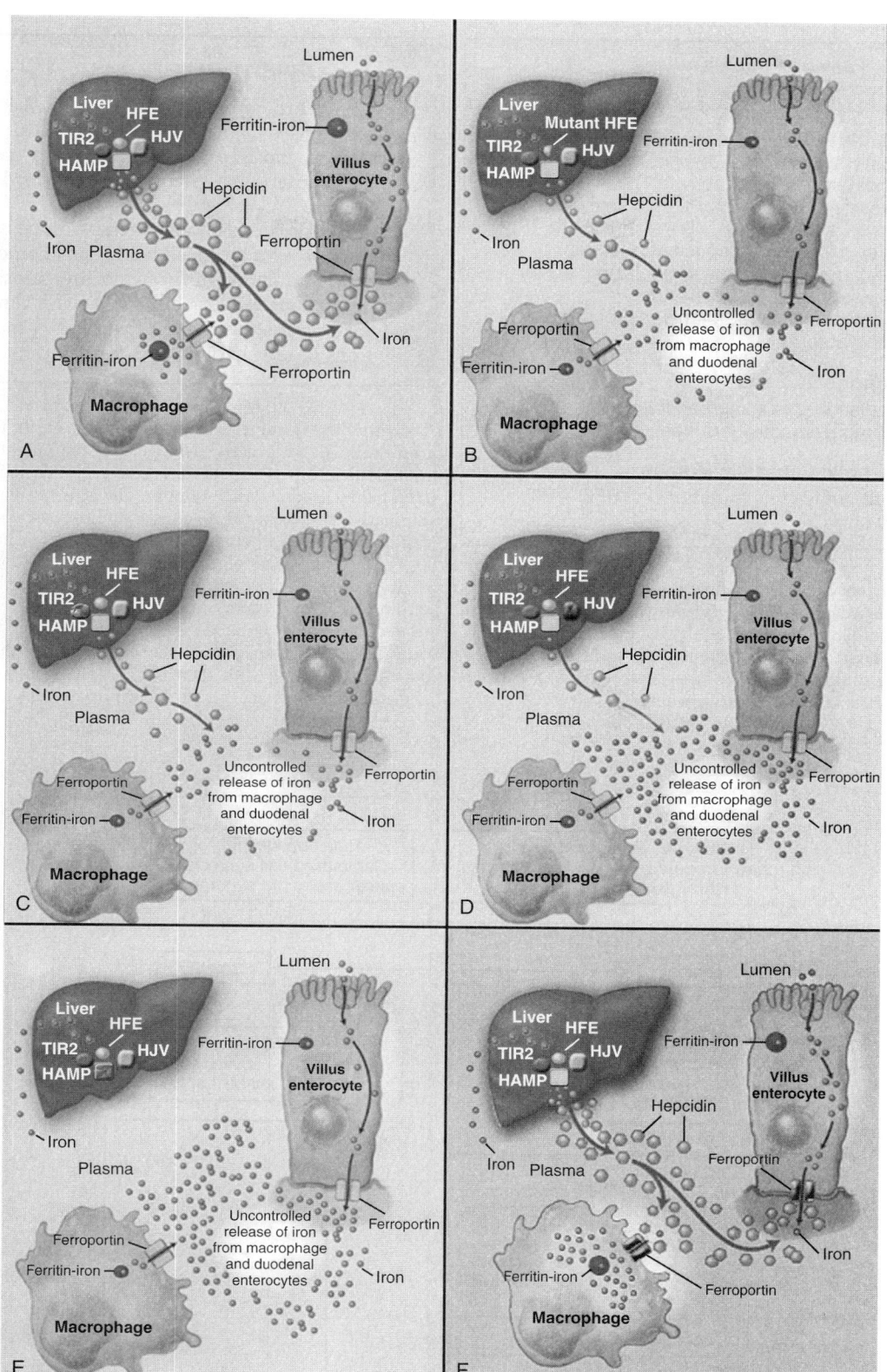

FIGURE 1. Hepcidin as the central pathogenic factor in hemochromatosis. **A,** In normal subjects, hepcidin secreted by the liver modulates the extent and rate of iron release from macrophages and enterocytes. *HFE, TfR2,* and *HJV* are required for hepcidin activation in response to the circulatory iron signal. Lack of one of the hepcidin regulators leads to unrestricted release of iron from macrophages and enterocytes followed by progressive expansion of the plasma iron pool, tissue iron overload, and organ damage (see text for details). **B** through **E,** Depending on the role of the regulators in the control of hepcidin expression, the extent of circulatory iron overload is marginal or massive. The role is marginal in *HFE* hemochromatosis **(B)** and *TfR2*-hemochromatosis **(C)** and massive in *HJV* hemochromatosis **(D)** and *HAMP* hemochromatosis **(E).** This leads to milder (*HFE* or *TfR2* associated) or more-severe forms of hemochromatosis (*HJV* or *HAMP* associated). **F,** The picture is different in the ferroportin disease, where lack-of-function mutations of *FPN* prevent iron export from macrophages and enterocytes, resulting in reticuloendothelial cell iron overload, hyperferritinemia, and low-normal transferrin saturation. (Modified with permission from Pietrangelo A., N Engl J Med 2004;350:2383–97.)

BOX 2   Main Features of Hereditary Hemochromatosis

Distinguishing Features

Hereditary (usually autosomal recessive) trait
Defective hepcidin synthesis or activity
Early and progressive expansion of the plasma iron compartment
Progressive parenchymal iron deposition that can cause severe damage and disease involving the liver, endocrine glands, heart, and joints
Unimpaired erythropoiesis and optimal response to therapeutic phlebotomy

Postulated Pathogenic Basis

Gene mutations leading to inappropriately low hepatic synthesis or impaired activity of hepcidin

Recognized Genetic Causes in Humans

Polymorphism or pathogenic mutations of *HFE, TfR2, HJV, HAMP,* or *FPN*

 CURRENT DIAGNOSIS

- Hemochromatosis is a genetic disease with multisystem involvement.
- The diagnosis of hemochromatosis has both phenotypic criteria of systemic iron overload and genotypic criteria.
- Approximately 80% of patients with "classic" hemochromatosis (European ethnicity) are homozygous for the C282Y mutation of the hemochromatosis gene *(HFE)*.
- Approximately 20% of patients with clinical hemochromatosis are not C282Y homozygotes: many carry mutations in distinct non-*HFE* hemochromatosis genes.

Symptomatic subjects with clear signs of circulatory and tissue iron overload but negative *HFE* gene testing might carry pathogenic mutations in other hemochromatosis genes. Genetic testing for non-*HFE* hemochromatosis is complex and it is not widely available. An alternative approach for diagnosis in these cases is based on biopsy demonstration of a hemochromatotic pattern of hepatic iron load.

Figure 2 shows an algorithm to diagnose hemochromatosis.

In patients with symptoms or signs suggesting hemochromatosis, serum iron parameters should be determined. If symptoms are related to hemochromatosis or iron overload, the transferrin saturation and serum ferritin will be elevated. On the other hand, in patients presenting with increased serum ferritin concentrations, it is mandatory to search first for common causes of hyperferritinemia,

for liver biopsy to rule out hepatic fibrosis or cirrhosis. Liver iron content can be assessed noninvasively by MRI over a wide range of iron concentrations. Considering the higher prevalence of C282Y homozygosity and higher phenotypic penetrance in family members, biochemical testing should be done in first-degree relatives, particularly siblings, and *HFE* testing should be offered.

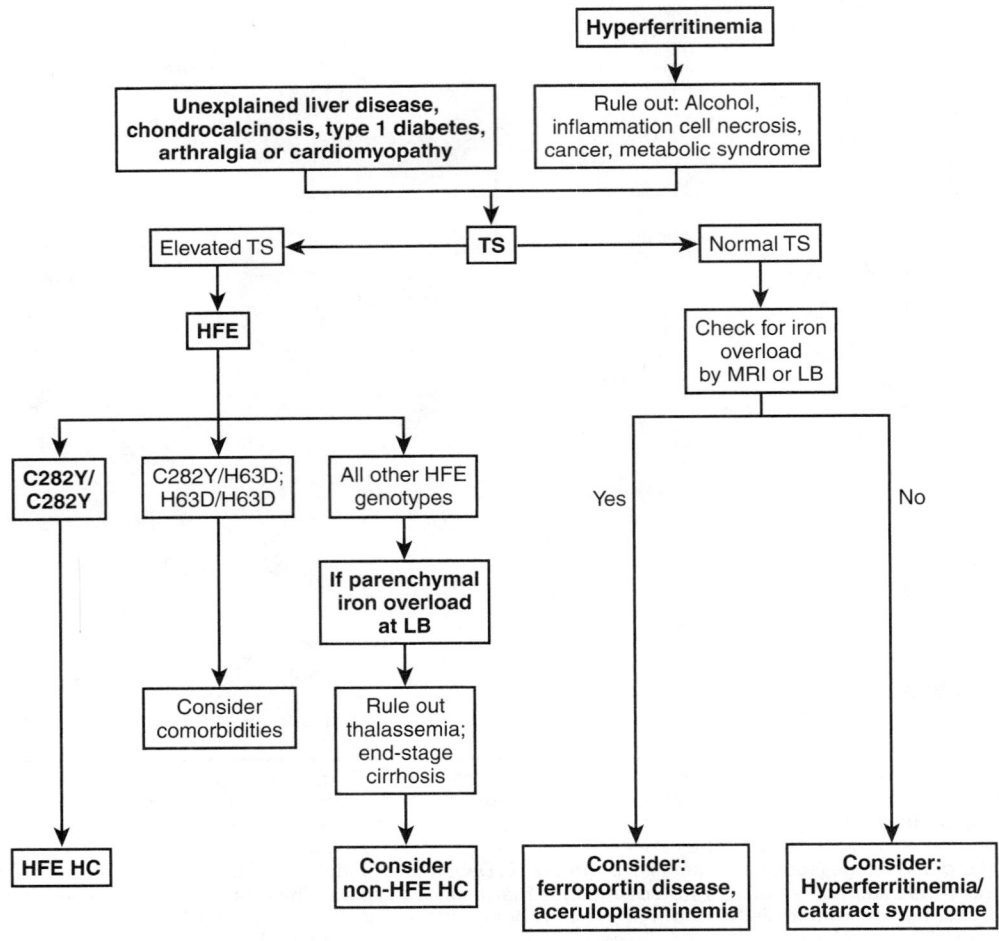

FIGURE 2. A diagnostic algorithm for hemochromatosis. TS, Transferrin saturation; LB, lever biopsy.

such as inflammatory states, alcohol abuse, cancer metabolic syndrome, and decompensated diabetes before genetic testing is carried out. In the absence of such conditions or when hyperferritinemia persists despite treatment of the underlying cause, transferrin saturation should be determined. After confirmation of elevated transferrin saturation, *HFE* gene testing should be ordered. If the patient is a C282Y homozygote, the diagnosis of *HFE* hemochromatosis is established. Patients with compound heterozygosity for the C282Y and H63D or homozygosity for H63D usually present with mild iron overload, which is associated with comorbid factors such as obesity and chronic alcohol consumption.

If symptomatic patients carry other *HFE* genotypes (e.g. C282Y heterozygosity or H63D heterozygosity) or are *HFE* wild-type, the presence of hepatocellular iron overload must be confirmed before suspecting rarer forms of hemochromatosis (see Fig. 2). If a liver biopsy demonstrates parenchymal iron overload and common causes of hepatocellular iron excess are excluded (e.g., compensated iron loading anemia—such as thalassemia intermedia associated with ineffective erythropoiesis and increased intestinal iron absorption—or end-stage liver cirrhosis), non-*HFE* hemochromatosis can be considered and genetic testing for *HJV*, *HAMP*, *TfR2*, and *FPN* mutations can be performed.

If patients present with hyperferritinemia but transferrin saturation is normal or low, the presence or absence of iron overload will guide further diagnostic work-up (see Fig. 2). Assessment of liver iron stores by direct means (MRI or liver biopsy) is recommended. If the liver iron concentration is increased, nonhemochromatosis hereditary iron overload diseases can be considered (e.g. ferroportin disease, aceruloplasminemia). If liver iron concentration is normal, genetic testing for L ferritin gene mutations (to investigate the hyperferritinemia-cataract syndrome) can be carried out.

Differential Diagnosis

The hallmark of hemochromatosis is circulatory and parenchymal cell iron overload. Serum iron concentration and transferrin saturation do not quantitatively reflect body iron stores and should not be used as surrogate markers of tissue iron overload. The most widely used biochemical surrogate for iron overload is serum ferritin. Normal serum ferritin concentrations essentially rule out iron overload. However, ferritin suffers from low specificity because elevated values can be the result of a range of inflammatory, metabolic, and neoplastic conditions such as diabetes mellitus, alcohol consumption, and hepatocellular necrosis. Therefore, in clinical practice, hyperferritinemia may be considered indicative of iron overload in C282Y homozygotes in the absence of the confounding factors listed earlier. In the presence of elevated serum ferritin, the diagnosis of hemochromatosis requires the coexistence of increased transferrin saturation and C282Y homozygosity or, in the case of non-*HFE* hemochromatosis, the presence of tissue iron overload and pathogenic mutations of other hemochromatosis genes.

In patients with hepatic iron deposition at liver biopsy, further diagnostic considerations depend on the cellular and lobular distribution of iron and on the presence or absence of associated lesions including fibrosis, steatosis/steatohepatitis, and chronic hepatitis. Iron deposits in hemochromatosis, as assessed by Perls' stain, typically involve the parenchymal cells, and Kupffer cells are spared until late in the disease (Fig. 3). Iron usually accumulates as fine granules predominating at the biliary pole of parenchymal cells. Iron is distributed throughout the lobule with a decreasing gradient from periportal to centrolobular areas. Mesenchymal iron deposits may be found, but at a later stage when hepatocytic iron is high enough to induce cell necrosis. In patients with pure hepatocellular iron overload, the two main diagnoses in the differential are end-stage cirrhosis, in which iron distribution is heterogeneous from one nodule to another and there are no iron deposits in fibrous tissue or in biliary and vascular walls, and compensated iron loading anemia with inefficient erythropoiesis.

Two other extremely rare hereditary disorders can lead to severe hepatic iron overload, namely aceruloplasminemia and a(hypo)

transferrinemia (see Box 1). In both instances clinical symptoms and signs are very informative for the differential diagnosis: aceruloplasminemia invariably has neurologic manifestations such as progressive extrapyramidal signs, cerebellar ataxia, and dementia. A (hypo)transferrinemia can result in life-threatening anemia.

In the absence of appreciable liver disease, iron deposition predominantly in nonparenchymal cells of the liver in adults is typical of the *ferroportin disease*. Ferroportin disease is caused by loss-of-function mutations of *FPN*. The ferroportin disease is the most common cause of hereditary hyperferritinemia beyond classic hemochromatosis (Table 2). It is an autosomal dominant inherited disorder of iron metabolism that causes progressive iron retention predominantly in reticuloendothelial cells of the spleen and liver. It is characterized by steadily increasing serum ferritin, which is inappropriately high compared to the extent of serum transferrin saturation. Patients are marginally anemic and suffer mild organ disease.

The disorder, clinically recognized in 1999 and linked to ferroportin mutations in 2001, has been now reported worldwide in different ethnic groups. It is thought that loss-of-function mutations of *FPN* impair iron recycling, particularly by reticuloendothelial macrophages, thereby leading to tissue iron accumulation (reflected in high serum ferritin) and decreased availability of iron for circulating transferrin (reflected in low-normal transferrin saturation). This can also lead to iron-restricted erythropoiesis and anemia in certain settings, such as during aggressive phlebotomy regimens. Recent studies suggest that a subgroup of patients with ferroportin disease might carry mutations that result in enhanced iron release from enterocytes and macrophages and a phenotype similar to that of classic hemochromatosis (see Table 2).

Treatment and Monitoring

Phlebotomy is the standard treatment of all forms of hemochromatosis. Phlebotomy is generally regarded as a safe and effective means for removing iron from tissues and preventing complications, although this has never been validated in controlled studies for obvious ethical reasons. One unit (400-500 mL) of blood contains approximately 200 to 250 mg of iron. There are no studies from which to give an evidence base to the optimal time to start therapeutic venesection. Threshold serum ferritin is currently empirically chosen as above the normal range. The goal of bloodletting during the iron-depletion stage is generally the induction of a mildly iron-deficient state. Weekly phlebotomy can restore safe blood levels of iron (reflected by serum ferritin levels of less than 20-50 µg/L and transferrin saturation below 30%) within 1 to 2 years. Maintenance therapy, which typically involves removing 2 to 4 units a year, must then be continued to keep serum ferritin normal. Despite its nonspecificity, serum ferritin should always be monitored during phlebotomy.

Nonexpressing C282Y homozygotes should be monitored by serum ferritin once a year. If the serum ferritin is increasing, a full clinical work-up should be implemented and phlebotomy should be started.

Blood taken from patients with hemochromatosis at phlebotomy should be made available for national blood transfusion services, if there is no medical contraindication and the patient has given consent. It is recognized that many patients with *HFE* hemochromatosis have clinical features that exclude them from being accepted as donors (e.g. elevated liver function tests, diabetes, medications). But in the absence of these, there appears to be no reason, other than administrative and bureaucratic, why the blood taken may not be used.

If phlebotomy is contraindicated or poorly tolerated, other strategies can be considered, such as iron chelation.

Complications

Patients with classic hemochromatosis are at risk for developing serious organ diseases and complications, including hepatocellular carcinoma (2- to 2.5-fold higher risk than in other liver diseases).

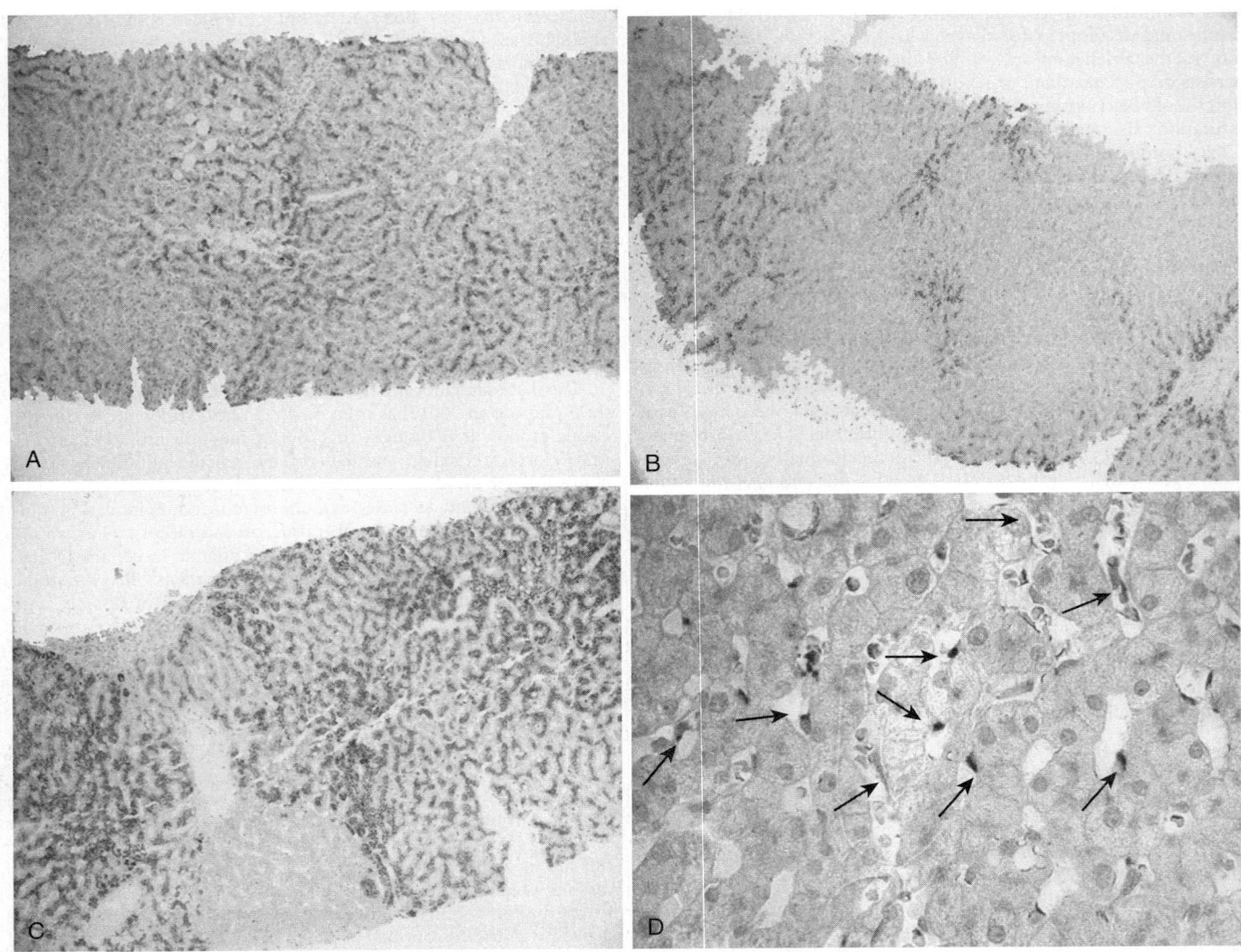

FIGURE 3. Histopathologic pictures of patients with hemochromatosis (Perls' Prussian blue stain for iron). **A,** Patient with *HFE* hemochromatosis presenting with pure parenchymal iron overload and portocentral iron gradient. **B,** Patient with *TfR2* hemochromatosis. The histopathologic picture is identical to *HFE* hemochromatosis, with iron accumulation in periportal parenchymal cells. **C,** Patient with *HJV* hemochromatosis, with massive parenchymal iron overload. **D,** Patient with classic ferroportin disease presenting with predominant Kupffer cell iron overload *(arrows).*

There are no randomized studies addressing survival in genotyped C282Y homozygous hemochromatosis patients. Survival of treated hemochromatosis patients without cirrhosis and diabetes seems equivalent to that of the normal population, whereas those with these complications have significantly reduced survival. The reported Kaplan-Meier analysis of survival at 5 years was 93% in adequately phlebotomized patients, compared with 48% for patients inadequately phlebotomized (10-year survival, 78% v 32%).

Elevated transaminases, skin pigmentation, and hepatic fibrosis seem to improve after phlebotomy. In studies of patients with biopsy-proven liver fibrosis, phlebotomy has been associated with improvement of liver fibrosis in 13% to 50% of treated patients, particularly those with the mildest fibrosis at baseline. It is recognized, however, that several clinical features are unlikely to improve with iron depletion, particularly arthralgia. Hypogonadism, cirrhosis, destructive arthritis, and insulin-dependent diabetes associated with hemochromatosis are usually irreversible, although phlebotomy can improve certain aspects of these diseases, such as daily insulin requirements, elevated aminotransferase levels, weakness, lethargy, and abdominal pain. End-stage liver disease or hepatocellular carcinoma secondary to hemochromatosis is often treated by orthotopic liver transplantation, but survival after liver transplantation might be expected to be reduced when compared to non–iron-loaded patients.

Prevention and Screening

Data emphasize the importance of early diagnosis of hemochromatosis and early initiation of iron removal. Genetic testing for C282Y polymorphism is a powerful tool for early diagnosis of hemochromatosis, but a positive test alone does not diagnose the disease, due to the unpredictable phenotypic penetrance of the polymorphism. This is the main argument against genetic screening for hemochromatosis in the general population. However, owing to the high prevalence of the polymorphism in patients with liver disease, porphyria cutanea tarda, or chondrocalcinosis or in distinct geographic areas (e.g., northern European countries), hemochromatosis screening by biochemical and eventually genetic testing should be reconsidered for early detection and prevention in selected populations.

TABLE 2 Hereditary Hemochromatosis in Humans

Affected Gene	Gene Name	Location	Known or Postulated Gene Product Function	Epidemiology	Genetics	Clinical Onset (Decade)	Main Clinical Manifestation	Clinical Course
Adult Onset								
Hemochromatosis gene	HFE	6p21.3	Interaction with transferrin receptor 1 Hepcidin regulator as component of the iron-sensor system involving BMPs	Whites of northern European descent C282Y polymorphism highly prevalent: 1/200-300	AR	3rd to 5th	Liver disease	Mild to severe
Transferrin-receptor 2	TfR2	7q22	Hepcidin regulator as component of the iron-sensor system involving BMPs	Any ethnicity Rare	AR	3rd to 5th	Liver disease	Mild to severe
Solute carrier family 40 (iron-regulated transporter), member 1/ Ferroportin	SLC40A1	2q32	Iron export from cells including macrophages, enterocytes, hepatocytes, and placental cells	Any ethnicity Very rare	AD	3rd to 5th	Liver disease	Mild to severe
Juvenile Onset								
Hepcidin antimicrobial peptide	HAMP	19q13.1	Downregulation of iron efflux from macrophages, through internalization and degradation of ferroportin	Any ethnicity Very rare	AR	2nd to 3rd	Hypogonadism and cardiac disease	Severe
Hemojuvelin	HJV	1p21	Coreceptor for BMPs Hepcidin transcriptional regulator	Any ethnicity Rare Most prevalent mutation: 230V	AR	2nd to 3rd	Hypogonadism and cardiac disease	Severe

Abbreviations: AD = autosomal dominant; AR = autosomal recessive; BMP = bone morphogenic protein.

CURRENT THERAPY

- Phlebotomy is the standard treatment of all forms of hemochromatosis.
- Threshold serum ferritin levels to start therapy in C282Y homozygotes are currently empirically chosen as above the normal range.
- Weekly phlebotomy of 500 mL can restore safe blood levels of iron (reflected by serum ferritin levels of <20-50 µg/L and transferrin saturation <30%) within 1 or 2 years.
- Maintenance therapy, which typically involves removal of 2 to 4 units a year, must then be continued to keep serum ferritin normal.
- Survival in adequately iron-depleted noncirrhotic and nondiabetic patients is not different from that of normal persons.
- If phlebotomy is contraindicated or poorly tolerated, iron chelators may be used.
- Mild hepatic fibrosis is reversible; fatigue, elevated transaminases, and skin pigmentation improve after phlebotomy.
- Arthralgia is unlikely to improve; destructive arthritis, hypogonadism, cirrhosis, and insulin-dependent diabetes associated with hemochromatosis are usually irreversible.
- In patients on an adequate phlebotomy program, dietary iron restrictions are not necessary.

REFERENCES

Allen KJ, Gurrin LC, Constantine CC, et al. Iron-overload-related disease in HFE hereditary hemochromatosis. N Engl J Med 2008;358(3):221–30.

Feder JN, Gnirke A, Thomas W, et al. A novel MHC class I–like gene is mutated in patients with hereditary haemochromatosis. Nat Genet 1996;13:399–408.

Merryweatherclarke AT, Pointon JJ, Shearman JD, Robson KJH. Global prevalence of putative haemochromatosis mutations. J Med Genet 1997;34(4):275–8.

Nemeth E, Tuttle MS, Powelson J, et al. Hepcidin regulates iron efflux by binding to ferroportin and inducing its internalization. Science 2004;306(5704):2090–3.

Papanikolaou G, Samuels ME, Ludwig EH, et al. Mutations in HFE2 cause iron overload in chromosome 1q-linked juvenile hemochromatosis. Nat Genet 2004;36:77–82.

Pietrangelo A, Montosi G, Totaro A, et al. Hereditary hemochromatosis in adults without pathogenic mutations in the hemochromatosis gene. N Engl J Med 1999;341:725–32.

Pietrangelo A. Hereditary hemochromatosis—a new look at an old disease. N Engl J Med 2004;350:2383–97.

Pietrangelo A. The ferroportin disease. Blood Cells Mol Dis 2004;32:131–8.

Sheldon J. Haemochromatosis. London: Oxford University Press; 1935.

Simon M, Pawlotsky Y, Bourel M, et al. Idiopathic hemochromatosis associated with HL-A 3 tissular antigen. Nouv Presse Med 1975;4:1432.

von Recklinghausen FD. Über Haemochromatose. Taggeblatt der (62) Versammlung deutscher Naturforscher und Ärzte in Heidelberg 1889;324–5.

Hodgkin's Lymphoma

Method of
Ralph M. Meyer, MD, and
David C. Hodgson, MD, MPH

Current estimates of the incidence and mortality of Hodgkin's lymphoma in the United States come from American Cancer Society statistics, which predicts approximately 7800 diagnoses and 1800 deaths in 2006. This mortality-to-incidence rate ratio of 0.19 reflects the high potential for cure of this disease and emphasizes that long-term issues of survivorship are important for these patients, but it also demonstrates that curative potential is not achieved in an important fraction of patients. Historically, understandings of the biology and management of Hodgkin's lymphoma have played pivotal roles in developing broader understandings of cancer; this continues to be the case. In this article, we describe these principles and review current management strategies.

Histologic Classification

The diagnosis of Hodgkin's lymphoma requires an adequate tissue biopsy and expert interpretation. The histologic classification of Hodgkin's lymphoma, and lymphomas in general, exemplifies how new understandings of biology, including advances in molecular oncology, require that categorization schema be continuously updated to accommodate new discoveries. Since the initial description of this lymphoma by Thomas Hodgkin in 1832 and the reporting of the hallmark features of the Reed-Sternberg cell in 1902, the classification of Hodgkin's disease has undergone sequential updating. Landmark schemata include those described by Jackson and Parker in 1943 and Lukes and Butler in 1966. This latter classification system was modified at the 1966 Rye Conference and included four separate entities: lymphocyte predominant, nodular sclerosing, mixed cellularity, and lymphocyte deplete. It is this classification system that has been used in the vast majority of clinical trials that have determined current treatments.

The most current classification schema was determined as part of the Revised European American Lymphoma (REAL) classification of 1994 and was updated in the World Heath Organization classification described in 1997 (Fig. 1). Major changes include recognition of nodular lymphocyte predominant disease as a distinct clinical entity that is separate from the other forms of Hodgkin's lymphoma, which are now grouped under the umbrella term of classic Hodgkin's lymphoma. Within classic Hodgkin's lymphoma are four entities: lymphocyte rich, nodular sclerosing, mixed cellularity, and lymphocyte deplete. As we describe later, the new clinical ramifications of incorporating recent biological findings into the WHO classification system are that an entity that is associated with a different clinical course and might require a different form of therapy has been defined (i.e., nodular lymphocyte predominant disease), and criteria that separate Hodgkin's from non-Hodgkin's lymphomas have been made more explicit. It is crucial that evaluation of biopsy material be performed by an expert pathologist, with necessary ancillary studies such as immunohistochemistry, flow cytometry, and molecular studies completed as appropriate to ensure that the Hodgkin's and non-Hodgkin's lymphomas have been distinguished and that subtypes of lymphoma have been properly characterized.

Staging and Risk Categorization

As with histologic classifications, the variables that determine the extent of disease and prognosis of patients with Hodgkin's lymphoma have evolved to account for new biological understandings and the relevance of these variables within the context of current therapies. Beginning with the initial observations of Peters in 1950, risk categorization of patients with Hodgkin's lymphoma has historically emphasized the anatomic spread of the disease. Subsequently, the Ann Arbor Staging Classification was devised in 1971; this was modified at the Cotswold meeting in 1989. The Cotswold criteria continue to be applied to newly diagnosed cases (Table 1).

Current management strategies for patients with classic Hodgkin's lymphoma involve collapsing the Ann Arbor and Cotswold classifications into two or three categories. These categories include at least limited-stage and advanced-stage disease. In North America, cooperative group clinical trials have defined limited-stage disease as clinical stage I to IIA and an absence of bulky disease. Bulky disease is defined as a mass that is at least 10 cm in diameter or that measures more than one third of the maximum transthoracic diameter on a standard posteroanterior chest radiograph. Other factors that have been considered of potential prognostic importance, such as erythrocyte sedimentation rate (ESR) and histologic subtype within classic Hodgkin's lymphoma, are no longer deemed to be important in defining therapy, because the prognostic properties of these factors have been obviated by current therapies. Patients with stages IIB,

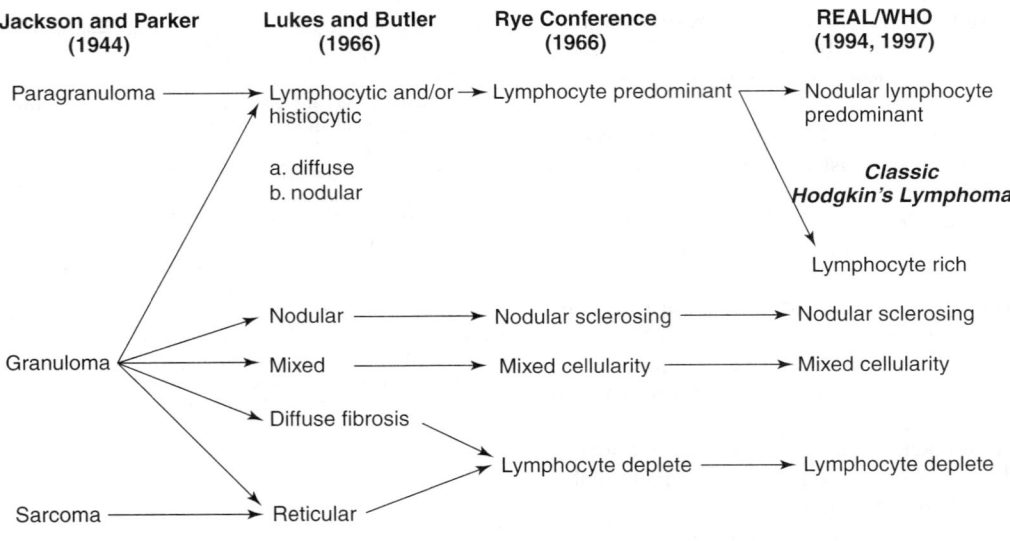

FIGURE 1. Histologic classifications of Hodgkin's lymphoma. REAL = Revised European American Lymphoma; WHO = World Health Organization.

TABLE 1 Ann Arbor Staging System Including Cotswold Modifications

Stage	Disease Involvement
I	Single lymph node region (I) or one extralymphatic site (I_E)
II	Two or more lymph node regions, on the same side of the diaphragm (II) or local extralymphatic extension plus one or more lymph node regions on the same side of the diaphragm (II_E)
III	Lymph node regions on both sides of the diaphragm (III), which may be accompanied by local extralymphatic extension (III_E)
IV	Diffuse involvement of one or more extralymphatic organs or sites
A	No B symptoms
B	Presence of at least one of unexplained weight loss >10% baseline during 6 mo before staging, recurrent unexplained fever >38°C, recurrent night sweats
X	Bulky tumor: either a single mass exceeding 10 cm in largest diameter or a mediastinal mass exceeding one third of the maximum transverse transthoracic diameter measured on a standard posteroanterior chest radiograph

TABLE 2 The International Prognostic Index*

Variable	Risk Level
Serum albumin	<40 g/L
Hemoglobin	<105 g/L
Sex	Male
Stage	Stage IV
Age	≥45 y
White cell count	$\geq 15 \times 10^9$/L
Lymphocyte count	$<0.6 \times 10^9$/L or <8% of total while cell count

*The number of factors present is totaled.

III, IV, and bulky disease associated with any stage are considered to have advanced-stage disease. Within this article, these definitions of limited and advanced-stage disease will be used to describe treatment practices. For the purposes of determining prognosis, and for designing clinical trials, patients with advanced-stage disease may be further assessed through use of the International Prognostic Index (IPI), which includes anatomic stage as a variable, but also includes six other parameters that have been shown to be prognostic through evaluation of large databases (Table 2).

Cooperative group practices in Europe use schemata that have considerable overlap with those used in North America. Patients who in North America would be classified in Europe as having limited-stage disease may be classified as having *favorable early-stage* disease. A separate category of *intermediate-stage* or *unfavorable early-stage* disease is used to include patients with stage I, IIA, or IIB disease and presence of one or more predefined risk factors, such as the presence of bulky disease, elevation of the ESR, or an increased number of nodal sites of disease. *Advanced stage* includes those with stage III or IV disease. Despite these minor variations, these classification systems result in similar stage-related treatment practices in both geographic regions.

Clinical Presentation and Initial Investigations

Patients with Hodgkin's lymphoma are typically young, with the peak incidence of disease occurring in those in late adolescence to their early 40s. The median age observed in most clinical trials is approximately 35 years. Although a bimodal age distribution has been

CURRENT DIAGNOSIS

- The most common age of patients is late adolescence to the early 40s.
- Many patients present with painless adenopathy that is often in the neck or axilla and is asymmetrical.
- Due to the frequency of mediastinal lymph node involvement, a chest radiograph can be helpful in evaluating patients with persistent symptoms for which an etiology has not been discovered.
- The diagnosis requires an adequate biopsy with expert review to confirm the diagnosis, distinguish Hodgkin's lymphoma from non-Hodgkin's lymphoma, and determine the histologic subtype of the disease.

historically described, with a second age peak occurring in elderly patients, recent revisions of lymphoma histologic classification have resulted in changing the diagnosis in many older patients from Hodgkin's disease to non-Hodgkin's lymphoma.

The presentation of patients with Hodgkin's lymphoma typically falls into two major categories: those who present with painless lymphadenopathy and those who present with other symptoms. Usually those with painless adenopathy present with supradiaphragmatic disease, with an enlarged lymph node in the neck or axilla. The lymph nodes are typically described as firm, hard, or rubbery as opposed to the softer or fleshy nodes in patients with lymphadenopathy that is reactive to an inflammatory condition. Nodes that are anatomically asymmetrical (unilateral) and that are present in the posterior triangle of the neck, as opposed to the internal jugular chain, are more suspicious for lymphoma, as opposed to a reactive condition. Only 5% of Hodgkin's lymphoma patients present with disease that is confined to the subdiaphragmatic regions; typically these patients present with adenopathy in the inguinal or femoral region and disproportionately may have the nodular lymphocyte–predominant histologic subtype. Symptoms can relate to local disease or be constitutional. Patients with mediastinal disease may present with chest fullness and cough. Constitutional symptoms often include fatigue, lethargy or the prognostic B symptoms of fevers, night sweats, or weight loss. Unusual, but potentially distinct, symptoms can include intractable pruritus or pain in a region affected by adenopathy associated with alcohol intake.

Evaluation of patients with suspected Hodgkin's lymphoma includes a thorough history and physical examination with particular attention to the presence of the above-described symptoms and of lymphadenopathy, hepatosplenomegaly, or a pleural effusion on physical examination. In patients with chest symptoms, a chest x-ray can be extremely valuable. The definitive diagnosis requires an adequate tissue biopsy; although cytologic evaluations of material obtained from a fine-needle aspirate might suggest a diagnosis of Hodgkin's lymphoma, at present, this technology is not consistently reliable to ensure a correct diagnosis. Material for histologic evaluation obtained from an adequate large-bore core biopsy might, in select circumstances, be sufficient for diagnosis, but in general, an excisional biopsy should be expected to achieve a definitive diagnosis.

Once a diagnosis of Hodgkin's lymphoma is confirmed, patients require systematic evaluation to assess prognostic features that will influence therapy and determine whether complications of the disease are present. Standard investigations are listed in Box 1. At present, the role of ^{18}F-fluorodeoxyglucose positron emission tomography (FDG-PET scanning) is under evaluation. Potential roles might include pretreatment disease staging, evaluation during therapy for purposes of prognosis or prediction of benefit with specific therapy, and determination of remission status at the completion of therapy. Currently, the utility of PET scanning is least well defined as a pretreatment staging tool and cannot yet be considered a standard test for this purpose.

Treatment

Treatment of patients with Hodgkin's lymphoma can be subdivided into categories that are determined by the histologic subtype and the stage of disease with the added potential that risk factors, such as those identified in the Hodgkin's lymphoma IPI, might further influence treatment options. Principles of management include careful balancing of the desire to maximally control the underlying disease, while minimizing the risks of long-term treatment-related toxicities (also referred to as late effects). Late effects include increased risks of developing acute leukemia, which is associated with use of chemotherapy regimens that include alkylating agents or epipodophyllotoxins, and second cancers and cardiovascular events, which are associated with radiation therapy. In addition, chemotherapy regimens that include alkylating agents are associated with dose-dependent risks of gonadal failure and infertility.

LIMITED-STAGE CLASSIC HODGKIN'S LYMPHOMA

The management of patients with limited-stage Hodgkin's lymphoma has changed dramatically over the past 15 to 20 years. As recently as 1990, standard management included a staging laparotomy with splenectomy followed by treatment with subtotal nodal radiation. With this treatment, other prognostic factors were identified and used to refine therapy; these included ESR, number of disease sites, and histologic subtype (e.g., nodular sclerosing vs mixed cellularity). These practices have been improved on by advances in diagnostic imaging and through the availability of more-efficacious and less-toxic systemic chemotherapy. Further improvements should be expected as other technologies, such as PET scanning, become validated.

Based on current data, patients and physicians have two main options for the treatment of limited-stage Hodgkin's lymphoma. These options are associated with specific trade-offs.

The first option is treatment with combined modality therapy that includes two cycles of doxorubicin (Adriamycin), bleomycin (Bleoxane), vinblastine (Velban) and dacarbazine (DTIC-Dome) (ABVD), and radiation therapy to the involved field. The advantage of this approach is that long-term disease control is maximized with initial therapy; this is expected in approximately 95% of patients. The disadvantage relates to use of radiation therapy and the associated risks of late effects such as second cancers and, with mediastinal radiation, cardiovascular events. Advances in radiation technology, such as conformal treatment, use of PET scanning for planning, and limiting the treatment field to the affected nodes as opposed to nodal regions, significantly reduces the radiation dose to normal tissues compared with radiation treatments given in the 1970s to the 1990s. Further data are required before we can confidently conclude that important long-term risks do not remain.

The second option is therapy with four to six cycles of ABVD alone. The advantage of this approach is avoidance of radiation therapy and the associated risks of late effects, with the disadvantage being a decrement in long-term disease control with initial therapy that is estimated to be about 7% (i.e., to approximately 88%). To date, no differences in long-term overall survival have been detected between these options. Ongoing randomized trials that assign use of radiation according to patients' early response to chemotherapy might clarify which patients can be treated with chemotherapy alone without increasing the risk of relapse. In the meantime, balancing these options requires careful discussions with patients about their preferences.

 CURRENT THERAPY

Limited Stage Classic Hodgkin's Lymphoma

- Option 1: Combined modality therapy consisting of two cycles of ABVD and involved-field radiation therapy. The advantage is long-term disease control with initial therapy in more than 90% of patients.
- Option 2: Treatment with ABVD (4–6 cycles). The advantage is that, although long-term disease control with initial therapy is about 7% less than with combined modality therapy, the risks of late effects of radiation therapy are avoided.

Advanced Stage Classic Hodgkin's Lymphoma

- Option 1: Treatment with ABVD (6–8 cycles). The advantage is that long-term disease control with initial therapy in at least 65% of patients. Gonadal function and fertility are preserved.
- Option 2: Treatment with escalated BEACOPP. The advantage is that long-term disease control with initial therapy is approximately 10% better than that associated with ABVD, but treatment is associated with more toxicity, including high rates of infertility (see text).

Refractory or Recurrent Classic Hodgkin's Lymphoma

- Usual initial treatment is with high-dose chemotherapy and autologous stem cell transplantation.
- Subsequent treatments require individualized approaches.

Nodular Lymphocyte–Predominant Hodgkin's Lymphoma

- The most common option is involved-field radiation therapy.
- Numerous new options, including use of rituximab and observation have been described.
- Advanced-stage disease is treated the same as classic Hodgkin's lymphoma.

ADVANCED-STAGE CLASSIC HODGKIN'S LYMPHOMA

The management of patients with advanced-stage disease has also evolved over the past 15 to 20 years. In 1990, standard therapy would have included six to eight cycles of nitrogen mustard, vincristine (Oncovin), prednisone, and procarbazine (Matulane) in combination with ABVD (± dacarbazine) (MOPP-ABVD or MOPP-ABV). Recent randomized, controlled trials have demonstrated that these regimens and ABVD all provide long-term disease control in approximately 65% of patients. However, there is less short-term toxicity with ABVD, and importantly, this regimen avoids the long-term risks of infertility and leukemogenesis associated with nitrogen mustard and procarbazine. Treatment with ABVD is therefore considered a standard.

An alternative strategy is to intensify therapy with use of the bleomycin, etoposide (Vepesid),[1] doxorubicin (Adriamycin), cyclophosphamide (Cytoxan), vincristine (Oncovin), prednisone, and procarbazine (BEACOPP) regimen. Use of this regimen, particularly in its escalated-dose form, has been associated with superior disease control and an improvement in overall survival that is in the range of 8% to 10% at 5 years (i.e., 91% with escalated BEACOPP versus 83% with ABVD). In comparison with ABVD, the magnitude of disease-control benefits associated with the BEACOPP regimens may be greatest in patients who have more than three IPI risk factors. However, the BEACOPP regimens are associated with more severe toxicities, including more severe myelosuppression and risks of infection during the treatment period, and a greater risk of acute leukemia and myelodysplasia as a late effect. Furthermore, risks of infertility are markedly increased: Preliminary reports suggest that escalated BEACOPP is associated with gonadal failure in 85% to 90% of all men and women who are older than 30 years and in 50% of female patients younger than 30 years.

Another strategy uses weekly chemotherapy that is administered over a shorter time course than ABVD. The prototype of this therapy is the Stanford V regimen. Although this treatment has shown promising results in a phase II trial, in three randomized, controlled trials testing this concept, outcomes were inferior in comparison with ABVD or an equivalent regimen. A large North American Intergroup study has completed accrual to a randomized comparison of Stanford V and ABVD. Until the results of this trial are known, use of regimens based on this concept should be limited to clinical trials testing.

The role of combining radiation therapy with chemotherapy has been studied in a number of randomized trials and an individual patient-data meta-analysis. A summary of these results shows that no differences in overall survival are detected, and particularly in patients with stage III or IV disease who are treated with ABVD or BEACOPP, there are also no differences in disease control. At present, there continues to be a role for combined modality therapy for patients with stage I or II disease who are considered to have advanced-stage disease because of the presence of a bulky mediastinal mass. The need for all of these patients to receive radiation therapy will require reevaluation as the utility of PET scanning is better understood.

Therefore, as with limited-stage disease, practitioners and patients are faced with a decision involving trade-offs as the treatment associated with the best long-term disease control is also associated with the greatest long-term risk. At an individual patient level, the risks of infertility associated with BEACOPP should be regarded as likely. Provided patients are aware of these trade-offs, treatment with either escalated BEACOPP or ABVD is a reasonable option.

RELAPSED OR REFRACTORY DISEASE

Unfortunately, an important number of patients have disease that is refractory to initial therapy or that is associated with subsequent recurrence. The vast majority of these patients present with advanced-stage disease and receive a full course of chemotherapy with ABVD. Based on the results of two randomized trials that have shown significant improvements in progression-free or event-free survival, treatment with high-dose chemotherapy and autologous stem cell transplantation is considered standard. Autologous transplantation is particularly recommended for patients with primary refractory disease and disease that recurs within 1 year of completing initial therapy; it is also a reasonable option for most other patients who experience disease recurrence after a longer disease-free interval. Patients with recurrent disease that includes a site of bulky disease, such as the mediastinum, should also receive radiation therapy to that site following confirmed stem cell engraftment.

Treatment options for recurrent Hodgkin's lymphoma in patients who initially present with limited-stage disease are poorly characterized due to the uncommon occurrence of this event. The choice of therapy is strongly influenced by specifics of the pattern of disease recurrence. Options for patients with recurrent disease after receiving combined modality therapy include receiving a full course of a standard regimen (e.g., ABVD) or, more commonly, stem cell transplantation. For patients whose disease recurs after receiving ABVD alone, and particularly when this recurrence is confined to the initial sites of disease, the option of treatment with combined-modality therapy that includes involved-field radiation is preferred over stem cell transplantation.

The treatment of patients with recurrent disease after stem cell transplantation has been poorly evaluated; there are no randomized, controlled trials. Management must be individualized and should account for the demographic features of the patient, the temporal profile, burden and symptoms associated with the disease, and natures of the previous therapies. A common option includes single-agent vinblastine for purposes of palliation, but additional options can include radiation therapy, including wide-field radiation, use of other standard-dose chemotherapy regimens, and for select patients, observation. For very select patients, the option of allogeneic stem cell transplantation, including with reduced-intensity conditioning regimens, has been described.

NODULAR LYMPHOCYTE–PREDOMINANT HODGKIN'S LYMPHOMA

There are now robust data indicating that nodular lymphocyte–predominant Hodgkin's lymphoma is a distinct biological entity and is associated with a clinical course that differs from classic Hodgkin's lymphoma. Most patients present with limited-stage disease and have an indolent clinical course; extensive mediastinal involvement is rare. An important biological feature is expression by the malignant cell of the CD20 antigen, which raises the opportunity for potential treatment with immunotherapy using the monoclonal antibody rituximab.

The uncommon incidence of this disease means that the clinical trials that inform current practices generally consist of case series, many of which are retrospective, and small subset analyses from larger randomized trials that evaluate patients with all histologic subtypes. From these data, a commonly preferred therapy is with involved-field radiation therapy as a single modality. An alternative option is combined-modality therapy as given for patients with limited-stage classic Hodgkin's lymphoma, but the curative potential of this option is uncertain. Small case series have evaluated observation alone or rituximab treatment, but sufficient data do not yet exist to permit recommending these as standard therapies. Patients with advanced-stage disease should receive the same therapy as patients with classic Hodgkin's lymphoma.

SPECIAL CIRCUMSTANCES

Special circumstances can arise that require modification of these treatment strategies. For each of these circumstances, the data on which current recommendations are based are limited and largely consist of case reports, case series, and generalizations from other diseases or biological principles.

A first circumstance is managing older patients with Hodgkin's lymphoma. As with the therapy of older patients with non-Hodgkin's lymphoma, the treatment plan must initially account for the presence of any comorbidities or specific patient preferences

---

[1]Not FDA approved for this indication.

related to individual values. When no additional factors are identified, treatment that incorporates the principles for managing younger patients should be followed. For these patients, the BEACOPP regimens are associated with excessive toxicity and should not be used. For patients with cardiac compromise who cannot receive doxorubicin, treatment with chlorambucil, vinblastine, prednisone, and procarbazine (ChlVPP) may be considered.

A second circumstance is management of female patients in whom Hodgkin's lymphoma is diagnosed during pregnancy. Diagnostic staging of these patients should include replacement of computed tomography with ultrasound examination. Provided that the disease is sufficiently indolent, many patients can be carefully observed until the postnatal period and then complete standard staging tests and therapy. For patients who must receive therapy before delivery, a common option is treatment with single-agent vinblastine, which is not teratogenic, followed by postnatal therapy with a full course of standard chemotherapy. In very select circumstances, patients who have rapidly progressing disease after their first trimester of pregnancy may, after thorough consideration and discussion of options, be treated with ABVD.

A third special circumstance is management of the HIV patient who develops Hodgkin's lymphoma. These patients might not be as profoundly immunosuppressed as HIV patients who develop non-Hodgkin's lymphoma, but unfortunately risks of infection associated with standard chemotherapy are increased. These patients should receive optimal antiretroviral therapy and ideally treatment that is otherwise considered standard for their stage of disease. Due to insufficient data, therapy with BEACOPP is not recommended and these patients should receive ABVD.

Issues of Survivorship

Studies of survivors have shown that delayed morbidity and excess mortality not directly attributable to Hodgkin's lymphoma is an important problem. For patients whose disease was diagnosed in the 1960s to 1980s, deaths from other causes exceeded deaths due to Hodgkin's lymphoma after 15 years of follow-up. A major cause of other deaths is the occurrence of a second cancer. A man whose disease was diagnosed at age 30 and who was treated with historical approaches, the 30-year cumulative incidence of developing a solid-tumor cancer is approximately 15% to 20%, which is 10% higher than expected in the gender- and age-matched general population. Comparable values for a 30-year-old woman include a 30-year cumulative incidence of a subsequent solid cancer of 25%, which is 15% higher than expected. The incremental risk of solid cancers among younger female patients is even more pronounced, largely due to the excess risk of breast cancer related to radiation therapy to the mediastinum.

A second major cause of late morbidity and mortality is cardiovascular diseases. These may be related to doxorubicin, which produces free radicals that are directly toxic to the myocardium, and mediastinal radiation to a field that includes the heart. The cumulative incidence of significant cardiac morbidity 10 years after treatment is approximately 2% to 6% and increases to 15% to 20% by 20 years. This represents a 1.5- to 3-fold increased relative risk and is largely related to the radiation therapy. Technical interventions that reduce the dose of radiation to the heart reduce this risk.

The persistence of symptoms associated with nonfatal complications is also common. Even following modern therapy, many survivors experience persistent fatigue; its cause is uncertain. Although persistent anemia and hypothyroidism are known late effects of treatment, these do not usually provide the reason for fatigue.

Specifically focused follow-up of survivors can reduce the morbidity of late treatment effects. Among patients who receive neck or mediastinal radiation, thyroid function should be evaluated at least annually to detect preclinical hypothyroidism. Female patients treated with mediastinal radiation should undergo annual breast cancer screening beginning 8 years after this treatment or beginning at age 25 years. Due to the suboptimal performance of mammography in women with dense breast tissue, which includes most young women, this screening should include magnetic resonance imaging (MRI) for women younger than 30 years. For women ages 30 to 50 years, mammography can be initiated and the adequacy of mammographic images can guide decisions regarding the appropriate screening modality. For those with good mammographic images (i.e., predominantly fatty breast tissue) mammography alone is recommended, whereas those with dense breast tissue should be screened with MRI plus mammography. Mammographic screening alone is recommended for women older than 50 years.

Recommendations for colorectal cancer screening for patients who have received abdominal radiation therapy are less clear. Some recommendations include initiation of colorectal cancer screening 15 years after treatment, or by age 35 years, whichever comes later. The evidence supporting this recommendation is indirect and there are no data to indicate whether colonoscopy or fecal occult blood testing is superior.

Most cardiac morbidity occurs in survivors who have conventional cardiac risk factors. Consequently, blood pressure and serum lipids should be monitored and, if elevated, treated aggressively. Similarly, strong efforts should be made to help survivors quit smoking, because the smoking-related risks of heart disease and lung cancer appear to be even greater than among the general population. Young survivors who experience progressive fatigue or chest pain require cardiac evaluation; these symptoms should not be attributed to noncardiac causes until heart disease has been excluded. Preliminary data suggest that screening stress echocardiography can detect clinically important valvular or coronary artery disease among long-term survivors who received mediastinal radiation to doses greater than 35 Gy; future studies are required to clarify the value of routine screening of all asymptomatic patients. Female survivors who become pregnant, however, should undergo cardiac evaluation because of the significant cardiac stress associated with pregnancy and childbirth.

Persistent fatigue among survivors can be a challenging management problem. Depression or dysthymia, hypothyroidism, impaired cardiac function, and anemia should be considered as potential causes. Regular exercise can significantly reduce fatigue and in severe cases, referral to a mental health professional should be considered for cognitive behavior therapy or short-term pharmacotherapy.

Given the nature of these and other survivorship issues, standard oncology clinics might not be well suited to deal with the types of issues that patients who have been otherwise successfully treated for Hodgkin's lymphoma. Specialized clinics for survivors, which focus on these late-effect issues as opposed to the less likely potentials of disease recurrence, are now more common and may be a preferred way to provide this health care.

REFERENCES

Connors JM. State-of-the-art therapeutics: Hodgkin's lymphoma. J Clin Oncol 2005;23(26):6400–8.

Diehl V, Franklin J, Pfreundschuh M, et al. Standard and increased-dose BEACOPP chemotherapy compared with COPP-ABVD for advanced Hodgkin's disease. N Engl J Med 2003;348(24):2386–95.

Duggan DB, Petroni GR, Johnson JL, et al. Randomized comparison of ABVD and MOPP/ABV hybrid for the treatment of advanced Hodgkin's disease: Report of an Intergroup trial. J Clin Oncol 2003;21(4):607–14.

Gospodarowicz MK, Meyer RM. The management of patients with limited-stage classical Hodgkin lymphoma. Hematology 2006;2006(1):253–8.

Harris NL, Jaffe ES, Diebold J, et al. World Health Organization classification of neoplastic diseases of the hematopoietic and lymphoid tissues: Report of the Clinical Advisory Committee Meeting, Airlie House, Virginia, November 1997. J Clin Oncol 1999;17(12):3835–49.

Harris NL, Jaffe ES, Stein H, et al. A revised European–American classification of lymphoid neoplasms: A proposal from the International Lymphoma Study Group. Blood 1994;84(5):1361–92.

Hasenclever D, Diehl V, Armitage JO, et al. A prognostic score for advanced Hodgkin's disease. N Engl J Med 1998;339(21):1506–14.

Hodgson DC, Gilbert ES, Dores GM, et al. Long-term solid cancer risk among 5-year survivors of Hodgkin's lymphoma. J Clin Oncol 2007;25(12):1489–97.

Lister TA, Crowther D, Sutcliffe SB, et al. Report of a committee convened to discuss the evaluation and staging of patients with Hodgkin's disease: Cotswolds meeting. J Clin Oncol 1989;7(11):1630–6.

Meyer RM, Gospodarowicz MK, Connors JM, et al. Randomized comparison of ABVD chemotherapy with a strategy that includes radiation therapy in patients with limited-stage Hodgkin's lymphoma: National Cancer Institute of Canada Clinical Trials Group and the Eastern Cooperative Oncology Group. J Clin Oncol 2005;23(21):4634–42.

Nogova L, Rudiger T, Engert A. Biology, clinical course and management of nodular lymphocyte–predominant Hodgkin lymphoma. Hematology 2006;2006(1):266–72.

Ralleigh G, Given-Wilson R. Breast cancer risk and possible screening strategies for young women following supradiaphragmatic radiation for Hodgkin's disease. Clin Radiol 2004;59:647–50.

Hodgkin's Disease: Radiation Therapy

Method of
Steve Carpenter, MD, and Ali Mazloom, MD

Hodgkin's disease (HD), or Hodgkin's lymphoma (HL), is an important disease for the primary care physician that was first described by Thomas Hodgkin in 1832. HD has a unique behavior. It usually manifests with painless lymphadenopathy and then spreads in a relatively predictable manner to the adjacent lymphatic regions. Next, the patient may have systemic manifestations such as B symptoms, and only much later does the disease spread to organs beyond the lymph nodes and spleen. HD has a high overall cure rate of greater than 80% for early-stage disease and greater than 50% for advanced-stage disease. In addition, recurrent HD often responds to salvage therapy. HD requires careful follow-up to discover late effects of therapy as well as second malignancies.

Epidemiology

HD is diagnosed in more than 7000 people in the United States each year. HD has a slight male predominance and can occur at almost any age. The incidence has a bimodal distribution, with the largest peak occurring in the third decade and a second peak appearing after the age of 50 years. Epstein-Barr virus infection may predispose to development of HD. Familial or genetic associations may also play a role in the development of this disease. The incidence of HD does not appear to be increased by immunosuppression.

Natural History

Early clinicians characterized the spread of HD from one contiguous nodal region to the next. These observations were enhanced by improvements in imaging modalities and by the systematic use of surgical staging with staging laparotomy. One result was an improved cure rate due to the prophylactic use of irradiation of contiguous uninvolved sites. Hematogenous spread occurs primarily as a late event in stage III disease. Bone marrow involvement is rare, occurring mainly in patients with advanced-stage disease or systemic symptoms, whereas hepatic spread does not usually occur without prior splenic disease.

Some patients report systemic symptoms that are referred to as B symptoms. These include unexplained fevers, drenching night sweats, and weight loss. Other systemic symptoms include fatigue, generalized pruritus, and alcohol-induced pain at affected sites.

The most common sites of disease are the cervical nodes, followed by the mediastinal nodes. Patients with HD also have an increased risk for development of other lymphomas. This can occur before or after the diagnosis of HD.

Pathology

Needle biopsies are not adequate for the diagnosis of HD, and tissue obtained for diagnosis should be from a nodal or mass excision. HD is divided into two types: classic Hodgkin's lymphoma and nodular lymphocyte predominance Hodgkin's lymphoma (NLPHL). NLPHL is a more indolent disease with a unique pattern of involvement that usually spares the mediastinum. NLPHL comprises 5% of HD cases. It usually manifests at an early stage, has a high cure rate with irradiation alone, and only rarely transforms to a diffuse large B-cell lymphoma. The pathologic types of HD, as listed by the World Health Organisation, are given in Box 1.

Immunnophenotyping is used to distinguish HD from other lymphomas and also to distinguish among the subtypes. Some groups have included grading for nodular sclerosis HL, and eosinophilic infiltrate of the specimen may be a high-risk feature. Mixed-cellularity HL more commonly involves the abdomen and spleen. The lymphocyte-depleted type is rare and usually manifests in an advanced stage involving the bone marrow.

Evaluation and Staging

A detailed history should be obtained to evaluate for systemic (B) symptoms. A careful physical examination is performed with attention to nodal areas, Waldeyer's ring, liver, and spleen. Bone marrow biopsy is advised for stages IB, IIB, III, and IV. Suspicious extranodal abnormalities may also require biopsy. Radiologic examinations should include chest radiography, computed tomography (CT) of chest and abdomen, and a CT/positron-emission tomographic (PET) scan. A CT of the neck is added if there is cervical adenopathy on examination. Laboratory tests should include a complete blood count, sedimentation rate, and kidney and liver function tests. Any effusion should be sent for cytologic examination.

A clinical stage is assigned based on the findings of these studies. The Ann Arbor Staging Classification has been used for several decades. It has received slight changes with the more recent Cotswold's modification, described in Table 1.

Treatment

The current preferred therapy for nonbulky stage IA and IIA classic HL consists of four cycles of ABVD chemotherapy (doxorubicin [Adriamycin], bleomycin [Bleoxane], vinblastine [Velban], and dacarbazine [DTIC-Dome]) followed by 30 Gy of involved-field irradiation. Involved-field irradiation consists of radiation given to the region of the body initially involved on pretreatment imaging. This includes the discernable tumor as well as the general anatomic area. As an example, for any abnormal lymph node on one side of the neck, involved-field irradiation would include the entire ipsilateral neck (from C1 down to below the clavicle).

BOX 1   Hodgkin's Disease: World Health Organisation Classification of Pathologic Types

Nodular lymphocyte predominance HL (NLPHL)
Classic Hodgkin's lymphoma (HL)
- Nodular sclerosis HL
- Mixed cellularity HL
- Lymphocyte-rich HL
- Lymphocyte-depleted HL
- Unclassifiable classic HL

CURRENT DIAGNOSIS

History

- Systemic (B) symptoms: unexplained fevers, drenching night sweats, and weight loss (>10% of weight in 6 months)
- Other symptoms: fatigue, generalized pruritus, alcohol-induced pain at affected sites
- Performance status

Physical Examination

- Examine lymphoid regions, spleen, liver

Laboratory Studies

- Complete blood count with differential
- Erythrocyte sedimentation rate
- Lactate dehydrogenase, liver function tests, albumin
- Blood urea nitrogen, creatinine
- Pregnancy test for women of childbearing age

Imaging Studies

- Chest radiography
- Computed tomography of chest, abdomen, pelvis; computed tomography of the neck if cervical adenopathy is present
- Positron-emission tomographic scan

Biopsy

- Excisional biopsy (core needle biopsy and fine-needle aspiration are insufficient)
- Immunohistochemistry
- Classic Hodgkin's lymphoma (HL): CD3, CD15, CD20, CD30, CD45
- Nodular lymphocyte predominance HL: CD3, CD15, CD20, CD21, CD30, CD57

Bone Marrow Biopsy: Stages IB-IIB, III, IV

TABLE 1 Cotswolds Staging of Hodgkin's Lymphoma

Stage	Description
I	Involvement of a single lymph node region or lymphoid structure
II	Involvement of two or more lymph node regions on the same side of the diaphragm or involvement of a single extralymphatic organ and one or more lymph node regions on the same side of the diaphragm; the number of sites is given with a numerical subscript
III	Involvement of lymph node regions or structures on both sides of the diaphragm
IV	Involvement of one or more extranodal sites beyond that designated as an E site (diffuse or disseminated)

Additional Designations

III-2	With involvement of paraaortic, iliac, and mesenteric nodes
A	No symptoms
B	Fever (>38°C), drenching night sweats, unexplained loss of >10% body weight within 6 mo
X	Bulky disease
E	Involvement of a single extranodal site that is contiguous or proximal to the known nodal site
CS	Clinical stage
PS	Pathologic stage

Only two cycles of chemotherapy may be sufficient in favorable cases. Restaging is performed after chemotherapy and before irradiation. Two cycles (8 weeks) of the Stanford V regimen (doxorubicin, vinblastine, mechlorethamine [nitrogen mustard, Mustargen], etoposide [Vepesid],[1] vincristine [Oncovin], bleomycin, and prednisone) may be substituted for ABVD. Six cycles of ABVD is a less acceptable alternative to combined-modality therapy (chemotherapy and irradiation).

Bulky disease is defined as any mass greater than 10 cm in diameter. Bulky mediastinal adenopathy can also be defined as a mediastinal mass greater than 35% of the intrathoracic diameter at T5–6 or greater than one third of the maximum intrathoracic diameter (near the level of the diaphragm). Bulky early-stage disease is treated with four to six cycles of ABVD followed by involved-field irradiation. Restaging is performed after four cycles of chemotherapy. Alternatively, Stanford V may given for three cycles (12 weeks), followed by involved-field irradiation.

For stage IB, IIB, III, and IV disease, ABVD chemotherapy is given for six to eight cycles, or an escalated dose of BEACOPP (bleomycin, etoposide,[1] doxorubicin, cyclophosphamide [Cytoxan], vincristine, procarbazine [N-methylhydrazine, Matulane], and prednisone) is given for eight cycles. Involved-field irradiation is given to disease sites greater than 5 cm or to residual abnormalities on PET scan at restaging. Stanford V for three cycles plus involved-field irradiation may also be used. The use of involved-field irradiation (consolidation) for bulky or residual sites in stages III and IV disease is currently being explored in a German Hodgkin's Study Group randomized trial (HD 12).

For those patients who are intolerant of chemotherapy or have medical conditions preventing chemotherapy, subtotal lymphoid irradiation may be used alone with a high cure rate. Subtotal lymphoid irradiation consists of radiation to the nodal sites above the diaphragm (mantle field) followed by radiation to the spleen and paraaortic nodes. Vaccinations for encapsulated organisms are given before irradiation of the spleen.

In NLPHL, radiation therapy alone is given for clinical stages IA and IIA. The literature for chemotherapy alone and for combination therapy is very limited. The mediastinum is usually not included in the radiation fields. For those with B symptoms or advanced stage, a variety of chemotherapy regimens, including ABVD or CHOP (cyclophosphamide, doxorubicin, vincristine, and prednisone), may be used. The regimen should include an alkylating agent. However, some patients have a chronic or indolent course requiring little treatment. A variety of effective second-line chemotherapy regimens exist. High-dose therapy or allotransplantation may be used for relapse or progressive disease, along with radiation to residual sites.

ACUTE EFFECTS OF RADIATION

A variety of acute effects are common and are largely self-limited. Reassurance and occasionally medications are helpful. Fatigue is common but is very rarely severe. Most patients can function normally and work full-time during radiation treatments. Mild exercise programs, increased caloric intake, and extra rest are advised. Xerostomia may occasionally occur to a mild degree if the neck is treated. Significant dryness occurs only with irradiation of very high cervical disease or Waldeyer's fields. Often, the dryness resolves completely after many months. Chronic dryness predisposes to dental decay, so daily prescription fluoride application and frequent professional cleaning are advised. Mild pharyngitis or dysphagia may occur at about 20 Gy, but this is minimal or absent in many patients. Topical agents are available to minimize and treat these symptoms, which usually resolve soon after irradiation. Hair loss may occur, but only inside the radiation field. Temporary hyperpigmentation or mild erythema of the skin may occur. Sunscreen should be applied during and after radiation therapy.

Pericarditis may occur during or after radiation therapy. Pneumonitis may occur in the first month after irradiation. These effects occur in fewer than 5% of patients and are even rarer with modern techniques and doses. Rare reports of acute pericarditis exist with limited cardiac volumes of radiation after prior exposure to doxorubicin.

---

[1]Not FDA approved for this indication.

CURRENT THERAPY

Stage IA-IIA

- Four cycles of ABVD + 30 Gy involved-field radiotherapy (IFRT)
- Stanford V for 8 weeks (two cycles) may be used as a substitute for ABVD, followed by IFRT
- Restaging is done with positron-emission tomography/computed tomography (PET/CT) before administration of IFRT
- ABVD for six cycles without IFRT is a less acceptable alternative

Stage I-II Bulky

- Four to six cycles of ABVD + 30–36 Gy IFRT
- Stanford V for 12 weeks (three cycles) may be used as a substitute for ABVD, followed by IFRT
- Restaging is done with PET/CT after four cycles of chemotherapy with ABVD or completion of therapy with Stanford V

Stage IB-IIB, III-IV

- Six to eight cycles of ABVD + 30–40 Gy IFRT for stage I-II disease and initial bulky disease
- Escalated-dose BEACOPP for eight cycles may be used as an alternative to ABVD, followed by IFRT
- Restaging is done with PET/CT after four cycles of chemotherapy with ABVD or BEACOPP
- IFRT is administered to initial sites >5 cm in diameter

Lhermitte's sign is an electrical shock-like sensation that radiates down the legs. It is precipitated by forward flexion of the trunk. This is very uncommon but can be alarming to the patient; the impact can be minimized if the patient is properly educated about the possibility of having these symptoms. It occurs 3 to 12 weeks after radiation and may be related to transient demyelinization of the cord. This syndrome does not predict for any permanent neurologic sequelae and resolves spontaneously after a few months.

Hematologic changes are usually minimal when radiation therapy is given after chemotherapy. These effects can be significant with larger volumes of radiation, especially with the use of irradiation alone with extended fields.

LATE EFFECTS

Pulmonary complications may occur from bleomycin chemotherapy or from excessive radiation volumes. Care should be exercised with radiation volumes after prior treatment with bleomycin. The large mantle fields treated in earlier regimens are rarely used now, so pulmonary toxicity is reduced. Acute symptomatic radiation pneumonitis typically occurs within 6 to 12 weeks after completion of radiation therapy. A subacute fibrotic phase may occur at 6 months. This acute syndrome is characterized by cough, dyspnea on exertion, and low-grade temperature elevation. The cough can usually be eliminated with oral steroids, but such drugs should be tapered slowly to prevent recurrence of symptoms. Although steroids improve the acute symptoms, they do not prevent the late fibrosis. Fibrotic changes may be seen on chest radiography or lung windows of CT studies without symptoms. The changes usually conform to the pattern of the radiation field.

Chronic cardiomyopathy increases as the dose of doxorubicin accumulates to greater than 400 mg/m^2. The magnitude of the effect of using lower doses and the interactions with radiation are unknown. Irradiation of cardiac vessels probably leads to accelerated arteriosclerosis. Currently used limited radiation fields may treat little or no cardiac vessels compared with previous mantle fields.

Additionally, current radiation doses of 20 to 30 Gy may be below a threshold for induction of arteriosclerosis. Chemical hypothyroidism occurs in about one third of patients when the thyroid is included in the radiation field. Patients should routinely be tested for hypothyroidism, and replacement hormone should be given if the thyroid-stimulating hormone concentration is elevated. Herpes zoster (shingles) may occur after radiation therapy. Sepsis may occur with chemotherapy-induced neutropenia or from pneumococcal organisms after splenic irradiation.

Treatment-related secondary malignancies can also occur. Acute myeloid leukemia or myelodysplastic syndrome may occur after chemotherapy. Non-Hodgkin's lymphomas occur more commonly in these patients than in the general population. The incidence of solid tumors is increased after irradiation. Smokers should be advised to discontinue smoking after thoracic irradiation to reduce the increased risk of lung cancer. Breast cancer may be increased after thoracic irradiation in women younger than 30 years of age. The risk is related not only to age but also to the dose and volume of exposed breast. Current progress in lowering the dose of radiation and reducing the field size should dramatically decrease the risk of secondary solid tumors. Women receiving thoracic irradiation should begin breast examinations and mammography at an earlier age. Approximately 5% of patients develop thyroid cancer after exposure to therapeutic levels of radiation to the thyroid gland. This is usually of the well-differentiated type and has a high cure rate.

Infertility may occur after treatment for HD. In males, azoospermia may occur after pelvic irradiation. The magnitude of this effect can significantly be reduced with proper gonadal shielding, allowing for near-complete recovery in most men. Sperm banking is recommended as a precaution for all young men receiving pelvic irradiation. Chemotherapy with MOPP (mechlorethamine, vincristine, procarbazine, and prednisone), MOPP-like regimens that include procarbazine, or BEACOPP causes sterility in most men. Male fertility is usually preserved with ABVD and Stanford V regimens. Elimination of ovarian function often occurs with pelvic irradiation of women older than 30 years of age. Younger women may be protected from pelvic irradiation by oophorpexy, with placement of the ovaries in the midline behind the uterus. Ovarian function is also affected by alkylating agents in women older than 30 years of age.

REFERENCES

DeVita VT, Lawrence TS, Rosenberg SA. DeVita, Hellman, and Rosenberg's Cancer: Principles and Practice of Oncology. 8th ed. Philadelphia: Wolters Kluwer/Lippincott Williams & Wilkins; 2008.

Diehl V, Engert A, Mueller RP, et al. HD 10: Investigating reduction of combined modality treatment intensity in early stage Hodgkin's lymphoma. Interim analysis of a randomized trial of the German Hodgkin Study Group (GHSG). J Clin Oncol 2005;23(16S):561S.

Dores GM. Second malignant neoplasms among long-term survivors of Hodgkin's disease: A population-based evaluation over 25 years. J Clin Oncol 2002;20:3484–94.

Engert A, Franklin J, Eich HT, et al. Two cycles of doxorubicin, bleomycin, vinblastine and dacarbazine plus extended field radiotherapy is superior to radiotherapy alone in early favorable Hodgkin's lymphoma: Final results of the GHSG HD7 trial. J Clin Oncol 2007;25:3495–502.

Engert A, Schiller P, Josting A, et al. Involved-field radiotherapy is equally effective and less toxic compared with extended-field radiotherapy after four cycles of chemotherapy in patients with early-stage unfavorable Hodgkin's lymphoma: Results of the HD8 trial of the German Hodgkin's Lymphoma Study Group. J Clin Oncol 2003;21:3601–8.

Halperin EC, Perez CA, Brady LW. Perez and Brady's Principles and Practice of Radiation Oncology. 5th ed. Philadelphia: Wolters Kluwer Health/Lippincott Williams & Wilkins; 2008.

Hancock SL, Tucker MA, Hoppe RT. Factors affecting late mortality from heart disease after treatment of Hodgkin's disease. JAMA 1993;270:1949–55.

Hoppe RT, Advani RH, Ambinder RF, et al. Hodgkin disease/lymphoma. J Natl Compr Cancer Netw 2008;6:594–622.

NCCN Clinical Practice Guidelines in Oncology. Hodgkin Disease/Lymphoma. Version 2, Available at http://www.nccn.org/professionals/physician_gls/PDF/hodgkins.pdf; [accessed November 13, 2008].

Acute Leukemia in Adults

Method of
Meir Wetzler, MD, FACP

Acute Myeloid Leukemia

EPIDEMIOLOGY

The age-adjusted incidence rate for acute myeloid leukemia (AML) is 3.5 per 100,000 men and women per year. The incidence increases with age and the median age at diagnosis is 67 years.

RISK FACTORS

Exposure to chemicals including benzene, petroleum products, herbicides, pesticides, and tobacco are associated with increased risk of AML. About 10% of patients exposed to chemotherapy or radiotherapy eventually develop therapy-related AML. Warfare and occupational exposure to ionizing radiation predispose to AML.

PATHOPHYSIOLOGY

The pathophysiology of AML consists of maturation arrest at the blast level and activation of genes through several mechanisms (e.g., epigenetic silencing). One of the reasons for treatment failure in AML is the inability of current chemotherapy to kill the leukemia stem cells. These cells are quiescent, can self-renew, and have extensive proliferative capacity and the ability to give rise to differentiated progeny in a hierarchical pattern. Most of the chemotherapeutic agents traditionally used to treat AML are cell-cycle–active agents that primarily target dividing cells. These agents are highly unlikely to be effective against the quiescent leukemia stem cells. Therefore, new agents are being studied that target the leukemia stem cell.

Secondary AML, defined as AML following antecedent hematologic disorder or therapy for another disease, is associated with very poor outcome.

PREVENTION

Smoking cessation and avoiding exposure to offending agents, such as benzene, can prevent AML.

CLINICAL MANIFESTATIONS

Patients might complain of fatigue or weakness, anorexia, or weight loss. Patients can also present with fever with or without source of infection, bleeding tendency, and sometimes bone pain, cough, or diaphoresis. Seldom patients present with soft tissue masses, called myeloid sarcoma, with or without bone marrow involvement.

On physical examination, fever, hepatosplenomegaly, lymphadenopathy, and evidence of infection and hemorrhage can be detected. Bleeding because of disseminated intravascular coagulopathy is more characteristic of **acute promyelocytic leukemia**. Infiltration of the gingiva, soft tissues, skin or meninges is more characteristic of monocytic leukemia. Patients with very high numbers of circulating blasts can develop signs of leukostasis such as headache, confusion, and dyspnea.

DIAGNOSIS

AML is diagnosed if at least 20% blasts are present in the blood or bone marrow; except in patients with t(8;21)(q22;q22), inv(16)(p13q22), t(16;16)(p13;q22), or t(15;17)(q22;q12), where the diagnosis is made even with less than 20% blasts. Increased promyeloblasts are associated with t(15;17) and dysplastic eosinophils are characteristics of inv(16)/t(16;16). Auer rods, representing abnormal condensation of cytoplasmic granules, may be observed in myeloblasts.

CURRENT DIAGNOSIS

Acute Myeloid Leukemia

- Diagnosis is made on 20% blasts or more; in patients with t(8;21)(q22;q22), inv(16)(p13q22) or t(16;16)(p13;q22), or t(15;17)(q22;q12) AML diagnosis is made even with less than 20% blasts.
- Separate entities are recognized based on specific chromosomal/molecular abnormalities.
- Presence of increased promyeloblasts facilitates diagnosis of acute promyelocytic leukemia.
- Presence of dysplastic eosinophils assists in the diagnosis of acute myeloid leukemia with inv(16)/t(16;16).
- Acute myeloid leukemia presentation is grouped based on presence of myelodysplastic changes, prior exposure to chemotherapy or radiotherapy, the presence of myeloid sarcoma, or Down syndrome.
- Acute myeloid leukemia with multilineage dysplasia is divided into subgroups based on prior history of myelodysplastic syndrome.

AML presentation is grouped based on presence of myelodysplastic changes, prior exposure to chemotherapy or radiotherapy, the presence of myeloid sarcoma, or Down syndrome. AML with multilineage dysplasia is grouped into specific subtypes with or without the presence of prior multilineage dysplasia.

The AML blasts are characteristically myeloperoxidase-positive. If they are negative, expression of myeloid markers on their surface such as CD13 and CD33 is diagnostic. Blasts carrying t(8;21) often express lymphoid markers (e.g., CD19, PAX5, and cytoplasmic CD79a) and promyeloblasts with t(15;17) commonly express CD2.

DIFFERENTIAL DIAGNOSIS

The main alternative diagnosis is acute lymphoblastic leukemia (ALL).

PROGNOSIS

Factors associated with worse outcome include older age (inability to survive induction either due to comorbidities or because of chemoresistance due to multidrug-resistance proteins), secondary presentation (prior chemotherapy for an unrelated disease or history of antecedent hematologic disorder), elevated white blood cell count (WBC $>100 \times 10^9$/L), and poor performance status.

Karyotype aberrations (structural and numerical) assign patients into favorable, intermediate, and unfavorable subgroups (Table 1). In patients with normal karyotype, submicroscopic genetic aberrations further assign subgroups. *NPM1* mutations are found in 46% to 62% of AML patients, and they are associated with improved outcome if they are solely present. Detection of internal tandem duplications within the juxtamembrane domain of the *FLT3* gene, reported in about a third of the normal karyotype AML patients, predict poor outcome, especially if the *FLT3-ITD/FLT3*-wild type allelic ratio is high. The prognostic significance of *FLT3* point mutations is still unclear. Additional, less frequent, aberrations such as biallelic mutations of *CEBPA*, are associated with improved outcome, and partial tandem duplication of the *MLL* gene, *WT1* mutations, and overexpression of *BAALC*, *ERG* and *MN1* genes are associated with worse outcome in normal karyotype AML. Submicroscopic genetic aberrations in the *KIT* gene adversely affect the outcome of t(8;21) and inv(16)/t(16;16).

Complete remission is defined as less than 5% blasts in the marrow, blood neutrophil count of at least 1×10^9/L, and platelet count at least 100×10^9/L without circulating blasts and disappearance of extramedullary disease, if such was present. Complete remission is necessary to achieve long-term survival or cure.

TABLE 1 Karyotype Risk Groups in Acute Myeloid Leukemia

Risk Group	Aberration
Favorable	t(8;21)
	inv(16)/t(16;16)
	t(15;17)
Intermediate: normal karyotype	-Y,
	del(7q)
	del(9q)
	del(11q)
	isolated +8, +11, +21
	del(20q)
Unfavorable: complex karyotype*	inv(3)/t(3;3)
	-7
	t(6;9)
	t(6;11)
	t(11;19)
	-5
	del(5q)

*Complex karyotype is defined as three or more aberrations.

TREATMENT

Induction therapy for patients younger than 60 years with newly diagnosed AML, in the absence of a clinical trial, consists of the combination of ara-C (Cytosar) at 100 to 200 mg/m^2/day for 7 days as continuous infusion along with an anthracycline (e.g., daunorubicin [Cerubidine] or idarubicin [Idamycin]) administered intravenously over the first 3 days. Attempts to escalate ara-C during induction results in longer disease-free survival in some studies, and escalating anthracyclines improves complete remission rate and overall survival. Adding etoposide (Toposar)[1] can improve remission duration.

Multilumen right atrial catheters should be used to administer medications, fluid, and transfusions and to draw blood. Induction treatment can result in tumor lysis syndrome, characterized mainly by elevated uric acid. Therefore, allopurinol (Zyloprim) and hydration should be initiated early.

Patients who are allergic to allopurinol, who are unable to take oral medications, or who have uric acid nephropathy may be treated with rasburicase (recombinant uric acid oxidase, Elitek) or hemodialysis. Aggressive supportive care during the period of granulocytopenia and thrombocytopenia are necessary for the success of this treatment. Using recombinant growth factors has been reported to shorten median time to neutrophil recovery, but it has not resulted in improved outcome. Therefore, their use is controversial and should be restricted to clinical trials or according to published guidelines.

---

[1]Not FDA approved for this indication.

CURRENT THERAPY

Acute Myeloid Leukemia

- Treatment is divided into induction and post-remission therapy.
- Standard induction therapy for patients who have de novo acute myeloid leukemia and are younger than 60 years include combination therapy with cytarabine (cytosine arabinoside, ara-C [Cytosar]) and an anthracycline.
- All-*trans*-retinoic acid (tretinoin [Vesanoid]) and an anthracycline is standard induction treatment for acute promyelocytic leukemia.

Platelet transfusions should maintain a platelet count greater than 10×10^9/L unless the patient has active bleeding or disseminated intravascular coagulation, when it may be necessary to maintain higher platelet counts. Similarly, red blood cell transfusions should maintain hemoglobin of greater than 8 g/dL unless patients have active bleeding, disseminated intravascular coagulopathy, or history of cardiovascular disease. All blood products should be leukodepleted by filtration and irradiated to prevent alloimmunization, fever, and transfusion-associated graft-versus-host disease.

Infections remain the most important cause of morbidity and mortality. Prophylactic antibiotics should be based on institutional antibiograms, and prophylactic antifungal and antiviral medications are highly recommended. Fever should be treated as resulting from bacterial and fungal infections.

After achieving complete remission, further treatment depends on the patient's age and prognostic factors. For example, high-dose ara-C is more effective than standard-dose ara-C in younger AML patients, especially for those with t(8;21) and inv(16)/t(16;16) and those with normal karyotype AML.

Acute Promyelocytic Leukemia

Acute promyelocytic leukemia (APL), characterized by t(15;17) and its product *PML/RARα*, should be treated with all-*trans* retinoic acid (tretinoin [Vesanoid]), which induces differentiation of the leukemic blasts. During this differentiation process, the promyeloblasts lose their characteristic granules that can release enzymes causing disseminated intravascular coagulopathy. The most important side effect of tretinoin is the retinoic acid syndrome, characterized by increasing leukocyte counts, fever, shortness of breath, chest pain, pulmonary infiltrates, pleural and pericardial effusions, and hypoxia. Treatment for this complication includes steroids, chemotherapy, and supportive care.

Tretinoin and an anthracycline is standard induction treatment for APL. The role of ara-C (Cytosar)[1] during induction remains controversial. Approximately 90% of APL patients achieve complete remission and then undergo consolidation therapy with arsenic trioxide (Trisenox) and additional courses of tretinoin and an anthracycline. Maintenance treatment with tretinoin, with or without chemotherapy, results in prolonged disease-free survival, though it is unclear whether it is beneficial to all patients or only a subgroup of them. Approaches devoid of chemotherapy are now being studied to evaluate which patients will benefit from those.

Relapse

Once relapse occurs, patients are rarely cured with standard chemotherapy. Patients should be offered allogeneic stem cell transplantation in either first relapse or second remission; the outcome following second remission seems better. Second complete remission is more likely if the first remission lasted longer than 12 months and patients achieved complete remission following one induction course. The long-term disease-free survival following an allogeneic stem cell transplant in relapsed patients is about 40%.

Relapse in APL, in the absence of clinical trials, can respond to the combinations of tretinoin, arsenic trioxide, and an anthracycline.[1]

Novel Approaches and Future Directions

Novel approaches and future directions include targeted therapies for patients with *FLT3* and *KIT* mutations with specific tyrosine kinase inhibitors and targeting aberrant DNA methylation or histone deacetylation (or both) resulting in epigenetic silencing of structurally normal genes. Current hypomethylating agents approved for myelodysplastic syndromes (5-azacitidine [Vidaza][1] and decitabine [Dacogen][1]) are being studied in AML. The proteasome inhibitor bortezomib (Velcade)[1] is also being explored in AML. Nonspecific chemotherapy agents (cloretazine[5] and clofarabine [Clolar][1]) have encouraging results in preliminary clinical trials in older or in relapsed or refractory AML.

Allogeneic stem cell transplantation reduces the relapse risk but this beneficial effect is offset by its treatment-related mortality.

---

[1]Not FDA approved for this indication.

Therefore, this approach should be reserved for patients with high-risk features and those in second remission and beyond.

MONITORING

Detection of minimal residual disease following complete remission by reverse-transcriptase polymerase chain reaction (PCR) of *PML/RARα* transcript predicts relapse. Therefore, sequential monitoring of *PML/RARα* is standard in APL. Detection of minimal residual disease in other types of AML is lagging behind, even though other fusion genes, such as t(8;21) and inv(16)/t(16;16), are available.

COMPLICATIONS

The main risk following successful AML treatment is late development of secondary myelodysplastic syndromes and AML.

Acute Lymphoblastic Leukemia

EPIDEMIOLOGY

The age-adjusted incidence rate is 1.6 per 100,000 population per year. The median age at diagnosis is 13 years of age; about 60% of cases are diagnosed in patients younger than 20 years.

RISK FACTORS

Genetic predisposition to ALL is associated with Down syndrome, Fanconi's anemia, Bloom syndrome, neurofibromatosis type 1, and ataxia telangiectasia.

PATHOPHYSIOLOGY

The theories about the origin of the leukemia-initiating cell in ALL vary. Some relate it to an already committed B- or T-lineage cell, and others propose that—at least in some ALL subtypes—the leukemia blasts might arise from a more phenotypically primitive hematopoietic stem cell. The most recent challenge to the leukemia-initiating cell theory is the report that B precursor blasts in various stages of differentiation displayed self-renewal capability, suggesting that leukemic lymphoid progenitors might not lose their self-renewal capability with maturation or are able to "move backward" in differentiation.

Secondary ALL, defined as ALL following another malignancy, irrespective whether patients received prior therapy, is rare. As in secondary AML, the outcome is extremely poor.

PREVENTION

Data suggest that early aspects of lifestyle and environment are associated with a decreased risk for ALL in children. For example, prolonged breast-feeding, daycare attendance, and early community-acquired infections are associated with a reduced incidence of childhood ALL. In the United States, ALL incidence rates are lower in rural communities compared with metropolitan areas. Finally, some data suggest that *Haemophilus influenzae* type b vaccine might reduce ALL risk.

CLINICAL MANIFESTATIONS

The symptoms are not significantly different from those of patients with AML. Central nervous system (CNS) involvement is detected in approximately 10% of the cases and is more prevalent in T-cell ALL.

DIAGNOSIS

The blasts range in size from homogeneous small cells with a high nuclear-to-cytoplasmic ratio and inconspicuous nucleoli to more-pleomorphic cells. Burkitt's leukemia is characterized by medium-sized homogeneous cells with dispersed chromatin, multiple nucleoli, and a moderate amount of deep blue cytoplasm with clearly defined vacuoles. The "starry sky" appearance is composed of the tinted body macrophages (the stars) scattered among sheets of dark blue blasts (the sky).

---

[1]Not FDA approved for this indication.
[5]Investigational drug in the United States.

CURRENT DIAGNOSIS

Acute Lymphoblastic Leukemia

- There is no agreed-upon lower limit of blast percentage required for diagnosing acute lymphoblastic leukemia. Many treatment protocols use 25% blasts as the cut-off for diagnosis and in general, a diagnosis of acute lymphoblastic leukemia should be avoided if there are less than 20% blasts.
- The diagnosis includes B-lineage, T-lineage, and unspecified acute lymphoblastic leukemia.
- B-lineage, but not T-lineage categories are recognized as separate entities based on the presence of specific chromosomal or molecular abnormalities.

ALL is characterized by blasts that are myeloperoxidase-negative and terminal deoxynucleotide transferase (TdT)-positive. CD10, CD19, cytoplasmic CD22, cytoplasmic CD79a, and PAX5 with variable expression of CD20 characterize B-lineage ALL, whereas CD1a, cytoplasmic CD3, CD7, CD4, and CD8 characterize T-lineage ALL. The presence of myeloid markers does not exclude the diagnosis of ALL.

Burkitt's leukemia is characterized by B-cell–associated antigens and moderate to strong levels of membrane immunoglobulin M (IgM) with light chain restriction; the cells are TdT-negative and more than 99% Ki-67 positive. Burkitt leukemia is a subtype of ALL whose hallmark is the t(8;14)(q24;q32) and its variants, t(2;8)(p12;q24) and t(8;22)(q24;q11). In these cases, *MYC*, located on 8q24, is activated and expressed at high levels, leading to uncontrolled cell proliferation. However, *MYC* translocations are not specific for Burkitt's leukemia.

DIFFERENTIAL DIAGNOSIS

The main diagnosis in the differential is AML. The leukemia blasts can resemble hematogones, the normal lymphoid progenitors. Morphologic distinction between hematogones and residual ALL can be difficult. However, hematogones display the continuum of B-cell markers whereas the leukemic blasts overexpress or underexpress specific markers. For example, ALL with myeloid markers can be relatively easily distinguished from hematogones because the latter lack myeloid markers. Leukemia of ambiguous lineage includes biphenotypic leukemia, describing a single blast population expressing antigens from more than one lineage, and bilineage leukemia describing separate populations of blasts from more than one lineage. The two most common examples are those with t(9;22) and 11q23/*MLL* translocations.

PROGNOSIS

Several factors are associated with worse outcome such as older age (inability to survive induction either owing to comorbidities or because of chemoresistance due to multidrug resistance proteins), secondary presentation (prior chemotherapy for an unrelated disease), elevated WBC count ($>30 \times 10^9$/L in B-cell ALL; $>100 \times 10^9$/L in T-cell ALL), immunophenotype (B-cell) and elevated lactate dehydrogenase, associated with CNS disease. Interestingly, persistence of normal residual hematopoiesis and intense leukemia cell mitotic index are associated with favorable outcome.

Recurring chromosomal abnormalities divide ALL into favorable, intermediate and unfavorable subgroups (Table 2). Submicroscopic genetic aberrations further characterize the disease. For example, in T-cell ALL, activating somatic mutations in *NOTCH1* are described in about 50% of cases. NOTCH1 protein, either normal or aberrant, is cleaved by the γ-secretase complex, leading to its translocation to the nucleus where it induces *NOTCH1*-target gene transcription. This pathway is currently being targeted in clinical trials with γ-secretase inhibitors. Lack of *HOX11* expression and high *ERG* and *BAALC* expression predict adverse outcome in T-lineage ALL.

TABLE 2 Karyotype Risk Groups in Acute Lymphoblastic Leukemia

Risk Group	Aberration
Favorable	Del(12p) or t(12p), t(14)(q11-q13), hyperdiploid
Intermediate	Normal Karyotype, +21, del(9p) or t(9p)
Unfavorable	t(9;22), -7, +8, t(4;11), hypodiploid, t(1;19)

As in AML, achievement of complete remission is necessary to achieve long-term survival or cure. In addition, lack of cytoreduction on day 7 or 14 correlates with adverse prognosis in ALL.

TREATMENT

The two most commonly used approaches in ALL include the BFM (Berlin-Frankfurt-Munster) and the hyper-CVAD (cyclophosphamide, vincristine, doxorubicin (Adriamycin), and dexamethasone) regimens.

BFM-like regimens include induction with vincristine, prednisone,[1] daunorubicin, and l-asparaginase (Elspar); early intensification with cyclophosphamide (Cytoxan), ara-C (Cytosar), 6-mercaptopurine (Purinethol), and vincristine; CNS prophylaxis with either cranial radiation or high-dose methotrexate and ara-C; late intensification with doxorubicin, vincristine, dexamethasone,[1] cyclophosphamide, 6-thioguanine (Tabloid),[1] and ara-C; and maintenance with prednisone, vincristine, 6-mercaptopurine, and methotrexate (POMP) for a total of 24 months.

The hyper-CVAD regimen consists of eight alternating courses of CVAD with methotrexate and high-dose ara-C. CNS prophylaxis includes intrathecal methotrexate and maintenance with POMP for a total of 24 months.

The outcome following these different approaches results in approximately 30% to 40% 5-year survival. Supportive care guidelines are similar to those described in the AML section.

A major breakthrough occurred with the introduction of imatinib mesylate (Gleevec) for the treatment of t(9;22) ALL and its product *BCR/ABL*. Imatinib functions though competitive inhibition at the adenosine triphosphate (ATP) binding site of the ABL kinase in the inactive conformation, which leads to inhibition of tyrosine phosphorylation of proteins involved in BCR/ABL signaling. It shows a

---

[1]Not FDA approved for this indication.

CURRENT THERAPY

Acute Lymphoblastic Leukemia

- The two most commonly used approaches include the Berlin-Frankfurt-Munster (BFM)-like and the hyper-cyclophosphamide (Cytoxan), vincristine (Oncovin), doxorubicin (Adriamycin) and dexamethasone (Decadron)[1] (CVAD) regimens
- Imatinib mesylate (Gleevec) has significantly improved the outcome of t(9;22) acute lymphoblastic leukemia.
- Relapsed T-cell acute lymphoblastic leukemia benefits from the addition of nelarabine (Arranon).
- The use of pediatric regimens to treat adolescents and young adults has improved the outcome of these patients.
- Including anti-CD20 antibody in Burkitt's leukemia has improved this disease's outcome.

---

[1]Not FDA approved for this indication.

---

high degree of specificity for BCR/ABL, the receptor for platelet-derived growth factor and KIT tyrosine kinases. Imatinib does not affect the normal hematopoietic progenitor cells. Combining imatinib with chemotherapy, either sequentially (aiming to reduce toxicity) or concurrently, resulted in a significant improvement in disease-free survival over chemotherapy-alone approaches.

Four mechanisms of resistance to imatinib have been described to date: gene amplification, mutations at the kinase site, decreased intracellular imatinib levels, and alternative signaling pathways functionally compensating for the imatinib-sensitive mechanisms. Unique to ALL, kinase domain mutations can precede imatinib-based therapy and give rise to relapse in patients with de novo t(9;22) ALL. Alternating signaling pathways such as Src family kinase members—Lyn, Hck, and Fgr—have been shown to be elevated in hematopoietic cells of mice with t(9;22) ALL. Even in the presence of suppressed BCR/ABL, t(9;22) ALL cells can proliferate in the presence of stromal support.

Approaches to overcome these mechanisms of resistance include introduction of dasatinib (Sprycel), which is almost 300-fold more potent than imatinib, binds to the kinase domain in the open conformation, is resistant to most mutations, and is active against Src kinases. Dasatinib, as a single agent and in combination with chemotherapy, was tested in imatinib-resistant and imatinib-naïve t(9;22) ALL with encouraging results. Dasatinib and prednisone alone have been studied as front-line therapy in newly diagnosed t(9;22)[1] ALL with encouraging results. Similarly, nilotinib (Tasigna)[1] is about 30-fold more potent than imatinib, binds to the kinase domain in the inactive formation, and is resistant to most mutations. Nilotinib has promising activity in imatinib-resistant ALL as monotherapy.

Nelarabine (Arranon) is a purine analogue shown to have significant activity in T-lineage ALL patients whose disease has not responded to or has relapsed following treatment with at least two chemotherapy regimens. In the adult clinical trial, the rate of complete remission was 31% and the overall response rate was 41%. The main toxicity was grade 3 to 4 neutropenia and thrombocytopenia. It is now going to be studied in newly diagnosed T-lineage ALL.[1]

Pediatric Regimens for Adolescents and Adults

Adolescents and young adults represent a challenging group for both pediatric and adult oncologists. Several groups have evaluated the outcome of patients aged 16 to 21 years based on their treatment on adult or pediatric protocols. Despite an assortment of treatment approaches among the different groups, the results of these retrospective analyses consistently demonstrated that adolescents and young adults treated on pediatric protocols had significantly better 5-year survival than those treated on adult protocols. Several reasons were suggested for these differences, including more-intensive use of non-myelosuppressive agents (e.g., steroids, l-asparaginase, vincristine), earlier CNS prophylaxis, and longer maintenance in the pediatric protocols. Moreover, protocol adherence and compliance, by both treating physicians and patients, was raised as a contributing factor to outcome differences. Therefore, several groups have started offering pediatric regimens to adolescents and young adults (up to age 30 year and beyond) with encouraging results.

The treatment of adult Burkitt's leukemia underwent significant improvement when pediatric regimens, including repetitive cycles of fractional alkylating agents and aggressive CNS therapy, were employed. Because Burkitt's leukemia is characterized by strong CD20 expression, two groups successfully included anti-CD20 antibody, rituximab (Rituxan),[1] in their treatment regimens. In addition to the favorable outcome in these patients, concerns about increased infectious complications, due to the use of rituximab, were dismissed by these studies.

Allogeneic stem cell transplantation continues to represent an effective treatment approach for adult ALL. It is usually recommended to high-risk ALL patients in first remission and those in second remission and beyond. Offering allogeneic stem cell transplantation for standard-risk ALL is controversial.

---

[1]Not FDA approved for this indication.

MONITORING

Minimal residual disease in ALL is one of the most powerful and informative parameters to guide clinical management. Two methods have been established to detect minimal residual disease: Flow cytometry relies on immunologic markers to identify residual leukemic cells, and PCR amplifies fusion transcript or uses antigen-receptor genes as targets to detect minimal residual disease.

COMPLICATIONS

The main risk following successful treatment of ALL is late development of secondary myelodysplastic syndromes and AML. Another complication is avascular necrosis due to steroid use.

REFERENCES

Abutalib SA, Wetzler M, Stock W. Looking toward the future: Novel strategies based on molecular pathogenesis of acute lymphoblastic leukemia. Hematol Oncol Clin North Am 2009;23:1099–119 vii.

Campana D. Role of minimal residual disease monitoring in adult and pediatric acute lymphoblastic leukemia. Hematol Oncol Clin North Am 2009;23: 1083–98 vii.

DeAngelo DJ. Nelarabine for the treatment of patients with relapsed or refractory T-cell acute lymphoblastic leukemia or lymphoblastic lymphoma. Hematol Oncol Clin North Am 2009;23:1121–35 vii–viii.

Dohner H, Estey EH, Amadori S, et al. Diagnosis and management of acute myeloid leukemia in adults: Recommendations from an international expert panel, on behalf of the European LeukemiaNet. Blood 2010;115:453–74.

Forman SJ. Allogeneic hematopoietic cell transplantation for acute lymphoblastic leukemia in adults. Hematol Oncol Clin North Am 2009;23:1011–31 vi.

Jeha S. Recent progress in the treatment of acute lymphoblastic leukemia: clofarabine. Hematol Oncol Clin North Am 2009;23:1137–44 viii.

Jeha S, Pui CH. Risk-adapted treatment of pediatric acute lymphoblastic leukemia. Hematol Oncol Clin North Am 2003;23:973–90 v.

Mrozek K, Harper DP, Aplan PD. Cytogenetics and molecular genetics of acute lymphoblastic leukemia. Hematol Oncol Clin North Am 2009; 23:991–1010 v.

Nathan PC, Wasilewski-Masker K, Janzen LA. Long-term outcomes in survivors of childhood acute lymphoblastic leukemia. Hematol Oncol Clin North Am 2009;23:1065–82 vi–vii.

NCCN. Acute myeloid leukemia. Clinical Practice Guidelines in Oncology: National Comprehensive Cancer Network; 2010.

Ravandi F, Kebriaei P. Philadelphia chromosome-positive acute lymphoblastic leukemia. Hematol Oncol Clin North Am 2009;23:1043–63 vi.

Ribera JM, Oriol A. Acute lymphoblastic leukemia in adolescents and young adults. Hematol Oncol Clin North Am 2009;23:1033–42 vi.

Sanz MA, Grimwade D, Tallman MS, et al. Management of acute promyelocytic leukemia: recommendations from an expert panel on behalf of the European LeukemiaNet. Blood 2009;113:1875–91.

Swerdlow SH, Campo E, Harris NL, et al. WHO Classification of Tumours of Haematopoietic and Lymphoid Tissues. In: Swerdlow SH, Campo E, Harris NL, et al., eds. WHO Classification of Tumours of Haematopoietic and Lymphoid Tissues. Lyon: IARC Press; 2008.

Thomas DA, O'Brien S, Kantarjian HM. Monoclonal antibody therapy with rituximab for acute lymphoblastic leukemia. Hematol Oncol Clin North Am 2009;23:949–71 v.

Wetzler M, Stock W. Preface: acute lymphoblastic leukemia–quo vadis? Hematol Oncol Clin North Am 2009;23:xi–xviii.

Acute Leukemia in Children

Method of
Patrick Brown, MD, and Stephen P. Hunger, MD

The word "leukemia" is derived from the Greek roots *leukos* (white) and *haima* (blood). Leukemia, cancer of the blood-forming cells, is characterized by a marked proliferation of abnormal leukocytes in the bone marrow and blood that may be associated with widespread infiltration in extramedullary sites including the central nervous system (CNS), testes, thymus, liver, spleen, and lymph nodes.

Classification

The first level of classification of leukemia is *acute* versus *chronic*. Acute leukemia is characterized by the predominance of very immature white blood cell precursors, or blasts, and is an aggressive, rapidly fatal disease if left untreated. Chronic leukemia is characterized by proliferation of relatively mature white blood cells and is typically an indolent disease.

The second level of classification is *lymphoid* versus *myeloid*, depending on whether the leukemic cells display characteristics of lymphocyte precursors or myelocyte (granulocyte, erythrocyte, monocyte, or megakaryocyte) precursors. Acute lymphoblastic leukemia (ALL) and acute myeloid leukemia (AML) account for the overwhelming majority of pediatric leukemias. Chronic leukemias are uncommon in pediatrics.

ALL and AML are further subclassified by morphology and expression of cell surface antigens using flow cytometry. For ALL, classification is largely based on cell surface and cytoplasmic marker expression (Table 1). AML cases are classified by characteristic chromosomal abnormalities (if present) or by light microscopic morphology in cases where these specific chromosomal changes are absent (Box 1).

Epidemiology

The incidence of childhood cancer is 14 cases per 100,000 children younger than 16 years of age per year, which translates into approximately 11,000 new cases per year in the United States. Leukemia accounts for approximately 30% of childhood cancers, making it the most common form of childhood cancer. The distribution of the major forms of leukemia is vastly different in children than in adults (Fig. 1). In general, children are far more likely to have acute leukemia, and ALL is much more common than AML. In adults, most cases of leukemia are chronic, and AML is much more common than ALL.

The incidence of the various forms of leukemia varies by age in both children and adults (Fig. 2). This is especially true for childhood ALL, for which there is a marked incidence peak in the 2- to 4-year-old age group. This ALL age peak is primarily found in children living in industrialized nations, leading to speculation that a common environmental exposure, coupled with age-related immunologic susceptibility, is at least partially responsible for many cases of ALL. Except for a small peak in infants, the incidence of AML is fairly constant in childhood but rises quickly in later adulthood.

Prognosis

One of the most dramatic success stories in modern medicine is the improvement in survival of children with ALL over the past four decades. Leukemia was once a uniformly fatal diagnosis, with less than a 5% to 10% cure rate until the mid to late 1960s. Today, approximately 85% of children with ALL are cured. The improved prognosis has been built on pioneering observations on the efficacy of multiagent systemic therapy and the importance of presymptomatic CNS treatment in the late 1960s and early 1970s. Further successive, incremental improvements in outcome have been achieved due to clinical trials conducted by large single centers and national and international cooperative groups that have successfully enrolled a high percentage of eligible children.

Similar approaches have unfortunately not been quite so successful in improving the prognosis of children with AML. Although approximately one half of children with AML are cured today, this has been accomplished by intensifying therapy to the point that the toxic death rate in the early phases of therapy is about 10%. Current research in AML is therefore focusing on developing novel molecularly targeted agents that hold the promise of improving efficacy and limiting toxicity.

TABLE 1 Classification of Childhood Acute Lymphoblastic Leukemia

ALL Subtype	Phenotypic Marker				%	Comment
	CD19	CD10	clg	slg		
Pre-pre B	+	−	−	−	5	Mostly infants, poor prognosis, frequent *MLL* 11q23 rearrangements
Early pre-B	+	+	−	−	63	Common ALL, young children, good prognosis
Pre-B	+	+	+	−	16	Older children, good prognosis with intense therapy
B-cell	+	+	+	+	4	Burkitt's leukemia, *MYC/Ig* fusion genes, good prognosis with lymphoma-type therapy
T-cell	−	−	−	−	12	Adolescents, anterior mediastinal mass, CNS involvement, good prognosis with intense therapy

ALL = acute myeloid leukemia; clg = cytoplasmic immunoglobulin; slg = surface immunoglobulin; CNS = central nervous system.

BOX 1   Classification of Childhood Acute Myeloid Leukemia (World Health Organization Criteria)

Acute Myeloid Leukemia with Recurrent Genetic Abnormalities

Acute myeloid leukemia with t(8;21)(q22;q22), (AML1/ETO)

Acute myeloid leukemia with abnormal bone marrow eosinophils and inv(16)(p13q22) or t(16;16)(p13;q22), (CBFβ/MYH11)

Acute promyelocytic leukemia with t(15;17)(q22;q12), (PML/RARα), and variants

Acute myeloid leukemia with 11q23 (MLL) abnormalities

Acute Myeloid Leukemia, Not Otherwise Categorized

Acute myeloid leukemia, minimally differentiated (FAB M0)

Acute myeloid leukemia without maturation (FAB M1)

Acute myeloid leukemia with maturation (FAB M2)

Acute myelomonocytic leukemia (FAB M4)

Acute monoblastic/acute monocytic leukemia (FAB M5)

Acute erythroid leukemia (FAB M6)

Acute megakaryoblastic leukemia (FAB M7)

FAB = French–American–British classification.

Etiology

The question, "What is the cause of leukemia?" can be considered on a few different levels. First, what is wrong with *this child* that caused the child to develop leukemia? Second, what is wrong with *the leukemia cell* that causes it to behave so badly? Third, what is wrong with *the leukemia cell's genes* that cause the cell to behave that way?

PREDISPOSITIONS

The answer to the first question is unknown in the vast majority of cases. Attempts to correlate various genetic features or environmental or infectious exposures with risk of childhood leukemia have been largely uninformative. It is presumed that children are particularly susceptible to ALL because of the marked expansion and genetic rearrangement of lymphocytes that occurs during early childhood as the result of exposure to a multitude of immunogenic antigens for the first time. The proliferation required to meet the constant demand for granulocytes, erythrocytes, and platelets is likely a setup for the development of AML in children.

Although a number of constitutional and single-gene disorders are known to confer an increased risk of childhood leukemia (Table 2), in total, these are involved in only a very small minority of cases. The most common of these is Down syndrome. Children with Down syndrome have a 10- to 20-fold increased risk of leukemia, with an approximately equal incidence of ALL and AML. The peak age at onset of leukemia for children with Down syndrome is earlier than for other children. Approximately 30% of Down syndrome children with AML have the megakaryoblastic form (M7AML), a subtype that is extremely rare in children without Down syndrome. In the newborn period, Down syndrome patients can

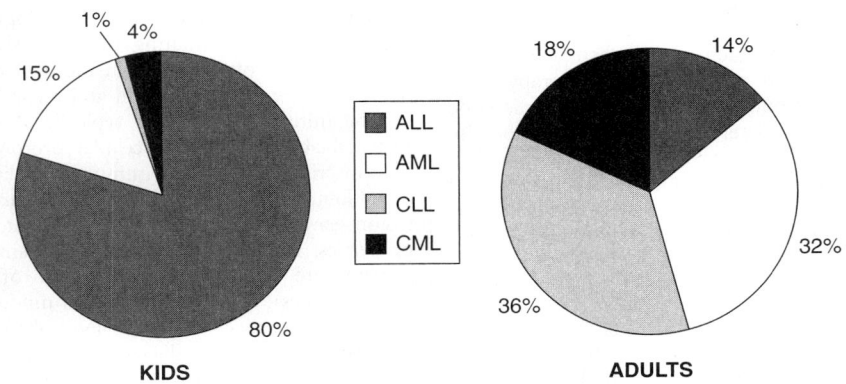

FIGURE 1. Relative incidence of four major leukemia subtypes in children and adults. ALL = acute lymphoblastic leukemia; AML = acute myeloid leukemia; CLL = chronic lymphoblastic leukemia; CML = chronic myeloid leukemia.

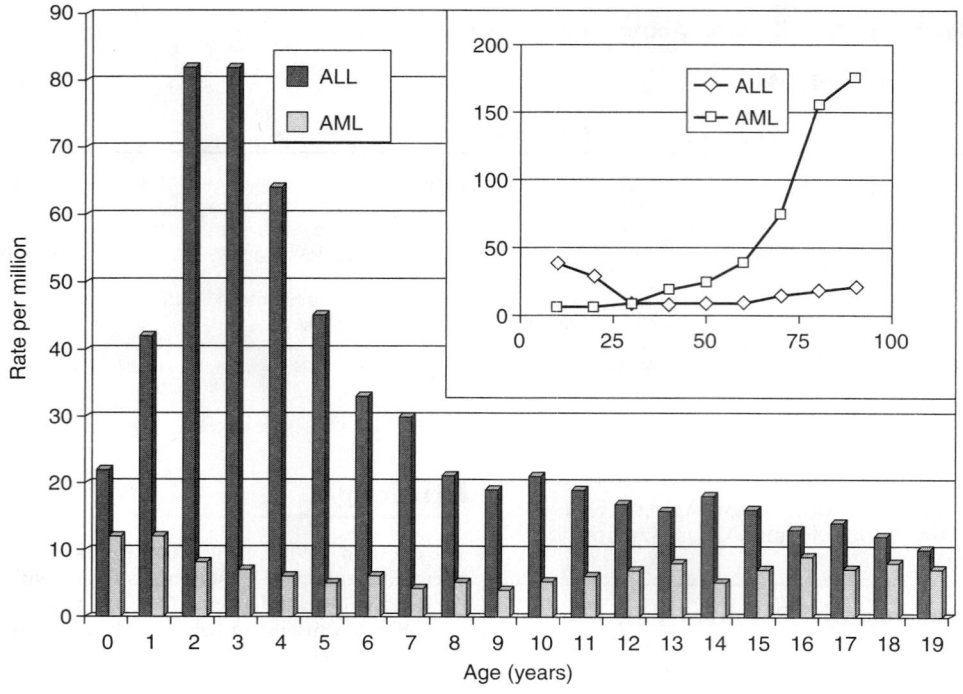

FIGURE 2. Age-specific incidence of acute lymphoblastic leukemia (ALL) and acute myeloid leukemia (ALL) in children and in adults *(inset)*.

TABLE 2 Summary of Known Constitutional and Heritable Childhood Leukemia Predispositions

Disorder	Inheritance	Malignancy Type	Comments
Ataxia-telangiectasia	AR	ALL, NHL	*ATM* gene mutations lead to defective DNA repair
Bloom's syndrome	AR	AML, ALL	Chromosomal instability, sister chromatid exchanges
Down syndrome	Sporadic	AML, ALL	See text
Li-Fraumeni syndrome	AD	AML, ALL, many others	*p53* mutations; leukemias less common than solid tumors
Fanconi's anemia	AR	AML	Chromosomal instability, increased sensitivity to DNA damage
Kostmann's syndrome	AR	AML	G-CSF receptor mutations lead to agranulocytosis
Neurofibromatosis type 1	AD	AML, JMML, MPNST	*NF1* gene mutations lead to enhanced *RAS* signaling

AD = autosomal dominant; ALL = acute lymphoblastic leukemia; AML = acute myeloid leukemia; AR = autosomal recessive; G-CSF = granulocyte colony-stimulating factor; JMML = juvenile myelomonocytic leukemia; MPNST = malignant peripheral nerve sheath tumor; NHL = non-Hodgkin's lymphoma.

present with transient myeloproliferative disease, a disorder distinguishable from congenital AML primarily by its spontaneous resolution within 3 months. Children with Down syndrome tend to present with biologically favorable subtypes of leukemia, but they also suffer increased toxicity from therapy. On balance, the prognosis of leukemia in Down syndrome patients is similar to that in other children.

The only environmental exposures that are known to predispose to leukemia are ionizing radiation (such as was seen with atomic bomb survivors) and prior exposure to certain chemotherapy drugs (cyclophosphamide [Cytoxan], etoposide [Vepesid]). There is good evidence that in utero exposure to maternal diagnostic radiation also increases the risk of childhood cancer (including leukemia), particularly if the exposure is in the first trimester. Other environmental or infectious exposures remain unproved as risk factors for childhood leukemia, including electromagnetic fields from power lines.

CELLULAR PATHOGENESIS

Three major characteristics of leukemia cells distinguish them from normal hematopoietic cells. They proliferate rapidly, they do not differentiate, and they have defects in apoptosis. This results in a growth advantage for leukemia cells, leading to progressive replacement of the normal bone marrow with a massive clonal population of poorly differentiated leukemic blasts. Another characteristic of leukemia cells

is their tendency to spread throughout the body and infiltrate organs other than the bone marrow. This is discussed in more detail in the section on clinical presentation.

MOLECULAR PATHOGENESIS

As is true of most human cancers, development of leukemia is a multihit process. The initiating or permissive mutation (first hit) in childhood ALL often occurs in utero or early infancy, which is the peak of lymphocyte expansion and recombinase activity.

The initiating events are typically chromosomal rearrangements that activate expression of cellular proto-oncogenes by fusing them to transcriptionally active immunoglobulin or T-cell receptor genes or by joining two genes from different chromosomes to create a new fusion gene that encodes a chimeric protein with unique functional properties. The most common of these sentinel chromosomal rearrangements are translocations (exchanges of genetic material between chromosomes), which can serve as a unique marker of the malignant clone. Retrospective studies of blood obtained at birth and preserved on filter paper used for diagnosis of genetic disorders (Guthrie cards) of children who developed leukemia in early childhood have shown that leukemia-associated fusion genes were present at birth in a large percentage of children, including some who did not develop leukemia for one or more years.

TABLE 3 Summary of Common Leukemogenic Genetic Events

Acute Lymphoblastic Leukemia	Acute Myeloid Leukemia
Chimeric Transcription Factors	
t(12;21): *TEL-AML1* fusion	t(8;21): *AML1-ETO* fusion
t(1;19): *E2A-PBX1* fusion	t(15;17): *PML-RAR* α fusion
t(4;11), et al: *MLL* fusions	t(9;11), et al: *MLL* fusions
t(8;14), t(8;22), t(2;8): *Ig-MYC* fusions	inv(16): MYH11-CBFB
T-cell receptor fusions	
Mutationally Activated Oncogenes	
t(9;22): *BCR-ABL* fusion	*FLT3* mutation
PTPN11 mutation	*RAS* mutation
FLT3 mutation	*KIT* mutation
Altered *Rb/p53* Tumor-Suppressor Network	
p16INK4a/p14ARF deletion or silencing	Nucleophosmin mutations
p21CIP1 silencing	*p53* mutations
HDM2 overexpression	HDM2 overexpression

In ALL, the promotional mutation (second hit) likely occurs during the proliferative stress generated by immune responses to exogenous antigens. Because these are maximal in the 2- to 4-year-old age group, this is thought to explain the age peak of childhood ALL during these years. The lack of such a peak in AML suggests that the promotional mutations can occur at any time or are not triggered by immune stimulation. Examples of specific genetic hits known to be associated with the development of childhood leukemia are summarized in Table 3.

Clinical Presentation

Most symptoms and signs of childhood leukemia are the result of the propensity of leukemia cells to replace the bone marrow and infiltrate multiple other organs throughout the body. It is estimated that approximately 10^9 (1 trillion) leukemia cells are present in the child's body at diagnosis.

The replacement of normal bone marrow is responsible for the characteristic abnormal blood counts, which in most cases include the triad of neutropenia, anemia, and thrombocytopenia. Depending on the number of circulating leukemic blasts in the peripheral blood, the total white blood cell count may be low, normal, or high. The neutropenia is often profound (absolute neutrophil count <500/μL), and is associated with an increased risk of serious infection. Blood cultures and broad-spectrum intravenous antibiotic coverage are indicated in any patient with newly diagnosed leukemia and fever. Anemia is often manifested by fatigue, lethargy, headache, pallor, and, in extreme cases, congestive heart failure that may be precipitated by vigorous transfusion or intravenous hydration. Thrombocytopenia often leads to bruising and petechiae; however, clinically significant hemorrhage is uncommon in industrialized countries. Platelet transfusion is indicated for bleeding or for very low platelet counts (<10,000–20,000/μL).

Infiltration of organs other than the bone marrow with leukemia cells is responsible for additional presenting clinical features. Box 2 summarizes the organ systems most often involved in leukemia and the typical clinical manifestations.

Medical Emergencies in Childhood Leukemia

Newly diagnosed leukemia in a child is a medical emergency. There are several potentially life-threatening complications that may be present at diagnosis or can develop within a short time after diagnosis. The need to diagnose and treat potential infection in patients who are febrile and neutropenic was discussed earlier.

BOX 2 Summary of Clinical Manifestations of Childhood Leukemia*

Bone Marrow
Pancytopenia, bone pain

Reticuloendothelial System
Lymphadenopathy
Hepatosplenomegaly

Thymus
Anterior mediastinal mass (T-cell leukemia)

Bones
Bone pain is common
Fractures and chloromas are rare

Gums
Gingival hypertrophy (M4 and M5 AML)

Skin
Leukemia cutis and chloromas (M2, M4, and M5 AML, infant ALL)

Central Nervous System
Meningitis
Cranial nerve palsies
Rarely intracranial epidural or orbital chloromas (M4 and M5 AML, T-cell ALL)

Kidneys
Often infiltrated or enlarged
Rarely acute renal failure (except in tumor lysis syndrome)

Genitourinary
Testicular enlargement (T-cell ALL)

---

*See Box 1 for descriptions of classifications.
ALL = acute lymphoblastic leukemia; AML = acute myeloid leukemia.

Tumor lysis syndrome (TLS) is a complication resulting from the rapid lysis of large numbers of tumor cells, releasing intracellular contents. Although TLS is seen most often after initial treatment with chemotherapy, it can also be present before therapy is initiated due to spontaneous lysis. Risk factors include high white blood cell (WBC) count, lymphadenopathy, hepatosplenomegaly, high mitotic index, and a diagnosis of ALL (especially Burkitt's leukemia or lymphoma and T-cell ALL). TLS is characterized by the triad of hyperuricemia (from breakdown of purines by xanthine oxidase), hyperkalemia, and hyperphosphatemia (with secondary hypocalcemia). Renal insufficiency can develop due to the nephrotoxic effects of precipitated urate crystals in the renal tubules; in severe cases, dialysis may be necessary.

Management consists of aggressive hydration to reduce tubular uric acid concentration and alkalinization of urine to promote solubility of urate crystals. The xanthine oxidase inhibitor allopurinol (Zyloprim) is routinely used during the first 3 to 7 days of leukemia treatment to decrease uric acid production. Rasburicase (Elitek) (recombinant urate oxidase) is a new agent used in severe cases of TLS to almost instantaneously convert uric acid to the more soluble allantoin. Frequent electrolyte monitoring with standard management of abnormal levels is essential.

Hyperleukocytosis becomes a potential clinical problem when the WBC count rises above 100,000/μL. Markedly elevated WBCs lead to increased blood viscosity that can produce sludging of blood in the brain, lungs, kidneys, and other organs, causing clinical features such as depressed level of consciousness, stroke, intracranial hemorrhage, respiratory distress, hypoxia, diffuse pulmonary infiltrates, and renal insufficiency. The risk of hyperviscosity is higher with AML than ALL, because myelolasts are generally larger and stickier than lymphoblasts (likely due to increased expression of integrins and other mediators of cell–cell adherence on the surface of myeloblasts). Management consists of treating the leukemia as soon as possible and performing exchange transfusion or leukopheresis in cases where symptoms are prominent.

Life-threatening bleeding is another potential complication of leukemia. Although all patients with thrombocytopenia are at risk, patients with concomitant coagulopathy due to disseminated intravascular coagulation (DIC) are at particularly high risk. The leukemia subtype most commonly complicated by DIC and serious bleeding is acute promyelocytic leukemia (APL). This association results from the release of thromboplastin from the cytoplasmic granules in promyelocytic blasts. Aggressive blood product support and early treatment with the differentiation-inducing agent all-*trans* retinoic acid (ATRA) has been shown to decrease the risk of bleeding in APL. Despite these measures, up to 10% of patients die of bleeding complications during the initial weeks of therapy, and additional patients suffer lasting morbidity from retinal hemorrhages and nonfatal central nervous system hemorrhages.

Tracheal compression and superior vena cava syndrome can result from large anterior mediastinal masses, which are commonly present in T-cell ALL but are rare in other forms of leukemia. Patients can present with respiratory distress, cough, orthopnea, headaches, syncope, dizziness, facial swelling, or plethora. A chest x-ray should be performed to assess the mediastinum in any patient suspected to have ALL. If the mediastinum is enlarged, a CT is indicated to assess airway patency. This evaluation must precede any attempts at sedation for diagnostic procedures, because even light sedation can precipitate acute airway collapse. Diagnostic material should be obtained by the least invasive method possible before treatment. If necessary, emergent airway compromise can be treated with radiation or steroids, or both.

Differential Diagnosis

Although leukemia should be considered in cases of isolated neutropenia, anemia, or thrombocytopenia, the vast majority of leukemia patients present with depressions in more than one cell line. In suspected cases of immune thrombocytopenic purpura (ITP), for example, a careful review of the peripheral blood smear should be performed to rule out the presence of circulating leukemic blasts. Routine bone marrow aspiration is not necessary for children with ITP, but it should be performed in patients with atypical features, such as concomitant anemia or neutropenia, hepatosplenomegaly, bone pain, or significant weight loss. Treatment of ITP with corticosteroids should only be instituted after evaluation by an experienced hematologist.

Pancytopenia can be caused by diseases other than leukemia. Some viral infections have a propensity to suppress bone marrow function and cause low peripheral blood cell counts, including Epstein-Barr virus (EBV), herpes simplex virus (HSV), influenza, hepatitis viruses, and HIV. Infectious mononucleosis from EBV infection can be particularly difficult to differentiate from leukemia, because patients often have hepatosplenomegaly and circulating atypical lymphocytes (which can appear very similar to leukemic blasts). Pancytopenia on the basis of bone marrow failure (from acquired aplastic anemia or rare inherited bone marrow failure syndromes) can be distinguished from leukemia by bone marrow biopsy for assessment of overall marrow cellularity. Certain solid tumors have a tendency to metastasize to the bone marrow and cause cytopenias, including neuroblastoma, rhabdomyosarcoma, and retinoblastoma, but it is rare for pancytopenia to be the primary presenting feature in these cases.

Joint pain, fever, hepatosplenomegaly, and pallor are common presenting features in both systemic-onset juvenile rheumatoid arthritis (JRA) and leukemia. A bone marrow aspirate should be performed to rule out leukemia before treatment with steroids in suspected cases of systemic-onset JRA.

Risk Stratification

In the last several years, treatment decisions for children with newly diagnosed acute leukemia have been based on the concept of risk stratification. Using factors identified during clinical trials to predict a high or low risk of relapse, patients are separated into risk groups before the start of treatment or at the end of the first month of induction therapy. The treatment plan is then tailored to the degree of risk. The desired result is that patients with relatively low-risk disease can be treated with less toxic therapy without compromising cure rates, and patients with high-risk disease receive more-intensive, potentially toxic therapy. The risk groups are currently defined based on several criteria and differ for ALL and AML. Different centers and cooperative groups typically employ different risk-stratification strategies.

In ALL, the initial risk assessment is based on two simple clinical parameters that are available immediately at the time of diagnosis (the National Cancer Institute [NCI] or Rome criteria): WBC count (>50,000/μL is high risk), and age (<1 year or >9 years is high risk). Further refinement of risk assignment is often based on a combination of leukemia phenotype (B- vs T-lineage), the presence of certain sentinel cytogenetic lesions, and how quickly the patient's leukemia responds to the first few weeks of therapy (rapid clearance of leukemia cells from the blood or marrow is associated with a lower risk of relapse).

Low-risk cytogenetic features include hyperdiploidy (≥50 chromosomes in the leukemia cells) or trisomies of specific chromosomes and the presence of a t(12;21) that results in *TEL/AML1* fusion. High-risk cytogenetic features include hypodiploidy (<44 chromosomes in the leukemia cells) and the presence of either an 11q23 (*MLL* gene) rearrangement or a t(9;22), or Philadelphia chromosome, that creates a *BCR/ABL* fusion gene.

Early response has historically been measured by the response to a prednisone prophase that includes a single dose of intrathecal methotrexate and 7 days of prednisone, or by the percentage of blast cells remaining in the bone marrow after 7 to 14 days of multiagent therapy. Over the past 10 to 15 years, measures of tumor burden remaining in the marrow at the end of induction therapy (minimal residual disease) have been shown to be highly predictive of outcome and have been integrated into risk-stratification schemata of all of the major leukemia cooperative groups.

In AML, risk stratification is based largely on cytogenetics. Low-risk features include a t(8;21), which results in the *AML1/ETO* fusion, and either inv(16) or a t(16;16), both of which create the *CBFβ/MYH11* fusion. High-risk features include monosomy 7 and abnormalities in the long arm of chromosome 5. In addition to these cytogenetic abnormalities, failure to achieve remission with induction chemotherapy is another high-risk feature in AML. All other cytogenetic abnormalities, as well as normal cytogenetics (which are seen in approximately 60% of cases), are considered intermediate risk. More recently, a specific type of genetic mutation in the tyrosine kinase gene *FLT3* has been identified as another high-risk feature. This type of *FLT3* mutation (called an internal tandem duplication [ITD]) occurs in 10% to 15% of childhood AML.

Treatment

There are significant differences in the specific treatments for ALL and AML, so they will be discussed separately. Table 4 summarizes the most salient features of the treatment for each.

ACUTE LYMPHOBLASTIC LEUKEMIA

Treatment for ALL generally occurs in four phases: remission induction, CNS preventive therapy, consolidation, and maintenance. Remission induction in ALL typically lasts 4 to 6 weeks and includes three to five systemic agents. Common to almost all regimens are a corticosteroid (either prednisone [Deltasone] or dexamethasone [Decadron]), vincristine [Vincasar], and L-asparaginase [Elspar],

TABLE 4 Summary of Treatment for Childhood Leukemia

Characteristics	Acute Lymphoblastic Leukemia	Acute Myeloid Leukemia
Remission Induction		
Chemotherapy	4 wk with prednisone or dexamethasone, vincristine, L-asparaginase, doxorubicin (not all cases)	Two courses (6–8 wk) with cytarabine (Ara-C), doxorubicin, others (e.g., etoposide, thioguanine)
Toxic death rate	Low (<3%)	High (>10%)
Remission rate	>98%	75%–85%
CNS Preventive Therapy		
Intrathecal chemotherapy	Methotrexate	Cytarabine
Cranial irradiation	For high risk (blasts in CSF at diagnosis and/or high WBC count)	None
Consolidation		
Chemotherapy	Combinations of various drugs (not cross-resistant) Intensity/duration based on risk stratification	Based on cytogenetic risk group Low risk: 2–3 additional courses Intermediate risk: BMT for patients with HLA-matched related donors High risk: BMT for patients with any suitable donor (including unrelated)
Maintenance		
Chemotherapy	Low-dose oral (6-mercaptopurine and methotrexate) Total duration of therapy 2–3 y	No maintenance therapy (does not improve survival)

BMT = bone marrow transplant; CNS = central nervous system; CSF = cerebrospinal fluid; HLA = human leukocyte antigen; WBC = white blood cell.

which compose the three-drug induction. An anthracycline, typically doxorubicin (Adriamycin), is also included in many regimens (four-drug induction), with other agents such as cyclophosphamide (Cytoxan) or etoposide (VePesid) used in a small minority of centers. More than 98% of children enter remission by the end of 4 weeks of induction therapy, and the mortality rate from toxicity during induction therapy is generally less than 2% to 3% in industrialized countries.

The concept that the CNS could be a sanctuary site for leukemia emerged in the mid 1960s when the introduction of multiagent systemic chemotherapy led to high remission rates, but a majority of patients relapsed within 6 to 12 months, with many of these recurrences being limited to the CNS. Routine introduction of presymptomatic CNS radiation in the late 1960s and early 1970s led to substantial increases in cure rates to approximately 50%. Modern CNS preventive therapy includes periodic administration of intrathecal chemotherapy (usually methotrexate) starting at the time of the first diagnostic lumbar puncture. Systemic agents with improved CNS penetration (dexamethasone rather than prednisone, higher doses of intravenous methotrexate) might also play an important role in CNS control. Cranial irradiation is currently reserved for patients at the highest risk for CNS relapse (e.g., those with high diagnostic WBC count or leukemic blasts in CSF at diagnosis). Over time, CNS radiation has been given to fewer and fewer ALL patients; some groups believe that it can be eliminated for all patients. With these modern strategies, the risk of isolated CNS relapse is less than 5%.

Following the induction of remission, patients receive additional chemotherapy designed to consolidate the remission. The intensity and duration of the consolidation phase are risk based, and alternating cycles of non–cross-resistant chemotherapy drugs are typically used. These consolidation or intensification phases typically last about 6 months and often include a reinduction phase similar to the first month of treatment.

It has been clearly demonstrated that the risk of relapse in ALL can be reduced with an extended phase of continuous low-dose chemotherapy (maintenance) that lasts until 2 to 3 years from the time of diagnosis. Oral 6-mercaptopurine (Purinethol) and methotrexate are used universally, with variable administration of intrathecal chemotherapy. Some centers or groups also employ periodic doses of vincristine and 5- to 7-day pulses of prednisone or dexamethasone. The optimal frequency of intrathecal chemotherapy treatments and vincristine and steroid pulses is uncertain and might depend on the intensity of therapy delivered during the induction and consolidation phases.

ACUTE MYELOID LEUKEMIA

Remission induction in AML typically consists of two courses of very intensive chemotherapy with cytarabine (Tarabine) and doxorubicin, often combined with thioguanine (Tabloid) or etoposide. Remission rates are 75% to 85%, with about one half of the failures due to resistant leukemia and the others to mortality from toxicity (usually infection).

Similar to ALL, CNS preventive therapy in AML begins at diagnosis with intrathecal chemotherapy (usually cytarabine) and continues with additional periodic intrathecal treatments during consolidation. High-dose cytarabine, which is a key component of most AML treatment regimens, also contributes to CNS treatment. Cranial radiation is not typically administered by most groups to children with AML, except for treatment of chloromas (solid masses of leukemia cells) that do not resolve with chemotherapy.

Consolidation in AML is risk dependent. For intermediate-risk patients, most groups have reported the best results using allogeneic bone marrow transplant (BMT) with a histocompatible (i.e., human leukocyte antigen (HLA)-identical or matched) sibling donor. However, only about 25% to 30% of children with AML with have a matched sibling donor. For the remaining intermediate-risk patients, consolidation consists of two to three additional chemotherapy courses that are slightly less intense and usually consist of cytarabine combined with drugs not used in induction such as mitoxantrone (Novantrone) and L-asparaginase. High-risk patients can be identified who have a less than 20% to 25% chance of cure with intensive chemotherapy. Most groups consider these patients to be candidates for BMT. If a matched sibling is unavailable, then alternative donor sources (e.g., matched unrelated bone marrow or umbilical cord blood) are usually offered. For low-risk patients, for whom the cure rate with chemotherapy alone approaches 70%, BMT is usually not offered in first remission, even for patients with a matched sibling donor. In addition, relapses in low-risk patients, unlike relapses in intermediate-risk or high-risk patients, can often be successfully treated with BMT in second remission, justifying reserving BMT for use as a salvage therapy for low-risk patients. Unlike ALL, most groups have found no benefit to extended maintenance therapy in children with AML.

TABLE 5 Summary of Late Effects of Leukemia Treatment

Late Effect	Treatment-Related Risk Factors	Diagnostic Approach
Bone	Avascular necrosis, osteonecrosis	X-ray and/or MRI of major joints for persistent pain
Cardiac dysfunction	Anthracyclines: cardiomyopathy (risk related to cumulative dose, higher risk in AML)	ECG or echocardiogram every 3 y (cardiomyopathy can occur decades after treatment)
Cataracts	CNS RT	Yearly eye exam
CNS and psychosocial	CNS RT, IT chemotherapy: learning problems, neurocognitive dysfunction	Yearly educational assessment, neurocognitive testing
Dental abnormalities	CNS RT	Dental exam at age 5
Endocrine and reproductive	CNS RT: pituitary dysfunction	Yearly growth curves, TSH, LH, FSH
	Alkylators: primary gonadal failure	LH, FSH, estradiol or testosterone, semen analysis
Hepatic dysfunction	Methotrexate, 6-mercaptopurine, 6-thioguanine: late hepatic fibrosis	Yearly LFTs
Secondary neoplasms	CNS RT: brain tumors	MRI for symptoms
	Alkylators or epipodophyllotoxins: secondary AML	Yearly CBC

ALL = acute lymphoblastic leukemia; AML = acute myeloid leukemia; CNS = central nervous system; ECG = electrocardiogram; FSH = follicle stimulating hormone; IT = Intrathecal; LFT = liver function test; LH = luteinizing hormone; MRI = magnetic resonance imaging; RT = radiation therapy; TSH = thyroid-stimulating hormone.

Relapse

The most common site of relapsed leukemia is the bone marrow (with or without concomitant CNS involvement). Less common are isolated extramedullary relapses (CNS or testicular relapse in ALL, chloromas in AML). For both ALL and AML, a critical determinant of outcome following relapse is the time from diagnosis to relapse.

ALL patients who relapse within 18 months of initial diagnosis have a dismal outcome, with only about one half able to attain a second remission and less than 10% overall cure rate; the outcome is marginally better for those who relapse between 18 and 36 months after diagnosis. ALL patients with such early relapses are typically treated with 3 to 4 months of intensive therapy in an attempt to achieve a second remission and attain further cytoreduction, followed by BMT using a matched sibling or unrelated donor. In contrast, children with ALL who relapse more than 3 years after initial diagnosis have an approximately 95% chance of entering a second remission, and 40% to 45% can be cured with intensive chemotherapy; these patients are generally considered to be candidates for matched sibling, but not unrelated donor, BMT in second remission.

Overall, relapsed AML has a dismal outcome (long-term survival approximately 20%), and the approach is to attempt to reinduce remission and then proceed to BMT or investigational treatments. Even in this setting, there is clearly an improved outcome for patients who relapse after a prolonged initial remission (>12 months from the end of remission-induction therapy) compared with patients who have refractory disease or who relapse after a shorter period of remission.

New treatment strategies are urgently needed for patients with relapsed ALL and AML, because the current regimens produce poor results and are associated with a great deal of toxicity. The major clinical trial groups are testing novel and targeted therapies in these patient populations.

Late Effects

Approximately 70% of children with leukemia are cured of their disease. As the numbers of long-term survivors of childhood leukemia has grown, there has been increasing interest in assessing the late effects of leukemic therapy. In childhood ALL, with cure rates of 85%, a major effort is being made in ongoing clinical trials to reduce the intensity of therapy for lower-risk patients, with the hope of reducing late effects of therapy without compromising high cure rates. The most common late effects of leukemia therapy, with the known treatment-related risk factors and recommended diagnostic approach for each, are summarized in Table 5. Many pediatric oncology centers have developed late-effects programs to conduct surveillance for the development of these problems and provide follow-up care to patients who develop late complications of therapy.

REFERENCES

Brown P, Small D. FLT3 inhibitors: A paradigm for the development of targeted therapeutics for paediatric cancer. Eur J Cance 2004;40:707–21.

Gaynon PS, Qu RP, Chappell RJ, et al. Survival after relapse in childhood acute lymphoblastic leukemia: Impact of site and time to first relapse—the Children's Cancer Group Experience. Cancer 1998;82:1387–95.

Gibson BE, Wheatley K, Hann IM, et al. Treatment strategy and long-term results in paediatric patients treated in consecutive UK AML trials. Leukemia 2005;19:2130–8.

Greaves MF, Wiemels J. Origins of chromosome translocations in childhood leukaemia. Nat Rev Cancer 2003;3:639–49.

Hitzler JK, Zipursky A. Origins of leukaemia in children with Down syndrome. Nat Rev Cancer 2005;5:11–20.

Meshinchi S, Alonzo TA, Stirewalt DL, et al. Clinical implications of FLT3 mutations in pediatric AML. Blood 2006;108:3654–61.

Moghrabi A, Levy DE, Asselin B, et al. Results of the Dana—Farber Cancer Institute ALL Consortium Protocol 95–01 for children with acute lymphoblastic leukemia. Blood 2007;109:896–904.

Mrozek K, Heinonen K, Bloomfield CD. Clinical importance of cytogenetics in acute myeloid leukemia. Best Pract Res Clin Haematol 2001;14:19–47.

Pinkel D, Simone J, Hustu HO, Aur RJ. Nine years' experience with "total therapy" of childhood acute lymphocytic leukemia. Pediatrics 1972;50:246–51.

Pui CH, Cheng C, Leung W, et al. Extended follow-up of long-term survivors of childhood acute lymphoblastic leukemia. N Engl J Med 2003;349:640–9.

Pui CH, Evans WE. Treatment of acute lymphoblastic leukemia. N Engl J Med 2006;354:166–78.

Pui CH, Mahmoud HH, Rivera GK, et al. Early intensification of intrathecal chemotherapy virtually eliminates central nervous system relapse in children with acute lymphoblastic leukemia. Blood 1998;92:411–5.

Pui CH, Sandlund JT, Pei D, et al. Improved outcome for children with acute lymphoblastic leukemia: Results of Total Therapy Study XIIIB at St Jude Children's Research Hospital. Blood 2004;104:2690–6.

Ries LAG, Melbert D, Krapcho M, et al. SEER Cancer Statistics Review, 1975–2004. Bethesda, Md: National Cancer Institute; 2007.

Schrappe M, Reiter A, Zimmermann M, et al. Long-term results of four consecutive trials in childhood ALL performed by the ALL-BFM study group from 1981 to 1995. Berlin–Frankfurt–Munster. Leukemia 2000;14:2205–22.

Stahnke K, Boos J, Bender-Gotze C, et al. Duration of first remission predicts remission rates and long-term survival in children with relapsed acute myelogenous leukemia. Leukemia 1998;12:1534–8.

Wakeford R, Little MP. Risk coefficients for childhood cancer after intrauterine irradiation: A review. Int J Radiat Biol 2003;79:293–309.

Woods WG, Kobrinsky N, Buckley JD, et al. Timed-sequential induction therapy improves postremission outcome in acute myeloid leukemia: A report from the Children's Cancer Group. Blood 1996;87:4979–89.

Woods WG, Neudorf S, Gold S, et al. A comparison of allogeneic bone marrow transplantation, autologous bone marrow transplantation, and aggressive chemotherapy in children with acute myeloid leukemia in remission. Blood 2001;97:56–62.

Chronic Leukemias

Method of
Katarzyna Jamieson, MD

Chronic Myelogenous Leukemia

Chronic myelogenous leukemia (CML) is a chronic myeloproliferative disorder defined by the presence of a chimeric gene, *bcr-abl*, encoded by translocation between chromosomes 9 and 22, the Philadelphia chromosome. Discovered in 1960, the Philadelphia chromosome was the first chromosomal abnormality implicated in carcinogenesis. This was followed by decades of unraveling of leukemogenic process, which culminated in a development of the *bcr-abl* inhibitor imatinib mesylate (Gleevec). As a result, in 2001 CML became the first human neoplasm in which the rationally designed therapeutic agent to target a carcinogenic pathway demonstrated great clinical efficacy.

EPIDEMIOLOGY AND RISK FACTORS

CML accounts for 7% to 15% of all cases of leukemia in adults. The median age at diagnosis is 45 to 55 years. The disease is extremely rare in children and the overall incidence increases with age. There is slight male predominance, with a male-to-female ratio of 1.4 to 1.0. There is no association with geographic distribution or race. The etiology of CML is unknown. High-dose radiation exposure is the only well-established environmental risk factor. No genetic predisposition is thought to play any role in pathogenesis of CML.

PATHOGENESIS

bcr-abl is created by a reciprocal translocation of genetic material between the long arm of chromosome 9 (containing the protooncogene *c-abl*) and the long arm of chromosome 22 (containing the *bcr* gene). This is the Philadelphia chromosome, and it is correctly annotated t(9;22)(q34.1;q11.21). The translocation results in constitutive upregulation of tyrosine kinase activity of *abl*, which triggers downstream transduction pathways of a signaling cascade of oncogenic events.

The natural course of CML is one of inevitable progression from an initial chronic phase to a more-aggressive accelerated phase and eventually to a rapidly fatal myeloid or lymphoid blast phase. It is thought that the transformation proceeds as a consequence of the accumulation of additional molecular changes in genetically unstable *bcr-abl*–containing cells. Supportive of this hypothesis, up to 80% of patients with advanced CML have secondary cytogenetic abnormalities.

CLINICAL AND LABORATORY CHARACTERISTICS

CML is a clonal myeloproliferative disorder that develops through accumulation of maturing cells of myeloid, erythroid, and megakaryocytic origin. CML has a biphasic or triphasic clinical course. Patients usually present in the initial chronic phase, exhibiting a cluster of specific clinical and laboratory features (listed in the Current Diagnosis box). More than half of patients with CML diagnosed in the chronic phase are asymptomatic, and the diagnosis is established following the incidental discovery of elevated white blood cell (WBC) count on a routine screening test.

The median time to the development of terminal blast phase is 3 to 6 years. The disease typically progresses through slow evolution into an accelerated phase and then blast phase, but it can transform rapidly directly into the blast phase. The detection of a change in the pace of the disease may be difficult and therefore definitions of accelerated phase vary and are imprecise. The blast phase is defined by the presence of extramedullary disease or at least 30% blasts or blasts and promyelocytes in the bone marrow or peripheral blood. Leukemic cells in blast phase are characterized by arrested maturation, and they proliferate rapidly, similar to acute leukemia cells. The symptoms of blast phase are also those typically seen in acute leukemia.

DIAGNOSIS

The diagnosis of CML can be usually made with reasonable certainty based on the results of peripheral blood cell counts and examination of the peripheral blood smear (see the Current Diagnosis box). The detection of the Philadelphia chromosome or *bcr-abl* by cytogenetic analysis, fluorescent in situ hybridization (FISH) or polymerase chain reaction (PCR) confirms the diagnosis: all patients positive for the Philadelphia chromosome by standard cytogenetic analysis will have a *bcr-abl* fusion gene detectable by FISH or PCR; however, in approximately 5% of patients with *bcr-abl* detectable by FISH or PCR, Philadelphia chromosome could not be appreciated by standard cytogenetics. The bone marrow biopsy is usually not necessary for diagnosis but should be performed for staging purposes in all patients with newly diagnosed CML.

DIFFERENTIAL DIAGNOSIS

At presentation, the differential diagnosis of CML usually involves distinction from leukemoid reaction. Among hematologic malignancies, CML may be difficult to differentiate from other myeloproliferative disorders (essential thrombocytosis, polycythemia vera, and mutagenic myeloid metaplasia), chronic neutrophilic leukemia, chronic myelomonocytic leukemia, juvenile chronic myeloid leukemia, and eosinophilic leukemia. In most cases, the detection of *bcr-abl* is sufficient to make the distinction. However, the differentiation between CML presenting in lymphoid-blast phase and Philadelphia chromosome–positive acute lymphoblastic leukemia might not be possible.

CURRENT DIAGNOSIS

Chronic Myelogenous Leukemia

- Clinical symptoms
  - Constitutional symptoms
  - Splenomegaly (abdominal discomfort, early satiety)
- Laboratory parameters
  - Increased white blood cell count, commonly >100,000/μL, with differential counts showing granulocytes in all stages of differentiation, and two peaks involving neutrophils and myelocytes
  - Absolute basophilia
- Genetic parameters
  - Demonstration of *bcr-abl* by standard cytogenetic analysis, fluorescent in situ hybridization, or polymerase chain reaction

Chronic Lymphocytic Leukemia

- Clinical symptoms
  - B symptoms (fever, night sweats, and weight loss)
  - Lymphadenopathy and organomegaly
  - Recurrent infections
- Laboratory parameters
  - Increased white blood cell count with absolute lymphocytosis
  - Anemia, thrombocytopenia
- Immunophenotypic analysis (flow cytometry)
  - Demonstration of monoclonal population of light chain–restricted mature B lymphocytes expressing CD19, CD20 (dim), and CD23 and coexpressing pan-T cell antigen CD5

Abbreviation: FISH = fluorescence in situ hybridization

PROGNOSIS

Before the effective therapies became available, the expected median survival of patients with CML was 39 to 47 months, with less than 20% surviving longer than 8 years. Allogeneic stem cell transplantation (SCT) and interferon (IFN) alfa-2b (Intron A)[1] and IFN alfa 2a (Roferon) in 1990s produced modest improvement in median survival to 60 to 65 months. The 5-year update of the IRIS trial (International Randomized Study of Interferon and STI-571) published in 2006 suggested that the survival of patients who received imatinib as first-line therapy was 89%, which appeared significantly improved in comparison to historical controls. Patients who are suboptimal responders, who are poor responders, or whose disease is refractory to imatinib have poorer prognosis than patients who met expected response criteria (Table 1). The Sokal prognostic score, originally derived from 800 patients treated in the early 1960s and 1970s, helps to identify patients who are at high risk for failure.

DEFINITIONS OF RESPONSE AND MONITORING OF THERAPEUTIC EFFICACY

The goal of CML therapy is the maximum possible reduction of leukemia burden. The status of the response is routinely evaluated by peripheral blood counts, cytogenetic analysis and FISH, and real-time quantitative PCR (RQ-PCR). The uniform criteria for hematologic, cytogenetic, and molecular responses have been developed to guide therapy and facilitate meaningful analysis of efficacy data across clinical trials (Tables 1 and 2). Selective testing for bcr-abl kinase domain mutations and drug-level testing might have a role in some settings.

[1]Not FDA approved for this indication.

TREATMENT

Chronic Phase

Throughout most of the 20th century CML was considered incurable. The principal options for treating CML included busulfan (Myleran, Busulfex) or hydroxyurea (Hydrea).[1] Such therapy, although successful in alleviating symptoms, did not alter the natural course of the disease. Introduction of allogeneic SCT in 1980s for the first time offered CML patients a prospect of cure. However, the high treatment-related morbidity and mortality associated with this procedure greatly limited its use to patients who were young and fit and for whom an HLA-identical donor could be identified. The alternative was treatment with IFN alfa 2b[1] or IFN alfa 2a, which offered prolongation of survival but generally only to a minority of patients who could tolerate it.

First-Line Therapy

In 2001, imatinib mesylate, a potent selective bcr-abl tyrosine kinase inhibitor, was introduced into clinical practice. The trial that established imatinib as the treatment of choice for newly diagnosed CML in the chronic phase was the International Randomized Study of Interferon Alpha Versus STI571 (IRIS). Between June 2000 and January 2001 IRIS accrued and randomized 1106 patients to imatinib 400 mg daily versus what was then the standard of care, interferon alfa plus subcutaneous cytarabine (Cytosar). After a median of 5 years, 382 of the 553 patients (69%) randomized to imatinib were still receiving it. The estimated progression-free survival was 83% were 83% and overall survival was 89%. The responding patients whose disease did not progress in any way in their first 3 years were unlikely to relapse and unlikely to suffer from late-onset side effects.

[1]Not FDA approved for this indication.

TABLE 1 European LeukemiaNet Definitions of Failure or Suboptimal Response after Treatment with Imatinib 400 mg/day

Time after Diagnosis	Reason for Failure	Suboptimal
3 mo	No hematologic response	Less than complete hematologic response
6 mo	Less than complete hematologic response; no CgR (Ph+ >95%)	Less than PCgR (Ph+ >35%)
12 mo	Less than PCgR (Ph+ >35%)	Less then CCgR
18 mo	Less than CCgR	Less than MMR
Anytime	Less than complete hematologic response; mutation	Additional chromosome abnormalities in Ph+ cells; loss of MMR; mutation

Reprinted with permission from Baccarani M, Saglio G, Goldman J, et al: Evolving concepts in the management of chronic myeloid leukemia: Recommendations from an expert panel on behalf of the European LeukemiaNet. Blood 2006;108:1809-1820.
Abbreviations: CCgR = complete cytogenetic response; MMR = major molecular response; PCgR = partial cytogenetic response; Ph = Philadelphia chromosome.

TABLE 2 European LeukemiaNet Definitions and Monitoring Recommendations

Hematologic Response	Cytogenic Response	Molecular Response*
Definitions		
Complete:	Complete: Ph+ 0%	Complete: transcript nonquantifiable and nondetectable
Platelet count <450 × 10⁹/L	Partial: Ph+ <35%	Major: ≤0.10
WBC count <10 × 10⁹/L	Minor: Ph+ 36-65%	
Differential without immature granulocytes and with <5% basophils	None: Ph+ >95%	
Nonpalpable spleen		
Monitoring		
Check every 2 wk until complete response is achieved and confirmed, then every 3 mo unless otherwise required	Check at least every 6 mo until complete response achieved and confirmed; thereafter at least every 12 mo	Check every 3 mo; conduct mutational analysis in case of failure, suboptimal response, or increase in transcript level

Reprinted with permission from Baccarani M, Saglio G, Goldman J, et al: Evolving concepts in the management of chronic myeloid leukemia: Recommendations from an expert panel on behalf of the European LeukemiaNet. Blood 2006;108:1809-1820.
Abbreviations: Ph = Philadelphia chromosome; WBC = white blood cell.

The recommended dose of imatinib for patients with CML in the chronic phase is 400 mg orally once daily. The drug is well tolerated by the majority of patients; the most common side effects are nausea, vomiting, edema (fluid retention), muscle cramps, skin rash, diarrhea, heartburn, and headache. Hematologic toxicity is quite common, particularly in patients with advanced CML, and the package insert contains exact guidelines for its management. Occasional severe hepatotoxicity has been reported.

Most patients with CML in the chronic phase today achieve and maintain excellent disease control with imatinib and seem to enjoy near-normal survival and quality of life. Unfortunately, continuation of therapy seems necessary to maintain the remission, and it is unclear if imatinib as a single agent is capable of curing CML.

Other Therapeutic Options

Despite the impressive efficacy of imatinib, approximately 30% of patients do not tolerate this drug or develop resistance to it. Therefore, close monitoring, particularly in the first 18 to 36 months, is crucial to the success of therapy. Consensus indicates that patients failing imatinib should be screened for compliance as well as *abl* mutations, and they should be considered for imatinib dose escalation to 800 mg a day, for the second-generation tyrosine kinase inhibitors dasatinib (Sprycel) or nilotinib (Tasigna), or for allogeneic SCT.

Advanced Phase

Imatinib mesylate is the treatment of choice for advanced CML in accelerated phase and blast phase. The recommended dosages are higher: 600 mg daily for CML accelerated phase and 800 mg daily for CML in the blast phase. Patients who satisfy criteria for acceleration are a heterogeneous group, because the disease biologically varies from slightly more advanced than late chronic phase to verging on blast phase. Up to 80% of patients achieve a hematologic remission, and approximately 40% achieve a complete cytogenetic response, which is considered a prerequisite to long-term survival.

Patients presenting in blast phase require a more-aggressive approach and are generally treated either with a combination of imatinib and chemotherapy or with a second-generation tyrosine kinase inhibitor with or without chemotherapy. Patients who achieve responses are immediately evaluated for an allogeneic SCT. The outcome of allogeneic SCT in advanced CML is much worse than in chronic phase, but a minority of patients can definitely be cured.

Allogeneic Stem Cell Transplantation

The curative potential of allogeneic SCT is well established, and transplantation remains the widely accepted regimen for patients who failed imatinib. Historically, in the pre-imatinib era the allogeneic SCT has been reported to produce long-term survival between 50% and 60%—and even as high as 80% for larger more experienced centers—in patients who underwent transplantation in the chronic phase.

Chronic Lymphocytic Leukemia

CLL has historically been considered an indolent disease of older patients. The general approach to treatment was conservative and the few therapies available were only marginally effective; since the 1990s, new treatments have dramatically changed the face of this disease. Intensive research provided great insight into the pathogenesis of CLL and brought about an appreciation for its heterogeneity. The availability of novel treatment strategies that are less toxic and more effective has rekindled hope that treatments with higher curative potential can be developed.

EPIDEMIOLOGY AND RISK FACTORS:

The median age at diagnosis is 70 years. The incidence is higher in men, and the male-to-female ratio is 1.7:1. It is the most common leukemia in the Western world; it is rare is Asian people and remains rare in people of Japanese origin who live in Hawaii, suggesting a genetic rather than environmental predisposition. An increased risk of developing the disease has been described in first-degree relatives of patients with CLL.

PATHOGENESIS

CLL develops by progressive accumulation of genetically altered mature lymphocytes in the blood, bone marrow, and lymphoid tissue. The CLL cell of origin is a B cell arrested in its pathway of differentiation, intermediate between a pre-B cell and mature B cell. One of the most important genetic parameters defining clinical behavior and prognosis is the mutation status of the variable segments of immunoglobulin heavy chain *VH* gene: CLL with unmutated *VH* shows an unfavorable course with rapid progression, whereas CLL with mutated *VH* typically shows slow progression and long survival.

FISH detects genetic aberrations in more than 80% of patients with CLL. The FISH CLL panel typically includes probes for 13q, 11q, 17p, and 6q deletions and for 12q duplication. The most common abnormality is deletion of 13q, which occurs in more than 50% of patients. Persons showing 13q14 abnormalities have a relatively benign disease that usually manifests as stable or slowly progressive isolated lymphocytosis. Trisomy 12 is associated with atypical morphology and progressive disease. Deletions of bands 11q22-q23 are associated with extensive lymph node involvement, aggressive disease, and shorter survival. Deletion of 17p results in loss of function of *p53* and is associated with a particularly poor prognosis.

CLINICAL MANIFESTATIONS

The clinical features of CLL are variable and depend on the stage of the disease. Up to 30% of patients with CLL are asymptomatic, and the diagnosis is established following the incidental discovery of leukocytosis and/or absolute lymphocytosis on routine screening tests. The remaining patients present with lymphadenopathy, splenomegaly, or B symptoms (fever, night sweats, and weight loss), alone or in combination. Anemia and thrombocytopenia are considered late signs of the disease but can be present at the time of diagnosis. Due to their immunocompromised state, patients can present with recurrent or persistent infections.

DIAGNOSIS

The diagnosis of CLL requires demonstration of absolute lymphocytosis of greater than 5000/mL and an immunophenotypic evidence of monoclonal population of mature B cells expressing CD19, CD20 (dim), and CD23 and coexpressing pan–T-cell antigen CD5. The malignant cells express low density of monoclonal surface immunoglobulin (IgM or IgD) with either κ or λ light chain. Patients are evaluated and grouped prognostically based on physical examination and complete blood count. The bone marrow biopsy and CT scans are not required for diagnosis but may be indicated based on symptoms.

DIFFERENTIAL DIAGNOSIS

The immunophenotypic profile of CLL is quite characteristic, but at times it has to be differentiated from other low-grade lymphoproliferative disorders: hairy cell leukemia, prolymphocytic leukemia, (splenic) marginal zone lymphoma, and lymphoplasmacytic lymphoma. Most importantly, CLL needs to be differentiated from mantle cell lymphoma, which also coexpresses CD5 but is characteristically CD23 negative and cycline D1 positive by immunohistochemical staining.

PROGNOSIS

The natural history of CLL is extremely variable, with survival times ranging from 2 to 20 (or more) years. Clinical staging using the Rai or Binet system provides a good estimate of prognosis but is not very reliable in an individual patient; for example, among patients presenting with early clinical stage disease, up to 30% never progress and eventually die of causes unrelated to CLL, and another 30% progress much more rapidly than expected. A number of additional prognostic factors are considered in estimating prognosis in an individual case: clinical characteristics such as age, sex, and performance status; laboratory parameters reflecting the tumor burden or disease activity such as lymphocyte count, lactate dehydrogenase (LDH), bone marrow infiltration pattern, or lymphocyte doubling time; serum markers such as soluble CD23 and β_2-microglobulin; and genetic markers such as genetic aberrations (see earlier), the *VH* mutation status, or its surrogate markers (CD38, ZAP-70).

TREATMENT

CLL is considered incurable, and no treatment strategy to date—short of allogeneic stem cell transplantation—has been demonstrated to prolong survival. Asymptomatic patients are followed expectantly. The treatment is initiated upon progression of the disease or appearance of symptoms such as rapid lymphocyte doubling time, bulky lymphadenopathy or organomegaly, disease-related B symptoms, and autoimmune or nonautoimmune cytopenias. CLL is quite sensitive to many chemo- and immunotherapeutic agents. However, remissions are rarely durable. The disease follows a remitting and relapsing pattern, and most patients receive at least a few different regimens throughout the course of their disease.

First-Line Therapy

The first-line treatment usually consists of purine analogue fludarabine (Fludara)-based chemotherapy in combination with the anti-CD20 monoclonal antibody rituximab (Rituxan). FR (fludarabine and rituximab) and FCR (fludarabine, cyclophosphamide [Cytoxan], and rituximab) are the chemoimmunotherapy combinations used most commonly. The overall response rates for these regimens are respectively 90% and 95%. FCR offers a higher complete remission rate of 70% vs 47% for FR; however, FR offers a more acceptable toxicity profile. Median overall survival with each of these regimens seems comparable: approximately 5 years. A choice between the regimens is made based upon the patient's characteristics and the goals of therapy. The treatment cycles are administered every 28 days for up to 6 cycles.

Other treatment options used in the newly diagnosed progressive disease setting include PCR (deoxycoformycin (Pentostatin [Nipent]),[1] cyclophosphamide, and rituximab); bendamustine (Treanda); the anti-CD25 antibody alemtuzumab (Campath); or chlorambucil (Leukeran).

Deoxycoformycin is another purine analogue, and the PCR regimen offers an alternative to FCR. The fludarabine-based regimens are only marginally effective in high-risk disease defined by the presence of del (17p) or del(11q). Patients carrying these abnormalities either do not respond to initial treatment or relapse soon after achieving remission. Therefore, other therapies, including investigational therapies, are often offered in this setting. Alemtuzumab is the only FDA-approved agent that has demonstrated activity in cells lacking *p53* function, as seen in patients with deletion of chromosome 17p.

Bendamustine is a new alkylating agent approved for treatment of CLL in March 2008. Based on the results of a randomized trial, like fludarabine, it offers a higher response rate and progression-free survival in comparison to single agent chlorambucil. However a survival benefit compared to chlorambucil has yet to be confirmed. Chlorambucil, which was the mainstay of treatment until it fell out of favor to fludarabine, remains a viable treatment option, particularly in older patients who are not good candidates for more-aggressive combination chemoimmunotherapy regimens. Alternatively, these patients can be treated with lower-dose fludarabine.

Other Therapeutic Options

Relapsed disease occurs in a patient who achieved at least a partial remission that lasted more than 6 months after completion of treatment. Many of those patients can be re-treated successfully with the same medications or can be switched to an alternative strategy. Specifically, it has been demonstrated that patients initially treated with fludarabine often achieve another durable response upon re-treatment. Whether patients treated with fludarabine-containing combination regimens or other newer therapies such as alemtuzumab or bendamustine will respond to re-treatment equally well is not yet known.

Patients who fail to achieve at least a partial remission or whose disease progresses within 6 months from completion of treatment have refractory disease, which is associated with a poor prognosis. Patients refractory to fludarabine have expected median survival of 48 weeks and only an 11% likelihood of responding to other therapies. The ideal approach to treating refractory CLL is unknown. Patients are encouraged to participate in clinical trials. Those who are potential transplant candidates are considered for an allogeneic stem cell transplant.

Allogeneic stem cell transplantation remains the only potentially curative treatment modality. Unfortunately, data on the use of allogeneic stem cell transplantation is limited to small case series. Allogeneic stem cell transplantation is associated with considerable treatment-related morbidity and mortality and is usually not considered until definitive evidence of poor prognosis.

COMPLICATIONS

Major complications of CLL include cytopenias and immune dysfunction. Anemia and thrombocytopenia can result from direct infiltration of the bone marrow and hypersplenism, in which case response to treatment usually results in improvement. Splenectomy obtained either surgically or via splenic irradiation is clinically useful in patients with splenomegaly and profound cytopenias unresponsive to chemotherapy. Autoimmune hemolytic anemia and thrombocytopenia seen in a significant percentage of patients often respond to steroids. Danazol,[1] high-dose intravenous immunoglobulin (IVIg) (Gammagard),[1] cyclosporine (Neoral),[1] and rituximab[1] have all also been used in this setting.

Infections are the major cause of mortality in CLL. They result from hypogammaglobulinemia, impaired T-cell function, and neutropenia. Patients with repeat major bacterial infections are candidates for treatment with high-dose IVIg.[1] Patients treated with purine analogues and alemtuzumab are at high risk for opportunistic infections by herpes simplex virus and herpes zoster virus, *Listeria monocytogenes*, *Pneumocystis jiroveci*, and cytomegalovirus and should be offered prophylaxis with acyclovir (Zovirax),[1] trimethoprim-sulfamethoxazole

---

[1]Not FDA approved for this indication.

[1]Not FDA approved for this indication.

(Bactrim), or aerosolized pentamidine (NebuPent) and antifungal agents. Patients receiving alemtuzumab should be monitored for cytomegalovirus reactivation or disease.

Patients with CLL have been reported to have a higher risk of developing other hematologic and solid malignancies. It is unknown how much of this increased risk is due to the underlying disease and accompanying chronic immunosuppression and how much is due to the treatments given. In 5% to 10% of patients with CLL, the disease transforms into an aggressive large-cell lymphoma (Richter's transformation) or prolymphocytic leukemia.

REFERENCES

Baccarani M, Saglio G, Goldman J, et al. Evolving concepts in the management of chronic myeloid leukemia: Recommendations from an expert panel on behalf of the European LeukemiaNet. Blood 2006;108:1809–20.

Byrd JC, Rai K, Peterson BL, et al. Addition of rituximab to fludarabine may prolong progression-free survival and overall survival in patients with previously untreated chronic lymphocytic leukemia: an updated retrospective comparative analysis of CALGB 9712 and CALGB 9011. Blood 2005;105:49–53.

Deininger MW, O'Brien SG, Ford JM, Druker BJ. Practical management of patients with chronic myeloid leukemia receiving imatinib. J Clin Oncol 2003;21:1637–47.

Druker BJ, Guilhot F, O'Brien SG, et al. Five-year follow-up of patients receiving imatinib for chronic myeloid leukemia. N Engl J Med 2006;355:2408–17.

Goldman JM. Initial treatment for patients with CML. Hematology Am Soc Hematol Educ Program 2009;453–60.

Hallek M. State-of-the-art treatment of chronic lymphocytic leukemia. Hematology Am Soc Hematol Educ Program 2009;440–9.

Keating MJ, Chiorazzi N, Messmer B, et al. Biology and treatment of chronic lymphocytic leukemia. Hematology Am Soc Hematol Educ Program 2003;153–75.

Lee SJ. Chronic myelogenous leukaemia. Br J Haematol 2000;111:993–1009.

Lozanski G, Heerema NA, Flinn IW, et al. Alemtuzumab is an effective therapy for chronic lymphocytic leukemia with p53 mutations and deletions. Blood 2004;103:3278–81.

Sokal risk score calculator. Available at: http://www.roc.se/sokal.asp; [accessed 10.07.10].

Tam CS, O'Brien S, Wierda W, et al. Long-term results of the fludarabine, cyclophosphamide, and rituximab regimen as initial therapy of chronic lymphocytic leukemia. Blood 2008;112:975–80.

Non-Hodgkin's Lymphoma

Method of
Andrew M. Evens, DO, MSc

The term malignant lymphoma was originally introduced by Billroth in 1871 to describe neoplasms of lymphoid tissue. Generally speaking, lymphomas are neoplasms of the immune system. Traditionally lymphomas are divided into Hodgkin's lymphoma (HL) and non-Hodgkin's lymphoma (NHL).

There are many different clinicopathologic subtypes of NHL (>50). By cell of origin, the majority of NHLs are of B-cell origin (85%-90%); T-cell lymphoma account for 10% to 15% of lymphomas, and natural killer cell or histiocytic lymphomas are rare (<1).

NHLs most often manifest clinically with involvement of lymph nodes, spleen, and bone marrow, but they can involve other extranodal sites (e.g., stomach, skin, liver, bone, brain). Peripheral blood involvement rarely occurs (leukemic phase of lymphoma). The natural history and prognosis vary greatly among the different subtypes of NHL from indolent and slow-growing types (over many years) to very aggressive and rapidly fatal (within weeks) types.

Epidemiology

Currently, NHL represents approximately 4.6% of all cancer diagnoses (4.8% in men and 4.4% in women), being the fifth most common cancer in women and the sixth in men. Estimates from the American Cancer Society indicate that in 2009 approximately 66,000 new cases of NHL were diagnosed in the United States and approximately 19,500 people died of the disease.

GEOGRAPHIC DISTRIBUTION

The incidence of NHL varies throughout the world, in general being more common in developed countries, with rates in the United States of more than 15 per 100,000 in the United States compared with 1.2 per 100,000 in China. In the United States, the incidence rates of NHL more than doubled between 1975 and 1995 (Fig. 1), representing one of the largest increases of any cancer. The increases have been more pronounced in whites, males, the elderly, and those with NHL diagnosed at extranodal sites. Similar findings have been reported in other developed countries. The overall incidence rates of NHL began to stabilize in the late 1990s, although the temporal trends varied by histologic subtype. Some of the increase may be related to improved diagnostic techniques and access to medical care and the development of NHL with HIV infection. However, additional factors must be responsible for this unexpected increase in incidence.

AGE

Overall, NHL incidence rises exponentially with increasing age. In persons older than 65 years, the incidence is 88.2 per 100,000 population compared with 7.1 per 100,000 population for persons aged 20 to 49 years (Fig. 2). Except for high-grade lymphoblastic and Burkitt's lymphomas (the most common types of NHL seen in children and young adults), the median age at presentation for all subtypes of NHL exceeds 50 years.

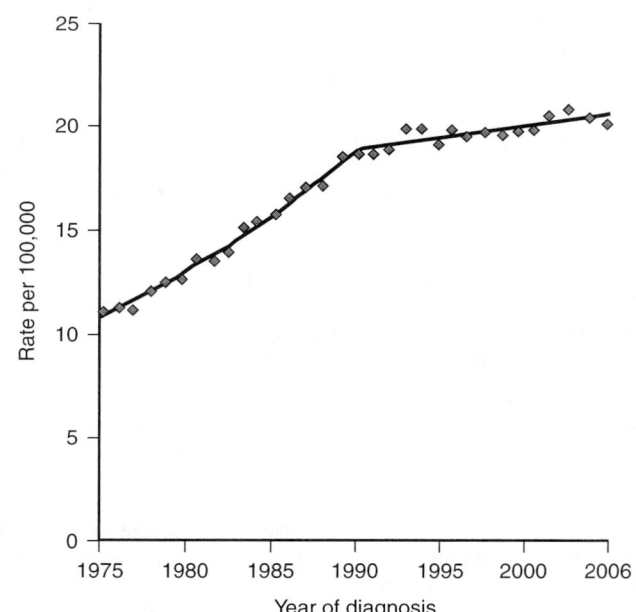

FIGURE 1. Surveillance Epidemiology and End Results (SEER) incidence rates for non-Hodgkin's lymphoma since 1975. Incidence rates are from nine areas (San Francisco, Connecticut, Detroit, Hawaii, Iowa, New Mexico, Seattle, Utah, and Atlanta) for 1975-2006. Rates are per 100,000 population and are age adjusted to the 2000 U.S. standard population age groups (19 age groups, Census P25-1130). Regression lines are calculated using the Joinpoint Regression Program Version 3.3.2 (June 2008, National Cancer Institute). Data available at http://seer.cancer.gov/csr/1975_2007/browse_csr.php?section=19&page=sect_19_table.05.html (accessed July 10, 2010).

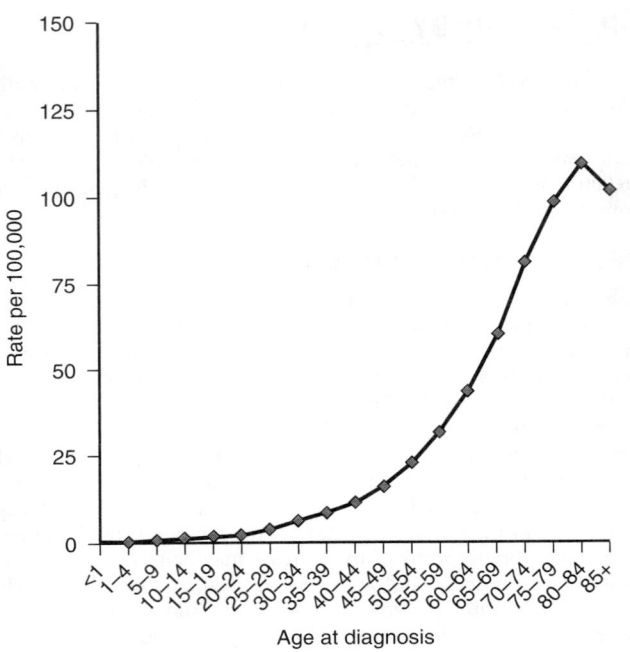

FIGURE 2. Surveillance Epidemiology and End Results (SEER) age-specific incidence rates for non-Hodgkin's lymphoma. Incidence rates are from 17 areas (San Francisco, Connecticut, Detroit, Hawaii, Iowa, New Mexico, Seattle, Utah, Atlanta, San Jose-Monterey, Los Angeles, Alaska Native Registry, Rural Georgia, California excluding SF/SJM/LA, Kentucky, Louisiana and New Jersey) for 2002-2006. Rates are per 100,000 population. Data available at http://seer.cancer.gov/csr/1975_2007/browse_csr.php?section=19&page=sect_19_table.07.html (accessed July 10, 2010).

RACE AND ETHNICITY

Incidence varies by race and ethnicity, with whites at higher risk than African Americans and Asian Americans (incidence rates increased 40% to 70% in whites compared with blacks). Most histologies, particularly low-grade lymphomas, are more common in whites than in blacks. Only peripheral T-cell lymphoma, mycosis fungoides, and Sézary syndrome are more common in blacks than in whites.

Etiology and Risk Factors

CHROMOSOMAL TRANSLOCATIONS AND MOLECULAR REARRANGEMENTS

Nonrandom chromosomal and molecular rearrangements play an important role in the pathogenesis of many lymphomas and correlate with histology and immunophenotype. These chromosomal changes often result in oncogenic gene products; for example, t(11;14)(q13;q32) translocation results in overexpression of *bcl-1* (cyclin D1 in mantle-cell lymphoma, while translocations involving 8q24 lead to c-*myc* deregulation in Burkitt's lymphoma. Research to discover more information regarding the prognostic and pathogenic importance of these oncogenes continues, although they are currently used in clinical practice now primarily for diagnostic purposes. In addition, these genes serve as potential targets for novel therapeutics.

ENVIRONMENTAL FACTORS

Environmental factors also may play a role in the development of NHL, such as particular occupations (e.g., chemists, painters, mechanics, machinists) and chemicals (solvents and pesticides). Patients who receive chemotherapy or radiation therapy for any indication are also at increased risk for developing NHL as a secondary cancer as discussed later.

VIRUSES

Several viruses have been implicated in the pathogenesis of NHL, including Epstein-Barr virus, human T-cell lymphotropic virus 1 (HTLV-1), Kaposi's sarcoma–associated herpesvirus (KSHV, also known as human herpesvirus 8 [HHV-8]), and hepatitis C virus. Meta-analyses have shown 13% to 15% seroprevalence of hepatitis C virus in certain geographic regions among persons with B-cell NHL. HTLV-1 is a human retrovirus that establishes a latent infection through reverse transcription in activated T-helper cells. A minority (5%) of carriers develop adult T-cell leukemia lymphoma. KSHV-like DNA sequences are often detected in primary effusion lymphomas in patients with HIV infection and in those with multicentric (plasma cell variant) Castleman's disease. Hepatitis C virus infection is associated with the development of clonal B-cell expansions and certain subtypes of NHL, particularly in the setting of essential (type II) mixed cryoglobulinemia.

BACTERIAL INFECTIONS

Gastric mucosa-associated lymphoid tissue (MALT) lymphoma is seen most often, but not exclusively, in association with *Helicobacter pylori* infection. Infection with *Borrelia burgdorferi* has been detected in about 35% of patients with primary cutaneous B-cell lymphoma in Scotland. Studies indicate that *Campylobacter jejuni* and immunoproliferative small intestinal disease are related. A report noted an association between infection with *Chlamydia psittaci* and ocular adnexal lymphoma. The infection was found to be highly specific and does not reflect a subclinical infection widespread among the general population. Remissions to antibiotics have been reported. Attempts to confirm this association in the Western hemisphere have been unsuccessful.

IMMUNODEFICIENCY

Patients with some congenital conditions of immunosuppression are at increased risk. These conditions include ataxia-telangiectasia, Wiskott-Aldrich syndrome, X-linked lymphoproliferative syndrome, and severe combined immunodeficiency. Acquired immunodeficiency states, such as HIV infection, and iatrogenic immunosuppression. Relative risk of NHL is increased 150- to 250-fold among patients with AIDS, usually high grade and extranodal disease. The incidence of posttransplantation lymphoproliferative disorders after solid organ transplantation is 1% to 2% in kidney transplant recipients and 10% to 12% in heart transplant recipients, the latter whom require more potent immunosuppressive therapy.

AUTOIMMUNITY

An increased incidence of gastrointestinal lymphomas is seen in patients with celiac (nontropical) sprue and inflammatory bowel disease, particularly Crohn's disease. An aberrant clonal intraepithelial T-cell population can be found in up to 75% of patients with refractory celiac sprue before overt T-cell lymphoma develops. Sjögren's disease is associated with a 6-fold increased risk of NHL overall with risk varying in part on severity of disease (5 to 200 times). Moreover, the risk specifically of parotid marginal zone lymphoma is increased 1000-fold. Additionally, systemic lupus erythematosus and rheumatoid arthritis have been associated with slightly increased risk of B-cell lymphoma.

GENETIC SUSCEPTIBILITY

Several reports have implicated a role for genetic variants in the risk of NHL, including genes that influence DNA integrity and methylation, genes that alter B-cell survival and growth, and genes that involve innate immunity, oxidative stress, and xenobiotic metabolism.

Signs and Symptoms

Fever, weight loss, and night sweats, referred to as B symptoms are more common in advanced and aggressive subtype NHLs, but they may be present at all stages and in all histologic subtypes.

LOW-GRADE OR INDOLENT LYMPHOMAS

Painless, slowly progressive peripheral adenopathy is the most common clinical presentation in patients with low-grade lymphomas. Patients sometimes report a history of waxing and waning adenopathy before seeking medical attention. Spontaneous regression of enlarged lymph nodes can occur and can cause a low-grade lymphoma to be confused with an infectious condition. Primary extranodal involvement and B symptoms are uncommon at presentation; however, both are more common in advanced or end-stage disease and in particular indolent NHL subtypes (e.g., gastric MALT and nongastric extranodal MALT). Bone marrow is frequently involved, sometimes in association with cytopenias. Splenomegaly is seen in about 40% of patients, but the spleen is rarely the only involved site at presentation besides the specific subtype of splenic marginal zone lymphoma.

HIGH-GRADE OR AGGRESSIVE LYMPHOMAS

The clinical presentation of high-grade lymphomas is more varied. Although the majority of patients present with adenopathy, more than one third present with extranodal involvement alone or with adenopathy, the most common sites being the gastrointestinal tract (including Waldeyer's ring), skin, bone marrow, sinuses, genitourinary tract, thyroid, and central nervous system. B symptoms are more common, occurring in about 30% to 40% of patients. Lymphoblastic lymphoma often manifests with an anterior superior mediastinal mass, superior vena cava syndrome, and leptomeningeal disease. American patients with Burkitt's lymphoma often present with a large abdominal mass and symptoms of bowel obstruction. In addition, certain histologic NHL subtypes manifest with symptoms unique to that particular lymphoma; for example, angioimmunoblastic T-cell lymphoma (AITL) in addition to lymphadenopathy manifests with disease features such as organomegaly, skin rash, pleural effusions, arthritis, eosinophilia, and varied immunologic abnormalities including positive Coombs' test, cold agglutins, hemolytic anemia, antinuclear antibodies, and polyclonal hypergammaglobulinemia.

Screening

No effective methods are currently available for screening patients or populations for NHL.

Diagnosis

A definitive diagnosis can be made only by biopsy of pathologic lymph nodes or tumor tissue. It is critical to perform an *excisional* lymph node resection to avoid false-negative results and inaccurate histologic classification; fine-needle aspirations or core biopsies are typically insufficient for diagnostic purposes. When clinical circumstances make surgical biopsy of involved lymph nodes or extranodal sites prohibitive, a core biopsy obtained under CT or ultrasonographic guidance might suffice, but it often requires the integration of histologic examination and immunophenotypic and molecular studies for diagnosis. A formal review by an expert hematopathologist is mandatory. In addition to morphologic review and immunostaining of tissue, other studies such as detailed cellular immunophenotyping and genotyping for relevant oncogenes are often needed to complete the diagnosis.

In addition to a detailed history and physical examination, baseline staging studies are warranted. These consist of blood tests (complete blood count with differential, complete metabolic panel including liver function tests, and lactate dehydrogenase), CT of chest, abdomen, and pelvis, and bilateral bone marrow biopsy and aspirate (Box 1). For aggressive NHL histologies, functional imaging is advocated (i.e., FDG-PET [fluorodeoxyglucose (^{18}F) positron emission tomography]), as is assessment of ejection fraction in anticipation of anthracycline-based chemotherapy. Testing for history of hepatitis B virus is recommended, especially before starting anti-CD20 antibody therapy; evidence suggests that anti-CD20 antibody therapy (e.g., rituximab) increases the risk of HBV reactivation above the

CURRENT DIAGNOSIS

- The etiology of non-Hodgkin's lymphoma (NHL) is not known, although several risk factors and conditions are associated with an increased risk of developing lymphoma, including congenital immunosuppression conditions (ataxia-telangiectasia, Wiskott-Aldrich syndrome, and X-linked lymphoproliferative syndrome), acquired immunodeficiency states (e.g., HIV and following any solid organ transplantation), viruses (e.g., human T-lymphotrophic virus (HTLV)-1 and hepatitis C virus), and autoimmune disorders (e.g., Sjögren's syndrome, celiac sprue, and systemic lupus erythematosus).

- Patients most commonly present clinically with enlarged lymph nodes, splenomegaly, and bone marrow involvement, but they may also present with other extranodal sites (e.g., stomach, skin, liver, bone, brain).

- NHL has many different clinicopathologic subtypes—more than 50 types are included in the WHO classification of lymphoid neoplasms. The natural history and prognosis of these vary greatly from indolent and slow-growing types (over many years) to aggressive and potentially fatal (within weeks) types.

- Excisional lymph node resection is the gold standard procedure in establishing the exact NHL histology. Expert hematopathology review incorporating morphologic, immunophenotypic, and genetic features is essential for an accurate diagnosis.

BOX 1   Initial Assessment and Work-up for Non-Hodgkin's Lymphoma

Excisional tissue resection
Detailed history and physical examination
CBC with differential, metabolic panel (including liver function), and LDH
CT scans (chest, abdomen, pelvis)
Nuclear functional imaging (i.e., FDG-PET)*
Bone marrow biopsy and aspirate
Heart function (e.g., MUGA)
EGD, colonoscopy, or both†
HIV and HBV testing (when applicable or with risk factors)
Consider TB testing (i.e., PPD with anergy panel) with history of exposure
Assessment of CSF (when applicable or with risk factors)‡
Consider early institution of TLS prophylaxis (e.g., intravenous fluids, allopurinol [Zyloprim])*

---

*For aggressive NHL subtypes.
†With clinical suspicion of involvement and EGD for NHL head and neck involvement (e.g., tonsil, base of tongue, nasopharynx), and consider colonoscopy for MCL (if symptomatic).
‡For aggressive histologies with >1 extranodal site and elevated LDH and for particular unique lymphoma locations (e.g., testicular, sinus, breast, paraspinal).
Abbreviations: CBC = complete blood count; CSF = cerebrospinal fluid; CT = computed tomography; EGD = esophagogastroduodenoscopy; FDG-PET = fluorodeoxyglucose (^{18}F) positron emission tomography; HBV = hepatitis B virus; LDH = lactate dehydrogenase; MCL = mantle-cell lymphoma; MUGA = multigated acquisition [scan]; NHL = non-Hodgkin's lymphoma; PPD = purified protein derivative [tuberculosis test]; TB = tuberculosis; TLS = tumor lysis syndrome.

known rate of chemotherapy-associated reactivation. HIV serology should be obtained in patients with relevant risk factors, especially for diffuse large B cell lymphoma (DLBCL) and Burkitt's lymphoma. HTLV-1 serology is recommended in patients who present with cutaneous T-cell lymphoma lesions, especially if they have hypercalcemia.

Examination of the cerebrospinal fluid and consideration of intrathecal chemotherapy prophylaxis is applicable for patients with DLBCL with bone marrow, epidural, testicular, paranasal sinus, breast, or multiple extranodal sites (especially when in conjunction with elevated lactate dehydrogenase); testing is mandatory for high-grade lymphoblastic lymphoma and Burkitt's lymphoma and its variants and primary central nervous system lymphoma if there is no evidence of increased intracranial pressure. Upper gastrointestinal endoscopy or gastrointestinal series with small bowel follow-through is recommended in patients with head and neck involvement (tonsil, base of tongue, nasopharynx) and those with a gastrointestinal primary. Mantle cell lymphoma is associated with a high incidence of occult gastrointestinal involvement. MRI of the complete craniospinal axis is advocated with any brain or leptomeningeal disease in part to rule out multifocal disease.

Classification

The 1965 Rappaport's Classification of malignant lymphomas was based solely on architecture and cytology. Since then, with the help of advanced cellular and genetic technologies, numerous new unique NHL entities have emerged. The latest classification is that of the World Health Organization (WHO) of 2008, which emphasizes immunophenotyping, genotyping, and clinical features (Box 2). Another way to group the many different lymphoma histologies is by clinical presentation and prognosis (Table 1).

BOX 2 WHO Classification of the Mature B-Cell, T-Cell, and Natural Killer–Cell neoplasms (2008)

Mature B-Cell Neoplasms
Chronic lymphocytic leukemia, small lymphocytic lymphoma
B-cell prolymphocytic leukemia
Splenic marginal zone lymphoma
Hairy cell leukemia
Splenic lymphoma/leukemia, unclassifiable*
• Splenic diffuse red pulp small B-cell lymphoma*
• Hairy cell leukemia-variant*
Lymphoplasmacytic lymphoma
Waldenström macroglobulinemia
Heavy chain diseases
• Alpha heavy chain disease
• Gamma heavy chain disease
• Mu heavy chain disease
Plasma cell myeloma
Solitary plasmacytoma of bone
Extraosseous plasmacytoma
Extranodal marginal zone lymphoma of mucosa-associated lymphoid tissue (MALT lymphoma)
Nodal marginal zone lymphoma
Pediatric nodal marginal zone lymphoma*
Follicular lymphoma
Pediatric follicular lymphoma*
Primary cutaneous follicle center lymphoma
Mantle cell lymphoma
Diffuse large B-cell lymphoma (DLBCL), NOS
• T-cell histiocyte rich large B-cell lymphoma
• Primary DLBCL of the central nervous system
• Primary cutaneous DLBCL, leg type
• EBV+ DLBCL of the elderly*
• DLBCL associated with chronic inflammation
Lymphomatoid granulomatosis
Primary mediastinal (thymic) large B-cell lymphoma
Intravascular large B-cell lymphoma
ALK+ large B-cell lymphoma
Plasmablastic lymphoma
Large B-cell lymphoma arising in HHV-8–associated multicentric Castleman disease
Primary effusion lymphoma
Burkitt's lymphoma
B-cell lymphoma, unclassifiable, with features intermediate between diffuse large B-cell lymphoma and Burkitt's lymphoma
B-cell lymphoma, unclassifiable, with features intermediate between diffuse large B-cell lymphoma and classic Hodgkin's lymphoma

Mature T-Cell and Natural Killer–Cell Neoplasms
T-cell prolymphocytic leukemia
T-cell large granular lymphocytic leukemia
Chronic lymphoproliferative disorder of NK cells*
Aggressive NK cell leukemia
Systemic EBV+ T-cell lymphoproliferative disease of childhood
Hydroa vacciniforme-like lymphoma
Adult T-cell leukemia/lymphoma
Extranodal NK/T-cell lymphoma, nasal type
Enteropathy-associated T-cell lymphoma
Hepatosplenic T-cell lymphoma
Subcutaneous panniculitis-like T-cell lymphoma
Mycosis fungoides
Sézary syndrome
Primary cutaneous CD30+ T-cell lymphoproliferative disorders
• Lymphomatoid papulosis
• Primary cutaneous anaplastic large cell lymphoma
• Primary cutaneous gamma-delta T-cell lymphoma
• Primary cutaneous CD8+ aggressive epidermotropic cytotoxic T-cell lymphoma*
• Primary cutaneous CD4+ small/medium T-cell lymphoma*
Peripheral T-cell lymphoma, NOS
Angioimmunoblastic T-cell lymphoma
Anaplastic large cell lymphoma, ALK+
Anaplastic large cell lymphoma, ALK−

Hodgkin's Lymphoma
Nodular lymphocyte-predominant Hodgkin lymphoma
Classic Hodgkin lymphoma
• Nodular sclerosis classic Hodgkin lymphoma
• Lymphocyte-rich classic Hodgkin lymphoma
• Mixed cellularity classic Hodgkin lymphoma
• Lymphocyte-depleted classic Hodgkin lymphoma

Posttransplantation Lymphoproliferative Disorders
Early lesions
Plasmacytic hyperplasia
Infectious mononucleosis-like
Polymorphic
Monomorphic (B- and T/NK-cell types)†
Classic Hodgkin's lymphoma type†

---

*Provisional entities for which the WHO Working Group felt there was insufficient evidence to recognize as distinct diseases at this time.
†These lesions are classified according to the leukemia or lymphoma to which they correspond.
Abbreviations: EBV = Epstein-Barr virus; HHV = human herpesvirus; NK = natural killer; NOS = not otherwise specified; WHO = World Health Organization.

TABLE 1 Clinical Prognostic Classification of Adult Non-Hodgkin's Lymphomas*

Lymphoma Type	Percentage of All Non-Hodgkin's Lymphomas
Indolent or Low-Grade Non-Hodgkin's Lymphomas	
Follicular lymphoma	20-25
Small lymphocytic lymphoma	7
MALT-type marginal zone lymphoma	7
Nodal-type marginal zone lymphoma	<2
Lymphoplasmacytic lymphoma	<2
Aggressive or High-Grade Non-Hodgkin's Lymphomas	
Diffuse large B-cell lymphoma	30
T-cell lymphomas: peripheral or systemic, multiple subtypes	10-12
Mantle cell lymphoma	6
Lymphoblastic lymphoma	<2
Burkitt's lymphoma	<1

Abbreviation: MALT, mucosa-associated lymphoid tissue.
*Subtypes are listed in order of most to least common.

Prognosis

INTERNATIONAL PROGNOSTIC INDEX

The International Prognostic Index was developed as a prognostic factor model for aggressive NHLs treated with doxorubicin-containing regimens (Box 3). In the pre-rituximab era, persons with no risk factors or one risk factor have a predicted 5-year overall survival of 73%, compared with 26% for high-risk patients with four or five risk factors. In the post-rituximab era, the survival rates have improved (see Box 3). The International Prognostic Index also appears to be useful in predicting outcome in patients with low-grade lymphoma or mantle cell lymphoma and in patients who have relapsed or refractory large B-cell lymphoma and are undergoing autologous stem-cell transplantation.

MOLECULAR PROFILING

DNA microarray technology for gene expression profiling has identified distinct prognostic subgroups in DLBCL and follicular NHL. Patients with germinal center B-like DLBCL have a significantly

improved overall survival compared with the other molecular profiles. Recent studies in follicular NHL have identified gene expression signatures that also predicted survival. Interestingly, the genes that defined the prognostic signatures were not expressed in the tumor cells but were expressed by the nonmalignant tumor-infiltrating cells—primarily T cells, macrophages, and dendritic cells.

Treatment

The therapeutic approach for NHL differs for each clinicopathologic subtype. Chemotherapy remains the most important modality. However, in some instances, radiation therapy or, rarely, surgical resection plays a role. Biological approaches, including monoclonal antibodies and antibody-drug conjugates have shown significant activity and are now incorporated into treatment paradigms. Autologous and allogeneic stem-cell transplantation are traditionally reserved for recurrent or refractory disease.

INDOLENT B-CELL NON-HODGKIN'S LYMPHOMAS

Indolent lymphomas are low-grade and represent slow-growing NHLs that may be stable with low tumor burden and might not warrant therapy for several years. The disease is responsive to treatment (high rates of remission), although the clinical course is characterized by repeated relapses. Outside of early-stage disease and therapy with an allogeneic stem cell transplant, low-grade NHLs are not curable. The median survival of patients with advanced-stage follicular lymphoma in the pre-rituximab era was 9 to 10 years, although that is likely longer now. Transformation to a high-grade NHL occurs in 30% to 50% (3%-4% of patients each year) of follicular lymphoma patients (less common in other indolent subtypes) and is typically heralded by an aggressive change in the patient's clinical condition.

BOX 3 International Prognostic Index Adverse Risk Factors and Associated Approximate Diffuse Large B-Cell Lymphoma Cure Rates in the Post-Rituximab Era

Factors

Age ≥60 years
Ann Arbor stage III or IV
Serum lactate dehydrogenase level above normal
Two or more extranodal sites of involvement
Performance status ECOG 2 or more (or equivalent)

Four-Year Progression-Free Survival Rates Based on Number of Factors Present at Diagnosis

0 factors: 94%
1 or 2 factors: 80%
3, 4, or 5 factors: 53%

Abbreviation: ECOG = Eastern Cooperative Oncology Group.

CURRENT THERAPY

- Indolent lymphomas are low-grade and represent slow-growing non-Hodgkin's lymphoma (NHL) that may be stable and with a low tumor burden that does not warrant therapy for several years. The disease is responsive to treatment with a variety of treatment options (high rates of remission), although the clinical course is characterized by repeated relapses. Outside of early-stage disease and therapy with allogeneic stem cell transplantation, low-grade NHLs are not curable.
- Transformation of follicular lymphoma to a high-grade NHL occurs in 30% to 50%, or 3% to 4% of patients each year; it is less common in other indolent subtypes. Transformation is typically heralded by an aggressive change in the patient's clinical condition.
- Diffuse large B-cell lymphoma (DLBCL), the most common aggressive NHL, is curable in all stages in the majority of patients with rituximab (Rituxan)-based chemotherapy. A variety of primary extranodal DLBCL clinical subtypes warrant specialized therapy, such as primary central nervous system lymphoma.
- Long-term survivors are at increased risk for second cancers. The highest relative risk of developing a secondary malignancy is 21 to 30 years after the original diagnosis. Patients who received an anthracycline (e.g., doxorubicin [Adriamycin]) as part of therapy are at a long-term increased risk for cardiovascular disease.

General Principles

Only a minority of patients present with early-stage disease (i.e., stage I or II). Radiotherapy is a treatment option for these patients (especially stage I), and associated 15- to 20-year disease-free survival rates are greater than 50%. Treatment for patients with advanced-stage disease ranges from observation (i.e., watchful waiting) to anti-CD20 monoclonal antibody therapy (rituximab) with or without chemotherapy. Treatment choice depends on tumor burden and the patient's characteristics. Treatment with frontline rituximab chemotherapy (outpatient therapy given once every 3-4 weeks typically for 6-8 cycles) is associated with median progression-free survival rates of approximately 4 to 5 years.

Treatment options for relapsed indolent lymphoma include repeating rituximab without or without a different chemotherapy regimen, radioimmunotherapy, or stem-cell transplantation. Autologous stem-cell transplantation is an option for patients with relapsed disease, although an improvement in overall survival is debated. Allogeneic stem cell transplantation is a potential curative modality for patients with relapsed or refractory disease, although patient selection is critical owing to potential morbidity and mortality related to this treatment.

Special Considerations

Localized gastric MALT lymphoma cases often may be managed with therapy for *H. pylori* infection; radiation is typically reserved for failure to eradicate *H. pylori*. Patients with lymphoplasmacytic lymphoma (Waldenström's macroglobulinemia) can present clinically with hyperviscosity or cryoglobulinemia, which can be managed acutely with plasmapheresis, but ultimately they are managed with systemic therapy similar to that for other indolent NHLs.

AGGRESSIVE OR HIGH-GRADE NON-HODGKIN'S LYMPHOMAS

High-grade B- and T-cell NHLs are typically aggressive lymphomas that are fatal in weeks to a few months if not treated. However, many of these NHLs are curable with multiagent chemotherapy.

General Principles

DLBCL, the most common aggressive NHL, is curable in all stages in the majority of patients (60%-70%). A key to treatment is anti-CD20 monoclonal antibody combined with anthracycline-based chemotherapy: rituximab-CHOP (R-CHOP) (cyclophosphamide, doxorubicin, vincristine, prednisone). The number of treatment cycles depends on stage of disease and response to treatment. Standard for advanced-stage disease is 6 to 8 R-CHOP cycles, and patients with early-stage disease may receive 3 or 4 cycles followed by involved field radiation. Standard therapy for relapsed DLBCL includes abbreviated salvage non–cross resistant chemotherapy followed by autologous stem-cell transplantation (autoSCT), which is curative in approximately 30% to 40% of patients.

Mantle cell lymphoma is a B-cell NHL with poorer outcomes, and it is difficult to cure. With standard chemotherapy regimens (e.g., R-CHOP), the median progression-free survival rates are only 18 to 20 months. With more-intensive chemotherapy regimens (e.g., R-hyperCVAD/R-MA [rituximab, cyclophosphamide, vincristine, doxorubicin, dexamethasone/rituximab, methotrexate]), 5-year progression-free survival rates are near 70%. Other groups advocate aggressive high-dose cytarabine[1] (Cytosar-U)-based chemotherapy followed by consolidative autologous stem-cell transplantation in first remission.

Burkitt's lymphoma and related high-grade NHLs (e.g., lymphoblastic lymphomas) are often rapidly growing malignancies with a doubling times of 24 hours. Prompt initiation of therapy, including aggressive supportive care measures, is often warranted. With aggressive chemotherapy regimens, including prophylactic intrathecal chemotherapy, the majority of patients younger than 50 years are cured (>70%-80%).

Systemic (i.e., non-cutaneous) T-cell NHLs are treatable, however cure rates are lower compared with most aggressive B-cell NHLs. Standard therapy consists typically of CHOP chemotherapy although +/− autologous SCT long-term disease-free survival rates are approximately 20% to 30%.

Special Considerations

There are several clinical subtypes of DLBCL that present as primary extranodal manifestations such as primary testicular DLBCL and primary gastric DLBCL. If these lymphomas are localized, treatment typically consists of abbreviated cycles (3-4) of R-CHOP followed by involved field radiation.

Primary central nervous system lymphoma is typically DLBCL; high-dose methotrexate chemotherapy is a key component of therapy.

A long-standing therapeutic maneuver for posttransplantation lymphoproliferative disorders has been reduction of immunosuppression, although using this approach alone, mortality rates have ranged from 50% to 60% in most series. However, recent evidence with use of initial rituximab-based therapy suggests significantly improved outcomes in the modern era.

The majority of AIDS-related NHLs are aggressive or high-grade types: DLBCL or Burkitt's lymphoma. Response to therapy, including cure rate, has improved significantly with better control of opportunistic infections and highly active antiretroviral therapy (HAART).

Mycosis fungoides and Sézary syndrome are cutaneous T-cell lymphomas that initially might show eczematous lesions. It is often difficult to establish diagnosis, but eventually the lesions develop into plaques and tumors. Lymph nodes, spleen, and visceral organs may be involved. Sézary syndrome is a variant of mycosis fungoides and shows peripheral blood involvement; patients usually have diffuse erythroderma. Skin-targeted modalities for treatment of early-stage mycosis fungoides include psoralens with ultraviolet A light (PUVA), narrowband-ultraviolet light, skin electron-beam radiation, and topical steroids, retinoids, carmustine (BiCNU), and nitrogen mustard (Mustargen).[1] Treatment goals in advanced stages are to reduce tumor burden and to relieve symptoms. Treatment options include mono- or polychemotherapy including CHOP, extracorporeal photopheresis, interferons, retinoids, monoclonal antibodies, and recombinant toxins.

During therapy for aggressive/high-grade NHLs, attention should be paid to preventing tumor lysis syndrome. Measures to prevent this complication include aggressive hydration, allopurinol (Zyloprim), alkalinization of the urine, and frequent monitoring of electrolytes, uric acid, and creatinine. Rasburicase (Elitek), a recombinant urate oxidase enzyme, is an expensive but potent agent for treating hyperuricemia.

NOVEL TREATMENT OPTIONS AND MODALITIES

Many new agents targeting specific molecular targets such as the ubiquitin-proteasome pathway have shown promise in the treatment of lymphoma. Novel agents in lymphoma include bortezomib (Velcade), which is approved for relapsed or refractory mantle-cell lymphoma, and histone deacetylase inhibitors for cutaneous T-cell lymphoma.[1] Other new agents are also showing activity include the immunomodulatory drugs (e.g., lenalidomide [Revlimid][1]) and a mammalian target of rapamycin (Rapamune)[1] (mTOR) inhibitor. Novel targeted antibodies and combinations of antibodies with immune toxins have also shown promise.

Follow-Up of Long-Term Survivors

RELAPSE

Among patients with aggressive lymphomas, such as DLBCL, most recurrences are seen within the first 2 years after the completion of therapy, although later relapses occur. Physical examination and

---

[1]Not FDA approved for this indication.

[1]Not FDA approved for this indication.

laboratory testing at 2- to 3-month intervals and follow-up CT scans at 6-month intervals for the first 2 years following diagnosis are recommended. Early detection of recurrent disease is important in part because these patients may be candidates for potentially curative therapy (e.g., stem-cell transplantation). Patients with advanced low-grade NHL are at a constant risk for relapse, as discussed before.

SECONDARY MALIGNANCIES

Long-term survivors are at increased risk for second cancers. Generally, the risk is increased with history of radiation use, but it is also seen with chemotherapy. In a survey of 28,131 Dutch registry patients with NHL who survived 2 years or longer, second cancers were reported in 2,829 subjects, with significant excesses seen for nearly all solid tumors as well as acute myelogenous leukemia (AML) and Hodgkin's lymphoma. The standardized incidence ratio (SIR) for solid tumors after NHL was 1.65. The SIRs for solid tumors increased for up to 30 years after NHL diagnosis, with the highest relative risk of developing a secondary malignancy occurring at 21 to 30 years after original diagnosis.

LATE TREATMENT COMPLICATIONS

There has been more selective use of radiation as part of therapy for NHL. Therefore, the risk of certain radiation-induced complications has been reduced in patients treated more recently. Nevertheless, total-body irradiation may be used as a component of myeloablative conditioning regimens. Transplant recipients are at increased risk for secondary myelodysplasia and AML, regardless of whether they received radiation. All chemotherapy agents have their own long-term morbidity; in particular, patients who received an anthracycline (e.g., doxorubicin [Adriamycin]) are at a long-term increased risk of cardiovascular disease. Among 476 Dutch and Belgian NHL patients treated with at least six cycles of doxorubicin-based chemotherapy, cumulative incidence of cardiovascular disease was 12% at 5 years and 22% at 10 years. Risk of coronary artery disease matched that of the general population, and risk of chronic heart failure was significantly increased (SIR, 5.4) as was stroke (SIR, 1.8). Risk factors associated with excess cardiovascular risk included younger age at start of NHL treatment (<55 years), preexisting hypertension, any salvage treatment, and use of radiotherapy; risk relating to radiotherapy was dose-dependent.

REFERENCES

Coiffier B, Lepage E, Briere J, et al. CHOP chemotherapy plus rituximab compared with CHOP alone in elderly patients with diffuse large B cell lymphoma. N Engl J Med 2002;346:235–42.

Dave SS, Wright G, Tan B, et al. Prediction of survival in follicular lymphoma based on molecular features of tumor-infiltrating immune cells. N Engl J Med 2004;351:2159–69.

Dave SS, Fu K, Wright GW, Lam LT, et al. Molecular diagnosis of Burkitt's lymphoma. N Engl J Med 2006;354:2431–42.

Evens AM, David KA, Helenowski IB, et al. Multicenter analysis of 80 solid organ transplant recipients with posttransplantation lymphoproliferative disease (PTLD): Outcomes and prognostic factors in the modern era. J Clin Oncol 2010; Feb 20; 28(6):1038–1046. Epub Jan 19, 2010.

Feugier P, Van Hoof A, Sebban C, et al. Long-term results of the R-CHOP study in the treatment of elderly patients with diffuse large B-cell lymphoma: a study by the Groupe d'Etude des Lymphomes de l'Adulte. J Clin Oncol 2005;23:4117–26.

Hemminki K, Lenner P, Sundquist J, Bermejo JL. Risk of subsequent solid tumors after non-Hodgkin's lymphoma: Effect of diagnostic age and time since diagnosis. J Clin Oncol 2008;26(11):1850–7.

Moser EC, Noordijk EM, van Leeuwen FE, et al. Long-term risk of cardiovascular disease after treatment for aggressive non-Hodgkin lymphoma. Blood 2006;107:2912–9.

Rizvi MA, Evens AM, Tallman MS, et al. T-cell non-Hodgkin's lymphoma. Blood 2006;107:1255–64.

Romaguera JE, Fayad L, Rodriguez MA, et al. High rate of durable remissions after treatment of newly diagnosed aggressive mantle-cell lymphoma with rituximab plus hyper-CVAD alternating with rituximab plus high-dose methotrexate and cytarabine. J Clin Oncol 2005;23(28):7013–23.

Sehn LH, Berry B, Chhanabhai M, et al. The revised International Prognostic Index (R-IPI) is a better predictor of outcome than the standard IPI for patients with diffuse large B-cell lymphoma treated with R-CHOP. Blood 2007;109:1857–61.

Shipp MA, for The International Non-Hodgkin's Lymphoma Prognostic Factors Project: A predictive model for aggressive non-Hodgkin's lymphoma. N Engl J Med 1993;329:987–94.

Swerdlow SH, Campo E, Harris NL, et al. WHO Classification of Tumours of Haematopoietic and Lymphoid Tissues. 4th ed. Lyons, France: International Agency for Research on Cancer; 2008.

Multiple Myeloma

Method of
Robert A. Kyle, MD, and S. Vincent Rajkumar, MD

Multiple myeloma is characterized by the neoplastic proliferation of a single clone of plasma cells producing a monoclonal (M) protein in the serum or urine.

Epidemiology

In the United States, multiple myeloma constitutes 1% of all malignant diseases and slightly more than 10% of hematologic malignancies. The annual incidence is 4 to 5 per 100,000; the incidence in African Americans is twice that in whites. The apparent increase in rates is probably caused by increased availability and use of medical facilities and improved diagnostic techniques, particularly in the older population. The median age at diagnosis is approximately 70 years, and only 2% of patients are younger than 40 years.

Risk Factors

The cause of multiple myeloma is unclear. Exposure to radiation from the atomic bomb explosion might play a role. Persons in agricultural occupations who are exposed to pesticides, herbicides, or fungicides might have an increased risk of multiple myeloma. Benzene and petroleum products, hair dyes, engine exhaust, furniture worker products, obesity, and chronic immune stimulation might also be risk factors. The risk of developing multiple myeloma is higher for patients with a first-degree relative with the disease. Clusters of two or more first-degree relatives or identical twins have been recognized.

Clinical Manifestations

Weakness, fatigue, bone pain, recurrent infections, and symptoms of hypercalcemia or renal insufficiency should alert the physician to the possibility of multiple myeloma. Anemia is present in 70% of patients at the time of diagnosis. An M protein is found in the serum or urine in 97% of patients with multiple myeloma by immunofixation studies. Lytic lesions, osteoporosis, or fractures are present at diagnosis in 80%. Technetium bone scanning is inferior to conventional radiography and should not be used. Magnetic resonance imaging (MRI) or positron emission tomography/computed tomography (PET/CT) is helpful in patients who have skeletal pain but no abnormality on radiographs or when spinal cord compression is suspected. Hypercalcemia is present in 15% of patients, and the serum creatinine value is 2 mg/dL or greater in almost 20% of patients at diagnosis.

Diagnosis

If multiple myeloma is suspected, the patient should have, in addition to a complete history and physical examination:

- Determination of values for hemoglobin, leukocytes with differential count, platelets, serum creatinine, calcium, and uric acid
- A radiographic survey of bones, including humeri and femurs
- Serum protein electrophoresis with immunofixation
- Quantitation of immunoglobulins, serum free light chain assay
- Bone marrow aspirate and biopsy
- Routine urinalysis
- Electrophoresis and immunofixation of an adequately concentrated aliquot from a 24-hour urine specimen
- Cytogenetics and fluorescence in situ hybridization (FISH); if available, a plasma cell labeling index is useful.
- Measurement of β_2-microglobulin, C-reactive protein, and lactate dehydrogenase.

Box 1 lists the criteria for diagnosis of myeloma. Metastatic carcinoma, lymphoma, leukemia, and connective tissue disorders can resemble multiple myeloma and must be considered in the differential diagnosis. Patients with multiple myeloma must be differentiated from those with monoclonal gammopathy of undetermined significance (MGUS) and smoldering (asymptomatic) multiple myeloma because they may remain stable for long periods (Box 1). The plasma cell labeling index is helpful in differentiating MGUS or smoldering multiple myeloma from multiple myeloma. The patient's symptoms, physical findings, and all laboratory and radiographic data must be considered in the decision to begin therapy. If there are doubts about whether to begin treatment, therapy should be withheld and the patient should be reevaluated in 2 to 3 months. No evidence indicates that early treatment of multiple myeloma is advantageous.

Treatment

Patients with symptomatic multiple myeloma may be classified as having high-risk or standard-risk disease. High-risk disease is defined as the presence of hypodiploidy or deletion of chromosome 13 [del (13)] with conventional cytogenetics or the presence of t(4;14), t (14;16), t(14;20), or del(17p) with FISH. Lactate dehydrogenase and β_2-microglobulin levels are additional important risk factors. Approximately 25% of patients with symptomatic multiple myeloma have high-risk disease.

If clinical trials are not available, one may separate patients into those who are eligible for an autologous stem cell transplant (SCT) or not eligible. An autologous SCT adds about 1 year of survival when compared with patients treated with alkylating agents.

CURRENT DIAGNOSIS

Newly Diagnosed Symptomatic Myeloma

- Eligible for stem cell transplantation
  - Lenalidomide (Revlimid) plus low-dose dexamethasone (Decadron)
  - Bortezomib (Velcade) plus dexamethasone
- Ineligible for stem cell transplantation
  - Lenalidomide plus low-dose dexamethasone
  - Melphalan (Alkeran), prednisone, bortezomib
  - Melphalan, prednisone, thalidomide (Thalomid)

Refractory or Relapsed Myeloma

- Lenalidomide or thalidomide plus low-dose dexamethasone
- Bortezomib and dexamethasone
- Alkylator-based therapy
- Clinical trials

Eligibility for autologous SCT in multiple myeloma varies from country to country. In the United States, decisions are made on a patient-by-patient basis depending on the physiologic age rather than the chronologic age. In most institutions, patients older than 70 years or with serum creatinine greater than 2.5 mg/dL, Eastern Cooperative oncology Group (ECOG) performance status of 3 or 4, or New York Heart Association (NYHA) functional status class III or IV are considered ineligible for autologous SCT. Although patients with kidney failure may have an autologous SCT, the morbidity and mortality are higher.

CURRENT THERAPY

- Do not begin treatment until symptomatic multiple myeloma develops (CRAB: *c*alcium elevated, *r*enal failure, *a*nemia, *b*one lesions).
- Decide whether an autologous stem cell transplant is feasible. If it is, one must avoid prolonged melphalan (Alkeran) therapy as initial treatment.
- Induction therapy for patients eligible for transplant is typically lenalidomide (Revlimid) or bortezomib (Velcade) combined with low-dose dexamethasone (Decadron).
- Initial therapy for patients not eligible for transplantation is typically melphalan and prednisone plus either thalidomide (Thalomid) or bortezomib, with thalidomide preferred in standard-risk patients and bortezomib in high-risk patients. Lenalidomide plus low-dose dexamethasone is a third option.
- Relapsed or refractory myeloma should be treated with one of the active classes of drugs given alone or in combination. Active agents include thalidomide, lenalidomide, bortezomib, corticosteroids, anthracyclines, and alkylators.

INITIAL THERAPY FOR TRANSPLANT-ELIGIBLE PATIENTS

Lenalidomide (Revlimid) is an analogue of thalidomide and is an immunomodulatory agent. Lenalidomide 25 mg daily on days 1 to 21 plus dexamethasone (Decadron) 40 mg weekly for each 28-day cycle is an effective regimen. The 1-year survival was 96%, and the 2-year survival probability was 87%. Bortezomib (Velcade) 1.3 mg/m^2 twice weekly for 2 weeks every 3 weeks plus dexamethasone 40 mg on the day of and the day after bortezomib produces a high response rate and is another effective regimen for initial therapy, particularly for high-risk patients and for patients with acute renal failure. One useful regimen is thalidomide (Thalomid) plus dexamethasone; another is bortezomib, thalidomide, and dexamethasone. There have been no phase III trials comparing any of these regimens. We prefer lenalidomide plus low-dose dexamethasone in standard-risk patients and bortezomib plus dexamethasone in high-risk patients.

AUTOLOGOUS STEM CELL TRANSPLANTATION

Following 3 to 4 months of induction therapy with one of the initial regimens, one must collect the stem cells in patients eligible for transplantation. There is suggestive evidence that induction therapy associated with a greater depth of response (very good partial remission [VGPR] or complete response [CR]) before transplantation translates into superior progression-free survival. The stem cells must be collected before the patient is exposed to prolonged melphalan (Alkeran) therapy. Granulocyte colony-stimulating factor (G-CSF, Neupogen) with or without cyclophosphamide (Cytoxan) is used for mobilizing stem cells. G-CSF plus cyclophosphamide is preferred in patients who are treated with lenalidomide plus dexamethasone induction, who are older than 65 years, or who have received such therapy for over 4 months. It is advisable to collect 6×10^6 CD34$^+$ cells/kg, which is sufficient for two transplants.

The timing of autologous SCT takes into account the patient's wishes, and it may be done early (when the patient recovers from stem cell collection) or delayed until relapse. There is no difference in overall survival among patients who receive an autologous SCT immediately following collection of stem cells and those who receive it at first relapse. In general, we prefer an early transplant because this provides a better quality of life and time without therapy.

Melphalan[3] 200 mg/m^2 is the preferred conditioning regimen for autologous SCT. This regimen has fewer adverse side effects than melphalan[3] 140 mg/m^2 plus total body irradiation. If a patient obtains a VGPR or CR with the first transplant, little benefit results from a second (tandem) transplant.

The mortality rate with autologous SCT is approximately 1%. Unfortunately, multiple myeloma is not eradicated, and the autologous peripheral stem cells are contaminated by myeloma cells or their precursors.

Bone marrow transplantation from an identical twin donor (syngeneic) is the treatment of choice if a donor is available. Results are superior to allogeneic transplantation.

Maintenance Therapy Following Autologous Stem Cell Transplantation

In a large prospective study, multiple myeloma patients were given a tandem transplant and then randomized to no maintenance, pamidronate (Aredia) maintenance, or pamidronate plus thalidomide maintenance. Although thalidomide improved the response rate and overall survival, it often resulted in peripheral neuropathy. However, the overall survival benefit was lost with longer follow-up. Interferon alfa 2b (Intron-A)[1] has produced benefit in progression-free survival and overall survival, but the benefit is modest. We recommend that patients who have obtained a response from autologous SCT be followed without maintenance therapy unless they are part of a clinical trial. Maintenance, usually for a fixed duration, is considered in high-risk patients and in patients who fail to achieve a VGPR following autologous SCT.

ALLOGENEIC TRANSPLANTATION

Allogeneic bone marrow transplantation is advantageous in that the graft contains no tumor cells and there is a graft-versus-tumor effect. However, subsequent graft-versus-host disease is troublesome. Only 5% to 10% of patients with multiple myeloma are eligible because a human leukocyte antigen (HLA)-compatible donor is available to only one third of patients, and 90% of patients are 50 years of age or older. Allogeneic transplantation currently is associated with a high mortality and cannot be recommended.

Nonmyeloablative allogeneic (mini-allo) transplant following autologous SCT is being pursued. It is hoped that the benefits of an allograft may be realized and the toxicity associated with the procedure may be decreased. The mortality is 10% to 15%, and graft-versus-host disease remains troublesome. Efforts are being made to reduce the toxicity of this approach. Currently, we believe that non-myeloablative approaches should be limited to clinical trials.

INITIAL THERAPY FOR PATIENTS WHO ARE INELIGIBLE FOR AUTOLOGOUS STEM CELL TRANSPLANTATION

Since the 1960s, alkylating agent–based chemotherapy with oral administration of melphalan and prednisone (MP) has been the standard of therapy, producing an objective response in 50% to 60% of patients and a median survival of 2 to 3 years. Various combinations of alkylating agents have been developed, but a large meta-analysis, based on data from 6633 patients in 30 trials comparing MP with various combinations of alkylating agents, was performed by the Myeloma Trialists' Collaborative Group. Although the response rate was higher with combination chemotherapy, there was no survival benefit over melphalan.

The addition of thalidomide 100 mg daily to MP (MPT regimen) produced a response rate of 76% and CR in 16% compared to 48% and 2%, respectively, for MP. The 3-year survival was 80% versus 64% favoring the MPT regimen. However, side effects were more common, and with longer follow-up, the survival advantage was lost. In another randomized study, MPT given for 1 year produced a longer progression-free survival (28 vs. 18 months) and overall survival (52 vs. 33 months). In a prospective randomized trial, melphalan, prednisone, and lenalidomide was superior to MP.

Another option for patients who are not candidates for transplantation is bortezomib (Velcade) 1.3 mg/m^2 IV on days 1, 4, 8, 11, 25, 29, and 32 during cycles 1 through 4 and bortezomib 1.3 mg/m^2 on days 1, 8, 22, and 29 during cycles 5 through 9 plus melphalan 9 mg/m^2 and prednisone 60 mg/m^2 days 1 through 4 of each cycle or MP in the same dose and schedule (VMP regimen). The CR plus VGPR was 45% for VMP compared to 10% for MP. Peripheral neuropathy occurred in 44% of the VMP patients and in 5% of those given MP. Currently, we prefer MPT for standard-risk myeloma patients, whereas VMP is recommended for patients with high-risk disease. It appears that VMP overcomes the adverse effect of chromosomal abnormalities.

We continue the initial chemotherapy regimen until the patient reaches a plateau state. There is no evidence that continued chemotherapy with MP, MPT, or VMP is of benefit after achieving a plateau state. In addition, there is risk of myelodysplasia from continued treatment with alkylating agents. The role of thalidomide, bortezomib, and lenalidomide for maintenance therapy has not been proved.

Lenalidomide plus low-dose dexamethasone is an excellent alternative for elderly patients who are not candidates for autologous SCT. If lenalidomide or thalidomide is used with low-dose dexamethasone or prednisone, aspirin[1] 81 mg or 325 mg daily is recommended as prophylaxis against deep venous thrombosis. If lenalidomide or thalidomide is given with high-dose dexamethasone, doxorubicin (Adriamycin), liposomal doxorubicin (Doxil), or erythropoietin (Epogen, Procrit),[1] then full-dose warfarin (Coumadin)[1] or low-molecular-weight heparin should be given. Anticoagulation is also recommended for patients who have a history of previous thromboembolic events, are on bed rest, are obese, or have any other risk factors for thrombosis. Bortezomib does not produce a higher risk of thromboembolic events.

RELAPSED OR REFACTORY MULTIPLE MYELOMA

Almost all patients with multiple myeloma who survive eventually relapse. If relapse occurs more than 6 months after treatment is discontinued, the initial chemotherapy regimen should be reinstituted. Most patients respond again, but the duration and quality of response are usually inferior to the initial response. Since the turn of the century, thalidomide, bortezomib, and lenalidomide have been introduced and have revolutionized the treatment of patients with relapsed or refractory disease. Objective responses occur in approximately a third of patients and have a median duration of approximately 12 months. The addition of dexamethasone increases the response rate.

Thalidomide

Thalidomide is usually instituted in a dose of 50 to 100 mg daily and, if necessary, escalated to 200 mg daily if tolerated. The duration of response is approximately 1 year. Side effects from thalidomide include sedation, fatigue, constipation, rash, deep venous thrombosis, edema, bradycardia, and hypothyroidism. Virtually all patients develop a sensorimotor peripheral neuropathy. The use of thalidomide in pregnancy is contraindicated, and the STEPS program (System for Thalidomide Education and Prescribing Safety) must be followed to prevent teratogenic effects.

Bortezomib

Bortezomib is a proteasome inhibitor that produces a response rate of approximately 35% in patients with relapsed or refractory myeloma. The median duration of response is 12 months. The response to bortezomib is rapid and usually occurs within 1 to 2 months.

Adverse effects include fatigue, anorexia, nausea, vomiting, fever, diarrhea, constipation, anemia, asthenia, neutropenia, and thrombocytopenia. The most troublesome side effect is peripheral neuropathy, which occurs in 35% to 40% of patients. The neuropathy is often painful, but does improve in most patients after discontinuing bortezomib.

Lenalidomide

Lenalidomide produces an objective response in approximately 30% of patients with relapsed or refractory multiple myeloma. The major side effects are cytopenias, and the dose needs to be modified accordingly.

The median survival of Mayo Clinic myeloma patients seen between 1971 and 1996 was 30 months; survival was 45 months in those whose multiple myeloma was diagnosed after 1996. The improved survival was due to autologous SCT or the three novel agents (thalidomide, bortezomib, or lenalidomide). In a retrospective study from the Mayo Clinic, patients who relapsed following an autologous transplant and received one of the novel agents had a median survival of 31 months compared with 15 months for those who relapsed and did not receive a novel agent.

Other New Drugs

New drugs that are in clinical trials include pomalidomide (Actimid),[5] vorinostat (Zolinza)[1](SAHA; a histone deacetylase inhibitor), and carfilzomib[5] (a proteasome inhibitor), as well as multiple other agents.

SUPPORTIVE THERAPY

Radiotherapy

Palliative radiation in a dose of 20 to 30 Gy should be limited to patients who have disabling pain and a well-defined focal process that has not responded to chemotherapy. Analgesics in combination with chemotherapy usually can control the pain. This approach is preferred to local radiation because pain often occurs at another site, and local radiation does not benefit the patient with systemic disease. In addition, the myelosuppressive effects of radiotherapy and chemotherapy are cumulative and can restrict future therapy. Radiation is required for spinal cord compression from plasmacytoma. Postsurgical radiation after stabilization of fractures or impending fractures is rarely needed.

Hypercalcemia

Hypercalcemia must be suspected if the patient has anorexia, nausea, vomiting, polyuria, increased constipation, weakness, confusion, stupor, or coma. If it is untreated, renal insufficiency usually develops. Hydration, preferably with isotonic saline and prednisone (25 mg orally four times daily), is effective in most patients with mild to moderate hypercalcemia (calcium <13 mg/dL). If more-severe hypercalcemia occurs, zoledronic acid (Zometa) at a dose of 4 mg intravenously over 15 minutes or pamidronate 90 mg given intravenously over at least 2 hours is indicated. Calcitonin (Miacalcin) may be used if rapid reduction of calcium levels is needed. Hemodialysis may be necessary for extremely severe hypercalcemia. The dosage of prednisone must be reduced and discontinued as soon as possible.

Renal Insufficiency

Approximately 20% of patients with multiple myeloma have a serum creatinine level of 2.0 mg/dL or more at diagnosis. Myeloma kidney (cast nephropathy) and hypercalcemia are the two major causes. Myeloma kidney is characterized by the presence of large, waxy, laminated casts in the distal and collecting tubules. Some light chains are very nephrotoxic, but no specific amino acid sequence of the nephrotoxic light chain has been identified.

Dehydration, infection, nonsteroidal antiinflammatory agents, and radiographic contrast media can contribute to acute kidney failure. Hyperuricemia or amyloid deposition can produce renal insufficiency. Nephrotic syndrome rarely occurs in multiple myeloma unless amyloidosis is present.

Maintenance of a high fluid intake producing 3 L of urine per 24 hours is important for preventing kidney failure in patients with Bence Jones proteinuria. IV pyelography or preparation for barium enema can be performed with little risk if dehydration is avoided. If hyperuricemia occurs, allopurinol (Zyloprim) in doses of 300 mg daily provides effective therapy.

Acute kidney failure should be treated promptly with appropriate fluid and electrolyte replacement. Patients with kidney failure should be treated with bortezomib and dexamethasone to reduce the tumor mass as quickly as possible. A trial of plasmapheresis is reasonable in an attempt to prevent chronic dialysis, but it is not a proven therapy. Hemodialysis and peritoneal dialysis are equally effective and are necessary for patients with symptomatic azotemia. Kidney transplantation for myeloma kidney is often followed by prolonged survival.

Anemia

Almost every patient with multiple myeloma eventually becomes anemic. Increased plasma volume from the osmotic effect of the M protein can produce hypervolemia and can spuriously lower the hemoglobin and hematocrit values. Patients with significant symptoms should be considered for red blood cell transfusion. If a transfusion is indicated, irradiated leukocyte-reduced red cells are preferred.

In patients with newly diagnosed myeloma, induction chemotherapy is often associated with a prompt improvement in hemoglobin levels, so it is better to avoid the use of erythropoietin. Erythropoietin should be seriously considered in relapsed patients receiving chemotherapy who have a hemoglobin level of 10 g/dL or less.

Erythropoietin (200 μg every 2 to 3 weeks) reduces the transfusion requirement and increases hemoglobin concentration in more than half of patients. Those with low serum erythropoietin values are more likely to respond. Most physicians proceed with a trial of erythropoietin 150 U/kg three times weekly, or 40,000 U once a week. Darbepoetin, a long-lasting erythropoietin (Aranesp), may be given weekly or biweekly.

---

[1]Not FDA approved for this indication.
[5]Investigational drug in the United States.

Skeletal Lesions

Bone lesions manifested by pain and fractures are a major problem. A skeletal radiographic survey should be repeated at 6-month intervals or sooner if pain develops. Patients should be encouraged to be as active as possible because confinement to bed increases demineralization of the skeleton. Trauma must be avoided because even mild stress can result in a fracture. Fixation of long bone fractures or impending fractures with an intramedullary rod and methyl methacrylate gives excellent results.

All patients with multiple myeloma who have lytic lesions, pathologic fractures, or severe osteopenia should receive an IV bisphosphonate. Pamidronate 90 mg IV over 2 hours every 4 weeks or zoledronic acid (Zometa) 4 mg IV over 15 minutes every 4 weeks are equally efficacious. The dosage of bisphosphonates should be reduced with renal insufficiency. Because renal insufficiency or nephrotic-range proteinuria can occur, serum creatinine and 24-hour urine protein monitoring is necessary. One should seriously consider stopping the IV bisphosphonate in patients who have responsive or stable disease after 2 years of therapy.

Bisphosphonates should be resumed upon relapse with new-onset skeletal-related events. Osteonecrosis of the jaw can occur in patients receiving bisphosphonates. Although the relationship is unclear, it is essential to obtain a complete dental evaluation and perform preventive dental treatment prior before beginning bisphosphonates. The patient should practice good oral hygiene during therapy. Invasive procedures (especially dental extractions) should be avoided during bisphosphonate therapy. Osteonecrosis of the jaw should be managed conservatively.

Vertebroplasty or kyphoplasty may be helpful for patients with an acute compression fracture of the spine. Both have been associated with pain relief. Results appear to be better when the procedure is performed shortly after the compression fracture. Leakage of the methyl methacrylate is a potential adverse event. A choice between vertebroplasty and kyphoplasty depends upon the expertise of the physician performing the procedure.

Infections

Bacterial infections are more common in patients with myeloma than in the general population. All patients should receive pneumococcal and influenza immunizations despite their suboptimal antibody response. Substantial fever is an indication for appropriate cultures, chest radiography, and consideration of antibiotic therapy. The greatest risk for infection is during the first 2 months after chemotherapy is initiated. The use of prophylactic antibiotics is controversial. Antiviral prophylaxis (acyclovir [Zovirax] 400 mg twice daily or valacyclovir [Valtrex] 500 mg once daily) should be given to all patients receiving bortezomib because of the increased risk of herpes zoster. Intravenous immunoglobulin (IVIg, Gammagard)[1] may be helpful in selected patients who have recurrent serious infections despite the use of prophylactic antibiotics. It is inconvenient, associated with side effects, and very expensive. Consequently, few of our patients receive intravenous gammaglobulin.

Hyperviscosity Syndrome

Symptoms of hyperviscosity can include oronasal bleeding, gastrointestinal bleeding, blurred vision, neurologic symptoms, or congestive heart failure. Most patients have symptoms when the serum viscosity measurement is more than 4 cP, but the relationship between serum viscosity and clinical manifestations is not precise. The decision to perform plasmapheresis, which promptly relieves the symptoms of hyperviscosity, should be made on clinical grounds rather than serum viscosity levels. Hyperviscosity is more common in immunoglobulin (Ig)A myeloma than in IgG myeloma.

[1]Not FDA approved for this indication.

Extradural Myeloma (Cord Compression)

The possibility of cord compression must be excluded if weakness of the legs or difficulty in voiding or defecating occurs. The sudden onset of severe radicular pain or severe back pain with neurologic symptoms suggests compression of the spinal cord. MRI or CT of the entire spine must be performed immediately. Radiation therapy in a dose of approximately 30 Gy is beneficial in about one half of patients. Dexamethasone should be administered in addition to radiation therapy. Surgical decompression is necessary only if the neurologic deficit does not improve.

Venous Thromboembolism

Patients with multiple myeloma have an increased risk of venous thromboembolism. This is due to the malignancy itself as well as therapy with lenalidomide or thalidomide with corticosteroids. Aspirin[1] given prophylactically is beneficial. If there is a history of previous thromboembolic events or if other risk factors are present, anticoagulation with full-dose warfarin or low-molecular-weight heparin is indicated.

Emotional Support

All patients with multiple myeloma need substantial and continuing emotional support. The physician's approach must be positive in emphasizing the potential benefits of therapy. It is reassuring for patients to know that some survive for 10 years or more. It is vital that the physician caring for patients with multiple myeloma has the interest and capacity for dealing with incurable disease over the span of years with assurance, sympathy, and resourcefulness.

[1]Not FDA approved for this indication.

REFERENCES

Facon T, Mary JY, Hulin C, et al. Melphalan and prednisone plus thalidomide versus melphalan and prednisone alone or reduced-intensity autologous stem cell transplantation in elderly patients with multiple myeloma (IFM 99-06): A randomised trial. Lancet 2007;370:1209–18.

Hulin C, Facon T, Rodon P, et al. Efficacy of melphalan and prednisone plus thalidomide in patients older than 75 years with newly diagnosed multiple myeloma: IFM 01/01 trial. J Clin Oncol 2009;27:3664–70.

Kumar SK, Mikhael JR, Buadi FK, et al. Management of newly diagnosed symptomatic multiple myeloma: updated Mayo Stratification of Myeloma and Risk-Adapted Therapy (mSMART) consensus guidelines. Mayo Clin Proc 2009;84:1095–110.

Kumar SK, Rajkumar SV, Dispenzieri A, et al. Improved survival in multiple myeloma and the impact of novel therapies. Blood 2008;111:2516–20.

Kyle RA, Rajkumar SV. Epidemiology of the plasma-cell disorders. Best Pract Res Clin Haematol 2007;20:637–64.

Kyle RA, Yee GC, Somerfield MR, et al. American Society of Clinical Oncology 2007 clinical practice guideline update on the role of bisphosphonates in multiple myeloma. J Clin Oncol 2007;25:2464–72.

Niesvizky R, Jayabalan DS, Christos PJ, et al. BiRD (Biaxin [clarithromycin]/Revlimid [lenalidomide]/dexamethasone) combination therapy results in high complete- and overall-response rates in treatment-naive symptomatic multiple myeloma. Blood 2008;111:1101–9.

Palumbo A, Bringhen S, Caravita T, et al. Oral melphalan and prednisone chemotherapy plus thalidomide compared with melphalan and prednisone alone in elderly patients with multiple myeloma: randomised controlled trial. Lancet 2006;367:825–31.

Rajkumar SV, Jacobus S, Callander NS, et al. Lenalidomide plus high-dose dexamethasone versus lenalidomide plus low-dose dexamethasone as initial therapy for newly diagnosed multiple myeloma: an open-label randomised controlled trial. Lancet Oncol 2010;11(1):29–37.

San Miguel JF, Schlag R, Khuageva NK, et al. Bortezomib plus melphalan and prednisone for initial treatment of multiple myeloma. N Engl J Med 2008;359:906–17.

Polycythemia Vera

Method of
Peter R. Duggan, MD

Polycythemia vera (PV) is a clonal stem cell disorder characterized by an increase in red cell production independent of the stimulation by erythropoietin. PV is the most common of the chronic myeloproliferative diseases, occurring in approximately 2 to 3 people per 100,000 annually. The median age at diagnosis is 70 years, and it is rare in patients younger than 40 years.

A mutation of the tyrosine kinase Janus kinase 2 (JAK2) is consistently found in PV. This sheds some light on the pathogenesis of the disease and is useful in the diagnosis of PV and other myeloproliferative disorders. A single acquired mutation (V617F) of the gene for the JH-2 domain of JAK2 can be found in 90% to 95% of PV patients. The JH-2 domain functions to inhibit JAK2 activity. In normal erythropoiesis, binding of erythropoietin to its receptor lifts this inhibition and allows JAK2 stimulation of cell division and differentiation. In mutated JAK2, this inhibitory function is absent, leading to constitutive activity of the tyrosine kinase. This mutation is also present in about half of patients with essential thrombocytosis and primary myelofibrosis. The small number of patients with PV who are negative for the common JAK2 mutation have another functionally similar mutation.

Presentation

Many patients with PV are asymptomatic, and the PV is diagnosed after the incidental finding of an elevated hemoglobin on routine complete blood count. Up to half of patients experience such non-specific symptoms as weight loss, sweating, headache, fatigue, epigastric discomfort, visual disturbances, and dizziness. Many of these symptoms are likely caused by decreased blood flow due to an increased blood viscosity from polycythemia.

Generalized pruritus is often described, often after a warm bath or shower. Although the cause of this is unknown, it is thought to be due to the degranulation of increased numbers of mast cells in the skin of patients, releasing histamine and other inflammatory mediators. However, the symptom responds poorly to antihistamines, and it does not always resolve with treatment of PV.

Venous and arterial thromboembolic events are a major cause of morbidity and mortality in PV. Thrombosis at presentation occurs in up to 40% of patients. Ischemic stroke, transient ischemic attack, and myocardial infarction are common, especially among elderly patients. These, along with deep venous thrombosis and pulmonary embolus, are the most common thrombotic events and often result in serious morbidity, disability, and even death. Thrombotic events that are considered unusual in the general population, such as Budd-Chiari syndrome and portal, mesenteric, and other abdominal vein thrombosis and cerebral venous thrombosis, occur more among PV patients. The possibility of an underlying myeloproliferative disorder should be considered when a patient presents with such an event.

PV can manifest with symptoms of peripheral vascular disease. Patients with erythromelalgia describe a painful burning sensation of the hands and feet; pallor, erythema, or cyanosis of the extremities; and sometimes cutaneous ulceration. Erythromelalgia results from microvascular thrombosis and ischemia due to platelet activation and aggregation and responds well to platelet reduction and antiplatelet agents such as aspirin (acetylsalicylic acid [ASA]).[1]

---

[1]Not FDA approved for this indication.

Almost all patients with PV are iron deficient at diagnosis, even before the onset of therapeutic phlebotomy. Other manifestations include acute gouty arthritis, peptic ulcer disease, erosive gastritis, and hypertension.

Diagnosis and Differential Diagnosis

The 2008 World Health Organization (WHO) diagnostic criteria for PV are shown in Box 1. The JAK2 V617F mutation is present in about 95% of cases of PV. Erythropoietin level is decreased in more than 90% and is rarely elevated. Most JAK2 assays are negative in the few PV patients with a mutation of exon 12 of the *JAK2* gene instead of the more common JAK2 V617F mutation. A JAK2 mutation can also be found in about half of patients with essential thrombocytosis and primary myelofibrosis.

Leukocytosis and thrombocytosis are present in the majority of cases of PV. Red cell mass is increased. A nuclear medicine study measuring red cell mass and plasma volume is rarely required with the availability of JAK2 testing, but it may be useful when relative polycythemia is suspected. Bone marrow biopsy and aspiration are not often needed for a diagnosis of PV, but they remain minor diagnostic criteria in the WHO classification. Bone marrow examination can be important for diagnosing PV in the rare cases where JAK2 is negative and to differentiate PV from other JAK2-positive myeloproliferative disorders when the distinction cannot be made based on peripheral blood counts.

Erythrocytosis can occur as a result of a number of other conditions in the absence of PV (Box 2). A careful history and physical with selected investigations can usually distinguish PV from secondary polycythemia and relative polycythemia (see Current Diagnosis). In relative (apparent, spurious) polycythemia, there is usually only a modest increase in the hematocrit, because of a decrease in plasma volume rather than a true increase in red cell mass. Thrombocytosis, leukocytosis, and splenomegaly should be absent. Causes include smoking, dehydration, and use of diuretics, and it is also described in middle-aged, obese, hypertensive men (Gaisböck's syndrome).

Red cell mass can be elevated owing to increased stimulation of erythropoiesis by high levels of erythropoietin. Erythropoietin can be increased as an appropriate response to chronic hypoxia (sleep apnea, right-to-left cardiac shunts, chronic lung diseases, high altitude, smoking, methemoglobinemia), and it can be inappropriately

---

BOX 1   **2008 World Health Organization Diagnostic Criteria for Polycythemia Vera**

Diagnosis requires two major criteria and one minor criterion, or one major criterion with at least two minor criteria.

Major Criteria

Hemoglobin >18.5 g/d/L in men, 16.5 g/dL in women, or other evidence of increased red cell volume*
Presence of JAK2 V617F or mother functionally similar mutation such as JAK2 exon 12 mutation

Minor Criteria

Bone marrow biopsy showing hypercellularity for age with trilineage proliferation
Low serum erythropoietin level
Endogenous erythroid colony formation in vitro

---

*Unexplained, sustained increase in hemoglobin of at least 2 g/dL, to >17 g/dL in men or >15 g/dL in women, or elevated red cell mass >25% above normal.

BOX 2 Differential Diagnosis of Polycythemia

Normal Red Cell Mass
Relative polycythemia
Gaisböck's syndrome

Elevated Red Cell Mass
Primary Polycythemia
Polycythemia vera

Secondary Polycythemia
Congenital
• EPO receptor mutations
• Chuvash polycythemia
• High-affinity hemoglobin
Appropriately elevated EPO (hypoxia driven)
• Chronic hypoxic lung disease
• Cardiac shunts or cyanotic heart disease
• Sleep apnea
• Methemoglobinemia
• High altitude
• Chronic carbon monoxide poisoning
• Cigarette smoking
• Renal artery stenosis
Inappropriately elevated EPO
• Renal cell carcinoma
• Hepatocellular carcinoma
• Hemangioblastoma
• Uterine fibroids
Other causes
• EPO (Epogen) administration
• Androgens (testosterone)
• Kidney transplant

Abbreviation: EPO, erythropoietin.

CURRENT DIAGNOSIS

- Polycythemia vera should be considered when there is persistent elevation of hemoglobin (>185 g/L in men and >165 g/L in women).
- *JAK-2* mutation testing and erythropoietin levels should be performed when polycythemia suspected.
- Bone marrow biopsy and aspiration may be necessary in some cases to confirm the diagnosis of polycythemia and to distinguish polycythemia from other myeloproliferative disorders.
- Polycythemia is highly likely when *JAK2* mutation is present and erythropoietin level is low. When *JAK2* mutation is seen with normal erythropoietin level, polycythemia is possible; bone marrow biopsy is recommended to differentiate polycythemia from other myeloproliferative diseases. When *JAK2* is normal and erythropoietin is low, polycythemia vera is less likely; consider congenital polycythemia. Unmutated *JAK2* and normal or high erythropoietin level make polycythemia very unlikely, and patients should be investigated for secondary causes of erythrocytosis.
- Secondary causes of polycythemia should be ruled out, especially when *JAK2* is not mutated or erythropoietin level is high. Investigations for secondary polycythemia that may be indicated include:
  - Red cell mass and plasma volume measurement
  - Chest x-ray
  - Pulse oximetry
  - Arterial blood gas including carboxyhemoglobin and methemoglobin levels
  - Kidney and liver function tests
  - Abdominal imaging studies (ultrasound or CT scan)
  - Oxyhemoglobin dissociation curve
  - Sleep studies

elevated owing to erythropoietin-secreting tumors (renal cell carcinoma, hepatocellular carcinoma, cerebellar hemangioma, uterine fibroids) or decreased kidney perfusion (renal artery stenosis). Familial causes of polycythemia include high-affinity hemoglobins, erythropoietin receptor mutations, and Chuvash polycythemia. Polycythemia occurs in 10% to 15% of patients following kidney transplantation, and this may be due to erythropoietin secretion by the native kidneys or increased sensitivity to erythropoietin. Polycythemia can be drug induced, such as with the use of performance-enhancing drugs (erythropoietin [Epogen], androgens) in athletes and testosterone replacement in men.

Prognosis

When PV is left untreated, the outlook for patients is poor, with median survival reported to be as low as 18 months. This improves considerably with treatment, though annual mortality remains almost twice as high as in the general population.

Despite therapy, thrombosis remains an important cause of mortality. Cardiac disease, ischemic stroke, pulmonary embolus, and other thrombotic events account for 40% of deaths among PV patients. Nonfatal thrombosis is common, occurring in almost 4% of patients annually. Age and a history of prior thromboembolic events are independent risk factors for thrombosis and can be used to predict a patient's risk of future events (Box 3). Low-risk patients are younger than 60 years and have no history of thrombosis. They experience new events at a rate of 2% per year. For patients older than 60 years or with a past history of thrombosis this rate is 5% annually, but it can be as high as 11% when both risk factors are present.

The contribution of other cardiovascular risk factors (smoking, diabetes, hypertension, hyperlipidemia) to thrombotic risk in PV has been studied, with inconclusive results. However, because these are major contributors to the development of cardiovascular disease in the general population, they should also be considered when assessing risk in patients with PV.

BOX 3 Thrombotic Risk in Polycythemia Vera

Low Risk
Age younger than 60 years
No history of thromboembolism
No cardiovascular risk factors
Less than 2% risk per year for thrombotic events

Intermediate Risk
Age younger than 60 years
No history of thromboembolism
Presence of cardiovascular risk factors

High Risk
Age older than 60 years
Prior thrombosis
Risk is 5% per year for thrombotic events, 11% if both risk factors are present

The risk of major hemorrhage is low, with fatal bleeding causing less than 5% of all deaths. However, there is considerable excess mortality from malignancy, in particular transformation to a myelodysplastic syndrome, myelofibrosis, or acute leukemia. The risk of transformation is highest in those older than 70 years and in patients treated with cytoreductive agents other than hydroxyurea (Hydrea)[1] or interferon alfa-2b (Intron A).[1]

Treatment

The goals of treatment in PV are to lower the risk of thrombosis while minimizing toxicity. This is achieved by a combination of phlebotomy, aspirin,[1] and hydroxyurea[1] or other cytoreductive agents. The use of these therapies can be individualized based on a patient's risk of developing future thromboembolic events.

PHLEBOTOMY

As the hematocrit increases in PV, there is a dramatic increase in blood viscosity. Phlebotomy is the fastest, most effective way to normalize a patient's hematocrit, and it should be initiated immediately in those with newly diagnosed or suspected PV. Blood volume should be reduced as rapidly as possible. Usually, 500 mL of blood is removed every 1 or 2 days until the hematocrit is less than 45%. The frequency of phlebotomy or volume of blood removed can be decreased in elderly patients, those with cardiovascular disease, or others who do not tolerate this schedule. The optimal target hematocrit has not been established, though it is generally accepted that that it should be maintained at less than 45%. Once this target is reached, phlebotomy should continue on a regular basis to maintain this result. Regular phlebotomy eventually results in iron deficiency, at which point most patients' phlebotomy needs decrease dramatically. Iron replacement should be avoided.

---

[1]Not FDA approved for this indication.

CURRENT THERAPY

- All patients should undergo regular phlebotomy with target hematocrit less than 45%.
- Low-dose aspirin[1] should be used in all patients without a contraindication.
- In patients with high-risk polycythemia vera, hydroxyurea (Hydrea)[1] should be used, with dose titrated to maintain a white blood cell count greater than 3.0×10^9/L and platelets in the normal range.
- Alkylating agents should be avoided as cytoreductive therapy owing to the risk of acute leukemia.
- Conventional cardiovascular risk factors (diabetes, hypertension, hyperlipidemia) should be aggressively managed, and cigarette smoking should be discouraged.
- Thromboembolic events should be managed according to accepted management guidelines. Thromboprophylaxis should be used after surgery and in other high-risk situations.

---

[1]Not FDA approved for this indication.

ASPIRIN

Previous studies did not support the routine use of aspirin to prevent thrombosis in PV. However, high doses of aspirin were used, resulting in excess bleeding in the treatment arm. The results of a recent large randomized trial show that low-dose aspirin reduces major thrombotic events (nonfatal myocardial infarction, nonfatal stroke, pulmonary embolism, major venous thrombosis). This was accomplished without an increase in bleeding risk. Although there was a trend suggesting more minor bleeding events in those receiving aspirin, the rates of major bleeding were identical for those receiving aspirin or placebo. The benefit from aspirin was seen even though this study included many low-risk patients without a prior history of thromboembolism. Low-dose aspirin (75-100 mg daily) should be started in all patients without a contraindication to the drug (history of bleeding or intolerance). Because of the risk of bleeding from acquired von Willebrand's disease that can occur with extreme thrombocytosis, aspirin should be held when platelets are more than 1500×10^9/L until the count can be lowered with hydroxyurea.

CYTOREDUCTIVE THERAPY

Hydroxyurea is the cytoreductive agent most commonly used to treat PV. Hydroxyurea can safely control blood counts and decreases spleen size in PV and other myeloproliferative disorders. Randomized data are limited, but hydroxyurea also appears to reduce thrombotic complications. It is recommended for patients with high-risk PV and should be considered in those with intermediate-risk disease. A starting dosage of 15 to 20 mg/kg daily (1000-1500 mg daily) is used. Occasional phlebotomy is still required to maintain hematocrit less than 45%, but the frequency usually decreases. Myelosuppression is the main toxicity. The lowest dosage that provides therapeutic effect should be used, and excess myelosuppression should be avoided. The dosage can be titrated to ensure that the white cell count remains higher than 3.0×10^9/L, neutrophils are higher than 2.0×10^9/L, and platelets are in the normal range.

Hydroxyurea has been associated with leg ulcers and other skin changes, especially after long-term use. There is growing evidence that hydroxyurea does not contribute to the excess rates of acute leukemia seen in PV; rates are no different than in those treated with phlebotomy alone. However, transformation is clearly associated with the use of other chemotherapeutic agents such as chlorambucil (Leukeran),[1] busulfan (Myleran),[1] and pipobroman (Vercyte),[2] accounting for one third of the deaths among PV patients treated with these agents. The use of these agents should be avoided.

OTHER TREATMENT ISSUES

Hyperuricemia is common in myeloproliferative disorders and occasionally results in kidney stones or gout. Allopurinol (Zyloprim) 300 mg daily can be used to reduce uric acid levels in patients with these complications. For those with intractable pruritus, several agents have been used with variable success. Some patients respond to aspirin,[1] hydroxyurea,[1] cimetidine (Tagamet),[1] or cyproheptadine (Periactin).[1] Interferon alfa-2b, 3 million units subcutaneously three times per week, is successful in the majority of cases, and success is also reported with paroxetine (Paxil)[1] 20 mg daily.

Less than 60% of pregnancies occurring in PV patients are successful. First trimester loss is the most common complication, and third trimester fetal loss, preterm birth, and intrauterine growth restriction are also common. Phlebotomy should be used to keep the hematocrit at less than 45%. Interferon alfa-2b[1] is recommended for those requiring cytoreductive therapy; other cytoreductive agents are contraindicated due to possible teratogenic effects. There is some evidence that the use of low-dose aspirin[1] throughout pregnancy improves live birth rate. It is recommended that prophylactic low-molecular-weight heparin (LMWH) be used for 6 weeks after delivery.

---

[1]Not FDA approved for this indication.
[2]Not available in the United States.

Surgery in patients with PV has a high risk of both operative bleeding and postoperative thromboembolism. Elective surgeries should be delayed until cytoreductive measures and phlebotomy can be used to achieve good control of blood counts. Aspirin should be held for 1 week before surgery to reduce the risk of hemorrhage. LMWH should be given after surgery to prevent deep venous thrombosis. Mechanical compression stockings are an option for patients with bleeding that prevents the use of anticoagulation.

Because cerebrovascular and cardiovascular disease are among the main causes of morbidity and mortality for these patients, careful attention should be paid to the management of conventional cardiovascular risk factors. Hypertension, diabetes, and hyperlipidemia should be controlled with standard measures, and patients should be encouraged to stop smoking.

When thromboembolic events do occur, treatment should be according to current management guidelines. Venous thromboembolism is treated with LMWH and warfarin (Coumadin). Indefinite anticoagulation should be considered because of the high risk of recurrent events. Low-dose aspirin is indicated in those with a history of arterial events such as stroke and myocardial infarction.

REFERENCES

Baxter EJ, Scott LM, Campbell PJ, et al. Acquired mutation of the tyrosine kinase JAK2 in human myeloproliferative disorders. Lancet 2005;365:1054–61.

Finazzi G, Barbui T. How I treat patients with polycythemia vera. Blood 2007;109:5104–11.

Finazzi G, Caruso V, Marchioli R, et al. for the ECLAP Investigators: Acute leukemia in polycythemia vera: An analysis of 1638 patients enrolled in a prospective observational study. Blood 2005;105(7):2664–70.

Fruchtman SM, Mack K, Kaplan ME, et al. From efficacy to safety: A polycythemia vera study group report on hydroxyurea in patients with polycythemia vera. Semin Hematol 1997;34:17–23.

Landolfi R, Marchioli R, Kutti J, et al. Efficacy and safety of low-dose aspirin in polycythemia vera. N Engl J Med 2004;350:114–24.

Marchioli R, Finazzi G, Landolfi R, et al. Vascular and neoplastic risk in a large cohort of patients with polycythemia vera. J Clin Oncol 2005;23(10):2224–32.

Najean Y, Mugnier P, Dresch C, Rain JD. Polycythemia vera in young people: An analysis of 58 cases diagnosed before 40 years. Br J Haematol 1987;67:285–91.

Robinson S, Bewley S, Hunt BJ, et al. The management and outcome of 18 pregnancies in women with polycythemia vera. Haematologica 2005;90 (11):1477–83.

Ruggeri M, Rodeghiero F, Tosetto A, et al. Postsurgery outcomes in patients with polycythemia vera and essential thrombocythemia: a retrospective survey. Blood 2008;111:666–71.

Silver RT. Long-term effects of the treatment of polycythemia vera with recombinant interferon-alpha. Cancer 2006;107(3):451–8.

Swerdlow S, Campo E, Lee Harris N, et al, editors. WHO Classification of Tumors of Hematopoietic and Lymphoid Tissues. 4th ed. Lyon, France: IARC; 2008.

Porphyrias

Method of
Claus A. Pierach, MD

The *porphyrias* present a group of mostly inherited diseases where disturbances along the biosynthetic pathway to heme lead to accumulations of metabolic intermediaries. Porphyria cutanea tarda usually occurs without discernible inheritance; it can also be induced by chemicals. All steps of heme synthesis are enzymatically regulated and all porphyrias are a result of specific impasses along these transitions. Not all enzymatic defects result in clinically relevant or recognizable disease manifestations in every patient. On the one hand, the severity of the enzymatic defect plays a role. On the other, some poorly understood revealing or unveiling cofactors are operational; enzyme cofactors are likely contributing as well. The prevalence of the porphyrias is not known and fluctuates in different parts of the world; for example, variegate porphyria is most common in South Africa, whereas porphyria cutanea tarda is the most common porphyria in the United States.

The porphyrias can be divided between neurovisceral (acute) and cutaneous manifestations. Two types, the very rare delta-aminolevulinic acid-dehydratase deficiency porphyria and acute intermittent porphyria (AIP), have only neurologic symptoms (acute attacks and possibly chronic manifestations). Hereditary coproporphyria and variegate porphyria can have both neurologic and dermatologic signs and symptoms. Congenital erythropoietic porphyria, porphyria cutanea tarda, and erythropoietic protoporphyria exhibit only skin lesions but can be complicated by other problems, such as anemia or hepatic insufficiency.

Heme Synthesis

Succinyl coenzyme-A and glycine are the initial building blocks, subsequently transformed through eight enzymatic steps to the end product, heme, in itself essential not only for hemoglobin but also for other hemoproteins such as cytochromes, myoglobin, and other enzymes including catalase, nitric oxide synthase, and tryptophan pyrrolase. Heme synthesis happens in all cells but mostly in the liver and in the bone marrow. It is controlled by heme through feedback inhibition of the first step, delta-aminolevulinic acid synthase. Figure 1 shows the various steps, intermediaries, and resulting porphyrias. Porphyrins and their precursors, delta-aminolevulinic acid

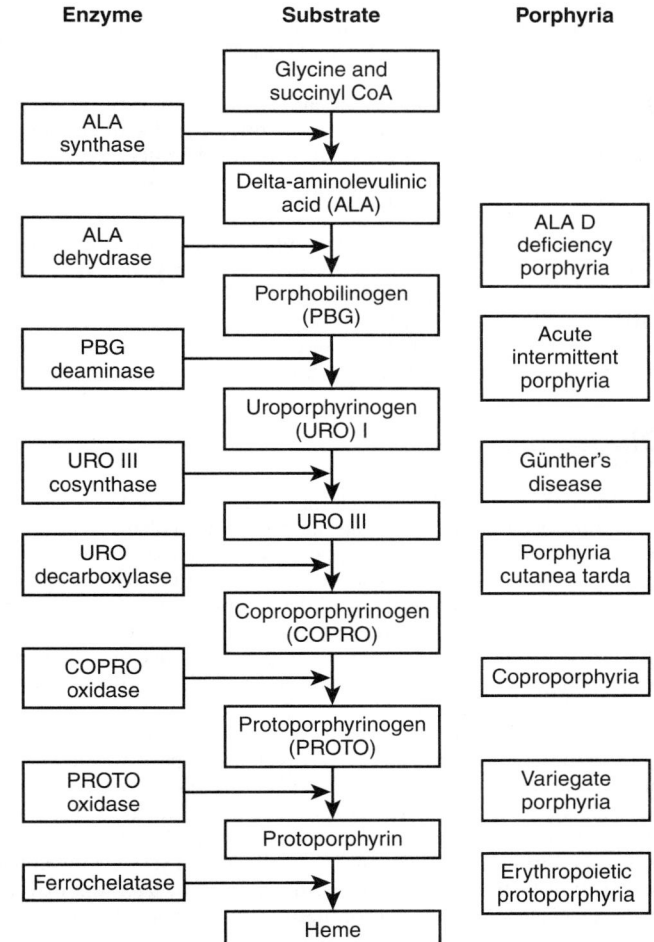

FIGURE 1. Heme biosynthetic pathway. Enzymes that have defects or deficiencies that cause the various porphyries are listed on the left side, heme and precursors are in the middle, and the resulting porphyrias are on the right side. *Abbreviation:* CoA = coenzyme A.

(ALA) and porphobilinogen (PBG), are only generated during heme synthesis and not during heme catabolism toward bilirubin.

Specific enzymatic defects result in specific patterns of heme precursors and are of high diagnostic value when determining the type of porphyria. The ultimate step in ruling in or out if a person has the genetic defect for a specific porphyria is DNA testing, currently offered by the Mount Sinai Genetic Testing Laboratory (porphyria@mssm.edu). However, these specific tests are not necessary in the clinical evaluation of a patient in whom porphyria is suspected. Here, quick and simple tests are sufficient. The excretory pattern of heme precursors is influenced by their water solubility, which decreases toward heme; ALA and PBG are highly water soluble and measured in urine, whereas protoporphyrin is so hydrophobic that it is only excreted in stool and not in urine.

There is no single test that can reveal all types of porphyrias. The porphyric symptomatology can differ from type to type and there is considerable overlap among the various porphyrias. For this reason, highly specific and sensitive laboratory tests are necessary. All porphyrias with acute manifestations manifest with similar attacks and respond to similar treatment, but they exhibit different biochemical patterns according to their specific enzyme defect. A clinically useful grouping splits the porphyrias between acute (neurovisceral) and cutaneous.

The Acute Porphyrias

There are four types of acute porphyria to consider:

- The very rare ALA-dehydratase deficiency porphyria is inherited in an autosomal recessive fashion.
- AIP, an autosomal dominant disorder, is the most common of the acute porphyrias (except in South Africa where variegate porphyria is more common).
- Hereditary coproporphyria, an autosomal dominant disease, is commonly misdiagnosed because coproporphyrin is often moderately and nonspecifically increased in many disorders.
- Variegate porphyria is autosomal dominant and probably the mildest of the acute porphyrias.

All acute porphyrias are sensitive to a multitude of drugs and circumstances (a short list is included in Box 1). Hereditary coproporphyria and variegate porphyria can also have skin lesions resembling porphyria cutanea tarda. Skin lesions and acute attacks can happen at the same time or one after the other, or only one manifestation may ever be present in a given patient.

Diagnosis

Diagnosis of the porphyric attack hinges mainly on a keen sense of suspicion. Any inexplicable symptom complex involving abdominal pain, tachycardia, and psychological findings should be suspect for porphyria. However, no clinical presentation can be called *porphyric* without biochemical support. Small deviations from the narrow normal range for heme precursors are fairly common and nonspecific. PBG or ALA must be markedly elevated, at least fivefold above the normal range, and, if not, porphyria is an unlikely explanation for a patient's acute symptoms.

Older screening mechanisms such as the Watson-Schwartz test and the Hoesch test have been replaced by easier, more specific, semiquantitative tests such as the Trace PBG kit (Thermo Fisher Scientific), but they still rely on the color reaction with Ehrlich's aldehyde. This or a similar test must be available in all emergency departments and in all acute care hospitals. A *random* urine sample is sufficient for the initial diagnostic evaluation, and if it is positive it must be later followed up by more-detailed tests such as quantitative measurements of porphyrins and precursors in a 24-hour urine collection. Fecal porphyrin measurements may also be called for. Enzyme measurements and genetic testing are rarely indicated, but they are used when more routine tests fail. Because the porphyrias are almost always hereditary, family studies are highly appropriate. The proper interpretation of any test result is best done in the context of available clinical information.

 CURRENT DIAGNOSIS

- There is not just one porphyria; there are at least six types (and a few very rare ones because of homozygosity and dual porphyrias).
- There is not one single test covering all porphyrias. For suspected acute porphyria, screening for excessive porphobilinogen in the urine is the test of choice.
- If cutaneous porphyria is in the differential diagnosis, quantitative measurements of porphyrins in urine and stool are recommended.
- Family studies and genetic counseling are always indicated in these hereditary diseases.

Clinical Presentation

Clinical presentations of porphyric attacks vary so much that the term *the little imitator* has been used. Not all signs or symptoms are always present, but severe and poorly localized abdominal pain and unexplained tachycardia are so prevalent that their absence further complicates the diagnosis of an acute porphyric attack. The genesis of the attack is not well understood, but acutely increased demand for heme and production of toxic intermediary products are considered to be the culprit. Increased demand for heme and increased production of intermediary products can be due to a wide variety of circumstances, from drugs through hormones (premenstrual phase) to stress, infection, fasting, and starvation. However, most carriers of the genetic defect for an acute porphyria remain asymptomatic all their lives. Some have only one or two attacks, and only a few suffer from many attacks.

The clinical picture with pain, fast heart rate, and neurovisceral symptoms can be complicated by, at times, severe hyponatremia, heralding seizures with therapeutic dilemmas (see Box 1) and respiratory paralysis necessitating ventilatory support. Death is rare nowadays, especially when the diagnosis is made early. The recovery is usually complete, but at times it is prolonged, up to 1 year after a severe attack.

Superb nursing care, initially preferable in an intensive care unit, is necessary, and meticulous attention has to be paid to *all* problems. Dehydration from vomiting is common and ileus and urinary retention are not infrequent; hyponatremia occurs in approximately half of the porphyric attacks. Muscle strength must be tested frequently. Twice-daily measurement of vital capacity helps to assess the necessity for respiratory assistance. High blood pressure and tachycardia deserve careful attention and, if appropriate, cautious treatment with a β-blocker. A negative caloric balance must be avoided, and if present initially it is best treated with carbohydrates (if necessary, intravenously with glucose, up to 300 g/day), and then later with a balanced diet.

Treatment

Therapy must always start with a careful look at the drugs recently taken by the patient. It is best to discontinue as many drugs as possible, especially those deemed unsafe (see Box 1). Appropriate lists of safe and unsafe drugs in porphyria are readily available from websites (www.porphyriafoundation.com and www.porphyria-europe.com). An infection must be diligently searched for and treated at once. Seizure precautions are especially indicated if hyponatremia is found. Analgesics should be adequately dispensed; opiates are often necessary in fairly large doses.

Specific therapy was introduced a generation ago in the form of hematin (hemin, Panhematin), available from Lundbeck Inc. (847-282-1000 or www.lundbeckinc.com). This has largely replaced glucose (300 g/day), which had the main advantages of availability, relatively low cost, and the possibility of curbing an early or mild attack.

CURRENT THERAPY

- Prophylaxis is mandatory and depends on the type of porphyria.
- Abstinence from alcohol is always indicated.
- The drug list should be respected in the acute porphyrias.
- Glucose therapy for the acute attack has been superseded by the more effective, definitive treatment with hematin (hemin, Panhematin), to be instituted as soon as possible once the diagnosis has been ascertained.

But one must not wait for quick improvement in a patient's condition and should at once take steps to obtain the definitive medication, hematin. This represents the equivalent to the end product, heme, and exerts its beneficial effect through repression of the deranged, and in the porphyric attack, markedly activated pathway to heme. It is still unclear whether the quick suppression of potentially toxic heme precursors (in 1-2 days) or a postulated replenishment of an assumed heme deficiency is the effective mechanism. *Early* administration of hematin is strongly advocated because the course of a porphyric attack is unpredictable, and a point of no return can unfortunately be reached quickly. Thus, the infusion of hematin must start as soon as possible.

A daily dose of 2 to 4 mg/kg body weight is recommended for up to 4 days. Longer treatment periods are of questionable value but may be tried in severe cases for up to 2 weeks. The infusion must be strictly intravenous and with ample flushing because hematin can cause thrombosis and phlebitis. Because it is a procoagulant and anticoagulant, frequent measurements of coagulation parameters are advisable. Anticoagulants such as warfarin (Coumadin) should if possible be avoided. Admixture of 5% human serum albumin (Albuminar-5) has been advocated to stabilize the final hematin solution and to lessen side effects. Hematin is available in many countries as heme arginate (Normosang).[2]

A beneficial clinical effect can be expected in 1 to 2 days, accompanied by a decrease in all heme precursors, most notably ALA and PBG. Many patients have received many treatment courses with hematin without apparent loss of effectiveness. Prophylactic use of hematin can be helpful in the treatment of women with frequent premenstrual exacerbations of their acute porphyria. Hematin should never be given as a diagnostic test to see if unexplained symptoms reminiscent of porphyria lessen. The diagnosis of a porphyric attack must be as quick, precise, and certain as possible, especially in new cases.

Partial liver transplantation has been successfully undertaken and found to be curative in patients with unrelenting porphyric attacks.

Prophylaxis of porphyric attacks is of great importance and can be accomplished to a large extent by avoidance of unsafe drugs, by stable caloric intake, and by prompt attention to intercurrent illnesses. It is a difficult decision if unsafe drugs have to be administered for a vital indication such as seizures. Here, consultation with an expert in porphyria is strongly advised.

The Cutaneous Porphyrias

The symptomatology of cutaneous porphyrias is mainly photosensitivity, often combined with skin fragility and blisters. All these findings occur because of porphyrin toxicity, resulting in cutaneous light absorption at the wavelength of 400 to 410 nm and subsequent formation of damaging reactive oxygen species. Thus, two therapeutic approaches are plausible: decrease of porphyrins and protection of the skin from sunlight. The usual sunscreens are, however, ineffective, and reflective agents containing zinc or titanium, although better, are less popular because of their appearance.

In three porphyrias—porphyria cutanea tarda, hereditary coproporphyria, and variegate porphyria—the skin lesions are rather similar, but erythropoietic protoporphyria and congenital erythropoietic porphyria can lead to very painful nonblistering skin lesions, and, in congenital erythropoietic porphyria, even to mutilations.

PORPHYRIA CUTANEA TARDA

Porphyria cutanea tarda is the most common porphyria and occurs because of uroporphyrinogen-decarboxylase deficiency and accumulation of mostly uroporphyrin. It can be inherited autosomal dominantly but more often occurs sporadically. It can also be due to toxins such as halogenated aromatic hydrocarbons.

---

[2]Not available in the United States.

The most prominent skin manifestations are seen on the dorsa of the hands and on the face, consisting of blisters filled with mostly clear fluid; shallow, slow-healing ulcers; whitish plaques; and tiny inclusion bodies, *milia*. Hypertrichosis and hyperpigmentation are often seen.

Unveiling factors promote the manifestation of the disease and consist mainly of liver disease, often due to alcohol. Hepatitis, often type C, and HIV infections are also common revealers. The drug list (see Box 1) is *not* applicable to the cutaneous porphyrias. The diagnosis is easily suspected at inspection and confirmed by measurement of urinary uroporphyrin excretion, typically manifold increased above the normal range.

There are two treatment options with different principles but rather similar effectiveness. Repeat phlebotomies of 350 to 450 mL at 1- to 2-week intervals are performed and followed by hemoglobin and ferritin measurements. Overt anemia should be avoided. Ferritin usually reaches the lower end of the normal range after approximately 8 to 10 phlebotomies, and clinical remission can be expected after approximately half a year. Remission can be long lasting, especially when unveiling factors are avoided; total abstinence from alcohol is advocated. Patients should not take iron-enriched vitamins because iron plays a critical role in porphyria cutanea tarda.

If phlebotomies are contraindicated (due to anemia or pulmonary or cardiac disease) or are very inconvenient, low-dose chloroquine (Aralen)[1] (125 mg twice weekly) can be given orally. This flushes porphyrins from the liver and can be continued until remission is reached. In such low doses, the drug is virtually free from side effects.

Patients on chronic dialysis can develop porphyria cutanea tarda and also *pseudoporphyria*. Here, plasma porphyrin measurements establish the correct diagnosis. Patients with porphyria cutanea tarda and end-stage renal disease respond well to erythropoietin (Epogen, Procrit),[1] probably via iron depletion through incorporation of iron into hemoglobin. Pseudoporphyria is also seen as a side effect of many drugs, mostly nonsteroidal antiinflammatory drugs and diuretics. Although it is phenotypically identical to porphyria cutanea tarda, pseudoporphyria does not respond to phlebotomies or chloroquine.

Patients with porphyria cutanea tarda have a much higher incidence of hepatocellular carcinoma and should be checked twice annually with hepatic imaging and measurement of alpha fetoprotein.

CONGENITAL ERYTHROPOIETIC PORPHYRIA (GÜNTHER DISEASE)

Congenital erythropoietic porphyria (Günther disease), a rare autosomal recessive disorder, is usually apparent shortly after birth when brick-colored urine in diapers is observed because of excessive amounts of uroporphyrin (even more impressive under UV light). This porphyria and the rare homozygous porphyria cutanea tarda, hepatoerythropoietic porphyria, can be progressive and severely mutilating. Therapy is limited to sun protection and blood transfusion if hemolytic anemia is present.

ERYTHROPOIETIC PROTOPORPHYRIA

Erythropoietic protoporphyria is an autosomal dominant disorder due to a deficiency of ferrochelatase, the last enzyme in heme biosynthesis. Urinary porphyrins are normal, but protoporphyrin is markedly elevated in red cells and in stool. These patients suffer from instantly painful sun sensitivity, followed by edema and wrinkles in the thickened, light-exposed skin. In contrast to porphyria cutanea tarda, blisters are not seen here. Approximately one fifth of these patients develop progressive liver disease secondary to hepatic accumulation of protoporphyrin. Liver transplantation can become necessary.

Therapy is often beneficial with oral β-carotene[1] (up to 400 mg/day for adults). This leads to a harmless slight orange-yellow discoloration of the skin and often effective sun protection. Ideally, the β-carotene dose should be adjusted to a plasma level between 11 and 15 mmol/L.

---

[1]Not FDA approved for this indication.

REFERENCES

American Porphyria Foundation. Home page. Available at: http://www.porphyriafoundation.com; [accessed 10.07.10].

Anderson KE, Bonkovsky HL, Bloomer JR, Shedlofsky SI. Reconstitution of hematin for intravenous infusion. Ann Intern Med 2006;144:537–8.

Anderson KE, Bloomer JR, Bonkovsky HL, et al. Recommendations for the diagnosis and treatment of the acute porphyrias. Ann Intern Med 2005;142:439–50.

Anderson KE, Sassa S, Bishop DF, et al. Disorders of heme biosynthesis: X-linked sideroblastic anemia and the porphyrias. In: Scriver CR, Beaudet AL, Sly WS, et al, editors. The Molecular and Metabolic Bases of Inherited Disease, vol. 1. 8th ed. New York: McGraw-Hill; 2001. pp. 2961–3062.

Badminton MN, Elder GH. Management of acute and cutaneous porphyrias. Int J Clin Pract 2002;56:272–8.

Chemmanur AT, Bonkovsky HL. Hepatic porphyrias: Diagnosis and management. Clin Liver Dis 2004;8:807–38.

European Porphyria Initiative. Home page. Available at: http://www.porphyria-europe.com/; [accessed 10.07.10].

Kauppinen R. Porphyrias. Lancet 2005;365:241–52.

Puy H, Gouya L, Deybach JC. Porphyrias. Lancet 2010;375:924–37.

Therapeutic Use of Blood Components

Method of
Peter A. Millward, MD, and Mark E. Brecher, MD

The transfusion of blood was the first successful transplantation of living tissue in humans. Today, transfusion is so commonplace that it is rarely thought of as a transplant. In 2001, for allogeneic transfusions within the United States alone, it is estimated that 13,898,000 units of whole blood or red blood cells, 2,614,000 units of whole blood–derived platelets, 1,264,000 units of apheresis platelets, and 3,926,000 units of plasma were administered. For red blood cell–containing products alone, this equates to 1 unit transfused every 2.3 seconds. A basic understanding of indications for blood component therapy is essential to optimally treat patients.

Red Blood Cells

Red blood cells are collected via whole blood donation or automated erythrocytapheresis. Both collection techniques employ a sterile closed system for blood collection. The blood is collected into plastic blood bags containing a sufficient formulation of anticoagulant and preservative solution.

The components of the anticoagulant solution determine the maximum shelf life (ranging from 21 to 35 days) of collected blood and blood components. The solution can contain citrate (trisodium citrate and citric acid), dextrose, phosphate (monobasic sodium phosphate), and adenine. Citrate is for anticoagulation, dextrose and adenine are for metabolic energy, and phosphate is for buffering pH.

Shelf life of red cells may be extended to 42 days with the addition of an preservative-additive solution, such as Adsol (AS-1), Nutricel (AS-3), or Optisol (AS-5). This additive solution must be added within 72 hours from primary collection. Additive solution contains dextrose, adenine, and sodium chloride and contains either monobasic sodium phosphate or mannitol.

Even with anticoagulant and preservative-additive solutions, biochemical changes, called storage lesions, develop with stored red blood cells. These biochemical changes are decreased pH, adenosine triphosphate (ATP), and 2,3-diphosphoglycerate (DPG) and increased plasma potassium and plasma hemoglobin (Hb). Even in massively transfused patients, storage lesions do not routinely cause significant clinical consequences when transfused.

The standard collection volume for a whole blood donation is 450 mL ± 45 mL. Because whole blood is rarely indicated, centrifugation is used to separate a whole-blood donation into various components, which maximizes this limited resource. One red blood cell (RBC) unit, also known as *packed RBCs*, is made by removing a significant portion of plasma from a whole-blood donation. Using apheresis technique, one or two RBC units can be specifically collected with each donation. With either technique, an RBC unit volume is approximately 300 mL. Based on the preservative-additive solution used, an RBC unit averages a hematocrit of 60% to 80%.

After initial processing of whole blood, an RBC unit is composed of RBCs, white blood cells (WBCs), platelets, and plasma. An erythrocytapheresis RBC unit is composed of RBCs with decreased platelets and plasma and are *leukocyte reduced* ($<5 \times 10^6$ leukocytes per component) due to intraprocedural leukocyte filtration.

RBC units can be further modified for specific needs of the patient to leukoreduced RBCs, washed RBCs, irradiated RBCs, and frozen deglycerolized RBCs.

LEUKOREDUCED RED BLOOD CELLS

In the United States, a leukoreduced RBC unit must have less than 5 million leukocytes per unit. This decrease in leukocytes is achieved using a leukocyte filter that extracts leukocytes based on their relative larger size and propensity to adhere to certain fiber types. Current leukoreduction filters remove between 3 and 5 log of leukocytes in an RBC unit. Leukocyte filtration can occur during or immediately after collection (prestorage leukocyte reduction) or at the time of transfusion (poststorage leukocyte reduction).

Common indications for leukoreduced RBCs are multiple febrile, nonhemolytic transfusion reactions (FNHTR), prevention of HLA alloimmunization, and reduction of cytomegalovirus (CMV) transmission.

An FNHTR is defined by a greater than 1°C (2°F) temperature rise occurring up to 2 hours after transfusion and unexplained by the patient's underlying medical condition; it may be accompanied by chills, rigors, nausea, vomiting, malaise, and headache. Two mechanisms of FNHTR with RBC transfusion have been proposed: recipient anti-HLA or antigranulocyte antibodies react with donor leukocytes and induce cytokine release, or donor leukocytes form an antigen-antibody complex resulting in recipient monocytes to release cytokines. Both mechanisms depend on the presence of donor leukocytes, and therefore leukoreduction effectively decreases the incidence of FNHTR associated with red blood cell transfusions.

The formation of HLA antibodies (also known as HLA alloimmunization) can lead to platelet transfusion refractoriness, which is especially problematic for patients requiring substantial platelet transfusion support (e.g., hematology-oncology patients). All potential candidates for bone marrow (BMT) or solid organ transplantation should receive leukoreduced RBCs to minimize the formation of HLA antibodies.

Transfusion-transmitted CMV (TT-CMV) infections in high-risk populations, such as CMV-negative neonates, AIDS patients, and BMT candidates or patients, are associated with considerable mortality and morbidity. CMV is latent in leukocytes, specifically in the monocyte-macrophage lineage. Based on Bowden and colleagues' findings in 1995, leukoreduced RBCs offer a CMV-safe blood product that is an equivalent alternative to providing blood from a CMV-seronegative donor. These findings and other confirming studies led to numerous institutions using leukoreduced RBCs as their sole method for providing CMV-safe blood products and abandoning a CMV-seronegative inventory. Recently, Nicholas and colleagues questioned the equivalence of leukoreduced blood products versus CMV-seronegative blood products and called for further investigation.

WASHED RED BLOOD CELLS

The objective of washing RBCs is to effectively remove 99% of antibodies, plasma proteins, and electrolytes contained within the RBC component. The washing process involves repetitive steps of infusion of normal (0.9%) saline and centrifugation, with final resuspension of washed RBCs in normal saline. Because this process is an open system and the anticoagulant-preservative solution is removed, washed red cells must be transfused within 24 hours. This process can be automated or achieved with a manual technique, leading to up to 20% red cell loss. Approximately 20% to 90% of the platelets and 90% of the leukocytes are removed during this procedure. This decrease in leukocytes is not effective enough to render the component leukoreduced ($<5 \times 10^6$ leukocytes per unit).

Common indications for washed RBCs are recurrent severe allergic reactions not controlled with antihistamines and immunoglobulin A (IgA) deficiency. Washed RBCs also reduce the potassium load of the product. IgA-deficient patients can develop anti-IgA antibodies that react to donor IgA in plasma and lead to anaphylaxis. Potassium accumulates in the plasma during storage of the RBC unit or following irradiation.

IRRADIATED RED BLOOD CELLS

The goal of irradiation is to prevent proliferation of transfused immunocompetent T lymphocytes. This goal is accomplished by using cesium-137 or cobalt-60 as a radiation source, which administers a dose of 2500 cGy (25 Gy or 2500 rad) to the central portion of the RBC unit and a minimum of 1500 cGy to all other areas of the component. Due to decreased survival and viability of the RBCs and increased potassium leakage, irradiated RBCs expire on their original assigned outdate or 28 days after irradiation, whichever occurs first.

The only indication for the irradiated RBCs is to prevent transfusion-associated graft-versus-host disease (TA-GVHD). TA-GVHD is a rare, fatal complication (mortality >90%) caused by the engraftment and proliferation of donor T lymphocytes in the transfused recipient. Irradiated RBCs are indicated for patients receiving hematopoietic stem cell or bone marrow transplantation, patients with congenital immunodeficiency syndromes, intrauterine transfusions, neonates, HLA-matched platelet transfusions, patients with Hodgkin's disease, and patients with chronic lymphocytic leukemia treated with purine analogues (e.g., fludarabine [Fludara]).

Patients receiving transfusions from first-degree relatives require irradiation because of the increased risk of TA-GVHD due to HLA similarity of donor and recipient.

FROZEN RED BLOOD CELLS

The purpose of frozen RBCs is to store units with rare blood types and autologous units for extended periods of time (routinely up to 10 years, but storage may be extended for certain circumstances). Before freezing the RBCs, glycerol, a cryoprotective agent, is added to the system, which allows freezing of the red cells without damage. Based on the concentration of glycerol used (~20% or ~40%), the storage temperatures vary. Most commonly in the United States, 40% glycerol is used, and therefore the frozen RBCs are stored at −65°C.

Frozen RBCs must be deglycerolized before transfusion. Washing the product in saline solutions of progressively decreasing osmolarity achieves glycerol removal. During the process, 99.9% of the plasma along with the vast majority of WBCs and platelets are removed. Depending on the technique used to deglycerolize the RBCs, once deglycerolized, these units have a 24-hour (open system) or 14-day (closed system) shelf life.

Frozen RBCs are indicated for heavily alloimmunized patients (e.g., multiple clinically significant RBC antigens) who require rare phenotypic RBCs for compatible transfusions.

Due to the multiple washing steps in the deglycerolized procedure, these units can be considered equivalent to a washed RBC unit.

INDICATIONS FOR RED BLOOD CELL TRANSFUSION

The purpose of RBC transfusions is to provide oxygen-carrying capacity and to maintain tissue oxygenation when the intravascular volume and cardiac function are adequate for perfusion. In a 70-kg recipient, 1 unit of transfused RBCs should increase the hemoglobin by 1 g/dL and the hematocrit by 3%. To obtain the same expected response in a pediatric patient, the RBC transfusion dose should be

15 mL/kg. RBC transfusions should only be used when time or underlying pathophysiology precludes other management (e.g., iron, erythropoietin, folic acid [folate]).

Criteria for administering RBC transfusions include:

- Hb <8 g/dL in an otherwise healthy patient
- Hb <11 g/dL in cases of increased risk of ischemia (e.g., pulmonary disease, coronary artery disease, cerebral vascular disease)
- Acute blood loss >15% of total blood volume (e.g., 750 mL in 70-kg man) or with evidence of inadequate oxygen delivery (e.g., electrocardiographic signs of cardiac ischemia, tachycardia, cyanosis)
- Symptomatic anemia in a normovolemic patient (e.g., tachycardia, mental status changes, electrocardiographic signs of cardiac ischemia, angina, shortness of breath, lightheadedness or dizziness with mild exertion)
- Regular predetermined therapeutic program for severe hypoplastic or aplastic anemia or for bone marrow suppression for hemoglobinopathies

The post-transfusion hemoglobin should not exceed 11.5 g/dL (12.5 g/dL in cases of increased risk of organ or tissue ischemia). Attempts to increase wound healing or merely to take advantage of available predonated autologous blood without a valid medical indication are not acceptable uses for RBC transfusions.

Platelets

Platelets are often a limited resource because of their relatively short shelf life and the inability to stockpile this product through freezing techniques. Temperature, pH, and gas exchange are critical issues for platelet viability and function, and they all determine the storage shelf life. Platelets remain viable for up to 7 days after collection, but the current 5-day shelf life has been instituted because of increased rates of clinically significant bacterial contamination on days 6 and 7. At a temperature lower than 20°C, platelets can be damaged and become nonfunctional. Platelets must be maintained at room temperature (20°–24°C) with gentle agitation in gas-permeable bags. Gas-permeable bags are required for platelet storage to ensure proper oxygenation and facilitate removal of carbon dioxide buildup. Constant gentle agitation is required to facilitate this gas exchange.

At present, two methods to obtain platelets are employed in the United States. First, platelets may be prepared from whole blood donations via centrifugation separation. These platelets are commonly referred to as *platelet concentrates, random donor platelets*, or *whole blood–derived platelets*. One platelet concentrate can be manufactured from a single whole blood donation. This platelet concentrate should have 5.5×10^{10} platelets per unit in 40 to 70 mL of plasma. One platelet concentrate should increase the platelet count by 7 to 10×10^9/L in a 70-kg recipient. Therefore, general platelet-concentrate dosing consists of a pool of 4 to 6 platelet concentrates, also known as a *four-pack* or *six-pack*, respectively. Second, platelets may be prepared using apheresis technology. These products are called *apheresis platelets, single-donor platelets*, or *platelet pheresis*.

Due to current apheresis technology, most apheresis platelets are leukoreduced at the time of collection. Apheresis platelets should have 3.0×10^{11} platelets per unit in 300 to 500 mL of plasma. One apheresis unit should increase the platelet count by 40 to 60 $\times$ 10^9/L in a 70-kg recipient.

One apheresis platelet product has an equivalent dose of a six-pack of platelet concentrates. In the United States, the use of apheresis platelets has been increasing annually. In 2004, it was estimated that 77% of all therapeutic doses of platelets transfused were apheresis platelets.

Once a platelet component is collected, it may be further modified in the same manner as RBCs: leukoreduced, washed, or irradiated.

LEUKOREDUCED PLATELETS

As with leukoreduced RBCs, common indications for leukoreduced platelets are multiple FNHTRs, prevention of human leukocyte antigen (HLA) alloimmunization, and reduction of CMV transmission.

The proposed mechanisms by which leukoreduction prevents these conditions are discussed in the leukoreduced RBCs section. These mechanisms are the same with one exception. FNHTRs with RBCs are associated with an active release of cytokines induced by leukocyte-antibody interaction. The mechanism of FNHTRs with platelets differs and is due to passively transfused cytokines. At room temperature, residual donor leukocytes release cytokines that accumulate during storage. Therefore, prestorage leukocyte reduction is the only effective way to prevent FNHTR with platelet transfusions because the leukocytes are removed before releasing their cytokines.

It has been determined that cytokine accumulation does not occur if a blood product is refrigerated, which explains why both prestorage and poststorage RBC leukoreductions prevent FNHTRs.

WASHED PLATELETS

As with RBCs, the goal of washing platelets is to effectively remove 99% of antibodies, plasma proteins, and electrolytes contained within the component. The process involves washing platelets with normal saline or saline buffered with ACD-A (acid citrate dextrose) or citrate. This process can be achieved via automated or manual technique, leading to approximately 33% platelet loss. Once a platelet component is washed, it must be transfused within 4 hours because it is now an open system with removed anticoagulant-preservative solution at room temperature. This differs from washed RBCs that have a 24-hour shelf life after washing.

The two most common indications for washed platelets are recurrent severe allergic or anaphylactic reactions and IgA-deficiency in patients with IgA antibodies.

IRRADIATED PLATELETS

As with RBCs, the objective of irradiating platelets is to prevent immunocompetent T lymphocytes from proliferating and leading to TA-GVHD in the transfused recipient. The current dose (2500 cGy to the central portion of the unit and 1500 cGy to other portions of the unit) inactivates the T lymphocytes within the product and achieves this goal without significantly altering platelet function during their maximum shelf life.

Indications for irradiated platelets are the same as for irradiated RBCs: hematopoietic stem cell or BMT patients, congenital immunodeficiency syndrome patients, intrauterine transfusions, neonates, HLA-matched platelet transfusions, Hodgkin's disease patients, and chronic lymphocytic leukemia patients treated with purine analogues (e.g., fludarabine).

Patients receiving transfusions from first-degree relatives require irradiation because of the increased risk of TA-GVHD due to HLA similarity of donor and recipient.

INDICATIONS FOR PLATELET TRANSFUSION

Criteria for instituting a platelet transfusion include:

- Platelet count $<10 \times 10^9$/L for prophylaxis in a stable, nonfebrile patient
- Platelet count $<20 \times 10^9$/L for prophylaxis with fever or instability
- Platelet count $<50 \times 10^9$/L in a patient with documented hemorrhage or rapidly decreasing platelet count or planned invasive or surgical procedure
- Diffuse microvascular bleeding in a patient with disseminated intravascular coagulation or following a massive blood loss (>1 blood volume) with a platelet count not yet available
- Bleeding in a patient with platelet dysfunction

It is unacceptable to empirically transfuse platelets for a massively transfused patient not exhibiting a clinical coagulopathy or for extrinsic platelet dysfunction (e.g., renal failure, hyperproteinemia, or von Willebrand's disease). Platelet transfusion is contraindicated in thrombotic thrombocytopenic purpura (TTP), hemolytic-uremic syndrome (HUS), or idiopathic thrombocytopenic purpura (ITP) unless the patient is experiencing life-threatening bleeding or coagulopathy.

PLATELET REFRACTORINESS

Both nonimmune and immune causes lead to poor platelet increment following transfusion. To accurately assess response to platelet transfusion, a post-transfusion platelet count should be obtained 10 to 60 minutes after the transfusion is complete. If the patient does not respond appropriately, platelet refractoriness must be considered.

Platelet refractoriness is defined as failure to achieve an appropriate post-transfusion response on more than one occasion. A post-transfusion corrected count increment (CCI) can be calculated to more accurately assess refractoriness. The CCI is calculated as follows:

$$CCI = \frac{(\text{Post-transfusion count} - \text{Pretransfusion count}) \times \text{Body surface area}}{\text{Platelets tranfused} \times 10^{11}}$$

where platelet counts are in microliters and body surface area is in square meters. A CCI less than 5000 (using a 10- to 60-minute post-transfusion platelet count) on two separate occasions is consistent with platelet refractoriness.

The most common causes for poor platelet increments are nonimmune causes, including splenomegaly, bleeding, fever, sepsis, and disseminated intravascular coagulation (DIC). If refractoriness is determined to be nonimmune in etiology, management often consists of increasing the dose or frequency (or both) of transfused platelets. HLA alloimmunization is the primary cause of immune-mediated platelet refractoriness. Other immune-mediated causes for poor platelet increment are anti–platelet-specific antibodies, drug-induced antibodies, and immune or idiopathic thrombocytopenia purpura (ITP). If HLA alloimmunization is the cause, three common treatment options can be employed:

- Give platelets that are platelet crossmatch compatible with recipient plasma
- Provide HLA antigen-negative platelets (for the identified HLA antibodies)
- Give HLA matched (class I: HLA A and HLA B) platelets

Plasma

FROZEN PLASMA

Platelet-poor plasma is obtained by centrifugation and separation of a whole-blood donation or direct collection with apheresis technique. If this plasma is frozen at −18°C within 8 hours of original collection, the product contains adequate levels of all labile (factor V and factor VIII) and nonlabile coagulation factors and is called *fresh frozen plasma* (FFP). If this plasma is frozen at −18°C for more than 8 hours but within 24 hours from original collection, the product contains adequate levels of all nonlabile and decreased levels of labile coagulation factors and is called *plasma frozen within 24 hours*. Both types of plasma units have a volume of approximately 220 mL, and both can be stored for 12 months at −18°C.

These products are indicated for the correction of multiple or specific coagulation factor deficiencies or for the empiric treatment of TTP or HUS. The usual starting dose is 5 to 15 mL/kg (2 to 4 units in a 70-kg recipient).

INDICATIONS FOR PLASMA TRANSFUSION

Criteria for implementing a plasma infusion include:

- Treatment or prophylaxis of multiple or specific coagulation factor deficiencies (PT and/or PTT >1.5 times the mean normal value)
- Congenital coagulation factor deficiencies (antithrombin III; factors II, V, VII, IX, X, and XI; plasminogen; antiplasmin)
- Acquired coagulation factor deficiencies related to warfarin (Coumadin) therapy, vitamin K deficiency, liver disease, massive transfusion (>1 blood volume in 24 h), and disseminated intravascular coagulation
- Patients with a suspected coagulation deficiency (PT/PTT pending) who are bleeding, or at risk of bleeding, from an invasive procedure

Unacceptable criteria are empiric use during massive transfusion in which the patient does not exhibit clinical coagulopathy, nutritional supplementation, or volume replacement. There is little evidence to support prophylactic plasma infusion in patients with mild prolongation of the prothrombin time (<1.5 times the mean normal value).

CRYOPRECIPITATE

Cryoprecipitate is a cold insoluble fraction of FFP that precipitates when FFP is thawed at 4°C. A unit of cryoprecipitate contains approximately 10 mL, which can be stored for 12 months at −18°C. Each unit contains approximately 80 to 100 U of factor VIII and 250 mg of fibrinogen, along with factor XIII, von Willebrand's factor, and fibronectin.

The usual starting dose is one unit per 7 to 10 kg, and therefore multiple units must be pooled for a therapeutic dose. Once pooled, cryoprecipitate must be transfused within 4 hours. In a 70-kg man, 14 units would be expected to raise the fibrinogen 100 mg/dL. Cryoprecipitate (2–4 units) may also be applied topically, with an equal volume of bovine thrombin, taking advantage of its adhesive, hemostatic, and sealant properties.

Appropriate indications for cryoprecipitate include:

- A bleeding patient with congenital or acquired hypofibrinogenemia, dysfibrinogenemia, or afibrinogenemia (fibrinogen <150 mg/dL)
- Treatment or prevention of bleeding associated with certain known or suspected clotting factor deficiencies (factor VIII, von Willebrand's, factor XIII, or factor I)
- Treatment of surface oozing and maintenance of tissues in tight apposition to each other or sealing of leaking spaces (fibrin glue)

Rather than cryoprecipitate, factor concentrates are mostly used to treat hemophilia A and type I von Willebrand's disease. Desmopressin acetate (DDAVP) may be used as an alternative treatment for these patients and for patients with certain platelet dysfunctional disorders.

Granulocytes

Using apheresis techniques, granulocytes contain approximately 20 to 30×10^9 granulocytes per collection, 200 to 400 mL of donor plasma, 10 to 30 mL of donor RBCs, and some donor platelets. Like platelets, this product is stored at room temperature but without agitation. Granulocytes have a 24-hour shelf life, but they should be transfused as soon as possible because of rapid decline of function and viability of the leukocytes.

There are several special considerations for this product. Granulocytes must be ABO compatible with the recipient because of significant RBC contamination. This is an Rh-specific product for female patients of childbearing age. CMV-negative donors must be used for CMV-negative recipients because the product cannot be leukoreduced. It is an HLA-matched product for alloimmunized patients. Granulocytes should be irradiated to prevent TA-GVHD.

Granulocyte infusions are indicated for adult neutropenic patients (granulocyte count <500/μL) who have fever for 24 to 48 hours due to bacterial or fungal sepsis that is unresponsive to appropriate antibiotic or antifungal treatment. In infants, granulocyte therapy should be considered in bacterial septicemic patients with a granulocyte count less than 3000/μL. Daily granulocyte transfusion should be continued until infection resolves or the granulocyte count remains greater than 500/μL for 48 hours.

REFERENCES

Bowden RA, Slichter SJ, Sayers M, et al. A comparison of filtered leukocyte-educed and cytomegalovirus (CMV) seronegative blood products for the prevention of transfusion-associated CMV infection after marrow transplant. Blood 1995;86:3598–603.

Brecher ME. Technical Manual, 15th ed. Bethesda, MD: American Association of Blood Banks; 2005.

British Committee for Standards in Haematology, Blood Transfusion Task Force. Guidelines for the use of platelet transfusions. Br J Haematol 2003;122:10–23.

Development Task Force of the College of American Pathologists. Practice parameters for the use of fresh frozen plasma, cryoprecipitate and platelets. JAMA 1994;271:777.

Goodnough LT, Brecher ME, Kanter MH, AuBuchon JP. Transfusion medicine. First of two parts—blood transfusion. N Engl J Med 1999;340:438–47.

Goodnough LT, Brecher ME, Kanter MH, AuBuchon JP. Transfusion medicine. Second of two parts—blood conservation. N Engl J Med 1999;340:525–33.

Menitove JE, McElligott MC, Aster RH. Febrile transfusion reaction: What blood component should be given next? Vox Sang 1978;5:101–6.

Nichols WG, Price TH, Corey L, Boeckh M. Transfusion-transmitted cytomegalovirus infection after receipt of leukoreduced blood products. Blood 2003;101:4195–200.

Strauss R. Neutrophil (granulocyte) transfusions in the new millennium. Transfusion 1998;38:710–2.

The Trial to Reduce Alloimmunization to Platelets Study Group. Leukocyte reduction and ultraviolet B irradiation of platelets to prevent alloimmunization and refractoriness to platelet transfusions. N Engl J Med 1997;337:1861–9.

Wandt H, Frank M, Ehninger G, et al. Safety and cost effectiveness of a 10×10^9/L trigger for prophylactic platelet transfusions compared with the traditional 20×10^9/L trigger: A prospective comparative trial in 105 patients with acute myeloid leukemia. Blood 1998;91:3601–6.

Adverse Effects of Blood Transfusion

Method of

Chelsea A. Sheppard, MD, and
Christopher D. Hillyer, MD

Although blood transfusion is a beneficial and not uncommonly lifesaving therapy, it carries inherent risks or adverse effects. These adverse effects are commonly classified either as *transfusion reactions* (Table 1), which occur immediately or shortly following the transfusion event, or as *transfusion-related complications*, which can occur up to many years following transfusion. These latter complications are commonly divided into *infectious* (Table 2) and *noninfectious*

(Table 3) categories. Indeed, 0.5% to 3% of all transfusions result in an adverse event; however, the majority of these are minor reactions with no long-term sequelae.

Herein we describe a large number of adverse events so that the physician can determine if his or her patient has had an adverse effect from a transfusion, assign a diagnosis, and consider if an intervention is needed. For a complete discussion of all of the adverse events related to transfusion, as well as more detailed references, the reader is referred to *Blood Banking and Transfusion Medicine* (see References).

Transfusion Reactions

When a patient experiences an immediate reaction to a transfusion, the most important question to answer is whether hemolysis is occurring. Thus, transfusion medicine specialists usually classify transfusion reactions as either *hemolytic* or *nonhemolytic*.

Hemolytic reactions are caused by recipient antibodies targeted against donor red cell antigens and the resultant response, which attempts to destroy or clear those foreign cells. These antibodies may be naturally occurring (e.g., a recipient with group A blood has antibodies to B-group red cells) or they can occur after exposure to foreign blood from past transfusion, pregnancy, or transplantation. This process is termed *alloimmunization.*

Nonhemolytic reactions occur via a variety of mechanisms usually involving recipient response to donor leukocytes or their byproducts, including inflammatory cytokines.

HEMOLYTIC TRANSFUSION REACTIONS

Acute Hemolytic Transfusion Reaction

Clinical Description

Arguably, the most devastating transfusion reaction is an acute hemolytic reaction caused by the mistransfusion of ABO incompatible blood. *Mistransfusion* is defined as failure to give the right blood product to the right person at the right time and for the right reason. The severity of the reaction is dose dependent; however, infusion of even a small amount of incompatible blood can cause intravascular hemolysis, resulting in a range of signs and symptoms including pain at the infusion site, back, or flank; fever; chills or rigors; hemoglobinuria or hemoglobinemia; chest pain; circulatory collapse or shock;

TABLE 1 Transfusion Reactions

Type	Frequency	Common Signs and Symptoms	Laboratory Diagnosis	Therapy
Hemolytic				
AHTR	Rare	Pain at the infusion site, back, or flanks Fever, chills, rigors Hemoglobinuria or hemoglobinemia Chest pain Circulatory collapse and shock Vasoconstriction resultant end-organ ischemia Activation of the coagulation system, resulting in microangiopathic thrombosis	Schistocytes on peripheral smear Indirect bilirubinemia and jaundice Decreased haptoglobin Elevated LDH and reticulocyte count	Stop the transfusion Maintain IV fluids (1 L NS over 1–2 h) to maintain urine flow >1 mL/kg/h Diuresis with furosemide or mannitol Support cardiovascular and respiratory function with vasopressors Intubate if necessary
Bacterial contamination	Rare	Fever, chills, rigors Hypotension Intravascular hemolysis	Positive blood cultures Similar organism found in product and recipient	Antibiotics Treat shock if appropriate
DHTR	Rare	Intra- or extravascular hemolysis	Same as AHTR, with spherocytes on peripheral smear if hemolysis is predominantly extravascular	Monitor renal function; forced diuresis or dialysis may be required to support renal function if extravascular hemolysis is severe Transfuse with antigen-negative blood if anemia is symptomatic

Continued

TABLE 1 Transfusion Reactions—Cont'd

Type	Frequency	Common Signs and Symptoms	Laboratory Diagnosis	Therapy
Nonhemolytic				
Allergic	Common	Itching, urticaria, generalized flushing or rash, angioedema Wheezing, cough	No abnormal laboratory tests	Diphenhydramine 25–50 mg PO or IV May premedicate for future transfusions if recurrent
Anaphylactic	Rare	Shortness of breath, vasomotor instability, bronchospasm	No abnormal laboratory tests	Epinephrine 1:1000 0.3 mL IM Secure airway
FNHTR	Common	Fever, chills, rigors Absence of hemolysis	No abnormal laboratory tests; r/o hemolysis	Acetaminophen 650 mg PO if not contraindicated May premedicate for future transfusions if recurrent
TA-GVHD	Rare	Fever, mucositis, dermatitis, hepatitis, enterocolitis, pancytopenia	Low blood counts, low reticulocyte count, elevated liver enzymes, elevated inflammatory markers	Treatment is usually ineffective High dose steroids, OKT3, cyclosporine A, and antithymocyte globulin may be helpful Irradiate blood for high-risk patients to prevent TA-GVHD
TRALI	Rare	Noncardiogenic pulmonary edema with dyspnea, acute hypoxemia, hypotension, occasionally fever Bilateral infiltrates on CXR Signs of congestive heart failure (increased jugular venous pressure and/or a third heart sound) absent Normal pulmonary capillary wedge pressure	HLA/HNA antibody or antigen cognates between recipient and donor can support diagnosis	Respiratory support High-dose steroids Avoid diuretics in hypotensive patients

Abbreviations: AHTR = acute hemolytic transfusion reaction; CXR = chest x-ray; DHTR = delayed hemolytic transfusion reaction; FNHTR = febrile nonhemolytic transfusion reaction; HLA = human leukocyte antigen; HNA = human neutrophil antigen; LDH = lactate dehydrogenase; NS = normal saline; OKT3 = muromonab CD3; r/o = rule out; TA-GVHD = transfusion-associated graft-versus-host disease; TRALI = transfusion-related acute lung injury.

495

TABLE 2 Infectious Complications of Transfusion

Type	Risk of Transfusion Transmitted Infection from Screened Units
Viruses	
CMV	Leukoreduction has made transfusion transmission rare (~1% remaining risk)
EBV	Rare
HAV	Rare
HBV	~1:200,000
HCV*	~1:2 million
HHV	
HIV*	~1:2 million to 4 million
HTLV	<1:3 million
WNV*	Rare
Parasitic Infections	
Babesia spp.	Rare
Plasmodium spp.	1:4 million
Trypanosoma cruzi	Rare
Prions	
CJD, BSE	Rare

*Risk after nucleic acid testing was implemented.
Abbreviations: BSE = bovine spongiform encephalopathy; CJD = Creutzfeldt-Jakob disease; CMV = cytomegalovirus; EBV = Epstein-Barr virus; HAV = hepatitis A virus; HBV = hepatitis B virus; HCV = hepatitis C virus; HHV = human herpesvirus; HTLV = human T-cell lymphotropic virus; WNV = West Nile virus.

1 in 12,000 and 1 in 19,000 transfused units. The fatality rate ranges from 1 in 800,000 to 1 in 2,000,000 transfused units. However, these numbers do not take into account the large number of near misses, which have been reported to be as common as 1 in 3000 to 4000 units transfused per year.

Diagnosis

The first signs of an acute hemolytic transfusion reaction (AHTR) are usually fever and pain. However, a decrease in blood pressure, tachycardia, and hemoglobinuria may be the only signs in an anesthetized patient.

Laboratory studies can help confirm a diagnosis of intravascular hemolysis. Red cell abnormalities including schistocytes on peripheral smear, increased indirect bilirubin and jaundice, and decreased haptoglobin are signs of increased red cell destruction. Elevated lactate dehydrogenase (LDH) and reticulocyte count indicate increased red cell turnover. It is important to maintain adequate renal function; therefore, it is necessary to monitor blood urea nitrogen (BUN), creatinine, and urine output.

Occasionally, patients with severe intravascular hemolysis can develop disseminated intravascular coagulation (DIC). Serial measurements including prothrombin time (PT), activated partial thromboplastin time (aPTT), D-dimer, fibrinogen, antithrombin, and platelet count can be used to evaluate for the presence of an ongoing consumptive process. After the transfusion is stopped, the unit itself and a post-transfusion sample should be immediately sent to the blood bank for further analysis. The blood bank will perform a clerical check for correct patient identification, look for the presence of visible hemolysis in the post-transfusion plasma, and compare direct Coombs' test results from the pre- and post-transfusion samples for evidence of in vivo antibody adsorption on the red cells.

Treatment and Prevention

If an acute hemolytic transfusion reaction is suspected, the transfusion should be stopped immediately. Intravenous fluids should be given to maintain an adequate blood pressure and to aid the kidneys

vasoconstriction with resultant end organ ischemia; and activation of the coagulation system, resulting in microangiopathic thrombosis.

The annual incidence of ABO-mismatched transfusion according to observed errors in the New York State database and the FDA database of transfusion-associated fatalities has been reported at between

TABLE 3 Noninfectious Complications of Transfusion

Type	Frequency	Common Signs and Symptoms	Laboratory Diagnosis	Therapy
Massive Transfusion Reactions				
Coagulopathy	Common in massive transfusion	Hemorrhage usually described as mucosal bleeding or oozing from suture lines	Prolonged PT, PTT Fibrinogen <100 mg/dL Rapidly decreasing platelet count and antithrombin level	Replace clotting factors with FFP In massive transfusion, RBC/FFP ratio should be 1:1–2 If fibrinogen <100 mg/dL, transfuse 1 cryoprecipitate pool and recheck fibrinogen Transfuse platelets if count <50,000/L
Citrate toxicity	Rare	Muscle cramping, shortness of breath secondary to bronchospasm, tetanic contractions, distal extremity numbness, tingling sensations, seizures	Decreased ionized calcium Monitor for hypomagnesemia	Calcium gluconate 2 g/250 mL NS Replete magnesium if indicated
Hyperkalemia	Rare	Generalized fatigue, weakness, paresthesias, paralysis, palpitations ECG changes: peaked T waves, shortened OT interval, ST segment depression	Elevated serum potassium Monitor for evidence of metabolic alkalosis Monitor for ECG changes	Replete with oral or IV potassium preparations if indicated
Iron overload	Rare	Iron deposition with end-organ damage in heart, liver, lungs, pituitary, thyroid, adrenals, exocrine pancreas	Elevated iron, ferritin (~10–20 g in patients with SCD is typical), and transferrin saturation	Phlebotomy or iron chelators if indicated
Transfusion-Related Immunomodulation				
Platelet refractoriness (HLA)	Occasional in highly sensitized patients	FNHTR No response or inadequate response to platelet transfusion	Corrected count increment (see text), flow cytomtery, or ELISA screen for anti-HLA antibodies or platelet-specific antibodies	Consider appropriateness of HLA-matched or crossmatched platelets, contact transfusion medicine specialist
Post-transfusion purpura (HPA)	Rare	Severe thrombocytopenia 5–10 d after transfusion Bruising and petechiae Can result in severe hemorrhage	Flow cytomtery or ELISA screen for anti-platelet-specific antibodies Must r/o other causes of thrombocytopenia, including HIT and DIC	Self-limited IVIg Efficacy of antigen-negative platelets is controversial
Other				
Volume overload	Common	Cardiogenic pulmonary edema with dyspnea, acute hypoxemia, hypertension Bilateral infiltrates on CXR Signs of congestive heart failure, increased jugular venous pressure, and/or absent third heart sound Elevated pulmonary capillary wedge pressure	BNP can help distinguish volume overload from TRALI	Diuresis If transfusion is required, slow the rate

Abbreviations: BNP = brain natriuretic peptide; CXR = chest x-ray; DIC = disseminated intravascular coagulation; ECG = electrorcardiogram; ELISA = enzyme-linked immunosorbent assay; FNHTR = febrile nonhemolytic transfusion reaction; FFP = fresh frozen plasma; HIT = heparin-induced thrombocytopenia; HLA = human leukocyte antigen; HPA = human platelet antigen; IVIg = intravenous immunoglobulin; NS = normal saline; PT = prothrombin time; PTT = partial thromboplastin time; RBC = red blood cells; r/o = rule out; SCD = sickle cell disease; TRALI = transfusion-related acute lung injury.

in expelling circulating hemoglobin. Some experts recommend furosemide (Lasix) or mannitol (Osmitrol) to induce diuresis; however, this has not been studied in a randomized fashion. A patient who develops signs of shock should be treated accordingly. Vasopressors and mechanical ventilation may be required in cases of circulatory collapse and respiratory failure.

Most cases of mistransfusion are the result of human error. More than one half of these errors occur from misidentification of the patient at the bedside. Approximately one third of these errors occur in the blood bank as a result of either a clerical misprint or the misidentification of a specimen. Despite strict transfusion procedures and protocols, the use of hospital identification wrist bands, and multiple redundant check systems, mistransfusions still occur at an alarming rate. Therefore, systems including the use of bar codes, barrier technology (Blood-Loc), and radiofrequency identification (RFID) systems are under investigation.

Delayed Hemolytic Transfusion Reaction

Clinical Description

Red blood cell antibodies acquired through exposure to foreign antigen can cause a delayed hemolytic transfusion reaction (DHTR). These patients can develop signs and symptoms of intra- or extravascular hemolysis approximately 2 weeks after transfusion due to the formation of a de novo alloantibody. Alternatively, symptoms appearing 3 to 4 days after transfusion support previous exposure to the antigen and a robust amnestic response on reexposure to antigen-positive blood.

Diagnosis

Patients with a history of a recent transfusion and signs and symptoms of hemolysis should be evaluated for a possible DHTR. Laboratory studies for intra- and extravascular hemolysis are described earlier. However, in delayed hemolytic transfusion reactions, extravascular hemolysis is more common; thus, spherocytes rather than schistocytes may be the predominant abnormal morphologic red cell type on peripheral smear.

Alloantibodies are usually detected during the antibody screen carried in blood banks as a "type and screen." If the screen is positive, the specificity of the antibody is determined. For patients with multiple antibodies, this can significantly lengthen the time it takes for the pretransfusion work-up. If the patient has not recently received a transfusion, antibody titers may be too low to be detected at the time of screening. However, if the patient is rechallenged with the antigen, an amnestic antibody response can cause destruction of the transfused cells. Intravascular and extravascular hemolysis can be severe and life threatening.

Treatment and Prevention

Treatment of intra- and extravascular hemolysis is discussed under acute hemolytic transfusion reactions.

The inherent immunogenicity of the antigen, antigen concentration per erythrocyte, transfused cell dosage, and individual patient factors determine the rate of alloimmunization. Patients with sickle cell disease are at greater risk, and immunosuppressed patients may be at less risk. Highly immunogenic antigens such as Kell, Duffy, and Kidd are generally associated with more severe reactions. These antigens are also commonly implicated in hemolytic disease of the newborn because these antibodies can cross the placenta.

Antibody screening is required before transfusion in any patient who has received a transfusion or been pregnant in the last 30 days; thus, it is important to take a thorough transfusion history. Additionally, hospitalized patients receiving transfusions should be rescreened every 3 days because antibodies that are initially too low in titer to be detected might be identified later.

Bacterial Contamination of Blood Products

Clinical Description

Bacterial contamination at the time of collection usually occurs through one of three mechanisms: asymptomatic donor bacteremia, introduction of skin flora to the unit, or manufacturing processes and manipulation of the unit. Initially, the amount of bacteria present is low; however, during storage the bacteria can proliferate to levels of 10^6/mL or greater. This amount of bacteria transfused over a short time can result in a spectrum of clinical signs and symptoms including bacteremia, fever, chills, hypotension, nausea, vomiting, diarrhea, and oliguria, which can progress to sepsis and ultimately multisystem organ failure and death.

Pathophysiology

The most common bacteria identified in 70% to 80% of contaminated platelets are gram-positive skin flora introduced to the unit during collection; however, 40% to 80% of fatalities are due to endotoxin-producing gram-negative organisms. The severity of the reaction depends on the species of bacteria present, the inoculum, the rate of bacterial propagation, and patient factors including underlying disease, including leukocyte count, the status of the immune system, and use of concomitant antibiotics in the recipient.

Diagnosis

Blood cultures should be obtained both from the recipient (cultures should not be drawn from the same line used for the transfusion) and from the blood product in question. Confirmation requires that the same organism be cultured from both sites. False negatives can occur in patients taking antibiotics. False-positive cultures are common due to improper collection of the sample.

Additional laboratory tests can help evaluate for end-organ damage including tests of renal and liver function. Endotoxin-induced DIC is a common complication; therefore, serial measurements of the PT, APTT, D-dimer, fibrinogen, antithrombin, and platelet count may be useful in evaluating for the presence of an ongoing consumptive process.

Treatment and Prevention

Sepsis caused by transfusion of a bacterially contaminated unit can be fatal. Antibiotics should be given empirically as soon as symptoms appear. The patient can develop septic shock and should be treated accordingly.

Bacterial contamination is the third most common cause of transfusion-associated fatality reported to the FDA. Improved phlebotomy practices (strict arm preparation standards and diversion of the first 10 mL containing the skin plug), donor questioning for recent illnesses or travel to endemic areas, better materials used in product collection and storage, and implementation of platelet culturing have helped reduce the incidence of fatality as a result of bacterial contamination of blood products. Red cell units and plasma, which are stored refrigerated or frozen, are less often implicated in bacteria-related transfusion reactions. However, platelets, which are stored at room temperature in a large volume of plasma and in a bag that allows oxygen diffusion, are most commonly implicated.

Prior to 2004 and the implementation of American Association of Blood Banks (AABB) Standard 5.1.5.1, which charged blood banks with the responsibility of limiting and detecting bacterial contamination, the infectious risk of receiving a contaminated unit was estimated at 1 in 2000 to 1 in 3000 platelet units per year. Risk of death was 1 in 60,000 to 1 in 85,000 units transfused. Since implementation of the AABB standard, many of the nation's blood collection systems have begun culturing platelet units using automated systems, which detect CO_2 generation or O_2 consumption by bacteria for 24 hours prior to hospital distribution. The American Red Cross reported that the incidence of a confirmed positive platelet pheresis unit between 2006 and 2008 was 1:6,015; however, 1:86,882 units had negative culture results but were associated with a septic transfusion reaction due to improvements in inlet-line diversion and increased culture volume. Despite a marked reduction in the number of cases of transfusion-transmitted bacterial infections, rare fatal consequences have been reported.

Pathogen reduction technology aims at eradicating pathogens without harming the blood cells or generating toxic chemical agents. Several methods under investigation include a number of photodynamic processes that use psoralen-based chemicals, pheno-thiazine dyes (methylene blue [urolene blue]), or riboflavin (vitamin B_2) followed by ultraviolet light to inactivate bacteria and viruses by degrading nucleic acids. Other methods include solvent-detergent treatment and treatment with FRALEs (frangible anchor linker effectors). The appeal of pathogen reduction is that it is proactive and may be able to prevent new and emerging infections. Nonetheless, serious regulatory hurdles remain before these methods are approved for use in the United States.

NONHEMOLYTIC TRANSFUSION REACTIONS

Transfusion-Related Acute Lung Injury

Clinical Description

Transfusion-related acute lung injury (TRALI) has now become the most common cause of transfusion-associated death *reported* to the FDA, with an incidence that ranges widely from 1 case per 432 whole blood units transfused to 1 case per 557,000 red blood cell units transfused. Because it was not until 2004 that standardized criteria were widely accepted for defining and diagnosing TRALI, these previous figures might not reflect current incidence, and thus most authorities agree that the true incidence of TRALI is unknown. Nonetheless, it is becoming increasingly clear that platelets and FFP are the most commonly implicated blood products due to the large plasma volume of these products and the likelihood of alloantibodies being passively transferred (see later).

TRALI is a clinical syndrome characterized by noncardiogenic pulmonary edema with dyspnea, acute hypoxemia, hypotension, and occasionally fever. Bilateral infiltrates in a white-out pattern are commonly described on chest x-ray. Signs of congestive heart failure (increased jugular venous pressure and/or a third heart sound) are usually absent. The pulmonary capillary wedge pressure is typically normal. Symptoms usually appear 1 to 6 hours after transfusion and resolve in 96 hours.

Diagnosis

Until recently, accepted criteria allowing standardized diagnosis of TRALI were lacking, thus complicating the ability to make accurate diagnoses and hindering attempts at determining true incidence rates. In April 2004, a consensus conference convened in Toronto, Ontario, and attempted to further adapt and improve previously proposed definitions of TRALI. The consensus panel recommended criteria for *TRALI* and *possible TRALI*.

TRALI was defined as a new occurrence of acute-onset acute lung injury (ALI) with hypoxemia and bilateral infiltrates on chest x-ray, but no evidence of left atrial hypertension. The ALI cannot have been preexisting, but it must emerge during or within 6 hours of the end the transfusion and have no temporal relation to an alternative ALI risk factor. *Possible TRALI* included cases in which there was a temporal association with an alternative ALI risk factor.

These proposed definitions continue to suffer the limitations inherent in the American-European Consensus Conference definition of ALI (including the subjectivity of certain findings, including chest x-ray and volume status and the influence of PEEP on measurements of the PaO_2/FiO_2 ratio). Brain natriuretic protein (BNP) might help to distinguish cardiogenic from noncardiogenic pulmonary edema.

Pathophysiology

The events and mechanisms that cause TRALI are incompletely understood. They have been described as antibody-mediated and non–antibody-mediated. Antibody-mediated mechanisms implicate alloantibodies directed toward human leukocyte antigen (HLA) or human neutrophil antigen (HNA) on leukocytes or lung tissue, which lead to granulocyte activation and pulmonary injury. In approximately 90% of TRALI cases where antibodies are identified, the antibodies are of donor origin and react with recipient leukocyte epitopes. Multiparous women and recipients of previous transfusions are more likely to be alloimmunized. Many investigators have suggested that a number of hits may be required to cause a full-blown case of TRALI.

The two-hit model of TRALI may be antibody- or non–antibody-mediated. In this model, the first hit is usually described as an underlying illness that primes recipient pulmonary endothelial cells and leukocytes. *Priming* refers to the development of a heightened stage of (cellular) activation. The second hit is delivered by the transfusion, which contains factors (either antibodies or biological response modifiers [BRMs], such as cytokines or certain lipids) capable of inducing complete activation of the presequestered primed neutrophils in the recipient's lungs. This results in the release of cytotoxic compounds in the pulmonary vasculature, leading to endothelial damage, capillary leak, and noncardiogenic pulmonary edema, namely, TRALI.

Treatment and Prevention

Treatment is primarily respiratory support until the injury resolves (usually in 24–96 hours); however, high-dose intravenous steroids may be beneficial. Approximately 20% of patients with TRALI require 1 week or more to fully recover. Death is estimated to occur in 6% to 23% of cases; survivors have no permanent sequelae.

Without a simple laboratory test to prospectively eliminate high-risk blood products, recommended strategies to prevent TRALI are currently based on deferral of donors implicated in TRALI cases. The United Kingdom has preemptively deferred all women from donating plasma. In the United States, recent mitigation strategies have also included the predominate use of male-only plasma. Eder et al, report the successful ARC experience of transition to predominately male-only plasma between 2006-2008 with a reducton in the rate of fatal and non-fatal cases of TRALI involving plasma only transfusions to roughly the rate of TRALI caused by RBC transfusions.

Febrile Nonhemolytic Transfusion Reaction

Clinical Description

Febrile nonhemolytic transfusion reaction (FNHTR) is defined as an increase in the recipient's temperature of at least 1°C or 2°F during transfusion in the absence of another cause of fever. Some patients develop chills or rigors. FNHTRs are very common, occurring in 0.1% to 0.5% of all leukodepleted transfusions occurring per year in the United States. The incidence is significantly higher in nonleukoreduced blood products. Additionally, transfusion reactions such as FNHTRs and allergic reactions are believed to be underreported in patients with frequent febrile episodes due to underlying diseases such as cancer and sepsis. Other causes for transfusion-associated fever, including hemolysis or bacterial contamination, must be excluded before a diagnosis of FNHTR can be made.

Pathophysiology

FNHTRS are attributed to white blood cells (WBCs) in blood products that synthesize and release proinflammatory cytokines during storage. Preformed recipient antibodies that target donor WBCs can also lead to cytokine release after transfusion.

Treatment and Prevention

Antipyretics are often used to treat these reactions. Patients prone to FNHTRs can require premedication with antipyretics. Many transfusion medicine services have implemented universal leukoreduction protocols to prevent FNHTRs.

Allergic Reactions

Clinical Description

Allergic transfusion reactions are very common. Allergic reactions are variably severe and result in a spectrum of clinical signs and symptoms. Uncomplicated or simple reactions manifest as itching, urticaria, generalized flushing or rash, or local swelling, also known as *angioedema*. However, recipients can also develop anaphylactoid reactions in which wheezing, cough, shortness of breath, vasomotor instability, and bronchospasm are typically observed. IgA-deficient patients with circulating anti-IgA antibodies can develop life-threatening anaphylaxis and cardiovascular collapse requiring emergent therapy. Most reactions are afebrile. The incidence of uncomplicated allergic reactions is 1% to 3%; however, anaphylactic reactions are very rare (0.002%–0.005% of all transfusions).

Pathophysiology

Simple allergic reactions occur when donor plasma proteins are targeted by preformed IgE antibodies on recipient mast cells, leading to histamine release. More severe reactions have been attributed to antibodies against IgA, C4 determinants, or other nonbiological elements (ethylene oxide used for sterilization of tubing sets). The presence of anti-IgA antibodies in IgA-deficient patients cannot predict the occurrence of allergic reactions.

Treatment and Prevention

Most simple allergic reactions can be treated with antihistamines or anticholinergic medications (e.g., diphenhydramine). Patients with more severe reactions can require IV steroids or epinephrine. Patients with respiratory failure require supportive therapy. In patients with recurrent allergic reactions, prophylactic antihistamine therapy administered 30 minutes before transfusion may be helpful. In patients with simple allergic reactions involving only the skin, the transfusion may be restarted 15 to 30 minutes after the administration of antihistamines; however, transfusions should never be restarted in patients with more severe reactions.

Transfusion-Associated Graft-Versus-Host Disease

Clinical Description

Transfusion-associated graft-versus-host disease (TA-GVHD) is a rare but uniformly fatal complication of blood transfusions in severely immunosuppressed patients in which donor lymphocytes escape immune clearance in the recipient and engraft. Following clonal expansion, these cells cause immune destruction of host tissues including the skin, gastrointestinal (GI) tract, liver, and bone marrow. These patients develop fever, mucositis, dermatitis (starting as a blistering rash on the palms, soles, and face, which then can generalize), hepatitis, enterocolitis with large volumes of secretory diarrhea, and pancytopenia, 1 to 2 weeks after transfusion. Infections are the most common cause of death, which generally occurs within 3 to 4 weeks of the transfusion.

The degree of immunosuppression and the dose of T lymphocytes are factors in determining an individual patient's risk of developing TA-GVHD. Patients with hematologic malignancy, patients with congenital immunodeficiency, premature infants weighing less than 1200 g, bone marrow transplant recipients, and patients receiving fludarabine (Fludara) (see Box 1 for a complete list) are susceptible. Patients with HIV, healthy newborns, and patients who are neutropenic due to sepsis are generally considered to be at low risk. There is a minimally increased risk associated with solid tumor transplants (especially heart and liver) or solid tumor malignancies. There have been reports of TA-GVHD associated with neuroblastomas, rhabdomyosarcomas, bladder tumors, and small cell lung cancer. It is possible that more immunosuppressive and myeloablative chemotherapy protocols are responsible for these cases.

The degree of HLA similarity between the donor and recipient is also an important determinant of a patient's risk of developing TA-GVHD. These patients may be immunocompetent heterozygotes of an HLA haplotype for which the donor is homozygous. Therefore, patients receiving transfusions from first-degree relatives or populations in which there is a great deal of HLA homology (including some Asian populations) might also require irradiated blood products.

Treatment and Prevention

The mortality rate of TA-GVHD approximates 100%. Currently, there is no effective treatment; however, high-dose steroids, muromonab-CD3 (OKT-3), cyclosporine A (Neoral, Sandimmune) and antithy-mocyte globulin (Atgam, Thymoglobin) have been used with few successes.

Prevention of TA-GVHD via irradiation of blood products in at-risk populations is absolutely required. A minimum dose of 25 Gy delivered to the midline of the container (with a minimum of 15 Gy to the distal parts of the bag) cross-links the DNA of T cells, thereby preventing replication and potential engraftment and expansion.

BOX 1 Risk Factors for the Development of TA-GVHD

Significantly Increased Risk
- Bone marrow transplantation
  - Allogeneic and autologous
  - HLA-matched platelet transfusions
  - Hodgkin's disease
  - Intrauterine transfusions
  - Patients treated with purine analogue drugs
  - Transfusions from blood relatives
- Congenital immunodeficiency syndromes

Minimally Increased Risk
- Acute leukemia
- Exchange transfusions
- Non-Hodgkin's lymphoma
- Preterm infants (<1200 g)
- Solid organ transplant recipients
- Solid tumors treated with intensive chemotherapy or radiotherapy

Perceived but No Reported Increased Risk
- Healthy newborns
- Patients with AIDS

Modified from Schroeder ML: Transfusion-associated graft-versus-host disease. Br J Haematol 2002;117:275–287.
Abbreviations: HLA = human leukocyte antigen; TA-GVHD = transfusion-associated graft-versus-host disease.

Transfusion-Related Complications

INFECTIOUS COMPLICATIONS

Viral Transmission

Clinical Description

A large number of viruses, including HIV-1 and HIV-2; hepatitis A, B, and C (HAV, HBV, HCV); human T-lymphotrophic viruses (HTLV) 1 and 2; cytomegalovirus (CMV); and West Nile virus can be transmitted via transfusion. These viruses, with the exception of CMV, are acquired from cellular and noncellular blood and blood products including plasma-derived clotting factors, intravenous immunoglobulin (IVIg), and anti-D immunoglobulin. CMV remains latent in monocytes and is essentially therefore transmitted only in cellular products. Other viruses that are potentially transmitted via transfusion are HAV, transfusion-transmitted virus (TTV), Epstein-Barr virus (EBV), human herpesvirus 8 (HHV 8), and parvovirus B19.

Hepatitis

Hepatitis viruses (especially B and C) are readily transfusion transmissible. About 70% of patients infected with HCV develop chronic infections resulting in chronic active hepatitis, cirrhosis, or hepatocellular carcinoma (HCC). A smaller but significant fraction of patients infected with HBV develop chronic disease proceeding to cirrhosis. Hepatitis viruses A and E are rarely transmitted through blood transfusion. Hepatitis G, TTV, and SEN viruses emerged as candidates for non–A to E type post-transfusion hepatitis, but no clear association has been demonstrated.

Human Immunodeficiency Virus

The annual risk of transfusion-transmitted HIV with the addition of nucleic acid testing is reported to be less than 1 in 2,000,000 units in the United States (1:4,000,000 in Canada). However, despite the implementation of this very sensitive testing, cases of transfusion-transmitted HIV have been reported. The average survival after diagnosis for adults and children with transfusion-transmitted HIV is approximately 5.6 months and 13.7 months, respectively.

West Nile Virus and Other Flaviviruses

In 2002, there was an emergence of West Nile virus in the United States, and several cases of transfusion-transmitted disease were identified. Infected elderly and immunocompromised patients developed a severe flulike illness rarely resulting in death. Other flaviviruses including dengue are transfusion transmissible and could threaten the blood supply if an epidemic were to emerge in the United States.

Parvovirus B19

Parvovirus B19 has been transmitted through plasma-derived products including clotting factors. Immunocompromised patients can develop erythema infectiosum, arthralgias, and aplastic crises with chronic anemia after infection with parvovirus B19.

Cytomegalovirus

Transfusion transmission of CMV to immunocompetent patients usually causes an asymptomatic infection or rarely an infectious mononucleosis. However, in seronegative immunocompromised patients, transfusion transmission can lead to lethal CMV disease. Seronegative immunocompromised patients include premature low-birth-weight infants (<1500 g) born to seronegative mothers and seronegative recipients of autologous or seronegative allogeneic bone marrow or peripheral blood stem cell transplantation.

Following primary infection, CMV remains latent and can reactivate, with subsequent production of progeny virus in macrophages. Transfusion-transmitted CMV can be mitigated through the transfusion of leukoreduced or seronegative blood. The rate of infectivity with either leukoreduced or seronegative blood is approximately the same (1%). Box 2 lists the indications for which many hospital blood banks dispense CMV seronegative blood or leukoreduced blood.

Parasitic and Emerging Infections

Clinical Description

Trypanosoma cruzi, *Plasmodium* spp., and *Babesia* spp. can be transmitted by blood transfusion. *T. cruzi* can cause fatal cardiac and GI disease (Chagas' disease). Malaria, the disease caused by *Plasmodium*, can cause fatal intravascular hemolysis and DIC. Human babesiosis generally causes a mild flulike syndrome, but it can be lethal in the elderly and in immunocompromised patients. In 2007 most ARC and ABC blood centers began screening donors for Chagas. There is an FDA approved EIA; however, at the time of this writing there is still no FDA approved confirmatory assay.

TRYPANOSOMA CRUZI

There have been fewer than 10 cases of transfusion-transmitted *T. cruzi* reported in the United States and Canada since 1990. Many of these patients were immunocompromised as a result of hematologic malignancy, AIDS, or bone marrow transplantation. Some of these recipients received platelets only, others received multiple blood products. A majority of the patients developed Chagas' disease. At least one case was fatal. Others did respond to nitrofurtimox[2] (Nifurtimox), interferon-γ[1] (Actimmune), and benznidazole,[1] followed by itraconazole[1] (Sporanox) and fluconazole[1] (Diflucan). In endemic areas, transfusion transmission of Chagas' disease is more common. In the United States, 1 in 25,000 donors are estimated to be seropositive, and as many as one half of these donors are actively parasitemic.

PLASMODIUM SPECIES AND BABESIA SPECIES

Annually, approximately two cases of transfusion-transmitted *Plasmodium* infections are reported in the United States. Donors who have traveled to malaria-endemic countries are deferred from donation for a period of 1 year. Red cell exchange may be helpful in patients with high parasitemia loads and intravascular hemolysis; however, this is controversial.

Between 2004 and 2008, 63 cases of transfusion-transmitted babesiosis have been reported. Currently, there are no licensed tests for screening the blood supply. However, a broad-based, region specific approach to blood donor testing for Babesia infection is currently being proposed by the FDA using nucleic-acid testing and/or antibody-based testing. Human babesiosis is treated with antibiotics.

PRIONS

The agent of variant Creutzfeldt-Jakob disease (vCJD), a novel human prion disease that results in a rare and fatal human neurodegenerative condition, can be transmitted via blood transfusion. Although this agent has no nucleic acids, the transmission results

in the conversion of normal prion protein to the abnormal β-sheet amyloid responsible for the clinical disease.

Since 2003, it has been established that prion infection could be transmitted via blood transfusion in animals. Additionally, in 2003 the first case of probable transfusion-transmitted vCJD was reported. The recipient received a transfusion in 1996 from a donor now known to have been incubating vCJD. The recipient died in 1996 from complications of vCJD.

In 2006, the National CJD Surveillance Unit (NCJDSU) and the UK Blood Services (UKBS) released the Transfusion Medicine Epidemiology Review (TMER), a look-back investigation that confirmed three separate incidents of probable transfusion transmission of vCJD infection. Two of these patients died less than 7 years after infection. At this time, sporadic CJD and familial CJD have still not been shown conclusively to be transfusion transmitted.

To date there is no known treatment for transmissible spongiform encephalopathy. The AABB Standard 5.4.1A Requirements for Allogeneic Donor Qualification states that donors with a risk of vCJD as defined by the FDA Guidance for Industry (January 2002) should be indefinitely deferred from giving blood. Currently those donors include anyone who has traveled to or resided in the United Kingdom for a cumulative period of 3 or more months between 1980 and the end of 1996, those with a history of 5 or more years of cumulative residence or travel in France since 1980, and current and former U.S. military personnel, civilian military personnel, and their dependents who were stationed at European bases for 6 months or more between 1980 and 1996.

NONINFECTIOUS COMPLICATIONS

Transfusion-Related Immunomodulation

Clinical Description

Transfusion-related immunomodulation (TRIM) describes the immunosuppression that occurs after transfusion. TRIM was first recognized in the 1960s and 1970s in renal allograft recipients who had less rejection and improved graft survival after receiving blood transfusions from their donors. Since then, TRIM has been implicated in the development of postoperative infections, the recurrence of resected malignancies (especially colorectal cancer), spontaneous abortions, and inflammatory bowel disease. TRIM has been suggested to cause reactivation of latent viruses such as CMV.

Pathophysiology

Most authorities agree that TRIM exists, although the mechanisms and magnitude are unclear. However, it is believed that donor WBCs, BRMs, and soluble HLA antigens that have accumulated during storage exert an effect on cell-mediated immunity. TRIM appears to be dose dependent, and thus conservative transfusion triggers might decrease the incidence.

Treatment and Prevention

There is no known treatment for TRIM. Leukoreduction and washing might reduce the incidence of TRIM.

Alloimmunization

Alloimmunization is the development of an antibody to a foreign donor antigen after exposure through blood transfusion, pregnancy, or transplantation. These antibodies, if directed against RBC antigens, can cause DHTRs and AHTRs. Anti-HLA antibodies can cause FNHTRs and platelet refractoriness. These patients may be difficult to match for bone marrow or solid organ transplants. Thrombocytopenia can result in patients who develop platelet-specific antigens either in utero (neonatal alloimmune thrombocytopenia) or after transfusion (post-transfusion purpura).

Refractoriness to Platelet Transfusions

Patients who become refractory to platelet transfusion can do so by several different mechanisms including immune-mediated and non–immune-mediated mechanisms. Immune-mediated refractoriness

---

[1]Not FDA approved for this indication.
[2]Not available in the United States.

occurs in highly sensitized patients with anti-HLA or anti–platelet-specific antibodies to donor-specific antigens. Alternatively, patients with sepsis, DIC, fever, splenomegaly, or portal hypertension and persons taking certain drugs can also appear refractory to platelet transfusion due to the sequestration or accelerated clearance of the transfused platelets.

Diagnosis

The expected corrected count index (CCI) can help distinguish between immune-mediated and non–immune-mediated platelet refractoriness. The CCI is calculated 15 minutes to 1 hour after transfusion using the following equation:

$$CCI = \frac{(\text{Post-transfusion platelet count} - \text{Pretransfusion platelet count}) \times \text{Body surface area}}{\text{Number of platelets tranfused} \times 10^{11}}$$

A CCI less than 5000 after two sequential platelet transfusions suggests immune-mediated platelet refractoriness. These patients should be screened for anti-HLA and anti–platelet-specific antibodies if other causes of non–immune-mediated refractoriness have been excluded.

Pathophysiology

HLA antibodies are not routinely tested for in most clinical laboratories and blood banks. Additionally, because platelets are not cross-matched prior to transfusion, the only clue to a significant HLA antibody may be FNHTR or the lack of response to a platelet transfusion. Patients who develop multiple HLA antibodies can become refractory to platelet transfusion. Rarely, patients develop platelet-specific antibodies, causing platelet refractoriness.

Treatment and Prevention

Treatment depends on the etiology of platelet refractoriness. Patients with non–immune-mediated refractoriness (including those with splenic sequestration, sepsis, or DIC) require treatment of the underlying disease. If an immune-mediated mechanism is more likely, HLA-matched or crossmatched platelets can be supplied on request. Leukoreduction can potentially reduce HLA-alloimmunization.

Post-transfusion Purpura

Post-transfusion purpura (PTP) is a rare disorder caused by alloantibodies to platelet-specific glycoprotein, most commonly human platelet antigen (HPA)-1a, resulting in destruction of both transfused platelets and the patient's own platelets, leading to severe thrombocytopenia and risk of life-threatening hemorrhage. Thrombocytopenia can last 1 to 2 weeks after transfusion. IVIg is the first-line treatment. The use of washed antigen-negative platelets is controversial.

Volume Overload

Clinical Description

The development of cardiogenic pulmonary edema and other signs of congestive heart failure after transfusion suggest volume overload. The annual reported incidence in the United States of volume overload secondary to transfusion is greatly variable, anywhere from 1 in 100 to 1 in 15,000 units, and largely depends on patient population. The elderly and newborn, as well as patients with cardiac disease, renal insufficiency, and anemia with expanded plasma volumes, are at greater risk for developing volume overload, especially with massive transfusions.

Diagnosis

Diagnosis depends on establishing a cardiac etiology for the resulting dyspnea and pulmonary edema. Elevated central venous pressures or pulmonary wedge pressures, chest x-ray consistent with pulmonary edema, and response to diuretics are used to confirm the suspected diagnosis. It is important to rule out TRALI and other etiologies of acute respiratory distress syndrome (ARDS). BNP may be a useful adjuvant marker in establishing a diagnosis of volume overload secondary to transfusion.

Treatment and Prevention

Some patients respond simply to slowing the rate of the transfusion. Others require diuretics and supportive therapy.

Massive Transfusion Coagulopathy

Clinical Description

Massive transfusion is usually defined as transfusion of 10 or more units of RBCs in less than 24 hours. Massive transfusion usually occurs in the setting of trauma and can be complicated by coagulopathy secondary to dilution of clotting factors and platelets, hypothermia, and hypofibrinogenemia. Patients often receive crystalloid fluids and numerous uncrossmatched group O packed red cells in transit to the hospital or in the emergency department to correct hypovolemia before receiving plasma (which requires at least 30 minutes' thawing time) or platelets. This results in dilution of platelets, clotting proteins, and fibrinogen. Additionally, as the patient's blood pressure is normalized, bleeding becomes brisker resulting in further losses of platelets and clotting factors.

Treatment and Prevention

Ideally, patients with massive bleeding are transfused with whole blood, thereby minimizing the complications of dilution. Additionally, current guidelines are based on whole-blood transfusion and wash-out equations, simple mathematical models that calculate exponential decay of blood components during bleeding, assuming that the blood volume of the patient is stable and the replacement rates are constant and equal. Blood volumes and bleeding rates are usually quite variable, and replacement tends to lag behind blood loss; therefore, these guidelines and equations tend to underestimate needs. Computer modeling has demonstrated that patients with penetrating traumas have generally lost 2500 mL (or one half the average blood volume) by the time they arrive in the emergency department, 3200 mL (or two thirds the average blood volume) by the start of surgery, and 11,000 mL (or more than two blood volumes) at the end of surgery. PT will be prolonged (>1.5 times normal) after a loss of less than one blood volume. Fibrinogen is next, dropping below 0.8 g/L, in a little over one blood volume. Platelets stay above $50,000 \times 10^9$/L until after losses of more than two blood volumes.

Various massive transfusion protocols have been reviewed extensively in the literature. Early plasma replacement at higher plasma–to–red cells ratios (∼1:1) is gaining popularity in this clinical setting despite the fear that some patients may be overtransfused. However, there are few studies comparing conservative with liberal plasma and platelet transfusion with regard to outcome.

Hypothermia due to massive transfusion of refrigerated and recently thawed products contributes to the coagulopathy associated with massive transfusion. For this reason, many products are transfused through blood warmers. The use of cryoprecipitate for fibrinogen replacement is often necessary and more efficient than use of plasma.

OTHER ADVERSE EVENTS

Less frequent adverse events of transfusion include hypocalcemia due to large infusions of citrate anticoagulant, hyperkalemia due to RBC leakage during storage, mechanical hemolysis, and iron overload. These events are rare and typically affect infants receiving large amounts of old blood or patients receiving chronic transfusions; thus they are outside of the scope of this article. However, it is important to be aware of their existence and to monitor patients accordingly for signs of their development.

REFERENCES

Allain JP, Bianco C, Blajchman MA, et al. Protecting the blood supply from emerging pathogens: The role of pathogen inactivation. Transfus Med Rev 2005;19(2):110–26.

Blumberg N. Deleterious clinical effects of transfusion immunomodulation proven beyond a reasonable doubt. Transfusion 2005;45(Suppl.):33S–39S.

Blumberg N, Heal JM, Gettings KEJ. WBC reduction of RBC transfusions is associated with decreased incidence of RBC alloimmunization. Transfusion 2003;43:945–52.

Dodd RY, Notari IV, Stramer SL. Current prevalence and incidence of infectious disease markers and estimated window-period risk in the American Red Cross blood donor population. Transfusion 2002;42(8):975–9.

Eder AF, Kennedy JM, Dye B, et al. Limiting and detecting bacterial contamination of apheresis platelets: Inlet-line diversion and increased culture volume improve component safety. Transfusion 2009;49:1554–63.

Eder AF, Herron RM, Strupp A, et al. Effective reduction of transfusion-related acute lung injury risk with male predominant plasma strategy in the American Red Cross (2006–2008). Transfusion 2010;50:1732–42.

Goldman M, Webert KE, Arnold DM, et al. TRALI Consensus Panel: Proceedings of a consensus conference: Towards an understanding of TRALI. Transfus Med Rev 2005;19(1):2–31.

Hillyer CD, Silberstein LE, Ness PM, et al, editors. Blood Banking and Transfusion Medicine. 2nd ed. Philadelphia: Churchill Livingstone; 2007.

Hirschberg A, Dugas M, Banez E, et al. Minimizing dilutional coagulopathy in exsanguinating hemorrhage: A computer simulation. J Trauma 2003; 54:454–63.

Kleinman S, Caulfield T, Chan P, et al. Toward an understanding of transfusion-related acute lung injury: Statement of a consensus panel. Transfusion 2004;44(12):1774–89.

Lee D. Perception of blood transfusion risk. Transfus Med Rev 2006;20(2): 141–8.

Linden JV, Wagner K, Voytovich AE, Sheehan J. Transfusion errors in New York State: An analysis of 10 years' experience. Transfusion 2000;40: 1207–13.

Luban NC. Transfusion safety: Where are we today? Ann N Y Acad Sci 2005;1054:325–41.

Schroeder ML. Transfusion-associated graft-versus-host disease. Br J Haematol 2002;117:275–87.

Sheppard CA, Roback JD, Hillyer CD. Transfusion-transmitted cytomegalovirus infection: Consideration toward an optimal plan for its mitigation. Blood Ther Med 2005;5(1):6–14.

Zhou L, Giacherio D, Cooling L, Davenport RD. Use of B-natriuretic peptide as a diagnostic marker in the differential diagnosis of transfusion-associated circulatory overload. Transfusion 2005;45:1056–63.

Zou S, Dodd RY, Stramer SL, Strong DM, for the Tissue Safety Group. Probability of Viremia with HBV, HCV, HIV and HTLV among tissue donors in the United States. N Engl J Med 2004;351(8):751–9.

Myelodysplastic Syndromes

Method of
Jamile M. Shammo, MD

Epidemiology

The myelodysplastic syndromes (MDS) represent a group of heterogeneous clonal stem cell disorders that affect the elderly. The reported annual incidence of approximately 3.3 per 100,000 of the general U.S. population is highest among whites and non-Hispanics. The onset of MDS before the age of 50 years is rare; the incidence rises with age such that in patients older than 70 years, the incidence exceeds 20 per 100,000 persons. Men are nearly twice as likely to be affected as women (4.5 vs. 2.7 per 100,000 per year).

Risk Factors

De novo or primary MDS refers to cases in which no prior toxic exposure can be documented. Therapy-related MDS, on the other hand, occurs in patients who have been treated with chemotherapy or radiotherapy or both. Median onset of therapy-related MDS varies with the agents used and is usually 2 to 5 years after initial exposure to chemotherapy.

Tobacco use and occupational exposure to solvents and agricultural chemicals have also been associated with the development of MDS. A minority of MDS cases might have evolved from an antecedent hematologic disorder such as aplastic anemia or paroxysmal nocturnal hemoglobinuria. Several rare and inherited genetic disorders have been associated with a higher risk of developing MDS, such as Fanconi's anemia, dyskeratosis congenita, Diamond-Blackfan syndrome, and Shwachman-Diamond syndrome.

Pathophysiology

A variety of pathophysiologic processes have been described in association with MDS, resulting in ineffective hematopoiesis and peripheral cytopenias. These processes include excessive apoptosis of myeloid progenitors, abnormal responses to cytokines and growth factors, epigenetic aberrations resulting in gene silencing, chromosomal abnormalities, and a defective bone marrow microenvironment. However, the initiating mutation or molecular pathway is unknown.

Clinical Manifestations

Some patients with MDS are asymptomatic, but the majority present with peripheral blood cytopenias of which anemia is the most common. Patients might complain of fatigue, weakness, and exercise intolerance. Those with significant neutropenia and thrombocytopenia can present with infections or bleeding. Systemic symptoms are less common, but when present they can herald disease progression to more-advanced forms. Similarly, the presence of Sweet's syndrome (acute febrile neutrophilic dermatosis) can herald transformation to acute leukemia. Organomegaly and lymphadenopathy are uncommon. Infection is the cause of death in approximately 20% to 35% of cases. Transformation to acute leukemia occurs in about 30% of all patients.

Diagnosis

The diagnosis of MDS can be challenging, because its clinical and pathologic characteristics can overlap with other disorders such as aplastic anemia, myeloproliferative neoplasms, and acute leukemia.

A thorough history and physical examination should be performed on every patient with one or more peripheral blood cytopenias, along with basic laboratory tests such as iron studies, vitamin B_{12}, and folic acid levels. However, many disorders can cause pancytopenia; therefore, consideration for a hematology referral should be entertained for the evaluation of pancytopenia or persistent otherwise-unexplained cytopenias, in which case a bone marrow biopsy may be necessary.

The diagnosis of MDS requires an evaluation of the peripheral blood smear, a bone marrow biopsy and aspirate to ascertain the presence of myeloid dysplasia; iron stains, which are necessary for the detection of ring sideroblasts; and cytogenetic studies to detect abnormal clones. Bone marrow dysplasia involving at least 10% of the cells of a specific myeloid lineage is the hallmark of MDS. Cytogenetic abnormalities can be found in up to 70% of patients with de novo MDS and 95% of of patients with therapy-related MDS, and their presence can aid in making the diagnosis, particularly when dysplastic features are not prominent.

 CURRENT DIAGNOSIS

- Myelodysplastic syndromes are diseases of the elderly.
- Chronic unexplained cytopenias should be evaluated to rule out myelodysplastic syndromes.
- Bone marrow biopsy with cytogenetic exam is necessary to make the diagnosis.
- The international prognostic scoring system is an important tool for risk stratification and choice of therapy.

Differential Diagnosis

MDS should be distinguished from a broad number of disorders including megaloblastic anemia, aplastic anemia, large granular lymphocyte leukemia, myelofibrosis, copper deficiency, and HIV infection, which can cause anemia and dysplastic features in the bone marrow. Exposure to certain drugs and toxins can result in marrow dysplasia. These include mycophenolate mofetil (Cellcept), ganciclovir (Cytovene), lead, and excess zinc. Such changes are reversible once the offending agent is discontinued. The diagnosis of MDS can be made by performing a bone marrow biopsy to detect dysplasia and rule out other disorders that can also cause pancytopenia.

Classification and Risk Stratification

Since 1982, there have been various proposals for the classification and risk stratification of MDS. The French-American-British (FAB) classification scheme was the first attempt developed to address the broad range of morphologic features and clinical outcomes in MDS. It identified five subtypes based on morphology and percentage of marrow blasts: refractory anemia (RA), refractory anemia with ringed sideroblasts (RARS), refractory anemia with excess blasts (RAEB), refractory anemia with excess blasts in transformation (RAEB-t), and chronic myelomonocytic leukemia (CMML). This classification allowed MDS to be separated into distinct subsets relative to their survival and acute leukemia evolution.

The World Health Organization (WHO) revised the FAB system to further refine MDS subsets by adding a category of refractory cytopenia with multilineage dysplasia, recognizing 5q-deletion syndrome as a separate clinical and pathologic entity, and lowering the blast percentage from 30% to 20% to diagnose acute myelogenous leukemia (AML). The WHO system was revised in 2008 to recognize the entity of refractory cytopenia with unilineage dysplasia, among other changes, (Table 1).

The International Prognostic Scoring System (IPSS) was introduced to address the variability in prognosis within the FAB subtypes. It predicts survival and risk of evolution to acute leukemia based on scores assigned to three variables: blast cell count, cytogenetics, and number of cytopenias, thereby identifying four distinct groups (Table 2). The IPSS is the most widely used clinical tool to predict the prognosis and clinical behavior of patients with various forms of MDS and to guide choice of therapy (Table 3).

Treatment

A variety of therapeutic options exist for the treatment of MDS patients spanning the spectrum from supportive care to allogeneic stem cell transplantation. Choice of therapy should take into account the patient's age, comorbidities, and the IPSS score.

CURRENT THERAPY

- Myelodysplastic syndromes are divided into two broad categories, low-risk and high-risk disease.
- Patients with low-risk disease s should receive supportive care and hematopoietic growth factors; those with del 5q abnormality should be treated with lenalidomide (Revlimid).
- Patients with high-risk disease should be treated with a hypomethylating agent and should be considered for allogeneic stem cell transplantation.

TABLE 1 Classification and Risk Stratification of Myelodysplastic Syndromes

Disease	Blood Findings	Bone Marrow Findings
Refractory cytopenias with unilineage dysplasia (RCUD) Refractory anemia (RA) Refractory neutropenia (RN) Refractory thrombocytopenia (RT)	Unicytopenia or bicytopenia* No or rare blasts (<1%)[†]	Unilineage dysplasia: ≥10% of the cells in one myeloid lineage <5% blasts <15% of erythroid precursors are ring sideroblasts
Refractory anemia with ring sideroblasts (RARS)	Anemia No blasts	>15% of erythroid precursors are ring sideroblasts Erythroid dysplasia only <5% blasts
Refractory cytopenia with multilineage dysplasia (RCMD)	Cytopenia(s) No or rare blasts (<1%)[†] No Auer rods <10^9/L monocytes	Dysplasia in ≥10% of the cells in ≥2 myeloid lineages (neutrophils, erythroid precursors, megakaryocytes) <5% blasts in marrow No Auer rods ±15% ring sideroblasts
Refractory anemia with excess blasts-1 (RAEB-1)	Cytopenia(s) <5% blasts[2] No Auer rods <10^9/L monocytes	Unilineage or multilineage dysplasia 5 5-9% blasts[2] No Auer rods
Refractory anemia with excess blasts-2 (RAEB-2)	Cytopenia(s) 5%-19% blasts ±Auer rods[‡] <10^9/L monocytes	Unilineage or multilineage dysplasia 10%-19% blasts ±Auer rods[‡]
Myelodysplastic syndrome, unclassified (MDS-U)	Cytopenias ≤1% blasts[2]	Unequivocal dysplasia in <10% of cells in one or more myeloid cell lines when accompanied by a cytogenetic abnormally considered as presumptive evidence for a diagnosis of MDS <5% blasts
MDS associated with isolated del(5q)	Anemia Usually normal or increased platelet count No or rare blasts (<1%)	Normal to increased megakaryocytes with hypolobated nuclei <5% blasts Isolated del(5q) cytogenetic abnormality No Auer rods

*Bicytopenia is occasionally observed. Cases with pancytopenia should be classified as MDS-U.
[†]If the marrow myeloblast percentage is <5% but there are 2%-4% myeloblasts in the blood, the diagnostic classification is RAEB 1. Cases of RCUD and RCMD with 1% myeloblasts in the blood should be classified as MDS, U.
[‡]Cases with Auer rods and <5% myeloblasts in the blood and <10% in the marrow should be classified as RAEB 2.

TABLE 2 Survival and Acute Myelogenous Leukemia Evolution

| Prognostic Variable | Score Value | | | | |
	0	0.5	1.5	1.0	2.0
Marrow blasts(%)	<5	5-10	—	11-20	21-30
Karyotype*	Good	Intermediate	Poor		
Cytopenia†	0/1	2/3			

*Cytogenetics: Good = normal, -Y alone, del(5q) alone, del(20q) alone; Poor = complex (≥3 abnormalities) or chromosome 7 anomalies; Intermediate = other abnormalities. This excludes karyotypes t(8;21), inv16 and t(15;17), which are considered to be AML, not MDS.
†Cytopenias: neutrophil count <1800/μL, platelets <100,000/μL, Hb <10 g/dL.

TABLE 3 Survival and Progression by IPSS Risk Category

Risk Category	% IPSS Pop.	Overall Score	Median Survival (y) in the Absence of Therapy	25% AML Progression (y) in the Absence of Therapy
Low	33	0	5.7	9.4
Intermediate 1	38	0.5-1.0	3.5	3.3
Intermediate 2	22	1.5-2.0	1.1	1.1
High	7	≥2.5	0.4	0.2

Abbreviation: IPSS = International Prognostic Scoring System.

The treating physician should consider the ultimate goal of therapy and whether it is intended to cure, extend survival, or merely palliate symptoms. In the first decade of the 21st century, several novel therapeutic options for MDS have emerged.

SUPPORTIVE CARE

Supportive care has been the cornerstone of MDS therapy for decades; it includes red blood cell transfusion for symptomatic anemia, platelet transfusion to reduce the risk of or to treat bleeding, and use of hematopoietic growth factors such as erythropoiesis stimulating agents (ESA) and colony-stimulating factors such as granulocyte colony-stimulating factor (G-CSF) (Filgrastim [Neupogen])[1] and granulocyte-macrophage colony-stimulating factor (GM-CSF) (Sargramostim [Leukine]).[1]

There are two currently available ESAs: a recombinant human erythropoietin (rhu-EPO; epoetin alfa [Epogen, Procrit])[1] and a super-sialylated form of EPO (darbepoetin alfa [Aranesp]).[1] These are considered the standard of care for the treatment of anemia in patients with low-risk MDS. A predictive model for response to such treatment has been developed by the Nordic MDS study group to guide patient selection. In general, patients with a serum EPO level less than 500 mU/mL and low transfusion burden are likely to respond by improving their hemoglobin level and reducing their need for transfusions.

IMMUNOMODULATORY DRUGS

The novel class of immunomodulatory drugs includes thalidomide (Thalomid)[1] and lenalidomide (Revlimid). Thalidomide was investigated initially with some success in patients with low-risk disease. However, its use was compromised because of poor tolerability. Lenalidomide has been approved for the treatment of patients with low-risk MDS who harbor deletion 5q abnormality, because it was shown in clinical trials to result in transfusion independence in about two thirds of such patients.

HYPOMETHYLATING AGENTS

Currently, two hypomethylating agents are approved for the treatment of MDS: 5-azacitidine (Vidaza) and decitabine (Dacogen).

These agents are cytosine analogues known to inhibit and deplete DNA methyltransferase, which typically adds a methyl group to cytosine residues in newly formed DNA, resulting in the formation of a hypomethylated DNA in vitro. The exact mechanism of action in vivo has not yet been identified.

Results of randomized clinical trials with these agents have demonstrated a statistically significant improvement in hematologic parameters when compared with best supportive care alone in the treatment of MDS patients. It has been shown for the first time that treatment with 5-azacitidine, when compared to other conventional therapies in MDS, can prolong survival in patients with high-risk disease by the IPSS. Both drugs have myelosuppressive properties and result in comparable response rates.

IMMUNOSUPPRESSIVE THERAPY

Immunosuppressive therapy with antithymocyte globulin (Thymoglobulin)[1] or cyclosporine (Neoral)[1] (or both) was evaluated in several clinical trials and shown to result in durable hematological responses in a subset of MDS patients, namely, younger patients with low-risk disease, hypocellular marrows, human leukocyte antigen (HLA)-DR 15 phenotype, and low transfusion need.

HEMATOPOIETIC STEM CELL TRANSPLANTATION

Allogeneic stem cell transplantation is the only curative therapy for MDS patients; this option is feasible for a small subset: typically, younger patients with good performance status and an available HLA-matched donor. Approximately 40% of patients can be cured with this modality. The recent introduction of reduced-intensity conditioning regimens and nonmyeloablative transplants has resulted in expanding the age limit for performing the procedure, reducing transplant-related complications and mortality. However it has been associated with a higher risk of relapse. Because stem cell transplantation is associated with a high rate of treatment-related death—estimated at 39% at 1 year—and the development of acute and chronic graft versus host disease, such treatment is recommended only for those with advanced or high-risk disease.

[1]Not FDA approved for this indication.

[1]Not FDA approved for this indication.

Conclusion and Future Direction

MDS is a chronic disease characterized by features reminiscent of bone marrow failure states with a variable propensity for leukemic evolution. It is curable only by allogeneic stem cell transplantation, which is feasible in only a small subset of patients. For all others, the treatment goal is aimed at improving quality of life and prolonging survival. A variety of clinical trials are evaluating novel agents and combinations of drugs to further optimize the outcome of patients with this disease. Meanwhile, a great deal of research is focused on understanding the molecular underpinning of this disease to enhance our understanding of the biology of this complicated disorder.

REFERENCES

Bennett JM, Catovsky D, Daniel MT, et al. Proposals for the classification of the myelodysplastic syndromes. Br J Haematol 1982;51:189–99.

Brunning RD, Porwit A, Orazi A, et al. Myelodysplastic syndromes/neoplasms. In: Swerdlow S, Campo E, Lee Harris N, et al, editors. WHO Classification of Tumors of Hematopoietic and Lymphoid Tissues. 4th ed. Lyon, France: IARC; 2008. pp. 88–103.

Cutler CS, Lee SJ, Greenberg P, et al. A decision analysis of allogeneic bone marrow transplantation for the myelodysplastic syndromes: Delayed transplantation for low-risk myelodysplasia is associated with improved outcome. Blood 2004;104(2):579–85.

Fenaux P, Mufti GJ, Hellstrom-Lindberg E, et al. Efficacy of azacitidine compared with that of conventional care regimens in the treatment of higher-risk myelodysplastic syndromes: A randomized, open-label, phase III study. Lancet Oncol 2009;10:223–32.

Godley LA, Larson RA. Therapy-related myeloid leukemia. Semin Oncol 2008;35:418–29.

Greenberg PL. The smoldering myeloid leukemic states: Clinical and biologic features. Blood 1983;61:1035–44.

Greenberg P, Cox C, LeBeau MM, et al. International scoring system for evaluating prognosis in myelodysplastic syndromes. Blood 1997;89:2079–88.

Hellstrom-Lindberg E, Negrin R, Stein R, et al. Erythroid response to treatment with G-CSF plus erythropoietin for the anaemia of patients with myelodysplastic syndromes: Proposal for a predictive model. Br J Haematol 1997;99(2):344–51.

Kantarjian H, Issa JP, Rosenfeld CS, et al. Decitabine improves patient outcomes in myelodysplastic syndromes: Results of a phase III randomized study. Cancer 2006;106(8):1794–803.

List A, Dewald G, Bennett J, et al. Lenalidomide in the myelodysplastic syndrome with chromosome 5q deletion. N Engl J Med 2006;355(14):1456–65.

Ma X, Does M, Raza A, Mayne ST. Myelodysplastic syndromes: Incidence and survival in the United States. Cancer 2007;109(8):1536–42.

Martino R, Iacobelli S, Brand R, et al. Retrospective comparison of reduced-intensity conditioning and conventional high-dose conditioning for allogeneic hematopoietic stem cell transplantation using HLA-identical sibling donors in myelodysplastic syndromes. Blood 2006;108:836–46.

Molldrem J, Leifer E, Bahceci E, et al. Antithymocyte globulin for treatment of the bone marrow failure associated with myelodysplastic syndromes. Ann Intern Med 2002;137(3):156–63.

Nisse C, Lorthois C, Dorp V, et al. Exposure to occupational and environmental factors in myelodysplastic syndromes: Preliminary results of a case-control study. Leukemia 1995;9:693–9.

Owen C, Barnett M, Fitzgibbon J. Familial myelodysplasia and acute myeloid leukaemia—a review. Br J Haematol 2008;140:123–32.

Rollison DE, Howlader N, Smith MT, et al. Epidemiology of myelodysplastic syndromes and chronic myeloproliferative disorders in the United States, 2001–2004 using data from the NAACCR and SEER programs. Blood 2008;112:45–52.

Silverman LR, Demakos EP, Peterson BL, et al. Randomized controlled trial of azacitidine in patients with the myelodysplastic syndrome: A study of the Cancer and Leukemia Group B. J Clin Oncol 2002;20(10):2429–40.

Soppi E, Nousiainen T, Seppa A, Lahtinen R. Acute febrile neutrophilic dermatosis (Sweet's syndrome) in association with myelodysplastic syndromes: A report of three cases and a review of the literature. Br J Haematol 1989;73(1):43–7.

Tefferi A, Vardiman JW. Myelodysplastic syndromes. N Engl J Med 2009;361 (19):1872–85.

Vardiman JW, Harris NL, Brunning RD. The World Health Organization (WHO) classification of myeloid neoplasms. Blood 2002;100:2292–302.

The Digestive System

Cholelithiasis and Cholecystitis

Method of
Grant R. Caddy, MD

Cholelithiasis

Gallstones affect 10% to 12% of people in Western populations, and the prevalence increases with age. The majority of patients with gallstones (approximately 80%) remain asymptomatic. The risk of complications, mainly that of acute cholecystitis, occurs in around 2% of patients with symptomatic gallstones.

Gallstones can be classified depending on their composition. The commonest stones are cholesterol or cholesterol-predominant stones (mixed stones), which make up around 80% to 85% of all gallstones. Mixed stones can be multiple, of varying sizes, and faceted. Most are radiolucent but 10% are radiopaque. Pure cholesterol stones are commonly solitary but may be multiple and are radiolucent. Pigment stones are less common in Western populations and are associated with hemolytic disorders such as hemolytic anemias, malaria, and cirrhosis.

Risk factors for cholesterol-predominant stone formation are shown in Box 1. Female patients have a 2 to 8 times greater risk of developing gallstones than male patients. This increased risk appears to decline following menopause. High intake of carbohydrate, high

glycemic load, and high glycemic index foods increase the risk of symptomatic gallstone disease by approximately 1.5 times. Other risk factors include a high body mass index (BMI), rapid weight loss (>1.5 kg/week), and history of dieting or gastric bypass surgery. In a 10-year follow-up study, patients who were overweight (defined as BMI >25) were approximately twice as likely to develop gallstones compared with controls. It has also been documented that following antiobesity surgery, 20% to 35% of patients develop gallstones in the postoperative period.

Complications of symptomatic gallstones are shown in Box 2.

Acute Cholecystitis

Acute cholecystitis is suspected when patients present with pain localized to the right upper quadrant (RUQ), pain aggravated by palpation in the RUQ (with or without a positive Murphy's sign), and an inflammatory response (e.g., fever and elevation in white blood cell count, C-reactive protein, and/or erythrocyte sedimentation rate). The exact mechanism of acute cholecystitis is uncertain, but blockage of the cystic duct in addition to irritation to the gallbladder mucosa result in further recruitment of inflammatory mediators such as prostaglandins (PG) I_2 and E_2. Secondary infection develops in approximately 20% of patients, usually with *Escherichia coli*, *Klebsiella* species, or *Streptococcus faecalis*. Mild elevations in bilirubin, aspartate aminotransferase (AST), alkaline phosphatase (ALP), and γ-glutamyl transpeptidase (GGT) are not uncommon (in up to one third of patients), but high levels often indicate concomitant choledocholithiasis, cholangitis, or Mirizzi's syndrome (see later).

DIAGNOSIS

First-line radiologic investigation should be a transabdominal ultrasound (TUS), which has a high specificity for cholecystitis (>98%). In addition to identifying gallstones, gallbladder thickening

---

BOX 1   Risk Factors for Developing Gallstones

- Age >50 years (relative risk, 2.5; $P < .001$)
- Bile salt loss (e.g., terminal ileal disease)
- Diabetes mellitus
- Female gender
- First-degree relative with symptomatic gallstone disease
- Gallbladder dysmotility and stasis
- Genetic factors
- High intake of carbohydrates and high glycemic load
- Hyperlipidemia
- Overweight and obesity
- Positive family history of previous cholecystectomy in a first-degree family member
- Pregnancy
- Starvation
- Total parenteral nutrition

BOX 2   Complications of Gallstones

- Acalculous cholecystitis
- Acute cholecystitis
- Biliary colic
- Cholecystoenteric fistulas
- Choledocholithiasis ± ascending cholangitis
- Chronic cholecystitis
- Gallstone ileus
- Gallstone pancreatitis
- Gangrenous gallbladder and gallbladder perforation
- Mirizzi's syndrome

CURRENT DIAGNOSIS

- The majority of patients with gallstones (approximately 80%) remain asymptomatic. The risk of complications, mainly acute cholecystitis, occurs in around 2% of patients with symptomatic gallstones.
- Mild elevations in bilirubin, AST, ALP, and GGT occur in approximately one third of patients but high levels often indicate concomitant choledocholithiasis or cholangitis.
- TUS has a high specificity for cholecystitis (>98%). A HIDA scan has a sensitivity of >95% and a specificity of 90%.
- Approximately 10% to 18% of patients undergoing cholecystectomy have coexisting bile duct stones.
- In choledocholithiasis, TUS is particularly sensitive if there is biliary dilatation (sensitivity is 96%) but is less sensitive in detecting stones within the duct (sensitivity is 63%).
- EUS, MRCP, and ERCP are equivalent in accuracy rates for detecting choledocholithiasis, but because of the complication rate of ERCP, this procedure should be reserved for patients with a high probability of choledocholithiasis.

Abbreviations: ALP = alkaline phosphatase; AST = aspartate aminotransferase; ERCP = endoscopic retrograde cholangiopancreatography; EUS = endoscopic ultrasound; GGT = γ-glutamyl transpeptidase; HIDA = hepatobiliary iminodiacetic acid; MRCP = magnetic resonance cholangiopancreatography; TUS = transabdominal ultrasound.

(>4–5 mm), edema, adjacent pericolic fluid, and tenderness with the transducer strongly suggest cholecystitis. Hepatobiliary iminodiacetic acid (HIDA) scan should be reserved for second-line investigation if the diagnosis remains in doubt. If the cystic duct is patent, HIDA will be taken up by the gallbladder and will be evident on scanning the abdomen after 1 hour. A positive test fails to detect any localization of HIDA within the gallbladder due to obstruction of the cystic duct. The test has a sensitivity of greater than 95% but a specificity of 90%.

TREATMENT

Patients should receive supportive care as first-line treatment with intravenous hydration and analgesia. There is evidence that nonsteroidal antiinflammatory drugs (NSAIDs) have additional benefits other than their analgesic properties, due to their antagonist effect on prostaglandins, which are central to the inflammation of cholecystitis. NSAIDs reduce intraluminal pressure in the gallbladder, which is increased in acute cholecystitis. In addition, NSAIDs have been shown to reduce the rate of progression of biliary colic to acute cholecystitis. Due to the risk of secondary infection, antibiotics such as cephalosporin (Zinacef) and metronidazole (Flagyl) are generally recommended, but in uncomplicated cholecystitis, the routine use of antibiotics does not appear to reduce the risk of gallbladder empyema.

Laparoscopic cholecystectomy remains the most common surgical treatment for acute cholecystitis and is considered the treatment of choice for most patients. The advantages of laparoscopic cholecystectomy over open cholecystectomy are well documented and include reduced mortality, reduced postoperative pain, better cosmetic result, and a reduction in hospital stay. Studies investigating the optimal timing of laparoscopic cholecystectomy following acute cholecystitis suggest that early cholecystectomy (within 72 hours) compared with delayed cholecystectomy results in a reduction in hospital stay

and readmission rate but no overall differences in operation time, conversion rate, or complication rates. Patient symptom scores (diarrhea, indigestion, and abdominal pain) at 4 weeks are significantly better in patients undergoing early cholecystectomy versus supportive treatment followed by delayed cholecystectomy.

There is evidence supporting mini-laparotomy cholecystectomy (usually defined as open cholecystectomy through an incision of 4 to 7 cm) with similar overall results to laparoscopic cholecystectomy. In one prospective study, laparoscopic cholecystectomy took a longer time to perform but produced a slightly shorter postoperative hospital stay and a smoother postoperative course than mini-laparotomy. The choice of which operation to perform is often determined by the experience of individual surgical centers.

COMPLICATIONS

Emphysematous Cholecystitis

Acute emphysematous cholecystitis is characterized by the presence of gas within the wall or lumen of the gallbladder caused by the gas-forming organisms (e.g., *Clostridium welchii* or *E. coli*). Symptoms can be identical to those of acute cholecystitis. In contrast to acute cholecystitis, emphysematous cholecystitis occurs more commonly in elderly and diabetic patients. Its importance lies in the increased rates of early gangrene and perforation of the gallbladder. Treatment is with empiric antibiotic therapy and early cholecystectomy.

Gangrenous Cholecystitis

Gangrenous cholecystitis occurs in 2% to 20% of patients admitted with acute cholecystitis. The risk factors for gangrenous cholecystitis is increased in male patients older than 50 years; in patients with diabetes, history of cardiovascular disease, or white blood cell count greater than 15,000/mm^3; and in those who delay seeking medical treatment. The risk of gallbladder perforation and mortality is increased with gangrenous cholecystitis. Treatment is with empiric antibiotic therapy and early cholecystectomy.

Gallbladder Perforation

Gallbladder perforation can occur following gangrenous cholecystitis. It is estimated to occur in 3% to 10% of patients with acute cholecystitis. Like gangrenous cholecystitis, patients with gallbladder perforations have similar characteristics including older age and cardiovascular disease. In addition, perforations were associated with more postoperative complications that required more ICU admissions and longer hospital stays. Perforations may be localized, resulting in a pericholecystic abscess, or, less commonly, free perforations may occur into the peritoneum. Diagnosis is often difficult preoperatively.

Acalculous Cholecystitis

Acalculous cholecystitis occurs in 5% to 10% of cases of cholecystitis. It is often associated with critically ill patients, severe trauma, burns, and cardiovascular surgery but is also associated with patients who have diabetes, cardiovascular disease, or AIDS and in patients on total parenteral nutrition or opiates. Without treatment, the mortality rate is 30% to 50%.

Characteristic features on TUS are thickened gallbladder wall, absence of gallstones, gallbladder distention, Murphy's sign induced by probe, and emphysematous cholecystitis with or without perforation. Treatment is initially with supportive therapy with antibiotics and urgent referral for laparoscopic cholecystectomy. In patients with high operative risk, percutaneous cholecystostomy (insertion of a drain into the gallbladder) under radiologic guidance is an alternative treatment.

Other complications of cholelithiasis include gallstone ileus, cholecystoenteric fistulas, and Mirizzi's syndrome (obstruction of the bile duct secondary to extrinsic compression from an impacted stone in the cystic duct).

Acute Cholecystitis in Pregnancy

Overall acute cholecystitis in pregnancy is relatively uncommon. The optimal treatment remains controversial. Conservative management of a pregnant patient results in resolution of symptoms in approximately 90% of patients. However, up to 60% of patients have recurrent symptoms (readmission with acute cholecystitis, biliary colic, and premature delivery). Due to concerns of fetal loss, a conservative approach is often adopted. However, studies have supported the role of laparoscopic cholecystectomy as a safe procedure in pregnant patients with acute cholecystitis, resulting in decreased hospital stay, reduced rate of labor induction, and reduced preterm deliveries.

Chronic Cholecystitis

Chronic cholecystitis refers to recurrent episodes of gallbladder inflammation usually due to stones. These episodes may be asymptomatic but they can also result in recurrent episodes of pain. However, there does not appear to be any correlation of symptoms and degree of fibrosis and thickening of the gallbladder wall. Patients with symptomatic gallstones with recurrent biliary colic should be referred for laparoscopic cholecystectomy.

Biliary Sludge

Biliary sludge is usually diagnosed on ultrasonography. Its appearance on ultrasonography is of layered echoes in the dependent portion of the gallbladder, with no associated acoustic shadows. It is often made up of cholesterol crystals and calcium salts.

Precipitating factors include total parenteral nutrition, rapid weight loss, pregnancy, prolonged fasting, bone marrow and solid organ transplants, and drugs such as octreotide (Sandostatin) and ceftriaxone (Rocephin). In one study, 50% of patients presenting with symptomatic biliary sludge had complete resolution of gallbladder sludge on repeat imaging. In the remaining group, in 50% the sludge remained but patients were asymptomatic and in 50% further symptoms developed.

The management of biliary sludge should be managed similar to gallbladder stones. Asymptomatic sludge should be managed conservatively. Symptomatic patients should be considered for laparoscopic cholecystectomy.

Choledocholithiasis

PRESENTATION

Approximately 10% to 18% of patients undergoing cholecystectomy have coexisting bile duct stones. The symptoms of choledocholithiasis are varied and include biliary colic, jaundice, cholangitis, and pancreatitis. Conversely, a portion of patients with choledocholithiasis are asymptomatic, with a prevalence estimated to be up to 12%. In patients who present with symptoms of retained bile duct stones, the risk of subsequent symptoms is up to 50%, and the risk of complications is up to 25% if the stones are left untreated.

Patients with choledocholithiasis often present with biliary colic—pain that is often located in the RUQ and lasting between 30 minutes and several hours. There is often associated nausea and vomiting. If there is partial or complete obstruction of the common bile duct, then patients develop jaundice with associated pale stools and dark urine. Infection often occurs, resulting in a cholangitis. Approximately three fourths of patients with cholangitis have Charcot's triad of jaundice, fever, and pain. However, in 10% of patients pain may be the only feature of cholangitis. Due to bacterial translocation from the bile duct to the bloodstream, 20% of patients with cholangitis have a bacteremia, usually with gram-negative organisms.

Smaller bile duct stones (up to 8 mm) are more likely to pass spontaneously through the ampulla into the duodenum. However, it is the passage of smaller stones through the ampulla that is more likely to result in gallstone pancreatitis compared with larger stones. For example, one study found that patients who presented with gallstone pancreatitis had a mean stone diameter of 4 mm compared with patients presenting with obstructive jaundice, who had a mean stone diameter of 9 mm.

DIFFERENTIAL DIAGNOSIS

The differential of choledocholithiasis will depend on the clinical presentation. Differentials are shown in Box 3.

DIAGNOSIS

Patients presenting with symptomatic choledocholithiasis often have elevations in serum GGT and ALP (increased in 94% and 91% of cases, respectively). Bilirubin levels may be increased depending on if obstruction of the bile duct has occurred.

BOX 3 Differential Diagnosis of Choledocholithiasis by Presentation

Jaundice with or without Pain
- Alcoholic liver disease
- Benign stricture
- Bile duct injuries
- Drug induced
- Malignant stricture
- Parasitic infection of the biliary tree
- Primary biliary cirrhosis
- Sclerosing cholangitis
- Viral hepatitis

Biliary Colic
- Acute pancreatitis
- Cholecystitis
- Duodenitis
- Esophageal spasm
- Inferior myocardial infarction
- Peptic ulcer disease
- Sphincter of Oddi dysfunction

Pancreatitis
- Appendicitis
- Biliary colic
- Dissecting aneurysm
- Diverticulitis
- Ectopic pregnancy
- Hematoma of abdominal muscles
- Inferior myocardial infarction
- Mesenteric infarction
- Perforated gastric or duodenal ulcer

Cholestatic Liver Function Tests
- Alcoholic liver disease
- Ampullary carcinoma
- Biliary strictures
- Drugs
- Granulomatous hepatitis
- Malignant infiltration of the liver
- Nonalcoholic fatty liver disease (NAFLD)
- Primary biliary cirrhosis
- Sclerosing cholangitis

TUS is the commonest method of imaging the gallbladder and biliary tree in choledocholithiasis. TUS is particularly sensitive if there is biliary dilation (sensitivity up to 96%). It is less sensitive in detecting stones within the duct (sensitivity up to 63%) but has high specificity (specificity 95%). Therefore, a negative TUS does not rule out suspected choledocholithiasis.

Other radiologic investigations include computed tomography (CT), endoscopic ultrasound (EUS), magnetic resonance cholangio-pancreatography (MRCP), and endoscopic retrograde cholangio-pancreatography (ERCP). A National Institutes of Health (NIH) consensus statement found that EUS, MRCP, and ERCP were equivalent in accuracy rates. However, due to the risks of ERCP (pancreatitis, bleeding, perforation, infection), ERCP is recommended in patients with a high probability of choledocholithiasis. In patients with an intermediate probability, other imaging modalities, such as MRCP or EUS, should be considered.

TREATMENT

Generally, patients with symptomatic choledocholithiasis should be offered treatment because of the high risk of recurrent symptoms and complications if stones are left in situ as already discussed. In some special circumstances, adopting a conservative approach may be appropriate such as severe end-stage dementia or severe comorbid factors that make removal hazardous.

The two main methods of bile duct stone removal are at ERCP or, in patients with an intact gallbladder, laparoscopic cholecystectomy and bile duct exploration (LC+BDE). Current practice in choosing between the two methods depends on center preference and local expertise in laparoscopic bile duct exploration. A recent Cochrane Database of systematic review comparing LC+BDE and ERCP found that both methods were equally effective, with no significant difference in morbidity and mortality. However, shorter hospital stay was achieved in patients undergoing LC+BDE.

There is a limited role for other techniques, such as extracorporeal shockwave lithotripsy and endoscopic laser lithotripsy, and these techniques should be reserved for bile duct stones that cannot be removed at ERCP or LC+CBE due to technical or safety reasons.

CURRENT THERAPY

- Patients with symptomatic gallstones should undergo laparoscopic cholecystectomy if there is no contraindication.
- For acute cholecystitis, first-line treatment is supportive care with intravenous hydration, analgesia (NSAIDs), and antibiotics. If there are no contraindications, patients should undergo laparoscopic cholecystectomy within 72 hours.
- Percutaneous cholecystostomy is an alternative option in patients with acalculous cholecystitis who are too unwell to undergo cholecystectomy.
- Treatment options for patients with choledocholithiasis include ERCP and stone removal followed by laparoscopic cholecystectomy or, in patients with an intact gallbladder, cholecystectomy and bile duct exploration. Overall, there are no differences in morbidity and mortality between the two procedures.
- There is a limited role for other techniques such as extracorporeal shockwave lithotripsy and endoscopic laser lithotripsy or oral dissolution therapy.

Abbreviation: ERCP = endoscopic retrograde cholangio-pancreatography.

REFERENCES

Al-Waili N, Saloom KY. The analgesic effect of intravenous tenoxicam in symptomatic treatment of biliary colic: A comparison with hyoscine *N*-butylbromide. Eur J Med Res 1998;3(10):475–9.

Field AE, Coakley EH, Must A, et al. Impact of overweight on the risk of developing common chronic diseases during a 10-year period. Arch Intem Med 2001;161(13):1581–6.

Johansson M, Thune A, Blomqvist A, et al. Impact of choice of therapeutic strategy on acute cholecystitis on patient's health-related quality of life. Results of a randomized, controlled clinical trial. Dig Surg 2004;21(5–6):359–62.

Lau H, Lo CY, Patil NG, Yuen WK. Early versus delayed-interval laparoscopic cholecystectomy for acute cholecystitis: A meta-analysis. Surg Endosc 2006;20(1):82–7.

Lu EJ, Curet MJ, El-Sayed YY, Kirkwood KS. Medical versus surgical management of biliary tract disease in pregnancy. Am J Surg. 2004;188(6):755–9.

Martin DJ, Vernon DR, Toouli J. Surgical versus endoscopic treatment of bile duct stones. Cochrane Database Syst Rev 2006;(2):CD003327.

Miller K, Hell E, Lang B, Lengauer E. Gallstone formation prophylaxis after gastric restrictive procedures for weight loss: A randomized double-blind placebo-controlled trial. Ann Surg 2003;238(5):697–702.

NIH state-of-the-science statement on endoscopic retrograde cholangiopancreatography (ERCP) for diagnosis and therapy. NIH Consens State Sci Statements 2002;19(1):1–26.

Papi C, Catarci M, D'Ambrosio L, et al. Timing of cholecystectomy for acute calculous cholecystitis: A meta-analysis. Am J Gastroenterol. 2004;99(1):147–55.

Ros A, Gustafsson L, Krook H, et al. Laparoscopic cholecystectomy versus mini-laparotomy cholecystectomy: A prospective, randomized, single-blind study. Ann Surg 2001;234(6):741–9.

Thornell E, Nilsson B, Jansson R, Svanvik J. Effect of short-term indomethacin treatment on the clinical course of acute obstructive cholecystitis. Eur J Surg 1991;157(2):127–30.

Tsai CJ, Leitzmann MF, Willett WC, Giovannucci EL. Dietary carbohydrates and glycaemic load and the incidence of symptomatic gall stone disease in men. Gut 2005;54(6):823–8.

Cirrhosis

Method of
Harmit Kalia, DO; Priya Grewal, MD; and Paul Martin, MD

Cirrhosis is the 12th most common cause of death in the United States; it is responsible for more than 27,000 deaths and 421,000 hospitalizations annually. Cirrhosis reflects the consequences of chronic hepatic necroinflammatory activity with an incomplete repair response. This involves collagen deposition and nodule formation, leading to disruption of the normal lobular arrangement of hepatocytes, blood vessels, and lymphatics. Although, strictly speaking, the diagnosis of cirrhosis is based on histology, in the absence of a liver biopsy its presence can be inferred in the appropriate setting by complications such as portal hypertension or radiologic appearances consistent with the diagnosis. Cirrhosis can result from any cause of chronic liver disease (Table 1). Most manifestations of advanced cirrhosis, such as portal hypertension and coagulopathy, reflect the consequences of extensive distortion of the hepatic architecture and impaired hepatocellular function. However, some symptoms may also reflect the specific etiology of cirrhosis—most notably, pruritus in patients with cholestasis and malabsorption of fat-soluble vitamins in patients with primary biliary cirrhosis or primary sclerosing cholangitis.

An important distinction among individual patients is whether the cirrhosis is compensated or decompensated. Cirrhosis that remains compensated implies the absence of an index complication such as onset of ascites or variceal hemorrhage, whereas overt hepatic decompensation indicates that a major complication has supervened

TABLE 1 Common Causes of Cirrhosis

Cause	Examples
Infection	Hepatitis B
	Hepatitis C
	Hepatitis D
Toxins	Alcohol, drugs
Cholestasis	Primary biliary cirrhosis
	Secondary biliary cirrhosis
	Primary sclerosing cholangitis
Autoimmune	Autoimmune hepatitis
Vascular	Cardiac cirrhosis
	Budd-Chiari syndrome
	Sinusoidal obstruction syndrome
Metabolic	Hemochromatosis
	Wilson's disease
	α_1-Antitrypsin deficiency
	Nonalcoholic steatohepatitis
Cryptogenic	

and the patient now has evidence of frank hepatic failure. A patient with compensated cirrhosis can continue to have a good prognosis. However, once an initial manifestation of cirrhosis has occurred, the patient's likelihood of long-term survival diminishes in the absence of liver transplantation. The diagnosis of cirrhosis per se does not suggest the need for evaluation for liver transplantation, but transplantation needs to be considered once a major complication such as a variceal hemorrhage, onset of ascites, or hepatic encephalopathy has supervened. Less florid evidence of cirrhosis may include a hyperdynamic circulation reflecting peripheral vasodilation with a resting tachycardia. However, many patients with cirrhosis are completely asymptomatic until a major complication of their liver disease supervenes. Clues to underlying cirrhosis are thrombocytopenia or coagulopathy not related to a primary hematologic disorder or biochemical dysfunction with hyperbilirubinemia and elevated serum aminotransferases or alkaline phosphatase.

In patients with well-compensated cirrhosis, the physical signs of liver disease may be subtle. The liver span may be somewhat diminished on percussion, with a firm edge and with splenic dullness due to splenomegaly. Cutaneous signs of cirrhosis other than jaundice include palmar erythema and spider nevi. In cirrhotic male patients, gynecomastia results from altered metabolism of sex hormones with testicular atrophy; it also reflects the antigonadal effects of alcohol in some patients. The catabolic effects of cirrhosis often result in a diminished muscle mass, obvious on physical examination. More florid evidence of cirrhosis on physical examination includes varying degrees of disturbed mentation along with asterixis, indicative of hepatic encephalopathy. Other key findings include ascites and peripheral edema. Additional physical findings may provide some clues to the underlying etiology of liver disease. For instance, xanthelasmata are frequent in patients with cholestatic liver disease, whereas patients with alcoholic cirrhosis may have other end-organ injury such as peripheral neuropathy.

Laboratory findings suggestive of portal hypertension are a low platelet count and a low leukocyte count due to hypersplenism. Impaired hepatic synthetic and secretory functions are reflected in a diminished serum albumin, elevated serum bilirubin, and prolonged prothrombin time.

Transition from compensated to decompensated cirrhosis occurs at a rate of 5% to 7% per annum. Various models have been developed to predict the likelihood of hepatic decompensation in individual patients. They typically incorporate a combination of routine blood tests, including the platelet count, which is depressed in portal hypertension mainly because of hypersplenism and diminished thrombopoietin. The development of hepatocellular carcinoma (HCC) accelerates the progression of cirrhosis as a result of the tumor mass and vascular invasion, most typically of the portal vein. However, the morbidity and mortality in chronic liver disease are related to a large extent to the severity of portal hypertension.

The median survival time in patients with compensated cirrhosis is 12 years, whereas in those with decompensated cirrhosis it is 1.5 years. Recently, there has been an increasing emphasis on anticipating the complications of cirrhosis, such as variceal hemorrhage (discussed in the chapter on bleeding esophageal varices), HCC, and spontaneous bacterial peritonitis (SBP), in an effort to enhance survival and allow appropriate intervention with liver transplantation.

Cirrhotic patients are immunocompromised and therefore are at increased risk for bacterial infections. The pulmonary complications of cirrhosis are relatively uncommon and include portopulmonary hypertension (PPHTN) and hepatopulmonary syndrome (HPS).

Ascites

Cirrhosis is the underlying cause for ascites in 85% of patients. Ascites is the most common complication of cirrhosis and carries a 2-year survival rate of only 50% after its onset. The pathogenesis of ascites in cirrhosis mainly reflects increased intrahepatic resistance due to fibrosis, which raises portal pressures. Compensatory mechanisms cause splanchnic vasodilation, resulting in a decrease in effective arterial blood volume. This results in a compensatory activation of the neurohumoral (renin-angiotensin) system and increased retention of sodium by the kidneys. The imbalance of elevated hydrostatic pressure due to portal hypertension and decreased oncotic pressure (low albumin) causes ascites. Therefore, sodium retention is key to the development of ascites. Other mechanisms can include disruption of normal lymphatic drainage in the liver due to extensive fibrosis.

Physical examination may reveal a bulging abdomen with shifting dullness; this sign is reliable when the volume of ascites is greater than 1500 mL. Ultrasound of the abdomen is helpful in locating smaller amounts of ascites (as little as 100 mL). Once ascites is found, a diagnostic paracenteses should be performed to determine whether it is exudative or transudative, a determination that narrows the differential diagnosis of ascites (Table 2). The fluid is tested for white blood cell count, culture, and albumin to calculate serum-ascites albumin gradient (SAAG). This must be done on initial paracenteses and accurately distinguishes ascites related to portal versus nonportal hypertensive causes. A SAAG of 1.1 g/dL or higher accurately predicts portal hypertension. Once the diagnosis of ascites is made, it is important to mitigate aggravating factors for fluid retention. Dietary indiscretion, noncompliance with diuretics, therapeutic volume expansion after gastrointestinal bleeding volume expansion, and renal toxicity from use of nonsteroidal antiinflammatory drugs are common causes.

TABLE 2 Diagnostic Tests on Ascites

Test	Comments
Cell count	If PMN $\geq$250 cells/mm^3, infection is presumed
Culture	High sensitivity if infected
Albumin	Necessary to calculate SAAG
Total protein	Assists in determining cause of ascites
Gram stain	Assists in infectious/inflammatory work-up
LDH	High in malignant ascites
Amylase	Elevated in ascites secondary to pancreatitis
TB smear, culture, PCR	If TB is suspected
Cytology	Assists in diagnosis of malignant ascites
Triglycerides	Chylous ascites if >110 mg/dL
Bilirubin	To confirm leakage of bile in peritoneum

Abbreviations: LDH = lactate dehydrogenase; PCR = polymerase chain reaction; PMN = polymorphonuclear neutrophils; SAAG = serum-ascites albumin gradient; TB = tuberculosis.

The mainstay of management of ascites is sodium restriction and judicious diuresis. Patients should be encouraged to stay on a sodium-restricted diet of 2 g/day. A sodium-to-potassium concentration ratio greater than 1 on a random urine sample correlates well with a 24-hour sodium excretion greater than 78 mmol/day and implies patient compliance with salt restriction. In reality, dietary restriction of sodium is efficacious in only 10% of patients; more typically, diuretics are needed. Mild to moderate ascites is controlled best by the use of diuretics with different modes of action, such as spironolactone (Aldactone) 100 mg (an aldosterone antagonist) and furosemide (Lasix) 40 mg (a loop diuretic) taken once daily. Serum electrolytes need to be monitored to avoid hypokalemia or hyperkalemia. Doses of spironolactone and furosemide can be increased in a 100:40 ratio every 3 to 5 days until an adequate diuresis is achieved. Doses greater than spironolactone 400 mg and furosemide 160 mg are generally not recommended, to lessen the risk of electrolyte imbalance or renal insufficiency. Fluid restriction is recommended if the serum sodium concentration is less than 120 to 125 mmol/L, because hyponatremia in this circumstance reflects an excess of free water rather than sodium depletion. Hospitalized patients can be weighed daily to help guide management. Ideally, the patient should shed about 1 pound of weight every day; failure to do so implies inadequate diuretic dosing or lack of compliance with fluid restriction. Excessive weight loss should also be avoided, to forestall precipitation of hepatorenal syndrome. Diuretic therapy should be withheld if a patient presents with encephalopathy, infection, renal insufficiency, or a serum sodium concentration of 120 mmol/L or greater.

Refractory ascites, defined as inability to obtain a diuresis with high-dose diuretics without inducing renal dysfunction, occurs in 10% of cirrhotic patients with ascites; the resultant 1-year survival rate is only 25%. Serial large-volume paracenteses (LVP) of greater than 5 L of fluid is safe and effective in controlling ascites. Continued dietary restriction of sodium is necessary to avoid overly frequent paracenteses. Patients requiring LVP more frequently than every 2 weeks are probably not complying with a sodium-restricted diet. The use of albumin as colloid replacement is controversial, but it is generally accepted for use with ascitic fluid removal of greater than 5 L, to prevent postparacentesis circulatory dysfunction leading to renal insufficiency.

A patient who requires frequent LVP may be a candidate for a transjugular intrahepatic portosystemic shunt (TIPS). This vascular shunt is placed under fluoroscopic guidance and bridges a branch of the hepatic vein with a branch of the portal vein to reduce portal pressures. It is effective in about 90% of patients with refractory ascites. Diuretic therapy needs to be continued in many patients after institution of TIPS. There is generally no survival advantage for TIPS compared with LVP in cirrhotic patients, although it may simplify patient management by removing the need for large-volume paracenteses.

The Model of End-Stage Liver Disease (MELD) score assesses the severity of liver disease and is based on the natural logarithms (base e) of the concentrations of bilirubin and creatinine (in milligrams per deciliter) and the international normalized ratio (INR):

$$\text{MELD} = [3.8 \times ln \,(\text{Bilirubin})] + [11.2 \times ln \,(\text{INR})] + [9.6 \, ln \,(\text{Creatinine})]$$

TIPS should be avoided in patients with a MELD score greater than 18 or Child-Pugh grade C disease (Table 3). These patients have a poor outcome because of deterioration in hepatocellular function secondary to this form of therapeutic portosystemic shunting. Not surprisingly, there is a high frequency (up to 40%) of portosystemic hepatic encephalopathy (PSE) after TIPS, which can be disabling and may even necessitate reduction in the shunt diameter to alleviate symptoms. TIPS occlusion was frequent in the past, but with newer covered stents the patency is maintained. As part of the evaluation for TIPS placement, patients should undergo echocardiography to confirm that the cardiac ejection fraction is greater than 60%. This is done to prevent heart failure precipitated by an increased venous return after shunt placement. Since the availability of TIPS, peritoneovenous shunting has fallen out of favor. Given the invasive nature of the procedure, along with its potential complications (disseminated intravascular coagulation, infection of the shunt, bleeding), this intervention is no longer considered in most centers. Despite available modalities for the management of ascites, the presence of ascites implies poor long-term survival, and referral to a transplant center is indicated.

Spontaneous Bacterial Peritonitis

SBP is infection of the ascitic fluid with enteric aerobic organisms in the absence of a primary discrete source of infection such as a perforated viscus. Cirrhotic patients with ascites have a 10% annual incidence of SBP. It is the most common bacterial infection in cirrhotics with ascites, with a mortality rate of 30% in older series. The mortality rises when SBP is complicated by renal failure.

Patients may be asymptomatic (Table 4), and on admission or readmission of a cirrhotic patient with ascites, diagnostic paracentesis is essential to exclude unrecognized SBP. A high index of suspicion is also necessary in cirrhotic patients with unexplained fever, worsening hepatocellular function, nonspecific abdominal pain, or unexplained PSE. SBP is defined as positive ascitic fluid culture (one organism) and a polymorphonuclear neutrophil (PMN) count of 250 cells/mm^3 or higher. Treatment with antibiotics is also indicated if the culture is negative but the PMN count is 250 cells/mm^3 or greater, or if the culture is positive with one organism and the PMN count is 250 cells/mm^3 or greater in a symptomatic patient. Diagnostic paracentesis revealing PMNs greater than 250 cells/mm^3 and multiple enteric organisms suggests secondary bacterial peritonitis, and treatment should include antibiotics with further evaluation to exclude bowel perforation.

TABLE 3   Child-Pugh Classification*

Factor	Points Assigned		
	1	2	3
Ascites	Absent	Slight	Moderate
Bilirubin	<2 mg/dL	2–3 mg/dL	>3 mg/dL
Albumin	>3.5 g/dL (35 g/L)	2.8–3.5 g/dL	<2.8 g/dL
Prothrombin time			
Seconds over control	<4	4–6	>6
International normalized ratio	<1.7	1.7–2.3	>2.3
Encephalopathy	None	Grade 1–2	Grade 3–4

*A total score of 5–6 is considered grade A (well-compensated disease); 7–9 is grade B (significant functional compromise); and 10–15 is grade C (decompensated disease).

TABLE 4   Frequency of Signs and Symptoms in Patients with Spontaneous Bacterial Peritonitis

Sign or Symptom	Frequency (%)
Fever	68
Abdominal pain	49
Abdominal tenderness	39
Rebound	10
Altered mental status	54

Adapted from Feldman M, Friedman LS, Brandt LJ (eds): Sleisenger & Fordtran's Gastrointestinal and Liver Disease, 8th ed. Philadelphia: Saunders Elsevier, 2006.

Treatment of SBP involves the empiric administration of third-generation cephalosporins (e.g., cefotaxime [Claforan]) before the bacterial culture results become available. The organisms most commonly involved are *Escherichia coli*, *Streptococcus* species, and *Klebsiella pneumoniae*. Ascitic fluid cultures are positive in only 50% to 60% of cases. Culture sensitivity is improved by immediate inoculation of aerobic and anaerobic blood culture bottles. For patients with an allergy to cephalosporins, alternatives include amoxicillin-clavulanate (Augmentin) and ciprofloxacin (Cipro). A 5-day antibiotic regimen is used, with resolution in 90% of cases. Repeat paracentesis 48 hours after starting antibiotics is useful to confirm the clinical response of the infection, especially if the initial ascitic white blood cell count was in the thousands. Paracentesis should also be repeated after 5 days of antibiotics to confirm the response before withdrawing antibiotic therapy. If the typical clinical response to antibiotics does not occur, important considerations include secondary bacterial peritonitis, intraabdominal abscess formation, and bacterial resistance. Plasma volume expansion with albumin in addition to antibiotics decreases the incidence of renal dysfunction and improves survival. Albumin, unlike other volume expanders, improves cardiac function by decreasing arterial vasodilation. The recommended dose of albumin is 1.5 g/kg at the time of diagnosis of SBP and 1.0 g/kg after 72 hours of treatment with antibiotics.

After a single episode of SBP, there is a 70%, 1-year cumulative probability of further SBP episodes; therefore, prophylaxis with antibiotics is appropriate. Oral norfloxacin (Noroxin)[1] 400 mg daily or ciprofloxacin[1] 750 mg weekly can reduce the risk of SBP to 20% over 1 year. For patients with a fluoroquinolone allergy, trimethoprim-sulfamethoxazole (one Bactrim DS daily)[1] may be administered. Primary prophylaxis for SBP is beneficial in patients with a low ascitic protein concentration (<1.0 g/dL). Other settings in which antibiotics are helpful include cirrhotic patients admitted with gastrointestinal bleeding. Antiobiotic therapy lowers the infection rate, decreases the rate of further variceal bleeding, and improves survival. Improvements in earlier detection and treatment of this infection have had a major impact on reducing mortality. In addition, prophylaxis against SBP has lowered its incidence in cirrhotics at risk.

Portosystemic (Hepatic) Encephalopathy

PSE is a syndrome of reversible neuropsychiatric dysfunction of varying severity that occurs on a background of portal hypertension with shunting of blood from the portal system into the systemic circulation. Despite its frequency in cirrhotic patients, there is continuing controversy about its exact pathogenesis. Nitrogenous products from the gut are clearly implicated. Pathologically, there may be evidence of swelling of astrocyte cells in the brain. Ammonia and other toxins accumulate in the blood to impair cognitive and motor function.

PSE is classified into three types (Table 5). The most common type has a gradual onset in cirrhotic patients and is referred to as type C. Type A is associated with acute liver failure, and type B is associated with portosystemic bypass (portocaval shunt) in the absence of cirrhosis. The clinical features of type C PSE include a wide range of neuropsychiatric symptoms. Stage 1 is characterized

---

[1]Not FDA approved for this indication.

TABLE 5 Types of Hepatic Encephalopathy

Type	Description
A	Acute liver failure
B	Portosystemic bypass without cirrhosis (portocaval shunt)
C	Chronic liver disease (cirrhosis)

by alterations in consciousness and behavioral changes (inversion of sleep/wake pattern, forgetfulness); stage 2 can include confusion and disorientation; stage 3 includes more profound symptoms, with lethargy and a stuporous state; and stage 4 is frank coma. The physical examination may elicit subtle findings such as mild tremor, as well as the more classic asterixis. Fetor hepaticus is a sweetish breath odor found in some patients with PSE. The diagnosis of PSE remains clinical. Serum ammonia levels correlate poorly with the severity of encephalopathy. An increased level of serum ammonia per se is not an indication to treat a patient with liver disease in the absence of clinical evidence of PSE. Minimal PSE is subclinical and is present in up to 70% of cirrhotics. It is diagnosed by psychomotor and neuropsychological tests only. Its progression to overt PSE seems to be related to deterioration of hepatocellular function.

When a cirrhotic patient presents with overt PSE, management includes identification of a precipitating cause, which is present in more than 80% of cases. Key precipitants include infection, noncompliance with medications, gastrointestinal bleeding, dehydration, electrolyte abnormalities, use of narcotics or sedatives, constipation, TIPS, and increased protein intake. Treatment of the precipitating cause, in addition to inducing a catharsis, is associated with improved cognitive and motor function. Upper gastrointestinal bleeding should be excluded by rectal examination and nasogastric lavage. An absence of improvement in mentation within 48 hours should lead to a further search for unrecognized precipitants (e.g., ongoing sepsis) or a separate neurologic diagnosis (e.g., subdural hematoma). Repeated admissions to hospital with easily reversible PSE suggest noncompliance with lactulose therapy, which remains the mainstay for its treatment.

Available therapies for overt PSE counteract the effects of gut-derived bacterial neuroactive toxins. Therapy for overt PSE includes the induction of a catharsis with lactulose (Cephulac) or lactitol. Lactulose 45 to 90 g/m^3 should be given via nasogastric tube every 2 hours (in severe PSE) until loose bowel movements are observed, and thereafter to obtain two to three loose bowel movements daily. Lactulose enemas may be given in a less alert patient. Cathartics used for PSE have frequent and troublesome common side effects, including abdominal cramping, diarrhea, and flatulence.

Outpatient therapy is initially with lactulose or lactitol titrated to obtain two to three soft bowel movements daily. These medications alter the pH in the colon and may promote ionization of ammonia, making it impossible for the drug to cross the mucous barrier in the colon. A more acidic gut pH always reduces bacterial replication and production of nitrogenous products. The use of spironolactone along with furosemide decreases the incidence of hypokalemia, which increases renal ammonia production. Traditionally, dietary protein restriction has been recommended in cirrhotics, often even in the absence of PSE, but rigorous evidence is lacking to support this strategy. It is more important for a patient with decompensated cirrhosis to maintain adequate nutrition. A nutritional evaluation is key in maintaining muscle mass in these patients.

If the cathartic effects of lactulose are poorly tolerated, nonabsorbable antibiotics can be used to inhibit bacterial toxin production. Neomycin has been used longest, but its ototoxicity and nephrotoxicity limit its long-term use. Other antibiotics, such as metronidazole (Flagyl)[1] and rifaximin (Xifaxan),[1] are now being used to treat PSE. Ongoing clinical trials are attempting to clarify the role of rifaximin. Antibiotics may be used in addition to lactulose if it alone does not improve symptoms.

In patients with intractable and severe post-TIPS PSE, reduction or occlusion of the shunt may be necessary if pharmacologic treatment is not efficacious. Type A PSE associated with acute liver failure does not respond to standard medical therapy, which is futile in this circumstance, and urgent referral for liver transplantation is indicated. Cerebral edema, a frequent and often lethal complication of acute liver failure, may lead to cerebral herniation or intracranial hemorrhage, precluding liver transplantation.

---

[1]Not FDA approved for this indication.

Hepatorenal Syndrome

There are several potential explanations for renal dysfunction in patients with cirrhosis. Renal dysfunction can reflect glomerulonephropathy (hepatitis B, hepatitis C, immunoglobulin A nephropathy, diabetes mellitus), whereas the differential for acute renal dysfunction includes hypovolemia (diuretics, gastrointestinal bleed, diarrhea), nephrotoxic drugs (aminoglycosides, nonsteroidal antiinflammatory drugs, contrast dye), sepsis, and hepatorenal syndrome (HRS).

The incidence of HRS in cirrhotic patients with ascites is up to 18% per annum. The pathogenesis of HRS in cirrhosis results from the marked splanchnic and systemic vasodilation and decreased cardiac function, which lead to a decrease in effective arterial blood volume typical of more advanced portal hypertension. Although the renal parenchyma is preserved, there is severe renal arterial vasoconstriction, low renal perfusion, and a decrease in the glomerular filtration rate. Clinically, the diagnosis of HRS is suspected when there is an increase in the creatinine level to greater than 1.5 mg/dL in the absence of shock, dehydration, infection, or nephrotoxic drugs. Clinically, there are two types of HRS (Box 1). Type 1 HRS is defined as a severe, rapidly progressive increase in creatinine to greater than 2.5 mg/dL in less than 2 weeks. It is often precipitated by SBP, alcoholic hepatitis, or gastrointestinal hemorrhage. These patients tend to have floridly decompensated cirrhosis with tense ascites, PSE, and coagulopathy. The median survival time is 2 weeks. Type 2 HRS, with a median survival time of 6 months, is defined as a moderate and steady decline in renal function to a creatinine level greater than 2.5 mg/dL.

Evaluation of renal dysfunction in patients with liver disease should include an ultrasound study to determine the presence of ascites. If ascites is not present, the diagnosis of HRS is unlikely, and prerenal or intrinsic renal causes should be sought. If ascites is present, a work-up for sepsis (urinalysis, diagnostic paracenteses, and blood cultures) is indicated. Discontinuing all diuretics and nephrotoxic agents along with plasma volume expansion (intravenous fluids or albumin) is the initial intervention to correct renal dysfunction in cirrhotic patients. If renal function does not improve, HRS is likely. Additional clues that are helpful in the diagnosis of HRS are urine volume less than 500 mL/day, urine sodium concentration less than 10 mEq/L (despite plasma volume expansion), urine osmolality greater than that of plasma, protein secretion of less than 500 mg/day, and serum sodium concentration less than 130 mEq/L.

Treatment of HRS is mainly limited to establishing whether a reversible component in the renal dysfunction is present. Most data on the efficacy of therapeutic interventions are based on small retrospective and pilot comparative studies. Realistically, patients with severe HRS require either an improvement in liver function or liver transplantation for renal function to recover. Medical therapy may result in modest improvement in renal function. In a small study, combination of an α-agonist, midodrine (ProAmatine),[1]

---

[1]Not FDA approved for this indication.

| **BOX 1** | **Diagnostic Criteria for Hepatorenal Syndrome** |

Cirrhosis with ascites
Serum creatinine >1.5 mg/dL
No improvement of serum creatinine after at least
   2 days with diuretic withdrawal and volume expansion
Absence of shock
No current or recent treatment with nephrotoxic drugs
Absence of parenchymal kidney disease

Adapted from Salerno F, Gerbes A, Ginès P, et al: Diagnosis, prevention and treatment of hepatorenal syndrome in cirrhosis. Gut 2007;56;1310–1318.

---

with octreotide (Sandostatin)[1] and albumin[1] resulted in improvement in three of five patients with HRS. Another trial of albumin and octreotide infusion failed to show benefit. Vasoconstrictors such as terlipressin (Glypressin)[2] and norepinephrine (Levophed)[1] have been shown to improve renal function, with a decrease in serum creatinine to less than 1.5 mg/dL demonstrated in two thirds of patients with HRS in one study. Albumin has typically been administered with these medications and seems to aid in vasoconstriction as well as plasma volume expansion. A retrospective study suggested improved survival for patients with HRS type 1 who had received terlipressin. However, a meta-analysis of 154 patients indicated no improvement in overall survival. Terlipressin is expensive and is not available for use in the United States.

TIPS has been advocated as a means to improve renal function in patients with HRS. In a small prospective study of 14 patients, 10 patients who had initially responded to medical therapy (midodrine, octreotide, and albumin) and subsequently underwent TIPS had improvement in renal function. This study supported the possible use of this combination. In one study, TIPS was shown to improve survival to an average of 5 months, much better than the otherwise expected survival time of 2 weeks. TIPS may provide short-term benefit, but more studies are needed with TIPS and HRS. TIPS may cause a precipitous deterioration in hepatocellular function in patients with more floridly decompensated liver disease, and its use should be entertained only in collaboration with a liver transplant center.

In patients with confirmed SBP, administration of albumin[1] on days 1 and 3 reduced the incidence of HRS from 33% to 10%. Also, the use of pentoxifylline (Trental)[1] 400 mg three times daily in patients with alcoholic hepatitis reduced the incidence of HRS from 35% to 8%.

Portopulmonary Hypertension

The prevalence of this complication of cirrhosis varies from 2% to 12.5% in candidates awaiting liver transplantation. Before making a diagnosis of PPHTN, other causes of pulmonary arterial hypertension, such as recurrent pulmonary emboli, collagen vascular disease, intracardiac shunts, and medications, need to be excluded. The criteria for diagnosis of pulmonary arterial hypertension by right heart catheterization are mean pulmonary artery pressure greater than 25 mm Hg at rest or greater than 30 mm Hg with exercise; pulmonary capillary wedge pressure lower than 15 mm Hg; pulmonary vascular resistance greater than 120 dynes/sec/cm^5; and transpulmonary gradient (pulmonary arterial diastolic pressure minus pulmonary capillary wedge pressure) greater than 10 mm Hg. The pathogenesis of PPHTN may relate to the effects of vasoconstrictive substances produced in the splanchnic circulation that bypass metabolism by the liver. Candidate substances include serotonin, interleukin 1, glucagon, thromboxane B_2, endothelin 1, and vasoactive intestinal peptide. All these have been detected in increased concentrations in patients with PPHTN.

Symptoms of PPHTN include dyspnea on exertion, syncope, chest pain, fatigue, hemoptysis, and orthopnea. On physical examination, an accentuated pulmonic component of the second heart sound, right ventricular heave, and lower extremity edema are common. More than 60% of patients are asymptomatic at the time of diagnosis. Transthoracic echocardiography is used to estimate pressures. Patients who have right ventricular systolic pressures greater than 50 mm Hg or symptoms of right-sided heart failure should undergo right heart catheterization. In one third of these patients, the pulmonary vascular resistance is normal. Treatment should be initiated in those patients who are symptomatic and have mean pulmonary arterial pressure greater than 35 mm Hg and increased pulmonary vascular resistance.

---

[1]Not FDA approved for this indication.
[2]Not available in the United States.

Several drugs have been used to treat PPHTN with variable success. Epoprostenol (Flolan),[1] a prostacyclin (which directly dilates peripheral vessels), has been frequently used. Other agents have been used, such as bosentan (Tracleer), an endothelin receptor antagonist; sildenafil (Revatio), a phosphodiesterase inhibitor; and iloprost (Ventavis),[1] a vasodilator. β-Blockers should be used cautiously in patients with PPHTN because of the cardiac depressant and pulmonary vasoconstrictive effects of these medications. Anticoagulation therapy should be considered, given the risk of venous stasis and pulmonary vascular thrombosis. These treatments should be attempted in concert with an evaluation for liver transplantation, which can arrest PPHTN. More severe PPHTN is a contraindication to liver transplantation, especially if it does not improve with pharmacologic therapy. Liver transplantation can be delayed if patients have a good clinical response to medical therapy.

Hepatopulmonary Syndrome

In patients with liver disease, hypoxemia (increased alveolar-arterial gradient while breathing on room air) and vascular dilations in the lung suggest the diagnosis of HPS. Its prevalence has been reported to be from 8% to 20% in transplantation candidates. The clinical features of HPS include the insidious onset of dyspnea, platypnea (shortness of breath exacerbated in upright position), orthodeoxia (hypoxemia in upright posture), clubbing, and cyanosis. Cutaneous spider nevi may reflect analogous vascular dilations in the lungs. A widened alveolar-arterial oxygen gradient on room air (>15 mm Hg, or >20 mm Hg in patients older than 64 years of age) should prompt evaluation for HPS in a patient with liver disease. A pulse oximetry reading of less than 97% on room air and an arterial partial pressure of oxygen (PaO_2) lower than 70 mm Hg on blood gas analysis indicate HPS in the absence of intrinsic cardiopulmonary diseases.

The diagnosis of HPS can be confirmed with contrast echocardiography. Agitated saline is injected intravenously, and bubbles are observed in the left side of the heart during the study. Normally, the bubbles from the agitated saline should be visualized on the left side of the heart. Bubbles resulting from vascular dilations in HPS appear 3 to 6 heartbeats after the appearance of contrast in the right side of the heart. If bubbles appear within 3 beats after injection, intracardiac shunting (e.g., atrial septal defect, patent foramen ovale) should be considered. If intrinsic cardiopulmonary disease is present, a technetium-labeled macroaggregated albumin scan can distinguish HPS. Normally, 20 μg of radiolabeled albumin gets trapped in the lung, but in a patient with pulmonary vascular dilations, the tracer escapes to elsewhere in the body. A shunt fraction of greater than 6% confirms the presence of HPS. Pulmonary angiography may be considered to rule out alternative causes of hypoxemia if noninvasive studies are nondiagnostic.

Patients with HPS have a median survival time of 10.6 months, compared with 40.8 months for cirrhotic controls. Therapeutic attempts with various modalities such as acetylsalicylic acid,[1] garlic powder,[7] indomethacin (Indocin),[1] methylene blue,[1] almitrine bismesylate (Duxil),[2] somatostatin analogues (Octreotide),[1] and plasma exchange have been tried, but currently none of these is recommended for use. Results of TIPS have been variable in HRS. Supplemental oxygen therapy has been shown to improve exercise tolerance and quality of life. Patients with HPS should be referred for a liver transplantation evaluation, because transplantation increases survival, with impressive improvement in hypoxemia in about 85% of patients who undergo the procedure. However, resolution of symptoms can take up to 1 year. The 1-year survival after transplantation in HPS is 71%, compared with 90% in patients without HPS.

---

[1]Not FDA approved for this indication.
[2]Not available in the United States.
[7]Available as dietary supplement.

Hepatic Hydrothorax

The manifestation of portal hypertension known as hepatic hydrothorax is defined as a pleural effusion of greater than 500 mL in a cirrhotic patient without evidence of a cardiopulmonary cause. Although patients can tolerate a large amount (>5 L) of ascites before becoming symptomatic, a hepatic hydrothorax greater than 1 L can cause shortness of breath and hypoxemia. It develops on the right side about 85% of the time, is left-sided in 13% of the cases, and is bilateral in 2%. Accumulation of a transudate in the pleural space is caused by portal hypertension with leakage of fluid from the peritoneal space through small defects in the diaphragm. With inspiration, there is an increase in negative intrathoracic pressure, facilitating fluid movement from the peritoneal space to the pleural space.

The clinical presentation includes dyspnea, nonproductive cough, chest discomfort, and even hypoxemia. Ascites is not always present, because it tends to be drawn into the pleural space. Less commonly, patients present dramatically, with severe dyspnea and hypotension, in the presence of tension hydrothorax. In patients with fevers and pleuritic chest pain, infection of the pleural fluid needs to be excluded; its incidence in patients with hepatic hydrothorax is 13%.

Spontaneous bacterial empyema is defined as a PMN count greater than 500 cells/mm[3] or a positive bacterial culture in the absence of parapneumonic effusion. Like most bacterial infections in patients with cirrhosis, It is associated with a high mortality rate of 20% despite therapy. Spontaneous bacterial empyema should be promptly treated with antibiotics (Ceftriaxone 1–2 g daily) to cover organisms such as *E. coli*, *Streptococcus*, *Enterococcus*, *Klebsiella*, and *Pseudomonas*. After an effusion is recognized on chest radiography in a cirrhotic patient, especially when there has been a change in clinical status, a diagnostic thoracentesis should be performed with analysis of fluid cell count, pH, Gram stain, culture, protein, and lactate dehydrogenase. Hepatic hydrothorax is typically transudative in nature. In the absence of infection, white cells should be scarce, fewer than 500 cells/mm[3] (PMNs <250 cells/mm[3]); pH greater than 7.4; and total protein less than 2.5 g/dL. If atypical features of hepatic hydrothorax cause concern, such as an exclusively left-sided effusion, other nonhepatic causes of pleural effusion (e.g., pleural infection, congestive cardiac failure) need to be excluded. A confirmatory test for hepatic hydrothorax is the nuclear-tagged colloid albumin study. If hepatic hydrothorax is the source of pleural fluid, the nuclear-tagged albumin injected in the peritoneum should migrate and be identified in the thoracic cavity in the study. Alternative diagnoses should be sought if the tracer does not demonstrate this behavior.

The management of hepatic hydrothorax in essence is similar to management of ascites, as discussed earlier. For severely symptomatic patients and those whose disease is refractory to diuretics, frequent therapeutic thoracentesis is necessary. A need for frequent thoracentesis in a patient who is compliant with medical therapy should lead to consideration of TIPS, which is effective in up to 80% of patients with hepatic hydrothorax. The usual considerations regarding TIPS in any patient need to be addressed.

Indwelling chest tubes should not be used, because they frequently lead to complications, including protein and electrolyte loss, infection, and fistula formation. Pleurodesis is ineffective in ablating the space between the parietal and the visceral pleura in patients with hepatic hydrothorax, and it can be associated with a variety of complications (e.g., fever, empyema, chest pain, pneumonia, incomplete expansion). Surgical repair of diaphragmatic defects has been reported in small case series, but clearly this is a major undertaking in a patient with decompensated cirrhosis.

Hepatocellular Carcinoma

HCC is one of the most common fatal malignancies worldwide, with a rising incidence in the United States reflecting the disease burden of the hepatitis C and B viruses as well as an increasing incidence of

HCC related to nonalcoholic steatohepatitis. The incidence of HCC in patients with cirrhosis is 1% to 4% per year.

The diagnosis is increasingly made radiologically. If two imaging techniques show that a mass in a cirrhotic liver (excluding patients with hepatitis B) has the characteristic features of HCC, with an arterial blood supply and rapid washout, a confident diagnosis can be made. An α-fetoprotein (AFP) level greater than 200 ng/mL is specific for HCC, although AFP is not produced in up to 40% of HCCs, limiting the sensitivity of this test. A radiographically guided biopsy of the mass may be necessary if noninvasive testing is inconclusive.

The prognosis and treatment of HCC are related to tumor stage, liver function, and the patient's performance status. Surgical resection or ablative therapy is an initial option for those with Child-Pugh grade A cirrhosis, a single mass smaller than 5 cm, a normal bilirubin level, and no portal hypertension. Liver transplantation is effective treatment, especially for patients who meet the Milan criteria (HCC with up to three tumors not more than 3 cm in size or one tumor not larger than 5 cm), provided that there is no vascular invasion of the tumors and no metastasis. Transplantation within the Milan criteria results in long-term survival equivalent to that seen in cirrhotic patients without HCC. Although these patients are given priority for liver transplantation, they may be undergo ethanol or radiofrequency ablation if the waiting time will be longer than 6 months, in an effort to prevent tumor progression while awaiting transplantation.

Transarterial chemoembolization may prolong survival in patients who are believed not to be candidates for resection or transplantation, and it can lead to a modest increase in survival time. For symptomatic patients with inoperable tumors and marginal liver function, survival is poor, and systemic chemotherapy is of little value, although sorafenib (a tyrosine kinase inhibitor) has shown some survival benefit compared with supportive care alone.

In order to detect and treat HCC at an early stage, screening and surveillance strategies are recommended. The following groups of patients are at high risk for HCC and should be in a surveillance program (Box 2 and Box 3): Asian males who are carriers of the hepatitis

---

BOX 2 Surveillance for Hepatocellular Carcinoma in High-Risk Patients: Hepatitis B Carriers*

Asian males ≥40 years of age
Asian females ≥50 years of age
All cirrhotic hepatitis B carriers
Family history of hepatocellular carcinoma
Africans >20 years of age

*For noncirrhotic hepatitis B carriers not listed here, surveillance is based on disease activity and clinical judgment.

BOX 3 Surveillance for Hepatocellular Carcinoma in High-Risk Patients: Non-Hepatitis Carriers

Hepatitis C
Alcoholic cirrhosis
Genetic hemochromatosis
Primary biliary cirrhosis
Consider surveillance based on disease activity and clinical judgment:
  α₁-Antitrypsin deficiency
  Nonalcoholic steatohepatitis
  Autoimmune hepatitis

Adapted from Bruix J, Sherman M; Practice Guidelines Committee, American Association for the Study of Liver Diseases: Management of hepatocellular carcinoma. Hepatology 2005;42:1208–1236.

B virus (HBV) and are 40 years of age or older; Asian female HBV carriers who are 50 years of age or older; all cirrhotic HBV carriers with a family history of HCC or cirrhosis of any etiology. Patients deemed to be at increased risk of HCC should be screened with twice-yearly ultrasound and measurement of AFP. If there is reason to suspect development of an HCC, such as rising AFP levels despite absence of a mass on ultrasound, additional abdominal imaging with magnetic resonance imaging or contrast computed tomography is necessary.

Vaccination

Cirrhotic patients have increased morbidity and mortality if they contract viral or bacterial infections. All patients with chronic liver disease should be vaccinated against hepatitis A virus (HAV), HBV, pneumococcus, and influenza. At initial evaluation for chronic liver disease, total hepatitis A antibody and total hepatitis B core antibody should be ordered to determine preexisting immunity against HAV and HBV, and appropriate vaccines should be administered to nonimmune patients.

Osteopenia

The prevalence of osteopenia is high in patients with chronic liver disease, and there is a particularly high risk of osteoporosis in patients with primary biliary cirrhosis, primary sclerosing cholangitis, hepatitis C, or alcoholic liver disease. Management of osteopenia can reduce morbidity before and after transplantation. All transplantation candidates should undergo screening for bone mineral density by dual-energy x-ray absorptiometry (DEXA), initially and repeated every 1 to 2 years. Hypothyroidism and disordered calcium and vitamin D metabolism should be excluded, and regular exercise should be encouraged. Concern about gastrointestinal irritation and bleeding from use of the oral bisphosphonates can be obviated by parenteral administration.

Liver Transplantation

With improvements in immunosuppression, surgical techniques, anesthesia, prophylaxis of common posttransplantation infections, and patient selection, liver transplantation has become the definitive intervention for decompensated cirrhosis, acute liver failure, and a subset of unresectable hepatic malignancies. Mean 1-year and 3-year survival rates after transplantation in the United States are about 90% and 80%, respectively. Liver transplantation should be considered once a cirrhotic patient has an index complication such as onset of ascites, and a timely referral should be made before the patient becomes debilitated from recurrent complications of cirrhosis.

The most common indication for transplantation is decompensated cirrhosis (Box 4). Other important indications are HCC, acute liver failure, and metabolic liver disease. Most donor organs come from brain-dead donors and are allocated based on the severity of liver disease in the potential recipient. The organ allocation system is now based on the MELD score (see earlier discussion), which ranges from 6 to 40 (Fig. 1). The higher the MELD score, the lower the likelihood that the patient will be alive 3 months later, and the higher the patient's rank on the transplant list. Other determinants regarding allocation of organs are blood type, the patient's weight, and waiting time (for patients with identical MELD scores). Patients with fulminant hepatic failure, posttransplantation primary graft nonfunction, and hepatic artery thrombosis are given highest priority, independent of MELD. Only a few conditions (e.g., HCC HPS) make patients eligible for higher MELD scores (priority), because reduced waiting times for those patients would be likely to increase mortality in other patients due to the finite supply of donor organs. The most frequent example of this situation is the cirrhotic patient with well-preserved hepatocellular function and a low MELD score

BOX 4 Indications for Liver Transplantation

Chronic noncholestatic liver disorders (decompensated disease)
Chronic hepatitis C
Chronic hepatitis B
Autoimmune hepatitis
Alcoholic liver disease
Cholestatic liver disorders (decompensated disease)
Primary biliary cirrhosis
Primary sclerosing cholangitis
Biliary atresia
Alagille's syndrome
Non-syndromic paucity of the intrahepatic bile ducts
Cystic fibrosis
Progressive familial intrahepatic cholestasis
Metabolic disorders causing cirrhosis
α_1-Antitrypsin deficiency
Wilson's disease
Nonalcoholic steatohepatitis and cryptogenic cirrhosis
Hereditary hemochromatosis
Tyrosinemia
Glycogen storage disease type IV
Neonatal hemochromatosis
Metabolic disorders causing severe extrahepatic morbidity
Amyloidosis
Hyperoxaluria
Urea cycle defects
Disorders of branched-chain amino acids
Primary malignancies of the liver
Hepatocellular carcinoma
Hepatoblastoma
Fibrolamellar hepatocellular carcinoma
Hemangioendothelioma
Fulminant hepatic failure
Miscellaneous conditions
Budd-Chiari syndrome
Metastatic neuroendocrine tumors
Polycystic disease
Retransplantation

Adapted from Murray KF, Carithers RL Jr: AASLD practice guidelines: Evaluation of the patient for liver transplantation. Hepatology 2005;41:1407–1432.

BOX 5 Contraindications for Liver Transplantation

Absolute:
  Irreversible severe cardiopulmonary disease
  Extrahepatic malignancy
  Active substance abuse
  Morbid obesity
Relative (varies by transplant center and experience):
  Age
  HIV
  Irreversible brain damage

whose indication for liver transplant is an HCC that meets Milan criteria. The organ allocation system under these circumstances awards extra MELD points to expedite transplantation, hopefully before metastatic spread has occurred. Specific etiologies of liver disease may be eligible for the highest priority for listing (status 1). An example is Wilson's disease with an acute presentation, because copper chelating therapy is ineffective and may even lead to further deterioration. Any patient with acute liver failure with onset of hepatic encephalopathy within 26 weeks after recognition of liver disease of any etiology is also eligible for status 1.

Expansion of the organ donor pool to reduce deaths on the waiting list for transplantation has been possible with live donor transplantation, in which a healthy adult donates a major portion of his or her liver to another adult (right lobe) or to a child (left lobe). This remains a somewhat controversial approach because of the risk to the donor, especially with right lobe donation, because of the larger volume of hepatic tissue required for an adult patient.

There are several important contraindications in liver transplantation (Box 5). Irreversible brain damage, as frequently occurs due to cerebral edema in acute liver failure, and advanced cardiopulmonary disease are absolute contraindications. PPHTN is not an absolute contraindication unless mean pulmonary pressures are greater than 50 mm Hg. In HPS, a Pao_2 of less than 50 mm Hg and a pulmonary artery shunt fraction greater than 30% are contraindications, because they are associated with a high mortality rate after transplantation. Extrahepatic malignancy or a history of malignancy with a disease-free period of less than 2 years, uncontrolled infection, and active alcohol intake or substance abuse are all contraindications. HIV infection is not a contraindication as long as it is well controlled on antiretroviral therapy. Advanced age is a relative contraindication, but biologic rather than chronologic age is more pertinent, with particular attention to key comorbidities such as cardiovascular disease and diabetes mellitus.

The transplantation evaluation process typically involves a multidisciplinary team. Key components of the evaluation consist of separate medical and surgical evaluations; assessment of the severity of comorbid medical conditions, if any; identification of psychosocial aspects requiring intervention; and determination of financial and insurance status. Other important issues, such as the patient's willingness to undergo transplantation, a history of compliance with medical care, and the availability of a dependable support network, are also evaluated. In patients with a history of drug or alcohol abuse, a commitment to long-term sobriety and a drug-free lifestyle is an important prerequisite for acceptance for transplantation. The management of complications of cirrhosis is challenging. Given the disparity between supply and demand for donor organs, physicians care for increasingly tenuous cirrhotic patients. Anticipation and prevention of complications of end-stage liver disease affect the ability of cirrhotic patients to survive until liver transplantation and to enjoy its benefits.

REFERENCES

Arroyo V, Fernandez J, Ginès P. Pathogenesis and treatment of hepatorenal syndrome. Semin Liver Dis 2008;28(1):81–95.
Boyer TD, Haskal ZJ. The role of transjugular intrahepatic portosystemic shunt in the management of portal hypertension. Hepatology 2005;41(2):386–400.

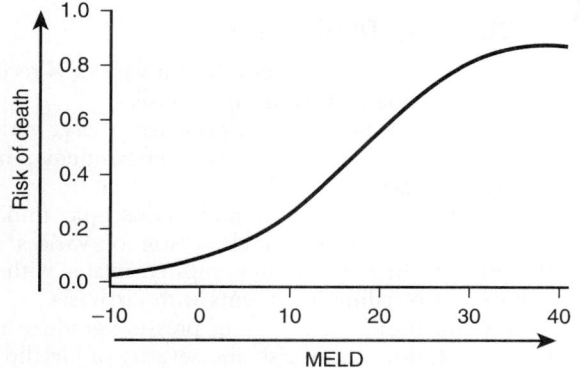

FIGURE 1. The Model for End-Stage Liver Disease (MELD) score predicts the risk of death over 3 months. See text for details.

Bruix J, Hessheimer AJ, Forner A, et al. New aspects of diagnosis and therapy of hepatocellular carcinoma. Oncogene 2006;25(27):3848–56.

Cárdenas A, Arroyo V. Management of ascites and hepatic hydrothorax. Best Pract Res Clin Gastroenterol 2007;21(1):55–75.

Golbin JM, Krowka MJ. Portopulmonary hypertension. Clin Chest Med 2007;28(1):203–18.

Lopez PM, Martin P. Update on liver transplantation: Indications, organ allocation, and long-term care. Mt Sinai J Med 2006;73(8):1056–66.

Mandell MS. The diagnosis and treatment of hepatopulmonary syndrome. Clin Liver Dis 2006;10(2):387–405.

Morgan MY, Blei A, Grüngreiff K, et al. The treatment of hepatic encephalopathy. Metab Brain Dis 2007;22(3–4):389–405.

Runyon BA. Management of adult patients with ascites due to cirrhosis. Hepatology 2004;39(3):841–56.

Bleeding Esophageal Varices

Method of
Cecilio Azar, MD, and Ala I. Sharara, MD

Epidemiology

Bleeding of esophageal varices is a major complication of portal hypertension, usually in the setting of liver cirrhosis, accounting for 10% to 30% of all cases of upper gastrointestinal hemorrhage. More than any other cause of gastrointestinal bleeding, this complication results in considerable morbidity and mortality, prolonged hospitalization, and increased affiliated costs. Variceal bleeding develops in 25% to 35% of patients with cirrhosis and accounts for up to 90% of upper gastrointestinal bleeding episodes in these patients. About 10% to 30% of these episodes are fatal, and as many as 70% of survivors rebleed following an index variceal hemorrhage. Following such events, the 1-year survival is 34% to 80%, being inversely related to the severity of the underlying liver disease.

Treatment of patients with esophageal varices includes preventing the initial bleeding episode (primary prophylaxis), controlling active variceal hemorrhage, and preventing recurrent bleeding after a first episode (secondary prophylaxis). Data on the optimal management of gastric varices are much more limited, and this topic is not covered in this article.

Pathophysiology

Chronic liver disease leading to cirrhosis is the most common cause of portal hypertension. The level of increased resistance to flow varies with the level of circulatory breach and can be divided into prehepatic, hepatic or sinusoidal, and posthepatic. In cirrhosis, several organ systems are involved in the pathophysiology of portal hypertension. At the splanchnic vascular bed level there is marked vasodilatation and increase in angiogenesis, leading to increase in portal blood flow and formation of collateral circulation, such as gastroesophageal varices, along with decrease in response to vasoconstrictors. At the systemic circulation level, there is an increase in cardiac output, decrease in vascular resistance, and hypervolemia. This hyperkinetic syndrome leads to an effective hypovolemia, with a resultant increase in vasoactive factors to maintain a normal arterial blood pressure.

Varices represent portosystemic collaterals derived from dilatation of preexisting embryonic vascular channels, such as those between the coronary and short gastric veins and the intercostal, esophageal, and azygous veins. In the distal esophagus, over an area extending 2 to 5 cm from the gastroesophageal junction, veins are found more superficially in the lamina propria rather than the submucosa. This results in reduced support from surrounding tissues owing to the predominant intraluminal location of these varices and might explain the predilection for bleeding at this site. The opening and dilation of portosystemic collaterals appears to depend on a threshold portal pressure gradient (measured as hepatic venous pressure gradient [HVPG]) of 12 mm Hg, below which varices do not form. This pressure gradient is necessary but not sufficient for the development of gastroesophageal varices.

Diagnosis

The current consensus states that every patient with liver cirrhosis should undergo an upper endoscopy to detect gastroesophageal varices. The main aim behind screening for gastroesophageal varices is to identify patients requiring prophylactic treatment or further surveillance. Several invasive and noninvasive procedures help in detecting portal hypertension and can, with variable accuracy, predict the presence of gastroesophageal varices. Unfortunately, none are sensitive enough to replace endoscopy. Endoscopic videocapsule is a new modality introduced for visualizing the esophagus; it allow correct identification of varices in 80% of cases but can have poor accuracy in identifying the presence of hypertensive gastropathy and gastric varices.

Not all esophageal varices bleed; hemorrhage occurs in only 30% to 35% of patients with cirrhosis. Variceal rupture is directly related to physical factors such as the radius, thickness, and elastic properties of the vessel in addition to intravariceal and intraluminal pressure and tension. Endoscopic findings that predict a higher risk of bleeding include larger size of varices and the presence of endoscopic red signs (described as red wale markings) on the variceal wall, indicating dilated intraepithelial and subepithelial superficial veins. A combination of clinical and endoscopic findings including the Child-Pugh class, size of varices, and the presence or absence of red wale markings was found to correlate highly with the risk of first bleeding in patients with cirrhosis. Hemodynamic parameters examined as predictors of bleeding include HVPG, azygous blood flow, and direct measurement of intravariceal pressure.

HVPG calculated by the gradient of wedged and free hepatic vein pressure (normal value, 5 mm Hg) is used most often and provides reliable measurement of portal pressure in patients with cirrhosis. The extent of elevation of HVPG may be the best indicator of risk of bleeding, severity of bleeding, and survival. A rise in pressure in a patient with known varices increases the risk of bleeding, and the extent of portal pressure elevation has an inverse relationship to prognosis after hemorrhage has occurred. In general, however, a linear relationship between the degree of portal hypertension and the risk of variceal hemorrhage or formation of varices does not exist, so that this technique cannot be used routinely to identify individual patients at high risk for bleeding.

CURRENT DIAGNOSIS

- Endoscopic screening for esophageal varices is recommended in patients with liver cirrhosis.
- Noninvasive predictors of the presence of large varices, such as splenomegaly and thrombocytopenia, have limited accuracy.
- A combination of clinical and endoscopic findings including the Child-Pugh class, size of varices and the presence of red wale markings correlates with the risk of first bleeding in patients with cirrhosis.
- Measurement of hepatic venous pressure gradient may be the best indicator of risk and severity of bleeding in patients with varices. It is an invasive test and is not widely available or used routinely in practice.

Treatment

PRIMARY PROPHYLAXIS

The natural evolution of gastroesophageal varices without treatment is characterized by an increase in size from small to large varices, which eventually rupture and bleed. The progression rate ranges from 5% to 30% per year. The incidence of bleeding from small esophageal varices is estimated to be 4% per year, and it is as high as 15% per year for medium to large varices. In a randomized, controlled trial, the nonselective β-blocker timolol (Blocadren)[1] failed to reduce the development of varices or variceal bleeding in patients without varices. Adverse events were more common in the timolol group. Therefore, it is not recommended to start β-blockers in patients who do not yet have esophageal varices.

Based on prospective studies of cirrhotic patients with varices identified at endoscopy and of untreated groups in randomized, controlled trials, the risk of bleeding from esophageal varices has been estimated at 25% to 35% at 1 year. Therapy for primary prophylaxis against variceal bleeding (prevention of a first variceal bleeding) is summarized in Table 1.

Pharmacologic Therapy

The general objective of pharmacologic therapy for variceal bleeding is to reduce portal pressure and consequently intravariceal pressure. Drugs that reduce portocollateral venous flow (vasoconstrictors) or intrahepatic vascular resistance (vasodilators) have been used and include β-blockers, nitrates, β_2-adrenergic blockers, spironolactone (Aldactone),[1] pentoxifylline (Trental),[1] molsidomine (Corvaton),[2] and simvastatin (Zocor).[1] Because varices do not bleed at an HVPG less than 12 mm Hg, reduction to this level is ideal, but substantial reductions in HVPG (i.e., by >20%) are also clinically meaningful.

---

[1]Not FDA approved for this indication.
[2]Not available in the United States.

CURRENT THERAPY

- Nonselective β-blockers and endoscopic band ligation are both effective first-line therapy in the primary prophylaxis of esophageal varices.
- The management of acute variceal hemorrhage consists of prompt resuscitation and correction of coagulation abnormalities, followed by endoscopic and pharmacologic therapy with vasoactive agents. Antibiotic prophylaxis is given to decrease the risk of infection and of rebleeding. Transjugular intrahepatic portosystemic shunt (TIPS) is reserved for refractory, uncontrolled, acute variceal bleeding.
- Strategies for secondary prophylaxis of variceal bleeding include endoscopic band ligation, pharmacologic therapy with nonselective β-blockers with or without nitrates, TIPS, and surgical shunts.
- Comparative cost-effectiveness of secondary prophylaxis strategies is unknown but should take into consideration the cost of failed therapy (e.g., rebleeding, shunt revision) and that of treatment related-complications (e.g., encephalopathy, esophageal stricture).

β-Blockers exert their beneficial effect on portal venous pressure by diminishing splanchnic blood flow and consequently gastroesophageal collateral and azygous blood flow. The effectiveness of β-blockers for primary prophylaxis against variceal bleeding has been demonstrated in several controlled trials. Meta-analyses have revealed a 40% to 50% reduction in bleeding and a trend toward improved survival. The estimated overall response rate is 49%, with bleeding

TABLE 1 Summary of Therapy for Esophageal Varices

	First-Line Therapy	Comments	Alternative Therapy	Comments
Primary prophylaxis*	β-Blockers or band ligation	In advanced cirrhosis, the best therapy is unclear (probably band ligation) Transplantation should be considered for these patients		The effectiveness of combined β-blockers and band ligation is unknown Neither TIPS nor sclerotherapy is recommended for primary prophylaxis
Active variceal bleeding	Somatostatin, octreotide (Sandostatin),[1] vapreotide (Octastatin),[5] or terlipressin (Glypressin)[2] *plus* Endoscopic therapy	Vasoconstrictors should be continued for ≥2 days after endoscopic therapy Band ligation is superior to endoscopic sclerotherapy Antibiotic prophylaxis should be initiated	Balloon tamponade TIPS Shunt surgery	Tamponade is indicated primarily as a temporizing measure if first-line treatment fails TIPS is reserved for refractory or recurrent early bleeding but should also be considered when basal HVPG >20 mm Hg Surgery is reserved for patients with compensated liver disease in whom TIPS fails or is not technically feasible
Secondary prophylaxis	β-Blockers ± nitrates *or* Band ligation	The combination of band ligation and β-blockers ± nitrates may be more effective than either alone Nitrates alone are not recommended Patients with advanced liver disease are often intolerant of β-blockers	TIPS Shunt surgery	TIPS is best used after failure of first-line therapy or as a bridge to transplantation in patients with advanced liver disease Shunt surgery is reserved for selected patients with compensated cirrhosis in whom TIPS fails or is not feasible

*Upon documentation of varices, variceal hemorrhage occurs in 25%-30% of patients by 2 years. β-Blockers reduce the risk to 15%-18%, and combination β-blockers plus nitrates reduce the risk to 7.5%-10%.
Abbreviations: HVPG = hepatic venous pressure gradient; TIPS = transjugular intrahepatic portosystemic shunt.

rates of 6% in responders and 32% in nonresponders, with number needed to treat (NNT) of 10.

The nonselective β-blockers, such as propranolol (Inderal)[1] and nadolol (Corgard),[1] are preferred because of the dual benefit of β$_1$- and β$_2$-receptor blockade. In the absence of HVPG determination, β-blockers are titrated to achieve a reduction in resting heart rate to 55 beats/min or 25% of baseline. Propranolol is generally given as a long-acting preparation and titrated to a maximum dose of 320 mg/day. Nadolol is initiated at 80 mg daily up to a maximum daily dose of 240 mg. Carvedilol (Coreg)[1] is initiated at 6.25 mg daily and increased if tolerated to 12.5 mg/day. The portal pressure–reducing effects of β-blockers are, however, unpredictable, and neither the resultant reduction in heart rate nor the reduction in drug blood levels are good indicators of response to therapy. For example, portal venous pressure is reduced in about 60% to 70% of patients who receive propranolol therapy, but only 10% to 30% of these patients show a substantial response (i.e., >20% reduction). Additionally, approximately 20% to 25% of patients have no measurable decline in portal pressure despite increasing dosage of propranolol.

In addition to β-blockers, a number of vasodilators have been investigated in patients with portal hypertension and in animal models of portal hypertension, most notably isosorbide mononitrate (Imdur).[1] The exact mechanism of action of nitrates is unclear but is thought to be mediated primarily by reducing intrahepatic resistance and possibly by splanchnic arterial vasoconstriction induced in response to venous pooling and vasodilation in other regional vascular beds. Monotherapy with nitrates is ineffective in primary prophylaxis and can have detrimental effects, particularly in cirrhotic patients with ascites, and should not be used.

The addition of isosorbide mononitrate to β-blockers, however, has been shown to result in an enhanced reduction in portal pressure in humans. In a randomized, controlled trial involving 42 patients with cirrhosis and esophageal varices, a reduction of greater than 20% in HVPG was documented in only 10% in the propranolol group compared to 50% in the combination therapy group. In patients with Child-Pugh class A and B cirrhosis, the addition of isosorbide mononitrate to nadolol has been shown, in a randomized trial, to result in a greater than 50% additional reduction in variceal bleeding rate when compared with nadolol monotherapy (12% versus 29%). However, a large subsequent double-blind, placebo-controlled study failed to confirm these results. Based on the existing evidence, the combination of β-blockers and isosorbide is not recommended in primary prophylaxis.

Endoscopic Therapy

Endoscopic therapies play a prominent role in treatment of esophageal varices. Endoscopic band ligation (EBL) is the endoscopic procedure of choice in the management of esophageal varices. As of 2010, 16 randomized, controlled trials have compared EBL to β-blockers in the primary prevention of variceal bleeding. These studies suffered from significant heterogeneity, and a large number were published in abstract form. Two meta-analyses of these trials showed a slight advantage of EBL over β-blockers in terms of primary prevention of variceal bleeding, but there were no differences in mortality.

β-Blockers are cheaper and much easier to administer but are associated with issues of noncompliance and a higher incidence of adverse events (e.g., hypotension, impotence, insomnia) than EBL. However, most of these side effects are easy to manage and none require hospitalization or result in direct mortality. On the other hand, adverse events related to EBL, such as bleeding from band-related ulcers, albeit infrequent, are more significant, often requiring hospitalization and blood transfusion and may rarely be associated with death.

According to the Baveno consensus conference, nonselective β-blockers should be considered as a first choice for preventing first variceal bleeding in high-risk patients who have not bled, and EBL should be provided for patients with contraindications or intolerance to β-blockers. The recent guidelines by the American College of Gastroenterology (ACG) and American Association for the Study of Liver Diseases (AASLD) recommend using β-blockers in low-risk patients who have medium to large varices but suggest both EBL and β-blockers for high-risk patients as first-line therapy. The optimal primary prophylaxis in patients with decompensated cirrhosis remains unclear and is arguably expedited liver transplantation. The combination of pharmacologic plus endoscopic therapy has been investigated in such patients with conflicting results. In one study, EBL plus β-blockers offered no benefit in terms of prevention of first bleeding when compared to EBL alone. In a more-recent study, combination therapy significantly reduced the occurrence of the first episode of variceal bleeding and improved bleeding-related survival in a group of cirrhotic patients with high-risk esophageal varices awaiting liver transplantation.

MANAGEMENT OF ACUTE VARICEAL HEMORRHAGE

Variceal hemorrhage is usually an acute clinical event characterized by rapid gastrointestinal blood loss manifesting as hematemesis (which can be massive), with or without melena or hematochezia. Hemodynamic instability (tachycardia, hypotension) is common. Although variceal bleeding is common in patients with cirrhosis presenting with acute upper gastrointestinal hemorrhage, other causes of bleeding, such as ulcer disease, must be considered. Urgent initiation of empiric pharmacologic therapy with vasoactive agents is indicated in situations where variceal hemorrhage is likely. Subsequently, direct endoscopic examination is critical to establish an accurate diagnosis and to provide the rationale for immediate and subsequent therapies. The immediate steps in the management of acute variceal bleeding include: volume resuscitation, prevention of complications, ensuring hemostasis, and initiating measures to prevent early and delayed rebleeding.

Patients with variceal hemorrhage and ascites are at increased risk for bacterial infections, particularly spontaneous bacterial peritonitis. This risk appears to be increased in the setting of uncontrolled hemorrhage or as a result of transient bacteremia following endoscopic sclerotherapy or variceal ligation. Short-term systemic antibiotics (e.g., third-generation cephalosporins or fluoroquinolones for 4-10 days) have been shown to decrease the risk of bacterial infections and to reduce rebleeding as well as mortality in cirrhotic patients with gastrointestinal bleeding.

The role of platelet transfusion or fresh frozen plasma administration has not been assessed appropriately. The use of recombinant activated coagulation factor VII (rFVIIa [Novoseven]),[1] which corrects prothrombin time in cirrhotic patients, has been assessed in two randomized, controlled trials. The first trial showed, in a post hoc analysis, that rFVIIa administration might significantly improve the results of conventional therapy in patients with moderate and advanced liver failure (Child-Pugh B and C) without increasing the incidence of adverse events. A more recent trial tested rVIIa in patients with active bleeding at endoscopy and with a Child-Pugh score 8 points or higher. This trial failed to show a benefit of rVIIa in terms of decreasing the risk of 5-day failure, but it did show improved 6-week mortality.

Pharmacologic Therapy

Pharmacologic therapy can be administered early, requires no special technical expertise, and is thus a desirable first-line option for managing acute variceal hemorrhage. Drugs that reduce portocollateral venous flow (vasoconstrictors) or intrahepatic vascular resistance (vasodilators) or both have been used to achieve this effect. Vasoconstrictors work by decreasing splanchnic arterial flow, and vasodilators are used in combination with vasoconstrictors to reduce their systemic side effects, but they can also exert an added beneficial effect on intrahepatic resistance (see Table 1).

---

[1]Not FDA approved for this indication.

Vasopressin and Terlipressin

Vasopressin (Pitressin)[1] is a nonselective vasoconstricting agent that causes a reduction of splanchnic blood flow and thereby a reduced portal pressure. Vasopressin, which is associated with severe vascular complications, has been largely replaced by other vasoconstrictors such as its synthetic analogue, triglycyl-lysine vasopressin (terlipressin [Glypressin]).[2] Terlipressin has fewer side effects and a longer biological half-life, allowing its use as a bolus intravenous injection (2 mg every 4 hours for the initial 24 hours, then 1 mg every 4 hours for the next 24 to 48 hours). Terlipressin has been shown in numerous placebo-controlled trials to control bleeding in about 80% of cases and is the only pharmacologic therapy proved, as of 2010, to reduce mortality from acute variceal hemorrhage. Terlipressin is not currently available in the United States.

Somatostatin, Octreotide, and Vapreotide

Somatostatin, a naturally occurring peptide, and its analogues, octreotide (Sandostatin)[1] and vapreotide (Octastatin),[5] stop variceal hemorrhage in up to 80% of patients and are generally considered equivalent to vasopressin (Pitressin), terlipressin (Glypressin), and endoscopic therapy for the control of acute variceal bleeding. Their precise mechanism of action is unclear but might result from an effect on the release of vasoactive peptides or from reduction of postprandial hyperemia. Somatostatin is used as a continuous intravenous infusion of 250 µg/hour following a 250-µg bolus injection. Octreotide is used as a continuous infusion of 50 µg/hour and does not require a bolus injection. Side effects are minor, including hyperglycemia and mild abdominal cramps. The addition of octreotide or vapreotide to endoscopic sclerotherapy or banding improves control of bleeding and reduces transfusion requirements, with no change in overall mortality. A continuous infusion of octreotide or vapreotide is therefore recommended for 2 to 5 days following emergency endoscopic therapy.

Endoscopy

Endoscopic sclerotherapy stops variceal hemorrhage in 80% to 90% of cases. Its drawbacks include a significant risk of local complications including ulceration, bleeding, stricture, and perforation. Rare systemic complications have been reported including bacteremia with endocarditis, formation of splenic or brain abscesses, and portal vein thrombosis. Randomized trials in patients with acute variceal bleeding have shown that EBL is essentially equivalent to endoscopic sclerotherapy in achieving initial hemostasis with lesser complications. These include superficial ulcerations, transient chest discomfort, and, rarely, stricture formation.

Balloon Tamponade

The use of the Sengstaken-Blakemore or Minnesota tube for hemostasis of variceal bleeding is based on the principle of the application of direct pressure on the bleeding varix by an inflatable—esophageal or gastric—balloon fitted on a rubber nasogastric tube. When properly applied, balloon tamponade is successful in achieving immediate hemostasis in almost all cases. However, early rebleeding following balloon decompression is high. Complications of balloon tamponade include esophageal perforation or rupture, aspiration, and asphyxiation from upper airway obstruction. Balloon tamponade is generally not recommended and should largely be reserved for rescue of cases of hemorrhage uncontrolled by pharmacologic and endoscopic methods and as a temporary bridge to more definitive therapy.

Transjugular Intrahepatic Portosystemic Shunt

Treatment with a transjugular intrahepatic portosystemic shunt (TIPS) consists of the vascular placement of an expandable metal stent across a tract created between a hepatic vein and a major intrahepatic branch of the portal system. TIPS can be successfully performed in 90% to 100% of patients, resulting in hemodynamic changes similar to a partially decompressive side-to-side portocaval shunt while avoiding the morbidity and mortality associated with a major surgical procedure. TIPS has been shown to be effective in treating refractory, uncontrolled, acute variceal bleeding. Patients with advanced liver disease and multiorgan failure at the time of TIPS have a 30-day mortality that approaches 100%.

Surgery

Surgery is generally considered in the setting of continued hemorrhage or recurrent early rebleeding—uncontrolled by repeated endoscopic or continued pharmacologic therapy—and when TIPS is not available or is not technically feasible. Surgical options include portosystemic shunting or esophageal staple transection alone or with esophagogastric devascularization and splenectomy (Sugiura procedure). Devascularization procedures may be useful in patients who cannot receive a shunt because of splanchnic venous thrombosis. Regardless of the choice of surgical technique, morbidity is high and the 30-day mortality for emergency surgery approaches 80% in some series. Understandably, rescue liver transplantation is not a practical option in patients with uncontrolled variceal hemorrhage.

SECONDARY PROPHYLAXIS

Variceal hemorrhage recurs in approximately two thirds of patients, most commonly within the first 6 weeks after the initial episode. Patients with advanced liver disease (MELD [model for end-stage liver disease] score ≥18) have an increased risk of early rebleeding and death. Early rebleeding (within the first 5 days) is reduced by the adjuvant use of octreotide[1] or vapreotide[5]—and possibly terlipressin[2] and somatostatin—after initial endoscopic or pharmacologic control of hemorrhage.

The severity of portal hypertension correlates closely with the severity and risk of rebleeding as well as actuarial probability of survival following an index episode. In a cohort of patients presenting with variceal hemorrhage, those with an initial HVPG greater than 20 mm Hg had a 1-year mortality of 64% compared to 20% for patients with lesser elevations in portal pressure. Given the high risk of recurrent hemorrhage and its associated morbidity and mortality, strategies aimed at prevention should be rapidly instituted following the index episode. The choice of preventive therapy should, therefore, take into consideration the efficacy of therapy, the side effects of the selected treatment, the patient's expected survival, and overall cost. Preventive strategies include pharmacologic, endoscopic, and surgical methods and are listed in Table 1. Relative effectiveness of these strategies is shown in Figure 1.

Pharmacologic Therapy

Reducing the portal pressure by more than 20% from the baseline value pharmacologically results in a reduction in the cumulative probability of recurrent bleeding from 28% at 1 year, 39% at 2 years, and 66% at 3 years to 4%, 9%, and 9%, respectively. Although adjustment of medical therapy based on portal pressure measurement would be ideal, HVPG determination might not be readily available, and treatment must be adjusted using empiric clinical parameters. Several randomized, controlled trials, including a meta-analysis, have demonstrated that β-blockers prevent rebleeding and prolong survival. The addition of isosorbide mononitrate (ISMO)[1] to β-blockers appears to enhance the protective effect of β-blockers alone for preventing recurrent variceal bleeding but offers no survival advantage and reduces the tolerability of therapy. Compared with either sclerotherapy or endoscopic band ligation, combination medical therapy is superior in reducing the risk of recurrent bleeding in patients with esophageal variceal hemorrhage, primarily in patients with Child-Pugh class A and B cirrhosis. Notably, in patients who show a significant hemodynamic response to therapy (defined as a reduction in the hepatic venous pressure gradient to <12 mm Hg or >20% of the baseline value), the risk of recurrent bleeding and of death is significantly reduced.

---

[1]Not FDA approved for this indication.
[2]Not available in the United States.
[5]Investigational drug in the United States.

[1]Not FDA approved for this indication.
[2]Not available in the United States.
[5]Investigational drug in the United States.

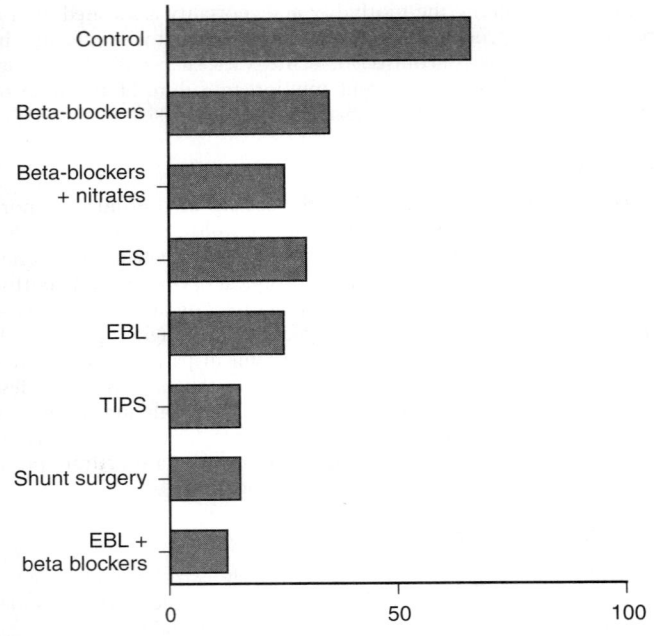

FIGURE 1. Relative effectiveness of available therapies for preventing recurrent variceal bleeding. The estimates shown are based on the cumulative data available in the literature for recurrent bleeding at 1 year. *Abbreviations:* EBL = endoscopic band ligation; ES = endoscopic sclerotherapy; TIPS = transjugular intrahepatic portosystemic shunt.

Endoscopy

Endoscopic therapy has been established over the past decade as a therapeutic cornerstone for preventing esophageal variceal rebleeding. Gastric varices, however, are not effectively treated by sclerotherapy or ligation. Patients with recurrent gastric variceal hemorrhage are best treated by *N*-butyl-2-cyanoacrylate injection[1] or by non-endoscopic means such as TIPS. On the other hand, EBL is highly effective at obliterating esophageal varices and is considered the endoscopic therapy of choice for secondary prophylaxis.

Combination modality approaches, usually including an endoscopic and pharmacologic treatment, are pathophysiologically attractive and may be more effective than single therapy. Two randomized, controlled trials have shown that adding β-blockers to EBL reduces the risk of rebleeding and variceal recurrence, suggesting that if EBL is used, it should be used in association with β-blockers. One randomized, controlled trial has evaluated whether EBL could improve the efficacy of the combined administration of nadolol[1] plus isosorbide.[1] In this study, adding band ligation to nadolol plus isosorbide was shown to be superior to nadolol plus isosorbide alone in preventing variceal rebleeding, but there were no significant differences in mortality. The combination of the best endoscopic treatment (EBL) and the best pharmacologic treatment (β-blockers plus isosorbide) may be the best choice in preventing rebleeding but needs further studies for confirmation.

Transjugular Intrahepatic Portosystemic Shunt

Transjugular shunting is more effective than endoscopic therapy for preventing variceal rebleeding but offers no survival benefit. The cumulative risk of rebleeding following TIPS placement is 8% to 18% at 1 year. The trade-off, however, is that TIPS is associated with a higher incidence of clinically significant hepatic encephalopathy (new or worsened portosystemic encephalopathy was noted in about 25% of patients after TIPS). Advanced liver disease is the main determinant of poor outcome following TIPS. Consequently, in patients with advanced liver disease, TIPS is best used as a bridge to liver transplantation.

TIPS, using bare stents, has been compared with surgical shunts in two studies (8 mm portocaval H-graft shunt in one and distal splenorenal shunt in the second). Although the first study showed a

significantly lower rebleeding rate in the surgical group, the second and larger trial did not find any differences in rebleeding rates, hepatic encephalopathy, or mortality, but it found a significantly higher reintervention rate in the TIPS group. However, the obstruction and reintervention rates are markedly decreased with the recent use of polytetrafluoroethylene (PTFE)-covered stents. According to these data, TIPS using PTFE-covered stents represents the best rescue therapy for failures of medical and endoscopic treatment.

Surgery

Portosystemic shunt surgery is the most effective means by which to reduce portal pressure. Although effective at eradicating varices and preventing rebleeding, nonselective portocaval shunts are associated with a significant incidence of hepatic encephalopathy, portal vein thrombosis, and occasionally liver failure. Commonly used shunts include the distal splenorenal shunt and the low-diameter (mesocaval or portocaval) interposition shunt. Rates of recurrent bleeding are on the order of 10%, with the highest risk of bleeding occurring in the first month after surgery. Devascularization procedures (i.e., esophageal transection and gastroesophageal devascularization) are usually considered in patients who cannot receive shunts because of splanchnic venous thrombosis and should be performed only by experienced surgeons. Surgical therapy has been largely supplanted by TIPS.

COST EFFECTIVENESS OF AVAILABLE THERAPIES

Data examining the cost of variceal bleeding and the cost-effectiveness of commonly used therapies are limited. The treatment cost of an episode of variceal bleeding has been estimated at $15,000 to $40,000. The cost-effectiveness of diagnostic methods used to guide therapy is unclear. For example, HVPG determination, which can accurately predict pharmacologic response to therapy, is an attractive, although invasive, adjunct in the management of patients with variceal bleeding, but its cost-effectiveness remains in question. Further, screening endoscopy for detecting large varices, while recommended, has not been demonstrated to be cost-effective.

There are areas in which management is controversial and not standardized. For example, given the right expertise, secondary prophylaxis with surgical shunts or TIPS may be more effective than medical or endoscopic therapy in Child-Pugh class A patients. On the other hand, patients with advanced cirrhosis are often intolerant of β-blockers—let alone in combination with nitrates—and therefore the use of combination therapy remains controversial in such patients. Arguably, the preferred treatment for such patients is TIPS as a bridge to early liver transplantation.

Therefore, when choosing a specific treatment plan, the clinician must take into consideration the direct costs of health care utilization, as well as the efficacy and morbidity of therapy. The treatment chosen should be tailored to fit the patient's clinical condition while also taking into account the possibility that the patient's liver disease can progress and thus necessitate transplantation. The cost-effectiveness of various treatment modalities should factor in the cost of failed therapy (e.g., rebleeding, shunt revision) and that of treatment-related complications (e.g., encephalopathy, esophageal stricture).

Summary

Esophageal variceal hemorrhage is a common and devastating complication of portal hypertension and is a leading cause of morbidity and mortality in patients with cirrhosis. Because the clinical outcomes are poor once variceal bleeding has occurred, primary prophylaxis with β-blockers or EBL should be considered in high-risk patients. The treatment of acute variceal hemorrhage is aimed at volume resuscitation and ensuring hemostasis with pharmacologic agents and endoscopic techniques as well as prevention of complications such as by the use of prophylactic antibiotics.

A high risk of rebleeding after an index episode mandates the institution of preventive strategies. Wedge pressure-guided medical therapy may be the preferred mode of secondary prophylaxis in patients with Child Pugh class A or B cirrhosis, but is invasive and not widely available. Patients at high risk for rebleeding, including

---

[1]Not FDA approved for this indication.

those with decompensated or advanced liver disease, should be considered for TIPS followed by liver transplantation when applicable. Treatment with a combination of methods is pathophysiologically attractive, but the choice of therapy should ultimately be tailored to fit the patient's clinical condition, risk factors, and prognosis, taking into account issues of risk-to-benefit ratio, compliance, and cost.

REFERENCES

Bambha K, Kim WR, Pedersen R, et al. Predictors of early rebleeding and mortality after acute variceal haemorrhage in patients with cirrhosis. Gut 2008;57:814–20.

Feu F, Garcia-Pagan JC, Bosch J, et al. Relation between portal pressure response to pharmacotherapy and risk of recurrent variceal haemorrhage in patients with cirrhosis. Lancet 1995;346:1056–9.

Garcia Pagan JC, De Gottardi A, Bosch J. Review article: the modern management of portal hypertension—primary and secondary prophylaxis of variceal bleeding in cirrhotic patients. Aliment Pharmacol Ther 2008;28:178–86.

Garcia-Pagan JC, Feu F, Bosch J, Rodes J. Propranolol compared with propranolol plus isosorbide-5-mononitrate for portal hypertension in cirrhosis. A randomized controlled study. Ann Intern Med 1991;114:869–73.

Laine L, Cook D. Endoscopic ligation compared with sclerotherapy for treatment of esophageal variceal bleeding. A meta-analysis. Ann Intern Med 1995;123:280–7.

Merkel C, Marin R, Sacerdoti D, et al. Long-term results of a clinical trial of nadolol with or without isosorbide mononitrate for primary prophylaxis of variceal bleeding in cirrhosis. Hepatology 2000;31:324–9.

Moitinho E, Escorsell A, Bandi JC, et al. Prognostic value of early measurements of portal pressure in acute variceal bleeding. Gastroenterology 1999;117:626–31.

North Italian Endoscopic Club for the Study and Treatment of Esophageal Varices. Prediction of the first variceal hemorrhage in patients with cirrhosis of the liver and esophageal varices: A prospective multicenter study. N Engl J Med 1988;319:983–9.

Poynard T, Cales P, Pasta L, et al. β-Adrenergic-antagonist drugs in the prevention of gastrointestinal bleeding in patients with cirrhosis and esophageal varices. An analysis of data and prognostic factors in 589 patients from four randomized clinical trials. Franco-Italian Multicenter Study Group. N Engl J Med 1991;324:1532–8.

Polio J, Groszmann RJ. Hemodynamic factors involved in the development and rupture of esophageal varices: a pathophysiologic approach to treatment. Semin Liver Dis 1986;6:318–31.

Sharara AI, Rockey DC. Gastroesophageal variceal hemorrhage. N Engl J Med 2001;345:669–81.

Villanueva C, Minana J, Ortiz J, et al. Endoscopic ligation compared with combined treatment with nadolol and isosorbide mononitrate to prevent recurrent variceal bleeding. N Engl J Med 2001;345:647–55.

Dysphagia and Esophageal Obstruction

Method of
Philip O. Katz, MD, and Girish Anand, MD

Dysphagia refers to a subjective sensation of the delayed passage of food from the mouth through the esophagus to the stomach. It derives its origin from Greek *dys*, meaning "difficulty," and *phagia*, meaning "eat."

Dysphagia has been reported in about 2% of healthy adults older than 65 years. The incidence increases to 12% to 13% in the hospitalized elderly. Dysphagia has been reported in about 50% to 60% of patients in nursing homes and other chronic care facilities.

There may be associated pain with swallowing (odynophagia) if there is coexistent inflammation. Most patients describe dysphagia as a feeling of food getting "stuck" or "not going down right." The history plays an important role in understanding the anatomic location and the severity of the symptoms. Key questions like the exact location where the food is getting stuck, associated regurgitation, types of foods causing dysphagia, and presence of weight loss or heartburn are crucial in assessing the symptom of dysphagia.

Pathophysiology

In the swallowing process, the oropharyngeal and esophageal phases transport solid or liquid boluses rapidly from the mouth to the stomach. *Primary peristalsis* is the classic coordinated motor pattern of the esophagus, combined with almost simultaneous upper and lower esophageal sphincter relaxation initiated by the act of swallowing. The food bolus is transferred by a progressive pharyngeal contraction through the relaxed upper esophageal sphincter (UES) into the esophagus. The UES closure is followed by a progressive circular contraction beginning in the upper esophagus and proceeding distally along the esophageal body to propel the bolus through the relaxed lower esophageal sphincter (LES), which subsequently closes with a prolonged contraction.

Secondary peristalsis is a progressive contraction in the esophageal body occurring in response to its distention by stimulation of sensory receptors in the esophageal body. It usually begins at or above a level corresponding to the location of the stimulus and is limited to the esophagus. A local intramural mechanism can at times take over as a reserve mechanism to produce peristalsis in the smooth muscle segment of the esophagus. This has been called *tertiary peristalsis*.

Any problem with either the strength or coordination of the musculature causes difficulty with movement of food, leading to obstruction. Similarly, any narrowing in the path of transit causes obstruction and distention of the lumen, leading to the sensation of dysphagia. The motility abnormalities might not be constant, thus giving intermittent dysphagia. The extent of luminal obstruction guides the diagnosis. Partial obstruction might initially give only solid food dysphagia related to large food boluses (e.g., steak). When the extent of obstruction progresses to near total occlusion, the symptoms involve both solid and liquid dysphagia. The extent of associated inflammation (esophagitis) determines whether or not odynophagia is an associated symptom.

Diagnosis

A careful history helps to localize the site of abnormality, and this forms the basis of further work-up. The evaluation of dysphagia begins with a complete history. A problem initiating a swallow and associated coughing or choking indicates a more proximal or oropharyngeal cause for the symptoms. Pure solid food dysphagia suggests a structural lesion, stricture, ring, or malignancy. A problem initially with solids progressing later to liquids suggests a benign or malignant stricture.

Rapidly progressive dysphagia is concerning for malignancy. The presence of other medical problems such as stroke or scleroderma might point to a systemic cause of the symptoms. A careful history of medications is important, because many drugs have been implicated in pill esophagitis and can cause dysphagia as well as odynophagia. The history can also differentiate dysphagia from globus sensation (feeling of a lump in the throat), which has a different evaluation from dysphagia.

Dysphagia for all practical purposes can be classified into oropharyngeal and esophageal dysphagia.

OROPHARYNGEAL DYSPHAGIA

Difficulty in transferring a food bolus from the hypopharyngeal area to the esophageal body across the upper esophageal sphincter gives rise to the suspicion of oropharyngeal or transfer dysphagia. Several clues in the patient's history help to establish the cause.

The onset of symptoms in oropharyngeal dysphagia is almost immediate. The patient describes the feeling of choking or coughing on initiation of swallowing and frequently points to the cervical region as the site of dysphagia. Patients might describe regurgitation of food, aspiration, or halitosis, which can point to a structural abnormality such as a Zenker's diverticulum.

Patients might have to resort to certain physical maneuvers, such as extending their arms and neck and using their fingers to move the bolus. There may be associated speech abnormalities such as hoarseness, nasal quality, or dysarthria, which points to a neuromuscular cause for the oropharyngeal dysphagia. The various causes of oropharyngeal dysphagia are listed in Box 1.

CURRENT DIAGNOSIS

- Differentiate between oropharyngeal and esophageal dysphagia.
- Pure solid food dysphagia implies a mechanical (obstructive) cause.
- Mixed solid and liquid dysphagia suggests functional (motility) abnormality.
- Eosinophilic esophagitis should be considered in any patient with dysphagia.
- Barium swallow (with solid bolus) and endoscopy are complementary.
- Esophageal function testing (manometry) should be performed for nonobstructive dysphagia.

In patients with oropharyngeal dysphagia, the oral cavity, head, and neck should be carefully examined. Special attention should be paid to the neurologic examination, especially the nerves involved in the act of swallowing, namely cranial nerves V, VII, IX, X, XI, and XII. Clues in the physical examination might suggest polymyositis or dermatomyositis as the cause of symptoms.

Video fluoroscopy (barium swallow) is a good first test that permits visualization of the swallowing mechanism. It can identify aspiration, pooling, and abnormal motor activities. This examination concentrates on the cervical esophageal region. A barium swallow can delineate the anatomic anomalies and also can show the remainder of the esophagus. The study starts with liquid barium, progressing to a solid phase. Different consistencies of food are used to assess the oropharynx, UES, and proximal esophagus.

A structural abnormality found on the barium examination generally requires an endoscopy for confirmation or treatment. Endoscopy is not the first test to use to evaluate oropharyngeal dysphagia, because the chances of missing an abnormality in the upper part of esophagus are higher than in the distal esophagus.

A nasopharyngeal laryngoscopy performed by the otolaryngologist provides detailed information of the hypopharynx, larynx, and oropharynx. It also allows a clear visualization of the vocal cords, valleculae, and the pyriform sinuses to assess any pooling of secretions.

Patients with oropharyngeal dysphagia who have an unrevealing barium study or endoscopy might need an esophageal manometry study with careful attention to the UES. Incoordination between UES opening and pharyngeal contractions can cause relaxation (opening) or shortening opening may be associated with dysphagia as well.

Zenker's diverticulum is an outpouching of the mucosa through an area of muscular weakness between the transverse fibers of the cricopharyngeus and the oblique fibers of the lower inferior constrictor. These generally occur in older adults and can show symptoms of pulmonary aspirations, gurgling, or regurgitation. Rarely, they become large enough to manifest as a mass and even cause esophageal obstruction.

ESOPHAGEAL DYSPHAGIA

Esophageal dysphagia occurs either from mechanical or motility causes. The abnormality lies within the body of the esophagus or the lower esophageal sphincter. Patients often complain of symptoms localizing to the upper epigastric region or lower sternum although the association is less significant than in oropharyngeal dysphagia. The type of food producing symptoms and its temporal progression help to identify the cause of symptoms. Dysphagia progressing from solids to liquids usually indicates a mechanical cause, and dysphagia to both solids and liquids from the outset favors a motility disorder. Symptoms of associated heartburn, weight loss, anemia, and regurgitation further narrow the differential diagnosis. Other medical conditions such as radiation therapy and medication use may be associated with dysphagia, as may infectious esophagitis. Both are often associated with odynophagia as well. Opportunistic infections—especially in the setting of HIV disease and AIDS—such as candida, cytomegalovirus, and herpes virus, are the most common and can be managed adequately with medical therapy.

The various causes of esophageal dysphagia are listed in Box 2.

BOX 1   Causes of Oropharyngeal Dysphagia

Structural (Mechanical)
- Carcinoma
- Cervical and proximal esophageal webs
- Cricopharyngeal bar
- Osteophytes and other skeletal abnormalities
- Prior surgery or radiation therapy

Neuromuscular
- Amyotrophic lateral sclerosis
- Brainstem tumors
- Dermatomyositis, polymyositis
- Head trauma
- Idiopathic upper esophageal sphincter dysfunction
- Multiple sclerosis
- Myasthenia gravis
- Myotonic dystrophy
- Paraneoplastic syndromes
- Parkinson's disease
- Postpolio syndrome
- Sarcoidosis
- Stroke

Infection
- Botulism
- Diphtheria
- Lyme disease
- Syphilis

BOX 2   Causes of Esophageal Dysphagia

Structural (Mechanical)
Intrinsic
- Benign tumors
- Carcinoma: Adenocarcinoma and squamous cell cancer
- Diverticula
- Eosinophilic esophagitis
- Esophageal rings and webs: Schatzki's ring
- Foreign body
- Infections: Herpes, CMV, EBV, MAI, *Candida, Pneumocystis*
- Peptic strictures
- Pill esophagitis
- Radiation strictures or esophagitis

Extrinsic
- Cervical osteophytes
- Mediastinal masses
- Vascular compression: Dysphagia lusoria

Motility (Neuromuscular)
- Achalasia
- Diffuse esophageal spasm (DES)
- Hypertensive lower esophageal sphincter
- Ineffective esophageal motility disorder
- Nutcracker esophagus
- Secondary causes like scleroderma, Sjögren's syndrome, Chagas' disease

Functional
- Functional dysphagia

Abbreviations: CMV = cytomegalovirus; EBV = Epstein-Barr virus; MAI = *Mycobacterium avium-intracellulare.*

The most common initial diagnostic approach to esophageal dysphagia is to perform endoscopy. In addition to the diagnostic value, endoscopy affords an opportunity to obtain tissue samples and do therapeutic intervention. A barium swallow with a solid bolus challenge is a reasonable alternative, especially with patients in whom oropharyngeal causes are a possibility or when the history suggests a complex stricture or achalasia. An endoscopy is required if a structural abnormality is discovered on the barium study.

STRUCTURAL CAUSES

Patients reporting only solid food dysphagia typically have a mechanical cause for their symptoms. This can progress to both solid and liquid dysphagia in cases of a high-grade obstruction. These patients tend to develop food impaction and might regurgitate. Benign causes for these symptoms include an esophageal web or a distal esophageal ring. The rings, also called Schatzki's rings, are smooth, thin mucosal structures at the gastroesophageal junction covered by squamous mucosa above and columnar epithelium below. Muscular rings, on the other hand, are characterized by hypertrophic esophageal musculature and are generally located about 2 cm above the gastroesophageal junction. Nonprogressive, episodic dysphagia is a characteristic of esophageal rings. Dysphagia becomes prominent when the diameter is smaller than 13 mm. Rings can manifest with acute dysphagia associated with impaction of a piece of meat, often referred to as "steakhouse syndrome." Esophageal webs, often asymptomatic, have been associated with iron deficiency anemia (Plummer-Vinson syndrome).

Peptic strictures occur in 8% to 10% of patients with symptomatic gastroesophageal reflux disease (GERD). Peptic strictures are associated with a long duration of reflux symptoms, male sex, and older age. Symptoms of dysphagia occur when the luminal diameter narrows to 13 mm or less.

Radiation-related strictures or esophagitis are seen in persons undergoing radiotherapy for thoracic or head or neck tumors. In the acute setting esophagitis is the predominant finding and can progress to fibrosis and strictures in the chronic phase.

Malignancy is the primary concern in patients with rapidly progressive solid food dysphagia associated with weight loss and anorexia. The staging of esophageal cancer involves CT scanning of the chest and abdomen and endoscopic ultrasonography (EUS). EUS provides the most accurate estimate of disease stage and assists with management decisions. The 5-year survival rate for patients with advanced esophageal cancer continues to be less than 5%.

Eosinophilic esophagitis is seen more often as a cause of dysphagia, particularly in young adults. Extensive diffuse eosinophilic infiltration (>15 per high-power field), particularly in the proximal esophagus, is seen. The disease can manifest for the first time as a food impaction requiring emergency endoscopic therapy. Feline esophagus, concentric mucosal rings, or ringed esophagus is the classic endoscopic description of eosinophilic esophagitis.

Pill-induced esophagitis has been shown to occur with a variety of medications including bisphosphonates, doxycycline, potassium chloride, quinidine, nonsteroidal antiinflammatory drugs (NSAIDs), aspirin, and iron preparations.

Vascular anomalies such as double aortic arch or aberrant right subclavian artery can cause dysphagia.

MOTILITY CAUSES

Patients reporting both solid and liquid dysphagia are more likely to have a motility disorder. Achalasia is a disease in which there is a loss of peristalsis in the distal esophagus and a failure of LES relaxation. These patients complain of chest pain, regurgitation, heartburn, and weight loss in addition to dysphagia. A barium swallow is the primary screening test when achalasia is suspected and manometry is confirmatory. The characteristic features on manometry include elevated resting LES pressure, incomplete LES relaxation, and aperistalsis.

Spastic motility disorders also manifest with dysphagia and often associated chest pain. The group of spastic motility disorders includes distal esophageal spasm, nutcracker esophagus, and hypertensive LES. The clinical relevance of these abnormalities identified during esophageal manometry is debated, and their management can be challenging.

Treatment

OROPHARYNGEAL DYSPHAGIA

Surgical and endoscopic therapeutic options are available, and these should be based on the patient's age and surgical risk. Surgery has been the mainstay of symptomatic Zenker's diverticulum. These involve cricopharyngeal myotomy with or without diverticulectomy or diverticulopexy. The efficacy of myotomy has been observed to be in excess of 80%. More recently, endoscopic techniques involving coagulation or cutting of the bridge, especially the cricopharyngeal muscle, between the esophagus and the diverticulum have been used. This approach is especially good for patients who are poor surgical risks and is now being used widely by experts in this technique.

Botulinum toxin injection might be an alternative to cricopharyngeal myotomy, although results are variable. Injection is usually performed under electromyographic guidance and has been shown to relieve dysphagia in small trials.

The presence of other structural abnormalities such as proximal strictures, can require endoscopic measures such as dilatation. A neoplasm requires appropriate intervention with surgical resection, chemotherapy, or radiation therapy.

If the oropharyngeal dysphagia is believed to be from nonstructural causes, swallowing rehabilitation may be the best option available. Swallowing rehabilitation is carried out by trained speech and language therapists, who teach patients maneuvers to overcome the risks of aspiration and improve dysphagia. These can involve proper positioning of the head and neck during swallowing, oral motor exercises, and deliberate multiple swallows. Certain diet modifications can improve swallowing and prevent aspirations.

The risk of malnutrition or recurrent aspiration can require placement of gastrostomy tubes for managing long-term nutritional needs.

ESOPHAGEAL DYSPHAGIA

The treatment of peptic strictures can involve dilatation, biopsies to rule out malignancy, and medical therapy for reflux. Proton pump inhibitor therapy has been shown to reduce the development of these strictures and the need for future dilatation.

Radiation-related strictures or esophagitis may be difficult to treat and require frequent esophageal dilatation.

The treatment of esophageal cancer depends on the stage of the cancer at the time of diagnosis. The various options available include surgery, chemotherapy, radiation therapy, palliative intraluminal stenting, and, more recently, photodynamic therapy.

Eosinophilic esophagitis is treated with topical steroid therapy with fluticasone[1] (Flovent), oral methylprednisolone, or montelukast in addition to dietary restrictions. These treatments have been studied in small series and have been shown to be beneficial. Dilatation may be helpful but must be done with care.

Treatment of pill-induced esophagitis involves stopping the offending agent and dilatation of strictures as needed.

Treatment modalities for achalasia include pneumatic dilatation of the LES, laparoscopic myotomy, botulinum toxin injection, and medical therapy with nitrates and calcium channel blockers. Medical therapy should be considered only for people who are not candidates for other modalities. Good to excellent relief of dysphagia can be achieved in patients with achalasia whether treated with pneumatic dilatation or myotomy. Many patients require multiple approaches and should be managed by experts in the field. Minimally invasive (laparoscopic or thoracoscopic) myotomy is gaining popularity, and in some centers it has become the procedure of choice.

Proposed treatments for distal esophageal spasm, nutcracker esophagus, and hypertensive LES include proton pump inhibitors, nitrates, calcium channel blockers, phosphodiesterase inhibitors, and tricyclic antidepressants or selective serotonin reuptake inhibitors.[1] Botulinum toxin[1] application and endoscopic dilatation have been tried in small series with varying results.

[1]Not FDA approved for this indication.

CURRENT THERAPY

- Treat the underlying disorder (e.g., GERD).
- Dilatation and antireflux therapy manage most peptic strictures.
- Multimodality therapy should be considered for malignant dysphagia.
- Achalasia can be effectively treated with pneumatic dilatation or surgery.
- Swallowing rehabilitation is helpful for oropharyngeal dysphagia following stroke.
- Eosinophilic esophagitis may respond to topical corticosteroids.

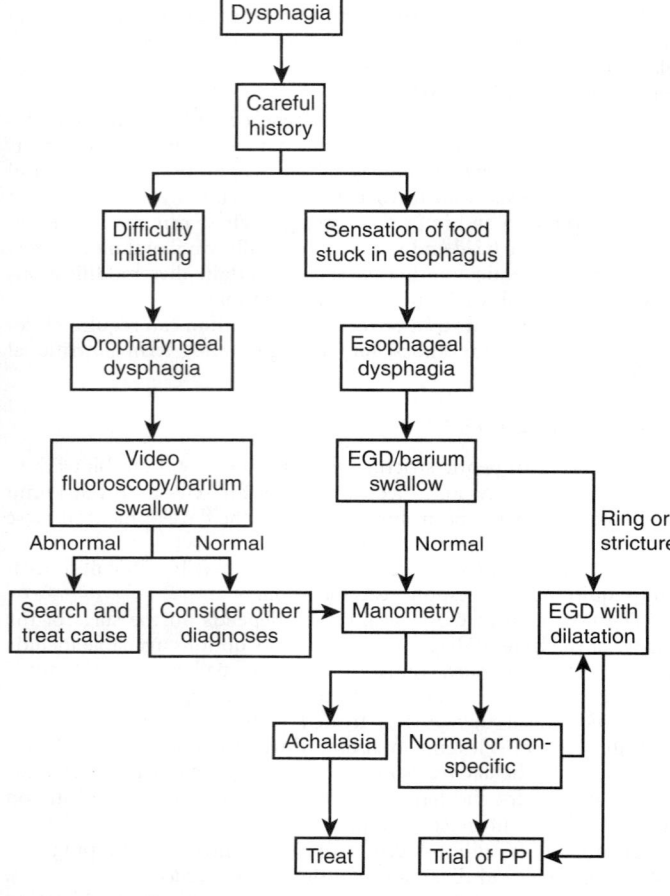

FIGURE 1. Diagnostic algorithm for patients with dysphagia. *Abbreviations:* EGD = esophagogastroduodenoscopy; PPI = proton pump inhibitor.

Summary

This review outlines the various causes and management of dysphagia. A careful history and examination with use of certain diagnostic tests help in establishing the reason for the symptom of dysphagia. Most of the conditions can be managed by medical therapy, endoscopic therapy, or surgery. A possible approach is outlined in Figure 1.

REFERENCES

Cook IJ, Kahrilas PJ. AGA technical review on management of oropharyngeal dysphagia. Gastroenterology 1999;116(2):455–79.

Furuta GT, Liacouras CA, Collins MH, et al. Eosinophilic esophagitis in children and adults: a systematic review and consensus recommendations for diagnosis and treatment. Gastroenterology 2007;133(4):1342–63.

Katz PO, Gilbert J, Castell DO. Pneumatic dilatation is effective long-term treatment for achalasia. Dig Dis Sci 1998;43(9):1973–7.

Khazanchi A, Katz PO. Strategies for treating severe refractory dysphagia. Gastrointest Endosc Clin N Am 2001;11(2):371–86 viii.

Spechler SJ. American Gastroenterological Association medical position statement on treatment of patients with dysphagia caused by benign disorders of the distal esophagus. Gastroenterology 1999;117(1):229–33.

Trate DM, Parkman HP, Fisher RS. Dysphagia: Evaluation, diagnosis and treatment. Prim Care 1996;(3):417–32.

Tutuian R, Castell DO. Esophageal motility disorders (distal esophageal spasm, nutcracker esophagus, and hypertensive lower esophageal sphincter): Modern management. Curr Treat Options Gastroenterol 2006;9(4):283–94.

Yan BM, Shaffer EA. Eosinophilic esophagitis: A newly established cause of dysphagia. World J Gastroenterol 2006;12(15):2328–34.

Diverticula of the Alimentary Tract

Method of
Alexander Perez, MD; Christopher R. Mantyh, MD; and Danny O. Jacobs, MD, MPH

A diverticulum is an abnormal saccular protrusion from the wall of the intestinal tract. It may be classified as a true diverticulum if the protrusion is composed of all of the layers of the intestinal wall or as a false diverticulum, or pseudodiverticulum, if it lacks the entirety of these layers. Although many diverticula are asymptomatic, some cause symptoms according to their anatomic location and the underlying process (obstruction, inflammation, or bleeding).

Esophagus

ZENKER'S DIVERTICULUM

Zenker's diverticulum, also known as a pharyngoesophageal pseudo-diverticulum, is the most common type of esophageal diverticulum. It arises because of muscular discoordination (in the area between the inferior pharyngeal constrictors and the cricopharyngeal muscle) that creates transmural pressure gradients within the esophagus, resulting in mucosal herniation through the esophageal muscular layer. This diverticulum typically manifests in older patients as dysphagia, aspiration, and regurgitation of undigested food. If this pathology is suspected, the diagnosis can be made by barium swallow (Fig. 1). If endoscopy is employed during the work-up, care must be taken to avoid perforation of the diverticulum.

Asymptomatic and incidentally encountered Zenker's diverticula may be managed with observation alone. Patients presenting with symptoms and a diverticulum of 2 cm or larger should undergo surgical resection of the diverticulum and myotomy of the cricopharyngeal muscle; those with smaller symptomatic diverticula may undergo myotomy alone. Patients undergoing surgical management have demonstrated symptomatic improvement more than 90% of the time. Although the diverticulum has traditionally been approached surgically via a cervical incision along the anterior border of the sternocleidomastoid muscle, an endoluminal approach is also available.

EPIPHRENIC DIVERTICULA

Epiphrenic diverticula are rare and are located in the distal third of the esophagus. It is thought that these diverticula are also associated with muscular dysmotility and gastroesophageal reflux. Symptoms include

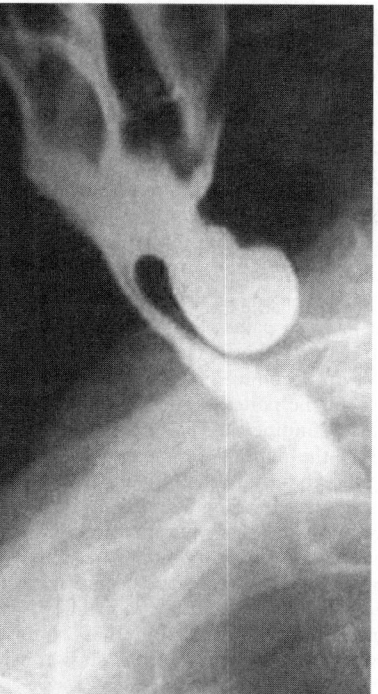

FIGURE 1. Zenker's diverticulum. (Image courtesy of Gastrolab—The Gastrointestinal Site. Available at http://www.gastrolab.net [accessed June 30, 2009].)

dysphagia, spasmodic chest pain, and reflux. The work-up consists of barium swallow, esophageal manometry, upper endoscopy, and 24-hour pH probe studies. Other disease processes, such as malignant obstruction, achalasia, and peptic stricture, should be ruled out.

Management includes resection of the diverticulum together with contralateral myotomy extending proximally through all regions of the esophagus documented to have abnormal motility and distally several millimeters on to the stomach. A partial fundoplication should be employed if reflux is identified during the preoperative work-up. Most recently, a laparoscopic approach has been employed successfully to address this pathology.

TRACTION DIVERTICULUM

A traction diverticulum, which is a true diverticulum (composed of all layers of the esophageal wall), results from inflammation in neighboring lymph nodes during processes such as tuberculosis and histoplasmosis.

These diverticula are usually small and asymptomatic and do not require surgical management. Rare cases of fistulization have been reported and have been managed with excision of the inflammatory mass and closure of the esophageal defect by a thoracotomy.

Stomach

Diverticula of the stomach are rare, with an incidence of 0.02% in autopsy studies. These diverticula may manifest with abdominal pain, dyspepsia, emesis, bleeding, and perforation. Diagnosis is made with an upper gastrointestinal contrast study, endoscopy, or contrast-enhanced computed tomography of the abdomen. Precise localization of the diverticulum is required preoperatively to plan the best operative approach.

Abdominal pain may be controlled with a proton pump inhibitor; however, those patients with persistent symptoms may require resection of the gastric diverticulum. A laparoscopic approach to resection of gastric diverticula is becoming more popular.

Small Intestine

DUODENAL DIVERTICULA

Both true and false diverticula may be found in the duodenum. Most are located in the second portion of the duodenum. Although the majority are asymptomatic, because of their location they may be associated with biliary obstruction or pancreatitis. Associated sphincter of Oddi dysfunction may also be present. Duodenal diverticula may be identified on barium swallow, contrast-enhanced computed tomography, or endoscopic retrograde cholangiopancreatography (Fig. 2).

Incidentally found duodenal diverticula should be left alone. In the rare instance that a duodenal diverticulum produces significant symptoms such as biliary obstruction or bleeding, an approach using endoscopic stenting, angiographic embolization, or surgical resection may be required.

JEJUNAL AND ILEAL DIVERTICULA

Jejunal and ileal diverticula occur throughout the length of the small intestine, predominately on the mesenteric side of the intestine where the blood vessels penetrate the muscular wall of the bowel. They are classified as false diverticula. Many are found incidentally, and some manifest with symptoms secondary to bleeding, obstruction, or infection. These symptoms may be a result of the bacterial overgrowth that occurs within these diverticula. Preoperative diagnosis may be made with a small bowel follow-through contrast study or capsule endoscopy.

Incidentally encountered jejunal and ileal diverticula should not be resected. Bacterial overgrowth may respond to antibiotic and intestinal promotility therapy. Resection may be required for refractory symptomatic diverticula. Laparoscopic approaches are feasible in this setting.

MECKEL'S DIVERTICULUM

A Meckel's diverticulum is a congenital anomaly that results from incomplete obliteration of the vitelline duct. It has a prevalence of approximately 1% to 2% in the population, is usually asymptomatic, is usually located within 2 feet of the ileocecal valve, and may contain ectopic gastric and pancreatic tissue. Symptoms may occur secondary to bleeding or obstruction associated with ectopic gastric mucosa and fibrous attachments to the umbilicus. A technetium 99m (Tc^{99})-pertechnetate scan will identify ectopic gastric mucosa in those presenting with ulceration and bleeding.

Resection of a Meckel's diverticulum is warranted in symptomatic patients. Patients with a Meckel's diverticulum found incidentally should not undergo resection, because there is a significantly higher

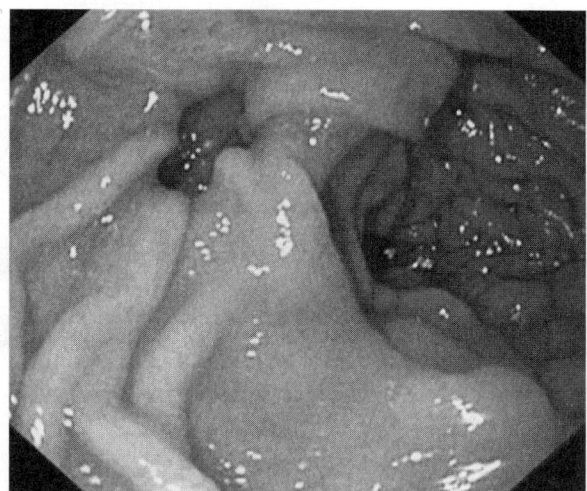

FIGURE 2. Duodenal diverticulum (Image courtesy of Gastrolab—The Gastrointestinal Site. Available at http://www.gastrolab.net [accessed June 30, 2009].)

rate of complications, such as infection and bowel obstruction (5.3% versus 1.3%, $P < 0.0001$), after resection in asymptomatic patients. Some have advocated a selective approach, with resection of incidentally found Meckel's diverticula in male patients, in patients younger than 50 years of age, if the diverticulum is longer than 2 cm, and if the diverticulum contains ectopic tissue.

Colon

The colon is most common site for diverticula of the alimentary tract. Colonic diverticula are of the false type and are composed primarily of mucosa protruding through the intestinal muscular layers (Fig. 3). Their presence is referred to as diverticulosis or diverticular disease. If these diverticula become inflamed or infected, the term diverticulitis is employed. If this acute process progresses to abscess, perforation, fistulization, or stenosis, then the term complicated diverticulitis is used.

Whereas the pathogenesis of diverticulosis remains uncertain, it is clear that its incidence increases with age, with the prevalence after age 80 years estimated to be 50% to 70%. The majority of colonic diverticula are located in the sigmoid colon, but approximately 50% of patients have disease that extends to other segments. The sigmoid is the narrowest portion of the colon and the location at which the highest intraluminal pressure may exist, according to Laplace's Law: $T = (P \times R)/M$, where T = wall tension, P = pressure across the wall, R = wall radius, and M = wall thickness. The pressure across the colonic wall (P) increases as the radius of the wall (R) decreases and the thickness of the wall (M) increases. The sigmoid is the narrowest portion of the colon, and patients with diverticular disease have a striking hypertrophy of the muscular wall that precedes the appearance of the diverticula. These diverticula appear at the site where arterioles penetrate the muscularis on the mesenteric side of the antimesenteric tenia. It is this anatomic relationship and the erosion into these blood vessels that is associated with 50% of all cases of lower gastrointestinal bleeding.

A reason for the predilection of the sigmoid colon to develop diverticula may be its relatively small diameter and increased intraluminal pressure. Other factors that may be associated with the development of diverticula are a low fiber, high fat, and highly refined carbohydrates in the diet.

Evaluation

The clinical presentation of diverticulitis spans the spectrum from mild, predominately left-sided, lower abdominal pain, fever, and leukocytosis to septic shock with diffuse peritonitis. The disease severity at presentation relates directly to the extent of inflammation, perforation, and the expected response to medical management.

The diagnosis of diverticulitis is made by physical examination, laboratory testing, and imaging. Physical findings may include mild left lower quadrant pain on palpation. However, pain may be elicited at the other sites because of the sigmoid colon's redundancy. If a perforation is present, it may produce signs of localized or generalized peritonitis, depending on the patient's ability to wall off the inflammatory process. Laboratory findings are nonspecific and reflect the degree of inflammation that the patient is experiencing. The most commonly employed imaging studies are plain abdominal radiography, ultrasonography, and computed tomography. The degrees of sensitivity and specificity are almost 100% for computed tomography with the use of intravenous and water-soluble oral contrast. Free air, free fluid, areas of inflammation, and abscesses may be detected with these modalities. Once the acute phase is over, additional modalities, such as colonoscopy and contrast enemas, should be used to establish the extent of disease and rule out the presence of other diseases such as cancer.

Treatment

A mild episode of diverticulitis may be managed on an outpatient basis with oral broad-spectrum antibiotics with coverage of anaerobic microorganisms. More severe episodes require hospitalization and stabilization with bowel rest, analgesia, intravenous fluids, and intravenous broad-spectrum antibiotics.

Localized abscesses may be successfully drained percutaneously under computed tomographic guidance, allowing resolution of symptoms and planning for future elective surgical resection of the involved segment and primary anastomosis of the remaining intestinal ends (Fig. 4). An elective resection should be delayed at least

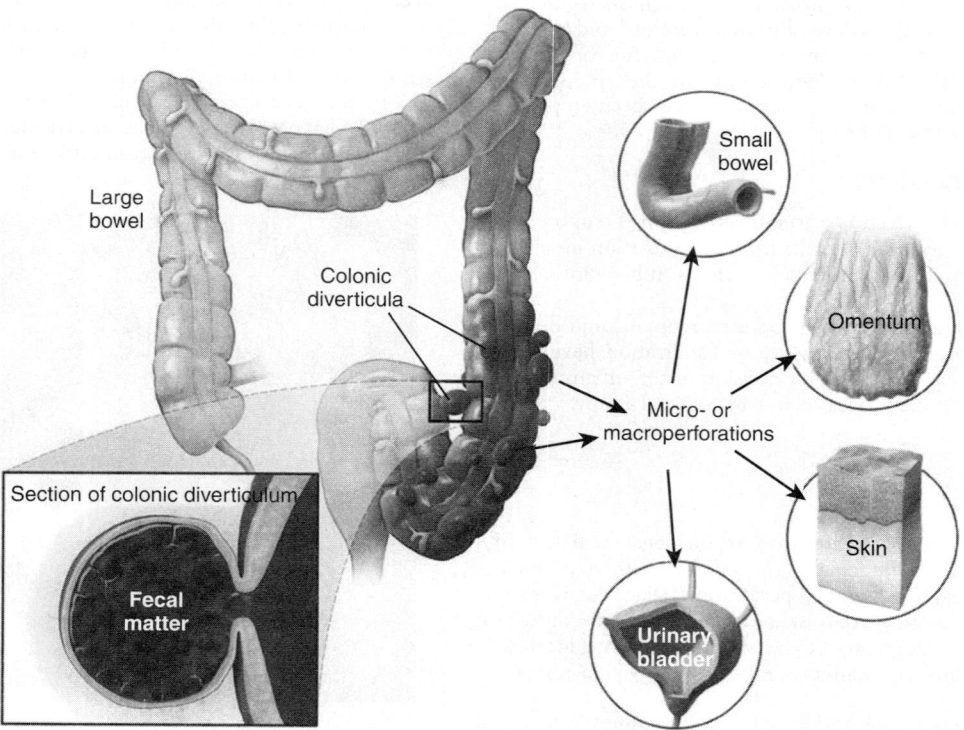

FIGURE 3. Colonic diverticula. Colonic diverticula have narrow necks that can be obstructed by fecal matter. Obstruction may produce distention of the sac, bacterial overgrowth, vascular compromise, and perforation. Some perforations are localized and contained, whereas others may invade the skin or erode into adjacent viscera, causing fistulas. (Image from Jacobs DO: Diverticulitis. N Engl J Med 2007;357:2058, courtesy of New England Journal of Medicine.)

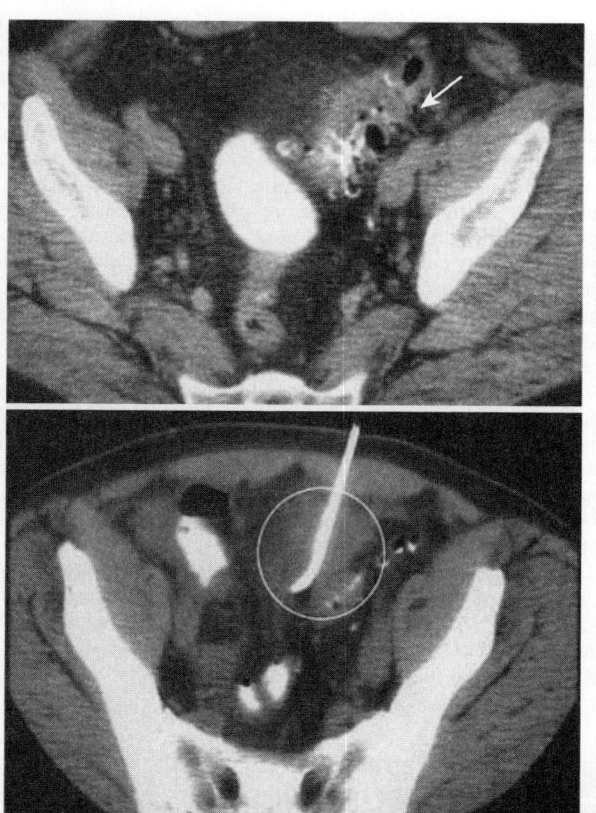

FIGURE 4. Computed tomographic findings of diverticulitis. The upper panel shows evidence of inflammation and wall thickening *(arrow)*. The bottom panel shows a diverticular abscess with a percutaneously placed drain. (Images courtesy of Dr. Erik Paulson, Department of Radiology, Duke University Medical Center.)

6 weeks to allow for resolution of inflammation and to lower the likelihood of conversion to an open procedure if a laparoscopic approach is attempted. Elective laparoscopic resection may prove to be superior to the traditional open resection in terms of reduction of morbidity and length of hospital stay.

Emergent surgical intervention may be required if the patient fails to improve or worsens clinically, which occurs approximately 10% of the time. Surgical intervention in this acute setting typically consists of a two-staged procedure beginning with resection of the involved segment, lavage, end colostomy, and oversewing of the distal rectal stump (Hartmann's procedure). During the second stage, the end colostomy is taken down, and intestinal continuity is reestablished in an elective fashion (Fig. 5). It is important that the margin of resection include the entire sigmoid colon, to reduce the risk of recurrence. In long-term quality-of-life studies, surgical management has provided a significant advantage compared with nonsurgical management for complicated diverticulitis.

Special Problems

Special circumstances worthy of further evaluation include diverticulitis in young patients, primary resection and anastomosis (single-stage approach) in cases of perforated diverticulitis, and nonoperative management of recurrent diverticulitis.

Controversy exists as to whether diverticulitis in the younger patient is more virulent than in their older counterparts. Some argue that diverticula in these young patients should be managed more aggressively, with surgical resection, whereas others believe that younger and older patients are at equal risk and should receive equivalent therapy.

Although most surgeons would consider a two-stage approach for perforated diverticulitis, there have been studies showing that a single-stage approach may be feasible in appropriately selected patients.

Controversy exists concerning the need and timing of surgical resection after recurrent diverticulitis. Some advocate elective resection after the second episode; others prefer to wait until after the fourth episode; and still others suggest that surgery can be avoided in uncomplicated recurrent diverticulitis regardless of the number of previous episodes.

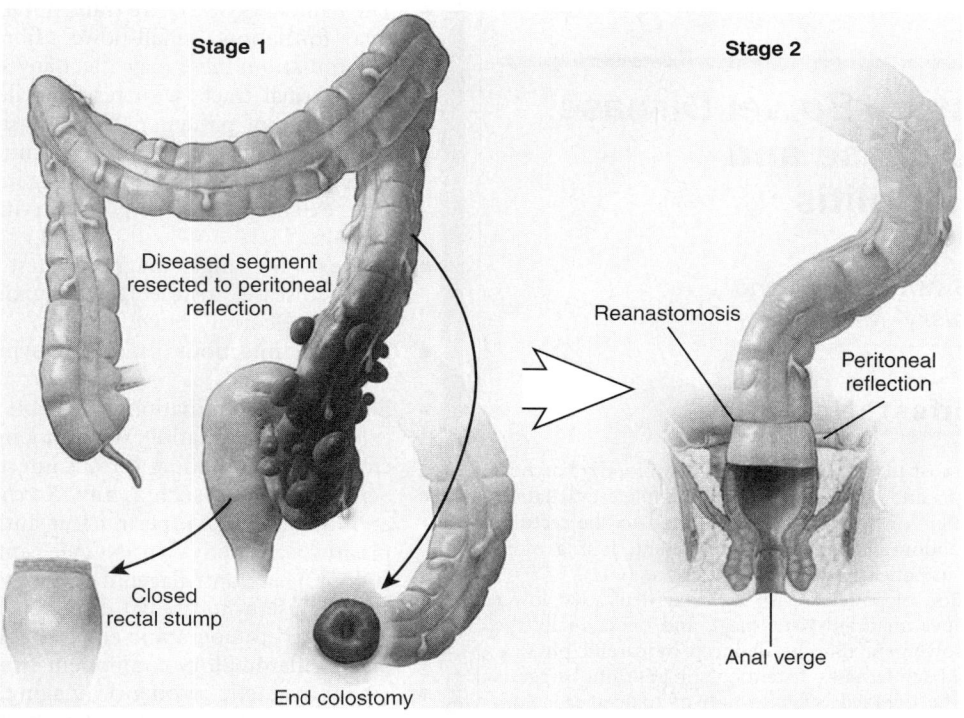

FIGURE 5. Two-staged operative approach to diverticulitis. In stage 1, the diseased segment of bowel is resected, an end colostomy is performed, and the distal rectal stump is oversewn (Hartmann's procedure). In stage 2, performed during a second procedure, colonic continuity is reestablished. (Image from Jacobs DO: Diverticulitis. N Engl J Med 2007;357:2063, courtesy of New England Journal of Medicine.)

REFERENCES

Alves A, Panis Y, Slim K, et al. French multicentre prospective observational study of laparoscopic versus open colectomy for sigmoid diverticular disease. Br J Surg 2005;92(12):1520–5.

Bordeianou L, Hodin R. Controversies in the surgical management of sigmoid diverticulitis. J Gastrointest Surg 2007;11(4):542–8.

Cassivi SD, Deschamps C, Nichols FC 3rd, et al. Diverticula of the esophagus. Surg Clin North Am 2005;85(3):495–503.

Donkervoort SC, Baak LC, Blaauwgeers JL, et al. Laparoscopic resection of a symptomatic gastric diverticulum: A minimally invasive solution. J Soc Laparoendosc Surgeons 2006;10(4):525–7.

Jacobs DO. Clinical practice: Diverticulitis. N Engl J Med 2007;357 (20):2057–66.

Mäkelä JT, Kiviniemi HO, Laitinen ST. Elective surgery for recurrent diverticulitis. Hepatogastroenterology 2007;54(77):1412–6.

Nelson RS, Velasco A, Mukesh BN. Management of diverticulitis in younger patients. Dis Colon Rectum 2006;49(9):1341–5.

Pautrat K, Bretagnol F, Huten N, et al. Acute diverticulitis in very young patients: A frequent surgical management. Dis Colon Rectum 2007;50 (4):472–7.

Richter S, Lindemann W, Kollmar O, et al. One-stage sigmoid colon resection for perforated sigmoid diverticulitis (Hinchey stages III and IV). World J Surg 2006;30(6):1027–32.

Salem L, Veenstra DL, Sullivan SD, et al. The timing of elective colectomy in diverticulitis: A decision analysis. J Am Coll Surg 2004;199(6):904–12.

Scarpa M, Pagano D, Ruffolo C, et al. Health-related quality of life after colonic resection for diverticular disease: Long-term results. J Gastrointest Surg 2008;13(1):105–12.

Schilling MK, Maurer CA, Kollmar O, et al. Primary vs. secondary anastomosis after sigmoid colon resection for perforated diverticulitis (Hinchey Stage III and IV): A prospective outcome and cost analysis. Dis Colon Rectum 2001;44(5):699–703.

Zani A, Eaton S, Rees CM, et al. Incidentally detected Meckel diverticulum: To resect or not to resect? Ann Surg 2008;247(2):276–81.

Zingg U, Pasternak I, Guertler L, et al. Early vs. delayed elective laparoscopic-assisted colectomy in sigmoid diverticulitis: Timing of surgery in relation to the attack. Dis Colon Rectum 2007;50(11):1911–7.

530

Inflammatory Bowel Disease: Crohn's Disease and Ulcerative Colitis

Method of
Prabhakar P. Swaroop, MD, and
Daniel K. Podolsky, MD

Clinical Manifestations

The cardinal symptom of ulcerative colitis (UC) is bloody diarrhea. Symptoms of tenesmus and the sensation of incomplete evacuation may dominate in patients who have disease limited to the rectum. Although cramping abdominal pain is often present, it is a more prominent symptom in patients with Crohn's disease (CD).

Physical examination of patients with UC may detect left lower quadrant and left upper quadrant tenderness, and occasionally the extent of colonic involvement may be deduced by careful physical examination. Rebound tenderness, distention, or guarding suggests the development of the dreaded complication of toxic megacolon, which may supervene in patients with severe UC.

Patients with CD have more widely varying symptoms as a result of the highly variable sites of involvement and the range of phenotypic forms. Disease manifestations may be dominated by inflammatory activity per se, by fistula formation (fistulizing or perforating disease), or by stricture formation (stricturing disease). Perianal fistulas can be a distressing manifestation and may parallel clinical flares. The symptom complex of right lower quadrant pain, nonbloody diarrhea, and weight loss is most common because of the frequent involvement of the ileum. However, in CD with colonic involvement (with or without more proximal disease), symptoms may be indistinguishable from those of UC. Intestinal narrowing may be caused by edema due to inflammation, fibrosis from chronic inflammation, or a combination of these factors. The presence of a mass in the right lower quadrant suggests inflammatory ileal disease (and probably abscess formation), whereas right lower quadrant pain in conjunction with obstructive symptoms in the absence of a mass may be suggestive of stricture formation. Fistula disease can manifest with especially variable symptoms because of the many anatomic structures that can be involved (e.g., fecaluria and pneumaturia in those with fistulas to the bladder). Rectovaginal fistulas may lead to passage of air from the vagina. Patients with upper gastrointestinal CD may present with dysphagia, early satiety, and fear of food leading to weight loss.

Diarrhea is common but not universal in CD. Inflammation of the ileum or of the colon can cause diarrhea. Occasionally, diarrhea is caused by small intestinal bacterial overgrowth, especially in patients with fistulizing disease, or it may be induced by bile salts in those with ileal disease (or after ileal resection).

CURRENT DIAGNOSIS

- The most common clinical symptom of ulcerative colitis (UC) is bloody diarrhea, which is often associated with cramping abdominal pain.
- Clinical manifestations of Crohn's disease (CD) are highly variable, but the most common constellation is right lower quadrant abdominal pain and nonbloody diarrhea, often accompanied by weight loss and other constitutional symptoms.
- The hallmarks of CD are transmural inflammation, fistula formation, small-bowel fibrosis, and patchy inflammation; these may affect any segment of the gastrointestinal tract (with terminal ileal involvement in two thirds of patients). In contrast, inflammation in UC is limited to mucosa and submucosa and is diffuse, with the rectum most commonly involved. Inflammation extends proximally to varying degrees among patients.
- There is no single diagnostic test for inflammatory bowel disease; instead, the diagnosis is made based on several corroborative features.
- Potential infectious causes of symptoms should be ruled out.
- Endoscopic examination is valuable in establishing the extent of inflammation, obtaining mucosal biopsy specimens, and excluding certain infectious agents.
- Serology studies, such as anti–*Saccharomyces cerevisiae* antibodies (ASCA), perinuclear antineutrophilic cytoplasmic antibody (pANCA), anti-porin antibody (OmpC), and anti-flagellin antibody (CBir1), are occasionally useful to predict disease behavior.
- Computed tomographic enterography can help distinguish inflammatory component from fibrosis.
- Rectal magnetic resonance imaging, endoscopic ultrasound, or examination under anesthesia can be used to fully delineate perianal fistulizing disease.

Diagnosis

Diagnosis of inflammatory bowel disease (IBD) is based on the combination of clinical features, laboratory abnormalities, imaging studies (e.g., upper gastrointestinal series with small bowel follow-through and abdominal computed tomography or magnetic resonance imaging or both), and endoscopic findings including examination of mucosal biopsies. None of these tests alone is diagnostic of IBD. In a patient with new symptoms and in those patients with flares if appropriate, infectious agents should be ruled out. Common pathogens that can mimic IBD are *Salmonella, Shigella, Aeromonas, Campylobacter, Yersinia, Clostridium difficile, Plesiomonas*, and parasites such as *Giardia lamblia* and *Entamoeba*; these should be ruled out. In an immunocompromised host (including patients with established IBD receiving immunosuppressive therapy), viral infections such as cytomegalovirus and herpes simplex virus may cause ulcers suggestive of IBD. Endoscopic imaging is often very useful. The constellation of findings in endoscopy and other studies, together with the histologic and clinical features, usually allows a reliable distinction between UC and CD. However, in as many as 10% of patients, it may not be possible to make the distinction with confidence, and such patients are said to have indeterminate colitis. The distinguishing features of UC and CD are presented in Table 1.

Hematologic abnormalities include evidence of microcytic anemia, elevated white blood cell count in peripheral blood, and thrombocytosis. Markers of inflammation such as erythrocyte sedimentation rate (ESR) and high-sensitivity C-reactive protein (hsCRP) may also be elevated, the latter more commonly in CD than in UC. Very high hsCRP may be associated with infections such as cytomegalovirus or *Clostridium difficile*.

Serologic measurements of perinuclear antineutrophilic cytoplasmic antibody (pANCA), anti–*Saccharomyces cerevisiae* antibodies (ASCA—immunoglobulin G and immunoglobulin A), anti-porin antibody (OmpC), and anti-flagellin antibody (CBir1) are occasionally helpful as corroborative evidence and to help identify patients who are at higher risk for complicating events. They may also be useful in differentiating between CD and UC in patients for whom colectomy is being considered when diagnostic ambiguity remains.

Hypoalbuminemia can be a sign of poor nutritional status, and these patients should be considered for total parenteral nutrition, particularly if surgery is being planned.

Among the imaging modalities commonly used in diagnosis and management of IBD, computed tomography of the abdomen and pelvis can alert physicians to perforation, bowel obstruction, and extent of inflammation. Computed tomographic enterography can be used

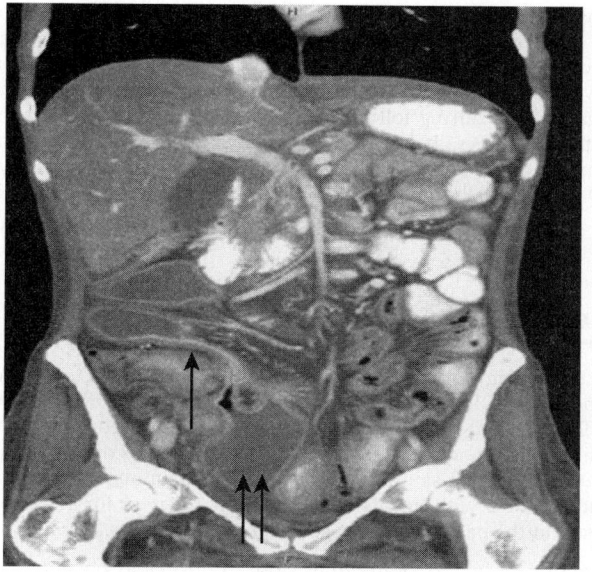

FIGURE 1. Computed tomographic enterography. Mural stratification; ileal wall thickening *(arrow)* suggestive of active inflammation; dilated loops of small bowel *(double arrow)* consistent with partial obstruction; and diffuse increased density of the subcutaneous and intraperitoneal fat compatible with anasarca are seen in this image. (Courtesy of Dr. Cecelia Brewington, MD.)

to evaluate the degree and extent of inflammation in the small bowel (Fig. 1). In cases of stenotic lesions of the small bowel, it can be especially helpful in identifying the inflammatory component, as evidenced by mural stranding. Lack of mural stranding in stenotic portions of small bowel suggests fibrosis, and if there is evidence of proximal dilation in a symptomatic patient, resection or strictureplasty should be considered.

Magnetic resonance imaging can be a helpful adjunct, along with examination under anesthesia and rectal endoscopic ultrasonography in cases of perianal fistulizing disease.

Endoscopic examination is helpful to establish the extent of disease and obtain tissue for histologic examination. Esophagogastroduodenoscopy should be done if upper gastrointestinal CD is suspected. Single-balloon and double-balloon enteroscopy have

TABLE 1 Distinguishing Features: Crohn's Disease and Ulcerative Colitis

Features	Crohn's Disease	Ulcerative Colitis
Location	Any part of gastrointestinal tract	Colonic
Inflammation	Transmural	Mucosal/submucosal
Smoking	Smokers higher than expected	Appears to be protective
Risk of colorectal cancer	Elevated in colonic Crohn's	Elevated
Risk of intestinal cancer	Elevated in small-bowel Crohn's disease	NA
hsCRP	Elevation common	Elevation not common
Serology	ASCA, OmpC, CBir1	pANCA
Surgery	Recurrence common	Total proctocolectomy may be curative
Fistulas	Common	Very rare
FDA-approved biologic agents	Infliximab (Remicade), adalimumab (Humira), certolizumab pegol (Cimzia), natalizumab (Tysabri)	Infliximab
Immunomodulator therapy	Azathioprine (AZA, Imuran),[1] 6-mercaptopurine (6MP, Purinethol),[1] methotrexate (MTX, Trexall)[1]	AZA, 6MP, cyclosporine (Sandimmune, Neoral)[1]
Endoscopic features	Skip lesions	Contiguous involvement
Strictures	Common	Colorectal cancer unless proven otherwise
Genetic markers*	NOD2, ATG16L1, IRGM, IL23R, IL12B, STAT3, NKX2-3	IL12B, STAT3. NKX2-3

*Not approved for diagnosis.
[1]Not FDA approved for this indication.
ASCA = anti–*Saccharomyces cerevisiae* antibodies; CBir1 = anti-flagellin antibody; FDA = U.S. Food and Drug Administration; hsCRP = high-sensitivity C-reactive protein; OmpC = anti-porin antibody; NA = not applicable; pANCA = perinuclear antineutrophilic cytoplasmic antibody.

allowed gastroenterologists to obtain tissue samples from jejunum and proximal ileum. Capsule endoscopy can be a useful alternative, although it does not allow tissue sampling and should not be used if even limited obstruction is suspected. Colonoscopy is helpful in diagnosis and during follow-up to assess response to various therapeutic modalities. It can also be used to obtain biopsy specimens from the colon and terminal ileum to be examined for findings of IBD or potentially confounding processes, including some infections.

Treatment

Once the diagnosis is confirmed, the treatment of IBD is based on manifestation, location, patient history, and severity of symptoms.

Treatment algorithms for IBD are usually divided into management of mild, moderate, and severe disease. The roles of various agents have evolved, and as more data are being accumulated, patients are treated earlier with agents that had been reserved for more severe disease in the past. Treatment goals for these patients are:

- Improving quality of life to as close to normal as possible
- Maintaining remission
- Avoiding surgery
- Minimizing the risk of steroid dependence
- Minimizing the risk of treatment-associated complications

CURRENT THERAPY

- Mesalamine products in adequate dosage and appropriate formulation can be effective therapy for mild to moderately active ulcerative colitis (UC) and in maintaining remission.
- Mesalamine products may be effective in mild Crohn's disease (CD), and the formulation selected should be determined by disease location.
- Steroids are useful in patients with moderate to severe CD or UC, but their use should be limited as much as possible because of frequent side effects and complications.
- Immunomodulators such as Azathioprine (Imuran)[1] and 6-mercaptopurine (Purinethol)[1] may be used as an adjunct therapy to minimize steroid use in patients who are steroid dependent and to minimize formation of neutralizing antibodies in patients receiving antibody-based biologic agents.
- Anti–tumor necrosis factor (anti-TNF) biologic agents such as infliximab (Remicade) and adalimumab (Humira) are effective in patients with moderate to severe inflammatory CD or UC that is unresponsive to conventional treatments. Certolizumab pegol (Cimzia) may be used to maintain remission. Immunomodulators and biologic agents may be used independently or in combination for treatment of inflammatory bowel disease and for maintaining surgically induced remission in CD.
- The proven role of antibiotics is limited to septic complications, perianal disease, small intestinal bacterial overgrowth, and pouchitis.
- Nataluzimab (Tysabri), an anti-α_4 agent, is effective in some patients with refractory CD, including those for whom anti-TNF therapy has failed.

[1]Not FDA approved for this indication.

ULCERATIVE COLITIS

In the initial evaluation of UC patients, it is important to establish the extent and degree of inflammation and the concomitant presence of extraintestinal manifestations. Extent and severity of UC are judged on clinical symptoms, basic laboratory parameters (complete blood count and albumin level), and colonoscopic findings. Disease limited to the rectum and distal colon may be treated with local mesalamine therapy, in a suppository (Canasa), foam (Salofalk),[2] or enema (Rowasa) formulation. Newly diagnosed patients with mild to moderate disease activity should be given an appropriate oral formulation of mesalamine (Asacol). Antidiarrheal agents may provide symptomatic relief once infectious causes of colitis have been excluded.

If remission is achieved with a mesalamine formulation, the same dose of mesalamine is continued for maintenance of remission. For an occasional flare suggested by symptoms of recurrence and documented by sigmoidoscopy or colonoscopy, steroids may be used. For patients who have frequent flares (more than two per year), initiation of therapy with a conventional immunomodulator or infliximab (Remicade) should be considered.

For patients with moderate disease unresponsiveness to mesalamine or severe disease, a topical, oral, or intravenous corticosteroid (depending on extent and severity) may be necessary, but it should be used for as short a period as possible, and, if it is not possible to taper and discontinue the steroid within 6 weeks, an immunomodulator should be added.

Surgical intervention should be considered for patients who have no response to therapy with infliximab, steroids, and/or cyclosporine (Neoral).[1] Patients who have high-grade dysplasia or colorectal cancer are also candidates for surgery.

CROHN'S DISEASE

Optimal treatment of CD is based on many factors, including location, severity, specific clinical manifestation and complications, prior clinical course intervention, whether fistulas are present, potential fibrostenotic strictures, history of steroid dependence, history of failure with other agents, and contraindications (e.g., malignancy, opportunistic infections, tuberculosis, intolerance to medications). Before deciding on treatment options, it is important to delineate behavior (fistulizing, stricturing, or inflammatory), location (ileal, colonic, or ileocolonic), and severity and to assess for the presence of extraintestinal complications and nutritional deficiencies.

In patients with mildly active, localized ileocecal disease, treatment has historically begun with a suitable mesalamine product (although effectiveness of this approach remains uncertain).[1] More recently, oral budesonide (Entocort EC, a steroid targeted to the ileum that undergoes extensive first-pass metabolism to minimize systemic steroid effects) has been used. For those with more extensive or severe disease, conventional systemic steroids (prednisone) may be used, but if it is not possible to wean the patient off steroids within 6 weeks, an immunodulatory agent should be started, typically 6-mercatopurine (Purinethol)[1]/azathioprine (Imuran)[1] or, in those unable to tolerate these agents, low-dose methotrexate (Trexall).[1] For patients with moderate to severe disease, treatment should include an anti-tumor necrosis factor (anti-TNF) agent with or without immunomodulator therapy. Natalizumab (Tysabri), an anti-α_4 integrin, is an alternative and may be used if anti-TNF therapy fails.

Before starting therapy with a biologic agent, patients should have a purified protein derivative (PPD) test and a hepatitis B surface antibody determination. Once biologic therapy begins, patients should continue to have an annual PPD test.

Perianal fistulizing disease, in the absence of abscess, can be treated with a combination of antibiotics, seton placement, immunomodulator therapy, and biologic agents. Complex perianal fistulizing disease may require a diverting ostomy.

[1]Not FDA approved for this indication.
[2]Not available in the United States.

Therapeutic Options

MESALAMINE PREPARATIONS

Aminosalicylate preparations have been used for the treatment of UC and CD. Some data suggest that mesalamine has limited efficacy in patients with CD.

In patients with limited distal UC (e.g., proctitis), treatment may be begun with a mesalamine enema (Rowasa) or suppository (Canasa). For more extensive disease, oral therapy (Asacol) should be used.

Combination therapy (oral administration as well as enemas/suppositories) has been shown to be more effective in inducing remission than either modality alone. In general, the dosage that induces remission is used for maintenance of remission (Table 2).

STEROIDS

The National Co-operative Crohn's Disease Study and the European Co-operative Crohn's Disease Study demonstrated that steroids are efficacious in inducing remission but ineffective in maintaining remission. Among patients who have received steroids, about 26% will have a partial response, and 16% will have no response; among those who have had a complete or partial response, about 28% will become steroid dependent. The requirement for surgery is high in the latter group of patients; about 38% require surgery by the end of 1 year.

The adverse effects of steroids are many and varied and can be classified as early effects and delayed effects associated with prolonged use (>12 weeks). Acne, moon facies, mood changes, sleep disturbances, gastrointestinal intolerance, hyperglycemia, hypertension, weight gain, and ulcers of the gastrointestinal tract can be seen early. Formation of cataracts, aseptic necrosis, suppression of the hypothalamic-pituitary axis, and myopathy are associated with prolonged used. Loss of bone density, previously thought to occur only with chronic use, may be evident in bone density studies after as little as 2 weeks of therapy.

Budesonide (Entocort EC) is used for ileal inflammatory and right-sided colonic CD, with lower expected incidences of acne, moon facies, adrenal suppression, and loss of bone mineral density. Alternative therapies (immunomodulators, biologic agents) should be discussed with the patient if there has been no response to steroids in a few weeks.

IMMUNOMODULATORY THERAPY

Azathioprine[1] and 6-mercaptopurine[1] are immunomodulators used as steroid-sparing agents for both CD and UC. Immunomodulators have been shown to modestly reduce the incidence of postsurgical

[1]Not FDA approved for this indication.

recurrence in CD. The onset of action of these agents is slow, up to 3 to 4 months. Some toxicities are associated with genetic variants in the enzymes responsible for catabolism of azathioprine and 6-mercaptopurine, most notably thiopurine methyl transferase (TPMT). Most (89%) patients have wild-type TPMT (full TPMT enzyme activity), 11% have intermediate enzyme activity, and 0.3% have none. In patients with full TPMT enzyme activity, therapy should be started with 1.5 mg/kg/day of 6-mercaptopurine or 2.5 mg/kg/day of azathioprine; those with intermediate activity should have the dosage reduced by half. Those who do not have any TPMT expression should not be started on these agents because of the high risk of bone marrow toxicity.

Some complications, including pancreatitis, hepatotoxicity, and serum sickness–like syndrome, cannot be predicted. It is recommended that patients starting these medications have a complete blood count and liver function tests performed every other week while their medications are being adjusted. Once they are on a stable dosage, these tests should be done every 2 to 3 months.

Parenteral methotrexate[1] 15 to 25 mg/week can be used to induce remission in patients with CD that has not responded to conventional agents. Once remission has been achieved, oral methotrexate[1] 15 mg can be used to maintain remission. Methotrexate is absolutely contraindicated in pregnancy. Leukopenia, hepatic fibrosis, nausea and vomiting, and hypersensitivity reactions are potential side effects. Risk of hepatic fibrosis is associated with a cumulative dose of more than 1.5 g, diabetes, and concomitant use of alcohol.

CYCLOSPORINE

In patients with severe UC, intravenous cyclosporine (Sandimmune)[1] at a dose of 2 to 4 mg/kg/day has been shown to be effective in inducing remission. A significant proportion of these patients may still require colectomy within 1 year. Those patients who have achieved response and remission on intravenous cyclosporine should be started on oral cyclosporine (Neoral)[1] for a few months, together with prophylaxis against *Pneumocystis*. 6-Mercaptopurine or azathioprine can also be used as maintenance agents.

Side effects commonly seen with cyclosporine include renal dysfunction, seizures (particularly in patients with hypocholesterolemia), hypertension, gingival hyperplasia, electrolyte abnormalities, and hirsutism.

BIOLOGIC AGENTS

Infliximab is a chimeric (murine-human) monoclonal anti-TNF antibody that has been approved for induction and maintenance of remission in both CD and UC. It was initially approved for the treatment of fistulizing CD, and subsequent studies showed it to be effective in maintenance therapy as well. In several other studies, it was found to be efficacious in reducing steroid use, length of hospital stay, and surgical intervention and achieving mucosal healing. Infliximab is administered intravenously with or without premedication to avoid allergic reactions.

For induction, infliximab 5 mg/kg is administered at weeks 0, 2, and 6, and maintenance is begun at 5 mg/kg every 8 weeks. Some patients require dose escalation because of diminution of response or failure to maintain remission. In these patients, depending on the clinical scenario, the dose should be increased to 10 mg/kg or the interval reduced to every 6 weeks. In the past, infliximab was routinely used with concomitant immunomodulator therapy to reduce the possibility of infliximab antibodies, but this practice has been associated with a higher risk for a rare hepatosplenic T-cell lymphoma (predominantly in the pediatric population), leading to reconsideration of the need for concomitant immunomodulators in some patients. However, results from the recently released Study of Biologic and Immunomodulator Naive Patients in Crohn's Disease (SONIC) trial demonstrated the superiority of combination therapy over either immunomodulator or infliximab alone, especially in patients with elevated C-reactive protein and ulcers in their baseline colonoscopy. Because reactivation of latent tuberculosis has been

[1]Not FDA approved for this indication.

TABLE 2 Mesalamine Products Indicated for Ulcerative Colitis

Aminosalicylate Product	Daily Dosage	Frequency
Azulfidine (sulfasalazine tablet)	0.5 g–4 g	qid
Asacol (mesalamine delayed-release tablet)	1.6–2.4 g	tid
Pentasa (mesalamine controlled-release tablet)	2–4 g	qid
Colazal (balsalazide capsule)	6.75 g	tid
Dipentum (olsalazine capsule)	1 g	bid
Lialda (mesalamine delayed-release tablet)	2.4–4.8 g	qd
Canasa (mesalamine rectal suppository)*	1 g	qd
Rowasa (mesalamine rectal enema)†	4 g	qd
Apriso (mesalamine delayed and extended-release capsule)	1.5 g	qd

*Indicated for ulcerative proctitis.
†Indicated for distal ulcerative colitis.

reported, patients should undergo a PPD test and chest radiography before beginning therapy.

OTHER ANTI–TUMOR NECROSIS FACTOR ANTIBODIES

Adalimumab

Recently, adalimumab (Humira), a recombinant fully human immunoglobulin targeting TNF, was approved for use in CD. In the CLASSIC and CHARM trials, adalimumab was demonstrated to be an effective agent in inducing and maintaining remission. It has also been shown to be effective in patients who have lost response to infliximab or are intolerant to it, but it has not yet been approved for treatment of UC. Serious reactions, reactivation of tuberculosis, allergic reactions, lupus-like reactions, and demyelinating diseases are some of the concerns.

For induction, adalimumab 160 mg is given subcutaneously at week 0, 80 mg at week 2, and then, for maintenance of remission, 40 mg every other week.

Certolizumab

Certolizumab (Cimzia) is a polyethylene glycolated Fab fragment of humanized anti-TNF monoclonal antibody approved for use in CD. In the PRECISE 1 and 2 studies, certolizumab was shown to result in modest improvement in response but no clinically significant improvement in remission.

ANTI-α_4 THERAPY

Natalizumab

Natalizumab (Tysabri) is a humanized monoclonal antibody against the α_4 integrin subunit, a molecule involved in cellular adhesion that is required for recruitment of key immune cells to sites affected by IBD. In several studies, it has been shown to be efficacious in inducing remission and maintaining response in CD patients. Enthusiasm has been tempered by the apparent risk for progressive multifocal leukoencephalopathy, a rare but fatal opportunistic infection.

The treatment regimens for UC and CD are summarized in Box 1.

BOX 1 Summary of Treatment Regimen

Ulcerative Colitis

Proctitis
- Initial treatment choices
  - Mesalamine suppositories (Canasa) or enemas (Rowasa) to induce remission
  - Steroid foam enemas (Cortifoam) to induce remission
  - Mesalamine suppositories or enemas to maintain remission
- Second-line treatment choices
  - Oral mesalamine (Asacol) in combination with local therapy
  - Adjunctive treatment with antibiotics: ciprofloxacin (Cipro),[1] metronidazole (Flagyl),[1] or rifaximin (Xifaxan)[1]
  - Probiotics

Left-Sided Colitis
- Initial treatment choices
  - Oral mesalamine product with or without local therapy
- Second-line treatment choices
  - Oral or intravenous steroids
  - Immunomodulator therapy
  - Infliximab (IFX, Remicade)
  - Cyclosporine (Sandimmune)[1] on an inpatient basis (avoid cyclosporine after IFX therapy due to risk of severe immunosuppression)

Pancolitis
- Initial treatment choices
  - Oral mesalamine with a short course of oral or intravenous steroids
- Second-line treatment choices
  - Immunomodulator therapy
  - Infliximab
  - Cyclosporine on an inpatient basis (avoid cyclosporine after IFX therapy due to risk of severe immunosuppression)

Crohn's Disease

Ileocecal Inflammatory Crohn's Disease
- First-line treatment
  - Oral mesalamine (Asacol for ileal disease; Pentasa for more proximal small-bowel disease)[1]
  - Budesonide (Entocort EC) 9 mg PO qd
  - Immunomodulator therapy
  - Biologic agents with or without concomitant immunomodulators

Ileal Stricturing Disease
- No proximal dilation
  - Trial with budesonide or biologic agents (patients with elevated hsCRP are more likely to respond)
- Proximal small-bowel dilation
  - Consider surgical approach

Internally Fistulizing Disease without Intraabdominal Abscess
- Stricture immediately distal to fistula
  - Surgical approach
- No stricture
  - Biologic agents with or without concomitant immunomodulators

Externally Fistulizing Disease without Intraabdominal Abscess
- Biologic agents with or without concomitant immunomodulators

Fistulizing Disease with Intraabdominal Abscess
- Intravenous antibiotics as appropriate
- Percutaneous drainage if appropriate
- Surgical drainage if indicated
- Biologic agents with or without concomitant immunomodulators once infectious process has been treated

Perianal Crohn's Disease without Abscess Formation
- Antibiotics: Ciprofloxacin (Cipro),[1] metronidazole (Flagyl),[1] rifaximin (Xifaxan)[1]
- Immunomodulators
- Biologic agents with or without concomitant immunomodulators
- Seton placement
- Diverting ostomy

Colonic Crohn's Disease
- Oral steroids to induce remission
- Immunomodulator therapy
- Biologic agents with or without concomitant immunomodulator therapy

---

[1]Not FDA approved for this indication.
hsCRP = high-sensitivity C-reactive protein.

REFERENCES

Booya F, Akram S, Fletcher JG, et al. CT enterography and fistulizing Crohn's disease: Clinical benefit and radiographic findings. Abdom Imaging 2009; 34(4):467–75.

Feagan BG, Panaccione R, Sandborn WJ, et al. Effects of adalimumab therapy on incidence of hospitalization and surgery in Crohn's disease: Results from the CHARM study. Gastroenterology 2008;135(5):1493–9.

Ghosh S, Goldin E, Gordon FH, et al. Natalizumab for active Crohn's disease. N Engl J Med 2003;348(1):24–32.

Hanauer SB, Sandborn WJ, Kornbluth A. Delayed-release oral mesalamine at 4.8 g/day (800 mg tablet) for the treatment of moderately active ulcerative colitis: The ASCEND II trial. Am J Gastroenterol 2005;100(11):2478–85.

Lichtenstein GR, Yan S, Bala M. Infliximab maintenance treatment reduces hospitalizations, surgeries, and procedures in fistulizing Crohn's disease. Gastroenterology 2005;128(4):862–9.

Podolsky DK. Inflammatory bowel disease. N Engl J Med 2002;347(6):417–29.

Thomsen OO, Cortot A, Jewell D, et al. A comparison of budesonide and mesalamine for active Crohn's disease. International Budesonide-Mesalamine Study Group. N Engl J Med 1998;339(6):370–4.

Thukral C, Travassos WJ, Peppercorn MA. The role of antibiotics in inflammatory bowel disease. Curr Treat Options Gastroenterol 2005;8(3):223–8.

Xavier RJ, Podolsky DK. Unraveling the Pathogenesis of Inflammatory Bowel Disease. Nature 2007;448(7152):427–34.

Irritable Bowel Syndrome

Method of
Brenda R. Velasco, MD, and
Robert S. Fisher, MD

Epidemiology

Irritable bowel syndrome (IBS) is one of the most common functional gastrointestinal disorders, with a worldwide prevalence estimated to be between 10% and 20%. It is a syndrome characterized by chronic abdominal pain or discomfort and irregular bowel habits that has a significant impact on affected individuals and society. The diagnosis of IBS is based on the absence of detectable structural or biochemical causes and the presence of a constellation of symptoms as outlined by the so-called Rome III criteria (Box 1).

Bloating or visible abdominal distention often is present in patients with IBS but is not considered essential for diagnosis. The Rome III diagnostic criteria divide IBS into subgroups based on stool form and not frequency. Each of the top three IBS subgroups constitutes approximately one third of all IBS patients (Box 2).

Gender differences have been documented in terms of both prominent symptoms and response to treatment. In the community, the ratio of women to men with IBS is estimated to be between 2:1 and 4:1; this difference is greater in the population of IBS patients who seek health care. Women with IBS report greater overall IBS symptom severity, greater intensity of abdominal pain and bloating, greater impact of symptoms on daily life, and lower health-related quality of life, compared to men with IBS. The estimated prevalence of IBS in children is similar to that in adults, and newly diagnosed adults frequently report symptoms of IBS (or other related functional gastrointestinal symptoms) dating back to childhood. The most common age group seen by physicians for treatment of IBS is 20- to 50-year-olds. Patients with a diagnosis of IBS are at increased risk for other, nongastrointestinal functional disorders, such as fibromyalgia, chronic pelvic pain, interstitial cystitis, and migraine headaches.

IBS is associated with substantial economic costs, including the direct costs of excess physician visits, diagnostic testing, medications, hospitalizations, and surgeries and indirect costs from absenteeism and decreased productivity at work (presenteeism). Patients with IBS have been reported to miss three times as many days from work compared to those without bowel symptoms. In 2006, there were at least 2.4 to 3.5 million U.S. physician visits annually for IBS. The annual direct and indirect costs of IBS were recently estimated to be at least $1.6 billion and $19 billion, respectively.

Pathophysiology

The pathophysiology of IBS is multifactorial and complex (Box 3). Altered bowel motility, visceral hypersensitivity, central nervous system effects, and an imbalance in neurotransmitters have all been considered. In addition, roles for infection, small-bowel bacterial overgrowth, abnormal colonic bacterial flora, genetics, and environmental and psychosocial factors have been proposed.

In about 10% of patients the onset of IBS-like symptoms can be attributed to a preceding episode of acute viral or bacterial gastroenteritis that was associated with a significant life stressor. The duration of the infectious gastroenteritis is also a factor in predisposing patients to the development of IBS: the longer the duration of the acute illness, the higher the risk of eventually developing IBS. Altered contractility of the colon and small bowel has been described in patients with IBS and may be related to ingestion of food and

---

BOX 1 Rome III Criteria for the Diagnosis of Irritable Bowel Syndrome

Recurrent abdominal pain or discomfort (with onset at least 6 months before diagnosis) that
- Occurred on at least 3 days per month in the last 3 months, and
- Is associated with two or more of the following:
  - Improvement with defecation
  - Onset associated with a change in frequency of stool
  - Onset associated with a change in form (appearance) of stool

Adapted from Longstreth GF, Thompson WG, Chey WD, et al: Functional bowel disorders. In Drossman DA, Corazziari E, Delvaux M, et al. (eds): Rome III: The functional gastrointestinal disorders, 3rd ed. McLean, VA, Degnon, 2006, pp 487–555.

BOX 2 Subgroups of Irritable Bowel Syndrome (IBS)

- IBS with diarrhea (more common in men)
- IBS with constipation (more common in women)
- IBS with mixed bowel habits (previously known as IBS with alternating bowel habits based on Rome II criteria)
- IBS unsubtyped (not enough stools are abnormal to meet criteria for any other subtype)

Adapted from Longstreth GF, Thompson WG, Chey WD, et al: Functional bowel disorders. In Drossman DA, Corazziari E, Delvaux M, et al. (eds): Rome III: The functional gastrointestinal disorders, 3rd ed. McLean, VA, Degnon, 2006, pp 487–555.

BOX 3 Pathophysiologic Factors of Irritable Bowel Syndrome

- Altered bowel motility
- Visceral hypersensitivity
- Central nervous system effects
- Neurotransmitter imbalance (i.e., serotonin)
- Infection
- Psychosocial factors
- Genetics

psychological or physical stress. For example, there have been reports of an exaggerated contractile response of the colon (gastrocolic reflex) and small intestine to a high-fat meal.

In addition, pain is more commonly perceived by IBS patients in association with irregular motor activity of the small bowel than by patients with inflammatory bowel disease or normal control subjects. There are documented studies using balloon distention of the rectosigmoid and the ileum that suggest that patients with IBS have a central defect in the ability to process visceral pain, characterized by the perception of pain and bloating at balloon volumes and pressures significantly lower than those required by normal subjects to elicit similar symptoms. Functional magnetic resonance imaging and positron emission tomography of the brain have revealed different levels of activity in the thalamus and the anterior cingulate cortex after balloon distention of the rectum in patients with IBS compared to normal subjects. This phenomenon is referred to as visceral hypersensitivity.

Both altered motility and visceral hypersensitivity could be mediated by imbalances of neurotransmitters. Serotonin has received the most attention given its significant presence in the gastrointestinal tract and its previously reported association with symptoms of nausea, vomiting, abdominal pain, and bloating. Increased concordance of IBS in monozygotic versus dizygotic twins and familial aggregation in IBS may support a genetic component to IBS. As always, the role of nature versus nurture is addressed and the idea that learned behavior plays a part in the manifestation of IBS has been contemplated. It has been observed that children of parents with IBS tend to actively seek medical care for gastrointestinal symptoms more than children of non-IBS patients (hypervigilance). There are reports that IBS is more frequent and more severe in women with a history of physical and/or sexual abuse.

Evaluation

Current clinical guidelines recommend that IBS can generally be diagnosed without additional testing beyond careful history taking, a general physical examination, and routine laboratory studies to exclude other organic causes in patients who have symptoms that meet the Rome criteria and who do not have alarm warning signs (red flags).

The red flags include, but are not limited to, blood in the stool (gross or occult), anemia, anorexia, weight loss, fever, family history of colon cancer, inflammatory bowel disease or celiac disease, onset of the first symptom after 50 years of age, nocturnal symptoms that awaken the patient from sleep, and a major change in symptoms. Routine laboratory tests have been suggested to include a complete blood count (CBC), thyroid function studies, stool studies for ova and parasites, and a comprehensive metabolic panel. In addition, it has recently been proposed that patients being evaluated for IBS-like symptoms who have a predominance of diarrhea be screened with serologic tests for celiac disease.

If the patient meets the Rome III criteria and does not have any red flags, classification of the IBS into one of the subcategories is recommended to guide and facilitate empiric therapy. If a red flag is present, diagnostic tests should be performed as appropriate based on the presenting symptoms, signs, and laboratory findings. The differential diagnosis for IBS-like symptoms is significant and should always be considered when evaluating patients (Box 4).

Treatment

Treatment of IBS involves a multilevel approach. One of the most important components is the establishment of a strong physician-patient relationship; this is done by being nonjudgmental and allowing for a patient-centered interview. Be sure to acknowledge the patient's symptoms, identify whether any of them are stress-related, and determine whether comorbid psychological symptoms exist. Addressing psychosocial factors may improve health status and treatment response. The second component of treatment involves an attempt to identify foods that precipitate or exacerbate symptoms. Recommendations to avoid agents such as caffeine, alcohol, fatty foods, gas-producing vegetables, or products containing sorbitol are valid. In addition, if constipation is a key symptom, it may be beneficial to encourage consumption of 20 to 30 g of fiber per day (as part of the diet or as a supplement). Pharmacotherapy is guided by the predominant symptom; placement of each patient into an IBS subcategory is useful (Table 1). In addition, alternative therapies, including complementary medicines and psychotherapy, are often coupled with the available FDA-approved pharmacotherapy in an effort to treat IBS (Box 5).

Table 1 lists most of the agents that have been employed to treat IBS. Although almost all of these agents have been tested in randomized, controlled studies, only three—alosetron, lubiprostone, and tegaserod—have received FDA approval for treatment of IBS. Alosetron is a serotonin 5-HT$_3$ antagonist that received FDA approval for treatment of IBS with diarrhea in adult women at a dose of 1.0 mg twice daily. Because of reports of ischemic colitis and bowel perforations, it was removed from the market. It has now been reintroduced for use in patients with refractory disease. The recommended dosing is to begin with 0.5 mg once daily and slowly increase the dose to 1.0 mg twice daily if necessary. Tegaserod, a 5-HT$_4$ agonist, was approved by the FDA for the treatment of IBS with constipation in adult women at a dose of 6 mg twice daily. It, too, was removed from the market because of cardiovascular side effects. Currently, it is available only in a compassionate use protocol. The third FDA-approved agent for IBS is lubiprostone, which is approved at a dose of 8 mg with breakfast and dinner to treat IBS with constipation in adult women; there are no restrictions on duration of use. Lubiprostone stimulates C-2 chloride channels to secrete chloride into the lumen of the small intestine and the colon.

TABLE 1 Pharmacotherapy for Irritable Bowel Syndrome According to Symptom

Symptom	Initial Dose	Target Dose
Diarrhea		
Loperamide (Imodium)	2 mg/d	2–8 mg/d
Diphenoxylate and atropine (Lomotil)[1]	5 mg	up to 20 mg/d
Alosetron (Lotronex)*	0.5 mg bid	up to 1 mg bid
Constipation		
Fiber (over-the-counter products)		
Laxatives and secretory stimulants		
Polyethylene glycol 3350 (MiraLAX)[1]	17 g/d	up to 34 g bid
Lactulose (Cephulac)[1]	10–20 g/d	up to 40 g/d
Lubiprostone (Amitiza)	8 μg bid	24 μg bid[3]
Osmotic laxatives		
Stimulant laxatives		
Prokinetics		
Tegaserod (Zelnorm)[2]	6 mg bid	
Bloating		
Rifaximin (Xifaxan)[1]		400 mg tid[3]
Probiotics (*Bifidobacterium infantis* 35624; Bifantis)[7]		1 capsule per day
Pain		
Dicyclomine (Bentyl)	10 mg qid	40 mg qid
Hyoscyamine (Levsin)[1]	0.25 mg SL/PO q4h prn	maximum 1.5 mg/d
Tricyclic antidepressants[1]		
Amitriptyline (Elavil)	10 mg qhs	10–75 mg qhs
Desipramine (Norpramin)	10 mg qhs	10–75 mg qhs
Nortriptyline (Pamelor)	10 mg qhs	10–75 mg qhs
Selective serotonin-reuptake inhibitors[1]		
Paroxetine (Paxil)	10 mg qhs	10–60 mg qhs
Citalopram (Celexa)	5 mg qhs	5–20 mg qhs
Fluoxetine (Prozac)	20 mg qhs	20–40 mg qhs

[1]Not FDA approved for this indication.
[2]Not available in the United States.
[3]Exceeds dosage recommended by the manufacturer.
[7]Available as dietary supplement.
*Available only to physicians enrolled in the Prescribing Program for Lotronex.

BOX 5 Alternative Management of Irritable Bowel Syndrome

Complementary Medicines
- Herbal medicines
- Megavitamins
- Folk remedies
- Microbial food supplements (prebiotics, probiotics, fungi)

Psychotherapy
- Cognitive behavioral therapy
- Relaxation therapy
- Contingency management
- Biofeedback
- Hypnosis

REFERENCES

Gershon MD, Tack J. The serotonin signaling system: From basic understanding to drug development for functional GI disorders. Gastroenterology 2007;132:397–414.
Horwitz BJ, Fisher RS. The irritable bowel wyndrome. N Engl J Med 2001;344:1846–50.
Longstreth GF, Thompson WG, Chey WD, et al. Functional bowel disorders. In: Drossman DA, Corazziari E, Delvaux M, et al, editors Rome III: The functional gastrointestinal disorders. 3rd ed. McLean, VA: Degnon; 2006. p. 487–555.
Mayer EA. Irritable bowel syndrome. N Engl J Med 2008;358:1692–9.
Park M, Camilleri M. Genetics and genotypes in irritable bowel syndrome: Implications for diagnosis and treatment. Gastroenterol Clin North Am 2005;34:305–17.
Quigley EM, Flourie B. Probiotics and irritable bowel syndrome: A rationale for their use and an assessment of the evidence to date. Neurogastroenterol Motil 2007;19:166–72.
Videlock EJ, Chang L. Irritable bowel syndrome: Current approach to symptoms, evaluation, and treatment. Gastroenterol Clin North Am 2007;36:665–85.

Hemorrhoids, Anal Fissure, and Anorectal Abscess and Fistula

Method of
Genevieve B. Melton, MD, MA

A number of conditions cause anorectal symptoms, but the majority of patients present with a complaint of "hemorrhoids." Most anorectal conditions can be diagnosed with a focused history and physical examination. Treatment is aimed at relief of symptoms, education of the patient, and prevention of further symptoms. Although most anorectal complaints are caused by a benign process, it is important for clinicians to be mindful that in some cases the etiology can be malignancy or other serious medical conditions, such as anorectal Crohn's disease.

History

A thorough, focused history is often the most helpful diagnostic tool for patients with anorectal complaints. Clinicians should inquire about pain, itching, discharge, extra tissue or a lump, and bleeding. It is particularly important to understand the patient's bowel habits with respect to constipation or diarrhea, as well as any change in defecatory habits. Other relevant history items include previous anorectal procedures and related medical conditions such as Crohn's disease, malignancy, sexually transmitted diseases, or immunosuppression.

Pain is an important symptom to elicit from patients. In most cases, pain is the predominant symptom with anal fissure, thrombosed external hemorrhoids, and anorectal abscess. Although discomfort from internal hemorrhoids can cause aching, soreness, or itching in the setting of tissue prolapse, internal hemorrhoid disease is most often painless. In contrast, external hemorrhoids that are acutely thrombosed cause pain that is acute in onset, severe, and constant. Fissure pain is often described as a tearing sensation or the feeling of "razor blades" with bowel movements that can continue for more than an hour following defecation. Patients with anal fissures might also express a fear of having bowel movements because of pain. Anorectal abscess is often associated with pain, and patients can also present with an acute lump and sometimes fever.

Anal discharge and difficulty with anorectal hygiene are also common complaints. The discharge associated with prolapsing internal hemorrhoids might contain mucus or small amounts of stool. In contrast, an anorectal fistula or abscess can spontaneously drain with associated purulent output.

When a patient has bleeding, specific details to inquire about include color (bright red versus dark blood), amount, frequency, and length of time. When no etiology for bleeding is found, further screening should be performed. Patients who are younger than 50 years and who have no other risk factors should undergo flexible sigmoidoscopy. Colonoscopy should be done when patients are 50 years of age or older, have abdominal pain, anemia, change in bowel habits, family history of polyps or colon cancer, or personal history of polyps or colon cancer.

Diagnosis

Although the prone jack-knife position allows the greatest exposure, the left lateral decubitus position with the knees up is preferred by patients and usually allows adequate exposure for anorectal examination. It is important to have sufficient lighting with a self-lighted anoscope or a headlight, as well as adequate instrumentation to perform anoscopy. An adjunctive test that can also be helpful in patients where mucosal (hemorrhoidal) or full-thickness rectal prolapse is suspected to have patients bear down on the commode and then to examine externally.

The perianal skin is the skin immediately surrounding the anal verge (Fig. 1). Perianal inspection includes careful examination of the surrounding skin for excoriation, an external orifice in the case of an anorectal fistula, lichenified skin with chronic irritation, other dermatitis, and presence of perianal lesions. The anal verge is the entrance to the anal canal. Inspection of the anal verge is best accomplished with

careful retraction of the buttocks to expose the anal verge. This maneuver can help to visualize an anal fissure located at the anal verge and extending into the anal canal.

Digital rectal examination is helpful for assessing resting and squeeze anorectal tone, palpating the prostate in men, assessing for rectocele in women, detecting any palpable anorectal lesions, and evaluating for tenderness within the anal canal or at the level of the levator ani muscles at the anorectal ring. Anoscopy is used to visually examine the anal canal, which is between 4 and 5 cm in length starting at the anal verge and extending to the top of the anorectal ring (top of external sphincter and levator ani muscles). Within the anal canal is the dentate line, which acts as a landmark anatomically and is located approximately 2 cm from the anal verge. The dentate line represents the transition from epithelial lining to the columnar lining of the rectum. Sensation above the dentate line is mediated by autonomic fibers and results in a relative lack of sensation in comparison to the highly sensitive somatically innervated tissue below the dentate line. The dentate line is also the location of the crypt anal glands from which anorectal abscesses and fistulas originate.

Hemorrhoids

Hemorrhoids are the anal vascular cushions that are present as normal structures in everyone. In the case of internal hemorrhoids, these cushions are arteriovenous channels that have overlying mucosa and submucosal smooth muscle and supportive fibroelastic connective tissue. It is believed that internal hemorrhoids function by aiding with fine control of fecal continence of liquids and gases. Internal hemorrhoids enlarge and become symptomatic as fixation by submucosal smooth muscle and connective tissue becomes disrupted and loosens. This results in a sliding or prolapsing of the anal canal lining and further engorgement of the internal hemorrhoid tissues. Common exacerbating factors include constipation, diarrhea, aging, and increased abdominal pressure that can occur with chronic straining, pregnancy, heavy lifting, and decreased venous return. Internal hemorrhoids are typically staged on a scale from I to IV based upon the extent of prolapse (Table 1).

CURRENT DIAGNOSIS

- While most anorectal complaints are caused by a benign process, it is important to be mindful that the etiology can be malignancy or other serious medical condition, such as anorectal Crohn's disease
- A thorough, focused history is often the most helpful diagnostic tool for patients with anorectal complaints.
- In patients where no etiology for bleeding is found or if there has been a change in bowel movements, further diagnostic work-up should be performed.
- Pain is the predominant symptom with anal fissure, thrombosed external hemorrhoids, and anorectal abscess but not prominently featured with internal hemorrhoids.

CURRENT THERAPY

- External thrombosed hemorrhoids are treated with evacuation in their early development (<72 hours) but in their subacute phase are treated with expectant, supportive management only.
- Most internal hemorrhoids can be treated with outpatient treatments including measures to normalize bowel movements and hemorrhoidal banding or injection therapy.
- Anal fissures are treated conservatively with medical therapy but require operative therapy in a minority of cases.
- Anal fistula repair techniques have variable success rates and can require multiple procedures to treat this condition effectively.

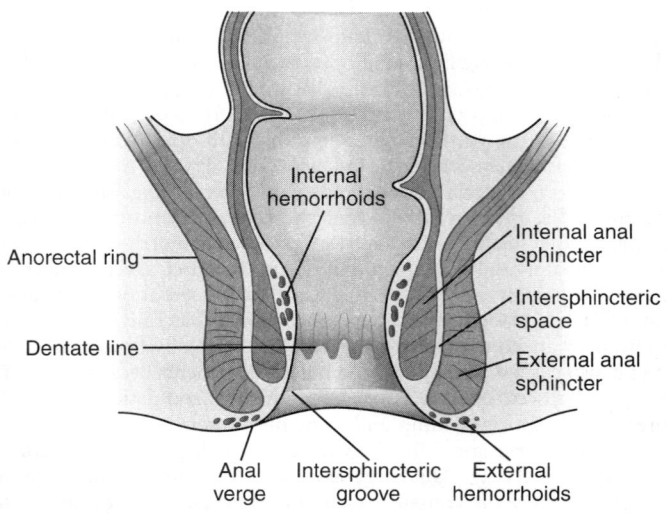

FIGURE 1. Anatomy of the anal canal.

TABLE 1 Staging of Hemorrhoidal Disease	
Grade	Description
I	Protrude only inside the lumen; seen only with the anoscope
II	Protrude during defecation; reduce spontaneously
III	Protrude during defecation; require manual reduction
IV	Permanently prolapsed and irreducible

Internal hemorrhoids, when symptomatic, most commonly occur with painless bleeding with bowel movements or prolapsing tissue. Patients often describe bright red blood in the toilet bowl or on the toilet paper. Other important symptoms include itching and leakage of mucus in the setting of tissue prolapse. Pain is rarely a prominent symptom except in the case of mixed hemorrhoid disease, when there is a thrombosed external component or in the case of stage IV incarcerated hemorrhoids.

The central principles for conservative treatment of internal hemorrhoids and for long-term prevention of worsening symptoms are normalization of bowel habits and avoidance of straining. Ideal bowel habits include having regular, soft, and formed stool resulting in minimal straining with elimination. An ideal diet should have high fiber content with fruits, vegetables, and whole grains along with sufficient fluid intake. A total of at least 30 g of fiber is generally recommended. For the majority of patients, this is most easily achieved with the addition of a fiber supplement. Other medical treatment of hemorrhoids includes local anesthetic topical ointments, which relieve symptoms but do not improve the hemorrhoids, and steroid ointments, which symptomatically improve itching and irritation but also thin and atrophy the overlying tissue if used regularly.

Internal hemorrhoids might benefit from further treatment in the setting of persistent prolapse or bleeding. Injection sclerotherapy works by shrinking and scarring the internal hemorrhoid by injecting a sclerosing agent (most commonly phenol in olive oil). Alternatively, infrared coagulation may be administered at the apex of the hemorrhoid. Both procedures have moderate effectiveness but are considered to be less effective than rubber-band ligation, which is widely used in the office setting with good results.

Rubber-band ligation requires the use of a rubber band ligator (either suction type or ligator with clamp) and is performed by placing a rubber band around excess hemorrhoidal tissue at the apex of the hemorrhoid. Rubber band ligation works by strangulating and cutting off blood flow to the hemorrhoid and by creating a scar that helps to fix tissue into place. The band must be placed well above the dentate line to prevent pain. Most patients experience a sensation of pressure with the procedure. Rarely, this procedure can cause significant pain, bleeding, or a vasovagal reaction. In general, only one or two band applications are performed in the same setting to prevent excessive pain or a vasovagal reaction.

Surgical treatment for hemorrhoidal disease should be considered in patients with stage III or IV internal hemorrhoids. Surgery is also a consideration in cases where office procedures and conservative treatment have been ineffective or when internal hemorrhoids are circumferential. In the United States, most hemorrhoidectomies continue to be performed using a closed technique, where the hemorrhoid is excised and the defect sutured closed. More recently, stapled hemorrhoidectomy (sometimes called hemorrhoidopexy) has been introduced. The stapled technique appears to work best in cases where patients have more circumferential disease and is performed by excising the rectal mucosa and disrupting blood flow, thereby shrinking hemorrhoidal tissue and lifting the prolapsing tissue into the anal canal. Although stapled hemorrhoidectomy has been demonstrated to be effective and on average less painful, it does not address any external hemorrhoidal component, costs significantly more money, and has been associated with rare but severe complications including pelvic sepsis.

External hemorrhoids are generally painless except in the case of thrombosis, and they normally appear as more prominent external perianal tissue or painless skin tags. Thrombosed external hemorrhoids, in contrast, are associated with severe pain and a prominent external lump but not with bleeding or fever. On examination, an external thrombosed hemorrhoid appears as a prominent, blue, and firm perianal lump. It is also not uncommon for multiple hemorrhoids to thrombose. Patients who present within 72 hours of the onset of symptoms benefit from an evacuation of the thrombosed clot using local anesthetic (Fig. 2). In contrast, patients who present after 72 hours should be treated expectantly with conservative supportive care, including sitz baths, normalization of bowel habits with fiber or stool softener, and pain management. The natural history in these cases is for the thrombosed clot to gradually be reabsorbed within several weeks.

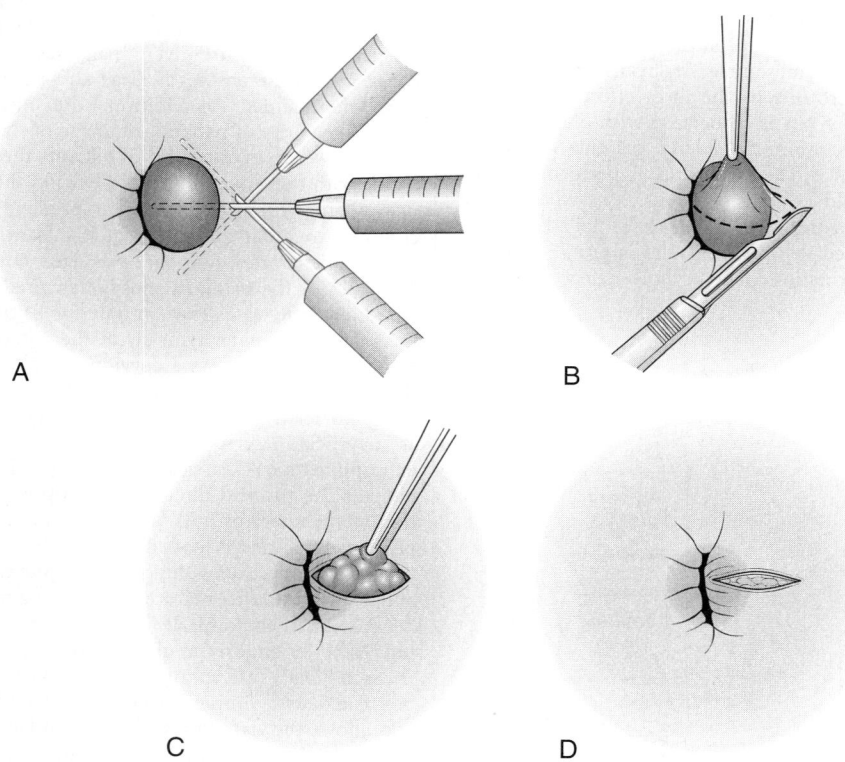

A

B

C

D

FIGURE 2. Incision and evacuation of an external thrombosed hemorrhoid. **A,** Local anesthetic is injected into the subcutaneous surrounding tissue and at the base of the hemorrhoid. **B,** Skin over the hemorrhoid is lifted and a small elliptical excision of skin is made. **C,** Thrombotic clot is evacuated. Additional dissection is sometimes needed in the subcutaneous tissue to extract the clot. **D,** Appearance of the evacuated area. Incision is left open and skin heals by secondary intention.

Anal Fissure

An anal fissure is a tear in the anoderm extending proximally into the anal canal and initially resulting from trauma. Fissures typically occur in the setting of constipation or frequent bowel movements. Although most superficial fissures resulting from trauma to the anorectal region will heal, some patients have prolonged symptoms, causing them to seek medical attention. The pathophysiology of anal fissures is still not completely understood but is related to local ischemia caused by hypertonia of the internal sphincter. The great majority of anal fissures are located at the posterior midline, and some also occur at the anterior midline (Fig. 3). Lateral fissures are rare and can be associated with anal malignancy, anorectal Crohn's disease, HIV, syphilis, or tuberculosis. In these cases, a biopsy should be strongly considered to confirm the diagnosis.

Patients who present with anal fissure most often have pain that is associated with bowel movements and that continues after defecation, bright red bleeding with bowel movements, and sometimes extra tissue or a lump at the anus. Physical examination demonstrates the fissure with retraction of the buttocks, as well as a sentinel tag overlying the fissure in more chronic cases. Chronic cases also demonstrate rolled edges around the fissure and exposed internal sphincter muscle fibers.

Conservative treatment for acute anal fissures includes normalization of bowel habits to minimize recurrent trauma to the anoderm and sitz baths for comfort. In cases where the fissure is chronic or unresponsive to conservative treatment, local therapy to relax the internal sphincter (i.e., a "chemical sphincterotomy") is prescribed. Classically, nitroglycerin ointment (0.2-0.4%)[1,6] has been used but is associated with significant headaches and lightheadedness. Diltiazem ointment (2%)[1,6] is a commonly used alternative without associated side effects. Either ointment can be applied topically two to three times per day for approximately 8 weeks. Reported healing rates are similar and range from 40% to 100%. An alternative agent that can be used for chemical sphincterotomy is botulinum toxin A (Botox),[1] which can be injected with a single application in the office or operating room into the internal sphincter. Although botulinum toxin A appears to be as effective as topical therapy, it is significantly more expensive and often is not reimbursed by insurance companies.

Surgical internal sphincterotomy is the most effective treatment for resolution of anal fissures but is associated with a risk of fecal incontinence, particularly in women, elderly patients, or others at risk for impaired continence. This procedure is performed in the outpatient setting and should be considered in cases where more-conservative dietary and medical treatments have failed. Internal sphincterotomy is performed by dividing the internal sphincter laterally, which prevents formation of a keyhole defect with stool

---

[1]Not FDA approved for this indication.
[6]May be compounded by pharmacists.

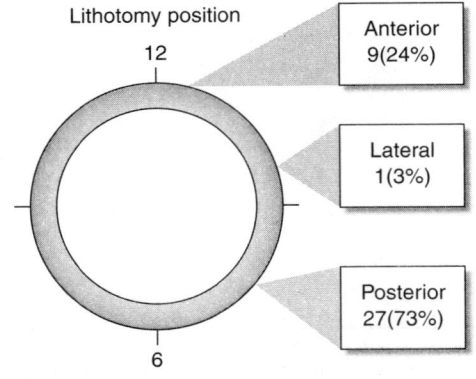

FIGURE 3. Distribution of the location of anal fissures.

---

leakage, which can occur with posterior division of the internal sphincter muscle. This procedure can be performed with an open approach (incising mucosa and exposing muscle) or a closed approach (using landmarks and then blindly dividing muscle) and can be full-thickness (entire internal sphincter) or tailored (partial thickness and length). Most surgeons perform a tailored sphincterotomy from the level of the top of the fissure distally, with partial division of the internal sphincter muscle to decrease the risk of postoperative fecal incontinence.

Anorectal Abscess and Fistula

Anorectal abscess is most commonly a self-limited process thought to result from obstruction and infection of anal glands located in the crypts along the dentate line. Clinicians should be aware that perianal Crohn's disease, trauma, and malignancy can cause anorectal abscess or fistula. Anorectal abscesses typically manifest with acute pain in the perianal area, acutely painful defecation, an indurated painful area, or fever. Most anorectal abscesses are superficial and manifest with pain and swelling at the anal verge or deeper within the ischiorectal fossa. These patients have obvious tenderness, induration, or fluctuance on physical examination. In contrast, patients with intersphincteric abscesses have severe pain but minimal findings on physical examination, except with palpation within the anal canal on digital rectal examination.

The mainstay of therapy is surgical drainage. Superficial abscesses can be drained using local anesthesia, but more-extensive infections typically require general anesthesia. When the abscess is fluctuant and appears easily accessible, an incision and drainage with local anesthetic can be considered in a motivated patient. Important principles in draining an anorectal abscess include keeping the patient comfortable, using aspiration with a large-bore (14- or 16-gauge) needle to help in the event of difficult localization, using a cruciate incision to ensure adequate drainage, and keeping the incision near to the anus to keep any potential fistula tract as short as possible. After the abscess is drained, the area is allowed to heal by secondary intention. Patients are given analgesics and encouraged to take sitz baths. When the abscess is large and extensive, sometimes drainage tubes, débridement, or additional dressing changes are required.

In a majority of patients, drainage of the anorectal abscess is sufficient. However, in one third of patients these do not heal and form a fistula with the external opening beyond the anal verge and the internal opening within an infected crypt gland at the dentate line. These continue to drain purulent material from the external opening and some patients continue to have signs and symptoms of infection. The tract of the fistula is most often predicted with Goodsall's rule. Goodsall's rule states that an anterior fistula follows a radial tract to the internal opening, typically at the anterior midline. In contrast, a posterior fistula follows a curvilinear path to the internal opening at the posterior midline. Anorectal fistulas are defined by their anatomy and path relative to the sphincter muscles and are classified typically as superficial, intersphincteric, transsphincteric, suprasphincteric, and extrasphincteric as classically described by Parks (Fig. 4). In most cases, patients can proceed directly to the operating room for initial definition of the anatomy and placement of a seton (a length of suture or other material that is looped through the fistula), which helps to allow drainage of infection within the tract, prevents recurrent infection, and allows the fistula to mature. Recurrent and complex fistulas may be better defined anatomically with the use of magnetic resonance imaging (MRI) or endorectal ultrasound.

Superficial, intersphincteric, or low transsphincteric fistulas can be treated with simple fistulotomy, which opens up the fistula tract and allows the tissue to heal by secondary intention. This, however, can result in impaired fecal continence, particularly if the fistula involves a significant amount of sphincter muscle. Initial treatment involves examination under anesthesia to define the anatomy and to place a draining seton.

Following this, a variety of methods can be used to repair the fistula. One classic technique is the use of a cutting seton, where a taut

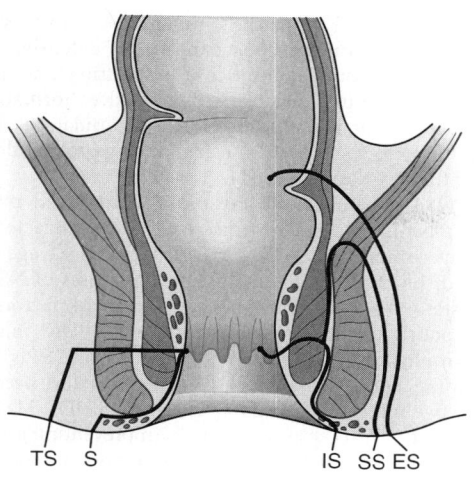

FIGURE 4. Classification of anal fistulas. ES = extrasphincteric; IS = intersphincteric; S = superficial; SS=suprasphincteric; TS = transsphincteric.

seton is progressively tightened over several weeks or months to form scar in place of the fistula and muscle. A cutting seton may be painful, and the scar is associated with impaired continence in some cases. Fibrin glue has been proposed as a method to repair a fistula but the long-term recurrence rate is high (>85%). Fistula plugs have also been proposed as a method to heal the fistula tract by repairing the internal opening and providing a scaffolding for fibrosis to occur. Although short- and medium-term success is reported to be approximately 30%, long-term results are not known.

Endorectal advancement flaps are the most well-established method to repair an anal fistula. With this technique, the internal orifice is closed and healthy tissue is brought down over the internal fistula opening to allow the area to heal. This procedure can be technically difficult, and failure most commonly results from ischemia of the flap, and repeat flap procedures are often not anatomically feasible owing to scar and fibrosis. Success rates have been reported between 50% and 80%.

A new procedure has been developed for transsphincteric and suprasphincteric fistulas called ligation of intersphincteric fistula tract (LIFT) procedure. This has been reported in a handful of centers as a method to treat complex fistulas and is performed by closing the internal opening and then ligating and removing the tract using an intersphincteric approach. Although long-term results are not known, initial reports are favorable for this technique in selected cases, and a multicenter trial is under way.

REFERENCES

Bleier JI, Moloo H, Goldberg SM. Ligation of the intersphincteric fistula tract: An effective new technique for complex fistulas. Dis Colon Rectum 2010;53(1):43–6.

Christoforidis D, Etzioni DA, Goldberg SM, et al. Treatment of complex anal fistulas with the collagen fistula plug. Dis Colon Rectum 2008;51 (10):1482–7.

Jayaraman S, Colquhoun PH, Malthaner RA. Stapled versus conventional surgery for hemorrhoids. Cochrane Database Syst Rev 2006;(4):CD005393.

Nelson R. Nonsurgical therapy for anal fissure. Cochrane Database Syst Rev 2006;(4):CD003431.

Nelson RL. Operative procedures for fissure in ano. Cochrane Database Syst Rev 2010;(1):CD002199.

Parks AG, Gordon PH, Hardcastle JD. A classification of fistula-in-ano. Br J Surg 1976;63(1):1–12.

Shanmugam V, Thaha MA, Rabindranath KS, et al. Rubber band ligation versus excisional haemorrhoidectomy for haemorrhoids. Cochrane Database Syst Rev 2005;(3):CD005034.

Wang JY, Garcia-Aguilar J, Sternberg JA, et al. Treatment of transsphincteric anal fistulas: Are fistula plugs an acceptable alternative? Dis Colon Rectum 2009;52(4):692–7.

Gastritis and Peptic Ulcer Disease

Method of
Robert C. Lowe, MD, and Michael Wolfe, MD

Peptic ulcer disease (PUD) affects 200,000 to 400,000 people each year, with estimated total annual costs of $3 billion to $4 billion. Although the incidence of PUD in the developed world has been steadily decreasing since the 1960s, it remains an important cause of morbidity worldwide. The discovery of *Helicobacter pylori* in the early 1980s and its association with peptic ulcer disease have significantly altered our approach to the management of this condition. Despite the importance of *H. pylori* infection, however, gastric acid continues to play a critical role in the pathogenesis of ulcers, and Schwarz's dictum, loosely translated as "no acid, no ulcer," remains a valid principle.

Epidemiology

Peptic ulcer disease has an overall point prevalence in the U.S. population of 1.8%, affecting men and women equally. One large study of male physicians reported a 10% lifetime risk of developing a duodenal ulcer. The most common risk factors for the development of an ulcer are infection with *H. pylori* and the use of nonsteroidal antiinflammatory drugs (NSAIDs). Cigarette smoking also plays a role in the development of ulcers, but other factors such as alcohol, stress, and spicy foods have not been proved to promote formation of ulcers. Although a family history of duodenal ulcer is reported in 20% to 50% of patients in published series, it is possible that intrafamilial transmission of *H. pylori* or a genetic predisposition to *H. pylori* infection is the cause of this apparent familial clustering. There does appear, however, to be a genetic predisposition to hypersecretion of gastric acid in some patients that contributes to the pathogenesis of duodenal ulcer. The incidence of PUD is also increased in patients with a number of comorbid conditions, including chronic obstructive pulmonary disease, kidney failure, and hepatic cirrhosis.

Pathophysiology

In the past, acid and pepsin had been considered the sole determinants of ulcer pathogenesis. Interestingly, patients with gastric ulcers tend to have normal or *reduced* levels of acid secretion, whereas patients with duodenal ulcers are, on the average, hypersecretors of acid. These patients secrete approximately 70% more acid during the day (meal-stimulated) and about 150% more acid at night (basal secretion), when compared with controls. Gastric acid secretion during the day is regulated mainly by the postprandial release of gastrin and subsequent inhibition of gastrin secretion after acidification of the gastric lumen. This inhibition is mediated by somatostatin-secreting D cells in the gastric antrum. Persons infected with *H. pylori* have been shown to have a diminished number of antral D cells, which decreases the magnitude of the somatostatin response during acidification of the gastric lumen. This decrease in somatostatin action blunts the negative feedback inhibition of gastrin release, resulting in higher postprandial gastrin levels and subsequent hypersecretion of acid.

Although the daytime rate of acid secretion in duodenal ulcer patients is increased, the presence of food in the stomach acts as a buffer that helps protect the gastric mucosa from acid-induced injury. At night, however, acid bathes the "bare" mucosa, and in patients with duodenal ulcers the increase in nocturnal acid secretion amplifies this effect. In addition, duodenal bicarbonate secretion is decreased in patients with duodenal ulcers, as well as in those infected with *H. pylori*, further increasing the mucosal exposure to acid. Vagal activity is the primary stimulus for acid secretion at night, explaining why surgical vagotomy provides an effective means of healing duodenal ulcers and preventing recurrence.

Factors other than acid and pepsin are involved in the pathogenesis of PUD because only 30% of patients with duodenal ulcers and a small number with gastric ulcers are hypersecretors of acid. Another important element is the balance between aggressive factors, which act to injure the gastroduodenal mucosa, and defensive factors that normally protect against noxious agents; when this balance is disrupted, ulcers can develop. The aggressive factors include primarily acid, as described, along with pepsin and bile salts. The mucosal defensive factors include mucus secretion, which traps H^+ ions; bicarbonate secreted by surface epithelial cells that titrate gastric acid; mucosal blood flow, which delivers oxygen and nutrients while removing metabolites; intercellular tight junctions that prevent transepithelial penetration of H^+ ions; and cell restitution and epithelial renewal, which permits the mucosa to repair itself following injury. These defensive properties appear to be mediated to a large extent by endogenous prostaglandins; when prostaglandin synthesis is diminished by the use of NSAIDs, the ability of the gastroduodenal mucosa to resist injury is significantly decreased, and even normal quantities of acid secretion may be sufficient to injure the mucosa and produce gastroduodenal ulcers.

Etiology

The vast majority of gastric and duodenal ulcers are caused by three factors: *H. pylori* infection, NSAID use, or acid hypersecretory states (e.g., Zollinger-Ellison syndrome).

HELICOBACTER PYLORI

As outlined earlier, chronic infection of the gastric antrum with *H. pylori* results in increased postprandial acid secretion caused by increased and prolonged gastrin release, occurring as a result of a marked decrease in the number of antral D cells, which decreases somatostatin activity and consequently attenuates its feedback inhibition of gastrin expression and secretion. As a result, persons infected with *H. pylori* appear to secrete more acid in response to gastrin compared to *H. pylori*–negative controls. Thus, duodenal ulcer patients who are infected with *H. pylori* not only release more gastrin but also are more responsive to the hormone.

It is important to recognize that *both* pH and *H. pylori* are integral to the pathogenesis of ulcers. It appears that unknown genetic factors can also lead to gastric acid hypersecretion, which can produce gastric metaplasia of the duodenum. Owing to a predilection for infection of gastric-type mucosa, the duodenum can be secondarily colonized with *H. pylori*, which can, in turn, incite an immune response leading to duodenitis and duodenal ulcer. Nonetheless, despite the clear epidemiologic association between *H. pylori* and PUD, there is mounting evidence that the actual percentage of ulcers associated with *H. pylori* might not be 90% to 95% but may be as low as 32% in nonreferral-based populations. Thus, peptic ulceration is clearly not caused solely by *H. pylori*, but rather involves the participation of several factors, most notably the erosive properties of acid and pepsin.

NONSTEROIDAL ANTIINFLAMMATORY DRUGS

The use of NSAIDS is clearly associated with peptic ulcer disease, and nearly 15% to 20% of persons who chronically use NSAIDs develop gastric or duodenal ulcers. It appears that NSAIDS damage the gastric mucosa more commonly than the duodenal mucosa; however, the mechanisms of injury are the same, and they involve the disruption of mucosal defensive factors by both topical and systemic effects. The topical effects of NSAIDs are seen primarily in the stomach and are due to a direct toxic insult to the gastric mucosal surface by these agents or their metabolites. The systemic effects are mediated by the inhibition of cyclooxygenase activity in the gastric epithelium and a subsequent decrease in the production of mucosal prostaglandins.

The diminished prostaglandin levels impair gastric mucus secretion, mucosal blood flow, ion transport, and other defensive properties inherent to the gastroduodenal mucosa, permitting acid and pepsin to induce mucosal injury that can result in ulcer formation. Thus, even enteric-coated or intravenous NSAID formulations, which are not directly toxic to the stomach, can induce gastroduodenal ulcers by virtue of their systemic effects.

Because NSAIDs are among the most widely used medications, numerous studies have been performed to identify risk factors for ulcer disease and its complications. Clear risk factors include age older than 65 years, prior history of PUD, the use of high doses of NSAIDs, and concurrent steroid use. Patients who have these risk factors, or those who would poorly tolerate any complications of PUD, might benefit from ulcer prophylaxis. Both proton pump inhibitors (PPIs) and misoprostol (Cytotec, a prostaglandin [PG]E_1 analogue) have been shown to provide effective ulcer prophylaxis in users of NSAIDs. Misoprostol is clearly superior to H_2-receptor antagonists in preventing gastric ulcers, and the two agents are equally effective in preventing duodenal ulcers. Famotidine (Pepcid)[1] in high doses (40 mg twice daily[3]) can also offer some degree of protection against gastric ulcers, but it does not appear to be as effective as misoprostol or PPIs and is quite costly at this dosage. Studies have shown that PPIs may be as effective as misoprostol in the prevention of gastroduodenal ulcers due to NSAIDs.

In addition to the use of prophylactic agents, several NSAIDs have been developed that might be less ulcerogenic than earlier preparations. Agents such as celecoxib (Celebrex) and rofecoxib (Vioxx)[2] preferentially or selectively inhibit inducible cyclooxygenase (COX) 2, which is responsible for inflammation, while having a minimal effect on constitutively expressed COX 1, the enzyme that plays a key role in preserving mucosal integrity. Unfortunately, the presence of cardiovascular side effects of these medications has limited their use, and their role in preventing NSAID ulcers remains to be determined.

HYPERSECRETORY STATES

Hypersecretory states such as Zollinger-Ellison syndrome, antral G-cell hyperplasia, and systemic mastocytosis are also associated with peptic ulcer disease. Zollinger-Ellison syndrome has been estimated to cause approximately 0.1% of all duodenal ulcers; thus, although it is uncommon, this syndrome needs to be considered in patients with PUD. Classically, these disorders are associated with multiple duodenal ulcers, ulcers in unusual locations (beyond the first portion of the duodenum), or ulcers that fail to respond to standard therapy. More commonly, however, they behave like typical ulcers associated with *H. pylori*, but they can have additional symptoms such as heartburn, diarrhea, and cutaneous flushing.

A significant number of patients with PUD are *H. pylori* negative, and the appropriate evaluation of such patients is at present unclear. Many of these patients are taking NSAIDs (57% to 75% in studies), whereas others have an underlying hypersecretory state or another illness associated with gastroduodenal ulceration, such as Crohn's disease. The remaining patients with truly idiopathic ulcers might have a disorder of gastric motility; delayed gastric emptying can predispose to gastric ulceration by increasing the contact time between acid and the mucosa, and overly rapid gastric emptying can have similar consequences for the duodenal mucosa. Most authorities recommend that patients with PUD who are *H. pylori* negative and who do not use NSAIDs should be evaluated with a fasting serum gastrin level (to identify a hypergastrinemic syndrome) and a biopsy of the ulcer to look for granulomatous infiltration or evidence of neoplasia (adenocarcinoma or lymphoma).

Clinical Features

The most common symptom of peptic ulcer disease is epigastric pain. The pain of duodenal ulcer is classically described as occurring 2 to 3 hours after a meal, improving with food or antacids, and at

---

[1]Not FDA approved for this indication.
[2]Not available in the United States.
[3]Exceeds dosage recommended by the manufacturer.

times awakening patients at night several hours after retiring. Gastric ulcer pain has been said to worsen with food intake, but the response to a meal cannot reliably distinguish between gastric and duodenal ulcers. Other symptoms of PUD include nausea and vomiting, which occurs more commonly in patients with prepyloric or pyloric channel ulcers. Unfortunately, the classic symptom complex occurs only in a minority of patients with ulcer disease, and it is difficult even to determine the percentage of patients who experience pain, because a significant number of patients with PUD lack any symptoms; in one study of patients presenting with a complication of ulcer disease (perforation or hemorrhage), 10% reported an absence of prior symptoms. The incidence of pain may be even lower with NSAID-induced ulcers, with studies reporting that in patients with hemorrhage from NSAID-induced gastroduodenal ulcers, as many as 50% to 60% had no antecedent symptoms. In patients who do present with epigastric pain, it appears that the relief of pain is not a reliable indicator of a successful response to therapy, because some patients have continued pain after ulcer healing, and others report relief of their symptoms despite the presence of a persistent ulcer.

The physical examination in patients with uncomplicated ulcer disease is typically unrevealing, with most patients having mild epigastric tenderness and no additional findings. When complications supervene, however, the range of clinical presentations includes an acute abdomen following perforation, hematemesis and melena after hemorrhage, and nausea and vomiting from gastric outlet obstruction.

Diagnosis

Establishing the diagnosis of PUD solely on the basis of history and physical examination is usually difficult and uncertain. Given the nonspecific symptoms and signs of peptic ulcer disease, the differential diagnosis is broad and includes gastroesophageal reflux disease, gastric cancer, gastroduodenitis, cholecystitis, biliary tract disease, pancreatic cancer, pancreatitis (acute or chronic), intestinal ischemia, pain associated with ischemic heart disease, and nonulcer dyspepsia. The diagnosis of PUD is typically made by endoscopy, although radiologic upper gastrointestinal (GI) series may be used when endoscopy is not readily available. These two modalities tend to correlate well, though reported sensitivities and specificities depend largely on the expertise of the examiners and might not be applicable to all centers. In the *best* hands, using double contrast fluoroscopic technique, upper endoscopy and upper GI series correlate 80% to 90% of the time in diagnosing duodenal ulcers. However, an upper GI series is not as effective in detecting small ulcers (<0.5 cm) and does not allow biopsy. Therefore, if endoscopic evaluation is available, it is clearly preferred for patients in whom peptic ulcer disease is suspected.

CURRENT DIAGNOSIS

- The most common causes of ulcer disease are *Helicobacter pylori* infection and use of nonsteroidal antiinflammatory drugs (NSAIDs).
- Hypersecretory states (e.g., Zollinger-Ellison syndrome) should be considered if a patient has multiple duodenal ulcers or if peptic ulcer disease is accompanied by severe gastroesophageal reflux symptoms or chronic diarrhea.
- Serologic testing for *H. pylori* is adequate for making the diagnosis of infection, but the most accurate tests include urea breath testing, stool antigen testing, or examination of endoscopic biopsy specimens. These tests are recommended for the confirmation of *H. pylori* eradication in patients with complicated peptic ulcer disease.

CURRENT THERAPY

- The treatment of *Helicobacter pylori* consists of combined antibiotic and antisecretory therapy; the most common regimen consists of a proton-pump inhibitor, amoxicillin (Amoxil), and clarithromycin (Biaxin), taken twice daily for 14 days.
- The treatment of nonsteroidal antiinflammatory drug (NSAID)-associated ulcers consists of antisecretory therapy and discontinuation of the NSAID. Patients who need to continue NSAIDs should be maintained on antisecretory therapy to decrease the risk of ulcer recurrence.
- Nonulcer dyspepsia is a common cause of ulcer-like symptoms. Empiric therapy may be considered if the patient lacks warning signs of structural disease, which include age older than 50 years, dysphagia, anorexia or weight loss, overt gastrointestinal bleeding, guaiac-positive stools, or anemia. The presence of any of these signs should prompt an early endoscopic examination.
- For patients with dyspeptic symptoms and no warning signs, current recommendations advocate testing for *H. pylori* and treating if the test is positive. If symptoms persist after treatment, then further work-up with endoscopy is recommended. Alternatively, an empiric trial of antisecretory therapy may be administered, and serologic testing may be reserved for patients whose symptoms do not improve.

Laboratory tests are generally of little help in evaluating patients with uncomplicated peptic ulcer disease. At times, a fasting serum gastrin level to evaluate for the presence of Zollinger-Ellison syndrome may be of use in patients with duodenal ulcer in whom a reasonable index of suspicion exists. Measurement of gastric acid secretion is generally helpful only in patients with elevated serum gastrin levels. In these patients, a gastric pH measurement at the time of endoscopy is useful in distinguishing atrophic gastritis or other causes of decreased acid secretion from Zollinger-Ellison syndrome. A pH greater than 2.5 in the absence of antisecretory medication (off H_2-antagonists for 24 hours or PPIs for 10-14 days) virtually excludes the diagnosis of Zollinger-Ellison syndrome.

Laboratory tests play an important role is the diagnosis of *H. pylori* infection. The serologic determination of anti–*H. pylori* IgG antibodies in peripheral blood is more than 90% sensitive and more than 90% specific for *H. pylori* infection. The use of ^{13}C and ^{14}C urea breath tests also provide an excellent means for establishing the presence of *H. pylori* infection and is the most sensitive method for determining successful eradication of the organism after antibiotic therapy.

In the urea breath tests, the patient ingests urea labeled with ^{13}C or ^{14}C. If *H. pylori* is present, bacterial urease converts the urea into ammonia and radiolabeled CO_2, which is absorbed into the bloodstream and exhaled. Breath samples are collected at intervals after urea ingestion and are analyzed using either mass spectroscopy (^{13}C) or a liquid scintillation counter (^{14}C). Urea breath testing is 95% sensitive and 98% specific for *H. pylori* infection. The diagnostic accuracy and the noninvasive nature of the test make it a superior means of documenting *H. pylori* and confirming eradication of the organism at 4 to 6 weeks after the cessation of treatment.

For patients undergoing upper endoscopy, testing for *H. pylori* can be performed on gastric biopsy specimens. Direct histologic examination of biopsy specimens represents a sensitive and specific means of diagnosing *H. pylori* infection and remains the gold standard. The rapid urease test provides a faster and less expensive way of establishing the presence of *H. pylori* infection from a biopsy specimen. These tests use a gel matrix impregnated with urea and a pH-sensitive color indicator. Gastric biopsies are placed into the gel, and in the presence of *H. pylori*–associated urease, ammonia is generated from urea and the gel turns red as the pH becomes increasingly alkaline. Rapid urease testing is 92% sensitive when read at 3 hours and 98% sensitive at 24 hours, with 100% specificity.

Treatment

The treatment of peptic ulcer disease has changed significantly since the discovery that ulcer recurrence rates decrease dramatically after eradication of *H. pylori* infection, compared with annual recurrence rates of 50% to 80% when antisecretory therapy alone is used. Thus, determining whether a patient with PUD is infected with *H. pylori* is essential for the appropriate management of ulcer disease. In patients who are not infected with *H. pylori*, an alternative etiology must be sought, such as NSAID use, hypersecretory states, or one of the other less-common causes of ulcer disease.

NONMEDICAL THERAPY

Historically, modification of diet was the mainstay of treatment for PUD. Bland diets rich in milk were advocated along with recommendations to eat smaller, more frequent meals in order to decrease gastric distention and subsequent acid secretion. These treatments were never evaluated in controlled clinical trials, and it was later discovered that milk itself was a potent stimulus of gastric acid secretion. Modification of diet is thus no longer advised apart from counseling patients to avoid any specific foods that precipitate dyspepsia. There are, however, a few general measures recommended in the treatment of ulcer disease, including the cessation of smoking and alcohol and, if possible, the discontinuation of NSAID use.

MEDICAL THERAPY

Antacids

Antacids are effective in relieving the symptoms of peptic ulcer disease, and a 1977 controlled, double-blind study demonstrated that antacids were superior to placebo in healing duodenal ulcers. Later studies evaluated the dosage and dose intervals of antacids and found that as little as a single antacid tablet before meals or at bedtime was effective in healing ulcers with a minimum of side effects. The toxicity of antacids is generally low. The predominant side effect is diarrhea with preparations that contain magnesium hydroxide.

H$_2$-Receptor Antagonists

The first clinically useful selective type 2 histamine receptor antagonist, cimetidine (Tagamet) was introduced in the 1970s and revolutionized the treatment of peptic ulcer. Later formulations (ranitidine [Zantac], famotidine, and nizatidine [Axid]) retained the basic structure of cimetidine with minor modifications affecting potency, bioavailability, and side-effect profile. All the H$_2$-receptor antagonists (H$_2$RAs) are equally effective in healing duodenal ulcers, with 90% to 95% healing rates achieved after 8 weeks of therapy. A single evening dose of H$_2$RA has replaced the previous twice-daily dosing regimen, which is consistent with the observation that ulcer healing is proportional to the effectiveness of *nocturnal* acid inhibition. Given the equivalent efficacy and improved compliance with the single-dose regimen, it has become the preferred dosing scheme for H$_2$RAs in the treatment of PUD.

Although H$_2$RAs are generally well tolerated, they can cause mild central nervous system (CNS) effects, including drowsiness, agitation, and headache by virtue of their ability to cross the blood-brain barrier and react with CNS histamine receptors. Cimetidine and ranitidine both interact with the hepatic cytochrome P-450 mixed oxidase system (ranitidine has fivefold to tenfold less avidity than

cimetidine), and can thereby alter the metabolism of a number of different drugs. However, only patients receiving warfarin (Coumadin), theophylline (Uniphyl), or phenytoin (Dilantin) are at risk for developing a clinically significant alteration in drug levels. Because monitoring of drug levels and coagulation parameters is routine in these patients, this interaction rarely has clinical relevance. Other reported side effects of H$_2$RAs include gynecomastia (cimetidine only) and rarely thrombocytopenia.

Sucralfate

Sucralfate ([Carafate], an aluminum salt of sucrose octasulfate) has been used since the 1980s to treat peptic ulcer disease and demonstrates healing rates similar to those of antacids and H$_2$RAs. Sucralfate does not inhibit gastric acid secretion, but rather it is thought to protect the gastroduodenal mucosa via adhesion to the ulcer base, adsorption of bile acids, inactivation of pepsin, and stimulation of bicarbonate and mucus secretion. It may be used as primary therapy for PUD (at a dose of 1 g orally four times daily), but sucralfate is also effective in preventing duodenal ulcer relapse (at a dose of 1 g twice daily). Sucralfate is generally well tolerated and has an excellent safety profile because less than 5% of a single dose is absorbed into the circulation. In patients with kidney disease, however, sucralfate must be used with caution, because even this small systemic dose can (uncommonly) lead to aluminum toxicity.

Prostaglandin Analogues

Analogues of prostaglandins have been used in the treatment of PUD. Misoprostol, a PGE$_1$ analogue, is the only prostaglandin available in the United States. These agents protect the gastroduodenal mucosa by promoting the secretion of bicarbonate and mucus and by augmenting mucosal blood flow and cell restitution in the gastric mucosa. At higher dosages, these drugs also exhibit an antisecretory effect. These agents are effective in healing peptic ulcers[1] and in preventing ulcer recurrence,[1] but only when administered at antisecretory doses. Thus, the relative contributions of mucosal protection and acid inhibition are difficult to distinguish clinically. Prostaglandin analogues require frequent dosing (for misoprostol, 200 µg two to four times daily) and are associated with significantly more side effects than H$_2$RAs. For this reason, they are generally not used in the treatment of PUD. The primary indication for these agents at present is to prevent NSAID-induced gastroduodenal ulceration.

Diarrhea, the most commonly reported side effect of these agents, occurs in up to 20% to 30% of patients. The diarrhea is dose-dependent and is due to an increase in cyclic adenosine monophosphate (cAMP) levels in intestinal mucosal cells, inducing a secretory diarrhea. Prostaglandin analogues also possess abortifacient properties and should not be used during pregnancy or in women of childbearing age.

Proton Pump Inhibitors

The PPIs are the most potent inhibitors of gastric acid secretion available. These agents are substituted benzimidazoles that inhibit the activity of H$^+$,K$^+$-ATPase, the acid pump located on the apical surface of gastric parietal cells. Administered as prodrugs with a pKa of approximately 4.0, they become concentrated in the secretory canaliculus of the *activated* parietal cell, where the local pH is less than 1.0. In this acidic environment, these agents are protonated to form thiophilic sulfenamides, which then bind covalently with cysteine residues within H$^+$,K$^+$-ATPase. PPIs are most effective after a prolonged fast and when the parietal cell is subsequently stimulated to secrete acid in response to a meal. These drugs thus should *only* be taken before a meal, optimally breakfast, and should *not* be used

---

[1]Not FDA approved for this indication.

TABLE 1 Healing Rates with Pharmacologic Treatments of Peptic Ulcer

Medication	Dose	Healing Rate
Antacids	200 mEq of neutralizing capacity	70%-80% at 4 wk
Sucralfate (Carafate)	4 g qd (1 g qid)	70%-80% at 4 wk
H₂-receptor antagonists		
Famotidine (Pepcid)	40 mg qd	
Ranitidine (Zantac)	300 mg qd	70%-80% at 4 w,
Nizatidine (Axid)	300 mg qd	87%-94% at 8 w,
Cimetidine (Tagamet)	800-1200 mg qd	
Proton Pump Inhibitor		
Omeprazole (Prilosec)	20 mg qd	80%-100% at 4 wk

in conjunction with H₂RAs or other antisecretory agents, including prostaglandins. They are extremely potent inhibitors of acid secretion, and in addition to their use in PUD, they are the agent of choice for the treatment of Zollinger-Ellison syndrome. Their safety profile is similar to that of H₂RAs, but PPIs heal peptic ulcers more rapidly than the H₂RAs do. In one study, lansoprazole (Prevacid) at a dose of 30 mg daily healed 74% of duodenal ulcers after 2 weeks compared with 51% of with ranitidine; at 4 weeks, however, healing rates were comparable (95% and 89%, respectively). PPIs are best administered when parietal cells are stimulated (i.e., with meals, optimally before breakfast).

In summary, all peptic ulcers eventually heal, but antisecretory therapy accelerates the healing process and allows more rapid relief of symptoms. Antacids, sucralfate, H₂RAs, PGE analogues, and PPIs have similar healing rates when given for at least 4 weeks (Table 1). The PPIs, however, appear to heal ulcers more rapidly than the others. Moreover, because they are commonly used in *H. pylori* eradication regimens and because they heal gastroduodenal ulcers in patients continuing NSAIDs, PPIs have become the mainstay of therapy for healing peptic ulcers.

TREATMENT OF *H. PYLORI* INFECTION

The basic issues germane to patient care are the determination of which patients should be treated for *H. pylori* infection and the choice of an effective therapeutic regimen out of the many available to the practicing physician.

It is clear that patients with a duodenal ulcer should be treated for *H. pylori*, because recurrence of duodenal ulcers in patients infected with *H. pylori* decreases significantly after the organism is eradicated. This decrease is evident in patients with active ulcers and in those with a past history of duodenal ulcer who remain *H. pylori* positive. Patients with gastric ulcer and *H. pylori* infection should also be treated, even when use of NSAIDs is thought to be a contributing factor in the pathogenesis of the ulcer, because *H. pylori* infection remains a risk factor for ulcer recurrence in these patients. The diagnosis of a gastric MALT (mucosa-associated lymphoid tissue) lymphoma in an *H. pylori*-infected patient is also an indication for treatment, because eradication of the infection can promote regression of the malignant lesion.

H. pylori infection has been associated with an increased incidence of gastric adenocarcinoma, but population screening and eradication

---

[1]Not FDA approved for this indication.

of infection as a preventive strategy is currently not recommended. Eradication of infection in patients with a strong family history of gastric cancer, however, would appear to be reasonable. Patients with type B antral gastritis and *H. pylori* infection might also benefit from treatment, but this issue is as yet unresolved. The treatment of *H. pylori* infection in patients with nonulcer dyspepsia is the subject of controversy and is discussed in detail later.

Once the decision to treat *H. pylori* infection is made, a regimen should be chosen that meets two key criteria: It must be effective in eradicating the organism, and it must be simple enough or inexpensive enough to ensure the patient's compliance. The first therapies against *H. pylori* combined bismuth subsalicylate (Pepto-Bismol)[1] with two antimicrobial agents, tetracycline (Sumycin)[1] and metronidazole (Flagyl).[1] In clinical trials, eradication rates of 77% to 89% were reported. This therapy was inexpensive, but it has a complex dosing regimen that decreases compliance outside the setting of clinical studies. Currently, the rising rate of metronidazole resistance among strains of *H. pylori* further decreases the efficacy of this regimen, and the need for concurrent antisecretory therapy during treatment of active ulcer disease increases both its cost and complexity.

Two-drug therapies consisting of a proton pump inhibitor and an antibiotic have the advantage of simplicity and resulting high rates of compliance. Unfortunately, the combination of amoxicillin (Amoxil)

---

[1]Not FDA approved for this indication.

TABLE 2 FDA-Approved *Helicobacter pylori* Eradication Regimens

H₂ Receptor Antagonist Therapy		Antibiotic	
Drug	Dosage	Drug	Dosage
Omeprazole (Prilosec)	20 mg PO bid	Clarithromycin (Biaxin) *or*	500 mg PO bid × 10-14 d
		Metronidazole (Flagyl)[1] *plus*	500 mg PO bid × 10-14 d
		Amoxicillin (Amoxil)	1 g PO bid
Lansoprazole (Prevacid)	30 mg PO bid	Clarithromycin *or*	500 mg PO bid × 10-14 d
		Metronidazole[1] *plus*	500 mg PO bid × 10-14 d
		Amoxicillin (Amoxil)	1 g PO bid
Esomeprazole (Nexium)	40 mg PO bid	Clarithromycin *plus*	500 mg PO bid × 10 d
		Amoxicillin (Amoxil)	1 g PO bid
Rabeprazole (Aciphex)	20 mg PO bid	Clarithromycin *plus*	500 mg PO bid × 7 d
		Amoxicillin (Amoxil)	1 g PO bid
Helidac			
Bismuth subsalicylate	525 mg PO qid	Metronidazole *plus*	250 mg PO qid × 14 d
		Tetracycline	500 mg PO qid × 4 wk

[1]Not FDA approved for this indication.

and omeprazole (Prilosec) has an eradication rate of only 30% to 50%, and the combination of clarithromycin (Biaxin) and omeprazole has eradication rates in U.S. studies of only 70% to 74%. These low rates of successful clearance of *H. pylori* make these regimens suboptimal for the treatment of *H. pylori*–associated PUD.

At present, three-drug regimens consisting of clarithromycin, a PPI, and either metronidazole[1] or amoxicillin are the most commonly used therapies for *H. pylori*. The three agents are dosed twice daily, which improves compliance. The duration of treatment has a significant effect on eradication rates. Although European studies reported clearance rates of 90% to 95% using 7-day regimens, clinical trials in the United States have shown rates less than 90% for 7-day regimens, whereas clearance with 14-day regimens has been as high as 92%, even though compliance decreases with increasing duration of therapy. Currently, the FDA has approved several regimens for treatment of *H. pylori*; these are provided in Table 2. In practice, any PPI may be used as part of a triple-therapy regimen, and metronidazole 500 mg orally twice daily may be used in place of amoxicillin, although eradication rates are lower in areas where metronidazole-resistant *H. pylori* is prevalent.

ROLE OF MAINTENANCE THERAPY

The practice of prolonging antisecretory therapy following ulcer healing was developed from observations regarding the natural history of peptic ulcer disease. Studies published during both the pre- and postendoscopy eras reported that up to 82% of patients with duodenal ulcers had persistent symptoms after the initial diagnosis. Bardhan and colleagues found that only 26% of patients with an untreated duodenal ulcer were free of symptoms at 1 year after diagnosis. The natural history of peptic ulcer disease has, however, changed with the recognition that the eradication of *H. pylori* infection in duodenal ulcer patients greatly diminishes the relapse rate. Graham and colleagues demonstrated that after a median follow-up of 38 weeks, only 12% of patients who underwent *H. pylori* eradication relapsed, compared with 95% of patients who received H₂RAs alone. Other studies report similar relapse rates after *H. pylori* therapy, so that the maxim "once an ulcer, always an ulcer" no longer holds true.

The role of maintenance antisecretory therapy has evolved in recent years. Before prescribing long-term therapy, attention must be paid to the elimination of the most important risk factors for ulcer recurrence: *H. pylori* infection and continued NSAID use. The cost-effectiveness of *H. pylori* eradication compared to maintenance antisecretory therapy has been clearly demonstrated, because antisecretory medications can cost up to $1200 per year. The American College of Gastroenterology currently recommends that only high-risk ulcer patients receive maintenance antisecretory therapy. This group includes patients with a history of ulcer complications, those who suffer frequent recurrences, those who are *H. pylori* negative, and those who fail to clear *H. pylori* infection despite appropriate therapy. Some experts, however, recommend that even patients who have had a complication of peptic ulcer disease do not require maintenance therapy provided *H. pylori* infection is cured. Although maintenance therapy plays a role in these situations, the most important principles in treating PUD are to diagnose and treat *H. pylori* infection and to discontinue or, if possible, minimize the use of NSAIDs.

Complications

Although the incidence of PUD is decreasing, there has been no change in the incidence of the major complications of ulcer disease: hemorrhage, perforation, and obstruction.

---

[1]Not FDA approved for this indication.

HEMORRHAGE

Upper GI bleeding is the most common complication of PUD. Peptic ulcer bleeding typically occurs with melena or hematemesis, though a very brisk hemorrhage can occur with bright red rectal bleeding along with signs of acute hypovolemia. Patients with ulcer bleeding might or might not have a prior history of ulcer pain. Asymptomatic hemorrhage is particularly common in patients with NSAID-induced ulcers, with studies reporting no antecedent symptoms in 50% to 60% of patients presenting with acute hemorrhage.

The detailed management of ulcer bleeding is beyond the scope of this chapter, but basic recommendations can be made. After appropriate resuscitation with fluid or blood products (or both), an upper endoscopy is indicated to determine the etiology of bleeding and possibly to perform therapeutic maneuvers aimed at controlling active bleeding or preventing recurrent hemorrhage. Before endoscopic evaluation, the patient should be given an intravenous proton pump inhibitor by continuous infusion, which has been shown to improve outcomes in acute ulcer bleeding. Once the hemorrhage has been controlled and the source of the bleeding is determined to be a peptic ulcer, oral antisecretory therapy should be started to promote ulcer healing, and the etiology of the ulcer (i.e., *H. pylori* or NSAIDs) should be investigated and treated as detailed earlier. Because of the low prevalence of cancer in patients with duodenal ulcers, repeat endoscopic evaluation is not recommended. Gastric ulcers, however, carry a more significant risk of malignancy, and it is recommended that ulcer healing be confirmed with repeat endoscopy after 8 to 12 weeks of treatment. Unhealed ulcers should be biopsied extensively, and brush cytology should be obtained to rule out malignancy.

PERFORATION

Perforation of a gastric or duodenal ulcer occurs most often in the fifth or sixth decade of life, with an approximate incidence of 7 to 10 cases per 100,000 person-years. The use of NSAIDs in particular is associated with a high risk of complications from PUD (hemorrhage and perforation), and although the use of steroids alone is not considered a risk factor for peptic ulcer, the combined use of systemic steroids and NSAIDS carries a significant risk of ulcer complications. Gastric or duodenal ulcer perforation most commonly manifests with severe abdominal pain, which is sudden in onset and most severe in the epigastrium and commonly radiates to the back. With time the pain can become more diffuse and radiate to the lower quadrants or be referred to the shoulders owing to diaphragmatic irritation. Nausea and vomiting can occur, and 10% to 15% of patients present with concomitant gastrointestinal hemorrhage. A history of prior peptic ulcer disease is reported in 60% to 75% of patients.

On examination, patients might have a low-grade fever, and tachycardia and tachypnea are common. The abdomen is usually diffusely tender, with signs of peritonitis (guarding, rebound tenderness, or rigidity). Laboratory examination often reveals a mild leukocytosis. Serum amylase is usually normal, but it is elevated to greater than 200 Somogyi units in up to 15% of patients, indicating possible pancreatic penetration. Radiographs of the chest and abdomen reveal free air under the diaphragm in 70% of cases. It is thus recommended that patients remain upright or in the decubitus position for 10 to 15 minutes before these films are obtained to allow intraperitoneal air to percolate to the highest point. In cases where the diagnosis is unclear, an upper GI series using *water-soluble contrast material* may be helpful.

The treatment of a perforated peptic ulcer is surgical in nearly 95% of cases, and consultation with an experienced surgeon is essential, even if medical management is contemplated. Medical therapy may be considered in patients who meet the following criteria: long-standing perforation (>24 hours), evidence of a contained perforation on upper GI contrast study, the absence of peritoneal signs, and the presence of comorbid illness that significantly increases the risk of operative repair. These criteria apply only to perforated *duodenal* ulcers, whereas gastric ulcer perforation should always be managed surgically. Medical management consists of nasogastric suction, intravenous hydration, and the continuous intravenous infusion of a proton pump inhibitor.

OBSTRUCTION

Gastric outlet obstruction is a relatively more common complication of peptic ulcer disease, with an incidence in several studies of 6% to 21.5%. The incidence of ulcer-induced gastric outlet obstruction has decreased significantly since the introduction of effective antisecretory therapy, and gastric carcinoma has surpassed PUD as the leading cause of this syndrome. Patients with gastric outlet obstruction form PUD typically have a long history of peptic ulcer pain. The obstruction is marked by the onset of nausea and vomiting, which is present in roughly 90% of cases. Additional symptoms include early satiety, bloating, and a sense of fullness in the epigastrium. Patients report progressive weight loss if the obstruction develops slowly, but an acute presentation with dehydration and electrolyte disturbances can occur. Physical examination is remarkable for signs of weight loss and the presence of a "succussion splash" heard with the stethoscope over the epigastrium while the abdomen is shaken from side to side. This sign is present in 25% to 49% of patients with outlet obstruction from any cause. The diagnosis can be confirmed with *barium* contrast radiography, which reveals a markedly dilated stomach and delayed emptying of contrast from the stomach. Endoscopy is recommended in order to visualize the gastric outlet and biopsy the obstructed region to look for malignancy.

Initial treatment of gastric outlet obstruction consists of nasogastric suction, intravenous hydration, antisecretory therapy, and, depending on the nutritional status of the patient, hyperalimentation. Once a diagnosis of ulcer-induced benign obstruction is established, a treatment plan should be formulated in consultation with both a gastroenterologist and a gastrointestinal surgeon. Medical therapy alone often relieves edema-related obstruction in the short term, though recurrence is common. More-definitive therapy can be performed via endoscopic dilation of the stenotic region or though a surgical drainage procedure.

Gastritis

Gastritis refers to inflammation of the gastric mucosa; it is a nonspecific lesion that is observed in a number of unrelated disorders. Most episodes of gastritis are probably caused by *H. pylori* infection. Acute infection with *H. pylori* causes gastric mucosal inflammation that is often asymptomatic, though it can at times be associated with mild epigastric discomfort. Persistent infection induces a chronic inflammatory state that had in the past been termed *type B gastritis*. This inflammatory process is usually confined to the antrum, but with time it can extend proximally to involve the body and fundus of the stomach as well. *H. pylori* gastritis can also progress to gastric atrophy, which, in a minority of patients, is associated with an increased risk of gastric adenocarcinoma.

Acute gastritis can also be caused by other infectious agents, with a majority of such infections occurring in immunocompromised hosts. Among patients with HIV disease, gastritis due to herpes simplex or cytomegalovirus infection has been recognized, as has gastritis caused by mycobacterial infections and syphilis. In immunocompetent hosts, bacterial gastritis is uncommon, but it can be life-threatening and associated with systemic sepsis. Predominant organisms in these cases include streptococcal and staphylococcal species, as well as enteric gram-negative rods. In all such cases, treatment consists of appropriate intravenous antimicrobial therapy, with gastric resection reserved for the most severe cases of bacterial gastritis.

Noninfectious gastritis comprises the majority of chronic gastritis not attributable to *H. pylori*. The classic type A gastritis is characterized by involvement of the fundus and body, in contrast to the antral predominance of the type B lesion. Type A gastritis is considered to be autoimmune in origin, because it is often associated with circulating antibodies to parietal cells or intrinsic factor and, in many cases, with frank pernicious anemia. This form of gastritis usually progresses to mucosal atrophy, resulting in decreased acid secretion and subsequent hypergastrinemia. Atrophic changes predispose to gastric carcinoma and possibly other gastrointestinal malignancies, and persistent high gastrin levels are associated with the development of carcinoid tumors.

Other types of chronic gastritis include the eosinophilic and lymphocytic gastritis, as well as granulomatous gastritis from fungal, mycobacterial, or treponemal infection and, uncommonly, from gastric Crohn's disease or sarcoidosis.

Nonulcer Dyspepsia

The term *dyspepsia* refers to a group of symptoms that includes upper abdominal pain or discomfort, often accompanied by bloating, abdominal distention, nausea, or early satiety. Dyspepsia, despite its vague definition, is a common problem, with a 14% to 26% prevalence reported in recent studies. Up to 5% of office visits to primary care physicians are for dyspeptic symptoms. The differential diagnosis of dyspepsia is similar to that of peptic ulcer disease. Several medications can induce dyspepsia, including NSAIDs, antibiotics (most commonly macrolides and metronidazole), estrogens, narcotics, and digoxin (Lanoxin). Systemic illnesses can manifest with dyspepsia, including hyperthyroidism, hyperparathyroidism, and several of the collagen-vascular diseases.

Functional or *nonulcer* dyspepsia refers to dyspeptic symptoms without a definable organic cause. This condition applies to 40% to 60% of cases of dyspepsia in medical practice. The pathogenesis of this disorder is incompletely understood, but it appears to involve heightened visceral sensitivity to painful stimuli, abnormal gastric and duodenal motility, and psychological factors. The role of *H. pylori* infection in functional dyspepsia is controversial, but well-designed studies show no clear relationship between *H. pylori* infection and the presence of dyspeptic symptoms. Moreover, *H. pylori* eradication provides little, if any, benefit in alleviating dyspepsia, especially in the long term.

DIAGNOSIS

The diagnostic evaluation of dyspepsia should commence with a thorough history and physical examination. The clinician should be cognizant of the alarm symptoms and signs that would necessitate an early endoscopic examination. These include age older than 50 years, weight loss, dysphagia, significant vomiting, a palpable epigastric mass, or guaiac-positive stools. The presence of any of these signs, or the finding of iron deficiency anemia on laboratory examination, is associated with a greater risk of structural gastrointestinal disease (malignancy, PUD) and warrants prompt endoscopy.

Several strategies have been proposed for evaluating dyspepsia in patients younger than 50 years and without alarm symptoms. A recent clinical guideline proposed a practice algorithm in which patients with dyspepsia first undergo serologic testing for *H. pylori* infection. Patients with documented infection receive empiric treatment; if symptoms do not resolve within 4 to 8 weeks, endoscopy is then performed. In patients who are initially *H. pylori* negative, an empiric trial of an H_2RA or PPI for 4 to 8 weeks is recommended; endoscopy is reserved for patients who fail to improve or who relapse after completion of therapy. This strategy is aimed at treating peptic ulcer disease, the cause of dyspepsia in 15% to 20% of patients, while minimizing invasive testing. However, most of the

APPROACH TO ULCER-LIKE DYSPEPSIA

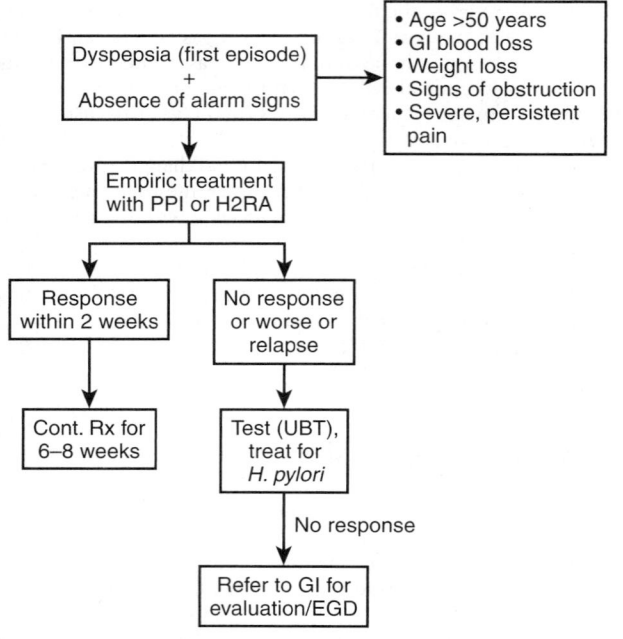

FIGURE 1. Approach to ulcer-like dyspepsia.

benefit that was demonstrated in a meta-analysis was derived from one study that employed a controversial definition of nonulcer dyspepsia. With the inclusion of that one study, 11 patients (number needed to treat) would have to be successfully treated for one to derive benefit in the form of symptom relief. If the one study were removed from consideration, the number needed to treat would be nearly 20 patients for one to enjoy symptom relief. Interestingly, 1 month after the position paper was published, a large-scale study that examined the relief of symptoms after 10 years reported no benefit.

In contrast, the eradication of *H. pylori* in patients with ulcer-like, rather than motility-like, dyspepsia has proven beneficial. Moreover, the widespread use of antibiotics in dyspeptic patients will likely increase the development of antibiotic-resistant strains of *H. pylori*, as well as other bacteria. In addition, as the prevalence of *H. pylori* decreases, this infection will be responsible for fewer peptic ulcers, further decreasing the effectiveness of empiric therapy. An alternative approach to dyspepsia is outlined in Figure 1. An empiric trial of PPI or H$_2$RA therapy may be given initially; if symptoms improve, then antisecretory therapy should be maintained for a 6- to 8-week trial. If symptoms do not resolve, then *H. pylori* testing should be considered.

TREATMENT

Pharmacologic treatment of nonulcer dyspepsia is not well established, and clinical studies have been hampered by small patient numbers and high placebo response rates. Antisecretory agents (H$_2$RAs and PPIs) can improve dyspeptic symptoms in patients with ulcer-like symptoms but not in those with dysmotility-type symptoms (nausea, bloating, early satiety). Prokinetic agents have been shown, in small studies, to confer a benefit in dyspeptic patients, with response rates of 65% to 90% compared with 13% to 42% for placebo. Tricyclic antidepressants, effective in a number of pain syndromes and in irritable bowel syndrome, have not been adequately studied in dyspepsia, but low doses of desipramine

(Norpramin)[1] or amitriptyline (Elavil)[1] may be effective in ameliorating symptoms.

Because drug therapy is not reliably effective in treating nonulcer dyspepsia, the focus of treatment is the maintenance of a supportive physician-patient relationship. After ruling out structural disease and medication-induced symptoms, the physician should explain to the patient that nonulcer dyspepsia is not a "psychological" condition, but is in fact a real disorder likely related to abnormal pain sensitivity and abnormal motility in the gastrointestinal tract. Patients should be reassured that their illness is not life-threatening, and the physician and patient should collaborate to develop a plan for symptomatic relief while minimizing the use of invasive diagnostic tests. Stress management, dietary modification to avoid symptom-inducing foods, and attention to the psychological factors that might contribute to dyspepsia are important components of long-term therapy. Pharmacologic agents may be used with the recognition that placebo response rates are high and symptoms can recur over time; if a medication proves ineffective, the patient should be changed to another agent, because stacking of medications is ineffective and expensive.

---

[1]Not FDA approved for this indication.

REFERENCES

Del Valle J. Zollinger-Ellison syndrome and other neuroendocrine tumors. In: Wolfe MM, editor. Therapy of Digestive Disorders. New York: Elsevier; 2006. p. 469–84.

Ford AC, Forman D, Bailey AG, et al. A community screening program for *Helicobacter pylori* saves money: 10-year follow-up of a randomized controlled tria. Gastroenterology 2005;129:1910–7.

Lowe RC, Wolfe MM. Acid peptic disorders, gastritis, and *Helicobacter pylori*. In: Noble J, editor. Textbook of Primary Care Medicine. 3rd ed. St. Louis: Mosby; 2000. p. 910–20.

Moayyedi P, Delaney BC, Vakil N, et al. The efficacy of proton pump inhibitors in nonulcer dyspepsia: A systematic review and economic analysis. Gastroenterology 2004;127:1329–37.

Talley NJ. American Gastroenterological Association medical position statement: Evaluation of dyspepsia. Gastroenterology 2005;129:1753–5.

Talley NJ, Vakil NB, Moayyedi P. American Gastroenterological Association technical review on the evaluation of dyspepsia. Gastroenterology 2005; 129:1756–90.

Wolfe MM, Lichtenstein DR, Singh G. Gastrointestinal toxicity of nonsteroidal antiinflammatory drugs. N Engl J Med 2004;340:1888–99.

Wolfe MM, Sachs G. Acid suppression: Optimizing therapy for gastroduodenal ulcer healing, gastroesophageal reflux disease, and stress-related erosive syndrome. Gastroenterology 2000;118:S9–31.

Acute and Chronic Viral Hepatitis

Method of
John Garber, MD, and Daniel Pratt, MD

The progress achieved in understanding viral hepatitis over the past decade has been dramatic. There are better diagnostic tools and rapidly evolving therapies, most particularly for hepatitis B. This improved therapy has made it critical that physicians effectively screen for chronic hepatitis B and identify all appropriate candidates for treatment. Hepatitis C therapy is also improving, and a percentage of patients can be cured—a proportion that will only increase as newer drugs become available.

Hepatitis A Virus

Hepatitis A virus (HAV), a member of the Picornaviridae family, exists as a single positive-stranded RNA virus of 7474 nucleotides, which encodes four structural proteins (capsids V1, V2, V3, and V4) and seven nonstructural proteins (e.g., protease, RNA-dependent polymerase). Four distinct genotypes exist. Despite intergenomic sequence variation of up to 20%, the genotypes are immunologically indistinguishable, so infection with one strain of HAV confers lifelong immunity to all strains.

EPIDEMIOLOGY

The virus is extremely stable in the environment and is shed in the stool of infected persons at a very high titer. It spreads within a population predominantly via the fecal-oral route, most commonly through ingestion of contaminated food or water. In the United States, the likelihood of having serologic evidence of past exposure is associated with age; it is approximately 11% at the age of 5 years and increases to almost 75% in those older than 50 years.

DIAGNOSIS

The presence of anti-HAV antibodies of the immunoglobulin M (IgM) class is diagnostic of acute HAV infection. Positive anti-HAV IgG antibodies along with negative anti-HAV IgM antibodies indicates immunity, from either prior infection or vaccination. Clinical laboratories often report the total anti-HAV antibodies, which is a mixture of IgG and IgM. To distinguish acute HAV infection from prior exposure, it is important to specifically test for the presence of anti-HAV IgM.

NATURAL HISTORY

HAV causes an acute hepatitis only; it never results in chronic hepatitis, and lifelong immunity is expected in all patients who recover. Once the virus is orally ingested, it reaches the liver via the portal vein. Viral shedding occurs when the replicating virus is excreted from hepatocytes through the bile duct into the intestine. Shedding continues until the prodromic phase and begins to decline once jaundice develops. However, infectious virions can be detected in the feces up to 2 weeks after the onset of jaundice.

The severity of symptoms associated with HAV depends in part on the age of the patient at the time of exposure: 90% of those infected before 5 years of age are asymptomatic, whereas 70% to 80% of those infected as adults have symptoms. HAV has an incubation period of approximately 25 days. This is followed by a prodromal phase of variable severity, characterized by weakness, anorexia, nausea, abdominal pain, and, less often, fevers, arthralgias, and diarrhea. The levels of the serum aminotransferases are elevated during this time, often to values greater than 500 U/L, and their peak usually coincides with intense nausea, vomiting, and anorexia. Jaundice typically occurs 1 to 2 weeks later and is associated with a lessening of the prodromal symptoms. The serum bilirubin level peaks later than the aminotransferases, rarely exceeds 10 mg/dL, and normalizes more slowly than the aminotransferases. In most patients, jaundice lasts less than 2 weeks. Complete normalization of the serum biochemical abnormalities is observed in 60% of patients by 2 months and in almost 100% by 6 months.

TREATMENT

There is no specific therapy for hepatitis A; treatment is largely supportive. Dehydration is common during the symptomatic phase and requires administration of intravenous fluids. A rare complication of acute HAV is the development of acute liver failure marked by encephalopathy and coagulopathy. The risk of developing acute liver failure is higher in older patients; those infected after the age of 50 years have a case-fatality rate of 2.7%. Patients with coexisting chronic HBV or HCV infection are also at higher risk for a more severe clinical course. Vaccination for HAV should be offered to all patients who have chronic viral hepatitis or cirrhosis and negative HAV antibodies.

Three vaccines containing inactivated HAV are currently licensed for use: HAVRIX (GlaxoSmithKline), VAQTA (Merck), and TWINRIX (GlaxoSmithKline). All are highly effective at generating antibody responses, with approximately 95% of recipients developing protective levels of anti-HAV antibodies within 1 month after the first dose, and 100% after the second dose. The Advisory Committee on Immunization Practices recommends HAV immunoprophylaxis for all children at the age of 1 year. Vaccination is also recommended for adults who travel to areas of high or intermediate endemicity (Fig. 1), men who have sex with men, people with underlying chronic liver disease, and users of injection drugs.

Passive immunization, in the form of pooled human anti-HAV immunoglobulins (IG; IGIM; GamaSTAN) can be given to patients who have been exposed to HAV. HAV IG is 80% effective in preventing HAV infection if given within 2 weeks after exposure, and a single intramuscular dose of 0.02 mL/kg confers protection for 3 to 5 months. Although the concurrent administration of HAV IG with the first dose of anti-HAV vaccine somewhat reduces the immunogenicity of the vaccine, patients develop antibody levels well above those considered to be protective. There are growing data suggesting that vaccination is as effective as HAV IG for postexposure prophylaxis.

Hepatitis E Virus

Hepatitis E virus (HEV) is an enterically transmitted RNA virus that causes an acute, self-limited hepatitis which varies in severity from an asymptomatic infection to acute liver failure. Its genome consists of a single, positive-stranded RNA that encodes several structural and nonstructural proteins using overlapping open reading frames. As with HAV, there are multiple genotypes but only one serotype. Major protection epitopes are common to all HEV isolates, and exposure to one strain confers immunity to all strains.

EPIDEMIOLOGY

Geographically, endemic regions of high HEV prevalence include Central America, Africa, the Middle East, Southeast Asia, and India. In nonendemic regions, HEV accounts for fewer than 1% of reported cases of acute viral hepatitis, and most of these occur in patients who have recently traveled to endemic areas.

DIAGNOSIS

The diagnosis of HEV is made by serologic detection of anti-HEV IgM and IgG antibodies. Anti-HEV IgM is the hallmark of acute HEV infection. Anti-HEV IgM is usually undetectable by 6 months after infection. Anti-HEV IgG appears during the convalescent phase and is a serologic marker for past infection.

NATURAL HISTORY

Infection with HEV is typically a self-limited disease, and patients are often anicteric. An incubation period of 2 to 8 weeks is followed by a classic prodromal phase. The symptoms usually resolve within 6 weeks. For reasons that are not well understood, women in the second and third trimesters of pregnancy are at risk for a more severe clinical course. Mortality due to acute liver failure from HEV ranges from 20% to 25% in pregnant woman.

TREATMENT

There is no specific treatment for HEV infection; therapy is strictly supportive. There are currently no commercially available vaccines for HEV. Phase II trials of a recombinant anti-HEV vaccine are under

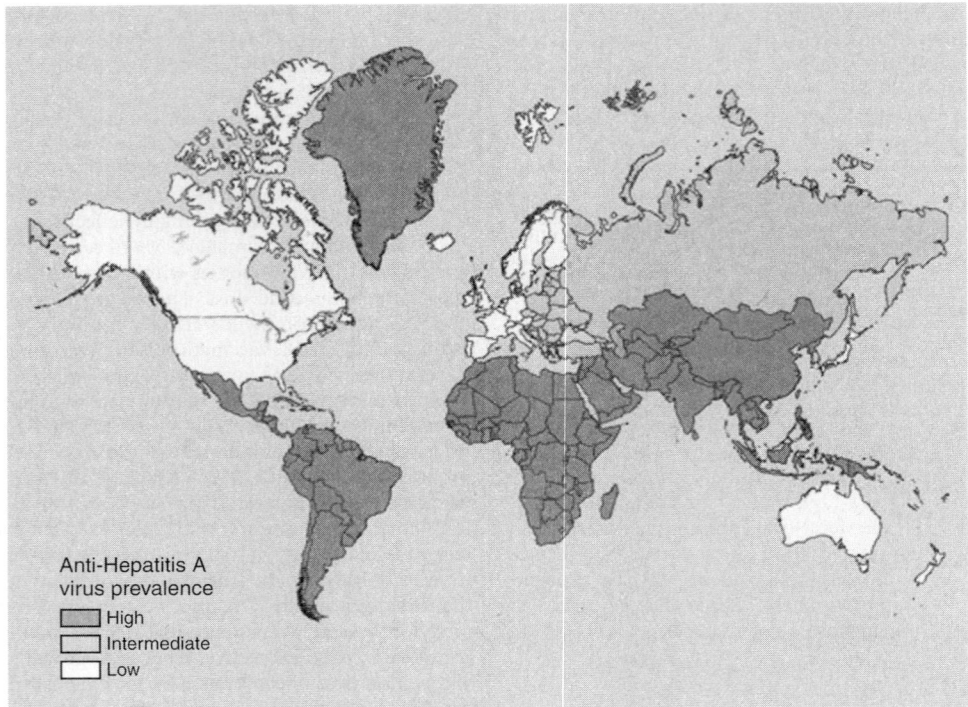

FIGURE 1. Prevalence of antibody to hepatitis A virus, by country, 2006. (From http://wwwn.cdc.gov/travel/yellowBook Ch4-HepA.aspx [accessed June 30, 2009].)

way and have shown promising results. Monoclonal antibodies against HEV have been produced and have proved effective for protecting nonhuman primates from HEV infection, but these preparations are not yet commercially available.

Hepatitis B Virus

Hepatitis B virus (HBV) is a partially double-stranded DNA virus in the Hepadnaviridae family with a 3200 base pair genome that uses multiple overlapping reading frames to encode surface, core, polymerase, and X proteins. Proteins of clinical importance include hepatitis B surface antigen (HBsAg), hepatitis B core antigen (HBcAg), and hepatitis B e antigen (HBeAg). Serum HBsAg is a marker of HBV infection, and HBeAg is a marker of active viral replication.

EPIDEMIOLOGY AND MODE OF TRANSMISSION

HBV infects an estimated 1.25 million people in the United States and 460 million people globally. Areas with a low prevalence of HBV (<2%) include North America, western and northern Europe, Australia, New Zealand, and southern South America; all other parts of the world have an intermediate prevalence (2%–8%) or high prevalence (>8%) in the general population (Fig. 2). Alaska is the only region in the United States considered to have a high prevalence of HBV, with a rate of 6.4% in the native population.

HBV is transmitted more efficiently than either HCV or HIV. The likelihood of transmission increases with the level of HBV DNA in serum. It is transmissible through perinatal, sexual, or percutaneous exposure; close person-to-person contact with open cuts and sores; and sharing of household items such as razors and toothbrushes. In high-prevalence areas, HBV is most often vertically transmitted. In the United States, the route is primarily horizontal; sexual transmission accounts for approximately 30% of cases.

In 2008, the CDC significantly expanded its recommendations for screening for chronic HBV (Box 1) to include all persons from inter-mediate-prevalence areas in addition to those from areas of high

prevalence. Those recommendations also now include patients who require treatment with immunosuppressive medications.

DIAGNOSIS

The presence of HBsAg in serum is the hallmark of infection with hepatitis B. Patients who recover from hepatitis B clear the HBsAg and develop an antibody to it, HBsAb. The presence of HBsAg for longer than 6 months indicates chronic HBV infection. Hepatitis B core antibody (HBcAb) is found in patients with both acute and chronic HBV. The acute illness is marked by the presence of HBcAb of the IgM class, whereas patients with chronic disease have HBcAb of the IgG class.

Appropriate testing for patients with suspected acute hepatitis B includes HBsAg, HBcAb IgM, HBeAg, and HBV DNA. Appropriate testing for patients with suspected chronic HBV includes HBsAg, HBcAb, and HBsAb. Patients found to have chronic HBV should undergo additional testing to assess their viral replication status by checking the levels of HBV DNA, HBeAg, and hepatitis B e antibody (HBeAb). This information allows the physician to determine whether a patient with chronic HBV is a candidate for antiviral therapy.

NATURAL HISTORY

Symptoms of acute HBV infection appear after an incubation period that ranges from 60 to 180 days. The presentation of acute HBV ranges from asymptomatic disease to acute liver failure. Markers of infection and viral replication—HBsAg, HBeAg, and HBV DNA—appear approximately 6 weeks after exposure. Their appearance is followed shortly by a rise in serum aminotransferases; the serum alanine aminotransferase (ALT) level is greater than the serum aspartate aminotransferase (AST) level, and both are generally higher than 500 U/L. During this time, anti-hepatitis B core antibody (HBcAb) of the IgM class, the only marker of acute infection, appears and may persist for many months.

Aminotransferase levels correspond well with the degree of necroinflammation. The liver injury results from a cytotoxic T lymphocyte–induced apoptosis of virally infected hepatocytes. Acute liver failure occurs when the severity of the injury results in

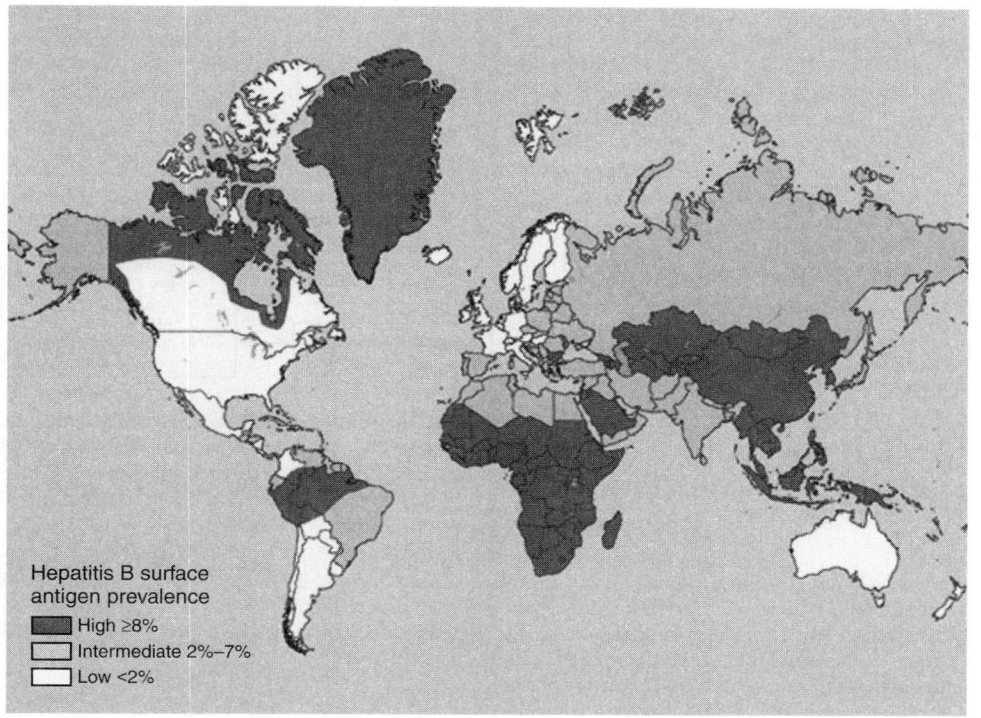

FIGURE 2. Prevalence of chronic hepatitis B virus infection, by country, 2006. (From http://wwwn.cdc.gov/travel/yellow BookCh4-HepB.aspx [accessed June 30, 2009].)

BOX 1   Populations for Whom Screening for Chronic Hepatitis B Virus Infection Is Recommended

- Persons born in areas with intermediate or high disease prevalence (>2%)*
- U.S.-born persons who were not vaccinated at birth and have parents from areas of high disease prevalence
- Injection-drug users*
- Men who have sex with men*
- Persons who require immunosuppressive therapy*
- Persons with unexplained elevation of the serum aminotransferases*
- Hemodialysis patients
- Pregnant women
- Infants born to HBsAg-positive mothers
- Household, needle-sharing, or sex contacts of HBsAg-positive persons
- Persons infected with the human immunodeficiency virus
- Persons who are the source of blood or body fluid exposures who might require postexposure prophylaxis

From Recommendations for identification and public health management of persons with chronic hepatitis B virus infection. MMWR Morb Mortal Wkly Rep 2008;57(RR08):1–20. Available at http://www.cdc.gov/mmwr/preview/mmwrhtml/rr5708a1.htm (accessed June 30, 2009).
*New recommendations.
HBsAg = hepatitis B virus surface antigen.

---

insufficient residual hepatic mass and function. Patients who clear the virus have normalization of aminotransferases by 4 months, followed by a slower resolution of hyperbilirubinemia. The likelihood of progression to chronicity (defined as persistence of HBsAg for >6 months) depends on the age at exposure. Whereas 90% of those perinatally infected progress to chronic infection, this rate decreases to 20% to 50% in those infected between age 1 to 5 years, and is less than 5% in persons infected with HBV as an adult.

It is useful to conceptualize the natural history of chronic HBV infection as a spectrum encompassing an immunotolerant stage, an immunoactive stage, an inactive carrier stage, a resolution stage, and an e antigen–negative chronic hepatitis (Fig. 3). This is particularly useful in patients infected via vertical transmission.

In addition to the testing needed to assess viral replication, the serum albumin level and prothrombin time should be checked to assess synthetic function, and a complete blood count should be performed to assess for thrombocytopenia and leukopenia, which are potential indicators of hypersplenism. Careful interpretation of these data allows proper placement of patients with chronic HBV on the natural history continuum and identifies patients who are candidates for therapy.

The immunotolerant stage of disease is characterized by very high HBV DNA levels, normal aminotransferases, and no hepatic necroinflammation. These patients are not currently thought to be candidates for therapy. At an undefined and variable point in time, these immunotolerant patients progress to the immunoactive stage, which is characterized by high serum HBV DNA levels, elevated aminotransferases, and hepatic necroinflammation. They are then at increased risk for disease progression and hepatocellular carcinoma and are candidates for therapy.

The next transition is from the immunoactive stage to the inactive carrier stage; this occurs spontaneously at a rate of 8% to 12% per year. The inactive carrier stage is marked by HBeAg seroconversion (i.e., loss of HBeAg and development of HBeAb). This event carries with it a number of beneficial effects, including a significant reduction in serum HBV DNA levels, resolution of necroinflammation, prevention of histologic progression, reduced risk of hepatocellular carcinoma, and decreased mortality.

Patients in the inactive stage require continued attention, because 10% to 25% will have flares of hepatitis, with or without e antigen reversion. The rate of reversion for patients who achieve e antigen seroconversion through treatment is higher than for those who seroconvert spontaneously. Patients in the inactive carrier stage can develop precore or core promoter mutations that allow for viral

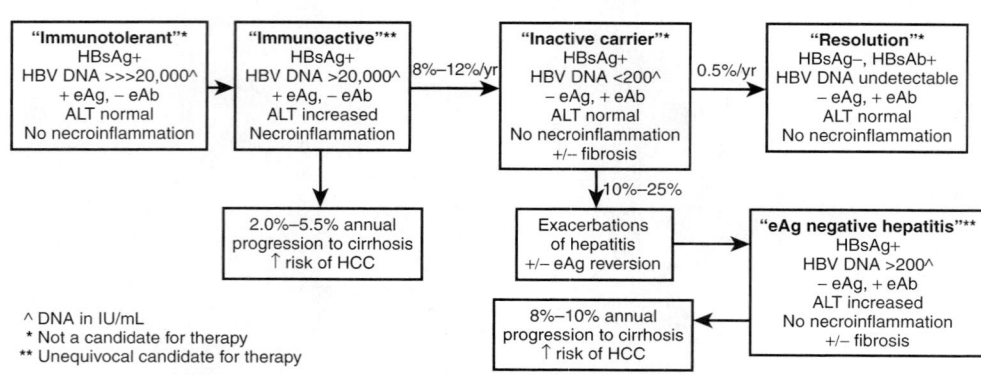

FIGURE 3. Natural history of chronic hepatitis B. ALT = alanine aminotransferase; eAb = hepatitis B e antibody; eAg = hepatitis B e antigen; HBsAb = hepatitis B surface antibody; HBsAg = hepatitis B surface antigen; HBV = hepatitis B virus; HCC = hepatocellular carcinoma. (Adapted from Pratt DS: Evaluation and management of hepatitis B virus infection. J Clin Outcomes Manage 2008;15:147–153.)

replication in the absence of e antigen. Like patients in the immunoactive stage, these patients with e antigen–negative hepatitis have elevated serum aminotransferases levels and necroinflammation on liver biopsy but lower levels of serum HBV DNA, compared with those in the immunoactive stage. They are at increased risk for histologic progression and for hepatocellular carcinoma and are candidates for therapy.

Patients in the inactive stage move into the resolution stage at a rate of 0.5% per year. The resolution stage is marked by surface antigen seroconversion (i.e., loss of surface antigen and development of surface antibody).

TREATMENT

Seven therapies approved by the U.S. Food and Drug Administration (FDA) for the treatment of HBV:

- Interferon: interferon alfa-2b (Intron A) and pegylated interferon alfa-2a (Pegasys)
- Nucleoside analogues: lamivudine (Epivir-HBV), telbivudine (Tyzeka), and entecavir (Baraclude)
- Nucleotide analogues: adefovir (Hepsera) and tenofovir (Viread)

The interferons are prescribed for a defined period (48 weeks), whereas the nucleoside and nucleotide analogues are continued until a specific end point of therapy is reached. The end point of therapy in immunoactive patients is loss of HbeAg and development of HbeAb, which is generally associated with sustained viral suppression. In HBeAg-negative patients, no such marker of treatment success exists, and there is a high likelihood of relapse when therapy is discontinued. These patients are usually treated indefinitely or until surface antigen seroconversion occurs.

Hepatitis D Virus

The hepatitis D virus (HVD) is a subviral particle composed of a single-stranded RNA genome complexed with hepatitis D antigen (HDAg) and enclosed in an outer lipoprotein envelope derived from HBsAg. It is believed that HDV uses some of the same pathways for attachment and entry into host cells as HBV; HDV infection requires the presence of HBV for infectivity. Immunity to HBV also protects against infection with HDV.

EPIDEMIOLOGY

HDV is a blood-borne pathogen with the same modes of transmission as HBV. Co-infection occurs when an individual is infected with both HBV and HDV at the same time. In contrast, HDV infection of a chronically HBV-infected individual is referred to as superinfection and carries a much higher risk of precipitating fulminant hepatic

failure. Chronic carriers of both HBV and HDV tend to have more rapid progression of liver disease, compared to those infected with HBV alone. It is estimated that 20 million HBV-infected people also have chronic HDV.

DIAGNOSIS

HDV elicits specific IgM and IgG antibody responses. Anti-HDV IgM is the only specific marker of acute HDV infection, although assays for IgM detection are not in clinical use in the United States. High titers of anti-HDV IgG often characterize chronic infections, but can also be seen in patients with prior infection, and therefore are not useful in distinguishing carriers from those who have cleared the virus. HDV RNA detection via polymerase chain reaction is commercially available in the United States and has a lower limit of detection (10 copies per milliliter). The diagnosis of HDV infection also requires evidence of concurrent HBV infection, and the presence of anti-HBV IgM suggests acute co-infection.

NATURAL HISTORY

HDV infection can produce a broad spectrum of liver injury, ranging from an asymptomatic carrier state to acute liver failure.

TREATMENT

The goal of treatment is suppression of HDV replication. The only drug shown to be of benefit in treating chronic HDV is interferon-alfa.[1] However, although interferon-alfa is capable of suppressing viral replication, its antiviral effect is not sustained after withdrawal of therapy.

Hepatitis C Virus

Hepatitis C virus (HCV) is a single minus-strand RNA virus of 9.6 kb whose genome encodes a core protein, envelope proteins, and several nonstructural proteins.

EPIDEMIOLOGY

Almost 170 million people are chronically infected with HCV worldwide. In the United States, there are an estimated 2.7 million individuals chronically infected, although the number of new cases per year has appreciably declined since 1990.

DIAGNOSIS

The initial test in diagnosing HCV infection is the presence of anti-HCV antibodies. The current serologic test uses a combination of the core protein and several nonstructural proteins in an

---

[1]Not FDA approved for this indication.

immunoassay that can detect reactive antibodies within 4 to 10 weeks of infection. As a screening test, the detection of anti-HCV antibodies is very sensitive, and it is estimated that only 0.5% to 1.0% of cases will be missed in a low-prevalence population. HCV RNA is used to confirm positive serologic testing and to assess the response to therapy. Measurement of HCV RNA can be either quantitative or qualitative. The quantitative assay is best for determining large changes in viral load and is therefore useful for monitoring the response to therapy; commercially available quantitative assays have a lower limit of detection, approximately 600 copies/mL. In contrast, qualitative tests for HCV RNA can detect as few as 10 copies/mL blood and are useful for confirming the presence of the virus, either when the titer is very low or at the end of therapy.

NATURAL HISTORY

Acute HCV infection is often asymptomatic; patients are rarely diagnosed at this stage. After an average incubation period of 6 weeks, a minority (15%–20%) of patients manifest a clinical syndrome of variable severity. Symptoms include fevers, malaise, nausea and anorexia, abdominal pain, and muscle aches. This period is anicteric, can last for 2 weeks to 3 months, and may be followed by the development of jaundice along with detectable serum HCV RNA. In asymptomatic infection, serum HCV RNA and aminotransferase elevations are usually detectable within 1 to 3 weeks of infection, and anti-HCV antibody becomes positive 3 weeks to 5 months after acute infection.

In approximately 30% of patients, acute HCV infection is self-limited and is followed by the resolution of aminotransferase elevations and disappearance of serum HCV RNA. Most patients who spontaneously clear HCV do so within 12 weeks after infection. Patients who do not clear the acute infection progress to chronic HCV infection, which is most often characterized by an asymptomatic elevation of serum aminotransferases. Approximately 30% of patients with chronic HCV infection have normal ALT levels.

TREATMENT

Because of the high likelihood that acute HCV infection will lead to chronic infection, treatment should be considered in all patients with evidence of acute HCV. Small studies have demonstrated high rates of viral clearance in patients with detectable HCV RNA who are treated within 3 months of infection. Although clear guidelines do not exist for treating this group of patients, a 24-week course of standard-dose pegylated interferon alfa-2b and ribavirin (Rebetol) is an accepted approach.

The decision to treat chronic HCV infection is based on multiple viral and host factors, including viral genotype and load, histology, likelihood of disease progression, and medical comorbidities. Patients with persistently detectable virus and histologic evidence of fibrosis or severe inflammation are at high risk for progression should be treated in the absence of contraindications. The indications for therapy are less clear in patients with no evidence of fibrosis and only minimal inflammation despite many years of infection. These patients have a lower risk of progression and may be observed with monitoring of serum liver enzymes and repeat liver biopsy in 4 to 5 years.

The mainstay of HCV therapy is pegylated interferon alfa-2a or alfa-2b (Intron A)[1] in combination with a weight-based dose of ribavirin. The duration of therapy is determined by the viral genotype: type 1 is treated for 48 weeks and types 2 and 3 for 24 weeks. Response to therapy is monitored by quantitative measurement of HCV RNA after 4 and 12 weeks of therapy. An undetectable HCV RNA level at 4 weeks is defined as a rapid virologic response; a greater than 2 log reduction in viral load at week 12 is defined as an early virologic response (EVR); and an undetectable HCV RNA at week 12 is a complete EVR. A rapid virologic response is the strongest positive predictor of sustained virologic response, which is defined as an undetectable HCV RNA 6 months after completion of treatment. At least an EVR is required to justify continuing therapy beyond 12 weeks, because patients with a less than 2 log reduction in viral load at week 12 have almost no chance of achieving a sustained virologic response. Patients who achieve an EVR but still have detectable virus after 24 weeks of therapy also have a very small chance of achieving SVR and therapy should be discontinued.

Treatment for hepatitis C will change dramatically in 2011 with the anticipated approval by the Food and Drug Administration of the first direct-acting antivirals—the protease inhibitors telaprevir and boceprevir. Once these new drugs are available, the standard of care for treating hepatitis C will be triple therapy with a protease inhibitor being used in combination with pegylated interferon and ribavirin.

REFERENCES

Dalton HR, Brendall R, Ijaz S, Banks M. Hepatitis E: An emerging infection in developed countries. Lancet Infect Dis 2008;8:698–709.
Dienstag JL. Hepatitis B virus infection. N Engl J Med 2008;359:1486–500.
Ghany MG, Strader DB, Thomas DL, Seeff LB. Diagnosis, management, and treatment of hepatitis C: An update. Hepatology 2009;49:1335–74.
Pratt DS. Evaluation and management of hepatitis B virus infection. J Clin Outcomes Manage 2008;15:147–53.
Wasley A, Fiore A, Bell BP. Hepatitis A in the era of vaccination. Epidemiol Rev 2006;28:101–11.
Wrinbaum CM, Williams I, Mast EE, et al. Recommendations for identification and public health management of persons with chronic hepatitis B virus infection, MMWR Morb Mortal Wkly Rep 2008;57(RR08):1–20. Available at http://www.cdc.gov/mmwr/preview/mmwrhtml/rr5708a1.htm [accessed June 30, 2009].

Malabsorption

Method of
Lawrence R. Schiller, MD

Every day the average human being consumes 2000–3000 kcal of food, much of it in the form of polymers or other complex molecules that must be digested and absorbed by the gut. The processes of digestion and absorption are complex and are readily disturbed by pathologic processes. More than 200 conditions have been described that can adversely affect nutrient absorption.

Strictly speaking, *maldigestion* refers to impaired hydrolysis of nutrients, usually due to lack of luminal factors, such as bile acids and pancreatic enzymes, and *malabsorption* refers to impaired mucosal transport. For clinical purposes, "malabsorption" is used to describe both processes.

Malabsorption can be generalized (panmalabsorption) or limited to a specific category of nutrients. Generalized malabsorption is usually due to maldigestion or to extensive mucosal dysfunction. Specific malabsorption occurs when a single transporter is disabled.

The causes of malabsorption can be divided into three categories: impaired luminal hydrolysis, impaired mucosal function (mucosal hydrolysis, uptake, packaging, and excretion), and impaired removal of nutrients from the mucosa (Box 1).

Diagnosis

SYMPTOMS AND SIGNS

Most patients with panmalabsorption have changes in their stools (Box 2). Steatorrhea (excess fat in stools) is characterized by pale color, bulkiness, greasiness, and a tendency to float (probably because of incorporated gas). Occasionally patients with malabsorption present with watery stools due to the osmotic effects of unabsorbed carbohydrates and short-chain fatty acids.

Abdominal distention and excess flatus also commonly occur due to fermentation of unabsorbed carbohydrate by colonic bacteria. This can occur not only with panmalabsorption but also with specific malabsorption of carbohydrate (e.g., lactase deficiency).

Weight loss is typical with severe panmalabsorption, but it might not be very prominent with lesser degrees of malabsorption due to

[1]Not FDA approved for this indication.

CURRENT DIAGNOSIS

- Recognize the presence of generalized malabsorption by the combination of typical symptoms: diarrhea, greasy stools, flatulence, weight loss, fatigue, edema.
- Recognize the presence of specific malabsorption by associated symptoms and those symptoms particular to deficiency states of the malabsorbed substance: flatus, diarrhea, anemia, dermatitis, glossitis, neuropathy, paresthesias, tetany, ecchymosis.
- Documentation of generalized malabsorption is best done by stool analysis demonstrating steatorrhea and acid stools (reflecting carbohydrate malabsorption). Diagnosis depends on visualization of the small bowel by endoscopy or radiography and small bowel biopsy. Additional tests may be needed.
- Documentation of specific malabsorption is best done by demonstrating low blood levels of the malabsorbed substance or by tests designed to measure absorption of that substance. Diagnosis depends on studies designed to identify the likely diagnosis for a given situation.

BOX 1   Causes of Malabsorption or Maldigestion

- Impaired luminal hydrolysis or solublization
  - Bile acid deficiency
  - Impaired mucosal hydrolysis, uptake, or packaging
  - Pancreatic exocrine insufficiency
  - Postgastrectomy syndrome
  - Rapid intestinal transit
  - Small bowel bacterial overgrowth
  - Zollinger-Ellison syndrome
- Brush border or metabolic disorders
  - Abetalipoproteinemia
  - Glucose-galactose malabsorption
  - Lactase deficiency
  - Sucrase-isomaltase deficiency
- Mucosal diseases
  - Amyloidosis
  - Chronic mesenteric ischemia
  - Crohn's disease
  - Celiac sprue
  - Collagenous sprue
  - Eosinophilic gastroenteritis
  - Immunoproliferative small intestinal disease (IPSID)
  - Lymphoma
  - Nongranulomatous ulcerative jejunoileitis
  - Radiation enteritis
  - Systemic mastocytosis
- Infectious diseases
  - AIDS enteropathy
  - *Mycobacterium avium-intracellulare*
  - Parasitic diseases
  - Small bowel bacterial overgrowth
  - Tropical sprue
  - Whipple's disease
- After intestinal resection
- Chronic mesenteric ischemia
- Impaired removal of nutrients
  - Lymphangiectasia

BOX 2   Symptoms and Signs of Malabsorption or Maldigestion

- Changes in stool characteristics
  - Floating stools
  - Pale, bulky, greasy stools
  - Watery diarrhea
- Increased colonic gas production
  - Abdominal distention
  - Borborygmi
- Vitamin and mineral deficiencies
  - Anemia
  - Cheilosis
  - Glossitis
  - Dermatitis
  - Neuropathy
  - Night blindness
  - Osteomalacia
  - Paresthesia
  - Tetany
- Ecchymosis
- Fatigue, weakness
- Edema
- Weight loss, muscle wasting

---

compensatory hyperphagia. Weight loss is most prominent early in the course of the illness, but body weight usually stabilizes as calorie absorption and body weight come into balance again. This is in contrast to illnesses like cancer or tuberculosis that produce continuing weight loss. If a patient with malabsorption has continuing weight loss, inflammatory bowel disease or lymphoma should be considered.

Abdominal pain is usually not present with malabsorption, although some cramping may be associated with diarrhea. Severe pain should bring chronic pancreatitis, Zollinger-Ellison syndrome, lymphoma, Crohn's disease, or mesenteric ischemia to mind.

Constitutional symptoms of fatigue and weakness commonly occur, even early in the course. In contrast, appetite is impaired only late in the course of most malabsorption states. Edema is uncommon until late in the course unless protein-losing enteropathy is present.

Vitamin and mineral deficiencies can lead to several symptoms or signs. Glossitis and cheilosis are common in patients with water-soluble vitamin deficiencies. Florid beriberi, pellagra, and scurvy are not commonly seen unless malabsorption has been particularly severe or long-lasting. Fat-soluble vitamin deficiencies also are unlikely to develop except when malabsorption has been long-standing because of substantial body stores.

Miscellaneous findings occasionally seen in patients with malabsorption can provide clues to the diagnosis. Aphthous ulcers in the mouth may be seen with celiac disease, Behçet's syndrome, or Crohn's disease. Hyperpigmentation is seen in Whipple's disease, and dermatitis herpetiformis (pruritic, blistering skin lesions) is seen in celiac disease. Scleroderma can manifest with tight skin, digital ulceration, nail changes, and Raynaud's phenomenon. Chronic sinusitis, bronchitis, and recurrent pneumonia suggest cystic fibrosis or IgA deficiency. Several systemic diseases can be associated with malabsorption syndrome (Box 3).

TESTS

Routine Laboratory Tests

Routine laboratory tests (Box 4) commonly are abnormal in patients with established malabsorption syndrome. Anemia is common but not universal. Iron deficiency anemia may be the only finding in some patients with celiac disease. Microcytic anemia may be present in Whipple's disease (due to occult blood loss) and in lymphomas manifesting with malabsorption. Macrocytic anemia due to folate or vitamin B_{12} deficiency can occur in short bowel syndrome, small bowel bacterial overgrowth, or ileal disease. Lymphopenia may be present in patients with AIDS or lymphangiectasia.

BOX 3 Systemic Diseases Associated with Malabsorption or Maldigestion

Endocrine Diseases
- Addison's disease
- Diabetes mellitus
- Hypoparathyroidism
- Hyperthyroidism, hypothyroidism

Collagen-Vascular and Miscellaneous Diseases
- AIDS
- Amyloidosis
- Scleroderma
- Vasculitis (systemic lupus erythematosus, polyarteritis nodosa)

CURRENT THERAPY

- Once a diagnosis is reached, therapy can be directed toward that specific problem:
  - Gluten-free diet for celiac disease
  - Antibiotics for bacterial overgrowth
  - Lactose-free diet for lactase deficiency

Electrolyte abnormalities may be due to a combination of poor intake and excess loss in stool. Renal function usually is well maintained in malabsorption syndrome, but blood urea nitrogen may be low due to poor protein absorption, and serum creatinine concentration may be low due to depletion of muscle mass. Serum calcium levels may be low due to malabsorption, vitamin D deficiency, or intraluminal complexing of calcium by fatty acids. Hypomagnesemia can produce hypocalcemia or hypokalemia that is resistant to intravenous repletion. Serum phosphorus, cholesterol, and triglyceride levels may be reduced due to poor intake or malabsorption. Liver tests may be abnormal due to fatty liver. Serum protein and albumin levels are well preserved in patients with malabsorption unless protein-losing enteropathy or an acute illness is present.

Prothrombin time is normal unless vitamin K malabsorption (typically associated with steatorrhea), anticoagulant therapy, antibiotic therapy, or colectomy is present.

Assays are available for several potentially malabsorbed substances, including iron, vitamin B_{12}, folate, 25-hydroxyvitamin D, and β-carotene. Malabsorption tends to lower blood levels, but substantial body stores of many of these can mitigate the reduction in concentration that otherwise might occur. Thus, the sensitivity and specificity of these assays for malabsorption are poor.

Tests for Malabsorption

Fat Malabsorption

The simplest test for fat malabsorption is a qualitative microscopic examination of stool using a fat-soluble stain, such as Sudan III. The finding of more than 5 stained droplets per high power field is abnormal and correlates well with quantitative measurement of fecal fat excretion. The test is subject to false-positive results with some drugs and food additives, such as mineral oil, orlistat, and olestra.

A more precise estimate of fat absorption is obtained by a quantitative analysis of a timed stool collection (48 or 72 hours). During the collection, a diary of dietary intake should be maintained so that fat excretion can be assessed as a percentage of intake. Normal fat excretion is <7% of intake when stool weight is normal, but it can be twice as high due to voluminous diarrhea without indicating defective mucosal transport of fat. Thus, fat excretion must be judged against stool weight. Stool fat concentration (grams of fat

BOX 4 Laboratory Tests for Evaluation of Malabsorption or Maldigestion

Routine Blood Tests
- Complete blood count
- Hemoglobin/hematocrit
- Platelet count
- WBC differential count

Biochemistry Tests
- Blood urea nitrogen
- Potassium
- Prothrombin time
- Serum albumin
- Serum calcium
- Serum creatinine

Blood Levels of Potentially Malabsorbed Substances
- Serum iron, vitamin B_{12}, folate, 25-OH vitamin D, carotene

Fat absorption
- Qualitative fecal fat
- Quantitative fecal fat

Protein Absorption and Protein-Losing Enteropathy
- α_1-Antitrypsin clearance
- Fecal nitrogen excretion

Carbohydrate Absorption
- Osmotic gap in stool water
- Quantitative excretion (anthrone)
- Stool pH < 5.5
- Stool reducing substances
- D-Xylose absorption test
- Oral glucose, sucrose, and lactose tolerance tests
- Breath hydrogen tests

Vitamin B_{12} Absorption
- Schilling test with intrinsic factor

Bile Acid Malabsorption
- ^{14}C-glycocholic acid breath test
- Fecal bile acid excretion
- Radiolabeled bile acid excretion
- ^{75}SeHCAT retention

Small Bowel Bacterial Overgrowth
- ^{14}C-glycocholic acid breath test
- ^{14}C-xylose breath test
- Glucose breath hydrogen test
- Quantitative culture of jejunal aspirate

Exocrine Pancreatic Insufficiency
- Dual-labeled Schilling test
- Secretin/CCK test
- Stool chymotrypsin concentration

Serologic Testing for Celiac Disease
- Anti-tissue transglutaminase antibody (IgA)
- Anti-endomysial antibody (IgA)

Abbreviations: CCK = cholecystokinin; SLE = systemic lupus erythematosus; ^{75}SeHCAT = selenium-75-labeled taurohomocholic acid.

per 100 grams of stool) also is of value. Pancreatic exocrine insufficiency is associated with high fecal fat concentration (>10 g/100 g stool) because unlike hydrolyzed fat, unhydrolyzed fat does not stimulate colonic water and electrolyte secretion that would dilute fecal fat concentration.

Protein Malabsorption

Fecal nitrogen excretion can be employed as a marker of protein malabsorption, but is not often used in clinical medicine because it adds little to the evaluation. If protein-losing enteropathy is suspected, an α_1-antitrypsin clearance study can be done. In this study, *fecal* excretion of α_1-antitrypsin, a serum protein that is relatively resistant to hydrolysis by luminal enzymes, is divided by *serum* concentration of α_1-antitrypsin, and the volume of serum leaked into the lumen can be calculated. Values of more than 180 mL/day are associated with hypoalbuminemia.

Carbohydrate Malabsorption

Carbohydrate malabsorption is difficult to measure directly because fermentation of malabsorbed carbohydrate by colonic bacteria reduces the amount of intact carbohydrate that can be recovered in stool. Indirect estimates of carbohydrate malabsorption can be made by examining fecal pH (<5.5 with carbohydrate malabsorption) or fecal osmotic gap (> 100 mOsm/kg with osmotic diarrhea). Oral carbohydrate tolerance tests may be used to evaluate absorption of sugars, such as lactose or fructose. Following an oral load of a given sugar, blood glucose levels are monitored; failure of blood glucose to increase suggests malabsorption.

Another test for carbohydrate malabsorption is the D-xylose absorption test. In this test, a 25-gram dose of D-xylose is given orally; blood xylose levels are measured 1 and 3 hours later, and urinary excretion of xylose is measured for 5 hours. Failure of blood xylose to rise above 20 mg/dL at 1 hour or above 22.5 mg/dL at 3 hours or failure of urinary excretion to exceed 5 g in 5 hours suggests malabsorption. In addition, because xylose does not require pancreatic enzymes or bile acids for absorption, an abnormal D-xylose test suggests a mucosal problem as the cause for malabsorption. The results of this test can be misleading if the patient is dehydrated or has ascites, if renal function is compromised, or if bacterial overgrowth is present in the upper small bowel.

Breath hydrogen testing is another method to assess carbohydrate absorption. If substrates such as lactose or sucrose are not absorbed in the small intestine, they pass into the colon, where bacterial fermentation produces hydrogen gas. The hydrogen is absorbed into the bloodstream and then is exhaled. The concentration of hydrogen in exhaled breath can be measured easily; a rise of more than 10 to 20 ppm after ingestion of a specific substrate is consistent with malabsorption. False-positive results can be seen in patients with small bowel bacterial overgrowth, and false-negative results can be seen in patients who lack hydrogen-producing flora or who have been on antibiotics recently.

Vitamin B₁₂ Malabsorption

The Schilling test can be used to measure vitamin B_{12} absorption. For purposes of a malabsorption evaluation, part II of the Schilling test (measurement of radiolabeled B_{12} absorption *with* intrinsic factor) is all that is needed. Recovery of less than 9% of the radiolabel in the urine is abnormal and suggests ileal dysfunction. The test may be falsely positive in patients with pancreatic exocrine insufficiency, small bowel bacterial overgrowth, or renal failure.

Bile Acid Malabsorption

Tests for bile acid malabsorption are not widely available in the United States. Direct measurement of bile acid excretion has been used mainly in research studies. Retention of a radioactive taurocholic acid analogue (SeHCAT, selenium-75-labeled taurohomocholic acid) is used in Europe to assess bile acid malabsorption. A breath test using ¹⁴C-glycocholic acid has been used for evaluating small bowel bacterial overgrowth, but it may have application for assessing bile acid malabsorption as well.

Small Bowel Bacterial Overgrowth

The gold standard method used to test for small bowel bacterial overgrowth in the upper intestine is quantitative culture of jejunal fluid. The sample can be obtained during endoscopy and sent to the laboratory with instructions to quantitate the aerobic and anaerobic flora. Finding more than 10^5 bacteria per mL confirms bacterial overgrowth. Breath tests using glucose, ¹⁴C-xylose, and lactulose also have been described for this purpose.

Pancreatic Exocrine Insufficiency

Tests for pancreatic exocrine insufficiency are not commonly used. The gold standard test is a secretin test. This study requires duodenal intubation, injection of secretin, and measurement of bicarbonate output. A tubeless test, the bentiromide test, had average clinical utility; it is no longer available in the United States. Measurement of fecal chymotrypsin or elastase activity is only moderately useful in predicting the presence of exocrine pancreatic insufficiency. For most situations, a therapeutic trial using a high dose of pancreatic enzymes with monitoring of the effect on steatorrhea is the best that can be done.

Evaluation of Suspected Malabsorption

When malabsorption is suspected because of the history, physical findings, and setting, the physician must decide if the malabsorption involves a specific nutrient or represents a generalized process (Figure 1). If the malabsorption seems to be specific, a diet and symptom diary, breath tests using the presumptively malabsorbed substrate, and stool pH to identify acid stools seen with carbohydrate malabsorption are reasonable diagnostic maneuvers.

Suspected generalized malabsorption requires a more intense evaluation. Steatorrhea should be confirmed with either a qualitative fecal fat test (e.g., Sudan stain) or a quantitative stool collection for measurement of fat excretion. If steatorrhea is confirmed, the small bowel should be visualized with either capsule endoscopy or radiography (small bowel follow-through examination or computed

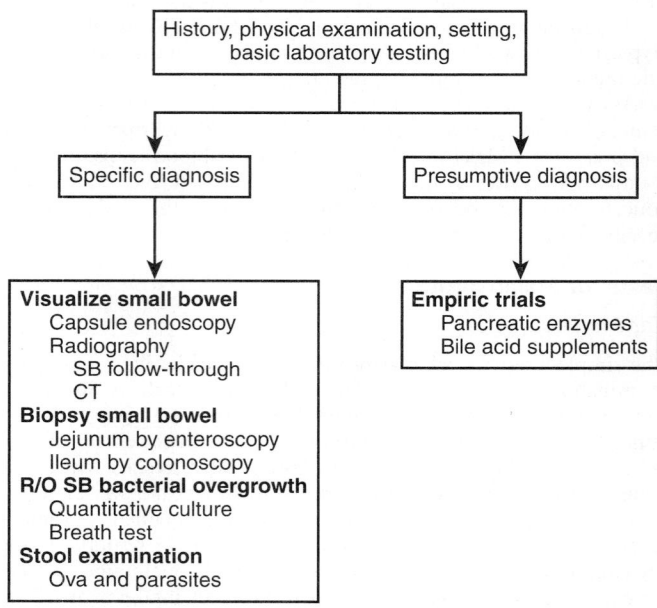

FIGURE 1. Flow chart for evaluation of malabsorption or maldigestion. *Abbreviations:* CT = computed tomography; R/O = rule out; SB = small bowel.

tomography) and biopsied from above by enteroscopy and from below by colonoscopy. During enteroscopy, an aspirate of small bowel contents can be obtained for quantitative culture to look for small bowel bacterial overgrowth. An alternative method to detect small bowel bacterial overgrowth is breath testing (see earlier). Stool samples also should be examined with microscopy or immunoassay for the presence of parasites that may be associated with malabsorption.

This sequence of evaluation often leads to a specific diagnosis. When it does not, empiric trials of pancreatic enzyme replacement or bile acid supplementation can lead to a presumptive diagnosis of pancreatic exocrine insufficiency or bile acid deficiency. Hard endpoints (e.g., quantitative fat excretion) should be used to assess the effectiveness of these empiric trials.

Specific Disorders Associated with Malabsorption

MALABSORPTION OF SPECIFIC NUTRIENTS

Disaccharidase Deficiency

Ingested disaccharides such as lactose and sucrose and starch-digestion products such as maltotriose and α-limit dextrins must be hydrolyzed by brush border enzymes into monosaccharides for absorption by the mucosa. If these brush border enzymes are not active or if the brush border is damaged, malabsorption of the specific carbohydrate substrate results. This can result in gaseousness or osmotic diarrhea when those substrates are ingested. This rarely occurs on a congenital basis, but it commonly occurs as an acquired disorder.

Lactase deficiency is the most common acquired disaccharidase deficiency. Infant mammals all rely on lactose as the carbohydrate source in milk, but lactase activity is shut off after weaning in most species. Most human populations lose lactase activity during adolescence as a normal part of maturation. Members of the northern European gene pool might maintain lactase activity into adult life, but lactase activity declines gradually in many. At some point the amount of lactose ingested might exceed the ability of the remaining enzyme to hydrolyze it, resulting in lactose malabsorption and symptoms. This also can occur with acute conditions such as gastroenteritis that can disturb the mucosa and temporarily reduce lactase activity. Patients might not recognize lactose ingestion as a cause of their problem because they have not had difficulty tolerating lactose in the past. Restriction of lactose in the diet (or use of products that have predigested lactose) mitigates symptoms. Use of exogenous lactase as a tablet may only be partially effective because of incomplete hydrolysis of ingested lactose.

Transport Defects at the Brush Border

Glucose-galactose malabsorption is a rare congenital disorder resulting from an inactive hexose transporter in the brush border. Hydrolysis of lactose is intact, but transport across the apical membrane of the enterocyte fails to occur. Fructose absorption, which is mediated by a different carrier, is unaffected.

In all human beings the ability to absorb fructose is limited by the availability of carriers in the brush border and may be overwhelmed when excess fructose is ingested. This can occur relatively easily nowadays, because high-fructose corn syrup is used frequently as a sweetener in commercial products such as soda pop. Limiting the amount of fructose ingested will reduce symptoms.

Abetalipoproteinemia is a rare condition that prevents absorption of long-chain fatty acids due to failure to form chylomicrons. Use of medium-chain triglycerides that do not require transport in chylomicrons can bypass this defect.

Pernicious anemia develops when failure to secrete intrinsic factor in the stomach prevents vitamin B_{12} absorption by the ileal mucosa. Parenteral replacement with cyanocobalamin by injection (Cyanoject) or nasal spray (Nascobal) is necessary.

GENERALIZED MALABSORPTION

Celiac Disease

Celiac disease (also known as celiac sprue) is a disorder in which the mucosa of the small bowel is damaged due to activation of the mucosal immune system by ingestion of gluten, a protein component found in wheat, barley, and rye. People who have HLA-DQ2 or DQ8 are susceptible to this condition because these specific antigen-presenting proteins produce particularly strong reactions by interacting with a unique peptide digestion product of gluten. Tissue transglutaminase, an enzyme produced in the mucosa, is an important cofactor in pathogenesis by amplifying the immunogenicity of gluten peptide fragments and is the target of autoantibodies that are characteristic of this disease. The condition produces generalized malabsorption by destroying the villi of the small intestine, reducing the surface area available for absorption.

In addition to malabsorption syndrome with diarrhea and weight loss, celiac disease can produce a host of nonspecific symptoms, including abdominal pain, fatigue, muscle and joint pains, and headaches and seemingly unrelated problems such as iron deficiency anemia, abnormal liver tests, and osteoporosis. These protean manifestations mean that celiac disease must be considered in the differential diagnosis of many conditions. The clinical course is quite variable, with symptoms coming and going. Symptoms can develop during childhood and produce growth retardation or first become manifest in adulthood.

Testing for celiac disease has been simplified by the development of an assay for anti–tissue transglutaminase antibodies. This test largely supplants measurement of antigluten antibodies, although these remain of some use in evaluating adherence to a gluten-free diet. IgA antibodies are the most useful for diagnosis, but IgA deficiency is common enough that an IgA level should be measured concomitantly.

Although serologic tests have high sensitivity and specificity, the implications of adhering to a gluten-free diet are so extreme that the diagnosis of celiac disease should be confirmed whenever possible by small bowel mucosal biopsy, now obtained routinely by endoscopy. An empiric trial of a gluten-free diet may be difficult to interpret because many persons with gastrointestinal symptoms improve with dietary carbohydrate restriction. Wheat starch is particularly hard to digest (due to gluten coating wheat starch granules), and ordinarily 20% of wheat starch are not absorbed by the small bowel and enter the colon.

Treatment of celiac disease at present involves strict lifetime exclusion of gluten from the diet. This is a difficult regimen that excludes most processed foods. Assistance of a dietitian is most helpful. The prognosis with effective treatment is very good. Symptoms should respond to the diet within weeks; failure to do so should prompt an examination of compliance with the diet or reconsideration of the diagnosis. Failure to respond may be seen when lymphoma or adenocarcinoma complicate the course of celiac disease or in cases of "refractory sprue" or "collagenous sprue" which can have a different autoimmune basis from classic celiac disease and which might respond to immunosuppressive drugs such as corticosteroids or azathioprine (Imuran).[1] Persistent diarrhea may be observed in patients with celiac disease who have concomitant microscopic colitis, another condition that is linked to HLA-DQ2 and HLA-DQ8.

Inflammatory Diseases

Diseases that produce extensive mucosal damage by inflammation cause generalized malabsorption by reduction of mucosal surface area, by promotion of small bowel bacterial overgrowth, by ileal dysfunction, or by development of enteroenteral or enterocolic fistulas. Examples include jejunoileitis due to Crohn's disease, nongranulomatous ulcerative jejunoileitis, radiation enteritis, and chronic mesenteric ischemia. With Crohn's disease, previous resection can

---

[1]Not FDA approved for this indication.

add to the problem (see later). Therapy aimed at the underlying process can improve absorption; in some cases (e.g., radiation enteritis) no effective therapy is available for the underlying problem, and symptomatic management is all that is possible. This includes use of antidiarrheal drugs to prolong contact time between luminal contents and the small bowel mucosa, ingestion of a reduced fat diet to reduce steatorrhea, and use of vitamin and mineral supplements to prevent deficiency states.

Infiltrative Disorders

Several conditions involve infiltration of the intestinal mucosa with cells or extracellular matrix that impede absorption or modify mucosal function by secretion of cytokines and other regulatory substances. These include eosinophilic gastroenteritis, systemic mastocytosis, immunoproliferative small intestinal disease (IPSID), lymphoma, and amyloidosis. These conditions are diagnosed by mucosal biopsy, but special stains might have to be employed to identify the infiltrating cells or matrix accurately.

Treatment of the underlying processes can improve absorption, but it is not uniformly effective. For eosinophilic gastroenteritis, a hypoallergenic (elimination) diet and corticosteroids may be useful. Mild systemic mastocytosis is treated with the mast cell-stabilizer sodium chromoglycate, H_1- and H_2-receptor antagonists, and low-dose aspirin. More advanced disease might respond to interferon or cytotoxic chemotherapy. IPSID initially is treated with antibiotics because small bowel bacterial overgrowth may be a causative factor. Once malignant change has occurred, it is treated like lymphoma with cytotoxic chemotherapy. Amyloidosis affecting the gut is not amenable to therapy and is usually fatal.

Infectious Diseases

Small Bowel Bacterial Overgrowth

Small bowel bacterial overgrowth in the jejunum can produce generalized malabsorption. It can occur whenever the mechanisms that reduce overgrowth are compromised. These situations include achlorhydria or hypochlorhydria, motility disorders of the small intestine (e.g., diabetes mellitus or scleroderma), and anatomic alterations (e.g., diverticulosis, gastrocolic fistula, or blind loops postoperatively). Fat malabsorption is attributed to bacterial deconjugation of bile acid. Bacterial toxins or free fatty acids can produce patchy mucosal damage, leading to less efficient carbohydrate and protein absorption. Bacteria also can compete with the mucosa for uptake of certain nutrients such as vitamin B_{12}.

Diagnosis of small bowel bacterial overgrowth can be difficult (see earlier). Treatment consists of antibiotic therapy unless a surgically correctable anatomic defect is discovered. Tetracycline is no longer uniformly effective; amoxicillin–clavulinic acid (Augmentin), cephalosporins, ciprofloxacin (Cipro), metronidazole (Flagyl), and rifaximin (Xifaxan) may be employed. Therapy should be given for 1 to 2 weeks initially and then discontinued. It should be restarted when symptoms recur. If this occurs quickly, longer treatment periods should be considered. Continuous antibiotic therapy is needed rarely.

Tropical Sprue

Tropical sprue is a progressive, chronic malabsorptive condition occurring in both the indigenous population and in visitors residing in certain tropical countries for extended periods. The prevalence of tropical sprue seems to be decreasing for uncertain reasons. The disease starts as an acute diarrheal disease that becomes a persistent diarrhea associated with substantial weight loss and typically megaloblastic anemia. Villi become shortened and thickened (partial villous atrophy), but the flat mucosa of celiac disease is not usually present. Enterocytes have disrupted brush borders and can have megaloblastic changes; the submucosa has a chronic inflammatory infiltrate. Intestinal biopsy is required for diagnosis.

Currently, tropical sprue is believed to represent a form of bacterial overgrowth with organisms that secrete enterotoxins. Most patients have evidence of excessive gram-negative bacterial colonization of the jejunum. The declining prevalence of tropical sprue may be due to improved nutrition, better sanitation, or prompt treatment of acute diarrhea with antibiotics. Treatment consists of pharmacologic doses of folic acid (folate) (5 mg daily[3]), injection of cyanocobalamin (if deficient), and antibiotic therapy for 1 to 6 months. Tetracycline 250 mg four times a day or sulfonamide is the treatment of choice. Newer antibiotics have not been tested extensively in this condition. Improvement should be noted after a few weeks. The prognosis with treatment is excellent; without treatment, tropical sprue can be fatal. Recurrence can occur.

Whipple's Disease

Whipple's disease is a rare chronic bacterial infection with multisystem involvement. The small bowel typically is heavily infiltrated with foamy macrophages containing periodic acid–Schiff (PAS)-positive material, distorting the villi. Small bowel biopsy with special stains or electron microscopy or a specific polymerase chain reaction (PCR) is diagnostic. Foamy macrophages and bacteria can be found outside the intestine in lymph nodes, spleen, liver, central nervous system, heart, and synovium. Accordingly, symptoms are protean. The bacterium has been identified as *Tropheryma whippelii*, a relative of *Acinetobacter*. It does not appear to be very contagious, and no direct person-to-person transmission has been demonstrated. Presumably differences in host resistance allow proliferation within macrophages without clearance of the bacteria.

Whipple's disease occurs mainly in older white men, but women and all ethnic groups are susceptible. Patients can present with malabsorption syndrome or with symptoms related to the extraintestinal disease (arthritis, fever, dementia, headache, or muscle weakness). Gross or occult gastrointestinal bleeding can occur. Protein-losing enteropathy may be present.

Treatment with any of several antibiotics (penicillin, erythromycin, ampicillin, tetracycline, chloramphenicol, or trimethoprim-sulfamethoxazole [TMP-SMX]) produces excellent symptomatic responses within days to weeks, but it should be continued for months to years. Even with protracted courses, relapses are common.

Other Infections

Mycobacterium avium–intracellulare is another chronic bacterial infection that can cause malabsorption, particularly in patients with AIDS. Mucosal biopsy with special stains to distinguish it from Whipple's disease is essential. Antibiotic therapy can reduce the intensity of infection; clearance depends on immunologic reconstitution with antiretroviral therapy. Clarithromycin (Biaxin) and ethambutol (Myambutol) are recommended as initial therapy.

Parasitic diseases can produce malabsorption by competing for nutrients and causing mechanical occlusion of the absorptive surface and epithelial damage. Protozoa that may be associated with malabsorption include *Giardia lamblia*, *Isospora belli*, *Cryptosporidium*, and *Enterocytozoon bieneusi*. Tapeworms associated with malabsorption include *Taenia saginata* (beef tapeworm), *Hymenolepis nana* (dwarf tapeworm), and *Diphyllobothrium latum* (fish tapeworm).

Giardia lamblia is a cosmopolitan parasite acquired from contaminated water or from another person by fecal-oral transmission. Cysts are relatively hardy, and ingestion of as few as 10 cysts is sufficient to establish infection. Patients with dysgammaglobulinemia (especially IgA deficiency) are likely to become infected. Diagnosis depends on finding the organism (cysts or trophozoites) in stool by microscopy (sensitivity ~50% for a single specimen), or detection of giardia antigens by immunologic testing of stool (sensitivity >90%), or discovery of the organism on small bowel biopsy.

Therapy consists of a single dose of tinidazole (Tindamax) (2 g), metronidazole (Flagyl)[1] (250 mg three times a day for a week), nitazoxanide (Alinia) (500 mg twice a day for three days), or quinacrine[2] (100 mg three times a day for a week).

---

[1]Not FDA approved for this indication.
[2]Not available in the United States.
[3]Exceeds dosage recommended by the manufacturer.

Isospora belli and *Cryptosporidium* spp. are coccidia, protozoa that disrupt the epithelium by intracellular invasion *(Isospora)* or by attaching to the brush border, destroying microvilli *(Crptosporidium)*. Stool examination or small bowel biopsy can identify the organism. *Cryptosporidium* antigen can be discovered by immunoassay on stool with excellent sensitivity. *Isospora* can be treated with TMP-SMX[1] or furazolidone.[2] *Cryptosporidium* can be treated by nitazoxanide.

Microsporidia are intracellular organisms now believed to be most closely related to fungi and are implicated in diarrhea and malabsorption in patients with AIDS and other immunodeficiency states. Small bowel biopsy can show partial villous atrophy, and electron microscopy displays characteristic changes. Stool examination occasionally is helpful. No treatment is of proven value.

Tapeworms compete with their hosts for nutrients in the lumen. *Diphyllobothrium latum* can produce vitamin B_{12} deficiency. The others can result in more extensive nutritional deficiencies. Diagnosis is based on stool examination, and treatment depends on the particular organism identified.

Luminal Problems Causing Malabsorption

Pancreatic Exocrine Insufficiency

Pancreatic exocrine insufficiency is the most common luminal problem that results in maldigestion. Patients develop symptoms of malabsorption when pancreatic enzyme secretion is reduced by >90%. There are several clinical features that distinguish pancreatic exocrine insufficiency from mucosal disorders, such as celiac disease. When fat is not digested, it is transported through the gastrointestinal tract as intact triglyceride, which can appear as oil in the stool. In contrast, if fat is digested but not absorbed, it is in the form of fatty acids that can produce secretory diarrhea in the colon, resulting in more voluminous, even watery stools. This has two important ramifications: Fecal fat concentration is lower with mucosal disease (typically <9% by weight), and hypocalcemia due to formation of soaps (calcium plus 2 fatty acids) is seen with mucosal disease but not with pancreatic exocrine insufficiency. In addition, patients with mucosal disease tend to have more problems with water-soluble vitamin deficiencies than those with pancreatic exocrine insufficiency. In some patients with pancreatic exocrine insufficiency, carbohydrate malabsorption can produce substantial bloating, flatulence, and watery diarrhea.

Tests to document pancreatic exocrine insufficiency are not widely available or are nonspecific (see earlier), and so diagnosis usually hinges on a consistent history, demonstration of anatomic problems in the pancreas (calcification or abnormal ducts), and documentation of a response of steatorrhea to empiric treatment with a large dose of exogenous enzymes.

Bile Acid Deficiency

Bile acid deficiency is a less common cause of maldigestion, and malabsorption in this setting is limited to fat and fat-soluble vitamins. The usual setting is a patient with an extensive ileal resection (see later), but this also occurs in certain cholestatic conditions in which bile acid secretion by the liver is markedly compromised, such as advanced primary biliary cirrhosis, or complete extrahepatic biliary obstruction. As with pancreatic exocrine insufficiency, stools tend to have high fat concentrations (>9% by weight) when bile acid secretion is limited by hepatic or biliary disorders.

Zollinger-Ellison Syndrome

Zollinger-Ellison syndrome produces several abnormalities that can affect absorption. High rates of gastric acid secretion produce persistently low pH in the duodenum, which precipitates bile acid and inactivates pancreatic enzymes. In addition, excess acid can damage the absorptive cells directly.

Postoperative Malabsorption

Substantial malabsorption can result from gastric surgeries. Weight loss can result from inadequate intake due to early satiety or symptoms of dumping syndrome. Malabsorption can result from impaired mechanical disruption of food, mismatching of chyme delivery and enzyme secretion, rapid transit, or small bowel bacterial overgrowth due to loss of the gastric acid barrier. In addition, gastric surgery sometimes brings out latent celiac disease.

Short intestinal resections are well tolerated, but more extensive resections produce diarrhea and malabsorption of variable severity. When these symptoms are associated with weight loss or dehydrating diarrhea, short bowel syndrome is said to exist. In general, nutrient absorptive needs can be met if at least 100 cm of jejunum are preserved, but fluid absorption will be insufficient and diarrhea may be profuse. The process of intestinal adaptation permits improved absorption with time; it depends on exposure of the absorptive surface to nutrients. Absorption of specific substances, such as bile acids or vitamin B_{12}, is reduced permanently by resection of the terminal ileum.

Malabsorption in short bowel syndrome is not due solely to loss of absorptive surface area. Gastric acid hypersecretion, bile acid deficiency, rapid transit (due to loss of the ileal brake), and bacterial overgrowth may be present. These conditions are amenable to treatment and therapy with antisecretory drugs, exogenous bile acids, opiate antidiarrheals, or antibiotics can produce substantial improvement. Injection of growth hormone in combination with glutamine and a special diet has been approved as treatment for short bowel syndrome; it can reduce the volume of parenteral fluid or nutrients required. Results with small bowel transplantation are improving with the use of better immunosuppressive regimens, and it remains the only cure for select patients with postresection malabsorption.

Attention to nutrition is vital in any patient with malabsorption. If adequate nutrition cannot be maintained by oral intake, nutritional therapy is needed. Because of impaired bowel function, success with enteral nutrition may be impossible; parenteral nutrition may be needed. It is important to distinguish between the need for supplemental fluid and electrolytes and the need for nutrients; total parenteral nutrition is not a good choice for patients who only require fluids and electrolytes.

REFERENCES

Batheja MJ, Leighton J, Azueta A, Heigh R. The Face of Tropical Sprue in 2010. Case Rep Gastroenterol 2010;4:168–72.

Catassi C, Fasano A. Celiac disease diagnosis: simple rules are better than complicated algorithms. Am J Med 2010;123:691–3.

DiMagno MJ, DiMagno EP. Chronic pancreatitis. Curr Opin Gastroenterol 2010;26:490–8.

Fernández-Bañares F, Esteve M, Viver JM. Fructose-sorbitol malabsorption. Curr Gastroenterol Rep 2009;11:368–74.

Lagier JC, Lepidi H, Raoult D, Fenollar F. Systemic Tropheryma whipplei: Clinical presentation of 142 patients with infections diagnosed or confirmed in a reference center. Medicine (Baltimore) 2010;89:337–45.

Rubio-Tapia A, Murray JA. Celiac disease. Curr Opin Gastroenterol 2010;26: 116–22.

Schiller LR. Diarrhea and malabsorption in the elderly. Gastroenterol Clin North Am 2009;38:481–502.

Shatnawei A, Parekh NR, Rhoda KM, Speerhas R, Stafford J, Dasari V, Quintini C, Kirby DF, Steiger E. Intestinal failure management at the Cleveland Clinic. Arch Surg 2010;145:521–7.

Tack GJ, Verbeek WH, Schreurs MW, Mulder CJ. The spectrum of celiac disease: epidemiology, clinical aspects and treatment. Nat Rev Gastroenterol Hepatol 2010;7:204–13.

Wales PW, Nasr A, de Silva N, Yamada J. Human growth hormone and glutamine for patients with short bowel syndrome. Cochrane Database Syst Rev 2010;6(6):CD006321.

Wedlake L, A'Hern R, Russell D, Thomas K, Walters JR, Andreyev HJ. Systematic review: the prevalence of idiopathic bile acid malabsorption as diagnosed by SeHCAT scanning in patients with diarrhoea-predominant irritable bowel syndrome. Aliment Pharmacol Ther 2009;30:707–17.

---

[1] Not FDA approved for this indication.
[2] Not available in the United States.

Acute and Chronic Pancreatitis

Method of
William E. Fisher, MD

Acute Pancreatitis

Acute pancreatitis is an inflammatory disease of the pancreas that is associated with little or no fibrosis of the gland. It can be initiated by several factors including gallstones, alcohol, trauma, and infections, and in some cases it is hereditary (Box 1). Very often patients with acute pancreatitis develop additional complications such as sepsis, shock, and respiratory and renal failure, resulting in considerable morbidity and mortality

EPIDEMIOLOGY

The annual incidence is of acute pancreatitis is probably about 50 cases per 100,000 population in the United States. Roughly 3000 of these cases are severe enough to lead to death.

RISK FACTORS

Biliary tract stone disease accounts for 70% to 80% of the cases of acute pancreatitis. Alcoholism accounts for another 10%, and the remaining 10% to 20% is accounted for either by idiopathic disease or by a variety of iatrogenic and miscellaneous causes including trauma, endoscopy, surgery, drugs, heredity, infection, and toxins.

PATHOPHYSIOLOGY

Pancreatitis begins with the activation of digestive zymogens inside acinar cells, which cause acinar cell injury. Digestive zymogens are colocalized with lysosomal hydrolase, and cathepsin-B catalyzed trypsinogen activation occurs, resulting in the acinar cell injury and necrosis. This triggers acinar cell inflammatory events with the secretion of inflammatory mediators. Studies suggest that the ultimate severity of the resulting pancreatitis may be determined by the events that occur subsequent to acinar cell injury. These include inflammatory cell recruitment and activation, as well as generation and release of cytokines, reactive oxygen species, and other chemical mediators of inflammation, ultimately leading to ischemia and necrosis. Early mortality in severe acute pancreatitis is caused by a systemic inflammatory response syndrome with multiorgan failure. If the patient survives this critical early period, a septic complication caused by translocated bacteria, mostly gram-negative microbes from the intestine, leads to infected pancreatic necrosis. Late deaths are caused by infected necrosis, leading to septic shock and multiorgan failure.

BOX 1   Common Causes of Acute Pancreatitis

Gallstones
Alcoholism
Hereditary
Hypertriglyceridemia
Trauma (including iatrogenic: ERCP or surgery)
Drugs: azathioprine, furosemide, mercaptopurine, opiates, pentamidine, steroids, sulfasalazine, sulindac, tetracycline, trimethoprim-sulfamethoxazole, valproic acid
Tumor
Infection (parasitic and viral)
Idiopathic

Abbreviation: ERCP = endoscopic retrograde cholangiopancreatography.

PREVENTION

Gallstones are present in about 15% to 20% of patients older than 60 years, but only a fraction become symptomatic. Although gallstone pancreatitis can rarely be the first symptom of gallstones, most patients have symptoms of cholecystitis before developing pancreatitis. Thus early and prompt referral of patients with symptomatic cholelithiasis for laparoscopic cholecystectomy to prevent life-threatening complications such as acute pancreatitis is important.

CLINICAL MANIFESTATIONS

All episodes of acute pancreatitis begin with severe pain, generally following a substantial meal. The pain is usually epigastric, but it can occur anywhere in the abdomen or lower chest. It has been described as penetrating through to the back, and it may be relieved by the patient's leaning forward. It precedes the onset of nausea and vomiting, with retching often continuing after the stomach has emptied. Vomiting does not relieve the pain, which is more intense in necrotizing than in edematous pancreatitis.

On examination the patient may show tachycardia, tachypnea, hypotension, and hyperthermia. The temperature is usually only mildly elevated in uncomplicated pancreatitis. Voluntary and involuntary guarding can be seen over the epigastric region. The bowel sounds are decreased or absent. There are usually no palpable masses. The abdomen may be distended with intraperitoneal fluid. There may be pleural effusion, particularly on the left side. With increasing severity of disease, the intravascular fluid loss may become life-threatening as a result of sequestration of edematous fluid in the retroperitoneum. Hemoconcentration then results in an elevated hematocrit. However, there also may be bleeding into the retroperitoneum or the peritoneal cavity. In some patients (about 1%), the blood from necrotizing pancreatitis can dissect through the soft tissues and manifest as a bluish discoloration around the umbilicus (Cullen's sign) or in the flanks (Grey Turner sign). The severe fluid loss cany lead to prerenal azotemia, with elevated blood urea nitrogen and creatinine levels. There also may be hyperglycemia, hypoalbuminemia, and hypocalcemia sufficient in some cases to produce tetany.

DIAGNOSIS

Although serum amylase is often elevated in acute pancreatitis, there is no significant correlation between the magnitude of serum amylase elevation and severity of pancreatitis. Other pancreatic enzymes also have been evaluated to improve the diagnostic accuracy of serum measurements. Specificity of these markers ranges from 77% to 96%, the highest being for lipase. Measurements of many digestive enzymes have methodologic limitations and cannot be easily adapted for quantitation in emergency laboratory studies. Because serum levels of lipase remain elevated for a longer time than total or pancreatic amylase, it is the serum indicator of highest probability of the disease.

Abdominal ultrasound examination is the best way to confirm the presence of gallstones in suspected biliary pancreatitis. It also can detect extrapancreatic ductal dilations and reveal pancreatic edema, swelling, and peripancreatic fluid collections. However, in about 20% of patients, the ultrasound examination does not provide satisfactory results because of the presence of bowel gas, which can obscure sonographic imaging of the pancreas.

 CURRENT DIAGNOSIS

- Acute pancreatitis is usually caused by gallstones, and chronic pancreatitis is usually caused by alcohol abuse.
- Other less-common causes of acute and chronic pancreatitis are considered only when gallstones and alcohol are definitively ruled out.
- Pancreatic cancer and chronic pancreatitis can sometimes be difficult to distinguish.

A computed tomographic (CT) scan of the pancreas is more commonly used to diagnose pancreatitis. CT scanning is used to distinguish milder (nonnecrotic) forms of the disease from more severe necrotizing or infected pancreatitis, in patients whose clinical presentation raises the suspicion of advanced disease (Figs. 1 and 2).

DIFFERENTIAL DIAGNOSIS

The clinical diagnosis of pancreatitis is one of exclusion. Hyperamylasemia can also occur as a result of conditions not involving pancreatitis. The other upper abdominal conditions that can be confused with acute pancreatitis include perforated peptic ulcer and acute colecystitis, and occasionally a gangrenous small bowel obstruction. Because these conditions often have a fatal outcome without surgery, urgent intervention is indicated in the small number of cases in which doubt persists. A tumor should be considered in a nonalcoholic patient with acute pancreatitis who has no demonstrable biliary tract disease. Approximately 1% to 2% of patients with acute pancreatitis have pancreatic carcinoma, and an episode of acute pancreatitis can be the first clinical manifestation of a periampullary tumor.

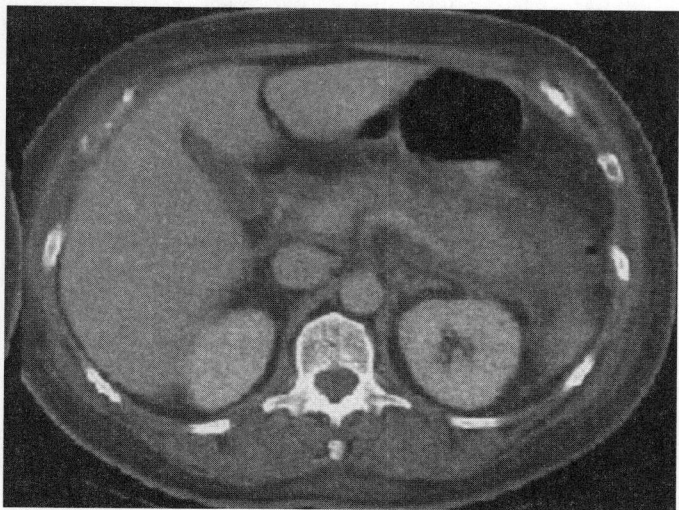

FIGURE 1. Computed tomographic scan confirming acute edematous pancreatitis.

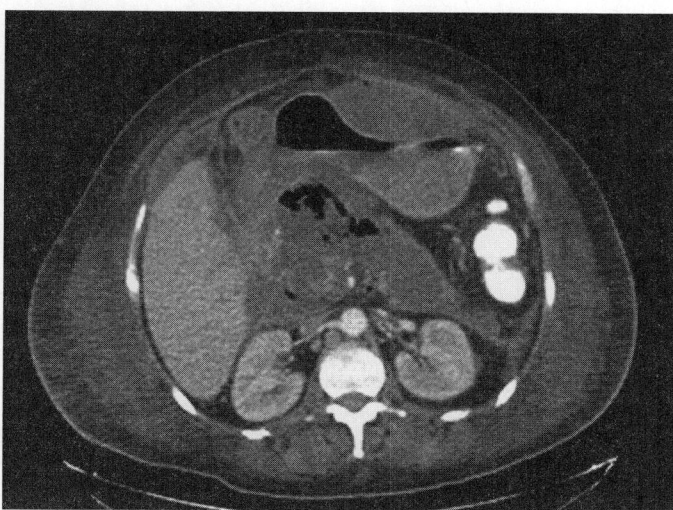

FIGURE 2. Computed tomographic scan confirming acute necrotizing, emphysematous pancreatitis.

TREATMENT

The severity of acute pancreatitis covers a broad spectrum of illness, ranging from the mild and self-limiting to the life-threatening necrotizing variety. Some cases are so mild they can be treated in an outpatient setting. However, most cases require hospitalization for observation and diagnostic study. A conservative approach has been advocated in the treatment of acute pancreatitis (Box 2). Severity is assessed with imaging results and clinical parameters and is quantitated with scores such as Ranson's criteria (Box 3), the Atlanta classification, and the APACHE II (Acute Physiology And Chronic Health Evaluation) score. Severe acute pancreatitis is defined by associated organ dysfunction. The Atlanta classification is based on an international concensus conference held in Atlanta in 1992 and has been updated. APACHE II was designed to measure the severity of disease for adult patients admitted to intensive care units. Though not

---

BOX 2 Treatment of Acute Pancreatitis

Assessment of severity
Fluid resuscitation and oxygenation
Early nasojejunal feeding
Avoid prophylactic antibiotics (reserve antibiotic therapy
   for specific infections)
Avoid or postpone necrosectomy if possible
Options for necrosectomy
- Open anterior approach with closed lavage
- Open anterior approach with packing and reoperation
- Open retroperitoneal approach
- Laparoscopic anterior approach with closed lavage
- Video-assisted retroperitoneal débridement (VARD)

BOX 3 Ranson's Criteria

There are 11 Ranson signs. Five of the signs are evaluated when the patient is admitted to the hospital and the remaining six are evaluated 48 hours after admission. The signs are added to reach a score:
- If the score <3, severe pancreatitis is unlikely.
- If the score ≥3, severe pancreatitis likely.

or
- Score 0-2: 2% mortality
- Score 3-4: 15% mortality
- Score 5-6: 40% mortality
- Score 7-8: 100% mortality

At Admission

Age in years >55 years
White blood cell count >16,000 cells/mm^3
Blood glucose >11 mmol/L (>200 mg/dL)
Serum AST >250 IU/L
Serum LDH >350 IU/L

At 48 Hours

Calcium (serum calcium) <2.0 mmol/L (<8.0 mg/dL)
Hematocrit fall >10%
Oxygen (hypoxemia Po_2 <60 mm Hg)
BUN increased by ≥1.8 mmol/L (≥5 mg/dL) after IV
   fluid hydration
Base deficit (negative base excess) >4 mEq/L
Sequestration of fluids >6 L

Abbreviations: ALT = alanine aminotransferase; AST = aspartate aminotransferase; BUN = blood urea nitrogen.

CURRENT THERAPY

- There has been a recent trend toward conservative medical therapy for acute and chronic pancreatitis, reserving surgery as a last resort.
- In acute pancreatitis, try to avoid necrosectomy except in the setting of infected necrosis with organ failure.
- Asymptomatic pseudocysts can generally be observed.
- Persistent symptomatic pseudocysts can often be addressed endoscopically.
- Medical therapy for chronic pancreatitis includes pain management, nutrition, diabetes control, and cessation of drinking alcohol and smoking.
- Surgical treatment for chronic pancreatitis currently favors strict patient selection and parenchyma-preserving techniques.

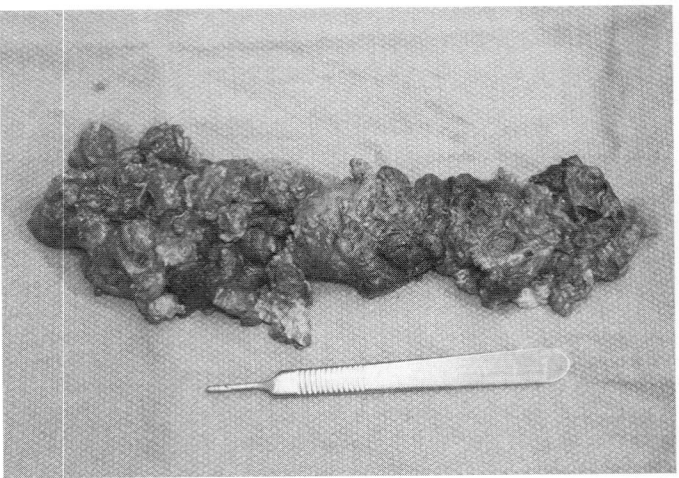

FIGURE 3. Necrotic material débrided from the retroperitoneum in a case of acute necrotizing pancreatitis.

specific to pancreatitis, APACHE II can be used in an effort to differentiate patients with mild and severe acute pancreatitis. APACHE II scores of 8 points or more correlate with a mortality rate of 11% to 18%.

Upon confirmation of the diagnosis, patients with severe disease should be transferred to the intensive care unit for observation and maximum support. Adequate fluid resuscitation optimizing organ perfusion and oxygenation is essential. The use of prophylactic intravenous antibiotics in the initial stages of severe acute pancreatitis is not proved to be useful. Two randomized, controlled studies failed to show any benefit from antibiotics. Prophylactic antibiotics did not decrease the incidence of infected pancreatic necrosis or lower mortality. Data from these well-designed trials refutes prior data from less-rigorous studies suggesting prophylactic antibiotics were useful. Additional studies are required, but there is increasing concern that the prolonged use of potent antibiotics might result in an increased prevalence of fungal infections and possibly increased mortality. Currently, antibiotic therapy should be reserved for treatment of specific infections such as positive blood, sputum, and urine cultures or percutaneous or operative cultures of necrotic tissue.

Randomized clinical trials have also shown a benefit from early nasojejunal feeding compared to total parenteral nutrition. Gastric decompression with a nasogastric tube is selectively used in patients with severe ileus and vomiting but is not necessary in a majority of cases.

In biliary pancreatitis, the gallbladder must eventually be removed or recurrent acute pancreatitis will occur in 30% to 60%. The timing of the cholecystectomy depends on the severity of the pancreatitis. Usually laparoscopic cholecystectomy is performed during the index admission as soon as the attack of acute pancreatitis has resolved. In more-severe cases, the cholecystectomy is delayed and often combined with interventions for late complications of acute pancreatitis. In cases with severe comorbidity, endoscopic sphincterotomy has been considered as an alternative to cholecystectomy. However, if the patient has a postinflammatory fluid collection, bacteria can be introduced during endoscopic retrograde cholangiopancreatography (ERCP) and sphincterotomy should be delayed.

Currently, there is no role for routine early laparotomy and necrosectomy or resection in the setting of acute necrotizing pancreatitis. If the necrotic pancreas becomes infected and the patient fails to respond to treatment, then necrosectomy may be warranted. Patients with infected necrosis are rarely managed conservatively without surgical intervention. However, even in the setting of infected necrosis, there has been consideration for antibiotic therapy until the acute inflammatory response has subsided if possible, with the view that surgery that is deferred for several weeks is more easily accomplished with one intervention. Patients who suffer from infected necrosis without having clinical signs of sepsis or other systemic complications might not need immediate surgical necrosectomy.

A nonsurgical alternative for the treatment of infected necrosis is percutaneous catheter drainage. This is considered a temporary measure to allow stabilization of the patient so that a safer surgical necrosectomy can be done at a later time. Multiple large drains are required, and patients frequently undergo repeat CT and revision of the drains. Current recommendations are to postpone surgery for as long as possible, usually beyond the second or third week of the disease or later, when necrotic tissue can be easily distinguished from viable pancreas and débridement without major blood loss can be performed. When surgery is performed, tissue-preserving digital necrosectomy is the usual technique rather than a classic surgical resection of the pancreas (Fig. 3).

Necrosectomy can be performed by an open anterior approach with closed lavage or with leaving the abdomen open and packing. The packing is replaced at intervals of 24 to 72 hours. Sometimes a left lateral retroperitoneal approach is helpful. Newer approaches are the video-assisted retroperitoneal débridement (VARD). This procedure is a combination of percutaneous drainage and the open lateral retroperitoneal approach. An anterior laparoscopic approach has also been described and mimics the open anterior approach using laparoscopic ports. Surgical necrosectomy is indicated in patients with sepsis caused by infected necrosis and in selected patients with extended sterile necrosis causing severe systemic organ dysfunction and sepsis without a septic focus.

In some cases, the acute inflammatory process can lead to erosion into retroperitoneal vessels, and acute hemorrhage occurs. This acute emergent complication is best managed with immediate angiography to determine the exact site of bleeding and can often be treated with embolization rather than surgery (Fig. 4).

MONITORING

Despite a conservative operative approach, endocrine and exocrine insufficiency develop in as many as half of the patients and is determined by the extent of pancreatic necrosis. Therefore, patients must be monitored with blood glucose measurements and stabilization of body weight and proper nutrition.

COMPLICATIONS

The most common complication after successful management of acute pancreatitis is a pseudocyst. The management of pseudocysts has also followed a minimally invasive trend. Most pseudocysts resolve spontaneously, even beyond 6 weeks, so asymptomatic pseudocysts are usually observed. Endoscopic cystogastrostomy is the approach of choice for symptomatic fluid-predominant pseudocysts when there is minimal necrosis. If there is significant necrotic debris or a solid-predominant pseudocyst, surgical drainage with laparoscopic cystogastrostomy is preferred (Fig. 5). This can also be performed with the traditional open technique. Cystjejunostomy (laparoscopic or open) is used in cases in which the site of the pseudocyst precludes drainage into the posterior aspect of the stomach.

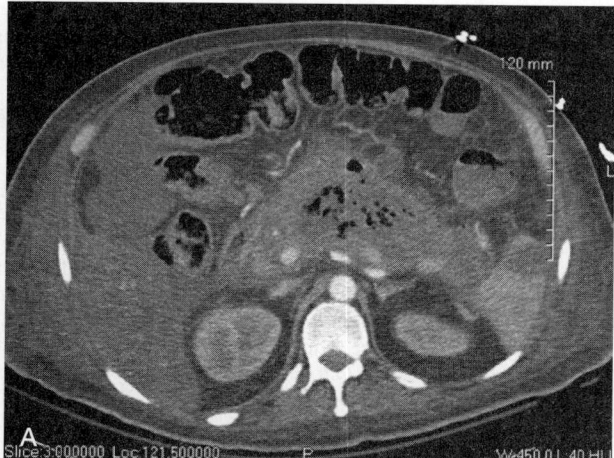

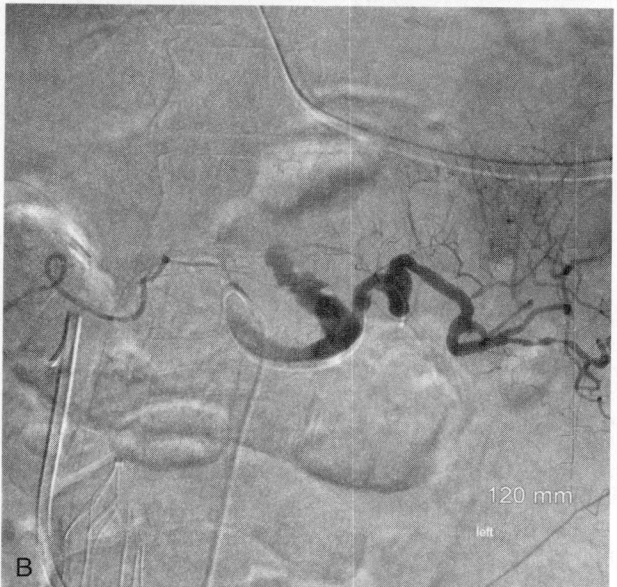

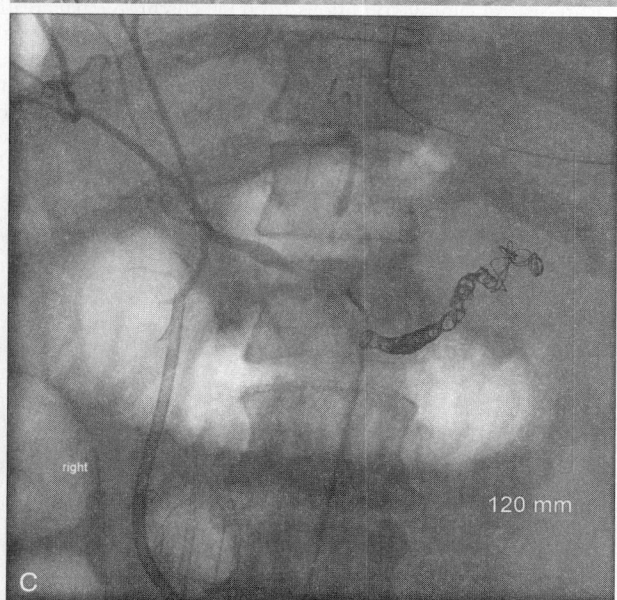

FIGURE 4. Acute necrotizing pancreatitis. **A,** Erosion into the splenic artery as seen on computed tomography. **B,** Erosion into the splenic artery as seen on angiogram. **C,** This complication of acute pancreatitis is best treated with angiographic embolization.

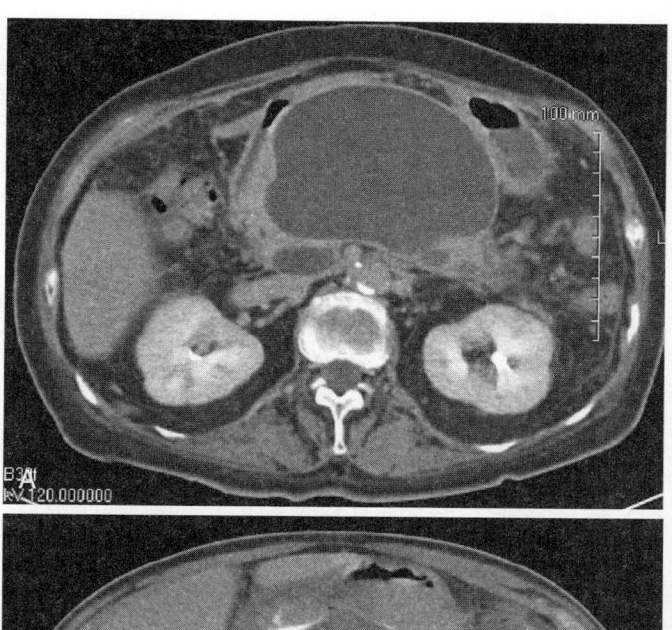

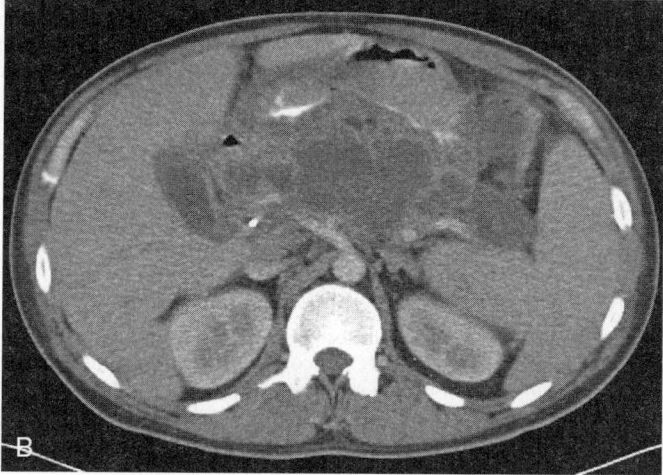

FIGURE 5. Computed tomographic scan showing fluid-predominant **(A)** and solid-predominant **(B)** pseudocysts. The former can be treated with endoscopic cystogastrostomy, and the latter is best treated with laparoscopic cystogastrostomy.

Chronic Pancreatitis

Chronic pancreatitis is a chronic inflammatory diesease of the pancreas characterized by irreversible morphologic changes that typically are associated with pain or permanent loss of function, or both.

EPIDEMIOLOGY

Population studies suggest a prevalence of chronic pancreatitis that ranges from 5 to 27 persons per 100,000 population, with considerable geographic variation. Autopsy data are difficult to interpret because a number of changes associated with chronic pancreatitis, such as fibrosis, duct ectasia, and acinar atrophy, are also present in asymptomatic elderly patients. Differences in diagnostic criteria, regional nutrition, alcohol consumption, and medical access account for variations in the frequency of the diagnosis, but the overall incidence of the disease has risen progressively since the 1960s. Chronic pancreatitis in the United States currently results in more than 120,000 outpatient visits and more than 50,000 hospitalizations per year.

RISK FACTORS

Alcohol consumption and alcohol abuse are associated with chronic pancreatitis in up to 70% of cases. Other major causes include tropical (nutritional) and idiopathic disease, as well as hereditary causes. There is a linear relationship between exposure to alcohol and the development of chronic pancreatitis. The incidence is highest in heavy drinkers (15 drinks/day or 150 g/day). However, chronic pancreatitis can occur in patients who drink very little, and it occurs in less than 15% of documented alcoholics. The duration of alcohol consumption is definitely associated with the development of pancreatic disease. The onset of disease typically occurs between ages 35 and 40 years, after 16 to 20 years of heavy alcohol consumption. Recurrent episodes of acute pancreatitis are typically followed by chronic symptoms after 4 or 5 years.

PATHOPHYSIOLOGY

Multiple episodes (or a prolonged course) of pancreatic injury ultimately leading to chronic disease is widely accepted as the pathophysiologic sequence. Most investigators believe that alcohol metabolites such as acetaldehyde, combined with oxidant injury, result in local parenchymal injury that is preferentially targeted to the pancreas in predisposed persons. Repeated or severe episodes of toxin-induced injury activate a cascade of cytokines, which in turn induces pancreatic stellate cells to produce collagen and cause fibrosis.

The pain caused by chronic pancreatitis is thought to be due to increased pressure in the pancreatic ducts and tissue. Neural and perineural inflammation is also thought to be important in pathogenesis of pain in chronic pancreatitis. Neuropeptides released from enteric and afferent neurons and their functional interactions with inflammatory cells might play a key role.

PREVENTION

Because alcohol is the cause of most cases of chronic pancreatitis, cessation of alcohol consumption is recommended to prevent progression to chronic pancreatitis. Unfortunately, the majority of patients are not able to recover from alcoholism, and relapse is common.

CLINICAL MANIFESTATIONS

Symptoms of chronic pancreatitis may be identical to those of acute pancreatitis, typically midepigastric pain penetrating through to the back. Patients with chronic pancreatic pain typically flex their abdomen and either sit or lie with their hips flexed, or lie on their side in a fetal position. Unlike ureteral stone pain or biliary colic, the pain causes the patient to be still. Nausea or vomiting can accompany the pain, but anorexia is the most common associated symptom. Patients with continuous pain can have a complication of chronic pancreatitis, such as an inflammatory mass, a cyst, or even pancreatic cancer. Other patients have intermittent attacks of pain with symptoms similar to those of mild to moderate acute pancreatitis. The pain sometimes is severe and lasts for many hours or several days.

As chronic pancreatitis progresses, endocrine and exocrine insufficiency begin to appear. Patients describe a bulky, foul-smelling, loose (but not watery) stool that may be pale and float on the surface of toilet water. Patients often describe a greasy or oily appearance to the stool or describe an "oil slick" on the water's surface. In severe steatorrhea, an orange, oily stool is often reported. As exocrine deficiency increases, symptoms of steatorrhea are often accompanied by weight loss. Patients might describe a good appetite despite weight loss, or they might have diminished food intake due to abdominal pain. The combination of decreased food intake and malabsorption of nutrients usually results in chronic weight loss. As a result, many patients with severe chronic pancreatitis are below ideal body weight. Usually islet cells are spared early in the disease process despite being surrounded by fibrosis, but eventually the insulin-secreting beta cells are also destroyed, gradually leading to diabetes.

DIAGNOSIS

The diagnosis of chronic pancreatitis depends on the clinical presentation, a limited number of indirect measurements that correlate with pancreatic function, and selected imaging studies. Diagnosis is usually simple in the late stages of the disease because of the presence of structural and functional alterations of the pancreas. Early in the disease, the diagnosis is more difficult. Various classification systems have been developed. The Cambridge classification uses imaging tests such as ERCP, CT and ultrasound to grade severity. The Mayo Clinic system is based on functional as well as imaging results. Tests of pancreatic function include the secretin-cerulein test, Lundh test, fecal excretion of pancreatic enzymes and quantitation of fecal fat.

Chronic pancreatitis can be classified as calcifying (lithogenic), obstructive, inflammatory, autoimmune, tropical (nutritional), hereditary, or idiopathic. Autoimmune and hereditary pancreatitis have recently been better understood and diagnosed more than before. Autoimmune pancreatitis is associated with fibrosis, a mononuclear cell (lymphocyte, plasma cell, or eosinophil) infiltrate, and an increased titer of one or more autoantibodies. It is usually associated with autoimmune diseases such as Sjögren's syndrome. Increased levels of serum β-globulin or immunoglobulin (Ig)G_4 are often present. This disease can be mistaken for chronic pancreatitis, with an inflammatory mass in the head of the pancreas suspicious for pancreatic cancer (Fig. 6). Diagnosis is important because steroid therapy is uniformly successful in ameliorating the disease, including any associated bile duct compression.

Hereditary pancreatitis first occurs in adolescence with abdominal pain, and patients develop progressive pancreatic dysfunction, and the risk of cancer is greatly increased. The disease follows an autosomal dominant pattern of inheritance with 80% penetrance and variable expression. Recent mutational analysis has revealed a missense mutation resulting in an Arg to His substitution at position 117 of the cationic trypsinogen gene, or *PRSS1*, one of the primary sites for proteolysis of trypsin. This mutation prevents trypsin from being inactivated by itself or other proteases, and it results in persistent and uncontrolled proteolytic activity and autodestruction within the pancreas. Similarly, *PSTI*, also known as *SPINK1*, has been found to have a role in hereditary pancreatitis and some cases of sporadic chronic pancreatitis. *SPINK1* specifically inhibits trypsin action by competitively blocking the active site of the enzyme.

It is likely that many of the "idiopathic" forms of chronic pancreatitis, as well as some patients with the more common forms of the disease, will be found to have a genetic linkage or predisposition.

DIFFERENTIAL DIAGNOSIS

There are several clinical conditions from which chronic pancreatitis needs to be distinguished. Other causes of upper abdominal pain, such as peptic ulcer disease, biliary tract disease, mesenteric vascular disease, or malignancy must be excluded. The major difficulty in the differential diagnosis of chronic pancreatitis is distinguishing it from pancreatic ductal adenocarcinoma. Chronic pancreatitis can closely

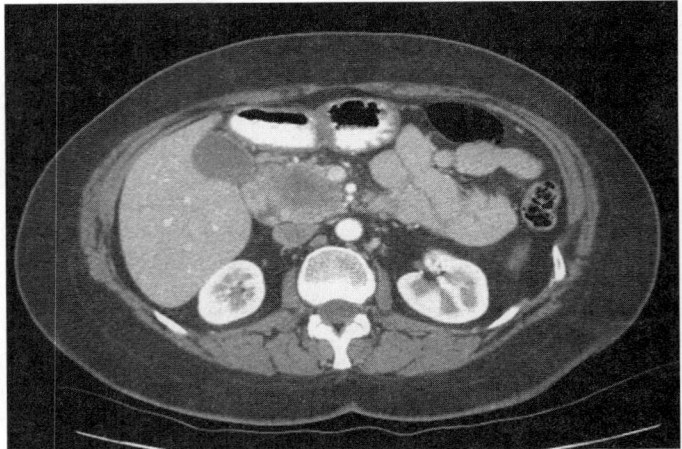

FIGURE 6. Computed tomographic scan of a patient with autoimmune pancreatitis and an inflammatory mass in the head of the pancreas. Preoperative diagnosis is not always possible, but surgery should be avoided because this disease often responds to steroid therapy.

mimic pancreatic cancer, both clinically and morphologically. In addition, chronic pancreatitis is a risk factor for the development of pancreatic cancer. Although in pancreatic resection specimens this problem may be finally resolved, distinguishing these two diseases preoperatively in small (needle) biopsy specimens is a formidable challenge for the pathologist. Therefore, especially in the setting of an inflammatory mass in the head of the pancreas, consideration of pancreatic cancer and surgical referral is important.

Treatment

Therapy for chronic pancreatitis is aimed at managing associated digestive dysfunction and relieing pain (Box 4). It is important to first address malabsorption, weight loss, and diabetes. When pancreatic exocrine capacity falls below 10% of normal, diarrhea and steatorrhea develop. Lipase deficiency tends to manifest itself before trypsin deficiency, so the presence of steatorrhea may be the first functional sign of pancreatic insufficiency. As pancreatic exocrine function deteriorates further, the secretion of bicarbonate into the duodenum is reduced, which causes duodenal acidification and further impairs nutrient absorption. Frank diabetes is seen initially in about 20% of patients with chronic pancreatitis, and impaired glucose metabolism can be detected in up to 70% of patients.

The medical treatment of chronic or recurrent pain in chronic pancreatitis requires the use of analgesics, a cessation of alcohol use, oral enzyme therapy, and endoscopic stent thearpy. Administration of pancreatic enzyme (e.g., Pancrease MT, Pancrelipase, Creon) serves to reverse the effects of pancreatic exocrine insufficiency and might also reduce or alleviate the pain[1] experienced by patients. Interventional procedures to block visceral afferent nerve conduction or to treat obstructions of the main pancreatic duct are also an adjunct to medical treatment. It has been taught that the pain of chronic pancreatitis decreases with increasing duration of the disease, the so called burn-out phase, where endocrine and exocrine insufficiency occurs and the pain decreases. However, recent studies have called this concept into question, demonstrating continued pain in patients with chronic pancreatitis despite long-standing disease and pancreatic insufficiency. Cessation of alcohol abuse, if possible, causes the pain to stop in about half of the patients.

Pain relief usually requires the use of narcotics, but these should be titrated to achieve pain relief with the lowest effective dose. Opioid addiction is common, and the use of long-acting analgesics by transdermal patch together with oral agents for pain exacerbations slightly reduces the sedative effects of high-dose oral narcotics. Celiac plexus neurolysis has been an effective form of analgesic treatment in patients with pancreatic carcinoma. However, its use in chronic pancreatitis has been disappointing, with about half of the patients deriving a benefit that lasts 6 months or less.

Pancreatic duct stenting is used for treatment of proximal pancreatic duct stenosis, decompression of a pancreatic duct leak, and drainage of pancreatic pseudocysts that can be catheterized through the main pancreatic duct. Pancreatic duct stones can also be removed

---

[1]Not FDA approved for this indication.

BOX 4   Treatment of Chronic Pancreatitis

Pancreatic enzyme replacement
Proper nutrition and vitamin supplementation
Blood sugar control
Long-acting narcotic analgesics at lowest effective
    doses
Cessation of alcohol and tobacco
Endotherapy (pancreatic duct stenting and removal of
    stones)
Parenchymal preserving surgery (Frey, Beger) in
    carefully selected patients

---

endoscopically. Stent therapy in chronic pancreatitis definitely plays a role and cany help select patients for successful operative therapy. However, the duration of success with stent therapy for chronic pancreatitis is probably less than with surgical therapy.

Major pancreatic resections for chronic pancreatitis have a high complication rate, both early and late. Patients with large duct disease, who can have nutrition restored, are working, are not drinking alcohol, and have a supportive family structure fare better. Failure to carefully select patients leads to disappointing results. The surgical management of pancreatic duct stones and stenoses has been shown to be superior to endoscopic treatment in randomized clinical trials. Beger introduced the duodenum-preserving pancreatic head resection (DPPHR) in the early 1980s. Later in the decade, Frey and Smith described the local resection of the pancreatic head with longitudinal pancreaticojejunostomy, which included excavation of the pancreatic head including the ductal structures in continuity with a long ductotomy of the dorsal duct. This operation is basically a hybrid of the Beger and Puestow (Partington-Rochelle modification) procedures and is more popular in the United States (Figs. 7 and 8).

Recent randomized prospective studies have compared the Whipple, Beger, and Frey procedures for chronic pancreatitis. Patients who had a Beger procedure had a shorter hospital stay, greater weight gain, less postoperative diabetes, and exocrine dysfunction than standard Whipple patients over a 3- to 5-year follow-up. Pain control was similar between the two procedures. In a study comparing the pylorus-preserving Whipple to the Frey procedure, there was a lower postoperative complication rate associated with the Frey procedure (19%) compared to the pylorus-preserivng Whipple group (53%), and the

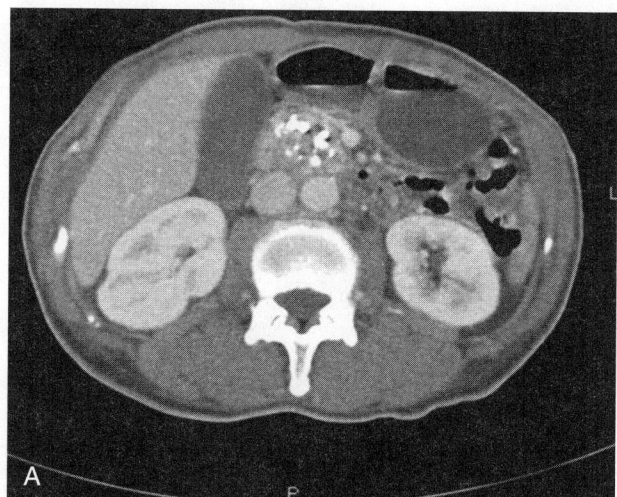

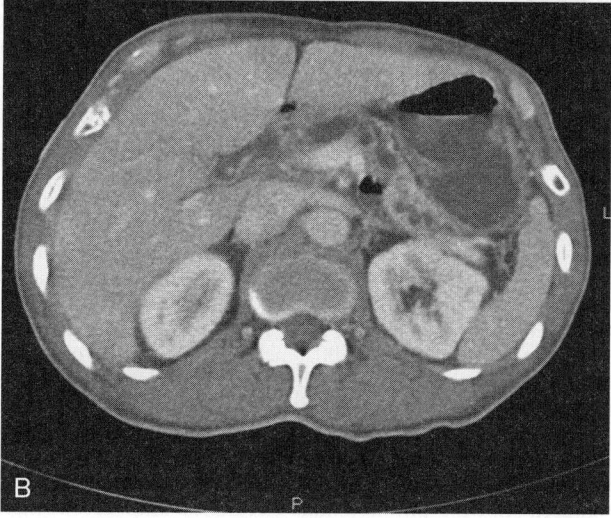

FIGURE 7. Computed tomographic scan of a patient with chronic calcific pancreatitis and a massively dilated pancreatic duct.

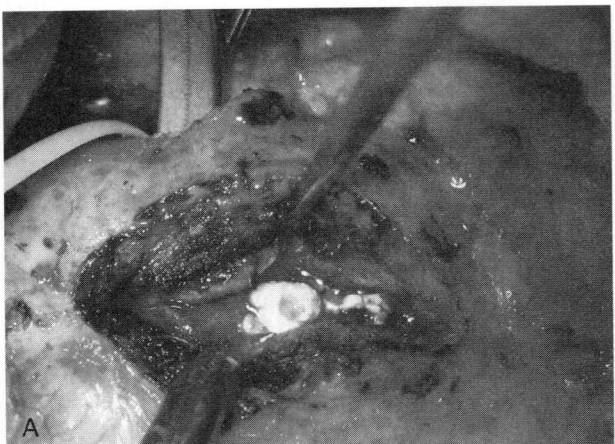

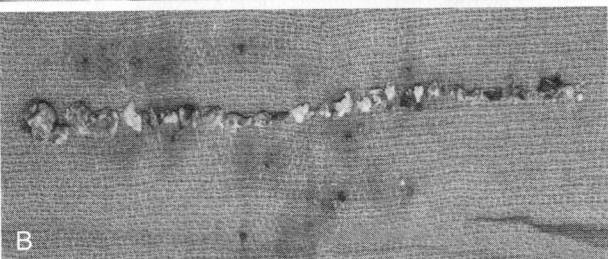

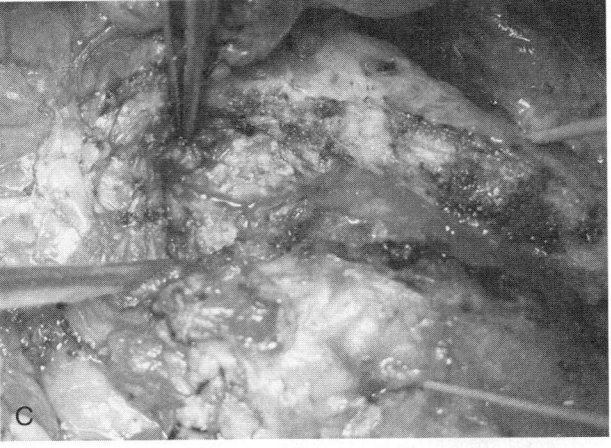

FIGURE 8. A, The pancreatic duct is opened to reveal a preoperatively placed pancreatic duct stent. **B,** The residual stones removed from the pancreatic duct. **C,** In the Frey procedure, the head of the pancreas is cored out in addition to a longitudinal pancreatic ductotomy. The pancreas is drained with a Roux-en-Y limb of jejunum.

sufficient quantity of islets from a sclerotic gland depends on the degree of disease present, so the selection of patients as candidates for autologous islet transplantation is important. As success with autotransplantation increases, patients with nonobstructive, sclerotic pancreatitis may be considered for resection and islet autotransplantation earlier in their course, because end-stage fibrosis bodes poorly for transplant success. As the necessary expertise with islet transplantation becomes more widespread, this therapy could become routine in the treatment of chronic pancreatitis.

MONITORING

Chronic pancreatitis is of course a chronic disease, so continued monitoring and maintenance therapy is essential after an acute exacerbation of chronic pancreatitis. Pain control, proper nutrition, and alcohol and smoking cessation must be maintained as an outpatient. The clinician must also be looking for the development of common complications.

COMPLICATIONS

Pseudocysts in the setting of chronic pancreatitis are less likely to resolve without intervention. Often, the pancreatic duct and bile duct are compressed, and the compression might need to be addressed at the same time as the pseudocyst. A trend toward minimally invasive management remains appropriate, with endoscopic drainage preferred over laparoscopic cystogastrostomy unless additional procedures are required. Resection of a pseudocyst is sometimes indicated for cysts located in the pancreatic tail, or when a midpancreatic duct disruption has resulted in a distally located pseudocyst. Distal pancreatectomy for removal of a pseudocyst, with or without splenectomy, can be a challenging procedure in the setting of prior pancreatitis. An internal drainage procedure of the communicating duct, or of the pseudocyst itself, should be considered when distal resection is being contemplated.

Pancreatic ascites results from a disrupted pancreatic duct with extravasation of pancreatic fluid that does not become sequestered as a pseudocyst but drains freely into the peritoneal cavity. Occasionally, the pancreatic fluid tracks superiorly into the thorax, causing a pancreatic pleural effusion. Both complications are seen more often in patients with chronic pancreatitis, rather than after acute pancreatitis. Paracentesis or thoracentesis reveals noninfected fluid with a protein level greater than 25 g/L and a markedly elevated amylase level. Paracentesis is critical to differentiate pancreatic from hepatic ascites.

ERCP is most helpful to delineate the location of the pancreatic duct leak and to elucidate the underlying pancreatic ductal anatomy. Pancreatic duct stenting may be considered at the time of ERCP. Paracentesis and antisecretory therapy with the somatostatin analogue octreotide acetate, together with bowel rest and parenteral nutrition, is successful in more than half of patients. Reapposition of serosal surfaces to facilitate closure of the leak is considered a part of therapy, and this is accomplished by complete paracentesis. For pleural effusions, a period of chest tube drainage can facilitate closure of the internal fistula. Surgical therapy is reserved for those who fail to respond to medical treatment.

REFERENCES

Acute Pancreatitis Classification Working Group. Revision of the Atlanta Classification of Acute Pancreatitis. PDF available for download at: http://www.pancreasclub.com/resources/AtlantaClassification.pdf; [accessed 14.07.10].

Beger HG, Matsuno S, Cameron JL. Diseases of the pancreas: Current surgical therapy. Berlin: Springer-Verlag; 2008.

Beger HG, Warshaw AL, Buchler MW, et al., The pancreas: An integrated textbook of basic science, medicine, and surgery. 2nd ed Malden, MA: Blackwell Publishing; 2008.

Dellinger EP, Tellado JM, Soto NE, et al. Early antibiotic treatment for severe acute necrotizing pancreeatitis: A randomized, double-blind, placebo-controlled study. Ann Surg 2007;245:674–83.

Fisher WE, Anderson DK, Bell RH, Saluja AK, Brunicardi FC. Pancreas. In: Brunicardi FC, Andersen DK, Billiar TR, et al., Schwartz's Principles of Surgery. 9th ed. New York: McGraw-Hill; 2010. p. 1167–243.

Isenmann R, Runzi M, Kron M, et al. Prophylactic antibiotic treatment in patients with predicted severe acute pancreatitis: A placebo-controlled, double-blind trial. Gastroenterology 2004;126:997–1004.

global quality-of-life scores were better (71% versus 43%, respectively). Both operations were equally effective in controlling pain over a 2-year follow-up. Operation times, intraoperative blood loss, and transfusion requirements have been shown to be decreased with the Frey and Beger procedures compared to the Whipple procedure. In long-term (>8 years) follow-up, there was no difference between the Beger and Frey procedures in pain relief, pancreatic insufficiency, quality of life, and late mortality. Compared to the Whipple procedure, the Beger and Frey procedures seem to produce a lower incidence of immediate complications and diabetes but no significant differences in pain relief. Although these limited pancreatic procedures have a lower initial rate of endocrine dysfunction, the long-term risk of diabetes is more related to the progression of the underlying disease than to the effects of operation.

Recent refinements in the methods of harvesting and preserving pancreatic islets, and standardization of the methods by which islets are infused into the portal venous circuit for intrahepatic engraftment, has improved the success and rekindled interest in islet autotransplantation for chronic pancreatitis. The ability to recover a

Gastroesophageal Reflux Disease

Method of
Jason R. Roberts, MD, and
Donald O. Castell, MD

Gastroesophageal reflux disease (GERD) is a motility disorder of the lower esophageal sphincter (LES). The definition of this disease has evolved over time, reflecting better understanding of the roles that transient LES relaxations and acid/pepsin contact with esophageal mucosa play, as well as the ability to identify these events. The diagnosis of GERD has changed from identification of a hiatal hernia, to identification of erosive esophagitis, to the currently accepted patient-centered definition: any symptom or injury to esophageal mucosa resulting from reflux of gastric contents into the esophagus. GERD should not be confused with physiologic gastroesophageal reflux, which is not associated with symptoms or esophageal mucosal injury.

The prevalence of GERD is difficult to ascertain, although several studies have indicated it to be as high as 50% of adults in Western countries, with 10% to 18% experiencing heartburn on a daily basis. Studies using health care utilization data may underestimate the prevalence because of self-treatment by individuals in the community, whereas population surveys may overestimate it because of inaccurate assessment of symptoms and absence of objective data. Regardless of the real number, the management of this disease costs more than $10 billion annually in the United States. GERD has been called a disease of white males, although recent data suggest increasing prevalence in Asia and Pacific regions.

Pathophysiology

GERD is a motility disorder of the LES characterized by inappropriate or transient relaxations that allow gastric contents to reflux into the esophagus. The LES is a tonically contracted ring of smooth muscle fibers innervated by the vagus nerve. Vagal stimulation during swallowing produces physiologic LES relaxation and is a likely source for transient LES relaxations. Gastroesophageal reflux occurs most frequently during postprandial periods, at a rate of 6 reflux episodes per hour, but averages 2 episodes per hour over the entire day. Increasing frequency of reflux in the postprandial period results from gastric distention after a meal and stimulation of tension receptors in the proximal stomach leading to transient LES relaxations (Box 1). A chronically hypotensive LES is not a major mechanism for GERD in most patients but can be seen in cases of severe erosive esophagitis.

Reflux of acidic gastric contents can lead to injury of the esophageal mucosa, including inflammation, ulceration, stricturing, Barrett's metaplasia, and adenocarcinoma. Peristaltic clearance, tissue resistance, and salivary bicarbonate make up host defense mechanisms that work by clearing reflux and neutralizing the acid residue on the mucosa. Erosive esophagitis or strictures result in the most severe form of GERD, which includes nocturnal reflux with longer acid contact times, decreased salivary production, and lower frequency of swallowing during sleep.

Complications

Acid reflux can lead to significant morbidity if it is not recognized and treated appropriately. Habitual contact of acid and activated pepsin with the stratified squamous epithelium, along with impaired defense mechanisms, results in tissue injury (Box 2). The end result of this process can be ulceration, fibrosis with stricture formation, Barrett's esophagus, or adenocarcinoma. These complications can produce alarm symptoms (Box 3). Patients presenting with alarm symptoms should undergo immediate diagnostic evaluation with an esophagogastroduodenoscopy (EGD).

EROSIVE ESOPHAGITIS

The endoscopic finding of erosive esophagitis is seen in fewer than 50% of patients with heartburn. The severity is stratified according to the Los Angeles Classification of Esophagitis. Treatment with a proton pump inhibitor (PPI) for 4 to 12 weeks heals erosive esophagitis in 78% to 95% of cases. The healing effect of antisecretory therapy, and particularly PPIs, demonstrates the important role of acid reflux in causing tissue injury. The recurrence rates for erosive esophagitis are high after discontinuation of PPI maintenance therapy (75%–92%), necessitating continuation of gastric acid suppression.

BOX 1   Factors That Modulate Transient Lower Esophageal Sphincter Relaxation

Stimulants
- Gastric distention
- Pharyngeal intubation
- Upright orientation
- Foods (fatty foods, caffeine, alcohol)
- Tobacco

Inhibitors
- Recumbency
- Lateral decubitus (left side)
- Anesthesia
- Sleep

BOX 2   Esophageal Tissue Defense Mechanisms

Preepithelial
- Mucous layer
- Unstirred water layer
- Surface bicarbonate concentration

Epithelial Structures
- Cell membranes
- Intercellular junctional complexes (tight junctions, glycoconjugates/lipid)

Cellular
- Epithelial transport (Na^+/H^+ exchanger, Na^+-dependent Cl^-/HCO_3^- exchanger)
- Intracellular and extracellular buffers
- Cell restitution
- Cell replication

Postepithelial
- Blood flow
- Tissue acid-base status

BOX 3   Alarm Symptoms of Gastrointestinal Esophageal Reflux Disease (GERD)

Presence of any of the following symptoms requires immediate evaluation:
- Dysphagia
- Odynophagia
- Weight loss
- Spontaneous resolution of GERD symptoms
- Iron deficiency anemia
- Gastrointestinal bleeding

STRICTURES

Most strictures caused by GERD are peptic in origin and are located at the squamocolumnar junction. Patients with GERD and strictures, compared to those without strictures, are more likely to have a hypotensive LES, abnormal peristalsis, and prolonged acid clearance time. Stricture formation decreases the luminal diameter, resulting in solid food dysphagia. Dysphagia in these patients is often a combination of decreased luminal diameter and dysmotility of the distal esophageal body with low-amplitude peristalsis. Patients with GERD who develop dysphagia should have immediate barium radiography and an endoscopic evaluation.

BARRETT'S ESOPHAGUS

Barrett's esophagus is a premalignant condition that may evolve into esophageal adenocarcinoma. The histologic abnormality involves intestinal-like metaplasia of the stratified squamous epithelium. Epidemiologic studies show Barrett's to be more common among Caucasians, males, and the elderly (mean age, 60 years). A finding of Barrett's esophagus portends a 30- to 125-fold increased risk of eventual adenocarcinoma, with an incidence of 0.5% per year. Despite the prevalent use of PPIs in the treatment of GERD, the incidence of adenocarcinoma has been increasing. Current guidelines encourage endoscopic surveillance for patients with Barrett's esophagus, yet there are sparse data showing the cost-effectiveness or mortality benefit of this strategy.

ADENOCARCINOMA

Approximately 50% of esophageal cancers are adenocarcinomas. Since the 1970s, the incidence has been rising for reasons that are still unknown. GERD is a risk factor for esophageal adenocarcinoma, and the risk increases with the duration and severity of GERD symptoms. There is a suggestion that cagA strains of *Helicobacter pylori* are protective against development of Barrett's esophagus and adenocarcinoma. The declining incidence of *H. pylori* may be a possible explanation for the rising incidence of adenocarcinoma.

Diagnosis

GERD is largely a clinical diagnosis under the current definition (i.e., any symptom or tissue injury resulting from reflux of gastric contents into the esophagus). Patients with the typical symptoms of heartburn and regurgitation most often associated with meals have a high pretest probability of having GERD. A well-obtained history and symptom questionnaire are usually sufficient to form a presumptive diagnosis and are more cost-effective than ambulatory reflux testing or EGD. An empiric trial of PPI therapy that leads to a significant reduction or resolution of symptoms likely confirms the diagnosis.

The pathophysiology of GERD is much more complex than previously thought. It involves more than acid reflux, because nonacid reflux with a pH greater than 4 can be a common source of symptoms. This entity is unmasked when PPI therapy is found to control gastric acid secretion and impedance-pH testing identifies a temporal relationship between symptoms and episodes of nonacid reflux.

Direct-to-consumer marketing and the availability of over-the-counter PPI medications (Prilosec OTC) have led to self-treatment of GERD-type symptoms and a consequent change in the type of patients seeking medical care for their symptoms. Patients with typical GERD symptoms that do not completely respond to therapy with PPIs, including over-the-counter and prescription PPIs, warrant a more detailed evaluation of their symptoms. A separate population requiring earlier diagnostic evaluation includes patients with exclusively atypical GERD symptoms such as cough, hoarseness, throat clearing, asthma attacks, and chest pain. Less commonly, patients presenting with signs or symptoms of tissue injury, such as solid food dysphagia, should also be more rigorously tested for GERD (Box 4).

Patients who have symptoms associated with GERD, whether typical or atypical, are frequently treated empirically with PPI therapy. With a lack of discrimination regarding symptom types, this population is very heterogeneous and comprises patients with symptoms that

---

BOX 4   Clinical Spectrum of Gastroesophageal Reflux Disease–Related Symptoms and Tissue Injury

Esophageal
Symptomatic Syndromes
- Typical reflux syndrome
- Reflux chest pain syndrome

Syndromes with Tissue Injury
- Reflux esophagitis
- Reflux stricture
- Barrett's esophagus
- Adenocarcinoma

Extraesophageal
Established Association
- Reflux cough
- Reflux laryngitis
- Reflux dental erosions

Proposed Association
- Sinusitis
- Reflux asthma
- Pulmonary fibrosis
- Pharyngitis
- Recurrent otitis media

---

are truly associated with GERD, not at all associated with GERD, and a combination of both. The pretest probability of GERD in this group is diluted, and nonresponders to empiric therapy are numerous. Partial responders and nonresponders to PPI therapy should undergo ambulatory reflux testing using combined multichannel intraluminal impedance (MII)-pH or standard pH. MII-pH catheters measure both esophageal pH changes and impedance changes that occur as an ion-rich refluxate passes a pair of ring electrodes, resulting in a drop in the resistance to a low-voltage current between the electrodes. The change in impedance can detect gastroesophageal reflux regardless of the acid content and can distinguish reflux types as liquid, gas, or mixed.

The goals of ambulatory reflux testing are to determine whether the esophageal acid contact time is abnormal, whether there are an abnormal number of reflux episodes, and whether a relationship between reflux and symptoms exists. The advantage of combined MII-pH is its ability to identify both acid and nonacid reflux, so that testing can be done while the patient is on acid-suppression therapy and the artifact of acidic food or beverage ingestion is eliminated; pH-only testing is affected by both of these conditions. The major disadvantage is that MII-pH testing is less available than conventional pH testing.

EGD is specific for detecting reflux-related tissue injury but is not sensitive, because fewer than 50% of patients with GERD-related heartburn have endoscopic findings of reflux. If erosive esophagitis or Barrett's esophagus is found on endoscopy, aggressive antisecretory therapy with a PPI is warranted.

A barium esophagram is unlikely to add useful diagnostic information in patients with GERD symptoms without dysphagia. It is a useful tool in distinguishing obstructive from nonobstructive dysphagia and may even be more sensitive than EGD in detecting causes of obstructive dysphagia. Achalasia is often mistaken for GERD during the onset of symptoms, and early use of esophagography may help make this diagnosis.

Management

GERD is predominantly a postprandial event involving transient LES relaxations. The primary focus in management of this disease is to eliminate or improve symptoms and prevent tissue injury. In most patients with recurrent GERD symptoms, this can be accomplished by controlling gastric acid secretion with antisecretory therapy. PPIs are the most effective pharmacologic therapy for improving symptoms and preventing tissue injury from acid reflux. Individuals with only occasional heartburn may successfully treat symptoms with a combination of lifestyle modifications and over-the-counter antacids, histamine 2 receptor antagonists, or a PPI.

Patients presenting with typical symptoms and a history consistent with GERD should be given a trial of PPI once daily for at least 4 weeks. A validated GERD symptom assessment questionnaire such as the Reflux Disease Questionnaire should be used as an initial screening tool, because symptom response is the primary outcome measure and subsequent questionnaire responses are useful in comparison with the initial responses for measuring treatment efficacy. If symptoms have not responded or have responded only partially after this trial, then the dosing or frequency of the PPI should be increased over another 4-week period. If the response is still unsatisfactory, diagnostic testing with ambulatory combined MII-pH or pH-only monitoring is indicated.

PPIs are an effective maintenance therapy for most patients with GERD and may be stepped down or used on demand, but GERD is a chronic condition with a high recurrence rate of symptoms without some form of maintenance therapy. This creates a large population of patients on antisecretory therapy for a disease with a low mortality rate, which raises the question of drug safety. There are insufficient data available that would warrant a recommendation against long-term PPI therapy. Clinical judgment in specific patient populations should be used to determine the optimal PPI regimen.

At present, pharmacologic reflux reduction therapy consists solely of the use of baclofen (Lioresal),[1] which has been shown to reduce transient LES relaxations and associated gastroesophageal reflux. The drawback of this medication is its unwanted side effects, which include somnolence and dizziness, limiting its tolerability and clinical utility as a stand-alone therapy.

Antireflux surgery is another alternative that is effective in limiting GERD symptoms in patients with a positive reflux-symptom relationship. Candidates for surgery include younger patients who do not want to continue chronic PPI therapy and patients with symptomatic nonacid reflux. Today, most antireflux surgery is performed laparoscopically with a 360-degree Nissen fundoplication. The associated mortality rate is small (0.5%–1%), and this approach is preferred to open laparotomy. Traditional predictors for surgical success have included the presence of typical symptoms (heartburn and regurgitation), symptom response to a trial of PPIs, and an abnormal ambulatory pH study. These criteria exclude the important group of patients with atypical symptoms or symptoms related to nonacid reflux. However, such patients should be considered candidates for antireflux surgery if a positive reflux-symptom relationship can be demonstrated.

Patients with alarm symptoms and those who are partial responders to PPI therapy should also undergo EGD to aid in determining the cause of the symptoms, such as obstructive dysphagia from peptic strictures, adenocarcinoma, and bleeding esophageal ulcers (which can cause anemia). EGD findings that suggest GERD are a result of acid reflux. However, the incidence of these findings has declined with the use of PPIs.

Nonerosive reflux disease is increasingly common as more patients are converted from acid refluxers to nonacid refluxers with PPI therapy. By definition, these patients have no findings on endoscopy to suggest ongoing GERD. Absence of endoscopic findings does not exclude GERD, however, because tissue injury can occur at the microscopic as well as the macroscopic level. Patients with either erosive esophagitis or nonerosive reflux disease have dilated intercellular spaces on electron microscopy.

As previously discussed, patients with GERD may develop Barrett's esophagus. The metaplastic transformation from normal stratified squamous epithelium to an intestinal-type, columnar-lined epithelium creates a premalignant lesion with a 0.5% per year risk of progression to adenocarcinoma. Screening for Barrett's esophagus remains controversial. There is no evidence that screening results in a mortality

---

[1]Not FDA approved for this indication.

benefit due to early detection of esophageal adenocarcinoma. Screening of all patients with GERD for Barrett's esophagus is clearly not cost-effective, but it is reasonable to target the highest-risk populations, such as Caucasian men older than 50 years of age. Current American College of Gastroenterology guidelines recommend surveillance endoscopy in patients with known Barrett's esophagus at intervals determined by the degree of dysplasia. Because there have been no long-term, controlled studies, it is a grade C recommendation.

REFERENCES

Bonino J, Sharma P. Barrett's esophagus. Curr Opin Gastroenterol 2005;21: 461–5.

Castell DO, Richter JE. The Esophagus. 4th ed. Philadelphia: Lippincott Williams & Wilkins; 2003.

Frye J, Vaezi M. Extraesophageal GERD. Gastroenterol Clin North Am 2008;37:845–58.

Hila A, Agrawal A, Castell D. Combined multichannel intraluminal impedance and pH esophageal testing compared to pH alone for diagnosing both acid and weakly acidic gastroesophageal reflux. Clin Gastroenterol and Hepatol 2007;5:172–7.

Kahrilas PJ, Shaheen N, Vaezi M. American Gastroenterological Association Institute technical review on the management of gastroesophageal reflux disease. Gastroenterology 2008;135(4):1392–413.

Mainie I, Tutuian R, Agrawal A, et al. Combined multichannel intraluminal impedance-pH monitoring to select patients with persistent gastro-oesophageal reflux for laparoscopic Nissen fundoplication. Br J Surg 2006; 93:1483–7.

Mainie I, Tutuian R, Castell D. Comparison between the combined analysis and the DeMeester score to predict response to PPI therapy. J Clin Gastroenterol 2006;40:602–5.

Mainie I, Tutuian R, Shay S, et al. Acid and non-acid reflux in patients with persistent symptoms despite acid suppressive therapy: A multicentre study using combined ambulatory impedance-pH monitoring. Gut 2006;55:1398–402.

Savarino E, Zentilin P, Tutuian R, et al. The role of nonacid reflux in NERD: Lessons learned from impedance-pH monitoring in 150 patients off therapy. Am J Gastroenterol 2008;103:2685–93.

Vakil N, Van Zanten SV, Kahrilas P, et al. The Montreal definition and classification of gastroesophageal reflux disease: A global evidence-based consensus. Am J Gastroenterol 2006;101:1900–20.

Vakil N. Review article: Test and treat or treat and test in reflux disease. Aliment Pharmacol Ther 2003;17(Suppl. 2):57–9.

Wang KK, Sampliner RE. Updated guidelines 2008 for the diagnosis, surveillance and therapy of Barrett's esophagus. Am J Gastroenterol 2008;103:788–97.

Tumors of the Stomach

Method of
Scott A. Hundahl, MD

Gastric Adenocarcinoma

Thanks to happy accident rather than specific planning, over the past 80 years, gastric adenocarcinoma has changed from the most-common solid organ malignancy in the United States to a relatively uncommon disease. Worldwide, however, it remains a scourge second only to lung cancer.

CLASSIFICATION AND EPIDEMIOLOGY

Several classification schemes exist. Two are commonly used. Bormann's morphologic classification relies on gross characteristics of the tumor. The histologic classification of Lauren, first described by Jarvi and Lauren in 1951, divides gastric adenocarcinomas into intestinal (gland-forming) and diffuse (discohesive) types, based on their microscopic appearance. Several other classification schemes have been proposed, including Broder's classification of differentiation, the WHO (World Health Organization) classification, the Nagayo–Komagome classification, the Ming classification, and the Goseki classification, but none eclipses the Lauren classification.

Epidemiologically, three patterns of disease can be discerned, with *Helicobacter pylori* infection playing an important role in the first two patterns: intestinal-type tumors arising from the lesser curve and distal stomach, related to *H. pylori*–associated atrophic gastritis and intestinal metaplasia; diffuse-type tumors involving the body of the stomach, often associated with intense *H. pylori*–associated inflammation but not associated with significant intestinal metaplasia; and intestinal-type tumors of the gastroesophageal junction.

In high-incidence regions of the world, such as Japan and Korea, up to two thirds of gastric adenocarcinomas are of the first type and are strongly associated with chronic multifocal atrophic gastritis and intestinal metaplasia from chronic *H. pylori* infection. The process usually begins at the antrum–corpus junction along the lesser curvature and predisposes to cancers of the intestinal type occurring in the sixth or seventh decades of life. The second type of gastric adenocarcinoma, also associated with *H. pylori*, afflicts younger persons in the fourth and fifth decades of life. The last type, seen in lower-incidence regions of the world such as the United States, is associated with chronic gastroesophageal reflux and Barrett's esophagitis.

Epidemiologists and public health experts estimate that more than 40% of gastric adenocarcinomas worldwide can be attributed to chronic. *H. pylori* infection. Strains containing the *cagA* gene appear more dangerous. The infection usually starts by the second or third decade, and unless it is successfully treated, it gives rise to chronic inflammation, atrophic gastritis, and eventually intestinal metaplasia, which is a premalignant histologic condition. Dietary factors such as high salt and high nitrates can accentuate this progression as well as the march to cancer. As the condition progresses, acid-producing oxyntic mucosa is progressively wiped out, gastric pH increases, and bacterial overgrowth with non–*H. pylori* bacteria is facilitated. The original *H. pylori*, which requires an acid environment to thrive, often disappears at this point.

Once intestinal metaplasia is established, dietary factors become particularly important in mitigating the risk of cancer development. Protective factors include intake of vitamin C, fresh fruits and vegetables, and antioxidants. The association of *H. pylori* infection with the development of intestinal metaplasia suggests that early detection and elimination of this infection might prevent gastric cancer. Unfortunately, in high-incidence areas, reinfection from contaminated water supply and other sources is common, thus undermining the strategy. Also, in prevention trials to date, benefit appears restricted to the subgroups without preexisting intestinal metaplasia.

RISK FACTORS

Risk factors other than *H. pylori* infection include low socioeconomic status, smoking, a diet deficient in fresh fruits and vegetables or high in salt-preserved high-nitrate foods, previous gastric ulcer, ionizing radiation, family history, and previous gastric resection. Blood group A is associated with higher risk of developing a diffuse-type tumor. Predisposing genetic conditions include the Lynch's syndrome (hereditary nonpolyposis colorectal cancer [HNPCC], a condition with microsatellite instability due to deficient DNA repair enzymes), as well as dominantly inherited germline mutations in the E-cadherin gene.

DIAGNOSIS

In Western populations, by the time gastric cancer causes symptoms, the disease is often relatively advanced. In a large National Cancer Data Base survey of U.S. patients, presenting ascribable symptoms included weight loss (62%), abdominal or epigastric pain (52%), nausea (34%), anorexia (32%), early satiety (32%), dysphagia (26%), and melena (18%).

Mass screening combining upper GI series, endoscopy, and serum pepsinogen I/II ratio have proved beneficial in high-incidence areas such as Japan, but they cannot be justified in the United States, where incidence is low. However, for defined risk groups, such as those with established atrophic gastritis and established intestinal metaplasia, strong family history, and those with HNPCC syndrome, surveillance screening should definitely be considered. For those with hereditary E-cadherin mutations associated with gastric cancer, prophylactic total gastrectomy is recommended.

In the United States, diagnosis is usually made by upper endoscopy. One should be aware that diffuse-type cancers manifesting as linitis plastica are often associated with minimal visible mucosal changes, and deep biopsies are often required for establishing the diagnosis. Furthermore, small, early gastric cancers (defined by the Japanese as in situ and T-1 cancers, with or without node involvement) can be associated with particularly subtle mucosal changes, presenting a challenge for even the most experienced endoscopist. Chromoendoscopy and other sophisticated mucosal imaging techniques have been used to identify such changes but are not yet standard.

Extent-of-disease studies for gastric adenocarcinoma include endoscopic ultrasound (good for estimating depth of tumor and visualizing immediately adjacent nodes), and helical CT scanning, which is good for evaluating extraluminal extent of disease, intraabdominal or mediastinal extension or spread, and liver or lung metastases. Because even high-resolution CT scanning can miss small peritoneal implants, extraregional nodal spread, and small liver metastases, staging laparoscopy or minilaparotomy are valuable adjuncts and should be considered mandatory if any preoperative chemotherapy is considered.

CURRENT DIAGNOSIS

- Intestinal metaplasia, which predisposes to cancer, results from chronic *Helicobacter pylori* infection.
- In the United States, screening studies are reserved for those with definite risk factors.
- Pretreatment staging drives subsequent treatment and involves endoscopy, endoscopic ultrasound, helical computed tomography, and often laparoscopy or mini-laparotomy.
- Mucosal abnormalities can be largely absent in early gastrointestinal stromal tumors, small carcinoids, and even diffuse-type linitis plastica. Deep endoscopic biopsies are required.

CURRENT THERAPY

Adenocarcinoma

- To ensure complete surgical resection, resection should be customized (e.g., gross margin, use of endoscopic mucosal resection for certain mucosal tumors).
- Survival is highest with low Maruyama Index surgery.
- Adjuvant therapy options include preoperative chemotherapy (± postoperative treatment), or postoperative chemoradiation

Gastrointestinal Stromal Tumors

- Node dissection is not indicated.

Gastric Lymphoma

- For aggressive diffuse-type lymphomas, chemotherapy with or without radiation therapy is now the mainstay of treatment. Surgery is reserved for complications such as acute perforation.
- Superficial mucosa-associated lymphoid tissue tumors can sometimes be treated by simply eliminating *Helicobacter pylori* infection. It comes back if reinfection occurs, however.

STAGING

Although a long-established, much-modified Japanese staging system, the General Rules, finds widespread use in many areas of the world, the AJCC/UICC (American Joint Committee on Cancer/International Union Against Cancer) TNM (tumor, nodes, metastases) system is by far the dominant staging system used. T stage is defined a bit differently than that for colorectal cancer: Muscularis propria penetration short of serosal penetration is still considered T2 disease, a serosal breach is required for T3 disease, and a T4 designation requires direct involvement of adjacent structures. Optimally, accurate nodal designation requires that more than 15 nodes be examined by the pathologist. N1 disease means metastases in 1 to 6 regional nodes, N2 disease means metastases in 7 to 15 regional nodes, and N3 disease means metastases in more than 15 nodes. Any N3 disease, any node-positive T4 disease, any M1 distant metastatic disease, and any involved extra-regional M1 nodes translate in the staging matrix to stage IV disease. The reader is referred to the AJCC staging manual referenced at the end of this chapter.

TREATMENT

Curative treatment of gastric cancer involves, as main therapy, complete negative-margin surgical resection of disease. For select tumors, such resection sometimes follows up-front chemotherapy. For localized in situ and select T1 tumors, endoscopic mucosal resection and minimally invasive techniques have been successfully employed. Unfortunately, most tumors in the United States are discovered at a stage where formal open surgery is required.

To secure a histologically negative mural margin of resection, a gross margin of 2 cm is usually adequate for exophytic, noninfiltrating tumors, and a margin of at least 5 to 6 cm of grossly normal tissue is recommended for ulcerated or infiltrating tumors or diffuse histology. Closest mural margins are generally checked by frozen section at the time of surgery to confirm adequacy of resection. Total gastrectomy is not indicated as a routine procedure, except in diffuse-type tumors involving most of the stomach (linitis plastica), but it is warranted whenever required for a negative-margin resection.

Routine splenectomy in the treatment of gastric cancer, as well as routine distal pancreatectomy (performed in the past to clear splenic nodes), should be avoided unless definitely required for complete resection of visible or palpable disease.

The optimal extent of lymph node dissection in this disease has generated—and continues to generate—international controversy. Although several prospective randomized trials to date in non-Asian populations—none perfect—fail to demonstrate that routine extensive lymphadenectomy increases survival, it has also been shown that insufficient lymphadenectomy definitely compromises survival. A prospective randomized single-institution trial in Taipei has documented survival benefit associated with radical lymph node dissection. The adequacy of lymphadenectomy for a given case can be quantified using the Maruyama Index of Unresected Disease. In both a large U.S. adjuvant chemoradiation trial and in a blinded reanalysis of a large Dutch surgical trial, low Maruyama Index score correlates with survival. Moreover, a dose–response effect is seen for the extent of surgical clearance of node groups at risk. Using the Maruyama computer program to predict the extent of nodal spread for a given cancer case before surgery is one way to facilitate a low Maruyama Index operation.

Sentinel node biopsy, an established technique in the treatment of other cancers, has largely failed to win support in cancer of the stomach owing to the organ's lymphatic complexity and relatively high reported false-negative rates.

A large North American prospective randomized trial of postoperative adjuvant 5-fluorouracil–based chemoradiation in completely resected gastric cancer revealed a significant increase in disease-free and overall survival with this treatment. The postoperative nature of this trial thwarted implementation of surgical guidelines, and the extent of node dissection for most patients in the trial was suboptimal. Practitioners in some countries, such as Japan, dismiss the necessity of adjuvant postoperative adjuvant chemoradiation with the (unproved but reasonable) argument that this is only a salvage technique for inadequate surgery. A separate Korean chemoradiation series has shown benefit even for radically treated cases, however. For patients with good postoperative performance status, good organ function, and adequate nutrition, postoperative adjuvant chemoradiation therapy remains the standard in North America.

A recent U.K. study of preoperative plus postoperative ECF (epirubicin [Ellence],[1] cis-platinum, and continuous-infusion 5-fluorouracil [Adrucil]) chemotherapy versus surgery alone has shown encouraging results for ECF, with a significant improvement in survival. Previous preoperative chemotherapy trials, using other regimens, have been negative, however. Preoperative ECF chemotherapy is now recommended by some, and this is especially the case for localized advanced tumors considered borderline resectable.

In Korea, a positive trial of adjuvant perioperative intraperitoneal chemotherapy has been reported. Considerable morbidity and mortality are associated with this adjuvant treatment, however, and it is unlikely it will be implemented without refinement and successful independent duplication of results.

For localized disease deemed not resectable to negative margins, both chemotherapy and chemoradiation have been used to convert such tumors to potentially resectable status. With successful negative-margin resection, some of these patients indeed survive free of disease long term. When localized unresected disease is documented to exist, administering chemoradiation with 5-fluorouracil as a radiation sensitizer can also result in some degree of 5-year survival (per reports, >10%).

Gastrointestinal Stromal Tumors

Gastrointestinal stromal tumors (GISTs) manifest as submucosal spindle cell tumors in the sarcoma family. In contrast to leiomyosarcomas and other spindle cell sarcomas, they express the antigen CD117 and most (>80%) tumors have activating mutations of c-KIT. Formerly considered rare, approximately 5000 of these tumors per year are now diagnosed in the United States. Owing to pattern of growth in the gastric wall, deep to the mucosa, early symptoms are unusual and these tumors often grow to massive size before mucosal ulceration and hemorrhage (or other major symptoms) finally develop. GISTs are classified as sarcomas. Even low-risk GISTs (<5 cm and <1 mitosis per 10 high-power fields) can metastasize, and no GIST can be considered truly benign.

Treatment of localized primary GISTs consists of complete surgical resection, and a 2-cm margin of grossly normal tissue usually accomplishes this. Specific lymph node dissection is not indicated for this histology. Surgical series indicate that approximately 50% of primary gastric tumors metastasize and recur within 5 years. For patients with widespread metastases, generally located in the peritoneal cavity or the liver, first-line therapy is now a well-tolerated oral agent, imatinib mesylate (Gleevec or STI-571) at an initial dose of 400 mg daily, which generates partial responses in more than 50% of cases and stable disease in an additional 25% of cases. Side effects are minimal, and 1-year survival in treated patients is approximately 85%. On the basis of a completed American College of Surgeons Oncology Group (ACOSOG) trial, patients who have all disease completely resected should receive postoperative adjuvant therapy for 1 year.

For tumors resistant to imatinib, SU11248, sunitinib malate (Sutent), is now used as effective second-line therapy. Additional targeted biological agents are under active investigation.

Carcinoid Tumors

Carcinoid tumors of the stomach are similar in behavior to small bowel carcinoids. When small (<1 cm), and unassociated with invasion of the muscularis propria, local excision to negative margins is generally deemed sufficient. For such tumors, endoscopic resection has an established role. However, even small tumors can metastasize to lymph nodes. Wider gastrectomy with lymph node dissection is generally recommended for gastric tumors larger than 1 cm. Many of these

---

[1]Not FDA approved for this indication.

tumors are associated with serum hypergastrinemia; those without this finding tend to be more aggressive. When metastatic to the liver or other organs, surgical cytoreduction (or other means of tumor ablation) can offer considerable palliation to those with carcinoid syndrome, and this should always be considered. Octreotide therapy is now a palliative mainstay in all patients with carcinoid syndrome.

Gastric Lymphomas

Gastric lymphomas encompass most of the lymphoma subtypes, but low-grade, mucosa-associated B-cell lymphomas (B-cell MALT lymphomas) deserve special mention because they are strongly associated with *H. pylori* infection. Indeed, localized cases can be controlled simply by treating the *H. pylori* infection. In such cases, molecular studies indicate persistence of the offending lymphoid clone in about one half of cases. However, and, particularly if *H. pylori* infection recurs, the lymphoma in such cases returns.

Aggressive high-grade diffuse-type B-cell gastric lymphomas, stage IE and IIE, once treated with multimodal therapy, are now treated with chemotherapy alone as the primary treatment, with or without radiotherapy. Surgical intervention is now reserved for emergencies, such as perforation.

For further information on this and other gastrointestinal lymphomas, please see the chapter on lymphoma.

REFERENCES

Cunningham D, Allum WH, Stenning SP, et al. Perioperative chemotherapy versus surgery alone for resectable gastroesophageal cancer. N Engl J Med 2006;355(1):11–20.

Ferrucci PF, Zucca E. Primary gastric lymphoma pathogenesis and treatment: What has changed over the past 10 years? Br J Haematol 2007;136 (4):521–38.

Hundahl SA, Macdonald JS, Benedetti J, et al. Surgical treatment variation in a prospective, randomized trial of chemoradiotherapy in gastric cancer: The effect of undertreatment. Ann Surg Oncol 2002;9(3):278–86.

Hundahl SA, Peeters KC, Kranenbarg EK, et al. Improved regional control and survival with "low Maruyama Index" surgery in gastric cancer: Autopsy findings from the Dutch D1-D2 Trial. Gastric Cancer 2007;10(2):84–6.

Macdonald JS, Smalley SR, Benedetti J, et al. Chemoradiotherapy after surgery compared with surgery alone for adenocarcinoma of the stomach or gastroesophageal junction. N Engl J Med 2001;345(10):725–30.

Modlin IM, Kidd M, Latich I, et al. Current status of gastrointestinal carcinoids. Gastroenterology 2005;128(6):1717–51.

Siehl J, Thiel E. C-kit, GIST, and imatinib. Recent Results. Cancer Res 2007;176:145–51.

Tumors of the Colon and Rectum

Method of
Pinckney J. Maxwell IV, MD, and
Gerald A. Isenberg, MD

Background, Epidemiology, and Etiology

Colorectal cancer is the third most common cancer in men and women, after prostate and lung/bronchus cancer in men and breast and lung/bronchus cancer in women. The American Cancer Society estimates that there will be 102,900 new diagnoses of colon cancer and 39,670 new diagnoses of rectal cancer in the United States in 2010. The incidence of colorectal cancer has been decreasing since the mid-1980s, with a more dramatic decrease occuring in the most recent decade. This decrease is likely related to an increase in screening with removal of precancerous polyps. The American Cancer Society expects an estimated 51,370 deaths from colorectal cancer in 2010, accounting for 9% of all cancer deaths. The mortality rate of colorectal cancer has similarly decreased since the mid-1980s, again with a sharper decline in the past decade most likely related to improved screening. Colorectal cancer is a highly treatable and frequently curable malignancy when it is detected early, highlighting the need for better screening.

The development of colorectal cancer is related to a number of factors, including age, diet, activity, environmental exposures, family history, and genetics. Ninety percent of colorectal cancers are diagnosed after the age of 50 years, and fewer than 5% of cases are diagnosed before the age of 40. The peak incidence of diagnosis is in the seventh decade of life. Dietary factors play a role in carcinogenesis. Western diets, containing high fat and low fiber, have been associated with increased rates of colorectal cancer, as has the intake of red or processed meats and alcohol. It is likely that the low-fiber Western diet slows transit time, leading to increased exposure to carcinogens. Activity level also can play a role in carcinogenesis: studies have shown an increase in cancer among those with sedentary jobs and a decreased incidence among those who exercise regularly. Exposure to cigarette smoke increases the risk of colorectal adenomas and cancers. The American Cancer Society Cancer Prevention Study II revealed that 12% of colorectal cancer deaths in the general U.S. population can be attributed to smoking. Family history and genetics also play a significant role in carcinogenesis, because approximately 10% of patients diagnosed have a first-degree relative with colorectal cancer.

ADENOMATOUS POLYPS

The progression from normal mucosa to an adenomatous polyp and then to an invasive colorectal cancer proceeds through a well-defined process over many years. Aberrant crypt foci develop into microadenomas and then into adenomatous polyps. Dysplastic cells develop within the polyp, continue to multiply, become a tumor and then break through the subepithelial barrier and invade the layers of the bowel wall, eventually spreading to pericolic tissues or to lymph nodes and distant sites. A number of genes have been implicated in carcinogenesis, including protooncogenes (*KRAS*, *SRC*, *MYC*), tumor-suppressor genes (*APC*, *DCC*, *TP53*, *MCC*, *DPC4*), and DNA-mismatch repair genes (*HMSH2*, *MLH1*, *PMS1*, *PMS2*, *GTBP*). Sporadic colorectal cancers develop as a result of several cumulative genetic insults involving these genes (Fig. 1).

FAMILIAL COLORECTAL CANCER SYNDROMES

Familial adenomatous polyposis (FAP) is an inherited, non–sex-linked, mendelian dominant disease that accounts for approximately 1% of all colorectal cancers. The high penetrance of FAP means that there is a 50% chance of development of colorectal cancer among members of affected families. However, 20% of FAP patients have no family history, and their cases most likely represent new, spontaneous mutations. The disorder is caused by mutations in the tumor-suppressor *APC* gene, which is located on chromosome 5 (5q21–q22), or in the *MUTYH* gene, which is located on chromosome 1 (1p34.3–p32.1). FAP is characterized by the progressive development of hundreds or thousands of adenomatous polyps located throughout the entire colon. The clinical diagnosis is based on histologic confirmation of at least 100 adenomas. All patients eventually develop colorectal cancer. The adenomas typically appear by the mid-twenties, and cancers by the late thirties.

An attenuated form of FAP is recognized in which fewer adenomas (20–100) are identified. Adenomas and cancers develop somewhat later, at average ages of 44 and 56 years, respectively. FAP also exhibits extracolonic manifestations, including gastric, duodenal, and small-bowel polyps; osteomas and desmoid tumors (Gardner's syndrome); eye lesions (congenital hypertrophy of retinal pigment epithelium [CHRPE]); epidermoid cysts; and brain neoplasms (Turcot's syndrome).

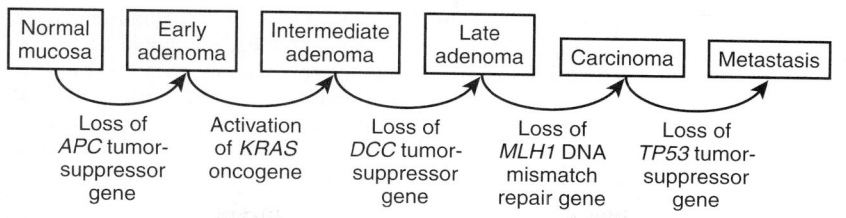

FIGURE 1. Sequence of progression from adenoma to carcinoma.

Hereditary nonpolyposis colon cancer (HNPCC), also called Lynch syndrome, is an inherited, non–sex-linked, mendelian dominant disease with virtually complete penetrance. HNPCC is caused by a defect in any of a number of DNA-mismatch repair genes (*MLH1, MSH2, MSH6, PMS, PMS2*) that leads to high-level microsatellite instability (MSI-H). A number of criteria have been generated for the diagnosis of HNPCC, including the Amsterdam I and II criteria and the Bethesda guidelines (Box 1). According to the EPICOLON study, the revised Bethesda guidelines are the most discriminating set of clinical parameters for diagnosis of HNPCC.

HNPCC is subdivided into Lynch syndrome types I and II. Lynch type I refers to site-specific nonpolyposis colon cancer, and Lynch type II (formerly called familial cancer syndrome) refers to cancers that develop in the colon and related organs such as the endometrium, ovaries, stomach, pancreas, and proximal urinary tract, among others. Lynch syndrome differs from sporadic colorectal cancer in a number of important ways. It has an autosomal dominant inheritance, a predominance of proximal lesions (75% are found in the right colon), an excess of multiple primary colorectal cancers (18%), an early age at onset (average, 44 years), a significantly improved survival rate with right-sided lesions (53% at 5 years, compared with 35% for distal colorectal cancer in family members), and an increased risk for development of metachronous lesions (24%). Patients and family members of those diagnosed with HNPCC or FAP should undergo genetic testing to help improve future diagnosis and treatment options.

CURRENT DIAGNOSIS

- Screening of asymptomatic, average-risk patients should begin at 50 years of age.
- Colonoscopy should be performed if any screening test result is positive.
- Colonoscopy should be performed for any patient with signs or symptoms of colorectal cancer.
- Screening of high-risk patients—those with inflammator bowel disease, familial adenomatous polyposis, or hereditary nonpolyposis colorectal cancer) and those with a significant positive family history—should begin at an earlier age and occur more frequently.

INFLAMMATORY BOWEL DISEASE

Both Crohn's disease and ulcerative colitis are associated with an increased risk of colorectal cancer; with the latter conferring approximately double the risk of the former. The duration and severity of Crohn's disease and the duration and extent (left-sided colitis versus pancolitis) of ulcerative colitis contribute to cancer risk in patients with inflammatory bowel disease. Cancer in Crohn's disease

---

BOX 1   Diagnosis of Hereditary Nonpolyposis Colon Cancer (HNPCC)

Amsterdam I Criteria, 1990
- Three or more family members with histologically verified colorectal cancer, one of whom is a first-degree relative (parent, child, sibling) of the other two
- Two successive affected generations
- One or more colon cancers diagnosed before age 50 years
- Familial adenomatous polyposis has been excluded.

Amsterdam II Criteria, 1999
- Three or more family members with histologically verified HNPCC-related cancers (endometrium, ovary, stomach, small intestine, hepatobiliary, upper urinary tract, brain, or skin), one of whom is a first-degree relative (parent, child, sibling) of the other two
- Two successive affected generations
- One or more colon cancers diagnosed before age 50 years
- Familial adenomatous polyposis has been excluded.

Revised Bethesda Guidelines, 2002
- Colorectal cancer diagnosed in a patient who is younger than 50 years of age.
- Presence of a synchronous, metachronous colorectal or other HNPCC-related malignancy, regardless of age
- Colorectal cancer with the high-level microsatellite instability (MSI-H) histology diagnosed in a patient who is younger than 60 years of age
  - Presence of carcinoma infiltrating lymphocytes, Crohn's-like lymphocytic reaction, mucinous/signet-ring differentiation, or medullary growth pattern
  - No general consensus based on this age
- Colorectal cancer diagnosed in one or more first-degree relatives with an HNPCC-related neoplasm
  - With one or more neoplasms being diagnosed before age 50 years
- Colorectal cancer diagnosed in two or more first- or second-degree relatives with HNPCC-related malignancies, regardless of age

typically occurs in a stricture or bypassed segment. Neoplasia in ulcerative colitis does not follow the adenoma-carcinoma development sequence seen in sporadic colorectal cancer, and this has important screening and treatment implications.

Evaluation

SCREENING AVERAGE-RISK PATIENTS

Patients with no personal history of colorectal polyps or cancers, no personal history of inflammatory bowel disease, no symptoms suspicious for colorectal cancer, no family history of colorectal polyps or cancers, and no evidence of a familial or genetic syndrome may be screened as having average risk. The two main categories of screening tests are those that detect adenomatous polyps and cancers (flexible sigmoidoscopy, colonoscopy, double-contrast barium enema, and computed tomographic [CT] colonography) and those that primarily detect cancer (fecal occult blood testing, fecal immunohistochemical testing, and stool DNA testing). The goal of screening is to reduce mortality by reducing the incidence of advanced disease. It seems intuitive that tests that detect polyps, the premalignant phase of colorectal cancer, would be preferred to tests that detect only cancers. However, testing for polyps and cancers is usually procedure related, whereas testing for only cancers can be conducted on stool samples alone. Screening with simple stool samples has the potential to more easily increase overall screening.

Regardless of the method employed, testing in the average-risk, asymptomatic patient should begin at age 50 years. A total colonoscopy is required only every 10 years but involves oral bowel preparation and carries a small risk of perforation (approximately 1/1000). A flexible sigmoidoscopy is required every 5 years, in combination with annual fecal occult blood testing. Flexible sigmoidoscopy requires only enemas for preparation and carries a lower risk of perforation. Air-contrast barium enemas may be used for screening every 5 years, but they also require oral bowel preparation and are only diagnostic. CT colonography is an evolving method for screening every 5 years and offers the opportunity for more accessible screening; however, the procedure is limited in regard to identification of polyps smaller than 1 cm, also requires oral bowel prepation, and is only diagnostic. Fecal occult blood testing and fecal immunohistochemical testing are done annually. The interval for stool DNA testing is uncertain, and it tests only for a limited number of mutations. The most complete screening test, which allows removal of any precancerous lesions that are identified, remains the total colonoscopy.

SCREENING HIGH-RISK PATIENTS

High-risk patients include those with a personal history of colorectal polyps or cancers, a family history of colorectal cancer in a first-degree relative, Crohn's disease or ulcerative colitis, or a personal or family history of FAP or HNPCC. Screening in these patients has been adjusted for changes in incidence and age at onset of neoplasia (Table 1).

TABLE 1 Screening High-Risk Patients for Colorectal Cancer

Risk Category	Age to Begin	Recommended Test	Comment
Personal history of <3 adenomas with low-grade dysplasia	5–10 y after the initial polypectomy	Colonoscopy	Exam interval should be based on other clinical factors, such as prior findings, family history, or endoscopist or patient preference.
Personal history of 3–10 adenomas, or 1 adenoma >1 cm, or any adenoma with villous features or high-grade dysplasia	3 y after the initial polypectomy	Colonoscopy	Adenomas require compete excision. If the follow-up is normal, the next examination should be in 5 y. Presence of >10 adenomas should raise suspicion of a familial syndrome.
Personal history of colorectal cancer	1 y after resection	Colonoscopy	Patients should undergo high-quality preoperative clearance. Follow-up after normal examinations should be extended to 3 y and then to 5 y.
Family history of adenomas or cancer in a first-degree relative <60 y of age or in 2 first-degree relatives at any age	Age 40 y, or 10 y before the age at onset of youngest affected family member	Colonoscopy	Every 5 y
Family history of adenomas or cancer in a first-degree relative >60 y of age or in 2 second-degree relatives with cancer	Age 40 y	Colonoscopy	Screening should be initiated at an earlier age. Intervals are based on findings or on the average-risk patient.
FAP or suspected FAP	Age 10–12 y	Annual FS, counseling for genetic testing if showing polyps	Colectomy should be considered for positive genetic testing.
HNPCC or risk for HNPCC	Age 20–25 y, or 10 y before the age at onset of youngest affected family member	Colonoscopy, counseling for genetic testing	Every 1–2 y. Genetic testing should be offered to first-degree relatives of persons with a known DNA-mismatch repair gene defect or with 1 of the first 3 Bethesda criteria.
IBD, Crohn's disease, or chronic UC	8 y after the onset of pancolitis, or 12–15 y after the onset of left-sided colitis	Colonoscopies with random four-quadrant biopsies every 10 cm for dysplasia	Screening should be offered every 1–2 y, and patients are best referred to a center with experience in the surveillance and management of IBD.

FAP = familial adenomatous polyposis; FS = flexible sigmoidoscopy; HNPCC = hereditary nonpolyposis colorectal cancer; IBD = inflammatory bowel disease.

CURRENT THERAPY

- Patients with familial adenomatous polyposis or hereditary nonpolyposis colorectal cancer should undergo early, prophylactic colon resection.
- Colon tumors should be treated with segmental laparoscopic or open resection.
- Chemotherapy is offered for colon cancers with locally advanced, nodal (stage III), or metastatic (stage IV) disease.
- Rectal tumors that are small (<3 cm), involve <25% of the rectal circumference, are superficial (Tis or T1), lack nodal involvement, and have favorable pathologic characteristics should be removed by transanal techniques.
- Rectal tumors that are larger, are locally invasive, or have nodal involvement should be removed by formal open resection, with sphincter-preservation if possible.
- Combination chemotherapy and radiation therapy is offered for advanced (stage II), nodal (stage III), or metastatic (stage IV) rectal cancer.
- Postoperative surveillance includes frequent office evaluations, measurements of carcinoembryonic antigen, endoscopy, and imaging.

SYMPTOMS AND DIAGNOSIS

Symptoms of colorectal cancer include bleeding (85%), a change in bowel habits, abdominal pain, malaise, and obstruction. Frequently, anemia is the only sign a patient exhibits. Patients with symptoms suspicious for colorectal cancer should undergo a colonoscopy. An anorectal source of bleeding should not preclude a complete colonic evaluation.

Management

PREOPERATIVE MANAGEMENT

Before operative intervention is undertaken, a complete evaluation should occur, including a careful history and physical examination, routine laboratory testing, and measurement of the level of carcinoembryonic antigen. A complete evaluation of the colon is essential, including colonoscopy with biopsy, or barium enema or CT colonography if colonoscopy is incomplete. Bowel preparation is no longer indicated as a routine preoperative measure for colonic surgery.

Preoperative staging should be undertaken for colorectal cancers. CT scanning of the abdomen and pelvis are indicated to aid in evaluating the extent of localized or metastatic disease and the presence of enlarged lymph nodes. Staging of rectal cancers includes determining the distance from the anal verge, frequently with the use of a rigid proctoscope; the depth of invasion; and the presence of enlarged lymph nodes, using endorectal ultrasound or endoanal coil magnetic resonance imaging. Metastatic disease mandates neoadjuvant chemotherapy in the absence of acute symptoms of obstruction or exsanguination. Rectal cancers with evidence of local invasion into perirectal fat or adjacent structures or evidence of enlarged metastatic lymph nodes may benefit from neoadjuvant chemotherapy and irradiation. Preoperative staging allows for the application of neoadjuvant therapy in selected candidates, which can downstage and downsize tumors and can decrease rates of local recurrence in rectal cancer. Neoadjuvant therapy can also allow for sphincter-preserving procedures in patients with previously bulky or very low rectal tumors.

SURGERY FOR COLONIC TUMORS

The primary therapy for tumors of the colon is operative. The basic principles of surgery for colon cancer are the following:

- Exploration: adequate visual, tactile, and potentially intraoperative hepatic ultrasound staging at the time of primary resection
- Removal of the entire cancer with enough proximal and distal bowel to encompass the possibility of submucosal lymphatic tumor spread
- Removal of the regional mesenteric pedicle, including draining lymphatics, based on the predictable lymphatic spread of the disease and the potential for regional mesenteric involvement without concurrent distant involvement
- En bloc resection of involved structures (T4 tumors).

Segmental colonic resections (right, transverse, left, or sigmoid colectomy) are undertaken based on the tumor location and blood supply with lymphatic drainage, specifically the ileocolic, middle colic, and left colic arteries. These arteries define a convenient anatomic boundary for standard colonic resection and also provide for adequate regional lymph node clearance, because the major draining lymphatics follow these blood vessels in the mesentery. Locally invasive tumors (T4) require en bloc resection of involved structures. Metastatic colonic tumors (M1) may require neoadjuvant chemotherapy before resection or palliation.

Numerous studies have verified that laparoscopic surgery is appropriate, and perhaps preferred, for colon cancer in experienced hands. The landmark Clinical Outcomes of Surgical Therapy (COST) trial in 2004 established that laparoscopic resection is equivalent to open resection for colon cancer.

SURGERY FOR RECTAL TUMORS

Two approaches for rectal tumors are local excision and formal rectal resection. Local excision is the treatment of choice for a select, small group (3%–5% of all patients diagnosed with rectal cancer). Tumors amenable to transanal excision are small (<3 cm), involve less than 25% of the rectal circumference, are confined to the mucosa or submucosa (Tis or T1), lack nodal involvement by preoperative imaging, and have favorable pathologic characteristics (well or moderately differentiated with no lymphovascular invasion). Tumors in the lower or middle third of the rectum are accessible by simple transanal excision, but tumors of the upper rectum require the use of transanal endoscopic microsurgery (TEMS) techniques for resection. Local excision requires a 1-cm normal margin, but the defect usually does not require closure.

Tumors staged at T2 or greater require a formal resection, the type of which depends on the location of the tumor. Upper and middle rectal tumors can usually be managed with a low or very low anterior resection. Lower rectal tumors frequently require a proctectomy with coloanal anastomosis or an abdominoperineal resection. The goal of resection is to obtain a 5-cm distal margin, but lower tumors can be managed with a 2-cm distal margin. Very low tumors and those involving the sphincter mechanism require an abdominoperineal resection.

Rectal tumors with greater depth of rectal wall invasion (T3), evidence of fixation or local invasion (T4), or evidence of lymph nodal (N1–2) or metastatic (M1) disease mandates neoadjuvant chemoradiation therapy. Proctectomy requires a specimen-appropriate total mesorectal excision. This involves complete excision of all mesorectal tissue located behind the rectum with no carcinoma at the lateral or circumferential margins. The goal is to remove all malignant tissue, so as to reduce or eliminate the possibility of locally recurrent disease.

Locally advanced rectal tumors may preclude an effective or safe resection. Some indications for likely inoperability include extensive pelvic disease, invasion of ileofemoral vessels, extensive lymphatic involvement or significant lower extremity lymphedema, bony involvement, and life expectancy less than 3 to 6 months.

Laparoscopy is being performed for rectal malignancies in advanced centers, and studies are under way to verify the efficacy and safety of laparoscopic rectal resection in comparison with traditional open resection.

COMPLICATED DISEASE

Colorectal tumors may manifest with complications such as obstruction, perforation, or significant bleeding. These presentations are generally related to more advanced disease and may preclude a complete staging work-up or potential neoadjuvant therapy. Unless patients are unstable or critically ill or the tumor is unresectable, the tumor should be appropriately resected. An ostomy is usually performed, whether as an end ostomy or as a proximal loop diversion for a primary anastomosis. Colonic stenting is an attractive option for obstructing lesions as palliation or as a bridge to resection after medical stabilization and staging for potential neoadjuvant therapy.

SURGERY FOR HIGH-RISK CONDITIONS

High-risk conditions for the development of colorectal malignancies include FAP, HNPCC, and chronic ulcerative colitis. Surgical management may be prophylactic or possibly therapeutic after a malignancy has been diagnosed. The mainstay of operative management in FAP and chronic ulcerative colitis is a total proctocolectomy. Reconstructive options include an ileal pouch–anal anastomosis, a continent ileostomy (Kock pouch), or an end ileostomy. A total abdominal colectomy with ileorectal anastomosis may be performed for temporary preservation of rectal function in selected cases of chronic ulcerative colitis with rectal sparing and FAP with few rectal polyps, but this requires aggressive surveillance of the remaining rectal mucosa because of the risk of malignancy. Patients with HNPCC should also undergo subtotal colectomy with ileorectal anastomosis; because of the prevalence of associated gynecologic malignancies, a total hysterectomy with bilateral salpingo-oophorectomy should be offered to women as well.

PATHOLOGIC STAGING AND ADJUVANT THERAPY

Excellent pathologic sampling and review of the operative specimen provide important prognostic and therapeutic information. Current standards recommend that at least 12 lymph nodes be removed for adequate staging of colon cancer. The decision for adjuvant chemotherapy or radiation therapy or both is based on the pathologic staging. This information also provides prognostic information in terms of survival for the patient and family. A number of staging systems have been developed, but the tumor-node-metastasis (TNM) system is the one most commonly used in the United States (Table 2).

Chemotherapy is offered for patients who have colorectal cancers with locally advanced, nodal (stage III), or metastatic (stage IV) disease. The combination of chemotherapy and radiation therapy for advanced rectal cancer (stage II–IV) has decreased local recurrence and increased survival. Numerous protocols are available for treatment, with the standard of care being FOLFOX: oxaliplatin (Eloxatin), 5-fluorouracil (5-FU [Adrucil]), and leucovorin. Elderly patients and those with multiple comorbidities who may not be able to tolerate full-dose chemotherapy may be candidates for capecitabine (Xeloda) or 5-FU and leucovorin. Numerous study protocols are available at specialized centers evaluating other medications. Newer technologies continue to evolve, such as antiangiogenesis agents and immunomodulatory agents.

METASTATIC DISEASE

Surgical therapy is also available for metastatic disease in certain situations. Metastatic liver lesions amenable to resection can be addressed at the time of colon resection or after the patient has healed from colectomy. The lesions could be resected or treated with radiofrequency ablation, a newer technology that allows in situ destruction of liver lesions. Similarly, selected pulmonary metastases can be resected, possibly with the use of minimally invasive thoracoscopic techniques.

SURVEILLANCE

Surveillance for colon and rectal cancer is a lifelong process. Patients are seen and examined in the office every 3 months for 2 years, then every 6 months for 3 years, and then yearly for 5 years. Levels of carcinoembryonic antigen are measured at each office visit, but current literature recommends obtaining levels every 3 months for 3 years as a marker for tumor recurrence in stage II–III patients. Colonoscopy should be performed at 1 year postoperatively, assuming a high-quality preoperative study has cleared the rest of the colon. A normal colonoscopy at 1 year postoperatively would allow the next surveillance colonoscopy to be performed 3 years later. If that one is normal, subsequent examinations should be performed every 5 years. After the examination at 1 year postoperatively, the subsequent intervals should be shortened if there is evidence of HNPCC or if additional adenomas are found. As an addition to formal colonoscopies, flexible sigmoidoscopies are performed with each office visit for patients with rectal cancer. Routine imaging utilizing CT scans of the chest, abdomen, and pelvis is performed annually for 3 years in patients with colorectal cancer. Patients with increased or rising CEA levels, as noted by routine surveillance checks, or evidence of recurrent disease, as noted by history and physical examinations or routine surveillance imaging studies, can be evaluated with the use of positron emission tomography (PET), an emerging sensitive test for tumor recurrence.

REFERENCES

American Cancer Society. Cancer Facts and Figures 2010, Atlanta, GA: American Cancer Society; 2010. Available at: http://www.cancer.org/Research/CancerFactsFigures/CancerFactsFigures/cancer-facts-figures-2010 [accessed September 8, 2010].

Beart RW, Steele Jr GD, Menck HR, et al. Management and survival of patients with adenocarcinoma of the colon and rectum: A national survey of the Commission on Cancer. J Am Coll Surg 1995;181:225–36.

Bentrem DJ, Okabe S, Wong WD, et al. T1 Adenocarcinoma of the rectum: Transanal excision or radical surgery? Ann Surg 2005;242:472–9.

TABLE 2 Pathologic Staging Systems for Colorectal Cancer

Pathologic Features	Stage	TNM	Dukes	Astler-Coller	5-yr Survival (%)
Depth of Invasion					
Lamina propria, muscularis mucosa	0	T0/Tis	A		>90
Submucosa	I	T1	A	B1	
Muscularis propria	I	T2	A	B1	
Subserosa, pericolic fat	II	T3	B	B1	70–85
Adjacent organs, perforation	II	T4	B	B2	55–65
Lymph Nodal Involvement					
None		N0			
1–3 nodes	III	N1	C	C1, C2	45–55
>3 nodes	III	N2	C	C1, C2	20–30
Distant Metastatic Disease					
Absent		M0			
Present	IV	M1	D		<5

TNM = tumor-node-metastasis system.

Clinical Outcomes of Surgical Therapy Study Group. A comparison of laparoscopically assisted and open colectomy for colon cancer. N Engl J Med 2004;350:2050–9.

Desch CE, Benson AB 3rd, Somerfield MR, et al. Colorectal cancer surveillance: 2005 update of an American Society of Clinical Oncology Practice Guideline. J Clin Oncol 2005;23(33):8512–9.

Floyd ND, Saclarides TJ. Transanal endoscopic microsurgical resection of pT1 rectal tumors. Dis Colon Rectum 2005;49:164–8.

Lan Y-T, Lin J-K, Li AFY, et al. Metachronous colorectal cancer: Necessity of postoperative colonoscopic surveillance. Int J Colorectal Dis 2005;20:121–5.

Levin B, Lieberman DA, McFarland B, et al. Screening and surveillance for the early detection of colorectal cancer and adenomatous polyps, 2008: A joint guideline from the American Cancer Society, the US Multi-Society Task Force on Colorectal Cancer, and the American College of Radiology. For the American Cancer Society Colorectal Cancer Advisory Group, the US Multi-Society Task Force, and the American College of Radiology Colon Cancer Committee. Gastroenterology 2008;134:1570–95.

Maetani I, Tada T, Ukita T, et al. Self-expandable metallic stent placement as palliative treatment of obstructed colorectal carcinoma. J Gastroenterol 2004;39:334–8.

Pinol V, Castells A, Andreu M, et al. Accuracy of Revised Bethesda Guidelines, microsatellite instability, and immunohistochemistry for the identification of patients with hereditary nonpolyposis colorectal cancer. JAMA 2005;293:1986–94.

Rex DK, Kahi CJ, Levin B, et al. Guidelines for colonoscopy surveillance after cancer resection: A consensus update by the American Cancer Society and the US Multi-Society Task Force on Colorectal Cancer. Gastroenterology 2006;130:1865–71.

Sauer R, Becker H, Hohenberger W, et al. for the German Rectal Cancer Study Group: Preoperative versus postoperative chemoradiotherapy for rectal cancer. N Engl J Med 2004;351:1731–40.

Stipa F, Chessin DB, Shia J, et al. A pathologic complete response of rectal cancer to preoperative combined-modality therapy results in improved oncological outcome compared with those who achieve no downstaging on the basis of preoperative endorectal ultrasonography. Ann Surg Oncol 2006; 13(8):1047–53.

Winawer SJ, Zauber AG, Fletcher RH, et al. Guidelines for colonoscopy surveillance after polypectomy: A consensus update by the US Multi-Society Task Force on Colorectal Cancer and the American Cancer Society. CA Cancer J Clin 2006;56:143–59.

Intestinal Parasites

Method of

Nathan Thielman, MD, MPH, and Elizabeth Reddy, MD

Intestinal parasites are a diverse group of pathogens with local and global significance. Immigration, international adoption, travel, and the frequency of HIV, AIDS, and other immune-compromising conditions (e.g., malignancy, organ transplantation) have all contributed to a need for ongoing or increased awareness of parasitic infections in the United States. Persons who reside in chronic care facilities, children in daycare, and persons whose sexual practices increase the likelihood of fecal–oral contact are also at risk for acquiring intestinal parasitic infection.

Globally, intestinal parasites are responsible for an enormous burden of disease. Although these pathogens are rarely fatal, ongoing exposure to intestinal parasites among persons in endemic areas exacerbates malnutrition, carries multiple morbidities, and causes stunting of growth and development in children, all of which have far-reaching consequences.

Patients who present with diarrheal illness (especially prolonged or travel-associated), unexplained eosinophilia, or expulsion of worms should be evaluated for intestinal parasites. In such cases, a careful history should focus on the patient's country of origin, detailed travel and recreational activities, dietary habits and new or unusual food exposures, occupation, sexual history, sick contacts,

and risks for or known immunodeficiency. Some specialists advocate obtaining a complete blood count with differential to assess eosinophil count in all international adoptees and immigrants from areas where parasitic infections are common. If eosinophilia is present, antibody testing for schistosomiasis and strongyloidiasis—two chronic parasitic infections with potentially serious consequences—should be performed, and appropriate therapy should be administered if infection is discovered. For key features of common intestinal parasitic infections, see the Current Diagnosis box.

Diagnosis of intestinal parasites has improved recently with the advent of quick, simple, and accurate stool antigen tests for some major pathogens, such as *Entamoeba, Giardia* and *Cryptosporidium* species. However, the fecal examination for ova and parasites is still the mainstay of diagnosis in many cases. Whenever possible, stool specimens should be sent to a laboratory with clinical expertise in parasitology, where wet preparation, concentration, or staining can identify most pathogens. Evaluation of fresh specimens and repeated examinations improve diagnostic sensitivity. Key diagnostic points are summarized in the Current Diagnosis box.

This review focuses on basic understanding, recognition, diagnosis and treatment of common intestinal parasites in the United States and throughout the world. Within each section, parasites are listed in order of relative clinical significance.

Protozoa: Amoebae, Flagellates, Ciliates

ENTAMOEBA HISTOLYTICA

Entamoeba histolytica, the cause of amoebic dysentery and amebic liver abscess, is a worldwide pathogen of major clinical significance. Approximately 10% of the world's population and up to 60% of children in highly endemic areas show serologic evidence of infection, and *E. histolytica* is estimated to cause 100,000 deaths per year globally. In the United States, infection is almost exclusively found among returned travelers, immigrants from endemic areas (especially Mexico and Central and South America), men who have sex with men (MSM), and institutionalized persons. *E. histolytica* exists in only two forms, the hardy cyst characterized by four nuclei, and the trophozoite, which has a single nucleus and survives poorly outside the human body. It is important to note that *Entamoeba dispar* and *Entamoeba moshkovskii*, which are morphologically identical to *E. histolytica* in stool microscopy, are now known to be nonpathogenic species. Other *Entamoeba*, including *Entamoeba hartmanni, Entamoeba coli, Entamoeba polecki* and others can be individually identified on microscopy but are of uncertain pathogenicity and thought to be benign.

E. histolytica infection is acquired by ingestion of cysts in contaminated water or food or by fecal–oral contact, as can occur in chronic care facilities or with anal–oral sexual practices. Acquisition of the parasite can result in asymptomatic infection (most common), diarrheal illness, or extraintestinal infection, the latter most commonly manifest as amebic liver abscess. An appropriately robust layer of colonic mucin may be protective against symptomatic infection, whereas attachment to intestinal epithelium results in penetration of the organism into the submucosal layer, where extensive tissue destruction can take place in the form of apoptosis and lysis of cells, hence the name "histolytica."

Symptoms of classic amebic dysentery begin insidiously 1 to 2 weeks after infection. Diarrhea is almost universal and typically consists of numerous small-volume stools that can contain mucus or frank blood, or both. Stools are almost always heme positive if not grossly bloody. Abdominal pain and tenesmus are common; fever is present in approximately 30% of cases. Some persons have a chronic course characterized by weight loss, intermittent loose stools, and abdominal pain. Rare presentations of amebic dysentery include amebomas, which can mimic malignancy, and perianal ulcerations or fistulae. Severe disease can occur in the form of fulminant colitis or toxic megacolon; the latter almost universally requires colectomy.

Young age, pregnancy, and corticosteroid use predispose to severe infection. Although persons with HIV infection or AIDS can develop invasive disease, *E. histolytica* does not appear to be a common opportunistic infection, and infection is curable in this population.

Amebic liver abscess is the most common extraintestinal complication of *E. histolytica*; cerebral and ocular amebiasis have also been reported. Amebic liver abscess affects children of both sexes equally, but it is up to nine times more common in men, indicating that hormonal milieu likely plays a role. Amebic liver abscess almost always manifests within 3 to 5 months of initial infection, but it can surface years later. Illness is characterized by fever and abdominal tenderness that worsen over several days to weeks. Weight loss, jaundice, and cough from diaphragmatic irritation can also occur. Symptoms of dysentery usually are not present, and diarrhea is reported in less than one third of cases. Laboratory abnormalities include leukocytosis, transaminitis, elevated alkaline phosphatase, and elevated sedimentation rate. Chest radiograph often demonstrates elevation of the right hemidiaphragm, and pleural effusion may be present. Rupture of the abscess can occur into the abdomen or pleuropulmonary space, manifesting as acute abdomen or empyema.

Diagnosis of intraintestinal *E. histolytica* infection has classically relied on stool microscopy, and this remains the only available method in much of the world. At least three stool specimens should be examined to improve sensitivity. Cysts visualized in stool might or might not indicate active infection and cannot be distinguished from *E. dispar* and *E. moshkovskii*. Presence of trophozoites with ingested red blood cells on stool preparation is diagnostic of dysentery secondary to *E. histolytica*, as are mobile amebae if seen within freshly examined biopsy material.

Diagnosis of *E. histolytica* infection has improved greatly with the advent of antigen tests, now available as enzyme-linked immunosorbent assays (ELISAs) and immunoflorescent probes. The Techlab ELISA antigen test is highly sensitive and specific and can be used on a freshly passed stool specimen, serum, or hepatic abscess material. It becomes positive with onset of symptomatic disease and resolves on treatment of infection. Other available antigen tests appear to function well but have not been as rigorously studied. Aspirate of liver abscess material may be necessary to distinguish from pyogenic liver abscess; a negative stool examination for *E. histolytica* does not preclude amebic liver abscess. In a patient at high risk for amebic liver abscess (e.g., young male immigrants), a trial of antimicrobial therapy can help in diagnosis because infection typically responds rapidly.

All patients who have confirmed *E. histolytica* infection and reside in nonendemic areas should be treated regardless of whether they are symptomatic, because invasive disease can develop in the future. Asymptomatic cyst passers may be treated with an intralumnal agent alone, such as paromomycin (Humatin) or iodoquinol (Yodoxin). In the United States, the most readily available effective treatment for patients with amebic colitis or liver abscess is metronidazole (Flagyl). It can be given intravenously for patients unable to tolerate oral medications. Experts recommend that a course of therapy with an intraluminal agent be given following the completed course of the systemic agent for all cases of invasive *E. histolytica*. See Table 1 for medications and doses.

GIARDIASIS

Giardia lamblia, also known as *Giardia intestinalis* or *Giardia duodenalis*, is the most commonly identified diarrheal parasitic infection in the United States, with an estimated 100,000 to 2.5 million cases per year. It is globally distributed and found in fresh water throughout mountainous regions of the United States and Canada. The organism is a flagellated aerotolerant anaerobe that exists in a cyst and trophozoite form. Cysts can survive for several weeks in cold water. Contaminated food and water are the most common sources of infection, but the organism can also be passed by person-to-person contact. In the United States, giardiasis is primarily diagnosed among international travelers, persons with recreational water exposure, institutionalized persons and children in day care, and persons with anal–oral sexual practices.

CURRENT DIAGNOSIS

Signs and Symptoms

- Watery diarrhea—Most protozoal infections: *Giardia, Blastocystis, Dientamoeba, Cryptosporidium, Cyclospora, Isospora, Microsporidia*
- Dysentery—Most commonly *Entamoeba histolytica*; less commonly *Balantidium coli, Trichuris trichuria* (whipworm)
- Eosinophilia—Throughout chronic infection: *Strongyloides*, schistosomiasis, *Isospora*; usually only in early infection: *Ascaris*, hookworm, whipworm
- Prolonged or severe diarrhea in HIV infection—Spore-forming protozoal infections: *Cryptosporidium, Cyclospora, Isospora, Microsporidia*
- Visible worms passed in stool—*Ascaris, Taeniasis, Diphyllobothrium*

Diagnosis of Parasitic Infections

- Stool antigen assay—*Entamoeba histolytica, Giardia, Cryptosporidium*
- Serology*—Strongyloides, schistosomiasis
- Stool for ova and parasites—All intestinal parasites. Sensitivity increased with repeat exams if necessary. Concentration, preservation, and staining improve diagnosis of certain pathogens.

Note: Key features of intestinal parasitic infection may overlap with other conditions, including nonparasitic infections, and extra-intestinal parasites.

*Optimal method of diagnosis in returned travelers and immigrants from endemic to nonendemic areas. Does not distinguish between active and resolved infections.

Illness can result from ingestion of as few as 10 to 25 cysts, which transform into trophozoites in the small intestine and attach to and damage the small bowel wall. Symptomatic disease begins insidiously over approximately 2 weeks in 25% to 50% of persons who ingest *Giardia* cysts. Others become asymptomatic cyst passers (5%–15%) or have no signs of infection (35%–50%). Hallmarks of infection are watery diarrhea, bloating, gas, abdominal pain, and weight loss; less commonly, patients have nausea, vomiting, or low-grade fever. Steatorrhea and malabsorption, particularly secondary to *Giardia*-induced lactase deficiency, can be observed. Chronic *Giardia* infection should be considered in the differential diagnosis for a long-standing diarrheal illness, especially if there is history of exposure to possibly contaminated water. Patients with common variable immune deficiency, X-linked agammglobulinemia, and IgA deficiency syndromes are at risk for fulminant and sometimes incurable disease, suggesting a significant role for humoral immunity in control of infection. Persons with HIV infection or AIDS have symptoms similar to those in patients without HIV and typically can be cured of infection with standard therapy.

Diagnosis of giardiasis is made by examination of fresh or preserved stool or by stool antigen assays. In the case of fecal examination, trophozoites may be directly visualized in fresh liquid stool; semiformed and preserved stool should be stained before examination. Currently, there are immunochromographic, direct fluorescence antibody, and ELISA tests for diagnosis of *Giardia*, including the ImmunoCard STAT! Cryptosporidium/Giardia Rapid Assay (Meridian Bioscience, Cincinnati, Ohio), which tests for both pathogens simultaneously. Although it is rarely necessary, the diagnosis can sometimes be made on duodenal biopsy.

For details of treatment options, see Table 1. Metronidazole is the most commonly prescribed treatment in the United States and should be given for a 10-day course. Tinidazole (Tindamax), recently approved in the United States, appears to have excellent efficacy and improved tolerability over metronidazole. Nitazoxanide (Alinia) has

TABLE 1 Pharmacologic Treatment of Major Protozoan Infections

Clinical Situation	Drug	Adult Dose	Pediatric Dose	Comments
Amebiasis				
Entamoeba histolytica				
Asymptomatic	Recommended: Paromomycin (Humatin) *or*	25–35 mg/kg/d in 3 doses × 7 d	25–35 mg/kg/d in 3 doses × 7 d	
	Iodoquinol (Yodoxin)	650 mg tid × 20 d	30–40 mg/kg/d (max 2g) in 3 doses × 20 d	
	Alternative: Diloxanide furoate (Furanmide)[2,*]	500 mg tid × 10 d	20 mg/kg/d in 3 doses × 10 d	
Mild to moderate intestinal disease	Recommended: Metronidazole (Flagyl) *or* Tinidazole (Tindamax)[§]	500–750 mg tid × 7–10 d 2 g once daily × 3 d	35–50 mg/kg/d in 3 doses × 7–10 d 50 mg/kg once daily (max 2 g) × 3 d	Treatment should be followed by a course of iodoquinol or paromomycin in the dosage used to treat asymptomatic amebiasis.
Severe intestinal or extraintestinal disease*	Metronidazole *or*	750 mg tid × 7–10 d	35–50 mg/kg/d in 3 doses × 7–10 d	
	Tinidazole	2 g once daily × 5 d	50 mg/kg once daily (max 2 g) × 5 d	A nitroimidazole similar to metronidazole, tinidazole is FDA approved and appears to be as effective and better tolerated than metronidazole. It should be taken with food to minimize GI adverse effects. For children and patients unable to take tablets, a pharmacist may crush the tablets and mix them with cherry syrup. The syrup suspension is good for 7 d at room temperature and must be shaken before use. Ornidazole, a similar drug, is also used outside the United States.
Balantidiasis				
Balantidium coli				
Symptomatic and asymptomatic disease	Recommended: Tetracycline[1,†,‖]	500 mg qid × 10 d	40 mg/kg/d (max 2 g) in 4 doses × 10 d[5]	
	Alternatives: Metronidazole[1] *or* Iodoquinol[1]	750 mg PO tid × 5 d 650 mg tid × 20 d	35–50 mg/kg/d in 3 doses × 5 d 30–40 mg/kg/d (max 2 g) in 3 doses × 20 d	
Blastocystis hominis				
Symptomatic disease only				Organism's pathogenicity is uncertain.[‡]
Cryptosporidiosis				
Cryptosporidium parvum				
Immune competent	Nitazoxanide	500 mg bid × 3 d	1–3 y: 100 mg bid × 3 d 4–11 y: 200 mg bid × 3 d	FDA approved as a pediatric oral suspension for treating Cryptosporidium in immunocompetent children <12 y and for *Giardia*. It might also be effective for mild to moderate amebiasis. Nitazoxanide is available in 500-mg tabs and an oral suspension; it should be taken with food.
HIV-infected	No optimal therapy available			All HIV-infected patients with cryptosporidiosis should receive HAART whenever possible. Limited data suggest nitazoxanide might have some benefit in patients with CD4 counts >50. Recent meta-analysis showed no efficacy over placebo for any antiparasitic therapy for cryptosporidiosis.
Cyclosporiasis				
Cyclospora cayetanensis	Recommended: TMP-SMX (Bactrim, Septra)[1]	160 mg TMP, 800 mg SMX (1 DS tab) bid × 7–10 d	5 mg/kg TMP, 25 mg/kg SMX bid × 7–10 d	In immunocompetent patients, usually a self-limited illness. Immunosuppressed patients might need higher doses, longer duration (TMP-SMX qid × 10 d, followed by bid × 3 wk) and long-term maintenance. For isosporiasis in sulfonamide-sensitive patients, pyrimethamine 50–75 mg qd in divided doses (*plus* leucovorin 10–25 mg/d) is effective.

Continued

TABLE 1 Pharmacologic Treatment of Major Protozoan Infections—Cont'd

Clinical Situation	Drug	Adult Dose	Pediatric Dose	Comments
Dientamoebiasis				
Dientamoeba fragilis Symptomatic disease only	Iodoquinol[1] *or*	650 mg tid × 20 d	30–40 mg/kg/d (max 2g) in 3 doses × 20 d	
	Paromomycin[1] *or*	25–35 mg/kg/d in 3 doses × 7 d	25–35 mg/kg/d in 3 doses × 7 d	
	Tetracycline[1] *or*	500 mg qid × 7–10 d	40 mg/kg/d (max 2g) in 4 doses × 10 d[5]	
	Metronidazole	500–750 mg tid × 10 d	20–40 mg/kg/d in 3 doses × 10 d	
Giardiasis				
Giardia lamblia	Recommended:	250 mg tid × 5–7 d	15 mg/kg/d in 3 doses × 5 d	
All symptomatic disease and asymptomatic carriage in nonendemic areas	Metronidazole[1] or Nitazoxanide *or*	500 mg bid × 3 d	1–3 y: 100 mg bid × 3 d 4–11 y: 200 mg bid × 3 d	
	Tinidazole	2 g once	50 mg/kg (max 2 g) once	Treatment should be followed by a course of iodoquinol or paromomycin in the dosage used to treat asymptomatic amebiasis.
	Alternatives: Quinacrine[1],* *or*	100 mg tid × 5 d	2 mg/kg/d (max 300 mg/d) tid × 5 d	Albendazole, 400 mg daily × 5 d alone or in combination with metronidazole may also be effective. Combination treatment with standard doses of metronidazole and quinacrine for 3 wk is effective for a small number of refractory infections. In one study, nitazoxanide was used successfully in high doses to treat a case of *Giardia* resistant to metronidazole and albendazole.
	Furazolidone (Furoxone) *or*	100 mg qid × 7–10 d	6 mg/kg/d in 4 doses × 10 d	
	Paromomycin[1]	25–35 mg/kg/d in 3 doses × 7 d	25–35 mg/kg/d in 3 doses × 7 d	Nonabsorbed luminal agent; may be useful for treating giardiasis in pregnancy
Isosporiasis				
Isospora belli[‡]	Recommended: TMP-SMX[1]	160 mg TMP, 800 mg SMX bid × 7–10 d	5 mg/kg TMP, 25 mg/kg SMX bid × 7–10 d	
Microsporidiosis				
Enterocytozoon bineusi				
Diarrheal or disseminated disease	Fumagillin[2]	60 mg/d PO × 14 d		Oral fumagillin (Sanofi Recherche, Gentilly, France) is effective in treating *E. bieneusi* but is associated with thrombocytopenia. HAART can lead to microbiological and clinical response in HIV-infected patients with microsporidial diarrhea. Octreotide (Sandostatin) has provided symptomatic relief in some patients with large-volume diarrhea.
Encephalocytozoon intestinalis				
Diarrheal or disseminated disease	Albendazole[1]	400 mg bid × 21 d		

Adapted from Drugs for parasitic infections. Med Lett Drug Ther, Volume 5 (Suppl) 2007.
[1]Not FDA approved for this indication.
[2]Not available in the United States.
[5]Investigational drug in the United States.
*The drug is not available commercially, but as a service it can be compounded by Panorama Compounding Pharmacy, 6744 Balboa Blvd., Van Nuys, CA 91406 (800-247-9767) or Medical Center Pharmacy, New Haven, CT (203-688-6816).
[†]An approved drug, but considered investigational for this condition by the FDA.
[‡]Clinical significance of these organisms is controversial; metronidazole 750 mg tid × 10 d, iodoquinol 650 mg tid × 20 d, or TMP-SMX11 double-strength tab bid × 7 d are effective. Metronidazole resistance may be common. Nitazoxanide is effective in children.
[§]Dosing recommendations only available for children ≥ to 3 y.
[||]Contraindicated in pregnant and breastfeeding women and children <8 y.
DS = double strength; GI = gastrointestinal; HAART = highly active antiretroviral therapy; max = maximum; tab = tablet; TMP-SMX = trimethoprim-sulfamethoxazole.

also been shown to eradicate infection well and can be used as an alternative or in patients who fail a first course of treatment. Patients who fail first-line therapy might have a persistent source of infection (contaminated water source, close contact with an infected person), immune deficiency predisposing to difficult eradication, or persistence of cysts. Once possible sources of reinfection have been investigated and eliminated, relapsed infections should either be re-treated with a longer course of therapy (21–28 days) or treated with a different agent. Patients who fail more than one course of therapy should undergo immunologic work-up.

Prevention of *Giardia* infection, as with other parasitic infections, involves primarily close attention to personal hygiene, hand washing, and avoidance of ingestion of fresh unfiltered water. Boiling water or use of a 0.2- to 1-μm water filter offer optimal protection against *Giardia* and other parasitic pathogens, although such filters still might not protect against *Cryptosporidium*.

BLASTOCYSTIS HOMINIS

Blastocystis hominis is a protozoan with worldwide distribution found most commonly in tropical regions; it is present in humans and several other animals. In temperate regions, *B. hominis* is detected at a high rate among MSM. *B. hominis* was long thought to cause only asymptomatic colonization, but there is some evidence to suggest a role in human disease, although this remains controversial. Ongoing molecular analysis might elucidate subtypes of *B. hominis* with varying degrees of pathogenicity in humans.

B. hominis has four forms: vacuolated, ameba-like, granular, and cyst, the latter of which is likely to be the infectious form. It appears to be transmitted via the fecal–oral route, possibly from waterborne sources.

As suggested previously, the majority of infections appear to be entirely asymptomatic, and number of organisms does not appear to accurately predict severity of illness. Symptoms consist mainly of watery diarrhea, bloating, and abdominal cramps. There are typically no pathologic findings on colonoscopy and there are no reports of invasive disease. Infection is diagnosed by stool microscopy with use of a trichrome or hematoxylin-stained preserved specimen. The organism is susceptible in vitro to numerous antimicrobials. Bactrim[1] or metronidazole is the treatment of choice; details are listed in Table 1.

DIENTAMOEBA FRAGILIS

Dientamoeba fragilis was originally classified as an amoeba, but it is more closely related to the flagellates such as *Trichomonas vaginalis*. It is distributed worldwide, including in Western nations, and has only recently been recognized as a clinically significant pathogen, possibly because it is difficult to visualize without specific staining techniques. Illness has commonly been found in travelers and MSM, but it can affect anyone.

The parasite exists only in the trophozoite form. Despite its genetic relationship to the flagellates, *D. fragilis* does not have a flagellum and is immotile. Trophozoites range in size from 4 to 20 μm and are binucleate. Patients in the United States who have *D. fragilis* were found in some studies to harbor other intestinal parasites as well, such as *E. vermicularis* and *B. hominis*, and in general *D. fragilis* is more prevalent in areas of the world with limited public sanitation. These features support a fecal–oral mode of transmission for *D. fragilis*.

Most patients are asymptomatic; however, numerous case reports and small series describe patients with no other organisms identified to cause their symptoms who improve significantly after treatment and documented clearance of *D. fragilis* from their stool. Illness is typically subacute to chronic, characterized by abdominal pain, watery diarrhea, anorexia, fatigue, and malaise. Diagnosis can be difficult, because the parasite is fastidious. If *D. fragilis* is suspected, stool should be preserved with polyvinyl alcohol and quickly stained with iron–hematoxylin and trichrome. Polymerase chain reaction (PCR) has been used for diagnosis as well, but it is not readily available for use in most clinical settings.

For full treatment information, see Table 1. Iodoquinol (Yodoxin) and metronidazole have both been used successfully to treat *D. fragilis*.

BALANTIDIUM COLI

Balantidium coli is the largest protozoan that infects humans, and the only ciliate. Balantidiasis is a relatively rare cause of illness and is found primarily in rural agrarian communities in Southeast Asia, Central and South America, and Papua New Guinea. *B. coli* is highly associated with animal farming, in particular, pigs; humans are incidental hosts. The parasite is transmitted by direct contact with animals or on ingestion of water or food contaminated by animal excrement. Persons with malnutrition or immune deficiency are particularly susceptible to infection.

B. coli invades the intestinal mucosa from the terminal ileum to the rectum. About one half of infections are asymptomatic; the other one half result in a subacute or chronic diarrheal illness with abdominal cramping, nausea, vomiting, weight loss, and occasional low-grade fever. Fewer than 5% of patients present with severe or even fulminant dysentery, and rare cases of colonic penetration with peritonitis, mesenteric lymphadenitis, or hepatic infection have been reported.

Diagnosis is made by visualization of trophozoites in fresh stool specimens or preserved and permanently stained samples. The trophozoite is large and ciliated; cysts are difficult to distinguish. It displays a distinct spiraling motility that can be seen under low power. On stained sample, visualization of *B. coli*'s characteristic macronucleus and spiral micronucleus can help confirm the diagnosis. All patients should be treated regardless of symptoms. Tetracycline (Sumycin and others) is the therapy of choice; the infection also responds to metronidazole[1]; see Table 1 for dosing information.

Spore-Forming Protozoa and Microsporidia

CRYPTOSPORIDIOSIS

Cryptosporidium is a pathogen with worldwide distribution that is endemic to the United States. Humans are most commonly infected by the recently reclassified *Cryptosporidium hominis*, but *Cryptosporidium parvum*, primarily a bovine pathogen, also causes human disease. *Cryptosporidium* has caused multiple waterborne out-breaks in the United States and can be acquired secondary to recreational water exposure (e.g., swimming pools, water parks). The best-known outbreak occurred secondary to heavy rains that brought farm runoff into the drinking water supply in Wisconsin in 1984. It resulted in 430,000 documented cases of cryptosporidiosis and contributed to the deaths of dozens of persons with advanced HIV infection or malignancy.

Cryptosporidium is a coccidian, part of a group of spore-forming protozoa with a complex life cycle and a structure that allows mechanical penetration into host cells. *Cryptosporidium* can mature and reproduce entirely within human hosts, thereby enabling infection to occur both from environmental sources and by direct person-to-person contact. Its oocysts, the source of infection on ingestion, are markedly hardy; they can withstand heavy chlorination, survive for months in cold water, and are small enough to occasionally evade even the smallest available water filtration systems.

All persons are susceptible to infection, which usually is self-limited. Fulminant or chronic infection, or both, can be seen among patients with immune compromise secondary to HIV infection or AIDS (especially those with CD4 <50), in patients with malignancy, and in malnourished children. As few as 100 oocysts can cause infection, which results when the parasite penetrates small bowel epithelium and replicates just beneath its surface. Villous flattening and small bowel wall edema are seen on pathologic examination from infected persons.

Asymptomatic infections occur but are relatively rare. Symptoms begin within several days to 1 week of ingestion of oocysts. The

---

[1]Not FDA approved for this indication.

---

[1]Not FDA approved for this indication.

hallmark of infection is explosive watery diarrhea, which can be so voluminous as to resemble cholera and can cause significant dehydration and electrolyte imbalance. Abdominal discomfort, nausea, vomiting, fever, malaise, and myalgia can also be present, and weight loss is common. Illness lasts 1 to 2 weeks, but a substantial percentage of patients report a relapse of symptoms after initial improvement. The biliary tract can be involved, particularly in patients with HIV infection, and infection at other distant sites, such as the lungs, has rarely been reported.

Diagnosis of *Cryptosporidium* has improved dramatically in recent years with the advent of antigen tests, which are highly sensitive and specific and can be used on a single sample of fresh stool. The ImmunoCard STAT! Cryptosporidium/Giardia Rapid Assay is useful because it can detect both pathogens. When such tests are not available, stools submitted for examination should be fixed in formalin and stained for trophozoites or cysts; multiple stool specimens improves the diagnostic sensitivity. Luminal fluid or biopsy specimens obtained during endoscopy can also reveal the organism.

Infection with *Cryptosporidium* is typically a self-limited illness in otherwise healthy persons, but symptoms can be improved and the course shortened with the antiparasitic nitazoxanide. *Cryptosporidium* remains an extremely challenging and potentially devastating infection in immunocompromised patients, especially those with HIV and a low CD4 count (counts <200 increase risk of severe illness, and counts < 50 markedly increase risk). Although anticryptosporidial therapies in this population have shown very limited efficacy, restoration of immune function with HAART often effects cure. Limited data suggest a trial of nitazoxanide may be reasonable in this circumstance as well. Appropriate supportive measures are also crucial in all patients with *Cryptosporidium*, including fluid and electrolyte replacement; avoiding lactose products is likely to be beneficial during the first 2 weeks after infection as the brush border regenerates. Appropriate treatment doses for nitazoxanide are listed in Table 1.

Prevention of *Cryptosporidium* infection requires a highly developed public water purification system including flocculation, sedimentation, and filtration. Use of 0.2- to 1-μm personal water filters for campers and hikers greatly reduces but does not eliminate risk of infection, whereas boiling water before drinking kills oocysts. Close attention to hygiene and avoidance of fecal–oral contact is the mainstay of prevention in the settings of institutional and community outbreaks.

CYCLOSPORA SPECIES

Cyclospora cayetanensis is a coccidian with structure similar to that of *Cryptosporidium*. Unlike *Cryptosporidium*, *C. cayetanensis* requires a period of development outside the human body, thereby eliminating the possibility of close person-to-person contact as a means of acquiring the infection. *C. cayetanensis* is distributed worldwide, most commonly in the tropics and subtropics where infection tends to exhibit seasonality. It has also been associated with food (e.g., raspberries) and waterborne outbreaks in temperate regions, including the United States, and in recent years it has become increasingly recognized as a cause of infectious diarrhea in returned travelers.

All persons are susceptible to infection, but those with HIV are at risk for more severe and prolonged disease, as seen with cryptosporidiosis and isosporiasis. Symptomatic disease appears to be most common in adults who do not have previous exposure to *Cyclospora*, such as travelers or persons who have relocated to endemic areas. Illness begins about a week after ingestion of sporulated oocysts and is characterized by watery diarrhea, abdominal cramping, bloating, anorexia, and weight loss. Low-grade fever can occur; marked fatigue is common and can last weeks or even months, and untreated infections can relapse after apparent resolution. Biliary involvement can occur in patients with HIV coinfection, as with cryptosporidiosis. Cyclosporiasis, similar to infection with other coccidians, causes damage to the small bowel epithelium, with resultant crypt flattening, edema, and inflammatory infiltrate. Lactose deficiency can remain for months following initial infection.

Diagnosis is made by stool examination. As with diagnosis of other parasitic infections, multiple stool specimens improve

sensitivity. In the case of *Cyclospora*, concentration of the stool specimen also increases yield. If cyclosporiasis is suspected, specific testing should be requested, because the organism exhibits unique properties. Organisms are about two times the size of *Cryptosporidium* and can be seen with Kinyoun acid-fast stain. They also autofluoresce and can be visualized under ultraviolet microscopy. Currently there is no stool antigen assay, but PCR testing has been used in experimental and limited clinical settings to assist in diagnosis.

Cyclosporiasis is best treated with trimethoprim-sulfamethoxazole (Bactrim)[1]; ciprofloxacin[1] may be effective for patients who have a sulfa allergy. Patients with HIV infection can require longer courses of treatment or chronic suppressive therapy; appropriate antiretroviral therapy is also important in the treatment of severe or relapsing infections. See Table 1 for details.

ISOSPORA SPECIES

Isospora belli is a large coccidian native to tropical areas. Similar to *Cyclospora*, it requires a period of maturation outside the human body and therefore cannot be spread directly from person to person. It appears to cause largely asymptomatic or mild infection in tropical areas to which it is endemic; the exception is among patients coinfected with HIV and particularly those with AIDS, in which it is a very common cause of chronic diarrhea in the Caribbean and Central America. Currently in wealthy countries it is found primarily in travelers returning from endemic areas.

Illness is typically mild and self-limited, consisting primarily of watery diarrhea. However, some immunocompetent persons can develop a chronic spruelike syndrome with malabsorption, and those with HIV infection or AIDS often have severe and prolonged diarrhea. *Isospora* can invade to the lamina propria and can cause eosinophilia, which is different from other coccidian infections.

Diagnosis is made by observation of cysts in stool. As with *Cyclospora*, they can be visualized with acid-fast stains or ultraviolet microscopy. Stool may also contain Charcot–Leiden crystals. Infection in immunocompetent hosts responds well to antimicrobials; persons coinfected with HIV can require longer courses of therapy or chronic suppression, and appropriate antiretroviral therapy may be helpful as well. Trimethoprim-sulfamethoxazole (Bactrim)[1] is the treatment of choice. Ciprofloxacin (Cipro)[1] or pyrimethamine (Daraprim)[1] may be used in cases of sulfa allergy. Doses are listed Table 1.

MICROSPORIDIOSIS

Microsporidia are eukaryotic organisms that have been recently reclassified as fungi based on molecular genotyping. They are distributed globally, and more than 100 genera have been identified, seven of which contain species known to be pathogenic in humans: *Encephalitozoon, Enterocytozoon, Trachipleistophora, Pleistophora, Nosema, Vittaforma,* and *Microsporidium*. These pathogens cause a wide variety of systemic and focal illness throughout the world.

Many immunocompetent patients in wealthy nations exhibit positive serology for certain types of microsporidial infections without a history of disease or travel. Microsporidia are most commonly associated with systemic infection in immunosuppressed persons, particularly those with HIV and a CD4 count of less than 100 or patients with organ transplants. Mode of transmission is not entirely clear, but the pathogen likely is spread both from water sources and possibly from close household contact.

Encephalitozoon intestinalis and *Enterocytozoon bieneusi* are responsible for intestinal microsporidial infections. *E. bieneusi* has been associated with self-limited diarrheal illness; *E. intestinalis* is commonly found in stool specimens throughout the developing world, but its pathogenicity is often not certain. Symptomatic infections, most often in patients coinfected with HIV, typically include a gradual onset of watery diarrhea, which may be worse in the morning and after oral intake. Significant volume and electrolyte depletion can occur, as well as fatigue, anorexia, weight loss, and malabsorption.

---

[1]Not FDA approved for this indication.

E. intestinalis can disseminate and cause acute abdomen with peritonitis, cholangitis, nephritis, and keratoconjunctivitis, and *E. bieneusi* infection can result in cholangitis and nephritis as well as rhinitis, bronchitis, and wheezing. Other microsporidia are implicated in a wide variety of illness both in previously healthy and immunosuppressed hosts and include several ocular pathogens.

Diagnosis of microsporidiosis is attained by visualization of spores in stool or in tissue specimens. As suggested by their name, microsporidial spores are much smaller than those produced by spore-forming protozoal infections; most are approximately 1 μm in length and can easily be confused with bacteria or debris on slides. Special staining techniques have been described, but electron microscopy is required for species identification. See Table 1 for details of treatment. Albendazole (Albenza)[1] is the treatment of choice for *Encephalocytozoon intestinalis*.

Treatment of *Enterocytozoon bieneusi* is more challenging. Although some response to albendazole has been reported, oral fumagillin[2] may have more efficacy. Unfortunately, it is not currently commercially available in the United States. Use of appropriate antiretroviral therapy is perhaps the most important treatment for patients with HIV infection or AIDS and chronic microsporidial infections.

Helminths

NEMATODES

Nematodes (roundworms) are cylindrical nonsegmented organisms that are found throughout the world both as free-living species and as human and animal pathogens. Nematodes are the most common type of human parasitic infestation, found in approximately one quarter of the world's population; often susceptible hosts carry multiple different pathogenic nematodes. There are at least 60 species that have been shown to infect humans and 10 times that many that cause disease in other animals, but a few pathogens account for the bulk of human infections, in particular *Ascaris*, hookworm, and whipworm. These three organisms all require a period of maturation outside the human body—typically in warm, moist soil—underscoring the fact that repeated contact with fecally contaminated soil or food and water is necessary to sustain the cycle of infestation. *Strongyloides* and *Enterobius* are unique in that they can both complete their life cycle on or within human hosts and therefore can cause chronic infection and be transmitted directly by close person-to-person contact where there is the possibility of fecal–oral contamination.

Ascaris

Ascaris lumbricoides, the most common human helminthic infection, is estimated to affect 20% to 25% of the world's population. Up to 80% of community members are infected in heavily endemic areas, namely in Africa, Asia, and Central and South America. Cases of *Ascaris* infestation are also seen in rural areas in the southeastern United States. *A. lumbricoides* are white to pinkish worms that range from 10 to 40 cm in length; the infectious eggs are oval white bodies with an adherent mucopolysaccharide capsule that clings to multiple surfaces and aids in transmissibility of the parasite. Eggs are also remarkably durable, capable of surviving up to 6 years in moist soil and able to weather brief droughts and periods of freezing.

Fecal contamination of water, food, and environmental surfaces such as doorknobs and countertops provide the means of transmission for *Ascaris*, and recurrent infection occurs as long as living conditions that predispose people to infection remain unchanged. Lack of adequate public sanitation, use of human feces as fertilizer (night soil), and frequent contact with soil or shared contaminated surfaces among close household members are risk factors for infection. Persons who move to environments with improved sanitation typically lose their infection within 2 years as all the adult worms die. Eggs excreted by an infected person must mature outside the human body for approximately 2 weeks. On ingestion by a susceptible host, mature eggs hatch in the small intestine and release larvae, which penetrate the intestinal wall and travel through the venous circulation to the lungs, where they are coughed up and swallowed. They then undergo maturation into adult worms in the intestine and produce eggs by 2 to 3 months after initial infection, which are excreted in the feces and mature outside the body to continue the cycle.

Most persons with *Ascaris* infection are asymptomatic. Approximately 15% of people have morbidity as a result of infection, which is associated with young age, large burden of worms, coinfection with other intestinal parasites, and genetic predisposition. In children, infection contributes to malabsorption of protein, fat, and vitamins A and C, and treatment of heavily infected children can improve their nutritional status. *Ascaris* infection can also cause intestinal, pancreatic, or biliary obstruction as a result of worm mass or worm migration. Despite the low incidence of obstructive complications per infected person, the *Ascaris*-related acute abdomen is a significant problem on a global level given the enormous number of people infected. Some patients with intestinal *Ascaris* infection report vague abdominal complaints, such as abdominal discomfort, nausea, vomiting or diarrhea, but these are relatively rare. Pulmonary migration of a large quantity of worms can produce Loeffler's syndrome, or eosinophilic pneumonitis.

Diagnosis is easily attained with standard saline stool preparation, and large numbers of eggs are typically seen. Larvae or worms can also sometimes be seen in sputum or stool samples. In cases of intestinal obstruction, worms may be visualized on upper gastrointestinal series, computed tomography, and even ultrasound. Eosinophilia with *Ascaris* infection is found only during the larval migratory phase, but not at all times. Chronic eosinophilia in an at-risk person suggests another parasitic infection, often *Strongyloides*.

All persons documented to carry *Ascaris* who have migrated to nonendemic areas should be treated to prevent complications in the future; in endemic areas, adults need only be treated if they are symptomatic. Children have been shown to benefit from intermittent anthelminthic therapy in heavily affected areas of the world.

For patients with intestinal obstruction, bowel rest and intravenous hydration are usually sufficient to relieve the obstruction, at which time anthelminthic therapy can be administered. In such cases, gastroenterology consultation should be obtained. In rare cases, surgical intervention is required. Treatment of pulmonary infection is controversial; however, most experts recommend steroid therapy for severe infections followed 2 to 3 weeks later (at the time full-grown worms will have migrated to the intestine) by administration of anthelminthic therapy.

The benzimadazoles (mebendazole [Vermox], albendazole,[1] levamisole,[2] and pyrantel [Pin-X]) all exhibit excellent activity against *Ascaris*. Doses and other options are listed in Table 2. Although albendazole and mebendazole carry a pregnancy class B label, they have been used in pregnant women, adolescent girls, and women of reproductive age without demonstrable effects on fetuses; most experts recommend holding treatment until the second trimester whenever possible.

Sanitary conditions that allow for proper management of human feces are crucial in control and prevention of *Ascaris* infection; boiling water kills the eggs.

Whipworm (Trichuriasis)

Trichuris trichuria has become recognized in recent years as a worldwide pathogen with a scope similar to that of *Ascaris*. Sanitary conditions that predispose to ingestion of food and water contaminated with human feces place people at risk for infection; in many communities infection is hyperendemic, with almost universal carriage of the pathogen.

The adult organism is a small worm about 4 cm in length with a unique whip-like structure that allows its thin tail to become embedded in colonic crypts. Whipworm eggs have a characteristic barrel shape with mucous plugs at either end. Infection is acquired by ingesting *Trichuris* eggs that have undergone embryonation in the soil for 2 to 4 weeks after excretion from a previous host. Larvae emerge from eggs in the intestine and migrate into crypts, where they begin to mature. Egg production begins approximately 3 months later.

Most persons with whipworm carry few worms (approximately 20) and are asymptomatic. As with many other intestinal parasites, children are at greater risk for symptomatic infection, which can cause failure to thrive, anemia, clubbing, inflammatory colitis, and rectal prolapse. Adults with a high worm burden can also experience inflammatory colitis characterized by frequent—often bloody—diarrhea and tenesmus. Infection has been shown to result in production of tumor necrosis factor (TNF)-α by lamina propria cells in the colon, which can contribute to poor appetite and wasting that can be seen with significant infection.

Diagnosis is made by standard stool microscopy without a need to concentrate stool, because large numbers of eggs are excreted. Worms can also be seen on colonoscopy, or they can be visualized grossly in cases of rectal prolapse. Eosinophilia may be seen.

Treatment of symptomatic infections can be accomplished with mebendazole, albendazole,[1] or ivermectin (Stromectal)[1]; see Table 2 for details.

Hookworm (*Necator americanus* and *Ancylostoma duodenale*)

Like other helminthic infections, hookworm affects a substantial portion of the world's population, particularly in rural subtropical and tropical communities where human feces is used as a component of fertilizer. Infection results primarily from parasite penetration into the skin; therefore persons with an agrarian lifestyle and significant soil contact are at greatest risk.

Two species are responsible for the majority of human hookworm: *Necator americanus* and *Ancylostoma duodonale. Ancylostoma braziliense*, a canine intestinal pathogen, causes cutaneous larval migrans in humans because the pathogen cannot penetrate the human dermis. Of the two common forms of human hookworm, *N. americanus* is smaller and a less aggressive pathogen with a longer life span than *A. duodenale*. Both parasites are found in warm climates throughout the world; *A. doudenale* exists in smaller pockets, whereas *N. americanus* is widely distributed throughout impoverished rural areas of the tropics in the Americas, Asia, and Africa.

Hookworms are small helminths, between 0.5 and 1 cm in length. Infection results from larval penetration of the skin on contact with contaminated soil. An intensely pruritic, erythematous, papulovesicular rash called *ground itch* can develop at the site of entry. Parasites then enter the venous or lymphatic circulation and travel to the lungs, at which point an urticarial rash with cough can develop. The larvae are swallowed and migrate to the small intestine, where they attach to the bowel wall with teeth or biting plates and take a continuous blood meal by sucking with strong esophageal muscles. As the hookworms lodge in the small intestine, peripheral eosinophilia peaks, and gastrointestinal discomfort with or without diarrhea can result. Large oral ingestion of *A. duodenale* can cause Wakana syndrome, characterized by cough, shortness of breath, nausea, vomiting, and eosinophilia. The most important clinical manifestation of hookworm infection is iron-deficiency anemia, which can be mild or severe and may be accompanied by malabsorption of protein in hosts with heavy burden of disease. Infants and pregnant women can become extremely ill or even die as a result of the anemia.

Hookworm may be difficult to diagnose because light infections often do not produce enough eggs to be readily seen on stool examination; stool should therefore be concentrated if infection is suspected. Eggs do not appear in stool until approximately 2 months after infection, so patients with pulmonary complaints will not yet have a positive stool examination.

Hookworm infection can be eradicated with benzimidazole anthelminthics; see Table 2 for details. Prevention of hookworm infection, as with other parasites, lies in improved sanitary conditions; wearing shoes is especially important because the majority of infections are acquired through the skin. Mass anthelminthic treatment campaigns have shown some efficacy in reducing disease in children; however, reinfection and concern for development of resistance continue to present significant challenges. Candidate vaccines are currently under investigation.

Strongyloides

Strongyloides stercoralis is a global pathogen that is estimated to affect as many as 100 million people, mostly in tropical regions of the world. In recent years, it has become more commonly recognized in the United States among immigrants as a cause of chronic eosinophilia as well as symptomatic infection.

Strongyloides infection results when filariform larvae dwelling in fecally contaminated soil penetrate the skin or mucous membranes of a susceptible host. Larvae move to the lungs and subsequently to the trachea, where they are coughed up and swallowed. Females, about 2 cm in length, lodge in the lamina propria of the duodenum and proximal jejunum where they begin to oviposit. Rhabdiform larvae emerge from these eggs and either repenetrate the intestinal wall or are passed into the feces, at which point they can begin a free-living cycle and reproduce sexually, or can molt directly into an infectious form ready to enter a subsequent susceptible host.

Persons infected with *Strongyloides* are typically asymptomatic. Those who have symptoms might report abdominal discomfort, diarrhea alternating with constipation, or rarely blood-tinged stool. Severe intestinal infections can occur and are manifest by chronic watery or mucousy diarrhea. In such cases, colonoscopy reveals excessive bowel wall thickening and copious secretions, or edema (catarrhal enteritis or edematous enteritis). Parasite migration through the dermis can manifest as serpiginous, erythematous, and pruritic patches along the buttocks, perineum, and thighs, known as *larvae currens*.

Strongyloides appear to attain a balanced state in their host, with similar numbers of adult worms throughout the many years of infection. During periods of host immunocompromise, in particular in patients taking corticosteroids, *Strongyloides* can enter into a state of rapid autoinfection and rampant reproduction called *hyperinfection syndrome*, which results in devastating illness. Persons with HIV infection do not seem to be at particular risk for symptomatic disease or hyperinfection, but hyperinfection has been linked to HTLV-1 infection. *Strongyloides* has also caused hyperinfection in organ transplant patients whose donor had been infected asymptomatically with the parasite. Although it has long been thought that steroid-induced immune compromise was the major trigger for hyperinfection, growing evidence suggests that steroids themselves may be the culprit by directly inducing the accelerated life cycle in the parasite.

The hyperinfection syndrome is characterized by systemic illness with fever, cough, hypoxia, patchy or diffuse pulmonary infiltrates with alveolar microhemorrhages, and dermatitis; it can include myocarditis, hepatitis, splenic abscess, meningitis and cerebral abscess, and endocrine organ involvement. Larvae migrating out of the intestines can drag bacteria with them, resulting in gram-negative or polymicrobial sepsis. The prognosis of *Strongyloides* hyperinfection syndrome is grave even with highly effective anthelminthic treatment given the diffuse nature of this disease. However, earlier recognition and intensive supportive care result in cure.

Diagnosis of uncomplicated *Strongyloides* infection in endemic areas can be challenging because few larvae are passed in stool, and numerous examinations may be necessary to detect them. ELISA is available and is highly sensitive, but it does not distinguish between active and past infections. It is, however, the test of choice for persons who have migrated to nonendemic areas, and all persons in this setting should be treated. Ivermectin is the treatment of choice; see Table 2 for dosing. During the first days of treatment, patients can experience intense dermal pruritis as parasites die. Eosinophilia and positive ELISA can persist for months even after effective therapy.

Enterobius vermicularis

Human pinworm infection, caused by the thread-like nematode *Enterobius vermicularis*, is found throughout the world and continues to be diagnosed commonly in the United States, especially in

---

[1]Not FDA approved for this indication.

TABLE 2 Pharmacologic Treatment of Nematode, Trematode, and Cestode Infections

Clinical Situation	Drug	Adult Dose	Pediatric Dose	Comments
Anisakiasis				
Anisaka spp. or *Pseudoterranova decipiens*	No recommended medical therapy Surgical or endoscopic removal of worm	—	—	Successful treatment of a patient with *Anisakiasis* with albendazole has been reported.
Ascariasis				
Ascaris lumbricoides	Albendazole (Albenza)[1,†] or	400 mg once	400 mg PO × 1	
	Mebendazole* (Vermox) or	100 mg bid × 3 d or 500 mg once	100 mg bid × 3 d or 500 mg once	
	Ivermectin[1] (Stromectol)	150–200 µg/kg once	150–200 µg/kg once	In heavy infection, therapy may be given for 3 d.
Enterobiasis (Pinworm)				
Enterobius vermicularis	Pyrantel pamoate or	11 mg/kg base (max 1 g) once; repeat in 2 wk	11 mg/kg base (max 1 g) once; repeat in 2 wk	Because all family members are usually infected, treatment of the entire household is recommended.
	Mebendazole* or	100 mg once, repeat in 2 wk	100 mg once, repeat in 2 wk	
	Albendazole[1]	400 mg once, repeat in 2 wk	400 mg once, repeat in 2 wk	
Hookworm				
Ancylostoma duodenale, Necator americanus	Albendazole[1] or Mebendazole or	400 mg once 100 mg bid × 3 d or 500 mg once	400 mg once 100 mg bid × 3 d or 500 mg once	
	Pyrantel pamoate[‡]	11 mg/kg (max 1 g) × 3 d	11 mg/kg (max 1 g) × 3 d	
Schistosomiasis				
Schistosoma haematobium, Schistosoma mansoni	Praziquantel or	40 mg/kg/d in 2 doses × 1 d	40 mg/kg/d in 2 doses × 1 d	
S. mansoni only	Oxamniquine[2]	15 mg/kg once	20 mg/kg/d in 2 doses × 1 d	Effective in some patients in whom praziquantel is less effective Contraindicated in pregnancy
Schistosoma japonicum, Schistosoma mekongi	Praziquantel	60 mg/kg/d in 3 doses × 1 d	60 mg/kg/d in 3 doses × 1 d	
Strongyloidiasis				
	Recommended: Ivermectin	200 µg/kg/d × 2 d	200 µg/kg/d × 2 d	In immunocompromised patients or in patients with disseminated disease, it may be necessary to prolong or repeat therapy or use other agents. Veterinary parenteral and enema formulations of ivermectin are used in severely ill patients unable to take oral medications.
	Alternative: Albendazole[1]	400 mg bid × 7 d	400 mg bid × 7 d	
Tapeworm				
Taenia solium (intestinal disease), *Taenia sanguinata, Diphyllobothrium latum*	Praziquantel[1,‡] (Biltricide) or	5–10 mg/kg once	5–10 mg/kg once	
	Niclosamide[‡] (Yomesan)	2 g once	50 mg/kg once	Available in the United States only from the manufacturer
Trichuriasis (Whipworm)				
Trichuris trichuria	Recommended: Mebendazole	100 mg bid × 3 d or 500 mg once	100 mg bid × 3 d or 500 mg once	
	Alternatives: Albendazole or	400 mg daily × 3 d	400 mg daily × 3 d	
	Ivermectin	200 µg/kg daily × 3 d	200 µg/kg daily × 3 d	

Adapted from Drugs for parasitic infections. Med Lett Drug Ther, August 2004.
[1] Not FDA approved for this indication.
[2] Not available in the United States.
*The drug is not available commercially, but as a service it can be compounded by Panorama Compounding Pharmacy, 6744 Balboa Blvd., Van Nuys, CA 91406 (800-247-9767) or Medical Center Pharmacy, New Haven, CT (203-688-6816).
[†] An approved drug, but considered investigational for this condition by the FDA.
[‡] Limited or no availability in the United States.
Max = maximum.

children. Its persistence is likely related to the fact that pinworm does not require a period of maturation outside the human body, and autoinfection or transmission by very close contact sustains the parasite within communities. *E. vermicularis* is at maximum 1 cm long with a tapered tail, and dwells in the cecum, appendix, and adjacent colon. At night, female worms travel to the anus and lay small (25–50 μm), double-walled oval eggs in the perianal skin. Within 6 hours, the eggs embryonate within their capsule and are infectious. In scratching the perianal area and subsequently bringing his or her hand to the mouth, the host ingests the embryos, which then hatch in the bowel about 2 months later and continue the cycle of infection. Embryonated eggs can also attach to bedclothes, thereby placing other household members with close contact at risk for infection. In family groups, infection is associated with close living quarters, poor hand washing, and infrequent washing of clothes and sheets. It can also be prevalent in among institutionalized persons.

Infection is often asymptomatic, but it can cause perianal itching, which helps to facilitate persistent infection by encouraging frequent touching of the perianal area. Rarely, worms migrate into ectopic foci and produce painful genitourinary tract disease with granulomatous inflammation; pinworm infection rarely results in pain that mimics acute appendicitis.

Pinworm infestation is best diagnosed by the classic Scotch tape test, which involves placing and immediately removing a piece sticky tape firmly across the perianal area early in the morning when the eggs have been deposited. The tape can then be brought into a physician's office or laboratory, where it is placed sticky-side down for microscopic examination to detect the eggs. Three specimens should be examined if necessary to improve the sensitivity. It is also sometimes possible to see the worms directly on the perianal region, although they are so small that they may easily be mistaken for residual bits of toilet paper. *E.vermicularis* is susceptible to standard anthelminthic therapies as listed in Table 2. All household contacts should be empirically treated with the same regimen to avoid reintroducing infection from family members who may be asymptomatically carrying the parasite. Careful laundering of all bedclothes is recommended as well.

Anisakiasis

Anisakiasis is a descriptive term for human infection with parasites of two distinct genuses: *Anisakis* and *Pseudoterranova*. Humans are incidental hosts for these roundworms that inhabit multiple species of fish and other marine animals (tuna, mackerel, hake, cod, sardines, and cephalopods) as intermediate hosts, and marine mammals such as whales, seals, sea lions, and walruses as final hosts. Humans acquire the parasite in its larval stage by eating raw fish (e.g., sushi, ceviche), and therefore the condition predominates in cultures where uncooked fish is consumed. Cases are most commonly reported from Japan but are seen throughout the world in other coastal nations and among restaurateurs.

On consumption of fish with anisakid larvae embedded in its musculature, humans can experience immediate symptoms in the form of itching or burning in the throat, which can provoke coughing that expels the parasite. If the parasite is swallowed, the larva attempts to embed in the gastric musculature at the pylorus. This can produce acute, short-lived epigastric abdominal pain and possibly immediate vomiting, at which point the parasite might again be ejected. If the larva does manage to penetrate gastric tissue, it dies because it is incapable of further tissue invasion in humans. An intense inflammatory response to the dead pathogen can then result, with gastric pain, nausea, and occasionally diarrhea with blood or mucus if a gastric ulcerative lesion has resulted.

Rare cases have been reported in which the larva penetrates the peritoneum, causing focal peritonitis and abscess formation. *Pseudoterranova* appears to cause milder symptoms and less tissue invasion, and the worm might simply be vomited several days after initial ingestion and presented to a physician, often by an alarmed patient. Because the vast majority of infections are caused by a single organism, vomiting of the parasite results in a definitive cure and patients can be reassured. Diagnosis in patients with ongoing symptoms related to an embedded parasite is ultimately endoscopic. Effective cure results on endoscopic or surgical removal of the worm.

TREMATODES

Schistosomiasis

Schistosomes are freshwater pathogens with areas of endemicity in Africa, South America, Southeast Asia, and parts of the Middle East. These small trematodes cause varied, often chronic infections that can carry significant morbidity, although some species cannot invade beyond the dermis in humans and result strictly in cercarial dermatitis or swimmer's itch. There are five species of schistosomes known to cause disease in humans: *Schistosoma haematobium*, found through much of Africa and parts of the Middle East; *Schistosoma mansoni*, also native to Africa and the Middle East as well as Latin America; *Schistosoma japonicum*, present in China, Southeast Asia, and the Philippines; *Schistosoma mekongi*, found only in the Mekong River basin in Southeast Asia; and *Schistosoma intercalatum*, endemic only in West Africa.

All persons who come in contact with schistosomes are at risk for infection, even after only very brief exposure to fecally contaminated freshwater in which the intermediate hosts of the pathogen (snails) reside. Frequency and degree of infection tend to be highest in children in endemic areas and then levels off in the early teenage years, likely secondary to level of environmental exposure and possibly to host immunity. *S. hematobium* causes disease in the genitourinary system; the others cause intestinal, hepatic, and sometimes pulmonary diseases.

Infection is acquired rapidly on contact with freshwater (including brief swims or by repeated splashing, as can occur during river rafting), when free-living fork-tailed schistosomal larvae penetrate human skin and lose their tail. These schistomorulae can cause intense itching and a papulovesicular, pruritic rash at the site of penetration, swimmer's itch. Invasive schistomorulae then enter the venous bloodstream and ultimately lodge in gut mesenteric and portal venules, where maturation occurs, and male and female forms join and mate for life. Females begin to oviposit, and the resultant inflammatory response to the eggs can cause either acute illness or chronic fibrosis and granulomatous inflammation of the tissues in which they reside.

Acute illness, called *Katayama fever*, is more common among hosts who have not been previously exposed to the organism and can be quite severe, even fatal. Katayama fever begins 4 to 8 weeks after exposure to the schistosomes, with fever, cough, abdominal pain, hepatomegaly, and lymphadenopathy. Eggs might not yet be present in the stool at the time of diagnosis. Chronic schistosomiasis is a slowly progressive illness. *S. haematobium* infection is manifest by gross or microscopic hematuria, urinary symptoms, and chronic bacterial urinary tract infections; ultimately ureteral fibrosis, hydronephrosis, and granulomatous genital lesions also can ensue. In infection with other invasive schistosomes, chronic illness can manifest as abdominal pain and diarrhea, which is often bloody, with associated iron-deficiency anemia. Hepatomegaly is often the first clinical finding in chronic intestinal schistosomiasis. Over many years, hepatic congestion and fibrosis can result in liver failure, and the pulmonary vasculature can be involved as well, which causes pulmonary hypertension and cor pulmonale.

Diagnosis of schistosomiasis is by observation of eggs in stool (intestinal disease), urine (urinary tract disease), or biopsy specimens, or by serum antibody testing. Concentration of stool may be necessary to detect the pathogen. The eggs of the three most common species of schistosomes can be readily identified microscopically: *S. haematobium* has an inferior spine, *S. mansoni* an inferolateral spine, and *S. japonicum* lacks a spine. Eosinophilia is a hallmark of chronic infection and is a common cause of asymptomatic eosinophilia among immigrants from schistoendemic regions of the world. Serology is highly sensitive and specific but cannot distinguish acute, chronic, or cleared infection; it is very useful when attempting to diagnose infection in returned travelers.

All patients with schistosomiasis should be treated, and those with chronic manifestations might experience significant regression of even late-stage organ-specific disease. Treatment of choice is with praziquantel; see Table 2 for details.

Prevention of schistosomiasis involves improving access to treated water and exploration of avenues to eliminate the intermediate snail hosts. Host immunity does appear to occur, and efforts are under way to better understand and induce such immunity in the form of a vaccine.

CESTODES

Taeniasis

Human tapeworm infection has long been implicated in North American oral folklore as a cause of insatiable appetite and excessive weight loss. In reality, despite their impressive size of up to 12 meters, tapeworm infection tends to be minimally symptomatic.

Taenia solium, pork tapeworm, and *Taenia sanguinata*, beef tapeworm, are the two most common flatworm infections of humans worldwide and occur in any setting in which raw or undercooked meat is served and cattle and pigs have access to feed contaminated with human feces. *T. sanguinata* is still found in areas of North America and Europe, as well as in Central and South America and Africa; *T. solium* is common throughout Mexico, Central and South America, Africa, China, and the Indian subcontinent. Although humans are the definitive hosts for both parasites, *T. solium* is best known for its pathogenicity in the form of cysticercosis. Cysticercosis is not an intestinal parasitic infection.

Domesticated animals acquire infection on ingestion of eggs excreted by humans; the eggs mature in their musculature and develop a scolex. When humans consume infected meat, the scolex attaches in the small intestine, and the adult tapeworm develops over approximately 2 months. Adult tapeworms are made up of hundreds to thousands of gravid proglottids and can live for up to 25 years. Symptoms tend to be mild or absent but can include nausea, abdominal pain, loose stools, anal pruritus, and occasionally weakness or increased appetite, especially in children. Serious illness rarely results when a tapeworm becomes lodged in the biliary or pancreatic ducts or is coughed up and aspirated. Some patients come to medical attention when the worm is noted emerging from the anus or on extrusion of proglottids in the stool.

Diagnosis of taeniasis can be made on visualizing the round eggs in stool; however, the species cannot be determined unless a segment of the worm is examined. Serum antibody and antigen tests, as well as stool PCR, have been developed for diagnosis but are not widely used in clinical practice. Eosinophilia and elevated IgE levels may be present. Single dose praziquantel[1] (see Table 2) is curative in almost all cases, but infectious eggs can still be released in the feces for a time; ingestion of these could result in the subsequent development if cysticercosis, so patients should be counseled to avoid fecal–oral contact.

Proper cooking of meat is the mainstay of prevention; disposal of human waste away from animals would also be effective in interrupting the life cycle.

Diphyllobothriasis

Diphyllobothrium latum is the longest parasite known to infect humans (10 to 12 m). It is found in freshwater lakes in areas of the Americas, Northern Europe, Africa, China, and Japan and has a complex life cycle involving two intermediate hosts: crustaceans and

---

[1]Not FDA approved for this indication.

---

small fish. Humans and other fish-eating mammals are the definitive hosts and acquire the infection on ingestion of raw fish or roe.

The organism attaches within the small intestine, and hosts are usually asymptomatic. Infected persons might complain of increased appetite, nausea, or abdominal discomfort. Many present after passage of portions of the tapeworm in stool, as with taeniasis; in others, diagnosis is on stool examination done for other purposes or during screening colonoscopy. As with other worms, the parasite occasionally migrates into biliary ducts or causes intestinal obstruction. Attachment of the parasite higher in the intestine can result in decreased levels of vitamin B_{12}. Rarely, pernicious anemia develops as a result (tapeworm anemia).

Diagnosis is made either by seeing eggs in unconcentrated stool or by encountering the adult worm. Eosinophilia is present in a minority of cases. Treatment with praziquantel[1] is curative; see Table 2. Vitamin B_{12} supplementation is necessary in cases of severe or symptomatic deficiency, but it will not recur once the tapeworm is eliminated. Prevention involves not ingesting undercooked fish.

---

[1]Not FDA approved for this indication.

REFERENCES

Abubakar I, Aliyu SH, Hunter PR, Usman NK. Prevention and treatment of cryptosporidiosis in immunocompromised patients. Cochrane Database Syst Rev 2007;(1) CD004932.

Bethony J, Brooker S, Albonico M, et al. Soil-transmitted helminth infections: Ascariasis, trichuriasis, and hookworm. Lancet 2006;367(9521):1521–32.

Boggild A, Yohanna S, Keystone J, Kain K. Prospective analysis of parasitic infections in Canadian travelers and immigrants. J Travel Med 2006;13:138–44.

Boulware DR, Stauffer WM, Hendel-Paterson RR, et al. Maltreatment of Strongyloides infection: Case series and worldwide physicians-in-training survey. Am J Med 2007;120:545.e1–545.e8.

Concha R, Hartington Jr W, Rogers AI. Intestinal strongyloidiasis: Recognition, management, and determinants of outcome. J Clin Gastroenterol 2005;39(3):203–11.

Drugs for parasitic infections. The Medical Letter [serial online]. 2004. p. 46. Available at: www.medicalletter.org [Accessed June 17, 2007].

Goodgame RW. Understanding intestinal spore-forming protozoa: Cryptosporidia, microsporidia, isospora, and cyclospora. Ann Intern Med 1996;124(4):429–41.

Guerrant R, Walker D, Weller P, editors. Tropical Infectious Diseases: Principles, Pathogens, and Practice. Philadelphia: Churchill Livingstone; 1999.

Huang DB, White AC. An updated review on Cryptosporidium and Giardia. Gastroenterol Clin North Am 2006;35:291–314.

Mandell G, Bennett J, Dolin R, editors. Mandell, Douglas and Bennett's Principles and Practice of Infectious Diseases. 5th ed. Philadelphia: Churchill Livingstone; 2005.

Pardo J, Carranza C, Muro A, et al. Helminth-related eosinophilia in African immigrants, Gran Canaria. Emerg Infect Dis 2006;12(10):1587–9.

Stark D, Beebe N, Marriott D, et al. Dientamoebiasis: Clinical importance and recent advances. Trends Parasitol 2006;22(2):92–6.

Metabolic Disorders

Diabetes Mellitus in Adults

Method of
*Anthony L. McCall, MD, PhD, and J. Terry
Saunders, PhD*

Epidemiology

The Centers for Disease Control and Prevention (CDC) estimated that in 2007 the prevalence of diabetes in the United States was 23.6 million. Diabetes is diagnosed in 17.9 million persons and undiagnosed in 5.7 million. Type 2 diabetes mellitus (T2DM) is 90% to 95% of prevalent diabetes, and type 1 diabetes (T1DM) is about 5% to 10%. There are fewer persons with secondary or monogenic forms of diabetes, called *maturity-onset diabetes of the young* (MODY). About 57 million people in the United States are believed to have prediabetes.

The focus of this article is T2DM because it is the most prevalent form and is increasing rapidly in the United States and worldwide. A few comments are made on adult T1DM. This chapter emphasizes both lifestyle and pharmacologic treatments.

Diagnosis and Classification of Diabetes and Prediabetes

DIAGNOSIS

Most diabetes is diagnosed by random or fasting glucose (Table 1). Symptoms should be present if random glucose criteria are used, but surprisingly, many people with diabetes are relatively asymptomatic. In the elderly, cognitive changes can occur and atypical symptoms such as prostatism can appear. The American Diabetes Association (ADA) screening recommendations suggest screening every 3 years starting at age 45 for the general population, but they suggest earlier and more frequent screening in those with high risk. Recently, a case has been made for using elevated Alc as an adjunct combined with glucose measurement or as a sole criterion when >7% for screening and diagnosis of diabetes.

Patients from diabetes-prone ethnic groups (e.g., Latin Americans, African Americans, Native Americans) or with a strong family history, polycystic ovary syndrome (PCOS), or gestational diabetes should have early and frequent screenings. High-risk persons include those with prediabetes (impaired glucose tolerance, impaired fasting glucose) or who meet the National Cholesterol Education Program (NCEP) criteria for the metabolic syndrome or its individual components (dyslipidemia, hypertension, central obesity, prediabetes). The metabolic syndrome as defined by the NCEP is criticized as flawed,

but such critique does not reduce the importance of fully documenting and treating cardiometabolic risk components in those with or at risk for T2DM in a targeted manner (see Box 1). The metabolic syndrome concept is useful to teach patients and clinicians about these risks and the response of the overweight and sedentary to a healthier lifestyle.

CLASSIFICATION

The classification of diabetes into its two most prominent types (T1DM and T2DM) seems straightforward in theory but in practice is increasingly confusing as more Americans become overweight. Although T1DM patients are traditionally lean, many now are overweight and some have metabolic syndrome characteristics. About 80% to 90% of persons with T2DM are overweight or have metabolic syndrome characteristics, but some are leaner and more active and do not have the metabolic syndrome. C-peptide measurements are not very helpful for those who are difficult to classify, but measuring three antibodies—including IA-2 (islet cell antigen 512), anti-GAD$_{65}$ (glutamic acid decarboxylase), and anti-insulin antibodies in high titers—can clarify a diagnosis of latent autoimmune diabetes. Younger age at onset, lean body habitus, severe loss of glycemic control with or without ketonemia, and weight loss all suggest insulin deficiency but might not be definitive.

Pathophysiology

The primary causes of most adult diabetes are insulin resistance and lack of compensatory insulin secretion. Insulin resistance is typically longstanding and begins at a young age because of heredity combined with environmental causes (sedentary lifestyle and calorie overconsumption with resultant overweight). Insulin secretory defects usually start about 10 years before diagnosis, and no therapy is proven so far to prevent progressive loss of insulin secretion. A few patients develop diabetes associated with malnutrition, but this is much less common. Longstanding insulin resistance is associated with dyslipidemia, central obesity, hypertension, and hyperglycemia. This long prodrome accounts for the common coexistence of cardiovascular disease and diabetes.

CARDIOVASCULAR RISK MANAGEMENT

Cardiovascular risk management in diabetes starts with lifestyle counseling and education. It is paramount that patients understand the intimate and direct links among diabetes, glycemic control, and cardiovascular disease. Drug interventions are ultimately needed for glycemia, lipid risks, and blood pressure in most patients. Women have higher relative risk and similar overall risk as men and are often undertreated. Specific recommended targets of therapy for diabetes in glycemia, blood pressure, dyslipidemia, and lifestyle are shown in Box 1.

589

TABLE 1 Diagnosis and Classification of Diabetes and Prediabetes

Diagnosis	Glucose Test	Diagnostic Level	Comments
Diabetes	Random	>200 mg/dL	Plus classic symptoms*
Diabetes	Fasting	>126 mg/dL	8-hour fast; need confirmation
Diabetes	Postglucose load (75 g in nonpregnant adults)	>200 mg/dL at 2 h	Need confirmation
Diabetes	HbA1c	≥6.5%	New
Prediabetes IFG	Fasting	>100 mg/dL	Decreased insulin secretion
Prediabetes IGT	Postglucose load (75 g)	140–199 mg/dL at 2 h	Increased insulin resistance
Prediabetes	HbA1c	5.7–6.4%	New

*Polyuria, polydipsla, unexplained weight loss.
Abbreviations: IFG = impaired fasting glucose; IGT = impaired glucose tolerance.

BOX 1 Summary of Goals for Treatment

Lifestyle
Medical Nutrition Therapy (individualized)
- Appropriate calories
- Low saturated and *trans* fats
- Moderate, consistent carbohydrates (whole grains, vegetables, fruits)
- Healthy fats and proteins (decreased saturated and trans fats, increased monosaturated fat; reduced consumption of animal protein)

Activity
- Consistent, regular activity tailored to complications and safety (ECG or stress test may be needed before starting an exercise program)

Glycemia
- Best possible without frequent or severe hypoglycemia
- HbA1c <7% minimally; 6% or less if possible in selected patients early in disease course

Self-Monitored Blood Glucose
- Preprandial 70–130* mg/dL; <110 ideally
- Postprandial (1 to 2 h) <180 minimal; <140 ideally

Lipids
- LDL <100 mg/dL; optional <70 mg/dL (ACS, clinical ASCVD)
- Non-HDL <130 mg/dL; optional <100 mg/dL
- HDL >40 mg/dL (men); >50 mg/dL (women)
- Triglycerides <150 mg/dL

Blood Pressure
- Systolic <130 mm Hg
- Diastolic <80 mm Hg

Abbreviations: ACS = acute coronary syndrome, ASCVD = atherosclerotic cardiovascular disease (also multiple severe risk factors that are difficult to control); HDL = high-density lipoprotein; LDL = low-density lipoprotein.
*70 mg/dL is too low for patients with high risk of hypoglycemia.

DOCUMENTING AND FOLLOWING COMPLICATIONS

Patients should have a thorough examination and evaluation for complications at the time of diabetes diagnosis. About one half of patients with newly diagnosed T2DM have established chronic complications, indicating delayed recognition of this disorder.

Neuropathy and circulatory signs and symptoms on foot examination should be assessed. Risk of ulcer and amputation can be gauged by 10-g Semmes-Weinstein monofilaments that test for severe

CURRENT DIAGNOSIS

- Screening for diabetes should be done in high-risk populations, especially:
  - Those with prediabetes or the metabolic syndrome.
  - High-risk ethnic groups (e.g., Native American, Latino American, African American).
  - Gestational diabetes.
  - Patients might present with atypical symptoms.
  - Most diabetes is type 2 in adults, but type 1 does occur in adults, and delayed diagnosis is common.
- Cardiovascular risk should be aggressively screened for and treated.
- Complications should be documented and tracked.
  - Check fasting lipids.
- Check renal function and albuminuria yearly.
  - Have a low threshold for stress testing, with imaging for all patients.
  - Refer for yearly eye examinations.
  - Check feet for sensation, deformity, and circulation at regular visits.
- All patients should receive an educational assessment and training in self-management and self-monitoring of blood glucose.
- Take a diet history; this is especially important for patients on insulin.
- Get a baseline HbA1c and repeat 2 to 4 times per year (twice yearly if at glycemic goal).

neuropathy and attendant risk of ulceration. Retina examinations should be done by skilled eye professionals likely to pick up significant eye disease. High-risk patients (poor glycemic control, established retinopathy, especially if preproliferative or worse) should be referred promptly to an eye specialist. Pregnancy counseling should be given to all women of childbearing age with diabetes. Microalbumin-to-creatinine ratio in the urine should be assessed and kidney function (serum creatinine and blood urea nitrogen [BUN]) should be tracked yearly.

Home glucose monitoring should be taught to patients so they understand the effects of food, stress, and exercise on glycemic patterns. Diabetes education should be arranged for all patients, preferably by a diabetes educator. Diabetes is unique in being a self-managed condition where patient knowledge and skills are critical to avoiding complications.

Treatment

BEHAVIORAL SELF-MANAGEMENT

Self-management of behavioral factors, including eating, physical activity, and psychological stress, is essential to good diabetes self-care. Ideally, professional support for behavioral self-management should

CURRENT THERAPY

- Diabetes requires nutrition and behavioral self-management counseling as well as drug therapy.
- Repeatedly encourage healthy eating and an active lifestyle.
- Prediabetes diagnosis represents an opportunity for behavioral and drug interventions.
- Metformin (Glucophage) is usually the first drug therapy.
- Don't expect one drug to do the job for very poorly controlled glycemia, especially if >9%.
- Dual defects (insulin resistance and secretion) should be addressed in most patients.
- Very insulin resistant patients might need a dual insulin resistance strategy.
- Therapy goals for both HbA1c and self-monitored blood glucose can be achieved in most patients.
- Cardiovascular risk reduction therapy is a very high priority—statins and BP control best.
- When patients have not met goals on dual oral agent therapy, basal insulin is often the most appropriate choice, particularly when patients are not near glycemic goals.
- For oral agent therapy, add don't switch unless side effects require it.
- When adding basal insulin, continue oral agent therapies.
- Threatening patients with insulin therapy is counterproductive.
- Follow the 3F rule: Fix the fasting glucose first, especially in patients with poor glycemic control.
- Prompt recognition of the need for meal insulin is critical to achieve glycemic goals.
- Balance meal and basal insulin; check post-meal BP.

be a coordinated, multidisciplinary effort involving expertise appropriate to a given patient from the areas of nutrition, nursing, exercise training, and behavioral counseling. The provider should develop a referral network of available multidisciplinary resources and make regular use of any appropriate community-based resources (e.g., local hospitals and health departments, lifestyle modification programs, YMCAs, local fitness facilities, community colleges, universities, extension services, and parks and recreation departments). Unfortunately, multidisciplinary resources are often in short supply or difficult to pay for. Therefore, it is essential that the provider develop basic skills and techniques for working with patients on behavior change.

Behavior change is slow and is inherently a multisession activity. Quick, one-shot interventions seldom change longstanding patterns of behavior. Initial sessions should be scheduled closely together (1–2 weeks), then further apart as the patient gains momentum and confidence. If multiple one-on-one sessions are impossible, other options such as group meetings, telephone support, or e-mail messaging should be considered.

Behavior change interventions should be highly individualized and specific. General advice about diet and exercise does not address the life experience or problems of a given patient and is often perceived as insensitive or unhelpful. Arriving at individualized objectives for behavior change can be accomplished using a simple three-step process composed of initial assessment, setting behavioral objectives, and follow-up and reassessment.

Initial Assessment

Initial assessment includes identifying salient features of social and family history that can affect efforts to change behavior. A nutrition assessment should be performed, including an appraisal of usual food intake, the patient's perception of problem eating behavior, and weight history. A physical activity assessment should also be conducted, focusing on past and current physical activity, preferences, perceived barriers, and general attitudes. Readiness to make changes in behavior should be assessed by asking how important a patient thinks it is to change a given area of behavior and how confident she or he is that she or he can succeed in making changes (on a 1 to 10 scale). Discussion of specific objectives for behavioral change should occur in areas where the patient indicates a definite readiness to begin. Other areas of change should be discussed, but not forced or driven by the provider. Finally, ask patients about current levels and sources of stress. Because depression is common with diabetes, patients should be screened for possible depression.

Behavioral Objectives

Setting behavioral objectives is initiated and facilitated by the provider, but the patient is responsible for selecting his or her own behavioral objectives. Resist the temptation to take over responsibility for this function. Objectives should be FIRM: *f*ew (1–3 at a time is plenty), *i*ndividualized to the patient's specific behavioral challenges, *r*ealistic (beware of trying to make big strides quickly), and *m*easurable. For measurement, the patient should be given a tracking form (such as the example in Figure 1) to use in recording daily progress on each objective. Note that although the patient might have long-term goals in the areas of weight loss, calorie intake, or general fitness, specific behavioral objectives such as eating a bowl of cereal for breakfast or walking one-half hour on five mornings each week are the means to achieving those outcomes. The primary focus of provider-patient discussions of progress should be on behavioral objectives, not outcomes. The ADA offers a web-based continuing medical education program to assist health care professionals in acquiring more detailed knowledge and skills in setting behavioral objectives for lifestyle change.

Follow-up and Reassessment

Follow-up and reassessment occur during each return visit, following a period of patient efforts to carry out mutually agreed on behavioral objectives. Reassessment focuses on the behavioral records kept by patients as well as on their verbal reports of difficulties and successes. Praise and encouragement are the order of the day. Efforts to initiate behavior change are highly responsive to external positive reinforcement, and the patient will need maximum external reinforcement until new behavior becomes self-sustaining. After review and discussion of patient records, new behavioral objectives or incremental changes in existing objectives are selected by mutual agreement, with the patient taking the lead.

A modest weight loss of 5% to 10% has a positive impact on cardiovascular risk factors and progression of diabetes. Reassure patients that medical goals for weight loss are achievable and worth the effort.

When discussing changes in eating with patients, distinguish dieting from gradual behavioral changes that result in a lasting pattern of healthy eating. Diets are impermanent and run the risk of large weight losses followed by even larger weight gains. Gradual behavioral changes offer the possibility of permanent lifestyle changes.

Prohibiting or demonizing foods is counterproductive. It leads patients to think of food in moral extremes (e.g., "sugar is bad for my diabetes") rather than along a continuum of nutritional benefit and blood glucose control. Food prohibition also casts the provider as withholding and overly controlling. These traps can be avoided by exploring very small changes that are not perceived as significant losses.

Patients may be extremely confused about the role of carbohydrates in weight loss and weight maintenance because of popular myths about sugar and the controversy surrounding low-carbohydrate diets. Low-carbohydrate diets (<130 g/day) are not recommended as an approach to weight loss. Carbohydrates should be included as an important part of a healthy diet for people with diabetes. Recommendations for achieving consistent, appropriate carbohydrate intake at meals are based on controlling postprandial blood glucose (<180 mg/dL 1 to 2 hours after beginning a meal). Carbohydrate counting and blood glucose pattern management are complicated and time consuming to teach. Referral to a dietitian for medical nutrition therapy (MNT) or nutrition education through an ADA-recognized diabetes patient education program is recommended.

FIGURE 1. Example of a behavioral goals tracking form.

The best place to begin setting behavioral objectives for nutrition and exercise is where the patient is currently. Obtaining a 3-day food record (2 work days and one nonwork day) and a baseline for activity (we generally use a week of daily steps measured with a pedometer) provide a solid baseline for setting objectives.

An irregular pattern of eating often underlies unhealthy food choices. For example, staying up late encourages late-night snacking, which in turn can suppress interest in eating breakfast. Eating tends to be deferred to the afternoon or evening, perpetuating the cycle.

A modest reduction in caloric consumption of around 250 to 500 kcal/day and moderate physical activity on the order of at least 150 minutes a week are the recommended approaches to weight loss. Reducing calories through decreased food consumption is more effective for weight loss than increasing energy expenditure through physical activity. Box 2 contains a checklist of healthy eating behaviors that can be used to stimulate patients' thinking about places they might like to make changes. Physical activity plays an important role in weight maintenance, but higher levels of activity (200 min/week) may be required to prevent long-term weight regain. Box 3 lists ways that patients can become more active. It is worth repeating that the point of these and other suggestions is not to direct patients but to expand their thinking about what might work for them.

Stress reduction is important in controlling blood glucose, but it can also play a role by helping patients achieve a mental focus on their behavior-management efforts. We encourage patients to sit calmly for a period of 5 to 10 minutes each day, focusing on slow deep breathing and muscle relaxation. Activities such as yoga or tai chi also reduce stress and support awareness of body and mind. Box 4 contains suggestions for coping behaviors that may be useful to patients in dealing with stress.

PHARMACOLOGIC THERAPY

Overview

Eventually, most patients with T2DM require drug treatment, often with multiple agents (combination therapy). Progressive insulin secretory loss probably is the primary explanation for the need to advance treatment. A resultant general rule with all therapies is *add, don't switch*. Table 2 lists major types of pharmacotherapeutic interventions with their usual hemoglobin (Hb) Alc lowering, balance of preprandial versus postprandial effects, and some comments on their actions and side effects. Table 3 lists classes of drugs, commonly used agents, and typical doses.

Recently the ADA and European Association for the Study of Diabetes (EASD) have issued a joint consensus algorithm on controlling hyperglycemia in T2DM. In our practice, we similarly initiate behavioral self-management along with medication, typically metformin unless there are contraindications or intolerance. Commonly, ineffective early attempts by physicians to change behavior (e.g., giving general advice) lead to abandonment of this therapy. A second oral medication may be initiated if patients cannot achieve glycemic goals. Commonly, we favor insulin secretagogues especially glimepiride (Amaryl) or extended-release glipizide (Glucotrol XL) for their relatively low risk of hypoglycemia, convenient once-daily dosing, and low expense. An alternative treatment strategy for heavier, more insulin-resistant patients is use of a thiazolidinedione, effectively a dual insulin-resistance strategy (see thiazolidinediones).

More reliably effective is the use of basal insulin treatment as a second agent to achieve control. Insulin initiation should be preceded by an open discussion of the patient's attitudes, beliefs, and possible fears regarding insulin. Insulin therapy should never be used as a

BOX 2 Checklist of Healthy Eating Behaviors

☑ **Eat meals and snacks at set times to promote health.**
Examples:

- I will eat breakfast within 1 hour of getting up.
- I will not skip meals.
- Other: ....
....

☑ **Eat healthy carbohydrates.**
Examples:

- I will avoid regular soft drinks and choose water or diet soft drinks instead.
- I will eat 5–7 servings of fruits and vegetables every day.
- I will choose whole-grain breads and cereals.
- Other: ....
....

☑ **Decrease serving sizes.**
Examples:

- I will keep a record of the food I eat and drink.
- I will know what counts as a serving size.
- When I am eating out, I will share or split an entrée and eat a salad.
- Other: ....
....

☑ **Eat less fat and choose healthy fats.**
Examples:

- I will bake, broil, roast, grill, or boil instead of fry food.
- I will have a meatless meal at least once a week.
- I will choose fried or high-fat foods no more than once a week.
- I will drink fat-free or low-fat milk.
- I will use healthy oils (olive oil, canola oil) and buy tub margarine.
- Other: ....
....

☑ **Make other healthy choices.**
Examples:

- I will drink plenty of fluids (at least 8 glasses of water or low-calorie fluid per day).
- I will limit how much alcohol I drink. (Women should drink no more than 1 alcoholic drink per day. Men should drink no more than 2 alcoholic drinks per day.)
- Other: ....
....

Unpublished source: Virginia Center for Diabetes Professional Education, University of Virginia; Virginia Diabetes Council.

threat or possible negative consequence for failure to carry out behavioral management. Many patients associate insulin with serious diabetes complications and mortality. A positive attitude about the value of insulin therapy and a reassuring, educational approach can help to reduce initial fears enough to begin. Self-demonstration of injection technique using saline is also useful in overcoming fear of injections. Improvement in blood glucose control with insulin generally makes patients feel better, which further reinforces its perceived value. Use of insulin pens may increase acceptance of insulin treatment, patient convenience, and dosing accuracy.

It should be noted that an alternative algorithm for glycemic control therapy is proposed by the American College of Endocrinology.

Oral Agents

Secretagogues

These drugs enhance insulin secretion. There are first- and second-generation oral sulfonylureas; the latter are most commonly used. They are inexpensive, are moderately effective, and often can be dosed once daily. First-generation agents such as tolbutamide, chlorpropamide (Diabenese), and tolazamide (Tolinase) are less often used than the second-generation agents glyburide (Diabeta, Glynase), glipizide (Glucotrol), and glimepiride (Amaryl).

The dose-response characteristics of sulfonylureas suggest that one half the approved maximum dose achieves maximum HbA1c

BOX 3 Checklist for Physical Activity

☑ **Do something that you enjoy.**
Examples:

- I will take the stairs.
- I will park my car farther away and walk.
- I will walk.
- I will swim or do water exercises.
- I will ride a bike.
- I will use an exercise video.
- I will do yoga.
- Other: ....
....

☑ **How often?**
Examples:
❏ Every day
❏ 3x/week
❏ 5x/week
❏ ....

☑ **How long?**
Examples:
❏ 10 minutes
❏ 15 minutes
❏ 20 minutes
❏ 30 minutes
❏ 60 minutes
❏ ___ minutes

☑ **Limit inactivity.**
Examples:

- I will watch no more than 1 hour of television per day.
- I will spend no more than 2 hour(s) per day on the computer.
- Other: ....
....

Unpublished source: Virginia Center for Diabetes Professional Education, University of Virginia; Virginia Diabetes Council.

BOX 4 Checklist of Coping Behaviors

Examples:

- Talk about how you feel to people you trust.
- Decide one small way to change your mood or old habit, and do it.
- Write down 10 good things about your life and think about and appreciate them.
- Organize your day with a "To Do" list.
- Learn how to relax through yoga, meditation, biofeedback, tai chi, deep breathing, or visual imagery.
- Take 30 minutes each day to relax through music, yoga, bath, writing, etc.
- Take time to have fun every day by exploring a new interest, watching a funny movie, going shopping, playing with a pet, etc.
- Get in touch with your spiritual side to help you feel better about yourself.
- Keep a stress diary to see what triggers your stress and discover better ways to react.
- Exercise every day to help you focus your energy on a more positive path.
- Keep your sleep cycle as regular as possible.
- Develop a favorite hobby.
- Other:

....

....

Unpublished source: Virginia Center for Diabetes Professional Education, University of Virginia; Virginia Diabetes Council.

TABLE 3 Dosing Used for Various Agents

Agent	Dose
Thiazolidinediones	
Pioglitazone (Actos)	15, 30, 45 mg
Rosiglitazone (Avandia)	2, 4, 8 mg
α-Glucosidase Inhibitors	
Acarbose (Precose)	25, 50, 100 mg ac
Miglitol (Glycet)	25, 50 mg ac
Biguanides	
Metformin (Glucophage) IR	500, 850, 1000 mg
Metformin SR	500, 750 mg
Glinides	
Nateglinide (Starlix)	60–120 mg ac
Repaglinide (Prandin)	0.5–4 mg ac
Sulfonylureas (Second Generation)	
Glimepiride (Amaryl)	1–4 mg
Glipizide (Glucotrol) IR	2.5–20 mg
Glipizide SR	2.5–10 mg
Glyburide (Glynase)	1.25–10; 1.5–6 mg
Incretins	
Exenatide (Byetta)	5, 10 µg
Liraglutide (Victoza)	0.6, 1.2, 1.8 mg
Saxagliptin (Onglyza)	2.5 mg, 5 mg*
Sitagliptin (Januvia)	25, 50, 100 mg*
Amylin Agonists	
Pramlintide (Symln)	15, 30, 60, 90, 120 µg
Bile Acid Sequestrant	
Colesevelam	1875–3750 mg
Insulin	
Aspart (Novolog)	No dose limit
Detemir (Levemir)	No dose limit
Glargine (Lantus)	No dose limit
Glulisine (Apidra)	No dose limit
Inhaled powder insulin (Exubera)	No dose limit
Lispro (Humalog)	No dose limit
NPH	No dose limit
Regular	No dose limit

*Based on renal function.
Abbreviations: ac = before meals; IR = immediate release; NPH = neutral protamine Hagedorn; SR = sustained release.

lowering, typically 1 to 1.5 percentage points. If the patient is not at goal with half-maximum doses, it is more effective to add a second agent than raise the dose. Common side effects include hypoglycemia, weight gain of about 2 kg, and, more rarely, hematologic or skin reactions.

Rapid secretagogues, the glinides (repaglinide [Prandin] and nateglinide [Starlix]), are more expensive and should be considered for patients who are sulfonylurea allergic, extremely erratic in eating, or at high risk for hypoglycemia.

TABLE 2 Overview and Characteristics of Therapy Interventions

Drug Type	HbA1c Lowering (Percentage Points)	Effect on Glycemia Levels Preprandial	Postprandial	Actions	Side Effects
SUs and non-SU rapid secretagogues**	1.5–2*	++	+	Direct and indirect secretagogue	Hypoglycemia, weight gain
Biguanides	1.5–2*	+++	0	↓ hepatic glucose output	GI, lactic acidosis, weight neutral
Thiazolidinediones	0.7–1.5	+++	0	↓ muscle insulin sensitivity	Edema, CHF, fractures
Incretin agonists	0.9–1.1	+	++	Strong GLP-1 effects, ↑ insulin ↓ glucagon	Nausea, vomiting, weight loss
DPP-4 inhibitors	0.6–0.8	+	++	Moderate GLP-1 effects, ↑ insulin ↓ glucagon	Weight neutral
Basal insulin	1.5–2.5	+++*	0*	↓ hepatic glucose output, ↑ muscle glucose disposal	Hypoglycemia, weight gain
Meal insulin	1.0–2.0	0-+*	++*	↓ hepatic glucose output, ↑ muscle glucose disposal	Hypoglycemia, weight gain
Pramlintide	0.5–0.7	0-+	++	↑ insulin ↓ glucagon	Nausea, vomiting
Colesevelam	0.4–0.8	+	+	Unknown	Constipation, hypertriglyceridemia

*Older drugs may be less effective in well-controlled patients.
**Rapid secretagogues have more postprandial effects and less preprandial effects.
Abbreviations: CHF = congestive heart failure; DPP = dipeptidyl peptidase; GI = gastrointestinal; GLP = glucagon-like peptide; Hb = hemoglobin; PFT = pulmonary function test; SU = sulfonylurea.

Biguanides

Metformin is the only available agent in this class. It is useful in both obese and normal weight T2DM patients. HbA1c lowering is typically about 1.5 percentage points in monotherapy or in combination therapy. Maximum efficacy is achieved with 2000 mg daily. The sustained-release preparation will last 24 hours if given with the evening meal.

Metformin's hypoglycemic mechanism is primarily by reduction of liver glucose production. It is cleared by the kidney, and the risk of lactic acidosis, a rare side effect with 50% mortality, may be increased in renal dysfunction. Serum creatinine should be less than 1.4 mg/dL in women and less than 1.5 mg/dL in men, and glomerular filtration rate (GFR) should be assessed in patients 80 years and older. It is also an increased lactic acidosis risk in patients with drug-treated congestive heart failure (CHF) or respiratory insufficiency. Intravascular contrast administration should prompt holding the drug for 24 to 48 hours until renal function is assured to be adequate. GI side effects are common initially and are dose dependent but wane; they can require gradual titration. Sustained-release preparations have fewer GI side effects. Weight gain is less with this drug than with many others for diabetes. The United Kingdom Prospective Diabetes Study (UKPDS) found that risk of MI and death was reduced, making it a first choice for pharmacotherapy in most patients.

Thiazolidinediones

Two drugs of the thiazolidinedione (TZD) class are available, rosiglitazone (Avandia) and pioglitazone (Actos). Both have similar glycemic-lowering effects and side effects. These drugs work by increasing the sensitivity of muscle tissue and fat to insulin action, probably through action of adipokines like adiponectin and muscle effects on adenosine monophosphate–activated protein kinase (AMPK), a fuel sensor enzyme. HbA1c lowering varies considerably, dependent on whether patients are very insulin resistant (central adiposity, often hypertriglyceridemia) and whether there is adequate endogenous insulin secretion (short diabetes duration or secretagogues) or insulin is given.

Diabetes may be prevented with rosiglitazone, and this is being tested for pioglitazone. Both TZDs can precipitate edema, weight gain due to obesity, and occasionally congestive heart failure even absent a prior heart failure history. It is thus wise to track weight in all patients and limit it to 5 or 6 pounds. The risk of heart failure is increased when TZDs are combined with insulin. Both TZDs have beneficial effects on some lipid parameters, but pioglitazone appears more effective in reducing hypertriglyceridemia. Recent analyses suggest, but do not prove, increased coronary ischemic events with rosiglitazone. Because of concerns about increased ischemic risk, the FDA has placed additional warnings. We do not recommend it be started, because better alternatives are available. Pioglitazone studies suggest reduced ischemic risk (stroke or myocardial infarction). Both medicines may increase heart failure, and new studies suggest more self-reported fractures in women, which will need further study.

Incretins

Incretins are gut hormones that enhance food-induced insulin secretion. Incretin drugs either are receptor agonists (e.g., exenatide) for glucagon-like peptide-1 (GLP-1), perhaps the most important incretin, or they enhance endogenous levels for both GLP-1 and gastrointestinal insulinotropic polypeptide (GIP).

Exenatide (Byetta) is one of two available GLP-1 receptor agonists—the other is liraglutide (Victoza), with the primary difference of once daily dosing for the liraglutide vs. twice daily for exenatide. Their actions increase meal insulin, decrease meal hyperglucagonemia, decrease rate of stomach emptying, and suppress appetite, which may cause a moderate weight loss. They work rapidly on injection. They have substantial GI side effects including nausea, vomiting, and diarrhea in a large minority of patients. Despite this, many patients favor it, probably because the side effects generally wane within weeks and there can be substantial weight loss in some very overweight patients. Typically, exenatide is given in doses of 5 µg twice daily at meals, advancing after a month to 10 µg twice daily.

Liraglutide is usually started at 0.6 mg once daily and advanced to 1.2 and then 1.8 mg as needed and tolerated. Patients might report that nausea is more tolerable if they have a little food in their stomach at the time of dosing. Pancreatitis may rarely occur (case reports).

Because incretin drugs all have a glucose-dependent insulin secretion and glucagon suppression, there is little tendency for hypoglycemia used alone or when they are combined with metformin and TZDs in comparison with sulfonylureas. HbA1c lowering with exenatide has been 0.9 to 1.1 percentage points, and liraglutide has similar or slightly more efficacy in lowering HbA1c but equal weight effects.

Dipeptidyl Peptidase-4 Inhibitors

Dipeptidyl peptidase-4 (DPP-4) is the peptidase that normally rapidly degrades the incretins GLP-1 and GIP to inactive proteolytic products. Inhibitors of DPP-4 have been shown to enhance GLP-1 and GIP levels to high physiologic levels and thereby reduce HbA1c concentrations, typically about 0.6 to 0.8 percentage points. At this writing, one of two drugs, sitagliptin (Januvia), has been approved and appears to be effective in doses of 100 mg once daily. This drug is excreted by the kidney largely unchanged and therefore should be given in lower doses (50 mg once daily) for those with moderate renal insufficiency (GFR 30–50 mL/min) and further reduced (25 mg) for those with severe renal dysfunction (GFR <30 mL/min).

Because DPP-4 inhibitors are oral, they may be preferred to the injectable exenatide. The side effects for these drugs are relatively minor and cause little nausea, vomiting, or diarrhea. They also do not cause significant weight loss but, like metformin, appear to be weight neutral. Recently, rare but serious allergic reactions such as angioedema and Stevens-Johnson syndrome have been reported in a few patients.

Amylin Agonists

Insulin is cosecreted with another beta cell hormone called amylin. The effects of amylin appear to be to help lower glycemia, reduce excess glucagon levels, curb appetite, and possibly reduce the rate of gastric emptying. A synthetic analogue of amylin, pramlintide (Symlin), is available as an injectable agent for treating both T1DM and T2DM as an adjunct to insulin. It lowers HbA1c about 0.5 to 0.7 percentage point. It also appears to have some weight loss effect, typically around 1 to 2 kg. Its action primarily controls glucose postprandially. Nausea and vomiting can occur in patients with either T2DM or T1DM but are worse in T1DM patients who require low doses at first (15 µg or less with meals) and slower titration. Those with T2DM usually start with 60 µg and can usually advance to 90 to 120 µg at meals.

Insulin

Barriers to Insulin Use

Insulin deficiency underlies the genesis of both T1DM and T2DM. Progression of therapy to use of insulin typically with oral agents in T2DM also seems predicated on progressive loss of insulin secretion. Nonetheless, it is often started too late, and patients often are in very poor control when this is done. Reluctance by patients and physicians alike might underlie this. Physicians should understand that exogenous insulin in T2DM is needed, does not negatively alter life quality, and is more likely to achieve therapeutic targets. Moreover, exogenous insulin does not worsen insulin resistance, does not cause excess cardiovascular disease, and has a low frequency of severe hypoglycemia, especially when used relatively early in the disease. Table 4 lists common insulin preparations and some notes about kinetics and timing.

Starting Insulin: Use of Basal Insulin in Type 2 Diabetes

How should insulin be started? Practitioners should use temporary insulin for patients whose glycemia is initially poorly controlled or when patients temporarily have worse control due to illness or

TABLE 4 Insulin Preparations

Insulin Type	Pharmacokinetics			Comments
	Onset (h)	Peak (h)	Duration (h)	
Basal Insulin				
NPH (Humulin N, Novolin N)	0.5	4–10	18	Kinetics is dose dependent Peak effects exert meal action Dose at breakfast, bedtime, supper*
Glargine[†] (Lantus)	2–4	none	24*	Up to 1/3 of C-peptide-negative T1DM need bid administration Dose can be given at any time of day if consistent
Detemir[†] (Levemir)		Less peak activity than NPH		Kinetics is dose dependent Dose at breakfast, bedtime, supper*
Meal Insulin				
Regular (Humulin R, Novolin R)	15–30	2–3	5–8	Give 1/2 hour before meals
Lispro (Humalog)	0.1–0.2	1.5–2.0	4	Dose at mealtime or immediately after
Aspart (Novolog)	0.1–0.2	1.5–2.0	4	Dose at mealtime or immediately after
Glulisine (Apidra)	0.1–0.2	1.5–2.0	4	Dose at mealtime or immediately after
Mixed Preparations				
NPH/regular (Humulin, Novolin)	70/30 dual kinetics based on components			Dosing 1/2 hour before meals Should not be dosed at bedtime
Lispro/NPLispro (Humalog Mix 75/25)	25/75 dual kinetics			Dosing at mealtime; should not be dosed at bedtime
Lispro/NPLispro Humalog Mix 50/50)	50/50 dual kinetics			Dosing at mealtime, should not be dosed at bedtime
Aspart/NPAspart (NovoLog Mix 70/30)	30/70 dual kinetics			Dosing at mealtime; should not be dosed at bedtime

*Bedtime dosing may be preferred for some patients, especially those on low doses.
[†]Should not be mixed with other insulins or used in the same syringe that other insulin has been in.
Abbreviation: NPH = neutral protamine Hagedorn.

medications, such as glucocorticoids. It is unwise to use insulin as a threat because it creates a sense of personal failure and dread of insulin use. When therapy progresses but there is failure to achieve glycemic goals after one or two oral medications, use of basal insulin is often the best way to achieve euglycemia, especially if patients are much more than 1 percentage point from HbA1c goal (< 7%).

The Treat-to-Target Trial offers a good example of how to initiate insulin therapy. In this study, as often in our practice, patients start with a basal insulin either with NPH insulin or insulin glargine (Lantus). Insulin detemir (Levemir) represents another new option to be used similarly. Insulin is instituted as 10 U once daily, commonly in the evening near bedtime, followed by weekly increases between 2 and 8 units depending on proximity to glucose goals, focusing on the fasting glucose.

This strategy is sometimes called the *fix the fasting first* rule. Average doses in that study were around 45 to 50 units for patients whose BMI was about 31 kg/m². An alternative initial dosing might be 0.2 U/kg body weight, but whatever the starting dose, a forced titration guided by patient self-monitoring with clear communication of target fasting glucose (90–130 mg/dL), size of increment (or decrement in case of hypoglycemia; usually 10%–20% of dose), and frequency of change (every 3–7 days) is necessary to get most patients to overall glycemic (HbA1c) goal. This strategy is referred to as *pattern management.* The intent is to use monitoring to adjust the insulin dose likely to affect the fasting glucose for basal insulin therapy. NPH and detemir usually can be used once daily, typically at bedtime. Patients using glargine may choose any time of the day as long as it is reasonably consistent, usually within an hour. Occasionally, twice-daily NPH or detemir is used.

At some point, basal insulin therapy alone may be insufficient for glycemic control for T2DM patients. Usually this is a consideration in patients whose HbA1c values are over 9% to 9.5% or where the fasting goal is met but HbA1c or daytime glycemia remains elevated. The need for meal insulin is particularly likely to occur with larger meals, such as supper. Diagnostically, what is important is to have patients check either both before and after large meals or, if they are unwilling to check frequently, simply check about 2 to 3 hours after meals. Self-monitored glucose values that exceed even minimum postprandial glycemic guidelines (<180 mg/dL) indicate the need for meal insulin. A common mistake made in practice is to treat fasting hyperglycemia only with increases in basal insulin, when in some patients, the cause is overeating or lack of meal insulin the previous evening. This can be discerned by observing the pattern of glycemia, with lows often between meals or overnight and highs occurring after meals or at bedtime.

FIXED-RATIO COMBINED INSULINS

A commonly employed strategy is to use fixed-ratio combination short-acting (either regular or rapid analogue) insulin combined with intermediate insulin (NPH or neutral protamine modified rapid analogue that mimics NPH timing). Examples of these preparations include 70/30 NPH and regular insulin, 75/25 neutral protamine lispro and lispro insulin (Humalog), and 70/30 neutral protamine aspart and aspart insulin (Novolog). These have the advantage of being able to achieve control very conveniently in T2DM patients who have quite poor control (HbA1c of 9.5% or more) with a simple twice-daily injection regimen. They also offer the advantage of greater dosing accuracy, especially when used with insulin pens. Important to the success of these formulations is consistent eating and carbohydrate intake with meals. Unfortunately, when such consistency is not advised or followed, patterns of glycemia can be erratic and hypoglycemia can be significantly increased due to both components of the combination. Patients who skip meals are poor candidates for such treatments and should either switch to individual dosing of an insulin mixture or, even safer, use a basal bolus insulin regimen.

Colesevalem hydrochloride (WelChol) in doses of 3.8 g/day altogether or in divided doses has been shown to reduce hyperglycemia when compared with placebo in patients with type 2 diabetes mellitus. A1c reductions range from 0.4% to 0.8% in comparison with placebo when used alone, with patients on metformin alone or in combination with other oral agents, with sulfonylureas, on sulfonylureas and other oral agents and when used with insulin and other oral agents. Although this drug has already been approved for hyperlipidemia, it is now FDA approved also for type 2 diabetes. It has the potential, however, to increase triglycerides, and thus baseline fasting lipid values should be obtained and tracked, especially in hypertriglyceridemic patients. There is little reason to justify its use alone or with thiazolidinediones but may be appropriate for some patients with type 2 diabetes not at goal on other therapies.

ADULTS WITH TYPE 1 DM

A significant minority of patients with a diagnosis of T2DM actually have a late onset of T1DM and typical autoimmunity (IA-2 antibodies, GAD-65 antibodies, and insulin antibodies). The diagnosis should certainly be suspected in patients who rapidly fail combination oral agent therapy. Nonobese body habitus, marked weight loss, extremely elevated glucose values, or a family or personal history of autoimmune disease (e.g., Hashimoto's or Graves' thyroid problems) should lead to diagnostic evaluation for such signs of autoimmunity.

T1DM patients need combined mealtime and basal insulin therapy. Although it is tempting to do so in a convenient fashion with combined preparations such as those with analogue fixed ratios, it usually is far preferable to use a better basal insulin, such as glargine or detemir combined with a rapid-acting analogue (separately injected) before meals. Sometimes an insulin pump is the best way for patients who have frequent hypoglycemia or marked variability to achieve good glycemic control safely. T1DM patients should preferably be seen by an endocrine specialist or other practitioner with extensive experience in T1DM management. Ready access to diabetes educators is an important key to success with both T1DM and T2DM.

ADULTS WITH TYPE 2 DM

Many T2DM patients eventually need mealtime insulin. For those on insulin alone, incretin mimetics[1] can be successfully used for mealtime control, because they effectively lower prandial hyperglycemia. If using exenatide, then additional injections will be required at the two major meals of the day. If using an incretin-enhancer drug such as sitagliptin, injections are not required. There are no published data yet to provide guidelines for this strategy, but we have occasionally used this approach with exenatide in patients who need to lose weight, who gain considerable weight with meal insulin, or who experience poor control despite attempts to regulate meal glycemia with short-acting insulins.

---

[1]Not FDA approved for this indication.

REFERENCES

American Diabetes Association. Diabetes care 2010;33:S11–61.

American Diabetes Association. Diabetes care 2010;33(Suppl. 1):S62–9.

American Diabetes Association. Facilitating Behavior Change: Key Strategies for Empowering Your Patients. http://www.facilitatingbehaviorchange.org/2009.

Diabetes Prevention Program Research Group. The Diabetes Prevention Program (DPP): Description of lifestyle intervention. Diabetes Care 2002; 25:2165–71.

Grundy SM, Cleeman JI, Daniels SR, et al. Diagnosis and management of the metabolic syndrome. An American Heart Association/National Heart, Lung, and Blood Institute Scientific Statement. Executive summary. Circulation 2005;112:2735–52.

Kahn R, Buse J, Ferrannini E, Stern M. The metabolic syndrome: Time for a critical appraisal. Joint statement from the American Diabetes Association and the European Association for the Study of Diabetes. Diabetes Care 2005;8:2289–304.

Knowler WC, Barrett-Connor E, Fowler SE, et al. Reduction in the incidence of type 2 diabetes with lifestyle intervention or metformin. N Engl J Med 2002;346:393–403.

Monnier L, Lapinski H, Colette C. Contributions of fasting and postprandial plasma glucose increments to the overall diurnal hyperglycemia of type 2 diabetic patients: Variations with increasing levels of HbA1c. Diabetes Care 2003;26:881–5.

Nathan DM, Buse JB, Davidson MB, et al. Management of hyperglycemia in type 2 diabetes: A consensus algorithm for the initiation and adjustment of therapy. A consensus statement from the American Diabetes Association and the European Association for the Study of Diabetes. Diabetes Care 2006;29:1963–72.

Nathan DM, Buse JB, Davidson MB, et al. Medical management of hyperglycemia in type 2 diabetes: A consensus algorithm for the initiation and adjustment of therapy. Diabetes Care 2009;32:193–203.

Nesto RW, Bell D, Bonow RO, et al. Thiazolidinedione use, fluid retention, and congestive heart failure. A consensus statement from the American Heart Association and American Diabetes Association. Diabetes Care 2004;27:256–63.

Pihoker C, Gilliam LK, Hampe CS, Lernmark A. Autoantibodies in diabetes. Diabetes 2005;54:S52–61.

Riddle MC, Rosenstock J, Gerich J. The treat-to-target trial: Randomized addition of glargine or human NPH insulin to oral therapy of type 2 diabetic patients. Diabetes Care 2003;26:3080–6.

Rodbard HW, Jellinger PS, Davidson JA, et al. Statement by an American Association of Clinical Endocrinologists/American College of Endocrinology consensus panel on type 2 diabetes mellitus: an algorithm for glycemic control. Endocr Pract 2009;15(6):540–59.

Saudek CD, Herman WH, Sacks DB, et al. A new look at screening and diagnosis of diabetes mellitus. J Clin Endocrinol Metab 2008; May 6, [epub ahead of print].

Diabetes Mellitus in Children and Adolescents

Method of
Lori M.B. Laffel, MD, MPH, and
Jamie R.S. Wood, MD

Diabetes mellitus is a group of metabolic disorders that have hyperglycemia as a common feature caused by inadequate insulin secretion, insulin action, or both. Chronic hyperglycemia and its numerous downstream effects lead to micro- and macrovascular complications involving the eyes, kidneys, nerves, and blood vessels. Childhood and adolescent years are periods of rapid physical growth and psychosocial change, and these two factors make the care of children and adolescents with diabetes both challenging and rewarding. The health care professional must balance the important goals of optimal glycemic control and normal growth and development along with the risks of hypoglycemia and the challenges of expected glycemic excursions during childhood. Multidisciplinary care is the hallmark of successful diabetes management for the child and adolescent with diabetes and for family members.

The American Diabetes Association (ADA) classifies diabetes mellitus into four main types: type 1 diabetes (T1D), type 2 diabetes (T2D), other specific types, and gestational diabetes mellitus (Table 1). T1D is caused by insulin deficiency, which results from the autoimmune destruction of the pancreatic β cells. There are multiple genetic loci in the major histocompatibility region of chromosome 6 that predispose (DR 3/4, DQ 0201/0302, DR 4/4, and DQ 0300/0302) or protect against (DQB1*0602, DQA1*0102) the development of T1D. T2D is caused by the combination of insulin resistance and relative insulin deficiency.

Genetic forms of diabetes include maturity-onset diabetes in the young (MODY), mitochondrial diabetes, and certain syndromes of insulin resistance. MODY is characterized by young age of onset, autosomal dominant inheritance, the lack of association with obesity, and a variable phenotype. The most common disease of the exocrine pancreas that causes diabetes in children and adolescents is cystic fibrosis. Glucocorticoids used in the treatment of systemic illnesses are also commonly associated with hyperglycemia and diabetes. Certain genetic syndromes, such as Down syndrome, Klinefelter's syndrome, and Turner's syndrome, increase the risk for diabetes.

TABLE 1 Classification of Diabetes Mellitus*

Type 1 diabetes
Type 2 diabetes
Other specific types:
- Genetic defects of β-cell function
  - MODY 1: chromosome 20, HNF-4α
  - MODY 2: chromosome 7, glucokinase
  - MODY 3: chromosome 12, HNF-1α
  - MODY 4: chromosome 13, IPF-1
  - MODY 5: chromosome 17, HNF-1β
  - MODY 6: chromosome 2, NeuroD1
  - Mitochondrial diabetes
- Genetic defects in insulin action
  - Leprechaunism
  - Rabson-Mendenhall syndrome
- Diseases of the exocrine pancreas
  - Pancreatitis
  - Cystic fibrosis
  - Pancreatectomy
- Endocrinopathies
  - Acromegaly
  - Cushing's syndrome
  - Glucagonoma
  - Pheochromocytoma
- Drug or chemical induced
  - Glucocorticoids
- Infections
  - Congenital rubella
  - Cytomegalovirus
- Other genetic syndromes associated with diabetes
  - Down's syndrome
  - Klinefelter's syndrome
  - Turner's syndrome
Gestational diabetes mellitus (GDM)

*Table is not all-inconclusive and gives examples of each subtype of diabetes mellitus. For complete list, see American Diabetes Association: Diagnosis and classification of diabetes mellitus. Diabetes Care 2005;28 (Suppl 1):S37–S42.
Abbreviations: MODY = maturity-onset diabetes in the young.

Diagnosis

The diagnosis of T1D in children and adolescents is typically straightforward. The classic symptoms of polyuria, polydipsia, polyphagia, and weight loss over a several-week period are common. A thorough history and physical exam may reveal perineal candidiasis or thrush. Such symptoms may be followed by nausea, abdominal pain, vomiting, lethargy, and Kussmaul respirations if diabetic ketoacidosis (DKA) and lactic acidosis develop. The presentation of T2D in children and adolescents can be more subtle and sometimes even clinically silent. However, approximately a third of adolescents with T2D have ketosis and a quarter have ketoacidosis at presentation.

The Current Diagnosis box outlines the diagnosis of diabetes mellitus. In the asymptomatic child or adolescent, diabetes is diagnosed when a fasting plasma glucose is 126 mg/dL or more, a 2-hour plasma glucose during an oral glucose tolerance test (OGTT) is 200 mg/dL or more, or a random plasma glucose is 200 mg/dL or more with confirmation on a second day. The symptomatic child or adolescent with a random plasma glucose of 200 mg/dL or more does not need repeat testing to confirm the diagnosis. Measurement of islet cell autoantibodies consistent with T1D (GAD, insulin, IA2) at diagnosis may help distinguish between type 1 and T2D. Care must be taken to avoid delay in the diagnosis and initiation of treatment because of the risk of rapid metabolic deterioration with insulin deficiency.

CURRENT DIAGNOSIS

ADA Recommendations for the Diagnosis of Diabetes

- Symptoms (polyuria, polydipsia, unexplained weight loss) and a casual plasma glucose (any time of day without regard to time since last meal) >200 mg/dL (11.1 mmol/L) *or*
- Fasting (no caloric intake for at least 8 h) plasma glucose >126 mg/dL (7.0 mmol/L) *or*
- 2-hour plasma glucose >200 mg/dL (11.1 mmol/L) during an oral glucose tolerance test (glucose load of 75 g anhydrous glucose dissolved in water or 1.75 g/kg body weight if weight <43 kg).

Note: Criteria 2 and 3 should be confirmed on a second day if child/adolescent is asymptomatic. The OGTT is not recommended for routine clinical use and should be reserved for the asymptomatic child with incidental glucosuria/hyperglycemia or in the child with suspected diabetes but normal fasting plasma glucose.

Adapted from American Diabetes Association: Care of children and adolescents with type 1 diabetes. Diabetes Care 2005;28(1):186–212.

Initial Management

The goals of initial management of the child or adolescent newly diagnosed with diabetes mellitus are to correct fluid and electrolyte imbalances, reverse hepatic gluconeogenesis and ketogenesis by halting lipolysis with insulin replacement, and begin the process of diabetes education. The location of this initial management depends on the severity of the clinical presentation, the age of the patient, the psychosocial assessment of the child or adolescent and caregiver, and the diabetes-related resources available in the family's geographic location (availability of an outpatient education program).

Diabetic Ketoacidosis

Approximately 30% of children with newly diagnosed T1D present with diabetic ketoacidosis (DKA). Children who are younger (less than 4 years), without a first-degree relative with T1D, and from a family of lower socioeconomic status are at higher risk of DKA at onset of T1D. The majority of DKA episodes occur in patients with established diabetes, not in those newly diagnosed. Children or adolescents with established T1D are at higher risk for DKA if they are in poor metabolic control, have had a previous episode of DKA, are peripubertal/adolescent girls, have a psychiatric disorder, or are from a disadvantaged background.

Management of DKA in children and adolescents is based on the same principles used in adults and therefore is covered in a separate chapter in this book. The development of cerebral edema, however, warrants discussion because this complication is seen primarily in children and is associated with both high morbidity and mortality. Risk factors for the development of cerebral edema include lower initial partial pressure of carbon dioxide, higher initial serum urea nitrogen concentrations, treatment with bicarbonate, and an attenuated rise in measured serum sodium concentrations during therapy. In addition, children who are younger (less than 5 years), have new-onset T1D, and longer duration of symptoms may also be at an increased risk. A high index of suspicion is needed with mannitol (Osmitrol) at the bedside to allow for timely intervention.

Initiation of Insulin Replacement Therapy

Subcutaneous insulin is initiated in the patient who does not present in DKA or following intravenous insulin therapy in the child with resolved DKA who is tolerating oral intake (pH of >7.3, tCO$_2$ >18, anion gap 12 ± 2 mEq/L). The starting dose of insulin replacement therapy depends on the age, weight, and pubertal status of the patient, as well as the presence or absence of DKA. For the prepubertal child without DKA, the starting dose is usually 0.25 to 0.5 U/kg/day. For the prepubertal child with resolved DKA, the usual starting dose is 0.5 to 0.75 U/kg/day. For the pubertal child without DKA, the starting dose is 0.5 to 0.75 U/kg/day and for the pubertal child with resolved DKA, 0.75 to 1 U/kg/day. This total daily dose (TDD) of insulin is typically divided into either two or three injections per day, with the latter the preference toward implementation of intensive therapy (Figure 1). The twice-daily regimen may be selected for the younger (less than 4 years) child or if the psychosocial assessment determines that fewer injections per day would be beneficial. The use of an insulin pump at diagnosis remains within the research realm currently.

When the patient is metabolically stable, the focus turns to the psychosocial assessment of the child or adolescent and caregiver(s) and the initiation of diabetes education. A licensed social worker or other mental health professional evaluates each family and screens for circumstances that might complicate diabetes management: family composition, alternative caregiver(s), financial concerns, lack of health insurance, psychiatric or medical illness in a family member, or severe emotional distress of caregiver secondary to the diabetes diagnosis.

Diabetes education is provided by a certified diabetes nurse educator (DNE) and focuses on the set of essential skills needed to keep a child or adolescent with diabetes safe at home and school. These survival skills include techniques of blood glucose monitoring, urine or blood ketone measurement, drawing up and administration of subcutaneous insulin and glucagon, recognition and treatment of hypoglycemia and hyperglycemia, basics of sick day management, and indications for and methods of contacting the child's diabetes team. In addition to the survival skills, the child or adolescent and family should meet with a registered dietician who will assist them in developing an individualized meal plan and introduce the family to the concept of carbohydrate counting or exchanges. Once the child or adolescent (if developmentally appropriate) and caregiver(s) demonstrate the knowledge and skills needed, they are discharged with the expectation of daily phone contact with a member of their diabetes team to further titrate insulin doses and answer questions. When available and clinically indicated, a visiting nurse may assist with ongoing home-based education and support in the short term.

Outpatient Diabetes Care

The management of children and adolescents with diabetes requires a multidisciplinary team approach. Members of this team include either a pediatric endocrinologist or pediatrician with training in diabetes, a pediatric DNE, a dietician, and a mental health professional (social worker and psychologist). Members of this team need to be easily accessible to the family in times of illness or metabolic crisis. Another member of the child/adolescent's team is a pediatrician or family doctor who will continue to provide routine well child care including anticipatory guidance, immunizations, and general medical care.

In the first few months of outpatient diabetes care, patients are seen frequently by members of the diabetes team to assess the family's adaptation to the new diagnosis, reinforce skills and knowledge learned during the first few days, and expand on the skills and knowledge needed for intensive diabetes management. Patients are subsequently seen at a minimum frequency of every 3 months, alternating between their DNE and their pediatric endocrinologist. Visits with the dietician are recommended yearly or more frequently if circumstances warrant (e.g., young child or toddler, desired weight loss, initiating pump therapy, etc.).

Diabetes Education

Diabetes education is an ongoing process with continuous need for review of previously learned material and introduction of new concepts as the family develops a more sophisticated understanding of intensive diabetes management. The educator should evaluate the patient and his or her caregiver's knowledge and skills regularly. In addition, age-appropriate issues need to be discussed as the patient matures (e.g., driving guidelines, issues related to alcohol and smoking, etc.). Diabetes education needs to be tailored to each family taking into account their educational level and cultural practices. The educator must be sensitive to the age and developmental stage of the child or adolescent, and shift his or her educational efforts from the caregiver(s) to the adolescent when it is developmentally appropriate. Continued parental involvement and supervision of the adolescent with diabetes is crucial to good metabolic control.

The health care provider should complete a focused interval history at each visit that includes recent illnesses, visits to the emergency department, hospitalizations, medications prescribed other than insulin, types of insulin and current doses, daily routine including meal plan and activity level, self-care behaviors and identifying who performs them, episodes of hypoglycemia and their precipitants, school performance, emotional health, and a review of systems focusing on symptoms of hyperglycemia (polyuria, polydipsia, polyphagia,

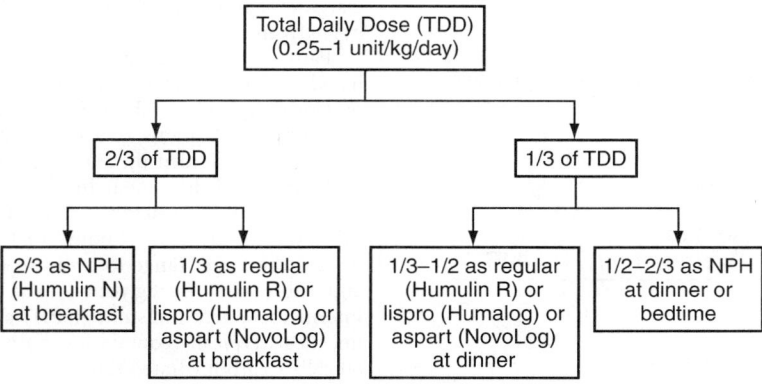

FIGURE 1. Initiation of Insulin Replacement Therapy. Two thirds of the total daily dose (TDD) is given at breakfast and further divided into NPH (two thirds) and short/rapid-acting insulin (one third). The remaining one third is either given in one injection at dinner (in a twice-daily regimen) or divided between dinner and bedtime (in a thrice-daily regimen), and should also be divided into NPH (two thirds) and short/rapid-acting insulin (one third). Short/rapid-acting insulin can be regular (Humulin R), lispro (Humalog), or aspart (NovoLog).

weight loss, candidal infections) and the possible development of other autoimmune disorders. If appropriate, a history of tobacco, alcohol, recreational drugs, and sexual activity should be elicited. A focused physical examination that includes measurement of blood pressure and heart rate, weight, height, body mass index (BMI), and examination of the thyroid gland, sites of blood glucose monitoring, and insulin injections should be completed at each visit. A more thorough physical examination including Tanner staging should be performed once per year or more frequently if indicated.

The hemoglobin A1C, the fraction of hemoglobin that has glucose attached to it, is a measure of the average level of blood glucose over the preceding 2 to 3 months. It should be measured every 3 months and serves as an objective measure of blood glucose control. A discrepancy between the hemoglobin A1C and the average blood glucose levels from self-monitoring records suggests that the patient needs to monitor at different times of day, may benefit from a review of blood glucose monitoring technique and equipment, or there may be fabrication of results. Obtaining computer downloaded data helps eliminate the latter possibility.

Goals of Therapy

The Diabetes Control and Complications Trial (DCCT) demonstrated that the incidence of microvascular complications was reduced with improved blood glucose control (hemoglobin A1C approximately 7%). The reduction in complications, however, was accompanied by an increased risk of severe hypoglycemia. Because young children are more vulnerable to hypoglycemia (reduced catecholamine response to hypoglycemia, decreased ability to communicate symptoms of hypoglycemia, and risk for neuropsychologic impairment from hypoglycemia), the ADA has developed age-specific glycemic targets (Table 2).

Insulin Therapy

The ideal insulin replacement therapy would be one that mirrors the basal and prandial insulin secretion in individuals without diabetes. Numerous insulin preparations are available that vary in time to onset, peak, and duration of action (Table 3). No single regimen is superior to another; thus individualization of the insulin regimen to the child or adolescent and family remains a major determinant. Important factors for consideration include blood glucose monitoring frequency, number of daily injections the family can perform, the need for flexibility in meal planning, and the unique family schedule. Regimens range in intensity from twice-a-day injections with a set dose of premixed insulin to intensive diabetes management with multiple injections per day of two or more types of insulin or use of an insulin pump (continuous subcutaneous insulin infusion [CSII]).

TABLE 2 Blood Glucose and A1C Goals for Type 1 Diabetes by Age Group

| Age Group | Plasma Blood Glucose Range (mg/dL) | | A1C |
	Before Meals	Bedtime/ Overnight	
<6 y	100–180	110–200	7.5%–8.5%
6–12 y	90–180	100–180	<8%
13–19 y	90–130	90–150	<7.5%

Adapted from American Diabetes Association: Care of children and adolescents with type 1 diabetes. Diabetes Care 2005;28(1):186–212.
Goals should be individualized; lower goals may be reasonable and achievable without hypoglycemia.
Goals should be higher in patients with frequent hypoglycemia or hypoglycemia unawareness.

CURRENT THERAPY

Examples of Insulin Regimens

Injections bid:
- Premixed insulin (70/30, 75/25) given at breakfast and dinner
- NPH and rapid- or short-acting insulin given at breakfast and dinner

Injections tid:
- NPH and rapid- or short-acting insulin given at breakfast, rapid- or short-acting insulin given at dinner, and NPH given at bedtime
- NPH and rapid- or short-acting insulin given at breakfast, rapid- or short-acting insulin given at dinner, and NPH or glargine (Lantus) given at bedtime

Injections qid:
- NPH and rapid-acting insulin given at breakfast, rapid-acting insulin given at lunch and dinner, and rapid-acting insulin and NPH given at bedtime
- NPH and rapid-acting insulin given at breakfast and lunch, rapid-acting insulin given at dinner, and NPH given at bedtime
- Rapid-acting insulin given at breakfast, lunch, and dinner, and glargine (Lantus) given at breakfast, dinner, or bedtime

Continuous subcutaneous insulin infusion (CSII)
- Rapid-acting insulin given for basal requirements and as bolus at every meal/snack and periodically to correct hyperglycemia (no more frequent than q2–3h)

The typical regimen that children or adolescents begin at diagnosis was described previously (Figure 1). Some centers initiate a basal-bolus regimen in which insulin is replaced in a manner that attempts to mimic physiologic insulin release. Basal-bolus regimens include the insulin pump and glargine (Lantus) given once a day with rapid-acting insulin (lispro [Humalog] or aspart [NovoLog]) before each meal/snack and as needed for correction of hyperglycemia. The school-age child who hopes to avoid an injection at lunch often benefits from a regimen of glargine (Lantus) at dinner or bedtime, along with NPH (Humulin N) and a rapid-acting insulin at breakfast, plus a rapid-acting insulin at dinner. The peak of the NPH covers carbohydrate intake at lunch. The use of basal insulin analogue glargine (Lantus) in the evening is associated with less nocturnal hypoglycemia.

Patients on a basal-bolus regimen determine their insulin doses based on an insulin-to-carbohydrate ratio and a correction factor or sensitivity index (CF or SI). The insulin-to-carbohydrate ratio is the number of grams of carbohydrate covered by 1 U of insulin (roughly 450 divided by TDD) for each meal and snack. The CF/SI is the expected decrement in glucose following 1 U of rapid-acting insulin (roughly 1650 divided by TDD). The CF/SI is applied no more than every 2 to 3 hours to lower an elevated blood glucose toward the target range to avoid so-called stacking of insulin action and subsequent hypoglycemia. For patients on a combination of intermediate-acting insulin (NPH) and rapid- or short-acting insulin, meals typically contain a certain amount of carbohydrates (e.g., 60 g or 4 carbohydrate exchanges) and require consistency in timing to avoid hypoglycemia.

The CSII, otherwise known as insulin pump therapy, comes the closest to mimicking the basal and prandial insulin secretion of an individual without diabetes. The insulin pump is steadily becoming a commonly used method to replace insulin, especially in the pediatric population. There are many advantages to the insulin pump

TABLE 3 Insulin Analogues

Insulin Preparation	Onset of Action	Peak Action	Effective Duration
Rapid Acting			
Insulin lispro	5–15 min	30–90 min	2–4 h
Insulin aspart	5–10 min	60–180 min	3–5 h
Insulin glulisine	5–15 min	30–90 min	3–5 h
Short Acting			
Regular	30–60 min	2–3 h	3–6 h
Intermediate Acting			
NPH (isophane insulin)	2–4 h	4–10 h	10–16 h
Long Acting			
Insulin glargine	1.1 h	None	24 h
Insulin detemir	2–3 h	6–14 h	16–24 h
Insulin Mixtures			
70/30 human mix* (70% NPH, 30% regular)	30–60 min	dual	10–16 h
70/30 aspart analog mix (70% intermediate, 30% aspart)*	5–15 min	dual	10–16 h
75/25 lispro analog mix* (75% intermediate, 25% lispro)	5–15 min	dual	10–16 h
50/50 lispro analog mix (50% intermediate, 50% lispro)	30–60 min	dual	10–16 h

In many countries, including the United States, insulin preparations contain 100 U/mL and are referred to as U-100 insulin. Highly concentrated U-500 short-acting insulin is available and used primarily in adults with severe insulin resistance.

Profiles for each insulin preparation are reasonable estimates only, based on data from adult study participants. There is variation between individuals, and time of onset, peak, and duration are also affected by size of dose, site and depth of injection, dilution, exercise, and temperature.

*Typically used in fixed doses in twice-a-day insulin regimens.

including the elimination of multiple daily injections, increased flexibility in meal planning, ease of decreasing insulin for physical activity, fewer hypoglycemic events, and the ability to deliver very small amounts of insulin. The disadvantages are more frequent blood glucose monitoring, always being tethered to the pump, and increased risk for the development of DKA. Because only rapid-acting insulin (lispro [Humalog] or aspart [NovoLog]) is used in the insulin pump, discontinuation of insulin delivery can result in ketone production within hours. Increased vigilance, therefore, is necessary to ensure proper functioning of the insulin pump with frequent blood glucose monitoring and checking for ketones if hyperglycemia develops.

Self-Monitoring

One of the main goals of diabetes education is to teach and empower the patient and family in the self-management of diabetes. Self-management of diabetes includes measuring blood glucose and blood/urine ketone levels, recording the results along with amount of carbohydrate intake and amount of insulin administered, and the ability to make insulin dosing decisions based on the interpretation of these records. Monitoring blood glucose four or more times daily is recommended in children with T1D. Additional monitoring may be necessary postprandially, overnight, or during periods of increased physical activity to help optimize control and prevent severe hypoglycemia. Preschool or early school-age children may require more frequent monitoring because of their inability to recognize symptoms or to communicate during episodes of hypoglycemia. In addition, children and adolescents using the insulin pump typically check their blood sugar six or more times per day. Ketone measurements should be done whenever the blood glucose is greater than 250 to 300 mg/dL and/or if the patient is ill, especially with nausea, vomiting, or abdominal pain. Ketones can be measured either in the urine (acetoacetate and acetone) or blood (β-hydroxybutyric acid). Measurement of blood ketones is now available on a home meter and is the preferred method in the current era stressing blood glucose monitoring. The key to successful intensive diabetes management is frequent blood glucose monitoring, good record keeping, and communication of these results with the diabetes team at frequent intervals so that timely modifications can be made to the insulin regimen and/or meal plan.

Medical Nutrition Therapy

The meal plan remains an important component of management aimed at good glycemic control, although it is often the most difficult aspect of intensive diabetes management for families. A dietician trained in pediatric nutrition and diabetes should meet with the family at the time of T1D diagnosis and periodically thereafter. The dietician should help develop a meal plan that is individualized to the patient's daily schedule, food preferences, cultural influences, and physical activity. The meal plan is more likely to be successful if it is designed to fit into the family's already established schedule and preferences. The patient and family should also be instructed on carbohydrate counting so that either carbohydrate exchanges or insulin-to-carbohydrate ratios can be used. Like the child without diabetes, the total number of recommended calories follows the child's growth requirements along with consideration of the need for weight gain or loss. Growth velocity, weight gain, and BMI should be monitored at every visit to ensure that the meal plan is sufficient to meet the energy requirements of the patient. Unexpected weight loss or poor weight gain should prompt consideration of suboptimal metabolic control, as well as eating disorders, thyroid dysfunction, or gastrointestinal disease.

The ADA does not have pediatric specific guidelines for medical nutrition therapy, but the recommendations for adults can be extrapolated to children. The ADA recommends that carbohydrates provide 45% to 65% of total calories, with protein and fat contributing 15% and 30%, respectively. The patient and family should be educated to avoid foods high in cholesterol, saturated fat, and concentrated sweets and select foods high in complex carbohydrate and dietary fiber.

All children and adolescents are recommended to have three meals per day. If they receive intermediate-acting insulin preparations, they should also receive three snacks per day (morning, afternoon, and bedtime) to match anticipated peaks of insulin action. If the child or adolescent is on a basal-bolus regimen, snacks are optional and require insulin coverage based on insulin-to-carbohydrate ratios.

Exercise

Exercise, or periods of sustained physical activity, can be beneficial to the patient by contributing to a sense of well-being, helping achieve the recommended BMI, improving glycemic control (exercise enhances insulin sensitivity), improving the lipid panel (increasing HDL), and lowering blood pressure and improving cardiovascular fitness. All children and adolescents, especially those with diabetes, should be encouraged to participate in routine physical activity.

The child or adolescent with diabetes needs to take precautions to avoid hypoglycemia during periods of increased physical activity. The patient and family need to check blood glucose before the initiation of activity, every hour during sustained activity, and at the completion of physical activity. For the first several days of increased activity, the child should also check his or her blood sugar frequently during the 12-hour postexercise period because there is often a delayed drop in the blood glucose following exercise (i.e., the lag effect). Some children require additional carbohydrate before, during, and after activity; lower insulin doses on the days of increased physical activity; or both. It is suggested that the child take 5 to 15 g of carbohydrates, depending on age and exercise intensity, before exercise if the blood sugar is below target, and repeat the 5 to 15 g of carbohydrate for every 30 minutes of sustained activity. Rapid-acting carbohydrate should be readily available, and coaches and trainers should be aware of the diagnosis of diabetes and trained in the treatment of hypoglycemia.

Psychosocial Support

The mental health professional is an important member of the diabetes team. A thorough family assessment generally accompanies the diabetes diagnosis with appropriate referrals for additional services as needed. Thereafter, children or adolescents should be referred back to a mental health professional if social, emotional, or economic barriers to the achievement of good glycemic control are identified. Family conflict, especially conflict over diabetes care, can be associated with deterioration in glycemic control. Encouragement of ongoing family teamwork in the management of childhood diabetes promotes successful outcomes with respect to glycemic control, reducing diabetes-specific conflict, and preventing acute complications and emergency assessments.

Sick Day Management

The goals for the management of children and adolescents during sick days are never omit insulin, prevent dehydration and hypoglycemia, monitor blood glucose frequently (every 2 to 4 hours), monitor for ketosis, provide supplemental rapid- or short-acting insulin doses (5% to 20% of TDD) depending on degree of hyperglycemia and ketosis, treat underlying illness, and have frequent contact with the diabetes team. The majority of DKA among children or adolescents with established diabetes is caused by insulin omission or errors in administration of insulin. Inadequate insulin therapy in the context of an intercurrent illness accounts for the remaining small percentage. Although it is more common for children to require more insulin during illnesses, some children require a reduction of the basal and/or rapid-acting insulin dose if he or she is unable to eat and the blood glucose is less than 200 mg/dL.

Families need to be educated about symptoms that warrant immediate medical attention, including signs of dehydration (dry mouth, sunken eyes, cracked lips, weight loss, dry skin), persistent vomiting for more than 2 to 4 hours, persistence of blood glucose levels greater than 300 mg/dL or ketones for more than 12 hours, or symptoms of DKA (nausea, abdominal pain, chest pain, vomiting, ketotic breath, hyperventilation, or altered consciousness). It is helpful for the diabetes team to review sick day management annually with the family (can accompany flu immunization) to avoid metabolic decompensation during intercurrent illness.

Hypoglycemia

Fear of hypoglycemia can be a common occurrence in the management of childhood diabetes, especially among caregivers, and can be a barrier to optimal glycemic control. Recognition and treatment of hypoglycemia are important topics for diabetes education. Families are trained to treat hypoglycemia with 10 to 15 g of rapid-acting carbohydrate, recheck blood glucose in 15 minutes, repeat treatment with 10 to 15 g if blood sugar remains below target, and follow with a protein-containing snack if a meal will not follow within 1 to 2 hours. This technique avoids the natural tendency to overtreat low blood glucose levels. Caregivers should also receive glucagon training (20 to 30 µg/kg; maximum 1 mg) for severe hypoglycemia and low-dose glucagon (1 U on an insulin syringe for every year of life up to 15 years) for impending hypoglycemia, for example, in the context of a gastrointestinal illness or inadvertent insulin administration (lispro given instead of NPH). A member of the diabetes team should assess frequency, treatment, awareness, and circumstances of hypoglycemia at each visit.

Screening for Diabetes-Related Complications

Patients, families, and caregivers worry about the risk of diabetes-related complications, and therefore the diabetes team must educate families and screen for complications with sensitivity and optimism, emphasizing prevention of complications and the maintenance of health. Screening for nephropathy, hypertension, dyslipidemia, and retinopathy are indicated.

Microalbuminuria (MA) is the first sign of diabetic nephropathy, and patients who develop persistent MA are at increased risk of progression to macroalbuminuria. Poor glycemic control, smoking, and a family history of essential hypertension are risk factors for the development of MA and nephropathy. Identification of persistent MA provides an opportunity for intervention and prevention of progressive renal disease through improvements in glycemic control and/or therapy with angiotensin-converting enzyme (ACE) inhibitors. There are currently no pediatric data on the use of angiotensin receptor blockers (ARBs). Table 4 outlines definitions, screening recommendations, and treatment.

Hypertension is an important predictor of the progression of diabetic nephropathy to end-stage renal disease. Hypertension in children and adolescents may go unrecognized because providers are not familiar with the gender-, age-, and height-specific definitions. Blood pressure should be measured every 3 months with standardized technique, using the proper size cuff. If elevated blood pressures are detected and confirmed, the first step is to exclude causes not related to diabetes. Table 4 outlines the definitions, screening recommendations, and treatment.

Dyslipidemia and diabetes are established risk factors for cardiovascular disease, and recent research suggests that a significant proportion of adolescents with diabetes already have evidence of atherosclerosis. Low-density lipoprotein (LDL) cholesterol is most closely associated with cardiovascular disease, and therefore, the ADA has developed guidelines for LDL cholesterol. Screening may be delayed until puberty if family history is negative for cardiovascular disease. A lipid profile should be performed on prepubertal children with diabetes who are older than 2 years if there is a positive family history of cardiovascular disease or if the family history is unknown. If the LDL cholesterol is less than 100 mg/dL, screening

TABLE 4 Screening for Diabetes-Related Complications

Complication	How to Screen	Definition	When to Screen	Therapy
Microalbuminuria	Spot urine sample timed overnight or 24-h collection	Spot urine albumin/creatinine ratio 30–299 µg/g or AER 20–199 µg/min from timed collection	Annual screening begins at 10 y or after >5 y duration of diabetes	Optimize glucose control, smoking cessation, normalize BP
Persistent microalbuminuria		2/3 of urine samples meet above criteria		Above, plus addition of ACE inhibitor
High-normal BP	Manual BP measurement with standard technique	Systolic or diastolic BP within the 90th–95th percentile for age, gender, and height	At every clinic visit	Dietary intervention, weight control, and exercise; if target BP not reached within 3–6 mo, then initiate pharmacologic therapy
Hypertension		Systolic or diastolic BP above the 95th percentile for age, gender, and height, or >130/80 on >3 occasions (whichever is lower)		Above, plus pharmacologic therapy titrated to achieve target BP

Note: Urine collection should not be performed following vigorous exercise, during an acute infection, during a female patient's menstrual cycle, or following an episode of severe hypoglycemia. Once angiotensin-converting enzyme (ACE) inhibitor is started, microalbumin excretion should be monitored q3–6 mo. Target BP is <130/80 or <90th percentile for age, gender, and height. Initial drug treatment is ACE inhibition.
Abbreviations: AER = albumin excretion rate; BP = blood pressure.

can be repeated every 5 years. The mainstay of therapy for dyslipidemia is dietary management (saturated fat less than 7% of calories and less than 200 mg/day of cholesterol). Children with levels between 130 and 159 mg/dL should be started on medication if diet and lifestyle modification are unsuccessful after 6 months or if the child has additional risk factors for cardiovascular disease, such as obesity or hypertension. Pharmacotherapy is recommended if the LDL cholesterol is more than 160 mg/dL. The LDL goal for children with diabetes is less than 100 mg/dL.

Diabetic retinopathy is a feared complication because it is the leading cause of vision loss. According to the ADA, the first ophthalmologic exam should be requested when the child is 10 years or older and has had diabetes for more than 3 to 5 years. Examinations with an eye care professional with expertise in diabetic retinopathy should occur early.

Screening for Other Autoimmune Diseases

Children and adolescents with T1D are at an increased risk for other autoimmune diseases and should be screened accordingly. Approximately 15% of patients with T1D also have autoimmune thyroid disease. All children and adolescents should be screened for autoimmune thyroid disease at the time of diabetes diagnosis once metabolic control is established. TSH measurement is a useful initial screen, with and without measuring the presence of thyroid autoantibodies. Screening should be repeated yearly or if there is any clinical suspicion of thyroid disease (abnormal growth rate, symptoms of hypo- or hyperthyroidism, goiter on examination, erratic blood glucose control).

Another commonly associated disorder is celiac disease. Nearly 6% of patients with T1D have elevated levels of circulating autoantibodies to tissue transglutaminase. Celiac disease can cause diarrhea, weight loss or failure to gain weight, abdominal pain, fatigue, and unexplained hypoglycemia or erratic blood glucose secondary to malabsorption. Patients with T1D should be screened with circulating IgA autoantibody to tissue transglutaminase. A quantitative serum IgA level should be drawn at the same time to rule out IgA deficiency as a cause for falsely low IgA tissue transglutaminase levels. Positive antibodies should be confirmed with a second measurement, and if positive, a referral should be made to a gastroenterologist for small bowel biopsy. If the diagnosis is confirmed, celiac disease is treated with a gluten-free diet with recommendations and support from a registered dietician with pediatric expertise in diabetes and celiac management.

Type 2 Diabetes Mellitus in Youth

With the increasing prevalence of childhood obesity during the last two decades, there is an increased occurrence of T2D in youth. Based on National Health and Nutrition Examination survey data, the prevalence of overweight children (defined as a body mass index greater than the 95th percentile for children and youth) increased from 5% in the 1970s to more than 15% by 1999. The epidemic of obesity follows the increased consumption of fast foods, increased consumption of soft drinks, increased sedentary behavior with more television watching, and decreased physical activity. Mirroring this epidemic of childhood obesity is the occurrence of T2D in children and adolescents. Before 1990, T2D in youth was a rare occurrence. By 2000, between 8% and 45% of all newly diagnosed cases of childhood diabetes were caused by T2D. T2D occurs most commonly in those with a family history of T2D; individuals from certain racial and ethnic minority groups including Native Americans, Hispanics, African Americans, and Asian and Pacific Islanders; those with obesity falling above the 85th percentile for BMI based on age and gender; and in association with markers of insulin resistance (Table 5). Markers of insulin resistance include the occurrence of acanthosis nigricans and polycystic ovarian syndrome (PCOS). In addition, other well-known risk factors include hypertension and hyperlipidemia.

As noted earlier, the diagnosis of T2D is based on fasting plasma glucose (FPG), 2-hour glucose value during an OGTT, or a casual glucose level. Because T2D often goes without symptoms, individuals who are overweight, have a positive family history of T2D, come from one of the high-risk racial and ethnic minority groups, and/or have markers of insulin resistance warrant screening for T2D. Screening can be performed with a FPG or OGTT when clinical concerns are high and the FPG is normal.

Currently one oral medication is approved for the treatment of T2D in youth. This medication is metformin (Glucophage), which is also available in a liquid formulation. The maximum recommended daily dose of metformin (Glucophage) in youth is 2000 mg/day divided as 1000 mg twice daily. Often patients with

TABLE 5 Risk Factors and Screening for Type 2 Diabetes in Children

Criteria	Age of Initiation	Frequency	Method
Overweight (BMI >85th percentile for age and gender), weight for height >85th percentile, or weight >120% of ideal for height Plus 2 of the following risk factors: Family history of T2D in 1st- or 2nd-degree relative Race/ethnicity (American Indian, African American, Hispanic, Asian/ Pacific Islander) Signs of or conditions associated with insulin resistance (acanthosis nigricans, PCOS, HTN, dyslipidemia)	10 y or at pubertal onset if puberty occurs at a younger age	q2y	Fasting plasma glucose

Adapted from American Diabetes Association: Type 2 diabetes in children. Diabetes Care 2000;23(3):381–389.
Note: Clinical judgment should be used to test for diabetes in high-risk patients who do not meet these criteria.
Abbreviations: BMI = body mass index; T2D = type 2 diabetes; HTN = hypertension; PCOS = polycystic ovarian syndrome.

TABLE 6 Medications to Treat Type 2 Diabetes

Class	Mechanism of Action	Adverse Effects
Biguanides (metformin)*	Decrease hepatic glucose production Increase peripheral glucose disposal	Gastrointestinal upset Lactic acidosis
Sulfonylureas (glimepiride, glyburide, glipizide)	Insulin secretagogues	Hypoglycemia Weight gain
Meglitinides (repaglinide, nateglinide)	Insulin secretagogues	Hypoglycemia Weight gain
α-Glucosidase inhibitors (acarbose)	Decrease gut carbohydrate absorption	Gastrointestinal upset
Thiazolidinediones (rosiglitazone† and pioglitazone)	Decrease hepatic glucose production Increase peripheral glucose disposal	Weight gain Edema Increased liver enzymes Anemia

*Metformin (Glucophage) is the only medication with FDA approval for use in children.
†FDA has required restrictions for use.

T2D present in ketoacidosis and require initial insulin therapy. The goal of management of the child with T2D is initial stabilization often with insulin therapy, metformin (Glucophage) directed at managing the insulin resistance, and education. Once glucose levels are stabilized, insulin dosage may be lowered along with continued treatment with metformin (Glucophage) and approaches to lifestyle management. Lifestyle management involves a healthy diet, increasing exercise, and decreasing sedentary behaviors.

Other medications used to treat T2D include second-generation sulfonylureas, meglitinides, thiazolidinediones, and α-glucosidase inhibitors, none of which is currently approved for use in pediatric patients. There is ongoing studies to assess the efficacy and safety of these medications (Table 6).

REFERENCES

American Diabetes Association. Diagnosis and classification of diabetes mellitus. Diabetes Care 2005;28(Suppl 1):S37–42.
American Diabetes Association. Type 2 diabetes in children. Diabetes Care 2000;23(3):381–9.
Barroso I. Genetics of type 2 diabetes. Diabet Med 2005;22:517–35.
Dunger DB, Sperling MA, Acerini CL, et al. ESPE/LWPES consensus statement on diabetic ketoacidosis in children and adolescents. Arch Dis Child 2004;89:188–94.
Fox LA, Buckloh LM, Smith SD, et al. A randomized controlled trial of insulin pump therapy in young children with type 1 diabetes. Diabetes Care 2005;28:1277–81.
Glaser N, Barnett P, McCaslin 1, et al. The Pediatric Emergency Medicine Collaborative Research Committee of the American Academy of Pediatrics. N Engl J Med 2001;344(4):264–9.
Goodwin G, Volkening LK, Laffel LM. Younger age at onset of type 1 diabetes in concordant sibling pairs is associated with increased risk for autoimmune thyroid disease. Diabetes Care 2006;29(6):1397–8.
Hannon TS, Rao G, Arslanian SA. Childhood obesity and type 2 diabetes mellitus. Pediatrics 2005;116(2):473–80.
Hirsch IB. Insulin analogues. N Engl J Med 2005;352:174–83.
Laffel LM, Vangsness L, Connell A, et al. Impact of ambulatory, family-focused teamwork intervention on glycemic control in youth with type 1 diabetes. J Pediatr 2003;142(4):409–16.
Rosenbloom AL. Cerebral edema in diabetic ketoacidosis and other acute devastating complications: Recent observations. Pediatr Diabetes 2005;6:41–9.
Silverstein J, Klingensmith G, Copeland K, et al. American Diabetes Association: Care of children and adolescents with type 1 diabetes. Diabetes Care 2005;28(1):186–212.
Wysocki T, Harris MA, Mauras N, et al. Absence of adverse effects of severe hypoglycemia on cognitive function in school-aged children with diabetes over 18 months. Diabetes Care 2003;26(4):1100–5.

Diabetic Ketoacidosis

Method of
David E. Trachtenbarg, MD

The diagnostic criteria for diabetic ketoacidosis (DKA) are a blood glucose greater than 250 mg/dL and an arterial pH less than 7.30. The most common precipitating causes are infection and lack of prescribed insulin. Treatment requires careful administration of fluids; electrolytes including potassium, bicarbonate, phosphorus, and sodium; and insulin. After the DKA has resolved care involves transition to a home regimen appropriate for each patient and a plan to prevent recurrence.

Epidemiology and Pathophysiology

There are more than 100,000 hospitalizations for diabetic ketoacidosis (DKA) every year and more than 2000 deaths. DKA is caused by decreased insulin levels and increased gluconeogenesis from counter-regulatory hormones. Inflammatory factors such as cytokines are also increased. Although it is more common in patients with type 1 diabetes, DKA also occurs in patients with type 2 diabetes.

Diagnosis and Differential Diagnosis

The diagnosis of diabetic ketoacidosis is usually straightforward. The American Diabetes Association's criteria are a blood glucose of greater than 250 mg/dL and an arterial pH less than 7.30 (Figure 1). Severity is linked to the arterial pH and symptoms (Table 1). Alcoholic ketosis, lactic acidosis, methanol ingestion, and starvation ketosis are other conditions in the differential diagnosis. DKA may be distinguished from the hyperglycemic hyperosmolar state (HHS) by a glucose greater than 600 mg/dL, pH greater than 7.30, and normal or only mildly elevated ketones.

Clinical Manifestations

Patients usually report polyuria, polydipsia, and polyphagia. Dry mucous membranes and other signs of dehydration are common. Other common symptoms include nausea, vomiting, and abdominal pain. If abdominal pain is present, it must be differentiated from an acute abdominal problem precipitating DKA. Other signs include a fruity breath odor, decreased skin turgor, Kussmaul breathing, confusion, and coma in severe cases.

CURRENT DIAGNOSIS

- The diagnosis of diabetic ketoacidosis (DKA) is generally straightforward, but each patient needs to be evaluated for precipitating causes.
- The severity of DKA is related to the degree of acidosis and symptoms, not the glucose level.
- Other causes of acidosis, including lactic acidosis, alcoholic ketosis, and methanol ingestion, generally do not cause the glucose elevation present with DKA.
- Patients in a hyperglycemic hyperosmolar state have a glucose greater than 600 mg/dL, pH greater than 7.30, and normal or only mildly elevated ketones.

PRECIPITATING FACTORS

The most common cause is infection, followed by not taking prescribed insulin. If required insulin is stopped, DKA can develop within 24 hours. Other causes include insulin pump failure and new-onset diabetes. Underlying diseases that can cause DKA include myocardial infarction, pancreatitis, acute abdomen, and hyperthyroidism. Medications can contribute to hyperglycemia, including steroids, β-agonists, and atypical antipsychotic drugs.

INITIAL LABORATORY EVALUATION

Glucose, electrolytes, phosphorus, blood urea nitrogen (BUN), and creatinine should be checked in all patients. An elevated anion gap is invariably present. Serum β-hydroxybutyrate testing is best for evaluating the degree of ketosis because it accounts for 75% of the ketones. If β-hydroxybutyrate testing is not available, serum ketone

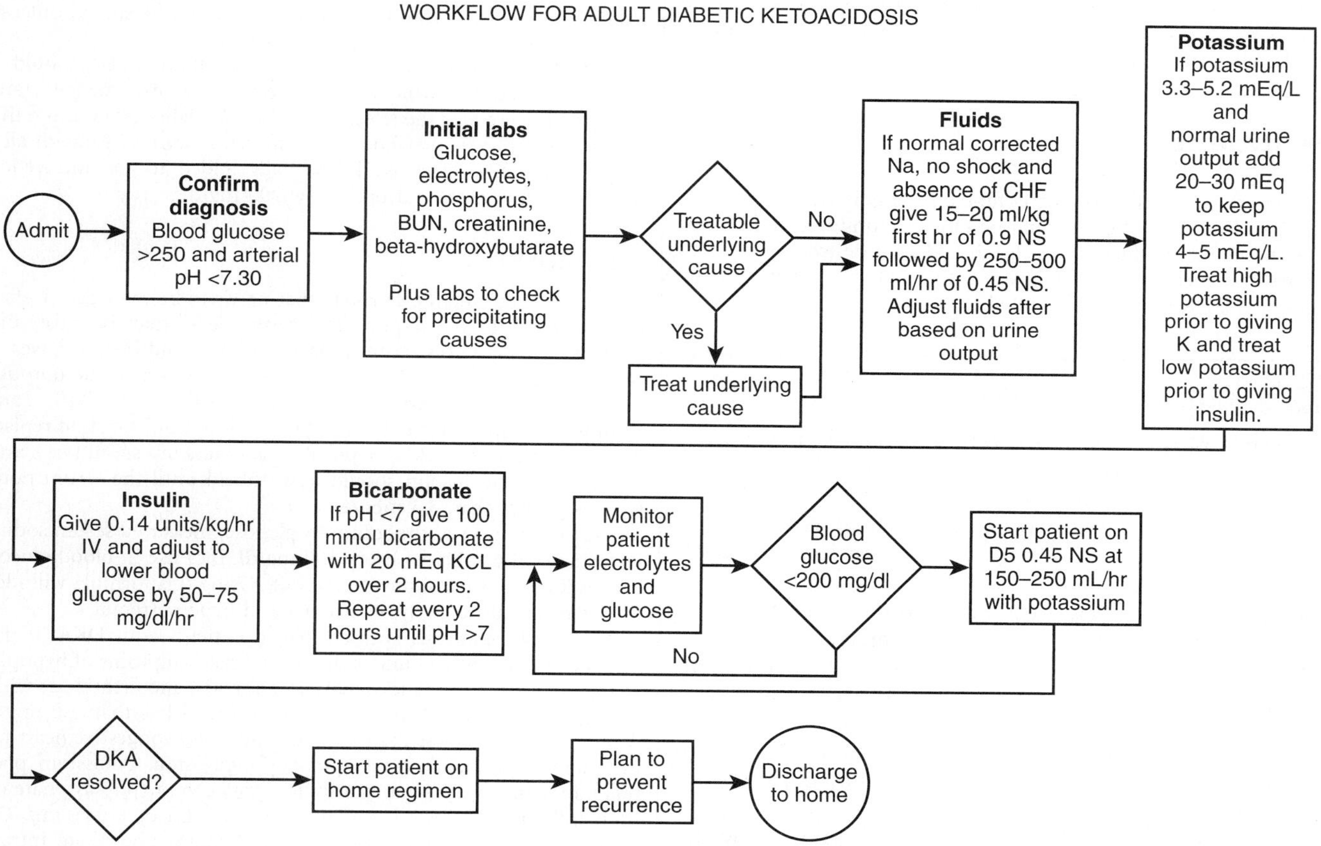

WORKFLOW FOR ADULT DIABETIC KETOACIDOSIS

FIGURE 1. Algorithm for diagnosing and treating adult diabetic ketoacidosis.

TABLE 1 Key Characteristics of Mild, Moderate, and Severe Diabetic Ketoacidosis

Severity	Glucose (mg/dL)	pH	Serum Bicarbonate (mEq/L)	Symptoms
Mild	>250	7.25-7.30	15-18	Alert
Moderate	>250	7.00-7.24	10-14.9	Alert to drowsy
Severe	>250	<7.00	<10	Stupor or coma

All patients have positive serum ketones or β-hydroxybutyrate
Adapted from Sabatini S, Kurtzman NA: Bicarbonate therapy in severe metabolic acidosis. J Am Soc Nephrol 2009;20(4)692-695.

testing may be substituted. An arterial blood gas (ABG) is useful to document the degree of acidosis. To screen for underlying causes consider a complete blood count (CBC), complete urinalysis, blood cultures, and chest x-ray. Leukocytosis of 10,000 to 15,000 is typically present. Fever, significant left shifts, and a white count greater than 25,000 indicate infection. A serum osmolality greater than 320 mOsm/kg is associated with mental status changes. A serum magnesium test may be helpful for patients on diuretics or who have signs of low magnesium.

Tests may be helpful for selected patients to rule out a precipitating cause, including troponin to rule out myocardial infarction. Because amylase is commonly elevated in DKA, it cannot be used to diagnose pancreatitis. Serum lipase can also be elevated in DKA, and it is more specific for pancreatitis than amylase. If pancreatitis is suspected, an imaging study of the pancreas may be helpful.

For patients with new-onset diabetes, measurement of C-peptide and islet cell antibodies are often helpful. Low C-peptide levels indicate type 1 diabetes and the need for insulin. A normal C-peptide with islet cell antibodies indicates that overt type 1 diabetes is likely to develop eventually. Patients with a normal C-peptide and absence of islet cell antibodies are most likely to respond to oral hypoglycemic therapy.

Measurement of hemoglobin A_{1C} helps to determine the degree of control of diabetes before the event and often affects follow-up care after the DKA has resolved.

Treatment

Initial treatment consists of giving fluids, managing electrolytes, and giving insulin. The patient should be closely monitored until he or she is stable. Blood glucose initially should be monitored every 1 to 2 hours and metabolic panels every 2 to 6 hours. Any underlying causes of the DKA should be treated.

CURRENT THERAPY

- The average fluid deficit for adults is 6 L. Fluid rehydration corrects dehydration and lowers glucose levels.
- Potassium is usually elevated from acidosis. Potassium replacement is normally started as soon as the potassium is in the normal range and appropriate urine output is ensured.
- Other electrolytes, including sodium, chloride, and phosphorus, also need to be monitored.
- Insulin is usually given intravenously, but equivalent results may be obtained with administration of short-acting insulin subcutaneously every 2 hours.
- After the DKA has resolved, the patient should have a regimen started that provides a smooth transition to home care.
- Every patient should be evaluated for opportunities to prevent recurrent DKA.

FLUIDS

The fluid deficit for the patient with DKA averages 100 mL/kg with 4% to 8% dehydration. The typical adult has a fluid deficit of 6 L. Most adult patients should be given isotonic saline (0.9%, normal saline) at 15 to 20 mL/kg for the first hour. This is usually followed by half-normal saline (0.45%) if the corrected sodium is high or by normal saline if the corrected sodium is low at a rate of 250 to 500 mL/hour. Patients with shock are typically given isotonic saline at 1 L/hour until they are out of shock before starting a standard regimen. Patients with congestive heart failure, kidney failure, and other critical diseases require modification of the standard fluid regimen. For adults, fluid replacement should correct the deficit within 24 hours. Patients using the new insulin analogues may be less dehydrated than those using regular insulin because the new insulin analogues have a shorter duration of action and DKA can develop more rapidly. Studies have found that rehydration may account for up to 80% of the decline in glucose during the first 4 hours of rehydration.

For children, initial volume expansion should be with isotonic solutions. A recent weight is very helpful in estimating degree of hydration because clinical evaluation can overestimate the degree of dehydration. To reduce the chance of cerebral edema in pediatric patients, subsequent volume replacement should be spread out over at least 48 hours using at least 0.45% saline.

For adults and children, adjustment of fluid intake should be modified based on urine output, electrolytes, and mental status. One goal is to reduce the effective serum osmolality by no more than 3 mOsm/hour. Patients who are able to drink can take some or all of their fluid orally. Dextrose is normally added to the intravenous fluids when the glucose drops below 200 mg/dL.

ELECTROLYTES

Potassium is the main electrolyte that needs to be managed. Deficits are usually 3 to 5 mEq/kg. The serum level may be misleading because acidosis raises serum potassium levels and insulin lowers it. Intravenous potassium should be started as soon as urine output is documented and the serum potassium is less than 5.2 mEq/L. Potassium is commonly given at 20 to 30 mEq/L of fluid for fluid replacement. Owing to the risk of hypokalemia, potassium should be started immediately and insulin should be withheld until the serum potassium is greater than 3.3 mEq/L.

Due to dilution of the serum by glucose, measured serum sodium is decreased 1.6 mEq for every 100 mg/dL increase in blood glucose. This is known as pseudohyponatremia. Using this formula will identify patients with true hyponatremia and hypernatremia.

Serum phosphorous is often low in patients with DKA. It does not need to be replaced unless the patient has symptoms of hypophosphatemia such as weakness, malaise, anorexia, and arthralgias with a blood level less than 2 mg/dL or a serum level less than 1.0 mg/dL. A phosphorus level less than 1 mg/dL can cause congestive heart failure, hemolytic anemia, or respiratory depression. Potassium phosphate may be given intravenously to correct the hypophosphatemia. Each millimole of phosphate contains 1.5 mEq of potassium. One regimen is to give 0.08 mmol/kg of potassium phosphate intravenously over 6 hours for phosphate levels between 1 and 2 mg/dL and 0.16 to 0.24 mmol/kg of potassium phosphate over 4 to 6 hours for a serum phosphorus level less than 1 mg/dL. The initial dose may be increased by 25% to 50% if the patient is symptomatic and lowered by 25% to 50% if the patient is hypercalcemic. Calcium should be monitored with the phosphorus.

Bicarbonate is only advised for severe acidosis. Give bicarbonate if the pH is below 7.0. One protocol is to give two ampoules of bicarbonate (100 mmoL sodium bicarbonate) in 400 mL sterile water with 20 mEq KCl at a rate of 200 mL/hour and repeat every 2 hours until the venous pH is greater than 7.0.

INSULIN

Although intravenous insulin is the most widely used insulin treatment for DKA, there is no evidence this route produces better outcomes than subcutaneous or intramuscular insulin. When giving intravenous insulin, there is no difference in outcome between regular insulin and the new insulin analogues. When using an insulin drip, start at 0.1 U/kg/hour if an initial intravenous bolus of 0.1 U/kg has been given and 0.14 U/kg/hour if no bolus was given. If the insulin does not decrease the glucose by 50 to 75 mg/dL/hour, the insulin dose should be increased. Recent studies have found that giving short-acting insulin every 2 hours subcutaneously is equal in outcome with an insulin drip. If short-acting insulin is given subcutaneously, the total dose is the same as the dose for an intravenous drip. A simple conversion is to administer the amount of insulin delivered during two hours of insulin drip every 2 hours subcutaneously.

Long-acting insulins and insulin pumps are generally stopped during treatment of DKA. Most patients are not given meals during initial DKA treatment. Once the blood glucose is controlled, short-acting insulin can be given subcutaneously with a meal based on the meal's carbohydrate content. If the carbohydrate ratio for a patient is not known, 1 unit of insulin for every 15 grams of carbohydrate is usually used as a starting point.

Complications

Common complications include hypoglycemia, hypokalemia, and recurrent hyperglycemia. If hyperchloremia develops, it usually resolves on its own.

The most feared complication is cerebral edema. This is most common in children. Although not proved, limiting fluids and gradual glucose lowering might help prevent it. However, cerebral edema can develop even before therapy is started. Signs and symptoms include headache, lethargy, and confusion. Fever, papilledema, hypertension, and diabetes insipidus can also occur. Magnetic resonance imaging (MRI) or computed tomography (CT) study can help confirm the diagnosis. If cerebral edema symptoms develop, fluids should be reduced and mannitol 0.25 to 1.0 g/kg should be given intravenously over 20 minutes. If there is no response, mannitol should be repeated in 2 hours. Limited experience suggests that if mannitol is not available, 3% hypertonic saline (5-10 mL/kg over 30 min) may be used. Once severe symptoms develop there is a 70% mortality rate, and only 10% of patients recover without sequelae.

Transition

Criteria for resolution of DKA are glucose less than 200 mg/dL, bicarbonate 15 mEq/L or greater, and an anion gap of 12 mEq/L or less. Even if the patient has type 2 diabetes that might eventually be controlled with oral medications, insulin is commonly used for initial treatment after the DKA has resolved.

Customizing the insulin regimen to match the patient's anticipated home regimen speeds recovery and hospital discharge. With a patient who can comply, regimens with long-acting insulin and multiple shots of short-acting insulin (basal-bolus regimen) are less likely to produce hypoglycemia. However, many patients are unable to

follow or afford a basal-bolus regimen. If the patient has a documented insulin regimen that has provided good control previously, it can be restarted.

If no information is available on prior insulin regimens, one standard for total daily insulin dose is 0.4 U/kg/day for thin patients with new-onset DKA, 0.6 U/kg/day for obese patients with new-onset DKA, and 0.8 units/kg/day for obese patients with a history of type 2 diabetes. If a basal-bolus regimen is used, typically half of the dose is given as long-acting insulin such as glargine (Lantus) or detemir (Levemir) and half is given in three divided doses for meals as short-acting insulin. Another method of calculating the basal insulin dose is to take 80% of the total daily insulin dose needed to keep the blood glucose under control with an intravenous insulin drip. For example, if 1.5 units of insulin per hour keeps the glucose in a stable target range, the basal insulin dose would be $24 \times 1.5 \times 0.8 = 28.8$ units of long-acting insulin a day. To get the best basal insulin estimate, the drip rate should be stable for at least 6 hours. When long-acting insulin is started subcutaneously, the insulin drip should be continued for 2 hours until the serum level of the injected insulin is stabilized. If twice-daily neutral protamine Hagedorn (NPH) and regular insulin regimen in used, such as 70/30, typically two thirds of the insulin is given in the morning and one third is given in the evening.

Most patients also need a correction scale. Ideally this should be based on the patient's insulin sensitivity. Clinically, insulin sensitivity means how many milligrams of glucose per deciliter of blood each unit of insulin lowers the patient's blood glucose toward the patient's target glucose (e.g., 1 unit of insulin for each 25 mg/dL the blood glucose is above 120 mg/dL). If the patient's sensitivity to insulin is not known, an initial scale may be constructed using the 1500 rule to calculate insulin sensitivity (Tables 2 and 3).

TABLE 2 Calculating a Correction Scale Using the 1500 Rule

Step	Example*
1. Calculate the daily insulin dose.	40 units of basal glargine per day plus 35 total units for meals equals 75 units per day.
2. Estimate the patient's sensitivity to insulin by dividing 1500 by the total daily insulin dose.	1500/75 = 20
3. The sensitivity estimates how much 1 unit of insulin will lower the blood glucose.	Each unit of insulin lowers glucose by 20 mg/dL.
4. Pick an appropriate target for the patient to correct to.	140 mg/dL
5. Develop a scale giving 1 unit of insulin for each unit of sensitivity (see Table 3).	Give 1 unit for every 20 mg/dL the glucose is higher than 140 mg/dlL.
6. Caution: This formula usually underestimates the final insulin dosage needed for type 2 diabetes, and it can overestimate the amount needed for some patients with type 1 diabetes.	Review the patient's history to verify the scale is reasonable.
7. The patient can test the scale when stable by giving a correction, not eating, and testing 4 hours later.	If the patient's starting blood glucose is 240 and the glucose drops to 100 with 5 units, the sensitivity should be changed to 28: 240 − 100 = 140 140/5 = 28

*This is an example. Every patient's calculations and targets are different.

TABLE 3 Sample Hyperglycemia Correction Scale

Blood Glucose (mg/dL)	Units of Insulin to Correct Hyperglycemia
<140	0
140-159	1
160-179	2
180-199	3
200-219	4
220-239	5
240-259	6
260-279	7
280-299	8
300-319	9
320-339	10
340 or higher	Give 11 units and call

Prevention of Recurrence

Blood glucose monitoring, diabetes education, sick day management education, financial support, and providing open access to care will help prevent recurrences of DKA. In addition to monitoring blood glucose, home monitoring of ketone bodies in the urine or the blood can aid in early detection and treatment of DKA. Careful attention to treatment, transition to home, and prevention of recurrence produce the best outcome.

REFERENCES

Centers for Disease Control and Prevention. Diabetes data and trends: Diabetes complications, http://www.cdc.gov/diabetes/statistics/complications_national.htm; [accessed 21.07.10].

Cooke DW, Plotnick L. Management of diabetic ketoacidosis in children and adolescents. Pediatri Rev 2008;29(12):431–5.

Dhatariya K. People with type 1 diabetes using short acting analogue insulins are less dehydrated than those with using human soluble insulin prior to onset of diabetic ketoacidosis. Med Hypotheses 2008;71(5):706–8.

Fagan MJ, Avner J, Khine H. Initial fluid resuscitation for patients with diabetic ketoacidosis: How dry are they? Clin Pediatr (Phila) 2008;47(9):851–5.

Karabachos AE, Miles JM, Umpierrez GE, Fisher JN. Hyperglycemic crises in adult patients with diabetes. Diabetes Care 2000;32(7):1335–43.

Kitabchi AE, Murphy MG, Spencer J, et al. Is a priming dose of insulin necessary in low-dose insulin protocol for the treatment of diabetic ketoacidosis? Diabetes Care 2008;31(11):2081–205.

Mazer M, Chen E. Is subcutaneous administration of rapid-acting insulin as effective as intravenous insulin for treating diabetic ketoacidosis? Ann Emerg Med 2009;53(2):259–63.

Morales AE, Daniels KA. Cerebral edema before onset of therapy in newly diagnosed type 2 diabetes. Pediatr Diabetes 2009;10(2):155–7.

Potassium phosphate: Drug information. Available at http://www.uptodate.com/online/content/topic.do?topicKey=drug_l_z/207137&source=see_link (subscription only).

Sabatini S, Kurtzman NA. Bicarbonate therapy in severe metabolic acidosis. J Am Soc Nephrol 2009;20(4):692–5.

Samuelsson U, Ludvigsson J. When should determination of ketonemia be recommended? Diabetes Technol Ther 2002;4(5):645–50.

Schade DS, Eaton RP. Diabetic ketoacidosis—pathogenesis, prevention and therapy. Clin Endocrinol Metab 1983;12(2):321–38.

Trachtenbarg DE. Diabetic ketoacidosis. Am Fam Physician 2005;71(9):1705–14.

Umpierrez GE, Jones S, Smiley D, et al. Insulin analogs versus human insulin in the treatment of patients with diabetic ketoacidosis.: A randomized controlled trial. Diabetes Care 2009;32(7):1164–9.

Weber C, Kocher S, Neeser K, Joshi SR. Prevention of diabetic ketoacidosis and self- monitoring of ketone bodies: An overview. Cur Med Res Opin 2009;25(5):1197–207.

Hyponatremia

Method of
Beejal Shah, MD, and
Susan L. Samson, MD, PhD

Homeostasis maintains the concentration of sodium in the serum between 138 and 142 mEq/L (normal, 135–145 mEq/L) despite variations in water intake. Hyponatremia is defined as a serum sodium concentration of less than 135 mEq/L. It is one of the most common electrolyte abnormalities found in the inpatient setting, occurring in up to 2.5% of patients, and it is a significant marker for mortality, associated with a 60-fold higher risk of death. It is not clear whether hyponatremia itself is the cause of a more adverse prognosis or whether it echoes the degree of stress caused by illness. In the outpatient setting, chronic hyponatremia is most prevalent among the elderly and nursing home residents. The approach to management of hyponatremia is highly dependent on the underlying process. Establishing the correct etiology is critical, because inappropriate treatment can worsen hyponatremia. Therapy must be administered judiciously because of the risk of severe neurologic sequelae, including central nervous system demyelination. However, with a systematic approach to the differential diagnosis of hyponatremia, the correct diagnosis can be made and therapy initiated.

Clinical Presentation

Acute hyponatremia is defined as hyponatremia of less than 48 hours in duration. Mild symptoms include headache, nausea, vomiting, confusion, and weakness, which usually occur with a sodium level of less than 129 mEq/L. More severe neurologic manifestations—seizure and coma—are seen usually below a threshold of 120 mEq/L, although there currently is no evidence-based critical sodium level above which neurologic sequelae do not occur. The neurologic manifestations of acute or recurrent symptomatic hyponatremia can be delayed, so continued monitoring is important.

In contrast, patients with chronic hyponatremia more often are asymptomatic or have blunted symptoms. In elderly patients with mild chronic hyponatremia, subtle neurocognitive manifestations can occur, with decreased balance, lowered reaction speed, memory loss, and directed gait. Mild hypoosmolar hyponatremia is not independently associated with increased morbidity and mortality. Even so, the underlying etiology needs to be determined because of the potential for other factors (e.g., new medications, dehydration, occult illness) to contribute to the development of more severe hyponatremia with its potential for neurologic injury.

Regulation of Water Balance

Approximately two thirds of total body water is contained in the intracellular fluid (ICF) and one third as extracellular fluid (ECF). Plasma osmolality is tightly regulated between 280 and 290 mOsm/kg and reflects the osmolality of the ECF. A change in plasma osmolality results in a shift of total body water between the ECF and the ICF to maintain their osmolar equivalence. Because sodium is the major osmole in the ECF, hyponatremia most often is a manifestation of decreased osmolality, so-called hypoosmolar or hypotonic hyponatremia.

RENAL HANDLING OF WATER

The major osmoregulatory hormone is arginine vasopressin, also called antidiuretic hormone, which is synthesized in the paraventricular and supraoptic nuclei of the hypothalamus. It is transported along axons to the posterior pituitary, where it is processed and stored in vesicles. Vasopressin secretion is regulated by osmotic and nonosmotic stimuli. Secretion occurs with a 1% to 2% rise in osmolality (>288 mOsm/kg), as detected by receptors in the antero-lateral walls of the hypothalamus adjacent to the third ventricle. Vasopressin secretion is inhibited when the plasma osmolality is lower than 280 mOsm/kg. The major nonosmotic stimulus is a decrease in effective circulating volume, which is detected by baroreceptors in the aortic arch and carotid sinuses. Although this mechanism requires a large drop (10%-15%) in blood pressure, the secretory response is more robust than for increases in osmolality. As such, acutely lowered blood pressure can override the inhibitory signal of low osmolality because of the need to maintain perfusion. Other physiologic nonosmotic stimuli include catecholamines and angiotensin II, but there is a long list of hormones and pharmacologic agents that induce or repress vasopressin secretion (Table 1).

The renal site of action of vasopressin is the V_2 receptors on the basolateral membrane of collecting duct cells in the distal nephron. The hormone-receptor interaction initiates intracellular signaling via cyclic adenosine monophosphate–dependent pathways, resulting in translocation of cytoplasmic aquaporon-2 channels to the surface of the collecting duct luminal membrane. These channels allow movement of water back into the cell for later reabsorption into the circulation. This results in a net concentration of urine and decreased plasma osmolality.

RENAL HANDLING OF SODIUM

In addition to renal water handling, sodium reabsorption and excretion are important for maintenance of water homeostasis. The renin-angiotensin-aldosterone system is activated by reduced arterial perfusion pressure sensed by the juxtaglomerular apparatus of the afferent renal arteriole. Reduced arteriole effective volume (low or perceived) is sensed by the juxtaglomerular apparatus, which secretes renin, activating the renin-angiotensin system. This cascade of events ultimately stimulates aldosterone secretion, which acts at the distal nephron to cause reabsorption of filtered sodium via Na^+, K^+-adenosine triphosphatase (ATPase)–dependent sodium channels.

Central Nervous System Response to Hyponatremia/ Hypoosmolality

Osmolar equivalence between the ECF and ICF is closely maintained by shifts in water between the two compartments. The major symptoms and signs of hyponatremia are neurologic in nature and are a clinical manifestation of swelling of the cells in the central nervous system, which results in cerebral edema. The most devastating consequence is herniation due to anatomic limitations on brain volume within the confines of the skull. Premenopausal women are at the highest risk for brain injury from hyponatremia.

A major compensatory mechanism in the central nervous system is the extrusion from the cells of intracellular solutes, which prevents further water influx. In the first few hours, inorganic ions (potassium, sodium, chloride) move out of the cell. After a few days of persistent hypoosmolality, the cells further compensate by extruding organic osmoles (glutamate, taurine, inositol). The clinician must be aware of this protective adaptation, because it necessitates a slower time course of correction during treatment. A rapid rise in plasma osmolality from aggressive treatment causes water to rapidly shift out of the cells, resulting in demyelination of neurons. In the past, this was termed pontine demyelinosis, but it has also been reported for extrapontine neurons and is now referred to as osmotic demyelination. The sequelae are permanent and devastating. There is clinical progression from lethargy to a change in affect, to mutism and dysarthria, and finally to spastic quadriparesis and pseudobulbar palsy.

Classification and Differential Diagnosis of Hyponatremia

Initial evaluation of hyponatremia requires a systematic and sequential approach. First, a thorough history and physical examination are required. It is important to identify any history of brain injury, stroke, mental illness, or chronic illness and the patient's current medication usage. On examination, special attention should be paid to mental status and neurologic abnormalities; manifestations of cardiac, hepatic, or renal disease; and signs of adrenal insufficiency or hypothyroidism. From the assessment of volume status, the hyponatremia should be classified as hypervolemic, euvolemic, or hypovolemic; each of these conditions leads in a different direction for diagnosis and treatment of the underlying cause (Figs. 1 and 2). Finally, it should be determined whether the hyponatremia is acute (<48 hours) or chronic, because this can determine the time course of treatment.

CURRENT DIAGNOSIS

- Perform a thorough history and physical examination with focus on the accurate assessment of volume status, neurologic symptoms and signs, current medications, and concurrent illnesses.
- Classify the hyponatremia as hypovolemic, euvolemic, or hypervolemic.
- Determine whether the hyponatremia is acute or chronic, based on the history and the clinical manifestations.
- Order the key laboratory tests, including a basic metabolic panel (serum sodium, glucose, blood urea nitrogen, and creatinine), plasma osmolality, urine osmolality, and urine sodium.

TABLE 1 Molecules That Regulate Vasopressin Secretion

Stimulate Vasopressin Release	Inhibit Vasopressin Release
Hormones and Neurotransmitters	
Acetylcholine (nicotinic)	Atrial natriuretic peptide
Histamine (H_1)	γ-Aminobutyric acid
Dopamine (D_1 and D_2)	Opioids (κ receptors)
Glutamine	
Aspartate	
Cholecystokinin	
Neuropeptide Y	
Substance P	
Vasoactive inhibitory peptide	
Prostaglandin	
Angiotensin II	
Pharmacologic Agents	
Vincristine (Oncovin)	Ethanol
Cyclophosphamide (Cytoxan)	Phenytoin (Dilantin)
Tricyclic antidepressants	Low-dose morphine
Selective serotonin reuptake inhibitors	Glucocorticoids
	Fluphenazine (Prolixin)
Nicotine	Haloperidol (Haldol)
Adrenaline (epinephrine)	Promethazine (Phenergan)
High-dose morphine	Butorphanol (Stadol)

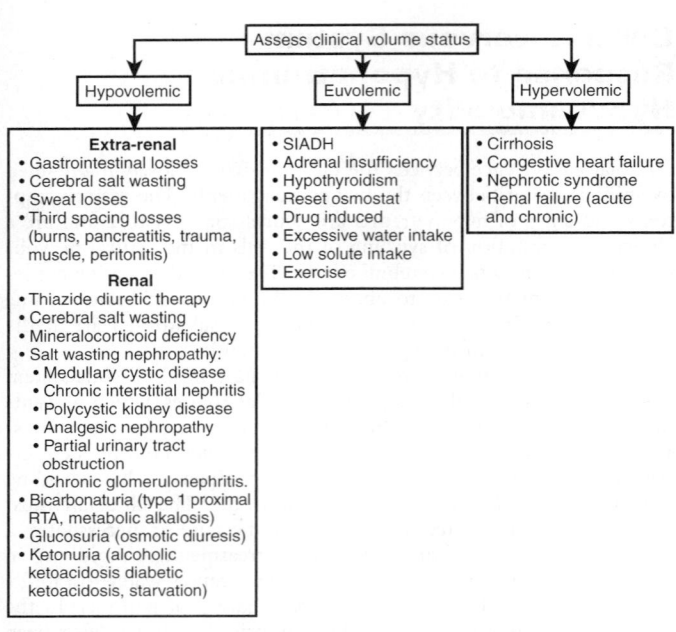

FIGURE 1. The differential diagnosis of hypoosmolar hyponatremia. *Abbreviations:* RTA, renal tubular acidosis; SIADH, syndrome of inappropriate antidiuretic hormone.

For the laboratory work-up, essential basic tests are the serum sodium and potassium levels, renal function tests with blood urea nitrogen (BUN) and creatinine, and liver function tests. It is likely that these tests have already been performed, motivating the assessment of hyponatremia. After this, the plasma osmolality (P_{Osm}), urine osmolality (U_{Osm}), and urine sodium concentration are key diagnostic tests. P_{Osm} is directly measured in the laboratory and also can be calculated. Calculated osmolality is the sum of the concentrations of the known major osmoles—sodium and glucose—in the ECF and the BUN:

$$P_{Osm} = (2 \times Na) + (glucose) + (BUN)$$

The calculation is done in SI units. For sodium, mEq/L is the same as the SI unit, mmol/L; if glucose and BUN values were reported in mg/dL, they must be divided by 18 and 2.8, respectively, to convert to SI units (mmol/L). The directly measured osmolality should be within 10 to 12 mOsm/kg of the calculated value; an increased osmolar gap compared with the calculated value points toward the presence of additional osmoles in the plasma that are causing hypertonicity.

Because hyponatremia usually is a reflection of plasma osmolality, most patients also have a low P_{Osm}, and the clinician often can proceed to the differential diagnosis of hypoosmolar (or hypotonic) hyponatremia after excluding pseudohyponatremia (which usually has normal osmolality) and hyperosmolar hyponatremia. Pseudohyponatremia can occur if the plasma lipid or protein content is greatly increased in the plasma (usually to >6%–8% of volume), as in extreme hypertriglyceridemia and paraprotein disorders. These extra components decrease the aqueous portion of the plasma volume and thereby interfere with the laboratory measurement of sodium by dilutional, indirect methods such as flame photometry. Most laboratories now use direct measurement of sodium to avoid this problem.

Hyperosmolar hyponatremia can occur if there are additional osmoles present that cause water movement from the ICF into the ECF, resulting in ECF expansion and dilutional hyponatremia. Overall, the total body water and total body sodium are unchanged in this situation. An important clinical example occurs with hyperglycemia, and the reported sodium value should be corrected for high glucose by the clinician, by adding 1.6 mEq/L to the measured Na for every 100 mg/dL rise in glucose above 200 mg/dL. Because glucose is included in the calculation of osmolality, there will be no significant osmolar gap.

Other osmotically active solutes encountered clinically are mannitol, which is used to manage increased intracranial pressure, and glycine, which is used for irrigation in urologic procedures. Mannitol and glycine are retained in the ECF and are not part of the calculated osmolality, so their presence results in an osmolar gap. High levels of alcohol or ethylene glycol also increase the osmolality, but these substances are so quickly metabolized that an osmolar gap may not be apparent by the time testing is performed.

Once pseudohyponatremia and hypertonicity have been ruled out, the diagnosis is narrowed to hypoosmolar hyponatremia. The combined physical examination and laboratory results allow classification of the patient as having hypervolemic hyponatremia with excess total body sodium, hypovolemic hyponatremia with a deficit of total body sodium, or euvolemic hyponatremia with near-normal total body sodium.

HYPOVOLEMIC HYPONATREMIA

The causes of hypovolemic hyponatremia can be classified as extrarenal or renal (see Fig. 1). Signs of volume contraction are apparent on examination, including poor skin turgor, skin tenting (forehead), decreased or undetectable jugular venous pressure, dry mucous membranes, and orthostatic changes in blood pressure and pulse rate. If the volume status is not completely clear from the examination, laboratory values can be helpful (see Fig. 2), but they need to be interpreted in the context of renal function tests. If the urine osmolality is less than maximally concentrated (<500 mOsm/kg), an infusion of 0.5 to 1 L of isotonic saline over 24 to 48 hours may

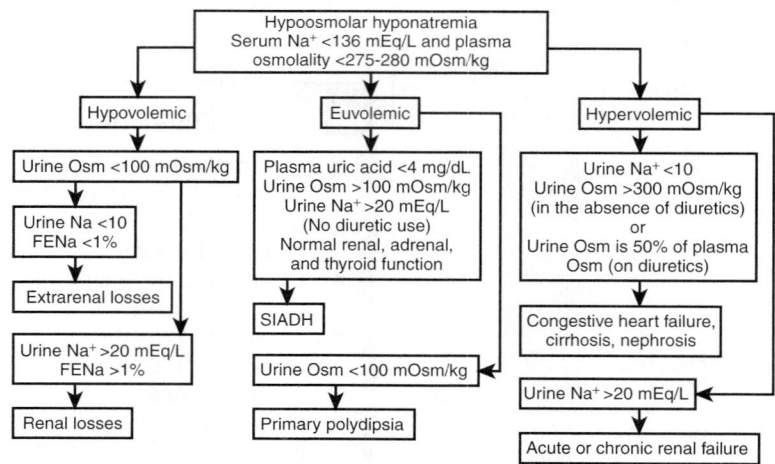

FIGURE 2. Laboratory findings in hypoosmolar hyponatremia. *Abbreviations:* FENa, fractional excretion of sodium; Osm, osmoles; SIADH, syndrome of inappropriate antidiuretic hormone.

help with differentiation. With hypovolemia, the sodium will begin to correct and the patient should improve clinically. Conversely, if the patient is actually euvolemic, such as with syndrome of inappropriate antidiuretic hormone (SIADH), discussed later, the serum sodium level will remain constant or decrease due to retention of free water with a concomitant increase in urinary sodium.

Extrarenal causes of hyponatremia include gastrointestinal losses and third-space losses such as in severe burns and pancreatitis. In the volume-depleted state, with intact renal function, the urine sodium is low (<10 mEq/L) reflecting a normal response by the kidney to maximally reabsorb sodium in response to volume depletion.

The renal causes of hypovolemic hyponatremia involve the inappropriate loss of sodium into the urine, and this is reflected by a urine sodium concentration of greater than 20 mEq/L.

Thiazide diuretics cause renal sodium loss, so the urine sodium is high. However, they also impair the kidney's diluting capacity, decreasing free water excretion and concentrating the urine. Only certain patients may be susceptible to hyponatremia while on thiazides. These patients may have an abnormally sensitive thirst response to the mild hypovolemia induced by the diuretics, causing increased water intake. Elderly women are the most susceptible, and hyponatremia can occur within days after initiation of thiazide therapy. Additional laboratory results reveal hypokalemia and a metabolic alkalosis. It is appropriate to stop the diuretic and restore potassium levels and volume status. Patients often have a recurrence of hyponatremia if rechallenged with thiazides. Loop diuretics, such as furosemide, are a less frequent cause of hyponatremia, which occurs only after long-term therapy.

In the absence of diuretic use, a urine sodium concentration greater than 20 mEq/L with hypovolemia is evidence for underlying renal pathology. Patients with salt-wasting nephropathy, from a number of causes (see Fig. 1), usually have significant renal failure, with a creatinine value in the range of 3 to 4 mg/dL. Because of the large net sodium loss, this condition is treated with salt tablets. Renal tubular acidosis causes bicarbonaturia, which requires a compensatory excretion of urinary cations, mainly Na^+ and K^+, to maintain electroneutrality. Similarly, excretion of ketones into the urine also demands additional electrolyte losses in spite of ECF volume depletion, leading to a loss of sodium.

Cerebral salt wasting (CSW), although it could be considered an extrarenal cause, also involves the renal loss of sodium (>20 mEq/L). The biochemical presentation is very similar to that of SIADH, but the diagnosis of CSW is restricted to cases involving extreme central nervous system pathology. CSW is most commonly associated with subarachnoid hemorrhage but also has been reported with stroke, brain trauma, infection, metastases and after neurosurgery. Onset of CSW is usually within first 10 days after the neurologic event.

CSW may be a protective mechanism against increased intracranial pressure. The proposed pathophysiologic mechanism of CSW is controversial, but one hypothesis is that the initiating event is a primary natriuresis, with renal loss of sodium, caused by the secretion of natriuretic peptides. Clinical studies have found both increased brain natriuretic peptide and increased atrial natriuretic peptide in neurosurgical patients with hyponatremia. Both hormones are vasodilators that increase the glomerular filtration rate while suppressing the renin-angiotensin system. This increases renal sodium losses as well as water excretion, resulting in volume depletion. Vasopressin levels rise in response to low volume, so that it becomes biochemically difficult differentiate CSW from SIADH, with a urine sodium level greater than 20 mEq/L, low uric acid, and high urine osmolality. It is helpful if CSW patients have signs of volume depletion in combination with the laboratory results. Also, the hyponatremia of CSW responds to normal saline, whereas SIADH worsens with normal saline. CSW is relatively rare in most case series, and it is important to rule out other causes for natriuresis.

HYPERVOLEMIC HYPONATREMIA

There are a variety of causes of hypervolemic hyponatremia (see Fig. 1), all of which are a result of decreased effective circulating volume. To correct this imbalance, the ECF expands, leading to fluid retention and hyponatremia. In spite of the increased total body water

and low serum sodium on testing, all of these patients have some degree of total body sodium excess. In many cases, volume overload is clinically evident from the presence of subcutaneous edema, ascites, elevated jugular venous pressure, or pulmonary edema.

In congestive heart failure (CHF), patients can develop hyponatremia with only 2 to 3 L of fluid intake per day despite normal renal function. The decreased filling pressures and cardiac output of CHF are perceived as volume depletion, detected by the baroreceptors. This stimulates vasopressin secretion, overriding the signal of low osmolality detected by the hypothalamic osmoreceptors. This lack of inhibition of vasopressin secretion is believed to be the most important contributing factor to the development of hyponatremia. In addition, decreased right atrial pressures result in inhibition of secretion of atrial natriuretic peptide, contributing to the water and sodium gain. With the low perfusion pressure, there is a decrease in the glomerular filtration rate, which is sensed by the juxtaglomerular apparatus, causing neurohumoral activation of the renin-angiotensin system and sympathetic nervous system. This leads to increased circulating levels of catecholamines, angiotensin II, and aldosterone, further stimulating tubular sodium and water reabsorption. In the absence of diuretics, the urine sodium level is very low (<10 mEq/L) in patients with CHF because of activation of the renin-angiotensin-aldosterone system and maximal tubular reabsorption of sodium. Also, there is less than maximally dilute urine (usually >300 mOsm/kg) in the absence of diuretic therapy. An elevated brain natriuretic peptide concentration helps to confirm the hypervolemia.

A similar mechanism is at work in cirrhotic patients, in whom the incidence of hyponatremia is even higher and is a strong predictor of poor outcome. In cirrhosis, low albumin results in third-spacing and decreased effective circulating volume. In addition, portal hypertension leads to splanchnic vasodilation, which also decreases the effective circulating volume. This serves to activate vasopressin secretion and the renin-angiotensin-aldosterone system.

Hyponatremia is less common in acute and chronic renal failure, but it can occur with a significant decrease in glomerular filtration rate accompanied by severe hypoalbuminemia. Interpretation of the laboratory results may be confounded by a high urine sodium concentration (>20 mEq/L) that reflects the concomitant presence of tubular dysfunction. Hyponatremia can develop in stage IV or V renal failure when fluid intake is in excess of 3 L/day.

EUVOLEMIC HYPONATREMIA

Euvolemic hyponatremia is caused by impaired excretion of free water by the kidney. The differential diagnosis is more limited (see Fig. 1) and the majority of cases are due to SIADH (Table 2). However, this often is a diagnosis of exclusion, and hypothyroidism and adrenal insufficiency must be ruled out clinically or biochemically in patients with euvolemic hyponatremia.

Hypothyroidism leads to reduced glomerular filtration rate and decreased flow to the distal nephron, causing maximal reabsorption of water to maintain arterial volume. Hypothyroidism has to be severe to cause hyponatremia and usually is obvious on examination. However, in the elderly population, apathetic hypothyroidism may be difficult to diagnose. Hypothyroidism can be confirmed by the presence of a high level of thyroid-stimulating hormone and a low level of free T_4 (thyroxine). Treatment involves thyroid hormone replacement and supportive care.

In primary adrenal insufficiency (Addison's disease), the concomitant aldosterone deficiency results in hyponatremia combined with hyperkalemia, prerenal azotemia, a urine sodium concentration greater than 20 mEq/L, and a urine potassium level lower than 20 mEq/L. In secondary or central adrenal insufficiency, the adrenal zona glomerulosa remains intact for the secretion of aldosterone. However, glucocorticoid deficiency still causes impaired water excretion, which can lead to dilutional hyponatremia. Vasopressin release may be stimulated by the nausea, vomiting, and orthostatic hypotension that occurs with adrenal insufficiency. Finally, corticosteroids normally inhibit vasopressin release, so their deficiency leads to enhanced vasopressin release, causing retention of free water that further contributes to the hyponatremia. The appropriate diagnostic test

TABLE 2 Causes of SIADH

CNS Disorders	Pulmonary Disorders	Medications	Other
Mass lesions	Viral/bacterial pneumonia	Vasopressin analogues (Desmopressin	Pain
Tumors	Positive-pressure ventilation	[DDAVP])	Nausea
CNS abscess	Bronchogenic carcinoma	NSAIDs	AIDS
Intracranial hemorrhage or hematoma	(small cell)	Tricyclic antidepressants	Prolonged exercise
Stroke	Acute respiratory failure	Phenothiazines	Idiopathic
CNS infections or inflammatory diseases	COPD	Butyrophenones	
Spinal cord lesions	Tuberculosis	SSRIs	
Acute psychosis	Aspergillosis	Morphine	
Pituitary stalk lesions	Pulmonary abscess	Opiates	
Hydrocephalus		Chlorpropamide (Diabinese)	
Dementia		Clofibrate (Atromid-S)[2]	
Guillain-Barré syndrome		Cyclophosphamide (Cytoxan)	
Head trauma		Vincristine (Oncovin)	
		Nicotine	
		Tolbutamide (Orinase)	
		Barbiturates	
		Acetaminophen (Tylenol)	
		ACE inhibitors	
		Carbamazepine (Tegretol)	
		Omeprazole (Prilosec)	

[2]Not available in the United States.
Abbreviations: ACE, angiotensin-converting enzyme; AIDS, acquired immunodeficiency syndrome; CNS, central nervous system; COPD, chronic obstructive pulmonary disease; NSAIDs, nonsteroidal antiinflammatory drugs; SSRIs, selective serotonin reuptake inhibitors.

is a 250-µg ACTH (cosyntropin, Cortrosyn) stimulation test, although an extremely low 8 AM cortisol level (<3 µg/dL) can be diagnostic. Treatment consists of glucocorticoid replacement.

Syndrome of Inappropriate Antidiuretic Hormone

SIADH is the most common cause of euvolemic hypoosmolar hyponatremia. Edema, ascites, and orthostasis are absent, and thyroid, adrenal, and renal functions are normal. Recent diuretic use should be ruled out. The primary event is the release of vasopressin, which results in water retention. The increased intravascular volume stimulates a natriuresis, which actually is appropriate, but the resulting loss of sodium compounds the hyponatremia. There is an extensive list of causes of SIADH, usually involving pulmonary or central nervous system pathology (see Table 2). A number of medications also are known to stimulate vasopressin release or to potentiate its antidiuretic properties at the level of the kidney (see Tables 1 and 2).

The diagnosis of SIADH is suggested by a low P_{Osm} (<280 mOsm/kg) with a high U_{Osm} (>100 mOsm/kg), confirming water retention and an inappropriately concentrated urine. A spot urine sodium level will be greater than 20 mEq/L, and usually greater than 30 mEq/L. Other helpful laboratory findings include low plasma uric acid (<4 mg/dL) which has a positive predictive value of 73% to 100% for SIADH in this setting. In complicated cases confounded by use of diuretics, the fractional excretion of uric acid has a positive predictive value of 100% for SIADH when the calculated excretion is greater than 12%.

Reset osmostat can be considered a form of SIADH, but the hyponatremia is usually chronic, mild, and asymptomatic. Vasopressin release continues to be regulated, but at a lower threshold of plasma osmolality. The thirst threshold may be altered as well. Interventions to raise the sodium usually have short-lived effects, and the sodium resets at its previous value over time. Therefore, treatment is not recommended if the sodium level is stable and the patient is asymptomatic. A physiologic example of reset osmostat is seen in pregnancy, when the normal sodium range is lowered by 5 mEq/L.

Other Causes of Euvolemic Hypoosmolar Hyponatremia

Primary or psychogenic polydipsia should be considered in patients presenting with hyponatremia and a history of psychiatric illness and treatment. Almost 6% to 7% of psychiatric inpatients are at risk for hyponatremia from increased water intake. The polydipsia may be related to a lowered osmolar threshold for thirst, below the threshold

of suppression of vasopressin secretion. This can be further complicated by the side effect of dry mouth caused by many psychiatric medications, which compounds the increased thirst and water intake. Because the kidney is capable of excreting up to 15 to 20 L/day of dilute urine, the fact that hyponatremia develops in these patients may point toward an additional and inappropriate increase in vasopressin release or sensitivity. These patients are clinically euvolemic because of renal excretion of the excess water and have otherwise normal laboratory results except for a dilute urine (<100 mOsm/kg), which is caused by vasopressin suppression and helps differentiate primary polydipsia from SIADH. However, some patients have mildly concentrated urine (>100 mOsm/kg), in which case the psychiatric history helps with the diagnosis.

Exercise-induced hyponatremia (e.g., from marathon running) is a form of euvolemic hypoosmolar hyponatremia primarily caused by excessive fluid intake during exercise. Vasopressin levels also may be inappropriately high, secondary to pain or the use of NSAIDs, which remove prostaglandin inhibition of vasopressin release. Low solute intake combined with high fluid intake also can cause hyponatremia, as is with beer potomania or a low-protein "tea and toast" diet in elderly patients. In both cases, the lack of solute in the urine does not allow retention of water in the filtrate, so the excess water is not excreted.

Hyponatremia also is common after pituitary surgery (transsphenoidal or by craniotomy) and may be a result of damage to the hypothalamic-pituitary tract that causes release of preformed vasopressin from damaged neurons. Often, hyponatremia occurs as the second phase of the classic triphasic response: transient diabetes insipidus, transient SIADH, followed by permanent diabetes insipidus. Hyponatremia can be delayed up to 1 week postoperatively, and sodium should be monitored during the second week as well. Contributions by central adrenal insufficiency and hypothyroidism also are considerations after pituitary surgery, although with these conditions there will be obvious clinical manifestations in addition to the hyponatremia.

Management

The major considerations for choosing the type and time course of treatment for hyponatremia are the duration of hyponatremia (acute or chronic) and the presence of neurologic signs and symptoms, especially severe manifestations such as altered mental status or seizure (see Table 2). Treatment options for hyponatremia include fluid

CURRENT THERAPY

- Severe and symptomatic hyponatremia should be treated with hypertonic saline (3%) at 1 to 2 mL/kg per hour. Neurologic status and serum sodium should be monitored every 2 to 4 hours. The objective is to raise sodium by 2 mEq/L per hour (or to >125 mEq/L) until deleterious neurologic symptoms improve. After this, the rate of infusion should be titrated to increase the serum sodium by 0.5 to 1.0 mEq/L per hour, with a maximum increase of 10 to 12 mEq/L over 24 hours and no more than 18 mEq/L over 48 hours, to avoid precipitating osmotic demyelination.

- As a general rule, the treatment of hyponatremia should be adjusted so that the serum sodium increases by 0.5 to 1.0 mEq/L per hour with a maximum increase of 10 to 12 mEq/L over 24 hours and no more than 18 mEq/L over 48 hours. Acute hyponatremia (<48 hours) may be treated more rapidly than chronic hyponatremia if dictated by neurologic findings. Treat SIADH with fluid restriction, medications, or observation; rule out adrenal insufficiency and hypothyroidism.

- Most cases of euvolemic hyponatremia are caused by the syndrome of inappropriate antidiuretic hormone (SIADH), which usually can be managed with fluid restriction, salt tablets, and demeclocycline (Declomycin)[1] in refractory cases.

- Discontinue thiazide diuretics in all cases of hypoosmolar hyponatremia.

- Hypovolemic and hypervolemic hyponatremia require therapy to correct the underlying cause (e.g., heart failure) and restore status to euvolemia.

- Conivaptan (Vaprisol) is a vasopressin receptor antagonist that is approved for inpatient management of euvolemic and hypovolemic hyponatremia. The same parameters apply for rate of sodium correction and monitoring as in conventional therapy.

[1]Not FDA approved for this indication.

restriction, saline infusion (hypertonic or isotonic), vasopressin receptor antagonists (Conivaptan, [Vaprisol]), and demeclocycline (Declomycin).[1] Also, treatment of the underlying abnormality, such as CHF or salt wasting, and correction of volume status are important for hypovolemic or hypervolemic patients. Autocorrection may occur after initiation of therapy, especially in cases of hypovolemia, adrenal insufficiency, or thiazide use. Once treatment is started, the contribution of the nonosmotic stimulation of vasopressin secretion is removed, and the patient is able to raise the sodium level by 2 mEq/L per hour over 12 hours.

ACUTE SEVERE SYMPTOMATIC HYPONATREMIA

Acute severe hyponatremia is defined as a rapid fall in sodium in less than 48 hours to less than 120 mEq/L. Under these circumstances, most patients develop neurologic symptoms because of the rapid fluid shifts between the ECF and the ICF in the brain. If left untreated, it can result in irreversible neurologic damage and death. Because of the acute drop in sodium, initial rapid correction is acceptable and should not lead to osmotic demyelination. Treatment is aimed at raising the sodium enough to resolve the neurologic signs and symptoms. The goal is to raise the serum sodium by 1 to 2 mEq/L per hour or to greater than 125 mEq/L until symptoms resolve. Hypovolemic patients will respond to infusion of isotonic saline (normal saline 0.9%), especially if the urine sodium concentration is less than 30 mEq/L. If the neurologic findings are severe, hypertonic saline (3%) may be infused at rate of 1 to 2 mL/kg per hour, or even up to 4 to 6 mL/kg per hour if the imbalance is life-threatening. A loop diuretic can be combined with the saline to enhance solute-free water excretion. Sodium levels should be monitored every 2 to 4 hours in patients undergoing hypertonic infusion. Once symptoms resolve, the rate of correction should be reduced to 0.5 to 1 mEq/hour, and the total rise in sodium should not exceed 8 to 12 mEq in 24 hours and no more than 18 mEq in 48 hours. No benefit has been observed for faster rates of correction of hyponatremia, whether acute or chronic. Useful formulas to determine the rate of infusion for fluids is provided in Figure 3. The formulas can only estimate the rate of correction, and sodium should be measured frequently.

[1]Not FDA approved for this indication.

Hyponatremia

613

Parameters for acute or chronic hyponatremia:
Do not increase serum Na by more than 10 to 12 mEq/L in 24 hours, or 18 mEq/L in 48 hours

Symptomatic hyponatremia with severe neurologic symptoms (acute <48 hours or chronic >48 hours)
1. Correct serum Na at a rate of 1–2 mEq/L per hour (for 2–4 hours) until symptoms have resolved
2. After symptoms have resolved, correct Na at a rate of 0.5 to 1 mEq/L per hour, maximum 10–12 mEq/24 h

Acute hyponatremia with mild symptoms
1. Correct at rate of 0.5 to 1 mEq/L per hour

Chronic hyponatremia with mild symptoms or asymptomatic
1. Correct at rate of 0.5 mEq/L per hour with fluid restriction
2. Treat underlying cause

Calculation of the rate of infusion of saline to correct hyponatremia
1. Change in serum sodium per liter infusate (# mEq/L) = $\dfrac{\text{Infusate [sodium]} - \text{Serum [sodium]}}{\text{TBW} + 1}$

2. Amount of infusate (L) required in 24 hours = $\dfrac{\text{Desired change in sodium over 24 hours}}{\text{Change in Na/L (from 1)}}$

3. Rate of infusate to raise serum Na by approximately 1 mEq/h

$\text{mL/hr} = \dfrac{\text{L/24 hr (from 2)} \times 100 \text{ mL/L}}{24 \text{ h}}$

4. (simplified) Hypertonic saline infused at 1–2 mL/kg per hour

Monitoring:
1. Monitor for improvement or worsening of symptoms
2. If on hypertonic saline or severely symptomatic, check sodium q2–4h

Infusate	Infusate [Na] mEq/L
5% sodium chloride in water	855
3% sodium chloride in water	513
Isotonic saline (0.9%)	154
Ringer's Lactate solution	130
0.45% sodium chloride in water	77
0.2% sodium chloride in water	34
5% dextrose in water	0

Total Body Water (TBW) is equal to 60% of body weight in young adult men and 50% in young adult women. Older patients have less TBW. In elderly males, TBW is equal to 50% of body weight and in elderly females it is 45%.

FIGURE 3. Treatment of hyponatremia. *Abbreviation:* TBW, total body water.

CHRONIC HYPONATREMIA

Chronic hyponatremia is defined as a gradual fall in sodium over more than 48 hours. By this time, the brain has begun to compensate for hypoosmolality by extrusion of solutes. However, the patient is at risk of osmotic demyelination if hyponatremia is treated too aggressively. If the duration of hyponatremia is unknown, the recommendation is to assume that it is chronic. However, as with acute hyponatremia, severe neurologic symptoms and signs need to be treated with hypertonic saline until they resolve, after which the rate of correction can be slowed to 0.5 to 1 mEq/L per hour. Most cases of osmotic demyelination occur with correction rates of greater than 12 mEq/L in 24 hours, but there are cases reported with increases of 9 or 10 mEq/day. Asymptomatic hyponatremia can be treated with an infusion of isotonic saline calculated to raise the sodium by 0.5 to 1 mEq/hour. If the patient has a dilute urine (<200 mOsm/kg), water restriction may be sufficient.

SYNDROME OF INAPPROPRIATE ANTIDIURETIC HORMONE

The mainstays of treatment of SIADH are fluid restriction and treatment of the underlying cause. Mild SIADH usually can be controlled with fluid restriction alone.

In most cases of SIADH, the degree of fluid restriction required can be calculated. It is dependent on three factors: the daily osmolar load, the minimum U_{Osm}, and the patient's maximum urine volume. A typical diet has a daily osmolar load of 10 mOsm/kg of body weight. For a 70 kg person, this would be 700 mOsm/day. With SIADH, the urine osmolality is held constant for that particular patient, as revealed by a spot U_{Osm}. If the U_{Osm} is 500 mOsm/kg and the solute load is 700 mOsm, the fluid load has to be less than 700/500 or 1.4 L/day just to maintain the serum sodium level. Fluid intake above this amount will cause the sodium to decrease.

When needed, salt tablets (sodium chloride tablet 1 g taken once to three times daily) can help to make up for renal loss of sodium in SIADH. With symptoms and severe hyponatremia, short-term use of hypertonic saline may also be instituted to restore sodium to the ECF compartment. Loop diuretics (e.g., furosemide [Lasix]) can increase free water clearance when given with solute (e.g., hypertonic saline or salt tablets). In refractory cases, demeclocycline (300–600 mg PO twice daily) can be used. Demeclocycline (Declomycin)[1] antagonizes the actions of vasopressin by inhibiting formation of cyclic adenosine monophosphate in the collecting duct. Long-term use is limited by the side effect of photosensitivity and by nephrotoxicity in patients with underlying liver disease. The vasopressin receptor antagonist, conivaptan (Vaprisol), is an important new adjunct treatment (see later discussion). A less favored treatment is urea (powder or capsules)[1,6] which causes an osmotic diuresis and increased free water excretion.

CEREBRAL SALT WASTING

Management of CSW involves treatment of the underlying neurologic problem as well as volume replacement. CSW often is difficult to differentiate biochemically from SIADH, but the rise in vasopressin in CSW is secondary to volume depletion. As a result, CSW responds to volume replacement with isotonic saline, suppressing release of vasopressin, whereas SIADH worsens with this therapy. The recommended correction rate is 0.7 to 1.0 mEq/L per hour, with a maximum of 8 to 10 mEq per 24 hours. Salt tablets may also be given to replete total body sodium. Fludrocortisone (Florinef[1] 0.05 to 0.1 mg every 12 hours), an aldosterone receptor agonist, is a third-line treatment to encourage volume expansion and sodium retention, but the potassium concentration and blood pressure should be monitored. Fluid restriction is inappropriate for CSW and should be avoided, especially in patients with subarachnoid hemorrhage, because volume depletion can exacerbate cerebral vasospasm and cause infarction. The duration of CSW is usually 3 to 5 weeks.

---

[1]Not FDA approved for this indication.
[6]May be compounded by pharmacists.

VASOPRESSIN RECEPTOR ANTAGONISTS

Vasopressin receptor antagonists, or vaptans, are a new class of nonpeptide drugs that have great potential for the treatment of dilutional hyponatremia. They block the binding of vasopressin to its receptors in the distal nephron, thereby inhibiting the insertion of aquaporin-2 channels into the membrane, increasing excretion of solute-free water by the kidneys, and resulting in a rise in serum sodium content. Currently, conivaptan (Vaprisol) is FDA approved for clinical use in euvolemic and hypervolemic hyponatremia in hospitalized patients, with the exception of patients with CHF or cirrhosis. Obviously, it is contraindicated in hypovolemic hyponatremia because of the water excretion that is induced. Conivaptan is given intravenously with a bolus of 20 mg over 30 minutes in 100 mL of 5% dextrose in water (D5W). After this, the drug (20 mg in 100 mL of D5W) is infused over 24 hours. Sodium is monitored every 2 to 4 hours, and the dose may be titrated to 40 mg per 24 hours to obtain an increase in sodium of 0.5 to 1.0 mEq/L per hour. During Vaprisol treatment, fluid restriction is liberal at 1.5 to 2.0 L/day. An oral formulation tolvaptan (Samsca) also is approved for outpatient treatment of hyponatremia associated with SIADH, CHF, and cirrhosis if it is clinically significant and Na is <125 mEq/L, or is resistant to other treatments. Tolvaptan is first initiated in the hospital setting, for careful monitoring of potassium and the rate of rise of sodium, at a dose of 15 mg once daily. It is titrated up with >24h between increased doses to a maximum of 60 mg once daily. The vasopressin receptor antagonists with caution in patients with renal or hepatic impairment. Inhibitors of the cytochrome P-450 3A4 isoenzyme (CYP3A4) are contraindicated, including ketoconazole (Nizoral), itraconazole (Sporanox), clarithromycin (Biaxin), ritonavir (Norvir), and indinavir (Crixivan). Additionally, the "vaptans" will alter the hepatic metabolism of other drugs that interact with Cyp 3A4 so that all concurrent medications should be checked carefully for potential interactions.

Summary

Hyponatremia is a common electrolyte abnormality and is usually caused by decreased plasma osmolality. Accurate assessment of volume status is a key to determining the underlying cause and choosing the correct treatment approach. The biggest risk of hyponatremia and its treatment is the possibility of severe neurologic sequelae, including fatal cerebral edema and osmotic demyelination. Therefore, more aggressive initial treatment is needed in patients with neurologic manifestations (hypertonic saline), but a more conservative approach (e.g., fluid restriction) is needed for less symptomatic patients. The new availability of the vasopressin receptor antagonists conivaptan, for euvolemic or hypervolemic hyponatremia is a welcome step forward for the treatment of hyponatremia in the inpatient setting.

REFERENCES

Androgué HJ. Consequences of inadequate management of hyponatremia. Am J Nephrol 2005;25:240–9.

Androgué HJ, Madias NE. Hyponatremia. N Engl J Med 2000;342(21):1581–9.

Cerdà-Esteve M, Cuadrado-Godia E, Chillaron JJ, et al. Cerebral salt wasting syndrome: Review. Eur J Intern Med 2008;19:249–54.

Ellison DH, Berl T. Clinical practice: The syndrome of inappropriate antidiuresis. N Engl J Med 2007;356:2064–72.

Fenske W, Störk S, Koschker A. Value of fractional uric acid excretion in differential diagnosis of hyponatremia patients on diuretics. J Clin Endocrinol Metab 2008;93:2991–7.

Hew-Butler T, Jordaan E, Stuempfle KJ. Osmotic and nonosmotic regulation of arginine vasopressin during prolonged exercise. J Clin Endocrinol Metab 2008;93:2072–8.

Palm C, Pistrosch F, Herbrig K, Gross P. Vasopressin antagonists as aquaretic agents for the treatment of hyponatremia. Am J Med 2006;119(Suppl. 1):S87–93.

Vaprisol conivaptan hydrochloride injection: Prescribing information. Deerfield, Ill: Astellas Pharma US, Inc; 2007.

Verbalis JG, Goldsmith SR, Greenberg A, et al. Hyponatremia treatment guidelines 2007: Expert panel recommendations. Am J Med 2007;120(11 Suppl. 1):S1–21.

Zada G, Liu CY, Fishback D, et al. Recognition and management of delayed hyponatremia following transphenoidal pituitary surgery. J Neurosurg 2007;106:66–71.

Hyperuricemia and Gout

Method of
Saima Chohan, MD

Epidemiology

Gout, or monosodium urate crystal deposition disease, is the most common inflammatory arthritis of men and is an increasingly common problem among postmenopausal women. It is a chronic disorder, affecting nearly 5 million people in the United States and increasing in both prevalence and incidence, especially in persons older than 65 years. Gout is often accompanied by serious comorbid disorders (hypertension, cardiovascular and chronic kidney disease, and all of the component features of the metabolic syndrome) and it is managed in primary care practice in about 90% of affected persons; therefore, identifying risk factors, optimizing diagnosis, and choosing appropriate treatment for gout are important skills for a wide array of caregivers.

The initial symptoms and signs of gout are most often those of an acute attack of arthritis occurring after many years of asymptomatic hyperuricemia. In untreated or inadequately treated patients, the course of the disease often involves acute attacks at increasing frequency, with shortening of asymptomatic periods (called intercritical gout) and, ultimately, development of chronic joint disease (gouty arthropathy) and tophi (masses of urate crystals in a chronic inflammatory matrix) in bone, joints, skin, and even solid organs (Fig. 1).

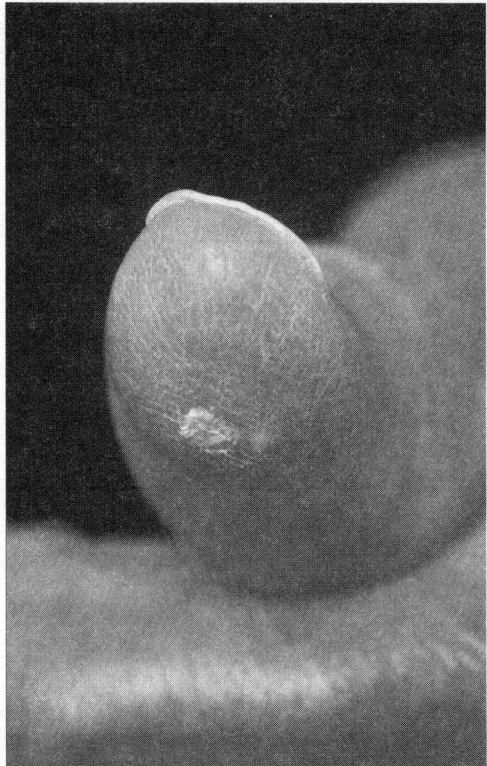

FIGURE 1. Intradermal urate deposit (tophus). (Reprinted with permission from Mandell BF: Gout and crystal deposition disease. In Weisman MH, Weinblatt ME, Louie JS, Van Vollenhoven R (eds): Targeted Treatment of the Rheumatic Diseases. Philadelphia, Saunders, 2010, pp 293-302.)

Pathophysiology and Risk Factors

Uric acid is the end product of purine metabolism in humans. Hyperuricemia, a serum urate concentration exceeding urate solubility (6.8 mg/dL), is an invariable accompaniment of gout, though serum uric acid levels might not be elevated during an acute attack. Hyperuricemia predisposes affected persons to urate crystal formation and deposition, which lead to the inflammatory responses underlying the symptoms of gout. Thus, treatment of gout is aimed at reducing and maintaining serum urate concentration at subsaturating levels, usually set at less than 6.0 mg/dL.

Risk factors for hyperuricemia include obesity, hypertension, hyperlipidemia, insulin resistance, renal insufficiency, and use of diuretics. Diets rich in certain foods are also associated with increased risk for gout. Many studies support the view that hyperuricemia is an integral part of the metabolic syndrome and that both hyperuricemia and gout increase the risk for myocardial infarction and other cardiovascular events.

Diagnosis

Acute gout is characterized by abrupt onset of joint pain, erythema and swelling, usually of one joint, but less commonly more than one. The arthritis most often occurs first in a lower extremity joint, especially the first metatarsophalangeal (MTP) joint at the base of the great toe. The predilection for this site is thought to be secondary to cooler acral temperature or repeated trauma and pressure on this joint.

The gold standard for diagnosis of gout is demonstration of monosodium urate crystals by polarized light microscopy either in joint fluid aspirated during an acute attack or between attacks, or from material aspirated from suspected tophi. To aspirate the first MTP joint, the joint is first identified by palpating the space at the base of the metacarpal on the dorsal aspect while flexing and extending the toe, then the needle is inserted perpendicularly into the joint space to avoid the extensor hallucis tendon. Synovial fluid from affected joints should immediately be examined under polarized microscopy to confirm the diagnosis of needle-shaped crystals with negative birefringence. If polarized microscopy is unavailable, then fluid should be sent in a sterile tube for crystal confirmation to an appropriate laboratory.

Unfortunately, the equipment and analytical expertise necessary to make this diagnosis are not widely available to primary care physicians. As a result, the diagnosis of acute gout is commonly made on clinical grounds, often using clinical and laboratory criteria established by organizations such as the American College of Rheumatology and the European League Against Rheumatism. These diagnostic guidelines emphasize the presence of signs of inflammation (swelling, warmth, redness, tenderness, and loss of joint function), abrupt onset, monoarticular involvement, occurrence in the first MTP joint and presence of tophi.

Indications for Treatment

Early in gout, patients might have attacks that are separated by years and manageable over the course of a few days with antiinflammatory medications and adjuncts such as joint rest and application of ice. Over time, the attacks usually become more frequent, prolonged, and disabling, eventually requiring long-term urate-lowering treatment aimed at preventing urate crystal deposition and eventually abolishing acute flares and resolving tophi. Indications for urate-lowering (antihyperuricemic) therapy are listed in Box 1.

BOX 1 Indications for Urate-Lowering Therapy

Frequent and disabling gouty attacks, often defined as two or three flares annually, though this is not evidence based. The decision to treat is based on both number of flares and the consequent disability resulting from flares.
Chronic gouty disease: clinically or radiographically evident joint erosions
Tophaceous deposits: subcutaneous or intraosseous
Gout with renal insufficiency
Recurrent kidney stones
Urate nephropathy
Urinary uric acid excretion exceeding 1100 mg/day (6.5 mmol), when determined in men younger than 25 years or in premenopausal women

CURRENT DIAGNOSIS

- Gout is the most common inflammatory arthritis of men and is increasing in prevalence.
- Definitive diagnosis of gout requires demonstration of monosodium urate crystals in synovial fluid or tophi.
- Gouty arthritis often begins in lower extremity joints.
- Septic arthritis, rheumatoid arthritis, and calcium pyrophosphate disease (pseudogout) can mimic gout and should be ruled out.

Treatment

ACUTE GOUT

Gouty arthritis occurs suddenly, and attacks are often very painful and disabling. Patients describe acute onset of exquisite pain, swelling, erythema, and inability to bear weight on the afflicted joint. Occasionally patients have constitutional symptoms including fevers and chills, with elevation of sedimentation rate and white blood cell count. To terminate an attack, nonsteroidal antiinflammatory drugs (NSAIDs), colchicine, or corticosteroids can be offered. If given at full antiinflammatory dosage, NSAIDs have a rapid onset and are quite efficacious in relieving pain and shortening the duration of an attack. The utility of this class of drugs may be limited by renal insufficiency, cardiovascular risk factors, and gastrointestinal bleeding. While indomethacin (Indocin), sulindac (Clinoril) and naproxen (Naprosyn) are all FDA approved for treating acute attacks of gout, nearly every drug in this class and the selective cyclooxygenase (COX) 2 inhibitors also have considerable efficacy. High-dose salicylate therapy lowers serum uric acid by interfering in renal urate transport, and low-dose aspirin has the opposite effect, but it is often continued in gout patients because of its overriding importance in managing coronary artery disease.

Oral colchicine has been used to treat gout for many years as an unproven drug with no FDA dosage recommendations or prescribing information. In July 2009, however, the FDA approved Colcrys, a single-ingredient colchicine product, for the first day of treatment of acute gout attacks at a low-dose regimen of 1.2 mg followed by 0.6 mg in 1 hour (total 1.8 mg). With this regimen, colchicine can be used to abort an attack if taken immediately after the development of the first symptom of gout flare. Higher colchicine doses (0.6 mg every hour, until symptoms improve or until gastrointestinal symptoms of diarrhea, nausea, or vomiting develop, for a total of 4.8 mg over 6 hours) have traditionally been recommended. A randomized, placebo-controlled trial comparing the low-dose and high-dose regimens showed both approaches had equivalent efficacy in pain relief at 24 hours (compared with placebo). However, adverse gastrointestinal events were significantly less common with the low-dose regimen. In subjects warranting additional flare treatment, continued use of colchicine 0.6 mg twice daily

CURRENT THERAPY

- The goal of successful gout treatment includes terminating the acute attack, preventing intermittent attacks, and taking long-term therapy to avoid chronic arthritis.
- Indications for chronic treatment of gout include frequent attacks, recurrent arthritis, and kidney disease.
- A serum urate level of less than 6.0 mg/dL is the goal when using urate-lowering therapy.
- Nonpharmacologic treatment includes lifestyle modification and dietary changes.
- The mainstay of urate-lowering therapies remains xanthine oxidase inhibition.

(reducing to once daily as the flare subsides) is appropriate in persons with normal renal and hepatic function.

Gastrointestinal symptoms are generally the first clinical signs of colchicine toxicity in patients with normal renal and hepatic function. More serious toxicities do occur and include neuromyopathy, aplastic anemia, and worsening renal and hepatic function. Care should be used in patients with renal or hepatic impairment, and because of potentially serious drug-drug interactions, colchicine should be avoided in patients receiving cyclosporine (Neoral), clarithromycin (Biaxin), verapamil (Calan), and amlodipine (Norvasc). Intravenous colchicine[2] is not available in Europe and is only available in limited settings in the United States.[6] This formulation should be avoided because of significant risk of fatal toxicity.

Corticosteroids provide a safe alternative for patients with contraindications to NSAIDs or colchicine. For isolated monoarticular attacks, especially of medium or large joints, aspiration of joint fluid and intraarticular injection with triamcinolone acetonide (Kenalog) 20 to 40 mg can quickly terminate an attack. For polyarticular attacks or attacks in smaller joints, systemic corticosteroids (oral or intramuscular) may be employed. Oral prednisone starting at 20 mg twice daily with a taper over 10 to 14 days is very effective. Patients can have rebound attacks if oral steroids are terminated too quickly, and thus methylprednisolone (Medrol) dose packs should be avoided. If intramuscular injection is used, a single dose of triamcinolone 40 mg may be employed.

There is interest in agents blocking the action of interleukin 1 (IL-1), a cytokine believed to play a major role in initiating and sustaining acute gouty inflammation. Anakinra (Kineret),[1] rilonacept (Arcalyst),[1] and canakinumab (Ilaris)[1] are each potent injectable or infusible IL-1 inhibitors, and studies are ongoing to assess the utility of these agents to mitigate acute attacks.

INTERCRITICAL GOUT

After an attack subsides, management is directed at preventing recurrent attacks. During acute attacks of gout, normal serum urate concentration is reported in up to 40% of affected patients, and thus it is not an accurate reflection of the true urate pool. Confirmation of hyperuricemia is best achieved either before or 2 to 4 weeks after resolution of an attack for an accurate serum urate concentration. There is a generalizable correlation between the serum urate level and risk for recurrent attack.

Prophylaxis of future attacks during early urate-lowering therapy can consist of colchicine at doses of 0.6 mg once or twice a day (based on renal function) or NSAIDs. If chronic NSAIDs are used, acid-reducing medications such as proton pump inhibitors or histamine-2 blockers may be employed for patients at risk for gastrointestinal bleeding.

[1]Not FDA approved for this indication.
[2]Not available in the United States.
[6]May be compounded by pharmacists.

LONG-TERM URATE-LOWERING (ANTIHYPERURICEMIC) THERAPY

The aim of urate-lowering therapy is to reduce and maintain serum urate at concentrations below those at which extracellular fluids are saturated with monosodium urate. In general, a goal of serum urate concentration of less than 6.0 mg/dL is advised. Urate lowering can be achieved either by increasing urinary excretion or by decreasing production of urate.

Nonpharmacologic urate-lowering treatment begins with lifestyle changes. Diet and weight loss must be addressed. Obesity and weight gain are risk factors for gout, and weight loss has been shown to decrease the risk of gout. A purine-restricted diet has often been recommended to patients but is often unpalatable and impractical. Reduction in alcohol intake, namely beer and liquor, can effectively reduce urate levels. Similarly, reduced intake of red meat and shellfish also lowers the risk of recurrent gouty attacks. Studies have shown increased frequency of attacks in patients who consume soft drinks containing high-fructose corn syrup, an ingredient not found in diet drinks.

Once the decision is made to institute serum urate–lowering therapy, the duration of treatment is indefinite and must be long term to be effective. The majority of patients with gout and tophaceous disease will continue to have attacks if therapy is discontinued, and thus education is a key part of the treatment plan. Patients should be instructed that with initiation of any urate-lowering therapy, they will be at increased risk for a flare and thus must continue regular use of prophylactic agents as outlined above. At least 80% to 95% of cases of hyperuricemia and gout are attributable to impaired urate excretion, which is reflected in diminished urate clearance or fractional excretion of uric acid, but not usually in low daily urine uric acid excretion. In practice, 24-hour urine collections are rarely performed. Patients are preferentially treated with xanthine oxidase inhibitors because of the easier dosing schedule and because many patients have contraindications to uricosurics such as renal insufficiency and kidney stones.

Uricosurics

Relative to medications aimed at urate synthesis, uricosurics are relegated to second-line treatment of patients with elevated urate burden or tophaceous disease. The most commonly used uricosuric agent in the United States is probenecid. This is a very effective drug that concentrates and promotes urinary excretion of urate. Its utility is limited in patients with renal insufficiency, and probenecid is not recommended as first-line therapy in patients with nephrolithiasis or uric acid overexcretion. The maintenance dose of probenecid required to achieve and maintain serum urate concentration at less than 6.0 mg/dL is 0.5 to 3 g[3] per day, administered in two or three daily doses. Once goal serum urate concentration is achieved with a uricosuric agent, the risk of uric acid calculi is diminished, because urinary uric acid excretion becomes normal.

Other drugs found to have uricosuric effects include fenofibrate (Tricor),[1] a fibric acid derivative used to treat hyperlipidemia, and the antihypertensives losartan (Cozaar)[1] and amlodipine.[1] Consumption of vitamin C[1] at 500 mg/day has also been found to be effective in lowering serum urate concentration. These agents have mild uricosuric properties and may be useful adjuncts to urate-lowering therapy.

Xanthine Oxidase Inhibitors

Allopurinol (Zyloprim) and febuxostat (Uloric) are the only FDA-approved xanthine oxidase inhibitors for the treatment of gout. Allopurinol, introduced in 1966, is approved in doses of 100 to 800 mg/day. More than 90% of patients with gout treated with urate-lowering medication in the United States are given allopurinol, but dosages of more than 300 mg/day are infrequently employed, and often patients do not achieve serum urate concentrations of 6.0 mg/dL or less. Appropriate use of allopurinol is limited for several reasons. There are genuine concerns about allopurinol drug interactions, gastrointestinal intolerance, rashes (ranging from mild to life-threatening), and the rare but sometimes fatal hypersensitivity syndrome. Allopurinol should be avoided with the immunosuppressives azathioprine and 6-mercaptopurine because it can increase the risk of bone marrow toxicity, because these medications are partially metabolized by xanthine oxidase. Allopurinol should not be taken with ampicillin owing to increased risk of rash.

Effective dosing of allopurinol is often not achieved because of compliance with published but recently disputed recommendations for allopurinol dose reduction in states of renal impairment. Allopurinol should be initiated at 100 mg daily in patients with creatinine clearance of 40 mL/min or greater, and it should be titrated in 100-mg increments every 2 to 4 weeks, with the endpoint of dosing determined by achievement of serum urate concentration of 6.0 mg/dL or less.

The FDA approved febuxostat in 2009. Unlike allopurinol, this is a nonpurine analogue and selective xanthine oxidase inhibitor that is not incorporated into purine nucleotides and does not appear to affect pyrimidine metabolism. Febuxostat is primarily metabolized by oxidation and glucuronidation in the liver, with little renal excretion of drug; this contrasts with the renal elimination of oxypurinol, the main allopurinol metabolite. The recommended starting dose of febuxostat is 40 mg daily, with an increase to 80 mg daily if serum urate concentrations do not reach goal urate levels in 2 weeks in patients with normal renal function. In Europe, higher doses have received approval (80-120 mg daily), and studies have affirmed the efficacy and safety of dosing in this range. In the FOCUS trial, a 5-year study of efficacy and safety, febuxostat was shown to have durable maintenance of serum urate concentration at 6.0 mg/dL or less, nearly complete elimination of gouty flares, and resolution of baseline tophi in subjects. An advantage of febuxostat over allopurinol is that it can safely be taken by patients with creatinine clearance greater than 30 mL/min.

Potential New Therapies

Pegloticase (pegylated porcine recombinant uricase, Krystexxa) has been studied in patients with severe progressive and previously treatment-refractory gout and is under review by the FDA. Humans lack the enzyme uricase, which converts uric acid to allantoin, a more-soluble purine-degradation product. Replacement of this missing enzyme allows direct conversion of urate to allantoin, with eventual depletion of increased body urate pools and control of disease, including resolution of tophi. Recombinant uricase therapy profoundly lowers serum urate concentration, as was demonstrated in a phase II study.

A number of other novel agents with new therapeutic targets for the treatment of gout and hyperuricemia are under investigation.

REFERENCES

Becker MA, Chohan S. We can make gout management more successful now. Curr Opin Rheum 2008;20:167–72.

Dalbeth N, Stamp L. Allopurinol dosing in renal impairment: Walking the tightrope between adequate urate lowering and adverse events. Semin Dial 2007;20(5):391–5.

Schumacher HR, Becker MA, Lloyd E, et al. Febuxostat in the treatment of gout: 5-year findings of the FOCUS efficacy and safety study. Rheumatology 2009;48:188–94.

Stamp L, O'Donnell JL, Frampton C, et al. Increasing allopurinol dose above the recommended range is effective and safe in chronic gout, including in those with renal impairment—a pilot study [abstract]. Philadelphia: American College of Rheumatology Scientific Meeting; 2009. October 17-21, Available at http://acr.confex.com/acr/2009/webprogram/Paper12049.html; [accessed 20.07.10].

Sundy JS, Becker MA, Baraf HS, et al. Reduction of plasma urate levels following treatment with multiple doses of Pegloticase (polyethylene glycol–conjugated uricase) in patients with treatment-failure gout: Results of a phase II randomized study. Arthritis Rheum 2008;58(9):2882–91.

Terkeltaub R, Furst DE, Bennett K, et al. Colchicine efficacy assessed by time to 50% reduction of pain is comparable in cow dose and high dose regimens: secondary analysis of the AGREE trial [abstract],

---

[1]Not FDA approved for this indication.
[3]Exceeds dosage recommended by the manufacturer.

Philadelphia: American College of Rheumatology Scientific Meeting; 2009. October 17–21. Available at http://acr.confex.com/acr/2009/webprogram/Paper15030.html; [accessed July 20, 2010].

Zhang W, Doherty M, Pascual E, et al. EULAR evidence based recommendations for gout. Part I: Diagnosis. Report of a task force of the standing committee for international clinical studies including therapeutics (ESCIT). Ann Rheum Dis 2006;65:1301–11.

Dyslipoproteinemias

Method of
Kerem Ozer, MD, and Lawrence Chan, MD

All cells need lipids to survive, and lipids are essential for maintenance of tissue structure and function. Lipids comprise an essential component of biologic membranes, and molecular communication within and between cells relies heavily on lipids. Not surprisingly, an imbalance in lipid metabolism has the potential to cause serious malfunction in multiple systems. In addition, abnormal accumulation of excess lipids in cells or tissues can lead to a severe disruption of normal organ structure and function. Among the many organ systems that are affected by lipid excess and imbalance, the cardiovascular system is the most susceptible; specifically, atherosclerotic cardiovascular disease continues to exert a heavy toll on human health. Indeed, atherosclerosis and its complications are the foremost causes of death and disability for men and women in the Western world. Atherosclerosis is a chronic, multifactorial disease with a complex pathogenesis. Insulin resistance and dyslipidemia are predominant risk factors in many patients with atherosclerosis. High among these risk factors are disorders of lipid and lipoprotein metabolism. Such dyslipoproteinemias encompass a wide spectrum of monogenic and polygenic conditions that are strongly modulated by environmental factors.

Dynamics of Lipid Metabolism and Its Contribution to Atherosclerosis

Lipids have two main points of entry into the circulation: the gut (exogenous pathway) and the liver (endogenous pathway). The exogenous and endogenous pathways are further interconnected by intermediate pathways (reverse cholesterol transport pathway and others). These pathways are outlined in Figure 1.

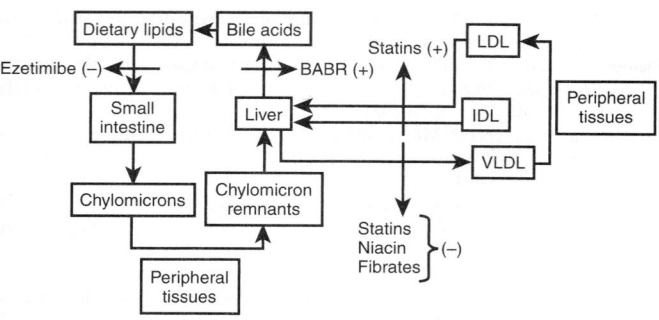

FIGURE 1. Overview of lipid metabolism showing points of therapeutic intervention by available pharmaceutical agents. High-density lipoprotein (HDL) is not shown because there is no approved agent that directly targets HDL, which can be raised indirectly by aerobic exercise, weight loss, and niacin. (+), stimulate; (−), inhibit; BABR, bile acid–binding resins; IDL, intermediate-density lipoprotein; LDL, low-density lipoprotein; VLDL, very-low-density lipoprotein.

EXOGENOUS PATHWAY

Dietary fat constitutes the sole source of exogenous lipids to the body. Triglycerides in food are hydrolyzed by pancreatic lipases within the intestinal lumen. They are then incorporated into micelles through interaction with bile acids acting as emulsifiers. Cholesterol, monoglycerides, free fatty acids, and phospholipids are absorbed through the intestinal brush border via carriers on the enterocyte membrane. Cholesterol molecules are turned into cholesteryl esters in intestinal epithelial cells by the addition of a fatty acid. Long-chain fatty acids (>12 carbons) are esterified to triglycerides and packaged with apolipoprotein (Apo) B48, cholesteryl esters, phospholipids, and cholesterol into the largest-sized lipoprotein particles, known as chylomicrons (>100 nm in diameter, more than 98% lipids, 1%–2% protein), which are secreted into intestinal lymph and delivered to the systemic circulation. Here, they function as a major source of lipids for cells. At the peripheral cell level, chylomicrons are acted on by lipoprotein lipase, which hydrolyzes the triglycerides, releasing the free fatty acids that are taken up by tissues for further metabolism or storage. Apo CII is an important cofactor for lipoprotein lipase. During their transit through the bloodstream, chylomicrons continue to lose lipids, and they also transfer cholesterol and phospholipids to high-density lipoproteins (HDL); they shrink in size and finally are taken up by the liver through chylomicron remnant receptors that use Apo E as a ligand. As a result of this extremely efficient process, normally within hours of eating, chylomicrons are no longer detectable in the circulation.

ENDOGENOUS PATHWAY

The endogenous pathway starts in the liver, which produces another species of triglyceride-rich lipoprotein particles called very-low-density lipoproteins (VLDL), which have a diameter of 30 to 70 nm and contain 85% to 90% lipids and 10% to 15% protein. The major apolipoprotein in VLDL is Apo B100. These particles also contain E and C apolipoproteins. Especially in muscle and adipose tissue, VLDL, like chylomicrons, undergo processing by lipoprotein lipase, which also hydrolyzes VLDL triglycerides, releasing free fatty acids. Catabolism of VLDL by lipoprotein lipase produces smaller particles, known as intermediate-density lipoprotein (IDL), which are enriched in cholesterol. The liver removes about half of the IDL (also known as VLDL remnants) through the action of apo E. The remaining IDL is further processed into low-density lipoproteins (LDL) by hepatic lipase. This process involves further triglyceride hydrolysis. All apoproteins except Apo B100 are removed and transferred to other lipoproteins, and LDL become further enriched in cholesterol. Normally, LDLs carry about 70% of the cholesterol in circulation. Liver cells recognize Apo B100 on LDL, which is taken up via the LDL receptor.

REVERSE CHOLESTEROL TRANSPORT

A major control mechanism by which the body maintains lipid homeostasis in mammals is reverse cholesterol transport. Because all cells synthesize cholesterol but only hepatocytes can metabolize and excrete it, excess cholesterol needs to be carried from peripheral tissues to the liver, where it can be eliminated by secretion into bile after conversion into bile acids. HDLs are the major lipoproteins involved in the transport of cholesterol from peripheral tissues back to the liver. HDLs are synthesized by both hepatocytes and enterocytes, initially in the form of small discoidal particles containing Apo AI and phospholipids. Nascent HDL rapidly accumulates unesterified cholesterol and phospholipids through the action of the membrane protein ABCA1 and the enzyme lecithin-cholesterol acyl transferase (LCAT). As additional lipids are transferred from VLDL to HDL, the latter become more spherical. HDLs are taken up directly in the liver by class B type I scavenger receptor (SR-BI) molecules. Lipids are also transported to the liver via Apo B–containing lipoproteins through the action of cholesteryl ester transfer protein.

PLASMA LIPIDS AND ATHEROSCLEROSIS

Although the physiologic function of the cholesterol-rich lipoproteins, IDL and LDL, is to deliver cholesterol to peripheral tissues, high circulating levels of these particles have long been known to be associated with an increased risk of atherosclerosis. These lipoproteins

CURRENT DIAGNOSIS

- Dyslipidemia encompasses a wide range of inherited and acquired conditions.
- The initial diagnosis should be followed by a complete fasting lipid profile and a thorough search to identify and treat secondary causes of dyslipidemia, such as hypothyroidism, alcoholism, diabetes mellitus, and nephrotic syndrome.
- The importance of early recognition and treatment of dyslipidemia lies in its role as a major risk factor for atherosclerosis and for pancreatitis (with high triglycerides).
- A comprehensive global risk assessment for cardiovascular disease should be carried out to stratify risk and guide treatment.

can pass through endothelial barriers and therefore have the potential to accumulate in the subendothelial space. Once trapped in the extracellular space of the intima, their lipid components are susceptible to biochemical modifications, including oxidation, the products of which become molecular targets for macrophages within the subendothelial space. Macrophages undergo upregulation of their scavenger receptors and take up and accumulate lipids, turning into lipid-engorged macrophages or foam cells, which are key constituents of fatty streaks, the earliest phase of the atherosclerotic plaque. Such early fatty streak plaques may regress, or they may progress to more advanced lesions. Macrophage activation leads to the recruitment of other inflammatory cells, with secretion of inflammatory cytokines initiating a vicious cycle of inflammatory cells and mediators culminating in lesion progression and instability.

As opposed to the atherogenic potential of IDL and LDL, HDL particles are protective against atherosclerotic plaque formation; high HDL levels are associated with a lower incidence of coronary artery disease. This is a result of the capacity of HDL to act in clearing cholesterol from peripheral tissues to the liver for elimination and locally as antiinflammatory and antioxidative mediators.

Assessment of the Patient with Dyslipoproteinemia

Given the strong epidemiologic evidence, supported by animal and cell experiments, for a proatherogenic role of VLDL, IDL, and LDL and a protective role of HDL in atherosclerotic cardiovascular disease risk in numerous populations, various societies and professional organizations have established clinical guidelines to aid the physician in reducing risk in people without heart disease (primary prevention) and to treat patients with known atherosclerotic disease (secondary prevention). Among the most widely used set of recommendations is the National Cholesterol Education Program (NCEP) Adult Treatment Panel III (ATP III) guidelines.

The NCEP ATP III defined stratified risk levels and treatment goals for each level. Risk stratification is based on consideration of cardiovascular risk factors. Smoking, HDL cholesterol (abbreviated HDL) concentration less than 40 mg/dL, hypertension or use of antihypertensive agents, family history of premature coronary artery disease, and age greater than 45 years in men or 55 years in women are positive risk factors, whereas an HDL level greater than 60 mg/dL is considered to be a negative risk factor. If two or more risk factors are present, a Framingham risk score is calculated (http://hp2010.nhlbihin.net/atpiii/calculator.asp?usertype=prof [accessed June 30, 2009]). The National Heart, Lung and Blood Institute (NHLBI) has provided this and other excellent clinical tools online to calculate risk and guide treatment. For purposes of primary prevention, the presence of zero or only one risk factor is defined as low risk for atherosclerotic vascular disease; two or more risk factors constitute moderate risk, and higher numbers constitute high risk. In patients with moderate risk, a 10-year risk for CHD of >20% qualifies one as "high risk." An optimal LDL cholesterol (abbreviated LDL) goal is 100 mg/dL for all patients. Also

of note is the introduction of LDL 100 mg/dL as a goal for people with known coronary artery disease. More recently, the committee has added consideration of 70 mg/dL as a goal for LDL in patients with very high risk (recent acute coronary syndrome or multiple poorly controlled risk factors, especially diabetes mellitus).

Using these goals as guidelines, a practicing physician aims to achieve therapeutic targets through early and consistent implementation of lifestyle changes along with pharmacologic therapy in appropriately selected patients according to the following general principles.

Lifestyle Changes

All patients with dyslipidemia should be counseled on lifestyle modifications. Dietary modification is an essential component, given that the main source of lipids is exogenous dietary fat. In a patient with dyslipidemia, dietary intake of saturated fatty acids should be limited, and a reduction in dietary total lipids is necessary. Other important goals include weight loss in overweight patients. Exercise and the use of plant stanols (e.g., Benecol) or omega-3 fatty acids may also be helpful. The dietary component to be restricted depends also in the component of lipid profile that is high. Patients with triglyceride levels in the >1000 mg/dL range should severely limit total fat intake, not only to reduce cardiovascular risk but also to prevent acute pancreatitis. In patients for whom the goal is to achieve LDL reduction, dietary changes emphasizing certain fatty acid classes, as detailed later, provide a better starting point. The addition of soy products to the diet also may contribute to lowering of LDL.

The American Heart Association heart-healthy diet recommendations are commonly used to guide patients in their dietary practices. The previously used step I and step II dietary recommendations have given way to the therapeutic lifestyle change (TLC) diet, which can be summarized as follows:

- Total dietary fat should be limited to 25% to 35% of total caloric intake, and saturated fats should constitute less than 7% of this fraction.
- Polyunsaturated fats should be less than 10% of energy intake, whereas monounsaturated fats (mainly olive and canola oil) may constitute up to 20% of energy intake.
- Carbohydrates are allocated 50% to 60% and proteins approximately 15% of energy intake.
- Cholesterol intake should be limited to less than 200 mg/day.
- Total caloric intake should balance energy intake and expenditure to maintain desirable body weight and prevent weight gain.

CURRENT THERAPY

- Dyslipidemia is a modifiable risk factor and one of the major risk factors for atherosclerotic cardiovascular disease.
- First-line therapy is therapeutic lifestyle modification.
- Therapy depends on risk stratification, as does the timing of initiation of treatment with pharmacologic agents in addition to lifestyle changes.
- Therapy should be guided based on goals which are in turn based on risk stratification.
- The main problem should be identified as high cholesterol (high LDL), high triglycerides, or a combined lipid problem.
  - High LDL: start with statin add ezetimibe (Zetia) if necessary.
  - High triglycerides: start fibrates; consider adding orlistat (Xenical, Alli)[1]; also, limit fat intake.
  - High LDL and triglycerides: consider combining statins and fibrates.
- Manage all other risk factors appropriately.

[1]Not FDA approved for this indication.

TABLE 1 LDL-Cholesterol Goals and Levels for Initiating Lifestyle and Pharmacologic Interventions (NCEP ATP III)

Risk Category*	LDL Goal (mg/dL)	LDL Level at Which To Initiate TLC (mg/dL)	LDL Level at Which To Initiate Drug Therapy (mg/dL)
CAD or CAD risk equivalents (risk >20%)	<100	>100	>130 (>100 optional)
2+ risk factors (risk 10%–20%)	<130	>130	>130
2+ risk factors (risk 5%–10%)	<130	>130	>160
0–1 risk factor (risk 0%–5%)	<160	>160	>190

*Number of risk factors and 10-year risk for atherosclerotic cardiovascular disease.
Abbreviations: CAD, coronary artery disease; LDL, low-density lipoprotein; NCEP ATP III, National Cholesterol Education Program Adult Treatment Panel III guidelines; TLC, therapeutic lifestyle changes.

If present, obesity should be aggressively treated. Treatment of obesity has a favorable effect on lipid levels. Obese patients who succeed in losing weight tend to show a decrease in triglycerides and LDL and an increase in HDL. The benefit of TLC usually becomes measurable within 6 to 12 months. There is a large amount of heterogeneity in the response to lifestyle changes, which is in part genetically based. Referral to a dietitian may lead to greater success in the short term. The benefits attained by dietary modifications tend to be short-lived in most patients, and diet compliance tends to decrease over time, especially after 1 year. Therefore, the physician should be ready to institute drug therapy concurrent with starting dietary modifications in patients who fulfill criteria for pharmacologic interventions (Table 1) and should be ready to add lipid-lowering agents for patients who have not responded to TLC or who display worsening lipid levels.

Drug Therapy for Dyslipoproteinemia

GENERAL CONSIDERATIONS

The decision to initiate pharmacotherapy should be based on a patient's risk status. The approach used in this chapter is largely based on the NCEP ATP III recommendations and as outlined in Table 1. The main goal in lipid reduction in most cases is to reduce the risk of atherosclerotic cardiovascular disease. The currently available lipid-lowering agents can be classified based on their structure and mechanism of action into statins (3-hydroxy-3-methylglutaryl coenzyme A [HMG-CoA] reductase inhibitors), cholesterol absorption inhibitors such as ezetimibe (Zetia), fibric acid derivatives (fibrates), bile acid sequestrants, and nicotinic acid (niacin). These classes differ with regard to degree and type of lipid lowering, and drugs within each group may differ in efficacy and side effects. Conventional dosing regimens and common adverse effects are summarized in Table 2. The choice of drug depends on the specific lipid abnormality and concurrent medical conditions.

Statins are usually the first choice in patients with high cholesterol levels for reduction of primary or secondary cardiovascular risk. If the LDL goal cannot be reached with statins only, addition of an agent from another class should be considered. The recommended goals for treatment are summarized in Table 1. For patients who cannot tolerate one specific statin because of myopathy, it may be appropriate to try pravastatin (Pravachol), which has a lower risk of myopathy. For patients who cannot tolerate statins, a combination of other agents can be started, and the patient can be referred to a lipid specialist.

STATINS

Statins have been in clinical use for more than 2 decades. They work through inhibition of HMG-CoA reductase, the rate-limiting enzyme in cholesterol biosynthesis. Among all lipid-lowering agents, statins achieve the highest degree of LDL reduction. In addition to decreasing cholesterol biosynthesis, statins also increase the clearance of IDL and LDL by upregulation of LDL receptors on hepatocytes.

Stimulation of Apo AI expression and increased hepatic HDL secretion have also been observed. In addition to their direct effects on lipid homeostasis, statins have been reported to have other, largely beneficial pleiotropic effects, which are thought to involve reductions in a wide range of atherogenic events (e.g., reduced formation of reactive oxygen species, inhibition of platelet reactivity, decreased vasoconstriction).

Statins are the only class of lipid-lowering agents that have been shown in multiple randomized clinical trials to have a direct effect on, and to produce clear improvement in, overall mortality in primary and secondary prevention. Statins decreased rates of myocardial infarction, stroke, coronary mortality, and all-cause mortality in both primary and secondary prevention studies. Furthermore, risk reduction was apparent in a wide range of patients, including men, women, smokers, patients with diabetes, and those with hypertension, as well as in older populations.

Atorvastatin (Lipitor) and rosuvastatin (Crestor) are the most potent statins. They cause an LDL reduction of 60% at doses of 80 and 40 mg/day, respectively. These agents also have the advantage of decreasing triglyceride levels. Rosuvastatin increases HDL cholesterol levels better than atorvastatin, simvastatin (Zocor), or pravastatin (Pravachol).

Statins are well tolerated, and usually they are taken in tablet form once daily. Potential common side effects include nonspecific gastrointestinal side effects such as dyspepsia. Headaches, fatigue, and muscle or joint pain have also been reported. Two important, albeit rare, side effects about which the patient should be informed are myopathy and hepatitis; the physician should monitor for these effects. Myopathy risk is increased in patients with renal insufficiency and in those who are taking multiple agents because of drug interactions. Commonly used drugs that can decrease statin metabolism include erythromycin, antifungal agents, immunosuppressive agents, and fibrates.

The risk of hepatotoxicity is less than 1%, and that of myopathy is less than 0.1%. Patients should be advised to report muscle pain of unexplained origin, and creatine kinase (CK) should be measured. Patients who develop muscle pain and CK elevations 10 times the upper limit of normal should be taken off the statin. CK elevations that are between 3 and 10 times the upper limit of normal require close clinical and biochemical monitoring. It is therefore valuable to determine a baseline CK level at initiation of therapy; however, serial CK measurements are of limited value, because myopathy and rhabdomyolysis can occur suddenly without antecedent CK elevation. The potential for hepatotoxicity does require follow-up of liver transaminases (alanine and aspartate aminotransferase) before the start of treatment, at 2 months, and every 6 months thereafter. Substantial elevation (>3 times the upper limit of normal) should prompt discontinuation. Severe elevations are very rare and resolve after discontinuation of the drug. When using statins in combination with a fibrate, especially in patients with elevations in both cholesterol and triglycerides, it is advisable to use lower doses of the statin.

EZETIMIBE

Ezetimibe (Zetia) is the first in a new class of agents that act through inhibition of absorption of sterol transporters in the gut lumen. LDL reduction is approximately 15% when the drug is used

TABLE 2 Major Drugs for Management of Dyslipidemia

Drug	Indications	Dose (Starting-Maximum)	Mechanism	Side Effects
Statins				
Atorvastatin (Lipitor)	Elevated LDL	10–80 mg qhs	Decreased cholesterol synthesis, increased hepatic LDL receptors, decreased VLDL release	Myalgias Arthralgias High liver enzymes Dyspepsia
Fluvastatin (Lescol)		20–80 mg qhs		
Lovastatin (Mevacor)		20–80 mg daily		
Pravastatin (Pravachol)		40–80 mg qhs		
Rosuvastatin (Crestor)		10–40 mg qhs		
Simvastatin (Zocor)		20–80 mg qhs		
Cholesterol Absorption Inhibitors				
Ezetimibe (Zetia)	Elevated LDL	10 mg daily	Decreased intestinal cholesterol absorption	High liver enzymes
Bile Acid Sequestrants				
Cholestyramine (Questran)	Elevated LDL	4–32 g daily	Increased bile acid excretion, increased LDL receptors	Bloating Constipation Elevated triglycerides
Colestipol (Colestid)		5–40 g daily		
Colesevelam (Welchol)		3750–4375 mg daily		
Fibrates				
Fenofibrate (Tricor)	Elevated TG Elevated remnants	160 mg daily 50–160 mg daily	Increased LPL activity, decreased VLDL synthesis	Dyspepsia, myalgia, gallstones, high liver enzymes
Gemfibrozil (Lopid)		600 mg bid		
Other				
Niacin (Niaspan, generic)	Elevated LDL, low HDL, elevated TG	100 mg-2g tid (rapid tab) 0.5–2 g qhs (ER tab, Niaspan)	Decreased VLDL synthesis	Flushing, high glucose, uric acid, liver enzymes
Fish oils (omega-3 fatty acids,[7] omega-3 acid ethyl esters [Lovaza])	Severely elevated TG	3–12 g daily 4 g daily (Lovaza)	Decreased chylomicron	Dyspepsia

[7]Available as dietary supplement.
Abbreviations: ER, extended release; LDL, low-density lipoprotein; LPL, lipoprotein lipase; TG, triglycerides; VLDL, very-low-density lipoprotein.

as monotherapy. Ezetimibe may be considered a good agent to add to statin therapy in a patient not achieving goal levels. As an added benefit, it may be possible to use a lower dose of statin and reduce potential statin toxicity. A recent study raised the issue of ezetimibe effectiveness in reducing adverse cardiovascular events; this should be resolved by ongoing research on this relatively new medication.

BILE ACID–BINDING RESINS

This class of agents has been in clinical use for many decades. They work by binding to bile acids in the intestine and promoting their fecal excretion. This causes the liver to integrate more cholesterol into bile acid synthesis, so as to maintain a stable bile acid pool. The consequent decrease in hepatic cholesterol causes LDL receptor upregulation and enhances LDL clearance from the plasma, leading to a net decrease in LDL levels. LDL can decrease 15% to 30%, and HDL can go up 3% to 5%. HMG CoA synthase activity can increase, so combination therapy with statin would be synergistic, especially in patients with a suboptimal response.

Available agents are colestipol (Colestid), cholestyramine (Questran), and colesevelam (Welchol). Most side effects involve the gastrointestinal tract, with constipation and bloating being the most common. These agents may interfere with the absorption of warfarin (Coumadin), phenobarbital, levothyroxine (Synthroid), and digoxin (Lanoxin), among other medications. Patients on multiple medications should be advised to take bile acid–binding resins 1 hour before or 4 hours after their other medications.

Because these drugs are not systemically absorbed, they may be preferred when systemic absorption is to be avoided, such as during pregnancy or lactation.

FIBRATES

Fibrates are effective in lowering plasma triglyceride levels; they are especially valuable in patients who have a combination of high triglycerides and low HDL. The Veterans Affairs High-Density Lipoprotein Intervention Trial (VA-HIT), one of the early secondary prevention lipid-lowering studies, showed that men with coronary artery disease and low HDL who were treated with gemfibrozil (Lopid) experienced a 6% increase in HDL and a 31% decrease in triglycerides, with no change in LDL, compared with similar subjects treated with placebo; there was also a 22% decrease in all-cause mortality and nonfatal myocardial infarction. Fibrates have multiple favorable metabolic effects, including activation of peroxisome proliferator–activated receptor-α (PPARα) (which contributes to the regulation of both lipid and carbohydrate metabolism), stimulation of lipoprotein lipase (increasing triglyceride hydrolysis), and downregulation of Apo CIII (improved lipoprotein remnant clearance, because Apo CIII inhibits lipoprotein lipase). An enhanced VLDL-to-LDL conversion may lead to mild LDL elevation in some patients. This effect may decrease over weeks as LDL receptor upregulation occurs.

Fibrates are generally well tolerated. The most common side effect is dyspepsia. Other side effects include low rates of myopathy and hepatic enzyme elevation. Fibrates increase the risk of gallstones, and patients on warfarin may need dose adjustment. Monitoring of liver enzymes is recommended every 6 months.

Patients with high triglycerides should start with a low-fat diet and a fibrate. Patients, especially those with familial high triglycerides, may benefit from the addition of orlistat (Xenical, Alli),[1] a pancreatic lipase inhibitor that decreases fat digestion and absorption, or omega-3 fatty acids,[7] or both.

[1]Not FDA approved for this indication.
[7]Available as dietary supplement.

NIACIN

Niacin or nicotinic acid (Niaspan, generic) is a B_3 vitamin that effectively increases HDL levels by blocking HDL uptake by the liver. Hepatic VLDL secretion is decreased due to inhibition of flux from adipocytes to the liver and inhibition of diacylglyceryl acyl transferase in the liver. It also increases Apo B100 catabolism. In the HDL Atherosclerosis Study (HATS), high-dose niacin combined with statins decreased cardiovascular mortality.

Patient education and monitoring of therapy are key to successful treatment with niacin. The most common side effect is flushing. This can be avoided or improved by initiating therapy with a low dose of niacin, taking an aspirin 1 hour before niacin, and avoiding hot foods or beverages at the time the niacin is taken. Other side effects include pruritus and increased uric acid levels. Mild elevations in liver enzymes can occur in 15% of subjects and rarely require discontinuation of the niacin.

REFERENCES

Ballantyne CM. Treatment of dyslipidemia to reduce cardiovascular risk in patients with multiple risk factors. Clin Cornerstone 2007;8(Suppl. 6):S6–13.

Ballantyne CM, Grundy SM, Oberman A, et al. Hyperlipidemia: Diagnostic and therapeutic perspectives. J Clin Endocrinol Metab 2000;85:2089–112.

Broedl UC, Geiss HC, Parhofer KG. Comparison of current guidelines for primary prevention of coronary heart disease. J Gen Intern Med 2003;18:190–5.

Grundy SM, Balady GJ, Criqui MH, et al. When to start cholesterol-lowering therapy in patients with coronary heart disease: A statement for healthcare professionals from the American Heart Association Task Force on Risk Reduction. Circulation 1997;95:1683–5.

Jones P, Kafonek S, Laurora I, et al. for the CURVES investigators: Comparative dose efficacy study of atorvastatin versus simvastatin, pravastatin, lovastatin, and fluvastatin in patients with hypercholesterolemia. Am J Cardiol 1998;81:582–7.

Otvos JD, Collins D, Freedman DS, et al. Low-density lipoprotein and high-density lipoprotein particle subclasses predict coronary events and are favorably changed by gemfibrozil therapy in the Veterans Affairs High–Density Lipoprotein Intervention Trial. Circulation 2006;113:1556–63.

Probstfield JL, Hunninghake DB. Nicotinic acid as a lipoprotein-altering agent: Therapy directed by the primary physician. Arch Intern Med 1994;154:1557–9.

Randomised trial of cholesterol lowering in 4444 patients with coronary heart disease: The Scandinavian Simvastatin Survival Study (4S). Lancet 1994;344:1383–9.

Sacks FM, Pfeffer MA, Moye LA, et al. The effect of pravastatin on coronary events after myocardial infarction in patients with average cholesterol levels: Cholesterol And Recurrent Events trial investigators. N Engl J Med 1996;335:1001–9.

Shepherd J, Cobbe SM, Ford I, et al. Prevention of coronary heart disease with pravastatin in men with hypercholesterolemia. N Engl J Med 1995;33:1301–7.

Third Report of the National Cholesterol Education Program (NCEP) Expert panel on detection, evaluation and treatment of high blood cholesterol in adults (Adult Treatment Panel III). Circulation 2002;106:3143–421.

Wilson PW. Established risk factors and coronary artery disease: The Framingham Study. Am J Hypertens 1994;7(7 Pt 2):7S–12S.

Obesity

Method of
Nicole Nader, MD, and Seema Kumar, MD

Epidemiology

Obesity is a complex disease that represents a growing epidemic in the United States and worldwide. According to current estimates, more than 33.5% of adult men, 35.3% of adult women, and 16.3% of children and adolescents age 2 to 19 years in the United States are obese. Between 1976–1980 and 2003–2004, the prevalence of obesity among adults almost doubled. There are disparities in the prevalence of obesity between ethnic groups, especially among women. In the United States, the prevalence of obesity is highest in non-Hispanic black women. Obesity is no longer a cosmetic issue; it has been found to be associated with several comorbidities and increased mortality.

Diagnosis

Obesity is a condition marked by the accumulation of excess body fat. The body mass index (BMI) is the most practical way to evaluate the degree of excess weight. It is calculated from the weight (in kilograms) and the square of the height (in meters), as follows:

$$BMI = Weight \div Height^2$$

The World Health Organisation (WHO) and National Institutes of Health (NIH) define overweight as BMI between 25 and 24.9 kg/m^2 and obesity as a BMI greater than 30 kg/m^2 (Table 1). These guidelines apply to whites, Hispanics, and blacks. Because Asians can have higher percentage of body fat at a lower BMI, overweight for this particular ethnic group is a BMI between 23 and 29.9 kg/m^2, and obesity is a BMI equal to or greater than 30 kg/m^2. Because BMI normative values are age and gender specific during childhood, BMI values greater than or equal to the 95th percentile for age and sex are used to define obesity in children and adolescents. The BMI correlates with percentage of body fat and body fat mass, as well as with mortality. However, for a given BMI, the degree of body fatness tends to be higher in women compared with men, and it is higher in older compared with younger people. Additionally, the BMI may overestimate the degree of body fat in athletes. The relationship between BMI and mortality appears to form a J- or U-shaped curve, with the lowest mortality rate seen in those with a BMI of about 25 kg/m^2 (Fig. 1).

Because people with abdominal (central) adiposity are more likely to develop many of the health conditions associated with obesity, waist circumference is an important adjuvant measurement to obtain when screening for obesity. Waist circumference is measured at the level of the top of the iliac crest with the measuring tape snug against the skin. A waist circumference of more than 102 cm (40 in) in men or 88 cm (35 in) in women is considered high and confers an increased risk for comorbidities such as type 2 diabetes, hypertension, and coronary heart disease (see Table 1). More precise measurement of abdominal fat can be made with abdominal computed tomography or magnetic resonance imaging. Alternative methods to assess body composition and degree of fatness include measurements of skin fold thickness, hydrostatic weighing, bioelectric impedance, and scanning by dual-energy x-ray absorptiometry (DEXA). These methods require specialized equipment and trained personnel, and they are not used routinely in clinical practice.

CURRENT DIAGNOSIS

- Body Mass Index (BMI) is calculated as weight in kilograms divided by height in meters squared (kg/m^2). BMI is currently the preferred method for determining whether a patient is obese.
- Patients with a BMI of 30 or greater are considered obese.
- Abdominal circumference should also be measured when screening for obesity.
- A waist circumference of greater than 102 cm (40 in) in men or 88 cm (35 in) in women is considered indicative of abdominal obesity.

TABLE 1 Classification of Overweight and Obesity by BMI, Waist Circumference, and Associated Health Risk

| Classification | BMI (kg/m²) | Disease Risk* | |
		Waist ≤102 cm (≤40 in) in men or ≤88 cm (≤35 in) in women	Waist >102 cm (>40 in) in men or >88 cm (>35 in) in women
Underweight	<18.5	—	—
Normal†	18.5–24.9	—	—
Overweight	25.0–29.9	Increased	High
Obesity—class I	30.0–34.9	High	Very high
Obesity—class II	35.0–39.9	Very high	Very high
Extreme obesity—class III	>40	Extremely high	Extremely high

Reproduced from Clinical Guidelines on the Identification, Evaluation, and Treatment of Overweight and Obesity in Adults: The Evidence Report. National Institutes of Health. Obes Res 1998;6(Suppl 2):51S-209S.
*Disease risk for type 2 diabetes, hypertension, and cardiovascular disease relative to normal weight and waist circumference.
†Increased waist circumference can also be a marker for increased risk even in persons of normal weight.

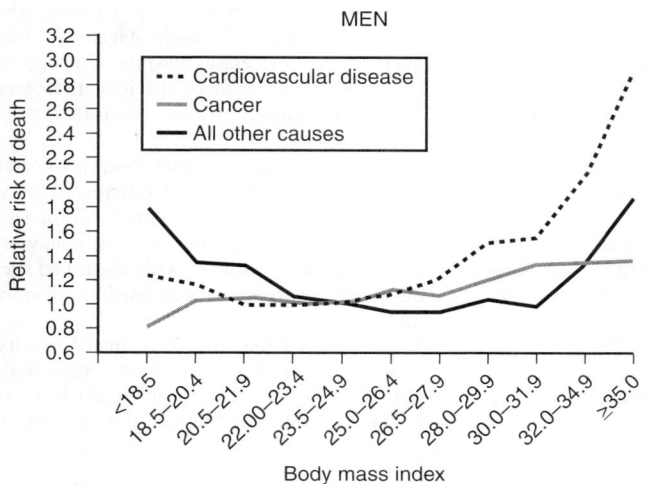

MEN

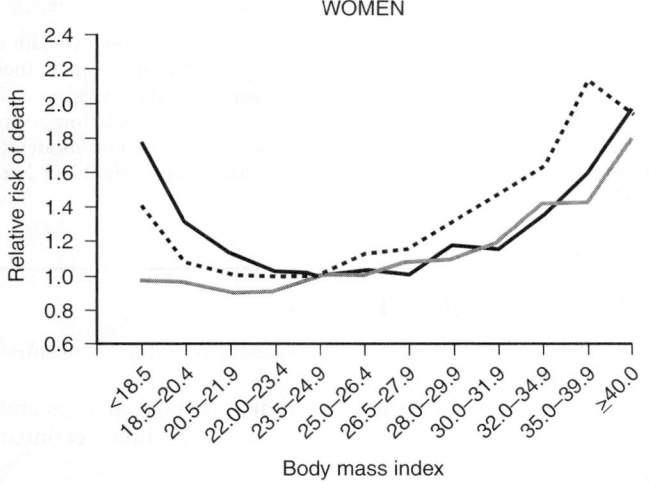

WOMEN

FIGURE 1. Correlation between mortality risk and increasing body mass index. (Data from Calle EE, Thun MJ, Petrelli JM, et al: Body-mass index and mortality in a prospective cohort of U.S. adults. N Engl J Med 1999;341:1097–1105.)

Etiology and Pathophysiology

Obesity is a complex, multifactorial disease characterized by excessive caloric consumption and inadequate caloric expenditure. Many factors, including genetic and environmental influences, can contribute

TABLE 2 Medications That May Promote Weight Gain

Drug Class	Examples
Antipsychotics	Risperidone (Risperdal), olanzapine (Zyprexa), clozapine (Clozaril)
Antidepressants	Imipramine (Tofranil), amitriptyline (Elavil), doxepin (Sinequan), tranylcypromine (Parnate)
Lithium	
Anticonvulsants	Valproic acid (Depakene), carbamazepine (Tegretol)
Antidiabetics	Insulin, rosiglitazone (Avandia), pioglitazone (Actos), glipizide (Glucotrol), glyburide (Diabeta, Micronase), glimepiride (Amaryl)
Antihistamines	Diphenhydramine (Benadryl)
α-Blockers	Doxazosin (Cardura), prazosin (Minipress), terazosin (Hytrin)
Steroids	Glucocorticoids
β-Blockers	Propranolol (Inderal), metoprolol (Lopressor), atenolol (Tenormin)

to the development of obesity. However, personal decisions regarding food choices, portion sizes, and level of activity also contribute to body size.

When evaluating a patient with obesity, it is important to rule out disorders such as Cushing's syndrome and hypothyroidism. Because many medications promote weight gain, including several antipsychotics, antidepressants, antiepileptics, sulfonylureas, and steroids (Table 2), it is prudent to obtain a complete medication history from any patient who is being evaluated for obesity. Single-gene mutations (e.g., in the leptin gene) and congenital syndromes (e.g., Prader-Willi, Bardet-Biedel, Cohen) typically cause early-onset obesity before 5 years of age.

Associated Comorbidities

Obesity is associated with a variety of other medical conditions that can increase morbidity and mortality. Comorbidities associated with obesity include metabolic syndrome and insulin resistance, type 2 diabetes, dyslipidemia, hypertension, coronary artery disease, degenerative joint disease, nonalcoholic fatty liver disease (NAFLD), and obstructive sleep apnea.

INSULIN RESISTANCE AND METABOLIC SYNDROME

Insulin resistance is defined as a subnormal response to endogenous insulin. This results in pancreatic B-cell compensation with hypersecretion of insulin. Insulin resistance leads to various components of the metabolic syndrome, including low HDL cholesterol, high trigly-cerides, elevated blood pressure, and hyperglycemia. Patients may also manifest acanthosis nigricans and skin tags.

TYPE 2 DIABETES

The increasing prevalence of obesity has resulted in an increasing prevalence of type 2 diabetes as well. More than 80% of type 2 diabetes can be attributed to obesity, but other factors, such as family history, are also involved. Criteria for diagnosis of type 2 diabetes include a fasting glucose level greater than 125 mg/dL or glucose levels greater than 200 mg/dL during a 2-hour oral glucose tolerance test.

HYPERTENSION

Hypertension is a common chronic disease, and it has been estimated that obesity is associated with approximately 30% to 50% of the cases of hypertension in the United States. Hypertension is associated with an increased risk for stroke, myocardial infarction, heart failure, and kidney disease. Even a modest weight loss (5%–10% of initial weight) can lead to a significant fall in blood pressure and, often, decreased need for antihypertensive medications.

DYSLIPIDEMIA

A variety of blood lipid abnormalities are seen frequently in obese patients. These include elevated levels of total cholesterol, LDL cholesterol, and triglycerides and decreased levels of HDL cholesterol. Patients with central adiposity are at particularly high risk for the development of hypertriglyceridemia and low HDL. Screening for dyslipidemia should be done with a fasting lipid profile. However, if the testing opportunity is nonfasting, the total cholesterol and HDL values can still be measured.

CORONARY HEART DISEASE

Comorbidities associated with obesity such as hypertension, insulin resistance, type 2 diabetes, and dyslipidemia lead to increased risk of cardiovascular disease in obese adults. Obesity is also associated with increased risk of coronary heart disease, heart failure, cardiovascular mortality, and all-cause mortality.

RESPIRATORY ABNORMALITIES

Obstructive sleep apnea is the most important respiratory problem associated with obesity. It is often underrecognized and inadequately treated. Patients may present with snoring, apneic episodes, excessive daytime somnolence, fatigue, irritability, and erectile dysfunction. Consequent nocturnal hypoxemia may result in arrhythmias, pulmonary hypertension, and right-sided heart failure. Treatment includes weight loss and use of continuous positive airway pressure at night.

HEPATOBILIARY DISEASE

Obesity increases the risk of cholelithiasis and of NAFLD. The spectrum of NAFLD ranges from steatosis with mild disruption of the liver architecture by fat to steatohepatitis with varying degrees of fibrosis and cirrhosis. Increased liver transaminase levels and findings of steatosis on ultrasonography are both suggestive of NAFLD in obese patients. However, the definitive diagnosis remains histologic.

OSTEOARTHRITIS

The incidence of osteoarthritis is increased in obese subjects. Osteoarthritis commonly develops in the knees and ankles but can also affect non–weight-bearing joints. Weight loss results in decreased risk of osteoarthritis.

CANCER

For both men and women, increased BMI is associated with increased mortality from several cancers, such as those of the esophagus, colon and rectum, liver, gallbladder, pancreas, kidney, as well as non-Hodgkin's lymphoma and multiple myeloma. Additionally, obese men are at increased risk of death from stomach and prostate cancer, and obese women are at increased risk of death from cancers of the breast, uterus, cervix, and ovary.

Treatment

Patients must undergo a detailed history and physical examination before a treatment plan is initiated. Secondary causes of obesity, such as Cushing's syndrome and hypothyroidism, should be considered in the evaluation. A complete medication history is crucial to determining whether any medications may have promoted weight gain.

Laboratory studies should be directed at ruling out secondary causes in selected patients and ruling out comorbidities (fasting glucose, lipid profile, liver function tests). It is important that practitioners assess each patient's willingness to change and expectations for weight loss. Treatment should be based on the patient's BMI, risk factors, and willingness to lose weight (Fig. 2). Patients who are in the precontemplative phase (i.e., in the early stages of thinking about it) are not likely to be successful despite appropriate counseling. Health care providers must enforce the idea that even a modest weight loss improves complications associated with obesity.

Treatment of obesity requires a multidisciplinary team approach. Lifestyle modifications, including dietary change and increased physical activity, represent first-line treatment for patients with obesity. Self-efficacy, which is a feeling of being able to perform the behaviors required, and positive coping skills are associated with improved success. Pharmacotherapy and bariatric surgery may be used as adjuvant therapies in certain patients.

The goal of treatment is to prevent the complications of obesity. The initial target goal of weight loss therapy is to decrease body weight by 10%. Once this target is achieved, further weight loss can be attempted if indicated. The rationales for this initial goal of moderate weight loss are that:

- It can decrease the severity of obesity-associated risk factors.
- It can set the stage for further weight loss, if indicated.
- It is realistic and can be achieved and maintained over time.

A reasonable timeline for a 10% reduction in body weight is 6 months of therapy. A period of weight maintenance should then occur. Further weight loss may be considered if the initial goal is achieved and then maintained for at least 6 months. It is important to inform patients that it is preferable to maintain a moderate amount of weight loss over time than to lose more weight but later regain it.

CURRENT THERAPY

- Treatment of patients with obesity requires a multidisciplinary team approach.
- Lifestyle modifications, including dietary changes and increased physical activity, remain first-line treatment for patients with obesity.
- Adjuvant pharmacotherapy may be considered for patients with a BMI greater than 30 kg/m^2 or a BMI of 27 to 30 kg/m^2 with concomitant weight-related complications.
- Bariatric surgery should be considered for patients with a BMI of 40 kg/m^2 or greater and for those with a BMI of 35 kg/m^2 or greater who have significant comorbidities such as severe diabetes, sleep apnea, or joint disease after nonsurgical weight loss attempts have failed.

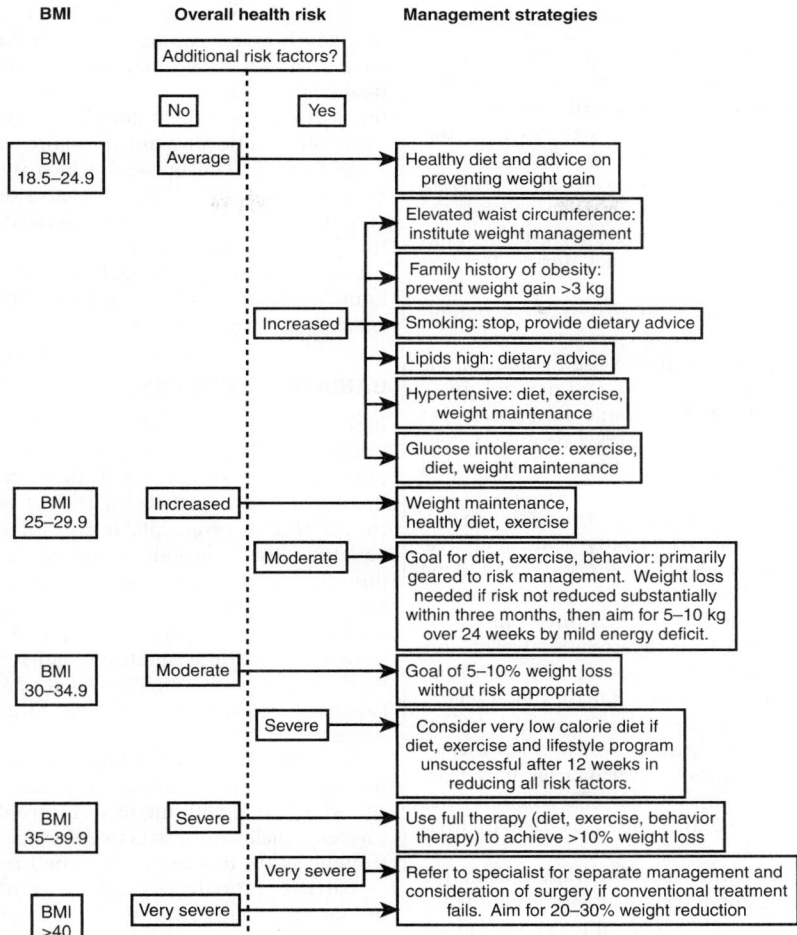

The figure columns are labeled **BMI**, **Overall health risk**, and **Management strategies**.

Additional risk factors? — No / Yes

- **BMI 18.5–24.9** — Average → Healthy diet and advice on preventing weight gain
- Increased →
  - Elevated waist circumference: institute weight management
  - Family history of obesity: prevent weight gain >3 kg
  - Smoking: stop, provide dietary advice
  - Lipids high: dietary advice
  - Hypertensive: diet, exercise, weight maintenance
  - Glucose intolerance: exercise, diet, weight maintenance
- **BMI 25–29.9** — Increased → Weight maintenance, healthy diet, exercise
- Moderate → Goal for diet, exercise, behavior: primarily geared to risk management. Weight loss needed if risk not reduced substantially within three months, then aim for 5–10 kg over 24 weeks by mild energy deficit.
- **BMI 30–34.9** — Moderate → Goal of 5–10% weight loss without risk appropriate
- Severe → Consider very low calorie diet if diet, exercise and lifestyle program unsuccessful after 12 weeks in reducing all risk factors.
- **BMI 35–39.9** — Severe → Use full therapy (diet, exercise, behavior therapy) to achieve >10% weight loss
- Very severe → Refer to specialist for separate management and consideration of surgery if conventional treatment fails. Aim for 20–30% weight reduction
- **BMI ≥40** — Very severe

FIGURE 2. Assessment of health risk and management of obesity. BMI, body mass index. (Reproduced with permission from World Health Organisation: Obesity: Preventing and managing the global epidemic. Report of a WHO consultation. World Health Organ Tech Rep Ser 2000;894: i. Copyright 2000 World Health Organisation.)

DIETARY THERAPY

Obese patients should be counseled to follow a hypocaloric and balanced meal plan. These typically provide 1200 to 1800 calories per day, with 20% to 30% of calories from fat, 50% to 55% from carbohydrates, and 15% to 20% from protein. In general, women should be advised to consume approximately 1000 to 1200 kcal/day and men 1200 to 1600 kcal/day during the weight loss phase of treatment. It has been recommended that total fat intake not exceed 30% of total daily calories, that saturated fat account for not more than 8% to 10% of total calories, and that cholesterol intake be limited to 300 mg/day. A healthy diet should also contain 20 to 30 g of fiber daily. Patients should be counseled to avoid unnecessary calories from alcohol and sugary beverages such as soda and juice. These diets result in losses of approximately 1 to 2 lb per week or 4 to 8 lb per month.

Several alternative diets have been tried over the years. Recent data suggest that the so-called Mediterranean diet and low-carbohydrate diets may represent effective alternatives to the low-fat diet for weight loss. The long-term efficacy and safety of these diets remains unknown at this time.

Very-low-calorie diets contain less than 800 kcal/day and are usually administered in the form of liquid supplements. Although these diets do produce significant and rapid weight loss, results are difficult to maintain in the long term. These diets require close monitoring by a health care professional. Side effects associated with very-low-calorie diets include fatigue, constipation, hair loss, and gallstones. These diets are strictly contraindicated in children and in pregnant and lactating women and are generally reserved for patients who require rapid weight loss for a specific purpose such as surgery.

PHYSICAL ACTIVITY

Physical activity is an integral component of therapy for obese patients and is most important in the prevention of weight regain. Physical activity also decreases the risks for cardiovascular disease and type 2 diabetes. Sedentary obese patients need to start their exercise program slowly and may require supervision from a health care professional. Initially, patients may be encouraged to increase their activities of daily living. For example, it may be suggested that they take the stairs instead of the elevator or that they park farther away from work or shopping. The intensity and duration of exercise should be increased gradually over time, with a goal of achieving 150 minutes of moderate-intensity aerobic activity (e.g., brisk walking) or 75 minutes of vigorous-intensity exercise (e.g., running) every week. It is acceptable to achieve these goals by breaking up the time into smaller chunks of at least 10 minutes per session.

Ideally, adults should also perform muscle strengthening exercises on two or more days per week. Patients should be encouraged to choose activities that they enjoy and to build these activities into their daily schedule. Sedentary activities, such as watching television, sitting in front of a computer screen, and playing video games, should be discouraged.

BEHAVIOR MODIFICATION

Behavior modification is an integral part of any weight loss program. This requires the availability of trained personnel such as psychologists and therapists. The behavioral strategies taught are aimed at decreasing caloric intake and increasing physical activity in the long term.

PHARMACOTHERAPY

Pharmacotherapy (Table 3) is usually reserved for patients with a BMI greater than 30 kg/m² without complications or a BMI greater than 27 to 30 kg/m² with concomitant weight-related complications. Pharmacotherapy typically is initiated if the patient has been unsuccessful in attaining goal weight loss after 6 months of lifestyle modifications, but it must be used in conjunction with a program that includes dietary changes and physical activity. In general, the use of medication promotes only a modest weight loss, in the range of 2 to 10 kg. The effects are generally maximal during the first 6 months of therapy.

Sibutramine is an anorexiant medication that inhibits norepinephrine, serotonin, and, to a lesser degree, dopamine reuptake into nerve terminals. Side effects associated with the use of sibutramine include increases in systolic and diastolic blood pressure and pulse. In October 2010, the manufacturer of sibutramine announced that the drug was being withdrawn from the U.S. market because of concerns about minimal efficacy and increased risk for heart attacks and stokes.

Orlistat alters fat absorption by inhibiting pancreatic lipases. Ingested fat is not completely hydrolyzed to fatty acids, and fecal fat excretion increases. The recommended dose for adults is 120 mg PO three times daily with meals. There is also an over-the-counter preparation (Alli), for which the dose is 60 mg PO three times daily with meals. Orlistat has been shown to be effective for weight loss and prevention of weight regain. Side effects associated with orlistat are mostly gastrointestinal and include cramping, flatus, fecal incontinence, oily spotting, and flatus with discharge. These side effects tend to decrease over time as patients learn to restrict their dietary intake to less than 30% fat. Severe cases of liver damage have been reported in patients taking orlistat. Orlistat may also interfere with the absorption of fat-soluble vitamins, so the use of a daily multivitamin supplement is recommended.

Other medications approved for weight loss therapy include the sympathomimetics phentermine (Adipex) and diethylpropion (Tenuate); however, these medications have the potential for abuse and are approved only for short-term use. The use of ephedra[2] with or without caffeine is not approved for the treatment of obesity.

---

[2]Not available in the United States.

Although not approved by the FDA, antidepressants such as fluoxetine (Prozac), sertraline (Zoloft), and bupropion (Wellbutrin) have been used to promote weight loss. The use of these drugs for treatment of obesity is not recommended; however, they may be the preferred treatment for depression in obese patients, because many other antidepressants promote weight gain.

Metformin (Glucophage), which is used for treatment of insulin resistance and type 2 diabetes, also tends to promote weight loss and may be preferable to other antidiabetic medications, which tend to result in weight gain. Many over-the-counter dietary and herbal supplements are also available to obese patients. However, there are limited efficacy and safety data to support their use, and they are generally not recommended.

BARIATRIC SURGERY

Bariatric surgery should be considered for patients with a BMI greater than 40 kg/m² or a BMI greater than 35 kg/m² with significant comorbid conditions. Patients should be well informed and motivated and have failed a trial of nonsurgical weight loss. They should also be of acceptable risk for surgery. Contraindications to bariatric surgery include untreated major depression, binge eating disorders, active drug or alcohol abuse, and a history of noncompliance. A comprehensive preoperative evaluation and close extended follow-up after surgery are required. Bariatric surgery has been shown to result in a significant and sustained weight loss, as well as resolution of many obesity-related complications, in most patients. Patients may lose more than 60% of their excess weight after bariatric surgery.

Bariatric surgery for children and adolescents remains highly controversial. However, surgery on patients between 12 and 18 years of age who had significant medical problems related to their obesity (diabetes mellitus, obstructive sleep apnea, reactive airway disease, steatohepatitis, metabolic syndrome) resolved their comorbidities.

Bariatric procedures can be divided into three types: restrictive procedures, which decrease gastric volume and limit food intake; malabsorptive procedures, which alter digestion of food and decrease the effectiveness of nutrient absorption; and mixed procedures, which have components of both restriction and malabsorption. Currently, the most common procedures performed in the United States are the Roux-en-Y gastric bypass (a mixed procedure) and the laparoscopic adjustable band (a restrictive procedure) (Fig. 3).

Roux-en-Y Gastric Bypass

A Roux-en-Y bypass is performed by making a small pouch at the superior portion of the stomach. The pouch is then connected to the jejunum, bypassing the duodenum, where the majority of calories are absorbed. Roux-en-Y bypasses are now being performed laparoscopically at several centers. The mortality rate associated with gastric bypass is low (<1%), but patients can have significant postoperative complications, including pulmonary emboli, deep vein thromboses, leaks from the gastrointestinal tract, gastric remnant distention, stomal stenosis, ulcers, gallstones, and hernias. Patients are required to take lifelong vitamin and mineral supplementation, because absorption of iron, vitamin B_{12}/folate, and others are affected.

Laparoscopic Adjustable Gastric Band

The vertical-banded gastroplasty was the restrictive procedure performed routinely in the past (see Fig. 3). It is not routinely performed any longer and has been superceded by the laparoscopic adjustable band. An adjustable band is placed around the entrance to the stomach. The band is connected to an infusion port that is placed in the subcutaneous tissue. The port can be accessed with a needle and syringe, and injection or removal of saline into the port may be used to manipulate the size of the band diameter, leading to greater or lesser degrees of restriction. Although weight loss with banding tends to be slower than with other weight loss procedures, the procedure is popular because it is performed laparoscopically and is reversible. The band is currently not approved by the FDA

TABLE 3 Drugs Approved by the FDA for Treatment of Obesity

Drug	Trade Names	Dosage
Pancreatic Lipase Inhibitor Approved for Long-Term Use		
Orlistat	Xenical	120 mg tid before meals
Noradrenergic Drugs Approved for Short-Term Use		
Phentermine	Adipex	15–37.5 mg/d
	Ionamin (slow-release resin)	15–30 mg/d
Diethylpropion	Tenuate	25 mg tid
	Tenuate Dospan	75 mg every morning
Benzphetamine	Didrex	25–50 mg tid
Phendimetrazine	Bontril	17.5–70 mg tid
	Prelu-2	105 mg/d

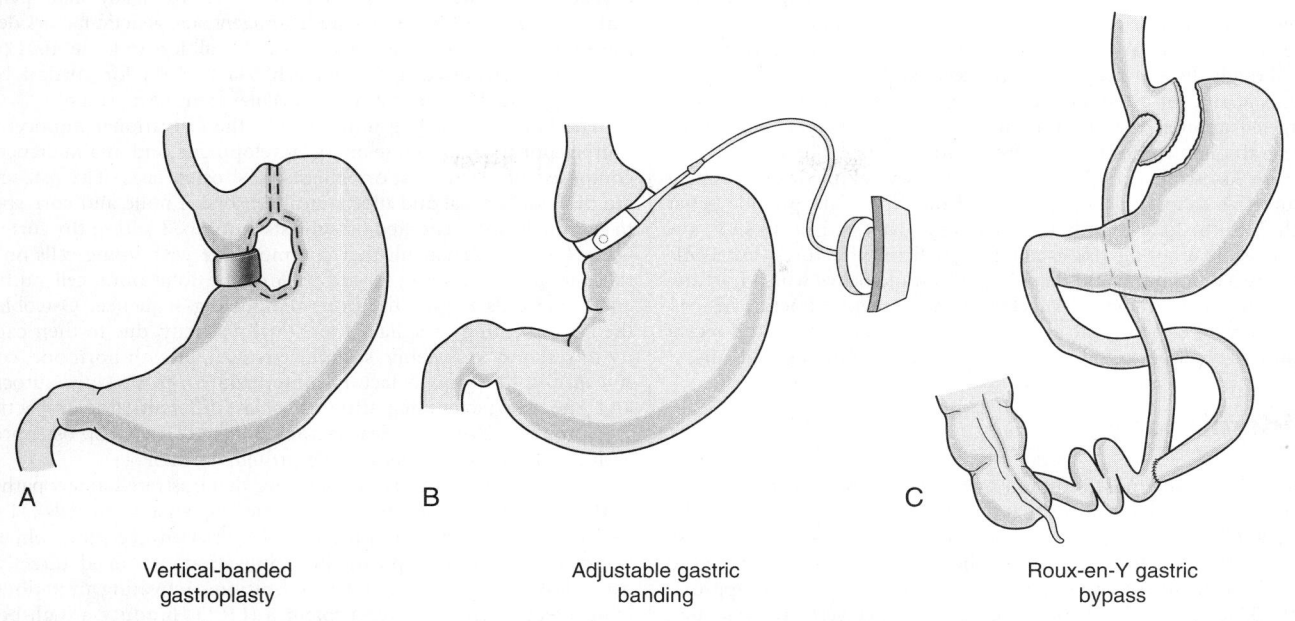

FIGURE 3. Techniques commonly used for the surgical treatment of obesity: vertical-banded gastroplasty (**A**), adjustable laparoscopic band (**B**), Roux-en-Y gastric bypass (**C**).

for adolescents younger than 18 years of age. Laparoscopic banding can also be associated with side effects such as stomal obstruction; band erosion, slippage, or prolapse; port malfunction, pouch or esophageal dilation; and infection.

Future Directions

Many genes, gene products, and hormones such as leptin,[5] peptide YY, and melanocortin 4 receptors that potentially have a role in the development of obesity have been identified. These discoveries point to potentially novel therapies for obesity.

In conclusion, obesity is a growing public health problem that has significant short- and long-term consequences. Lifestyle modification with or without adjuvant therapies should be used to achieve a goal of modest weight loss. With modest weight loss, patients experience a decreased risk of mortality and improvement of obesity-related complications.

---

[5]Investigational drug in the United States.

REFERENCES

Apovain C. The medical management of obesity and the role of pharmacotherapy: An update. Nutr Clin Pract 2000;15:5–12.

Aronne LJ. Classification of obesity and assessment of obesity-related health risks. Obes Res 2002;10:105S–115S.

Buchwald H, Avidor Y, Braunwald E, et al. Bariatric surgery: A systematic review and meta-analysis. JAMA 2004;292(14):1724–37.

Hedley AA, Ogden CL, Johnson CL, et al. Prevalence of overweight and obesity among US children, adolescents, and adults, 1999–2002. JAMA 2004;291:2847–50.

National Institutes of Health; National Heart, Lung and Blood Institute: North American Association for the Study of Obesity. The Practical Guide to the Identification, Evaluation, and Treatment of Overweight and Obesity in Adults. Bethesda, Md: National Institutes of Health; 2000. Available at http://www.nhlbi.nih.gov/guidelines/obesity/ob_home.htm [accessed June 30, 2009].

Yanovski SZ, Yanovski JA. Obesity. N Engl J Med 2002;346:591–602.

Osteoporosis

Method of
Francisco J.A. de Paula, MD, PhD,* and
Clifford J. Rosen, MD

The World Health Organization (WHO) defines osteoporosis as a systemic skeletal disease characterized by low bone mass and micro-architectural deterioration of bone tissue with a consequent increase in bone fragility and susceptibility to fracture. Its clinical importance rests not only with emerging fracture rates in developing countries but also the associated morbidity and mortality associated with these occurrences. The signs and symptoms of osteoporosis such as back pain, height loss, and thoracic kyphosis are usually late manifestations of previous unrecognized vertebral fractures but are also important risk indicators for future fractures. The overwhelming challenge to primary care clinicians is to develop methods to accurately identify patients at the highest risk for fracture before the onset of clinical manifestations and to target those who would benefit the most from a preventive or therapeutic intervention.

The WHO has further defined osteoporosis as a condition in which a bone mineral density (BMD) is less than −2.5 standard deviations (SD) below normal peak bone masses assessed by dual energy X-ray absorptiometry (DEXA). Osteopenia, which signifies a milder degree of bone loss, is defined as a T-score between −1.0 and −2.5 SD. Although the risk of fracture increases significantly with decreasing BMD, large observational studies have demonstrated that osteoporotic fractures can occur across a wide spectrum of BMDs. In all probability, these events are related not only to bone quantity but also to bone quality, a component not captured by DEXA measurements. Qualitative determinants of bone strength include trabecular perforation, microcracks, mineralization defects,

---

*Francisco J.A. de Paula receives financial support from the National Council for Scientific and Technological Development (CNPq, Brazil), 201650/2008-8.

bone geometry, cell death, changes in bone size, and changes in bone turnover. Thus, even though low BMD defines osteoporosis, this diagnosis should not be excluded in susceptible persons, particularly those with a personal or family history of a fragility fracture.

Although there is no universally accepted policy for screening for patients at risk for osteoporotic fracture, some guidelines recommend a targeted approach to the prevention of osteoporosis based on the 10-year absolute risk of major osteoporotic fracture. The FRAX (Fracture Risk Assessment) tool, which considers several major independent fracture risk factors, including BMD of the hip, might provide better insight into the long-term fracture risk of a given patient. In sum, low bone mass is a strong risk factor for predicting fractures, but BMD values are a continuum and there is no threshold below which fractures occur. Other independent risk factors such as previous fracture history, age older than 65 years, glucocorticoid use, alcohol abuse, and recent weight loss must be considered in the clinical evaluation of patients.

Epidemiology

Osteoporosis is the most common metabolic disorder of the skeleton. Worldwide, 200 million women suffer from osteoporosis, with a lifetime risk of fracture between 30% and 40%. In men, the lifetime risk of osteoporotic fracture is currently about 13%, but it is projected to rise with an increased life expectancy. In the United States, approximately 350,000 hip fractures, close to 1 million vertebral fractures, and 200,000 wrist fractures occur every year. Population-based surveys show a bimodal curve for the incidence of fracture, with the peaks occurring in adolescents and in elders. The former represents the occurrence of long bone fractures associated with trauma in young subjects. The latter peak clearly reflects the weakening process that takes place in the skeleton during aging. After the fourth decade, fracture rates in women are twice that in men. In addition, hip fracture has a seasonal influence, with an increase during winter months in temperate countries. Ethnicity also influences the incidence of skeletal failure: adult African Americans have fewer fractures than whites or Asians.

Risk Factors

Assessment of fracture risk should be part of the clinical evaluation of persons older than 50 years. Several clinical risk factors for osteoporosis have been identified and should be considered on routine patient visits. Nonmodifiable risk factors include genetic background, advancing age, female sex, Asian or white ethnicity, personal history of fracture, family history of fracture in a first-degree relative, and rheumatoid arthritis. Modifiable risk factors consist of low body weight, hormonal deficiencies, long-term use of medications that affect skeletal homeostasis (e.g., glucocorticoids, immunosuppressive medications), smoking, alcohol abuse, an inactive lifestyle, and a lifetime diet low in calcium and vitamin D.

In attempts to identify persons at a high risk for fracture, algorithms have been developed that combine BMD and clinically identifiable independent risk factors to estimate a treatment-naïve person's absolute fracture risk over a defined time interval. The World Health Organization's FRAX incorporates many of these risk factors for previously untreated persons to provide a 10-year absolute fracture risk. This more holistic approach targets the recognition of persons susceptible to fracture whose BMD might not be in the osteoporotic range. Cost and easy applicability are inherent advantages of these algorithms.

Pathophysiology

The risk of fracture for adults of any population is determined by the interaction among genetic, environmental, and hormonal factors throughout life. Adult BMD is determined both by the acquisition of peak bone mass and by the degree of subsequent bone loss after maturity. Actually, three distinct phases of BMD are found in the human life cycle. The period of bone mass accrual occurs during the first 2 decades

of life and the phase of bone catabolism begins at the end of the fifth decade; these two are separated by a short steady-state period. Although causes of bone loss are heterogeneous, genetic factors determine 60% to 80% of peak bone mass. Overall loss of bone mass from 25 years to advanced age can reach 5% to 15% for cortical bone (e.g., hip) and 15% to 45% for trabecular bone (e.g., spine).

The bone remodeling unit (BMU), the operational multicellular unit responsible for bone mass development and maintenance, is composed of osteocytes, osteoblasts, and osteoclasts. The osteocytes are the biochemical and mechanical sensors of bone and correspond to terminally differentiated osteoblasts entombed within the cortex of bone, but with canaliculi that communicate with lining cells on the skeletal surface. Osteocytes are 95% of the total bone cell number, and these cells trigger the bone-remodeling sequence. Osteoblasts, the bone-forming cells, have functional plasticity, due to their capacity to respond to systemic stimuli (estrogen, growth hormone, cortisol, insulin-like growth factor I, interleukins) to produce autocrine and paracrine factors that affect osteoclast differentiation and activity (receptor activator of nuclear factor κB ligand [RANKL], osteoprotegerin, and monocyte chemotactic protein-1 [MCP-1]).

Advances in osteoblast biology have demonstrated a new pathway in the commitment of bone marrow mesenchymal stem cells (MSCs) to osteoblasts. The Wnt protein-LRP5-Frizzled receptor, which is necessary to promote β-catenin stabilization, is linked directly to osteoblast differentiation and proliferation. Activating mutations of lipoprotein receptor-related protein 5 (LRP5) produce a high-bone-mass phenotype, whereas inactivating mutations lead to bone fragility and blindness (osteoporosis pseudoglioma syndrome). Osteoclasts, unique bone resorbing cells, originate from the monocyte-macrophage lineage. The discovery and subsequent elucidation of RANKL, which belongs to the tumor necrosis factor (TNF) and TNF receptor superfamily, provided important insight into the interaction between osteoblasts and osteoclasts. RANKL is expressed on the surface of osteoblasts and its receptor, RANK, on the surface of osteoclasts. The interaction between RANKL and RANK stimulates preosteoclast differentiation and osteoclast activity. Osteoprotegerin is a decoy receptor produced by osteoblasts to inactivate RANKL. Thus, during activation of remodeling, osteoblasts stimulate osteoclasts through the RANK-RANKL system. This allows synchronization between formation and resorption.

Bone fragility in osteoporosis reflects the predominance of bone resorption over formation in conditions of high bone turnover (e.g., after menopause and during early phases of glucocorticoid use) or low bone turnover (e.g., senescence and after long-term glucocorticoid use). In states of high bone turnover, bone loss occurs owing to the relatively short period needed by osteoclasts to resorb bone (2 weeks) relative to the 3 to 4 months necessary for bone formation and optimal mineralization.

The imbalance in bone remodeling most commonly results from the deprivation of estrogen and/or the aging process, which have been didactically classified as primary or idiopathic osteoporosis. But, osteoporosis can be secondary to a large number of common disorders. Hormonal disorders (most commonly hypogonadism, but also hypercortisolism, thyrotoxicosis, and growth hormone deficiency), weight loss, metabolic disturbances (renal osteodystrophy, hepatic osteodystrophy, and type 1 diabetes mellitus) and rarer causes of secondary osteoporosis are associated with low BMD. In other conditions, such as obesity and type 2 diabetes mellitus, bone fragility can occur despite normal or even high BMD. Alterations in bone quality resulting from glycation of collagen crosslinks in type 1 diabetes and increased susceptibility to falls in obesity and type 2 diabetes are other causes for bone fragility.

Prevention

Limitations in the accrual of peak bone mass during adolescence might determine bone strength decades later. Hence, osteoporosis has been considered a pediatric disorder with repercussions for the elderly. Prevention starts with the creation of conditions that optimize bone mass during puberty, extending the period of bone mass stability in adulthood, and attempting to reduce bone loss in aging. General measures (see later) for preventing osteoporosis should be directed to all subjects, and particularly those at highest risk for fracture by BMD and those who have a 10 year risk of hip fracture greater than 3% or greater than 20% for major osteoporotic fractures estimated from the FRAX tool. For patients with a prevalent osteoporotic fracture, the secondary prevention of a new fracture requires active pharmacologic intervention in addition to general measures that are applied to those with very low BMD.

Clinical Manifestations

The symptoms and signs associated with osteoporosis correspond to direct or indirect manifestations of fractures, the end result of skeletal fragility. Fractures of long bones are medical emergencies and almost always require medical intervention. Vertebral fractures are clinically less conspicuous and manifest as height loss, back pain, and thoracic kyphosis, which can be associated with respiratory limitation and intestinal constipation. Previous vertebral or long bone fractures are strong risk factors for new fracture events, but medical awareness of these powerful predictors is not common. Fractures can also be the first manifestation of a systemic disease associated with osteoporosis, as well as a predictable complication of medical intervention such as glucocorticoid therapy or solid organ transplantations.

Vitamin D deficiency is now recognized as a widespread problem in the world, affecting elderly persons living in regions of high latitude and those with social customs preventing sunlight exposure to the skin. Bone loss, muscle tenderness, and greater susceptibility to falls are clinical manifestations of severe vitamin D deficiency. Whether modestly reduced levels of serum 25-OH vitamin D are also associated with fracture risk and clinical symptomatology is still debated. The incidence of vitamin D deficiency in hospitalized patients with osteoporotic fracture is as high as 70%.

Diagnosis

Clinically, the diagnosis of osteoporosis can be established after the occurrence of a bone fracture with low trauma in appendicular or axial bones, excluding the skull. However, secondary causes of osteoporosis should always be excluded. Since the 1990s, the use of BMD measurements of the lumbar spine, femoral neck, or total hip has grown exponentially, facilitating the diagnosis of osteoporosis. There is no consensus about the target population for osteoporosis screening using BMD. Bone mass measurements by DEXA must be interpreted in relation to the patient's age, ethnicity, fracture history, family background, previous medications, timing of menopause, and other concomitant disorders. Notwithstanding the significant advances following widespread introduction of DEXA screening for identifying persons at risk for fracture, it is clear that some portion of the population is highly susceptible to fracture despite a normal or slightly low BMD.

CURRENT DIAGNOSIS

- Evaluation of risk factors for osteoporosis and related fractures is always recommended.
- Recommend routine bone mineral density to evaluate women aged 65 years and older.
- In postmenopausal women younger than 65 years, bone mineral density testing may be indicated depending on evaluation of fracture risk.
- Determination of bone mineral density is indicated for those with osteoporotic fractures to determine the severity of the disorder.
- Pursue clinical and laboratory evidences of secondary causes of osteoporosis in all patients with osteoporosis.

The development of the FRAX Internet tool has made prediction of long-term fracture risk an important and easy tool for evaluating patients. Attempts to further refine the algorithms have become available, such as the recent QFracture Score developed for women and men in England and Wales. This includes variables such type 2 diabetes, cardiovascular disease, asthma, use of hormone replacement therapy (HRT), and use of tricyclic antidepressants in addition to all the traditional variables of FRAX.

Several techniques are available for measuring bone mass, besides DEXA of the lumbar spine, hip, radius, and total body. These include ultrasound of the calcaneus, wrist, and finger and computed tomography (CT) of the spine and peripheral quantitative CT of the wrist and tibia. Magnetic resonance imaging (MRI) of the calcaneus and radius, virtual MRI using computerized reconstructions of trabecular bone, and high-resolution CT imaging of the radius are currently in testing for future clinical application. Still, the most precise and least expensive tool for assessing risk is DEXA, which is currently the preferred method for measuring BMD. The disadvantages of other techniques, such as the insensitivity of ultrasound scanning for discerning changes with treatment and the radiation exposure and minor precision errors associated with CT, preclude large-scale application of these techniques.

DEXA results are expressed as a T-score and a Z-score. The T-score is the number of standard deviations the patient's BMD differs from the peak reference population for the same ethnic group and sex. The Z-score is the number of standard deviations the patient's BMD differs from a that of a reference population of the same age, sex, and ethnicity. The T-score provides an indication of the risk for developing fractures, and this risk increases exponentially with decreasing T-scores. BMD measurements often are discordant across various bone sites in the same patient. These discrepancies most likely are related to differences in skeletal compartments (trabecular vs cortical) at distinct sites. Vertebral bones consist predominantly of trabecular bone, whereas total hip and forearm sites have a preponderance of cortical bone. Estrogen deficiency affects trabecular bone first and cortical bone later, wand primary hyperparathyroidism affects predominantly cortical bone (especially captured on the 1one-third section of the forearm site by the DEXA examination).

Biochemical markers reflect the activity of the bone remodeling unit. Markers of bone resorption such as urinary pyridinoline and deoxypyridinoline, as well as serum or urinary cross-links of the C- and N-terminal peptides of type I collagen, derive from the breakdown of collagen. Osteocalcin, bone-specific alkaline phosphatase, type I procollagen amino-terminal propeptide, and type I procollagen carboxy-terminal propeptide correspond to biochemical markers of bone formation. Previous studies on large cohorts showed that high levels of bone markers predict fractures in elderly women. These markers are independent of BMD and imply that accelerated bone turnover itself is a risk for fracture. However, bone turnover markers have substantial day-to-day variability and do not differentiate between trabecular and cortical bone; furthermore, their circulatory levels depend on production and clearance rates. These issues have limited the use of these biochemical markers for determining risk and for following up patients treated with active drugs.

Differential Diagnosis

A comprehensive evaluation of osteoporosis comprises the search for secondary causes of osteoporosis, starting with a careful clinical assessment, which should be complemented by routine laboratory tests. Although primary osteoporosis is much more common than other diseases associated with osteopenia, the diagnosis of idiopathic osteoporosis should be made only after the causes of secondary osteoporosis have been excluded.

Secondary osteoporosis is associated with a substantial minority of osteoporotic fractures in women, but that differs in men: More than 50% of men with vertebral crush fractures have secondary causes of osteoporosis. The most prominent causes are long-term use of glucocorticoids, hypogonadism, alcohol abuse, myeloma, and gastrointestinal, thyroid, and parathyroid disorders. Routine assessment of thyroid, renal, and hepatic function should be checked. Urinary calcium to exclude idiopathic hypercalciuria and serum calcium levels to detect asymptomatic hyperparathyroidism are also mandatory. High or high normal serum calcium values require the additional measurement of intact parathyroid hormone. Complete blood count (CBC), erythrocyte sedimentation rate (ESR), and multichannel chemistries are useful tools for detecting multiple myeloma, and these tests can be complemented with protein electrophoresis when indicated. The measurement of 25-hydroxy vitamin D should be considered in elderly people (especially in those living in high latitude regions), institutionalized persons, and osteoporotic patients with or without muscle weakness or tenderness. The evaluation of hypercortisolism is reserved for patients presenting clinical clues of Cushing's syndrome, although often this diagnosis can be very difficult to ascertain.

Treatment

GENERAL MEASURES

Nutrients are essential for bone health. Although there are specific requirements for bone tissue to achieve and maintain strength, a balanced diet to provide energy support and maintenance of normal weight are the initial steps in the nutrition management of osteoporosis. Calcium and vitamin D are the most important for peak bone acquisition and maintenance. The efficiency of calcium absorption declines with age, most likely owing to the decreased intestinal sensitivity to $1,25(OH)_2D$ (the calcitriol form of vitamin D) and reduced

CURRENT THERAPY

- A comprehensive nutritional orientation targeting normal body weight is recommended. Additionally, healthy bone orientation requires adequate ingestion of calcium and vitamin D. Calcium intake should be at least 1200 mg/day, including supplements, when necessary. Vitamin D should be prescribed for persons at risk of insufficiency at doses of 800 to 1000 IU.
- Weight-bearing and muscle-strengthening exercise are important tools to reduce the risk of falls and fracture.
- Pharmacologic therapy is indicated for those with clinical or morphometric vertebral fracture or hip fracture.
- Pharmacologic therapy is indicated for those with bone mineral density T-scores −2.5 standard deviations or less at the lumbar spine, at the femoral neck, and of the total hip, after proper evaluation.
- Pharmacologic therapy is indicated for postmenopausal women and men aged 50 years and older who have lower bone mass (T-score −2.5 to −1.0) at the femoral neck, of total hip, and of the lumbar spine if the 10-year hip fracture probability is 3% or more or if the 10-year probability of a major osteoporosis-related fracture is 20 or more based on the US-adapted WHO absolute fracture risk model.
- The drugs currently approved by the FDA for preventing or treating osteoporosis include bisphosphonates (alendronate, ibandronate, risedronate, and zoledronate), calcitonin, estrogens or hormone therapy, raloxifene, and parathyroid hormone (1-34) (teriparatide).
- The assessment of therapeutic response can be monitored by bone mineral density. Normally, bone mineral density is repeated every 2 years after starting pharmacotherapy. However, in some conditions (e.g., glucocorticoid therapy) 1-year intervals may be warranted.

circulating levels in part related to lower creatinine clearance. However, evidence that calcium and vitamin D reduce fracture risk in the osteoporotic patient remains somewhat controversial, although several meta-analyses support the complementary role of calcium and vitamin D supplementation as a preventive measure in persons older than 65 years. Currently, an average daily total calcium intake of 1200 to 1500 mg is recommended for postmenopausal women. Concerns about renal adverse events, particularly nephrocalcinosis, exist when ingestion is greater than 2000 mg per day for dietary plus supplemental sources.

Severe vitamin D deficiency (i.e., serum 25-hydroxyvitamin D [25(OH)D] levels <10 ng/mL) causes impaired mineralization and osteomalacia. This is accompanied by proximal muscle weakness, bone pain, and very low bone mass. With lesser degrees of vitamin D insufficiency (10-20 ng/mL), bone loss often follows. Less reliable is the correlation between baseline serum levels of 25(OH)D and BMD values or parathyroid hormone (PTH) levels. Vitamin D receptors are found in muscle cells, and it is believed that vitamin D insufficiency can contribute to falls and subsequent fractures. Meta-analyses by Bischoff-Ferrari suggest that a serum level of at least 30 ng/mL is needed to reduce falls and improve physical function in the elderly. However, large randomized trials with dose escalation in this vulnerable population have not been done.

Notwithstanding, for most osteoporotic patients, 800 to 1000 IU/day of vitamin D is prescribed to maintain normal 25(OH)D serum levels. In patients with vitamin D insufficiency—25(OH)D <20 ng/mL—or deficiency—25(OH)D <10 ng/mL—administration of 50,000 IU of ergocalciferol (vitamin D_2 [Drisdol])[1] or cholecalciferol (vitamin D_3)[1] given once weekly is a safe and effective way to restore vitamin D. Currently, vitamin D analogues are not recommended for the routine treatment of osteoporosis, in part due to potential long-term effects on renal function.

Immobilization has a devastating effect on bone mass comparable to the microgravity environment of spaceflight. Merely returning to an upright position or to normal gravity can partially reverse this process. On the other hand, intensive physical activity has limited additional effect on bone mass gain in comparison to a regular practice of exercise. Regular physical activity, performing aerobic, weight-bearing, and resistance exercises are effective in increasing spine BMD, although the magnitude of increase is relatively modest. Changes in bone quality may be more pronounced with exercise, but large-scale trials have not been done with the newer technologies. Smoking and alcohol abuse are independent risk factors for fracture. In addition, alcohol consumption contributes to the risk of falls.

PHARMACOLOGIC INTERVENTION

All drugs approved by the FDA for osteoporosis therapy reduce fracture risk at least at the spine. Most of the antifracture effects of these medications are not due to an increase in BMD, but rather to an improvement in qualitative measures of bone strength. Two main classes of medications are available for osteoporosis: antiresorptives, which decrease bone resorption, and anabolics, which promote bone formation.

The antiresorptive drugs approved by FDA to treat or prevent osteoporosis are noted in Table 1: bisphosphonates, including alendronate (Fosamax), risedronate (Actonel)], zoledronic acid (Reclast) and ibandronate (Boniva); estrogen therapy; the selective estrogen receptor modulator (SERM) raloxifene (Evista); and calcitonin (Miacalcin). The bisphosphonates impair osteoclastic resorption through the inhibition of farnesyl diphosphate synthase, a key enzyme that supports osteoclast activity. Estrogen and raloxifene inhibit osteoclastogenesis by stimulating synthesis of osteoprotegerin and inhibiting RANKL expression in osteoblasts. Calcitonin acts directly on osteoclasts, inhibiting their activity through the calcitonin receptor.

There are different approved indications for these drugs in osteoporosis. Alendronate is indicated for the prevention (5 mg PO daily) and treatment (10 mg PO daily or 70 mg PO weekly) of postmenopausal osteoporosis, treatment of osteoporosis in men, and glucocorticoid-induced osteoporosis. Risedronate is approved for the treatment of osteoporosis in men (5 mg PO daily, 35 mg PO weekly) and for

---

[1]Not FDA approved for this indication.

TABLE 1 Efficacy of Approved Drugs for Osteoporosis Treatment on Fracture Risk

Medication	Route	Dose	Vertebral	Hip	Nonvertebral
Alendronate (Fosamax)	Oral	10 mg qd or 70 mg weekly	+	+	+
Risedronate (Actonel)	Oral	5 mg qd or 35 mg weekly	+	+	+
Zoledronic acid (Reclast)	IV	5 mg yearly	+	+	+
Ibandronate (Boniva)	Oral	150 mg monthly	+	−	−
	IV	3 mg q3mo	+	−	−
Raloxifene (Evista)	Oral	60 mg qd	+	−	−
Calcitonin (Miacalcin)	Nasal	200 IU qd	+	−	−
	SC	100 IU qd		−	−
Conjugated equine estrogen (Premarin)	Oral	0.624 mg qd	+	+	NR
Medroxyprogesterone (Provera)	Depot	2.5 mg qd	+	+	NR
Teriparatide (Forteo)	SC	20 μg qd	+		+

Abbreviations: HRT = hormone replacement therapy; NR = not reported.

prevention (5 mg PO daily or 35 mg PO weekly) and treatment of postmenopausal osteoporosis (5 mg PO daily, 35 mg PO weekly, or 150 mg PO monthly) and glucocorticoid-induced osteoporosis. Ibandronate (Bonvia) (150 mg PO monthly, or 3 mg IV every 3 months) and raloxifene (60 mg PO daily) are approved for prevention and treatment of postmenopausal osteoporosis. Zoledronic acid 5 mg IV is approved for once-yearly treatment of postmenopausal osteoporosis, and 5 mg IV administered once every other year is approved to prevent osteoporosis. Calcitonin (200 IU nasally daily, or 100 IU SC daily) is approved for treating postmenopausal osteoporosis. Estrogen is approved only for the prevention of osteoporosis.

Side effects of oral bisphosphonates include esophageal and gastric irritation and musculoskeletal pain. Intravenous bisphosphonates are associated with hyperthermia, episcleritis, uveitis, and hypocalcemia; hypocalcemia can be prevented by prior administration of oral calcium and vitamin D. Alendronate and risedronate have been evaluated for up to 10 and 7 years of treatment, respectively, and their long-term safety profile is well established. There have been reports of subtrochanteric fractures during prolonged treatment with bisphosphonates, particularly alendronate. Although the mechanism is not clearly delineated, oversuppression, particularly when the drug is used with other antiresorptives, likely causes localized changes in the subtrochanteric region. Young women are particularly prone to these fractures, which can be devastating and often require surgical intervention. Prodromal symptoms that have been linked to this syndrome include proximal femur pain and evidence of previous stress fracture or cortical thickness on x-ray. Osteonecrosis of the jaw is a serious rare complication observed in patients treated with bisphosphonates. Usually, these patients are on higher doses of an intravenous regimen to treat bone metastases associated with malignancy.

Raloxifene, a SERM given daily, improves BMD and reduces the risk of spine fractures. However, it can exacerbate the climacteric symptoms. Although raloxifene increases serum levels of high-density lipoprotein (HDL) cholesterol, it is also associated with thromboembolic events. Studies suggest that raloxifene reduces the risk of breast cancer in high-risk women.

PTH (1-34) (teriparatide [Forteo]) has recognized antifracture effects on vertebral and nonvertebral sites, and it is the only anabolic option available for treating postmenopausal osteoporosis in the United States. PTH (1-34) inhibits osteoblast apoptosis, stimulates terminal differentiation, and subsequently increases bone formation. Currently, it is recommended that PTH (1-34) therapy (20 μg SC daily) should be limited to 2 years for the treatment of postmenopausal women and hypogonadal men with osteoporosis. More recently, recombinant human PTH (1-84)[2] has become available in Europe and has similar effects on bone as teriparatide, although with more transient hypercalcemia. Other side effects from PTH therapy include a greater risk of renal stones, prolonged hypercalcemia, and increases in uric acid.

No evidence indicates that the combination of anticatabolic and anabolic classes of drug provides additive results. However, after a period of 2 years of intermittent PTH (1-34), antiresorptives should be introduced to avoid post-treatment bone loss.

Strontium ranelate (Protelos)[2] is an orally administered medication that is capable of stimulating bone formation and inhibiting bone resorption. After 3 years of treatment, strontium ranelate preserves or enhances trabecular microarchitecture and increases cortical thickness. Strontium is not approved for the treatment of osteoporosis in the United States.

NEW AGENTS

Two new SERMs, bazedoxifene (Conbriza)[5] and lasofoxifene (Fablyn),[5] are in clinical development, and both have demonstrated antifracture effects but neither has won FDA approval. Denosumab (Prolia),[5] a synthetic RANKL antibody administered twice-yearly over 3 years, also has demonstrated strong antifracture efficacy. Long-term safety studies are pending, but approval is likely by 2011. Finally, an inhibitor of cathepsin K,[5] which is an osteoclast enzyme required for resorption of bone matrix, is under clinical investigation and currently is in phase III trials.

[2]Not available in the United States.
[5]Investigational drug in the United States.

REFERENCES

Bilezikian JP. Efficacy of bisphosphonates in reducing fracture risk in postmenopausal osteoporosis. Am J Med 2009;122(2 Suppl):S14–21.

Bischoff-Ferrari HA, Dawson-Hughes B, Staehelin HB, et al. Fall prevention with supplemental and active forms of vitamin D: A meta-analysis of randomised controlled trials. BMJ 2009;339:b3692.

Hippisley-Cox J, Coupland C. Predicting risk of osteoporotic fracture in men and women in England and Wales: prospective derivation and validation of QFracture Scores. BMJ 2009;339:b4229.

Khosla S, Melton LJ. Clinical practice. Osteopenia. N Engl J Med. 2007;356 (22):2293–230.

Rosen CJ. Bone remodeling, energy metabolism, and the molecular clock. Cell Metab 2008;7:7–10.

Sambrook P, Cooper C. Osteoporosis. Lancet 2006;367:2010–8.

Schousboe JT, Taylor BC, Fink HA, et al. Cost-effectiveness of bone densitometry followed by treatment of osteoporosis in older men. JAMA 2007;298:629–37.

Uitterlinden AG, Ralston SH, Brandi ML, et al. The association between common vitamin D receptor gene variations and osteoporosis: A participant-level meta-analysis. Ann Intern Med 2006;145:255–64.

U.S. Department of Health and Human Services. Bone health and osteoporosis: A report of the Surgeon General. Rockville, MD: U.S. Department of Health and Human Services, Office of the Surgeon General; 2004.

Wells GA, Cranney A, Peterson J, et al. Alendronate for the primary and secondary prevention of osteoporotic fractures in postmenopausal women. Cochrane Database Syst Rev 2008;(1):CD001155.

[2]Not available in the United States.

Paget's Disease of Bone

Method of
Ian R. Reid, MD

Paget's disease is a focal skeletal condition in which one or more bones has a clearly circumscribed area of increased turnover (Fig. 1A). Either osteoblasts or osteoclasts may predominate at a given time, resulting in sclerosis or lysis, respectively. Areas that are initially lytic often become sclerotic later, and it is common to see both changes within the same bone (see Fig. 1B). Unaffected areas of the skeleton are completely normal, in marked contrast to some rare congenital conditions which are sometimes (inappropriately) referred to as early-onset or juvenile Paget's disease. Such conditions (e.g., familial expansile osteolysis, idiopathic hyperphosphatasia) have different etiologies, clinical presentations, and responses to treatment when compared to Paget's disease.

Etiology

Within pagetic bone, there is a loss of the usual tight control of bone cell function, and the bone-resorbing cells (osteoclasts) and bone-forming cells (osteoblasts) both exhibit overactivity. In the case of osteoclasts, this leads to local areas of bone loss, which can result in deformity or fracture. Osteoblast overactivity leads to the random laying down of new bone, which is disorganized in its structure, mechanically inadequate, and prone to deformity. Osteoblast overactivity can also lead to bone expansion, resulting in bone pain, premature arthritis (if it affects articular surfaces), and nerve compression (e.g., in the spine or skull). Figure 1B shows the effects of osteoblast

and osteoclast overactivity on the structure of an affected tibia. The disease progresses along a long bone at a rate of about 1 cm per year, so most patients have had active disease for 1 or more decades before presentation. Typically, the disease progresses until the entire bone is involved. However, Paget's disease does not spread from one bone to another, so the number of affected bones remains constant throughout the disease course.

Paget's disease sometimes runs in families, and about 10% of patients are reported to have an affected relative. This observation has led to much work seeking genetic associations of the condition. It is now apparent that mutations of the gene for sequestosome 1 are associated with Paget's disease in some families. Other research has focused on possible environmental causes, and a slow viral infection has been suggested. Evidence that the prevalence of Paget's disease has decreased in recent decades would be consistent with altered exposure to an environmental agent. However, both the genetic and environmental hypotheses fail to account for the focal nature of the condition, which in some ways resembles a benign neoplasm.

Altered gene expression in osteoblasts and bone marrow stromal cells from pagetic bone has been demonstrated recently, including increased levels of dickkopf-1, interleukin-1, and interleukin-6. These changes are likely to result in stimulation of osteoclast proliferation and inhibition of osteoblast growth, leading to development of the characteristic lytic bone lesions. This work suggests that the key abnormality may reside in the osteoblast, rather than the osteoclast, as was assumed in the past. Uncertainties remain regarding the primary abnormality giving rise to this condition.

Epidemiology

Paget's disease is classically a condition of older adults, most patients being older than 60 years of age at diagnosis. There is a male preponderance in some studies. It is overwhelmingly a condition of individuals with European forebears, particularly from the United Kingdom and Western Europe (excluding Scandinavia), where about 6% to 7% of the older population is affected. Among older white Americans, the prevalence is about 2%. There is some evidence that prevalence and disease severity are both declining, possibly reflecting change in an environmental etiologic factor. It is extremely uncommon in individuals with predominantly Asian or Polynesian ancestry, although it is observed in some black populations.

Clinical Presentation

The most common symptoms attributable to Paget's disease are bone and joint pain. The bone pain is typically worse at rest and may trouble patients particularly at night. With skull involvement, pounding

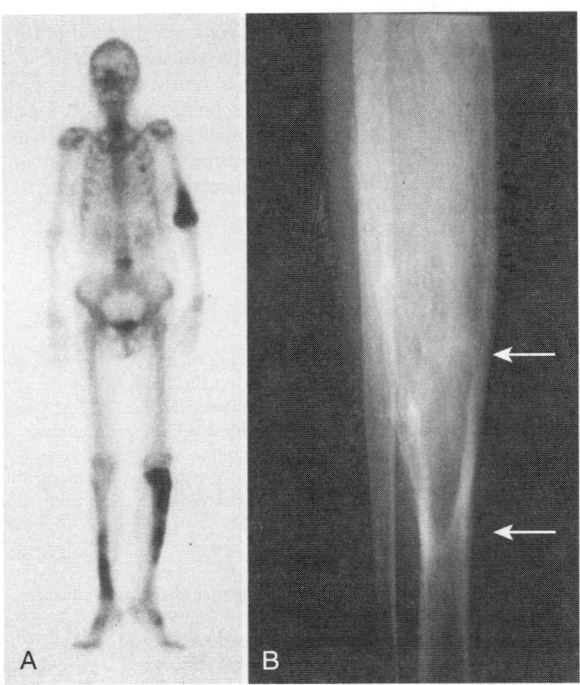

FIGURE 1. A, Bone scintigram in a patient with Paget's disease, demonstrating the multifocal nature of the condition and the presence of normal bone at other sites. **B,** Tibia affected by Paget's disease. The upper tibia is of increased density and width as a result of osteoblast overactivity, whereas the lower part of the affected bone shows a lytic region *(between arrows)* resulting from osteoclastic bone resorption. Below this, the bone is normal. (Copyright I. R. Reid, used with permission.)

CURRENT DIAGNOSIS

- Suspect the presence of Paget's disease in those patients with bone pain, bone deformity, isolated elevation of alkaline phosphatase, or lytic/sclerotic lesions on radiographs.
- Paget's disease is diagnosed from plain radiographs.
- Bone scintigraphy identifies the affected bones and allows some assessment of disease activity.
- Biochemical markers of bone turnover allow more precise assessment of turnover and response to therapy.
- Serum total alkaline phosphatase activity is the most cost-effective marker, although bone-specific alkaline phosphatase and procollagen type I N-terminal propeptide (PINP) are marginally more sensitive.

headaches can result. If Paget's disease leads to deformity of joint surfaces, premature arthritis occurs. This is particularly common at the hips. Deformity in long bones can occur, and involvement of the radius or weight-bearing bones of the lower limb often manifests in this way. Microfractures, which can be very painful, sometimes occur over the convexity of a deformed, weight-bearing bone. These can progress to complete fractures. Fractures can also occur through an area of active lytic disease in a weight-bearing bone.

Deafness is a common manifestation of Paget's disease and is caused by involvement of the bones of the middle ear or compromise of the eighth cranial nerve. More rarely, other neurologic syndromes can arise from nerve entrapment, including paraplegia as a result of spinal cord involvement.

Some pagetic patients are asymptomatic and are diagnosed because of an incidental finding of elevated circulating levels of alkaline phosphatase. The diagnosis may also result from an incidental radiographic finding, such as in studies of the urinary tract. Commonly, only one or two bones are involved, although disease may be more widespread. The pelvis, vertebral bodies, long bones, and skull are the most common sites, but almost any bone can be involved.

Diagnosis

Serum alkaline phosphatase, the most widely available marker of osteoblast activity, is usually elevated; however, if only one bone is involved, this test can be normal. In any patient with an elevation of alkaline phosphatase, it is important to determine whether this is coming from liver or bone. This question is usually addressed by measuring other liver function tests, although assays of bone-specific alkaline phosphatase and of other osteoblast-specific markers (e.g., procollagen type I N-terminal propeptide [PINP]) are available. If the elevation of alkaline phosphatase is bony in origin, it is important to rule out other bone conditions such as metastatic cancers (e.g., breast, prostate). This is usually done by identifying the sites of skeletal abnormality on a bone scintigram and then obtaining plain radiographs of the abnormal areas.

Paget's disease has a characteristic appearance on plain radiographs, showing either bony rarefaction or sclerosis (depending on whether the osteoclastic or osteoblastic phase is predominating), disorganization of trabecular architecture, and the other abnormalities already discussed (e.g., deformity). Bone biopsy is not usually necessary to confirm the diagnosis.

Other biochemical markers of osteoblast or osteoclast activity, such as breakdown products of bone collagen, have been used in Paget's disease. Total alkaline phosphatase, bone alkaline phosphatase, PINP or N-terminal telopeptide of type I collagen (NTX) identified more than 95% of pagetic subjects in one cohort of pagetic subjects, although the poorer precision of NTX reduced its utility in monitoring the effects of treatment. Osteocalcin, C-telopeptide of type I collagen, and urinary free deoxypyridinoline are less useful for assessment of baseline activity and monitoring response to therapy. Total alkaline phosphatase remains the most widely used test because of its low cost and wide availability.

CURRENT THERAPY

- Zoledronate (zoledronic acid, Reclast) 5 mg given as a single infusion over 15 minutes; retreatment is seldom required within 5 years.
- Alendronate (Fosamax) 40 mg/day for 6 months; retreatment may be required between 2 and 6 years.
- Risedronate (Actonel) 30 mg/day for 2 months; retreatment may be required between 1 and 5 years.

Treatment

Treatment of Paget's disease almost always relies on the potent bisphosphonates. These compounds have a very high affinity for the bone surface, where they remain for years. They are ingested by osteoclasts when bone is resorbed and inhibit a key enzyme in the mevalonate pathway, farnesyl pyrophosphate synthase. This results in disruption of the osteoclast cytoskeleton and cell death. Bisphosphonates are preferentially taken up at sites of high bone turnover, which accounts for their utility as bone scintigraphy agents, and therefore target active pagetic bone.

The injectable bisphosphonate pamidronate (Aredia) has been used for many years in the treatment of Paget's disease. It is typically given as a series of infusions of 60 to 90 mg, each administered over a period of 1 to 2 hours. Pamidronate produces partial or complete remissions of disease activity that last for up to several years. The first administration of the drug may be accompanied by mild flu-like symptoms, which settle over 24 to 48 hours and usually do not recur. Their resolution can be hastened by the use of paracetamol (acetaminophen, Tylenol) or similar agents.

More recently, potent oral bisphosphonates such as alendronate (Fosamax) and risedronate (Actonel) have become widely used. These are administered daily over periods of 2 to 6 months and produce good disease control. The duration of treatment chosen in the pivotal clinical trials was arbitrary to some extent, and individual patients may require longer or shorter initial courses to achieve remission. Oral bisphosphonates have a very low bioavailability. Therefore, they must be taken in a fasting state, with a glass of water, and at least 30 minutes before consumption of food or other fluids. Positively charged ions (including calcium supplements, antacids, and mineral supplements) bind avidly to bisphosphonates and impair their absorption, so they must be taken at a different time of day. Potent bisphosphonates can cause irritation to the upper gastrointestinal tract and should not be prescribed to patients with inflammation or ulceration in that region. Patients should remain upright for 30 minutes after taking oral bisphosphonates to minimize the risk of reflux and associated esophagitis or ulceration.

The latest addition to the therapeutic armamentarium in managing Paget's disease is the more potent intravenous bisphosphonate zoledronate (Reclast), which is administered in a single dose of 5 mg over 15 minutes. It was recently compared with the standard 2-month course of risedronate in two randomized, controlled trials. At 6 months, 96% of patients receiving zoledronate had a therapeutic response, compared with 74% of those randomized to risedronate ($P < 0.001$). Alkaline phosphatase levels normalized in 89% of patients in the zoledronate group and in 58% of those in the risedronate group ($P < 0.001$). Zoledronate showed a more rapid onset of action and superior effects on quality-of-life measures. Perhaps the most impressive data with zoledronate have been those from the open follow-up of responders in these studies. Two years after drug administration, therapeutic response was found to be maintained in 98% of those receiving zoledronate but in only 57% of risedronate-treated patients. Therefore, zoledronate produces much more sustained responses to therapy than have hitherto been possible.

Potent bisphosphonates can cause mild hypocalcemia, which is usually asymptomatic and not a cause for concern. However, in patients with vitamin D deficiency, hypocalcaemia can be more severe and sustained. Therefore, it is important to ensure that patients are vitamin D sufficient before receiving these drugs—a serum 25-hydroxyvitamin-D level greater than 50 nmol/L is more than adequate. Many physicians prescribe calcium to patients receiving bisphosphonate therapy (given in the evening if the oral bisphosphonate is given in the morning), as a further protection against hypocalcemia.

In the past, the weak bisphosphonate etidronate (Didronel) was used to treat Paget's disease. This is much less effective than the agents discussed previously. If used in high doses or for more than a few months, it carries the risk of producing osteomalacia, which can lead to bone pain and fractures. Therefore, it no longer has a place in the treatment of Paget's disease. Calcitonin (Miacalcin

Injection) has also been relegated to an historical role only, because its efficacy is much less than that of the potent bisphosphonates, and its effects are rapidly reversed after cessation of therapy.

There are several philosophical approaches to Paget's disease management, none of which is strictly evidence based. There is general agreement that patients with symptoms attributable to Paget's disease should receive treatment. This is clear-cut in patients who have bone pain at the site of a pagetic lesion, but it is a common observation that antipagetic drugs can produce variable degrees of improvement in pain from joints adjacent to pagetic bone. Patients with neurologic complications from spinal cord or other nerve entrapments also improve with antipagetic therapy.

Treatment aimed at preventing complications of Paget's disease is variably endorsed, because there is no clinical trial evidence that treatment prevents the progression of deformity, the development of pagetic symptoms, or fracture. However, it is clear that treatment leads to a restoration of normal bone histology (Fig. 2) and radiographic healing of lytic lesions and that, in the absence of such intervention, both bone lysis and deformity progress. It seems unreasonable to withhold safe therapies that are able to halt histologic and radiologic disease progression. Therefore, many experienced physicians endorse the provision of antipagetic therapy for individuals with lytic lesions in long bones, lesions at sites that are likely to lead to neurologic complications, arthritis or deformity, or involvement of the skull that could compromise hearing. Expert opinion also supports the use of antipagetic therapy before elective surgery on pagetic bone, because this approach reduces the vascularity of pagetic bone and results in less perioperative blood loss. On the other hand, Paget's disease in asymptomatic patients whose future risk of complications is thought to be low (e.g., with involvement of the ilium) is commonly managed without specific pharmaceutical intervention, although the availability of a safe, single-dose treatment with zoledronate is increasing the inclination to treat.

When providing treatment targeted at these goals, it is important to consider how adequacy of therapy can be judged. In the case of patients with pain, maximal relief of pain is an important endpoint. Lytic lesions should be treated and monitored with sequential radiographs until healing is apparent. Activity at other sites can be assessed indirectly with biochemical markers of bone turnover, although these are much less sensitive in patients with monostotic disease. In this context, there can be considerable residual activity at a single affected site without the markers' being abnormal. Bone scintigrams provide the most sensitive method of assessing local disease activity.

In the past, Paget's disease caused substantial morbidity in the elderly population. However, it is now possible to achieve adequate and sustained disease control with use of the potent bisphosphonates. Prompt use of these agents, when indicated, can be expected to halt disease progression and to effectively prevent the development of significant complications from this condition.

REFERENCES

Kanis JA. Pathophysiology and Treatment of Paget's Disease of Bone. London: Martin Dunitz; 1991.

Lyles KW, Siris ES, Singer FR, et al. A clinical approach to diagnosis and management of Paget's disease of bone. J Bone Miner Res 2001;16:1379–87.

Miller PD, Brown JP, Siris ES, et al. A randomized, double-blind comparison of risedronate and etidronate in the treatment of Paget's disease of bone. Am J Med 1999;106:513–20.

Ralston SH, Langston AL, Reid IR. Pathogenesis and management of Paget's disease of bone. Lancet 2008;372:155–63.

Reid IR, Davidson JS, Wattie D, et al. Comparative responses of bone turnover markers to bisphosphonate therapy in Paget's disease of bone. Bone 2004;35:224–30.

Reid IR, Miller P, Lyles K, et al. Comparison of a single infusion of zoledronic acid with risedronate for Paget's disease. N Engl J Med 2005;353:898–908.

Reid IR, Nicholson GC, Weinstein RS, et al. Biochemical and radiologic improvement in Paget's disease of bone treated with alendronate: A randomized, placebo-controlled trial. Am J Med 1996;101:341–8.

Selby PL, Davie MWJ, Ralston SH, et al. Guidelines on the management of Paget's disease of bone. Bone 2002;31:366–73.

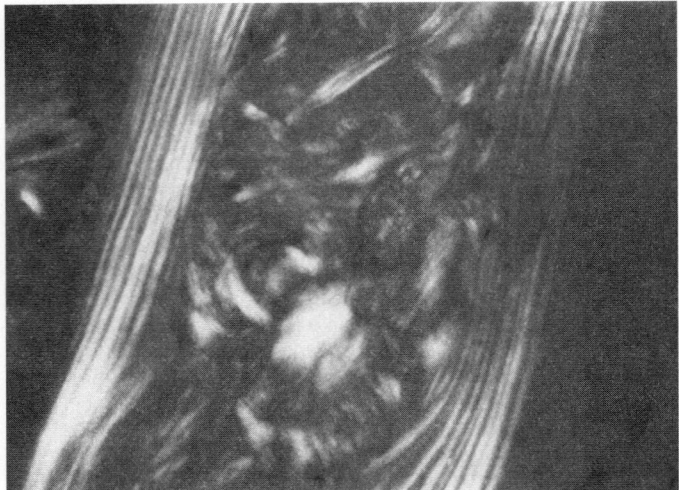

FIGURE 2. Section of a bone trabecula affected by Paget's disease, viewed under polarized light to show orientation of lamellae. In the center of the trabecula, the collagen fibers are chaotically laid down (woven bone), consistent with active Paget's disease. Over the outer surfaces, collagen is organized in parallel lamellae, indicating the restoration of normal bone microarchitecture after treatment with alendronate. (Reprinted with permission from: Reid IR, Nicholson GC, Weinstein RS, et al: Biochemical and radiologic improvement in Paget's disease of bone treated with alendronate: A randomized, placebo-controlled trial. Am J Med 1996;101:341–348.)

Parenteral Nutrition in Adults

Method of
Elaine B. Trujillo, MS, RD, and
Malcolm K. Robinson, MD

Since the inception of parenteral nutrition (PN) in the 1960s, the science of PN has matured in a number of ways. The initial excitement of being able to feed basic nutrients, vitamins, and trace elements intravenously has been tempered by the realization that indiscriminant use of PN can be harmful. Although PN can still be lifesaving, it is imperative that it be used judiciously and only as long as necessary. This chapter discusses the current use of PN in adult patients.

Indications and Contraindications

Enteral nutrition is the preferred method of nutrition support, primarily because it is associated with fewer infectious and metabolic complications. However, total PN (TPN), which is the provision of all nutrient requirements intravenously, may be indicated when feeding through the gastrointestinal (GI) tract is not possible. PN may be appropriately initiated in those who cannot receive enteral nourishment and are malnourished or at risk for developing malnourishment. Malnourishment can be defined as unintentional loss of more than 10% of usual body weight or greater than 7 to 10 days of inadequate nutrient intake. The body stores of well-nourished persons are generally sufficient to provide the essential nutrients, resist infection, promote wound healing, and support other necessary physiologic functions for this time period. In patients who are anticipated not to be able to receive adequate enteral nutrition for longer than 10 days, it is not necessary to wait 10 days before initiating

PN. This may include patients with short-bowel syndrome and others who are expected to have prolonged GI dysfunction.

According to the American Society of Parenteral and Enteral Nutrition guidelines, enteral nutrition is contraindicated in conditions such as diffuse peritonitis, intestinal obstruction, early stages of short-bowel syndrome, intractable vomiting, paralytic ileus, severe GI bleeding and severe diarrhea and malabsorption syndromes. Other relative contraindications to enteral nutrition include pancreatitis and enterocutaneous fistulae, although depending on the clinical circumstances, enteral nutrition may be indicated. PN and enteral nutrition may be provided concomitantly, although in patients who are critically ill, PN should not be started until all strategies to maximize enteral feeding (such as the use of postpyloric feeding tubes and motility agents) have been attempted. PN support is unlikely to benefit a patient who will be able to take enteral nutrition within 4 or 5 days after the onset of illness or who has a relatively minor injury (Fig. 1).

There are four key steps to consider before initiating PN, including assessing nutritional status, determining energy needs, evaluating GI function, and estimating the length of time a patient will require PN (Box 1).

Assessment of Nutritional Status

Nutrient depletion is associated with increased morbidity and mortality, and the prevalence of malnutrition in hospitalized patients is approximately 50%. Therefore, it is imperative to identify patients who have or are at risk for developing protein-energy malnutrition or specific nutrient deficiencies. A patient's risk of developing malnutrition-related medical complications needs to be quantified, and it is necessary to monitor the adequacy of nutritional therapy.

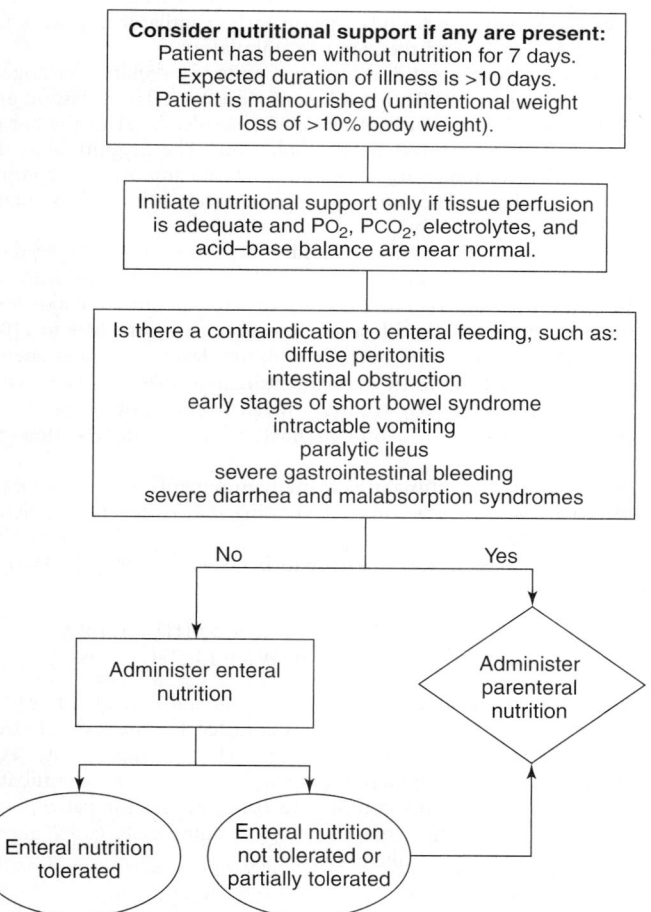

FIGURE 1. Determining route of feeding.

Nutrition assessment begins with a thorough history and physical examination in conjunction with select laboratory tests aimed at detecting specific nutrient deficiencies in patients who are at high risk for future abnormalities. The nutrition assessment should establish whether the patient will need maintenance therapy or nutrition repletion and should assess the status of the patient's GI tract, especially if nutrition support will be required.

A thorough history includes an assessment of recent weight changes, dietary habits, GI symptoms, and changes in exercise tolerance or physical abilities that would indicate functional capacity deficiencies. The physical examination includes inspecting for a loss of subcutaneous fat and muscle wasting, which indicate a loss of body energy and protein stores; edema and ascites, which can also indicate altered energy demands or decreased energy intake; and signs of vitamin and mineral deficits such as dermatitis, glossitis, cheilosis, neuromuscular irritability, and coarse, easily pluckable hair.

Several laboratory measurements have been used as nutritional biomarkers to aid the nutritional assessment. The serum proteins prealbumin, transferrin, and retinol binding protein have a rapid turnover rate and short half-lives and therefore may be used as indicators of recent nutritional intake. However, these proteins are affected by the metabolic responses to stress and illness, as well as other conditions, including iron status (transferrin) and renal status (retinol binding protein, prealbumin). This can limit their usefulness during acute illness states.

Prealbumin is least affected by fluctuations in hydration status and by liver and renal function compared with other plasma proteins. However, prealbumin levels drop in acute inflammatory conditions during which the liver switches to acute phase protein production and decreases prealbumin synthesis. A rise in C-reactive protein, a protein synthesized by the liver as part of the acute-phase response, indicates inflammatory states. Thus, C-reactive protein, when measured along with prealbumin, can help differentiate a low prealbumin due to nutritional inadequacy versus low prealbumin due to an acute-phase response.

The serum albumin concentration has traditionally been used as an indicator of nutritional status. Although it is a good preoperative predictor of outcome for patients undergoing surgery, it is affected by too many variables in the acute care setting to make it a reliable marker of nutritional status under such conditions or in the immediate postoperative period.

A simple and practical index of malnutrition is the degree of weight loss. Unintentional weight loss of greater than 10% within the previous 6 months indicates protein-energy malnutrition and is a good prognosticator of clinical outcome. Weight can also be compared with an ideal or desirable weight, or an index of body weight relative to height. The body mass index (BMI) is the best known such index and can be used to detect both undernutrition and overnutrition: BMI equals weight in kilograms divided by height in meters squared. This index is independent of height, and the same standards apply to both men and women. A BMI of 18.5 to 25 is considered normal, 25 to 29.9 is considered overweight, and greater than 30 is considered obese. Patients with a normal or high BMI can still have nutrient deficiencies and therefore can be malnourished if they have recently lost a significant amount of weight. In addition, a BMI of 18 kg/m^2 or less in an adult indicates moderate malnutrition and a BMI less than 15 kg/m^2 is associated with increased morbidity.

Another practical tool for evaluating nutritional status is the subjective global assessment (SGA) that encompasses historical, symptomatic, and physical parameters. The SGA technique determines if nutrient assimilation has been restricted because of decreased food intake, maldigestion, or malabsorption; if any effects of malnutrition on organ function and body composition have occurred; and if the patient's disease process influences nutrient requirements. The findings of the history and physical examination are subjectively weighted to rank patients as being well-nourished, moderately malnourished, or severely malnourished and are used to predict their risk for medical complications (Box 2).

BOX 2   Subjective Global Assessment

Select the appropriate category with a checkmark, or enter a numeric value where indicated by #.

History
1. Weight change
   Overall loss in past 6 months: amount = # _____ kg; % loss = # _____.
   Change in past 2 weeks: _____ increase, _____ no change, _____ decrease.
2. Dietary intake change (relative to normal)
   _____ No change
   _____ Change _____ duration = # _____ weeks.
   _____ Type: _____ suboptimal solid diet, _____ full liquid diet, _____ hypocaloric liquids, _____ starvation.
3. Gastrointestinal symptoms (that persisted for >2 weeks)
   _____ None, _____ nausea, _____ vomiting, _____ diarrhea, _____ anorexia.
4. Functional capacity
   _____ No dysfunction (e.g., full capacity),
   _____ Dysfunction _____ duration = # _____ weeks.
   _____ Type: _____ working suboptimally, _____ ambulatory, _____ bedridden.
5. Disease and its relation to nutritional requirements
   Primary diagnosis (specify) _____
   Metabolic demand (stress): _____ no stress, _____ low stress, _____ moderate stress, _____ high stress.

Physical (for each trait specify: 0 = normal, 1+ = mild, 2+ = moderate, 3+ = severe)
_____ Loss of subcutaneous fat (triceps, chest)
_____ Muscle wasting (quadriceps, deltoids)
_____ Ankle edema
_____ Sacral edema
_____ Ascites

SGA Rating (select one)
_____ A = Well nourished
_____ B = Moderately (or suspected of being) malnourished
_____ C = Severely malnourished
_____

Reprinted with permission from Detsky AS, McLaughlin JR, Baker JP, et al: What is subjective global assessment of nutritional status? JPEN 1987;11:8–13.

Estimating Nutritional Requirements

Historically, TPN often provided nutrients in excess of actual requirements. This was based on the assumption that patients requiring nutritional intervention were severely depleted and required aggressive repletion, hence the misnomer "hyperalimentation." Overfeeding is associated with increased carbon dioxide production and difficulty weaning from a ventilator as well as metabolic complications, such as hyperglycemia, which can lead to increased infection, morbidity, and mortality. Thus, nutritional support should be titrated to match actual metabolic requirements.

ENERGY REQUIREMENTS

There are four components of daily energy requirement. The first component is the basal metabolic rate (BMR), which is the amount of energy expended under complete rest, shortly after awakening and in a fasting state (12–14 hours). BMR varies with age, sex, and body size, correlates roughly with body surface area, and is proportional to lean tissue mass. This relationship holds true even among persons of different ages and sexes. Resting metabolic rate or resting energy expenditure (REE) represents the amount of energy expended 2 hours after a meal under conditions of rest and thermal neutrality. However, although it is often used synonymously with BMR, the REE is typically 10% higher.

The second component of daily energy expenditure is the thermic effect of exercise or the energy used in physical activity. The contribution of this component increases markedly during intense muscular work, and admission to a hospital generally results in a marked decrease in physical activity. Hospital activity in ambulatory patients accounts for a 20% to 30% increase in BMR. Critically ill patients who are on a ventilator generally have low activity levels (BMR increases by only 5% to 10%) because the ventilator performs the work of breathing, and they are not ambulatory.

The third component of energy expenditure is dietary thermogenesis, the increase in BMR that follows food intake. The digestion and metabolism of exogenous nutrients, whether delivered to the gut or vein, result in an increase in metabolic rate. The magnitude of the thermic effect of food varies depending on the amount and composition of the diet and accounts for approximately 10% of daily energy expenditure.

Finally, acute illness adds an additional stress factor to the daily energy expenditure and correlates with disease severity. For example, a patient's metabolic rate increases by 10% to 30% after a major fracture, from 20% to 60% with severe infection, and from 40% to 110% with a severe third-degree burn. In addition, fever accelerates chemical reactions and the BMR rises approximately 10% for each degree Celsius increase in temperature. Alternatively, cooling of febrile patients produces a reduction in BMR of approximately 10% per degree Celsius.

The first step of estimating calorie requirements is to estimate the BMR. This is usually accomplished using one of several predictive equations. The most commonly used method is based on the predictive equations reported by Harris and Benedict in 1909. The Harris–Benedict equations are as follows:

$$\text{BMR (men)} = 66.47 + 13.75(W) + 5.0(H) - 6.76(A)$$
$$\text{BMR (women)} = 655.1 + 9.56(W) + 1.85(H) - 4.68(A)$$

where W is weight in kg, H is height in cm, and A is age in years.

After the BMR is calculated, it is adjusted for the level of stress induced by injury or the disease process (Fig. 2) and activity level. Activity factors for hospitalized patients are 1.0 to 1.1 for intubated patients, 1.2 for patients confined to bed, and 1.3 for patients out of bed. Therefore, the patient's energy requirements (total energy expenditure [TEE]) are finally calculated:

$$\text{TEE} = \text{BMR} \times \text{Activity factor} \times \text{Stress factor}$$

The thermic effect of feeding is generally not included in the calculation of energy requirements for hospitalized patients.

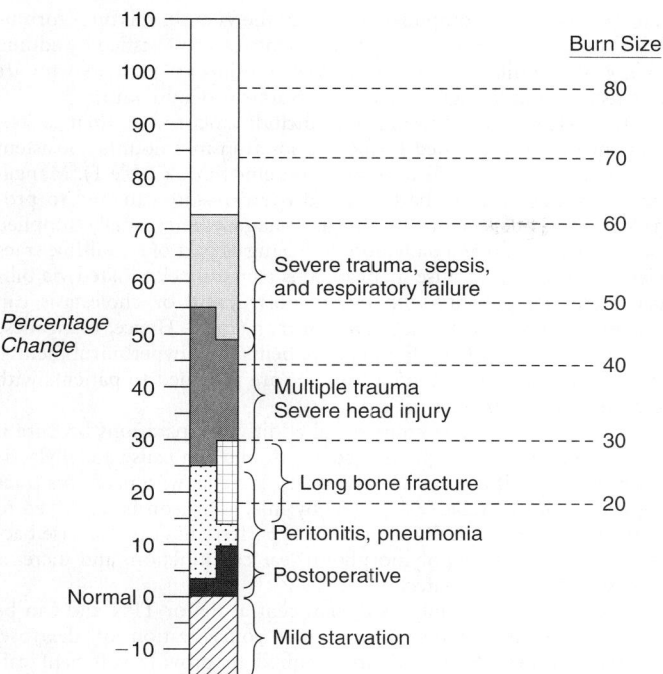

FIGURE 2. Percentage change in metabolic rate due to injury. (Adapted from Wilmore DW: The Metabolic Management of the Critically Ill, New York: Plenum Medical Books, 1977.)

TABLE 1 Recommended Daily Doses of Parenteral Vitamins and Trace Elements

Micronutrient	Parenteral Dose
Vitamins	
Vitamin A	3300 IU
Vitamin D	200 IU
Vitamin E	10 IU
Vitamin K	150 µg
Ascorbic acid (Vitamin C)	200 µg
Folic acid	600 µg
Niacin	40 mg
Riboflavin (Vitamin B_2)	3.6 mg
Thiamine (Vitamin B_1)	6 mg
Pyridoxine (Vitamin B_6)	6 mg
Cyanocobalamin (Vitamin B_{12})	5 µg
Pantothenic acid	15 mg
Biotin	60 µg
Trace Elements	
Zinc	2.5–5 mg
Copper	0.3–0.5 mg
Chromium	10–15 µg
Manganese	60–100 µg
Selenium	20–60 µg

Data from American Medical Association, Department of Foods and Nutrition: Multivitamin preparations for parenteral use. A statement by the Nutrition Advisory Group, JPEN J Parenter Enteral Nutr 1979;3:258–262; Food and Drug Administration: Parenteral multivitamin products: Drugs for human use: Drug efficacy study implementation: Amendment, Federal Register 2000;65(77):21200–21201.

Alternatively, some clinicians estimate energy requirements based on actual body weight. Thus, 20 to 25 calories (kcal)/kg is administered to the critically ill intubated patient and 30 kcal/kg is given to nonventilated patients in whom excessive intake is not a major concern.

Predicting energy expenditure in obese patients can be difficult, because using predictive formulas with current body weight can lead to high TEE and potentially to overfeeding. A factor of 18 to 21 kcal/kg has been validated in obese patients, and the Harris–Benedict equation using the average of actual and ideal weight and a stress factor of 1.3 accurately predicts REE in acutely ill obese patients with a BMI of 30 to 50 kg/m².

Indirect calorimetry is a more precise, clinically practical and individualized method to determine energy expenditure, particularly in patients in whom estimating requirements through predictive equations are difficult, such as those who continue to lose weight despite what appears to be an adequate caloric intake, who are critically ill, or who have rapidly changing energy needs.

Indirect calorimetry measures changes in oxygen consumption and carbon dioxide production to calculate the REE. Including a stress factor to account for injury is not necessary with indirect calorimetry because the measured energy expenditure accounts for the effects of disease state, stress, and trauma. However, the measurement occurs at rest, and therefore an activity factor of 1.0 to 1.3, depending on whether the patient is intubated, bedridden, or ambulatory, must be applied.

NUTRIENT REQUIREMENTS

The recommended daily protein allowance for most healthy persons who are not hospitalized is 0.8 g/kg or about 60 to 70 g of protein each day. The stressed, critically ill patient generally needs a higher dose of protein in the range of 1.0 to 1.5 g/kg/day. For most patients, providing protein beyond 1.5 g/kg/day is not beneficial. In fact, providing excess protein does not enhance uptake and can lead to increased ureagenesis, which can cause renal injury in some patients.

The calorie-to-nitrogen ratio for most PN solutions typically is around 150:1, with an acceptable range of 100:1 to 180:1. Nitrogen content is used as a marker for protein, and hence the two terms are used interchangeably. Usually, 6.25 g of protein is equal to 1.0 g of nitrogen. The conversion factor is slightly higher (6.4) for PN solutions, such as those with higher concentrations of crystalline amino acids.

Vitamin and mineral requirements are altered in certain disease states due to increased losses, greater use or both. Guidelines for parenteral vitamin and trace elements, developed by the Nutrition Advisory Group of the American Medical Association, were approved by the U.S. Food and Drug Administration (FDA) in 1979 and amended in 2000 (Table 1).

Composition of Central and Peripheral Venous Solutions

Central venous access is required for providing TPN because of the hypertonicity of the formulas infused (1900 mOsm/kg). The infusion of a hypertonic solution into a peripheral vein, known as *peripheral parenteral nutrition* (PPN), can result in thrombophlebitis and venous sclerosis unless the PN is drastically diluted to lower the tonicity. To minimize the hypertonicity of PPN solutions, dextrose is limited to 5% to 10% and amino acids are limited to 2.5% to 3.5%. Lipids are isotonic and therefore provide a significant portion of the caloric substrate of PPN formulas.

Central venous solutions, which are prepared by the hospital's pharmacy, typically combine carbohydrate in the form of dextrose, protein as crystalline amino acids, and lipids from polyunsaturated long-chain triglycerides such as soybean oil or a safflower/soybean oil mixture. Vitamins, electrolytes, and trace elements are added to the formulation as needed. Typical substrate profiles of carbohydrate, protein, and lipids in central PN are shown in Table 2. A usual PN prescription administers 1 to 2 L of a solution each day. Administration of 500 mL of a 20% fat emulsion 1 day each week is sufficient to prevent essential fatty acid deficiency. Alternatively, if additional calories from lipids are needed on a daily basis, they can be administered as a separate infusion or most commonly as part of the mixture of dextrose and amino acids, a technique known as *triple mix* or *three-in-one*.

TABLE 2   Central Versus Peripheral Parenteral Nutrition

Property	Central Nutrition	Peripheral Nutrition
Daily calories	2000–3000	1000–1500
Protein	Variable	56–87 g
Volume of fluid required	1000–3000 mL	2000–3500 mL
Duration of therapy	>7 d	5–7 d
Route of administration	Dedicated central venous catheter	Peripheral vein or multi-use central catheter
Substrate profile	55%–60% carbohydrate 15%–20% protein 25% fat	30% carbohydrate 20% protein 50% fat
Osmolarity	~2000 mOsm/L	~600–900 mOsm/L

Including intravenous fat emulsion into a parenteral admixture changes the conventional nutritional solution into an emulsion. Various electrolytes and micronutrients can adversely influence emulsion stability, and therefore their concentration in three-in-one solutions is limited to prevent cracking of the TPN solution, in which microscopic or macroscopic precipitates are formed. The higher the cation valence, the greater the destabilizing influence to the emulsifier. Therefore, trivalent cations such as ferric ion (iron dextran) are more disruptive than divalent cations such as calcium or magnesium ions, which are more disruptive than monovalent cations such as sodium or potassium. No concentration of iron dextran is safe in triple-mix formulations. In-line filtration is necessary for all PN solutions, including triple-mix solutions because it is impossible to visually detect precipitates until they are grossly incompatible and unsafe for infusion.

Once the basic solution is created, electrolytes are added as needed (Table 3). Sodium or potassium salts are given as chloride or acetate depending on the patient's requirements. Normally, equal amounts of chloride and acetate are provided. However, if chloride losses from the body are increased, such as can occur in patients who have nasogastric tubes, then most of the salts should be given as chloride. Similarly, more acetate should be given to patients when additional base is required because acetate generates bicarbonate when it is metabolized. Sodium bicarbonate is incompatible with PN solutions and so cannot be added to the mixture. Phosphate may be given as the sodium or potassium salt. Lipid emulsions contain an additional 15 mmol/L of phosphate.

Commercially available preparations of fat-soluble and water-soluble vitamins, minerals, and trace elements are added to the nutrient mix unless they are contraindicated. Adequate thiamine is essential for patients receiving PN and can be provided separately.

Vitamin K is not a component of any of the vitamin mixtures formulated for adults. Maintenance requirements can be satisfied by adding 10 mg of vitamin K weekly in the PN solution for patients who are not receiving anticoagulants such as warfarin (Coumadin).

Trace element preparations that include zinc, copper, manganese, and chromium are added to the PN solution in amounts consistent with the American Medical Association guidelines (Table 1). Manganese accumulation can be toxic, and overexposure can lead to progressive neurodegenerative damage. Manganese is usually supplied in the PN solution at a daily dose of 0.5 mg as part of a multiple trace element additive. Because manganese is primarily eliminated via biliary excretion, patients with biliary obstruction or cholestasis can accumulate potentially toxic levels of manganese. Hence, manganese should be removed from the PN of patients with hyperbilirubinemia. Higher doses, 10 to 15 mg/day, of zinc are provided to patients with excessive GI losses.

Iron is not a part of commercial additive preparations because it is incompatible with triple mix solutions and can cause anaphylactic reactions when it is given intravenously. Patients who need this trace element should receive it orally or by injection. Iron is not given to patients who are critically ill because hyperferremia can increase bacterial virulence, alter polymorphonuclear cell function, and increase host susceptibility to infection.

PPN is less commonly used than central PN or TPN and can be disadvantageous. Because of the low concentration of dextrose, greater volumes (>2 L/day) are required to provide sufficient calories, which might not be feasible in fluid-restricted patients. PPN generally does not approximate a patient's energy needs, because PPN provides only 1000 to 1500 kcal/day and a large percentage of the calories (50%) are derived from fat. High-fat infusions are undesirable because they are associated with impaired reticuloendothelial system function and are potentially immunosuppressive. There is no evidence that IV lipids improve outcomes or significantly decrease nitrogen losses. Generally, PPN should be avoided unless it is combined with enteral feeding in patients who can not tolerate full enteral feeding, patients who cannot get a central venous catheter, or patients with low body weights in whom PPN can meet at least two thirds of estimated needs.

Administration and Venous Access

Typically, central PN solutions are administered into the superior vena cava. Access to this vein can be achieved by cannulation of the subclavian or internal jugular veins. Peripherally inserted central venous catheters (PICC) (typically inserted via an antecubital vein and advanced into the superior vena cava) are the most commonly used central venous access devices for providing PN. PICC placement offers the advantage of central venous access while avoiding the risks associated with accessing the subclavian or jugular veins, such as hemothorax, pneomothorax, and arterial injury.

TABLE 3   Electrolyte Concentrations in Parenteral Nutrition

Electrolyte	Recommended Central PN Doses	Recommended Peripheral PN Doses	Usual Range of Doses
Potassium (mEq/L)	30	30	0–120 (CVL) 0–80 (PV)
Sodium (mEq/L)	30	30	0–150
Phosphate (mmol/L)	15	5	0–20
Magnesium (mEq/L)	5	5	0–16
Calcium (mEq/L) (as gluconate)	4.7	4.7	0–10
Chloride (mEq/L)	50	50	0–150
Acetate (mEq/L)	40	40	0–100

CVL = central venous line; PN = parenteral nutrition; PV = peripheral vein.

Tunneled catheters or catheters with indwelling ports should be considered for patients who will need prolonged central venous nutrition (e.g., >6 weeks). Patients who will be using their catheters solely for daily central PN and who require home IV feeding may be best served by a tunneled catheter rather than an indwelling port. Tunneled catheters may be more easily manipulated and cared for, which can minimize the risk of infection.

Inserting a dedicated line for infusing hypertonic solutions requires strict aseptic technique or maximal barrier protection: Hat, mask, gown, and gloves must be worn. The position of the catheter tip in the superior vena cava is confirmed by chest x-ray before any concentrated solutions are administered. Once the position of the tip has been confirmed, the line should be used exclusively for administering the hypertonic nutrient solution based on the Centers for Disease Control and Prevention (CDC) guidelines.

Multiple-lumen central venous catheters are most commonly used. Although at least one lumen is dedicated to the infusion of the PN solutions, the other(s) may be used for monitoring, blood drawing, or medication. The rate of catheter sepsis associated with multiple-port catheters may be the same as or slightly greater than the rate associated with the use of single-port catheters. However, multiple-port PICCs are used to infuse PN solutions for a shorter time, which can minimize their inherent risk. Multiple-port catheters should be carefully maintained, including dressing changes, maintaining the dedicated lumen, careful handling of the other lumens, and removing the catheter as soon as it is no longer needed.

Infusion and Patient Monitoring

It is advisable to start with 1 L of central PN and increase the volume as needed, depending on the patient's metabolic stability. Blood sugar levels should be closely monitored and maintained at 80 to 110 mg/dL, tissue perfusion should be adequate, and Po_2, Pco_2, electrolytes (especially potassium, phosphate, and magnesium) and acid–base balance should be near normal before starting or advancing to the goal solution. The solutions should be administered using a volumetric pump set at a constant rate. It is important not to modify the infusion rate during any given day to try to compensate for excess or inadequate administration of the PN solution, such as when the PN solution arrives later than expected. A cyclic schedule (10–16 h/day) for patients requiring long-term PN can be initiated once the patient is metabolically stable. In situations when the central PN solution must be suddenly discontinued, a 10% dextrose solution may be given at the same infusion rate as was used for the PN unless the patient is severely hyperglycemic. PN solutions may be administered at one half the infusion rate to patients who are undergoing surgical procedures because circulating glucose and electrolyte levels are easier to control.

In addition to hyperglycemia, metabolic complications include hyper- and hypophosphatemia, hyper- and hypokalemia, hyper- and hypomagnesemia, and hyper- and hypocalcemia. Thus, it is important to monitor the patient's serum electrolytes closely, especially when initiating TPN. Once the patient has stabilized on the individual nutritional prescription, serum chemistries should be obtained at least twice weekly to measure chloride, CO_2, potassium, sodium, blood urea nitrogen, creatinine, calcium, and phosphate levels and once weekly for a full profile that includes liver function, magnesium, and triglyceride levels.

Patients with Special Needs

GLUCOSE INTOLERANCE

Hyperglycemia is the most common metabolic complication related to PN, and glucose regulation may be especially difficult in patients who have diabetes mellitus or who develop insulin resistance in response to severe stress or infection. Control of blood glucose levels is important for all patients who receive PN because uncontrolled hyperglycemia may be associated with complications such as fluid and electrolyte disturbances and increased infection risk due to impairment of host defenses, including decreased polymorphonuclear leukocyte mobilization, chemotaxis, and phagocytic activity. Evidence suggests that maintaining tight blood glucose concentrations between 80 and 110 mg/dL decreases morbidity and mortality in critically ill surgical patients. Intensive insulin therapy minimizes derangements in normal host defense mechanisms and modulates release of inflammatory mediators.

Patients with difficult glycemic control may best be managed by continuous insulin infusion, which is safe, effective, and more timely than subcutaneous insulin therapy. Hypoglycemia that occurs during this type of infusion generally is short lived and more easily corrected than hypoglycemia resulting from subcutaneous insulin administration. A separate IV insulin infusion can be used rather than adding incremental doses of insulin to the PN bag every 24 hours in patients in whom glycemic control is difficult. Many intensive care units (ICUs) have an insulin drip infusion protocol in which there are frequent checks of serum glucose and adjustments of the insulin infusion drip (e.g., every 1–2 hours) to maintain tight control of glucose levels. The conventional approach of using sliding scale insulin to cover high blood glucose levels may be unsafe and ineffective, and repetitive doses of subcutaneous insulin in the edematous patient can have a cumulative effect leading to prolonged hypoglycemia. In addition, adjusting insulin in the TPN bag every 24 hours might not achieve the desired rapid correction of hyperglycemia deemed appropriate based on the literature, which indicates worse outcomes for those with poor glucose control. See Table 4 for guidelines for managing hyperglycemia in critically ill patients receiving PN.

Abrupt discontinuation of PN can lead to hypoglycemia and should be avoided. Instead, it is recommended to decrease the PN infusion rate by one half before discontinuation to prevent rebound hypoglycemia.

TABLE 4 Management of Hyperglycemia in Critically Ill Patients Receiving Parenteral Nutrition

Blood Glucose	Treatment
Before Parenteral Nutrition or Insulin Infusion	
>220 mg/dL	Start insulin infusion at 2–4 U/h
110–220 mg/dL	Start insulin infusion at 1–2 U/h
<110 mg/dL	Do not start insulin infusion
	Check BG every 4 h
During Insulin Infusion	
Above Normal Range	
>140 mg/dL	Increase insulin infusion by 1–2 U/h
	Monitor BG every 1–2 h until in normal range
110–140 mg/dL	Increase insulin infusion by 0.5–1 U/h
	Monitor BG every 1–2 h until in normal range
Normal Range	
80–110 mg/dL	No change
	Monitor BG every 4 h
Below Normal Range	
60–80 mg/dL	Reduce insulin dosage
	Monitor BG every 4 h
	Recheck BG within 1 h
40–60 mg/dL	Stop insulin, ensure adequate baseline glucose intake
	Recheck BG within 1 h
<40 mg/dL	Stop insulin, ensure adequate baseline glucose intake, give 10 g IV glucose bolus
	Recheck BG within 1 h
Steeply Falling	
Any	Reduce insulin dosage by one half
	Monitor BG every h

Adapted from Butler SO, Btaiche IF, Alaniz C: Relationship between hyperglycemia and infection in critically ill patients. Pharmacotherapy 2005;5(7):963–976.
BG = blood glucose.

PANCREATITIS

Most cases of pancreatitis are mild, and nutritional support is not needed. However, 10% to 20% of patients with pancreatitis develop severe disease that results in a hypermetabolic, hyperdynamic, systemic inflammatory response syndrome that creates a highly catabolic stress state. Although the usual care of pancreatitis had been gut rest, with or without PN, an evidence-based review found a trend toward reductions in the adverse outcomes of acute pancreatitis after administration of enteral nutrition. Hence, if feasible, enteral nutrition should be used in patients with pancreatitis because it is associated with a significant reduction in infectious morbidity and hospital length of stay compared with PN.

Initiation of PN should be delayed in patients with acute pancreatitis who cannot tolerate enteral nutrition even though they might eventually require PN. Providing PN within 24 hours of admission has been shown to worsen outcome, and providing PN after resuscitation and abatement of the acute inflammatory process appears to improve outcome compared with standard therapy. Consequently, if enteral nutrition is not feasible, the initiation of PN should be delayed for at least 5 days after admission to the hospital, when the peak period of inflammation has abated.

ACUTE RENAL FAILURE

Acute renal failure (ARF) is associated with severe nutritional deficits. Most patients with ARF are catabolic and have energy requirements of 50% to 100% greater than resting requirements, likely the result of other coexisting conditions such as sepsis, trauma, and burns. Calories are provided to patients with ARF in sufficient quantities to minimize protein degradation, generally in the range of 25 to 35 kcal/kg/day. Lipid emulsions can be used as a source of concentrated energy in patients who are on fluid restriction.

Protein loss is accelerated and protein synthesis is impaired in patients with ARF. Loss of amino acids in the dialysate and renal replacement therapies add to the protein deficit and increase individual protein needs. Approximately 10 to 12 g of amino acids are lost with each dialysis therapy, depending on the type of dialyzer membrane, blood flow rate, and dialyzer reuse procedure, and approximately 10 to 16 g/day of amino acids are lost through continuous renal replacement therapies (CRRT). The provision of protein 1.0 to 1.4 g/kg/day and 1.5 to 2.5 g/kg/day is recommended for ARF patients receiving hemodialysis and CRRT, respectively.

Protein is provided with a standard solution containing both essential and nonessential amino acids. Traditionally, formulas designed for renal failure contained predominantly essential amino acids. These formulas often were insufficient in calories and protein for metabolic needs and further compromised the patient's nutritional status. They also increase the risk for hyperammonemia and metabolic encephalopathy when used for longer than 2 to 3 weeks. The current recommendations are to provide adequate protein while treating the patient aggressively with dialysis to prevent the accumulation of nitrogenous waste products.

Fluid and electrolyte balance are often impaired in patients with ARF. The amount of fluid from the PN might need to be adjusted daily, depending on the phase of ARF, whether the patient is receiving dialysis, and whether dialysis is continuous or intermittent. Serum potassium and phosphate levels typically rise in patients with ARF until dialysis is initiated, at which time levels might drop, especially with the provision of PN. Potassium, phosphate, and magnesium levels need close monitoring and adjusting to correct imbalances. Acetate salts of potassium or sodium can be administered to help correct a metabolic acidosis.

Standard doses of the water-soluble vitamins and additional folic acid (1 mg/day total) and pyridoxine (vitamin B_6) (10 mg/day) might need to be added to the solution for patients who are being dialyzed because these vitamins are lost from the body in the dialysate bath. The dose of vitamin C might need to be restricted to 100 mg/day to prevent oxalate deposits. The supplementation of fat-soluble vitamins is usually not required, especially in patients who also are eating, because excretion of fat-soluble vitamins is reduced in renal failure. For example, serum vitamin A levels may be elevated in ARF due to enhanced hepatic release of retinol and retinol-binding protein, decreased renal catabolism, and decreased degradation of vitamin A transport protein by the kidneys. Vitamin D levels may be decreased because of impaired activation of 1,25-dihydroxycholecalciferol in the kidneys. In anuric patients, trace elements may be withheld from the PN solution; however, for prolonged PN, trace elements and fat-soluble vitamins should be monitored and replaced accordingly.

Patients with chronic renal failure (CRF) also have nutritional deficits due to anorexia, amino acid losses into the dialysate, concurrent illness, metabolic acidosis, and endocrine disorders. However, unlike those suffering from ARF, patients with CRF have normal energy requirements. Protein intake generally is restricted in predialysis patients to 0.5 to 0.6 g/kg/day but required in higher amounts in patients on dialysis, depending on the type of dialysis (1.2 g/kg/day for hemodialysis; 1.2 to 1.5 g/kg/day for peritoneal dialysis). Predialysis patients who become acutely ill should be given protein 1.2 to 1.5 g/kg/day even if this precipitates the need for dialysis. Starvation from insufficient calories or protein in the patient with renal dysfunction increases the risk of nutritionally related complications and should be avoided in the severely ill patient regardless of the potential need for dialysis.

Intradialytic PN is the provision of IV amino acids, carbohydrates, and fat directly into the venous drip chamber of the hemodialysis unit during treatment. It is a method of providing additional calories and protein in malnourished chronic hemodialysis patients. It is associated with significant increases in body weight and serum albumin in patients with chronic renal failure. However, intradialytic PN is expensive and the benefits have not been fully elucidated. A typical solution contains about 1100 kcal and 50 g of protein, which is provided three times per week with dialysis. For example, intradialytic PN provides a patient with energy and protein requirements of 2500 kcal and 70 g of protein/day, respectively, only 20% of the weekly calorie and 30% of the weekly protein needs. Thus, intradialytic PN is reserved for patients with CRF who cannot ingest sufficient nutrients by mouth and who are not candidates for nutritional support via enteral nutrition on PN due to GI intolerance or venous access problems or for other reasons. Appropriate use of intradialytic PN should be limited to a very small fraction of people who are on dialysis.

HEPATIC DYSFUNCTION AND LIVER FAILURE

Hepatic dysfunction is associated with a variety of abnormalities including metabolic abnormalities, malabsorption, maldigestion, anorexia, and early satiety due to ascites. Dietary restrictions also can contribute to malnutrition.

Protein intake in patients with stable chronic liver disease depends on the patient's nutritional status and protein tolerance. Nutritionally depleted patients can require as much protein as 1.5 g/kg estimated dry weight. In a minority of patients who have protein-sensitive hepatic encephalopathy, protein intake might need to be decreased to 0.5 to 0.7 g/kg/day and gradually increased to 1.0 to 1.5 g/kg/day, as tolerated. These patients have deranged plasma amino acid profiles, with increased concentrations of aromatic amino acids (phenylalanine, tyrosine, and tryptophan) and methionine and decreased branched-chain amino acids (valine, leucine, and isoleucine). Randomized, controlled trials that provided parenteral or enteral formulas enriched with branched-chain amino acids have been inconsistent and have had results including no benefit, improved morbidity, no change in mortality, and improvement in encephalopathy. These specialty products should be reserved for patients with disabling encephalopathy who do not tolerate standard proteins and have not responded to other therapies, such as lactulose or neomycin administration.

Energy requirements are difficult to predict in patients with liver failure. Whereas most patients have a normal metabolic rate, up to one third may be hypermetabolic. Although providing 25 to 30 kcal/kg/day is a guideline for providing energy needs, basing requirements on indirect calorimetry is often recommended.

Fluid restriction due to ascites and edema often necessitates increasing the dextrose concentration in the PN so as to maintain sufficient calories in a restricted volume. Sodium is reduced in the formula because liver-failure patients excrete nearly sodium-free urine. Vitamin and mineral deficiencies often occur as a result of suboptimal nutrient intake, decreased absorption, decreased storage, and in some cases alcohol use, which decreases thiamine (vitamin B_1) and folate absorption. Copper and manganese may be contraindicated because a major route of excretion for these substances is the biliary system. Zinc deficiency is common in cirrhotic patients, and supplementation of this mineral may be necessary, especially if there are excessive GI losses.

ACUTE RESPIRATORY DISTRESS SYNDROME

Patients with protein-calorie malnutrition have an increased incidence of pneumonia, respiratory failure, and acute respiratory distress syndrome (ARDS). Nutritional support is indicated in patients with ARDS, and underfeeding and overfeeding can be detrimental to pulmonary function.

Overfeeding calories, and particularly glucose, can lead to increased minute ventilation, increased dead space, and increased carbon dioxide production and ultimately to difficulty weaning from a ventilator. Hypercapnia from increased carbon dioxide production is the result of glucose combustion causing more carbon dioxide production and excess calories triggering lipogenesis. A healthy person increases ventilation in response to increased calories and thus avoids hypercapnia. However, patients with compromised ventilatory status might not be able to compensate with increased ventilation and can develop respiratory distress, acute respiratory failure, and difficulty weaning from mechanical ventilation. Thus, the use of indirect calorimetry measurements to determine respiratory quotient and energy expenditure is imperative in patients with ARDS.

OTHER CONDITIONS AND NUTRITIONAL TREATMENTS

The catabolic response to major surgery, trauma, burn, and sepsis is characterized by a net breakdown of body protein stores to provide substrates for gluconeogenesis and acute-phase protein synthesis. Adequate nutrition can attenuate whole-body catabolism but rarely, if ever, prevents or reverses the loss of lean body mass during the acute phase of injury. Several strategies to prevent the loss of lean body mass have been investigated, including growth hormone, growth factors, and conditionally essential amino acids, such as glutamine.

Growth hormone is a potent anabolic agent, and administration to humans increases the rate of wound healing, decreases rates of wound infection, and decreases the catabolism and muscle wasting of critical illness. However, a large European trial found increased morbidity and mortality in patients with prolonged critical illness who received high doses of growth hormone. Thus, the use of growth hormone in patients who are in the acute phase of critical illness is not recommended.

Alternative anabolic agents, such as oxandrolone (Oxandrin) and testosterone[1] are being pursued to induce positive nitrogen balance and enhance wound healing in critically ill patients. These anabolic steroid hormones increase protein synthesis and can reduce the rate of protein breakdown. In a study of patients with alcoholic hepatitis, administration of oxandrolone was associated with lower mortality compared with patients receiving placebo. The patients receiving oxandrolone had improvements in the severity of their liver injury and the degree of malnutrition. Several studies have demonstrated a benefit of oxandrolone use in the burn patient population. Other anabolic steroid hormones, such as methandieone and nandrolone decanoate, have been shown to increase protein anabolism and nitrogen balance in hospitalized patients.

Growth factors should be reserved for patients with major burns and documented impaired healing, patients who have large wounds or enterocutaneous fistulae and who have impaired healing, and patients with muscle wasting and weakness associated with AIDS, other failure to thrive conditions, and in general, patients who have

not responded to aggressive nutritional support but whose underlying disease processes are controlled. Growth factors have not been shown to decrease length of time on a respiratory in ICU patients. In fact, such factors can increase ventilator time and worsen outcome.

Glutamine-supplemented PN solutions administered to trauma or stressed patients can improve overall nitrogen balance, enhance muscle protein synthesis, improve intestinal nutrient absorption, decrease gut permeability, improve immune function, and decrease hospital stays and costs in some patient populations. A review of 14 randomized trials in surgical and critically ill patients found that glutamine supplementation was associated with reduced mortality, lower rates of infectious complications, and a decreased hospital stay. The greatest benefit was in patients receiving high-dose (>0.29 g/kg/day) parenteral glutamine.

Patients with intestinal dysfunction requiring PN, such as those with short bowel syndrome, mucosal damage following chemotherapy, irradiation, or critical illness might benefit from glutamine-containing PN. Glutamine-containing PN might also be beneficial in patients with immunodeficiency syndromes, including AIDS, immune-system dysfunction associated with critical illness, and bone marrow transplantation; patients with severe catabolic illness, such as major burns; patients with multiple trauma; and patients with other diseases associated with a prolonged ICU stay. Glutamine-supplemented solutions should not yet be considered routine care and should not be used in patients with significant renal insufficiency or in patients with significant hepatic failure.

Common Complications and Management

CATHETER SEPSIS

Central venous catheter–related bloodstream infection ranges from 3% to 20% in hospitalized patients and is the most common complication of central venous catheters. The migration of microorganisms along the external surface of the catheter is likely the most common cause, followed by intraluminal contamination from manipulation of the catheter hub or IV connectors. The most common organisms associated with catheter-related bloodstream infections include *Staphylococcus epidermidis*, *Staphylococcus aureus*, *Enterococcus* spp, *Candida albicans*, and *Enterobacter* spp as well as resistant strains such as methicillin-resistant *S. aureus* and vancomycin-resistant enterococci. Primary catheter sepsis occurs when there are signs and symptoms of infection and the indwelling catheter is the only anatomic focus of infection. Secondary catheter infections are associated with another focus or multiple infectious foci that cause bacteremia and seed the catheter.

Management of patients with catheter infection depends on their clinical condition. With extremely ill patients with high fevers who are hypotensive or who have local signs of infection around the catheter site, the catheter should be removed, its tip cultured, and peripheral and central venous blood cultures obtained. The organisms that grow from the catheter tip are the same as the ones that are identified in the peripheral blood culture and typically greater than 10^3 organisms are grown from cultures of the catheter tip.

Specific therapy should be initiated against the primary source in patients in whom a source of infection, other than the catheter tip, is present. Peripheral blood cultures should be obtained and blood cultures should not be taken from the central venous catheter port dedicated for PN because this increases the risk of contaminating the line. If the infection resolves, central venous feedings can be continued. If a secondary source is not identified and the symptoms persist, the catheter should be removed and its tip should be cultured. If the culture of the catheter tip returns positive or if the index of suspicion is high, appropriate antibiotic therapy is initiated. Central venous feeding can be resumed, maintaining euglycemia.

Occasionally, the situation arises in which a site of infection, other than the catheter, is identified, but signs and symptoms persist despite what is assumed to be adequate therapy. Again, if blood cultures are positive, the safest course of action may be to remove the

---

[1]Not FDA approved for this indication.

catheter. If peripheral blood cultures are negative, the catheter may be changed over a guidewire and the catheter tip cultured to determine if it was contaminated. Central venous feedings may be continued during this interval if the patient is stable. If the catheter tip returns positive, a new catheter should be inserted at a different site. Changing the central venous catheter over a guidewire can also facilitate the diagnosis of primary catheter infections. Changing the site of catheter location, rather than guidewire exchange, is recommended in patients in whom infection is suspected.

OTHER COMPLICATIONS

Common complications, their etiologies, and treatments are outlined in Table 5. Prolonged administration of PN can result in altered hepatic function and changes in liver pathologic conditions that can lead to liver failure. One to 2 weeks after initiating PN, transaminases may be elevated, but this often resolves without any change in the composition of PN or rate of administration. However, in patients receiving long-term PN (>20 days), prolonged elevations of alkaline phosphatase followed by elevated levels of serum transaminases can occur, even after therapy is discontinued.

Serum levels of alkaline phosphatase and bilirubin initially remain normal, but they rise in many patients who receive long-term PN. Patients who do not receive lipids in the PN solution have more

> ### BOX 3   Management of Parenteral Nutrition–Related Liver Dysfunction
>
> Have the patient eat, if possible.
> Avoid administering large amounts of glucose or protein calories.
> Supply lipid emulsions (up to 30% of total calories).
> Cycle the parenteral nutrition, infusing for 10–12 hours per day.
> Reevaluate caloric needs; reduce caloric intake if liver dysfunction persists.

frequent and severe hepatic abnormalities, most likely due to higher carbohydrate loads. Excess glucose increases insulin secretion, which stimulates hepatic lipogenesis and results in hepatic fat accumulation. Fatty infiltration is the initial histopathologic change; it is readily reversible and might not be accompanied by altered liver function tests.

Longer PN therapy may be associated with cholestasis, cholelithiasis, steatosis, and steatohepatitis and can progress to active chronic hepatitis, fibrosis, and eventual cirrhosis. The management of PN-related liver dysfunction is summarized in Box 3.

TABLE 5   Possible Etiologies and Treatment of Common Complications of Central Parenteral Nutrition

Problem	Possible Etiology	Treatment
Glucose		
Hyperglycemia, glycosuria, hyperosmolar nonketotic dehydration, or coma	Excessive dose or rate of infusion, inadequate insulin production, steroid administration, infection	Decrease the amount of glucose given, increase insulin, administer a portion of calories as fat
Diabetic ketoacidosis	Inadequate endogenous insulin production and/or inadequate insulin therapy	Give insulin Decrease glucose intake
Rebound hypoglycemia	Persistent endogenous insulin production by islet cells after long-term high-carbohydrate infusion	Give 5%–10% glucose before parenteral infusion is discontinued
Hypercarbia	Carbohydrate load exceeds the ability to increase minute ventilation and excrete excess CO_2	Limit glucose dose to 5 mg/kg/min Give greater percentage of total caloric needs as fat (up to 30%–40%)
Fat		
Hypertriglyceridemia	Rapid infusion Decreased clearance	Decrease rate of PN infusion Allow clearance (~12 h) before testing blood
Essential fatty acid deficiency	Inadequate essential fatty acid administration	Administer essential fatty acids in doses of 4%–7% of total calories
Amino Acids		
Hyperchloremia metabolic acidosis	Excessive chloride content of amino acid solutions	Administer Na^+ and K^+ as acetate salts
Prerenal azotemia	Excessive amino acids with inadequate caloric supplementation	Reduce amino acids Increase the amount of glucose calories
Miscellaneous		
Hypophosphatemia	Inadequate phosphorus administration with redistribution into tissues	Give 15 mmol phosphate/1000 IV kcal Evaluate antacid and Ca^{2+} administration
Hypomagnesemia	Inadequate administration relative to increased losses (diarrhea, diuresis, medications)	Administer Mg^{2+} (15–20 mEq/1000 kcal)
Hypermagnesemia	Excessive administration; renal failure	Decrease Mg^{2+} supplementation
Hypokalemia	Inadequate K^+ intake relative to increased needs for anabolism; diuresis	Increase K^+ supplementation
Hyperkalemia	Excessive K^+ administration, especially in metabolic acidosis; renal decompensation	Reduce or stop exogenous K^+ If ECG changes are present, treat with calcium gluconate, insulin, diuretics, and or Kayexalate
Hypocalcemia	Inadequate Ca^{2+} administration; reciprocal response to phosphorus repletion without simultaneous calcium infusion	Increase Ca^{2+} dose
Hypercalcemia	Excessive Ca^{2+} administration; excessive vitamin D administration	Decrease Ca^{2+} and/or vitamin D administration
Elevated liver transaminases or serum alkaline phosphatase and bilirubin	Enzyme induction secondary to amino acid imbalances or overfeeding	Reevaluate nutritional prescription Cycle TPN Avoid overfeeding calories Consider administering carnitine

ECG = electrocardiogram; PN = parenteral nutrition; TPN = total parenteral nutrition.

Complications are minimized and nutritional therapy maximized when the care of patients who require specialized nutritional support is supervised by a nutrition support team. Ideally, the nutrition support team consists of a pharmacist, dietitian, nurse, and physician.

REFERENCES

ASPEN Board of Directors. Guidelines for the use of parenteral and enteral nutrition in adult and pediatric patients. JPEN J Parenter Enteral Nutr 2002;26(1 Suppl.):1SA–138SA.

Bistrian BR, McCowen KC. Nutritional and metabolic support in the adult intensive care unit: Key controversies. Crit Care Med 2006;34:1525–31.

Butler SO, Btaiche IF, Alaniz C. Relationship between hyperglycemia and infection in critically ill patients. Pharmacotherapy 2005;25:963–76.

Heyland DK, Dhaliwal R, Drover JW, et al. Canadian clinical practice guidelines for nutrition support in mechanically ventilated, critically ill adult patients. JPEN J Parenter Enteral Nutr 2003;27:355–73.

Heyland DK, Dhaliwal R, Suchner U, Berger MM. Antioxidant nutrients: a systematic review of trace elements and vitamins in the critically ill patient. Intensive Care Med 2005;31:327–37.

Heyland DK, MacDonald S, Keefe L, Drover JW. Total parenteral nutrition in the critically ill patient: A meta-analysis. JAMA 1998;280:2013–9.

Kochevar M, Guenter P, Holcombe B, et al. ASPEN statement on parenteral nutrition standardization. JPEN J Parenter Enteral Nutr 2007;31:441–8.

McClave SA, Chang W-K, Dhaliwal R, Heyland DK. Nutrition support in acute pancreatitis: A systematic review of the literature. JPEN J Parenter Enteral Nutr 2006;30:143–56.

Novak F, Heyland DK, Avenell A, et al. Glutamine supplementation in serious illness: A systematic review of the evidence. Crit Care Med 2002;30:2022–9.

O'Grady NP, Alexander M, Dellinger EP, et al. Guidelines for the prevention of intravascular catheter-related infections. MMWR Recomm Rep 2002;51 (RR-10):1–29.

Parenteral Fluid Therapy in Children

Method of
Aaron Friedman, MD

Children receive three types of parenteral fluid therapy: maintenance therapy, restoration therapy, and replacement therapy. Maintenance fluid therapy provides the typical anticipated fluid and electrolyte losses seen in otherwise normal, euvolemic children. Restoration fluid therapy restores fluid volume previously lost. Replacement fluid therapy keeps up with ongoing abnormal fluid losses, such as ongoing losses from the gastrointestinal tract or abnormal urinary losses.

Maintenance Fluid Therapy

In 1957, Holliday and Segar proposed an approach to providing parenteral fluids and electrolytes to hospitalized children who are not permitted to eat or drink. The formulation was based on calories expended, presumed the patient did not have previous fluid losses (was euvolemic), and had normal kidney function. The surrogate for calories is weight because calories expended correlates to weight in grams. Therefore, the anticipated fluid losses for the upcoming 24 hours would come from urine excreted, water lost during breathing, and fluids lost from sweating. The prescription includes two components: water and electrolytes. Table 1 describes the approach recommended by Holliday and Segar to determine parenteral fluids and electrolytes for a 24-hour period. It includes determining the amount of water to be provided based on weight as a surrogate for calories expended and it includes electrolytes to be provided. The electrolytes are sodium and potassium. Sodium is given at 2 to 3 mmol per 100 mL water provided, and potassium is given at 2 mmol per 100 mL water provided, with each provided as the chloride salt. Once the amount is calculated, the hourly rate can be determined by dividing the final calculation by 24.

The prepared solution that most closely resembles this maintenance prescription is 0.2 NS (0.2 normal saline, or 154 mmol sodium and chloride per liter) with 20 mEq KCl/L of fluid. Often glucose is added at 50 g/L (D_5W) or 5 g/100 mL. This provides some readily available calories to reduce catabolism. Note also that D_5W has an osmolality of nearly 300 mOsm/kg H_2O, essentially the same as plasma. This allows safe administration of the solution, because a markedly hypotonic solution administered into a vein could result in lysis of cells (especially red cells) in the vicinity of the infused hypotonic solution.

Another approach for calculating the water with the appropriate electrolytes to be provided is 1500 mL/m^2/24 hours. This approach requires measuring the child's height and weight to determine square meters and is less convenient. The volume provided by the approach in Table 1 and the 1500 mL/m^2 calculation are equivalent.

Another approach is to determine the hourly need of water bearing the electrolytes to be provided, the same as Holliday and Segar. The hourly approach to determining volume is shown in Table 2. Using this approach, maintenance fluid therapy for a 15-kg child would be infused at a rate of 50 mL/hour:

$$(4 \text{ mL/kg/h} \times 10 \text{ kg}) + (2 \text{ mL/kg/h} \times 5 \text{ kg})$$

Maintenance fluid therapy was designed to provide water and electrolytes to cover *future* (anticipated) loss, particularly from urine, expired air, and sweat. Unfortunately, since the publication of maintenance fluid therapy guidelines by Holliday and Segar, the formulation has often been misused. Maintenance fluid therapy should *not* be used as a fluid prescription for *restoring* extracellular fluid volume previously lost, for example, as a result of vomiting, diarrhea, or burns. It is almost always *not* an appropriate solution for *replacing* abnormal losses from the gastrointestinal tract, urinary tract, and so on. The volume calculation and the electrolyte concentrations are *not* appropriate to calculate a restoration solution or replacement solution.

The primary reason that a hypotonic solution such as maintenance fluids, as described by Holliday and Segar, is problematic for use as a restoration solution is the nonosmotic release of antidiuretic hormone (ADH, also called AVP [arginine vasopressin]). Since the mid 1950s it has been known that ADH is released from the hypothalamus under two different physiologic stimuli. One is an increase in serum and extracellular osmolality, usually greater than 290 mOsm/kg H_2O, termed *osmotic stimulus*. The other is a nonosmotic stimulus, usually

TABLE 1 Approach to Determine Parenteral Fluids and Electrolytes for a 24-Hour Period

Weight (kg)	Water (mL)	Na (mEq/L)	K (mEq/L)
0-10	100/kg	3/100 mL	2/100 mL
11-20	1000 + 50/kg 11-20 kg	3/100 mL	2/100 mL
>20	1500 + 20/kg >20 kg	3/100 mL	2/100 mL
Examples			
15-kg child	1250	37 mEq/1250 mL	25 mEq/1250 mL
30-kg child	1700	51	34

Note: For sodium, potassium, and chloride, milliequivalents (mEq) and milliosmoles (mOsm) are the same.

TABLE 2 Hourly Administration of Fluids

Child's Weight (kg)	Volume of Water per Hour
≤10	4 mL/kg
11-20	40 mL + 2 mL/kg for every kilogram 11-20
>20	60 mL + 1 mL/kg for every kilogram >20

the result of a fall in extracellular fluid volume or the perception of such a fall by volume receptors mainly in the thorax.

Since the 1950s we have come to learn that a large number of other stimuli can act as a nonosmotic stimulus to ADH release. These include, but are not limited to, a wide range of medications (antihypertensives, some antineoplastics, barbiturates), stress, central nervous system (CNS) injury or surgery, positive pressure ventilation, malignancy, and intrathoracic infection or malignancy. Under these conditions, ADH levels will be high and the administration of a hypotonic solution even at calculated maintenance doses could result in a fall in serum sodium and serum osmolality, on occasion to levels that might cause serious CNS injury, seizures, and even CNS herniation and death. Even in the early 1960s, when the precise reasons for the nonosmotic release of ADH were not well known, the risk of developing hyponatremia when providing the full volume prescribed in maintenance fluid therapy in the face of a concentrated urine and low urine volumes (signaling ADH release) was well known. The recommendation was to reduce the volume of fluid provided to approximately 50% of the standard calculated amount.

More recently, some have recommended, to prevent the development of hyponatremia, that all maintenance fluid therapy should be delivered as isotonic (normal) saline. The volume portion of the Holliday–Segar formulation is not altered, but the solution recommended in this approach is isotonic saline. The full impact of this approach on all types of hospitalized children is still unknown. It seems clear that patients in the perioperative period should receive normal saline in anticipation of the potential need for extracellular volume restoration. This approach does not guarantee that hyponatremia or hypernatremia will be totally prevented.

Restoration Fluid Therapy

Many children require parenteral fluids because of an inability to take fluids by mouth or due to abnormal fluid losses, such as from vomiting and diarrhea, excessive urinary losses, burns (excessive fluid losses from skin), or third spacing (the extravasation of fluid from the extracellular spaces such as the abdominal or thoracic cavity). In these situations, patients are at risk for serious extracellular volume depletion and even plasma volume depletion, which, left untreated, can result in hypotension or shock.

 CURRENT DIAGNOSIS

- Maintenance fluid therapy is designed to replace the next 24 hours' anticipated losses from sensible and insensible losses in an otherwise healthy, euvolemic patient with normal kidney function.
- In a patient with extracellular volume loss, the percentage of body weight lost should be used as a guide to the volume needed for restoration.
- Serum sodium in patients with dehydration should be measured at the time of presentation and also after restoration fluid has been provided. The further correction of serum sodium will be much easier in a patient with a normalized extracellular volume.

 CURRENT THERAPY

- Maintenance fluid therapy should not be used as a restoration or replacement fluid.
- Restoration fluid therapy can be given over short periods with a plan for complete restoration, in the majority of patients, within 24 hours.
- When treating hyponatremia or hypernatremia, the goal should be to change the serum sodium by *no more than* 10 mmol/L in a 24-hour period.
- When calculating how much water (in the case of hypernatremia) or how much sodium (in the case of hyponatremia) to provide a patient in order to restore sodium into the normal range, remember the calculation is based on the *total body water,* which is 60% of body weight, and the aim is to get to the closest serum sodium considered normal; for example, sodium 135 mmol/L for hyponatremia and sodium 145 mmol/L for hypernatremia.
- Replacement fluid therapy for patients with abnormal losses—gastrointestinal or urinary losses—should be based on measurement of the lost fluid volume and fluid electrolyte content.

The parenteral fluid therapy for volume depletion should aim to first replace extracellular volume depletion. How much fluid to provide can be estimated by a long-standing approach using clinical signs to estimate the percentage of reduction in body weight associated with fluid losses (Table 3). In general, these losses can be replaced with a solution that restores extracellular fluid (isotonic saline or lactated Ringer's solution). In situations of prolonged fluid losses (more than 7 days), partial replacement with isotonic saline followed by a slower replacement with a more hypotonic solution with added potassium may be warranted. Table 3 outlines the clinical approach to assessing a patient's degree of volume depletion as a percentage of body weight.

Once the percentage of volume depletion is determined and the decision is made to use parenteral fluids based on moderate to severe volume depletion and ongoing vomiting, thus decreasing the effectiveness of oral rehydration, then rapid parenteral volume repletion is usually safe and effective. Replacing 50% of the determined volume depletion in 1 to 4 hours is appropriate, with the remaining replacement in the subsequent 4 to 16 hours. This should result in restored volume and improvement in the signs and symptoms demonstrated or reported by the patient. Often, partial restoration of extracellular

TABLE 3 Signs of Volume Depletion

Sign	Degree of Depletion		
	Mild (1-4%)	Moderate (5-7%)	Severe (>7%)
Skin	Normal	Cool	Cool, mottled
Capillary refill	Normal	Decreased	Markedly decreased
Skin turgor	Normal	Loose	Tenting
Buccal mucosa	Slightly dry	Dry	Parched
Eyes	Normal	Sunken	Markedly sunken
Fontanel*	Normal	Sunken	Markedly sunken
Pulse	Normal (full)	Rapid	Rapid, thready
Urine output	Normal	Decreased	Oliguria (<1 ml/kg/hr)
Systolic blood pressure	Normal	Normal, low	Low, shock

*Infants <9 mo of age.

volume depletion improves gastrointestinal symptoms and allows a switch to the oral route for completing volume restoration.

Example: A 15-kg patient presents with a 3-day history of vomiting and diarrhea. Physical examination suggests 5% volume depletion. The patient has ongoing vomiting, and parenteral fluids will be started. Volume depletion of 5% is 750 mL of fluid:

$$0.5 \times 15 \text{ kg (body weight)}$$

A commonly used volume expansion technique is to provide isotonic saline, 20 mL/kg, in a bolus (over 30 minutes to 1 hour). This amount of 300 mL (15 kg × 20 mL/kg) is approximately 2% of body weight and in this example is less than 50% of the determined volume depletion. The plan, therefore, is 375 mL (50%) over 1 to 2 hours of isotonic saline (or lactated Ringer's solution) parenterally, then 375 mL of the same solution over the next 4 to 6 hours.

Replacement Fluids

As a general rule of thumb, unusual losses—gastrointestinal or renal, for example—should be replaced with a solution of comparable electrolyte concentration and of comparable volume. The most precise way to determine the needed solution is to measure the concentration of solutes such as sodium, potassium, chloride, or bicarbonate lost in emesis, diarrhea, or urine. Emesis contains sodium at 10 to 40 mmol/L and even less potassium (5-20 mmol/L) but large amounts of chloride (90-150 mmol/L). Diarrheal fluid typically contains sodium at 40 to 90 mmol/L, potassium at 10 to 50 mmol/L, and up to 40 or 50 mmol/L of bicarbonate. Cholera patients can excrete sodium up to 140 mmol/L. When possible, the volume of loss should be measured so a replacement fluid solution volume can be planned.

The safe approach to the patient with ongoing losses is first to restore extracellular volume to normal using normal saline or lactated Ringer's solution as noted earlier. During extracellular volume restoration, measure the output and electrolyte content of abnormal losses, preferably over a 12- to 24-hour period. Once this is known, then replacement of ongoing losses should be provided as a separate solution, the volume and electrolyte concentration determined by the measurements of each. Provide the replacement solution over the next 12 to 24 hours. For example, a patient with diarrhea is found to be producing 300 mL of diarrheal fluid over 12 hours. The measured sodium concentration is 80 mmol/L, potassium is 20 mmol/L, and bicarbonate is 40 mmol/L. The solution that will nearly approximate the losses is 0.2 NS (34 mmol/L of sodium and of chloride) with 20 mmol/L of potassium and 40 mmol/L of sodium bicarbonate. The solution will contain 74 mmol/L of Na, 20 mmol/L of K and 40 mmol/L of bicarbonate. The solution would be infused at a rate of 25 mL/hour. The advantage of providing this separately from maintenance or restoration fluids is that the rate of infusion or even the electrolyte content can be changed to address just the replacement needs without having to change all the intravenous solutions.

Hyponatremia and Hypernatremia

Hyponatremia (serum sodium <135 mmol/L) and hypernatremia (serum sodium >145 mmol/L) are often associated with volume depletion. Hypernatremia is nearly exclusively associated with volume depletion, and hyponatremia can be seen in situations of volume expansion such as vasopressin excess (syndrome of inappropriate antidiuretic hormone [SIADH]) or congestive heart failure, kidney failure, or liver failure. At times, the need to normalize the serum sodium concentration requires parenteral intervention.

APPROACH TO HYPONATREMIA

Symptomatic hyponatremia can occur if the serum sodium falls rapidly, but usually not until the serum sodium falls below 125 mmol/L. The symptoms associated with hyponatremia include anorexia, anxiety, agitation, ataxia, weakness, lethargy, disorientation, depressed deep tendon reflexes, seizures, coma, and death (usually the result of CNS herniation).

In situations where hyponatremia is associated with volume depletion, restoration of volume with isotonic saline often raises the serum sodium. When extracellular fluid volume is normal or expanded (such as situations when SIADH is at play), a four-fold approach to hyponatremia should be considered:

1. Treat the underlying condition.
2. Reduce water intake. In particular, if parenteral fluids are being provided, reduce or eliminate the use of hypotonic fluids.
3. Increase water excretion. This is usually done with loop diuretics such as furosemide (Lasix), (0.5-1 mg/kg IV) to achieve a more rapid response.
4. Hypertonic saline IV is a step reserved for symptomatic patients. The most readily available hypertonic saline solution is 3% normal saline (sodium concentration of 513 mmol/L or approximately 0.5 mmol/mL). The desired outcome is to raise the serum sodium sufficiently to improve symptoms, but never more than 10 mmol/L in a 24-hour period. There is no need to raise the serum sodium beyond the lower limit of normal or 135 mmol/L. The desired increase in the serum sodium concentration should not exceed a maximum of 10 mmol/L.

The addition of sodium into the extracellular space will result in a shift of water from the intracellular to the extracellular space. Thus, the entire water space will be affected. The following example demonstrates how to calculate the amount of hypertonic saline to infuse in the face of severe hyponatremia:

A patient weighing 15 kg has a serum sodium of 125 mmol/L and experiences a seizure. The patient is felt to be euvolemic. Thus, hypertonic saline infusion is being considered. How should this be prescribed? Raise the serum sodium to 135 mmol/L from 125 mmol/L:

$$\text{Change in serum sodium(mmol/L)} \times \text{body weight(kg)}$$
$$\times 0.6\text{(total body water space)}$$
$$= 10 \times 15 \times 0.6 = 90 \text{ mmol}$$

Because hypertonic saline is approximately 0.5 mmol/mL, if 90 mmol is the amount of sodium calculated to raise the serum sodium and osmolality, then 180 mL of 3% saline is needed.

An alternative way to calculate the maximum 3% saline to use is: The maximum change in serum sodium is 10, the body weight is 15 kg, the water space is 1.2 (0.6 × 2 = 1.2; i.e., 2 mL/mmol sodium in 3% saline), so:

$$10 \times 15 \times 1.2 = 180 \text{ mL of 3\% saline}$$

Once the amount is calculated, the rate of administration should be no more than 2 to 4 mL/kg/hour, with measurements of the serum sodium at 2-hour intervals. Usually symptoms improve before there is a full 10-mmol rise in serum sodium. This rate should not result in a change of greater than 1 to 2 mmol/hour. If a change faster than this is seen, slow or stop the infusion immediately.

APPROACH TO HYPERNATREMIA

Hypernatremia (serum sodium >145 mmol/L) is seen with volume depletion. The extremely rare situation of pure salt overload is seen in babies receiving improperly mixed formula or intensive care patients receiving concentrated blood products and IV solutions. In these situations the patients do not show evidence of volume depletion, and urinary sodium excretion (and fractional excretion of sodium) is very high. In the overwhelming majority of patients who are volume depleted, hypernatremia signals volume losses of *at least* 10% of body weight. The classic teaching is that hypernatremic patients appear less-severely volume depleted than they actually are. This is attributed to the increased osmolality protecting the extracellular space at the cost of intracellular space. Intracellular volume contains two thirds of total body water, and the decreased volume in the intracellular space means nearly all cells in the body (importantly, including in the brain) are smaller than normal.

The approach to hypernatremia is first to restore volume using isotonic saline. Providing 40 to 50 mL/kg of isotonic saline over 4 hours will improve extracellular volume and is unlikely to markedly reduce the serum sodium. Restoring extracellular volume will improve organ perfusion, especially perfusion of the gut and the kidney. This will improve the likelihood of being able to use the gut for fluid replacement and improve glomerular filtration rate and overall kidney function so as to be able to restore volume and safely return serum sodium and osmolality to normal. The major consequence of a too-rapid fall in serum sodium or osmolality is cerebral edema, the result of smaller-than-normal cell volume too rapidly expanded by IV (especially hypotonic) fluids.

Following the first infusion, as noted earlier, consider providing 30 to 40 mL/kg of isotonic fluid over the next 20 hours (to complete a 24-hour treatment plan) to continue replenishing extracellular volume. Check the serum sodium and serum osmolality frequently, at 2- to 4-hour intervals in the first 24 to 48 hours if the serum sodium is greater than 155 mmol/L at presentation. As with hyponatremia, it is important not to change (in this case, drop) the serum sodium by more than 10 mmol/L in 24 hours or to change the serum osmolality by more than 20 mOsm/kg H_2O in 24 hours. To determine how much water is necessary to lower the serum sodium, the following formula is often used:

Actual serum sodium − desired serum sodium (not to exceed 10)
  × body weight in kg × 4 mL

For a 15-kg child with a serum sodium of 155:

$$10 \times 15 \times 4 = 600 \text{ mL of water}$$

The safe approach to reducing the water deficit is to provide no more than half of the water deficit in the first 24 hours as a solution of 5% dextrose (D_5W) with potassium of 20 to 30 mmol/L. The intracellular fluid compartment is rich in potassium, and patients with hypernatremic dehydration have had considerable intracellular volume loss and have lost potassium, usually through urinary losses. The same approach may be considered in day 2 and following. Certain caveats are important here. First, as noted earlier, frequent measurements of serum sodium and serum osmolality are necessary to prevent too rapid a decline. Because the maintenance prescription is very hypotonic in the first 24 hours, at least, replacing volume loss should be the first priority. Once the patient approaches a normal volume status and serum sodium, providing maintenance *may* be appropriate. Patients with hypertonicity (hypernatremic dehydration) are very thirsty. Any fluid they consume by mouth must be measured and monitored lest their oral consumption along with parenteral fluids exceed the safe amount recommended.

Intravenous Electrolyte Replacements

At times, IV replacement of other electrolytes may be necessary. The IV replacement of potassium, in situations where the serum potassium concentration falls below 2.5 mmol/L or where oral replacement cannot be used, can be given as potassium chloride or potassium phosphate at a dose of no more than 0.5 mmol/kg/hour. The concentration of potassium in the solution infused should not exceed 40 mmol/L in a peripheral vein because potassium infusions are painful and sclerosing. Higher concentrations under the appropriate circumstances could be given through a central vein.

On occasion, IV administration of calcium or phosphate (or both) is clinically indicated. IV calcium is considered in patients with tetany, usually a serum calcium <6.5 mg/dL with a normal serum albumin. For IV calcium administration to correct symptomatic hypocalcemia, in older children the recommendation is 10 to 20 mL of a 10% calcium gluconate solution over 15 minutes to reduce or stop symptoms such as tetany or seizures. In neonates and young children, 10 to 20 mg/kg or 1 to 2 mL/kg of a 10% calcium gluconate solution administered at a rate of 1 mL/min with cardiac monitoring is recommended. For more chronic administration, 50 to 75 mg/kg/24 hours of calcium gluconate is recommended. Rapid calcium administration temporarily lowers the serum phosphate and can lead to arrhythmia, hence the cardiac monitoring.

Hypophosphatemia might require parenteral administration of phosphate. This approach is usually reserved for patients with a serum phosphate less than 1 mg/dL. The recommended dosage of elemental phosphorus is 2.5 to 5 mg/kg (0.08 to 0.16 mmol/kg) over 6 to 8 hours. This administration can lower serum calcium, so frequent testing of both the serum phosphorus and calcium is appropriate.

Finally, bicarbonate may be given intravenously. Usually the IV solution of bicarbonate should not exceed a concentration of 45 mmol/L. For example, in certain clinical conditions alkalinization of the urine is desired to prevent crystal or stone formation. The usual prescription is 1 to 2 mmol/kg body weight in 24 hours. Higher infused concentrations of bicarbonate (seen in patients with proximal tubule disease or injury as noted with certain chemotherapeutic agents) should be given into a central vein under careful monitoring. Calcium and bicarbonate should not be given in the same solution.

REFERENCES

Feld LG, Friedman AL, Massengil SF. Disorders of water metabolism in fluid and electrolytes. In: Feld LG, Kaskel FJ, editors. Pediatrics. Totowa, NJ: Humana Press; 2010. p. 3–47.

Friedman AL, Ray PE. Maintenance fluid therapy. What it is and what it is not. Pediatr Nephrol 2008;23:677–80.

Gauer OH, Henry JP. Circulatory basis of fluid volume control. Physiol Rev 1963;43:423–81.

Holliday MA, Segar WE. The maintenance need for water in parenteral fluid therapy. Pediatrics 1957;19:823–32.

Moritz ML, Ayus JC. Prevention of hospital acquired hyponatremia, a case for using isotonic saline. Pediatrics 2003;111:227–30.

Nelville KA, Sondeman DJ, Rubenstein A, et al. Prevention of hyponatremia during maintenance intravenous fluid administration: A prospective, randomized study of fluid type versus fluid rate. J Pediatr 2010;156:313–9.

Robertson GL. Antidiuretic hormone. Normal and disordered function. Endocrinol Metab Clin North Am 2001;30:671–84.

The Endocrine System

Acromegaly

Method of
Moises Mercado, MD

Acromegaly is a disorder resulting from an excessive secretion of growth hormone (GH), with a prevalence of 40 to 60 cases per million and an annual incidence of 3 to 4 per million.

Physiology, Biochemistry and Regulation of the GH/IGF-1 Axis

GH secretion is regulated at the hypothalamus (Fig. 1). The pulsatile secretion of GH-releasing hormone (GHRH) stimulates somatotroph proliferation and GH gene transcription, whereas somatostatin, which is secreted tonically, inhibits GH synthesis. These two hypothalamic signals result in the pulsatile secretion of pituitary GH, with most pulses occurring during the night. GH is also stimulated by ghrelin, a hypothalamic and gastrointestinal orexigenic hormone that binds specific receptors in the somatotroph known as GH-secretagogue receptors. GH exerts its actions through a specific membrane receptor located predominantly in the liver and cartilage. One molecule of GH interacts with two molecules of GH receptor, resulting in functional dimerization and conformational changes that lead to the phosphorylation of several kinases and eventually the interaction with target genes such as the insulin-like growth factor (IGF)-1 gene.

IGF-1 is closely related to proinsulin and circulates in plasma bound to six binding proteins (IGFBPs) that are synthesized and released by the liver. IGFBP3 is the most important of these binding proteins and is also GH dependent; it forms a heterotrimeric complex composed of BP3, IGF-1, and the acid-labile subunit (ALS). IGF-1 is responsible for most of the trophic and growth-promoting effects of GH. Blood levels of IGF-1 are increased during puberty, coinciding with the acceleration of somatic growth, and decline with aging. Malnutrition, poorly controlled type 1 diabetes, hypothyroidism, and liver failure all result in diminished IGF-1 concentrations. IGF-1 is the main player in GH negative feedback regulation and it acts at both the pituitary and the hypothalamic levels. Glucose regulates GH release by increasing (hypoglycemia) or decreasing (hyperglycemia) somatostatin synthesis in the hypothalamus. Exercise and amino acids such as arginine also stimulate GH secretion.

Etiopathogenesis of Growth Hormone–Secreting Tumors

The molecular pathogenesis of pituitary tumors includes the inactivation of tumor suppressor genes, the activation of oncogenes, and the trophic effect of factors such as the hypothalamic releasing hormones. Approximately 40% of GH-producing tumors in whites harbor somatic point mutations of the α subunit stimulatory G protein coupled to the GHRH receptor (GSPα mutations). This molecular alteration causes constitutive activation of the GHRH receptor, resulting in an increased transcription of the GH gene and the promotion of somatotroph proliferation. Acromegalic patients whose tumors harbor GSPα mutations usually have a more benign clinical course and appear to be more susceptible to management with somatostatin analogues. Nonwhite acromegalic populations, including persons of Japanese, Korean, and Mexican heritage, have a much lower prevalence of GSPα mutations.

Other molecular events should be present in GSPα-negative somatotrophinomas. Menin is a protein encoded by a tumor suppressor gene located on the short arm of chromosome 11. Inactivating mutations of menin are the molecular basis of type 1 multiple endocrine neoplasia (MEN1); however, GH-secreting tumors occurring out of this context do not have such genetic abnormalities. Inactivating mutations of other putative tumor-suppressor genes located relatively close to the menin locus have been described in several kindreds with familial acromegaly; however they do not seem to play an important oncogenic role in the sporadic form of the disease. Other genetic alterations such as underexpression of GADD 45γ (growth arrest and DNA damage-inducible protein) and overexpression of the securing molecule PTTG (pituitary tumor transforming gene) have also been shown to be involved in the molecular pathogenesis of acromegaly. Although hereditary acromegaly is rare (less than 2% of the cases) familial somatotrophinomas account for 30% of the tumors seen in the syndrome of familial isolated pituitary adenomas. Patients with isolated familial somatotrophinomas are younger and usually have more aggressive tumors than subjects with sporadic acromegaly. Affected members do not show any molecular alterations in the MEN1 gene. However, 15% of 73 tested families harbor inactivating, germline mutations of the AIP gene (Aryl Hydrocarbon Interacting Protein) located on chromosome 11q13.3.

In more than 90% of cases, acromegaly is caused by a sporadic pituitary adenoma. In approximately 70% of these patients, these benign epithelial neoplasms are larger than 1 cm in diameter and are known as *macroadenomas*, whereas one third of the patients harbor lesions smaller than 1 cm or *microadenomas*. One third of the patients have tumors that cosecrete GH and prolactin (PRL) (mammosomatoroph cell adenomas). Real pituitary GH-secreting carcinomas, with

647

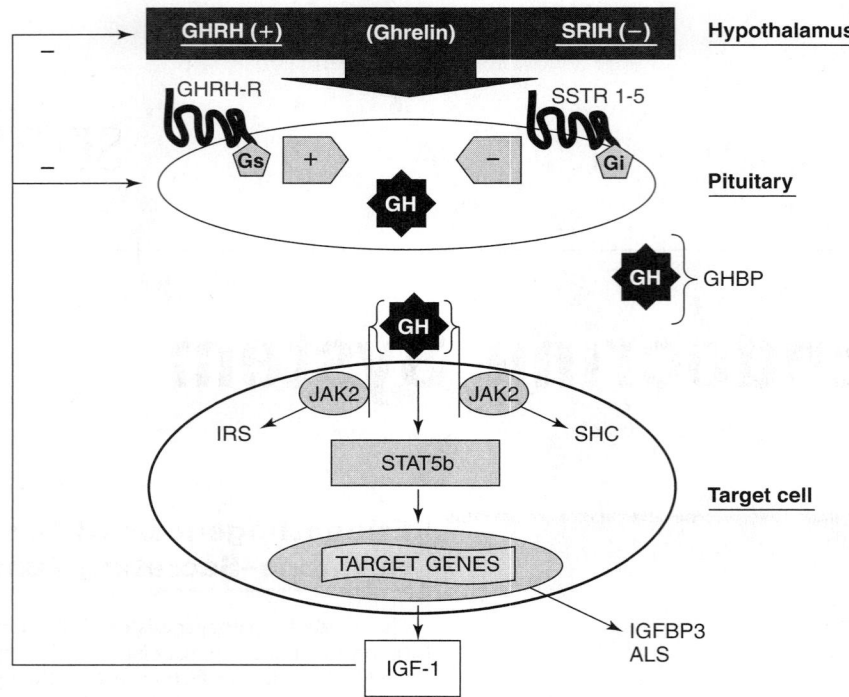

FIGURE 1. GH is regulated positively by GHRH and negatively by somatostatin. Fifty percent of circulating GH is bound to the GH binding protein, which represents the extracellular portion of the GH receptor. One molecule of GH dimerizes two molecules of GH receptor, and the ensuing signal transduction results in IGF-1 synthesis and secretion, which exerts negative feedback on GH secretion at the hypothalamic and pituitary levels. ALS = acid-labile subunit; GH = growth hormone; GHRH = growth hormone–releasing hormone; IGF = insulin-like growth factor; IGFBP3 = insulin-like growth factor binding protein 3; IRS = insulin receptor S; SRIH = somatostatin; SSTR = somatostatin receptor.

documented metastasis as the irrefutable malignancy criterion, are exceedingly rare. On rare occasions, acromegaly results from GHRH-secreting neuroendocrine tumors, usually located in the lungs, thymus, or endocrine pancreas. In this scenario, the ectopically produced GHRH leads to hyperplasia of the somatotroph, with the consequent excessive production of GH. Even less common are GH-secreting tumors arising in ectopic pituitary tissue, usually located in the sphenoid sinus. A case of GH-secreting lymphoma has been reported.

Clinical Manifestations

Acromegaly develops insidiously over many years. An 8- to 10-year delay in diagnosis has been estimated from the beginning of the first symptom. Clinical characteristics are often attributed to aging. Symptoms and signs can be divided into those resulting from the compressive effects of the pituitary tumor and those that are a consequence of the GH and IGF-1 excess.

LOCAL TUMOR EFFECTS

Headache results from an increase in intracranial pressure and from the effects of GH itself; it is usually described as a dull pain that persists throughout the day. Occasionally, large tumors invading laterally into the cavernous sinuses give rise to cranial nerve syndromes, usually third and sixth. Visual field defects are relatively common with macroadenomas extending superiorly and compressing the optic chiasm. This usually results in different combinations of bitemporal homonymous hemianopia or quadrontopia.

CONSEQUENCES OF THE GH/IGF-1 EXCESS

Skeletal Growth and Skin Changes

A GH excess developing before the pubertal closure of epiphyseal bone leads to an acceleration of linear growth, and this results in gigantism. Once the patient is in adulthood, the GH/IGF-1 excess results in acral enlargement, which is manifested by increases in ring and shoe sizes as well as enlargement of the nose, supracilliary arches, frontal bones and mandible. There is thickening of soft tissues of the hands and feet; hands are fleshy and bulky and the heel pad is increased. The skin is thickened due to the deposition of glycosaminoglycans and excessive collagen production. Hyperhidrosis and seborrhea occur in 60% of patients; skin tags (previously associated with colon cancer) and acanthosis nigricans are common.

Musculoskeletal System

Generalized arthralgias are present in the majority (80%) of patients. Degenerative osteoarthritis is more common than in the general population. Paresthesias of the hands and feet and a proximal painful myopathy are often reported. Nerve entrapment syndromes such as the carpal tunnel syndrome occur in nearly one half of patients.

Cardiovascular System

Arterial hypertension is found in 30% of patients, and when associated with diabetes it contributes to the increased mortality rate of the disease. Hyperaldosteronism with low renin levels and the resulting sodium retention play an important role in the pathogenesis of hypertension, but other contributors such as an increased sympathetic tone are also present. Echocardiographic findings include left ventricular and septal hypertrophy with varying degrees of diastolic dysfunction. Symptomatic cardiac disease develops in 15% of patients and is usually due to coronary artery disease, heart failure, and arrhythmias. Although the existence of an acromegalic cardiomyopathy is still controversial, there are patients without hypertension and with angiographically normal coronaries, who develop severe congestive heart failure, in whom histologic evidence of subendocardial, subepicardial, and myocardial fibrosis and necrosis has been documented.

Respiratory Abnormalities

The majority of patients with acromegaly are affected by loud snoring. A significant fraction of these have sleep apnea (with both central and obstructive components) with significant drops in oxygen saturation, which can be complicated by arrhythmias, daytime somnolence, and chronic fatigue.

Abnormalities in Glucose Metabolism

Chronic GH hypersecretion creates a state of insulin resistance, and glucose intolerance has been reported in 30% to 50% of patients with acromegaly; the percentage with fasting hyperglycemia can be close to 30%, depending on the population. Hyperglycemia has correlated with GH concentrations in some studies and with IGF-1 levels in others.

Abnormalities in Lipid Metabolism

The classic lipid profile consists of diminished total cholesterol, along with elevated triglyceride concentrations. Intermediate-density lipoprotein (IDL) particles and Lipoprotein(a) might also be elevated, and there is a higher percentage of the more atherogenic type II low-density lipoprotein (LDL).

Bone and Calcium Metabolism

Acromegaly is associated with hypercalciuria and hyperphosphatemia. High serum 25-hydroxyvitamin D_3 and urinary levels of hydroxyproline can be found, reflecting a state of increased bone turnover. Cortical bone mineral density is elevated, whereas trabecular bone mass is diminished.

Neoplasia

Retrospective studies suggested that colonic adenomatous polyps and adenocarcinoma were more frequent in acromegalic patients than in the general population. Prospective studies have demonstrated that the risk, albeit smaller than previously thought, is real and probably justifies screening colonoscopy in these patients. Patients with uncontrolled acromegaly have a higher risk of recurrence of premalignant polyps and a higher mortality rate from colon cancer compared with subjects with biochemically controlled disease and the general population.

Associated Endocrine Abnormalities

A euthyroid goiter is often found but seldom requires specific treatment. Hypopituitarism occurs variably, depending on the size and extension of the tumor and whether the patient has undergone surgery or radiation therapy. Hypogonadotropic hypogonadism is the most common pituitary deficiency, occurring in 20% of patients. A decreased libido is a common presenting complaint in both male and female patients with acromegaly; women often have menstrual and ovulatory disturbances and men complain of impotence.

Although an elevated PRL is common, it does not always reflect cosecretion of this hormone by the somatotrophinoma, but rather an interruption of the descending dopaminergic tone by the tumor compressing the pituitary stalk. Central hypocortisolism and hypothyroidism are less common.

GH-secreting pituitary adenomas are the second, after prolactinomas, pituitary tumor occurring in the context of MEN1 (multiple parathyroid adenomas, pituitary adenoma, and pancreatic islet cell tumors). Acromegaly can also develop in patients with the McCune-Albright syndrome (polyostotic fibrous dysplasia, café au lait spots, and endocrinopathies such as sexual precocity and autonomous thyroid nodules).

Mortality

Life expectancy in patients with acromegaly is decreased by about 10 to 15 years, and the standardized mortality ratio is 1.5 to 2. Most patients die of cardiovascular causes, followed by cerebrovascular events, respiratory abnormalities, and neoplastic diseases. Hormonal control has a definite impact on survival. Lowering serum GH to less than 2.5 ng/mL results in reduction of the mortality rate to levels comparable with the general population. These safe GH levels were obtained using old radioimmunoassays, and there are no equivalent studies using ultrasensitive GH assays. IGF-1 levels have not been as good as GH as independent predictors of mortality. Other factors associated with an increased mortality include advanced age and the presence of hypertension and diabetes. A recent meta-analysis including 16 series from 1970 to 2005 reveals a 72% increase in all-cause mortality in patients with acromegaly. Although the mortality rate has decreased in the past decade, likely due to modern treatment strategies, there is still a 32% increase in mortality risk.

Biochemical Diagnosis

Due to the pulsatile nature of GH secretion, random determinations of this hormone are not useful in the diagnosis of acromegaly. The gold standard for the diagnosis is the measurement of GH after an oral glucose load of 75 g; current guidelines state that suppression to less than 0.3 ng/mL (using ultrasensitive assays), reliably excludes the diagnosis. Situations associated with decreased suppression of GH by glucose include puberty, pregnancy, use of oral contraceptives, uncontrolled diabetes, and renal and hepatic insufficiency.

IGF-1 levels reflect the integrated concentrations over 24 hours of GH and correlate well with clinical activity. Blood IGF-1 concentrations decrease with age, reflecting the parallel decline of the somatotropic axis. There is a gender difference in IGF-1 (premenopausal women have lower levels than age-matched male subjects). Other conditions that lower IGF-1 levels include malnutrition, uncontrolled diabetes, and hepatic and renal failure. Normal ranges for IGF-1 should be established in each particular center based on age and sex. The determination of other GH-dependent peptides such as IGFBP3 and ALS has not proved to be superior to IGF-1.

Imaging

Pituitary magnetic resonance imaging (MRI) with gadolinium enhancement allows visualization of lesions as small as 2 or 3 mm in diameter. High-resolution computed tomography (CT) is a reasonable alternative, although it is much less sensitive. An ectopic source of GHRH should be suspected when the MRI is completely normal. In these rare cases, serum GHRH should be measured and the ectopic tumor should be sought, usually with high-resolution CT of the chest and abdomen.

Treatment

The decision as to what therapeutic modality should be used has to take into account medical issues (cardiopulmonary comorbidities, size, and extension of the tumor) as well as the local characteristics of the treating center. The latter refers to the availability of pituitary surgeons and radiotherapeutic technologies as well as the economic feasibility of pharmacologic therapy.

SURGERY

Transsphenoidal surgery has been the traditional treatment for acromegaly and achieves biochemical cure (normalization of IGF-1 and a glucose-suppressed GH <1 ng/mL) in 80% to 90% of microadenomas. Cure rates for macroadenomas are much lower (40%–50%), and invasive lesions have a very slight chance (<10%) of being cured by surgery. Even though surgery often fails to achieve a full biochemical cure, debulking the pituitary adenoma relieves optic chiasm compression and can result in a sufficient decrement of tumor mass (and therefore of GH production) to allow better results with either pharmacologic or radiotherapeutic regimens.

CURRENT DIAGNOSIS

Clinical

- Headaches, visual field defects
- Coarse features, increased size of hands (rings) and feet (shoes)
- Thick, oily skin, skin tags, acanthosis nigricans
- Arthralgias, osteoarthritis
- Paresthesias, carpal tunnel syndrome
- Hypertension, arrhythmia, heart failure
- Glucose intolerance, diabetes, hypertryglyceridemia
- Snoring, sleep apnea
- Risk of colon polyps or colon cancer

Biochemical

- Glucose-suppressed growth hormone >0.3 ng/mL by ultrasensitive assays or >1 ng/mL by old radio-immunoassays
- Elevated age- and sex-matched insulin-like growth factor 1
- Other growth hormone–dependent peptides: insulin-like growth factor binding protein 3, acid-labile subunit

Imaging

- Computed tomography
- Magnetic resonance imaging

 CURRENT THERAPY

- If a pituitary surgeon is available: Transsphenoidal surgery for microadenomas, intrasellar macroadenomas, and debulking or decompressing surgery in invasive macroadenomas
- Somatostatin analogues as secondary treatment for patients failing surgery or waiting for radiotherapy effect to occur and as a primary treatment for patients with inaccessible lesions, contraindications for surgery, or preference
- Dopamine agonists: Bromocriptine (Parlodel) is ineffective; cabergoline (Dostinex)[1] may be added to patients resistant to somatostatin analogues
- Growth hormone receptor antagonists: Pegvisomant (Somavert) for patients resistant or intolerant to somatostatin analogues and who have tumors >5 mm from the optic chiasm
- Radiotherapy for patients resistant or intolerant to pharmacologic therapy, with clinically and biochemically active disease and a tumor remnant on MRI
- Radiosurgery might be better than external-beam radiotherapy

[1]Not FDA approved for this indication.

PHARMACOLOGIC THERAPY

Somatostatin analogues are the most commonly used medical treatment for acromegaly. Somatostatin inhibits GH secretion and somatotroph cell growth via its interaction with five different somatostatin receptor (SSTR) subtypes. The development of long-acting somatostatin analogues such as octreotide (Sandostatin) and lanreotide (Somatuline) overcame the pharmacologic difficulties of native somatostatin (short half-life, rebound GH secretion, and need for IV administration) and resulted in a more potent inhibition of GH secretion. The most commonly used preparations are intramuscular octreotide LAR (long-acting repeatable) and subcutaneous lanreotide autogel, which are administered every 4 weeks. Doses of octreotide-LAR range from 10 to 40 mg and those of lanreotide autogel from 60 to 120 mg, both administered every 4 weeks; although in specific patients the interval of injection can be increased to every 6 or even 8 weeks, thus diminishing the cost of therapy. Octreotide and lanreotide have very high affinities for SSTR-2 and to a lesser extent SSTR-5, which are precisely the most commonly expressed somatostatin receptors in GH-secreting adenomas.

When used after surgery has failed, somatostatin analogues can achieve a safe and a normal IGF-1 in 50% to 60% of patients. Primary treatment with somatostatin analogues is increasingly being used in patients with invasive tumors, when cardiopulmonary contraindications are present, and more recently as a result of the patient or treating physician's preference. In these settings, biochemical success rates (achievement of safe GH levels and normalization of IGF-1) have ranged between 50% and 80%, and more than 80% report significant relief of symptoms. Tumor shrinkage occurs in 70% of primarily treated patients. Overall, treatment success is directly related to the abundance of SSTR-2 and SSTR-5 in the tumor. Lower pretreatment GH levels are also associated with a better response to somatostatin analogues. Side effects of somatostatin analogues, including nausea, abdominal pain, alopecia, and biliary sludge, occur in 20% of subjects.

Pegvisomant is a GH mutant that prevents functional dimerization of the GH receptor, thus acting as an antagonist. Its use results in normalization of IGF-1 in more than 90% of patients, while increasing GH levels. Concern about adenoma growth due to the abolition of IGF-1 negative feedback on the tumoral somatotroph, prevents its use in patients with very large lesions in close proximity to the optic chiasm. Transient elevations of liver aminotransferases can occur, although this seldom requires drug discontinuation. Pegvisomant does not compromise insulin secretion, as somatostatin analogues do. GH-receptor antagonists are expensive and should not be used as primary treatment; they are currently indicated in patients who are intolerant or have failed somatostatin analogue therapy.

Few patients respond marginally to difficult-to-tolerate large doses of bromocriptine. Newer dopamine agonists, such as cabergoline, are better tolerated and more efficacious, particularly in tumors that cosecrete PRL. Combination treatment with cabergoline and octreotide appears to be promising in cases resistant to somatostatin analogues.

RADIATION THERAPY

Both external-beam radiotherapy and radiosurgery are indicated in patients with persistent disease and a demonstrable tumor remnant who are either intolerant or resistant to pharmacologic treatment. Biochemical success occurs in 20% to 60% and requires many years to become apparent. Hypopituitarism, involving at least two axes, develops in more than 50% of patients within 10 years. Serious adverse effects such as brain necrosis and optic nerve damage seldom occur with the currently used techniques that minimize radiation to the normal surrounding tissues.

Novel pharmacologic therapies are being developed, some of which will likely become useful particularly in patients who do not respond to current somatostatin analogues. These include the so-called "universal" somatostatin analogue pasireotide, which is capable of interacting not only with the sstrs 2 and 5, but also with subtypes 1 and 3. At earlier stages of development are "chimeric" compounds which behave as somatostatin analogues and dopamine agonists at the same time.

REFERENCES

Beckers A, Daly AF. The clinical, pathological and genetic features of familial isolated pituitary adenomas. Eur J Endocrinol 2007;157:371–82.

Bevan JS. Clinical review: The antitumoral effects of somatostatin analog therapy in acromegaly. J Clin Endocrinol Metab 2005;90:1856–63.

Colao A, Ferone D, Marzullo P, Lombardi G. Systemic complications of acromegaly: Epidemiology, pathogenesis and management. Endocr Rev 2004; 25:102–52.

Dekkers OM, Biermasz NR, Pereira AM, et al. Mortality in acromegaly: A metaanalysis. J Clin Endocrinol Metab 2008;93:61–7.

Espinosa-de-Los-Monteros AL, Sosa E, Cheng S, et al. Biochemical evaluation of disease activity after pituitary surgery in acromegaly: A critical analysis of patients who spontaneously change disease status. Clin Endocrinol 2006;64:245–9.

Freda P. Current concepts in the biochemical assessment of the patient with acromegaly. Growth Horm IGF Res 2003;13:171–84.

Freda P, Katznelson L, van der Lely AJ, et al. Long-acting somatostatin analog therapy of acromegaly: A meta-analysis. J Clin Endocrinol Metab 2005; 90:4465–73.

Growth Hormone Research Society. Pituitary Society. Biochemical assessment and long term monitoring in patients with acromegaly: statement from a joint consensus conference of the Growth hormone Research Society and the Pituitary Society. J Clin Endocrinol Metab 2004;89:3099–102.

Holdaway IM, Rajasoorya RC, Gamble GD. Factors influencing mortality in acromegaly. J Clin Endocrinol Metab 2004;89:667–74.

Kopchick JJ, Parkinson C, Stevens EC, Trainer PJ. Growth hormone receptor antagonists: Discovery, development, and use in patients with acromegaly. Endocr Rev 2002;23:623–46.

Melmed S. Acromegaly: Pathogenesis and treatment. J Clin Invest 2009;119: 3189–202.

Melmed S, Colao A, Barkan A, et al. Guidelines for acromegaly management: An update. J Clin Endocrinol Metab 2009; February, published ahead of print.

Vance ML, Laws ER. Role of medical therapy in the management of acromegaly. Neurosurgery 2005;56:877–85.

Adrenocortical Insufficiency

Method of
Joseph M. Hughes, MD

Adrenocortical insufficiency, also referred to as Addison's disease, is an uncommon endocrine disorder. The presentation varies from the nonspecific symptoms of anorexia, nausea, and weight loss to the dramatic hypotensive crisis. The original description by Thomas Addison in 1849 was of a patient with adrenocortical destruction, and the term Addison's disease typically is reserved for those with primary adrenocortical failure. The challenge for the clinician is to establish not only the diagnosis but also the etiology. Patients may present with either primary adrenocortical failure or secondary adrenal insufficiency—disruption of hypothalamic-pituitary function. The long-term treatment with glucocorticoids and mineralocorticoids is effective but differs depending on the etiology. Finally, special attention must be given to the unique problem of patients with potential adrenal insufficiency from chronic pharmacologic doses of glucocorticoids.

Clinical Presentation

The presenting symptoms are often nonspecific, which frequently delays the diagnosis. The clinician often thinks of patients with adrenal insufficiency as presenting in crisis with vomiting, diarrhea, dehydration, and life-threatening hypotension. However, most patients have had a chronic course with symptoms present for a prolonged period. The prominent ones are anorexia, weight loss, fatigue, nausea, diarrhea, and abdominal pain. The symptoms, when associated with physical findings and laboratory clues, should prompt evaluation.

There may be a paucity of findings on physical examination. The clinician may be struck when reviewing the vital signs by weight loss and hypotension, particularly orthostatic hypotension. Examination of the skin may help to distinguish primary from secondary causes. The patients with primary causes, resulting from increased levels of plasma corticotropin (ACTH) and the subsequent stimulation of melanocytes, are described as having bronzing of the skin and increased pigmentation of the buccal mucosa, gingiva, palmar creases, scars, and pressure points (e.g., the elbows). A further clue to the etiology may be the finding of vitiligo, which is associated with autoimmune adrenalitis.

There are characteristic findings on routine laboratory testing—electrolytes, blood urea nitrogen, glucose, creatinine, and hematology profile—which further suggest the diagnosis to the clinician. The most common of these is hyponatremia, which is seen in both primary and secondary forms, although the etiology is different. With secondary causes, excess antidiuretic hormone has been proposed as an explanation; with primary causes, because of the destruction of the adrenal cortex, there is aldosterone deficiency. The finding of hyperkalemia due to hypoaldosteronism often prompts the investigation for adrenal insufficiency and is specific for primary adrenal insufficiency. Azotemia develops because of dehydration. Hypercalcemia is reported. Hypoglycemia is uncommon and is most often seen with secondary forms. The complete blood count demonstrates eosinophilia in up to 20% of patients. Less common findings are anemia and neutropenia.

Evaluation

The diagnosis can usually be made by three tests: random cortisol levels, plasma ACTH levels, and the synthetic corticotropin stimulation test. The random cortisol can be a helpful test as a first step. A value less than the lower limit of normal may be diagnostic and provides enough data to initiate therapy in patients with clinical signs and known pathology (e.g., a hypothalamic-pituitary lesion). The converse is also true: a random cortisol level greater than 20 μg/dL, unless the patient's presentation is highly suspicious for adrenal insufficiency, makes the diagnosis unlikely. It is important to remember that patients with adrenal insufficiency can have a random cortisol level within the laboratory's normal range, and further testing would be required to establish the diagnosis.

The rapid synthetic corticotropin stimulation test is the principal investigation for the diagnosis of adrenal insufficiency. Synthetic tetracosactrin (Synacthen,[2] cosyntropin [Cortrosyn]) contains the the first 24 amino acids of the human ACTH sequence. The traditional dose has been 250 μg given intravenously or intramuscularly. Plasma cortisol levels are measured at time 0 and at 30 and 60 minutes and can be drawn at any time during the day. Various criteria have been used to determine a normal response. Typically, the baseline, the peak, and the delta from baseline to peak have been used. However, careful study by various authors has shown that a peak level at any time greater than 20 μg/dL is a normal response. Lower levels indicate adrenal insufficiency but do not distinguish between primary and secondary failure.

There has been a great deal of discussion recently about the recommended dose of tetracosactrin. There is agreement that the standard dose, 250 μg, delivers pharmacologic concentrations. Newer protocols have advocated the use of 1 μg, a more physiologic concentration. The hypothesis is that a low-dose protocol allows the diagnosis of borderline or mild cases of adrenal insufficiency. Previously, when only the high-dose test was used, some patients with normal tests became adrenally insufficient, especially during times of extreme stress. This is a concern, especially if the etiology is secondary adrenal insufficiency. The experience with both tests at our hospital shows that normal patients can have inadequate stimulation with the low-dose test. Our protocol is to use the high-dose test almost exclusively, except in the special situation in which one expects possible borderline secondary adrenal insufficiency.

The clinician is simultaneously diagnosing and establishing the etiology. The now-accurate measurement of plasma ACTH levels

---

[2]Not available in the United States.

has proved to be very helpful in distinguishing primary from secondary failure. In primary failure, the pituitary is intact, and one anticipates elevated ACTH levels, typically greater than 100 pg/mL. ACTH levels should be low in patients with secondary failure. However, the concentrations may also be in the normal range in these patients.

After it is determined that the patient has either primary or secondary insufficiency, radiologic studies provide important information. With primary failure, the computed tomography scan may show atrophied adrenal glands in autoimmune adrenalitis. Enlarged glands with high-density areas or calcification suggest hemorrhage, granulomatous disease, or neoplasm. The magnetic resonance scan of the hypothalamic-pituitary region in patients with secondary insufficiency is often diagnostic.

Infrequently, other studies can be helpful if the diagnosis of adrenal insufficiency or the cause is in question. The gold standard for diagnosing secondary adrenal insufficiency is the insulin tolerance test. Because the patient must become hypoglycemic and the test has, rarely, been implicated in fatalities, it is best performed by those familiar with the protocol. Several prolonged ACTH protocols to distinguish primary from secondary insufficiency have been published. Finally, with the availability of corticotropin-releasing hormone (CRH) for testing, measurement of ACTH levels after CRH localizes secondary insufficiency to a lesion in either the hypothalamus or the pituitary.

Etiology

After the diagnosis of primary adrenal insufficiency has been established, the clinician is confronted by multiple possible causes (Table 1). The most common (80%–90% of patients) is autoimmune adrenalitis, which is often associated with other autoimmune diseases (Box 1). Evidence of these diseases should be sought and may be present at the time of diagnosis or may appear months or years later. The diagnosis of autoimmune adrenalitis may be the first finding in a patient with an autoimmune polyendocrine syndrome. Tuberculosis has been reported as the second most common cause of primary adrenal insufficiency. Although they are rare, adrenoleukodystrophy and adrenomyeloneuropathy should be considered in a young man who presents with adrenal insufficiency.

Secondary adrenal insufficiency may also be caused by a number of diseases (Box 2), but it is most commonly a result of chronic glucocorticoid therapy, pituitary tumors, or iatrogenic causes. Radiation-induced adrenal failure may present 5 or more years after

---

BOX 1 Autoimmune Diseases Associated with Adrenal Insufficiency

Thyroid disease (Hashimoto's thyroiditis or Graves' disease)
Type 1 diabetes mellitus
Pernicious anemia
Primary ovarian or testicular failure
Vitiligo
Gastrointestinal (celiac disease, inflammatory bowel disease, chronic hepatitis)
Rheumatologic (Sjögren's syndrome)
Alopecia
Neurologic (multiple sclerosis)
Hypoparathyroidism
Chronic candidiasis

---

therapy. If the patient is found to have secondary adrenal insufficiency, other hypothalamic-pituitary hormonal deficiencies should be sought, because isolated ACTH deficiency is rare. Initiation of therapy for growth hormone deficiency or hypothyroidism may uncover previously clinically inapparent adrenal insufficiency.

Treatment

When considering the treatment of adrenal insufficiency, one must understand the management of adrenal crisis, long-term glucocorticoid and mineralocorticoid therapy, and stress-dose glucocorticoids at the time of acute illness. In adrenal crisis, the goal is to reverse the hypovolemia with normal saline, 2 to 3 L infused rapidly, and to administer parenteral glucocorticoids. The choice of glucocorticoid is critical. If the diagnosis of adrenal insufficiency has not been established and diagnostic testing is required, then 4 mg of dexamethasone (Decadron) should be given intravenously every 12 hours. Dexamethasone does not interfere with the cortisol assay, and corticotropin stimulation can be performed as the patient is receiving dexamethasone. Preferably, the ACTH level is obtained and the corticotropin stimulation tests are performed close to the time of initiation of therapy. If the diagnosis and etiology of adrenal insufficiency are known, then either dexamethasone or hydrocortisone (Solu-Cortef) 100 mg IV every 6 to 8 hours may be used. Intravenous glucocorticoid on a tapering dose may be required for several days until oral replacement therapy is begun. Mineralocorticoids are not required for acute management. After the patient is stable, oral therapy is initiated.

All patients with adrenal insufficiency require glucocorticoids. I usually prescribe hydrocortisone (Cortef). Even though the plasma concentrations rise and fall rapidly after oral administration, most patients respond well to a single morning dose and a second dose

---

TABLE 1 Causes of Primary Adrenal Insufficiency

Type	Examples
Autoimmune	
Infectious	Tuberculosis, histoplasmosis, blastomycosis, coccidioidomycosis, cryptococcosis, HIV, cytomegalovirus
Hemorrhage	Sepsis, anticoagulation
Metastatic disease	Lung, breast
Drugs	Ketoconazole (Nizoral), aminoglutethimide (Cytadren)
Infiltrative diseases	Sarcoid, hemochromatosis, amyloidosis
Familial	Adrenoleukodystrophy, adrenomyeloneuropathy, familial glucocorticoid deficiency
ACTH resistance syndromes	
Congenital adrenal hypoplasia	

Abbreviation: ACTH, adrenocorticotropic hormone (corticotropin).

BOX 2 Causes of Secondary Adrenal Insufficiency

Steroid therapy
Iatrogenic (pituitary or adrenal adenoma surgery, radiation therapy)
Pituitary tumors, adenoma, craniopharyngioma, Rathke cleft cyst
Infiltrative (sarcoid)
Pituitary infarction
Lymphocytic or granulomatous hypophysitis
Isolated corticotropin (ACTH) deficiency
Metastasis
Tuberculosis

in the early afternoon. Individualizing the dose is important to prevent long-term complications from overreplacement. The calculation, 12 mg/m²/day, is helpful in determining the total dose of hydrocortisone. For example, if the total daily calculated dose is 25 mg, then 20 mg could be given in the morning and 5 mg in the early afternoon. In the long term, the patient may find that only the morning dose is required.

Some experts prescribe the longer-acting preparations prednisone or dexamethasone. The rationale is a more prolonged pharmacologic effect as opposed to what is seen with hydrocortisone or cortisone acetate (Cortone). The usual doses are 5 mg for prednisone and 0.5 mg for dexamethasone. Because of the prolonged action and an attempt to mimic the circadian rhythm, these medications are given in the morning or at bedtime.

Patients with primary adrenal failure are unable to produce aldosterone. In patients with secondary adrenal insufficiency, the renin-angiotensin-aldosterone system is intact, and aldosterone is infrequently required. Mineralocorticoid is prescribed as fludrocortisone (Florinef); the usual dose is 0.1 mg/day. The patient should obtain a medical alert bracelet and be instructed in the use of stress-dose steroid at times of acute illness. For example, the patient may double or triple the dose of glucocorticoids for 3 days if he or she has a febrile illness. There is no need to taper the dose. If vomiting or profuse diarrhea occurs, the patient should be instructed to seek emergency care. Some patients are capable of giving intramuscular injections of glucocorticoids (Decadron, Solu-Cortef) at home in an attempt to prevent the need for an emergency department visit. For outpatients having procedures, administration of 50 to 100 mg of hydrocortisone (Solu-Cortef) IV beforehand, then converting to oral stress doses afterward, is appropriate. The adrenal cortex is also a source of androgens. For patients, especially women, with decreased libido and persistent fatigue, dehydroepiandrosterone (DHEA)[7] 25 to 50 mg daily may be added.

After glucocorticoids and mineralocorticoids have been prescribed, the clinician constantly monitors the adequacy of the treatment. There is equal concern for insufficient as for excessive doses, particularly glucocorticoids. Through the history, the clinician learns about symptoms of low-grade adrenal insufficiency, particularly fatigue and orthostatic hypotension. On examination, one looks for evidence of Cushing's syndrome, particularly weight gain, striae, and facial plethora, indicating possible overreplacement. Osteoporosis is always a concern. On laboratory testing, the sodium and potassium levels and the plasma renin or plasma renin activity levels should be normal if the patient is receiving adequate doses of fludrocortisone. Finally, by its inhibitory effects on release of arginine vasopressin and renal effects, glucocorticoid treatment may uncover quiescent central diabetes insipidus.

Adrenal Suppression and Chronic Glucocorticoid Therapy

Chronic glucocorticoid (prednisone) therapy causes secondary adrenal insufficiency. There is generalized consensus about the doses and duration of prednisone therapy that cause suppression. If prednisone at doses greater than 20 mg/day for more than 3 weeks is prescribed, then the dose of prednisone should be tapered. Also, patients who have required prednisone at doses greater than 5 mg/day for months to years are presumed to be suppressed. If there is a question about the integrity of the hypothalamic-pituitary-adrenal axis in patients taking prednisone 5 mg/day or less, then a corticotropin stimulation test can be helpful. After suppression is established, a prolonged taper is required, because 6 to 12 months is needed for the axis to recover.

The tapering of prednisone must be gradual, especially after the 5-mg dose is reached. An approach to the patient on high-dose prednisone is to decrease the dose by increments of 5 to 10 mg every

[7]Available as dietary supplement.

2 weeks until the 20-mg dose is reached. Afterward, the dose should be adjusted by 5 mg or less every 2 weeks until the 5-mg dose is established. At that point, decreasing the dose by 1 mg per month is a conservative approach. After the patient reaches the dose of 1 or 2 mg/day, a corticotropin stimulation test can be helpful. Also, a fasting cortisol measurement before the dose of prednisone that is greater than 10 ng/dL usually predicts normal adrenal function. Often, the limitation in tapering prednisone is the activity of the underlying disease, not the integrity of the hypothalamic-pituitary-adrenal axis. Stress-dose steroids for major illness, surgery, or trauma should be provided for the first year after a patient has successfully stopped prednisone.

REFERENCES

Barbetta L, Dall'Asta C, Re T, et al. Comparison of different regimens of glucocorticoid replacement therapy in patients with hypoadrenalism. J Endocrinol Invest 2005;28:632–7.

Crown A, Lightman S. Why is the management of glucocorticoid deficiency still controversial: A review of the literature. Clin Endocrinol 2005; 63:483–92.

Hughes J, Whelan MA, Deringer P. Adrenoleukodystrophy: An important cause of adrenal insufficiency. Endocrinologist 2000;10:271–6.

Cushing's Syndrome

Method of
Madson Q. Almeida, MD, and Constantine A. Stratakis, MD, PhD

Definition and Epidemiology

Cushing's syndrome remains one of the most difficult diagnoses in endocrinology. By definition, Cushing's syndrome is a multisystem disorder that develops in response to glucocorticoid excess. Iatrogenic Cushing's syndrome is common, but endogenous Cushing's syndrome is a rare condition, with an estimated incidence of 0.7 to 2.4 per million population per year. The etiology of Cushing's syndrome may be excessive adrenocorticotropic hormone (ACTH) production from the pituitary gland, ectopic ACTH secretion by nonpituitary tumors, or autonomous cortisol hypersecretion from adrenal hyperplasia or tumors (Table 1). Cushing's disease refers to the subset of Cushing's syndrome cases caused by an ACTH-producing pituitary adenoma. Cushing's disease is the most common cause of spontaneous Cushing's syndrome in almost all ages, including older children and adolescents. Approximately 20% to 30% (with the exception of very young children) of endogenous Cushing's syndrome is caused by primary adrenocortical diseases that are not ACTH dependent. Cushing's disease and adrenocortical adenomas occur more commonly in women, with a female-to-male ratio of 3-5:1.

Pathophysiology

Cortisol inhibits the biosynthesis and secretion of corticotropin-releasing hormone (CRH) and ACTH in a negative-feedback loop that is tightly controlled. The hallmark of Cushing's syndrome is the absence of suppression of cortisol levels after low-dose dexamethasone (Decadron) administration owing to autonomous ACTH secretion by a tumor or autonomous glucocorticoid production by a primary adrenocortical disease. It is essential to understand that all diagnostic testing in Cushing's syndrome relies on the disturbance of this feedback mechanism, as revealed by dexamethasone, CRH [corticorelin ovine trifluate [Acthrel]), and all related testing.

TABLE 1 Etiology of Cushing's Syndrome in Older Children, Adolescents, and Young adults*

Syndrome	% of Total
ACTH-dependent	
Cushing's disease	60-70
Ectopic ACTH-syndrome	5-10
Ectopic CRH-syndrome	<1
ACTH-independent	
Adrenocortical adenoma	10-15
Adrenocortical carcinoma	5
Bilateral adrenocortical disease	5-10

*In infants and younger children, the distribution is different.
Abbreviations: ACTH = adrenocorticotropic hormone; CRH = corticotropin-releasing hormone.

ACTH-producing pituitary adenomas are microadenomas (<1 cm in diameter) in 80% to 90% of cases. Macroadenomas are rare and often invasive, with extension outside of the sella turcica. Chronic ACTH hypersecretion commonly leads to secondary adrenocortical hyperplasia.

Ectopic ACTH secretion is most often associated with small cell lung carcinoma, which accounts for half of the cases in adult patients with Cushing's syndrome. The ectopic ACTH syndrome causes severe hypokalemia and is usually underdiagnosed in patients during advanced stages of neoplasia. Other tumors causing the syndrome are bronchial, thymic, and pancreatic carcinoids; medullary thyroid carcinoma; pheochromocytoma; or other rare neuroendocrine tumors, especially in pediatric patients.

Adrenocortical tumors are more often adenomas that are usually smaller than 5 cm. Adrenocortical carcinomas are rare but very aggressive neoplasms; they most commonly occur as large nonsecreting abdominal masses at diagnosis, and only rarely does Cushing's syndrome develop.

Up to recently, only two types of primary adrenal hyperplasias that are ACTH-independent and cause Cushing's syndrome were known: primary pigmented nodular adrenocortical disease (PPNAD) and ACTH-independent macronodular adrenocortical hyperplasia, also known as massive macronodular adrenocortical disease.

Table 2 lists no fewer than six types of bilateral adrenocortical hyperplasias. They are divided into two groups of disorders, macronodular and micronodular hyperplasias, on the basis of the size of the associated nodules. In macronodular disorders, the greatest diameter of each nodule exceeds 1 cm; in the micronodular group nodules are less than 1 cm. Although nodules less than 1 cm can occur in macronodular disease (especially the form associated with McCune-Albright syndrome), and single large tumors may be encountered in PPNAD (especially in older patients), the size criterion has biological relevance, because we rarely see a continuum in the same subject: most patients have either macronodular or micronodular hyperplasia. We use two additional basic characteristics in this classification of bilateral adrenocortical hyperplasias: presence of tumor pigment and status (hyperplasia or atrophy) of the surrounding cortex.

Pigment in adrenocortical lesions is rarely melanin; most of the pigmentation in adrenocortical adenomas and bilateral adrenocortical hyperplasias that produce cortisol is lipofuscin. The accumulation of lipofuscin-like material results from the progressive oxidation of unsaturated fatty acids by oxygen-derived free radicals in lysosomes. Lipofuscin pigmentation appears macroscopically as light brown to occasionally dark brown or even black discoloration of the tumor or hyperplastic tissue. Lipofuscin can be seen with a light microscope, but it is better detected by electron microscopy.

TABLE 2 Bilateral Adrenal Hyperplasias Causing Cushing's Syndrome

Lesion	Age Group	Histopathology	Genetics	Gene, Locus
Macronodular Hyperplasias (Multiple Nodules >1 cm Each)				
Bilateral macroadenomatous hyperplasia	Middle age	Distinct adenomas (usually 2 or 3) with internodular atrophy	MEN1, FAP, MAS, HLRCS; isolated (AD); other	Menin, *APC*, *GNAS*, FH, ectopic GPCRs
Bilateral macroadenomatous hyperplasia of childhood	Infants, very young children	Distinct adenomas (usually 2 or 3) with internodular atrophy; occasional microadenomas	MAS	*GNAS*
ACTH-independent macronodular adrenocortical hyperplasia, also known as massive macronodular adrenocortical disease	Middle age	Adenomatous hyperplasia (multiple) with internodular hyperplasia of the zona fasciculata	Isolated, AD	Ectopic GPCRs; WISP-2 and Wnt-signaling; 17q22-24, other
Micronodular Hyperplasias (Multiple Nodules <1 cm Each)				
Isolated primary pigmented nodular adrenocortical disease	Children; young adults	Microadenomatous hyperplasia with (mostly) internodular atrophy and nodular pigment (lipofuscin)	Isolated; AD	*PRKAR1A*, *PDE11A*; *PDE8B*; 2p16; other
Carney complex–associated primary pigmented nodular adrenocortical disease	Children; young and middle aged adults	Microadenomatous hyperplasia with (mostly) internodular atrophy and (mainly nodular) pigment (lipofuscin)	CNC (AD)	*PRKAR1A*, 2p16; other
Isolated micronodular adrenocortical disease	Mostly children; young adults	Microadenomatous, with hyperplasia of the surrounding zona fasciculata and limited or absent pigment	Isolated, AD; other	*PDE11A*, *PDE8B*; other; 2p12-p16, other

Abbreviations: ACTH = adrenocorticotropic hormone; AD = autosomal dominant; *APC* = adenomatous polyposis coli gene; cAMP = cyclic adenosine monophosphate; CNC = Carney complex; FAP = familial adenomatous polyposis; FH = fumarate hydratase; *GNAS* = gene coding for the stimulatory subunit alpha of the G-protein (Gsα); GPCR = G-protein-coupled receptor; HLRCS = hereditary leiomyomatosis and renal cancer syndrome; MAS = McCune–Albright syndrome; MEN1 = multiple endocrine neoplasia type 1; *PDE8B* = phosphodiesterase 8B gene; *PDE11A* = phosphodiesterase 11A gene; *PRKAR1A* = protein kinase, cAMP-dependent, regulatory, type I, alpha gene; WISP2 = Wnt1-inducible signaling pathway protein 1; Wnt = wingless-type MMTV integration site family.

Massive macronodular adrenocortical disease is a bilateral disease and may be caused by abnormal hormone receptor expression or activating mutations of $G_S\alpha$, which leads to stimulation of steroidogenesis. Another cause of ACTH-independent Cushing's syndrome is primary pigmented nodular adrenocortical disease, usually associated with a syndrome of cardiac myxomas, lentigines, and schwannomas (Carney's complex).

Clinical Manifestations

The clinical presentation of Cushing's syndrome is variable and differs in severity (Table 3). Truncal obesity is the most common clinical sign and is usually the initial manifestation in most patients. Growth failure in children is the most reliable sign of Cushing's syndrome, especially when combined with continuing weight gain. Other symptoms include central fat deposition, supraclavicular fat accumulation, buffalo hump, plethora, rounded face, purple striae, thin skin, proximal muscle weakness, hypertension, impaired glucose metabolism and diabetes, gonadal dysfunction, and hirsutism (see Table 3). Diabetes mellitus and hypertension also develop. Osteoporosis, mood disorders, emotional liability, and cognitive deficits are commonly observed. Proximal myopathy is common, especially in older patients. Ectopic ACTH syndrome caused by small cell lung cancer can have an unusual presentation characterized by rapid onset, severe weakness, and associated hypokalemia without classic symptoms of Cushing's syndrome. In contrast, ACTH-secreting carcinoids manifest with typical clinical manifestations.

Diagnosis

CONFIRMATION OF THE DIAGNOSIS

The initial evaluation should always include a careful clinical history and physical examination. Reliable symptoms and signs of Cushing's syndrome (see Table 3) should be present in any patient who undergoes evaluation for Cushing's syndrome; patients with no reliable symptoms and signs of Cushing's syndrome should not be investigated, as this often leads to unnecessary, extensive, and expensive testing. It is essential to investigate the use of exogenous glucocorticoids and other conditions, which may be associated with mild hypercortisolism, such as alcoholism, anorexia nervosa, severe depression, and morbid obesity; these are pseudo-Cushing's states and are often difficult to exclude, especially in older or chronically ill patients.

TABLE 3 Clinical Manifestations of Cushing's Syndrome

Signs and Symptoms	Incidence (%)
Central obesity	97
Plethora	89
Moon facies	89
Decreased libido	86
Atrophic skin and easy bruising	75
Decreased linear growth	70-80
Menstrual irregularities	80
Hypertension	76
Hirsutism	56
Depression or emotional lability	67
Glucose intolerance/diabetes mellitus	70
Purple striae	60
Buffalo hump	54
Osteoporosis	50
Headache	10

CURRENT DIAGNOSIS

- Cushing's syndrome remains one of the most challenging diagnoses in endocrine medicine.
- Cushing's disease is caused by corticotropin (ACTH)-producing pituitary adenomas (corticotropinomas) and constitutes the most common cause of endogenous Cushing's syndrome, although its prevalence varies across different age groups.
- Growth failure in children, facial plethora and rounded face, central fat deposition, supraclavicular fat accumulation, buffalo hump, purple striae, thin skin, and proximal myopathy are relatively sensitive clinical features of Cushing's syndrome.
- Ectopic ACTH syndrome occasionally has an unusual presentation of rapid onset, severe weakness, and hypokalemia without classic symptoms of Cushing's syndrome.
- A urinary free cortisol test is the most cost-effective and reliable outpatient screening test.
- A 1-mg overnight dexamethasone screening test is less useful and more expensive than the urinary free cortisol test, but it provides a good alternative for patients in whom urinary collection is impossible or unreliable.
- Midnight salivary cortisol levels greater than 3.6 nmol/L (0.13 µg/dL) have a sensitivity and specificity of approximately 95% for the diagnosis of Cushing's syndrome.
- Undetectable ACTH levels (<1 pmol/L or <5 pg/mL) indicate a primary autonomous adrenocortical disease.
- Postcontrast spoiled gradient-recalled acquisition (SPGR) magnetic resonance imaging (MRI) is superior to conventional MRI for the localization of corticotropinomas in children and adults.
- Computed tomography (CT) is used to investigate adrenal disease in patients with ACTH-independent Cushing's syndrome. Usually, conventional MRI is less useful owing to motion artifacts.

The first task in the work-up of any patient is documentation of hypercortisolism. On an outpatient basis, this is typically done through the urinary free cortisol test. This is the most cost-effective and reliable outpatient screening test. We typically recommend collections over two or three consecutive days so that we avoid errors due to over- or undercollection that are not uncommon with single 24-hour studies. The results of the test need to be corrected for body surface area, as long as total creatinine excretion is normal. A 1-mg overnight dexamethasone test is less useful and more expensive, but it provides a good alternative for patients in whom urinary collection is impossible or unreliable. During these screening tests for hypercortisolism, patients should avoid any activation of the hypothalamic-pituitary-adrenal axis by stress, especially physical. The baseline measurements may be repeated as needed, because cyclic hypercortisolism often precedes overt Cushing's syndrome (Fig. 1).

A 24-hour urinary free cortisol excretion of greater than 250 nmol per 24 hours (90 µg/24 hours measured by radioimmunoassay) is highly specific for the diagnosis of hypercortisolism. However, pseudo-Cushing's states are often associated with abnormal levels of 24-hour urinary free cortisol. Administration of 1 mg dexamethasone (15 µg/kg for children) at 11 pm results in suppression of the hypothalamic-pituitary-adrenal axis in normal persons and a fall in plasma and urinary cortisol levels: At 8 am, serum cortisol should be less than 50 nmol/L (1.8 µg/dL). Unfortunately, dexamethasone is primarily metabolized by the cytochrome P-450 (CYP) system;

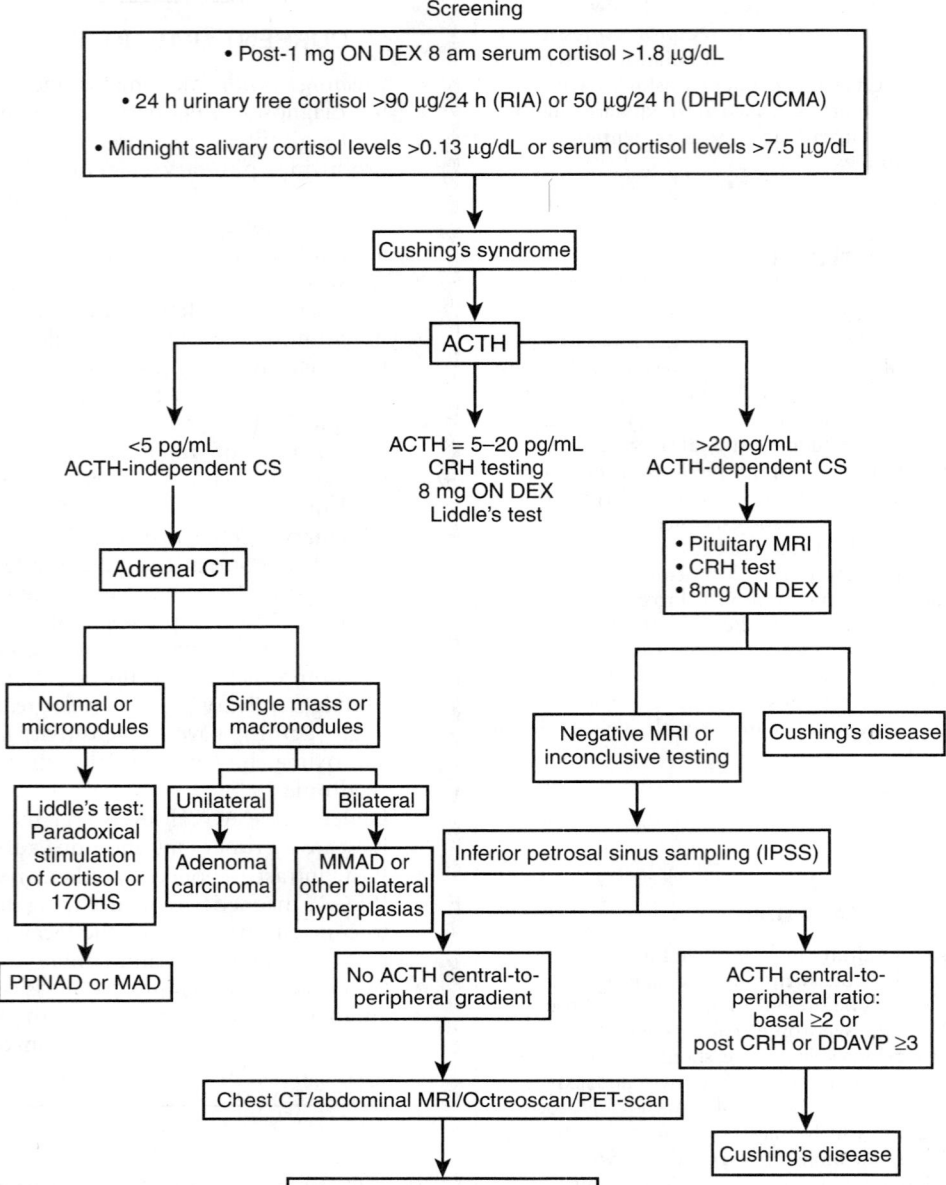

FIGURE 1. Algorithm for evaluating patients with Cushing's syndrome. *Abbreviations:* ACTH = adrenocorticotropic hormone; CRH = corticotropin-releasing hormone; CS = Cushing's syndrome; CT = computed tomography; DDAVP = desmopressin; DHPLC = denaturing high-performance liquid chromatography; ICMA = immunochemiluminometric assay; MAD = micronodular disease; MMAD = massive macronodular adrenocortical disease; MRI = magnetic resonance imaging; 17OHS = 17-hydroxysteroids; ON DEX = overnight dexamethasone; PPNAD = primary pigmented nodular adrenocortical disease; RIA = radioimmunoassay.

several drugs, such as phenobarbital, carbamazepine (Tegretol), and rifampicin (Rifadin), which induce the activity of CYP3A4 can lead to false-positive tests. Oral contraceptives also interfere with serum cortisol levels owing to an increase in corticosteroid-binding globulin and by increasing dexamethasone metabolism. The test can only be interpreted if the serum dexamethasone levels reach the expected range; however, this additional requirement can make the test significantly more cumbersome and expensive.

Once hypercortisolism is suspected by the urinary free cortisol or the overnight dexamethasone test, the patient may undergo testing of the cortisol diurnal rhythm. The lack of circadian rhythm of cortisol is the earliest consistent biochemical abnormality of Cushing's syndrome, even in situations of cyclic or other atypical forms of Cushing's syndrome. Serum or salivary cortisol levels at midnight may be used for this test. Normally, the level of serum cortisol begins to rise at 3 to 4 am and reaches a peak at 7 to 8 am, falling during the day. A sleeping midnight serum cortisol level lower than 50 nmol/L (1.8 µg/dL) excludes the diagnosis of Cushing's syndrome, whereas a midnight serum cortisol higher than 207 nmol/L (7.5 µg/dL) is highly suggestive of Cushing's syndrome. This test does require inpatient admission, and the blood sample needs to be drawn within 5 to 10 minutes of waking up the patient. Salivary cortisol levels have an excellent correlation with serum cortisol levels and offer an easy and convenient outpatient way of evaluating circadian rhythm; saliva is also stable at room temperature (for up to 7 days). Midnight salivary cortisol levels greater than 3.6 nmol/L (0.13 µg/dL) have a sensitivity and specificity of approximately 95% for the diagnosis of Cushing's syndrome (see Fig. 1).

After the biochemical confirmation of hypercortisolism, the next step is to investigate the source (see Figure 1). Baseline ACTH plasma levels greater than 2 to 5 pmol/L (>20-25 pg/mL) are diagnostic of ACTH-dependent Cushing's syndrome. On the other hand, undetectable ACTH levels (<1 pmol/L or 5 pg/mL) indicate a primary autonomous adrenocortical disease. Values in between should be further investigated with dynamic testing.

High-Dose Dexamethasone Testing

Oral dexamethasone is administrated as 2 mg every 6 hours for 48 hours or as a single 8 mg (120 µg/kg for children) overnight dose. Urinary and serum cortisol levels are suppressed by more than 50% in most patients with Cushing's disease.

Corticotropin-Releasing Hormone Testing

Synthetic ovine CRH (corticorelin ovine trifluate [Acthrel]) or human[1] CRH is administered intravenously (100 µg), and plasma ACTH and cortisol levels are measured at 15-minute intervals during the next 60 minutes. Patients with Cushing's disease typically have an increase in ACTH or cortisol level of 35% and 22%, respectively. This test has a sensitivity of approximately 85% for the diagnosis of Cushing's disease, but it is often falsely positive in patients with adrenal, ACTH-independent Cushing's syndrome, who do not have a fully suppressed hypothalamic-pituitary-adrenal axis.

Inferior Petrosal Sinus Sampling

None of the noninvasive tests are 100% accurate in distinguishing pituitary (Cushing's disease) from ectopic sources of ACTH. Inferior petrosal sinus sampling (IPSS) is indicated in all cases where an ACTH-dependent source of hypercortisolism is expected but the diagnosis of Cushing's disease versus an ectopic source remains uncertain. Typically, IPSS is done when the ovine CRH and dexamethasone tests are in disagreement or when the pituitary imaging by magnetic resonance imaging (MRI) is negative. An ACTH gradient of central-to-peripheral ACTH levels of 2 or more suggests Cushing's disease. When ovine CRH, human CRH, or desmopressin (DDAVP) testing is performed during IPSS, the diagnostic accuracy of IPSS increases. After ovine CRH stimulation, a central-to-peripheral ratio of ACTH levels of 3 or more suggest the diagnosis of Cushing's disease with specificity and sensitivity greater than 95%. The test is less useful for suggesting the tumor location (right versus left side of the pituitary gland).

IMAGING STUDIES

Pituitary Magnetic Resonance Imaging

Unfortunately, less than 50% of ACTH-producing pituitary adenomas are detectable with MRI, even with the use of contrast enhancement. Typically, we recommend against obtaining an MRI until ACTH dependency is established, because as many as 20% of the patients have an incidental pituitary microadenoma. To avoid false-negative and false-positive imaging, several centers have sought improved methods for MRI detection of ACTH-producing tumors. Our studies demonstrated that postcontrast spoiled gradient-recalled acquisition (SPGR) MRI in addition to the conventional T1-weighted spin echo was superior to conventional MRI for the diagnostic evaluation of corticotropinomas in both children and adults.

Adrenal Imaging

Computed tomography (CT) and MRI are used to investigate adrenal disease in patients with ACTH-independent Cushing's syndrome. Adrenal tumors larger than 6 cm are highly suspicious for adrenocortical carcinomas. The fat content contributes to the differentiation between benign and malignant adrenal tumors. Measurement of Hounsfield units (HU) in unenhanced CT is of great value in differentiating malignant from benign adrenal lesions. Adrenal lesions with an attenuation value of more than 10 HU in unenhanced CT or an enhancement washout of less than 50% and a delayed attenuation of more than 35 HU (on 10- to 15-min delayed enhanced CT) are suspicious for malignancy. MRI with dynamic gadolinium-enhanced and chemical shift technique is as effective as CT in distinguishing malignant from benign lesions. However, MRI is much less useful for detecting adrenal nodularity owing to motion artifacts. Thus, especially for detecting small unilateral adrenocortical adenomas or bilateral micronodular hyperplasia, we recommend CT rather than MRI.

Ectopic Adrenocorticotropic Hormone Syndrome

Chest high-resolution CT and abdominal MRI are the recommended imaging procedures in patients with an IPSS that indicates a nonpituitary ACTH-producing source. Additionally, somatostatin receptor scintigraphy is a useful and complimentary tool in the evaluation of patients with ectopic ACTH-dependent Cushing's syndrome. Recent studies have demonstrated a higher sensitivity of somatostatin receptor scintigraphy in comparison to CT or MRI for diagnosing occult ectopic tumors.

Treatment

Untreated chronic hypercortisolism is associated with high morbidity and mortality owing to diabetes mellitus, hypertension, cardiovascular disease, thromboembolism, and suppression of the immune system. Cushing's syndrome should be treated effectively; patients should be closely monitored to rapidly detect recurrent disease.

TREATMENT OF PITUITARY CORTICOTROPINOMAS

Transsphenoidal Pituitary Surgery

The initial therapy of choice for patients with Cushing's disease is transsphenoidal surgery. This procedure is associated with low mortality and morbidity, but complications can include cerebrospinal fluid leaks, meningitis, hypopituitarism, and venous thromboembolism.

CURRENT THERAPY

- The initial therapy of choice for patients with Cushing's disease is transsphenoidal surgery of the pituitary gland to remove the responsible adenoma.
- Transsphenoidal surgery has a success rate greater than 80% in most experienced centers. Lower success rates and higher incidence of relapse are recorded in less-experienced centers.
- Laparoscopic adrenalectomy has become the treatment of choice for benign adrenal lesions with a diameter of less than 6 cm.
- In stages I to III adrenocortical carcinoma, complete tumor resection offers the best chance for cure.
- Mitotane, an adrenolytic agent, is used in the treatment of metastatic adrenocortical carcinoma and also as an adjuvant for tumors with a high risk of recurrence.
- Medical treatment with ketoconazole,[2] metyrapone,[1] aminoglutethimide, and mitotane[1] may be used to control hypercortisolism in preparation for surgery; medical adrenalectomy may also be used in cases of cyclic Cushing's syndrome.
- The most effective treatment option for ectopic ACTH syndrome is resection of the tumor. Somatostatin analogues and various chemotherapeutic regimens have been used in the treatment of metastatic tumors.

[1]Not FDA approved for this indication.
[2]Not available in the United States.

[1]Not FDA approved for this indication.

The success rate for transsphenoidal surgery varies between 60% and 80%, but in experienced centers can be as high as 90% to 95%. Relapses are rare when surgery is performed in an experienced tertiary care center; it can be as high as 30% in less-experienced centers. Postoperative morning serum cortisol levels of less than 50 nmol/L (2 µg/dL) are highly predictive of remission and a low recurrence rate of less than 10% at 10 years.

After successful transsphenoidal surgery, glucocorticoid replacement therapy (hydrocortisone at 12-15 mg/m²/day; 20-30 mg daily in adults) is mandatory until the hypothalamic-pituitary-adrenal axis recovers from the chronic exposure to glucocorticoid excess; this usually takes place within a year after surgery. For recurrent disease, the choice of second-line therapy remains controversial. Repeat surgery can be successful when residual tumor is detectable on MRI imaging, but it carries a high risk of hypopituitarism. Irradiation is recommended in most cases where a tumor is not seen on MRI.

Radiotherapy

Radiotherapy has been used to suppress pituitary secretion of ACTH, but its success rate is variable (50% in some series). It can take as long as 5 years for a full effect; hypopituitarism develops in more than 70% of the patients over a period of 10 to 20 years after the therapy is completed. Stereotactic radiosurgery with gamma knife is associated with a more-rapid effect and a lower risk of hypopituitarism, but it has not been extensively studied.

Medical Treatment to Control Secretion of Adrenocorticotropic Hormone

Cushing's disease responds to the dopamine agonist cabergoline (Dostinex)[1] with a normalization of cortisol production in as many as 40% of the cases. The peroxisome proliferator-activated receptor γ (PPAR-γ) agonist rosiglitazone (Avandia) was demonstrated to be effective in animal models, but it was unsuccessful in controlling ACTH oversecretion in patients with Cushing's disease. A new agent, SOM-230 (pasireotide),[2] blocks both type 2 and type 5 somatostatin receptors and reduces ACTH secretion in vitro. However, the first controlled trial in humans did not show a high efficacy in Cushing's disease.

Bilateral Adrenalectomy

Bilateral adrenalectomy offers a definitive treatment that provides immediate control of hypercortisolism, but this surgery should be reserved for patients with Cushing's disease who have failed all other treatments. Bilateral adrenalectomy in active Cushing's disease often leads to Nelson's syndrome, a condition characterized by unabated progression of a corticotropinoma (owing to the lack of negative feedback by cortisol), very high ACTH levels, and high morbidity.

TREATMENT OF ADRENAL DISEASE

Adrenocortical Tumors

For adrenocortical tumors, the recommended treatment is surgical. Laparoscopic adrenalectomy has become the treatment of choice for benign adrenal lesions with a diameter of less than 6 cm. In stages I to III adrenocortical carcinoma, complete tumor removal by a well-trained surgeon offers by far the best chance for cure. Surgery often needs to be extensive, with en bloc resection of invaded organs, and regularly includes lymphadenectomy. Surgery for local recurrences or metastatic disease is accepted as a valuable therapeutic option and was associated with improved survival in retrospective studies. The overall 5-year survival in different series ranged between 16 and 38%. Median survival for metastatic disease (stage IV) at the time of diagnosis is still consistently less than 12 months.

Radiotherapy has been considered ineffective for treatment of adrenocortical cancer, but it can be indicated to control localized disease not amenable to surgery.

Mitotane (o,p′-DDD [Lysodren]) is the only adrenal-specific agent available for treating adrenocortical cancer. Mitotane is indicated in metastatic adrenocortical carcinoma and can also be used as an adjuvant for tumors with a high risk of recurrence. Mitotane exerts a specific cytotoxic effect on adrenocortical cells, leading to focal degeneration of the fascicular and particularly the reticular zone. In most patients, treatment should be initiated with a dose that does not exceed 1.5 g/day; this is then rapidly increased, depending on gastrointestinal symptoms, to 5–6 g/day. This high-dose regimen requires measurement of mitotane blood levels 14 days after initiation of therapy. The dose is then adjusted according to the medicine's plasma concentrations (which should be greater than 14 mg/L) and tolerance of the side effects. Because mitotane treatment induces adrenal insufficiency and increases the metabolic clearance of glucocorticoids, glucocorticoid replacement is indicated, often at higher than normal doses owing to increased clearance.

Cytotoxic Chemotherapy

Cytotoxic chemotherapy includes etoposide (VePesid),[1] doxorubicin (Adriamycin),[1] and cisplatin (Platinol),[1] or streptozocin (Zanosar)[1] plus mitotane. Chemotherapy has limited efficacy for advanced adrenocortical cancer and is associated mainly with partial responses.

Bilateral Adrenal Hyperplasias

The treatment of choice for bilateral adrenal hyperplasias associated with ACTH-independent Cushing's syndrome is bilateral adrenalectomy. Patients require life-long replacement therapy with glucocorticoids and mineralocorticoids, and they should be adequately educated about the risk of acute adrenal insufficiency.

TREATMENT OF ECTOPIC CORTICOTROPIN SYNDROME

The choice of treatment for ectopic ACTH syndrome depends on tumor identification, localization, and classification. The most effective treatment option is surgical resection, although this is not always possible in metastatic disease or in the case of occult tumors. Because the ectopic ACTH syndrome is usually severe and occult tumors can become evident at imaging studies only during the follow-up, medical treatment to control hypercortisolism is often necessary. Bilateral adrenalectomy may be an option to be considered, when the hypercortisolism cannot be controlled by other treatment options.

MEDICAL ADRENALECTOMY

Several drugs that inhibit steroid synthesis are often effective for rapidly controlling hypercortisolism in preparation for surgery, after unsuccessful TSS or removal of an adrenal tumor such as extensive cancer, or while awaiting the full effect of radiotherapy in recurrent Cushing's disease (Table 4).

Most experience with inhibitors of steroidogenesis has been with metyrapone (Metopirone)[1] and ketoconazole (Nizoral),[1] two medications that appear to be more effective and better tolerated than aminoglutethimide (Cytadren). Metyrapone reduces cortisol and aldosterone production by inhibiting 11β-hydroxylation in the adrenal cortex. Ketoconazole is a broad-spectrum antifungal drug, which inhibits C17-20 desmolase, cholesterol side-chain cleavage, and 11β-hydroxylation. Ketoconazole is also associated with inhibition of testosterone biosynthesis and gynecomastia.

RU-486, or mifepristone (Mifeprex),[1] is an antagonist of the progesterone and glucocorticoid receptors. Unexpectedly, the treatment of Cushing's disease with this glucocorticoid antagonist has been associated with increased ACTH secretion and consequent stimulation of cortisol production. RU-486 may be more useful in ectopic ACTH-producing tumors and in adrenal Cushing's syndrome, but its efficacy and potential side effects when administered chronically are currently unknown.

---

[1]Not FDA approved for this indication.
[2]Not available in the United States.

[1]Not FDA approved for this indication.

TABLE 4 Medical Treatment for Hypercortisolism

Medication	Initial Dose	Maximum Dose	Adverse Effects
Ketoconazole (Nizoral)[1]	100-200 mg bid/tid	1200 mg	Nausea, vomiting, abdominal pain, weakness, hypothyroidism, gynecomastia, hepatotoxicity, hypertriglyceridemia
Metyrapone (Metopirone)[1]	250 mg qid	6000 mg	Headache, alopecia, hirsutism, acne, nausea, abdominal discomfort, hypertension, weakness, leucopenia
Mitotane (Lysodren)[1]	500 mg tid	9000 mg	Nausea, vomiting, anorexia, diarrhea, ataxia, confusion, skin rash, hepatotoxicity
Aminoglutethimide (Cytadren)	250 mg qid	2000 mg/d	Lethargy, nausea, anorexia, hypothyroidism, somnolence

[1]Not FDA approved for this indication.

REFERENCES

Allolio B, Fassnacht M. Clinical review: Adrenocortical carcinoma: Clinical update. J Clin Endocrinol Metab 2006;91:2027–37.

Batista D, Courkoutsakis NA, Oldfield EH, et al. Detection of adrenocorticotropin-secreting pituitary adenomas by magnetic resonance imaging in children and adolescents with Cushing disease. J Clin Endocrinol Metab 2005;90:5134–40.

Batista DL, Riar J, Keil M, Stratakis CA. Diagnostic tests for children who are referred for the investigation of Cushing syndrome. Pediatrics 2007;120:e575–86.

Bertagna X, Guignat L, Groussin L, Bertherat J. Cushing's disease. Best Pract Res Clin Endocrinol Metab 2009;23:607–23.

Biller BM, Grossman AB, Stewart PM, et al. Treatment of adrenocorticotropin-dependent Cushing's syndrome: A consensus statement. J Clin Endocrinol Metab 2008;93:2454–62.

Boscaro M, Arnaldi G. Approach to the patient with possible Cushing's syndrome. J Clin Endocrinol Metab 2009;94:3121–31.

Newell-Price J, Trainer P, Besser M, Grossman A. The diagnosis and differential diagnosis of Cushing's syndrome and pseudo-Cushing's states. Endocr Rev 1998;19:647–72.

Terzolo M, Angeli A, Fassnacht M, et al. Adjuvant mitotane treatment for adrenocortical carcinoma. N Engl J Med 2007;356:2372–80.

Diabetes Insipidus

Method of
Kerem Ozer, MD, and
Ashok Balasubramanyam, MD

Physiology of Antidiuretic Hormone

Antidiuretic hormone (ADH), a nine–amino acid peptide produced by the supraoptic and paraventricular nuclei of the hypothalamus, increases urine concentration by decreasing renal water excretion. ADH, released in response to increased plasma tonicity, binds to G-protein coupled V_2 receptors on the cells lining the distal tubules and medullary collecting ducts of the kidney. In the absence of ADH, these cells are relatively impermeable to water and the osmolality of the filtrate changes very little as it travels through the nephron, resulting in hypotonic polyuria. ADH causes the translocation of water channels called aquaporins into the luminal membranes of these cells, thereby increasing permeability to water. The resultant increase in water reabsorption decreases urine volume, concentrates the urine, and dilutes the plasma. Dilution of the plasma switches off hypothalamic ADH secretion.

Pathophysiology

When the effective action of ADH is reduced (by approximately 75%) through decreased hormone production or action, the concentrating ability of the kidneys is reduced significantly and polyuria ensues. In most cases, increased urine volume causes a small decrease in total body water (<3%), increased plasma osmolarity, and mild hypernatremia. This stimulates thirst, and the resultant increase in water intake prevents excess loss of body water and only a mild increase in the serum sodium concentration. Consequently, unless there is a concomitant defect in thirst regulation, or water intake is limited for other reasons such as dementia, immobility, or physical restraint, signs or symptoms of severe dehydration do not develop.

Etiology

Diabetes insipidus may be due to deficiency of ADH secretion (central diabetes insipidus) or a lack of response to the hormone at the target organ (nephrogenic diabetes insipidus) (Box 1).

Central diabetes insipidus, also known as neurogenic, vasopressin-responsive, pituitary, neurohypophyseal, or cranial diabetes insipidus, is characterized by hypotonic polyuria secondary to insufficient or absent secretion of ADH despite appropriate physiologic stimuli in the setting of a normal renal response to the hormone. Depending on the severity of hormonal deficiency, some investigators distinguish complete central diabetes insipidus (absolute lack of hormone secretion) from partial central diabetes insipidus (insufficient hormone secretion).

Whether complete or partial, central diabetes insipidus can be caused by congenital malformations, hereditary disorders, or acquired conditions. Congenital malformations associated with diabetes insipidus include midline craniofacial defects, septo-optic dysplasia, and hypogenesis of the posterior pituitary. Hereditary central diabetes insipidus is most commonly as result of mutations in the AVP-neurophysin II gene *(AVP-NPII)*. This is generally an autosomal dominant trait (e.g., OMIM 192340) associated with onset of symptoms within the first several years after birth. Onset in later childhood suggests slower degeneration of the magnocellular neurons of the supraoptic and paraventricular nuclei as a result of a variety of other gene mutations. Autosomal recessive and X-linked recessive forms have also been described.

Nephrogenic diabetes insipidus comprises various disorders of defective ADH action. The usual causes are drugs, vascular insults, or genetic mutations. Genetic mutations are generally loss-of-function mutations of the V_2 receptor gene or occasionally mutations of aquaporin-2. Vasopressin receptor antagonists, such as conivaptan, have been recently approved for the treatment of the syndrome of inappropriate ADH secretion. If used without careful clinical and biochemical monitoring, they could cause iatrogenic diabetes insipidus.

Clinical Spectrum

Diabetes insipidus is a clinical syndrome characterized by excretion of large volumes of dilute urine in the face of concentrated plasma. The spectrum of disorders comprising diabetes insipidus result from

BOX 1   Causes of Diabetes Insipidus

Central Diabetes Insipidus
Malformations
Midline defects
Pituitary hypogenesis

Hereditary
Autosomal dominant (AVP-neurophysin)
Autosomal recessive
- AVP-neurophysin
- Wolfram syndrome
X-linked recessive

Acquired
Trauma
Neoplasms (primary or metastatic)
Infections
- Meningitis
- Encephalitis
Granulomatous disease
Vascular
- Aneurysms
- Hypotension
Idiopathic

Nephrogenic Diabetes Insipidus
Hereditary
AVP receptor-2 gene (AVPR2)
Aquaporin-2 gene

Acquired
Drugs
- Lithium (Eskalith)
- Demeclocycline (Declomycin)
- Cisplatin (Platinol)
- Aminoglycosides)
- Vasopressin receptor antagonists
Vascular (ischemia)
Infiltrative (amyloid)
Electrolyte disorders
- Low or high calcium
- Low potassium
Obstruction

Primary Polydipsia
Psychiatric disorders
Schizophrenia
Obsessive-compulsive disorder

Disorders of thirst regulation
Trauma
Neoplasms
Infections
Granulomatous disease

Abbreviation: AVP = arginine vasopressin.

either decreased secretion or blunted action of ADH. In patients with diabetes insipidus, total 24-hour urine volume is generally greater than 30 mL/kg/day and urine osmolality is usually less than 300 mOsm/L. The symptoms are polyuria and thirst. If the patient is able to drink sufficient quantities of fluid to compensate for the fluid loss, overt dehydration is uncommon. Otherwise, signs and symptoms of dehydration may be present.

Clinical Manifestations

Patients with central diabetes insipidus typically present with polyuria and polydipsia, with symptoms occurring during both day and night. Many patients tend to prefer cold drinks. Urine output can exceed 20 liters a day in complete central diabetes insipidus. The metabolic and plasma electrolyte status depends on the availability of water and the ability of the patient to respond to thirst. This is of special concern if diabetes insipidus occurs following hypothalamic or pituitary surgery, when the patient may be drowsy or unable to respond to thirst, or in nursing home patients with stroke or dementia.

Familial nephrogenic diabetes insipidus is usually of very early onset and can manifest with excessive urination and lethargy or somnolence. Timely diagnosis, based on close monitoring of fluid and electrolyte status, is critical for survival. Presentation of diabetes insipidus secondary to acquired causes depends on the timing and intensity of the insult.

Diagnosis

The first step is objective documentation of polyuria with dilute urine. The patient's complaint of "urinating too much" may be due to dysuria, urgency, or enuresis with or without excessive thirst. These symptoms, if persistent, should prompt attempts to document 24-hour urine volume and osmolality. If urine output is more than 30 mL/kg/day and urine osmolality is less than 300 mOsm/L, evaluation for causes of water diuresis should begin. Specific instances

CURRENT DIAGNOSIS

- Diabetes insipidus is a clinical syndrome comprising excretion of large volumes of dilute urine in the face of concentrated plasma. Patients with diabetes insipidus usually have a total 24-hour urine volume of greater than 30 mL/kg/day and urine osmolality less than 300 mOsm/L.
- Diabetes insipidus may be due to deficiency of antidiuretic hormone (ADH) secretion (central diabetes insipidus) or a lack of response to the hormone at the target organ (nephrogenic diabetes insipidus).
- Plasma ADH level is not helpful in differentiating among the various etiologies.
- Dipsogenic polydipsia and psychogenic polydipsia can mimic the symptoms of diabetes insipidus.
- Rule out other common causes of polyuria such as hyperglycemia or cystitis. This is usually simple, because the urine in these conditions is concentrated rather than dilute.
- Check serum sodium level during free fluid intake.
- If hypernatremia is present while concurrent urine osmolality is less than 300 mOsm/kg of water, inject desmopressin.
- If urine osmolality 1 to 2 hours later is at least two times greater than at baseline, the patient most likely has central diabetes insipidus.
- If the urine osmolality response to desmopressin is less, the patient likely has nephrogenic diabetes insipidus.
- If serum sodium is within normal range with concurrent urine osmolality less than 300 mOsm/kg of water, a formal water deprivation test with desmopressin stimulation helps establish the diagnosis.

might point to a cause including hypotonic polyuria in the setting of psychiatric disease (psychogenic polydipsia) and sudden onset of polyuria after surgery or trauma to the skull base (central diabetes insipidus). More often, features in the history and physical examination are of low sensitivity and specificity; although they are useful in prompting suspicion of the condition, they are unhelpful in differentiating between the various causes of diabetes insipidus.

The next step is to confirm the diagnosis of diabetes insipidus. This can be done in some instances by checking to see if the serum sodium is at the upper end of the normal range or frankly elevated in the face of a dilute urine. The assessment can start by checking the sodium level during free fluid intake. If hypernatremia is present while concurrent urine osmolality is less than 300 mOsm/kg of water, desmopressin (DDAVP) should be injected and a urine osmolality measured in 1 to 2 hours. If urine osmolality is at least two times greater than baseline, the patient most likely has central diabetes insipidus. If the response is less, the patient most likely has nephrogenic diabetes insipidus.

In many cases, the serum sodium is within normal limits, and concurrent low urine osmolality and dynamic testing is indicated. The test of choice is the water deprivation test. Following the general endocrine axiom for a suspected hormonal deficiency, the initial phase of this test is a stimulation test. The general steps of this test and their rationale are as follows:

1. Start the test in the morning. Withhold all fluids. The goal is to cause dehydration and induce the most potent stimulus for maximal ADH secretion.
2. Check plasma osmolality, urine volume and osmolality, and body weight hourly.
3. If fluid deprivation does not result in urine concentration greater than 300 mOsm/L before the body weight decreases by 5%, or if plasma osmolality or serum sodium concentration increase significantly, primary polydipsia or partial diabetes insipidus are unlikely. Complete diabetes insipidus is likely, so proceed to an acute trial of hormone replacement to differentiate between central diabetes insipidus and nephrogenic diabetes insipidus.
4. Administer desmopressin 10 μg by nasal route or 0.03 μg/kg SC or IV. Check urine osmolality 1 to 2 hours later. If there is an increase of the urine osmolality of more than 50%, severe central diabetes insipidus is the diagnosis. A smaller response or no response at all suggests nephrogenic diabetes insipidus.

Imaging can help with diagnosis or localization of the defect, but the findings should be interpreted with caution and in conjunction with clinical information and the results of biochemical testing. Briefly, the hyperintense signal emitted by the posterior pituitary in most healthy subjects on T1-weighted mid-sagittal MRI imaging ("bright spot") is absent in more than 95% of patients with central diabetes insipidus but present in 85% of patients with primary polydipsia.

Differential Diagnosis

Two important conditions that mimic the symptoms of diabetes insipidus are dipsogenic polydipsia and psychogenic polydipsia. In dipsogenic polydipsia, the patient has a normal threshold for ADH release but a malfunctioning thirst mechanism. The osmotic threshold for thirst is lower than that for ADH release, which reverses the normal sequence of physiologic responses to plasma concentration. As a result of early thirst stimulation and water ingestion, serum osmolality is maintained at a level below the threshold for ADH release, with constant hypotonic polyuria. The main feature of psychogenic polydipsia is compulsive and excessive water drinking due to psychiatric disorders, without changes in the threshold for thirst.

Treatment

Management of diabetes insipidus should address amelioration of signs and symptoms, as well as treatment directed at the main etiologic factors, if possible. Polyuria and polydipsia are best treated

CURRENT THERAPY

Desmopressin

- Control of polyuria and associated fluid and electrolyte perturbations is best achieved with desmopressin (DDAVP).
- The available pharmacologic preparations are rhinal tube solution, nasal spray, oral tablets and injectable preparations for subcutaneous or intravenous use (see Table 1)

Other Agents

- Rarely, treatment of partial diabetes insipidus or problems with obtaining or using desmopressin may warrant the use of agents such as Chlorpropamide (Diabinese),[1] Carbamazepine (Tegretol),[1] Clofibrate (Atromid-S),[2] and thiazide diuretics that directly or indirectly augment or mimic the action of desmopressin.

---

[1]Not FDA approved for this indication.
[2]Not available in the United States.

by agents that replace or augment the action of ADH. In addition, replacement of fluid losses, especially in patients with faulty thirst mechanisms, is important. The current treatment of choice for central diabetes insipidus is desmopressin, a synthetic analogue of ADH. Its action is selective for the V_2 receptor in the distal regions of the renal tubular system, with negligible effects on the V_1 receptor that mediates vasoconstriction. An added advantage of desmopressin is its longer half-life compared to ADH. Dose requirements vary widely. A rough guide for an effective dose range for the different preparations (Table 1) would be 0.5 to 3 μg once or twice daily[3] by the subcutaneous or intravenous routes, 5 to 25 μg two or three times daily[3] by nasal administration, and 50 to 500 μg two or three times daily[3] orally.

Education of the patient regarding fluid intake and urine output is crucial. Medications such as chlorpropamide (Diabinese),[1] carbamazepine (Tegretol),[1] clofibrate (Atromid-S),[2] and thiazides may be used in patients with partial diabetes insipidus or in settings where desmopressin availability is limited. These medications are less potent and less predictable and they are more likely to produce adverse effects than desmopressin. Chlorpropamide[1] most likely acts through direct effects on the kidney; carbamazepine[1] enhances the response to ADH, and clofibrate[2] increases ADH release.

The treatment for nephrogenic diabetes insipidus is usually achieved through a combination of thiazides or amiloride (Midamor)[1] and dietary salt restriction. The approach should be guided by the severity of symptoms and the patient's ability to tolerate them, because the thirst mechanism is usually intact and can keep fluid-electrolyte balance at a near-normal status. Salt restriction can regulate urine volume to some extent by limiting the solute load of the filtrate that enters the distal nephron. Because nephrogenic diabetes insipidus is characterized by a constant level of urine osmolality, overall urine volume is closely linked to solute load. Restriction to ≤2.3 g of sodium per day is required, but compliance is difficult and highly variable.

Thiazides may be effective by causing a gentle volume depletion and consequent increased reabsorption of both solutes and water in the proximal tubule. Hydrochlorothiazide (Hydrodiuril)[1] (25 mg once or twice daily) can induce a 2- to 3-lb weight loss and up to 60% decrease in urine volume. Amiloride can synergize with

---

[1]Not FDA approved for this indication.
[2]Not available in the United States.
[3]Exceeds dosage recommended by the manufacturer.

TABLE 1 Treatment of Central Diabetes Insipidus: Most Commonly Used Pharmacologic Preparations

Name	Concentration	Available as
Desmopressin rhinal tube	100 µg/mL	Bottle with rhinal tube
Desmopressin nasal spray	100 µg/mL	Bottle with spray pump
Desmopressin tablets (oral)	n/a	0.1, 0.2 mg tablets
Desmopressin injection (SC, IV)	4 µg/mL	1 and 10 mL vials
Arginine vasopressin (AVP, Petressin) injection (SC, IV)	20 U/mL	0.5, 1, and 10 mL vials

thiazides and may be added to the regimen for patients who do not respond optimally to hydrochlorothiazide alone.

Finally, it is often reasonable and worthwhile to try desmopressin at moderate to relatively high doses, because this may be able to overcome partial resistance to ADH at the receptor or postreceptor level. Several authors have demonstrated 40% to 50% increase in urine osmolality in patients with nephrogenic diabetes insipidus with the use of desmopressin; addition of indomethacin (Indocin)[1] may improve the response to desmopressin.

Monitoring, Prognosis and Potential Complications

Most patients with central diabetes insipidus can be treated with a relatively stable dose of desmopressin that eliminates their symptoms and reestablishes fluid-electrolyte balance. Patients should be instructed to report any significant changes in fluid intake and urine output, so that the ADH axis can be reinvestigated and the dose of desmopressin adjusted as necessary.

In patients with nephrogenic diabetes insipidus for which a precipitating agent has been identified, resistance to ADH may be reversible if the culpable factor is eliminated in a timely manner. Reversal of metabolic causes such as hypercalcemia is usually followed quite rapidly by partial or complete normalization of urine volume and osmolality. Early recognition and treatment is especially important in lithium-induced nephrogenic diabetes insipidus, because the resistance to ADH may be irreversible if severe tubular injury has occurred.

---

[1]Not FDA approved for this indication.

REFERENCES

Abu Libdeh A, Levy-Khademi F, Abdulhadi-Atwan M, et al. Autosomal recessive familial neurohypophyseal diabetes insipidus: onset in early infancy. Eur J Endocrinol 2010;162(2):221–6.

Adrogue HJ, Madias NE. Hypernatremia. N Engl J Med 2000;342:1493–9.

Birnbaumer M, Gilbert S, Rosenthal W. An extracellular congenital nephrogenic diabetes insipidus mutation of the vasopressin receptor reduces cell surface expression, affinity for ligand, and coupling to the Gs/adenylyl cyclase system. Mol Endocrinol 1994;8(7):886–94.

De Bellis A, Colao A, Di Salle F, et al. A longitudinal study of vasopressin cell antibodies, posterior pituitary function, and magnetic resonance imaging evaluations in subclinical autoimmune central diabetes insipidus. J Clin Endocrinol Metab 1999;84(9):3047–51.

Fjellestad-Paulsen A, Laborde K, et al. Water-balance hormones during long-term follow-up of oral DDAVP treatment in diabetes insipidus. Acta Paediatr 1993;82(9):752–7.

Mutig K, Saritas T, Uchida S, et al. Short-term stimulation of the thiazide-sensitive Na^+-Cl^- cotransporter by vasopressin involves phosphorylation and membrane translocation. Am J Physiol Renal Physiol 2010;298(3):F502–9.

Primary Hyperparathyroidism and Hypoparathyroidism

Method of
John P. Bilezikian, MD

Primary Hyperparathyroidism

INCIDENCE AND GENERAL CHARACTERISTICS

Primary hyperparathyroidism (PHPT) is a relatively common endocrine disease with an incidence as high as 1 in 500 to 1 in 1000. The high visibility of PHPT today marks a dramatic change from several generations ago when it was considered rare. The increased incidence is undoubtedly due to widespread use of the multichannel autoanalyzer. PHPT occurs in individuals of all ages but occurs most frequently in the sixth decade of life. Women are affected more often than men by a ratio of 3:1. PHPT in children is an unusual event. It might be a component of one of several endocrinopathies with a genetic basis, such as multiple endocrine neoplasia (MEN), type I or II. PHPT is caused by excessive secretion of parathyroid hormone (PTH) from one or more parathyroid glands. A benign, solitary adenoma is found in 80% of patients. Less commonly, in 15% to 20% of subjects, all four glands are hyperplastic. Four-gland parathyroid disease may occur sporadically or in association with the MEN syndromes. The most uncommon presentation of PHPT is parathyroid cancer, occurring in less than 0.5% of patients with PHPT.

DIFFERENTIAL DIAGNOSIS

The major diagnostic distinction to be made is between PHPT and malignancy, the other most common cause of hypercalcemia. These two etiologies account for more than 90% of all patients with hypercalcemia (Table 1). A much longer, complete list of potential causes of hypercalcemia is considered after these two etiologies are ruled out or if there is reason to believe that a different cause is likely. Today, PHPT presents most often as an asymptomatic disorder. In contrast, malignancy-associated hypercalcemia is usually found at a later stage of the malignant process and is associated with symptoms. Besides a major difference in clinical presentation between these two most common causes of hypercalcemia, the PTH immunoassay is a helpful distinguishing point. In patients

TABLE 1 Differential Diagnosis of Hypercalcemia

Primary hyperparathyroidism
Malignancy
Other endocrinopathies
   Hyperthyroidism
   Pheochromocytoma
   Adrenal insufficiency
   VIPoma
Medications
   Lithium
   Thiazides
   Thyroid hormone
   Vitamin D
   Vitamin A
Granulomatous diseases
Familial hypocalciuric hypercalcemia
Immobilization

with PHPT, the PTH level will be elevated or in the upper range of normal, whereas in malignancy, the PTH level is invariably suppressed.

PATHOPHYSIOLOGY, MOLECULAR GENETICS, AND PATHOLOGY

The pathophysiology of PHPT relates to the loss of normal feedback control of PTH by extracellular calcium. Why the parathyroid cell loses its normal sensitivity to calcium is not known. Genetic abnormalities that could be linked to sporadic parathyroid tumors have been described. A rearrangement of the cyclin D1/(PRAD1) protooncogene has been seen in some patients with PHPT. The rearrangement associates the PTH gene with the growth promoter cyclin D1. Only a small number of parathyroid tumors have been demonstrated to harbor this defect. Tumor suppressors, such as the gene associated with MEN-I, have generated interest, as have potential abnormalities in the gene for the calcium-sensing receptor. Although the gene for the calcium receptor has been implicated in familial hypocalciuric hypercalcemia and neonatal severe hyperparathyroidism, there is little evidence for this genetic abnormality in the sporadic form of PHPT. Even the vitamin D receptor has been implicated in pathogenetic abnormalities associated with parathyroid neoplasia.

The typical parathyroid adenoma is an enlarged, oval-shaped, smooth, red-brown gland. A visible rim of normal yellow-brown parathyroid tissue is sometimes seen. The typical parathyroid adenoma is between 300 and 500 mg, much larger than a normal gland that generally weighs 35 to 50 mg. Microscopically, the parathyroid adenoma consists of a network of cells arranged alongside a capillary network, resembling classic endocrine microanatomy. Fat cells are reduced or absent. The form of PHPT characterized by four-gland hyperplasia is seen grossly as enlarged glands that may be of equal size. Microscopically, solid masses of chief cells are seen in the absence of fat cells. In contrast to the adenoma, in which a rim of normal tissue can sometimes be seen, normal tissue is absent in hyperplastic disease.

SIGNS AND SYMPTOMS

PHPT is associated classically with skeletal and renal complications. In severe cases, the skeleton can be involved in a process called *osteitis fibrosa cystica*. Subperiosteal resorption of the distal phalanges, tapering of the distal clavicles, a "salt and pepper" appearance of the skull, bone cysts, and brown tumors of the long bones are all overt manifestations of hyperparathyroid bone disease. This form of hyperparathyroid bone disease is now most unusual, occurring in fewer than 5% of patients with PHPT. Much less severe, but nevertheless significant, skeletal involvement in PHPT is detected by dual energy x-ray absorptiometry (see later). Similar to the reduced incidence of gross skeletal disease, the kidney is also involved in PHPT much less commonly than before. From an incidence of approximately 33% in the 1960s, most series place the incidence of nephrolithiasis now to be no more than 15% to 20%. Nephrolithiasis, nevertheless, is still the most common complication of PHPT. Other renal features of PHPT include diffuse deposition of calcium–phosphate complexes in the parenchyma (nephrocalcinosis). The frequency of this complication is unknown. Hypercalciuria (daily calcium excretion of >250 mg in women or >300 mg in men) is seen in 30% to 40% of patients. PHPT may be associated with a reduction in creatinine clearance, in the absence of any other cause. Classic associations exist between PHPT and other organs, such as the neuromuscular system, the gastrointestinal tract, and the cardiovascular and articular systems, but such panopleistic features of PHPT are rarely seen today. More vexing are nonspecific elements associated with PHPT, such as easy fatigability, a sense of weakness, and a feeling that the aging process is advancing faster than it should be. This is sometimes accompanied by an intellectual weariness and a sense that cognitive faculties are less sharp. Whether these nonspecific features of PHPT are truly part of the disease process, reversible upon successful parathyroid surgery, remains under active investigation.

CLINICAL FORMS OF PRIMARY HYPERPARATHYROIDISM

Asymptomatic PHPT with serum calcium levels within 1 mg/dL above the upper limits of normal is the most common clinical presentation. Most patients do not have specific complaints and do not show evidence of any target organ complications. In parts of the world where severe vitamin D deficiency is common, more symptomatic PHPT is seen. Unusual clinical presentations of PHPT include MEN-I and MEN-II, familial PHPT not associated with any other endocrine disorder, familial cystic parathyroid adenomatosis, jaw tumor syndrome, and neonatal PHPT. Another presentation of PHPT is being described, namely, in individuals with normal serum calcium concentrations but elevated PTH levels. Potential secondary causes of elevated PTH levels are considered but have not been found. It is considered likely that these patients represent the earliest stage of PHPT, when there is glandular overproduction of hormone, before hypercalcemia becomes evident.

DIAGNOSIS AND EVALUATION

Hypercalcemia and elevated levels of PTH establish the diagnosis. The serum phosphorus concentration tends to be in the lower range of normal. Serum alkaline phosphatase activity may be elevated. More specific markers of bone formation (bone-specific alkaline phosphatase, osteocalcin) and bone resorption (urinary deoxypyridinoline, N or C-telopeptide of collagen) tend to be in the upper range of normal. In some patients, the actions of PTH in altering renal acid-base handling leads to a small increase in the serum chloride concentration and a concomitant small decrease in the serum bicarbonate concentration. Urinary calcium excretion, when elevated, is not generally excessively high. The circulating 25-hydroxyvitamin D concentration is low, and the 1,25-dihydroxyvitamin D concentration is high in some patients.

ROLE OF BONE MASS MEASUREMENT

Dual-energy x-ray absorptiometry shows a pattern of skeletal involvement that is consistent with the physiologic actions of PTH, that of eroding cortical bone while sparing cancellous sites. The typical patient with PHPT shows reductions in bone density that are most marked in the distal third of the forearm, a cortical site, with much less involvement of the lumbar spine, a cancellous site. The hip region, a mixture of cortical and cancellous bone, shows changes that are intermediate between changes in the forearm and the lumbar spine.

CURRENT DIAGNOSIS

Primary Hyperparathyroidism

- Most common cause of hypercalcemia.
- Diagnosis established by elevated serum calcium concentration and parathyroid hormone level that is frankly elevated or is in the upper range of normal.
- In some patients, the parathyroid hormone level is elevated but the serum calcium concentration is normal.

Hypoparathyroidism

- Much less common than primary hyperparathyroidism.
- Most often due to autoimmune destruction or removal of the parathyroid glands.
- Diagnosis is established by hypocalcemia and low parathyroid hormone levels.

CURRENT THERAPY

Primary Hyperparathyroidism

- When symptoms are present, parathyroid surgery is indicated.
- In the absence of symptoms, surgery is recommended if any one of four criteria is met (see Table 2).
- Preoperative localization testing prior to surgery has become routine.
- Medical management is reserved generally for those who do not meet surgical criteria in whom it is intended to lower the serum calcium or to increase the bone mineral density.
- Prudent use of calcium and vitamin D is recommended, and ambulation is encouraged.
- Pharmacologic agents, such as bisphosphonates and calcimimetics, show promise.

Hypoparathyroidism

- Acute management of hypocalcemia is a medical emergency and requires intravenous administration of calcium.
- Chronic treatment is based upon adequate calcium, vitamin D, and, in some cases, the active vitamin D metabolite 1,25-dihydroxyvitamin D.

TREATMENT

Localization Tests Prior to Surgery

Imaging of abnormal parathyroid tissue is accomplished most accurately with technetium-99m sestamibi. Sestamibi is taken up by both thyroid and parathyroid tissue, but it persists in the parathyroid glands. Various approaches to the use of technetium-99m sestamibi include using the imaging agent alone, and thereby depending upon a difference in uptake kinetics between thyroid and parathyroid tissue, or in combination with iodine 123 (^{123}I). Some believe that use of dual isotopic methods provides better definition of the thyroid from which the image obtained with sestamibi can be subtracted. Even more sophisticated approaches have been developed using sestamibi imaging with single-photon emission computed tomography. Ultrasound, computed tomography, and magnetic resonance imaging are also used to localize abnormal parathyroid tissue. Invasive localization tests with arteriography and selective venous sampling for PTH are used when noninvasive studies have not been successful. In the past, parathyroid imaging was reserved for patients who had undergone neck surgery. With greater success in parathyroid imaging and the increasing popularity of minimally invasive parathyroid surgery, preoperative imaging is becoming routine in all patients.

Guidelines for Surgical Management of Primary Hyperparathyroidism

The Third International Workshop on the Management of Asymptomatic Primary Hyperparathyroidism was held in 2008, the proceedings of which were published in 2009. The Workshop reviewed new data since the previous workshop in 2002 and suggested revised guidelines for surgical management (Table 2). The major changes are summarized here. Since the urinary calcium excretion does not predict stone disease in patients with primary hyperparathyroidism who do not have nephrolithiasis or nephrocalcinosis, it has been removed as a guideline. However, the collection of a 24-hour urine for calcium determination is routinely performed and still recommended. The other major change in the guidelines relates to the cut-point of creatinine clearance below which surgery is recommended. A creatinine clearance <60 mL/min

TABLE 2 2008 Guidelines for Parathyroid Surgery in Asymptomatic PHPT

Measurement	Surgery Recommended if
Serum calcium	>1.0 mg/dL (0.25 mmol/L) above normal
Creatinine clearance (calculated)	Reduced to less than 60 mL/min/1.73 m^3
Bone mineral density	T score less than −2.5 SD at spine, hip (total or femoral neck), and radius (distal 1/3 site predominantly cortical bone) or presence of fragility fracture
Age	Patient age less than 50 years

is associated with an increase in PTH levels in individuals without primary hyperparathyroidism. In primary hyperparathyroidism, therefore, if the creatinine clearance is reduced to below this level, it seems likely that PTH levels will increase further. The Workshop Panel recommends that surgery be considered in these individuals.

SURGERY

PHPT is cured when abnormal parathyroid tissue is removed. Asymptomatic patients are advised to have surgery if they meet current guidelines (see Table 2). Symptomatic patients are always advised to undergo parathyroid surgery. At the present time, a number of different surgical procedures can be performed. The standard four-gland parathyroid gland exploration is performed under general or local anesthesia. The single adenoma is removed, and the other glands are ascertained to be normal but not removed. In the case of multiglandular disease, the approach is to remove all tissue except for a remnant that is left in situ or autotransplanted in the nondominant forearm. A popular recent advance in parathyroid surgery is the minimally invasive parathyroidectomy. This procedure depends upon preoperative localization by an imaging technology and confirmation of the success of parathyroid surgery with intraoperative PTH measurements. The circulating PTH level should fall to less than 50% of the preoperative value within minutes after removal of the parathyroid adenoma. Minimally invasive parathyroid surgery, this latter approach, has become a standard for many parathyroid surgeons now.

MEDICAL MANAGEMENT

In patients who do not meet surgical guidelines or who, for other reasons, will not undergo parathyroid surgery, the following medical principles apply. Adequate hydration and ambulation are always encouraged. Thiazide diuretics are to be avoided because they may lead to worsening hypercalcemia. Dietary intake of calcium should be moderate, avoiding both high- and low-calcium diets. Low-calcium diets theoretically could fuel abnormal parathyroid tissue to secrete more PTH. High-calcium diets could be detrimental by worsening hypercalcemia, especially if the 1,25-dihydroxy vitamin D level is elevated. Monitoring with annual measurements of the serum calcium and annual or every-other-year measurements of bone mass by dual-energy x-ray absorptiometry are recommended. In patients whose 25-hydroxyvitamin D level is low, careful replacement seems reasonable. The serum calcium concentration must be monitored to guard against the potential for worsening hypercalcemia in some patients.

Oral phosphate will lower the serum calcium concentration in PHPT by approximately 0.5 to 1 mg/dL, but concerns about ectopic calcium–phosphate deposition limit its utility. Prior to the results of the Women's Health Initiative, estrogen was an option in postmenopausal women. The serum calcium concentration would fall by about 0.5 mg/dL; estrogens are no longer advised for this specific reason. Preliminary observations suggest that raloxifene, a selective estrogen receptor modulator, may have calcium-lowering effects similar to those of estrogen in postmenopausal women with PHPT.

The bisphosphonate alendronate (Fosamax) has shown promise in patients with PHPT. Lumbar spine bone density improves by as much as 5% in the first year of therapy. Neither the serum calcium concentration nor the PTH level falls significantly. Patients who will not undergo parathyroid surgery but in whom lumbar spine bone density is reduced may benefit from bisphosphonate therapy.

An early clinical experience with hyperparathyroid postmenopausal women has shown that, in principle, a calcimimetic can significantly reduce PTH and serum calcium levels in patients with the disease. By binding to a site on the calcium-sensing receptor, the calcimimetic increases the affinity of the calcium receptor for extracellular calcium. The result is an increase in intracellular calcium and thus reductions in PTH synthesis and secretion. Even though the drug has not yet been approved for use for PHPT in the United States, early data are promising. The serum calcium concentration typically becomes normal and remains within normal limits for as long as the drug is used. Interestingly, the serum PTH level falls only modestly and continues to be elevated despite correction of the hypercalcemia by the drug.

Hypoparathyroidism

Hypoparathyroidism is much more uncommon than is PHPT. It results from the destruction, removal, or dysfunction of all parathyroid tissue.

ETIOLOGY

The most common causes of hypoparathyroidism are neck surgery and an autoimmune process (Table 3). Surgical hypoparathyroidism can follow the operation by many years and can occur after any neck surgery. Autoimmune destruction of the parathyroid glands can occur in an isolated fashion or in connection with a variety of polyglandular syndromes. The two major forms are type I (multiple endocrine gland failure along with candidiasis, pernicious anemia, and/or alopecia) and type II (with adrenal or thyroid failure and/or diabetes mellitus). Activating mutations of the calcium-sensing receptor or of the parathyroid gene itself can be associated with hypoparathyroidism. Parathyroid gland destruction is rarely due to infiltration of the glands by iron, copper, granulomas, or malignancy. In severe magnesium deficiency, parathyroid secretion is impaired along with a peripheral resistance to the actions of PTH. Mild hypoparathyroidism can become symptomatic in the presence of a potent bisphosphonate such as alendronate.

TABLE 3 Causes of Hypoparathyroidism

Parathyroid gland destruction
Postsurgical
Autoimmune
Sporadic
Polyglandular syndromes
Activating antibodies against the calcium-sensing receptor
Infiltration
Iron, copper
Malignancy
Granulomatous
Genetic
Activating mutations of the calcium-sensing receptor
Inactivating mutations in the PTH gene
DiGeorge syndrome
Impaired secretion and/or action of PTH
Hypomagnesemia
Pseudohypoparathyroidism

Abbreviation: PTH = parathyroid hormone.

CLINICAL FEATURES

Increased neuromuscular irritability is the clinical hallmark of hypoparathyroidism. Features of hypoparathyroidism can range from mild paresthesias around the mouth, fingers, and toes to muscle cramping, and, at their worst, carpal, pedal, or laryngospasm. Central nervous system seizure activity is also seen as a severe manifestation of hypocalcemia. These symptoms are due, in part, to the actual serum calcium level but also to the rate at which the serum calcium level falls. Rapid declines in the serum calcium concentrations are more likely to be associated with symptoms than to situations in which the serum calcium concentration has fallen gradually. If respiratory or metabolic alkalosis is present, symptoms can worsen because the partition between bound and free calcium is shifted to the bound state when the blood pH rises. Signs of hypocalcemia include the Chvostek sign (evoked facial nerve irritability), the Trousseau sign (carpal spasm when the blood pressure cuff is inflated to pressures above systolic), and a prolonged QT interval on the electrocardiogram. When severe hypocalcemia is present, impaired cardiac contractility, unresponsive to inotropic agents until the hypocalcemia is corrected, has been reported. Pseudopapilledema and subcapsular cataracts can be seen. In some individuals, hypoparathyroidism is detected only by an asymptomatic reduction in the serum calcium concentration. Pseudohypoparathyroidism is a group of genetic disorders of the PTH receptor/G-protein transduction system responsible for PTH action. In the type I variant, subjects have a classic phenotype (Albright's hereditary osteodystrophy) with short stature, brachydactyly, subcutaneous and basal ganglia calcifications, rounded facies, shortened neck, seizures, and below-average intelligence. Other endocrine glands, such as the thyroid and gonads, can also be dysfunctional. In the type II form of pseudohypoparathyroidism, PHT resistance is present in the absence of the clinical phenotype.

DIAGNOSIS

Hypocalcemia and an elevated serum phosphorus concentration in association with absent PTH levels confirm the diagnosis of hypoparathyroidism. In pseudohypoparathyroidism, PTH levels are elevated, reflecting the PTH-resistant state, but otherwise the biochemical findings of hypocalcemia and hyperphosphatemia are similar to those of hypoparathyroidism. The urinary calcium concentration is usually not elevated because the filtered load of calcium is low, but actually renal handling of calcium is impaired in this setting because of the lack of PTH. Such individuals have an increase in urinary calcium for the given filtered calcium load, even though the actual amount of urinary calcium excretion might not be excessive.

TREATMENT

The goals of treatment are to establish a serum calcium concentration that is not associated with symptoms or signs and to prevent long-term complications of hypocalcemia. Acute, symptomatic hypocalcemia is a medical emergency and must be treated urgently. The management of chronic hypocalcemia follows a different set of guidelines.

Acute Management

The initial approach is to infuse intravenously 1 to 2 ampules of calcium gluconate (90–180 mg of elemental calcium), diluted in 50 to 100 mL of 5% dextrose over a 10- to 15-minute period. If the acute symptoms are not quickly ameliorated, another 1 to 2 ampules can be administered. To raise the serum calcium concentration further, but more gradually, an infusion of 15 mg/kg of calcium gluconate in 1 L of 5% dextrose over 8 to 10 hours will raise the serum calcium concentration by 2 to 3 mg/dL. Because 1 ampule of calcium gluconate contains 90 mg of elemental calcium, 9 to 11 ampules of calcium gluconate are required for an average-size adult (60–70 kg). The serum calcium concentration should be monitored frequently. If the hypocalcemia is due to magnesium deficiency, these measures are also appropriate while magnesium is being replaced. Acute administration of magnesium without calcium will not immediately correct hypocalcemia because peripheral resistance to PTH, one component of hypocalcemia induced by magnesium deficiency, is not corrected for several days. Intravenous replacement of magnesium is 2.4 mg/kg, up to 180 mg, over a 10-minute period or a continuous infusion of 576 mg of magnesium over 24 hours.

Chronic Management

Oral calcium supplementation is required in virtually all patients. The amount varies but is generally in the range of 1 to 3 g in divided doses. The carbonate or citrated form of calcium is most commonly used. Calcium carbonate is generally preferred because it contains the highest amount of elemental calcium. When calcium preparations are given with meals, both the carbonate and the citrated form of calcium are equally bioavailable. The presence of food obviates the need for gastric acid when calcium carbonate is used.

Most patients also require vitamin D. The amount of ergocalciferol (vitamin D_2) or cholecalciferol (vitamin D_3) ranges from 25,000 to 200,000 IU daily (1.25–10 mg). These large amounts are required because the absence of PTH and hyperphosphatemia both limit the amount of vitamin D that ultimately is converted to 1,25-dihydroxy-vitamin D, the active metabolite in the kidney. Because activation of vitamin D is impaired, much more vitamin D is required. There is no impairment of the first activation step in the liver, namely, from vitamin D to 25-hydroxyvitamin D, the storage form. Because there is no impairment in this step, large amounts of 25-hydroxyvitamin D can accumulate in fat tissues. At times and unpredictably, these stores can be mobilized and lead to hypercalcemia. Sometimes, the hypercalcemia is severe, requiring emergent treatment. Other times, a simple adjustment in the amount of calcium and/or vitamin D is sufficient. In any event, patients receiving large doses of vitamin D should always be regularly monitored for serum calcium concentrations approximately every 3 to 6 months.

Although many patients with hypoparathyroidism can be adequately managed with oral calcium and vitamin D, other patients also require therapy with 1,25-dihydroxyvitamin D, the active metabolite of vitamin D. 1,25-Dihydroxyvitamin D is used in addition to, but not in place of, vitamin D because 1,25-dihydroxyvitamin D alone does not provide for smooth control. Perhaps this is because 1,25-dihydroxyvitamin D is not stored to any appreciable extent in fat tissue. The half-life of 1,25-dihydroxyvitamin D is as short as 6 hours. Therefore, patients managed without parent vitamin D but with 1,25-dihydroxyvitamin D as the only source of vitamin D are more likely to have unpredictable fluctuations in serum calcium concentration. The amount of 1,25-dihydroxyvitamin D ranges from 0.5 to 1.0 μg/day. Some patients require more. Enhanced gastrointestinal absorption of calcium with 1,25-dihydroxyvitamin D can lead to hypercalciuria because in hypoparathyroidism there is no PTH to facilitate calcium reabsorption in the renal tubule. Urinary calcium should be checked on a regular basis. If hypercalciuria occurs, the dose of 1,25-dihydroxyvitamin D and/or vitamin D should be adjusted downward. In this situation, a thiazide diuretic such as hydrochlorothiazide[1] can be used to reduce urinary calcium excretion. In pseudohypoparathyroidism, hypercalciuria is less likely to occur because PTH is present and does have some renal effects in reabsorbing filtered calcium.

Another reason for variability in the control of serum calcium concentration in hypoparathyroidism is a change in medications. For example, if a thiazide or loop diuretic is started for hypertension, the serum calcium concentration may increase or decrease, respectively. Glucocorticoids can lead to a reduction in the serum calcium concentration because glucocorticoids interfere with vitamin D action in the gastrointestinal tract. Bile-sequestering resins can interfere with vitamin D absorption. Midcycle changes in estrogen levels in premenopausal women can lead to altered control.

Hypoparathyroidism is one of the few endocrine disorders for which the replacement hormone, namely, PTH, is not yet available, but it is being studied in some clinical trials.

---

[1]Not FDA approved for this indication.

REFERENCES

Arnold A, Shattuck TM, Mallya SM, et al. Molecular pathogenesis of primary hyperparathyroidism. J Bone Miner Res 2002;17(Suppl. 2):N30–6.

Bilezikian JP, Khan AA, Potts JT Jr. 2009 Guidelines for the Management of Asymptomatic Primary Hyperparathyroidism: Summary Statement from the Third International Workshop. J Clin Endocrinol Metab 2009;94: 335–9.

Bilezikian JP, Silverberg SJ. Primary hyperparathyroidism. In: Rosen C, editor. Primer on the Metabolic Bone Diseases and Disorders of Calcium Metabolism. 7th ed. Am Soc Bone Min Research. 2008. p. 302–6.

Eastell R, Arnold A, Brandi ML, et al. 2009 Diagnosis of Asymptomatic Primary Hyperparathyroidism: Proceedings of the Third International Workshop. J Clin Endocrinol Metab 2009;94:340–50.

Grey A, Lucas J, Horne A, et al. Vitamin D repletion in patients with primary hyperparathyroidism and coexistent vitamin D insufficiency. J Clin Endocrinol Metab 2005;90:2122–6.

Khan AA, Bilezikian JP, Kung AWC, et al. Alendronate in primary hyperparathyroidism: a double-blind, randomized, placebo-controlled trial. J Clin Endocrinol Metab 2004;89:3319–25.

Lowe H, McMahon DJ, Rubin MR, et al. Normocalcemic primary hyperparathyroidism: further characterization of a new clinical phenotype. J Clin Endocrinol Metab 2007;92:3001–5.

Marx SJ. Hyperparathyroid and hypoparathyroid disorders. N Engl J Med 2000;343:1863–75.

Peacock M, Bilezikian JP, Klassen PS, et al. Cinacalcet hydrochloride maintains long-term normocalcemia in patients with primary hyperparathyroidism. J Clin Endocrinol Metab 2005;90:135–41.

Rubin MR, Bilezikian JP, McMahon DJ, et al. The natural history of primary hyperparathyroidism with or without parathyroid surgery after 15 years. J Clin Endocrinol Metab 2008;93:3462–70.

Rubin MR, Dempster DW, Zhou H, et al. Dynamic and structural properties of the skeleton in hypoparathyroidism. J Bone Miner Res 2008;23: 2018–24.

Silverberg S, Bilezikian JP. The diagnosis and management of asymptomatic primary hyperparathyroidism. Nat Clin Practice Endocrinol Metab 2006; 2:494–503.

Silverberg SJ, Lewiecki EM, Mosekilde L, et al. 2009 Presentation of Asymptomatic Primary Hyperparathyroidism: Proceedings of the Third International Workshop. J Clin Endocrinol Metab 2009;94:351–65.

Primary Aldosteronism

Method of
Beejal Shah, MD, and Lawrence Chan, MD

Primary Aldosteronism

Aldosterone was first discovered in 1952, and Jerome W. Conn described the first case of primary aldosteronism (PA) in 1954. PA is a state of excess aldosterone secreted autonomously of the renin-angiotensin system. It is the most common cause of secondary hypertension, and recent reports suggest that 5% to 20% of hypertensive patients have PA, a result of increased awareness and screening. It is a curable form of hypertension but, if left untreated, can result in renal, cardiovascular, and cerebrovascular morbidity greater than that seen in age-matched controls with essential hypertension.

CAUSES OF PRIMARY ALDOSTERONISM

The most common cause of PA is an adrenal adenoma autonomously producing aldosterone or hyperfunctioning adrenal nodules (usually bilateral) producing aldosterone. Less common causes of PA are listed in Box 1.

CLINICAL PRESENTATION

The classic clinical presentation of a patient with PA in the past was hypertension and hypokalemia; however, most patients with PA (60%) are hypertensive and normokalemic with inappropriate

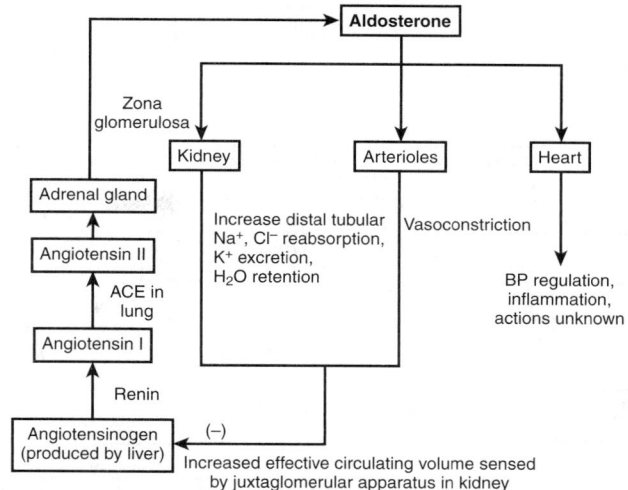

FIGURE 1. The renin-angiotensin-aldosterone system (RAAS). *Abbreviations:* ACE = angiotensin-converting enzyme; BP = blood pressure.

BOX 1 Causes of Primary Aldosteronism

Most Common
- Aldosterone-producing adenoma
- Bilateral adrenal hyperplasia or idiopathic hyperaldosteronism

Less Common
- Unilateral hyperplasia or primary adrenal hyperplasia
- Familial hyperaldosteronism type 1 or glucocorticoid remedial aldosteronism
- Familial hyperaldosteronism type 2
- Aldosterone-producing adrenocortical carcinoma
- Ectopic aldosterone-secreting tumor (ovary, kidney)
- Multiple endocrine neoplasia type 1

aldosterone excess. All patients with PA have hypertension, which can be severe but is rarely malignant. If a patient does present with hypokalemia, then aldosterone excess may be severe and the patient may have symptoms of hypokalemia (if <2.5 mEq/L), such as muscle weakness and disorientation. Patients with PA usually do not develop edema, because there is preserved hormonal balance of sodium wasting with sodium retention (mineralocorticoid escape). Less often, patients present with left ventricular hypertrophy, albuminuria, or retinopathy. PA patients have greater cardiovascular morbidity and mortality than patients with essential hypertension; however, once their condition is appropriately treated, they have no excess cardiovascular risk beyond the general population.

PATIENT SCREENING CRITERIA

Any patient who fulfills any of the following profiles should be screened for PA (reported prevalence included when known):

- Joint National Commission (JNC) 7 stage 2 hypertension (≥160–179 mm Hg systolic, ≥100–109 mm Hg diastolic), prevalence 8%
- JNC 7 stage 3 hypertension (≥180/110 mm Hg), prevalence 13%
- Drug-resistant hypertension, prevalence 17% to 23%
- Hypertension and spontaneous or diuretic-induced hypokalemia
- Hypertension and family history of early-onset hypertension or cerebrovascular accident at a young age (<40 years)
- Family members with PA
- Adrenal incidentaloma and hypertension, median prevalence 2%

Patients with essential hypertension who are not included in these criteria should not be routinely screened for PA.

PATHOPHYSIOLOGY

Aldosterone is a hormone produced by the zona glomerulosa in the adrenal gland. It is part of the renin-angiotensin-aldosterone system (RAAS). Normally, low plasma volume, reduction in effective circulation volume, or a low glomerular filtration rate (GFR) is sensed by the zona glomerulosa and stimulates renin production, which initiates the RAAS cascade (Fig. 1). Aldosterone acts at the distal nephron, where it stimulates sodium reabsorption and potassium excretion. Mineralocorticoid receptors are present at high levels in the distal nephron, but they also occur in other tissues, including the heart.

A negative feedback mechanism exists in the kidney at the juxtaglomerular apparatus, which responds to volume expansion and vasoconstriction by decreasing renin secretion and consequently decreasing aldosterone production. PA is therefore a low-renin state, as opposed to secondary aldosteronism, which is a high-renin state as seen in cases of renovascular hypertension and diuretic therapy. Under abnormal physiology, there is autonomous adrenal production of aldosterone despite an appropriately suppressed renin, which results in excess sodium reabsorption, hypokalemia, water retention, and hypertension.

HYPOKALEMIA

The prevalence of hypokalemia in PA is vastly overestimated. It is found in fewer than 40% of patients with PA, with APA being the subtype majority. The etiology of hypokalemia in PA is threefold. First, hyperaldosteronism causes potassium secretion from principal cells into the lumen of the cortical collecting tubule, resulting in urinary potassium wasting. Second, increasing sodium intake exacerbates hypokalemia, because the associated volume expansion does not appropriately suppress aldosterone production. Third, many PA patients are not hypokalemic under basal conditions, probably because a new steady state may occur wherein the potassium-wasting effect of hyperaldosteronism (due to increasing sodium absorption) is counterbalanced by the physiologic potassium-retaining effect of hypokalemia itself. PA also causes metabolic alkalosis, mild hypernatremia, hypomagnesemia, and increased urinary albumin excretion, which in two case series resolved with treatment of PA but not in patients with essential hypertension.

BIOCHEMICAL TESTS

An early-morning (8–9 AM) plasma aldosterone level is most accurate. Measurement of urine aldosterone excretion over 24 hours (from 8–9 AM to the next morning) is also useful. The aldosterone secretion rate has many drawbacks and therefore is not clinically useful.

Renin cleaves circulating angiotensinogen into angiotensin and is measured in terms of this enzymatic activity, called plasma renin activity (PRA). Current assays are very sensitive; the normal range is laboratory dependent but usually very low. All normal ranges for any assay are dependent on hydration, posture, and salt intake. Angiotensin I and II assays are neither sensitive nor specific and are rarely used.

Screening Test for Primary Aldosteronism

A quick and inexpensive screening test for PA is the ratio of plasma aldosterone concentration (PAC) to the PRA. A positive test is a PAC/PRA ratio equal to or greater than 20, or 30 for greater specificity. The PAC should be greater than 15 ng/dL to avoid a false-positive result, because the PRA is almost always very low or undetectable, which can raise the PAC/PRA ratio. If the PRA is greater than 1 ng/mL/hour, then PA is very unlikely.

The sensitivity of the PAC/PRA ratio is about 87%, and the specificity is 75%, when the patient is off medications that affect the ratio. There is no consensus on cutoff values for PRA, PAC, or the PAC/PRA ratio, so the sensitivity and specificity of this test change

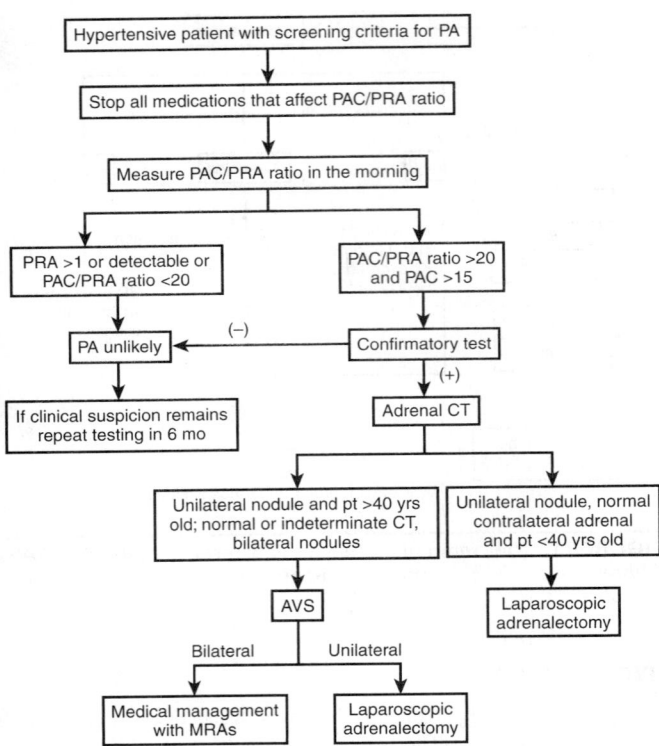

FIGURE 2. Evaluation of primary aldosteronism (PA). *Abbreviations:* AVS = adrenal vein sampling; CT = computed tomography; MAs = mineralocorticoid receptor antagonists; PAC = plasma aldosterone concentration; PRA = plasma renin activity; pt = patient.

depends on the cutoff values used. Inconclusive results should be repeated, and once a positive screening test establishes hyperaldosteronism, a confirmatory test should be performed (Fig. 2).

Protocol for the PAC/PRA Screening Test

Performing the screening test under correct conditions is the most important step in establishing the diagnosis of PA. The following drugs should be withdrawn at least 4 weeks, and ideally 6 weeks, before testing: spironolactone (Aldactone), eplerenone (Inspra), amiloride (Midamor), triamterene (Dyrenium), potassium-losing diuretics, and licorice-derived products.[7] Angiotensin-converting enzyme inhibitors (ACEIs), angiotensin receptor blockers (ARBs), and renin inhibitors should be withdrawn 2 weeks before testing. If ACEIs, ARBs, or diuretics are continued, the PRA will be falsely elevated. In this situation, a detectable PRA or a low PAC/PRA ratio does not exclude PA. However, if the PRA is undetectable while the patient is on ACEIs, ARBs, or diuretics, suspicion of PA is increased. If needed, hypertensive medications that do not affect the RAAS system can be substituted (Box 2).

Before testing, the hypokalemia is corrected and liberal salt intake is encouraged. Hypokalemia decreases aldosterone levels, and a low salt diet increases aldosterone levels. For utmost accuracy, PAC and PRA should be measured between 8 and 10 AM (because aldosterone has a diurnal variation), with the patient ambulatory just before the venipuncture and recumbent for the blood draw. If the PAC/PRA is nondiagnostic, the test is repeated with the following drugs also withdrawn for at least 1 to 2 weeks: β-blockers, central α₂-agonists, nonsteroidal antiinflammatory drugs, and dihydropyridine calcium channel blockers.

Imperative to diagnostic testing and its interpretation is understanding of the factors that can affect the aldosterone and renin levels (see Box 2). All medications that affect the ratio should be stopped.

Low sodium intake and upright posture increase PRA and increase PAC, whereas high sodium intake and supine posture decrease both PRA and PAC.

The elimination of factors that affect the PAC/PRA ratio pertains most to patients who in actuality do not have PA despite clinical suspicion. A false-positive or false-negative result can lead to diagnostic and therapeutic misadventures. In patients with PA, the aldosterone secretion is autonomous from RAAS, regardless of influencing factors, so the PAC/PRA ratio should remain high despite elimination of such factors. However, because the physician does not know which patients ultimately have true disease, the screening protocol must be followed.

Confirmatory Testing for Primary Aldosteronism

The confirmatory test is aimed at suppressing aldosterone, which rules out PA. However, there is no gold standard confirmatory test. To confirm PA, patients undergo an oral salt loading test, a saline suppression test, or, more rarely, a fludrocortisone (Florinef)[1] suppression test or a captopril (Capoten)[1] challenge test.

Oral Sodium Loading Test

PROTOCOL

The protocol for the oral sodium loading test is as follows:

1. Hold all pertinent blood pressure medications (see Box 2).
2. Place the patient on a high-sodium diet (2 g NaCl tablets every 6 hours) for 3 days.
3. Replace potassium to compensate for the kaliuresis induced by the high-sodium diet.
4. Collect a 24-hour urine sample (morning to morning) for determination of aldosterone, sodium, and creatinine. The urine collection is adequate if the urine sodium over 24 hours is greater than 200 mmol/day.

INTERPRETATION OF RESULTS

PA is confirmed if the 24-hour urine aldosterone concentration is greater than 33 nmol or 12 to 14 µg. PA is ruled out if the 24-hour urine aldosterone is less than 10 ng, and the test is equivocal if the value falls in between 10 and 12 ng/24 hr. This test has a sensitivity of 96% and a specificity of 93%. Alternatively, an 8 AM aldosterone level can be determined in place of a 24-hour urine collection on the morning of day 3, and a cut off value of 7 ng/dL or higher confirms PA. An 8 AM aldosterone level greater than 7 ng/dL has a sensitivity of 88% and a specificity of 100% if the screening PAC/PRA ratio is greater than 40, although this varies.

PRECAUTION

Do not perform this test in patients with severe uncontrolled hypertension, renal failure, cardiac failure, cardiac arrhythmias, or severe hypokalemia.

Intravenous Saline Infusion Test

PROTOCOL

1. Hold all pertinent blood pressure medications (see Box 2).
2. Place the patient supine 1 hour before drawing blood for morning baseline fasting levels of renin, aldosterone, cortisol, and potassium.
3. Start an infusion of 2 L 0.9% sodium chloride over 4 hours, keeping the patient supine.
4. Monitor for increased blood pressure and heart rate.
5. After 4 hours, draw a blood sample for measurement of renin, aldosterone, cortisol, and potassium.

INTERPRETATION OF RESULTS

PA is ruled out if the PAC is suppressed to less than 5 ng/dL or 139 pmol/L. PA is biochemically confirmed if the PAC after saline infusion is greater than 10 ng/dL or 277 pmol/L. If the PAC falls between these values, the test is equivocal.

---

[7]Available as dietary supplement.

[1]Not FDA approved for this indication.

BOX 2 Medications and Factors That Affect Aldosterone and Renin Levels

Decrease Renin Level
- β-Blockers
- Central α_2-agonists
- NSAIDs
- Renin inhibitors (when renin is measured as PRA)
- Potassium loading (or no change)
- High-sodium diet
- Aging (>65 y)
- Renal failure
- Prolonged supine posture

Increase Renin Level
- Potassium-wasting diuretics
- ACE inhibitors
- ARBs
- Dihydropyridines (mild elevation)
- Hypokalemia (or no change)
- Pregnancy
- Low-sodium diet
- Renovascular hypertension
- Malignant hypertension
- Prolonged upright posture

Decrease Aldosterone Levels
- β-Blockers
- Central α_2-agonists
- NSAIDs
- ACE inhibitors
- ARBs
- Dihydropyridines (or no change)
- Renin inhibitors
- Hypokalemia
- High-sodium diet
- Aging (>65 y)
- Prolonged supine posture

Increase Aldosterone Levels
- Potassium-wasting diuretics (or no change)
- Potassium-sparing diuretics

- Dihydropyridones (or no change)
- High-potassium diet
- Low-sodium diet
- Pregnancy
- Malignant hypertension
- Renovascular hypertension
- Prolonged upright posture

Suppression of PAC/PRA Ratio
- ACE inhibitors
- ARBs
- Potassium-sparing diuretics
- Potassium-wasting diuretics
- Hypokalemia
- Dihydropyridines
- Low-sodium diet
- Pregnancy
- Renovascular hypertension
- Malignant hypertension
- Prolonged supine posture

Elevation of PAC/PRA Ratio
- β-Blockers (or no change)
- Central α_2-agonists
- NSAIDs
- Renin inhibitors
- High-potassium diet
- High-sodium diet
- Renal failure
- Upright posture
- Aging (>65 y)

Minimal Effect on PAC/PRA Ratio
- Verapamil slow release (Calan SR)
- Hydralazine (Apresoline)
- Prazosin (Minipress)
- Doxasozin (Cardura)
- Terazosin (Hytrin)

Abbreviations: ACE = angiotensin converting enzyme; ARBs = angiotensin receptor blockers; NSAIDs = nonsteroidal antiinflammatory drugs; PAC = plasma aldosterone concentration; PRA = plasma renin activity.

PRECAUTION

Do not conduct this test in patients with severe uncontrolled hypertension, renal failure, cardiac failure, cardiac arrhythmias, or severe hypokalemia.

Fludrocortisone Suppression Test

PROTOCOL

1. Give 0.1 mg fludrocortisone (Florinef)[1] every 6 hours for 4 days, with the potassium level checked every 6 hours to be sure that it is greater than 4 mmol/L. Encourage a liberal sodium diet to keep urinary sodium excretion greater than 3 mmol/kg/day.
2. On day 4, draw blood for an upright 7 AM plasma cortisol level and a 10 AM upright plasma aldosterone, renin, and cortisol levels.

INTERPRETATION OF RESULTS

PA is confirmed if the 10 AM PAC is greater than 6 ng/dL, as long as PRA is less than 1 ng/mL/hour and the plasma cortisol at 10 AM is less than at 7 AM.

PRECAUTION

Because of its risky nature, the test may require hospitalization. Risks include severe hypokalemia, QT changes on electrocardiography, worsening of left ventricular function, hypertension, and consequences of the frequent blood draws for potassium levels.

Captopril Challenge Test

PROTOCOL

1. The patient remains upright throughout the test.
2. Give 25 to 50 mg captopril (Capoten)[1] after the patient has been upright for 1 hour.
3. Draw blood for measurement of plasma renin, aldosterone, and cortisol at time 0, at 1 hour, and at 2 hours.

INTERPRETATION OF RESULTS

Normally, captopril suppresses PAC by more than 30% from baseline. PA is confirmed if there is no suppression of PAC. The false-negative rate for this test is high, because suppression occurs in more than

---

[1]Not FDA approved for this indication.

[1]Not FDA approved for this indication.

CURRENT DIAGNOSIS

- Screen patients with the following criteria: Joint National Commission (JNC) 7 stage 2 or 3 hypertension, young age, hypertension and spontaneous or diuretic-induced hypokalemia, significant family history for hypertension or primary aldosteronism (PA), or adrenal incidentaloma and hypertension.
- Measure a morning plasma aldosterone concentration (PAC, in ng/dL) and plasma renin activity (PRA, in ng/mL/hour) with the patient in a sodium- and potassium-repleted state and off spironolactone (Aldactone), eplerenone (Inspra), amiloride (Midamor), triamterene (Dyrenium), potassium-losing diuretics, and licorice-derived products[7] for at least 4 to 6 weeks.
- A positive screening test result is a PAC/PRA ratio equal to or greater than 20 to 40 with a PRA <1 ng/mL/hr and a PAC equal to or greater than 15 ng/dL.
- Perform a confirmatory test for PA with a saline suppression, oral salt loading, fludrocortisone (Florinef)[1] suppression, or captopril (Capoten)[1] challenge test.
- If the confirmatory test is positive, proceed to computed tomography (CT) of the adrenal glands to subtype the PA, which most often is caused by an aldosterone-producing adrenal adenoma or bilateral adrenal hyperplasia, and to exclude adrenal cortical carcinoma.
- Perform adrenal vein sampling on all patients with biochemically confirmed PA unless the patient is younger than 40 years of age and has a CT-confirmed adrenal nodule larger than 1 to 2 cm and a normal contralateral adrenal on imaging.

---

[1]Not FDA approved for this indication.
[7]Available as dietary supplement.

30% of PA patients. A slight decrease in aldosterone can suggest bilateral adrenal hyperplasia or idiopathic hyperaldosteronism (a subtype of PA). Overall, this is a poor confirmatory test because of the high proportion of false-negative or equivocal results.

Summary of Confirmatory Tests

In summary, there is insufficient evidence-based data to support one PA confirmatory test over another. Therefore, factors such as cost, accessibility, feasibility, patient compliance, local expertise, and accuracy of assay testing at the institution should play a role in determining which test is best.

DETERMINING THE CAUSE OF PRIMARY ALDOSTERONISM

The two most common causes of PA are BAH, also known as idiopathic hyperaldosteronism, and aldosterone-producing adenomas (APAs). These entities cannot be differentiated biochemically or clinically. The next step in the workup of biochemically positive PA is adrenal imaging to determine the etiology or subtype of PA.

Imaging Studies

Computed Tomography and Magnetic Resonance Imaging

Radiologic studies are critical to differentiate unilateral from bilateral adrenal nodules or APA from BAH. The next test after a positive confirmatory test for PA is computed tomography (CT). In most institutions, CT is the test of choice for reasons of cost and availability,

compared to magnetic resonance imaging (MRI). CT can confirm an adrenal adenoma and can place BAH as a diagnosis of exclusion, but there is significant variation in sensitivity with both imaging modalities. The sensitivity of adrenal CT is only 53% to 73%, whereas MRI has a sensitivity of 70% to 100%. The lack of sensitivity in CT is a result of the 5-mm cuts, which often miss very small adenomas. Up to 20% of adenomas in series of 143 cases were smaller than 1 cm. Specificity is limited because of a high prevalence of adrenal incidentalomas, the possibility of a dominant nodule in macronodular BAH, and increasing adrenal nodularity with age and hypertension.

The results of a CT or MRI scan of the adrenals can lead to one of five conclusions: normal adrenals, unilateral macroadenoma (>1 cm), minimal unilateral adrenal limb thickening, unilateral microadenoma (≤1 cm), and bilateral macroadenomas and/or microadenomas. Adenomas are typically smaller than 2 cm, and BAH exhibits either normal or nodular adrenals on CT. However, adrenal hyperplasia could be misread as microadenomas, which could lead to an unnecessary surgery. Also, nonfunctioning unilateral adrenal adenomas are radiologically indistinguishable from APA on CT. Although imaging criteria exist for an adrenal adenoma, no study has conclusively established specific criteria that differentiate a nonfunctioning from a hyperfunctioning adenoma.

One study using CT or MRI suggested measurement of mean adrenal limb width as a differentiating criterion for BAH. Mean adrenal limb width was found to be larger in BAH compared with APA and normal adrenals. Lingam and colleagues recently proposed that a measured mean adrenal limb width of 5 mm or greater confirms BAH regardless of whether a nodule was seen on imaging. If the CT or MRI showed a nodule and the mean adrenal limb width is 3 mm or less, APA is confirmed. If the mean adrenal width is between 3 and 5 mm, then adrenal vein sampling (AVS) should be done, regardless of the presence of a nodule on imaging. In Lingam's study, this algorithm had a 100% specificity and 100% sensitivity for BAH. However, it was a small study, most patients still required AVS, and the results need confirmation by larger studies.

NP-59 Adrenal Scintigraphy

The NP-59 (iodocholesterol) nuclear medicine scan assesses adrenal hyperfunction, but its use should only be supplementary to CT, MRI, and AVS in difficult cases, to differentiate functioning from nonfunctioning adenomas, or if there are bilateral nodules on CT. After stopping all pertinent medications and 7 days before the scan, dexamethasone (Decadron) suppression (1 mg every 6 hours) is given to enhance sensitivity. Adrenal imaging begins on day 4 and can continue to day 10, until the NP-59 is taken up by the adrenal glands. Early (<5 days) unilateral uptake is consistent with APA. Symmetrical early uptake (<5 days) suggests BAH, whereas symmetrical late uptake (>5 days) suggests normal adrenal glands. A negative adrenal scintigraphy scan does not rule out BAH or APA. Sensitivity of the test for functional adenomas varies widely, and smaller adenomas (<1.5 cm) can be missed by NP-59, because its uptake correlates with adrenal volume.

Summary of Imaging

A multimodality approach can be used to diagnose the cause of PA; however, to date no specific imaging algorithm has established proven superiority.

Adrenal Vein Sampling

AVS is the gold standard for diagnosing the cause of PA and is often essential, given the limited sensitivity and specificity of imaging. In more recent years, its popularity and usefulness have dramatically increased due to greater operator skill. It should be performed only by physicians experienced with AVS. Complications of AVS include adrenal hemorrhage, adrenal infarction, adrenal vein perforation, and adrenal vein thrombosis, which all occur only rarely in the hands of a skilled physician.

Indications for Adrenal Vein Sampling

It is important to include patients who would otherwise have unnecessary adrenalectomies without AVS, as well as those who otherwise would be excluded from surgery if CT or the biochemical work-up pointed toward BAH. Debate still exists as to whether bilateral AVS should be performed on all patients. The only situation in which a PA patient can go directly to adrenalectomy without AVS is if the patient meets all of the following criteria: solitary, unilateral, small, hypodense macroadenoma (>1 cm); normal contralateral adrenal on CT; and age less than 40 years.

AVS should be performed only after biochemical confirmation of inappropriate aldosterone excess. There are several indications for AVS, including CT/MRI scan showing normal adrenals, unilateral nodules smaller than 1 cm, bilateral macronodules, minimal unilateral adrenal limb thickening on CT/MRI, and age older than 40 years (because older patients have a higher incidence of nonfunctioning adrenal adenomas).

Performing the Adrenal Vein Sampling Test

RECOMMENDED PROTOCOL

1. After both adrenal veins have been cannulated, draw baseline samples for PAC, adrenocorticotropic hormone (ACTH), cortisol, and PRA from the inferior vena cava (IVC), right adrenal vein, and left adrenal vein.
2. Inject 250 µg ACTH (cosyntropin, Cortrosyn) after cannulation, or infuse 50 µg cosyntropin per hour beginning 30 minutes before adrenal vein cannulation. This reduces stress-related fluctuations in aldosterone and cortisol values and augments the biochemical gradients. This step is optional but is recommended.
3. Draw blood for aldosterone and cortisol levels at 5, 15, and 30 minutes from the peripheral site and each adrenal vein.

INTERPRETATION OF RESULTS

The use of cosyntropin stimulation is still controversial, and some believe that it has no effect on AVS accuracy. If cosyntropin stimulation is performed, a ratio of aldosterone to stimulated cortisol is used to confirm proper cannulation and stimulation. If cosyntropin is not used, then AVS should be done in the morning, after overnight recumbency, to avoid postural changes in the aldosterone level and to obtain benefit from circadian aldosterone secretion.

Interpreting the Results of Adrenal Vein Sampling

First, determine whether the procedure was done correctly. If cosyntropin was given, the adrenal vein-to-IVC cortisol ratio should be greater than 10:1. Without cosyntropin, the adrenal vein-to-IVC cortisol ratio should be greater than 3:1. If the ratios are significantly less than these, improper cannulation is implied. Next, divide the PAC values for the right and left adrenal veins by their respective cortisol values; this is termed the cortisol-corrected aldosterone (A/C) ratio.

RESULTS THAT CONFIRM UNILATERAL ALDOSTERONE EXCESS

If the cosyntropin-stimulated A/C ratio in the vein of the affected side is at least fourfold higher than the ratio for the contralateral gland, or if the contralateral gland has a suppressed ratio, unilateral excess or APA is confirmed. The mean A/C ratio for APA is 18:1.

If cosyntropin stimulation was not done, unilateral aldosterone excess is confirmed if the A/C ratio on one side is 2.5-fold higher than in the periphery and the contralateral side is not higher than the periphery, indicating suppression of the contralateral side (Table 1).

RESULTS THAT CONFIRM BILATERAL ALDOSTERONE EXCESS

BAH is confirmed if the A/C ratio in each adrenal vein is greater than the A/C ratio in the IVC. If cosyntropin stimulation was used, an A/C ratio of less than 3:1 (i.e., the higher adrenal gland value is less than 3 times that of the lower adrenal gland) is suggestive of BAH. The mean comparison from the high to the low side is 1.8:1. If the comparison ratio is between 3:1 and 4:1, then it is unclear whether aldosterone excess production is bilateral or unilateral.

Without cosyntropin stimulation, a comparison of A/C ratios from the high side to the low side of less than 2:1 confirms BAH (see Table 1).

INTERPRETATION OF RESULTS WITH ONE ADRENAL VEIN CATHETERIZED

AVS results can still be interpreted if only one adrenal vein was catheterized. If the A/C ratio of the catheterized adrenal vein divided by the IVC A/C ratio is less than 1 or suppressed, an APA or primary adrenal hyperplasia on the contralateral side (noncatheterized side)

TABLE 1 Interpretation of Dynamic Testing

Test	Findings
Screening Test	
PAC/PRA ratio	Positive if >20–30 with PAC >15 ng/dL and PRA <1 ng/mL/h
Confirmatory Test for PA	
Oral sodium loading test	Positive if 24-h urine aldosterone excretion is >12–14 µg
Saline infusion test	Positive if PAC after infusion is >10 ng/dL
Fludrocortisone (Florinef)[1] suppression test	Positive if upright PAC is >7 ng/dL on day 4 at 10 AM
Captopril (Capoten)[1] challenge test	Positive if PAC does not decrease by 30% and PRA remains suppressed
Adrenal Vein Sampling	
After cosyntropin (Cortrosyn) stimulation	A/C ratio from high to low side >4:1: unilateral aldosterone excess
	A/C ratio 3:1 to 4:1: overlap zone
	A/C ratio <3:1: bilateral aldosterone excess
Without cosyntropin stimulation	A/C ratio in one adrenal vein is 2.5 times higher than in the peripheral vein (and in the contralateral adrenal vein is less than in the periphery): unilateral aldosterone excess
	A/C ratio from high to low side is <2:1: bilateral aldosterone excess
Diagnostic Tests if AVS Is Equivocal	
Recumbent 18-hydroxycorticosterone	A level >100 ng/dL is consistent with APA
Postural stimulation test	PAC falls or fails to rise by 30%: consistent with APA
	PAC increases by at least 33%: consistent with BAH
NP-59 iodocholesterol scintigraphy	Unilateral early uptake (<5 d): consistent with unilateral excess
	Bilateral early uptake (<5 d): consistent with bilateral aldosterone excess
	Negative scan does not rule out either etiology

[1]Not FDA approved for this indication.
Abbreviations: A/C ratio = cortisol-corrected aldosterone ratio; APA = aldosterone-producing adenomas; BAH = bilateral adrenal hyperplasia; PA = primary aldosteronism; PAC = plasma aldosterone concentration; PRA = plasma renin activity.

is confirmed. If the result is greater than 1, an adenoma or hyperplasia on the ipsilateral side or on both sides is confirmed. In the setting of only one catheterized vein, AVS results are not 100% accurate and should be placed in the context of the prior findings from the biochemical and imaging work-up.

FOLLOW-UP OF INCONCLUSIVE RESULTS

If the AVS results are inconclusive, there are three options: repeat AVS, treat medically, or obtain another diagnostic test, such as the postural stimulation test or a plasma 18-hydroxycorticosterone level.

Postural Stimulation Test. The postural stimulation test is a supplementary test for diagnosing the cause of PA. Aldosterone levels in APA have a preserved diurnal variation because APAs are ACTH responsive, but APA is not affected by angiotensin II. In contrast, BAH has increased sensitivity to angiotensin II that occurs with standing, causing a rise in the aldosterone level.

The protocol for the postural stimulation test is as follows:

1. With the patient supine, draw blood for measurement of 8 AM cortisol, renin, and aldosterone.
2. Ambulate the patient for 4 hours.
3. After 4 hours, with the patient upright, draw blood for measurement of upright plasma cortisol, renin, and aldosterone.

APA is diagnosed if the aldosterone level falls or fails to rise by 30% after 4 hours of ambulation. An aldosterone level that increases with standing (usually by 33%) is consistent with BAH.

The postural stimulation test has some important shortcomings. This test is valid only if the cortisol decreases between 8 AM and 12 PM, and its sensitivity is only 65% to 85% for APA. Moreover, some APAs are also angiotensin II sensitive, and some cases of BAH exhibit diurnal variation in aldosterone.

Plasma 18-Hydroxycorticosterone Level. Measured plasma 18-hydroxycorticosterone level can be a useful blood test if the results of prior testing are equivocal. 18-Hydroxycorticosterone is an immediate precursor of aldosterone or an end product formed after 18-hydroxylation of corticosterone.

A recumbent plasma 18-hydroxycorticosterone level greater than 100 ng/dL at 8 AM is consistent with APA. A level lower than 100 ng/dL is consistent with BAH. Again, the accuracy is less than 80%.

CHARACTERISTICS OF APA VERSUS BAH

Besides testing there are a few characteristic features of each disease that can be helpful towards establishing the cause of PA.

Patients with APA tend to be younger (<40 years), are predominantly female, are very hypertensive with marked hypokalemia (<3 mmol/L), have a very high PAC (>25 mg/dL), and have no change in the PAC after 4 hours of standing. Pathologically, APAs are distinct. They are typically yellowish, round, and smaller than 2 cm. It is important to pursue high specificity for diagnosing APA, to minimize false positive findings and subsequent unnecessary surgery. Unilateral primary adrenal hyperplasia is biochemically like unilateral adenoma but histologically like nodular hyperplasia. Both APA and primary adrenal hyperplasia are treated surgically.

In BAH, patients are older (>40 years), are moderately hypertensive with mild hypokalemia and modest elevations of aldosterone (<25 mg/dL), and their aldosterone level increases after 4 hours of standing. In BAH, the saline infusion test is more likely to be indeterminate. The adrenal glands are grossly enlarged and can be smooth, micronodular, or macronodular. Given this variability, some experts suggest that there is a spectrum to PA, with a solitary adrenal nodule at one end and BAH at the other end. In most cases, diagnosis is not straightforward and requires a combination of tests and imaging to confirm the source of PA.

TREATMENT OF PRIMARY ALDOSTERONISM

Treatment of PA is more straightforward than establishing its diagnosis. APA and unilateral adrenal hyperplasia are managed surgically with an adrenalectomy of the respective side, and BAH is managed medically with mineralocorticoid receptor antagonists (MRAs).

 CURRENT THERAPY

- If the adrenal vein sampling (AVS) result lateralizes, with a cortisol-corrected aldosterone ratio (A/C ratio) from the high to the low side greater than 4:1, perform a laparoscopic adrenalectomy.
- If there is no lateralization on AVS, treat medically with a mineralocorticoid receptor antagonist, spironolactone (Aldactone), or eplerenone (Inspra).[1]
- Spironolactone: 12.5 to 25 mg/day titrated to a maximum dose of 400 mg/day to achieve normokalemia. Side effects are increased serum creatinine, gynecomastia, menstrual irregularities, erectile dysfunction, and hyperkalemia.
- Eplerenone: 25 mg once or twice daily titrated to a maximum dose of 100 mg/day to achieve normokalemia. Side effects are increased creatinine, hyperkalemia, hypertriglyceridemia, increased liver enzymes, headache, and fatigue.
- Other useful antihypertensive agents include thiazide diuretics, triamterene (Dyrenium),[1] and amiloride (Midamor).[1] The Ca^{+2} channel blockers, angiotensin-converting enzyme inhibitors, and angiotensin receptor blockers have not been as effective in lowering aldosterone levels but are an option for blood pressure control.

[1]Not FDA approved for this indication.

Aldosterone-Producing Adenomas and Unilateral Adrenal Hyperplasia

Adrenalectomy, usually laparoscopic, is the only successful treatment for APA and unilateral adrenal hyperplasia, but surgery alone is often not totally curative. After adrenalectomy, blood pressure improves in all patients, but 30% to 60% of patients have persistent hypertension.

MRAs, mainly spironolactone and eplerenone,[1] can be used to control blood pressure in patients awaiting adrenalectomy. Preoperatively, the patient should be normokalemic, and MRAs should be discontinued. Postoperatively, all MRAs, potassium supplements, and intravenous fluids should be discontinued. Also postoperatively, the serum potassium level should be kept at 3 mmol/L or higher and monitored weekly for 4 weeks. The patient is kept on a generous sodium diet to avoid hyperkalemia of hypoaldosteronism due to chronic suppression of the axis.

To confirm a biochemical cure, the PAC and PRA are checked every 3 to 5 days after surgery. If the surgery is successful and the patient indeed had an APA and not some element of BAH, the hypertension should resolve in 1 to 3 months. Risk factors for persistent hypertension after adrenalectomy include older age, duration of hypertension (>5 years), use of two or more antihypertensive agents preoperatively, blood pressure higher than 165/100 mm Hg, low PAC/PRA ratio preoperatively, low urine aldosterone, poor response to spironolactone preoperatively, family history of more than one first-degree relative with hypertension, and a raised serum creatinine concentration.

A few cases of successful CT-guided ablation and transarterial embolization of a presumed aldosteronoma have been reported. Side effects can be serious and include transient increase in blood pressure, fever, flank pain, pneumothorax, adrenal hematoma, and adrenal infarction. Also, in both procedures, the ablated lesion cannot be confirmed histologically.

Bilateral Adrenal Hyperplasia

Antihypertensive medications are the only treatment modality for BAH. However, there have been no randomized, double-blinded, placebo-controlled trials to evaluate the efficacy of drugs in the treatment of PA. The mainstay of treatment is MRAs.

[1]Not FDA approved for this indication.

Spironolactone is the most widely used MRA. It is very effective in decreasing blood pressure in PA. The medication is dosed initially at 12.5 to 25 mg daily and can be titrated to 400 mg/day, with most patients needing at least 200 mg daily. The patients should attain normokalemia without use of potassium supplements. Use of spironolactone is limited by side effects. In men, its antiandrogenic effects can cause gynecomastia, decreased libido and energy, galactorrhea, and hyperkalemia. In women, its progesterone effect can cause menstrual irregularities and hyperkalemia. Spironolactone increases the half-life of digoxin and should be taken separately from salicylates, because the latter decrease the effectiveness of spironolactone.

Eplerenone[1] is a steroid-based antimineralocorticoid that is competitive and selective for the aldosterone receptor; it was approved by the FDA in 2003 for children and adults. It has lower binding affinity to androgen and progesterone receptors than spironolactone. This leads to less antiandrogenic and progestational side effects. However, there are no trials comparing eplerenone with spironolactone. Dosing is started at 25 mg twice daily, with a maximum dose of 100 mg/day. Blood pressure, potassium, and creatinine are monitored. Possible side effects include dizziness, headache, fatigue, diarrhea, hypertriglyceridemia, and elevated liver enzymes. All MRAs are contraindicated in patients with hyperkalemia, a creatinine concentration greater than 2.0 mg/dL in men or 1.8 mg/dL in women, diabetes with microalbuminuria, or concomitant administration of strong cytochrome P-450 isoenzyme 3A4 inhibitors such as ketoconazole (Nizoral) or itraconazole (Sporanox).

Other useful antihypertensive agents are amiloride,[1] which is dosed at 10 to 20 mg PO daily in divided doses to normalize potassium. Side effects are dizziness, fatigue, and impotence. Triamterene (Dyrenium)[1] is dosed at 200 to 300 mg PO daily in divided doses, and its side effects are mainly dizziness and nausea. Patients with BAH may have hypervolemia, and addition of a thiazide diuretic (12.5–50 mg daily) is helpful. If blood pressure remains uncontrolled, other antihypertensive agents may be used. Potassium levels should be maintained at the upper limits of normal, with supplementation used only if MRAs are unable to maintain normokalemia. Potassium levels are monitored frequently the first 4 to 6 weeks after initiation of treatment, especially in renal and diabetic patients.

Nonpharmacologic treatment for both subtypes of PA includes aerobic exercise, smoking cessation, weight loss, and a low-sodium diet (<100 mEq/day).

Diagnosis and Treatment of Less Common Causes of Primary Aldosteronism

Glucocorticoid remedial aldosteronism (GRA) is a rare disease caused by a mutation of the aldosterone synthase gene. In GRA, aldosterone is ectopically produced in the zona fasciculata and regulated by ACTH (as opposed to normal production in the zona glomerulosa and regulation by angiotensin II). Clinically, most patients present with childhood hypertension, and 50% are normokalemic; the morning cortisol level is elevated, but patients are not cushingoid. Biochemically, elevated serum 18-hydroxycortisol and 18-oxocortisol concentrations are diagnostic for GRA. Genetic testing for GRA is recommended for PA patients who are younger than 20 years of age or have a family history of PA or stroke at a young age. Treatment for GRA is physiologic cortisol replacement in children, usually as a long-acting glucocorticoid given at bedtime to suppress morning ACTH, and MRAs can be given in place of steroids to avoid disruption of growth. The target blood pressure is age specific in children.

Familial hyperaldosteronism II is another rare cause of PA. It is an autosomal dominant, possibly genetically heterogeneous, disease. The aldosterone level does not suppress with dexamethasone, and the GRA mutation is absent. Patients with familial hyperaldosteronism II are clinically indistinguishable from those with APA or BAH.

---

[1]Not FDA approved for this indication.

REFERENCES

Auchus RJ, Chandler DW, Singeetham S, et al. Measurement of 18 hydroxysterone during adrenal vein sampling for primary aldosteronism. J Clin Endocrinol Metab 2007;92:2648–51.

Funder JW, Carey RM, Fardella C, et al. Case detection, diagnosis, and treatment of patients with primary aldosteronism: An Endocrine Society clinical practice guideline. J Clin Endocrinol Metab 2008;93:3266–81.

Ganguly A. Primary aldosteronism. N Engl J Med 1998;339:1828–34.

Lau JH, Drake W, Matson M. The current role of venous sampling in the localization of endocrine disease. Cardiovasc Intervent Radiol 2007;30:555–70.

Mulatero P, Bertello C, Rossato D, et al. Roles of clinical criteria, computed tomography scan, and adrenal vein sampling in differential diagnosis of primary aldosteronism subtypes. J Clin Endocrinol Metab 2008;93:1366–71.

Mulatero P, Milan A, Fallo F, et al. Comparison of confirmatory tests for the diagnosis of primary aldosteronism. J Clin Endocrinol Metab 2006;91:2618–23.

Patel SM, Lingam RK, Beaconsfield TI, et al. Role of radiology in the management of primary aldosteronism. Radiographics 2007;27:1145–57.

Schirpenbach C, Reinke M. Primary aldosteronism: Current knowledge and controversies in Conn's syndrome. Nat Clin Pract Endocrinol Metab 2007;3:220–7.

Tiu SS, Choi CH, Shek CC, et al. The use of aldosterone-renin ratio as a diagnostic test for primary hyperaldosteronism and its test characteristics under different conditions in blood sampling. J Clin Endocrinol Metab 2005;90:72–8.

Young WF. Primary aldosteronism: Renaissance of a syndrome. Clin Endocrinol 2007;66:607–18.

Hypopituitarism

Method of
Mary Lee Vance, MD

Definition

Hypopituitarism is target endocrine gland failure resulting from insufficient hypothalamic or pituitary hormone stimulation of the target gland or tissue. Loss of hypothalamic or pituitary hormone production can cause secondary adrenal insufficiency, secondary hypothyroidism, secondary gonadal failure, growth hormone (GH) deficiency, and diabetes insipidus, alone or in combination. Regardless of the etiology, replacement of glucocorticoid and thyroid hormone is necessary to sustain life; replacement of gonadal steroids, GH, and antidiuretic hormone is necessary for normal function and to prevent morbidity. Loss of all pituitary function is termed *panhypopituitarism;* loss of one or more pituitary hormones is termed *partial hypopituitarism.*

Etiology

The most common causes of hypopituitarism are pituitary lesion or infiltrative disease (Box 1). Pituitary lesions include pituitary adenoma (Fig. 1), craniopharyngioma, and Rathke's cleft cyst; infiltrative diseases include lymphocytic hypophysitis, sarcoidosis, and metastatic tumor. In general, the larger the pituitary lesion, the greater the likelihood of loss of pituitary function. Infiltrative disease often causes permanent loss of pituitary function. Selective removal of a pituitary adenoma, taking care to avoid damage to remaining normal pituitary tissue, can result in recovery of pituitary function.

Hypopituitarism also occurs as a result of any type of pituitary radiation for a pituitary lesion, total brain radiation for a brain lesion, or head and neck radiation for carcinoma because the radiation field often involves the pituitary gland. Head trauma can cause

BOX 1 Causes of Hypopituitarism

Hypothalamic Disease

Histiocytosis
Eosinophilic granuloma
Sarcoidosis
Hypothalamic tumor
- Gangliocytoma
- Hamartoma
- Optic nerve glioma
- Third-ventricle tumor
Metastatic tumor
Congenital midline defects

Pituitary Disease

Pituitary adenoma
Craniopharyngioma
Rathke's cleft cyst
Pilocytic astrocytoma
Infiltrative disease
- Giant cell granuloma
- Sarcoidosis
- Lymphocytic hypophysitis
- Lymphoma
- Plasmacytoma
- Metastatic tumor
Chordoma with pituitary involvement
Parasellar ro suprasellar meningioma
Pituitary apoplexy
- Hemorrhage into pituitary adenoma
- Postpartum hemorrhage
Congenital pituitary hypoplasia

Radiation

Cranial
Pituitary
Head and neck

Infection

Tuberculosis
Mycoses

Miscellaneous

Head trauma
Empty sella
Carotid-cavernous aneurysm
Iatrogenic adrenal insufficiency

CURRENT DIAGNOSIS

- Diagnosis is biochemical in association with clinical features.
- Diagnosis can require a stimulation test to determine the need for replacement of glucocorticoid, growth hormone, or both.
- Initial evaluation should include measurement of concentrations of early-morning serum cortisol, adrenocorticotropic hormone, free thyroxine T_4, gonadotropins (luteinizing hormone, follicle-stimulating hormone, insulin-like growth factor-1, and testosterone (in men).
- Menstrual history should be obtained from premenopausal women.

loss of pituitary function. Less commonly, developmental defects of the hypothalamus or pituitary cause loss of pituitary function. A common cause of secondary adrenal insufficiency is not pituitary disease but exogenous administration of steroid medications for conditions such as asthma, rheumatologic disorders, and chronic pain syndrome resulting in iatrogenic secondary adrenal insufficiency. Patients who receive intra-articular injections for joint pain might not be aware that the medication administered is a steroid with depot release characteristics and long-lasting systemic effects. Iatrogenic secondary adrenal insufficiency is caused by exogenous steroid treatment that suppresses hypothalamic-pituitary stimulation of the adrenal glands.

Diagnosis

The diagnosis of pituitary deficiency is often straightforward but sometimes requires a definitive stimulation test to assess hypothalamic-pituitary-adrenal function and GH reserve. In a patient who presents with a large pituitary lesion such as a macroprolactinoma, the most critical determination is whether there is a need for glucocorticoid and thyroid hormone replacement before recommending surgical resection or medical treatment. A subnormal morning serum cortisol or subnormal free thyroxine (T_4) concentration indicates the need for immediate replacement. In a patient who has undergone pituitary surgery, it is important to review the operative note to assess the amount of resection and to make an estimate of remaining pituitary gland. Unfortunately, this estimate is not always mentioned in the operative report.

A history of frequent nocturia, polyuria, and excessive thirst indicates diabetes insipidus. Diabetes insipidus most commonly occurs in patients with a craniopharyngioma, Rathke's cleft cyst, or infiltrative disease such as lymphocytic hypophysitis or sarcoidosis. Extensive surgical resection in a patient with one of these lesions can damage the pituitary stalk, resulting in a high probability of permanent diabetes insipidus. The diagnosis of diabetes insipidus is made clinically in a patient with a pituitary lesion and does not usually require a formal water deprivation test. Serum sodium concentration is usually normal in diabetes insipidus patients who have normal thirst sensation. Serum osmolality usually is normal and urine osmolality usually is low. A subnormal morning serum cortisol or free T_4 level concentration requires prompt glucocorticoid or thyroxine (Synthroid) replacement.

A patient who has a large pituitary lesion commonly has loss of some or all anterior pituitary hormone production. This loss is less common in a patient with a small pituitary lesion but still requires evaluation and replacement as indicated. Pituitary function might recover after surgical removal of the lesion, but it is not common; approximately 6% of patients have recovery of some pituitary function after surgery. Postoperative or postradiation assessment should include clinical history (menses in premenopausal women, sexual function in men, symptoms of hypothyroidism, adrenal insufficiency, diabetes insipidus) and basal and dynamic endocrine testing. In general, a stimulation test to assess for hypothalamic-pituitary-adrenal function to determine the need for cortisol replacement and for GH deficiency should be conducted after surgical removal of the lesion.

A subnormal morning serum cortisol concentration (without administration of steroid for 2 to 3 days) is usually adequate to diagnose secondary adrenal insufficiency. The serum adrenocorticotropic hormone (ACTH) concentration may be low or in the normal range. A normal morning serum cortisol concentration does not provide information regarding the ACTH-cortisol response to stress; the definitive study is an insulin hypoglycemia test in which the serum glucose concentration decreases to 40 mg/dL or less and the serum cortisol concentration increases to 18 µg/dL or greater to exclude secondary impaired hypothalamic-pituitary-adrenal reserve. This test is also the most rigorous test of GH reserve to determine the need for GH replacement. A hypoglycemia stimulated serum GH concentration less than 5 ng/mL indicates GH deficiency.

Cortisol stimulation with ACTH (cosyntropin [Cortrosyn]) test may be misleading in patients with recent ACTH deficiency. The cortisol response may be normal but the ACTH response to stress is impaired. For this reason, an ACTH stimulation test should not be

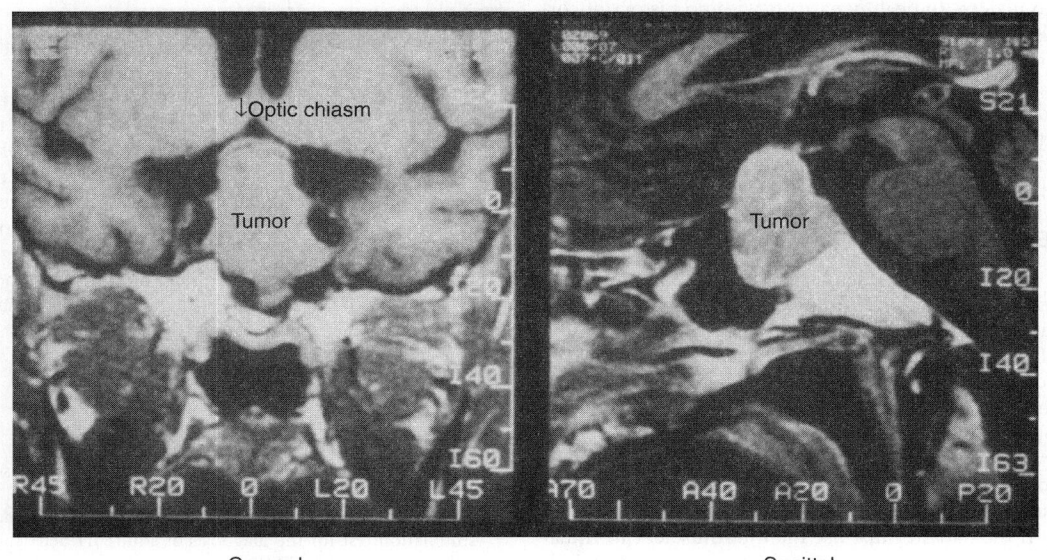

Coronal

Sagittal

FIGURE 1. Magnetic resonance image of a pituitary macroadenoma.

performed in the immediate postoperative period. It is prudent to wait 4 to 6 weeks after surgery before performing this test.

A subnormal serum free T_4 concentration, often in the setting of a "normal" serum thyroid-stimulating hormone (TSH) concentration, indicates the need for thyroid hormone replacement.

SECONDARY GONADAL FAILURE

The diagnosis of secondary gonadal failure is straightforward. Chronic amenorrhea in a premenopausal woman indicates gonadotropin insufficiency. In premenopausal women with secondary gonadotropin insufficiency, serum LH and FSH concentrations are typically either low or "normal" and the estradiol level is usually low or in the follicular phase range.

In men, a low serum testosterone concentration indicates gonadal insufficiency. Low serum testosterone concentration with LH and FSH concentrations within the "normal" range indicate secondary gonadal failure.

GROWTH HORMONE DEFICIENCY

The diagnosis of GH deficiency is more complicated, usually requiring an insulin hypoglycemia stimulation test. In a patient with three or four other pituitary hormone deficiencies, the probability of GH deficiency is 96% and 99%, respectively. Three or four pituitary hormone deficiencies and a serum insulin-like growth factor 1 (IGF-1) concentration less than 84 μg/L reliably predicts GH deficiency in more than 95% of patients. Despite this finding, many third-party payers (insurance companies) require the results of a stimulation test confirming GH deficiency because of the cost and misuse of GH. The most rigorous test for determining GH deficiency is the insulin hypoglycemia test; the next "best" test is the arginine–growth hormone-releasing hormone test. Other tests of GH reserve, such as arginine or clonidine (Catapres),[1] are less reliable.

Treatment

Treatment of hypopituitarism requires replacement of all hormone deficiencies with adjustment of hormone doses based on both hormone levels and clinical response. Optimal hormone replacement is the goal. Optimal hormone replacement often requires a great deal of time and effort; "one dose" is not suitable for all patients.

---

[1]Not FDA approved for this indication.

 CURRENT THERAPY

- All hormone deficiencies require replacement. Optimal replacement often requires dosage adjustments.
- Dosage adjustments for thyroid hormone replacement and growth hormone replacement can be made at 6-week intervals.
- Thyroid hormone dosage adjustment may be necessary in pregnant patients.
- Estrogen supplementation can require growth hormone dosage adjustments.
- Growth hormone replacement is not approved during pregnancy.

Glucocorticoid replacement exemplifies the "art of medicine": No blood test accurately assesses the adequacy or insufficiency of a glucocorticoid replacement dose. In general, a daily dose of hydrocortisone (Cortef) 15 mg on awakening and 5 mg at 6 pm or prednisone 5 mg on awakening and 2.5 mg at 6 pm should be adequate replacement. However, patients who gain weight on this regimen might feel better with a lower dose of hydrocortisone, such as 10 mg on awakening and 5 mg at 6 pm or 5 mg of prednisone on awakening without an evening dose. Rarely, a patient receiving hydrocortisone replacement requires dosing three times daily.

Glucocorticoid replacement with dexamethasone (Decadron) is discouraged because of the long biologic half-life and cumulative effect causing symptoms of Cushing's syndrome and bone loss. Mineralocorticoid therapy (fludrocortisone [Florinef]) is not required in a patient with secondary adrenal insufficiency because mineralocorticoid (aldosterone) secretion is not regulated chronically by pituitary ACTH secretion. Patients should be instructed to double the glucocorticoid dose during intercurrent illness (such as flu, urinary tract infection) and to always wear a medical alert necklace or bracelet.

THYROID HORMONE REPLACEMENT

Thyroid hormone replacement with l-thyroxine should be monitored by measuring free T_4, not TSH. Because the TSH level in patients with hypopituitarism is often low, basing hormone replacement therapy on TSH level could result in an inappropriate reduction of the thyroid hormone dose. In healthy patients with no history of coronary artery disease or angina, a beginning dose of 0.088 or 0.1 mg of l-thyroxine daily is reasonable, with dose adjustment after 1 month of therapy according to the serum free T_4 concentration and clinical response. Thyroid hormone replacement in the elderly or in patients with coronary artery disease should be initiated with a smaller dose (e.g., 0.025 mg/day) and gradually increased to achieve a normal serum free T_4 concentration.

GONADAL STEROID REPLACEMENT

Gonadal steroid replacement in men is most often accomplished physiologically with either a testosterone gel (AndroGel, Testim) or a testosterone patch (Androderm) that delivers a physiologic dose over 24 hours. Intramuscular testosterone, testosterone enanthate (Delatestryl), and testosterone cypionate (Depo-Testosterone) are not physiologic and often result in supraphysiologic levels soon after injection and subphysiologic levels before the next injection. Depending on the interval after injection, intramuscular testosterone can cause mood swings, irritability, and depression. Intramuscular formulations can cause erythrocytosis and elevated hemoglobin and hematocrit levels. If the patient must use the intramuscular formulation, hemoglobin and hematocrit levels should be monitored periodically. A buccal formulation of testosterone (Striant) is available, requires multiple daily doses, and can cause irritation of the gums. Men should undergo a prostate examination and determination of serum prostate-specific antigen concentration yearly. Testosterone replacement does not cause prostate cancer but can promote growth of an undiagnosed carcinoma.

Premenopausal women requiring gonadal hormone replacement should receive cyclic estrogen and progesterone replacement for its beneficial effect on bone physiology and libido and to prevent hot flushes. This can be accomplished with an oral contraceptive or cyclic estradiol and progesterone treatment. Annual gynecologic and breast examinations are necessary.

HORMONE REPLACEMENT FOR DIABETES INSIPIDUS

Hormone replacement for diabetes insipidus with desmopressin acetate (DDAVP) can be administered as an oral formulation or as a nasal spray. Because the duration of biologic activity varies among patients, the beginning dose should be low (0.1-mg tablet at bedtime), and dosing frequency should be changed according to the duration of activity. In some patients, control is achieved with a single bedtime dose, whereas others require dosing two or three times daily. The patient can sense when the effect of desmopressin wears off because of frequent urination and return of increased thirst. Desmopressin is available as a generic formulation, and clinical experience has shown that not all formulations are equally efficacious, sometimes resulting in the need to prescribe higher-than-usual doses to control the polyuria.

GROWTH HORMONE REPLACEMENT

Growth hormone (somatropin [Genotropin, Humatrope, Norditropin, Nutropin]) replacement is indicated in GH-deficient adults. The recommendation is to begin with a small dose (0.3 mg/day by subcutaneous injection) and then titrate the dose every 4 to 6 weeks according to the serum IGF-1 level and symptoms. An optimal serum IGF-1 level is at the middle or a little above the middle of the age-adjusted normal range. Women usually require a higher final dose than do men, and women receiving oral estrogen replacement usually require a higher final dose to achieve an optimal serum IGF-1 level than do women not receiving oral estrogen. Patients should be informed that a beneficial effect on energy, endurance, body composition, and serum lipid levels might not be noted for several months Patients receiving GH replacement should be monitored every 6 months with a serum IGF-1 measurement, to determine the adequacy of the dose, and yearly serum lipid measurements.

Summary and Conclusions

Loss of pituitary function is common in patients with a hypothalamic or pituitary lesion, resulting either from the lesion or the treatment; these patients require regular monitoring and treatment as indicated. Patients who have undergone pituitary or cranial radiation therapy are always at risk for developing a new pituitary deficiency. Knowing if, or when, a new pituitary deficiency will occur is not possible, thus emphasizing the need for regular endocrine assessment. Optimal hormone replacement is similar to the best possible management of a patient with diabetes mellitus: frequent monitoring and adjustment of hormone doses based on hormone measurements and clinical response. The goal is accurate diagnosis and optimal replacement to prevent risk of premature mortality. With hormone replacement, a patient can lead a normal and productive life.

REFERENCES

Cook DM, Ludlam WH, Cook MB. Route of estrogen administration helps to determine growth hormone (GH) replacement dose in GH-deficient adults. J Clin Endocrinol Metab 1999;84:3956–60.

Hartman ML, Crowe BJ, Biller BM, et al. Which patients do not require a GH stimulation test for the diagnosis of adult GH deficiency? J Clin Endocrinol Metab 2002;87:477–85.

Kelly KF, Gonzalo IT, Cohan P, et al. Hypopituitarism following traumatic brain injury and aneurysmal subarachnoid hemorrhage: A preliminary report. J Neurosurg 2000;93:743–52.

Lieberman SA, Oberoi AL, Gilkison CR, et al. Prevalence of neuroendocrine dysfunction in patients recovering from traumatic brain injury. J Clin Endocrinol Metab 2001;86:2752–6.

Vance ML. Hypopituitarism. N Engl J Med 1994;330:1651–62.

Hyperprolactinemia

Method of
Janet A. Schlechte, MD

Epidemiology

Prolactin-secreting adenomas are the most common functioning pituitary tumors and are more common in women. Hyperprolactinemia occurs in about one third of patients with chronic kidney disease and resolves after successful transplantation. About 10% of patients with primary hypothyroidism have a small increase in serum prolactin, and hyperprolactinemia is reported in about 30% of women with polycystic ovarian syndrome. About 5% to 20% of patients with cirrhosis have elevated prolactin levels. Occasionally no cause of hyperprolactinemia can be identified (idiopathic hyperprolactinemia), and these patients might have pituitary adenomas too small to detect on magnetic resonance imaging (MRI).

Risk Factors

Estrogen can increase serum prolactin and hyperprolactinemia is often detected after discontinuation of an oral contraceptive, but case control studies have shown no relation between the use of estrogen and the formation of prolactinomas.

Pathophysiology

The secretion of prolactin from pituitary lactotrophs is regulated by hypothalamic dopamine. Prolactin secretion is episodic and serum levels are usually less than 25 ng/mL in women and less than

20 ng/mL in men. During pregnancy, estrogen induces hyperplasia of pituitary lactotrophs, which leads to a progressive increase in prolactin and a 10-fold elevation at term. In lactating women, prolactin levels remain elevated until about 6 weeks after delivery. The primary action of prolactin is to stimulate mammary tissue, but it is the prolactin-induced suppression of gonadotropins and sex steroids that brings patients to clinical attention.

Clinical Manifestations

In both sexes, hyperprolactinemia is associated with hypogonadism, infertility, and bone loss. In women galactorrhea is also commonly observed. Prolactin-secreting tumors in women are usually small and are rarely associated with pituitary hypofunction. Men with prolactinomas usually have large tumors and present with headaches, neurologic deficits, visual loss, and hypopituitarism in additional to gonadal dysfunction.

Diagnosis

A single measurement of serum prolactin obtained at any time of day is usually adequate to make the diagnosis of hyperprolactinemia. Stress can increase prolactin, and minimally elevated levels should be repeated before the diagnosis of hyperprolactinemia is confirmed. A history and physical examination; assessment of thyroid, liver, and kidney function; and a pregnancy test will exclude most causes of hyperprolactinemia. Provocative tests using thyrotropin-releasing hormone, levodopa (L-dopa), domperidone (Motillium),[5] nomifensine (Merital),[2] and insulin-induced hypoglycemia are not useful or necessary. When other causes of hyperprolactinemia have been excluded, gadolinium-enhanced MRI should be used to visualize the pituitary. In general, serum prolactin levels parallel tumor size. Prolactinomas larger than 1 cm are typically associated with prolactin levels greater than 250 ng/mL, and levels can exceed 1000 ng/mL.

Differential Diagnosis

Medications are the most common cause of hyperprolactinemia other than tumor (Box 1). By blocking dopamine receptors, metoclopramide (Reglan), phenothiazines, and risperidone (Risperdal) lead to prolactin levels greater than 200 ng/mL, but tricyclic antidepressants, verapamil (Calan), and estrogen cause only mild elevation. In general, medication-induced hyperprolactinemia is associated with prolactin levels between 25 and 100 ng/mL. Other causes of hyperprolactinemia include pregnancy, chest trauma, nipple stimulation, and hypothalamic disease.

Treatment

Medication-induced hyperprolactinemia is reversible, and it usually takes 3 to 4 days for prolactin to normalize after drug withdrawal. It is not always possible to discontinue a drug causing elevated

CURRENT DIAGNOSIS

- A history and physical examination; assessment of thyroid, liver, and kidney function; and a pregnancy test will exclude many causes of hyperprolactinemia.
- A single prolactin measurement is usually adequate for diagnosis.
- In patients with prolactinomas, prolactin levels generally parallel tumor size.

---

[2]Not available in the United States.
[5]Investigational drug in the United States.

BOX 1 Causes of Hyperprolactinemia

Prolactinomas
Pregnancy
Medications
- Phenothiazines
- Metoclopramide (Reglan)
- Estrogen
- Verapamil (Calan)
- Butyrophenones
- Risperidone (Risperdal)
- Tricyclic antidepressants
Primary hypothyroidism
Renal failure
Nonfunctioning pituitary tumors
Hypothalamic disease
Nipple stimulation
Idiopathic

CURRENT THERAPY

- Medication-induced hyperprolactinemia is reversible upon discontinuation of the drug.
- A dopamine agonist is the treatment of choice for a prolactinoma.
- Discontinuation of therapy is usually associated with recurrence of hyperprolactinemia.

---

prolactin. For example, in a patient with hyperprolactinemia, an antipsychotic agent should not be changed or discontinued without consulting the patient's psychiatrist. If a medication cannot be safety discontinued in a patient with medication-induced hyperprolactinemia, radiographic evaluation of the pituitary may be necessary to exclude a pituitary tumor.

The goals in treating a prolactinoma are to normalize prolactin, restore gonadal function and fertility, and reduce tumor size. The preferred treatment is a dopamine agonist, and the drugs approved for use in the United States are bromocriptine (Parlodel) and cabergoline (Dostinex). Both bind to pituitary dopamine receptors, thereby decreasing prolactin and reducing tumor size. Prolactin levels normalize within days of drug administration, and tumor shrinkage or disappearance is usually apparent 3 to 6 months after instituting therapy. Bromocriptine is less expensive, has a half-life of 8 hours, and must be given twice daily. Cabergoline has a half-life of about 24 hours and can be administered once or twice weekly. Both drugs are available in generic form.

Bromocriptine should be initiated at bedtime with a dose of 0.625 mg and a snack. After 1 week, twice-daily dosing should be initiated by adding a morning dose of 1.25 mg. At weekly intervals the dosage should be increased to a total of 5 mg daily, and after 6 to 8 weeks of therapy a prolactin level should be repeated. Most patients require 5 mg of bromocriptine daily. The starting dose of cabergoline is 0.25 mg weekly. After 1 week, twice-weekly dosing should be initiated by adding 0.25 mg. At weekly intervals the dose should be increased to a total of 0.5 mg twice weekly. After 6 to 8 weeks of therapy a prolactin level should be repeated. Most patients will require 1 mg of cabergoline *weekly*. Treatment with either drug can restore gonadal function without normalizing prolactin. If this occurs, it is not necessary to increase the dosage just to normalize the prolactin. The lowest dosage possible should always be used.

The major disadvantage of both dopamine agonists is that discontinuation usually leads to tumor regrowth and recurrence of hyperprolactinemia. Recent reports suggest that discontinuing therapy may be feasible in selected patients, but the optimal length of therapy has not been established and there are no precise criteria to predict which patients will benefit from drug withdrawal. I recommend a minimum of 2 years of therapy before considering withdrawal of therapy. Drug withdrawal is more likely to be successful if the prolactin has normalized and no tumor is visible on MRI before the drug is discontinued.

When fertility is the goal, bromocriptine is the treatment of choice. After starting bromocriptine a woman should use mechanical contraception until at least two regular menstrual cycles have occurred, and the drug should be discontinued as soon as pregnancy is confirmed. When administered in this fashion, bromocriptine has not been associated with an increased incidence of congenital malformations. Although cabergoline has *not* been associated with an increased risk of congenital malformations, it is not currently recommended because less information about its safety is available. It is not necessary to measure prolactin levels during pregnancy because rising levels do not reliably correlate with tumor enlargement. The risk of clinically significant tumor growth during pregnancy is less than 2%, so it is not necessary to perform serial MRI scans or visual field examinations during pregnancy in women who have small tumors. In contrast, there is a 15% to 30% risk of tumor enlargement during pregnancy in women with macroadenomas (>1 cm). With large or invasive tumors there is no single therapeutic option, and treatment must be individualized.

Monitoring

Small prolactinomas rarely progressively increase in size, so prevention of tumor growth is not an indication for treatment. It is crucial, however, to treat prolactin-induced gonadal dysfunction. When fertility is not desired, one option is to administer a dopamine agonist. Another option when fertility is not an issue is to use estrogen or testosterone *instead* of a dopamine agonist. Sex steroids are better tolerated and less expensive than either dopamine agonist and effectively treat hypogonadism and protect the skeleton. Short-term use of estrogen in women with prolactinomas has not been associated with tumor growth, but it should be used with caution in women with very large tumors. With either option, prolactin levels should be monitored yearly. Tumor growth is usually preceded by an elevation of serum prolactin, so it is not necessary to perform yearly MRI examinations. An MRI is indicated if clinical symptoms of tumor expansion occur or if the prolactin increases substantially.

Complications

Both dopamine agonists can cause nasal stuffiness, nausea, and orthostatic hypotension, but fewer women taking cabergoline demonstrate drug intolerance. Pleural thickening, retroperitoneal fibrosis, and cardiac valve regurgitation have been noted in patients who have Parkinson's disease and are taking high doses (3 mg daily) of cabergoline.[1] Long-term therapy of hyperprolactinemia with bromocriptine has not been associated with pulmonary complications, and clinically relevant valvular regurgitation has not been seen in patients who have prolactinomas and are taking 1 to 2 mg of cabergoline weekly.

Pituitary surgery may be necessary for occasional patients who cannot tolerate either of the dopamine agonists. When performed by an experienced neurosurgeon, transsphenoidal surgery normalizes prolactin in about 70% of patients with microadenomas and about 30% with macroadenomas, but recurrence of hyperprolactinemia is common.

[1]Not FDA approved for this indication.

REFERENCES

Gillam MP, Molitch ME, Lombardi G, Colao A. Advances in the treatment of prolactinomas. Endocr Rev 2006;27:485–534.
Kilbanski A. Prolactinoma. N Engl J Med 2010;362:1219–26.
Molitch ME. Medication-induced hyperprolactinemia. Mayo Clin Proc 2005; 80:1050–7.
Molitch ME. Prolactinomas and pregnancy. Pituitary 2005;8:31–8.

Hypothyroidism

Method of
William J. Hueston, MD

Epidemiology

Hypothyroidism is second only to diabetes in the prevalence of endocrine disorders in adults in the United States. Hypothyroidism occurs in up to 18/1000 population, with women outnumbering men by approximately 10:1. Rates of hypothyroidism increase dramatically with older age, so that about 2% to 3% of all older women have hypothyroidism, and the prevalence is up to 5% in nursing home populations.

Risk Factors

Thyroid conditions are more common in patients who have a family history of thyroid disorders. In addition, hypothyroidism as well as thyroid cancers are more common in patients who had neck irradiation in childhood. However, most cases of hypothyroidism occur in people who have no risk factors.

Pathophysiology

Several conditions can lead to hypothyroidism (Box 1). Two categories, hypothyroidism following thyroiditis and iatrogenic hypothyroidism secondary to treatment of Graves' disease, account for the overwhelming majority of cases of hypothyroidism in the United States.

The most common non-iatrogenic conditions causing hypothyroidism in the United States is Hashimoto's thyroiditis. Most idiopathic hypothyroidism also represents Hashimoto's thyroiditis that has followed an indolent course. Hashimoto's thyroiditis, also called chronic lymphocytic thyroiditis, is the most common of the inflammatory thyroid disorders and the most common cause of goiter in

---

BOX 1 Conditions Causing Hypothyroidism

Thyroiditis
Hashimoto's thyroiditis
Subacute granulomatous thyroiditis (de Quervain's thyroiditis)
Subacute lymphocytic thyroiditis (silent or painless thyroiditis)

Iatrogenic Hypothyroidism
Radioactive iodine treatment of Graves' disease
Thyroidectomy

Secondary Hypothyroidism (Pituitary Dysfunction)
Pituitary surgery
Intercranial radiation
Congenital panhypopituitarism

Other Causes
Infiltratative diseases (sarcoidosis, amyloidosis, hemochromatosis)
Drugs (lithium, interferon, amiodarone [Cordarone])
Iodine deficiency

the United States. The prevalence of Hashimoto's thyroiditis has been increasing dramatically since the 1960s in the United States, but the cause for this rise is unknown. In patients with acute thyroiditis, either subacute granulomatous (also known as de Quervain's) and subacute lymphocytic (also known as silent or painless), transient hypothyroidism is common following an acute attack, and 10% of these patients also develop long-term hypothyroidism.

Another common cause of hypothyroidism is a medical intervention to treat Graves' disease or thyroidectomy for chronic fibrocytic thyroiditis (Riedel's struma). Radioactive iodine ablation of the thyroid for Graves' disease often results in underproduction of thyroxine in the remaining tissue, necessitating thyroid replacement.

A third uncommon cause of hypothyroidism that should not be overlooked is secondary hypothyroidism due to hypothalamic or pituitary dysfunction. These conditions are seen primarily in patients who have received intracranial irradiation or surgical removal of a pituitary adenoma.

Finally, a variety of other conditions including infiltration of the thyroid (amyloidosis, sarcoidosis), iodine deficiency, or medications (such as amiodarone [Cordarone] or interferon) can cause hypothyroidism.

Prevention

There are no known interventions to prevent hypothyroidism. According to their 2004 analysis, the U.S. Preventive Services Task Force found insufficient evidence to support early detection through routine screening of asymptomatic persons.

Clinical Manifestations

Individual who have hypothyroidism can present with a variety of symptoms, many of which are not specific. Consequently, clinicians must have a high index of suspicion for hypothyroidism when patients come in with any one or combination of the symptoms that could signal hypothyroidism.

Symptoms of hypothyroidism include lethargy, weight gain, hair loss, dry skin, constipation, poor concentration, trouble thinking or forgetfulness, and depression (Box 2). In older patients, hypothyroidism easily can be confused with Alzheimer's disease or other conditions that cause dementia. Patients who present with depression also should have their thyroid function assessed.

The thyroid examination in most patients with hypothyroidism is completely normal. Patients might have a painless goiter; tenderness in the thyroid is generally a sign of active inflammation consistent

---

CURRENT DIAGNOSIS

- Hypothyroidism is more common in women as they age.
- The signs and symptoms of hypothyroidism are non-specific and can mimic other diseases found in the elderly, so clinicians need to have a high index of suspicion.
- The key diagnostic test is to find a low free T_4. The presence of an elevated TSH indicates primary hypothyroidism, and a low TSH indicates secondary hypothyroidism.
- There is insufficient evidence for screening for hypothyroidism in asymptomatic adults.

---

with acute thyroiditis. Once the thyroid inflammation has subsided, thyroid function might return to normal. Other physical findings that can occur with hypothyroidism include low blood pressure, bradycardia, nonpitting edema, generalized hair loss especially along the outer third of the eyebrows, dry skin, and a lag in the relaxation phase of reflexes that can be assessed most easily in the ankle jerk reflexes.

Diagnosis

The diagnosis of hypothyroidism is based on finding a low free thyroxine (T_4) level, usually with an elevation in the thyroid stimulating hormone (TSH) levels. For patients with hypothyroidism due to pituitary dysfunction, also called secondary hypothyroidism, both the free T_4 and the TSH levels are low.

One situation where clinicians need to be wary is evaluating thyroid status in patients who are severely ill. During times of acute physiologic stress, patients may have mildly elevated TSH levels that suggest hypothyroidism but are, in fact, euthyroid. This condition, called euthyroid sick syndrome, does not require treatment with thyroid replacement and resolves within a few weeks after recovery, but it may be difficult to distinguish from preexisting or new-onset hypothyroidism. Clinicians need to use other clinical symptoms to try to differentiate euthyroid sick syndrome from hypothyroidism. Even though it does not require treatment, the presence of euthyroid sick syndrome in a critically ill patient is a poor prognostic sign.

In contrast to hyperthyroidism, there is no role for thyroid scans or iodine uptake testing in patients with hypothyroidism. The only exception to this is when the clinician identifies a mass on physical examination. In that situation, scanning or other imaging is essential to determine the malignancy potential of the mass.

Differential Diagnosis

The differential diagnosis for hypothyroidism is broad and depends on the primary complaints given by patients. For patients with slowed mentation, depressed affect, or confusion, clinicians should suspect depression. Patients with lethargy and a slow pulse and low blood pressure might have adrenal insufficiency. Patients with constipation need to have colonic obstruction from a mass considered as well. In the elderly, common drugs that can cause depression (such as centrally acting antihypertensive agents), bradycardia (such as β-blockers or calcium channel blockers), constipation (calcium channel blockers), hair loss, or confusion also should be considered.

In patients with pituitary failure, other pituitary hormones are likely to be deficient as well, so clinicians should look for evidence of adrenal and gonadotropic failure.

BOX 2   **Symptoms and Signs of Hypothyroidism**
Common Symptoms
Lethargy
Weight gain
Constipation
Slowed mentation, forgetfulness
Depression
Hair loss
Dry skin
Neck enlargement or goiter
Physical Examination Findings
Goiter
Low blood pressure and slow pulse
Hair thinning or loss
Dry skin
Confusion
Depressed affect
Non-pitting edema

Treatment

The treatment for hypothyroidism is thyroxine replacement (Synthroid, Levoxyl). The usual dose required to achieve full replacement is between 100 μg and 150 μg, although patients who are treated with radioactive iodine and have some remaining thyroid activity might require lower doses. For patients with known heart disease or at risk for heart problems, doses should be initiated at 25 to 50 μg with increases of 25 μg every 4 to 6 weeks guided by TSH levels. Young patients who are at low risk for cardiac problems can be started at doses of 100 μg.

In choosing an agent to use for thyroid replacement, there is good evidence that generic substitutes are just as effective as brand-name drugs. A detailed study examining the metabolic effectiveness of a variety of generic drugs compared to a brand-name medication demonstrated no clinical or subclinical differences among preparations. So even though clinicians often hear that they should use a brand name drug to maintain the stability of the replacement dose, this is not supported by the evidence.

One area of uncertainty is whether the addition of triiodothyronine (T_3, Cytomel) adds additional benefit to thyroid replacement with thyroxine. In some studies with elderly patients, subjects with continued neurocognitive dysfunction benefited from the addition of T_3 at a dose of 125 μg, with a concomitant decrease in the T_4 dose of 50 μg. However, subsequent studies of younger patients (aged 29 to 44 years) failed to find any benefits of partial T_3 substitution. Furthermore, studies of patients on doses of T_4 adequate to restore TSH levels to normal have been found to have normal T_3 levels. At this time, routine use of T_3 cannot be recommended; however, for selected elderly patients who have lingering confusion, depression, or slow mentation on adequate doses of T_4, a trial of T_3 partial substitution might be tried.

Another situation where there is controversy is the use of thyroid replacement in patients with a mildly elevated TSH and a normal free T_4. This condition, called subacute hypothyroidism or mild hypothyroidism, is more common in white elderly women. Some studies have shown clinical improvement in symptoms when low doses of T_4 are given to these patients, although the patient populations tend to be those with preexisting thyroid disease (such as Graves' disease), and studies have had only a small number of patients. An expert panel has suggested using the TSH level as an indication for therapy.

CURRENT THERAPY

- Thyroxine replacement with l-thyroxine (Synthroid, Levoxyl) is the treatment for hypothyroidism. Medication should be titrated to normalize the thyroid-stimulating hormone (TSH) level, which is usually achieved at an overall dose of 100 to 150 μg.
- Initial dosing for those with potential cardiac disease should be started low (25-50 μg/day) and advanced slowly every 6 to 8 weeks.
- Partial substitution of triiodothyronine (Cytomel) for thyroxine should be reserved for elderly patients with persistent neurocognitive dysfunction despite normalization of their TSH.
- Patients who have subclinical hypothyroidism with a TSH greater than 10.0 should be considered for treatment. Patients with a TSH lower than this do not require therapy.

Patients with a TSH less than 10 do not require any therapy. Treatment is reasonable in those with a TSH level of 10.0 because these patients may be most symptomatic and have a progression to overt hypothyroidism of 5%.

Monitoring

In general, once a patient receives a full replacement dose of T_4 (usually between 100 and 150 μg) and has a TSH consistently in the normal range, there is little likelihood that their thyroid requirement will change over time. Although many advocate annual retesting of TSH to ensure patients are euthyroid, there is no evidence to show this is necessary.

Some conditions do warrant closer monitoring of the TSH level. Because T_4 and T_3 are highly protein bound, any conditions where a patient's serum protein status changes should prompt additional testing. This includes conditions that lower serum protein levels, such as liver disease, nephrotic syndrome, or malnutrition, as well as those where serum proteins are increased, such as pregnancy or initiation of estrogen therapy. Because patients' dietary protein usually decreases with advancing age, older patients whose diet declines can also require monitoring and a lowering of their T_4 dose over time.

Patients with subclinical hypothyroidism also might benefit from annual retesting of their free T_4 levels. Approximately 10% of patients with subacute hypothyroidism progress to hypothyroidism within 3 years of diagnosis. Because of this, yearly testing is recommended. Also, 50% of patients with subacute hypothyroidism have positive anti-thyroid antibodies; however, routine testing for these is not recommended.

Complications

Most of the complications of hypothyroidism are associated with undertreatment or overtreatment. Patients with inadequately treated hypothyroidism are at higher risk for cardiac disease. On the other hand, over-replacement of thyroxine increases the risk of both atrial fibrillation and osteoporosis.

In addition, Hashimoto's thyroiditis is associated with other endocrine autoimmune diseases such as Addison's disease and pernicious anemia. Clinicians should be aware of these associations and not overlook new endocrine disorders that might have clinical features similar to hypothyroidism.

Finally, patients with Hashimoto's hypothyroidism also are at higher risk for the future development of lymphoma. Clinicians should educate patients about the need to have new enlarged lymph nodes evaluated and be aggressive about evaluating symptoms or signs consistent with the development of a lymphoma.

REFERENCES

Bunevicius R, Kazanavicius G, Zalinkevicius R, Prange AJ. Effects of thyroxine as compared with thyroxine plus triiodothyronine in patients with hypothyroidism. N Engl J Med 1999;340:424–9.

Dong BJ, Hauck WW, Gambertoglio JG, et al. Bioequivalence of generic and brand-name levothyroxine products in the treatment of hypothyroidism. JAMA 1997;277:1205–13.

Helfand M, Crapo LM. Screening for thyroid disease. Ann Intern Med 1990; 112:840–9.

Sawin CT, Chopra D, Azizi F, et al. The aging thyroid. Increased prevalence of elevated serum thyrotropin levels in the elderly. JAMA 1979;242:1386–8.

Surks MI, Ortiz E, Daniels GH, et al. Subclinical thyroid disease: Scientific review and guidelines for diagnosis and management. JAMA 2004;291(2):228–38.

U.S. Preventive Services Task Force: Screening for thyroid disease. Available at http://www.ahrq.gov/clinic/uspstf/uspsthyr.htm; [accessed July 24, 2010].

Hyperthyroidism

Method of
William J. Hueston, MD

Epidemiology

Hyperthyroidism is relatively uncommon and usually caused by three conditions: Graves' disease, toxic nodular goiter, or acute thyroiditis. Graves' disease is the most common cause of hyperthyroidism in the United States and usually affects younger patients from the teens to the 40s. Like other autoimmune diseases, women are at higher risk (seven to eight times) than men. Toxic nodular goiter accounts for 15% to 30% of hyperthyroid diagnoses. It usually occurs after age 50 years, is more common in women, and follows several decades of multinodular thyroid disease. A less-common cause is administration of amiodarone. Amiodarone is about one third iodine and can cause hyperthyroidism either through iodine-induced thyroid damage or from increased thyroxine synthesis owing to excessive iodine.

Risk Factors

There are no known environmental or reversible risk factors for any of the causes of hyperthyroidism. Graves' disease is associated with a specific human leukocyte antigen (HLA) region on chromosome 6 (*CTLA 4*).

Pathophysiology

The most common causes of hyperthyroidism are shown in Box 1.

Graves' disease is an autoimmune disorder caused by antibodies against thyroid-stimulating hormone (TSH) receptors on the thyroid gland. Graves' disease is associated with many other autoimmune diseases, including pernicious anemia, vitiligo, type 1 diabetes mellitus, autoimmune adrenal disease, Sjögren's syndrome, rheumatoid arthritis, and lupus. As with these other disorders, the etiology is unknown.

Toxic nodular goiter, also known as Plummer's disease, results from the development of autonomous thyroid adenoma. Patients who develop a toxic nodular goiter usually have a long history of many other nodules that spontaneously burn out over time, but then develop a single large nodule (usually 2.5 cm or greater) that continues to produce thyroid hormone of such large quantities that patients become hyperthyroid. No clear cause is known for the development of the nodules.

BOX 1 Conditions Causing Hyperthyroidism

Graves' disease
Autonomous thyroid nodule (toxic nodular goiter)
Acute thyroiditis
- Hashimoto's thyroiditis
- Subacute granulomatous thyroiditis (de Quervain's thyroiditis)
- Subacute lymphocytic thyroiditis (silent or painless thyroiditis)
- Suppurative thyroiditis (bacterial infection of thyroid)
Excessive exogenous thyroid use
- Over-replacement after thyroid ablation or for hypothyroidism
- Thyroxine (Synthroid) abuse for weight loss
Iodine overconsumption
Amiodarone administration

Acute thyroiditis can also produce hyperthyroidism. Several different conditions can cause thyroiditis (see Box 1). The inflammation resulting in thyroiditis is thought to be related to subacute viral infections or autoimmune reactions; suppurative thyroiditis is a rare bacterial thyroid infection, usually caused by *Staphylococcus aureus*. During the acute period of thyroid inflammation, damage to the gland leads to the release of stored thyroxine from thyroid lakes, producing hyperthyroidism. However, after the initial release of thyroid hormone from the stored lakes, damage to the gland inhibits production of new thyroxine. After the initial surge in thyroid hormone levels, thyroxine levels drop, often to levels that can result in transient hypothyroidism. Most patients return to the euthyroid state after the thyroid gland heals, but about 10% of patients with acute thyroiditis remain chronically hypothyroid.

Other, less-common causes of hyperthyroidism include excessive exogenous administration of thyroid medications. This is most commonly the result of over-replacement of thyroxine (Levoxyl, Synthroid) in patients with hypothyroidism, but it may be intentional for weight loss. Because thyroxine and triiodothyronine (T_3) are highly protein bound, over-replacement is most common if patients experience hypoproteinemia, such as in nephrotic syndrome, cirrhosis, or malnutrition.

Excessive iodine consumption can also lead to thyrotoxicosis.

Prevention

There are no known strategies to prevent hyperthyroidism. For patients with hypothyroidism, annual monitoring of TSH levels is recommended to ensure that patients receive the appropriate replacement dose and not over-replacement.

Clinical Manifestations

Patients with hyperthyroidism complain of a variety of symptoms that can include anxiety, tachycardia, wide-pulse pressure hypertension, palpitations, fine tremor, weight loss, heat intolerance, and, particularly in the elderly, confusion or delirium. Patients with Graves' disease also have opthalmopathy characterized by lid retraction and exophthalmoses that can lead to optic nerve damage. In contrast, older patients can have few of the classic signs of hyperthyroidism and instead might complain of fatigue or weakness (apathetic hyperthyroidism), unexplained delirium, weight loss, heart failure, or isolated atrial fibrillation.

Some patients have a rapid escalation of symptom severity (thyroid storm) that is life-threatening if not identified and treated promptly. These patients usually have underlying thyrotoxicosis from Graves' disease complicated by a secondary physiologic stressor such as infection, surgery, or trauma. This is a medical emergency and needs immediate attention, including hospitalization with close observation.

On physical examination, patients with hyperthyroidism due to Graves' disease or thyroiditis might have a diffusely enlarged and mildly tender thyroid gland. In suppurative thyroiditis, the thyroid gland is red, hot, and very tender and accompanied by a fever and other systemic signs of severe infection. Patients with toxic nodular goiter can have palpable nodules in their thyroid gland and often have a single palpable nodule.

Diagnosis

Hyperthyroidism is diagnosed by finding an elevation in the free thyroxine (T_4) level accompanied by a low TSH level. Patients with Graves' disease often have positive anti–thyroid receptor antibody titers. Only anti-thyroglobulin receptor antibody testing is helpful because it can help differentiate Graves' disease from other causes. No other anti-thyroid tests are clinically indicated. Once the thyroid level abnormalities are found, a definitive diagnosis of the cause for the hyperthyroidism is needed to select the appropriate treatment strategy.

CURRENT DIAGNOSIS

- Hyperthyroidism or thyrotoxicosis is most often caused by Graves' disease, toxic nodular goiter (Plummer's disease), or acute thyroiditis.
- Common symptoms in hyperthyroidism are tachycardia, elevated systolic blood pressure, tremor, and anxiety. Patients with Graves' disease also might exhibit exophthalmos. In contrast, elderly patients can present with apathetic hyperthyroidism, which can be confused with hypothyroidism.
- Hyperthyroidism should be suspected in all patients who present with atrial fibrillation, palpitations, panic disorder, or unexplained tremors.
- Thyroid storm is an acute life-threatening condition usually occurring in patients with undiagnosed or untreated hyperthyroidism placed under physiologic stress.
- An elevated free T_4, usually with a low thyroid stimulating hormone is the hallmark of hyperthyroidism, and anti–thyroid stimulating hormone antibodies can help identify Graves' disease.
- Ultimately, a thyroid scan and uptake are usually necessary to differentiate the cause of hyperthyroidism.

Other conditions can produce a depressed TSH but have normal free T_4 levels. These include T_3 toxicosis and subclinical hyperthyroidism. T_3 toxicosis refers to situations where triiodothyronine (T_3) is produced in excess rather than thyroxine (T_4); this can occur in any of the conditions that can cause hyperthyroidism as well as in surreptitious triiodothyronine (Cytomel) ingestion.

Thyroid scanning and radiolabel uptake are usually necessary to differentiate the causes of hyperthyroidism. Thyroid scanning and uptake rely on the thyroid gland to concentrate radioactive molecules, such as iodine-131 (^{131}I) or technetium. Because of the risk of thyroid storm with iodine administration, patients should be treated with antithyroid drugs for 2 to 8 weeks before a scan and the drugs should be stopped at least 4 days before the test. Patients with Graves' disease show increases in uptake and diffuse distribution of the tracer throughout the thyroid gland. Patients with toxic nodular goiter also have increased uptake, but the isotope is concentrated in a one or a few focal areas, with the remainder of the thyroid gland suppressed. In contrast, patients with thyroiditis have decreased uptake of the radiolabel and a washed-out or mottled distribution on scanning.

Differential Diagnosis

Symptoms of hyperthyroidism also occur in patients with panic disorder and other anxiety conditions. These patients can have sinus tachycardia, tremor, and nervousness that mimic hyperthyroidism.

Treatment

Treatment depends on the cause of the hyperthyroidism (Table 1). In Graves' disease, immediate goals of treatment include reducing thyroid hormone production and blocking the peripheral effects of the excessive thyroid hormone. About 30% to 60% of patients, mostly adolescents, enter remission spontaneously, and the remission may be permanent. Remission rates are highest for those with a small goiter, no ophthalmopathy, thyroglobulin levels less than 50 μg/mL, and thyroxine levels less than 20 μg/dL. Signs of remission include a decreased ratio of T_3 to T_4, lower thyroid-stimulating thyroglobulin levels, and decreased radioactive iodine uptake on rescanning. When remissions do occur, it is usually within a year of starting antithyroid medications.

TABLE 1 Treatment Strategies for Hyperthyroidism

Treatment	Drug	Dosage
Graves' disease and Toxic Nodular Goiter		
Thyroid hormone suppression	Propylthiouracil	Initial: 300-400 mg/d Maintenance: 100-300 mg/d
	Methimazole	initial: 30-40 mg/d
β-Blockade	Propranolol[1]	10 mg qid
	Metoprolol (Lopressor)[1]	50-100 mg bid
Thyroid gland removal	Radioactive iodine ablation Thyroidectomy	
Acute Thyroiditis		
β-Blockade transiently		
May need thyroid replacement long-term		
Thyroid Storm		
Thyroid hormone suppression	Propylthiouracil	300-400 mg/d
β-Blockade	Propranolol[1]	1 mg/min IV to max 10 mg[3]
Iodine	Lugol's solution	1-2 gtt mixed in water tid
	Dexamethasone (Decadron)[1]	2 mg q6h
Cardiac and fluid monitoring		

[1]Not FDA approved for this indication.
[3]Exceeds dosage recommended by the manufacturer.

CURRENT THERAPY

- In patients with Graves' disease or autonomous thyroid nodules (toxic nodular goiter), short-term treatment includes thyroid suppression medications (such as methimazole [Tapazole]) and β-blockers (such as propranolol [Inderal][1]). Long-term management with radioiodine thyroid gland ablation is often pursued once symptoms are controlled.
- Patients with acute thyroiditis might need transient β-blockade but can often be managed expectantly until symptoms abate and thyroid hormone levels normalize. A small number of patients (~10%) have persistent hypothyroidism following an episode of illness.
- Thyroid storm is a medical emergency that requires close monitoring along with an antithyroid drug, β-blockers, corticosteroids, and iodine-potassium solution (Lugol's solution).

[1]Not FDA approved for this indication.

For those who do not undergo spontaneous remission, which includes most adults, consideration should be given to thyroid gland ablation to permanently treat this condition. Although the dosage can be calculated to attempt to leave patients euthyroid, permanent hypothyroidism occurs in about half of all patients treated with radioactive iodine ablation.

The initial approach to toxic nodular goiter is similar to that for symptom control, but thyroid ablation should be recommended routinely because remissions are very rare.

Thyroid gland production of hormone can be reduced rapidly with either methimazole (Tapazole) or propylthiouracil. Propylthiouracil is preferred in early pregnancy because it does not cross the placenta, but it has been associated with a higher risk of liver failure and is not used routinely for long periods. For chronic therapy, methimazole is preferable and has the advantage of less-frequent dosing, which improves compliance. With both drugs, clinicians need to be aware of drug-associated agranulocytosis, which can result in life-threatening bacterial infections. In patients on either of these medications who develop a sore throat, fever, or other signs of infection, a white blood count should be done immediately to ensure that they are not neuropenic. Additionally, antithyroid drugs are associated with drug-induced lupus syndromes and other forms of vasculitis.

In addition to reducing production of thyroid hormone, initial therapy for patients with Graves' disease and toxic nodular goiter should include a β-blocker to reduce the tachycardia, tremor, hypertension, and anxiety. A β-blocker that crosses the blood-brain barrier, such as propranalol (Inderal)[1] or metoprolol (Lopressor),[1] is the best choice in this situation because these also reduce the central nervous system effects such as anxiety as well as the vascular problems caused by thyroid hormones.

Thyroid storm requires immediate attention and should be managed in the hospital setting, especially in older patients where tachycardia and hypertension can lead to cardiac instability. Prompt administration of β-blockers and propylthiouracil along with cardiac monitoring for dysrhythmias and appropriate fluid management are essential for managing this life-threatening condition. Once antithyroid drugs have been administered, iodine-potassium solution (Lugol's solution) at a dose of 1 or 2 drops three times a day should be administered, which will further reduce thyroid hormone production and reduce peripheral conversion of T_4 to T_3. Finally, corticosteroids also have been shown to rapidly reduce thyroid hormone levels in thyroid storm.

For long-term management, thyroid ablation with radioactive iodine (sodium iodide, ^{131}I) can restore patients to a permanent euthyroid state. However, radioactive iodine thyroid ablation often results in destruction of more thyroid than optimal, causing hypothyroidism. Radioactive iodine thyroid ablation is contraindicated in pregnancy. For patients in whom radioactive iodine is either contraindicated or not acceptable, thyroidectomy is an option. Thyroidectomy almost always results in permanent hypothyroidism as well as having other risks inherent in surgery including hypoparathyroidism and recurrent laryngeal nerve damage.

In patients with hyperthyroidism associated with acute thyroiditis, symptoms often resolve by the time the evaluation is complete. In the interim, symptoms can be managed with β-blockers. β-Blocker therapy can be discontinued fairly rapidly (2 to 3 weeks) after the initial onset of symptoms.

Monitoring

In patients on antithyroid drugs, thyroid hormone levels should be monitored frequently until they reach a stable euthyroid state. Any change in the patient's underlying health, especially changes that could alter protein levels, should prompt reevaluation. In addition, patients who have thyroid ablation need follow-up testing of TSH and free T_4 levels to ensure that sufficient thyroid tissue has been destroyed to reverse their hyperthyroidism but not make them hypothyroid. This should be done 6 to 8 weeks following ablation therapy.

Complications

Complications of hyperthyroidism include acute and chronic conditions. Acutely, the most concerning complications are cardiac dysrhythmias, especially atrial fibrillation. Chronically, excessive thyroxine is associated with cardiomyopathy and osteoporosis. In patients with opthalmopathy, untreated Graves' disease can lead to progressive vision loss and blindness.

[1]Not FDA approved for this indication.

REFERENCES

Cooper DS. Antithyroid drugs for the treatment of hyperthyroidism caused by Graves' disease. Endocrinol Metab Clin North Am 1998;27:225–47.

Kharlip J, Cooper DS. Recent developments in hyperthyroidism. Lancet 2009;373:1930–2.

Lazarus JH. Hyperthyroidism. Lancet 1997;349:339–43.

Nayak B, Hodak SP. Hyperthyroidism. Endocrinol Metab Clin North Am 2007;36(3):617–56.

Zimmerman D, Lteif AN. Thyroxicosis in children. Endocrinol Metab Clin North Am 1998;27:109–26.

Thyroid Cancer

Method of
Richard A. Prinz, MD, and Emery Chen, MD

Thyroid cancer is the most common malignancy of the endocrine system. It affects more women than men by a ratio of 3:1. The National Cancer Institute (NCI) estimates that in 2009, 37,200 new cases of thyroid cancer were diagnosed in the United States and 1630 patients will die of thyroid cancer.

From 1997 to 2006, the incidence of thyroid cancer has increased by about 6% per year. This may be due, in part, to the frequent use of imaging modalities that have been detecting increasing numbers of incidental thyroid nodules. The mortality associated with thyroid cancer has not increased appreciably despite its rising incidence. The biological behavior of thyroid cancers, as a group, covers a broad spectrum. The overall 5- and 10-year survival rates of patients with papillary thyroid cancer, the most common type, remain approximately 97% and 90% respectively. Patients with anaplastic thyroid cancer, the least common type, rarely survive beyond 1 year.

The five subtypes of thyroid cancer are papillary, follicular, Hürthle cell, medullary, and anaplastic. Surgery is the initial treatment for all of these; however, the extent of surgery and subsequent adjuvant therapy depend on the clinical features and characteristics of each type.

Causes and Risk Factors

The causes of most sporadic forms of thyroid cancer remain unclear. Persons who have a family history of thyroid cancer or are older than 40 years are at greater risk for developing the disease. The incidence of malignancy in thyroid nodules is higher in children than adults, varying from 15% to 20% versus 5% to 6%, respectively.

The link between prior radiation exposure of the thyroid gland and cancer is clear. In the past, children and adults were sometimes treated with radiation for acne, fungal infections of the scalp, enlarged thymus, tonsils and adenoids, and other benign conditions. Numerous studies have linked these treatments to a higher risk of developing thyroid cancer, especially in patients with a thyroid nodule where the likelihood may be as high as 30% to 50%. Population studies of those affected by the Chernobyl accident showed a dramatic spike in the incidence of thyroid cancer, especially in children. Radiation exposure in adulthood carries a lesser risk of developing thyroid cancer than in children but it is still higher than in the general population.

A diet low in iodine is a risk factor for follicular thyroid cancer, the most common type of thyroid cancer in parts of the world where iodine deficiency is endemic. A low-iodine diet also seems to increase the risk of papillary thyroid cancers in those exposed to radiation.

Diagnosis

Most patients with thyroid cancer present with a nodule, which is extremely common in the general population. Sonographic screening of populations without thyroid disease shows that 33% of adults have at least one thyroid nodule. The number of detected nodules increases with age, with the highest prevalence in the seventh decade. Cancer is rare, occurring in 5% to 6% of those with a palpable thyroid nodule.

The best way to determine the nature of a thyroid nodule is by fine needle aspiration (FNA) for cytology. Some cancers are diagnosed after surgical excision for presumed benign disease (an indeterminate nodule, symptomatic multinodular goiter, or Graves' disease). These occult thyroid cancers are of uncertain biological behavior. Retrospective studies with long-term follow-up suggest that death resulting from papillary or follicular thyroid cancers detected in this fashion is uncommon with appropriate treatment.

Evaluation of a patient with a thyroid nodule (Box 1) should include a detailed review of their risk factors and symptoms, and a thorough neck examination that notes the characteristics of the nodule, and the presence or absence of cervical lymphadenopathy. Serum thyroid stimulating hormone (TSH) level should be measured to determine the patient's thyroid function. If the patient is euthyroid or hypothyroid by clinical evaluation or by having a normal or high TSH level, we proceed directly to FNA biopsy. We also start these patients on a TSH-suppressive dose of levothyroxine (Synthroid), beginning with 25 μg daily and titrating it to a TSH level just below 1 mIU/L to halt or reverse the growth of the nodule. However, there is no consensus as to the effectiveness of this approach. If the TSH level is suppressed below normal, a thyroid scan can determine if the nodule is a hyperfunctioning adenoma. Increased isotope uptake confirms a toxic or hot nodule. The risk of a hot nodule harboring a malignancy is less than 1%. We recommend thyroid lobectomy for definitive treatment of toxic adenomas; others favor radioiodine if the adenoma is less than 4 cm in diameter.

FNA biopsy is the gold standard test to separate benign disease from malignant disease. This can be guided by direct palpation of the nodule or with ultrasound to increase accuracy. It is a rapid, safe, sensitive, and inexpensive test that can be performed in the office and is well tolerated by patients. Its false-positive rate of 1% to 2% and false-negative rate of 2% to 5% have been well validated.

There are four possible cytopathologic results from an FNA biopsy specimen: malignant, benign, suspicious or indeterminate, and nondiagnostic. Treatment options for the first two possibilities are clear. Malignant lesions mandate thyroidectomy. Benign lesions should be followed unless they are associated with symptoms or growth while under observation. In addition, we recommend a second FNA biopsy in 6 to 12 months to decrease the possibility of a false-negative result.

CURRENT DIAGNOSIS

- A history of thyroid irradiation or family history of thyroid cancer increases the likelihood that a patient with a thyroid nodule will have thyroid cancer.
- Thyroid nodules in children are more likely to be cancers.
- Plasma thyroid-stimulating hormone level should be measured to assess thyroid function.
- A hyperfunctioning thyroid nodule is unlikely to harbor a malignancy.
- Ultrasound evaluation of the thyroid and neck can aid in the diagnosis and treatment of thyroid cancer.
- Fine needle aspiration (FNA) biopsy is the gold standard diagnostic test to detect most thyroid cancers.
- Follicular and Hürthle cell neoplasms require thyroid lobectomy because histopathologic evidence of capsular or vascular invasion is required to diagnose malignancy.

Suspicious or indeterminate lesions are mainly follicular and Hürthle cell neoplasms. These encapsulated tumors can be either benign or malignant. The differentiation cannot be made on the cytologic appearance of individual or even clusters of cells. The diagnosis of malignancy can only be made by finding direct tumor invasion into the capsule or vasculature. Therefore, thyroid lobectomy with definitive histologic examination of the specimen is recommended. There is conflicting evidence about the accuracy of intraoperative frozen section evaluation to guide surgical treatment. We use it because it is available and can be helpful when the pathologist makes a diagnosis of malignancy, but quite often the diagnosis must be deferred to permanent sections. If the final pathologic diagnosis reveals malignancy, a second procedure for completion thyroidectomy is recommended. For Hürthle and follicular neoplasms larger than 4 cm, total thyroidectomy is advised because of the greater risk of cancer. If the FNA is nondiagnostic, a repeat aspiration should be performed under ultrasound guidance. Patients with nodules that continue to yield nondiagnostic results should be offered thyroidectomy to clarify the diagnosis.

Histologic Classification, Treatment, and Prognosis

Cytology and management of thyroid tumors are shown in Table 1.

PAPILLARY CANCER

Papillary thyroid cancers are the most common form of thyroid cancer, accounting for approximately 80% of thyroid malignancies. They typically appear as hard, white nodules on gross examination. They are characterized microscopically by cuboidal cells with intranuclear cytoplasmic inclusions, nuclear grooves, prominent nuclei with marginated chromatin (Orphan Annie eyes), and round collections of calcium (psammoma bodies). Generally, the tumors are not encapsulated, but if they are, it is usually a good prognostic sign. Multicentric disease is common in papillary cancers, occurring in up to 85% of patients.

The cancer spreads early within the thyroid gland and through the lymphatics of the central and lateral neck. Cervical lymph node metastases occur in 30% to 40% of patients. Hematologic spread to the lungs and bones is usually found only in advanced disease.

The best treatment for papillary thyroid cancer is total thyroidectomy followed by radioiodine ablation and TSH suppression. Central and lateral modified radical neck dissections should be performed when there are nodal metastases in these compartments. Some

---

BOX 1   Risk Factors, Signs, and Symptoms Associated with Thyroid Cancer

Risk Factors
Head and neck irradiation
Family history of thyroid cancer
Low-iodine diet

Signs
Hard, fixed mass in a thyroid lobe
Cervical lymphadenopathy
Rapidly enlarging thyroid mass

Symptoms
Generally asymptomatic except in advanced disease
New onset of dysphonia, dyspnea, or dysphagia
Pressure or pain is unusual

TABLE 1 Fine Needle Aspiration Cytology and Associated Management

FNA Cytology Result	Diagnosis	Treatment
Benign	Benign nodule	Observation with repeat FNA in 6–12 mo
Malignant	Papillary, medullary, or anaplastic thyroid cancer	Total thyroidectomy with TSH suppression and ± adjuvant radioiodine
Indeterminant or suspicious	Follicular or Hürthle cell neoplasm	Thyroid lobectomy; return to surgery for completion thyroidectomy if final pathology shows cancer
Nondiagnostic	N/A	Repeat FNA with ultrasound guidance Lobectomy if still nondiagnostic

FNA = fine needle aspiration; N/A = not applicable; TSH = thyroid-stimulating hormone.

surgeons advocate routine central compartment lymph node sampling or dissection, which can upstage papillary thyroid cancers without substantially increasing operative morbidity. External beam radiation is reserved for those rare patients who cannot tolerate an operation, have recurrent disease not amenable to resection or who do not concentrate radioiodine, or for treatment of bony metastases. Overall 10-year survival after suitable treatment is greater than 90%.

FOLLICULAR CANCER

Follicular thyroid cancers macroscopically appear as a firm, solitary nodule that is usually encapsulated. Microscopically, they have a well-formed follicular structure composed of well-differentiated cells that are indistinguishable from their benign counterpart, follicular adenoma.

CURRENT THERAPY

- Total thyroidectomy is the initial treatment for most thyroid cancers.
- Therapeutic neck dissections are performed when evidence of lymph node involvement exists.
- Radioactive iodine and thyroid-stimulating hormone suppression are effective adjuvant therapies in patients with well-differentiated thyroid cancers.
- When final pathology proves a follicular or Hürthle cell neoplasm to be malignant, completion thyroidectomy is recommended if only a lobectomy has been performed.
- Patients with medullary thyroid cancer should be screened for pheochromocytoma, which should be treated before thyroidectomy.
- External beam irradiation and multidrug chemotherapy are adjuvant therapies for patients with anaplastic thyroid cancer.
- Most thyroid cancer patients require long-term follow-up after treatment.

Diagnosis of malignancy requires histologic confirmation of vascular or capsular invasion. Metastases are hematogenous, and lymphatic spread develops late in the disease.

The optimal management for a preoperative diagnosis of follicular neoplasm smaller than 4 cm is thyroid lobectomy and isthmusectomy. If there is histologic evidence of malignancy at operation, a total thyroidectomy should be performed followed by radioactive iodine therapy and TSH suppression. If the diagnosis must be deferred to permanent sections and the final pathology identifies a follicular thyroid cancer, a second procedure for a completion thyroidectomy followed by radioiodine is usually recommended. Lymph node dissection is rarely indicated and is reserved for patients with clinical evidence of nodal metastases. The 10-year survival rate following appropriate treatment is approximately 75% to 85%.

HÜRTHLE CELL CANCER

The American Thyroid Association and the World Health Organization classify Hürthle cell carcinomas, which account for up to 5% of thyroid malignancies, as a subtype of follicular thyroid cancer. Hürthle cell cancers are often more aggressive than the typical follicular cancer, with an increased likelihood of multicentricity and lymphatic spread and a decreased tendency to concentrate radioactive iodine. Microscopically, the eosinophilic granular cytoplasm, large clear nuclei, and trabecular architecture distinguish them from typical follicular thyroid cancers.

Treatment is the same as that described for follicular thyroid cancers. Some surgeons recommend routine central-compartment lymph node sampling or dissection due to the tumor's propensity for lymphatic spread, but there is no consensus on this because good evidence of benefit is lacking. The overall 10-year survival is approximately 60% to 70% following treatment.

MEDULLARY CANCER

Medullary thyroid carcinomas (MTCs) arise from the parafollicular C-cells. These neuroendocrine cells typically secrete calcitonin and can also secrete carcinoembryonic antigen (CEA), which can be used as tumor markers for both diagnosis and monitoring response to treatment. MTCs make up approximately 5% of thyroid cancers.

Grossly, MTC appears as a hard, unencapsulated nodule in the thyroid gland. Microscopically, the tumor's round, polyhedral, and spindle-shaped cells form a variety of patterns that range from trabecular to glandlike. Sheets of amyloid are also commonly found. MTCs tend to metastasize early through the lymphatics but can also spread through the bloodstream to the liver and lungs.

MTC is usually sporadic but approximately 25% are familial. Familial MTC is an autosomal dominant disorder due to mutations in the RET (rearranged during transfection) proto-oncogene. Identification of RET mutations in family members should prompt consideration for early prophylactic thyroidectomy to avert the certain development of medullary thyroid cancer. This is usually done between the ages of 6 months and 10 years, depending on the aggressiveness of the specific RET mutation.

MTC is also one of the endocrinopathies, along with pheochromocytoma and hyperparathyroidism, that make up the multiple endocrine neoplasia (MEN) type 2 syndromes. Patients with MTC should be screened for pheochromocytoma before thyroidectomy. If pheochromocytoma is present, it should be removed before thyroidectomy.

There is widespread agreement that total thyroidectomy with routine central compartment lymph node dissection is the best treatment for MTC. A lateral neck dissection is reserved for patients with clinically involved lymph nodes in the jugular chain. Radioiodine therapy is not an option because parafollicular cells do not take up iodine. Therapy with tyrosine kinase receptor inhibitors that selectively target pathways for tumor growth and angiogenesis is under investigation.

The overall 10-year survival after treatment is approximately 70% to 80% when the disease is confined to the thyroid gland and 30% to 40% when distant metastases are present.

ANAPLASTIC CANCER

Anaplastic thyroid cancers are exceptionally aggressive and lethal. They result in more than one half the deaths attributed to thyroid malignancy every year. They are rare, accounting for up to 2% of all thyroid cancers.

Anaplastic thyroid cancers arise from dedifferentiation of papillary thyroid cancer and usually manifest as a rapidly growing central neck mass. Most patients are elderly, with locally advanced disease and nodal and distant metastases at presentation.

The three main conditions that can occur in a similar fashion are Riedel's thyroiditis, thyroid lymphoma, and parapharyngeal sarcoma. FNA cytology is often insufficient to establish a firm diagnosis and early open wedge biopsy may be needed.

Aggressive therapy with surgery, radiation, and chemotherapy is recommended. However, complete surgical resection is usually not possible, and there is no effective chemotherapy. Tracheostomy should be considered for impending obstruction rather than prophylaxis. Prognosis is poor, and median survival varies from 2 to 12 months. One-year survival after multimodality therapy is less than 3%.

Follow-up

Papillary, follicular, and Hürthle cell thyroid cancers are grouped together and referred to as *well-differentiated thyroid cancers* (WDTC). They are all derived from thyroid follicular cells, respond well to surgical and adjuvant therapies, and are associated with generally favorable outcomes (Table 2). A small minority of patients, however, eventually succumbs to WDTC.

Many prognostic factors have been used to classify patients with WDTC into high-risk and low-risk groups. They include the patient's age and sex, tumor size and extent of invasion or metastasis, and completeness of surgical resection. Using these prognostic factors, several scoring systems were devised to reliably predict individual patient prognosis. Among the first was the AGES scoring system (*age*, histologic *grade* of the tumor, *extrathyroidal* invasion and distant metastases, tumor *size*), which was later refined to the MACIS scoring system (*metastases*, *age*, *completeness* of resection, extrathyroidal *invasion*, tumor *size*). The DeGroot classification consists of class I (intrathyroidal), class II (cervical node metastases), class III (extrathyroidal extension), and class IV (distant metastases) groups. The AMES system (*age*, *metastases*, *extrathyroidal* invasion, primary tumor *size*) is easy to use, but does not accurately distinguish low-risk from high-risk patients with FTC. Arguably the most widely used is the TNM staging system (*tumor* size, *nodal* status, distant *metastases*). None of the scoring systems can be used to guide the extent of surgical resection because the only factors known preoperatively are age and sex.

The rate of recurrence in low-risk patients with WDTC is about 10%, whereas in high-risk patients it is about 45%. Among the low-risk patients who have a recurrence, 33% to 50% die from their disease. Traditionally, radioactive iodine whole body scans (WBS) have been performed every 6 to 12 months to detect recurrent disease. However, the usefulness of serum thyroglobulin assays combined with routine neck ultrasound has decreased the need for frequent WBS.

Serum thyroglobulin is a useful marker for follow-up of patients with WDTC, because most of these tumors synthesize thyroglobulin. After successful treatment, thyroglobulin levels should be undetectable. Thyroglobulin levels that are elevated more than 10 ng/mL in the absence of thyroglobulin antibodies indicate residual thyroid tissue or persistent or recurrent thyroid cancer. Further imaging studies are then used to localize the residual tissue or cancer. For medullary thyroid cancer, elevated serum calcitonin or CEA levels after thyroidectomy should prompt appropriate imaging studies to localize persistent or recurrent disease. Persistent and recurrent disease that is detectable with imaging should be resected if it can be done with minimal morbidity.

There are no useful tumor markers for anaplastic thyroid cancer.

Summary

Thyroid cancer is increasing in frequency. The majority of thyroid cancers are slow growing and indolent, but a small minority can be aggressive and fatal. Thyroid cancer treatment depends on the characteristics of each histopathologic type. FNA biopsy can be useful in detecting the presence and type of thyroid cancer prior to the initiation of therapy. Thyroidectomy is the first step in the successful treatment of most thyroid cancers; however, the extent of surgery and subsequent adjuvant therapy varies with the subtype of thyroid cancer. Serial measurement of tumor markers coupled with neck imaging studies is useful in the long-term follow-up of patients treated for thyroid cancer.

REFERENCES

Ball DW. Medullary thyroid cancer: Therapeutic targets and molecular markers. Curr Opin Oncol 2007;19:18–23.

Chabre O, Piolat C, Dyon JF. Childhood progression of hereditary medullary thyroid cancer. N Engl J Med 2007;356:1583–4.

Cooper DS, Doherty GM, Haugen BR, et al. Management guidelines for patients with thyroid nodules and differentiated thyroid cancer. Thyroid 2006;16:109–42.

D'Avanzo A, Ituarte P, Treseler P, et al. Prognostic scoring systems in patients with follicular thyroid cancer: A comparison of different staging systems in predicting the patient outcome. Thyroid 2004;14:453–8.

Fialkowski EA, Moley JF. Current approaches to medullary thyroid carcinoma, sporadic and familial. J Surg Oncol 2006;94:737–47.

Kebebew E, Clark OH. Differentiated thyroid cancer: "Complete" rational approach. World J Surg 2000;24:942–51.

Kim AW, Maxhimer JB, Quiros RM, et al. Surgical management of well-differentiated thyroid cancer locally invasive to the respiratory tract. J Am Coll Surg 2005;201:619–27.

Lang BH, Lo CY. Surgical options in undifferentiated thyroid carcinoma. World J Surg 2007;31:969–77.

Mazzaferri EL, Robbins RJ, Spencer CA, et al. A consensus report of the role of serum thyroglobulin as a monitoring method for low-risk patients with papillary thyroid carcinoma. J Clin Endocrinol Metab 2003;88:1433–41.

Pacini F, DeGroot LJ. Thyroid neoplasia. In: DeGroot LJ, Jameson JL, editors. Endocrinology. 5th ed. Philadelphia: Saunders; 2006. p. 2147–80.

Phitayakorn R, McHenry CR. Follicular and Hürthle cell carcinoma of the thyroid gland. Surg Oncol Clin N Am 2006;15:603–23.

Sanders Jr EM, Livolsi VA, Brierley J, et al. An evidence-based review of poorly differentiated thyroid cancer. World J Surg 2007;31:934–45.

TABLE 2 Long-Term Follow-Up

Type	Tumor Marker(s)	Imaging	Frequency
WDTC	Tg (basal and stimulated with ↑TSH levels)	Neck U/S, ^{131}I whole body scan	6–12 mo or when Tg > 10 ng/mL
Medullary	Calcitonin, CEA	CT of neck, thorax, abdomen; consider PET scan	6–12 mo or when calcitonin is newly elevated
Anaplastic	None	Neck U/S	1–3 mo

CEA = carcinoembryonic antigen; CT = computed tomography; PET = positron emission tomography; Tg = thyroglobulin; TSH = thyroid stimulating hormone; U/S = ultrasound; WDTC = well-differentiated thyroid cancer.

Pheochromocytoma

Method of
Tobias Engel, MD, and Karel Pacak, MD, PhD, DSc

Pheochromocytomas are catecholamine-producing neuroendocrine tumors arising from chromaffin cells of the adrenal medulla or extra-adrenal paraganglia. Tumors from extra-adrenal chromaffin tissue are referred to as extra-adrenal pheochromocytomas or paragangliomas. The term *paraganglioma* is also used for tumors derived from parasympathetic tissue in the head and neck, the head and neck paragangliomas. For the purpose of this chapter, a discussion of pheochromocytomas includes paragangliomas.

Extra-adrenal pheochromocytomas mainly arise in the abdomen from chromaffin tissue neighboring sympathetic ganglia. Less often, they originate from the pelvis and infrequently from the mediastinum (2%) and neck (1%). In the abdomen, they often derive from the organ of Zuckerkandl, a collection of chromaffin tissue around the origin of the inferior mesenteric artery (Fig. 1).

Epidemiology

Pheochromocytoma can occur at any age, including childhood, but most often they are detected in the fourth and fifth decades. There is no gender preference. In western countries the prevalence of pheochromocytoma is estimated between 1:4500 and 1:1700, with an annual incidence of 3 to 8 cases per 1 million per year in the general population. About 15% to 20% of pheochromocytoma are extra-adrenal, about 24% are familial, and 10% are malignant.

Genetics

There are no lifestyle-related risk factors that increase the risk of pheochromocytoma. However, the role of genetics has been growing over the last years. Up to 24% of pheochromocytomas are probably hereditary. One can conclude that gene mutations are the largest risk factor involved with pheochromocytoma.

Hereditary pheochromocytomas have been associated with multiple endocrine neoplasia (MEN) types 2A and 2B, neurofibromatosis type 1, von Hippel–Lindau syndrome, and familial paraganglioma syndromes caused by germline mutations of genes encoding succinate dehydrogenase (SDH) subunits B, C, and D. *SDHB* mutations mainly predispose patients to extra-adrenal paragangliomas and, to a lesser extent, adrenal paragangliomas, with a high malignant potential. *SDHB* mutations can also lead to head and neck paragangliomas. *SDHD* mutations are typically associated with multifocal head and neck paragangliomas or adrenal and extra-adrenal paragangliomas, which are usually benign. *SDHC* mutations are rare, mainly manifesting in head and neck paragangliomas.

In addition to *SDHB*, *SDHC*, and *SDHD*, a new gene has been associated with paraganglioma: *SDH5*. It is located on chromosome 11q13.1 and interacts with the SDH complex. The SDH complex is a component of both the electron transport chain and the tricarboxylic acid cycle. Studies indicate that *SDH5* mutations do not play an important role in the development of pheochromocytoma and only rarely cause head and neck paragangliomas.

Pheochromocytomas can occur as part of a syndrome, associated with additional clinical conditions (Box 2). The characteristics of hereditary pheochromocytomas are described in Table 1.

Although widespread genetic testing is debated, it would be neither appropriate nor cost-effective to test for each disease-causing gene in every patient with a pheochromocytoma. An algorithm that takes family history, clinical characteristics, and biochemical phenotype into consideration is shown in Figure 2. In cases of confirmation of a hereditary disorder, one should offer specific genetic tests to the patient's family members. Disease screening should be offered to presymptomatic relatives who have a diagnosed mutation.

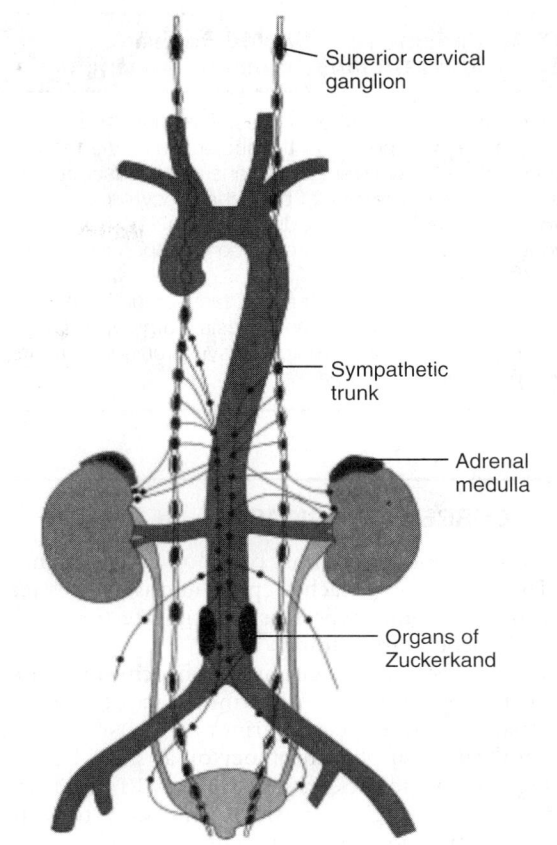

FIGURE 1. Anatomic distribution of chromaffin tissue. (Adapted from Lack E: Tumors of the adrenal gland and extra-adrenal paraganglia. In Armed Forces Institute of Pathology: Atlas of Tumor Pathology. Washington, DC, Armed Forces Institute of Pathology, 1997, pp 261-267.)

Clinical Manifestations

The signs and symptoms of pheochromocytoma are mostly the result of the hemodynamic and metabolic actions of the often inconsistent and disorderly secreted catecholamines on α- and β-adrenoreceptors. Most symptoms are nonspecific, but when the triad of headaches, palpitations, and sweating is accompanied by hypertension, pheochromocytoma should immediately be suspected. The typical episodic symptoms of catecholamine secretion seen in patients may be caused by manipulation of the tumor (e. g. palpitation, micturition, defecation, or an accident), endoscopy, anesthesia, ingestion of food or beverages that contain tyramine, and certain medications. However, very often these symptoms occur spontaneously. Psychological stress does not seem to provoke a hypertensive crisis. Many patients have no symptoms or only minor ones. The diagnosis can therefore be easily missed. This is especially true for elderly patients.

The primary clinical clues for the diagnosis of pheochromocytoma are summarized in Box 1.

Differential Diagnosis

Pheochromocytoma is often referred to as "the great mimic," because it has signs and symptoms that are common in numerous other clinical conditions. As a result, this often leads to the misdiagnosis of

Anyone with the triad of headaches, sweating, and tachycardia, whether or not the subject has hypertension
Anyone with a known mutation of one of the susceptibility genes or a family history of pheochromocytoma
Anyone with an incidental adrenal mass
Anyone whose blood pressure is poorly responsive to standard therapy
Anyone who has had hypertension, tachycardia, or an arrhythmia in response to anesthesia, surgery, or medications known to precipitate symptoms in patients with pheochromocytoma

 CURRENT DIAGNOSIS

- Hypertension is the most common clinical sign.
- The triad of headaches, palpitations, and sweating, with or without hypertension, indicate the possibility of a pheochromocytoma.
- The biochemical diagnosis of pheochromocytoma is mainly based on the determination of fractionated plasma or urine metanephrines.
- Localization of pheochromocytomas should consist of sensitive anatomic imaging (CT, MRI) and specific functional imaging (positron emission tomography [PET], meta-iodobenzylguanidine [MIBG]).
- Cost-effective genetic screening should be performed on patients. The identification of a causative mutation should lead to presymptomatic genetic testing in a patient's family.

pheochromocytoma. Consideration should be given to other conditions that are associated with sympathomedullary activation (e.g., hyperadrenergic hypertension, renovascular hypertension, panic disorders), because they mimic pheochromocytoma most closely. This overlap can be excluded by a normal response to the clonidine suppression test.

Biochemical Diagnosis

Missing a pheochromocytoma can have a fatal outcome. Therefore, tests with high sensitivity are needed to safely exclude a pheochromocytoma without using expensive and unnecessary biochemical follow-up or imaging studies.

After multiple studies at the National Institutes of Health (NIH), measurement of plasma free metanephrines showed superior combined diagnostic sensitivity (98%) and specificity (92%) over all other tests examined, including urinary and plasma catecholamines, urinary total and fractionated metanephrines, and urinary vanillyl-mandelic acid (VMA). However, the relative advantage of measuring plasma free metanephrines compared to fractionated urinary metanephrines is small. Therefore, expert recommendations for initial biochemical testing include measurement of fractionated metanephrines in urine or plasma, or both if possible. The decision to rule out pheochromocytoma should be based on nonelevated values of these tests.

The conditions under which blood samples are collected can be crucial to the reliability and interpretations of test results. The optimal circumstances are noted in Box 3. Besides these conditions, there are also numerous dietary constituents or medications that can cause direct or indirect interference in the measurement of epinephrines and metanephrines. This should be kept in mind when interpreting a positive test result. Tricyclic antidepressants, phenoxybenzamine (Dibenzyline) and other drugs interfere with test results. Tricyclic antidepressants and phenoxybenzamine lead to raised norepinephrine and normetanephrine levels. The future use of liquid chromatography tandem mass spectrometry (LC-MS/MS)

BOX 2 Main Clinical Features of Syndromes Associated with Pheochromocytoma

von Hippel–Lindau syndrome
Type 1 (no pheochromocytoma)
Renal cell cysts and carcinomas
Retinal and CNS hemangioblastomas
Pancreatic neoplasms and cysts
Endolymphatic sac tumors
Epididymal cystadenomas

Type 2 (with pheochromocytoma)
Type 2A: Retinal and CNS hemangioblastomas
- Pheochromocytomas
- Endolymphatic sac tumors
- Epididymal cystadenomas
Type 2B: Renal cell cysts and carcinomas
- Retinal and CNS hemangioblastomas
- Pancreatic neoplasms and cysts
- Pheochromocytomas
- Endolymphatic sac tumors
- Epididymal cystadenomas
Type 2C: Pheochromocytomas only

Multiple Endocrine Neoplasia Type 2
Type 2A (medullary thyroid carcinoma)
- Pheochromocytomas
- Hyperparathyroidism
- Cutaneous lichen amyloidosis

Type 2B (medullary thyroid carcinoma)
- Pheochromocytomas
- Multiple neuromas
- Marfanoid habitus
FMTC: familial medullary thyroid carcinoma only

Neurofibromatosis Type 1
Multiple benign neurofibromas on skin and mucosa
Café au lait skin spots
Iris Lisch nodules
Learning disabilities
Skeletal abnormalities
Vascular disease
CNS tumors
Malignant peripheral nerve sheath tumors
Pheochromocytomas

Paraganglioma Syndromes
Head and neck tumors
- Carotid-body tumors
- Vagal, jugular, and tympanic paragangliomas
Abdominal and/or thoracic paragangliomas
Pheochromocytomas
Renal cell carcinoma (SDHB)
Gastrointestinal stromal tumor (SDHB and SDHD)

Abbreviations: CNS = central nervous system; SDH = succinate dehydrogenase.
Adapted from Lenders JW, Eisenhofer G, Mannelli M, Pacak K. Phaeochromocytoma. Lancet 2005;366:665-675.

TABLE 1 Characteristics of Hereditary Pheochromocytoma

Disease	Mutation	Gene	Protein	Develop (%)	Bilateral	Malignant	Adrenal or Extra-adrenal	Peak Age (y)	Biochemical Phenotype
MEN2	10q11.2	*RET*	Tyrosine kinase receptor	50	70	Usually benign	Mainly adrenal	40	Adrenergic
VHL	3p25-26	*VHL*	pVHL19 and pVHL30	<30	50	Rarely malignant	Mainly adrenal	30	Noradrenergic
NF-1	17q11	*NF-1*	Neurofibromin	1-2	12	Rarely malignant	Mainly adrenal	50*	Adrenergic
SDHB	1p36	Gene encoding the B subunit of mitochondrial succinate dehydrogenase	Catalytic iron-sulfur protein	3-10	Has not been studied consistently	Often malignant	Mainly extra-adrenal	30	Mainly noradrenergic (and dopaminergic)
SDHC	1q21	Gene encoding the C subunit of mitochondrial succinate dehydrogenase	CybL	Has not been studied consistently	Has not been studied consistently	Rarely malignant	Mainly extra-adrenal	43	Has not been studied consistently
SDHD	11q23	Gene encoding the D subunit of mitochondrial succinate dehydrogenase	CybS (membrane-spanning subunit)	4-7	Has not been studied consistently	Rarely malignant	Adrenal and extra-adrenal	30	Dopaminergic

*Seldom seen in children.
Abbreviations: MEN = multiple endocrine neoplasia; NF = neurofibromatosis; SDH = succinate dehydrogenase; VHL = von Hippel-Lindau.

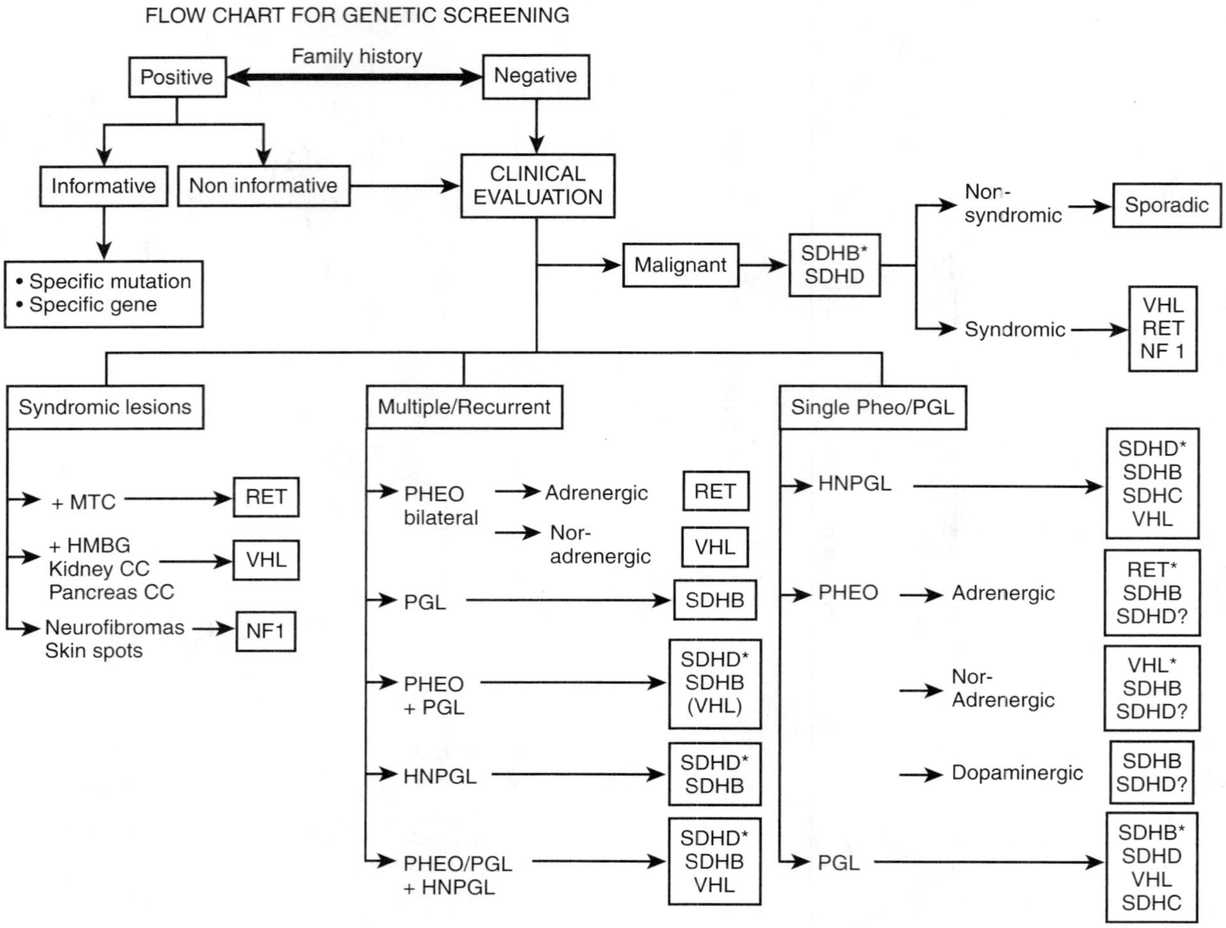

FLOW CHART FOR GENETIC SCREENING

Family history

Positive ◄──────► Negative

Positive → Informative | Non informative

Negative → CLINICAL EVALUATION

Informative → • Specific mutation • Specific gene

CLINICAL EVALUATION → Malignant → SDHB* SDHD → Non-syndromic → Sporadic

SDHB* SDHD → Syndromic → VHL RET NF 1

Syndromic lesions
- + MTC → RET
- + HMBG Kidney CC Pancreas CC → VHL
- Neurofibromas Skin spots → NF1

Multiple/Recurrent
- PHEO bilateral → Adrenergic → RET
- → Nor-adrenergic → VHL
- PGL → SDHB
- PHEO + PGL → SDHD* SDHB (VHL)
- HNPGL → SDHD* SDHB
- PHEO/PGL + HNPGL → SDHD* SDHB VHL

Single Pheo/PGL
- HNPGL → SDHD* SDHB SDHC VHL
- PHEO → Adrenergic → RET* SDHB SDHD?
- → Nor-Adrenergic → VHL* SDHB SDHD?
- → Dopaminergic → SDHB SDHD?
- PGL → SDHB* SDHD VHL SDHC

FIGURE 2. Flow chart suggested for genetic analysis in patients affected by pheochromocytomas or paragangliomas. The genes reported in the boxes are those more likely to be found mutated according to the clinical picture. First choice is denoted by the *asterisk. Abbreviations:* CC = cancer or cysts; HMGB = hemangioblastomas; HNPGL = head and neck paraganglioma; MTC = medullary thyroid carcinoma; PGL = paraganglioma; PHEO = pheochromocytoma. (Adapted from Mannelli M: Clinically guided genetic screening in a large cohort of Italian patients with pheochromocytomas and/or functional or nonfunctional paragangliomas. J Clin Endocrinol Metab 2009;94:1541-1547.)

BOX 3 Optimal Conditions for Blood Collection of Plasma Free Metanephrines or Catecholamines

Patient is supine for at least 15 minutes before sampling.
Samples are collected through a previously inserted IV, to avoid stress associated with the needle stick.
Patient has abstained from nicotine and alcohol for at least 12 hours.
Patient has fasted overnight before blood sampling.

---

will be useful, because it can remove potentially interfering substances. It is also faster, cheaper, and more specific than current detection methods.

Besides the initial biochemical tests, which can exclude the disease, follow-up tests are required to establish the diagnosis. This is necessary because although the initial tests are specific, the diagnosis of pheochromocytoma is so rare that there are many false-positive results. Options for biochemical follow-up testing are repeated plasma or urinary metanephrine tests, additional sampling for plasma or urinary fractionated catecholamines, and the clonidine (Catapres)[1]-suppression test. Biochemical follow-up testing is not necessary for patients with increases above four times the upper reference limit (URL) of plasma free metanephrines. The once-used glucagon[1] stimulation test should be abandoned, because this test offers insufficient sensitivity and can lead to hypertensive complications.

Based on these methods, the algorithm in Figure 3 for biochemical diagnosis was designed.

Localization of Pheochromocytoma

The localization and confirmation of pheochromocytoma should involve at least two imaging modalities. For optimal results, anatomic imaging studies with high sensitivity, such as CT and MRI, should be combined with high-specificity functional imaging studies. Currently, no consensus indicates whether CT or MRI is preferred for initial localization of a tumor. However, T2-sequenced MRI should be used as the initial imaging procedure in children and pregnant or lactating women. MRI scans are also preferred for localizing difficult-to-locate extra-adrenal tumors, for instance paraganglioma near the heart.

Initial imaging should be focused on the adrenals. Negative imaging of the adrenals should be followed by CT or MRI scans of the abdomen and pelvis, where extra-adrenal pheochromocytomas are

---

[1]Not FDA approved for this indication.

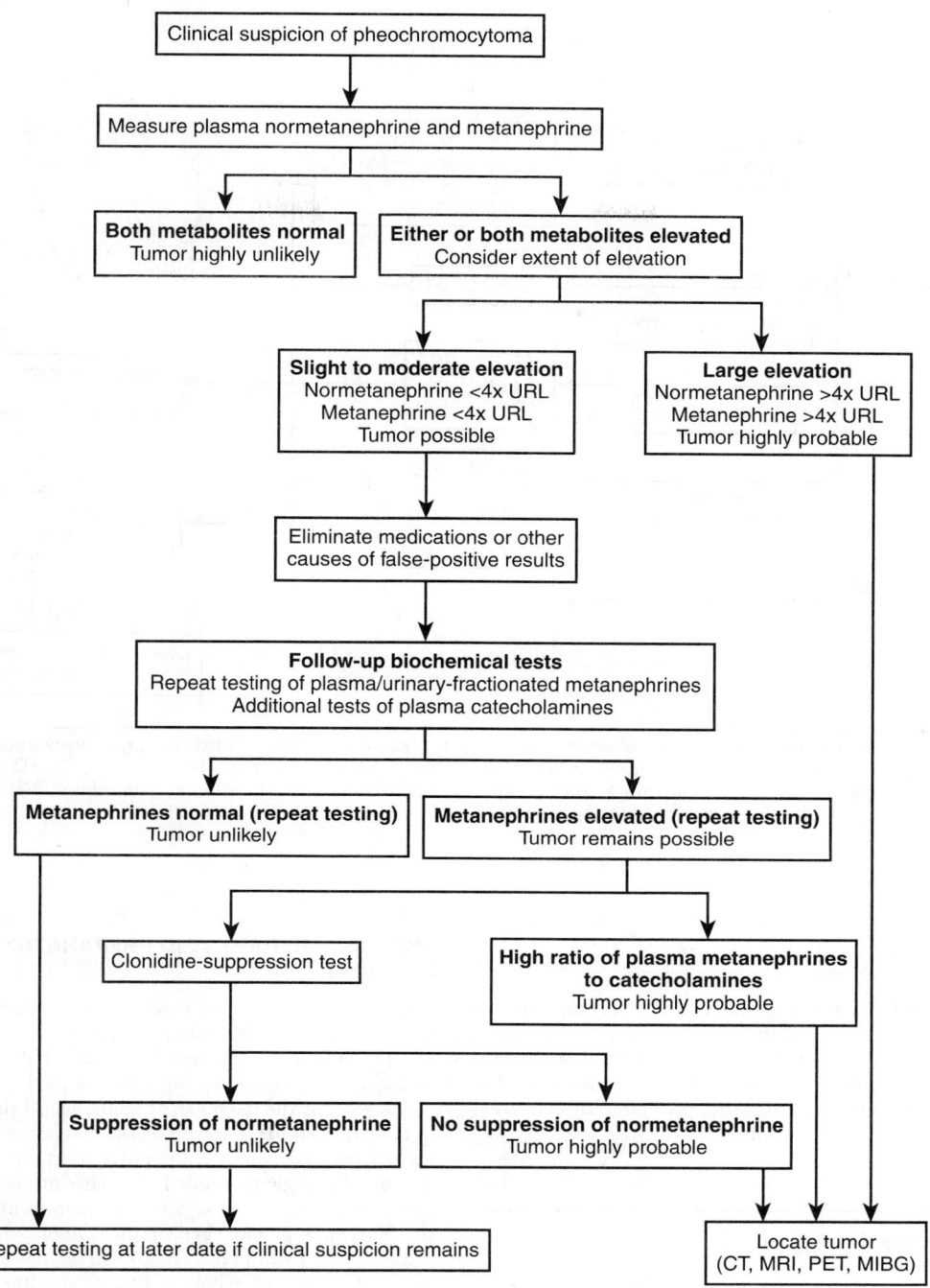

FIGURE 3. Algorithm for biochemical diagnosis. *Abbreviations:* MIBG = meta-iodobenzylguanidine; MRI = magnetic resonance imaging; PET = positron emission tomography; URL = upper reference limit.

most commonly located. If these scans are negative, chest and neck images should be obtained. Ultrasound is not recommended to localize pheochromocytoma. Exceptions include children and pregnant women when MRI is not available.

After anatomic imaging, which lacks the specificity to indisputably identify a mass as a pheochromocytoma, functional imaging methods can confirm a tumor as a pheochromocytoma. Functional imaging also detects most cases of metastatic and multifocal disease. They include ^{123}I-metaiodobenzylguanide (MIBG) scintigraphy (or ^{131}I-MIBG if ^{123}I-MIBG is not available), positron emission tomography (PET), and somatostatin receptor scintigraphy (Octreoscan). PET scanning is preferred for comprehensive localization of metastatic disease. The most commonly used radiopharmaceuticals in PET scanning are ^{18}F-fluorodopamine (^{18}F-FDA), ^{18}F-3,4-dihydroxyphenylalanine (^{18}F-FDOPA), and ^{18}F-fluorodeoxyglucose (^{18}F-FDG). Different circumstances require different radiopharmaceuticals (Fig. 4). The use of ^{123}I-MIBG scintigraphy in patients with known metastatic pheochromocytoma should be limited to the evaluation of whether a patient qualifies for ^{131}I-MIBG treatment. The algorithm described in Figure 4 provides the basis for diagnostic localization of pheochromocytoma.

If all tests return negative, it is advised to repeat noninvasive localization after 2 to 6 months.

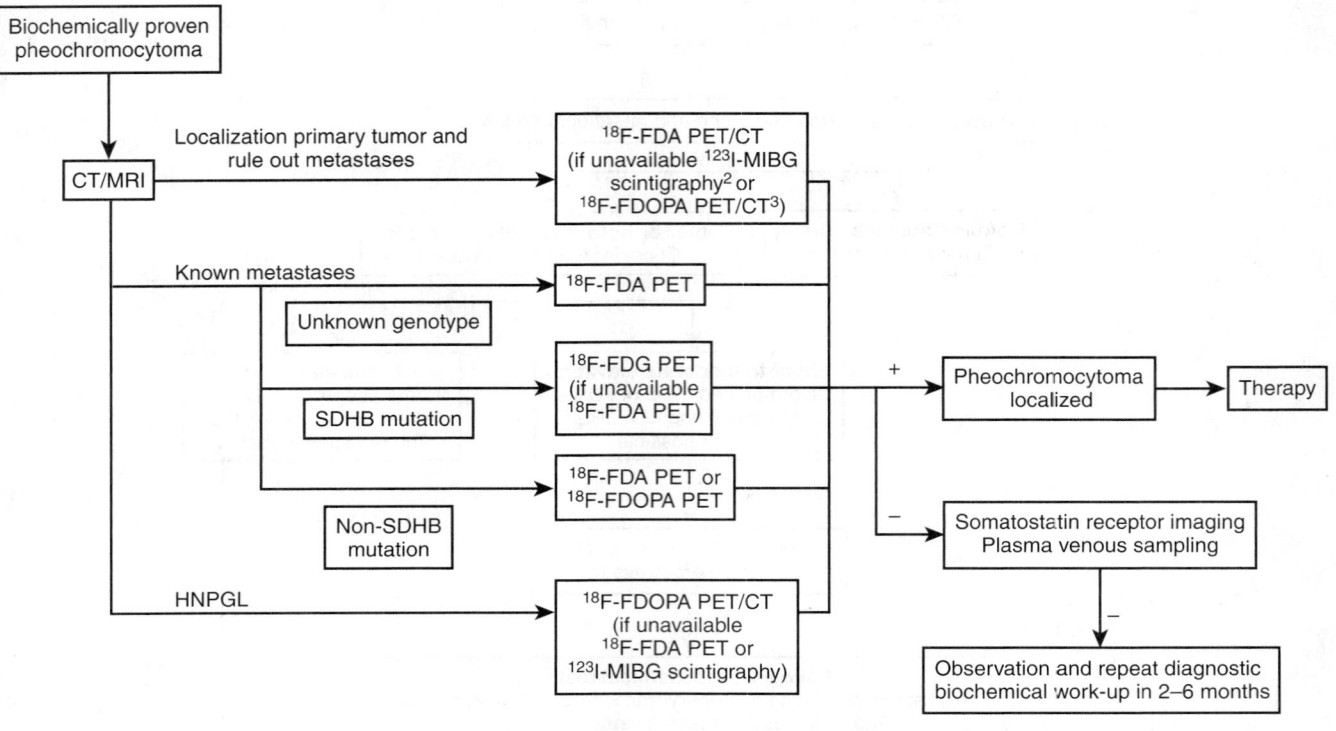

FIGURE 4. Flow chart for localization of pheochromocytoma. [2], second choice; [3], third choice. *Abbreviations:* CT = computed tomography; ^{18}F-FDA = ^{18}F-fluorodopamine; ^{18}F-FDOPA = ^{18}F-3,4-dihydroxyphenylalanine; ^{18}F-FDG = ^{18}F-fluorodeoxyglucose; HNPGL = head and neck paraganglioma; MIBG = meta-iodobenzylguanidine; MRI = magnetic resonance imaging; PET = positron emission tomography.

Treatment

The optimal therapy for a pheochromocytoma is prompt surgical removal of the tumor because an unresected tumor represents a time bomb waiting to explode with a potentially lethal hypertensive crisis. Safe surgical removal requires the efforts of a team made up of an internist, an anesthesiologist and a surgeon, preferably all with previous experience with pheochromocytoma.

 CURRENT THERAPY

- The optimal therapy for a pheochromocytoma is prompt surgical removal of the tumor.
- At least 2 weeks before the operation there should be adequate maintenance of blood pressure using mainly α-blockers and possibly β-blockers, calcium-channel blockers, and metyrosine (Demser).
- For most adrenal and extra-adrenal pheochromocytomas, laparoscopy has replaced laparotomy as the procedure of choice.
- Adrenal cortex–sparing surgery is advocated in patients with bilateral pheochromocytomas.
- Clinical follow-up should be lifelong, especially in cases of an underlying germline mutation.
- Management of malignant pheochromocytomas requires a multidisciplinary approach, in which pharmacologic treatment, targeted radiotherapy, chemotherapy, and surgery can all play a part.

MEDICAL THERAPY AND PREPARATION FOR SURGERY

The goal of preoperative medical treatment is to control hypertension, maintain stable blood pressure during surgery, minimize adverse effects during anesthesia, and reduce other clinical signs and symptoms caused by high plasma levels of catecholamines.

As soon as the diagnosis is made, blood pressure should be adequately treated for at least 2 weeks before the operation. With satisfactory pretreatment, perioperative mortality has fallen to less than 3%. α-Adrenergic blockade is the basis of medical management and preoperative preparation. The most commonly used α-adrenoreceptor blocker is phenoxybenzamine. Other α-blocking agents of use are prazosin (Minipress), terazosin (Hytrin), and doxazosin (Cardura). Though these have a shorter duration of action and more often cause hypotension when initially administered for preoperative blood pressure control, postoperative hypotension is more often seen with phenoxybenzamine. Besides α-blockers, one can use β-blockers, calcium-channel blockers, and α-methyl-l-tyrosine/metyrosine (Demser). β-Adrenoreceptor blockers should never be used until α-adrenoreceptor blockers have been administered for at least 2 to 3 days. This is because unopposed stimulation of α-adrenoreceptors and loss of β-adrenoreceptor–mediated vasodilatation can cause a serious and life-threatening elevation of blood pressure. A proposed algorithm for preoperative treatment is given in Figure 5.

OPERATIVE AND POSTOPERATIVE MANAGEMENT

After extensive preoperative preparation, surgery may be performed by an experienced surgeon.

To ensure adequate preoperative preparation, several criteria have been proposed: Blood pressure should be below 160/90mm Hg for at least 24 hours; orthostatic hypotension should be present, but not

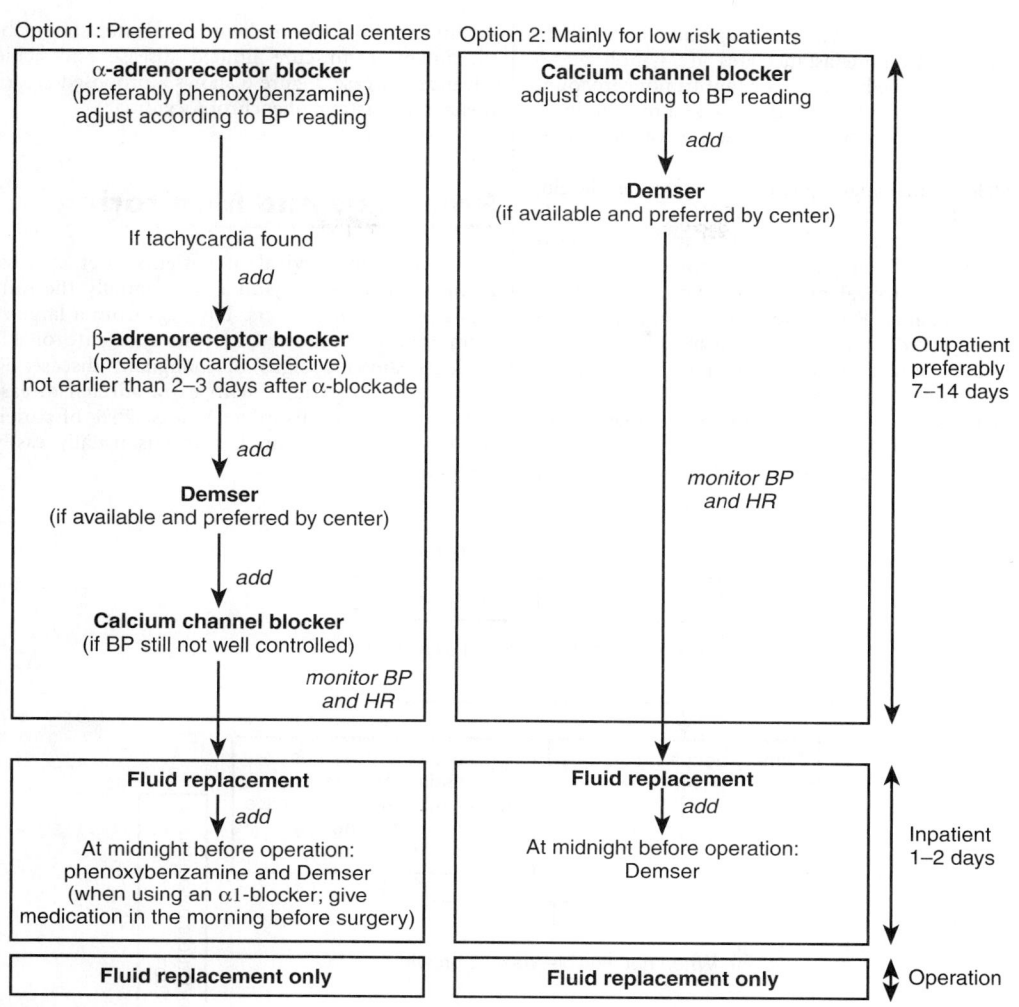

FIGURE 5. Current recommended preoperative treatment algorithms in patients with pheochromocytoma. *Abbreviations:* BP = blood pressure; HR = heart rate. (Adapted from Pacak K: Preoperative management of the pheochromocytoma patient. J Clin Endocrinol Metab 2007;92:4069-4079.)

below 80/45 mm Hg. There should be no more than one ventricular extrasystole every 5 min, and the electrocardiogram (ECG) should show no S-T segment changes and T-wave inversions for at least 1 week. In some cases, Doppler or conventional echocardiography are indicated in addition to ECG to detect the presence of cardiomyopathy or coronary artery disease. In patients with a large left adrenal pheochromocytoma, splenectomy is likely; therefore, vaccination against pneumococcus, *Haemophilus influenzae*, and meningococcus should be given preoperatively.

For most adrenal and extra-adrenal pheochromocytomas, laparoscopy has replaced laparotomy as the procedure of choice because of significant postoperative benefits. To prevent permanent glucocorticoid deficiency in patients with bilateral pheochromocytomas, adrenal cortex–sparing surgery is advocated.

There are multiple hazardous events and situations during surgery, including anesthesia induction, tumor manipulation, hypotension, and hypoglycemia. The treatment of hypotension with pressor agents is not recommended, especially when long-acting β-blockers or metyrosine (Demser) have been used, which paralyze the vascular bed in a dilated state. Instead, volume replacement is the treatment of choice.

Postoperative hypertension can indicate incomplete tumor resection. However, during the first 24 hours after surgery, hypertension is most likely attributed to pain, volume overload, or autonomic instability, all of which are treated symptomatically. If hypertension persists, any attempt to collect specimens for biochemical evidence of incompletely resected tumor should be delayed for at least 5 to 7 days after surgery to ensure that large increases in both plasma and urinary catecholamines produced by surgery have dissipated.

Hypertensive Crisis

The most dangerous complication of pheochromocytoma is the occurrence of a hypertensive crisis. Hypertensive crises can manifest as a severe headache, visual disturbances, acute myocardial infarction, congestive heart failure, or a cerebrovascular accident. It is treated with an intravenous bolus of 5 mg phentolamine (Regitine), a reversible nonselective α-adrenergic antagonist. Phentolamine has a very short half-life, and therefore the same dose can be repeated every 2 minutes until hypertension is adequately controlled. Phentolamine can also be given as a continuous infusion. Continuous intravenous infusion of sodium nitroprusside (Nitropress) or, in some cases, oral or sublingual nifedipine (Procardia)[1] can also be given to control hypertension.

Malignant Pheochromocytoma

Malignant pheochromocytoma is established by the presence of metastases at sites where chromaffin cells are normally absent.

Pheochromocytoma metastasizes via hematogenous or lymphatic routes, and the most common metastatic sites are lymph nodes, bones, lung, and liver. About one half of malignant tumors are found at original presentation, and the other half develop at a median interval of 5.6 years. Based on the localization of the metastatic lesions, there are short-term and long-term survivors.

Up to 80% to 90% of malignant pheochromocytomas develop owing to a germline mutation. Currently, an *SDHB* mutation is the greatest known risk factor for the development of malignant pheochromocytoma. *SDHB*-related malignant pheochromocytoma have been associated with lower survival more than non-*SDHB*–related malignant pheochromocytoma. Except for *SDHB* mutations, no other factors can strongly predict development of metastatic disease.

Successful management of malignant pheochromocytoma requires a multidisciplinary approach, where pharmacologic treatment, targeted radiotherapy, chemotherapy, and surgery can all play a part. Newly discovered, alternative options such as targeted therapies and radiolabeled somatostatin analogues should also be considered.

Treatment should be individualized and should be performed with the intention to cure limited disease and achieve palliation for advanced disease. Figure 6 shows a proposed algorithm for the treatment of metastatic pheochromocytoma.

Prognosis and Monitoring

The long-term survival of patients after successful removal of a benign pheochromocytoma is essentially the same as that of age-adjusted normal subjects. Findings from a large study with a long-term follow-up showed a recurrence rate of 17%, with half the patients showing signs of malignant disease. Recurrences occur more often in patients with extra-adrenal disease and in patients with a hereditary disorder. At least 25% of patients remain hypertensive after treatment, but this is usually easily controlled with medication.

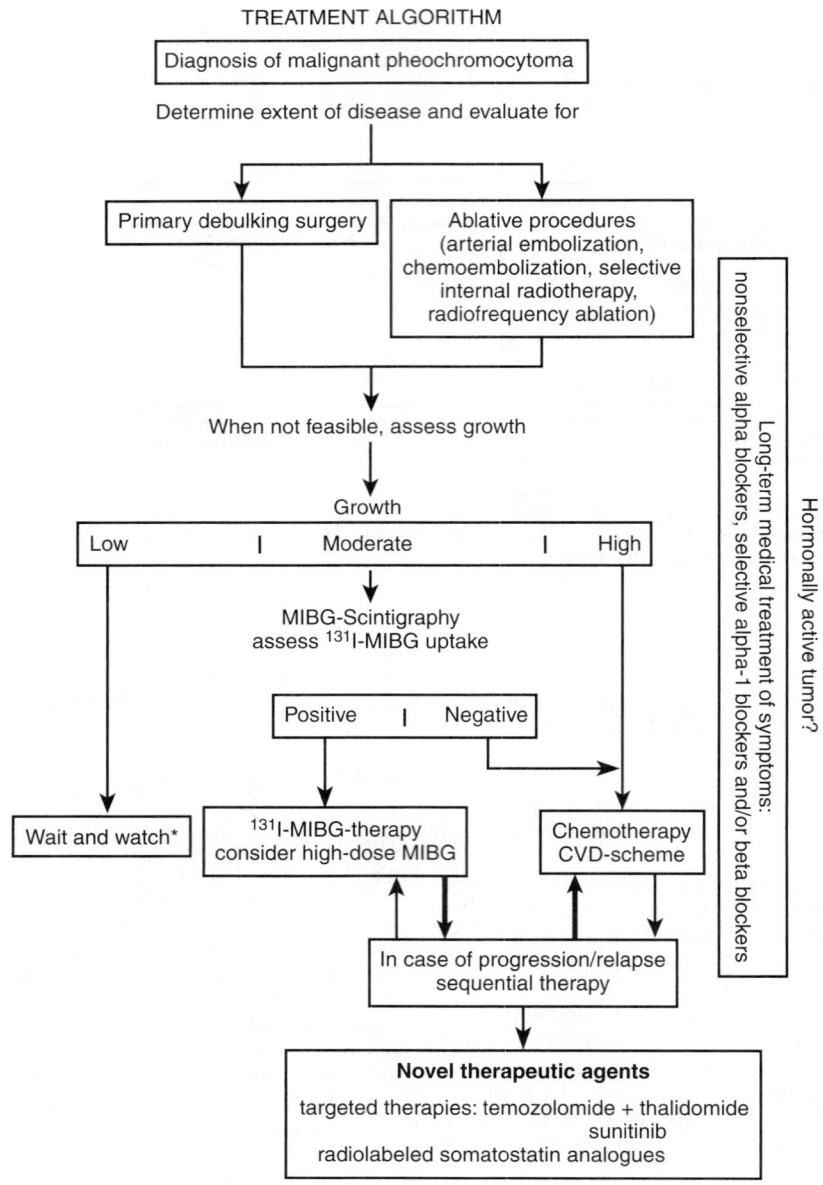

FIGURE 6. Treatment algorithm for metastatic pheochromocytoma. *Asterisk* indicates that the risk of side-effects exceeds the chance of benefit. *Abbreviations:* CVD = cyclophosphamide, vincristine, and dacarbazine [chemotherapy]; MIBG = meta-iodobenzylguanidine. (Adapted from Adjallé R, Plouin PF, Pacak K, Lehnert H: Treatment of malignant pheochromocytoma. Horm Metab Res 2009;41:687-896.)

Clinical follow-up should be lifelong, especially in the case of an underlying hereditary disorder. The frequency of checkups, once a year or more often, and the kind of diagnostic measurements, only biochemical tests or also imaging studies, should depend on the characteristics of the pheochromocytoma. Follow-up must be more intensive in hereditary and malignant pheochromocytoma.

REFERENCES

Adjallé R, Plouin PF, Pacak K, Lehnert H. Treatment of malignant pheochromocytoma. Horm Metab Res 2009;41:687–96.

Amar L, Baudin E, Burnichon N, et al. Succinate dehydrogenase B gene mutations predict survival in patients with malignant pheochromocytomas or paragangliomas. J Clin Endocrinol Metab 2007;92:3822–8.

Bayley JP, Kunst HP. Cascon A, et al: *SDHAF2* mutations in familial and sporadic paraganglioma and phaeochromocytoma. Lancet Oncol 2010;11 (4):366–72.

Baysal BE. Screening: Correlation of genotype and phenotype in paraganglioma. Nat Rev Endocrinol 2009;5:594–5.

Lenders JW, Eisenhofer G, Mannelli M, Pacak K. Phaeochromocytoma. Lancet 2005; 366:665–75.

Mannelli M, Castellano M, Schiavi F, et al. Clinically guided genetic screening in a large cohort of Italian patients with pheochromocytomas and/or functional or nonfunctional paragangliomas. J Clin Endocrinol Metab 2009;94:1541–7.

Neumann HPH, Bausch B. McWhinney, et al: Germ-line mutations in nonsyndromic pheochromocytoma. N Engl J Med 2002;346:1459–66.

Pacak K. Preoperative management of the pheochromocytoma patient. J Clin Endocrinol Metab 2007;92:4069–79.

Pacak K, Eisenhofer G, Ahlman H, et al. Pheochromocytoma: Recommendations for clinical practice from the First International Symposium. Nat Clin Pract Endocrinol Metab 2007;3:92–102.

Pacak K, Eisenhofer G, Goldstein DS. Functional imaging of endocrine tumors: Role of positron emission tomography. Endocr Rev 2004; 25:568–80.

Timmers HJLM, Gimenez-Roqueplo A-P, Mannelli M, Pacak K. Clinical aspects of SDHx-related pheochromocytoma and paraganglioma. Endocr Relat Cancer 2009;16:391–403.

Timmers HJLM, Chen CC, Carrasquillo JA, et al. Comparison of ^{18}F-fluoro-l-dopa, ^{18}F-fluoro-deoxyglucose, and ^{18}F-fluorodopamine PET and ^{123}I-MIBG scintigraphy in the localization of pheochromocytoma and paraganglioma. J Clin Endocrinol Metab 2009;94:4757–67.

Thyroiditis

Method of
Anthony P. Weetman, MD, DSc

Thyroiditis simply means inflammation of the thyroid gland, and it arises from a number of different causes. Clinically these are best classified by the tempo of inflammation: acute, subacute, or chronic. Mild to moderate focal thyroiditis, in which there is a patchy infiltration of the thyroid gland by lymphocytes, is so common (in ~15% of all autopsy specimens) that it has little clinical significance; in only a small fraction of such patients does disease progress to a chronic thyroiditis and destruction of thyroid tissue. Similarly, a focal thyroiditis is often found adjacent to (or even within) benign or malignant neoplasms of thyroid.

Acute Thyroiditis

BACKGROUND

Acute (suppurative) thyroiditis is a rare condition caused by a suppurative infection of the thyroid through the bloodstream, lymphatics, trauma, a persistent thyroglossal duct, or most commonly, extension

CURRENT DIAGNOSIS

- Thyroiditis can be classified as acute, subacute, or chronic, with pain as a hallmark of the first two types.
- Silent thyroiditis occurs after pregnancy or following drug treatment.
- A combination of thyroid function testing and thyroid peroxidase antibody measurement, supplemented by erythrocyte sedimentation rate and thyroid radionuclide uptake is sufficient to establish a diagnosis in most cases.
- Thyrotoxicosis in patients with thyroiditis is transient, and subsequent hypothyroidism should be anticipated.

from nearby infection. The latter typically arises through the piriform sinus, an anomalous remnant of the fourth branchial pouch, usually on the left side. This is the main cause of acute thyroiditis in children and young adults; a long-standing goiter, degeneration in a carcinoma, and immunosuppression are additional risk factors.

Virtually any bacterium can cause acute thyroiditis. The most common are *Staphylococcus aureus*, *Streptococci* species, *Klebsiella pneumoniae*, and *Escherichia coli*. In immunosuppressed patients, including those with AIDS, unusual organisms can invade the thyroid, including *Aspergillus*, *Candida*, and *Coccidioides* species and *Pneumocystis jiroveci*. In rare instances, tuberculosis can affect the thyroid, but the picture then is usually one of subacute thyroiditis.

The dominant clinical features are pain in the thyroid radiating to the ear, tenderness and erythema over the gland, fever, dysphagia, respiratory symptoms, and malaise. Features of septicemia may be present, as may lymphadenopathy and a local thrombophlebitis. The differential diagnosis for thyroid pain includes subacute and, rarely, chronic thyroiditis, hemorrhage into a cyst, and lymphoma. Clinical features help in the diagnosis, and simple investigations usually confirm the clinical suspicion.

TREATMENT

Treatment is with high-dose antibiotics selected on the basis of the microbiology results from fine-needle aspiration biopsy. Surgical drainage of any abscess is indicated when pus cannot be fully removed by aspiration. Complications of acute thyroiditis include tracheal obstruction, retropharyngeal abscess, mediastinitis, and internal jugular venous thrombosis. Any piriform sinus should be located (usually by barium swallow study 2 months after the acute episode) and excised to prevent a recurrence; a thyroid lobectomy is usually needed for this.

Subacute Thyroiditis

BACKGROUND

Subacute thyroiditis (de Quervain's, viral, or granulomatous thyroiditis) has a variable incidence, depending on region. In North America the incidence is 5 cases per 100,000 population per year. It is possible that it is overlooked in areas of apparently low incidence. Three times more women are affected than men, with a median incidence around the age of 45 years, and HLA-B35 is a predisposing genetic factor.

Many viruses have been implicated, especially coxsackievirus, influenza, measles, mumps, and Epstein-Barr virus. There is no need to attempt identification serologically.

The main clinical features are a painful and tender goitrous thyroid with fluctuating thyroid hormone levels. The pain can be in one or both thyroid lobes. Occasionally, a nodular form can be detected on palpation.

Patients usually have a phase of thyrotoxicosis (caused by release of stored hormone from the damaged gland) lasting up to 4 weeks, followed by a phase of hypothyroidism of 1 to 3 months and then recovery. Many patients describe a prodromal phase of systemic upset or upper respiratory tract infection. The diagnosis is confirmed by the high erythrocyte sedimentation rate (ESR) and low isotope uptake.

TREATMENT

Mild cases do not require treatment except analgesics, usually nonsteroidal antiinflammatory drugs. Severe disease (around one third of cases) warrants treatment with prednisolone at a dose of 30 to 40 mg/day initially. Depending on the clinical response and sedimentation rate, this is gradually tapered after 1 to 2 weeks so that steroids are stopped after 4 to 6 weeks. Patients' thyroid function should be monitored closely (every 1 to 2 weeks).

During a phase of symptomatic thyrotoxicosis, propranolol (Inderal),[1] 20 to 40 mg three to four times a day, is useful for controlling the symptoms. Antithyroid drugs (methimazole [Tapazole], propylthiouracil [PTU]) are not effective in this situation. Subsequent symptomatic hypothyroidism is treated with levothyroxine (Synthroid, Levothroid, Levoxyl) 50 to 100 µg/day, but this should be withdrawn after 6 to 8 weeks because the phase is typically transient. However, patients with preexisting thyroid abnormalities can develop permanent hypothyroidism after subacute thyroiditis (5%–10% of cases), and therefore full recovery of thyroid function must be established by testing.

Recurrences occur in around 5% of cases and are dealt with in the same way as the initial attack, although prolonging prednisolone treatment by 2 to 4 weeks may be useful.

Silent Thyroiditis

A similar pattern of subacute thyroid dysfunction without thyroid pain is called _silent thyroiditis_. This has an autoimmune etiology and occurs most distinctly 3 to 6 months after pregnancy in women with thyroid peroxidase antibodies before delivery. Treatment for thyroid dysfunction is again with propranolol for thyrotoxicosis and levothyroxine for the usually transient hypothyroidism; steroids are not needed. Thyroxine treatment is discontinued 1 year after delivery and the TSH is checked after 6 weeks to verify the patient is euthyroid.

Postpartum thyroiditis is a risk factor for the development of future permanent hypothyroidism. Affected women should therefore be screened annually for this and should be warned that the disease may well recur in future pregnancies. The appropriateness of screening all pregnant women for thyroid peroxidase antibodies in the first trimester is not yet clear except in women with type 1 diabetes mellitus, who are at particular risk of developing postpartum thyroiditis. In such women, the presence of thyroid antibodies

_____

before delivery should lead to careful monitoring of postpartum thyroid function.

Chronic (Autoimmune) Thyroiditis

BACKGROUND

Hypothyroidism caused by autoimmunity affects approximately 1% of women and 0.1% of men. However, there is a much higher prevalence of subclinical autoimmune thyroiditis shown by the presence of sustained, elevated circulating thyroid-stimulating hormone (TSH) levels with normal free thyroxine levels, with or without accompanying thyroid peroxidase or thyroglobulin antibodies. This condition often comes to light during screening for nonspecific symptoms such as fatigue or weight gain.

Some patients have a goiter of variable size that is usually hard and often irregular (bosselated); this is Hashimoto's, or goitrous, thyroiditis. At the opposite end of the pathologic spectrum is atrophic thyroiditis or primary myxedema in which the thyroid is replaced by fibrous tissue and the only clinical sign of the destructive process is the development of hypothyroidism. These patients may have antibodies that block the TSH receptor, but these are neither frequent nor unique in atrophic thyroiditis.

TREATMENT

Overt hypothyroidism resulting from chronic thyroiditis is treated with levothyroxine. There is no role normally for thyroid extract or for liothyronine (triiodothyronine, T$_3$) supplementation (Thyrolar, liotrix) or substitution (Cytomel), inasmuch as levothyroxine is converted smoothly and physiologically to T$_3$, whereas the short half-life of liothyronine leads to peaks and troughs of circulating T$_3$. Several recent trials have failed to confirm initially promising results from the addition of triiodothyronine to levothyroxine, and such current formulations of treatment can lead to excessive T$_3$ levels, with the potential for adverse effects on bone and the heart.

In otherwise healthy patients younger than 60 years with overt hypothyroidism, I start levothyroxine at 50 to 100 µg a day, but in those older than 60 years or with ischemic heart disease, the usual starting dose is 12.5 to 25 µg a day, increasing every 2 weeks by 25-µg increments. In all cases, the aim is to normalize the TSH level, although rarely this proves impossible in patients whose angina is worsened by thyroxine replacement. Propranolol[1] or other β-blockers help minimize this adverse effect.

If the TSH is maintained in the reference range, there are no adverse effects. I check TSH levels only 2 to 3 months after changing dose because it can take this length of time for symptoms and TSH levels to normalize. The same applies if the commercial preparation of levothyroxine is changed. Once the desired dose is achieved, TSH levels need to be checked only annually. It is unusual for patients to need more than 200 µg of levothyroxine a day. In my experience an elevated (and usually fluctuating) TSH level in patients taking higher doses usually indicates poor compliance, although malabsorption syndromes and certain drugs—such as colestipol (Colestid), cholestyramine sucralfate (Questran), ferrous sulfate (Feosol), aluminum hydroxide (Amphojel), phenytoin (Dilantin), activated charcoal (CharcoAid), rifampicin (rifampin, Rifadin), and hormone replacement therapy—can interfere with absorption or metabolism.

There is controversy about the optimal management of subclinical hypothyroidism. The risk of progression to overt hypothyroidism is highest in patients with both an elevated TSH and positive thyroid antibodies, and in my view it is worth treating these patients and those whose TSH is higher than 10 mU/L with levothyroxine (usually 25–50 µg initially) from the outset. In those with an elevated TSH but no thyroid antibodies, one option is a 3-month trial of levothyroxine, and if any symptomatic improvement occurs, to continue with this. If there is no improvement or the

_____

patient chooses not to have treatment, an annual check of thyroid function should be arranged to deal with the risk of progression to overt hypothyroidism.

The goiter of Hashimoto's thyroiditis usually shrinks with levothyroxine. Surgery is only rarely needed to control the goiter. Any focal irregularity in the goiter raises the suspicion of malignancy; such hard nodules are sometimes found in Hashimoto's thyroiditis and should be investigated, initially by aspiration biopsy. Pain suggests lymphoma, which is a rare complication of autoimmune thyroiditis. Very rarely is the thyroid tender in uncomplicated Hashimoto's thyroiditis, and this may be associated with an elevated ESR. Corticosteroids may be used but are sometimes unhelpful, and surgery may be needed in extreme cases.

Drug-Induced Thyroiditis

Autoimmune thyroiditis can be precipitated by lithium, excess iodide, or recombinant cytokines such as interferon (IFN)-α, interleukin-2, and granulocyte-macrophage colony-stimulating factor (GM-CSF). Such patients usually have thyroid peroxidase and other thyroid antibodies before treatment, and screening for these, as well as measuring serum TSH, should be undertaken before starting these drugs. Regular monitoring of TSH thereafter is also indicated.

Thyroxine replacement should be given and adjusted to maintain a normal TSH level. Treatment with amiodarone (Cordarone), lithium, and IFN-α can be continued. Amiodarone can cause both hypothyroidism, readily managed by levothyroxine, and thyrotoxicosis, the latter resulting either from a destructive process or from excess iodide supply that precipitates hyperthyroidism. Amiodarone-induced thyrotoxicosis can be very difficult to manage and necessitates specialist advice. Corticosteroids, potassium perchlorate, antithyroid drugs, and even surgery might be needed to control the disease, whereas stopping amiodarone has no immediate impact because of the long half-life of the drug. A painful but transient thyroiditis can occur 1 to 2 weeks after radioiodine for hyperthyroidism. It responds to simple analgesics, or corticosteroids if severe.

Riedel's Thyroiditis

Riedel's thyroiditis is a rare condition of unknown etiology that is caused by fibrosis of the thyroid, leading to a woodlike, hard mass often extending outside the thyroid and involving any of the adjacent structures. There is an association with idiopathic fibrosis elsewhere (retroperitoneum, orbit, mediastinum, biliary tree, lung). The condition is often detected because of suspicion of thyroid malignancy. Aspiration biopsy typically yields no specimen, and diagnosis requires open biopsy. Thyroxine is useful only if there is hypothyroidism, and corticosteroids are ineffective. The condition runs an unpredictable course, with a slow progression in many cases, and surgery should be reserved only for patients with esophageal or tracheal compression. Tamoxifen (Soltamox)[1] treatment 20 mg twice daily has been successful in individual cases; due to the rarity of the disease, there have been no controlled trials of treatment.

---

[1]Not FDA approved for this indication.

REFERENCES

Basaria S, Cooper DS. Amiodarone and the thyroid. Am J Med 2005; 118:706–14.

Escobar-Morreale HF, Botella-Carretero JI, Escobar del Rey F, Morreale de Escobar G. Treatment of hypothyroidism with combinations of levothyroxine plus liothyronine. J Clin Endocrinol Metab 2005;90:4946–54.

Fatourechi V, Aniszewski JP, Fatourechi GZ, et al. Clinical features and outcome of subacute thyroiditis in an incidence cohort: Olmsted County, Minnesota, study. J Clin Endocrinol Metab 2003;88:2100–5.

Jung YJ, Schaub CR, Rhodes R, et al. A case of Riedel's thyroiditis treated with tamoxifen: Another successful outcome. Endocr Pract 2004;10:483–6.

Nicholson WK, Robinson KA, Smallridge RC, et al. Prevalence of postpartum thyroid dysfunction: A quantitative review. Thyroid 2006;16:573–82.

Surks MI, Ortiz E, Daniels GH, et al. Subclinical thyroid disease: Scientific review and guidelines for diagnosis and management. JAMA 2004; 291:228–38.

Weetman AP. The thyroid gland and disorders of thyroid function. In: Warrell DA, Cox TM, Firth JD, Benz EJ, editors. Oxford Textbook of Medicine, vol. 2. Oxford: Oxford University Press; 2003. p. 209–24.

The Urogenital Tract

Bacterial Infections of the Male Urinary Tract

Method of
John N. Krieger, MD

Urinary tract infections (UTIs) include a wide clinical spectrum whose common denominator is bacterial invasion of the genitourinary organs and tissues. Any portion of the urinary tract may be involved from the renal cortex to the urethral meatus. UTI can predominate at a single site, such as the bladder (cystitis), prostate (prostatitis), epididymis (epididymitis), kidneys (pyelonephritis), or perinephric space (perinephric abscess). When any of its parts has become infected, the entire urinary tract is placed at risk for bacterial invasion.

The great majority of UTIs occur by the ascending route. Bacteria from the fecal flora colonize the perineum and then ascend via the urethra to involve the bladder, the ureter, and the kidneys. On occasion, hematogenous dissemination can result in bacterial seeding of the urinary tract. Classic examples of such hematogenous infection are genitourinary tuberculosis or staphylococcal infection of a renal cyst (historically known as a *renal carbuncle*). On rare occasions, the urinary tract may be involved by infection from contiguous structures. For example, patients with diverticulitis or appendicitis occasionally develop abscesses or fistulae that involve the urinary tract.

Distinguishing Complicated from Uncomplicated Infections

The first step in evaluating a patient is to distinguish uncomplicated (medical) infections from complicated (surgical) infections. An uncomplicated UTI occurs in the absence of underlying structural, functional, or neurologic disorders of the urinary tract. Uncomplicated UTIs usually respond promptly to appropriate antimicrobial therapy. Anatomic evaluation and imaging studies are seldom indicated in patients with uncomplicated UTIs.

In contrast, complicated UTIs occur when the urinary tract has been repeatedly invaded by bacteria, leaving residual inflammation or—in cases accompanied by obstruction—stones, foreign bodies, or neurologic conditions that interfere with urinary drainage. Antimicrobial therapy alone is markedly less effective in complicated UTIs than in uncomplicated UTIs. Managing patients with complicated infections often requires anatomic evaluation and imaging studies. An important differential point is that patients with complicated UTIs tend to have persistence of bacteria within the urinary tract in the face of antimicrobial agents to which the bacteria appear to be sensitive in laboratory tests. Often, it is necessary to correct an underlying obstructive lesion or voiding problem to clear the infection.

The ideal goal of UTI therapy is total elimination of the infecting organism from the urinary tract. This is a realistic goal for patients with uncomplicated UTIs. However, achieving this goal can prove difficult in patients with complicated UTIs whose underlying abnormalities cannot be corrected. For example, it is often impossible to achieve long-standing resolution of bacteriuria in patients who require indwelling catheters or who have functional obstruction of their voiding mechanisms. In such cases, resolution of symptoms directly related to UTI is the only practical therapeutic goal.

Natural History

During infancy, the incidence of symptomatic UTIs is higher in boys than in girls. In part, this has been related to male circumcision status. It appears that bacteria can adhere to the prepuce of uncircumcised boys, providing access to the urinary tract. Neonatal circumcision appears to reduce the UTI rate in boys by about 90%. After the neonatal period, symptomatic UTIs in boys and men are distinctly uncommon until middle age. This contrasts dramatically with UTI rates in girls and women, who experience increasing rates of both symptomatic and asymptomatic infections with a marked increase following initiation of sexual activity, then a continued gradual rise with increasing age. Asymptomatic bacteriuria is also distinctly unusual in male patients compared with female patients.

Well-documented UTIs in boys mandate thorough urologic investigation. This is because of the high prevalence of structural urinary tract abnormalities in boys with UTIs. Often, UTI represents the key diagnostic presentation for major abnormalities of the urinary tract. For example, vesicoureteral reflux of urine, posterior urethral valves, and other major structural abnormalities often manifest initially with bacterial UTIs. Early diagnosis and appropriate therapy offer the best chance for preservation of maximal renal function. Unfortunately, the developing kidneys are very susceptible to continued renal scarring, which may be progressive despite appropriate treatment.

Structural urinary tract abnormalities remain a major cause of renal failure in children. Morbidity may be minimized by appropriate evaluation and therapy. The traditional choice for evaluation of a boy with a urinary tract infection is the combination of renal ultrasound to evaluate the upper urinary tract plus a voiding cystourethrogram to evaluate the lower urinary tract. Voiding cystourethrography should be obtained after resolution of the initial infection, because dilation of the upper urinary tract may be exaggerated after a recent UTI. More recent data suggest that a nuclear medicine scan is an attractive and accurate initial evaluation.

Because UTIs are unusual in young men, there are few well-done natural history studies in this population. In young men with UTIs who have no obvious neurologic or structural abnormalities, sexual intercourse, particularly among homosexual men or heterosexual men who practice insertive anal intercourse, may be a risk factor. The overall contribution of these practices to bacterial UTIs in men is uncertain.

Traditional urologic teaching is to carry out a thorough evaluation for structural abnormalities in such patients, including radiographic studies and cystourethroscopy. However, our published experience suggests that previously healthy college-age men with well-documented UTIs have a low rate of structural genitourinary tract abnormalities. A uroflow study and postvoid residual urine determination by ultrasound are adequate to screen for structural abnormalities in young men whose UTIs resolve. We reserve cystoscopy for patients whom we determine to be at risk for significant abnormalities on the basis of these screening studies and a thorough physical examination. The other major risk factors for UTIs in men are instrumentation of the urinary tract and bacterial prostatitis.

Diagnosis and Localization

Accurate diagnosis is prerequisite for appropriate UTI therapy. Therefore, we recommend culture and sensitivity testing of urine specimens from any male patient with symptoms or signs suggesting a UTI. In patients who do not have obstructive lesions, stasis, stones, or foreign bodies, recurrent and persistent bacterial UTIs are often related to bacterial prostatitis. Segmented localization cultures can be used to differentiate cystitis and urethritis from bacterial prostatitis. The procedure should be carried out at a time when the patient does not have bacteriuria.

My procedure for lower urinary tract localization is outlined briefly. After cleaning the glans with sterile water, the first-void urine (initial 5–10 mL of voided urine) is collected in a sterile container. Next, a midstream specimen is obtained. The patient is asked to stop voiding. Prostatic fluid is expressed by digital rectal prostate massage. The post–prostate massage urine (next 5–10 mL voided after the massage) is then collected. Culture and sensitivity testing are then carried out on each of these four specimens. It is critical to ensure that the clinical microbiology laboratory is aware of the purpose of these studies so that they will evaluate low concentrations of uropathogens that may be present in the localization cultures.

Diagnosis of chronic bacterial prostatitis can be made if the post–prostate massage urine specimen or the expressed prostatic secretion contains a 10-fold or greater increase in the concentration of the uropathogen compared with that in the first-void urine specimen. In patients with well-documented bacterial prostatitis, the causative organism is identical to the uropathogen causing recurrent UTI episodes.

It is important to recognize that only a small minority of men presenting with symptoms of prostatitis fit into the acute or chronic bacterial prostatitis categories. The great majority of patients with symptoms of prostatitis are classified in the chronic prostatitis/chronic pelvic pain category. In contrast to the recognized benefit of therapy for patients with acute and chronic bacterial prostatitis, the role of antimicrobial therapy and other treatments has not been defined for men with symptoms of chronic prostatitis/chronic pelvic pain syndrome.

Treatment

There are three keys to successful UTI therapy. First, eliminate or control predisposing factors, if possible. For example, we are often asked to manage resistant urinary infections in long-term care patients with indwelling catheters. One approach is to change their bladder management from a chronic indwelling catheter to an intermittent self- or assisted-catheterization program. Other examples include removal or correction of obstructing lesions, stones, or strictures to improve drainage of the urinary tract. These measures may be successful in eliminating the focus of infection, even with no antimicrobial therapy. Second, eradicate the infection as soon as possible to prevent colonization of the prostate and other structures. Third, ensure resolution of the UTI by obtaining cultures during or immediately after therapy and at follow-up 1 to 2 months after therapy.

UNCOMPLICATED INFECTIONS

Uncomplicated infections generally manifest with symptoms of bacterial cystitis, such as the combination of urinary frequency, urgency, dysuria, nocturia, suprapubic discomfort, low-back pain, or hematuria. Systemic symptoms of fever, chills, and rigor are absent. Urine culture confirms the diagnosis, with *Escherichia coli* being the most common pathogen. Uncomplicated infections, including those introduced by a single or short course of indwelling urethral catheterization, generally respond promptly to a short course of antimicrobial therapy. The infection can persist and become difficult to eradicate if the prostate becomes colonized or if the patient has a stone or structural abnormality of the urinary tract. Thus, an effort should be made to eliminate predisposing factors while routine therapy is guided by in vitro susceptibility tests.

I prefer oral therapy with one of the agents listed in Table 1. In the Pacific northwest, bacteria causing urinary tract infections have developed substantial resistance to trimethoprim-sulfamethoxazole (Bactrim). Therefore, I usually initiate empiric therapy with a quinolone. Nitrofurantoin (Macrodantin) remains highly effective and is an attractive alternative drug. In general, I recommend that the duration of therapy be at least 2 weeks, although only limited data address this point in male patients.

 CURRENT DIAGNOSIS

- UTIs include a wide clinical spectrum.
- Infection at any site in the urinary tract places the entire system at risk.
- The critical clinical issue is to distinguish uncomplicated (medical) from complicated (surgical) infections.
- Anatomic evaluation and imaging studies are seldom indicated for patients with uncomplicated UTIs.
- Well-documented UTIs in boys require thorough urologic investigation because of the high prevalence of structural urinary tract abnormalities.
- We recommend culture and sensitivity testing of urine specimens for any male patient with symptoms or signs suggesting a UTI.
- In contrast, we discourage routine screening urine cultures in long-term care patients who have no localizing signs or symptoms suggesting a UTI.

UTI = urinary tract infection.

CURRENT THERAPY

- The optimal goal of therapy is to eliminate the infecting organism from the urinary tract.
- Antimicrobial therapy alone is less effective for patients with complicated UTIs than for patients with uncomplicated UTIs.
- Managing patients with complicated UTIs often requires anatomic evaluation and imaging studies.
- For patients with complicated UTIs it is often necessary to eliminate or control predisposing factors.
- Rapid eradication of the infection can limit the potential for infection of adjacent structures.
- Ensure elimination of the infection by repeating urine cultures.
- A prolonged course of antimicrobial therapy may prove necessary for patients with persistent infections.

UTI = urinary tract infection.

TABLE 1 Oral Antimicrobial Agents Prescribed for Urinary Tract Infections In Men

Agent	Dosage
Fluoroquinolones	
Ciprofloxacin (Cipro)	250–500 mg bid
Ciprofloxacin (CiproXR)	500–1000 mg qd
Lomefloxacin (Maxaquin)*	400 mg qd
Levofloxacin (Levaquin LEVA-pak)	500–750 mg qd
Ofloxacin (Floxin)	200–400 mg bid[3]
Norfloxacin (Noroxin)	400 mg bid
Combination Agents	
Trimethoprim-sulfamethoxazole (Bactrim, Septra, Bactrim DS, Septra DS)	160 mg trimethoprim, 800 mg sulfamethoxazole bid
Amoxicillin-clavulanate (Augmentin)	500–875 mg amoxicillin, 125 mg clavulanate bid
Other Antimicrobials	
Nitrofurantoin (Macrobid)	100 mg bid
Nitrofurantoin (Macrodantin)	50–100 mg qid

[3]Exceeds dosage recommended by the manufacturer.
*Discontinued in the United States.

COMPLICATED INFECTIONS

Patients with systemic signs or those with a history of structural or neurologic abnormalities merit anatomic and functional investigation of the urinary tract. Antimicrobial therapy alone might fail to cure infection and urosepsis can develop unless there is specific management of the underlying problem. My initial choice for evaluating these patients is either computed tomography (CT) with contrast or an excretory urogram with postvoid film. If a renal or retroperitoneal abscess is suspected, computed tomographic scanning has proved superior to the other modalities for diagnosis. In contrast, I prefer transrectal ultrasound for evaluation of possible prostatic abscesses.

Prolonged courses of therapy are indicated for patients with persistent infections. Often, I have used 3 to 4 months of therapy in this situation. In patients with chronic bacterial prostatitis, elderly patients, or those in nursing homes, continuous therapy may be necessary to suppress bacteriuria, even though eradication can prove impossible. Thus, for patients with recurrent or complicated infections, I recommend an attempt to eradicate the focus of infection, following thorough evaluation of the urinary tract. The therapy is usually with the drugs listed in Table 1. My first choice for curative therapy is usually a quinolone. For patients with persistent or frequently relapsing infections, I consider long-term therapy (months or years) using low dosages of antimicrobial drugs for prophylaxis or suppression. In this situation, my choice is usually either trimethoprim-sulfamethoxazole (Bactrim) or nitrofurantoin (Macrodantin).

PROSTATITIS

Acute and chronic bacterial prostatitis can manifest with local urinary tract symptoms characteristic of bacterial cystitis or with systemic signs and symptoms. Acute bacterial prostatitis can manifest with the sudden onset of chills, fever, malaise, and low back and perineal pain, as well as difficulty with urination. On rectal examination, the prostate is tense and exquisitely tender. Excessive palpation can induce septicemia.

For patients who require hospitalization, my initial choice is the combination of a β-lactam drug and an aminoglycoside until the results of antimicrobial sensitivity testing are available. Following parenteral therapy, the patient is managed with continued antimicrobial therapy for at least 4 weeks, usually employing a quinolone. Patients with acute bacterial prostatitis usually respond well to a variety of antimicrobial agents that penetrate an acutely inflamed prostate. Many of these agents are not effective in chronic bacterial prostatitis.

In contrast to acute bacterial prostatitis, chronic bacterial prostatitis is often insidious in onset. Patients usually have recurrent symptomatic UTIs and, sometimes, recurrent episodes of acute prostatitis. Between symptomatic episodes, patients may be totally asymptomatic. Diagnosis depends on the localization cultures described earlier. Treatment must be prolonged, because diffusion of many antimicrobial agents into the uninflamed prostate is poor.

My initial choice is usually a quinolone, with trimethoprim-sulfamethoxazole (Septra, Bactrim) as a second-choice agent. Carbenicillin indanyl sodium (Geocillin) is also approved for this indication, but it has not been particularly effective in my hands.

It is important to avoid confusing bacterial prostatitis with chronic prostatitis/chronic pelvic pain syndrome. This is the most common category of symptomatic prostatitis. A critical distinguishing point is that patients with chronic prostatitis/chronic pelvic pain syndrome do not have bacteriuria and they have negative bacterial localization cultures.

LONG-TERM CARE PATIENTS

My approach to managing UTI differs in long-term care patients, including those with incontinence and indwelling urinary catheters or other devices. In such patients, chronic asymptomatic bacterial colonization should not be treated. It is impossible to sterilize the urine permanently in such men. Furthermore, resistant organisms will likely emerge, making subsequent therapy difficult. I treat such patients only if they develop acute symptoms referable to the urinary tract or before genitourinary tract procedures. I strongly recommend against obtaining screening cultures in long-term care patients because these cultures often lead to unnecessary therapy that selects resistant bacterial flora. Further, there is evidence that bacterial colonization with relatively benign strains can inhibit establishment of symptomatic infections caused by more virulent bacteria.

REFERENCES

Abarbanel J, Engelstein D, Lask D, et al. Urinary tract infection in men younger than 45 years of age: Is there a need for urologic investigation? Urology 2003;62:27–9.

Andrews SJ, Brooks PT, Hanbury DC, et al. Ultrasonography and abdominal radiography versus intravenous urography in investigation of urinary tract infection in men: Prospective incident cohort study. BMJ 2002; 324:454–6.

Bjerklund Johansen T. Diagnosis and imaging in urinary tract infections. Curr Opin Urol 2002;12:39–43.

Craig JC, Knight JF, Sureshkumar P, et al. Effect of circumcision on incidence of urinary tract infection in preschool boys. J Pediatr 1996;128:23–7.

Griebling TL. Urologic diseases in America project: Trends in resource use for urinary tract infections in men. J Urol 2005;173:1288–94.

Hummers-Pradier E, Ohse AM, Koch M, et al. Urinary tract infection in men. Int J Clin Pharmacol Ther 2004;42:360–6.

Johansen TE. The role of imaging in urinary tract infections. World J Urol 2004;22:392–8.

Krieger JN, Nyberg L, Nickel JC. NIH consensus definition and classification of prostatitis. JAMA 1999;282:236–7.

Krieger JN, Ross SO, Simonsen JM. Urinary tract infections in healthy university men. J Urol 1993;149:1046–8.

Naber KG. Levofloxacin in the treatment of urinary tract infections and prostatitis. J Chemother 2004;16(Suppl. 2):18–21.

Nicolle LE SHEA Long-Term-Care Committee. Urinary tract infections in long-term-care facilities. Infect Control Hosp Epidemiol 2001;22:167–75.

Sunden F, Hakansson L, Ljunggren E, et al. Bacterial interference—is deliberate colonization with Escherichia coli 83972 an alternative treatment for patients with recurrent urinary tract infection? Int J Antimicrob Agents 28 Suppl 2006;1:S26–9.

Ulleryd P, Zackrisson B, Aus G, et al. Selective urological evaluation in men with febrile urinary tract infection. BJU Int 2001;88:15–20.

Wagenlehner FM, Naber KG. Current challenges in the treatment of complicated urinary tract infections and prostatitis. Clin Microbiol Infect 2006;12(Suppl 3):67–80.

Urinary Tract Infections in Women

Method of
Burke A. Cunha, MD

General Concepts

Urinary tract infections (UTIs) are common in adult women. The two major clinical manifestations of UTIs in adult women are cystitis or pyelonephritis. Young adult women may also present with so-called dysuria pyuria syndrome (abacteriuric cystitis), previously known as acute urethral syndrome, as outpatients. Hospitalized compromised female hosts with cystitis may be complicated by bacteremia or ascending infection. Renal abscess may complicate pyelonephritis in normal or compromised female hosts.

Cystitis Versus Pyelonephritis

The therapeutic approach to UTIs in adult women depends on accurate localization of the site of infection in the urinary tract. The most common clinical problem is differentiating cystitis from pyelonephritis. Patients with acute bacterial cystitis present with dysuria and frequency, which may or may not be accompanied by suprapubic discomfort or lower back pain. The fever accompanying cystitis is ≤ to 38.9°C (102°F) and is not usually associated with chills. The clinical manifestation of cystitis is confirmed by finding pyuria and significant bacteriuria, (i.e., $\geq 10^6$ CFU/mL) in such patients. The urinalysis in acute cystitis is not usually accompanied by microscopic hematuria.

Staphylococcus saprophyticus is the only uropathogen in the ambulatory setting that is responsible for the majority of cases of UTIs accompanied by microscopic hematuria. Microscopic hematuria in a urinalysis in a patient with an apparent UTI should be carefully observed and should disappear after therapy of the UTI. If the microscopic hematuria disappears, then the physician can safely assume it was related to the UTI. Particularly in elderly patients, if the microscopic hematuria persists after eradication of the UTI, then the patient should be investigated for a bladder or renal source of the microscopic hematuria.

Dysuria-Pyuria Syndrome

In sexually active young women, dysuria-pyuria syndrome manifests with the symptoms of cystitis but with negative urine cultures, or if organisms are cultured, they are present in low numbers (i.e., *E. coli*) ($\leq 10^3$ CFU/mL). Most cases of dysuria-pyuria syndrome are caused by *Chlamydia trachomatis*. In patients with dysuria-pyuria syndrome, if the urine is cultured for *Chlamydia*, cultures are frequently positive.

Catheter-Associated Bacteriuria (CAB)

Hospitalized patients with indwelling Foley catheters often acquire bacteriuria as a function of time that the Foley catheter is in place. Pyuria is often in the urine of patients with indwelling Foleys because the catheter elicits inflammation of the urinary tract. The presence of pyuria and bacteriuria in a patient with an indwelling Foley suggests either UTI or CAB. The majority of such patients are asymptomatic and afebrile. More than 95% of the time these patients have colonization of the urinary tract without infection. The urinalysis in patients with indwelling Foley catheters is helpful if either bacteria without pyuria or pyuria without bacteria is demonstrated. Bacteriuria without pyuria signifies colonization of the urinary tract, whereas pyuria without bacteriuria indicates inflammation of the urinary tract. In non–Foley catheter patients, the presence of pyuria plus significant bacteriuria is diagnostic of a UTI. This is not the case with CAB. In normal hosts with a Foley catheter, CAB, i.e., bacteriuria plus pyuria, represents colonization and not a UTI.

Benign Bacteriuria of the Elderly

In elderly female patients, varying degrees of relaxation of the pelvic musculature are common. Patients often have varying degrees of cystocele of rectocele, which changes anatomic relationship and the angularity of the urethra as it enters the bladder and predisposes to colonization of the bladder urine by the introital flora, such as coliform flora derived from the colon. For this reason, elderly female patients often have bacteriuria with few or no symptoms of a UTI. The presence of bacteriuria/pyuria is often discovered on a routine urinalysis obtained as part of either admission laboratory work or an outpatient workup/screening test battery. The presence of bacteriuria/pyuria in an elderly female patient without underlying genitourinary (GU) disease or impaired host defenses has been appropriately termed *benign bacteriuria of the elderly*, it has been shown that these patients do not go on to have symptomatic UTIs, ascending infection (e.g., pyelonephritis/renal abscess), or bacteremia from the urinary tract.

Recurrent Urinary Tract Infections: Reinfection Versus Relapse

Most UTIs in women are acute. CAB is often incorrectly considered a chronic UTI because in most cases it represents colonization rather than infection. Recurrent UTIs are chronic in the sense that they persist over a long period of time, but are really episodic infections. However, the approach to recurrent UTIs is based on determining whether the recurrence is on the basis of reinfection or relapse. The reinfection variety of recurrent UTIs is defined as a recurrent UTI because of different organisms being cultured during each UTI episode. The relapse form of recurrent UTIs is defined as demonstrating the same organism during repeated bouts of UTIs. The reinfection form of recurrent UTIs is usually because of rapid colonization of the vaginal introitus/entry into the urethra, usually following sexual intercourse. The relapse variety of recurrent UTI by the same organism recovered during each episode suggests an underlying structural abnormality of the GU tract. The correct diagnostic approach to recurrent UTIs because of relapse is a thorough investigation of the GU tract from the urethra to the kidneys, which determines a possible source for the focus for the organisms to periodically reappear as a relapsing UTI. Relapse UTIs cannot be successfully approached therapeutically without correcting the underlying condition predisposing to relapse (i.e., bladder calculi, kinked ureters, renal stones, renal abscesses).

Acute Pyelonephritis

Acute pyelonephritis is most common in pregnancy and as a complication of an ascending infection from cystitis/GU instrumentation. An acute episode of pyelonephritis may occur in patients who have chronic pyelonephritis; the acute episode is superimposed on the chronic condition. Renal abscess may complicate acute and chronic pyelonephritis. Renal cortical abscesses are often caused by gram-positive cocci (e.g., staphylococci acquired hematogenously), whereas medullary abscesses are usually caused by aerobic gram-negative bacilli (e.g., coliforms or enterococci).

Acute pyelonephritis may be differentiated from cystitis by the presence of unilateral costovertebral angle (CVA) tenderness (otherwise unexplainable) and a temperature of ≥38.9°C (102°F). Bilateral pyelonephritis is unusual, and the presence of bilateral CVA tenderness should suggest an alternative diagnosis. Pyelonephritis is often bilateral pathologically, but clinically it is almost always unilateral in its presentation with CVA tenderness. The urinalysis in pyelonephritis is the same as in cystitis, for example with significant pyuria/bacteriuria in addition to the findings suggestive of pyelonephritis. The clinical presentation of renal abscess may resemble pyelonephritis if CVA tenderness is present, but this is not an invariable finding. The urinalysis in renal abscess may reveal pyuria and bacteria if the abscess is medullary but only pyuria if the renal abscess is cortical. Renal imaging studies are usually unnecessary in cystitis or pyelonephritis. If there is confusion regarding the presence or absence of chronic pyelonephritis, then a computed tomography/magnetic resonance imaging (CT/MRI) scan of the abdomen or renal ultrasound is appropriate.

Chronic Pyelonephritis

Chronic pyelonephritis results in shrunken and distorted kidneys with a distorted collecting system. If the patient presents with *chronic pyelonephritis* and has kidneys of normal or large size, then an alternate explanation should be sought. The only way to diagnose a renal abscess with certainty is with renal imaging studies. For this purpose, the CT/MRI of the kidneys is vastly superior in picking up small lesions than is the renal ultrasound. For the purposes of excluding a renal abscess, a negative renal ultrasound should never be used to rule out the diagnosis. A negative renal ultrasound should always be followed with a renal CT/MRI of the kidneys if a renal abscess is in the differential diagnosis.

CURRENT DIAGNOSIS

- Acute uncomplicated cystitis is the most common type of UTI in adult women.
- The initial peak incidence of cystitis occurs with sexual intercourse and gradually increases through adulthood.
- Cystitis may occur as a single event or may be recurrent because of reinfection or relapse.
- Cystitis is usually caused by coliform or enterococci from the fecal flora or by *Staphylococcus saprophyticus* from the skin flora.
- Clinically, cystitis is marked by low-grade fever (≤38.9°C [102°F]) with lower abdominal/suprapubic discomfort, and/or dysuria.
- *Staphylococcus aureus*, *Streptococcus pneumoniae*, groups A, C, G streptococci, and *Bacteroides fragilis* are not uropathogens in cystitis.
- In elderly women, *cystitis* manifests as pyuria and bacterluria without fever or dysuria, which is termed *benign bacteriuria of the elderly*.
- A variant of cystitis, the so-called *dysuria/pyuria syndrome*, is also known as *abacteriuric cystitis*.
- Dysuria/pyuria syndrome, most common in young adult women, manifests as cystitis, but urine cultures are negative for bacteria or uropathogens such as *Escherichia coli* are present in low numbers. *Chlamydia trachomatis* is frequently isolated if the urine is cultured for *Chlamydia*.
- Pyelonephritis in women may occur as an uncommon complication of cystitis or during pregnancy.
- It is not possible to predict the uropathogen of cystitis from clinical features except for *S. saprophyticus*.
- *S. saprophyticus* cystitis is characterized by a fishy urine odor, microscopic hematuria, and an alkaline urinary pH.
- Cystitis with alkaline urine suggests infection secondary to *S. saprophyticus*, *Ureaplasma urealyticum*, or a struvite stone with associated infection caused by a urea-splitting organism such as *Proteus*.
- Microscopic hematuria is common with *S. saprophyticus* cystitis but is uncommon with other uropathogens. If a patient with cystitis and microscopic hematuria fails to promptly resolve with antimicrobial therapy, work up the patient for a bladder/renal neoplasm or renal TB.
- The diagnosis of cystitis in women is made by demonstrating pyuria and significant bacteriuria (≥10^6 col/mL) in the setting of cystitis symptoms.
- Cystitis symptoms with gross hematuria should suggest a viral hemorrhagic cystitis or a renal lesion.
- Pyuria without bacteriuria indicates urinary tract inflammation. Persistent pyuria without bacteriuria should suggest interstitial cystitis or renal TB.
- With cystitis, the specific gravity of the urine is not decreased in contrast to pyelonephritis where the specific gravity is decreased.
- Urinary concentration returns to normal with treatment in pyelonephritis.
- Pyelonephritis may be differentiated from cystitis by the presence of fever ≥38.9°C (102°F) and otherwise unexplained unilateral CVA tenderness.
- The urine analysis/culture findings in pyelonephritis and cystitis are the same. Bacteremia frequently occurs with pyelonephritis but is not a feature of cystitis in normal hosts.
- Nonleukopenic compromised hosts, such as diabetes mellitus, systemic lupus erythematosus, multiple myeloma, cirrhosis, and so on, with cystitis may be complicated by pyelonephritis or bacteremia.
- Pyelonephritis is caused by the same uropathogens that cause cystitis; however, *S. saprophyticus* occurs only in cystitis.
- Acute pyelonephritis clinically improves unless complicated by renal abscess.
- Clinically, pyelonephritis is almost always unilateral, but pathophysical findings may be bilateral.
- Bilateral CVA tenderness should suggest an alternate diagnosis.
- In pyelonephritis, radiologic studies typically show unilateral renal involvement characterized by cortical scarring, medullary abnormalities, and renal shrinkage.
- Bilateral, normal-sized, or enlarged kidneys should suggest an alternate diagnosis to pyelonephritis.

Abbreviations: CVA = costovertebral angle; TB = tuberculosis; UTI = urinary tract infection.

CURRENT THERAPY

- Virtually all cases of initial uncomplicated cystitis will resolve spontaneously with or without treatment. No urine analysis/culture is needed with the initial episode of cystitis.
- For the dysuria of cystitis, phenazopyridine (Pyridium), which has no antibacterial properties but relieves pain and relative urinary obstruction from muscle spasm, may be used. Relief of spasm promptly clears the bacteriuria.
- Recurrent cystitis of the reinfection variety is because of different uropathogens with each episode that the urine is cultured. Reinfection is related to vaginal introital colonization following sexual intercourse and may be treated with a postcoital/HS of an appropriate antibiotic.
- Although the initial attack of cystitis resolves in virtually all patients without treatment, those who prefer to treat may use single-dose therapy with nitrofurantoin (Macrodantin), TMP-SMX (Bactrim), or amoxicillin (Amoxil).
- Cystitis in a nonleukopenic compromised host (discussed previously) should be treated for 1 to 2 weeks to prevent bacteremia/ascending infection, such as pyelonephritis/renal abscess.
- Ampicillin should be avoided because of its high resistance potential. Amoxicillin should be used instead, which has not been associated with resistance and is effective against the common coliforms and enterococci (*Enterococcus faecalis*).
- Nitrofurantoin has no resistance potential, is effective against all common uropathogens and all enterococci, such as *E. faecalis* (non-VRE) and *Enterococcus faecium*

(VRE). Nitrofurantoin (Macrodantin) is useful in cystitis or catheter-associated bacteremia but is not to be used in pyelonephritis/bacteremia.
- Recurrent UTI of the relapse variety is caused by the same uropathogen with each occurrence. The problem in relapse UTIs is not therapeutic but diagnostic. Relapsing UTIs have an underlying structural abnormality or ureteral shunts that do not permit antimicrobial therapy to be effective.
- The treatment of pyelonephritis is with IV or PO antibiotics, depending on the severity of the clinical manifestation. Treatment is for 2 to 4 weeks with an effective antibiotic.
- For pyelonephritis, parenteral agents useful against coliforms are cephalosporins, aztreonam (Azactam), aminoglycosides, TMP-SMZ (Bactrim), or renally eliminated quinolones. Against enterococci (most of which are non-VRE), parenteral ampicillin, antipseudomonal penicillins, and meropenem (Merrem) are useful.
- Oral antibiotics useful against coliform causes of pyelonephritis include renally eliminated quinolones, amoxicillin (Amoxil), antipseudomonal penicillins, or TMP-SMZ (Bactrim).
- Linezolid (Zyvox) may be used for pyelonephritis caused by enterococci (non-VRE), amoxicillin (Amoxil), or for VRE.
- Patients with acute pyelonephritis become afebrile/nearly afebrile within 72 hours with or without treatment. Persistence of high fevers for greater than 72 hours should be considered as representing a renal abscess until proved otherwise.

Abbreviations: HD = half dose; IM = intramuscular; IV = intravenous; TMP-SMZ = trimethoprim-sulfamethoxazole; UTI = urinary tract infection; VRE = vancomycin-resistant *Enterococcus*.

Therapeutic Considerations

ACUTE CYSTITIS

The initial episode of acute complicated cystitis in a normal host without GU abnormalities/preexisting renal disease need not be treated with antimicrobial therapy. Usually treatment with phenazopyridine (Pyridium), which has no antibacterial effect, is sufficient to relieve bladder spasm and the relative urine obstruction because of the bladder spasm, and the bacteria will spontaneously clear itself without antimicrobial therapy. Repeated episodes of acute cystitis should have appropriate diagnostic studies, for example, a urinalysis and urinary culture with sensitivities with each episode to differentiate reinfection from relapse. If cystitis occurs in a nonleukopenic compromised host (e.g., with diabetes mellitus, systemic lupus erythematosus, multiple myeloma, cirrhosis, etc.), then a 7-day course of therapy is recommended with an oral agent such as nitrofurantoin (Macrodantin), trimethoprim-sulfamethoxazole (TMP-SMX) (Bactrim), fosfomycin (Monurol), or amoxicillin (Amoxil). Ampicillin should be avoided because of its resistance potential with coliform bacteria.

DYSURIA-PYURIA SYNDROME

The dysuria-pyuria syndrome because of *Chlamydia* should be treated with a 2-week course of doxycycline (Vibramycin). Patients unable to tolerate doxycycline (Vibramycin) may be treated with a

macrolide for the same period of time. A grossly hemorrhagic cystitis suggests a viral etiology for which no specific therapy is available. Patients with cystitis and microscopic hematuria are often infected with *S. saprophyticus*.

Fortunately, *S. saprophyticus* is susceptible to a wide range of antibiotics and virtually any agent selected to treat a UTI will be effective. Antimicrobial resistance has not been a problem in *S. saprophyticus* UTIs. Chronic interstitial cystitis is not an infectious disorder and therefore antimicrobial therapy is unnecessary.

CATHETER-ASSOCIATED BACTERIURIA

CAB in hospitalized patients who are normal hosts without structural abnormalities need not be treated, because virtually all of these patients are colonized and not infected. CAB in nonleukopenic compromised hosts (with diabetes mellitus, systemic lupus erythematosus, multiple myeloma, cirrhosis, and so forth), should be treated to prevent ascending infection/bacteremia from the lower urinary tract. Such individuals should be treated with an oral agent such as amoxicillin (Amoxil), nitrofurantoin (Macrodantin), or TMP-SMX (Bactrim) for 1 to 2 weeks.

Nonleukopenic compromised hosts with enterococci CAB are best treated with oral nitrofurantoin (Macrodantin), which is effective against enterococcal strains such as *E. faecalis* (non-vancomycin-resistant *Enterococcus* [non-VRE]) as well as *E. faecium* [VRE]). *Enterococcus faecalis* strains may also be treated with oral amoxicillin (Amoxil). These instances represent prophylaxis/early therapy because the majority of patients who are nonleukopenic-compromised hosts will have colonization of the urinary tract prior to catheterization or rapidly develop it soon thereafter. Therefore, prevention of ascending infection/bacteremia is the primary aim of therapy in patients with CAB who are compromised on the basis of their host defenses or GU tract abnormalities (e.g., ureteral stents).

ACUTE PYELONEPHRITIS

Acute pyelonephritis may be caused by aerobic gram-negative bacilli, such as coliforms or enterococci (almost always *E. faecalis*). The empirical treatment of pyelonephritis is based on a Gram stain of the urine, which, if the diagnosis is pyelonephritis, will show significant pyuria and a single predominant organism. In a patient with presumed pyelonephritis, the absence of bacteria in the Gram stain of the urine in an acutely ill patient essentially eliminates the diagnosis of pyelonephritis from further consideration, and an alternate explanation for the patient's fever and CVA tenderness should be sought (e.g., renal imaging studies).

Because acute pyelonephritis is often accompanied by bacteremia (urosepsis), parenteral agents may be used initially followed by oral agents; or in mild-to-moderate cases, oral agents may be used for the entire course of therapy. The parenteral agents useful in the treatment of acute pyelonephritis because of aerobic gram-negative bacilli include aminoglycosides, aztreonam (Azactam), antipseudomonal penicillin (e.g., ticarcillin [Ticar]), piperacillin (Pipracil), or a renally excreted respiratory quinolone. Patients presenting with acute pyelonephritis, who have streptococci in the Gram stain of the urine indicating enterococci, may be treated empirically with ampicillin and antipseudomonal penicillin, ticarcillin (Ticar), piperacillin (Pipracil), or meropenem (Merrem). In the rare instance where there is enterococcal urosepsis complicating acute pyelonephritis because of VRE, then linezolid (Zyvox), quinupristin-dalfopristin (Synercid), or daptomycin (Cubicin) may be used. In patients presenting with acute pyelonephritis where a Gram stain is unobtainable or unavailable, then empirical coverage for both aerobic gram-negative bacilli and enterococci (*E. faecalis*), may be achieved with antipseudomonal penicillins, nonrenally eliminated respiratory quinolones, or meropenem (Merrem). After the organism responsible for the pyelonephritis is subsequently identified by urine/blood culture, then the patient may be switched to one of the agents mentioned. Similarly, if the patient is shown to have enterococci as the cause of the urosepsis, it may be treated initially as non-VRE, as indicated previously in the article. Patients with pyelonephritis are usually treated for 1 to 2 weeks.

Particularly in critically ill patients, initial therapy is often started parenterally. Patients may be switched to an oral agent as soon as the patient clinically defervesces or treated entirely by an oral agent for the duration of therapy. The ideal oral antibiotic has the same spectrum as its parenteral counterpart and has excellent bioavailability; blood/tissue levels are approximately the same after intravenous/oral (IV/PO) administration. For example, by giving 1 g of amoxicillin (Amoxil) every 8 hours, the same blood/tissue levels are achieved as by giving ampicillin by intramuscular injection (IM). Nonrenally eliminated respiratory quinolones, such as levofloxacin (Levaquin) and gatifloxacin (Tequin), achieve the same blood and tissue levels when given either by the IV or PO route. This permits completion of therapy at home and does not require 2 to 4 weeks of inpatient hospitalization for intravenous drug therapy. There is some rationale for treating acute pyelonephritis for an extended period, such as 2 to 4 weeks, to prevent chronic pyelonephritis.

CHRONIC PYELONEPHRITIS

Patients with chronic pyelonephritis are a therapeutic challenge because of the distorted intrarenal architecture and decreased blood supply to the kidney, which limits access of white blood cells (WBCs), impairs host defenses, and limits penetration of the antibiotic into the infected/diseased areas of the kidney. Treatment of chronic pyelonephritis should be based on susceptibility testing of the isolates that are present in the urine. In chronic pyelonephritis, bacteriuria is intermittent but is present over a long period of time

and will persist after short or inadequate treatment. The antibiotic selected should be effective against the isolate recovered from the urine in patients with chronic pyelonephritis and possess the ability to penetrate into diseased kidneys. The ideal oral agents for therapy are TMP-SMX (Bactrim), doxycycline (Vibramycin), or a nonrenally eliminated respiratory quinolone.

RENAL ABSCESS

Acute pyelonephritis treated appropriately results in a rapid defervescence of temperature and decrease in CVA tenderness within 72 hours. If the temperature does not decrease after 72 hours of appropriate therapy, suggest a renal abscess until proved otherwise. Renal abscesses should be treated for the presumed organism based on the location of the abscess by renal imaging studies. If sensitivities from an isolate available from the urine or percutaneous aspiration of the abscess are unavailable, then empirical treatment directed against aerobic gram-negative bacilli for medullary abscesses is indicated. Treatment is the same as for pyelonephritis except is more prolonged and should be given until the abscess is drained or it resolves. For cortical abscesses in the absence of culture and sensitivity data, antibiotic therapy should be directed against *Staphylococcus aureus* and *E. faecalis*, and treated in the same manner as pyelonephritis but for an extended period of time. Acute pyelonephritis with or without acteremia is usually treated for 7 days.

RECURRENT UTIs

Reinfection may be treated with nitrofurantoin (Macrodantin), TMP-SMX (Bactrim), or amoxicillin (Amoxil) as a single postcoital dose. Therapeutic approach to relapse is to remove the underlying condition responsible for perpetuating the bacteriuria. Antimicrobial therapy may be selected based on the susceptibility of the organism, but antimicrobial therapy alone will not eradicate the relapsing form of recurrent UTI.

REFERENCES

Cunha BA. Clinical concepts in the treatment of urinary tract infections. Antibiotics for Clinicians 1999;3:88–93.

Cunha BA. Nosocomial catheter-associated urinary tract infections. Hosp Physician 1986;22:13–6.

Cunha BA. *Staphylococcus saprophyticus* urinary tract infections. Intern Med 1985;19:35–7.

Cunha BA. Urosepsis in the Critical Care Unit. In: Cunha BA, editor. Infectious Diseases in Critical Care Medicine. 3rd ed. New York, NY: Informa Healthcare USA, Inc; 2009.

Cunha BA. Antibiotic Essentials. 8th ed. Sudbury, MA: Jones and Bartlett; 2009.

Cunha BA. Urinary tract infections: Therapy. Postgrad Med 1981;70:149–57.

Hooton TM. The current management strategies for community-acquired urinary tract infection. Infect Dis Clin North Am 2003;17:303–32.

Kahan E, Kahan NR, Chinitz DP. Urinary tract infection in women—Physician's preferences for treatment and adherence to guidelines: A national drug utilization study in a managed care setting. Eur J Clin Pharmacol 2003;59:663–8.

Kraft JK, Stamey TA. The natural history of symptomatic recurrent bacteriuria in women. Medicine (Baltimore) 1977;56:55.

Meiland R, Geerlings SE, Hoepelman LI. Management of bacterial urinary tract infections in adult patients with diabetes mellitus. Drugs 2002;62: 1859–68.

Miller LG, Tang AW. Treatment of uncomplicated urinary tract infections in an era of increasing antimicrobial resistance. Mayo Clin Proc 2004;79: 1048–53.

Nicolle LE. Urinary tract infection: Traditional pharmacologic therapies. Am J Med 2002;113(Suppl. 1A):35S–44S.

Nicolle LE, Ronald AR. Recurrent urinary tract infection in adult women: Diagnosis and treatment. Infect Dis Clin North Am 1987;1:793.

Ronald AR, Conway B. An approach to urinary tract infection in women. Infection 1992;20(Suppl. 3):S203.

Schaeffer AJ, Stuppy BA. Efficacy and safety of self-start therapy in women with recurrent urinary tract infections. J Urol 1999;161:207.

Wong ES, McKevitt M, Running K, et al. Management of recurrent urinary tract infections with patient administered single-dose therapy. Ann Intern Med 1985;102:302.

Urinary Tract Infections in Infants and Children

Method of
Ellen R. Wald, MD

The urinary tract is the most common site for serious bacterial infections in infants and young children. Urinary tract infections (UTIs) are more common than bacterial meningitis, bacterial pneumonia, and bacteremia.

Infection of the urinary tract may involve only the bladder, or only the kidney, or both. In general, infections of the bladder (cystitis), while causing substantial morbidity, are not regarded as serious bacterial infections. In contrast, infections that involve the kidney (pyelonephritis), can cause acute morbidity and lead to scarring with the consequences of hypertension, preeclampsia, and chronic renal disease.

Diagnosis

The diagnosis of UTI may be suggested by certain signs and symptoms, but culture of the urine is the gold standard. Because culture results are not available for at least 24 hours, there has been considerable interest in evaluating tests that may predict the results of urine culture, so that appropriate therapy can be initiated at the first encounter with the symptomatic patient. The tests that have received the most attention are urine microscopy for white cells and bacteria and biochemical analysis of leukocyte esterase and nitrite, which can be assessed rapidly by dipstick.

Several studies have concluded that both the presence of any bacteria on Gram staining of an uncentrifuged urine sample and dipstick analysis for leukocyte esterase and nitrite perform similarly in children from birth through 12 years of age and are helpful in identifying individuals with UTI. Other recent studies done involving young infants (<2 months of age) and older infants (<12 months and 1–24 months) concluded that a hemocytometer white blood cell count of 10 or more cells per microliter provides the most valuable cutoff point for identifying infants for whom urine culture is warranted.

The definition of a positive urine culture depends on the method used to collect the specimen. This variable definition reflects the fact that urine which has passed through the urethra may be contaminated by bacteria present in the distal urethra. If the urine is obtained by the clean-catch method, a positive culture is defined as equal to or greater than 10^5 colony-forming units (CFU)/mL. If the specimen is obtained by catheterization of the urethra, a positive culture is defined as equal to or greater than 5×10^4 CFU/mL. Finally, if a urine culture is obtained by suprapubic aspiration, a method that bypasses the potential source of contamination, a positive culture is defined as recovery of any bacteria from the urine.

Imaging

Imaging studies have been the standard of care for young children with a first UTI for the past decade. Commonly, a renal ultrasound study is performed to evaluate the gross anatomy of the urinary tract (size and shape of the kidneys, duplication or dilatation of the ureters). A voiding cystourethrogram (VCUG) is done to determine whether vesicoureteral reflux is present. This practice has rested on the assumption that continuous prophylactic antimicrobial therapy is effective in reducing the incidence of reinfection of the kidney and renal scarring that may occur in children with vesicoureteral reflux. This remains a controversial issue, because it is only the few children with high degrees of reflux who benefit from antimicrobial prophylaxis (approximately 15%).

Treatment

In general, there are many choices for the antibiotic treatment of UTIs in children. If a child is toxic in appearance or vomiting (thereby precluding oral antimicrobials), admission to the hospital for parenteral therapy is appropriate. Many would recommend a third-generation cephalosporin, such as ceftriaxone (Rocephin) 50 mg/kg/day given once daily or cefotaxime (Claforan) 50 mg/kg/dose every 6 hours, until the emesis has resolved and the patient can be treated orally. Otherwise, children, even those with presumed pyelonephritis, do well on oral therapy.

For the child who is to receive oral therapy, the choices are amoxicillin potassium clavulanate (Augmentin) 30 mg/kg/dose given every 12 hours[3]; a second- or third-generation cephalosporin such as cefuroxime (Ceftin) 50 mg/kg/dose twice daily,[3] cefpodoxime (Vantin)[1] 5 mg/kg/dose given twice daily, cefdinir (Omnicef)[1] 7 mg/kg/dose given twice daily, or cefixime (Suprax)[1] 10 mg/kg/dose once daily[3]; or sulfamethoxazole-trimethoprim (Bactrim) 6 mg/kg/day[3] or trimethoprim given once daily. There has been a tendency during the past several years for the prevalence of antimicrobial resistance to increase. The overall resistance to antibiotics varies geographically, and it is essential for the practitioner to be familiar with local antibiotic resistance patterns. In patients with suspected acute pyelonephritis, amoxicillin (Amoxil), cephalexin (Keflex), and sulfamethoxazole-trimethoprim should be avoided because of the potentially high rate of antibiotic resistance.

The optimal duration of therapy for children with UTI has been somewhat controversial. If the diagnosis of pyelonephritis is known or suspected, 10 days of treatment is conventional. Shorter courses of therapy have been successful in adult women with infection of the lower urinary tract. A recent meta-analysis conducted by the Cochrane Database of Systematic Reviews evaluated 10 trials (652 children) with lower-tract UTI. There was no significant difference in frequency of positive urine cultures between short-term (2–4 days) and standard (7–14 days) duration of oral antibiotic therapy for cystitis in children, either early after treatment or at 1 to 15 months after treatment. Furthermore, there was no difference between groups in the development of resistant organisms at the end of treatment or in the incidence of recurrent UTIs. Accordingly, in cases in which the diagnosis of cystitis is assured, 4 days of antimicrobial therapy is sufficient.

Voiding Dysfunction

Voiding dysfunction is a broad term indicating a voiding pattern that is abnormal for the child's age. This is a condition that should be considered in all children who are diagnosed as having a UTI after toilet training has been accomplished. Constipation plays a significant role in some children with voiding dysfunction, and attention to this comorbidity sometimes results in resolution of recurrent UTIs.

Prophylaxis

For children who are considered to be at risk for recurrent UTIs and potential scarring, prophylactic treatment with sulfamethoxazole-trimethoprim or nitrofurantoin (Macrodantin) is recommended. These groups include children with high degrees of reflux, vesicoureteral reflux, those with frequent and closely spaced UTIs without reflux, and, occasionally, those who have urologic abnormalities or who have just sustained an episode of acute pyelonephritis.

The latest Cochrane Review of the effectiveness of long-term antibiotics for preventing recurrent UTIs in children indicated that most published studies to date have been poorly designed without proper blinding. There is no question of the biologic plausibility of

---

[1]Not FDA approved for this indication.
[3]Exceeds dosage recommended by the manufacturer.

prophylactic antimicrobial therapy in preventing recurrent UTI; however, adverse effects and difficulties with long-term adherence to prophylactic strategies present barriers to effectiveness.

REFERENCES

Gorelick MH, Shaw KN. Screening tests for urinary tract infection: A meta-analysis. Pediatrics 1999;104:e54.

Hellerstein S, Linebarger JS. Voiding dysfunction in pediatric patients. Clin Pediatr 2003;42:43–9.

Hellerstein S, Nickell E. Prophylactic antibiotics in children at risk for urinary tract infection. Pediatr Nephrol 2002;17:506–10.

Hoberman A, Charron M, Hickey RW, et al. Imaging studies after a first febrile urinary tract infection in young children. N Engl J Med 2003;348:195–202.

Hoberman A, Keren R. Antimicrobial prophylaxis for urinary tract infection in children. N Engl J Med 2009;361:1804–6.

Hoberman A, Wald ER, Hickey RW, et al. Oral versus initial intravenous therapy for urinary tract infections in young febrile children. Pediatrics 1999;104:79–86.

Hoberman A, Wald ER, Reynolds EA, et al. Pyuria and bacteriuria in urine specimens obtained by catheter from young children with fever. J Pediatr 1994;124:513–9.

Huicho L, Campos-Sanchez M, Alamo C. Metaanalysis of urine screening tests for determining the risk of urinary tract infection in children. Pediatr Infect Dis J 2002;21:1–11, 88.

Lin D-S, Huang F-Y, Chui N-C, et al. Comparison of hemocytometer leukocyte counts and standard urinalyses for predicting urinary tract infection in febrile infants. Pediatr Infect Dis J 2000;19:223–7.

Michael M, Hodson EM, Craig JC, et al. Short versus standard duration oral antibiotic therapy for acute urinary tract infection in children. Cochrane Database Syst Rev 2009;(1):CD003966 [First published in 2003].

Williams GJ, Wei L, Lee A, Craig JC. Long-term antibiotics for preventing recurrent urinary tract infection in children. Cochrane Database Syst Rev 2003;(2):CD001534 [First published in 2001].

Childhood Incontinence

Method of
Walid A. Farhat, MD, and Kristin Kozakowski, MD

Urinary incontinence is defined by the International Continence Society as "involuntary loss of urine, objectively demonstrable, and constituting a social or hygienic problem." In contrast to adults, in whom incontinence is always considered pathologic, pediatric urinary incontinence must be evaluated in the context of the child's developmental age.

An infant voids approximately 20 times a day via a vesicovesical reflex mechanism mediated by the spinal cord. As the child develops, the neural pathways in the spinal cord mature. In the first 18 to 24 months of life, this primitive voiding reflex is gradually inhibited, bladder capacity increases, and voiding becomes less frequent. Eventually, the more complex voiding reflex develops, and the coordination of voiding control becomes mediated by the pons and midbrain, the pontine micturition center. By the age of 2 years, children become consciously aware of bladder fullness, which leads to the ability to postpone voiding.

Although most children are toilet trained by 3 years of age, there can be a wide variation. Bloom and associates found that the mean age ranged from 0.75 to 5.25 years, with girls being trained earlier (2.25 years) than boys (2.56 years). In two other studies, Wnydaele and colleagues found that 12% of Belgian schoolchildren aged 10 to 14 years had incontinence episodes, and Dahm and colleagues found that 29% of 7- to 8-year-old Danish children had symptoms of underdeveloped bladder control. However, by the age of 5 years and entry into school, children can be expected to have developed volitional urinary control. Therefore, urinary incontinence after age 5, specifically daytime urinary incontinence, is a matter of both social and clinical concern.

Classification of Pediatric Urinary Incontinence

Clinical management of pediatric urinary incontinence is often complicated by a lack of standardized definitions as to what exactly constitutes different types of incontinence in children. This stems from the fact that a large percentage of wetting in children is sporadic and can be considered a variation of normal behavior. Parents and children are often embarrassed or desensitized to the incontinence and fail to bring it to their doctor's attention. It is also important to recognize that urinary incontinence is frequently related to an underlying disease process (organic urinary incontinence). This is distinct from functional urinary incontinence, in which no anatomic or neurologic abnormality is present. Organic incontinence is subdivided into structural and neurologic causes. Structural incontinence includes all congenital, traumatic, and iatrogenic factors that interfere with the bladder's ability to store and empty urine. Neurologic causes include congenital or acquired conditions that interfere with the innervation of the bladder and urinary sphincter (Fig. 1).

To address this problem, the International Children's Continence Society (ICCS) published a report in 1997 that attempted to standardize and define lower urinary tract dysfunction in children; this was updated in 2006. They defined incontinence as the uncontrollable leakage of urine, which can be broadly classified as continuous or intermittent (Fig. 2). Continuous urinary incontinence is constant urine leakage with no dry periods. This is almost exclusively associated with organic urinary incontinence. Intermittent incontinence is urine leakage in discrete amounts, which can occur day or night and is applicable to children older than 5 years of age. Bedwetting, also termed "enuresis," is intermittent incontinence that occurs at night. Accidents that occur during the day are classified as daytime incontinence. Patients with both daytime incontinence and bedwetting have two separate diagnoses; the term "diurnal incontinence" is now obsolete.

ENURESIS

Enuresis, often termed "nocturnal enuresis," is a normal void that occurs while the child is sleeping, usually without the child's being aroused by the wetting. Bedwetting is usually not considered pathologic before the age of 7 years, and it is an extremely common occurrence. In a recent large-scale, longitudinal study, at least 20% of children in the first grade occasionally wet the bed, and 4% wet the bed two or more times per week. Bedwetting is more common in boys and can often show a familial tendency. The ICCS subdivides enuresis into two types: monosymptomatic enuresis (no other lower urinary tract symptoms) and non-monosymptomatic enuresis (other lower urinary tract symptoms are present). Primary enuresis means that the child never had any dry periods at night; children who had at least 6 months of nighttime dryness are said to have secondary enuresis.

Most cases of enuresis resolve with time and when the child becomes more focused on changing the behavior. The treatment of enuresis begins with behavioral modification, including reducing evening fluid intake, increasing daytime voiding frequency, and the use of alarm therapy to condition the child to awaken with wetting. Pharmacologic therapy with desmopressin (DDAVP), which reduces overnight production of urine, is usually reserved for situations such as overnight visits and summer camp; this is no longer considered acceptable as a

COMMON CAUSES OF ORGANIC INCONTINENCE

Structural	Neurologic
Ectopic ureter	Spina bifida
Exstrophy/epispadias complex	Tethered cord
Posterior urethral valves	Sacral agenesis
	Cerebral palsy
	Spinal cord injury

FIGURE 1. Common causes of organic incontinence.

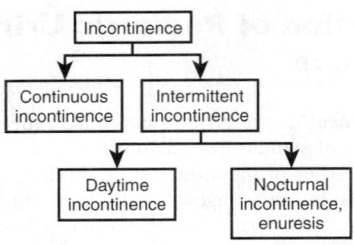

FIGURE 2. Terminology of lower urinary tract function in children and adolescents. (Reprinted with permission from Nevéus T, von Gontard A, Hoebeke P, et al: The standardization of terminology of lower urinary tract function in children and adolescents: Report from the Standardisation Committee of the International Children's Continence Society. J Urol 2006;176:314–324.)

first-line agent or for regular usage. Tricyclic antidepressants are no longer used because of their adverse side-effect profiles.

DAYTIME WETTING CONDITIONS

The classification of daytime wetting conditions is difficult, because children often have overlapping symptoms that can change as they age. The ICCS recommends that clinicians focus on four symptom parameters when assessing children with wetting accidents: incontinence (presence, absence, and frequency), normal voiding frequency, voided volumes, and fluid intake. There are several recognized syndromes that affect the pediatric population, and incontinence may occur in any of them.

Overactive Bladder and Urge Incontinence

The hallmark symptom of overactive bladder is urgency, the imperative urge to void is usually accompanied by holding maneuvers such as squatting and often results in the socially inappropriate loss of urine. Urgency is caused by overactive detrusor contractions early in the bladder filling phase; these are then countered by voluntary pelvic floor contractions or maneuvers to compress the urethra. In these children with overactive bladder, normal voiding frequency may be high, and bladder capacity is often small for age. This type of incontinence occurs more commonly in girls and can progress to a very severe form of dysfunctional voiding.

Urge incontinence is treated with a combination of behavioral therapy, specifically timed voiding programs, and anticholinergic agents such as oxybutynin (Ditropan), which can help to reduce bladder overactivity. Oxybutynin can have side effects such as constipation, dry mouth, drowsiness, and flushing, which lead to discontinuation of its use in approximately 10% of children.

Voiding Postponement

Children who continuously postpone the urge to urinate at normal voiding intervals experience wetting accidents because they do not void unless their bladder is full and contracts involuntarily due to overcapacity. These children infrequently void and are often observed performing holding maneuvers. Children who routinely postpone the need to void often do so because of aversion to public bathrooms or because of not being allowed to use the bathroom during class. These children also may have comorbid psychological or behavioral disturbances.

Management consists of behavioral modification, and specifically of strictly timed voiding bladder retraining programs. In extreme cases in which the child refuses to void, clean intermittent catheterization becomes necessary to empty the bladder.

DYSFUNCTIONAL VOIDING

Dysfunctional voiding patterns, specifically staccato and fractionated voiding, involve some form of overactivity of pelvic floor musculature during voiding, with an uncoordination between the detrusor and the musculature of the external sphincter or pelvic floor or both. These children habitually contract the urethral sphincter during voiding, but the condition is not related to any dysfunction of bladder storage.

Staccato voiding is a pattern characterized by periodic contractions of the pelvic floor musculature during voiding and interruptions in the flow of urine, leading to prolonged voiding time and residual urine. Fractionated voiding is characterized by small voided volumes with incomplete bladder emptying and an underactive detrusor muscle. Some children augment this voiding pattern with Valsalva maneuvers. These patients usually have large-capacity bladders and detrusor hypoactivity. Dysfunctional voiding can have serious long-term consequences, including high-pressure voiding, chronic urinary tract infections, vesicoureteral reflux, and decompensation of the detrusor muscle.

These dysfunctional voiding patterns are often very difficult to treat. Behavioral modification and biofeedback therapy are the most useful tools.

UNDERACTIVE BLADDER

Children with underactive bladder typically void only once or twice per day. They have increased bladder capacity and diminished bladder sensation to void and carry a high postvoid residual. They also typically need to strain to urinate and show decreased detrusor activity. The leakage that occurs is due to overflow incontinence.

The first line of therapy for these patients is timed-voiding and double-voiding bladder retraining programs. If this treatment fails, clean intermittent catheterization must be used to empty the bladder.

NON-NEUROGENIC NEUROGENIC BLADDER SYNDROME

Non-neurogenic neurogenic bladder, also called Hinman-Allen syndrome, is the most severe form of dysfunctional voiding. This occurs when there is chronic voluntary tightening of the external sphincter during an overactive detrusor contraction, resulting in learned failure to relax the external sphincter during voluntary voiding. This pattern results in bladder-sphincter dyssynergy and eventually leads to detrusor decompensation. These children present with symptoms of daytime and nighttime wetting, overflow and urge incontinence, and recurrent urinary tract infections, and their bladders show severe trabeculations and high postvoid residuals. Often, they have acquired vesicoureteral reflux and hydronephrosis from the decreased bladder compliance. Despite the abnormal findings, they are neurologically normal.

The treatment for these children is a combination of behavioral modification, biofeedback therapy, and possibly prophylactic antibiotics and anticholinergic medications. These patients need aggressive treatment.

GIGGLE INCONTINENCE

Giggle incontinence, which occurs most commonly in girls, is a large-volume loss of urine that happens exclusively with laughter. Patients have no other voiding symptoms, and their bladder is otherwise completely normal.

Treatment is a combination of timed-voiding programs and use of anticholinergic medications to suppress the bladder contraction. For patients in whom excessive muscle relaxation is thought to be the cause, α-sympathomimetic agents or methylphenidate (Ritalin)[1] has been used.

VAGINAL VOIDING

Patients with vaginal reflux present with urine leakage that occurs within 10 minutes after voiding, usually after standing up; foul-smelling urine; and frequent nonfebrile urinary tract infections. It occurs because of urine backflow into the vagina caused by labial fusion or failure to adequately separate the legs while voiding due to obesity or improper voiding posture.

---

[1]Not FDA approved for this indication.

Vaginal voiding is treated by mechanical or pharmacologic (hormonal cream) separation of labial fusion or by adjusting the voiding position.

CONSTIPATION

Treatment of underlying constipation is vital in the management of pediatric urinary incontinence. The combination of a high-fiber diet and agents such as polyethylene glycol (MiraLax) has been shown to maintain a regular bowel routine and help in addressing urinary incontinence.

Clinical Assessment

MEDICAL HISTORY

In addition to a thorough overall medical history, the focused voiding history should include information about urinary frequency, urgency, wetting accidents, urinary tract infections, dysuria, voiding postures, and, importantly, associated constipation. Patients should be asked to keep a voiding diary and to record urinary frequency, bowel activity, wetting accidents, and fluid intake. It is also important to ask about any developmental delay, impaired motor skills, traumatic birth history, prenatal diagnoses, and mental disorders. In addition, a family history of voiding dysfunction, particularly enuresis, and any stressful social situation, whether at home or at school, is very useful in the assessment of pediatric incontinence.

PHYSICAL EXAMINATION

A focused physical evaluation should include examination of the abdomen, genitalia, perineum, and spine and a directed neurologic examination of the lower pelvis and extremities. Specifically, the abdomen is palpated for a full bladder or possible fecal impaction. The female perineum must be examined for possible labial adhesions, ectopic ureter, vaginal irritation, and abnormal position of the urethral meatus. The male genitalia should be examined for possible phimosis or abnormal urethral meatus. The lower back must be inspected for a sacral dimple or hair tuft, absence of the sacrum, or asymmetry.

LABORATORY AND IMAGING STUDIES

A basic urinalysis can provide valuable information about the presence of infection, hematuria, glucose, and protein and urine concentrating ability.

A renal and bladder ultrasound study provides information about possible structural abnormalities of the urinary tract, thickness of the bladder wall, and the presence of kidney or bladder stones. Based on a history of febrile urinary tract infections or structural abnormality found on ultrasonography, a voiding cystourethrogram may be indicated. Spinal radiography or magnetic resonance imaging may be necessary to diagnose a suspected underlying neurologic abnormality. Basic uroflowmetry and measurement of postvoid residuals provides information about voided volumes, strength of flow, and whether the bladder can empty—all indirect ways of investigating bladder and sphincter function. More invasive urodynamic testing is reserved for complex cases such as non-neurogenic neurogenic bladder syndrome.

REFERENCES

Bauer SB. Special considerations of the overactive bladder in children. Urology 2002;60:43–9.
Bloom DA, Seely WW, Ritchey ML, McGuire EJ. Toilet habits and continence in children: An opportunity sampling in search of normal parameters. J Urol 1993;149:1087–90.
Butler RJ, Heron JA. The prevalence of infrequent bedwetting and nocturnal enuresis in childhood: A large British cohort. Scand J Urol Nephrol 2008;42:257–326.
Chin-Peuckert L, Pippi Salle JL. A modified biofeedback program for children with detrusor-sphincter dyssynergia: 5 year experience. J Urol 2001;166:1470–5.
Feldman AS, Bauer SB. Diagnosis and management of dysfunctional voiding. Curr Opin Pediatr 2006;18:139–47.
Hinman Jr F. Nonneurogenic neurogenic bladder (the Hinman syndrome): 15 years later. J Urol 1986;136:769–77.
Loening-Baucke V. Urinary incontinence and urinary tract infection and their resolution with threatment of chronic constipation in childhood. Pediatrics 1997;100:228–32.
Nevéus T, von Gontard A, Hoebeke P, et al. The standardization of terminology of lower urinary tract function in children and adolescents: Report from the Standardisation Committee of the International Children's Continence Society. J Urol 2006;176:314–24.
Nijman RJM. Role of antimuscarinics in the treatment of nonneurogenic daytime urinary incontinence in children. Urology 2004;63:45–50.
Norgaard JP, van Gool JD, Hjalmas K, et al. Standardization and definitions in lower urinary tract dysfunction in children. Br J Urol 1998;81(Suppl. 3):1–16.
Sher P, Reinberg Y. Successful treatment of giggle incontinence with methylphenidate. J Urol 1996;156:656–8.

Urinary Incontinence

Method of
E. Ann Gormley, MD

Urinary incontinence is a significant problem that affects millions of Americans. Patients may not report incontinence to their primary care providers because of embarrassment or misconceptions regarding treatment. Because incontinence is often treatable, it behooves the health care professional to identify patients who might benefit from treatment. Given that the treatment of incontinence varies depending on the etiology, the aim of evaluation is to identify the etiology.

Etiology

Urinary incontinence is generally the result of either bladder or urethral dysfunction (Table 1). Incontinence also may result from a nonurologic cause and is usually reversible when the underlying problem is treated (Table 2). More uncommon causes of incontinence are urinary fistulae and ectopic ureteral orifices.

BLADDER DYSFUNCTION

Bladder dysfunction causes urge or overflow incontinence. *Urge incontinence* occurs when the bladder pressure is sufficient to overcome the sphincter mechanism. Elevated bladder or detrusor pressure tends to

---

TABLE 1 Etiology of Incontinence

Bladder Dysfunction
1. Urge incontinence
   - Detrusor overactivity
     - Idiopathic
     - Neurogenic origin
   - Poor compliance
2. Overflow incontinence

Urethral Dysfunction
3. Stress incontinence
   - Anatomic
   - Intrinsic sphincter deficiency

TABLE 2 Transient Causes of Incontinence *(DIAPPERS)*

Cause	Comment
Delirium	Incontinence may be secondary to delirium and will often stop when acute delirium resolves.
Infection	Symptomatic infection may prevent a patient from reaching the toilet in time.
Atrophic vaginitis	Vaginitis may cause the same symptoms as an infection.
Pharmacologic	
• Sedatives	Alcohol and long-acting benzodiazepines may cause confusion and secondary incontinence.
• Diuretics	A brisk diuresis may overwhelm the bladder's capacity and cause uninhibited detrusor contractions, resulting in urge incontinence.
• Anticholinergics	Many nonprescription and prescription medications have anticholinergic properties. Side effects of anticholinergics include urinary retention with associated frequency and overflow incontinence.
• α Adrenergics	Tone in the bladder neck and proximal sphincter is increased by α-adrenergic agonists and can cause urinary retention, particularly in men with prostatism.
• α Antagonists	Tone in the smooth muscles of the bladder neck and proximal sphincter is decreased with α-adrenergic antagonists. Women treated with these drugs for hypertension may develop or have an exacerbation of stress incontinence.
Psychological	Depression may be occasionally associated with incontinence.
Excessive urine production	Excessive intake, diabetes, hypercalcemia, congestive heart failure, and peripheral edema can all lead to polyuria, which can lead to incontinence.
Restricted mobility	Incontinence may be precipitated or aggravated if the patient cannot get to the toilet quickly enough.
Stool impaction	Patients with impacted stool can have urge or overflow urinary incontinence and may also have fecal incontinence.

From Resnick NM: Urinary incontinence in the elderly. Med Grand Rounds 1984;3:281–290.

open the bladder neck and urethra. An elevation in detrusor pressure may occur from intermittent bladder contractions (detrusor overactivity) or because of an incremental rise in pressure with increased bladder volume (poor compliance). Detrusor overactivity may be idiopathic, or it may be associated with a neurologic disease (detrusor overactivity of neurogenic origin). Detrusor overactivity is common in the elderly and may be associated with bladder outlet obstruction. Poor bladder compliance results from loss of the viscoelastic features of the bladder or because of a change in neuroregulatory activity. The patient with urge incontinence may appreciate a sudden sensation to void but then is unable to suppress the urge fully. In severe cases, the patient may not be aware of the sensation of needing to void until he or she is actually leaking. The amount of leakage in patients with urge incontinence is variable, depending on the patient's ability to suppress the contraction. Patients with urge incontinence will often have frequency and nocturia in addition to urgency and urge incontinence. They may also have nocturnal enuresis.

Overactive bladder is a newer term that describes patients with frequency and urgency with or without urge incontinence.

Overflow incontinence occurs at extreme bladder volumes or when the bladder volume reaches the limit of the bladder's viscoelastic properties. The loss of urine is driven by an elevation in detrusor pressure. Overflow incontinence is seen in the case of incomplete bladder emptying caused by either obstruction or poor bladder contractility. Obstruction is rare in women but can result from severe pelvic prolapse or following surgery for stress incontinence. Patients with overflow incontinence complain of constant dribbling, and they may also describe extreme frequency.

URETHRAL-RELATED INCONTINENCE

Urethral-related incontinence, or *stress incontinence,* occurs because of either urethral hypermobility or intrinsic sphincter deficiency (ISD). Incontinence associated with urethral hypermobility has been called *anatomic incontinence* because the incontinence is due to malposition of the sphincter unit. Displacement of the proximal urethra below the level of the pelvic floor does not allow for transmission of abdominal pressure that normally aids in closing the urethra. Some women with mobility of the bladder neck or urethra do not experience incontinence. ISD was initially believed to occur after failure of one or more operations for stress incontinence. Other causes of ISD include myelodysplasia, trauma, and radiation. Some authors have theorized that all incontinent patients must have an element of ISD in order to actually leak. The patient with stress incontinence leaks urine with any sudden increase in abdominal pressure. In patients with severe ISD, the increase in abdominal pressure required to cause leakage is small, so patients may leak urine with minimal activity.

Evaluation of the Incontinent Patient

The evaluation of the incontinent patient includes a history, physical examination, laboratory tests, and possibly urodynamic testing. The onset, frequency, severity, and pattern of incontinence should be sought, as well as any associated symptoms such as frequency, dysuria, urgency, and nocturia. Incontinence may be quantified by asking the patient if he or she wears a pad and how often the pad is changed. Obstructive symptoms, such as a feeling of incomplete emptying, hesitancy, straining, or weak stream, may coexist with incontinence, particularly in males and in female patients with previous incontinence procedure, cystoceles, or poor detrusor contractility. Female patients should be asked about symptoms of pelvic prolapse, such as recurrent urinary tract infection, a sensation of vaginal fullness or pressure, or the observation of a bulge in the vagina. All incontinent patients should be asked about bowel function and neurologic symptoms. Response to previous treatments, including drugs, should be noted. Important features of the history include previous gynecologic and urologic procedures, neurologic problems, and past medical problems. A list of the patient's current medications, including over-the-counter medications, should be obtained.

Although the history may define the patient's problem, it may be misleading. Urge incontinence may be triggered by activities such as coughing, so according to the patient's history, he or she seems to have stress incontinence. A patient who complains only of urge incontinence may also have stress incontinence. Mixed incontinence is very common; at least 65% of patients with stress incontinence have associated urgency or urge incontinence.

A complete physical examination is performed, with emphasis on the neurologic assessment and on the abdominal, pelvic, and rectal examinations. In females, the condition of the vaginal mucosa and the degree of urethral mobility are determined. Simple pelvic examination with the patient supine is sufficient to determine if the urethra moves with straining or coughing. The degree of movement is not as important as the determination of whether movement occurs. The presence of associated pelvic organ prolapse should be noted because it can contribute to the patient's voiding problems and may have an impact on diagnosis and treatment. A rectal examination in both males and females includes the evaluation of sphincter tone and perineal sensation.

A urinalysis is performed to determine if there is any evidence of hematuria, pyuria, glucosuria, or proteinuria. A urine specimen is sent for cytologic examination if there is hematuria and/or irritative voiding symptoms. The urine is cultured if there is pyuria or bacteriuria. Infection should be treated prior to further investigations or interventions. Hematuria consisting of more than three red cells per high-power field warrants further investigation.

CURRENT DIAGNOSIS

Urge Incontinence

Symptoms
- Urgency
- Frequency
- Nocturia
- Unable to reach the toilet with urge

Stress Incontinence

Symptoms
- Leakage with physical activity

Signs
- Bladder neck mobility
- Positive stress test

Mixed Incontinence

Symptoms
- Urgency
- Frequency
- Nocturia
- Unable to reach the toilet with urge
- Leakage with physical activity

Signs
- Bladder neck mobility
- Positive stress test

Overflow Incontinence

Symptoms
- Frequency
- Nocturia
- Urgency
- Leakage with physical activity

Signs
- High postvoid residual

A postvoid residual (PVR) should be measured either with pelvic ultrasound or directly with a catheter. A normal PVR is less than 50 mL, and a PVR greater than 200 mL is abnormal. A significant PVR urine may reflect either bladder outlet obstruction or poor bladder contractility. The only way to distinguish outlet obstruction from poor contractility is with urodynamic testing.

Urodynamic testing is used to accurately diagnose the etiology of a patient's incontinence; however, many patients can be successfully treated without urodynamic testing. The purpose of urodynamic testing is to examine compliance, diagnose stress incontinence, and rule out obstruction as a cause of either overflow or urge incontinence. Urodynamic testing should ideally be performed prior to invasive therapies and certainly in patients who are undergoing repeat procedures following failed procedures.

Treatment of Urinary Incontinence

URGE INCONTINENCE

Patients with urge incontinence need to understand that they leak urine because their bladder contracts with little or no warning. The first line of treatment is timed voiding. Often, reminding patients to void every 1 to 2 hours during the day, before they get an urge to void, will result in them staying dry. Other behavioral interventions, such as modification of fluid intake, avoidance of bladder irritants, and bladder retraining, where the patient attempts to consciously delay voiding and to increase the interval between voids, may also have a role in the treatment of urge incontinence.

Anticholinergics are the mainstay of medical therapy in achieving continence. The side effects of anticholinergics include urinary retention, dry mouth, constipation, nausea, blurred vision, tachycardia, drowsiness, and confusion. They are contraindicated in patients with narrow-angle glaucoma. Anticholinergics are also used to decrease bladder pressure in patients with poor compliance. Anticholinergics are combined with clean intermittent catheterization in patients who have a significant PVR prior to treatment and in patients who develop retention while taking anticholinergics.

Patients with intractable detrusor overactivity may require surgical intervention, consisting of neuromodulation with a sacral nerve stimulator or various forms of bladder augmentation.

The primary goal in caring for the patient with poor compliance is treating the high bladder pressure. Complete bladder emptying with clean intermittent catheterization combined with anticholinergics will often lower bladder pressure to a safe range. Some patients may require a combination of anticholinergics and α agonists. Bladder augmentation is required when medical management fails.

OVERFLOW INCONTINENCE

Overflow incontinence is treated by emptying the bladder. If the cause of overflow is obstruction, then relieving the obstruction should lead to improved emptying. Anatomic obstruction in males derives from either urethral stricture disease or prostatic obstruction. Depending on the severity of urethral stricture disease, the patient may require urethral dilation, internal urethrotomy, or urethroplasty. Prostatic obstruction may be treated in a variety of ways, but transurethral resection remains the gold standard. If a woman is obstructed from previous surgery or from pelvic prolapse, she may benefit from urethrolysis or surgical correction of the prolapse. Clean intermittent catheterization is an option in the obstructed patient who does not want or could not tolerate further surgery.

The patient with overflow incontinence secondary to poor detrusor contractility is best treated with clean intermittent catheterization.

Indwelling catheters are not an optimum treatment modality for treatment of incontinence. All patients with indwelling catheters will have infected urine, which predisposes them to bladder calculi and ultimately to squamous cell carcinoma of the bladder. Any foreign object in the bladder can cause or exacerbate elevated bladder pressure that is associated with hydronephrosis, ureteral obstruction, renal stones, and eventually renal failure.

STRESS INCONTINENCE

The amount of incontinence and how it affects the patient often determines the aggressiveness of treatment. The patient who is severely restricted because of severe leakage with minimal movement may not want to try medical therapy but may opt for surgical treatment, whereas the patient who leaks small amounts infrequently may choose conservative treatment. Pelvic floor exercises can improve anatomic stress urinary incontinence by augmenting closure of the external urethral sphincter and by preventing descent and rotation of the bladder neck and urethra. To benefit from the exercises, women must be taught to do the exercises properly, and they must do them. Adjuncts to learning pelvic floor exercises include weighted vaginal cones, a perineometer, and electrical stimulation.

α Agonists such as phenylpropanolamine[1] and pseudoephedrine (Sudafed)[1] can be used for treatment of stress incontinence. The bladder neck and proximal urethra have abundant α receptors. Activation of these receptors by α agonists leads to an increase in smooth muscle tone. The usual dose is twice daily, but some women who are incontinent with exercise may benefit from taking an α agonist 1 hour before exercise. Tricyclic antidepressants, such as imipramine (Tofranil),[1] have both α-agonist and anticholinergic properties.

---

[1]Not FDA approved for this indication.

CURRENT THERAPY

Urge Incontinence

Behavioral Changes
- Avoidance of bladder irritants
- Timed voiding
- Pelvic muscle exercises

Anticholinergics—Antimuscarinics—Nonselective for M3 Receptor
- Propantheline (Pro-Banthine)[1] 7.5 to 30 mg orally, three to five times daily
- Tolterodine (Detrol LA) 4 mg orally, daily
- Trospium (Sanctura) 20 mg orally, two times daily
- Solifenacin (Vesicare) 5–10 mg orally, daily

Anticholinergics—Antimuscarinics—Selective for M3 Receptor
- Darifenacin (Enablex) 7.5–15 mg orally, daily

Anticholinergics—Antimuscarinics/Smooth Muscle Relaxants
- Oxybutynin
- Regular (Ditropan) 2.5–5 mg orally, one to three times daily
- Extended-release (Ditropan XL) 5–30 mg orally, daily
- Transdermal (Oxytrol) 3.9-mg patch, twice per week
- Hyoscyamine (Levsin) 0.125–0.375 mg orally, two to four times daily

Anticholinergics/α Agonists—For Urge or Mixed Incontinence
- Imipramine (Tofranil)[1] 10–25 mg, once to three times daily

Stress Incontinence

Behavioral Changes
- Weight loss
- Quitting smoking
- Pelvic muscle exercises

α Agonists
- Pseudoephedrine (Sudafed)[1] 30–60 mg, up to four times daily

Surgery
- Anatomic
  - Retropubic suspensions
    - Burch
    - Marshall-Marchetti-Krantz
  - Slings
  - Pubovaginal
  - Midurethral
  - Obturator
- Intrinsic Sphincter Deficiency
  - Slings
    - Pubovaginal
    - Midurethral
    - Obturator
  - Artificial sphincter
  - Submucosal Injections with Bulking Agents
  - Collagen (Contigen)
  - Carbon-coated zirconium oxide beads (Durasphere)
  - Ethylene vinyl alcohol copolymer (Tegress)

[1]Not FDA approved for this indication.

Surgical therapy for stress incontinence is indicated when a patient does not wish to pursue nonsurgical therapy, or if such therapy has failed. The type of surgical therapy depends on the diagnosis. Patients who have anatomic stress incontinence can benefit from a

---

BOX 1   Overview of Treatments

Behavioral Changes
- Avoidance of bladder irritants
- Weight loss
- Quitting smoking
- Pelvic muscle exercises

Medical Therapy
- α Agonists
  - Stress incontinent patients
  - Mixed incontinent patients
- Anticholinergics
  - Urge incontinent patients
- Anticholinergics/α agonists
  - Mixed incontinent patients

Surgical Therapy
- Stress incontinent patients
- Rare patients with urge incontinence

---

variety of surgical repairs that restore the bladder neck to its normal retropubic position or improve urethral support. Patients with ISD usually have a well-supported bladder neck. These patients require a procedure that will close or coapt the proximal urethra. Coaptation may be achieved with a variety of bulking agents that are injected into the bladder neck or proximal urethra. A pubovaginal sling is the ideal procedure for the patient with both ISD and anatomic stress incontinence, as a sling will coapt the proximal urethra and restore the bladder neck to its normal location.

Synthetic midurethral slings are ideal for the patient with anatomic stress incontinence who wishes surgery with minimal recovery time. In one of the rare randomized surgical trials for stress incontinence, the result with tension-free vaginal tape has been shown to be comparable to that of a Burch colposuspension at 6, 12, and 24 months. The newest sling is a transobturator sling that is placed transversely underneath the urethra from one obturator foramina to the other. The advantage of this sling is that the retropubic space is avoided, with low risk of bladder, bowel, and major vessel injury. Randomized trials comparing midurethral or transobturator slings to pubovaginal slings have not been performed.

MIXED INCONTINENCE

Stress and urge incontinence often coexist. Burgio et al. advocate pelvic muscle exercises with biofeedback for treatment of stress and urge incontinence. Behavioral therapy can result in a reduction in incontinence episodes and patient-perceived improvement.

Imipramine (Tofranil)[1] is beneficial in patients with mixed (stress and urge) incontinence. The recommended dose is 10 to 25 mg, three times daily.

Seventy percent of patients with combined incontinence (stress and urge) will be relieved of urge incontinence following a procedure for stress incontinence. Patients whose urge incontinence does not respond to anticholinergics preoperatively may have a good response to anticholinergics once their stress incontinence is treated. Box 1 provides an overview of treatments.

---

[1]Not FDA approved for this indication.

REFERENCES

Blaivas JG, Groutz A. Urinary incontinence: Pathophysiology, evaluation, and management overview. In: Walsh PC, Retik AB, Vaughan Jr ED, Wein AJ, editors. Campbell's Urology. 8th ed., vol. 2. Philadelphia: WB Saunders; 2002. p. 1027.

Burgio KL, Locher JL, Goode PS, et al. Behavioral vs drug treatment for urge urinary incontinence in older women: A randomized controlled trial. JAMA 1998;280:1995–2000.

Leach GE, Dmochowski RR, Appell RA, et al. Female Stress Urinary Incontinence Clinical Guidelines Panel summary report on surgical management of female stress urinary incontinence. The American Urological Association. J Urol 1997;158:875.

Ward KL, Hilton P. A randomized trial of colposuspension and tension-free vaginal tape (TVT) for primary genuine stress incontinence: 2 year followup. Int Urogynecol J Pelvic Floor Dysfunct 2001;12(Suppl. 2):S7–8.

Epididymitis

Method of
David M. Quillen, MD

Epididymitis by definition is inflammation of the epididymis and can be classified by the cause of inflammation. Epididymitis can be infectious (bacterial or nonbacterial) or noninfectious. One can further separate epididymitis into acute (lasting less than 6 weeks) or chronic (lasting more than 3 months).

Anatomy and Physiology

The epididymis is a narrow, tightly coiled tube connecting the testicle to the vas deferens. The epididymis has three basic functions: transit, storage, and maturation of sperm.

Definition and Classification

There are three types of epididymitis: bacterial, nonbacterial infectious, and nonbacterial noninfectious epididymitis.

Bacterial epididymitis generally manifests with a gradual occurrence of pain and swelling of the epididymis associated with inflammation. It can be secondary to urinary tract infection, usually in older men and occasionally in infants. Bacterial epididymitis can occur secondary to a sexually transmitted disease, most commonly chlamydia.

Nonbacterial infectious epididymitis is uncommon. The infectious agent can be viral, fungal, or parasitic.

Nonbacterial noninfectious epididymitis can result from an autoimmune cause, can be associated with a known syndrome, such as Behçet's disease, or can be induced by medication, such as amiodarone. It can be related to trauma, including from exercise, direct trauma, or sexual activity. Epididymitis that does not result from one of these causes is considered idiopathic.

Definition

Chronic epididymitis is defined as a 3-months or longer history of symptoms of discomfort or pain in the scrotum, testicle, or epididymis that are localized to one or both epididymides on clinical examination.

In inflammatory chronic epididymitis, the patient has pain and discomfort associated with abnormal swelling and induration. The types are infective (e.g., chlamydia, gonorrhea), postinfective (e.g., after acute bacterial epididymitis), granulomatous (e.g., tuberculosis), drug-induced (e.g., amiodarone), associated with a known syndrome (e.g., Behçet's disease), or idiopathic (no identifiable etiology for inflammation).

In obstructive chronic epididymitis, the patient has pain or discomfort associated with congenital, acquired, or iatrogenic obstruction of epididymis or vas deferens, such as congenital obstruction or surgical scarring after vasectomy.

Chronic epididymalgia is pain or discomfort in a normal-feeling epididymis associated with no identifiable etiology. The epididymis is normal but it tender on palpation.

Epidemiology

Epididymitis can effect men of all ages, but it is most common among men between the ages of 18 and 35 years. Based upon the National Ambulatory Medical Care Survey of 2002, there are around 600,000 cases a year.

Different patient populations have different risk factors. The most common cause across all patient populations is a sexually transmitted chlamydia infection usually in 18- to 35-year-old men. Coliform bacteria can also be sexually transmitted cause when associated with anal intercourse in homosexual men. In young children or infants, bladder infections and coliform bacteria are usually the cause. In older men, hypertrophy of the prostate, prostatitis, surgery, catheterization, and bladder infections are common causes.

Subacute infections (less-acute pain, few voiding symptoms) are generally associated with sexual activity (without sexually transmitted diseases), heavy physical activity, or bicycle or motorcycle riding. Uncommon and rare causes of epididymitis include medications (amiodarone [Cordarone]), viral infections, fungal infections, and autoimmune disease.

Diagnosis

Patients with epididymitis generally present with a gradual increase in scrotal pain and discomfort that is usually unilateral to start. Frequently painful urination and lower abdominal pain are often present. A normal cremasteric reflex is present, and pain relief can occur with testicular elevation (Prehn sign). Symptoms generally increase gradually with noninfectious causes than with infectious ones. The physical examination usually localizes the tenderness to the epididymis and often demonstrates testicular pain. The spermatic cord is also commonly tender and swollen. Very early on in the presentation, only the tail of the epididymis may be tender, but the inflammation can quickly spread to the rest of the epididymis, to the testicle, and to the other epididymis and testicle.

CURRENT DIAGNOSIS

History

- In men 18 to 35 years, risk factors include unprotected sexual activity and anal intercourse. Signs and symptoms include gradual onset of unilateral pain and dysuria or urethra discharge.
- In men older than 35 years, causes can include urologic abnormality or infection resulting from prostatitis, surgery, catheterization, and urinary tract infection. Other causes are heavy lifting, bicycle riding, and direct trauma.
- In children or infants, look for a urinary tract infection and genital or urinary abnormality.

Physical Examination

- Unilateral pain and swelling
- Urethral discharge
- Structural abnormality
- Normal cremasteric reflex (decreases possibility of torsion)

Laboratory Tests and Ultrasonography

- Perform a urethral swab for white blood cell count, gonococcal and chlamydial infection, and DNA testing.
- Urine should be collected for culture and analysis.
- Consider ultrasonography of the scrotum to rule out torsion.

Both acute infectious and acute noninfectious epididymitis present in much the same way as do acute infectious and acute noninfectious orchitis. Orchitis typically manifests with acute pain, testicular swelling, and a normal cremasteric reflex. Orchitis is much less common than epididymitis, but it should be included in the differential.

Testicular torsion manifests abruptly, with more-severe pain than either epididymitis or orchitis. It is almost always unilateral, and the cremasteric reflex is abnormal. Testicular torsion is a medical emergency and needs quick surgical consultation if considered. Unfortunately, occasionally acute bacterial epididymitis or orchitis can manifest with similar symptoms.

Patients with chronic epididymitis and epididymalgia usually present with a long-standing history of pain (waxing and waning or constant) localized to the epididymis and by definition for at least 3 months. Chronic orchitis manifests similarly, and both can have a significant impact on the patient's quality of life.

Common laboratory tests can include a urethral smear (Gram stain and culture, DNA probe for *Neisseria gonorrhoeae* or *Chlamydia trachomatis*) and a midstream urine specimen for analysis and culture. When epididymitis is diagnosed in an infant or young boy, the child should be further evaluated with abdominopelvic ultrasound to assess urinary tract abnormality and should have a urology referral or urologic work-up.

Imaging with ultrasound is often an important tool to confirm the diagnosis and help eliminate the possibility of testicular torsion. On ultrasound, epididymitis is characterized by an enlargement and thickening of epididymis with an increase in blood flow on color Doppler. Orchitis is characterized by normal epididymis, testicular mass, or swollen testicles with hypoechoic and hypervascular areas. Testicular torsion is characterized by normal-appearing testes, but with decreased blood flow on one side.

Treatment

The Centers for Disease Control and Prevention (CDC) recommends in young men at risk for chlamydia or gonorrhea empiric treatment after obtaining cultures and DNA probe. Ceftriaxone (Rocephin) 250 mg

CURRENT THERAPY

- For men 18 to 35 years who have sexually transmitted diseases or are at risk for them, empiric therapy includes ceftriaxone (Rocephin) 250 mg IM once (can substitute cefixime (Suprax) 400 mg PO once) plus doxycycline (Vibramycin) 100 mg bid for 10 days or azithromycin (Zithromax) 1 g PO for one dose.
- For men older than 35 years in whom the suspected cause is coliform bacteria and *not* gonococcal or chlamydial infection, therapy includes ofloxacin (Floxin) 300 mg bid for 10 days or levofloxacin (Levaquin) 500 mg qd for 10 days. Treat for 21 days if prostatitis is suspected.
- Children and infants should be treated for urinary tract infection and should have a urologic work-up for anatomic abnormality.
- All patients should take antiinflammatory medications and pain medications, should decrease their activity, and should wear supportive undergarments.
- Follow-up includes reevaluation if treatment fails to improve over 2 to 3 days. Consider rare causes, including viral infection, tuberculosis, autoimmune disease, and abscess.
- If cultures are obtained (urethral or urinary), results should be followed and antibiotic adjusted (if necessary) to optimize coverage.
- Patient and sexual partner should be educated (if indicated) to prevent future incidents.

intramuscular injection or cefixime (Suprax) 400 mg orally once and 10 days of oral doxycycline (Vibramycin) are first-line treatment. Azithromycin [Zithromax] 1 g orally once is an acceptable alternative for doxycycline. The one-dose quinolone regimen for gonorrhea is no longer recommended owing to widespread resistance. For older men, empiric treatment with levofloxacin (Levaquin) 500 mg once daily or ofloxacin (Floxin) 300 mg twice daily for 10 days and obtaining urine cultures is acceptable. If prostatitis is suspected, treatment with either levofloxacin or ofloxacin should be extended to 21 days.

REFERENCES

Centers for Disease Control and Prevention (CDC). Update to CDC's sexually transmitted diseases treatment guidelines, 2006: fluoroquinolones no longer recommended for treatment of gonococcal infections. MMWR Morb Mortal Wkly Rep 2007;56(14):332–6.

Centers for Disease Control and Prevention, Workowski KA, Berman SM. Sexually transmitted diseases treatment guidelines, 2006. MMWR Recomm Rep 2006;55(RR-11):1–94.

Lee JC, Bhatt S, Dogra VS. Imaging of the epididymis. Ultrasound Q 2008;24(1):3–16.

Nickel JC. Chronic epididymitis: A practical approach to understanding and managing a difficult urologic enigma. Rev Urol 2003;5(4):209–15.

Trojian TH, Lishnak TS, Heiman D. Epididymitis and orchitis: an overview. Am Fam Physician 2009;79(7):583–7.

Yagil Y, Naroditsky I, Milhem J, et al. Role of Doppler ultrasonography in the triage of acute scrotum in the emergency department. J Ultrasound Med 2010;29(1):11–21.

Primary Glomerular Diseases

Method of
Manuel Praga, MD, and Enrique Morales, MD

Clinical Presentation and Diagnosis

The clinical manifestations of primary glomerular diseases are very variable, ranging from asymptomatic urinary abnormalities to severe forms of rapidly progressive glomerulonephritis. The different clinical presentations are summarized and defined in Box 1.

Most milder forms of glomerular diseases are diagnosed by a positive dipstick test for microhematuria or proteinuria. All these patients should have quantitative estimations of proteinuria (24-hour proteinuria or protein-to-creatinine ratio in a random sample of urine), urinary microscopic examination, and serum creatinine. Glomerular disorders can be the renal manifestation of systemic diseases of different causes (e.g., malignancies, infections, autoimmune disorders), as discussed later. Therefore, medical history and physical examination should carefully investigate data suggesting such diseases. In addition to general laboratory analysis and assessment of renal morphology (renal echography), more specific determinations should be performed in all patients with suspected glomerular diseases: protein electrophoresis, serum levels of immunoglobulins, serum complement fractions C3 and C4, antinuclear antibody (ANA), anti-DNA antibodies, antineutrophilic cytoplasmic antibodies (ANCA), and tests for hepatitis B virus (HBV), hepatitis C virus (HCV), and HIV infections.

Renal biopsy is the conclusive method for establishing the diagnosis and classification of primary glomerular disorders. Indications for renal biopsy include the nephrotic syndrome in adults (except cases attributed to diabetic nephropathy) and steroid-resistant nephrotic syndrome in children, rapidly progressive nephritis, persistent nephritic syndrome with deteriorating renal function, and, usually, recurrent macroscopic hematuria. The need for renal biopsy in patients with asymptomatic urinary abnormalities should be individualized. The most characteristic pathologic findings of the main primary glomerulonephritis are summarized in Box 2, and their commonest clinical presentations are summarized in Box 3.

BOX 1 Clinical Presentations of Glomerular Diseases

Nephrotic Syndrome
- Proteinuria >3.5 g/d in adults and >40 mg/h/m^2 in children
- Hypoalbuminemia
- Hyperlipidemia
- Edema

Nephritic Syndrome
- Hypertension
- Oliguria
- Edema
- Hematuria (usually macroscopic)
- Red cell casts
- Non-nephrotic proteinuria
- Mild and nonprogressive GFR decrease

Rapidly Progressive Glomerulonephritis
- Acute or subacute progressive worsening of renal function
- Hematuria (usually macroscopic)
- Red cell casts
- Proteinuria (usually <3.5 g/d)
- Blood pressure often normal

Persistent Asymptomatic Urinary Abnormalities
- Non-nephrotic proteinuria (<3.5 g/d in adults and <40 mg/h/m^2 in children)
- Persistent microscopic hematuria

Recurrent Macroscopic Hematuria
- Bouts of gross hematuria, usually triggered by infections
- Persistent microhematuria between the episodes of gross hematuria

Chronic Renal Insufficiency
- Persistent proteinuria and/or microhematuria
- Hypertension
- Small kidneys

Hypocomplementemia

The C3 and C4 fractions of serum complement are characteristically reduced in some types of glomerular diseases. This is an important clue for diagnosis.

Abbreviation: GFR = glomerular filtration rate.

BOX 2 Main Histologic Findings of Primary Glomerular Diseases

Minimal Change Disease
- Normal glomeruli on light microscopy
- Negative immunofluorescence and diffuse effacement of epithelial foot processes on electron microscopy

Focal and Segmental Glomerulosclerosis
- Focal (some glomeruli) and segmental (parts of affected glomeruli) scarring of the glomerular tuft

Membranous Nephropathy
- Thickening of glomerular capillary walls with projections of glomerular basement membrane ("spikes")
- Subepithelial immune deposits detected by immunofluorescence and electron microscopy

Membranoproliferative Glomerulonephritis
- Increase of mesangial cells and mesangial matrix
- Widening (double contoured appearance) of capillary loops
- IgG, C3, and IgM on immunofluorescence and subendothelial (type I) or intra-GBM (type II) deposits on electron microscopy

IgA Nephropathy
- Predominant deposition of mesangial IgA on immunofluorescence
- Proliferation of mesangial cellularity and mesangial matrix on light microscopy
- Mesangial electron-dense deposits on electron microscopy

Acute Postinfectious (Diffuse Proliferative) Glomerulonephritis
- Marked hypercellularity due to mesangial and endothelial cell proliferation and glomerular influx of neutrophils
- Hump-like subepithelial dense deposits on electron microscopy

Crescentic Glomerulonephritis
- Cellular or fibrocellular crescents in a variable percentage of glomeruli
- Immunofluorescence pattern distinguishes the main three types:
  - Type I: Linear IgG staining of the GBM (anti-GBM disease)
  - Type II: Granular deposits along GBM (immune complex deposition)
  - Type III: Negative immunofluorescence (pauci-immune glomerulonephritis)

Abbreviations: GBM = glomerular basement membrane; Ig = immunoglobulin.

CURRENT DIAGNOSIS

- Clinical presentations of glomerular diseases range from asymptomatic urinary abnormalities (proteinuria, microhematuria) to severe forms of rapidly progressive glomerulonephritis (gross hematuria, edema, acute renal function worsening, hypertension).
- Secondary causes of glomerular disease should be excluded by means of history, physical examination, and appropriate laboratory tests.
- Renal biopsy establishes the diagnosis and classification of primary glomerular diseases.

Treatment

CONSERVATIVE THERAPY

Hypertension is a common finding in patients with primary glomerulonephritis. Current guidelines recommend blood pressure targets lower than 130/80 mm Hg in these patients and lower than 125/75 mm Hg in patients with proteinuria greater than 1 g/24 hours. Any antihypertensive drug or drug combinations are useful, and they should be selected on the basis of the patient's characteristics.

BOX 3   Commonest Presentations of the Main Primary Glomerular Diseases

Minimal Change Disease
- Nephrotic syndrome

Focal and Segmental Glomerulosclerosis
- Nephrotic syndrome in more than two thirds of patients
- Non-nephrotic proteinuria in the remaining patients
- Renal insufficiency (20%–40%), hypertension (50%), and microhematuria (40%)

Membranous Nephropathy
- Nephrotic syndrome in >80% of patients
- Non-nephrotic proteinuria in the remaining patients

Membranoproliferative Glomerulonephritis
- Nephrotic syndrome in 50%
- Nephritic syndrome in 20%–30%
- Asymptomatic urinary abnormalities in 20%–30%
- Hypocomplementemia is common.

IgA Nephropathy
- Asymptomatic urinary abnormalities (microhematuria ± proteinuria) in >75%
- Intercalated recurrent or isolated episodes of macroscopic hematuria in >40%
- Nephritic or nephrotic syndrome in <10%

Acute Postinfectious Glomerulonephritis
- Nephritic syndrome
- Hypocomplementemia

Crescentic Glomerulonephritis
- Rapidly progressive glomerulonephritis

Abbreviation: Ig = immunoglobulin.

CURRENT THERAPY

- Appropriate treatment should be instituted as early as possible.
- Blood pressure should be lower than 130/80 mm Hg (<125/75 mm Hg in patients with proteinuria >1 g/24 h).
- Angiotensin-converting enzyme inhibitors and angiotensin receptor blockers are indicated in most cases of chronic proteinuric glomerular diseases due to their antiproteinuric, antihypertensive, and renoprotective effects.
- Specific therapy of primary glomerular diseases includes steroids, anticalcineurinic agents, and cytotoxics. Due to the potential risks of these therapies, the likelihood of progression and the presence of chronic irreversible parenchymal damage must be carefully assessed.
- Primary or idiopathic glomerular diseases comprise a wide variety of glomerular histologic lesions, with different clinical presentations and variable prognosis. Although some entities portend a favorable long-term prognosis, a considerable fraction of untreated patients who have other glomerular entities reach end-stage renal failure.

However, blockade of the renin-angiotensin system either with an angiotensin-converting enzyme inhibitor (ACEI) or an angiotensin receptor blocker (ARB) should be the main basis of antihypertensive treatment because of their demonstrated renoprotective effect (slowing or preventing loss of renal function) in patients with chronic renal diseases. The beneficial effects of ACEIs and ARBs appear to be similar and are also observed in proteinuric patients with normal blood pressure. Renal protection induced by ACEIs and ARBs is closely related to the significant reduction in proteinuria that these agents induce. The level of proteinuria is the best way to monitor the efficacy of ACEIs and ARBs. Recent studies in primary glomerular diseases have shown that a combination of ACEI and ARB is more beneficial in terms of proteinuria decrease than either drug alone. Aldosterone antagonists (spironolactone, eplerenone) have also shown a remarkable antiproteinuric efficacy. Nevertheless, serum creatinine and potassium should be monitored after ACEI, ARB, or antialdosteronic agents are initiated, particularly in patients with reduced renal function.

Hyperlipidemia is a common finding in patients with glomerular diseases, particularly in those with the nephrotic syndrome. Prospective clinical studies have demonstrated that treatment of hyperlipidemia decreases proteinuria and prevents renal function loss. Statins such as atorvastatin (Lipitor) (10–40 mg after the evening meal) are the most commonly used lipid-lowering drugs. A level of LDL cholesterol lower than 100 mg/dL is recommended. Weight loss in obese patients induces a significant reduction in proteinuria, and smoking should be strictly forbidden, because smoking is associated with a more rapid progression toward renal failure in any type of renal disease.

All these measures (blood pressure lowering, treatment with ACEIs and ARBs, treatment of hyperlipidemia, weight loss, cessation of smoking) are also beneficial for the global cardiovascular risk that is significantly higher in proteinuric patients (mainly in those with renal insufficiency) than in the normal population.

The complications of the nephrotic syndrome require specific treatment. Edema is usually managed with a low-sodium diet plus furosemide (Lasix) in doses carefully adjusted to the severity of edema. Daily weight measurement is very important, because excessive diuretic doses can lead to volume depletion and functional worsening of renal function. In resistant cases, combinations of different types of diuretics (furosemide plus a thiazide diuretic, or furosemide plus a potassium-sparing diuretic such as spironolactone [Aldactone] in patients with hypokalemia) are needed. More severe cases require albumin infusions followed by high-dose intravenous furosemide (although intravenous albumin [Albuminar][1] increases proteinuria) or even removal of fluids by hemodialysis. Nephrotic patients are at increasing risk for thrombotic events. Prophylactic treatment (subcutaneous low-molecular-weight heparin) is indicated in conditions of high risk, such as immobilization.

SPECIFIC THERAPY

Box 4 summarizes the immunosuppressive treatment of primary glomerular diseases.

Minimal Change Disease

Minimal change disease (MCD) is most common in children but also causes 10% to 15% of nephrotic syndrome in adults. Corticosteroid therapy is a very effective treatment for MCD. For children, the dose of prednisone is 60 mg/m^2/day and for adults 1 mg/kg/day (up to 80 mg/day). About 75% of patients respond (complete proteinuria disappearance) within 2 weeks, and more than 90% respond within 8 weeks, but adults show in general a slower response than children. Initial steroid dose is continued for 4 weeks and then changed to alternate-day prednisone (40 mg/m^2 on alternate days) or to daily prednisone, slowly tapering off over 6 to 10 weeks. Keeping patients on steroids for more than 3 months is associated with a lower 1-year relapse rate.

[1]Not FDA approved for this indication.

BOX 4 Immunosuppressive Treatment of Primary Glomerular Disease

Minimal Change Disease
First Line
- Steroids

Second Line
- Cytotoxics (frequent relapsers)
- Anticalcineurinics or mycophenolate mofetil (CellCept)[1] (steroid-dependent)

Focal Segmental Glomerulosclerosis
First Line
- Steroids
- ACEIs
- ARBs

Second Line
- Anticalcineurinics
- Mycophenolate mofetil[1]

Membranous Nephropathy
First Line
- Anticalcineurinics
- Steroids plus cytotoxics
- ACEIs
- ARBs

Second Line
- Mycophenolate mofetil
- Intramuscular ACTH (Synacthen)[1,2]
- Rituximab (Rituxan)[1]

Membranoproliferative Glomerulonephritis
- Steroids
- ACEIs
- ARBs

IgA Nephropathy
First Line
- ACEIs
- ARBs

Second Line
- Steroids
- Fish oil
- Cytotoxics

Acute Postinfectious Glomerulonephritis
- Conservative therapy

Crescentic Glomerulonephritis
Type I (anti-GBM)
- Steroids
- Cyclophosphamide (Cytoxan)[1]
- Plasmapheresis

Type II and III
Induction
- Steroids
- Cyclophosphamide[1]
- Plasmapheresis in severe acute renal failure

Maintenance
- Low-dose steroids
- Azathioprine (Imuran)[1]

[1]Not FDA approved for this indication.
[2]Not available in the United States.
Abbreviations: ACEI = angiotensin-converting enzyme inhibitor; ACTH = adrenocorticotropic hormone; ARB = angiotensin receptor blocker; GBM = glomerular basement membrane; Ig = immunoglobulin.

Up to 75% of children and many adults have nephrotic syndrome relapses. Isolated relapses are re-treated with steroids as in the first episode. Frequent relapsers (two or more relapses within a 6-month period) are treated with a low-dose steroid course plus cyclophosphamide (Cytoxan) (1.5–2 mg/kg/day) or chlorambucil (Leukeran)[1] (0.1–0.2 mg/kg/day) in an 8-week course. After these short-term cytotoxic courses, a considerable fraction of patients remain free of proteinuria for prolonged periods, with a low rate of serious complications. Longer or repeated courses can induce severe side effects and are not recommended.

The response of steroid-dependent patients (reappearance of the nephrotic syndrome during or immediately after steroid withdrawal) to cytotoxics is poorer than that of frequent relapsers. Steroid-dependent patients and frequent relapsers unresponsive to cytotoxics are commonly treated with cyclosporine (Neoral)[1] given in an initial dose of 3–4 mg/kg in two divided doses, then adjusting for serum levels of 100–175 ng/mL. Most steroid-dependent patients transform into cyclosporine-dependent, and the risk of cyclosporine-induced nephrotoxicity should be considered. Mycophenolate mofetil (MMF, CellCept)[1] (600 mg/m^2/12 h in children, 500–1000 mg/12 h in adults) is a very useful alternative. Rates of response and relapse are similar to those of cyclosporine, but tolerance is better and there

is no risk of nephrotoxicity. Therapy with cyclosporine or MMF if the patient responds is continued for up to 12 months before slow and careful tapering.

Less than 10% of MCD patients are steroid resistant. Because most of them subsequently have focal segmental glomerulosclerosis (FSGS) on biopsy, their therapeutic approach is the same as for FSGS.

Focal and Segmental Glomerulosclerosis

Causes of secondary FSGS (obesity, reflux nephropathy, reduction in renal mass) should be carefully excluded. Treatment with an ACEI or ARB (or both) is the first option in patients with non-nephrotic proteinuria or in patients with nonaggressive nephrotic syndrome (proteinuria <5 g/day, serum albumin >3 g/dL, normal renal function), mainly if hypertension coexists. Patients with severe nephrotic syndrome or nephrotic proteinuria after ACEI or ARB introduction should be treated with prednisone 1 mg/kg/day. Several retrospective studies have shown that steroid treatment maintained for at least 6 months is followed by more than 50% partial or complete remissions. However, in responsive patients, proteinuria starts to decrease after 2 to 3 months of treatment.

If proteinuria did not show significant changes within this period, introduction of an anticalcineurinic agent together with steroid tapering is recommended. Cyclosporine (doses and blood levels as in MCD) has been the most commonly used drug, and prospective studies have

[1]Not FDA approved for this indication.

shown more than 70% partial or complete remission after 6 months of treatment. Tacrolimus (Prograf)[1] (0.05–0.10 mg/kg/day in two divided doses, then adjusted for serum levels of 4–7 ng/mL) is proved to be effective in some cyclosporine-resistant FSGS cases.

In patients with complete or partial response to cyclosporine or tacrolimus, these drugs should be maintained at the lowest effective doses for at least 1 year before slowly tapering off. In some patients resistant to steroids and cyclosporine, or in those with mild degrees of renal insufficiency, MMF[1] (same doses as in MCD) has decreased proteinuria and stabilized renal function for prolonged periods. Sirolimus (Rapamune)[1] has induced complete (19%) or partial (38%) remission in a series of patients, although other studies have failed to confirm these beneficial effects and have shown a remarkable number of serious side effects.

About 20% to 25% of children with aggressive forms of FSGS have mutations in the genes coding for several podocyte proteins, mainly podocin. Most of these patients are unresponsive to any kind of treatment.

Membranous Nephropathy

More than one third of MGN patients have a spontaneous remission, and most remissions take place during the first 2 years of the disease. Conservative therapy should be maintained during the first 9 to 12 months, unless renal function starts to deteriorate. ACEIs or ARBs, or both, can induce partial remission (non-nephrotic proteinuria) in a considerable percentage of cases.

In patients with an aggressive presentation (massive nephrotic syndrome and deteriorating renal function) a 6-month course of alternating monthly prednisone 0.5 mg/kg/day with a month of chlorambucil[1] 0.2 mg/kg/day is recommended. Other clinicians simultaneously use prednisone starting with 1 mg/kg/day and tapering off over 6 months plus chlorambucil 0.15 mg/kg/day for 14 weeks. Another regimen is prednisone 0.5 mg/kg/day every other day for 6 months plus cyclophosphamide[1] 1.5 mg/kg/day for 12 months.

In patients maintaining normal renal function and persistent nephrotic proteinuria beyond 9 to 12 months, immunosuppressive therapy should be initiated, mainly in the presence of markers of poor outcome, which include male gender, older age, and proteinuria persistently higher than 8 g/day after ACEI or ARB treatment. Alternating prednisone and chlorambucil (as indicated earlier), prednisone and cyclophosphamide, and cyclosporine[1] 3–4 mg/kg/day, targeting blood levels of 100–175 ng/mL are beneficial, inducing complete or partial remission in most patients.

Side effects (diabetes, bone necrosis, infections) are more serious with steroids plus cytotoxic treatments; trimethoprim-sulfamethoxazole (TMP-SMX, Bactrim) (80 mg/400 mg/day) should be concurrently administered for *Pneumocystis jiroveci* prophylaxis. Cyclosporine, administered for 6 months, is followed by approximately 50% of recurrences after drug withdrawal.

No studies comparing anticalcineurinic and cytotoxics have been published for MGN. Tacrolimus,[1] another anticalcineurinic agent, can also induce partial response in more than 80% of treated patients, although recurrence after withdrawal is the same (50%) as with cyclosporine. A recent randomized pilot trial reported that tetracosactide (Synacthen),[1,2] an analogue of ACTH (1 mg IM twice a week for 1 year) induced remissions in the same percentage as a regimen of steroids plus cyclophosphamide.

Uncontrolled studies reported that MMF[1] (1000–2000 mg/day) reduced proteinuria and stabilized renal function in some MGN patients unresponsive to other therapies. Rituximab (Rituxan),[1] a monoclonal antibody against CD20-lymphocytes, has induced complete (15%–20%) or partial (35%–40%) remission in several series of patients, although no prospective controlled studies have been published. On the other hand, rituximab has been effective to avoid nephrotic syndrome relapse after tacrolimus withdrawal in patients successfully treated with this drug but showing anticalcineurin dependence.

Membranoproliferative Glomerulonephritis

The incidence of idiopathic membranoproliferative glomerulonephritis (MPGN) has progressively decreased over the last decades, being currently an uncommon disease in developed countries. Most cases of MPGN are now secondary to HCV infection and concurrent cryoglobulinemia. No prospective studies about the treatment of idiopathic MPGN have been carried out in the last several years. Uncontrolled series of patients suggested that prolonged (>2 years) prednisone treatment is beneficial in terms of proteinuria reduction and renal survival. Prospective randomized trials with aspirin[1] and dipyridamole (Persantine)[1] showed a significant reduction in proteinuria some decades ago, but later analysis did not demonstrate long-term benefits on renal survival.

Conservative therapy, including ACEIs and ARBs, should be prescribed in all cases. In patients with the nephrotic syndrome after an observation period or in those with more aggressive presentations (deteriorating renal function, crescents), a 6- to 12-month course of prednisone could be indicated. Some small series of patients suggested that cyclophosphamide[1] is effective in aggressive cases of MPGN, but conclusive evidence is lacking.

Immunoglobulin A Nephropathy

As in all types of primary glomerular diseases, the aggressiveness of therapeutic approaches in patients with immunoglobulin A (IgA) nephropathy should be graded according to the severity of the presentation. In patients with microhematuria and normal renal function, only regular follow-up is required. If slowly increasing proteinuria appears, an ACEI or ARB, or a combination of both drugs, should be started, even in the absence of hypertension, targeting for proteinuria less than 1 g/day and blood pressure lower than 125/75 mm Hg.

In patients with increasing proteinuria greater than 1–1.5 g/day in spite of these measures, other therapies should be contemplated. Steroids were proven to be beneficial in patients with normal renal function and proteinuria greater than 1 g/day in a prospective randomized trial: methylprednisolone (Solu-Medrol) pulses, 1 g/day for 3 days in the beginning of months 1, 3, and 5, and oral prednisone 0.5 mg/kg every other day for 6 months reduced proteinuria and increased renal survival in comparison with untreated patients.

Treatment with fish oil supplements[1] in this type of patient remains controversial. Although eicosapentaenoic acid (1.8 g/day) or docosahexaenoic acid (1.2 g/day) demonstrated beneficial effects in some trials, these effects were not reproduced in others.

In patients with more aggressive presentations (proteinuria and deteriorating renal function), a prospective trial demonstrated that prednisone 40 mg/day tapering to 10 mg/day within 2 years plus cyclophosphamide[1] 1.5 mg/kg/day for 3 months followed by azathioprine (Imuran)[1] 1.5 mg/kg/day for at least 2 years significantly improved renal survival in comparison with untreated patients.

After initial suggestions of the benefits of MMF[1] 1000 to 2000 mg/day in IgA nephropathy patients unresponsive to other therapies, recent prospective and controlled trials have failed to demonstrate these good results, although the number of study subjects was small and many of them had advanced renal insufficiency.

Acute Postinfectious (Diffuse Proliferative) Glomerulonephritis

As in MPGN, the incidence of diffuse proliferative glomerulonephritis has drastically decreased in recent years in developed countries. The prognosis is generally good, and signs and symptoms of the disease (nephritic syndrome) resolve sporadically within 2 to 6 weeks in a great majority of cases. Treatment should be focused on adequate control of blood pressure, salt restriction, and diuretics to prevent fluid excess and the risks of cardiac failure. The triggering infection should be investigated and treated if it has not disappeared spontaneously.

---

[1]Not FDA approved for this indication.
[2]Not available in the United States.

---

[1]Not FDA approved for this indication.

Some patients present with more aggressive courses, developing progressive renal insufficiency. In these cases, crescents involving a large proportion of glomeruli can be observed in a second biopsy. No controlled studies have been carried out in these aggressive cases, but some series of patients recommend high-dose intravenous pulse steroid, followed by oral prednisone 1 mg/kg/day, tapering off over 2 to 3 months. There is no evidence that more aggressive immunosuppressive therapy is beneficial.

Crescentic Glomerulonephritis

Treatment of crescentic glomerulonephritis (CGN) should be promptly instituted because of the rapid transformation of cellular crescents into irreversible fibrotic crescents that collapse the glomerular tufts. Prognosis of type I (anti-GBM disease) CGN is poorer than that of types II and III, particularly in the presence of oligoanuria, dialysis requirement, or a large fraction of glomeruli with crescents.

Treatment of type I CGN includes steroids, cyclophosphamide,[1] and plasmapheresis. Pulse intravenous methylprednisolone (500–1000 mg daily for 3–4 days) is followed by oral prednisone (1 mg/kg/day for 3–4 weeks, then slowly tapering off over 6 months). Oral cyclophosphamide (2 mg/kg/day) is usually maintained for 2 to 3 months. Plasmapheresis (daily or alternate-day 4-liter exchanges) using albumin as replacement fluid or fresh frozen plasma if bleeding risk is high, is usually performed for 2 to 3 weeks. The duration of plasmapheresis, as well as the intensity and the duration of immunosuppressive therapy, should be guided by the clinical status and the titers of anti-GBM antibodies. In patients without pulmonary hemorrhage and with very advanced renal involvement (massive presence of glomerular fibrotic crescents), aggressive immunosuppression is not indicated.

The precise etiology of type II CGN (e.g., systemic lupus erythematosus, cryoglobulinemia) should be identified and the therapy guided by the diagnosis. If no apparent diagnosis is available, treatment is similar to that for type III (pauci-immune) CGN.

Induction treatment of type III CGN consists of steroids (oral prednisone, 1 mg/kg/day for 3–4 weeks, slowly tapered to a maintenance dose of 10–20 mg), and intravenous monthly pulses of cyclophosphamide (initial dose 0.5 to 1 g/m^2, adjusted for renal function and age), which has proved to be as effective and less toxic than oral administration. Once remission is achieved (recovery of renal function, absence of extrarenal symptoms), usually within 3 to 6 months, cyclophosphamide is replaced by azathioprine[1] 1 to 2 mg/kg/day for 12 to 18 months plus prednisone 5 to 10 mg daily or every other day. Positive titers of ANCA, particularly p-ANCA, can indicate more prolonged, low-dose, maintenance treatment, because the risk of recurrence is high. Plasmapheresis (similar to that in type I CGN) is proven to add benefits in type III CGN manifesting with severe renal failure. Although not tested in prospective trials, MMF[1] (1500–3000 mg/day) has been shown effective and well tolerated, even as induction therapy in some series of patients.

---

[1]Not FDA approved for this indication.

REFERENCES

Cattran DC, Appel GB, Hebert LA, et al. A randomized trial of cyclosporine in patients with steroid-resistant focal segmental glomerulosclerosis. Kidney Int 1999;56:2220–6.

Cattran DC, Appel GB, Hebert LA, et al. Cyclosporin in patients with steroid-resistant membranous nephropathy: A randomized trial. Kidney Int 2001;59:1484–90.

Jayne D, Rasmussen N, Andrassy K, et al. A randomized trial of maintenance therapy for vasculitis associated with antineutrophil cytoplasmic autoantibodies. N Engl J Med 2003;349:36–44.

Nakao N, Yoshimura A, Morita H, et al. Combination treatment of angiotensin-II receptor blocker and angiotensin-converting-enzyme inhibitor in nondiabetic renal disease (COOPERATE): A randomized controlled trial. Lancet 2003;361:117–24.

Ponticelli C, Altieri P, Scolari F, et al. A randomized study comparing methylprednisolone plus chlorambucil versus methylprednisolone plus cyclophosphamide in idiopathic membranous nephropathy. J Am Soc Nephrol 1998;9:444–50.

Pozzi C, Bolasco PG, Fogazzi GB, et al. Corticosteroids in IgA nephropathy: A randomised controlled trial. Lancet 1999;13:883–7.

Praga M, Gutiérrez E, González E, et al. Treatment of IgA nephropathy with ACE inhibitors: A randomized and controlled trial. J Am Soc Nephrol 2003;14:1578–83.

Torres A, Domínguez-Gil B, Carreño A, et al. Conservative versus immunosuppressive treatment of patients with idiopathic membranous nephropathy. Kidney Int 2002;61:219–27.

Pyelonephritis

Method of
Patricia D. Brown, MD

Acute pyelonephritis (APN) is a urinary tract infection (UTI) that involves the renal parenchyma, also referred to as *upper tract UTI*. Most episodes of APN occur as a result of ascending infection from the bladder; patients with APN might or might not have symptoms of concomitant cystitis. Rarely, pyelonephritis occurs secondary to hematogenous seeding of the kidney as a result of infection elsewhere, most commonly endocarditis due to *Staphylococcus aureus* or disseminated fungal infection.

Epidemiology

Surprisingly little is known about the epidemiology of APN. Similar to cystitis, APN (and hospitalization for APN) is more common in women than men; men have been reported to have higher in-hospital mortality. In contrast to cystitis, risk factors for pyelonephritis are not well defined. One recent study of nonpregnant women 18 to 49 years of age found risk factors for APN included factors known to be risk factors for acute cystitis, including frequency of sexual intercourse, recent UTI, diabetes, and maternal UTI history. The incidence of bacteremia in patients with APN is reported to be 11% to 53% in various studies; risk factors for bacteremia are not well established.

Similar to lower UTI, APN can be further classified into complicated or uncomplicated infection. The factors that make an episode of APN a complicated UTI are outlined in Box 1.

BOX 1   Factors Associated with Complicated Pyelonephritis

- Diabetes
- Foreign body (catheter, stent)
- Health care–associated infections
- Immunocompromise
- Incomplete voiding (detrusor muscle dysfunction due to neurologic disease or medications)
- Infections due to multidrug-resistant pathogens
- Obstruction (including stones)
- Pregnancy
- Recent history of instrumentation
- Renal transplant recipient
- UTI in a male patient
- Vesicoureteral reflux

Abbreviation: UTI = urinary tract infection.

Clinical Presentation

The classic presenting features of APN include abrupt onset of fever, flank pain, and costovertebral angle tenderness with or without symptoms of lower UTI including dysuria, urgency, and frequency. Unfortunately, there is no single constellation of signs or symptoms that is pathognomonic for APN. When localization studies have been performed on patients with symptoms of acute cystitis, 30% to 50% have been shown to have APN. Women who present with symptoms that have been present more than 7 days and those with a recent history of UTI are more likely to have APN. Flank pain is reported in approximately one half of patients with APN but also occurs in almost 20% of patients with cystitis. Fever is present in one half of patients with APN, but less than 5% of patients with cystitis. Nausea, vomiting, and diarrhea occur commonly in patients with APN, and gastrointestinal (GI) symptoms can dominate the presenting complaints.

In general, patients who present with lower urinary tract symptoms or laboratory evidence of urinary tract infection accompanied by fever, flank pain or tenderness, or signs of systemic toxicity, such as GI symptoms, should be treated for APN.

The diagnosis can be particularly challenging in the frail elderly patient, because symptoms such as frequency, urgency, and incontinence are often chronic in this patient population and unrelated to active UTI. Change in mental status may be the only presenting complaint. Because the prevalence of bacteriuria in this patient population is high, particularly among those with chronic indwelling catheters, UTI must be a diagnosis of exclusion.

Acute pelvic inflammatory disease can have a presentation similar to APN. Pelvic examination should be performed on all sexually active women to exclude this diagnosis.

The differential diagnosis of APN is outlined in Box 2.

Diagnosis

Urinalysis, ideally with microscopic examination, using a clean-catch, midstream specimen, should be performed in all patients with suspected APN. Pyuria is a key finding in the diagnosis of UTI, and the absence of pyuria is strong evidence against a diagnosis of APN. Direct microscopic examination under high power of the urinary sediment from a centrifuged specimen should reveal more than 10 leukocytes per high-powered field. The presence of white blood cell (WBC) casts is highly specific for localization of the infection to the kidney, but it is inadequately sensitive to exclude the diagnosis of APN. The dipstick test for leukocyte esterase is used as a rapid screening test to detect significant pyuria; the sensitivity is reported to be 75% to 96%, with a specificity of 94% to 98%. Because of the lower range of the reported sensitivity of the dipstick test, microscopic examination to exclude significant pyuria should be obtained in patients with suspected APN.

CURRENT DIAGNOSIS

- Abrupt onset of fever, flank pain, and costovertebral angle tenderness with or without symptoms of cystitis are classic presenting features.
- Patients with lower UTI symptoms or laboratory evidence of UTI accompanied by flank pain, fever, or signs of systemic toxicity such as GI complaints should be managed as having APN.
- Urinalysis with microscopic examination should be performed in all patients with suspected APN. Absence of pyuria is strong evidence against the diagnosis.
- A urine culture should be obtained in all patients with APN. Blood cultures should be obtained in those who are hospitalized.
- Patients should be categorized into those with uncomplicated and those with complicated infections.

Abbreviations: APN = acute pyelonephritis; GI = gastrointestinal; UTI = urinary tract infection.

The presence of nitrite in the urine, detected by a dipstick test, has a reported sensitivity of 35% to 85% and a specificity of 92% to 100% for UTI. Microscopic examination of a Gram-stained, centrifuged urine specimen revealing at least one bacterium per oil-immersion field correlates with more than 10^5 colony-forming units (cfu)/mL of bacteria, with a sensitivity of 95%. Although this is the standard definition of significant bacteriuria, it has been shown that women with UTI can have levels of bacteriuria as low as 10^2 cfu/mL.

Although the microbiology of APN has remained predictable, significant changes in antimicrobial susceptibility patterns have occurred. Therefore, in contrast to recommendations for acute uncomplicated cystitis, a urine culture should be obtained in all patients with suspected APN. The need to obtain blood cultures has been debated, because blood cultures rarely yield a pathogen different from what was isolated from the urine. Bacteremia has been reported in 11% to 53% of patients hospitalized with APN. Bacteremic patients have a longer length of stay, and one recent report suggests that this is due to a longer time to resolution of fever. Many experts continue to recommend that blood cultures be obtained as part of the diagnostic evaluation of patients who are ill enough to require hospitalization; blood cultures are not necessary for those who will be managed as outpatients.

The role of diagnostic imaging in the management of APN is discussed later. In some cases with an atypical presentation, imaging may be helpful to confirm the diagnosis of APN. In this setting, pre- and postcontrast computed tomography (CT) is the imaging procedure of choice in adults.

Microbial Etiology

Most cases of APN are caused by *Escherichia coli*. Other enterobacteriaceae, including *Klebsiella* species and *Proteus* species, are also occasionally implicated. Other gram-negative pathogens such as *Pseudomonas, Serratia, Enterobacter*, and *Acinetobacter* should be considered in health care–associated infections. *Enterococcus* is an uncommon pathogen in community-acquired infections, but it must be considered in health care–associated infections, including vancomycin-resistant enterococci. Other gram-positive pathogens include *Streptoccocus agalactiae* and *Staphylococcus* species. Although a common cause of acute cystitis in young women, *Staphylococcus saprophyticus* is a rare cause of pyelonephritis; the finding of *Staphylococcus aureus* in a urine culture should always prompt a search for an extrarenal source of infection that might have served as a source of hematogenous seeding. A Gram stain of the urine is a simple and rapid test to exclude a gram-positive pathogen as the etiology of APN and guide the initial selection of empiric therapy.

BOX 2   Differential Diagnosis of Acute Pyelonephritis

- Appendicitis
- Cholecystitis
- Diverticulitis
- Gastroenteritis
- Herpes zoster
- Musculoskeletal pain, including vertebral disorders
- Ovarian cysts, tumors
- Pancreatitis
- Perforated viscus
- Pelvic inflammatory disease
- Pneumonia
- Renal stones, renal vein thrombosis, renal infarction

The emergence of resistance to trimethoprim-sulfamethoxazole (TMP-SMX [Bactrim]) among *E. coli* has had a major impact on the approach to initial empiric antimicrobial therapy for APN. It is clear that the prevalence of resistance varies depending on geographic region, and clinicians often do not have access to meaningful local resistance data. Recent reports of increasing fluoroquinolone resistance among uropathogens are of great concern, although overall resistance rates in North America remain low.

Treatment

The first decision in the management of patients with APN is whether or not the patient requires hospitalization. Although prospective randomized trials are lacking, several retrospective studies as well as several prospective nonrandomized trials suggest that outpatient management is safe for many patients. Hospitalization should be considered for patients who cannot tolerate oral intake or who have severe pain or signs of severe sepsis. A strategy of initial management in the emergency department or an observation unit with an initial dose of parenteral antibiotic therapy, intravenous fluids, and symptomatic treatment of nausea and pain may be used in select patients to avoid hospital admission. Patients who will be treated as outpatients should have a stable social situation and the ability to contact the physician and return promptly if their symptoms worsen. Hospitalization is generally recommended for patients with complicated infections. Most experts believe that pregnant women with APN should always be hospitalized.

There are surprisingly few prospective randomized trials of the treatment of pyelonephritis. For patients who require hospitalization, parenteral therapy with an aminoglycoside, a third-generation cephalosporin, or a fluoroquinolone is recommended. At my institution, we discourage fluoroquinolones for this indication because there are other effective alternatives and we wish to minimize the use of these very broad-spectrum agents in the hospital setting. Although resistance to TMP-SMX among uropathogenic *E. coli* appears to have leveled off and might actually be decreasing, this agent should not be used for empiric therapy of APN.

If a gram-positive pathogen is suspected or suggested by the results of urine Gram stain, ampicillin or ampicillin-sulbactam (Unasyn) with or without an aminoglycoside can be used. Patients should receive intravenous therapy until they are clinically improving and able to reliably tolerate oral intake; oral therapy can be chosen based on the results of urine culture and susceptibility data. TMP-SMX, a fluoroquinolone, and ampicillin are all potential candidates for oral switch therapy. The narrowest spectrum, least expensive agent to which the isolated pathogen is susceptible should be chosen. Despite in vitro susceptibility data, first- and second-generation cephalosporins have a poor track record in the treatment of APN and are generally not recommended, with the exception of pyelonephritis in pregnancy.

CURRENT THERAPY

- Hospitalization is recommended for patients unable to tolerate oral intake, those with severe pain, and those with signs of severe sepsis. Hospitalization is generally recommended for patients with complicated infections and for all pregnant women.
- Parenteral regimens for hospitalized patients include an aminoglycoside, third-generation cephalosporin, or fluoroquinolone, with oral switch therapy selected on the basis of culture and susceptibility data.
- Initial empiric therapy for outpatients is a fluoroquinolone.
- Imaging is not recommended for patients with uncomplicated infections. Pre- and postcontrast computed tomographic scans should be obtained in those who fail to respond within 72 hours to appropriate antibiotic therapy.

BOX 3   Antimicrobial Therapy for the Management of Acute Pyelonephritis

Parenteral Regimens
- Ampicillin 2 g q4h–q6h
- Ampicillin-sulbactam (Unasyn) 3 g q6h
- Ceftriaxone (Rocephin) 1–2 g q24h
- Ciprofloxacin (Cipro) 400 mg q12h
- Gentamicin (Garamycin) 3–5 mg/kg q24h
- Levofloxacin (Levaquin) 500 mg q24h

Oral Regimens
- Amoxicillin 500 mg q8h
- Ciprofloxacin 500 mg q12h
- Ciprofloxacin XR 1000 mg q24h
- Levofloxacin 250 mg q24h
- Trimethoprim-sulfamethoxazole DS (Bactrim DS) 160/800 mg q12h

---

Bacteremic patients might take longer to respond but do not require more prolonged parenteral therapy. The total duration of therapy for pyelonephritis is generally 14 days. Seven days of therapy with ciprofloxacin for uncomplicated APN has been shown to be effective as has 5 days of therapy with high-dose (750 mg daily) levofloxacin. Longer courses of therapy may be required for select patients with complicated pyelonephritis. For outpatients, initial empiric therapy with a fluoroquinolone is recommended, with adjustment of therapy, if needed, based on the results of urine culture. All of the currently available fluoroquinolones can be used, with the exception of moxifloxacin (Avelox), which does not achieve adequate levels in the urine. Although it is useful in the treatment of cystitis, norfloxacin (Noroxin) is not recommended for the treatment of APN because it does not achieve sustained tissue or serum levels. Suggested antimicrobial dosing regimens for APN are outlined in Box 3.

Imaging

Imaging is generally not needed in patients with uncomplicated APN. For patients with complicated infections (e.g., history of stones, prior renal surgery), renal ultrasound with abdominal plain films is considered an acceptable alternative to excretory urography. For patients with diabetes or other immunocompromise and for patients who fail to respond after 72 hours of appropriate antibiotic therapy, pre- and postcontrast CT is the imaging procedure of choice.

Follow-up

Most patients will respond to appropriate antibiotic therapy. Follow-up urine cultures to document microbiological response are not recommended in patients who have responded clinically.

REFERENCES

Foxman B, Klemstine KL, Brown PD. Acute pyelonephritis in US hospitals in 1997: Hospitalization and in-hospital mortality. Ann Epidemiol 2003; 13:144–50.

Pappas PG. Laboratory in the diagnosis and management of urinary tract infections. Med Clin North Am 1991;75:313–25.

Sandler CM, Amis ES Jr, Bigongiari LR, et al. Imaging in acute pyelonephritis. American College of Radiology. ACR appropriateness criteria. Radiology 2000;215(Suppl):677–81.

Scholes D, Hooton TM, Roberts PL, et al. Risk factors associated with acute pyelonephritis in healthy women. Ann Intern Med 2005;142:20–7.

Talan DA, Stamm WE, Hooton TM, et al. Comparison of ciprofloxacin (7 days) and trimethoprim-sulfamethoxazole (14 days) for acute uncomplicated pyelonephritis in women: A randomized trial. JAMA 2000;283:1583–90.

Warren JW, Abrutyn E, Hebel JR, et al. Guidelines for antimicrobial treatment of uncomplicated acute bacterial cystitis and acute pyelonephritis in women. Clin Infect Dis 1999;29:745–58.

Trauma to the Genitourinary Tract

Method of
Sean P. Elliott, MD, and Bahaa S. Malaeb, MD

The genitourinary tract is involved in 3% to 10% of trauma cases. The kidney, followed by the bladder and urethra, are the most commonly involved genitourinary organs. In most cases, injury to the genitourinary tract is not isolated, and the initial evaluation of the urologic injuries should emphasize the context of the patient's associated injuries that might be more pressing or life-threatening. Still, early involvement of the urologist is prudent to help plan further interventions. The spectrum of genitourinary injuries is widespread, and management can range from immediate repair to temporization with delayed reconstruction. The goal of a urologist in the trauma setting is to establish urinary drainage in order to optimize kidney function, minimize hemorrhage, and control urinary extravasation to reduce associated complications such as infection or ileus.

Renal Trauma

Renal injury occurs in 1% to 5% of all trauma cases. Blunt impact accounts for the majority of renal injuries (90%–95%) and causes damage secondary to direct organ injury or disruption of the kidney from its attachments (e.g., renal hilum and ureteropelvic junction). Penetrating trauma most commonly is caused by stabbing or gunshot wounds. The damage from penetrating injury can be limited to the tract of the stab wound, or it can be more extensive secondary to necrosis from energy transfer and the blast effect of high-velocity bullets. The history is crucial in the diagnosis of renal injury and should include the mechanism of trauma as well as any preexisting kidney disease or condition that might contribute to worsening renal function. Hematuria has a very poor correlation with degree of injury, because disruption of the ureteropelvic junction, arterial disruption or thrombosis, and other severe injuries can exist in a setting with no hematuria.

The American Association for the Surgery of Trauma (AAST) classifies renal injuries into five grades (Figs. 1 and 2):

- Grade 1: Nonexpanding subcapsular hematoma/contusion with absence of parenchymal injury

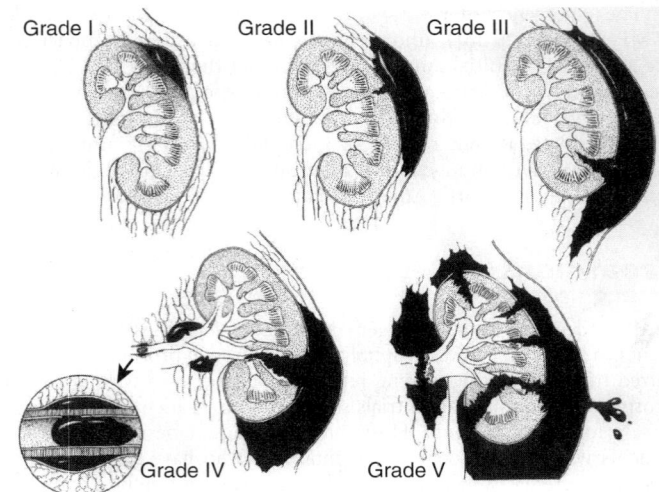

FIGURE 2. American Association for the Surgery of Trauma grading system for traumatic renal injuries: grade I, renal contusion and subcapsular hematoma; grade II, cortical laceration and perirenal hematoma; grade III, laceration into medulla or segmental renal artery thrombosis without a parenchymal injury; grade IV, laceration involving the collecting system, with or without a devascularized segment and contained vascular injury; grade V, renal artery thrombosis, avulsion of the renal pedicle, and shattered kidney. (From McAninch JW [ed]: Traumatic and Reconstructive Urology. Philadelphia, WB Saunders, 1996.)

- Grade 2: Less than 1 cm laceration into the renal cortex, not extending into the collecting system, with a nonexpanding hematoma confined to the perirenal fascia
- Grade 3: Greater than 1 cm laceration, extending through the renal cortex and medulla but not the collecting system
- Grade 4: Laceration extending to the collecting system with urinary extravasation or a segmental vascular injury with contained hematoma; renal artery thrombosis
- Grade 5: Shattered kidney or renal pedicle avulsion

Renal injury should be suspected in any trauma patient who has a penetrating injury with gross or microscopic hematuria (>2 red blood cells per high-power field), a blunt injury with gross hematuria, or a blunt injury with microscopic hematuria and shock (systolic blood pressure <90 mm Hg). In addition, imaging of the urinary tract should be obtained in children who have more than 50 red blood cells per high-power field even in the absence of hypotension.

In a stable patient, radiographic evaluation should consist of computed tomographic (CT) scanning with intravenous contrast and delayed images showing opacification of the collecting system and ureters. In the absence of a CT scan in a patient who is transported directly to the operating room for exploration, an intraoperative single-film intravenous pyelogram can be performed to confirm that two functioning kidneys are present; however, the poor quality of the images makes them unreliable for staging purposes.

Kidney exploration is indicated for the unstable patient in whom renal injury is thought to be the reason for a life-threatening and persistent hemorrhage. Another absolute indication for renal exploration and revascularization is renal artery hilar avulsion or renal artery thrombosis, if bilateral or in a solitary kidney. In patients undergoing exploratory laparotomy for associated injuries, renal exploration should be performed only in the presence of an expanding or pulsatile hematoma. Exploration of a nonexpanding, nonpulsatile hematoma is associated with a higher rate of nephrectomy and should be avoided. Almost all other injuries can be managed conservatively or with minimally invasive methods.

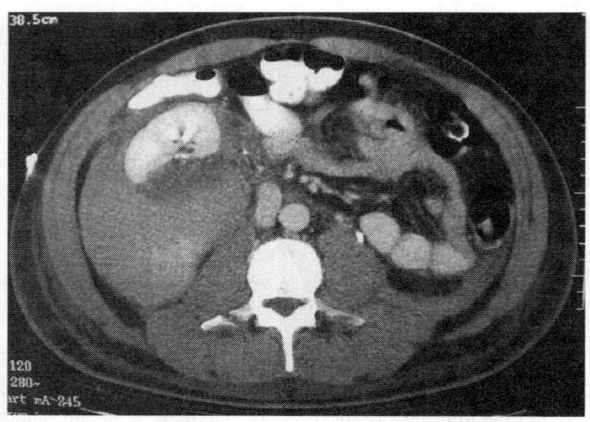

FIGURE 1. Computed tomography scan demonstrating large right perirenal hematoma and thrombosed posterior segmental artery. This was classified as a grade IV renal injury.

Nonoperative management consists of supportive care with intravenous hydration, antibiotics, bedrest, and serial measurements of hemoglobin and hematocrit. Patients can ambulate after they are clinically stable, gross hematuria has resolved, and the hemoglobin and hematocrit have been relatively constant over 24 hours.

Routine early follow-up imaging for grades 1 to 3 blunt renal injury is unnecessary. Any imaging should be motivated by a change in the patient's clinical situation or laboratory values. Grade 4 renovascular injuries can be followed up clinically. Follow-up imaging is indicated for patients with grade 4 or 5 injuries with urinary extravasation to assess for worsening urinoma or hematoma that might require further intervention.

Ureteral Trauma

Trauma to the ureter is rare, most likely because of its retroperitoneal and bony pelvis location, its relatively small caliber, and its mobility. The etiology of ureteric trauma is mostly iatrogenic (75% of all ureteric injuries); 73% of iatrogenic injuries occur secondary to gynecologic procedures, and the remainder are divided between general surgery and urologic procedures. Ureteral injury should be suspected in all cases of penetrating trauma to the abdomen, especially with high-velocity projectiles, because of the blast effect.

The AAST has classified ureteric injuries into five grades of severity:

- Grade 1: Hematoma only
- Grade 2: Injury involving less than 50% of the circumference of the ureter
- Grade 3: Injury involving more than 50% of the circumference of the ureter
- Grade 4: Complete transsection with less than 2 cm of devascularization
- Grade 5: Complete transsection with more than 2 cm of devascularization

The diagnosis usually is made intraoperatively if a high suspicion of ureteric injury is present or postoperatively by imaging obtained for investigation of fistula formation or clinical signs of upper tract obstruction. For noniatrogenic injuries, imaging should be obtained in patients who had rapid deceleration or penetrating injuries to the flank. Imaging modalities used are usually intravenous pyelography, CT scanning with intravenous contrast and delayed images, and retrograde pyelography. Findings indicative of ureteral injury include contrast extravasation, ureteral narrowing, and delayed peristalsis (Fig. 3). Alternatively, the ureters may be interrogated intraoperatively by using direct inspection, by injecting intravenous methylene blue[1] and watching for leakage of dye, or by passing a ureteral catheter (if it passes easily, an injury is unlikely).

Grade 1 and 2 injuries can be managed initially by placement of a ureteral stent. If grade 2 or 3 injuries are identified immediately during exploration for a suspected ureteric injury, they can be managed by primary closure of the ureteric injury over an internal stent and placement of a nonsuction abdominal drain, as long as there is no associated thermal injury or necrosis. Grade 3 to 5 injuries usually require débridement of nonviable ends with reanastomosis over an internal ureteral stent or more complicated surgical procedures involving mobilization of the bladder and reimplantation of the ureter into the bladder. The type of ureteral repair depends on the amount of devitalized tissues and the location of the injury (proximal, middle, or distal ureter). Ureteroureterostomy, transureteroureterostomy, ureterocalicostomy, renal autotransplantation, ureteroneocystostomy with or without Boari flap or psoas hitch, and bowel interposition are all treatment options for various degrees of ureteral injuries.

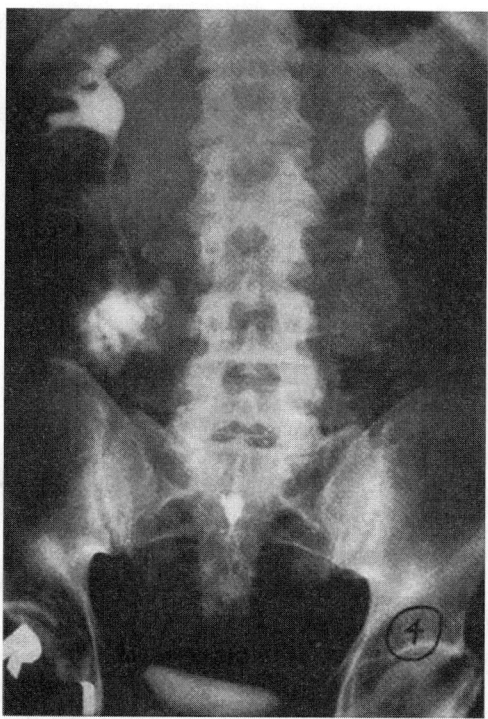

FIGURE 3. Intravenous pyelogram demonstrating extravasation of urine from right mid-ureter.

Bladder Trauma

Blunt trauma accounts for 67% to 86% of bladder injuries resulting from external trauma, and up to 97% of those patients have associated pelvic fractures. The most common cause of blunt trauma is motor vehicle crashes. Penetrating trauma accounts for 14% to 33% of traumatic bladder injuries. The incidence of iatrogenic injury varies by procedure but is highest for hysterectomy and other obstetric and gynecologic procedures (up to 61 per 1000 cases). In cases of blunt trauma, injury should be suspected in patients who have pelvic fractures, suprapubic pain and inability to void, ileus, absent bowel sounds, or abdominal distention. For iatrogenic injuries, any urine in the field, visible laceration in bladder, or gas distention of the urinary drainage bag in laparoscopic surgery warrants further investigation. It is important to delineate whether a bladder injury involves intraperitoneal or extraperitoneal rupture. Intraperitoneal rupture occurs at the level of the bladder dome, where the muscular support is weakest (Figs. 4 and 5).

The diagnostic test of choice is a CT cystogram, in which the bladder is filled with contrast to capacity (350–400 mL instilled by gravity). In children, the volume instilled is 60 mL plus 30 mL per year of age up to a maximum of 300 mL. Passive filling of the bladder by clamping of the catheter is associated with unacceptably high rates of false-negative tests. Plain film cystography is an alternative, but a single anteroposterior film is insufficient; postdrainage films and, preferably, oblique views should be obtained as well. In both settings, retrograde urethrography should be performed, if there is a suspicion of urethral injury, before placement of a Foley catheter.

Most extraperitoneal bladder ruptures can be managed with Foley catheter drainage for 7 to 10 days. Bladder neck involvement, concomitant vaginal or rectal injuries, presence of bone fragments in the bladder, or bladder wall entrapment necessitates surgical intervention. Intraperitoneal ruptures should be managed with surgical exploration because of the associated ileus and peritonitis caused by urine leak. In contrast, all penetrating bladder injuries should be explored and repaired because of the risk of necrosis and nonhealing. Bladder repair is performed with a multiple-layer closure and catheter drainage for 7 to 10 days.

---

[1]Not FDA approved for this indication.

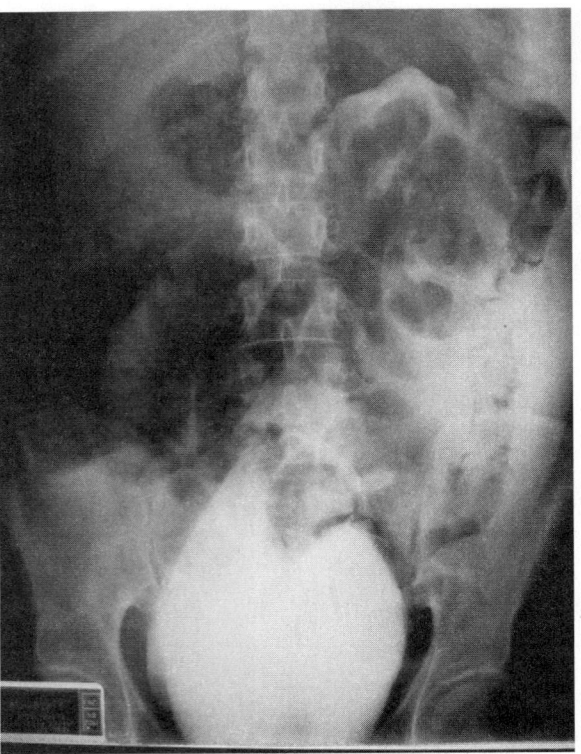

FIGURE 4. Intraperitoneal bladder rupture. Note contrast extravasating from the dome of the bladder and outlining the small intestine as well as the left colon.

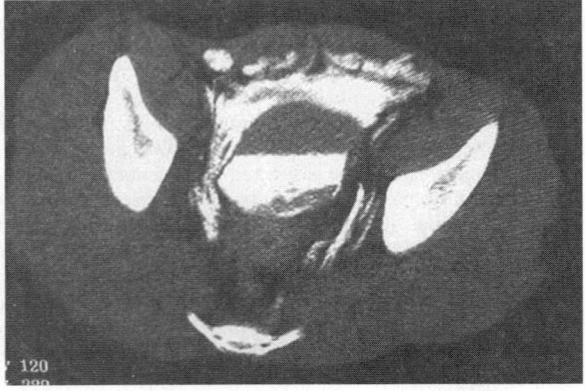

FIGURE 5. Extraperitoneal bladder rupture seen on computed tomographic cystogram.

Urethral Trauma

Traumatic injury to the urethra occurs in 10% of patients who sustain a pelvic fracture. Female urethral injuries are very rare. The male urethra is anatomically divided into a posterior part (prostatic and membranous urethra) and an anterior part (bulbous urethra, penile/pendulous urethra, and fossa navicularis). Injury to the anterior urethra occurs mostly from blunt trauma, penetrating injuries, or instrumentation. Posterior urethral injuries are usually associated with pelvic fractures but can occur secondary to blunt, penetrating, or iatrogenic injury.

Classic signs of urethral injury include blood at the meatus, a high-riding prostate on rectal examination, and perineal or scrotal ecchymosis. Imaging is indicated with any of these signs. The imaging study of choice is a retrograde urethrogram, and it should be

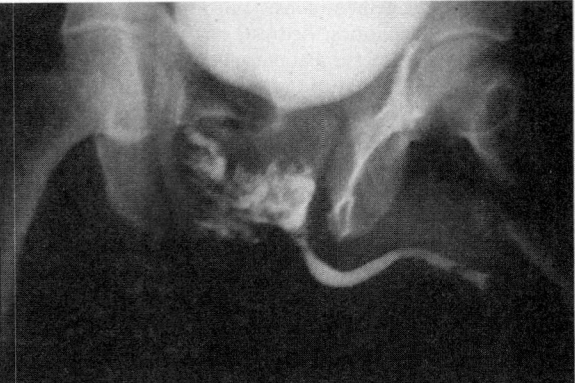

FIGURE 6. Retrograde urethrogram diagnostic of partial bulbar urethral transaction resulting from straddle injury.

performed before placement of a urethral catheter is attempted. In the absence of any signs, the diagnosis is most frequently made when retrograde urethrography is performed to investigate difficulty with urethral catheter placement (Fig. 6).

The AAST grading system does not distinguish between anterior or posterior injury but classifies urethral injuries as follows:

- Grade 1: Contusion and blood at the meatus with normal urethrogram
- Grade 2: Stretch injury with no extravasation of contrast
- Grade 3: Partial disruption with contrast extravasating at the injury site but still reaching the bladder
- Grade 4: Complete disruption with contrast not reaching the bladder; urethral defect of less than 2 cm
- Grade 5: Complete disruption with urethral defect greater than 2 cm or complex injury involving the bladder neck, prostate, rectum, or vagina

Grade 1 and 2 injuries can be managed conservatively by placement of a urethral catheter. Management of grade 3 urethral injury should initially emphasize stabilization of the patient, because extensive bleeding could be present in cases of severe injury to the pelvis. Placement of a catheter may be attempted even if there is a suspicion of partial urethral injury. If this is met with difficulty, a suprapubic tube may be placed.

In cases of complete disruption, evidence supports early endoscopic realignment performed within the initial hospitalization if the patient is stable. This involves endoscopic passage of a guidewire across the defect and placement of a catheter over the guidewire, with the purpose of reestablishing urethral continuity. An alternative method is placement of a suprapubic tube and delayed reconstruction; the latter approach is associated with a 100% rate of stricture formation. Early endoscopic alignment has been shown to decrease the rate of stricture formation and the severity of strictures when they do occur, compared with suprapubic tube placement and delayed urethral reconstruction. Immediate open repair is rarely indicated unless complex injury extends into the bladder, rectum, or vagina and the patient is undergoing surgery for associated injuries. Immediate exploration is recommended for anterior urethral injuries associated with penetrating trauma or penile fractures.

Trauma to the External Genitalia

Injury to the scrotum is most frequently secondary to blunt trauma and can cause subcutaneous hematoma, hematocele, or testicular injury. Scrotal swelling and patient discomfort can make separation of testicular injury from extratesticular scrotal trauma difficult on physical examination. Therefore, one should have a low threshold for further investigation with ultrasound. A heterogeneous echo pattern in the testicular parenchyma on ultrasonography suggests

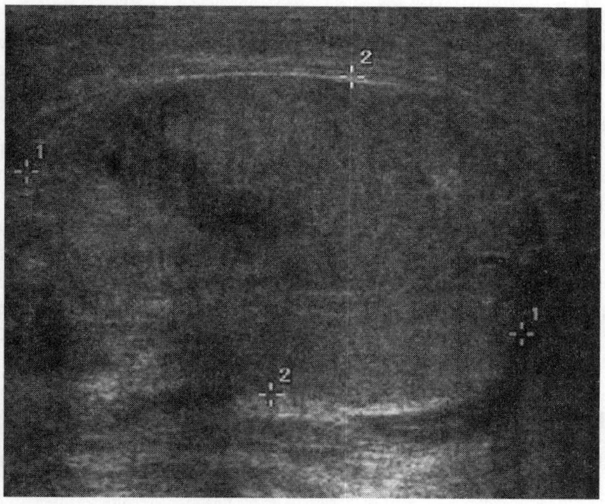

FIGURE 7. Testis ultrasound image demonstrating heterogeneous architecture characteristic of testicular rupture.

testicular injury (Fig. 7). Visualization of a tear in the tunica albuginea is less accurate. Ultrasound studies additionally provide information about any compromise in testicular blood flow.

Scrotal exploration should be performed whenever testicular injury is suspected. If the tunica is ruptured and there is extrusion of seminiferous tubules, the extruded tubules should be débrided, hemorrhage controlled, and the tunica closed. Testicular salvage rates are high (90%) when the scrotum is explored acutely but drop by half if exploration is delayed. Another indication for scrotal exploration is a large hematocele; evacuation of the hematoma can decrease the morbidity associated with protracted recovery and resolution of the hematoma and can occasionally identify a manageable source of bleeding. Scrotal exploration should also be performed in cases of inconclusive ultrasound findings or whenever the clinical suspicion for testicular injury is high.

Trauma to the penis can range in severity from a contusion to complete amputation. In cases of penile amputation, stabilization of the patient is important, and the need for transfusion should be addressed. Immediate microreimplantation is the management technique of choice if available. Penile fracture occurs after blunt injury to the erect penis, usually incurred during sexual intercourse. Patients often report a "crack" or a "pop" followed by severe pain and detumescence. Penile fractures involve rupture of the tunica albuginea. The hematoma is usually limited to the penis, unless the injury also involves Buck's fascia, causing ecchymosis and bruising that involves the scrotum as well. It is important to rule out associated urethral injury, which occurs in 10% of the cases. Surgical exploration, closure of the fascial defect, and repair of any associated urethral injury should be done acutely.

In females, blunt trauma to the vulva is rare. Injuries to genitalia can be associated with sexual assault and must be evaluated in that context. Consequently, vaginal smears should be taken, and the vagina should be thoroughly inspected with a speculum and with the patient under anesthesia.

Trauma resulting in skin loss, such as burns, large abrasions, and avulsions, the lesions should be explored and débrided in an effort to stage the injury and decrease the risk of complications such as Fournier's gangrene and urinoma. Delayed reconstruction can be performed after stabilization and proper delineation of viable versus nonviable tissues. The reconstructive options include mobilization of local flaps or skin grafts.

Conclusion

An understanding of the mechanism of injury is important to establish clinical suspicion of urologic trauma. Radiologic imaging is essential in making the correct diagnosis and managing it appropriately. Early diagnosis minimizes patient morbidity.

Studies of prospective design are clearly lacking for urologic trauma. Consolidation of the experience of major trauma institutions nationwide in a consortium for multi-institutional protocols could be the answer to this lack of prospective data.

REFERENCES

Brandes S, Coburn M, Armenakas N, McAninch J. Diagnosis and management of ureteric injury: An evidence-based analysis. BJU Int 2004;94(3):277–89.

Chapple C, Barbagli G, Jordan G, et al. Consensus statement on urethral trauma. BJU Int 2004;93(9):1195–202.

Gomez RG, Ceballos L, Coburn M, et al. Consensus statement on bladder injuries. BJU Int 2004;94(1):27–32.

Lynch TH, Martínez-Piñeiro L, Plas E, et al. European Association of Urology: EAU guidelines on urological trauma. Eur Urol 2005;47(1):1–15.

Malcolm JB, Derweesh IH, Mehrazin R, et al. Nonoperative management of blunt renal trauma: Is routine early follow-up imaging necessary? BMC Urol 2008;8:11.

Morey AF, Metro MJ, Carney KJ, et al. Consensus on genitourinary trauma: External genitalia. BJU Int 2004;94(4):507–15.

Phonsombat S, Master VA, McAninch JW. Penetrating external genital trauma: A 30-year single institution experience. J Urol 2008;180(1):192–5; discussion 195–196.

Santucci RA, Fisher MB. The literature increasingly supports expectant (conservative) management of renal trauma: A systematic review. J Trauma 2005;59(2):493–503.

Santucci RA, Wessells H, Bartsch G, et al. Evaluation and management of renal injuries: Consensus statement of the renal trauma subcommittee. BJU Int 2004;93(7):937–54.

Prostatitis

Method of
Louis Kuritzky, MD

Definitions

A classification scheme developed by the National Institutes of Health (NIH) is the most widely recognized, and it is also included in the most recent British National Guidelines for the Management of Prostatitis. This categorization recognizes three main clinical entities: acute bacterial prostatitis, chronic bacterial prostatitis, and chronic prostatitis & chronic pelvic pain syndrome.

Acute Prostatitis

PRESENTATION

Men with acute prostatitis usually present with signs of genitourinary inflammation and systemic toxicity. Lower urinary tract symptoms (LUTS), most commonly dysuria, frequency, and urgency, are prominent. Patients often report aching pain in the genitorectal area, which can manifest as perineal, penile, or even low back pain. Bacteremia can produce a toxic state with fever and generalized malaise. Gentle examination of the prostate generally reveals a gland that is markedly tender but unusually pliable owing to inflammatory swelling. Vigorous prostate palpation should be avoided lest additional load of prostatic bacteria be delivered to the bloodstream.

DIAGNOSIS

Acute onset of LUTS with signs of systemic toxicity should prompt urinalysis and genitourinary examination. The presence by urinalysis of pyuria and bacteriuria, coupled with distinct prostatic tenderness and bogginess, should be sufficient to arrive at a provisional diagnosis of acute bacterial prostatitis.

CURRENT DIAGNOSIS

- A diagnosis of acute prostatitis is usually made on a clinical basis when typical lower urinary tract symptoms such as dysuria and frequency are coupled with the corroborative physical findings of a tender, boggy prostate and urinalysis revealing pyuria. If the presentation is less typical, the literature suggests that the diagnosis may be missed.
- Chronic prostatitis is a little-understood malady with diverse presentations ranging from chronic pelvic pain syndromes to intermittent flares of lower urinary tract symptoms. Although the pathophysiology that allows lower urinary tract symptoms to persist and recur is obscure, some pharmacologic interventions have been shown to provide symptomatic relief.
- The inflammatory changes seen in bacterial prostatitis typically involve the anatomic central zone of the prostate, giving credence to the likely ascending urethral origin of most prostatitis episodes.

DIFFERENTIAL DIAGNOSIS

Dysuria, frequency, and urgency mimic simple cystitis, but systemic symptoms, especially fever, should be absent from either urethritis or cystitis. Although upper urinary tract infection (e.g., pyelonephritis) might have some similar symptoms, localization of pain in pyelonephritis is distinctly different.

Urethritis can cause dysuria and—if incomplete bladder emptying ensues—frequency, but because it is most likely initiated secondary to a sexually transmitted infection (especially gonorrhea or chlamydia), history of a new sexual partner is typical. Urethritis and associated prostatic tenderness should not be associated with systemic symptoms. Overactive bladder causes frequency and urgency, but it is not associated with pain, and the symptoms are not acute in onset. A kidney stone is usually unilateral, and it causes prominent hematuria and colicky rather than constant pain. Pain is the most prominent and acute feature of kidney stone, and it might be better described as a second tier complaint in prostatitis.

LABORATORY EVALUATION

Standard urinalysis is fundamental to the diagnosis. Absence of pyuria should generate reconsideration of the diagnosis. Because of bacteremia associated with acute bacterial prostatitis, both urine and blood cultures should be obtained.

TREATMENT

The most common organism that causes acute prostatitis is *Escherichia coli,* but other gram-negative species (e.g., *Proteus, Klebsiella, Pseudomonas*) are sometimes responsible. Less commonly, *Enterococcus* species, *Staphylococcus aureus* (usually following instrumentation or catheterization), or even *Bacteroides* species can cause acute prostatitis. Presumptive treatment for acute prostatitis should provide coverage for these organisms. Hence, it is reasonable to initiate treatment with a broad-spectrum cephalosporin (e.g., cefuroxime [Zinacef], cefotaxime [Claforan], ceftriaxone [Rocephin]) or a quinolone *plus* gentamicin (Garamycin) pending results of urine and blood cultures. Although oral quinolones provide effective coverage for the majority of organisms causing acute bacterial prostatitis, the toxic state of many men with acute prostatitis as well as risk from bacteremia suggest that intravenous antibiotics be administered on an inpatient basis. When a confirmed pathogen and its sensitivity are defined, specific oral treatment can be initiated when evidence of toxicity (e.g., fever, elevated white blood cell count) is resolved.

Once acute toxicity is resolved, a long-term regimen of an oral quinolone is suggested, unless specific organisms or sensitivities preclude it. Regimens include 4 weeks of either ciprofloxacin (Cipro) 500 mg twice daily or ofloxacin (Floxin) 200 mg twice daily. For patients intolerant of quinolones, the combination of trimethoprim-sulfamethoxazole 800 mg/160 mg twice daily or even trimethoprim (Proloprim) 200 mg twice daily[3] alone for 28 days are reasonable alternatives.

Not all antibiotics penetrate into the prostate with equal efficacy, and it has been suggested that pharmacologic permeability of the blood-prostate barrier is greatest during acute inflammation, becoming progressively less as inflammation resolves. Nonetheless, experience has suggested that penetration of quinolone antibiotics is substantial even as infection dissipates.

PARTNER TREATMENT

Prostatitis is not generally considered a sexually transmitted infection. There is no need for partner treatment.

FOLLOW-UP

Most patients with acute prostatitis do well, though a substantial minority go on to have chronic or recurrent episodes. Once the patient has recovered, many experts suggest evaluation of the genitourinary tract, seeking abnormalities that might lend themselves to bacterial colonization, such as urethral stricture, bladder diverticulum, prostate stones, or urinary obstruction. In only a small percentage of patients, however, is a definitive pathogenetic defect that leads to acute bacterial prostatitis identified.

NONRESPONDERS

Infrequently, acute prostatitis does not respond with prompt relief of symptoms and defervescence. Assuming that an antibiotic has been chosen to appropriately match organism sensitivity, clinicians should seek consultation from colleagues with special knowledge of male genitourinary health or infectious disease, because secondary pathology involving the genitourinary tract may be involved. For instance, prostatic abscess, identifiable by transrectal ultrasound or CT of the prostate, can manifest as acute bacterial prostatitis but be refractory to antibiotic intervention unless the abscess itself is surgically drained.

Chronic Bacterial Prostatitis

Although some patients enjoy freedom from future episodes of prostatitis after an acute episode, many go on to have chronic recurrences. Fortunately, the intensity of recurrences is much less than an initial acute attack, and because patients learn to recognize signs of recurrence early and intervene with antibiotics, hospitalizations for second episodes of acute bacterial prostatitis are uncommon. Unfortunately, the constellation of symptoms associated with chronic prostatitis is diverse and includes both the typical LUTS symptoms seen with acute attacks (frequency, urgency, and dysuria) and additional symptoms such as perineal pain and ejaculatory pain. The precipitant of recurrent symptoms after widely varying intervals is unknown. It appears that not all organisms responsible for acute bacterial prostatitis have the same proclivity to produce chronic bacterial prostatitis; the majority of cases are caused by *E. coli, S. aureus,* or *Enterococcus faecalis,* with other causative organisms being distinctly less common.

PRESENTATION

Because of prior episodes of prostatitis, recurrences are usually readily recognized by both the clinician and patient. There is, however, a fairly broad diversity in presentation, ranging from typical symptoms

---

[3]Exceeds dosage recommended by the manufacturer.

of urinary tract infection to vague pelvic pain. In between recurrences, patients are most often asymptomatic. However, mild LUTS can become chronic, and I have seen men who date the onset of erectile dysfunction to establishment of a pattern of chronic prostatitis. Similarly, I have seen men complaining of ejaculatory pain, new-onset urinary frequency, or urgency as symptoms of recurrence during the course of chronic bacterial prostatitis. Such symptoms usually promptly remit with antibiotic treatment (see later).

Patients with chronic bacterial prostatitis are not generally systemically ill or toxic, so that blood cultures are rarely necessary. Occasionally, a recurrence of bacterial prostatitis is as acute and systemically toxic as the initial case, in which circumstance it is appropriate to approach the management in a similar fashion as for acute bacterial prostatitis.

DIAGNOSIS

Initial evaluation should include rectal examination and urinalysis. The prostate may be enlarged or tender, but it lacks the dramatic sensitivity to palpation seen in acute bacterial prostatitis. When pyuria is present with typical symptoms, suspicion for a recurrence of prostatitis should be strong. Some clinicians prefer to confirm localization of infection to the prostate (as opposed to kidneys, bladder, or urethra), by performing the four-glass urine test. The theory of this test is that by measuring different consecutive urine specimens, a comparison of bacterial counts can support localization of the infected tissue.

In the four-glass test, the patient is asked to provide a small amount of urine, and then stop urinating (glass 1). Glass 1 colony counts are thought to reflect proportionately greater urethral content than other subsequent specimens. Glass 2 is obtained from midstream urine, and is thought to reflect bladder concentrations of bacteria more than urethral. Glass 3 is obtained after prostatic massage to induce prostatic secretions. Glass 4 is obtained by urinating immediately after prostatic massage. Higher bacterial counts in glass 4 than glass 1 or glass 2 corroborate contribution of prostatic fluid to the increased colonies, and hence likely prostatitis. The clinical utility of this methodology is uncertain, because most patients are treated similarly regardless of results, and differential colony counts are not always straightforward and convincing. Nonetheless, in challenging cases this method may be helpful.

TREATMENT

As in acute bacterial prostatitis, provisional treatment should be guided by the knowledge of typical pathogens (E. coli, S. aureus, E. faecalis), and revised once confirmation of pathogen and sensitivity are obtained. Because patients are generally not toxic, oral antibiotics are appropriate, such as 4 weeks of a quinolone: ciprofloxacin 500 mg twice daily, levofloxacin 500 mg once daily, or ofloxacin 200 mg twice daily. No particular advantage for one quinolone over another has been demonstrated. Because patients with chronic bacterial prostatitis might need to receive multiple courses of antibiotics over time, it is suggested that clinicians advise patients about the tendinopathy uncommonly induced by quinolones. For patients intolerant to quinolones, minocycline (Minocin)[1] 100 mg twice daily for 28 days or trimethoprim[1] (200 mg twice daily[3] for 28 days are reasonable alternatives.

Such long courses of antibiotics are intended to eradicate the prostatic nidus of infection. If, however, recurrences are very frequent, some patients prefer to take shorter courses of antibiotics, which often resolve symptoms equally effectively. I suggest that if, after an initial recurrence has been treated for 28 days, another recurrence appears, brief antibiotic trials be offered (3-7 days), rather than expose the patient to unnecessarily protracted courses.

Prostatic irritability manifesting as urinary frequency and dysuria may be modulated by use of α-blockers. Although not indicated as primary therapy, for persons with substantial residual LUTS (especially frequency and urgency), α-blocker treatment is worth considering. All α-blockers (alfuzosin [Uroxatral]),[1] doxazosin [Cardura],[1] prazosin [Minipress],[1] silodosin [Rapiflo],[1] terazosin [Hytrin],[1] tamsulosin [Flomax],[1]) are considered essentially equivalent for efficacy in relieving prostatic symptoms. Because of associated symptoms of hypotension, and the need to titrate the first-generation α-blockers, I suggest preferential consideration of second-generation agents such as alfuzosin, silodosin, or tamsulosin.

FOLLOW-UP

If an evaluation of the genitourinary tract has not been done, recurrences suggest that it be done. Nonetheless, in my experience, an etiologic source for prostatitis is rarely found. It is suggested that all patients with chronic bacterial prostatitis receive at least a one-time urology consultation, if available.

Chronic Prostatitis & Chronic Pelvic Pain Syndrome

PRESENTATION

Chronic pelvic pain syndrome can include one or more of genitourinary and musculoskeletal symptoms including abdominal pain, perineal aching, penile pain, back pain (very low), ejaculatory pain, LUTS, and testicular pain. The cause(s) of chronic prostatitis & chronic pelvic pain syndrome remain obscure, although abnormalities in neuromuscular function, autoimmune dysfunction, and infection are but a few of the suggested contributors. Symptoms are not acute, and they can occur individually or in combination. Symptoms can be constant or can wax and wane.

DIAGNOSIS AND DIFFERENTIAL DIAGNOSIS

There is no specific laboratory test to confirm chronic prostatitis & chronic pelvic pain syndrome. Rather, the diagnosis is suggested by prototypical symptoms combined with an absence of confirmatory findings such as normal urinalysis, normal—albeit sometimes tender—prostate examination, and normal urine culture. The critical part of evaluation is to exclude other important pathology. Hence a prostate-specific antigen (PSA) test to rule out prostate cancer, urine cytology to rule out bladder cancer, urocystometry to look for abnormal neuromuscular function of the bladder, and transrectal ultrasonography to seek anatomic abnormalities of the genitourinary system, abscess, or cyst are considerations. Because of the potential depth of evaluation needed, urologic referral is usually required.

Exhaustive investigations have sought potential urinary tract pathogens without consistent success, including Chlamydia, Mycoplasma, and Ureaplasma species. Pyuria is not a reliable sign.

Because the symptom profile of chronic prostatitis & chronic pelvic pain syndrome is consonant with other categories of prostatitis, it is likely that many men who carry a diagnosis of prostatitis instead have chronic prostatitis & chronic pelvic pain syndrome. Some experts suggest that chronic prostatitis & chronic pelvic pain syndrome is actually more common than acute bacterial prostatitis and chronic bacterial prostatitis combined.

TREATMENT

There is no definitive treatment. Symptomatic treatment trials are appropriate. For instance, α-blockers might provide symptom relief from typical LUTS symptoms. If urgency is a primary complaint, antimuscarinic agents might be useful, such as darifenacin (Enablex),[1] fesoterodine (Toviaz),[1] oxybutynin (Ditropan),[1] solifenacin (Vesicare),[1] tolterodine (Detro)],[1] or trospium (Sanctura).[1]

Some data suggest modest symptom improvement with nonsteroidal antiinflammatory drugs (NSAIDs). However, long-term use of NSAIDs has been associated with substantial gastrointestinal toxicity, renal toxicity, increased risk of cardiovascular disease, and retention of sodium, potassium, and water.

Although the symptom burden may be substantial, patients should be reassured about the absence of any progressive pathologic process. Indeed, symptoms spontaneously improve or even resolve in as many as one third of sufferers in long-term observational studies.

REFERENCES

Clinical Effectiveness Group. United Kingdom national guideline on the management of prostatitis, London: British Association for Sexual Health and HIV (BASHH); 2008. Available at http://www.guideline.gov/summary/summary.aspx?ss=15&doc_id=14278&nbr=7154; [accessed July 26, 2010].

Nickel JC, Downey JA, Nickel KR, Clark JM. Prostatitis-like symptoms: One year later. Br J Urol Int 2002;90:678–81.

Pontari M: Chronic prostatitis/chronic pelvic pain syndrome. UpToDate (subscription only).

Propert KJ, McNaughton Collins M, et al. A prospective study of symptoms and quality of life in men with chronic prostatitis/chronic pelvic pain syndrome: The National Institutes of Health chronic prostatitis cohort study. J Urol 2006;175:619–23.

Scofield S, Kaplan SA. Voiding dysfunction in men: Pathophysiology and risk factors. Int J Impot Res 2008;20(Suppl 3):S2–10.

Benign Prostatic Hyperplasia

Method of
Judd W. Moul, MD

Epidemiology

Benign prostatic hyperplasia (BPH) was generally a topic only of interest to urologists up to about 20 years ago, when several classes of medical therapy became available. Once widespread direct-to-consumer medical advertising hit the airwaves, the public's lexicon included "BPH" and men and their families were being educated about it. When combined with the aging population, the obesity epidemic, and subsequent health consequences, we have a very important disease process. As other countries improve their standards of living, BPH has become one of the most common health conditions of the aging man worldwide.

From a practical standpoint, BPH and its symptoms are very uncommon before the age of 40 years. By ages 60 years and 85 years, the histologic prevalence of BPH at autopsy is 50% and 90%, respectively. The symptoms of BPH are now referred to as lower urinary tract symptoms (LUTS). At age 70 years, about 40% of men report LUTS and by age 75 years, the incidence of LUTS increases to 50%.

The diagnosis and treatment of BPH has always been in the realm of the specialty of urology, and this remains the case. However, as more medical therapies have been introduced and prostate-specific antigen (PSA) testing for prostate cancer has become commonplace, urologists are working more closely with internists, family physicians, generalists, and physician extenders to jointly manage these patients.

Pathophysiology

Even though BPH is common, we know very little about the true pathophysiology. However, we do know that men who were castrated before puberty do not develop BPH, and we also know that it is a progressive disease of aging. Before the 1980s, BPH was generally thought of as a static condition of a gradually growing prostate gland that caused progressive bladder outlet obstruction. In fact, it was common to use the "donut hole" analogy with patients, explaining to them that the prostate is like a donut surrounding the bladder neck and outlet. With aging and prostate growth, the donut hole gets smaller, causing progressive obstruction. In the era when transurethral resection of the prostate (TURP) was the only effective treatment, this simple static explanation was sufficient.

However, from the 1980s onward, our understanding has advanced to recognize that BPH has both a static, obstructive and a dynamic component under neural control. The donut hole now has to have electrical wires attached to it with the ability to adjust the current. In addition, the contribution of the bladder to LUTS has been well recognized as a key contributor to the dynamic component of BPH and LUTS.

The static growth and proliferation of the periurethral tissue into BPH is under androgenic stimulation. Specifically, the main male hormone testosterone is converted to the more active metabolite dihydrotestosterone by the enzyme 5α-reductase in the prostatic stromal and epithelial cells of the prostate. 5α-Reductase occurs in two forms, type 1 and type 2. Only type 2 is present in the prostate and genitalia. This is critical for the understanding of one of the two main classes of medical therapy for BPH, the 5α-reductase inhibitors (5-ARIs).

The dynamic component of BPH and LUTS is based on autonomic input to the smooth muscles in the lower urinary tract, including the bladder, prostate, and urethra. These areas have a large concentration of α_1-adrenergic receptors that when stimulated by various stressors cause increasing smooth muscle tone. This increased smooth muscle tone leads to increased urethral resistance and contributes to the bladder outlet obstructive symptoms of BPH. This physiology leads to the basis for the other main class of drugs to treat BPH, the α_1-adrenergic blockers.

Symptoms

Lower urinary tract symptoms (LUTS) include urinary frequency, decreased force and caliber of the urinary stream, hesitancy, straining, urgency, and nocturia. The severity can range from the stoic man who refuses to acknowledge any symptoms to the man in frank urinary retention. Most urologists now use a standardized patient-self-administered questionnaire, such as the International Prostate Symptom Score (IPSS) (Fig. 1). This is very useful to elicit symptoms and bother in a typical male population with suboptimal health-seeking behavior.

It is now very common for men to be referred to urology for a collection of age-related issues including elevated PSA, LUTS, BPH, or erectile dysfunction. Commonly, the PSA or the erectile dysfunction brings the patient to the attention of the health care system for the first time in years and may be the first opportunity to influence men on healthy living and health maintenance as they enter middle or older vulnerable ages. Recognizing this, all health care providers should keep this in mind and try to perform a broader men's health assessment while the patient is captive.

Diagnosis

The diagnosis of BPH is generally made based on symptoms or the IPSS standardized patient-self-administered questionnaire combined with a digital rectal examination, PSA blood test, urinalysis, and, in some cases, a cystoscopy. The differential diagnosis can include urinary tract infection (UTI), prostatitis, urinary stones in the lower urinary tract, urethral stricture disease, neurogenic or overactive bladder, prostate or bladder cancer, and even congestive heart failure. Some common medications, such as over-the-counter cold medicines containing α-adrenergic agents, can exacerbate LUTS and can even put a man into acute urinary retention if he has underlying BPH.

International Prostate Symptom Score (I-PSS)

Patient Name: _____ Date of birth: _____ Date completed _____

In the past month:	Not at all	Less than 1 in 5 times	Less than half the time	About half the time	More than half the time	Almost always	Your score
1. Incomplete emptying How often have you had the sensation of not emptying your bladder?	0	1	2	3	4	5	
2. Frequency How often have you had to urinate less than every two hours?	0	1	2	3	4	5	
3. Intermittency How often have you found you stopped and started again several times when you urinated?	0	1	2	3	4	5	
4. Urgency How often have you found it difficult to postpone urination?	0	1	2	3	4	5	
5. Weak stream How often have you had a weak urinary stream?	0	1	2	3	4	5	
6. Straining How often have you had to strain to start urination?	0	1	2	3	4	5	
	None	**1 Time**	**2 Times**	**3 Times**	**4 Times**	**5 Times**	
7. Nocturia How many times did you typically get up at night to urinate?	0	1	2	3	4	5	
Total I-PSS score							

Score   1–7: *Mild*   8–19: *Moderate*   20–35: *Severe*

Quality of life due to urinary symptoms	Delighted	Pleased	Mostly satisfied	Mixed	Mostly dissatisfied	Unhappy	Terrible
If you were to spend the rest of your life with your urinary condition just the way it is now, how would you feel about that?	0	1	2	3	4	5	6

FIGURE 1. International Prostate Symptom Score (IPSS) questionnaire. (Available from the Urological Sciences Research Foundation at http://www.usrf.org/questionnaires/AUA_SymptomScore.html [accessed July 26, 2010].)

A properly performed digital rectal examination is critical to master in the diagnosis of BPH. Because the posterior prostate gland is located adjacent to the rectum and about 3 to 5 cm internal to the anus, the experienced clinician can gain valuable information. I prefer the patient to bend over the examining table with toes pointed slightly inward, the knees bent slightly forward and the forehead and arms resting on the table. The examiner uses a liberally lubricated gloved index finger to palpate the posterior side of the prostate for size estimate and for any induration or nodularity that might indicate the presence of prostate cancer. In this case, referral to an urologist is mandatory.

The size of the prostate is measured either by estimating the weight in grams or the volume in cubic centimeters. Models have been developed to teach clinicians how to gauge size and consistency. In general, a normal size prostate is 20 to 25 g (or cm³) in middle-aged men. A size of 25 to 30, 30 to 50, and greater than 50 g (or cm³) is a general guide to mild, moderate, and severe BPH. However, size does not necessarily correlate to symptoms, and both symptom score and size estimate should be reported. The size gauges the histologic condition and the symptoms indicate the LUTS and the bother index, which are both important for individualized treatment.

The laboratory assessment should include a urinalysis to rule out hematuria. Like an abnormal digital rectal examination, a urinalysis that shows persistent red blood cells should prompt referral to a urologist for cystoscopic and upper urinary tract assessment.

A urinalysis suggesting urinary tract infection should be followed up with a urine culture. If the patient presents in acute or chronic urinary retention and especially if there is a high postvoid or postcatheter residual bladder volume, a serum creatinine and blood urea nitrogen should be obtained. Severe BPH sometimes causes hydronephrosis and renal insufficiency, and rarely it causes renal failure. In-office bladder ultrasound scanners are very useful to quickly assess residual urine.

Contemporary diagnosis of BPH involves obtaining a PSA result. The latest guidelines from the American Urological Association regarding the use of PSA testing are very helpful (http://www.auanet.org/content/guidelines-and-quality-care/clinical-guidelines.cfm?sub=bph&CFID=2798600&CFTOKEN=24474979&jsessionid=843087b6ce7b4a4c6000302623b1d48497b4). While the traditional upper limit of normal for PSA testing has been 4.0 ng/mL, recent guidelines base more on changes in PSA levels over time, considering that most men with BPH will have prior PSA results. In the specific setting of using PSA to help manage BPH, the best data come from the PLESS trial (Proscar Long-Term Efficacy and Safety Study), where a PSA of 0 to 1.3 ng/mL, 1.4 to 3.2 ng/mL, and greater than 3.2 ng/mL was associated with small, medium, and large prostate glands (assuming prostate cancer has been ruled out) and predicted therapeutic response to finasteride (Proscar) (see later section).

Treatment

Treatment of BPH is always individualized to the patient and involves evaluation of symptoms and bother along with objective findings from examination and laboratory results. Current treatments range from periodic monitoring without treatment to treatment of extreme cases with open enucleative surgery.

ACTIVE SURVEILLANCE AND WATCHFUL WAITING

For many men, especially those with lower symptom scores and little bother, annual monitoring with digital rectal examination, PSA, urinalysis and symptom assessment is all that is required. Many men are happy to be reassured that they do not have clinically significant prostate cancer and are glad to hear that no immediate treatment is necessary.

COMPLEMENTARY AND ALTERNATIVE MEDICINE

The use of complementary and alternative medicine supplements is very common and physicians should ask patients about their use just as they ask about prescription medications. There are now many "prostate" and "men's health" supplements containing a variety of chemicals that include zinc, saw palmetto, vitamin E,[1] vitamin D,[1] and selenium, among others. Aside from a few European clinical trials of saw palmetto, the use of supplements to help BPH is speculative. One challenge is quality assurance of dose and ingredients of these agents that are not FDA-regulated. Although not for BPH, the NIH-funded SELECT trial (Selenium and Vitamin E Cancer Prevention Trial) to determine whether vitamin E or selenium, or both, would prevent prostate cancer is illustrative. Neither supplement had any effect on prostate cancer (or BPH to my knowledge). With the lack of robust trial data for the plethora of supplements, the evidence-based medicine answer to patients is clear.

MEDICAL THERAPY

α-Blocker Medications

The use of α-adrenergic blocking oral agents to treat BPH has been commonplace since the 1980s. These agents are directed at the dynamic component of BPH and LUTS by relaxing the smooth muscle tissue in the bladder neck and prostate. In simple terms, they relax the bladder outlet, resulting in better urinary flow.

Initial agents, such as prazosin (Minipress),[1] were not selective blockers and were also used to treat hypertension. Furthermore, these early agents were not long-acting and had to be taken multiple times per day, which severely limited their practical clinical utility. The next generation in the class were doxazosin (Cardura) and terazosin (Hytrin), which were longer-acting agents only dosed once a day. However, they were not selective and also lowered blood pressure, so titration was necessary. The third and current generation agents are selective blockers that treat BPH but do not lower blood pressure when used at recommended doses. The two in this class are tamsulosin (Flomax) and alfuzosin (Uroxatral).

In general, clinicians use α-blockers in men with smaller prostate glands ($\leq$30-35 g or cm^3), in younger men, and in patients where rapid effect is needed. Side effects of this class include headache, dizziness, asthenia, drowsiness, and retrograde ejaculation. Alfuzosin is reported to have the lowest rate of retrograde ejaculation. α-Blockers lower urinary tract muscular relaxation properties and are also now employed for ureteral urinary calculi (kidney stones) to facilitate spontaneous passage. α-Blockers are often used to treat prostatitis as well. In this setting, the agents can relieve dysfunctional voiding that contributes to some cases of prostatitis.

5α-Reductase Inhibitors

The 5α-reductase inhibitors have been available since the early 1990s. Finasteride (Proscar) was the first agent in this class (5 mg/daily) and is a type 1 inhibitor. Dutasteride (Avodart; 0.5 mg/daily) is a type 1 and type 2 inhibitor and was approved in 2002. Both drugs prevent the conversion of testosterone to the more active metabolite dihydrotestosterone in the prostate. This inhibition results in involution of BPH tissue and prostate shrinkage. On average, most men achieve 20% to 40% reduction in prostate size after at least 6 months of use. In general, these agents are most effective in men with prostate glands more than 30 g (or cm^3). Both drugs lower PSA levels by about 50% after 6 months of use. This is critical to take into account when screening for prostate cancer. If the PSA level does not fall by one half and the patient has been compliant with medication, the patient should be referred to a urologist for a work-up. In follow-up of men, PSA is generally doubled in assessing risk for prostate cancer. However, the use of PSA velocity or doubling-time and other prostate cancer screening tools are still valid as long as the effect on PSA is appreciated.

There are two key clinical trials that are important. The MTOPS trial (Medical Therapy of Prostate Symptoms) showed that the combination of an α-blocker (doxazosin) and a 5α-reductase inhibitor (finasteride) was more effective than either alone or placebo in treatment of BPH and LUTS. The PCPT (Prostate Cancer Prevention Trial) showed that finasteride[1] lowered the rate of prostate cancer by 25% over placebo in a large 7-year study. Recently, the REDUCE trial (Reduction by Dutasteride of Prostate Cancer Events) confirmed the prostate chemoprevention benefit of this class of drugs showing, that dutasteride[1] also lowered the rate of prostate cancer by 23% over placebo.

Urologists also use 5α-reductase inhibitors to treat chronic hematuria due to an enlarged prostate and sometimes prescribe these agents before transurethral resection of the prostate (TURP) to lessen surgical bleeding.

MINIMALLY INVASIVE PROCEDURES

Since the 1980s, a series of transurethral procedures have been evaluated to shrink or non-obstruct the prostate using heat, pressure, or direct pharmacotherapy. Balloon dilation of the prostate was the first

---

[1]Not FDA approved for this indication.

[1]Not FDA approved for this indication.

to come and go as it was proved not to be durable. Then came microwave energy delivered either transurethrally (transurethral microwave thermotherapy [TUMT]) or via the rectum using transrectal ultrasound guidance. The microwaves create heat in the prostate gland, which can shrink the prostate and improve BPH and LUTS symptoms and flow rates. A number of these therapies are FDA approved; however, their popularity has waned a bit because long-term follow up is lacking and results are thought not to be as durable as the gold standard TURP.

Heat energy to the prostate can also be delivered via radiofrequency energy in the form of the transurethral needle ablation (TUNA) procedure. A transurethral cystoscope-like device deploys several radiofrequency needles into the prostate to deliver the heat and shrinkage or cavitation effect. Clinical trials were also conducted with transurethral ethanol injection into the prostate to cause shrinkage; however, this therapy has yet to be FDA approved. High-intensity focused ultrasound (HIFU) is also used in some countries to treat prostate cancer, but it is not approved in the United States to treat cancer or BPH as of 2010.

SURGICAL THERAPY

Surgical therapy for BPH was the mainstay of treatment until about 1990, when medical and minimally invasive treatments came on the scene. Currently, surgical therapy, mostly consisting of TURP, is generally reserved for men who fail medical or minimally invasive therapy or men who present with advanced or complicated BPH. The classic indications to proceed directly to TURP include bladder calculi, severe BPH causing renal insufficiency, or urinary retention in cases of severe BPH. It is also reasonable to proceed to TURP in the man who does not desire medical therapy.

A TURP has become safer in the era of improved fiberoptic and endoscopic equipment now employed by urologists. This new generation of equipment allows improved visualization during the operation, especially when combined with microchip endoscopic cameras and large flat-screen technology available in modern endoscopic suites. The removal of prostate tissue has traditionally been accomplished using resectoscopes equipped with electrocautery. Today, this tissue removal can also be accomplished using laser technology, including the Green-Light laser system of tissue vaporization and other lasers that employ laser enucleation of tissue.

A variation of TURP is the transurethral incision of the prostate (TUIP). In this operation, the laser or resectoscope is used to make longitudinal cuts or incisions along the course of the prostate urethra from the bladder neck out to the apex of the prostate. This effective treatment can be used in men with smaller prostate glands who have significant LUTS.

Finally, for men with severe BPH and gland sizes 80 to 100 g/mL or more, open prostatectomy is still a valuable and highly effective surgical treatment. A small suprapubic incision is used to remove the prostate adenoma. As with radical prostatectomy used for prostate cancer, open prostatectomy for BPH should be performed by urologic surgeons who are experienced in this area.

REFERENCES

Burnett AL, Wein AJ. Benign prostatic hyperplasia in primary care: What you need to know. J Urol 2006;175(3 Pt 2):S19–24.

Donnell RF. Minimally invasive therapy of lower urinary tract symptoms. Urol Clin North Am 2009;36(4):497–509.

Emberton M, Zinner N, Michel MC, et al. Managing the progression of lower urinary tract symptoms/benign prostatic hyperplasia: Therapeutic options for the man at risk. BJU Int 2007;100(2):249–53.

Harkaway RC, Issa MM. Medical and minimally invasive therapies for the treatment of benign prostatic hyperplasia. Prostate Cancer Prostatic Dis 2006;9(3):204–14.

Hoffman RM, Monga M, Elliot SP, et al. Microwave thermotherapy for benign prostatic hyperplasia. Cochrane Database Syst Rev 2007;(4):CD004135.

Neal RH, Keister D. What's best for your patient with BPH? J Fam Pract 2009;58(5):241–7.

Roehrborn CG. BPH progression: Concept and key learning from MTOPS, ALTESS, COMBAT, and ALF-ONE. BJU Int 2008;101(Suppl 3):17–21.

Roehrborn CG. Pathology of benign prostatic hyperplasia. Int J Impot Res 2008;(Suppl 3):S11–8.

Erectile Dysfunction

Method of
Luciano Kolodny, MD

The term *erectile dysfunction* (ED) is relatively new, having replaced *impotence* approximately a decade ago. ED is defined as the "inability of the male to attain or maintain an erection sufficient for satisfactory sexual intercourse." ED affects millions of men worldwide with implications that go far beyond sexual activity alone. ED is now recognized as a sentinel event in cardiovascular disease, diabetes mellitus (DM), and depression. It can also be damaging to interpersonal relationships and self-esteem.

Epidemiology

The Massachusetts Male Aging Study is one of the pivotal studies on the prevalence of ED. Between 1987 and 1989, men between the ages of 40 and 70 years received questionnaires inquiring about several aspects of their sexual health. Of the 1790 men who received the questionnaires, 1290 responded. They revealed that 52% of them had some degree of dysfunction, 17% with minimal, 25% with moderate, and almost 10% with complete absence of erectile function. It also showed the extremely detrimental link between coronary artery disease (CAD), DM, and ED. A few years later another group used the same patient database and followed up on these subjects. The risk of ED was 26 cases per 1000 men annually, which increased with age, lower education, DM, heart disease, and hypertension.

Physiology of Erection

The penile erection requires intact vascular, neuronal, and hormonal systems. The intricate details of this process are beyond the scope of this article, but in summary, after any sensorial stimulation, which can be visual, tactile, auditory, or olfactory, nitric oxide (NO) and other neurotransmitters are released at the cavernous nerve terminals. The endothelial cells then release vasoactive relaxing factors, which lead to vasodilatation of the penile blood vessels and increased blood flow. As blood flow increases, compression of the subtunical venular plexuses will substantially decrease venous outflow and finally cause the penis to change from flaccid to erect (Figure 1).

NO is the principal neurotransmitter involved in penile erection, but other vasoactive substances such as vasoactive intestinal peptide, neuropeptide Y, calcitonin gene-related peptide (CGRP), substance P, and serotonin also play roles. High levels of intrapenile NO facilitate the relaxation of intracavernosal trabeculae, thereby maximizing blood flow and penile erection. Nonadrenergic, noncholinergic neurons have been found to release NO, leading to increased production of cyclic guanosine monophosphate (cGMP). Through a series of reactions, cGMP will lead to relaxation of the smooth muscle, directly impacting the ability to go from a flaccid to an erect penile

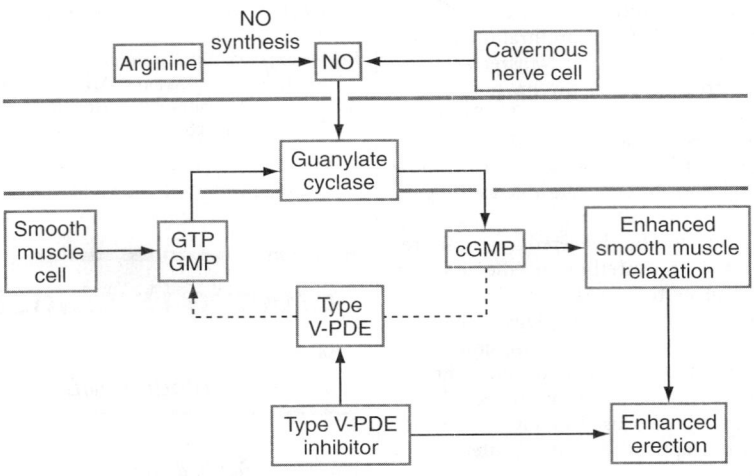

FIGURE 1. The biochemical process involved in erections and the mechanism of action of sildenafil citrate (Viagra). The cavernous nerves (S2-S4) innervate the penis and release NO. NO stimulates the production of cGMP in the smooth muscle cells of the penis. cGMP is directly responsible for increasing smooth muscle relaxation, which leads to increased arterial inflow and an erection. When cGMP is metabolized by PDE5, the penis undergoes detumescence. Sildenafil citrate (Viagra) inhibits PDE5 and increases the available cGMP, thereby leading to an enhanced erection. cGMP = cyclic guanosine monophosphate; NO = nitric oxide; PDE5 = phosphodiesterase 5.

state. The return from erect to flaccid requires the hydrolysis of cGMP to guanosine monophosphate (GMP) by phosphodiesterase 5 (PDE5) (see Figure 1).

Testosterone and Erectile Function

Testosterone provides intrapenile nitrous oxide synthase (NOS), which has an important role in enhancing the production of NO, subsequent local vasodilatation, and penile erection. There is no correlation between serum testosterone levels and the degree of ED. However, hypogonadal men may experience significantly reduced libido. Hypogonadism is associated with decreased self-esteem, depression, osteoporosis, insulin resistance, increased fat mass, decreased lean body mass, and cognitive dysfunction.

Pathophysiology of Erectile Dysfunction

ED can be classified as psychogenic, organic (hormonal, vascular, drug-induced, or neurogenic), or mixed psychogenic and organic. Up to 80% of ED cases have an organic origin. The most common cause of ED is vascular disease (Box 1).

Atherosclerosis is the most common cause of vasculogenic ED, whereas endothelial damage is the most common mechanism. Aging is a well-known risk factor for ED, and it is hypothesized that there are alterations in the levels of NO that occur as a consequence of the aging endothelium. Additionally, chronic illness, depression, and lack of a sexual partner are all prevalent in this age population.

Chronic tobacco use is a major risk factor for the development of vasculogenic ED because of its effects on the vascular endothelium. Additionally, blood nicotine levels rise after smoking, which increases sympathetic tone in the penis and leads to nicotine-induced, smooth-muscle contraction in the cavernosal body. Chronic smoking also leads to decreased penile NOS activity and neuronal NOS content.

DM is a major risk factor for ED. In the Massachusetts Male Aging Study, the diabetic subset had a threefold increased prevalence

---

BOX 1   Classification of Erectile Dysfunction

Endocrine
- Hypogonadism
- Hyperprolactinemia

Drug Induced
- β-Blockers
- Calcium channel blockers
- Alcohol
- Nicotine
- Antiandrogens
- Cocaine
- Heroin
- Marijuana
- Cimetidine
- Metoclopramide
- Antidepressant medications
- Antipsychotic medications

Vascular
- Coronary artery disease
- Peripheral vascular disease
- Hypertension
- Diabetes mellitus

Psychogenic
- Depression
- Performance anxiety

Neurogenic
- Spinal cord injury
- Neuropathy (diabetic, hypertensive)
- Cerebrovascular disease
- Radical prostatectomy
- Pelvic surgery

Multifactorial
- Aging
- End-stage renal disease
- Pelvic trauma (neurogenic and vasculogenic)
- Diabetes mellitus (neurogenic, vasculogenic, drug induced)

BOX 2   Tools Used to Quantify Erectile Dysfunction Severity

Tools used in the quantification of the severity of erectile dysfunction (ED) include the International Index of Erectile Function (IIEF), the Sexual Encounter Profile (SEP), and the Global Assessment Question (GAQ).

International Index of Erectile Function

The IIEF is a standardized questionnaire designed to measure ED and detect treatment-related changes. It is a 15-item questionnaire addressing five different domains: erectile function, orgasmic function, sexual desire, intercourse satisfaction, and overall satisfaction. The IIEF is the most frequently used efficacy measurement employed in ED drug trials. Using a scale from 1 (never/almost never) to 5 (almost always/always), men grade each domain. It is very sensitive and specific, and has been validated in 20 languages to assess treatment-related changes in sexual function. The questions 1–5 and 15 are used to quantify erectile dysfunction severity and are as follows:

1. How often were you able to get an erection during sexual activity?
2. When you had erections with sexual stimulation, how often were your erections hard enough for penetration?
3. When you attempted sexual intercourse, how often were you able to penetrate (enter) your partner?
4. During sexual intercourse, how often were you able to maintain your erection after you had penetrated (entered) your partner?
5. During sexual intercourse, how difficult was it to maintain your erection to completion of intercourse?
6. How do you rate your confidence that you could get and keep an erection?

And it is scored as follows:

26–30	Normal ED
22–25	Mild ED
17–21	Mild to moderate ED
11–16	Moderate ED
≤10	Severe ED

Sexual Encounter Profile

SEP is a five-question survey provided to patients with ED in clinical studies of oral therapies. The survey is completed after each sexual attempt. The questions are as follows:

1. Were you able to achieve at least some erection?
2. Were you able to insert your penis into your partner's vagina?
3. Did your erection last long enough to have successful intercourse?
4. Were you satisfied with the hardness of your erection?
5. Were you satisfied with the overall sexual experience?

Answers to questions 2 and 3 are the ones most often used in the literature.

Global Assessment Questions

GAQ is usually administered at the end of the treatment period during efficacy studies.
Question 1: Has the treatment taken during the study improved your erections?
Question 2: If yes, has the treatment improved your ability to engage in sexual activity?
This is very subjective, and its responses tend to be valued less than SEP and IIEF.

---

of ED compared with nondiabetic subjects (28% versus 9.6%). In the same study, the overall incidence rate of ED was 26 cases per 1000 man-years in nondiabetics and 50 cases per 1000 man-years in the diabetic population. The pathogenesis of ED in the diabetic patient is related to accelerated atherosclerosis, alterations in the corporal erectile tissue, and neuropathy.

Hypertension is another major risk factor for ED. Whether ED in patients with hypertension is related to the disease itself or to the use of antihypertensive medications has been debated for years. In a study looking at 104 subjects, the differences in incidence or severity of ED were minor between distinct types of antihypertensive medications or the number of agents being used simultaneously. This favors the concept that antihypertensive agents as well as the disease itself contribute to the appearance of ED. There are, however, classes of antihypertensive medications that are notorious for their negative impact on erectile function such as thiazides and β-blockers. The only β-blocker not associated with significant incidence of ED is carvedilol (Coreg).

Hyperlipidemia is another etiologic factor for ED. It is believed to contribute to ED by its relationship to endothelial dysfunction. One study showed that decreasing total cholesterol to less than 200 mg/dL by using atorvastatin (Lipitor) led to significant improvement of ED as measured by the International Index of Erectile Function (IIEF). A number of clinical studies with PDE5 inhibitors have shown significant improvement of erectile function in men with ED and hyperlipidemia.

ED may be a sentinel manifestation of vascular disorders. In a study of 980 subjects seeking ED advice, 18% were suffering from undiagnosed hypertension, 16% had DM, 5% had ischemic heart disease, 15% had benign prostatic hyperplasia, 4% had prostate cancer, and 1% had depression. ED can itself be an independent marker for CAD. In addition, the extent of CAD correlates with the prevalence of ED.

Cardiovascular risk reduction alleviates ED in patients with type 2 DM. In a study in which patients received interventions to improve hemoglobin A1C, blood pressure, and total cholesterol, there was significant improvement in the International Index of Erectile Function-5 (IIEF-5), suggesting that improved glycemic control in men with diabetes may lead to an improvement in ED. A study by Thompson revealed significant trends regarding the association of ED and subsequent cardiovascular disease in a retrospective analysis of data from 9457 men. A study published in 2009 looked at the association between ED and the long-term risk of CAD. Results showed that when ED occurred in a younger man, it was associated with a marked increase in the risk of future cardiac events, whereas in older men it appeared to be of little prognostic significance.

Quantification of the Severity of Erectile Dysfunction and Improvement

There are several tools designed to assess the severity of ED, as well as to measure the efficacy of different treatments. We discuss three different measures, the IIEF, the Sexual Encounter Profile (SEP), and the Global Assessment Question (GAQ) (Box 2).

PATIENT HISTORY

When assessing sexual dysfunction, it is important to inquire about a number of issues:

1. Differentiate between decreased libido and ED: assess whether the patient has one or both
2. Tobacco use: type, amount, duration
3. Alcohol intake
4. History of depression or anxiety disorder
5. Presence of social/relationship stressors

6. Ability to have erections while masturbating versus when with partner
7. List of all prescription, over-the-counter, and herbal medications
8. Knowledge of whether nocturnal erections are present
9. History of drug use: marijuana, cocaine, other recreational drugs
10. History of genitourinary trauma
11. History of prostatic disease, or possible related symptoms
12. History of hypertension, hyperlipidemia, CAD, peripheral vascular disease, cerebrovascular disease
13. History of DM
14. History of spinal cord injury
15. History of penile plaques: possible Peyronie's disease
16. Frequency of intercourse or attempted intercourse
17. Ability to ejaculate

PHYSICAL EXAMINATION

The physical examination should include a careful testicular examination to assess testicular size, asymmetries, presence of hernias, or varicoceles. Additionally, a digital rectal examination to assess the prostatic size, consistency, and presence of nodules is warranted. Penile inspection and palpation should be performed, with special attention to possible fibrotic plaques. Palpation and auscultation of femoral arteries for possible bruits is another important part of the examination.

LABORATORY STUDIES

Laboratory workup on a patient with ED should include total and bioavailable testosterone levels drawn in the morning, prolactin, prostate-specific antigen, fasting glucose, and fasting lipid panel. Further studies may be warranted depending on the results of the aforementioned.

Management of Erectile Dysfunction

The landscape of ED was revolutionized with the introduction of sildenafil citrate (Viagra), the first oral medication for the treatment of this condition. Since then, oral agents have become the preferred mode of treatments by patients in surveys worldwide. There are three oral agents that inhibit PDE5 currently on the market:

1. Sildenafil citrate (Viagra)
2. Vardenafil (Levitra)
3. Tadalafil (Cialis)

All three drugs work by inhibiting PDE5, which maintains intracavernosal levels of cGMP, subsequently producing vasodilatation and penile erection (see Figure 1).

SILDENAFIL CITRATE (VIAGRA)

Sildenafil citrate (Viagra) is an orally active, potent, and selective inhibitor of cGMP-specific PDE5. The predominant phosphodiesterase isoform in the penile tissue is type 5. The selectivity of sildenafil citrate (Viagra) for PDE5 is approximately 4000-fold greater than its selectivity for phosphodiesterase 3 (PDE3), the isoform involved in the control of cardiac contractility. Sildenafil citrate (Viagra) is absorbed rapidly after oral administration, with an absolute bioavailability of 40%. The time of maximal (T-max) plasma after oral dosing in the fasting state is between 30 and 120 minutes. A high-fat meal increases the time to peak plasma concentration by 60 minutes and reduces the peak plasma concentration by 29%. The half-life of the drug is from 3 to 5 hours. Sildenafil citrate (Viagra) is metabolized by hepatic microsomal cytochrome P450 isoenzyme 3A4 for the most part. Cytochrome P450 3A4 inhibitors, cimetidine (Tagamet), erythromycin, ketoconazole (Nizoral), and protease inhibitors may retard the metabolism of sildenafil citrate (Viagra).

The recommended dose is from 25 to 100 mg as needed approximately 1 hour before sexual activity. In some individuals, the onset of activity may be seen as early as 11 to 19 minutes, but this is not the norm. The usual starting dose is 50 mg.

The maximum recommended dose is 100 mg, and the maximum dosing frequency is once daily. A starting dose of 25 mg can be considered for patients older than age 65 years as well as for patients with severe hepatic cirrhosis or severe renal impairment.

There are more than two dozen, randomized, double-blind, placebo-controlled studies involving this agent. It produces positive results regardless of the etiology of ED. It has been studied in patients with DM, CAD, postcoronary artery bypass graft (post-CABG), spinal cord injury, depression, hypertension, prostate cancer post-prostatectomy, benign prostate enlargement post-transurethral resection of the prostate (TURP), patients on hemodialysis, as well as recipients of renal transplants. Results vary according to the underlying condition causing ED in the first place, ranging from 50% to 85%.

The most common side effects of sildenafil citrate (Viagra) include vasodilatory effects such as headaches, flushing, and nasal congestion caused by hyperemia of the nasal mucosa, as well as dyspepsia. Up to 30% of patients may get at least one side effect. Another side effect that presents on occasion is blurred or blue-green vision because of inhibition of phosphodiesterase 6 (PDE6) in the retina. It is absolutely contraindicated in men taking long-acting or short-acting nitrate drugs, and men taking any form of nitrates should be informed about the dangerous interaction.

Do not prescribe sildenafil citrate (Viagra) to patients with unstable CAD who need nitrates. Assess the need for ordering treadmill testing in select patients. Initial monitoring of blood pressure (BP) after the administration of sildenafil citrate (Viagra) may be indicated in men with complicated congestive heart failure (CHF). α-Blockers should not be used in combination with sildenafil citrate (Viagra) because of possible orthostatic hypotension.

VARDENAFIL (LEVITRA)

Vardenafil (Levitra) is a highly potent inhibitor of PDE5. It was approved for use in the United States in late 2003. It is a more selective PDE5 inhibitor than sildenafil citrate (Viagra). The absorption of vardenafil (Levitra) is delayed by a fatty content of more than 30% in a meal. However, that does not seem to affect its effectiveness in different trials. The half-life of vardenafil (Levitra) is 4.4 to 4.8 hours, and the clinical effectiveness may be as long as 12 hours. The time for maximum plasma concentration is between 42 and 54 minutes. The first trial using the agent included 580 patients, excluding patients with spinal cord injury, radical prostatectomy, hypogonadism, thyrotoxicosis, or DM.

The successful rates of intercourse were 71% to 75% on patients taking 5 or 10 mg at a time. Those taking 20 mg had a success rate of 80%. The placebo groups had an average success rate of 30%.

Vardenafil (Levitra) has been tested in patients with type 2 DM; 452 patients were enrolled in a double-blind, placebo-controlled trial. The success rate in the vardenafil (Levitra) group ranged from 57% to 72%.

In a different study involving 736 subjects including men with DM and stable CAD, the success rates were 28% for the placebo group, 65% for those taking 5 mg, 80% for those taking 10 mg, and 85% for the 20-mg group.

Patients who were unresponsive to sildenafil citrate (Viagra) at a dose of 100 mg on several attempts were given vardenafil (Levitra) in doses of 10 and 20 mg (proved in trial). Vardenafil (Levitra) produced statistically and clinically significant results compared with placebo in men who were historically unresponsive to sildenafil citrate (Viagra). The dose that offers the best clinical results is 20 mg. It should not be taken more than once every 24 hours. Safety studies have shown no deleterious effects with long-term daily use of this drug for up to 12 months.

The most common side effects include headaches (10% to 21%), flushing (5% to 13%), rhinitis (9% to 17%), and dyspepsia (1% to 6%) because vardenafil (Levitra) does not inhibit PDE6. Unlike sildenafil citrate (Viagra), it does not produce problems of blurred vision or blue-green visual disturbances. The same warning regarding the use of nitrates as sildenafil citrate (Viagra) applies to vardenafil (Levitra). Patients taking vardenafil (Levitra) may use α-blocking agents with caution.

TADALAFIL (CIALIS)

The third oral agent of this class is tadalafil (Cialis). It has a half-life of 17.5 hours, with two thirds of patients experiencing clinical benefits of this drug up to 36 hours after its use. The clinical onset of action occurs in less than 1 hour. There is no interaction between food and alcohol on the absorption of the drug.

There have been numerous phase II and III studies in Europe, Canada, and the United States using doses of 2, 5, 10, and 25 mg of the drug in comparison with placebo. The average success rates on these studies averaged 17% for placebo, 51% for the 2-mg dose, and 80% for the other doses, as well as up to 88% on the 25-mg dose in one study. In one study looking at 216 subjects with type 2 DM, improved erections were reported in 56% to 64% of the patients.

A recent article looking at all the previously published patient data showed that among 2102 men studied in 11 randomized placebo-controlled trials lasting 12 weeks, each mean improvement in IIEF at 20 mg of tadalafil (Cialis) was 8.6. Mean positive Sexual Encounter Profile Diary Question 3 (SEP3) response was 68% versus 31% in placebo groups. Mean GAQ was 84% versus 33% in placebo group.

In a multicenter, randomized, double-blind, crossover study looking at 181 men who received either sildenafil citrate (Viagra) or tadalafil (Cialis), 73% (132) preferred tadalafil (Cialis) at 20 mg instead of sildenafil citrate (Viagra) at 50 or 100 mg.

The most clinically effective dose of tadalafil (Cialis) is 20 mg. It should be taken at least 30 minutes before intercourse. It may be used with caution in patients using α-blocking agents. Nitrates are absolutely contraindicated for use in patients taking tadalafil (Cialis). The most common side effects include headaches, dyspepsia, back pain, rhinitis, and flushing. There are no visual side effects reported. Tadalafil has most recently been studied for use on a daily basis, with doses ranging from 2.5 to 5 mg, and showed favorable results.

Use of PDE5 Inhibitors and Cardiovascular Safety

The safety and efficacy of the three currently available PDE5 inhibitors (sildenafil, tadalafil, vardenafil) have been evaluated extensively in patients with ED and concomitant CVD, hypertension, hyperlipidemia, or diabetes, with or without additional risk factors. Overall, these studies have shown similar efficacy for the three agents, resulting in significant improvement of erectile function in patients with any of these comorbid conditions, and there was no evidence of cardiovascular risk from using any of these agents. However, because ED is known to be a harbinger of cardiovascular events in some men, the presence of ED should prompt investigation and intervention for cardiovascular risk factors.

APOMORPHINE (UPRIMA)[1]

Apomorphine (Uprima)[1] is a potent emetic that acts on central dopaminergic receptors. The stimulation of central dopaminergic receptors transmits excitatory signals down the spinal cord to the sacral parasympathetic nucleus, stimulating activity of the sacral nerves supplying the penis. It has been used successfully in up to 67% of patients when administered through a sublingual preparation. Subcutaneous

injections[2] of apomorphine (Uprima)[1] produce almost a 100% erectile response, but nausea and vomiting are limiting factors to this mode of administration.

The most common side effects are headache, nausea, and dizziness. Rare syncopal episodes have been reported.

PHENTOLAMINE (REGITINE)

Phentolamine (Regitine) is an α_1- and α_2-adrenergic receptor antagonist.

The sympathetic system via the release of noradrenaline (NA) is the primary determinant of cavernosal smooth muscle contraction and detumescence. A relative predominance of NA-induced contraction over NO-induced smooth muscle relaxation may contribute to ED.

In large phase III studies, 55% to 59% of patients receiving 40 and 80 mg were able to achieve vaginal penetration. Adverse effects include nasal congestion (10%), headaches (3% to 5%), dizziness (3% to 5%), tachycardia (3%), and nausea.

TRAZODONE (DESYREL)[1]

Trazodone (Desyrel)[1] is a serotonin reuptake inhibiting agent. Its action in ED is believed to be the result of central serotonergic and peripheral α-adrenolytic activity. The efficacy of trazodone is poorly demonstrated; however, it may have a place in those with performance anxiety. Side effects include drowsiness, insomnia, headaches, and weight loss.

DIETARY SUPPLEMENTS AND ERECTILE DYSFUNCTION

Yohimbine[1] is an α_2-adrenoreceptor antagonist with short duration of action. It is administered orally, and it is believed to have a central effect at adrenergic receptors in brain centers associated with libido and penile erection. A meta-analysis of seven studies established that it is superior to placebo, although results can be very erratic. Side effects include palpitations, tremors, and anxiety. Yohimbine should *not* be recommended as part of the management of ED.

A study with 60 patients who had failed papaverine[1] injections (50 mg or less) were treated with an extract of *Ginkgo biloba*, 60 mg for 12 to 18 months. After 6 months, 50% of the patients reported improvement in erectile function. A placebo-controlled randomized trial using 240 mg of *Ginkgo biloba* extract daily for 24 weeks in patients with vasculogenic ED did not demonstrate significant differences between the groups.

L-Arginine[1] is an amino acid that is the precursor to NO. Three small studies are looking at this drug. There are encouraging results in one study.

Zinc is found in high concentrations in seminal fluid. Anecdotal reports of improvement in ED.

ALPROSTADIL (PROSTAGLANDIN E1, CAVERJECT, MEDICATED URETHRAL SYSTEM FOR ERECTION)

Prostaglandin E1 (PGE_1) exerts a number of pharmacologic effects including systemic vasodilatation, inhibitory actions on platelet aggregation, and relaxation of smooth muscle. PGE_1 binds to PGE receptors and causes a relaxation response mediated by cyclic adenosine monophosphate (cAMP). It can be administered intracavernosally or intraurethrally.

It has been used in combination with papaverine,[1] and the combination was superior to PGE_1 alone. The intracavernosal administration seems to be more effective than transurethral (medicated urethral system for erection [MUSE]). MUSE should be administered in 1-mg doses, applied intraurethrally. Responses to intracavernosal

---

[1]Not FDA approved for this indication.
[2]Not available in the United States.

---

[1]Not FDA approved for this indication.

injections (Caverject) as high as 80% may be expected in patients with organic ED with a dose of 20 µg, and much lower to MUSE (35% to 43%). Injections are given with 27- to 30-gauge needles. The administration of PGE_1 is usually relegated as an alternative in patients who have contraindications to the use of phosphodiesterase 5 (PDE5) inhibitors. The possible side effects include penile fibrosis, priapism, urethral bleeding, hypotension, or syncopal episodes.

Papaverine[1] is a nonspecific phosphodiesterase inhibitor that increases cAMP and cGMP levels in penile erectile tissue. It produces smooth muscle relaxation and vasodilatation. It decreases the resistance to arterial inflow and increases the resistance to venous outflow. It is highly effective in psychogenic and neurogenic ED but not vasculogenic. It has been commonly used in combination with phentolamine (Regitine). Major side effects include priapism, corporeal fibrosis, and possible elevation of liver transaminases.

Moxisylyte chlorohydrate[2] is an α-blocking agent. In a study where 156 subjects received either alprostadil or moxisylyte in a dose-escalating fashion, alprostadil had much better success rates (46% versus 81%).

Chlorpromazine (Thorazine)[1] is useful when given in combination with alprostadil or papaverine. It has α-blocking properties, and it is cheaper than phentolamine (Regitine).

Decreased concentration of vasoactive intestinal polypeptide (VIP)* has been reported in the penile tissue of men with ED. VIP is believed to play a role in the erectile process. It is ineffective when administered alone but can be quite effective in combination with phentolamine (Regitine). In a small study of 52 subjects with organic ED, 100% of them achieved an erection sufficient for intercourse. Further studies into the effectiveness of VIP may be needed.

PENILE PROSTHESES

This surgical approach used to be quite common before the advent of oral agents. The use of prostheses is still a suitable alternative for those who are unresponsive to less invasive treatments. Prostheses can be classified as rod, one-piece inflatable, two-piece inflatable, and three-piece inflatable. Postsurgical infections and malfunctions are the most common complications. Patients are usually satisfied with the results of prosthetic placement.

---

[1]Not FDA approved for this indication.
[2]Not available in the United States.
*Investigational drug in the United States.

CURRENT DIAGNOSIS

- The risk factors for ED include tobacco, alcohol, and drug use, as well as DM, hypertension, hyperlipidemia, and prostate disease.
- ED is widely prevalent, and incidence sharply increases with age.
- ED is a cardiovascular sentinel event, and its occurrence warrants a cardiac workup.
- The workup of ED should include checking testosterone levels, prolactin, glucose, and lipid levels.
- First-line therapies include the use of PDE5 inhibitors such as sildenafil citrate (Viagra), vardenafil (Levitra), and tadalafil (Cialis).

Abbreviations: DM = diabetes mellitus; ED = erectile dysfunction; PDE5 = phosphodiesterase 5.

CURRENT THERAPY

- PDE5 inhibitors
  Sildenafil citrate (Viagra) 25–100 mg
  Vardenafil (Levitra) 10–20 mg
  Tadalafil (Cialis) 10–20 mg
- Alprostadil (PGE_1) intracavernosal injections (Caverject) 20 µg
  Intraurethral application (MUSE) 1-mg pellet
- Papaverine injections[1] 30–60 mg
- Agents not yet approved for use by the FDA:
  Apomorphine (Uprima)[1] 3, 4, 6 mg
  Phentolamine (oral)[1] 40, 60, 80 mg

---

[1]Not FDA approved for this indication.
Abbreviations: MUSE = medicated urethral system for erection; PDE5 = phosphodiesterase 5; PGE_1 = prostaglandin E1.

Vacuum Constrictive Device

Vacuum constrictive device is a plastic cylinder that is placed over the penis and connected to a pump that creates a partial vacuum. After achieving penile rigidity, a band is placed around the base of the penis to maintain the erection. This is a safe, noninvasive, and effective method of treating ED. It requires an understanding partner and the quality of the erection is not ideal, but patients are usually satisfied.

Testosterone

Patients who have low testosterone levels may benefit substantially from replacement. Men may expect significant improvements in libido, self-esteem, and overall energy levels. Additionally, testosterone is necessary for NO generation in the penile tissue.

The different testosterone preparations include injections such as testosterone enanthate (Delatestryl), cypionate (Depo-Testosterone) given as an intramuscular (IM) injection in doses of 100 to 200 mg, every 2 weeks on average. They also include transdermal testosterone patches (Androderm and Testoderm, 5 mg/d) or transdermal gel (AndroGel 5-g packets, one daily; or Testim 1% testosterone gel, one packet daily). Testosterone gel preparations provide physiologic replacement of testosterone and are preferred more than depot IM injections.

REFERENCES

Archer SL. Potassium channels and erectile dysfunction. Vascul Pharmacol 2002;38:61–71.

Burchardt M, Burchardt T, Baer L, et al. Hypertension is associated with severe erectile dysfunction. J Urol 2000;164(10):1188–91.

Carson CC, Rajfer J, Eardley I, et al. The efficacy and safety of tadalafil: An update. BJU Int 2004;93:1276–81.

Crowe SM, Streetman DS. Vardenafil treatment for erectile dysfunction. Ann Pharmacother 2004;38:77–85.

Donatucci CF, Wong DG, Giuliano F, et al. Efficacy and safety of tadalafil once daily: Considerations for the practical application of a daily dosing option. Curr Med Res Opin 2008;24(12):3383–92.

Feldman HA, Goldstein I, Hatzichristou DG, et al. Impotence and its medical and psychosocial correlates: Results of the Massachusetts Male Aging Study. J Urol 1994;151(1):54–61.

Inman BA, St. Sauver JL, Jacobson DJ, et al. A population-based, longitudinal study of erectile dysfunction and future coronary artery disease. Mayo Clin Proc 2009;84(2):108–13.

Jackson G, Betteridge J, Dean J, et al. A systematic approach to erectile dysfunction in the cardiovascular patient: A consensus statement—Update 2002. Int J Clin Pract 2002;56(9):663–71.

Jaynat D, Shepherd MD. Evaluation and treatment of erectile dysfunction in men with diabetes mellitus. Mayo Clin Proc 2002;77(3):276–82.

Johannes CB, Araujo AB, Feldman HA, et al. Incidence of erectile dysfunction in men ages 40 to 69 years old: Longitudinal results from the Massachusetts Male Aging Study. J Urol 2000;163(2):460–3.

Khatana SAM, Taveira TH, Miner MM, et al. Does cardiovascular risk reduction alleviate erectile dysfunction in men with type II diabetes mellitus? Int J Impotence Res 2008;20:501–6.

Kirby M, Jackson G, Betteridge J, et al. Is erectile dysfunction a marker for cardiovascular disease? Int J Clin Pract 2002;55(9):614–8.

Lue TF. Drug therapy: Erectile dysfunction. N Engl J Med 2000;342 (24):1802–13.

Michelakis E, Tymchak W, Archer S. Sildenafil: From the bench to the bedside. CMAJ 2000;163(9):1171–5.

Nehra A. Erectile dysfunction and cardiovascular disease: Efficacy and safety of phosphodiesterase type 5 inhibitors in men with both conditions. Mayo Clin Proc 2009;84(2):139–48.

NIH Consensus Development Panel on Impotence. Impotence (NIH Consensus Conference). JAMA 1993;270(1):83–90.

Padma-Nathan H. Intra-urethral and topical agents in the management of erectile dysfunction. In: Carson CC III, Kirby RS, Goldstein I, editors. Textbook of Erectile Dysfunction. Oxford: Isis Medical Media; 1999. p. 323–6.

Rhoden EL, Teloken C, Mafessoni R, et al. Is there any relation between serum levels of testosterone and the severity of erectile dysfunction? Int J Impot Res 2002;14:167–71.

Shokeir AA, Alserafi MA, Mutabagani H. Intracavernosal versus intraurethral alprostadil: A prospective randomized study. BJU Int 1999;83:812–5.

Spahn M, Manning M, Juenemann KP. Intracavernosal therapy. In: Carson CC III, Kirby RS, Goldstein I, editors. Textbook of Erectile Dysfunction. Oxford: Isis Medical Media; 1999. p. 345–53.

Sullivan ME, Thompson CS, Dashwood MR, et al. Nitric oxide and penile erection: Is erectile dysfunction another manifestation of vascular disease? Cardiovasc Res 1999;43:658–65.

Thompson IM, Tangen CM, Goodman PJ, et al. Erectile dysfunction and subsequent cardiovascular disease. JAMA 2005;294(23):2996–3002.

Acute Renal Failure

Method of
Kevin Schroeder, MD

Epidemiology and Definitions

Acute renal failure (ARF), increasingly called acute kidney injury, is a clinical syndrome that can include decreased urine output, retention of nitrogenous metabolic waste products normally excreted by the kidney, retention of sodium and extracellular fluid resulting in peripheral and sometimes central edema, and various electrolyte and acid-base disturbances that may be associated with elevations in the blood urea nitrogen (BUN) and serum creatinine concentrations. Typically these changes occur rapidly over hours to days. Acute renal failure may further be described by the decrement in urine output: polyuric failure, indicating greater than 3 L urine output per 24 hours; nonoliguric failure, indicating 0.4 to 3L urine output per 24 hours; oliguric failure, indicating less than 400 mL urine output per 24 hours; and anuric failure, with less than 50 mL urine output per 24 hours.

Currently accepted definitions of ARF include a rise in the serum creatinine concentration by more than 0.5 mg/dL or a relative increase in the serum creatinine concentration by more than 25% for patients with preexisting chronic kidney disease (CKD) and a reduction in the glomerular filtration rate (GFR) by 50%. Note that these definitions are very operational and based on laboratory data readily available to practicing physicians, but consensus regarding a single, more sensitive measure of ARF is lacking.

Traditionally, ARF has been subclassified mechanistically into three categories. *Prerenal azotemia* refers to conditions that cause a fall in GFR because of reduced glomerular perfusion pressure. *Intrinsic renal failure* refers to conditions that directly damage any of the four main structural components of the kidney, including the afferent and efferent arterioles, glomeruli, tubules, and interstitium. *Postrenal failure* commonly refers to any condition that causes obstruction of either the upper or lower urinary tract. From a practical standpoint, clinicians must also consider the situation in which ARF occurs (in an ambulatory patient, at hospital admission, during hospitalization, or after discharge) and the rapidity of deterioration, because some diagnoses are more likely depending on the clinical context.

The reported incidence of ARF varies by clinical situation and patient population, occurring in about 2% of all inpatient admissions. Varying definitions of disease and methodologic characteristics of epidemiologic studies also affect the reported incidence. General surgical patients undergoing nonemergent, noncardiac surgery had ARF at a reported incidence of 0.8%, and critically ill surgical patients undergoing noncardiac surgery experienced ARF at a rate nearly 80 times higher. Several scoring systems have been developed to predict the risk of ARF in patients undergoing cardiac surgery, which can vary from 5% to 25%. General medicine patients can experience ARF during a hospitalization at a rate of up to 7%, but the incidence may be in the 30% to 50% range for patients in critical care units. It may be possible that the true incidence of ARF in the United States will increase substantially as the baby boom generation enters its seventh decade.

Despite advances in medical technology, pharmacotherapeutics, and dialysis modalities in the critical care setting, mortality associated with ARF remains largely untouched at 20% to 80%. Recent studies have detected an increased mortality with even a slight rise in serum creatinine (increase <0.5 mg/dL). ARF adds to length of stay by about 4 days and can easily increase the cost of admission by more than $10,000.

Classification

Causes of ARF (Box 1) are elucidated chiefly from the history and physical examination. In particular, the history should focus first on symptoms causing volume depletion, second on symptoms relating to obstruction, and third on systemic symptoms including unexplained malaise, weight loss, fever, sinopulmonary bleeding, joint pain or swelling, rashes, myalgias, and neuropathies. All these factors must be considered in light of the patient's comorbid conditions, especially cardiovascular disease, hypertension, diabetes, liver disease, and peripheral vascular disease. Medications including antihypertensives, diuretics, analgesics, and over-the-counter supplements should be reviewed carefully. The physical examination serves to confirm the patient's volume status (e.g., frank hypotension or orthostatic change in blood pressure with tachycardia), to identify signs of cardiovascular disease and cardiopulmonary decompensation, to assess the status of the urinary bladder, and to detect signs of systemic disease. In addition to routine serum chemistries, BUN, and serum creatinine levels, all patients with nonanuric ARF must have a urinalysis. The clinician must observe the urine sediment for the presence of protein, blood, dysmorphic red cells, and cellular and noncellular casts. Finally, for oliguric patients, calculation of the fractional excretion of sodium (FE_{Na}) might prove useful. Serologic testing regarding acute glomerulonephritis should be obtained when the history and physical examination suggest sufficient pretest probability.

PRERENAL AZOTEMIA

Prerenal azotemia is the most common cause of ARF among patients admitted to general medicine services. It is commonly observed in cases of volume depletion or decreased effective arterial blood volume. These include profuse emesis or diarrhea, hemorrhage, and overzealous diuresis, especially in the face of poor oral intake. In these cases, peripheral and central edema is often absent. Decompensated CHF, decompensated cirrhosis leading to the hepatorenal syndrome, and the nephrotic syndrome all lead to effective decreases in circulating arterial volume. Commonly, patients with these conditions have peripheral edema and sometimes central edema with

BOX 1 Causes of Acute Renal Failure

Prerenal Azotemia
Effective Arterial Blood Volume and Hypotension
Emesis or diarrhea
Hemorrhage
Nephrotic syndrome
Sepsis
Third spacing
- Acute abdomen
- Bowel infarct
- Burns
- Cirrhosis or hepatorenal syndrome
- *Clostridium difficile* colitis
- Pancreatitis
- Peritonitis
- Postoperative abdomen

Pump Failure
- Acute myocardial infarction
- Congestive heart failure
- Tamponade

Overmedication
- Anesthetics
- Diuretics
- Nonsteroidal antiinflammatory drugs (including cyclooxygenase-2 inhibitors)

Intrinsic Acute Renal Failure
Acute Tubular Necrosis
Toxins
- Aminoglycosides
- Cyclosporine (Neoral)
- Ethylene glycol
- Heavy metals
- Hemoglobinuria
- Iodinated dye
- Myoglobinuria
- Nonsteroidal antiinflammatory drugs (including cyclooxygenase-2 inhibitors)
- Pentamidine (Pentam)
- Tumor lysis syndrome
Ischemia
- Cardiovascular surgery
- Dissection
- Embolism

- Severe hypotension
- Trauma
Septic
- Gram-positive or gram-negative sepsis

Interstitial Nephritis
Allopurinol (Zyloprim)
Antibiotics
- Cephalosporins
- Penicillins
- Rifampin (Rifadin)
- Sulfonamides
Diuretics
Nonsteroidal antiinflammatory drugs
Phenytoin (Dilantin)

Macrovascular Disease
Atheroembolic disease
Malignant hypertension

Microvascular Disease
HELLP syndrome
Hemolytic-uremic syndrome and thrombotic thrombocytopenic purpura
Hepatorenal syndrome
Rapidly progressive glomerulonephritis
Vasculitis

Postrenal Obstruction
Intratubular Obstruction
Crystals
Myeloma casts

Ureteral Obstruction
Ligation
Retroperitoneal fibrosis
Stones/papillae
Tumor compression

Bladder Outlet Obstruction
Anticholinergic medicines
Benign prostatic hyperplasia
Diabetic autonomic dysfunction
Stones and papillae
Urethral valves

HELLP = hemolysis, elevated liver enzymes, low platelets.

low albumin states. In the former case, diuretics often improve not only the heart failure but also the renal dysfunction concomitantly. Recalling the principles of vascular autoregulation (Fig. 1), the clinician must realize that the kidneys of elderly patients and patients with chronic hypertension are especially susceptible to intravascular volume changes. This is particularly true when patients are medicated with angiotensin converting enzyme inhibitors and angiotensin receptor blockers, nonsteroidal antiinflammatory drugs and cyclooxygenase-2 inhibitors, and calcineurin inhibitors, all of which effectively paralyze the kidney's ability to regulate glomerular perfusion.

Typical laboratory findings in prerenal azotemia include an elevated BUN:creatinine ratio (>20:1) and a FE_{Na} of less than 1%. However, if the patient had been taking diuretics, the FE_{Na} may be falsely elevated. Metabolic alkalosis and hypokalemia might or might not be present. The urinalysis is expected to show a high specific gravity with no blood, no protein, and bland sediment except may be a few hyaline casts. Clinically, pure prerenal azotemia often responds quickly to restoration of euvolemia with increased urine output and a falling creatinine within 24 hours. Therapy for prerenal azotemia should be aimed at restoring clinical euvolemia and eliminating the cause of the azotemia. Infusion of isotonic saline is the norm, with supplemental oral rehydration where possible, and use of colloids or blood products when needed. In the case of decompensated left heart failure with pulmonary embarrassment, it is often necessary to employ an inotrope (e.g., dobutamine [Dobutrex]) in combination with a diuretic, whereas with hepatorenal syndrome, combinations of midodrine (Proamatine)[1] and octreotide (Sandostatin)[1] have been employed with some success.

[1]Not FDA approved for this indication.

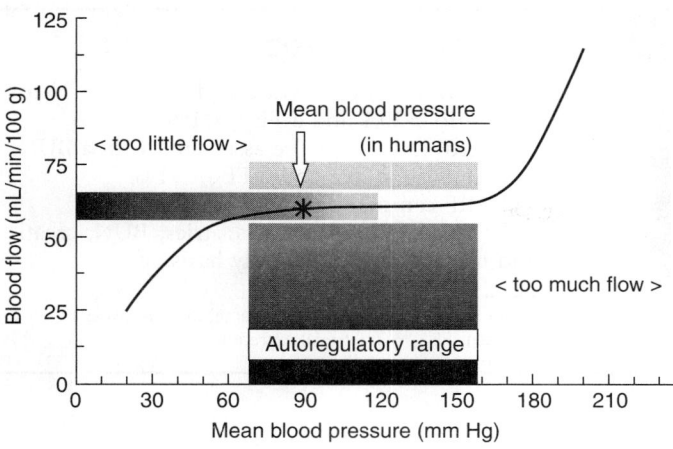

FIGURE 1. Principle of vascular autoregulation.

Intrinsic renal failure may be subdivided into diseases that affect the renal microvasculature, glomeruli, tubules, and interstitium. Although the pharmacologic effects of certain medications (e.g., angiotensin-converting enzyme inhibitors [ACEIs] and nonsteroidal antiinflammatory drugs [NSAIDs]) directly affect the renal microvasculature, renal dysfunction associated with their use physiologically produces a prerenal picture. However, cholesterol emboli syndrome and small vessel vasculitis represent two diseases whose impact on the renal microvasculature is pathologic. In the former case, cholesterol-laden debris dislodged from the abdominal aorta or aortic arch showers distal vascular beds. The classic scenario involves a patient who, having recently undergone an endovascular procedure, presents with abdominal colic, ARF, livedo reticularis, and evidence of ischemic toes. Depending on the size of the embolus, the patient can have frank intestinal or renal infarction or an acutely ischemic lower extremity, necessitating emergent intervention. Eosinophiluria and hypocomplementemia may be noted. The elevation in creatinine can progress in a stepwise fashion for several days to weeks after the original event. Magnetic resonance imaging (MRI) can show evidence of wedge-shaped infarcts in the renal parenchyma. Optimal therapy with regard to antiplatelet agents versus anticoagulants remains uncertain.

GLOMERULAR DISEASE

Glomerular disease accounts for roughly 10% of ARF among hospitalized patients. The hallmarks of rapidly progressive acute glomerulonephritis (RPGN) include an active urine sediment (dysmorphic red blood cells (RBCs) and cellular casts), hypertension, some edema, and a rapid decline in renal function over days. World Health Organization (WHO) class IV systemic lupus erythematosus (SLE) nephritis, anti-neutrophil cytoplasmic antibodies (ANCA)-mediated disease, and anti-GBM (glomerular basement membrane) disease are examples. Serologic testing is often useful, but a renal biopsy is almost always indicated for definitive diagnosis. Treatment usually involves some combination of corticosteroids and cytotoxic medications. Because of the severe increase in morbidity and mortality when these diseases are untreated, RPGN should be considered a medical emergency, with prompt attempts to diagnose and treat. It is important to recognize that whereas diseases that primarily manifest as the nephritic syndrome commonly cause ARF, entities associated more with a nephrotic-syndrome picture—including membranous disease, minimal change disease, or focal sclerosis—can certainly produce ARF as well. This usually occurs in the setting of massive nephrotic-range proteinuria (10–20 g/24 hours) and associated marked hypoalbuminemia.

ACUTE TUBULAR NECROSIS

Acute tublar necrosis (ATN) accounts for fully 50% of ARF among hospitalized patients; depending on the scenario, this figure can rise to as much as 75%. ATN has three common causes: ischemic, toxic, and septic. ATN has been described by its phases: Injury, during

which time the insult causes direct damage to the tubules, is manifested as a progressive increase in the serum creatinine and possibly the development of oliguria. In the plateau phase, the creatinine, urinary output, and volume status are relatively stable. Recovery is marked by a spontaneous decline in serum creatinine and increase in urinary output, perhaps even into a polyuric range. The time course of ATN from injury to recovery is variable. Depending on the severity of the injury and the preexistence of renal disease, ATN can reverse within 1 to 3 weeks, although a small percentage of patients with ATN remain dialysis dependent after months. ATN is typically associated with a loss of urinary concentration, elevated urinary sodium excretion, and an elevated FE_{Na} of greater than 2%. The BUN and creatinine tend to rise proportionally. The urinary sediment can reveal tubular epithelial cell casts that have a coarsely granular or muddy brown appearance.

Ischemic ATN typically occurs during periods of prolonged hypotension and represents an evolution of prerenal azotemia. Ischemic ATN is commonly observed to varying degrees after cardiovascular and major orthopedic or trauma surgery. Careful attention must be paid to urine output and volume status. High-dose diuretics may be employed to avoid pulmonary edema, and if a suboptimal response is seen, the dosage should be doubled after the first dose. Patients who rapidly become oliguric have a high mortality rate, which is unaffected by diuretics and can therefore require early initiation of dialysis. Specific risk factors for developing ischemic ATN in the postoperative setting include advanced age (older than 70 years), preexisting CKD, diabetes, emergent surgery, preexisting vascular disease, and the need for valvular, particularly aortic valve, heart surgery in addition to bypass grafting. The degree and duration of intraoperative hypotension as well as time spent on cardiopulmonary bypass can also play roles.

Toxic ATN is proximal tubular cell death as a consequence of drugs or other endogenous chemicals. Drugs that classically cause toxic ATN include aminoglycosides, amphotericin B (Fungizone), radiocontrast, platinum-based chemotherapy, and NSAIDs. Endogenous chemicals known to cause toxic ATN include uric acid, myoglobin, and heme. Clinically, it is worthwhile noting that although the onset of ATN after a single dose of NSAID or iodinated radiocontrast material may be rapid (24–72 hours) especially in volume-depleted patients, in the case of aminoglycosides the onset of injury may be a bit slower, consistent with cumulative dose exposure. In general, ATN is best avoided by limiting the dose of potentially toxic medications (e.g., once-daily dosing of aminoglycosides), maintenance of adequate volume status, and close attention to the serum creatinine and urinary output.

In the case of radiocontrast agents, low osmolar and isosmolar agents are thought to be less toxic, and dose limitation (or elimination) to less than 100 mL are helpful strategies. Although prospective randomized, controlled trial data are inconclusive, and meta-analyses are equivocal, in cases of elective contrast exposure it remains common practice at many centers to administer *N*-acetylcysteine (Mucomyst)[1] in a dosage of 600 mg orally every 12 hours on the day before and the day of exposure. This, along with intravenous fluid administration for up to 6 hours before elective procedures (some authors use bicarbonate-containing solutions) seem to be reasonably safe, low-cost measures that can offer some protection against ATN in patients with known renal disease. After contrast-enhanced procedures, serum creatinine should be measured daily in hospitalized patients and at 48 hours after the procedure in outpatients.

Septic ATN often manifests in the critical care setting in patients with multisystem organ failure. Patients are typically hypotensive with either gram-positive or gram-negative bacteremia and anuria, often with severe acidemia. Unlike patients with prerenal azotemia whose urine output responds to volume resuscitation, patients with septic ATN do not produce urine in response to substantial volume resuscitation (Table 1). The clinical picture is difficult to distinguish from ischemic ATN because the two disease processes can coexist. Clinically, ischemic and toxic ATN are thought to show signs of

---

[1]Not FDA approved for this indication.

TABLE 1 Laboratory Differentiation of Prerenal Azotemia from Acute Tubular Necrosis

	Result	
Test	Prerenal Azotemia	Acute Tubular Necrosis
U_{Na}	<10–20	>40
FE_{Na}	<1	>1
Urine SG	>1.020	<1.010
BUN:Cr	>20:1	≈10:1
Fe_{Ur}	>60:1	<20:1
U_{Cr}:P_{Cr}	>40:1	<10:1

BUN = blood urea nitrogen; Cr = creatinine; FE_{Ur} = fractional excretion of urea; FE_{Na} = fractional excretion of sodium; SG = specific gravity; U_{Cr}:P_{Cr} = ratio of urine creatinine to serum creatinine; U_{Na} = urine sodium.

resolution within 14 days of removal of the insult, whereas the sequelae of septic ATN can persist for one or several months after the infection requiring prolonged hospitalization and dialysis support. Mortality in this setting can be as high as 80%, and patients who survive their initial illness are particularly susceptible to nosocomial infections, catheter-related bacteremia, and malnutrition.

INTERSTITIAL DISEASE

Interstitial disease represents the third most common cause of ARF among hospitalized patients after prerenal azotemia and ATN. Acute interstitial nephritis is usually the effect of either drugs or pyelonephritis. In the case of medications, key diagnostic points include a delayed onset after medication exposure, as much as 7 days, and the co-incidence of fever and a central rash in about 30% of patients. The diagnosis may be suspected in the presence of sterile pyuria, eosinophiluria, and eosinophilia. Because the disease is of nonglomerular and nontubular origin, the urine sediment should be relatively bland, with minimal hematuria or proteinuria. Renal biopsy confirming the presence of increased numbers of eosinophils in the interstitium remains the gold standard. Antibiotics that are particularly notorious for causing acute interstitial nephritis include penicillins, particularly methicillin (Staphcillin); sulfa-containing drugs; rifampin (Rifadin); and quinolones. Typically, cessation of the suspected agent results in improved renal function within 5 days; however, in severe, prolonged cases, a course of corticosteroids can hasten improvement. Importantly, if the patient is re-exposed to the offending agent, acute interstitial nephritis can develop much more rapidly.

OBSTRUCTIVE DISEASE

Obstructive renal disease, although relatively uncommon, should be highly suspected in any patient with otherwise unexplained anuria, especially in those with a known pelvic malignancy or recent pelvic surgery. Obstruction of the lower tract and bladder outlet is more prevalent among elderly men with prostatic hypertrophy and diabetics with autonomic nervous dysfunction. Upper-tract obstruction can be seen in cases of retroperitoneal fibrosis, uroepithelial malignancy, and nephrolithiasis. Certain systemic processes including tumor lysis syndrome, myeloma cast nephropathy, and ethylene glycol overdose can all cause an intratubular obstruction due to massive crystal and cast deposition within the kidney.

Clinically, obstruction of the bladder outlet may be diagnosed and treated via placement of a Foley catheter. Bladder scans, ultrasounds, and measurement of the pre- and postvoid residual bladder volumes are also important but not always immediately necessary. Bilateral upper tract obstruction requires intervention in the form of bilateral percutaneous nephrostomy tubes or internal double-J stent placement via cystourethroscopy. Patients with severe obstruction may be significantly hyperkalemic at presentation, requiring prompt treatment. Fortunately, if the obstruction is relieved in a timely fashion, the hyperkalemia usually dissipates without emergent dialysis.

 CURRENT DIAGNOSIS

- Prerenal azotemia may be associated with a BUN-to-creatinine ratio >20:1 and a FE_{Na} <1%.
- Intrarenal ARF (ATN) may be associated with a BUN-to-creatinine ratio <20:1 and a FE_{Na} >1%.
- Postrenal ARF can manifest with frank anuria.
- Follow the trends of serum chemistries, BUN, creatinine, and urine output on a daily basis.

ARF = acute renal failure; ATN = acute tubular necrosis; BUN = blood urea nitrogen; FE_{Na} = fractional excretion of sodium.

Treatment

Management of hospitalized patients is generally supportive. Specific measures include a thorough daily review of the medication list to ensure that all possible toxic medications have been eliminated and that all drugs excreted via the kidneys have been dose adjusted for the level of renal dysfunction. The patient's volume status should be assessed frequently, with appropriate adjustments in intravenous fluids or diuretics. Similarly, electrolytes, BUN, and creatinine should be checked daily. In general, hospitalized patients should remain hospitalized until the clinical course has at least stabilized and close outpatient follow-up is ensured. Outpatients with acute renal failure can require urgent hospitalization if the cause is not immediately apparent and reversible, or if significant hyperkalemia or volume overload exists, or if the patient has significant comorbidities.

The decision to initiate renal replacement therapy is made by the nephrologist on a patient-by-patient basis. Some absolute clinical indications for dialysis exist, such as severe hyperkalemia; peaked T waves or prolongation of the QRS complex by electrocardiogram; volume overload or acidosis refractory to medical therapy; certain intoxications or electrolyte abnormalities; and symptomatic uremia with pericarditis, neurologic changes, or bleeding diatheses. Depending on the clinical setting, the two most common are hyperkalemia and volume overload; rarely will the nephrologist let ARF with either of these conditions progress to the point of cardiac arrhythmia or intubation undialyzed.

Patients who require urgent or emergent dialysis can typically be dialyzed via standard intermittent hemodialysis. This method is more effective for acute correction of electrolyte, toxin, and acid–base aberrations as well as pulmonary edema. Controversy exists as to the proper dose of dialysis for patients with ARF, particularly those in the critical care setting. Clinical practice varies by center, but studies have shown a survival benefit favoring daily hemodialysis to keep the BUN less than 100 mg/dL.

Continuous renal replacement therapy (CRRT) or continuous veno-venous hemofiltration is usually reserved for critically ill patients, particularly those with hypotension requiring vasopressor support or those with sufficiently poor cardiac performance and volume overload who cannot tolerate acute intravascular volume shifts associated with conventional hemodialysis.

Acute peritoneal dialysis, although certainly a viable modality, is practiced much less commonly in the United States partly due to the widespread availability of hemodialysis.

Emerging Issues

In clinical practice, the diagnosis and treatment of ARF rest on the ability to recognize it in a timely fashion. The two universally available indicators—urinary output and serum creatinine measurement—are limited in their sensitivity and specificity; however, new urinary and

CURRENT THERAPY

- Hemodynamic support and maintenance of euvolemic state
- Correction of electrolyte and acid–base imbalances
- Removal of all offending agents and correction of underlying causes
- Adjustment of all medications for decreased glomerular filtration rate
- Renal replacement when needed on an individual basis

plasma biomarkers are emerging that can allow earlier identification of ARF. Urinary neutrophil gelatinase–associated lipocalin (NGAL), kidney injury molecule-1 (KIM-1), and interleukin-18 (IL-18), in combination with plasma NGAL and cystatin C measurements, are all currently being evaluated in ARF clinical trials. These assays hold the promise of earlier detection and perhaps more specific anatomic localization of the injury within the kidney. Whether these biomarkers are used alone, serially, or in combination as an acute kidney injury panel remains to be seen as they transition from primarily clinical trial–based application to widespread clinical use. Questions regarding their ability to help predict which patients with ARF will spontaneously recover renal function and which will require dialysis remain to be answered.

Nephrotoxicity associated with gadolinium-containing contrast media has risen to the front of discussion among radiologists and nephrologists. Originally thought to be non-nephrotoxic, gadolinium has been implicated in a number of well-documented cases. Perhaps more striking are the mounting reports of gadolinium-related nephrogenic systemic fibrosis, which is characterized by brawny epidermal fibrotic plaques developing over several weeks after exposure. It is important to recognize that other organs including the subcutaneous tissues, skeletal musculature, lungs, and heart may be involved. Although the pathogenesis of this disease has not been fully elucidated, epidemiologically, 90% of cases have been described among end-stage renal disease patients requiring dialysis, and fully 10% have occurred among patients with CKD stages 3 and 4. Because there is no cure for this disease and its clinical consequences are potentially devastating, clinicians now must consider the risk-to-benefit ratio of exposing a patient to gadolinium-enhanced MRI procedures and weigh that risk against the well-established risk of iodinated contrast used in CT scans.

REFERENCES

Coca SG, Peixoto AJ, Garg AX, et al. The prognostic importance of a small acute decrement in kidney function in hospitalized patients: A systematic review and meta-analysis. Am J Kidney Dis 2007;50(5):712–20.

Dennen P, Parikh CR. Biomarkers of acute kidney injury: Can we replace serum creatinine? Clin Nephrol 2007;68(5):269–78.

Devarajan P. Proteomics for biomarker discovery in acute kidney injury. Semin Nephrol 2007;27(6):637–51.

Eachempati SR, Wang JC, Hydo LJ, et al. Acute renal failure in critically ill surgical patients: Persistent lethality despite new modes of renal replacement therapy. J Trauma 2007;63(5):987–93.

Greenberg A, Cheung A, Coffman T, et al. editors. Primer on Kidney Diseases. 2nd ed. San Diego: Academic Press; 1998.

Johnson J, Feehally J. Comprehensive Clinical Nephrology. 1st ed. St Louis: Mosby; 2000.

Kheterpal S, Tremper KK, Englesbe MJ, et al. Predictors of postoperative acute renal failure after noncardiac surgery in patients with previously normal renal function. Anesthesiology 2007;107(6):892–902.

Nagle PC, Warner MA. Acute renal failure in a general surgical population: Risk profiles, mortality, and opportunities for improvement. Anesthesiology 2007;107(6):869–70.

Rakel R, Bope E, editors. Conn's Current Therapy 2007. Philadelphia: Elsevier; 2007.

Chronic Renal Failure

Method of
Jeffrey A. Kraut, MD

Chronic renal failure is defined as a reduction in glomerular filtration rate (GFR) below the normal values of approximately 120 to 130 mL/minute developing over months to years. Its incidence has increased significantly over the last several years, but this probably reflects more accurate estimations of GFR. However, there is an increased prevalence of type II diabetes mellitus, a frequent cause of renal disease, in Western societies that could contribute to a higher incidence of chronic renal failure. When renal failure is severe (GFR <10 mL/minute), renal replacement therapy, either dialysis or renal transplantation, is required to preserve life. However, even before several renal failure ensues, the presence of chronic renal failure has an important impact on organ function and can contribute to the development of significant electrolyte derangements, important hormonal abnormalities, and anemia. Also, its presence can alter the metabolism and therefore the blood concentrations and tissue concentrations of drugs administered for the treatment of various diseases. Moreover, a reduced GFR is associated with an increased risk of death, increased incidence of cardiovascular events, and hospitalizations independent of known risk factors or a history of cardiovascular diseases. Finally, the mortality of several surgical procedures is substantially increased by the presence of chronic renal failure. Therefore, detecting and treating patients with chronic renal failure is extremely important.

Causes of Chronic Renal Failure

Many disorders can cause chronic renal failure. However, epidemiologic studies indicate that diabetes mellitus and hypertension account for the majority of cases (>60%). Chronic glomerulonephritis, polycystic kidney disease, obstructive uropathy, and ischemic nephropathy caused by atherosclerotic renal artery stenosis are less common, but important causes of renal impairment. The latter disorder is postulated to be more frequent than previously believed and is an important undiagnosed cause of chronic renal impairment.

Recent studies have indicated that a reduction in GFR occurs with aging in the absence of factors known to produce renal injury such as hypertension or diabetes. Indeed, the average GFR of subjects in the 8th decade of life in one large study was 40 to 50 mL/minute. Pathologic examination of these individuals, when available, may reveal only benign nephrosclerosis.

Importantly, because a majority of individuals older than 60 years of age have lower muscle mass, the reduced GFR is not accompanied by a rise in serum creatinine concentration. Therefore, renal failure is not detected unless the physician considers other variables such as the patient's age and muscle mass in assessing GFR (see the following section).

Approach to the Diagnosis of Chronic Renal Failure

The first step in the diagnosis of chronic renal failure is, of course, to detect a reduction in GFR. In the past, estimations of GFR were based on the measurement of serum creatinine concentration alone. In adults, the normal serum creatinine ranges between 0.6 and 1.3 mg/dL. Individuals with values greater than this are said to have renal failure. However, there is a wide range of normal values. Also, creatinine production, which is dependent on muscle mass, is a critical variable affecting serum creatinine concentration. Thus, a large group of individuals with reduced muscle mass can have serum creatinine values within the normal range, but a decreased GFR.

The most common situation in which this paradox is encountered is in the elderly and in individuals with malignancy or chronic liver disease.

Precise measurement of GFR is accomplished by calculating the clearance of creatinine in a timed urine collection, generally 24 hours in duration:

$$\text{Creatinine clearance (mL/minute)} = \text{Ucr (mg/dL)} \times \text{volume (mL)}/\text{Scr (mg/dL)}/1440.$$

where Ucr = urine creatinine concentration,
Scr = plasma creatinine concentration

However, timed urine collections are often inaccurate because of errors in collection. Moreover, as renal function progresses and serum creatinine rises, or in the presence of nephrotic range proteinuria, GFR tends to be overestimated by creatinine clearance. Most recently, formulas derived from studies of large groups of patients—such as those by Cockroft and Gault and the Modification of Diet in Renal Disease (MDRD) in which GFR was correlated with other factors (e.g., body weight, age, and serum albumin)—are sufficiently accurate to use for clinical purposes:

$$\text{Cockroft} - \text{Gault}: \text{CrCl (mL/minute)}$$
$$= \{(140 - \text{age}) \times \text{wt} \times [1 - (0.15 \times \text{gender})]\}/(0.814 \times \text{Scr})$$

$$\text{MDRD}: \text{GFR} = 170 \times [\text{PCr}]^{-0.999} \times [\text{Age}]^{-0.176}$$
$$\times [0.762 \text{ female}] \times [1.180 \text{ if patient is black}]$$
$$\times [\text{SUN}]^{-0.170} \times [\text{Alb}]^{+0.318}$$

Once renal function is depressed, the physician determines whether this represents acute or chronic renal failure, When previous measurements of GFR are available, it is relatively easy to determine if the renal failure is chronic in nature. However, if these studies are not available, demonstration that the kidneys are small in size (less than 8 to 9 cm when they are normally approximately 10 to 12 cm) by renal ultrasound will confirm the chronicity of the disease. Evidence of increased echogenicity reflecting augmented fibrous deposits is also suggestive of chronic disease. However, several disorders associated with chronic renal failure have normal kidney size such as diabetes mellitus, polycystic kidney disease, and amyloidosis. Therefore, normal kidney size does not exclude chronic renal failure. If individuals have normal kidney size, the presence of anemia and/or certain abnormalities of divalent ion metabolism can also suggest the disease is chronic in nature.

Once impaired renal function is recognized, measurements of blood urea nitrogen (BUN), sodium, potassium, chloride, bicarbonate, hemoglobin and hematocrit, and calcium and phosphorus are obtained. A urinalysis is obtained looking for increased excretion of protein, presence of blood in the urine, and abnormal cellular elements. In patients with diabetes, studies to find microalbuminuria (albumin urine concentrations less than 300 mg per day) are important to detect the early stages of renal disease. A 24-hour or spot urine protein and creatinine determination to assess the urine's protein-to-creatinine ratio is obtained to quantitate the amount of protein being excreted. Urine protein excretion in excess of 3.5 g daily indicates the presence of glomerular pathology, whereas interstitial disease is characterized by values below 2 g. However, urine protein excretion can vary with glomerular disease so values below 3.5 g are still consistent with this diagnosis. Assessment of urine protein excretion is important for diagnostic purposes, but also because urine protein excretion is often followed to assess effectiveness of therapy.

Obstruction uropathy, an important cause of chronic renal failure and exacerbation of renal failure, can be excluded in the majority of cases by ultrasound of the kidneys. Doppler ultrasound of the renal arteries performed at the same time is helpful in excluding obstruction of the renal arteries. The necessity of obtaining other diagnostic studies such as measurement of serum complement, blood and urine eosinophils, serum and urine and protein electrophoresis, antiglomerular basement membrane antibodies, anti–double-stranded DNA (dsDNA) antibodies, hepatitis B and C antibodies, sedimentation rate, and HIV studies depends on the context of the renal failure.

CURRENT DIAGNOSIS

The following lists the optimal care of patients with chronic kidney disease:

- Test for albuminuria and estimate glomerular filtration rate using MDRD formula yearly for early diagnosis and stratification of CKD.
- If possible, determine cause of kidney disease.
- Initiate treatment to delay or prevent progression of disease including use of converting enzyme inhibitors and/or angiotensin receptor blockers to reduce BP to less than 130/80 mm Hg and urine protein excretion to as low as possible but at least less than 1 g/24 hours.
- Control or prevent biochemical or clinical abnormalities including those of serum potassium, serum bicarbonate, serum phosphorus, parathyroid hormone, and hemoglobin.
- Evaluate patients for presence of and treat important co-morbid conditions, particularly heart disease.
- If the GFR is less than 30 mL/min, consider referral to a nephrologist.

Abbreviations: BP = blood pressure; CKD = care of patients with chronic kidney disease; GFR = glomerular filtration rate; MDRD = modification of diet in renal disease.

Finally, a renal biopsy may be required in certain situations to make a definitive diagnosis. Because treatment of specific diseases can vary, making a precise pathologic diagnosis can be extremely important for proper management. Unfortunately, once the renal failure is moderate to severe in nature, renal pathologic examination may not always be helpful in determining the cause.

Clinical and Laboratory Abnormalities in Chronic Renal Failure

Because the kidney plays a critical role in the regulation of the serum concentrations of sodium, potassium, bicarbonate, chloride, calcium, and phosphorus as well as the levels of hemoglobin and hematocrit, blood pressure and extracellular volume, chronic renal injury can lead to derangements in these parameters as summarized in Table 1.

TABLE 1 Clinical and Electrolyte Abnormalities Noted with Chronic Renal Failure

Clinical or Laboratory Disorder	GFR or Stage of Renal Failure*
Hypertension	GFR <60 mL/min (stage 3)
Hyponatremia or hypernatremia	GFR <30 mL/min (stage 4)
Hyperkalemia*	GFR <30 mL/min (stage 4)
Hyperphosphatemia*	GFR <30 mL/min (stage 4)
Metabolic acidosis	GFR <30 mL/min (stage 4)
Anemia	GFR <60 mL/min (stage 3)
Uremic symptoms	GFR <15 mL/min (stage 5)
Nausea, vomiting, disturbances in sleep	

*Descriptions of the various stages are presented in the text. These electrolyte abnormalities can be seen at higher levels of GFR.
Abbreviation: GFR = glomerular filtration rate.

HYPONATREMIA AND HYPERNATREMIA

The kidney plays an essential role in excreting water by producing a dilute urine (less than 1/6 plasma osmolality) or retaining water by producing a concentrated urine (three to four times plasma osmolality). The ability to concentrate or dilute the urine in the majority of cases is usually retained until GFR falls to less than 30% of normal, and therefore hyponatremia or hypernatremia are uncommon until that time. If the disease is primarily interstitial in nature, alterations in urine concentrating ability can appear prior to significant reductions in GFR. However, even with higher levels of GFR the patient can be at risk for either of these electrolyte abnormalities should they ingest large quantities of fluid or be deprived of appropriate fluid intake.

HYPERKALEMIA

The kidney plays the most critical role in the regulation of potassium balance. Adaptive changes in renal tubular function and possible colonic function enable the kidney to maintain serum potassium within the normal range until GFR falls below 20% to 25% of normal (serum creatinine of 4 mg/dL or greater). Recent studies indicate a tendency for elevations in serum potassium to appear at even modest reductions in GFR (<60 mL/min). When disease of the kidney involves the medullary portion or hormonal derangements such as hyporeninemic hypoaldosterinism are present, hyperkalemia can be observed prior to significant declines in GFR. In addition, patients with even moderate renal failure have a reduced reserve to eliminated potassium and therefore can develop hyperkalemia if potassium load is increased dramatically.

METABOLIC ACIDOSIS

A fall in plasma bicarbonate concentration in association with a reduced blood pH (metabolic acidosis) is frequently observed when GFR falls below 20% to 25% of normal. The acidosis results from acid excretion falling below acid production leading to positive proton balance. Recent studies have documented that a tendency to the development of metabolic acidosis can be seen with mild reductions in GFR (<60 mL/min).

The electrolyte pattern seen with the metabolic acidosis of renal failure is often of the high anion gap variety, but frequently a hyperchloremic (normal anion gap) or combined anion gap and hyperchloremic pattern can be observed. The degree of acidosis is usually mild to moderate with plasma bicarbonate concentration ranging from 12 to 22 mEq/L. Of interest, at any given level of GFR, the acidosis is often not progressive, but plasma bicarbonate concentration remains stable unless renal function declines further or there is an increment in acid production.

ABNORMAL DIVALENT IN METABOLISM

Serum phosphorus is regulated by the kidney but in most cases remains within the normal range until GFR falls below 20% to 25% of normal. This stabilization of serum phosphorus is attributed to increased tubular excretion of phosphorus as a result of increased parathyroid hormone secretion. As with potassium and bicarbonate, recent studies demonstrate a tendency for elevation in serum phosphorus can be observed with mild renal failure (<50 to 60 mL/min). Serum calcium is usually in the normal range, but varies receiprocally with serum phosphorus. Because of derangements in divalent ion metabolism bone disease with increased tendency to fractures and disordered soft tissue structures can be observed.

Hyperparathyroidism is a common occurrence in patients with renal failure, the values usually being higher with a greater degree of renal impairment. The elevated PTH values are usually induced by hypocalcemia, although increased serum phosphorus concentrations independent of serum calcium values can also play a role. The increased parathyroid hormone levels can induce damage to bone and soft tissue structures, but also may affect other functions such as cardiac function and the production of red blood cells.

ANEMIA

The kidney is the source of erythropoietin, the hormone that regulates bone marrow production of red blood cells. Thus, with the development of renal impairment, there is a fall in red blood cell production. A fall in red cell survival also contributes to development of anemia. Anemia generally appears when GFR falls below 60 mL/minute. There is a rough correlation between the severity of renal failure and the degree of anemia: the more severe the renal failure the greater the degree of anemia. However, this relationship is not invariable, and many patients have only mild reductions in hemoglobin and hematocrit.

Anemia initially was believed to contribute only to changes in oxygen delivery. However, recent studies show that anemia can contribute to the genesis of left ventricular hypertrophy and other cardiomyopathies noted with chronic renal failure and can raise mortality in patients with chronic renal failure.

HYPERTENSION

Recent studies emphasize the importance of the kidneys in the regulation of blood pressure, and the bulk of patients with diabetes or other glomerular disease will develop hypertension in the course of their renal failure. In many instances, hypertension does not develop until GFR is below 40% to 50% of normal. The type of renal disease underlying chronic renal failure appears to be important, as hypertension is less common with pyelonephritis. Hypertension might be observed earlier in the course of renal failure, however, in patients with polycystic kidney disease or ischemic nephropathy. Because hypertension is one of the most critical factors in the genesis of cardiovascular disease and can accelerate the progression of renal failure, careful attention of control of hypertension is important.

VOLUME OVERLOAD

Salt retention often accompanies chronic renal failure even when GFR is not severely compromised. The degree of salt retention can be profound if significant albuminuria with resultant hypoalbuminemia is seen and is more severe as GFR falls below 20% to 25% of normal. Salt retention is a critical factor in the development of hypertension and can promote congestive heart failure.

Symptoms and Signs of Renal Failure

Patients with chronic renal failure are often asymptomatic with little evidence of disease other than laboratory abnormalities until late in the course of renal failure. If anemia is present, patients may complain of fatigue; and if significant elevations in parathyroid hormone levels are noted, bone pain, ruptured tendons or other disorders of soft tissue structures can be noted. Once moderate to severe renal failure appears, symptoms of the electrolyte abnormalities can be observed. Hyperkalemia, if severe, can lead to arrhythmias or heart block and muscle weakness. Metabolic acidosis can contribute to fatigue. Anemia can contribute to fatigue and changes in mentation and physical stamina. Weight loss related to metabolic acidosis and or retention of various uremic toxins may occur. Sexual dysfunction characterized by reduced libido and reduced fertility are common with moderate to severe renal failure.

Once severe renal failure develops (stage 4 or 5), the uremic syndrome can be observed characterized by a decreased appetite, nausea, vomiting, and subtle changes in mental status including changes in sleep patterns. However, even with severe renal failure many patients feel surprisingly well.

Management of Chronic Renal Failure

STAGING OF CHRONIC RENAL FAILURE

As noted earlier, within the last several years, a great deal of effort has been expended into developing guidelines for the evaluation, monitoring, and treatment of patients with chronic renal failure. To this end, experts working with the National Kidney Foundation have divided chronic renal failure into different states based on measurements or estimations of GFR. The value of staging to the physician is that the studies necessary to monitor patients and the complications of chronic renal failure are often different depending on the stage of renal failure.

Stage 0 (GFR Greater Than 90 mL/Minute with Risk Factors for Renal Disease)

Patients at stage 0 have increased risk for development of chronic renal failure, such as those with diabetes or hypertension but who have GFR greater than 90 mL/minute in the absence of proteinuria or urinary sedimentary abnormalities. These patients should have their blood pressure and diabetes controlled. Estimates of GFR should be obtained approximately every 6 months from measurement of serum creatinine, and qualitative tests for urine protein excretion should be obtained. In diabetics measurement of microalbumin should also be obtained. Because control of disease may forestall progression glycosylated hemoglobin (HbA1C) values should also be obtained.

Stage 1 (GFR Greater Than 90 mL/Minute with Albuminuria)

Once evidence of renal damage is obtained, as reflected by microalbuminuria or proteinuria, but GFR is either normal or increased, patients are said to be in stage 1. These individuals should be monitored more closely and strict attention must be given to maintain blood pressure below 130/80. Furthermore, angiotensin converting enzyme inhibitor (ACEI) or angiotensin receptor blocker (ARB) should be given to prevent evolution of microalbuminuria to fullblown proteinuria (see the following). No clinical or laboratory abnormalities are observed at this stage.

Stage 2: Mild Renal Failure (GFR 60 to 90 mL/Minute)

When GFR is mildly reduced to values from 60 to 90 mL/minute, patients are in stage 2. These patients should also be carefully monitored and blood pressure tightly controlled. If diabetes is present, strict attention to maintaining HbA1C within recommended guidelines should be given. Again, it is rare at this stage for any significant clinical abnormalities other than hypertension to be present.

Stage 3: Moderate Renal Failure (GFR 30 to 59 mL/Minute)

When GFR ranges between 30 to 59 mL/minute, patients are in stage 3. At this point hypertension may appear, mild abnormalities in serum phosphorus might be observed, and anemia can be seen. Also in some patients an elevation in serum potassium can be noted, particularly if they are ingesting a relatively high potassium diet. These patients need to be followed more closely, and it is recommended that patients at the lower end of this stage (i.e., close to 30 mL/min) be monitored by a nephrologist.

Stage 4: Moderate to Severe (GFR from 15 to 29 mL/Minute)

Once GFR falls to values from 15 to 29 mL/minute, patients have severe renal failure, or stage 4 disease. At this level of GFR, significant electrolyte abnormalities such as metabolic acidosis, hyperkalemia, and hyperphosphatemia are frequent. Anemia is common and the patient may begin to note reductions in appetite and have a fall in muscle mass. However, there is great variability in the appearance of symptoms or laboratory derangements.

Stage 5: Severe (GFR Less Than 15 to 29 mL/Minute)

When GFR falls below 15 mL/minute, severe electrolyte abnormalities are often present, anemia is common. Clinical symptoms can develop. Renal replacement therapy, either dislysis or transplantation, is usually required at this stage.

Recommendations for treatment of patients are summarized below. The frequency of patient visits, of course, largely depends on the complications of renal disease present and co-morbid conditions. Therefore, these are only general recommendations for frequency of examination.

When patients are in stage 0, they should be seen once per year for renal evaluation. When GFR remains normal or elevated, but proteinuria is present, renal evaluation should be performed every 6 months. When stage 3 develops, we usually repeat renal evaluation every 3 months. Patients in stage 4 are seen more frequently, usually at the minimum of once per month. Patients with end-stage disease require renal replacement therapy.

GENERAL APPROACH TO TREATMENT OF CHRONIC RENAL FAILURE

Treatment of chronic renal failure can be divided into the modalities that are specific to the underlying disorder and those that are used to treat all patients with chronic renal failure. Thus, patients with systemic lupus erythematosus or other immune-mediated or inflammatory disease may benefit from treatment with steroids and immunosuppressive agents. Treatments specific for individual disorders are beyond the scope of this article.

The physician treating the patient with renal failure has two goals: preventing or delaying progression of renal failure, and alleviating the electrolyte and hormonal abnormalities that can lead to symptoms or complications of the disease. Understanding the methods to accomplish the former requires knowledge of those factors that are integral to progression of the disease.

FACTORS CAUSING PROGRESSION OF CHRONIC RENAL FAILURE

It has been recognized for several years that once renal failure has developed, renal function can decline at a predictable rate in the absence of further insults to the kidney. Essential to the optimal approach used to treat chronic renal failure, therefore, is an understanding of those factors that can cause progression of renal failure, including:

- Systemic and intraglomerular hypertension
- Glomerular hypertrophy
- Intrarenal precipitation of calcium and phosphorus
- Hyperlipidemia
- Altered metabolism of prostanoids
- Metabolic acidosis
- Anemia
- Tubulointerstitial disease
- Proteinuria

Intraglomerular Hypertension and Glomerular Hypertrophy

As nephrons are lost, changes are induced in the kidney to preserve GFR such as renal vasodilatation, an increase in glomerular capillary pressure, and an increment in size of individual glomeruli raising wall stress. These adaptive mechanisms probably induce damage by causing endothelial cell damage with detachment of epithelial cells allowing enhanced flux of water and solutes that might cause narrowing of capillary lumens. Also, strain on mesangial cells causes them to produce cytokines and extracellular matrix with resultant expansion of the mesangium and glomerular sclerosis.

Proteinuria

Although proteinuria has traditionally been a marker of glomerular injury, with greater amounts of urinary protein excretion being associated with more severe injury, recent studies indicate that proteinuria, can induce mesangial and tubular damage. Therefore, treatments to reduce proteinuria, may be beneficial in limiting further renal damage.

Tubulointerstitial Disease

Some component of tubulointerstitial disease is generally found in individuals with chronic renal failure even when the primary process affects the glomerulus. It has been postulated that the tubulointerstitial disease can produce atrophy of tubules or obstruction destroying individual nephrons. Even when tubular inflammation is treated, progressive scarring can continue unabated. Thus, treatments designed to reduce interstitial fibrosis may be important for preventing progression of disease. At present, only experimental drugs not available for human use have been examined for this purpose.

Hyperlipidemia

Hyperlipidemia is frequently observed in disorders associated with nephrotic range proteinuria, but is also noted in a large percentage of the general population without renal disease. Experimental evidence obtained from animal studies shows hyperlipidemia can promote progression of renal failure. Thus, loading with cholesterol augments renal injury and treatment with cholesterol-lowering drugs slows the rate of progression. This effect is synergistic to that achieved by lowering blood pressure.

The mechanisms underlying the effects of lipids are not well understood, but possible explanations include mesangial lipid deposition leading to glomerular injury or tubular injury. A few studies performed in human subjects have demonstrated benefit from lipid lowering on the progression of renal injury, although they are not conclusive. Because patients with chronic renal failure have a high prevalence of cardiovascular disease, it is reasonable to inititate therapy with statin drugs to lower serum cholesterol and lipid levels.

Calcium-Phosphate Deposition

A rise in serum phosphorus, usually seen at the later stages of renal failure, can lead to precipitation of calcium phosphate in the renal interstitium. The deposits can then induce an inflammatory response producing interstitial fibrosis and tubular atrophy. Some have indicated that the deposits may form prior to detectable elevations in serum phosphorus concentrations.

Increased Glomerular Prostaglandin Production

An increment in glomerular prostaglandin production has been found in several studies of chronic renal failure. The increased prostanoids produce renal vasodilatation and a rise in intraglomerular pressure, factors that augment progression of disease.

METABOLIC ACIDOSIS

Metabolic acidosis commonly develops in the course of chronic renal failure. Recent studies in humans have demonstrated that correction of the acidosis by administration of base slows the progression of renal failure and delays the development of end-stage renal failure.

SPECIFIC TREATMENT MEASURES

Treatment of patients with chronic renal failure should be designed to ameliorate those factors that can cause progression of renal injury, treat or prevent important complications, and normalize important laboratory abnormalities that contribute to symptoms of the disease.

Measures Designed to Reduce the Rate of Progression of Renal Failure

CONTROL OF SYSTEMIC AND INTRAGLOMERULAR HYPERTENSION

Experimental and human studies demonstrate that control of systemic hypertension can slow the rate of progression of renal disease substantially. Recent evidence indicates that target blood pressure levels should be lower than recommended for the general population (<130/80 mmHg). Control of hypertension with the use of myriad agents can benefit the patient with renal failure. However, as indicated previously,

reduction in intraglomerular hypertension may be the most important factor underlying the benefits from blood pressure control. Therefore, when possible, treatment with ACEIs, ARBs, or the combination of these agents should be first-line antihypertensive therapy in these patients. Patients who do not tolerate these drugs might benefit from administration of non-dihydropyridine calcium channel blockers. In patients with proteinuria, even if blood pressure is controlled or they are normotensive, the doses of ACEIs or ARBs should be raised to levels even greater than recommended to reduce urine protein excretion to levels less than 500 mg. This reduction in proteinuria is the most optimal in protecting the kidney.

Potentially serious complications with ACEIs or ARBs include acute reduction in GFR and hyperkalemia. If these complications occur, a reduction in dose or even discontinuation of these agents might be required. It is recommended that these agents be continued even when GFR is less than 20 mL/min. Given the potential severity of these complications, patients should be monitored closely.

PROTEIN RESTRICTION

The benefits of protein restriction in preventing progression are unclear, but it has suggested that reducing protein intake to 0.8 to 1.0 g/kg body weight of high biologic value is beneficial. Others have indicated that 0.6 g/kg body weight should be used. In patients with substantial proteinuria, the quantity of protein recommended will have to be adjusted to prevent hypoalbuminemia. Once patients reached later stage 4, protein restriction may be useful to prevent expression of uremic symptoms. Reducing protein intake will have the added benefit of decreasing acid, potassium, and phosphate production.

CONTROL OF LIPIDS

Control of cholesterol with statins may help prevent progression and should reduce the burden of cardiovascular disease, which remains the most lethal disorder for patients with chronic renal failure. Adherence to the newly proposed aggressive recommendation appears reasonable.

Measures Designed to Treat Significant Laboratory Abnormalities

ANEMIA

Patients with renal anemia should be treated with erythropoietin (Procrit). Although this requires subcutaneous injection once per week, newer, long-lasting forms (darbepoetin [Aranesp]) enable patients to be treated every 3 weeks. Because iron stores need to be repleted for anemia to be successfully treated, these should be monitored and iron given. Because of the vagaries of ferritin measurements, we use serum iron and iron binding capacity with the goal of maintaining saturation above 20% and near 30%. At present, the target hemoglobin and hematocrit vary between 11 mg/dL and 12 mg/dL 33 and 36, respectively. Given the recent concern about vascular complications with EPO therapy, the clinican must be vigilant in preventing Hg values from exceeding 12 mg/dL.

METABOLIC ACIDOSIS

Controversy exists as to the target value of bicarbonate for patients with chronic renal failure. Some experts recommend raising plasma bicarbonate to levels above 20 mEq/L, whereas others recommend complete normalization of plasma bicarbonate. To properly raise plasma bicarbonate concentration, the deficit should be calculated from the formula:

Desired − prevailing level of plasma bicarbonate
× 50% body weight = Total bicarbonate deficit

The deficit should be corrected slowly over several days.

CURRENT THERAPY

The recommendations for the treatment of patients with renal failure is as follows:

Recommendation	Goal
Control BP.	130/80 mm Hg
Reduce proteinuria by administering angiotensin converting enzyme inhibitors or angiotensin receptor blockers. In some cases both agents may have to be given concomitantly.	Decrease urine protein excretion as low as possible but at least less than 1 g per day.
Control phosphate concentrations with phosphate binders with noncalcium containing binders when possible.	Serum phosphate <4.5 mg/dL
Maintain vitamin D by administration of ergocalciferol.	Maintain 25 OH vitamin D levels at 30 ng/mL by administration of ergocalciferol
Prevent hyperparathyroidism with vitamin D or calcimimetics.	Maintain PTH <150 pg/mL
Correct anemia with erythropoietin and iron replacement as needed.	Maintain Hg between 11 and 12 mg/dL
Administer diuretics to control hypertension and volume overload.	Maintain euvolemia when possible
Control serum potassium with dietary restriction, diuretics, and/or potassium exchange resin as necessary.	Maintain serum potassium <5.0 mEq/L
Keep protein intake at 0.6 to 0.8 g/kg body weight per day.	Slow progression of renal disease while preventing protein depletion
Control metabolic acidosis with administration of sodium citrate (Citra pH).	Maintain serum HCO$_3$ >20 mEq/L

Abbreviations: BP = blood pressure; HCO$_3$ = bicarbonate; Hg = mercury; PTH = parathyroid hormone.

Because patients experience gas when the base is given as bicarbonate, the base is usually administered as Shohl's solution sodium citrate,* the citrate being metabolized to bicarbonate in the liver. Each milliliter of Shohl's solution represents 1 mEq of the base.

DIVALENT ION METABOLISM

Serum phosphorus is controlled by administration of phosphate binders usually starting with calcium citrate (Citracal) or acetate (PhosLo). If these are not successful or if patients have elevated serum calcium levels, then sevelamar (Renagel) or lanthanum (Fosrenol) can be used alone or in combination with calcium binders. Physicians should aim to maintain serum phosphorus levels below 5 mg/dL and keep serum calcium phosphorus product below 60.

Parathyroid hormone (PTH) levels should be maintained below 150 pg/mL, or less depending on stage; levels associated with proper

_____
*Investigational drug in the United States.

bone remodeling but not to values observed in patients without kidney disease. Suppression of parathyroid hormone secretion can be achieved by administration of various vitamin D analogues. The recent recognition of the calcium-sensing receptor and development of calcimimetic drugs that are extremely effective in lowering PTH secretion may make using vitamin D compounds obsolete in the future.

Low 25 OH D levels have been documented in a large number of individuals both with and without renal failure. In patients with renal impairment this can contribute to the abnormal 1,25 OH vitamin D levels. Measurement of 25-hydroxy vitamin D levels should be obtained in all patients with CKD and EGFR <60 mL/min. If levels are below 30 ng/mL they should be supplemented with ergocalciferol sufficient to maintain levels above this level.

HYPERKALEMIA

As this is the most serious electrolyte disorder encountered, patients should be monitored closely. Serum potassium concentrations should be maintained below 5 mEq/L. If hyperkalemia develops during treatment with ACEIs or ARBs, the doses of these agents should be reduced or discontinued. Diuretic administration, often given for control of hypertension, can help control hyperkalemia, but if it should develop, particularly when GFR falls below 20% of normal, it can be treated with the potassium exchange resin, sodium polystyrene sulfonate (Kayexalate).

ELEVATED BLOOD UREA NITROGEN CONCENTRATION

The precise solutes that are retained, which are important for the pathogenesis of the uremic syndrome, are not clear. However, BUN is a marker for other retained solutes and is roughly correlated with development of uremic symptoms. When the BUN is greater than 100 mg/dL and serum creatinine concentration is greater than 8 mg/dL uremic symptoms may develop. These symptoms will often abate merely with protein restriction and reduced production of these compounds. Protein restriction is usually not instituted until GFR is less than 15% to 20% of normal. Prior to that time, it is important to maintain protein intake to keep serum albumin within the normal range.

VOLUME OVERLOAD

Because salt retention is an essential component of the development of hypertension and underlies volume overload, diuretic administration is usually necessary in the treatment of chronic renal failure. Thiazides frequently used in the treatment of hypertension or volume overload in subjects with normal renal function may not be efficacious once GFR is less than or equal to 33% of normal. Therefore, loop diuretics, such as furosemide (Lasix) or a combined loop and proximal tubule diuretic such as metolozone (Zaroxolyn), are generally indicated. Because the effectiveness of both agents requires access to the tubule lumen, the effective dose is often higher than in those with normal renal function. Once patients are in stage 4 renal failure, use of diuretics is hampered by worsening of renal failure and often must be used cautiously.

REFERENCES

Beco JA, Bansal VK. Medical nutrition therapy in chronic kidney failure: Integrating clinical practice guidelines. J Am Diet Assoc 2004;104:404–9.

Clase CM, Garg AX, Kiberd BA. Prevalence of low glomerular filtration rate in nondiabetic Americans: Third National Health and Nutrition Examination Survey (NHANES III). J Am Soc Nephrol 2002;13.

Cleveland DR, Jindal KK, Hirsch DJ, et al. Quality of pre-referral care in patients with chronic renal insufficiency. Am J Kidney Dis 2002;40:30–6.

Curtin RB, Becker B, Kimmel PL, Schatell D. An integrated approach to care for patients with chronic kidney disease. Semin Dial 2003;16:399–402.

Djamali A, Kendziorski C, Brazy PC, Becker BN. Disease progression and outcomes in chronic kidney disease and renal transplantation. Kidney Int 2003;64:1800–7.

Fox CH, Voleti V, Khan LS, Murray B, Vassalotti J. A quick guide to evidence-based chronic kidney disease care for the primary care physician. Postgrad Med 2008;120:E01–6.

James MT, Hemmelgarn BR, Tonelli M. Early recognition and prevention of chronic kidney disease. Lancet 2010;10(375):1296–309.

KDOQI. Clinical practice guidelines and clinical practice recommendations for diabetes and chronic kidney disease. Am J Kidney Dis 2007;49:S1–154.

Kopple JD. National Kidney Foundation K/DOQ1 clinical practice guidelines for nutrition in chronic renal failure. Am J Kidney Dis 2001;37:S66–S70.

Maschio G, Alberti D, Janin G, et al. Effect of the angiotensin-converting-enzyme inhibitor benazepril on the progression of chronic renal insufficiency. N Engl J Med 1996;334:939–45.

Tonelli M, Gill J, Pandeya S, et al. Slowing the progression of chronic renal insufficiency. Can Med Assoc J 2002;166:906–7.

Malignant Tumors of the Urogenital Tract

Method of
Peter E. Clark, MD

Carcinoma of the Prostate

Prostate cancer is the most common noncutaneous solid malignancy among men in the United States, and it is second only to lung cancer with respect to cancer-related mortality. In 2008, there were an estimated 186,320 new cases of prostate cancer and 28,660 deaths due to this disease. Because prostate cancer is predominantly a disease of the elderly, its incidence may be expected to rise over time as the U.S. population ages.

There is a familial predisposition to prostate cancer, which is more common among those with a first-degree relative who also has the disease, and it appears to be more common among African American men than among Caucasian men. Environmental factors that have been associated with an increased risk of prostate cancer include a high-fat Western-style diet, as compared with a high-soy Asian diet, and low levels of vitamin D.

Hereditary prostate cancer is relatively rare but may account for up to 40% of tumors among young men with the disease. One of several genes found in families with hereditary prostate cancer is hereditary prostate cancer 1 (*HPC1*), which is located on the long arm of chromosome 1. Translocations leading to fusion of two genes (TMPRSS2:ERG gene fusion) has also been implicated in a large number of sporadic prostate cancers.

DIAGNOSIS

The vast majority of prostate cancers are adenocarcinomas. There is a large discrepancy between the risk of finding incidental prostate cancer at autopsy (estimated to be as high as 75% by age 80 or older) and the risk of having the disease clinically diagnosed (lifetime risk, approximately 1 in 6). Most men with early-stage prostate cancer diagnosed in the modern era have no specific disease-related symptoms. Benign prostatic hypertrophy is often found in association with prostate cancer and is also more common in men as they age, but there is no known causal relationship between the two. Prostate cancer can rarely manifest with pelvic pain, bladder outlet obstruction, or ureteral obstruction from locally advanced disease or with bone pain from distant metastatic disease.

The advent and widespread use of the serum prostate-specific antigen (PSA) test as a screening tool for prostate cancer has resulted in a stage migration, with most men now diagnosed with early-stage disease. This has been associated with better recurrence-free survival rates after definitive local therapy. Certain groups, such as the American Urologic Association and the American Cancer Society, have advocated that physicians offer annual screening with a serum PSA determination and digital rectal examination for all men older than 50 years of age and for African American men and those with a family history of prostatic cancer starting at age 40 years. However, these recommendations are not uniformly accepted; the U.S. Preventive Services Task Force continues to state that the available evidence is insufficient to recommend routine screening with PSA for prostate cancer. It is generally accepted that the decision to screen for prostate cancer should be made in individuals with at least 10 years of life expectancy.

Serum PSA is specific for the prostate but is not specific for cancer. It is secreted by both benign and malignant prostatic epithelial cells. The PSA may be elevated in men with a variety of prostate-related conditions, such as prostatitis, benign prostatic hypertrophy, urinary tract infection, or prostatic cancer. Until recently, a PSA level lower than 4.0 ng/mL was considered normal, and in younger men a value of greater than 2.5 ng/mL could perhaps be considered abnormal. More recently, it has become clear that there is no true cutoff value for PSA. Instead, the association between PSA and prostate cancer risk is a continuum. Even at a PSA of essentially zero, there is still a 6% chance of having prostate cancer on biopsy.

The majority of the serum PSA is bound to protease inhibitors such as α_1-antichymotrypsin, whereas a fraction is unconjugated or free. The relative proportion of free serum PSA can be used to improve the specificity of PSA for diagnosis of prostate cancer by biopsy. Benign prostatic hypertrophy is associated with a higher proportion of free PSA, and patients with greater 25% free serum PSA are less likely to harbor prostate cancer. The precise cutoff point associated with prostate cancer is controversial and ranges from 10% to 20% or higher. Development of new tests to improve PSA specificity, such as measurement of complexed PSA or early pro-forms of PSA, is an area of ongoing investigation.

The most common method used to diagnose prostate cancer is a transrectal ultrasonography (TRUS)-guided prostate biopsy. TRUS allows for accurate localization of the zonal anatomy of the prostate and can accurately measure its size. It therefore acts as a guide for the biopsy, because prostatic cancers typically reside in the peripheral zone, and biopsies are concentrated within that zone. Although prostate cancer can manifest as hypoechoic lesions on TRUS, the tumors usually are not visible. TRUS lacks both sensitivity and specificity and should not be used as a screening test.

The most common grading system used to estimate the degree of tumor differentiation is the Gleason grading system. The two most common Gleason grade patterns (on a scale of 1 to 5) are summed to give a score between 2 and 10. Tumors with Gleason scores between 2 and 6 are well differentiated and have a better prognosis, whereas those with Gleason scores between 8 and 10 are poorly differentiated and have a worse prognosis. Gleason score 7 is associated with intermediate differentiation and prognosis. The majority of cancers found in the modern era are well to intermediately differentiated (Gleason score 5 to 7).

Staging of prostatic cancer defines the local, regional, and distant extent of disease. The tumor-node-metastasis (TNM) staging system is the most commonly used method. The most common clinical stage in the modern era is that of nonpalpable tumors detected because of a concerning PSA result (stage T1c). The primary staging modality for local disease is the digital rectal examination. This may be supplemented by pelvic magnetic resonance imaging in selected cases where there is significant concern for locally advanced disease based on the digital rectal examination. Although PSA only roughly correlates with the overall disease burden, bone metastasis is quite uncommon among patients whose PSA value is less than 20 ng/mL. Therefore, a radionucleotide bone scan in the absence of symptoms is not required routinely if the PSA value is less than 10 ng/mL and the Gleason sum is 7 or less. Computed tomography (CT) scanning is not routinely used, because grossly positive nodes are detected rarely with a clinically localized tumor.

Lymph node staging is important in selecting patients for therapy. CT scanning may show enlarged lymph nodes in patients with high-volume or high-grade primary tumor but has poor sensitivity and specificity. Laparoscopic pelvic lymphadenectomy can provide adequate sampling of the pelvic lymph nodes in those patients not selecting surgery. More commonly, lymph node dissection is performed concomitantly at the time of radical prostatectomy.

TREATMENT

There is no one optimal treatment for clinically localized prostatic cancer, so therapy must be individualized. Among men with a life expectancy of less than 10 years, observation alone may be appropriate. Carefully selected men with low-risk prostate cancer may choose active surveillance rather than curative treatment but must be rigorously monitored for evidence of worsening disease.

Surgery and radiation therapy are the most commonly used curative modalities. For low-risk, organ-confined tumors, the 15-year disease-free survival rates are greater than 90% among patients treated with surgery. Moreover, the survival outcome is similar after radiation therapy and after surgery. However, properly done prospective, randomized comparisons among similarly staged patients have not been done. Radiation therapy can be delivered as external-beam radiotherapy or as brachytherapy using radioactive seeds (iodine 125 or palladium 103) implanted directly into the prostate. Cryotherapy (i.e., freezing of the prostate) is another approved treatment for men with prostatic carcinoma that is becoming more widely accepted as an alternative treatment option.

Radical prostatectomy, or surgical removal of the prostate, may be performed via an open incision or by a laparoscopic technique. Traditionally, an open surgery is performed through an anterior, retropubic approach or, less commonly, through a perineal incision. Laparoscopic and, in particular, robot-assisted radical prostatectomy is being performed with increasing frequency. The benefits of a robot-assisted approach may include reduced blood loss, sooner return to normal function, and possibly better functional outcomes and better surgical margin rates (although the latter two have not been definitively demonstrated to this point). In patients who were sexually active before therapy, preservation of the neurovascular bundles is often undertaken in an attempt to maintain postoperative sexual function. For patients with organ-confined disease, the prognosis is excellent, with a life expectancy similar to that of men without prostatic cancer. For those patients with positive surgical margins or positive lymph nodes on final pathology, consideration can be given to delivering, respectively, adjuvant irradiation or androgen-deprivation therapy (ADT).

Serum PSA should rapidly become undetectable after radical prostatectomy, because, in theory, all PSA-producing tissue has been removed. After radiation therapy or cryotherapy, the PSA is expected to reach low levels over time and then remain stable. An increasing serum PSA is evidence of tumor recurrence. There is controversy about when to initiate ADT in men with a rising PSA level after treatment.

Prostatic cancer, at least initially, is an androgen-sensitive disease. Therefore, the primary first-line treatment for metastatic prostate cancer is ADT. Suppression of serum testosterone can be achieved by orchiectomy (i.e., surgical castration). Alternatively, medical castration may be considered. Luteinizing hormone–releasing hormone analogues effectively suppress testosterone to the castrate range within 1 month after administration by suppressing central nervous system secretion of luteinizing hormone. There is increasing awareness that ADT can be associated with significant long-term morbidity, including vasomotor reflex changes (hot flushes), loss of libido, erectile dysfunction, osteoporosis, anemia, muscle wasting, gynecomastia, and possibly cognitive changes and increased risk of cardiovascular disease. The choice to use ADT must, therefore, be carefully balanced based on the individual patient's overall risk of prostate cancer–related morbidity and mortality versus ADT-related morbidity.

Most patients with metastatic disease initially respond to ADT, but almost inexorably the disease progresses despite ongoing ADT, to become castrate-resistant prostate cancer (CRPC). At that point, the median survival time is less than 2 years. The standard chemotherapy for CRPC is docetaxel (Taxotere) plus prednisone, and prospective randomized trials have demonstrated a modest survival benefit among patients so treated. Another approved drug is mitoxantrone (Novantrone) for palliative relief of symptomatic bone pain from CRPC. Radiation therapy can be used effectively to palliate focal sites of bone metastases. The mechanisms by which prostatic carcinoma escapes hormonal control and becomes castrate resistant represent an area of ongoing intensive research.

Tumors of the Renal Parenchyma

Malignant tumors of the renal parenchyma are of either primary or metastatic origin. Primary renal tumors may be benign or malignant. The most common tumor is primary renal cell carcinoma (RCC);

other tumor types, such as papillary, chromophobe, collecting duct, and medullary carcinomas and sarcomas, occur infrequently. The most common benign renal tumors are angiomyolipomas and oncocytomas. The latter, in particular, are generally indistinguishable from malignant lesions on radiographic imaging. Metastatic lesions (e.g., from lung, breast, melanoma, or ovary) may occur, and primary lymphoma may be present in the kidney.

RENAL CELL CARCINOMA

RCC is the most common primary neoplasm of the kidney, accounting for more than 85% of all primary renal tumors. There were an estimated 54,390 newly diagnosed cases of RCC in the United States in 2008, and an estimated 13,010 people died of this disease. RCC represents approximately 3% of all adult malignancies and usually manifests between 40 and 60 years of age, although it can be found in younger age groups. It has a 2:1 male-to-female preponderance and in both sporadic and familial forms is associated with aberrations of the von Hippel–Lindau (VHL) gene and protein.

RCC is thought to arise from cells of the proximal convoluted tubule. The most consistent genetic aberration found in most cases of sporadic, conventional RCC are aberrations in the *VHL* gene. No specific agent has been implicated as the cause of RCC, although tobacco products are associated with an approximately twofold increased risk of being diagnosed with the disease. Patients, and particularly younger patients, with end-stage renal disease who develop acquired cystic disease of the kidney also have an increased risk of RCC. Between 1% and 2% of these patients develop RCC, so annual renal ultrasonography is reasonable as a screening tool in this population, with confirmatory studies such as CT for complex or suspicious lesions.

Diagnosis

The most common sign associated with RCC in 29% to 60% of cases is hematuria. The classic triad of flank pain, hematuria, and a palpable abdominal mass is relatively rare, occurring in fewer than 10% of cases. Other common symptoms and signs include fever, anemia, hypercalcemia, thrombocytosis, and elevated erythrocyte sedimentation rate, lactate dehydrogenase, or alkaline phosphatase. Currently, there are no reliable, commercially available tumor markers for RCC. Most often, these tumors are incidentally diagnosed on radiographic imaging performed for unrelated or nonspecific purposes.

The most commonly used staging system for RCC is the TNM staging system. It allows for a distinction between venous involvement and nodal invasion and stratifies the extent of each stage. RCC can involve the renal vein and vena cava and may even extend into the right atrium. Locally, it can directly invade surrounding structures such as the adrenal gland and colon. Five-year survival rates range from 80% to 90% for stages T1 N0 M0 (<7 cm) and T2 N0 M0 (>7 cm), 40% to 60% for stage T3 N0 M0, and 10% to 20% for N1–3 and M1 disease.

Treatment

Surgical excision of the tumor is the primary treatment for RCC. The classic procedure was a radical nephrectomy, in which the kidney was removed en bloc within Gerota's fascia and the ipsilateral adrenal gland and lymph nodes. This was routinely performed as an open procedure (flank, transabdominal, or thoracoabdominal incision). Adrenalectomy is now generally reserved for upper-pole tumors, very large tumors, or lesions that directly extend into the adrenal gland. Although these operations are increasingly performed through a laparoscopic approach, an open approach is usually preferred if there is extensive involvement of the inferior vena cava. In rare cases with supradiaphragmatic tumor extension within the cava, cardiopulmonary bypass may be required for tumor extraction.

A partial nephrectomy has become a standard approach for surgical excision of renal parenchymal tumors, particularly for individuals with solitary kidneys, those with bilateral masses, and those with compromised renal function. It has become the preferred operation for patients who have lesions of 4 cm or smaller and a normal contralateral kidney, because local recurrence rates are less than 5%, and partial (rather than radical) nephrectomy is associated with a lower long-term risk of chronic renal failure. As with radical nephrectomy, there is a growing experience with laparoscopic approaches to partial nephrectomy. There are also several investigational, minimally invasive approaches that are being explored including radiographically guided, percutaneous thermal tumor ablation using radiofrequency ablation or cryotherapy. Final acceptance of these modalities awaits more long-term data on their oncologic efficacy.

Up to 25% of patients initially present with metastatic disease. Sites of metastasis of RCC, in decreasing frequency of occurrence, include lung, lymph nodes, liver, bone, and adrenal gland. Chemotherapy and irradiation have little to no survival benefit, with radiation therapy only palliating painful metastases. The mainstay of treatment in the past was immunotherapy, with 5-year survival rates of 10% to 20%. Modern therapies for advanced or metastatic RCC now include the so-called targeted therapies, such as the oral tyrosine kinase inhibitors, sunitinib (Sutent) and sorafenib (Nexavar), and the mammalian target of rapamycin (mTOR) inhibitor, temsirolimus (Torisel). Evidence suggests improved survival among those patients who undergo nephrectomy before systemic immunotherapy.

BENIGN RENAL TUMORS

Although they are not as frequent as malignant tumors, benign solid masses are also seen in the kidney. Angiomyolipomas can often be diagnosed radiographically based on the appearance of fat by CT scan. They can occur sporadically or as part of an inherited familial syndrome, tuberous sclerosis. The latter entity is characterized by mental retardation, benign tumors of the cerebellum, epilepsy, adenoma sebaceum, and angiomyolipomas. Approximately 50% of patients with tuberous sclerosis develop angiomyolipomas, most of which are bilateral and multifocal. The management of angiomyolipoma is controversial and should be individualized. Asymptomatic tumors smaller than 4 cm can generally be observed with annual radiographic imaging. Symptomatic lesions (bleeding, pain, rapid growth) and lesions larger than 4 cm should be considered for surgical excision, although angioembolization is another option. Acute hemorrhage from an angiomyolipoma can often be managed or at least stabilized by angioembolization.

Oncocytomas are the most common solid, benign renal tumors and account for 5% to 10% of solid renal lesions. Although these lesions tend to have a more uniform density than RCC and can have a characteristic central scar or spoke-wheel appearance on CT, there is no radiographic feature that reliably distinguishes an oncocytoma from a malignant renal lesion. Oncocytoma is therefore a diagnosis that should be made only on histologic analysis. The tumors characteristically exhibit eosinophilic, granular cells packed with mitochondria. Oncocytomas are thought to arise from the distal portion of the renal tubule.

METASTATIC RENAL LESIONS

The most common primary malignancy to metastasize to the kidney is lung cancer, although cancers of the ovary, breast, or bowel, melanoma, and lymphoma can do so as well. Lymphoma of the kidney is almost always a manifestation of systemic disease. The management is therefore grounded in systemic chemotherapy, with surgery reserved for palliative symptom relief. However, approximately 15% of renal lymphomas manifest with a solitary renal mass as the sole radiographic manifestation. These lesions can be challenging to manage and difficult to distinguish from RCC preoperatively.

Tumors of the Renal Pelvis and Ureter

Approximately 10% of all renal tumors originate in the renal pelvis rather than the renal parenchyma. These account for 5% of all urothelial carcinomas (the majority of which arise in the bladder). Of the upper tract urothelial carcinomas, approximately one fourth arise in the ureter and the remainder in the renal pelvis. Urothelial carcinoma of the upper urinary tract is more common in men than in women and more common in whites than in blacks. Environmental exposures associated with

a higher risk of developing upper tract urothelial carcinoma include analgesic abuse, cyclophosphamide (Cytoxan), and a strong association with tobacco abuse.

Among patients with bladder cancer, approximately 3% to 5% develop upper tract urothelial carcinoma. This can increase to as high as 20% among those with carcinoma in situ (CIS) or high-grade disease. Conversely, approximately 30% to 70% of patients with a history of upper tract urothelial carcinoma go on to develop bladder cancer. As a consequence, these patients require ongoing periodic cystoscopic surveillance. The incidence of bilateral upper tract tumors is 2% to 5%. Other histologic tumor types that can manifest in the upper urinary tract include squamous cell carcinoma (SCC) and adenocarcinoma. Although they are rare, the risk is increased among patients with a history of recurrent, refractory urinary tract infections or staghorn calculi.

DIAGNOSIS

The most common presenting symptom for upper tract urothelial tumors is hematuria. For patients with adequate renal function, the evaluation for hematuria includes CT urography, urinary cytology (or another urinary-based tumor marker), and cystoscopy. Urinary cytology has a high specificity but a generally poor sensitivity, particularly for low-grade disease. Other urinary tumor markers, such as NMP-22, and fluorescent in situ hybridization approaches typically have better sensitivity but are not as specific. A retrograde ureteropyelogram may be helpful in patients with poor renal function who cannot receive intravenous contrast agents. In general, if a suspicious mass is seen on CT or other imaging, a ureteroscopy is typically performed with biopsy or brushings to establish the diagnosis. The TNM system is the standard for staging.

TREATMENT

Disease isolated to the distal ureter is most often managed with distal ureterectomy and ureteroneocystostomy. High-grade or high stage disease and multifocal disease isolated to one side are optimally managed in most cases by excision of that upper tract system via a radical nephroureterectomy, including excision of the distal portion of the ureter and complete excision of the ureteral orifice together with a cuff of bladder. Traditionally, these procedures were done via open incisions (one or two separate incisions, depending on the surgeon), but laparoscopy is increasingly being used to decrease patient morbidity and improve surgical recovery. In selected patients who have low-grade, low-stage disease with a small overall disease burden, an endoscopic approach using laser or electrocautery to destroy the tumors may be considered. This is also a strong consideration for those patients with bilateral disease or involvement of a functionally solitary renal unit. Most often, retrograde endoscopic approaches via ureteroscopy are employed, although in highly selected cases antegrade percutaneous approaches have been reported.

Carcinoma of the Bladder

UROTHELIAL CARCINOMA OF THE BLADDER

Bladder carcinoma is the fifth most common malignancy in the United States, with more than 68,810 new cases diagnosed annually. It is almost three times more common in men than in women, in whom it is the fourth most common cancer. Because of its propensity to recur, particularly in patients with superficial disease, it is the second most prevalent cancer. High-grade bladder cancer is a deadly disease and is the fifth most common cause of cancer deaths among men. There is a well-established relationship between the development of bladder cancer and a variety of carcinogens. Perhaps the most widespread factor is tobacco abuse. Cigarette smoking is thought to account for up to half of all bladder cancers in men. Bladder cancer is also associated with other, less frequent occupational exposures, such as in the rubber and oil refinery industries. It is also associated with exposure to the chemotherapeutic agent, cyclophosphamide (Cytoxan); exposed patients have up to a ninefold increased risk of developing bladder cancer, most likely related to a urinary metabolite of cyclophosphamide, acrolein.

CURRENT DIAGNOSIS

Carcinoma of the Prostate

- Average-risk patients are offered screening with prostate-specific antigen (PSA) testing and digital rectal examination (DRE) at 50 years of age, high-risk patients with a strong family history, and African American patients at age 40 years.
- Patients with an elevated PSA or abnormal DRE are referred for discussion regarding risks, benefits, and alternatives to biopsy of the prostate.
- Diagnosis is made with transrectal ultrasound-guided biopsy of the prostate.
- Staging with bone scan is done for patients with high-grade tumors (Gleason grade 4 or 5), PSA levels greater than 20 µg/mL, elevated alkaline phosphatase levels, or bone pain.

Renal Cell Carcinoma

- Hematuria is the single most common sign, occurring in up to 60% of cases. Flank pain and a palpable mass can also occur, but the classic triad of hematuria, flank pain, and a palpable abdominal mass is present in only 10% of cases. Other common signs and symptoms are fever, anemia, thrombocytosis, hypercalcemia, and an elevated sedimentation rate.
- Most tumors are asymptomatic and are detected incidentally on radiographic imaging (renal ultrasonography, computed tomography [CT] scanning, or magnetic resonance imaging).

Benign Renal Tumors

- Angiomyolipomas have a characteristic appearance of fat within the lesion on CT scans.
- Angiomyolipomas may occur sporadically or as part of the tuberous sclerosis complex.
- Tuberous sclerosis is characterized by benign tumors within the cerebellum, mental retardation, epilepsy, and adenoma sebaceum. Angiomyolipomas occur in half of these patients and are typically bilateral and multifocal, making management more challenging.
- Oncocytomas are benign renal tumors that account for 5% to 10% of solid renal lesions.
- Oncocytomas can be more round and of uniform density, or they may have a central scar or spoke-wheel appearance on CT scan. However, no feature can reliably distinguish these tumors from a malignant renal tumor.
- Oncocytomas should be diagnosed only histologically; they are characterized by eosinophilic granular, mitochondria-laden cells.
- In general, a non–fat-containing, solid renal mass should be considered malignant until proven otherwise.

Tumors of the Renal Pelvis and Ureter

- Tumors arising in the renal pelvis account for 10% of all renal tumors and approximately 5% of all urothelial carcinomas.
- Ureteral tumors account for 25% of upper tract urothelial carcinomas.
- These tumors are more common in men than in women.
- Cigarette smoking is strongly associated with an increased risk, as are analgesic abuse and cyclophosphamide (Cytoxan).
- The most common presenting symptom is hematuria.

- Diagnostic work-up usually includes CT urography, urinary cytology, and cystoscopy.
- Cytologic examination of the urine has a high specificity but poor sensitivity, particularly for low-grade lesions.
- Between 3% and 5% of patients with bladder cancer have associated upper tract urothelial carcinoma. This risk is increased in patients with carcinoma in situ (CIS) or high-grade disease, in whom the risk can be as high as 20%.
- Patients with upper tract urothelial carcinoma have a 30% to 70% risk of developing bladder cancer.

Urothelial Carcinoma of the Bladder

- Painless, gross hematuria is the most common presenting symptom.
- Twenty percent of patients present with only microscopic hematuria.
- Irritative voiding symptoms such as frequency, urgency, or dysuria may also suggest a malignancy, particularly CIS.
- Patients with suspected bladder cancer should undergo an evaluation of their upper tracts (typically by CT), cystoscopy, and cytologic examination of the urine (or another urine-based tumor marker study).
- Transurethral biopsy or resection confirms the diagnosis.
- Ninety percent of bladder cancers are urothelial carcinoma, and 75% are non–muscle-invasive (superficial) at presentation.

Urethral Carcinoma

- Urethral carcinoma is the only urologic malignancy that is more common in females than in males.
- Fifty percent of cases are associated with urethral stricture.
- Urethral carcinoma may manifest as hematuria, obstructive voiding, or a palpable mass.
- Transurethral biopsy is usually required for diagnosis.

Penile Cancer

- Squamous cell carcinoma of the penis occurs most commonly in the sixth decade of life.
- Symptoms are related to ulceration, necrosis, suppuration, and hemorrhage of the penile lesion.
- The diagnosis is established by biopsy.
- Clinical evaluation of patients with penile cancer includes physical examination with palpation of the inguinal region, chest radiography, CT of the abdomen and pelvis, and bone scan.

Testicular Cancer

- Testicular cancer is relatively rare overall, but it is the most common malignancy in men between the ages of 15 and 35 years, with 8090 new cases occurring annually.
- Testicular cancer often manifests as a painless, enlarging testicular mass.
- Malignant tumors of the testis can be divided into those originating from the germinal cells (seminomatous and nonseminomatous germ cell tumors), rare tumors from the supporting cells (Leydig cells and Sertoli cells), and rare metastases from another primary site.
- Ninety-five percent of tumors originating in the testis are germ cell tumors. Fewer than 10% of all germ cell tumors arise from extragonadal primary sites such as the mediastinum or retroperitoneum.
- Human β-chorionic gonadotropin and α-fetoprotein are accurate and relatively specific tumor markers for testicular cancer.

Approximately 90% of bladder malignancies are urothelial carcinomas. Of these, the majority (70%) are papillary, 10% are sessile, and 20% demonstrate mixed morphology. Although roughly three quarters of bladder cancer patients present with superficial disease, approximately 20% to 25% progress to muscle invasion over time. Nevertheless, 80% to 90% of patients with muscle-invasive disease had it at initial presentation. A strong correlation exists between tumor grade and stage; most well-differentiated tumors are superficial, and most poorly differentiated tumors are invasive. CIS is a poorly differentiated urothelial carcinoma that grows as a sheet confined to the urothelium. CIS may be found as a solitary or multifocal process and is associated with invasive carcinoma in 25% of cases, where it portends a poor prognosis. Between 10% and 20% of patients treated with cystectomy for diffuse or refractory CIS are found to have microscopic muscle-invasive disease.

Diagnosis

Gross painless hematuria is the most common presenting sign of bladder cancer. However, approximately 1 in 5 patients have only microscopic hematuria. Other symptoms that can be indicative of urothelial carcinoma (in particular, CIS) include irritative voiding symptoms such as frequency, urgency, and dysuria. Patients who present with symptoms and signs concerning for urothelial carcinoma should undergo an evaluation that includes cystoscopy, urinary tumor marker study (typically, urinary cytology), and evaluation of the upper tracts (typically by CT urography). The diagnosis is usually confirmed at the time of transurethral resection or biopsy.

Treatment

The management options for urothelial carcinoma are heavily dependent on the stage and grade of disease. The TNM system is recommended for staging. For most superficial, low-grade tumors, transurethral resection, with or without a single, immediate instillation of a chemotherapeutic agent such as mitomycin-C (Mutamycin),[1] is all that is required. This must then be followed by careful, ongoing surveillance by cystoscopy, urinary tumor studies (typically cytology), and periodic upper tract imaging. For patients with high-grade disease (including CIS) and tumors that superficially invade the lamina propria (stage T1) or are rapidly recurrent tumors, adjuvant treatment with intravesical agents such as thiotepa (Thioplex), doxorubicin (Adriamycin), and mitomycin-C (Mutamycin)[1] or intravesical bacillus Calmette-Guérin (Tice BCG) may be indicated. In the United States, the most frequently used agent for this purpose, particularly for CIS, is intravesical BCG.

Patients with superficial disease must undergo regular surveillance, because the recurrence rate is as high as 50% at 5 years. Surveillance protocols vary but typically include cystoscopy and urinary tumor studies (usually urinary cytology) every 3 months for 2 years, then every 6 months for 3 years, and annually thereafter. Periodic evaluation of the upper tracts, typically by CT urography, is warranted, because there is a 3% to 5% incidence of development of upper tract urothelial carcinoma among patients with bladder urothelial carcinoma.

The risk of disease progression in patients with low-grade, low-stage (Ta) urothelial carcinoma is less than 5% to 10%. This risk increases as the stage and grade of the tumor increase. Patients who have muscle-invasive disease (stage T2 or higher), either at presentation or with progression after therapy for superficial disease, are best treated by radical cystectomy and urinary diversion. A thorough pelvic lymphadenectomy should be performed at the time of surgery. The precise limits of dissection for the lymphadenectomy remain somewhat controversial, although the latest data suggest that patients who have more lymph nodes removed fare better.

High-grade bladder cancer is a potentially lethal disease. There are an estimated 14,100 deaths due to bladder cancer annually. Among patients with organ-confined (pT2a-pT2b), muscle-invasive disease

who undergo cystectomy, the 5-year recurrence-free survival rates are between 60% and 85%. For patients undergoing radical cystectomy who have extravesical extension of their disease (pT3-pT4 disease), the 5-year recurrence-free survival rates are lower, 40% to 60%. Patients with lymph node–positive disease fare the worst, with 5-year recurrence-free survival rates of 20% to 30%.

Patients with muscle-invasive bladder cancer should be considered for multimodal therapy (i.e., chemotherapy in addition to surgery). The standard regimen over the past decade has been MVAC: methotrexate (Trexall),[1] vinblastine (Velban),[1] doxorubicin (Adriamycin), and cisplatin (Platinol). This can be delivered either before surgery (neoadjuvant) or in the postsurgery setting (adjuvant). There is level 1 evidence to support MVAC chemotherapy combined with cystectomy for muscle-invasive bladder cancer, although the survival benefit across studies is only on the order of 5% to 10%. Newer agents, such as gemcitabine (Gemzar)[1] along with cisplatin, appear to offer similar response rates and reduced toxicity and are often used currently in lieu of MVAC. Cytotoxic chemotherapy produces response rates of 50% to 70% in patients with advanced or metastatic disease; however, the durable, long-term, complete response rates at 5 years are no more than 15% across series.

Urinary diversion may be accomplished after cystectomy in several ways, but the fundamental categories are incontinent and continent forms. Incontinent forms of diversion include ileal and colon conduits, both of which require that the patient wear an external collection appliance. Continent forms of diversion include the continent cutaneous diversion, which requires creation of a low-pressure reservoir (often of colon) and a catheterizable efferent limb with an associated valve mechanism to prevent urine leakage. More recently, emphasis has shifted to continent diversions in which the low-pressure reservoir is anastomosed to the native urethra. These orthotopic neobladders may be crafted from colon or ileum and offer the opportunity to avoid any external collection devices and, usually, any need for catheterization. Such devices may improve patients' quality of life after surgery, although this has not been formally demonstrated in a randomized trial.

ADENOCARCINOMA OF THE BLADDER

Adenocarcinomas account for fewer than 2% of bladder cancers. They can be found in three settings: as primary lesions in the bladder, as metastases or local extensions from another site, or as primary urachal carcinomas. They are typically invasive and poorly differentiated and carry a poor prognosis. Adenocarcinomas may be found in association with bladder augmentation cystoplasties and are the most common form of bladder cancer in patients born with bladder exstrophy. The treatment of choice is typically radical cystectomy, pelvic lymphadenectomy, and urinary diversion.

SQUAMOUS CELL CARCINOMA OF THE BLADDER

SCC accounts for approximately 6% of bladder cancers in the United States but more than 75% of bladder cancers in Egypt. SCC is associated with chronic bladder inflammation from a variety of sources. These include chronic indwelling Foley catheters, recurrent or refractory bladder infections, and bladder diverticula or stones. In Egypt, approximately 80% of SCCs are associated with *Schistosoma haematobium* infestation. These bilharzia-associated SCCs of the bladder tend to occur in patients 10 to 20 years earlier than in the United States.

SCC of the bladder often carries a poor prognosis and is usually best treated by radical cystectomy. After surgery, this form of bladder cancer has a higher propensity for local recurrence, compared with urothelial carcinomas. SCC of the bladder is typically resistant to cytotoxic chemotherapy, particularly the regimens frequently used for urothelial carcinoma. The benefit of neoadjuvant radiation therapy before cystectomy remains to be proven, at least for the non-bilharzial SCC typically found in the United States.

---

[1]Not FDA approved for this indication.

[1]Not FDA approved for this indication.

Urethral Carcinoma

DIAGNOSIS

Urethral carcinoma is unusual in that it is more common in women than in men. It is a disease of the elderly, typically occurring after 60 years of age. The etiology remains to be determined, but approximately half of the cases are associated with urethral stricture disease. In women, there is an association with urethral malakoplakia and urethral caruncles. The usual presenting symptom in this circumstance is a papillary or fungating urethral mass and hematuria. A number of scenarios warrant a more thorough evaluation for possible urethral carcinoma, including a palpable urethral mass, an obstruction that does not respond to conventional management, development of a urethral abscess or fistula, presence of microscopic or gross hematuria, and the development of inguinal adenopathy.

TREATMENT

The primary treatment of urethral carcinoma is most often surgical excision, with the approach and the extent of surgery driven by both gender and the location of the mass relative to the sphincteric complex (likelihood of postoperative continence). For example, cystectomy with en bloc urethrectomy and anterior vaginectomy along with pelvic lymphadenectomy is usually required for tumors located in the proximal urethra or tumors with extension into adjacent structures. In selected cases, radiation therapy can provide local control. In locally advanced disease, multimodality treatment with chemotherapy and either surgical excision or radiation therapy provides the optimal chance for long-term cure, although there is no standard regimen to date.

Penile Cancer

DIAGNOSIS

Penile cancer is relatively rare in the United States. Penile carcinoma has been associated with retained phimotic foreskin and poor personal hygiene. It is rare among men who are circumcised before puberty and occurs most commonly in the sixth decade of life. The symptoms relate directly to the mass itself and can include ulceration, pain, necrosis, foul odor, hemorrhage, and suppuration of the lesion. The clinical evaluation of patients with penile cancer involves a thorough physical examination including of the phallus and careful attention to palpation of the inguinal lymph nodes. Additional studies include radiographic testing with chest radiography, CT scan of the abdomen and pelvis, and bone scan.

TREATMENT

Treatment is usually dictated by the tumor stage (TNM system), size, and location. Small tumors that are confined to the prepuce can often be managed by circumcision alone. Smaller tumors on the distal shaft can be treated by partial penectomy, provided that a 1-cm normal tissue margin can be achieved and there is enough penile length remaining to permit voiding in the standing position. Among patients treated by partial penectomy, the 5-year recurrence-free survival rate is 70% to 80%. Large lesions and tumors on the proximal shaft may require total penectomy and perineal urethrostomy to achieve adequate local tumor control. If there is involvement of local structures such as the scrotum or pubis, radical en bloc resection may be required. Achieving negative margins is critical, because local recurrence of the disease can rarely be salvaged by radiation or chemotherapy.

Although many patients have inguinal lymphadenopathy at presentation, inguinal lymph node enlargement before excision of the primary tumor may be the result of infection and not metastatic disease. Clinical assessment of the inguinal region is therefore typically delayed for 4 to 6 weeks, during which time the patient receives antibiotic treatment. Lymphadenopathy that persists or develops de novo raises the strong possibility of lymph node metastases, and an ilioinguinal lymphadenectomy should be performed. If inguinal lymphadenopathy resolves on antibiotics, prophylactic lymph node dissection may not be necessary. It is often necessary to perform bilateral inguinal lymphadenectomy, particularly in patients with high-risk disease, for whom this should be considered regardless of the presence or absence of palpable nodes. Radiation of the primary tumor and regional lymph nodes is an alternative to surgery in carefully selected patients with small (≤2 cm), low-stage tumors. Similarly, Mohs' surgery is an option for small tumors, particularly ones at the base that otherwise might require a total penectomy.

Testicular Cancer

Malignant tumors of the male gonads can be divided into neoplasms originating from the germinal cells, rare tumors from the supporting cells (Leydig cells and Sertoli cells), and rare metastases from another primary site. The germinal neoplasms include seminomatous and nonseminomatous germ cell tumors (NSGCTs). Ninety-five percent of tumors originating in the testis are germ cell tumors. Fewer than 10% of all germ cell tumors arise from extragonadal primary sites such as the mediastinum and retroperitoneum. Testicular cancer is relatively rare overall, but it is the most common malignancy in men between the ages of 15 and 35 years, with 8090 new cases occurring annually.

Testicular cancer represents one of the great success stories in modern medicine. The mortality rates for testis cancer have decreased from more than 50% before the 1970s to less than 10% in the modern age. This is the result of a variety of advances, including more effective multiagent chemotherapy, improved surgical techniques, and better methods to diagnose and monitor the disease (e.g., CT scans, tumor markers). Testicular cancer currently serves as a paradigm for the multimodal treatment of malignancies.

Germ cell tumors are substantially more prevalent in Caucasians than in African Americans, by a margin of at least 5:1. Indeed, a report from the U.S. military indicated a relative incidence of 40:1. The exact etiology of germ cell tumors is not fully understood. Familial clustering has been demonstrated, particularly among siblings. Two conditions associated with a higher risk for germ cell tumors are cryptorchidism and Klinefelter's syndrome, the latter associated with disease arising from the mediastinum. Orchidopexy for cryptorchidism does not appear to reduce the risk of neoplasia, but it does improve the ability to monitor the testis.

DIAGNOSIS

A painless testicular mass in a patient of the appropriate age group should be considered a primary testicular tumor until proven otherwise. A substantial number of testicular tumors manifest with less specific symptoms, including diffuse testicular pain, swelling, hardness, or some combination of these findings. A tumor can be difficult to distinguish from an infectious epididymo-orchitis. However, because the latter is more common than a testicular tumor, a short trial of antibiotics is often undertaken. If symptoms do not abate or the findings do not revert to normal within 2 to 4 weeks, testicular sonography is indicated to identify any underlying testicular mass. A radical inguinal orchiectomy with early, high ligation of the spermatic cord at the internal ring is required for all patients with a suspected testicular tumor.

Testicular cancers typically first spread to regional, retroperitoneal lymph nodes below the level of the renal vessels. The primary nodal landing zone for right-sided tumors lies between the aorta and the inferior vena cava (interaortocaval nodes), whereas for left-sided tumors it is lateral to the aorta (para-aortic). Other frequent sites of metastases include the left supraclavicular lymph nodes and the lungs. Standard initial metastatic evaluation should include a CT scan of the abdomen and pelvis and chest radiography.

Enlarged lymph nodes (>1–2 cm) in the primary lymphatic drainage areas (landing zones) of the affected side are involved by metastatic disease in approximately 70% of cases. CT imaging of the chest is required if mediastinal, hilar, or lung parenchymal disease is suspected. Serum tumor markers should be measured before orchiectomy and should include human β-chorionic gonadotropin (β-hCG), α-fetoprotein (AFP), and the less specific marker, lactate dehydrogenase.

TREATMENT

All suspected testicular tumors should be treated with a radical orchiectomy through an inguinal approach and early, high ligation of the spermatic cord. β-hCG and AFP are relatively specific tumor markers for testicular cancer. They have substantially improved the ability to monitor the disease and to intervene early in the event of recurrence. They, along with lactate dehydrogenase, should be measured before orchiectomy. AFP production is restricted to NSGCTs, specifically tumors that contain at least a component of embryonal carcinoma or yolk sac tumor. Patients with an increased AFP and pure seminoma on pathologic examination of the orchiectomy specimen are still considered to have an NSGCT. Increased serum β-hCG can occur with seminomatous and nonseminomatous tumors. Increased concentrations of β-hCG are seen in 40% to 60% of patients with metastatic NSGCT and in 15% to 20% of patients with metastatic seminomas. Lactate dehydrogenase is less specific but has independent prognostic value in patients with advanced germ cell tumors. Serum lactate dehydrogenase is increased in approximately 60% of patients with NSGCT and in 80% of those with seminomatous germ cell tumors.

Persistently elevated concentrations of AFP and β-hCG, even in the absence of radiographic or clinical findings, implies active disease and is sufficient cause to initiate systemic therapy, provided that false-positive elevations have been ruled out. The serum half-life of β-hCG is 5 to 7 days, and that for AFP is 30 hours. A slow decrease in serum levels after orchiectomy also implies metastatic disease.

Seminoma is the most common histologic form of germ cell tumor and generally carries a better prognosis than other variants. Standard therapy for low-stage (T1, 2a, or 2b) disease is orchiectomy with consideration of radiation therapy to the retroperitoneal and possibly the ipsilateral pelvic lymph nodes. Relapse is relatively rare, occurring in 4% of patients with stage 1 and 10% of patients with stage 2 disease. Relapses after radiation therapy can be salvaged in more than 90% of cases by systemic chemotherapy. The long-term cure rate for low-stage seminoma is approximately 99%.

NSGCTs include embryonal cell carcinomas, choriocarcinomas, yolk sac carcinomas, teratomas, and mixed germ cell tumors. As with pure seminoma, the cure rate is high (>95%) in patients with stage 1 disease. Retroperitoneal lymphatic metastases may be found in 20% of patients who have no lymphatic or vascular invasion or invasion into the tunica albuginea, spermatic cord, or scrotum at the time of orchiectomy, even if CT scans are negative for lymphadenopathy. There are two options for low-stage NSGCT after orchiectomy in the absence of radiographic evidence of lymphadenopathy and with normalized serum tumor markers: surveillance and nerve-sparing retroperitoneal lymph node dissection (RPLND). Patients with clinical stage 1 disease but embryonal histology or the presence of lymphovascular invasion or extension beyond the tunica albuginea have a higher risk of relapse (>30%) with surveillance and should be considered for primary RPLND.

Although RPLND is a major abdominal operation, it offers the best way to control disease within the retroperitoneum. Lymph nodes are removed from the level of the renal hilum caudad to the level of the aortic bifurcation. The lateral margins are the ureters. Historically, this operation was associated with loss of ejaculatory function due to ligation of the sympathetic nerve fibers in the region. With modern, nerve-sparing techniques, ejaculatory function can be preserved in more than 95% of patients. Patients with persistently elevated AFP or β-hCG after orchiectomy most likely have metastatic disease, even in the absence of radiographically detectable lesions.

These patients usually should go on to systemic chemotherapy first, rather than RPLND.

Clinical stage 2 NSGCTs can be managed by either RPLND or primary chemotherapy, depending on several factors. Those patients who are without marker elevation, are asymptomatic, and have small-volume retroperitoneal-only disease can be offered primary RPLND. Those with persistently elevated tumor markers, symptomatic disease, or more bulky retroperitoneal disease usually undergo systemic chemotherapy. Local recurrence in the retroperitoneum after a properly performed RPLND is rare (<10%).

Adjuvant chemotherapy after RPLND should be considered if any lymph node is more than 2 cm in diameter, if six or more nodes are involved, or if there is extranodal invasion. Cure rates are not different in those who do or do not receive adjuvant chemotherapy, but the former group require fewer cycles of chemotherapy and fewer additional surgeries.

Approximately one third of patients require up-front chemotherapy. Those patients with clinical stage 2c disease (or higher), primary retroperitoneal germ cell tumor, or mediastinal seminomas treated with radiation therapy should all undergo systemic, cisplatin-based, multiagent chemotherapy.

Postchemotherapy RPLND for seminoma is typically reserved for patients with residual masses more than 3 cm in size. For NSGCT, this issue is more controversial. Some groups reserve this treatment for patients who do not have substantial tumor shrinkage (>90% shrinkage of retroperitoneal nodes and no residual nodes >1.5 cm) and for those with teratomatous elements in the primary tumor. Others advocate surgery for all patients with initial bulky retroperitoneal disease, regardless of the response to chemotherapy. All agree that a clear residual mass after chemotherapy in the setting of NSGCT warrants a postchemotherapy RPLND.

The first successful combination chemotherapy regimens for testicular cancer included cisplatin, vinblastine, and bleomycin (Blenoxane) and resulted in complete remission in 70% to 80% of patients with metastatic disease. Studies have shown that prolonged maintenance chemotherapy is unnecessary, and etoposide (VePesid) has largely replaced vinblastine (because it is less toxic and probably more efficacious). Serious adverse effects of chemotherapy include neuromuscular toxic affects, myelosuppression, bleomycin-induced pulmonary fibrosis, Raynaud's phenomenon, and secondary malignancy.

Leydig cell tumors are generally benign tumors that make up between 1% and 3% of all testicular tumors. The majority of cases occurs in men aged 20 to 60 years old, although roughly one fourth are diagnosed before puberty. After radical orchiectomy, the prognosis is usually good, with recurrences rarely reported.

Gonadoblastoma is a rare tumor that occurs almost exclusively in patients with a history of gonadal dysgenesis. They account for fewer than 1% of all testicular neoplasms and can occur at any age from infancy to beyond 70 years, although most patients are diagnosed before age 30. Initial management is with radical orchiectomy. Because of a 50% incidence of bilateral disease, a contralateral gonadectomy is generally warranted. The prognosis after orchiectomy is usually excellent.

Lymphoma is the most common secondary neoplasm of the testicle and the most common testicular neoplasm in men older than 50 years of age, with a median age at presentation of 60 years. Although survival is often poor for patients with bilateral disease and those presenting with lymphoma at other sites who later experience a testicular relapse, the prognosis is substantially better for patients presenting with primary testicular lymphoma confined to the testicle.

Disclaimer

The views expressed in this article are those of the author and do not reflect the official policy or position of the United States Army, the Department of Defense, or the U.S. government.

Carcinoma of the Prostate

- Potentially curative treatment is generally offered to men with at least a 10-year life expectancy.
- Treatment options for clinically localized T1c and T2 tumors include active surveillance/watchful waiting, radiation therapy (external irradiation and brachytherapy), cryotherapy, and surgery (open and laparoscopic).
- Treatments for locally advanced tumors (T3/T4) or high-risk cancer patients include surgery and external irradiation in combination with androgen-deprivation therapy (ADT).
- Treatment for patients with metastatic disease (N1–2 or M1) is generally palliative with ADT.
- Follow-up includes history, physical examination, and monitoring of prostate-specific antigen at least every 6 months for 2 years and then annually. Any abnormalities may be more fully evaluated with appropriate imaging.

Renal Cell Carcinoma

- Treatment for localized masses is almost always surgical excision via radical or partial nephrectomy. Both operations may be performed with an open or a laparoscopic approach.
- Partial nephrectomy should be attempted in patients who have a solitary kidney, bilateral disease, or renal insufficiency. Partial nephrectomy is the preferred operation for patients who have lesions 4 cm or larger and a normal contralateral kidney, with local recurrence rates of less than 5%.
- Minimally invasive approaches including percutaneous radiofrequency ablation and cryotherapy are under investigation, although more long-term data are needed.
- Up to 25% of patients have metastatic disease at diagnosis. Sites of metastasis, in decreasing frequency, include lungs, lymph nodes, liver, bone, and adrenal gland.
- Chemotherapy and radiation therapy provide little to no survival benefit, with radiation only palliating painful metastases.
- The mainstay of treatment in the past was immunotherapy, with 5-year survival rates of 10% to 20%.
- Modern therapies for advanced or metastatic RCC include targeted therapies such as the oral tyrosine kinase inhibitors, sunitinib (Sutent) and sorafenib (Nexavar), and the mammalian target of rapamycin (mTOR) inhibitor, temsirolimus (Torisel).
- Evidence suggests improved survival for those undergoing nephrectomy before systemic immunotherapy for metastatic disease.

Benign Renal Tumors

- For angiomyolipomas, management should be individualized. With asymptomatic lesions smaller than 4 cm, observation with annual imaging is reasonable.
- For patients with a symptomatic angiomyolipoma or one larger than 4 cm, surgical excision should be considered, although angioembolization is another option. Angioembolization can be used to stabilize a patient with acute hemorrhage secondary to an angiomyolipoma.

Tumors of the Renal Pelvis and Ureter

- Distal ureteral tumors can be managed with distal ureterectomy and ureteroneocystostomy.
- High-grade, multifocal, or high-stage tumors are optimally treated by nephroureterectomy with removal of a cuff of bladder at the ureteral orifice.
- Laparoscopic (with or without hand assist) nephroureterectomy is the preferred surgical approach, allowing for complete tumor removal and often quicker convalescence.
- Carefully selected patients, especially those who have bilateral disease or a functionally solitary kidney, can be managed with endoscopic tumor ablation.

Urothelial Carcinoma of the Bladder

- Treatment depends on tumor stage.
- Superficial (Ta) low-grade cancers are managed with transurethral resection, with or without a single, immediate postresection instillation of a chemotherapeutic agent, typically mitomycin-C (Mutamycin).
- Carcinoma in situ or high-grade stage Ta tumors that involve the lamina propria (stage T1) and recurrent tumors are managed with transurethral resection and intravesical agents such as thiotepa (Thioplex), doxorubicin (Adriamycin), and mitomycin-C[1] or intravesical bacillus Calmette-Guérin (Tice BCG).
- Bladder surveillance is mandatory, because the recurrence rate in the bladder can be as high as 50% at 5 years.
- Surveillance protocols vary but typically include cystoscopy and urinary tumor studies (usually cytology) every 3 months for the first 2 years, semiannually in years 3 to 5, and annually thereafter.
- Periodic evaluation of the upper tracts should be performed, usually by computed tomographic (CT) urography.
- Superficial disease that progresses or is refractory to conservative management, as well as tumors that invade the bladder muscle (stages T2–4), is best managed by radical cystectomy and urinary diversion.
- Urinary diversion may be either incontinent (conduit) or continent (orthotopic or continent cutaneous).
- Five-year recurrence-free survival rates are 60% to 85% after cystectomy for organ-confined disease (stages T2a–T2b). For extravesical disease (stages T3a to T4), the 5-year survival decreases to 40% to 60%, for node-positive disease it is less than 30%.
- Patients with T2–T4 disease should be strongly considered for combination therapy with surgery plus chemotherapy, either in the neoadjuvant or the adjuvant setting. Recent randomized trials have suggested an approximately 5% survival advantage for neoadjuvant chemotherapy plus surgery, compared with surgery alone.
- Patients with M1 disease are usually treated with chemotherapy.
- The standard regimen over the past decade has been MVAC: methotrexate (Trexall),[1] vinblastine (Velban),[1] doxorubicin (Adriamycin), and cisplatin (Platinol); however, durable complete response rates are less than 15%.
- Newer agents such as gemcitabine (Gemzar)[1] along with cisplatin appear to offer similar response rates and reduced toxicity.

---

[1]Not FDA approved for this indication.

Urethral Carcinoma

- Treatment of the primary tumor is surgical excision and varies based on the location and stage of the tumor.
- In men, urethrectomy can be performed via a perineal incision.
- Proximal tumors of the bulbar urethra are often managed with cystoprostatectomy and en bloc urethrectomy.
- Among women, for tumors of the proximal urethra and tumors with extension into adjacent structures, cystectomy with en bloc urethrectomy and anterior vaginectomy along with pelvic lymphadenectomy is usually required.
- Radiation therapy is also reported to provide local control in selective cases.

Penile Cancer

- Small penile cancers limited to the prepuce can be treated by circumcision alone.
- Partial penectomy with at least a 1-cm margin of normal tissue is used to treat smaller (2–5 cm) distal penile tumors. The remaining penis should be long enough to permit voiding in the standing position. The 5-year cure rate for patients treated with partial penectomy is 70% to 80%.
- Larger distal penile lesions and proximal tumors require total penectomy and perineal urethrostomy. If the scrotum, pubis, or abdominal wall is involved, radical en bloc excision may be necessary.
- Many patients have inguinal lymphadenopathy at presentation. However, inguinal lymph node enlargement before excision of the primary tumor may be the result of infection and not metastatic disease. Therefore, clinical assessment of the inguinal region should be delayed 4 to 6 weeks, during which time the patient is treated with antibiotics.
- If inguinal lymphadenopathy persists or develops, there is a high likelihood of metastatic disease, and ilioinguinal lymphadenectomy should be performed. The procedure is performed on the contralateral side if the initial side contains tumor and could be simultaneously performed or staged.
- Irradiation of the primary tumor and regional lymph nodes is an alternative to surgery in patients with small (≤2 cm), low-stage tumors.
- Mohs' surgery is another alternative for small lesions (≤2 cm).

Testicular Cancer

- All patients with suspected testicular tumors should undergo a radical orchiectomy through an inguinal approach and early, high ligation of the spermatic cord.
- Serum tumor markers should be measured before surgery and are used for disease staging and to monitor for recurrence.
- Radiographic staging should include, at a minimum, a CT scan of the abdomen and pelvis and chest radiography.
- Seminoma is the most common histologic form of germ cell tumor and generally carries a better prognosis than other variants. Standard therapy for low-stage (T1, 2a, or 2b) disease is orchiectomy with consideration of radiation therapy to the retroperitoneal and possibly the ipsilateral pelvic lymph nodes. Relapse is relatively rare, occurring in 4% of patients with stage 1 and 10% of patients with stage 2 disease. Relapses after radiation therapy can be salvaged in more than 90% of cases through systemic chemotherapy. The long-term cure rate for low-stage seminoma is approximately 99%.
- Nonseminomatous germ cell tumors (NSGCTs) include embryonal cell carcinomas, choriocarcinomas, yolk sac carcinomas, teratomas, and mixed germ cell tumors. As with pure seminoma, the cure rate for low-stage NSGCTs is high (>95%) in patients with stage 1 disease.
- Surveillance and retroperitoneal lymph node dissection (RPLND) are both standard treatment options for stage 1 NSGCT. Twenty percent of these patients have lymph node involvement, and those with vascular invasion or predominance of embryonal cell carcinoma are at increased risk (>30%).
- RPLND is a major abdominal operation in which lymph nodes from the retroperitoneum are removed, from the renal hilum down to the level of the common iliac artery, with lateral margins being confined by the ureters.
- Adjuvant chemotherapy after RPLND should be considered if any lymph node is larger than 2 cm in diameter, if at least six nodes are involved, or if there is extranodal invasion.
- Patients with persistently increased concentrations of α-fetoprotein, human β-chorionic gonadotropin, or both but without other clinical evidence of disease after orchiectomy usually have systemic disease and are treated with chemotherapy.
- Approximately one third of patients require up-front chemotherapy. Those with clinical stage 2c disease (or higher), primary retroperitoneal germ cell tumors, or mediastinal seminomas treated with radiation therapy should undergo systemic, cisplatin-based, multiagent chemotherapy.
- Postchemotherapy RPLND for seminoma is typically reserved for patients with residual masses larger than 3 cm. For NSGCT, some groups reserve postchemotherapy RPLND for patients who do not have substantial tumor shrinkage (>90% shrinkage of retroperitoneal nodes and no residual nodes >1.5 cm) and those with teratomatous elements in the primary tumor. Others advocate surgery for all patients with initial bulky retroperitoneal disease. All agree that a clear, residual mass after chemotherapy in the setting of NSGCT warrants postchemotherapy RPLND.
- Multimodal therapy has allowed 90% to 95% of testicular cancer patients to be cured, even in the face of metastatic disease.

REFERENCES

Barocas DA, Clark PE. Bladder cancer. Curr Opin Oncol 2008;20:307–14.

Damber JE, Aus G. Prostate cancer. Lancet 2008;371:1710–21.

Flechon A, Rivoire M, Droz JP. Management of advanced germ-cell tumors of the testis. Nat Clin Pract Urol 2008;5:262–76.

Jemal A, Siegel R, Ward E, et al. Cancer statistics, 2008. CA Cancer J Clin 2008;58:71–96.

Rini BI, Rathmell WK, Godley P. Renal cell carcinoma. Curr Opin Oncol 2008;20:300–6.

Urethral Strictures

Method of
Brian J. Flynn, MD, and David Hadley, MD

Urethral stricture occurs when scar tissue in the epithelium contracts and subsequently narrows the urethral lumen. The scarring process is induced by trauma, inflammation, or ischemia, with more severe strictures involving progressive fibrosis into the corpus spongiosum (spongiofibrosis). By definition, urethral strictures may involve the anterior urethra (fossa navicularis, pendulous urethra, and bulbous urethra), the posterior urethra (membranous or prostatic urethra), or both. Anterior urethral injuries commonly result from direct penile or perineal trauma, instrumentation, catheterization, infections, or lichen sclerosis. Posterior urethral strictures may represent an actual defect in the membranous urethra after a distraction injury or a complication from prostate cancer treatment (surgery, irradiation, cryosurgery, or brachytherapy).

The prevalence of urethral strictures has been reported to be as high as 0.6% in the male population, and they have been a recognized problem throughout history, usually in relation to trauma and infection. Antibiotics for gonococcal urethritis have significantly reduced the incidence of strictures after infection, but iatrogenic injuries from urologic instrumentation and urethral catheterization have significantly increased as a cause of urethral stricture disease.

Evaluation and Diagnosis

Men with a urethral stricture may present acutely in the emergency department with urinary retention or may be referred to the clinic with chronic obstructive voiding symptoms. Patients complain of decreased force of the urinary stream, hesitancy, inability to empty, nocturia, postvoid dribbling, and difficulty emptying the bladder. Irritative symptoms can also occur, including frequency, urgency, and dysuria. Patients are typically 16 to 40 years of age and tend to live an active lifestyle (e.g., mountain biking, riding motorcycles or all-terrain vehicles, horseback riding), which may cause chronic perineal trauma. Often a hallmark event such as urethral trauma or urethral instrumentation resulting in blood per urethra occurs immediately before the onset of symptoms.

CURRENT DIAGNOSIS

- Retrograde urethrography is essential in the diagnosis and management of urethral stricture disease.
- Obstructive voiding complaints are the most common presentation in patients with urethral stricture disease.
- Patients with recurrent urinary tract infections, prostatitis, or epididymitis should be evaluated for urethral stricture.

Physical examination should include a standard genital examination for any abnormalities, specifically evaluating the meatus for stenosis and the penile shaft for any fibrosis or stigmata of lichen sclerosis. Laboratory evaluation should include urinalysis, urine culture for infection, and a basic metabolic panel for renal function. Basic urodynamic studies, including simple uroflowmetry and measurement of the postvoid residual with ultrasound, can assess for obstruction and ability to empty. Inability to pass a catheter should further raise suspicion for a urethral stricture and prompt an evaluation of the urethra with endoscopy and retrograde urethrography.

Retrograde urethrography remains the gold standard for diagnosis and evaluation of urethral strictures, defining the length, location, caliber, and number of strictures. A voiding cystourethrogram (VCUG) obtained by means of a suprapubic cystotomy tube should outline the proximal urethra in cases of complete urethral occlusion. Alternative imaging modalities include magnetic resonance imaging and ultrasonography. These studies are better able to image a urethral cancer or diverticulum.

Cystourethroscopy complements the radiologic findings, confirming the anatomic location of the stricture and its caliber, and can rule out other urethral pathology such as stones, necrosis, fistula, or cancer. Urethral dilation, if planned, can also be performed by initially placing a wire under direct vision across the stricture and into the bladder.

Management

Once the diagnosis has been made, the first step is to treat the acute issues such as urinary retention and concomitant genitourinary infections. Urinary retention is treated with urethral catheterization or with a suprapubic cystotomy tube if urethral catheterization is unsuccessful. Once the acute issues are resolved, future management is based on the length, location, degree, and cause of the stricture and patient preference. Absolute indications for intervention include urinary retention, azotemia, recurrent infections, stone formation, and pain.

URETHROTOMY AND DILATION

Urethral dilation or urethrotomy is often the initial treatment, because it is less invasive than open surgical management. Dilation may be performed with filiforms and followers, serial dilators, or a balloon in the clinic or the emergency room. Urethrotomy is performed in the operating room with the patient under general regional anesthesia, with the use of an endoscopic knife or a laser to incise the scar under direct vision.

Strictures amenable to dilation are short (<1.0 cm) and are associated with minimal spongiofibrosis. Typically, dilation is performed initially, and urethrotomy is reserved for denser strictures in the bulbar or posterior urethra. In general, there is no statistical difference in success rate between dilation and urethrotomy. Recurrent strictures, long strictures, and those associated with significant fibrosis reoccur in more than 80% of cases and therefore require self-dilation or open urethral reconstruction (urethroplasty).

STENTS

Urethral stents such as the UroLume (American Medical Systems, Minnetonka, MN) are made with titanium and are considered permanent. Introduced with much enthusiasm, stents have fallen out of favor secondary to problems of migration, encrustation, postvoid dribbling, and perineal and penile pain. Overall, long-term success is less than 30%, and these devices are best reserved for patients who are not candidates for open reconstruction.

OPEN RECONSTRUCTION

Surgical excision of the diseased segment with primary anastomosis (EPA) remains the gold standard for short strictures in the bulbous or posterior urethra, with long-term success rates greater than 95% in most studies. Keys to a successful repair include complete excision of the spongiofibrosis and a widely spatulated, tension-free anastomosis. Typically, strictures smaller than 2 cm are amenable to EPA, although longer stricture repair has been reported, especially in the

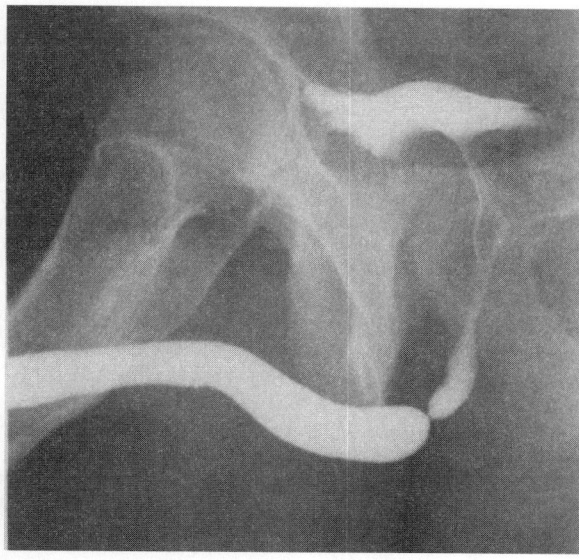

FIGURE 1. Retrograde urethrogram demonstrating a short bulbar urethral stricture amenable to excision with primary anastomosis.

posterior urethra (Fig. 1). Whereas significant bulbar urethral mobilization can create length in men with longer strictures, this may compromise penile length and cosmesis.

If the stricture is located in the pendulous urethra or its length exceeds the limits of EPA (>2 cm), substitution urethroplasty with a graft or a flap may be performed (Figs. 2 and 3). The graft or flap is onlayed ventrally or dorsally after a longitudinal incision is made in the diseased segment, thereby increasing the urethral caliber. A hybrid technique involves stricture excision of the worst disease with onlay to the less severe adjacent segments. If there are long obliterative segments, a two-stage repair is necessary.

Multiple sources of graft material have been successfully used in urethroplasty, including preputial skin, split-thickness skin from the thigh, bladder epithelium, rectal mucosa, and buccal mucosa. Buccal mucosa has emerged as the graft of choice, with excellent short-term results. Buccal mucosa has the ideal histologic characteristics, is non–hair bearing, leaves no visible scar, and is water resistant and hence does not appear to have has much contracture as other graft materials.

Posterior urethral distraction injuries are a result of pelvic fracture and occur in up to 10% of cases. At the time of pelvic fracture, if there

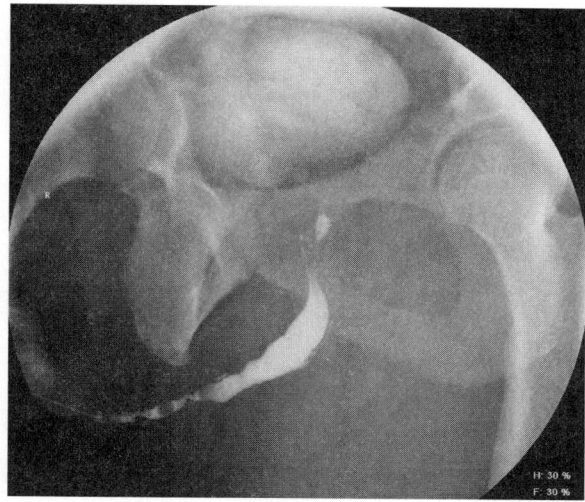

FIGURE 3. Retrograde urethrogram showing a panurethral stricture from lichen sclerosis. These may be repaired with complex staged reconstruction or perineal urethrostomy.

is blood at the meatus, a high index for suspicion, or inability to void, a RUG should be performed (Fig. 4). In some cases, a partial disruption may have occurred, with a small portion of epithelium left intact. An endoscopically placed urethral catheter can facilitate stricture-free healing. If complete transection has occurred or a urethral catheter cannot be placed, the patient can be taken to the operating room, where a suprapubic cystotomy tube is placed. An antegrade-retrograde two-team approach using cystoscopy and fluoroscopy is then performed in an effort to place a catheter across the defect. Recent literature has suggested that early realignment decreases the need for subsequent urethroplasty without compromising erectile or sphincter function. However, if a primary realignment is not feasible, a suprapubic catheter is used for drainage, and delayed repair (3 months after the injury) is indicated. A progressive perineal anastomotic repair in these cases has a success rate of more than 95%. Complex posterior urethral injuries (e.g., with a concomitant bladder neck injury, rectal injury, or fistula) usually require an abdominal-perineal approach.

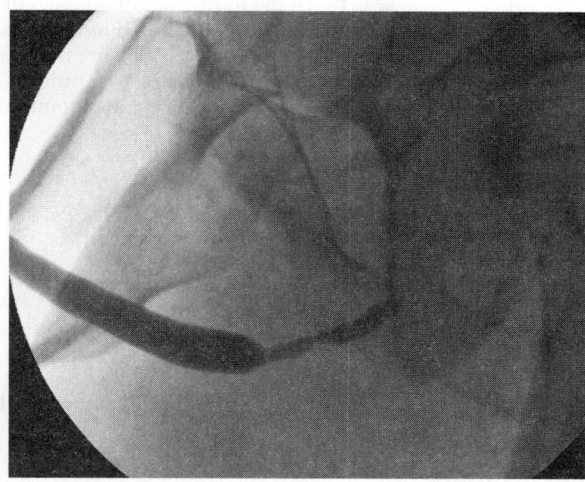

FIGURE 2. Retrograde urethrogram demonstrating a longer bulbar urethral stricture requiring excision of the most significant area of stricture and onlay of the remaining stricture: the excisional, augmented anastomotic urethroplasty.

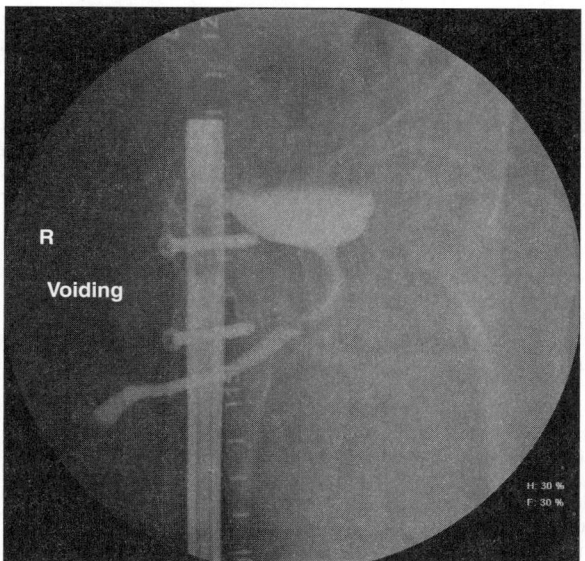

FIGURE 4. Retrograde urethrogram may be combined with a voiding cystourethrogram (the bladder is filled via a suprapubic catheter) to demonstrate a posterior urethral disruption due to pelvic fracture. These defects are usually amenable to excision with primary anastomosis.

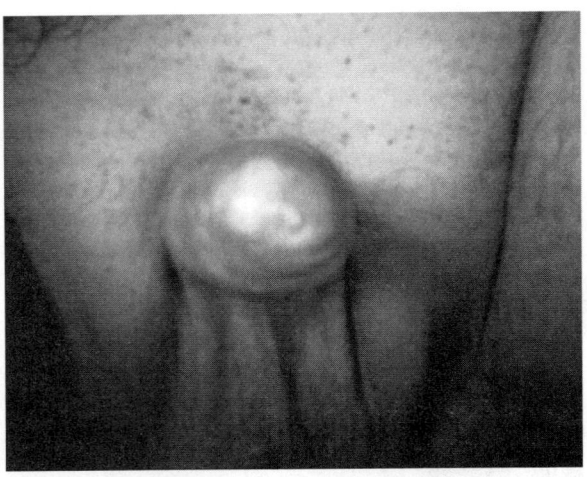

FIGURE 5. Picture of the glans penis afflicted with lichen sclerosis.

CURRENT THERAPY

- The patient and doctor should have a good understanding of the goals, limitations, and definitions of success before treatment of urethral stricture disease is undertaken.
- Office-based dilation is the most common and accepted initial treatment for urethral strictures.
- Dilation and urethrotomy are equivalent in terms of long-term success and are more likely to succeed in short, bulbar strictures with minimal fibrosis.
- Open surgical therapy is based on the length, location, and cause of the urethral stricture.

A variant of lichen sclerosis, balanitis xerotica obliterans, is an idiopathic, lymphocyte-mediated inflammatory skin disease that affects the anogenital region. A sclerotic white ring around the prepuce or glans penis is diagnostic in the early stage (Fig. 5) and can lead to phimosis or meatal stenosis and urethral stricture in as many as 20% of patients. The use of genital tissue for reconstruction is contraindicated because it has a failure rate of more than 90%. Surgical options include a two-stage repair with buccal mucosa or extended meatotomy and perineal urethrostomy for more severe disease. In some cases, penile biopsy for diagnosis and to rule out squamous cell carcinoma is necessary preoperatively.

REFERENCES

Abouassaly R, Angermeier KW. Augmented anastomotic urethroplasty. J Urol 2007;177(6):2211–5; discussion 2215–16.

Armitage JN, Cathcart PJ, Rashidian A, et al. Epithelializing stent for benign prostatic hyperplasia: A systematic review of the literature. J Urol 2007;177(5):1619–24.

Dubey D, Vijjan V, Kapoor R, et al. Dorsal onlay buccal mucosa versus penile skin flap urethroplasty for anterior urethral strictures: Results from a randomized prospective trial. J Urol 2007;178(6):2466–9.

Eltahawy EA, Virasoro R, Schlossberg SM, et al. Long-term followup for excision and primary anastomosis for anterior urethral strictures. J Urol 2007;177(5):1803–6.

Flynn BJ, Webster GD. Urethral stricture and disruption. In: Graham SD, Keane TE, Glenn J, editors. Glenn's Urologic Surgery. 6th ed. Philadelphia: Lippincott Williams & Wilkins; 2003. p. 394–407.

Heyns CF, Steenkamp JW, Kock MLSD, et al. Treatment of male urethral strictures: Is repeated dilation of internal urethrotomy useful? J Urol 1998;160 (2):356–8.

Jordan GH. Imaging of the penis and male urethra. AUA Update Series 2008;27: [Lesson 23].

Jordan GH, Schlossberg SM. Surgery of the penis and urethra. In: Wein AJ, Kavoussi LR, et al., editors. Campbell-Walsh Urology. 9th ed. Philadelphia: Saunders/Elsevier; 2007. p. 1054–87.

Levine LA, Strom KH, Lux MM. Buccal mucosa graft urethroplasty for anterior urethral stricture repair: Evaluation of the impact of stricture location and lichen sclerosis on surgical outcome. J Urol 2007;178(5):2011–5.

Mouraviev VB, Coburn M, Santucci RA. The treatment of posterior urethral disruption associated with pelvic fractures: Comparative experience of early realignment versus delayed urethroplasty. J Urol 2005;173(3):873–6.

Pugliese JM, Morey AF, Peterson AC. Lichen sclerosis: Review of the literature and current recommendations for management. J Urol 2007;178(6): 2268–76.

Santucci RA, Joyce GF, Wise M. Male urethral stricture disease. J Urol 2007;177(5):1667–74.

Renal Calculi

Method of
Vahan Vartanian, BS, and Sangtae Park, MD, MPH

In the United States, upper urinary tract stones are responsible for significant morbidity, loss of work, and medical cost. The prevalence of urinary stone disease is estimated at 5% to 12%, and the lifetime chance of being diagnosed with a stone is 1 in 8. In the United States, the annual medical expenditure for a diagnosis of nephrolithiasis approaches $2.1 billion. Furthermore, long-term effects such as renal function loss are significant. A recent study of more than 1300 new cases of end-stage renal disease requiring dialysis found that, in 3.2% of the cases, renal failure was a direct result of stone disease.

In addition to the morbidity of an acute stone event, at least 50% of patients ultimately require surgical intervention. As such, the goal of medical treatment is to prevent disease progression and recurrence and, potentially, to reduce stone burden. Nonetheless, the recurrence rate of urinary calculi is roughly 50% within 5 years.

Epidemiology

Most kidney stones occur in patients between 20 and 50 years old, with peak onsets of disease between the third and fifth decades of life. Kidney stones are more prevalent in Caucasians, Latinos, and Asians than in African Americans or Native Americans. Men are more commonly affected with kidney stones than women, by a ratio of 2:1. Geographic analysis demonstrates that stones are more common in hot and dry areas.

Pathophysiology

Calcareous stones, including calcium oxalate, calcium apatite, and brushite stones, represent approximately 75% of upper tract stones, and the remaining 25% are struvite, cystine, uric acid, and other stones (Table 1). Supersaturation of urine by urinary constituents such as calcium, oxalate, and uric acid is necessary for stone formation. Supersaturation is defined as concentration of an ion to a level beyond which it is not soluble.

HYPERCALCIURIA

Hypercalciuria is classified as absorptive, renal, or resorptive based on the underlying pathophysiologic abnormality. Absorptive hypercalciuria is caused by intestinal overabsorption of calcium. It is classified as type II if urinary calcium normalizes with dietary calcium

TABLE 1 Classification of Nephrolithiasis

Condition	Metabolic or Environmental Defect	Prevalence (%)
Hypercalciuria		
Absorptive hypercalciuria	Increased gastrointestinal calcium absorption	20–40
Renal hypercalciuria	Impaired renal calcium reabsorption	5–8
Resorptive hypercalciuria	Primary hyperparathyroidism	3–5
Hyperuricosuric calcium nephrolithiasis	Dietary purine excess, uric acid overproduction	10–40
Hypocitraturic calcium stone		10–50
Chronic diarrhea	Gastrointestinal alkali loss	
Distal RTA	Impaired renal acid excretion	
Thiazide-induced	Hypokalemia and intracellular acidosis	
Hyperoxaluric calcium stone		2–15
Primary hyperoxaluria	Genetic oxalate overproduction	
Dietary hyperoxaluria	Excessive dietary intake	
Enteric hyperoxaluria	Increased gastrointestinal oxalate absorption	
Gouty diathesis	Low urinary pH	15–30
Cystinuria	Impaired renal cystine reabsorption	<1
Infection stones	Urinary infection with urease-producing bacteria	1–5

restriction or type I if it is unresponsive to diet. In renal hypercalciuria, impaired renal tubular reabsorption of calcium results in elevated urinary calcium levels. Resorptive hypercalciuria is an uncommon abnormality that is most often associated with primary hyperparathyroidism and calcium resorption from bone stores.

HYPERURICOSURIA

Hyperuricosuria is present in up to 10% of calcium stone formers. Hyperuricosuria predisposes to calcium or uric acid stone formation by causing supersaturation of the urine with respect to monosodium urate. At urinary pH values lower than 5.5, the undissociated form of uric acid predominates, leading to uric acid stone formation. At pH values greater than 5.5, sodium urate formation promotes development of calcium oxalate stones through heterologous nucleation. The most common cause of hyperuricosuria is increased dietary purine intake because uric acid is the end product of purine metabolism. However, acquired and hereditary diseases, such as gout and hematologic disorders, can cause hyperuricosuria.

CYSTINURIA

Cystinuria is an autosomal recessive disorder characterized by a defect in intestinal and renal tubular transport of dibasic amino acids, resulting in excessive urinary excretion of cystine. Cystine is poorly soluble in urine, so its precipitation and subsequent stone formation occur at physiologic urine conditions.

INFECTION STONES

Struvite stones (magnesium ammonium phosphate) occur only in association with urinary infection by urea-splitting bacteria. Under these conditions, urinary urea is hydrolyzed to ammonia by bacterial urease, resulting in alkaline urine that further promotes phosphate dissociation and allows formation of the stones.

Diagnosis

Patients with urinary calculi can present with pain, fever, dysuria, or hematuria. Nonobstructive intrarenal calculi do not usually cause pain, in contrast to ureteral calculi. As ureteral calculi move distally through the ureter, pain migrates from the flank to the abdomen, then to the groin, and finally to the scrotal or labial area. Staghorn calculi are kidney stones that occupy the renal pelvis and calyceal system. These stones are often asymptomatic, and if they do manifest, it is usually with hematuria and infection rather than acute onset of pain.

During history-taking, it is important to ask about the presence of fever, nausea, or vomiting and the location and duration of pain. A history of recurrent urinary tract infections, previous renal calculi,

medications, a family history of calculi, and the presence of a solitary or transplanted kidney are informative.

On physical examination, the patient is usually in significant distress, and costovertebral angle tenderness is common. Patients do not present with peritoneal signs. The presence of fever, tachycardia, or hypotension is a sign of impending or frank urosepsis from an obstructing calculus, and this is a bona fide surgical emergency requiring ureteral stenting or percutaneous nephrostomy tube placement.

Laboratory and Radiographic Studies

All patients should be evaluated with urinalysis, urine culture, a complete blood count, and a chemistry profile. Urinalysis assesses for pH, microhematuria, and crystalluria. An elevated white blood cell count may reflect renal or systemic infection. The chemistry profile, including measurements of serum electrolytes, creatinine, calcium, parathyroid hormone, and uric acid, assesses the patient's renal and metabolic function. Patients who are recurrent stone formers and those who are high-risk first-time stone formers (age <30 years, multiple bilateral calculi, pediatric calculi, intestinal disease, or solitary or transplanted kidney) warrant a more extensive laboratory evaluation, including 24-hour urine collections. Elevation of the 24-hour excretion of calcium, oxalate, or uric acid indicates predisposition to stone formation. Decreased urinary volume and a decreased urinary citrate level suggest stone-forming propensity, because citrate is the most common stone inhibitor.

The plain abdominal radiograph is mandatory in assessing total stone burden and the size, shape, and location of urinary calculi. Although the sensitivity and specificity are in the range of 70% to 80%, radiography is a cheap and simple means of monitoring the course of the stone if it is visible. Ultrasonography is useful for detecting hydronephrosis and hydroureter but is limited because of the inability to visualize ureteral calculi and small intrarenal calculi. Intravenous pyelography is an historical study that has been replaced by the current diagnostic gold standard test, the noncontrast abdominopelvic computed tomography scan.

Treatment

MEDICAL CARE

Once renal colic has been diagnosed, pain is usually well controlled with nonsteroidal anti-inflammatory drugs such as ketorolac (Toradol) and opiates. Outpatient management is possible if none of the

TABLE 2 Summary of Medical Expulsive Therapy for Distal Ureteral Calculi

Medicine	Dose
Nifedipine extended-release (Procardia XL)[1]	30 mg PO daily
Tamsulosin (Flomax)[1]	0.4 mg PO daily
Terazosin (Hytrin)[1]	5–10 mg PO daily

[1]Not FDA approved for this indication.

following clinical signs and symptoms exists: fever, intractable nausea and vomiting, uncontrolled pain, solitary kidney, acute renal failure, or sepsis. Outpatient medical care includes the use of analgesics, antinausea medications, and expulsive therapy (α-blocker or calcium channel blocker) for small (<5 mm) distal ureteral calculi. Urologic follow-up is critical to prevent obstructive renal failure from untreated renal or ureteral calculi. Medical expulsive therapy (Table 2) has been shown to be effective in randomized controlled trials for α-blockers such as tamsulosin (Flomax)[1] and calcium channel blockers such as nifedipine (Procardia).[1]

For prevention of stone recurrence, randomized clinical trials have demonstrated that the most important factor is increased fluid intake so that urine output is more than 2 L/day. Excessive intakes of salt, oxalate, and animal protein should be avoided. Empiric dietary restriction of calcium is not necessary in most patients, and it can have adverse effects on bone mineralization, especially in women and in patients with osteoporosis.

SURGICAL CARE

Endoscopic surgery is the mainstay of treatment for nephrolithiasis. Indications for surgery are intractable pain, active infection, and obstruction. Renal obstruction lasting longer than 1 month leads to permanent renal dysfunction; for this reason, medical expulsive therapy should be limited to that period, with surgical therapy instituted thereafter. Treatment for most renal calculi is noninvasive (e.g., extracorporeal lithotripsy), and open or laparoscopic surgical excision is limited to rare, atypical cases. In an obstructed and infected collecting system secondary to a stone, emergent relief of obstruction is necessary by ureteral stenting or percutaneous nephrostomy placement.

---

[1]Not FDA approved for this indication.

Almost 85% of kidney and ureteral stones requiring intervention are treated with extracorporeal shock-wave lithotripsy (ESWL) under general anesthetic or monitored anesthetic care. Shocks are generated and are focused on the calculus. As the stone is hit by the shockwave, it breaks into smaller fragments that can pass in the urine. ESWL is less successful if the stone is larger than 1.5 cm or is in the lower pole of the kidney. Absolute contraindications to ESWL include pregnancy, ureteral obstruction distal to the stone, and uncorrected coagulopathy.

Ureteroscopic management is the second most common management option. With the patient under anesthesia, a flexible 7F or rigid scope is passed through the bladder and up the ureter to visualize the stone. The stone is either extracted with a stone basket or fragmented with the use of a Holmium laser. Complete ureteral and renal endoscopy is performed to ensure stone-free status and to treat any concomitant obstructive disease. Percutaneous nephrostolithotomy is reserved for stones larger than 2 cm. In this operation, a percutaneous nephrostomy tract is created, followed by insertion of a sheath 1 cm in diameter. Ultrasonic or pneumatic lithotripsy is performed under direct vision of the calculi. Because of the rather invasive nature of this operation, morbidity can reach 20%; therefore, this modality is reserved for large, infectious stones that are not appropriate for ESWL or ureteroscopy.

REFERENCES

Borghi L, Meschi T, Amato F, et al. Urinary volume, water and recurrences in idiopathic calcium nephrolithiasis: A 5-year randomized prospective study. J Urol 1996;155:839–43.

Borghi L, Schianchi T, Meschi T, et al. Comparison of two diets for the prevention of recurrent stones in idiopathic hypercalciuria. N Engl J Med 2002;346:77–84.

Clark JY, Thompson IM, Optenberg SA. Economic impact of urolithiasis in the United States. J Urol 1995;154:2020–4.

Grover PK, Ryall RL. Urate and calcium oxalate stones: From repute to rhetoric to reality. Miner Electrolyte Metab 1994;20:361–70.

Jungers P, Joly D, Barbey F, et al. ESRD caused by nephrolithiasis: Prevalence, mechanisms, and prevention. Am J Kidney Dis 2004;44:799–805.

Ng CS, Streem SB. Contemporary management of cystinuria. J Endourol 1999;13:647–51.

Pak CY. Kidney stones. Lancet 1998;351:1797–801.

Pak CY, Britton F, Peterson R, et al. Ambulatory evaluation of nephrolithiasis: Classification, clinical presentation and diagnostic criteria. Am J Med 1980;69:19–30.

Rahman NU, Meng MV, Stoller ML. Infections and urinary stone disease. Curr Pharm Des 2003;9:975–81.

Shekarriz B, Stoller ML. Uric acid nephrolithiasis: Current concepts and controversies. J Urol 2002;168:1307–14.

The Sexually Transmitted Diseases

Genital Ulcer Disease: Chancroid, Granuloma Inguinale, and Lymphogranuloma

Method of
Todd Stephens, MD

Chancroid, granuloma inguinale, and lymphogranuloma venereum (LGV) are important genital ulcer diseases that should be included in the differential diagnosis of patients presenting with anal or genital ulcers with or without inguinal adenopathy. Syphilis and herpes simplex virus testing should be considered on all such patients because of similarities in clinical presentation. Testing or treatment for other potential sexually transmitted infections (STIs), including HIV, should be considered given the high risk for concomitant infection.

Chancroid

HISTORY

Chancroid, also called soft sore, was first distinguished from the hard chancre of syphilis by Ricord in 1838. Ducrey, in Naples, demonstrated that inoculation of material from the chancroid ulcer into the skin of the forearm could reproduce the ulcer, and he went on to identify the causative organism, which bears his name.

EPIDEMIOLOGY

Chancroid is an important cause of genital ulceration in most countries of the developing world, accounting for about 10 million cases annually. Chancroid was diagnosed in 60% of patients who had genital ulcers and who presented to STI clinics in Africa before the HIV epidemic. Now, herpes simplex lesions represent a higher percentage. The prevalence of this disease is highest among commercial sex workers, and the presence of chancroid lesions significantly increases the risk of transmission of HIV. Although generally rare in industrialized countries, there have been several well-documented outbreaks in urban centers of North America, particularly among men who have sex with men.

ETIOLOGY

Chancroid is caused by *Haemophilus ducreyi*, a small anaerobic gram-negative bacillus that forms streptobacillary chains on Gram stain and grows only on enriched media.

CLINICAL FEATURES

After an incubation of 3 to 7 days, a papule appears that soon ulcerates, leaving a soft ulcer with an undermined edge and a purulent base. Vesicles are not seen. About half of patients develop unilateral inguinal adenopathy (Fig. 1). Both the adenopathy and the lesions are very painful. Lesions can be single or multiple, and atypical presentations occur. Kissing lesions often occur on adjacent cutaneous surfaces. Not infrequently, a giant ulcer develops with several smaller satellite ulcers around the periphery, which can mimic the ulcerative phase of herpes simplex. More than half of the lesions occur on the prepuce, particularly in uncircumcised men. In women, the majority of lesions are on the fourchette, labia, and perianal area. Adenopathy can progress to bubo formation with tender, overlying erythema. These buboes can rupture and produce inguinal abscesses.

DIAGNOSIS

Gram stain of smears obtained from the ulcer base has been advocated in the past for diagnosis, but this lacks both sensitivity and specificity. The preferred diagnostic modality is swabs for culture from the ulcer base or undermined edge. These are plated directly on enriched media (GC agar and Mueller-Hinton agar base) and incubated for 72 hours in an atmosphere of 5% carbon dioxide at 33°C. Polymerase chain reaction (PCR) and immunochromatography tests are also available.

TREATMENT

The Centers for Disease Control and Prevention (CDC) recommend a syndromal management approach in which a positive diagnosis is suggested if the patient has one or more painful ulcers and no evidence of syphilis or herpes simplex virus. Ulcers with painful adenopathy are pathognomonic (Table 1 lists antimicrobial treatment). The safety and efficacy of azithromycin (Zithromax) for pregnant and lactating women have not been established. Ciprofloxacin (Cipro)[1] is contraindicated during pregnancy and lactation. No adverse effects of chancroid on pregnancy outcome have been reported. Serologic testing for syphilis, HIV, and other appropriate STIs should be performed. Chancroidal ulcers should be kept clean with regular washing in soapy water and kept dry. Fluctuant buboes might require incision and drainage, which is preferable over needle aspiration. Treatment of all sexual partners within

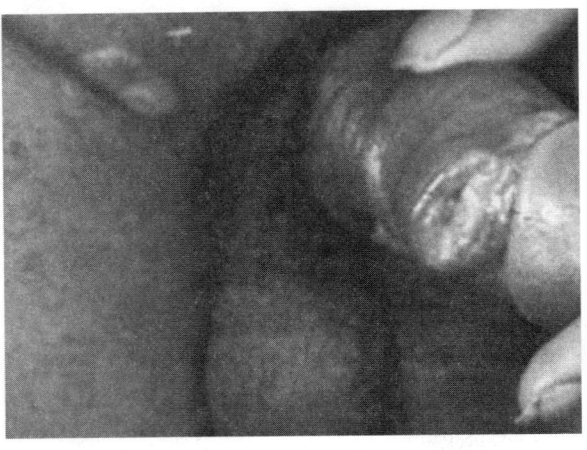

FIGURE 1. Chancroid. This photo shows an early chancroid ulcer on the penis along with accompanying regional inguinal adenopathy. (Courtesy of Dr. Pirozzi, Centers for Disease Control and Prevention.)

60 days should be pursued, and treatment is similar to that for the source patient. Patients should not engage in sexual activity until the ulcers are healed.

Granuloma Inguinale (Donovanosis)

HISTORY

Granuloma inguinale was first recognized in India, where Donovan observed the bodies that bear his name in an oral lesion of the disease. There is considerable confusion about terminology

---

[1]Not FDA approved for this indication.

between this disease and LGV, because various similar synonyms have been used inconsistently. Adding to the confusion, Donovan's name is associated with two tropical diseases that he discovered: Leishmaniasis, with the discovery of intracellular protozoan inclusions that bear his name (Leishman-Donovan bodies), and granuloma inguinale (whose intracellular inclusions were believed to be caused by protozoa but are now known to be caused by bacteria).

EPIDEMIOLOGY

Endemic areas are localized to a few specific areas of the tropics, particularly India, Papua New Guinea, Brazil, and the eastern part of South Africa, particularly Durban. Commercial sex workers and men are primarily involved.

ETIOLOGY

The disease is caused by an encapsulated gram-negative coccobacillus *Klebsiella granulomatis* (previously known as *Calymmatobacterium* or *Donovania granulomatis*).

CLINICAL FEATURES

A firm, painless papule or nodule is the presenting sign of granuloma inguinale. The incubation period is variable from 3 to 40 days from inoculation. This nodule quickly ulcerates, and the base is highly vascular, is beefy red, and bleeds easily. Lymphadenopathy is not part of the clinical presentation of this disease, distinguishing granuloma inguinale from chancroid and LGV. However, the ulcer can be easily confused with chancroid, condyloma lata, ulcerated verrucous warts, and squamous carcinoma. Untreated, the ulcers slowly expand, particularly along skin folds toward the inguinal region or anus (Fig. 2). The ulcers are flat and raised and have slightly hypertrophic margins, but the bases are typically free of pus and necrotic debris. Less-common presentations include extragenital lesions involving the neck and mouth; cervical lesions that resemble carcinoma; and involvement of the uterus, tubes, and ovaries, producing hard masses, abscesses, or frozen pelvis.

TABLE 1 Clinical Features and Treatment Summary of Chancroid, Granuloma Inguinale, and Lymphogranuloma Venereum

Features and Treatment	Chancroid	Granuloma Inguinale	Lymphogranuloma Venereum
Clinical Features			
Incubation period	11-14 days	3-42 days	1-28 days
Primary lesion	Papule	Papule	Papule or vesicle
Ulcerative lesion painful	Yes	No	No
Lymphadenopathy	Yes (unilateral)	No	Yes (unilateral)
Base	Purulent	Raised, easily bleeds	Nonvascular
Border	Round, raised, undermined edges	Irregular, expansion along skin folds	Irregular, ragged
Treatment			
Treatment of choice (any of the options listed)	Azithromycin (Zithromycin) 1 g Ciprofloxacin (Cipro)[1] 500 mg bid × 3 d Ceftriaxone (Rocephin)[1] 250 mg IM once	Azithromycin[1] 1 g weekly* Doxycycline (Vibramycin) 100 mg bid*	Azithromycin[1] 1 g weekly × 3 wk Doxycycline 100 mg bid × 3 wk
Alternative treatment (any of the options listed)	Erythromycin (Ery-Tab)[1] 500 mg qid × 7 d	Erythromycin[1] 500 mg* Ciprofloxacin[1] 750 mg* Tetracycline 500 mg*	Erythromycin[1] 500 mg qid × 3 wk Doxycycline 100 mg bid × 3 wk Tetracycline 500 mg qid × 3 wk

*Continue until lesions are re-epithelialized.
[1]Not FDA approved for this indication.

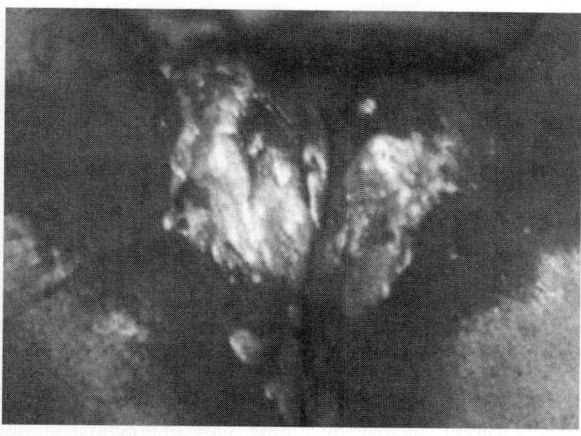

FIGURE 2. Granuloma Inguinale. (Source: NEHC http://www.nhec.med.navy.mil/hp/sharp/std_pictures.htm)

DIAGNOSIS

Diagnosis requires the demonstration of intracellular Donovan bodies from Giemsa or Wright staining of smears taken from a swab of the ulcer base or from biopsy material.

TREATMENT

See Table 1 for antimicrobial treatment. Treatment should be continued until lesions are resolved and, if possible, a little longer to reduce the risk of relapse.

Lymphogranuloma Venereum

HISTORY

LGV was first differentiated from syphilis in 1906 by Wasserman, though the first full description of the disease was given by Durand, Nicolas, and Favre in 1913. In 1925, Frei developed an intradermal skin test that gave positive responses in most LGV patients. The term "tropical bubo" was associated with the disease later.

EPIDEMIOLOGY

LGV is largely confined to the tropics and is not a common STI. The global overall incidence is in a decline. It is seen more commonly in men, but since 2004, there has been a resurgence manifesting as proctitis in North America and Europe among HIV-positive men who have sex with men.

ETIOLOGY

LGV is a chlamydial infection caused by the invasive L1, L2, and L3 serovars of *Chlamydia trachomatis*, an intracellular gram-negative bacterium.

CLINICAL FEATURES

LGV is essentially a systemic disease whose natural course is divided into three distinct phases. The initial phase of LGV is normally an inconspicuous genital lesion beginning as a typically small, painless papule or vesicle occurring 1 to 28 days after inoculation. This papule or vesicle quickly ulcerates and heals without a scar, and it often goes unrecognized by the patient (Fig. 3). However, the second phase of LGV is the development of increasingly painful lymphadenopathy, often with fever and malaise. The lymphadenopathy progresses to bubo formation over 1 to 2 weeks. When a sexually active adult patient presents with an inguinal bubo not associated with genital ulcers, LGV is an important diagnosis to consider. The infected nodes are usually unilateral (bilateral in a third of cases) and often coalesce into a matted mass that can project outwards above or below the inguinal ligament, producing the pathognomonic groove sign present in 20% of patients with LGV. The buboes are likely to rupture, forming multiple sinuses. Untreated, LGV can cause extensive lymphatic damage, resulting in elephantiasis of the genitalia. Anal involvement,

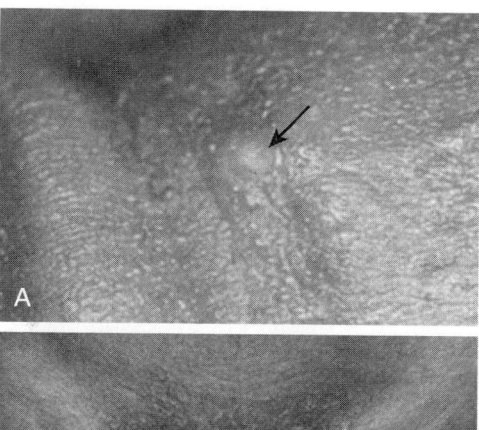
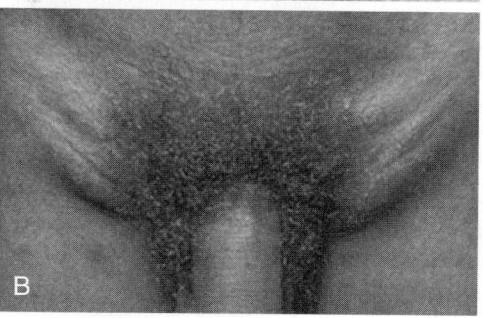

FIGURE 3. Lymphogranuloma venereum. **A,** Small ulcerative lesion near corona of penis *(arrow)*. **B,** Bilateral inguinal adenopathy, with developing groove sign as adenopathy expands above and below the inguinal ligament. (**A** Courtesy of Ronald Ballard, Reproduced with permission from The Diagnosis and Management of Sexually Transmitted Infections in South Africa, 3rd ed., Johannesburg, South African Institute for Medical Research, 2000. **B** courtesy of Connexions, [http://cnx.org/content/m14883/latest/Case_10-pres1-1.jpg])

likewise, can lead to perirectal abscesses, fistulas, and rectal strictures. These complications represent the late phase of LGV.

DIAGNOSIS

The diagnosis of LGV can only be confirmed using PCR methods of smears, scrapings, or aspirated material. Alternatively, the ability to perform micro-immunofluorescence serology testing using a fluorescein-conjugated monoclonal antibody and viewing the slide with a fluorescence microscope can demonstrate the inclusion bodies within the cytoplasm of macrophages. Gram staining by itself lacks appropriate sensitivity or specificity. Additional laboratory findings include leukocytosis, elevated erythrocyte sedimentation rate, and increases in immunoglobulin G and cryoglobulins.

TREATMENT

Antimicrobial treatment is summarized in Table 1. Needle aspiration or incision and drainage of fluctuant buboes may be required for symptomatic relief but are not routinely recommended for treatment because drainage can delay healing. Fistula openings should receive sterile dressings. One of the primary goals of treatment of LGV is to prevent long-term complications such as anogenital strictures or fistulas. Plastic surgical operations may be of benefit in cases with extensive rectal strictures or elephantiasis of the genitalia. However, these surgical interventions should only be performed after a prolonged course of antibiotics. Scars should be monitored to detect malignant change.

REFERENCES

Centers for Disease Control and Prevention, Workowski KA, Berman SM. Sexually transmitted diseases treatment guidelines, 2006, MMWR Recomm Rep Aug 4;2006;55(RR-11):1–94. Available at http://www.cdc.gov/std/treatment/default.htm; [accessed 28, 2010].

Habif T. Clinical Dermatology. 4th ed. Philadelphia: Mosby; 2004. p. 325–9.

Leppard B. An Atlas of African Dermatology. Oxon, UK: Radcliffe Medical Press; 2002. p. 69 151,237.

Ndinya-Achola JO, Kihara AN, Fisher LD, et al. Presumptive specific clinical diagnosis of genital ulcer disease (GUD) in a primary health care setting in Nairobi. Int J STD AIDS 1996;7(3):201–5.

Richens J, Mabey DC. Sexually transmitted infections (excluding HIV). In: Cook GC, Zumla AI, editors. Manson's Tropical Diseases. 22nd ed London: Saunders; 2009. p. 403–34.

Ronald A. Chancroid. In: Hunter GW, Strickland GT, Magill AJ, editors. Hunter's Tropical Medicine and Emerging Infectious Diseases. 8th ed Philadelphia: WB Saunders; 2000. p. 367–9.

Gonorrhea

Method of
Khalil G. Ghanem, MD, PhD

Gonorrhea is caused by the gram-negative diplococcus *Neisseria gonorrhoeae*, an obligate parasite of humans that has no other natural host and to which no animal is naturally susceptible. In 2007, 355,991 cases were reported to the Centers for Disease Control and Prevention (CDC). This number is likely an underestimate because many cases are asymptomatic and others go unreported. Rates of gonorrhea in the United States declined sharply starting in the 1970s after the institution of gonorrhea control programs. It remains, however, the second most commonly reported communicable disease. Worldwide, more than 60 million new cases are estimated to occur every year.

In 2007 in the United States, the gonorrhea rate among women was 123.5 and the rate among men was 113.7 cases per 100,000 people in the general population; the rate among African Americans was 19 times greater than the rate for whites, although this is a decrease from 2001, when there was a 26-fold difference. Risk factors for infection include young age, unprotected intercourse, multiple sexual partners, new sexual partners, and sexual activity associated with illicit drug use. Gonococcal infection increases the rate of HIV transmission fivefold.

N. gonorrhoeae infects noncornified epithelia, including urethral, endocervical, rectal, oropharyngeal, and conjunctival cells. It is transmitted through contact with infected secretions, most often sexually, although vertical transmission from mother to infant is well described. Sexual transmission is efficient; a man who has intercourse 2.5 times with an infected female partner has a 22% chance of becoming symptomatically infected. The transmission from men to women is thought to be even more efficient.

Clinical Manifestations

Asymptomatic urethral infections occur in at least 10% of men and asymptomatic cervical infections occur in about 40% to 50% of women. More than 50% of rectal and up to 90% of pharyngeal gonorrhea in men and women may be asymptomatic. These numbers highlight the importance of a thorough sexual history in all at-risk patients that focuses on a history of exposure rather than symptoms.

In men, urethritis is the most common manifestation of gonococcal infection. Urethral discharge and dysuria are the most frequent signs occurring 2 to 5 days after exposure. Acute epididymitis manifesting as unilateral scrotal pain is the most common local complication. In young men, 30% of cases of acute epididymitis are caused by *N. gonorrhoeae*. Rarely, cellulitis, lymphangitis, or periurethral abscesses may complicate local infections. Differential diagnosis of urethritis in men includes *Chlamydia trachomatis*, *Mycoplasma genitalium*, and *Trichomonas vaginalis* infections.

Among women, the most common manifestation of local gonococcal infection is cervicitis, which tends to occur 5 to 10 days after exposure. When patients are symptomatic, common complaints include a vaginal discharge, dysuria, and genital itching. Concomitant infection of the urethra may occur in up to 90% of women and accounts for some of these symptoms. *N. gonorrhoeae* may also infect Skene's and Bartholin's glands. The differential diagnosis of cervicitis includes infection with *C. trachomatis*, *T. vaginalis*, *M. genitalium*, or herpes simplex virus and bacterial vaginosis. An important complication of gonococcal infections in women is pelvic inflammatory disease (PID). PID is the result of ascending infection involving the uterus, fallopian tubes, ovaries, or peritoneum. Sequelae of PID include infertility, ectopic pregnancy, and chronic pelvic pain. All women presenting with cervicitis should undergo a bimanual examination. The diagnosis of PID is made when one or more of the following signs are present: uterine tenderness, cervical motion tenderness, or adnexal tenderness.

Among men and women with rectal gonorrhea, those who are symptomatic may complain of rectal discharge, pain, and tenesmus. Most cases of rectal gonorrhea in men result from receptive anal intercourse; some cases in women may result from perineal contamination. The differential diagnosis includes *C. trachomatis* (including lymphogranuloma venereum strains), *Treponema pallidum*, and herpes simplex virus infections. Most cases of pharyngeal gonorrhea are asymptomatic; when present, signs and symptoms may include acute pharyngitis, tonsillitis, and cervical lymphadenopathy.

The pharynx may be the only infected site in up to 10% of patients. A careful history, including past oral-genital contact, is mandatory. Conjunctivitis is rare in adults and usually is a result of self-inoculation from anogenital infections.

Disseminated gonococcal infections may occur in up to 2% of untreated patients. Certain gonococcal strains are more likely to cause disseminated gonococcal infections. Although patients are bacteremic, many appear nontoxic. Symptoms and signs may include fevers, myalgias, arthralgias, asymmetrical polyarthritis, and a characteristic dermatitis consisting of a small number (<30) of skin lesions on the distal extremities that begin as papules and progress to pustules and ulcerations. Rarely, meningitis and endocarditis may occur.

Vertical transmission to neonates may result in ophthalmia neonatorum, sepsis, arthritis, meningitis, rhinitis, vaginitis, urethritis, and inflammation at the sites of fetal monitoring. Gonococcal infections diagnosed in preadolescent children usually indicate sexual abuse.

Diagnosis

Gram's stain of urethral discharge among symptomatic men is 90% sensitive and 95% specific. It is only 70% sensitive in asymptomatic men. Endocervical Gram's stain is only 50% to 70% sensitive, and anal swabs are only 60% sensitive. Culture (usually on Thayer-Martin medium) is 95% sensitive in symptomatic men but is less so for asymptomatic men and women (80%–90%). The sensitivity of culture in detecting gonococcal infections from urine is low. Culture is the most common test used to diagnose pharyngeal and rectal infections (despite low sensitivity) and is the only FDA-approved test to diagnose gonococcal infections in children. Antibiotic susceptibility testing can be performed only on cultured specimens.

Definitive diagnosis of gonorrhea by culture from any genital or extragenital site requires confirmation of isolates by biochemical, enzymatic, serologic, or nucleic acid testing (e.g., carbohydrate use, rapid enzyme substrate tests, serologic methods such as coagglutination or fluorescent antibody tests) supplemented with additional tests that can ensure accurate identification of isolates or a DNA probe technique for confirmation. After the culture is submitted, this type of identification is usually performed by the laboratory without requesting it, and when these methods are used, there should be no pitfalls in interpreting the extragenital culture data.

Nonamplified molecular tests (e.g., GenProbe Pace II) are the most common tests used in the United States. The sensitivity is 85% to 90%, and the specificity is more than 95%. The tests can be performed only on urethral or endocervical specimens. Nucleic acid amplification tests (e.g., polymerase chain reaction, transcription-mediated amplification) are the most sensitive (>95%) and specific (>95%), and most can be performed on urethral or cervical specimens in addition to urine and self-collected vaginal swabs. Among women, vaginal swabs are the preferred collection specimen. Nucleic acid amplification tests are not FDA cleared for pharyngeal and rectal specimens, although data increasingly suggest that some are far more sensitive than culture in detecting gonococcal infections at these sites. Many commercial laboratories now offer testing of extragenital specimens using nucleic acid amplification. Serologic tests

CURRENT DIAGNOSIS

- Gonorrhea is caused by the gram-negative diplococcus *Neisseria gonorrhoeae*.
- Asymptomatic genital gonococcal infections are common in men and women.
- Most cases of rectal and pharyngeal infections are asymptomatic.
- Culture and molecular tests are available for diagnosis, depending on the specimen type and anatomic site tested.
- All patients diagnosed with gonorrhea should be tested for other sexually transmitted infections, including HIV.

CURRENT THERAPY

- Ceftriaxone (Rocephin) 125 mg IM × 1 *or* cefixime (Suprax) 400 mg PO × 1 is the first-line treatment for gonorrhea.
- In the United States, fluoroquinolones should no longer be used to treat gonorrhea.
- Patients treated for gonorrhea also should be treated for concomitant *Chlamydia trachomatis* infection.

have been used for epidemiologic studies, but they should not be used for diagnosis. All patients tested for gonorrhea should also be tested for *Chlamydia trachomatis*, syphilis, and HIV.

ANTIMICROBIAL RESISTANCE AND THERAPY

For 40 years, penicillin was the drug of choice for treating gonorrhea. Tetracyclines were also highly effective. By the 1980s, widespread resistance to both of these drug classes rendered them all but useless. Subsequently, drug resistance to aminoglycosides, spectinomycin,[2] macrolides, trimethoprim-sulfamethoxazole (Bactrim),[1] and fluoroquinolones has made the treatment of gonorrhea more challenging.

Fluoroquinolone-resistant *N. gonorrhoeae* (FQRNG) strains emerged in the 1990s, and high rates have been reported in Asia, Africa, and the Middle East. In April 2007, the CDC recommended that fluoroquinolones not be used to treat gonococcal infections in the United States.

Table 1 summarizes the current CDC recommendations for treating uncomplicated and complicated gonococcal infections. Since 1997,

---

[1]Not FDA approved for this indication.
[2]Not available in the United States.

TABLE 1 Centers for Disease Control and Prevention 2006 Treatment Recommendations for Complicated and Uncomplicated Gonorrhea

Disease	Treatment
Uncomplicated infections of the cervix, urethra, and rectum*	Ceftriaxone (Rocephin) 125 mg IM × 1 *or* Cefixime (Suprax) 400 mg PO × 1 *plus* Treatment for *Chlamydia trachomatis* if not ruled out: Azithromycin (Zithromax) 1g PO × 1 *or* Doxycycline (Vibramycin) 100 mg PO bid × 7 d
Infections of the pharynx	Ceftriaxone (Rocephin) 125 mg IM × 1 *plus* Treatment for *Chlamydia trachomatis* if not ruled out
Epididymitis	Ceftriaxone (Rocephin) 250 mg IM × 1 *plus* Doxycycline (Vibramycin) 100 mg PO bid × 10 d
Gonococcal conjunctivitis	Ceftriaxone (Rocephin) 1g IM × 1
Disseminated gonococcal infections[†]	Ceftriaxone (Rocephin) 1g IM or IV q24h

*Alternate agents include spectinomycin 2 g IM × 1, if available.
[†]Should be treated with a parenteral regimen until 24 hours after clinical improvement; can complete a 7-day course of therapy with oral cefixime.

---

there have been no reports of ceftriaxone-resistant strains in the United States. Cephalosporins are the most reliable and only recommended first-line agents to treat gonorrhea. Ceftriaxone (Rocephin) is given intramuscularly and is effective for infections at all sites. Cefixime (Suprax) is effective for anogenital infections, but it may have lower efficacy than ceftriaxone for pharyngeal infections. Cephalosporins are safe to use in pregnancy. Patients should be treated for presumed *C. trachomatis* co-infection unless it is ruled out. All sexual contacts in the preceding 60 days of index patients should also be treated.

For penicillin-allergic patients, treatment of gonorrhea has become more challenging. Initially, spectinomycin was recommended as a second-line agent. Spectinomycin has only 80% efficacy in treating pharyngeal gonococcal infections, but spectinomycin is no longer available in the United States.

Alternate agents include a single dose of azithromycin (Zithromax) 2 gm PO. The gastrointestinal side effects associated with this high dose and concern about increasing drug resistance resulted in the CDC dropping it as a second-line agent in its 2006 treatment guidelines. However, if tolerated by the patient, this regimen has excellent activity against anogenital and pharyngeal infections. Azithromycin has been used in pregnant women without evidence of teratogenicity.

To prevent gonococcal ophthalmia neonatorum, 1% silver nitrate aqueous solution, 0.5% erythromycin ophthalmic ointment (Ilotycin), or 1% tetracycline ophthalmic ointment[1] should be instilled into the eyes of all newborns. Treatment of gonococcal ophthalmia requires hospitalization, evaluation for evidence of disseminated infection, and ceftriaxone (Rocephin) 25 to 50 mg/kg IM or IV × 1 dose.

Several drugs are being tested for the treatment of gonorrhea. They include cefpodoxime (Vantin), ertapenem (Invanz),[1] telithromycin (Ketek),[1] tigecycline (Tygacil),[1] and newer-generation fluoroquinolones (e.g., gemifloxacin [Factive][1]). None is currently recommended by the CDC.

Prevention and Screening

Abstinence from sexual intercourse is the single most reliable method of preventing infection. Male condoms, when used correctly and consistently, are highly effective in preventing infection. Diaphragms may help prevent gonococcal infections in women. There have not been any successful vaccine candidates.

The CDC does not recommend universal screening for *N. gonorrhoeae*. High-risk women (e.g., multiple sexual partners, illicit drug use, history of gonorrhea or other sexually transmitted infection, commercial sex worker, inconsistent condom use) should be screened. Up to 20% of heterosexual men and women diagnosed

---

[1]Not FDA approved for this indication.

with gonorrhea become reinfected in the next few months. High-risk pregnant women should be screened during the first prenatal visit. Repeat testing during the third trimester for those at continued risk is recommended.

REFERENCES

Centers for Disease Control and Prevention. Update to CDC's sexually transmitted diseases treatment guidelines, 2006: Fluoroquinolones no longer recommended for treatment of gonococcal infections. MMWR Morb Mortal Wkly Rep 2007;56(14):332–6.

Newman LM, Moran JS, Workowski KA. Update on the management of gonorrhea in adults in the United States. Clin Infect Dis 2007;44: S84–101.

Schachter J, Moncada J, Liska S, et al. Nucleic acid amplification tests in the diagnosis of chlamydial and gonococcal infections of the oropharynx and rectum in men who have sex with men. Sex Transm Dis 2008;35 (7):637–42.

Workowski KA, Berman SM, Douglas Jr JM. Emerging antimicrobial resistance in Neisseria gonorrhoeae: Urgent need to strengthen prevention strategies. Ann Intern Med 2008;148(8):606–13.

Workowski KA, Berman SM. for the Centers for Disease Control and Prevention. Sexually transmitted diseases treatment guidelines, 2006. MMWR Morb Mortal Wkly Rep 2006;55(RR-11):1–94.

Nongonococcal Urethritis

Method of
John N. Krieger, MD

Urethritis is defined as inflammation of the urethra and is commonly caused by urogenital infection. Urethritis is classified as either gonococcal, in patients whose inflammation is caused by *Neisseria gonorrhoeae*, or nongonococcal (NGU), in patients with inflammation that is not related to infection with *N. gonorrhoeae*.

Clinical Presentation

More than 4 million NGU cases are estimated to occur among men in the United States every year. Urethritis is characterized by symptoms of urethral discharge and dysuria, often accompanied by increased urinary frequency or pruritus. Signs of urethritis include urethral discharge that can occur spontaneously or after stripping of the urethra, erythema, and urethral tenderness.

Although the clinical presentation varies, the incubation of NGU averages 7 to 14 days from exposure to an infected partner. Typically the onset is gradual, with mild dysuria and mucoid discharge. In some high-risk populations, up to 50% of infections are asymptomatic.

Etiology

NGU should be considered infectious until proven otherwise. Most infectious cases of urethritis are sexually transmitted.

Chlamydia trachomatis remains the most important pathogen, accounting for 15% to 40% of NGU cases. The prevalence of *C. trachomatis* is lower in older patients and in referral populations. Other infectious causes of NGU include *Mycoplasma genitalium*, *Trichomonas vaginalis*, and herpes simplex virus. The etiologic roles are less well defined for other infectious agents including *Ureaplasma urealyticum*, enteric bacteria, anaerobes, and *Candida* species.

CURRENT DIAGNOSIS

- Documenting urethral inflammation is critical for diagnosis of urethritis. One or more of the following techniques can provide documentation:

  - Physical examination showing urethral discharge, either present spontaneously at the meatus or after stripping the urethra. This discharge may be either mucoid or purulent in character.
  - Gram stain of urethral exudate showing five or more WBCs per oil immersion field ($\times 1000$). The Gram stain is the preferred rapid diagnostic test.
  - Urine leukocyte esterase dip stick test positive on first-void urine
  - First-void urine sediment microscopic examination demonstrating 10 or more WBCs per high-power field ($\times 400$).

Abbreviation: WBC = white blood cell.

Occasionally, patients with other urologic conditions (e.g., prostatitis, urethral stricture disease, or, rarely, bacterial urinary tract infection) present with symptoms of NGU. Other unusual causes of NGU include chemical, allergic, and autoimmune processes.

Diagnosis

It is important to document the presence of urethral inflammation. This may be done by finding mucoid or mucopurulent discharge on physical examination or by diagnostic testing. The Gram stain is the preferred rapid diagnostic test. Urethral inflammation may also be documented by a positive leukocyte esterase test on first-void urine or by finding pyuria on microscopic examination of the first-void urine sediment.

Diagnostic testing for both *N. gonorrhoeae* and *C. trachomatis* organisms is strongly recommended. Specific etiologic diagnosis may guide therapy and can improve compliance and partner notification. These infections are both reportable to state health departments. Patients at risk for *N. gonorrhoeae* and *C. trachomatis* should receive appropriate counseling and should receive testing for HIV and syphilis. Clinical evaluation and treatment of sex partners are critical for preventing complications and interrupting sexual transmission. Pathogens responsible for NGU are associated with cervicitis, pelvic inflammatory disease, and tubal infertility.

The Gram stain is the preferred rapid diagnostic test for evaluating urethritis because it provides high sensitivity and specificity. Gonococcal infection can be established by documenting the presence of white blood cells (WBCs) containing intracellular gram-negative diplococci. Presence of gram-negative rods should raise the suspicion for enteric bacteria.

Confirmatory tests should be employed to identify a specific etiology. *N. gonorrhoeae* and *C. trachomatis* can be detected using culture, DNA hybridization tests on a urethral specimen, or nucleic acid amplification tests on a urethral or urine specimen. Because of their increased sensitivity, nucleic acid amplification tests are recommended for diagnosing chlamydial infection. For urine testing, 10 to 15 mL of first-void urine is collected then evaluated using nucleic acid amplification testing.

Diagnostic tests for the genital mycoplasmas (*M. genitalium*, *U. urealyticum*, and other genital mycoplasmas) are available in research settings. Such tests are usually unavailable for routine clinical use. *T. vaginalis* may be cultured, but specific media are necessary for isolation. To increase sensitivity, cultures of both a urethral swab sample and a urine specimen are recommended.

Treatment

If gonorrhea cannot be ruled out by Gram stain of urethral secretions, potentially noncompliant patients should be treated for both gonorrhea and chlamydial infection. Both azithromycin (Zithromax) and doxycycline (Vibramycin) are highly effective for treating chlamydial NGU. Azithromycin also provides convenient single dosing and the opportunity for directly observed therapy. Doxycycline is inexpensive but requires twice-daily dosing for a full week. Alternatives include erythromycin and fluoroquinolone regimens.

For patients with erratic health care–seeking behavior in whom poor compliance is anticipated, azithromycin offers the easiest administration. Further, *M. genitalium* appears to respond better to macrolides than to tetracyclines. Patients should be advised to abstain from sex until therapy is completed, symptoms have resolved, and sex partners have been treated.

Follow-up

Routine follow-up is not recommended for patients whose symptoms resolve after therapy. Patients with persistent or recurrent symptoms should return for reevaluation.

Symptoms alone should not prompt a second course of therapy unless the patient has documented urethritis or a positive test for a urogenital pathogen. Patients should return for evaluation and treatment if their symptoms persist or recur after completion of therapy. Patients with NGU should refer all sex partners in the past 60 days for evaluation and treatment.

Chronic Urethritis

Chronic urethritis is defined as persistent or recurrent urethritis within 6 weeks following treatment. An estimated 20% to 40% of NGU cases do not respond to first-line therapy. Although up to 20% of men with chlamydial NGU develop chronic urethritis, up to 50% of men with nonchlamydial NGU develop chronic urethritis. Noncompliance and reinfection are important considerations. Other causes include organisms that do not respond to the standard treatment regimens, such as *T. vaginalis*, tetracycline-resistant mycoplasmas, viral etiologies, and other bacteria.

CURRENT THERAPY

Recommended Regimens

- Azithromycin (Zithromax) 1 g PO in a single dose
- Doxycycline (Vibramycin) 100 mg PO bid × 7 days

Alternative Regimens

- Erythromycin base (E-Mycin, ERYC, E-Base) 500 mg PO qid × 7 days
- Erythromycin ethylsuccinate (EES) 800 mg PO qid × 7 days
- Ofloxacin (Floxin) 300 mg PO bid × 7 days
- Levofloxacin (Levaquin)[1] 500 mg PO qd × 7 days
- If an erythromycin regimen is the only possibility and the patient cannot tolerate high-dose schedules, then one of the following regimens should be considered:
- Erythromycin base (E-Mycin, ERYC, E-Base) 250 mg PO qid × 14 days
- Erythromycin ethylsuccinate (EES) 400 mg PO qid × 14 days

---

[1]Not FDA approved for this indication.

Up to 30% of NGU has no identifiable infectious etiology. These cases can involve allergy and postinfectious immunologic responses. Before administering therapy, presence of urethral inflammation should be documented. Patients with persistent or recurrent urethritis who did not comply with therapy or who had exposure to an untreated sex partner should be re-treated with the initial drug regimen. Otherwise, recommended treatment regimens include metronidazole (Flagyl),[1] 2 g orally in a single dose, plus either erythromycin base (E-Base), 500 mg orally four times a day for 7 days, or erythromycin ethylsuccinate (EES), 800 mg orally four times a day for 7 days.

Complications

For infected men, complications of untreated NGU include epididymitis in less than 3% of cases and, rarely, Reiter's syndrome. Patients with a history of NGU also appear to be at increased risk for developing chronic prostatitis/chronic pelvic pain syndrome.

Female sex partners are at risk for pelvic inflammatory disease, tubal infertility, and ectopic pregnancy. Prompt and appropriate therapy and treatment of sexual partners decrease the risk of complications substantially.

REFERENCES

Aydin D, Kucukbasmaci O, Gonullu N, Aktas Z. Susceptibilities of *Neisseria gonorrhoeae* and *Ureaplasma urealyticum* isolates from male patients with urethritis to several antibiotics including telithromycin. Chemotherapy 2005;51:89–92.

Bradshaw CS, Tabrizi SN, Read TR, et al. Etiologies of nongonococcal urethritis: Bacteria, viruses, and the association with orogenital exposure. J Infect Dis 2006;193:336–45.

Centers for Disease Control and Prevention. Screening tests to detect *Chlamydia trachomatis* and *Neisseria gonorrhoeae* infections. MMWR Recomm Rep 2002;51(RR-15):3–19.

Centers for Disease Control and Prevention. Sexually transmitted disease treatment guidelines 2002. MMWR Recomm Rep 2002;51(RR-6):30–42.

Deguchi T, Yoshida T, Miyazawa T, et al. Association of *Ureaplasma urealyticum* (biovar 2) with nongonococcal urethritis. Sex Transm Dis 2004; 31:192–5.

Falk L, Fredlund H, Jensen JS. Symptomatic urethritis is more prevalent in men infected with *Mycoplasma genitalium* than with *Chlamydia trachomatis*. Sex Transm Infect 2004;80:289–93.

Geisler WM, Yu S, Hook EW 3rd. Chlamydial and gonococcal infection in men without polymorphonuclear leukocytes on Gram stain: Implications for diagnostic approach and management. Sex Transm Dis 2005;32:630–4.

Jensen JS. *Mycoplasma genitalium*: The aetiological agent of urethritis and other sexually transmitted diseases. J Eur Acad Dermatol Venereol 2004;18:1–11.

Kaydos-Daniels SC, Miller WC, Hoffman I, et al. The use of specimens from various genitourinary sites in men, to detect *Trichomonas vaginalis* infection. J Infect Dis 2004;189:1926–31.

Leung A, Eastick K, Haddon LE, et al. *Mycoplasma genitalium* is associated with symptomatic urethritis. Int J STD AIDS 2006;17:285–8.

O'Mahony C. Adenoviral non-gonococcal urethritis. Int J STD AIDS 2006;17:203–4.

Ozgül A, Dede I, Taskaynatan MA, et al. Clinical presentations of chlamydial and non-chlamydial reactive arthritis. Rheumatol Int 2006;26:879–85.

Pontari MA, McNaughton-Collins M, O'Leary P, et al. A case-control study of risk factors in men with chronic pelvic pain syndrome. BJU Int 2005;96:559–65.

Swygard H, Sena AC, Hobbs MM, Cohen MS. Trichomoniasis: Clinical manifestations, diagnosis and management. Sex Transm Infect 2004;80:91–5.

Taylor SN. *Mycoplasma genitalium*. Curr Infect Dis Rep 2005;7:453–7.

Taylor-Robinson D, Gilroy CB, Thomas BJ, Hay PE. *Mycoplasma genitalium* in chronic non-gonococcal urethritis. Int J STD AIDS 2004;15:21–5.

Yasuda M, Maeda S, Deguchi T. In vitro activity of fluoroquinolones against *Mycoplasma genitalium* and their bacteriological efficacy for treatment of *M. genitalium*–positive nongonococcal urethritis in men. Clin Infect Dis 2005;41:1357–9.

---

[1]Not FDA approved for this indication.

Syphilis

Method of
Jennifer Frank, MD

Epidemiology

Primary and secondary syphilis rates have increased since 2000. The initial rise was seen primarily in men, with an increase in women starting in 2003 and in congenital syphilis starting in 2007. Men who have sex with men (MSM) accounted for 65% of cases of primary and secondary syphilis in 2007. Almost one half of primary and secondary syphilis occurs in the South.

Risk factors

MSM and HIV-positive persons are at highest risk for primary and secondary syphilis. Other risk factors include living in the southern part of the United States or an urban area, young age (20 to 29 years), and being born to a mother infected with syphilis.

Pathophysiology

Syphilis is caused by infection with the spirochete *Treponema pallidum* subspecies *pallidum* (Fig. 1). Primary infection manifests with signs and symptoms at the site of infection; secondary and tertiary syphilis manifest with systemic signs and symptoms. Syphilis is primarily sexually transmitted but may be transmitted perinatally or through nonsexual cutaneous transmission.

Prevention

Prevention includes both avoiding initial infection and preventing disease progression through early detection and treatment. Transmission of syphilis can be reduced (although not eliminated) by using condoms. Screening for syphilis in pregnancy combined with treatment of infected women reduces perinatal transmission.

Clinical Manifestations

Primary syphilis manifests as a chancre at the site of inoculation. The chancre, a painless ulcer with sharp borders, is usually solitary and associated with regional lymphadenopathy. Atypical presentations

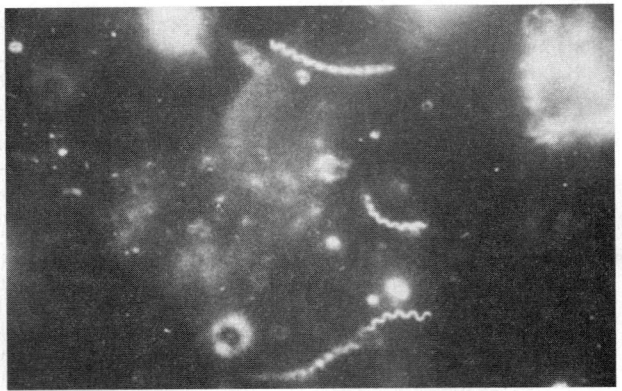

FIGURE 1. *Treponema pallidum* on darkfield microscopy.

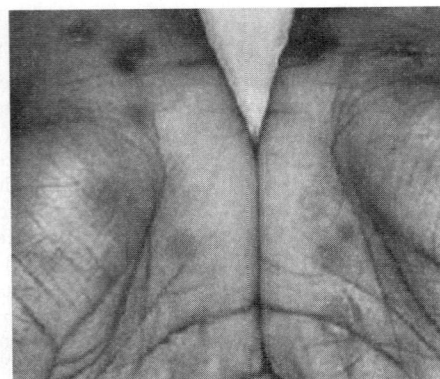

FIGURE 2. Syphilis skin lesion.

include extragenital location (most commonly oral or anal) and the presence of pain or multiple lesions. Secondary syphilis characteristically manifests with a generalized rash with variable features (Fig. 2). The palms and soles are affected in the majority of patients. Typically, the rash is maculopapular or papulosquamous and nonpruritic. Other clinical manifestations include highly infectious flat lesions (condyloma lata), fever, malaise, sore throat, headache, myalgias, alopecia, and, rarely, renal, bone, eye, or liver involvement. Latent syphilis, by definition, has no clinical manifestations.

Tertiary syphilis is a late manifestation in untreated people and includes neurosyphilis, cardiovascular, and gummatous disease. Gummas are nodular lesions that vary in size and location. They can ulcerate and cause local tissue destruction. Other skin lesions include granulomas and plaque formation. Cardiovascular syphilis most commonly manifests as aortitis of the ascending aorta. The clinical manifestations of neurosyphilis are numerous and include meningitis with or without vascular involvement, dementia, tabes dorsalis (posterior column involvement with ataxia and bowel and bladder dysfunction), and ocular or otologic involvement.

Congenital syphilis has early (birth to 2 years) and late (2 to 20 years) clinical manifestations. Early signs include hepatosplenomegaly, rash, fever, neurosyphilis, pneumonitis, rhinitis, generalized lymphadenopathy, hepatitis, ascites, hematologic disease, renal disease, periostitis, and osteochondritis. Late manifestations (present in 40% of untreated patients) include skeletal deformities, neurologic disease (deafness), dental abnormalities, and ocular abnormalities.

Diagnosis

Diagnostic evaluation of syphilis depends on the stage and location of suspected infection. Darkfield microscopy or direct fluorescent antibody testing is done on tissue or exudates obtained from an ulcer or chancre (primary infection). Serologic testing is done using nontreponemal (VDRL or RPR) and treponemal testing (FTA-ABS or TP-PA) because both tests have limitations. Nontreponemal testing may be falsely positive with other medical conditions, but antibody titers correlate with disease activity and therefore can indicate response to treatment. Nontreponemal tests usually become nonreactive after successful treatment. A serofast reaction can occur in which the nontreponemal test stays reactive. Treponemal tests are specific for syphilitic infection but usually stay reactive regardless of treatment or disease status. Treponemal test antibody titers do not match the level of disease activity and therefore cannot be used to monitor treatment response.

Neurosyphilis is diagnosed using laboratory testing and clinical evaluation. Laboratory testing includes reactive serologic testing; cerebrospinal fluid (CSF) VDRL (Venereal Disease Research Laboratory) testing, which is specific but not sensitive; and CSF positive for white blood cells or protein, or both. The CSF FTA-Abs (fluorescent treponemal antibody absorption) test is sensitive but less specific than CSF VDRL testing.

CURRENT DIAGNOSIS

- Serologic testing includes both nontreponemal-specific testing (VDRL and RPR) and treponemal-specific testing (FTA-Abs [fluorescent treponemal antibody absorption] and TP-PA [*Treponema pallidum* particle agglutination]).
- Cerebrospinal fluid testing (VDRL [Venereal Disease Research Laboratory], protein, cell count) is performed to diagnose neurosyphilis.

Differential Diagnosis

Syphilis, which can affect every organ system, has historically been called the great mimicker. Syphilis is on the differential diagnosis of, most commonly, conditions causing genital ulcers or lesions, conditions causing systemic rashes affecting the palms and soles, conditions causing ocular and otologic manifestations (uveitis, sudden visual changes, hearing loss), and conditions causing dementia, meningitis, or ataxia.

Treatment

Penicillin G is the preferred treatment for all stages of syphilis. The stage and extent of clinical disease determine which preparation is used, the dosage, and the length of treatment (Table 1). In penicillin-allergic patients, antibiotic alternatives exist for all types and stages of syphilis except for syphilis in pregnancy and congenital syphilis.

Neurosyphilis is ideally treated with penicillin. Alternative treatment of primary and secondary syphilis and early latent syphilis

CURRENT THERAPY

- Penicillin is first-line therapy for all types and stages of syphilis.
- Penicillin is the only recommended treatment for pregnant women and for congenital syphilis. Penicillin-allergic patients should undergo desensitization.

includes doxycycline (Vibramycin) 100 mg orally twice a day or tetracycline 500 mg orally four times daily for 14 days or ceftriaxone (Rocephin)[1] 1 g daily IM or IV for 8 to 10 days. Azithromycin (Zithromax)[1] 2 g orally as a single dose may be used, although treatment failures have been reported. Late latent or tertiary syphilis can be treated with doxycycline 100 mg orally twice daily or tetracycline 500 mg orally four times daily for 28 days. Ceftriaxone[1] 2 g given IV or IM daily for 10 to 14 days has been described for the treatment of neurosyphilis in penicillin-allergic patients.

The Jarisch-Herxheimer reaction is an acute febrile reaction (with accompanying headache, myalgias, and other symptoms) occurring within 24 hours of treatment of syphilis. It is more common in early stages of syphilis and rare in newborns.

Monitoring

No definite criteria exist for either cure of syphilis or treatment failure. It is recommended that nontreponemal antibody titers be followed

---

[1]Not FDA approved for this indication.

TABLE 1 CDC Recommendations for Treatment of Syphilis

Stage	Recommended Penicillin Treatment	
	Penicillin	Dosage
Primary and secondary syphilis	Benzathine penicillin G (Bicillin LA)	2.4 million U IM once
Early latent syphilis (acquired within previous 12 mo)	Benzathine penicillin G	2.4 million U IM once
Late latent syphilis	Benzathine penicillin G	2.4 million U IM weekly × 3 doses
Tertiary syphilis	Benzathine penicillin G	2.4 million units IM weekly × 3 doses
Neurosyphilis	Aqueous crystalline penicillin G *or*	3-4 million U q4h
	Continuous infusion *or*	18-24 U daily IV × 10-14 d (preferred)
	Procaine penicillin (Wycillin) *plus*	2.4 million U IM
	Probenecid	500 mg PO qid
Congenital Syphilis		
Proven or highly probable disease	Aqueous crystalline penicillin G *or*	100,000-150,000 U/kg/d (divided 50,000 units/kg/dose) IV q12h × first 7 d of life, then q8h for total of 10 d of treatment
	Procaine penicillin G	50,000 U/kg/dose IM daily × 10 d
Normal examination but mother inadequately treated	Aqueous crystalline penicillin G *or*	100,000-150,000 U/kg/d (divided 50,000 U/kg/dose) IV q12h × first 7 d of life, then q8h for total of 10 days of treatment
	Procaine penicillin G *or*	50,000 U/kg/dose IM daily × 10 d
	Benzathine penicillin G	50,000 U/kg/dose IM once
Normal examination, serologic titers ≤4× the maternal titer, and mother adequately treated during pregnancy	Benzathine penicillin G	50,000 U/kg/dose IM once

Abbreviation: CDC = Centers for Disease Control and Prevention.

every 6 months, and patients should be periodically reexamined for clinical signs or symptoms of syphilitic infection. Treatment failure is probable in patients with either persistent or recurrent clinical signs or symptoms or a sustained fourfold increase in nontreponemal antibody titer (compared to maximum titer at time of treatment). Treatment failure is possible if nontreponemal antibody titers fail to decline fourfold within 6 months after treatment. Suspected treatment failure warrants retesting for neurosyphilis and HIV infection. Patients with HIV infection, with congenital syphilis, who are pregnant, or who have neurosyphilis warrant closer and more-specific laboratory and clinical follow-up. Full recommendations can be found in the Centers for Disease Control and Prevention (CDC) treatment guidelines (http://www.cdc.gov/std/treatment/default.htm).

Complications

Complications of syphilis are primarily related to neurologic involvement, tertiary syphilis, or late manifestations of congenital syphilis.

REFERENCES

Centers for Disease Control and Prevention. Sexually transmitted diseases surveillance, 2007, Syphilis, Available at: http://www.cdc.gov/std/stats07/syphilis.htm; [accessed July 28, 2010].

Centers for Disease Control and Prevention, Workowski KA, Berman SM. Sexually transmitted diseases treatment guidelines, 2006. MMWR Recomm Rep Aug 4;2006;55(RR-11):1–94. Available at http://www.cdc.gov/std/treatment/default.htm; [accessed July 28, 2010].

Kent ME, Romanelli F. Reexamining syphilis: An update on epidemiology, clinical manifestations, and management. Ann Pharmacother 2008;42:226–36.

Koss CA, Dunne EF, Warner L. A systematic review of epidemiologic studies assessing condom use and risk of syphilis. Sex Trans Dis 2009;36:401–5.

Lautenschlager S. Cutaneous manifestations of syphilis. Am J Clin Dermatol 2006;7:291–304.

Marra CM. Update on neurosyphilis. Curr Infect Dis Rep 2009;11:127–34.

Woods CR. Congenital syphilis—persisting pestilence. Pediatr Infect Dis 2009; 28:536–7.

Contraception

Method of
Emily J. Herndon, MD

More than 15% of all primary care visits to an internist or family physician is for contraceptive counseling and care. Compared with the financial costs and mortality of pregnancy-related births and abortions, contraception saves money and lives. Despite these facts, 49% of the pregnancies in the United States are unintended, with almost one half of these ending in an elective abortion. In a study of women who had had an unintended pregnancy, 41% believed that they could not get pregnant at the time of conception. These statistics demonstrate the need for primary care providers educating patients regarding contraception.

The ideal contraceptive is one that is safe, highly effective, and rapidly reversible; provides good cycle control; and protects against sexually transmitted infections (STIs). Patients want a method that is user-friendly, is easily accessible, and has minimal side effects. Although no single contraceptive provides all these characteristics, primary care providers need to be aware of all the methods to help a patient choose one that is medically appropriate and best suits his or her needs.

Contraceptives can be categorized as hormonal and nonhormonal, as reversible or permanent, and as precoital or postcoital. The reversible, nonhormonal methods include the copper intrauterine device (IUD) (ParaGard), barrier methods, spermicides, withdrawal, abstinence, fertility awareness, and lactation amenorrhea (Table 1). Of these, male condoms are the most widely used reversible, nonhormonal method, with 18% of couples choosing this method for contraception. All other methods combined are used less frequently (<10% of choices).

Combined Hormonal Methods

The hormonal methods of contraception can be divided into two categories: those with combined estrogen and progesterone and those with progesterone only. The combined estrogen and progesterone methods all work by suppressing ovulation and thickening the cervical mucus, and only their delivery systems are different. The estrogen and progesterone methods available in the United States include combined oral contraceptive pills (COCPs), the vaginal ring, and the contraceptive patch.

The noncontraceptive benefits of combined hormonal therapy include excellent cycle control[1] and decreased rates of ectopic pregnancy,[1] pelvic inflammatory disease,[1] and endometrial and ovarian cancer.[1] They are also used to treat dysfunctional uterine bleeding,[1] dysmenorrhea,[1] mittelschmerz,[1] ovarian cysts,[1] and acne[1] (except Ortho Tri-Cyclen and Estrostep). Likewise, the side effect profile and contraindications are similar and usually result from the estrogen component of the methods. Higher estrogen doses are associated with nausea, headache, breast tenderness, and chloasma, whereas breakthrough bleeding occurs more commonly with the lower estrogen methods. With the exception of chloasma, most of these side effects are seen in the first few cycles, and they tend to improve with time. Combined hormonal methods should not be used if the patient has a history of liver or breast cancer or has a significant history of liver or gallbladder disease. Because estrogen can interfere with lactation, it is also contraindicated in the first 6 months after delivery if a woman is breast-feeding.

The most serious concerns about using combined hormonal methods are the potential cardiovascular complications. Although rare, the use of estrogen has been associated with the development of deep vein thrombosis, myocardial infarction, hypertension, and stroke. Combined hormonal methods are contraindicated if the patient has a history of any of these conditions or has other factors that may increase the risk of these complications. Factors include age older than 35 years combined with smoking, uncontrolled hypertension, coronary artery disease, having diabetes for more than 20 years, having a positive family history of deep vein thrombosis, or having a known hypercoagulable condition. Studies have also shown that patients who have a history of migraine headaches associated with focal neurologic findings or auras are at higher risk for stroke when using combined hormonal methods.

COMBINED ORAL CONTRACEPTIVE PILLS

Of the hormonal therapies, COCPs are the most widely used, with 31% of all couples choosing this method. COCPs have a failure rate of 0.3% with perfect use and 8% when used typically. The difference in these rates largely results from incorrect use of the pills. Patients must take the COCP daily, ideally at the same time each day. If the patient accidently misses a pill, she should take the missed pill as soon as possible. If she misses two or more pills, the patient should double up on the pills daily until the missed tablets are taken and use a backup form of contraception for 7 days.

COCPs come in monophasic (i.e., same dose of hormones in each active tablet) and multiphasic (i.e., active tablets with different doses) combinations, and they are available in various cycle lengths. A 28-day cycle, with 21 active tablets and 7 placebo tablets, is the most commonly used form. Extended cycle forms (84 active pills and 7 placebo pills) are monophasic, and they are ideal for patients who have problems associated with menstruation such as endometriosis, dysmenorrhea, or menstrual headaches. Patients should be warned that breakthrough bleeding is more likely with extended cycles. COCPs that contain drospirenone as the progesterone component

---

[1]Not FDA approved for this indication.

TABLE 1 Reversible Nonhormonal Methods of Contraception

Method	Percent Failure (%)*	Advantages	Disadvantages	Comments
Abstinence	0 (unknown)	Can be started or restarted at any time; decreases risk of STIs and cervical cancer; no cost	Requires commitment, self-control, and communication between patient and partner	Patient needs to establish ground rules and be aware of back-up methods if changes mind
LAM	0.5 (2)	No cost; helps postpartum weight loss; decreases risk of ovarian and endometrial cancers	Contraindicated if patient is HIV+; offers no protection against STIs; return of ovulation unpredictable	Effectiveness sharply decreases after 6 mo; return of fertility often precedes menses
Withdrawal	4 (2.7)	No cost	Not adequate protection against STIs; contraindicated if history of premature ejaculation; male partner must be very disciplined	Couples must be able to communicate during intercourse, and men must be able to predict ejaculation in time
FAM	1–9 (25)	May be only method acceptable to couples for religious or cultural reasons	Not useful if patient's periods are irregular; no protection against STIs; need good discipline and documentation of cycles	Use back-up form of contraception during fertile times
Barriers				Consider having EC at home
Condom, male	2 (15)	Low cost and easily available; protects against STIs	Need to use consistently; may interrupt love making	Third most common method used in the United States
Condom, female	5 (21)	Same as for male condom	More difficult to use than male condom	
Diaphragm	6 (16)	Can insert several hours earlier; no need to remove for multiple acts of intercourse up to 24 h	Needs a doctor visit and prescription; does not protect against HIV; may increase risk of UTIs; patient must be comfortable with inserting and removing device	Contraindicated in cases of latex allergy
Cervical cap	9–26 (16–32)	Same as for diaphragm; can stay in for 48 h	Same as for diaphragm	Two cervical caps available in the United States; both types latex free
Cervical sponge	18 (29)	Easily available; relatively low cost	Same as for diaphragm	Made of polyurethane foam prefilled with spermicide
Spermicide	15 (29)	Easily available and easy to use	N-9 contraindicated if at high risk for HIV	Some studies suggest increased risk of HIV transmission with N-9
Copper IUD	0.6 (0.8)	Highest level of user satisfaction; long duration of action; rapidly reversible	Requires office procedure; may increase cramps and menstrual bleeding; no protection against STIs	Most cost-effective reversible method; increased infection risk in first 20 d after insertion

*Percent failure is defined as the percentage of women experiencing an unintended pregnancy in the first year, when the method is used perfectly (% with typical use).
Abbreviations: CA = cancer; EC = emergency contraception; FAM = fertility awareness combined with periodic abstinence; HIV = human immunodeficiency virus; IUD, intrauterine device; LAM = lactation amenorrhea; N-9 = nonoxynol-9 spermicide; STI = sexually transmitted infection; UTI = urinary tract infection.

(Yaz) have an antimineralocorticoid-like activity with decreased rates of bloating and premenstrual weight gain. Potassium levels should be monitored if these patients are also taking other potassium-sparing drugs.

Intermenstrual spotting is a common problem for COCP users, and it may lead to discontinuation of the pill by patients. Patients should be counseled that spotting is more likely in the first two cycles and that 70% to 90% of women have no further breakthrough bleeding by the third cycle. Because incorrect or inconsistent use of the pill is one of the most common reasons for intermenstrual bleeding, the patient must be instructed on how to take the pill and what she should do and expect if a pill is missed. Other causes of vaginal bleeding, such as pregnancy, cervicitis, vaginitis, and medications that interfere with the hormones, should be ruled out. If persistent spotting continues after 2 or 3 months, changing to a different formulation of pill may help. Patients who report spotting before they complete their active pills usually need higher progesterone levels, and changing to a different monophasic pill or to a triphasic formulation, which usually has a higher progesterone content in the last active pills, is a good option. Patients who report continued bleeding after their normal withdrawal bleeding usually need a higher estrogen-to-progesterone ratio. Options for these patients include changing to a higher-dose estrogen pill or changing to a formulation that has lower progesterone levels in the early part of the cycle.

CONTRACEPTIVE PATCH

The contraceptive patch (Ortho Evra) delivers 20 µg of ethinyl estradiol and 150 µg of progesterone (norelgestromin) per day and is ideal for patients who want to avoid daily pill taking. It has a failure rate similar to COCP, although it is much less effective in women weighing more than 90 kg. The patch is applied weekly on the same day of the week (i.e., the patch change day) for 3 weeks, followed by a patch-free week. Recommended application sites include the upper arms, buttocks, lower abdomen, and upper torso, excluding the breasts. Patients should be told to rotate the application site to decrease the risk of pigment changes or skin irritation, an uncommon side effect that occurs in 1% of women. Adhesion rates are very reliable, with less than 2% of patches completely detaching. If a patch detaches and has been off for less than 24 hours, patients should apply a new patch but keep the previous patch change day. If it detaches and has been off for 24 hours or more, patients should apply a new patch, change the patch change day to that day, and use a backup form of contraception for 7 days. Because the patch has enough medicine to last for 9 days, the patient has 2 extra days during which it remains effective if left on too long. However, the patient should *not* extend the patch-free interval. If the patient has a late restart ($\geq$9 days), she should apply a new patch and use a backup form of contraception for 7 days.

The average estrogen concentration in women using the patch was higher than in those taking COCPs, raising the possibility of an increased risk of deep vein thrombosis and cardiovascular events. Epidemiologic data show conflicting results, and further studies are pending, but patients should be adequately counseled regarding this potential risk.

VAGINAL RING

The vaginal ring (NuvaRing) releases 15 µg of ethinyl estradiol and 120 µg of etonogestrel per day, and, in studies, it had the lowest steady-state level of hormones compared with other methods, making it ideal for patients who want good cycle control but are worried about estrogen-related side effects. The ring is placed in the vagina and left there for 3 weeks; it is then removed for 1 week to allow for withdrawal bleeding. Unlike barrier methods, the ring does not have to be in any particular position because transmucosal hormone absorption occurs as long as the ring is in the vagina. Like the patch, the ring also has enough medicine to last longer than the time recommended for use (up to 35 days for the ring), allowing some flexibility regarding insertion and removal times. Although not recommended, patients may take the ring out during intercourse, as long as the ring-free time is less than 3 hours/day. Although douching is discouraged, there are no contraindications to using intravaginal topical agents (e.g., antifungal creams) at the same time as the ring.

The rate of adverse effects that led to discontinuation of the ring was low (3.6%), and they included foreign body sensation, coital problems, and device expulsion. The ring should not be exposed to high temperatures outside the body for prolonged periods because this can activate premature release of the hormones. It may be stored for up to 4 months at room temperature or can be refrigerated if stored for longer periods.

Progesterone-Only Methods

For women who would like to use a hormonal method of contraception but cannot take estrogen, progesterone-only methods are an excellent choice. These methods provide a steady dose of progesterone daily, and they work by thickening the cervical mucus, thinning the endometrial lining, and inhibiting ovulation. Because there is no hormone-free interval, menstrual periods are often irregular, and amenorrhea is common. Like combined hormonal methods, progesterone-only methods have been shown to decrease dysmenorrhea and menstrual bleeding. Progesterone-only methods include mini-pills (Micronor), injections, the intrauterine system, and implants.

PROGESTERONE-ONLY PILLS

Mini-pills or progesterone-only pills have a failure rate similar to that for COCPs. On average, the cost of mini-pills is slightly more than that for COCPs. Because the dose of progesterone in each pill is very close to the therapeutic level needed for contraception, it is important to take the tablets at the same time each day. A backup form of contraception should be used if there is a delay of more than 3 hours in taking the pills or if the pill is missed altogether.

PROGESTERONE INJECTIONS

Depot medroxyprogesterone acetate (DMPA) injections are one of the most popular progesterone-only methods. The intramuscular injection (Depo-Provera) is given every 12 weeks and has a perfect-use failure rate of 0.3% and a typical-use failure rate of 3%. A lower dose of DMPA (104 mg in Depo-SubQ Provera 104) has been approved for subcutaneous injection and has the potential advantage of allowing the patient to administer the injection in the privacy of her home. Noncontraceptive benefits of DMPA include improvement of endometriosis and decreased rates of sickle cell crisis in patients with sickle cell anemia. It is also an ideal choice for women who are on anticonvulsants because there is no potential decrease in the contraceptive's effectiveness as there is with COCPs.

Disadvantages of DMPA injections include spotting, weight gain, a delayed return of fertility (average of 10 months), and a decrease in bone mineral density. The average weight gain is 5.4 pounds in the first year and 16.5 pounds at 5 years. The effect on bone mineral density was unique to DMPA, with an average decrease of 5% to 7% after 2 years of continuous use. This decrease returned to baseline by 2 to 3 years after stopping DMPA in women who were not menopausal. All women who use DMPA should be counseled to stop smoking, participate in weight-bearing exercise at least three times per week, and take 1000 to 1200 mg/day of calcium in the diet or as a supplement.

PROGESTERONE INTRAUTERINE SYSTEM

A levonorgestrel-releasing intrauterine system (Mirena) has been available in the United States since 2001. The device is effective for 5 years and has a failure rate of 0.1%. Unlike the copper IUD, which has side effects of dysmenorrhea and menorrhagia, the levonorgestrel-releasing intrauterine system decreases the incidence of both effects. Approximately 20% of women have reversible amenorrhea after 1 year of use, and that number increases to 47% at 5 years. Because of the bleeding pattern, the levonorgestrel-releasing intrauterine system is being studied as a treatment for other conditions that cause dysfunctional uterine bleeding.

Disadvantages of the system include a risk of expulsion (similar to that for the copper IUD) and increased rates of headache, acne, and breast tenderness during the first few months of use. The cost is also significantly higher compared with the copper IUD, which is the most cost-effective contraceptive over a 5-year period.

PROGESTERONE IMPLANTS

Subdermal implants have a long duration of action and are therefore very convenient and appealing to many patients. Both two-rod (Jadelle)[2] and single-rod systems (Implanon) are FDA approved, although only the single-rod system is marketed in the United States. The single-rod system releases etonogestrel at a rate of 60 µg/day in the first year, decreasing to 30 µg/day by the end of the third year, at which time it is removed and replaced. It has a failure rate of 0.2% with typical use and was well accepted, with a continuation rate of 87% after 2 years in one study. The rod is 4 cm long and 2 mm in diameter, and it is easily placed under the skin of the nondominant arm using a 16-gauge, disposable inserter. Removal is much easier than with the previous six-rod system, with an average removal time of 3 minutes. Irregular bleeding, although common, has not been as heavy as with the six-rod system (Norplant),[2] and amenorrhea occurs in 18% of women at 1 year. Patients should be counseled before insertion of the implant that these side effects are normal and to be expected while the implant is in place.

Initiating Hormonal Methods of Contraception

Traditionally, all hormonal methods of contraception were initiated after delivery, on the first Sunday of a patient's menses, or on the first day of her cycle. This made it less likely that she would be pregnant,

---

[2]Not available in the United States.

and if her periods had been regular, it allowed her to continue her usual cycle.

The quick-start method of initiating hormonal contraception has been gaining popularity. If a woman is reasonably sure that she is not pregnant and an in-office pregnancy test confirms this, she can begin the hormonal method on the same day as her office visit, as long as she uses a backup form of contraception for the next 7 days. The quick-start method is especially useful for women with oligomenorrhea and for women who may have trouble correctly remembering initiation instructions with a delayed start.

Emergency Contraception

Emergency contraception should not be used regularly as a form of contraception. It is meant to be used if unplanned intercourse occurs or a condom breaks. Worldwide, progesterone-only pills, COCPs, and copper IUDs have been used for emergency contraception. In the United States, progesterone-only pills are most commonly used and have the least side effects.

In 2006, the FDA ruled that Plan B, which contains two 750-μg pills of levonorgestrel and is packaged specifically for emergency contraception, could be sold without a prescription to women 18 years old or older. These pills should be taken as soon as possible after unplanned intercourse or condom breakage. The contraceptive effectiveness of this method is better if the first pill is taken before 12 hours, but it can be used as late as 120 hours. The second pill can be taken at the same time as the first pill or 12 hours later. Use of emergency contraception has not been shown to decrease compliance with other first-line methods. Plan B One-Step, a single progesterone-only emergency contraceptive is also available without a prescription for women 17 years or older.

Permanent Birth Control Methods

Permanent birth control methods include vasectomy and female sterilization by various procedures. Female sterilization is the second most popular form of birth control after COCPs, with 27% of all couples choosing this form. Male sterilization is chosen by 9% of couples. Each sterilization procedure has advantages and disadvantages that should be considered by the patient before choosing which one to use (Table 2).

Contraceptive Counseling

Although patients may not be concerned about contracting an infection as much as they are about preventing pregnancy, this is an ideal time to evaluate and discuss behavior that may put them at higher risk for disease. The contraceptives with the greatest efficacy for preventing pregnancy provide no protection against STIs, and the contraceptives that best protect against STIs have larger contraceptive failure rates for typical users. For patients at highest risk for STIs, it is prudent to stress barrier methods, specifically condoms, alone or in combination with another method.

When counseling patients about their contraceptive choices, it is important that providers are aware of their own biases. The only effective contraceptive is one that a patient is willing to use consistently and correctly, and the choice of contraception is ultimately the patient's decision. Providers must educate patients regarding the advantages and disadvantages of each method that is medically appropriate for them. If patients are not candidates for their first contraceptive choice, the physician should help them decide on another method that is medically appropriate and discuss how to correctly use it. Educational handouts should be given and reviewed, and counseling should be documented in the medical record.

TABLE 2 Permanent Birth Control Methods

Procedure	Percent Failure (%)*	Advantages	Disadvantages	Comments
Male sterilization	0.1 (0.15)	Office procedure; simpler, safer, and more cost-effective than female sterilization; allows man to take part in contraception	Short-term postoperative discomfort, bruising, and swelling; back-up method needed until confirmation of no sperm	No increased risk of postoperative sexual dysfunction, cancers, tumors, or masses; 1% of men choose reversal later
Female sterilization PP partial salpingectomy Bands or clips Bipolar cautery	0.5 (0.5)	Ease of surgery; does not extend hospital stay Easiest female method to reverse	Counseling must be done before onset of labor Higher risk of ectopic pregnancy	PP women most likely to regret sterilization
Transcervical tubal occlusion		Does not require an incision; can be done in an outpatient setting under local anesthesia; recovery time much faster	Requires back-up method for first 3 months; requires hysterosalpingogram to confirm blockage; not reversible	Bilateral placement successfully achieved after first attempt in 86%; only 4.6% unable to rely on the device

*Percent failure for male and female sterilization is defined as the percentage of women experiencing an unintended pregnancy in the first year when the method is used perfectly (% with typical use).
Abbreviation: PP = postpartum (within 48 hours of delivery).

CURRENT THERAPY

- Combined estrogen and progesterone methods (e.g., pills, patch, ring) provide excellent cycle control and decreased rates of ectopic pregnancy, pelvic inflammatory disease, and endometrial and ovarian cancer.
- Although rare, the use of estrogen has been associated with the development of deep vein thrombosis, myocardial infarction, hypertension, and stroke, and it should not be used in smokers older than 35 years; patients who have diabetes for more than 20 years; patients with uncontrolled hypertension, coronary artery disease, or migraines with aura; and patients with a family history of deep vein thrombosis or a known hypercoagulable condition.
- Combined oral contraceptive pills come in extended-cycle forms for patients who desire or for medical reasons need to have fewer periods (i.e., those with endometriosis, dysmenorrhea, or menstrual migraines).
- The patch (Ortho Evra) and ring (NuvaRing) work the same way as combined oral contraceptive pills, but they have a longer duration of action, making it easier for patients to adhere to the correct regimen.
- The patch is less effective in women weighing more than 90 kg.

Progesterone-only methods (i.e., mini-pills [Micronor], intrauterine device [Mirena], and subdermal implants) do not have any estrogen-related side effects, but they are associated with irregular periods and amenorrhea.

- Depot medroxyprogesterone acetate is available as an intramuscular or subcutaneous injection, and its use is associated with mild weight gain and a reversible decrease in bone mineral density.
- The single-rod subdermal progesterone implant (Implanon) is effective for 3 years and is easier to insert and remove than the six-rod system used previously.
- Patients can initiate hormonal methods on the same day as the office visit (i.e., quick-start method) if they are reasonably sure they are not pregnant and are willing to use a backup form of contraception for the first week.
- Emergency contraception (Plan B One-Step) in the form of one progesterone-only pill can be sold without a prescription to anyone 17 years old or older, and it can be used any time during the first 120 hours after unplanned intercourse or condom breakage.
- Transcervical tubal occlusion offers an outpatient alternative for female patients desiring permanent sterilization. A follow-up hysterosalpingogram should be done 3 months after the procedure, and a backup method must be used during that interval.
- Contraceptive counseling includes helping patients choose a method that is medically appropriate and educating them about its correct use. The only effective contraception is one that a patient is willing to use consistently and correctly.

REFERENCES

Bensyl DM, Iuliano D, Carter M, et al. Contraceptive Use—United States and Territories, Behavioral Risk Factor Surveillance System 2002. MMWR Surveill Summ 2005;18(6):1–72 54.

Hatcher RA, Trussell J, Nelson A, et al. Contraceptive Technology. New York: Ardent Media; 2007.

Herndon EJ, Zieman M. New contraceptive options. Am Fam Physician 2004;69:853–60.

Scholle S, Chang J, Harman J, McNeil M. Trends in women's health services by type of physician seen: Data from the 1985 and 1997–98 NAMCS. Womens Health Issues 2002;12(4):165–77.

Nettleman MD, Chung H, Brewer J, et al. Reasons for unprotected intercourse: Analysis of the PRAMS Survey. Contraception 2007;75:361–6.

Van den Heuvel MW, van Bragt AJM, Alnabawy AK, Kaptein MC. Comparison of ethinylestradiol pharmacokinetics in three hormonal contraceptive formulations: The vaginal ring, the transdermal patch and an oral contraceptive. Contraception 2005;72:168–74.

Westhoff C, Heartwell S, Edwards S, et al. Initiation of oral contraceptives using a quick start compared to a conventional start: A randomized controlled trial. Obstet Gynecol 2007;109(6):1270–6.

World Health Organization (WHO). Medical eligibility criteria for contraceptive use, http://www.who.int/reproductive-health/publications/mec/mec.pdf (accessed May 12, 2009).

Zieman M, Hatcher RA, Cwiak C, et al. A Pocket Guide to Managing Contraception. Tiger, GA: Bridging the Gap Foundation; 2007.

Diseases of Allergy

Anaphylaxis and Serum Sickness

Method of
Stephen F. Kemp, MD

Anaphylaxis

Anaphylaxis, an acute and potentially lethal multisystem allergic reaction, is virtually unavoidable in medical practice. Health care professionals must be able to recognize the signs of anaphylaxis, treat an episode promptly and appropriately, and be able to provide preventive recommendations. Epinephrine, which should be administered immediately, is the drug of choice for acute anaphylaxis.

Anaphylaxis is not a reportable disease, and both its morbidity and mortality are probably underestimated. A variety of statistics on the epidemiology of anaphylaxis have been published, but the lifetime risk per person in the United States is presumed to be 1% to 3%, with a mortality rate of 1%.

There is no universally accepted definition of anaphylaxis. An international and interdisciplinary group of representatives and experts from thirteen professional, governmental, and lay organizations proposed the following working definition: "Anaphylaxis is a serious allergic reaction that is rapid in onset and may cause death." Clinically, anaphylaxis is considered likely to be present if any one of the following three criteria is satisfied within minutes to hours: Acute onset of illness with involvement of skin, mucosal surface, or both, and at least one of the following: respiratory compromise, hypotension, or end-organ dysfunction; two or more of the following occurring rapidly after exposure to a likely allergen: involvement of skin or mucosal surface, respiratory compromise, hypotension, or persistent gastrointestinal symptoms; hypotension develops after exposure to a known allergen for that patient: age-specific low blood pressure or decline of systolic blood pressure of greater than 30% compared with baseline. In clinical practice, however, waiting until the development of multiorgan symptoms is risky because the ultimate severity of anaphylactic reaction is difficult to predict from the outset.

Anaphylaxis has varied clinical presentations, but respiratory compromise and cardiovascular collapse cause the most concern because they are the most frequent causes of fatalities. Urticaria and angioedema are the most common manifestations (more than 90% in retrospective series) but may be delayed or absent in rapidly progressive anaphylaxis. The previous severity of anaphylaxis is not predictive of the severity of a future reaction. The more rapidly anaphylaxis occurs after exposure to an offending stimulus, the more likely the reaction is to be severe and potentially life threatening.

Anaphylaxis often produces signs and symptoms within 5 to 30 minutes, but reactions sometimes may not develop for several hours.

PATHOPHYSIOLOGY

The chemical mediators that cause anaphylaxis are preformed and released from granules (histamine, tryptase, and others) or are generated from membrane lipids (prostaglandin D_2, leukotrienes, and platelet-activating factor) by the activated mast cell or basophil.

Tryptase is concentrated selectively in the secretory granules of all human mast cells. Its plasma levels during mast cell degranulation correlate with the clinical severity of anaphylaxis but need not be elevated in all forms of anaphylaxis (e.g., food-associated anaphylaxis).

Histamine exerts its pathophysiologic effects via both H_1 and H_2 receptors. Erythema (flushing), hypotension, and headache are mediated by both H_1 and H_2 receptors, whereas tachycardia, pruritus, bronchospasm, and rhinorrhea are associated with H_1 receptors alone.

Increased vascular permeability during anaphylaxis can produce a shift of 35% of intravascular fluid to the extravascular space within 10 minutes. This shift of effective blood volume causes compensatory catecholamine release, activates the renin-angiotensin-aldosterone system, and stimulates production of endothelin-1.

Mast cells accumulate at sites of coronary plaque erosion and rupture and they may contribute to coronary artery thrombosis. Because antibodies attached to mast cells can trigger mast cell degranulation, some investigators suggest that anaphylaxis may promote plaque rupture.

AGENTS THAT CAUSE ANAPHYLAXIS

Cause and effect often is confirmed historically in subjects who experience recurrent, objective findings of anaphylaxis upon inadvertent reexposure to the offending agent. Diagnostic testing, where appropriate, may confirm the presence of specific IgE and/or the degranulation of mast cells and basophils.

CURRENT DIAGNOSIS

- Cutaneous: urticaria, angioedema, diffuse erythema, generalized pruritus
- Respiratory: tachypnea, bronchospasm, laryngeal or tongue edema, dysphonia
- Cardiovascular: tachycardia, bradycardia, hypotension, angina, cardiac arrhythmias
- Gastrointestinal: nausea, emesis, diarrhea, abdominal cramps, dysphagia
- Other: rhinitis, conjunctivitis, uterine cramps, headache, dizziness, syncope, blurred vision, seizure

TABLE 1 Representative Agents That Cause Anaphylaxis

IgE dependent:
- Foods (such as peanuts, tree nuts, and crustaceans)
- Medications (such as antibiotics)
- Venoms (fire ants, yellow jackets, others)
- Allergen extracts
- Latex
- Exercise (where food or medication dependent)
- Hormones

IgE independent:
- Nonspecific degranulation of mast cells and basophils
  - Opioids
  - Muscle relaxants
  - Idiopathic
- Physical factors
  - Exercise
  - Cold, heat
- Disturbance of arachidonic acid metabolism
  - Aspirin and other nonsteroidal anti-inflammatory drugs (NSAIDs)
- Immune aggregates
  - Intravenous immunoglobulin
- Cytotoxic
  - Transfusion reactions to cellular elements (IgM, IgG)
- Multimediator complement activation/activation of contact system
  - Radiocontrast media
  - Angiotensin-converting enzyme (ACE) inhibitor administered during renal dialysis with selected dialysis membranes
  - Protamine (possibly)
- Other
  - c-kit mutation (D816V)

Modified and updated from Kemp SF, Lockey RF: Anaphylaxis: A review of causes and mechanisms. J Allergy Clin Immunol 2002;110:341–348.

Virtually any agent capable of activating mast cells or basophils may potentially precipitate anaphylactic or anaphylactoid reactions. Table 1 lists common causes of anaphylaxis classified by pathophysiologic mechanism. Idiopathic anaphylaxis, anaphylaxis with no identifiable cause, has accounted for approximately a third of cases in most retrospective studies of anaphylaxis. However, of 601 patients evaluated for more than two decades in a university-affiliated practice (the largest retrospective series), 59% of subjects were deemed to have idiopathic anaphylaxis.

Idiopathic anaphylaxis remains a diagnosis of exclusion, however. Serial histories and diagnostic tests for foods, spices, and vegetable gums occasionally identify a specific culprit in subjects previously presumed to have idiopathic anaphylaxis. The most common identifiable causes of anaphylaxis are foods, medications, insect stings, and immunotherapy injections. Anaphylaxis to peanuts and/or tree nuts causes the greatest concern because of its life-threatening severity, especially in subjects with asthma, and the tendency for subjects to develop lifelong allergic responsiveness to these foods.

RECURRENT ANAPHYLAXIS

Depending on the report, recurrent (biphasic) anaphylaxis occurs in 1% to 20% of subjects who experience anaphylaxis. Signs and symptoms experienced during the recurrent phase of anaphylaxis may be equivalent to or worse than those observed in the initial reaction and may occur 1 to 72 hours (most within 8 hours) after apparent remission. Thus, it may be necessary to monitor subjects up to 24 hours after apparent recovery from the initial phase. Observation periods after apparent recovery from the initial phase should be individualized and based on such factors as comorbid conditions and distance from the patient's home to the closest emergency facility, particularly because there are no reliable predictors of biphasic anaphylaxis.

DIFFERENTIAL DIAGNOSIS

Several systemic disorders share clinical features with anaphylaxis. The vasodepressor (vasovagal) reaction probably is the condition most commonly confused with anaphylactic reactions. In vasodepressor reactions, however, urticaria is absent, dyspnea is generally absent, the blood pressure is usually normal or elevated, and the skin is typically cool and pale. Tachycardia is the rule in anaphylaxis. Bradycardia may be underrecognized in anaphylaxis, however. Brown and others conducted sting challenges in 19 subjects known to be allergic to jack jumper ants (*Myrmecia*). All eight subjects who became hypotensive developed bradycardia after an initial tachycardia.

Systemic mastocytosis, a disease characterized by mast cell proliferation in multiple organs, usually features urticaria pigmentosa (brownish macules that transform into wheals upon stroking them) and recurrent episodes of pruritus, flushing, tachycardia, abdominal pain, diarrhea, syncope, or headache. Other diagnostic considerations include myocardial dysfunction, pulmonary embolism, foreign body aspiration, acute poisoning, seizure disorder, and psychogenic manifestations (no objective findings observed or documented).

MANAGEMENT OF ANAPHYLAXIS

Table 2 outlines a sequential approach to management. Assessment and maintenance of airway, breathing, circulation, and mentation are necessary before proceeding to other management steps. Subjects are monitored continuously to facilitate prompt detection of any treatment complications. The recumbent position is strongly recommended. In a retrospective review of prehospital anaphylactic fatalities in the United Kingdom, the postural history was known for 10 individuals. Four of the 10 were associated with assumption of an upright or sitting posture and postmortem findings consistent with "empty heart" and pulseless electrical activity.

Epinephrine is the treatment of choice for acute anaphylaxis. Aqueous epinephrine 1:1000 dilution 0.2 to 0.5 mL (0.01 mg/kg in children; maximum dose, 0.3 mg) administered intramuscularly every 5 minutes, as necessary, should be used to control symptoms and sustain or increase blood pressure. Comparisons of intramuscular injections to subcutaneous injections during acute anaphylaxis are not available. However, absorption is more rapid and plasma levels are higher in asymptomatic individuals who receive epinephrine intramuscularly in the anterolateral thigh.

All subsequent therapeutic interventions depend on the initial response to epinephrine and the severity of the reaction. Development of toxicity or inadequate response to epinephrine injections indicates that additional therapeutic modalities are necessary.

The α-adrenergic effect of epinephrine reverses peripheral vasodilation, which alleviates hypotension and also reduces angioedema and urticaria. It may also minimize further absorption of antigen from a sting or injection. The β-adrenergic properties of epinephrine increase myocardial output and contractility, cause bronchodilation, and suppress further mediator release from mast cells and basophils.

Fatalities during witnessed anaphylaxis usually result from delayed administration of epinephrine and from severe respiratory and/or cardiovascular complications. *There is no absolute contraindication to epinephrine administration in anaphylaxis.*

Oxygen should be administered to subjects with anaphylaxis who require multiple doses of epinephrine, receive inhaled β_2 agonists, have protracted anaphylaxis, or have preexisting hypoxemia or myocardial dysfunction.

Antihistamines (H_1 and H_2 antagonists) support the treatment of anaphylaxis. However, these agents act much slower than epinephrine and should never be administered alone as treatment for anaphylaxis. Antihistamines thus should be considered as *second-line* treatment.

Systemic corticosteroids have no role in the acute management of anaphylaxis because even intravenous administration of these agents may have no effect for 4 to 6 hours after administration. Although corticosteroids traditionally are used in the management of anaphylaxis, their effect has never been evaluated in placebo-controlled trials. Corticosteroids administered during anaphylaxis might provide additional benefit for patients with asthma or other conditions recently treated with corticosteroids.

TABLE 2 Management of Anaphylaxis

Immediate intervention:
- Assessment of airway, breathing, circulation, and adequacy of mentation.
- Administer aqueous epinephrine 1:1000 dilution, 0.2–0.5 mL (0.01 mg/kg in children; maximum dose, 0.3 mg) *intramuscularly* q5 min, as necessary, to control symptoms and blood pressure.

Possibly appropriate, subsequent measures depending on response to epinephrine:
- Place subject in recumbent position and elevate lower extremities.
- Establish and maintain airway.
- Administer oxygen.
- Establish venous access.
- Use normal saline IV for fluid replacement.

Specific measures to consider after epinephrine injections, where appropriate:
- An epinephrine infusion might be prepared. Continuous hemodynamic monitoring is essential (see reference for specific details).
- Diphenhydramine (Benadryl). Note: In the management of anaphylaxis, a combination of diphenhydramine and ranitidine (Zantac)[1] is superior to diphenhydramine alone.
- For bronchospasm resistant to epinephrine, use nebulized albuterol (Proventil).
- For refractory hypotension, consider dopamine (Intropin), 400 mg in 500 mL D_5W, administered IV at 2–20 μg/kg/min titrated to maintain adequate blood pressure. Continuous hemodynamic monitoring is essential.
- Where use of β-blockers complicates therapy, consider glucagon,[1] 1–5 mg (20–30 μg/kg; maximum: 1 mg in children), administered IV over 5 min followed by an infusion 5–15 μg/min. Aspiration precautions should be observed.
- For patients with a history of asthma and for those who experience severe or prolonged anaphylaxis, consider methylprednisolone (Solu-Medrol) (1.0–2.0 mg/kg/d).
- Consider transportation to the emergency department or an intensive care facility.

Interventions for cardiopulmonary arrest occurring during anaphylaxis:
- High-dose epinephrine and prolonged resuscitation efforts are encouraged, if necessary, because efforts are more likely to be successful in anaphylaxis where the subject (often young) has a healthy cardiovascular system (see reference for specific details).

Observation and subsequent outpatient follow-up:
- Observation periods after apparent resolution must be individualized and based on such factors as the clinical scenario, comorbid conditions, and distance from the patient's home to the closest emergency department. After recovery from the acute episode, patients should receive epinephrine syringes (EpiPen or TwinJect) and be instructed in proper technique. Everyone postanaphylaxis requires a careful diagnostic evaluation in consultation with an allergist-immunologist.

Modified from Lieberman P, Kemp SF, Oppenheimer J, et al (chief eds). Joint Task Force on Practice Parameters. The diagnosis and management of anaphylaxis: An updated practice parameter. J Allergy Clin Immunol 2005;115:S483–S523.
[1]Not FDA approved for this indication.
Abbreviation: IV = intravenous.

Numerous cases of unusually severe or refractory anaphylaxis are reported in subjects receiving β-blocking agents. Greater severity of anaphylaxis observed in usual doses of epinephrine administered during anaphylaxis to subjects taking β-blockers may not produce the desired clinical response. In such situations, both isotonic volume expansion and glucagon[1] administration are recommended. Glucagon may potentially reverse refractory hypotension and bronchospasm because it bypasses the β-adrenergic receptor and directly activates adenyl cyclase.

[1]Not FDA approved for this indication.

Persistent hypotension despite epinephrine injections should first be treated with intravenous crystalloid solutions. Saline is generally preferred. One to 2 L of normal saline might need to be administered to adults at a rate of 5 to 10 mL/kg in the first 5 minutes. Children should receive up to 30 mL/kg in the first hour. Large volumes (e.g., 7 L) are often required.

Vasopressors should be administered if epinephrine injections and volume expansion fail to alleviate hypotension. Dopamine (Intropin) frequently increases blood pressure while maintaining or enhancing renal and splanchnic perfusion. These agents would not be expected to work as well in patients already maximally vasoconstricted by their internal compensatory response to anaphylaxis.

PREVENTION OF ANAPHYLAXIS

Table 3 outlines the basic principles for the prevention of future anaphylactic episodes in high-risk individuals. An allergist-immunologist can provide comprehensive professional advice on these matters.

All subjects at high risk for recurrent anaphylaxis should carry epinephrine syringes and know how to administer them. An EpiPen (Dey Laboratories) is a spring-loaded, pressure-activated syringe with a single 0.3 mg dose (1:1000 dilution) of epinephrine. It is easy to use and injects through clothing. An EpiPen Jr, which delivers 0.15 mg (1:2000 dilution) epinephrine, is appropriate for children weighing less than 30 kg. The TwinJect (Sciele Pharma) is a pre-filled, pen-sized, epinephrine auto-injector with two doses of either 0.3 or 0.15 mg.

Serum Sickness

Serum sickness is a clinical syndrome of fever, malaise, and urticarial and/or morbilliform cutaneous eruption that is often preceded by generalized erythema and pruritus. Arthralgias or arthritis (mainly

TABLE 3 Preventive Measures for Subjects with Anaphylaxis

General measures:
- Obtain thorough history to diagnose life-threatening food or drug allergy.
- Identify cause of anaphylaxis and those individuals at risk for future attacks.
- Provide instruction on proper reading of food and medication labels, where appropriate.
- Patient should avoid exposure to antigens and cross-reactive substances.
- Manage asthma and coronary artery disease optimally.
- Employ a waiting period of 30 minutes after injections
- Consider office waiting period of 2 hours for oral medication patient has not taken previously.

Specific measures for high-risk subjects:
- Individuals at high risk for anaphylaxis should carry self-injectable syringes of epinephrine (EpiPen or TwinJect) at all times and receive instruction in proper use with placebo trainer.
- Individuals should wear a Medic Alert bracelet or chain.
- Other agents for β-adrenergic antagonists, angiotensin-converting enzyme (ACE) inhibitors, tricyclic antidepressants, and monoamine oxidase inhibitors should be substituted whenever possible.
- Agents suspected of causing anaphylaxis should be administered slowly, supervised, and orally if possible.
- Where appropriate, use specific preventive strategies, including pharmacologic prophylaxis, short-term challenge and desensitization and long-term desensitization.

Modified from Kemp SF: Office approach to anaphylaxis: sooner better than later. Am J Med 2007;120:664–668.

TABLE 4 Representative Agents That Cause Serum Sickness

Medications: β-lactam antibiotics, sulfonamides, ciprofloxacin (Cipro), metronidazole (Flagyl), rifampin (Rifadin), allopurinol (Zyloprim), carbamazepine (Tegretol), phenytoin (Dilantin), fluoxetine (Prozac), bupropion (Wellbutrin), methimazole (Tapazole), propylthiouracil, thiazide diuretics, captopril (Capoten), propranolol (Inderal), verapamil (Calan), streptokinase (Streptase), others.

Heterologous (animal-derived) antisera:
- Horse: snake and spider venom, tetanus, botulism, diphtheria
- Horse or rabbit: anti-lymphocyte globulin
- Mouse: monoclonal antibodies (muromonab-CD3 [Orthoclone OKT3], rituximab [Rituxan], infliximab [Remicade])

Homologous (human-derived) antisera: cytomegalovirus, hepatitis B, rabies, tetanus, perinatal $RH_0(D)$

large joints), neuropathy, lymphadenopathy, nephritis, abdominal pain (emesis or melena are possible), or vasculitis (cutaneous or systemic) may occur in some cases. Cutaneous vasculitis, also known as hypersensitivity vasculitis, is often manifested by palpable purpura, which most commonly are found on the lower extremities of ambulatory individuals or on the sacral or gluteal region of patients with restricted mobility. These purpura reflect vascular leakage from inflamed postcapillary venules. Systemic vasculitis may occur in association with autoimmune diseases, infection, or malignancy.

Many agents may produce serum sickness or serum sickness–like reactions (Table 4). *Serum sickness* classically refers to the immune complex syndrome caused by immunization with heterologous serum proteins (often equine or murine). The most frequent cause is immune complex-mediated drug hypersensitivity. A serum sickness–like drug reaction generally develops 6 to 21 days after the culprit medication is started, but it can occur within 12 to 48 hours in previously sensitized individuals.

PATHOGENESIS AND LABORATORY ABNORMALITIES

Healthy individuals regularly generate low levels of circulating immune complexes, which are either excreted by the kidneys or extracted in the liver and spleen by monocytes and macrophages. It is hypothesized that serum sickness results when a drug (hapten) binds to plasma protein and antibodies are generated in response to the drug-protein complex. Complement activation occurs when large quantities of soluble antigen-antibody (immune) complexes fix to vascular endothelial receptors. Complement fragments attract and activate neutrophils, which release proteases that induce tissue injury. The urticaria in serum sickness probably results from immune complex necrotizing vasculitis and complement activation that induces mast cell degranulation. IgE-dependent mechanisms likely are also contributory in some individuals. Laboratory abnormalities include elevated erythrocyte sedimentation rate, leukopenia (acute phase), occasional plasmacytosis, and decreased total hemolytic complement (CH50), C3, and C4. Slight albuminuria, hyaline casts, and microscopic hematuria may also occur.

TREATMENT

Stoppage of the culprit agent, when identified, is recommended. Serum sickness is usually self-limited and rarely life threatening when the offending drug or protein is stopped or removed. Symptoms generally improve over 2 to 4 weeks as patients clear their immune complexes. Evidence-based treatment recommendations for serum sickness are very limited. Long-acting, less-sedating H_1 antihistamines such as cetirizine (Zyrtec), desloratadine (Clarinex), fexofenadine (Allegra), or loratadine (Claritin) generally control urticaria. Systemic corticosteroids (e.g., prednisone, 0.5 to 1.0 mg/kg/day)

may help severe symptoms. Fever and arthralgias typically resolve within 48 to 72 hours of treatment, and the formation of new cutaneous eruptions usually ceases within the same time frame. Antihistamine therapy is continued for 1 week after apparent resolution of symptoms and then slowly discontinued. Skin testing with heterologous antisera is performed routinely to avoid anaphylaxis to future administration of heterologous serum.

REFERENCES

American Heart Association in collaboration with International Liaison Committee on Resuscitation. 2005 American Heart Association guidelines for cardiopulmonary resuscitation and emergency cardiovascular care. Anaphylaxis. Circulation 2005;112(Suppl. 4):143–5.

Brown SGA, Blackman KE, Stenlake V, Heddle RJ. Insect sting anaphylaxis: Prospective evaluation of treatment with intravenous adrenaline and volume resuscitation. Emerg Med J 2004;21:149–54.

Kemp SF, Lockey RF, Simons FE. World Allergy Organization Ad Hoc Committee on Epinephrine in Anaphylaxis. Epinephrine: The Drug of Choice for Anaphylaxis. A statement of the World Allergy Organization. Allergy 2008;63:1061–70.

Kemp SF, Palmer GW. Anaphylaxis. emedicine from WebMD. Updated April 29, 2009. Available at http://emedicine.medscape.com/article/135065-overview.

Lieberman P. Biphasic anaphylactic reactions. Ann Allergy Asthma Immunol 2005;95:217–26.

Lieberman P, Nicklas RA, Oppenheimer J, Kemp SF, Lang DM, chief editors. Joint Task Force on Practice Parameters. The diagnosis and management of anaphylaxis parameter: 2010 update. J Allergy Clin Immunol 2010;126:477–80.e42.

Project Team of the Resuscitation Council (UK). Emergency medical treatment of anaphylactic reactions. J Accid Emerg Med 1999;16:243–7.

Pumphrey RSH. Fatal posture in anaphylactic shock. J Allergy Clin Immunol 2003;112:451–2.

Pumphrey RSH. Fatal anaphylaxis in the UK, 1992–2001. Novartis Found Symp 2004;257:116–28.

Sampson HA, Muñoz-Furlong A, Campbell RL, et al. Second symposium on the definition and management of anaphylaxis: Summary report—second National Institute of Allergy and Infectious Disease/Food Allergy and Anaphylaxis Network symposium. J Allergy Clin Immunol 2006;117:391–7.

Simons FER. Anaphylaxis: recent advances in assessment and treatment. J Allergy Clin Immunol 2009;124:625–36.

Simons FER, Gu X, Simons KJ. Epinephrine absorption in adults: Intramuscular versus subcutaneous injection. J Allergy Clin Immunol 2001;108:871–3.

Simons FER, Roberts JR, Gu X, Simons KJ. Epinephrine absorption in children with a history of anaphylaxis. J Allergy Clin Immunol 1998;101:33–7.

Wener M. Serum sickness and serum sickness-like reactions. In: Rose BD, editor. UpToDate. www.uptodateonline.com, Version 18.2 (current through January 2010). Wellesley, Ma.

Asthma in Adolescents and Adults

Method of
Michael Schatz, MD, MS

Asthma is an extremely common chronic medical condition that causes substantial morbidity among its sufferers. In addition to discomfort, asthma can cause sleep disruption, missed school and work, limitations of recreational activities, and acute episodes requiring emergency hospital care. Although the past 30 years have seen the introduction of increasingly effective and convenient medications, recent surveys continue to suggest that asthma remains suboptimally controlled in a substantial proportion of patients. The purpose of this article is to describe an approach to assessment and therapy that leads to optimal asthma control. It is based on the National Asthma Education and Prevention Program (NAEPP) Expert Panel Report 3: Guidelines for the Management of Asthma (http://www.nhlbi.nih.gov/guidelines/asthma/asthgdln.pdf).

Diagnosis

The first step in evaluating a patient with asthma is to confirm the diagnosis. This is particularly important in patients with atypical symptoms or a poor response to asthma therapy. Asthma is confirmed by the demonstration of reversible airways obstruction, which most commonly is an increase in forced expiratory volume in 1 second (FEV_1) by 12% or more and at least 200 cc after an inhaled bronchodilator. For some patients, 2 to 4 weeks of chronic inhaled asthma therapy or 2 weeks of oral corticosteroid therapy is necessary to demonstrate reversibility. The latter is particularly important in adults with a history of smoking in whom chronic obstructive pulmonary disease (COPD) is a diagnostic consideration. In patients with normal pulmonary function, asthma can also be confirmed by means of methacholine (Provocholine) or exercise challenge.

Particularly important masqueraders of asthma include vocal cord dysfunction, panic attacks, hyperventilation, and cough due to post-nasal drip, reflux, or angiotensin-converting enzyme (ACE) inhibitor therapy. All of these can also coexist with asthma, so their presence does not exclude asthma. Even when these conditions coexist with asthma, their diagnosis and appropriate therapy usually reduce the patient's respiratory symptoms.

Assessment

Assessment of asthmatic patients involves assessment of past severity, identification of aggravating factors, and definition of current status regarding treatment and clinical severity or control.

PAST SEVERITY

Asthma can be a mild, infrequent illness or a daily severe one. Certain severity markers identify patients who are more likely to experience severe exacerbations or to have symptoms that are more difficult to control and who thus require more careful surveillance. These include histories of asthma hospitalization, especially requiring intensive care or intubation, past requirement for oral corticosteroids, and exacerbation by aspirin or other NSAIDs. In patients with prior severe exacerbations, the rapidity of the onset of the exacerbation should be ascertained.

AGGRAVATING FACTORS

Factors that appear to trigger asthma symptoms should be assessed because they may be targets for avoidance therapy. Certain aspects of the patient's *environment* that can contribute to asthma triggering should be specifically ascertained, including occupational exposures, age of the home, pets, carpeting, visible mold, passive smoke, and cockroach exposure. Patients with persistent asthma should have in vitro or skin tests to identify *allergic sensitization* to pollens, house dust mites, mold spores, animal dander, and cockroaches that can contribute to the maintenance of asthma inflammation or can trigger episodes. The presence of *comorbidities* that can aggravate asthma, including cigarette smoking, obesity, rhinitis, sinusitis, reflux, and COPD, should be identified and treated. Finally, *psychosocial factors* to assess include a history or symptoms of anxiety or depression, attitudes toward asthma and asthma therapy, adherence to therapy, and social support. These may be targets for therapy or may be necessary to understand in order to create an effective therapeutic plan and therapeutic alliance.

CURRENT STATUS

Assessment of the current therapy the patient is actually taking is necessary for understanding the asthma's severity and to appropriately initiate or change therapy. It is particularly important to determine if the patient is taking long-term control medications, such as inhaled corticosteroids, long-acting β-agonists, leukotriene modifiers, cromolyn (Intal), nedocromil (Tilade), or theophylline (Theo-Dur). If the patient is not taking controllers, *severity* should be assessed,

CURRENT DIAGNOSIS

- Confirm the diagnosis by demonstrating an increase in FEV_1 by 12% or more after asthma therapy.
- Assess past severity by a history of exacerbations requiring hospitalization, intubation, or oral corticosteroids.
- Identify environmental exposures, allergic sensitization, and comorbidities that may be aggravating asthma.
- Assess current *severity* in patients not taking long-term control medications and assess *control* in patients who are taking long-term control medications based on symptom frequency, nocturnal awakenings, rescue therapy use, activity limitation, spirometry, and recent exacerbation history.

Abbreviation: FEV_1 = forced expiratory volume in 1 second.

as described in Table 1, based on symptom frequency, nocturnal awakenings, rescue therapy use, activity limitation, spirometry, and exacerbation history. If the patient is already taking controllers, *control* should be assessed (Table 2). Normal FEV_1/FVC (forced vital capacity) by age is shown in Table 3.

Long-Term Management

The goals of long-term management are to achieve and maintain well-controlled asthma. Both nonpharmacologic and pharmacologic therapy must be considered.

NONPHARMACOLOGIC THERAPY

The first tenet of nonpharmacologic therapy in the long-term management of asthma is *education*. Patients need to understand the inflammatory pathophysiology of asthma and the relationships among airway inflammation, bronchospasm, and symptoms. Patients should be informed that the cause of asthma is unknown and there is no cure but that triggers can be identified and asthma can be controlled. They should receive education regarding self-assessment, either based on symptoms or peak flow monitoring, and regarding the recognition of early signs of an impending exacerbation.

The next step is to discuss and agree on the *goals of therapy*. The NAEPP has defined the following goals:

- Prevent chronic and troublesome daytime and nighttime symptoms.
- Maintain optimal pulmonary function for that patient.
- Maintain normal activity, including work, school, leisure activity, and exercise.
- Prevent recurrent exacerbations, especially those requiring urgent medical visits.
- Provide pharmacotherapy with minimal or no adverse effects.
- Achieve patient and family satisfaction with asthma care.

The physician should let the patient know that these are the expectations of optimal management and confirm that those are the patient's goals as well.

A very important component of nonpharmacologic therapy is reduction of relevant *environmental triggers*. Information should be given regarding environmental control of pollen, mite, mold, animal dander, and cockroach antigens (Box 1) that appear to be relevant based on the history and results of skin or in vitro specific IgE tests. Inhalant allergen *immunotherapy* should be considered for patients who have persistent asthma when there is clear evidence of a relationship between symptoms and exposure to an allergen to which the patient is sensitive.

TABLE 1 Classifying Asthma Severity and Initiating Treatment in Patients 12 Years and Older Not Currently Taking Long-Term Control Medications

| | Classification of Severity* | | | |
| | | Persistent | | |
Components of Severity	Intermittent	Mild	Moderate	Severe
Impairment				
Symptoms	≤2 d/wk	>2 d/wk but not daily	Daily	Throughout the d
Nighttime awakenings	≤2 ×/mo	3–4 ×/mo	>1 ×/wk but not nightly	Often 7 ×/wk
Short-acting β_2-agonist use for symptom control (not prevention of EIB)	≤2 d/wk	>2 d/wk but not daily, and not more than 1 time on any d	Daily	Several times per d
Interference with normal activity	None	Minor limitation	Some limitation	Extremely limited
Lung function[†]	Normal FEV_1 between exacerbations FEV_1 >80% predicted FEV_1/FVC normal	FEV_1 >80% predicted FEV_1/FVC normal	FEV_1 >60% but <80% predicted FEV_1/FVC reduced 5%	FEV_1 <60% predicted FEV_1/FVC reduced >5%
Risk				
Exacerbations requiring oral systemic corticosteroids	0–1/y[‡]	≥2/y[‡]		

Consider severity and interval since last exacerbation.
Frequency and severity may fluctuate over time for patients in any severity category.

Relative annual risk of exacerbation may be related to FEV_1.

Recommended Step for Initiating Treatment[§]

Initiation	Step 1	Step 2	Step 3[¶]	Step 4 or 5[¶]
Follow-up	In 2–6 wk, evaluate level of asthma control and adjust therapy accordingly.			

Data from the National Asthma Education and Prevention Program (NAEPP) Expert Panel Report 3: Guidelines for the Management of Asthma.

*Level of severity is determined by assessment of both impairment and risk. Assess impairment domain by patient's/caregiver's recall of previous 2–4 weeks and spirometry. Assign severity to the most severe category in which any feature occurs.

[†]See Table 3 for normal FEV_1/FVC.

[‡]At present, there are inadequate data to correspond frequencies of exacerbations with different levels of asthma severity. In general, more frequent and intense exacerbations (e.g., requiring urgent, unscheduled care, hospitalization, or ICU admission) indicate greater underlying disease severity. For treatment purposes, patients who had ≥2 exacerbations requiring oral systemic corticosteroids in the past year may be considered the same as patients who have persistent asthma, even in the absence of impairment levels consistent with persistent asthma.

[§]See Table 6 for treatment steps. The stepwise approach is meant to assist, not replace, the clinical decision making required to meet individual patient needs.

[¶]And consider short course of oral systemic corticosteroids.

Abbreviations: EIB = exercise-induced bronchospasm; FEV_1 = forced expiratory volume in one second; FVC = forced vital capacity; ICU = intensive care unit.

Finally, *psychosocial* issues should be considered and addressed. For many patients, the education and therapeutic alliance described earlier adequately addresses psychosocial concerns. For other patients, poor past adherence requires identifying the barriers to adherence and finding solutions together. Resources for patients with poor social support should be identified. Clinically significant anxiety or depression that can make asthma harder to control should be treated.

PHARMACOLOGIC STEP THERAPY

The main principle of asthma pharmacologic step therapy is to add therapy in steps until control is achieved (step up) and decrease therapy in reverse steps (step down) to established the lowest effective dose necessary to maintain control.

There are two types of asthma medications: quick-relief medications (Table 4) and long-term control medications (Table 5). Systemic corticosteroids can be used either short-term to treat an exacerbation (see Table 4) or as long-term maintenance therapy for patients with severe disease (see Table 5). The generally recommended steps of pharmacologic therapy are shown in Table 6. Definitions of low, medium, and high dose inhaled corticosteroids for each of the available preparations are given in Table 7. At each therapeutic step level, the NAEPP Expert Panel has indicated *preferred* medications, which generally identify medications with the best balance of efficacy and

safety in clinical trials for patients at that level of severity. However, these recommendations are based on population data and must be tailored to individual patient needs, circumstances, and responsiveness to therapy.

All patients with asthma should have an action plan that describes their pharmacologic self-management. Aspects of pharmacologic self-management include the maintenance medication schedule, rescue therapy doses for increased symptoms, when and how to increase control medication therapy, when and how to use prednisone, how to recognize a severe exacerbation, and when and how to seek urgent or emergency care. Control medications should be increased with an upper respiratory infection or with symptoms requiring more than two doses of rescue therapy in 12 hours. Although doubling the dose of inhaled corticosteroids does not appear to generally be sufficient to provide clinical benefit under these circumstances, higher-fold increases may be effective (e.g., three- or fourfold increases). The increased dose of control medications should be maintained at least until increased symptoms resolve. Prednisone is usually needed for patients with incomplete or temporary responses to adequate doses of β-agonists (4 puffs with a spacer, waiting at least 1 minute between puffs), substantial interference with sleep every night, requirement for 12 or more puffs of β-agonist in a 24-hour period, or a peak flow less than 60% predicted. Home treatment of exacerbations is further discussed later.

TABLE 2 Assessing Asthma Control and Adjusting Therapy in Patients 12 Years and Older

Components of Control	Classification of Control*		
	Well Controlled	**Not Well Controlled**	**Very Poorly Controlled**
Impairment			
Symptoms	≤2 d/wk	>2 d/wk	Throughout the d
Nighttime awakenings	≤2 ×/mo	1–3 ×/wk	≥4 ×/wk
Short-acting β₂-agonist use for symptom control (not prevention of EIB)	≤2 d/wk	>2 d/wk	Several times per d
Interference with normal activity	None	Some limitation	Extremely limited
FEV₁ or peak flow	>80% predicted or personal best	60%–80% predicted or personal best	<60% predicted or personal best
Validated Questionnaires[b]			
ACQ	≤0.75[†]	≥1.5	N/A
ACT	≥20	16–19	≤15
ATAQ	0	1–2	3–4
Risk			
Exacerbations requiring oral systemic corticosteroids	0–1/y	≥2/y[a] ————————————————→	
Progressive loss of lung function	Evaluation requires long-term follow-up care		
Treatment-related adverse effects	Medication side effects can vary in intensity from none to very troublesome and worrisome. The level of intensity does not correlate to specific levels of control, but it should be considered in the overall assessment of risk.		
Recommended action for treatment[‡]	Maintain current step. Regular follow-up at every 1–6 mo to maintain control. Consider step down if well controlled for ≥3 mo	Step up 1 step and reevaluate in 2–6 wk. For side effects, consider alternative treatment options	Consider short course of systemic oral corticosteroids. Step up 1–2 steps and reevaluate in 2 wk. For side effects, consider alternative treatment options

Data from the National Asthma Education and Prevention Program (NAEPP) Expert Panel Report 3: Guidelines for the Management of Asthma.

[a]At present, there are inadequate data to correspond frequencies of exacerbations with different levels of asthma control. In general, more frequent and intense exacerbations (e.g., requiring urgent, unscheduled care, hospitalization, or ICU admission) indicate poorer disease control. For treatment purposes, patients who had ≥2 exacerbations requiring oral systemic corticosteroids in the past year may be considered the same as patients who have not-well-controlled asthma, even in the absence of impairment levels consistent with not-well-controlled asthma.

[b]Validated questionnaires for the impairment domain (the questionnaires do not assess the risk domain). Minimal important difference. 0.5 for the ACQ, 1.0 for the ATAQ and 3.0 for the ACT.

*The level of control is based on the most severe impairment or risk category. Assess impairment domain by patient's recall of previous 2–4 weeks and by spirometry or peak flow measures. Symptom assessment for longer periods should reflect a global assessment, such as inquiring whether the patient's asthma is better or worse since the last visit.

[†]ACQ values of 0.76–1.4 are indeterminate regarding well-controlled asthma.

[‡]See Table 6 for treatment steps. The stepwise approach is meant to assist, not replace, the clinical decision making required to meet individual patient needs. Before a step up in therapy, review adherence, inhaler technique, environmental control, and comorbid conditions. If an alternative treatment option was used in a step, discontinue it and use the preferred treatment for that step.

Abbreviations: ACQ = Asthma Control Questionnaire; ACT = Asthma Control Test; ATAQ = Asthma Therapy Assessment Questionnaire; EIB = exercise-induced bronchospasm; FEV₁ = forced expiratory volume in one second; N/A = not applicable.

For patients not on long-term control medications, assess *severity* and select the level of treatment that corresponds to the patient's level of severity (see Table 1). Persistent asthma is most effectively controlled with daily long-term control medications, specifically anti-inflammatory therapy. For patients receiving long-term control medications, identify their current *step of therapy*, based on what they are actually taking (see Table 6), and their level of *control* (see Table 2). In general, step up one step for patients whose asthma is not well controlled. For patients with very poorly controlled asthma, consider increasing by two steps, a course of oral corticosteroids, or both. Before increasing pharmacologic therapy, consider adverse environmental exposures, poor adherence, or comorbidities as targets for intervention. For patients with troublesome or debilitating side effects from asthma therapy, explore a change in therapy.

TABLE 3 Normal FEV₁/FVC by Age

Age Range (y)	Normal FEV₁/FVC (%)
8–19	85
20–39	80
40–59	75
60–80	70

Data from the National Asthma Education and Prevention Program (NAEPP) Expert Panel Report 3: Guidelines for the Management of Asthma.
Abbreviations: FEV₁ = forced expiratory volume in one second; FVC = forced vital capacity.

Follow-up

Patients whose asthma is not controlled should be seen every 2 to 6 weeks (depending on their initial level of severity or control) until control is achieved. Once control is achieved, follow-up contact at 1- to 6-month intervals is recommended. These checkups should ensure continued control, identify other changes in the patient's status, and update the patient's action plan.

When well-controlled asthma has been maintained for at least 3 months, a step down in therapy can be considered to determine the minimal amount of medication required to maintain control or reduce the risk of side effects. Reduction in therapy should be gradual

BOX 1   Measures to Control Environmental Factors That Can Make Asthma Worse

ALLERGENS

Reduce or eliminate exposure to the allergen(s) the patient is sensitive to:

Animal Dander

- Remove animal from house or, at a minimum, keep animal out of the patient's bedroom and keep the bedroom door closed.

Dust Mites

- Recommended
  - Encase mattress in a special dust-proof cover
  - Encase pillow in a special dust-proof cover or wash it weekly in hot water.
  - Wash sheets and blankets on the patient's bed in hot water weekly. Water must be hotter than 130°F to kill the mites. Cooler water used with detergent and bleach can also be effective.
- Desirable
  - Reduce indoor humidity to 60% or less.
  - Remove carpets from the bedroom.
  - Avoid sleeping or lying on cloth-covered cushions or furniture.
  - Remove carpets that are laid on concrete.

Cockroaches

- Keep all food out of the bedroom.
- Keep food and garbage in closed containers.
- Use poison baits, powders, gels or paste (e.g., boric acid). Traps can also be used.
- If a spray is used to kill cockroaches, stay out of the room until the odor goes away.

Pollens (from Trees, Grass, or Weeds) and Outdoor Molds

- Try to keep windows closed
- If possible, stay indoors, with windows closed, during periods of peak pollen exposure, which are usually during the midday and afternoon.

Indoor Mold

- Fix all leaks and eliminate water sources associated with mold growth.
- Clean moldy surfaces.
- Dehumidify basements if possible.

TOBACCO SMOKE

- Advise patients and others in the home who smoke to stop smoking or to smoke outside the home.
- Discuss ways to reduce exposure to other sources of tobacco smoke, such as from daycare providers and the workplace.

INDOOR AND OUTDOOR POLLUTANTS AND IRRITANTS

- If possible, do not use a wood-burning stove, kerosene heater, fireplace, unvented gas stove, or heater
- Try to stay away from strong odors and sprays, such as perfume, talcum powder, hair spray, paints, new carpet, or particle board.

Data from the National Asthma Education and Prevention Program (NAEPP) Expert Panel Report 3: Guidelines for the Management of Asthma.

---

because asthma can deteriorate at a highly variable rate and intensity. Doses of inhaled corticosteroids may be reduced about 25% to 50% every 3 months to the lowest dose possible to maintain control. Most patients with persistent asthma relapse if inhaled corticosteroids are totally discontinued.

Patients should be encouraged to contact their asthma physician for signs of loss of asthma control, such as nocturnal symptoms, increasing β-agonist use, or activity limitation. The Expert Panel recommends consultation with an asthma specialist if the patient has difficulties achieving or maintaining control of asthma, immunotherapy or omalizumab (Xolair) is being considered, the patient requires step 4 care or higher, or the patient has had an exacerbation requiring hospitalization.

Treatment of Exacerbations

Asthma exacerbations are acute or subacute episodes of progressively worsening shortness of breath, cough, wheezing, or chest tightness associated with decreases in expiratory airflow.

HOME MANAGEMENT

Patients' action plans should direct their home therapy of asthma exacerbations according to the following recommendations.

Initial therapy should be with inhaled short-acting β-agonists (2–6 puffs by metered-dose inhaler [MDI] or nebulizer). This may be repeated in 20 minutes. With a good response (minimal or no symptoms and peak expiratory flow (PEF) ≥80% predicted or personal best), the patient may continue β-agonists every 3 to 4 hours for 24 to 48 hours. If repeated β-agonists are needed, a short course of oral corticosteroids should be considered.

With an incomplete response to initial therapy (persistent wheezing and dyspnea and PEF 50% to 79% predicted or personal best), oral corticosteroids should be added, β-agonists should be repeated, and the clinician should be contacted that day.

With a poor response (marked wheezing and dyspnea at rest, PEF <50% predicted or personal best), oral corticosteroids should be added, the β-agonist should be repeated immediately, and the patient should call the clinician and usually proceed to the emergency department. For signs of severe distress (e.g., difficulty talking in full sentences, diaphoresis, drowsiness, confusion, or cyanosis), 911 should be called. Patients with histories of rapid-onset severe exacerbations should have self-injectable epinephrine (EpiPen)[1] at home to use at the onset of increased symptoms.

---

[1]Not FDA approved for this indication.

CURRENT THERAPY

- Nonpharmacologic therapy includes asthma education (especially regarding inhaler technique, self-monitoring, and self-management), reduction in environmental triggers, addressing any relevant psychosocial issues, and immunotherapy for select patients.
- Preferred step therapy for long-term asthma management is (in order): low-dose inhaled corticosteroids; medium-dose inhaled corticosteroids or low-dose inhaled corticosteroids plus long-acting β-agonists; medium-dose inhaled corticosteroids plus long-acting β-agonists; high-dose inhaled corticosteroids plus long-acting β-agonists; and oral prednisone.
- Asthma exacerbations should be treated with high-dose inhaled β-agonists and early use of systemic corticosteroids.

TABLE 4 Usual Dosages for Quick-Relief Medications for Patients 12 Years and Older

Medication	Dosage Form	Adult Dose	Comments
Inhaled Short-Acting β₂-Agonists (SABA)			
Metered-Dose Inhaler		*Applies to all three SABAS*	
Albuterol HFA (Proventil, Ventolin)	90 µg/puff, 200 puffs/canister	2 puffs 5 min before exercise	An increasing use or lack of expected effect indicates diminished control of asthma.
Pirbuterol CFC (Maxair)	200 µg/puff, 400 puffs/ canister	*or*	Not recommended for long-term daily treatment. Regular use exceeding 2 d/wk for symptom control (not prevention of EIB) indicates the need for additional long-term control therapy.
Levalbuterol HFA (Xopenox)	45 µg/puff, 200 puffs/canister	2 puffs q4–6h prn	Differences in potencies exist, but all products are essentially comparable on a per puff basis.
			May double usual dose for mild exacerbations.
			For levalbuterol, should prime the inhaler by releasing 4 actuations prior to use. For HFA, periodically clean HFA activator, as drug may block/plug orifice.
			Nonselective agents (epinephrine [Primatene Mist], isoproterenol [Isopro Aerometer], metaproterenol [Alupent]) are not recommended due to their potential for excessive cardiac stimulation, especially in high doses.
Nebulizer Solutions			
Albuterol (Accuneb, Proventil)	0.63 mg/3 mL 1.25 mg/3 mL 2.5 mg/3 mL 5 mg/mL (0.5%)	1.25–5 mg in 3 mL saline q4–8h prn	May mix with budesonide (Pulmicort) inhalant suspension, cromolyn (Intal) or ipratropium (Atrovent) nebulizer solutions. May double the dose for severe exacerbations.
Levalbuterol (R-albuterol) (Xopenex)	0.31 mg/3 mL 0.63 mg/3 mL 1.25 mg/0.5 mL 1.25 mg/3 mL	0.63 mg–1.25 mg q8h prn	Compatible with budesonide (Pulmicort) inhalant suspension. The product is a sterile-filled, preservative-free, unit-dose vial.
Anticholinergics			
Metered-Dose Inhalers			
Ipratropium HFA (Atrovent)	17 µg/puff, 200 puffs/canister	2–3 puffs q6h	Multiple doses in the emergency department (not hospital) setting provide additive benefit to short-acting beta agonists. Treatment of choice for bronchospasm due to β-blocker. Does not block EIB Reverses only cholinergically mediated bronchospasm; does not modify reaction to antigen. May be alternative for patients who do not tolerate short-acting beta-agonist. Evidence is lacking for anticholinergics producing added benefit to β₂ agonists in long-term control asthma therapy.
Ipratropium with albuterol (Combivent)[1]	18 µg/puff of ipratropium bromide and 90 µg/puff of albuterol, 200 puffs/ canister	2–3 puffs q6h	
Nebulizer Solutions			
Ipratropium bromide	0.2 mg/mL (0.2%)	0.5 mg q6h	
Ipratropium bromide with albuterol (DuoNeb)[1]	0.5 mg/3 mL ipratropium bromide and 2.5 mg/3 mL albuterol	3 mL q4–6h	Contains EDTA to prevent discoloration of the solution. This additive does not induce bronchospasm.
Systemic Corticosteroids			
Methylprednisolone (Medrol)	2, 4, 6, 8, 16, 32 mg tab	Short course (burst): 40–60 mg/d as single or 2 divided doses for 3–10 d	Short courses (bursts) are effective for establishing control when initiating therapy or during a period of gradual deterioration. Action may be begin within an hour. The burst should be continued until symptoms resolve. This usually requires 3–10 d but can require longer. There is no evidence that tapering the dose following improvement prevents relapse in asthma exacerbations.
Prednisolone (Delta-Cortef, Prelone)	5 mg tabs; 5 mg/5 mL, 15 mg/5 mL		
Prednisone (Deltasone, Orasone)	1, 2.5, 5, 10, 20, 50 mg tabs; 5 mg/mL, 5 mg/5 mL		
Repository Injection			
Methylprednisolone acetate (Depo-Medrol)	40 mg/mL 80 mg/mL	240 mg[3†] IM once	May be used in place of a short burst of oral steroids in patients who are vomiting or if adherence is a problem.

Data from the National Asthma Education and Prevention Program (NAEPP) Expert Panel Report 3: Guidelines for the Management of Asthma.
[1]Not FDA approved for this indication.
[3]Exceeds dosage recommended by the manufacturer.
[†]80–120 mg per package insert.
Abbreviations: CFC = chlorofluorocarbon; EIB = exercise-induced bronchospasm; HFA = hydrofluoroalkane; PEF = peak expiratory flow; tab = tablet.

TABLE 5 Usual Dosages for Long-Term Control Medications for Patients 12 Years and Older

Medication	Dosage Form*	Adult Dose	Comments
Systemic Corticosteroids			
Methylprednisolone (Medrol)	2, 4, 8, 16, 32 mg tab	7.5–60 mg qd in a single dose in AM or qod as needed for control	For long-term treatment of severe persistent asthma, administer single dose in AM either daily or on alternate d (alternate-day therapy may produce less adrenal suppression).
Prednisolone (Delta-Cortef, Prelone)	5 mg tab 5 mg/5 mL, 15 mg/5 mL	Short-course (burst) to achieve control, 40–60 mg/d as single or 2 divided doses for 3–10 d	Short courses (bursts) are effective for establishing control when initiating therapy or during a period of gradual deterioration. There is no evidence that tapering the dose following improvement in symptom control and pulmonary function prevents relapse.
Prednisone (Deltasone, Orasone)	1, 2.5, 5, 10, 20, 50 mg tab 5 mg/mL, 5 mg/5 mL		
Inhaled Long-Acting β_2-Agonists			Should not be used for acute symptoms relief or exacerbations. Use only with ICS.
Salmeterol (Serevent)	DPI 50 µg/blister	1 blister q12h	Decreased duration of protection against EIB may occur with regular use.
Formoterol (Foradil)	DPI 12 µg/single-use capsule	1 cap q12h	Each cap is for single use only; additional doses should not be administered for at least 12 h. Caps should be used only with the Aerolizor inhaler and should not be taken orally.
Inhaled Combined Medications			
Fluticasone and salmeterol (Advair)	DPI 100 µg/50 µg, 250 µg/50 µg, or 500 µg/50 µg	1 inhalation bid†	100/50 DPI or 45/21 HFA for patients not controlled on low-to-medium dose ICS.
	HFA 45 µg/21 µg 115 µg/21 µg 230 µg/21 µg	2 puffs bid†	250/50 DPI or 115/21 HFA for patients not controlled on medium-to-high dose ICS.
Budesonide and formoterol (Symbicort)	HFA MDI 80 µg/4.5 µg 160 µg/4.5 µg	2 inhalations bid†	80/4.5 for patients not controlled on low-to-medium dose ICS. 160/4.5 for patients not controlled on medium-to-high dose ICS.
Mometazone and formoterol (Dulera)	100 mcg/5 mcg 200 mcg/5 mcg	2 inhalations bid	100/5 for patients not controlled on low-to-medium dose ICS 200/5 for patients not controlled on medium-to-high dose ICS
Inhaled Cromolyn and Nedocromil			
Cromolyn (Intal)	MDI 0.8 mg/puff	2 puffs qid	One dose before exercise or allergen exposure provides effective prophylaxis for 1–2 h. Not as effective for EIB as SABA.
	Nebulizer 20 mg/ampule	1 amp qid	4–6 wk trial of cromolyn or nedocronil may be needed to determine maximum benefit. Dose by MDI may be inadequate to affect hyperresponsiveness.
Nedocromil (Tilade)	20 mg/ampule MDI 1.75 mg/puff	2 puffs qid	Once control is achieved, the frequency of dosing may be reduced.
Leukotriene Modifiers			
Leukotriene Receptor Antagonists			
Montelukast (Singulair)	4 mg or 5 mg chewable tab 10 mg tab	10 mg qhs	Montelukast exhibits a flat dose-response curve. Doses >10 mg do not produce a greater response in adults.
Zafirlukast (Accolate)	10 or 20 mg tab	40 mg/d (20 mg tab bid)	For zafirlukast: Administration with meals decreases bioavailability; take at least 1 h before or 2 h after meals. Zafirlukast is a microsomal p450 enzyme inhibitor that can inhibit the metabolism of warfarin. Doses of this drug should be monitored accordingly. Monitor for signs and symptoms of hepatic dysfunction.
5-Lipoxygenase Inhibitor			
Zileuton (Zyflo)	600 mg tab	2400 mg daily (600 mg qid)	Monitor hepatic enzymes (ALT). Zileuton is a microsomal p450 enzyme inhibitor that can inhibit the metabolism of warfarin and theophylline. Doses of these drugs should be monitored accordingly.

Continued

TABLE 5 Usual Dosages for Long-Term Control Medications for Patients 12 Years and Older—Cont'd

Medication	Dosage Form*	Adult Dose	Comments
Methylxanthines			
Theophylline (Slophyllin, Theobid, TheoDur)	Liquids, sustained-release tab, cap	Starting dose 10 mg/kg/d up to 300 mg max Usual max 800 mg/d	Adjust dosage to achieve serum concentration of 5–15 µg/mL at steady-state ($\geq$48 h on same dosage). Due to wide interpatient variability in theophylline metabolic clearance, routine serum theophylline level monitoring is essential. Patient should be told to discontinue if they experience symptoms of toxicity. Various factors (diet, food, febrile illness, age, smoking, and other medications) can affect serum concentration.
Immunomodulators			
Omalizumab (Anti-IgE)	Subcutaneous (SQ) injection 150 mg/1.2 mL following reconstitution with 1.4 mL sterile water for injection	150–375 mg SQ every 2–4 wk, depending on body weight and pretreatment serum IgE level	Do not administer more than 150 mg per injection site. Monitor patient following injections; be prepared and equipped to indentify and treat anaphylaxis that may occur. Whether patients will develop significant antibody titers to the drug with long-term administration is unknown.

Data from the National Asthma Education and Prevention Program (NAEPP) Expert Panel Report 3: Guidelines for the Management of Asthma.
*See Table 7 for estimated comparative daily dosages for inhaled corticosteroids.
[†]Dose depends on level of severity or control.
Abbreviations: ALT = alanine aminotransferase; amp = ampule; cap = capsule; DPI = dry powder inhaler; EIB = exercise-induced bronchospasm; HFA = hydrofluoroalkane; ICS = inhaled corticosteroid; LABA = long-acting β2-agonist; max = maximum; MDI = metered-dose inhaler; SABA = short-acting β2-agonist; tab = tablet.

TABLE 6 Stepwise Approach For Managing Asthma in Patients 12 Years and Older[a]

Step	Preferred Therapy	Alternative Therapy
1	Short-acting β-agonist prn	—
2	Low-dose ICS	Cromolyn (Intal), LTRA, nedocromil (Tilade), theophylline (Theo-Dur)
3	Low-dose ICS *plus* LABA *or* Medium-dose ICS	Low-dose ICS *plus* LTRA *or* theophylline *or* zileuton (Zyflo)
4	Medium-dose ICS *plus* LABA	Medium-dose ICS *plus* LTRA *or* theophylline *or* zileuton
5	High-dose ICS *plus* LABA Consider omalizumab (Xolair) for patients who have allergies	—
6	High-dose ICS *plus* LABA *plus* oral corticosteroid[b] Consider omalizumab for patients who have allergies	—

Data from the National Asthma Education and Prevention Program (NAEPP) Expert Panel Report 3: Guidelines for the Management of Asthma.
[a]The stepwise approach is meant to assist, not replace, the clinical decision making required to meet individual patient needs.
[b]In step 6, before oral corticosteroids are introduced, a trial of high-dose ICS + LABA + either LTRA, theophylline or zileuton may be considered, although this approach has not been studied in clinical trials.
Abbreviations: ICS = inhaled corticosteroid; LABA = long-acting β agonist; LTRA = leukotriene receptor antagonist.

TABLE 7 Estimated Comparative Daily Dosages for Inhaled Corticosteroids for Patients 12 Years and Older

Drug	Dosage Form	Daily Dose		
		Low (µg)	Medium (µg)	High (µg)
Beclomethasone HFA (QVAR)	40 or 80 µg/puff	80–240	>240–480	>480
Budesonide DPI (Pulmicort)	90, 180, or 200 µg/inhalation	180–600	>600–1200	>1200
Ciclesonide (Alvesco)	80 or 160 µg/actuation	160–320	>320–640	>640
Flunisolide (AeroBid)	250 µg/puff	500–1000	>1000–2000	>2000
Flunisolide HFA (AeroSpan)	80 µg/puff	320	>320–640	>640
Fluticasone-HFA (Flovent HFA, Flovent Diskus)	MDI: 44, 110, 220 µg/puff DPI: 50, 100, 250 µg/inhalation	88–264 100–300	>264–440 >300–500	>440 >500
Mometasone DPI (Asmanex)	110 or 220 mcg/actuation	220	440	>440
Triamcinolone acetonide (Azmacort)	75 µg/puff	300–750	>750–1500	>1500

Data from the National Asthma Education and Prevention Program (NAEPP) Expert Panel Report 3: Guidelines for the Management of Asthma and *Ann Pharm* 2009;43:519.
Abbreviations: DPI = dry powder inhaler; HFA = hydrofluoroalkane.

EMERGENCY DEPARTMENT AND HOSPITAL MANAGEMENT

Assessment should rapidly determine the severity of the exacerbation based on intensity of symptoms, signs (heart rate, respiratory rate, use of accessory muscles, chest auscultation), peak flow (unless the patient is too dyspneic to perform), and pulse oximetry. Treatment should begin immediately following recognition of an exacerbation severe enough to cause dyspnea at rest, peak flow less than 70% predicted or personal best, or pulse oximetry oxygen saturation less than 95%. While treatment is being given, a brief focused history and physical examination pertinent to the exacerbation can be obtained.

In patients with *mild-moderate exacerbations* (PEF >40% predicted), initial therapy is oxygen to achieve oxygen saturation greater than 90% and inhaled short-acting β-agonist by nebulizer or MDI (4–8 puffs) with holding chamber, which may be repeated up to three times in the first hour. Oral corticosteroids (prednisone 40–80 mg) are recommended if there is no immediate response to therapy or if the patient had been recently treated with oral corticosteroids.

In patients with *severe exacerbations* (PEF <40% predicted), initial therapy is oxygen as above, inhaled high-dose short-acting β-agonist (e.g., albuterol 5 mg) and ipratropium (0.5 mg) by nebulizer every 20 minutes or continuously for 1 hour, and oral or intravenous corticosteroids (prednisone or methylprednisolone 80 mg).

Repeated assessments of symptoms, signs, PEF, and oxygen saturation determine the responsiveness of the exacerbation to therapy. Such assessments should be made in patients presenting with severe exacerbations after the initial bronchodilator treatment and in all patients after three doses of bronchodilator therapy (60–90 min after initial treatment). In patients who are improving, short-acting β-agonists may be repeated every hour until a good response is achieved (no distress, PEF >70%). When this response is sustained at least 60 minutes after the last treatment, the patient may usually be discharged on a course of oral corticosteroids (generally prednisone 40–60 mg for 5–10 days), initiation or continuation of medium-dose inhaled corticosteroids, and arrangement for outpatient follow-up.

In patients who are not improving with the above therapy, adjunctive therapy, such as with intravenous magnesium sulfate[1] (2 g) or heliox, may be considered. Intubation and mechanical ventilation may be required for patients with respiratory failure in spite of treatment.

Summary

Asthma is a very common problem with the potential to cause substantial interference with quality of life. Although there is no cure for asthma, asthma can be well controlled in the majority of patients with proper management and an effective patient-physician relationship. I hope that the method described herein for assessing and managing asthma will help physicians help their patients to achieve well-controlled asthma.

---

[1]Not FDA approved for this indication.

Asthma in Children

Method of
Gerald B. Kolski, MD, PhD

Asthma is the most common cause of significant childhood morbidity. This includes school absenteeism, hospitalizations, emergency department visits, and acute care visits. Its prevalence has been increasing throughout the 1990s and into this century. An estimated 5 million children younger than 15 years have asthma as identified by the National Health Interview Survey of 2003. According to this survey, the prevalence of asthma in the general population is somewhere between 6% and 10%. Prevalence in inner-city populations and especially in African Americans is closer to 14% to 15%. Pediatricians and family practitioners are often reluctant to make the diagnosis because of difficulty with giving prognostic information to parents. Wheezing during the first few years of life can often be associated with acute viral infections, especially respiratory syncytial virus (RSV) and rhinovirus (RV). Longitudinal studies suggest there are three patterns to wheezing in children. There are a group of children who wheeze during infancy associated with viral infections, a second group that wheeze during infancy and also as they get older, and a third group that only develops wheezing later after sensitization with allergens. Because of these groups it is oftentimes difficult to give prognostic information to parents until you have seen the pattern that a child will follow.

Despite tremendous improvement in medications and treatments for asthma, deaths from asthma continue to occur. Most recently, however, the mortality rates seem to have leveled off or decreased slightly.

One theory for the high prevalence of asthma is the "hygiene hypothesis." Studies done in homogeneous populations in Europe and Scandinavian countries have noted less asthma and allergies in rural populations versus those that live in urban environments. Attempts have been made to correlate this with endotoxin exposure during infancy and/or infections during this period of time that turn on immune responses that do not promote allergies. This concept favors an immune response, which postulates that certain infections and endotoxin exposure promote a T_H1 T cell response in which interferon gamma and interleukin(IL)-2 predominate, whereas a lack of these infections promotes a T_H2 response where there is an IL-4, IL-13, and IL-5 predominance with increased IgE production.

Pathophysiology

Over the last several decades the idea that reversible bronchoconstriction is the main element in asthma has changed. It has become apparent that in addition to bronchoconstriction there is considerable inflammation involving increased mucus production, inflammatory cell infiltrates, and airway thickening. With longitudinal studies it has become apparent that there may in fact be some fibrosis that leads to "airway remodeling." The increased inflammatory infiltrates lead to increasing airway reactivity characterized by hyperresponsiveness to various stimuli. The inflammatory cell infiltrates can include eosinophils, lymphocytes, basophils, neutrophils, and macrophages depending on the stimulus. Unchecked inflammation is believed to be the cause of the fibrosis. Clearly it is important to try and identify the triggers in an individual patient that are causing the inflammation as well as treating the inflammation.

Differential Diagnosis

Determining the cause of wheezing in infancy can often be difficult. During the first year of life if the wheezing is associated with a viral infection, a diagnosis of bronchiolitis is often made. A clinical response to bronchodilators might be helpful in assessing whether this is going to be a child with asthma. Recurrent wheezing in an atopic child with a strong family history of asthma would strongly suggest that the child has underlying asthma. An association with eczema and/or other allergic manifestations might also be suggestive of asthma. Because of the difficulty in doing pulmonary functions during the first few years of life, clinical assessment is the key. In addition to asthma, Table 1 lists the other diagnoses that have to be considered. Cystic fibrosis, gastroesophageal reflux disease, and foreign body aspiration probably are the most common diagnoses that have to be entertained. Recurrent infiltrates should make you worry about immune deficiencies including hypogammaglobulinemia and ciliary defects such as immotile cilia syndrome.

TABLE 1 Differential Diagnosis of Wheezing	
Infants	**Older Children**
Laryngomalacia	Asthma
Tracheomalacia	Cystic fibrosis
Vascular rings	Gastroesophageal reflux disease
Subglottic stenosis	Foreign body aspiration
Airway congenital masses	Airway tumors
Gastroesophageal reflux	Viral infections (RSV, adenovirus)
Bronchiolitis	Tuberculosis
Pneumonia	

Abbreviation: RSV = respiratory syncytial virus.

Diagnostic tests such as a sweat test, immunoglobulins, skin or radioallergosorbent assay test (RAST), barium swallow, bronchoscopy, or chest radiograph may be indicated.

In older children asthma may be diagnosed by doing pulmonary functions. Spirometry can often be done in the office and can be a reproducible way to measure the extent of airway disease in known asthmatics as well as diagnostic by looking at pre- and postbronchodilator responses. The forced expiratory volume at 1 second (FEV_1) is often thought to be a measure of large airway obstruction. The FEF_{25-75} or expiratory flow between the 25th and 75th percentile of the forced vital capacity (FVC) is often thought to be a measure of small airway disease. A 15% increase in FEV_1 pre- and postbronchodilator or 25% increase in FEF_{25-75} is thought to be diagnostic of asthma. Inhalation challenges with methacholine (Provocholine) or histamine are often used to measure airway reactivity in experimental studies. Bronchoconstriction with these inhalation challenges can determine the degree of airway hyperreactivity. Similar results can also be obtained with exercise challenges or cold air challenges. These tests are often used to diagnose asthma in children whose pulmonary functions at baseline are not significantly depressed. In children with asthma, peak expiratory flow rates (PEFRs) are often used to monitor the asthma as well as the management. This test is effort dependent.

Key Diagnostic Points Consistent with Asthma

- Recurrent wheezing responding to bronchodilators
- Coughing or wheezing shortly after exercise
- Pulmonary functions that show obstruction responding to bronchodilators
- Strong family history of asthma
- Associated allergic symptoms including seasonal rhinitis, eczema, or urticaria

History

Once a diagnosis of asthma is made, it is important to determine the trigger for this individual's asthma symptoms or exacerbations. The history is very important in determining treatment. Box 1 lists the most common causes for asthma exacerbations.

The most common perennial allergens are dust mites, cockroaches, mold, and pets. In the inner cities, cockroaches and dust mites are very common causes for allergic sensitization. They are extremely common and very difficult to control. Dust mites need moisture and thus are much more common in humid areas. With increased humidity, molds also can play a significant role. Children are often treated with humidifiers or vaporizers for upper respiratory infections, which may exacerbate dust mite and mold exposure. In drier climates, pets, especially indoor animals, are often exacerbating causes. Recent studies have indicated that more than two or three

BOX 1 Asthma Triggers
- Allergies: perennial or seasonal
- Viral infections
- Irritants, especially cigarette smoke and air pollution
- Exercise
- Weather changes
- Gastroesophageal reflux
- Medications including aspirin and nonsteroidal anti-inflammatory drugs (NSAIDs)
- Sinusitis

pets decreased the likelihood of sensitization, whereas an isolated pet is more likely to be associated with the development of allergy. This may have to do with endotoxin and the previously discussed hygiene hypothesis.

Children who only have difficulty with their asthma in the spring and fall may have sensitization to the pollens. This is very regional and often associated with being outdoors. Pollination and dissemination is most problematic with dry windy days. Keeping the windows closed at night as well as air conditioning may benefit individuals with seasonal allergies. These children may need medications at particular times of the year but not throughout the year. Airway reactivity often continues even 4 to 6 weeks after the allergen is no longer present.

Children who have trouble with viral infections may also have increased reactivity from perennial or seasonal exposures that exacerbate the asthma with infection. It is often helpful to reduce allergy exposure in these individuals so as to reduce their response to viral infections. Parents may be alerted to signs of upper respiratory infection so that they can increase asthma treatment at those times.

At all times cigarette smoke causes increased mucus production as well as decreases mucociliary clearance. Children with asthma thus are especially prone to having difficulty around cigarette smoke. During infancy, cigarette smoke exposure is associated with a two- to threefold increase in risk of asthma as well as upper respiratory infections, ear infections, and pneumonia. Smoking during pregnancy is also associated with a sustained decrease in infant pulmonary functions. Smoke is a form of indoor air pollution. Outdoor air pollution, especially small particles, ozone, nitrogen dioxide, and sulfur dioxide, all can be exacerbating factors in asthma.

Exercise is associated with asthma exacerbations because of the inhalation of cold dry air. Exercise is often associated with mouth breathing. The nose normally moisturizes, filters, and warms the air. Nasal congestion secondary to allergies, viral infections, or nasal obstruction can all lead to more difficulty with exercise as well as with breathing cold dry air at any time.

Weather changes are often a problem secondary to what is in the air or the changes in temperature of the air. Children who have trouble with weather changes are often responding to changes in pollen distribution or other allergens or irritants.

Children who have reflux as the exacerbating cause of their asthma often have difficulty at night when they lie down, shortly after meals, or when ingesting very acidic substances. Often there will be

 CURRENT DIAGNOSIS

- Always focus on the ABCs (airway, breathing, and circulation).
- Start prescription early and aggressively (titrate β-agonist to effect).
- Reevaluate frequently (try to avoid intubation at all cost).
- Lack of wheezing is not always a good thing.
- Plan ahead in case things go bad.
- Ensure adequate hydration.

considerable coughing and if the child is old enough to talk some significant heartburn. Reflux is often worse when the asthma is a problem because the lower esophageal sphincter tone decreases with hyperinflation at that time.

Children with sensitivity to aspirin or nonsteroidal anti-inflammatory drugs (NSAIDs) often have associated sinusitis, nasal polyps, and profuse rhinorrhea with aspirin exposure. It often goes undiagnosed until adulthood. Nasal polyps should always raise this possibility in addition to a diagnosis of cystic fibrosis.

Sinusitis can be associated with significant exacerbations of asthma. Often treating the sinusitis treats the asthma exacerbation. Purulent nasal discharge for 5 to 7 days associated with significant coughing and maxillary tenderness may be suggestive of underlying sinusitis. In children with allergic rhinitis, complications of sinusitis often occur.

In all children with asthma it is very important that you try and assess severity of disease. There should be questions asked about whether the patient has ever been intubated or had an intensive care unit admission. In addition questions about recent use of oral corticosteroids should be asked to determine the recent course of asthma. Children with underlying seizure disorders are also important to identify because they are at greater risk for mortality. Signs of mental illness or depression should also be noted because this predisposes children to significant morbidity and mortality.

Physical Examination

In examining a patient with asthma, the complete physical is extremely helpful. Children with skin findings of eczema or hives associated with an exacerbation of asthma may often lead to a search for an allergy exposure that is responsible for symptoms. Nasal examination may show boggy turbinates suggestive of allergy or erythematous turbinates suggestive of infection. Purulent discharge associated with sinus tenderness may suggest sinusitis. Nasal polyps should also be looked for to ascertain whether the patient may have underlying cystic fibrosis or aspirin-sensitive asthma. Enlarged tonsils and adenoids may predispose to mouth breathing and exacerbate underlying asthma. Examination of the chest may show whether there is a pectus suggesting chronic disease or whether there is hyperinflation with a barrel chest. Supraclavicular, intercostal, and subcostal muscular activity give information as to the work of breathing. The cardiac examination should focus on heart rate as well as any sign that might indicate this is cardiac wheezing instead of asthma. Abdominal examination is important to evaluate any signs of liver or spleen enlargement that might indicate evidence of pulmonary hypertension or cardiac disease. Examination of the extremities is important to look for clubbing and/or cyanosis. The neurologic exam is especially important acutely to ascertain whether the patient is having any change in mental status secondary to hypoxia.

Treatment

Treatment for asthma has changed considerably since the mid 1990s. The chronic management of asthma has focused on assuring that the patient functions as normally as possible with the following goals of asthma management:

- No nocturnal asthma
- Full exercise activity
- No emergency department visits or hospitalizations
- No lost time from school or work
- No or minimal side effects from medication

Asthma treatment has focused on the anti-inflammatory nature of the disease to eliminate long-term damage to the lungs. Asthma treatment has followed the National Heart, Lung, and Blood Institute (NHLBI) guidelines with assessment of asthma severity and management based on the classifications (Table 2). We developed

a color-coded questionnaire that gives an indication of asthma control. The new guidelines for 2008 put out by NHLBI focus on asthma control and asthma control questionnaires.

Medications

Asthma medications are classified according to medications that are used for acute relief of symptoms called *relievers* and those that are used for chronic control of symptoms characterized as *controllers.* This classification was established to give patients a better understanding of the role of their individual medications. It is also a better way to educate patients as to why they have to continue to take medications even when they are not having symptoms. It is important to discuss these individual classifications and medications for both acute and chronic management.

RELIEVERS

Various bronchodilators are used for acute management of asthma. These bronchodilators are predominantly β-agonists such as albuterol (Proventil), pirbuterol (Maxair), levalbuterol (Xopenex), and terbutaline (Brethine) that are selective for β_2-receptors. Table 3 gives the generic as well as trade names for these medications. The short-acting β-agonists are used for acute relief in most circumstances. In children anticholinergics such as ipratropium bromide (Atrovent) are often used in the emergency department and hospital setting acutely but are rarely given chronically. Chronic use of β-agonists is avoided because of a decrease in effectiveness as well as an increase in airway reactivity with their chronic use. With chronic use there is also a decrease in both the number and affinity of β-receptors for these bronchodilators. The affinity as well as number of β-receptors is increased with the use of corticosteroids.

In the management of acute episodes of asthma, an algorithm is used (see Current Therapy box). β-agonists are given either by nebulizer or inhaler. In addition to albuterol, a selective stereoisomer levalbuterol (Xopenex) is also available but is more expensive. This isomer may cause fewer side effects and have a slightly longer duration of action. In the acute setting, treatments are often given every 20 minutes times three and then are continued every 2 to 3 hours for hospitalized patients. In critical situations, albuterol may also be given continuously. It is during the acute situation where ipratropium bromide is beneficial for the first 24 to 48 hours of treatment. It can be given by nebulizer every 4 to 6 hours.

Injectable epinephrine is still recommended especially in the acute attack if it is thought to be secondary to allergies or anaphylaxis. It also can be used in the acute situation to make sure that inhaled drugs can reach the lower airway.

Magnesium sulfate[1] is used intravenously in severe asthmatics for its bronchodilator properties to prevent intubation or respiratory failure. This is outlined again in the acute management algorithm (Current Therapy box).

Theophylline (Theolair) was often the mainstay of asthma management in the 1980s, but its toxicity and the difficulty in having to monitor levels has reduced its use. Nausea, vomiting, abdominal pain, and an increase in hyperactivity often lead to noncompliance. With the selective β-agonists their use has been minimal. They can be used for chronic management in patients to decrease corticosteroid need.

Oral or systemic corticosteroids are always indicated in acute management of episodes of asthma exacerbation. The usual recommended starting dose is 2 mg/kg and should be continued during the episode. Prolonged use of corticosteroids may require a taper, but a short course of 4 to 5 days does not usually require a taper. Any patient who was admitted for an acute exacerbation of asthma should go home on a controller with an action plan for future attacks.

---

[1]Not FDA approved for this indication.

CURRENT THERAPY

- **Severe:** ABCs, oxygen, monitors, POX, IV, isotonic fluids to maintain volume.

Start with (consider SC epinephrine if really tight):

- Albuterol, 0.5% inhalation solution, 0.5 mL (<20 kg), 0.75 mL (>20 kg) q20min × 3 (may give as mini-Nebs or start continuous at 2–3 mL/h). After initial stabilization patient will likely need q2h Nebs or continuous albuterol.
- Methylprednisolone (Solu-Medrol), 2 mg/kg IV (maximum, 125 mg) then start 1 mg/kg q6h (maximum, 80 mg/dose).
- Ipratropium bromide (Atrovent), 250 μg (<5 y), 500 μg (>5 y) × 2, then q4h.

If minimal improvement:

- Magnesium sulfate,[1] 45 mg/kg IV over 20 min (maximum, 2 g).

If still severe, consider terbutaline drip:

- Terbutaline (Brethine), 2–10 μg/kg loading dose, then start infusion at 0.1–0.4 μg/kg/min (maximum, 6 μg/kg/min). **Needs pediatric intensive care unit (PICU).**

At any time if minimal air entry, use:

- Epinephrine (1:1000), 0.01 mL/kg SC (maximum, 0.3 mL) or
- Terbutaline, 0.01 mg/kg SC (maximum, 0.25 mg)

Note: Adequate volume can be critical in maintaining circulatory volume (preload), so use volume freely. Also buffering with THAM for severe acidosis can be useful. These two strategies may help you avoid intubation.

If you really need to intubate (impending respiratory failure), use atropine, 0.02 mg/kg IV (minimum), 0.1 mg (maximum, 1 mg); ketamine (Ketalar), 1–2 mg/kg IV; or vecuronium (Norcuron), 0.1–0.2 mg/kg IV.

- **Moderate:** ABCs, POX, oxygen, monitors. ± IV

Start with

- Albuterol, 0.5 mL (<20 kg), 0.75 mL (>20 kg) q20 min × 3 (may start with mini Nebs or continuous). Then patient will likely need q2h Nebs or continuous albuterol (2 mL/h <10 kg, 3 mL/hr >10 kg)
- Ipratropium bromide, 250 μg (<5 y), 500 μg (>5 y) × 2, then q4h
- Prednisone, 2 mg/kg (maximum, 80 mg) if tolerating PO or
- Methylprednisolone, 2 mg/kg (maximum, 80 mg) (continue steroids for 5 d, 2 mg/kg/d)

If minimal improvement:

Consider magnesium sulfate as above.

- **Mild:** ABCs, POX

Start with

- Albuterol Nebs or MDI with spacer q2–4h
- Prednisolone, 2 mg/kg loading dose (maximum, 80 mg), then 2 mg/kg/d divided bid × 5 d

For mild to moderate exacerbation, discharge home may be considered if patient shows good improvement, is no longer dyspneic or hypoxic, tolerates Nebs q4h, and has good supervision at home.

CXR: Consider for a first-time wheezer; a condition other than asthma (i.e., FB); a febrile child with clinical signs of pneumonia; or no clinical improvement or worsening condition (pneumothorax, pneumomediastinum).

Continuous albuterol: To calculate the total amount of albuterol and normal saline, remember that the total amount of solution per hour must equal 30 mL.

Example: For a child >10 kg, the albuterol dose for continuous Nebs is 3 mL/h so you need to add 27 mL of NSS to run for 1 h (to set it up for 4 h, total mL = 120 with 12 mL albuterol + 108 mL NSS).

---

[1]Not FDA approved for this indication.

Abbreviations: ABCs = airway, breathing, and circulation; CXR = chest radiograph; FB = foreign body; IV = intravenous; Nebs = nebulization; NSS = normal saline solution; POX = pulse oximeter; SC = subcutaneous; THAM = tromethamine.

In the chronic management of asthma, albuterol is still the mainstay of acute attacks, pre-exercise, and for any reduction in peak flow or pulmonary functions. Albuterol (Proventil or Ventolin) is usually given by metered-dose inhaler and for most patients it is recommended that it be given with a spacer. Spacers increase the deposition in the lower airway and increase the effectiveness of inhaled drugs. In the chronic management of asthma, the NHLBI guidelines recommend that if albuterol is being used more than two or three times a week a step up in controller medications is suggested (Table 2).

CONTROLLERS

Inhaled corticosteroids are established as the mainstay of chronic management of asthma. Various preparations are available either by dry powder inhaler or metered-dose inhaler. Table 2 outlines the doses and route. Side effects of growth suppression and decreases in bone mineralization are dose related as well as preparation dependent. Individuals on any of the corticosteroids need to have their growth monitored and also to have instructions on mouth rinsing after inhalation to reduce fungal colonization in the oropharynx.

Leukotriene antagonists are available in oral preparations. These offer some advantage in pediatric patients in that they do not require good inhalation technique and can be given once a day. This may improve compliance and offer benefit in asthma as well as allergic rhinitis. They are not as effective as inhaled corticosteroids but offer some benefit in mild disease or as an adjunct to inhaled corticosteroids.

Cromolyn (Intal) and nedocromil (Tilade) are available as inhaled medications. Both of these drugs are mast cell stabilizers and appear to be most effective in allergic patients. These drugs should be taken three to four times a day, which makes their compliance more difficult. There are no significant side effects to these medications, however, and they are used in children because of their safety profile. They are used primarily in the mildest of patients and as pretreatment before allergy exposure.

Long-acting β-agonists are characterized as controllers, but these medications cannot be taken as anti-inflammatory agents. They have an increased risk of mortality when taken alone. For this reason only the preparations that are in combination with inhaled corticosteroids should be used in children. The drug preparations contain varying doses of inhaled corticosteroid with one standard dose of long-acting β-agonist.

TABLE 2 Stepwise Approach for Managing Asthma in Children

Classify Severity: Clinical Features Before Treatment or Adequate Control			Medications Required to Maintain Long-Term Control
	Symptoms/Day	*PEF or FEV$_1$*	
	Symptoms/Night	*PEF Variability*	*Daily Medications*
Step 4 Severe persistent	Continual Frequent	<60% >30%	**Preferred treatment:** • High-dose inhaled corticosteroids, *and* • Long-acting inhaled β$_2$-agonists (combination preferred) *and*, if needed, • Corticosteroid tablets or syrup long term (2 mg/kg/d, generally do not exceed 60 mg/d). (Make repeat attempts to reduce systemic corticosteroids and maintain control with high-dose inhaled corticosteroids.)

Step 3
Moderate persistent
	Daily
	>1 night/wk
		>60% – <80%
		>30%
			• **Preferred treatment:**
			  • Low- to medium-dose inhaled corticosteroids.
			• **Alternative treatment** (listed alphabetically):
			  • Increase inhaled corticosteroids within medium-dose range
			  or
			  • Low to medium–dose inhaled corticosteroids and either leukotriene modifier or theophylline.
			
			If needed (particularly in patients with recurring severe exacerbations):
			• **Preferred treatment:**
			  • Increased inhaled corticosteroids within medium-dose range and add long-acting inhaled β$_2$-agonists (combination inhaler preferred).
			• **Alternative treatment** (listed alphabetically);
			  • Increase inhaled corticosteroids within medium-dose range, and add either leukotriene modifier or theophylline.

Step 2
Mild persistent
	>2/wk but <1/d
	>2 nights/mo
		>80%
		20% – 30%
			• **Preferred treatment:**
			  • Low-dose inhaled corticosteroids.
			• **Alternative treatment** (listed alphabetically):
			  • Cromolyn (Intal).
			  • Leukotriene modifier.
			  • Nedocromil (Tilade) *or* sustained-release theophylline (Slo-bid Gyrocaps) to serum concentration of 5–15 µg/mL.

Step 1 Mild intermittent	<2d/wk <2 nights/mo	>80% <20%	• **No daily medication needed.** • Severe exacerbations may occur, separated by long periods of normal lung function and no symptoms. A course of systemic corticosteroids is recommended.

Note: Children <5 y cannot do adequate peak flows.

Quick relief All patients	• Short-acting bronchodilator: 2–4 puffs short-acting inhaled β$_2$-agonists as needed for symptoms. • Intensity of treatment depends on severity of exacerbation; up to 3 treatments at 20-min intervals or a single nebulizer treatment as needed. Course of systemic corticosteroids may be needed. • Use of short-acting β$_2$-agonists >2 times/wk in intermittent asthma (daily, or increasing use in persistent asthma) may indicate the need to initiate (increase) long-term-control therapy.

↓ **Step down** Review treatment q1–6 mo; a gradual stepwise reduction in treatment may be possible.	↑ **Step up** If control is not maintained, consider step up. First, review patient medication technique, adverse effects from medications.

Notes:
The stepwise approach is meant to assist, not replace, the clinical decision making required to meet individual patient needs.
Classify severity: Assign patient to most severe step in which any feature occurs (PEF is percentage of personal best; FEV$_1$ is percentage predicted).
Gain control as quickly as possible (consider a short course of systemic corticosteroids); then step down to the least medication necessary to maintain control.
Minimize use of short-acting inhaled β$_2$-agonists. Overreliance on short-acting inhaled β$_2$-agonists (e.g., use of approximately 1 canister/mo even if not using it every day) indicates inadequate control of asthma and the need to initiate or intensify long-term control therapy.
Provide education on self-management and controlling environmental factors that make asthma worse (e.g., allergens and irritants).
Refer to an asthma specialist if there are difficulties controlling asthma or if step 4 care is required. Referral may be considered if care at level step 3 is required.

Continued

TABLE 2 Stepwise Approach for Managing Asthma in Children—Cont'd

Usual Dosages for Long-Term-Control Medications

Medication	Dosage Form	Child Dose
Systemic Corticosteroids		
Methylprednisolone (Medrol)	2-, 4-, 8-, 16-, 32-mg tablets	0.25–2 mg/kg daily in single dose in AM or qod as needed for control
Prednisolone (Prelone) (Orapred)	5-mg tablets 5 mg/5 mL, 15 mg/5 mL	Short-course "burst": 1–2 mg/kg/d, maximum
Prednisone (Orasone)	1-, 2.5-, 5-, 10-, 20-, 50-mg tablets: 5 mg/5 mL, 5 mg/mL	60 mg/d for 3–10 d
Long-Acting β₂-agonists		
(Do not use for symptom relief or for exacerbations.)		
Salmeterol (Serevent)	DPI 50 μg/blister	1 blister q12h
Formoterol (Foradil)	DPI 12 μg/single-use capsule	1 capsule q12h
Combine Medication		
Fluticasone/ salmeterol (Advair)	DPI 100, 250, or 500 μg/50 μg	1 inhalation bid; dose depends on severity of asthma
Budesonide/ formoterol	80 or 160/4.5	
Mast Cell Stabilizer		
Cromolyn (Intal)	MDI 800 μg/puff Nebulizer 20 mg/ampule	1–2 puffs tid–qid 1 ampule tid–qid
Nedocromil (Tilade)	MDI 1.75 mg/puff	1–2 puffs bid–qid
Leukotriene Modifiers		
Montelukast (Singulair)	4- or 5-mg chewable tablet 10-mg tablet	4 mg qhs (2–5 y) 5 mg qhs (6–14 y) 10 mg qhs (>14 y)
Zafirlukast (Accolate)	10- or 20-mg tablet	20 mg daily (5–11 y) (10-mg tablet bid)
Methylxanthines		
(Serum monitoring is important.)		
Theophylline (Slo-Phyllin)	Liquids, sustained-release tablets and capsules	Starting dose 10 mg/kg/d; usual maximum: <1 y: 0.2 (age in wks) + 5 = mg/kg/d >1 y: 16 mg/kg/d

Estimated Comparative Daily Dosages for Inhaled Corticosteroids

Drug	Low Daily Dose	Medium Daily Dose	High Daily Dose
Beclomethasone HFA (QVAR) 40 or 80 μg/puff	80–160 μg	160–320 mcg	>320 μg
Budesonide DPI (Pulmicort) 200 μg/inhalation	200–400 μg	400–800 mcg	>800 μg
Budesonide inhalation suspension for nebulization (Pulmicort Respules)	0.5 mg	1.0 mg	2.0 mg
Flunisolide (AeroBid) 250 μg/puff	500–750 μg	1000–1250 μcg	1250 μg
Fluticasone (Flovent)	88–176 μg	176–440 μg	>440 μg
MDI: 44, 110, or 220 μg/puff	100–200 μg	200–400 μg	>400 μg
DPI: 50, 100, or 250 μg/inhalation			
Triamcinolone acetonide (Azmacort) 100 μg/puff	400–800 μg	800–1200 μg	>1200 μg
Mometasone fumarate (Asmanex) 220 mg	220 μg	440 μg	880 μg

Abbreviations: DPI = daily permissible intake; FEV₁ = forced expiratory volume at 1 second; MDI = metered-dose inhaler; PEF = peak expiratory flow (rate).

Oral corticosteroids have been used for asthma since they were developed. They were used for patients with severe or chronic asthma before inhaled steroids were available. Because oral corticosteroids have significant side effects they should be used with caution. Prolonged use of systemic steroids leads to adrenal suppression, osteoporosis, and growth suppression. With prolonged use the dose should be reduced gradually. Inhaled corticosteroid effects can be similar to the systemic corticosteroids, especially if they are used at doses higher than recommended.

OMALIZUMAB

Omalizumab (Xolair) is a monoclonal antibody that is humanized and was developed against IgE. It is expensive and requires monthly injections. It is most effective when allergies are the main trigger for asthma. It is also used in patients with severe anaphylaxis.[1] It is indicated for children with moderate to severe persistent asthma that is exacerbated by significant documented allergies. Because it is nonspecific it does not reduce specific allergies and cannot be used in patients who have no significant atopy.

IMMUNOSUPPRESSIVE AGENTS

Various experimental studies in patients with chronic steroid-dependent asthma have used immunosuppressive agents such as methotrexate[1] (Trexall), IV gammaglobulin[1] (Gamimune N), and anti-inflammatory

---

[1]Not FDA approved for this indication.

TABLE 3 Medications for the Acute Relief of Symptoms

Generic β-agonist	Brand Name*
Albuterol	Ventolin, Ventolin HFA, Proventil HFA, Proventil
Pirbuterol	Maxair, Maxair Autohaler
Terbutaline	Brethaire, Brethine, Bricanyl
Metaproterenol	Alupent
Levalbuterol	Xopenex

Albuterol is also available in an inhaler in combination with ipratropium bromide (Combivent).
*Many of these drugs are available in liquid, tablet, inhalation aerosol, as well as metered-dose inhalers.

monoclonal antibodies against cytokines. None of these produced dramatic results, and none is available or can be recommended at this time.

IMMUNOTHERAPY

Specific injections of extracts of allergens to which the patient is allergic is effective for allergic rhinitis that is secondary to certain allergens. Therapy with allergy extracts is effective for pollens, and by reducing allergic rhinitis symptoms it can affect nasal breathing and therefore benefit asthma. Because of the risk of reactions to immunotherapy it should be used cautiously when the patient is having significant asthma symptoms at the time of injection. Studies in Europe suggest that in the future sublingual immunotherapy may be effective. Well-documented studies in this country have not been done and it is not approved as an FDA procedure.

Education and Environmental Control

Education of the individual asthmatic is important. Action plans in which treatment of acute episodes is outlined is recommended. Parents and patients should be taught about the patient's triggers as well as steps they should take to increase or decrease their medications depending on symptoms. Environmental precautions such as dust mite avoidance, focusing on reducing humidity, and limiting tobacco smoke exposure have had some success. Pet avoidance has not worked unless the pet is totally eliminated.

The NHBLI Guidelines as put forth in NAEPP Expert Panel 3 has been updated. It focuses on asthma control and uses asthma control questionaries.[1] In addition, it recommends that asthmatics on being discharged from the hospital or after being seen by their primary care physician be sent home with an action plan. In addition to assessing severity of asthma and outlining an action plan, a risk assessment is suggested with an emphasis on removing triggers, controlling the environment, and assessing comorbidities. The characteristic of the new guidelines focuses on the severity at the initial assessment, but in subsequent evaluations focuses on assessing control. The recommendation is to step up treatment if there is inadequate control and step down on treatment if it can be achieved with continued excellent control. Periodic assessment and monitoring are recommended, especially using spirometry, when possible.

REFERENCES

Castro-Rodriguez JA, Holberg CJ, Wright AL, Martinez FD. A clinical index to define risk of asthma in young children with recurrent wheezing. Am J Respir Crit Care Med 2000;162:1403–6.

National Institutes of Health/National Heart, Lung, and Blood Institute. NAEPP expert panel report 2: Guidelines for the diagnosis and management of asthma. Publication no. 97–4051. Bethesda, Md: The Institutes; 1997.

National Institutes of Health/National Heart, Lung, and Blood Institute. NAEPP expert panel report 3: Guidelines for the diagnosis and management of asthma. Publication no. 08–4051 Bethesda, Md: The Institutes; 2007.

O'Connor GT. Allergen avoidance in asthma: What do we do now? J Allergy Clin Immunol 2005;116:26–30.

Romagnani S. Immunologic influences on allergy and the TH1/TH2 balance. J Allergy Clin Immunol 2004;113:395–400.

Spahn JD, Szefler SJ. Childhood asthma: New insights into management. J Allergy Clin Immunol 2002;109:3–13.

Allergic Rhinitis Caused by Inhalant Factors

Method of
David M. Quillen, MD

Rhinitis is characterized by one or more of the following nasal symptoms: congestion, anterior and posterior rhinorrhea, sneezing, and nasal itching. Rhinitis has significant morbidity and is not a trivial disease. Rhinitis has several causes (Box 1). The most common form is allergic rhinitis (AR), which is rhinitis caused primarily by inhaled allergens. The three main AR subgroups are *seasonal* (i.e., hay fever), *perennial* (i.e., chronic allergic rhinitis), and *occupational*. Among the atopic diseases of AR, asthma, and dermatologic reactions, AR is the most common. Depending on the source of information, AR affects between 10% and 30% of all adults and as many as 40% of children (40 million Americans). Most patients who present with rhinitis symptoms have AR, but several other causes should be considered as part of the evaluation (see Box 1).

Pathophysiology and Morbidity

AR involves inflammation of the upper respiratory tract mucosa (i.e., nasal mucosa, eustachian tubes, and sinuses) and eyes. In severe cases, patients can also have systemic symptoms. Complex interactions among inhaled allergens and irritants, immunoglobulin E (IgE), and inflammatory mediators are the cause of the inflammation. Genetics play a role in the tendency for an individual to develop atopic disease such as AR and asthma. AR usually develops in childhood and is slightly more common in boys than girls. By adulthood, the incidence is equal between men and women. Susceptible individuals produce specific IgEs in response to inhaled proteins. The IgEs cause the mast cells to release a variety of mediators, such as histamine, tryptase, chymase, kinins, leukotrienes, prostaglandins, and heparin. The inflammatory mediators cause immediate vasodilatation, nasal congestion, sneezing, and itching. The mediators also cause recruitment of other inflammatory cells (i.e., macrophages, eosinophils, neutrophils, and lymphocytes), which lead to a delayed response that can last for hours or days and occasionally include systemic symptoms (e.g., malaise, fatigue).

AR is not a life-threatening disease, but the effects on an individual's quality of life are high. Societal costs from AR are also high and have been estimated at more than $5 billion per year in lost productivity, time away from work, and other expenses. AR predisposes affected individuals to otitis media and sinusitis. Those with AR frequently have associated atopic conditions (e.g., asthma, atopic dermatitis, nasal polyps), and there is some evidence that poorly controlled AR can worsen asthma.

---

[1]Not FDA approved for this indication.

BOX 1 Differential Diagnosis of Rhinitis Symptoms

Allergic rhinitis
  Seasonal
  Perennial
  Episodic
  Occupational (may be nonallergic)
Nonallergic rhinitis
  Infectious
    Acute (usually viral)
    Chronic (rhinosinusitis)
  Nonallergic rhinitis with eosinophilia syndrome (NARES)
  Perennial nonallergic rhinitis (vasomotor rhinitis)
  Other types
    Ciliary dyskinesia syndrome
    Atrophic rhinitis
    Hormone induced
      Hypothyroidism
      Pregnancy
      Oral contraceptives
      Menstrual cycle
    Exercise induced
    Drug induced
      Rhinitis medicamentosa
      Oral contraceptives
      Antihypertension medications
      Aspirin
      Nonsteroidal antiinflammatory drugs
    Reflux induced
      Gustatory rhinitis
      Chemical or irritant
      Postural reflexes
      Nasal cycle
      Emotional cause
    Occupational (may be allergic)
Conditions that may mimic symptoms of rhinitis
  Structural or mechanical causes
    Deviated septum
    Hypertrophic turbinates
    Enlarged adenoids
    Foreign bodies
    Choanal atresia
  Inflammatory or immunologic
    Wegener's granulomatosis
    Midline granuloma
    Sarcoidosis
    Systemic lupus erythematosus
    Sjögren's syndrome
    Nasal polyposis
  Cerebrospinal fluid rhinorrhea

Modified from Dykewicz MS, Fineman S, Skoner DP, et al: Diagnosis and management of rhinitis: Complete guidelines of the Joint Task Force on Practice Parameters in Allergy, Asthma and Immunology. American Academy of Allergy, Asthma, and Immunology. Ann Allergy Asthma Immunol 1998;81(Pt 2):478–518.

Diagnosis

DIFFERENTIAL DIAGNOSIS

Differentiating AR from the other forms of rhinitis is important. Nonallergic rhinitis (NAR) is a common cause of rhinitis and can be difficult to differentiate from AR. The ratio of AR to NAR is approximately 3:1. However, preliminary data suggest that up to two thirds of patients with AR may have mixed rhinitis, a combination of AR and NAR. Understanding that many patients have some component of NAR explains why many have mixed symptoms.

In many cases, a thorough history suggests the diagnosis. Infectious causes of rhinitis (i.e., viral upper respiratory infections, influenza, or sinusitis) usually produce more acute symptoms with limited durations, unlike the more chronic nature of AR and NAR. Vasomotor rhinitis and NAR usually do not have historical triggers or seasonal patterns. Endocrine and hormonal conditions such as hypothyroidism and pregnancy can cause chronic congestion, as can a variety of medications. Systemic disease such as Wegener's granulomatosis, Sjögren's syndrome, and nasal polyposis can also cause similar symptoms. Unilateral symptoms suggest an obstruction, and, particularly in children, a foreign body must be excluded.

PATIENT EVALUATION

A comprehensive history usually suggests the correct diagnosis. Occasionally, the diagnosis may be elusive because of the many different causes of rhinitis (Fig. 1). Areas to focus on include symptoms (i.e., duration, exposures, magnitude of reaction, patterns, and chronicity), triggers, seasonal variation, environmental influences, history of allergies, medical history, and family history. Eighty percent of patients with AR first develop symptoms before the age of 20 years. Eliciting a positive family history is helpful, because allergic symptoms and asthma tend to run in families. The success of past and current treatments can help to identify the cause and help to direct future treatment.

A focused physical examination should follow the history. Patients with chronic allergic symptoms may have dark circles under the eyes (i.e., allergic shiners) or be obvious mouth breathers. Conjunctivitis and an acute viral upper respiratory infection may be components of AR. A careful examination of the nose is important to identify structural abnormalities, obvious polyps, mucosal swelling, and discharge. Examining the pharynx for enlarged tonsils and postnasal drip can help support viral causes or chronic drainage from chronic rhinitis. Lymphadenopathy with associated symptoms can help support the diagnosis of viral or bacterial rhinitis, and findings of other atopic diseases (e.g., wheezing from asthma, eczema) support an allergic cause.

In most cases, the history and physical examination provide enough information to make the diagnosis or at least initiate a treatment program with periodic follow-up. Specific testing should be used when the diagnosis is in question or attempts are being made to tailor therapy. The two most common tests are percutaneous skin testing and allergen-specific IgE antibody testing (i.e., radioallergosorbent test [RAST]). Intradermal skin testing is less common.

CURRENT DIAGNOSIS

- Appropriate history
  - Perennial or seasonal symptoms
  - Identified triggers
  - History of asthma or eczema
  - Supported by family history of atopy
  - Previous response to treatment
- Nonallergic causes
  - Hormones
  - Medications
  - Systemic disease
  - Obstruction
  - Nonallergic rhinitis
- Physical examination
  - Rhinorrhea
  - Nasal congestion
  - Allergic facial changes
- Diagnostic testing
  - Percutaneous test (prick test)
  - Radioallergosorbent test (RAST)
  - Allergen-specific IgE antibody testing

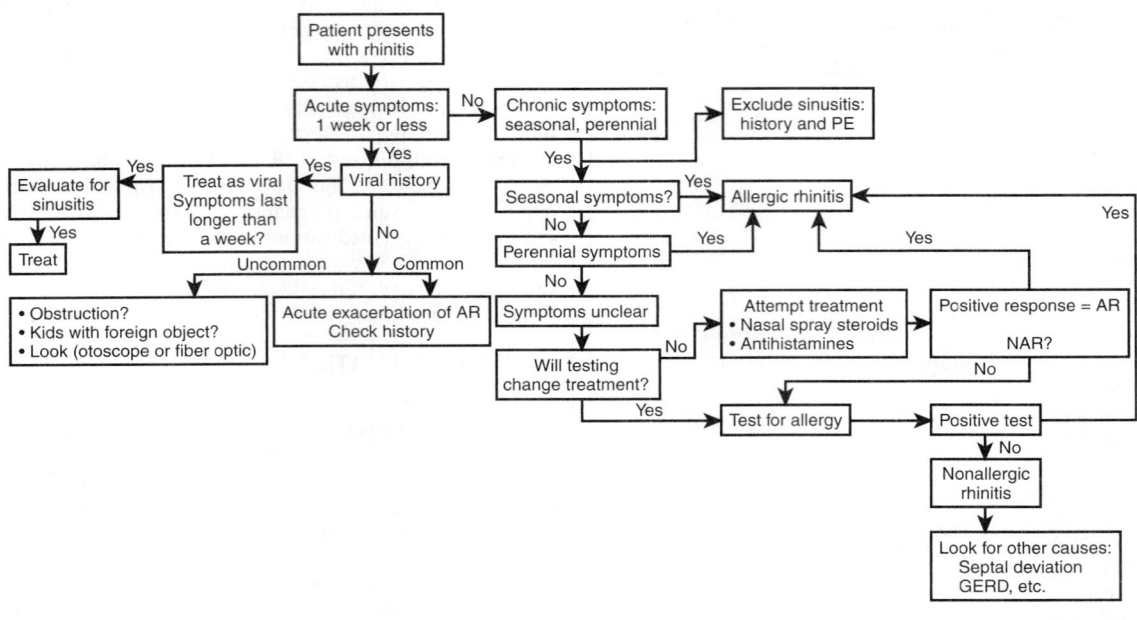

FIGURE. 1. Rhinitis algorithm. *Abbreviations:* AR = allergic rhinitis; GERD = gastroesophageal reflux disease; NAR = nonallergic rhinitis; PE = physical examination.

Percutaneous skin testing (i.e., prick test) is specific and cost effective, but it is not always available and may require referral. RAST testing, a blood test, usually is available and is useful for common allergens, such as pet dander, dust mites, grass pollen, and common molds, but is not very specific for food, venom, or drug allergies. Intradermal skin testing is an alternative option and historically considered to be more sensitive but with a lower specificity. Controversy remains about which test is superior, but there does appear to be increased safety concerns with intradermal testing. If available, we recommend percutaneous testing and RAST testing to local allergens.

Treatment

Treatment for allergic rhinitis is relatively straightforward (Box 2). General principles include using the minimum medication for relief, combination treatment (i.e., nasal spray steroids and antihistamines work better together than either alone), and continuously reevaluating

---

BOX 2 Treatment Strategy for Allergic Rhinitis

- Confirm the diagnosis with a history and physical examination; if in doubt, consider allergy testing.
- Reduce exposure to allergens.
- Start an oral antihistamine; use a second-generation drug before a first-generation drug if possible or use nasal spray steroid for a 2-week trial.
- Select a second agent, an antihistamine or nasal spray steroid, if relief has been inadequate.
- If results are not satisfactory, consider testing (if not already done).
- Consider a leukotriene receptor antagonist.
- Treat ocular symptoms with a nonsteroidal antiinflammatory drug, antihistamine, or mast cell stabilizer (use one at a time).
- Other options include use of a nasal spray antihistamine, a nasal spray mast cell stabilizer, or a nasal spray anticholinergic.
- If relief is inadequate, consider testing to confirm sensitivity to specific allergens and institution of immunotherapy.

---

when treatment is not working. Testing is not required initially if the history and physical examination findings are consistent. However, if standard treatment is not working, testing is important to eliminate the many other diagnoses that cause rhinitis symptoms.

Pharmacotherapy, environmental modification, and immunotherapy are the primary treatment modalities. Pharmacotherapy is usually tried first, and oral antihistamines are the most commonly selected agent. Oral antihistamines have been around for more than 50 years and are used in numerous over-the-counter (OTC) cold and allergy preparations. Overall efficacy of the oral antihistamines is good, but they are not as effective as nasal spray steroids.

The older first-generation antihistamines (H_1-blockers) are effective against the symptoms of rhinorrhea, itching, and sneezing. There are many OTC first-generation antihistamines available in generic form. The antihistamines are not very effective against congestion, which is why many OTC preparations are combined with an oral decongestant (pseudoephedrine or phenylephrine). Common side effects of antihistamines include sedation and anticholinergic effects, and they require dosing several times per day.

Second-generation H_1-blockers include loratadine (Claritin, Alavert), fexofenadine (Allegra), and cetirizine (Zyrtec). All are available as generic preparations, and loratadine and cetirizine are available OTC. All three have less anticholinergic and sedative side effects than first-generation antihistamines. All can be taken once daily. Cetirizine is the active metabolite of the first-generation H_1-blocker hydroxyzine (Atarax). Of the three second-generation H_1-blockers, cetirizine has more potential for sedation.

Topical treatments include nasal spray antihistamines, nasal spray mast cell stabilizers, ophthalmic antihistamines, ophthalmic nonsteroidal antiinflammatory drugs (NSAIDs), nasal spray anticholinergics, and nasal spray steroids. Azelastine (Astelin) is an H_1-antagonist, and it can be used in a nasal spray twice daily for nasal symptoms and in an ophthalmic solution (Optivar) for allergic conjunctivitis. Patient acceptance is limited because of the bitter taste associated with the nasal spray. Many types of ophthalmic drops can be used for ocular symptoms associated with AR or for allergic conjunctivitis alone. Olopatadine (Patanol) is an H_1-antagonist that is approved for allergic conjunctivitis. Ketorolac (Acular 0.5%) is an NSAID and available in an ophthalmic solution for allergic conjunctivitis, although only the 0.5% drop is approved for this indication.

Cromolyn is a specific mast cell stabilizer that inhibits degranulation. For AR, cromolyn is available in a nasal spray (Nasalcrom) and in an ophthalmic solution (Crolom).[1] It is well tolerated and has minimal side effects; however, its efficacy is limited due to frequency of administration (3–6 times daily). Ipratropium (Atrovent nasal spray) is the only available anticholinergic for nasal administration, and it produces a localized parasympatholytic effect on the nasal mucosa. Ipratropium antagonizes the action of acetylcholine by blocking muscarinic cholinergic receptors, which reduces watery hypersecretion from mucosal glands of the nose. This provides symptomatic relief by reducing rhinorrhea associated with the common cold or allergic or nonallergic perennial rhinitis.

Topical or nasal spray steroids are by far the most effective single medication for AR, and they are effective for long-term and short-term treatment. Corticosteroids exhibit antiinflammatory, antipruritic, and vasoconstrictive properties. Early antiinflammatory effects of topical corticosteroids include the inhibition of macrophage and leukocyte activity in the inflamed area and reversal of vascular dilation and permeability. Nasal spray steroids are generally well tolerated; however, side effects may include epistaxis, headaches, sinus infection, coughing, musculoskeletal pain, and dysmenorrhea. Rare reports of nasal septum perforation are most likely related to improper dosing or administration techniques. Results of clinical trials have not supported concerns about long-term exposure to nasal steroids and growth retardation in children.

Available nasal spray preparations include fluticasone (Flonase), budesonide (Rhinocort Aqua), mometasone (Nasonex), beclomethasone (Beconase), flunisolide (Nasalide [available only as a generic]), and triamcinolone (Nasacort). Although there are variations in potency and systemic bioavailability among the different preparations, most differences are not clinically important.

The practice of using oral or intramuscular injections of steroids to manage AR is not advised. The efficacy, side effects, and potential risks do not justify the treatment.

The leukotriene receptor antagonist montelukast (Singulair) has been FDA approved for AR. Its efficacy is comparable to that of antihistamines, but it is less effective than the nasal spray steroids. The expense of this treatment is a major drawback, but it is well tolerated and has few side effects. The addition of montelukast to the treatment regimen is probably best done after a trial of antihistamines or nasal spray steroids, or both.

There is evidence that topical saline wash is beneficial in the treatment of the symptoms of chronic rhinorrhea and rhinosinusitis when used as a sole modality or for adjunctive treatment. When to use this treatment for patients with AR is unclear. The side effects and risks of saline washes are minimal, and they therefore can be used at any point in a treatment plan.

Avoiding specific allergens can be difficult and impractical. The most common allergic triggers are pollens, molds, dust mite excrement, furry animal dander, and insect emanations (e.g., cockroaches). The types of pollen responsible for rhinitis symptoms vary widely with locale, climate, and introduced plantings. Depending on the region of the United States or world, pollen seasons vary in length and by time of year. Fungi and molds can produce clinically important allergens. Reduction of indoor fungi requires removal of moisture sources and replacement of contaminated materials. The use of dilute bleach solutions on nonporous surfaces can help. Humidity control helps to retard mold and fungus growth and can help to control dust. Dust mite control requires covers for bedding, high-efficiency particulate air (HEPA) filter vacuuming of carpeting or removal to nonporous floors. Avoidance is the most effective way to manage sensitivity to animals. Cockroaches are a significant cause of nasal allergy, particularly in inner-city populations and warm climates.

For patients who fail to get adequate results with medications and avoidance measures, allergen injection immunotherapy is an effective treatment for AR. Exactly how injection therapy works is unclear. High doses of systemic allergens are thought to change humeral and cellular components of the immune process, resulting in modulation of the immune response. Successful injection therapy can result in up to a 50% reduction in symptom scores and an 80% reduction in medication use. The effects of injection treatment can persist for at least 3 years after discontinuation of treatment. However, there are reports of severe systemic reactions, including a few fatalities. Weekly injection treatments with observation up to an

[1]Not FDA approved for this indication.

CURRENT THERAPY

- Allergen avoidance
- Nasal spray steroids (most effective single agent, less patient acceptance than antihistamines)
  - Triamcinolone (Nasacort AQ)
  - Fluticasone (Flonase)
  - Budesonide (Rhinocort Aqua)
  - Mometasone (Nasonex)
  - Flunisolide (Nasalide)
  - Beclomethasone (Beconase AQ)
- Oral antihistamines (first-line or second-line agent after nasal spray steroids)
  - Cetirizine (Zyrtec) (nonsedating second generation)
  - Fexofenadine (Allegra) (nonsedating second generation)
  - Loratadine (Claritin, Alavert) (nonsedating second generation)
  - Diphenhydramine (Benadryl)
  - Hydroxyzine (Atarax)[1]
  - Chlorpheniramine (Chlor-Trimeton)
  - Many other generics
- Topical antihistamines (add-on treatment)
  - Azelastine (Astelin intranasal spray)
- Topical ophthalmic drops (allergic conjunctivitis symptoms)
  - Antihistamines (e.g., azelastine [Optivar], olopatadine [Patanol])
  - NSAIDs (e.g., ketorolac [Acular 0.5%])
  - Mast cell stabilizer (e.g., cromolyn [Crolom][1])
- Oral leukotriene receptor antagonist (add-on treatment, confirm AR with testing)
  - Montelukast (Singulair)
- Nasal saline irrigation (add-on therapy)
- Oral decongestants (better for congestion rather than rhinorrhea)
  - Pseudoephedrine* (Sudafed and combined with many antihistamines)
  - Phenylephrine (alone or combined with antihistamines)
- Immunotherapy (requires testing)
  - Injection therapy
  - Sublingual therapy

[1]Not FDA approved for this indication.
*Federal and state restrictions limit the purchase of pseudoephedrine to discourage illegal conversion to methamphetamine.

hour afterward make injection therapy time consuming and expensive. Because of the risks and expense associated with injection therapy, alternate routes of treatment have been investigated.

Immunotherapy by nasal spray and sublingual administration has been investigated, with sublingual immunotherapy being the most successful route. Meta-analysis of 22 studies of sublingual administration has demonstrated efficacy. The buildup process (i.e., increasing dose over time) appears to be faster than injection. The availability of sublingual immunotherapy is limited partially because of insurance coverage taking time to catch up to clinical science.

Management Overview

AR is a common condition that has a significant negative impact on the quality of life for those who suffer. Diagnosis is usually straightforward with the option for specific testing if needed. Treatment is usually pharmacologic, and antihistamines and nasal spray steroids are the most commonly used agents. Making lifestyle changes to avoid specific allergens can help. Second-generation antihistamines have fewer anticholinergic side effects and require less frequent dosing than first-generation antihistamines. Combination therapy using nasal spray steroids with antihistamines works better than either medication alone. For patients who do not get adequate relief, there are other medication options, and reevaluating to confirm diagnosis should be explored. Immunotherapy can help those with severe disease who do not respond to standard treatments.

REFERENCES

Agency for Healthcare Research and Quality. Evidence report/technology assessment no. 54. Management of allergic and nonallergic rhinitis, May 2002. Available at http://www.ahrq.gov/clinic/tp/rhintp.htm (accessed June 3, 2009).

Plaut M, Valentine MD. Clinical practice. Allergic rhinitis. N Engl J Med 2005;353:1934–44.

Quillen DM, Feller DB. Diagnosing rhinitis: Allergic vs. nonallergic. Am Fam Physician 2006;73(9):1583–90.

Settipane RA, Lieberman P. Update on nonallergic rhinitis. Ann Allergy Asthma Immunol 2001;86:494–507.

Wallace DV, Dykewicz MS, Bernstein DI, et al. The diagnosis and management of rhinitis: An updated practice parameter. J Allergy Clin Immunol 2008;122(2 Suppl.):S1–84.

Wilson DR, Lima MT, Durham SR. Sublingual immunotherapy for allergic rhinitis: Systematic review and meta-analysis [review]. Allergy 2005;60(1):4–12.

Allergic Reactions to Drugs

Method of
Donald McNeil, MD

Drug allergic reactions fall under the broader category of adverse drug reactions (ADRs), which also include toxic drug effects, drug interactions, drug intolerance, and, finally, allergic (or immunologic) drug reactions. Adverse drug reactions are common and often result in only trivial consequences. Some may be severe and life-threatening, and may result from both allergic and nonallergic causes.

The incidence of adverse drug effects is unknown but estimates of 20% of hospital admissions are not unreasonable. A skin rash is the most common manifestation; more importantly, however, severe life-threatening reactions occur, of which only a small portion have an allergic etiology. Most drug reactions are the result of unknown mechanisms. Drug intolerance, drug overdose, and side effects of drugs, as well as drug interactions, all play a significant role. These reactions should be considered both common and predictable.

Although allergic drug reactions are potentially severe, they are also the least common and least predictable. Allergic drug reactions are given particular attention because of the unpredictable, costly, and severe consequences that occasionally arise.

Several mechanisms may play a role in the underlying etiology of immunologic drug reactions. Immediate IgE-mediated reactions represent the classic allergic reaction. This is well characterized and the best understood, but other mechanisms also exist, for example, a cytotoxic reaction in which drug-induced antibodies result in hemolytic anemia. Another example is immune complex formation resulting in organ damage. This is commonly referred to as a "serum sickness" reaction and is characterized by fever, rash, and arthralgia beginning 2 to 4 weeks after initiation of drug. Finally, a delayed-type hypersensitivity reaction occurs when drug-specific T-lymphocytes react. This completes the picture of the four types of immunologic-mediated drug reactions according to the original Gell and Coombs classification. These are referred to as Type I, II, III, or IV reactions, respectively.

Cutaneous reactions comprise the most frequent type of allergic drug reaction. Approximately 94% cause a morbilliform rash and only 5% cause an urticarial reaction. Idiosyncratic reactions are still the most likely cause for a rash and occur much more frequently than a true drug-induced allergic reaction. Ampicillins in conjunction with a viral hepatitis or sulfa drugs taken in the AIDS population are common examples.

Both allergic and nonallergic reactions are known to be associated with severe reactions, including fatalities. Contrast media agents, allergic extracts, anesthetics, and antibiotics are the most commonly implicated drugs. Penicillin remains the most common cause of fatal drug reactions and accounts for up to 75% of these severe drug reactions in the United States.

An allergy to penicillin is the most frequently reported, but as many as 90% of patients labeled "penicillin allergic" are able to tolerate penicillin. This allergy is often mislabeled because of underlying illness or interaction between antibiotic and illness. Unfortunately one third to half of vancomycin (Vancocin) prescriptions in hospitals are given because of a history of "penicillin allergy." This raises the incidence of drug-resistant bacteria because of broad-spectrum antibiotic overuse. The economic impact of treating antibiotic-resistant infections is roughly $4 billion annually.

Pathophysiology

Some drugs are capable of reacting in the body without further alteration in chemical structure, whereas others must first be metabolized to become immunogenic. Many drugs are too small to be immunogenic alone and are incapable of eliciting an immune allergic response. These drugs require binding to a high-molecular-weight protein followed by antigen processing and presentation by the macrophage in the presence of major histocompatibility complex (MHC)-specific antigen to appropriate T-cell receptors.

Penicillin is capable of inducing an allergic reaction in more than one manner. Benzylpenicilloyl, the major penicillin determinant, is able to produce a strong antigenic response. A commercially available product, benzylpenicilloyl-polylysine (PPL) (Pre-Pen), provides the means to reproduce the same allergic response by simple skin testing. Minor determinants are metabolic derivatives of penicillin that may also produce an immune response. The diagnostic capabilities of a penicillin allergy are strengthened by including some measure of the allergic response to the minor determinants when skin testing is conducted for penicillin (Figure 1).

Patients with a history of penicillin allergy but negative skin testing to PPL and the minor determinants rarely experience allergic reactions on re-exposure. If they should occur, these are not fatal, but rather mild and self-limited.

PPL alone will potentially miss a significant percentage of allergic reactions to penicillin. Allergy testing with fresh benzylpenicillin G, aged penicillin (reconstituted more than 24 hours) as well as skin testing with the specific penicillin in question will greatly enhance the likelihood of uncovering of penicillin allergy in a patient with a positive history.

Cephalosporins do not provide the same degree of certainty with respect to an allergic evaluation. Cross-reactivity with penicillin allergy patients is known to exist, and although uncommon, it is also unpredictable. To err on the side of safety, a patient with a known penicillin allergy should not be treated with a cephalosporin. A patient with a previous cephalosporin reaction with a negative penicillin skin test cannot safely receive penicillin or another cephalosporin unless further diagnostic measures are taken. This patient may be allergic to a side chain on the cephalosporin that has not been identified by penicillin skin testing. Others recommend a graded oral challenge using a cephalosporin with a different side chain. The latter should be done realizing that standardized procedures have not been developed for this and therefore false negative results may occur.

Successful desensitization to penicillin has permitted a similar approach with other drugs. If the drug in question is required, either intravenous or oral drug administration is possible by incremental doses given usually every 15 minutes. A 10,000-fold dilution of the initial dose is usually sufficient to begin, followed by higher doses,

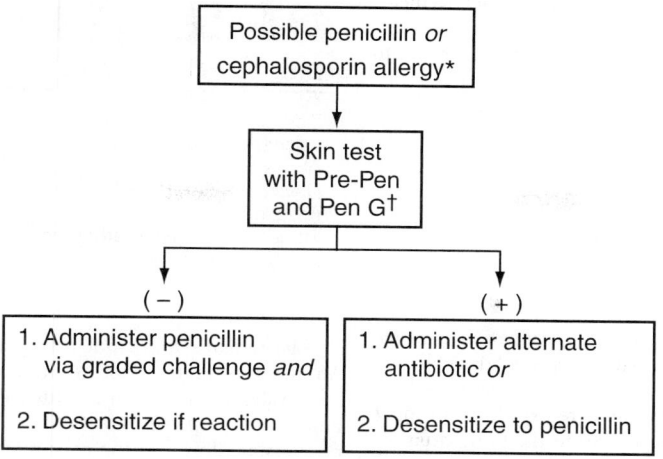

Possible penicillin *or*
cephalosporin allergy*

Skin test
with Pre-Pen
and Pen G†

(−)

1. Administer penicillin
via graded challenge *and*

2. Desensitize if reaction

(+)

1. Administer alternate
antibiotic *or*

2. Desensitize to penicillin

*Only 10%–20% of patients who report a penicillin allergy are actually allergic.
†Benzylpenicilloyl-polylysine (Pre-Pen) and penicillin G (Pen G) will not include all potential
penicillin derivatives. The additional benefit of testing with the minor determinant mixture is
impractical and usually not available.

FIGURE 1. Penicillin allergy evaluation.

2-fold or greater. The vital signs are monitored throughout the procedure with timely medical intervention if problems arise.

Sulfonamides typically cause cutaneous reactions, infrequently in healthy individuals but extremely common in AIDS patients. Reactions may be relatively benign in nature such as urticaria or fixed-drug eruption, but may also cause more serious reactions (Stevens-Johnson syndrome, toxic epidermal necrolysis). A variety of mechanisms may exist, alone or in combination, using IgE antibody response, T-lymphocytes, and inflammatory cytokines. Because of our inadequate understanding of these mechanisms, there are no universally acceptable means of evaluating sulfonamide hypersensitivity. Unless there has been previously severe reaction, a graded challenge with the drug in question is considered a reasonable alternative (Box 1). Although a theoretical risk exists between sulfonamides and drugs with sulfonamide derivatives (diuretics, COX-2 inhibitors), little data show this is actually true.

Radiographic contrast media (RCM) produce an anaphylactoid reaction by an unknown mechanism. Conventional RCM is hypertonic. The newer nonionic RCM with lower osmolarity are associated with fewer anaphylactoid or allergic-like reactions. Complement system activation, which is capable of causing histamine release, is thought to be the method by which this reaction occurs.

In the continuum of adverse drug effects with suspected hypersensitivity, exposure to *aspirin* and other nonsteroidal antiinflammatory drugs (NSAIDs) rarely exhibits features that are IgE mediated and allergic in nature, and are more often nonimmunologic mediated. A non-IgE-mediated event must still be approached with caution because the consequences are potentially life-threatening.

More commonly, NSAIDs are associated with the asthma triad syndrome associated with nasal polyps or rhinitis, and severe asthma. This is not an allergic drug reaction, but it represents a largely unrecognized subpopulation of asthmatics who will benefit by avoiding the use of NSAIDs.

The antibiotic *vancomycin* (Vancocin) causes a reaction referred to as *red man syndrome*. Histamine and other mast cell mediators are released, but not through vancomycin-induced IgE antibody (rare cases have been reported). Most, but not all, cases of the red man syndrome are related to the rate of the infusion, and most will subside once the medication is stopped. A graded challenge with the drug or a full course of desensitization usually permits resumption of treatment.

Angiotensin-converting enzyme (ACE) inhibitors are well known to be associated with cough and angioedema, but like NSAIDs, the mechanism is unknown. Newer ACE inhibitors have been described to cause similar reactions but at a much lower incidence. The symptoms of cough and angioedema may continue to recur for several months and up to a year after the discontinuation of the drug.

As seen from the discussion above, IgE-mediated allergic drug reactions represent only a portion of immune-mediated drug reactions. To assist in the diagnosis, a 7- to 10-day delay in the appearance of the drug reaction after initial treatment or immediate reactivation on re-exposure suggests an immunologic etiology. Oftentimes, only the history will provide this index of suspicion. Confirmation by positive skin testing with the drug in question is highly predictive of IgE-mediated hypersensitivity.

Attempts to label reactions as either IgE- or non-IgE-mediated may prove to be costly, time-consuming, and of no immediate benefit. Non-IgE reactions are capable of eliciting changes in vital signs, pulmonary function, and cutaneous effects similar to anaphylaxis and are referred to as anaphylactoid. These need to be regarded with the same degree of caution as IgE-mediated reactions. Narcotics, radiographic contrast media, and chemotherapeutic agents may directly affect mast cell mediator release with the consequences listed above. Antihistamines and corticosteroids given prior to administration of these drugs are usually sufficient to prevent a reoccurrence, or at least to minimize these reactions.

Drug desensitization is indicated for those patients with positive skin tests who must receive the drug, but should not be assumed to be universally safe or protective. Some chemotherapeutic agents, such as etoposide (VePesid) and teniposide (Vumon), have a much higher incidence of anaphylactoid reactions. Readmministration of these drugs

---

BOX 1 Graded Challenge

1. Cautious administration of medications to patient not likely allergic to drug.
2. Not to be considered equivalent to desensitization.
3. Used when insufficient evidence available to exclude drug allergy.
4. Medication administered in incremental doses beginning at 1:100 dilution of final dose.
5. Adequate medical resources exist to treat allergic reaction.

in the face of a previous reaction and in spite of prophylactic measures often leads to disappointing results.

Current biologic response modifier agents, as well as others soon to arrive, are associated with adverse reactions. Monoclonal antibodies, T- and B-cell inactivators, and others may prove to have adverse immunologic effects that will only become more apparent with the experience of increased use.

Evaluation of Drug Allergy in Practice

The importance of a reliable history in a medical evaluation is never more evident than during the initial workup of a suspected drug allergy. The timing of exposure, with the first allergic reaction occurring within days of the priming dose or immediately upon re-exposure, strongly points to an allergic etiology. Multiple exposures to the same drug on previous occasions do not preclude an allergic reaction de novo. Similarly, a previous history of an allergic drug reaction does not by itself predict a reoccurrence on re-exposure. The allergic diathesis may wane over time for drugs just as it may occur for other allergens.

Armed with this suggestive drug history and clinical findings such as a rash, fever, bronchospasm, or anaphylaxis, the evaluation becomes more straightforward. In the appropriate clinical setting, eosinophilia will also support a drug-allergic reaction.

Avoiding the implicated drug may be the simplest approach because confirmation of the diagnosis with appropriate skin testing is often unavailable. (Standardized skin testing exists only for penicillin, but even this does not provide 100% reliability.) Skin testing with the drug is questionable, but using both a positive and negative control of histamine and saline may still provide useful information. A positive skin test would certainly discourage use of this drug unless adequate precautions were taken.

If a non-life-threatening history of a reaction exists and the drug cannot be appropriately substituted, the option exists for a graded oral challenge to confirm the diagnosis. This should not be considered to be the same as desensitization because it involves higher doses and exposure over a shorter period of time than would be considered safe in a truly allergic individual. A challenge such as this should be conducted in suitable medical facilities under close medical supervision.

If the drug in question has been shown to cause an allergic reaction but still must be used, then a carefully monitored drug desensitization program should be considered. Under medical supervision, the drug should be administered orally or intravenously beginning with doses that are tenfold more dilute than the final strength. Incrementally higher doses of the drug should be administered every 15 minutes, increasing the dose twofold each time.

Drug-induced skin reactions are common and warrant particular attention. Early recognition is necessary to avoid an incorrect diagnosis and to institute appropriate interventional measures as soon as possible.

The following points will assist the physician in arriving at a correct diagnosis. The *timing of the onset* of the reaction in relation to the time the drug was given provides an important clue. Often signs and symptoms develop 1 to 2 weeks after time of initial drug exposure. Symptoms may develop rapidly on repeat exposure. *Pruritic urticarial lesions* strongly suggest an adverse drug reaction. A *symmetrical or truncal distribution* or a rash that occurs only in sun-exposed areas (polymorphous light eruption) also supports an ADR finding. The morphology of the reaction is helpful, although many types occur (lichenoid, morbilliform, eczematous). The histopathology of the lesion on skin biopsy may reveal eosinophils, which may also be detected in the peripheral blood.

Drugs that commonly cause ADRs tend to be antibiotics. The most common is the morbilliform rash when ampicillin is given in the presence of a viral infection such as infectious mononucleosis or cytomegalovirus. Rarely is this IgE mediated and it should not be regarded as a basis for a history of penicillin allergy. It should also be noted that not all ADRs are caused by prescription medications. A patient may fail to disclose over-the-counter medications that might be responsible (e.g., St. John's wort).

TABLE 1 Drugs Used to Treat AIDS/HIV

Drug	Reaction
Zidovudine, AZT (Retrovir)	Hyperpigmentation
Zalcitabine, ddC (Hivid)	Oral ulcers
Abacavir (Ziagen)	Severe rash/anaphylaxis
Nevirapine (Viramune)	Toxic epidermal necrolysis
Foscarnet	Urethral ulceration
Trimethoprim-sulfamethoxazole (TMP-SMX) (Bactrim)	Morbilliform rash or erythema multiforme

The *response to treatment* may aid in the recognition of an ADR. An incomplete response to topical steroids is typical of an ADR and systemic steroids may turn out to be the therapy of choice. Finally, the *response to withdrawal* of drug may range from a rapid recovery to slow clearing over many weeks, but a favorable response nonetheless.

Table 1 lists several drugs used to treat AIDS/HIV that are worthy of mention. Not all should be considered to be an allergic cause of ADR.

A careful and systematic approach to the patient with a suspected drug allergy will provide valuable information for both the immediate and the long-term management of the patient. A suspected drug allergy that is disproved will facilitate good medical care because unnecessary expense and the risk of further sensitizing the patient to a new medication will be spared if the patient is not allergic. On the other hand, a positive screen for a suspected drug allergy will result in a safe alternative. It should be emphasized, however, that neither a family history of a drug allergy nor a patient requesting a "test" for a possible drug allergy without other reason is an indication for further drug allergy evaluation because of the risk of false-negative results.

Allergic Reaction to Stinging Insects

Method of
Theodore M. Freeman, MD

Most stinging insects belong to the order Hymenoptera. They include species of bees (genus *Apis*, including honey bees and bumblebees), wasps (genus *Polistes*), yellow jackets (genus *Vespula*), hornets (genus *Dolichovespula*), and fire ants (genus *Solenopsis*).

Diagnosis

There are two important historical points to ascertain when seeing a patient with an allergic reaction to a stinging insect. The first is the type of insect that caused the sting. The physician may not rely on the patient's identification. Clues about the type of insect can be obtained from the circumstances of the sting.

Bees are herbivores and not aggressive. Stings from these insects often occur in fields with flowering plants when a barefoot patient steps or accidently sits on them. Bees have a barbed stinger and attached venom sac, which may be left in place after a sting. These should be removed immediately with a scraping motion; any pinching of the sac may inject additional venom.

Yellow jackets are aggressive scavengers and are found wherever food is left in the open. Stings from these insects usually occur in picnic areas or around open garbage containers. Like bees, yellow jackets occasionally leave a stinger in place, so this historical feature is not definitive. Wasps usually are not aggressive, except in defense of their nests. However, they tend to build these nests under the eaves and overhangs of our homes, and people stung by wasps are usually entering or exiting their homes.

Hornets are not as aggressive, except in defense of their nest. Because the nests are built in trees, stings by these insects are rarer.

Fire ants are very aggressive in defense of their nests, which are low mounds built above ground with extensive tunnels beneath the surface. In endemic areas (mostly southeastern United States), they swarm and attack as a group when disturbed. Patients stung by fire ants are usually outdoors and accidently stand in a mound or disturb a mound while working or playing in their yard or garden. Fire ant workers do not fly. They bite only to get a grip and then sting from the abdomen and inject a toxic alkaloid venom. Because they attack as a group, they are usually seen and clearly identified by the patient. The size of the fire ants means their venom is injected less deeply than that of other hymenoptera, which leads to the usual development of a pseudopustule about 24 hours after a sting. These pseudopustules contain necrotic cellular material but are sterile because fire ant venom has antibiotic properties that can kill bacteria and fungi. The pseudopustules should be left alone; opening and draining them only increases the risk of secondary infection.

The second historical point is the type of reaction by the patient to the sting. The active venom components produce immediate swelling, redness, and tenderness with fairly intense pain at the site of the sting that slowly resolves over several hours. Sometimes, the immediate reaction progresses, and swelling (>10 cm) continues for 1 to 2 days and extends across several contiguous joints from the site of the sting. This large local reaction may take 5 to 10 days to fully resolve, and it may be difficult to differentiate this from a secondary infection. Large local reactions peak in 1 to 2 days and then slowly recede, whereas secondary infections continue to get worse. Large local reactions do not cause systemic fever or lymphangitis, which should be treated with antibiotics if they occur.

The reaction of most concern is anaphylaxis. Unfortunately, many of the symptoms are similar to those of anxiety, which also may occur in a concerned patient: feelings of impending doom, a rapid heartbeat, shortness of breath, and nausea. Other symptoms that should not be seen in anxiety include a metallic taste, pruritus, and abdominal or uterine cramping. Signs of anaphylaxis include flushing, urticaria, angioedema, vomiting, diarrhea, bronchospasm, hypotension, and shock. Involvement of the upper airway and cardiopulmonary systems is associated with death, and hymenoptera stings are the cause of about 40 deaths per year in the United States. Documentation of the type of reaction is essential for future risk assessment and determination of whether prophylactic therapy should be offered.

The risk for a systemic reaction after hymenoptera sting in the general population is estimated to be 3% to 5%. In patients who have a documented large local reaction to an insect sting, the risk of systemic reactions increases slightly to about 10%. Patients suffering large local reactions may be referred to a specialist for specific IgE testing. For patients who have suffered anaphylaxis, the risk of systemic reactions after a sting is 50% to 60%. However, children (<16 years old) who have only cutaneous signs and symptoms of anaphylaxis (e.g., pruritus, flushing, urticaria, angioedema) do not seem to have a tendency for life-threatening anaphylaxis, and their risk for more than cutaneous anaphylaxis is only about 10%. If a patient has suffered an anaphylactic event after a hymenoptera sting and has specific IgE to that hymenoptera as determined by in vivo (skin testing) or in vitro methods and is then placed on immunotherapy for that insect, the risk of systemic reaction after another sting is only 2% to 3%. Immunotherapy entails the use of specific venom products for each species, with the exception of fire ants. Because of the difficulty in extracting venom from fire ants, the only commercially available product for fire ants is the whole-body extract. Although whole-body extract is not effective therapy for other hymenoptera, it has been shown to be effective for fire ants.

CURRENT DIAGNOSIS

- Determine the insect involved by recording circumstances of sting event.
- Determine the type of reaction: usual (expected), large local, or systemic (anaphylaxis).

Treatment

Immediate therapy for insect stings depends on the type of reaction. For the expected short-duration local reaction, treatment includes cold compresses; antihistamines, such as diphenhydramine (Benadryl 25 to 50 mg for adults; 1 mg/kg [up to 50 mg] for children) or cetirizine (Zyrtec 10 mg for adults and children older than 6 years; 5 mg for children younger than 6 years); and analgesics, such as acetaminophen (Tylenol) or ibuprofen (Motrin). Avoidance of future stings may be discussed with the patient. Recommendations include the following:

- Avoid looking or smelling like a flower—avoid flower-printed clothing and flowery or fruity colognes and perfumes.
- Remove wasps' nests from around the home, especially near doorways.
- Avoid areas near open garbage.
- Do not leave open food or drinks during outdoor eating.
- Wear shoes, socks, and work gloves when working in the yard or garden.

Large local reactions may be treated as described for short-duration local reactions, with the addition of a short course (5–7 days) of oral steroids (e.g., Medrol dose pack), especially if there is significant morbidity associated with the site of the reaction. For instance, if a hand or foot is involved, a patient may not be able to write, work, or walk for up to a week. Avoidance measures should be discussed. Epinephrine autoinjectors (e.g., EpiPen, EpiPen Jr, Twinject) may be given, depending on the patient's anxiety about future stings. Epinephrine autoinjectors are simple devices with instructions clearly printed on them, but mistakes in usage do occur. The most common include "bouncing" the injector off the leg, which ejects the epinephrine onto the leg instead of delivering it intramuscularly, and putting the thumb over the end of the injector, which if the injector is reversed leads to no delivery of epinephrine and thumb trauma. Demonstration pens and videos of proper technique may be obtained from the manufacturers (e.g., Dey, Sciele).

The primary treatment of anaphylaxis is epinephrine (1:1000 concentration), with 0.3 to 0.5 mL given intramuscularly in adults or 0.01 mL/kg in children every 5 to 15 minutes as needed. The patient should be placed in a recumbent position with the feet elevated. Supplemental therapy includes antihistamines (i.e., H_1-receptor antagonists); H_2-blockers (e.g., ranitidine [Zantac[1]] 150 mg PO) for cutaneous signs and symptoms; β-adrenergics (e.g., albuterol [Proventil, AccuNeb]) administered by metered-dose inhaler or nebulizer for bronchoconstriction; oxygen for hypoxia; intravenous fluids and possibly vasopressors for hypotension; and intubation for compromise of the upper airway.

Physicians must avoid the tendency to treat cutaneous-only anaphylaxis with antihistamines alone, because cutaneous signs and symptoms often develop rapidly into life-threatening events. The appropriate therapy, even for only cutaneous signs and symptoms, is epinephrine. Most anaphylaxis responds quickly to a single dose of epinephrine, although up to 30% of anaphylaxis cases require two or more doses. Because anaphylaxis may be prolonged and last hours and epinephrine has a short duration of action (1 hour), patients should be observed for 4 to 6 hours after the last epinephrine dose. They should remain symptom free during that time before being released from the clinic or emergency department. In 3% to 20% of patients, a biphasic reaction occurs with recurrence of signs and symptoms 4 to 6 hours (range, 1 to 72 hours) after the initial reaction. For patients with prolonged or severe reactions, which are more often associated with a recurrence, overnight admission for observation should be considered.

---

[1]Not FDA approved for this indication.

CURRENT THERAPY

- Treatment for usual reactions
  - H₁-antihistamines, analgesics, cold compresses
  - Discussion of avoidance measures
- Treatment of large local reactions
  - H₁-antihistamines, analgesics, cold compresses
  - Discussion of avoidance measures and possible prescription of epinephrine autoinjectors (e.g., EpiPen, Twinject)
- Treatment of systemic reactions
  - Epinephrine
  - Supplemental therapy, including antihistamines, β-adrenergics, oxygen, intravenous fluids, and perhaps vasopressors
  - Patients on β-blockers may require glucagon (e.g., Glucagon Emergency Kit, GlucaGen HypoKit)
  - Discussion of avoidance measures, medical alert accessories, prescription for epinephrine autoinjectors
  - Referral to allergist-immunologist to evaluate for specific IgE and possible institution of immunotherapy

Oral (prednisone 1 mg/kg up to 50 mg daily) or intravenous (methylprednisolone [Solu-Medrol] 1 to 2 mg/kg every 6 hours) steroids are sometimes given to minimize recurrences. Many patients are on β-blocking agents, which may make patients suffering anaphylaxis refractory to treatment with epinephrine. In this case, glucagon (e.g., GlucaGen HypoKit, Glucagon Emergency Kit[1]) at a dose of 1 to 5 mg (20 to 30 μg/kg [maximum 1 mg] in children)[3] may be tried intravenously over 5 minutes, followed by infusions (5 to 15 μg/min)[3] titrated to clinical response. Patients who have suffered anaphylaxis must be given instructions on avoidance of future stings, epinephrine pen autoinjectors (EpiPen), and information on medical alert accessories (e.g., necklaces, bracelets). They should also be referred to an allergist-immunologist to evaluate them for the presence of specific IgE, counseling, and consideration of immunotherapy, which may significantly reduce their future risk.

REFERENCES

Freeman TM, Hylander RD, Ortiz AA, Martin MF. Imported fire ant immunotherapy: Effectiveness of whole body extracts. J Allergy Clin Immunol 1992;90:210–5.

Freeman TM. Hypersensitivity to hymenoptera stings. N Engl J Med 2004;351:1978–84.

Hunt KJ, Valentine MD, Sobotka AK, et al. A controlled trial of immunotherapy in insect hypersensitivity. N Engl J Med 1978;299:157–61.

Moffitt JE, Golden DBK, Reisman RE, et al. Stinging insect hypersensitivity: A practice parameter update. J Allergy Clin Immunol 2004;114:869–86.

Sampson HA, Munoz-Furlong A, Campbell RL, et al. Second symposium on the definition and management of anaphylaxis: Summary report—Second National Institute of Allergy and Infectious Disease/Food Allergy and Anaphylaxis Network symposium. J Allergy Clin Immunol 2006;117:391–7.

Schuberth KC, Lichtenstein LM, Kagey-Sobotka A, et al. Epidemiologic study of insect allergy in children. II. Effects of accidental stings in allergic children. J Pediatr 1983;102:361–5.

[1]Not FDA approved for this indication.
[3]Exceeds dosage recommended by the manufacturer.

Diseases of the Skin

Psychocutaneous Medicine

Method of
Ladan Mostaghimi, MD

Psychocutaneous medicine explores the interactions between mind and skin. The spectrum of patients ranges from those who are delusional and refuse to see a psychiatrist to those who are depressed because of chronic disfiguring skin problems. The relationship between chronic skin diseases and psychological factors has been known for many years. In the first reference to it from 1200 BC, the physician to the Prince of Persia speculated that his patient's skin disease (possibly psoriasis based on the description) was related to his anxiety about succeeding his father. Research in psychoneuroimmunology has better defined the relationship between skin and mind. This chapter discusses common psychodermatologic disorders and their treatment.

Classification

The five general categories of psychocutaneous medicine, as adapted from *Psychocutaneous Medicine*, are as follows:

- Psychophysiologic disorders: Emotional factors can exacerbate a skin disorder, such as psoriasis.
- Primary psychiatric disorders: Patients have no primary skin disorder, and the cutaneous signs are self-induced, such as delusions of parasitosis.
- Secondary psychiatric disorders: A chronic, disfiguring skin disorder causes psychological problems.
- Cutaneous sensory disorders: Patients have a purely sensory complaint, such as pruritus, burning, stinging, or biting, without a visible primary skin disease or an underlying medical condition.
- Use of psychotropic medications for dermatologic conditions such as urticaria or postherpetic neuralgia.

Another way to classify psychocutaneous conditions is based on the underlying psychopathology, such as depression, anxiety, delusional disorders, and impulse control disorders. Standardized self-rating questionnaires are available for different conditions. These questionnaires can be administered and rated by office staff before the appointment with the physician. This classification system can also help with treatment choices and follow-up plans.

Delusions of Parasitosis

Delusions of parasitosis falls under the *Diagnostic and Statistical Manual of Mental Disorders*, fourth edition, text revision (DSM-IV-TR), category of delusional disorder, somatic type. These patients have false fixed beliefs that they are infested by parasites. To meet the diagnostic criteria, the problem should last at least for a month, and it should not be part of schizophrenia manifestations. Apart from the impact of the delusions, the patient's functioning is not markedly impaired, and behavior is not always odd or bizarre. Other delusional disorders for which a patient would seek dermatologic advice are delusion of bromhidrosis (i.e., patients are convinced they have a foul odor that no one else can perceive) and the delusion of dysmorphosis (i.e., patients are convinced that they have a defect in appearance that no one else can appreciate).

Another group of patients with delusions of parasitosis are those with psychotic mood disorders such as depression or bipolar disorder and false fixed somatic beliefs. If the patient has mood symptoms in addition to delusional symptoms, treatment of the mood problem may correct the delusional beliefs. For about 12% of patients, the delusion of parasitosis is shared by a family member or significant other. This condition is called folie à deux (i.e., madness of two) or folie partagé (i.e., shared delusions).

The patient with delusions of parasitosis usually has multiple superficial excoriations due to manipulating the skin to try to remove the parasites. Patients come to the clinic with many boxes and bags of skin samples, which is known as the matchbox sign. They can become very agitated when the physician denies presence of any infestation after physical examination or assessment of the samples collected and brought in.

Physicians should rule out substance abuse disorders. Some substances, especially amphetamines, cocaine, and phencyclidine (PCP), can cause formication and organic delusional syndrome in some patients. Organic reasons such as temporal lobe epilepsy or other brain pathology, neurosyphilis, pernicious anemia, hypothyroidism or hyperthyroidism, and systemic lupus erythematosus should be investigated, especially in older patients and if any neurologic symptoms are identified during the physical examination.

Treatment consists of antipsychotic or neuroleptic medications. For patients with psychotic mood disorder, treatment of the mood disorder usually improves the delusional symptoms. Depending on the amount of distress that the delusions are causing, treatment may start with combination of a neuroleptic medication and an antidepressant and later taper off the neuroleptic and continue only the antidepressant. To facilitate acceptance of the treatment, it is important for the physician to have a good rapport with patients and address their concerns; at the same time, the physician must not accept or feed into their delusions by giving the impression that the delusion is believed to be real. Statements such as the following may help to encourage patients to accept treatment: "I'll be very honest with you; what you are telling me is very unusual. In most cases of infectious diseases, the doctors are able to easily identify the culprit. In your case, we have not found anything. Although we will keep looking to find the culprit, if any, I know it is difficult to live with this condition, and we have medications that can help to alleviate the symptoms you are experiencing."

TABLE 1 Recommended Monitoring for Patients on Atypical Antipsychotics According to the American Diabetic Association Consensus Statement on Diabetes Care, 2004

Characteristic	Baseline	4 Weeks	8 Weeks	12 Weeks	Quarterly	Annually	Every 5 Years
Personal and family history	+					+	
Weight (BMI)	+	+	+	+	+		
Waist circumference	+					+	
Blood pressure	+			+		+	
Fasting plasma glucose	+			+		+	
Fasting lipid profile	+			+			+

Modified with permission from The American Diabetes Association. Diabetic Care 2004;27:596–601. Copyright 2004 American Diabetes Association.

 CURRENT DIAGNOSIS

Delusions of Parasitosis

- The patient has false fixed beliefs about being infested.
- Look for the matchbox sign: Many samples of excoriated pieces of skin, scabs, clothing lint, or other debris are kept in plastic wrap, on adhesive tape, or in matchboxes by the patient and brought to the physician's office for examination to detect suspected parasites.
- Determine the type of delusional disorder: primary or secondary, such as mood disorder with delusional features.
- Determine possible causes and contributing factors, such as substance abuse, organic brain pathology, pernicious anemia, hypothyroidism or hyperthyroidism, and systemic lupus erythematosus.
- Determine the extent of damage to the skin and history of skin infections.

Dermatitis Artefacta, Neurotic Excoriations, and Acne Excoriée

- Determine the type of problem: need to assume sick role (dermatitis artefacta), secondary gain (malingering), impulsive skin picking (neurotic excoriations and acne excoriée).
- Assess the degree of scarring, which may require intensive treatment.

Prurigo Nodularis and Lichen Simplex Chronicus

- Hard nodules that are 1 to 5 cm in diameter with hyperpigmentation and warty or excoriated surface in prurigo nodularis
- Lichenification (thickening) of the skin in lichen simplex chronicus
- Different histopathology for prurigo nodularis and lichen simplex chronicus

- Complete blood cell count to rule out lymphoma and polycythemia rubra vera
- Renal function tests (BUN, creatinine, and electrolytes) to rule out renal failure
- Liver function tests to rule out chronic obstructive biliary disease
- Serology for hepatitis
- Test for diabetes mellitus
- Levels of thyroid and parathyroid hormones
- Total serum IgE levels for atopy
- Patch test if allergies are suspected
- HIV test and PPD (if indicated)
- Skin biopsy and direct and indirect immunofluorescence assays to rule out immunobullous diseases
- Stool check for parasites
- Gastrointestinal testing to rule out malabsorption and gluten sensitivity
- Psychological evaluation

Trichotillomania

- Hair loss is caused by repeated hair pulling, producing oddly shaped patches of alopecia with broken hair and no signs of inflammation.
- Other areas beside the scalp may be affected.
- The age of onset and underlying psychopathology should be determined.
- If patient denies hair pulling, rule out other causes of alopecia.

Cutaneous Sensory Disorders

- Patients have a sensation of burning and itching in different areas of skin and mucous membranes, with no signs and symptoms of inflammation.

Pimozide (Orap)[1] is a first-generation antipsychotic that dermatologists have traditionally used for delusions of parasitosis. However, most antipsychotic medications can help this condition. Physicians should be familiar with the first- and second-generation antipsychotics (Table 2) and their side effect profile to select the treatment that is best tailored to each patient. Please notice the FDA warning about increased risk of stroke with the use of neuroleptics in elderly patients with Alzheimer's disease.

---

[1]Not FDA approved for this indication.

Dermatitis Artefacta, Neurotic Excoriations, and Acne Excoriée

DERMATITIS ARTEFACTA OR FACTITIOUS DERMATITIS

Dermatitis artefacta (i.e., factitious dermatitis) refers to intentional production of skin lesions to satisfy a psychological need. This may be achieved by different methods, such as excoriation, burning, or injection of toxic substances. Patients usually deny the self-induced nature of the problem. If the motivation for production of skin lesions is unconscious (e.g., assuming sick role), it falls under the category of factitious disorder. If the motivation is apparent and

CURRENT THERAPY

Delusions of Parasitosis

- Treatment of main problem in cases of secondary delusional disorder helps to clear the delusions.
- Psychosocial intervention is warranted; work with families, and provide a good support system.
- Evaluate and monitor safety for the patient, family members, and health care providers.
- Some patients may try to get rid of parasites by burning their belongings or their body or by using toxic substances to treat parasites, damaging their skin and causing serious toxicity, which must be treated.
- Treatment may include psychoeducation and cognitive-behavioral therapy (CBT).
- Neuroleptic and antipsychotic medications may be used:
    Pimozide (Orap)[1] is a first-generation antipsychotic frequently used by dermatologists.
    There are case reports of second-generation antipsychotics working well in these situations.
- Treatment must be customized based on each patient's profile and the medications' side effects.

Dermatitis Artefacta, Neurotic Excoriations, and Acne Excoriée

- For dermatitis artefacta and malingering, the patient should be confronted in a nonjudgmental, empathetic way. Provide supportive dermatologic care for the skin and refer the patient for appropriate psychological interventions.
- For acne excoriée and neurotic dermatitis, rule out underlying psychopathology, and use a combination of therapy (cognitive-behavioral therapy or behavioral therapy) and medications that help impulsive behavior, such as selective serotonin reuptake inhibitors (SSRIs), serotonin-norepinephrine reuptake inhibitors (SNRIs), buspirone (Buspar),[1] anticonvulsants, naltrexone (ReVia),[1] and neuroleptics, depending on the extent of the problem and scarring.
- There are no FDA-approved medications for these impulse control problems, and use of the suggested medications should be based on the risk-benefit assessment for each patient.

Prurigo Nodularis and Lichen Simplex Chronicus

- Topical antipruritic creams
- Topical steroids

- Topical capsaicin (Zostrix)[1]
- Cryosurgical treatment for a small number of Prurigo nodularis lesions
- For lichen simplex chronicus, some reports of efficacy of tacrolimus (Protopic)[1]
- Narrow-band ultraviolet B (UVB) light
- Psychosocial and therapy interventions to break the itch/scratch cycle
- Psychotropic medications to help with itching and sleep: mirtazapine (Remeron),[1] doxepin (Sinequan),[1] or trazodone (Desyrel)[1]
- In resistant cases, other treatments such as naltrexone (ReVia),[1] cyclosporine (Sandimmune),[1] or thalidomide (Thalomid)[1]

Trichotillomania

- In children, trichotillomania is usually self-limited, and parents should be reassured. Psychotherapeutic interventions are helpful.
- In adolescents and adults, first-line treatment is psychotherapy: cognitive-behavioral therapy or behavioral therapy and habit reversal. Improving coping mechanisms with stress is helpful.
- Case reports and small double-blind studies have shown the efficacy of clomipramine (Anafranil)[1] and SSRIs.
- Depending on the extent of the problem, augmentation with neuroleptics can be considered, but because of the important side effects profile of these medications, their risks and benefits should be carefully considered.
- Before using antidepressants, patients should be screened for a family history of bipolar disorder or personal history of previous manic episodes.

Cutaneous Sensory Disorders

- Rule out possible causes of abnormal sensations: infection, allergic reactions (e.g., dental fillings), vitamin and minerals deficiencies, diabetes, Sjögren's syndrome, nerve injuries, medications, and neoplasia.
- Treat the primary cause of the abnormal sensation if found.
- In cases of idiopathic abnormal sensations, some medications may help: Tricyclic Antidepressant, gabapentin (Neurontin),[1] pregabalin (Lyrica),[1] SNRIs, and SSRIs.

[1]Not FDA approved for this indication.

---

conscious (e.g., legal gain, disability), it falls under the category of malingering. Clinically, the lesions are located in reachable areas of the skin and can mimic any skin disease.

Factitious dermatitis usually occurs in patients with underlying psychopathology. After a diagnosis is made, the physician needs to discuss it with the patient in a nonjudgmental, empathetic way. Supportive dermatologic care should be provided for wounds, and the patient should be referred for psychological evaluation. Antidepressant and antianxiety medications can help to treat underlying depression and anxiety. Supplementary therapies include biofeedback, relaxation, acupuncture, hypnosis, cognitive behavioral therapy, and behavioral therapy.

ACNE EXCORIÉE AND NEUROTIC EXCORIATIONS

Patients with acne excoriée create excoriations by repetitive scratching or skin picking. Women are affected more than men. Patients scratch and pick at their acne, an insect bite, or other bumps or rough spots on the skin, and any part of the skin that is not smooth can be a target. However, the patient may inflict neurotic excoriations without the trigger of any skin pathology because the condition is a psychological process with dermatologic manifestations. Patients usually have ritualistic picking habits and report building of tension before picking and release of tension afterward.

For any self-injurious behavior, patients must be screened for underlying psychopathologies such as personality disorders. However, in many patients, the behavior results from an impulse control problem.

In addition to treating the underlying psychopathology, treatment includes a combination of behavioral therapy and medications that help with impulsive behavior. The success of treatment depends on patients' motivation to avoid scarring and to replace the self-injurious behavior with better behavior, including gentle skin care. Patients need to replace picking with other relaxing behaviors that are not harmful to skin, such

TABLE 2 Medications Used in Psychocutaneous Disorders

Drug Class	Drug Name	Dosage Range*	Side Effects to Monitor
Neuroleptics			
First-generation neuroleptics	Pimozide (Orap)[†]	1 mg daily in divided doses, gradually increase up to maximum dose of 10 mg/d	Multiple drug-drug interactions due to metabolism through CYP-450 1A2 and CYP 3A4; prolonged QT interval; torsades de pointes; GI, hematologic, hepatic, and neurologic (tardive dyskinesia, neuroleptic malignant syndrome, extrapyramidal symptoms, akathisia) effects; drug-induced SLE and priapism
	Haloperidol (Haldol)[†]	0.5–3 mg bid or tid	Neurologic side effects (tardive dyskinesia, NMS, etc.); QT prolongation; drug-drug interactions
Second-generation neuroleptics	Olanzapine (Zyprexa)[†]	2.5–max 20 mg/d	QT prolongation; neurologic side effects (extrapyramidal symptoms, tardive dyskinesia, neuroleptic malignant syndrome) less with second-generation neuroleptics (least for quetiapine) but still exist; metabolic syndrome (needs regular monitoring; see Table 1); drug-drug interactions, blood dyscrasias
	Risperidone (Risperdal)[†]	1–4 mg/d, max 8 mg/d	
	Aripiprazole (Abilify)[†]	2–max 30 mg/d	
	Quetiapine (Seroquel)[†]	25–max 800 mg/d in divided doses	
	Ziprasidone (Geodon)[†]	20–80 mg bid	
Antidepressants and Antianxiety Medications			
Antidepressants/ antianxiety SSRIs	Sertraline (Zoloft)[†]	50–200 mg/d	Each SSRI has own side effect profile (e.g., fluoxetine may prolong QT interval, Luvox may cause Stevens-Johnson syndrome); watch for sweating, GI symptoms, sexual side effects, myalgia, sleep problems, tremor, dizziness, bleeding tendencies, hyponatremia (rare), seizure (rare), manic episode, and suicidal ideation and suicide (rare); watch for drug-drug interactions
	Citalopram (Celexa)[†]	20–60 mg/d	
	Escitalopram (Lexapro)[†]	10–20 mg/d	
	Fluoxetine (Prozac)[†]	20–60 mg/d	
	Paroxetine (Paxil)[†]	20–50 mg/d	
	Fluvoxamine works best in OCD	50–300 mg/d in divided doses (bid)	
Antidepressants/ antianxiety SNRIs (help for peripheral neuropathies)	Venlafaxine (Effexor),[†] extended-release form available	37.5–225 mg/d	Hypertension, sweating, GI symptoms, blurred vision, sexual side effects, hyponatremia, bleeding tendencies, neuroleptic malignant syndrome, serotonin syndrome, hepatitis (rare), drug-drug interactions
	Duloxetine (Cymbalta), also for treatment of fibromyalgia	30–60 mg/d	Sweating, GI symptoms, sleep problems, bleeding tendencies, hepatotoxicity, fatigue, drug-drug interactions; not recommended for patients with end-stage renal disease or hepatic impairment
Antidepressants/ antianxiety other	Trazodone (Desyrel), helps insomnia[†] and sometimes itching[†]	50–400 mg/d	Sweating, weight change, GI symptoms, neurologic symptoms, blurred vision, hypertension, hypotension (rare), cardiac dysrhythmia (rare), priapism, seizure, drug-drug interactions
	Mirtazapine (Remeron), helps insomnia[†] and itching[†] with higher affinity for histamine receptors than doxepin (Sinequan)	15–45 mg/d	Increased appetite, hyperlipidemia, somnolence, neurologic disorders, agranulocytosis and neutropenia (rare), seizure, drug-drug interactions
	Bupropion (Wellbutrin),[†] sustained-release and extended-release forms available	100–450 mg/d in divided doses	Hypertension, tachycardia, arrhythmia, pruritus, urticaria, GI symptoms, arthralgia, myalgia, neurologic symptoms, agitation, anger outbursts, menstrual problems, Stevens-Johnson syndrome, anaphylaxis, drug-drug interactions
	Buspirone (BuSpar), works for anxiety problems	5–60 mg/d in divided doses	Nausea, blurred vision, nervousness, angry behavior, neurologic symptoms, CHF (rare), MI (rare), CVA (rare), drug-drug interactions
Tricyclic antidepressant for pruritus	Doxepin (Sinequan)	10–300 mg/d single and divided doses for depression 10–25 mg/d for pruritus[†]	Weight gain, GI symptoms, neurologic symptoms, blurred vision, urinary retention, arrhythmia (rare), blood pressure changes, bleeding tendencies, hematologic changes, drug-drug interactions
Tricyclic antidepressant for trichotillomania	Clomipramine (Anafranil)[†]	25–250 mg/d	Weight gain or loss, GI symptoms, blurred vision, neurologic symptoms, urinary retention, MI, orthostatic hypotension, hematologic side effects, hepatotoxicity
Neuropathic Pain Treatments			
Tricyclic antidepressant	Amitriptyline[†]	10–150 mg/d	Weight gain, GI symptoms, neurologic symptoms, blurred vision, cardiac dysrhythmia, hematologic symptoms, hepatic symptoms, CVA, drug-drug interactions
Antiepileptic medications	Gabapentin (Neurontin), for postherpetic neuralgia	100 mg at night, gradually increase to up to 1800 mg daily in divided doses if needed	Myalgia, peripheral edema, neurologic symptoms, angry behavior, mood swings, problems with thinking, Stevens-Johnson syndrome, seizure, pruritus, drug-drug interactions
	Pregabalin (Lyrica), for postherpetic neuralgia and treatment of fibromyalgia	50 mg tid, with gradual increase up to 600 mg/d in divided doses	Peripheral edema, weight gain, GI symptoms, ataxia, somnolence, blurred vision, euphoria, problems with thinking, angioedema

Continued

TABLE 2 Medications Used in Psychocutaneous Disorders—Cont'd

Drug Class	Drug Name	Dosage Range*	Side Effects to Monitor
	Carbamazepine (Tegretol), for trigeminal neuralgia Screen patients for HLA-B*1502 allele prior to treatment[§]	50–1200 mg/d in divided doses for blood levels of 4–12 µg/mL	Hyponatremia, severe blood dyscrasias (rare but needs regular CBC monitoring), toxicity over therapeutic ranges, atrioventricular block, cardiac dysrhythmia, CHF, syncope, hypertension or hypotension, GI symptoms, hepatitis, SLE, rash, Stevens-Johnson syndrome, TEN, psoriasis, acne, angioedema, nephrotoxicity, drug-drug interactions
	Lamotrigine (Lamictal), helps impulsive behavior[†] and neuropathic pain[†]	25–400 mg/d in divided doses; do not increase to more than 50 mg/wk Needs dose adjustment if used with valproate or enzyme-inducing AEDs	Headaches, sleep problems, diplopia, ataxia, GI symptoms, rhinitis, photosensitivity, rash, Stevens-Johnson syndrome, TEN, angioedema, memory problems, hypersensitivity reactions, neutropenia, DIC, hematologic problems, hepatic failure, pancreatitis, rhabdomyolysis, teratogenicity, drug-drug interactions
Various treatments for intractable pruritus	Thalidomide (Thalomid),[†] also used in Behçet's syndrome[†]	50–400 mg/d	Severe birth defects in pregnancy, edema, skin rash, GI symptoms, leukopenia, thrombotic disorder, peripheral neuropathy, Stevens-Johnson syndrome, TEN, seizure, pulmonary embolism, hypocalcemia, tremor, somnolence, drug-drug interactions
	Naltrexone (ReVia)[†]	50 mg/d	GI symptoms, headaches, anxiety, hepatic damage, opioid withdrawal (rare), drug-drug interactions
	Cyclosporine (Sandimmune)[†]	4–5 mg/kg/d	Hirsutism, pruritus in some patients, GI symptoms, neurologic symptoms, hepatotoxicity, nephrotoxicity, infectious disease, hyperkalemia, hypomagnesemia, hypertension, anaphylaxis, lymphoproliferative disorder, drug-drug interactions
Benzodiazepines (sometimes used for burning mouth syndrome)	Clonazepam (Klonopin)[†]	0.25 mg at night, with gradual increase to 1 mg at night if needed	Sialorrhea, ataxia, dizziness, somnolence, impaired cognition, aggravation of seizure, depression, behavioral problems, respiratory depression

Note the FDA black box warning suggesting an increased risk of mortality with use of antipsychotics in the elderly, suicidality with antidepressants in those under age 25, and increased suicidality with antiepileptic medications.

*Because of a lack of clinical trials in psychocutaneous disorders, these medications do not have specific FDA approval for these disorders, and their use is based on case reports and my experience. The dosage in the table is adult dosing. For pediatric dosing and for a complete list of side effects, consult other medication databases such as the *Physicians' Desk Reference* (PDR). Always begin with the smallest dose and increase gradually. After the symptoms are controlled, decrease the dose to the minimum effective dose for maintenance. Give each dose 1–2 weeks before increasing.

[†]Not FDA approved for this indication.

[§]Strong association between severe dermatologic reaction and HLA-B*1502 allele.

Abbreviations: AED = antiepileptic drugs; CBC = complete blood cell count; CHF = congestive heart failure; DIC = disseminated intravascular coagulopathy; FDA = U.S. Food and Drug Administration; GI = gastrointestinal; MI = myocardial infarction; OCD = obsessive-compulsive disorder; SLE = systemic lupus erythematosus; SNRI = serotonin-norepinephrine reuptake inhibitor; SSRI = selective serotonin reuptake inhibitor; TEN = toxic epidermal necrolysis.

as breathing relaxation or using a stress ball, Chinese exercise balls, Greek worry beads, stuffed animals, or Silly Putty. In finding appropriate replacement behavior, the physician should remember that tactile stimulation is important for these patients' anxiety relief.

Another therapy model for skin pickers is to consider chronic picking as an addiction and apply the addiction therapy models to picking. Self-help groups and web sites such as Pickers Anonymous could help with treatment.

There is no FDA-approved medication for this condition, and the use of different classes of medications is mostly based on case reports. The first step is to use an SSRI, such as fluoxetine (Prozac),[1] sertraline (Zoloft),[1] paroxetine (Paxil),[1] or citalopram (Celexa),[1] or use an SNRI, such as venlafaxine (Effexor)[1] or duloxetine (Cymbalta).[1] Dosage and side effect profiles are provided in Table 2. If this is insufficient, the physician can add antianxiety medications, such as buspirone (Buspar),[1] and some of the newer anticonvulsant medications, such as lamotrigine (Lamictal).[1] In the case of severe picking, multiple infections, and scarring, such as in patients with Prader-Willi syndrome, other medications such as the opioid antagonist naltrexone (ReVia)[1] and sometimes the use of neuroleptics such as aripiprazole (Abilify)[1] and quetiapine (Seroquel)[1] can help to break the cycle of scratching and give time for behavioral treatments to take effect. After the patient has improved, medications can be tapered and discontinued, but he or she may need to stay on a maintenance dose of medications.

Prurigo Nodularis and Lichen Simplex Chronicus

PRURIGO NODULARIS

Clinically, prurigo nodularis (i.e., chronic circumscribed nodular lichenification or picker's nodules) is a chronic, severe itch accompanied by 1- to 5-cm, hard nodules with smooth or warty surfaces surrounded by hyperpigmentation. The new lesions are usually red and inflamed, whereas old lesions are pigmented. The lesions may also be excoriated. The lesions are mostly located in extensor surfaces of limbs, but they can be located on the face and trunk. Histopathologic evaluation shows lichenification, a dense infiltrate in dermis and neural hyperplasia, and proliferation of Schwann cells.

Computed tomography scans and chest radiographs are obtained if lymphoma is suspected.

Topical treatments with antipruritic creams are not very helpful. Potent topical steroids such as betamethasone dipropionate (Diprosone)[1] ointment under occlusion or intralesional injection of steroids such as triamcinolone acetonide (Kenalog-10)[1] may be successful, but they have the risk of skin atrophy. Topical capsaicin (0.025% to 0.1% Zostrix),[1] a component of red pepper, can help in the early stages.

---

[1]Not FDA approved for this indication.

[1]Not FDA approved for this indication.

For diffuse and resistant forms of prurigo nodularis, broadband and narrowband ultraviolet B (UVB) and ultraviolet A (UVA) can be effective. Narrowband UVB is more effective and has fewer side effects than UVA.

For resistant forms, cyclosporine (Sandimmune)[1] at the dosage of 4 mg/kg/day can help. It should be continued at least for 6 months (see Table 2).

Thalidomide (Thalomid)[1] at the dose of 200 to 400 mg in different studies has been an effective treatment for prurigo nodularis. It is difficult to obtain because of its teratogenicity, and it does have serious side effects, such as irreversible peripheral neuropathies. Naltrexone (ReVia),[1] an opioid antagonist, at the dosage of 50 mg/day is effective in some cases. Another treatment that had some success was the synthetic retinoid etretinate (Tegison), but it was removed from the U.S. market because of the high risk of birth defects.

Psychological intervention is important in breaking the itch/scratch cycle. Help can be obtained with techniques such as biofeedback, in which patients learn how to consciously control their autonomic responses; hypnosis; cognitive-behavioral therapy; and supportive counseling.

Some psychotropic medications can help with excessive itching and compulsive scratching, including doxepin[1] (10 mg at bedtime, which can be increased up to 25 mg; the recommended dose for pruritus is lower than the dose for the treatment of depression, anxiety, or alcoholism, in which case it can be increased up to a maximum of 300 mg daily in divided doses); mirtazapine (Remeron)[1] (15 to 45 mg at night); and trazodone (50 to 400 mg at night). Doxepin is a tricyclic medication, and because it has the potential to cause cardiac arrhythmias, it should not be used in patients with recent myocardial infarction. Patients need to have periodic cardiovascular evaluations if they use tricyclic medications long term. Antidepressants should not be used in patients with bipolar disorder without a mood stabilizer because of the risk of triggering a manic episode.

LICHEN SIMPLEX CHRONICUS

Lichen simplex chronicus (i.e., circumscribed neurodermatitis) is characterized by lichenification of skin due to chronic, excessive scratching. Clinically, it appears as plaques of thickened skin with hyperpigmentation and accentuated skin lines. The most commonly affected areas are the occipital scalp, sides of the neck, ankles, genital areas, and extensor forearms. Itching is the main symptom. The histopathologic pattern in lichen simplex chronicus is different from that of prurigo nodularis and does not show the neural hyperplasia.

The physician must rule out underlying diseases that may cause pruritus. The treatment for lichen simplex chronicus is similar to that for prurigo nodularis. In addition to other treatments, topical tacrolimus (Protopic)[1] has been effective in some cases of lichen simplex chronicus.

Trichotillomania

Trichotillomania is partial hair loss caused by repeated hair pulling. Clinically, the patient has patches of alopecia with broken hair and different hair lengths without any inflammation of the scalp. The affected area has an unusual shape. A hair pull test result is negative. It can involve areas other than the scalp, and patients may pull hair in many sites. Trichotillomania occurs in any age group. In children, it is usually benign and self-limited, but in adults, it usually accompanies other psychopathologies and requires psychological intervention.

Trichotillomania is classified with impulse control disorders in the DSM-IV-TR. If a patient denies hair pulling, other causes of alopecia, especially alopecia areata, need to be ruled out.

In children, trichotillomania may occur during periods of increased stress, such as the arrival of a new sibling or parent's divorce. It is usually self-limited, and parents should be reassured. In preadolescents and young adults, the diagnosis needs to be established first, followed by psychotherapeutic interventions; behavioral modification usually works well. Psychopharmacologic treatments should be reserved for last. Because of the FDA black box warning about the increased risk of suicide and suicidal behavior with use of antidepressants in children, adolescents, and young adults, these patients should be referred to a psychiatrist for medication, if needed.

In adults, trichotillomania often accompanies other psychopathology, and the treatment of the underlying illness helps to resolve the condition. Habit reversal therapy usually works better than negative feedback. Habit reversal therapy teaches the patient to monitor the behavior and the triggering factors and to replace the harmful habit with another habit. Working on increasing coping skills for stress is also helpful. Relaxation and other stress-relief techniques are helpful, especially in patients with underlying anxiety. The Trichotillomania Learning Center (www.trich.org) is a good source of information for patients.

Psychotropic medications can be used if psychotherapy alone is not enough. Most reports of effective medications are based on open-label studies. Clomipramine (Anafranil)[1] at a dosage of 180 mg to 250 mg/day in a small, double-blind comparison with desipramine (Norpramin)[1] showed greater efficacy with a significant decrease in symptoms. There have been some open-label studies showing efficacy of fluoxetine (Prozac),[1] but this result was not reproduced in double-blind, placebo-controlled trials. Other SSRIs, such as sertraline (Zoloft),[1] fluvoxamine (Luvox),[1] and paroxetine (Paxil),[1] have shown efficacy in case reports and open-label studies. In some augmentation trials, adding haloperidol (Haldol),[1] pimozide (Orap),[1] or olanzapine (Zyprexa)[1] has been beneficial for patients taking fluoxetine or clomipramine. Small studies on using haloperidol or lithium (Eskalith) have shown some efficacy. Because of important side effects such as tardive dyskinesia with haloperidol and the narrow therapeutic window with lithium, it is best to leave these treatments to psychiatrists. Before these patients use antidepressants, it is important to screen them for bipolar disorder.

Cutaneous Sensory Disorders

Cutaneous sensory disorders are part of chronic pain syndromes, with pain occurring in different parts of the skin or mucous membranes. Disorders include burning mouth syndrome and vulvodynia (i.e., burning and itching of the vagina).

Burning mouth syndrome is a burning sensation that happens more frequently in middle-aged women. It affects the tongue more frequently, but other parts of the mouth also may be affected. It can be associated with dry mouth and a metallic taste in the mouth.

The physician should rule out local problems (e.g., dental problems, allergic reactions, infection) and systemic problems (e.g., vitamin B, folate, iron, and zinc deficiencies; diabetes; autoimmune problems such as Sjögren's syndrome; nerve injury; side effects of antivirals, antiretrovirals, antiseizure medications, hormones, and angiotensin-converting enzyme [ACE] inhibitors). The diagnosis needs a thorough physical examination and laboratory work-up, as well as screening for depression and anxiety. Mood problems may result from chronic pain issues.

The primary cause needs to be treated. In idiopathic cases, therapy to help relaxation, coping skills training, and biofeedback may help. There is no FDA-approved medication for this condition, but medications used to treat neuropathies may help. Gabapentin[1] can be started at 100 mg at night, for 3 days and gradually increased to 100 mg three times a day. The dosage can be adjusted to 300 to 600 mg three times a day as tolerated up to a maximum of 1800 mg. Tricyclics such as amitriptyline (Elavil) (10 to 35 mg PO at bedtime[1]) may increase every week to a maximum dosage of 150 mg/day. SNRIs such as venlafaxine (Effexor extended-release capsule)[1] can be given at a dosage of 37.5 mg in the morning with a gradual weekly increase to the maximum of 225 mg daily, and duloxetine (Cymbalta)[1] can be given as 60 mg daily. Clonazepam (Klonopin)[1] given

---

[1]Not FDA approved for this indication.

in small doses at night may help in some cases. Up to two thirds of patients report spontaneous partial recovery within 6 to 7 years of onset.

Vulvodynia is burning and pain in vulvar area. It should be evaluated by a gynecologist. Infectious, neoplastic, and inflammatory causes need to be ruled out. Depression and the impact on quality of life should be evaluated. Biofeedback and gabapentin[1] or amitriptyline[1] have been helpful in some cases. Depression and anxiety lower the pain threshold, and their treatment can help patients with chronic pain syndromes to better cope with their pain and have a higher pain threshold.

Medications for Pain and Itching

Some of the psychotropic medications can be used for various dermatologic conditions, such as urticaria or postherpetic neuralgia. The older tricyclic medications have specific effects on pain or itching.

When itching is the main symptom, doxepin[1] has a much higher affinity for histamine receptors than conventional antihistamines. It has a long half-life, and taking it once at night can control daytime itching. The effective antipruritic dosage is usually 10 to 25 mg at night, but it can be increased at weekly intervals as needed. Amitriptyline (Elavil)[1] works best for disorders with pain as the main symptom, such as burning mouth syndrome or postherpetic neuralgia. The usual dosage is 10 to 35 mg taken orally at bedtime, but it may be increased every week to a maximum dosage of 150 mg/day. Because tricyclic medications can affect cardiac conduction, patients need to have stable cardiovascular status and a normal electrocardiogram. Periodic testing is required during long-term treatment. These drugs should not be used with other medications that prolong the QT interval, such as cisapride (Propulsid).[2] They should not be prescribed during the immediate recovery period after myocardial infarction, and they should not be used at the same time as monoamine oxidase inhibitors. Patients need to be instructed to avoid driving due to drowsiness side effects of tricyclics.

Other medications can help with pain symptoms:

- Gabapentin is started at 100 mg at night, increased every 3 days to 300 mg at night, and then increased weekly to 900 to 1800 mg daily in three to four divided doses as tolerated.
- Pregabalin is started with 50 mg taken orally three times daily and increased to 100 mg three times daily within 1 week based on efficacy and tolerability. If patients with postherpetic neuralgia do not experience sufficient pain relief in 2 to 4 weeks and are tolerating the medication well, the dosage can be increased to 300 mg twice daily or 200 mg three times daily (600 mg/day).
- SNRIs such as duloxetine (60 mg daily) have FDA approval for diabetic neuropathy and fibromyalgia.[1]
- Venlafaxine,[1] which has a mechanism of action similar to that of duloxetine at the dosage of 37.5 mg in the morning, with a gradual weekly increase to the maximum of 225 mg daily, may help pain symptoms, but it is not FDA approved for pain treatment.
- There are some reports that SSRIs can help pain symptoms.

---

[1]Not FDA approved for this indication.
[2]Not available in the United States.

REFERENCES

Epocrates database. Available at http://www.epocrates.com [accessed September 19, 2009].
Grant JE, Odlaug BL, Kim SW. Lamotrigine treatment of pathologic skin picking: An open-label study. J Clin Psychiatry 2007;68:1384–91.
Koo JY, Lee CS. Psychocutaneous Medicine. New York: Marcel Dekker; 2003.
Koo JY, Lee CS. Psychocutaneous diseases. In: Bolognia JL, Jorizzo JL, Rapini RP, editors. Dermatology. 2nd ed. Philadelphia: Elsevier; 2008.
Koo JY. Psychotropic agents in dermatology. Dermatol Clin 1993;11:215–24.
Lotti T, Buggiani G, Prignano F. Prurigo nodularis and lichen simplex chronicus. Dermatol Ther 2008;21:42–6.
Micromedex database. Available at http://www.micromedex.com/products/ under Physicians Drugdex® System [accessed May 13, 2009].
Sah DE, Koo J, Price V. Trichotillomania. Dermatol Ther 2008;21:13–21.
Shafii M, Shafii SL. Exploratory psychotherapy in the treatment of psoriasis. Twelve hundred years ago. Arch Gen Psychiatry 1979;36:1242–5.
Shah M. Burning mouth syndrome. In: Ferri FF, editor. Ferri's Clinical Advisor. St Louis: Mosby; 2009.

Acne Vulgaris and Rosacea

Method of
*Steven R. Feldman, MD, PhD, and
Alan B. Fleischer, Jr., MD*

Acne and rosacea are common conditions that share a propensity to cause red follicular papules of the face. Nonetheless, they are distinct disorders.

Acne is associated with comedones, a noninflammatory plugging of follicular orifices. Comedones may become inflamed, at least partially due to the inflammatory activity induced by the action of bacterial skin flora (*Pityrosporum* species) on lipids produced by sebaceous glands. There is a distinct tendency toward development of acne nodules with scarring.

The pathogenesis of rosacea is less well understood. Vascular dilatation and inflammation are important components of the process, with prominent flushing and blushing. Although telangiectasia can become permanent, scarring is rare. Another feature distinguishing rosacea from acne is a tendency for ocular involvement.

Acne Vulgaris

CLINICAL FEATURES

Acne is a common disorder of teenagers and young adults but occurs in middle age as well. The manifestations of acne are diverse. The face is characteristically involved, and the upper trunk is involved in some patients. The individual lesions can consist of comedones, inflammatory papules, pustules, and deeper inflammatory nodules mistakenly termed *cysts*. There might or might not be resulting scarring. Genetics contributes to the pattern of involvement. Environmental exposures seem less important, although some oil-based cosmetic products can induce acne comedones.

TREATMENT

Treatments for acne address several different components of the pathogenesis of the disorder. Topical retinoids appear to have a primary effect on normalizing keratinization of the follicular ostia, reducing comedones and inflammatory papules and pustules. Topical and oral antibiotics reduce bacteria counts on the skin and can have intrinsic anti-inflammatory activity. Hormonal treatments in women reduce the production of sebaceous gland lipids. Oral retinoids (isotretinoin in particular), the most effective therapy for acne, reduces sebaceous gland activity as well.

There are no well-established evidence-based guidelines for acne treatment. There are, however, generally accepted patterns of treatment based on the type and extent of the clinical lesions. At its simplest, topical retinoids are the foundation of treatment because of their effect on comedones, the primary lesion of acne, as well as their effect on inflammatory acne papules and pustules. With increasing microbial resistance, retinoid agents work independently of direct effects on skin flora and are excellent long-term agents. Topical antibiotics, prescribed singly, in combination with antimicrobial products, or in combination with topical retinoids, are used for superficial inflammatory lesions. Oral antibiotics are used when the inflammation and potential scarring are more severe. Hormonal treatment (in the form of oral contraceptives) is used for female patients when the acne is unresponsive to both topical retinoids and topical and oral antibiotics or if there are menstrual abnormalities that suggest the acne is secondary to a primary hormonal process.

Topical Retinoids

Topical retinoids are used for nearly all patients with acne because of their comedolytic effect and their activity on papules and pustules, as well as to spare the use of antibiotics in an age of growing antibiotic resistance. The first topical retinoid was topical tretinoin (Retin-A). It is available in cream, gel, solution, and newer slow-release particle vehicles. The main side effect of topical retinoids is the potential for drying and irritation of the skin. This is less of a problem with lower strengths of topical tretinoin (0.025% and 0.05% cream) and more of a problem with the stronger strengths (0.01% and 0.025% gel and the 0.1% cream). The drying effect may be beneficial for patients who feel their skin is too oily.

Topical tretinoin is easily oxidized and photodegraded. With the growing use of benzoyl peroxide as an anti-acne treatment, there is greater concern about the lability of topical tretinoin. Stabilized tretinoin in the form of microsphere (Retin A Micro 0.04% and 0.1%) and in the combination with clindamycin 1.2% (Ziana) are stable in the presence of benzoyl peroxide. Topical adapalene (Differin) gel or cream can be used as an alternative. It is equally effective as tretinoin, but it has far less potential to cause irritation. Less irritation can lead to greater compliance. It also is a robust molecule that is stable when combined with other agents, including benzoyl peroxide. Topical tazarotene (Tazorac) is another retinoid that is more effective than tretinoin and adapalene, but it is much more irritating than the other agents.

Adapalene and tazarotene may be used at any time of the day, but tretinoin should be used at night because of its photodegradation. This recommendation probably started with topical tretinoin because of the potential for photoinactivation of tretinoin.

Topical Antimicrobial Agents

The most widely used topical antimicrobial agent is benzoyl peroxide. This biocide is available in a wide variety of inexpensive and expensive over-the-counter and prescription acne products. Benzoyl peroxide is very effective at reducing bacterial counts on the skin, and it is probably far more effective than the traditional topical antibiotics such as erythromycin (Akne-Mycin), clindamycin (Cleocin), and sulfacetamide (Klaron).

Benzoyl peroxide (in 2.5%–10% formulations) is often used in conjunction with topical retinoids or with other topical antibiotics. Combined use of benzoyl peroxide with topical erythromycin (Benzamycin) or clindamycin (BenzaClin) helps prevent development of bacterial strains resistant to the antibiotics. A combined benzoyl peroxide–erythromycin product was once widely used, but it needed to be kept refrigerated, and had a short shelf life. Newer benzoyl peroxide–clindamycin preparations (Acanya, Benzaclin, Duac) are more stable, can be used once or twice daily, and have excellent efficacy. A combination of 2.5% benzoyl peroxide plus 0.1% adapalene (Epiduo Gel) is more effective than either of its components and provides an option for simplifying the treatment regimen in patients who would otherwise require separate topical antimicrobial and retinoid products.

All benzoyl peroxide products bleach clothing, bed linens, and towels. Not all vehicles are appropriate for all patients, and excellent vehicle choices can enhance compliance and clinical outcomes.

Topical azelaic acid is a useful adjunct, especially in the 15% gel formulation (Finacea). It is antimicrobial and antiinflammatory, and it can promote pigmentary normalization. Azelaic acid can be simultaneously combined with many other agents and does not appear to be subject to microbial resistance.

A combination clindamycin–tretinoin product is now available in the United States (Ziana). Topical dapsone (Aczone) has recently entered the market as the first new molecule approved for treating acne. In an elegant and nonirritating vehicle this product is a useful antiinflammatory adjunct to other treatment. Sulfacetamide is occasionally used and many forms are available (e.g., Klaron), either alone or combined with precipitated sulfur. Sulfacetamide and dapsone chemically react with benzoyl peroxide, and these two agents should not be used simultaneously with a stay on benzoyl peroxide preparation.

Oral Antibiotics

Oral antibiotics remain widely used for acne, sometimes for short courses, other times for more prolonged periods. There are growing efforts to limit the course of these drugs in order to limit side effects and antibiotic resistance. Commonly used antibiotics include tetracycline (Sumycin), doxycycline (Doryx), and minocycline (Dynacin).

Of these, minocycline may be the most effective, although it has potential for uncommon and rare side effects. Common side effects include vestibular symptoms; rare ones include altered cutaneous pigmentation and lupus-like syndromes. Minocycline, in extended-release tablets (Solodyn), is the only FDA-approved antibiotic for acne treatment and has fewer vestibular side effects than other agents. This agent has an established dose-response relationship and is most effective with least toxicity at 1 mg/kg/day. It is available in 45-mg, 90-mg, and 135-mg doses.

None of the tetracycline agents should be used during pregnancy or in children younger than 12 years, because tetracycline can stain developing teeth. Erythromycin may be used in these situations; however, there are often poor gastrointestinal tolerance and marginal efficacy. Other antibiotics such as cephalexin (Kelex),[1] ampicillin,[1] or trimethoprim-sulfamethoxazole (Bactrim)[1] are alternatives that are occasionally used.

Birth Control Pills

Oral contraceptives are somewhat effective antiacne treatments that can be used in women. Three products (Tri-Cyclen, Estrostep, and Yaz) are FDA approved for the treatment of acne. The former two are combinations of norethindrone acetate and ethinyl estradiol, although other formulations are probably also effective. Yasmin and Yaz, for instance, have an effective antiandrogenic agent, drospirenone, combined with the ethinyl estradiol. Oral contraceptives should be considered as a treatment for moderate to severe acne in women (along with topical agents and oral antibiotics) before isotretinoin is used. If effective, it can spare the need to expose a woman of childbearing potential to the teratogenic isotretinoin. If this approach is not effective, the woman will already be taking an oral contraceptive when isotretinoin is started.

Isotretinoin

Isotretinoin (Accutane, Sotret, and others) is a highly effective oral agent that can cure even very severe acne. It is given in doses of 0.5 to 2.0 mg/kg/day for 4 to 5 months. It is a potent teratogen and must be used with great caution in women of childbearing potential. Although evidence is lacking, it has been reported to cause depression in rare instances, and true informed consent is required. Other potential side effects include hair loss, decreased night vision, xerophthalmia, epistaxis, cheilitis, xerosis, arthralgias, hepatic dysfunction, and elevated cholesterol and triglycerides. Oral retinoids should not be used in conjunction with tetracycline agents because of the possible increased risk of pseudotumor cerebri.

Behavioral Issues

Perhaps the most important environmental exposure affecting acne is behavioral: patients' tendency to pick at their acne lesions, resulting in excoriation, infection, and scarring. Psychological fixation on facial appearance is not uncommon. Patients often perceive that their follicular ostia (pores) are too large. They can manipulate their skin,

---

[1]Not FDA approved for this indication.

resulting in excoriated lesions that mimic acne. This type of acne is not uncommon and is termed acne excoriée. The severity and extent of the lesions vary. Some patients have few lesions, others have many with considerable scarring.

Treatment of acne excoriée is difficult. Some patients respond to the suggestion that they "are spreading the infection by manipulating the skin," For other patients with more severe psychological issues, oral psychotropic medication and psychotherapy may be warranted.

Another key factor affecting outcomes of acne treatment is adherence. Patients' adherence to even short-term oral medication regimens is often poor. Adherence to topical treatment is generally worse, and adherence to chronic topical treatment is probably severely limited. Involvement of the patient in treatment planning, choosing regimens of limited complexity, and psychological interventions to promote better adherence can lead to improved treatment outcomes. Whenever possible, agents that can be administered in combination and may be used once daily are likely to promote compliance and increase efficacy.

Rosacea

DIAGNOSIS AND DIFFERENTIAL DIAGNOSIS

Rosacea is a common cause of a red face in adults. It must be distinguished from other conditions causing a red face, particularly seborrheic dermatitis, irritant dermatitis, and lupus. Seborrheic dermatitis, another common condition, is typically more scaly than rosacea. Seborrheic dermatitis involves the scalp (a cause of dandruff), eyebrows, nasal bridge, nasolabial and melolabial folds, and central chest. Rosacea does not typically have scale or scalp involvement of seborrhea and typically involves the cheeks and nose, sparing the fold in between. Irritant dermatitis may be confused as well, because rosacea patients report burning and stinging. Lupus is a far less common disorder and may be associated with scarring lesions of the face or a malar pattern of erythema.

CLASSIFICATION

Rosacea is divided into four subtypes, papulopustular, erythematotelangiectatic, phymatous, and ocular. Papulopustular rosacea responds best to topical and oral therapies, ocular disease responds best to oral therapy, and erthematotelangiectatic and phymatous types respond best to physical modalities. None of these subtypes or treatment modalities is mutually exclusive. Rosacea patients with papulopustular and erythematotelangiectatic subtypes should receive counseling about gentle cleansing and use of moisturizers and sunscreens, because these improve outcomes.

TREATMENT

Topical Antibiotics

Most patients with papulopustular rosacea benefit from topical antibiotic therapies. There are three agents in widespread use: metronidazole, azelaic acid, and sodium sulfacetamide and sulfur preparations. Metronidazole is widely used and is available in gel, lotion (Metrolotion), and cream (Metrocream) for twice-daily use at 0.75%, and cream (Noritate) and gel (Metrogel) for once-daily use at 1%. The gel vehicle is likely the preferred for facial use, and this is a generally well-tolerated agent. The 1% product offers the advantage of single daily dosing. Some patients report mild irritation from the use of these agents. Topical azelaic acid 15% (Finacea) gel is more effective than metronidazole gel 0.75%, but appears to be equal in effectiveness to metronidazole 1% gel. Like metronidazole, it can cause mild irritation and appears slightly more irritating than metronidazole.

Sodium sulfacetamide and sulfur compounds are available as washes and topical gels and may be additional agents that can improve outcomes in treating rosacea. One product, with sodium sulfacetamide 10% and 5% sulfur with sunscreen (Rosac) was found to be at least as effective as metronidazole cream 0.75%. Small reports of the efficacy of topical clindamycin and erythromycin appear in the dermatology literature.

As with acne therapy, combinations of topical agents are more effective than monotherapy. Thus, combinations of metronidazole, azelaic acid, and sodium sulfacetamide and sulfur compounds in various combinations and permutations improve outcomes. Most patients, when counseled about appropriate use of combinations of products, with good soap-free cleansing and moisturizing products, can tolerate these agents.

Oral Antibiotics

Oral tetracycline agents are commonly used to treat rosacea. Some employ antimicrobial doses such as tetracycline 500 mg twice daily or doxycycline 100 mg twice daily. Then the dose is tapered to the lowest dose that maintains control of the disease. A sub-antimicrobial dose doxycycline product (Oracea) has been FDA approved as a rosacea treatment. This product reduces the inflammation of rosacea and can help prevent development of organisms resistant to the antibiotic. When oral therapies are employed, efficacy of topical therapies is increased, which can decrease the need for or duration of the systemic agent.

Isotretinoin

Isotretinoin is an effective agent in treating papulopustular rosacea, and lower doses than those employed for acne can be highly effective. With increasing difficulty in using isotretinoin due to the iPLEDGE program, physicians might find other therapeutic alternatives more appealing.

Physical Modalities

Although there has been a report of a series of patients with erythematotelangiectatic rosacea responding well to azelaic acid 15% gel, most patients are likely to require optical vascular destructive modalities, including vascular laser or intense pulsed light. These approaches often require multiple treatment sessions, but they do decrease erythema, flushing and blushing, and telangiectasia. Phymatous disease responds well to surgical approaches, including use of high-frequency electrosurgery with a wire loop, CO_2 laser, or scalpel surgery.

REFERENCES

Gollnick H, Cunliffe W, Berson D, et al. Global Alliance to Improve Outcomes in Acne: Management of acne: A report from a Global Alliance to Improve Outcomes in Acne. J Am Acad Dermatol 2003;49(1 Suppl.):S1–37.

James WD. Clinical practice. Acne. N Engl J Med 2005;352(14):1463–72.

Leyden JJ, Shalita A, Thiboutot D, et al. Topical retinoids in inflammatory acne: A retrospective, investigator-blinded, vehicle-controlled, photographic assessment. Clin Ther 2005;27(2):216–24.

Leyden JJ, Thiboutot DM, Shalita AR, et al. Comparison of tazarotene and minocycline maintenance therapies in acne vulgaris: A multicenter, double-blind, randomized, parallel-group study. Arch Dermatol 2006;142(5):605–12.

Margolis DJ, Bowe WP, Hoffstad O, Berlin JA. Antibiotic treatment of acne may be associated with upper respiratory tract infections. Arch Dermatol 2005;141(9):1132–6.

Ozolins M, Eady EA, Avery AJ, et al. Comparison of five antimicrobial regimens for treatment of mild to moderate inflammatory facial acne vulgaris in the community: Randomised controlled trial. Lancet 2004;364(9452):2188–95.

Sanchez J, Somolinos AL, Almodovar PI, et al. A randomized, double-blind, placebo-controlled trial of the combined effect of doxycycline hyclate 20-mg tablets and metronidazole 0.75% topical lotion in the treatment of rosacea. J Am Acad Dermatol 2005;53(5):791–7.

Thevarajah S, Balkrishnan R, Camacho FT, et al. Trends in prescription of acne medication in the U.S.: Shift from antibiotic to non-antibiotic treatment. J Dermatolog Treat 2005;16(4):224–8.

Diseases of the Hair

Method of
Dirk M. Elston, MD

Epidemiology

Hair disorders are common, with more than half of the population affected by pattern alopecia and the prevalence of hirsutism varying significantly by ethnicity.

Risk Factors

Most causes of alopecia and hirsutism are genetically determined.

Pathophysiology

Pattern alopecia relates to increased sensitivity to dihydrotestosterone. Telogen effluvium relates to an alteration in the normal hair cycle, with many hairs shedding synchronously. Alopecia areata represents an inflammatory insult directed against melanocytes in the hair bulb. There is strong evidence that the disease is mediated by T_H1 lymphocytes. Polycycstic ovarian syndrome is an insulin-resistance syndrome resulting in excess production of androgens.

Prevention

Little can be done to prevent hair disorders, so the focus is generally on diagnosis and treatment.

Clinical Manifestations

Pattern alopecia manifests with apical scalp thinning. In men, receding of the hairline at the temples is typical, whereas women demonstrate widening of the part but retain the anterior hairline. Telogen effluvium manifests with diffuse shedding of telogen hairs (hairs with a nonpigmented bulb). Alopecia areata typically occurs with patchy hair loss. Shed hairs demonstrate tapered fracture at the base. Syphilitic alopecia resembles alopecia areata but often affects smaller areas, with only partial hair loss, resulting in a moth-eaten appearance. Scarring alopecia shows permanent areas of smooth alopecia lacking follicular openings.

Polycystic ovarian syndrome manifests with evidence of anovulation and excess androgen production. Signs of virilization suggesting a possible tumor include new onset of hirsutism, deepening of the voice, change in body habitus, and clitoromegaly.

Diagnosis

ALOPECIA

The first step is to determine if a hair shaft abnormality exists (Box 1). This is particularly important in black patients, in whom trichorrhexis nodosa is a common cause of hair loss. Trichorrhexis nodosa results from overprocessing of the hair. Hair density is normal at the level of the scalp, but hairs break off, leaving patches of short hair.

The next step is to determine if telogen effluvium exists. Telogen effluvium manifests with increased shedding of hairs with a blunt nonpigmented bulb (Fig. 1), and it commonly follows an illness, surgery, delivery, or crash diet by 3 to 5 months. Hairs can often be easily extracted with a gentle hair pull or 1 minute of combing. The presence of tapered fracture suggests alopecia areata, syphilis, or heavy metal poisoning. Alopecia areata can result in diffuse hair loss, but it more commonly manifests with well-defined round patches of hair loss. The skin is either normal or salmon pink. Syphilis more often shows a moth-eaten pattern of alopecia (Fig. 2).

CURRENT DIAGNOSIS

- A sudden increase in shedding most commonly represents telogen effluvium.
- Hair thinning is more likely to represent pattern alopecia.
- Scarring alopecia generally requires a biopsy for diagnosis.
- Most medically significant hirsutism results from polycystic ovarian syndrome.
- New-onset virilization suggests the possibility of a tumor.

BOX 1   Diagnosis of Alopecia

Trichodystrophy

Types

Trichorrhexis nodosa
Inherited trichodystrophies
Fractures

Causes

- Alopecia areata
- Chemotherapy
- Heavy metal

Determine Type

Anagen Effluvium

Tapered fractures can be caused by
- Alopecia areata
- Chemotherapy
- Heavy metal

Loose anagen can be caused by
- Loose anagen syndrome
- Easily extractable anagen in scarring alopecia

Telogen Effluvium

Increased shedding of club hairs can be caused by
- Diet, illness
- Pregnancy

- Medication
- Papulosquamous disorders
- Pattern alopecia

Diagnosis

Laboratory Studies

Iron
Thyroid stimulating hormone
Endocrine studies in virilized women

Biopsy

Nonscarring types
- Telogen effluvium
- Pattern alopecia
- Alopecia areata

Scarring types
- Lupus erythematosus
- Lichen planopilaris
- Folliculitis decalvans

Other Permanent Alopecia

Idiopathic pseudopelade
Morphea

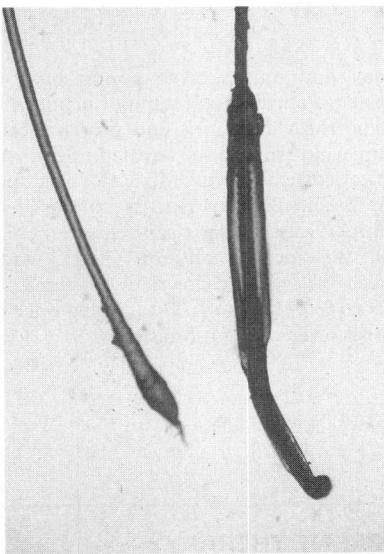

FIGURE 1. Telogen hair on *left,* anagen hair on *right* for comparison.

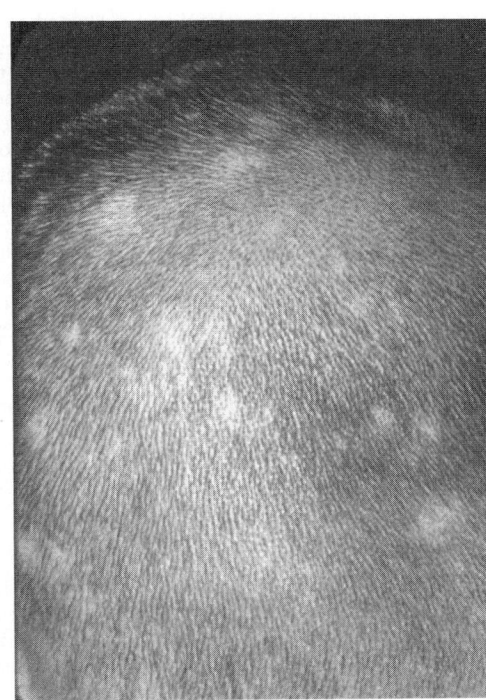

FIGURE 2. Moth-eaten syphilitic alopecia.

Most patients with hair loss need only limited laboratory testing or none at all. Thyroid disorders and iron deficiency are common, and testing for them is relatively inexpensive. I recommend them when telogen effluvium is present. Their presence can also accelerate the course of pattern alopecia, and it is reasonable to test for them in women with this disorder. Thyroid-stimulating hormone is the best screen for thyroid disorders. The role of iron deficiency in telogen hair loss is controversial, but iron deficiency is common, easily established, and inexpensive to correct. Iron status also serves as an indicator of overall nutritional status. Although a low ferritin level proves iron deficiency, ferritin behaves as an acute phase reactant and a normal level does not rule out iron deficiency. Therefore, I recommend measurement of ferritin, serum iron, iron binding capacity, and saturation.

A scalp biopsy is required in any patient with scarring alopecia. It may also be necessary in other patients if history and physical examination do not establish a diagnosis and the alopecia is progressive. The scalp biopsy should be performed with a 4-mm biopsy punch oriented parallel to the direction of hair growth. Gelfoam can be placed into the resulting hole to stop bleeding and eliminate the need for sutures. The biopsy should be done in a well-established, but still active area of inflammation if one can be identified.

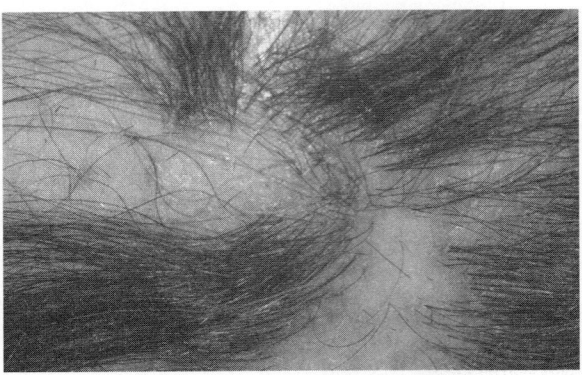

FIGURE 3. Scarring alopecia secondary to chronic cutaneous lupus erythematosus.

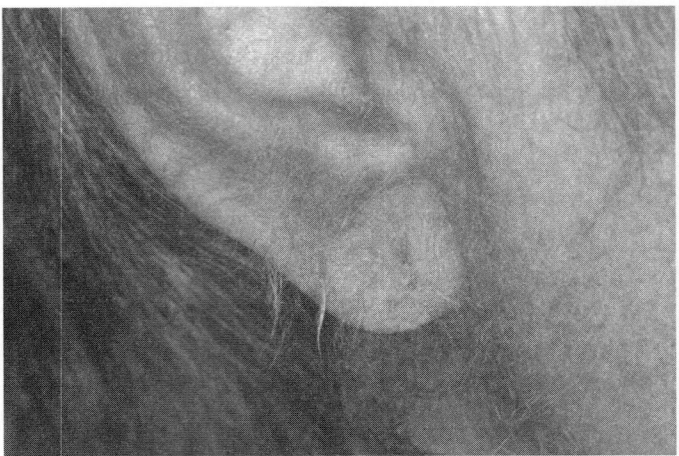

FIGURE 4. Malignant hypertrichosis secondary to ovarian cancer.

A combination of vertical and transverse sections increases the diagnostic yield and is usually recommended. In patients with scarring alopecia, half of the vertically bisected specimen should be sent for direct immunofluorescence. An additional biopsy of an end-stage scarred area can demonstrate characteristic patterns of scarring with an elastic tissue stain. This can help distinguish among causes of scarring alopecia such as lupus erythematosus (Fig. 3), lichen planopilaris, pseudopelade, and folliculitis decalvans.

HIRSUTISM

Patients with *new-onset* virilization should be evaluated to rule out an ovarian or adrenal tumor. Ovarian and adrenal imaging studies and a total testosterone level are the best screens. A total testosterone more than 200 ng/dL or dehydroepiandrostenedione sulfate (DHEAS) more than 8000 ng/dL suggests tumor. In patients with physical signs of Cushing's disease, a 24-hour urine cortisol should be obtained. Most patients with *chronic* medically significant hirsutism have polycystic ovarian syndrome (PCOS). The diagnosis is established by means of history and physical examination, and the most important laboratory tests are serum lipids and fasting glucose to establish associated cardiac risk factors. A clinical diagnosis of PCOS requires the presence of hirsutism, acne or pattern alopecia, and evidence of anovulation (fewer than 9 periods per year or cycles longer than 40 days). Ratios of luteinizing hormone (LH) to follicle-stimulating hormone (FSH) have poor sensitivity and specificity for diagnosing PCOS. Imaging for ovarian cysts seldom affects management.

Differential Diagnosis

Syphilis can mimic alopecia areata, and serologic testing should be performed in any sexually active patient with a new diagnosis of alopecia areata. Correct diagnosis of scarring alopecia depends of a thorough examination for other cutaneous signs of lupus erythematosus or lichen planus as well as the results of a skin biopsy.

Tinea capitis can occur as inflammatory boggy areas with hair loss (kerion) or with subtle seborrheic-type scale and black dot areas of hair loss. A KOH examination can be performed by rubbing the affected area with moist gauze and examining broken hairs that cling to the gauze.

Hirsutism should be distinguished from hypertrichosis. Hirsutism is a male pattern of hair growth occurring in a woman and is hormonal in nature. Hypertrichosis is excess hair growth that occurs outside of an androgen-dependent distribution. It can be found in metabolic disorders such as porphyria or may be a sign of internal malignancy (Fig. 4).

Nonclassic 21-hydroxylase deficiency accounts for up to 10% of patients with medically significant hirsutism. Screening with a baseline morning 17-OH-progesterone is associated with many false positive results. A stimulated 17-OH- progesterone is more specific, but the results of testing seldom affect management because outcomes with dexamethasone (Decadron)[1] are no better than with spironolactone (Aldactone).[1]

Treatment

ALOPECIA

Telogen effluvium commonly resolves spontaneously once the cause has been eliminated. Poor diet and papulosquamous diseases of the scalp such as seborrheic dermatitis and psoriasis can perpetuate a telogen effluvium and should be treated. Seborrheic dermatitis responds to topical corticosteroids. Medicated shampoos containing selenium sulfide (Selsun Blue) or zinc pyrithione (T-gel Daily Control) can be helpful. Scalp psoriasis can require more potent topical steroids such as fluocinonide solution (Lidex) and calcipotriene (Dovonex) applied on weekends or daily. Systemic agents such as methotrexate (Trexall) at doses of 7.5 to 20 mg once weekly may be required to control severe scalp psoriasis.

---

[1]Not FDA approved for this indication.

 CURRENT THERAPY

- Pattern alopecia in men is treated with oral finasteride (Propecia), topical minoxidil (Rogaine), or both.
- Pattern alopecia in women is treated with antiandrogens (such as spironolactone [Aldactone][1]), topical minoxidil, or both.
- Alopecia areata can require intralesional corticosteroid injections, topical immunotherapy, or systemic therapy with agents such as methotrexate (Trexall).[1]
- A scalp biopsy is critical to guide therapy in scarring alopecia.
- Hirsutism may be treated with laser epilation or systemic antiandrogens. Topical eflornithine (Vaniqa) can slow regrowth of hair.

---

[1]Not FDA approved for this indication.

Pattern alopecia in men is mediated by dihydrotestosterone (DHT). Men with pattern alopecia may be treated with daily topical minoxidil 2% to 5% (Rogaine) or oral finasteride (Propecia) at a dose of 1 mg daily. In women, the pathogenesis is complex, and adrenal androgens may play a larger role. Finasteride[1] is of no benefit to the majority of women with pattern alopecia. Spironolactone[1] 100 mg twice daily can be helpful. In women of childbearing potential, spironolactone should always be used in conjunction with an oral contraceptive. Side effects are uncommon but can include urinary frequency, irregular periods, and nausea. Most patients demonstrate a minor increase in serum potassium. Those with kidney failure are a risk for life-threatening potassium retention. Topical 2% minoxidil can also be of benefit, but women derive little added benefit from higher concentrations. All patients with pattern alopecia should be evaluated for superimposed causes of telogen effluvium such as inadequate diet and seborrheic dermatitis.

Tinea capitis is often overlooked in adults and black children, in whom the manifestations of inflammation can be subtle. Black dot and seborrheic tinea are common in black children. Patchy hair loss is an important clue to the diagnosis. Treatment is summarized in Table 1.

Localized patches of alopecia areata respond to intralesional injections of triamcinolone hexacetonide (Aristospan) (2.5-5 mg/mL) given once per month. Approximately 0.1 mL/cm² is injected to a maximum of 3 mL during any one session. Minoxidil[1] solution produces slow regrowth in some patients who cannot tolerate other treatments. Anthralin (Dritho-Scalp 0.5%)[1] is sometimes used in children. It is applied 30 minutes before showering. It can stain skin and anything else it touches.

Topical immunotherapy with dinitrochlorobenzene (DNCB),[1] squaric acid dibutylester (SADBE)[1] or diphenylcyclopropenone (DPCP)[1] is more effective than either minoxidil or anthralin. DNCB is mutagenic in the Ames assay and none of the topical immunotherapies are currently approved for human use. A 2% solution of the sensitizer is applied to the arm in acetone to induce initial sensitization. Subsequently, diluted solutions, starting at about 0.001%, are applied weekly to the scalp with a cotton-tipped applicator. Roughly 20% to 60% of patients have responded to this regimen in various studies.

Biologic agents have been disappointing, but methotrexate[1] in psoriatic doses (7.5-20 mg weekly for an adult) can be effective. Sulfasalazine (Azulfidine)[1] is sometimes effective in doses ranging from 500 to 1500 mg three times a day.[3] Patients should be encouraged to read about new therapies on the National Alopecia Areata Foundation website (www.naaf.org).

---

[1]Not FDA approved for this indication.
[3]Exceeds dosage recommended by the manufacturer.

TABLE 1 Treatment of Tinea Capitis

Antifungal agent	Dosage	Usual Duration of Therapy
Griseofulvin (Fulvicin U/F)	Required dosages are often higher than reflected in the product label; 4-10 mg/kg/d is a good starting dosage	1 mo or more
Fluconazole (Diflucan)[1]	5-6 mg/kg/d	1 mo or more
Itraconazole (Sporanox)[1]	3-5 mg/kg/d	1 wk, repeated monthly until cured
Terbinafine (Lamisil)	Patient <20 kg: 62.5 mg/d Patient 20-40 kg: 125 mg/d Patient >40 kg: 250 mg/d	1 mo or more

[1]Not FDA approved for this indication.

Early aggressive therapy for discoid lupus erythematosus is recommended to prevent permanent scarring. Topical corticosteroids are rarely sufficient. Intralesional injections are performed in a manner similar to that described above. Initial control of severe disease can be achieved with a single 3-week tapered course of oral prednisone at a dose of 60 mg daily for the first week, 40 mg daily for the second week, and 20 mg daily for the third week. Intralesional steroid injections or a systemic steroid-sparing agent are required for maintenance therapy. Systemic agents that can be effective include antimalarials, dapsone,[1] methotrexate,[1] mycophenolate mofetil (CellCept),[1] and thalidomide (Thalomid).[1] I generally begin treatment with hydroxychloroquine (Plaquenil) at a dose of 400 mg daily for an adult. Dapsone is used at a dose of 100 mg daily for an adult. Thalidomide has been used effectively at doses of 50 to 100 mg daily, but peripheral neuropathy and teratogenicity limit its use. Mycophenolate mofetil is used at a dose of 1 gram twice daily, and methotrexate is used at doses of 7.5 to 20 mg weekly.

End-stage cicatricial alopecia is best treated by scalp reduction and hair transplantation. The disease can flare in response to surgery, and it is best to plan a 3-week tapered course of prednisone[1] as described to help prevent the flare.

Lichen planopilaris is treated in a manner similar to lupus, except that hydroxychloroquine[1] is of less benefit and oral retinoids (Soriatane[1] at doses of 25 to 50 mg daily) are more likely to be successful. Mycophenolate mofetil 1 g twice daily is often effective when other treatments fail.

Folliculitis decalvans manifests with crops of pustules that result in permanent scarring. Patients respond to weekend applications of clobetasol (Clobex, Olux) together with prolonged use of antistaphylococcal antibiotics such as doxycycline (Doryx)[1] 100 mg twice daily.

HIRSUTISM

Treatment options include laser epilation, eflornithine (Vaniqa) cream to reduce the rate of hair growth, or spironolactone[1] at a starting dose of 100 mg twice daily as described for pattern alopecia. Cyproterone acetate is used in some countries but is not available in the United States. Other options that are less commonly used include insulin sensitizers, flutamide (Eulexin),[1] metformin (Glucophage),[1] and leuprolide (Lupron)[1] plus estrogen.

Monitoring

Patients treated with topical or intralesional corticosteroids should be monitored for cutaneous atrophy. Those on hydroxychloroquine should be monitored for ocular toxicity, including corneal deposits and retinal damage, although these are very rare at usual doses. They should also be monitored periodically for thrombocytopenia, agranulocytosis, and hepatitis. Patients beginning dapsone therapy should be screened for G6PD deficiency. Potential side effects include hemolysis, methemoglobinemia, and neuropathy. Monitoring includes periodic blood count assessment and measurement of strength and sensation. Mycophenolate mofetil can produce pancytopenia and blood counts should be monitored. Methotrexate is cleared by the kidneys, and kidney function should be assessed at baseline. Periodic assessment of liver-function tests and blood count is warranted, as is a yearly chest radiograph. I also monitor procollagen 3 terminal peptide levels quarterly to assess the risk of hepatic fibrosis.

Complications

Patients with pattern alopecia and polycystic ovarian syndrome have a greater risk of metabolic syndrome with cardiac complications. They should be evaluated for lipid abnormalities and glucose intolerance and treated appropriately.

---

[1]Not FDA approved for this indication.

REFERENCES

Avram M, Rogers N. Contemporary hair transplantation. Dermatol Surg 2009;35(11):1705–19.

Brown J, Farquhar C, Lee O, et al. Spironolactone versus placebo or in combination with steroids for hirsutism and/or acne. Cochrane Database Syst Rev 2009;(2):CD000194.

Chang KH, Rojhirunsakool S, Goldberg LJ. Treatment of severe alopecia areata with intralesional steroid injections. J Drugs Dermatol 2009;8(10):909–12.

Elston DM, Ferringer T, Dalton S, et al. A comparison of vertical versus transverse sections in the evaluation of alopecia biopsy specimens. J Am Acad Dermatol 2005;53(2):267–72.

Hawryluk EB, English 3rd JC. Female adolescent hair disorders. J Pediatr Adolesc Gynecol 2009;22(4):271–81.

Lowenstein EJ. Diagnosis and management of the dermatologic manifestations of the polycystic ovary syndrome. Dermatol Ther 2006;19(4):210–23.

Mukherjee N, Burkhart CN, Morrell DS. Treatment of alopecia areata in children. Pediatr Ann 2009;38(7):388–95.

Shah D, Patel S. Treatment of hirsutism. Gynecol Endocrinol 2009;25(4):205–7.

Tsuboi R, Arano O, Nishikawa T, et al. Randomized clinical trial comparing 5% and 1% topical minoxidil for the treatment of androgenetic alopecia in Japanese men. J Dermatol 2009;36(8):437–46.

Cancer of the Skin

Method of
Bernhard Ortel, MD, and Diana Bolotin, MD, PhD

Nonmelanoma skin cancer (NMSC) is a heterogeneous group of skin malignancies that includes basal cell cancer (BCC) and squamous cell cancer (SCC). These are the most common skin cancers and NMSC in the stricter sense of the definition (Fig. 1). The more-inclusive use of the term NMSC also includes malignant neoplasms of adnexal, fibrohistiocytic, and vascular origin, as well as Merkel cell carcinoma and metastatic tumors. The vast majority of NMSCs are slowly growing and locally invasive neoplasms that are often diagnosed and treated by dermatologists. Management of the more-aggressive tumors often requires a team approach to diagnosis, treatment, and clinical follow-up (Table 1).

Basal Cell Carcinoma

BCC accounts for the majority of NMSC seen in the United States and is increasingly diagnosed in younger patients. Light skin complexion and history of ultraviolet (UV) light exposure are the predominant risk factors for BCC in the majority of the population. Intermittent intense UV light exposures early in life, but not cumulative UV light exposure, pose the highest risk factor for developing BCC later in life. Other risk factors for BCC include exposure to ionizing radiation, psoralen photochemotherapy, arsenic, and smoking. A history of BCC also increases one's risk for developing a subsequent BCC. Immunosuppression, especially in recipients of solid-organ transplants, presents a significant risk factor for BCC. Inherited genodermatoses such as Gorlin's, Bazex's, and Rombo's syndromes, xeroderma pigmentosum, and some forms of albinism are predisposing factors for BCC as well. Mutations in *PTCH1* that are found in Gorlin's syndrome have been shown to be an early event underlying BCC pathogenesis.

Clinically, BCC is most commonly found on the head and neck region, though any part of the body can develop this tumor. The presentation varies depending on the histologic subtype of the tumor. Although many histologic variants of BCC exist, the most common subtypes are superficial, nodular and micronodular, morpheaform, and metatypic. The histologic heterogeneity results in variable clinical findings. Superficial BCC typically forms an erythematous scaly patch or plaque. Nodular BCC is the more classic-appearing lesion, a pink pearly nodule with or without central crust or ulcer. Unlike these subtypes, morpheaform BCC clinically resembles an ill-defined scar; it is the most histologically aggressive variant with a tendency for deep local invasion. Metatypic BCC is also known as basosquamous carcinoma, because it has histologic features of both BCC and SCC, though

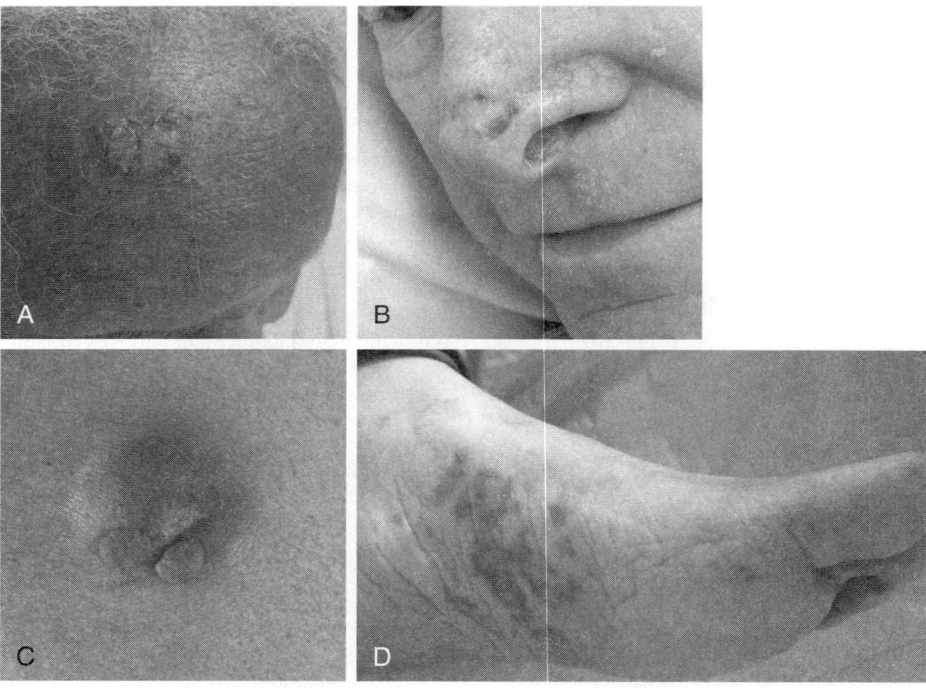

FIGURE 1. Clinical images of skin cancers. **A,** Squamous cell carcinoma in sun-exposed skin of a 102-year-old African American woman. **B,** Depressed scarlike appearance of a morpheiform basal cell carcinoma on the nose. **C,** This firm tumor on the abdomen is a dermatofibrosarcoma protuberans. **D,** Violaceous plaques on the instep in an elderly Greek man typical for endemic Kaposi's sarcoma.

TABLE 1 Overview of Therapeutic Modalities for the Management of Skin Cancers

Therapeutic Modality	Neoplasm	Comment
Cryotherapy	AK, SCC in situ Superficial BCC Kaposi's sarcoma	Versatile, but operator dependent
Topical 5-fluorouracil (Efudex)	AK, SCC in situ Superficial BCC	Will treat preclinical AK
Topical imiquimod (Aldara)	AK Superficial BCC	Flulike adverse effects can occur
Photodynamic therapy	AK, SCC in situ Superficial BCC	SCC and BCC are off-label uses
Electrodesiccation and curettage	AK, SCC BCC	
Excision	All	
Mohs' micrographic surgery	BCC, SCC MAC, sebaceous carcinoma DFSP, AFX Angiosarcoma EMPD, MCC	Preferred for certain types of invasive tumors (e.g. morpheaform BCC), on high-risk regions (e.g., nose, lip), and settings (e.g., recurrence, immunosuppressed patient)
Radiation therapy	BCC, SCC Kaposi's sarcoma, angiosarcoma MCC Inoperable tumors	Careful risk-to-benefit evaluation

Abbreviations: AFX, atypical fibroxanthoma; AK, actinic keratosis; BCC, basal cell carcinoma; DFSP, dermatofibrosarcoma protuberans; EMPD, extramammary Paget's disease; MAC, microcystic adnexal carcinoma; MCC, Merkel cell carcinoma; SCC, squamous cell carcinoma.

it is distinguished from the latter by molecular markers. This subtype also has a tendency for more-aggressive growth.

Although it is potentially locally destructive, BCC rarely metastasizes. Successful treatment of this tumor involves its local eradication. A number of treatment options exist and depend on the histologic subtype of the tumor. For small superficial tumors a nonsurgical approach can suffice, though nonsurgical treatment often carries a higher risk of recurrence than surgical treatment. Nonsurgical options include topical 5-fluorouracil (Efudex 5%), topical imiquimod (Aldara), liquid nitrogen cryotherapy, photodynamic therapy, and local radiation therapy.

Electrodesiccation and curettage (ED&C) is an option that has a high cure rate for small and superficial tumors (95% to 98%). Standard excision with adequate margins is an appropriate surgical treatment providing good cure rates, especially for tumors with nonaggressive histologic pattern. Mohs' micrographic surgery (MMS) offers the advantage of precise margin examination during excision and therefore carries the lowest overall rate of recurrence. This tissue-sparing procedure is also advantageous in terms of reconstruction on cosmetically sensitive regions. MMS is indicated to treat recurrent tumors, those in immunosuppressed patients, aggressive histologic variants, and BCCs located on certain areas of the face known to carry a higher risk of recurrence.

Squamous Cell Carcinoma

Cutaneous squamous cell carcinoma (SCC) is the second most common skin malignancy. Its incidence is rising among both men and women in the United States. Development of SCC is intimately linked to the cumulative ultraviolet radiation exposure of the patient via a mechanism that combines DNA damage with immunosuppression. History of ionizing radiation exposure is a risk factor as well.

Similar to BCC, occupational exposures such as arsenic can also predispose one to SCC. Patients with xeroderma pigmentosum or oculocutaneous albinism also are at higher risk for SCC.

Chronic inflammation or injury can predispose to epidermal malignant transformation. Examples of this phenomenon are SCC developing within scars from burns, in chronic ulcers and skin overlying osteomyelitis, and in persistent lichen sclerosus or lichen planus. These tumors have a more-aggressive behavior and higher rates of metastasis.

Human papilloma virus (HPV) predisposes to SCC. Verrucous carcinoma, a well-differentiated subtype of SCC, has a well-documented association with HPV types 6 and 11.

Transplant patients are at high risk for SCC that correlates with the degree of immunosuppression. In fact, SCC development is up to 250 times greater in the immunosuppressed compared to the general population, whereas BCC increases to a lesser extent with immunocompromise. A more common association between HPV and SCC has been noted in the immunocompromised population and might account for the disproportional increase of SCC over BCC in this population.

As with BCC, history of previous SCC has been found to be a risk factor for developing a subsequent SCC. This risk appears especially pronounced in smokers.

Unlike BCC, SCC often has a precursor lesion: actinic keratosis. Histologically, actinic keratosis demonstrates partial thickness atypia of the epidermis, and patient often describe it as waxing and waning. Full-thickness histologic atypia is seen in SCC in situ (Bowen's disease), whereas invasive SCC penetrates the basement membrane to invade underlying dermis. Histologically, the degree of differentiation of SCC tends to correlate with its clinical behavior. Well-differentiated lesions tend toward local invasion, as opposed to poorly differentiated SCC, which more commonly is infiltrative.

The typical clinical presentation of SCC is that of a hyperkeratotic pink plaque. More-advanced lesions may be nodular and can ulcerate. In most cases, SCC shows only local invasion; however, perineural invasion and rarely metastasis are more likely with SCC than BCC. The central face, temples, and scalp present high-risk zones for recurrence and metastasis.

Treatment of SCC involves modalities similar to those used for BCC. Cryotherapy is the mainstay of treatment for actinic keratosis. Topical treatment with 5-fluorouracil (Carac 0.5%, Fluoroplex 1%, Fluorouracil 2%, Efudex 5%), imiquimod (Aldara) or photodynamic therapy is often used as field therapy to depopulate large regions of the skin of actinic keratosis lesions. Continued sun protection has been shown to be of benefit to prevent progression from actinic keratosis to SCC, especially in the immunocompromised population. SCC in situ may be treated with ED&C. Excision with a clear surgical margin is often used in treatment of SCC on the trunk or extremities, but MMS yields the highest cure rates, especially in high-risk areas such as the face and scalp. Adjuvant radiotherapy may be used along with surgical excision for more-aggressive tumors. Overall, the prognosis for a patient with cutaneous SCC depends heavily on location, degree of histologic differentiation, invasion, and metastasis.

Neoplasms of Adnexal Origin

The adnexal structures of the skin include the pilosebaceous unit as well as apocrine and eccrine glands and ducts. A great number of benign and malignant tumors of adnexal origin occur in the skin. Most of the adnexal malignancies are rare. Sebaceous carcinoma and microcystic adnexal carcinoma (MAC) are two of the more common adnexal carcinomas that have an aggressive nature and may be subtle at presentation.

SEBACEOUS CARCINOMA

Sebaceous carcinoma is an aggressive malignancy that is most commonly found on the head and neck region. More specifically, it is one of the more common tumors of the eyelid and periocular area. Due to its nonspecific clinical presentation it is often treated as chalazion before biopsy and diagnosis. Population-based risk factors associated with development of sebaceous carcinoma include older age and European ethnicity. History of irradiation and immunosuppression predisposes to sebaceous carcinoma development, similar to BCC and SCC. Sebaceous carcinoma is one of the cutaneous neoplasms characteristic of Muir-Torre syndrome, which results from mutations in DNA mismatch repair genes and is associated with multiple sebaceous neoplasms and internal malignancy.

Clinical diagnosis of sebaceous carcinoma is difficult, and therefore progressive or nonresolving eyelid lesions require biopsy. Treatment of sebaceous carcinoma is primarily surgical. Wide local excision with 5- to 6-mm margins or MMS is indicated. A lower rate of recurrence with MMS (11.1%) has been shown as compared to local excision (32%). Close follow-up is indicated to monitor for recurrence and metastasis.

MICROCYSTIC ADNEXAL CARCINOMA

Microcystic adnexal carcinoma (MAC) is another adnexal malignancy with predilection for the head and neck. In the United States it is most prevalent in the white population and on the left side of the body, suggesting UV irradiation as a risk factor. Although it can be seen in a wide age range of patients, older patients have a higher risk of developing MAC. The low incidence of this tumor makes it difficult to evaluate other risk factors, though cases have been reported in immunosuppressed patients and those with a history of radiation therapy.

Clinically MAC occurs as a slowly growing, pink to flesh-colored ill-defined plaque. Paresthesia and/or numbness are common complaints and have been attributed to the high degree of perineural invasion by this tumor. MAC is a locally aggressive tumor with an unpredictable pattern of infiltrative growth. Histologically, MAC exhibits both pilar and sweat duct differentiation, deep invasion with a desmoplastic stromal response, and perineural invasion.

Surgical excision is the standard of care treatment for MAC, and radiation as an adjunct therapy is reported in a few cases. Because this tumor can extend for centimeters subclinically, MMS is favored as the first-line surgical treatment because it allows complete examination of the surgical margins intraoperatively and has been reported to have a lower recurrence rate than standard excision.

Fibrohistiocytic Malignancies

Fibrohistiocytic tumors of the skin are derived from the mesenchymal tissue and range from those of intermediate malignant potential to aggressive pleomorphic sarcomas. Of these overall rare malignancies, dermatofibrosarcoma protuberans (DFSP) and atypical fibroxanthoma are more frequently encountered.

DERMATOFIBROSARCOMA PROTUBERANS

DFSP is the most common fibrohistiocytic malignancy of the skin. It occurs at various ages ranging from infancy to older adulthood. The pathogenesis of DFSP involves a translocation between chromosomes 17 and 22 that fuses the collagen type 1 α1 gene (COL1A1) with the platelet-derived growth factor B-chain gene (PDGFB). This fusion gene results in overexpression of PDGFB, which acts as a potent growth stimulant for mesenchymal cells. In general slowly growing, DFSPs are locally invasive and infiltrative rather than metastatic. Therefore, treatment of this tumor is primarily surgical.

A high recurrence rate has been noted in a number of studies and is attributed to the infiltrative growth of the tumor. MMS reduces recurrence rates, and is often recommended. DFSP is thought to be a radiosensitive tumor, and adjunctive radiation therapy has been successful used both pre- and postoperatively. The discovery of COL1A1-PDGFB fusion has led to trials of imatinib (Gleevec) therapy as an adjunct to surgery for DFSP. So far, a limited number of clinical reports have demonstrated regression of DFSPs during treatment with imatinib. Larger studies and long-term follow-up are needed to determine whether this warrants a change to the current treatment recommendations.

ATYPICAL FIBROXANTHOMA

Atypical fibroxanthoma is a low-grade sarcoma of the skin. This locally invasive tumor favors sun-damaged skin of the head and neck region in older adults. Patients with xeroderma pigmentosum have a higher risk for developing atypical fibroxanthoma . It has a nonspecific clinical presentation, and a biopsy with histopathology is needed for diagnosis. Histologically, this tumor often exhibits marked pleomorphism and frequent mitoses. Often immunohistochemical staining is necessary for definitive diagnosis. Surgery is the treatment of choice for atypical fibroxanthoma . Either wide local excision or MMS may be used, though lower recurrence rates have been reported with MMS. Despite the pleomorphic microscopic appearance, this tumor rarely metastasizes, and the prognosis with appropriate treatment is favorable.

Vascular Malignancies

Vascular neoplasms of the skin are rare. Kaposi's sarcoma (KS) and angiosarcoma, both increasingly encountered in healthy older adults as well as immunosuppressed patients, are discussed here.

KAPOSI'S SARCOMA

Controversy exists regarding the nature of cell proliferation seen in KS. Some regard it as a true malignancy, and others view it as a reactive proliferation. Four types of KS exist: KS of elderly men of Jewish and Mediterranean origin, African endemic KS, immunosuppression-associated KS, and AIDS-associated KS. Infection with human herpesvirus 8 (HHV 8) is involved in the pathogenesis of all types of KS. Clinical findings include nonblanching purpuric patches and plaques that can progress to nodules with ulceration. KS can be isolated to the skin or can become disseminated to the lymph nodes and viscera. Diagnosis is established with histopathology and immunostaining. Management of KS is complex owing to the varied clinical course of the four subtypes. In cases of localized lesions, surgery, cryotherapy, or laser treatment may be useful. Radiotherapy can also be used for localized disease. Patients with disseminated KS are generally treated with chemotherapy. In AIDS-associated KS, institution of HIV medications has been shown to effect resolution of KS.

ANGIOSARCOMA

Angiosarcoma is a more rare but aggressive vascular cutaneous malignancy that tends to metastasize and carries a poor prognosis. Clinically, angiosarcoma favors the head and neck area of elderly men; it can also arise within sites of previous radiation therapy or chronic lymphedema. No association between angiosarcoma and HHV 8 has been found. Patients present with an asymptomatic enlarging purpuric plaque that can eventually develop a nodular component. Angiosarcoma may have multifocal involvement that is often not appreciated clinically. The treatment for angiosarcoma involves wide local excision and postoperative radiation. The overall prognosis is poor, and distant metastasis-free 5-year survival rates range between 20% and 37%.

Other Nonmelanoma Skin Cancers

MERKEL CELL CARCINOMA

Merkel cell carcinoma (MCC) is a rare but often fatal NMSC that derives from cutaneous neuroendocrine cells. Fair skin and a history of exposure to UV light are risk factors for developing MCC. Like many other NMSCs, MCC favors the head and neck and is much more common in the elderly. Immunosuppression appears to be a risk factor for MCC development because its incidence is significantly increased in patients with AIDS and recipients of organ transplants. Polyomavirus has been implicated in the pathogenesis of MCC.

This malignancy is often metastatic upon presentation. Clinically, it occurs as a nonspecific, red asymptomatic papule or nodule. A biopsy with immunohistochemical analysis is diagnostic. The therapy for MCC involves surgery with wide local excision or MMS. Sentinel lymph node biopsy can be performed for staging purposes but should be considered on a case-by-case basis. MCC is sensitive to radiation therapy, which is a recommended adjuvant treatment for patients with lymph node involvement. Palliative chemotherapy often produces a response; however, recurrence is common. Prognosis is poor for metastatic disease or lymph node involvement.

PAGET'S DISEASE

Paget's disease refers to intraepidermal spread of adenocarcinoma. Two types are seen in the skin: mammary Paget's disease and extramammary Paget's disease. Mammary Paget's disease is most commonly seen in women and has a strict association with adenocarcinoma of the breast. The lesions are usually unilateral scaly red plaques that favor the nipple. Often the underlying tumor is not clinically present but is detected through imaging. Other dermatoses of the nipple can resemble mammary Paget's disease, and therefore definitive diagnosis requires biopsy and immunohistochemistry. Surgical excision along with appropriate treatment of the breast cancer is the recommended treatment. Prognosis depends on the extent of breast cancer at diagnosis, though it appears to be worse for breast cancer patients with mammary Paget's disease than those without.

Extramammary Paget's disease consists of two types of disease: type I disease, which is associated with distant adenocarcinoma, and type II, primary cutaneous EMPD. Both are very rare but, like mammary Paget's disease, have a female predominance. Most commonly extramammary Paget's disease is found in the genital or perianal region; however, other areas of the skin can be affected less frequently. Clinically, extramammary Paget's disease manifests as a well demarcated red plaque that can become erosive. Long-standing disease can spread from the groin to the trunk, mimicking an inflammatory dermatosis. Definitive diagnosis is based on biopsy findings, and further work-up includes extensive screening for associated internal malignancy. Treatment relies on surgical excision with wide margins. MMS can be used to examine margins intraoperatively. Prognosis for type I extramammary Paget's disease depends on the extent of underlying tumor, but that for type II is favorable.

CUTANEOUS METASTASES

Metastasis to the skin often heralds the systemic spread of an internal malignancy. Primary malignancy underlying the skin metastasis tends to differ by sex and age. In men, lung cancer is the most common source of skin metastasis, whereas breast cancer is the more common primary tumor in women. The head and neck are favored as sites of skin metastasis in men but the trunk is favored in women.

CURRENT DIAGNOSIS

- Skin cancers are polymorphous in appearance, ranging from small papules and plaques to nodules and tumors of different colors, sizes, and consistencies.
- The surface may be smooth, scaly, ulcerated, or crusted.
- A common feature is that all of these skin neoplasms grow continuously and relapse when superficially treated.
- The distinction between skin cancers and benign neoplasms or inflammatory dermatoses may be difficult for the nondermatologist to make.

CURRENT THERAPY

- For the majority of nonmelanoma skin cancers, localized treatments are sufficient and include cryotherapy, immunotherapy, topical chemotherapy, and photodynamic therapy.
- Surgical techniques include electrodesiccation and curettage, simple excision, and Mohs' micrographic surgery, which offers intraoperative confirmation of complete tumor removal and maximal cure rates.
- The Mohs procedure is indicated for more-aggressive tumors, for tumors in certain anatomic locations, and in immunosuppressed patients.
- Rarely, sentinel lymph node dissection and adjuvant therapies, such as radiation and chemotherapy, are warranted.

The clinical presentation of skin metastasis is varied and often nonspecific. A new, asymptomatic cutaneous or subcutaneous nodule may be the reason for a biopsy that reveals metastasis of an unknown primary tumor. Diagnosis is made by histopathology and appropriate molecular staining. Specific clinical patterns of metastasis may be encountered. Inflammatory carcinoma can be seen with cutaneous breast cancer metastases. Occasionally, neoplastic infiltration leads to localized areas of alopecia. Zosteriform distribution of skin metastasis has been reported with breast, colon, or squamous cell cancer.

Leukemia cutis refers to skin involvement with acute myelogenous leukemia, chronic myelogenous leukemia, myelodysplastic syndromes, chronic lymphocytic leukemia, or adult T-cell lymphoproliferative diseases. In rare cases, skin involvement precedes bone marrow disease and is termed *aleukemic leukemia cutis*. In chronic leukemias, skin involvement tends to predict disease progression into the acute phase. Children appear to have a higher incidence of leukemia cutis as compared to adults but better overall prognosis.

Metastatic skin tumors are distinguished from primary cutaneous malignancies histologically. Treatment is always geared toward the primary malignancy. Regardless of type of neoplasm or site of metastasis, spread of an internal malignancy to the skin carries a poor prognosis.

REFERENCES

Alam M, Ratner D. Cutaneous squamous-cell carcinoma. N Engl J Med 2001;344(13):975–83.

Billings SD, Folpe AL. Cutaneous and subcutaneous fibrohistiocytic tumors of intermediate malignancy: An update. Am J Dermatopathol 2004;26(2):141–55.

Buitrago W, Joseph AK. Sebaceous carcinoma: The great masquerader: Emerging concepts in diagnosis and treatment. Dermatol Ther 2008;21(6):459–66.

Cho-Vega JH, Medeiros LJ, Prieto VG, Vega F. Leukemia cutis. Am J Clin Pathol 2008;129(1):130–42.

Christenson LJ, Borrowman TA, Vachon CM, et al. Incidence of basal cell and squamous cell carcinomas in a population younger than 40 years. JAMA 2005;294(6):681–90.

Cumberland L, Dana A, Liegeois N. Mohs micrographic surgery for the management of nonmelanoma skin cancers. Facial Plast Surg Clin North Am 2009;17(3):325–35.

Dasgupta T, Wilson LD, Yu JB. A retrospective review of 1349 cases of sebaceous carcinoma. Cancer 2009;115(1):158–65.

Dubina M, Goldenberg G. Viral-associated nonmelanoma skin cancers: A review. Am J Dermatopathol 2009;31(6):561–73.

Eisen DB, Michael DJ. Sebaceous lesions and their associated syndromes: Part I. J Am Acad Dermatol 2009;61(4):549–60.

Fan H, Oro AE, Scott MP, Khavari PA. Induction of basal cell carcinoma features in transgenic human skin expressing Sonic Hedgehog. Nat Med 1997;3(7):788–92.

Feng H, Shuda M, Chang Y, Moore PS. Clonal integration of a polyomavirus in human Merkel cell carcinoma. Science 2008;319(5866):1096–1100.

Hussein MR. Skin metastasis: A pathologist's perspective. J Cutan Pathol 2010;37(9):e1–320.

Kamino H, Jacobson M. Dermatofibroma extending into the subcutaneous tissue. Differential diagnosis from dermatofibrosarcoma protuberans. Am J Surg Pathol 1990;14(12):1156–64.

Kanitakis J. Mammary and extramammary Paget's disease. J Eur Acad Dermatol Venereol 2007;21(5):581–90.

Karagas MR, Stukel TA, Greenberg ER, et al. Risk of subsequent basal cell carcinoma and squamous cell carcinoma of the skin among patients with prior skin cancer. Skin Cancer Prevention Study Group. JAMA 1992;267(24):3305–10.

Lee DA, Miller SJ. Nonmelanoma skin cancer. Facial Plast Surg Clin North Am 2009;17(3):309–24.

Lehmann P. Methyl aminolaevulinate-photodynamic therapy: a review of clinical trials in the treatment of actinic keratoses and nonmelanoma skin cancer. Br J Dermatol 2007;156(5):793–801.

Lemm D, Mugge LO, Mentzel T, Hoffken K. Current treatment options in dermatofibrosarcoma protuberans. J Cancer Res Clin Oncol 2009;135(5):653–65.

Maddox JS, Soltani K. Risk of nonmelanoma skin cancer with azathioprine use. Inflamm Bowel Dis 2008;14(10):1425–31.

Marcet S. Atypical fibroxanthoma/malignant fibrous histiocytoma. Dermatol Ther 2008;21(6):424–7.

McGuire JF, Ge NN, Dyson S. Nonmelanoma skin cancer of the head and neck. I: Histopathology and clinical behavior. Am J Otolaryngol 2009;30(2):121–33.

Mendenhall WM, Mendenhall CM, Werning JW, et al. Cutaneous angiosarcoma. Am J Clin Oncol 2006;29(5):524–8.

Prieto VG, Shea CR. Selected cutaneous vascular neoplasms. A review. Dermatol Clin 1999;17(3):507–20, viii.

Rockville Merkel Cell Carcinoma Group. Merkel cell carcinoma: Recent progress and current priorities on etiology, pathogenesis, and clinical management. J Clin Oncol 2009;27(24):4021–6.

Rubin AI, Chen EH, Ratner D. Basal-cell carcinoma. N Engl J Med 2005;353 (21):2262–9.

Schwartz RA, Micali G, Nasca MR, Scuderi L. Kaposi sarcoma: a continuing conundrum. J Am Acad Dermatol 2008;59(2):179–206.

Smeets NW, Krekels GA, Ostertag JU, et al. Surgical excision vs Mohs' micrographic surgery for basal-cell carcinoma of the face: Randomised controlled trial. Lancet 2004;364(9447):1766–72.

Spencer JM, Nossa R, Tse DT, Sequeira M. Sebaceous carcinoma of the eyelid treated with Mohs micrographic surgery. J Am Acad Dermatol 2001;44 (6):1004–9.

Ulrich C, Jurgensen JS, Degen A, et al. Prevention of non-melanoma skin cancer in organ transplant patients by regular use of a sunscreen: A 24 months, prospective, case-control study. Br J Dermatol 2009;161(Suppl. 3):78–84.

Wetter R, Goldstein GD. Microcystic adnexal carcinoma: a diagnostic and therapeutic challenge. Dermatol Ther 2008;21(6):452–8.

Yu JB, Blitzblau RC, Patel SC, et al. Surveillance, Epidemiology, and End Results (SEER) Database analysis of microcystic adnexal carcinoma (sclerosing sweat duct carcinoma) of the skin. Am J Clin Oncol 2010;33(2):125–7.

Cutaneous T-Cell Lymphomas, Including Mycosis Fungoides and Sézary Syndrome

Method of
Gary S. Wood, MD

Cutaneous T-Cell Lymphomas

CLASSIFICATION

Virtually every subtype of T-cell lymphoma involves the skin primarily or secondarily. The principal types of primary cutaneous T-cell lymphomas (CTCLs) recognized in the World Health Organization and European Organization for Research and Treatment of Cancer classification include mycosis fungoides (MF) and its leukemic variant, the Sézary syndrome (SS); CD30$^+$ large cell lymphoma; CD30$^-$ large cell lymphoma; and pleomorphic CD4$^+$ small or medium cell variants (Table 1). All other primary CTCLs comprise only a few percent of the total. This discussion focuses on MF and SS because they account for up to 75% of primary cutaneous cases.

TABLE 1 Classification of Primary Cutaneous T-Cell Lymphomas

CTCL Type	Proportion of Primary CTCLs (%)	5-Year Survival Rate (%)
MF and variants	70	85
SS	<5	<50*
CD30$^+$ large cell	13	90
CD30$^-$ large cell	7	15
Pleomorphic small/medium cell	4	60
Miscellaneous	<1	Variable

*The 5-year survival rate depends on the criteria used to define SS, and it may be as low as 10%.
Abbreviations: CTCL = cutaneous T-cell lymphoma; MF = mycosis fungoides; SS = Sézary syndrome.

CURRENT DIAGNOSIS

For Cutaneous T-cell Lymphomas, Obtain the Following:

- History: duration and pace of lesion development
- Skin examination: extent of patches, plaques, tumors, and ulcers
- Extracutaneous examination: status of lymph nodes, liver, and spleen
- Laboratory: complete blood cell count, differential, and lesional biopsy results
- Imaging: CT or fused PET/CT scans of the chest, abdomen, and pelvis (not needed for early stage mycosis fungoides)

Standard Diagnosis and Staging Methods

The evaluation of CTCL patients begins with a thorough clinical history and physical examination. Key elements of the history include the pace and nature of disease development, the presence or absence of spontaneous regression of lesions, prior therapy, and ingestion of drugs (e.g., anticonvulsants, antihistamines, other agents with antihistaminic properties) that have been associated with pseudolymphomatous skin eruptions that can mimic CTCLs. The review of systems should establish the presence of lymphoma-associated constitutional symptoms (e.g., fever of unknown origin, night sweats, weight loss, fatigue). In addition to general aspects, the physical examination should document the type and distribution of skin lesions and whether there is lymphadenopathy, hepatosplenomegaly, or edema of extremities (i.e., potential sign of lymphatic obstruction).

Histopathologic analysis of representative lesional skin biopsy specimens is the primary means of confirming the clinical diagnosis. Biopsy specimens should be deep enough to include the deepest portions of the cutaneous lymphoid infiltrates because these areas often exhibit the most diagnostic features. Putative extracutaneous involvement should be confirmed by biopsy if it is relevant to clinical management.

Routine blood tests include a complete blood cell count, differential review, and general chemistry panel. A "Sézary prep" is used to assess peripheral blood involvement.

Internal nodal and visceral involvement by lymphoma usually is assessed with chest radiography, computed tomography (CT), or combined positron emission tomography and CT (PET/CT) scans of the chest, abdomen, and pelvis. These radiologic studies usually are not needed for patients with early forms of MF (i.e., nontumorous skin lesions without evidence of extracutaneous involvement assessed by physical examination); however, they are usually obtained during the work-up of other types of CTCLs. The role of immunopathologic and molecular biologic assays in the diagnosis and staging of CTCLs is discussed later.

An algorithm for the diagnosis of early MF has been proposed by the International Society for Cutaneous Lymphomas (ISCL) (see Pimpinelli et al. in References). It relies on a combination of clinical, histopathologic, immunopathologic, and clonality criteria. This differs from former approaches that have been based primarily on histopathologic criteria.

Mycosis Fungoides, Sézary Syndrome, and Variants

CLINICAL FEATURES

MF classically manifests as erythematous, scaly, variably pruritic, flat patches or indurated plaques, often favoring the most sun-protected areas. The patches or plaques may progress to cutaneous tumors and involvement of lymph nodes or viscera, although this usually does not occur as long as the skin lesions are reasonably well controlled by therapy. SS manifests as total-body erythema and scaling (i.e., erythroderma), generalized lymphadenopathy, hepatosplenomegaly, and leukemia. Large-plaque parapsoriasis is essentially the prediagnostic patch phase of MF. Lesions may exhibit poikiloderma (i.e., atrophy, telangiectasia, and mottled hyperpigmentation and hypopigmentation) and have then been referred to as *poikiloderma atrophicans vasculare*.

Follicular mucinosis refers to a papulonodular eruption in which hair follicles are infiltrated by T cells and contain pools of mucin. In hairy areas, this may result in alopecia. Follicular mucinosis may exist as a lesional variant of MF (i.e., follicular MF) or as a clinically benign entity (i.e., alone or associated with other lymphomas).

Granulomatous slack skin is a variant of MF that manifests with pendulous skin folds in intertriginous areas. Lesional skin biopsy specimens contain atypical T cells in a granulomatous background.

Pagetoid reticulosis manifests as a solitary or localized, often hyperkeratotic plaque containing atypical T cells that are frequently confined to a hyperplastic epidermis. Some authorities regard it as a variant of unilesional MF, whereas others think it is a distinct entity.

Other variants of MF include hypopigmented, palmoplantar, bullous, and pigmented purpuric forms. The latter form shows clinicopathologic overlap with the pigmented purpuric dermatoses. *Tumor d'emblée* MF is an outmoded concept used in the past to refer to supposed cases of MF that manifested as cutaneous tumors in the absence of patches or plaques. Most experts now prefer to classify such cases as other forms of CTCL, depending on their histopathologic features.

HISTOPATHOLOGIC AND CYTOLOGIC FEATURES

A well-developed plaque of MF contains a bandlike, cytologically atypical lymphoid infiltrate in the upper dermis that infiltrates the epidermis as single cells and cell clusters known as Pautrier's microabscesses. The atypical lymphoid cells exhibit dense, hyperchromatic nuclei with convoluted, cerebriform nuclear contours and scant cytoplasm. The term *cerebriform* comes from the brainlike ultrastructural appearance of these nuclei. In more advanced cutaneous tumors, the infiltrate extends diffusely throughout the upper and lower dermis and may lose its epidermotropism. In the earlier patch phase of the disease, the infiltrate is sparser, and lymphoid atypia may be less pronounced. In some cases, it may be difficult to distinguish early patch-type MF from various types of chronic dermatitis. The presence of lymphoid atypia and absence of significant epidermal intercellular edema (i.e., spongiosis) help to establish the diagnosis of early MF.

Involvement of lymph nodes by MF begins in the paracortical T-cell domain and may progress to complete effacement of nodal architecture by the same types of atypical lymphoid cells that infiltrate the skin. These cells can be seen in low numbers in the peripheral blood of many MF patients; however, those with SS develop gross leukemic involvement, usually defined as at least 1000 tumor cells/mm[3]. These cells are known as Sézary cells, and they are traditionally detected by manual review of the peripheral blood smear (the so-called Sézary prep). They may also be defined by various immunophenotypic criteria.

IMMUNOPHENOTYPING

Cellular antigen expression is usually assessed by immunoperoxidase methods for tissue biopsy specimens and by flow cytometry for blood specimens. Almost all cases of MF or SS begin as phenotypically and functionally mature $CD4^+$ T-cell neoplasms of skin-associated lymphoid tissue (SALT). They express the SALT-associated homing molecule cutaneous lymphocyte antigen (CLA) and most mature T-cell surface antigens, with the exceptions of CD7 and CD26, which are often absent. As disease progresses, the tumor cells often dedifferentiate and lose one or more mature T-cell markers, such as CD2, CD3, or CD5.

Cases typically express the α/β form of the T-cell receptor. At least in advanced cases, the cytokine profile is consistent with the T_H2 subset of $CD4^+$ T cells (i.e., production of interleukin [IL]-4, IL-5, and IL-10 rather than T_H1 cytokines such as IL-2 and interferon-γ). Expression of the high-affinity IL-2 receptor (CD25, TAC) ranges widely, with most cases showing a variable minority of lesional $CD25^+$ cells. Tumor cells can be induced to express a regulatory T-cell phenotype (Treg) in vitro. MF cases that express $CD8^+$ or other aberrant phenotypes occur occasionally but behave like conventional cases. They should not be confused with rare aggressive CTCLs exhibiting cytotoxic T-cell differentiation.

In addition to tumor cells, MF and SS lesions contain a minor component of immune accessory cells (i.e., Langerhans cells and macrophages) and $CD8^+$ T cells with a cytolytic phenotype. This presumed host response correlates positively with survival and tends to decrease as lesions progress. A favorable response to therapy such as photopheresis appears to correlate with normal levels of circulating $CD8^+$ cells.

MOLECULAR BIOLOGY

Well-developed MF or SS is a monoclonal T-cell lymphoproliferative disorder. Southern blotting or polymerase chain reaction (PCR) assays demonstrate monoclonal T-cell receptor gene rearrangements. The greater sensitivity of PCR assays allows the demonstration of dominant clonality in many early patch-type lesions of MF. These assays sometimes detect dominant clonality in lesional skin showing only chronic dermatitis histopathologically. These cases are called *clonal dermatitis* and may represent the earliest manifestation of MF because several have progressed to histologically recognizable MF within a few years. However, some cases of clinicopathologically defined early-phase MF lack a detectable monoclonal T-cell population until later in their clinical course.

In addition to aiding initial diagnosis, gene rearrangement analysis has facilitated staging and prognosis. Because some patients without MF or SS can have low levels of circulating Sézary-like cells and because not all cases of peripheral blood involvement in MF or SS exhibit morphologically recognizable tumor cells, the demonstration of dominant clonality that matches the clone in lesional skin has proved to be a useful diagnostic adjunct. The same holds true for assessing lymph node involvement. T-cell receptor gene rearrangement analysis of MF and SS lymph nodes is more sensitive than histopathology and possesses at least some prognostic relevance.

TNMB STAGING

Although several proposed methods have used a weighted extent approach to more accurately determine the MF or SS tumor burden, the preferred approach is the TNMB system, which is detailed in Tables 2 and 3. The original tumor (skin), lymph nodes, and metastasis (visceral organs) version of this system has been modified by the ISCL to incorporate the extent of blood involvement (B classification) into the staging process. Table 2 shows the TNMB classification relevant to MF and SS, and Table 3 shows how this information is used to determine the stage of disease. The prognostic relevance of this staging system has been supported by numerous studies, and use of the TNMB helps to guide the selection of therapies. For example, early-stage MF is the most amenable to control with topically

TABLE 2 TNMB Classification of Mycosis Fungoides and Sézary Syndrome

Skin (T)
T1	Patches and/or plaques; <10% body surface area
T2	Patches and/or plaques; ≥10% body surface area
T3	Tumors with/without other skin lesions
T4	Generalized erythroderma

Lymph Nodes (N)
N0	Not clinically enlarged; histopathology not required
N1	Clinically enlarged; histopathologically negative
N2	Clinically enlarged; histopathologically equivocal
N3	Clinically enlarged; histopathologically positive

Visceral Organs (M)
M0	No involvement
M1	Involvement

Peripheral Blood (B)
B0	Atypical cells ≤5% of leukocytes
B1	Atypical cells >5% of leukocytes
B2	Atypical cells ≥1000/mm^3

TABLE 3 TNMB Staging System for Mycosis Fungoides and Sézary Syndrome

Stage	Skin	Lymph Nodes	Viscera	Blood
IA	T1	N0	M0	B0–1
IB	T2	N0	M0	B0–1
IIA	T1–2	N1–2	M0	B0–1
IIB	T3	N0–2	M0	B0–1
IIIA	T4	N0–2	M0	B0
IIIB	T4	N0–2	M0	B1
IVA-1	T1–4	N0–2	M0	B2
IVA-2	T1–4	N3	M0	B0–2
IVB	T1–4	N0–3	M1	B0–2

Modified from Olsen E, Vonderheid E, et al: Revisions to the staging and classification of mycosis fungoides and Sézary syndrome: A proposal of the International Society for Cutaneous Lymphomas (ISCL) and the cutaneous lymphoma task force of the European Organization of Research and Treatment of Cancer (EORTC). Blood 2007;110(6):1713–1722.

directed treatments, whereas advanced MF or SS with extracutaneous involvement usually requires systemic therapies or topical plus systemic combinations.

TREATMENT

Rather than cure, which is attained in less than 10% of cases, the goal of MF and SS therapy is to reduce the impact of the skin disease on quality of life. For most patients, this is achieved by reducing pain, itch, and infection and improving clinical appearance. Appearance is affected by the disfigurement of the eruption and by the profound degree of scale shedding in some patients. Because the natural history of early-stage MF predicts a virtually normal life span, the goal of treatment must be directed at quality of life. For more advanced stages, prolongation of life expectancy may be a reasonable treatment goal.

Regardless of presentation, relief of symptoms should be addressed early. For dryness and scaling, the use of emollient ointments is indicated. These include petrolatum, Aquaphor, and commercially available shortening such as Crisco (an inexpensive alternative).[1] For modest dryness, creams (e.g., Nivea, Cetaphil, Eucerin) can be adequate and more acceptable to patients. Mild superfatted soaps such as Dove and Oil of Olay are recommended. Soap substitutes such as Cetaphil are also acceptable. Pruritus can be addressed with oral agents such as hydroxyzine (Atarax) or diphenhydramine (Benadryl)[1] 2 to

5 mg/kg/day and divided into four daily doses. Antipruritics work better when used on a regular basis rather than on an as-needed basis. Nonsedating antihistamines tend to be less effective. Measures to reduce dryness also help to reduce pruritus. Secondary infection needs to be treated with appropriate antibiotics. Their selection is guided by results of skin cultures but usually involves coverage of gram-positive organisms.

Phototherapy

Two main phototherapeutic regimens are used to treat CTCLs. Ultraviolet B radiation (290–320-nm broad band or 311-nm narrow band) can be used for patients with patches but not those with well-developed plaques or tumors. Seventy percent of patients achieve total clinical remission, usually within about 3 to 5 months. Another 15% achieve partial remission. Narrow-band UVB usually is more effective than broadband UVB and achieves maximal responses more rapidly.

Psoralen–ultraviolet A (PUVA) photochemotherapy uses oral 8-methoxypsoralen (8-MOP)[1] 0.6 mg/kg as a photosensitizer before UVA (320–400 nm) exposure. Sixty-five percent of patients with patch or plaque disease achieve complete remissions, and 30% have partial responses to this modality. For most patients, maximal responses are achieved within 3 months, and after 5 months, it is unlikely that further improvement will be gained. Limitations of these modalities include actinic damage, photocarcinogenesis, retinal damage (if eyes are not protected), and the inconvenience of getting to phototherapy centers. PUVA also has the risk of nausea and a theoretical risk of cataract induction without proper eye protection.

During the clearing phase of treatment, phototherapy treatments usually are administered three times per week. After resolution of skin lesions, treatment frequency is usually tapered gradually to once weekly for UVB and once every 4 to 6 weeks for PUVA. These maintenance regimens are often continued for months to years because abrupt cessation of phototherapy is commonly associated with rapid relapse, which is probably related to the persistence of microscopic disease after clinical clearing.

Topical Therapy

Like phototherapeutic regimens, topical therapies are appropriate for disease confined to the skin (stage I). Topical corticosteroids are frequently used for CTCLs, often before diagnosis. Low-potency formulations are useful on the face and skin folds. Medium-potency preparations are appropriate for the trunk and extremities. High-potency formulations are useful for recalcitrant lesions; however, prolonged use of such potent agents can cause local atrophy and adrenal suppression. Roughly one half of patients achieve complete remissions, and most others have partial remissions. Response duration varies widely with the individual pace of disease and patient compliance. Topical corticosteroids are particularly useful as a means to relatively quickly ameliorate severe signs and symptoms and as an adjuvant therapy in combination with other primary treatments.

Mechlorethamine (nitrogen mustard, HN$_2$, Mustargen)[1] is applied topically in an aqueous solution or in an ointment, such as Aquaphor. The aqueous form is prepared at home and involves a daily dose totaling 10 mg in 60 mL water. The ointment form is prepared by a pharmacist in 1-pound lots at a concentration of 10 mg of mechlorethamine per 100 g of ointment. Only the amount of ointment needed to apply a thin layer is used. Either formulation is usually applied at bedtime to lesional skin for limited disease or to the entire skin surface (excluding the head unless it is also involved) for more extensive disease. It is then showered off every morning using soap and water. Results are similar to those from PUVA. Advantages include therapy at home and availability in all regions of the country. Disadvantages are daily preparation (aqueous form only), daily application, and possible allergic contact dermatitis (more common with the aqueous preparation). Maximal efficacy is expected within 6 months. Mild flares of disease may occur during the first few months of treatment and probably represent inflammation of subclinical skin lesions,

---

[1]Not FDA approved for this indication.

[1]Not FDA approved for this indication.

analogous to the clinical accentuation of actinic damage during topical therapy with 5-fluorouracil (Efudex). As with phototherapy, topical mechlorethamine is tapered gradually after remission is achieved in an effort to delay clinical relapse.

Carmustine (BCNU, BiCNU)[1] is applied to the total skin surface as an alcohol/aqueous solution (10 to 20 mg in 60 mL).[6] Complete responses are seen in 85% of patients with stage IA disease (<10% involvement) and 50% of patients with stage IB disease (>10% involvement). Another 10% of patients obtain partial responses. Advantages include those described for nitrogen mustard and reports of success with application only to lesional skin. Disadvantages include skin irritation followed by telangiectasia formation and possible bone marrow suppression necessitating blood monitoring.

A topical gel formulation of the retinoid X receptor (RXR)–specific retinoid, bexarotene (Targretin), is useful for localized or limited skin lesions. The principal side effect is local irritation.

Radiotherapy

Conventional radiotherapy for mycosis fungoides therapy has been used for approximately 100 years. It is useful in the treatment of isolated, particularly problematic lesions such as recalcitrant tumors or ulcerated plaques. In addition to benefit from the photons delivered by radiotherapy, electron beam therapy (0.4 Gy per week for 8 to 9 weeks) is also useful for CTCL therapy. An approximately 85% complete response rate of skin disease with a median duration of 16 months is expected with electron beam therapy. An advantage is an excellent rate of complete response. Disadvantages include limited access to required equipment and expertise and cutaneous toxic effects, such as alopecia, sweat gland loss, radiation dermatitis, and skin cancers. As with other skin-directed therapy, the benefit for internal disease is limited. Cumulative toxicity also limits the number of courses a patient may receive. Localized electron beam therapy is also useful for treating cases of limited-extent MF and in treating selected problematic MF lesions in patients who are otherwise responding to therapy. After completion of total-skin electron beam therapy, patients require maintenance therapy such as topical mechlorethamine[6] or phototherapy to prolong remission.

Apheresis-Based Therapy

Leukapheresis and particularly lymphocytapheresis (6000 to 7000 mL of blood treated tiw initially, then according to response) have been used in the treatment of SS patients. Benefit has been reported in several case reports and small case series; however, response rates are not possible to determine. Photopheresis (i.e., extracorporeal photochemotherapy) describes an apheresis-based therapy in which circulating lymphocytes are first exposed to a psoralen (orally or extracorporeally) and then exposed to UVA extracorporeally. In contrast to leukapheresis, in which leukocytes are discarded, all cells are returned to the patient's circulation during photopheresis. Response rates in erythrodermic patients are 33% to 50%, and median survival for SS patients is prolonged from 30 months to more than 60 months. In recent years, extracorporeal photochemotherapy has been used increasingly in conjunction with one or more systemic therapies to enhance efficacy. The toxicity of the systemic agents is diminished because they are often used in combination at reduced doses.

Cytokine Therapy

Interferon alfa-2a (Roferon-A) or alfa-2b (Intron-A)[1] (1 to 100 × 10^6 units) is given subcutaneously or intralesionally every other day to once weekly. A standard starting dose is 3 × 10^6 units three times per week. Response rates are approximately 55%, with complete responses occurring in 17% of patients. Advantages include the relative ease of delivery. Disadvantages include anorexia, fever, malaise, leukopenia, and risk of cardiac dysrhythmia. Interferon alfa-2a or alfa-2b combined with narrow-band UVB or PUVA is effective for many patients with generalized skin lesions unresponsive to phototherapy alone.

Tumor-Associated Antigen-Directed Therapies

Various specific tumor-associated antigens have been targeted with antibody-based therapy. The response rate typically is low, and response durations are short. Less specific targets are CD4, CD5, and IL-2 receptors. Of this class of agent, the most promising is denileukin diftitox (Ontak, DAB389 IL-2) (9 to 18 µg per/kg/day IV on 5 consecutive days, every 3 weeks). This agent is a fusion protein combining IL-2 and diphtheria toxin. Cells bearing the IL-2 receptor (in the lesions of at least one half of MF patients) bind and internalize the drug. The drug also may destroy Treg cells that are CD25+ and suppress immune responses. Inside the cell, the toxin portion of the molecule disrupts protein synthesis, leading to cell death. Approximately 10% of patients achieve complete responses, and total response rates of near 40% have been reported. One half of responders and 20% of nonresponders experienced decreased pruritus. Adverse events include capillary leak syndrome, flulike symptoms, and allergic reactions. Combination therapy with denileukin diftitox and multiagent chemotherapy is being explored for advanced disease. Alemtuzumab (Campath)[1] is an antibody directed against CD52. It has shown benefit in advanced-stage disease. This agent can be used alone or in conjunction with multiagent chemotherapy.

Systemic Chemotherapy

Various regimens of single-agent and multiagent chemotherapy have been used in the treatment of MF and SS. Oral methotrexate, chlorambucil (Leukeran)[1] with or without prednisone,[1] and etoposide (VePesid)[1] have shown therapeutic activity. The best response has been in erythrodermic patients treated with methotrexate (5 to 125 mg weekly),[3] who have shown a 58% response rate. The combination of low-dose methotrexate and interferon alfa has been reported to yield a high response rate in advanced-stage MF and SS.

The use of multiagent regimens is controversial because of the small number of patients treated with any given regimen. There is even some evidence that for some populations of CTCL patients, survival may be reduced. For individual patients with advanced disease, however, cyclophosphamide (Cytoxan),[1] doxorubicin (Adriamycin),[1] vincristine (Oncovin),[1] and prednisone[1] (CHOP regimen) can provide some short-term palliation. In some cases, CHOP has successfully eradicated large cell transformation of MF and returned patients to their more clinically indolent patch or plaque baseline disease. Idarubicin (Idamycin)[1] in association with etoposide, cyclophosphamide, vincristine, prednisone, and bleomycin (Blenoxane)[1] (VICOP-B regimen) has demonstrated response rates of 80% (36% complete response rate) for patients with stage II through IV disease and 84% for MF patients, with a median duration of response longer than 8 months. Other regimens have been used with more modest success.

Several purine nucleoside analogues have been used for CTCL treatment, including erythrodermic variants. These include 2-chlorodeoxyadenosine (cladribine [Leustatin],[1] with a response rate of 28%), 2-deoxycoformycin (pentostatin [Nipent],[1] with a response rate of 39%), and fludarabine (Fludara).[1] Toxicities include pulmonary edema, bone marrow and immune suppression, and neurotoxicity.

Retinoids

Retinoids have therapeutic activity against MF and SS alone and in combination with other therapies, such as interferon alfa or PUVA (the latter combination is called Re-PUVA). Arotinoid,[5] acitretin (Soriatane),[1] and 13-cis-retinoic acid (isotretinoin [Accutane])[1] have various degrees of efficacy, and they typically are used in conjunction with other modalities. A newer RXR-specific retinoid, bexarotene, has an overall response rate of about 40% and can be used alone or in combination with phototherapy and other systemic agents such as interferon alfa-2. Disadvantages of bexarotene therapy include signs of hypothyroidism and vitamin A toxicity, particularly hyperlipidemia.

---

[1]Not FDA approved for this indication.
[6]May be compounded by pharmacists.

[1]Not FDA approved for this indication.
[3]Exceeds dosage recommended by the manufacturer.
[5]Investigational drug in the United States.

Enzyme Inhibitors

Vorinostat (Zolinza) is the first histone deacetylase inhibitor to be FDA approved for MF and SS. The overall response rate approaches 40% using a standard oral dose of 400 mg/day. Side effects include gastrointestinal symptoms, thrombocytopenia, and cardiac conduction abnormalities. Rhomidepsin (Isotodax) is an intravenously administered histone deacetylase inhibitor recently approved by the FDA for MF and SS. Forodesine[5] is a purine nucleoside phosphorylase inhibitor that preferentially affects T cells because they contain relatively high concentrations of this enzyme. Forodesine is undergoing clinical trials for MF and SS in the United States and appears to have a response rate of about 40%.

Miscellaneous Therapies

Various other therapies have been tried for MF and SS with modest success. Nonmyeloablative allogeneic stem cell transplantation has led to favorable responses in some patients; however, the total number treated is small. Cyclosporine (Sandimmune)[1] has been used for MF and SS. Transient improvement is followed by worsened survival due to immunosuppression, and it is not a recommended therapy. Thymopentin[5] has given excellent results in SS patients (i.e., 40% complete response rate and 35% partial response rate, with a median duration of response of 22 months). The lack of follow-up reports in recent decades leaves the status of this therapy in question.

Selection of Therapy

Initial choices among conventional treatments for MF and SS depend on the types of lesions and the stage of disease. Disease subsets are followed by recommended initial treatments in parentheses: unilesional or localized MF (local radiation therapy), patch MF (broad- and narrow-band UVB, PUVA, mechlorethamine), patch/plaque MF (PUVA, mechlorethamine), thick plaque/tumor MF (electron beam radiation therapy, interferon alfa-2, bexarotene, histone deacetylase inhibitors), erythrodermic MF/SS (photopheresis), and nodal or visceral MF or SS (interferon alfa-2, bexarotene, histone deacetylase inhibitors, denileukin diftitox, experimental systemic therapies, systemic chemotherapy).

Second-line therapeutic choices often involve interferons, retinoids, or histone deacetylase inhibitors, usually in combination with primary modalities. Multimodality combinations, often at reduced doses, are used commonly to treat patients with stage IIB or more advanced disease. Medium-potency topical corticosteroids, such as 0.1% triamcinolone cream or ointment (Kenalog),[1] are useful adjuncts to many different therapies. The optimal use of newer

[1]Not FDA approved for this indication.
[5]Investigational drug in the United States.

CURRENT THERAPY

GUIDELINES ARE PRIMARILY FOR MYCOSIS FUNGOIDES AND SÉZARY SYNDROME:

- Stages IA-IIA: skin-directed therapy with potent topical corticosteroids, topical mechlorethamine (Mustargen),[1] or phototherapy; radiation therapy or topical bexarotene (Targretin) in selected cases
- Stages IIB-IVB: skin-directed therapy plus one or more systemic therapies, such as interferon alfa-2a (Roferon-A) or alfa-2b (Intron A),[1] bexarotene (Targretin), vorinostat (Zolinza), denileukin diftitox (Ontak), or methotrexate; photopheresis for erythrodermic cases
- Combination therapies are often used in intermediate- and advanced-stage disease.
- Multiagent chemotherapy is usually not an effective long-term treatment strategy.

[1]Not FDA approved for this indication.

therapeutic agents in various subtypes and stages of MF and SS is still being established. Evidence-based guidelines for MF and SS therapy have been developed by the National Comprehensive Cancer Network (NCCN) (www.nccn.org).

Lymphoproliferative Disorders Associated with Mycosis Fungoides and Sézary Syndrome

TYPES AND CLINICAL FEATURES

Patients with MF or SS are at increased risk for large T-cell lymphomas, lymphomatoid papulosis, and Hodgkin's disease. Molecular biologic analysis has shown that these disorders and MF often share the same clonal T-cell receptor gene rearrangement when they arise in the same individual. As a consequence, they are considered to be subclones of the original MF tumor clone. The development of large T-cell lymphoma in a patient with MF or SS is referred to as *large cell transformation of MF.* This occurs in up to 20% of cases in some series and is associated with a median survival of only 1 to 2 years. One half of these large T-cell lymphomas are CD30[+]; however, the generally favorable prognosis of primary cutaneous CD30[+] anaplastic large cell lymphoma does not extend to these secondary forms of CD30[+] lymphoma. These patients are usually treated with systemic chemotherapy such as CHOP or with experimental systemic therapies appropriate for advanced-stage CTCL.

Lymphomatoid papulosis manifests as recurrent, usually generalized crops of spontaneously regressing, erythematous papules that can exhibit crusting or vesiculation before resolution. It is the clinically benign end of a disease continuum that has primary cutaneous CD30[+] anaplastic large cell lymphoma at its other extreme. Intermediate forms of disease can occur. Histopathologically, lesions contain a mixed-cell infiltrate, including large, atypical T cells that resemble Reed-Sternberg cells and their mononuclear variants (so-called type A) or large MF-type cells (so-called type B). Type A cells are CD30[+]. A type C form is also recognized. It has sheets of type A cells histologically mimicking CD30[+] large T-cell lymphoma but is different from it clinically. A type D variant containing CD8[+] CD30[+] large atypical cells has also been described recently. All types of lymphomatoid papulosis behave similarly. Patients with lymphomatoid papulosis sometimes respond to tetracycline or erythromycin (500 mg PO bid), presumably on the basis of antiinflammatory activity. Most cases improve within 1 month with low-dose methotrexate (10 to 20 mg PO every week). PUVA and narrow-band UVB given three times per week are other therapeutic options.

TREATMENT

In most cases, non-MF/SS CTCLs are treated with radiation therapy (with or without complete surgical excision) if they are localized or with various multiagent systemic chemotherapy regimens if they are generalized. The roles of other agents remain to be defined, except that studies have proved that methotrexate (10 to 40 mg PO every week) is effective therapy for most cases of primary cutaneous CD30[+] anaplastic large cell lymphoma. Therapies being investigated for this lymphoma include anti-CD30 antibodies, alone or conjugated to toxins. Denileukin diftitox has been reported to be effective against some subcutaneous panniculitic T-cell lymphomas.

REFERENCES

Olsen E, Vonderheid E, et al. Revisions to the staging and classification of mycosis fungoides and Sézary syndrome: A proposal of the International Society for Cutaneous Lymphomas (ISCL) and the cutaneous lymphoma task force of the European Organization of Research and Treatment of Cancer (EORTC). Blood 2007;110(6):1713–22.

Pimpinelli N, Olsen EA, Santucci M, et al. Defining early mycosis fungoides. J Am Acad Dermatol 2005;53(6):1053–63.

Richardson SK, Lin JH, Vittorio CC, et al. High clinical response rate with multimodality immunomodulatory therapy for Sézary syndrome. Clin Lymphoma Myeloma 2006;7(3):226–32.

Vonderheid EC, Bernengo MG, Burg G, et al. Update on erythrodermic cutaneous T-cell lymphoma: Report of the International Society for Cutaneous Lymphomas. J Am Acad Dermatol 2002;46(1):95–106.

Willemze R, Jaffe ES, Burg G, et al. WHO-EORTC classification for cutaneous lymphomas. Blood 2005;105(10):3768–85.
Wood GS, Greenberg HL. Diagnosis, staging, and monitoring of cutaneous T-cell lymphoma. Dermatol Ther 2003;16(4):269–75.

Papulosquamous Eruptions—Psoriasis

Method of
David Puchalsky, MD

Psoriasis is one of the papulosquamous (i.e., red, scaly, and noninfectious) skin diseases. The onset of psoriasis can occur at any age from birth to old age, but it usually occurs between the ages of 20 and 30 years. Both sexes are affected equally. The incidence is 2% to 3% of the population in North America. Psoriasis is chronic, and treatment controls but does not cure. The severity of untreated psoriasis tends to vary only slightly around each patient's baseline, which is established soon after onset. The appearance of psoriasis and its clinical variants are characteristic enough that a biopsy is usually not needed for diagnosis.

When a biopsy is needed, it is more often diagnostic if done to nonmanipulated and nontreated involved skin. Patients tend to have one dominant clinical variant, although some have more than one or shift from one to another. The cause of psoriasis is unknown, although certain genes are found to cluster in affected families and about 40% have a known family history of the disease. Symptoms of untreated psoriasis include itch, although this is severe in less than 50% of patients and often only when the skin is dry; discomfort, especially in the palms and soles when they are fissured or pustular; irritation, especially in skin folds; pain and stiffness in joints, ligaments, and tendons; and perception of social stigma.

Treatment

Current therapy is summarized in Figure 1. All psoriasis patients should be reassured that psoriasis is noncontagious and not cancerous. They should be informed that it is chronic and incurable but fortunately controllable. Baseline severity can be most safely reduced by a basic management approach (Box 1) that maximizes topical treatment and that should be continued long term, even if more aggressive treatment is added.

The objective and subjective severity of psoriasis should be carefully assessed to guide treatment choices. Objective severity for research purposes is assessed with a psoriasis area and severity index (PASI) score, which is a composite of measures of area involved as a percentage of the total-body surface area (TBSA) and severity (i.e., elevation, redness, and scale) of lesions in particular regions of the skin. In clinical practice, objective severity is more quickly assessed as a combination of percent of TBSA involved and general intensity of inflammation. TBSA involvement is often estimated using the patient's total hand and finger area as an approximation of 1% of the TBSA. Lesion inflammation is usually described in terms of degree of redness, elevation, scale, and the presence of pustules.

Subjective severity is best measured with a quality-of-life (QOL) tool (Box 2). Objective and subjective severity should be measured regularly to guide treatment decisions. A hypothetical patient can help make this point. Assume the presenting patient has a TBSA of 15% with moderately inflamed but nonpustular lesions and a QOL score of 80 of 110. If he has not been on any type of topical or other basic management, it would be reasonable to start such management alone. However, if on follow-up the TBSA is greater than 10%, lesions are still mildly inflamed, and the QOL score is higher than 50 despite reasonable compliance with basic psoriasis management (BPM), ultraviolet (UV) or systemic treatment should be strongly considered.

Compliance is difficult for psoriasis patients, as it is in any patient with a chronic disease. One study showed that primary adherence (i.e., filling prescriptions) is lower for psoriasis patients than for

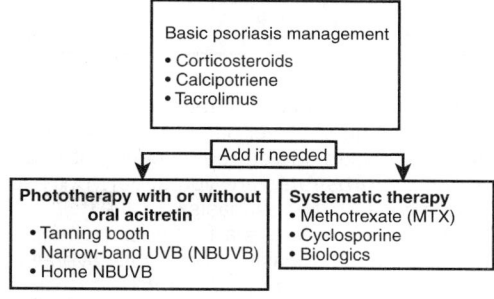

FIGURE 1. Algorithm for psoriasis management, including topical therapies (see Box 1).

CURRENT DIAGNOSIS

- Sharply demarcated, red, symmetrical plaques have a silvery scale (unless in skin folds).
- There are five clinical variants:
  - Plaque: silvery scale–topped, round or oval plaques on extensor surfaces, the torso, and often on the scalp
  - Guttate: <1-cm scaly papules, often occurring in children or young adults and often after streptococcal infection
  - Inverse: little scale, located in skin folds, often occurring in the obese, and occasionally occurring with secondary infection
  - Pustular: frank pustules with little scale, often localized to palms or soles or may be generalized, and often occurring with secondary infection
  - Erythrodermic: covering almost all of the skin
- Fifty percent of patients have nail findings, such as surface pits, lifting of the nail plate from the nail bed, and yellow discoloration under the nails, called *oil spots*.
- About 15% of patients develop psoriatic arthritis, most commonly asymmetrical oligoarthritis of the small joints of the hands and feet but rarely rheumatoid-like or spondylitis-like disease.

BOX 1 Basic Psoriasis Management

- Educate and support the patient (requires frequent visits).
- Reduce skin injury (koebnerization):
  No scratching, picking, or rubbing
  As-needed application of menthol or camphor creams
  Oral sedating antihistamines 2 hours before bed to decrease itch and scratch cycle
- Reduce or eliminate other exacerbating factors:
  Streptococcal and other infections
  Stress
  Alcohol consumption
  Smoking
  Obesity
- Use certain medicines (e.g., lithium, β-blockers, antimalarials).
- Repair dry skin or microinjury (see Box 3).
- Monitor for joint, tendon, and ligament involvement.
- Maximize topical therapy.
- Urge patient to seek natural sun exposure but avoid burning.

BOX 2 Quality-of-Life Tool

	Not at All			Somewhat			Very Much		
1. How much does psoriasis affect your *social life*?	0 1 2 3			4 5 6 7			8 9 10		
2. How *helpless* do you feel because of your psoriasis?	0 1 2 3			4 5 6 7			8 9 10		
3. How *embarrassed* do you feel because of your psoriasis?	0 1 2 3			4 5 6 7			8 9 10		
4. How *angry or frustrated* are you about your psoriasis?	0 1 2 3			4 5 6 7			8 9 10		
5. How *unsightly* is your psoriasis?	0 1 2 3			4 5 6 7			8 9 10		
6. How much does psoriasis affect your *clothing choices*?	0 1 2 3			4 5 6 7			8 9 10		
7. How much does psoriasis impact your *overall life enjoyment*?	0 1 2 3			4 5 6 7			8 9 10		
8. How much does your psoriasis *itch*?	0 1 2 3			4 5 6 7			8 9 10		
9. How much does your psoriasis *irritate or chafe*?	0 1 2 3			4 5 6 7			8 9 10		
10. How much does your psoriasis *hurt or cause pain*?	0 1 2 3			4 5 6 7			8 9 10		
11. I would be willing to take stronger medications that could carry significant risks to *control but not cure* my skin psoriasis.	0 1 2 3			4 5 6 7			8 9 10		

Total points: _____/110

those with other common skin diseases. Compliance with topical medications is especially poor, falling off soon after each visit and then rising before the next visit. I suggest frequent visits, good patient rapport, prescribing less-expensive generic medications, having the patient bring in unused medications to each visit, and carefully assessing compliance at each visit as methods to improve compliance and therefore treatment response.

TOPICAL THERAPY

Topical steroids are the first-line therapy for all psoriasis patients. They should be continued long term along with all other aspects of BPM. Adherence to BPM can lessen the required doses and therefore the toxicity of any added UV or systemic treatment. Topical steroids work on inflammation and hyperproliferation, the two key elements of psoriasis pathology. Topical steroid ointment preparations are preferable, because ointment vehicles repair the skin surface cracking, which perpetuates inflammation (i.e., the Koebner phenomenon). Petroleum jelly (Vaseline) alone improves psoriasis, whereas alcohol vehicles (in topical steroid solutions for scalp use) worsen psoriasis, and cream vehicles are often neutral. Ointments are the simplest vehicles, requiring fewer inactive ingredients that have the potential for irritation or contact sensitization. Ointment does not rub into the skin, and the patient should be instructed to apply the ointment gently in a thin film. The prescription amount should be based on the area treated, knowing that 20 g of ointment covers the entire skin once. For example, 4 g can cover 20% of TBSA once, and a 120-g tube of topical steroid ointment for once-daily use is a 30-day supply.

The timing of topical steroid application is important. To maximize efficacy and compliance, application should be done once daily after a hydrating bath in the evening (Box 3). After application, soft cotton clothing can be worn to keep the ointment from soiling home surfaces such as upholstery and sheets. Daytime application, although messy, is tolerated by many patients, and it can provide some additional control. Because steroid receptors are saturated at twice-daily applications, topical steroids can be applied more frequently without harm. One strategy is to allow patients to use topical steroids any time to help stop scratching behavior, because scratching is counterproductive and can be more of a habit than a response to a true itch. Alternatively, less messy nonsteroidal anti-itch creams can be used in this manner.

The potency of topical steroids is an important issue. Because psoriasis is a chronic disease, a safe but maximal potency is favored for each skin zone. Potency needs to match the thickness of the skin in each zone. There are seven potency groups, from group 1 (ultrapotent) to group 7 (least potent), and five skin-thickness zones. Box 4 provides the recommended generic topical steroid for each zone. Tachyphylaxis to topical steroids probably is minimal, with apparent decrease in potency over time resulting from declining compliance.

The physician should monitor for side effects, including adrenal suppression (avoid by following Box 4), skin thinning with prominent surface capillaries or stretch marks, infections, and rosacea-like facial eruptions. Topical steroids (even group 7) should be avoided near the eyelids, because they can increase risk of cataracts and glaucoma.

Occasionally, steroids can be injected intralesionally into resistant body plaques. This is best done by experienced clinicians. Triamcinolone typically is used at concentrations of 5 to 10 mg/mL (Aristospan Intralesional 5 mg/mL, Kenalog-10 10 mg/mL). Side effects are atrophy and secondary infection.

BOX 3 Evening Bath and Dry Skin Repair

- Take a *bath*—better than a shower.
- *Evening* bath is best so ointments can be applied generously.
- Use *warm* water, not hot, and do not use additives.
- Use only *mild* soap (near the end of the bath) only on skin folds and other necessary areas.
- *Do not scrub or scrape skin* (e.g., do not use a loofa, washcloth, or brush).
- Rinse soap off *thoroughly*.
- Pat dry—*no rubbing*.
- When skin is still slightly damp, apply medicated ointments to psoriasis.
- Apply plain Vaseline or plain mineral oil (may be warmed by prior immersion of bottle in bath water) to entire dry areas and psoriasis-prone areas.
- Wear loose-fitting cotton clothes (e.g., long johns, socks, gloves) after moisturizing and overnight.

BOX 4 Recommended Topical Steroids for Skin Thickness Zones*

- Palms or soles: group 1 ointment
  Clobetasol (Temovate), augmented betamethasone dipropionate (Diprolene)
  May be occluded under plastic for increased potency
- Body <30% TBSA: group 2 ointment
  Fluocinonide 0.05% (Lidex), desoximetasone 0.25% (Topicort)
- Body >30% TBSA: group 3 ointment
  Betamethasone valerate 0.1% (Valisone)
- Scalp: group 2 solution
  Fluocinonide 0.05% (Lidex)
- Folds: group 4 or 5
  Triamcinolone (Kenalog) 0.1% ointment or cream
- Face: group 7 ointment
  Hydrocortisone (Hytone) 1% or 2.5% (avoid eyelids)

TBSA = total body surface area.

Another major topical treatment in the armamentarium for psoriasis is calcipotriene (Dovonex), a vitamin D analogue. Unfortunately, it is available only in a cream vehicle, but it may be available soon as a generic drug and in the more effective ointment vehicle. It has no steroid side effects. Although it is not impressive as monotherapy, it does have additive efficacy with topical steroids, which can lower the mild irritancy of calcipotriene. Calcipotriene can be applied immediately before topical steroid ointments to all zones, although calcipotriene can occasionally be too irritating to use on the face. Use should be less than 400 g per month because of the risk of hypercalcemia. Calcipotriene is available in a very expensive, premixed combination with a group I steroid (i.e., betamethasone dipropionate), marketed as Taclonex ointment. Calcipotriene should not be used within 2 or 3 hours before UV treatment, because it decreases UV penetration.

Calcineurin inhibitors can be useful for psoriasis. Of the two available, tacrolimus, available only as brand-name Protopic,[1] is more effective because it is in an ointment vehicle. The 0.1% strength is more effective than the 0.03%. Tacrolimus ointment can be used on the face and even on the eyelids without fear of steroid side effects. Potency of tacrolimus 0.1% is somewhat unclear for psoriasis, but it is probably equivalent to a group 5 or 6 topical steroid. The FDA has put a black box warning on calcineurin inhibitors. This warning was based on giving mice and rats large systemic quantities and finding that lymphoma was more common and observing that tacrolimus did get absorbed through the skin in some pediatric patients with genetic deficiencies in skin barrier function. Most dermatologists think that calcineurin inhibitors are safe, although most avoid use in infants and toddlers and in patients with skin barrier function defects.

Many other topical medications have been used to treat psoriasis. Tazarotene (Tazorac) is a topical retinoid that has proved to be too irritating for routine use, except in some cases of localized pustular palm or sole psoriasis. Anthralin (Dritho-Scalp 0.5%, Psoriatec 1%) is also very irritating and stains surfaces, and it is rarely used. Tar (DHS Tar, Doak Tar) is of mostly historical interest because of poor efficacy, odor, and messiness, although it has mild efficacy in shampoos.

Topical adjuncts can be very useful. Camphor and menthol are ingredients that occupy skin temperature receptors and give an immediate cooling sensation that can provide instant relief of psoriasis pruritus. These products (e.g., Sarna Original Lotion, Eucerin, or Aveeno Anti-Itch Lotion) can be applied any time as a substitute behavior for scratching.

Topical antihistamines, such as those containing pramoxine (Prax),[1] can be helpful, although topical diphenhydramine (Benadryl)[1] can be sensitizing, as can topical doxepin (Zonalon[1]), which can also cause sedation. Oral sedating antihistamines taken before bed are preferred (see Table 1).

PHOTOTHERAPY AND ACITRETIN

Phototherapy with or without acitretin (Soriatane) is a natural next step if BPM is not effective enough. BPM must be continued to decrease the doses and toxicity of phototherapy. Phototherapy ages the skin and can cause skin cancer. Patients should be examined for precancerous or cancerous lesions before, during, and forever after this approach to controlling their psoriasis. Natural sun, which contains UV radiation in the range of 320 to 400 nm (UVA) and in the range of 280 to 320 nm (UVB), can be helpful. However, burning can trigger a flare of psoriasis through the Koebner phenomenon. In some climates, natural sun is practical only in summer or on vacation. Tanning booths, which emit largely UVA light (which tends not to burn but which causes tanning and some cutaneous immunosuppression) can help psoriasis but not as much as UVB light. UV therapy is not necessarily contraindicated by risk factors for skin cancer, including a history of skin cancer itself. First, improving the patient's

psoriasis by any means allows earlier detection of precancerous and cancerous growths, especially those in the nonmelanoma lineage, which can occasionally blend in with the psoriasis because they are also erythematous and often scaly. Second, systemic treatments are a concern because of their carcinogenicity, including that of the skin. The exception is acitretin, which has antineoplastic effects and is often paired with UV treatment.

Choice of provider-administered UV treatment has become simpler. First, narrow-band UVB (NBUVB) with a wavelength of 311 nm (the UVB wavelength most effective for psoriasis) has replaced broad-spectrum UVB. Second, NBUVB has largely replaced PUVA (i.e., psoralens PO [8 MOP, Oxsoralen-Ultra] or topically [Oxsoralen lotion] plus UVA). NBUVB is associated with easier compliance, better tolerance, reduced risk of burning, reduced risk of ocular damage, and equal or near-equal efficacy.

The NBUVB initial dose is based usually on an estimate of the patient's minimal erythematous dose and then steadily but carefully increased (e.g., by 5%) each treatment to achieve a mild and transient erythema the day after each treatment. Maximal treatment is usually four times per week. A consent form should be employed. It reviews risks and benefits of treatment and gives some responsibility to the patient to keep health care providers apprised of medication changes that could change the tendency to burn. Natural sun exposure should be limited because added UV can cause burning, and depending on the timing, a suntan can limit efficacy of the NBUVB. Most patients improve by 80% to 90% after 2 months of maximal treatment. Psoriasis clears completely in very few patients, except some who have guttate psoriasis. The scalp and skin fold areas are particularly resistant.

Many patients benefit from a maintenance protocol with a reduction of treatment to twice and then once per week after improvement is near-maximal. Most maintenance protocols hold the dose steady at an amount 50% to 75% of the maximal dose achieved. The dose is held steady because patients do not build an increasing tolerance to the NBUVB with less frequent treatments. One efficient approach in geographic locations with pronounced seasons is to treat aggressively in the winter, go to a maintenance protocol in the spring, and then consider maintenance with natural sun in the summer.

A home NBUVB unit is recommended for some patients who are experienced with provider-administered NBUVB, are located far from facilities, and are reliable about follow-up appointments.

Acitretin is a systemic treatment that can improve natural sun, tanning booth, or NBUVB efficacy. This oral retinoid does not cause immunosuppression, nor is it carcinogenic. It can reduce the number and the dose of UV treatments required for near-clearing efficacy. At the usual dose of 25 mg/day with food, this agent tends to be well tolerated. The minimal side effects include a slight and reversible increase in triglyceride or cholesterol levels, rare and mild increase in the levels of liver transaminases, and manageable mucocutaneous drying.

Acitretin does not work well without UV treatment, unless used for pustular psoriasis, in which case it works well for generalized or localized forms. Acitretin is a teratogen, and use is not advised in fertile women. The agent is stored in fat as a teratogenic metabolite for at least 3 years after the last dose. Storage may be increased with alcohol consumption. Alcohol consumption should be limited when using acitretin.

OTHER SYSTEMIC AGENTS

Systemic treatment of psoriasis is undergoing a constant evolution, especially with new biologic agents becoming available every few years. Although very expensive, these agents can help control moderate to severe psoriasis, and some work for psoriatic arthritis. Topical agents and the rest of BPM need to be continued to keep doses and toxicities low. These agents are to some extent immunosuppressive and thereby increase the risk of infection and neoplasia. Certain agents seem to increase the risk of some infections more than others or certain forms of cancer more than others. This is a controversial and evolving area as postmarketing studies continue to collect data. Each agent has specific risks in addition to immunosuppression.

---

[1]Not FDA approved for this indication.

The advisability of written informed consent when using these agents cannot be overstated. Systemic agents usually are reserved for those who fail to improve well enough on BPM and have other issues. These issues include inability to get UVB treatment because of distance from facilities; lack of candidacy for UV treatment because of UV-induced disease, such as lupus; resistance to UV treatment, such as severe skin fold psoriasis; long history of poor response to previous UV treatment; and significant psoriatic arthritis, preferably diagnosed by a rheumatologist.

Methotrexate (MTX; Trexall) is the systemic agent with the longest record of use. It is effective for all variants of psoriasis and helps psoriatic arthritis, although not as well for the spinal type. MTX is a dihydrofolate reductase inhibitor and has been found to work as an immune modulator. The major potential toxicity is hepatic. It is metabolized by the kidney, and renal dysfunction can increase the risk of hepatotoxicity. This drug is contraindicated in pregnancy; for patients with liver disease, renal dysfunction, some types of immunodeficiency or immunosuppression, and acute or chronic infection; and for those with malignancy. Alcohol abuse (>1 drink/day) is not allowed while on this hepatotoxic agent. Sulfa drugs cannot be used simultaneously, and nonsteroidal antiinflammatory drugs can be used only at low doses. Because of the rare but devastating possibility of agranulocytosis, MTX is often given at a 5- to 7.5-mg test dose, followed by a complete blood cell (CBC) count before dose progression.

This systemic agent is relatively inexpensive, because it is available generically. The least expensive option is to use injection solution MTX.[1] It can be given in preloaded syringes that patients can squirt into orange juice. Folic acid 1 g/day decreases nausea experienced by some and oral ulcerations experienced by few, and it does not decrease efficacy. Intramuscular weekly dosing rather than oral dosing is an option for those with gastrointestinal intolerance or poor efficacy because this mode of administration bypasses the portal circulation and some metabolism that occurs.

Monthly laboratory monitoring is best done 6 to 7 days after a weekly dose and should include levels of liver enzymes and creatinine, a CBC count with a differential, and any tests for infection that may be suggested by the patient's history. Patients should be checked monthly for efficacy as the dose is increasing. Doses start at 7.5 mg and can be steadily increased to 30 mg in a single once-weekly dose. After near-clearing has occurred, the dose can usually be held steady or decreased, and patients can be seen and blood tests drawn every 3 months.

Liver enzymes are not completely sensitive for MTX-induced liver damage. A liver biopsy done under ultrasound guidance is required at 1.5 g of cumulative MTX and should be done sooner if there are liver abnormalities. Some patients prefer not to get a liver biopsy, despite the documented excellent safety and tolerance of this procedure. They must be switched from MTX to another agent or approach. If the liver biopsy interpreted by an experienced pathologist shows no significant fibrosis, MTX can be continued up to another 3 g (cumulative) with monitoring until a repeat liver biopsy is advised. Even with a second normal liver biopsy result, I recommend a switch to another agent after 6 g of cumulative MTX. Patients can be switched to UV, if a candidate, or a nonhepatotoxic systemic agent. For example, at the common dose of 25 mg of MTX per week, this occurs at 5 years of treatment.

Oral cyclosporine (Neoral) is a potent immunosuppressive agent that has been used for the past 20 years for psoriasis. Its greatest strength is its speed in improving the skin. However, it has no significant effect on the symptoms or signs of psoriatic arthritis. It predictably raises blood pressure and decreases renal function, even in the low doses (≤4 mg/kg/day) used for psoriasis. It is contraindicated if there is known renal disease and dysfunction, hypertension that is newly diagnosed or under poor control, immunodeficiency or immunosuppression, infection, or malignancy. The creatinine level

must be checked twice before starting the medication, and blood pressure should be monitored closely in the first few weeks. Ultimately, blood pressure and creatinine levels should be checked at least once each month.

Cyclosporine is used mostly as an emergency drug to quickly decrease moderate to severe psoriasis over 1 to 3 months. It is a way to bridge to another approach that can maintain the improvement in a safer manner. Systemic steroids are never used for this purpose because they can cause a rebound severe or even pustular flare of psoriasis. This has been reported even after a relatively short course or a relatively long taper.

BIOLOGICALS

Biologic agents for psoriasis are proteins produced by recombinant DNA technology. There are four FDA-approved biologic agents for psoriasis: etanercept (Enbrel), adalimumab (Humira), infliximab (Remicade), and alefacept (Amevive). Efalizumab (Raptiva)[2] was withdrawn from the U.S. market as of June 8, 2009, because of the risk of progressive multifocal leukoencephalopathy. These are expensive and powerfully marketed agents. Most insurance carriers do not cover these biologicals unless patients have failed treatment with UV and MTX. Efficacy for the skin usually is no greater than that of MTX, cyclosporine, or NBUVB (especially NBUVB combined with acitretin). However, the tumor necrosis factor (TNF) blockers etanercept, adalimumab, and infliximab are as effective or more effective than MTX for psoriatic arthritis. Rheumatologists have much experience with the TNF blockers, and FDA approval has followed for moderate to severe skin psoriasis even without psoriatic arthritis.

Etanercept is a recombinant human TNF-α receptor (p75) protein fused with the Fc portion of IgG1 that binds to soluble and membrane-bound TNF-α. It is prescribed in a subcutaneous autoinjector that is easy to use for most patients. Dosage is 50 mg twice each week for the first 3 months, followed by once-weekly dosing thereafter.

Adalimumab binds specifically to soluble and membrane-bound TNF-α and blocks TNF-α interactions with the p55 and p75 cell surface TNF receptors. A dose of 80 mg is given by subcutaneous autoinjector, followed by 40 mg the next week and then every 2 weeks thereafter. Written consent forms should be used when prescribing adalimumab or etanercept. Both are contraindicated in patients with active infections or malignancy. Tuberculosis testing should be performed before starting them, because they can reactivate the disease. They should not be used with live vaccines. There may be an increased risk of lupus, multiple sclerosis, and new onset or worsening of congestive heart failure. Hepatitis B reactivation has been reported, and patients should be screened for hepatitis. Patients not uncommonly report injection-site reactions. Rarely, skin psoriasis can flare even after months of excellent control. Etanercept or adalimumab can be overlapped with MTX when there is a rotation from MTX to a TNF blocker or if rotating from TNF blocker to MTX. Long-term combined use may be needed for refractory severe disease. In these cases, there is added concern about infection and neoplasia plus the usual concern about MTX hepatotoxicity.

The third TNF blocker infliximab has been used more by gastroenterologists than by rheumatologists because it is used for inflammatory bowel disease. It is a chimeric antibody composed of a mouse variable region and a human IgG1-α constant region. It binds to the soluble and the transmembrane TNF-α molecules. Administration is by intravenous infusion of 5 mg/kg over 2 to 3 hours at weeks 0, 2, and 6 and then every 8 weeks for psoriasis and psoriatic arthritis. Infliximab has a rapid response and may work slightly better than other TNF blockers. However, some patients develop infusion reactions and serum sickness. Infusion reactions may need to be ameliorated by concurrent administration of MTX. Infliximab shares the same list of potential side effects as etanercept and adalimumab,

---

[1]Not FDA approved for this indication.

[2]Not available in the United States.

including infection and malignancy. All of the TNF blockers are pregnancy category B drugs.

Alefacept is less useful for a few reasons. The efficacy is probably somewhat less than that for the TNF blockers; medical experience is less because it has no activity against psoriatic arthritis or colitis; and it has some potential side effects that are worrisome. Alefacept binds to CD2 on memory-effector T lymphocytes, depleting these T cells. The lymphocytes must be measured before treatment and monitored every other week, with the medication withheld if the CD4 count falls below 250 cells/mL. The marketing claim for longer remissions than those from other biologicals is not convincing.

Only a very experienced dermatologist should prescribe biologic agents. Some patients are reluctant or unwilling to rotate off these medications and back to UV light or MTX. It is unknown whether these agents have some cumulative side effects. For etanercept and adalimumab, we have the rheumatologists' longer experience, but they tend to use the agents in lower doses for rheumatoid arthritis, and there may be some differences in the patient populations (e.g., psoriatic arthritis patients may have more side effects).

There is promise for future biologic agents directed against interleukins, which are involved in psoriasis inflammation. At least eight chromosomal loci have been identified as significantly linked to psoriasis. There is hope that identifying gene products will help the understanding of psoriasis and the development of better biologic treatments.

In summary, BPM has not been emphasized enough in treating patients with psoriasis, despite our knowledge that this is a chronic disease with no cure. Compliance has not been emphasized, with the result that many patients who would not need treatment beyond BPM are placed on more potentially harmful treatment. There are still many patients with good compliance with BPM who have severe enough skin psoriasis (measured objectively and subjectively) or who have significant psoriatic arthritis that requires more potent treatment. UV treatment, particularly NBUVB, is favored for skin disease before going to systemic treatment, but systemic treatment is needed for significant psoriatic arthritis. These patients still need BPM to minimize the doses and toxicities of their systemic agents. Patients should be followed especially carefully for side effects, many of which are arguably worse than the psoriasis itself. Long-term risks of biologic agents are still not clear, but the TNF blockers have established themselves as bona fide options and have probably replaced cyclosporine, even for skin psoriasis alone, except when cyclosporine is used for only 1 or 2 months to quiet a severe flare.

REFERENCES

Brown KK, Rehmus WE, Kimball AB. Determining the relative importance of patient motivations for nonadherence to topical corticosteroid therapy in psoriasis. J Am Acad Dermatol 2006;55(4):607–13.

Carroll CL, Feldman SR, Camacho FT, et al. Better medication adherence results in greater improvement in severity of psoriasis. Br J Dermatol 2004;151(4):895–7.

Feldman SR, Koo JY, Menter A, et al. Decision points for the initiation of systemic treatment for psoriasis. J Am Acad Dermatol 2005;53(1):101–7.

Gottlieb A, Korman NJ, Gordon KB, et al. Guidelines of care for the management of psoriasis and psoriatic arthritis: Section 2. Psoriatic arthritis: Overview and guidelines of care for treatment with an emphasis on the biologics. J Am Acad Dermatol 2008;58(5):851–64.

Gutman AB, Kligman AM, Sciacca J, et al. Soak and smear: A standard technique revisited. Arch Dermatol 2005;141(12):1556–9.

Menter A, Gottlieb A, Feldman SR, et al. Guidelines of care for the management of psoriasis and psoriatic arthritis: Section 1. Overview of psoriasis and guidelines of care for the treatment of psoriasis with biologics. J Am Acad Dermatol 2008;58(5):826–50.

National Psoriasis Foundation. About psoriasis and treatment overview for medical providers, Available at: http://www.psoriasis.org/NetCommunity/Page.aspx?pid=798 [accessed May 24, 2009].

Storm A, Andersen SE, Benfeldt E, et al. One in 3 prescriptions are never redeemed: primary nonadherence in an outpatient clinic. J Am Acad Dermatol 2008;59(1):27–33.

Autoimmune Connective Tissue Disease

Method of
Molly Hinshaw, MD, and Susan Lawrence-Hylland, MD

Lupus Erythematosus

Lupus erythematosus is an autoimmune connective tissue disease that may localize to the skin or involve several organ systems. A complete review of systems with evaluation of positive findings is necessary to thoroughly assess patients for signs of systemic lupus as defined by the American Rheumatism Association. Cutaneous lupus erythematosus manifests in chronic, subacute, and acute forms. A punch biopsy from within an erythematous lupus lesion is useful for confirming the diagnosis.

CLINICAL FEATURES

Discoid lupus and tumid lupus are the two forms of chronic cutaneous lupus erythematosus. Discoid lupus lesions are tender or pruritic, erythematous to violaceous, scaly plaques that typically occur on sun-exposed skin. The lesions resolve with scarring, and when the lesions affect the scalp, they cause scarring alopecia. Tumid lupus manifests as pruritic, erythematous to violaceous, nonscaly plaques that typically preferentially affect the face and trunk.

The lesions of subacute cutaneous lupus erythematosus occur as erythematous to violaceous, scaly macules and as annular or polycyclic patches. These lesions are commonly located on sun-exposed skin and heal without scarring.

Acute cutaneous lupus erythematosus is exemplified by malar erythema (i.e., butterfly rash) and by poikiloderma (i.e., hyperpigmentation, telangiectasias, and epidermal atrophy). It is a manifestation of systemic lupus erythematosus (SLE). Cutaneous lesions may be widespread. In addition to the American Rheumatism Association criteria, patients with SLE may also develop Raynaud's phenomenon, hypercoagulability, and overlap syndromes with Sjögren's disease, dermatomyositis, and other conditions.

Hydrochlorothiazide (HydroDIURIL), terbinafine (Lamisil), minocycline (Minocin), procainamide (Pronestyl), hydralazine (Apresoline), and isoniazid (Nydrazid) are a few of the pharmaceutical agents that cause drug-induced lupus. This disease manifests with synovitis, photosensitivity, and positive serology results, and it may have cutaneous lesions that do not necessarily abate with cessation of the medication.

MANAGEMENT

Prevention

All patients with lupus erythematosus should be counseled on photoprotection, including protecting skin from sunlight and avoiding sun exposure during peak hours (i.e., between 10 AM and 2 PM). Ultraviolet A and B wavelengths may cause lupus to flare. Broad-spectrum sunscreen with an SPF of 30 or higher and that contains titanium, zinc, Mexoryl (L'Oreal), or Helioplex (Neutrogena) should be used whenever patients are outdoors. Photoprotective clothing that is available from multiple vendors is useful for limiting sun exposure.

Patients with lupus are relatively immunosuppressed by their disease. Vaccinations should be kept up to date, although there is a debate about the necessity and safety of vaccination against meningococcal disease (*Neisseria meningitidis*) (Menactra, Menomune), varicella-zoster virus (Zostavax), and *Streptococcus* (Pneumovax).

Treatment of Cutaneous Lupus Erythematosus

Medium-potency topical corticosteroids should be used for lupus localized to the skin, and they are used as adjunct treatment for patients with systemic lupus. Use of triamcinolone 0.1% cream (Flutex) for lesions on the head and neck until symptoms subside or up to 2 weeks continuously is an appropriate starting strength. Ointment-based vehicles are useful for lesions on the trunk and extremities. They are also the vehicles of choice on the scalp of patients of African American descent. Foam or liquid- or lotion-based corticosteroids work well in the scalp of other ethnic groups and can be used on the trunk and extremities. If lesions persist, the corticosteroid can be occluded, or intralesional injections with triamcinolone can be repeated monthly as needed. Intralesional triamcinolone acetonide at concentrations of 5 mg/mL (Kenalog) can be injected into lesions on the face or neck and doses of 10 to 20 mg/mL (Kenalog-10, Kenalog) into lesions on the trunk or extremities. Intralesional corticosteroids may cause mild discomfort, atrophy of the skin or subcutis, or stretch marks. Topical calcineurin inhibitors such as pimecrolimus (Elidel)[1] or tacrolimus (Protopic)[1] may be used for maintenance treatment but are not recommended for new or active lesions because they do not work quickly. Recurrent or refractory cutaneous lesions require systemic treatment.

Treatment of Systemic Lupus Erythematosus

Antimalarials, including hydroxychloroquine (Plaquenil),[1] are disease-modifying agents that limit the progression of lupus. Hydroxychloroquine, chloroquine (Aralen),[1] and quinacrine[2] (at compounding pharmacies) raise the pH of inflammatory cells, inhibiting inflammatory pathways that cause end-organ damage in patients with SLE.

Hydroxychloroquine is typically used first at 200 mg daily for 2 weeks and then increased to 400 mg daily. Patients need laboratory monitoring and a baseline and then yearly eye examination because the medication may be deposited in the retina over time. Hydroxychloroquine exerts its effects within 2 to 3 months of beginning treatment. Its effects are diminished in smokers.

Depending on end-organ involvement in SLE, immunosuppression with systemic corticosteroids such as prednisone at doses of 1 mg/kg/day is appropriate. Steroid-sparing drugs such as methotrexate (Rheumatrex),[1] acitretin (Soriatane),[1] or mycophenolate mofetil (CellCept)[1] are added. After signs of inflammation subside, prednisone is tapered.

Treatment of Musculoskeletal Manifestations

Arthralgia is a common complaint that can usually be managed with acetaminophen or nonsteroidal antiinflammatory drugs (NSAIDs). For true arthritis unresponsive to the previously described measures, hydroxychloroquine[1] 200 mg twice daily can be added. After that, treatments similar to those used for rheumatoid arthritis can be added, although the antitumor necrosis factor agents usually are avoided in lupus. Methotrexate[1] 7.5 to 25 mg PO once weekly may be used along with folic acid[1] 1 mg daily to help limit side effects. Routine toxicity monitoring includes frequent complete blood cell counts and liver tests. Azathioprine (Imuran)[1] 0.5 to 2 mg/kg can be used with frequent monitoring of complete blood cell counts and liver tests. A sample for testing the thiopurine methyltransferase activity level should be drawn before initiating therapy because a genetic deficiency can lead to severe pancytopenia. Leflunomide (Arava)[1] 10–20 mg PO once daily can be used with frequent blood cell counts and liver tests. Low-dose glucocorticoids (prednisone 5 to 10 mg/day) may be used as a bridge to steroid-sparing therapy and to treat intermittent flares.

Treatment of Hematologic Manifestations

Autoimmune cytopenias are common and are often a defining feature of SLE. Lymphopenia (absolute lymphocyte count <1500 cells/microliter) does not require therapy. Hemolytic anemia in SLE is the result of antierythrocyte antibodies that activate complement, and it is treated with prednisone at a dose based on clinical severity. Typically, 1 mg/kg/day, or approximately 60 mg, is used for 4 to 6 weeks, with gradual tapering as long as the response is maintained. For severe hemolytic anemia, pulse methylprednisolone (Solu-Medrol) 1 g IV for 3 consecutive days can be tried, followed by the previously described standard dosing. For patients who do not respond to glucocorticoids or are unable to taper prednisone to low doses, other treatments can be used. They may include azathioprine[1] 1.5 to 2.5 mg/kg/day, mycophenolate mofetil[1] 1000 to 2000 mg/day in divided doses, danazol (Danocrine)[1] 300 to 600 mg/day in divided doses, intravenous immunoglobulin,[1] or rituximab (Rituxan)[1] 375 mg/m^2 weekly for four doses.

Immune thrombocytopenia results from antiplatelet antibodies that identify platelets for early destruction. Treatment is indicated when patients have signs or symptoms of spontaneous bleeding or when the platelet count drops below 50,000/mL. The initial treatment approach with glucocorticoids is similar to that used for hemolytic anemia. For patients with chronic thrombocytopenia or for those who cannot achieve an acceptable long-term dose of prednisone, steroid-sparing agents, including azathioprine,[1] mycophenolate mofetil,[1] danazol,[1] rituximab,[1] and intravenous immunoglobulin[1] can be used in doses similar to those used for hemolytic anemia. Dapsone,[1] cyclosporine (Sandimmune, Neoral),[1] and cyclophosphamide (Cytoxan)[1] have also been used.

Thrombotic thrombocytopenia purpura may occur in SLE, and it must be differentiated from immune thrombocytopenia because treatment requires emergent plasmapheresis. Manifestations of thrombotic thrombocytopenia purpura include fever, microangiopathic hemolysis, and central nervous system and renal abnormalities.

Antiphospholipid antibodies include the lupus anticoagulant, anticardiolipin antibodies, and β$_2$-glycoprotein. They are associated with coagulopathy, thrombocytopenia, late-trimester miscarriage, and heart valve abnormalities. Antiphospholipid antibodies that can be determined with blood testing but are not associated with thromboembolism do not require treatment. Low-dose aspirin[1] may be considered but has not been shown to prevent future thrombosis. Hydroxychloroquine[1] 200 mg twice daily has been shown to reduce the risk. Patients with antiphospholipid antibodies who develop thromboembolism need lifelong treatment with warfarin (Coumadin). A goal international normalized ratio (INR) remains controversial because different studies advocate for high-intensity warfarin (INR >3) or low-intensity therapy (INR >2). For women who have suffered a miscarriage determined to be related to antiphospholipid antibodies, low-dose aspirin and heparin 5000 units SQ twice daily may increase the likelihood of a successful pregnancy.

Treatment of Renal Manifestations

Many patients with SLE have mild to severe renal involvement. Diagnosis by renal biopsy is important to establish the type of kidney involvement. Lupus nephritis is considered one of the more severe manifestations of the disease, and treatment is aimed at preventing renal failure. Treatment should be coordinated with a rheumatologist or nephrologist.

Class I disease requires no specific therapy. The class IIb pattern with more than 1 g of proteinuria can be treated with moderate-dose prednisone (20 mg/day for 6 weeks to 3 months), followed by tapering. Class III and IV patterns of disease have the same prognosis and are treated similarly with high-dose prednisone (1 mg/kg/day) for at least 6 weeks before tapering based on clinical response by 10 mg a week to a maintenance of 10 to 15 mg/day. In addition to prednisone, cytotoxic therapy is initiated with cyclophosphamide[1] 0.5 to 1 g/m^2 of body surface area monthly for 6 months and tapered to every 3 months based on clinical response for a total of 2 to 3 years. Cyclophosphamide has serious toxicities, including hemorrhagic cystitis, bone marrow suppression, infertility, teratogenicity, and

---

[1]Not FDA approved for this indication.
[2]Not available in the United States.

---

[1]Not FDA approved for this indication.

increased risk of malignancy. 2-Mercaptoethane sulfonate sodium (Mesna)[1] can be given with each infusion to minimize bladder toxicity. Class V disease can be treated with prednisone alone, similar to class IIb disease, unless there are coexisting features of class III or IV disease, for which treatments outlined previously should be implemented.

An acceptable alternative to cyclophosphamide for class III and IV disease is mycophenolate mofetil[1] 2 to 3 g/day in divided doses combined with corticosteroids (dosing outlined earlier). This appears to be an effective therapy with fewer side effects than traditional therapy.

Treatment of Nervous System Manifestations

Neuropsychiatric involvement is common in patients with lupus. Symptoms can range from mild to severe and include headache, aseptic meningitis, neuropathy, myelopathy, cognitive dysfunction,

---

[1]Not FDA approved for this indication.

CURRENT DIAGNOSIS

Lupus Erythematosus

- The erythematous-violaceous and variably pruritic, tender, or scaly eruption is photosensitive.
- Mild to moderate systemic involvement may include arthritis and pleurisy.
- Severe systemic involvement may include nephritis, cerebritis, vasculitis, and severe cytopenias.
- Associated findings include antiphospholipid antibodies associated with thromboembolism or stroke, Raynaud's phenomenon, and sicca symptoms.

Dermatomyositis and Polymyositis

- Photosensitive, violaceous-erythematous, poikilodermatous, and variably scaly patches occur around eyes, on extensor extremities (especially over joints), upper back, scalp, and dystrophic nail folds with prominent telangiectasias.
- Patients may have or develop myositis or pulmonary involvement.
- Age-appropriate cancer screening is required for adults.

Scleroderma

- Patients have firm, variably pruritic, and indurated plaques.
- Localized scleroderma (i.e., morphea or asymmetric sclerotic plaques) may be seen.
- Limited systemic sclerosis is characterized by symmetric sclerosis of distal extremities, and patients may have systemic disease.
- Diffuse systemic sclerosis is characterized by symmetric sclerosis of the trunk and proximal extremities, and patients may have systemic disease.
- Sclerodactyly (i.e., thickening of skin of digits) may occur in patients with systemic sclerosis.
- Pulmonary, cardiac, and gastrointestinal screening should be done for patients with systemic sclerosis.
- Patients with systemic sclerosis should be evaluated and monitored for renal crisis.
- Raynaud's phenomenon may develop in patients with systemic sclerosis.

---

seizures, cerebritis, and stroke. A thorough evaluation is necessary to define the cause of nervous system dysfunction and differentiate it from a medication side effect. For seizures, antiepileptic therapy is used, preferably in coordination with a neurologist. Lupus cerebritis and transverse myelitis are two of the more serious manifestations that need to be treated emergently with aggressive immunosuppression in coordination with a rheumatologist or neurologist. Treatment includes high-dose corticosteroids and cyclophosphamide,[1] similar to treatment for lupus nephritis.

Dermatomyositis and Polymyositis

CLINICAL FEATURES

Dermatomyositis may affect skin and muscle. Cutaneous dermatomyositis manifests with violaceous erythema of characteristic areas, including the periorbital skin (i.e., heliotrope rash), upper back (i.e., shawl sign), dorsal hands (i.e., Gottron's papules), scalp, lateral thighs (i.e., holster sign), and periungual skin, where dilated capillary loops and erythema are observed. Patients may report muscle weakness. As in lupus, a punch biopsy of an actively inflamed cutaneous lesion shows characteristic features.

Evaluation of patients with cutaneous dermatomyositis is not complete without assessment for systemic involvement. Serum aldolase is the most specific marker for myositis, and it can be used as a measure of response to treatment. Creatinine kinase and alanine aminotransferase levels may be elevated but are not specific indicators. An electromyogram shows dampening of signals, and a muscle biopsy shows a characteristic pattern of myositis. Inflammatory lung disease, diagnosed by the characteristic pattern on chest computed tomography, bronchoalveolar lavage, or biopsy, may be life limiting and therefore should be treated aggressively, similar to lung disease in scleroderma. Adult patients should have age-appropriate cancer screening because dermatomyositis is a paraneoplastic phenomenon in 10% to 50%.

Some patients present with characteristic cutaneous dermatomyositis but no systemic involvement (i.e., dermatomyositis sine myositis). The risk of concurrent or subsequent cancer development is thought to be increased. These patients require monitoring for systemic involvement that may develop over time.

TREATMENT

Patients with dermatomyositis need photoprotection similar to patients with lupus. Periodic evaluation by clinical examination and review of systems allows for early intervention for developing visceral or muscle involvement.

Cutaneous dermatomyositis is treated the same as lupus (see earlier). Dermatomyositis with systemic involvement is initially treated with immunosuppression using prednisone at doses of 1 mg/kg/day. Steroid-sparing agents are incorporated early in the disease and include antimalarials, methotrexate,[1] azathioprine,[1] and mycophenolate mofetil)[1] at doses that are used in treating lupus.

Scleroderma

CLINICAL FEATURES

Scleroderma is a sclerosing condition of skin or viscera, or both. The cause is unknown, but transforming growth factor-β plays a role. Type I and III collagens are excessively produced, as are other substances, including glycosaminoglycans, tenascin, and fibronectin.

Cutaneous scleroderma without Raynaud's phenomenon or clinically relevant systemic involvement is also known as *morphea*. Morphea has different distribution patterns, including guttate, linear,

---

[1]Not FDA approved for this indication.

CURRENT THERAPY

Lupus Erythematosus

- Patients should be counseled on photoprotection measures.
- Localized cutaneous disease is treated with medium- to high-potency topical corticosteroids, and intralesional triamcinolone acetonide 10 mg/mL (Kenalog-10) is added if needed.
- Mild to moderate systemic involvement is treated with low- to medium-potency prednisone 5 to 20 mg/day and with antimalarials.
- Severe disease is treated with prednisone 1 mg/kg/day with a taper based on clinical response. Steroid-sparing agents include azathioprine (Imuran),[1] mycophenolate mofetil (CellCept),[1] methotrexate (Rheumatrex),[1] and cyclophosphamide (Cytoxan).[1]
- Thromboembolism or stroke is treated by anticoagulation with warfarin (Coumadin), aspirin, or heparin.
- Sicca syndrome is treated with frequent water intake, saliva replacement, artificial tears, routine dental care, and pilocarpine (Salagen).

Dermatomyositis and Polymyositis

- Patients should be counseled on photoprotection measures.
- Medium-potency topical corticosteroids and calcineurin inhibitors are used for cutaneous disease.
- Prednisone 1 mg/kg/day is first-line therapy for muscle or pulmonary disease.
- Methotrexate[1] 10 to 25 mg/week is a steroid-sparing agent used for muscle involvement.
- Hydroxychloroquine (Plaquenil)[1] 200 mg/day is used for persistent skin involvement.

Scleroderma

- For localized scleroderma, UVA[1] 20 to 60 J/cm² or psoralen plus UVA (PUVA) is used to resolve established lesions; high-potency corticosteroids and calcipotriene (Dovonex)[1] may help to reduce pruritus and inflammation in new lesions; and systemic prednisone[1] or methotrexate[1] may be used for rapidly progressive new lesions.
- Treatment of systemic sclerosis is primarily aimed at limiting complications.
- Physical therapy is used for contractures.
- Systemic sclerosis is treated with cyclophosphamide (Cytoxan),[1] mycophenolate mofetil (CellCept),[1] methotrexate[1] 10 to 25 mg/week, and photopheresis.
- Renal crisis is treated with captopril (Capoten)[1] 6.25 mg three to six times/day and titrated to effect.
- Raynaud's is treated with warming techniques, calcium channel blockers, antiadrenergic agents, antiplatelet drugs, and topical vasodilators.

---

[1]Not FDA approved for this indication.
[2]Not available in the United States.

---

segmental, or diffuse distribution, but it is always characterized by indurated plaques that are inflammatory initially, have an advancing inflammatory ("lilac") border as they progress, and then become hyperpigmented. The cutaneous lesions may restrict movement of joints and can cause restricted growth of underlying structures, particularly when they develop in childhood.

Systemic sclerosis may affect the respiratory, renal, cardiovascular, genitourinary, and gastrointestinal systems and vascular structures. Raynaud's phenomenon may be the first presenting symptom of systemic sclerosis, and it can be severe, leading to digital ulcerations and autoamputation. The American College of Rheumatology has defined criteria for the diagnosis.

Tests for antinuclear antibodies are positive in approximately 95% of patients, who typically present with a homogeneous or speckled pattern. A nucleolar pattern is more specific for systemic sclerosis. Anticentromere antibodies are present in 60% to 90% of patients with limited disease but are rare in diffuse disease. Topoisomerase I (Scl-70) antibodies are positive in 30% of patients with diffuse disease and are associated with pulmonary fibrosis. Anti-PM-Scl antibodies are present in overlap syndromes and are associated with myositis and renal involvement.

TREATMENT

Treatment of Limited Scleroderma

For limited scleroderma, treatment with topical medium-potency corticosteroids such as triamcinolone 0.1% ointment (Kenalog) plus calcipotriene (Dovonex)[1] 0.005% cream or intralesional triamcinalone[1] 20 mg/mL may slow progression of active lesions or improve the pruritus and cutaneous stiffness that typify cutaneous scleroderma. For rapidly evolving disease, prednisone[1] 1 mg/kg/day and methotrexate[1] 15 to 20 mg/week may help slow progression of disease. UVA[1] given over 36 treatments at doses of 30 to 60 mJ/cm² or PUVA (oral methoxsalen [8-MOP] 10 mg taken 2 hours before treatment with UVA light) can soften the existing plaques of morphea.

Treatment of Systemic Sclerosis: Raynaud's Phenomenon

First-line treatment for Raynaud's phenomenon is preventive, with cold avoidance and the use of warming techniques. If pharmacotherapy is required, extended-release calcium channel blockers such as nifedipine (Procardia XL)[1] starting at 30 mg/day or amlodipine (Norvasc)[1] starting at 5 mg/day may be useful. If this is not helpful, the α-blocker prazosin (Minipress)[1] 1 mg three times daily or the angiotensin receptor blocker losartan (Cozaar)[1] 50 mg daily may be helpful. Antiplatelet therapy with low-dose aspirin[1] (81 mg/day) or dipyridamole (Persantine)[1] 50 to 100 mg three or four times daily may be useful. Topical vasodilators such as nitroglycerin ointment (Nitro-Bid)[1] applied to the base of the affected finger three times daily can be helpful in refractory disease. Digit-threatening ischemia may be treated with an intravenous prostaglandin such as alprostadil (Prostin VR)[1] or iloprost (Ilomedine),[5] which require peripheral or central access. Patients with severe recurrent digital ischemia may ultimately benefit from surgical sympathectomy.

Treatment of Gastrointestinal Manifestations

The most common gastrointestinal manifestation is esophageal reflux caused by esophageal dysmotility. Proton pump inhibitors such as omeprazole (Prilosec)[1] 20 mg twice daily should be used and may prevent the development of esophageal strictures. Prokinetic drugs such as metoclopramide (Reglan)[1] 10 mg four times daily can be helpful. Erythromycin[1] 500 mg three or four times daily can help esophageal and gastric hypomotility. Small bowel hypomotility can lead to bacterial overgrowth, resulting in malabsorption and diarrhea. Rotating antibiotics that include metronidazole (Flagyl),[1] ciprofloxacin (Cipro),[1] and amoxicillin/clavulanate (Augmentin)[1] can be used.

Treatment of Pulmonary Manifestations

Inflammatory lung disease occurs commonly in patients with scleroderma and can be life limiting. Cyclophosphamide[1] at doses of up to 2 mg/kg/day for up to 2 years may slow progression of pulmonary disease. Pulmonary hypertension occurs more commonly in limited systemic sclerosis than in diffuse disease. Symptomatic patients may

---

[1]Not FDA approved for this indication.
[5]Investigational drug in the United States.

receive treatment with prostacyclin analogues, which require continuous infusions. The endothelin receptor antagonist bosentan (Tracleer)[1] can be given orally starting at 62.5 mg twice daily. Liver tests should be monitored frequently. At this point, care is typically coordinated with a cardiologist to monitor disease progression and treatment response. Anticoagulation for pulmonary hypertension may improve survival because of the frequent occurrence of pulmonary arterial thrombosis.

Treatment of Renal Manifestations

Angiotensin-converting enzyme (ACE) inhibitors (e.g., captopril [Capoten[1]] beginning at 6.25 mg three to six times daily and titrated for blood pressure control) have dramatically reduced the incidence of renal failure and death due to renal crisis. Avoidance of prednisone at doses greater than 15 mg/day is also important in reducing the risk of renal crisis.

---

[1]Not FDA approved for this indication.

REFERENCES

Atzeni F, Bendtzen K, Bobbio-Pallavicini F, et al. Infections and treatment of patients with rheumatic diseases. Clin Exp Rheumatol 2008;26(Suppl. 48):S67–73.

Dziadzio M, Denton CP, Smith R. Losartan therapy for Raynaud's phenomenon and scleroderma. Arthritis Rheum 1999;42(12):2646–55.

Ginzler EM, Dooley MA, Aranow C, et al. Mycophenolate mofetil or intravenous cyclophosphamide for lupus nephritis. N Engl J Med 2005;353 (21):2219–28.

Iorizzo LJ, Jorizzo JL. The treatment and prognosis of dermatomyositis: An updated review. J Am Acad Dermatol 2008;59:99–112.

Matucci-Cerinic M, Steen VD, Furst DE, et al. Clinical trials in systemic sclerosis: Lessons learned and outcomes. Arthritis Res Ther 2007;9(Suppl. 2):S7.

Nihtyanova SI, Denton CP. Current approaches to the management of early active diffuse scleroderma skin disease. Rheum Dis Clin North Am 2008;34:161–79.

Pisoni CN, Sanchez FJ, Karim Y, et al. Mycophenolate mofetil in systemic lupus erythematosus: Efficacy and tolerability in 86 patients. J Rheumatol 2005;32:1047–52.

Steen VD. The many faces of scleroderma. Rheum Dis Clin North Am 2008;34:1–15.

Subcommittee for Scleroderma Criteria of the American Rheumatism Association Diagnostic and Therapeutic Criteria Committee. Preliminary criteria for the classification of systemic sclerosis (scleroderma). Arthritis Rheum 1980;23:581–90.

Tan EM, Cohen AS, Fries JF, et al. The 1982 revised criteria for the classification of lupus erythematosus. Arthritis Rheum 1982;25:1271–2.

Wallace DD. Lupus Erythematosus. 7th ed. Philadelphia: Lippincott Williams & Wilkins; 2006.

Cutaneous Vasculitis

Method of
Molly Hinshaw, MD, and Susan Lawrence-Hylland, MD

Vasculitis is an inflammatory-mediated destruction of blood vessels. The systemic vasculitides have historically been differentiated by their involvement of small, medium, or large blood vessels. Names used to describe isolated cutaneous vasculitis have included hypersensitivity vasculitis and leukocytoclastic vasculitis (LCV). In 1990, the American College of Rheumatology proposed five criteria for the classification of hypersensitivity vasculitis: age older than 16 years, possible drug trigger, palpable purpura, maculopapular rash, and skin biopsy showing neutrophils around vessel. At least three out of five criteria yield a sensitivity of 71% and specificity of 84%. In 1994, a new nomenclature proposed at the Chapel Hill International Concensus Conference in North Carolina further classified vasculitis (Box 1).

BOX 1 Chapel Hill Consensus 1994 Classification of Vasculitis

Large-Vessel Vasculitis
Giant cell arteritis
Takayasu's arteritis

Medium-Vessel Vasculitis
Classic polyarteritis nodosa
Kawasaki's disease

Small-Vessel Vasculitis
Churg-Strauss syndrome
Cutaneous leukocytoclastic vasculitis
Essential cryoglobulinemia
Henoch-Schönlein purpura
Microscopic polyangiitis (polyarteritis)
Wegener's granulomatosis

The term "hypersensitivity vasculitis" was not used, because most vasculitides that would have previously been in this category fall into either microscopic polyangiitis or cutaneous LCV. LCV is vasculitis restricted to the skin without involvement of vessels in other organs. Cutaneous vasculitis may be a clue to systemic vasculitis and guides the clinician to a comprehensive evaluation (Table 1).

Vasculitis can affect almost any organ, and once affected, end organs can become dysfunctional. Such dysfunction may be as innocuous as cutaneous, tender, transient papules or as devastating as a stroke. A thorough evaluation of the patient with a complete review of systems, physical examination, laboratory evaluation, and clinical follow-up allows a distinction to be made between the different forms of vasculitis.

Leukocytoclastic Vasculitis

EPIDEMIOLOGY

LCV is common. The incidence and prevalence are unknown. Mean age of onset ranges from 34 to 49 years of age. The female-to-male ratio ranges from approximately 2:1 to 3:1.

RISK FACTORS

LCV is often secondary to a known trigger including infection, drug ingestion, or malignancy. LCV can also be a presenting feature of autoimmune disease.

PATHOPHYSIOLOGY

LCV is best characterized as immune complex–mediated inflammatory destruction of the postcapillary venules of any organ. The exact mechanisms of vascular destruction is unknown.

CLINICAL MANIFESTATIONS

LCV typically manifests as nonblanchable macules that evolve to papules or, less commonly, pustules and ulcers (Fig. 1). Clues to the diagnosis include a monomorphous, ruddy-brown appearance owing to leakage of hemosiderin pigment from vessels. Lesions measure a few millimeters to a few centimeters in diameter. LCV is often localized to the lower extremities but may be diffuse. Pruritus, pain, or burning of the skin lesions are indicators that the patient might have a vasculitis extending beyond LCV.

DIAGNOSIS

To confirm a clinical impression of LCV, perform a punch biopsy in the center of a nonulcerated cutaneous lesion that is less than 24 to 48 hours old and submit the sample in 10% formalin (standard medium). It is important to biopsy an intact, nonulcerated active lesion (Fig. 2) because ulcers can show histologic features simulating vasculitis regardless of whether the patient has true vasculitis or not.

TABLE 1 Diseases with Cutaneous Vasculitis as a Component of Their Presentation

Disease	Skin Lesions	Clues and Confirmation
Urticarial vasculitis	Individual lesions look like urticaria but last >24 h; typical urticaria last a few hours, always <24 h Pruritus, burning of skin lesions	May be associated with connective tissue disease, medications, low complement, viral infections (e.g., hep B, hep C, EBV) Skin biopsy
Henoch-Schönlein purpura	Wheals progress to petechia, ecchymoses and palpable purpura Lesions are in gravity-dependent or pressure-dependent areas such as legs or the buttocks in toddlers	Arthralgia or arthritis, hematuria, abdominal pain, melena Skin biopsy and DIF for IgA
Essential mixed cryoglobulinemia	Palpable purpura	Peripheral neuropathy, GN Hep C positive Serum cryoglobulins
Wegener's granulomatosis	Palpable purpura, hemorrhagic lesions, petechiae, skin ulcers	c-ANCA >80% Pulmonary hemorrhage, GN Biopsy affected organ
Churg-Strauss syndrome	Maculopapular rash, palpable purpura, hemorrhagic lesions, subcutaneous nodules, livedo reticularis or Raynaud's disease	ANCA (50%) Asthma, allergic rhinitis Eosinophilia >1.5 × 10⁹/L Pulmonary infiltrates, pulmonary neuropathy Biopsy affected organ
Microscopic polyangiitis	Palpable purpura, hemorrhagic lesions, petechiae, skin ulcers, splinter hemorrhages	p-ANCA >60% Pulmonary hemorrhage, GN Biopsy affected organ
Polyarteritis nodosa	Livedo reticularis, tender nodules, skin ulcers, bullae or vesicles	Hypertension, elevated creatinine, abdominal pain, constitutional symptoms (fever) Abnormal angiogram Biopsy affected organ

c-ANCA = classic antineutrophil cytoplasmic antibody; DIF = direct immunofluorescence; EBV = Epstein-Barr virus; GN = glomerulonephritis; hep = hepatitis; Ig = immunoglobulin; p-ANCA = protoplasmic-stainng antineutrophil cytoplasmic antibody.

FIGURE 1. Leukocytoclastic vasculitis: palpable, purpuric, non-blanching, erythematous to ruddy-brown thin papules. Additional secondary changes include small pustules (pustular vasculitis) or shallow, small ulcerations.

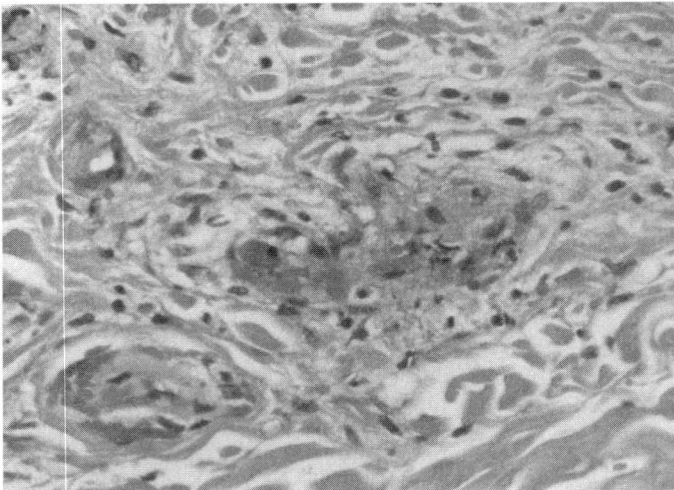

FIGURE 2. Biopsy of intact clinical lesion of leukocytoclastic vasculitis. Histology shows destruction of postcapillary venules with fibrin deposition, degenerate inflammatory cells, and extravasated erythrocytes.

Pathology reveals a mononuclear or polymorphonuclear inflammation of the small blood vessels (called LCV), most prominent in the postcapillary venules. The appearance may be necrotizing or non-necrotizing.

DIFFERENTIAL DIAGNOSIS

LCV manifests as erythematous papules or occasionally as papulopustules that can simulate a variety of entities (see Table 1). The review of systems and physical examination should be directed to

CURRENT DIAGNOSIS

- Cutaneous vasculitis can be limited to skin (leukocytoclastic vasculitis) or associated with systemic disease.
- Perform punch biopsy of intact, nonulcerated skin lesion.
- "Vasculitis" on skin biopsy describes vessel appearance and is not a clinical diagnosis.
- Thorough review of systems and physical examination are necessary to evaluate for systemic vasculitis.

evaluate for diseases that have cutaneous vasculitis as a component of their presentation (see Table 1). All patients with LCV should have a urinalysis to evaluate for hematuria as a sign of kidney involvement, with subsequent evaluation and management if identified.

TREATMENT

The primary goal in the management of LCV is to identify and treat instigating factors, including infection and medications. Supportive treatment includes resting, elevating legs, and wearing support hose. When review of systems, physical examination, and urinalysis do not reveal associated systemic diseases, treatment of LCV is generally not necessary. Lesions typically remit without treatment. In rare patients with symptomatic, extensively pustular, or progressive lesions, a short course of prednisone[1] dosed at 1 mg/kg/day initially and tapered over 3 to 6 weeks may be used, although no controlled trials have been performed using oral corticosteroids for isolated LCV. Rapid steroid taper can lead to rebound. Systematic evaluation of the use of other medications, such as colchicine[1] or dapsone,[1] to treat isolated LCV has not been performed.

MONITORING

Patients with LCV are at risk for recurrent or chronic vasculitis. In addition, apparent LCV can occur as a systemic disease that is not recognizable at the first episode. Patients with persistent or recurrent LCV require follow-up to ensure disease clearance, to monitor for medication side effects, and to evaluate for evolving disorders known to be associated with cutaneous vasculitis (see Table 1).

COMPLICATIONS

Isolated LCV generally resolves without sequelae. However, pustular or ulcerative LCV may be complicated by local sequelae such as cutaneous ulcerations and scars.

Cutaneous Vasculitis Associated with Systemic Vasculitis

Cutaneous vasculitis may be a component of the presentation of multiple diseases (see Table 1). When a clinician reads a pathology report from a biopsy of a skin lesion that states "vasculitis," it is important to realize that this term is a descriptor of the histopathology. It is the clinician's challenge to determine whether "vasculitis" is as potentially innocuous as LCV or part of a more severe systemic disease. Symptoms that are clues to a systemic process can include fever, arthralgias, myalgias, anorexia, abdominal pain, pulmonary abnormalities, or neurologic symptoms.

Skin biopsy may aid in the diagnosis of a systemic vasculitis (Henoch-Schönlein purpura), but biopsy of an affected end organ may be necessary to confirm a diagnosis. Pathology focuses on the confirmation of vasculitis in a small, medium, or large vessel.

Aside from Henoch-Schönlein purpura, treatment of systemic vasculitis is typically much more aggressive than treatment of LCV and

[1]Not FDA approved for this indication.

CURRENT THERAPY

Leukocytoclastic Vasculitis

- First identify instigating factors: infection, medications.
- Care is symptomatic. Lesions typically remit without treatment.
- If needed, short course of prednisone may be given and tapered over 3 to 6 weeks.

All Forms of Vasculitis

- Treat underlying systemic vasculitis.

should be pursued in conjunction with involvement of a rheumatologist, nephrologist, or pulmonologist. Systemic disease leads to severe complications including renal failure, pulmonary damage, permanent vascular disease, or neurologic insult depending on the viscera affected.

REFERENCES

Gayraud M, Guillevin L, le Toumelin P, et al. Long-term followup of polyarteritis nodosa, microscopic polyangiitis, and Churg-Strauss syndrome: Analysis of four prospective trials including 278 patients. Arthritis Rheum 2001;44:666–75.

Hannon CW, Swerlick RA. Vasculitis. In: Bolognia J, Jorizzo J, Rapini R, editors. Dermatology, vol. 1. St Louis: Mosby; 2003. pp. 381–402.

Hoffman GS, Kerr GS, Leavitt RY, et al. Wegener granulomatosis: An analysis of 158 patients. Ann Intern Med 1992;116:488–98.

Jennette JC, Thomas DB, Falk RJ. Microscopic polyangiitis (microscopic polyarteritis). Semin Diagn Pathol 2001;18:3–13.

Jennette JC, Falk RF, Andrassy K, et al. Nomenclature of systemic vasculitides. Proposal of an international consensus conference. Arthritis Rheum 1994;37(2):187–92.

Diseases of the Nails

Method of
Nathaniel Jellinek, MD, and Ralph C. Daniel, MD

Overview

The nail plate in humans has many functions. It facilitates scratching; it is used as a tool, a weapon, and a form of adornment (to the cost of approximately $6 billion per year in the United States); and most importantly it supports the underlying distal phalanx and soft tissue to maximize fine touch and manual dexterity.

The nail unit consists of the nail plate, an underlying nail bed, a germinative nail matrix, proximal and lateral nail folds, a cuticle and distal hyponychium (Fig. 1). The matrix exists under the proximal nail fold, beginning just distal to the insertion of the dorsal extensor tendon, and extends distally under the nail plate beyond the cuticle as the crescent-shaped lunula. The lunula is usually most apparent on the thumbnail, less so on each consecutive finger.

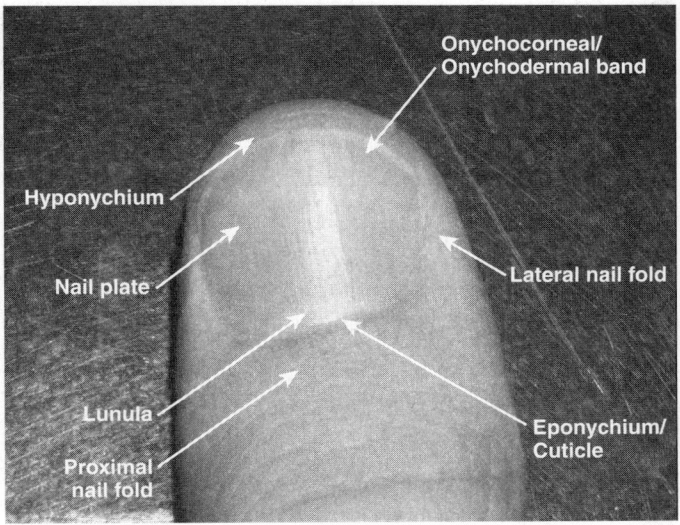

FIGURE 1. Surface anatomy of the nail.

The nail bed is contiguous with the matrix, tightly adherent to the overlying plate, to which it is connected in a tongue-and-groove pattern, ending distally at the onychocorneal (or onychodermal) band, the distal-most attachment point between the bed and plate. The onychocorneal band region provides the ventral barrier of the nail unit. When it is breached, onycholysis results.

Dorsally and laterally, the nail folds provide an anatomic barrier to the nail unit. When they are breached, moisture, yeast, bacteria, and contact irritants and allergens penetrate the normal barrier and cause paronychia, acute and chronic.

An understanding of normal nail anatomy facilitates comprehension of the pathology discussed here.

Lichen Planus

CLINICAL FEATURES AND DIAGNOSIS

Lichen planus is an inflammatory disorder that can involve the skin, hair, nails, and mucous membranes. Nail disease can accompany skin or mucosal disease or can manifest as isolated nail disease. It is characterized histologically by lichenoid inflammation and can involve any or all of the nail subunits. Onychorrhexis, longitudinal striations in the nail plate, and nail plate thinning or fragility, result from nail matrix involvement. Onycholysis (nail lifting) and nail thickening are caused by hyponychium and nail bed involvement. Nail pain can herald the onset of bullous lichen planus of the nail. This represents an urgent problem, because permanent scarring of the nail bed and matrix can result, manifesting clinically as dorsal pterygium. It is crucial to check all patients with suspected nail lichen planus with a complete skin and oral mucosal examination for lesions.

TREATMENT

Overt, repetitive, and incidental trauma to the nail apparatus worsens the nail disease and makes it more resistant to treatment (the Koebner phenomenon). The Koebner and Koebner-like phenomena are important in the diathesis of lichen planus. Therefore, trauma, contact irritants, and moisture must be minimized or avoided. The nails should be kept short. Intralesional triamcinolone 2.5 to 5 mg/mL monthly for several months and occasionally systemic corticosteroids may be required in more severe cases or with scarring.

Onychomycosis

CLINICAL FEATURES AND DIAGNOSIS

Approximately one half of all doctor visits relating to nail complaints are for onychomycosis. It is not only the most common nail diagnosis, however; it is also the most common misdiagnosis, and even experienced nail clinicians might not make an accurate diagnosis up to 50% of the time. It is therefore crucial to confirm the diagnosis by potassium hydroxide, fungal culture, or clipping for periodic acid–Schiff analysis before initiating any therapy, with its inherent risks and costs.

In the United States, 80% to 90% cases of onychomycosis are caused by dermatophyte fungi, most commonly *Trichophyton rubrum* or *Trichophyton mentagrophytes*. The tendency to acquire these infections appears to be inherited in an autosomal dominant fashion with incomplete or variable penetrance. The infection usually begins with tinea pedis; the nail barrier between plate and hyponychium or nail fold is compromised, often through repetitive trauma, and fungus enters the nail apparatus.

CURRENT DIAGNOSIS

Brittle Nails

- Brittle nails are present in approximately 20% of the North American population.
- They are more common in women, those who use nail cosmetics, and persons >50 years old.
- Diagnose with subjective complaint of brittle nails with observation of onychorrhexis (longitudinal nail plate ridging) and onychoschizia (lamellar splitting of nail plate).

Onychomycosis

- Make an objective diagnosis with KOH, culture or clipping for periodic acid–Schiff.
- Onychomycosis is much more common on the toenails than the fingernails.
- The most common organisms are *Trichophyton rubrum* or *Trichophyton mentagrophytes*.
- *Candida* only rarely causes onychomycosis. It is primarily a colonizer in the setting of barrier breakdown of the nail apparatus.
- Nondermatophyte molds (such as *Aspergillus, Fusarium, Penicillium* spp) are unusual causes of onychomycosis in the United States. Repeat tests showing the same organisms and ruling out other causes are mandated before initiating treatment.

Primary Onycholysis and Chronic Paronychia

- Primary onycholysis and chronic paronychia are diagnoses of exclusion. Onychomycosis, psoriasis, lichen planus, and drug reactions all must be ruled out before diagnosis.
- Both are more common on the fingernails than the toenails, in women, in adults, in those who use nail cosmetics, or and those who have recurrent exposure to moisture or chemicals.
- Both primary onycholysis and chronic paronychia represent breakdown in the normal barrier of the nail apparatus. Onycholysis results from breakdown of the onychocorneal band or nail bed–nail plate connection. Chronic paronychia results from breakdown of the cuticle and nail folds.
- In both scenarios, moisture, contact irritants, contact allergens, colonizing yeast, and bacteria invade the exposed nail apparatus and contribute to a cycle of inflammation.

Ingrown Nails

- Common risk factors include incorrect nail cutting, wide feet, narrow-toed shoes, lateral plate malalignment, and lateral nail fold hypertrophy.
- Neonates and infants demonstrate distal nail ingrowing, which is separate in pathogenesis and treatment from the disease in adolescents and adults.
- Ingrown nails can be graded on a scale from I to III, with I being erythema and swelling with drainage from the nail fold and III being associated with exuberant overgrowth of granulation tissue over and around the ingrown nail plate.

CURRENT THERAPY

Brittle Nails

- Treatment is frustrating and represents the limitations in our understanding of disease pathogenesis.
- Oral biotin, 2–3 mg (2000–3000 μg) (Appearex) daily, dosed for 4–6 months and then discontinued, is a reasonable trial. Patients will notice an effect during this period if it has helped, then may continue to treat if it is helpful.
- Topical moisturizers (petrolatum) or humectant agents (12% ammonium lactate, 20% urea) might help those with hard brittle nails.

Onychomycosis

- Topical treatment is disappointing, except in cases of superficial white onychomycosis.
- Oral treatment should be reserved for patients with symptomatic disease or who are at risk for complications (diabetics, immunosuppressed, at risk of secondary bacterial cellulitis).
- Oral treatment is more successful than topical treatment. Terbinafine (Lamisil) 250 mg PO qd × 90 days in adults is the first-line treatment. Itraconazole (Sporanox), dosed daily or pulsed 1 week per month, is the next most successful agent.
- Patients are at high risk for recurrence. Post-treatment prevention of tinea pedis is important to prevent reinfection.

Primary Onycholysis and Chronic Paronychia

- It is important not to misdiagnose the presence of yeast (especially *Candida*) as a primary infection or pathogen. It almost always represents a colonizer. Treatment of the yeast is therefore secondary.
- Avoidance is the mainstay of treatment. Avoid all wet work and exposure to acids, bases, and chemicals by wearing cotton gloves under heavy-duty vinyl gloves. Avoid all nail cosmetics and nail manipulation except for regular plate trimming. No nail salon. Keep the plate trimmed to its proximal-most attachment point. Avoid obvious triggers and traumas to the nail apparatus.
- It can take up to 6 months for the nail apparatus to normalize.

Ingrown Nails

- Infantile disease: Warm soaks followed by massage of the nail and distal phalangeal tuft.
- Adolescent and adult disease: Correct nail plate cutting and shoes. For mild disease, twice daily cold soaks, topical steroids, 20% to 40% topical urea cream (Keralac, Carmol), and cotton wisps or dental floss under the aggravating part of the lateral nail plate will decrease inflammation, improve symptoms, and normalize the nail plate without surgery.
- For more advanced cases, twice-daily warm soaks, oral antibiotics (with signs of infection), followed by lateral plate avulsion and lateral matricectomy (either chemical or surgical).

There are four main types of onychomycosis: distal and lateral subungual onychomycosis (DLSO, most common), occasionally leading to total dystrophic onychomycosis (TDO), superficial white onychomycosis (SWO), and proximal subungual onychomycosis (PSO). SWO is the most straightforward to diagnose; scraping the surface yields abundant fungi for examination. DLSO and TDO are best diagnosed by acquiring the proximal-most area of involved nail plate and subungual debris; this occasionally involves aggressive paring by the practitioner to remove the distal nail plate and debris, with lower diagnostic yield. PSO may be a marker for systemic immunosuppression and is therefore important to diagnose. A nail plate punch biopsy is the most direct and accurate way to make this diagnosis of the latter.

Candida only rarely causes onychomycosis. This fact is widely misunderstood, probably because *Candida* is commonly found as a colonizing organism in conditions such as primary onycholysis and chronic paronychia. The unusual situation of primary *Candida* onychomycosis is limited to those with inherited chronic mucocutaneous candidiasis or severe immunosuppression. The presence of this organism in the setting of onychomycosis should arouse doubt rather than confirm the diagnosis. In most cases, it is a colonizer rather than a pathogen.

The presence of an underlying disease with nail manifestations (such as psoriasis or lichen planus) does not rule out the concomitant presence of onychomycosis and can cause barrier breakdown of the nail apparatus, facilitating secondary fungal infection.

TREATMENT

Oral treatment should be reserved for patients who have symptomatic disease or who are at risk for complications, such as diabetics and immunocompromised patients, who are at risk for secondary bacterial cellulitis.

Confirm the diagnosis. The presence of *Candida* or nondermatophyte mold is unusual in the United States. Tests should be repeated and other diagnoses should be entertained before diagnosing onychomycosis and initiating treatment. If a dermatophyte is found, systemic terbinafine (Lamisil) offers the best systemic choice. Systemic itraconazole (Sporanox) is the next most effective agent and can be dosed in a pulsed fashion (off label) or daily like terbinafine. Topical ciclopirox (Loprox) clears the nails in less than 10% of cases; other topical agents are equally ineffective.

Because a person is often genetically predisposed to acquire onychomycosis, once the disorder is cleared by a systemic agent, then topical agents must be used indefinitely, with the goal being to avoid subsequent cases of tinea pedis. Powders and lotions are available over the counter and may be used on a regular basis.

Brittle Nails

CLINICAL FEATURES AND DIAGNOSIS

A simplistic view, but perhaps representing the best of our understanding about brittle nails, is that hard brittle nails are caused and worsened by too little moisture, and that soft brittle nails are associated with too much moisture. Both may be worsened by irritants. Older persons tend to have dry brittle nails, analogous to skin in the aging population. Although up to 20% of North Americans have brittle nails, our understanding of the pathogenesis is limited.

Brittle nails are diagnosed when subjective and objective criteria are met. Patients must complain of nail fragility and easy breaking with clinical signs of onychorrhexis (longitudinal ridging), onychoschizia (lamellar splitting), and occasionally dull, lusterless plate appearance.

TREATMENT

Biotin (vitamin H or B7) 2 to 3 mg (often dosed as 2000–3000 μg)][3,7] taken once daily improves brittleness in some cases. It is helpful to have the patient take this water-soluble vitamin for 4 to 6 months,

---

[3]Exceeds dosage recommended by the manufacturer.
[7]Available as a dietary supplement.

then discontinue it for a several months to evaluate for improvement, worsening, or no change. This initial trial therapy can prevent continued cost to the patient if he or she notices no improvement and then worsening when taking and discontinuing the vitamin, respectively. Irritant avoidance is also helpful. Application of petrolatum at bedtime under light white cotton gloves (apply ointment after soaking the nail in water for 5 minutes) increases the moisture content of the nail plate. Topical humectant agents include over-the-counter 12% ammonium lactate cream and 10% to 20% urea preparations.

Ingrown Nails

CLINICAL FEATURES AND DIAGNOSIS

Ingrown nails represent a foreign body reaction of the nail plate in the lateral nail fold. It is more common on toenails, particularly the great toenails, than fingernails. Predisposing factors include wide feet, ill-fitting or narrow-toed or high heeled shoes, lateral plate malalignment, hypertrophic lateral nail folds, cutting the nails incorrectly in a half-circle instead of straight across, and possibly hyperhidrosis. Secondary infection can occur after the plate pierces the nail fold skin.

In adolescents and adults, the nail fold embedding and spicule formation tends to be lateral, whereas in neonates and young children the embedding tends to be distal. The former group is predisposed to multiple episodes of ingrowing; procedural treatment is recommended and often required. The latter group often responds to conservative treatment; surgery is only occasionally required.

TREATMENT

Correct nail cutting and appropriate shoes are the main treatment. For mild disease, use of twice-daily cold soaks, topical steroids, 20% to 40% topical urea cream, and cotton wisps or dental floss under the aggravating part of the lateral nail plate can decrease inflammation, improve symptoms, and normalize the nail plate without requiring surgery. For more advanced cases, twice-daily warm soaks, oral antibiotics (with signs of infection), followed by lateral plate avulsion and lateral matricectomy (either chemical or surgical) represent standard of care. Infantile disease responds to warm soaks followed by massage of the nail and distal phalangeal tuft.

Subungual Hematoma

CLINICAL FEATURES AND DIAGNOSIS

Blood under the nail plate can appear red or black. Because the physiologic blood-metabolizing enzymes are not found in the nail plate, blood trapped between the plate and bed is not metabolized to the same evolving brown- and green-colored metabolites in the nail, and instead stays red-black and grows out with the nail plate. Nail plate growth is slow, approximately 3 mm/month for fingernails and about one half that rate for toenails, so that growing out of the hematoma will take several months and may be difficult to appreciate without photographs or serial measurements.

Diagnosis is usually straightforward. In ambiguous presentations, a urinalysis reagent strip efficiently and accurately tests for subungual blood. However, nail tumors are often preceded or first recognized after trauma, and they might even bleed spontaneously. Therefore, the presence of blood does not rule out a concomitant neoplasm.

TREATMENT

Any hematoma involving more than 50% of the nail plate carries a significant risk of underlying distal phalangeal fracture, and an x-ray should be ordered. For relief of acute symptomatic subungual hematomas, digital anesthesia followed by trephination using a sterilized hot paper clip, punch, #11 blade, or nail drill provides rapid relief and confirms the diagnosis. For most cases, however, no treatment is indicated, and the blood will grow out distally with the nail plate, albeit slowly.

Psoriasis

CLINICAL FEATURES AND DIAGNOSIS

Psoriasis commonly involves the nails in patients with cutaneous disease and occasionally occurs as a disease isolated to the nail unit. In those with psoriatic arthritis, nail disease is over represented, and may be present up to 90% to 95% of the time. Like lichen planus, psoriasis can involve any part of the nail unit; hyponychium and nail bed involvement manifest as onycholysis and subungual hyperkeratosis and a red nail bed or oil drop (salmon patch) change.

Nail pitting occurs from proximal matrix psoriasis, where parakeratotic columns lose attachment from the superficial plate, leaving a narrow depression behind in the nail plate. Any patient with these signs should have a detailed history (looking for family history) and complete skin examination, with particular attention given to the scalp, external auditory meatus, postauricular crease, umbilicus, intergluteal fold, groin, and flexural areas. Even without these helpful cutaneous signs, the combination of three nail signs is highly suggestive of nail psoriasis. In ambiguous cases, a nail clipping or nail bed biopsy can provide additional diagnostic information.

TREATMENT

Overt, repetitive, and incidental trauma to the nail apparatus worsens the nail disease and makes it more resistant to treatment (the Koebner phenomenon). Therefore, it is important to keep the nails trimmed short, use no nail cosmetics or artificial nails, and avoid aggressive nail manicuring or débridement of nail bed hyperkeratosis.

Topical treatment may be applied with a variety of agents, many of which represent off-label uses: corticosteroids, 5-fluorouracil (Efudex, Carac),[1] calcipotriene (Dovonex), tazarotene (Tazorac), cyclosporine (Sandimmune), and urea (Keralac, Carmol). Topical treatment is low risk but generally disappointing. Intralesional injection of triamcinolone 2.5 to 5 mg/mL is effective and can be dosed on a monthly basis and gradually tapered until the nails are free of disease; this therapy can provide a period of remission from nail disease. Systemic agents (methotrexate [Trexall], cyclosporine, or injectable therapies) used for severe psoriasis and psoriatic arthritis are inappropriate to use off label for isolated nail disease; however, in the case of widespread disease, they often improve concomitant nail psoriasis. Systemic corticosteroids, as with all forms of psoriasis, are contraindicated and can provoke an outbreak of widespread pustular (von Zumbush) psoriasis.

Primary (Simple) Onycholysis

CLINICAL FEATURES AND DIAGNOSIS

Onycholysis means separation of nail plate from nail bed or nail folds and represents a ventral or lateral break in the normal nail barrier. It can be graded from stage 1 (minimal involvement) to stage 4 or 5 (maximal involvement). The longer onycholysis is present, the less likely it is to resolve as the nail bed can pathologically cornify and develop a granular layer.

The most common causes are trauma and contact irritants or moisture. Other causes include psoriasis and onychomycosis; whereas onychomycosis tends to involve the toenails only and manifests with yellow nails, onycholysis nearly always involves the fingernails and

---

[1]Not FDA approved for this indication.

demonstrates classic physical signs. Primary onycholysis usually involves the fingernails, and might involve only one nail. Women, those who use nail cosmetics, and persons with prolonged irritant or moisture contact, are all at highest risk.

Monodactylous onycholysis should always raise the possibility of an underlying neoplasm. Yeast is commonly cultured but is usually an opportunistic colonizer rather than a pathogenic organism. Hence the presence of *Candida* does not mean a diagnosis of onychomycosis, but secondary colonization in the setting of onycholysis.

TREATMENT

Nails must be kept short. Patients must practice a strict irritant and moisture avoidance regimen, including avoidance of all nail cosmetics and artificial nails. They should use heavy cotton gloves for dry work and light cotton gloves under vinyl gloves for wet work. A topical antifungal solution, lotion, or lacquer may be added as an adjuvant agent but is considered secondary after the avoidance regimen. For monodactylous cases, x-ray and biopsy should always be considered.

Primary (Simple) Chronic Paronychia

CLINICAL FEATURES AND DIAGNOSIS

Chronic paronychia may be defined as inflammation of one or more nail folds, usually the proximal fold, lasting 6 weeks or longer. It represents a dorsal or lateral (or both) barrier breakdown of the nail unit, compared with onycholysis on the ventral of the nail plate. In both situations, irritants and moisture contribute to a chronic irritant contact dermatitis and yeast colonization. Women, persons who use nail cosmetics or work in the food industry, and persons with prolonged irritant or moisture contact are at risk. As with onycholysis, patients with single-digit involvement or refractory cases who fail to respond to treatment should bring to mind the possibility of an underlying neoplasm, and a biopsy is warranted.

TREATMENT

The same principles apply to treatment of chronic paronychia as for onycholysis. An irritant and moisture avoidance regimen, combined with an antifungal solution as an adjuvant, is central to therapy. Nail cosmetics and nail manipulation, with an orange stick, for example, are forbidden. A topical corticosteroid agent may be used to decrease inflammation for 3 to 4 weeks initially, combined with the avoidance regimen. Refractory cases might respond to intralesional corticosteroids 2.5 to 5 mg/mL or occasionally a surgical saucerization of the proximal nail fold.

REFERENCES

Daniel 3rd CR, Daniel MP, Daniel J, et al. Managing simple chronic paronychia and onycholysis with ciclopirox 0.77% and an irritant-avoidance regimen. Cutis 2004;73(1):81–5.

de Berker D. The physical basis of cosmetic defects of the nail plate. J Cosmet Dermatol 2002;1(1):35–42.

de Berker D. Management of nail psoriasis. Clin Exp Dermatol 2000;25 (5):357–62.

Gupta AK, Tu LQ. Onychomycosis therapies: Strategies to improve efficacy. Dermatol Clin 2006;24(3):381–6.

Haneke E. Ingrown and pincer nails: evaluation and treatment. Dermatol Ther 2002;15:148–58.

Rounding C, Bloomfield S. Surgical treatments for ingrowing toenails. Cochrane Database Syst Rev 2005;(2):CD001541.

Tosti A, Piraccini BM. Treatment of common nail disorders. Dermatol Clin 2000;18(2):339–48.

van de Kerkhof PC, Pasch MC, Scher RK, et al. Brittle nail syndrome: A pathogenesis-based approach with a proposed grading system. J Am Acad Dermatol 2005;53(4):644–51.

Keloids

Method of
Woraphong Manuskiatti, MD

Keloids are a common dermatologic condition, especially in dark-skinned persons. The incidence of keloids in persons of European descent is reported to be <1%, whereas the incidence in persons of sub-Saharan African ethnicity and Latin Americans varies from 4.5 to 16%. Persons of sub-Saharan African and Asian extraction develop keloids more often than those of European descent by a ratio ranging from 5:1 to 15:1.

Clinically, keloids appear as firm, bulbous nodules or markedly elevated plaques following the healing process of a skin injury that extends beyond the confines of the original wound, do not regress spontaneously, and tend to recur after excision. Histologically, keloids are characterized by foci of markedly thickened, brightly eosinophilic-staining collagen bundles arranged randomly and appear within the mass of fibrillary collagen. The presence of a keloid is often cosmetically unacceptable to the affected patient. It may be painful or pruritic and can restrict range of motion.

Pathogenesis

Keloids represent abnormal wound healing in response to cutaneous surgery, physical trauma, or inflammatory responses. The pathogenesis of keloids has yet to be determined and may be multifactorial. Studies have demonstrated both overproduction of collagen and increased procollagen levels, as well as decreased levels of collagenase in keloidal tissue. Proposed mechanisms for the cause of keloid formation include tension and vessel occlusion, as well as genetic, hormonal, and immune-mediated mechanisms. Currently, much of the research attention has focused on the immunoregulation of collagen production and deposition.

Prevention

Prevention should be the first rule of keloid therapy. Avoiding all unnecessary wounds in any patient, whether keloid-prone or not, remains an evident solution. Nonessential surgical and cosmetic procedures should not be performed in patients with histories of forming keloids and in anatomic sites prone to keloid formation including the mid-chest, shoulder, back, and posterior neck. All postoperative and cutaneous trauma sites should be treated with appropriate antibiotics to prevent infection. All surgical wounds should be closed with normal tension. If possible, incision should not cross joint spaces and skin excisions should be horizontal ellipses in the same direction as the skin tension lines.

Treatment

Several forms of treatment have been used with varying degrees of success. No single therapy has been shown to be superior. Often, use of multiple modalities is necessary to successfully treat the lesions. The selection of therapeutic options typically depends on the scar's size, location, and depth and on the patient's age, past responses to treatment, and economic status (Table 1).

CURRENT DIAGNOSIS

- Clinical characteristics: a raised, firm scar, possibly painful or pruritic, and extending beyond wound borders
- Histologic characteristics: thick bundles of hyalinized collagen arranged in dense swirls or nodules

TABLE 1 Common Therapeutic Regimens for Keloids

Treatment modality	Regimen	Treatment interval
Intralesional corticosteroids	TAC 10-40 mg/mL	Every 2-4 wk
Intralesional 5-FU plus TAC	5-FU 45 mg/mL mixed with TAC 1 mg/mL	Every 1-2 wk
Imiquimod (Aldara)[1]	Once every 3-4 d	8 wk
Onion extract (e.g., Mederma)	3-4 times/d	8 wk on new scars and 2-6 mo on old scars
Excision	Scalpel or CO_2 laser excision	Should be followed by another treatment modality
Cryosurgery	2 to 3 freeze–thaw cycles of 10-30 sec	Every 3-4 wk
Pressure therapy	Pressure maintained between 24 and 30 mm Hg, 18-24 h/d	Continue for at least 6-12 mo
Pulsed dye laser	7 mm spot size, 5-7 J/cm^2	Every 4-8 wk
Silicone gel sheeting	Apply for at least 12 h/d	Continue for at least 3 mo

[1]Not FDA approved for this indication.
Abbreviations: 5-FU = 5-fluorouracil; TAC = triamcinolone acetonide.

 CURRENT THERAPY

Medical Therapies

- Corticosteroid injections
- Interferon (INF-α [Intron-A], IFN-γ, [Actimmune])[1]
- 5-Fluorouracil (5-FU, Adrucil)[1]
- Imiquimod (Aldara)[1]
- Onion extract (Mederma)

Surgical Therapies

- Primary excision
- Cryosurgery

Physical Modalities

- Radiation therapy
- Pressure therapy
- Laser therapy

Silicone Gel Sheeting

Miscellaneous Therapies

- Topical vitamin E
- Retinoic acid (Retin A)[1] and tacrolimus (Protopic)[1]
- Intralesional verapamil (Isoptin)[1] and bleomycin (Blenoxane)[1]
- Colchicine[1]
- Ultraviolet A1 phototherapy

---

[1]Not FDA approved for this indication.

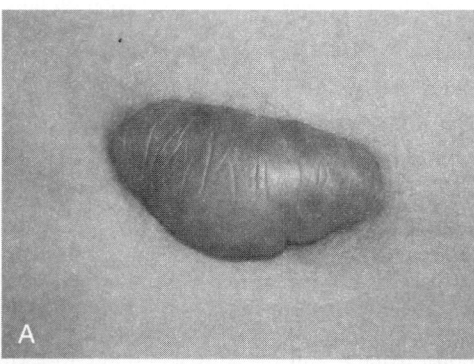

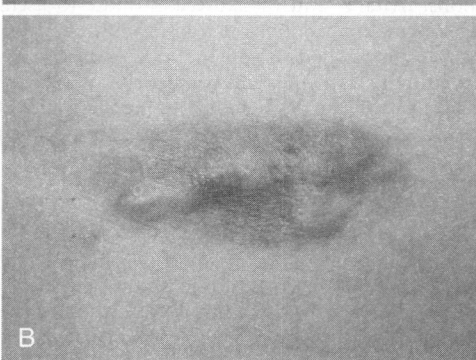

FIGURE 1. A, A keloid on the back. **B,** The scar after four intralesional injections of corticosteroid 10 mg/mL at 4 weeks apart. Note side effects of skin atrophy and hypopigmentation. (Reprinted with permission from Manuskiatti W. Current management of hypertrophic scars and keloids. *Siriraj Hosp Gaz* 2003;55:249–58.)

MEDICAL THERAPIES

Corticosteroid Injections

Intralesional corticosteroid injections have been the mainstay therapy for treatment of keloids. Corticosteroids decrease excessive scarring by reducing synthesis of collagen and glycosaminoglycan and by reducing inflammatory mediators and fibroblast proliferation during the wound-healing process. The most commonly used corticosteroid is triamcinolone acetonide (Kenalog, 10-40 mg/mL), which, depending on the size and location of the lesions, is administered intralesionally at 2- to 4-week intervals over the course of months to years. Response rates vary from 50% to 100%, with a recurrence rate of 50%. Intralesional corticosteroid injections also reduce symptoms of pruritus and tenderness. Results are improved when corticosteroids are combined with other therapies such as excision and cryosurgery. Complications of repeated corticosteroid injections include atrophy, telangiectasia, and hypopigmentation at and around the injection sites (Fig. 1).

Interferon

Interferon (IFN) causes a decrease in collagen I and III synthesis by reducing cellular messenger ribonucleic acid. Intralesional IFN-γ injection (Actimmune)[1] administered twice weekly for 4 weeks showed improved to complete resolution of keloids. However, injections tend to be exceedingly painful and are complicated by flulike symptoms.

5-Fluorouracil

Treatment of keloids with intralesional 5-FU injection (Adrucil)[1] combined with corticosteroids has been shown to be as effective as intralesional corticosteroids alone, but the latter is much more likely to cause adverse effects. 5-FU appears to work by decreasing keloid

---

[1]Not FDA approved for this indication.

fibroblast proliferation. Injections are given once a week at the beginning and then adjusted up or down according to the treatment response. Side effects of intralesional 5-FU include spots of purpura, burning sensation during injection, and localized superficial tissue slough.

Imiquimod

A study on the effect of postoperative application of imiquimod 5% cream (Aldara)[1] on the surgically excised keloids for a period of 8 weeks noted a lower recurrence rate than that of excision alone. Theoretically, imiquimod induces production of interferon and thus downregulates collagen synthesis. Reported side effects include local skin irritation and mild hyperpigmentation.

Onion Extract

Extract of *Allium cepa,* or onion extract, is an active ingredient in a number of topical scar treatment products (e.g., Mederma). Onion extract exhibits antiinflammatory, bacteriostatic, and collagen down-regulating properties and improves collagen organization. It is recommended that onion extract be applied three times daily for 8 weeks for new scars (after wound closure) and three times daily for 2 to 6 months on old scars. However, most of documented clinical studies of onion extract have shown that onion extract does not improve hypertrophic and keloid scarring.

SURGICAL THERAPIES

Primary Excision

Surgical excision of keloids without adjunctive therapy has persistently shown poor results, with a high rate of recurrence (45% to 100%). Decreased recurrence rates are consistently reported with excision in combination with other postoperative treatment modalities, such as intralesional corticosteroids, radiation, pressure therapy, silicone gel sheeting, or imiquimod cream. Surgical techniques to minimize tissue trauma, closing with minimal tension, and using buried sutures when necessary for layered closure are recommended in order to decrease the possibility of recurrence.

Cryosurgery

Freezing keloids with a cryogen such as liquid nitrogen affects the microvasculature and causes cell damage. This occurs via intracellular crystallization, leading to tissue anoxia with subsequent tissue necrosis and sloughing, followed by tissue flattening. Cryosurgery alone results in keloid flattening in 51% to 74% of the patients after two or more sessions performed at 3- to 4-week intervals. Limitations to this procedure include postoperative pain, slow healing, and hypopigmentation (especially in dark-skinned patients).

PHYSICAL MODALITIES

Radiation Therapy

Radiation may be used as a monotherapy or combined with surgery to prevent recurrence of keloids following excision. Radiation therapy is thought to work by inhibiting fibroblast proliferation and neoangiogenesis in wound healing. When used as a monotherapy, radiation is not very effective and the a recurrence rate of 50% to 100% is high. The risks of carcinogenicity associated with radiotherapy are controversial. Caution is advised when treating young children or when treating areas around the breasts and thyroid due to the increased radiosensitivities of these tissues.

Pressure Therapy

The mechanism involved in how pressure therapy reduces keloid formation is not well understood, but it is hypothesized that pressure induces tissue hypoxia, resulting in fibroblast degeneration and subsequent collagen degradation. It is generally recommended that the pressure be maintained between 24 and 30 mm Hg for 18 to 24 hours a day for at least 6 to 12 months for this therapy to be effective. Pressure therapy is commonly used in combination with other modalities such as silicone gel sheeting following surgical excision. The patient's compliance is the limiting factor because the success of the therapy requires long-term pressure application.

Laser Therapy

At present, the common use of lasers to treat keloids is based on two different approaches. One technique is an application of carbon dioxide (CO_2) laser for nonspecific destruction of keloids. Keloid vaporization or excision by CO_2 laser alone results in high (40% to 90%) recurrence rate and provides no distinct advantage over scalpel excision. The CO_2 laser is now reserved to use for debulking of large keloids before initiating other treatment modalities. Another method is 585-nm or 595-nm pulsed dye laser for selectively damaging the microvasculature of the keloids (Fig. 2). Multiple (more than two) pulsed dye laser treatment sessions have been shown to decrease scar height and erythema and to improve scar texture and dysesthesia.

SILICONE GEL SHEETING

The mode of action of silicone gel sheeting remains unclear but thought to occur through an increased scar hydration effect provided by the sheet, leading to antikeloidal effects. To be effective, the sheets must be applied for at least 12 hours daily for 2 to 3 months, with removal permitted for routine hygiene. Adverse events such as pruritus, rash, maceration, and odor can be managed by temporary interruption of treatment and regular washing of the sheet and the scar. The efficacy of silicone gel sheeting on hypertrophic and keloid scarring remains unclear and warrants rigorous evaluation. The ease of use of silicone gel sheeting and its lack of

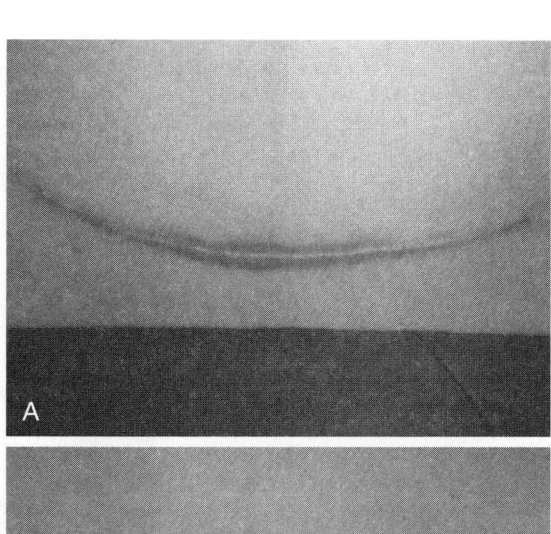

FIGURE 2. A, A scar developing after caesarian section. **B,** The scar after two pulsed-dye laser treatments 8 weeks apart.

---

[1]Not FDA approved for this indication.

serious adverse effects make it an attractive alternative to invasive treatments, such as intralesional injection of corticosteroids, radiation, laser treatment, surgical excision, cryotherapy, and pressure therapy. Silicone gel sheeting may be especially useful in children and others who cannot tolerate the pain associated with other treatment modalities.

MISCELLANEOUS THERAPIES

There are additional novel therapies; however, many treatments are anecdotal and require confirmation of the treatments' efficacy and safety through formal studies. Some of these therapies include topical vitamin E, retinoic acid (Retin-A)[1] and tacrolimus (Protopic),[1] intralesional verapamil (Isoptin)[1] and bleomycin (Blenoxane),[1] colchicine,[1] and ultraviolet A1 phototherapy.

CONCLUSIONS

Therapeutic management of keloids remains a challenge because of their high rate of recurrence and lack of curative treatment. The most important point concerning keloid formation is prevention. Treatment approaches to keloids is depend not only on the size of the lesion but also on the age, location, and economic status of the patient. The use of several approaches in combination or sequentially, based on the patient's individual requirements and responses, is recommended to maximize the therapeutic outcome.

---

[1]Not FDA approved for this indication.

REFERENCES

Al-Attar A, Mess S, Thomassen JM, et al. Keloid pathogenesis and treatment. Plast Reconstr Surg 2006;117:286–300.

English RS, Shenefelt PD. Keloids and hypertrophic scars. Dermatol Surg 1999;25:631–8.

Kelly AP. Update on the management of keloids. Semin Cutan Med Surg 2009;28:71–6.

Manuskiatti W, Fitzpatrick RE. Treatment response of keloidal and hypertrophic sternotomy scars: Comparison among intralesional corticosteroid, 5-fluorouracil, and 585-nm flashlamp-pumped pulsed-dye laser treatments. Arch Dermatol 2002;138:1149–55.

Mustoe TA, Cooter RD, Gold MH, et al. International clinical recommendations on scar management. Plast Reconstr Surg 2002;110:560–71.

Seifert O, Mrowietz U. Keloid scarring: Bench and bedside. Arch Dermatol Res 2009;301:259–72.

Slemp AE, Kirschner RE. Keloids and scars: A review of keloids and scars, their pathogenesis, risk factors, and management. Curr Opin Pediatr 2006;18:396–402.

Warts (Verruca)

Method of
Anne E. Rosin, MD

Warts are a nuisance. For the most part, they are benign and harmless skin growths caused by one of the more than 80 saprophytic human papillomaviruses (HPVs). These viruses are ubiquitous and spread by contact with an infected person or indirectly through fomites such as wet towels, swimming pools, and locker room floors. The conventional thinking is that the epidermis must be defective at the site of inoculation.

CURRENT DIAGNOSIS

- Common warts: rough, hyperkeratotic, firm papules on the hands, legs, or feet
- Flat warts: small, flat-topped, pink or flesh-colored papules on the face, arms, or legs
- Plantar and palmar warts: hard, thickened, callus-like lesions that disrupt skin lines
- Mosaic warts: large clusters of warts
- Filiform warts: small, finger-like lesions on the face
- Differential diagnoses: seborrheic keratoses, keratoacanthoma, squamous cell carcinoma, callus, and corns

Clinical Features

Nongenital warts affect 10% of the population and are among the three most common reasons for dermatologic visits. Warts are more common in adolescents and in immunosuppressed persons because of immature or compromised immune systems.

Several types of warts occur with variations in appearance, the site affected, and the virus involved. Common warts (i.e., verrucae vulgaris) are rough, hyperkeratotic, firm papules that most often occur on the hands and legs and that are caused by HPV types 1, 2, or 4. Flat warts (i.e., verrucae planae), caused by HPV 3 or 10, are small, flat-topped, and flesh-colored growths that occur in large numbers on the face, arms, or legs. Plantar and palmar warts (i.e., verrucae plantares et palmares) are hard, thickened, callus-like lesions that disrupt skin lines on the soles or palms. Mosaic warts are larger clusters of these warts. Filiform warts are small, digitate or finger-like lesions most commonly seen on the face, especially around the eyelids, nose, and mouth. Periungual warts are common warts impinging on and growing under fingernails or toenails. Genital warts are discussed in a separate chapter.

Differential diagnoses include seborrheic keratoses, keratoacanthoma, squamous cell carcinoma, callus, and corns. Paring the stratum corneum (outer layer of the skin) may reveal thrombosed or bleeding capillaries seen as black dots.

The manifestation of viral warts and various modes of therapy have been referenced throughout history. The word *condyloma* is of Greek origin and means "knuckle or knob"; *verruca* is Latin for "little hill." Warts are mentioned in early Hippocratic writings and in the Old and New Testaments of the Bible. In Arthurian legend, King Arthur was known by the diminutive nickname *wart* until he proved his royalty by pulling Excalibur from a stone. Chaucer described a distinctive wart on the Miller's nose in his *Canterbury Tales*. Shakespeare invokes warts as the result of a curse in *Hamlet*. The phrase "warts and all" is attributed to Oliver Cromwell, who gave specific instructions to his portraitist. Tom Sawyer was afflicted with common warts from "playing with frogs" (obviously not possible because HPV is species specific). Even "The King," Elvis Presley, had a wart removed from his right hand. It now resides in a velvet-lined box in a museum in Hawaii.

Treatment

ALTERNATIVE AND STANDARD APPROACHES

Because 40% of warts will spontaneously disappear within 2 years in healthy individuals, treatment is not always necessary. As a corollary, treatment of warts does not guarantee their complete resolution. Many patients are compelled to seek treatment of their warts because of the social embarrassment or physical discomfort that warts can cause. Patients with compromised immune systems due to immunodeficiency or immunosuppression are at higher risk for numerous warts, and treatment to prevent their progression to squamous cell carcinoma is important.

Popular reports and the medical literature are replete with descriptions of successful methods for treating warts. Whether anecdotal or evidence based, reports are largely without the support of randomized, controlled trials. No one therapy is always effective, and warts resolve, recur, shrink, or grow despite therapy. It is likely that all wart therapies work by triggering an immune response to the presence of papillomavirus in the skin.

Treatment methods fall into several broad categories, which include folk remedies, over-the-counter (OTC) treatments, and office-based therapies. Office-based treatments include destructive methods, surgical or laser procedures, immunologic intervention, and combination therapy.

Folk remedies for curing warts are espoused by Tom Sawyer and Huck Finn more than once in Mark Twain's classics. Tom recommended rubbing the warts with a split potato and then burying the potato, whereas Huck was certain that swinging a dead cat over his head and then burying it trumped the potato. They recited the wart chant:

Barley-corn, barley-corn, injun meal shorts,
Spunk-water, spunk-water, swaller these warts.

Both agreed that the wart chant spoken at midnight in the middle of the woods was the superior method, although neither was brave enough to prove the hypothesis.

The many alternative folk cures include transference, various prayers and incantations, hypnosis, and applications of garlic extract,[7] tea tree oil,[7] bacon fat, blood or entrails of various animals, and saliva of a loved one. Duct tape[1] application has received much attention. One study comparing cryotherapy with duct tape occlusion of common warts showed resolution in 85% of the children treated by occlusion, compared with 60% in the liquid nitrogen group. Another study found no statistically significant difference between duct tape and moleskin for the treatment of warts in an adult population.

Treatment of warts is often initiated by the patient, who most often uses one of the OTC salicylic acid products available. These keratolytic products, when used consistently and as directed, can be quite successful. Unfortunately, salicylic acid treatment, which destroys the infected epidermis and causes an immune reaction, can be irritating and tedious, prompting many patients to seek medical care.

Office-based treatments are largely destructive or immunomodulating, or both. The first line of therapy in the physician's office is usually cryotherapy. Liquid nitrogen is −196°C in the canister, and when applied by cotton-tipped application or cryospray, it effects a freeze that far surpasses a Wisconsin winter's frostbite. It is painful, unfortunately. Another destructive physician-applied treatment is cantharidin (Cantharone),[1,6] a chemical derived from blister beetles. It is painless on application and well tolerated by children. Acids, including bichloroacetic and trichloroacetic (Tri-Chlor), have risks, including pain on application, ulceration, and scarring.

Other destructive methods of wart removal usually are reserved for resistant or multiple lesions. Surgical removal followed by electrodesiccation and curettage is effective for large, solitary common warts but requires local anesthesia and results in scarring. Laser therapy, most often with pulsed-dye (PDL) or carbon dioxide (CO_2) lasers, has its place for selected patients. The PDL method is less aggressive and less painful than CO_2 vaporization, which is reserved for resistant common or plantar warts, multiple warts in immunosuppressed patients, or genital warts.

Immune modulation alone or in combination with destructive methods is helpful in treating resistant warts. The newest immunomodulator in the wart warrior's armamentarium is imiquimod (Aldara),[1] which was initially approved for treatment of genital warts but has since received FDA approval for treatment of nonmelanoma skin cancers. It is also frequently used to treat flat warts, acting through immune system modulation by inducing cytokines, including interferon-α. Other topical immunomodulators, such as squaric acid dibutylester (SADBE)[1,6] or diphencyprone[1,6] are contact sensitizers that induce an allergic dermatitis through type IV hypersensitivity reactions. Treatment with SADBE is well tolerated and a good choice for recalcitrant warts in children, although it is time consuming.

Intralesional immunotherapy by *Candida* antigen injection (Candin)[1] is effective in improving or clearing warts in up to 74% of patients. It is considered a first-line therapy in children with large or multiple warts and second-line therapy for warts resistant to standard therapies. It is well tolerated. Intralesional interferon alfa-2b (Intron A)[1] has been used successfully to treat genital warts and warts that have not responded to conventional therapies.

Oral immunomodulation with high-dose cimetidine (Tagamet)[1] has been proposed as a helpful adjunctive therapy in the treatment of multiple warts in children and adults. It is postulated to enhance cell-mediated immune response. Studies comparing cimetidine with placebo have not been convincing, but cimetidine is well tolerated, and anecdotal reports of its usefulness abound.

Other topical products available for off-label treatment of warts include retinoids, formaldehyde compounds, and 5-fluorouracil (Efudex).[1] These agents interfere with epidermal proliferation, effect a nonspecific antiviral action, or inhibit mitosis, leading to keratinocyte and therefore viral death.

Because photodynamic therapy (PDT) with 20% 5-aminolevulinic acid (ALA [Levulan Kerastick])[1] is all the rage in dermatology for the treatment of actinic keratoses, acne, nonmelanoma skin cancers, and aging, why not add warts to the list? Studies have shown various success rates, but most demonstrated improvement or resolution of recalcitrant warts treated by ALA-PDT.

Family medicine physicians, internists, and dermatologists are asked to treat warts on a regular basis. Almost 50% of visits to a dermatologist are for wart treatment. The choice of therapeutic modality depends on the wart, the patient, and the practitioner. As Lempriere stated in his treatise on the treatment of warts: "Of all the futile disorders of the skin, it would be hard to find any that are regarded with greater contempt by the lay public and yet capable of resisting a greater variety of treatment than the group of papillary lesions commonly known as warts."

The American Academy of Dermatology has established guidelines for the treatment of warts:

- Desire of the patient for therapy
- Symptoms of pain, bleeding, itching, or burning
- Disabling or disfiguring lesions
- Large numbers or large size of lesions
- Desire to prevent spread to unblemished skin of the patient or others
- Immunocompromised condition

The goal of all therapy, including treatment of the pesky wart, should be "First, do no harm." To ensure resolution and nonrecurrence of warts, however, the patient and practitioner must often make compromises that include inconvenience, discomfort, and scarring. Treatment choices depend on the patient's age and level of pain tolerance; the location, type, and size of the warts; and the comfort level of the practitioner with the specific treatment.

---

[1]Not FDA approved for this indication.
[6]May be compounded by pharmacists.

 CURRENT THERAPY

- Keratolytics such as salicylic acid
- Cantharidin (Cantharone)[1,6]
- Cryotherapy
- Surgical removal
- Pulsed-dye laser
- Immunotherapy: topical imiquimod (Aldara)[1], intralesional *Candida* antigen (Candin)[1]
- Photodynamic therapy

---

[1]Not FDA approved for this indication.
[6]May be compounded by pharmacists.

---

[1]Not FDA approved for this indication.
[6]May be compounded by pharmacists.
[7]Available as dietary supplement.

SELECTED TREATMENT METHODS

Over the years, I have used most of the office methods mentioned previously, often asking the patient to incorporate OTC methods as well. Simple methods are appropriate for warts that are small and few. In children, painless methods are preferred and usually successful. I tend to combine modalities of destruction and immune stimulation, such as cantharidin,[1,6] and cimetidine[1] in children or use liquid nitrogen and *Candida* antigen injection[1] in more mature patients.

Keratolytics, which are 40% salicylic acid plaster pads (OTC Mediplast), are an excellent first-line therapy for common hand warts and plantar warts in motivated patients. Repeated application, with pumice stone or callus file use, results in cure rates of up to 80%. This method can cause irritation if the pad slips out of place (patients should try duct tape over the plaster) and can take several weeks to work.

Cantharidin[1,6] in a 0.7% colloidal solution can induce a painless blister after application and occlusion for 8 hours. It is applied in the office and repeated every 4 weeks. It is useful for treatment of common, periungual, and plantar warts in children, and the cure rate approaches 80%. Unfortunately, an occasional "donut wart," a ring of new warts surrounding the cleared original, occurs.

Cryotherapy uses liquid nitrogen applied by cotton applicator or, better, by a cryospray gun, and it is the most commonly used office-based treatment. The wart and a 1- to 2-mm margin around it should be frozen for 10 to 20 seconds. The freeze should be repeated once after a thaw of 20 seconds. If the warts are thick, they can be pared first. The patient is told that a blister (sometimes hemorrhagic) will result and should be left intact if possible. Treatment should be repeated every 3 to 4 weeks until normal skin markings return. If warts persist beyond 3 months of therapy, another method of treatment should be selected.

Surgery is used for large warts. Large common warts of the hands or extremities are more easily treated if they are debulked. If the wart is solitary, this method is more direct and often more successful than others. The wart should be anesthetized, removed at its base using a blade, and then curetted and cauterized. This method is not recommended for plantar warts because of scarring.

Pulsed-dye lasers (585- to 595-nm wavelength) can provide selective photothermolysis of blood vessels within the wart, which compromises blood supply and results in necrosis. This technique results in destruction of blood vessels within the wart but minimal damage to normal skin. It is generally well tolerated, but local anesthesia can be used if necessary. I use the following parameters: 7-mm spot size, pulse duration of 1.5 msec, and fluence of 10 to 12 J/cm^2, with double pulses applied to achieve purpura. This method is useful for recalcitrant flat, periungual, common, and plantar warts and has a success rate of 50% to 90%.

Immunotherapy is an effective method of treating some patients. I often add oral cimetidine[1] at daily doses of 30 to 40 mg/kg to other painless therapies for wart treatment in children. If the patient tolerates injections, I am a fan of *Candida* antigen[1] as monotherapy in patients with multiple warts or in combination with a destructive method such as cryotherapy or PDL. I choose the largest wart and inject 0.2 to 0.3 mL of a commercially available 1:1000 dilution of *Candida* antigen directly into the wart using a 30-gauge needle and tuberculin syringe. Pretesting is unnecessary, side effects are minimal, and more than 75% of patients treated with a series of three injections have clearing of the injected and distant warts. Imiquimod[1] is effective as monotherapy for genital warts, and I agree with anecdotal reports of its efficacy in flat warts. However, it is expensive (gram for gram it costs as much as platinum), and I have not found it useful except as adjunctive therapy for common warts. Treatment protocol is a thin coat of imiquimod cream applied three times weekly and combined with cryotherapy or salicylic acid.

Photodynamic therapy is useful for patients with multiple recalcitrant warts, especially patients who are immunosuppressed due to organ transplantation and anti-rejection therapy or human immunodeficiency virus (HIV) disease. PDT, which involves a topically applied photosensitizer that is activated by visible light, results in tissue destruction, and studies of this method for treatment of warts have been promising. My protocol includes a 60-minute incubation of affected lesions with topically applied ALA[1] followed by a 15-minute exposure to blue light, repeated every 4 weeks as needed. Transplant recipients I have treated, who typically present with many warts and early squamous cell cancers, have shown remarkable improvement in their skin lesions.

Warts are a bane and frustration to the patient and the physician who treats them. The myriad treatments available are for the most part supported by anecdotal evidence rather than randomized control trials. There are few inclusive reviews of successful treatment methods, and until an effective HPV vaccine is developed for all strains that cause warts, we will have to limp along using methods that are comfortable and have produced results. Each treatment should be tailored to fit the wart, the patient, and the practitioner.

---

[1]Not FDA approved for this indication.

REFERENCES

Bigby M, Gibbs S, Harvey I, Sterling J. Warts. Clin Evid 2005;14:2091–103.

Drake LA, Ceilley RI, Cornelison RL. Guidelines of care for warts: Human papillomavirus. J Am Acad Dermatol 1995;32:98–103.

Gibbs S, Harvey I, Sterling J, Stark R. Local treatments for cutaneous warts: Systematic review. Br Med J 2002;325:461.

Johnson SM, Roberson PK, Horn TD. Intralesional injection of mumps or *Candida* skin test antigens: A novel immunotherapy for warts. Arch Dermatol 2001;137:451–5.

Leman JA, Benton EC. Verrucas. Guidelines for management. Am J Clin Dermatol 2000;1:143–9.

Lempriere WW. Treatment of warts. Aust J Dermatol 1951;1:34–8.

Massing AM, Epstein WL. Natural history of warts. A two-year study. Arch Dermatol 1963;87:306–10.

Oster-Schmidt C. Imiquimod: A new possibility for treatment-resistant verrucae planae. Arch Dermatol 2001;137:666–7.

Robson KJ, Cunningham NM, Kruzan KL, et al. Pulsed-dye laser versus conventional therapy in the treatment of warts: A prospective randomized trial. J Am Acad Dermatol 2000;43:275–80.

Stender IM, Na R, Fogh H, et al. Photodynamic therapy with 5-aminolaevulinic acid or placebo for recalcitrant foot and hand warts: Randomized double-blind trial. Lancet 2000;355:963–6.

Sterling JC, Handfield-Jones S, Hudson PM. for the British Association of Dermatologists. Guidelines for the management of cutaneous warts. Br J Dermatol 2001;144:4–11.

Yelverton CB. Warts. In: Arndt KA, Hsu JT, editors. Manual of Dermatologic Therapeutics. 7th ed. Philadelphia: Lippincott Williams & Wilkins; 2006. p. 233–40.

Condyloma Acuminata (Genital Warts)

Method of
Athena Daniolos, MD

Etiology

Genital warts, or condylomata acuminata, are the result of cutaneous human papillomavirus (HPV) infection. HPV is a member of the Papillomaviridae family. This virus is a non-enveloped DNA virus with an icosahedral capsid that is 50 to 55 nm in diameter and contains 72 capsomeres. More than 90 different types of HPV have been described, based on the results of DNA sequencing studies. This virus is epidermotropic, and different HPV types appear to have predilections for different anatomic sites.

---

[1]Not FDA approved for this indication.
[6]May be compounded by pharmacists.

Epidemiology and Pathogenesis

The Centers for Disease Control and Prevention (CDC) estimated the incidence of genital HPV infection to be 1% to 2% in the United States. This incidence appears to be increasing and is probably underestimated. The peak age of occurrence is between 15 and 29 years. The disease is primarily transmitted through sexual contact, and based on available data, the virus is easily transmitted. Condylomata acuminata are often caused by HPV genotypes 6 or 11. Viral infection of the squamous epithelial cells results in an increase in the epithelium and keratin production, ultimately producing a clinically evident wart. Anogenital HPV infection with the high-risk HPV genotypes (e.g., 16, 18, 31, 33, 35, 45) is associated with vulvar, vaginal, cervical, penile, and anorectal intraepithelial neoplasia and with invasive squamous cell carcinoma.

Clinical Presentation

Most anogenital warts are asymptomatic on presentation, although localized irritation, itching, or bleeding may occur. Typically, the flesh-colored, pink, brown, or whitish gray lesions are flat to exophytic "cauliflower" papules or plaques. The lesions may be single or multiple, and the size may range from 1 mm to several centimeters in diameter. The presence of anogenital condylomata externally should prompt an examination of the urethral meatus, vagina, cervix, anus, and oral mucosa, based on the patient's clinical and sexual history. Flat HPV lesions may not be grossly visible. Application of dilute acetic acid solution (5% acetic acid) to the skin surface with a Q-tip or applied with a 5- to 10-minute gauze soak may help to detect subtle HPV lesions. Acetic acid screening may have up to a

CURRENT DIAGNOSIS

- Mucocutaneous disease may affect the perineum, external genitalia, anus, perianal area, vagina, or urethra.
- Flat to raised lesions may be skin colored, pink, brown, or whitish gray.

25% false-positive rate because other keratinized skin lesions may appear "aceto-white," including dermatitis, lichen planus, psoriasis, and local infections (e.g., *Candida*, herpes simplex virus).

Diagnostic Tests

When the clinical appearance of the lesions is typical, no other confirmatory tests or investigations may be necessary. Pap smears of samples from the lesions may demonstrate degenerative cytoplasmic vacuolization and koilocytosis in the virus-infected epithelial cells. Tissue biopsy can provide histopathologic confirmation of the diagnosis. Although rarely indicated in the routine evaluation of an HPV-infected patient, HPV identification and DNA genotyping by polymerase chain reaction in situ hybridization is the most sensitive technique available.

Treatment and Management

The 2006 CDC guidelines state that treatment for subclinical HPV infections, in the absence of dysplasia, is not necessary. None of the current treatments for condylomata acuminata is specifically

TABLE 1 Treatments for Human Papillomavirus Infections Recommended by the CDC

| Treatment | Mechanism of Action | Methods | | Adverse Reactions | Studies |
		Patient Applied	Provider Applied		
Podophyllotoxin 0.5% gel or solution (Condylox)	Antimitotic agent; secondary cell necrosis	2×/d for 3 d, then 4 d off; repeat up to 4–6 cycles		Erythema, pain, erosion	CDC, Von Krogh, et al
Imiquimod 5% cream (Aldara)	Interferon-α and cytokine induction; cytolysis	3×/wk at bedtime, wash off in 6–10 h; can apply qhs if tolerated; repeat up to 16 wk		Erythema, pain, erosion, infection	CDC, Von Krogh, et al, Wiley, et al
Cryotherapy	Thermal injury, inflammatory reaction, and cell necrosis		Apply liquid nitrogen with cotton-tipped applicator; freeze time of 10–20 sec, depending on wart thickness; two freeze-thaw cycles; treat every 1–2 wk	Pain, blistering, scarring, pigmentary changes, infection	Beutner, et al, CDC
Podophyllin resin 10%–25% in tincture of benzoin (Podocon 25)	Antimitotic agent; secondary cell necrosis		Apply small amount; wash off in 4 h; treat every 1–2 wk	Erythema, pain, erosion, rare systemic toxicity	CDC, Von Krogh, et al, Wiley, et al
TCA (Tri-Chlor 80%) or BCA 80%–90%	Caustic chemical ablation and cell necrosis		Apply small amount every 1–2 wk	Pain, erythema, blistering, erosion, ulceration, pigmentary changes	CDC, Von Krogh, et al
Surgical—excision, curettage, electrosurgery	Physical removal or destruction		Office procedure	Pain, scarring, infection	CDC, Von Krogh, et al
Interferon, intralesional (Intron A)	Immunomodulatory cytokine		Injection 1–3×/wk, for up to 4 wk	Pain, flulike symptoms	CDC, Wiley, et al
Laser surgery	Physical ablation		Office procedure	Pain, scarring, pigmentary changes, infection	CDC, Von Krogh, et al

Abbreviations: CDC = Centers for Disease Control and Prevention; BCA = bichloroacetic acid; TCA = trichloroacetic acid.

TABLE 2 Other Treatments for Human Papillomavirus Infection

Treatment	Mechanism of Action	Methods Patient Applied	Methods Provider Applied	Adverse Reactions	Studies
5-Fluorouracil 5% cream (Efudex)[1]	Fluorinated pyrimidine antimetabolite; inhibits DNA and RNA synthesis	Thin coat at bedtime, 1–3×/wk as tolerated; repeat up to 6 wk		Pain, erythema, erosion, ulceration	Wiley, et al
5-Fluorouracil, intralesional (Adrucil)[1]	Fluorinated pyrimidine antimetabolite; inhibits DNA and RNA synthesis		Injection weekly for up to 6 wk	Pain, erythema, erosion, ulceration	Beutner, et al
Retinoids, oral— acitretin (Soriatane)[1] or isotretinoin (Accutane)[1]	Modify cell keratinization and proliferation	0.5–1 mg/kg/d PO for up to 12 wk		Erythema, xerosis, photosensitivity, teratogen, hypervitaminosis A syndrome	Cardamakis, et al, Tsambaos, et al
Cidofovir 1% gel or ointment[5]	Acyclic nucleoside phosphonate; broad anti-DNA virus activity	Thin coat daily for 5 d, every other week; repeat up to 12–16 wk		Erythema, pain, erosion	Snoek, et al
Photodynamic therapy (ALA-PDT, Levulan Kerastick)	Laser-induced photochemical cytotoxicity with free radical–mediated local cell destruction		Office procedure	Pain, erythema, pigmentary changes	Ross, et al

[1]Not FDA approved for this indication.
[5]Investigational drug in the United States.
Abbreviations: ALA = 5-aminolevulinic acid; PDT = photodynamic therapy.

antiviral, and none of these interventions can eradicate the virus from the host. The ultimate therapeutic goal is to treat and clear all clinically apparent HPV disease. Two clinically relevant areas are the treatment of sexual partners and the prevention of HPV disease.

The factors to consider when deciding on treatment include wart size and location, the patient's tolerance of the therapy, cost, and the clinician's preference and training. Data regarding the efficacy of using more than one treatment at a time are lacking. However, it is not uncommon for health care providers to combine more than one treatment modality when managing HPV-infected patients. Various therapeutic approaches are summarized in Tables 1 and 2.

Referral for consultation with a specialist should be considered in certain situations, as indicated in the treatment algorithm (Fig. 1).

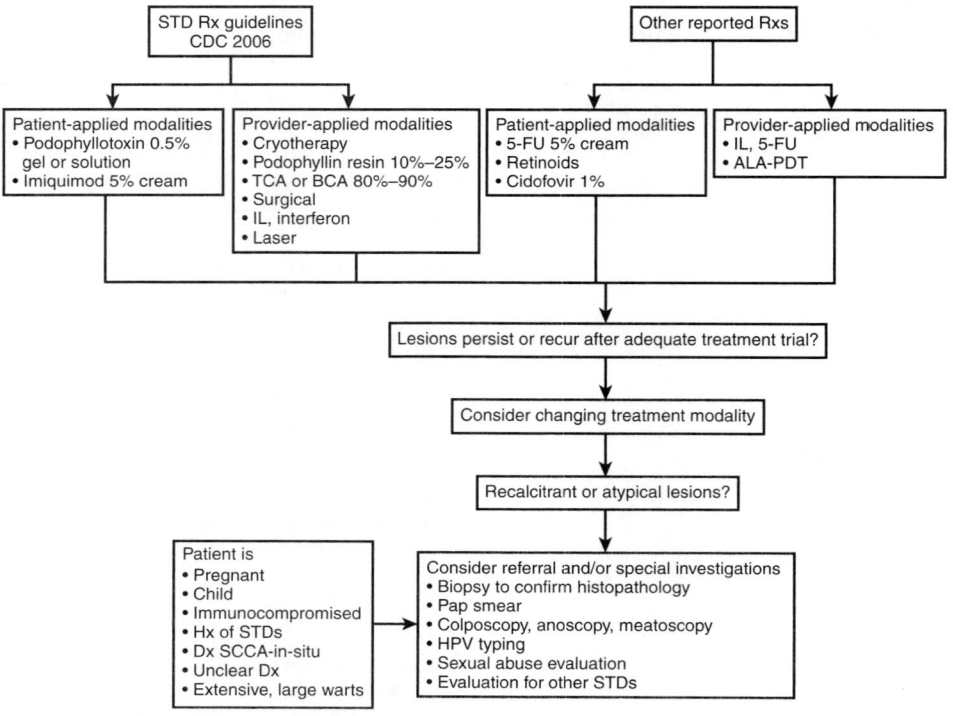

FIGURE 1. Algorithm for the treatment of anogenital warts. *Abbreviations:* ALA = 5-aminolevulinic acid; BCA = bichloroacetic acid; CDC = Centers for Disease Control and Prevention; Dx = diagnosis; 5-FU = 5-fluorouracil; HPV = human papillomavirus; Hx = history; IL = interleukin; PDT = photodynamic therapy; Rx = treatment; STD = sexually transmitted disease; TCA = trichloroacetic acid.

CURRENT THERAPY

- Treatment of subclinical HPV disease is not recommended by the 2006 STD Treatment Guidelines from the Centers for Disease Control and Prevention.
- No specifically antiviral and curative therapy exists for HPV infection.
- Recommended therapies include podophyllotoxin (podofilox [Condylox]), podophyllin resin (Podocon-25), imiquimod (Aldara), cryotherapy, trichloroacetic acid (TCA) or bichloroacetic acid (BCA), standard or laser surgery, and intralesional interferon alfa-2b (Intron A).

Advances in the treatment of HPV disease could include the development of a therapeutic HPV vaccine to boost the patient's antiviral immune response. Potential complementary medicine approaches may use green tea polyphenols.[7]

Counseling should be part of the comprehensive management of these patients. Education regarding the nature of HPV disease, prevention strategies, and screening of sexual partners are important components of quality health care.

---

[7] Available as a dietary supplement.

REFERENCES

Baker GE, Tyring SK. Therapeutic approaches to papillomavirus infections. Dermatol Clin 1997;15:331–40.

Beutner KR, Ferenczy A. Therapeutic approaches to genital warts. Am J Med 1997;102(5A):28–37.

Bonnez W, Reichman RC. Papillomaviruses. In: Mandell GL, Bennett JE, Dolin R, editors. Principles and Practice of Infectious Diseases. 6th ed. Philadelphia: Churchill Livingstone; 2005. p. 1841–51.

Buntin DM, Rosen T, Lesher JL, et al. Sexually transmitted diseases: Viruses and ectoparasites. J Am Acad Dermatol 1991;25:527–34.

Cardamakis E, Kotoulas IG, Relakis K, et al. Comparative study of systemic interferon alfa-2a plus isotretinoin versus isotretinoin in the treatment of recurrent condyloma acuminatum in men. Urology 1995;45:857–60.

Centers for Disease Control and Prevention (CDC). Sexually transmitted diseases treatment guidelines. MMWR Morb Mortal Wkly Rep 2006; 55:14–30.

Koutsky L. Epidemiology of genital human papillomavirus infection. Am J Med 1997;102(5A):3–8.

Ross EV, Romero R, Kollias N, et al. Selectivity of protoporphyrin IX fluorescence for condylomata after topical application of 5-aminolaevulinic acid: Implications for photodynamic treatment. Br J Dermatol 1997; 137:736–42.

Snoeck R, Bossens M, Parent D, et al. Phase II double-blind, placebo-controlled study of the safety and efficacy of cidofovir topical gel for the treatment of patients with human papillomavirus infection. Clin Infect Dis 2001;33:597–602.

Tsambaos D, Georgiou S, Monastirli A, et al. Treatment of condylomata acuminata with oral isotretinoin. J Urol 1997;158:1810–2.

Von Krogh G, Lacey CJ, Gross G, et al. European course on HPV associated pathology: Guidelines for primary care physicians for the diagnosis and management of anogenital warts. Sex Transm Infect 2000;76:162–8.

Wiley DJ, Douglas J, Beutner K, et al. External genital warts: Diagnosis, treatment, and prevention. Clin Infect Dis 2002;35(Suppl. 2):210–24.

Melanocytic Nevi

Method of
**Jane M. Grant-Kels, MD, and
Michael Murphy, MD**

Melanocytic nevi, or moles, are benign neoplasms composed of melanocytes. Melanocytic nevus cells are derived from melanocytes. Compared with melanocytes, nevus cells are not dendritic, are larger, and contain more abundant cytoplasm, often with coarse melanin granules. Nevus cells tend to aggregate into groups or nests. Melanocytic nevi are extremely common and can be found on almost everyone, anywhere on the cutaneous surface. This article discusses the most common types of melanocytic nevi: acquired melanocytic nevi, recurrent melanocytic nevi, halo melanocytic nevi, congenital melanocytic nevi, blue nevi, Spitz nevi, and dysplastic melanocytic nevi.

Acquired Melanocytic Nevi

Acquired melanocytic nevi are subdivided into junctional, compound, and intradermal types based on the location of the nevus cells. By definition, these lesions are not present at birth but can begin to appear in early childhood, usually after 6 to 12 months of age. Peak ages of appearance of melanocytic nevi are 2 to 3 years of age in children and 11 to 18 years in adolescents. Although nevi can appear at any age, it is relatively unusual for new melanocytic nevi to develop in middle-aged or older adults. With time, nevi can spontaneously regress. Consequently, patients in their ninth decade of life usually demonstrate few melanocytic nevi. An average white adult has 10 to 40 melanocytic nevi, but African Americans have far fewer, averaging only 2 to 8.

The number and location of melanocytic nevi have been shown to be associated with sun exposure, immunologic factors, and genetics. Consequently, melanocytic nevi are most numerous on the sun-exposed skin of the head, neck, trunk, and extremities, but they are only rarely found on covered areas such as the buttocks, female breasts, and scalp. Evidence suggests that patients with an increased number of melanocytic nevi (>50) might have an increased risk of melanoma.

Melanocytic nevi appear in a sequential fashion. Junctional melanocytic nevi arise during childhood as flat, dark macules. Histologically, an increase in single or nests of melanocytes are located at the dermoepidermal junction. With time, some of the junctional nests of melanocytes migrate into the dermis (compound melanocytic nevi). Clinically, compound melanocytic nevi are elevated and less heavily pigmented than junctional melanocytic nevi. Ultimately, all of the nevus cells migrate into the dermis (intradermal melanocytic nevi), resulting in the development of a tan or skin-colored dome-shaped papule. Melanocytic nevi can be flat or elevated and even polypoid, papillomatous, or verrucous and can demonstrate a range of color from skin-tone to black, but they are characteristically uniform in color, symmetrical, well marginated, and usually smaller than 6 mm in diameter.

All melanocytic lesions of clinical concern should be examined with a dermatoscope, a hand-held instrument with a magnified lens and a light source similar to an ophthalmoscope. This instrument allows evaluation of colors and microstructures not visible to the naked eye, helps distinguish whether pigmented lesions are melanocytic or nonmelanocytic, and helps distinguish whether melanocytic pigmented lesions are likely to be malignant. Used by an experienced dermatologist with proper training, the dermatoscope improves diagnostic accuracy by 20% to 30%.

It is unnecessary to surgically remove all melanocytic nevi because they are benign neoplasms of melanocytes. However, indications for removal include ABCD (*a*symmetry, irregular *b*order, variegation or change in *c*olor, or change in *d*iameter), symptoms (e.g., pruritus), evidence of inflammation or irritation, cosmetic issues, and patient anxiety. Melanocytic nevi on acral, genital, or scalp skin that appear benign do not require surgical removal. Shave biopsies are appropriate therapy for lesions considered clinically benign. However, if a lesion is being removed because of concern regarding the possibility of malignancy, an excisional biopsy (biopsy of choice) or incisional biopsy (including punch or deep scoop) that extends to the subcutaneous tissue is indicated. All melanocytic lesions should be submitted to a dermatopathologist for histologic review. A history of recent sun exposure or trauma should be conveyed to the dermatopathologist because such external trauma can induce reactive atypical histologic findings.

Recurrent Melanocytic Nevi

Recurrent melanocytic nevi are melanocytic nevi that have previously been incompletely removed (either iatrogenically or traumatically) and have recurred weeks to months later. Irregular brown pigmentation is clinically noted within the scar site. If the original biopsy demonstrated a benign melanocytic nevus, re-treatment is unnecessary unless the aforementioned indications are present. However, these nevi can demonstrate pseudomelanomatous histologic features. Therefore, if the repigmented area is excised, the dermatopathologist should be notified of the clinical history and, if possible, the slides from the original biopsy should be obtained and reviewed to ensure that the lesion is not histologically misdiagnosed.

Halo (Melanocytic) Nevi

Halo (melanocytic) nevi are melanocytic nevi in which a white rim or halo has developed. This phenomenon most commonly occurs around compound or intradermal nevi and is histologically associated with a dense, bandlike inflammatory infiltrate. The white halo area is histologically characterized by diminished or absent melanocytes and melanin. Approximately 20% of patients with halo nevi also exhibit vitiligo.

Although a halo can develop around many lesions in the skin, the most important differential diagnosis is between a halo nevus and melanoma with a halo. The halo and the central melanocytic nevus of halo nevi are symmetrical, round or oval, and sharply demarcated. Halo nevi most commonly occur in adolescence as an isolated event, but approximately 25% to 50% of affected persons have two or more.

The clinical course of halo nevi is variable. With time, the halo can repigment while the central nevus persists. Alternatively, the melanocytic nevus can regress completely and leave a depigmented macule that can persist or repigment over months or years.

Halo nevi do not require surgical excision unless atypical clinical features suggest the possibility of an atypical melanocytic lesion. It is advisable (particularly in adults, in whom halo nevi are less

common) to perform a complete cutaneous examination with and without the aid of a Wood's lamp to rule out any associated atypical pigmented or regressed lesions. All patients should be warned to use sunscreens or protective clothing because of the increased risk of sunburn in the depigmented halo region.

Congenital Melanocytic Nevi

By definition, congenital melanocytic nevi are present at birth. Arbitrarily, they have been classified into small (<1.5 cm), medium (1.5–20 cm) and large (>20 cm) lesions. Terms such as *bathing trunk* or *garment-type* nevi refer to CMN that cover a significant portion of the cutaneous surface.

The approximate incidence of small congenital nevi is 1% of all live births. Large congenital nevi are rare and reported in only 1 in 20,000 births. Histologically, some congenital nevi have distinguishing histologic features (melanocytic nevus cells that extend into the deeper dermis as well as the subcutis and melanocytic nevus cells arranged periadnexally, angiocentrically, within nerves, and interposed between collagen bundles). However, these features have been identified in some acquired melanocytic nevi and are absent in some congenital nevi (especially small ones). In addition, the history obtained from the patient or their parents is often inaccurate. Consequently, it can be very difficult in some cases to distinguish a small congenital nevus from an acquired nevus.

Congenital nevi can give rise to dermal or subcutaneous nodular melanocytic proliferations. The vast majority of these lesions, particularly in the neonatal period, are biologically benign, despite a worrisome clinical presentation and atypical histologic features. Genetic analysis has shown that benign melanocytic proliferations within congenital nevi express aberrations qualitatively and quantitatively different from those seen in melanoma.

The primary significance of congenital nevi is related to the potential risk for progression to melanoma. Essentially, the larger the nevus, the greater the risk of progression to melanoma. Historically, even small nevi were estimated to exhibit a lifetime melanoma risk of 5%. However, recent prospective studies suggest that small and medium congenital nevi are associated with a low risk that may approximate the risk of acquired nevi. Conversely, large congenital nevi have a lifetime risk of melanomatous progression of approximately 6.3%.

CURRENT DIAGNOSIS

Benign Melanocytic Lesions

- Symmetrical
- Sharply demarcated border
- Uniform color
- Diameter usually ≤6 mm and stable

Malignant Melanocytic Lesions

- Asymmetrical
- Poorly circumscribed border
- Variegated in color
- Diameter often ≥10 mm and increasing (changing or evolving)

CURRENT THERAPY

- Acquired melanocytic nevus: No treatment is required unless the lesion is asymmetrical or has an irregular border, change or variegated in color, or change in diameter. Symptomatic lesions should be biopsied.
- Recurrent melanocytic nevus: No treatment required if the original biopsy was benign.
- Halo melanocytic nevus: No treatment, but excision is recommended if atypical clinical features are identified.
- Congenital melanocytic nevus: Removal based on melanoma risk, cosmetics, and functional outcome. If not excised, routine follow-up with the use of photography, dermoscopy, and computer assistance is recommended.
- Blue nevus: No treatment, but excision is recommended if atypical clinical features are identified.
- Spitz nevus: If clinically unusual, a complete excisional biopsy is recommended.
- Dysplastic nevus: If only one lesion is present, excision is recommended. Patients with many dysplastic nevi require close surveillance with removal of any lesion suspicious for melanoma.

Up to two thirds of melanomas that arise in these giant congenital nevi have a nonepidermal origin, thus making clinical observation for malignant change difficult. Approximately 50% of these melanomas occur in the first 5 years of life, 60% in the first decade, and 70% before 20 years of age. Patients with large congenital nevi, especially those that involve posterior axial locations (head, neck, back, or buttocks) and are associated with satellite congenital nevi, are at increased risk for neurocutaneous melanosis (melanosis of the leptomeninges).

For large congenital nevi that involve a posterior axial location, magnetic resonance imaging (MRI) is indicated. If clinical symptoms or MRI indicate neurocutaneous melanosis, excision of the large nevus should be postponed until 2 years of age (the median age of neurologic symptoms). Patients with neurocutaneous melanosis have a greater than 50% mortality rate within 3 years. The risk and morbidity of multiple, staged excisions of a large congenital melanocytic nevus is not appropriate in patients with symptomatic neurocutaneous melanosis. All other large congenital melanocytic nevi are candidates for excision as soon as general anesthesia is considered a relatively safe risk. Other issues that need to be considered before undertaking staged excisions include cosmetic issues, functional outcome, and psychosocial issues. The staged excisions are usually started after 6 months of age for nevi on the trunk and extremities and later for those on the scalp to allow closure of the fontanelle. If removal is not undertaken, follow-up with monthly self-examination, photography, dermoscopy, confocal laser microscopy, and computer assistance are recommended.

For small congenital nevi, routine excision is not always recommended because the risk of melanoma is lower, and if it occurs, it usually arises within the epidermis after puberty. If the lesions are not excised, follow-up by alternating visits to a dermatologist and primary care physician along with serial photography are indicated. Inasmuch as small congenital nevi typically enlarge with the growth of the child and can change in appearance with time, educating families on benign, predictable changes in contradistinction to potentially alarming changes is extremely important. If a lesion enlarges or changes suddenly or if parental anxiety or cosmetic issues arise, excision should then be contemplated for even small congenital nevi. Elective excision is best done when the patient is approximately 8 years old. With the use of topical anesthetic cream EMLA (eutectic mixture of local anesthetics: 2.5% lidocaine plus 2.5% prilocaine) or topical 4% lidocaine (ELA-Max), children of this age are usually cooperative and unscathed by the procedure.

Blue Nevi

Blue nevi occur primarily on the face and scalp, in addition to the dorsal surfaces of the hands and feet, as well-circumscribed, slightly raised or dome-shaped bluish papules that are usually less than 1 cm in diameter. Although these lesions are usually acquired in childhood and adolescence, rare congenital lesions have been reported. Histologically, blue nevi demonstrate a combination of intradermal spindle or dendritic melanin-pigmented melanocytes and melanophages with dermal fibrosis. The blue appearance of these lesions is a function of both the depth of the melanin in the dermis and the Tyndall phenomenon: longer wavelengths of light penetrate the deep dermis and are absorbed by the lesional melanin, and shorter wavelengths (e.g., blue) are reflected back. Blue nevi that are clinically stable and that do not demonstrate atypical features do not require removal.

Spitz Nevi

Nevi of large spindle and epithelioid cells (Spitz nevi) are relatively uncommon. In Australia, an annual incidence of 1.4 per 100,000 people has been recorded. Most Spitz nevi are noted in children and adolescents: One third occur before the age of 10 years, one third between the ages 10 to 20 years, and one third past the age of 20 years. Rarely, lesions can occur in patients older than 40 years. Seven percent of SN have been reported as congenital.

Four clinical types of SN are recognized: light-colored soft Spitz nevi that can resemble a pyogenic granuloma; light-colored hard Spitz nevi that can resemble a dermatofibroma; dark Spitz nevi that must be distinguished from other melanocytic lesions, including melanoma; and disseminated or agminated Spitz nevi. Spitz nevi are typically smaller than 6 mm in diameter and dome shaped, with a smooth pink or tan surface and sharp borders. Although they can occur anywhere on the cutaneous surface except mucosal or palmoplantar areas, they are most commonly seen on the face (especially in children) and legs (especially in women). Spitz nevi in adults are usually more heavily melanized than those in children.

Dermatoscopy or epiluminescent microscopy (examination of lesions with enhanced light and a dermatoscope) helps magnify the images in vivo and can assist in establishing the clinical diagnosis of some Spitz nevi. Histologically, the lesion can demonstrate features similar to those of melanoma, which earned the lesion its original designation by Sophie Spitz as a melanoma of childhood. Because Spitz nevi can be histologically difficult to distinguish from melanoma, if a biopsy is performed on a lesion because of parental, cosmetic, or transitional concern, complete excision with clear margins is recommended. Spitz nevi show fundamental genomic differences compared with MM, consistent with the generally benign behavior of these lesions. Spitz nevi typically demonstrate no or only a very restricted set of chromosomal aberrations (i.e., 11p gain in a subset of Spitz nevi).

Dysplastic Melanocytic Nevi

Dysplastic melanocytic nevi, or Clark's nevi, or nevi with architectural disorder and cytologic atypia can occur sporadically as an isolated lesion or lesions or as part of a familial autosomal dominant syndrome. When such lesions occur sporadically, they are considered a marker for a patient who is at increased risk of melanoma (6% risk versus an approximate 0.6% risk in the normal white population in the United States). In association with a family history or personal past medical history of melanoma, patients with dysplastic melanocytic nevi should be considered to have a significant risk of melanoma. One first-degree family member with melanoma is associated with a lifetime risk of melanoma of 15% for the patient with dysplastic melanocytic nevi. Two or more first-degree family members with melanoma place a patient with dysplastic melanocytic nevi at a lifetime risk of developing melanoma that approaches 100%. Less commonly, dysplastic melanocytic nevi can progress to melanoma. Such progression has been documented by serial photography. However, these data are confounded by the fact that clinically and histologically, dysplastic melanocytic nevi may be difficult to distinguish from an early melanoma.

Dysplastic melanocytic nevi are clinically distinguished from common acquired melanocytic nevi by a diameter usually larger than 6 mm, irregular border, asymmetry, and variable color with possible shades of brown, red, pink and black; DMN can be flat with or without a raised center (fried egg appearance). The lesions begin to appear in mid-childhood and early adolescence. New lesions can appear throughout the patient's life. In addition to the back and extremities, these lesions can occur on sun-protected areas, including the scalp, buttocks, and female breasts. Dysplastic melanocytic nevi can be few or numerous, with hundreds of lesions.

Histologically, dysplastic melanocytic nevi show both architectural disorder: extension of the junctional component beyond the dermal component (shouldering); bridging between adjacent rete ridges; papillary dermal concentric and lamellar fibroplasia; and a variable lymphocytic infiltrate with vascular ectasias. They also show cytologic atypia of melanocytes: increased nuclear size, hyperchromasia, dispersion or variation of nuclear chromatin patterns, and presence of nucleoli. Although there is some discordance in the histologic grading of dysplastic melanocytic nevi among expert dermatopathologists, there is some evidence to support the use in clinical practice of a two-tier grading system: Grade A are dysplastic melanocytic nevi with mild or moderate cytologic atypia and grade B are dysplastic melanocytic nevi with severe cytologic atypia. The probability of having a personal history of melanoma in any given dysplastic melanocytic nevi patient correlates with the grade of cytologic atypia in dysplastic melanocytic nevi. In addition, the presence of severe cytologic atypia in dysplastic melanocytic nevi correlates with a significantly greater risk of melanoma development (19.7%) compared with moderate (8.1%) or mild (5.7%) cytologic atypia.

Management of these patients is difficult. Dysplastic melanocytic nevi are not uncommon. Reportedly, as many as 4.6 million people in the United States have one or more sporadic dysplastic melanocytic nevi. Familial dysplastic melanocytic nevi are estimated to involve 50,000 patients in the United States. The risk of melanoma for these patients is probably on a continuum and correlated with their family history of melanoma or dysplastic melanocytic nevi, personal history of melanoma, number of acquired melanocytic and dysplastic lesions, and history of sun exposure. Removal of all dysplastic melanocytic nevi is inappropriate inasmuch as the chance of any single lesion becoming malignant is small and, in addition, the melanoma can arise de novo.

Management includes patient education and total body photography for comparison at future skin examinations. Patients should avoid the sun and use sun screens and protective clothing. These patients should have regular biannual or quarterly examinations of the entire integument, including the oral, genital, and perianal mucosa, the scalp, and an ophthalmologic examination. Comparison with the previous total body photographs and use of the dermatoscope can be helpful. Any lesions that are suspicious for melanoma should be excised. Examination of first-degree family members (parents, siblings, and children) of patients with melanoma or dysplastic melanocytic nevi is recommended to identify other persons at high risk.

REFERENCES

Arumi-Uria M, McNutt NS, Finnerty B. Grading of atypia in nevi: Correlation with melanoma risk. Mod Pathol 2003;16:764–71.

Bauer J, Bastian BC. Distinguishing melanocytic nevi from melanoma by DNA copy number changes: Comparative genomic hybridization as a research and diagnostic tool. Dermatol Ther 2006;19:40–9.

Bett BJ. Large or multiple congenital melanocytic nevi: Occurrence of cutaneous melanoma in 1008 persons. J Am Acad Dermatol 2005;52:793–7.

de Snoo FA, Kroon MW, Bergman W, et al. From sporadic atypical nevi to familial melanoma: Risk analysis for melanoma in sporadic atypical nevus patients. J Am Acad Dermatol 2007;56:748–52.

Ferrara G, Soyer HP, Malvehy J, et al. The many faces of blue nevus: A clinicopathologic study. J Cutan Pathol 2007;34:543–51.

Kinsler VA, Chong WK, Aylett SE, Atherton DJ. Complications of congenital melanocytic naevi in children: Analysis of 16 years' experience and clinical practice. Br J Dermatol 2008;159:907–14.

Krengel S, Hauschild A, Schafer T. Melanoma risk in congenital melanocytic naevi: A systematic review. Br J Dermatol 2006;155:1–8.

Margoob AA, Borrego JP, Halpern AC. Congenital melanocytic nevi: Treatment modalities and management options. Semin Cutan Med Surg 2007;26:231–40.

Naeyaert JM, Brochez L. Dysplastic nevi. N Engl J Med 2003;349:2233–40.

Park HK, Leonard DD, Arrington JH 3rd, Lund HZ. Recurrent melanocytic nevi: Clinical and histologic review of 175 cases. J Am Acad Dermatol 1987;17:285–90.

Melanoma

Method of
Vesna Petronic-Rosic, MD, MSc

Melanoma is a malignancy of pigment-producing cells (melanocytes). Melanocytes are located predominantly in the skin, but they are also found in the eyes, ears, gastrointestinal tract, leptomeninges, and oral and genital mucous membranes.

Epidemiology

Even though melanoma accounts for less than 5% of skin cancer cases, it causes most skin cancer deaths. U.S. incidence figures estimate that there were about 108,230 new cases of melanoma in 2007: 48,290 in situ (noninvasive) and 59,940 invasive (33,910 in men and 26,030 in women). The American Cancer Society's most recent estimates for melanoma in the United States for 2009 are 68,720 new cases with 8,650 deaths. Overall, the lifetime risk for developing melanoma is about 1 in 50 for whites, 1 in 1000 for blacks, 1 in 200 for Latin Americans. At current rates, 1 in 63 Americans will develop an invasive melanoma over a lifetime.

Risk Factors

A large number of nevi is the strongest risk factor for melanoma in persons of European ancestry. Atypical mole syndrome is another risk factor. Exposure to ultraviolet light is a major risk factor, especially in persons who have fair hair and skin, who have solar damage, who had sunburns and short sharp bursts of sun exposure in childhood, and who used tanning beds. Tanning beds appear more detrimental when used before age 20 years. Familial risk factors include mutations in *CDKN2A*, which are associated with increased risks for both melanoma and pancreatic cancer. Organ transplant recipients have an increased risk for melanoma. Genodermatoses with a defect in DNA repair (such as xeroderma pigmentosum) increase risk for melanoma.

Pathophysiology

Transformation of normal melanocytes into melanoma cells likely involves a multistep process of progressive genetic mutations that alter cell proliferation, differentiation, and death and affect susceptibility to the carcinogenic effects of ultraviolet radiation. Primary cutaneous melanoma can develop in preexisting melanocytic nevi, but more than 60% of cases likely appear de novo.

Melanomas arising in skin that is chronically sun damaged show molecular features that distinguish them from melanomas arising in skin that is not sun-damaged. These features might determine tumor behavior and potential response to new targeted drugs. About 70% of melanomas arising in skin that is not sun damaged carry *BRAF* mutations. Genetic studies have shown that 50% of familial melanomas and 25% of sporadic melanomas may be due to mutations in the tumor suppressor gene *p16*. Linkage studies have identified chromosome 9p21 as the site of the familial melanoma gene.

Prevention

Early detection of thin cutaneous melanoma is the best means of reducing mortality. Patients with a history of melanoma should be educated regarding sun protective clothing and sunscreens, skin self-examinations for new primary melanoma, possible recurrence within the surgical scar, and screening of first-degree relatives, particularly if they have a history of atypical moles.

Clinical Manifestations

Early signs of melanoma include the ABCDEs:

- **A**symmetry of lesion
- **B**order irregularity, bleeding, or crusting
- **C**olor change or variegation
- **D**iameter larger than 6 mm or growing lesion
- **E**volving: surface changes or symptomatic

The "ugly duckling" sign is also useful to recognize lesions that look or feel different compared to surrounding moles.

Lentigo maligna (melanoma in situ) begins as an irregular tan-brown macule that slowly expands on sun-damaged skin of elderly persons. Long-term cumulative sun exposure confers the greatest risk. Progression to invasive lentigo maligna melanoma is estimated to be 30% to 50%.

Superficial spreading melanoma, the most common type in light skin, represents approximately 70% of all melanomas. Peak incidence is in the fourth and fifth decade. Superficial spreading melanoma can arise in a preexisting melanocytic nevus that slowly changes over several years; it most commonly affects intermittently sun-exposed areas with the greatest nevus density (upper backs of men and women and lower legs of women). Pigment varies from black and blue-gray to pink or gray-white, and the borders are irregular. Absence of pigmentation often represents regression.

Nodular melanoma represents 15% of all melanomas. The median age at onset is 53 years. Clinically, a uniform blue-black, blue-red, or red nodule usually begins de novo and grows rapidly. About 5% are amelanotic. The most common sites are the trunk, head, and neck.

Acral lentiginous melanoma accounts for 10% of melanomas overall but is the most common type among Japanese, African Americans, Latin Americans, and Native Americans. The median age is 65 years, with equal gender distribution. It occurs on the palms or soles or under the nails, and it is on average 3 cm in diameter at diagnosis. Clinically, the lesion is a tan, brown-to-black, flat macule with color variegation and irregular borders. It does not appear to be linked to sun exposure.

Diagnosis

Excisional biopsy with narrow margins is recommended for diagnosis. Incisional biopsy is acceptable when suspicion for melanoma is low, the lesion is large, or it is impractical to perform a complete excision. It is believed not to be detrimental if subsequent therapeutic surgery is performed within 4 to 6 weeks. Dermatoscopy and total body photography are adjunctive noninvasive diagnostic techniques. Routine laboratory tests and imaging studies are not required for asymptomatic patients with primary cutaneous melanoma 4 mm or less in thickness for initial staging or routine follow-up. Indications for such studies are directed by a thorough medical history and complete physical examination.

Histologic interpretation should be performed by a physician experienced in the microscopic diagnosis of pigmented lesions. Molecular analyses for evidence of gene mutations, DNA copy-number abnormalities, or changed protein expression are useful adjunctive tools in the assessment of histologically ambiguous primary melanocytic tumors.

CURRENT DIAGNOSIS

- ABCDEs:
  - Asymmetry of lesion
  - Border irregularity, bleeding, or crusting
  - Color change or variegation
  - Diameter larger than 6 mm or growing lesion
  - Evolving: surface changes or symptomatic
- The "ugly duckling" sign
- Total-body photography and dermatoscopy
- Excisional biopsy with narrow margins
  - Interpretation by physician experienced in the microscopic diagnosis of pigmented lesions
  - Molecular analyses (rarely)
- Appropriate staging work-up
- Genetic testing when appropriate (rarely)

TABLE 1 Tumor, Node, and Metastasis (TNM) Staging Categories for Cutaneous Melanoma

Tumor (T)

Classification	Thickness (mm)	Ulceration Status/Mitoses
Tis	NA	NA
T1	≤1.00	a: without ulceration and mitosis <1/mm^2 b: with ulceration or mitoses >1/mm^2
T2	1.01-2.00	a: without ulceration b: with ulceration
T3	2.01-3.00	a: without ulceration b: with ulceration
T4	≥4.00	a: without ulceration b: with ulceration

Nodes (N)

Classification	Number of Metastatic Nodes	Nodal Metastatic Burden
N0	0	NA
N1	1	a: Micrometastasis b: Macrometastasis
N2	3	a: Micrometastasis b: Macrometastasis
N3	4+ metastatic nodes or matted nodes or in transit metastases/ satellites with metastatic nodes	c: In transit metastases/ satellites without metastatic nodes

Metastases (M)

Classification	Site	Serum LDH
M0	No distant metastasis	NA
M1a	Distal skin, subcutaneous or nodal metastasis	Normal
M1b	Lung metastasis	Normal
M1c	All other visceral metastasis	Normal
	Any distant metastasis	Elevated

Note: Micrometastases are diagnosed after sentinel lymph node biopsy. Macrometastases are defined as clinically detectable nodal metastases confirmed pathologically.

Abbreviations: is = in situ; LDH = lactate dehydrogenase; NA = not applicable.

The new revised American Joint Committee on Cancer (AJCC) staging system (Tables 1 and 2) includes simplified tumor-thickness thresholds of 1.0, 2.0, and 4.0 mm. Although tumor thickness and ulceration continue to define T2, T3, and T4 categories, T1b melanomas are defined by a tumor mitotic rate of 1/mm^2 or greater or ulceration, rather than Clark level of invasion. N1 and N2 categories remain for microscopic and macroscopic nodal disease respectively, with sentinel node biopsy recommended for pathologic staging. M staging continues to be determined both by site of distant metastasis and serum concentration of lactate dehydrogenase, but in patients with regionally isolated metastases from an unknown primary site, disease will be categorized as stage III rather than stage IV, because the prognosis corresponds to that of stage III disease from a known primary site.

Five-year and 10-year survival rates based on the TNM classification range from 97% and 93% for patients with T1a N0 M0 melanomas to 53% and 39%, respectively for patients with T4b N0 M0 melanomas.

TABLE 2 Pathology Staging for Cutaneous Melanoma and Survival Rates

Stage	T	N	M	5-Year survival	10-Year survival
0	Tis	N0	M0		
IA	T1a	N0	M0	97%	95%
IB	T1b	N0	M0		88%
	T2a	N0	M0		
IIA	T2b	N0	M0	82%	
	T3a	N0	M0	79%	
IIB	T3b	N0	M0	68%	
	T4a	N0	M0	71%	
IIC	T4b	N0	M0	53%	39%
IIIA	T1-4a	N1a	M0		
	T1-4a	N2a	M0		
IIIB	T1-4b	N1a	M0		
	T1-4b	N2a	M0		
	T1-4a	N1b	M0		
	T1-4a	N2b	M0		
	T1-4a	N2c	M0		
IIIC	T1-4b	N1b	M0		
	T1-4b	N2b	M0		
	T1-4b	N2c	M0		
	Any T	N3	M0		
IV	Any T	AnyN	M1		

Pathology staging includes microstaging of the primary melanoma and pathologic information about the regional lymph nodes after partial (i.e., sentinel node biopsy) or complete lymphadenectomy. Pathologic stage 0 or stage IA patients are the exception; they do not require pathologic evaluation of their lymph nodes.
Adapted from Balch CM, Gershenwald JE, Soong SJ, et al: Final version of 2009 AJCC melanoma staging and classification. J Clin Oncol 2009;27 (36):6199-206.

Differential Diagnosis

The differential diagnosis includes melanocytic nevus, angioma, pigmented basal cell carcinoma, pyogenic granuloma, seborrheic keratosis, Kaposi's sarcoma, and hematoma (especially for acral lentiginous melanoma).

Treatment

Early diagnosis combined with appropriate surgical therapy is currently the only curative treatment. The recommended margins are:

- Melanoma in situ: 0.5 cm
- Melanoma <1 mm: 1 cm
- Melanoma 1-2 mm: 1-2 cm
- Melanoma >2 mm: 2 cm

The recommended deep margin is muscle fascia. Wider margins and Mohs micrographic surgery can reduce risk of contiguous subclinical spread for the desmoplastic variant of melanoma.

Sentinel lymph node biopsy provides accurate staging information for patients with clinically unaffected regional nodes and without distant metastases. In cases of positive sentinel node biopsy or clinically detected regional nodal metastases (palpable, positive cytology or histopathology), radical removal of lymph nodes of the involved basin is indicated. There is clinical trial evidence suggesting that the survival outcome for patients who are sentinel node positive is improved if immediate regional lymphadenectomy is done.

For resectable local or in-transit recurrences, excision with a clear margin is recommended. For numerous or unresectable in-transit metastases of the extremities, isolated limb perfusion or infusion with melphalan may be considered.

CURRENT THERAPY

- Early diagnosis and appropriate surgical therapy is the gold standard.
- Complete excision must be achieved with appropriate margins based on tumor thickness.
- Sentinel lymph node biopsy may be offered to patients with melanoma larger than 1 mm, with clinically unaffected regional nodes, and without distant metastases.
- Dissection of the lymph node basin may be offered to patients with micronodal or macronodal metastases.
- Adjuvant therapy may be considered for stage III disease.
- Stage IV treatment depends on location and extent of metastatic disease and may include surgical resection, chemotherapy, biological therapy, or radiation therapy.

Radiotherapy is indicated in select patients with lentigo maligna melanoma, as an adjuvant in select patients with regional metastatic disease, and for palliation, especially in bone and brain metastases.

Numerous adjuvant therapies have been investigated for the treatment of localized cutaneous melanoma following complete surgical removal. Adjuvant interferon (IFN) alfa-2b (Intron A) is the only adjuvant therapy approved by the FDA for high-risk melanoma that affects outcome after surgery. No survival benefit has been demonstrated for adjuvant chemotherapy, nonspecific (passive) immunotherapy, radiation therapy, retinoid therapy, vitamin therapy, or biologic therapy.

Various experimental melanoma vaccines show promise in the adjuvant setting, although caution is needed because four phase III trials (E1694, MMAIT-III [Canvaxin], MMAIT-IV, and EORTC 18961) showed a deleterious effect of the experimental vaccine compared with control intervention. Considerable effort is now being focused on selecting patients on the basis of molecular profiling and on combining agents targeting melanoma-specific aberrations in signaling and apoptotic pathways to overcome the many resistance mechanisms in melanoma cells.

Monitoring

Most metastases occur in the first 1 to 3 years after treatment of the primary tumor, and an estimated 4% to 8% of patients with a history of melanoma develop another primary melanoma, usually within the first 3 to 5 years following diagnosis. The risk of new primary melanoma increases in the setting of multiple dysplastic nevi and family history of melanoma. Consider cancer genetics consultation in patients with three or more melanomas in aggregate in first-degree or second-degree relatives on the same side of the family, families with three or more cases of melanoma or pancreatic cancer on same side of family, and (in low-incidence countries) patients with three or more primary melanomas.

Frequency of monitoring is as follows: For patients with melanoma smaller than 1 mm: every 3 months for 1 year, then every 6 to 12 months for 4 years, then annual examinations thereafter. For patients with melanoma larger than 1 mm: every 3 months for 1 to 2 years, then every 6 months until the fifth year, then annual examinations thereafter.

Follow-up visits for all patients should include a thorough history, review of systems, complete skin examination, and examination of lymph nodes. In patients at high risk for metastatic disease or with an abnormal examination, appropriate imaging studies, laboratory studies, or biopsies may be indicated. Evidence to support the use of routine imaging and laboratory studies in asymptomatic patients with a normal physical examination remains controversial and is left to the discretion of the physician.

Complications

Metastasis may occur locally in the regional lymph node basins, or they can occur distally in the skin (away from the melanoma scar), the remote lymph node(s), the viscera, and skeletal and central nervous system sites.

REFERENCES

Abbasi NR, Shaw HM, Rigel DS, et al. Early diagnosis of cutaneous melanoma: Revisiting the ABCD criteria. JAMA 2004;292(22):2771–6.

American Cancer Society. Overview: Skin cancer: Melanoma. Available at: http://www.cancer.org/docroot/CRI/CRI_2_1x.asp?dt=39; [accessed 12.08.10].

Balch CM, Gershenwald JE, Soong SJ, et al. Final version of 2009 AJCC melanoma staging and classification. J Clin Oncol 2009;27(36):6199–206.

Curtin JA, J Fridlyand J, Kageshita T, et al. Distinct sets of genetic alterations in melanoma. N Engl J Med 2005;353:2135–47.

Eggermont AM. Vaccine trials in melanoma—time for reflection. Nat Rev Clin Oncol 2009;6:256–8.

Leachman SA, Carucci J, Kohlmann W, et al. Selection criteria for genetic assessment of patients with familial melanoma. J Am Acad Dermatol 2009;61(4):677e1–4.

Sladden MJ, Balch C, Barzilai DA, et al. Surgical excision margins for primary cutaneous melanoma. Cochrane Database Syst Rev 2009;(4):CD004835.

Thompson JF, Scolyer RA, Kefford RF. Cutaneous melanoma in the era of molecular profiling. Lancet 2009;374(9687):362–5.

Premalignant Cutaneous and Mucosal Lesions

Method of
Juliet Gunkel, MD

Identification and clinical monitoring of premalignant skin lesions can reduce the morbidity and mortality of skin cancer for many patients with diverse histories and exposures. The link between precancerous and cancerous lesions and ultraviolet (UV) light exposure has been studied extensively. Some patients do not understand the importance of or choose not to adhere to sun-protection precautions and the prudent use of sunscreens. The cause of premalignant lesions also includes human papillomavirus (HPV) disease, arsenic exposures, and degeneration of benign nevi, birthmarks, and neoplasms.

Although certain exposures and conditions are associated with premalignant lesions, some groups of patients are at higher risk for precancerous and cancerous lesions. In many cases, these cancers are rapidly progressive, high grade, and aggressive. Patients who are at high risk are immunocompromised due to human immunodeficiency virus infection or acquired immunodeficiency syndrome, have heritable immunodeficiencies, have had effective immunosuppression of chronic lymphocytic leukemia, have undergone organ transplantation, or are on immunosuppressive medications. An increased susceptibility to infection with oncogenic HPV types may be important in the pathogenesis of malignancies in these patients. Genodermatoses associated with a higher risk of skin cancer include xeroderma pigmentosa, oculocutaneous albinism, Bazex syndrome, and nevoid basal cell carcinoma syndrome. A history of UV exposure and cigarette smoking further compounds the risk for many of these patients.

A variety of dermatoses and neoplasms have a demonstrated association with development of malignancies, although these benign conditions or lesions are not necessarily precancerous. In certain long-standing skin diseases, persistence or progression of characteristic lesions despite apparent appropriate treatment may herald development of skin cancer. Similarly, atypical appearance of or change in the classic lesion of a skin condition or in a previously stable neoplasm is suspicious. These conditions include Zoon balanitis or vulvitis, discoid lupus erythematosus, lichen planus, lichen sclerosus, lymphedema, and chronic radiodermatitis. The neoplasms include nevus sebaceus, plexiform neurofibromas, and leukoplakia or erythroplakia. Scars, epitomized by the persistent scarring seen in dystrophic epidermolysis bullosa, and nonhealing wounds (e.g., burns, chronic ulcers) also may provide sites for malignant growth.

By recognizing these risk factors, predispositions, special populations, and associations, the practitioner can identify premalignant lesions in at-risk patients and recommend appropriate follow-up evaluation and treatment. This approach is essential for prevention and early detection of various types of cancers of cutaneous and mucosal surfaces. Lesions that progress, become symptomatic, become locally destructive or disfiguring, do not respond to appropriate treatment, or change their clinical appearance or behavior should be evaluated for malignancy. Biopsy and referral to a dermatologist are recommended.

Actinic Keratoses or Cheilitis

CLINICAL MANIFESTATIONS

Precursors to squamous cell carcinoma in situ (SCCIS) and squamous cell carcinoma (SCC) can develop on cutaneous and mucosal surfaces subjected to intense, intermittent, or frequent sun exposure. They manifest as flesh-colored, red, or pigmented papules and plaques. Some are rather firm and indurated with a hard scale; others are thin and friable, with a more delicate scale or without scale, appearing shiny and atrophic.

Clinical diagnosis is facilitated by light palpation of sun-exposed sites with the fingertips because the characteristic, gritty, sandpaper-like scale can be very prominent. Involvement can range from multiple or few discrete lesions to an ill-defined zone or field. Occurrence on the lip, often exclusively the lower lip, may be associated with pain, swelling, and fissures. Most lesions remain stable for years without progression or degeneration. The absolute risk is not known but is estimated at 1 case in 1000 lesions per year. Lesions that persist after treatment or show rapid progression should raise suspicion for malignant degeneration. Suspicion should be elevated if mucosal lesions are ulcerated, and biopsy is recommended.

TREATMENT

Limited mechanical removal of discrete lesions is possible with curettage. Liquid nitrogen applied with a cotton-tipped applicator or spraying device is a common and effective treatment for cutaneous and mucosal lesions. Lesions can be treated until they appear white or frozen for 8 to 10 seconds on the lip and other delicate tissues. Thicker skin and thicker lesions require freeze times of 20 seconds or to the patient's tolerance. After this, a second cycle may be used immediately. Some lesions may require two or three such treatments separated by 4 to 12 weeks before resolution. Posttreatment pain, swelling, and blistering can be limiting. Because this modality is nonselective, normal and atypical cells are affected equally.

Treatment of individual lesions with chemical peeling agents such as glycolic acid 20% (e.g., Biomedic MicroPeel Solution)[1] and trichloroacetic acid 10% to 30%[1] can be effective and repeated as needed. These nonselective agents can also be applied to a wider field of involvement for broader effect (i.e., field treatment).

Field treatment also is available as a patient-delivered topical chemotherapy. Topical 5-fluorouracil (available as 0.5% [Carac], 1% [Fluoroplex], and 5% cream [Efudex] for cutaneous surfaces and 1% [Fluoroplex], 2% [Efudex], and 5% solution [Efudex] for mucosal surfaces) can be applied in various regimens, once or twice daily for 2 to 6 weeks as the patient tolerates. More delicate mucosal tissues should be treated once or twice daily for 1 to 3 weeks. Use is limited by development of irritation, pain, and skin breakdown. Because this is a selective chemical treatment, affected cells are targeted, and a more vigorous response should lead to more significant improvement. Inflammatory response is individual, and for patients who are not tolerating treatment well, application can be reduced to once to three times weekly.

---

[1]Not FDA approved for this indication.

Breaks or time off during a treatment course can be introduced. The treatment course can be abbreviated if needed. An effective treatment course also may treat early or in situ lesions of SCC or basal cell carcinoma (BCC) in the field.

Other topical chemotherapeutic field treatments include diclofenac sodium 3% gel (Solaraze) applied once or twice daily for 8 to 12 weeks. The inflammatory response is attenuated and therefore may be better tolerated by patients. Concomitantly, improvement is less dramatic. Imiquimod 5% cream (Aldara) may be applied daily for 3 to 6 weeks or twice daily for 3 days per week for 4 to 8 weeks. Another regimen is once or twice application per week for 4 to 8 months, used continuously or in alternating 1-month cycles. The daily dosing schedule and treatment course should be decreased by about one half for mucosal surfaces. The disadvantage is unpredictability of response. However, imiquimod also may treat early or in situ lesions of SCC and BCC in the field.

Photodynamic treatment is another selective treatment for individual lesions or field treatment. Application of 20% 5-aminolevulinic acid (ALA [Levulan Kerastick]) to affected areas is followed by activation by a light source. Treatment can be completed by the practitioner in 1 day. Before ALA application, scale should be removed with acetone, chemical peel, or microdermabrasion. Alternatively, the patient can apply 5-fluorouracil cream or solution for 5 days or any topical retinoid (tretinoin [Retin-A],[1] adapalene [Differin],[1] or tazarotene [Tazorac][1]) for 1 month. ALA is available as a stick or swablike applicator, and application is challenging on larger areas. After ALA application, absorption or incubation is required: 1 to 2 hours for the face and lips, 3 to 4 hours for the chest and upper extremities, and 5 to 24 hours for the lower extremities. The light source for activation can be laser (585 or 595 nm), intense pulsed light (560 to 1200 nm), or blue light (412 to 422 nm). Only the blue light source is conducive for field treatment. Like 5-fluorouracil and imiquimod, photodynamic therapy may treat early or in situ lesions of BCC or SCC in the field.

[1]Not FDA approved for this indication.

 CURRENT DIAGNOSIS

Actinic Keratoses or Cheilitis

- Flesh-colored, red, or pigmented lesions with thick or delicate keratotic scale
- Swelling, fissures, and scaling on lower lip
- Sun-exposed sites

Arsenical Keratoses

- Punctate, hyperkeratotic lesions of palms and soles
- Exposure to contaminated well water or medications

Porokeratoses

- Lesions with atrophic center and peripheral grooved ridge of hyperkeratosis
- Large and solitary; diffuse, small, and annular on sun-exposed sites; linear, segmental, or generalized; punctate on palms and soles without ridge

Human Papillomavirus Disease

- Verrucous, hyperkeratotic lesions on palms and soles
- Fleshy, hyperkeratotic lesions or shiny, atrophic lesions or erosions in the anogenital region
- White, adherent, keratotic lesions on mucosal surfaces; may become verrucous and exophytic

Atypia in Melanocytic Nevi

- "Fried egg" appearance with a papular center on a macular base
- Asymmetry, ill-defined borders, variegated color, diameter larger than 6 mm, ulceration, bleeding, pain, or pruritus in a new or previously stable pigmented lesion

---

Topical (tretinoin, adapalene, or tazarotene) and oral (acitretin [Soriatane][1]) retinoids can decrease development of actinic keratoses and nonmelanoma skin cancer in at-risk individuals. Efficacy is relatively mild, but any topical retinoid can be used each night indefinitely as tolerated by the patient. Acne and early signs of aging improve with this regimen. Oral retinoids can be used daily or every other day at the lowest dose (acitretin 10 mg) producing clinical improvement. The dose should be titrated up (to 50 mg maximum) as needed and as tolerated. Benefits are conferred only with maintenance of retinoid therapy.

Arsenical Keratoses

CLINICAL MANIFESTATIONS

The small, punctate, hyperkeratotic lesions of arsenical keratoses are seen on the palms and soles of patients exposed to arsenic through contaminated well water and various medications. Carcinoma may develop after 10 to 20 years and evolve from precancerous keratoses or on any skin surface.

TREATMENT

Although acute toxicity can be treated with chelation, it has little value in chronic exposure. As for actinic keratoses, treatment of arsenical keratoses includes cryotherapy, topical chemotherapy, photodynamic therapy, and retinoids.[1] Discrete lesions can be treated with surgery or curettage.

Porokeratoses

CLINICAL MANIFESTATIONS

The classic porokeratosis has a smooth, atrophic center surrounded by a grooved ridge of hyperkeratosis called a *cornoid lamella*. The plaque form (i.e., Mibelli's porokeratosis) is large and progressive, often appearing early in life. The disseminated superficial type favors sun-exposed sites and manifests as numerous, small, annular papules. The linear type may be generalized or segmental and often manifests very early in life. Only the punctate keratotic papules seen in *porokeratosis palmaris, plantaris et disseminate* have no clinically evident cornoid lamellae. Malignant transformation occurs mostly commonly in the linear type, followed by the Mibelli type. It is rare in the disseminated type and has not been reported in the punctate type.

TREATMENT

Treatment modalities include those described for actinic keratoses. Other destructive modalities may be beneficial for discrete lesions, including curettage, surgical excision, dermabrasion, and ablative lasers such as carbon dioxide (CO_2) and erbium yttrium-aluminum-garnet (Er:YAG) lasers.

Human Papillomavirus Disease

CLINICAL MANIFESTATIONS

The clinical manifestations of precancerous HPV infection on cutaneous and mucosal surfaces are diverse. The initial appearance and clinical behavior of verrucous carcinoma (i.e., Buschke-Lowenstein tumor on the genitals and oral florid papillomatosis) is as plantar, genital, and mucosal HPV disease; verrucous hyperkeratotic papules and plaques on the plantar surface; fleshy or hyperkeratotic papules in the anogenital region; and white, adherent keratotic plaques or leukoplakia of the mucosal surfaces. The clinically benign appearance and behavior change may signal malignant degeneration. Lower-risk types HPV-6 and -11 or high-risk HPV-16 may be implicated.

HPV-8, -16, -31, and -33 may be the causative agents in premalignant anogenital squamous intraepithelial lesions. The preferred terms

[1]Not FDA approved for this indication.

CURRENT THERAPY

Actinic Keratoses or Cheilitis

- Physical methods: curettage, liquid nitrogen
- Nonselective topical chemical agents: glycol acid 20%,[1] trichloroacetic acid 10% to 30%[1]
- Selective topical chemical agents: 5-fluorouracil (Carac, Efudex), diclofenac sodium (Solaraze), imiquimod (Aldara), 5-aminolevulinic acid (Levulan Kerastick) activated by a light source, and retinoids, including tretinoin (Retin-A),[1] adapalene (Differin),[1] and tazarotene (Tazorac)[1]
- Oral agents: retinoids[1]

Arsenical Keratoses

- Surgery and modalities used for actinic keratoses

Porokeratoses

- Surgery, dermabrasion, lasers (CO_2 and Er:YAG)
- Modalities for actinic keratoses

Human Papillomavirus Disease

- Blistering agents: liquid nitrogen, Cantharone (0.7% cantharidin),[1,6] podophyllin 25% in tincture of benzoin (Podocon-25), purified podophyllotoxin 0.5% solution or gel (Condylox)
- Keratolytics: topical salicylic acid products (e.g., Compound W, Wart-Off, Dr. Scholl's, Duofilm, Salactic, Mediplast, Sal-Acid), topical retinoids,[1] and topical urea 10% to 40% (Carmol, Gordon's)
- Physical methods: curettage, liquid nitrogen, surgery, ablative laser, electrofulguration, occlusive tapes such as duct tape
- Immunotherapy: imiquimod (Aldara), intralesional candida or mumps antigen injections[1]
- Oral agents: cimetidine (Tagamet)[1]

Atypia in Melanocytic Nevi

- Close clinical observation and mole mapping
- Surgery, curettage, ablative laser

---

[1]Not FDA approved for this indication.
[6]May be compounded by pharmacists.

---

vulvar intraepithelial lesions/neoplasia (VIL/N), *anal intraepithelial lesions/neoplasia* (AIL/N), and *penile intraepithelial lesions/neoplasia* (PIL/N) have replaced the confusing terminology Bowen's disease, erythroplasia of Queyrat, and bowenoid papulosis for these anogenital lesions. Dermatologists reserve the term *bowenoid papulosis* for discrete, fleshy, red-brown papules with a better prognosis that are seen in younger patients. Clinical appearance includes verrucous keratotic plaques, erosions, bowenoid-papulosis–type lesions, erosions, and erythematous, well-demarcated plaques, which may be shiny on the glans penis.

Progressive verrucous leukoplakia may appear as benign leukoplakia early—hyperplastic, thin, white plaques of the mucosal surface. These slowly progress to verrucous exophytic masses, many of which degenerate to SCC. HPV-16 infection has been associated with this multifocal premalignant condition.

Epidermodysplasia verruciformis (EDV) is a rare, inherited condition that predisposes to infection with the less common viral types of HPV-5, -8, -9, -12, -14, -15, -17, -19, -25 through -36, and -38 and with the more common types of HPV-3 and -10. This leads to flat verrucous papules on the extremities, face, and neck, which may be numerous and may coalesce. Lesions similar to tinea versicolor may develop over the trunk. SCC develops in 30% to 60% of these patients, and HPV-5, -8, and -47 are identified in 90% of the lesions.

TREATMENT

Eradication of HPV infection is challenging and often requires months of treatment. Observation may be reasonable for certain lesions with clinically benign appearance and behavior, and spontaneous resolution may occur.

Lesions of nonmucosal sites, including the plantar feet, can be treated by freezing with liquid nitrogen for 10 to 30 seconds for two cycles. This may need to be repeated every 3 to 6 weeks until resolution. Another blistering agent, Cantharone (0.7% cantharidin [Canthacur][1,6], can be applied under occlusion for 6 to 24 hours. The advantage is painless application, but individual responses are unpredictable. Hyperkeratotic lesions, such as those on the plantar surface, require more aggressive use of these modalities. Imiquimod (Aldara)[1] applied daily can be beneficial, but it may require 6 months of treatment. Constant use of occlusive tapes such as duct tape has demonstrated efficacy and may be combined with any treatments. Between liquid nitrogen treatments or as adjunctive therapy, use of keratolytics such as topical salicylic acid products (e.g., liquid [Compound W, Wart-Off, Dr. Scholl's, Duofilm], film [Salactic], plaster [Mediplast, Duofilm, Sal-Acid], compounded in ointment), topical retinoids, and topical urea 10% to 40% (Carmol, Gordon's), as well as mechanical paring, can reduce the size of the lesion. This approach is rarely effective as monotherapy. Oral cimetidine (Tagamet)[1] 30 to 40 mg/kg/day may be a helpful adjunctive therapy. In those demonstrating sensitivity, cure rates of 60% to 80% can be achieved with intralesional candidal (*Candida albicans* skin test antigen [Candin])[1] or mumps antigen (mumps skin test antigen)[1] injections. Surgical treatment, including excision, curettage, and ablative CO_2 laser, have relatively low efficacy and may result in painful scars.

For treatment of lesions in the anogenital region, liquid nitrogen may be used less aggressively. Imiquimod (Aldara) applied twice daily for 3 days of the week for 10 to 16 weeks is about 50% effective. Adjunctive treatment with cimetidine (Tagamet)[1] has a role as described earlier. Physician-applied podophyllin 25% in a tincture of benzoin (Podocon-25) is placed for 4 to 8 hours each week for 6 weeks. Alternatively, purified podophyllotoxin 0.5% solution or gel (podofilox [Condylox]) is applied by the patient over 3 consecutive days for 4 to 6 weeks. Electrofulguration may be the most effective treatment, with a cure rate of 70% at 3 months. Surgical treatment, including excision, curettage, and ablative CO_2 laser, have relatively low efficacy and may result in painful scars.

Lesions of the oral mucosa are best treated with cryotherapy as for anogenital lesions, curettage, surgical excision, electrofulguration, and ablative CO_2 laser.

Treatment recommendations for lesions of EDV include those for lesions on nonmucosal surfaces as described earlier. Although there is no particular treatment for patients with EDV, prevention (i.e., UV protection and smoking cessation) is important, as it is for all patients.

Atypia in Melanocytic Nevi

CLINICAL MANIFESTATIONS

Because almost one half of melanomas arise in benign, preexisting melanocytic nevi, these nevi can be considered premalignant lesions. Nevi manifest as acquired pigmented macules and papules in the first 3 decades of life. Dysplastic nevi are clinically and histologically atypical and therefore likely represent a higher risk. They have a "fried egg" appearance, with a papular center on a macular base, and they are 5 to 12 mm in diameter, larger than common nevi. Their shape is often irregular with indistinct borders and variegated tan, brown, and pink coloration.

The incidence of melanoma arising in a giant congenital melanocytic nevus (CMN) is 2% to 15%. Other associated sarcomas are rare. Giant CMN are pigmented plaques larger than 20 cm in diameter in

---

[1]Not FDA approved for this indication.
[6]May be compounded by pharmacists.

adults. They often cover most of an extremity, the trunk, the scalp, or even the entire dorsal surface in the neonate. They grow with the individual but do not spread. Often, satellites or smaller nevi are seen beyond the border of the primary lesion.

TREATMENT

Pigmented lesions should be monitored for changes such as development of asymmetry, irregular borders, change or variegation in color, and growth, especially greater than 6 mm. Ulceration, bleeding, pain, or pruritus can signal malignant degeneration. On a given individual, identification of the pigmented lesion clinically dissimilar to the others is known as the ugly duckling sign. Changes in a giant CMN or a satellite such as nodularity are worrisome. In these cases, biopsy or very close monitoring, including use of clinical photographs called mole mapping, is essential. For giant CMNs, in theory, decreasing the number of nevus cells should decrease the risk of malignant degeneration, and partial or serial excision using tissue expanders, curettage, and ablative laser treatment may be beneficial.

REFERENCES

Bolognia JL, Jorizzo J, Rapini RP, editors. Dermatology. New York: Mosby; 2003.
James WD, Berger TG, Elston DM, editors. Andrews' Diseases of the Skin—Clinical Dermatology. 10th ed. Philadelphia: WB Saunders; 2006.
McKenna WG, editor. Abeloff's Clinical Oncology. 4th ed. Philadelphia: Churchill Livingstone; 2008.
Morton CA, McKenna KE, Rhodes LE, et al. Guidelines for topical photodynamic therapy: Update. Br J Dermatol 2008;159:1245–66.
Robinson JK, Hanke CW, Sengelman RD, Siegel DM, editors. Surgery of the Skin—Procedural Dermatology. New York: Mosby; 2005.
Wood GS, Gunkel J, Stewart D, et al. Nonmelanoma skin cancers. In: Abeloff MD, Armitage JO, Niederhuber JE, Kastan MB, editors. Abeloff's Clinical Oncology. Philadelphia, 2008.

Bacterial Diseases of the Skin

Method of
Dennis L. Stevens, MD, PhD

The spectrum of bacterial diseases of the skin ranges from superficial, localized, easily recognized, and treated skin eruptions to deep, aggressive, gangrenous, or necrotizing infections that may appear innocuous at first but quickly become life threatening. The prompt recognition and treatment of these infections are paramount in limiting morbidity and mortality. A healthy respect for the aggressiveness of gangrenous and necrotizing infections of the skin and soft tissues is developed by first harboring a high index of suspicion to provide early recognition and appropriate treatment before overwhelming clinical infection occurs.

Common Infections

IMPETIGO

Impetigo is the most common bacterial infection of the skin. It is highly contagious and can occur at any age from infancy to adulthood, but it is most common in preschool-age children. There are two classic forms of impetigo: nonbullous and bullous. Both forms have a predominantly staphylococcal cause, but they manifest with different morphologic characteristics.

Nonbullous (crusted) impetigo can be recognized by the development of a serous, yellow-brown exudate, which dries into a golden crust. Lesions rarely elicit pain but can be associated with erythema and pruritus. They are most common on exposed areas such as the hands, feet, face, and legs and are often associated with a minor traumatic event such as an insect bite, abrasion, or laceration. Crusted impetigo is usually caused by a heavy mixed flora of staphylococci and streptococci. Streptococcal impetigo has been associated with the postinfectious sequelae of post-streptococcal glomerulonephritis.

The bullous variety usually manifests as a rapidly spreading papule, which may progress to a thin-walled vesicle if the lesion is infected with *Staphylococcus aureus*, an organism that produces an exfoliative toxin. These lesions occur most often in warm, moist areas of the body. Predisposing factors include warm ambient temperatures, humidity, poor hygiene, and crowded living conditions.

Treatment of impetigo begins with eradication or with the environmental factors thought to be influential in its development. Aggressive lesion débridement with mesh gauze sponges or brushes and antibacterial soap is encouraged. Special attention to hygiene and disinfection of towels and bedding are also necessary. Topical antibiotic treatment with mupirocin (Bactroban) or bacitracin[1] has been effective in mild to moderate cases. In more extensive cases, oral antibiotic therapy with a penicillinase-resistant synthetic penicillin (oxacillin) is the treatment of choice (Table 1). However, a high percentage of methicillin-resistant strains of *S. aureus* (MRSA) are isolated in institutional and community settings. Patients should be treated for at least 5 to 7 days. If no improvement is seen, lesions should be cultured and antibiotics adjusted appropriately.

Systemic complications from impetigo are very uncommon. Cellulitis has occurred but is usually susceptible to systemic antibiotic therapy. Septicemia and staphylococcal scaled skin syndrome are rare complications of impetigo. When they occur, systemic therapy is indicated.

FOLLICULITIS

Folliculitis is a pyoderma that arises within a hair follicle. The process is known as a furuncle (boil) when the infection extends beyond the hair follicle. These lesions occur most frequently in the moist areas of the body and in areas subject to friction and perspiration. Host factors known to predispose one to folliculitis include obesity, blood dyscrasias, defects in neutrophil function, immune deficiency states (e.g., diabetes, transplantation-related immunosuppression, acquired immunodeficiency syndrome [AIDS]), and treatment with corticosteroids or cytotoxic agents. The offending organism in most immunocompetent patients is *S. aureus*; however, when immunosuppression impairs host

---

[1]Not FDA approved for this indication.

TABLE 1 Suggested Antibiotic Therapy for Gram-Positive Bacterial Isolates

Isolate	Oral	Parenteral
GABHS	Penicillin G or V Erythromycin First-generation cephalosporin	Penicillin G Ampicillin/sulbactam (Unasyn) First-generation cephalosporin
Staphylococcus aureus (methicillin sensitive)	Penicillinase-resistant synthetic penicillin (Oxacillin)	First-generation cephalosporin Clindamycin (Cleocin) Oxacillin
Staphylococcus aureus (methicillin resistant)	Linezolid (Zyvox)	Vancomycin (Vancocin) Daptomycin (Cubicin) Linezolid (Zyvox)
Clostridial species	Penicillin G or V Clindamycin (Cleocin) Metronidazole (Flagyl)	Penicillin G Clindamycin Metronidazole

Abbreviation: GABHS = group A β-hemolytic *Streptococcus*.

defenses, gram-negative organisms (*Klebsiella*, *Enterobacter*, and *Proteus* species) can be involved. *Pseudomonas* species such as *aeruginosa* or *cepacia* are associated with hot-tub folliculitis, which involves numerous hair follicles. It is usually self-limited, resolving in 7 to 10 days.

Successful treatment of folliculitis depends on correcting the predisposing factors that promote the development of this condition. For patients with localized disease, topical wound care including antibiotics such as mupirocin (Bactroban) is effective. Patients with furunculosis or multiple lesions with surrounding erythema of more than 2.5 cm should be treated with orally administered systemic antibiotics that are effective against *S. aureus*. Any fluctuant nodules or abscesses should be incised and drained. Patients with recurrent furunculosis should have their nares cultured for methicillin-susceptible *Staphylococcus aureus* (MSSA) or MRSA because nose rubbing and self-inoculation are the usual means of developing infection. This not only determines which type of *Staphylococcus* is causing the infection, but illustrates to the patient the importance of self-inoculation. Intranasal bacitracin or mupirocin (Bactroban) and daily baths with chlorhexidine (Hibiclens) or hexachlorophene (PHisoHex) (adults only) may break the cycle of nasal colonization and reinfection.

CELLULITIS

Cellulitis is an acute infection of the skin and underlying soft tissues. It commonly begins as a hot, red, edematous, sharply defined eruption and may progress to lymphangitis, lymphadenitis, or in severe cases, necrotizing fasciitis and gangrene. Cellulitis usually occurs in local skin trauma caused by insect bites, abrasions, surgical wounds, contusions, or other cutaneous lacerations. Immunosuppressed patients are particularly susceptible to the progression of cellulitis to regional or systemic infections, and these patients should be treated aggressively with systemic antibiotics, drainage, and débridement when indicated. Cellulitis is 20-fold more common in patients with chronic venous stasis or lymphedema. Recurrent cellulitis may occur in patients at the exact site of saphenous donor site surgery.

Initial presentation is that of a rapidly expanding, tender, erythematous, indurated area of skin. An ascending lymphangitis may be present, especially in cellulitis involving an extremity often associated with regional lymphadenopathy. Systemic signs and symptoms can eventually evolve and when present, mandate hospitalization and treatment with systemic antibiotics. Offending organisms are most commonly group A β-hemolytic *Streptococcus* (GABHS) species and *S. aureus*. Cellulitis caused by *S. aureus* usually is associated with localized abscess, furuncles, or carbuncles. In diabetic patients, cellulitis can be caused by group B *Streptococcus*.

Localized processes are treated with oral antibiotics (see Table 1). If fever, septicemia, or other signs of advancement to deeper tissues are present, the patient should be admitted to the hospital for blood and wound cultures, parenteral antibiotics (see Table 1), and observation. If a prompt response is not observed after parenteral antibiotic treatment, surgical exploration of the involved area may be indicated to establish an etiologic diagnosis and rule out the presence of necrotic or gangrenous tissue. Immunosuppressed patients or patients with recurrent cellulitis should be extensively examined to exclude chronic sources of infection, and these patients should be treated with parenteral antibiotics until the cellulitis resolves, followed by 5 to 7 days of oral antibiotics.

ABSCESS

Local skin signs and symptoms such as pain (dolor), redness (rubor), warmth (calor), and swelling (tumor) often denote an abscess. Loss of function associated with fluctuation may also indicate abscess formation. Localization of purulent fluid necessitates surgical drainage and local wound care. The administration of oral or parenteral antibiotic therapy should not be used routinely after incision and drainage of localized abscesses. They should be administered only when clinically indicated, and antibiotic therapy should be based on culture and sensitivity testing.

CURRENT DIAGNOSIS

- Most infections are superficial and local and not associated with systemic toxicity.
- Deeper infections may involve many layers of the soft tissues, including fascia and muscle.
- Systemic toxicity is always present in deeper infections.
- Rapid advancement of the local infection with areas of necrosis indicates more serious infections, including necrotizing and gangrenous processes.
- Streptococci and clostridial microorganisms are the cause of most gangrenous infections.
- Mixed aerobic and anaerobic microflora cause most necrotizing infections.

Life-Threatening Infections

GROUP A β-HEMOLYTIC STREPTOCOCCAL GANGRENE

Group A β-hemolytic streptococcal gangrene is an extremely rapidly progressing skin and soft tissue infection commonly caused by *Streptococcus pyogenes*. These organisms secrete hemolysins and streptolysins O and S, which are cardiotoxic, leukocytic, and responsible for the characteristic hemolysis. Gangrene results when the cutaneous blood vessels thrombose, a finding that is often associated with intense local pain. The involved skin is initially erythematous and indurated and quickly evolves to hemorrhagic blebs with focal necrotic zones. The potential for extensive tissue loss and mortality exists, especially if treatment is delayed. Prompt, aggressive tissue débridement and antibiotic therapy are necessary for a favorable outcome (see Table 1).

SYNERGISTIC NECROTIZING CELLULITIS

Synergistic necrotizing cellulitis (SNC) is an extremely aggressive, often lethal, polymicrobial infection of the skin and soft tissues, which exhibits progressive invasion superficial to fascial planes. This condition may initially begin as a benign process with scant indication of its impending severity. The initial lesion is typically an erythematous, tender pustule or abscess with a small area of necrosis. The benign appearance of this lesion belies the widespread and aggressive tissue destruction that has occurred beneath it.

Direct inspection through skin incisions reveals extensive gangrene of the superficial tissues and fat that rarely involves the underlying fascia and muscles. These lesions characteristically exude a thin, brown, malodorous discharge, which manifests mixed flora with abundant polymorphonuclear leukocytes with a Gram stain. Crepitus, which is caused by the accumulation of gas in the tissue produced by facultative or obligate anaerobes, can be palpated in 25% of patients, and it mandates immediate surgical attention.

The most common site of involvement is the perineum, which is involved in 50% of patients with SNC. Predisposing factors include perirectal abscess and ischiorectal abscess, both of which may track to the deeper structures of the pelvis, leading to abscess formation and subsequent septicemia. The thigh and leg are involved in approximately 40% of patients. This infection can occur after amputation and is usually associated with diabetes mellitus (75% of cases) or peripheral vascular disease (50% of cases). The relative immunosuppression and poor circulation that accompany these significant causes of morbidity are also responsible for upper extremity and neck SNC, which account for the remaining 10% of cases.

Synergistic necrotizing cellulitis is commonly caused by mixed flora originating in the gastrointestinal tract. Coliforms are the most prevalent aerobes (*Escherichia coli*, *Klebsiella*, *Proteus*), and anaerobic flora include *Bacteroides*, *Peptostreptococcus*, *Clostridium*, and *Fusobacterium*. The primary treatment modality is aggressive

TABLE 2 Suggested Parenteral Antibiotic Therapy for Mixed Infections

Organisms	Primary Choice
Aerobic (must include an agent effective against anaerobic organisms)	Amikacin (Amikin) Aztreonam (Azactam) Ceftriaxone (Rocephin) Ciprofloxacin (Cipro) Gentamicin (Garamycin) Levofloxacin (Levaquin) Tobramycin (Nebcin)
Body ID: T13015002.100 Anaerobic (must include an agent effective against aerobic organisms)	Clindamycin (Cleocin) Metronidazole (Flagyl)
Body ID: T13015002.150 Aerobic and anaerobic coverage	Ampicillin/sulbactam (Unasyn) Imipenem/cilastatin (Primaxin) Meropenem (Merrem) Piperacillin/tazobactam (Zosyn) Tigecycline (Tygacil)

débridement of nonviable skin and subcutaneous tissues. This may involve several operations and dressing changes under general anesthesia, which should be performed until all necrotic tissue is removed. Rotation or free myocutaneous flaps and split-thickness skin grafting may cover areas of tissue loss when necessary. If the perineum is involved, fecal diversion by colostomy may be necessary to facilitate healing. Empiric parenteral antibiotics effective against polymicrobial gram-positive and gram-negative aerobic and anaerobic flora are also a mainstay of therapy. However, antibiotic coverage must be modified as soon as culture and susceptibility testing reveal specific offending organisms (Table 2) to reduce the emergence of resistant organisms.

CLOSTRIDIAL MYONECROSIS

Clostridial myonecrosis (i.e., gas gangrene) is a destructive infectious process of muscle associated with infections of the skin and soft tissues. It is often associated with local crepitus and systemic signs of toxemia, which are caused by the anaerobic, gas-forming bacilli of the *Clostridium* species. This infection most often occurs after abdominal operations on the gastrointestinal tract; penetrating trauma, such as gunshot wounds, and frostbite can also expose muscle, fascia, and subcutaneous tissues to these organisms. Common to all these conditions is an environment containing tissue necrosis, low oxygen tension, and sufficient amounts of amino acids and calcium to allow germination of clostridial spores and production of the lethal α toxin.

Clostridia are gram-positive, spore-forming, obligate anaerobes that are widely found in soil contaminated with animal excreta. They have also been isolated in the human gastrointestinal tract and skin, most importantly in the perineum and oropharynx. *Clostridium perfringens* is the most common isolate (in 80% of cases) and is among the fastest growing clostridial species, having a generation time under ideal conditions of approximately 16 minutes. This organism produces collagenases and proteases that cause widespread tissue destruction and produces α toxin, which is associated with the high mortality rate of clostridial myonecrosis. The α toxin, a phospholipase C, causes platelet-neutrophil complexes, vascular obstruction, and extensive compromised vascular perfusion, leading to necrosis of the muscle and overlying fascia, skin, and subcutaneous tissues.

Historically, clostridial myonecrosis was a disease associated with battle injuries, but 60% of current cases occur after trauma: 50% after automobile accidents and the remainder after crush injuries, industrial accidents, and gunshot wounds. Mortality can be the result of a failure to recognize that clostridial infection is under way, which leads to a delay in the débridement of devitalized tissues. Patients often complain of a sudden onset of pain at the site of trauma or

surgical wound, which increases rapidly in severity and extends beyond the original borders of the wound. The skin initially exhibits tense edema, but its pale appearance progresses to a magenta hue. Hemorrhagic bullae and a thin, watery, foul-smelling discharge are common. A Gram stain examination of wound discharge reveals abundant gram-positive rods with a paucity of leukocytes.

The diagnosis of gas gangrene is based on the appearance of the muscle on direct visualization by surgical exposure, because many changes are not apparent when inspected through a small traumatic wound. Initially, the muscle is pale, edematous, and unresponsive to stimulation. As the disease process continues, the muscle becomes frankly gangrenous, black, and extremely friable. This occurs as a late event and is often accompanied by septicemia and shock. Despite profound hypotension and impending organ failure, these patients may be remarkably alert and extremely sensitive to their surroundings. They feel their impending doom and often panic just before slipping into toxic delirium and eventually into coma.

The clinical features should arouse suspicion early in the course, so the disease can be recognized and treated with aggressive surgical débridement. Gas in the wound is a relatively late finding, and by the time crepitation is observed, the patient may be near death. Approximately 15% of blood cultures are positive, but this is also a late finding. Serum creatinine kinase levels, although relatively nonspecific, are always elevated in cases with muscle involvement.

The mortality rate for gas gangrene is as high as 60%. It is highest in cases involving the abdominal wall and lowest in those affecting the extremities. Among the signs that prognosticate a poor outcome are leukopenia, thrombocytopenia, hemolysis, and severe renal failure. Myoglobinuria is common and can contribute significantly to worsening renal function. Frank hemorrhage may also be present and indicates disseminated intravascular coagulation.

Successful treatment of this life-threatening infection depends on early recognition and débridement of devitalized and infected tissues. Hyperbaric oxygen and systemic antibiotics are important adjuncts. Surgical intervention should include wide débridement of all necrotic tissue and amputation if extremities are involved. Hyperbaric oxygen (100% O_2 at 3 atm) has been reported to reduce associated tissue loss and mortality; however, core treatment is surgical débridement, and it should never be delayed to arrange for hyperbaric oxygen treatments. In animal studies of gas gangrene, hyperbaric oxygen was not efficacious, whereas clindamycin (Cleocin) treatment had dramatic effects in reducing mortality. A parenteral antibiotic is directed toward the offending organism (see Table 1). Clindamycin is the treatment of choice because of its ability to suppress toxin production. Cardiovascular collapse mandates careful monitoring of intravenous fluid resuscitation, which may require large volumes. Failure to adequately resuscitate these patients compromises therapy by limiting oxygen delivery and antibiotic distribution to the affected tissues and may promote progression to multisystem organ failure.

A less life-threatening form of this disease is known as clostridial cellulitis. In this process, the bacterial tissue invasion is primarily superficial, extending to the fascial layer without muscle involvement. Prompt recognition and treatment can reduce morbidity and mortality. Spontaneous gas gangrene caused by *Clostridium septicum* can occur in the absence of trauma in patients with gastrointestinal lesions such as carcinoma of the colon.

NECROTIZING FASCIITIS

Necrotizing fasciitis is an aggressive soft tissue infection involving the fascia with extensive undermining and tracking along anatomic planes. This process usually occurs in patients with significant comorbidity, such as diabetes mellitus or peripheral vascular disease, but it is also seen in obese or malnourished patients and intravenous drug abusers. Cellulitis is a frequent occurrence, and progressive necrosis to subcutaneous tissue results from thrombosis of the perforating vessels. Necrotizing fasciitis can be caused by single organisms such as GABHS and staphylococci (MRSA), *Vibrio vulnificus* or *Aeromonas hydrophila*, or a combination of a variety of organisms, including aerobic streptococci, staphylococci, and coliforms, as well as anaerobic *Peptostreptococcus* and *Bacteroides*. Ninety percent of these infections have a polymicrobial cause, and it is common to culture up to five organisms from the fascial planes involved with this infection.

Polymicrobial necrotizing fasciitis most commonly evolves from a benign-appearing skin lesion (80% of cases). Minor abrasions, insect bites, injection sites, and perirectal abscesses have been implicated. Rare cases have been reported in women with Bartholin's gland abscess, from which the infection has spread to fascial planes of the perineum and thigh. The remaining 20% of patients have no visible skin lesion. Surgical procedures, especially bowel resections, and penetrating trauma can be complicated by superficial wound infections that evolve into necrotizing fasciitis. The infection commonly involves the buttocks and perineum, which results from untreated perirectal abscesses or decubitus ulcers; intravenous drug abusers commonly participate in *skin popping*, which leads to infections of the upper extremities.

Fifty percent of group A streptococcal necrotizing fasciitis patients have a portal of entry such as an insect bite, slivers, surgical procedures, or burns, whereas the other 50% have no portal of entry, and the infection begins at the exact site of nonpenetrating trauma, such as a muscle strain or bruise. This idiopathic form, commonly known as spontaneous necrotizing fasciitis, is particularly dangerous because of the frequent delay in diagnosis.

For those with a portal of entry, the initial presentation is a slowly advancing cellulitis that progresses to a firm, tense, woody feel of the subcutaneous tissues. This entity may be distinguished from other aggressive anaerobic soft tissue infections (e.g., SNC) by the brawny, pale, erythematous appearance of the skin overlying subcutaneous tissues that are unyielding, making fascial planes and muscle groups indistinguishable during palpation. Often, a broad, erythematous tract along the route of the underlying fascial plane can be discerned through the skin. If an open wound exists, probing the edges with a blunt instrument permits ready dissection of the superficial fascia well beyond the wound margins, and this is the most important diagnostic feature of necrotizing fasciitis. On direct inspection, the fascia is swollen and dully gray in appearance, with stringy areas of fat necrosis. A thin, brown exudate can be expressed from the wound, but frank purulent drainage is rare. These wounds are remarkably insensate when found and mandate immediate débridement.

As with other gangrenous soft tissue infections, the most important component of the treatment plan is aggressive, total débridement of all devitalized and necrotic tissue. This often necessitates frequent operations and dressing changes. Wide débridement and parenteral antibiotics have a profound effect on survival, and limited or staged débridement has no place in the treatment of this very aggressive, life-threatening infection. Parenteral antibiotics (see Table 2) should be directed against the polymicrobial aerobic and anaerobic microorganisms isolated from these infections. Every effort should be made to quickly identify the offending organisms, and antibiotic therapy should be changed accordingly.

CURRENT THERAPY

- Local care and oral antibiotics chosen for the suspected or culture-proven pathogens are the usual treatment for most limited skin infections.
- Infections that show evidence of rapid advancement associated with bullae, blebs, crepitus, or necrosis require parenterally administered antibiotics and prompt surgical débridement.
- Morbidity and mortality rates associated with the deeper infections increase with delays in antibiotic therapy and surgical débridement.
- Antibiotic therapy should be guided by clinical presentation and changed if necessary when culture and sensitivity studies are available.

In patients with no defined portal of entry, severe pain at the site of previous nonpenetrating trauma is common. Early in the course, there may be no cutaneous evidence of infection. Severe pain and fever may be the only presenting symptoms. These patients usually have a slightly elevated white blood cell count with a left shift and an elevated pulse. Later, erythema, induration, and warmth occur and may rapidly progress to violaceous skin, ecchymosis, and blister formation. A markedly elevated creatine phosphokinase levels in a patient with any erythematous rash may suggest a necrotizing process. By the time these late cutaneous findings are present, most patient have evidence of shock and organ failure. Misdiagnosis and delay in diagnosis are common and associated with significant morbidity and mortality. Surgical exploration with débridement of infected and necrotic tissue in addition to systemic antibiotic therapy directed toward the aerobic *Streptococcus* organism can result in decreased morbidity and mortality (see Table 1).

Special Circumstances

FOURNIER'S GANGRENE

Fournier's gangrene is a necrotizing fasciitis that originates as a necrotic black area on the scrotum of male patients or the labia of female patients, and it most often has a cryptogenic origin. In my experience, Fournier's gangrene occurs more commonly without a predisposing event or after routine, uncomplicated hemorrhoidectomy. Less commonly, this condition has occurred after urologic manipulation or as a late complication of deep anorectal suppuration.

Fournier's gangrene is characterized by necrosis of the skin and soft tissues of the scrotum or perineum and is associated with a fulminant, painful, and severely toxic infection. Definitive diagnosis is made by identification of a necrotic black area on the scrotum associated with local and systemic signs of infection. Left untreated, death ensues from uncontrolled, severe systemic sepsis and multiple-organ failure. Prompt recognition and treatment can minimize tissue loss, especially the skin and soft tissues of the scrotum, labia, and perineum, and may prevent complete loss of genitalia.

The infection is often polymicrobial, as with necrotizing fasciitis, with several species of aerobic and anaerobic bacteria predominating. Successful treatment is based on early recognition and vigorous surgical débridement, occasionally including diversion of the fecal stream. Empiric treatment is appropriate until results of culture and susceptibility testing are available (see Table 2). The therapeutic benefit of hyperbaric oxygen treatments has not been proved and, it should be used only as an adjunct to surgical débridement.

ECTHYMA GANGRENOSUM

Occasionally, hospitalized patients with overwhelming pseudomonal septicemia develop a patchy dermal and subcutaneous necrosis. Although sepsis caused by *Pseudomonas aeruginosa* is often indistinguishable from other types of gram-negative sepsis, a characteristic skin lesion may develop with erythematous macular eruptions that quickly become bullous with central ulceration and necrosis. This lesion may resemble a decubitus ulcer with the characteristic black eschar. There are usually multiple lesions occurring in different stages of development. They may concentrate on the extremities or the gluteal region. These lesions may be distinguished from the lesions of pyoderma gangrenosum (a noninfectious dermatosis) by their association with clinical signs of infection (i.e., fever and leukocytosis) in addition to the isolation of *P. aeruginosa* from culture of the lesion.

Treatment is primarily administration of antimicrobial therapy effective against the *Pseudomonas* organism and by débridement of the multiple lesions. This may lessen the bacterial burden, perhaps allowing greater antibiotic efficacy.

SEA AND FRESH WATER INFECTIONS

Infections caused by *V. vulnificus* and *A. hydrophilia* can be extremely aggressive, with necrosis often occurring within hours and necessitating rapid, wide débridement. Although infections caused by these organisms cannot be differentiated from those caused by mixed infections, a history of exposure to sea water (*V. vulnificus*) or fresh water (*A. hydrophila*) and the rapidity with which the infection spreads often suggest the cause of the infection. The antibiotics of choice for *V. vulnificus* infection are doxycycline (Vibramycin) or tetracycline and an aminoglycoside. In patients with impaired renal function, chloramphenicol (Chloromycetin) may be used. *A. hydrophila* is susceptible to cephalosporins such as ceftazidime (Fortaz), cefuroxime (Ceftin), and fluoroquinolones such as levofloxacin (Levaquin) and ciprofloxacin (Cipro).

Conclusions

The many types of soft tissue infections caused by bacteria may be distinguished by their presenting signs, symptoms, and body location and by the time course of the pathologic processes unique to each. Early recognition is of paramount importance to the effective treatment plan, which most often includes aggressive surgical débridement and specific antimicrobial therapy. This approach can often minimize tissue damage and promote recovery.

REFERENCES

Adinolfi MF, Voros DC, Moustoukas NM, et al. Severe systemic sepsis resulting from neglected perineal infections. South Med J 1983;76:746–9.
Craig ML, Hardin Jr WD, Fox LS, et al. Ecthyma gangrenosum: A deadly complication. Hosp Physician 1987;23:65–71.
Moustoukas NM, Nichols RL, Voros D. Clostridial sepsis: Usual clinical presentations. South Med J 1985;78:440–5.
Nichols RL, Florman S. Clinical presentations of soft-tissue infections and surgical site infections. Clin Infect Dis 2001;33(Suppl. 2):84–93.
Nichols RL. Postoperative infection in the age of drug-resistant gram-positive bacteria [review]. Am J Med 1998;104(Suppl. 5A):11S–16S.
Stevens DL, Bisno AL, Chambers HF, et al. Practice guidelines for the diagnosis and management of skin and soft-tissue infections. Clin Infect Dis 2005;41:1373–406.
Stevens DL. Necrotizing infections of the skin and fascia, UpToDate 2009;9.2 Available at: www.uptodate.com [accessed June 2009].

Viral Diseases of the Skin

Method of
Sylvia L. Brice, MD

Herpes Simplex Viruses 1 and 2

Herpes simplex virus types 1 and 2 (HSV-1 and HSV-2) are the most closely related members of the human herpesvirus family, and the skin lesions they produce are clinically indistinguishable. Clusters of tense blisters on an erythematous base often quickly evolve into erosions or ulcerations with associated crusting. Lesions can develop at any mucocutaneous site but are typically found in the perioral or anogenital regions. Both HSV-1 and HSV-2 are transmitted by direct mucocutaneous contact with an infected host. Following viral replication in the skin or mucosa, intact viral nucleocapsids travel via sensory neurons to the corresponding dorsal root ganglia to establish latency. Later, a variety of stimuli can trigger reactivation. The virus travels back along the sensory neurons to the mucocutaneous surface to replicate and induce active or subclinical infection. In the case of subclinical infection, no active skin lesions are evident, but infectious particles are present, a state known as asymptomatic shedding. Although the viral titer is much lower than during clinically active disease, asymptomatic shedding of the virus in oral and genital

secretions is thought to be responsible for the majority of cases of HSV transmission.

Primary, initial nonprimary (also known as first episode), and recurrent are terms used to further define the nature of the HSV infection. A *primary* infection refers to a patient's first infection with either type of HSV at any site. These patients are seronegative initially but subsequently develop HSV type-specific antibodies. A patient who is already infected with one HSV type and then develops an infection with the alternate type experiences an *initial nonprimary* or first-episode infection (e.g., the first episode of genital herpes in a patient with a prior history of orofacial herpes). These patients are seropositive for one type-specific HSV antibody (e.g., HSV-1) and later develop antibodies specific for the alternate HSV type (e. g., HSV-2). A *recurrent* infection is one that occurs at a site of prior infection. These patients are seropositive for HSV-1 or HSV-2, or both. Because most primary infections, whether oral or genital, are asymptomatic, the first evidence of disease often represents a recurrent or initial nonprimary infection.

OROFACIAL HERPES SIMPLEX VIRUS INFECTION

Orofacial HSV, also known as herpes labialis, fever blisters, or cold sores, is commonly acquired during childhood or adolescence. symptomatic primary disease usually takes the form of gingivostomatitis with or without additional lesions on the cutaneous perioral surfaces. Fever, malaise, and tender lymphadenopathy may also be present. In recurrent episodes, clusters of blisters erupt along the vermillion border of the lips, and subsequent erosions and crusting persist for several days up to 2 weeks. Lesions can develop anywhere in the perioral area, especially on the cheeks. In men, a viral folliculitis of the beard area (herpetic sycosis) may be mistaken for a bacterial process because it is often pustular. The presence of a prodrome and recurrence in the same site are clues to the correct diagnosis. Although recurrent intraoral lesions of HSV can occur, they are uncommon in immunocompetent persons. Exposure to ultraviolet light is a common trigger factor for herpes labialis, as is fever or intercurrent infection.

GENITAL HERPES SIMPLEX VIRUS INFECTION

When symptomatic, primary genital herpes often involves bilaterally distributed lesions in the anogenital area with associated fever, inguinal adenopathy, and dysuria or urinary retention. Aseptic meningitis can also occur. The lesions often persist for 2 to 3 weeks or longer. Nonprimary infections are usually less severe and have fewer constitutional symptoms. Recurrent episodes tend to be milder and shorter in duration. Often, there is a prodrome of tingling or burning followed by the development of localized vesicles that can quickly rupture, leaving nonspecific erosions or ulcerations. The lesions may be anywhere within the anogenital region but tend to recur close to the same area in subsequent episodes. The time between exposure and development of primary disease is estimated to be from 3 to 14 days. However, more often the first clinical indication of disease is a recurrence, which can occur weeks to years after the initial infection. Prior infection with HSV-1 provides some protection against acquisition of HSV-2.

Based on seroepidemiologic evidence, it is estimated that approximately 17% of the United States population aged 14 to 49 years is infected with HSV-2. In most of these persons, this disease has not been officially diagnosed and they are unaware that they are infected. Nevertheless, they experience asymptomatic shedding and unknowingly transmit the disease to sexual partners. Interrupting this cycle of transmission has become a major focus among health care providers who work with these patients. A combination of patient education and appropriate use of systemic antiviral agents may be gradually having some impact on this epidemic. Recommendations for patients with genital herpes include avoiding sex with uninfected partners when active lesions or prodromal symptoms are present and routinely using latex condoms to minimize transmission during periods of asymptomatic shedding. Chronic suppressive doses of oral antiviral agents (Table 1), including acyclovir (Zovirax), valacyclovir (Valtrex), and famciclovir (Famvir), significantly reduce the

TABLE 1 Recommendations for Systemic Antiviral Treatment of Mucocutaneous Herpes Simplex Virus Infection

Episode	Drug	Dosage
Genital Herpes Simplex Virus		
Primary or first episode	Acyclovir	Mild to moderate: 400 mg PO tid[3] or 200 mg PO 5 ×/d × 7-10 d
		Severe: 5 mg/kg IV q8h × 5 d
	Valacyclovir	1 g PO bid × 7-10 d
	Famciclovir[1]	250 mg PO tid × 10 d
Recurrent episode (start at prodrome)	Acyclovir	400 mg PO tid[3] or 200 mg PO 5 ×/d × 5 d
	Valacyclovir	500 mg PO bid × 3 d *or* 1 g daily × 5 d
	Famciclovir	1 g PO bid × 1 d *or* 125 mg PO bid × 5 d
Chronic suppression	Acyclovir	>6 outbreaks per year: 400 mg PO bid *or* 200 mg PO tid
		Adjust up or down according to response
	Valacyclovir	6-10 outbreaks per year: 500 mg PO qd
		≥10 outbreaks/year: 1 g PO qd
	Famciclovir	≥6 outbreaks/year: 250 mg PO bid
Orofacial Herpes Simplex Virus		
Primary or first episode	Acyclovir[1]	15 mg/kg 5 ×/d × 7 d
	Valacyclovir[1]	1 g bid × 7 d
	Famciclovir[1]	500 mg bid × 7 d
Recurrent episode (start at prodrome)	Acyclovir[1]	400 mg PO 5 ×/d × 5 d
	Valacyclovir	2 g PO bid × 1 d
	Famciclovir	1500 mg in 1 dose
Chronic suppression	Acyclovir[1]	400 mg PO bid-tid
	Valacyclovir[1]	500 mg-1 g PO qd
Orolabial or Genital Herpes Simplex Virus in Immunosuppressed Patients		
Recurrent or suppressive	Acyclovir[1]	400 mg PO tid *or* 5-10 mg/kg IV q8h
	Valacyclovir	500 mg-1 g PO bid
	Famciclovir	500 mg PO bid

[1]Not FDA approved for this indication.
[3]Exceeds dosage recommended by the manufacturer.

frequency of clinical recurrences as well as the rate of asymptomatic shedding and may be recommended together with these other practices to reduce the risk of transmission.

Although HSV-2 is the etiologic agent in a majority of cases of genital herpes infections, an increasing number of genital herpes infections are caused by HSV-1. Symptomatic recurrences and asymptomatic shedding are less frequent with genital HSV-1 infection than with genital HSV-2 infection, and this distinction becomes important for patient counseling and prognosis.

OTHER MUCOCUTANEOUS HERPES SIMPLEX VIRUS INFECTIONS

Eczema herpeticum, also known as Kaposi's varicelliform eruption, represents a cutaneous dissemination of HSV usually seen in patients with atopic dermatitis or other underlying skin disease. Herpetic vesicles develop over an extensive mucocutaneous surface, most often the face, neck, and upper trunk, presumably spreading from a recurrent oral HSV infection or asymptomatic shedding from the oral mucosa. Eczema herpeticum can also develop in the presence of genital HSV. As with other HSV infections, eczema herpeticum may be recurrent. In addition, patients can develop localized, recurrent HSV in previously involved areas. Because of the extensive and inflammatory nature of the process and the possible secondary bacterial infection, the underlying viral etiology may be obscured. A history of eczema and

recurrent HSV in the patient and careful observation for the grouped vesicles or erosions can be key to the correct diagnosis.

Herpetic whitlow refers to HSV infection of the hand, usually one or more distal digits. Previously thought to be limited to health care professionals with exposure to oral secretions of their patients, it is now recognized that autoinoculation from orolabial or genital HSV contributes to a significant number of cases.

Herpes gladiatorum is a problem seen most commonly in athletes who participate in close contact sports such as wrestling. Typically transmitted from active herpes labialis or asymptomatic shedding in oral secretions of an infected opponent, herpes gladiatorum often affects the head, neck, or shoulders and may be recurrent. In the wrestler with frequent outbreaks chronic suppressive therapy may be recommended.

DIAGNOSIS

Viral culture remains a common and acceptable method for diagnosing HSV infection. This method is sensitive when specimens are obtained from lesions that have not yet become too dry or crusted, usually during the first 2 to 3 days after onset. An adequate sample, obtained by unroofing the blister and swabbing the base, increases the likelihood of an accurate result. Antigen detection tests can remain positive even after lesions have dried, as long as the specimen includes epithelial cells and not just debris. For this method, a scraping from the lesion is usually smeared on a glass slide to be sent to the laboratory.

Not all antigen detection methods are designed to distinguish HSV-1 from HSV-2. The Tzanck smear (cytologic detection) is both insensitive

CURRENT DIAGNOSIS

Herpes Simplex Viruses 1 and 2

- Clinical: Grouped vesicles or erosions, especially in perioral or anogenital location
- Laboratory: Tzanck smear, viral culture, antigen detection, PCR, gG-based type-specific serology

Varicella-Zoster Virus

- Clinical: Papules, pustules, vesicles in diffuse (varicella) or dermatomal (herpes zoster) distribution
- Laboratory: Tzanck smear, antigen detection, viral culture

Hand-Foot-and-Mouth Disease

- Clinical: Papulovesicles on oral mucosa, hands, feet following fever, constitutional symptoms
- Laboratory: Viral culture, PCR, serology

Parvovirus B19

- Clinical: "Slapped cheeks" reticular erythema on trunk or extremities following fever, constitutional symptoms; arthralgias, arthritis, purpuric eruptions; transient aplastic crisis, fetal hydrops
- Laboratory: B19 specific IgM serology, PCR

Molluscum Contagiosum

- Clinical: Few to multiple 1- to 4-mm umbilicated flesh-colored papules
- Laboratory: Histopathology if clinical appearance atypical

Orf

- Clinical: One to several solid to vesicular nodules on hands, forearms; history of exposure to sheep, goats, cattle
- Laboratory: Histopathology if clinical appearance atypical; PCR

Abbreviations: gG = glycoprotein G; HSV = herpes simplex virus; IVIg = intravenous immunoglobulin; PCR = polymerase chain reaction.

and nonspecific but may be of use in some clinical settings. It does not differentiate HSV types or HSV from varicella-zoster virus (VZV). Polymerase chain reaction (PCR) is highly sensitive and has become more routinely available for diagnosis of mucocutaneous HSV infections.

Serologic testing for HSV was previously of limited use because it could not reliably differentiate HSV-1 from HSV-2. Because they share significant genetic homology, HSV-1 and HSV-2 code for a number of common proteins that are not antigenically distinct. However, they also code for type-specific proteins that can be used to differentiate them. Current tests based on detecting type-specific viral glycoprotein G (gG-based, type-specific assays) are accurate and should be requested for this purpose. A positive HSV-2 serology may be useful in confirming the diagnosis of genital herpes in a patient with a negative viral culture or with unrecognized or asymptomatic disease. Alternatively, a negative serology can help exclude the diagnosis of HSV in a patient with chronic, nonspecific oral or genital symptoms.

Varicella-Zoster Virus

VZV, another member of the human herpesvirus family, produces two specific patterns of disease in the skin. The primary infection results in varicella, also known as chickenpox, a widespread vesicular eruption usually seen in the pediatric population. Following the primary infection, VZV establishes latency in the dorsal root ganglia until some later point, when reactivation can occur. The ensuing unilateral dermatomal distribution of blisters, often preceded by neuralgic pain, is known as herpes zoster or shingles. Herpes zoster is especially common in patients older than 50 years, but it may be seen at any age. It is also seen more commonly in immunocompromised patients, such as organ-transplant recipients or patients infected with HIV. Herpes zoster is no longer considered a marker for underlying cancer, and evaluation for occult malignancy in an otherwise asymptomatic patient is not indicated. A single recurrence of herpes zoster, usually in the same dermatome, occurs in up to 4% of zoster patients. Additional recurrences, however, suggest a dermatomal form of HSV, and laboratory assessment for this possibility may be indicated.

The most common dermatomes involved with herpes zoster are in the thoracolumbar (T3-L2) and trigeminal (V1) regions. Skin lesions typically evolve from papules to vesicles and pustules, and then crusted erosions, before healing approximately 2 to 4 weeks after onset. The associated neuropathic pain commonly persists after the lesions have healed. Pain that continues for more than 3 months after the skin lesions resolve is referred to as postherpetic neuralgia, one of the most common and debilitating complications of this infection.

Several clinical presentations of herpes zoster deserve additional attention. Ophthalmic zoster, with lesions along the tip, side, or base of the nose indicating involvement of the nasociliary branch of the trigeminal nerve (Hutchinson's sign), may be associated with increased risk for ocular complications. Prompt initiation of a systemic antiviral agent (Table 2) and evaluation by an ophthalmologist are recommended. Disseminated zoster, with more than a few lesions outside the primary and immediately adjacent dermatomes, can indicate visceral involvement and its associated complications. The term zoster sine herpete describes patients with neuropathic pain resembling zoster but without any skin lesions. The diagnosis can be supported by demonstration of increased IgG antibody titers between the acute and convalescent phases. Chronic zoster is seen predominantly in HIV-infected persons. Single or multiple warty growths can persist for weeks or months in areas of skin previously involved by typical lesions of varicella or herpes zoster. Chronic zoster is often resistant to acyclovir. Tissue biopsy and viral cultures, with further testing for antiviral resistance, may aid in assessment.

Herpes Zoster

DIAGNOSIS

Diagnosis of herpes zoster is often made on clinical grounds alone. A Tzanck smear can provide additional support of the viral etiology. With atypical presentations, however, the diagnosis is best confirmed by either an antigen detection method or viral culture. Both differentiate VZV from HSV. Samples submitted for viral culture should be obtained from vesicular fluid because dried or crusted lesions are unlikely to yield positive results. Viral cultures are required if there is a need to assess possible antiviral resistance. PCR can be useful for detecting VZV in bodily fluids such as cerebrospinal fluid. Basic VZV serology is rarely useful for diagnosis, because a majority of the population is seropositive.

TREATMENT

There are three systemic antiviral agents routinely used for the treatment of HSV and VZV infections: acyclovir, valacyclovir, and famciclovir. All three are highly effective and generally well tolerated. Because they inhibit only actively replicating viral DNA, they have no impact on latent infection. Recommendations for antiviral treatment of mucocutaneous HSV infections and herpes zoster, localized topical measures, and available formulations are outlined in Tables 1 to 5. Optimal antiviral dosage schedules for less-common HSV infections, such as herpetic whitlow, have not been determined. The doses outlined in Table 1 for either episodic or chronic suppressive therapy can be used as a guideline in these cases.

CURRENT THERAPY

Herpes Simplex Viruses 1 and 2

- Acyclovir (Zovirax), valacyclovir (Valtrex), famciclovir (Famvir)
- For acyclovir resistance: foscarnet (Foscavir),[1] cidofovir (Vistide)[1]

Varicella-Zoster Virus

- Acyclovir, valacyclovir, famciclovir
- For acyclovir resistance: foscarnet,[1] cidofovir (Vistide)[1]

Hand-Foot-and-Mouth Disease

- Supportive care

Parvovirus B19

- Supportive care, IVIg (Gammagard)[1]

Molluscum Contagiosum

- Surgical or chemical methods of destruction
- Immunomodulators (imiquimod [Aldara],[1] cimetidine [Tagamet][1])

Orf

- Self-limited

---

[1]Not FDA approved for this indication.
Abbreviations: HSV = herpes simplex virus; IVIg = intravenous immunoglobulin.

TABLE 2 Recommendations for Systemic Antiviral Treatment of Herpes Zoster

Drug	Dosage	
	Immunocompetent Patients	Immunosuppressed Patients
Acyclovir	800 mg PO 5 × per d × 7-10 d	800 mg PO 5 × per d × 10 d* 10 mg/kg/dose IV q8h × 7-10 d*
Valacyclovir	1 g PO tid × 7 d	1 g PO tid × 10 d*
Famciclovir	500 mg PO tid × 7 d	500 mg PO tid × 10 d*

*Continue until there are no new lesions for 48 h.

TABLE 3 Topical Treatment Options for Mucocutaneous Herpes Simplex Virus and Varicella-Zoster Virus Infections

Treatment	Comment
Cool, moist compresses using tap water or aluminum acetate 1:20 to 1:40 (Burow's solution, Domeboro, Bluboro)	Good for moist, oozing lesions to accelerate drying. Apply wet dressing to involved skin and cover with a dry cloth to allow evaporation
Calamine lotion or similar shake lotion containing alcohol, menthol, and/or phenol; Aveeno colloidal oatmeal	Useful as drying and antipruritic agent. May be applied after wet dressing
Bacitracin,[1] Polysporin, mupirocin[1] (Bactroban)	Use if there is concern for localized secondary bacterial infection
2% Viscous lidocaine, compounded suspensions[1,6] (e.g., Kaopectate[1] or Maalox,[1] diphenhydramine,[1] lidocaine)	Useful for temporary pain relief of oral or genital mucosal involvement
Acyclovir ointment	Used together with systemic antiviral agents, may be of benefit to immunocompromised individuals for localized HSV
Penciclovir (Denavir) cream	Can decrease the duration of lesions in herpes labialis by half a day if applied every 2 h while awake for 4 days beginning at the first sign of disease

[1]Not FDA approved for this indication.
[6]May be compounded by pharmacists.
Abbreviation: HSV = herpes simplex virus.

TABLE 4 Formulations of Acyclovir, Valacyclovir, and Famciclovir

Drug	Oral	Topical	Intravenous
Acyclovir	200, 400, 800 mg 200 mg/5 mL suspension	5% Ointment (15 g) 5% cream (5 g)	Yes
Valacyclovir	500 mg, 1 g	No	No
Famciclovir	125, 250, 500 mg	No	No
Penciclovir (Denavir)	No	1% cream (1.5 g)	No

TABLE 5 Recommended Antiviral Dose Modification in Patients with Impaired Renal Function

Creatinine Clearance (mL/min)	Genital Herpes Simplex Virus			Herpes Zoster	Herpes Labialis
	Initial	Recurrent	Suppression		
Acyclovir (Zovirax)					
>25	200 mg 5 ×/d	200 mg 5 ×/d	400 mg q12h	800 mg 5 ×/d	
10-24	200 mg 5 ×/d	200 mg 5 ×/d	400 mg q12h	800 mg q8h	
<10	200 mg q12h	200 mg q12h	200 mg q12h	800 mg q12h	
Valacyclovir (Valtrex)					
>50	1 g q12h	500 mg q12h	500 mg-1 g q24h	1 g q8h	2 g PO bid for 1 d
30-49	1 g q12h	500 mg q12h	500 mg-1 g q24h	1 g q12h	1 g PO bid for 1 d
10-29	1 g q24h	500 mg q24h	500 mg q24-48h	1 g q24h	500 mg bid for 1 d
<10	500 mg q24h	500 mg q24h	500 mg q24-48h	500 mg q24h	500 mg single dose
Famciclovir (Famvir)					
>60		125 mg q12h	250 mg q12h	500 mg q8h	
40-59		125 mg q12h	250 mg q12h	500 mg q12h	
20-39		125 mg q12h	125 mg q12h	500 mg q24h	
<20		125 mg q24h	125 mg q24h	250 mg q24h	
>60		1 g bid × 1 d			1500 mg single dose
40-59		500 mg bid × 1 d			750 mg single dose
20-39		500 mg single dose			500 mg single dose
<20		250 mg single dose			250 mg single dose

Acyclovir became available more than 25 years ago and continues to be widely used. Inside an infected host cell, acyclovir must be phosphorylated—first by a virally encoded enzyme (thymidine kinase) and then by host-cell enzymes—to the active form of the drug, acyclovir triphosphate. As a nucleotide analogue, acyclovir triphosphate is incorporated into replicating viral DNA, abruptly terminating further synthesis of that viral DNA chain. Acyclovir triphosphate also interferes with viral DNA replication by directly inhibiting viral DNA polymerase. Valacyclovir is an oral prodrug of acyclovir and has a much higher bioavailability. After ingestion, valacyclovir is rapidly metabolized to acyclovir, and the subsequent mechanism of action is as just described. Famciclovir is an oral prodrug of penciclovir (Denavir), designed for greater bioavailability. Similar to acyclovir, penciclovir must first be phosphorylated by viral thymidine kinase and then by cellular enzymes to penciclovir triphosphate. In this active form, penciclovir triphosphate interferes with viral DNA synthesis and replication by inhibiting viral DNA polymerase. Famciclovir has greater bioavailability and a longer intracellular half-life than acyclovir. For all three agents, the required activation by viral thymidine kinase and the preferential inhibition of viral DNA synthesis contribute to the highly specific antiviral activity.

If taken as recommended, acyclovir, valacyclovir, and famciclovir are generally comparable in their safety and effectiveness. Valacyclovir and famciclovir offer the convenience of less-frequent dosing. Dosing for all three should be adjusted in the presence of renal insufficiency (see Table 5).

Although antiviral therapy does not decrease the incidence of postherpetic neuralgia, all three agents decrease the time for lesion healing and shorten the overall duration of pain if initiated within 48 to 72 hours after the onset of herpes zoster. Valacyclovir and famciclovir appear to be more effective than acyclovir for this purpose, presumably because of easier dosing. An otherwise healthy person younger than 50 years who has discrete involvement on the trunk and mild to moderate pain might benefit minimally or not at all from this intervention, especially if it is initiated after 72 hours of lesion onset. However, patients who are older than 50 years, are immunosuppressed, have involvement in the ophthalmic distribution, or have more-extensive lesions or severe pain should receive systemic antiviral therapy, even if the 72-hour deadline has expired. Adequate pain control, often requiring opiates, is also important.

The addition of systemic corticosteroids to the antiviral regimen remains controversial. There is evidence to suggest this can lessen the severity of the acute episode but does not decrease the incidence or duration of postherpetic neuralgia. Corticosteroids may be of benefit in herpes zoster complicated by facial paralysis or cranial polyneuropathy. Corticosteroids should not be used without concomitant systemic antiviral therapy.

In patients 60 years of age or older, the live-attenuated herpes zoster vaccine (Zostavax) was shown to substantially reduce the incidence of both herpes zoster and postherpetic neuralgia. It is recommended that this option be discussed with immunocompetent patients in this older age group.

Despite widespread use of these antiviral agents, antiviral resistance is rarely a problem in the immunocompetent population. However, it does arise in the setting of immunosuppression. The basis for the resistance is most commonly a mutation in the gene coding for thymidine kinase. Less often there is a mutation in the viral DNA polymerase. In either case, all three standard drugs become ineffective. Alternative antiviral agents available for treatment of acyclovir-resistant HSV and VZV infections include foscarnet (Foscavir)[1] and cidofovir (Vistide).[1]

Hand-Foot-and-Mouth Disease

Hand-foot-and-mouth disease is typically a disease of childhood. The most common etiologic agent is a nonpolio enterovirus, Coxsackie A16, and transmission is via the oral–oral or fecal–oral route. It is highly contagious. Several days after exposure, a prodrome of low-grade fever, malaise, abdominal pain, or respiratory symptoms can develop, followed by the appearance of papulovesicles on the palate, tongue, or buccal mucosa. Similar lesions can subsequently develop on the feet and hands. The eruption persists for 7 to 10 days and then resolves. Treatment is symptomatic.

Since 1997, outbreaks of hand-foot-and-mouth disease caused by enterovirus 71 have been reported in Asia and Australia. Although Hand-foot-and-mouth disease associated with Coxsackie A16 infection is typically a mild illness, Hand-foot-and-mouth disease caused by enterovirus 71 has shown a higher incidence of neurologic involvement, including fatal cases of encephalitis.

Parvovirus B19

Cutaneous manifestations of parvovirus B19 infection include the childhood exanthem known as erythema infectiosum (fifth disease) and, less commonly, petechial or purpuric eruptions. The virus is transmitted primarily via respiratory secretions and, to a much lesser extent, through blood or blood products. The host cells for viral replication are erythroid progenitor cells, which subsequently undergo cell lysis.

A child with erythema infectiosum typically develops a low-grade fever and nonspecific upper respiratory symptoms approximately 2 days before the onset of rash. The rash has been described as having a slapped-cheeks appearance, with prominent redness over the malar eminences. This is followed by a pink-to-red lacy or reticular eruption over the trunk and extensor surfaces of the arms and legs. The rash usually lasts a week to 10 days but can transiently recur over months in response to precipitating factors such as sunlight, exercise, and bathing. Diagnosis of erythema infectiosum is usually made on clinical grounds, and treatment is symptomatic. By the time the rash appears and the diagnosis has been made, the child is no longer infectious.

Infection with parvovirus B19 in older adolescents and adults often manifests with arthralgias or arthritis rather than a rash. In certain patient populations, parvovirus B19 infections may be associated with complications including transient aplastic crisis, chronic anemia, and hydrops fetalis. In these less-typical presentations, serology (anti-B19 IgM or documented seroconversion) may be needed for diagnosis. Intravenous immunoglobulin (IVIg [Gamimune N][1]) is used successfully for treatment of chronic or persistent infection in immunosuppressed patients.

Molluscum Contagiosum

Molluscum contagiosum are benign umbilicated papules caused by infection with the *Molluscipoxvirus*, a member of the poxvirus family. Lesions are limited to the mucocutaneous surface and typically appear in clusters on the face, trunk, and skin fold areas in children and on thighs, lower abdomen, and suprapubic areas in sexually active adults. Large numbers of lesions in an extensive distribution may be seen in the immunosuppressed population.

Transmission routinely occurs by skin-to-skin contact with an infected host, but transmission from contaminated fomites has been reported. Autoinoculation commonly occurs. Diagnosis is usually based on clinical examination, but histopathology of atypical lesions may be used for confirmation.

Because molluscum contagiosum tends to be self-limited, treatment is not always required, but it can reduce the risk of autoinoculation and transmission to others. Treatment modalities are primarily aimed at destroying the lesions, similar to those used for verruca vulgaris (Table 6). In the case of sexual transmission, evaluation for other sexually transmitted diseases may be indicated.

Orf and Milker's Nodules

Orf (also known as ecthyma contagiosum) and milker's nodules are caused by the closely related *Parapoxvirus*, a member of the poxvirus family. The virus responsible for orf is widespread in sheep and goats, whereas the virus causing milker's nodules is found in cattle. Transmission to humans is by direct contact with infected animals or recently vaccinated animals and is usually seen several days and up to 2 weeks after exposure. Preexisting skin trauma or other disruption of the normal cutaneous barrier enhances the risk of transmission. Barrier precautions and proper hand hygiene are important preventive measures.

Orf and milker's nodules most commonly appear as one to several nodules on the dorsal aspect of the hands or forearms. Lesions evolve through several clinical stages over a period of 3 to 5 weeks ranging from solid red nodules to vesicular, exudative, or wartlike tumors. As with other poxvirus infections, lesions of orf often demonstrate central umbilication. Regional lymphadenopathy and lymphangitis are commonly seen.

Diagnosis is based on a history of exposure and clinical examination. Tissue biopsy for histopathology or electron microscopy may

---

[1]Not FDA approved for this indication.

[1]Not FDA approved for this indication.

TABLE 6 Treatment Options for Molluscum Contagiosum

Treatment	Comment
Cryotherapy (liquid nitrogen)	Freeze individual lesions for 5-10 sec Repeat PRN in 2-3 wk
Curettage	Entire lesion may be removed using a curette; this results in bleeding Removal of central core with toothpick or other pointed instrument is also effective
Cantharidin (Cantharone)[1]	Blister-inducing agent: Apply to lesion with toothpick, air dry Cover with tape or adhesive bandage Patient to wash area after 24 h (or sooner if significant pain)
Podophyllin (25% in tincture of benzoin)[1]	Cytotoxic agent: Apply to lesion with toothpick Patient to wash off after 4-6 h Contraindicated in pregnancy
Podofilox (Condylox 0.5% gel or solution)[1]	Done by patient: Apply bid for 3 consecutive d/wk × 2-4 wk Contraindicated in pregnancy
Salicylic acid/lactic acid (Occlusal, Duofilm)[1]	Done by patient: Apply daily
Imiquimod (Aldara) 5% cream[1]	Done by patient: Apply daily 5 consecutive d/wk Leave on overnight Continue for 8-12 wk
Cimetidine (Tagamet)[1]	30 mg/kg/d PO × 6-12 wk Can boost cell-mediated immunity

[1]Not FDA approved for this indication.

---

also be used. Orf virus infection can resemble skin lesions associated with potentially life-threatening zoonotic infections such as tularemia, cutaneous anthrax, and erysipeloid. Should this be a concern, definitive diagnostic testing using PCR is available through the Centers for Disease Control and Prevention (CDC).

In general, the lesions of orf are self-limited, resolving within 4 to 6 weeks, and treatment is not routinely required. However, immunocompromised persons can develop more progressive and destructive lesions requiring therapeutic intervention such as topical cidofovir[1,6] or imiquimod (Aldara).[1]

---

[1]Not FDA approved for this indication.
[6]May be compounded by pharmacists.

REFERENCES

Bikowski Jr JB. Molluscum contagiosum: The need for physician intervention and new treatment options. Cutis 2004;73:202–6.

Centers for Disease Control and Prevention (CDC). Orf virus infection in humans–New York, Illinois, California, and Tennessee, 2004-2005. MMWR Morb Mortal Wkly Rep 2006;55(3):65–8.

Cernik C, Gallina K, Brodell RT. The treatment of herpes simplex infections: An evidence-based review. Arch Intern Med 2008;168:1137–44.

Corey L, Wald A. Maternal and neonatal herpes simplex virus infections. N Engl J Med 2009;361:1376–85.

Gupta R, Warren T, Wald A. Genital herpes. Lancet 2007;370:2127–37.

Harpaz R, Ortega-Sanchez IR, Seward JF. Prevention of herpes zoster. Recommendations of the Advisory Committee on Immunization Practices (ACIP). MMWR 2008;57:1–30.

Sampathkumar P, Drage LA, Martin DP. Herpes zoster (shingles) and postherpetic neuralgia. Mayo Clin Proc 2009;84:274–80.

Scott LA, Stone MS. Viral exanthems. Dermatol Online J 2003;9(3):4.

Servey JT, Reamy BV, Hodge J. Clinical presentations of parvovirus B19 infection. Am Fam Physician 2007;75:373–446.

Whitley RJ. A 70 year-old woman with shingles: review of herpes zoster. JAMA 2009;302:73–80.

Xu F, Sternberg MR, Kottiri BJ, et al. Trends in herpes simplex virus type 1 and type 2 seroprevalence in the United States. JAMA 2006;296:964–73.

Parasitic Diseases of the Skin

Method of
Andreas Katsambas, MD, PhD, and
Clio Dessinioti, MD, MSc

Diseases Caused by Protozoa

CUTANEOUS AMEBIASIS

Intestinal amebiasis is caused by *Entamoeba histolytica*, which may rarely invade the skin and cause cutaneous amebiasis. The disease is transmitted by ingestion of food or water contaminated with cyst forms of the parasite and through fecal exposure during sexual contact.

Cutaneous amebiasis develops at the site of the invasion of the parasites into the skin from an underlying amebic abscess, usually at the perianal area or the abdominal wall. Cutaneous findings include purulent, foul-smelling nodules, cysts, and sinuses, which are associated with regional adenopathy and dysentery. Skin lesions grow rapidly and may lead to death if left untreated.

Diagnosis of cutaneous amebiasis is confirmed by microscopic identification of *E. histolytica* in the stool and in aspirates or biopsy samples obtained during colonoscopy, during surgery, or from the border of an ulcer. Treatment of choice for extraintestinal amebiasis is oral metronidazole (Flagyl) 750 mg PO three times daily for 7 to 10 days or tinidazole (Tindamax). Tinidazole was FDA approved in 2004 for the treatment of intestinal amebiasis in adults (2 g/day for 3 days) and children older than 3 years, and it appears to be as effective as and better tolerated than metronidazole. Either treatment should be followed by iodoquinol (Yodoxin) 650 mg PO three times daily for 20 days or paromomycin 25 to 35 mg/kg/day PO divided in three doses for 7 days.

LEISHMANIASIS

Leishmaniasis results from the infection with intracellular protozoan parasites belonging to the genus *Leishmania*. Leishmania parasites are transmitted to humans and other mammalian hosts (e.g., dogs, rodents) during feeding by infected female phlebotomine sandflies that serve as vectors. The parasites exist as promastigotes in the midgut of sandflies and as amastigotes (i.e., Leishman-Donovan bodies) within macrophages of humans and other mammals. Based on the extent and the severity of involvement in the human host, leishmaniasis may be clinically classified as cutaneous leishmaniasis, diffuse cutaneous leishmaniasis, mucocutaneous leishmaniasis, and visceral leishmaniasis.

Cutaneous leishmaniasis (New World or Old World form) begins as a small erythematous papule at the site of the bite of the sandfly, which evolves into an ulcerated nodule with a raised and indurated border (i.e., volcano sign) (Fig. 1). The lesions gradually heal with

CURRENT DIAGNOSIS

Parasitic diseases are a common cause of morbidity and mortality, particularly in tropical and developing countries. They may be caused by protozoa, helminths, or arthropods. Because of the immigration of persons from tropical and subtropical countries worldwide and the travel of people from industrialized to tropical regions, parasitic diseases may be found in temperate climates. Skin lesions may provide important diagnostic clues for parasitic infections, and they are reviewed in the following sections, along with updated treatment guidelines.

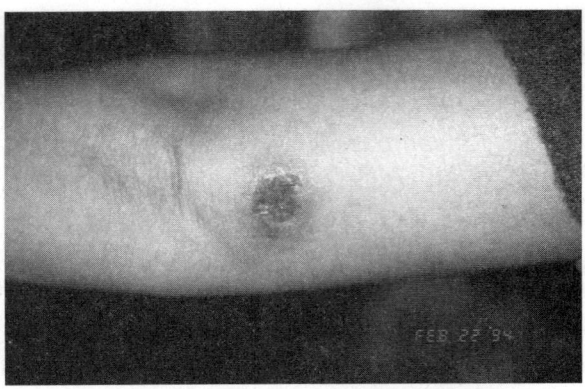

FIGURE 1. Cutaneous leishmaniasis is characterized by an ulcerated nodule with a raised and indurated border (i.e., volcano sign).

a depressed scar. Diffuse cutaneous leishmaniasis is characterized by widespread cutaneous involvement without visceralization. Mucocutaneous leishmaniasis (known as espundia in South America) affects the skin, the mucosa, and the cartilages of the upper respiratory tract (especially the nose and the larynx) and may result in severe disfigurement. Visceral leishmaniasis results from the involvement of the bone marrow, spleen, and the liver, and it may lead to death if left untreated. It manifests with fever, splenomegaly, pancytopenia, and wasting. Post–kala azar dermal leishmaniasis may appear within a year after visceral disease independent of treatment, and it is characterized by macules, papules, and nodules, which are usually hypopigmented.

Diagnosis of leishmaniasis is based on finding the parasites in the skin from the lesion aspirate or biopsy by direct examination or culture. The leishmanin (Montenegro) skin test shows past and current infections, and it detects the inflammatory response in the skin after injection of phenol-killed parasites into the dermis. A past or current infection is also documented by an in vitro lymphocyte proliferation assay that requires a drop of blood from a finger prick. Polymerase chain reaction (PCR) techniques may be used to identify different *Leishmania* species. Circulating antibody levels are not considered a useful diagnostic sign.

Cutaneous leishmaniasis is usually self-limited and may not require treatment. Treatment of cutaneous leishmaniasis is indicated in case of numerous lesions or when lesions affect the face to avoid scarring. Therapies include sodium stibogluconate (Pentostam)[10] 20 mg/kg/day IV or IM for 20 days. Meglumine antimoniate (Glucantime)[2] 20 mg/kg/day IV or IM for 20 days or miltefosine (Impavido)[2] 2.5 mg/kg/day PO (up to 150 mg/day) for 28 days may be used. Alternatively, intralesional injections of antimonials 1 mg/kg once weekly, cryotherapy, local heat, oral ketoconazole (Nizoral),[1] topical amphotericin B,[2] pentamidine (Pentam)[1] 2 to 3 mg/kg IV or IM daily or every second day for four to seven doses, or topical paromomycin[6] (applied twice daily for 10–20 days) may be used.

The production of antileishmanial antibodies does not correlate with resolution of the disease. Infection and recovery are associated with lifelong immunity to reinfection by the same species of *Leishmania*, although interspecies immunity may also exist.

TRYPANOSOMIASIS

There are three types of trypanosomiasis:

- American trypanosomiasis or Chagas' diseases, caused by *Trypanosoma cruzi*
- East African sleeping sickness, caused by *Trypanosoma brucei rhodesiense*
- West African sleeping sickness, caused by *Trypanosoma brucei gambiense*

[1]Not FDA approved for this indication.
[2]Not available in the United States.
[6]May be compounded by pharmacists.
[10]Available in the United States from the Centers for Disease Control and Prevention.

American trypanosomiasis (i.e., Chagas' disease) is caused by the parasite *T. cruzi*, and it is endemic in Central and South America. The disease is transmitted by the bite of infected "cone-nosed" insects, by transfusion of infected blood, by organ transplantation, and across the placenta. During the acute stage, Chagas' disease manifests with a painful erythematous nodule, known as chagoma, which is associated with regional adenopathy. The chronic stage manifests with cardiomyopathy, megaesophagus, and megacolon. Diagnosis is confirmed by microscopic identification of the parasite in fresh anticoagulated blood, in blood smears, by lymph node biopsy or skin biopsy, or by culture. Treatment includes benznidazole (Radanil, Rochagan)[2] 5 to 7 mg/kg/day PO in two doses for 60 to 90 days or nifurtimox (Lampit)[10] 8 to 10 mg/kg/day PO in three or four doses for 90 to 120 days.

African trypanosomiasis (i.e., East and West African sleeping sickness) occurs in Africa and is transmitted by the bite of infected male and female tsetse flies. It manifests with a highly inflammatory, painful, red or violaceous, indurated nodule surrounded by an erythematous halo, called trypanosome chancre, at the site of the inoculation of the parasites. There is regional adenopathy. Later, the chancre resolves spontaneously, and the patient has fever, malaise, a generalized pruritic eruption with erythematous annular plaques or urticarial lesions, and central nervous system (CNS) involvement with personality changes, apathy, somnolence, coma, and death. Diagnosis is based on the identification of trypanosomes by microscopic examination in chancre fluid, affected lymph node aspirates, blood, bone marrow, or in the late stages of infection, cerebrospinal fluid.

Treatment of East African sleeping sickness consists of suramin (naphthylamine sulfonic acid, Germanin)[10] 100 to 200 mg (test dose) IV and then 1 g IV on days 1, 3, 7, 14, and 21. For late disease with CNS involvement, melarsoprol B (a trivalent organic arsenical, Mel-B)[10] is used in the following dosage regimen: 2 to 3.6 mg/kg/day IV for 3 days; after 7 days, 3.6 mg/kg/day for 3 days; and the latter repeated after 7 days. For West African sleeping sickness, treatment of choice is pentamidine isethionate (Pentam 300)[1] 4 mg/kg/day IM for 10 days or suramin (Germanin) as used for East African sleeping sickness. For late disease with involvement of the CNS, eflornithine (Ornidyl)[2] 400 mg/kg/day IV in four doses for 14 days is used.

CUTANEOUS TOXOPLASMOSIS

Systemic toxoplasmosis (congenital or acquired) is caused by the parasite *Toxoplasma gondii*, and it usually is transmitted from contact with infected cats. The disease may also be acquired by eating raw or undercooked meats from infected animals. Cutaneous involvement is rare. It manifests with punctate macules or ecchymoses in the congenital form, and the acquired form manifests with roseola and erythema multiforme lesions, urticaria, prurigo-like nodules, and maculopapular lesions. Diagnosis of cutaneous toxoplasmosis is confirmed by isolation of the parasite in the skin. Treatment is not needed for healthy nonpregnant patients because symptoms resolve in a few weeks. Treatment for pregnant women or immunocompromised patients includes pyrimethamine (Daraprim) 25–100 mg/d PO for 3–6 wks together with sulfadiazine[1] 1–15 g PO qid for 3–6 wks. Leucovorin should be taken with each dose of pyrimethamine.

Diseases Caused by Helminths

ASCARIASIS

Ascariasis is caused by *Ascaris* species, mainly *Ascaris lumbricoides*. It is transmitted by the ingestion of eggs in soil contaminated with human feces. Skin involvement of ascariasis manifests with urticaria. Diagnosis is based on finding the adult worm or eggs in the feces. Treatment includes albendazole (Albenza)[1] 400 mg PO once or mebendazole (Vermox) 100 mg PO twice daily for 3 days (or 500 mg once) or ivermectin (Stromectol)[1] 150 to 200 μg/kg PO once.

[1]Not FDA approved for this indication.
[2]Not available in the United States.
[10]Available in the United States from the Centers for Disease Control and Prevention.

CUTANEOUS LARVA MIGRANS

Cutaneous larva migrans is also known as creeping eruption, with the first term describing a syndrome and the second a clinical sign found in various conditions. The syndrome cutaneous larva migrans is caused when various nematode larvae (i.e., hookworms, such as *Ancylostoma braziliense*, *Ancylostoma caninum*, *Bunostomum phlebotomum*) of dogs, cats, and other mammals penetrate and migrate through the skin. Cutaneous larva migrans is transmitted by skin contact to soil contaminated with animal feces. In humans, larvae are unable to reach internal organs and eventually die. Cutaneous larva migrans manifests with intensely pruritic, papular lesions, which evolve as the larvae migrate to a characteristic linear, minimally elevated, serpiginous tract that moves forward in an irregular pattern. Diagnosis is easily made clinically and is supported by a travel history or by possible exposure in an endemic area.

 CURRENT DIAGNOSIS

Cutaneous Amebiasis

- Purulent, foul-smelling nodules, ulcers, cysts, sinuses
- Microscopic identification of *Entamoeba histolytica* in stool or biopsy samples
- Molecular methods

Cutaneous Leishmaniasis

- Ulcerated nodule (i.e., volcano sign)
- Identification of *Leishmania* parasites by direct examination or culture from the lesion aspirate or biopsy
- Montenegro skin test
- In vitro lymphocyte proliferation assay
- Polymerase chain reaction

Trypanosomiasis

CHAGAS' DISEASE

- Chagoma: painful erythematous nodule
- Regional adenopathy
- Cardiomyopathy, megaesophagus, megacolon
- Microscopic examination of *Trypanosoma cruzi* in blood, lymph node biopsy, or skin biopsy or culture

AFRICAN SLEEPING SICKNESS

- Trypanosome chancre: painful, inflammatory nodule
- Regional adenopathy
- Fever, generalized pruritic eruption with erythematous annular plaques
- Central nervous system involvement
- Microscopic identification of *Trypanosoma brucei* in chancre fluid, lymph node aspirates, blood, bone marrow, cerebrospinal fluid

Cutaneous Toxoplasmosis

- Roseola, urticaria, prurigo-like nodules
- Isolation of *Toxoplasma gondii* in the skin

Ascariasis

- Urticaria
- Identification of adult worm or eggs in stool

Cutaneous Larva Migrans

- Creeping eruption
- Intense pruritus

Cysticercosis

- Subcutaneous nodules
- Isolation of *Taenia solium* in skin lesion
- Serologic tests

Dracunculiasis

- Ruptured blister with prolapsing worm

Filariasis

LYMPHATIC FILARIASIS

- Fever with lymphangitis and lymphadenitis
- Chronic pulmonary infection
- Progressive lymphedema leading to massive tissue thickening, especially of the legs and scrotum (i.e., elephantiasis)
- Microscopic identification of microfilariae in blood

ONCHOCERCIASIS (RIVER BLINDNESS)

- Subcutaneous nodules, dermatitis, "leopard skin," "lizard skin," lymphedema
- Identification of microfilariae in skin snips
- Blindness

LOIASIS (CALABAR SWELLINGS)

- Pruritus, localized subcutaneous swellings
- Serpiginous lesion on the conjunctivae
- Microscopic identification of microfilariae in blood

Schistosomiasis (Snail Fever)

- Pruritic papules, edema
- Fever, lymphadenopathy, diarrhea
- Bilharziasis cutanea tarda: pruritic, grouped papules
- Identification of the eggs in stool, urine, biopsy of affected tissues
- Enzyme-linked immunosorbent assay (ELISA) tests

Cercarial Dermatitis (Swimmer's Itch)

- Extremely pruritic erythematous macules, papules, vesicles on body areas exposed to infested water

Human Scabies

- Pruritus worsening at night
- Papules, excoriations, nodules, burrows on genitals, interdigital spaces, axillae, wrists
- Microscopic identification of mites or eggs or feces from burrows or papules

Pediculosis

PEDICULOSIS CAPITIS

- Intense pruritus of the scalp
- Nape dermatitis
- Identification of lice and nits on the hair

PEDICULOSIS CORPORIS (VAGABOND'S ITCH)

- Intense pruritus, erythema, urticarial lesions, papules, nodules, and excoriations
- Identification of lice and nits on clothing

PEDICULOSIS PUBIS

- Pruritus
- Blue macules
- Identification of lice and nits on pubic hair

Treatment of choice consists of ivermectin (Stromectol)[1] at a single dose of 200 μg/kg. In case of treatment failure, a second dose usually suffices. Ivermectin has an excellent safety profile, without any notable adverse events, and it has been used in millions of individuals in developing countries during onchocerciasis and filariasis control operations. It is contraindicated in children who weigh less than 15 kg (or are younger than 5 years) and in pregnant or breast-feeding women. Alternatively, repeated courses of oral albendazole (Albenza)[1] 400 mg daily for 3 days may be used. Treatment with oral thiabendazole (Mintezol) 50 mg/kg daily for 2 to 4 days has been associated with adverse events such as dizziness, nausea, vomiting, and intestinal cramps, and it is therefore not recommended. In the absence of multiple or widespread lesions, topical treatments may be considered, such as topical thiabendazole[6] 10% to 15%, applied three times daily for 5 to 7 days, which has similar efficacy with oral ivermectin and no adverse events.

CYSTICERCOSIS

Cysticercosis is caused by the larval stage (i.e., cysticerci) of the pork tapeworm Taenia solium, and it is the most common helminthic infection of the CNS. It is transmitted by ingesting eggs in food, water, or on hands contaminated with human feces. Cutaneous manifestations are subcutaneous nodules that occur mainly on the extremities and trunk. There may be involvement of the CNS (i.e., seizures), the eye, the intestines, the skeletal muscle, heart, kidneys, lung, and liver. Diagnosis is confirmed by isolation of the parasite in a nodule and by serologic tests.

Treatment options include surgery, albendazole (Albenza) 400 mg PO twice daily for 8 to 30 days, or praziquantel (Biltricide)[1] 100 mg/kg/day PO in three doses for 1 day and then 50 mg/kg/day in three doses for 29 days. Any cysticercocidal drug may cause irreparable damage when used in the presence of ocular or spinal cysts.

DRACUNCULIASIS

Dracunculiasis is caused by the nematode Dracunculus medinensis. It is transmitted by drinking water with copepods (i.e., tiny aquatic arthropods) infected with the larvae of D. medinensis. In the human stomach, copepods release the larvae that mature and migrate to the skin, causing an erythematous papule or blister. The blister ruptures, and the female worm can often be seen prolapsing through the skin. Treatment includes extraction of the worm combined with wound care. Metronidazole (Flagyl)[1] 250 mg PO three times daily for 10 days may be efficacious and facilitates removal of the worm.

FILARIASIS

Filariasis is caused by nematodes (i.e., roundworms) that inhabit the lymphatics and subcutaneous tissues. The most common filarial infections include lymphatic filariasis, onchocerciasis, and loiasis.

Lymphatic Filariasis

Lymphatic filariasis is caused by Wuchereria bancrofti, Brugia malayi, and Brugia timori, and it is transmitted by mosquitoes. Adult worms result in a chronic inflammatory cell infiltrate around lymphatic vessels, causing their dilatation, hypertrophy, and obstruction. Many patients are asymptomatic, but some may develop fever with lymphangitis and lymphadenitis, chronic pulmonary infection, and progressive lymphedema leading to massive tissue thickening, especially of the legs and scrotum (i.e., elephantiasis). The overlying skin is thickened. Diagnosis is based on microscopic identification of the microfilariae in the blood and affected tissues.

Treatment consists of diethylcarbamazine (DEC, Hetrazan)[10] in the following regimen: 50 mg on day 1, 50 mg three times daily on day 2, 100 mg three times daily on day 3, and 6 mg/kg in three doses on days 4 through 14. Prophylaxis with DEC 500 mg/day for 2 days each month is effective against W. bancrofti infection for travelers in endemic areas.

Onchocerciasis

Onchocerciasis (i.e., blinding filariasis) is caused by the filarial nematode Onchocerca volvulus, which is transmitted by the blackflies Simulium. It may manifest with subcutaneous onchocercid nodules, acute or chronic dermatitis, depigmentation (i.e., leopard skin), and skin atrophy (i.e., lizard skin), and in later stages, it may manifest with lymphadenopathy and lymphedema. The microfilariae have a predilection for the eyes, and the infection can lead to blindness (i.e., river blindness). Diagnosis is based on identification of microfilariae in skin snips.

Treatment consists of ivermectin (Stromectol) 150 μg/kg PO every 6 to 12 months until asymptomatic. DEC is contraindicated as it may lead to blindness.

Loiasis

Loiasis (i.e., Calabar swellings) is caused by the parasite Loa loa, which is transmitted by deerflies (Chrysops). Cutaneous manifestations include pruritus, urticaria, and Calabar swellings, which are erythematous, warm, subcutaneous swellings associated with the migration of the worm through the subcutaneous tissues. Occasionally, there is subconjunctival migration of the adult worm, producing a migrating serpiginous lesion on the conjunctivae. Diagnosis is confirmed by identification of microfilariae in the blood by microscopic examination.

DEC[10] is the treatment of choice in the following regimen: 50 mg on day 1, 50 mg three times daily on day 2, 100 mg three times daily on day 3, and 9 mg/kg/day in three doses on days 4 through 14. Ivermectin (Stromectol)[1] may cause encephalopathy in patients with a heavy L. loa infection. Prophylaxis with DEC is effective for L. loa in adults who travel in endemic areas.

SCHISTOSOMIASIS

Schistosomiasis (i.e., snail fever) in humans is caused mainly by the trematodes Schistosoma haematobium, Schistosoma japonicum, and Schistosoma mansoni. All trematodes have a life cycle that involves the snail as an intermediate host. The infective cercariae leave the snail, swim, and penetrate the human skin, causing a pruritic papular dermatosis. The disease is transmitted by exposure to contaminated water with live cercariae or by drinking infested water. Skin findings of acute schistosomiasis include pruritic schistosomal dermatitis due to a hypersensitivity response to the cercariae and edema of the face, extremities, genitals, and trunk. Schistosomal fever (i.e., Katayama fever), lymphadenopathy, and diarrhea may also develop. Late skin findings (i.e., bilharziasis cutanea tarda) appear in patients with visceral disease and include firm, pruritic, grouped papules. Secondary infection, ulceration, and development of squamous cell carcinoma may follow. Diagnosis is confirmed by identification of the eggs in the urine or stool, by biopsy of affected tissues, or by enzyme-linked immunosorbent assay (ELISA).

Treatment includes praziquantel (Biltricide)[3] 40 mg/kg/day in two doses for 1 day (for S. haematobium and S. mansoni) or 60 mg/kg/day in three doses for 1 day (for S. japonicum).

CERCARIAL DERMATITIS

Cercarial dermatitis (i.e., swimmer's itch) is caused by cercariae (i.e., larvae) of nonhuman schistosomes that penetrate the skin and die without invading other tissues. It is transmitted by contact with fresh or salt water contaminated with cercariae. It manifests with extremely pruritic, erythematous macules of sudden onset, which evolve into papules, vesicles, and urticarial lesions located on parts of the body directly exposed to the water, while sparing clothed areas. Cercarial dermatitis is a self-limited disease, and treatment is symptomatic with topical steroids and oral antihistamines.

[1]Not FDA approved for this indication.
[6]May be compounded by pharmacists.
[10]Available in the United States from the Centers for Disease Control and Prevention.

[1]Not FDA approved for this indication.
[3]Exceeds dosage recommended by the manufacturer.
[10]Available in the United States from the Centers for Disease Control and Prevention.

Diseases Caused by Arthropoda

HUMAN SCABIES

Scabies is a common skin infestation caused by the mite *Sarcoptes scabiei*, which is an obligate human parasite. Scabies is transmitted by direct contact with an infested individual or by contact with bedding and clothing. The incubation period for scabies is about 3 weeks, and reinfestation results in symptoms within 1 to 3 days. Scabies is characterized by pruritus that usually worsens at night. Papules, nodules, excoriations, and burrows may be found. Lesions are usually located on interdigital spaces, wrists, ankles, axillae, waist, and genitals. Scabies manifests as red-brown nodules that represent a hypersensitivity response. In adults, the head is usually spared, whereas the involvement of the scalp, palms, and soles is common in infants.

 CURRENT THERAPY

Cutaneous Amebiasis

- Metronidazole (Flagyl) 750 mg PO three times daily for 7 and 10 days, or
- Tinidazole (Tindamax) 2 g once PO daily for 5 days, followed by iodoquinol (Yodoxin) 650 mg PO three times daily for 20 days or paromomycin (Humatin) 25 to 35 mg/kg/day PO in three doses for 7 days

Cutaneous Leishmaniasis

- Sodium stibogluconate (Pentostam)[10] 20 mg/kg/day IV or IM for 20 days, or
- Meglumine antimoniate (Glucantime)[2] 20 mg/kg/day IV or IM for 20 days, or
- Miltefosine (Impavido)[2] 2.5 mg/kg/day PO (up to 150 mg/day) for 28 days, or
- Topical paromomycin, a formulation of 15% paromomycin and 12% methylbenzethonium chloride in soft white paraffin (Lesheutan)[1,6] applied twice daily for 10 days or
- Pentamidine (Pentam 300)[1] 2 to 3 mg/kg IV or IM daily or every second day for four to seven doses

Trypanosomiasis

CHAGAS' DISEASE (AMERICAN TRYPANOSOMIASIS)

- Nifurtimox (Lampit)[10] 8 to 10 mg/kg/day PO in three or four doses for 90 to 20 days, or
- Benznidazole (Radanil, Rochagan)[2] 5 to 7 mg/kg/day PO in two doses for 60 to 90 days

EAST AFRICAN SLEEPING SICKNESS

- Suramin (Germanin)[10] 100 to 200 mg (test dose) IV, then 1 g IV on days 1, 3, 7, 14, 21
- For late disease with involvement of the central nervous system, melarsoprol (Mel-B)[10] 2 to 3.6 mg/kg/day IV for 3 days; after 7 days, 3.6 mg/kg/day for 3 days; repeat after 7 days

WEST AFRICAN SLEEPING SICKNESS

- Pentamidine (Pentam 300)[1] 4 mg/kg/day IM for 10 days,[1] or
- Suramin (Germanin)[10] 100 to 200 mg (test dose) IV, then 1 g IV on days 1, 3, 7, 14, 21
- For late disease with involvement of the central nervous system, melarsoprol (Mel-B)[10] 2.2 mg/kg/day IV for 10 days, or
- For late disease with involvement of the central nervous system, eflornithine (Ornidyl)[2] 400 mg/kg/day IV in four doses for 14 days

Cutaneous Toxoplasmosis

- Self-limited disease; treatment not needed in healthy, nonpregnant persons
- For pregnant women or immunocompromised patients: pyrimethamine (Daraprim) 25 to 100 mg/day PO for 3 to 4 weeks (plus leucovorin 10 to 25 mg with each dose of pyrimethamine) and sulfadiazine[1] 1 to 1.5 g PO four times daily for 3 to 4 weeks

Ascariasis

- Albendazole (Albenza)[1] 400 mg PO once, or
- Mebendazole (Vermox) 100 mg PO twice daily for 3 days or 500 mg once, or
- Ivermectin (Stromectol)[1] 150 to 200 μg/kg PO once

Cutaneous Larva Migrans

- Ivermectin (Stromectol)[1] 200 μg/kg PO once; a second dose may be needed, or
- Albendazole (Albenza)[1] 400 mg daily PO for 3 days
- Topical thiabendazole[6] 10% to 15% applied three times daily for 5 to 7 days for a limited number of lesions

Dracunculiasis

- Slow extraction of the worm, which is facilitated by metronidazole (Flagyl)[1] 250 mg PO three times daily for 10 days

Filariasis

LYMPHATIC FILARIASIS

- Diethylcarbamazine (DEC, Hetrazan)[10] 6 mg/kg/day PO in three doses for 12 days, or
- Ivermectin (Stromectol)[1] 200 μg/kg PO once together with albendazole (Albenza)[1] 400 mg PO once; kills only the microfilaria, not the adult worms
- For patients with microfilaria in the blood, DEC as follows: day 1: 50 mg; day 2: 50 mg three times daily; day 3: 100 mg three times daily; days 4 through 14: 6 mg/kg in three doses

ONCHOCERCIASIS

- Ivermectin (Stromectol) 150 μg/kg PO once for 6 to 12 months, until asymptomatic
- DEC: contraindicated because it may lead to blindness

LOIASIS

- DEC[10] 6 mg/kg/day PO in three doses for 12 days
- For patients with microfilaria in the blood, DEC as follows: day 1: 50 mg; day 2: 50 mg three times daily; day 3: 100 mg three times daily; days 4 through 14: 9 mg/kg in three doses

Schistosomiasis

- Praziquantel (Biltricide) 40 mg/kg/day[3] in two doses for 1 day (*S. haematobium* and *S. mansoni*) and 60 mg/kg/day[3] in three doses for 1 day (*S. japonicum, S. mekongi*)

Human Scabies

- Permethrin (Acticin, Elimite) 5% cream rinse, applied for 10 hours; a second application 7 to 10 days later, or
- Benzyl benzoate 25% solution[6] applied topically; second application 7 to 10 days later, or

Continued

- Crotamiton 10% (Eurax) applied twice daily for 2 days; second application 7 to 10 days later
- Sulfur 6% to 10% ointment in petrolatum[6]
- Ivermectin (Stromectol)[1] 200 μg/kg PO once: treatment of choice for crusted scabies

Pediculosis

PEDICULOSIS CAPITIS

- Malathion (Ovide) 0.5% lotion, applied for 8 to 12 hours before being washed off; approved for children older than 6 years, or
- Permethrin (Nix) 1% lotion, applied to shampooed hair and washed off after 10 minutes; second application 7 to 10 days later; approved for children older than 2 years

- Pyrethrins with piperidyl butoxide (RID) applied for 10 minutes
- Benzyl benzoate 25% solution[6]
- Lindane shampoo: for recalcitrant disease, not to be used in children
- Ivermectin (Stromectol)[1] 200 μg/kg on days 1, 2, and 10[1]

PEDICULOSIS CORPORIS

- Disinfection of clothes

PEDICULOSIS PUBIS

- Same treatment as pediculosis capitis: three times daily

---

[1]Not FDA approved for this indication.
[2]Not available in the United States.
[3]Exceeds dosage recommended by the manufacturer.
[6]May be compounded by pharmacists.
[10]Available in the United States from the Centers for Disease Control and Prevention.

Crusted or Norwegian scabies manifests with hyperkeratotic papules or plaques of the hands and feet (often with nail involvement) and an erythematous scaly eruption on the face, neck, scalp, and trunk. Because pruritus is often absent, this disease can be misdiagnosed as psoriasis, eczema, or an adverse drug reaction. Lesions contain thousands of mites and are highly contagious. Crusted scabies mainly affects immunocompromised patients (e.g., patients with human immunodeficiency virus infection), mentally retarded persons, or debilitated patients.

Diagnosis is based on the microscopic identification of mites or their eggs or feces from burrows or papules. Treatment should be applied from the neck down in adults, and in infants, application should include the scalp and face (avoiding the eyes and mouth).

Treatment includes 5% permethrin (Elimite) applied for 10 hours and repeated after 1 week. A 25% benzyl benzoate solution[6] is also efficacious in adults, and because of low toxicity, it is recommended in a lower concentration (10%) for children older than 4 months and for women during pregnancy. Sulfur ointments in petrolatum[6] at concentrations of 6% to 10% may be used for scabies in children and pregnant women. Alternative treatments for scabies include crotamiton 10% (Eurax) applied once daily for 2 days, or ivermectin (Stromectol)[1] as a single- or two-dose regimen of 200 μg/kg/dose can be used. Aggressive treatment with ivermectin at a single dose of 200 μg/kg, repeated after 2 weeks with or without topical 5% permethrin cream (two applications, 1 week apart) and keratolytics (5% salicylic acid ointment[1] applied twice daily) is the treatment of choice for crusted scabies. All sexual and close personal and household contacts within the preceding 6 weeks should be treated simultaneously. Bedding and clothing should be decontaminated (i.e., machine washed and dried using the hot cycle or dry cleaned) or removed from body contact for at least 3 days, because the mite dies when separated from the human host.

PEDICULOSIS

Pediculosis (i.e., lice) is a contagious dermatosis, caused by lice, which are blood-sucking, wingless insects and are obligate human parasites. Two species of lice infest humans causing three clinical forms of infestation: *Pediculus humanus capitis* (i.e., head louse), *Pediculus humanus corporis* (i.e., body louse), and *Phthirus pubis* (i.e.,

pubic louse). The body louse is the only louse that can carry human disease, including rickettsioses and epidemic typhus.

Pediculosis Capitis

Pediculosis capitis is caused by *P. humanus capitis*, and it is transmitted by close contact or by fomites with combs, brushes, towels, and hats. It manifests with pruritus (due to the saliva of the louse), excoriations, nape dermatitis, secondary bacterial infection, and cervical and suboccipital lymphadenopathy. Diagnosis is based on identification of lice and eggs or nits on the hair and on fluorescence of nits with Wood's light. Visible nits are deposited on the hair shaft, close to the scalp. After adequate treatment, nits found at 1.0 to 1.5 cm from the scalp are not alive.

Treatment includes malathion (Ovide) 0.5% lotion applied for 8 to 12 hours or permethrin (Nix) 1% cream rinse applied to shampooed hair for 10 minutes. A second application with permethrin is recommended 1 week later to kill hatching progeny. Alternatively, pyrethrins with piperidyl butoxide (RID) can be applied and washed off after 10 minutes. Benzyl benzoate 25% solution[6] is mainly a scabicide, but it may also be used as a pediculicide. Ivermectin (Stromectol)[1] can be used at a dose of 200 μg/kg on days 1, 2, and 10. Vinegar[1] may be used to facilitate nit removal from the hair shaft, using a fine-toothed comb. Bedding, clothing, and headgear should be decontaminated (as for scabies) or removed from body contact for 2 weeks. Information for managing head lice can be found at the National Pediculosis Association Web site (http://www.headlice.org).

Pediculosis Corporis

Pediculosis corporis (i.e., vagabond's itch) is caused by *P. humanus corporis*, which lives and reproduces in the lining of clothes and leaves the clothing only for feeding from the skin. This disease is usually found among vagabonds. Transmission occurs mainly through contact with contaminated clothing or bedding. Clinical manifestations include pruritus, excoriations, and small, red macules that usually occur on the back. Clothes should be examined carefully for lice.

Treatment is the same as for pediculosis capitis. Dry heat or washing in hot water followed by ironing is effective in killing the lice and their ova in clothing. Items that cannot be washed should be removed from body contact for 2 weeks.

---

[1]Not FDA approved for this indication.
[6]May be compounded by pharmacists.

---

[1]Not FDA approved for this indication.
[6]May be compounded by pharmacists.

Pediculosis Pubis

Pediculosis pubis is caused by *P. pubis* and affects the pubic hair. However, if left untreated, it may also affect very hairy regions of the chest, abdomen, axillary region, and especially in children, the eyelashes, edge of the scalp, and eyebrows. Patients present with pruritus. Useful diagnostic signs include small, blue-gray macules on the trunk, thighs, and axillae (i.e., taches bleuâtres or maculae ceruleae) due to conversion of bilirubin to biliverdin by the saliva of the louse and a brown "dust" found on underclothing due to the excreta of the insects. *P. pubis* is transmitted mainly by sexual contact, but it also may be transmitted by clothing or from parents to children.

Patients with pubic lice should be evaluated for other sexually transmitted diseases. Treatment of pediculosis pubis is the same as for pediculosis capitis. Bedding and clothing should be decontaminated (as for scabies) or removed from body contact for 2 weeks. Attention should be paid to treating sexual partners within the previous month because they are a common cause of reinfestation. For infested eyelashes and eyebrows, ophthalmic-grade petrolatum ointment may be used two to four times daily for 10 days, and lice and nits should be carefully removed from the eyelashes with forceps.

REFERENCES

Centers for Disease Control (CDC). Disease exposure while traveling. Available at: http://www.cdc.gov/travel/ [accessed June 2009].

Gorkiewicz-Petkow A. Scabicides and pediculicides. In: Katsambas AD, Lotti TM, editors. European Handbook of Dermatological Treatments. 2nd ed. Berlin: Springer; 2003. pp. 775–9.

Goyal NN, Wong GA. Psoriasis or crusted scabies. Clin Exp Dermatol 2008;33:211–2.

Heukelbach J, Feldmeier H. Epidemiological and clinical characteristics of hookworm-related cutaneous larva migrans. Lancet Infect Dis 2008;8:302–9.

Klaus SN, Frankenburg S, Dhar AD. Leishmaniasis and other protozoan infections. In: Freedeberg IM, Eisen AZ, Wolff K, et al., editors. Fitzpatrick's Dermatology in General Medicine. 6th ed. New York: McGraw-Hill; 2003. pp. 2215–24.

Lucchina LC, Wilson ME. Cysticercosis and other helminthic infections. In: Freedeberg IM, Eisen AZ, Wolff K, et al., editors. Fitzpatrick's Dermatology in General Medicine. 6th ed. New York: McGraw-Hill; 2003. pp. 2225–59.

Paller AS, Mancini AJ. Bites and infestations. In: Hurwitz Clinical Pediatric Dermatology. 3rd ed. Philadelphia: WB Saunders; 2006. pp. 479–501.

Stone SP. Scabies and pediculosis. In: Freedeberg IM, Eisen AZ, Wolff K, et al., Fitzpatrick's Dermatology in General Medicine. 6th ed. New York: McGraw-Hill; 2003. pp. 2283–9.

Tsoureli-Nikita E, Campanile G, Hautmann G, et al. Pediculosis. In: Katsambas AD, Lotti TM, editors. European Handbook of Dermatological Treatments. 2nd ed. Berlin: Springer; 2003. pp. 775–9.

Fungal Diseases of the Skin

Method of
Robert Grossberg, MD

Fungal infections of the skin, hair, and nails are some of the most common infections worldwide, with special prominence among children, the elderly, men, and immunocompromised hosts such as those with diabetes, cancer, or HIV infection. Fungal infections of the skin can be divided into four general categories. Superficial fungal infections are caused by dermatophytes such as those from the *Trichophyton*, *Microsporum*, and *Epidermophyton* genera. Cutaneous infections include tinea corporis, candidiasis, and onychomycosis. Subcutaneous (e.g. mycetoma, sporotrichosis) and systemic fungal infections (cryptococcosis, blastomycosis) that manifest in the skin are less common.

Diagnosing superficial fungal infections is generally based on clinical characteristics and response to empiric treatment. In unclear or recalcitrant cases, confirmation of diagnosis can be attempted by potassium hydroxide (KOH) preparation or histologic examination of scrapings, examination of scrapings under Wood's light, or culture. Fungal elements, however, are sometimes difficult to detect by microscopy, and tinea species grow poorly on routine culture media. Growth of dermatophytes is best performed on specific mycologic media at laboratories experienced in fungal isolation. However, depending on the specific fungal disease, the optimal site to obtain scrapings varies and affects the yield on culture.

Differential diagnosis depends on the location of the suspected fungal infection and specific clinical characteristics. Most commonly, discrimination must be made from eczema, contact dermatitis, acneiform eruptions, folliculitis of other cause, skin maceration, psoriasis, lichen planus, or trauma.

Tinea Pedis

Tinea pedis (also called athlete's foot) is most commonly caused by *Trichophyton rubrum*. It is spread by contact with infected desquamated skin and is more prevalent among men than women or children. Infection may be asymptomatic or cause various degrees of interdigital itching and cracking, erythema, scaling, and rarely blisters. The scaling occasionally causes an extensive moccasin sole appearance, one manifestation of dry-type tinea pedis. The disease can become extensive in immunocompromised patients, especially those with AIDS.

Tinea Cruris

Tinea cruris (also called "jock itch") is most commonly caused by *T. rubrum* or *Epidermophyton floccosum*. Occurring more commonly during summer months, tinea cruris manifests with unilateral or bilateral medial thigh and/or scrotal redness, itching, and scaling, generally with a sharp border and occasionally with papules and pustules near the leading edge. There are no satellite lesions as with candidiasis of the skin.

Tinea Corporis

Also called ringworm, tinea corporis is now relatively uncommon in the United States, being seen more commonly in tropical parts of the world. However, cases still occur in this country, especially among the homeless, HIV-infected persons, and inner city children and their caregivers. Clusters have also occurred among athletes who have skin-to skin contact, such as wrestlers. Typical cases are caused by *T. rubrum* and appear ringlike, well demarcated, and scaly, with central clearing and little inflammation. Lesions may be hyperpigmented in darker-skinned persons. Less commonly, infection derives from animal sources such as cows, dogs, and cats and is caused by *Trichophyton verrucosum* or *Microsporum canis*. Animal-associated species tend to cause a more nodular and inflammatory form of tinea corporis that is especially seen in children. Kerions are characteristic large pustular lesions caused by these dermatophytes.

Tinea Manuum

Tinea infection of the hand usually involves only a single palm, and concurrent foot infection is typical. The appearance is of a diffuse, dry, scaly eruption, similar to the moccasin sole form of tinea pedis. *T. rubrum* is the most common cause.

Tinea Faciei and Tinea Barbae

Tinea infections of the face (tinea faciei) are typically caused by *T. rubrum* but appear different from infections by this organism at other sites. Lesions may be follicular, pruritic, and mildly red, with inexact margins. Highly inflamed and pustular lesions of the neck and beard (tinea barbae) are caused by the animal dermatophytes *T. verrucosum* or *Trichophyton mentagrophytes*, thereby being similar to tinea corporis lesions caused by these dermatophytes, and are mainly an occupational illness.

Tinea Capitis

Tinea capitis (scalp ringworm) is principally a disease of young children. After puberty, changes in fatty acid content of sebum are believed to inhibit dermatophyte growth and lead to a dramatic decline in disease incidence. Large geographic variation occurs in overall incidence as well as causative genera and species, but most infections are due to *Trichophyton* species. Characteristic features of tinea capitis include mild to severe scaling, itching, hair loss, erythema, and sometimes pustules or kerions. Ectothrix infections have dermatophyte arthrospores forming on the outside of the hair shaft and cause hair breakage just above the surface of the scalp. In endothrix infections, arthrospores form within the hair shaft, so hair breakage occurs at the skin surface. Favus is a particularly severe form of tinea capitis caused by *T. schoenleinii*, in which a thick inflammatory crust forms on the scalp and hair follicles. This can lead to scarring and permanent alopecia if untreated.

Onychomycosis

Onychomycosis, fungal infection of the nails (also called tinea unguum), usually occurs in the setting of chronic dermatophyte infection of adjacent skin. The disease is common in elderly, diabetic, and immunocompromised persons, but it also occurs commonly in those without predisposing conditions. Various forms of onychomycosis can occur, but the most common begins at the distal and lateral subungual margins of the nail, can extend to involve the whole nail, and is caused by *T. rubrum*. Affected nails are typically thickened and raised, with white or yellow discoloration and various degrees of cracking. Nail growth may be impaired, and at times the nail dislodges spontaneously or with minor pressure. Candidiasis of the nails almost exclusively involves the fingernails, sometimes inoculated by nail biting, and is usually less extensive than typical dermatophytic infection.

Tinea (Pityriasis) Versicolor

Tinea versicolor is not a true tinea infection as it caused by lipophilic skin commensals of the *Malassezia* family, most commonly *Malassezia furfur*. This common infection is characterized by hypo- or hyperpigmented macules of the trunk or proximal extremities, sometimes with scaling. Diagnosis is usually clinical, but it can be confirmed by a scraping that demonstrates numerous round yeasts with short hyphae. After treatment, pigmentation changes can persist for weeks or months, often until the area receives sun exposure.

Candidiasis

Candida species are normal flora of the mouth and vagina, especially in settings such as antibiotic exposure, dry mouth, excessive skin moisture, and extremes of age and in immunocompromised hosts, and can cause disease on skin and mucosal surfaces. In the mouth or vagina, candidiasis is suggested by white plaques, cheesy exudates, and erythema. Candidiasis of the mouth can also occur in other forms such as erythematous plaques, angular cheilitis, acute or chronic atrophic lesions (the latter in the setting of dentures), or chronic hypertrophic plaques. Candidiasis of the skin most commonly occurs in moist or occluded areas such as the groin, buttocks (especially under diapers), and axillae, but it can involve any area including the nails (described earlier). Satellite lesions help to differentiate skin candidiasis from tinea or other conditions.

Treatment

Treatments for fungal infections are shown in Table 1.

TABLE 1   Treatments of Choice for Fungal Infections of the Skin, Hair, and Nails

Infection	Preferred Agents and Regimens	Alternative Agents/ Regimens	Adjunctive Treatments/Comments
Tinea pedis	Topical terbinafine (Lamisil AT) or naftifine (Naftin)	Oral azole,[†] oral terbinafine (Lamisil),[1] griseofulvin (Grifulvin V)	Improve foot hygiene; Whitfield's ointment (benzoic acid/salicylic acid) may be applied for extensive disease; oral agents may be more effective for dry-type disease
Tinea cruris	Topical azole*	Oral azole,[†] terbinafine[1]	
Tinea corporis	Topical* or oral[†] azole	Terbinafine	Minimum 4-6 wk of treatment; oral if >1-2 lesions or large areas of skin involvement
Tinea manuum	Topical* or oral[†] azole	Terbinafine	
Tinea faciei	Oral azole[†] or terbinafine[1]		
Tinea barbae	Oral azole[†] or terbinafine[1]		
Tinea capitis	Griseofulvin (children), oral itraconazole (Sporanox),[1] oral terbinafine, fluconazole (Diflucan)[1]		Selenium sulfide shampoo (Selsun)[1] or ketoconazole shampoo (Nizoral)[1] is used only as an adjunct to oral therapy
Onychomycosis	Oral terbinafine or itraconazole	Pulse itraconazole: 200 mg PO bid for 1 wk of the mo, repeated 3-4 consecutive mo	Prolonged therapy needed (3-6 mo); topical therapy is usually ineffective alone, though success has been shown with some regimens including combined oral plus topical treatments
		Ciclopirox nail lacquer (Penlac)	Fingernails respond better than toenails Culture of deep specimens can help guide therapy Débridement or nail removal may be needed
Tinea versicolor	Oral azole,[†] selenium sulfide shampoo or lotion, ketoconazole shampoo	Topical azole* or terbinafine	Recurrence is common; hypopigmentation might persist despite treatment
Candidiasis	Topical azole* or nystatin (Mycostatin)	Oral[†] or IV azole, amphotericin B (Fungizone)	Improve underlying cause such as moisture, diabetes, etc.

*Topical azoles include clotrimazole (Lotrimin), econazole (Spectazole), ketoconazole (Nizoral), miconazole (Micatin), oxiconazole (Oxistat), and tioconazole (Vagistat).
[†]Oral azoles include ketoconazole (Nizoral), fluconazole (Diflucan), and itraconazole (Sporanox).
[1]Not FDA approved for this indication.

REFERENCES

Crissey JT, Lang H, Parish LC. Manual of Medical Mycology. Cambridge: Blackwell Science; 1995.

Havlickova B, Friedrich M. The advantages of topical combination therapy in the treatment of inflammatory dermatomycoses. Mycoses 2008;51(Suppl. 4):16–26. Erratum in: Mycoses 2009;52(1):96.

Schwartz RA. Superficial fungal infections. Lancet 2004;364(9440):1173–82.

Smith ES, Fleischer AB, Feldman SR, Williford PM. Characteristics of office-based physician visits for cutaneous fungal infections. An analysis of 1990 to 1994 National Ambulatory Medical Care Survey Data. Cutis 2002;69(3):191–8, 201–2.

Diseases of the Mouth

Method of
Gary C. Coleman, DDS, MS

The numerous diseases that affect the oral cavity can pose difficult diagnostic and therapeutic challenges. Some simplification can be attained by dividing oral diseases into three groups based on management perspective. The first group includes conditions such as dental caries and periodontitis that are directly associated with the teeth and are the dentist's treatment responsibility. The second group consists of conditions that do not cause symptoms, present little risk of adverse consequences, or are so rarely encountered that they represent more of a novelty than a clinically significant consideration. The third group consists of a relatively short list of conditions that produce pain or pose the risk of serious complications and require treatment other than dental care. The diseases of this third group are compared in the Current Diagnosis box and were selected to frame this therapeutic overview because patients may seek treatment from the physician rather than the dentist.

Disseminated Odontogenic Infection

With few exceptions, disseminated bacterial infections of odontogenic origin represent a dramatic, acute exacerbation of a chronic, asymptomatic infection. A variety of dental conditions are possible causes, such as a periodontal abscess, an abscess within the supportive bone resulting from the pulpal necrosis of a carious tooth, or an infection of the gingiva surrounding a partially erupted third molar. The patient often describes a history of one or more prior acute episodes of bacterial infection symptoms from the site followed by resolution. The degree of swelling, lymphadenopathy, pain, and fever is proportional to the risk of potential complications such as septicemia. Of particular concern is evidence of rapid progression of diffuse swelling into the floor of the mouth and neck because of the risk of respiratory distress (i.e., Ludwig's angina) or superiorly from the anterior portion of the maxilla because of the possibility of cavernous sinus thrombosis.

Definitive dental treatment to eliminate the underlying infectious source is the treatment goal after the acute, disseminated infection has been controlled. Penicillin is still considered the empiric antibiotic choice for disseminated odontogenic bacterial infections in individuals with no history of adverse reaction, and clindamycin (Cleocin) is used for those hypersensitive to penicillin. Many patients mistakenly assume that empiric antibiotic treatment can eliminate the infection in the same sense that antibiotic treatment can cure bacterial sinusitis or pharyngitis. The patient should be informed that improvement of an acute odontogenic infection after antibiotic treatment is not curative and that dental care to eliminate the underlying cause is necessary. One or more courses of antibiotics without elimination of the source increase the probability of the emergence of more virulent, antibiotic-resistant pathogens. More aggressive treatment, including intravenous antibiotics and surgical drainage in a hospital setting, must be considered in cases of rapid progression or extensive swelling, particularly if the anterior maxilla or submandibular areas are involved and in instances of compromised host resistance.

Suspicion of Oral Cancer

Primary malignant neoplasms originating from virtually every tissue type found in the oral cavity have been reported. However, more than 90% of intraoral malignancies are squamous cell carcinoma (SCC) originating from the lining oral epithelium. The typical features and clinical course of oral SCC heavily influence the differential diagnostic assessment of any oral lesions if malignant neoplasia is suspected. Careful consideration is critical because the 5-year survival probability for oral SCC is approximately 50%, and early diagnosis is one of the few favorable prognostic factors.

Several features that strongly correlate an eventual diagnosis of oral SCC are summarized in Table 1. The two most significant etiologic factors for intraoral SCC are the habitual use of tobacco and alcoholic beverages. Other potential causative factors, such as exposure to virulent human papillomavirus (HPV) subtypes, have shown some positive correlation, but by far the probability of oral cancer is greatest among heavy drinkers and smokers. The carcinogenic effect of the two substances appears to be synergistic. This process typically requires decades for the emergence of clinical lesions, as is shown by the observation that the initial diagnosis of more than 90% of oral SCCs is made after age 40, with a peak incidence in the sixth decade of life.

SCC of the exposed lower lip surface usually is included in oral cancer statistics, but important differences in cause and prognosis compared with intraoral SCC affect diagnosis and management. SCC of the exposed lower lip is primarily caused by actinic cellular damage and is comparable to actinic skin lesions in terms of appearance, a more positive prognosis, and low probability of metastasis. As with actinic skin cancers of the face, the possibility of SCC of the lower lip is greatest during the sixth or seventh decade for fair-skinned individuals with a vocation or avocation associated with prolonged sun exposure.

Premalignant dysplastic lesions and early intraoral SCC may manifest as a superficial white or red patch compared with the typical appearance of the mucosa. However, routine frictional irritation or incidental abrasion is the much more common cause of this

TABLE 1 Clinical Suspicion Factors for Oral Squamous Cell Carcinoma

Feature	More Suspicious	Less Suspicious
Causative factors	Alcohol and tobacco use	Frictional cause (e.g., sharp tooth)
Age	>40 years (younger much less likely)	<40 (probability increases if immunocompromised)
Surface appearance	Altered and heterogeneous	Unaltered or homogeneous
Peripheral delineation	Vague borders	Sharp borders
Distribution	Isolated	Multifocal
Pain (ulcers)	Painless or less pain than expected for lesion size	Pain (inflammatory)
Location	Tongue, oropharynx, floor of mouth	Gingiva, hard palate, buccal mucosa (less likely)
Palpation	Indurated, nontender	Compressible, tender
Clinical course	Unchanging (weeks), progressive (months)	Variable (within weeks), static (months or years)

appearance, and this is by far the most likely cause in areas prone to friction, such as the buccal mucosa. A white or red lesion of the soft palate or floor of the mouth is much more suspicious. Oral SCC may manifest primarily as an ulcer, although most oral ulcers are inflammatory. In contrast to asymptomatic white or red mucosal patches, the patient's history reveals valuable awareness of the duration and course of oral ulcers because of the pain they cause. Intraoral ulcers of SCC tend to be of long duration and much less painful compared with inflammatory ulcers of similar size. Palpation tends to demonstrate an indurated periphery to the malignant oral ulcer.

Most oral enlargements are benign neoplasms or inflammatory in origin. Enlargements that are benign tend to be sharply delineated and of long duration (many months or years) and have a normal surface appearance. Chronic inflammatory enlargements are somewhat tender and compressible to palpation with a shorter duration (days or weeks) or vary in size with time. The combination of induration, altered surface appearance, lack of tenderness to palpation, and progressive enlargement over a period of weeks or months suggests malignancy.

Definitive diagnosis of most oral lesions requires a biopsy, and this is indicated if oral SCC is considered a significant differential diagnostic possibility. Exfoliative cytology is much less reliable as a screening method in the assessment of malignant and premalignant oral disease compared with lesions of the uterine cervix. The harsh nature of the oral environment from food, tobacco use, and other habits limits the appreciation of cytologic features. The diagnosis of oral candidiasis and some viral lesions can be made by exfoliative cytology. Table 1 lists features that prompt increased suspicion of oral cancer and the need for definitive diagnosis by biopsy. As with any differential diagnosis, one or two corresponding features may not be compelling unless dramatic. A greater number of findings that suggest oral SCC indicate a stronger justification for biopsy. The decision to obtain a biopsy of an oral lesion should be made with consideration of the substantial positive impact that early detection has on a disease with an otherwise unfavorable prognosis.

Necrotizing Ulcerative Gingivitis

Necrotizing ulcerative gingivitis (NUG) is a characteristic, potentially destructive infection of the dental supportive tissues caused by a predominance of fusiform bacteria and spirochetes. Some combination of psychologic stress, compromised immune function, malnutrition, or other condition of diminished host resistance dramatically increases the risk of NUG. This is suggested by the colloquial phrase *trench mouth* used to refer to this infection, because it was frequently observed among debilitated soldiers during World War I. It has also been called Vincent's infection and acute NUG (ANUG).

Acute onset of poorly localized, severe dental pain and a putrid taste are typically the patient's chief complaints. Onset usually corresponds with a significant alteration in the general health or emotional status, although a more chronic course of variably pronounced symptoms can be expected with protracted conditions such as acquired immunodeficiency syndrome (AIDS). Visual features of NUG include necrotic deterioration of the gingiva with pronounced peripheral erythema and a superficial pseudomembrane. The tissue around the mandibular anterior teeth is most severely affected in most cases, and the gingiva often appears "punched out" from between the teeth. The gingival necrosis produces the characteristic fetid breath that is far more pungent than that caused by typical gingivitis. The putrid odor in combination with the acute onset and poor localization of pain is usually a more reliable basis for diagnosis than visual findings. Additional features, such as fever and cervical lymphadenopathy, are proportional to the severity of the oral findings.

Treatment of NUG consists of the combination of supportive care, antimicrobial measures, and improvement in the underlying compromising health conditions. Supportive care is nonspecific and includes rest, fluid intake, and a soft but nutritious diet. Warm saline, dilute hydrogen peroxide, and chlorhexidine gluconate (Peridex) are effective antimicrobial rinses. Penicillin and metronidazole (Flagyl) are the empiric systemic antibiotics of choice. Ultimately, the most

CURRENT DIAGNOSIS

High-Risk Conditions

- Acute exacerbation of odontogenic infections: rapid onset, swelling, purulence, obvious dental origin
- Suspicion of oral cancer: mucosal surface color change, nonhealing ulcer, enlargement, asymptomatic or incidental finding, use of tobacco and alcohol

Opportunistic Infections and Dry Mouth

- Necrotizing ulcerative gingivitis (trench mouth): compromised host resistance, generalized dental pain, usually acute onset, fetid odor
- Oral candidiasis: compromised host resistance, chronic or recurring course, poorly localized "burning" soreness, superficial change in mucosal appearance
- Salivary dysfunction (xerostomia): patient's perception of dry mouth, causative condition or associated findings

Acute-Onset Oral Ulcers with Focal Pain

- Aphthous stomatitis: recurring episodes, formation of one or more superficial oral ulcers, located on nonbound mucosa, healing in approximately 7 to 10 days
- Primary herpetic gingivostomatitis: acute onset of systemic viral infection features, including fever and multiple oral vesicles degenerating into ulcers, resolution in 7 to 10 days
- Recurrent herpes: recurring episodes, acute formation of vesicles collapsing to ulcers, located on exposed lip or bound mucosa, healing in 7 to 10 days
- Erythema multiforme: acute onset of oral ulcers, triggering event, mild systemic features such as fever, characteristic skin lesions, resolution in 2 to 4 weeks

Chronic Oral Ulcers

- Erosive lichen planus and lichenoid reaction: reticular appearance at periphery of ulcers, buccal mucosa affected, may cause desquamative gingivitis, skin lesions possible
- Mucous membrane pemphigoid: typically desquamative gingivitis presentation, possible eye and genital ulcers, skin lesions unlikely
- Pemphigus vulgaris: ulcers of irregular shape and jagged peripheral contour, possible skin lesions

effective antimicrobial treatment is the combination of thorough dental cleaning of the teeth with débridement of the necrotic soft tissue and improved oral hygiene. Resolution of NUG, including complete healing of the gingival tissue, is strikingly rapid in most instances if this is accomplished and underlying health status improves. Persistence or recurrence of NUG after débridement suggests the possibility of human immunodeficiency virus (HIV) infection or another undiagnosed compromising condition.

Oral Candidiasis

Oral candidiasis is a superficial fungal infection of the oral mucosa that is clinically similar to vaginal candidiasis in many respects. With isolated exceptions, the infection is caused by the fungus *Candida albicans*, which can be identified in the mouths of approximately 50% of healthy adults. The risk of oral candidiasis is increased by one or more factors of compromised host resistance: decreased local resistance, compromised immune function, or uncontrolled systemic disease. Frequently encountered examples of decreased local resistance include poor oral hygiene, xerostomia, wearing dentures that provide an organism reservoir or limit hygiene, and recent antibiotic therapy that has altered the normally competitive oral bacteria. The combination of one or more of these local factors with a systemic condition that causes compromised immune status or constitutional compromise dramatically increases the risk of clinical apparent infection. Common examples include AIDS, corticosteroid therapy, severe anemia, and poorly controlled diabetes mellitus.

Oral candidiasis lesions can have four distinct appearances. The most characteristic form is the pseudomembranous, curdlike globules of thrush that wipe off with cotton gauze, leaving a sore, erythematous mucosal surface. The erythematous or atrophic form of oral candidiasis produces a thin, "beefy" appearance often affecting the dorsum of the tongue or mucosa that supports a denture. The third type of lesion is the formation of fissures similar to those of tinea pedis that usually are at the corners of the mouth and are referred to as angular cheilitis. The fourth is a hyperplastic form that produces a patchy, white thickening of the surface epithelium that does not rub off and that appears similar to the hyperkeratosis of chronic frictional irritation. Oral candidiasis often produces more than one lesion form simultaneously in different areas of the mouth, which may be a confirmational finding. Patients often describe little discomfort or only a mild burning sensation from affected sites.

The clinical course of the infection may be acute, chronic, or cyclic in severity, depending on the nature of the underlying causes. The combination of clinical appearance, suspected compromised host status, and improvement after empiric treatment provides an adequate basis for the diagnosis. Exfoliative cytology provides definitive evidence of the infection in more equivocal situations.

Antifungal treatment eliminates oral candidiasis in most instances, but recurrences or a chronic, subclinical course can be expected if the predisposing condition remains unchanged. This implies that treatment of superficial oral candidiasis may not be justified in such instances if the affected individual is asymptomatic, because the only realistic treatment goal is elimination of symptoms. That decision must be weighed against the possibility of spread to the esophagus.

Options for routine topical treatment of oral candidiasis include clotrimazole (Mycelex) troches or nystatin (Mycostatin) pastilles, and use should continue for 1 week after resolution of symptoms. Several considerations can complicate effectiveness. Patients with xerostomia have difficulty dissolving the troches or pastilles and prefer a nystatin rinse. Concurrent management of the dry mouth (discussed later) increases the effectiveness of topical antifungal treatment for candidiasis. Limiting the *Candida* organism reservoir in the denture acrylic for those who wear dentures can be accomplished by soaking overnight in most commercial denture soaking solutions, mouthwashes such as Listerine, or chlorhexidine gluconate. These products are adequately fungicidal, and keeping the denture out overnight disrupts adherence and colonization of candidal organisms. Some patients are more compliant about managing the denture problem by applying a thin layer of nystatin ointment[1] or clotrimazole cream (Lotrimin)[1] to the denture before wearing. Direct application of these preparations also promotes rapid resolution of angular cheilitis. Systemic administration of ketoconazole (Nizoral) or fluconazole (Diflucan) is an alternative for patients who cannot manage topical treatment or for severely immunocompromised individuals in the interest of controlling oral symptoms and minimizing the risk of spread to the esophagus.

Xerostomia

Xerostomia is defined by the patient's subjective perception of "dry mouth" rather than by any objective parameter. The amount of saliva is decreased, and its character typically is altered to a more viscous, ropey consistency. The condition is common because salivary function is adversely affected by so many routinely encountered influences, including many frequently prescribed medications, smoking, methamphetamine abuse, several common systemic diseases, and tumoricidal

irradiation exposure. In addition to these influences, primary Sjögren syndrome is characterized by chronic dry eyes and dry mouth caused by autoimmune-mediated acinar degeneration. Secondary Sjögren syndrome is defined as oral and ocular dryness concurrent with an autoimmune connective tissue disorder such as rheumatoid arthritis.

The subjective response of different individuals to a mild or moderate degree of oral dryness varies considerably. Many patients who appear to produce adequate saliva complain of dryness, whereas others who seem unusually dry during oral examination have no complaints. Most patients with an advanced degree of dryness find the continual "cotton mouth" sensation and other consequences to be a significant quality-of-life issue. Decreased saliva production causes difficulty chewing and swallowing, as well as painful abrasion of the mucosa by coarse foods. Beyond the physical irritation, limited saliva alters the sense of taste and the enjoyment of food. Saliva contributes to oral health by providing antimicrobial components such as lactoperoxidase and IgE antibodies, and it has a significant flushing and cleansing function. Xerostomia causes a rampant and rapidly progressive pattern of dental decay that is particularly destructive even for previously caries-resistant individuals. This is compounded if the patient compensates for the dryness by drinking sucrose-rich soft drinks or sucking on hard candy. Similarly, periodontitis tends to progress rapidly despite normally effective treatment if saliva production is limited. Xerostomia is also associated with complaints of generalized soreness of the mouth caused by frequent and persistent episodes of oral candidiasis.

Management of xerostomia is challenging and often frustrating for the patient and the clinician. The treatment for severe, irreversible xerostomia, as in cases of head and neck radiotherapy, is essentially symptomatic. Different patients prefer different combinations of compensation methods. Sipping water throughout the day is the single most effective and simplest way to counter loss of saliva. Some patients report additional improvement with the use of commercially available saliva substitutes, although many do as well with water and ice chips. Most patients soon learn to avoid abrasive foods, irritating commercial mouth rinses that contain alcohol, and highly flavored toothpastes in favor of less irritating alternatives. Use of a humidifier at night is often beneficial. Comprehensive dental treatment should be recommended to limit the progression and severity of dental caries and periodontitis. Smoking and compensation by drinking sucrose-rich soft drinks, sports drinks, drinks that contain caffeine, and highly acidic citric juices should be discouraged.

Additional options beyond the previous recommendations are available for those who have some residual salivary function. Drinking ample water moistens the mucosa and maintains general hydration, which maximizes the residual saliva production. Sugar-free gum or hard candy significantly stimulates saliva flow. Alternate medications may be substituted in some cases to treat conditions such as hypertension that are equally effective therapeutically but are less likely to cause xerostomia.

Several cholinergic sialologs are available, including cevimeline (Evoxac), pilocarpine (Salagen), and bethanechol (Urecholine).[1] Titration of dosage is usually necessary to optimize saliva flow while minimizing frequent adverse effects such as excessive sweating and gastritis. Many patients discontinue treatment because of these and less common side effects that become more troublesome than the xerostomia. Contraindications such as glaucoma and the risk of serious complications such as arrhythmia must also be considered.

Aphthous Stomatitis

Recurrent aphthous stomatitis, colloquially known as *canker sores*, is a common condition of complex immune-mediated pathogenesis. Patients describe recurring episodes of painful ulcers that often follow triggering events such as minor tissue abrasion, eating certain foods, or episodes of emotional stress. The phrase *minor aphthous stomatitis* differentiates the most common, mild form of the disease from the more severe *major* and *herpetiform variations*. Most

[1]Not FDA approved for this indication.

[1]Not FDA approved for this indication.

authorities believe these categorizations are somewhat artificial distinctions within a continuum of a single process. Similar ulcers are a feature of Behçet's syndrome but are of minor diagnostic and treatment significance compared with the other manifestations of this rare, multisystem condition.

The clinical features of minor recurrent aphthous stomatitis are characteristic. One or more painful ulcers develop soon after a short prodromal period of burning or itching at the affected site. The superficial ulcers exhibit a uniform, yellowish white, pseudomembranous surface with an erythematous peripheral halo at the sharply delineated ulcer margin. Typical size is 1 to 2 cm, and lesions affect only unbound oral mucosal surfaces of the lips, cheeks, floor of the mouth, or soft palate. This distribution specifically excludes the bound surfaces of the gingiva, hard palate, and the dorsum of the tongue. This feature is valuable for differentiating aphthous stomatitis from the intraoral recurrent herpetic lesions (discussed later) that affect only bound surfaces.

Aphthous lesions typically heal within 7 to 10 days, and most patients describe a long clinical course of symptom-free periods of various durations interrupted by episodes of ulcer formation. Lesion-free periods of weeks, months, or even years typically distinguish recurrent aphthous stomatitis from autoimmune conditions such as erosive lichen planus (discussed later) that produce a continuous course of oral ulcers.

The major form of recurrent aphthous stomatitis produces ulcers of similar appearance, but the lesions are larger, require a longer healing time, often heal with scarring, and form so frequently that at least one ulcer is usually present. The herpetiform variant is characterized by a cluster of numerous smaller (1–3 mm) ulcers that often coalesce into a single, large lesion, and the ulcers are described as exceptionally painful. The clustering distribution explains the somewhat misleading herpetiform designation for this nonviral condition. This form of aphthous stomatitis may affect keratinized and nonkeratinized surfaces, which in addition to the clustering distribution may lead to confusion with recurrent herpes simplex lesions.

Minor recurrent aphthous stomatitis is more irritating than serious, and treatment beyond symptomatic management is usually not justified. Patients soon learn to avoid their particular trigger event as much as possible, and many find relief during outbreaks from over-the-counter preparations such as Orabase with benzocaine 20% or by rinsing with soothing, coating products such as bismuth subsalicylate (Kaopectate).[1] Rinses containing a variety of ingredients, such as tetracycline,[1] aloe,[7] and chlorhexidine gluconate,[1] have been reported to promote ulcer healing in some cases. Treatment with corticosteroids (see Current Therapy box), however, is more consistently effective and is justified for major and herpetiform variants, as well as for particularly severe or frequent outbreaks of minor aphthous lesions.

Orofacial Herpes Simplex Infection

Most herpes simplex infections of the oral mucosa are caused by herpes simplex virus type 1 (HSV-1). A much smaller proportion of oral cases results from the type 2 herpes simplex virus that typically causes genital lesions. Transmission occurs by direct contact or contaminated saliva, and serologic studies demonstrate that as much as 90% of the population has been infected by age 50.

The initial infection, referred to as acute herpetic gingivostomatitis or primary herpes, usually affects children and causes acute onset of cervical lymphadenopathy, chills, and fever similar to many acute viral infections. The distinguishing manifestation is the formation of multiple, painful oral vesicles that rapidly rupture. The resulting ulcers most prominently affect the gingiva, lips, and tongue but may occur on any oral surface. Primary herpes in adults is more likely to cause complaints of pharyngitis rather than oral ulcers, which makes distinguishing it from other systemic viral infections unlikely. The severity of primary herpes varies from virtually subclinical or

indistinguishable from nonspecific viral infections to debilitating. The distinguishing oral lesions are probably seen only in severe cases because relatively few seropositive individuals recall the oral ulcers of the primary infection when questioned. Symptoms resolve within 5 days to 2 weeks, depending on the severity of the manifestations, and significant complications such as encephalitis or keratoconjunctivitis are rare.

The HSV-1 virus becomes latent within the sensory neurons that supply the primary infection site. Episodes of recurrent lesions may develop after the primary infection, a pattern similar to the recurring genital lesions caused by HSV-2. The frequency, severity, and course of these outbreaks vary widely among individuals, and at least one half of HSV-1–seropositive individuals rarely or never suffer recurrent lesions. Those who do often associate occurrence with causative events, such as sun exposure of the exposed lip, abrasion of the surface, or an illness such as a nonspecific viral infection. This explains the colloquial terms *cold sore* and *fever blister* used to describe the most common presentation affecting the exposed lip, which is referred to as herpes labialis.

The typical episode begins with a prodromal sensation of burning or itching at the site near the vermillion border, followed by formation of one or more vesicles within 24 hours. The vesicles soon rupture, forming a coalesced crust that heals after 7 to 10 days. A few individuals suffer similar recurrent herpes lesions of the intraoral mucosa. Intraoral herpes lesions produce features of pain, onset, recurrent course, and healing time that are similar to those for aphthous stomatitis, which may present some differential diagnostic uncertainty. The diagnosis can be made in most cases based on the affected surface. Aphthous lesions are usually limited to the unbound mucosa of the lips, cheeks, soft palate, and floor of the mouth, whereas the intraoral ulcers of recurrent herpes simplex infection are limited to the bound mucosa of the gingiva and hard palate.

Treatment of primary herpes simplex infection for immunocompetent individuals is supportive and symptomatic, as for any acute systemic viral infection. In cases of significant oral discomfort, a rinse consisting of a 1:1 mixture of diphenhydramine (Benadryl)[1] elixir 12.5 mg/5 mL and Kaopectate[1] used as needed provides some relief by coating the ulcers. The FDA recommends that systemic antiviral medication such as acyclovir (Zovirax)[1] and valacyclovir (Valtrex)[1] be reserved for immunocompromised individuals, with the goal of decreasing the duration and severity of symptoms. Administration of the antiviral agent must be started during the initial stage of the infection to be effective.

Most individuals affected by secondary herpes lesions suffer relatively few episodes, and no treatment is warranted. Patients prone to frequent lip lesions after sun exposure soon learn the preventive value of sunscreen lip balms, but the advice may be helpful to those who have not made the association. For patients who experience numerous secondary herpetic episodes, topical antiviral treatment with penciclovir (Denavir) cream or docosanol 10% (Abreva) cream may limit the severity and duration of the lesions, but applications must begin during the prodromal stage to be effective. Systemic administration of valacyclovir (Valtrex) can be used therapeutically during the prodromal stage or prophylactically.[1] FDA recommendations limit the use of systemic acyclovir[1] for recurrent orofacial herpetic lesions to immunocompromised patients for prophylaxis and treatment of individual outbreaks at the onset of prodromal symptoms.

Erythema Multiforme

Erythema multiforme, which is discussed in greater detail elsewhere in this textbook, is characterized by shallow oral ulcers and characteristic "target" skin lesions. Outbreaks of secondary herpetic lesions have been implicated as a frequent trigger for erythema multiforme. A prodrome of mild fever, malaise, sore throat, and headache may precede the appearance of the oral ulcers and skin lesions. The shallow oral ulcers usually affect the lips, tongue, or soft palate and are less likely to develop on the gingiva or hard palate. Ulcers gradually heal after 2 to 4 weeks, and approximately 20% of affected individuals experience multiple episodes. Certain medications, especially

---

[1]Not FDA approved for this indication.
[7]Available as a dietary supplement.

---

[1]Not FDA approved for this indication.

antibiotics, have also been implicated as triggers for erythema multiforme. Medication exposure is the typical stimulus for the onset of Stevens-Johnson syndrome and toxic epidermal necrolysis, which by similar allergic mechanisms produce much more extensive, generalized epithelial sloughing.

Treatment of the oral lesions of erythema multiforme is somewhat controversial. Topical and systemic corticosteroids have been recommended in the past based largely on the presumed pathogenesis of the lesions. However, little evidence exists to demonstrate the effectiveness of this approach. Supportive care usually is adequate and includes a less abrasive diet, maintaining hydration, use of analgesics, and use of a soothing, coating rinse (1:1 mixture of Benadryl elixir and Kaopectate).[1] Patients who experience recurring episodes may benefit from herpes simplex virus suppression with acyclovir or valacyclovir. More extensive epithelial sloughing or rapid progression suggesting Stevens-Johnson syndrome or toxic epidermal necrolysis requires hospitalization.

Erosive Lichen Planus and Similar Autoimmune Ulcerative Conditions of the Oral Mucosa

Several diseases cause oral ulcers by autoimmune-mediated degeneration at or near the epithelial–connective tissue interface. In some patients, painful oral ulceration is the only presenting feature of the disease. For other patients, the oral pain is only an occasional or secondary complaint. With few exceptions, however, a chronic course of oral pain for months or years without complete remission is described by the patient. The location and severity may change over time with cyclic formation of new ulcers and concurrent healing of others, but the dominant trend is a chronic, protracted, or progressive course with little or no complete relief. This continuous course distinguishes the ulcers caused by autoimmune diseases from those of other conditions, such as aphthous stomatitis, which characteristically have an episodic pattern of occurrence. As with autoimmune diseases in general, the demographic pattern tends toward middle-aged women. Definitive diagnosis typically relies on biopsy results, but the differential diagnosis is often narrowed by the appreciation of additional findings, such as lesions of the skin or other mucous membranes, and by laboratory tests, such as obtaining an antinuclear antibody (ANA) titer.

Most patients presenting with a chronic course of oral ulcers are suffering from one of three conditions: erosive lichen planus (ELP), mucous membrane pemphigoid (MMP), or pemphigus vulgaris (PV). Because ELP is relatively common and the oral ulcers are a prominent feature of the condition, it is described in some detail. The clinical features that are of differential diagnostic value in distinguishing similar diseases are briefly compared.

The characteristic skin manifestations of lichen planus are a pruritic, papular eruption of flexor surfaces of the limbs and linear hyperkeratotic lesions known as Wickham's striae. These findings combined with the chronic course typically provide an adequate basis for the clinical diagnosis. Approximately 1% of the adult population is affected by lichen planus or the clinically indistinguishable adverse reaction to certain medications referred to as *lichenoid reaction*. Oral lesions affect a significant proportion of patients with skin lesions, and many individuals exhibit oral lesions without skin abnormalities. The oral lesions appear as a lacy network of white, hyperkeratotic lines that bilaterally affect the buccal mucosal surfaces, although any intraoral surface may be affected. This is referred to as the *reticular presentation* of oral lichen planus, and no treatment is warranted because the white lesions are asymptomatic. The erosive form of lichen planus is less common but is of greatest therapeutic concern because affected patients seek pain relief. Ulcers tend to form in the same oral sites for a given patient and cyclically vary in severity as ulcers concurrently heal somewhat in some areas and progress elsewhere. Buccal mucosa and gingiva are the typically affected sites, but any intraoral surface may be affected.

One helpful distinguishing visual feature of ELP lesions from other autoimmune oral ulcers is that the zone between the ulcer and unaffected mucosa often exhibits a fine pattern of white lines that suggests the reticular form of the disease. This appearance is enhanced by drying the saliva with cotton gauze. The term *desquamative gingivitis* is used to describe the clinical presentation if the erosive lesions most dramatically affect the gingiva, which is often the case. The gingiva appears uniformly erythematous and delicately thin, with isolated ulcers. Bulla formation after lateral pressure on this atrophic surface (i.e., Nikolsky's sign) results from the compromised epithelial-connective tissue interface. The patient often complains of sore, bleeding "gums," but the atrophic appearance and Nikolsky's sign are helpful in distinguishing similar complaints from the much more commonly encountered gingivitis and periodontitis caused by poor oral hygiene.

MMP has also been referred to as *cicatricial pemphigoid* and *benign MMP*. The typical presentation of MMP is a chronic course of primarily gingival vesicles and bullae that rapidly degenerate into ulcers that fit the desquamative gingivitis description, although any intraoral area may be affected. The white, hyperkeratotic striations seen at the periphery of the ulcers caused by ELP are absent or less conspicuous with MMP. In contrast to ELP, if nonoral lesions of MMP are present, they affect the conjunctiva and genital mucous membrane surfaces rather than the skin. Occurrence of ocular lesions eventually approaches nearly 25% of affected individuals during the protracted disease course, and these lesions may cause blindness in severe cases.

Of the four characteristic forms of pemphigus, only PV causes oral lesions to any clinically significant degree. Approximately one half of patients develop oral ulcers before the appearance of skin lesions. Oral ulcers may affect any intraoral surface and appear superficial with an irregular shape. Initial vesicle or bulla formation is unusual with oral PV, in contrast to MMP, and the peripheral striations described with ELP are absent. The oral ulcers caused by PV tend to show slow progression without healing over time, in contrast to the cyclic variation of concurrent healing and lesion formation characteristic of ELP and MMP.

Several less common conditions can cause oral ulcers with a protracted clinical course. Bullous pemphigoid typically develops after age 60, but the condition is uncommon, skin lesions are the prominent feature, and less than one third of patients exhibit oral ulcers. Lupus erythematosus can cause oral ulcers very similar to those of ELP, but this occurs infrequently and only well into the course of the disease after the diagnosis has been established. Approximately 20% of individuals affected by erythema multiforme experience recurrences, but the course of oral lesions is much more episodic than continuous, and the characteristic target skin lesions often suggest the diagnosis. Graft-versus-host disease produces oral lesions similar to those of ELP, but the cause is obvious.

The oral ulcers caused by all of the conditions in this group respond to corticosteroid medications in the recommended therapeutic approach as described in the Current Therapy box. Several pivotal issues about these conditions and treatment with corticosteroids are important for successful management:

- The possibility of candidiasis and recurrent herpes simplex infection should be excluded on the basis of clinical course and features before empiric treatment of oral ulcers because corticosteroids worsen these infectious conditions.
- The patient should understand that the therapeutic goal is to control the oral ulcers rather than to cure the disease. Optimal treatment for ELP using corticosteroids, for example, converts the ulcers to the asymptomatic reticular form. Neither the patient nor the clinician should expect treatment to yield a completely normal tissue appearance.
- Oral candidiasis is a frequent complication of corticosteroid treatment, and this risk is increased with any concurrent condition such as xerostomia. Candidiasis can be detected early with periodic recall evaluation and by exfoliative cytology in suspected situations. Understanding the typical oral candidiasis symptoms increases the patient's awareness of the need to return for treatment.
- Empiric topical corticosteroid treatment should be discontinued for 2 weeks if a biopsy becomes necessary for a definitive diagnosis.

---

[1]Not FDA approved for this indication.

Every effort should be made to identify and discontinue use of causative or irritating agents. Examples such as the link of acidic foods with aphthous ulcers are obvious to the patient, but many are more subtle. One example is cinnamon flavoring agents in many foods and toothpastes. Others are irritating to the mucosa but are mistakenly perceived as beneficial. Hydrogen peroxide, phenol preparations, and alcohol-based mouth rinses that "seem to be doing some good" because they are painful and consequently assumed to be killing bacteria are examples, and they should be avoided by patients with oral ulcers.

Corticosteroid Treatment of Immune-Mediated Oral Ulcers

Corticosteroid management of oral ulcers is similar to the approach for immune-mediated skin lesions. The therapeutic goal is lesion and symptom control, because disease cure or spontaneous remission is unlikely. This should be understood by the patient to avoid unreasonable expectations. Healing of ulcers should be achieved with as little corticosteroid medication as possible. Topical corticosteroids should be tried first, limiting systemic administration to "bursts" as needed to control outbreaks of refractory ulcers followed by maintenance with topical treatment. Long-term systemic corticosteroid administration should be considered only as a last resort. The severity of lesions in these conditions typically varies with time, which means that the need for treatment beyond topical control also varies. Understanding several issues unique to the oral cavity can increase treatment effectiveness:

- Application of the topical corticosteroid after eating and at bedtime and avoiding frequent snacks promote adherence, absorption, and effectiveness.
- Application of preparations with a cotton swab minimizes the risk of onychomycosis from routine application with the fingers.
- Low- and intermediate-potency topical corticosteroid preparations such as hydrocortisone (Hytone) and betamethasone valerate (Valisone) tend to be less than optimally effective in the oral environment. Initial trial with a higher-potency preparation is justifiable because significant systemic absorption through the oral mucosa is minimal. The use of ultrapotent topical corticosteroids is reserved for persistent ulcers if some systemic absorption is acceptable.

CURRENT THERAPY

Initial Management with Potent Corticosteroid Preparations

- Fluocinonide (Lidex)[1] gel 0.05%: apply thin film to affected area as needed after meals and at bedtime to control oral ulcers
- Dexamethasone (Decadron)[1] elixir 0.5 mg/5 mL: rinse with 1 teaspoon for 2 minutes and spit out after meals and at bedtime to control oral ulcers

Management of Resistant Ulcers with Ultrapotent Corticosteroid Preparations

- Clobetasol propionate (Temovate)[1] 0.05%
- Halobetasol propionate (Ultravate)[1] 0.05%

Management of Ulcers That Cannot Be Controlled with Topical Preparations

- Prednisone 5- to 20-mg tablets concurrent with topical preparations: as needed to control ulcers and then taper and maintain control with topical corticosteroids
- Prednisone minimum dose: alternate-day concurrent with topical preparation as needed to control ulcers

---

[1]Not FDA approved for this indication.

REFERENCES

Coleman GC. Oral cancer suspicion factors. Tex Dent J 2003;120(6):486–94.

Goldberg MH, Topazian RG. Odontogenic infections and deep fascial space infections of dental origin. In: Topazian RG, Goldberg MH, Hupp KR, editors. Oral and Maxillofacial Infections. 4th ed. Philadelphia: WB Saunders; 2002. p. 158–87.

Greenberg MS, Glick M. Burket's Oral Medicine Diagnosis & Treatment. 10th ed. Ontario, BC Decker, Hamilton; 2003.

Neville BW, Damm DD, Allen CM, Bouquot JE. Oral and Maxillofacial Pathology. 3rd ed. St Louis: Saunders Elsevier; 2009.

Silverman S, Eversole LR, Truelove EL. Essentials of oral medicine. Ontario, BC Decker, Hamilton; 2002.

Venous Ulcers

Method of
*Zuleika L. Bonilla-Martinez, MD, and
Robert S. Kirsner, MD, PhD*

Ulcers resulting from venous insufficiency are the most common cause of leg ulceration. Many definitions exist for a chronic wound, which ultimately reflect the demographics, incidence, and prevalence data available. For example, although sometimes referred to as stasis ulcers, patients actually have increased blood flow locally. The Wound Healing Society classifies wounds as *acute* if they sustain restoration of anatomic and functional integrity in an orderly and timely process and *chronic* if they do not. Some of the biologic events that affect the "orderly" process include inflammation, angiogenesis (i.e., new blood vessel formation), matrix regeneration, and remodeling. The "timely" process is affected by the environment, age, pathologic process, wound location, and other factors.

Epidemiology

Venous disease affects approximately 5% of the world's population, and about 2% of the American population. It was once thought to be a disease affecting solely the elderly. The incidence increases from middle age onward. Seventy percent of all leg ulcers result solely from venous disease, and an additional 20% of patients have mixed arterial and venous disease. The other 10% of leg ulcers result from a variety of causes, including neuropathy, prolonged pressure, and infectious, malignant, and inflammatory causes.

The high prevalence of venous disease directly affects patients' quality of life. Family history of venous disease, obesity, smoking, high cost of treatment, time off work, prolonged standing, and hypertension are among the factors that contribute to a strong socioeconomic impact of a country's health care. A retrospective study from Cleveland Clinic Foundation showed the average cost per month of care was approximately $2400, and the mean total cost per patient was between $9685 and $14,136 U.S. dollars.

PATHOPHYSIOLOGY

In the lower extremities, the venous system comprises the deep and superficial veins, which are connected by the perforating venous system. Blood flows from the superficial to the deep veins through the communicating veins to ultimately reach the heart. Veins contain valves that prevent blood reflux and allow the unidirectional flow. When a healthy individual contracts the calf muscles, a high pressure develops in the deep vein system, allowing blood flow to go from the deep to the superficial veins. During calf muscle relaxation, the pressure difference (high pressure in the superficial veins) allows blood flow from the superficial to deep veins. Venous ulcers are associated with venous hypertension, which is defined as sustained elevated venous pressures during ambulation. Venous hypertension results from failure of the calf muscle pump, which normally assists in venous return. Blood reflux from the deep to superficial veins creates the sustained high pressure in the superficial vein system and therefore increased cutaneous blood flow. Valvular incompetence, vein distention, muscular weakness, and a decreased in the range of motion of the ankle may lead to calf muscle pump failure. Alterations in the microcirculation because of calf muscle pump failure ultimately lead to ulceration.

How does the skin ulcerate in patients with venous insufficiency? The mechanism of cutaneous ulceration as a consequence of venous insufficiency remains unknown. Several hypotheses have been reported since the beginning of the 20th century. In the early 1980s, Browse and Burnard suggested that venous hypertension could lead to endothelial distention, causing extravasation of fibrinogen into the interstitial fluid, which results in "pericapillary fibrin cuff" formation around the capillary vessels. Fibrin cuffs act as a barrier to diffusion of oxygen and nutrients, causing ischemia and ulcer formation. A few years later, Coleridge and colleagues suggested that venous hypertension could lead to decreased capillary perfusion, resulting in leukocyte trapping. The trapped leukocytes release proteolytic enzymes, which result in free radical formation and capillary damage. The increased capillary permeability causes extravasation of fibrinogen and other metabolites, which leads to formation of a fibrin cuff around the capillaries and ultimately ischemia.

Further studies supported the presence of increased levels of monocyte aggregation. Claudy and colleagues showed that leukocyte activation caused release of tumor necrosis factor alpha (TNF-α), ultimately leading to pericapillary fibrin cuff formation. In 1993, Falanga and Eaglstein observed that fibrin cuffs were discontinuous around capillaries and therefore did not form a barrier to oxygen and nutrients causing ischemia. They also postulated the "trap" hypothesis, which suggests that venous hypertension causes endothelial cell distention leading to extravasation of macromolecules (i.e., α2-macroglobulin and fibrinogen) into the dermis. Moreover, α2-macroglobulin can bind to growth factors, such as TNF-α and transforming growth factor beta (TGF-β), making them unavailable for wound repair. Patients with venous disease may have other factors that contribute to venous ulcer formation, such as systemic alteration in fibrinolysis and arteriovenous shunting. Despite all previously conducted studies and hypotheses, further research is needed to explain the mechanism of cutaneous ulceration resulting from venous insufficiency.

Evaluation and Diagnosis

The typical location for a venous ulcer is around the medial aspect of the lower extremity near the ankle (medial malleolus) or the gaiter area. The ulcer usually begins as a blister or erosion on the skin. Ulcer borders are irregular and usually smooth. The base of the ulcer may be covered with granulation tissue or yellow slough, or both.

Venous ulcers are associated with presence of pigmentation, erythema, dermatitis, edema, and induration (i.e., lipodermatosclerosis) of the surrounding skin and with varicose veins in the lower leg. Hemosiderin deposition resulting from red blood cell extravasation causes the surrounding hyperpigmentation. Lipodermatosclerosis, commonly known as an inverted bottle shape, is caused by sclerosis of the dermis and subcutaneous tissue. The presence of lipodermatosclerosis has been associated with a greater impairment of fibrinolysis in patients with venous ulcers and may be a poor prognostic factor for restriction of leg movement. Other known prognostic factors are duration and size of the ulcer and history of venous surgery. Ulcers present for longer than 6 months and larger than 5 cm² in diameter tend to be more refractory to therapy. Duration (27 months) and size (15.9 cm²) were reported as poor prognostic factors.

A diagnosis of venous ulcers may be based on clinical presentation. The findings of a lower leg ulcer associated with lipodermatosclerosis or varicose veins, or both, suggest a venous ulcer. Other common findings include atrophie blanche (i.e., porcelain white scars with telangiectasia and dyspigmentation) and dermatitis. Venous

dermatitis is associated with erythema, eczema, pruritus, and scaling of the skin. Contact dermatitis surrounding the ulcer may result from the use of topical agents.

Venous disease can be confirmed by a variety of techniques, including duplex ultrasound or plethysmography. However, it is critical that arterial disease be excluded because treatment with compression bandages is the mainstay of therapy and should be used cautiously in patients with arterial disease. A simple, noninvasive measurement to assess peripheral vascular disease is the ankle brachial index (ABI). This value is calculated by dividing the systolic pressure in the ankle by the systolic pressure in the arm. An ABI of less than 0.9 indicates peripheral vascular disease and represents an independent risk factor for vascular disease in other vascular beds, such as the coronary arteries. Care must be taken with diabetic or elderly patients who may have a falsely negative ABI value. All patients with an abnormal ABI value should be further evaluated. Consider a vascular consultation, magnetic resonance angiography (MRA), angioplasty, and stent bypass.

To aid in the exclusion of any underlying disease (e.g., hematologic disease, diabetes), initial laboratory tests should include complete blood cell (CBC) count with a differential count, chemistry panel, hemoglobin A1C, prealbumin and albumin determinations, liver function tests, and levels of homocysteine, protein C and S, antithrombin III, and factor V Leiden.

Several vascular studies help in the diagnosis and severity of venous disease. Color duplex ultrasound is usually the initial study done to assess venous reflux in the lower extremities. Continuous-wave Doppler studies may yield false-negative results because it may be difficult to differentiate between the superficial and deep venous system. Air plethysmography and photoplethysmography are helpful in evaluating venous reflux and calf muscle dysfunction. Invasive venography is the gold standard to assess venous reflux, but it is used only as a last resort because of its invasive properties.

The CEAP classification was developed in 1994 by the American Venous Forum (AVF) to standardize the diagnosis and treatment of venous disease. It was based on clinical manifestations (C), etiologic factors (E), anatomic distribution of disease (A), and underlying pathophysiologic findings (P).

Complications

Main complications of long-term or chronic venous ulcers are osteomyelitis and squamous cell carcinoma. A finding of exposed tendon or bone, in addition to suggesting an underlying osteomyelitis, suggests an ulcer with a nonvenous cause.

Radiographs and biopsy for histology and culture are appropriate first steps in evaluation. Consult an orthopedic surgeon for further analysis and treatment, which may include a bone biopsy and bone débridement.

Treatment

Compression is the gold standard of treatment of venous disease. After arterial disease has been excluded, reversal of the effects of venous hypertension through compression bandages and leg elevation is the cornerstone of therapy.

The goal of compression therapy is to deliver sustained graded compression with 30 to 40 mm Hg at the ankle. These bandages are applied circumferentially from the toes to the knees (involving the heel) with the foot dorsiflexed. The optimal method to deliver this pressure is through multilayered elastic compression dressings. Elastic compression dressings deliver compression during ambulation (i.e., walking) and at rest, accommodate to reduction in edema, and are superior to single-layered dressings. Inelastic compression (short-stretch compression) may deliver similar results but appear to require greater sophistication by those applying them to accomplish this. Inelastic bandages, which do not deliver compression at rest, may be advantageous in patients with arterial disease or patients who do not tolerate full compression (e.g., elderly). Patients with associated lymphatic damage may also benefit from pneumatic compression.

Systemic medication as adjuvant therapy to compression bandages, such as pentoxifylline (Trental 400 to 800 mg three times daily[3]), aspirin,[1] or micronized purified flavonoid fraction (MPFF, Daflon 500[2] [diosmin[7] 90% and hesperidin[7] 10%]) may be superior to compression bandages alone with regard to the rate of healing. The use of pentoxifylline as adjuvant therapy to compression in venous ulcers has been shown to be very beneficial.

Wound bed preparation was proposed as a way to help the healing process. It is a multistep process that improves the wound bed by removing necrotic and fibrinous wound tissue, increasing the amount of granulation tissue, and decreasing edema, chronic wound fluid (i.e., exudate), and bacterial burden.

Local care is best accomplished with occlusive dressings. Occlusive dressings provide a moist environment for healing. A variety of types of occlusions may be used, and the choice depends on several factors, including the location of the wound and the amount of fibrinous slough and exudate present. A fear of excessive infection with the use of occlusive dressings is unfounded. Topical antiseptics and cleansing agents should be used with caution because they may prolong healing. Topical agents such as cadexomer iodine (Iodosorb), silver-impregnated dressings, and topical anesthetics are alternatives that do not prolong healing, but they should be applied directly to the wound because they may lead to skin sensitization.

---

[1]Not FDA approved for this indication.
[2]Not available in the United States.
[3]Exceeds dosage recommended by the manufacturer.
[7]Available as a dietary supplement.

CURRENT THERAPY

- Compression therapy is used to deliver a graded compression of 30 to 40 mm Hg at the ankle. Exclude arterial disease before using compression.
- Systemic medications as adjuvant therapy to compression bandages include aspirin,[1] pentoxifylline (Trental), or micronized purified flavonoid fraction (Daflon 500).[2]
- Other treatments, along with compression, include engineered skin, skin graft, electrical stimulation, locally derived growth factors, and venous surgery.
- The lifelong use of elastic compression stockings (30–40 mm Hg) is the mainstay of therapy.

---

[1]Not FDA approved for this indication.
[2]Not available in the United States.

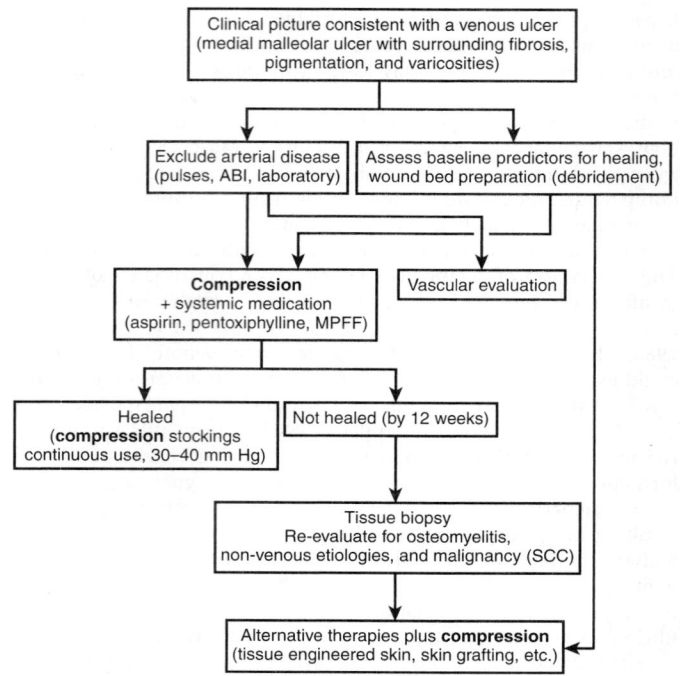

FIGURE 1. Simplified algorithm for the diagnosis and treatment of patients with venous ulcers. *Abbreviations:* ABI = ankle-brachial index; MPFF = micronized purified flavonoid fraction; SCC = squamous cell carcinoma.

Up to 50% of venous ulcers may be refractory to compression therapy alone. This refractory subset may be predicted by baseline characteristics (size and duration) and by a decrease in size with 2 to 4 weeks of treatment (Fig. 1). Other available treatments include tissue-engineered skin, autologous skin, electrical stimulation, treatment with locally delivered growth factors, and venous surgery. Three categories exist for skin grafts: autograft, allogeneic (cultured), and artificial (tissue-engineered skin). Two types of autografts are full-thickness (FTSG) and split-thickness (STSG) skin grafts. The latter is commonly used by expanding it with a meshing technique.

Apligraf, a bilayered engineered living skin composed of keratinocytes and fibroblasts from neonatal foreskin, is approved by the FDA for treatment of venous leg and diabetic neuropathic foot ulcers. Surgical treatment of incompetent superficial and perforator veins along with standard of care (i.e., compression) reduce the risk of recurrence.

After healing occurs, patients with venous insufficiency are at risk for recurrence. The lifelong use of elastic compression stockings (30–40 mm Hg) is the mainstay of therapy, but early intervention after recurrence is critical. Health professionals need to understand the importance of further research to ultimately minimize the psychological, physical, and socioeconomic impact that ulcers caused by venous insufficiency have on patients and society.

REFERENCES

Abbade LP, Lastória S. Venous ulcer: Epidemiology, physiopathology, diagnosis and treatment. Int J Dermatol 2005;44:449–56.

Browse NL, Burnand KG. The cause of venous ulceration. Lancet 1982;2:243–5.

Claudy AL, Mirshahi M, Soria C, et al. Detection of undegraded fibrin and tumor necrosis factor alpha in venous leg ulcers. J Am Acad Dermatol 1991;25:623–7.

Coleridge-Smith PD, Thomas P, Scurr JH, et al. Causes of venous ulceration: A new hypothesis? Br Med J 1988;296:1726–7.

Falanga V, Eaglstein WH. The trap hypothesis of venous ulceration. Lancet 1993;341:1006–8.

Jull A, Arroll B, Parag V, Waters J. Pentoxyphilline for treating venous leg ulcers. Cochrane Database Syst Rev 2007;(3) CD001733.

Kirsner R. Wound bed preparation. Ostomy Wound Manage 2003;(Feb, Suppl.):2–3.

Kirsner RS, Falanga V. Techniques of split-thickness skin grafting for lower extremity ulcerations. J Dermatol Surg Oncol 1993;19:779–83.

Kirsner RS, Pardes JB, Eaglstein WH, Falanga V. The clinical spectrum of lipo-dermatosclerosis. J Am Acad Dermatol 1993;28:623–7.

Lazarus GS, Cooper DM, Knighton DR, et al. Definitions and guidelines for assessment of wounds and evaluation of healing. Arch Dermatol 1994;130:489–93.

Olin JW, Beusterien KM, Childs MB, et al. Medical costs of treating venous stasis ulcers: Evidence from a retrospective cohort study. Vasc Med 1999;4:1–7.

Phillips TJ, Machado F, Trout R, et al. Prognostic indicators in venous ulcers. J Am Acad Dermatol 2000;43:627–30.

Trent JT, Falabella A, Eaglstein WH, Kirsner RS. Venous ulcers: Pathophysiology and treatment options. Ostomy Wound Manage 2005;51:38–54.

Pressure Ulcers

Method of
David R. Thomas, MD

A pressure ulcer is the visible evidence of pathologic changes in blood supply to the dermal and underlying tissues, usually because of compression of the tissue over a bony prominence.

A differential diagnosis of ulcer type is critical to treatment. Chronic ulcers of the skin include arterial ulcers, venous stasis ulcers, diabetic ulcers, and pressure ulcers. Pressure ulcers generally appear in soft tissue over a bony prominence. A classic presentation aids the diagnosis. For example, arterial ulcers occur in the distal digits or over a bony prominence, diabetic ulcers occur in regions of callus formation, and venous stasis ulcers occur on the lateral aspect of the lower leg. However, atypical presentations may occasionally obscure the etiology. The treatment of these various etiologies differs considerably. This discussion is limited to the treatment of pressure ulcers and should not be used to treat other types of ulcers.

Seven principles of management guide treatment of pressure ulcers. The chief cause of these ulcers is pressure applied to the tissues that compromises blood flow. Therefore, the first treatment principle is to relieve pressure. Pressure relief can be obtained by positioning the patient frequently at a fixed interval to relieve pressure over the compromised area. Turning and positioning may be difficult to achieve because of a patient's self-positioning or medical treatments that interfere with the ability to position the patient. Because of this difficulty, a number of medical devices are designed in an attempt to relieve pressure. These devices can be classified as static or dynamic. Static devices include air-, gel-, or water-filled containers that reduce the tissue–surface interface. Dynamic devices use a power source to fill compartments with air that support the patient's weight or alternate the pressure on different areas of the body. Choose a static device when the patient has good bed mobility. Choose a dynamic device when the patient cannot self-position in bed.

At the present time, results of reported clinical trials do not favor one device over another. The choice should be based on durability, ease of use, and patient comfort. A simple check for so-called bottoming out should be done for all devices. Your hand should be inserted palm upward under the patient's sacrum between the device and the bed surface. If there is not an air column between the patient and the bed surface, the device is ineffective and should be changed. No device is effective in reducing heel pressure, the second most common site for pressure ulcers. Bridging with pillows is effective in reducing heel pressure in immobile patients; patients with high bed mobility may require

boot devices to elevate the heel off the bed surface. Patients who fail to improve or who have multiple pressure ulcers should be considered for a dynamic-type device, such as a low-air-loss bed or air-fluidized bed. Studies in turning and positioning suggest an optimum interval of 4 hours while on a pressure-reducing device. More frequent turning schedules, including the often-suggested 2-hour interval, have not been demonstrated to prevent pressure ulcers.

The second principle of pressure ulcer therapy is to assess pain. Pressure ulcers do not always result in pain, particularly in insensate patients. However, some pressure ulcers do result in pain and should be treated aggressively. Oral or parenteral pain medications should be used to control symptoms.

The third principle of ulcer therapy is to assess nutrition and hydration. Pressure ulcers occur in sicker individuals in whom nutrient intake may be reduced by coexisting illness. Increased intake of protein (1.2 to 1.5 g/kg/day) is associated with higher healing rates. Achievement of high protein intake may be difficult because of anorexia of aging or anorexia associated with coexisting diseases. Adequate calories, adjusted for stress (30 to 35 kcal/kg/day), should be prescribed. Adequate dietary intake should provide adequate vitamins and minerals. No difference in healing rates is associated with supertherapeutic doses of vitamin C or zinc. If adequate dietary intake is compromised, a supplemental vitamin/mineral prescription at RDA (recommended daily allowance) doses should be considered. Adequate hydration can be maintained by 30 mL/kg/day of water. The decision to institute enteral feeding in patients with pressure ulcers who are unable to maintain adequate oral intake should not be undertaken lightly. The decision to use enteral feeding must consider the patient's wishes, overall goal of care, and the complications of enteral feeding. In several studies, the long-term result of enteral feeding was associated with poorer outcomes in patients with pressure ulcers.

The fourth principle of pressure ulcer management requires removing necrotic debris. Phagocytosis removes necrotic debris naturally. Accelerating the rate of removal may shorten healing time. Options include sharp surgical débridement, mechanical débridement with gauze dressings, application of exogenous enzymes, or autolytic débridement under occlusive dressings. Choose surgical débridement if the ulcer is infected. Surgical débridement is the fastest method but may remove some viable tissue, cause discomfort, and is the most expensive method, especially if done in an operating room. Applying moist gauze that is allowed to adhere to the ulcer bed by drying is a form of débridement. When the dry dressing is removed, nonselective tissue removal occurs. This method can be associated with discomfort, may delay healing while débridement is in progress, and is often defeated when the dressing is remoistened before removal. Enzymatic débridement can digest necrotic material. Only one enzymatic preparation is currently available in the United States: collagenase. Enzyme preparations are nonselective, possibly resulting in some damage to fibroblasts, epithelial cells, or granulation tissue. Enzymatic débridement is slower, can be associated with discomfort, and should be limited in duration until a clean wound bed is obtained. Autolytic débridement is achieved by allowing autolysis under an occlusive dressing. Both enzymatic and autolytic débridement may require 2 to 6 weeks to achieve a clean wound bed. A total of five clinical trials did not show that enzymatic agents increased the rate of complete healing in chronic wounds compared to control treatment. Unless clinically infected, heel ulcers are better left undébrided because they occur in poorly vascularized tissues.

CURRENT DIAGNOSIS

- Differentiate among pressure, diabetic, venous stasis, and arterial ulcers.

CURRENT THERAPY

Seven Principles of Pressure Ulcer Therapy

- Relieve pressure.
- Assess pain.
- Assess nutrition and hydration.
- Remove necrotic debris.
- Maintain a moist wound environment.
- Encourage granulation and epithelial tissue formation.
- Control infection.

The fifth principle of pressure ulcer management is to maintain a moist wound environment. Maintaining a moist wound environment is associated with more rapid healing rates compared to dressings that are allowed to dry. Continuously moist saline gauze is the historical standard dressing for stage II through IV pressure ulcers. Care must be taken to change the gauze frequently to prevent drying because this may delay healing. Newer wound dressings provide a low moisture vapor transmission rate (MVTR), a measure of how quickly the dressing allows drying. A MVTR of less than 35 g of water vapor per square meter per hour is required to maintain a moist wound environment. Woven gauze has a MVTR of 68 g/m^2/hour, and impregnated gauze has a MVTR of 57 g/m^2/hour. By comparison, hydrocolloid dressings have a MVTR of 8 g/m^2/hour. Dressings with low MVTR provide a healing environment that encourages granulation tissue formation and epithelialization.

The use of occlusive-type dressings is more cost effective than gauze dressings primarily because of a decrease in nursing time for dressing changes. A meta-analysis of five clinical trials comparing a hydrocolloid dressing with a dry dressing demonstrated that treatment with a hydrocolloid dressing resulted in a statistically significant improvement in the rate of pressure ulcer healing (odds ratio: 2.6).

Occlusive dressings can be divided into broad categories of polymer films, polymer foams, hydrogels, hydrocolloids, alginates, and biomembranes. Each has advantages and disadvantages. No single agent is perfect. The choice of a particular agent depends on the clinical circumstances. Nonpermeable polymers can be macerating to normal skin. Polymer films are not absorptive and may leak, particularly when the wound is highly exudative. Most films have an adhesive backing that may remove epithelial cells when the dressing is changed. Hydrogels are hydrophilic polymers that are insoluble in water but absorb aqueous solutions and are available in amorphous gels or sheet dressings. They are poor bacterial barriers and are nonadherent to the wound. Because of their high specific heat, these dressings are cooling to the skin, aiding in pain control and reducing inflammation. Most of these dressings require a secondary dressing to secure them to the wound. Hydrocolloid dressings are complex dressings similar to ostomy barrier products. They are impermeable to moisture and bacteria and highly adherent to the skin. Hydrocolloid dressings have an accelerated healing of 40% compared to moist gauze dressings. Hydrocolloid dressings are particularly suited for areas subject to urinary and fecal incontinence. Their adhesiveness to surrounding skin is higher than some surgical tapes, but they are nonadherent to wound tissue and do not damage epithelial tissue in the wound. The adhesive barrier is frequently overcome in highly exudative wounds. Hydrocolloid dressings should be used cautiously over tendons or on wounds with eschar formation. Alginates are complex polysaccharide dressings that are highly absorbent in exudative wounds. This high absorbency is particularly suited to exudative wounds. Alginates are nonadherent to the wound, but if the wound is allowed to dry, damage to the epithelial tissue may occur with removal. Alginates may be used under other dressings to absorb exudate. The biomembranes are very expensive and not readily available.

Stages I and II pressure ulcers can be managed with a polymer film or hydrocolloid dressing. Stages III and IV pressure ulcers may be treated with a film or hydrocolloid dressing. In addition, some stage III and IV wounds with dead space or tunneling may require a wound filler, such as a calcium alginate or an amorphous hydrogel, to obliterate dead space and decrease potential for anaerobic colonization.

Vacuum-assisted closure is used in both acute and chronic wounds. Only two randomized, controlled trials in pressure ulcers are reported. In both trials, vacuum-assisted closure was not superior to treatment with a hydrogel or moistened gauze, at a higher cost.

Electrotherapy is used for stages III and IV pressure ulcers unresponsive to conventional therapy. Several clinical trials suggest that electrotherapy is likely to be marginally effective. Hyperbaric oxygen, ultrasound, infrared, ultraviolet, and low-energy laser irradiation have insufficient data to recommend their use currently. No data support the use of a systemic vasodilator, hemorheologics, serotonin inhibitors, or fibrolytic agents in the treatment of pressure ulcers. Topical agents such as zinc, phenytoin,[1] aluminum hydroxide,[1] honey, sugar, yeast, aloe vera gel, or gold[1] were not effective in clinical trials.

---

[1]Not FDA approved for this indication.

Because the theory of augmenting ulcer healing under the newer dressings suggests that wound fluid contains favorable healing factors, it is important not to change the dressings too frequently. Unless the wound fluid seeps from under the dressing, it should not be changed more often than every 3 to 7 days.

The sixth principle of pressure ulcer treatment is to encourage granulation tissue formation and promote reepithelialization. Growth factors show promising early results, but the data do not suggest accelerated healing of pressure ulcers. It is important not to affect granulation and epithelial tissue negatively. A number of wound cleaners and antiseptics are toxic to fibroblasts and epithelial tissues, including benzalkonium chloride, povidone-iodine solution (Betadine), Dakin's solution, hydrogen peroxide, Granulex, Hibiclens, and pHisoHex. The use of these agents in a pressure ulcer should be limited to use in infected ulcers and strictly limited in duration.

The seventh principle of pressure ulcer management is to control infection. Quantitative microbiology alone is a poor predictor of clinical infection in chronic wounds. All pressure ulcers are colonized with bacteria, usually from skin or fecal flora. The presence of microorganisms alone (colonization) does not indicate an infection in pressure ulcers. The diagnosis of infection in chronic wounds must be based on clinical signs: erythema, warmth, pain, edema, odor, fever, or purulent exudate. In the presence of clinical signs of infection, enteral or parenteral antibiotics should be used. In ulcers that are not progressing toward healing, an empirical trial of topical antimicrobials may be considered, although the data are inconclusive.

REFERENCES

Thomas DR. The role of nutrition in prevention and healing of pressure ulcers. Geriatr Clin North Am 1997;13:497–512.

Thomas DR. Are all pressure ulcers avoidable? J Am Med Dir Assoc 2001;2:297–301.

Thomas DR. Improving the outcome of pressure ulcers with nutritional intervention: A review of the evidence. Nutrition 2001;17:121–5.

Thomas DR. Issues and dilemmas in managing pressure ulcers. J Gerontol Med Sci 2001;56:M238–340.

Thomas DR. Prevention and management of pressure ulcers. Rev Clin Gerontol 2001;11:115–30.

Thomas DR. The promise of topical nerve growth factors in the healing of pressure ulcers. Ann Intern Med 2003;139:694–5.

Thomas DR. Management of pressure ulcers. J Am Med Dir Assoc 2006;7:46–59.

Thomas DR. Managing pressure ulcers: Learning to give up cherished dogma. J Am Med Dir Assoc 2007;8:347–8.

Thomas DR. Prevention and management of pressure ulcers. Clin Rev Gerontol 2008;17:1–17.

Atopic Dermatitis

Method of
Peck Y. Ong, MD

Atopic dermatitis (AD) is a chronic inflammatory skin disease that is characterized by itch and a predilection of eczema on extensor areas in young infants or flexural areas in older children and adults. In the United States, AD affects about 15% of children and 2% of adults. For more than 85% of patients, AD begins during the first 5 years, but 50% of the children with AD improve significantly or outgrow the disease by age 7. The persistence of AD depends on various factors: early onset, severity, family history of AD, personal history of asthma, and food or inhalant allergies.

The itch associated with AD causes significant discomfort in these patients and often leads to sleep loss and to poor school or work performance. The quality of life of children with generalized AD is worse than that for children with diabetes, epilepsy, asthma, cystic fibrosis, or renal disease. The maternal stress in taking care of children with moderate to severe AD is equivalent to that associated with care of children with diabetes, Rett syndrome, profound deafness, or the need for enteral feeding.

Pathophysiology

AD is caused by a combination of genetic and environmental factors. Patients with AD have a defective skin barrier. This leads to a loss of skin hydration and susceptibility to environmental triggers. There is evidence that the skin barrier defects of AD are caused by genetic mutations. Studies have shown that many AD patients carry a genetic mutation in filaggrin, a protein with important barrier function.

Potential external triggers of AD include microbial pathogens and environmental allergens. Almost 100% of AD skin lesions are colonized by *Staphylococcus aureus*, which may produce toxins that trigger immune response in the skin. As a result, AD patients produce an increased amount of pro-allergic cytokines, such as interleukin-4 (IL-4), IL-5, and IL-13 in their skin. These cytokines lead to an increased infiltration of inflammatory T cells and eosinophils. IL-4 and IL-13 also are important for the production of serum IgE, the level of which is elevated in AD patients.

Diagnosis and Clinical Assessment

Most AD patients can be diagnosed by clinical history and physical examination. Typical presentation includes itch, dryness, flexural dermatitis, early age of onset, and atopy such as multiple food allergies. Patients with generalized eczema or adult-onset eczema can present as a diagnostic challenge. The differential diagnosis includes immunodeficiency (e.g., hyper-IgE syndrome, Omenn syndrome), malignancy (e.g., cutaneous T-cell lymphoma), zinc deficiency (i.e., acrodermatitis enteropathica), and celiac-associated dermatitis (i.e., dermatitis herpetiformis) (Table 1). AD children seldom present with failure to thrive, unless they are under severe dietary restriction. Failure to thrive should therefore prompt further investigation. Punch skin biopsies may be needed when the diagnosis is still unclear.

The prevalence of mild, moderate, and severe AD is 80%, 18%, and 2%, respectively. Most patients with mild to moderate disease have flexural, extensor, or facial involvement, whereas patients with severe disease often present with total-body involvement with or without erythroderma (Fig. 1). Validated scales for assessing the severity of AD include Scoring of Atopic Dermatitis (SCORAD) and Eczema Area and Severity Index (EASI). These scoring systems or a simplified diagram documenting the extent of dermatitis are useful for more objective follow-up of the patient's progress.

TABLE 1 Differential Diagnoses of Atopic Dermatitis

Disease Category	Differential Diagnoses
Dermatologic diseases	Contact dermatitis, seborrheic dermatitis, psoriasis, dyshidrotic eczema, eosinophilic pustular folliculitis, ichthyosis vulgaris
Neoplastic diseases	Cutaneous T-cell lymphoma, Langerhans cell histiocytosis
Immunodeficiencies	Hyper-IgE syndrome, severe combined immunodeficiency, Omenn syndrome, IPEX (immune dysregulation, polyendocrinopathy, enteropathy X-linked) syndrome
Infectious diseases	Scabies, cutaneous candidiasis, tinea versicolor
Nutritional deficiencies	Acrodermatitis enteropathica (zinc deficiency), essential fatty acid deficiency, biotin deficiency
Multisystemic disorders	Netherton syndrome, dermatitis herpetiformis

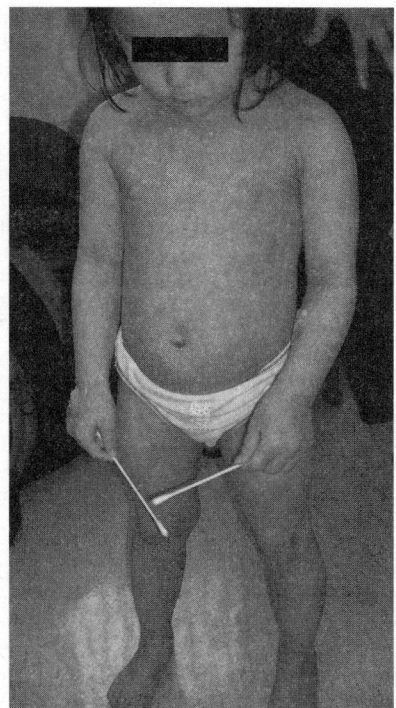

FIGURE 1. Generalized atopic dermatitis.

 CURRENT DIAGNOSIS

- Itch must be present for the diagnosis of atopic dermatitis. In addition, the diagnosis must include three or more of the following criteria (U.K. Working Party's Diagnostic Criteria for Atopic Dermatitis):

    - History of generalized dry skin
    - Visible flexural dermatitis
    - Onset of the skin condition before 2 years (not used for patients younger than 4 years)
    - History of itchy skin involving the following areas: elbows, behind knees, front of ankles, or around the neck
    - History of asthma or allergic rhinitis (or for children younger than 4 years, history of atopic disease in a first-degree relative)

Management of Atopic Dermatitis and Associated Conditions

DAILY MAINTENANCE CARE

Changes in humidity can adversely affect AD symptoms. Dry conditions lead to increased transepidermal water loss and dry AD skin. Extreme heat, humidity, and sweating may lead to irritation of AD skin. AD patients are at increased risk for contact or irritant dermatitis, which may occur with over-the-counter topical skin medications that contain multiple ingredients. Wool or synthetic acrylic fabrics may also be irritating to AD skin.

To improve barrier function, AD patients should bathe or shower for 10 to 20 minutes once or twice daily, followed immediately by gently drying the skin and applying an emollient on the unaffected areas and a topical antiinflammatory medication on the affected areas.

A petrolatum-based emollient is recommended in infants and young children because of its occlusive property. In older children and adults, the ointment may not be tolerated well because of its greasy feel, and another emollient or moisturizer may be chosen based on the patient's preference or experience.

Itch may continue to be a problem even if the rash has improved. The mechanisms of itch in AD are not fully understood but do not appear to be mediated solely by histamine. The use of first-generation antihistamines (diphenhydramine [Benadryl] and hydroxyzine [Vistaril]) in AD largely depend on their sedative effects and are best used at bedtime. The second-generation, nonsedating antihistamines such as loratadine (Claritin)[1] and cetirizine (Zyrtec)[1] have not proved helpful in treating AD.

TOPICAL AND SYSTEMIC MEDICATIONS

The first-line medication for AD is a topical corticosteroid (TCS). For mild AD, a TCS with group VI and VII potency (Table 2) may suffice. However, for moderate to severe AD, a TCS with at least group III to V potency is chosen to increase efficacy and to shorten the duration of need for these medications.

The use of TCS is confronted with various obstacles, including rare side effects such as skin atrophy, but mostly with patients' or parents' misunderstanding of TCS. Studies have shown that twice-daily use of fluticasone propionate (Cutivate) 0.05% cream (group V) and desonide (DesOwen, Tridesilon) 0.05% ointment or aqueous gel (group V and VI, respectively) continuously up to 1 month in young children with AD resulted in no significant adverse effect. It is therefore important to clarify for patients or parents the safety and side effects based on the potency of the TCS.

Topical calcineurin inhibitors (TCI) (pimecrolimus [Elidel] 1% cream and Protopic/tacrolimus ointment) are alternative nonsteroidal antiinflammatory medications for AD. Elidel is indicated for mild to moderate AD in patients older than 2 years, whereas 0.03% and 0.1% Protopic are indicated for moderate to severe AD in patients 2 to 15 years old and in patients 16 years old or older, respectively. Both Elidel and Protopic have an FDA black box warning saying that their long-term use may be associated with cancer risk. It is recommended that these medications be used on a short-term and as-needed basis in minimal amounts. They continue to be useful alternatives for skin areas that are prone to atrophy, including the face, axillae, and groins.

A new class of topical medications (so-called barrier creams) emphasize skin barrier repair. These medications include Atopiclair, MimyX, Eletone, and EpiCeram. Only EpiCeram has been compared directly with TCS. It was shown to be as effective as fluticasone propionate 0.05% cream in children with moderate to severe AD in a preliminary study. Atopiclair and MimyX may be effective for patients with mild to moderate AD. There is no published study on Eletone. These barrier creams have no age limitations, but they require a prescription because they have been approved as a medical device by the FDA.

Wet-wrap treatment, phototherapy, and systemic immunosuppressive therapies (e.g., cyclosporine [Sandimmune, Neoral],[1] azathioprine [Imuran],[1] methotrexate [Trexall],[1] and mycophenolate mofetil [CellCept][1]) are reserved for severe AD patients. Because of the potential serious adverse effects associated with these treatments, referral to an allergist or dermatologist is recommended before their initiation.

Systemic corticosteroids usually are not recommended for AD because of their known adverse effects, including stunted growth in children, adrenal suppression, osteoporosis, and cataracts. A rebound of AD symptoms is common after the medication is stopped. If a systemic corticosteroid is used, it should be tapered over a short period (e.g., a week) while topical antiinflammatory treatment is intensified.

The efficacy and side effects of the following medications have not been established in AD: intravenous immunoglobulin (IVIG), anti-IgE (omalizumab [Xolair][1]), probiotics,[7] montelukast (Singulair),[1] Chinese medicinal herbs,[7] and fish oils.[1]

FOOD ALLERGIES

At least 30% of children with moderate to severe AD have one or more food allergies, compared with 4% to 6% of the general population. Accurate diagnosis of food allergies in AD patients is crucial, because it can prevent life-threatening anaphylaxis or unnecessary food restriction.

The diagnosis of food allergy involves one or more of the following: history taking, skin tests, serum-specific IgE tests, and food challenge. History taking is helpful in the diagnosis of food allergy in most patients. It is often useful to begin by asking the patients whether they have any problems or reactions with any of the seven food allergens: milk, egg, peanut, wheat, soybean, seafood, and tree nuts. These foods account for more than 90% of food allergies. Almost all food allergic reactions occur in the first hour. AD patients may complain of immediate worsening of itching after ingestion. Symptoms of anaphylactic reactions include throat-clearing, cough, shortness of breath, vomiting, dizziness, fainting, and headache, which may be attributed to hypotension. Most food allergic reactions also manifest with skin symptoms, including hives, swelling, or generalized itching.

---

[1]Not FDA approved for this indication.

[1]Not FDA approved for this indication.
[7]Available as a dietary supplement.

TABLE 2   Classification of Topical Corticosteroids Based on Potency

Group	Topical Corticosteroids
I (most potent)	Clobetasol propionate 0.05% (Temovate) (cream, ointment, gel), betamethasone dipropionate, augmented 0.05% (Diprolene) (cream, ointment), diflorasone diacetate 0.05% (Psorcon) (ointment)
II	Amcinonide 0.1% (Cyclocort) (ointment), betamethasone dipropionate 0.05% (Diprosone) (ointment), mometasone furoate 0.1% (Elocon) (ointment), halcinonide 0.1% (Halog) (cream), fluocinonide 0.05% (Lidex) (gel, cream, ointment), desoximetasone (Topicort) (0.05% gel, 0.25% cream, 0.25% ointment)
III	Fluticasone propionate 0.005% (Cutivate) (ointment), amcinonide 0.1% (Cyclocort) (lotion, cream), diflorasone diacetate 0.05% (Florone) (cream), betamethasone valerate 0.1% (Valisone) (ointment)
IV	Flurandrenolide 0.05% (Cordran) (ointment), mometasone furoate 0.1% (Elocon) (cream), triamcinolone acetonide 0.1% (Kenalog) (cream), fluocinolone acetonide 0.025% (Synalar) (ointment), hydrocortisone valerate 0.2% (Westcort) (ointment)
V	Flurandrenolide 0.05% (Cordran) (cream), fluticasone propionate 0.05% (Cutivate) (cream), hydrocortisone butyrate 0.1% (Locoid) (cream), fluocinolone acetonide 0.025% (Synalar) (cream), desonide 0.05% (Tridesilon) (ointment), betamethasone valerate 0.1% (Valisone) (cream), hydrocortisone valerate 0.2% (Westcort) (cream), prednicarbate 0.1% (Dermatop) (cream)
VI	Alclometasone dipropionate 0.05% (Aclovate) (cream, ointment), fluocinolone acetonide 0.01% (Synalar) (solution, cream) (Derma-Smoothe/FS Oil), Desonide 0.05% (Tridesilon) (cream and aqueous gel)
VII (least potent)	Hydrocortisone 1%/2.5% (lotion, cream, ointment).

Data from Stoughton RB: Vasoconstrictor assay—specific applications. In Maibach HI, Surber C (eds): Topical Corticosteroids. Basel, Switzerland: Karger, 1992, p 42–53.

TABLE 3 Predictability of ImmunoCAP-Specific IgE

Reaction*	Milk	Soy	Egg	Wheat	Peanut	Fish	Tree Nuts
Reaction highly probable	>15 kU/L	>60 kU/L	>7 kU/L	>80 kU/L	>14 kU/L	>20 kU/L	>15 kU/L
Reaction highly probable (young children)	>5 kU/L (<1 y)		>2 kU/L (<2 y)				

*Because of their high positive predictive values, quantitative serum-specific IgE antibodies are used in the diagnosis of food allergies.

Skin tests are useful in the context of negative test results because they have a negative predictive value of more than 95%. A positive test result has only a 50% positive predictive value.

Quantitative serum-specific IgE antibodies (ImmunoCAP, Phadia) have become useful in the diagnosis of food allergies because of their high positive predictive values (Table 3). These tests are also useful for deciding whether a food challenge is necessary to confirm the diagnosis.

Although history, skin tests, and serum-specific IgE values are useful in the diagnosis of food allergy, a double-blind, placebo-controlled food challenge remains the gold standard in diagnosing food allergy. Food challenge should be done in consultation with an allergist because of the risk of anaphylaxis.

Patients with confirmed food allergy should avoid any amount of the food allergen. Parents or patients should be instructed to read food allergen labels carefully. All packaged foods in the United States are required to label the contents of milk, eggs, peanuts, wheat, soybeans, fish, shellfish, or tree nuts. Organizations, such as the Food Allergy and Anaphylaxis Network, can provide patients and parents with useful information on potential hidden food allergens and alternative food sources.

AD children often have multiple food allergies, including cow's milk and soy, and the use of a hydrolyzed or amino acid–based formula can provide an alternative source of nutrition. For these patients, consultation with a dietitian can be helpful in managing food avoidance and nutrition needs.

Patients or parents of children with anaphylactic reactions should be prescribed and instructed on the use of an epinephrine autoinjector (EpiPen or Twinject: 0.15 mg for patients who weigh more than 15 kg but less than 30 kg; 0.3 mg for patients who weigh 30 kg or more).

Delaying highly allergic foods in early childhood remains controversial. However, for infants who are at high risk for food allergy (e.g., children with AD and multiple food allergies), it is recommended that they avoid eggs, peanuts, tree nuts, fish, and shellfish in the first 3 years, unless there are major issues such as nutrition or social hindrance. Further studies are needed to confirm the role of this practice in preventing food allergies.

INFECTIONS

Most AD patients are colonized by *S. aureus* on their skin lesions or in their nostrils. The frequency of colonization increases with AD severity. Exacerbation of AD is frequently associated with secondary *S. aureus* skin infections. Other common skin pathogens in AD include group A β-hemolytic *Streptococcus* and herpes simplex virus (HSV), which causes eczema herpeticum (Fig. 2). Many reports have documented invasive *S. aureus* infections such as bacteremia, septic arthritis, osteomyelitis, and endocarditis in AD patients. Persistent fever or focal limb pain should alert the physician to the possibility of these infections.

The reasons for the high rate of bacterial colonization and skin infections in AD are not completely understood. A defective skin barrier and decreased cutaneous innate immunity (i.e., deficiency in natural skin antibiotics) likely contribute to the frequency of skin infections in patients with AD.

Because of the concern about increasing bacterial resistance, antibiotics are not recommended for treating *S. aureus* colonization in patients with AD. An area of active research involves the use of silver-coated fabrics or antimicrobial-coated silk fabrics to reduce *S. aureus* colonization and improve symptoms in AD patients.

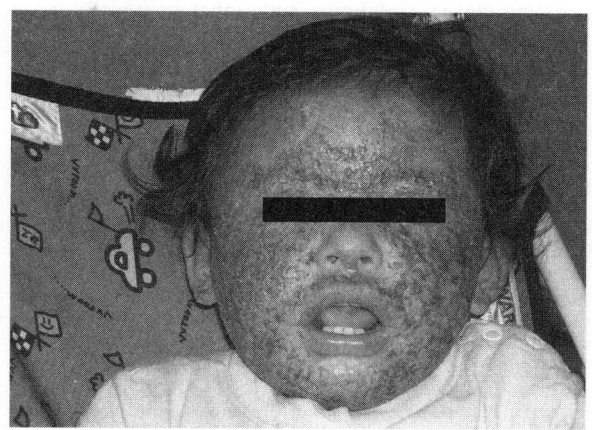

FIGURE 2. Eczema herpeticum.

 CURRENT THERAPY

- Bathe or shower for 10 to 20 minutes daily and pat dry gently.
- Follow immediately by applying an emollient on unaffected areas and an antiinflammatory medication on affected areas.
- Use topical corticosteroids as a first-line antiinflammatory medication; alternative medications are topical calcineurin inhibitors or barrier creams.
- Avoid environmental triggers such as extreme heat, humidity, or dryness.
- Avoid food allergens that may cause anaphylaxis. Consult an allergist regarding the interpretation of serum-specific IgE tests or food challenge.
- Treat skin infection only when clinical signs are present (e.g., oozing, impetigo).
- Severe, generalized infection or vesicular lesions may indicate herpes simplex virus infection; persistent fever may indicate invasive *S. aureus* infection.

INHALANT ALLERGIES AND ASTHMA

Eighty-five percent of AD infants have concurrent respiratory allergies or are at risk for allergic rhinitis or asthma. However, whether inhalant allergens lead to a worsening of AD remains controversial. Randomized, double-blind, placebo-controlled studies have shown positive and negative effects of house dust mites (HDM) as a trigger for AD symptoms. Because there is no serious side effect associated with the use of HDM-proof bed and pillow encasings, unless cost is an issue, these encasings are recommended for AD patients with HDM sensitization. Further research is needed to confirm the role of inhalant allergens, including furry pets and pollens as triggers for AD.

Investigational Treatments for Atopic Dermatitis

Because of the concern about potential side effects associated with existing therapies of AD, several agents are being investigated for the treatment of AD. They include a topical nuclear factor-κB decoy, phosphodiesterase 4 inhibitors, urocanic acid oxidation products, vitamin B$_{12}$,[1] rose bengal disodium,[1] *Vitreoscilla filiformis*, alefacept (Amevive),[1] and pitrakinra (Aerovant).[5] Subcutaneous and sublingual allergen immunotherapy may also be helpful in a subgroup of patients with HDM sensitization. Topical opioid receptor antagonists, systemic chymase inhibitors, and cannabinoid receptor agonists are potential anti-itch medications for AD.

------

[1]Not FDA approved for this indication.
[5]Investigational drug in the United States.

REFERENCES

Beattie PE, Lewis-Jones MS. A comparative study of impairment of quality of life in children with skin disease and children with other chronic childhood diseases. Br J Dermatol 2006;155:145–51.

Bewley A. Dermatology Working Group: Expert consensus: Time for a change in the way we advise our patients to use topical corticosteroids. Br J Dermatol 2008;158:917–20.

Bock SA. Diagnostic evaluation. Pediatrics 2003;111:1638–44.

Boguniewicz M, Zeichner JA, Eichenfield LF, et al. MAS063DP is effective monotherapy for mild to moderate atopic dermatitis in infants and children: A multicenter, randomized, vehicle-controlled study. J Pediatr 2008;152:854–9.

Eichenfield LF, Basu S, Calvarese B, et al. Effect of desonide hydrogel 0.05% on the hypothalamic-pituitary-adrenal axis in pediatric subjects with moderate to severe atopic dermatitis. Pediatr Dermatol 2007;24:289–95.

Elias PM. Barrier-repair therapy for atopic dermatitis: Corrective lipid biochemical therapy. Expert Rev Dermatol 2008;3:441–52.

Faught J, Bierl C, Barton B, Kemp A. Stress in mothers of young children with eczema. Arch Dis Child 2007;92:683–6.

Friedlander SF, Hebert AA, Allen DB. for the Fluticasone Pediatrics Safety Study Group: Safety of fluticasone propionate cream 0.05% for the treatment of severe and extensive atopic dermatitis in children as young as 3 months. J Am Acad Dermatol 2002;46:387–93.

Ong PY. Emerging drugs for atopic dermatitis. Expert Opin Emerg Drugs 2009;14:165–79.

Ong PY, Leung DYM. Immune dysregulation in atopic dermatitis. Curr Allergy Asthma Rep 2006;6:384–9.

Sampson HA. The evaluation and management of food allergy in atopic dermatitis. Clin Dermatol 2003;21:183–92.

Sugarman J, Parish L. A topical lipid-based barrier repair formulation (EpiCeram) cream is highly effective monotherapy for moderate-to-severe pediatric atopic dermatitis. J Invest Dermatol 2008;128(Suppl. 1):S54 [Abstract].

Erythema Multiforme, Stevens-Johnson Syndrome, and Toxic Epidermal Necrolysis

Method of
Erin Vanness, MD

Erythema multiforme (EM), Stevens-Johnson syndrome (SJS), and toxic epidermal necrolysis (TEN) were previously thought to represent a spectrum of one disorder and therefore have been traditionally grouped together. Current understanding of these disease entities allows us to separate EM from the latter two disorders. EM usually represents a hypersensitivity reaction to human herpes simplex virus type 1 or 2 (HSV-1, HSV-2) reactivation. SJS and TEN are severe, life-threatening drug hypersensitivity reactions that represent a spectrum of mucosal and cutaneous involvement. Exceptions are discussed in the following paragraphs.

Erythema Multiforme

DIAGNOSIS

EM is an abrupt, self-limited, but often recurrent eruption of symmetrically distributed papules, plaques, and targetoid erythematous to dusky red lesions that are fixed and have a predilection for the extensor and acral surfaces. Many patients also have oral erosions or targetoid lesions. Vesicles and bullae may evolve from the target lesions. Eye or genital involvement is not typical. Symptoms may include burning or pruritus. The skin heals without scarring, but transient hyperpigmentation is commonly seen.

Young adults are most commonly affected. EM is rare in the young and elderly. There should not be a prodrome or systemic illness associated with the eruption, although some patients report vague flulike symptoms. The eruption most commonly follows clinical or subclinical HSV-1 or HSV-2 reactivation. EM can uncommonly be associated with mycoplasma, histoplasmosis, or Epstein-Barr virus infection. An EM-like drug eruption and other similar clinical entities exist.

The clinician should consider the following in the differential diagnosis: subacute cutaneous lupus erythematosus; urticaria and urticarial vasculitis; gyrate erythema; multiple, fixed drug eruptions; granuloma annulare; polymorphous light eruption; and multiple forms of acute cutaneous small vessel vasculitis. Although EM is a clinical diagnosis, skin biopsy with interpretation by a dermatopathologist and appropriate laboratory work-up are helpful when indicated.

TREATMENT

Patients with isolated episodes or first episodes of erythema multiforme should be treated symptomatically, reassured, and educated about HSV and EM. HSV reactivation typically precedes the onset of EM by 3 to 14 days; antiviral medications are not beneficial after the eruption has commenced.

Symptomatic measures to reduce burning and pruritus include oral antihistamines (diphenhydramine [Benadryl] 25 to 50 mg PO every 6 hours as needed, weight-based dosage in children) and mid-potency topical corticosteroids (triamcinolone acetonide cream [Kenalog] 0.1% twice daily applied to affected skin; avoid the face). For oral involvement, gentle oral hygiene (saline rinses, very soft toothbrush, 0.2% chlorhexidine gluconate [Corsodyl] or the 0.12% concentration [Peridex] in the United States) and topical anesthetics (2% viscous lidocaine [Xylocaine Viscous] applied as pea-sized amount every 2 hours as needed) can help alleviate symptoms. A short burst of oral corticosteroids may be helpful for severe involvement of the oral mucosa (prednisone 0.5 to 1 mg/kg/day for 4 to 5 days).

CURRENT DIAGNOSIS

Erythema Multiforme

- Acute, symmetric, primarily extensor and acral eruption
- Oral lesions sometimes present
- Papules, plaques, targets, and blisters
- Preceding herpes simplex virus episode
- Young adults

Stevens-Johnson Syndrome and Toxic Epidermal Necrolysis

- Severe, potentially life-threatening hypersensitivity reactions
- Erythema and tenderness of skin and mucosa
- Subsequent extensive denudation of epithelium
- Associated prodrome and systemic illness

CURRENT THERAPY

Erythema Multiforme

- First episode: symptomatic care
- Recurrent episodes: prophylaxis with antivirals

Stevens-Johnson Syndrome and Toxic Epidermal Necrolysis

- Discontinue offending agents immediately
- Supportive care in intensive care unit or burn unit
- Skilled wound care (minimize manipulation, avoid débridement)
- Avoid and monitor for infection
- Pain control
- Ophthalmology consultation for eye involvement
- Consider intravenous immune globulin (IVIG, Baygam)[1] and cyclosporine (Sandimmune, Neoral)[1]

[1]Not FDA approved for this indication.

BOX 1 Drugs Commonly Associated with Stevens-Johnson Syndrome and Toxic Epidermal Necrolysis*

- Sulfonamide antibiotics (trimethoprim-sulfamethoxazole [Bactrim])
- Aminopenicillins
- Quinolones
- Cephalosporins
- Tetracyclines
- Acetaminophen (Tylenol)
- Carbamazepine (Tegretol)
- Phenobarbital
- Valproic acid (Depakene)
- Nonsteroidal anti-inflammatory drugs (NSAIDS, oxicam group)
- Allopurinol (Zyloprim)
- Corticosteroids

*Many other drugs are reported to induce Stevens-Johnson syndrome and toxic epidermal necrolysis.

Patients who suffer from multiple recurrences of EM may be treated prophylactically with oral antiviral medications. When patients can identify the onset of the preceding HSV reactivation, episodic treatment initiated at the onset of the HSV prodrome may significantly reduce the severity and duration of the following EM. Treat with valacyclovir (Valtrex) 500 mg twice daily for 7 days. When patients have multiple recurrences (>6 per year) or cannot identify the preceding HSV activation, treat with valacyclovir 500 mg daily or acyclovir (Zovirax) 400 mg twice daily for at least 6 months. Some patients may achieve a remission at this point, and some may require further suppressive therapy.

Stevens-Johnson Syndrome and Toxic Epidermal Necrolysis

DIAGNOSIS

SJS and TEN are rare, severe, potentially fatal drug hypersensitivity reactions characterized by extensive denudation of skin or mucosal epithelium, or both, and they are accompanied by systemic illness. These entities are best considered on a diagnostic spectrum: SJS has less than 10% body surface area (BSA) with epidermal detachment and two or more mucosal surfaces involved; SJS/TEN overlap has 10% to 30% BSA with detachment and mucosal surfaces typically involved; and TEN has more than 30% detachment, and mucosal surfaces are usually involved. SJS is characterized by an EM-like eruption of the skin of variable severity (see earlier description of EM) and extensive mucosal erosions of at least two sites (i.e., lips or oral tissue, ocular tissue, and genital mucosae). TEN has a skin eruption characterized by dusky red plaques that rapidly progress to denuded, coalescing plaques with a shiny red base. Epidermal detachment can be elicited by placing lateral pressure on a dusky plaque (i.e., Nikolsky's sign).

The accompanying systemic illness usually correlates with the severity of the overall clinical picture. SJS or TEN has an initial flulike prodrome followed by various degrees of fever, lymphadenopathy, systemic toxicity with dehydration and electrolyte imbalance, toxic hepatitis, leukocytosis, anemia, proteinuria, and microscopic hematuria. Less commonly, there is involvement of the nasal, esophageal, pulmonary, and gastrointestinal mucosae; arthritis; myocarditis; and nephritis.

A causal drug can usually be identified. The eruption follows drug exposure by 1 week to 2 months. It is crucial that all potential causative drugs be discontinued immediately (Box 1). Other factors are thought to less frequently induce SJS (Box 2).

The clinician should consider autoimmune bullous disease (i.e., pemphigus, pemphigoid, paraneoplastic pemphigus, and linear IgA bullous dermatosis [LABD]), staphylococcal scalded skin syndrome

---

BOX 2 Reported Causes of Stevens-Johnson Syndrome

- Drugs
- Bacterial infections
- Mycobacterial and mycoplasma infections
- Fungal infections (e.g., histoplasmosis, coccidioidomycosis)
- Viral infections
- Radiation therapy
- Inflammatory bowel disease
- Vaccines

(SSSS), bullous lupus Kawasaki disease, acute generalized exanthematous pustulosis, and acute graft versus host disease in the differential diagnosis. Biopsy of early lesional skin (with epidermis still attached) may reveal necrolysis and interface dermatitis and can help to rule out SSSS. Biopsy of perilesional, noninvolved skin for direct immunofluorescence can help to rule out autoimmune bullous disease.

TREATMENT

It is essential to immediately identify the offending agent and discontinue it. If several possible agents exist, they must all be immediately discontinued. Prompt discontinuation is associated with a 35% reduction in mortality per day (Table 1).

Supportive care is the mainstay of treatment of SJS or TEN. If systemic illness is significant or if the BSA involved exceeds 10% to 20%, the patient should be cared for in an intensive care unit or burn unit setting whenever possible.

Essential supportive care includes thermoregulatory equipment, monitoring, and replacement of fluid and electrolytes as indicated. A controlled-pressure thermoregulated bed is helpful. All care should be performed under sterile conditions, and isolation precautions are necessary to reduce infection risk. Wound care should be performed under the supervision of a dermatologist or burn specialist. Goals of wound care are to minimize manipulation and further denudation of skin, promote healing, reduce infection risk, and increase comfort. Isotonic saline can be used to cleanse involved skin once daily. Silicon or biologic dressings or skin equivalents may be left in place, but the surfaces and surrounding skin should be cleansed. Vaseline gauze may be used for limited BSA and in pressure sites. Mucosal surfaces, orifices, and crusts should be cleansed with saline several times daily, and mupirocin (Bactroban) ointment should be placed around orifices and in macerated areas twice daily.

TABLE 1 SCORTEN: Predicted Mortality in Stevens-Johnson Syndrome and Toxic Epidermal Necrolysis

Prognostic Factor	Present	Absent
Age >40 y	1	0
Heart rate >120 beats/min	1	0
Malignancy present	1	0
Day 1 BSA >10%	1	0
Serum urea >10 mmol/L	1	0
Serum HCO$_3$ <20 mmol/L	1	0
Serum glucose >14 mmol/L	1	0
SCORTEN sum*		

SCORTEN Value	Predicted Mortality
0–1	3.7%
2	12.1%
3	35.8%
4	58.3%
5 or higher	90%

*SCORTEN is a severity-of-illness score developed for toxic epidermal necrolysis (TEN).

An ophthalmologist should be consulted to manage ocular involvement and help prevent adhesions and scarring. Eyelids should be cleansed three times daily with saline and antibiotic ointment subsequently applied to the lids. Antibiotic drops should be instilled to protect the cornea. Gentle oral care with 0.2% chlorhexidine gluconate (0.12% in the United States) should be administered three to four times daily.

Pain control and nutritional support are imperative. Lines should be placed through noninvolved skin when possible and changed every 3 days with culture of the catheter tips. Routine cultures from involved skin and sputum can help to monitor for infection and guide treatment when necessary. Clinical infection should be treated quickly and aggressively.

There are no generally accepted evidence-based standards for specific therapy for SJS or TEN. When patients are stable with limited skin and mucosal involvement and do not seem to be progressing to worse disease, supportive care with close observation is most appropriate. If the patient has extensive or rapidly progressing disease, immunosuppressive therapy should be considered, weighing the risks and benefits, and started without delay if it is to be pursued.

Evidence from several case series and other reports supports the use of intravenous immunoglobulin (IVIG)[1] in TEN, but there also exists contradictory evidence from limited controlled trials that IVIG is not beneficial. If used, it should be started as early as possible in an attempt to halt progression to further BSA involvement. A dose of 1 g/kg for 3 consecutive days is recommended. Some case reports and a case series support the use of cyclosporine (Sandimmune, Neoral)[1] to reduce disease progression, but no randomized trials have been conducted to prove its efficacy. Although IVIG would usually be the drug of choice under current practice standards, cyclosporine may also be considered. Conflicting reports about the use of corticosteroids exist, and some evidence points to increased mortality associated with their use. However, evidence to the contrary was found in a retrospective analysis that showed reduced mortality associated with corticosteroid use. The rarity of SJS or TEN combined with the variability in patient and institutional factors and the bias inherent in retrospective studies has resulted in a paucity of evidence to support any specific therapy. Ultimately, treatment decisions must be made on an individual basis.

---

[1]Not FDA approved for this indication.

REFERENCES

Bachot N, Revuz J, Roujeau JC. Intravenous immunoglobulin treatment for Stevens-Johnson syndrome and toxic epidermal necrolysis; a prospective noncomparative study showing no benefit on mortality or progression. Arch Dermatol 2003;139:33–6.

Bastuji-Garin S, Fouchard N, Bertocchi M, et al. SCORTEN: A severity-of-illness score for toxic epidermal necrolysis. J Invest Dermatol 2000;115:149–53.

Craven N. Toxic epidermal necrolysis and Stevens-Johnson syndrome. In: Lebwohl M, et al., editors. Treatment of Skin Disease. London: Mosby; 2002. pp. 633–6.

French LE, Prins C. Toxic epidermal necrolysis. In: Bolognia JL, et al., editors. Dermatology. Edinburgh: Mosby; 2003. pp. 323–31.

Prins C, Kerdel FA, Padilla S, et al. Treatment of Toxic epidermal necrolysis with high-dose intravenous immunoglobulins: Multicenter retrospective analysis of 48 consecutive cases. Arch Dermatol 2003;139:26–32.

Roujeau JC, Kelly JP, Naldi L, et al. Medication use and the risk of Stevens-Johnson syndrome or toxic epidermal necrolysis. N Engl J Med 1995;333:1600–7.

Schneck J, Fagot J, Sekula P, et al. Effects of treatments on the mortality of Stevens-Johnson syndrome and toxic epidermal necrolysis: A retrospective study on patients included in the prospective EuroSCAR Study. J Am Acad Dermatol 2008;58:33–40.

Schofield JK, Tatnall FM, Leigh IM. Recurrent erythema multiforme: Clinical features and treatment in a large series of patients. Br J Dermatol 1993;128:542–5.

Weston WL. Erythema multiforme and Stevens-Johnson syndrome. In: Bolognia JL, et al., editors. Dermatology. Edinburgh: Mosby; 2003. pp. 313–21.

Bullous Diseases

Method of
Diya F. Mutasim, MD

Epidemiology

The primary lesion in bullous diseases is a vesicle or a bulla. Autoimmune bullous diseases result from immune dysregulation that increases with age, hence the incidence of autoimmune bullous diseases is higher in the elderly. This group of disorders is heterogeneous, and generalizations about the epidemiology cannot be made.

Risk Factors

In general, predisposition to autoimmune bullous diseases is genetic and manifests as loss of tolerance toward self antigens followed by a T-cell and B-cell response resulting in antibody production. Age may be a risk factor in the development of bullous pemphigoid and mucous membrane pemphigoid. Pemphigus vulgaris has a higher incidence among persons of Jewish ancestry.

Pathophysiology

Autoimmune bullous diseases result from an immune response against proteins of desmosomes or the epidermal (or other epithelial) basement membrane. The pemphigus group of diseases is associated with antibodies to different desmosomal proteins. There is strong direct experimental evidence that these antibodies cause acantholysis and blister formation directly without significant participation of cellular components of the immune system. The subepidermal autoimmune bullous diseases, however, result from antibodies against one or more components of the basement membrane that activate the complement system. The latter results in chemoattraction of inflammatory cells, particularly eosinophils and neutrophils, to the basement membrane, as well as activation of local mast cells with degranulation of their cytoplasmic granules, resulting in the release of mediators that further attract inflammatory cells. Both complement and inflammatory cells are required for blister formation. Experimental animals that lack complement or leukocytes fail to develop lesions when injected with patients' serum antibodies.

Prevention

There are no methods for preventing autoimmune bullous diseases. These disorders result from genetically controlled immune dysregulation.

Clinical Manifestations

Clinical manifestations are described for each disease separately under the section on therapy.

Complications

Severe blistering can lead to extensive erosions that heal slowly, especially in the elderly and in those with nutritional deficiencies or systemic disease. Slow healing of extensive erosions predisposes patients to considerable loss of fluids and electrolytes as well as secondary bacterial infection and sepsis. Superficial erosions can become ulcers owing to increased local pressure in immobile and bedridden patients. Temperature regulation can also be compromised following loss of large areas of epidermis. Over the past several decades, mortality from bullous disease has decreased significantly. At present, the common causes of death are complications of the pharmacologic agents used in the treatment.

Diagnosis

The diagnosis of autoimmune bullous diseases requires clinical evaluation, histopathology, direct immunofluorescence, and indirect immunofluorescence. The ideal specimen for direct immunofluorescence should be from normal-appearing skin immediately adjacent to a lesion (perilesional skin). Immunofluorescence tests are usually performed in specialized immunopathology laboratories and are best interpreted by a dermatopathologist with special expertise in the area of immunofluorescence and autoimmune bullous diseases.

Differential Diagnosis

An accurate diagnosis is essential for predicting the course and prognosis of a disease as well as for choosing therapy. Autoimmune bullous diseases overlap clinically and histologically, hence the need for immunofluorescence studies. For example, epidermolysis bullosa acquisita can have clinical and histologic overlap with both bullous pemphigoid and linear IgA disease. The three diseases, however, have different courses and therapeutic responses and may be easily differentiated on the basis of immunofluorescence tests.

Treatment

PRINCIPLES

Because autoimmune bullous disorders result from immune dysregulation, the principle of treatment is immune modulation. Immune modulation can be accomplished by several methods: blocking antibody production by B cells and plasma cells, eliminating antibodies

---

CURRENT DIAGNOSIS

- Clinical
- Histology (always required)
- Direct immunofluorescence (always required)
- Indirect immunofluorescence (sometimes required)
- Antibody specificity for the antigen by enzyme-linked immunosorbent assay (ELISA) (rarely required)

CURRENT THERAPY

- Topical steroids
- Systemic glucocorticoids
- Steroid-sparing (adjuvant) immunosuppressive agents
    - Azathioprine (Imuran)[1]
    - Mycophenolate mofetil (Cellcept)[1]
    - Methotrexate (Trexall)[1]
    - Cyclosporine (Neoral)[1]
    - Cyclophosphamide (Cytoxan)[1]
    - Dapsone
    - Tetracycline (Sumycin)[1]
- Other
    - Niacinamide, nicotinamide[1]
    - High-dose intravenous immunoglobulin (IVIg) (Gammagard)[1]
    - Rituximab (Rituxan)[1]
    - Plasmapheresis, immunoapheresis

---

[1]Not FDA approved for this indication.

---

from the circulation, suppressing inflammation, or inducing resistance of target epithelial cells to separation and blister formation. Antibody production by B cells and plasma cells may be blocked by destroying the B cell lineage or suppressing activation of T or B cells. The former is accomplished by the drug rituximab (Rituxan) and, to a lesser degree, cyclophosphamide (Cytoxan), and the latter may be accomplished by many immunosuppressive agents including corticosteroids, azathioprine (Imuran), cyclosporine (Neoral), cyclophosphamide, methotrexate (Trexall), and mycophenolate mofetil (Cellcept). Antibodies may be eliminated from circulation by plasmapheresis, high-dose intravenous immunoglobulin (IVIg, Gammagard), and immunoadsorption.

Inflammation that is required for blister formation, especially in subepidermal bullous diseases, may be suppressed by several agents. These include systemic and topical corticosteroids, dapsone, tetracyclines, erythromycin, nicotinamide, and etanercept (Enbrel). Although not yet available, agents that experimentally inhibit signal transduction and agents that inhibit apoptosis can induce resistance of the target epidermal or epithelial cell to separation (acantholysis) and blister formation.

The choice of agents in therapy of bullous diseases requires evaluation of both disease-specific parameters and patient-specific parameters. Disease-specific parameters include the pathophysiology of the disease and its severity; patient-specific parameters include age and concomitant illness such as diabetes, hypertension, active infection, or cancer. There are very few controlled studies that provide high-quality evidence for bullous disease therapy. This is primarily a result of the rarity of many of these disorders. Because of the relative frequency of bullous pemphigoid, some controlled studies have been performed on the disease in Europe. Most of the evidence for bullous disease therapy is available from case reports, case series, and personal experience.

PHARMACOLOGIC TREATMENT

Glucocorticoids

Glucocorticoids (prednisone, prednisolone) have both antiinflammatory and immunosuppressive effects. Long-term use of glucocorticoids is associated with well-known adverse effects.

Azathioprine

Azathioprine (Imuran)[1] interferes with de novo purine synthesis and hence DNA synthesis. This results in suppression of T-cell function and a decrease in B-cell antibody production. In low doses (1-2 mg/kg/day), azathioprine is usually well tolerated. In higher doses

---

[1]Not FDA approved for this indication.

(2-4 mg/kg/day), bone marrow may be suppressed, resulting in leukopenia (most commonly) and, less commonly, thrombocytopenia and anemia. Severe bone marrow suppression can occur in patients who are homozygous deficient for the enzyme thiopurine methyltransferase. Other adverse effects include hepatotoxicity and gastrointestinal toxicity as well as pancreatitis and are all dose related. Allopurinol (Zyloprim) is contraindicated in patients receiving azathioprine because it results in an increase in the blood level of azathioprine.

Mycophenolate Mofetil

Mycophenolate mofetil[1] is a purine analogue antimetabolite that inhibits inosine monophosphate dehydrogenase resulting in suppression of purine and DNA synthesis and hence suppression of both T and B cell function. Mycophenolate mofetil is usually well tolerated.

Methotrexate

Methotrexate[1] is an antimetabolite and a folic acid analogue. Its metabolites inhibit folate-dependent enzymes of de novo purine and thymidylate synthesis. This results in the suppression of DNA and RNA synthesis, which causes decreased lymphocyte function and hence immune modulation.

Cyclophosphamide

Cyclophosphamide[1] is an alkylating agent that binds DNA, resulting in cell cycle arrest, DNA repair, and cell death. The most susceptible cells reside in rapidly proliferating tissues. The toxicity of cyclophosphamide is significantly higher than that of azathioprine, mycophenolate mofetil, and methotrexate. Acute myelosuppression is common, with a nadir at 6 to 10 days and recovery in 2 to 3 weeks. Both cellular and humoral immunity are suppressed.

Cyclosporine

Cyclosporine[1] significantly suppresses cellular immunity and preferentially inhibits antigen-triggered signal transduction in T lymphocytes, which results in decreased expression of several lymphokines. Cyclosporine forms complexes with the receptor protein cyclophilin in the cytoplasm. The complex binds and inhibits calcineurin, resulting in failure of T cells to respond to antigenic stimulation.

Several drugs can interact with cyclosporine and influence its blood level. Agents that can increase cyclosporine blood level include calcium channel antagonists (diltiazem [Cardizem], nicardipine [Cardene], and verapamil [Calan]), systemic antifungal agents (fluconazole [Diflucan], itraconazole [Sporanox], and ketoconazole [Nizoral]), antibacterials (clarithromycin [Biaxin], erythromycin), methylprednisolone (Medrol), other drugs (allopurinol [Zyloprim], bromocriptine [Parlodel], danazol [Danocrine], metoclopramide [Reglan], colchicine [Colcrys], and amiodarone [Cordarone]), and grapefruit juice.

Dapsone

Dapsone is highly effective in neutrophil-mediated conditions. The mechanism of action of dapsone is not well understood. Its clinical benefit in inflammatory conditions probably results from inhibition of neutrophil chemotaxis. Dapsone is associated with multiple potential adverse effects that include dose-related hemolysis, methemoglobulinemia (which is common and may be severe in patients who are genetically predisposed), and agranulocytosis (not dose-related and usually occurs in the first 3 months of therapy).

Tetracycline

Tetracycline (Sumycin),[1] doxycycline (Vibramycin),[1] and minocycline (Minocin)[1] have been used interchangeably for the treatment of subepidermal, inflammation-mediated, bullous diseases. Their mechanism of action is not clear.

---

[1]Not FDA approved for this indication.

Niacinamide (Nicotinamide)

Niacinamide[1] is a vitamin whose mechanism of action in cutaneous disorders including autoimmune bullous diseases is not known.

High-Dose Intravenous Immunoglobulin

IVIg[1] is a purified human source of immunoglobulin that is given as a slow infusion over 6 to 8 hours. Treatment is repeated every 3 to 4 weeks. IVIg is highly expensive.

Rituximab

Rituximab[1] is a chimeric monoclonal antibody against CD20 on the surface of pre-B, mature B, and malignant B cells and is not expressed on stem, pro-B or plasma cells. B cells are depleted primarily by antibody-dependent cellular cytotoxicity and, to a lesser degree, by complement-dependent cytotoxicity or apoptosis. Rituximab is given in different regimens, including 375 mg/m^2/week (approximately 500 mg for an average-size adult) for 4 consecutive weeks, or 1000 mg once or on two occasions 2 weeks apart.

Plasmapheresis and Immunoapheresis

Plasmapheresis and immunoapheresis are procedures that aim to physically remove pathogenic antibodies. Plasmapheresis consists of withdrawing the patient's blood, filtering cellular elements from the plasma, and returning the cellular components to the patient. Immunoapheresis consists of exposing the patient's plasma to immunoglobulin-binding matrix that contains the disease-specific antigen. Plasmapheresis and immunoapheresis are usually used in patients who are resistant to other therapies. Plasmapheresis or immunoapheresis is accompanied by immunosuppressive drugs to prevent the rebound phenomenon of excessive antibody production.

TREATMENT OF INDIVIDUAL DISORDERS

Pemphigoid

There are three forms of pemphigoid: bullous pemphigoid (primary skin involvement); mucous membrane pemphigoid (primary mucosal disease), previously referred to as cicatricial pemphigoid; and pemphigoid gestationis (bullous pemphigoid in pregnant women), previously called herpes gestationis. The pemphigoid group of diseases shares the histology of a subepithelial vesicle with usually eosinophil-rich infiltrate, skin-bound IgG and C3 along the basement membrane, and circulating IgG antibodies against two hemidesmosomal proteins of the basement membrane.

Bullous Pemphigoid

Bullous pemphigoid affects primarily persons older than 60 years and is rarely reported in children. Lesions have a predilection for the inner thighs, groin, axillae, neck, and abdomen. The course of bullous pemphigoid is variable. The disease is self-limited within 5 years and the mortality from the disease is low.

Because blisters in bullous pemphigoid result from an abnormal immune response that is mediated by inflammatory cells, therapy for bullous pemphigoid should suppress inflammation or the immune response. Potent topical steroids may be considered for patients with localized disease. Although potent topical steroids lead to rapid resolution of a lesion at its earliest manifestation, they are impractical for patients with generalized disease because they do not prevent new lesions. Patients with generalized bullous pemphigoid require systemic therapy. Glucocorticoids are the most commonly used agents. Prednisone (or methylprednisolone) is sufficient as the only therapy in most cases. The dose varies between 0.2 and 0.5 mg/kg/day depending on the severity of the disease, the age of the patient, and the patient's general health status. A clinical response is usually obtained within 1 to 2 weeks and is manifested by healing of existing lesions and cessation of new blister formation. The dose

---

[1]Not FDA approved for this indication.

is then gradually decreased by relatively large amounts initially (approximately 10 mg) and smaller amounts (2.5-5 mg) subsequently. If the patient develops a flare of lesions during the tapering phase, the dose may be increased to the previous level or higher and maintained longer before further, slower tapering. In many patients, prednisone may be decreased to 5 mg every day or completely discontinued after 6 months.

For patients who require a high dose of steroid for either clearing or maintenance, adjuvant therapy with another agent should be considered in order to avoid the long-term adverse effects of corticosteroids. These drugs include azathioprine[1] (1-3 mg/kg/day in two equally divided doses), mycophenolate mofetil[1] (1000-3000 mg/day or 40 mg/kg/day in two divided doses), and methotrexate[1] (10-15 mg/week). The dose of the second drug may be decreased a few months after clinical remission, slowly tapered, and ultimately discontinued. Dapsone[1] and sulfapyridine[1] are used less commonly and may be effective. Dapsone may be commenced at 25 to 50 mg/day and increased as needed by 25 mg every week until a beneficial effect is obtained. The maximum dose of dapsone is 250 mg/day.

Plasmapheresis and high-dose IVIg[1] are reserved for more-resistant cases. Antibiotics of the tetracycline family as well as erythromycin[1] have been used alone or in combination with niacinamide[1] and have been shown to have some benefit. The dose of tetracycline[1] is 500 mg four times daily and niacinamide 500 mg three times daily. Minocycline[1] or doxycycline[1] in a dose of 100 mg twice daily may be substituted for patients who do not tolerate tetracycline. In my view, a tetracycline with niacinamide is indicated in two situations. In mild cases, the combination alone can lead to a clinical remission. In patients with extensive disease, the addition of this combination to prednisone can have a corticosteroid-sparing effect.

Mucous Membrane Pemphigoid

Therapy for mucous membrane pemphigoid varies with the disease location, extent, and severity. In limited oral disease, local therapy with topical anesthetic agents and topical glucocorticoids in addition to oral hygiene can suffice. The steroid may be applied under occlusion with a prosthetic device or may be injected intralesionally. Patients with extensive oral involvement can require systemic therapy.

Dapsone[1] is effective in some patients with oral mucous membrane pemphigoid. The drug may be started at 50 mg daily and increased gradually. Tetracyclines,[1] with or without niacinamide,[1] may be effective. In patients with severe oral disease and in patients with ocular, pharyngeal, or laryngeal involvement, systemic glucocorticoids, in combination with cyclophosphamide[1] are indicated. In my experience, most patients have an excellent response, with a prolonged remission after treatment with the combination of prednisone (1 mg/kg/day for 6 months) and cyclophosphamide (1-2 mg/kg/day for 18 to 24 months).

Azathioprine[1] and mycophenolate mofetil[1] are generally less effective but may be used if there are contraindications to steroid or cyclophosphamide use. High-dose IVIg[1] may be used for patients who are refractory to other therapy.

Patients with severe ocular scarring might benefit from cryotherapy ablation of eyelashes. Ocular surgery is contraindicated when the disease is active. Surgical intervention may cause severe flares of the disease.

Epidermolysis Bullosa Acquisita

Unlike bullous pemphigoid and other subepidermal autoimmune bullous diseases, epidermolysis bullosa acquisita is generally resistant to therapy. The disease waxes and wanes, with periods of exacerbation and remission. Trauma contributes to blister formation, especially in the classic form of epidermolysis bullosa acquisita. The inflammatory form of epidermolysis bullosa acquisita responds more easily to therapy than the classic form.

Because of the neutrophil predominance in the inflammatory form, patients might respond to dapsone.[1] The drug may be started at a dose of 50 mg daily and increased by 50 mg every week until

clinical remission (usually 100-250 mg). The dose is maintained for several months. If the patient remains in remission, the dose may be decreased slowly and ultimately discontinued. Colchicine[1] 0.6 mg two or three times daily is variably effective. Patients who do not tolerate or do not respond to colchicine and dapsone may be treated with oral glucocorticoids such as prednisone in a dose of 0.5-1 mg/kg/day in divided doses. The response is variable. If there is no response to glucocorticoids or the patient develops adverse effects, cyclosporine[1] 4-6 mg/kg/day may be initiated and is usually associated with a rapid response. Once disease activity is controlled, the dose may be slowly decreased. Cyclosporine should be discontinued if there is no response in a few weeks.

The duration of treatment varies with the course of the disease. The same agents used for the inflammatory form may be used for the classic form. The latter is generally more resistant to treatment. Patients who fail to respond may be treated with immunosuppressive agents such as azathioprine,[1] cyclophosphamide,[1] mycophenolate,[1] or methotrexate[1] in a manner similar to pemphigus vulgaris, bullous pemphigoid, or mucous membrane pemphigoid. Patients who are resistant to these agents may be treated with extracorporeal photochemotherapy or with IVIg[1] alone or in conjunction with plasmapheresis.

Dermatitis Herpetiformis

Dermatitis herpetiformis results from an immune response to gluten and manifests as pruritic papulovesicles over the elbows, knees, buttocks, and scalp. A gluten-free diet is extremely helpful and is often associated with a marked decrease in the requirement for pharmacologic therapy. A strict gluten-free diet can result in complete remission of the disease without requiring dapsone. Reinstitution of gluten-containing diet results in rapid recurrence of the disease.

Many patients find a strict gluten-free diet too restrictive and choose pharmacologic therapy. The drug of choice is dapsone. Treatment is initiated with dapsone 50 mg daily and is increased by 25 to 50 mg every week as needed and as tolerated. The average daily maintenance dose is 100 mg. Some patients require slowly increasing doses several years later, likely secondary to increased deposition of IgA in the skin that results in increased disease activity.

In patients who are intolerant or allergic to dapsone, therapy with sulfapyridine may be considered. The initial dose is 500 mg three times daily and may be increased slowly to 2 g three times daily. The response to sulfapyridine is not as predictable as that to dapsone. Patients who are allergic to dapsone often tolerate sulfapyridine.

Patients who are intolerant or allergic to dapsone and sulfapyridine may be treated with colchicine,[1] cholestyramine (Questran),[1] heparin,[1] tetracycline,[1] or nicotinamide.[1] These agents are much less effective than dapsone and sulfapyridine. Topical steroids are only minimally effective.

Linear Immunoglobulin A Disease

Linear IgA disease is mediated by neutrophils and clinically mimics bullous pemphigoid and dermatitis herpetiformis. Dapsone[1] is the first-line agent. The drug may be started at 25 to 50 mg daily and increased by 25 to 50 mg every 1 to 2 weeks until an effective dose is reached. Patients with early disease tend to respond to lower doses of dapsone.

Sulfapyridine[1] is an alternative agent for patients who cannot tolerate dapsone. The starting dose is 500 mg twice daily and may be increased by 1000 mg every 1 to 2 weeks until the disease is adequately controlled. Colchicine[1] 0.6 mg 2-3 times daily may also be used if a patient is allergic to dapsone. Glucocorticoids may be added if patients do not respond completely to these agents.

Tetracyclines in combination with niacinamide[1] have been reported to be effective. The dose of tetracycline[1] is 500 mg 4 times daily. Alternatively, doxycycline[1] or minocycline[1] 100 mg twice daily may be used. The dose of niacinamide is 500 mg three times daily. Cyclosporine[1] or high-dose IVIg[1] may be used in resistant cases.

---

[1]Not FDA approved for this indication.

[1]Not FDA approved for this indication.

Pemphigus

Pemphigus Vulgaris

Pemphigus vulgaris often manifests with erosions in the oral cavity that may be followed by skin blisters. Successful therapy suppresses the production of pathogenic autoantibodies. Therefore immunosuppressive drugs are used. A positive clinical response is associated with a decrease in or absence of pathogenic circulating autoantibodies in the serum and then absence of bound autoantibodies in the skin. There has been a dramatic decrease in the mortality of pemphigus vulgaris owing to the increasing availability of immunosuppressive drugs and glucocorticoids, as well as earlier diagnosis and treatment.

Unless there is an absolute contraindication, the initial therapy of pemphigus vulgaris is systemic glucocorticoid. Prednisone is the most commonly used agent. The initial dose is 1 mg/kg/day divided into two or three doses. Most patients obtain remission within 4 to 12 weeks. The dosage is maintained for 6 to 10 weeks, then decreased by 10 to 20 mg every 2 to 4 weeks. If there is no recurrence, the patient is maintained on 5 mg daily or every other day for several years. Pulsed-steroid therapy with intravenous methylprednisolone, 1 g daily for 3 consecutive days, is reserved for severe cases. The goal of this approach is to quickly achieve the immunosuppressive effects of glucocorticoids while avoiding the long-term side effects.

If prednisone fails to induce a remission, or if the patient develops serious adverse effects, adjuvant immunosuppressive drugs should be instituted. My practice is to initiate adjuvant therapy concomitant with steroid therapy to decrease the total dose of glucocorticoid used. The glucocorticoid is tapered rapidly and the patient is maintained on the steroid-sparing agent for 24 to 36 months. The most commonly used steroid-sparing immunosuppressive drugs are azathioprine[1] and mycophenolate mofetil.[1] Cyclophosphamide[1] is used for resistant cases at a dose of 2 to 3 mg/kg/day, azathioprine at a dose of 3 to 5 mg/kg/day, and mycophenolate at a dose of 2 to 3 g daily (or 40 mg/kg/day in two divided doses). Methotrexate[1] may also be used, but it is generally less effective than other treatments.

The response of pemphigus vulgaris to cyclosporine[1] is controversial. High-dose IVIg[1] has a rapid onset of action and appears most effective when used as an adjuvant to conventional therapy, especially as a steroid-sparing agent. Plasmapheresis is used in refractory cases. To avoid the rebound phenomenon (increased production of autoantibodies), immune suppression (usually with cyclophosphamide) is used concomitantly with plasmapheresis. Rituximab[1] has been used successfully in several cases of pemphigus vulgaris and other autoimmune bullous diseases. For resistant cases, extracorporeal photochemotherapy may be considered.

Pemphigus Foliaceous

The principles and practice of managing pemphigus foliaceous are similar to those for pemphigus vulgaris.

Paraneoplastic Pemphigus

Paraneoplastic pemphigus is a unique intraepidermal blistering disease associated with antibodies against a unique set of skin and internal organ antigens. The most common associated neoplasms are lymphoproliferative. The management of paraneoplastic pemphigus consists of the treatment of the underlying neoplasm as well as immune suppression. Surgical excision of benign neoplasms such as thymoma and Castleman's disease can result in clinical and serologic improvement. In patients with malignant neoplasms, treatment of the associated neoplasm might not result in remission. Generally, skin lesions respond more rapidly than mucosal lesions.

Systemic glucocorticoids are often used as the first-line agent in a dose of 1 to 2 mg/kg/day. Patients usually have a partial response and rarely have complete resolution of lesions. Other immunosuppressive drugs have been used with variable success. These include mycophenolate mofetil,[1] azathioprine,[1] and cyclosporine.[1]

---

[1] Not FDA approved for this indication.

Rituximab[1] has been reported to be effective in a case of paraneoplastic pemphigus associated with CD20-positive follicular lymphoma and in a case of paraneoplastic pemphigus associated with follicular non-Hodgkin's lymphoma. Immunoapheresis has been used successfully occasionally.

---

[1] Not FDA approved for this indication.

REFERENCES

Bystryn JC, Jiao D, Natow S. Treatment of pemphigus with intravenous immunoglobulin. J Am Acad Dermatol 2002;47:358–63.

Herron MD, Zone JJ. Treatment of dermatitis herpetiformis and linear IgA bullous dermatosis. Dermatol Ther 2002;15:374–81.

Kirtschig G, Middleton P, Hollis S, et al. Interventions for bullous pemphigoid. Cochrane Database Syst Rev 2005;(3):CD002292.

Kirtschig G, Murrell D, Wojnarowska F, Khumalo N. Interventions for mucous membrane pemphigoid and epidermolysis bullosa acquisita. Cochrane Database Syst Rev 2003;(1):CD004056.

Mutasim DF. Treatment considerations while awaiting the ideal bullous pemphigoid trial. Arch Dermatol 2002;138:404.

Mutasim DF. Management of autoimmune bullous diseases: Pharmacology and therapeutics. J Am Acad Dermatol 2004;51:859–77.

Mutasim DF. Autoimmune bullous dermatoses in the elderly: An update on pathophysiology, diagnosis and management. Drugs Aging 2010;7:1–19.

Nousari HC, Sragovich A, Kimyai-Asadi A, et al. Mycophenolate mofetil in autoimmune and inflammatory skin disorders. J Am Acad Dermatol 1999;40:265–8.

Rogers RS 3rd, Seehafer JR, Perry HO. Treatment of cicatricial (benign mucous membrane) pemphigoid with dapsone. J Am Acad Dermatol 1982;6:215–23.

Wojnarowska F, Kirtschig G, Highet AS, et al. Guidelines for the management of bullous pemphigoid. Br J Dermatol 2002;147:214–21.

Contact Dermatitis

Method of
James A. Yiannias, MD, and Genevieve L. Egnatios, MD

Dermatitis typically manifests as papules and vesicles with weeping and oozing that can become lichenified and scaly when chronic. When this clinical picture is secondary to an exogenous substance coming into contact with the skin, it is termed *contact dermatitis*. Further delineation leads to irritant versus allergic contact dermatitis, although in practice these often overlap.

Irritant contact dermatitis is not an allergic process. It represents damage to the skin from repeated and cumulative exposure to an agent. Irritants do not require prior sensitization. Decreased barrier function of the skin, for example with frequent hand washing, can predispose or exacerbate the condition. Examples include alkalis (in soaps, detergents, and cleansers), acids (in germicides, dyes, and pigments), hydrocarbons (in petroleum and oils), and solvents.

Allergic contact dermatitis is an immunologic process classified as a type IV cell-mediated delayed hypersensitivity reaction. Poison ivy is a classic example. It requires an initial exposure to the contactant in which sensitization occurs but without outward physical effect. Subsequent exposure can elicit a striking response that is independent of the amount of the contactant.

The most common contact allergens from 1994 to 2005 have changed very little. Based on studies performed by the North American Contact Dermatitis Group (NACDG) and the Mayo Clinic Contact Dermatitis Group (MCCDG), the allergens most consistently in the top ten were nickel sulfate, balsam of Peru, fragrance mix, quaternium-15, neomycin, bacitracin, formaldehyde, and cobalt chloride (Box 1). Common sources of exposure to nickel include costume jewelry, snaps, zippers, and other metal objects. Balsam of Peru and

BOX 1   Top 10 Most Common Allergens

North American Contact Dermatitis Group

Nickel sulfate
Balsam of Peru
Fragrance mix 1
Quaternium-15
Neomycin
Bacitracin
Formaldehyde
Cobalt chloride
Methyldibromoglutaronitrile
p-Phenylenediamine

Mayo Clinic Contact Dermatitis Group

Nickel sulfate
Balsam of Peru
Gold sodium thiosulfate
Neomycin
Fragrance mix
Cobalt chloride
Formaldehyde
Benzalkonium chloride
Bacitracin
Quaternium-15

Data from Zug KA, Warshaw EM, Fowler JF Jr, et al: Patch-test results of the North American Contact Dermatitis Group 2005-2006. Dermatitis 2009;20:149-160; and Davis MD, Scalf LA, Yiannias JA, et al: Changing trends and allergens in the patch test standard series: A Mayo Clinic 5-year retrospective review, January 1, 2001 to December 31, 2005. Arch Dermatol 2008;144:67-72.

fragrance mix 1 are markers for fragrance sensitivity. Sources of exposure to formaldehyde include skin-care products, household products, and the resins in plastics and clothing. Quaternium-15 is a formaldehyde releasing preservative and may be found in products such as skin care products, paper, inks, and photocopier toner. Neomycin and bacitracin are topical antibiotics available alone and in combination with polymyxin (Neosporin), antifungals, and corticosteroids. Cobalt is found with other metals, including zinc, and in items such as jewelry, crayons, hair dye, and antiperspirants.

Others in the top ten less consistently during that period were methyldibromo glutaronitrile, p-phenylenediamine, gold sodium thiosulfate, thiuram mix, benzalkonium chloride, and potassium dichromate. Methyldibromo glutaronitrile is a preservative and can be found in health care and personal products. Permanent hair dyes are the usual source of p-phenylenediamine. Clinically relevant sources of gold may be found in jewelry and dental appliances. Thiuram mix is in rubber and some personal products. Benzalkonium chloride is used commonly in the health care field as a cleanser, antiseptic, and preservative, but it is also found in personal care products and medications. Potassium dichromate is used in cement, leather, and steel surfaces.

Diagnosis

The evaluation of a patient with suspected contact dermatitis begins with the history. Specific questions directed at the patient's occupation, hobbies, and home routine will be helpful. Examination should note the location and pattern of the eruption. Although eyelid dermatitis may be seen in the atopic patient, it nail polish if often the source of the offending allergen. Dyshidrotic eczema occurs as vesicles along the lateral aspects of the fingers, whereas eczematous changes along the dorsal hands is more commonly due to an allergen. Other distributions as clues include post-auricular scalp (perfume), perioral area (chewing gum, toothpaste), trunk (dyes or clothing finish), wrist (nickel or chrome), waistline (rubber), feet (shoes), and history or presence of wounds (topical antibiotic ointment).

CURRENT DIAGNOSIS

Gather Detailed History on Skin Exposures

- Irritants
  - Alkalis: soaps, detergents, cleansers
  - Acids
  - Hydrocarbons: petroleum, oils
  - Solvents
- Allergens
  - Nickel sulfate
  - Balsam of Peru (fragrance)
  - Fragrance mix
  - Quaternium-15 (formaldehyde-releasing preservative)
  - Neomycin
  - Bacitracin
  - Formaldehyde
  - Cobalt chloride (metals, personal products)

Examine Skin for Location and Pattern of Eruption

- Eyelid: nail polish
- Postauricular scalp: perfume
- Perioral area: chewing gum, toothpaste
- Trunk: dyes, clothing finish
- Wrist: nickel, chrome
- Waistline: rubber
- Feet: shoes
- Wounds: topical antibiotic ointment

Perform Patch Testing

- TRUE Test with 29 allergens (note: four common allergens are not included in this panel)
- Customized series with 65 or more allergens

Patch testing can confirm or reveal a contact allergy. It involves placement of allergens against the skin of the patient's back for 48 hours. Then an initial reading is done with follow-up readings, typically at 96 hours. Prepared series include the thin-layer rapid-use epicutaneous test (TRUE Test), which consists of 29 allergens (www.truetest.com); customized series such as the NACDG Standard Series with 65 allergens and the Mayo Clinic's Standard series with 74 allergens must be manually assembled. The majority of dermatologists performing patch testing use the TRUE Test. Note that bacitracin, methyldibromo glutaronitrile, gold sodium thiosulfate, and benzalkonium chloride are not included in that panel.

In addition to ascertaining degree of positivity, relevance must be determined. This involves collaborating with patients to assess the likelihood that they are currently exposed to the positive antigen.

Treatment

Ideally, the allergen(s) will be identified and avoided. Realistically, compliance is a challenge. To assist patients in avoiding antigens in skin care products, the Contact Allergen Replacement Database (CARD) was created in 1999. It includes approximately 6500 ingredients and 3000 individual over-the-counter and prescription skin-care products. Once the patient's allergens have been identified with patch testing, they can be entered into the database, and a list of products free of those substances is generated. The patient should be reminded that even small and infrequent exposures can perpetuate the eczema.

Topical corticosteroids twice daily are helpful in hastening resolution and may also be used for disease control when the allergen is unknown. Low-potency corticosteroids such as 2.5% hydrocortisone (Hytone) are recommended for the thinner skin of the face, neck, axillae, groin, and intertriginous areas. Mid-potency steroids such as triamcinolone 0.1% (Kenalog, Kenonel) are appropriate for the

CURRENT THERAPY

- Avoidance of irritants and allergens using prepared patient handout
- CARD shopping list free of most common allergens (if patch testing is not performed)
- Customized CARD shopping list based on patch test results
- Topical corticosteroids
  - Hydrocortisone 2.5% bid for face, neck, axillae, groin, intertriginous areas
  - Triamcinolone 0.1% bid for body
  - Short-term, higher-potency steroids for severe reaction (e.g., clobetasol 0.05% bid)

- Sedating antihistamines: doxepin 10-20 mg nightly 2 hours before bed
- Steroid-sparing topical agents: tacrolimus 0.1%, pimecrolimus 1%
- Systemic corticosteroids: several-week tapering course for severe acute episodes (e.g., prednisone 60 mg for 5 days, 40 mg for 5 days, and 20 mg for 5 days)
- Longer-term systemic therapy for severe or recalcitrant disease
  - Phototherapy with narrowband ultraviolet B
  - Cyclosporine 2.5-5 mg/kg daily
  - Azathioprine 1-3 mg/kg daily

CARD = Contact Allergen Replacement Database

---

thicker skin of the body. Short-term use of higher-potency steroids may be necessary if the reaction is severe. If there is significant pruritus, sedating antihistamines such as doxepin (Sinequan)[1] 10 to 20 mg taken nightly 2 hours before bedtime can provide relief. Steroid-sparing topical immunosuppressants such as tacrolimus (Protopic)[1] and pimecrolimus (Elidel)[1] may be helpful adjuncts. Treatment for severe acute episodes can entail a several-week tapering course of systemic corticosteroids, especially if the eruption is widespread. Other longer-term systemic therapies for severe or resistant disease include phototherapy, or systemic immunosuppressants such as cyclosporine (Neoral)[1] or azathioprine (Imuran).[1]

It may take many weeks before the skin reverts to a normal appearance despite successful avoidance of antigens. A prepared handout with concrete recommendations for the patient on truly hypoallergenic skin is beneficial. A sample of that used at Mayo Clinic in Arizona is shown in Figure 1.

[1]Not FDA approved for this indication.

[1]Not FDA approved for this indication.

Introduction

Eczema, also known as Dermatitis, is an inflammation of the skin due to dryness irritation or possible external allergy. Eczema/Dermatitis is not contagious.

Some skin care products contain fragrance even though the package says "fragrance free" or "unscented." Therefore, please choose the skin care products as listed below by their exact brand name.

Suggestions

Soaps/Cleansing
- Vanicream Cleansing Bar®
- Free and Clear Liquid Cleanser®
- Aveeno® Moisturizing Bar for Dry Skin, Fragrance Free or Aveeno® Eczema Care Body Wash
- Oilatum Unscented Soap®
- Neutrogena Original Formula® Fragrance-Free® (bar or liquid)
- Any of the shampoos listed in this brochure may be used as your hand or body soap
- Aveeno® Therapeutic shave gel or Edge® unscented shave gel

Moisturizers
- Vanicream®, Vanicream Lite®
- Aveeno® Daily Moisturizing Lotion, Fragrance Free or Aveeno® Eczema Care Moisturizing Cream
- Plain Vaseline®
- DML unscented®
  - Use moisturizers twice daily
  - All of the above are OK to use on face
  - To assist with your applying the cream after shower, just blot water off with hand and apply cream. Do not use a towel to dry off.
- Robathol Bath Oil®

Deodorants
- Almay® unscented antiperspirants
- Mitchum® unscented cream antiperspirant and deodorant
- May use plain cornstarch from grocer

Shampoo
- Free and Clear Shampoo® and Conditioner
- DHS Clear Shampoo® and DHS Conditioner®
- If you have dandruff, use DHS Sal Shampoo or Neutrogena T-SAL Shampoo (not T-Gel)
- Conditioners can be used as "leave on" hair gel

Hairspray
- Fragrance-Free hairspray such as Free and Clear® Hairspray (Caution: Hairsprays labeled as "unscented" may not be fragrance free.)

Laundry and Home Care
- Unscented laundry detergents (Tide Free®, Cheer Free and Gentle®, All Free and Clear®, Arm & Hammer Unscented®, Wisk Free®, Purex Unscented®)
- Wash all new clothes and linens five times before using.
- Old clothes and fabrics are preferred.
- White vinegar in rinse cycle help to remove soap, and may be used as a general household cleaner.

Hand, Nail & General Skin Care Tips
- Wear cotton gloves under rubber/vinyl gloves for any activities where hand-wetting is expected.
- Trim nails short. Long nails are dangerous to skin especially when sleeping.

Sunscreens
- Vanicream Sunscreen # 30 or 60°

Avoid

Soaps/Cleansing
- No hot water (use lukewarm).
- Avoid hot tubs.
- No rubbing alcohol.

Moisturizers
- No creams, lotions, oils or powders other than those recommended in this brochure.
- No Neosporin® products.

Fragrances
- No perfumes, colognes, after-shave, pre-shave on any part of body/clothing.

Laundry and Home Care
- No fabric softener in washer.
- No fabric softener sheets in dryer.
- No washing machine water softener such as Calgon® (in-house water softeners are acceptable).

Hand, Nail & General Skin Care Tips
- No wetting of hands more than 5 times a day.
- No tight-fitting clothes
- No scrubbing! No Loofa! No pumice stone!
- Do not pull off dead skin. Snip with scissors instead.

FIGURE 1. Sample of prepared handout (used at Mayo Clinic, Arizona) with recommendations for the patient on hypoallergenic skin care products.

If patch testing is not performed, an initial approach may be to instruct the patient on avoiding the most common contact allergens via such a handout and prescribing symptomatic treatment including topical and oral therapies. CARD can generate a shopping list of products free of the top 10 allergens as identified by the NACDG and the MCCDG. Some physicians follow these measures for several months, especially if the eruption is mild, before pursuing formal patch testing.

An excellent primer for the physician interested in learning more about contact allergy diagnosis and management is *Contact and Occupational Dermatology*.

REFERENCES

Davis MD, Scalf LA, Yiannias JA, et al. Changing trends and allergens in the patch test standard series: A Mayo Clinic 5-year retrospective review, January 1, 2001 to December 31, 2005. Arch Dermatol 2008;144:67–72.

Marks JG, Elsner P, DeLeo VA. Contact and Occupational Dermatology. 3rd ed. St Louis: Mosby; 2002.

Nelson SA, Yiannias JA. Relevance and avoidance of skin-care product allergens: Pearls and pitfalls. Dermatol Clin 2009;27(3):329–36.

Thin-layer rapid-use epicutaneous test (TRUE-test). Available at: http://www.truetest.com/PatientPDF/File18.pdf; [accessed 12.08.10].

Zug KA, Warshaw EM, Fowler JF, et al. Patch-test results of the North American Contact Dermatitis Group 2005-2006. Dermatitis 2009;20:149–60.

Anogenital Pruritus

Method of

Lynne Margesson, MD, FRCPC, and F. William Danby, MD, FRCPC

Anogenital pruritus is a common symptom that affects the genitals or anus, or both. Pruritus ani affects 1% to 5% of the population and is more common in men. Pruritus vulvae is a common vulvar complaint affecting up to 10% of women. Genital pruritus in men is less common. Pruritus in these areas can be acute or chronic, and it can range from minor to debilitating.

Finding the cause of the pruritus is of utmost importance to manage these patients effectively. The most common causes are outlined in Box 1. Because the cause of pruritus is often multifactorial, always consider a combination of conditions.

In the vulvar area, the most common cause is acute candidiasis. Irritant contact dermatitis is next and often results from overzealous cleansing habits or exposure to topical irritants such as urine, feces, sweat, and topical medications. Among the chronic conditions, the most common causes are lichen simplex chronicus and lichen sclerosus. Psoriasis and lichen planus are seen less often. Patients may have a combination of infection, contact dermatitis (usually irritant), and dermatoses. Pruritus of the penis alone is unusual, and the most common causes are scabies and monilial balanitis. Scrotal itch may result from a primary irritant (often in atopics) or allergic contact dermatitis, scabies, and tinea cruris, even though the dermatophyte rarely involves the scrotum itself. Pubic lice cause pruritus of the entire hairy genital area.

In the anal area, dietary factors (through irritant contact dermatitis from fecal soiling) account for most cases of anal pruritus. As in the vulva, this is confounded by excessive cleansing and irritation and less frequently by allergic reactions to topical medications. Underlying anorectal diseases should be sought. Dermatologic diseases, infections, and infestations need to be considered. Concurrent conditions can confuse the picture. Anxiety and depression can further confuse the diagnosis.

BOX 1 Causes of Anogenital Pruritus

Acute Pruritus

Infections

- *Candida*, dermatophytosis
- Herpes simplex virus, human papillomavirus, molluscum contagiosum
- *Staphylococcus aureus, Streptococcus*

Dermatoses

- Contact dermatitis (irritant, allergic, enzymatic)
- Atopic dermatitis/eczema
- Psoriasis

Chronic Pruritus

Dermatoses

- Lichen simplex chronicus
- Contact dermatitis (irritant or allergic)
- Lichen sclerosus
- Lichen planus
- Psoriasis

Neuropathy
Malignancy

- Vulvar and anal intraepithelial neoplasia
- Squamous cell carcinoma, extramammary Paget's disease

Anal-Specific Causes

- Dietary factors
- Hemorrhoids
- Anal fissures and fistulae
- Proctitis
- Inflammatory bowel disease

Evaluation and Diagnosis

A complete history and careful full-surface physical examination of the skin is needed. The examiner should adequately detail information about all hygiene practices and all topical products (prescribed and proprietary) used. For vulvar pruritus, a complete vulvar and vaginal examination is essential. Telephone diagnosis is unacceptable. For anal pruritus, a digital examination with anoscopy, proctoscopy, or colonoscopy may be indicated. Consider appropriate potassium hydroxide (KOH) preparations, cultures, skin biopsies, and patch testing as indicated (Box 2).

Management

Support and education of the patient are important (Box 3). All excess washing, irritants, and protease-containing laundry detergents must be eliminated. Unnecessary topical agents must be stopped. Infection control is important. Use oral antibiotics, and for women, add fluconazole (Diflucan)[1] to prevent secondary yeast infection. Topical anesthetics such as lidocaine 5% ointment can help ease the need to scratch. Avoid benzocaine (Vagisil), because it can be a very strong irritant and allergen. Cooling the area is helpful, and this can be done with Sitz baths, gel packs (cold but not frozen), or compresses. Keep the gel packs or cool, moist clothes in self-sealing bags in the refrigerator. Avoid ice, which can cause frostbite of the area.

For anal pruritus, dietary factors may be important. Avoid foods, beverages, and medications that can exacerbate symptoms. Address dietary changes to improve bowel function. It is essential to control

---

[1]Not FDA approved for this indication.

BOX 2 Investigations for Anogenital Pruritus

- Culture—bacteria, *Candida*, dermatophyte
- Wet prep of vaginal secretions for *Candida*, bacterial vaginosis, trichomoniasis
- Culture all balanitis for yeast and bacteria
- Adhesive tape testing for pinworms
- Potassium hydroxide testing of skin and vaginal secretions for yeast, scabies, dermatophytes
- Patch testing for allergic contact dermatitis
- Skin biopsy for dermatoses, tumors
- Anal or gastrointestinal disease—anoscopy, proctoscopy, colonoscopy
- Prostate cancer—prostate-specific antigen (PSA) and digital rectal examination (DRE)

BOX 3 Treatment of Anogenital Pruritus

Non-Specific Measures
- Patient support and education
- Stop all irritants (e.g., overwashing, scratching, infection, unnecessary topical preparations)
- Topical anesthetics (e.g., 5% lidocaine ointment bid to qid [may sting]), avoid benzocaine (Vagisil).
- Cool compresses, soaks, gel packs (not frozen); keep in refrigerator in self-sealed plastic bag.
- Bland emollients (plain petrolatum or zinc oxide) ointment to soothe open fissured or eroded tissue.

Specific Measures
- Eliminate protease-containing laundry detergents
- Eliminate local secondary bacterial and yeast infection
- Stop scratching—use nighttime sedation (hydroxyzine [Vistaril]/doxepin [Sinequan] 10–100 mg)/citalopram (Celexa) 20–40 mg each morning
- Reduce inflammation—topical corticosteroid ointments once infection is controlled

Mild disease: 1% to 2.5% hydrocortisone ointment with or without pramoxine (Pramasone)
Moderate disease: triamcinolone 0.1% (Kenalog) ointment
Severe pruritus or thick skin areas: superpotent clobetasol (Temovate) or halobetasol (Ultravate) 0.05% ointment
For very severe pruritus—systemic prednisone or IM triamcinolone (Kenalog-40) 1 mg/kg up to maximum 80 mg/dose

- As steroid sparer, consider calcineurin inhibitors 1% pimecrolimus cream (Elidel) or 0.03% to 1% tacrolimus ointment (Protopic)
- Manage anxiety and depression

Specific for Pruritus Ani
- Implement dietary changes
- Control fecal leakage and constipation

Specific for Pruritus Vulvae
- Treat vaginitis
- Manage urinary incontinence and contributory menstrual flow

For Neuropathic Pruritus
- Amitriptyline (Elavil) 10–150 mg qhs
- Gabapentin (Neurontin) up to 3600 mg per day
- Venlafaxine (Effexor) up to 150 mg per day

fecal leakage and constipation. Consider the possibility of rectal or prostatic pathology. Use bland emollients such as plain petrolatum or zinc oxide ointment to coat eroded, fissured skin after careful cleansing.

For genital pruritus, manage urinary incontinence and any contributing irritation from menstrual flow. Adjustments can be made to minimize flow with medications. Consider tampons rather than pads.

Gentle hygiene is important. The patient should use a hypoallergenic cleansing bar with hands only and avoid washcloths and wipes. Use a small amount of mineral oil or Albolene cleanser on a tissue to remove fecal material. Scratching must be controlled with nighttime sedation such as hydroxyzine (Vistaril) or doxepin (Sinequan).[1] These patients have a tendency to scratch at night. They may be unaware of this. These medications assist with a deeper sleep to help stop the scratching. This is imperative for healing. Daytime sedation with citalopram (Celexa)[1] or fluoxetine (Prozac)[1] may be necessary.

Inflammation must be addressed. Classically, topical corticosteroid ointments are used. For mild disease, mild-potency hydrocortisone (Hycort) 1% to 2.5% ointment may be all that is necessary. A 1% hydrocortisone/1% iodoquinol cream (Vytone) used topically as an antimicrobial with mild antiinflammatory action can be effective for perianal pruritus and skin fold areas such as labiocrural and inguinal folds and the gluteal cleft. For more severe pruritus, especially if the skin is thickened with lichen simplex chronicus or lichen sclerosus or is severely involved with lichen planus, a superpotent corticosteroid is needed. Lichen sclerosus is treated with a superpotent steroid one or two times daily for 8 to 12 weeks and then three times per week, gradually decreasing to a maintenance regimen of one or two applications per week for the long term. Lichen simplex chronicus responds to superpotent steroid twice daily for 2 weeks, once daily for 2 weeks, and then three times per week. Consider switching to a calcineurin inhibitor such as pimecrolimus (Elidel)[1] or tacrolimus (Protopic)[1] twice daily as a steroid sparer. Ointments are suggested because they are more effective and less allergenic than creams. Use as a thin, invisible film. There is controversy about the use of calcineurin inhibitors in the treatment of lichen sclerosus and lichen planus. Calcineurin inhibitors can cause a burning sensation.

For severe intractable pruritus, a limited course of systemic corticosteroid may be indicated, using intramuscular triamcinolone acetonide (Kenalog 40), 1 mg/kg up to a maximum dose of 80 mg, or prednisone tapered over a three week course.

For perianal pruritus, a mild 1% to 2.5% hydrocortisone ointment may be all that is necessary. Because the skin is thin, strong corticosteroids should be used only for a limited time. The calcineurin inhibitors can be very helpful. For patients with intractable anal symptoms, cautious local injections of methylene blue (Urolene Blue)[1] have been beneficial.

For patients with neuropathy, management is like that for chronic pain conditions, with amitriptyline (Elavil),[1] gabapentin (Neurontin),[1] venlafaxine (Effexor),[1] or combinations of these drugs. Anxiety and depression need to be addressed in all of these patients.

Itching in these areas can be chronic and recurrent, and long-term follow-up will be needed. Treatment regimens must be used long enough to get adequate healing and completely break the itch, scratch, itch cycle. Otherwise, relapse is common.

---

[1]Not FDA approved for this indication.

REFERENCES

Al-Ghnaniem R, Short K, Pullen A, et al. 1% Hydrocortisone ointment is an effective treatment of pruritus ani: A pilot randomized controlled crossover trial. Int J Colorectal Dis 2007;22(12):1463–7.

Bohl TG. Overview of vulvar pruritus through the life cycle. Clin Obstet Gynecol 2005;48(4):786–807.

Cork MJ, Danby SG, Vasilopoulos Y, et al. Epidermal barrier dysfunction in atopic dermatitis. J Invest Dermatol. 2009;129(8):1892–908.

Farage MA, Miller KW, Berardesca E, Maibach HI. Incontinence in the aged: Contact dermatitis and other cutaneous consequences. Contact Dermatitis 2007;57(4):211–7.

Koca R, Altin R, Konuk N, et al. Sleep disturbance in patients with lichen simplex chronicus and its relationship to nocturnal scratching: A case control study. South Med J 2006;99(5):482–5.

Kranke B, Trummer M, Brabek E, et al. Etiologic and causative factors in perianal dermatitis: Results of a prospective study in 126 patients. Wien Klin Wochenschr 2006;118(3–4):90–4.

Lynch PJ. Lichen simplex chronicus (atopic/neurodermatitis) of the anogenital region. Dermatol Ther 2004;17(1):8–19.

Margesson LJ. Contact dermatitis of the vulva. Dermatol Ther 2004;17 (1):20–7.

Mentes BB, Akin M, Leventoglu S, et al. Intradermal methylene blue injection for the treatment of intractable idiopathic pruritus ani: Results of 30 cases. Tech Coloproctol 2004;8(1):11–4.

Weichert GE. An approach to the treatment of anogenital pruritus. Dermatol Ther 2004;17(1):129–33.

Weisshaar E. Successful treatment of genital pruritus using topical immunomodulators as a single therapy in multi-morbid patients. Acta Derm Venereol 2008;88(2):195–6.

Urticaria and Angioedema

Method of
Joyce M.C. Teng, MD, PhD

Urticaria, or hives, is a common cutaneous eruption that occurs in up to 25% of the general population sometime during their lives.[1] It is characterized by transient, circumscribed, pruritic, erythematous papules or plaques, often with central pallor. Individual lesions often coalesce into large wheals on the trunk and extremities that may resolve over a few hours without leaving any residual skin changes. The process is mediated by mast cells in the superficial dermis.

Angioedema is a similar process occurring in deep dermis or subcutaneous tissue. Angioedema may occur independently, accompanied by urticaria, or as a component of anaphylaxis. It is characterized by localized swelling that develops over minutes to hours and resolves within 24 to 48 hours. Common locations of angioedema include the mucosa and areas with loose connective tissue, such as the face, eyes, lips, tongue, and genitalia. Patients usually do not have pruritus, but they may have pain and a sensation of warmth. Angioedema is usually a benign process that resolves without sequelae unless it involves the larynx. African Americans are disproportionately affected, representing up to 40% of the hospital admissions for angioedema.[2]

Classification

Urticaria can be classified as acute or chronic, depending on the duration. Acute urticaria usually lasts for less than 6 weeks and is commonly triggered by infection, medication, insect bite, and food (Table 1). The chronic form, lasting more than 6 weeks, accounts for approximately 30% of cases of urticaria, and no clear causes can be identified in more than 80% of these cases. A significant number of patients with chronic urticaria may have persistent symptoms for more than 10 years.[3] Approximately 40% of patients with chronic urticaria have associated angioedema, although the incidence of laryngeal edema is low.

[1]Not FDA approved for this indication.
[2]Not available in the United States.
[3]Exceeds dosage recommended by the manufacturer.

TABLE 1 Mechanisms in Urticaria and Angioedema

Disorder	Causes
Immunoglobulin-mediated urticaria	Ig-E mediated: food, medication, insect bites, contact allergen, aeroallergens, other causes
	Urticaria associated with autoimmunity: antinuclear antibodies (ANAs), thyroid autoantibodies, other causes
Direct activation of mast cell degranulation	Physical stimuli: exercise, heat, cold, pressure, aquagenic, solar radiation, etc.
	Other agents: opiates, antibiotics (e.g., vancomycin [Vancocin]), radiocontrast, ACTH (Cortrosyn), muscle relaxants
Complement-mediated	Viral infections, parasites, blood transfusion
C1 inhibitor deficiency	Genetic and acquired angioedema, paraproteinemia
Reduced kinin metabolism	Angiotensin-converting enzyme (ACE) inhibitors
Reduced arachidonic acid metabolism	Aspirin

CURRENT DIAGNOSIS

- Acute and chronic urticaria have the same features, including erythematous, edematous papules or wheals with central pallor that last less than 24 to 48 hours.
- Laboratory assessments are not recommended for acute urticaria in the absence of evidence suggesting underlying systemic illness.
- Limited laboratory studies are indicated for chronic urticaria.
- Serum measurements of C4 and C1 are the recommended initial tests if hereditary or acquired angioedema are suspected.
- Skin biopsy should be considered to rule out urticarial vasculitis if an individual lesion is painful and persists for more than 2 to 3 days with accompanying ecchymosis or petechiae.

Diagnosis

Urticaria is diagnosed clinically in most cases. A detailed history, physical examination, and complete review of systems are essential for diagnosing patients with urticaria and angioedema. The history should include the distribution and characteristics of lesions (e.g., pain, pruritus), duration of skin eruption, accompanying angioedema, airway involvement and other associated systemic symptoms (e.g., fever, arthralgia, swelling joints, refusal to walk by children). Patients should also be questioned about changes in dietary habits, recent exposures, infection, and newly administered medications, including antibiotics, over-the-counter analgesia, and hormones.

Laboratory assessment is usually not helpful in diagnosing patients with acute urticaria who lack any history or clinical findings to suggest an underlying disease process. A limited number of diagnostic tests are indicated in the evaluation of patients with chronic urticaria, such as a complete blood cell count with differential white blood cell count, an erythrocyte sedimentation rate (ESR) or C-reactive protein (CRP) determination, a thyroid-stimulating hormone (TSH) level, antithyroglobulin and antimicrosomal antibodies, antinuclear antibodies (ANA), and hepatitis B and C serologies. A detailed review of systems may help to narrow the focus of the screening test.

CURRENT THERAPY

- Primary treatment of urticaria and angioedema is removal of triggering factors and initiation of therapy for symptomatic relief.
- Oral antihistamines are the cornerstones of therapy. The application of first-generation H_1-antihistamines may be limited by central nervous system and anticholinergic side effects.
- Nonsedating second-generation antihistamines are often used in combination and can be as effective as first-generation agents.
- Systemic corticosteroids and immunosuppressive therapy, especially cyclosporine (Neoral),[1] have been used successfully in cases that are refractory to the maximum dose of antihistamines.
- Fresh-frozen plasma infusions along with standard airway precautions have been recommended for angioedema patients with laryngeal edema.

[1]Not FDA approved for this indication.

A skin biopsy of an early lesion should be performed to rule out urticarial vasculitis if the affected individual has skin lesions that are painful and last for more than 2 to 3 days with residual ecchymosis or petechiae. In patients with angioedema, prominent edema of the interstitial tissue may be demonstrated by biopsy. Serum measurements of C4 and C1 are recommended initial tests if hereditary or acquired angioedema is suspected. A C1q level should be obtained to screen for the acquired form of angioedema if the affected individual is middle-aged.[3]

Treatment

More than two thirds of cases of urticaria are self-limited. Spontaneous remission of chronic urticaria and angioedema is also common. The primary objective of management is to identify and discontinue the offending trigger. A patient presenting with angioedema must first be assessed for signs of airway compromise. Medical therapy is indicated for those who are symptomatic.

Antihistamines remain the first-line therapy for most patients with urticaria, because the primary complaint of pruritus is predominantly mediated by histamine released from mast cells.[5,6] First-generation antihistamines such as hydroxyzine (Atarax or Vistaril 25 to 50 mg every 6 hours), diphenhydramine (Benadryl 25 to 50 mg every 6 hours), cyproheptadine (Periactin 4 mg three times daily), and chlorpheniramine (Chlor-Trimeton 4 mg every 6 hours) are potent and have the quickest onset of action. However, the treatments are often limited by their sedating and anticholinergic side effects. Many first-generation antihistamines are available over the counter, providing accessible first-line therapy for patients. Patients with urticaria that lasts for several days should be considered for treatment using second-generation antihistamines such as loratadine (Claritin[1] 10 mg twice daily[3]), desloratadine (Clarinex 5 mg twice daily[3]), cetirizine (Zyrtec 10 mg twice daily[3]), levocetirizine (Xyzal 5 mg daily), and fexofenadine (Allegra 180 mg twice daily[3]). Doxepin (Sinequan),[1] an H_1- and H_2-receptor antagonist, is seven times more potent than hydroxyzine in suppression of wheal and flare responses. Because of its central nervous system side effects, combined use of doxepin with a first-generation antihistamine should be restricted. Topical 5% doxepin cream (Zonalon)[1] may help to suppress pruritus in patients with localized urticaria.

[1]Not FDA approved for this indication.
[3]Exceeds dosage recommended by the manufacturer.
[5]Investigational drug in the United States.
[6]May be compounded by pharmacists.

Systemic prednisone at 30 to 40 mg in a single morning dose is sufficient to suppress urticaria in adults. Tapering should be gradual over a 3- to 4-week period by decreasing the dosage 5 mg every 3 to 5 days to minimize rebound. Alternate-morning dosing when reaching 20 mg daily may help to minimize the steroid side effects. Methylprednisolone (Solu-Medrol 40 mg) should be given intravenously as initial therapy to patients with angioedema. This may be followed by a tapering oral course. Three months of treatment with cyclosporine (Neoral)[1] at 3 to 5 mg/kg can be given safely to patients who are refractory to corticosteroid therapy or have difficulty tapering their therapy. Close monitoring for hypertension and renal insufficiency is necessary during the treatment.

Leukotriene inhibitors such as zileuton (Zyflo[1] 600 mg four times daily), zafirlukast (Accolate[1] 20 mg twice daily), and montelukast (Singulair[1] 10 mg once daily) may be effective for patients with autoimmune urticaria. Successful treatment of chronic urticaria with anti-IgE (omalizumab [Xolair][1]) has been reported but is not yet approved by the FDA.

Proper management of underlying autoimmune thyroid disease or autoimmune collagen vascular diseases has been beneficial for patients with associated urticaria. Life-threatening angioedema triggered by angiotensin-converting enzyme (ACE) inhibitors has been successfully treated with infusion of fresh-frozen plasma. Treatments with warfarin (Coumadin),[1] plasmapheresis, and intravenous immunoglobulin (Baygam)[1] have been reported for severe, refractory[1] urticaria. These treatments are administered only by specialists on an individual basis.

[1]Not FDA approved for this indication.

REFERENCES

Bailey E, Shaker M. An update on childhood urticaria and angioedema. Curr Opin Pediatr 2008;20(4):425–30.

Champion RH, Roberts SO, Carpenter RG, Roger JH. Urticaria and angioedema. A review of 554 patients. Br J Dermatol 1969;81(8):588–97.

Joint Task Force on Practice Parameters. The diagnosis and management of urticaria: A practice parameter. Part II. Chronic urticaria/angioedema. Ann Allergy Asthma Immunol 2000;85(2):521–44.

Kaplan AP, Joseph K, Maykut RJ, et al. Treatment of chronic autoimmune urticaria with omalizumab. J Allergy Clin Immunol 2008;122(3):569–73.

Lin RY, Cannon AG, Teitel AD. Pattern of hospitalizations for angioedema in New York between 1990 and 2003. Ann Allergy Asthma Immunol 2005;95 (2):159–66.

Nizami RM, Baboo MT. Office management of patients with urticaria: An analysis of 215 patients. Ann Allergy 1974;33(2):78–85.

Powell RJ, Du Toit GL, Siddique N, et al. BSACI guidelines for the management of chronic urticaria and angio-oedema. Clin Exp Allergy 2007;37 (5):631–50.

Pigmentary Disorders

Method of
Rebat M. Halder, MD, and Ahmad Reza Hossani-Madani, MD

Definition

The word *chromophore* is defined as elements that impart color to the skin. Hyperchromias describe abnormally darker skin, and hypochromias describe abnormally lighter skin. Pigmentation refers to melanotic causes of skin color change, differentiating it from skin color changes due to blood, carotene, bilirubin, or other causes. Hyperpigmentation refers to an increase in melanin production, melanocyte number, or both in the skin. Hypopigmentation refers to decrease of melanin, melanocytes, or both in the skin. Depigmentation refers to the absence of both melanin and melanocytes. Deposition of melanin in the epidermal layers visibly appears as a yellow to brownish hue. Dermal deposition appears as blue or blue-gray, with mixed epidermal and dermal melanin deposition appearing gray or blue-brown.

Evaluation

A thorough history and visual inspection of the pigmentary disorder can provide useful clues to the diagnosis, particularly recognition of pigmentary patterns (diffuse, circumscribed, linear, or reticulated). Further examination may be achieved by using the Wood's lamp to differentiate epidermal from dermal melanin.

General Recommendations for All Pigmentary Disorders

Broad-spectrum sunscreen with an SPF of 30 is recommended, in addition to wearing protective clothing. Avoiding prolonged sun exposure is also desired, if possible.

Hyperpigmentation

EPHELIDES

Description

Ephelides (freckles) are multiple, small (1-4 mm), light to dark brown macules with poorly defined margins that occur on sun-exposed areas of the body (face, upper back, arms). They are more commonly found in children (fading with age), fair-skinned persons,

CURRENT DIAGNOSIS

Hyperpigmentation

- Ephelides: Multiple, small (1-4 mm), light to dark brown macules with poorly defined margins that occur on sun-exposed areas of the body
- Solar lentigines: Light brown to black macular hyperpigmented lesions that are induced by natural or artificial sources of radiation and that can coalesce; they are located on face, neck, forearms, and hands
- Melasma: Arcuate or polycyclic brown to blue macules that coalesce into patches on face, neck, or forearms
- Postinflammatory hyperpigmentation: Dark patches or macules with indistinct margins at the location of an inciting inflammatory event

Hypopigmentation

- Pityriasis alba: 2 to 3 round, well-defined, paler macules with overlying powdery white scales, ranging in size from 0.5 to 5 cm in diameter, that transition to smooth, hypopigmented macules
- Vitiligo: Sharply demarcated, depigmented, milky white macules in a localized or generalized distribution
- Idiopathic guttate hypomelanosis: Multiple circular, smooth, small macules that have are porcelain white, with occasional black dots, found on sun-exposed areas of upper and lower extremities
- Postinflammatory hypopigmentation: Off-white or tan macules, with ill-defined borders at the site of an inciting inflammatory event

and those with red or blonde hair (especially those of Celtic ancestry). A relationship has been shown between painful sunburns in youth and development of ephelides, and the macules become darker with greater UV exposure. They are thought to be genetic in origin, following an autosomal dominant pattern, and are strongly associated with variants in the melanocortin-1-receptor (MC1R). Ephelides are significant because they are associated with an increased risk of melanoma and nonmelanoma skin cancer, perhaps serving as a marker for sun susceptibility.

Treatment

Although treatment is not necessary, modalities include either hydroquinone 4% (Claripel, Eldopaque Forte) or glycolic plus kojic acid combination (Brown Spot Night Gel) plus maximum ultraviolet A (UVA)-blocking sunscreen in the morning and tretinoin 0.1% cream (Retin-A)[1] in the evening. Other therapies have included cryotherapy, lasers, and chemical peels.

SOLAR LENTIGO (LENTIGO SENILIS ET ACTINICUS)

Description

Solar lentigines are pigmented spots that share morphologic similarities with ephelides, making differentiation difficult. They are defined as light brown to black macular hyperpigmented lesions induced by natural or artificial sources of radiation, which can coalesce. The incidence increases with age, and more than 90% of white persons older than 50 years demonstrate lesions. They appear most often on the face, neck, forearms, and hands. They can occur on nonclassic locations in those receiving phototherapy (such as the penis). Histologically, they differ from ephelides by the presence of epidermal hyperplasia, increased melanocyte number, and elongation of the rete ridges.

Treatment

Although treatment is not necessary, two different modalities have been used: physical therapies and topical therapies. Physical therapies include cryotherapy and lasers, and topical treatments include retinoids or combinations of agents. Liquid nitrogen may be used with a cotton swab for 5 to 10 seconds to induce lightening. Recurrence rates may be as high as 55% at 6 months. Side effects include atrophy with longer cryoprobe application, postinflammatory hyper- or hypopigmentation, and pain. The Q-switched Nd:YAG (532 nm), among others, has been used with success. An effective topical treatment includes hydroxyanisole (mequinol) 2% plus tretinoin 0.01% (Solage) applied twice daily. Side effects include erythema and burning or stinging.

MELASMA

Description

Melasma is a hypermelanosis of the face, neck, and forearms that occurs with a higher incidence in women of African American, Latin American, and Asian descent. It appears on sun-exposed areas as arcuate or polycyclic macules that coalesce into patches. Epidermal melanin deposition causes a brownish appearance, and dermal melanin appears bluish. Combined epidermal and dermal melanin deposition appears gray. It is distributed in a central facial (65%), malar (20%), or mandibular (15%) pattern. It is more commonly seen in women and those with darker skin, but it can also be found in men. Contributing factors include a genetic predisposition, pregnancy, oral contraceptive use, endocrine dysfunction, hormonal treatment, UV light exposure, cosmetics, and phototoxic drugs.

Treatment

First-line treatment for melasma consists of broad-spectrum sunscreen with greater than SPF 30 coverage in addition to monotherapy with hydroquinone 4% twice daily or tretinoin 0.1%[1] once daily. If that fails, triple therapy may be attempted, with fluocinolone

---

[1] Not FDA approved for this indication.

acetonide 0.01%, hydroquinone 4%, and tretinoin 0.05% (Tri-Luma) once daily being effective. Side effects of triple therapy include erythema, desquamation, burning, dryness, and pruritus at the site of application; telangiectasia; perioral dermatitis; acne breakouts; and hyperpigmentation. Chemical peels, superficial and medium depth, and erbium:YAG laser may also be used for patients whose topical treatments have failed.

POSTINFLAMMATORY HYPERPIGMENTATION

Description

Postinflammatory hyperpigmentation is a very common condition that occurs as a result of a previous or ongoing inflammatory process, most commonly acne vulgaris, atopic dermatitis, infections, and phototoxic reactions and as a result of treatment with topical medications, chemical peels, and lasers. Postinflammatory hyperpigmentation occurs more commonly in persons with darker skin pigmentation and appears as dark patches or macules with indistinct margins at the location of the inciting inflammatory event.

Treatment

Primary treatment is aimed at treating the inciting cause of the hyperpigmentation. Additional effective therapies include 4% hydroquinone alone or in combination with a topical steroid. Other combination treatments include mequinol 2% plus tretinoin 0.01% combination[1] twice daily or fluocinolone acetonide 0.01%, hydroquinone 4%, tretinoin 0.05%[1] once daily. Treatment must be temporarily stopped if irritation occurs. Broad-spectrum sunscreen should also be employed.

Hypopigmenation or Depigmentation

PITYRIASIS ALBA

Description

Pityriasis alba is a childhood or adolescent condition that affects all races. It begins as an erythematous macule with ill-defined borders. The erythema fades after a few weeks, leaving two or three round, well-defined, paler macules with overlying powdery white scale, ranging in size from 0.5 cm to 5 cm in diameter. These eventually transition to smooth, hypopigmented lesions, which are generally located on the face. The pathogenesis of this disorder is unknown.

Treatment

Pityriasis alba is thought to be a self-limited skin disease. However, general treatment guidelines include use of emollients and lubricant, use of sunscreen, and decreasing sun exposure. Lesions limited to the face may be treated with hydrocortisone 1% (Lanacort 10 Crème)[1] or other mild, nonfluorinated steroid. More-potent steroids may be used for lesions on the body, including hydrocortisone valerate 0.2% (Westcort)[1] or alclometasone dipropionate 0.05% (Aclovate).[1] However, these can lead to atrophy if used over an extended period. Newer, safer, effective alternatives include tacrolimus 0.1% ointment (Protopic)[1] twice daily. Side effects include a burning sensation that fades over time. Extensive disease that is not amenable to topical therapy might benefit from photochemotherapy (psoralen plus UVA [PUVA] or UVB alone).

VITILIGO

Description

Persons with vitiligo acquire sharply demarcated, depigmented macules in a localized or generalized distribution. These macules appear milky white as compared with the surrounding normally pigmented skin. Lesions can increase with size. There is no predilection for race or sex, and three quarters of patients generally present before the age of 30 years.

Treatment

General recommendations include the use of sunscreen, avoidance of the sun, and use of protective clothing. Treatments for localized vitiligo (<20% of body surface area) include cosmetics, a 2-month trial of topical treatment (potent or very potent corticosteroid or calcineurin inhibitor), excimer laser, or topical PUVA. Adults who have failed treatments for localized vitiligo may be considered for narrow-band UVB, oral PUVA, or surgical treatment, which includes split-skin grafting, transfer of suction blisters, or autologous epidermal suspensions added to dermabraded skin (followed by UVB). Surgical candidates should not demonstrate lesion enlargement or Koebner phenomenon for the past 12 months. Patients with more than 20% body involvement may be considered for narrow-band UVB (311 nm) or oral PUVA. Those with greater than 50% body involvement or disfiguring facial involvement may be considered for complete depigmentation with monobenzyl ether of hydroquinone (Benoquin 20%), 4-methoxyphenol, or the Q-switched ruby laser (694 nm). Children are generally not offered surgical treatment, and oral PUVA is relatively contraindicated in children younger than 10 years.

 CURRENT THERAPY

Hyperpigmentation

- Ephelides: Hydroquinone 4% (Claripel) or glycolic plus kojic acid combination (Brown Spot Night Gel) plus maximum UVA-blocking sunscreen in the morning and tretinoin 0.1% cream (Retin-A)[1] in the evening
- Solar lentigines: Hydroxyanisole (mequinol) 2% plus tretinoin 0.01% (Solage) applied twice daily; cryotherapy; laser therapy
- Melasma: Monotherapy with hydroquinone 4% twice daily or tretinoin 0.1%[1] once daily; double therapy; triple therapy with fluocinolone acetonide 0.01% plus hydroquinone 4% plus tretinoin 0.05% (Tri-Luma) once daily
- Postinflammatory hyperpigmentation: Treat inciting event; hydroquinone 4% alone or in combination with topical steroid; mequinol 2% plus tretinoin 0.01% combination[1] twice daily; fluocinolone acetonide 0.01% plus hydroquinone 4% plus tretinoin 0.05% combination[1] once daily

Hypopigmentation

- Pityriasis alba: Emollients, lubricants, sunscreen; tacrolimus 0.1% ointment (Protopic)[1] twice daily or mild nonhalogenated steroid for face and medium potency steroid for body; phototherapy (PUVA or UVB) for extensive disease
- Vitiligo: In patients with less than 20% body surface area (BSA) involvement, treat with cosmetics, topical (potent or very potent steroid or calcineurin inhibitor trial for less than 2 months), topical PUVA, or excimer laser. If local treatment fails, the surgical approach may be tried if the patient meets criteria or those with more than 20% BSA involvement. For patients with more than 20% BSA involvement, UVB is preferred over oral PUVA. For patients with more than 50% BSA or disfiguring facial involvement, treat with monobenzyl ether of hydroquinone (Benoquin 20%), 4-methoxyphenol or Q-switched ruby laser (694 nm).
- Idiopathic guttate hypomelanosis: Cryotherapy; dermabrasion; surgical minigrafting; intralesional steroids
- Postinflammatory hypopigmentation: Cosmetics; topical corticosteroids; topical PUVA

---

[1]Not FDA approved for this indication.

[1]Not FDA approved for this indication.

IDIOPATHIC GUTTATE HYPOMELANOSIS

Description

This is an acquired, asymptomatic leukoderma with multiple, circular, smooth, small macules that have a porcelain white color. Black dots are occasionally observed within the macules. They increase in number with age, but they generally do not increase in size. They are most commonly located on sun-exposed areas of the upper and lower extremities.

Treatment

Treatments have included cryotherapy, dermabrasion, surgical minigrafting, and intralesional steroids; however, none of these have shown consistent acceptable results. Phototherapy has not been shown to be effective.

POSTINFLAMMATORY HYPOPIGMENTATION

Description

Postinflammatory hypopigmentation is the result of an inciting inflammatory event leading to lesions that are off-white or tan, with ill-defined borders. This entity is noticed more commonly in those with darker skin.

Treatment

Hypopigmentation resolves with treatment of the underlying condition. Topical cosmetics may be useful. Topical corticosteroids may also be used in patients who have lesions in cosmetically distressing areas, as well as topical PUVA therapy.

REFERENCES

Cestari T, Arellano I, Hexsel D, Ortonne JP. Melasma in Latin America: Option for therapy and treatment algorithm. J Eur Acad Dermatol Venereol 2009;23:760–72.

Gupta AK, Gover MD, Nouri K, Taylor S. The treatment of melasma: A review of clinical trials. J Am Acad Dermatol 2006;55:1048–65.

Halder RM, Richards GM. Management of dyschromias in ethnic skin. Dermatol Ther 2004;17:151–7.

Halder RM, Richards GM. Topical agents used in the management of hyperpigmentation. Skin Therapy Lett 2004;9:1–3.

Hexsel DM. Treatment of idiopathic guttate hypomelanosis by localized superficial dermabrasion. Dermatol Surg 1999;25:917–8.

Lin RL, Janniger CK. Pityriasis alba. Cutis 2005;76:21–4.

Nordlund JJ, Boissy RE, Hearing VJ, et al., editors. The Pigmentary System: Physiology and Pathophysiology. 2nd ed. Malden, Mass: Blackwell Publishing; 2007.

Nordlund JJ, Cestari TF, Chan F, Westerhof W. Confusions about color: A classification of discolorations of the skin. Br J Dermatol 2007;156(Suppl. 1):S3–6.

Ortonne JP, Pandya AG, Lui H, Hexsel D. Treatment of solar lentigines. J Am Acad Dermatol 2006;54:S262–71.

Ploysangam T, Dee-Ananlap S, Suvanprakorn P. Treatment of idiopathic guttate hypomelanosis with iquid nitrogen: Light and electron microscopic studies. J Am Acad Dermatol 1990;23:681–4.

Rigopoulos D, Gregoriou S, Charissi C, et al. Tacrolimus ointment 0.1% in pityriasis alba: An open-label randomized, placebo-controlled study. Br J Dermatol 2006;155:152–5.

Taylor SC, Burgess CM, Callender VD, et al. Postinflammatory hyperpigmentation: evolving combination treatment strategies. Cutis 2006;78:S6–19.

Sunburn

Method of
Warwick L. Morison, MD

Sunburn is a common problem, particularly in fair-skinned white persons, caused by excessive exposure to ultraviolet (UV) radiation from sunlight or artificial sources such as sunlamps. When induced by sunlight, it is mainly due to UVB (280–320 nm) radiation plus a smaller contribution from UVA (320–400 nm) radiation. Sunburn is also described as erythema and it appears 3 to 4 hours after exposure, reaches a maximum at 12 to 18 hours, and usually settles after 72 to 96 hours. In severe reactions with blistering, complete resolution can take a week or more.

Sunburns are graded as pink, red, and blistering. In contrast, thermal burns are graded by degree (first, second, and third), but this classification should not be applied to sunburns because thermal burns have quite different sequelae, such as scarring and death, which are extremely rare consequences of a sunburn. Keratoconjunctivitis, or ocular sunburn, can also be caused by UV radiation and it follows a similar time course.

There are two facets to management of sunburn: prevention and treatment. Because there is no effective treatment for an established sunburn, most emphasis should be placed on prevention.

Prevention

Skin color and the capacity of a person to tan will determine how important it is for an individual person to take preventive measures. However, even dark-skinned people can sunburn provided the exposure dose is sufficiently high. Skin color, past history of sunburn, and likely exposure should therefore be used as a guide in advising people about protection. Protection from sunlight is often equated with use of sunscreens, but this approach is too narrow, and protection should consist of a package of measures: avoiding overexposure to sunlight, using sunscreens, and wearing protective clothing.

AVOIDANCE OF EXPOSURE

Simple avoidance of excessive exposure to a threshold dose of UV radiation is often the best advice for fair-skinned people. Scheduling outdoor activities for before 10 AM and after 4 PM will avoid the peak UV irradiance period and still permit enjoyment of the outdoors. This advice should be accompanied by several warnings. Sitting in the shade or under a beach umbrella only reduces exposure by about 70%. A cloudy day is often the setting for the worst sunburns because even complete white cloud cover reduces UV exposure by only about 50%.

Clothing is not always an effective protector. If it is possible to see through a fabric, UV radiation can also penetrate to a significant extent. The geographic location of exposure must also be considered because UV radiation may be twice as intense at the equator as compared with much of continental North America.

CURRENT DIAGNOSIS

- Sunburn appears 3 to 4 hours after exposure to sunlight or an artificial source of UV radiation such as a sunlamp.
- The redness of skin is diffuse and continuous, unlike rashes, which are often discontinuous.
- Sunburns are graded as pink, red, and blistering.

SUNSCREENS

There is now a great number of sunscreens on the market, and they contain numerous active ingredients. If this is not enough to cause confusion, some are not even labeled as sunscreens: sunblocks and tanning lotions are other terms. However, the informed physician need only know four properties of a sunscreen: the sun protection factor (SPF), the spectrum of protection, the base, and whether or not it is water resistant.

The SPF is a index of the amount of protection provided by the sunscreen. For example, a fair-skinned person who normally begins to sunburn after a 10-minute exposure to sunlight should be able to tolerate up to 150 minutes of exposure after application of an SPF 15 sunscreen.

There are several provisos for this statement. To provide the stated protection, a sunscreen must be applied 10 minutes before exposure to allow binding to skin proteins to occur, and it must be applied in an adequate amount. Several studies have shown that under ideal circumstances in which sunscreen is supplied freely and the subject is observed while making the application, most people only use one half the required amount. Ordinary use probably provides much less protection. As a rough guide, one ounce of sunscreen is necessary to cover a 70-kg adult in a bathing suit; in other words, a four ounce bottle of sunscreen only provides four applications.

Sunscreens vary in the amount of the solar spectrum for which they provide protection. All sunscreens provide protection against UVB radiation and the shorter end of UVA radiation. Some sunscreens claim to provide broad-spectrum protection against UVB and UVA radiation and contain avobenzone or titanium dioxide to protect against the longer wavelengths in the UVA spectrum. Ecamsule (Mexoryl SX), a recently approved sunscreen active, provides good absorption in the middle of the UVA spectrum so that a sunscreen containing this, avobenzone, and octocrylene, an absorber of UVB radiation, provides very good broad-spectrum protection.

The base of a sunscreen is also important because it often determines whether or not a sunscreen will be used. Men usually prefer alcohol-based lotions because they dry quickly and leave a dry and nongreasy film. Women usually prefer lotions or creams because they give a moisturizing feel to the skin.

Finally, a sunscreen may be labeled water resistant or very water resistant. Because almost all outdoor pastimes involve perspiring or contact with water, a very water-resistant sunscreen should be selected.

CURRENT THERAPY

- Prevention is the best approach to management and consists of a package of measures: avoiding overexposure, using sunscreens, and wearing protective clothing.
- Treatment of a sunburn consists of cool baths and use of moisturizing creams.
- Topical and systemic corticosteroids do not alter the course of a sunburn.

A fair-skinned person should always use a sunscreen with an SPF 15 or higher. People who tan well and never burn are probably adequately protected with an SPF of 8 to 10. People with black or brown skin probably do not need sunscreens except for extreme occupational or social exposure.

A few myths should be dismissed. There is no effective oral sunscreen. Many have been tested and all have failed. Self-tanning preparations are not sunscreens. They do provide the appearance of a tan and are safe to use but they provide no significant protection against UV radiation.

PROTECTIVE CLOTHING

There has been significant progress in recent years in the development, testing, and classification of UV-protective clothing. Akin to the SPF for sunscreens, such clothing is labeled with an ultraviolet protective factor (UPF), and a fabric with a UPF of 50 blocks transmission of 98% of UV radiation. A hat with a 3-inch brim all around completes the package of protection.

PROTECTIVE TANNING

The proliferation of suntan parlors has generated a lot of interest in protective tanning, with much misinformation provided by the commercial interests involved. Little scientific information is available to provide a guide as to whether protective tanning is of any value in preventing the long-term hazards of excessive exposure to sunlight, namely skin cancer and premature aging of the skin. Certainly, preventive tanning using multiple suberythemal doses of UV radiation can prevent sunburn, but the cost in terms of chronic damage is unknown.

Most tanning salons claim to use only UVA radiation in their tanning beds, but this claim is false. All so-called UVA tanning beds emit some UVB radiation, the most damaging wavelengths, and in addition, UVA radiation, especially in large doses can produce the same damaging effect as UVB radiation. Furthermore, a UVA-induced tan is not very protective and at most has an SPF of 6 to 8.

A person who tans well and never burns might gain some protection from sunlight by preventive tanning without incurring too much damage. However, the risk-to-benefit ratio for people who do sunburn is probably very unfavorable.

Treatment

When a person has a sunburn, general supportive measures are the only approach to treatment. Cold compresses and cool baths with bath oil provide some relief. Frequent application of moisturizing creams help alleviate dryness. Blistering of the skin can lead to secondary infection and require use of an antibiotic cream. Rarely, an extremely severe sunburn necessitates hospitalization and management as a thermal burn.

Topical corticosteroids reduce erythema by causing vasoconstriction, but this effect is temporary and does not reduce epidermal damage. Systemic corticosteroids, even in very large doses, do not alter the course of a sunburn. Nonsteroidal antiinflammatory drugs, if given at the time of exposure or beforehand, reduce the degree of erythema over the first 24 hours but do not change epidermal damage. Of course, few people lying on the beach anticipate an excessive exposure, so they are unlikely to embark on such preventive measures.

The Nervous System

Alzheimer's Disease

Method of
*Edmond Teng, MD, PhD, and
Mario F. Mendez, MD, PhD*

Dementia is an acquired impairment in cognitive abilities that results in significant functional decline. The most common dementing illness is Alzheimer's disease (AD), which accounts for 50% to 70% of demented patients. Globally, AD affects approximately 26.6 million people, and the annual worldwide societal costs of AD and other dementias are estimated to be $315.4 billion. The prevalence of AD is strongly associated with increasing age. The rapidly growing elderly populations in the United States and other industrialized countries suggest that AD may continue to consume a disproportionate share of health care resources and expenditures in the coming years.

Neuropathology

AD is a neurodegenerative disorder characterized by insidious onset and gradual progression. The underlying neuropathologic changes begin to develop many years before cognitive, behavioral, or functional deficits become clinically apparent and are typically quite advanced by the time a diagnosis is made.

The amyloid cascade hypothesis postulates that AD pathogenesis begins with the accumulation of β-amyloid (Aβ), which is derived from amyloid precursor protein (APP). β-Secretase and γ-secretase proteases sequentially cleave APP to produce neurotoxic $A\beta_{40}$ and $A\beta_{42}$ peptides, which subsequently aggregate into oligomers and fibrils that form extracellular amyloid plaques. These *senile plaques* are among the neuropathologic hallmarks of AD. Many experimental therapeutic agents for AD being evaluated in clinical trials target specific mechanisms along the Aβ pathway.

Although Aβ accumulation appears to be one of the earliest steps in the pathogenesis of AD, the extent of Aβ plaque deposition does not consistently correlate with clinical severity. These findings suggest that additional pathology precipitated by Aβ accumulation contributes to the progressive synaptic dysfunction, neuronal loss, and neurotransmitter deficits that produce the clinical symptoms of AD. These Aβ-induced pathologic changes include the hyperphosphorylation of tau protein to form intracellular neurofibrillary tangles (NFTs) and increased levels of inflammation, oxidative stress, and excitotoxicity.

Neuropathologic criteria for AD focus on plaque and NFT deposition, which is primarily seen in medial temporal lobe structures such as the entorhinal cortex and the hippocampus in the earliest stages of the disease. With disease progression, these changes extend to neighboring limbic structures, with later widespread deposition in other cortical regions. These microscopic changes are reflected by similar patterns of increasing regional brain atrophy.

Epidemiology

Epidemiologic studies have identified several genetic and environmental risk factors for AD. Increasing age is the strongest of these factors. Most patients are older than 60 years. By age 65, approximately 1% of the general population meets diagnostic criteria for AD. The prevalence roughly doubles with every 5 years thereafter, with estimates as high 35% to 40% for individuals older than 90 years.

A family history of AD is another major risk factor. Individuals with at least one first-degree relative diagnosed with AD are four times more likely to develop the disease themselves than people without a family history of AD. Genetic studies indicate that much of this increased risk may depend on apolipoprotein E (ApoE) genotype. Relative to the more common ApoE3 allele, the ApoE4 allele is associated in a copy-dependent fashion with a greater prevalence of AD and an earlier age of onset. Other variables associated with increased risk for AD include female gender, low levels of education, cardiovascular risk factors, and history of head trauma.

Clinical Presentation

The clinical presentation of AD is heterogeneous and related to disease severity. The primary symptoms fall into three categories: cognitive, behavioral, and functional. In mild cognitive impairment (which often represents incipient AD) or in mild AD, defined as a Mini-Mental Status Examination (MMSE) score >20, cognitive deficits are commonly seen in episodic memory, primarily for recall and recognition of recent events and other newly learned information, and in word-finding abilities. Behavioral abnormalities such as apathy, depression, and irritability start to emerge. In mild cognitive impairment, functional abilities remain essentially intact, but in mild AD, difficulties with employment and other complex instrumental activities of daily living (ADLs), such as finances and driving, begin to develop.

With moderate AD (MMSE score of 11–20), patients begin to experience increasing difficulty with remote memory, verbal communication, and getting around without getting lost. Agitation, aggression, and anxiety are frequently reported. They are no longer able to independently perform their instrumental ADLs, and they may need increasing assistance with some basic ADLs, such as dressing, bathing, and toileting.

With severe AD (MMSE score ≤10), patients have widespread deterioration in all cognitive domains, including near-mutism, which limits formal assessment. Agitation continues to worsen, and aberrant motor activity (i.e., pacing, restlessness, and wandering) becomes a major issue. They are no longer able to perform their basic ADLs and may develop urinary and fecal incontinence.

Diagnosis

The two most commonly used diagnostic criteria for AD, the *Diagnostic and Statistical Manual of Mental Disorders*, fourth edition (DSM-IV), and the National Institute of Neurological and Communicative Disorders and Stroke-Alzheimer's Disease and Related Disorders Association (NINCDS-ADRDA) criteria, share a common emphasis on gradual symptom onset and progression, impairments in memory and at least one additional cognitive domain, deficits in ADLs, and exclusion of delirium and other medical or psychiatric conditions as the primary cause of these deficits. Factors that make a diagnosis of AD less likely include sudden onset or the presence of focal neurologic or extrapyramidal signs, seizures, gait abnormality, and behavioral disturbances early in the disease course. The DSM-IV and NINCDS-ADRDA criteria exhibit accuracy ranging from 65% to 90% in clinicopathologic studies, but may be relatively insensitive to incipient AD. More recently proposed criteria focus on deficits in episodic memory supported by genetic, imaging, or cerebrospinal fluid biomarkers.

A diagnostic evaluation for AD should start with a comprehensive history, obtained from the patient and a knowledgeable informant, that focuses on the time course and progression of cognitive, behavioral, and functional symptoms; relevant medical history; and medication use. Mental status examination to confirm subjective cognitive deficits should be performed with instruments such as the MMSE, the Memory Impairment Screen, the Clock Drawing Test, or other brief screening tools. Patients with more subtle cognitive deficits or higher levels of premorbid functioning may perform well on these assessments and should be referred for formal neuropsychological testing if a clinical suspicion of cognitive impairment persists. Physical and neurologic examination results are typically normal aside from parkinsonism or frontal release signs that can be seen with more advanced disease.

Although there are no laboratory tests of sufficient accuracy to independently confirm a diagnosis of AD, several tests can rule out other conditions that can cause or contribute to the presenting symptoms: complete blood cell count, serum chemistries, glucose, thyroid function, vitamin B_{12}, rapid plasma reagin, and liver function. Structural neuroimaging by computed tomography (CT) or magnetic resonance imaging (MRI) can assess medial temporal lobe atrophy and rule out other potential etiologies. Additional assessments that are not routinely indicated but may be useful in more complicated cases include positron emission tomography (PET) to assess for glucose metabolism in temporal, parietal, and posterior cingulate regions; cerebrospinal fluid levels of $A\beta_{42}$ and tau; and genetic testing for early-onset autosomal dominant forms of AD. ApoE testing has no current diagnostic utility, but it may become more useful in the future; research is emerging that suggests genotype-specific responses to various therapeutic interventions.

Differential diagnosis for AD includes other common dementing conditions: vascular dementia (15% to 25% of dementia cases), dementia with Lewy bodies (10% to 20%), depression (5% to 10%), and frontotemporal lobar degeneration (5%). Vascular dementia can manifest with abrupt symptom onset, stepwise deterioration, focal neurologic signs or symptoms, multiple cardiovascular risk factors, and neuroimaging abnormalities consistent with cerebrovascular disease. Vascular dementia can be difficult to distinguish from AD because these conditions share similar risk factors and a significant proportion of vascular dementia cases exhibit comorbid AD pathology. The core features that distinguish dementia with Lewy bodies include spontaneous parkinsonism, visual hallucinations, and fluctuations in alertness and cognition. Severe depression can cause cognitive deficits in elderly patients, particularly on tasks that emphasize attention, information-processing speed, or effort. Depression-related dementia can resemble AD or vascular dementia because depressive symptoms are commonly seen in these conditions. Frontotemporal lobar degeneration results in prominent social, behavioral, and language impairment early in the course of the disease, and in most cases, manifests before age 65. Referral to a memory disorders specialist is appropriate if the patient exhibits atypical clinical features, rapid progression, or poor response to AD therapeutics.

CURRENT DIAGNOSIS

- Memory and other cognitive domains (e.g., language, visuospatial, executive, motor skills) are impaired.
- Declines are noticed in social or occupational function or in performance of usual activities of daily living.
- Symptoms are insidious in onset and exhibit a gradual and continuing progression.
- Symptoms do not occur solely in the context of a delirium syndrome.
- Symptoms are not better explained by other neurologic conditions (e.g., stroke, subdural hematoma, normal pressure hydrocephalus, brain tumor, traumatic brain injury, other neurodegenerative conditions); other systemic medical conditions (e.g., vitamin B_{12} deficiency, hypothyroidism, neurosyphilis, human immunodeficiency virus infection, sleep apnea, medication effects); or other psychiatric disorders (e.g., depression, bipolar disorder, schizophrenia, substance abuse).
- Factors suggesting other causes include sudden onset or prominent early neurologic signs, seizures, gait abnormality, and behavioral disturbances.
- Diagnosis may be supported by findings from structural neuroimaging (i.e., medial temporal lobe atrophy on MRI or CT); functional neuroimaging (i.e., reduced glucose metabolism in temporal, parietal, or posterior cingulate regions on PET); and cerebrospinal fluid biomarkers (i.e., decreased $A\beta_{42}$ and increased total and phosphorylated tau).

Treatment

At preclinical and clinical stages of drug development, investigators are assessing a plethora of pharmacologic interventions that target key steps in the pathophysiology of AD, including $A\beta$ and tau synthesis, aggregation, and deposition into plaques and NFTs. Although these strategies have shown much potential in animal and in vitro models of AD, several putative disease-modifying agents have produced disappointing results in phase III clinical trials.

Four FDA-approved medications are available for the treatment of AD (Table 1). Three are cholinesterase inhibitors (ChE-I): donepezil (Aricept), galantamine (Razadyne), and rivastigmine (Exelon). The fourth, memantine (Namenda), is an *N*-methyl-D-aspartate (NMDA) receptor antagonist. These medications demonstrate modest effects on slowing the progress of cognitive, behavioral, and functional symptoms of AD, but they do not appear to reverse or arrest the underlying neurodegenerative processes associated with the disease.

ChE-I therapy addresses the relative depletion of acetylcholine (ACh) levels in AD brains by preventing its metabolism and potentiating ACh-related neurotransmission. The utility of ChE-I therapy appears to be most robust in mild to moderate AD, although there appears to be some benefit with donepezil (Aricept) among subjects with incipient or severe AD. Although the ChE-Is that are available have slightly different enzymatic specificities, their overall efficacy appears to be similar. Treatment responses appear to be dose related, and dosing should be gradually titrated up every 4 weeks to the maximum recommended dosages or until limited by side effects. Recently, the maximum recommended dose of donepezil was increased from 10 mg to 23 mg daily, which may provide additional efficacy in moderate to severe AD, but is also is associated with a higher frequency of side effects. ChE-Is are reasonably well tolerated, and side effects are typically transient and dose dependent. The most common adverse reactions are gastrointestinal, such as nausea, vomiting, and anorexia. Other frequently encountered side effects include dizziness, bradycardia, insomnia, and vivid dreams. The use

TABLE 1 First-Line Pharmacologic Treatments for Alzheimer's Disease

Feature	Donepezil (Aricept)	Rivastigmine (Exelon)	Galantamine (Razadyne*)	Memantine (Namenda)
Mechanisms	AChE-I	AChE-I BuChE-I	AChE-I Nicotinic receptor modulator	NMDA receptor antagonist
Disease severity	Mild to moderate	Mild to moderate	Mild to moderate	Moderate to severe
Initial dose	5 mg daily	1.5 mg bid (oral) 4.6 mg daily (patch)	4 mg bid (standard) 8 mg daily (ER)	5 mg daily
Maximum dose	23 mg daily	6 mg bid (oral); 9.5 mg daily (patch)	12 mg bid (standard) 24 mg daily (ER)	10 mg bid
Plasma $t_{1/2}$	70 h	1.5 h	7 h	70 h
Common side effects	Nausea, vomiting, anorexia, diarrhea, bradycardia, syncope, insomnia, vivid dreams	Nausea, vomiting, anorexia, diarrhea, bradycardia, syncope, insomnia, vivid dreams	Nausea, vomiting, anorexia, diarrhea, bradycardia, syncope, insomnia, vivid dreams	Dizziness, headache, confusion, constipation
Significant drug-drug interactions	Bethanechol (Urecholine), ketoconazole (Nizoral), quinidine, succinylcholine (Anectine)	None	Amitriptyline (Elavil), fluoxetine (Prozac), fluvoxamine (Luvox), paroxetine (Paxil), ketoconazole, quinidine	Carbonic anhydrase inhibitors, cimetidine (Tagamet), ranitidine (Zantac), quinidine, hydrochlorothiazide (HCTZ), sodium bicarbonate

*Previously Reminyl.

Abbreviations: AChE-I = acetylcholinesterase inhibitor; BuChE-I = butyrylcholinesterase inhibitor; NMDA = *N*-methyl-D-aspartate; bid = twice daily; ER = extended release.

of once-daily oral or transdermal patch (Exelon Patch) formulations may minimize the incidence of these adverse effects. Oral formulations of galantamine or rivastigmine should be administered with food. Responses to ChE-Is are often idiosyncratic, and patients who report poor efficacy or tolerability on one medication may achieve better results when switched to another.

Memantine blocks NMDA receptor ion channels, but how this mechanism translates into clinical efficacy remains uncertain. Studies suggest that it is most effective for the treatment of moderate to severe AD, although weaker evidence also supports its use in mild AD. The starting dose is 5 mg daily, and it is typically titrated up by 5 mg per week to a final dose of 10 mg twice daily in patients with normal renal function and 5 mg twice daily for those with creatinine clearance rates less than 30 mL/min. Adverse events are less frequently reported with memantine than with the ChE-Is, and include dizziness, headache, confusion, and constipation. Memantine can be used as monotherapy, particularly in patients who cannot tolerate ChE-I therapy, but it may be more effective when administered in tandem with a ChE-I.

Earlier work indicated that high doses of vitamin E[1] (2000 IU/day) administered to patients with moderate AD significantly delayed progression to a composite end point of death, institutionalization, loss of basic ADLs, or severe AD. However, a later trial of this dosage of vitamin E in incipient AD showed no benefit, and a meta-analysis revealed that doses >400 IU/day result in an increase in all-cause mortality. The role of vitamin E in the treatment of AD therefore remains uncertain. Smaller studies of dietary supplements such as gingko biloba[1,7] and huperzine A[1,7] conducted in Europe and China demonstrate benefits similar to the ChE-Is, but larger studies in the United States have shown no benefit (gingko biloba) or are in progress (huperzine A). Likewise, other potential interventions such as coenzyme Q10,[1,7] selegiline (Eldepryl),[1] nonsteroidal antiinflammatory drugs (NSAIDs), statins, and hormone replacement therapy have yet to consistently demonstrate significant benefits in the treatment of AD and should not be routinely recommended for this purpose. The FDA has recently approved caprylidene (Axona), a prescription dietary supplement, for the treatment of mild to moderate AD, but currently there is relatively limited data supporting its efficacy.

Although cognitive complaints are the most common presenting symptoms of AD, behavioral symptoms are often the most problematic for caregivers, particularly with disease progression. Treatment with a ChE-I or memantine demonstrates modest reductions in many of the behavioral abnormalities associated with AD. However, adjunctive pharmacologic or nonpharmacologic therapy may be necessary. The wide spectrum of AD-related neuropsychiatric disturbances necessitates specific treatment strategies that are tailored to each patient's symptoms.

Nonpharmacologic approaches should be pursued before pharmacologic interventions. Although many such treatments have been proposed and investigated, most studies are not rigorously blinded or controlled, which limits the scope of evidence-based recommendations. Agitation and aggression may be most amenable to nonpharmacologic strategies, such as maintaining a consistent and predictable daily routine, providing frequent reassurance and reorientation to time and place, minimizing insufficient or excessive sensory and social stimulation, simplifying instructions and tasks, and distraction or redirection when such behaviors occur.

Adjunctive pharmacologic treatments that have demonstrated efficacy for treating behavioral disorders in AD include antipsychotics, anticonvulsants, anxiolytics, and antidepressants (Table 2). Studies investigating the use of these medications for AD-related psychopathology have not been uniformly supportive, and for some patients, the risks posed by their potential adverse effects may outweigh the expected therapeutic gains. To reduce risks associated with prolonged use of these psychotropic medications, treatments initiated for specific target symptoms should be administered at the lowest effective doses and discontinued on sustained symptom resolution.

Antipsychotics have demonstrated some utility for ameliorating agitation, aggression, psychosis, and insomnia. The most effective agents appear to be risperidone (Risperdal),[1] olanzapine (Zyprexa),[1] and to a lesser extent, quetiapine (Seroquel).[1] For acute agitation and aggression in patients who are unable or unwilling to take oral medications, intramuscular forms of olanzapine (Zyprexa IntraMuscular)[1] and haloperidol (Haldol)[1] are available. However, antipsychotic use in elderly dementia patients has been associated with a small increase in all-cause mortality. The FDA has issued a black-box warning highlighting this risk, and it emphasizes that the use of typical and atypical antipsychotics for behavioral symptoms in this population is not formally approved. Nevertheless, short-term use of these agents may be warranted in patients with behavioral

---

[1]Not FDA approved for this indication.
[7]Available as a dietary supplement.

---

[1]Not FDA approved for this indication.

TABLE 2 Adjunctive Pharmacologic Therapies for Behavioral Symptoms

Medication	Symptoms	Dose	Side Effects	Safety Issues
Antipsychotics				
Risperidone (Risperdal)[1]	Agitation, aggression, psychosis, insomnia	0.25–2 mg daily	Extrapyramidal symptoms, sedation, confusion, headache, weight gain	FDA black box warning for increased all-cause mortality when used in demented elderly patients
Olanzapine (Zyprexa)[1]	Agitation, aggression, psychosis, insomnia	2.5–10 mg daily (oral), 2.5–5 mg daily (IM)	Extrapyramidal symptoms, sedation, confusion, weight gain, psychosis	FDA black box warning for increased all-cause mortality when used in demented elderly patients
Quetiapine (Seroquel)[1]	Agitation, aggression, psychosis, insomnia	25–200 mg daily	Sedation, weight gain, dizziness, urinary symptoms	FDA black box warning for increased all-cause mortality when used in demented elderly patients
Haloperidol (Haldol)[1]	Agitation, aggression, psychosis, insomnia	0.25–1 mg daily (IM)	Hypotension, somnolence, extrapyramidal symptoms, tardive dyskinesia	FDA black box warning for increased all-cause mortality when used in demented elderly patients
Anticonvulsants				
Carbamazepine (Tegretol)[1]	Agitation, aggression	300–600 mg daily	Sedation, confusion, dizziness, ataxia, confusion, nausea, vomiting	Many drug-drug interactions
Anxiolytics				
Lorazepam (Ativan)	Anxiety, agitation,[1] aggression[1]	0.5–2 mg daily	Sedation, confusion, dizziness	Short-term use for acute symptoms only
Antidepressants				
Citalopram (Celexa)	Depression, anxiety,[1] irritability,[1] agitation,[1] aggression[1]	10–40 mg daily	Sedation, nausea, vomiting, dry mouth, diarrhea, sexual dysfunction	
Sertraline (Zoloft)	Depression, anxiety,[1] irritability,[1] agitation,[1] aggression[1]	25–150 mg daily	Sedation, insomnia, nausea, vomiting, dry mouth, dizziness, tremor, sexual dysfunction	Reduce dosing in patients with hepatic impairment
Mirtazapine (Remeron)	Depression, insomnia,[1] anorexia[1]	15–45 mg daily	Sedation, dizziness, headache, increased appetite, weight gain, edema	Rare agranulocytosis

[1]Not FDA approved for this indication.
Abbreviation: IM = intramuscular.

disturbances of appropriate severity that have not responded to other therapies and after a careful discussion of risks and benefits with the patient and the caregivers.

Alternatives to antipsychotics for the treatment of agitation and aggression include anticonvulsants and anxiolytics. Many studies indicate that the severity of these symptoms can be reduced with carbamazepine (Tegretol).[1] Factors that may limit the use of carbamazepine include the potential for side effects such as ataxia, dizziness, and sedation and drug-drug interactions caused by induction of hepatic enzymes. The efficacy of valproic acid (Depakene)[1] has been evaluated in other studies, but the results have been less encouraging. Anxiolytics, particularly benzodiazepines, may be indicated for short-term management of acute agitation and anxiety. However, prolonged use can be associated with tolerance, dependence, somnolence, and exacerbation of cognitive impairment.

Antidepressants also have a role in the management of a range of behavioral pathology in AD. Serotonin-specific reuptake inhibitors (SSRIs) such as citalopram (Celexa) or sertraline (Zoloft) significantly reduce mood symptoms such as depression, anxiety,[1] and irritability[1] with relatively few adverse effects or drug-drug interactions. Mirtazapine (Remeron), which blocks presynaptic α_2-adrenergic receptors and increases norepinephrine and serotonin release, is another attractive option, particularly because it exhibits antihistaminergic effects that can help address other common neuropsychiatric symptoms seen in AD, such as insomnia,[1] anorexia,[1] and weight loss.[1] Although its potential efficacy in this population is suggested by small preliminary studies, it has yet to be evaluated with more rigorous clinical trial methodologies. Treatment with citalopram has been associated with reductions in agitation[1] and aggression,[1] suggesting that the benefits of antidepressants in this population may extend beyond the treatment of mood disorders.

[1]Not FDA approved for this indication.

Community Support Services

Dedicated caregivers are an essential component for optimizing quality of life for AD patients. In particular, caregivers can encourage continued physical, mental, and social activities. Unfortunately, caregiver

CURRENT THERAPY

First-line pharmacologic treatments
- Cholinesterase inhibitors, including donepezil (Aricept), rivastigmine (Exelon), or galantamine (Razadyne [previously Reminyl]), which are primarily indicated for mild to moderate AD
- NMDA receptor antagonists, including memantine (Namenda), which are primarily indicated for moderate to severe AD; better efficacy when used in conjunction with a cholinesterase inhibitor

Adjunctive therapies for behavioral symptoms
- Nonpharmacologic interventions are used with emphasis on reorientation, reassurance, and redirection.
- Pharmacologic interventions include atypical antipsychotics for agitation, aggression, psychosis, or insomnia; anticonvulsants for agitation or aggression; anxiolytics for agitation, aggression, or anxiety; and antidepressants for depression, anxiety, or irritability.

Early referral to community organizations such as the Alzheimer's Association and Leeza's Place for additional caregiver support resources

stress and burnout often increases with disease severity. Early referral to community organizations such as the Alzheimer's Association (www.alz.org) or Leeza's Place (www.leezaplace.org) may help minimize caregiver distress and frustration and improve patient care and safety. These organizations frequently sponsor educational programs and support groups targeted toward caregivers of patients at various stages of the disease. Consultation is often available to assist with advance planning, such as establishing advance directives, durable power of attorney, and other legal considerations. As the disease progresses and patients become more difficult to manage, these organizations can provide referrals for additional support services, including adult day care programs, professional in-home caregivers, and assisted living or skilled nursing facilities.

REFERENCES

Buschke H, Kuslansky G, Katz M, et al. Screening for dementia with the memory impairment screen. Neurology 1999;52:231–8.

Cummings JL. Alzheimer's disease. N Engl J Med 2004;351:56–67.

Dubois B, Feldman HH, Jacova C, et al. Research criteria for the diagnosis of Alzheimer's disease: Revising the NINCDS-ADRDA criteria. Lancet Neurol 2007;6:734–46.

Farlow MR, Miller ML, Pejovic V. Treatment options in Alzheimer's disease: Maximizing benefit, managing expectations. Dement Geriatr Cogn Disord 2008;25:408–22.

Folstein MF, Folstein SE, McHugh PR. "Mini-mental state." A practical method for grading the cognitive state of patients for the clinician. J Psychiatr Res 1975;12:189–98.

Herrmann N, Lanctot KL. Pharmacologic management of neuropsychiatric symptoms of Alzheimer disease. Can J Psychiatry 2007;52:630–46.

Holsinger T, Deveau J, Boustani M, Williams Jr JW. Does this patient have dementia? JAMA 2007;297:2391–404.

McKhann G, Drachman D, Folstein M, et al. Clinical diagnosis of Alzheimer's disease: Report of the NINCDS-ADRDA Work Group under the auspices of Department of Health and Human Services Task Force on Alzheimer's Disease. Neurology 1984;34:939–44.

Sink KM, Holden KF, Yaffe K. Pharmacological treatment of neuropsychiatric symptoms of dementia: A review of the evidence. JAMA 2005;293:596–608.

US Food and Drug Administration. Information for healthcare professionals: Antipsychotics. Available at http://www.fda.gov/Drugs/DrugSafety/Postmarket DrugSafetyInformationforPatientsandProviders/DrugSafetyInformationfor HealthcareProfessionals/ucm084149.htm#note [accessed September 2009].

Sleep Disorders

Method of
Erik K. St. Louis, MD, and
Timothy I. Morgenthaler, MD

Sleep is a universal yet enigmatic biological imperative for all mammals. Experiments in rats have clearly demonstrated that total sleep deprivation, as well as selective deprivation of rapid eye movement (REM) and non-REM (NREM) sleep, can be fatal within 3 weeks. Insufficient sleep quantity in humans likewise appears to relate to a variety of health problems and to contribute to mortality. Adequate sleep quality is similarly necessary to ensure optimal daytime functioning, because basic vigilance, attention and cognitive performance, and overall quality of life are each substantially eroded by disordered sleep, and insufficient sleep and sleep-disordered breathing pose significant health hazards. Unfortunately, insufficient sleep quantity and quality is a widespread public health crisis in children and adults worldwide in the developed world, and primary sleep disorders are a highly prevalent cause of morbidity, an important contributor to mortality, and a public health hazard in raising risk of motor vehicle collisions and catastrophic injuries and accidents in safety-sensitive occupations.

The clinical specialty of sleep medicine initially emerged in earnest during the 1970s and 1980s, surrounding growing clinical application of diagnostic polysomnography. The main diagnostic use for polysomnography remains evaluation and initial treatment for sleep-disordered breathing, but this tool and related techniques have tremendous utility for evaluating selected patients with nocturnal events, suspected periodic limb movement disorder, narcolepsy, and related primary central nervous system (CNS) hypersomnias.

In this chapter, we review the classification of common sleep disorders, a practical bedside approach toward interviewing and examining patients with sleep problems, advantages and limitations of the diagnostic implements of the sleep laboratory, and we summarize diagnostic and therapeutic approaches to the most common sleep disorders.

The International Classification of Sleep Disorders

The International Classification of Sleep Disorders (ICSD) provides a common nomenclature and taxonomy for disorders of sleep for clinicians and researchers alike. The current ICSD, ICSD-2, divides sleep disorders into eight distinct categories. The ICSD-2 nomenclature is shown in Box 1, and the most common sleep complaints and disorders are presented and discussed in detail throughout this chapter.

Clinical Approach to the Sleep Medicine Patient

The three most common clinical presenting sleep-related patient complaints are hypersomnia, insomnia, and parasomnias (unusual behavior or events at night). Hypersomnia is present where there is excessive sleepiness during what ought to be waking hours. Insomnia may be regarded as a problem in initiating or maintaining sleep under conditions that are normally conducive to sleep. Parasomnias are disorders in which unusual or dangerous events occur during sleep.

Insomnia is a subjective complaint. To some patients it is not at all bothersome to require 20 minutes to fall asleep, whereas to others it seems very wrong. Although insomnia is fundamentally a subjective symptom, the manifestations follow common patterns. Sleep latency, the time taken to fall asleep, varies significantly, but initial sleep latency longer than 20 to 30 minutes may be considered prolonged, once proper conditions for sleep have been established: lights off, dark quiet sleep environment without distracting stimuli. Likewise, there is significant variation in what degree of subjective sleep disruption reflects sleep maintenance insomnia because normal persons can briefly awaken as often as 10 to 15 times each hour, although most such arousals are below the threshold of conscious awareness.

Multiple nocturnal awakenings that are disturbing to the patient, especially when there is difficulty reinitiating sleep, may be regarded as sleep-maintenance insomnia. Patients admitting to insomnia should be asked to ascribe what amount of their problem is ascribable to an active mind or worries, restless legs, or body pain. Disturbing influences in the sleep environment such as the ambient light, temperature, and noise conditions in the bedroom should be sought. A precise diagnosis is not possible without detailed knowledge of sleep and wake behavior over the entire circadian cycle as well as over a more protracted time, such as 1 to 2 weeks. A sleep log can be very helpful in gaining needed insights for diagnosis.

The patient and physician might at times have difficulty differentiating between hypersomnia and complaints of fatigue (poor energy and motivation without the tendency toward falling asleep inadvertently). A quick and incisive test is administration of the Epworth Sleepiness Scale (ESS), a short questionnaire asking the patient the likelihood of dozing inadvertently during usual daytime sedentary, permissive settings including reading, watching television, or traveling in a car. An online version of this tool is available at http://www.stanford.edu/~dement/epworth.html. Scores greater than

BOX 1   International Classification of Sleep Disorders, 2nd Edition (ICSD-2)

Insomnia and Inadequate Sleep Hygiene
Primary Insomnias

Idiopathic insomnia
Psychophysiological insomnia
Paradoxical insomnia

Secondary Insomnias

Insomnia due to mental disorder
Inadequate sleep hygiene
Behavioral insomnia of childhood
Adjustment insomnia
Insomnia due to drug or substance (alcohol)
Insomnia due to medical condition
Insomnia not due to substance or known physiologic
   condition, not organic
Physiologic (organic) insomnia, unspecified

Sleep-Related Breathing Disorders

Continuum of obstructive sleep-disordered breathing:
   snoring, upper airway resistance syndrome, and
   obstructive sleep apnea
Central sleep apnea
• Primary central sleep apnea
• Due to Cheyne–Stokes breathing pattern
• Due to high-altitude periodic breathing
• Due to medical condition not Cheyne–Stokes
• Due to drug or substance
Primary sleep apnea of infancy
Complex sleep apnea syndrome
Sleep-related hypoventilation
• Sleep related nonobstructive alveolar hypoventilation,
   idiopathic
• Congenital central alveolar hypoventilation syndrome
• Due to lower airways obstruction, neuromuscular and
   chest wall disorders, or pulmonary parenchymal or
   vascular pathology
• Unspecified

Narcolepsy and Primary CNS Hypersomnias

Narcolepsy
• With cataplexy
• Without cataplexy
• Due to medical condition
• Unspecified
Recurrent hypersomnia
• Kleine-Levin syndrome
• Menstrual-related hypersomnia
Idiopathic hypersomnia
• With long sleep time
• Without long sleep time
Behaviorally induced insufficient sleep syndrome
Hypersomnia due to medical condition, drug, or
   substance (alcohol)
Hypersomnia not due to substance or known physiologic
   condition
Physiologic hypersomnia (unspecified)

Circadian Sleep Disorders

Delayed sleep phase syndrome

Advanced sleep phase syndrome
Irregular sleep–wake type
Nonentrained type (free running)
Jet lag type
Shift work type
Circadian sleep disorder due to medical condition
Circadian sleep disorder due to drug or substance
(alcohol)

Parasomnias
Disorders of Arousal from NREM Sleep

Confusional arousals
Sleepwalking
Sleep terrors

Parasomnias Usually Associated with REM Sleep

REM sleep behavior disorder
Recurrent isolated sleep paralys s
Nightmare disorder

Other Parasomnias

Sleep-related dissociative disorders
Sleep enuresis
Sleep-related groaning (catathrenia)
Exploding head syndrome
Sleep-related hallucinations
Sleep-related eating disorder
Parasomnias due to drug or substance (alcohol)
Parasomnias due to medical condition

Sleep-Related Movement Disorders

Restless legs syndrome
Periodic limb movement disorder
Sleep-related leg cramps
Sleep-related bruxism
Sleep-related rhythmic movement disorder
Sleep-related movement disorder, unspecified, due to
   drug or substance, due to medical condition

Isolated Symptoms, Apparently Normal Variants, and Unresolved Issues

Long sleeper
Short sleeper
Snoring
Sleep talking
Sleep starts (hypnic jerks)
Benign sleep myoclonus of infancy
Hypnagogic foot tremor and alternating leg muscle
   activation during sleep
Propriospinal myoclonus at sleep onset
Excessive fragmentary myoclonus

Other Sleep Disorders

Physiologic sleep disorder, unspecified
Environmental sleep disorder
Fatal familial insomnia

Abbreviations: CNS = central nervous system; NREM = non–rapid eye movement [sleep]; REM = rapid eye movement [sleep].

10 are considered abnormal indicating a possible underlying primary sleep disorder, and suggest the need for further evaluation. Complaints of hypersomnia must be placed into the context of the sleep history, with particular emphasis on the quantity, timing, and quality of obtained sleep.

Patients can also present with complaints of disturbing or unusual activities during sleep (parasomnias). Key diagnostic points in determining the diagnosis for parasomnias include their onset, frequency, time of night, stereotypy, injuries sustained, and what behavior ensues following the parasomnia event.

Collateral history obtained from a bed partner may be particularly instructive. Patients should be asked whether they are reported to snore, whether the snoring is intermittent or constant and whether it is related to body positions such as sleeping supine, and whether there have been witnessed apneic episodes or self-awareness of arousals from sleep related to a snort or gasp. Symptoms such as morning dry mouth and sore throat, frequent morning headaches, or heartburn can indicate a higher likelihood of significant snoring and associated sleep-disordered breathing. Patients should be asked about awareness of restless legs symptoms or movements during sleep, and whether they have been told of peculiar sleep-related behavior or evidence of acting out their dreams, yelling or thrashing in sleep, or exhibiting sleep walking or other amnestic behavior during sleep.

In addition to a detailed sleep history, it is important to gather a general medical history because sleep disorders are often tightly linked to other diseases. Obstructive sleep apnea (OSA) is closely associated with hypertension, coronary artery disease, cerebrovascular disease, atrial fibrillation, obesity, and the metabolic syndrome. Congestive heart failure, even when well compensated, is often associated with central sleep apnea syndrome. Restless legs syndrome and periodic limb movements of sleep (PLMS) are commoner in patients with spinal cord or peripheral nerve pathologies. Hypoventilation is more prevalent in patients with neuromuscular disease, advanced obstructive lung disease, and kyphosis and in traumatic, vascular, neoplastic, or degenerative disorders that affect the medullary centers of the brain. Various genetic syndromes, such as trisomy 21, produce facies that predispose to OSA owing to anatomic narrowing of the upper airways.

Physical examination in sleep medicine focuses upon signs indicating predisposition to or associated sequelae of sleep-disordered breathing. Careful inspection of the oropharynx and nares is particularly crucial because significant oropharyngeal narrowing is the chief anatomic substrate for obstructive sleep-disordered breathing, whereas nasal septal deviation or other nasal obstruction, in addition to a thickened neck and overweight body habitus, can also be contributory substrates for sleep apnea. Careful inspection for signs of neuromuscular disease, such as fasciculations or thoracoabdominal paradox, can help detect the underlying cause for sleep-related hypoventilation. Elevated blood pressure, a cardiac gallop, wet rales, and peripheral edema may be present as signs of systemic hypertension, heart failure, or cor pulmonale associated with untreated sleep-disordered breathing.

Diagnostic Tools in the Sleep Laboratory

POLYSOMNOGRAPHY

Polysomnography is the gold standard for formal assessment of suspected sleep-disordered breathing, hypersomnia, or parasomnias. Polysomnography is a diagnostic test most often performed at a sleep laboratory, attended by trained technicians, combining evaluation of sleep, breathing, and movement. During polysomnography, several polygraphic physiologic variables are analyzed, including electroencephalography (EEG), electrooculography (EOG), and chin electromyography (EMG) to allow determination of sleep staging, limb EMG leads to analyze periodic leg or arm movements that may disrupt sleep, oronasal airflow measured by a thermistor and nasal pressure sensors, electrocardiography (ECG), and respiratory effort measured by inductance plethysmography monitors. Body position is also analyzed to delineate effects of sleeping position on breathing.

Each 30-second epoch of the polysomnogram is subsequently scored by a polysomnography technologist as either wake (W), light non-rapid eye movement (NREM) sleep (N1 or N2), slow-wave NREM sleep (N3), and rapid eye movement (REM) sleep according to well-defined guidelines. Sleep architecture, or the composition of sleep by different stages, varies greatly by age, but in middle-aged adults it is approximately 60% to 75% N1 and N2, 10% to 20% N3, and 15% to 25% REM sleep; children usually have higher, and elderly persons have lower, percentages each of N3 and REM. Arousals from sleep and their mechanisms, whether due to breathing, movement, or spontaneous causes, are determined. Accordingly, a precise determination of the duration of a patient's total sleep time, sleep efficiency (total time spent asleep divided by time in bed), and disrupting influences on sleep, such as abnormal respiration or movement, may be determined. The effects of confounding medical disorders and medications on sleep architecture must also be considered. Common medications that affect sleep include SSRI medications that suppress and delay REM sleep and benzodiazepines that reduce the amount of N3 and REM and lead to increased sleep stage shifting and heightened light NREM (N1 and N2).

Attended polysomnography is advantageous because it allows precise measurement of sleep and relevant cardiorespiratory and neurologic behavior and it allows intervention with therapeutic trials, if therapy is indicated. Disadvantages of polysomnography include inconvenience to the patient, the need to sleep in a foreign environment, and the expenses associated with the highly trained personnel and the technology. Polysomnography is currently the only way to actually measure sleep, but because the sleep state is currently defined by the variables measured in polysomnography (EEG, EMG, and electrooculography [EOG]), this is teleologic rather than technologic. The science of sleep medicine may develop new ways of marking the sleep state that are more convenient and more precise and that correlate even better with health and disease.

OUT-OF-LABORATORY TESTING

A wide variety of out-of-laboratory testing devices have been developed (Table 1). In a recent device classification (see Table 1), type I denotes attended laboratory polysomnography, and types II through IV may be out-of-laboratory devices. Type II devices are rarely used for clinical purposes. Type III and IV devices measure cardiorespiratory parameters (pulse oximetry, respiratory effort, airflow). Some add markers for sleep, such as actigraphy (see later) or pattern recognition of pulse or autonomic variability (PAT) to estimate sleep time (see Table 1). The validity and usefulness of such a wide variety of devices has been the subject of much debate, but most agree that there are two main uses for type III devices: as a diagnostic test in patients who have a high pretest probability of having moderate to severe OSA and as a means of reassessing treatment in patients in whom OSA has already been diagnosed. Type IV devices (pulse oximeters) are not a valid way to diagnose sleep apnea, but they may be useful adjuncts to diagnostic suspicion in deciding whether or not to pursue further testing or in assessing oxygenation during treatment of sleep-disordered breathing.

MULTIPLE SLEEP LATENCY AND MAINTENANCE OF WAKEFULNESS TESTING

The multiple sleep latency test (MSLT) provides an objective measure of sleepiness compared with normal persons lacking primary sleep disorders. Its chief clinical indication is for evaluating narcolepsy and related primary CNS hypersomnias such as idiopathic hypersomnia and Kleine-Levin syndrome. A MSLT is carried out during the daytime in a sleep laboratory following nocturnal polysomnography, with four or five nap opportunities at standard times and intervals, usually at 9:00 AM, 11:00 AM, 1:00 PM, 3:00 PM, and 5:00 PM. Careful inspection of each nap is subsequently performed to determine the timing of sleep onset relative to commencement of each nap and whether REM sleep occurs during each nap. A mean sleep latency is then calculated from the average initial sleep latency from each nap. Mean sleep latencies shorter than 8 minutes are considered

TABLE 1 Types of Sleep Monitors and Out-of-Laboratory Testing Devices

Type	Synonyms	Physiologic Measures	Indications
Type I	Attended polysomnography	7 parameters, including EEG, chin EMG, ECG, airflow, respiratory effort, oximetry	Suspected sleep-disordered breathing, hypersomnia, parasomnia, insomnia unexplained or unresponsive to treatment
Type II	Home polysomnography	7 parameters, including EEG, chin EMG, heart rate or ECG monitor, airflow, respiratory effort, oximetry	Suspected sleep-disordered breathing, hypersomnia, insomnia unexplained or unresponsive to treatment
Type III	Cardiorespiratory monitor	4 parameters, including ventilation or airflow ($\geq$2 channels of respiratory movement, or respiratory movement and airflow), heart rate or ECG, oximetry	Suspected sleep apnea (best validated for obstructive sleep apnea)
Type IV	Pulse oximetry	1 or 2 parameters, typically oximetry plus heart rate or airflow	Detect variability in oxygen saturation during sleep
PAT	WatchPAT (proprietary device)	Oximetry, peripheral arterial tonometry	Suspected sleep apnea (controversial)
Actigraphy	Actigraphy	Accelerometer to detect movement frequency, sometimes light detector	Determine sleep patterns and quantity in evaluation of hypersomnia or suspected circadian rhythm disorders, or to assess response of treatment in insomnia

Abbreviations: ECG = electrocardiogram; EEG = electroencephalogram; EMG = electromyogram; PAT = pulse or autonomic variability.

abnormal and indicate pathologic excessive daytime sleepiness. Whether or not a sleep-onset REM period (a SOREMP, i.e., reaching REM sleep within 15 minutes of sleep onset during a nap) is captured is also considered and tabulated. More than one SOREMP is abnormal and is consistent with the diagnosis of narcolepsy.

There are several considerations before performing and interpreting a valid MSLT. Patients should be instructed to sleep well for at least 2 weeks preceding the study, allowing at least 6 to 7 hours per night. Many sleep specialists document the quantity of sleep before the test with actigraphy monitoring or a sleep diary to ensure adherence to this recommendation and to exclude the contaminating influence of insufficient sleep quantity. If it is safe and practically possible to do so, patients should be instructed to taper or discontinue sedative, stimulant, or REM-suppressant medications (opiate analgesics, antidepressants, or other psychotropic or CNS-active drugs) with the oversight and permission of other relevant treating primary care, psychiatry, and pain physicians at least 1 to 2 weeks before the MSLT. Certain psychotropic drugs, such as fluoxetine (Prozac), with a long elimination half-life should be discontinued for at least 1 month before the MSLT to avoid a decrease in MSLT sensitivity for early REM latency. Patients should undergo full-night diagnostic polysomnography the night before the MSLT study to ensure that there is not another primary sleep disorder such as sleep-disordered breathing or periodic limb movement disorder that could provide an alternative reason for significant sleepiness and to ensure that sufficient sleep quantity of 6 hours or more is obtained.

The Maintenance of Wakefulness Test (MWT) is used to assess ability to remain awake. It is most useful as an objective measure of the effectiveness of treatment for disorders causing hypersomnolence. The patient is seated in a dim room in a comfortable semireclined position and asked to remain alert but passive for four 40-minute periods 2 hours apart. EEG, EOG, and chin EMG are measured, and the signals are analyzed to detect any epochs of unequivocal sleep during each 40-minute period. Normal patients have a mean time to epochs of unequivocal sleep of 30.4 minutes, but the data are not normally distributed and 42% of all patients remain awake for the entire 40 minutes on all four opportunities.

ACTIGRAPHY MONITORING

Wrist actigraphy monitoring provides an estimation of sleep quantity and its circadian pattern. The actigraphy monitor may be worn like a wrist watch and contains an accelerometer that detects movements, which are recorded over periods lasting up to weeks. The magnitude and pattern of movements may be analyzed and modeled to infer the sleep–wake pattern and provides a graphic representation of the patient's sleep schedule. The test is used to evaluate suspected circadian rhythm disorders, to assess response to treatment of insomnia, and to investigate patients with hypersomnia before PSG and MSLT to more accurately document the adequacy of sleep before the assessment for sleepiness.

Diagnostic and Therapeutic Approach to Common Sleep Disorders

INSOMNIA

The insomnia disorders all share three basic components: the insomnia itself, which can involve difficulties falling asleep or staying asleep, poor sleep quality, or waking undesirably early; an adequate time and opportunity for sleep; and daytime impairment resulting from inadequate sleep. Insomnia is the most common of sleep complaints, affecting nearly 45% intermittently within the past year in some large studies and affecting up to 15% with chronic insomnia disorders. Risks for insomnia include female sex, older age, and a psychiatric or medical comorbidity. Chronic insomnia should be distinguished from acute insomnia, which can occur in anyone occasionally (e.g., the night before an important job interview or during periods of increased stress). Some suggest a 3-month duration of these symptoms to define chronicity, but there is evidence to suggest that symptoms for a period as short as 30 days may be clinically significant.

Insomnia may be classified as primary or secondary, with secondary insomnia being far more common (see Box 1). Idiopathic insomnia begins in childhood, is lifelong, and appears to be a manifestation of neurologic hyperarousal, with demonstrable increases in cerebral metabolism via functional MRI, increases in beta and theta EEG activity, and generalized increased metabolism and production of stress hormones compared with normal persons in either wake or sleep states. To a lesser extent, these same markers for hyperarousability are seen in other causes of primary insomnia (see Box 1).

In the past, secondary insomnia was thought to be a result or accompaniment of an underlying illness. This may be incorrect. For example, it was previously thought that treatment of secondary insomnia ought to focus on treatment of the underlying disorder. Newer evidence indicates that this approach may be suboptimal because secondary insomnia does not reliably improve when the underlying disorder does. Secondary insomnia in general responds to treatment directed at insomnia, and in some cases the underlying disorder, such as depression, responds better to treatment when the insomnia is addressed directly and concurrently. In several illnesses such as depression, insomnia can predate the disorder by months, and insomnia is a risk factor for future development of many psychiatric illnesses. For these reasons, many now prefer the term *comorbid insomnia* to secondary insomnia.

Chronic insomnia may be preceded in predisposed persons by precipitating factors such as illness or stress, and it may be propagated by behavioral or maladaptive cognitive factors. Some persons, such as those with idiopathic insomnia, do not appear to require precipitating or propagating factors to develop chronic insomnia. They are prototypical for an underlying predisposition toward insomnia. These persons manifest insomnia from infancy, and the insomnia persists despite optimization of sleep hygiene and habit. However, in most cases of insomnia, precipitating or propagating influences may be found through careful interview, and they help to establish a secure diagnosis.

As a prototype of insomnia largely due to precipitating and propagating influences, adults with psychophysiologic insomnia not infrequently have identifiable precipitating causes that may be traumatic, stressful periods or struggles, medical illness, drugs, or toxins. However, even when the cause is removed, a conditioned response built upon associated and at times maladaptive sleep-related behavior ensues. Instead of beginning to relax for sleep under permissive circumstances, affected patients experience paradoxical arousal as they approach their sleep conditions. The patient under the influence of the precipitating cause might have spent many hours worrying, feeling uncomfortable, watching the clock, or otherwise raising anxiety levels. Propagating factors include these same behaviors that help to maintain sleeplessness once it has begun, and they additionally include irregular sleep schedules and the use of drugs. Abuse of alcohol may be contributory or secondary to the sleep disturbance.

Effective treatment strategies for insomnia focus on removing any residual precipitating influences and mitigating or eliminating propagating influences. The main therapies for insomnia are sleep hygiene, behavioral therapies, cognitive therapies, and pharmacologic treatment. It is increasingly clear that patients often respond best to combined modalities. There is very high-level evidence that cognitive-behavioral therapy (CBT) is at least as effective as pharmacologic therapy for most patients with insomnia. CBT also appears to have enhanced rates of remitting insomnia, so this approach ought generally to be employed first. The addition of sedative-hypnotic medications to CBT has resulted in more rapid remission in some studies.

In childhood, the most common causes of insomnia include limit-setting sleep disorder and sleep-onset association disorder. Limit-setting sleep disorder can occur when parents fail to establish and enforce an appropriate nightly bedtime, so that the child subsequently stalls and refuses to go to bed in a timely fashion. Sleep-onset association disorder results when a child cannot fall asleep until a usual condition is present such as being held, rocked, or fed. Appropriate advice and treatments include strict limit-setting for bedtime resistance, maintaining regular sleep schedules with avoidance of napping during the daytime, and curtailing disrupting influences such as television watching, gaming, and computer use. Suggesting a nightly cell phone check-in procedure is especially helpful in teenage children, and caffeinated soda and excessively stimulating activities should be avoided during the evenings. Selected children benefit from incentives such as a patient–parent contract that offers privileges for later bedtimes on weekends after the child adheres regularly to a specified sleep schedule during school nights.

Four considerations for restoring normal sleep hygiene to discuss with all insomnia patients in the office include these central concepts: Maintain a regular sleep schedule, avoid lying sleepless in bed, avoid watching the clock, and schedule thinking time early in the evening.

- Maintain a regular sleep schedule. Go to bed and arise at the same time each day. Ideally, the schedule should match the patient's biological clock, with nocturnal sleep and bedtime and rising time matching the patient's tendency for sleepiness and alertness (sleep education and sleep hygiene).
- Avoid lying sleepless in bed. After 15 to 20 sleepless minutes spent trying to fall asleep, the patient should be instructed to leave the bedroom to pursue a quiet distracting activity such as reading mundane material or watching a boring television program and waiting until he or she feels sleepy enough to return to bed. Patients should explicitly avoid reading in bed, listening to the radio, or watching television in bed if they are having difficulty initiating or maintaining sleep. This is a practical form of stimulus control (Table 2).
- Avoid watching the clock. Patients should be instructed to remove clocks from the bedroom or to hide the clock face so as to make the insomnia period timeless and of uncertain duration. Falling asleep should not be a race against time, and repetitive checking of the time only serves to reinforce anxiety and further activate

TABLE 2 Therapeutic Tools for Treating Insomnia

Specific Therapies and Components	Goals
Education and Sleep Hygiene	
Improve knowledge about behaviors that foster or hinder healthy sleep	Improve opportunity and environment for sleep
Behavioral Therapies	
Stimulus control: Unmodified extinction, graduated extinction, positive routines and faded bedtime with response cost, scheduled awakenings	Dissociate anxiety or conditioned autonomic response from the process or location of going to sleep
Sleep restriction	Increase pressure for sleep by decreasing the time allotted for sleep, increasing the probability of successful sleep attempts
Relaxation training: Progressive muscle relaxation, passive relaxation, autogenic training—biofeedback, imagery training, meditation, hypnosis	Reduce physiological and/or cognitive arousal that hinders or disrupts sleep
Paradoxical Intention	Reduce performance anxiety that confounds ability to successfully go to sleep
Cognitive Therapies	
Cognitive restructuring, decatastrophizing, reappraisal, attention shifting	Decrease unrealistic expectations about sleep, misconceptions, or misattributions regarding causes of insomnia, consequences of insomnia, ability to control sleep; produce a more appropriate and adaptive mind set
Pharmacologic Therapies	
Hypnotics, sedating antidepressants, herbal supplements	Enhance sleepiness at appropriate times, or to enhance convenience of sleep time and/or duration

the mind (stimulus control; see Table 2). For the same reason, when watching television, patients should not watch news shows with scrolling tickertape newsflashes with clock time shown.

- Schedule thinking time earlier in the evening well in advance of the sleep period. Patients who worry, plan, or think out their problems in bed should be encouraged to schedule a time earlier in the evening, well in advance of their normal bedtime, to attempt to work out these concerns instead of carrying them into bed. This "constructive worry" or "worry time" represents a practical form of cognitive and stimulus-control therapy.

Numerous other associated issues and types of behavior may be useful in selected patients, such as cutting down overall time in bed (sleep restriction), establishing a regular and relaxing bedtime routine (such as by taking a relaxing bath, listening to soothing music, or having a light snack before bed), avoiding daytime naps, avoiding caffeinated beverages after noon, establishing a regular morning exercise routine, and avoiding evening exercise. Importantly, the physician should avoid overloading the patient with too many considerations and tasks at once, because as the burden of implementing these suggestions can become obtrusive. One or two concepts to start with is sufficient, and once these are mastered and implemented, the patient can gradually phase in other ideas over time. Second-order therapies such as relaxation training and CBT can be very helpful in selected receptive patients who have failed the typical self-help measures, and as a last resort, periodic or even scheduled chronic pharmacotherapy can also be implemented.

Several highly effective, safe, and tolerable hypnotic medications are available for short-term, intermittent, or chronic use. The class of nonbenzodiazepine receptor agonists (the "Z" drugs: zolpidem [Ambien], zaleplon [Sonata], and eszopiclone [Lunesta]) are preferred by most sleep specialists, but they remain costlier than the older-generation choices including the benzodiazepines, which have adverse effects on sleep architecture, and diphenhydramine (Benadryl), and trazodone (Desyrel),[1] each of which has less-specific sleep-promoting effects and more adverse effects and potential for drug–drug interactions, especially in elderly patients. The clinical pharmacology of the most commonly prescribed and most useful hypnotic medications are summarized in Table 3.

---

[1]Not FDA approved for this indication.

SLEEP-DISORDERED BREATHING

Obstructive Sleep-Disordered Breathing: Snoring and Obstructive Sleep Apnea

Upper airway obstruction results in a continuum of sleep-disordered breathing that varies from mild snoring, to limited airflow resulting in reduced airflow and tidal volume or *hypopnea*, to cessation of airflow or *apnea*. Some patients demonstrate predisposing anatomy of a narrowed oropharynx, such as a low-lying palate or redundant soft palate tissue, a thickened tongue base, or a narrow hypopharynx, although nasal anatomy with septal deviation or chronic congestion can also aggravate the problem.

Snoring without other symptoms, signs, or polysomnographic evidence of upper airway obstructions such as hypersomnia, frequent associated arousals, or significant airflow limitation is termed primary snoring. Snoring may be a socially objectionable symptom or disruptive to the patient's sleep partner, but snoring in isolation is otherwise not considered to be abnormal, and such patients may be reassured if their bed partners are not bothered by their snoring. If treatment is desired, options include relieving nasal obstruction, using commercially available lubricant throat sprays, using maxillary-mandibular advancement devices, and undergoing nasal or upper airway surgery such as nasal septal repair or uvulopalatopharyngoplasty. An otorhinolaryngology consultation may be helpful in determining which surgical approaches may be most beneficial for the patient.

OSA is an extremely common health problem present in 2% to 4% of the general population. It is characterized by a history of loud disruptive snoring, with or without snort arousals, witnessed apneic periods during sleep, and daytime sleepiness. OSA has been associated with the development of hypertension, and it is a risk factor for incident development of stroke, coronary artery disease, congestive heart failure, and atrial fibrillation. OSA has been shown associated with a wide variety of endothelial and metabolic abnormalities that favor vascular disease, and when patients with moderate to severe OSA are compared to normal subjects or treated OSA patients, they appear to have a higher mortality and cardiovascular event incidence. Thus the two main reasons to detect and treat OSA are to improve symptoms and to decrease cardiovascular risks. There are good data to show that treatment of OSA improves symptoms and quality of life; data regarding the reversal of cardiovascular risk are not as firm and mostly consist of retrospective studies with

TABLE 3 Hypnotic Medications

Drug	Mechanism of Action	Dosage	Duration of Action ($t_{1/2}$)	Typical Adverse Effects	Interactions
Older Hypnotics					
Diphenhydramine (Benadryl)	H_1	25-50 mg	Intermediate (2.4-9.3 h)	Dry mouth, constipation, urinary retention	Not signifant
Trazodone (Desyrel)[1]	SRI	50-150 mg	Short (3-6 h)	Dry mouth, dizziness, rash	CYP substrate; several others
Triazolam (Halcion)	BRA	0.125-0.5 mg	Short (1.5-5.5 h)	Tolerance	CYP induction
Lorazepam (Ativan)[1]	BRA	0.5-2.0 mg	Intermediate (10-20 h)	Tolerance	CYP induction
Melatonin[7]	MT_1-MT_2	1-3 mg	Ultra-short (35-50 min)	Hangover type effect	None
Newer Hypnotics					
Zolpidem (Ambien)	NBRA	5, 10 mg	Short (2-2.6 h)	Amnestic behavior	Numerous
Zaleplon (Sonata)	NBRA	5, 10 mg	Short (1 h)	Headache, amnestic behavior	Several
Eszopiclone (Lunesta)	NBRA	1-3 mg	Intermediate (6 h)	Headache, amnestic behavior, rash possible	Not significant
Ramelteon (Rozerem)	MT_1-MT_2	8, 16 mg	Short (1-2.6 h)	Hyperprolactinemia	Ketaconazole (Nizoral), rifampin

[1]Not FDA approved for this indication.
[7]Available as a dietary supplement.
Abbreviations: BRA = benzodiazepine receptor agonist; CYP = cytochrome P-450; H_1 = antihistamine H_1 receptor blocker; MT_1-MT_2 = melatonin type 1 and type 2 receptor agonist; NBRA = nonbenzodiazepine benzodiazepine receptor agonist; SRI = serotonin reuptake inhibitor.

methodologic and biasing issues. Nonetheless, most experts agree that at least moderate and severe OSA ought to be treated, regardless of symptom severity.

Severity of OSA is rated by the polysomnographic apnea–hypopnea index (AHI), the hourly rate of apneas and hypopneas averaged over the total sleep time. An AHI of 4 per hour or less is considered normal. Mild OSA is diagnosed with an AHI of 5 to 14 per hour, moderate OSA with AHI 15 to 29 per hour, and severe OSA with AHI with 30 per hour or more. In most laboratories, the AHI is usually correlated with specific sleep stages and body positions to determine whether positional therapy may be offered, because many patients have OSA only in the supine sleep position (position-dependent OSA), and some manifest OSA only during REM sleep in the supine position.

A form of OSA called the upper airway resistance syndrome (UARS) is defined by a clinical complaint of hypersomnia, often accompanied by snoring, but without an abnormally high frequency of overt apneas or hypopneas resulting in significant decline in oxygen saturation. Polysomnography confirms repetitive arousals related to the increased respiratory effort (respiratory effort–related arousals, or RERAs, during polysomnography) required to overcome upper airway obstruction. Because of the similar pathogenesis and treatment response to relief of upper airway obstruction, this is considered a variant of OSA.

Treatment

Therapeutic options for snoring and sleep apnea include reducing nasal congestion or obstruction, positional therapy, nasal continuous positive airway pressure (nCPAP), oral appliances, or surgical management (Table 4).

Positional Therapy

Among the lifestyle or behavioral changes, positional therapy involves employing one or more simple strategies to enforce sleep only in nonsupine body positions, usually on the side. One method is the "tennis ball in the t-shirt" approach. The patient wears a snug-fitting t-shirt with a pocket sewn onto the back between the shoulder blades, and 2 or 3 tennis or Wiffle balls are inserted to discourage the patient from turning onto the back during sleep. Other options include similar commercially marketed shirts or vests (the "snoring backpack" and similar strategies), and body pillows propped or wedged behind the patient or hugged by the patient. Unfortunately, shoulder or hip pain often limits application of positional therapy, especially in elderly persons, and long-term adherence or compliance remains poor, with only about one third of patients able to perpetuate positional therapy strategies in long-term follow-up. Patients with position-dependent OSA should be counseled to be cautious for development of severe OSA problems during any

TABLE 4 Treatment of Sleep-Related Breathing Disorders

Treatment Modality	Goal
Obstructive Sleep Apnea	
Lifestyle and Behavior Modification	
Weight loss	Reduced weight can result in improved airway patency
Alcohol avoidance	Alcohol worsens OSA; avoidance of exacerbating factor
Positional therapy	Enhance airway patency by nonsupine sleeping
Positive Airway Pressure	
Continuous positive airway pressure	Counteract collapsing forces in upper airway, stent open the upper airway
Bi-level positive airway pressure	End expiratory pressure stents open the airway, inspiratory pressure enhances minute ventilation and decreases hypopneas
Autotitrating positive airway pressure	Uses feedback algorithms to adjust pressure in response to airway conditions to provide airway patency with minimal mean pressure
Oral Appliances	
Mandibular positioning devices, tongue-retaining devices	Enhance airway patency by stabilizing lateral pharyngeal walls and enhancing anteroposterior airway dimensions at the velopharyngeal level
Surgery	
Palatal surgeries (uvulopalatopharyngoplasty, others); maxillomandibular advancement	Enhance airway patency by reconfiguring soft tissues and/or skeletal structures
Central Sleep Apnea	
Correct Underlying Disorders (e.g., Heart Failure)	
Various	Reduce stimuli to ventilatory hyperresponsiveness
Gases	
Oxygen	Reduce responsiveness to variation in CO_2
Positive Airway Pressure	
Continuous positive airway pressure	Reduce stimulation to ventilate by decreasing lung water, improving $\dot{V}/\dot{Q}$ matching, reducing airway resistance
Noninvasive positive pressure ventilation	Provide ventilatory assistance to prevent hypercapnia and hypoxemia associated with central apneas or hypopneas, thus reducing hyperventilatory feedback
Adaptive servoventilation	Provide ventilatory assistance in proportion to needs, reducing or eliminating variability in ventilation and ventilatory drive; avoid hypercapnia and hypoxemia associated with central apneas or hypopneas, thus reducing hyperventilatory feedback
Hypoventilation Syndromes	
Positive Airway Pressure	
Noninvasive positive pressure ventilation	Provide ventilatory assistance to avoid hypercapnia and hypoxemia associated with central apneas or hypopneas
Tracheostomy with mechanical ventilation	Provide ventilatory assistance to avoid hypercapnia and hypoxemia associated with central apneas or hypopneas, protect or control airway

Abbreviation: OSA = obstructive sleep apnea.

future anticipated prolonged periods of supine sleep, such as postoperative recovery periods following surgery or following a major injury.

Weight Loss

Weight loss can reduce soft tissue in the neck, making the oropharynx less compressible. The improvement in lung volumes accompanied by weight loss also favor enhancement of longitudinal traction on the upper airway, the "tracheal tug." About 30% to 40% of patients who are able to achieve substantial weight loss are cured of their OSA. Careful follow-up is needed, because many remissions are not permanent. Alcohol and other substances that reduce upper airway tone or cause sedation or reduced responsiveness worsen OSA and should be avoided.

Positive Airway Pressure

The mainstay of treatment for OSA for the majority of patients remains positive airway pressure (PAP) therapy. The main components of PAP appliances are the blower unit, which delivers calibrated pressures to hold open the airway, tubing to conduct the pressurized air to the patient, an interface such as a nasal or oronasal mask, and a harness to hold the mask firmly to the patient's face during use. Of the PAP therapies, continuous PAP (CPAP), which delivers a continuous set pressure between 5 and 20 cm H_2O, is usually first tried in the setting of polysomnography, and in many sleep centers, the practice of performing split-night polysomnography (an initial diagnostic phase, followed by a treatment phase of CPAP titration toward an optimal pressure for the individual patient) allows diagnosis and treatment prescription to occur in an efficient manner. If an optimal pressure cannot be determined by laboratory titration or data is not available to guide prescription of a specific pressure for a patient, an autotitrating PAP device may be considered, offering flexibility for delivering a relatively wide range of self-adjusting treatment pressures as the patient changes sleep position and enters different sleep stages through the night with accordingly varying apnea severity.

CPAP is typically delivered through an interface chosen as most comfortable by the patient, either a nasal mask, nasal pillows, or a full face mask. Nasal pillows are most effective at lower treatment pressures and are favored by many patients with claustrophobia, but they tend to dislodge at higher pressures. Nasal masks of various types are used in many patients, but if mouth breathing and consequent leak is a problem, a chin strap may be added, or a full face mask may be substituted. Many newer PAP machines offer the feature of expiratory pressure relief (EPR), which can enhance tolerability at higher-level PAP pressures by giving way as the patient exhales. Bilevel positive airway pressure (BiPAP) may also be employed at higher treatment pressures if CPAP is not well tolerated. Setting a pressure delta of 3 to 4 cm between the inspired and expired pressure can also add a degree of positive pressure ventilation for patients with concurrent sleep-related hypoventilation from intrinsic pulmonary disease or neuromuscular respiratory muscle weakness.

Oral Appliances

Oral appliances may be fitted by a dental sleep specialist, and they provide a means of advancing the mandible, which pulls the tongue base forward slightly, opening the oropharyngeal airway to some degree and obviating some apnea and hypopnea events. The device is most effective for OSA of mild to moderate severity, but it is generally less predictably effective for most cases of severe OSA.

Surgery

Surgical options include palatal approaches, tongue-based procedures (genioglossus advancement, hyoid myotomy and suspension, lingualplasty), or maxillary-mandibular advancement (MMA). Palatal approaches such as uvulopalatopharyngoplasty performed by otorhinolaryngologists are effective for relief of snoring but mostly ineffective for treatment of OSA, especially if severity is moderate or greater. MMA appears to be quite effective in mild to moderate OSA and can even be applied with good effect even in selected severe OSA cases;

however, morbidity from perioperative pain is considerable and long-term outcomes remain unclear. There are several experimental approaches for OSA treatment currently in development in randomized controlled trials, including hypoglossal nerve stimulation, but the efficacy, safety, and tolerability of such approaches is currently unknown.

Central Sleep Apnea Syndrome

Central sleep apnea syndrome results from an unstable ventilatory drive during sleep, resulting in periods of insufficient ventilation and compromise of gas exchange despite a patent oropharyngeal airway. Clinically, patients can share similar symptoms with those of OSA including snoring, except patients with central sleep apnea more often complain of insomnia than hypersomnia. Central sleep apnea has a heterogeneous pathophysiology, and it may be idiopathic or due to high altitude induced periodic breathing, Cheyne-Stokes breathing, and narcotic-induced apnea. Neurologic causes such as brainstem infarction or neurodegenerative disorders including multiple systems atrophy can also cause central apnea. In heart failure, the presence of central sleep apnea syndrome or Cheyne-Stokes breathing imparts a poor prognosis.

A high-quality trial showed that CPAP did not reduce mortality, but central sleep apnea is often at least partially resistant to treatment with conventional nasal CPAP therapy, and although CPAP can effect improved mean oxygenation, frequent arousals that fragment sleep often continue. There is emerging evidence that alternative modes of PAP such as noninvasive positive airway pressure (NIPPV) therapy, particularly adaptive servoventilation (ASV), may be superior to conventional CPAP for treating the central sleep apnea syndrome. Trials to determine if these more-effective PAP therapies might reduce mortality in CSA patients with heart failure are under way. In the meantime, at least symptomatic patients with CSA ought to be treated.

Complex Sleep Apnea Syndrome

Complex sleep apnea syndrome is a subtype of central sleep apnea wherein patients have significant obstructive or anatomic problems with ventilation but also have the unstable ventilatory patterns noted in patients with central sleep apnea syndromes. These patients have clinical and PSG presentations of OSA, but once the upper airway is opened with CPAP, they experience frequent but physiologic postarousal central apneic events that can later resolve with continued exposure to PAP in the home setting. However, some patients clearly continue to manifest frequent central sleep apneic events more than five times per hour, leading to the suboptimal outcomes of persisting clinical complaints of hypersomnia and medical risk. Complex sleep apnea syndrome can occur in as many as 4% to 15% of those with OSA. There is emerging evidence that alternative modes of PAP such as bilevel positive airway pressure therapy, particularly ASV, may be superior to conventional CPAP for treating the complex sleep apnea syndrome. A randomized, controlled trial to determine which modality of PAP therapy is superior is currently in progress.

Sleep-Related Hypoventilation

The causes of hypoventilation during sleep include primary pulmonary parenchymal disorders, neuromuscular conditions affecting bellows musculature, or restrictive physiology of the chest wall accompanying kyphoscoliotic disorders. Each of these disorders can also ultimately cause daytime hypoventilation, but sleep recumbency, especially supine sleep positioning, and REM sleep stage (which leads to relative paralysis of the chest wall and sole dependency on diaphragmatic excursion to drive respiratory effort) often lead to exclusive or initial sleep-related hypoventilation, with subsequent medical risk consequent to suboptimal nocturnal oxygenation. Failure to treat significant nocturnal hypoventilation can result in sequelae of hypoxemia such as polycythemia, pulmonary hypertension, and right heart failure or sequelae of hypercapnic respiratory failure.

Treatment most often involves use of noninvasive positive pressure ventilation (NIPPV) (see Table 4). These therapies are best titrated in the context of a supervised overnight laboratory polysomnogram under the direction of a sleep or pulmonary medicine specialist. One must be careful not to resort to the potentially dangerous solution of added oxygen therapy alone in severe COPD or neuromuscular etiologies of sleep-related hypoventilation, becauase as ventilation fails and hypercapnia results, the hypoxic drive to breathe can become the chief factor leading to continued ventilatory effort, and oxygen in this context can precipitate acute respiratory failure in some patients. A morning arterial blood gas on room air following polysomnography is indicated to assess for potential hypercapnia and assess the impact of ventilatory support. In the context of severe hypercapnia (i.e., Pco_2 of 55 or greater), continuous transcutaneous CO_2 monitoring to monitor the effects of ventilatory support, oxygenation, and accumulating hypercapnia may be helpful to determine whether nocturnal mechanical ventilatory support is indicated.

NARCOLEPSY AND PRIMARY CENTRAL NERVOUS SYSTEM HYPERSOMNIAS

Narcolepsy is the prototypical and best-known disorder among the primary CNS hypersomnias. Narcolepsy is categorized further as narcolepsy with or without cataplexy. Cataplexy is a distinctive and highly specific symptom characterized by emotionally provoked muscle atonia intruding into wakefulness that is seen in a minority of patients overall and can precede but more often follows onset of the main symptom of hypersomnia. The full clinical tetrad of narcolepsy also includes the symptoms of sleep paralysis, the inability to move the body upon awakening, and commonly associated hypnagogic hallucinations, the intrusion of dream imagery and mentation into conscious awareness following awakening. However, narcolepsy is most commonly monosymptomatic, with the sole symptom being pervasive, enduring sleepiness and decreased vigilance with a tendency toward dozing off inadvertently in permissive settings, and the overwhelming desire to nap during the daytimes, especially in the afternoons. Naps are most often highly refreshing, and scheduled naps can be used to therapeutic advantage or indeed, in rare patients, as the sole treatment for those bent on avoiding stimulant pharmacotherapy.

Narcolepsy is relatively uncommon, affecting approximately 1 in 2000 of the general population. Although the etiology of narcolepsy remains unknown, most experts continue to favor a long-hypothesized autoimmune cause. Major advances in the understanding of the neurobiology of narcolepsy since the 1990s have included the clear linkage of the HLA DQB1*0602 haplotype in up to 90% patients having narcolepsy with cataplexy, discovery of wake-promoting hypocretin (orexin) peptides produced by the perifornical posterolateral hypothalamus, and low to unmeasurable CSF hypocretin in nearly 90% of patients who have narcolepsy with cataplexy. Unfortunately, these tantalizing discoveries have not yet yielded clear insight into pathogenic mechanisms or more-specific therapies for patients, and the mainstay of treatment for the condition remains use of older nonspecific stimulant medications. Supportive laboratory evidence for narcolepsy includes a relatively normal polysomnogram to exclude other causes of hypersomnia.

Idiopathic hypersomnia is a closely related condition often difficult to distinguish from narcolepsy without cataplexy, although a few differing clinical features tend to distinguish it from narcolepsy. Idiopathic hypersomnia is further subclassified as variants with or without prolonged sleep period. Other similar enigmatic and poorly understood primary CNS hypersomnias include posttraumatic hypersomnia when there is a history of temporally related antecedent substantial head injury, and recurrent hypersomnia, also known as the Kleine-Levin syndrome, which in addition to hypersomnia includes other neurovegetative sequelae including cognitive and behavioral changes such as hypersexuality and hyperphagia. Hypersomnia is also commonly associated with as many as 50% of those with myotonic dystrophy type 1.

The mainstay of treatment for each of these conditions is stimulant therapy with the goal of improved vigilance and psychomotor functioning. Stimulants range in intensity from lower to higher intensity and are more or less effective and tolerable. These include modafinil (Provigil) and armodafinil (Nuvigil) on the milder end of the spectrum, although selected narcolepsy patients respond quite selectively to these drugs. Methylphenidate (Ritalin) and the amphetamines are strong. Relevant clinical pharmacology of the stimulant medications commonly used in clinical practice is summarized in Table 5. Patients with uncontrolled hypersomnias should be cautioned against drowsy driving or operating dangerous machinery or engaging in other similarly dangerous activities or hobbies while drowsy because they may be prone to sudden and unpredictable sleep attacks.

TABLE 5 Clinical Pharmacology of Stimulant Medications

Drug	Mechanism of Action	Dosage	Duration of Action ($t_{1/2}$)	Typical Adverse Effects	Interactions
Modafinil (Provigil)	Unknown	100-600 mg	Intermediate (12-15 h)	Tremor, jitteriness, palpitations, hypertension	Oral contraceptives
Armodafinil (Nuvigil)	Unknown	150-450 mg	Intermediate (12-15 h)	Tremor, jitteriness, palpitations, hypertension	Oral contraceptives
Methylphenidate (Ritalin)	DNRI	15-100 mg[3]	Short (2-4 h)	Tremor, jitteriness, palpitations, hypertension	Nonsignificant
Methylphenidate SR (Concerta)[1]	DNRI	18-72 mg	Intermediate (3.5 h)	Tremor, jitteriness, palpitations, hypertension	Nonsignificant
Amphetamine/ dextroamphetamine (Adderall)	DNRI	15-100 mg[3]	Intermediate (10-13 h)	Tremor, jitteriness, palpitations, hypertension, QTc prolongation	Beware MAOIs, SSRIs, SNRIs, TCAs, bupropion (Wellbutrin)
Dextroamphetamine (Dexedrine)	DNRI	15-100 mg[3]	Long (10-28 h)	Tremor, jitteriness, palpitations, hypertension, QTc prolongation	Beware MAOIs, SSRIs, SNRIs, TCAs, bupropion
Lisdexamfetamine (Vyvanse)[1]	DNRI	20-100 mg[3]	Short (<1 h as prodrug, 10-28 h as dextroamphetamine)	Tremor, jitteriness, palpitations, hypertension, QTc prolongation	Beware MAOIs, SSRIs, SNRIs, TCAs, bupropion
Methamphetamine (Desoxyn)[1]	DNRI	15-100 mg[3]	Intermediate (9-15 h)	Tremor, jitteriness, palpitations, hypertension, QTc prolongation	Beware MAOIs, SSRIs, SNRIs, TCAs, bupropion

[1]Not FDA approved for this indication.
Abbreviations: DNRI = dopamine and norepinephrine monoamine reuptake inhibitor; MAOI = monoamine oxidase inhibitor; SNRI = selective norepinephrine reuptake inhibitor; SSRI = selective serotonin reuptake inhibitor; TCA = tricyclic antidepressant.

CIRCADIAN RHYTHM SLEEP DISORDERS

Etiology and Clinical Manifestations

Circadian rhythm sleep disorders result in misalignment of the timing of the sleep period relative to the desired bed and rise times, resulting in concurrent insomnia and hypersomnia symptoms despite normal total sleep time. The most common circadian rhythm disturbances are actually exogenous influences on the patient and his or her circadian axis, which in these cases is functioning normally but is unable to adjust rapidly enough to the required new temporal milieu. These exogenous disorders include jet lag syndrome and shift work sleep disorder, resulting either from imposed transmeridian travel or alternating work shifts, respectively, that disturb the patient's environmental entraining cues and homeostatic drives for sleep and wakefulness and result in misalignment of the patient's endogenous biological sleep drive and typical sleep schedule to the clock time and environment to which they must rapidly adapt.

Jet lag syndrome results when crossing across several time zones in a single day. Crossing one or two time zones is usually not too difficult for the traveler to accommodate to, but crossing three time zones typically causes symptoms of jet lag. Flying eastward is generally much more difficult than flying westward, because patients more easily accommodate phase delay then phase advance or "loss" of time. Treatments for jet lag syndrome usually involve efforts to rapidly re-entrain the patient to the new environment, and protocols for advance preparation include setting back (for eastward travel) or setting ahead (for planned westward travel) one's daily routine 2 to 3 weeks before the trip so that the traveler is already partially reset in the circadian routine before the trip. Attempting to rapidly adapt to the new time zone is also critical, such as seeking regular sunlight exposure during the daytime and avoiding light exposure in evenings. Brief use of a hypnotic medication and regular daily doses of melatonin[7] 0.5 to 5.0 mg at bedtime for the first few nights after arrival can aid resetting the sleep schedule in the new time zone.

Shift work sleep disorder results from workers who must constantly alter or rotate their work schedules regularly between different shifts (so called swing shifts) or workers who must accommodate to a regular scheduled second or third shift (i.e., shifts other than a day shift). Shift workers accordingly often have difficulty adapting and shifting their sleep–wake schedules, and they develop symptoms of insomnia or hypersomnia. Shift workers must be educated to regularly obtain a sufficient quantity of sleep regardless of their work circumstances. Swing shift workers should also be counseled to avoid working more than 5 night shifts in a row because night shift work often leads to a greater degree of sleep deprivation over time. Shift workers should also be counseled to avoid rotating and swing shifts whenever possible, to strictly avoid scheduling overtime duty, to avoid long commutes, and to exercise special caution to avoid drowsy driving. Judicious use of caffeinated beverages or prescribed stimulant therapy with modafinil (Provigil) may be helpful for enhancing vigilance in some patients but should be used with caution.

The two most common endogenous circadian disorders are delayed sleep phase syndrome and advanced sleep phase syndrome, which are most prevalent in opposite extremes of life. Delayed sleep phase syndrome is seen most often in adolescents and young adults, who are biologically night owls in their circadian preference, preferring a delayed bedtime and rise time: bedtimes well past midnight and subsequent arising times in the late morning or early afternoon. Patients with delayed sleep phase syndrome have an extreme and enduring form of this tendency, however, resulting in persisting misalignment of the patient to societal norms. Adolescent and young adult patients present with profound intractable initial insomnia due to their inability to fall asleep at a conventional bedtime as required for school or most daytime occupations, and profound daytime hypersomnia due to their inability to arise and function in the morning hours. Diagnosis is easily recognized by clinical history and sleep diaries, with or without adjunctive actigraphy to objectively verify the pattern of consistent phase delayed sleep periods.

Advanced sleep phase syndrome is more common in elderly persons, who are biological larks, preferring an early bedtime and early rise time by nature. However, elderly persons with advanced sleep phase syndrome are unable to stay awake for desired evening activities, are often even unable to go out to dinner with friends any longer, and awaken undesirably early in the morning and are not able to fall back asleep in early morning hours. The presentation can mimic depression, whose hallmark biological sign is often noted to be an early morning awakening; care should be taken to carefully distinguish these two diagnoses.

Treatment

Treatment of advanced or delayed sleep phase is difficult, and options include specifically timed bright light therapy, with or without light restriction, and timed low-dose melatonin.[7] The time of administration differs for the two disorders and is determined by the patient's own endogenous dim light melatonin onset and arise time and the phase-response curve for light and melatonin administration. Bright light therapy is administered at approximately 2500 lux for at least 30 minutes. The timing of bright light administration is first thing in the morning after arising in delayed sleep phase syndrome, where a phase-advancing influence is desired. For patients with advanced sleep phase disorder, bright light is prescribed in the late afternoon and early evening hours, where it will have a phase-delaying effect. Weeks to a few months of regular therapy are necessary to achieve effect, and adherence is difficult and compliance unable to be verified.

Specifically timed melatonin may be given at very low doses for this indication (contrary to its use in higher supraphysiolgic doses as a soporific by many patients in other contexts of insomnia or its use at high doses in REM sleep behavior disorder). Dosage and timing are complicated, and melatonin must be given in accordance with the circadian phase-response curve to have optimal effects and to prevent complicating the problem. For most patients with delayed sleep phase disorder, melatonin 0.5 mg should be administered at approximately 6 pm, or 8 hours following the usual rise time, when the phase-response curve shifts so that melatonin administration will have a phase-advancing effect. In advanced sleep phase disorder, melatonin is instead given before the time point of 8 hours following the patient's usual rise time so as to have a phase-delaying effect.

Adjunctive light restriction is recommended in the late afternoon and evenings for delayed sleep phase disorder to avoid precipitating additional phase delays, such as avoidance of working with luminescent computer screens or viewing video media from close distance in the late evenings. Some experts advocate commercially available blue light–restricting glasses as biologically reasonable because blue light stimuli in evening hours can exacerbate phase delay and confound other recommended treatment effects. However, efficacy of blue light restriction currently lacks explicit evidence from large clinical trials.

As a last resort, the measure of chronotherapy, a progressive delay of bedtime every few days, is prescribed and the bedtime and rise time are progressively and successively delayed until the desired bedtime and rise time are achieved. Attempts to then entrain the patient on this schedule with the aforementioned measures are again attempted with scheduled bright light and prescribed timed melatonin dosing. This is a lengthier process for patients with delayed sleep phase disorder and necessitates work restriction during the approximately 2 weeks necessary to adjust the patient's sleep–wake schedule.

PARASOMNIAS AND OTHER NOCTURNAL EVENTS

Parasomnias are nocturnal events that disrupt sleep but usually do not appreciably disturb sleep quality. Nocturnal events do not typically manifest with symptoms of insomnia or hypersomnia unless there are other comorbid primary sleep disorders such as OSA, which is a common comorbidity with the parasomnias, especially in adults.

Parasomnias can arise from either NREM or REM sleep. The NREM parasomnias are essentially all variations on the theme of

---

[7]Available as a dietary supplement.

[7]Available as a dietary supplement.

disorders of arousal, where the behavioral sleep state lingers into awakening, leaving arousal from sleep incomplete. Consequent clinical manifestations are surprisingly heterogeneous and often age-related, with specific syndromes such as night terrors in children, sleep walking and confusional arousals seen in children and adults, and sleep eating behavior seen almost exclusively in adults, especially those receiving zolpidem (Ambien) or other newer prescribed hypnotics. NREM disorders of arousal are especially common in children in the first decade of life, regarded as relatively normal and perhaps in some cases simply representing an exaggerated manifestation of the physiologic difficulty in arousing from the characteristically deeper N3 NREM sleep inherent in the developing brain. Pediatric parasomnias are often outgrown, but in many patients they do endure throughout life, albeit less frequently. In adult patients who present with newly evolved nocturnal events proved to be NREM disorders of arousal, one should be highly suspicious of comorbid primary sleep disorders serving to provoke the arousing events, such as sleep-disordered breathing or periodic limb movement disorder.

REM parasomnias include nightmares and REM sleep behavior disorder. Nightmares represent undesirable, disturbing dream content that leads to sudden arousal from sleep with heightened autonomic sequelae of sweating, hypervigilance, tachycardia, and tachypnea. Nightmares and vivid dreaming are present in 10% to 50% of normal young children and in about 50% of adults, but they become abnormally disturbing in content or frequency in a small subset of patients, and the true prevalence of nightmare disorder remains unknown. Patients who present with a chief complaint of frequent nightmares should be reassured as to their biological nature and receive a detailed physical and neurologic history and examination to exclude potential provoking comorbid causes such as a recent medication change in type or dosage, a mood or anxiety disorder, or a primary sleep disorder such as sleep-disordered breathing. If no certain readily reversible triggering cause can be identified, referral for consideration of hypnosis or pharmacotherapy with clonazepam (Klonopin)[1] is helpful in some cases.

In REM sleep behavior disorder (RBD) patients have frightening dreams (characteristically involving fighting off attackers or defending oneself against assailants) that they might or might not recall. Patients act out these dreams, manifested often by violent thrashing movements and screaming or shouting in sleep. RBD patients rarely leave the bed and sleepwalk, but falls or other injurious behavior to the patient or the bed partner are common. Importantly, elderly patients with newly diagnosed RBD harbor a 40% to 50% risk of developing parkinsonism within 10 to 15 years of symptom onset, so all patients with RBD require serial neurologic examinations and follow-up. RBD in young adults may be caused by antidepressant medications, especially the SSRIs, and discontinuing the offending drug can lead to complete resolution of dream enactment.

Diagnosis of RBD is by clinical history as well as confirmatory evidence for heightened muscle tone in the chin and limbs evident on EMG leads (REM sleep without atonia). Treatment options include melatonin,[7] initially at doses of 3 mg and gradually titrating toward 12 mg nightly as needed to suppress visible behavior, or clonazepam[1] 0.5 to 1.0 mg increased to 2 to 3 mg nightly. Great care should be taken to first exclude comorbid OSA in such patients before they use clonazepam, which is a potential respiratory and upper airway suppressant.

Nocturnal epilepsies or psychogenic nonepileptic spells can also arise from sleep or apparent sleep and are additional diagnostic considerations in the differential diagnosis of parasomnias. A high degree of stereotypy (one attack being essentially identical to the next) and multiple attacks within a single night are features that suggest organic partial extratemporal (frontal lobe) epilepsy, even in the absence of EEG changes between episodes or during an episode. In children, benign rolandic epilepsy can lead to stereotyped episodes of facial twitching and drooling, with or without secondary generalized tonic–clonic seizures. Children or adults with autosomal dominant nocturnal frontal lobe epilepsy can present with bizarre brief motor behavior (typically of 10 to 60 seconds duration) without postictal sleepiness. Autosomal dominant nocturnal frontal lobe epilepsy has recently been mapped in several kindreds as a channelopathy, producing a defect of the neuronal nicotinic acetylcholine receptor. Psychogenic nonepileptic spells are instead characterized by nonstereotypic and often prolonged attacks that arise from a behavior state of apparent sleep that is instead confirmed during video-EEG polysomnography to represent normal waking EEG background (alpha activity, a phenomena described as preictal pseudosleep). The differential diagnosis of nocturnal events is shown in Table 6.

---

[1]Not FDA approved for this indication.

[1]Not FDA approved for this indication.
[7]Available as a dietary supplement.

TABLE 6 Distinguishing Features of Nocturnal Events

Parasomnia	Premonitory Symptoms	Behavioral Characteristics	Duration	Frequency	EEG and PSG Findings
NREM Parasomnias					
Night terrors	None	Inconsolable screaming	Minutes	≥1/night	Arousal from N2-N3
Confusional arousals	None	Confused, amnestic	Seconds to minutes	≥1/night	Arousal from N3>N2
Sleepwalking	None	Ambulation, amnesia	Minutes	≥1/night	Arousal from N3>>N2
REM Parasomnias					
Nightmares	Dream recall	Arousal, frightened, palpitations	Seconds	≥1/night	Arousal from REM
REM behavior disorder	Variable dream recall	Thrashing, complex motor behavior	Seconds to minutes	≥1/night	REM sleep without atonia
Epilepsies					
BECTS	Facial twitching, hypersalivation	Focal motor or GTC, postictal	Seconds to minutes	≥1/night	Arousal from NREM, IEDs, ictal EEG pattern
ADNFLE	Bizarre stereotypes motor behavior	Focal motor, bizarre motor	Seconds, <1 min	≥1/night	Arousal from N2
TLE	Aura variable	CPS, postictal	1-2 min	≥1/night	Arousal from N2
Psychogenic spells	Variable	Variable	Often >5 min	≥1/night	Normal awake EEG

Abbreviations: ADNFLE = autosomal dominant nocturnal frontal lobe epilepsy; BECTS = benign epilepsy of childhood with centrotemporal spikes; EEG = electroencephalogram; IED = interictal epileptiform discharge; N2 = Stage 2 NREM sleep; N3 = Stage 3 NREM sleep; NREM = non–rapid eye movement sleep; PSG = polysomnogram; REM = rapid eye movement sleep; TLE = temporal lobe epilepsy.

SLEEP-RELATED MOVEMENT DISORDERS

Sleep-related movement disorders include restless legs syndrome, periodic limb movement disorder, leg cramps, bruxism, rhythmic movement disorder, and others.

Restless Legs Syndrome and Period Limb Movements in Sleep

Clinical Manifestations and Diagnosis

Diagnosis of RLS is based completely on the clinical history, and typically requires four central elements to the described symptoms: urge to move the legs, with or without uncomfortable leg sensations; temporary relief by movement; symptoms that occur solely or predominantly at rest; and nocturnal worsening of symptoms. About 50% of patients with RLS carry a positive family history of the disorder, but positive family history is not necessary for the diagnosis.

The nature of the symptoms as described by the patient may be quite variable with regard to the symptom quality, location or distribution, temporal occurrence, frequency, and severity. RLS symptoms are usually described as uncomfortable, although not really painful, with a sense of a creepy-crawly or prickling discomfort, often below the knees and centered about the shins or calves, but sometimes more proximally in the thighs, or even isolated to the feet and ankles. Symptoms can occur in the arms as well, especially proximally near the shoulders. The much feared but little understood phenomenon of augmentation involves a worsening of the symptoms in temporal expression, severity, and distribution, with symptoms changing from intermittent to constant, with growing intensity and frequency, occurring earlier in the day, and spreading up the legs to the trunk and arms.

Restless legs syndrome has been linked to deficient iron stores and dopaminergic neurotransmission in the brain. It is more common in patients with parkinsonism, multiple sclerosis, epilepsy, and chronic renal insufficiency.

Periodic limb movements of sleep are seen in 80% to 90% of RLS patients, but periodic limb movements (PLMs) are not necessary for the diagnosis of RLS. PLMs are also extremely common in the general population, seen in 5% to 15% of younger adults and as many as 45% of elderly persons. Periodic limb movement disorder is diagnosed when PLMs are thought to be the cause of daytime hypersomnia.

Treatment

Nonpharmacologic treatments including warm or cool baths, massage, stretching, or even application of spontaneous compression devices have been reported to be effective anecdotally and in small case series, but evidence for these measures remains poor, and most patients seeking medical care for the symptom have severe enough symptoms to merit pharmacologic treatment.

Iron and pharmacologic treatments for restless legs syndrome are outlined in Table 7. Iron deficiency, or even low normal body iron stores, can worsen or precipitate symptoms. Measuring a serum ferritin should be considered early in all patients with restless legs syndrome, with iron replacement therapy begun if serum ferritin values are less than 50 µg/L. Iron therapy can be constipating or cause gastrointestinal distress, and the formulation of ferrous gluconate with added vitamin C is often well tolerated by those who cannot stomach ferrous sulfate.

Carbidopa-levodopa (Sinemet)[1] may be used for patients with only intermittently disturbing symptoms, but chronic nightly use of carbidopa-levodopa, especially a dosage greater than 200 mg daily, can raise the risk of augmentation. For nightly use, the newer dopaminergic agonist medications pramipexole (Mirapex) or ropinirole (Requip) are the mainstay of treatment. Pramipexole may be initiated at 0.125 to 0.25 mg nightly and titrated every few days to the 0.375 to 0.50-mg range or beyond if needed to control symptoms. Doses greater than 1.0 mg[3] are typically not additionally effective. Ropinirole may be initiated at 0.5 to 1.0 mg with gradual upward titration to the 4- to 6-mg[3] range as needed and tolerated. Generally, dosing 1 hour before bedtime is sufficient, but if earlier evening or late afternoon symptoms emerge, the patient may take divided doses but must be warned that this can cause augmentation.

For patients intolerant or resistant to the dopaminergic drugs, gabapentin (Neurontin)[1] has become the preferred second-line medication, dosed 300 to 1200 mg at bedtime as needed and tolerated. Other alternatives include clonazepam[1] and tramadol (Ultram).[1] For patients unresponsive to these measures, opiate treatment with oxycodone (Roxicodone)[1] 5 to 15 mg at bedtime, hydromorphone (Dilaudid),[1] or methadone (Dolophine)[1] is often effective. Small case series suggest other alternatives for refractory cases of restless legs syndrome, including carbamazepine (Tegretol),[1] oxcarbazepine (Trileptal),[1] and lamotrigine (Lamictal).[1] The impact of comorbid OSA should also be considered, because optimization of treatment for sleep-disordered breathing can improve both subjective restless legs symptoms as well as the incidence of periodic limb movements in many patients.

Sleep-Related Cramps

Sleep-related leg cramps are a common and enigmatic problem affecting 7% to 10% of children and up to 70% of elderly adults. Unfortunately, although cramps are extremely common and affect the quality of life of cramp sufferers, little is known about the pathophysiology or treatment of this condition. Cramps are painful, involuntary sustained muscle contractions, lasting 2 to 10 minutes,

---

[1]Not FDA approved for this indication.

TABLE 7 Pharmacologic Treatments for Restless Legs Syndrome

Drug	Dosage	Typical Adverse Effects	Interactions
Iron Replacement			
Ferrous sulfate[1,7]	324 mg tid	Nausea, constipation	None
Ferrous fumarate and vitamin C[1,7]	200/125 mg tid	Nausea, constipation	None
Dopamine Agonists			
Carbidopa-levodopa (Sinemet)[1]	1 or 2 25/100 tabs prn	Nausea, dizziness, impulse-control disorder	None
Pramipexole (Mirapex)	0.125-1 mg[3] qhs	Nausea, dizziness, impulse-control disorder	None
Ropinirole (Requip)	1-6 mg[3] qhs	Nausea, dizziness, impulse-control disorder	None
Mu Opiate Receptor Agonists			
Tramadol (Ultram)[1]	50-400 mg qhs	Nausea, dizziness	None
Oxycodone (Roxicodone)[1]	5-15 mg	Nausea, dizziness	None
Other			
Gabapentin (Neurontin)[1]	300-1800 mg qhs	Nausea, dizziness, pedal edema, weight gain	None
Pregabalin (Lyrica)[1]	100-600 mg qhs	Nausea, dizziness, pedal edema, weight gain	None

[1]Not FDA approved for this indication.
[7]Available as a dietary supplement.

affecting unilateral or bilateral calves, thighs, or feet, with residual tenderness of the affected muscle lasting up to an hour or longer. The clinical approach to sleep-related leg cramps is to first determine whether they are also present during daytime in addition to sleep. If daytime cramping is prominent, exclusion of a precipitating neuromuscular disorder is paramount, including amyotrophic lateral sclerosis, peripheral neuropathy, myositis, or cramp-fasciculation syndrome. In elderly men, peripheral vascular disease and other systemic medical comorbidities are also common.

A neurologic examination should be conducted on all cramp sufferers, and those having sensorimotor findings, fasciculations, or pathologic reflex findings should be referred for electromyography, serum creatine kinase, or additional blood and urine tests for exclusion of symptomatic causes of neuropathy as appropriate. Additional testing for abnormal levels of electrolytes such as hypomagnesemia, hypocalcemia, hyponatremia, and hypokalemia can be considered, but they are of extremely low yield. When examination findings are normal and cramps are isolated to the sleep state, further diagnostic work-up can usually be avoided. Symptomatic treatment measures for sleep-related leg cramps include tonic water with lemon and advising adequate hydration and nightly stretching of the calves and thighs. For refractory cramps, prescription quinine sulfate (Qualaquin)[1] or a sodium-channel blocking anticonvulsant such as carbamazepine[1] or oxcarbazepine[1] may also be considered.

Sleep-Related Bruxism

Sleep-related bruxism, rhythmic grinding of the teeth during sleep, can lead to significant tooth wear and dental or jaw pain. The condition is usually idiopathic, although bruxism, especially if also present during the day, may be associated with psychiatric conditions such as mood or anxiety disorders. Treatment usually involves dental referral for consideration of a fitted mouth guard, although in extreme cases pharmacotherapy with clonazepam[1] may be necessary or botulinum toxin A (Botox)[1] may be considered.

Movement Disorders

Sleep-related rhythmic movement disorder usually occurs in patients with psychomotor maldevelopment and involves repetitive head and neck or axial body movements. This behavior is not strictly voluntary and often persists during polysomnography into deep drowsiness or light NREM sleep, so behavioral treatments alone are often ineffective. Head-banging behavior, sometimes into the headboard of the bed, can be injurious at times, so that a protective helmet or treatment with clonazepam[1] is advisable in some cases. Most other movement disorders such as organic tremors, myoclonus, or dyskinesias generated by the basal ganglia are suppressed during sleep but may reemerge during drowsiness or nocturnal awakenings.

ISOLATED SYMPTOMS, APPARENTLY NORMAL VARIANTS, AND UNRESOLVED ISSUES

Other conditions probably represent either normal variants or otherwise largely benign disorders. The definition of long and short sleepers is somewhat arbitrary, but long sleep may be considered as greater than 10 hours and short sleep as shorter than 5 hours of habitual sleep. Short or long sleep time are each assumed to be variants of normal behavior in the absence of hypersomnia or nighttime symptoms of insomnia.

Sleep talking, or somniloquy, in isolation is rarely of concern. History is often lifelong in such patients. When sleep talking is newly evolved in an elderly person or a younger patient receiving antidepressant therapy, RBD should be considered in the differential diagnosis, and the patient should be questioned about other potential evidence for dream enactment. A careful medication history and neurologic examination alone usually dictate whether further evaluation with polysomnography may be indicated, but in most cases isolated sleep talking is not a cause for concern.

Sleep starts, hypnic jerks, or physiologic myoclonus, are near universal and are often associated with recent excessive caffeine intake or emotional or physical stress. A history of occurrence of jerks limited to the arms, legs, or axial musculature causing arousal within the first 5 to 10 minutes of sleep and not recurring later during the night is typical. Reassurance and avoidance of precipitating factors is advised, but occasionally if hypnic jerks are excessive or recur later in the night, polysomnography is necessary to distinguish this benign diagnosis from periodic limb movement disorder or propriospinal myoclonus.

Propriospinal myoclonus at sleep onset is characterized by myoclonic jerks having their primary and earliest onset in abdominal and axial muscles before spreading to the limbs. They may be associated with thoracic spinal cord pathology, so that spinal imaging with MRI is advised. Treatment with clonazepam[1] is usual for this uncommon diagnosis.

OTHER SLEEP DISORDERS

Environmental sleep disorder results from undesirable influences in the patient's sleep environment that serve to regularly distract or disturb the patient from initiating or maintaining sleep. Typical influences include a bed partner who snores loudly or who causes bed motion due to restless or disturbed sleep, pets who sleep in bed with the patient and cause awakening, environmental noise from neighborhood dogs, car alarms, or neighboring freeway or railroad, too much outdoor ambient light, or undesirable household ambient temperature. There is considerable overlap in this category of problems with inadequate sleep hygiene because activating stimuli in the environment can lead the patient toward chronic insomnia and adapting undesirable sleep-related behavior that serves to further disrupt restful sleep.

Fatal familial insomnia is an extremely rare autosomal dominant variant form of familial Creutzfeld-Jakob disease, a prion disorder that leads to progressive insomnia and progressive cognitive impairment, with death inevitably occurring within 3 years of onset. Aggregate prion protein accumulates in the thalamus and other brain regions, and relentlessly progressive insomnia, panic disorder, hallucinosis, and dementia ensue. Unfortunately, no treatments are currently known for this rare disorder.

Conclusions

Sleep disorders are common and result in significant morbidity, daytime dysfunction, and impaired quality of life. Untreated sleep-disordered breathing also raises the risk for hypertension, vascular events, and mortality. The most common presenting symptoms of sleep disorders include insomnia, characterized by difficulty initiating and maintaining sleep and poor sleep quality, and hypersomnia, the symptom of excessive daytime sleepiness. Evaluation begins with a detailed history and physical examination, which in selected cases can require support and clarification by polysomnography and multiple sleep latency testing.

Fortunately, effective therapies are available for the majority of sleep disorders. Insomnia typically requires both behavioral and pharmacologic interventions, and sleep-disordered breathing may be effectively treated in most cases with PAP therapy. Primary CNS hypersomnias including narcolepsy require stimulant management in most cases, and most parasomnias benefit from clonazepam.[1] Circadian sleep disorders can require timed light and melatonin[7] therapies. Patients who have restless legs syndrome and periodic limb movement disorder should be evaluated for iron deficiency, and symptoms might be controlled by dopaminergic or other alternative symptomatic treatments. The majority of patients with sleep disorders benefit from a careful clinical evaluation and appropriately selected therapies.

Sleep Disorders

---

[1]Not FDA approved for this indication.

---

[1]Not FDA approved for this indication.
[7]Available as a dietary supplement.

REFERENCES

American Academy of Sleep Medicine. International classification of sleep disorders, 2nd ed: Diagnostic and coding manual. Westchester, IL: American Academy of Sleep Medicine; 2005.

Avidan AY. Parasomnias and movement disorders of sleep. Semin Neurol 2009;29(4):372–92.

Boeve BF, Silber MH, Saper CB, et al. Pathophysiology of REM sleep behaviour disorder and relevance to neurodegenerative disease. Brain 2007;130(Pt 11):2770–88.

Chesson AL, Anderson WM, Littner M, et al. Practice parameters for the nonpharmacologic treatment of chronic insomnia. Sleep 1999;22(8):1128–33.

Johns MW. A new method for measuring daytime sleepiness: The Epworth Sleepiness Scale, Sleep 1991;14(6):540–5. Also available online in a patient fillable version at: http://www.stanford.edu/~dement/epworth.html; [accessed 12.08.10].

Kushida CA, Littner MR, Morgenthaler T, et al. Practice parameters for the indications for polysomnography and related procedures: An update for 2005. Sleep 2005;28(4):499–521.

Littner MR, Kushida C, Anderson WM, et al. Standards of Practice Committee of the American Academy of Sleep Medicine: Practice parameters for the dopaminergic treatment of restless legs syndrome and periodic limb movement disorder. Sleep 2004;27(3):557–9.

Loube DI, Gay PC, Strohl KP, et al. Indications for positive airway pressure treatment of adult obstructive sleep apnea patients: A consensus statement. Chest 1999;115(3):863–6.

Morgenthaler TI, Lee-Chiong T, Alessi C, et al. Standards of Practice Committee of the American Academy of Sleep Medicine. Practice parameters for the clinical evaluation and treatment of circadian rhythm sleep disorders. An American Academy of Sleep Medicine report. Sleep 2007;30 (11):1445–59.

Wise MS, Arand DL, Auger RR, et al. American Academy of Sleep Medicine: Treatment of narcolepsy and other hypersomnias of central origin. Sleep 2007;30(12):1712–27.

Intracerebral Hemorrhage

Method of
Jonathan Rosand, MD, MSc

Epidemiology

Intracerebral hemorrhage (ICH) is most often the acute manifestation of a chronic progressive disorder of the blood vessels of the brain. With an estimated incidence rate of between 35 and 45 cases per 100,000 population in Europe and North America, ICH generally accounts for between 10% and 15% of acute strokes on those continents. The incidence is higher in East Asia, with estimates that ICH accounts for as many as 30% to 40% of acute stroke cases in those countries. Hospital-based series consistently reveal an acute mortality from ICH ranging between 35% and 65% and substantial permanent disability in at least 50% of survivors. Because mortality figures are all confounded by the fact that withdrawal of aggressive care by clinicians and families is a very common precipitant of death in these patients and often occurs in patients whose ICH is survivable, it is more useful to focus on rates of disability among survivors when discussing prognosis (see later).

Risk Factors

Risk factors for primary ICH include chronic conditions, chronic exposures, and acute physiologic derangements. Secondary ICH refers to hemorrhage that develops in the setting of vascular malformations including saccular aneurysms, brain tumor, cerebral venous thrombosis, or hemorrhagic conversion of an ischemic infarct.

Among patients older than 55 years, who account for the majority of cases, chronic hypertension, cerebral amyloid angiopathy, and chronic use of antithrombotic medication are the leading risk factors for primary ICH. History of a prior stroke, chronic alcohol use, and family history of ICH also contribute, and patients with severe coagulopathy, cocaine abuse, and liver disease are also at higher risk for ICH. Accumulating data suggest that aggressive lowering of serum cholesterol or chronic use of statin therapy can increase risk for ICH in the elderly. Although chronic hypertension has long been identified as contributing to the largest proportion of ICH cases, recent population-based studies demonstrate a substantial fall in hypertension-associated ICH. In parallel, however, the aging of the population has led to the broader use of antithrombotic medications as well as increases in the prevalence of amyloid angiopathy. The result is that ICH incidence rates have not fallen.

Pathophysiology

ICH arises when a blood vessel within the brain ruptures and blood leaks out to form a hematoma. Because the skull is fixed in volume and is completely filled by brain, blood, and CSF, any accumulation of blood within the brain must necessarily compress, distort, and disrupt surrounding brain structures. The result is that the damage caused by ICH is due the mass effect of the hematoma as well as the toxic effects of the blood itself. The volume of blood that leaks out is thus the most potent predictor of outcome from ICH. In addition, extravasated blood can enter the CSF drainage system, leading to hydrocephalus, another predictor of poor outcome.

Bleeding in ICH often occurs over hours, a phenomenon that can be documented with serial head computed tomography (CT) scans. The volume of ICH can be compared between a CT scan obtained at the time of presentation to the emergency department and one obtained several hours later. The shorter the time interval between symptom onset and presentation to the emergency department, the more likely the patient is to have ongoing bleeding and hematoma expansion after the initial CT scan.

Location of the ICH within the brain can be a clue to the underlying vessel abnormality responsible for the rupture. Among patients 55 years and older, hemorrhage in lobar locations, the junction of the cortical gray matter and underlying white matter, are most commonly a manifestation of underlying cerebral amyloid angiopathy, although other underlying conditions such as chronic hypertension and an underlying vascular malformation may instead be responsible. By contrast, hemorrhages centered in the deep gray structures of the basal ganglia, thalamus, and the brain stem arise most often as a complication of chronic hypertension, with amyloid angiopathy playing no role. Hemorrhages in the cerebellum can arise from any of these conditions.

ICH in the setting of chronic antithrombotic therapy is increasing in incidence as use of anticoagulants becomes increasingly widespread. Although it is likely that excessive doses of antithrombotic medication (e.g., supratherapeutic prothrombin times in patients receiving warfarin [Coumadin]) can cause ICH in the absence of an underlying chronic disorder of the blood vessels of the brain, the majority of ICH cases in patients receiving antithrombotic medication occur in the absence of an overdose. This suggests that the majority of cases of antithrombotic-associated ICH arise in patients with an underlying disorder of the cerebral vessels such as cerebral amyloid angiopathy or hypertensive vasculopathy.

Recurrent ICH is common among survivors of ICH. In particular, patients 55 years and older who survive a lobar hemorrhage have a risk of recurrent lobar ICH in the range of 10% per year. The explanation for this is likely the inexorable progression of the underlying blood vessel disease, amyloid angiopathy. On the other hand, whereas survivors of ICH in the nonlobar regions are also at high risk for recurrent ICH, adequate control of hypertension following the initial ICH appears to substantially reduce that risk, suggesting that hypertension-related disease of the cerebral blood vessels can be arrested.

Prevention

Adequate control of chronic hypertension reduces the incidence of ICH in addition to reducing the incidence of a broad range of cardiovascular and other conditions. Although no specific therapies are shown to be effective in preventing ICH in patients with cerebral amyloid angiopathy, recognition of this condition might become useful in selecting patients for long-term antithrombotic use. Chronic statin therapy can increase risk of ICH, but more studies are required to inform the decision to withhold statins from patients at high risk for ICH.

Clinical Manifestations

Symptomatic ICH manifests with an acute stroke syndrome such as the sudden development of impaired consciousness, language difficulty, disorientation, or weakness. Nausea and vomiting can be prominent, particularly in patients with cerebellar hemorrhages as well as those who rapidly develop substantial mass effect or hydrocephalus. Headache and seizure at the onset of symptoms are more common in ICH than in ischemic stroke.

Small asymptomatic ICH occurs in the setting of diseases like chronic hypertension and cerebral amyloid angiopathy. These hemorrhages, usually only detectable on magnetic resonance imaging (MRI) of the brain that includes susceptibility-weighted sequences sensitive to the permanent hemosiderin deposits left by all hemorrhages, are increasingly recognized as contributing to age-related deterioration in cognition and memory, as well as gait.

Diagnosis

ICH is a medical emergency. Rapid diagnosis and urgent critical care management (airway, breathing, circulation) are essential, particularly because ICH patients can deteriorate rapidly within hours of presentation. Noncontrast CT scan of the brain is the gold standard for confirming acute ICH, and all patients with suspected acute stroke or ICH should undergo an emergent noncontrast CT scan. In centers where emergent MRI is available, it can be substituted for noncontrast CT only if susceptibility-weighted sequences are performed. Angiographic imaging in the form of traditional catheter-based angiography or CT angiography should be performed in any patient younger than 55 years or in patients in whom underlying vascular malformation or ruptured saccular aneurysm is suspected. The history and laboratory evaluation, summarized in Box 1, should be focused on identifying possible contributing causes as well as targets for treatment.

Differential Diagnosis

Emergent neuroimaging can confirm the presence of ICH (Box 2). For patients in whom the history is not obtainable, or who have associated trauma, it is sometimes difficult to distinguish traumatic from nontraumatic ICH. It is therefore essential to examine head imaging for skull fractures and the presence of subdural or subarachnoid hemorrhage, which might be traumatic in origin.

CURRENT DIAGNOSIS

- Obtain a thorough history, including time of symptom onset
- Imaging of the cerebral vessels should be performed in all patients younger than 55 years and should be strongly considered in all patients in whom underlying aneurysm or arteriovenous malformation is suspected.
- Obtain contrast-enhanced neuroimaging if underlying cerebral mass or tumor is suspected.

BOX 1 — Focused Evaluation of Intracerebral Hemorrhage

Assess airway, breathing, circulation

History
Time of symptom onset (or when last seen well)
Recent trauma or surgery
Headache
Seizures
Alcohol or drug abuse
History of hypertension
Prior stroke
Liver disease
Cancer
Coagulopathy
Medications including antithrombotics

Physical Examination
General physical examination
Glasgow coma score
NIH stroke scale

Neuroimaging
Computed tomography, magnetic resonance imaging
Angiography for patients younger than 55 years or in whom an underlying vascular lesion is suspected
Venography if venous sinus thrombosis is suspected
Cervical spine imaging if trauma is suspected

Laboratory
Electrolytes
Complete blood count
Coagulation panel
Toxicology screen
Electrocardiogram

Abbreviations: NIH = National Institutes of Health.

BOX 2 — Differential Diagnosis of Intracerebral Hemorrhage

Primary Intracerebral Hemorrhage
Cerebral small-vessel disease
Cerebral amyloid angiopathy
Hypertensive vasculopathy

Secondary Intracerebral Hemorrhage
Vascular malformations
Cerebral venous thrombosis
Hemorrhagic conversion of an ischemic infarct
Moya moya disease
Cerebral vasculitis
Bacterial endocarditis
Brain tumor
Trauma

Treatment

After the focused evaluation (see Box 1) is completed, emergency care is devoted to preventing neurologic deterioration (Box 3). Blood pressure elevation is common in ICH; clinical trials are under way to investigate the benefit of blood pressure reduction, but accumulated data suggest it is safe.

BOX 3 Targeted Therapy to Prevent Deterioration in Acute Intracerebral Hemorrhage

Neck stabilization in any patient at risk for cervical spine injury

Anticoagulant-associated ICH: Correct prothrombin time as rapidly as possible using intravenous vitamin K and fresh frozen plasma or prothrombin complex concentrate

Severe thrombocytopenia or coagulation factor deficiency: Platelet and/or factor replacement. There are no data to support the use of platelet transfusion in ICH patients taking oral antiplatelet agents.

Blood pressure: For patients whose systolic BP is 150 to 220 mm Hg, reduce systolic BP to 140 mm Hg using intravenous agents. Reduce systolic BP to 180 mm Hg for patients whose systolic BP is >220 mm Hg.

Avoid hypoglycemia

Maintain euthermia

Anticonvulsant medication: Only in patients who have had a seizure

External ventricular drainage catheters: Consider for any patient with hydrocephalus or intraventricular hemorrhage

Emergent surgical clot removal: Indicated for cerebellar hemorrhage with brain stem compression or neurologic deterioration

Prevention of deep venous thrombosis: Intermittent pneumatic compression device and elastic stockings. Low-dose heparin should be started once serial CT scans confirm that bleeding has stopped and there is no longer any ICH expansion occurring.

Rehabilitation: Multidisciplinary rehabilitation should be offered to all ICH patients.

Abbreviations: BP = blood pressure; CT = computed tomography; ICH = intracerebral hemorrhage.

CURRENT THERAPY

- Maintain airway, breathing and circulation; stabilize the neck if fracture is considered.
- Detect and emergently correct coagulopathy.
- Arrange an emergent neurosurgical consultation for cerebellar hemorrhage.
- Maintain systolic blood pressure ≤140 mm Hg using intravenous agents. Reduce systolic blood pressure to 180 mm Hg for patients whose systolic pressure is greater than 220 mm Hg.

Because ICH is a devastating condition that most commonly affects the elderly, physicians and families are often confronted with the question of whether their patient or loved one would choose to survive the event. Accurate prediction of prognosis is essential to guide such decision-making. In this context, tools that predict mortality are of limited utility, as they do not give any guidance on the likelihood of functional recovery among survivors. The FUNC score (Table 1) enables prediction of the likelihood of recovering functional independence for patients with primary ICH. Tools such as the FUNC score calculator (http://www2.massgeneral.org/stopstroke/funcCalculator.aspx) can be useful in guiding decisions about aggressiveness of care, but their precision remains to be proved. Clinicians are therefore advised to provide care according to the principles outlined in this chapter for all patients at the outset, and to proceed to limitation of aggressive care no sooner than 48 hours after admission to an intensive care unit.

TABLE 1 FUNC Score

Component	FUNC Score Points
ICH Volume (cm³)	
<30	0
30-59	2
≥60	3
Age (y)	
<70	0
70-79	1
≥80	2
ICH Location	
Lobar	0
Deep	1
Infratentorial	2
Glasgow Coma Scale Score	
≥8	0
<8	2
Pre-ICH Cognitive Impairment	
No	0
Yes	1
Total FUNC score	0-10

Abbreviation: ICH = intracerebral hemorrhage.

Monitoring

Initial monitoring of the ICH patient is best provided by an intensive care unit with neurointensive care specialists available. Because subclinical seizures are common in ICH patients, EEG monitoring should be considered in any patient who has had a seizure or whose level of consciousness is altered. Invasive monitoring of intracranial pressure should be considered in patients with evidence of shift of the intracranial contents on neuroimaging.

Complications

Prevention of ICH, particularly recurrent ICH, is increasingly recognized as a priority in making decisions about whether or not to offer chronic anticoagulation to elderly patients with atrial fibrillation, prosthetic heart valves, and other conditions accompanied by high risk of thromboembolic ischemic stroke. Given the established benefit of antithrombotic therapy for preventing ischemic stroke, decision-analysis models suggest that only patients at very high risk for ICH might benefit from antiplatelet therapy rather than anticoagulation, or even neither therapy. Factors that must be considered include the patient's presumed risk for ICH, risk for thrombembolic stroke, expected outcomes from each should they occur, and the patient's preferences. At the present, patients who have survived a lobar ICH and are therefore at very high risk for recurrent ICH should be considered candidates for antiplatelet or no antithrombotic therapy at all.

REFERENCES

Becker KJ, Baxter AB, Cohen WA, et al. Withdrawal of support in intracerebral hemorrhage may lead to self-fulfilling prophecies. Neurology 2001;56:766–72.

Eckman MH, Rosand J, Knudsen KA, et al. Can patients be anticoagulated after intracerebral hemorrhage? A decision analysis. Stroke 2003;34:1710–6.

Eckman MH, Wong LK, Soo YO, et al. Patient-specific decision-making for warfarin therapy in nonvalvular atrial fibrillation: How will screening with genetics and imaging help? Stroke 2008;39:3308–15.

Kothari RU, Brott T, Broderick JP, et al. The ABCs of measuring intracerebral hemorrhage volumes. Stroke 1996;27:1304–5.

Morgenstern LB, Hemphill JC, Anderson C, et al. Guidelines for the management of spontaneous intracerebral hemorrhage in adults: 2010 update. Stroke 2010; Epub ahead of print.

Rost NS, Smith EE, Chang Y, et al. Prediction of functional outcome in patients with primary intracerebral hemorrhage: The FUNC score. Stroke 2008;39:2304–9.

Ischemic Cerebrovascular Disease

Method of
Alvaro Cervera, MD, and Geoffrey A. Donnan, MD

Treatment of ischemic stroke has improved significantly in the past few years, and mortality and disability rates due to this condition have decreased. The demonstration of efficacy of thrombolysis in the management of patients in stroke units has been crucial in this achievement. Control of vascular risk factors has been decreased the number and severity of events. Improved management has included high-quality rehabilitation, which is started as soon as possible to improve the recovery (i.e., functional independence) of stroke survivors.

The multidisciplinary management of stroke can be improved with specific educational programs aimed at increasing awareness of stroke in the general population and among professionals. The concept of *time is brain* has a great value in emphasizing that stroke is an emergency. Because the window for the available time-dependent treatments is very narrow, avoiding delay is the major goal in the prehospital phase of acute stroke care. All stroke patients must be transported as soon as possible to the closest hospital with a stroke unit. In rural or remote areas with no stroke unit facilities, telemedicine has proved to be a valid alternative.

Prevention

Lifestyle modification can be a major contributor to reducing the risk of ischemic stroke. Strategies to achieve this protection include avoiding smoking and excessive alcohol consumption, keeping a low-normal body mass index, practicing regular exercise, and having a diet low in salt and saturated fat, high in fruit and vegetables, and rich in fiber. There is no need to add vitamin supplements to the diet because they have not been found to affect stroke prevention.

Regular assessment of vascular risk factors (e.g., hypertension, diabetes, hypercholesterolemia) is important because their control can reduce significantly the incidence of vascular events. Blood pressure should be managed with diet and pharmacologic therapy, aiming at normal levels of 120/80 mm Hg. After an ischemic stroke, blood pressure should be lowered even in patients with normal blood pressure. Diabetes should be managed with lifestyle modification and pharmacologic therapy as required, and blood pressure needs to be more tightly controlled in these patients (<130/80 mm Hg). The best antihypertensive treatments for diabetics are angiotensin-converting enzyme (ACE) inhibitors or angiotensin receptor antagonists. Hypercholesterolemia should be managed with lifestyle modification and a statin. After a noncardioembolic ischemic stroke, statins are beneficial in all patients for secondary prevention.

Postmenopausal hormone replacement therapy should be avoided for the primary or secondary prevention of stroke because it can increase the risk of new vascular events. Other strategies to prevent stroke include the treatment of obstructive sleep apnea with continuous positive airway pressure (CPAP) breathing.

ANTITHROMBOTIC THERAPY

Low-dose aspirin can be used for the primary prevention of stroke in women or of myocardial infarction in men. Nevertheless, its effect is very small, and it cannot be recommended on a population-wide basis. Aspirin is beneficial for the prevention of stroke in patients with asymptomatic carotid stenosis.

In patients with atrial fibrillation, aspirin can prevent ischemic events in those younger than 65 years and free of vascular risk factors. In patients older than 65 years, anticoagulation is the first option, although aspirin is an alternative for those younger than 75 years without other risk factors (Table 1). In all patients with atrial fibrillation who have suffered a stroke, anticoagulation should aim for an international normalized ratio (INR) of 2.0 to 3.0. Patients with prosthetic heart valves

TABLE 1 Prevention of Stroke In Patients with Atrial Fibrillation

Prevention	Therapy
Primary prevention	
No risk factors	<65 years old: aspirin
	65–75 years old: aspirin or warfarin
	>75 years old: warfarin
Risk factors*	All age groups: warfarin
Secondary prevention	All groups: warfarin

*Previous systemic embolism, high blood pressure, or poor left ventricular function.

should also receive anticoagulation, and the target INR depends on the prosthesis type. Dabigatran, a direct thrombin inhibitor, has recently shown to be more effective than warfarin in non-valvular atrial fibrillation at high doses (150 mg twice daily) and is associated with a lower hemorrhagic risk at low doses (110 mg twice daily).

After ischemic stroke, all patients should receive antithrombotic therapy. Antiplatelet agents are the first choice unless anticoagulation is required. The most effective regimen is aspirin and extended-release dipyridamole combined (Aggrenox). However, after the PRoFESS trial failed to show the noninferiority criteria for aspirin plus dipyridamole compared with clopidogrel (Plavix), this superiority is not clear. Aspirin plus dipyridamole, clopidogrel, or aspirin alone are acceptable therapies for secondary stroke prevention. Triflusal,[2] or cilostazol (in Asian populations) are other alternatives. The combination of aspirin and clopidogrel is not recommended after stroke, except if there is an association with unstable angina or non-Q-wave myocardial infarction, or there has been a recent stenting.

Anticoagulation is usually indicated for secondary prevention if the stroke cause is cardioembolic and in specific situations such as aortic arch atheroma, fusiform aneurysms of the basilar artery, cervical artery dissection, or patent foramen ovale in the presence of proven deep venous thrombosis. However, level one evidence is lacking for these approaches.

Management of Carotid Stenosis

In patients with asymptomatic carotid stenosis (≥60%), surgery is indicated only if the risk of stroke is high. Endarterectomy is the treatment of choice if the stenosis is symptomatic (i.e., has been associated with an ipsilateral stroke or transient ischemic attack) and severe (70% to 99%). Surgery should be performed in centers with a perioperative complication rate of less than 6% and as soon as possible after the last ischemic event.

Endarterectomy may be indicated for certain patients with moderate stenosis (50% to 69%), although it should be performed only in centers with a perioperative complication rate of less than 3% to be effective. In cases of symptomatic carotid lesions, angioplasty plus stenting is recommended only for selected patients, mainly younger than 70 years old. If stenting is performed, a combination of clopidogrel and aspirin is required immediately before the procedure and for at least 1 month to prevent stent thrombosis.

In patients with intracranial atheromatosis and stroke recurrences despite appropriate antiplatelet therapy, endovascular treatment may be a reasonable choice.

Management of Acute Ischemic Stroke

All stroke patients should be treated in a stroke unit, because this is associated with a reduction of death, dependency, and the need for institutional care. This effect is seen for all types of patients,

---

[2]Not available in the United States.

irrespective of gender, age, stroke subtype, and stroke severity. Patients with stroke should have a careful clinical assessment, including a neurologic examination. The use of a stroke rating scale, such as the National Institutes of Health Stroke Scale (NIHSS), provides important information about the severity of stroke.

Urgent cranial computed tomography (CT) is mandatory after an ischemic stroke before starting any therapy. Alternatively, magnetic resonance imaging (MRI) can be performed and can provide additional information about the selection of patients for thrombolytic therapy beyond 3 hours. However, there is not enough evidence to recommend its routine use in the acute stroke setting.

For the detection and early management of the medical complications of stroke, neurologic status, pulse, blood pressure, temperature, and oxygen saturation should be monitored. Similarly, serum glucose levels need to be monitored and hyperglycemia treated with insulin accordingly. Normal saline is recommended for fluid replacement during the first 24 hours after stroke. If the patient has fever, treatment with paracetamol (acetaminophen) may be used while sources of infection are being sought. Reducing blood pressure is recommended only in patients with extremely high blood pressure or when indicated by other medical conditions. Blood pressure should be lowered gradually, avoiding abrupt changes.

THROMBOLYSIS

All patients with an ischemic stroke within 3 hours of onset should receive thrombolytic treatment with intravenous tissue plasminogen activator (tPA [Activase]) unless contraindicated, because it is effective in improving stroke outcome (Box 1). The ECASS III clinical trial showed that this effect could also be obtained over a longer period (4.5 hours). Based on the available evidence, thrombolysis with tPA can be given in ischemic stroke within 4.5 hours of onset, provided that it is approved by the local regulatory authorities. There is also evidence from phase II trials (e.g., EPITHET) that selecting patients with MRI to assess the penumbra can be an appropriate tool to extend the time to more than 3 hours, because tPA was associated with increased reperfusion in these patients and a trend toward better outcomes. Nevertheless, increasing the time window does not mean that treatment can be delayed. As evidenced by pooled analysis, earlier treatment results in a better outcome. There is little evidence that thrombolysis is effective in patients older than 80 years, but the available information indicates that it is safe.

Intraarterial administration of a thrombolytic agent within a 6-hour time can be an alternative therapy. Another treatment, which has been approved by some regulatory authorities, is the MERCI device. It mechanically removes the thrombus, which can be associated with thrombolytic therapy. However, no evidence for the clinical efficacy of mechanical devices has been derived from randomized clinical trials.

BOX 1   Treatment of Acute Ischemic Stroke: Intravenous Administration of Tissue Plasminogen Activator

- Infuse 0.9 mg/kg (maximum dose 90 mg) of tissue plasminogen activator (tPA) over 60 minutes, with 10% of the dose given as a bolus over 1 minute.
- Admit the patient to a stroke unit for monitoring. Perform neurologic assessment and blood pressure measurement every 15 minutes during the infusion, every 30 minutes thereafter for the next 6 hours, and then hourly until 24 hours after treatment. Administer antihypertensive medications to maintain systolic blood pressure ≤180 and diastolic ≤105.
- If intracranial hemorrhage is suspected, discontinue the infusion, and obtain an emergency CT scan.
- Obtain a follow-up CT scan at 24 hours before starting anticoagulants or antiplatelet agents.

ANTITHROMBOTIC DRUGS

All patients should receive a low dose of aspirin daily, and this should be started within 48 hours after stroke onset. The use of other antiplatelet agents during the acute phase of stroke cannot be recommended based on available evidence. Similarly, early administration of unfractionated heparin, low-molecular-weight heparin, or heparinoids is not indicated in acute ischemic stroke patients.

TREATMENT OF STROKE COMPLICATIONS

Brain edema develops between the second and fifth day after stroke onset and is the cause of early deterioration and death. In the case of a malignant infarction of the middle cerebral artery, the mortality rate is 80%. In patients younger than 60 years with this pattern of cerebral infarction, hemicraniectomy has been effective in reducing mortality and severe disability, as shown in the pooled analysis of the DECIMAL, DESTINY, and HAMLET trials. Surgery needs to be performed within 48 hours after symptom onset. Surgical decompression is also indicated in the case of large cerebellar infarctions that compress the brainstem.

Stroke-associated infections require appropriate antibiotics, but prophylactic administration is discouraged. Venous thromboembolism is a frequent complication after stroke, but its incidence can be reduced with appropriate hydration and graded compression stockings. If the risk of deep venous thrombosis or pulmonary embolism is high, the use of subcutaneous heparin or low-molecular-weight heparins is beneficial. Early mobilization is an effective way of preventing complications such as aspiration pneumonia or pressure ulcers. Anticonvulsants are administered only to prevent recurrent seizure but are not used prophylactically.

In stroke patients at risk for falls, hip fracture can be prevented with bisphosphonates. In case of urinary incontinence, specialist assessment and management are recommended. Dysphagia is common after stroke and is associated with a higher incidence of medical complications and increased mortality. Malnutrition also predicts a poor functional outcome and increased mortality, and it is important to assess the swallowing capacity and the nutritional status of the patient.

Rehabilitation should be started after admission to the stroke unit. The optimal timing of first mobilization is unclear, but mobilization within the first few days appears to be well tolerated. The AVERT study demonstrated that very early mobilization (i.e., within 24 hours of symptom onset) is safe and feasible. An ongoing study is assessing its efficacy and cost-effectiveness. It is important to assess cognitive deficits and depression during the patient's hospital stay, because this may require specific intervention, although evidence about the type is lacking.

REFERENCES

Adams Jr HP, del Zoppo G, Alberts MJ, et al. Guidelines for the early management of adults with ischemic stroke: A guideline from the American Heart Association/American Stroke Association Stroke Council, Clinical Cardiology Council, Cardiovascular Radiology and Intervention Council, and the Atherosclerotic Peripheral Vascular Disease and Quality of Care Outcomes in Research Interdisciplinary Working Groups: The American Academy of Neurology affirms the value of this guideline as an educational tool for neurologists. Stroke 2007;38:1655–711.

Bernhardt J, Dewey H, Thrift A, et al. A very early rehabilitation trial for stroke (AVERT): Phase II safety and feasibility. Stroke 2008;39:390–6.

Davis SM, Donnan GA, Parsons MW, et al. Effects of alteplase beyond 3 h after stroke in the Echoplanar Imaging Thrombolytic Evaluation Trial (EPITHET): A placebo-controlled randomised trial. Lancet Neurol 2008;7:299–309.

European Stroke Organisation (ESO). Executive Committee; ESO Writing Committee: Guidelines for management of ischaemic stroke and transient ischaemic attack 2008. Cerebrovasc Dis 2008;25:457–507.

Hacke W, Kaste M, Bluhmki E, et al. Thrombolysis with alteplase 3 to 4.5 hours after acute ischemic stroke. N Engl J Med 2008;359:1317–29.

Kent DM, Thaler DE. Stroke prevention—Insights from incoherence. N Engl J Med 2008;359:1287–9.

Sacco RL, Diener HC, Yusuf S, et al. Aspirin and extended-release dipyridamole versus clopidogrel for recurrent stroke. N Engl J Med 2008;359:1238–51.

Vahedi K, Hofmeijer J, Juettler E, et al. Early decompressive surgery in malignant infarction of the middle cerebral artery: A pooled analysis of three randomised controlled trials. Lancet Neurol 2007;6:215–22.

Rehabilitation of the Stroke Patient

Method of
Marlís González-Fernández, MD, PhD, and
Dorianne Feldman, MD, MSPT

According to the national center for health statistics, 5.6 million Americans live with the disability caused by a previous stroke. Stroke is the leading cause of permanent disability in adults. Conservative estimates suggest that about 45% of stroke patients have moderate to severe disabilities requiring rehabilitation.

The goals of stroke rehabilitation are to maintain and optimize medical management, to maximize functional recovery, to minimize disability, and to improve quality of life and participation in society. The rehabilitative approach endeavors to provide patient-centered care that is organized, comprehensive, and specific to the needs of the stroke patient. The concerted efforts of the patient, family, and the rehabilitation team are essential for achieving these goals. Recovery after stroke can be a long and challenging process for the patient and the family. Although functional gains occur most rapidly in the first year after a stroke, additional motor recovery is possible beyond 1 year when patients are involved in targeted rehabilitation programs.

The rehabilitation team is composed of rehabilitation physicians (physiatrists), other physicians such as neurologists and neurosurgeons, rehabilitation nurses, occupational therapists, physical therapists, speech and language pathologists, rehabilitation neuropsychologists, social workers, case managers, nutritionists, vocational counselors, and pharmacists. A goal of the acute inpatient rehabilitation team is discharging the patient to the least restrictive environment, ideally home. To accomplish this goal, it is critical to evaluate family support and the home environment.

Rehabilitation should start as part of the acute stroke inpatient stay. The decision-making process to determine the appropriate rehabilitation setting after discharge is described in Figure 1. Speech-language pathologists, physical therapists, and occupational therapists evaluate deficits in cognition, communication, deglutition, mobility, and activities of daily living. The severity of deficits in these major areas and the ability of the patient to tolerate therapy determine the appropriate rehabilitation setting.

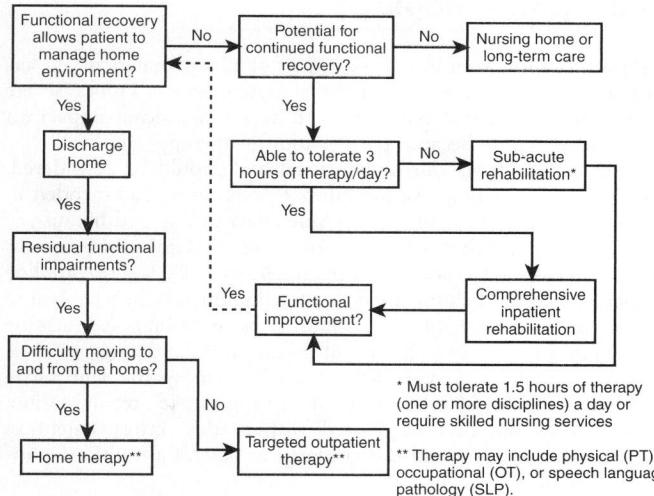

FIGURE 1. Determination of rehabilitation needs of patients being discharged after an acute stroke.

Stroke patients with mild deficits are able to return home with home or outpatient therapy services. Patients with moderate to severe strokes benefit from more intensive therapy in an institutional setting. Comprehensive inpatient rehabilitation is suitable for patients with moderate to severe deficits who can tolerate intensive rehabilitation (3 hours/day). If the severity of deficits or medical comorbidities limits the ability of the patient to participate in intensive therapy, alternate settings can be considered.

During the inpatient rehabilitation stage, medical management focuses on secondary stroke prevention: diet, exercise, smoking cessation, and reducing complications, including optimizing blood pressure control while maintaining cerebral perfusion, preventing and treating lipid disorders, and managing post-stroke pain, depression, and abnormal muscle tone. During this stage, much of the rehabilitation effort is directed toward educating stroke survivors about complications and the importance of adherence to medical recommendations.

Medical complications such as deep venous thrombosis and related thromboembolism, pneumonia (usually related to aspiration), skin breakdown, and urinary infections can hinder a patient's recovery. Early identification of these complications is necessary to maintain progress in the rehabilitation effort. Other complications, such as seizures and cardiac decompensation, are possible and should be monitored.

Stroke often causes significant impairment and activity limitations. Deficits in strength, swallowing, vision, balance, muscle tone, communication, comprehension, cognition, attention, sensory perception, and bladder function are common and can cause difficulty completing activities of daily living, walking, transferring to and from different surfaces, and getting in and out of the bed. Post-stroke depression, fatigue, and pain are common and should be addressed to maximize participation in rehabilitative efforts.

Transition to the chronic phase begins after the patient is medically stable and inpatient therapy goals are met. Outpatient therapy services are initiated in conjunction with physiatric, primary care, and neurologic follow-up.

Hemiparesis

Hemiparesis, or one-sided weakness, is one of the most frequent complications after stroke. Recovery of motor function varies. Often, it is limited by muscle atrophy, co-contraction of agonists and antagonists, and abnormal tone. Usually, motor recovery is preceded by the development of patterned muscle movements, or synergies. Synergies occur when select muscles contract in a predictable manner. In the paretic upper extremity, a flexion synergy pattern (i.e., humeral adduction, internal rotation, elbow flexion, forearm pronation, and wrist and finger flexion) is common. In the lower extremity, extension synergies (i.e., hip internal rotation, adduction, extension, knee extension, and ankle extension and inversion) predominate. These patterns can be regarded as functional and nonfunctional. For instance, extension synergy patterns of the lower limb can augment rehabilitation because this position fosters early ambulatory therapy. Conversely, flexion synergy patterns in the upper extremity can significantly impair arm function.

Rehabilitation of the patient with hemiparesis should concentrate on maintaining range of motion and improving strength and posturing. Exercise programs should incorporate functional use of the hemiparetic limb and weight bearing to promote limb recognition, better alignment, muscle elongation, and muscle tone reduction.

Hemiparesis can lead to contracture, particularly when profound weakness is present. and contracture occurs most commonly in the wrist and ankle. Resting hand splints and solid ankle-foot orthoses can be used to maintain the limb in a neutral position. These devices can be used to prevent loss of motion, control muscle tone, and aid in positioning, particularly when wheelchairs are necessary.

Functional electrical stimulation (FES) has gained increasing interest as a means of enhancing functional movement and strength. Muscle contraction is induced with electrical stimulation. Many products on the market incorporate FES technology for the treatment of footdrop and hand weakness.

Preservation of scapulohumeral positioning is a critical component of rehabilitation. With shoulder weakness, the scapula becomes downwardly rotated, causing the glenoid fossa to move vertically and resulting in humeral subluxation. Traditionally, shoulder slings have been prescribed for the hemiplegic shoulder, but their effectiveness in preventing subluxation is questionable.

FES has been used to augment motor return in the hemiplegic shoulder and prevent subluxation. Despite advances in the treatment of the hemiplegic shoulder, it is still unclear which therapeutic interventions should constitute the standard of care.

Constraint-induced therapy, a therapeutic approach in which the nonparetic limb is restrained, can improve functional movement of the paretic upper extremity in patients with residual hand and wrist movement, even in patients more than 1 year after a stroke.

Dysphagia

Dysphagia after stroke occurs acutely in approximately 50% of stroke patients. Identifying dysphagia in this population is essential for preventing associated morbidity and mortality. Stroke patients with dysphagia are at risk for dehydration, malnutrition, and aspiration pneumonia. As allowed by their overall clinical status and consciousness level, stroke patients should be evaluated as early as possible during their acute hospital stay. Trained clinicians (most commonly speech-language pathologists) should evaluate the patient to make recommendations regarding further dysphagia evaluation or testing and the need for diet modifications or dysphagia rehabilitation.

Hemiplegic Shoulder Pain

Stroke survivors with residual hemiparesis or weakness are at risk for pain syndromes (particularly in the upper extremity), which can significantly limit rehabilitation efforts. These pain syndromes are usually multifactorial. In the rehabilitation setting, prevention of shoulder pain is key, and interventions should focus on proper positioning, handling, and transfer techniques.

In severe cases, shoulder pain can be accompanied by hand swelling, tenderness, skin changes, erythema, hyperhidrosis, and allodynia. When this occurs, it is referred to as shoulder-hand syndrome, a subtype of complex regional pain syndrome (CRPS). Although the mechanism and cause are unclear, it has been suggested that this process is the result of an overreaction to a neurologic insult and may be inflammatory in nature. In some cases, the pain is severe, resulting in decreased and guarded movements of the limb that limit functional use. Shoulder pathology such as rotator cuff strains or tears, bicipital tendonitis, subacromial and subdeltoid bursitis, and glenohumeral subluxation or dislocation contribute to post-stroke shoulder pain and should be treated.

Nonpharmacologic treatment focuses on desensitization techniques, gentle range-of-motion exercises, and physical modalities (e.g., heat, cold, transcutaneous electrical nerve stimulation [TENS], functional electrical stimulation). Pharmacologic management includes medications typically used for neuropathic pain syndromes, such as anticonvulsants, tricyclic antidepressants, nonsteroidal antiinflammatory drugs, topical agents (e.g., lidocaine [Xylocaine],[1] clonidine [Catapres-TTS],[1] capsaicin [Zostrix][1]), and injections of steroid or local anesthetics. Antispasmodic medications have been used. When pain relief is not achieved with conservative treatment, sympathetic blocks can be considered. Sympathectomies and spinal cord stimulators can be considered as last resorts.

Spasticity

Spasticity after stroke can significantly impact rehabilitation. The classic upper extremity flexor synergy pattern (i.e., adducted shoulder with flexed elbow, wrist, and fingers) can markedly interfere with function of the affected arm. Conversely, the classic lower extremity extensor synergy pattern (i.e., extended hip and knee and ankle plantar flexion) can be advantageous for ambulation if plantar flexion can be controlled by physical or pharmacologic agents. If untreated, these patterns can lead to abnormal positioning and contracture.

Treatment of spasticity after stroke should address positioning and exacerbating factors. Splinting or bracing, appropriate wheelchair sitting position, and physical therapy techniques are important to prevent contracture and promote motor recovery. Painful or noxious stimuli can exacerbate spasticity. Shoulder pain, pressure sores, deep venous thrombosis, bladder distention, and constipation are examples of stimuli that can exacerbate spasticity. Pharmacologic treatment should take into account the presence of these triggers because spasticity is likely to improve after the stimuli are resolved or relieved.

Pharmacologic treatment of post-stroke spasticity presents some challenges. Effective antispasticity agents such as baclofen (Lioresal) or tizanidine (Zanaflex) can cause somnolence or weaken unaffected muscles, which can significantly affect rehabilitation. Localized treatments such as botulinum toxin injections[1] or phenol[1] blocks can be useful, because treatment can be directed toward muscles that are affecting functional use of the limbs. Surgical interventions can be used for patients with severe spasticity limiting functional positioning or for those with the potential for functional grip if tendon lengthening or transfer can be considered.

Cognitive Dysfunction

Stroke patients can experience many cognitive deficits, including visuospatial neglect, cognitive-linguistic deficits, apraxia, memory loss, and attention deficits. Cognitive rehabilitation should concentrate on treatment of the specific deficits of the patient. Visuospatial rehabilitation (including scanning training) is recommended for deficits associated with visual neglect after right stroke. Cognitive-linguistic therapies are recommended for left hemispheric stroke patients with language deficits. Treatment of apraxia should include specific gestural and strategy training.

The use of medications that may impair cognitive function should be limited. Medications that are commonly considered during a stay in a rehabilitative facility that may have a significant impact on cognition and rehabilitation are highlighted in Table 1.

Depression and Neuropharmacology

Depression can be seen in up to one half of all stroke patients. It has been associated with poor functional outcomes and more severe impairments. Vegetative symptoms can have a significant impact on rehabilitative efforts because participation in therapy is critical.

Psychoactive drugs can be beneficial and should be considered. Selective serotonin reuptake inhibitors (SSRIs) are recommended in this population because of a better side effect profile and because of the undesirable anticholinergic side effects of tricyclic antidepressants (TCAs). In cases unresponsive to treatment with SSRIs, nortriptyline (Pamelor) may be helpful. In the rehabilitation setting when rapid short-term improvement in symptoms is necessary to increase participation in therapy, the use of psychostimulants (e.g., methylphenidate [Ritalin][1]) may be indicated. Table 1 shows the neuropharmacologic agents commonly used during stoke rehabilitation. Psychotherapy has been associated with modest improvement in post-stroke depression and is considered as part of a multidisciplinary approach.

---

[1]Not FDA approved for this indication.

[1]Not FDA approved for this indication.

TABLE 1 Neuropharmacologic Agents Commonly Used During Stroke Rehabilitation

Drug Class	Drug Name	Indication	Potential Problems
Benzodiazepines	Diazepam (Valium) Lorazepam (Ativan)	Agitation,[1] spasticity Agitation,[1] seizures	Sedation, confusion, sundowning Sedation, paradoxical reactions, confusion, sundowning
Tricyclic antidepressants (TCAs)	Nortriptyline (Pamelor)	Depression, neuropathic pain,[1] central pain[1]	Anticholinergic effects, sedation
Selective serotonin reuptake inhibitors (SSRIs)	Sertraline (Zoloft) Escitalopram (Lexapro) Citalopram (Celexa)	Depression, stimulation[1]	Long titration period, suicidal ideations, serotonin syndrome, syndrome of inappropriate antidiuretic hormone (SIADH), somnolence, seizures
Stimulants	Modafinil (Provigil) Methylphenidate (Ritalin)	Drowsiness,[1] decreased alertness,[1] impaired concentration,[1] diminished attention[1]	Arrhythmia, seizures, hepatotoxicity, blood pressure changes

[1] Not FDA approved for this indication.

Bladder Dysfunction

Bladder dysfunction after stroke depends on the stroke's location. During the rehabilitation phase, the most common problem is urinary incontinence and urgency associated with uninhibited bladder contraction. Ultrasound bladder scans (usually every 4 hours and after voiding) should be ordered to detect bladder distention and urinary retention. It is standard practice to intervene when bladder volumes are greater than 500 mL. If volumes exceed this cutoff point, intermittent catheterization should be started. Intermittent catheterization is preferable to indwelling catheters because the risk of urinary tract infection is higher with the latter. Bladder scans are usually discontinued when post-voiding residual volumes at 3- to 4-hour intervals are low (<150 mL) for a period of 24 to 48 hours.

Mobility and Use of Adaptive Equipment

Activity limitations vary among stroke survivors and can include difficulties with bed mobility, wheelchair propulsion, transfers, gait, stairs, and basic activities of daily living. The goal of physical therapy and occupational therapy is to maximize functional independence. Addressing mobility limitations is fundamental in stroke rehabilitation because it is related to long-term care needs and independence.

Transfer training comprises learning how to maneuver from one surface or height to another. Ideally, patients should learn to roll and transfer toward the involved and uninvolved sides; however, early mobility efforts are directed to the uninvolved side to minimize the risk of injury.

CURRENT THERAPY

- Stroke rehabilitation improves functional outcomes.
- A comprehensive rehabilitation team composed of physicians, nurses, therapists, and community reintegration professionals can achieve the best outcomes.
- Early evaluation of family support and the home environment is critical to prevent unnecessary institutionalization.
- Evaluation and management of modifiable stroke risk factors, such as smoking, hypertension, and diabetes, are imperative during stroke rehabilitation to prevent stroke recurrence.
- Rehabilitation of the stroke patient can be hindered by conditions such as pneumonia (usually caused by aspiration), deep venous thrombosis, urinary tract infections, shoulder pain, depression, and spasticity. Early identification and treatment of these conditions are necessary to maximize functional outcomes.

Gait deviations are common after stroke and interfere with safety and efficiency of locomotion. If an assistive device is needed, the goal of physical therapy is to progress to the least restrictive device possible. Hemiwalkers and wide-based quad canes provide the most stability. An ankle-foot orthosis may be indicated for patients with decreased ankle control and footdrop.

Instruction in ascending or descending stairs depends on assistive device requirements. With weakness, stairs are ascended by initiating movement with the uninvolved or stronger lower extremity. This process is reversed when descending.

For some stroke survivors, functional ambulation is not a realistic goal. In these cases, the wheelchair becomes the primary means of locomotion. Wheelchair prescription requires considerable skill and training and must take into account posturing, body habitus, cognition, physical fitness level, and the home environment. An appropriate wheelchair prescription is required to maximize mobility and prevent complications such as shoulder pain. Physical and occupational therapists should evaluate the patient to provide wheelchair recommendations to vendors.

Hemi-wheelchairs (i.e., wheelchairs situated closer to the ground) and one-arm drive wheelchairs allow hemiplegic patients to use the uninvolved side for wheelchair propulsion. Lap boards with arm supports can be added to improve hemiparetic arm posturing and sitting symmetry.

For some stroke survivors, the ability to return to driving is considered one of the most important long-term rehabilitation goals. Formal driving rehabilitation programs are available to evaluate and improve driver safety. Driver rehabilitation specialists perform vision, cognitive, and perceptual examinations. Perception tests assess reaction times to visual and auditory stimuli. Values for vision and reaction times are standardized and state dependent. Specialists should also perform a behind-the-wheel assessment, beginning in a parking lot and progressing to negotiation of more complex traffic situations. Many modifications can increase independence and assist with return to driving, including a spinner knob, which can be attached to the steering wheel to allow one-arm control; hand controls for acceleration and braking; left foot pedals to substitute for right foot impairment; and wheelchair lifts.

Adaptive equipment, including bracing, shoe modification, and other tools, increase independence through completion of activities of daily living (e.g., long-handled sponge, reacher, shoe horn, mirror, sock aids) and are extremely beneficial for those with moderate to severe strokes, particularly if hemiparesis is dense (Fig. 2). Silverware, pens, and other utensils can be modified for easier maneuverability. Multipodus boots can be used to prevent plantar flexion contracture development in the hemiparetic limb.

Falls

Falls are common after moderate to severe strokes. In rehabilitation settings, fall prevention usually requires a multimodal approach. Strategies include use of bed-chair alarms, placing those at risk close

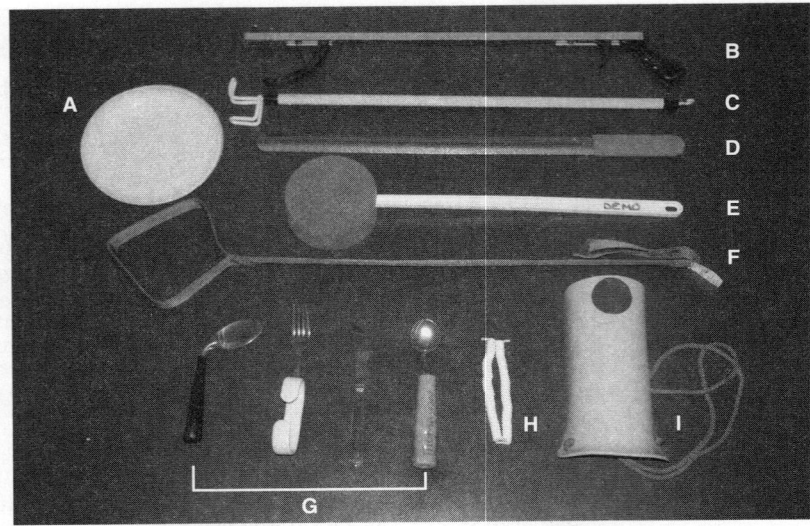

FIGURE 2. Adaptive equipment commonly used during stroke rehabilitation. The tapered front scoop dish (**A**) has non-skid feet to keep the plate from sliding. The curved edge simplifies scooping food. The dish is especially suited for individuals who have limited flexibility, have decreased motor coordination, or feed using one hand, such as a hemiparetic stroke patient. The reacher (**B**) is used to get items from the floor. The long-handled dressing aid (**C**) is used to reach clothes on the floor or to bring clothes up the paretic side. The long-handled shoe horn (**D**) aids with slipping into shoes. The long-handle sponge (**E**) is used for reaching the involved side while bathing or when the shoulder range of motion does not allow reaching. The leg lifter (**F**) and the sound upper limb can be used to assist in moving the paretic lower limb. Adapted feeding utensils (**G**) are used for patients with grip weakness or difficulties with upper limb range of motion; *left to right*: bent-handle spoon, no-grip fork, rocker bottom knife, and thick-handle spoon. No-tie laces (**H**) are elastic shoe-laces that do not require tying. When using the sock-donning aid (**I**), the sock slides onto the plastic portion of the device, and the strap is used to pull the sock with the device on the foot.

to the nursing station, wearing skid socks, limiting or refraining from polypharmacy, eliminating slick or irregular floors, and in some cases, providing a sitter for closer monitoring. Physical and occupational therapists must include general safety and fall recovery as part of the treatment plan.

Visual Impairment

Depending on the location of the stroke, the visual system may be involved. One of the most debilitating visual impairments is visuo-spatial neglect, a complication of right hemisphere strokes. Left-sided stimuli are not attended to or recognized, and affected individuals must learn to deal with this deficit. Other complications include gaze weakness or paralysis, diplopia, visual field loss, ptosis, tracking disorders, decreased visual acuity, and cortical blindness.

Screening for primary visual skills, including visual acuity, visual fields, and visual tracking, should be done by physiatrists, neurologists, and occupational therapists. If problems are identified, patients should be referred to neuro-ophthalmologists and low-vision rehabilitation programs. Visual acuity problems often can be addressed by incorporating the use of glasses into the therapy session or by changing the prescription. Eye movement disorders and visual field deficits usually lessen as time elapses and may respond to treatment with prisms, head positioning, and unilateral eye occlusion with tape or a patch technique. Those with continued visual field impairment should be taught eye movement techniques to expand the visual area.

Conclusions

Stroke rehabilitation requires the concerted efforts of the patient, family, and medical professionals. A multidisciplinary team with training to address the particular impairments and functional limitations of the stroke patient is critical. The physician's efforts should focus on preventing complications and treating stroke sequelae with the primary goal of improving overall function and participation in society.

REFERENCES

Bhakta BB. Management of spasticity in stroke. Br Med Bull 2000;56:476.

Cicerone KD, Dahlberg C, Malec JF, et al. Evidence-based cognitive rehabilitation: Updated review of the literature from 1998 through 2002. Arch Phys Med Rehabil 2005;86:1681.

Hackett ML, Anderson CS, House A, et al. Interventions for treating depression after stroke. Cochrane Database Syst Rev 2008;(4):CD003437.

Jones SA, Shinton RA. Improving outcome in stroke patients with visual problems. Age Ageing 2006;35:560.

Kelly-Hayes M, Beiser A, Kase CS, et al. The influence of gender and age on disability following ischemic stroke: The Framingham Study. J Stroke Cerebrovasc Dis 2003;12:119.

Lannin NA, Cusick A, McCluskey A, et al. Effects of splinting on wrist contracture after stroke: A randomized controlled trial. Stroke 2007;38:111.

Legg L, Drummond A, Leonardi-Bee J, et al. Occupational therapy for patients with problems in personal activities of daily living after stroke: Systematic review of randomised trials. BMJ 2007;335:922.

Pertoldi S, Di Benedetto P. Shoulder-hand syndrome after stroke. A complex regional pain syndrome. Eura Medicophys 2005;41:283.

Poole D, Chaudry F, Jay WM. Stroke and driving. Top Stroke Rehabil 2008;15:37.

Starkstein SE, Mizrahi R, Power BD. Antidepressant therapy in post-stroke depression. Expert Opin Pharmacother 2008;9:1291.

Stein J. Stroke. In: Frontera WR, Silver JK, editors. Essentials of Physical Medicine and Rehabilitation. Philadelphia: WB Saunders; 2002. pp. 778–83.

Stein J, Harvey RL, Macko RF, et al, editors. Stroke Recovery & Rehabilitation. New York: Demos Medical Publishing; 2009.

Umphred DA. Neurological Rehabilitation. St Louis: Mosby Elsevier Health Science; 1995.

van Wijk I, Algra A, van de Port IG, et al. Change in mobility activity in the second year after stroke in a rehabilitation population: Who is at risk for decline? Arch Phys Med Rehabil 2006;87:45.

Wolf SL, Winstein CJ, Miller JP, et al. Effect of constraint-induced movement therapy on upper extremity function 3 to 9 months after stroke: The EXCITE randomized clinical trial. JAMA 2006;296:2095.

Seizures and Epilepsy in Adolescents and Adults

Method of
Utku Uysal, MD, and Nathan B. Fountain, MD

With the advent of more sophisticated diagnostic tools and newer antiepileptic medications, the recognition and diagnosis of seizures and epilepsy has become more important in today's clinical practice. Because of their paroxysmal nature and varied presentation, seizures have a broad differential diagnosis. Therefore, a systematic approach to the diagnosis is paramount. The steps should include confirming that the paroxysmal symptom of concern is a seizure, determining the type of seizure present, classifying it as focal or generalized in onset, determining the neuroanatomic site of seizure onset to direct investigations toward identifying pathology at that site, identifying the etiology or determining the epilepsy syndrome if the etiology is not identifiable, and selecting the appropriate therapy.

A seizure is a change in behavior caused by transient, abnormal, self-limited paroxysmal hypersynchronous electrical activity of cortical neurons. Seizure symptoms depend on whether the seizure is focal or generalized, the spread of the discharge in the brain, and the function of the affected brain region. Epilepsy is a disorder of the brain characterized by an enduring predisposition to generate epileptic seizures, and diagnosis requires that at least one epileptic seizure has occurred. However this definition, which is different from the classic definition that mandates recurrent unprovoked seizures to diagnose epilepsy, is still controversial owing to various concerns such as inappropriate inclusion of acute symptomatic seizures and what defines the enduring predisposition to generate epileptic seizures.

Seizures sometimes result from transient brain problems that disturb normal neuronal physiology such as acute head trauma, metabolic abnormalities, intoxication, and overdose or withdrawal from substances. When due to transient brain problems, seizures are generally termed *acute symptomatic seizures* and do not constitute epilepsy because they do not have an enduring tendency to seizures. "Epilepsy" is only used when seizures result from an enduring underlying tendency to seizures, such as from structural brain abnormalities like tumors, stroke, vascular abnormalities, long-term sequelae of trauma, or a defined epilepsy syndrome.

Epilepsy syndromes are diseases that are characterized exclusively or primarily by the occurrence of seizures with few other systemic or neurologic symptoms. When the etiology of seizures is definitely known, for example when they are caused by a brain tumor or penetrating brain injury, then classification into an epilepsy syndrome is less important. However, when the etiology is not known because it is not identifiable or the evaluation is incomplete, then classification becomes useful. Patients grouped into a specific epilepsy syndrome are presumed to share a similar pathophysiology and therefore a similar natural history and response to therapy. Patients with classic named epilepsy syndromes have fairly homogeneous presentations.

Epidemiology

Epilepsy is a common chronic disease. Epilepsy occurs at some time of life in approximately 3% of people. In the majority of both prevalence and incidence studies, men seem to be effected more than women, but the difference is minimal. The incidence of epilepsy is highest in the very young and old in developed countries. In developing countries, the peak prevalence of epilepsy is seen in adolescents and young adults. Universally the incidence of epilepsy is high in infants and children.

Classification of Epileptic Seizures and Epilepsy Syndromes

To have a common language and facilitate communication among physicians, the International League Against Epilepsy (ILAE) developed a standardized classification system and terminology in 1981 for epileptic seizures and in 1989 for epilepsy syndromes (Fig. 1 and Table 1). According to the 1981 ILAE Classification of Epileptic Seizures, seizures are mainly divided into two categories: partial and generalized. *Partial seizures* arise from one discrete region of one cerebral hemisphere. Preservation or impairment of consciousness is an important factor in partial seizure classification. If

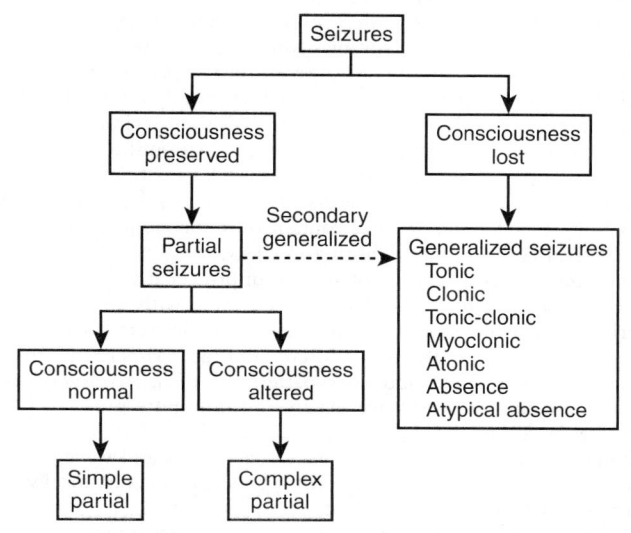

FIGURE 1. Algorithm of seizure classification.

TABLE 1 Examples of Epilepsy Syndromes in Adolescents and Adults

	Focal (localizaton related)	Generalized
Idiopathic	Benign childhood epilepsy with centrotemporal spikes	Childhood absence epilepsy
	Autosomal dominant nocturnal frontal lobe epilepsy	Juvenile absence epilepsy
		Juvenile myoclonic epilepsy
Symptomatic	Temporal lobe	Cortical malformations
	Frontal lobe	Cortical Dysplasias
	Parietal lobe	Metabolic abnormalities
	Occipital lobe	West's syndrome
		Lennox-Gastaut syndrome
Cryptogenic	Any occurrence of partial seizures without obvious pathology	West's syndrome (unidentified pathology)
		Lennox-Gastaut syndrome (unidentified pathology)

consciousness is preserved, the seizure is classified as *simple partial seizure,* and impairment of consciousness is present in *complex partial seizure.*

Simple partial seizures arise in a small region of cortex and give discrete symptoms, depending on the area from which they arise, without altering consciousness. For example, seizures arising in the primary motor cortex in the frontal lobe cause clonic jerking of the contralateral limb, usually the hand. The most common simple partial seizures are indescribable auras arising in the temporal lobe and causing autonomic symptoms or auras. Complex partial seizures are characterized by staring with a fixed gaze and lack of distractibility to examiners. Automatisms are common, especially picking or pulling at clothing, lip smacking, and swallowing.

Generalized seizures result from involvement of both cerebral hemispheres at the initiation of a seizure. Therefore, impaired consciousness is the first sign. The motor manifestations are bilateral, and an electroencephalogram (EEG) recorded during the seizure shows activity starting simultaneously over the entire scalp. Generalized seizures are classified based on the predominant motor activity. *Generalized tonic–clonic* (GTC) *seizures* begin with sudden tonic extension of the extremities, often with an expiratory scream, followed by clonic rhythmic jerking of the extremities. Postictally, patients are always unresponsiveness for at least a brief period and usually sleep for minutes to hours. *Tonic seizures* contain only the tonic phase and *clonic seizures* contain only the clonic phase. *Myoclonic seizures* are a brief lightning-like jerk, most commonly of the arms. *Atonic seizures* consist of sudden unprotected falling with loss of muscle tone. *Absence seizures* are associated with nondistractible staring, similar to complex partial seizures, but are very brief, are frequent, occur primarily in children, and are associated with a generalized 3-Hz spike-and-wave pattern on EEG. *Atypical absence seizures* are similar to absence seizures but are more prolonged and are often accompanied by brief myoclonic jerks or loss of tone, and the EEG shows a slow or atypical generalized spike-and-wave pattern. *Secondarily generalized seizures* occur when seizures start focally and spread to involve the whole brain.

The underlying pathology or etiology of seizures ultimately determines the natural history and, to some degree, the response to therapy. To help clinicians make appropriate decisions regarding the evaluation and treatment of patients with epilepsy, the ILAE has established a systematic approach to epilepsy classification (the epilepsy syndromes).

The most important division of epilepsy syndromes is into *focal (localization-related) epilepsies* in which there is pathology localized to one region of the brain, and *generalized epilepsies* in which the pathology is expressed throughout the whole brain. Focal epilepsies generally occur with simple partial, complex partial, or secondary GTC seizures. Generalized epilepsies typically occur with primary generalized seizures such as absence, primary GTC, atonic, or myoclonic seizures. The epilepsies can be further subdivided based on the type of etiology into three categories: syndromes that are *symptomatic* of an identified underlying brain lesion; *cryptogenic* syndromes, in which an anatomic lesion is suspected but cannot be identified with current technology; and *idiopathic* syndromes, in which an identifiable lesion is neither identified nor suspected. The idiopathic syndromes are primarily caused by inherited abnormalities of neurotransmission without an anatomic lesion. The importance of the latter distinction is that an aggressive search for underlying pathology is not necessary or indicated for idiopathic epilepsies, but it is necessary for cryptogenic cases.

Two common types of epilepsy encountered in the adult population are temporal lobe epilepsy and juvenile myoclonic epilepsy, which can be used to illustrate the difference between symptomatic focal epilepsies and idiopathic generalized epilepsies. Temporal lobe epilepsy is a focal epilepsy characterized by refractory complex partial seizures with occasional secondary generalization, originating in the temporal lobe. If neuroimaging is normal, the patient is said to suffer from "cryptogenic focal epilepsy," the most common type of epilepsy in adults. Quite often, however, MRI demonstrates atrophy and gliosis of the hippocampus in the temporal lobe. Histopathologically, this is represented by neuronal loss and gliosis of the hippocampus and

several mesial temporal structures, giving rise to the term "mesial temporal sclerosis." Mass lesions in the temporal lobe can occur in a manner similar to this and include malformations, tumors such as astrocytomas and dysembryoplastic neuroepithelial tumors (DNET), and other focal pathology. Patients with anatomic abnormalities on MRI are said to suffer from "symptomatic focal epilepsy." Temporal lobe epilepsy is important to recognize because temporal lobectomy renders more than 60% of patients essentially seizure-free. This contrasts with juvenile myoclonic epilepsy, an idiopathic generalized epilepsy, which begins in adolescence or early adulthood with myoclonic and GTC seizures that are well controlled with medications in 85% of patients, although the underlying tendency to seizures is life-long. Obviously, patients with juvenile myoclonic epilepsy, are not candidates for resective surgery.

Although it has been extensively useful and well accepted in daily practice and in research settings, the classification of epilepsies has come under review because of the advent of more-advanced diagnostic tools such as video EEG monitoring, neuroimaging, and better knowledge of pathophysiology of epilepsy in the last 20 years. Today the 1981 and 1989 classifications for epileptic seizures and epilepsy syndromes are still valid. However, revisions were proposed in 2001 to include ictal phenomenology, seizure type, syndrome, etiology, and impairment of consciousness and updated in 2006 to consider pathophysiologic mechanisms, neuronal substrates, response to antiepileptic drugs (AEDs), ictal EEG patterns, propagation patterns and postictal features.

Diagnosis

The evaluation of *a first seizure* is aimed at determining whether it was provoked by a transient cause or is the first seizure resulting from underlying epilepsy. It is also important to exclude acute life-threatening etiologies, such as infection, neoplasm, or hemorrhage. Most patients seek emergency care after the first seizure. At that time it is usually not possible to determine whether this represents epilepsy or an acute medical illness. Consequently, simple screening laboratory tests may be indicated including electrolytes, complete blood count, liver enzymes, and urine drug screen to rule out acute problems that might cause provoked seizures such as infections, electrolyte abnormalities, organ dysfunction, and intoxication or drug overdose. If CNS infection is suspected, then lumbar puncture should

---

 CURRENT DIAGNOSIS

Consider a Nonepileptic Origin for the Paroxysmal Event

- Syncope, migraine, transient ischemic attack, sleep disorder, movement disorder, hypoglycemia, psychiatric disease

Exclude General Medical Etiology for the First seizure

- Laboratory tests: complete blood count, electrolytes, glucose, liver enzymes, urine drug screen
- Perform lumbar puncture, if central nervous system infection is considered
- Neuroimaging, preferably magnetic resonance imaging (MRI). Computed tomography (CT) is acceptable in the acute setting to rule out hemorrhage (neoplasms may be missed by head CT)

Characterize Seizure Type and Etiology or Epilepsy Syndrome

- High-resolution MRI
- Routine electroencephalogram (EEG). If routine EEG is unrevealing, consider sleep-deprived EEG.
- Consider inpatient video EEG monitoring to capture the events if seizures occur at least once per week.

be performed. An EEG is always indicated in adults because it might reveal interictal epileptiform discharges of the type present in patients with epilepsy, but it is not needed acutely. Neuroimaging is always indicated in the evaluation of a partial-onset seizure to exclude acute or serious focal pathology. The imaging technique of choice is an MRI scan, but if MRI is not available, a noncontrast head CT may be substituted in the acute setting.

The evaluation of *recurrent seizures* is aimed at defining the underlying cause of the epilepsy syndrome, which is usually more subtle. An EEG is always indicated because it might reveal focal epileptiform discharges and assist in classifying the seizure type and epilepsy syndrome. However, a normal EEG does not exclude epilepsy. The first EEG is abnormal in only about 40% of patients with clinically definite epilepsy. The EEG remains normal in approximately 40% of these patients, even after as many as seven EEGs.

The diagnostic evaluation of intractable epilepsy is intertwined with the presurgical evaluation and is discussed later.

Differential Diagnosis of Paroxysmal Symptoms

Because epileptic seizures vary broadly in symptomatic presentation, there are many symptoms that can mimic an epileptic seizure, particularly syncope, migraine, transient ischemic attack (TIA), movement disorders, and psychogenic nonepileptic pseudoseizures. Detailed information from the patient and a witness about the triggering factors, prodromal symptoms, ictal phase, and postictal phase are of paramount importance. Common triggering factors are sleep deprivation, drug intake, and alcohol withdrawal. Prodromal symptoms can be déjà vu, an epigastric rising sensation, visual hallucinations, or altered smell or taste preceding the onset of the seizure. Witnesses should be questioned about altered consciousness, duration of each phase, automatism, or head turning; abnormal movements such as tonic, tonic–clonic, or myoclonic activity and the spread of the abnormal movements if they start focally; falling; urinary or bowel incontinence; and tongue biting. Duration of postictal confusion, tiredness, sleeping, focal neurologic signs, and muscle aches extending to the next day often, or usually, follow a GTC seizure; it is extremely rare for someone to recover full consciousness immediately after a GTC seizure.

Syncope is commonly accompanied by motor movements, especially clonic or brief tonic arm movements, termed *convulsive syncope* or a *syncopal seizure*, during which the EEG shows profound suppression of brain activity due to cerebral anoxia; it does not show seizure discharges. Convulsive syncope is not an epileptic seizure. Syncope is distinguished from an epileptic seizure by the presence of presyncopal symptoms (nausea, flushing, and lightheadedness), brief loss of consciousness, and the return of normal cognition within a few seconds after arousal. Motor symptoms such as clonic jerking or stiffening often accompany prolonged syncope and can resemble an epileptic seizure; however, consciousness returns immediately after syncope despite the motor symptoms but does not return for at least minutes after a GTC seizure.

Migraine headaches are occasionally accompanied by complex visual phenomena or sensorimotor symptoms, which could be confused with seizures. However, visual auras associated with seizures are usually shorter than 30 seconds whereas migraine auras tend to evolve over minutes. Postictal headaches may be confused with migraine. Complicated migraine with hemiparesis may be mistaken for a postictal paralysis. A history of migraine headaches and preservation of normal consciousness help identify the spells as migraine. Rarely, basilar migraines and acute confusional migraine may be accompanied by loss of consciousness.

TIAs should almost never be mistaken for seizures because TIAs of carotid artery territory origin usually cause focal negative phenomena, such as weakness, numbness, aphasia, or ataxia, whereas seizures usually cause positive phenomena such as jerking, tingling, automatisms, or movements. TIAs of vertebrobasilar artery territory origin occasionally cause loss of consciousness and falls that could be confused with seizures, but vertebrobasilar TIA is usually accompanied by neighborhood signs. Transient global amnesia, which is sudden-onset alteration of anterograde memory and confusion, can mimic seizures and nonconvulsive status epilepticus. Patients with transient global amnesia can perform complex tasks such as calculating, reading, and writing despite appearing confused, whereas patients with nonconvulsive status epilepticus cannot.

Some movement disorders, sleep disorders, and hypoglycemia also mimic seizures. Cataplexy attacks of narcolepsy precipitated by emotional stimuli manifest with sudden loss of muscle tone but preservation of consciousness. Other narcolepsy symptoms such as excessive daytime sleepiness, hypnagogic hallucinations, and sleep paralysis help to make the diagnosis. Parasomnias, arousal disorders, and periodic limb movements in sleep can rarely be confused with epileptic seizures.

Psychiatric disease can manifest with symptoms nearly identical to seizures. Anxiety attacks can be characterized by anxiety, palpitation, facial flushing, and incoherence, and so can seizure auras. Seizure auras usually progress to complex partial seizures at some point in the evolution of epilepsy, and seizure auras are usually more stereotyped than anxiety attacks. Pseudoseizures, which are also termed *psychogenic nonepileptic seizures*, may be identical to seizures in their presentation. However, pseudoseizures are more likely to be long in duration, involve bizarre or unusual symptoms and movements, have pelvic thrusting or thrashing, may be precipitated by psychologically stressful events, and persist despite treatment with AEDs. Unfortunately, epileptic seizures can also have these characteristics, and video/EEG monitoring may be the only way to definitively distinguish seizures from pseudoseizures. Surprisingly, as many as 30% of patients admitted to inpatient epilepsy units for the diagnosis of spells are found to have pseudoseizures.

Treatment

ANTIEPILEPTIC DRUG THERAPY

The clinician faces the challenge of choosing the best AED from among 14 AEDs available. This requires the clinician to consider the spectrum of efficacy, pharmacokinetic and pharmacodynamic properties, and the patient's comorbidities (Tables 2 and 3). The aim of treatment should be complete freedom from seizures and no side effects. When initiating therapy it is best to "start low and go slow." Most side effects are experienced at the initiation of therapy and can be avoided by starting with a low enough dose and increasing more slowly than recommended by the manufacturer. The maintenance doses cover a wide range because there is no set final dose for any of the AEDs (see Table 2).

CURRENT THERAPY

- Select an antiepileptic drug by seizure type and epilepsy syndrome.
- Consider side-effect profile, dosing schedule, drug interactions, and cost.
- "Start low and go slow" in starting antiepileptic drug therapy.
- Increase dose to maximum tolerated dose before changing.
- Substitute one drug at a time in an attempt to achieve monotherapy.
- Refer to an epilepsy center for consideration of surgery if seizures are refractory to two antiepileptic drugs.
- After a seizure-free period of at least 2 years, withdrawal of antiepileptic drugs may be considered for cryptogenic epilepsy or syndromes known to resolve.
- Risk of seizure recurrence upon withdrawal of antiepileptic drugs is lowest if magnetic resonance imaging and follow-up electroencephalogram are both normal and the etiology is cryptogenic.

TABLE 2 Dose and Side Effect Profile of Commonly Prescribed Antiepileptic Drugs

Drug	Half-life (hours)	Initial Dose (mg)	Maintenance Dose (mg)	Increment (mg)	Dosing Schedule	Adverse Effects
Carbamazepine (Tegretol)	12-17 h	200 mg bid	600-1800[3] mg	200 mg q wk	tid-qid	Hyponatremia, leukopenia, rare aplastic anemia and hepatitis
Gabapentin (Neurontin)	5-7 h	300 mg qd	1200-3600 mg	300 mg q3-7d	tid	60% removed by hemodialysis, prolonged half life to 51 h with hemodialysis. Dosed 300 mg after hemodialysis
Lacosamide (Vimpat)	13 h	50 mg qd	300-600[3] mg	100 mg q wk	bid	Extra 50% of dose after each hemodialysis. Can prolong PR interval at high doses
Lamotrigine (Lamictal)	25 h alone 60 h with VPA	6.25-12.5 mg qd to qod	400 mg alone 100 mg with VPA	12.5-25 mg q2wk	bid	Life-threatening rash, especially with rapid titration and VPA. Titration and maintenance doses vary based on other AEDs
Levetiracetam (Keppra)	7 h	500 mg qd	2000-4000[3] mg	500 mg q wk	bid	Decrease dose in chronic renal insufficiency, severe hepatic disease
Oxcarbazepine (Trileptal)	9-11 h	300 mg qd	900-2400 mg	300 mg q wk	bid	Hyponatremia. Fewer side effects than carbamazepine
Phenobarbital	80-100 h	30-60 mg qd	60-120 mg	30 mg q1-2wk	qd-bid	Sedation, Dupuytren's contractures, rebound seizures with rapid tapering
Phenytoin (Dilantin)	22 h	200 mg qd	200-300 mg	100 mg q wk	qd-bid	Gum hypertrophy, hirsutism, cerebellar ataxia or atrophy, peripheral neuropathy, rare hypersensitity, hepatitis
Pregabalin (Lyrica)	6 h	50 mg qd	150-600 mg	50 mg q 3-7d	bid-tid	Weight gain
Topiramate (Topamax)	21 h	25 mg qd	200-400 mg	25 mg q1-2wk	bid	Cognitive impairment at >400 mg/day, rare kidney stones, glaucoma, oligohidrosis
Valproic acid (Depakene)	9-16 h	250 mg qd	750-3000 mg	250 mg q 3-7 d	tid-qid	Tremor, weight gain, alopecia, thrombocytopenia. Rare hepatitis and pancreatitis. Risk of teratogenesis and neural tube defects
Zonisamide (Zonegran)	63 h	100 mg qd	200-400 mg	100 mg q 2 wk	bid	Kidney stones, oligohidrosis, rare blood dyscrasias

[3]Exceeds dosage recommended by the manufacturer.
Abbreviations: AED = antiepileptic drug; VPA = valproic acid.

TABLE 3 Choice of Antiepileptic Drug in Special Situations

Special Situation	Drug of Choice	Comments
Partial Seizures	Carbamazepine, lamotrigine, levetiracetam, oxcarbazepine, topiramate, gabapentin	
Refractory partial seizures	Lacosamide, pregabalin, zonisamide	Second-line treatment
Generalized epilepsies	Lamotrigine, topiramate, valproic acid,[1] zonisamide[1]	Avoid valproic acid in women
Absence seizures	Ethosuximide, lamotrigine,[1] valproic acid, topiramate[1]	Ethosuximide is the choice for only pure absence seizures and is insufficient in other associated generalized tonic–clonic or myoclonic seizures
Juvenile myoclonic epilepsy	Valproic acid,[1] topiramate,[1] lamotrigine,[1] zonisamide,[1] levetiracetam	Avoid valproic acid in women
Myoclonic seizures	Clonazepam, valproic acid,[1] levetiracetam	Lamotrigine occasionally exacerbates myoclonic seizures
Women of childbearing potential	Lamotrigine, topiramate, levetiracetam, oxcarbazepine	Avoid enzyme-inducing agents that alter steroid hormones and OCP levels; use OCPs with ≥50 µg of estrogen; OCPs increase the elimination of lamotrigine. Significant increased risk of teratogenicity with valproic acid
Elderly patients	Lamotrigine, gabapentin, levetiracetam, topiramate	Avoid polypharmacy and highly protein-bound AEDs and AEDs with high drug-drug interactions
Depression	Lamotrigine,[1] topiramate[1]	
Bipolar disorder	Valproic acid,[1] carbamazepine, lamotrigine, topiramate[1]	
Migraine	Valproic acid, topiramate	Consider the choice according to sex, side effect profile, and seizure type
Chronic pain	Pregabalin,[1] gabapentin[1]	
Neuropathic pain	Carbamazepine,[1] gabapentin,[1] pregabalin	

[1]Not FDA approved for this indication.
Abbreviations: AED = antiepileptic drug; OCP = oral contraceptive pill.

The only method to determine that a given AED dose is therapeutic is to determine that the seizure frequency has decreased. Serum drug levels are available for conventional and essentially all new AEDs, but the levels of new AEDs are of very limited utility because they are effective over a very wide range of serum levels. Most patients do not need routine monitoring of blood levels. In some instances drug levels can provide a general guide, but many patients will be on a therapeutic dose while their blood level is below the usual "normal" range. On the other hand, blood levels can help guide dosage increases by warning that toxic side effects might occur with further increases when the blood level is at the upper limit of the established therapeutic range. Nonetheless, it is important to increase each drug to the maximum tolerated dose before labeling it ineffective. This usually requires increasing the drug until side effects occur and then reducing the dosage by one step. Patients must be informed of this strategy or they might refuse to take the drug, even at a lower dose. If seizure control does not improve or side effects occur at low doses, then checking a serum level can help to uncover unexpectedly low levels due to fast metabolism or noncompliance, a problem especially common among adolescents.

When substituting one AED for another it is important to start the second drug and determine that it is effective before gradually withdrawing the first drug. This affords at least some protection from seizures at all times. After a 2-year seizure-free period, a trial of drug withdrawal should be considered in patients with cryptogenic epilepsy. The risk of seizure recurrence after drug withdrawal is lowest in patients who have a normal MRI and EEG and do not have adult-onset idiopathic epilepsy. Drug withdrawal is usually not logical in patients who have an epilepsy syndrome with a known life-long tendency to seizures, such as juvenile myoclonic epilepsy.

CHARACTERISTICS OF SPECIFIC ANTIEPILEPTIC DRUGS

Phenytoin

Phenytoin (Dilantin, Phenytek) is the most widely used and familiar AED despite having the most problematic side effects. Mechanism of action is thought to be through use-dependent sodium channel blockade. The metabolism of phenytoin is saturable, which means that it shows zero-order kinetics at high blood levels. Very steep elevations in the blood level can occur with even small dose increases when the blood level is near 20 µg/mL, despite the occurrence of a linear increase in the blood level with dose increases when blood levels are below 20 µg/mL. For example, the blood level may be 10 µg/mL with 200 mg/day and then increase to 15 µg/mL with 300 mg/day and then increase to 20 µg/mL with 400 mg/day but with an increase to 500 mg/day the level might skyrocket to more than 30 µg/mL if metabolism is saturated.

Phenytoin's idiosyncratic side effects of hepatitis and blood dyscrasias are rare. Cumulative side effects of phenytoin occur over many years, including gum hypertrophy, hirsutism, coarsening of features, ataxia due to cerebellar atrophy, peripheral neuropathy, and osteoporosis. All patients on phenytoin should receive supplemental calcium and vitamin D because phenytoin induces the metabolism of vitamin D, thus lowering its level and causing osteoporosis. Phenytoin is prone to drug-drug interactions, and it increases clearance of oral contraceptives and decreases their effectiveness.

Intravenous phenytoin solution is very basic (pH 11), which often causes venous irritation and can cause purple glove syndrome and severe acute necrosis leading to amputation. Intravenous phenytoin is mixed in polyethylene glycol, causing bradycardia and hypotension, which limits the rate of infusion to less than 50 mg/minute. This can be a significant problem in the treatment of status epilepticus or frequent seizures. Fosphenytoin (Cerebyx) is a phenytoin prodrug in which the phosphate group is rapidly cleaved off upon entering the bloodstream, yielding phenytoin. It is mixed in an aqueous solution and has a more neutral pH; thus it is much better tolerated and can be given as fast as 150 mg/min.

Carbamazepine

Carbamazepine (Carbatrol, Tegretol), like phenytoin, is metabolized by and induces hepatic metabolism. It also undergoes autoinduction, inducing its own metabolism for up to 3 weeks after initiating it, so that steady-state blood levels are not achieved for several weeks. Carbamazepine has a relatively narrow therapeutic window, with usual therapeutic blood levels of between 7 µg/mL and 12 µg/mL. It has a similar mechanism of action to phenytoin's. It is indicated for simple partial, complex partial, and GTC seizures. It commonly causes acute toxicity (ataxia, diplopia, and lethargy) with only a small increase in the dose.

Carbamazepine does not have cumulative side effects but rarely causes serious idiosyncratic side effects including blood dyscrasias, hepatitis and hyponatremia. Mild leukopenia is common and does not require intervention unless the white blood cell count falls below 3000 per mm³. Very rarely it can cause bone marrow suppression with aplastic anemia. Extended-release preparations, which can be dosed twice daily, are preferable to standard preparations, which must be dosed every 8 hours. Like phenytoin, it increases the clearance of oral contraceptives and decreases their effectiveness.

Valproic Acid

Valproic acid is available as valproic acid (Depakene) and sodium divalproex (Depakote) and in an extended-release form (Depakote ER). Valproic acid affects many systems and so has several potential mechanisms of action, including through sodium-channel blockade and augmenting γ-aminobutyric acid (GABA) inhibition. It is most commonly used for primary generalized seizures such as in juvenile myoclonic epilepsy[1] and syndromes with absence seizures, but it is also effective for focal seizures. It often causes dyspepsia and other gastrointestinal side effects. Sodium divalproex is immediately cleaved to valproate in the stomach, but this preparation has much better gastrointestinal tolerance. Valproate is usually dosed every 8 hours because of its relatively short half-life. Depakote ER was approved for once-daily dosing for migraine headaches, but it is actually released over less than 24 hours, so twice-daily dosing is more useful for the treatment of epilepsy. Valproate is available as an intravenous preparation (Depacon), dosed identical to the oral forms.

Valproate is usually well tolerated but it occasionally causes weight gain, alopecia, tremor, and thrombocytopenia. It can cause potentially fatal hepatitis and pancreatitis. Hepatitis occurs in only 1 in 40,000 adult patient exposures, but it is much more common in children (as many as 1 in 500) who are taking multiple AEDs and have mental retardation, possibly because they have an undiagnosed metabolic abnormality. It has been suggested that l-carnitine (levocarnitine, Carnitor)[1] supplementation might reduce the risk of hepatitis. Although this has not been demonstrated, it is prudent for children who have unknown causes of mental retardation and who are taking valproate to take carnitine.

The overall risk of birth defects associated with valproate is approximately 10%, and the rate is only approximately 2% in the general population and seemingly not more than approximately 4% for any other AED. Of even greater concern, is that valproate is more often associated with neural tube defects such as spina bifida. Folic acid supplementation at 4 mg/day is recommended because it reduces the risk of neural tube defects in all pregnant women. Valproate is a poor choice for women of childbearing potential, and if they are on valproate, they should use an effective method of birth control and take folic acid.

Phenobarbital

Phenobarbital has fallen out of favor as an AED because it occasionally induces lethargy, depression, and learning difficulties. However, it is usually well tolerated in adults, is effective for partial-onset and primary GTC seizures, is inexpensive, and can be given intravenously. It can be dosed once per day and has a very long half-life, which is an advantage in poorly compliant patients. Primidone (Mysoline) is an infrequently used prodrug of phenobarbital that also has its own antiseizure effects but less often causes lethargy.

Ethosuximide

Ethosuximide (Zarontin) is unique because it is the only AED that is effective exclusively for absence seizures and is not effective for other

---

[1]Not FDA approved for this indication.

types of seizures. It is usually well tolerated but occasionally causes nausea, anorexia, headache, and blood dyscrasias. It can be dosed once per day because of its very long half-life, but it is usually better tolerated dosed twice daily.

Felbamate

Felbamate (Felbatol) is highly effective for the most intractable epilepsies, such as the Lennox-Gastaut syndrome, as well as for partial-onset seizures despite frequent side effects of anorexia, insomnia, and agitation and the common occurrence of AED interactions. However, it can cause aplastic anemia and fulminant hepatitis so that it is only indicated for intractable epilepsy, in cases where the potential benefit outweighs the risk of potentially fatal side effects. Its use should probably be limited to epilepsy centers.

Gabapentin

Gabapentin (Neurontin) is very well tolerated and has no pharmacokinetic interactions because it is renally excreted unchanged. It is indicated for partial seizures with and without secondary generalization. It has engendered an unwarranted poor reputation as an AED because some have thought that it is ineffective. Clinical studies examined doses that statistically reduced the frequency of seizures with minimal side effects but were not high enough to determine the maximum tolerated dose; thus it was approved and initially used at relatively low doses of 900 to 1800 mg/day. However, clinical experience suggests that doses of as much as 3600 mg/day may be required to be effective for most patients. On the other hand, very high doses might not increase blood levels because drug absorption may be saturated at doses above 4000 mg/day.

Lamotrigine

Lamotrigine (Lamictal) is particularly useful because it is effective for partial seizures, generalized seizures, and Lennox-Gastaut syndrome. It is severely affected by hepatic enzyme–inducing or -inhibiting AEDs so that its dosing is drastically different depending on concomitant AEDs. When taken alone (or with a combination of an enzyme inducer and inhibitor), the half-life of lamotrigine is about 25 hours, but this is reduced to 12 hours when it is taken with enzyme inducers (such as phenytoin, phenobarbital, carbamazepine) and prolonged to as much as 60 hours when taken with valproate, an enzyme inhibitor. Oral contraceptives decrease the half life to 12 hours, necessitating dose adjustment.

The only potentially serious side effect of lamotrigine is rash. Mild rash is common and was present in as many as 1 in 50 children and 1 in 1000 adults during initial clinical studies. The rash can be life threatening in the form of Stevens-Johnson syndrome or toxic epidermal necrolysis, but the incidence of serious rash, as lamotrigine is used today, is probably only about 1 in 40,000. The rash is most likely to occur after the first 3 weeks of therapy but can occur at any time, and it is more common with high initial doses and titration rates and when taken with valproic acid. A slow titration rate decreases the risk of rash. As a matter of fact, the rate is so slow that patients are unlikely to see an effect for many weeks or months and can require encouragement from the physician. When a rash is reported, the patient must be examined immediately, and serious consideration must be given to stopping the drug.

Levetiracetam

Levetiracetam (Keppra) is very well tolerated and has not been associated with serious side effects. It occasionally causes significant irritability that necessitates stopping the drug. It can be titrated relatively rapidly so that its effectiveness in a patient can be determined in a few months. It is primarily excreted unchanged, so it does not have significant drug interactions.

Oxcarbazepine

Oxcarbazepine (Trileptal) is a derivative of carbamazepine, and its mechanism of action is similar to carbamazepine's. The primary CNS side effects of carbamazepine are due to epoxide-10,11-carbamazepine, a metabolite produced by oxidation. Oxcarbazepine cannot undergo this conversion and thus does not produce this metabolite. Therefore, it is better tolerated than carbamazepine and is less likely to cause diplopia and ataxia, although it is not clear whether it causes less sedation. The incidence of blood dyscrasias also appears lower than with carbamazepine, but hyponatremia seems more common than with carbamazepine. It does not induce AED-metabolizing liver enzymes (although it does affect other liver enzymes) or undergo autoinduction. The daily dose cannot be directly converted from the carbamazepine dose. It is effective as monotherapy, so it is likely that in the future oxcarbazepine will entirely replace carbamazepine.

Tiagabine

Tiagabine (Gabitril) is approved as add-on therapy for partial-onset seizures. It is the only AED that was designed for a specific mechanism of action; it inhibits the reuptake of GABA in the synaptic cleft. It has a very short serum half-life, but it affects the GABA transporter for at least 12 hours so that it can be dosed twice a day. Some patients require more frequent dosing. It is not associated with any end-organ toxicity, but it can exacerbate myoclonic and absence seizures and precipitate nonconvulsive status epilepticus in those who are predisposed, usually patients with generalized epilepsy. Thus, it is uncommonly prescribed.

Topiramate

Topiramate (Topamax) is effective for partial seizures and some types of generalized seizures, especially the Lennox-Gastaut syndrome. It has acquired an unwarranted reputation for causing cognitive side effects. The source of this is probably the design of clinical studies, which appropriately determined the maximum tolerated dose by finding the dose at which an unacceptable incidence of side effects occurs. Considering all topiramate clinical studies together, the incidence of subject dropout in those treated with more than 400 mg/day was twice that of the group treated with less than 400 mg/day, which was approximately equal to dropout in the placebo group. This indicates that the average maximum tolerated dose is about 400 mg/day and so it should usually be used at a dose lower than this. Topiramate is a weak carbonic anhydrase inhibitor and can cause kidney stones and metabolic acidosis; the use of other carbonic anhydrase inhibitors is relatively contraindicated. Acute narrow-angle glaucoma has been reported in a few cases and requires immediate discontinuation.

Zonisamide

Zonisamide (Zonegran) appears to be effective for both focal and some generalized[1] epilepsies. It is approved as adjunctive treatment of partial seizures in adults. Its pharmacology is not well described, but it is metabolized by multiple mechanisms and has a very long half-life, which might allow it to be dosed once per day. It rarely causes kidney stones. It also can cause oligohidrosis (reduced sweating) and has rarely been associated with blood dyscrasias.

Pregabalin

Pregabalin (Lyrica) is approved as adjunctive treatment of partial seizures in adults. It is not metabolized significantly so it is excreted unchanged in urine. It does not bind to plasma proteins. Common side effects are dizziness, weight gain, pedal edema, and somnolence.

Vigabatrin

Vigabatrin (Sabril) is approved for infantile spasms in children ages 1 month to 2 years and for adult use in combination with other medications to treat complex partial seizures that have not responded adequately to previous drug therapies. It irreversibly inhibits the major degradative enzyme for GABA (GABA-transaminase). It does not bind to plasma proteins. It is eliminated primarily by the kidneys. The side effects can be serious. Peripheral visual field defects can be seen in about 25% to 50 % of adults and about 15% of children. Psychotic disorders and hallucinations are rare but also can be seen. Therefore it is recommended to have cognitive and age-appropriate vision testing at baseline and repeated at intervals. If it is effective,

---

[1]Not FDA approved for this indication.

then it will be effective within 12 weeks. If there is significant reduction in seizures or the patient becomes seizure free, then the continuation of therapy depends on the risk-to-benefit ratio, and the patient or caregiver should be involved in decision making. If there is no benefit after 12 weeks of treatment, it should be discontinued. Its use should be limited primarily to epilepsy centers.

Rufinamide

Rufinamide (Banzel) is approved as adjunctive therapy for seizures associated with Lennox-Gastaut syndrome, a severe form of epilepsy. The proposed mechanism of action is the limitation of sodium-dependent action potential firing. There seems to be a good cognitive and psychiatric adverse effect profile with few drug interactions. Rufinamide use is most appropriate when Lennox-Gastaut patients have failed valproate,[1] topiramate, and lamotrigine, and it probably should be considered before felbamate, other newer AEDs, vagus nerve stimulation, or corpus callosotomy is considered.

SELECTION OF ANTIEPILEPTIC DRUGS

A systematic approach should be adopted in selecting an AED. The goal is freedom from seizures, with no side effects. To achieve this, the seizure type and etiology or epilepsy syndrome must be diagnosed accurately. Treatment should start with a single AED as monotherapy that is effective for all the seizure types that the patient experiences. The therapy can last years and sometimes is lifelong. Therefore, a medication that would minimally affect the patient's quality of life with minimal side effects should be chosen. If the patient has comorbidities, an AED that might be effective for that specific comorbidity should be chosen among the candidate AEDs, or if a specific side effect would be particularly problematic, then AEDs with that side effect should be avoided. There are no blinded, randomized clinical trials comparing the effectiveness of several different AEDs, and thus the selection of an AED depends primarily on the unique characteristics of each AED and the unique characteristics of the patient. Thus, selecting an AED for special populations is of particular importance. Nevertheless, some recommendations can be made based on common clinical experience and the SANAD (Standard and New Antiepileptic Drugs) open-label clinical trials that compared some AEDs in a large number of patients (see Table 2).

Special Patient Populations

ELDERLY PATIENTS

Elderly patients with epilepsy have several unique characteristics. Altered physiology during aging and possible polypharmacy for other medical conditions need to be considered when selecting an AED. The incidence of epilepsy is high among elderly people, increasing after the age of 75 years. The recognition of seizures may be difficult owing to atypical clinical presentations. The most common presumed cause is stroke. Alzheimer's disease and head injury are other common causes. Complex partial and simple partial seizures are the most common presentation, especially in the form of memory lapses, confusion, change in mental status, and staring.

When initiating an AED, lower doses are required owing to decreased renal and hepatic clearance. An age-related decrease in serum albumin increases the free fraction of the protein-bound AEDs. Phenytoin is particularly poorly tolerated in the elderly and in addition can have a prolonged half-life so that levels are unexpectedly high. Some new AEDs are better tolerated and less likely to cause drug interactions. Gabapentin is particularly desirable because it has no drug interactions. Lamotrigine, oxcarbazepine, and levetiracetam are also usually well tolerated and often selected as first-line agents in this age group.

WOMEN

The key considerations in epileptic women include the effect of treatment on hormonal function thereby influencing sexuality and reproductive function, potential teratogenicity in women of childbearing potential, and bone health. Enzyme-inducing drugs such as phenytoin,

carbamazepine, primidone, and phenobarbital and the enzyme-inhibitor drug valproic acid alter the endogenous steroids, oral contraceptives, and vitamins. Women with epilepsy have increased rates of infertility due to intrinsic hormone changes, anovulatory cycles, irregular menstrual cycles, and altered sexuality. This can be compounded by the effects of AEDs, especially valproate, which is associated with polycystic ovarian disease. Hepatic enzyme–inducing AEDs induce the metabolism of vitamin D, increasing the risk of osteoporosis. Therefore, supplemental vitamin D and calcium should be recommended.

All enzyme-inducing AEDs decrease the efficacy of oral contraceptives, which can lead to unwanted pregnancies. Valproic acid, gabapentin, levetiracetam, pregabalin, and zonisamide do not effect oral contraceptives. Oxcarbazepine has an inconsistent effect, and topiramate at higher doses (>200 mg) decreases oral contraceptives' efficacy. Lamotrigine levels are decreased by oral contraceptives, but oral contraceptives have only an inconsistent and mild effect on lamotrigine levels. Patients who are on one of the enzyme-inducing agents should use an oral contraceptive agent with a higher estrogen dosage.

The fear of birth defects caused by the AEDs is a major concern in women of childbearing potential. It is a general principle that the risk to the fetus from seizures is greater than the risk to the fetus from AEDs. It is generally recommended to continue AEDs at the lowest effective dose and use the fewest drugs during pregnancy.

Birth defects occur in 1.6% to 2.3% of all live births in the general population. The absolute risk is less than 4% for most of the AEDs except valproic acid, which has higher risk (6.2% to 10.7%). Carbamazepine has a risk (2.2% to 4.0%) comparable to that of second-generation drugs such as levetiracetam (2.7%), lamotrigine (1.4% to 2.3%), and topiramate (4.8%) according to the information from different pregnancy registries. Phenytoin and phenobarbital have higher risks (5.9% and 6.5%, respectively) compared to newer AEDs and carbamazepine. Therefore, with the exception of valproic acid, major congenital malformations rate for women on AEDs is about twice that of the general population. However, the absolute risk of birth defects is still less than about 4%, so women on AEDs should be reassured that they are likely to have a normal baby.

Valproic acid is the AED that clearly has a higher teratogenicity rate and causes neural tube defects. Therefore it should not be used as a first-line treatment in women of childbearing potential. If it is, the dosage should be limited to the lowest effective dosage. Also, to reduce the risk of major congenital malformations, AED polytherapy should be avoided during the first trimester of pregnancy, if possible. All women of childbearing potential should take folate supplements daily to decrease the risk of neural tube defects.

Enzyme-inducing AEDs can induce vitamin K deficiency, potentially causing bleeding in the neonate and fetus. Therefore, it is recommended to give 10 to 20 mg oral vitamin K (Mephyton)[1] daily in the last month of pregnancy and give 1 mg intramuscularly (Phytonadione)[1] to the infant at birth.

MIGRAINEURS

Migraine is a common neurologic disease affecting about 12% of the general population and has an even higher incidence in patients with epilepsy. Some AEDs are used as prophylaxis against migraine attacks separate from their use for seizures. Valproic acid and topiramate are effective in migraine prevention and are usually well tolerated, making them suitable for first-line clinical use in patients who have epilepsy and also have migraine headaches. Lamotrigine, oxcarbazepine, and vigabatrin have generally been shown to be not effective for migraine, and gabapentin[1] has had equivocal results. Other AEDs have not been studied systematically enough to routinely expect them to be useful for comorbid migraine.

PATIENTS WITH MOOD DISORDERS

Mood disorders are common, with major depressive disorder having a prevalence of more than 10% of the population. Depression may be seen in about 50% of patients with epilepsy, especially in temporal lobe epilepsy secondary to mesial temporal sclerosis and frontal lobe

---

[1]Not FDA approved for this indication.

epilepsy. Psychiatric disorders occur more often in patients with higher seizure frequency. Comorbid psychiatric disorders, depression and anxiety in particular, are an independent risk factor for a poor quality of life for patients with epilepsy. Therefore, it is extremely important to ensure that patients with epilepsy are assessed for depression and that depression is adequately treated. Fortunately, some AEDs have demonstrated or suggested antidepressant properties.

Carbamazepine, valproic acid, and lamotrigine have been found to have positive psychotropic properties. Indeed, carbamazepine, valproic acid, and lamotrigine have mood-stabilizing properties, and carbamazepine and valproic acid have antimanic effects and lamotrigine[1] has antidepressant effects in patients with bipolar depressive episodes. It has not been demonstrated that gabapentin[1] is more effective than placebo, and there are still very few results on levetiracetam,[1] oxcarbazepine,[1] pregabalin,[1] and zonisamide.[1] Overall, lamotrigine is an excellent choice in patients with epilepsy and depression, for whom lamotrigine is also a good choice to treat their epilepsy. Levetiracetam can rarely cause irritability, so some suggest not using it in patients for whom irritability would be a significant problem; however, it is not predictable who will get this uncommon side effect, so many clinicians use it even in this situation.

PATIENTS WITH NEUROPATHIC PAIN

Some AEDs are used in chronic pain treatment and should be selected when chronic pain, particularly neuropathic pain, is comorbid with epilepsy. According to the guidelines for pharmacologic treatment of chronic neuropathic pain and painful neuropathy, pregabalin and gabapentin[1] are among the first-line treatment options, whereas carbamazepine,[1] lamotrigine,[1] oxcarbazepine,[1] topiramate,[1] and valproic acid[1] are considered third-line options.

Gabapentin and pregabalin have established efficacy in postherpetic neuralgia, and carbamazepine and oxcarbazepine[1] are the two most widely used and recommended drugs for trigeminal neuralgia.

Refractory Epilepsy

EVALUATION OF INTRACTABLE SEIZURES

The definition of what constitutes refractory epilepsy has evolved. In statistical terms, patients who continue to have seizures after trying therapeutic doses of two AEDs are very unlikely to respond to additional AEDs, although some do. The definition is becoming increasingly important because patients with refractory epilepsy should be referred to an epilepsy center for diagnosis and consideration of the many therapeutic options now available, including epilepsy surgery to resect the seizure focus, palliative surgery to reduce the severity of some seizure types, unconventional AEDs, and experimental AEDs.

The evaluation of intractable seizures depends on a careful history and physical examination directed at elucidating the seizure type, neuroanatomic site of seizure origin, and the epilepsy syndrome or etiology. The most important diagnostic test is prolonged (24 hours per day) simultaneous video and EEG monitoring to capture seizures. Video EEG is vitally important to determine that the spells in question are indeed seizures, to define the seizure type, and to localize the site of origin. Video EEG might need to continue for days or weeks to capture enough spells to make a correct diagnosis. Magnetic resonance imaging (MRI) of the brain using special acquisition protocols to define fine brain anatomy often reveals abnormalities that are not obvious on routine MRI, especially in the temporal lobe, where seizures often arise. Positron emission tomography (PET) can reveal focal hypometabolism in the region of seizure onset. Interictal single photon-emission computed tomography (SPECT) occasionally reveals focal hypoperfusion at the focus. To perform an ictal SPECT scan, the radio tracer is injected within 90 seconds of the seizure's onset, and subsequent scanning often reveals focal hyperperfusion in the region of the seizure's onset. Magnetic resonance spectroscopy is primarily a research tool but can reveal focal changes in the region of the seizure focus. Neuropsychological testing may demonstrate lateralized or localized deficits.

EPILEPSY SURGERY

Surgery to resect the epilepsy focus is the only method of curing epilepsy available today. Successful surgery is, of course, heavily dependent on correctly localizing the seizure focus. Presurgical evaluation is usually carried out in three phases. Phase I consists of scalp (extracranial) video-EEG monitoring and the noninvasive tests noted earlier. If the findings yield a general area from which the seizures arise, but do not pinpoint the exact site of onset, then the patient may proceed to phase 2, which is intracranial EEG monitoring through electrodes placed on or into the brain. Phase 3 is the removal of the seizure focus. Fortunately, most patients do not require intracranial monitoring now because neuroimaging often identifies an anatomic abnormality to corroborate the EEG findings.

Any area of the brain is a candidate for resection, but in reality the vast majority of patients have temporal lobe epilepsy and undergo anterior temporal lobectomy to remove the anterior 3 to 4 cm of the temporal lobe containing the hippocampus and amygdala. Approximately 70% of patients are essentially seizure free after anterior temporal lobectomy, and the risk of stroke or other serious complication is less than 1%.

Extratemporal resections are more complicated than temporal lobe surgery. The seizure focus must be more precisely localized and electrical brain mapping or other methods must be used to ensure that important brain functions will not be removed during surgery. This usually requires intracranial monitoring. Approximately 50% of patients who undergo an extratemporal resection are essentially seizure free. The risk of complications, such as a motor deficit, is only slightly higher than with anterior temporal lobectomy. More-drastic surgeries, such as hemispherectomy or corpus callosotomy, are indicated in special circumstances.

Devices have an increasingly important role in treatment of refractory epilepsy. Vagus nerve stimulation is a well-established device used to reduce seizure frequency. A small generator is placed subcutaneously in the left chest wall and wire electrodes are led to the left vagus nerve. The generator supplies a few seconds of current every few minutes at predetermined settings. Its efficacy in blinded controlled trials is about the same as a new AED; it reduces the frequency of seizures by 50% in about half of the subjects.

Continuous deep brain stimulation was proved to be effective in a double-blind controlled trial but it is not FDA approved yet. The thalamus is stimulated by a stimulator placed in the chest wall that leads to electrodes placed into the thalamus. Responsive neurostimulation is a novel approach to aborting seizures. Electrodes are implanted at the seizure focus and lead to a microprocessor implanted in the skull. The microprocessor monitors brain wave activity and when it detects a seizure, it provides a small electrical stimulus to the seizure focus intended to stop the seizure. It has recently been submitted to the FDA for consideration.

REFERENCES

Azar NJ, Abou-Khalil BW. Considerations in the choice of an antiepileptic drug in the treatment of epilepsy. Semin Neurol 2008;28(3):305–16.

Banerjee PN, Filippi D, Hauser WA. The descriptive epidemiology of epilepsy—a review. Epilepsy Res 2009;85(1):31–45.

Commission on Classification and Terminology of the International League Against Epilepsy. Proposal for revised clinical and electroencephalographic classification of epileptic seizures. Epilepsia 1981;22:489–501.

Commission on Classification and Terminology of the International League Against Epilepsy. Proposal for revised classification of epilepsies and epileptic syndromes. Epilepsia 1989;30:389–99.

Harden CL, Meador KJ, Pennell PB, et al. Management issues for women with epilepsy—focus on pregnancy (an evidence-based review): II. Teratogenesis and perinatal outcomes: Report of the Quality Standards Subcommittee and Therapeutics and Technology Subcommittee of the American Academy of Neurology and the American Epilepsy Society. Epilepsia 2009;50(5):1237–46.

Harden CL, Pennell PB, Koppel BS, et al. Management issues for women with epilepsy—focus on pregnancy (an evidence-based review): III. Vitamin K, folic acid, blood levels, and breast-feeding: Report of the Quality Standards Subcommittee and Therapeutics and Technology Assessment Subcommittee of the American Academy of Neurology and the American Epilepsy Society. Epilepsia 2009;50(5):1247–55.

---

[1]Not FDA approved for this indication.

Jobst BC. Treatment algorithms in refractory partial epilepsy. Epilepsia 2009;50(Suppl. 8):51–6.

Marson AG, Al-Kharusi AM, Alwaidh M, et al. The SANAD study of effectiveness of carbamazepine, gabapentin, lamotrigine, oxcarbazepine, or topiramate for treatment of partial epilepsy: An unblinded randomised controlled trial. Lancet 2007;369:1000–15.

Marson AG, Al-Kharusi AM, Alwaidh M, et al. The SANAD study of effectiveness of valproate, lamotrigine, or topiramate for generalised and unclassifiable epilepsy: An unblinded randomised controlled trial. Lancet 2007;369:1016–26.

Wiebe S, Blume WT, Girvin JP, et al. A randomized, controlled trial of surgery for temporal-lobe epilepsy. N Engl J Med 2001;345:311–8.

Epilepsy in Infants and Children

Method of
Mary Zupanc, MD

Epilepsy is defined as two or more unprovoked seizures. A seizure is the result of an abnormal synchronous depolarization of a group of neurons. The clinical manifestations of a seizure depend on where in the brain the discharges begin and how they spread.

Epilepsy is a common medical condition, occurring in 0.5% to 1% of all children. Each year 150,000 children and adolescents in the United States have a single unprovoked seizure. One fifth of those, or 30,000, eventually develop epilepsy. The highest incidence of epilepsy is during the first year of life.

Appropriate classification of epilepsy is the cornerstone of therapy. Most children with epilepsy are seizure-free with the use of one antiepileptic drug (AED) without side effects. Some epileptic children, approximately 15%, have medically refractory seizures.

Classification

In any evaluation of a child who might have had a seizure, the first job of the physician is to determine whether the event was indeed an epileptic seizure or some other paroxysmal event. The history is the key to differentiating between these episodes and epileptic seizures.

There are many different types of paroxysmal events in children that can mimic seizures (Box 1). For example, pallid or cyanotic breath-holding spells can result in brief generalized tonic–clonic seizures. Pallid breath-holding spells are precipitated by excitement, surprise, or trivial head trauma, resulting in an exaggerated vasovagal event with concomitant bradycardia and central nervous system (CNS) ischemia. If the event is sufficiently prolonged, the child might have a brief seizure. Cyanotic breath-holding spells, on the other hand, are prolonged crying episodes, often stimulated by frustration or anger, resulting in an involuntary inability to breathe, with concomitant cyanosis, decreased oxygen concentration, and hypercapnia. This is typically followed by a brief loss of consciousness; sometimes a brief generalized tonic–clonic seizure follows. These episodes must be distinguished from the unprovoked seizures characteristic of epilepsy. Breath-holding spells do dissipate in the preschool years and do not need to be treated with AEDs.

Other paroxysmal events that can resemble seizures include motor tics; vasovagal syncope; shuddering attacks, a rare condition associated with tremor or shuddering of the upper trunk and shoulders with no alteration of consciousness, occurring in young toddlers and preschoolers; confusional migraines, which can mimic complex partial seizures; sleep disturbances; gastroesophageal reflux, which sometimes produces tonic posturing and can resemble tonic seizures (Sandifer's syndrome); and paroxysmal choreoathetosis or dystonia. There are also patients who have pseudoseizures. Their events can mimic seizures; sometimes they cannot be distinguished from clinical epileptic seizures without performing closed-circuit television electroencephalographic monitoring. Children with pseudoseizures often have complex psychosocial situations and may be victims of either physical or sexual abuse.

If it is determined that a child most likely has epilepsy, the primary physician must determine the appropriate seizure classification and epilepsy syndrome in order to make intelligent decisions with respect to diagnostic studies, treatment, and prognosis. The International League Against Epilepsy has established the International Classification of the Epilepsies and Epileptic Syndromes. This system is used as the foundation for decision making.

In the classification of epilepsy, seizures are divided into two categories, generalized and partial (Box 2). *Generalized seizure* indicates that the clinical seizure does not contain any focal features. Electrographically, the electroencephalogram (EEG) demonstrates generalized spike, polyspike, or sharp wave discharges (or some combination of these) without localizing features over both hemispheres. Clinical seizures of this type are myoclonic, tonic (episodes of tonic posturing), atonic (drop attacks), absence (formerly petit mal), and tonic–clonic (old terminology, grand mal). On the other hand, *partial seizures* are events that begin focally in one part of the brain. The clinical manifestations depend on where in the brain the epileptic discharge begins. A simple partial seizure is a seizure in which there is no associated alteration of consciousness. A simple partial seizure can constitute the aura that

---

BOX 1 Nonepileptic Events That Can Be Mistakenly Diagnosed as Epilepsy in Children

Benign paroxysmal vertigo
Breath-holding spells
• Classic (cyanotic)
• Pallid
Paroxysmal choreoathetosis or dystonia
Syncope
Migraine, especially acute confusional
Pseudoseizures
Shuddering spells
Sleep disorders
Tics

BOX 2 Classification of Epileptic Seizures

Partial Seizures
Simple partial seizures
• With motor signs, such as focal clonic activity
• With somatosensory or special-sensory symptoms such as lateralized numbness, tingling, visual or auditory hallucinations, abnormal odors or smells
• With automatic symptoms or signs such as tachycardia, diaphoresis
• With psychic symptoms such as fear, anxiety, déjà vu, jamais vu, confusion
Complex partial seizures
• With simple partial seizures (aura) at onset
• With impairment of consciousness at onset
Partial seizures evolving to secondarily generalized seizures

Generalized Seizures
Absence seizures
Myoclonic seizures
Clonic seizures
Tonic seizures
Tonic–clonic seizures
Atonic seizures

patients often refer to before they have more recognizable clinical seizures. As the electrical discharges progress, simple partial seizures typically transform into complex partial seizures. Complex partial seizures are defined as focally generated seizures that are associated with an alteration of consciousness. These seizures can, and often do, generalize to become generalized tonic–clonic seizures. Examples of simple partial seizures include olfactory hallucination, abdominal queasiness, déjà vu, jamais vu, or a tingling sensation in the hands. An example of a complex partial seizure is a paroxysmal episode that begins with staring, drooling, lip smacking automatism, and confusion, lasting 1 to 2 minutes.

In addition to seizure classification, the clinician should be aware of the International Classification of Epilepsy Syndromes. The epilepsy syndromes are determined by further classifying epileptic seizures on the basis of age at onset; seizure type; family history; risk factors for epilepsy; associated neurodevelopmental delays; neuroimaging results; EEG data, both ictal and interictal; other diagnostic tests, such as lumber puncture and metabolic testing; and physical examination. This information can more specifically identify an epileptic condition, resulting in more appropriate management and predictions with respect to prognosis.

Epilepsy Syndromes

The classification of epilepsy syndromes differentiates generalized, localization-related, and undetermined epileptic syndromes, in addition to special syndromes (Box 3). These syndromes are classified into *idiopathic*, implying normal neurologic status and a genetic predisposition; *symptomatic*, implying an underlying lesion or other CNS pathologic condition; and *cryptogenic*, implying that the epileptic condition is probably symptomatic but the exact cause cannot be pinpointed.

GENERALIZED EPILEPSY SYNDROMES

Examples of idiopathic generalized epilepsy syndromes include childhood absence epilepsy, juvenile absence epilepsy, and juvenile myoclonic epilepsy. Childhood absence epilepsy is probably genetically

---

BOX 3   Classification of Epileptic Syndromes

Localization Related (Focal, Local, Partial)
Benign rolandic epilepsy
Benign occipital epilepsy
Idiopathic
Symptomatic

Generalized
Idiopathic, Age Related
Benign idiopathic convulsions
Benign myoclonic epilepsy in infancy
Benign neonatal familial convulsions
Childhood absence epilepsy
Epilepsy with tonic–clonic seizures on awakening
Juvenile absence epilepsy
Juvenile myoclonic epilepsy

Idiopathic and/or Symptomatic
Epilepsy with myoclonic–astatic seizures
Epilepsy with myoclonic absences
Infantile spasms (West's syndrome)
Lennox–Gastaut syndrome
Symptomatic: early myoclonic encephalopathy

Focal or Generalized (Not Known)
Acquired epileptic aphasia (Landau–Kleffner syndrome)
Epilepsy with continuous spike waves during slow-wave sleep
Neonatal seizures
Severe myoclonic epilepsy in infancy

---

linked to juvenile absence epilepsy and juvenile myoclonic epilepsy. These epilepsy syndromes are most likely different phenotypic expressions of the same gene. These children have normal neurologic examinations and tend to have above-average intelligence. Depending on the age at onset, children and adolescents with these epilepsy syndromes can have a varied clinical manifestation: absence, myoclonic, or generalized tonic–clonic seizures.

Childhood and Juvenile Epilepsy

Childhood absence epilepsy accounts for 2% to 8% of all cases of childhood epilepsy. The age at onset is during elementary school age, and the peak is at 6 to 7 years of age. The seizure semiology is characterized by absence seizures, which are brief episodes of staring, often accompanied by eyelid fluttering, facial clonic activity, or upper extremity myoclonus. These seizures are very brief, lasting only 2 to 10 seconds, occurring multiple times per day and without a concomitant postictal phase. Absence seizures can be induced by hyperventilation. If the epilepsy begins before 9 years of age, the risk of having comorbid generalized tonic–clonic seizures is only 16%. If the epilepsy begins later, the risk of generalized tonic–clonic seizures is close to 50%. Myoclonic seizures are rare.

Juvenile absence epilepsy is associated with absence seizures and generalized tonic–clonic seizures. The age at onset is prepubertal, usually between 10 and 15 years of age. Absence seizures occur in all patients; generalized tonic–clonic seizures occur in almost 80%.

With juvenile myoclonic epilepsy, the age at onset is typically during adolescence, between 12 and 18 years of age. The characteristic clinical symptom is early morning sudden myoclonic jerks of the shoulders and arms. Ninety percent of patients have generalized tonic–clonic seizures, and 33% have absence seizures.

The interictal EEG in all cases demonstrates generalized spike and slow-wave discharges. With the earlier onset, the generalized spike and slow-wave discharges are at 3 cycles per second (cps). With juvenile myoclonic epilepsy, the generalized discharges consist of generalized polyspike, spike, and slow-wave discharges at 4 to 5 cps.

The treatment for these three epilepsy syndromes is similar. Valproate (Depakote) is the drug of choice for patients with both absence and generalized tonic–clonic seizures, except in girls of reproductive age (see later). Ethosuximide (Zarontin) can be used if the patient is having only absence seizures. There recently has been an NIH multicenter study that compared the efficacy of valproate, ethosuximide, and lamotrigine in the treatment of childhood absence epilepsy. It was a double-blinded, placebo-controlled study. It demonstrated that valproate and ethosuximide (as monotherapy treatments) are significantly more effective than lamotrigine monotherapy in the treatment of childhood absence epilepsy. Lamotrigine is approved as adjunctive therapy for generlized tonic–clonic seizures in children older than 2 years. It has been successfully used in the treatment of juvenile myoclonic epilepsy, as add-on therapy. Topiramate (Topamax) also shows promise in treating generalized tonic–clonic seizures and myoclonus but not with absence seizures. Levetiracetam (Keppra)[1] is also being studied to determine its efficacy with respect to absence seizures. Levetiracetam is approved as adjunctive therapy for myoclonic seizures in juvenile myoclonic epilepsy in adolescents 12 years and older. Levetiracetam is also approved as adjunctive therapy for primary generalized tonic clonic seizures in the idiopathic generalized epilepsy syndromes in children and adolescents 6 years and older.

The prognosis varies, depending on the age at onset. Juvenile myoclonic epilepsy requires lifelong treatment because of the high rate of relapse when AED therapy is discontinued. On the other hand, childhood absence epilepsy has a much better prognosis, with more than 50% of patients outgrowing their epilepsy by the age of puberty.

Infantile Spasms

Another generalized epilepsy syndrome is infantile spasms. The incidence of infantile spasms is 1 in 4000 to 6000 live births. The peak age at onset is 4 to 6 months. The seizures are characterized by flexor or extensor (or both) myoclonic spasms, usually occurring in clusters after the infant awakens in the morning or from a nap.

---

[1]Not FDA approved for this indication.

Infantile spasms can be divided into three categories: symptomatic, cryptogenic, and idiopathic. Improvements in neuroimaging and metabolic testing now enable better identification of a specific etiology for infantile spasms. Some of the most common causes of symptomatic infantile spasms include tuberous sclerosis (approximately 25% of patients with tuberous sclerosis have infantile spasms); malformations of cortical development, such as Aicardi's syndrome or malformations in the posterior quadrants of the brain; chromosomal abnormality, one of the most common abnormalities is trisomy 21; inborn errors of metabolism, aminoacidopathies, or mitochondrial cytopathies; asphyxia; meningitis or encephalitis; and trauma.

Interictally, the EEG demonstrates a hypsarrhythmia pattern. This is a markedly abnormal pattern with high amplitude slowing at 1 to 3 cps and multifocal polyspike, spike, and slow-wave discharges.

According to the new practice parameter published by the American Academy of Neurology, the mainstay of treatment for infantile spasms in the United States is corticotropin (ACTH [HP Acthar]).[1] It demonstrates "probable" efficacy, using current evidence-based medicine. The mechanism of action for ACTH remains unclear, but this drug does affect CNS concentration of various biogenic amines and increases γ-aminobutyric acid (GABA)-receptor affinity. It also reduces corticotropin-releasing hormone (CRH), which is elevated in patients with infantile spasms and is a potent proconvulsant. In Europe and Canada, vigabatrin (Sabril),[5] a structural analogue of GABA, is the drug of choice in treating infantile spasms, particularly in children with tuberous sclerosis. Vigabatrin appears to be about 89% to 90% effective in eliminating infantile spasms in children with tuberous sclerosis and infantile spasms. Vigabatrin has not been approved by the FDA because of reports of retinal changes and peripheral visual constriction after long-term use of this drug. Other drugs that have questionable efficacy (due to inadequate evidence) in treating infantile spasms include the benzodiazepines, valproate, zonisamide (Zonegran),[1] topiramate,[1] lamotrigine,[1] and felbamate (Felbatol).[1] The principal deterrent in the use of valproate in these children is the risk of hepatotoxicity.

Lennox–Gastaut Syndrome

Lennox–Gastaut syndrome (LGS) is another generalized epilepsy syndrome, predominantly confined to children. The criteria for the diagnosis of LGS include generalized, multiple seizure types, including tonic, atonic, absence, and myoclonic seizures; an electrographic signature of generalized slow spike and wave discharges at 1½ to 2½ cps; and cognitive impairment. The degree of cognitive impairment is correlated with the underlying substrate of epilepsy and seizure control. As with infantile spasms, LGS can be divided into categories of symptomatic, cryptogenic, and idiopathic. In 30% of patients, infantile spasms evolve to LGS. Therefore, it follows that the two epileptic syndromes have similar underlying etiologies. This epileptic syndrome is often medically intractable.

Relatively few AEDs have been shown to be effective in treating LGS. The ketogenic diet is one of the oldest known treatments for pediatric epilepsy and status epilepticus. It remains a reasonable alternative therapy for LGS. The ketogenic diet consists of a high ratio of fats to carbohydrates and protein. Every piece of food must be carefully weighed and measured for fat, carbohydrate, and protein content so that the proper ratios are maintained. Any deviation from the diet can result in a loss of ketosis and renewed seizures. The exact mechanism by which the ketogenic diet provides seizure control remains unknown. It is presumed that the ketones have anticonvulsant properties. One third to one half of children with LGS have an excellent response to the ketogenic diet, with either a significant reduction in or complete elimination of seizures. Phenobarbital[1] and phenytoin (Dilantin),[1] in part because of their sedative effects, have never been shown to be effective in treating LGS.

The introduction of valproate in the late 1970s provided one of the first effective antiepileptic drugs in treating LGS, based on empiric evidence. There has never been a double-blind, placebo-controlled trial of valproate in treating LGS. The AEDs that have evidence to support their use in treating LGS are felbamate, topiramate, lamotrigine, and the newly FDA-approved drug, rufinamide. Rufinamide is very effective in treating the tonic and atonic seizures associated with LGS, but it can cause nausea, vomiting, and somnolence. Felbamate, released in 1993, showed great promise in treating LGS. Unfortunately, it has been associated with an increased risk of aplastic anemia and liver failure. The risk of aplastic anemia is now known to be highest in women with known autoimmune disorders; it has never been reported in a child younger than 13 years. The collective risk is 20 to 207 per million patients treated with this drug. The risk of hepatotoxicity is no greater than that of any of the other AEDs. Felbamate is reserved for patients with severe, intractable epilepsy. It is probably the most effective AED in treating LGS. The benzodiazepines are occasionally helpful in patients with LGS, but only if given intermittently to abort seizure clusters. Otherwise they are too sedating, and many patients develop tachyphylaxis.

LOCALIZATION-RELATED EPILEPSIES

The localization-related epilepsies can also be divided into two categories: symptomatic and idiopathic. The symptomatic localization-related epilepsies are the result of an underlying CNS abnormality, such as tumor, stroke, encephalomalacia from head trauma, hemorrhage, or malformation of cortical development. It is thought that the idiopathic epilepsies have an underlying genetic predisposition.

The most common epilepsy syndrome of childhood is an idiopathic localization-related epilepsy (benign rolandic epilepsy or benign epilepsy of childhood) associated with central-temporal spikes (BECTS). It accounts for 24% of all epileptic seizures in children between the ages of 5 and 14 years. It is genetically determined, probably autosomal dominant with variable penetrance and age-limited expression. The children are neurologically normal. The seizure semiology is characterized by sensorimotor symptoms and clonic activity in the face, arm, or leg, usually with associated hypersalivation and speech arrest. The seizure frequency varies, but typically seizures are rare. They are usually nocturnal, occurring in children in the early morning hours before they awaken or soon after they fall asleep. One known precipitating factor is sleep deprivation.

In benign rolandic epilepsy, the interictal EEG demonstrates drowsiness and sleep-activated central temporal spikes that can be asymmetrical or have a wide field spread. AEDs are seldom used in patients with rare seizures. They may be indicated for patients who are experiencing more frequent seizures that disrupt sleep, school performance, or psychosocial well-being. This epilepsy condition is outgrown in virtually 100% of patients by the time of adolescence.

SPECIAL SYNDROMES

Neonatal Seizures

Neonatal seizures are commonly the result of hypoxic–ischemic injury, hypoglycemia, or hypocalcemia in the perinatal period. Sepsis can also result in seizures. Three rare causes of neonatal seizures include pyridoxine dependency, folinic acid deficiency, and glucose transporter deficiency.

Pyridoxine dependence causes seizures unresponsive to AEDs. It is related to an insufficient production of GABA, a primary inhibitory neurotransmitter. The glucose transporter deficiency is characterized by a low cerebrospinal glucose concentration. There is an enzymatic defect in glucose transport that disrupts facilitative diffusion of glucose across the blood–brain barrier. The seizure semiology is different from that in older children and adolescents. Because of the primitive synaptic network, neonatal seizures can be quite subtle. Examples of neonatal seizures include eye deviation with apnea or multifocal clonic activity. Neonates do not have generalized tonic–clonic seizures, although they can have tonic seizures. There is controversy over whether or not the bicycling movements and lip-smacking seen in neonates are subtle seizures or "brainstem release" phenomena.

The most important therapeutic intervention in neonatal seizures is recognition of the underlying cause, followed by its prompt treatment.

---

[1]Not FDA approved for this indication.
[5]Investigational drug in the United States.

---

[1]Not FDA approved for this indication.

This can, in itself, abort any further seizure activity without the use of chronic AEDs. A pyridoxine[1] challenge and treatment with folinic acid (Leucovorin)[1] should be given to any neonate with intractable seizures. For status epilepticus in neonates, the most effective initial therapy is 20 mg/kg of phenobarbital given twice if necessary. Fosphenytoin (Cerebyx)[1] [mcl] at 20 mg/kg can also be used if the phenobarbital is ineffective. However, even when both of these medications have been given for neonatal status epilepticus, the success rate is only 67%. Preliminary studies indicate that intravenous lidocaine (Xylocaine)[1] may be effective for refractory neonatal seizures. The benzodiazepines are less effective in neonates than in older infants and children because the GABA receptors are excitatory in neonates, not inhibitory.

Febrile Seizures

Febrile seizures denote a special developmental seizure disorder that is not highly correlated with the development of epilepsy. By definition, a febrile seizure is a generalized tonic–clonic seizure occurring in a child between the ages of 6 months and 5 years and associated with a high fever not related to an underlying CNS infection. Simple febrile seizures carry a low risk of epilepsy (only 1%–2%) compared with the general population's risk of 0.5% to 1%. There is an underlying genetic predisposition, with a positive family history in one third of first-degree relatives. The risk of febrile seizure recurrence is quite high, with 33% of children having at least one recurrence. If a child is younger than 12 months at the time of the first febrile seizure, the risk of recurrence is 50%.

If the history is clear, no diagnostic studies need to be performed, with the exception of a lumbar puncture in infants younger than 18 months. The physician should design the work-up in response to the most likely cause of the fever. If meningitis is suspected at all, a lumbar puncture should be performed. This is particularly true in infants younger than 18 months who present with high fever, because they might not have reliable clinical signs and symptoms of meningismus.

Although phenobarbital[1] was once used to prevent febrile seizure recurrence, this is no longer the standard of care. There is no evidence to suggest that phenobarbital treatment decreases the risk of the development of epilepsy. Furthermore, the side effects of phenobarbital in these children are significant, with more than 40% exhibiting hyperactivity, aggressive behavior, impulsivity, poor attention and concentration, or sleep disturbance. Oral or rectal diazepam (Valium, Diastat) therapy can be given to prevent recurrence of febrile seizures in predisposed children. The dosage of oral diazepam[1] is 0.33 mg/kg every 8 hours during the course of the febrile illness. This medication can produce side effects including sedation and irritability. The dosage of rectal diazepam for patients 2–5 years of age is 0.5 mg/kg. It is usually reserved for febrile seizure recurrence and prolonged febrile seizure (>5 min).

The prognosis for febrile seizures is excellent. Very few children develop epilepsy (1%–2%). Those who have a greater risk for developing epilepsy include children with focal or prolonged febrile seizures, children with a family history of epilepsy, and children with developmental delays and abnormal neurologic examinations. These risk factors suggest that an underlying substrate of epilepsy already exists and that the seizure threshold was simply lowered by the fever.

Landau–Kleffner Syndrome

Landau–Kleffner syndrome (acquired epileptic aphasia) is a poorly understood syndrome that is characterized by a regression in expressive and receptive language in association with an epileptiform EEG, either focal or multifocal. Overt clinical seizures occur in more than 70% of patents; in the remaining 30%, the only ictal manifestation is the deterioration in speech and language. The diagnosis of Landau–Kleffner syndrome is determined solely on the basis of clinical symptoms and EEG finding. Twenty-four-hour EEG monitoring may be helpful in establishing the diagnosis because there is generally activation of the epileptiform discharges during sleep.

The underlying pathophysiology of Landau–Kleffner syndrome remains unknown. The treatment of this syndrome is controversial,

in part related to our poor understanding of this disorder. The goal of therapy is normalization of the EEG and improvement in speech and language, although it has still not been determined if the epileptiform discharges produce the symptoms of Landau–Kleffner syndrome or if they simply represent an epiphenomenon. AEDs are used, particularly valproate (Depacon). Steroid therapy has also been tried with some reported success. In refractory cases, multiple subpial transections have been performed over the epileptogenic zone, with only a few reported cases in the literature. A multicenter, double-blind, placebo-controlled treatment trial is needed to determine appropriate and effective therapies. The prognosis for this disorder is variable.

Some clinicians have broadened the definition of Landau–Kleffner syndrome to include children with developmental aphasia and underlying epileptiform EEGs. As a result, some children with autism have been treated with AEDs and even steroids to see whether there would be an improvement in clinical symptoms. This remains an area of considerable controversy. Again, are the epileptiform discharges producing the clinical symptoms or are the epileptiform abnormalities merely an epiphenomenon pointing to an underlying, poorly understood CNS disorder?

Assessment

Appropriate classification of a paroxysmal event is the initial step in the evaluation of a child with a suspected seizure. The history is the key to the diagnosis. Care must be taken to elicit possible precipitating factors and risk factors for epilepsy. Precipitating factors that result in provoked seizures include an underlying CNS infection or head trauma. With breath-holding spells, as mentioned earlier, frustration, anger, surprise, excitement, or trivial head trauma can provoke a spell sometimes followed by a brief generalized tonic–clonic seizure. The risk factors for epilepsy include history of encephalitis or meningitis; history of significant head trauma–associated loss of consciousness, concussion, skull fracture, prolonged coma, or penetrating injury; history of a prolonged febrile seizure lasting longer than 20 minutes; developmental delays; abnormal neurologic examination; and history of asphyxia.

The seizure semiology and its evolution are also very helpful in determining the portion of the brain where the epileptogenic focus resides. Specifically, if the patient typically senses a funny taste or feels queasy before the episode of staring, drooling, and lip smacking automatism, one can surmise that the epileptogenic zone probably resides in either one of the temporal lobes. If the epileptogenic focus is near the sensorimotor cortex, the patient might first experience numbness and tingling in the contralateral extremity followed by rhythmic clonic activity of this same extremity as the epileptogenic discharges spread. Forced head version is a reliable indicator of a contralateral frontal epileptogenic focus.

Home videos of paroxysmal events have proved helpful in appropriately classifying both epileptic and nonepileptic events. An EEG—both awake and asleep—is especially helpful. The presence of focal or generalized epileptiform discharges in the context of an appropriate clinical history is usually sufficient for making the appropriate diagnosis. However, a normal awake and asleep EEG does not exclude the diagnosis of epilepsy, particularly in the face of a compelling history. If the epileptiform discharges are infrequent or deep-seated in the mesial temporal structures, the EEG might not reflect the underlying epileptogenic zone. Untreated generalized epilepsies, however, almost invariably are associated with generalized spike and slow-wave discharges on routine EEGs. Prolonged closed-circuit television EEG monitoring is reserved for patients whose diagnosis is unclear or whose seizures are sufficiently intractable to warrant an evaluation for epilepsy surgery.

If epilepsy is confirmed, depending on the nature of the epilepsy syndrome, further diagnostic studies may be necessary. If the diagnosis is clearly a known benign generalized epileptic syndrome such as childhood absence epilepsy, no further tests are needed and the child can begin AED therapy. If the diagnosis is a localization-related epilepsy, a neuroimaging study is indicated, preferably magnetic resonance imaging (MRI). Computed tomography is inadequate for

---

[1]Not FDA approved for this indication.

detecting the underlying substrates of epilepsy. If the epilepsy is thought to be the result of an underlying encephalopathy, metabolic testing and a chromosomal analysis might also need to be performed. In addition, the neurocutaneous syndromes, particularly tuberous sclerosis, are associated with epilepsy. In 25% of patients with tuberous sclerosis, the initial apparent symptom is infantile spasms.

Treatment

Epilepsy is a condition characterized by recurrent seizures. It is not necessary to treat the patient after the first seizure. The chance of seizure recurrence after the first seizure is approximately 30% to 40%. If the EEG demonstrates temporal epileptiform discharges or generalized spike and slow-wave discharges, the chance of recurrence is much higher, bordering on 90%. If a child has a second seizure, the risk of continued seizures is also much higher. Antiepileptic medication is generally recommended after a second seizure. There are exceptions to this, particularly if a benign epilepsy syndrome is identified (e.g., benign rolandic epilepsy). There are also epilepsy syndromes that are malignant. When these are identified, treatment should begin without delay, regardless of the seizure frequency.

When antiepileptic drug therapy is discussed, it is important to recognize the seizure type as well as the epileptic syndrome. This is the single most important criterion in making a decision about antiepileptic medication. There are basic principles to remember in choosing AED therapy:

- AED monotherapy is effective in most patients and avoids undesirable drug interactions.
- AEDs should be titrated slowly and only to the point of seizure control, if possible.
- Seizure control should not be achieved without trying to avoid side effects. If side effects develop, attempts should be made to reduce the dosage, change to a sustained-release formulation, or change AEDs.
- Drug compliance is enhanced when medication is given once or twice daily. Therefore, sustained-release medication should always be considered.
- Therapeutic blood levels are determined on the basis of trough levels and represent a statistical range of efficacy. They are not absolute levels.

The past few years have seen a rapid escalation in the marketing of AEDs. The drugs of choice for partial seizures now include a broad range of AEDs, including carbamazepine (Tegretol; Carbatrol [extended-release formulation]), oxcarbazepine (Trileptal), gabapentin (Neurontin), lamotrigine, topiramate, valproate, levetiracetam, zonisamide (not approved for children <16 years), phenobarbital, and phenytoin (Tables 1 and 2). The new AEDs have all been approved by the FDA as adjunctive therapy in treating partial seizures in adults. Topiramate has received approval for treating partial seizures in children as young as 2 years. Lamotrigine has been approved for treating both partial seizures and generalized tonic–clonic seizures, as adjunctive therapy, in children ages 2 or older. Levetiracetam is approved as adjunctive therapy for partial seizures and for myoclonic seizures. Phenobarbital and phenytoin are not currently being prescribed by pediatric neurologists nearly as often as they were in the past 10 years.

ANTIEPILEPTIC DRUGS

Carbamazepine

Carbamazepine is still the most widely used AED in treating partial seizures. Its mechanism of action is similar to that of phenytoin. Both drugs work by inhibiting the high-frequency repetitive firing of voltage-dependent sodium channels. Carbamazepine is generally tolerated well but should be introduced slowly. This reduces the risk of toxicity and enhances compliance. Autoinduction of carbamazepine metabolism via the cytochrome P-450 enzyme system occurs within the first month of therapy, often necessitating an increase in the total

dosage of carbamazepine. If at all possible, once the dosage has been adjusted, attempts should be made to change to a sustained-release preparation. Carbamazepine is available in a liquid formulation, chewable tablets, tablets, a sustained-release preparation, and sustained-release sprinkle capsules.

The toxic side effects of carbamazepine include dizziness, diplopia, sedation, ataxia, and nausea. Rare idiosyncratic reactions include aplastic anemia and hepatic dysfunction. Transient leukopenia occurs in 10% of children, usually during the first month of therapy. Allergic rash occurs in about 8% to 10% of patients; cases of Stevens-Johnson syndrome have been reported. Other rare side effects include irritability and dystonia. The antibiotic erythromycin alters the kinetics of carbamazepine, resulting in significant increases in carbamazepine levels.

Before carbamazepine therapy is initiated, a baseline complete blood cell count with differential and liver function tests should be obtained. These studies should be repeated monthly for the first 3 months of therapy or if there are signs or symptoms of liver dysfunction or blood dyscrasias.

Oxcarbazepine

Oxcarbazepine is related to carbamazepine and is approved as adjunctive therapy in treating localization related epilepsy. It does not induce the cytochrome P-450 enzyme system and is not metabolized to 10,11-epoxide, the known metabolite of carbamazepine thought to be responsible for teratogenicity and for many of carbamazepine's toxic side effects. It is formulated as a liquid (300 mg/5 mL suspension) or in pills (150 mg; 300 mg; 600 mg). It can be given twice daily. It has the same mechanism of action as carbamazepine and can produce the same side effects with toxicity. Patients can develop hyponatremia with this medication.

Valproate

Valproate is a broad-spectrum AED demonstrating efficacy for both partial and generalized seizures. Its mechanisms of action include reduction of T-type calcium channel currents, modulation of sodium channels, and, possibly, enhancement of GABA activity, the primary inhibitory neurotransmitter. Valproate comes in several formulations, including the liquid valproic acid, sodium divalproex tablets; and sodium divalproex sprinkle capsules.

The most common side effects of valproate include an increase in appetite with concomitant weight gain and tremor. Rarely, valproate causes an encephalopathy with sedation and cognitive impairment. Occasionally, this is due to hyperammonemia. At other times, the exact mechanism remains unclear. With high doses, tremor, transient alopecia, and thrombocytopenia (with easy bruising and bleeding) can occur. Another rare side effect of valproate is pancreatitis.

The most publicized and serious side effect of valproate is hepatotoxicity. There have been fatalities. The highest risk group is children younger than 2 years who have developmental delays and abnormal neurologic examination and who are on multiple AEDs. The risk of hepatic failure in these children is estimated at 1 in 500. The hepatotoxicity is an idiosyncratic reaction, is not dose related, and occurs in the first 6 months of therapy. The initial signs and symptoms of liver dysfunction are sedation, nausea, vomiting, and anorexia. Most pediatric neurologists and researchers agree that these cases of fatal hepatotoxicity probably occur in children with an underlying defect in the β-oxidation of fatty acids. Carnitine is an essential cofactor in this process. Therefore, carnitine supplementation[1] at 30 to 100 mg/kg/day is recommended for any child younger than 2 years. It is thought that carnitine provides protection against liver toxicity, aiding β-oxidation by bringing fatty acids across the mitochondrial membrane and binding to toxic valproate metabolites.

Literature has implicated valproate in the development of polycystic ovary syndrome. This syndrome is associated with infertility, dyslipidemia, and insulin-resistant diabetes mellitus. The exact mechanism by which this occurs is still being investigated, but the risk of polycystic

---
[1]Not FDA approved for this indication.

TABLE 1 Summary of Commonly Used Antiepileptic Drugs (Established Drugs)

Drug	Indications	Maintenance Dosage (mg/kg/d)	Starting Dosage	Half-Life (h)	Therapeutic Range (µg/mL)	Common Side Effects	Serious Idiosyncratic Side Effects
Carbamazepine (Tegretol)	Partial Partial w/secondary general, primary general, tonic–clonic	10–20	5–10 mg/kg/d	8–25	8–12	Diplopia, lethargy, blurred vision, ataxia, incoordination	Rashes, hepatic dysfunction, pancreatitis, aplastic anemia, leukopenia
Ethosuximide (Zarontin)	Absence	15–40; most children require 15–20	<6 y: 10 mg/kg/d >6 y: 250 mg/d	25–40	40–100	Gastrointestinal distress, hiccups, lethargy	Rashes, leukopenia, pancytopenia, systemic lupus erythematosus
Phenobarbital	Partial Partial w/secondary general, primary general, tonic–clonic	<1 y: 5–6 >1 y: 4–6 Teenagers, adults: 1–3	Same as maintenance	40–70	15–40	Irritability, hyperactivity, lethargy	Rashes
Phenytoin (Dilantin)	Partial Partial w/secondary general, primary general, tonic–clonic	5 (might need higher doses in children <5–6 y)	Same as maintenance	Depends on concentration	10–20	Lethargy, dizziness, ataxia, gingival hypertrophy, hirsutism	Rashes, hepatic dysfunction, lymphadenopathy, blood dyscrasias
Primidone (Mysoline)	Partial Partial w/secondary general, primary general, tonic–clonic	12–25	<6 y: 50 mg qhs <12 y: 100 mg qhs[3] >12 y: 100–125 mg qhs[3]	5–8 (phenobarbital 40–70)	5–12	Irritability, hyperactivity, lethargy, nausea	Rashes
Valproic Acid (Depakene)	Partial Partial w/secondary general, primary general, tonic–clonic Absence Myoclonic Tonic Atonic	15–60	5–15 mg/kg/d; incr by 10–15 mg/kg/d every 2 wk Max dosage 60 mg/kg/d	4–14	60–100	Lethargy, weight gain or loss, hair loss, tremor	Hepatic dysfunction, pancreatitis, anemia, thrombocytopenia

[3]Exceeds dosage recommended by the manufacturer.

TABLE 2 Summary of Commonly Used Antiepileptic Drugs (New Drugs)

Drug	Indications	Maintenance Dosage (mg/kg/d)	Starting Dosage	Half-Life (h)	Therapeutic Range (mg/mL)	Common Side Effects	Serious Idiosyncratic Side Effects
Felbamate (Felbatol)	Partial Partial w/secondary general Tonic Atonic	30–45, max 90[3]	15 mg/kg/d; incr in 10-mg/kg increments to 60 mg/kg/d[3] if necessary	13–24	30–100 (not well established)	Anorexia, insomnia, somnolence, tics	Aplastic anemia, hepatoxicity, rashes
Gabapentin (Neurontin)	Partial Partial w/secondary general	20–60[3]	10 mg/kg/d, incr in 5-mg/kg increments	5–8	Not established 2–6	Lethargy, dizziness, irritability	None
Lamotrigine (Lamictal)	Partial Partial w/secondary general Generalized tonic–clonic	5–15[3]; dosage depends on other drugs used: w/ enzyme inducers, use 10–15; w/valproate, use 2–3	12.5–25 mg/d, incr slowly; be cautious in patients on valproate	15–60 (highly dependent on concomitant AEDs)	Not established 5–15	Rashes, lethargy, irritability, movement disorder	Rashes
Levetiracetam (Keppra)	Partial Partial w/secondary general Myoclonic	30–60	10 mg/kg/d, incr in 10-mg/kg increments	6–8	3–40	Agitation, behavioral disinhibition	None
Oxcarbazepine (Trileptal)	Partial Partial w/secondary general	30–60	15 mg/kg/d,[3] incr by 10–15 mg/kg increments	8–10	10–35	Hyponatremia, somnolence, lethargy, dizziness, blurred vision	Rash
Rufinamide (Banzel)	Partial (See footnote.)	45 mg/kg/day	10 mg/kg/day	6–10	Not established	Nausea, vomiting, somnolence	None
Tiagabine (Gabitril)	Partial Partial w/secondary general (approved for ≤12 y)	0.5–1; dosage depends on other drugs used: w/ enzyme inducers, use 0.7–1.5; w/o enzyme inducers, use 0.3–0.4	0.1 mg/kg/d; incr weekly by 0.1 mg/kg/d	3–13	Not established 5–70 ng/mL	Lethargy, confusion, mental dullness, difficulties with concentration	None
Topiramate (Topamax)	Partial Partial w/secondary general	5–10[3]	1–2 mg/kg/d; incr weekly by 1 mg/kg/d	12–60	5–20	Irritability, hyperactivity, cognitive slowing, weight loss, renal stones, metabolic acidosis, oligohidrosis	Rash
Zonisamide (Zonegran)	Partial Partial w/secondary general (approved for ≤16 y)	5–10	2 mg/kg/d, incr by 1–2 mg/kg	48–65	10–40	Irritability, cognitive slowing, weight loss, renal stones, oligohidrosis	Rash

Banzel is approved as adjunctive therapy for the tonic and atonic seizures associated with Lennox–Gastaut syndrome.
[3]Exceeds dosage recommended by the manufacturer.
AED = antiepileptic drug; incr = increase.

ovaries, hyperandrogenism, and anovulatory menstrual cycles is definitely increased in women with epilepsy who are taking valproate. In addition, because of these findings and its teratogenic effects (increased risk of neural tube defects and possible neurocognitive effects in the fetus), the American Academy of Neurology and the American Epilepsy Society have both stated that valproate is relatively contraindicated in women with epilepsy who are in the reproductive age.

A baseline complete blood cell count with differential and liver function studies should be obtained before initiating valproate therapy. During the first 6 months of therapy; these blood parameters should be followed monthly or more often if signs and symptoms warrant a closer check.

Gabapentin

Gabapentin is one of the newer AEDs that is sometimes used in treating partial seizures. Its mechanism of action remains largely unknown although it is structurally related to GABA. Gabapentin has not been shown to be effective in treating generalized epilepsies. Gabapentin does not come in a chewable tablet but is available in an oral solution and in tablet and capsule form.

One of the biggest advantages of gabapentin is the lack of drug interactions. It is generally safe and tolerated well. There are no known fatal side effects. In the pediatric population, irritability, aggressiveness, agitation, and other behavioral side effects have been reported, particularly in children with underlying encephalopathy.

Unlike other AEDs, gabapentin is not metabolized by the liver, does not induce the cytochrome P-450 enzyme system, and is not highly protein bound. It is excreted via the kidneys.

Lamotrigine

Lamotrigine was released in 1994. The best known mechanisms of action for lamotrigine include an inhibition in the release of glutamate and an effect on voltage-sensitive sodium channels. It has been approved as adjunctive therapy for treating partial seizures and for treating generalized tonic–clonic seizures. It is probably another broad-spectrum AED, effective in treating partial and generalized seizures. Clinical research is ongoing to determine its efficacy in treating generalized epilepsies. Lamotrigine comes in several formulations including tablets and chewable dispersible tablets.

Lamotrigine has been associated with an allergic rash. Patients who take a combination of valproate and lamotrigine are at highest risk for an allergic rash. Valproate inhibits the metabolism of lamotrigine, resulting in an increase in the half-life from 12 to 72 hours. Therefore, the level of lamotrigine escalates considerably if valproate is added; the required dosage of lamotrigine when taken in combination with valproate is only 2 to 3 mg/kg/day as opposed to 4.5–7.5 mg/kg/day.[3] When lamotrigine therapy is initiated, the dosage must be increased very slowly, especially when it is used in combination with valproate. If a rash is reported, the patient should be seen immediately because the rash can progress rapidly. Patients who have reported skin allergies to other drugs, especially to carbamazepine, are also at high risk for an allergic rash from lamotrigine.

Other less common side effects of lamotrigine include dizziness, headaches, diplopia, sedation, and movement disorders, including choreoathetosis and dystonia. Positive behavioral side effects, including antidepressant effects, have been reported with lamotrigine.

Topiramate

Topiramate is another broad-spectrum AED. Topiramate appears to have a variety of mechanisms of action, including inhibition of voltage-sensitive sodium channels, enhancement of the inhibitory action of GABA, modest inhibitory effects on glutamate receptors, and weak inhibition of carbonic anhydrase. Drug interactions are minimal. It comes in several formulations including tablets and sprinkle capsules.

The major side effect of topiramate is cognitive dysfunction, including dysnomia, slowing of cognitive processing, and poor memory. These side effects can be minimized by a slow titration process, waiting to increase the dosage until habituation has taken place. Rare patients have an idiosyncratic reaction to topiramate, becoming encephalopathic on very small dosages of this medication. Topiramate can also cause renal stones, probably a result of its inhibition of carbonic anhydrase. Therefore, it should be used with caution in patients who are on the ketogenic diet or who have kidney dysfunction. Patients should be kept well hydrated.

Tiagabine

Tiagabine (Gabatril) is another antiepileptic drug that has been approved as adjunctive therapy by the FDA for treating partial seizures (for those ≤12 years of age). Its mechanism of action is via the inhibition of GABA reuptake in the synaptic cleft. There are no known drug interactions. It is formulated in pills only.

The major side effects of tiagabine include lethargy, irritability, aggressive behavior, dizziness, headache, and tremor. It is 96% protein bound and is metabolized by the liver.

Levetiracetam

Levetiracetam is also one of the newer antiepileptic medications. It has a novel mechanism of action that probably involves the synaptic vesicle protein. Levetiracetam has been approved as adjunctive therapy for partial seizures in children and adolescents 4 years and older, for myoclonic seizures in juvenile myoclonic epilepsy in adolescents 12 years and older, and for generalized tonic–clonic seizures in primary generalized epilepsy in children and adolescents 6 years and older.

Levetiracetam has no drug interactions; it is not toxic to the bone marrow or to the liver. It is excreted via the kidneys. Its major side effect is irritability and agitation. This is most prominent in those children who are already behaviorally disinhibited. Levetiracetam comes in a liquid preparation (500 mg/5 mL) or in tablets of 250 mg, 500 mg, 750 mg, or 1000 mg.

Zonisamide

Zonisamide is related to topiramate, with respect to its mechanisms of action. It is approved as adjunctive therapy in partial seizures in children and adolescents at least 16 years of age. In Japan, it is commonly used for myoclonic seizures associated with mitochondrial disorders. Preliminary studies indicate possible efficacy with infantile spasms,[1] myoclonic seizures,[1] and absence seizures.[1]

Its major side effects include lethargy, irritability, cognitive slowing, renal stones, and oligohidrosis. Therefore, it should be used with caution in patients who are on the ketogenic diet or who have kidney dysfunction. Patients should be kept well hydrated. Zonisamide comes in 25-mg, 50-mg, and 100-mg capsules.

ALTERNATIVES TO ANTIEPILEPTIC DRUGS

The ketogenic diet as a treatment for epilepsy has been known since biblical times. It was rediscovered in the modern era by Dr. Haddow Keith from the Mayo Clinic, who observed in a 1921 newsletter that children with status epilepticus usually experienced cessation of seizure activity once they were in ketosis. The ketogenic diet again fell out of favor with the advent of phenobarbital and phenytoin as AEDs. It has recently been repopularized by the Johns Hopkins Medical Center.

In appropriately chosen cases, the ketogenic diet can eliminate seizures in one third of patients and can decrease seizure frequency by more than 50% in another third, but it lacks efficacy in the final third. Patients with LGS have the best chance of responding to this diet. The diet requires that every piece of food and medicine be analyzed with respect to fat, carbohydrate, and protein content. All food and drink must be weighed and measured with respect to calories and type of food. The diet can be very difficult for children who already have dietary preferences.

---

[3]Exceeds dosage recommended by the manufacturer.

[1]Not FDA approved for this indication.

The vagal nerve stimulator (VNS) has been approved by the FDA for use as adjunctive therapy in treating medically refractory, localization-related epilepsy in adults and children older than 12 years. The vagal nerve stimulator is a pacemaker, implanted in the chest pocket below the clavicle, that delivers pulses from a bipolar electrode connected to the vagus nerve. The exact mechanism of action remains an enigma. The VNS influence over the EEG is probably mediated by the solitary tract nucleus–parabrachial nucleus ceruleus–thalamic pathways with concomitant cortical projections. High stimulation of the vagus nerve appears to result in EEG desynchronization, with the full effects gradually being seen over 6 months to 1 year.

Side effects include bleeding, infection, voice alteration or hoarseness when the VNS cycles on, cough, throat pain, dyspepsia, and nausea. There are no reports of cardiac arrhythmias with this device.

Preliminary research on the VNS in patients with symptomatic generalized epilepsies such as LGS indicates significant efficacy, especially over time.

IMMUNOTHERAPY

Immunotherapy has been used in treating a variety of rare and unusual epileptic syndromes, such as Rasmussen's syndrome and Landau–Kleffner syndrome. Rasmussen's syndrome is characterized by progressive hemiparesis, associated cognitive decline, and epilepsia partialis continua. Studies have suggested that autoimmune mechanisms play a role in the pathogenesis of Rasmussen's syndrome. The syndrome affects only one hemisphere. Immunotherapy appears to result in a transient improvement in seizure control.

Steroids are also used in treating infantile spasms and Landau–Kleffner syndrome, as described earlier.

EPILEPSY SURGERY

The five most important questions that must be asked before the consideration of a presurgical evaluation are as follows: is this an epileptic syndrome that is most likely going to continue without resolution? Are the epileptic seizures having a significant impact on the child's development or quality of life? Have the seizures been intractable to a variety of AEDs? Is the epileptogenic zone identifiable? Can the epileptogenic zone be resected without unacceptable neurologic deficits?

Certain children are possible candidates for epilepsy surgery. It can be effective for children with nonlesional localization-related epilepsy in whom standard AED therapy—two to three AEDs—has failed and in children with lesional localization-related epilepsy—the presence of a tumor or other structural lesion, whether or not controlled with AEDs. Children with catastrophic epilepsies in whom the continuation of the epileptic encephalopathy and clinical seizures would result in substantial morbidity in terms of development and quality of life can benefit from surgery. Examples include patients with infantile spasms; Sturge–Weber syndrome with progressive hemiparesis and intractable seizures; Rasmussen's syndrome with progressive encephalopathy, seizures, and hemiparesis; and malformations of cortical development (e.g., hemimegalencephaly). Surgery can be effective for children with medically refractory generalized or multifocal epilepsies in whom the clinical presentation, seizure semiology, EEG findings, MRI of the brain, or other ancillary tests suggest an underlying focal generator for the epileptic condition. Children with intractable generalized epilepsy who have tonic or atonic seizures may be candidates for corpus callosotomy.

The presurgical evaluation must consist of a multidisciplinary approach. The concept of convergence is very important. The identification of the epileptogenic zone requires the confluence of data accumulated by the medical history, seizure semiology, physical examination, EEG interictal and ictal MRI of the brain, and the newer neuroimaging techniques. One technique is MRI of the brain with thin contiguous cuts and FLAIR sequencing (fluid-attenuated inversion recovery technique, i.e., T2-weighted imaging with the cerebrospinal fluid signal subtracted out). Ictal SPECT scan determines cerebral blood flow using radiotracers. These compounds rapidly cross the blood–brain barrier and record the cerebral blood flow at the time of injection. Observations made a century ago document that there is increased cerebral blood flow at the site of the epileptogenic focus during an ictal event. The SPECT scan can, therefore, provide one with a snapshot of the epileptogenic zone. It becomes increasingly accurate if the ictal SPECT scan is subtracted from the interictal SPECT scan and coregistered with the MRI study, a technique termed SISCOM. Interictal positron-emission tomography (PET) scan is another noninvasive functional imaging technique used to identify cerebral metabolic rates using a radioisotope designed to measure glucose metabolism. Interictally, the epileptogenic zone is hypometabolic. Other experimental technologies include MRI (looking at dynamic metabolism of the brain), magnetoencephalography (looking at the flux of magnetic fields in the brain), and functional MRI mapping.

The type of epilepsy surgery performed depends on the localization of the epiletogenic zone. Some of the more common surgical procedures include temporal lobectomy with amgydalohippocampectomy, focal cortical resection, hemispherectomy, implantation of a VNS, corpus callosotomy, and multiple subpial transaction (a technique employed over eloquent cortex that one chooses not to resect because of the potential loss of functional tissue).

Epilepsy surgery can be very effective in eliminating seizures in carefully chosen patients. For example, if a patient has mesial temporal sclerosis and seizures emanating from the temporal lobe, the chance of surgery's producing a seizure-free outcome is as high as 85% to 90%.

REFERENCES

Baumann RJ, Duffner PK. Treatment of children with simple febrile seizures: The AAP practice parameter. Pediat Neurol 2000;23(1):11–7.

Donat JF. The age-dependent epileptic encephalopathies. J Child Neurol 1992;7:7–21.

Dreifuss FE, Rosman NP, Cloyd JC, et al. A comparision of rectal diazepam gel and placebo for acute repetitive seizures. N Engl J Med 1998;26:1869–75.

Freeman JM, Vining EP, Pillas DJ, et al. The efficacy of the ketogenic diet-1998: A prospective evaluation of intervention in 150 children. Pediatrics 1998;102(6):1358–63.

Genton P, Dravet C. Lennox–Gastaut syndrome and other childhood epileptic encephalopathies. In: Engel J Jr, Pedley TA, editors. Epilepsy: A Comprehensive Textbook, vol. 3. Philadelphia: Lippincott-Raven; 1997. pp. 2355–66.

Glauser TA, Pellock JM, Bebin EM, et al. Efficacy and safety of levetiracetam in children with partial seizures: An open-label trial. Epilepsia 2002;43 (5):518–24.

Hirtz D, Berg A, Bettis D, et al. Practice parameter: Treatment of the child with a first unprovoked seizure. Neurology 2003;60:166–75.

Levisohn PM. Safety and tolerability of topiramate in children. J Child Neurol 2000;15(Suppl. 1):S22–6.

Loiseau P. Benign focal epilepsies of childhood. In: Wyllie E, editor. The Treatment of Epilepsy: Principles and Practice. Philadelphia: Lea and Febiger; 1993. pp. 503–12.

Mackay MT, Weiss SK, Adams-Webber T, et al., for the American Academy of Neurology and Child Neurology Society. Practice parameter: medical treatment of infantile spasms. Report of the American Academy of Neurology and the Child Neurology Society. Neurology 2004;62(10):1668–81.

Messenheimer J, Ramsay RE, Willmore LJ, et al. Lamotrigine therapy for partial seizures: A multicenter, placebo-controlled, double-blind, cross-over trial. Epilepsia 1994;35:113–21.

Morrell MJ. Reproductive and metabolic disorders in women with epilepsy. Epilepsia 2003;44(Suppl. 4):11–20.

Murphy JV. Pediatric VNS Study Group. Left vagal nerve stimulation in children with medically refractory epilepsy. J Pediatr 1999;134:563–6.

Nordli DR, Bazil CW, Scheuer ML, Pedley TA. Recognition and classification of seizures in infants. Epilepsia 1997;38:553–60.

Shinnar S, Pellock JM, Berg AT, et al. Short term outcomes of children with febrile status epilepticus. Epilepsia 2001;42(1):47–53.

Tharp BR. Neonatal seizures and syndromes. Epilepsia 2002;43(Suppl 3):2–10.

Trevathan E. Seizures and epilepsy among children with language regression and autistic spectrum disorders. J Child Neurol 2004;19(Suppl 1):S49–57.

Zupanc ML. Infantile spasms. Expert Opin Pharmocother 2003;4(11):2039–48.

Zupanc ML. Early Onset Epilepsy. Pediatric Neurology Continuum: Lifelong Learning in Neurology. Philadelphia, Pennsylvania: American Academy of Neurology, Lippincott Williams and Wilkins; 1999.

Zupanc ML. Neuroimaging in the evaluation of children and adolescents with intractable epilepsy. I: MRI and substrates of epilepsy. Pediatr Neurol 1997;17:19–26.

Attention-Deficit/ Hyperactivity Disorder

Method of
Harris Strokoff, MD, and Craig L. Donnelly, MD

Attention-deficit/hyperactivity disorder (ADHD) is among the most commonly diagnosed illnesses in pediatric medicine. Approximately 4% to 8% of children are diagnosed with ADHD. ADHD is most commonly diagnosed in children between the ages of 6 and 12 years, but it is also diagnosed and treated in children as young as age 3. Although previously thought to largely abate in adolescence and adulthood, ADHD is now considered to be a chronic condition. More than 60% of children with ADHD have impairing symptoms well into adolescence and adulthood. ADHD can cause social problems, academic and learning problems, emotional problems, delinquency, and increased risk-taking behavior, including substance abuse.

ADHD is highly heritable. Approximately 10% to 35% of immediate family members of children with ADHD have ADHD themselves, and approximately 30% of siblings of children with ADHD also have the disorder. Parents of children with ADHD are at high risk for ADHD themselves, and appropriate assessment and potential treatment of ADHD in the parents can improve the child's environment. ADHD is thought to reflect decreased dopamine and norepinephrine transmission in the brain. Maternal smoking and alcohol use, low birth weight, and lead exposure are associated with increased rates of ADHD. Social factors are not thought to play a major role in the development of ADHD.

Diagnosis

Children with ADHD tend to have profound difficulties in maintaining or sustaining attention, and/or they are hyperactive or impulsive. The core inattentive and hyperactive/impulsive symptoms of ADHD are defined by the *Diagnostic and Statistical Manual of Mental Disorders*, fourth edition (DSM-IV). ADHD is classified according to three subtypes: predominantly inattentive type, predominantly hyperactive/impulsive type, and combined type, which is the most common subtype.

The predominantly inattentive type of ADHD is characterized by at least six of the inattention core symptoms but fewer than six of the hyperactive/impulsive symptoms (see Current Diagnosis box). The predominantly hyperactive/impulsive type of ADHD involves six of

CURRENT DIAGNOSIS

- Patients with ADHD have several impairing inattentive symptoms or hyperactive/impulsive symptoms, or both.
- The DSM-IV inattentive core symptoms of ADHD include difficulty sustaining attention, making careless mistakes, increased distractibility, forgetfulness, not seeming to listen when spoken to, not following through on instructions, difficulties with organization, reluctance to engage in schoolwork, and a tendency to lose things.
- The DSM-IV hyperactive/impulsive core symptoms of ADHD include being fidgety; running or climbing excessively; having difficulty awaiting a turn, staying seated, or being quiet; acting as if "driven by a motor"; talking excessively, blurting out answers, and interrupting others.

CURRENT THERAPY

- Stimulant medications (e.g., methylphenidate [Ritalin, Methylin, Concerta] and amphetamine preparations) and atomoxetine (Strattera) are the primary treatments for ADHD in children and adults.
- Medication should be implemented collaboratively, with the child's parents and teachers providing feedback about treatment efficacy and tolerability.
- Psychosocial therapies can add benefit to pharmacotherapy and may be necessary for patients who cannot use pharmacotherapy due to intolerability or preference.

nine hyperactive/impulsive symptoms but fewer than six of the inattention symptoms. If a patient has at least six of the inattention and six of the hyperactive/impulsive symptoms, the diagnosis is combined-type ADHD. These symptoms must also cause significant impairment in the child's life in more than one domain (e.g., in school and home settings) to meet the criteria for ADHD. Symptoms of ADHD must have been present before the age of 7 years to meet the full criteria, although lack of this specifier alone should not preclude treatment.

ADHD is diagnosed by clinical interviews of the child and parents and from information from outside sources, especially from the child's school or daycare. Standardized assessment tools and rating scales, such as the Medium SNAP IV (developed by Swanson, Nolan, and Pelham), the Behavior Assessment System for Children (BASC), the Achenbach Child Behavior Checklist (CBCL), the Achenbach Teacher Report Form (TRF), the Achenbach Youth Self-Report (YSR), and the Connor's rating scale are useful for the diagnosis of ADHD, for monitoring of symptoms over time, and as broader indicators of psychopathology in children and adolescents with ADHD. It is important to rule out underlying conditions (e.g., absence seizures, sleep apnea, learning disorder, anxiety) when making a diagnosis of ADHD.

Comorbidity is the rule in childhood ADHD. It is estimated that only 30% of children with ADHD have the disorder alone. Up to 60% of children with ADHD may have learning disorders, 30% to 40% of children with ADHD also have oppositional defiant disorder or conduct disorder, approximately 30% of children with ADHD have a comorbid anxiety disorder, and approximately 25% of these children have a comorbid major depressive disorder. ADHD is typically diagnosed three or four times more often in boys than in girls, and girls tend to have more predominant inattentive symptoms that may not be noticed as easily in classroom or home settings.

In adults with ADHD, hyperactivity commonly found in children tends to change into a sense of internal restlessness, and impaired attention and distractibility tend to evolve into difficulties with organization and planning. An estimated 4.4% of adults in the United States meet the diagnostic criteria for ADHD. Adults with ADHD tend to be underdiagnosed and have a higher incidence of criminal behavior, injuries, accidents, and employment and marital difficulties compared with adults without ADHD. Untreated symptoms of inattention or hyperactivity often cause or exacerbate anxious and depressive disorders, which may manifest in adulthood in complex comorbid patterns along with ADHD.

Treatment

The gold standard for treatment of ADHD is pharmacotherapy. Treatment with a stimulant medication or atomoxetine (Strattera) is most effective for ADHD, regardless of ADHD subtype. Psychosocial interventions can be a useful adjunct in many children with ADHD, especially those for whom poor tolerability or comorbid diagnoses could be better addressed with psychotherapy.

STIMULANTS

For approximately 75% of children with ADHD, treatment with stimulants decreases their symptoms. As a class, stimulants are fast acting (i.e., improvements are usually evident in the first few days of treatment) and usually well tolerated. Several types of stimulant medications are available. No stimulant has consistently proved to be more effective than another. Choice of a first stimulant medication for the treatment of ADHD is typically based on the desired duration of effect, frequency of dosing, percentage of short-acting medication versus long-acting medication, and the desired delivery system.

The two major classes of stimulant medications are methylphenidate (e.g., Ritalin, Methylin, Concerta) and amphetamine-type preparations. Figure 1 summarizes the medications FDA approved for the treatment of ADHD. Because the data equally support short-acting (immediate-release) and longer-acting stimulant preparations, most clinicians begin with longer-acting preparations, which are thought to offer a smoother level of medication effect and need to be dosed only once daily, which tends to improve compliance. Reasons to consider a shorter-acting medication include wanting to give a test dose before beginning a longer-acting stimulant, wanting to use a very low dose (e.g., in very young children or children with a pervasive developmental disorder), or attempting to minimize potential side effects, such as insomnia and anorexia. Stimulants given twice daily are typically given once in the morning and once at lunchtime. Stimulant medications are available in tablet, capsule, liquid, chewable, and transdermal patch forms.

Like all medications, stimulants have side effects. Stimulants commonly cause appetite suppression, which can lead to weight loss. Stimulants also can decrease linear growth rates, and children with ADHD who are managed with stimulant medication over time may have decreases in projected maximum height of approximately 0.4 to 1 inch. However, after stimulant pharmacotherapy is discontinued, children's linear growth velocity usually accelerates. In the past, drug holidays (e.g., having a child with ADHD off medication for the summer) were common, but it is currently thought that these holidays interrupt optimal treatment and that untreated symptoms during drug holidays can be difficult for the child psychologically and socially. If weight loss and decreased linear growth velocity remain concerns despite attempts at optimizing the psychopharmacologic regimen, drug holidays could be considered.

Stimulants can cause or exacerbate vocal and motor tics. Stimulants may also cause insomnia. α-Blocking agents such as clonidine (Catapres)[1] or guanfacine (Tenex)[1] are sometimes used in addition to stimulant medication to treat the side effects of insomnia or tics. Insomnia can sometimes be managed by decreasing the dose of the stimulant, changing the timing of the dose, or changing to a different stimulant preparation. Melatonin[1,7] is commonly used as an adjunct therapy for the treatment of stimulant-induced insomnia.

Headaches and stomachaches are side effects of stimulants, although they are usually transient in nature. In some patients, stimulants can cause or worsen anxiety in patients with comorbid anxiety disorders, and in these cases, switching to a more anxiety-neutral ADHD treatment (e.g., atomoxetine) or the addition of a selective serotonin reuptake inhibitor (SSRI) should be considered. Rarely, stimulants can cause mood changes and psychotic reactions.

Stimulant treatment in preschool-age children (3–5.5 years old) with ADHD is effective, but it is not as effective as using stimulants to treat school-age children with ADHD. Side effects commonly include emotional lability and aggression in this population, and stimulants should be dosed lower and monitored carefully.

Stimulants have the potential to exacerbate preexisting cardiac conditions, and children should be screened for cardiac disease and a history of premature cardiac death in the family. Patients on stimulant medication should have their heart rate and blood pressure monitored, although the average predictable increases in heart rate (1–2 beats/min) and blood pressure (3–4 mm Hg) are thought to be clinically insignificant. In April 2008, the American Heart Association (AHA) released a statement recommending that children receiving stimulant treatment for ADHD receive screening electrocardiograms (ECGs), and in May 2008, the AHA released a clarification stating that screening ECGs for patients with ADHD are reasonable to consider but not mandatory. In summary, children on stimulants should have their height, weight, blood pressure, and heart rate monitored while receiving therapy.

Stimulants are potential drugs of abuse and are class II schedule medications. Stimulant abuse can cause euphoria, enhance academic and athletic performance, cause weight loss, and induce desired insomnia. ADHD alone is associated with increased rates and severity of substance abuse, and most studies show no change in substance abuse rates in adolescents with ADHD treated with stimulants compared with those left untreated. Longer-acting and alternative formulations (e.g., patch, prodrug, osmotic pump mechanism) stimulants are more difficult to abuse (e.g., intranasally, intravenously) than are immediate-release agents.

NONSTIMULANTS

Atomoxetine is an FDA-approved medication used to treat children, adolescents, and adults with ADHD. Although the degree of effect tends to be somewhat lower than those found with stimulant treatments of ADHD, it is typically effective and well tolerated. Atomoxetine works less quickly than stimulants (peak effectiveness usually apparent around weeks 4 to 6), but it may provide longer duration (i.e., 24-hour) coverage. Atomoxetine is less likely to exacerbate anxiety or cause tics compared with stimulant medications. Atomoxetine has no abuse liability and is not a controlled substance.

Side effects include increased heart rate and blood pressure, and it should be used with caution in children with structural or conductive cardiac abnormalities. Atomoxetine carries an FDA black box warning recommending monitoring for the potential emergence of suicidality in patients taking this medication. Atomoxetine can markedly elevate hepatic enzymes and bilirubin, although hepatic failure is thought to be a rare event. Patients who exhibit symptoms such as jaundice or other indices of liver disease should stop taking this medication and receive medical work-up. Other potential side effects of atomoxetine include agitation, gastrointestinal upset, and headaches, although overall, this medication is thought to be well tolerated.

α-Adrenergic agonists such as clonidine[1] and guanfacine[1] are antihypertensive medications that have been used off-label for many years for the treatment of ADHD, lacking FDA approval for this purpose. Although these medications can improve functioning in patients with ADHD, clinical response is usually less robust than with stimulants. Clonidine and guanfacine are potentially useful in the treatment of hyperactive/impulsive symptoms and are most commonly used adjunctively with stimulants in children with ADHD to treat stimulant-induced tics and insomnia. Clonidine requires three to four doses throughout the day, and guanfacine is typically dosed twice daily. These medications should be used with caution because they carry risks of sedation, orthostasis, potential cardiac side effects, and rare reports of sudden cardiac death with overdose. They should be started at low doses and then titrated slowly. These medications should not be discontinued without a gradual taper over the course of 1 to 2 weeks because of the potential of rebound hypertension and irritability. The FDA has recently approved two long-acting versions of the α-adrenergic agents guanfacine (Intuniv) and clonidine (Kapvay).

Certain antidepressant medications are used to treat children and adults with ADHD, although they do not carry FDA approval for this purpose. Some studies have shown that the antidepressant bupropion (Wellbutrin)[1] improves symptoms of ADHD in children and adults, and it is efficacious in treating depression and ADHD in children and adults who suffer from these comorbid conditions. Potential side effects of bupropion include increases in pulse and blood pressure and potential lowering of a person's seizure threshold. Bupropion, like all antidepressants, carries an FDA black box warning about the potential of these medications to increase suicidality in youths and young adults.

Although rarely used for this purpose and not FDA approved, the tricyclic antidepressants desipramine (Norpramin),[1] imipramine (Tofranil),[1] and nortriptyline (Pamelor)[1] are thought to have some efficacy in the treatment of ADHD. These medications are used less commonly

---

[1]Not FDA approved for this indication.

[7]Available as a dietary supplement.

[1]Not FDA approved for this indication.

Drug	Dosing	Typical starting dose	Comments
Methylphenidate preparations			
Methylphenidate (generic name)			
(Brand name formulations)			
Ritalin	bid to tid	5 mg bid	
Methylin	bid to tid	5 mg bid	available in both liquid and chewable tablet forms
Methylin ER	once daily	10 mg qam	capsule can be opened and contents can be sprinkled into food, longer-acting formulation
Metadate ER	once daily	10 mg qam	capsule can be opened and contents can be sprinkled into food, longer-acting formulation
Metadate CD	once daily	20 mg qam	
Ritalin SR	once daily	10 mg qam	
Ritalin LA	once daily	20 mg qam	capsule can be opened and contents can be sprinkled into food, longer-acting formulation
Concerta	once daily	18 mg qam	uses osmotic pump mechanism, longer-acting formulation
Daytrana patch	apply once daily, then remove at end of the day	10 mg patch	
D-Methylphenidate (generic name)			
(Brand name formulations)			
Focalin	bid to tid	2.5 mg bid	
Focalin XR	once daily	5 mg qam	capsule can be opened and contents can be sprinkled into food, longer-acting formulation
Amphetamine preparations			
Mixed amphetamine salts [D-amphetamine and amphetamine] (generic name)			
(Brand name formulations)			
Adderall	qd to bid	3–5 y: 2.5 mg qam ≥6 y: 5 mg qd to bid	
Adderall XR	once daily	≥6 y: 10 mg qam	capsule can be opened and contents can be sprinkled into food, longer-acting formulation
D-Amphetamine (generic name)			
(Brand name formulations)			
Dexedrine	qd to bid	3–5 y: 2.5 mg qam ≥6 y: 5 mg qd to bid	capsule can be opened and contents can be sprinkled into food
Dextrostat	qd to bid	3–5 y: 2.5 mg qam ≥6 y: 5 mg qd to bid	capsule can be opened and contents can be sprinkled into food
Dexedrine Spansule	qd to bid	≥6 y: 5–10 mg qd to bid	capsule can be opened and contents can be sprinkled into food, longer-acting formulation
Lisdexamphetamine (generic name)			
(Brand name formulations)			
Vyvanse	once daily	30 mg qam	is a pro-drug, thus must be enzymatically cleaved in the gastrointestinal tract in order to yield active D-amphetamine. Not thought to be abusable intranasally
Non-stimulant medication			
Atomoxetine (generic name)			
(Brand name formulations)			
Strattera	once daily (also can be given divided bid)	patients <70 kg: 0.5 mg/kg/day for 4 days; then 1 mg/kg/day for 4 days; then 1.2 mg/kg/day	less likely to exacerbate anxiety in some children, not thought to be abusable
Guanfacine (generic name)			
(Brand name formulations)			
Intuniv	once daily	1 mg/day increasing by 1 mg each week to a max of 4 mg/day	little abuse potential, may cause somnolence
Clonidine (generic name)			
(Brand name formulations)			
Kapvay	once daily	1 mg/day	little abuse potential, may cause somnolence

FIGURE 1. Medications commonly used to treat ADHD. *Abbreviations:* bid = twice daily; ER = extended release; LA = long acting; qam = every morning; qd = once daily; SR = sustained release; tid = three times daily; XR = extended release.

because of significant side effects such as ECG changes (prolonged QTc), sedation, and risk of sudden cardiac death with overdose.

Modafinil (Provigil)[1] is FDA approved for the treatment of narcolepsy, shift-work sleep disorder, and obstructive sleep apnea/hypopnea syndrome, and it is thought to improve vigilance and decrease distractibility. It is sometimes used to treat ADHD. Modafinil is not thought to be as easily abused as the stimulant medications.

Stimulant pharmacotherapy should be the initial treatment for most cases of ADHD. Formal dosing guidelines of stimulants should be followed. Titration of the dose until sufficient improvement is gained or limiting side effects emerge is the best way to optimize stimulant treatment outcome. There is sufficient evidence to suggest switching to another stimulant if treatment with the initial agent is suboptimal (e. g., switching from an amphetamine preparation to a methylphenidate preparation), and if the second stimulant trial fails, consideration should be given to a third stimulant trial. If there is a partial response to a stimulant trial, consider augmentation with atomoxetine or the addition of an α-blocking agent if insomnia or tics are mitigating side effects.

Although ADHD tends to be a chronic condition, not all children with ADHD progress to become adults with ADHD. Children who are being treated for ADHD should be reassessed yearly to determine if treatment for ADHD is still indicated. In the treatment of adults with ADHD, the same treatment strategies apply, although adults may require higher doses of medication. Stimulants and atomoxetine are the primary treatments for adults with ADHD. Because of higher rates of substance abuse comorbidities in adults, the risks of potential stimulant abuse and diversion may be higher in this population.

PSYCHOSOCIAL TREATMENTS

Psychosocial therapies can be a useful and sometimes necessary adjunct to pharmacotherapy for the treatment of ADHD. Behavior therapy can be effective in helping to manage symptoms of ADHD, and parents and teachers are essential for implementing behavioral strategies and for continually assessing ADHD symptoms and treatment side effects. Parent training groups are effective at maximizing children's compliant behaviors, and several books (e.g., Barkley's *Your Defiant Child*, Forehand and Long's *Parenting the Strong-Willed Child*) are available for training parents and clinicians to teach and reinforce behavioral therapy.

Classroom management techniques are an important part of any psychosocial approach to the treatment of ADHD in children and adolescents. Teachers of students with ADHD have found it helpful to increase the structure in classrooms, use consistent rewards and punishments, and use daily report cards to communicate school performance to parents at home.

Psychosocial interventions alone are not highly effective for the treatment of children with ADHD. For children with uncomplicated ADHD, psychosocial interventions may not significantly add benefit to pharmacotherapy alone. Because of the high rates of comorbidity in children and adolescents with ADHD, additional psychotherapies (and sometimes pharmacotherapies) may be necessary to treat these more complex presentations.

---

[1]Not FDA approved for this indication.

REFERENCES

Adler LA. From childhood into adulthood: The changing face of ADHD. CNS Spectr 2007;12(Suppl. 23):12.

American Academy of Pediatrics/American Heart Association. Clarification of statement on cardiovascular evaluation and monitoring of children and adolescents with heart disease receiving medications for ADHD. Available at http://americanheart.mediaroom.com/index.php?s=43&item=422 [accessed July 2009].

American Psychiatric Association Task Force on DSM-IV. Diagnostic and Statistical Manual of Mental Disorders: DSM-IV-TR. Washington, DC: American Psychiatric Association; 2000.

Barkley R. Attention-Deficit Hyperactivity Disorder: A Handbook for Diagnosis and Treatment. 3rd ed. New York: Guilford Press; 2006.

Clinical Pharmacology Online Version 8.06. Drug and toxicology information. Available at http://www.clinicalpharmacology.com [accessed July 2009].

Gilchrist RH, Arnold EL. Long-term efficacy of ADHD pharmacotherapy in children. Pediatr Ann 2008;37:46.

Greenhill L, Kollins S, Abikoff H, et al. Efficacy and safety of immediate-release methylphenidate treatment for preschoolers with ADHD. J Am Acad Child Adolesc Psychiatry 2006;45:11.

Jensen PS, Arnold LE, Swanson JM, et al. 3-Year follow-up of the NIMH MTA study. J Am Acad Child Adolesc Psychiatry 2007;46:8.

Kessler RC, Adler L, Barkley R, et al. The prevalence and correlates of adult ADHD in the United States: Results from the National Comorbidity Survey Replication. Evid Based Ment Health 2006;9:116.

Newcorn JH. Nonstimulants and emerging treatments in adults with ADHD. CNS Spectr 2008;13(Suppl. 13):9.

Palumbo DR, Sallee FR, Pelham WE. Clonidine for attention-deficit/hyperactivity disorder. I. Efficacy and tolerability outcomes. J Am Acad Child Adolesc Psychiatry 2008;47:2.

Pliszka S. AACAP Work Group on Quality Issues: Practice parameter for the assessment and treatment of children and adolescents with attention-deficit/hyperactivity disorder. J Am Acad Child Adolesc Psychiatry 2007;46:7.

Towbin K. Paying attention to stimulants: Height, weight, and cardiovascular monitoring in clinical practice. J Am Acad Child Adolesc Psychiatry 2008;47:9.

Gilles de la Tourette Syndrome

Method of
Steve W. Wu, MD, and Donald L. Gilbert, MD, MS

Gilles de la Tourette syndrome, or Tourette syndrome, was named after French neurologist Georges Gilles de la Tourette, who in 1885 described a series of nine patients with chronic tics. Tourette syndrome is a neuropsychiatric illness that begins in childhood. It is characterized by multiple motor and vocal tics that last for longer than 1 year (see Current Diagnosis box). The prevalence of Tourette syndrome varies greatly among epidemiologic studies, ranging from 0.1% to 3.8%. The prevalence of tic disorders is even higher, especially in children requiring special education.

Simple motor tics are sudden, brief, patterned movements such as eye blinking, facial grimace, head jerk, or shoulder shrug. Complex motor tics can involve a series of simple tics or a seemingly purposeful action, such as jumping, touching, or copropraxia (i.e., performing obscene gestures). Simple vocal tics consist of sounds such as throat clearing, sniffing, and coughing. Patients with complex vocal tics may exhibit echolalia (i.e., repeating others' words), palilalia (i.e., repeating their own words), or coprolalia (i.e., utterance of foul language).

Older children and adolescents often describe a premonitory urge before their tics. Tics can usually be transiently suppressed and are often diminished during focused mental or physical activities. Unlike myoclonus or chorea, tics usually do not affect activities of daily living or occupational or recreational activities. After the brief suppression, the release of the tic often brings relief to the patient. Tic severity commonly worsens during times of emotional stress. Fatigue or illness may also increase tics. Parents often notice more tics when the child is bored or unoccupied with an activity. Tics can occur during light sleep and rapid eye movement (REM) sleep.

Clinical Course

The onset of tics can occur after children are 3 years old, but they usually begin in children 6 to 7 years old. Children often present with motor tics first, followed by the development of vocal tics. Tics often wax and wane in the course of Tourette syndrome. During the early school years, tics often can go unnoticed or be mislabeled as a habit. If tics are noticed by fellow students, bullying is typically not an issue at this age. However, when parents notice the tics, they are often distressed and frequently tell their children to stop the movements.

Tic severity usually increases in the later elementary school years and into adolescence. This is the time when social interference such as bullying begins to occur. By late adolescence and early adulthood, most patients with Tourette syndrome have minimal tics, and some may "outgrow" tics. Because of this pattern, most individuals presenting for medical attention for tics are children.

Patients with Tourette syndrome frequently present with comorbid attention-deficit/hyperactivity disorder (ADHD) and obsessive-compulsive disorder (OCD). They also tend to have more sleep problems, anxiety, and mood disorders.

Diagnosis and Differential Diagnosis

Diagnosis of tic disorders depends on correctly recognizing that the abnormal movements are tics by means of a careful history and thorough physical examination. Laboratory and imaging studies are rarely needed.

Tics may resemble other abnormal movements, such as stereotypy, chorea, ballism, dystonia, and myoclonus. *Stereotypies* are repetitive, simple movements that are suppressible and that usually occur when a child is excited. Stereotypies usually start when the child is younger than 3 years. *Chorea* consists of a sequence of random, continual, involuntary, nonpurposeful, nonrhythmic movements. Choreic movements often flow from one body part to another. *Ballism* is a large-amplitude choreic movement affecting the proximal limb. *Myoclonus* is an involuntary, sudden, shocklike movement. Chorea, ballism, and myoclonus cannot be volitionally suppressed. *Dystonia* is produced by co-contraction of agonist and antagonist muscles, leading to abnormal postures, and its twisting movements typically are slower than tics.

Vocal tics may sometimes lead to the misdiagnosis of asthma, chronic cough, or allergic rhinitis. Other primary tic disorders include transient tic disorder, chronic motor or vocal tic disorders, and tic disorder not otherwise specified. Persons with autistic spectrum disorders often have tics.

Tics are nonspecific and may occur in drug-induced movement disorders, after head trauma, and in a variety of neurodevelopmental and neurodegenerative disorders. Complex or atypical cases with multiple comorbidities or multiple abnormalities identified on a general or neurologic examination should be referred for specialist consultation.

A controversial diagnosis in which tics or OCD may occur is called pediatric autoimmune neuropsychiatric disorders associated with streptococcal infections (PANDAS). Criteria for this diagnosis classically include abrupt appearance in prepubertal children of tics or OCD on two or more occasions after documented group A β-hemolytic streptococcal (GABHS) infections. The paradigm for this diagnosis is rheumatic (Sydenham's) chorea; however, PANDAS has no arthritis, carditis, or nephritis and is not thought to be a rheumatic disease. Epidemiologic studies of PANDAS show mixed findings, with stress and other types of infections appearing to trigger exacerbations. The following interventions are not routinely recommended: diagnostic throat cultures and antistreptococcal antibody tests; therapeutic or preventive antibiotics; and immune-modulating therapies such as steroids, intravenous immunoglobulins, or plasmapheresis. Specialty consultation should be considered.

Treatment

There are many factors to consider when treating a patient with Tourette syndrome, including the presence of common symptoms such as inattentiveness, hyperactivity, obsessive or compulsive behaviors, depression, and anxiety (Box 1). When deciding to treat the patient, it is important to prioritize all the neuropsychiatric

---

CURRENT DIAGNOSIS

- Multiple motor and one or more vocal tics have been present for some time during the illness, although not necessarily concurrently.
- The tics occur many times per day (usually in bouts) almost every day or intermittently throughout a period of more than 1 year. During this time, there is not a tic-free period of more than 3 consecutive months.
- The disturbance causes marked distress or significant impairment in social, occupational, or other important areas of functioning.
- Onset occurs before age 18 years.
- The disturbance is not caused by the direct physiologic effects of a substance or a general medical condition.

BOX 1 Therapeutic Approach for Tourette Syndrome

- Educate the patient and family about tics and how tics often diminish spontaneously. Long-term reductions in tics may occur in the late teens, irrespective of pharmacologic therapy.
- Rank the tics, attention-deficit hyperactivity disorder (ADHD), obsessive-compulsive disorder (OCD), anxiety, mood problems, learning problems, and behavior problems in order of the patient's or the family's perception of severity.
- Consider nonpharmacologic and pharmacologic treatment for each symptom in the order of perceived severity or impairment.
- Provide information to educate teachers and classmates to reduce social impairment.
- If the patient has learning problems, encourage formal assessment through the school or a psychologist. These children may qualify for modified educational methods.
- If ADHD is the most concerning problem, consider treating with clonidine (Catapres),[1] guanfacine (Tenex),[1] atomoxetine (Strattera), or methylphenidate (Ritalin). Stimulants are *not* absolutely contraindicated in patients with Tourette syndrome. However, if symptoms of OCD, anxiety, or pervasive developmental disorder are present, ticcing or compulsions may escalate on stimulants. If a patient has done well for months to years on stimulants for ADHD before an exacerbation of tics, it usually is not necessary to discontinue stimulants.
- If behavior problems are the most concerning problem or if a first-degree family member has a bipolar or psychotic disorder, refer the patient to a psychologist or psychiatrist.
- Anxious parents often worsen tic severity. If the family's anxiety is excessive, refer family members to a psychologist.
- If OCD or generalized anxiety disorder is the most severe problem, treatment with a selective serotonin reuptake inhibitor may be considered.
- Do not begin treatment with more than one central nervous system drug simultaneously. Start one, wait 2 to 4 weeks, and then reassess all symptoms before starting the next medication.
- Monitor the benefits and side effects at regular intervals.
- Maintain stable dosing during the school year; consider tapering medications in the summer.
- Consider weaning tic-suppressing medications in the middle to late teen years if tics wane.

---

[1]Not FDA approved for this indication.

symptoms and provide accurate educational information. Tics may not always need to be treated medically, and if treatment is needed, tics may not be the first symptom to manage. Daily tic-suppressing medication is considered when there is functional interference, social interference, pain, or classroom or occupational disruption.

The first step in treating Tourette syndrome is educating the patient, parents, and other adult caregivers. Parents, teachers, and other adult caregivers are discouraged from telling the child to stop ticcing because this produces emotional anxiety that may worsen the tics. Educational materials for teachers often promote a conducive environment for the child at school. The patient is encouraged to openly talk about his or her disorder to classmates to promote understanding and minimize bullying. Newer cognitive-behavioral treatments for tic suppression appear to be helpful for children and adolescents, and they should be considered.

Clinical trials enrolling patients with Tourette syndrome are usually small and show small effect sizes. Most commonly used tic-suppressing medications belong to two classes: α_2-adrenergic agonists and dopamine receptor blocking agents (Table 1). Other agents may show modest benefit. Because Tourette syndrome is a chronic, nonfatal disorder, it is prudent to start treatment with medications that carry the least side effects. For this reason, α_2-adrenergic agonists are usually the first-line treatment. Although it is unclear what the second-line agents should be, it is reasonable in many cases to restrict dopamine receptor blocking agents to the most severe cases.

α_2-ADRENERGIC AGONISTS

Clonidine (Catapres)[1] and guanfacine (Tenex)[1] are α_2-adrenergic agonists often used to treat tics. Several randomized trials have shown that these agents reduce tic and ADHD symptoms. The main side effects are sedation and lightheadedness due to mild hypotension. Sedation is more common with clonidine. The clonidine patch (Catapres-TTS)[1] may produce less peak sedation, but it commonly produces local skin irritation.

DOPAMINE RECEPTOR BLOCKING AGENTS

Typical and atypical neuroleptics are dopamine receptor blocking agents that can be used to treat tics. Neuroleptics can be very effective in tic suppression, but they can cause acute akathisia, dystonic reactions, cognitive blunting, acute anxiety with somatizations and school refusal, sedation, weight gain, metabolic syndrome, and QT prolongation. Monitoring for tardive dyskinesia is also important. Some experts recommend baseline electrocardiograms, particularly for individuals with personal or family history of cardiac arrhythmias. Weight gain and metabolic syndrome should be considered when starting neuroleptics, particularly risperidone (Risperdal).[1]

[1]Not FDA approved for this indication.

Some experts recommend obtaining baseline values for weight, blood pressure, fasting glucose, and lipid profile, with follow-up monitoring every 3 months to detect drug-induced metabolic syndrome. Diet modification, routine exercise, or medical therapy may be needed.

OTHER TIC-SUPPRESSING MEDICATIONS

Several small, controlled studies show benefit for dopamine agonists, baclofen (Lioresal),[1] benzodiazepines, and botulinum toxin type A (Botox) injections for focal, strong tics. Tetrabenazine (Xenazine),[1] a drug approved by the FDA for use in Huntington disease, has been reported to reduce tics.

EVOLVING THERAPIES

A new form of cognitive-behavioral/habit reversal therapy, in which the patient learns to increase self-awareness of tics and premonitory urges and to apply antagonistic movements to compete with the tics, has shown early beneficial results. Transcranial magnetic stimulation therapy and deep brain stimulation have been reported anecdotally to reduce tics.

TREATMENT OF COMORBID CONDITIONS

ADHD and OCD are common comorbid conditions in Tourette syndrome. These comorbid symptoms are often more debilitating than the tics. Concern about stimulant therapy worsening tics was addressed by the Tourette Syndrome Study Group in the landmark Treatment of ADHD in Children with Tics (TACT) study. In this study, children treated with methylphenidate (Ritalin) had, on average, reduced tic severity, contrary to the widely held belief that stimulants exacerbate tics.

Medical treatment options for ADHD include psychostimulants and the selective norepinephrine reuptake inhibitor atomoxetine (Strattera). OCD management includes cognitive-behavioral therapy, clomipramine (Anafranil), and any of the selective serotonin reuptake inhibitors.

Summary

Tourette syndrome is a complex neuropsychiatric illness with many potential symptoms that may need medical and nonmedical therapies. Cooperation among the primary care physician, neurologist, psychiatrist, and psychologist is imperative for the comprehensive care of severely affected patients. If a patient has mild tics and few or no comorbid symptoms, medical therapy may not be needed. However, if the tics are severe in the presence of many neuropsychiatric symptoms, it is reasonable to refer patients to specialists.

[1]Not FDA approved for this indication.

TABLE 1 Therapy for Tics in Tourette Syndrome

Medication	Starting Dose	Titration	Goal Dose
Clonidine (Catapres)[1]	0.05 mg qhs	0.05 mg every 3–7 d	0.05–0.1 mg tid
Clonidine patch (Catapres-TTS)[1]	Catapres TTS-1 weekly*	Weekly as needed	Catapres TTS-1, -2, or -3 weekly*
Guanfacine (Tenex)[1]	0.5 mg qhs	0.5 mg every 3–7 d	1–4 mg divided bid
Baclofen (Lioresal)[1]	10 mg qhs	10 mg every 3–7 d	40–90 mg/d divided bid/tid
Clonazepam (Klonopin)[1]	0.5 mg qhs	0.5 mg every wk	1–2 mg bid
Pimozide (Orap)	1 mg qhs	1 mg every 3–5 d	1–4 mg/d divided daily or bid
Haloperidol (Haldol)	0.25–0.5 mg qhs	0.25–0.5 mg every 5–7 d	1–4 mg/d divided daily or bid
Fluphenazine (Prolixin)[1]	0.5 mg qhs	0.5 mg every 3–5 d	1–4 mg/d divided daily or bid
Risperidone (Risperdal)[1]	0.5 mg qhs	0.5 mg every 3–5 d	1–4 mg/d divided daily or bid
Ziprasidone (Geodon)[1]	20 mg qhs	20 mg every wk	20–80 mg/d divided daily or bid
Botulinum toxin type A (Botox)[1]	Not applicable	Not applicable	30–300 units in one or more focal sites, injected once every 3 mo

[1]Not FDA approved for this indication.
*The system areas are 3.5 cm^2 (Catapres TTS-1), 7.0 cm^2 (Catapres TTS-2), and 10.5 cm^2 (Catapres TTS-3), and the amount of drug released is directly proportional to the area.

REFERENCES

Gilbert DL. Treatment of children and adolescents with tics and Tourette syndrome. J Child Neurol 2006;21:690–700.

Kurlan R, Johnson D, Kaplan EL. Streptococcal infection and exacerbations of childhood tics and obsessive-compulsive symptoms: A prospective blinded cohort study. Pediatrics 2008;121:1188–97.

Piacentini J, Woods DW, Scahill L, et al. Behavior therapy for children with Tourette disorder: A randomized controlled trial. JAMA 2010;3:192–206.

Tourette Syndrome Study Group. Treatment of ADHD in children with tics: A randomized controlled trial. Neurology 2002;58:527–36.

Zinner SH. Tourette syndrome: Much more than tics. Contemp Pediatr 2004;21:22–49.

Headache

Method of
R. Michael Gallagher, DO

Headache is a disturbing and sometimes fearsome affliction that has plagued humankind throughout recorded history. It often is debilitating and particularly disturbing to the sufferer because the pain is located in the head, the very center of the body's cognitive and control functions. With its accompanying pain and debilitating symptoms, stress can mount and the headache can become all consuming.

Headache is experienced by all age groups from young children to the elderly. It is more common than asthma, diabetes, mental illness, and rheumatoid arthritis. In fact, the World Health Organization identifies severe migraine, along with psychosis and quadriplegia, as "one of the most debilitating chronic conditions." Although the majority of Americans experience tension-type headaches at some time in their lives, approximately 30 million experience migraine headache: 13% of women and 6% of men, predominantly in their most productive years between the ages of 13 and 55 years. Prepubescent boys and girls suffer equally; however, boys often outgrow their migraine attacks as they mature, and they are less subjected to hormonal influences. Smaller percentages of people, by comparison, suffer with other chronic headaches, such as cluster headache and chronic daily headache.

No sure diagnostic tests are available to differentiate headache types. The headache condition can progress over time in frequency, severity, and debilitation. Each sufferer can be different and may require a detailed evaluation and individualized treatment plan; more frequent or prolonged attacks often necessitate a more comprehensive treatment plan. Thus, the headache problem can be a challenge for both the sufferer and the clinician.

During the 20th century, dramatic advancements were made in medicine. Longevity and quality of life improved for many individuals. Unfortunately, for headache sufferers, most of these advances were for maladies that killed or maimed rather than for non-life-threatening conditions. It was not until the 1960s that even a reasonable preventive medication, propranolol (Inderal), was introduced, and by the 1980s only a handful of medications were available for wide use. Physicians had to improvise with medications and treatments that were originally designated for other medical conditions.

In the late 1980s and 1990s, epidemiologic, psychosocial, and pharmacologic research resulted in an increase in available headache information and treatment possibilities. The development of the triptans, serotonin agonists, brought a new awareness to both physicians and sufferers. Today, seven triptans and two relatively new preventive medications are available. In spite of this, a minority of migraine sufferers use these options, and more than 50% continue to self-treat without benefit of professional care.

In the past, patients wanted the physician to believe their headache problem was real. They hoped that they would be taken seriously and that the physician would make a sincere attempt to help them. The headache patient has changed. The headache sufferer who seeks treatment today is more knowledgeable and interested in rapid relief and tolerability of medication.

Evaluation and Diagnosis

An accurate diagnosis is essential for effective management of patients with the more commonly encountered headaches. Because no biologic markers or diagnostic tests exist to determine headache type, the history is the single most important element in the evaluation of the headache patient. Various headache types sometimes have similar initial presentations, or patients may suffer with more than one type of headache (e.g., migraine and tension-type headache), which can be confusing at first, but the careful history usually differentiates the headache type. In general, little in the way of diagnostic testing is needed unless a physical cause is suspected. Some physicians prefer to perform simple laboratory tests to establish a baseline for medication toleration and monitoring as necessary (Table 1).

The headache complaint on occasion can be a sign of a more serious medical condition, such as a tumor, infection, or aneurysm. For this reason, the clinician always must be cautious and diligent in establishing an accurate and timely diagnosis. Certain so-called red flags in the history require immediate attention. These include any complex of symptoms or history that does not fit a typical headache type; report of a significant neurologic deficit; significant or prolonged neurologic deficit with aura; late-onset migraine (patient older than 30 years); sudden onset of a new head pain without history of similar headaches; changes in headache character; headache associated with elevated temperature; or completely unresponsive attacks in the absence of analgesic or caffeine overuse. When any of these symptoms are present or physical examination reveals significant findings, further diagnostic evaluation with imaging studies and consultation is imperative.

The appropriate headache patient evaluation includes a thorough history, physical examination with special attention to the head and the neurologic, cardiovascular, and musculoskeletal systems, and

TABLE 1   Current Diagnosis

Symptoms	Frequency	Duration
Tension-Type Headache		
Bilateral variable pain	Variable	Hours to days
Squeezing or bandlike	Often related to	
Tightness of head and shoulders	known precipitant	
Migraine Headache		
Unilateral mostly	1–6 mo	Hours to days
Throbbing or constant pain	Sometimes cyclic	
Nausea, vomiting		
Photophobia/phonophobia		
Fluid disturbances		
Mood changes		
Can be associated with aura		
Cluster Headache		
Unilateral severe boring pain	Multiple daily	45–90 min
Ipsilateral lacrimation, scleral injection, rhinorrhea	Near-daily	Cycles of attacks
Eyelid droop		
Restlessness		

diagnostic tests when appropriate. The history should include headache onset, location, pain character (e.g., pressure, throb), frequency, duration, associated symptoms, aura or prodrome, triggers, previous treatment, and family history. Certain clues in the history may lean toward the diagnosis of migraine, such as motion sickness, absence of headache during pregnancy, and headache relationship to menses, sun glare, oversleep, fatigue, fasting, foods, or alcohol.

Various diagnostic screening questionnaires and tools have been developed over the years to assist busy clinicians in establishing the diagnosis of migraine. Most are long and cumbersome and do not easily become a part of routine patient evaluation. A simple three-question screener for migraine is helpful for generalist clinicians. A "yes" answer to all three questions indicates a strong possibility of the migraine diagnosis:

1. Do you experience headaches severe enough to see a physician?
2. Are your headaches accompanied by other symptoms?
3. Are your headaches intermittent (i.e., nondaily)?

Note: This screener should not be substituted for a complete history; it should be used only for screening purposes.

TENSION-TYPE HEADACHE

Tension-type headache (TTHA) is the most common of headaches and first was believed to be caused by sustained muscle contraction of the neck, jaw, scalp, or facial muscles. However, it is now thought that the sustained muscle contraction can, in fact, be an epiphenomenon to possible central disturbances rather than a primary process. Evidence suggests that altered levels of serotonin, substance P, and neuropeptide Y in the serum or platelets of patients with TTHA are responsible.

TTHA is characterized by intermittent or persisting bilateral pain, usually described as a squeezing pressure or a bandlike sensation around the head. Most patients experience their symptoms in the frontal, temporal, or occipital areas of the head. Location frequently varies with the attack, and tightness of the neck and shoulders is common. Intensity varies greatly. The attacks can last from hours to days, and in some extreme cases they may last for months. Aura, nausea, photophobia and phonophobia, and incapacitation are not typically associated with TTHA.

Many TTHA sufferers easily recognize the origin of their attacks. TTHA typically results from emotional upset, periods of stress, and major life changes. Anxiousness, poor adaptation skills, and anxiety and depression often are present. Physical causes, such as degenerative joint disease, trauma to the head or neck, poor posture, or temporomandibular joint dysfunction, also can precipitate attacks. Persons older than 50 years are prone to excessive muscle contraction because of arthritis of the neck and jaw, poor posture, or stress. TTHA that is consistently precipitated by tension or pathology of the neck frequently is referred to as a *cervicogenic headache*. In contrast to migraine headache, TTHA is more likely to begin in later life.

MIGRAINE HEADACHE

Migraine headache is a familial disease characterized by unilateral or bilateral paroxysmal headache lasting hours to days. Adult women experience attacks more than men by a ratio of 3:1. Children and the elderly experience migraine equally. Attacks occur from as infrequently as one or two per year to several times weekly. Associated symptoms usually occur and frequently include throbbing, nausea, vomiting, photophobia, phonophobia, fluid retention, and mood changes.

The two basic types of migraine headache are *migraine with aura* (previously called classic migraine) and *migraine without aura* (previously called common migraine). Migraine with aura is preceded by an aura, a transient neurologic symptom that usually is visual, such as scotoma, teichopsia, tunnel vision, or visual field deficit, lasting 10 to 30 minutes. However, aura can manifest as any neurological deficit. Migraine without aura is more commonly experienced and comes on gradually or is present on awakening from sleep. In some patients, these headaches are associated with a nonspecific prolonged prodrome, such as mood changes, food cravings, or fluid retention hours before the pain.

BOX 1 Migraine Dietary Triggers

- Dairy: Ripened cheese (cheddar, brie, camembert, half-cup of sour cream)
- Meats: Processed lunch meats, hot dogs, sausage, bologna, salami, chicken liver
- Fish: Pickled or dried herring
- Grains: Sourdough bread
- Fruits: Bananas, raisins, figs, avocado, half-cup limit of citrus
- Vegetables: Broad and fava beans, onions, snow peas
- Other: Chocolate, nuts, peanut butter, pickled foods, Chinese food with monosodium glutamate (MSG)
- Beverages: Most wines and alcohol, 200-mg daily limit of caffeine
- Additives: MSG, soy sauce, meat tenderizers, aspartame, sulfites, garlic

---

The underlying cause of migraine headache is not clearly established, and various theories are proposed. Migraine appears to be of genetic origin and to be an inflammatory disease that causes disturbances in serotonin use and activity. Strong evidence indicates the migrainous attack originates in the central nervous system by stimulation of the locus ceruleus and dorsal raphe nuclei. Resultant changes alter cerebral and extracranial blood flow, activate the trigeminovascular system, and cause vascular dilation, neurogenic inflammation, and pain. Various precipitants are known, and many sufferers report that migraine attacks frequently are associated with menstruation or are triggered by foods containing vasoactive amines, strong odors, too much or too little sleep, sun glare, stress, altitude, weather changes, exertion, or fasting (Boxes 1 and 2, Table 2).

Some physicians classify migraine according to its precipitant or description (e.g., menstrual migraine, exertional migraine, coital migraine, cervicogenic migraine, cyclic migraine, acephalic migraine). Regardless, the fundamentals of evaluation and treatment are the same.

CLUSTER HEADACHE

The cause of cluster headache is unknown, and little credible research is available. Various possibilities or theories are suggested and include, but are not limited to, disturbances in histamine production or use; hypothalamic biorhythm dysfunction; or serotonin and neurotransmitter mechanisms similar to those of migraine. Some authorities consider cluster headache one of the most severe pain conditions known to humankind.

Cluster headache predominantly affects men, with a male-to-female ratio of 6:1. It occurs in well under 0.5% of the population. Onset later in life (after age 30 years) is common, and patients

---

BOX 2 Migraine Triggers

- Altitude
- Alcohol
- Caffeine withdrawal
- Fluorescent or flickering lights
- Sun glare
- Weather changes
- Stress, stress letdown
- Foods
- Skipping meals
- Smoky environment
- Noisy environment
- Strong odors
- Lack of sleep, oversleep
- Exertion
- Hormonal changes

TABLE 2 Current Therapy

Headache Type	PRN	Prophylaxis
Tension	OTC*	Stress/precipitant avoidance
	NSAIDs	Stretching
	Muscle relaxants	Warm packs
	Combination analgesics	Relaxation techniques
		NSAIDs
		Muscle relaxants
		Antidepressants
Migraine	NSAIDs*	Biofeedback
	Triptans*	β-Blockers*
	Ergotamine*	Divalproex sodium*
	Dihydroergotamine*	
	Isometheptene*	Topiramate*
	Combination analgesics	TCA antidepressants
		Calcium channel blockers
Cluster	Oxygen	No alcohol
	Triptans	Calcium channel blockers
	Dihydroergotamine	Divalproex sodium
	Ergotamine	NSAIDs
		Lithium
		Steroids

*FDA indication.
Abbreviations: NSAID = nonsteroidal antiinflammatory drug; OTC = over-the-counter; TCA = tricyclic antidepressant.

sometimes report head injury or a traumatic event occurring months before onset. Attacks occur on a daily or near-daily basis for weeks or months at a time and mysteriously disappear for months to years regardless of treatment, only to recur and cycle again. Although non-specialist physicians only occasionally encounter the patient with cluster headaches, it is important to consider cluster headaches in the differential diagnosis.

The typical patient with a cluster headache experiences relatively brief attacks (45–90 minutes) of horrible unilateral head pain associated with ipsilateral lacrimation, scleral injection, rhinorrhea, or eyelid droop. The hallmark of the syndrome is its associated symptoms and its severe and intense pain. During attacks, most cluster patients move about, trying unsuccessfully to get more comfortable, similar to renal colic, in contrast to migraine sufferers, who prefer to lie quietly in a dark quiet room. Few triggers are identified, and alcohol almost always precipitates an attack during a cluster "on" cycle. A rare form of cluster headache, chronic cluster, does not cycle and continues on a daily or near-daily basis without cessation.

Treatment

The doctor–patient relationship frequently is the key to successful treatment in the headache patient. Although to some this statement seems an obvious truism, its importance cannot be overemphasized. Patients who experience frequent, near-daily, or daily headaches invariably require a comprehensive treatment program that necessitates good communication. Anxious patients sometimes do not comprehend medical explanations or instructions; busy doctors sometimes do not have or take the time to ensure that the patient understands.

The two elements of headache treatment are *abortive treatment,* directed at attacks once they have begun, and *prophylactic treatment,* directed at preventing or reducing the frequency of attacks. In general, the abortive approach is used for patients who suffer infrequent attacks and for those who experience breakthrough attacks while undergoing prophylactic therapy. Prophylactic therapy should be instituted when headaches are frequent, when headaches are unresponsive to abortive medication, or when there are contraindications to abortives (Table 2).

Headache treatment can include nonpharmacologic measures, such as physical exercise, stretching, stress avoidance, relaxation exercises, biofeedback, manipulation, massage, or cold/warm packs. Pharmacologic therapies can include a vast array of medicaments from over-the-counter (OTC) drugs to prescription drugs such as triptans, other vasoconstrictors, β-blockers, antiepileptic agents, antidepressants, nonsteroidal antiinflammatory drugs (NSAIDs), analgesics, muscle relaxants, anxiolytics, and others.

Treatment, whether prophylactic or abortive, should follow a definite plan incorporating the clinician and patient into a team focused on reducing the headache frequency, severity, and disability. As mentioned earlier, impressions and physical findings should be explained to the patient in as much detail as necessary to ensure the patient's complete understanding. The complexity of the headache condition needs to be explained, emphasizing its chronicity, rather than its curability, and that the goal of treatment is disease control.

The comprehensiveness of the treatment plan depends on the frequency of the patient's attacks. The more frequent and severe the attacks, the more detailed plan may be necessary. Patients experiencing infrequent attacks (e.g., once or twice monthly) may require only an abortive medication and little else. Patients with more frequent attacks may benefit from dietary restrictions, psychosocial intervention, biofeedback relaxation training, manipulation, and physical modality intervention, in addition to medication.

TENSION-TYPE HEADACHE TREATMENT

TTHA often is associated with emotional stress and muscle strain or tension of the shoulders and neck. Simple self-administered measures, such as stress avoidance, stretching, warm packs, or relaxation techniques, can be helpful in reducing or relieving attacks. More comprehensive professional intervention, such as manipulation, physical therapy, local injections, or biofeedback training, are considerations for more frequent or severe cases.

Prophylactically, the use of OTC or prescription medications can be considered in addition to nonmedicinal measures for reducing the frequency and duration of attacks. NSAIDs, muscle relaxants, or antidepressants (tricyclic antidepressant [TCA], selective serotonin reuptake inhibitor [SSRI]), at the lowest effective doses, are more commonly used.

Daily use of the longer-acting NSAIDs, such as naproxen[1] (Naprosyn) or celecoxib[1] (Celebrex), in the appropriately screened patient over a 2- to 3-week period, can be an effective preventative. TCAs, such as nortriptyline[1] (Pamelor) or amitriptyline[1] (Elavil), in low doses at night over 1 to 3 months, are frequently effective, especially in patients with anxiety or mild depression. The SSRI drugs, such as fluoxetine[1] (Prozac) or sertraline[1] (Zoloft), similarly can be useful. The muscle relaxant cyclobenzaprine[1] (Flexeril), at low doses, with a similar mechanism to the TCAs, can be administered at night for limited periods. Other muscle relaxants occasionally can be effective. Potential side effects can limit the use of NSAIDs (gastrointestinal irritation) and the TCAs (fatigue and weight gain).

Abortive or symptomatic treatment of TTHA can include simple OTC medications (e.g., aspirin or acetaminophen), NSAIDs (short-acting), muscle relaxants, combination analgesics, and, in some cases, opioid or opioidlike drugs. Caution should be exercised in prescribing potentially habituating drugs. Daily or near-daily use of analgesics can lead to analgesic rebound headache, Medication Overuse Headache, which can compound the patient's headache problem.

Botulism toxin[1] (Botox) reportedly is helpful in the treatment of tension-type and migraine headache, but controlled studies are limited. In this treatment, a diluted solution of botulism toxin is injected into various muscles of the face, scalp, neck, or shoulders. Because this treatment frequently is used in headache specialty and pain centers, simultaneous comprehensive measures and medication may contribute to positive results. Side effects from botulism toxin are low when injected properly.

---

[1]Not FDA approved for this indication.

MIGRAINE TREATMENT

Migraineurs are unique individuals, and the effectiveness and tolerance of medications can vary from patient to patient. Medication changes, combinations of medications, and trial and error may be necessary in the early stages of treatment.

Nonmedicinal measures for migraine sufferers include biofeedback stress reduction, caffeine and dietary restrictions, regimentation of meals and sleep, rest, exercise, stretching, and avoidance of work or activity overload. Limiting caffeine to less than 200 mg/day is important to prevent the caffeine headache (rebound headache) in most patients. Elimination of vasoactive foods, such as chocolate, aged cheese, and processed meats, and avoidance of fasting for more than 4 hours can be helpful for patients with more frequent attacks (Table 3). Regular exercise and stretching, planned relaxation, regular sleep schedules, and following a healthy lifestyle are frequently included in a comprehensive treatment regimen. In some patients, especially children and adolescents, biofeedback stress reduction or psychotherapeutic intervention may be necessary.

The more commonly used medications for prophylaxis are β-blockers, calcium channel blockers, antiepileptics (neurostabilizers), and the antidepressants. Treatment should be continued for a 4- to 8-week trial before discontinuation for ineffectiveness. Determination of which medication to use depends on comorbidities, interactions with concomitant medications, and tolerability.

β-Blockers such as propranolol (Inderal) and timolol (Blocadren) are nonselective and are approved by the Food and Drug Administration (FDA) for migraine prevention. Other β-blockers, such as nadolol[1] (Corgard), metoprolol[1] (Lopressor), and atenolol[1] (Tenormin), also can be effective. The mechanism of action in migraine is not wholly understood, but it is thought to involve anxiolytic effects as well as vascular changes and stabilization. The usual dosage is recommended (e.g., timolol 10–30 mg/day, propranolol 120–160 mg/day), and many consider the nighttime dose the more significant.

Calcium channel antagonists are well tolerated in general and can be as effective as the β-blockers. They are believed to alter serotonin release and inhibit platelet serotonin uptake and release within the brain. Verapamil[1] (Calan) is considered the more effective and is commonly recommended to patients. Dosage can vary from 120 to 480 mg/day. Nimodipine[1] (Nimotop) is equally effective, but it is rarely used in the United States because of its high cost.

Antiepileptic medications such as phenytoin[1] (Dilantin) and carbamazepine[1] (Tegretol) have been prescribed for migraine prevention over the years, with mixed results. Their use is now limited with the advent of newer, more easily tolerated agents, such as divalproex sodium (Depakote) and topiramate (Topamax).

Divalproex sodium is effective in reducing migraine attacks and is particularly useful in patients with coexisting head injury, seizure

---

[1]Not FDA approved for this indication.

TABLE 3 Triptans

Medication	Brand Name	Half-Life	Form/Strength
Sumatriptan	Imitrex	1.5 hr	Oral: 25, 50, 100 mg; NS: 20 mg; injection: 6 mg, 4 mg
Naratriptan	Amerge	6 hr	Oral: 2.5 mg
Zolmitriptan	Zomig	3 hr	Oral: 2.5, 5 mg; Melt: 2.5, 5 mg; NS: 5 mg
Rizatriptan	Maxalt	2–3 hr	Oral: 5, 10 mg; Melt: 10 mg
Almotriptan	Axert	3–4 hr	Oral: 6.25, 12.5 mg
Frovatriptan	Frova	25 hr	Oral: 5 mg
Eletriptan	Relpax	4 hr	Oral: 20, 40 mg

Abbreviations: Melt = oral disintegrating; NS = nasal steroid.

---

disorders, and bipolar disorders. It is thought to improve inhibitory and excitatory amino acid imbalance in the brain. It is best to start with a lower dose and to gradually increase as needed and tolerated. The dosage of 500 to 1000 mg/day is more frequently prescribed. A commonly experienced side effect is sedation, which can sometimes be used to the patient's advantage when anxiolytic effects are needed.

Topiramate is the most recent preventive medication approved by the FDA for migraine prophylaxis. It has multiple mechanisms of action, but its exact mechanism in migraine headache is unknown. Its effectiveness is believed to involve sodium ion channel stabilization, calcium ion channels, GABA (γ-aminobutyric acid) receptors, and neuronal membrane stabilization. The average daily dose is variable and ranges from 30 to 100 mg/day. A most unusual side effect of weight loss or appetite suppression can be used to the patient's advantage in preventing weight gain, which frequently accompanies migraine prophylactic medications.

The TCAs can be useful in patients who experience frequent attacks and in those who experience anxiety and depression. The TCAs inhibit synaptic reuptake of serotonin, thereby reducing neuron firing and release of neurotransmitters. Starting with a low dose in the evening and titrating up to efficacy and tolerability is recommended. Significant anticholinergic and sedation effects sometimes limit their use. The SSRIs[1] are reported helpful in some patients, but their use in migraine prevention is limited.

In general, prophylactic medications should be taken for 6 to 8 weeks to determine efficacy. If effective, a course of 4 to 6 months is recommended before an attempt is made to discontinue medication.

A variety of abortive treatment options are available for migraine sufferers. Although the triptans (Table 3) have generated much interest and are frequently prescribed, other medications continue to be used, including ergotamine and its derivatives, isometheptene, and NSAIDs. Many of the abortive medications carry significant prescribing limitations that must be taken into consideration. Vasoconstrictor medications are contraindicated in patients with cardiovascular or peripheral vascular disease. NSAIDs should not be used in those with gastrointestinal or bleeding disorders. As with all medications, the clinician must consider appropriate prescribing, contraindications, and side-effect information.

The vasoconstrictor ergotamine is available in oral, rectal (Ergocaff PB), and sublingual forms (Ergomar). Ergotamine has a relatively long half-life and duration of action (up to 3 days) and should be used no more frequently than every 4 to 5 days to avoid ergotamine rebound headache. The ergot derivative dihydroergotamine (DHE-45, Migranal NS) is available for intramuscular (IM), subcutaneous (SC), intravenous (IV), and intranasal use. IV dihydroergotamine (DHE-45) sometimes is used for intractable migraine (status migrainosus) in emergency departments and inpatient settings. The intranasal form (Migranal) is an effective treatment when administered correctly by the patient. Unfortunately, dihydroergotamine is not absorbed by the gastrointestinal tract, and, unlike other abortive nasal sprays, any swallowed medication will be wasted. Dihydroergotamine has a low headache recurrence rate of approximately 12%. All forms of ergotamine and dihydroergotamine are more effective when taken early in attacks.

Isometheptene is used in combination with dichloralphenazone and acetaminophen (Midrin, Duradrin). It is slow acting and more effective when taken early in attacks and when used for attacks preceded or accompanied by stress and muscle tension of the neck. Although isometheptene is considered less potent than ergotamine and triptans, it is preferred by many patients whose headaches have features of both migraine and TTHA.

At the present time, seven serotonin agonists (triptans) are approved for abortive migraine treatment in the United States (see Table 3). As a category, the triptans are approximately 65% to 70% effective in published clinical trials. Their similarities are greater than their differences, but each triptan is not necessarily effective for all patients, and familiarity with their differences can be helpful to the treating physician. Half-life, onset and duration of action, adverse

---

[1]Not FDA approved for this indication.

events, tolerability, recurrence of headache, and routes of administration may vary and allow the physician to match the medication to the individual patient. For example, a slower onset of action and longer-lasting triptan may be appropriate for slow-onset, longer-lasting migraine attacks.

Like other treatments, oral triptan tablets are more effective in the early phases of migraines. It is thought that peripheral sensitization—allodynia—is a sign of later phase migraine, and treating the attack before this phenomenon occurs is important. When treatment is delayed or the patient awakens with severe migraine, the injection, nasal spray, or rapidly acting triptans may be more beneficial. Although triptans as a group are very effective, recurrence of headache, after initial relief, requiring retreatment is common and can be as high as 40%. The recurrence rate tends to be less with triptans having a longer half-life.

The ergots and triptans are contraindicated in patients with ischemic heart disease, uncontrolled hypertension, and cerebrovascular disease. Physicians initially were extremely cautious about recommending triptans to their patients when the triptans were first introduced in the United States. However, significant human exposure to the triptans has revealed that catastrophic myocardial infarction or serious ischemia is rare. Chest pain following triptan use affects a small percentage of patients, and because the significance of this finding is not clear, refraining from future triptan use in these patients is recommended.

Sumatriptan (Imitrex), the first triptan approved in the United States, is available in nasal spray (20 mg), SC (6 mg, 4 mg), and oral formulations (25, 50, 100 mg). Its half-life is approximately 1.5 hours, and its duration of action is less than 4 hours. The injectable form produces rapid relief in 70% to 80% of patients, and it appears to be the most effective of all the available triptan forms. Conversely, it appears to cause the most side effects, and, for this reason, it should be used only for the more severe attacks. The oral forms are more favorable with regard to adverse effects, and their effectiveness is similar to that of other triptans (approximately 65%). Because of sumatriptan's short half-life and duration of action, recurrence of headache is common, necessitating repeat dosing.

Zolmitriptan (Zomig) is available in 2.5- and 5-mg oral and oral disintegrating tablets (ZMT) and as a 5-mg nasal spray. The efficacy of oral zolmitriptan is approximately 65% and that of the nasal form is 70%. The half-life of oral zolmitriptan is 3 hours, and its duration of action is longer than the nasal form, which improves on the need to remedicate. The nasal spray has a biphasic absorption curve, which accounts for its favorable adverse effect profile over the 5-mg oral tablet.

Naratriptan (Amerge) was the first to be approved of the gradual-onset, longer-acting triptans. It is available as oral 2.5-mg tablets and has a half-life of 6 hours. Naratriptan is well tolerated by patients and often is used by patients with slow-onset migraine. Some specialists prescribe daily naratriptan for limited periods for treatment of menstrual or intractable migraine attacks.

Rizatriptan (Maxalt) is available as oral 5- and 10-mg tablets and as an oral disintegrating form (MLT). It has a relatively rapid onset of action and a favorable one-dose 2-hour response rate. Patients who are undergoing concomitant treatment with propranolol should take the lesser 5-mg rizatriptan dose because of higher resultant rizatriptan plasma levels.

Almotriptan (Axert) is available in 6.25- and 12.5-mg tablets. It has a half-life of 3.5 hours and, because of a broad T_{max} (time of maximal concentration) range of 1.4 to 3.8 hours, a relatively rapid onset of action. Almotriptan has favorable adverse effect and headache recurrence profile. Chest pain symptoms after almotriptan use are similar to placebo in clinical trials.

Frovatriptan (Frova) is a long-acting triptan available in 2.5-mg oral tablets. It has the longest half-life of 25 hours and a favorable recurrence rate. Frovatriptan is frequently used for treatment of menstrual migraine and for attacks of longer duration. Some specialists prescribe daily frovatriptan for a limited period for menstrual and prolonged migraine attacks.

Eletriptan (Relpax) is the most recently approved triptan. It is available in 20- and 40-mg oral tablets and has a half-life of nearly 5 hours. Eletriptan has a relatively rapid onset but a longer duration of action and a favorable recurrence rate. In studies, some patients who were unresponsive to other triptans responded to eletriptan.

Various attempts have been made to compare triptans. Head-to-head trials mostly have compared one triptan to sumatriptan. A meta-analysis of 53 clinical trials published in 2001 compared the efficacy, recurrence, duration of action, and tolerability of all available triptans. Almotriptan and eletriptan were rated favorably across the major parameters of onset of action, efficacy, adverse events, and recurrence. In spite of efforts to adjust for variations in protocols and placebo response, specialists reached no clear consensus as to the validity or value of the meta-analysis or the preferability of one triptan over another.

NSAIDs frequently are recommended for treatment of acute migraine and can be effective when taken early. Their effects on the physiology of pain, inflammation, and platelets are believed to be the mechanisms responsible. Some physicians recommend taking a NSAID with the first dose of a triptan for added efficacy. Various agents are used, but none of the rapid-acting NSAIDs appears to have significant efficacy superiority. OTC ibuprofen (Motrin) and aspirin, in combination with caffeine and acetaminophen (Excedrin Migraine), is approved by the FDA for treatment of migraine.

Symptomatic treatment of pain may be necessary in patients who do not respond to recommended abortive treatment. Any effective analgesic can be appropriate, provided it is used infrequently and not on a daily or near-daily basis. In general, the more effective analgesics have anti-inflammatory and sedative properties.

CLUSTER HEADACHE TREATMENT

Cluster headache is one of the more unusual pain conditions occasionally encountered by physicians. Pain onset is rapid, and the duration of the attack is brief. For this reason, prophylactic treatment usually is the most practical. Abortive prescriptions frequently are given, but, for the most part, the cluster attack is resolving by the time medication is absorbed.

Nonmedicinal prophylactic measures are extremely limited. The reduction of cigarette smoking, the addressing of individual stress and hostility issues when appropriate, and the complete cessation of alcohol consumption during cluster periods should be part of any treatment program. Prophylactic medications include the calcium channel blockers verapamil[1] (Calan) and nimodipine[1] (Nimotop), the neurostabilizers valproate[1] (Depakote) and topiramate[1] (Topamax), various NSAIDs, ergotamine,[1] lithium[1] (Eskalith), cyproheptadine (Periactin) and, in extreme cases, short intervals of steroids.[1] These medications are used in average therapeutic doses, and combinations of medications are commonly needed (Table 4). The preventatives should be used during the cluster cycle and discontinued during off-cycle periods.

[1]Not FDA approved for this indication.

TABLE 4 Cluster Headache Prophylactic Medications

Medication	Brand	Average Daily Dose
Verapamil[1]	Calan, Isoptin, Verelan	240–420 mg
Divalproex[1]	Depakote	500–1500 mg
Topiramate[1]	Topamax	50–200 mg
Indomethacin[1]	Indocin	100–150 mg
Naproxen[1]	Naprosyn	1000–1500 mg
Lithium[1]	Lithobid	600–1200 mg*
Ergotamine[1]	Bellergal[1]	1 tablet bid†
Prednisone[1]	—	100 mg, decrease to 0
Cyproheptadine	Periactin	8–16 mg

[1]Not FDA approved for this indication.
*With serum level monitoring.
†Ergotamine 0.6 mg with phenobarbital 40 mg and 0.2 mg L-alkaloids of belladonna.

Abortive treatment is less preferred for cluster headache, as noted previously. However, inhalation oxygen via facial mask at 6 L terminates cluster attacks in 75% to 80% of sufferers within 12 minutes. Other possibilities include sumatriptans (Imitrex) SC or nasal spray,[1] zolmitriptan (Zomig ZMT) nasal spray,[1] ergotamine (Ergomar) sublingual, or dihydroergotamine injection (DHE-45) or nasal spray[1] (Migranal). The occasional patient reports relief with the oral triptans or analgesics. When triptans, ergotamine, or analgesics are used, appropriate prescribing and frequency guidelines should be followed. In general, with the exception of oxygen, daily as-needed medications should be avoided.

Headache continues to present a challenging problem for clinicians as well as for suffering patients. In spite of recent treatment advances and more public awareness, millions continue to needlessly endure pain and debilitation. At first glance, the headache problem appears complex and difficult when, in actuality, most sufferers experience straightforward, easily diagnosed headaches. The interested generalist or specialist who takes the time to elicit a careful history can establish the headache diagnosis and direct a simple treatment plan that can make a tremendous difference in the headache sufferer's life.

---

[1]Not FDA approved for this indication.

REFERENCES

Astin JA, Ernst E. The effectiveness of spinal manipulation for the treatment of headache disorders: A systematic review of randomized clinical trials. Cephalalgia 2002;22:617–23.

Diamond ML, Dalessio DJ, editors. Diamond and Dalessio's The Practicing Physician's Approach to Headache. 5th ed. Philadelphia: WB Saunders; 1999.

Ferrari MD, Roon KI, Lipton RB, et al. Oral triptans (serotonin 5HT-IB/ID-agonists) in acute migraine treatment: A meta-analysis of 53 trials. Lancet 2001;358:1668–75.

Gallagher RM, Kunkel R. Migraine medication attributes important for patient compliance: Concerns about side effects may delay treatment. Headache: J Head Face Pain 2003;43:36–43.

Goadsby PJ, Lipton RB, Ferreri MD. Migraine current understanding and treatment. N Engl J Med 2002;346:257–70.

Silberstein SD, Lipton EB, Dalessio DJ. Wolff's Headache and Other Head Pain. 7th ed. New York: Oxford University Press; 2001.

Vernon H, McDermaid C, Hagino C. Systematic review of randomized clinical trials of complementary/alternative therapies in the treatment of tension-type and cervicogenic headache. Complement Ther Med 1999;7:142–55.

Viral Meningitis and Encephalitis

Method of
Mark J. Abzug, MD

Viral meningitis is the most common cause of aseptic meningitis, an inflammatory process involving the meninges in which usual bacterial etiologies cannot be identified. Encephalitis is an inflammatory process that affects the brain parenchyma, typically producing more severe illness. Many viral infections of the central nervous system produce inflammation of both the meninges and brain tissue (meningoencephalitis). Encephalitis may result from acute viral invasion of the brain and a concomitant inflammatory response or from a postinfectious, autoimmune process characterized by demyelination following a viral illness or vaccination (acute disseminated encephalomyelitis). The majority of the approximately 8000 to 13,000 cases of aseptic meningitis and approximately 20,000 cases of encephalitis reported annually in the United States are caused by viral infections.

Clinical Features

Regardless of etiology, most cases of viral meningitis present similarly. Infants and young children display nonspecific symptoms, such as fever, irritability, lethargy, anorexia, and emesis. More specific findings suggestive of meningeal inflammation, such as nuchal rigidity, bulging fontanelle, and photophobia, are often absent. In older children and adults, nuchal rigidity and photophobia, along with fever, headache, and emesis, are more frequent. Focal neurologic findings and seizures are uncommon presenting findings in viral meningitis, although approximately 10% of children hospitalized with viral meningitis may develop acute complications such as obtundation, seizures, increased intracranial pressure, and inappropriate antidiuretic hormone secretion. Illness can last up to 1 to 2 weeks, with protracted headache not uncommon in adults.

Encephalitis is distinguished from meningitis by a change in sensorium and/or by focal neurologic findings. In younger children, encephalitis typically presents with irritability and/or lethargy, often after a febrile illness. Older children may manifest headache, disorientation, unusual behavior, abnormal speech, bizarre movements, and disorientation in addition to fever, nausea, emesis, myalgias, and photophobia. Generalized or, less commonly, focal neurologic abnormalities, including seizures and motor deficits, may be present. Progression to extreme lethargy, stupor, or coma may ensue.

Etiology

In recent studies, a specific etiologic agent was identified in 55% to 70% of presumed cases of viral meningitis and in only 25% to 65% of cases of encephalitis despite thorough investigation. The list of implicated viruses is extensive (Table 1). Enteroviruses (EVs) are the most common cause of both viral meningitis and encephalitis of proven etiology. Other important agents include arboviruses (transmitted by arthropod vectors such as mosquitoes or ticks), herpes simplex virus (HSV), influenza virus, Epstein-Barr virus, varicella-zoster virus, adenovirus, and rabies virus.

Diagnosis

Important diagnostic clues may come from history (respiratory or gastrointestinal symptoms, family exposures, seasonality, prevalent diseases, travel, animal and insect exposure, and recreational activities) and physical examination (see Table 1). The presence of a rash may suggest specific agents, such as varicella-zoster virus, or West Nile virus. Whereas identification of a mucocutaneous vesicle in a neonate may be key to the diagnosis of HSV infection, cold sores in older children and adults are *not* predictive of HSV encephalitis. The combination of findings of encephalitis and myelitis in the same patient is suggestive of infection with an EV (especially EV 71), West Nile virus, Japanese encephalitis virus, or rabies virus. Although focal signs are present in the majority of older children and adults with HSV encephalitis, the positive predictive value of focal findings for HSV is low.

Examination of the cerebrospinal fluid (CSF) is indicated in suspected meningitis or encephalitis unless contraindicated by concern for a space-occupying lesion or increased intracranial pressure. CSF in viral meningitis typically has a low-grade pleocytosis (100–1000 white blood cells [WBCs]/mm^3, range <100 to ≥2000 WBC/mm^3). Polymorphonuclear leukocytes may predominate early, with the profile becoming mononuclear within 8 to 48 hours. In general, CSF protein is normal or slightly increased, and the glucose concentration is normal or slightly decreased, although exceptions occur. The CSF in encephalitis typically has a predominantly mononuclear pleocytosis, increased protein, and normal glucose, although CSF may be normal in 3% to 5% or more of cases, especially early in the course. Certain viruses, including influenza and parvovirus B19, typically cause encephalopathies characterized by the absence of pleocytosis.

Imaging and electroencephalography (EEG) are useful adjuncts, particularly for encephalitis. Magnetic resonance imaging generally

TABLE 1 Epidemiology and Clinical Features of Viral Meningitis and Encephalitis

Enteroviruses
Epidemiology
- Most common proven cause of viral meningitis and encephalitis (up to 85%–95% of viral meningitis and 80% of viral encephalitis).
- Majority of meningitis and encephalitis occurs in children <1 year old; incidence of meningitis exceeds that of encephalitis.
- Epidemic in warm seasons in temperate climates.
- Poliovirus infection decreased with widespread immunization.
- Enterovirus 71 frequently occurs in regional outbreaks, e.g., Asia since the late 1990s. Severe disease occurs primarily in children <5 years old.

Clinical Features
- Meningitis and severe encephalitis more common in younger children, especially neonates. Encephalitis may be part of multisystem illness in newborns.
- Encephalitis typically generalized, although focal seizures and other abnormalities may occur, especially in neonates.
- May have biphasic febrile course; meningeal and encephalitic symptoms occur during second phase.
- Rash (macular, maculopapular, petechial, vesicular), enanthem, conjunctivitis, respiratory symptoms, pleurodynia, pericarditis, myocarditis, diarrhea, myalgias may accompany.
- Chronic meningoencephalitis with waxing and warning neurologic symptoms and high fatality rate occur in hypogammaglobulinemic patients.
- Enterovirus 71 associated with hand-foot-and-mouth disease, herpangina, and neurologic disease (meningitis, brainstem encephalitis, myelitis/acute flaccid paralysis, Guillain-Barré syndrome).
  - Signs of brainstem encephalitis include myoclonic jerks, tremors, ataxia, cranial nerve palsy, limb weakness, altered consciousness, seizures, increased intracranial pressure.
  - Imaging reveals high-intensity lesions in the midbrain, brainstem, and spinal cord anterior horn cells and ventral roots.
  - Pulmonary edema/hemorrhage, cardiac failure, shock may develop rapidly.

Herpes Simplex Virus
Epidemiology
- ~1%–3% of viral meningitis.
  - Predominantly associated with primary type 2 HSV genital infection and less frequently with primary type 1 HSV genital infection, nonprimary HSV genital infection (either type), or without recent genital disease.
  - Mollaret's meningitis (recurrent, benign aseptic meningitis) mostly associated with type 2 infection without signs of genital infection and occasionally with type 1 HSV or with Epstein-Barr virus.
- ~10%–20% of encephalitis in the United States.
  - Encephalitis primarily due to type 2 HSV in neonates and type 1 HSV in older age groups.
  - Encephalitis occurs in ~50% of neonatal HSV infections.
  - ~33%–50% of non-neonatal HSV encephalitis is caused by primary HSV infection and ~50%–67% is caused by HSV reactivation.
  - Cases linked to defects in interferon production or response in the central nervous system.
  - Most common focal viral encephalitis in nonepidemic settings; most common sporadic fatal encephalitis.

Clinical Features
- Neonatal encephalitis characterized by seizures (focal and generalized), lethargy, irritability, tremors, anorexia, temperature instability, bulging fontanelle.
  - Central nervous system–only disease frequently begins in temporal lobe and then becomes bitemporal.
  - Encephalitis with disseminated disease more commonly is diffuse.
- Non-neonatal encephalitis characterized by fever and focal encephalitis with necrosis and hemorrhage.
  - Tropism for temporal lobe: Aphasia, anosmia, temporal lobe seizures, other focal findings.
  - Findings include headache, emesis, altered consciousness, bizarre behavior, personality changes, disorientation, ataxia, hallucinations, hemiparesis.
  - Focal findings are not always present; bilateral disease, widespread disease, or brainstem encephalitis may occur.
  - Elevated red blood cell count may be present in CSF; CSF protein levels may be normal early and increase over time.
  - Focal abnormalities on imaging studies, especially involving one or both temporal lobes, are suggestive of HSV disease. However, focal disease may occur with other viruses, other regions of the brain may be affected by HSV, and imaging may be normal in early HSV.
  - Temporal lobe focality on electroencephalography, especially with periodic lateralizing epileptiform discharges, is characteristic of HSV but is not specific.
  - Rapid progression is common; however, atypical and mild, slowly progressive cases are increasingly being reported.

Arboviruses
Epidemiology
- ~5% of viral meningitis and important cause of encephalitis.
- Prevalent during warm and/or wet seasons; incidence related to mosquito or tick exposure.
- Leading agents in the United States:
  - West Nile virus: U.S. outbreaks since late 1990s; July to September predominance. Lower incidence and severity in children. Risk factors for severe neurologic disease include older age and immune compromise.
  - La Crosse virus: Central, eastern United States. Incidence of encephalitis exceeds that of meningitis; affects children more than adults.
- St. Louis encephalitis virus: Central, western, southern United States. Incidence of encephalitis less than that of meningitis; lower incidence and severity of encephalitis in children.
- Japanese encephalitis virus: Most common cause of epidemic encephalitis worldwide; causes encephalitis more than meningitis. Prevalent in Asia and Australia; affects children more than adults.
- Other important viruses:
  - Eastern equine encephalomyelitis virus: Causes encephalitis more than meningitis.
  - Western equine encephalomyelitis virus: Causes encephalitis more than meningitis.
  - Venezuelan equine encephalomyelitis: Causes encephalitis more than meningitis.
  - Colorado Tick Fever virus: Rocky Mountains; tickborne. Meningitis in up to 18% of cases; encephalitis uncommon.
  - Powassan, Rocio, Murray Valley, Kyasuma Forest, Jamestown Canyon, California encephalitis, tickborne encephalitis, Ilheus, Snowshoe Hare, Rift Valley viruses.

Clinical Features

- West Nile virus
  - ~20% of infections are symptomatic; West Nile fever in majority of these infections.
  - Neurologic illness in ~1/150 infected; of these, meningitis in ~30% and encephalitis in ~65%. Neurologic manifestations also include acute asymmetrical flaccid paralysis, polyradiculitis, transverse myelitis, Guillain-Barré syndrome, optic neuritis, and chorioretinitis.
  - Encephalitis is characterized by altered consciousness, cranial nerve palsies (brainstem involvement), generalized or focal motor deficits (weakness, tremor, myoclonus), movement disorders, sensory deficits, and ataxia. Focal temporal lobe disease may mimic HSV. Case fatality rate ~10%.
  - Fever, emesis, maculopapular rash (especially in children) frequently accompany neurologic disease.
- Japanese and Eastern equine encephalitides
  - Thalamic, midbrain, basal ganglia, brainstem lesions characteristic.

Influenza Virus
Epidemiology
- Rare cause of meningitis.
- Cause of 8%–10% of encephalitis.
  - More commonly associated with influenza A than with influenza B.
  - Encephalitis may be acute or postinfectious.
  - Acute necrotizing encephalopathy reported primarily in 1- to 5-year-old children in Asia since the late 1990s.
  - Mutations in Ran Binding Protein 2 associated with familial and recurrent acute necrotizing encephalopathy.
- Neurologic spectrum includes Reye's syndrome (influenza B), myelitis, Guillain-Barré syndrome.

Clinical Features
- Acute necrotizing encephalopathy
  - Fever, altered consciousness, prolonged seizures; rapid progression to coma.
  - Elevated CSF protein, usually without pleocytosis.
  - Magnetic resonance imaging: Bilateral thalamic lesions and multifocal symmetrical lesions (brainstem, putamina, medulla, pons, periventricular white matter, cerebellum).
  - Mortality ~30%; severe sequelae among survivors.

Varicella-Zoster Virus
Epidemiology and Clinical Features
- Chickenpox associated with cerebellar ataxia, meningitis, encephalitis, postinfectious encephalitis/ADEM, transverse myelitis, Guillain-Barré syndrome.
- Zoster associated with encephalitis, granulomatous hemiparesis, myelitis, cranial neuritis (including Bell's palsy). Neurologic complications may occur with rash, weeks to months after rash or without rash (especially in immune-compromised patients).

Epstein-Barr Virus
Epidemiology and Clinical Features
- Neurologic complications occur in 1%–5% of primary infections.
- Etiology of 2%–5% of acute viral encephalitis.
- Spectrum includes meningitis, encephalitis, ADEM, cranial nerve palsy (including Bell's palsy), transverse myelitis, and Guillain-Barré syndrome. Alice in Wonderland syndrome, consisting of visual seizures with metamorphopsia, may accompany encephalitis.
- Neurologic disease more frequent in immune-compromised hosts.
- Typical features of infectious mononucleosis, atypical lymphocytosis, and heterophile antibody often absent in Epstein-Barr virus neurologic syndromes.

Cytomegalovirus
Epidemiology and Clinical Features
- Encephalitis primarily in congenitally infected neonates and immune-compromised hosts.
- Insidious progression.

Human Herpesvirus 6
Epidemiology and Clinical Features
- Meningoencephalitis occasionally occurs with primary infection.
- Increased incidence of encephalitis in immune-compromised hosts.
- Confusion, headache, seizures may accompany encephalitis; disease may be focal and mimic HSV encephalitis.

Adenovirus
Epidemiology and Clinical Features
- Neurologic spectrum includes acute encephalitis, postinfectious encephalitis, Reye's syndrome-like encephalopathy, and transient encephalopathy.
  - Acute encephalitis is characterized by seizures, CSF pleocytosis, and severe disease.
  - Transient encephalopathy is characterized by obtundation, normal CSF, and complete recovery within several days.

Lymphocytic Choriomeningitis Virus
Epidemiology and Clinical Features
- Transmission by rodent secretions.
- Meningitis and encephalitis more commonly occur in developing countries.
- Spectrum includes encephalitis, hydrocephalus, transverse myelitis.

Human Immunodeficiency Virus
Epidemiology and Clinical Features
- Transient meningitis and, more rarely, encephalitis may accompany primary infection (acute retroviral syndrome).
- Chronic infection may be associated with subacute encephalopathy (loss of developmental milestones in young children, dementia).
- Acute encephalitis may accompany treatment failure during chronic infection (uncommon).

Continued

TABLE 1 Epidemiology and Clinical Features of Viral Meningitis and Encephalitis—Cont'd

Rabies Virus
Epidemiology and Clinical Features
- Relatively uncommon in United States; major sources are bats, raccoons, foxes, skunks.
- Important cause of encephalitis in developing countries; important sources are dogs and cats.
- Incubation period can vary from weeks to months to years. Pain, pruritus, or paresthesias at bite wound is followed by prodromal fever and anxiety and then by encephalitis.
- Rare reports of survivors and abortive cases.

Measles, Mumps, Rubella Viruses
Epidemiology and Clinical Features
- Meningitis occurs in ~30% of measles infections; measles also causes acute encephalitis, postinfectious encephalitis, and delayed subacute sclerosing panencephalitis.
- Mumps was the leading cause of meningitis in the prevaccine era.
- Meningitis and encephalitis due to each virus dramatically decreased with widespread immunization in developed countries.

Other Viral Agents
- Parainfluenza virus, respiratory syncytial virus, human metapneumovirus, rhinovirus, coronavirus, parvovirus B19, rotavirus, encephalomyocarditis virus, hepatitis C virus, simian herpes B virus, human T-lymphotropic virus, JC virus, Lassa fever virus, yellow fever virus, Hendra virus, Nipah virus, Australian bat Lyssavirus, parechoviruses.

Acute Disseminated Encephalomyelitis
Epidemiology
- Implicated in 10%–15% of cases of encephalitis in the United States.
- Increased incidence in infants and children.
- Onset days to weeks after respiratory tract infection (influenza, enteroviruses, measles, mumps, rubella, *Mycoplasma pneumoniae*, and others), gastroenteritis (rotavirus), and other infections (HSV, Epstein-Barr virus, varicella-zoster virus, human herpesvirus 6, cytomegalovirus).
- History of preceding infection or vaccination elicited in up to two thirds of cases.
- Winter–spring predominance in some series.

Clinical Features
- Diffuse, often multifocal symptoms reflecting regions of brain affected. Spectrum includes motor deficits, cranial nerve palsies, optic neuritis, cerebellar ataxia, altered consciousness, psychosis, seizures, transverse myelitis, peripheral neuritis.
- Multifocal, asymmetrical demyelinating lesions in imaging studies, with predilection for white matter.
- CSF cytology may be normal or show pleocytosis; CSF protein elevated in 50%–70%.
- Typically monophasic; occasionally relapses occur.
- Acute hemorrhagic leukoencephalitis is a rare entity representing the fulminant end of the spectrum. It primarily affects young adults and is characterized by seizures, coma, cerebral edema, and a rapid, often fatal course.

Abbreviations: ADEM = acute disseminated encephalomyelitis; CSF = cerebrospinal fluid; HSV = herpes simplex virus.

has better sensitivity than does computed tomography, especially early in disease. Characteristic imaging findings may suggest specific pathogens (see Table 1), and imaging can exclude alternative diagnoses, for example, a parameningeal focus or tumor. EEG is the most sensitive tool for confirming encephalitis and can distinguish infection from metabolic encephalopathy.

Viral culture, polymerase chain reaction (PCR), and serology are the major techniques for specific virologic diagnosis. Sensitivity of CSF viral culture is better for meningitis than for encephalitis. Sensitivity reaches 65% to 75% for EVs, and CSF culture may be positive in young infants lacking pleocytosis. CSF culture is positive in 25% to 40% of neonates with HSV encephalitis but in less than 2% of older children and adults. CSF PCR is generally more sensitive than culture in both meningitis and encephalitis. CSF PCR for EVs has greater than 95% sensitivity and specificity. Sensitivity and specificity of CSF PCR for HSV are between 75% and 100% in neonatal HSV encephalitis and 91% and 98% in older children and adults with HSV encephalitis. Importantly, HSV PCR may be falsely negative within the first 3 to 4 days of illness in up to 25% of cases; repeat testing 3 to 7 days later is generally positive. In many viral encephalitides, viral cultures, antigen detection tests, and PCR of non-CSF specimens have better yields than do CSF culture and PCR (e.g., throat and stool/rectum for EV 71, for which CSF culture and PCR are more often negative, and respiratory specimens for influenza, adenovirus, and other respiratory viruses). Detection of serum and CSF antibodies can be performed for many viruses (e.g., most arboviruses and lymphocytic choriomeningitis virus), frequently requiring acute and convalescent specimens. Serum and CSF IgM assays can be diagnostic for West Nile virus, Japanese encephalitis virus, Epstein-Barr virus, and EV 71. A brain biopsy should be considered in a patient with symptoms that are progressive or do not improve, with an uncertain diagnosis, and with a focal, accessible lesion.

Treatment

The mainstay of therapy for viral meningitis and encephalitis is supportive care. In patients in whom there is difficulty distinguishing between bacterial and viral meningitis (e.g., young children, especially those younger than 1 year), hospitalization and parenteral antibiotics (e.g., vancomycin [Vancocin] plus a third-generation cephalosporin such as cefotaxime [Claforan] or ceftriaxone [Rocephin]) are administered until bacterial cultures are negative and/or an alternative diagnosis is made. Additionally, newborns or other immune-compromised patients with EV meningitis may require supportive therapy for severe disseminated disease (e.g., hepatitis, coagulopathy, or myocarditis). A presumptive diagnosis of viral meningitis can often be made in older children and adults who are not very ill based on clinical and CSF examination (low-grade pleocytosis with mononuclear predominance initially or 8–24 hours later, normal to slightly depressed glucose concentration, normal to slightly increased protein level). Lumbar puncture may alleviate symptoms such as headache, irritability, and emesis. Therefore, in older children and adults, hospitalization and/or empirical antibiotic treatment are indicated for patients who appear ill, including those requiring parenteral hydration and/or analgesics, those in whom viral and bacterial infection cannot be readily distinguished, and those who manifest findings of encephalitis. Presumptive therapy for *Mycobacterium tuberculosis* may be indicated if the exposure history, clinical presentation, CSF examination, and imaging findings are suggestive of this agent.

There are few proven specific antiviral therapies for meningitis and encephalitis. Acyclovir[1] (Zovirax) can hasten recovery from HSV meningitis, although HSV meningitis without encephalitis generally has an excellent outcome without antiviral treatment. Valacyclovir[1] (Valtrex) and famciclovir[1] (Famvir) are also available for oral therapy of HSV meningitis associated with genital HSV in immune-competent patients.

---

[1]Not FDA approved for this indication.

CURRENT DIAGNOSIS

Differential diagnosis of viral meningitis and encephalitis is broad and includes:

- Bacteria: *Streptococcus pneumoniae, Neisseria meningitidis, Haemophilus influenzae, Listeria monocytogenes, Mycobacterium tuberculosis, Borrelia burgdorferi, Mycoplasma pneumoniae, Mycoplasma hominis, Bartonella henselae*, syphilis, leptospirosis, brucellosis, rickettsial and ehrlichial infections
- Parasites: Neurocysticercosis, toxoplasmosis, amebic encephalitis
- Fungi: *Cryptococcus neoformans, Coccidioides immitis*
- Parameningeal focus: Brain abscess or subdural or epidural empyema
- Kawasaki disease
- Sarcoidosis
- Autoimmune disease: Systemic lupus erythematosus, cerebral vasculitis, Wegener's granulomatosis, Hashimoto's encephalopathy, Anti-N-Methyl-D-Aspartate Receptor Encephalitis, other antibody-mediated encephalopathies
- Medication-induced meningitis: Nonsteroidal antiinflammatory drugs, sulfa antibiotics, immune globulin, cytosine arabinoside (Cytarabine), muromonab-CD3 (Orthoclone OKT3), carbamazepine (Tegretol)
- Metabolic derangements: Inborn errors of metabolism, leukodystrophy, uremia, hepatic encephalopathy, Reye's syndrome
- Cerebrovascular hemorrhage and/or infarct
- Malignancy
- Drug toxicity (e.g., neuroleptic malignant syndrome)
- Toxins

Historical information may suggest specific etiologic viruses:

- Respiratory symptoms: Influenza virus, adenovirus, other respiratory viruses
- Gastrointestinal symptoms: Rotavirus
- Family exposure: Influenza virus, EV
- Seasonality and prevalent diseases in the community: EV, West Nile virus, other arboviruses, influenza virus, other respiratory viruses
- Travel to areas with endemic or epidemic disease: West Nile virus, EV 71, Japanese encephalitis virus, other arboviruses
- Animal exposure: Rabies virus, lymphocytic choriomeningitis virus
- Mosquito exposure: West Nile virus, other arboviruses
- Tick exposure: Colorado tick fever virus, Powassan virus
- Recreational activities: Spelunking-associated bat exposure and rabies infection, hiking-associated mosquito and tick exposure and arbovirus infection

Useful laboratory evaluations for viral meningitis and encephalitis include CSF examination, imaging (especially magnetic resonance imaging), and electroencephalography. Imaging abnormalities may suggest certain pathogens (see Table 1). CSF PCR, serum and CSF IgM assays, and viral culture/antigen detection/PCR of mucosal specimens are especially useful specific diagnostic tests.

- CSF PCR is a more sensitive technique than viral culture for detection of viruses such as EVs; HSV; varicella-zoster virus, cytomegalovirus, human herpesvirus 6, Epstein-Barr virus, and JC virus in immune-compromised patients; measles virus; parvovirus B19; and human immunodeficiency virus. CSF PCR for other viruses, such as adenovirus, influenza virus, and arboviruses (including West Nile virus), has low or variable sensitivity. PCR of saliva has high sensitivity for rabies virus (other testing includes immunostain of a nape of neck biopsy, corneal impression, buccal mucosa, or brain tissue and serology).
- The etiology of encephalitis is elusive in many cases. Extensive investigations ultimately are able to identify a specific etiologic agent in only 25% to 65% of cases.

Abbreviations: CSF = cerebrospinal fluid; EV = enterovirus; PCR = polymerase chain reaction.

For children and adults with encephalitis, empirical therapy with acyclovir (30 mg/kg/day intravenously divided every 8 hours) should generally be initiated pending diagnostic studies, especially in the presence of fever and any evidence of focal neurologic abnormality (clinical examination, imaging, or electroencephalography). Treatment for 14 to 21 days* is indicated if HSV infection is confirmed or if clinical and diagnostic findings are strongly suggestive in the absence of other proven etiologies; a 21-day course is generally favored for more severe disease. Acyclovir (60 mg/kg/day intravenously divided every 8 hours) should be presumptively administered to newborns with encephalitis with focal or generalized findings. Treatment of proven or highly suspect neonatal HSV encephalitis is generally continued for 21 days and until an end-of-therapy CSF PCR is negative, although proof that extending therapy until the PCR is negative is beneficial is lacking in neonates, children, and adults. Whether higher doses (45–60 mg/kg/day) or longer courses (≥21 days) confer additional benefit and are safe outside the neonatal period is not established. Relapse within the first 1 to 3 months after therapy of neonatal and childhood/adult HSV encephalitis has been reported with variable incidence, in some cases correlated with lower daily dose and treatment duration. Whether relapses reflect active viral replication or an immune-mediated phenomenon is

controversial, although CSF PCR positivity in some cases suggests the former.

Whether encephalitis associated with varicella-zoster virus is due more often to direct viral infection or an immune-mediated parainfectious process is not established. Thus, although acyclovir is frequently recommended for varicella-zoster virus encephalitis, including cerebellar ataxia, the role of antiviral therapy is unproven. Ganciclovir (Cytovene) and/or foscarnet (Foscavir) are used for meningoencephalitis in immune-compromised hosts caused by cytomegalovirus and human herpesvirus 6.

Pleconaril (Picovir) is an experimental agent that has been studied for treatment of EV meningitis and encephalitis, including chronic meningoencephalitis in hypogammaglobulinemic patients, with some evidence of benefit; however, the agent is not currently available. Intraventricular, intrathecal, and intravenous administration of immune globulin[1] have been used to suppress or stabilize chronic EV meningoencephalitis in immune-compromised patients. The mainstays of management of severe EV 71 neurologic disease are close monitoring, fluid restriction, osmotic diuretics, and cardiorespiratory support. Various agents, including pleconaril, interferon α,[1] intravenous immune globulin, and corticosteroids have been tried, but none has been proven to be effective.

---

*Exceeds duration recommended by the manufacturer.

[1]Not FDA approved for this indication.

CURRENT THERAPY

- General supportive measures for patients with severe meningitis or encephalitis include:
  - Analgesics for headache, antiemetics, intravenous fluids and medications for patients with depressed consciousness, anticonvulsants for seizures, provision of a quiet environment
  - Intensive care for severely ill patients, including tracheal intubation for airway protection, respiratory support, cardiorespiratory monitoring
  - Mild fluid restriction for cerebral edema or inappropriate antidiuretic hormone secretion
  - Head of bed elevation, hyperventilation, osmotic (mannitol) and loop diuretics, and control of temperature, pain, and seizures for increased intracranial pressure
- Specific antiviral agents available for meningoencephalitis include acyclovir (Zovirax) for HSV and varicella-zoster virus, ganciclovir (Cytovene) for cytomegalovirus and human herpesvirus 6, foscarnet (Foscavir) for cytomegalovirus and human herpesvirus 6, amantadine (Symmetrel) for susceptible influenza A, rimantadine (Flumadine) for susceptible influenza A, and oseltamivir (Tamiflu) for susceptible influenza A and B.
- Rehabilitative therapy and neurodevelopmental follow-up are frequently necessary after the acute phase of encephalitis regardless of the etiologic agent.
- Prognosis for viral meningitis is generally favorable without long-term sequelae, although fatigue, decreased concentration, and irritability may last for several weeks.
- Prognosis for viral encephalitis is variable and may be difficult to predict, especially early in the course of illness. In general, a worse prognosis is associated with extremes of age (infants <1 year and older adults), specific etiologies (HSV, enterovirus 71, West Nile virus, Japanese encephalitis virus, rabies), more severe illness (lower Glasgow Coma Scale) and extensive brain involvement, and, in the case of HSV, longer duration prior to initiation of treatment.

Abbreviation: HSV = herpes simplex virus.

Influenzal encephalitis is frequently treated with oral antivirals, including amantadine (Symmetrel) for influenza A (if susceptible), rimantadine (Flumadine) for influenza A (if susceptible), and oseltamivir (Tamiflu) for influenza A (if susceptible), and B; corticosteroids and immune globulin[1] have also been tried. However, none of these agents has been proven to be effective for influenzal encephalitis. A combination of antiviral treatment, corticosteroids, and intravenous immune globulin has been suggested to reduce mortality due to influenzal acute necrotizing encephalopathy. There currently are no established therapies for West Nile virus encephalitis. Ribavirin (Rebetol),[1] interferon, high-titer immune globulin, and corticosteroids have been used, and therapeutic trials are currently ongoing. No specific therapies have been proven to be effective for encephalitis due to other arboviruses or for rabies; successful use of coma-inducing therapy plus the antivirals ribavirin and amantadine was reported in one patient with rabies encephalitis. Corticosteroids, intravenous immune globulin, and plasmapheresis have been used for acute disseminated encephalomyelitis, but efficacy trials have not been performed.

[1]Not FDA approved for this indication.

REFERENCES

Beaman MH, Wesselingh SL. Acute community-acquired meningitis and encephalitis. Med J Aust 2002;176:389–96.

Chang L, Hsia S, Wu C, et al. Outcome of enterovirus 71 infections with or without stage-based management: 1998–2002. Pediatr Infect Dis J 2004;23:327–31.

Glaser CA, Honarmond S, Anderson LJ, et al. Beyond viruses: Clinical profiles and etiologies associated with encephalitis. Clin Infect Dis 2006;43:1565–77.

Huang C, Morse D, Slater B, et al. Multiple-year experience in the diagnosis of viral central nervous system infections with a panel of polymerase chain reaction assays for detection of 11 viruses. Clin Infect Dis 2004;39:630–5.

Lindsey NP, Staples JE, Lehman JA, Fischer M. Centers for Disease Control and Prevention. Surveilance for human West Nile virus disease—United States, 1999–2008. MMWR Surveill Summ 2010;59:1–17.

Kennedy PGE. Viral encephalitis: causes, differential diagnosis, and management. J Neurol Neurosurg Psychiatry 2004;75(Suppl 1):i10–5.

Kimberlin DW. Herpes simplex virus infections of the central nervous system. Semin Pediatr Infect Dis 2003;14:83–9.

Rotbart HA. Viral meningitis. Semin Neurol 2000;20:277–92.

Sancho-Shumizu V, Zhang SY, Abel L, et al. Genetic susceptibility to herpes simplex virus 1 encephalitis in mice and humans. Curr Opin Allergy Clin Immunol 2007;7:495–505.

Tunkel AR, Glaser CA, Bloch KC, et al. The management of encephalitis: Clinical practice guidelines of the Infectious Diseases Society of America. Clin Infect Dis 2008;47:303–27.

Weitkamp J, Spring MD, Brogan T, et al. Influenza A virus-associated acute necrotizing encephalopathy in the United States. Pediatr Infect Dis J 2004;23:259–63.

Whitley RJ, Gnann JW. Viral encephalitis: Familiar infections and emerging pathogens. Lancet 2002;359:507–14.

Willoughby RE Jr, Tieves KS, Hoffman GM, et al. Survival after treatment of rabies with induction of coma. N Engl J Med 2005;352:2508–14.

Multiple Sclerosis

Method of
B. Mark Keegan, MD, FRCPC

Multiple sclerosis (MS) is an autoimmune inflammatory demyelinating disease of the central nervous system (CNS) that affects approximately 400,000 people in the United States alone.

Risk Factors

Women are at least twice as likely to develop MS as are men. Other known risk factors for developing MS include: ethnicity, genetic background, and environmental exposures. Persons of European ethnicity, particularly those born and reared in extreme northern or southern latitudes, are particularly susceptible to MS. African Americans are less likely to be diagnosed with MS than European Americans, but they have a more severe clinical course. Genetic susceptibility is associated with the major histocompatibility (MHC) allele HLA-DRB1 as well as interleukin-2 and interleukin-7 receptors. Low serum vitamin D levels are associated with an increased risk of development of MS in whites but are of unclear significance in the severity of its clinical course. There are intriguing but as yet unproven associations with infection with Epstein-Barr virus (infectious mononucleosis), particularly if this is contracted later in adolescence. Exposure to Epstein-Barr virus may be necessary but insufficient for developing MS. Cigarette smoking is associated with an increased risk of development of MS and likely is associated with an increased severity and clinical course of MS, including that of cognitive impairment.

Pathophysiology

The etiology and pathophysiology of MS as a whole remains uncertain. However, most evidence supports an inflammatory demyelinating disease induced by uncertain environmental factors in a genetically susceptible host. Animal studies including experimental allergic encephalomyelitis and Theiler's murine encephalomyelitis virus also point to an autoimmune inflammatory demyelinating etiology, possibly associated with viral infection. Studies that suggest chronic cerebrospinal vascular insufficiency has an important association with MS remain preliminary.

Pathophysiology likely varies among individual patients with MS. Four distinct pathologies in active demyelinating MS lesions have been described. Pattern 1 displays marked macrophage infiltration without humoral abnormalities. Pattern 2 shows distinct humoral abnormalities with complement activation and immunoglobulin (Ig) deposition. Pattern 3 involves primary oligodendrocyte degeneration and early loss of myelin-associated glycoprotein. Pattern 4 reveals oligodendrocyte dystrophy in periplaque white matter. Early studies suggest there could be a therapeutic advantage with different therapies for different types of demyelinating disease.

Prevention

Currently, there is no known way to prevent the development of MS. Patients with a single clinical attack of demyelination and abnormal magnetic resonance imaging (MRI) ("high risk" clinically isolated syndrome) have a delayed onset to MS diagnosis with immunomodulatory therapy; however, there is no evidence to support that this prevents the eventual development of MS.

Clinical Manifestations

The clinical course of MS is varied. Approximately 85% of patients present with a relapsing–remitting course. This entails an acute impairment within the CNS, depending on the area of inflammation. A demyelinating cause of a focal neurologic symptom is suggested by an onset over hours to days, with a plateau of impairment over a few weeks. Symptoms then improve either spontaneously or with the use of corticosteroids over a number of days to weeks or longer. Following this, however, symptoms might not completely resolve. Inflammation within the optic nerve (optic neuritis) is heralded by painful, unilateral, central monocular visual deficit (central scotoma). Symptoms of brain stem dysfunction include binocular diplopia, sensory deficits unilaterally on the face

and contralaterally on the arm and leg, significant dysarthria, and vertigo. Cerebellar dysfunction is seen with pure ataxia that is typically unilateral. Spinal cord inflammation is indicated by a distinctive usually gradually rising sensory level of deficit that commonly is accompanied by bowel and bladder impairment and paraparesis or quadriparesis, depending on a thoracic versus cervical level of the lesion.

Progressive forms of MS include secondary progressive MS and primary progressive MS. These are heralded by a slow (months to years), but steady and insidious, progressive neurologic deficit, usually a progressive myelopathy of upper motor neuron gait disorder with spasticity, neurogenic bladder and bowel impairment, and progressive weakness. Occasionally, patients with progressive MS have insidious cerebellar ataxia or dementia in isolation or in association with the myelopathy. Secondary progressive MS is diagnosed when a patient has had a history of at least one clinical attack (relapse) with improvement in the past. Primary progressive MS is diagnosed in the entire absence of any prior relapse but with progressive CNS disease consistent with MS and typical MRI brain or spinal lesions, often with cerebrospinal fluid (CSF) or visual evoked potential abnormalities that support the diagnosis.

Diagnosis

The diagnosis of MS is formalized by the revised McDonald criteria. This entails having two or more clinical attacks (relapses) in the accompaniment of two or more objective lesions seen on clinical examination or with evidence for dissemination in space and time diagnosed by further development of new MRI lesions. Progressive MS is diagnosed when there is progressive disease for at least 1 year and abnormal MRI scan of the brain and abnormal MRI scan of the spinal cord, with or without abnormal CSF and visual evoked potentials (Fig. 1). An abnormal CSF examination is defined as elevated oligoclonal IgG bands within CSF that are not present in serum with or without elevations in the IgG index. Occasionally, visual evoked potentials and somatosensory evoked potentials are used to further document dissemination of MS within the CNS. Serologic investigations are done primarily to rule out MS mimickers depending on and directed by any accompanying systemic symptoms and the clinical setting in individual patients. These may include antinuclear antibodies (ANA for lupus), erythrocyte sedimentation rate, anticardiolipin antibodies, vitamin B_{12}, Lyme serology, and chest imaging for CNS sarcoidosis.

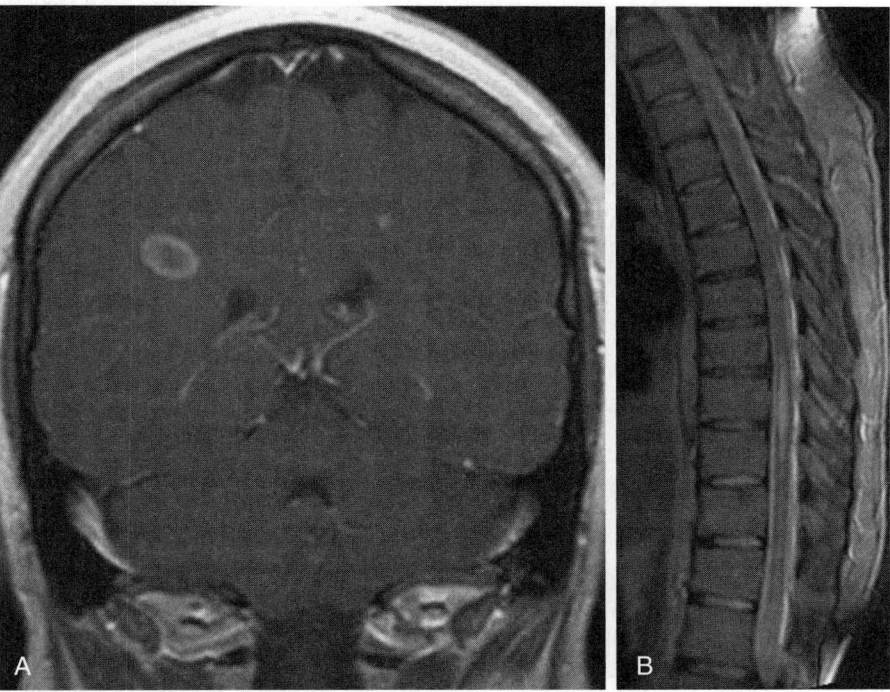

FIGURE 1. Magnetic resonance image showing brain T1 gadolinium-enhancing lesions **(A)** and T2 thoracic spine **(B)** typical of multiple sclerosis.

CURRENT DIAGNOSIS

- Multiple sclerosis (MS) is an autoimmune demyelinating disease of the central nervous system (CNS).
- Diagnosis is secured from having repeated CNS demyelinating attacks and/or new CNS demyelinating lesions on magnetic resonance imaging (MRI) or progressive neurologic dysfunction consistent with MS with no better alternative explanation.

Differential Diagnosis

Other CNS demyelinating diseases can mimic relapsing or progressive MS. Acute disseminating encephalomyelitis is an acute, typically monophasic, and postinfectious CNS inflammatory demyelinating disease. It may be severe; however, if recurrent episodes occur separated by at least 3 months, a diagnosis of relapsing–remitting MS is by far more likely.

Neuromyelitis optica is an autoimmune disease with severe acute attacks but is relatively restricted to the optic nerves and spinal cord. Other brainstem and deep cerebral structures, such as the area postrema, cerebral white matter, and hypothalamus, can also be affected by neuromyelitis optica. Brain MRI scan is usually not consistent with MS, at least early on in the disease, and a specific autoantibody (neuromyelitis optica IgG) directed against the aquaporin 4 water channel is found in more than 70% of cases.

Progressive myelopathies that mimic primary progressive MS or secondary progressive MS include a compressive myelopathy from cervical spondylosis, disk disease, or neoplastic infiltration; nutritional deficiencies (such as vitamin B_{12} or copper deficiencies); paraneoplastic disease (usually associated with CRMP-5 auto-antibodies); or a vascular progressive cause due to dural arteriovenous fistula.

Optic neuritis may be mimicked by acute ischemic optic neuropathy. This condition is typically painless, occurs suddenly, and occurs in patients with advanced age and preexisting vascular risk factors.

Treatment

Acute demyelinating MS attacks (relapses) may be treated with high doses of corticosteroids. These may be given orally or intravenously; however, high doses of corticosteroids are necessary and are superior to low doses. For example, a typical regimen is intravenous methylprednisolone (Solu-Medrol) 1000 mg once daily for 3 to 5 days without oral corticosteroid tapering doses. The oral equivalent to this intravenous regimen is prednisone 1250 mg orally once daily for 5 days with no oral corticosteroid taper following. Gastrointestinal intolerance occurs in some patients, and concomitant use of stomach-protecting agents such proton pump inhibitors may be recommended. Typical acute corticosteroid side effects include insomnia, irritability, and increased appetite as well as an extremely rare association with avascular hip necrosis. Chronic corticosteroid side effects such as diabetes mellitus, cataracts, and weight gain and cushingoid habitus are more associated with chronic corticosteroid use and not short courses of steroids.

CURRENT THERAPY

- Acute attacks of multiple sclerosis (MS) are treated with high-dose corticosteroids and, in severe cases, plasma exchange.
- Therapy is directed at relapsing–remitting disease with interferon β1, glatiramer acetate (Copaxone), and natalizumab (Tysabri). Therapy for secondary progressive MS (typically with ongoing relapses) is mitoxantrone (Novantrone).
- Novel MS medications, including oral medications, are currently under scientific evaluation.

Generally, only MS attacks that are associated with functional impairment (vision loss, diplopia, motor weakness, ataxia) are treated because clinical recovery is hastened but final clinical recovery is not found to be altered by this therapy. Rarely, patients have very severe acute attacks of MS or other demyelinating disease that does not improve with use of high-dose corticosteroids. In these rare patients, the use of plasma exchange (seven exchanges over approximately 14 days) is recommended. Approximately 45% of patients experience functional recovery within 1 month following plasma exchange. Side effects of plasma exchange therapy include paresthesias related to hypocalcemia, anemia, thrombocytopenia, or complications of central venous access that is required for many patients. Intravenous immunoglobulin (Gammagard)[1] has not yet been shown to improve severe clinical attacks of demyelinating disease.

Chronic therapy for relapsing–remitting MS includes the use of β1 interferon (IFN-β1), glatiramer acetate (Copaxone), natalizumab (Tysabri), or, for secondary progressive MS (typically with ongoing attacks or new inflammatory lesions on MRI), mitoxantrone (Novantrone) (Table 1). First-line therapy for patients with relapsing–remitting MS is one of three preparations of IFN-β1 or, alternatively, glatiramer acetate. The side-effect profile is well known for these agents (see Table 1), and they have been safely used for many years. Second-line therapy, if first-line medications are intolerable or if therapeutic response is suboptimal (continued MS attacks or marked ongoing and new inflammatory disease on MRI)includes agents such as natalizumab or mitoxantrone. The goal of chronic immunomodulatory therapy for MS is a reduction in clinical attacks of MS (somewhere between 30% and 60%, depending on the agent) and reduction in new inflammatory MRI lesions (somewhere between 40% and 90%, depending on the agent). Patients and health care professionals should realize that the medications are not a cure or for symptomatic benefit (making people feel better) but specifically for reduction in relapse-related disease.

Second-line immunomodulatory agents are effective in reducing MS attacks; however, they are rarely associated with serious side effects. Natalizumab, as monotherapy or in combination with other medications, is associated with the development of progressive multifocal leukoencephalopathy, a severely impairing, and often fatal, opportunistic brain infection caused by reactivation of dormant JC virus. It occurs in approximately 1 in 1000 patients treated with this agent. In North America, natalizumab is only available through the TOUCH (Tysabri outreach: unified commitment to health) prescribing program. Mitoxantrone is a chemotherapy agent that is the only approved medication for secondary progressive MS. It may be associated with pulmonary and urinary tract infections, alopecia, and cardiotoxicity. The lifetime cumulative dosing of mitoxantrone is restricted to no more than approximately 100 mg/m^2. Cases of acute myelogenous leukemia as well as acute or delayed cardiotoxicity are additional concerns to the use of mitoxantrone in MS patients, and close clinical and investigational (e.g., measuring ejection fraction by echocardiography) follow-up is needed.

Novel medications for MS are under therapeutic investigation. These include intravenous monoclonal antibodies that have a direct effect on inflammatory mediators such as alemtuzumab (Campath)[1] (anti-CD52; T and B cells), daclizumab (Zenapax)[1] (anti-CD25, IL2 receptor), and rituximab (Rituxan)[1] (anti-CD20 B cells). Orally administered immunomodulatory medications are also due to undergo approval review within a few years. These include cladribine (Leustatin)[1] (purine analogue), fingolimod[5] (sphingosine 1-phosphate [S1P] receptor agonist), and laquinimod.[5]

Monitoring

Most, if not all, MS patients should be followed by a neurologist at least occasionally. Recommendations for clinical assessment range from 6 to 18 months, depending on clinical activity of relapses and disability. The ideal scheduling of repeat brain MRI scans is

---

[1]Not FDA approved for this indication.
[5]Investigational drug in the United States.

TABLE 1 Approved Immunomodulatory Therapy for Relapsing–Remitting Multiple Sclerosis

Medication	Dosing	Side Effects	Monitoring	Additional Information
Interferon β1a (Avonex)	30 µg IM injection 1×/wk	Flulike symptoms (fever, chills, arthralgias, myalgias, and headaches), elevated liver function tests, anemia, leukopenia, thrombocytopenia, depression Localized injection-site rejections	CBC with differential, AST, ALT, ALP, and total bilirubin level every 3 mo while on therapy Thyroid function cascade upon initiation of therapy	Premedication with acetaminophen can ameliorate any postinjection flulike symptoms Ibuprofen and naproxen Pregnancy category C medication
Interferon β1a (Rebif)	44 µg SC injection 3×/wk	Flulike symptoms (fever, chills, arthralgias, myalgias, and headaches), elevated liver function tests, anemia, leukopenia, thrombocytopenia, depression Localized injection-site rejections	CBC with differential, AST, ALT, ALP, and total bilirubin level every 3 mo while on therapy Thyroid function cascade upon initiation of therapy	Premedication with acetaminophen can ameliorate any postinjection flulike symptoms Ibuprofen and naproxen Pregnancy category C medication
Interferon β1b (Betaseron, Extavia)	250 µg SC injection every other day	Flulike symptoms (fever, chills, arthralgias, myalgias, and headaches), elevated liver function tests, anemia, leukopenia, thrombocytopenia, depression Localized injection-site rejections	CBC with differential, AST, ALT, ALP, and total bilirubin level every 3 mo while on therapy Thyroid function cascade upon initiation of therapy	Premedication with acetaminophen can ameliorate any postinjection flulike symptoms Ibuprofen and naproxen Pregnancy category C medication
Glatiramer acetate (Copaxone)	20 mg SC injection once daily	Injection-site reactions (erythema, edema, pruritus, pain), transient chest pain, palpitations, facial flushing, anxiety, shortness of breath	None	Pregnancy category B medication
Mitoxantrone hydrochloride (Novantrone)	12 mg/m² IV once every 3 mo	Nausea, skin extravasation reactions, neutropenia, alopecia, amenorrhea, cardiotoxicity, acute myelogenous leukemia	CBC, AST, ALT, bilirubin, creatinine, BUN, and urinalysis at baseline, chest x-ray, PPD skin test, transthoracic echocardiogram before every infusion and annually following therapy	Approved for SPMS Delivered commonly in oncology setting Dose reduction may be needed for prolonged neutropenia Cardiotoxicity may be delayed Pregnancy category D medication
Natalizumab (Tysabri)	300 mg IV once every 28 d	Urticaria and anaphylaxis, headache, arthralgias, nausea, fatigue, depression, infections (urinary tract, pneumonia, herpes simplex or reactivation)	Before treatment: neurologic exam, MRI of head with and without gadolinium should be considered every 12 months while on therapy and if symptoms or signs of progressive multifocal leukoencephalopathy are present	Monotherapy approved Discontinue other immunomodulatory medications at least 1 mo before starting treatment Prescribing professional requires TOUCH enrollment Pregnancy category C medication

Abbreviations: ALP = alkaline phosphatase; ALT = alanine aminotransferase; AST = aspartate aminotransferase; BUN = blood urea nitrogen; CBC = complete blood count; MRI = magnetic resonance imaging; PPD = purified protein derivative; SPMS = secondary progressive multiple sclerosis; TOUCH = Tysabri Outreach: Unified Commitment to Health.

controversial and varies depending on MS clinical activity, but general recommendations are every 1 to 2 years.

Complications

MS is one of the main causes for impairment at a young age and trails only acute trauma. Often patients need gait assistance when impairment becomes more severe. This includes the use of a single gait aid, such as a cane or walking stick, or an ankle- foot orthosis for symptomatic foot drop.

Patients often experience symptoms of neurogenic bladder dysfunction. This includes symptoms of urgency and urge-related incontinence. Bladder stimulants such as caffeine need to be avoided. Patients with this symptom should be investigated for completeness of bladder emptying. If there is severe impairment in bladder emptying, urinary catheterization often is recommended. If bladder emptying is complete or only mildly impaired (<100 mL postvoid residual), use of medications such as oxybutynin (Ditropan) or tolterodine (Detrol) may be recommended for urge-related symptoms; however, ongoing monitoring of bladder emptying is recommended. Some patients require formal urodynamic evaluation for complex bladder symptoms.

Fatigue is a common MS-related symptom. A complete sleep history to ensure appropriate sleep hygiene is imperative. This includes initiating sleep promptly, maintaining sleep throughout the night, and awakening feeling refreshed. Encouragement of a formal exercise program to facilitate restful sleep and daytime vigor is important. Obstructive sleep apnea, restless legs syndrome, and other parasomnias need to be ruled out as additional contributing factors to fatigue. If sleep hygiene is entirely normal and late afternoon fatigue remains a problem, pharmacologic therapy for MS-related fatigue can proceed. Pharmacologic recommendations are limited but include amantadine hydrochloride (Symmetrel)[1] 100 mg by mouth twice daily. Modafinil (Provigil)[1] has been shown in some studies to have an effect on MS-related fatigue at a dose of 200 mg by mouth once daily. Limited early evidence suggests that high-dose aspirin[1] could be effective in some patients as well, 650 mg by mouth twice daily.

[1]Not FDA approved for this indication.

Spasticity associated with upper motor neuron weakness in the lower extremities may be treated with an active daily exercise program directed by physical therapists and physiatrists. Judicious use of baclofen (Lioresal) is helpful (starting at 10 mg once to three times by mouth daily no more than a maximum of 80 mg per day). Baclofen side effects include drowsiness and liver enzyme elevations. Some patients with significant lower extremity weakness are assisted in their gait by the leg support provided by spasticity, and if spasticity is reduced pharmacologically, this can in fact worsen their gait. Alternatives to baclofen include tizanidine (Zanaflex) and clonidine (Catapres).[1]

Summary

MS is a common CNS inflammatory demyelinating disease with heterogenous presentation and prognosis. Relapsing–remitting or attack-related MS is treated with corticosteroids to hasten resolution of acute relapses and chronic immunomodulatory medications such as IFN-β,[1] glatiramer acetate, or natalizumab to reduce the number of future clinical attacks and new MRI lesions. Mitoxantrone is the only medication approved for secondary progressive MS, but is appears to improve primarily those with ongoing attacks or continued inflammatory lesions. Purely progressive forms of primary progressive MS and secondary progressive MS are not responsive to immunomodulatory or immunosuppressive medications. Symptomatic care is important in those patients, including the treatment of gait disorder, spasticity, neurogenic bladder dysfunction, and fatigue.

[1]Not FDA approved for this indication.

REFERENCES

Cohen JA. Emerging therapies for relapsing multiple sclerosis. Arch Neurol 2009;66(7):821–8.

Compston A, Coles A. Multiple sclerosis. Lancet 2008;372(9648):1502–17.

Hartung HP, Gonsette R, König N, et al. Mitoxantrone in progressive multiple sclerosis: A placebo-controlled, double-blind, randomised, multicentre trial. Lancet 2002;360(9350):2018–25.

Keegan BM, Noseworthy JH. Multiple sclerosis. Ann Rev Med 2002;53(1):285–302.

Keegan M, König F, McClelland R, et al. Relation between humoral pathological changes in multiple sclerosis and response to therapeutic plasma exchange. Lancet 2005;366(9485):579–82.

Lublin FD, Reingold SC. Defining the clinical course of multiple sclerosis: Results of an international survey. Neurology 1996;46:907–11.

Lucchinetti C, Parisi J, Lucchinetti CF. The pathology of multiple sclerosis. Neurol Clin 2006;23(1):77–105.

Polman CH, O'Connor PW, Havrdova E, et al. A randomized, placebo-controlled trial of natalizumab for relapsing multiple sclerosis. N Engl J Med 2006;354(9):899–910.

Polman CH, Reingold SC, Edan G, et al. Diagnostic criteria for multiple sclerosis: 2005 revisions to the McDonald criteria. Ann Neurol 2005;58(6):840–6.

Wingerchuk DM, Lennon VA, Pittock SJ, et al. Revised diagnostic criteria for neuromyelitis optica. Neurology 2006;66(10):1485–9.

Myasthenia Gravis

Method of
Bryan Ho, MD

Epidemiology

Myasthenia gravis is often described as a disease of young women and old men. The disease most commonly occurs in women younger than 40 years and men between the ages of 50 and 70 years. However, it can certainly occur in men and women outside of these age ranges.

Risk Factors

Patients with immediate family members who have a history of autoimmune disease may be at higher risk for developing myasthenia gravis.

Pathophysiology

Myasthenia gravis may be the best understood of all the autoimmune disorders. Before discussing the pathophysiology, a brief overview of the neuromuscular junction may be useful.

The neuromuscular junction is the synapse between the motor unit axon and the motor end plate. An action potential arriving at the neuromuscular junction opens voltage-gated calcium channels, which trigger the release of acetylcholine into the synaptic cleft. The acetylcholine diffuses across the cleft and binds to receptors in the motor end plate, which leads to depolarization and ultimately to muscle activation. To prevent involuntary sustained muscle activation, the acetylcholine is rapidly broken down by acetylcholinesterase in the synaptic cleft.

In myasthenia gravis, autoantibodies bind to the acetylcholine receptors in the motor end plate but do not activate them. Thus, there is competitive inhibition with the endogenous acetylcholine released in the synaptic cleft, leading to reduced activation of the motor end plate.

The muscle tissue itself is healthy and a muscle biopsy is unremarkable.

Prevention

The primary disease itself is not preventable. However, myasthenic exacerbations can be triggered by many types of medications, particularly β-blockers, aminoglycosides, and neuromuscular junction–blocking agents, among many others (Box 1). These agents should be avoided if possible or used with extreme caution if they are medically necessary. Systemic medical illnesses can also trigger myasthenic crisis, particularly upper respiratory infections. These patients can deteriorate quickly, so close monitoring is essential.

Clinical Manifestations

The hallmark of myasthenia gravis is pure motor weakness involving ocular, bulbar, or skeletal muscles in any combination and that fluctuates over time. Ocular myasthenic symptoms generally include diplopia and ptosis. Patients can present with oculoparesis that can mimic isolated cranial nerve III, IV, or VI palsies in any combination and is a common feature in myasthenic patients. Bulbar symptoms include dysarthria and dysphagia. Skeletal muscle weakness is usually affected more in the proximal muscles than the distal muscles. A common complaint is difficulty walking up stairs owing to hip flexor weakness, but any muscle group can be affected. There also tends to be a diurnal variation of the symptoms, with the weakness tending to get worse towards the end of the day after exertion but improving with rest. About half of patients with only ocular symptoms on initial presentation develop more generalized symptoms later in life.

Diagnosis

The diagnosis of myasthenia can often be made based on a careful history and detailed neurologic examination demonstrating the pattern of weakness and its variable nature. Laboratory testing and electromyography help to confirm the diagnosis. If the patient is not presenting with any symptoms at the time of the examination, muscle fatigability can often be induced. Sustained upward gaze can induce ptosis and unmask oculoparesis leading to diplopia. Prolonged speech can induce slurring or a nasal quality to the voice. Repetitive muscle movements can lead to clinically detectable weakness.

BOX 1 Common Drugs that Can Exacerbate Myasthenia Gravis

Anesthetics

Halothane (Fluothane)
Ketamine (Ketalar)
Lidocaine (Xylocaine)
All neuromuscular blocking agents
Procaine

Antibiotics

Aminoglycosides
Fluoroquinolones
Tetracyclines
Erythromycin
Clarithromycin (Biaxin)
Clindamycin (Clecoin)

Antiepileptics

Gabapentin (Neurontin)
Phenytoin (Dilantin)

Antipsychotics

Chloropromazine (Thorazine)
Lithium (Eskalith, Lithobid)
Phenothiazines

Cardiovascular Agents

β-Blockers
Calcium channel blockers
Procainamide (Pronestyl)
Quinidine

Others

Anticholinergic agents
Cholinesterase inhibitors
Glucocorticoids
Narcotics
Statins

CURRENT DIAGNOSIS

- Myasthenia gravis is an autoimmune disease that affects the neuromuscular junction.
- Symptoms include fluctuating skeletal, ocular, or bulbar muscle weakness in any combination and of varying degrees of severity.
- Depending on the clinical severity, treatment can focus on controlling symptoms or can require chronic immunomodulating therapy. Thymectomy may also induce remission in many patients.
- Myasthenic crisis can be potentially life-threatening due to rapid respiratory compromise and can be triggered by a wide variety of medications and acute illness.

Another helpful bedside examination finding is the ice pack test. In a patient presenting with ptosis, applying an ice pack over the affected eye can lead to demonstrable improvement supporting the diagnosis of myasthenia gravis.

Another way to confirm the diagnosis clinically is a Tensilon (edrophonium) test. To do this, there needs to be a clear observable sign of weakness, preferably ptosis, because this is difficult for the patient to simulate factitiously. Because of the risk of bradycardia, this test needs to be done with telemetry monitoring, with atropine 1 mg on hand at the bedside. An initial test dose of edrophonium 2 mg is given intravenously and the patient is observed for any side effects. If the patient tolerates this dose, another 8 mg (10 mg total) is given. The patient is monitored for any clinical improvement in the weakness being observed; improvement supports the diagnosis of myasthenia. Some clinicians, if a skeletal muscle is observed, administer a placebo before the edrophonium. Improvement in symptoms with the placebo suggests a psychogenic component to the symptoms.

Serologic tests are available for confirming the clinical diagnosis of myasthenia gravis; the most useful are assays for detecting acetylcholine receptor antibodies (AChR-Ab). This test is very specific and has very low false-positive rates. It is fairly sensitive in generalized myasthenia (more than 80%) but less sensitive in detecting milder forms like ocular myasthenia (as low as 50%). In cases where clinical suspicion is high but the patient is AchR-Ab negative, another assay for antibodies to muscle-specific receptor tyrosine kinase (anti-MuSK) is available. Anti-MuSK is positive in up to 50% of AchR-Ab negative patients with myasthenia gravis. Up to 10% of patients with myasthenia gravis are seronegative for both assays.

Notably, patients who are AchR-Ab positive are more likely to have thymic abnormalities and thus can be predicted to benefit more from thymectomy. Conversely, patients who are seronegative or have anti-MuSK antibodies alone are less likely to have thymic pathology and may be expected to receive less benefit from thymectomy. Otherwise the medical approach to treatment is unchanged regardless of the presence or absence of serologic markers.

An autoimmune screen is also recommended in any patient being worked up for myasthenia gravis. Thus checking erythrocyte sedimentation rate, C-reactive protein, antinuclear antibodies, rheumatoid factor, and thyroid-stimulating hormone levels is advised.

Electromyography is very useful in confirming the diagnosis of myasthenia gravis as well as excluding other possible neuromuscular diagnoses. Electromyography should be viewed as an extension of the neurologic examination. If myasthenia gravis is suspected, the ordering physician should request that repetitive nerve stimulation and single-fiber electromyography (EMG) be done if the equipment is available. In repetitive nerve stimulation, a motor nerve to a clinically affected muscle is stimulated repeatedly at low frequencies. In myasthenia gravis, this test should demonstrate decrement in amplitude of the compound motor action potentials and has a sensitivity of roughly 75% of generalized myasthenia. Single-fiber EMG is a more time-consuming and technically difficult test that involves simultaneously measuring the motor action potentials of two muscle fibers innervated by the same motor nerve. The time between action potentials (referred to as "jitter") is measured, and increased jitter strongly suggests delayed neuromuscular transmission. Single-fiber EMG has a sensitivity up to 95%. Milder forms such as ocular myasthenia are more likely to have false negatives in either of these tests. However, even with single-fiber EMG, the sensitivity in these cases is greater than 90%.

In patients with a confirmed diagnosis of myasthenia gravis, a chest CT scan is recommended to evaluate for any gross thymic pathology. All myasthenic patients should be considered for thymectomy if there are no medical contraindications, even if there are no gross abnormalities on imaging.

Differential Diagnosis

Other neuromuscular junction disorders can manifest with features similar to myasthenia gravis, such as botulism, Lambert-Eaton syndrome, and cholinergic crisis. However, usually these conditions can be distinguished clinically, particularly by the presence of autonomic features that are not present in myasthenia gravis. Botulism is associated with ingestion of toxin from the bacteria *Clostridium botulinum*, usually from home-canned food, and generally occurs in infants rather than adults. In addition to oculobulbar and generalized weakness, these patients also present with dilated pupils, dry skin, and dry mucosal membranes. Lambert-Eaton myasthenic syndrome (LEMS) is due to autoantibodies to the presynaptic voltage-gated calcium channels and is often associated with underlying malignancy, usually small cell lung cancer. In contrast to myasthenia, weakness often spares the oculobulbar muscles and the weakness tends to improve rather than worsen with exercise. These patients are usually areflexic and also have other autonomic symptoms such as dry mouth and sexual dysfunction. Cholinergic crisis can occur with overdose of acetylcholine esterase inhibitors or exposure to pesticides with organophosphates, leading to excess cholinergic activity in the neuromuscular junction. In addition to bulbar, generalized, and respiratory weakness, these patients usually present with autonomic signs of cholinergic excess such as pupillary constriction, hypersalivation, and sweating.

Other neuromuscular conditions can lead to weakness that can mimic myasthenia gravis. Acute demyelinating polyneuropathy (Guillain-Barré syndrome), if severe, could appear similar to myasthenic crisis. However, the cerebrospinal fluid usually shows elevated protein, and EMG findings should show demyelination. Critical illness polyneuropathy and myopathy occur in patients with prolonged ICU courses, particularly if sepsis is part of the clinical picture, and EMG studies are helpful in clarifying the diagnosis. Inflammatory myopathies and motor neuron disease are also in the differential diagnosis, and EMG studies should be very helpful to elucidate the diagnosis in clinically uncertain cases.

In cases of pure ocular myasthenia, third, fourth, or sixth cranial neuropathies in any combination could be considered in the differential diagnosis. In the case of third nerve palsy, the pupil is usually involved as well and the affected eye is deviated down and outward. There can also be ptosis. In fourth nerve palsy, the affected eye is usually elevated compared to the normal eye, leading to a vertical diplopia. In sixth nerve palsies, the eye is deviated inward and there is clear weakness in abducting the affected eye. Conversely, myasthenia gravis should be considered in any patients with isolated ocular weakness.

Treatment

Treatment for myasthenia gravis can be divided into symptomatic control, immunosuppression, and, in selected patients, thymectomy, depending on the severity of the disease.

CURRENT THERAPY

- Mild symptoms respond very well to anticholinesterase inhibitors, with pyridostigmine (Mestinon) being the most commonly used.
- Chronic control of symptoms can require oral immunosuppressive agents such as steroids, azathioprine (Imuran),[1] or mycophenolate mofetil (Cellcept).[1] If necessary, plasmapheresis or IV immunoglobulin (IVIg; Gammagard)[1] can be helpful to treat worsening symptoms or as maintenance therapy.
- A diverse range of medications can exacerbate myasthenic symptoms. Clinicians need to be mindful of this with their prescriptions for myasthenic patients.
- Myasthenic crisis is a medical emergency and requires aggressive supportive care. Such patients need to be hospitalized in an intensive care setting with close respiratory monitoring and intubation if necessary. Such patients require acute immunologic treatment with plasmapheresis or IVIg[1] to accelerate recovery followed by chronic immunomodulating therapy.

[1]Not FDA approved for this indication.

Symptoms can be controlled in many patients with acetylcholinesterase inhibitors. Inhibition of acetylcholinesterase leads to prolonged action of acetylcholine in the synaptic cleft, partially overcoming the competitive inhibition with acetylcholine-receptor antibodies. This may be sufficient alone to address mild forms of the disease, such as in ocular myasthenia. The most commonly used agent in this class is pyridostigmine (Mestinon). Neostigmine (Prostigmin) is another alternative, though it is less often used.

PYRIDOSTIGMINE

Pyridostigmine is effective for controlling mild symptoms. It should not be relied on as therapy for suspected myasthenic crisis or if respiratory compromise is a concern.

The dose is 30 to 90 mg, generally used every 3 to 6 hours as needed, and tailored to clinical response. Maximum dose should not exceed 120 mg per single dose. Patients typically get a response within 30 minutes. It is also available in a long-acting formulation (Mestinon TS 180 mg). The long-acting form is generally not recommended for daytime use owing to a less-predictable onset of action. It may be useful as a bedtime dose for patients who have severe morning weakness on awakening.

Side effects for acetylcholine esterase inhibitors are mostly gastrointestinal, with abdominal cramping, nausea and vomiting, and diarrhea being most common. Patients might find it helpful to take the medicine with some food. Other symptoms of cholinergic excess such as miosis, sweating, and hypersalivation can also occur. Overdose can lead to cholinergic crisis, with severe weakness, bradycardia, and hypotension being potentially life-threatening, but these effects generally do not occur if the medication is taken within recommended parameters.

If necessary, side effects can be alleviated with certain anticholinergic medications with little or no activation of nicotinic receptors. A commonly used agent for this purpose is glycopyrrolate (Robinul)[1] 1 mg taken with each pyridostigmine dose or as a stand-alone dose three times a day.

In patients with baseline weakness beyond mild bulbar or ocular symptoms or with progressively worsening symptoms, chronic immunosuppression may be necessary. The most commonly used agents are prednisone,[1] azathioprine (Imuran),[1] mycophenolate mofetil (Cellcept),[1] and cyclosporine (Sandimmune, Neoral), each with its own advantages and disadvantages.

PREDNISONE

Prednisone[1] is often the first agent used in long-term management of generalized myasthenia. Prednisone has the advantage of having relatively quick onset of action compared to other immunosuppressive agents used for chronic myasthenia. Some clinicians favor starting patients on high doses (1.5 mg/kg to a maximum dose of 100 mg) to achieve a quick clinical response initially, then tapering to the lowest dose possible to maintain control of symptoms. Other immunosuppressive treatments can be used in conjunction as steroid-sparing agents. The disadvantage with this strategy is that for unclear reasons, prednisone can exacerbate symptoms in the short term, and this risk increases with higher doses. Thus this strategy is generally initiated in the inpatient setting. Most clinicians, if possible, favor avoiding the risk of exacerbating symptoms and instead start at a lower dose (15-20 mg) and titrate the dose slowly based on the patient's clinical response. The drawback is that it generally takes longer to achieve significant symptomatic improvement.

AZATHIOPRINE

Azathioprine[1] can be used for chronic immunosuppression as a steroid-sparing agent. Patients are started on 50 mg/day and then titrated 50 mg/week to a target dose of 2 to 3 mg/kg/day. During the first few weeks, some patients have to discontinue the medication

[1]Not FDA approved for this indication.

owing to a systemic reaction involving fever, abdominal pain, nausea, and vomiting. Patients also require weekly monitoring of complete blood counts and liver function during the titration phase. Upon reaching the target dose, monitoring can be extended to every 3 months. The medication can take up to 6 months to take effect.

MYCOPHENOLATE MOFETIL

Mycophenolate mofetil[1] is less well studied than azathioprine, but from clinical experience, it appears to be efficacious in chronic treatment of myasthenia and has become preferred owing to better side-effect profile, faster onset of action (usually within 3 months), and no need for regular monitoring of liver function. Patients start on 1 g twice a day, titrated by 500 mg a month until a target dose of 1.5 g twice a day is reached. Side effects include diarrhea, abdominal pain, and nausea. Less commonly, leukopenia can occur.

CYCLOSPORINE

Cyclosporine[1] is viewed by most clinicians as a second-line agent for patients who fail treatment with azathioprine and mycophenolate mofetil. Patients can start on 3 mg/kg daily divided in two doses, titrated up to 6 mg/kg daily. The dose should be adjusted to a trough cyclosporine level between 50 and 150 ng/mL. Kidney function also needs to be monitored. Cyclosporine tends to take effect within 2 to 3 months of drug initiation.

PLASMAPHERESIS AND INTRAVENOUS IMMUNOGLOBULIN

Plasmapheresis and intravenous immunoglobulin (IVIg, Gammagard)[1] have been shown to be effective in the acute management of myasthenia and are mainstays of treatment in myasthenic crisis. These treatments are also useful as bridging therapies in patients transitioning to chronic immunosuppression or as prophylaxis for patients at risk for myasthenic crisis. Plasmapheresis directly removes circulating acetylcholine receptor antibodies, leading to alleviation of symptoms. The mechanism of action of intravenous immunoglobulin is less clear. It may be due to the pooled immunoglobulin binding to the autoantibodies, in turn preventing them from binding to the acetylcholine receptors.

Plasma exchange typically involves five sessions spread over 1 to 2 weeks. Clinical response correlates with the reduction in acetylcholine receptor antibody levels, though it is not necessary to check levels routinely during exchanges. Patients often have a clinical response within a few days after initiation of treatment. The most common significant complication of the procedure is hypotension and other cardiac issues. Because the procedure requires catheter placement, infection and thrombosis are also potential risks.

IVIg therapy is typically given at a dose of 2 g/kg divided over 5 days. An IgA level should be checked before starting the therapy in a treatment-naïve patient because patients with IgA deficiency are at risk for developing an anaphylactic reaction to the infusion. Patients generally respond within a week of initiation. Complications of treatment are uncommon but include thrombotic events such as stroke and myocardial infarction. It should also be used with caution in patients with congestive heart failure owing to the fluid load. There is also a risk of acute renal failure. Aseptic meningitis can also occur.

Comparatively, plasmapheresis and IVIg have roughly equivalent efficacy, so the choice is based on the clinical scenario, preference of the treating physician, and available resources. If one treatment fails to confer any clinical improvement, it is perfectly reasonable to attempt the other.

THYMECTOMY

Thymectomy should be strongly considered in any patient who is younger than 60 years and has no medical contraindications for the surgery. It should also be considered in older patients with significant weakness beyond mild ocular or bulbar symptoms. A significant number of patients achieve significant improvement or full remission of symptoms after thymectomy, even if no thymic pathology is found at the time of surgery.

Myasthenic Crisis

Any myasthenic patient, regardless of how mild the baseline symptoms are, has a risk of developing myasthenic crisis at some point in his or her lifetime. Myasthenic crisis is often precipitated by systemic illness, particularly upper respiratory infections, and a wide variety of medications are also known to exacerbate myasthenia symptoms. Any myasthenic patient complaining of worsening symptoms, particularly dyspnea, should be evaluated urgently because the patient can quickly decompensate. Such patients also should not be managed by adjusting their cholinesterase inhibitor regimen alone because symptomatic control is insufficient to forestall further progression into crisis.

These patients require immunomodulating therapy with either plasmapheresis or IVIg.[1] They should also be monitored in an intensive care unit setting with frequent respiratory mechanics assessed at least two or three times a day. If forced vital capacity (FVC) is less than 20 mg/kg or the net inspiratory force (NIF) is less than -30 cm H_2O, elective intubation is strongly advised. Either plasmapheresis or IVIg therapy should be started. A thorough work-up should be done to search for the underlying trigger (e.g., infection, new medication), and any triggers that are found should be treated or removed. Once stabilized, the patient should also begin taking chronic immunomodulation, if this medication is not already used. Prednisone[1] is most commonly used initially because its onset of action is faster than the other options.

Monitoring

Patients should be monitored as outpatients on a regular basis to ensure stability of symptoms and adequate symptomatic response, as well as monitoring laboratory studies, depending on the chronic immunomodulating medication being used. Acute deterioration in symptoms needs to taken very seriously, with a low threshold for urgent evaluation and hospitalization.

Complications

The dreaded complication of myasthenia is myasthenic crisis leading to fulminant generalized weakness and respiratory failure, often precipitated by systemic illness or other medications. Because patients can deteriorate rapidly, patients in whom symptoms appear to be worsening acutely need to be evaluated urgently. See "Myasthenic Crisis" earlier for further discussion.

---

[1]Not FDA approved for this indication.

REFERENCES

Drachman DB. Myasthenia gravis. N Engl J Med 1994;330:1797–810.

Hoch W, McConville J, Helms S, et al. Auto-antibodies to the receptor tyrosine kinase MuSK in patients with myasthenia gravis without acetylcholine receptor antibodies. Nat Med 2001;7:365–8.

Keesey JC. Clinical evaluation and management of myasthenia gravis. Muscle Nerve 2004;29(4):484–505.

McConville J, Farrugia ME, Beeson D, et al. Detection and characterization of MuSK antibodies in seronegative myasthenia gravis. Ann Neurol 2004; 55:580–4.

Ropper AH, Brown RH. Adam and Victor's Principles of Neurology. 8th ed. New York: McGraw-Hill; 2005.

Saperstein DS, Barohn RJ. Management of myasthenia gravis. Semin Neurol 2004;24:41–8.

---

[1]Not FDA approved for this indication.

Trigeminal Neuralgia

Method of
Ronald F. Young, MD

Trigeminal neuralgia (TN) is one of the most devastating pain conditions that people endure. The pain is frequently misdiagnosed as being of dental or paranasal sinus origin. Unnecessary dental procedures, such as root canals and extractions or sinus surgery, are often performed in misguided attempts to treat the pain. The condition is also referred to as *tic douloureux* because of the sudden facial grimacing that may be seen as a reaction to the pain. The illness is estimated to affect about 1 in 20,000 people and becomes more frequent with advancing age. TN may be of primary (idiopathic) origin or secondary origin due to a variety of structural conditions, such as tumors (meningiomas and vestibular schwannomas in particular), multiple sclerosis (MS), vascular malformations, and cysts of the posterior cranial fossa. The exact etiology of TN is still debated, but it is generally accepted that most cases of idiopathic TN are due to compression of the trigeminal nerve root near its entry into the brainstem at the pons by adjacent blood vessels, most commonly arteries. Such compression is thought to result in segmental demyelination due to the constant pulsatile forces directed against the nerve root. The underlying pathology is thought to be related to the aging process wherein arteries (particularly the superior cerebellar artery) that normally course superior to, but not in contact with, the nerve root gradually come into contact and then compress and distort the nerve root as a result of constant pulsatile pressure. Such pressure causes localized demyelination and loss of the normal insulating function of the myelin. Ephaptic or nonsynaptic transmission and abnormal local depolarization are then postulated to result in ectopic impulse generation. Such impulses are thought to activate nerve fibers in the trigeminal nerve root that generate the pain of TN. Ephaptic transmission is also thought to account for the "triggering" of pain by usually innocuous stimuli, such as lightly touching the face or brushing the teeth.

Diagnosis

In spite of modern technology, TN is a diagnosis based almost exclusively on the medical history. Neither laboratory nor imaging studies establish the diagnosis conclusively, although properly formatted magnetic resonance imaging (MRI) scans recently have been thought to contribute to the correct diagnosis if they demonstrate arterial compression of the trigeminal nerve root. Three aspects of the history are critical to the diagnosis: (1) the type of pain, (2) the location of the pain, and (3) the factors that trigger or activate the pain. The pain of TN is sharp, sudden, severe, and brief in character, usually lasting only a few seconds but often occurring in repeated bursts. The pain is often described as feeling like an electric shock or ice pick jabbing into the face. Pains that are of longer duration and described as burning, aching, boring, or like pressure are not typical of TN; when such symptoms are described, an alternative diagnosis should be considered. The pain of TN is confined within one or more of the major three peripheral divisions of the trigeminal nerve: the first division encompassing the anterior two thirds of the scalp, the forehead, the eye, and the upper portion of the nose; the second division encompassing the edges of the nares, the upper lip and cheek, the upper teeth, gums, and mucosal lining of the mouth; and the third division encompassing the skin over the mandible, including the lower lip as well as the lower teeth, gums, and anterior two thirds of the tongue. Pain that is located in the mastoid or occipital region, deep within the ear canal, extending below the edge of the mandible onto the neck or traversing the midline is not trigeminal in origin. TN is almost exclusively a unilateral condition. Bilateral pain is estimated to occur in less than 1% of cases; when bilateral the pain on

CURRENT DIAGNOSIS

- Sudden, sharp, severe pain on one side of the face
- Confined to the cutaneous or intraoral distribution of the trigeminal nerve
- Triggered by otherwise innocuous stimulation of the face or mouth
- Usually due to arterial compression of the trigeminal nerve root but may be due to multiple sclerosis, tumors, or vascular malformations

the two sides is often different with regard to the age of the patient at onset and the location of the pain. Most cases of bilateral TN occur in patients with MS wherein the pain is due to demyelination in the trigeminal nerve root secondary to an MS plaque. One of the most characteristic historical features of TN is the triggering of jabs or jolts of pain by stimuli that usually are innocuous. Such triggers include a variety of light mechanical stimuli, such as touching the face lightly, brushing the teeth, talking, attempting to eat and drink, and even a light breeze blowing against the face. Light, gentle stimuli are often more effective in eliciting the pain than are more forceful ones. Facial pain, even severe pain, probably is not TN if trigger phenomena are not described. The time course of TN is marked by unexplained, erratic exacerbations and remissions that may last days, weeks, months, or even years. The exacerbations tend to be less severe and shorter in duration at the onset of the illness and tend to become more severe and longer in duration and marked by shorter interval remissions as the illness persists over time. Patients who complain of persistent, unremitting facial pain, often with durations of weeks, months, or even years, probably do not suffer from TN. TN is often misdiagnosed as being of dental or paranasal sinus origin, but conversely other forms of facial pain are often misdiagnosed as TN. Most commonly misdiagnosed is so-called atypical facial pain. Such pain, often seen in young or middle-aged women but seen in men as well, usually is described as a strong, unremitting pressure or burning sensation that encompasses an area of the head and/or neck outside of the distribution of the trigeminal nerve, unassociated with trigger phenomena, often of prolonged durations (years), and usually unresponsive to a variety of medical interventions. Patients with atypical facial pain often express feelings of depression and hopelessness. Such pain is unresponsive to surgical intervention, and ill-advised surgical procedures often aggravate the pain and may leave the patient with new medical problems due to complications of the surgical procedures.

Physical Examination

In classic, or idiopathic, TN due to vascular compression of the trigeminal nerve root, the physical examination is usually completely unremarkable. Specifically, at least by the usual clinical examination techniques, facial sensation including the corneal reflex is normal. When loss of facial sensation to innocuous or painful stimuli is detected, a structural cause of TN should be sought. Tumors, vascular malformations, and MS are usually accompanied by other abnormal neurologic examination findings, including double vision, unilateral hearing loss, and facial weakness. MRI scanning is recommended in all patients with a suspected diagnosis of TN because even in some cases of TN caused by structural lesions, the examination may be normal, and the diagnosis of TN may be strengthened if an MRI scan demonstrates arterial compression of the trigeminal nerve root. Occasionally, an MRI scan discloses a completely unexpected cause of TN, such as a tortuous vertebrobasilar artery complex compressing the nerve root or even a large contralateral tumor or cyst displacing the brainstem. Such findings may radically alter any surgical recommendations made for treatment of TN. Patients who are unable to undergo MRI scanning because they have a cardiac pacemaker, for instance, should undergo thin-section computed tomography scanning, which cannot detect arterial vascular compression and small tumors but can detect larger tumors, vascular malformations, and vertebrobasilar artery compression.

Treatment

MEDICAL TREATMENT

The anticonvulsant family of drugs is the mainstay of medical treatment of TN. Carbamazepine (Tegretol) and oxcarbazepine (Trileptal)[1] are the best drugs for initial medical treatment of TN. Both should be started in relatively low doses, for example, 100 to 200 mg once or twice daily and then increased gradually and slowly until either satisfactory control of the pain or intolerable side effects occur. Such side effects include drowsiness, weakness, difficulty with recent memory, and unsteadiness of gait. Older patients are particularly sensitive to such side effects, and the initial dose and maximum tolerable dose are usually lower in older patients, particularly those in their 70s and older. From 5 to 7 days should elapse between dosing increments in order to allow development of a stable blood level of medication. Additional increments of 100 to 200 mg/day are recommended. Laboratory tests of serum levels of the medications are of little or no help in the treatment of TN. In order to establish a consistent blood level of these medications and to provide the best chance for achieving lasting pain relief with minimum side effects, counseling of the patient by the physician regarding the correct dosing regimen is essential. Patients often regard these medications as analgesics and vary the dosage on an as-needed basis, some days taking little or no medication and other days taking large amounts. Because of their pharmacokinetics, these medications must be taken in a consistent dosage on a daily basis in order to maximize the chance of success. It is surprising how hard it may be for patients to understand and adhere to such a regimen, but maintaining the regimen is essential for successful pain relief. Gabapentin (Neurontin)[1] has become popular for the treatment of TN, but experience indicates it is a secondary medication only. It may be useful when pain control cannot be achieved with carbamazepine (Tegretol) or oxcarbazepine (Trileptal) or when those medications cannot be tolerated because of side effects. Other potential second-line medications include a variety of other anticonvulsants (e.g., lamotrigine [Lamictal],[1] phenytoin [Dilantin][1]) as well as baclofen (Lioresal) A variety of toxicities, including liver dysfunction, bone marrow suppression, and allergic reactions, may accompany use of these medications, so appropriate laboratory surveillance should be performed per manufacturers' recommendations.

SURGICAL TREATMENT

In the past, surgery was reserved for patients who did not respond to medical management of TN because the medication was ineffective or the side effects or toxicities were intolerable. However, some studies suggest that the longer the illness persists, the smaller the chance

----

[1]Not FDA approved for this indication.

CURRENT THERAPY

- Usually responds to oral anticonvulsant medications, such as carbamazepine (Tegretol) or oxcarbazepine (Trileptal).[1]
- Early radiosurgical treatment offers a good chance of curing the illness with minimal side effects.
- Microvascular decompression is the most effective surgical treatment of TN, but it is associated with the greatest risk of serious complications.

----

[1]Not FDA approved for this indication.

for lasting successful surgical relief of the pain. Many patients considered the potential side effects and complications of the surgical procedures unacceptable, and neurologists often referred patients for surgical procedures only as a last resort. With the advent of radiosurgery as a viable, successful, and safe surgical treatment of TN, consideration of surgical intervention earlier rather than later in the disease course may be better. Microvascular decompression (MVD) is the most effective, yet most dangerous, of the surgical procedures for TN. About 90% of patients will achieve immediate relief of TN after MVD, but this success rate drops to about 75% in long-term follow-up. MVD is the only surgical procedure that treats the putative cause of TN, namely, vascular compression of the trigeminal nerve root. In the MVD procedure, a small posterior fossa craniotomy is performed. The trigeminal nerve root is visualized using the operating microscope, any compressing vessels are dissected free of the nerve, and future contact is prevented by placing a shock-absorbing material, usually shredded Teflon felt, between the vessel and the nerve. Fatal complications may occur in up to 1% of patients undergoing the MVD procedures. From 15% to 20% of patients who undergo MVD experience some complication of the procedure, such as cerebellar edema, brainstem infarction, subdural and epidural hematomas, facial paralysis, unilateral hearing loss, cerebrospinal fluid leakage, meningitis, and infection. Percutaneous procedures (e.g., radiofrequency electrocoagulation, glycerol rhizolysis, balloon compression) are considerably safer than MVD, but loss of facial sensation usually accompanies such procedures. Loss of facial sensation should be avoided in order to prevent secondary complications such as anesthesia dolorosa and loss of the corneal reflex with subsequent corneal ulceration or loss of vision. The initial success rate is about 90% with the percutaneous procedures, but recurrences are frequent. Serious side effects, such as meningitis, brain abscess or hematoma, and carotid artery to cavernous sinus fistulas, occasionally occur. One of the attractive features of percutaneous procedures is that they can be repeated fairly easily if pain recurs. Radiosurgery is gaining increased acceptance as a surgical method for treating TN. Although considered a form of surgery, the procedure is accomplished without an incision, instead using either gamma rays (Gamma Knife, Elekta, Inc.) or high-energy x-rays (linear accelerator [LINAC]) that are focused on the trigeminal nerve root adjacent to the brainstem. The treatment is planned using MRI or computed tomography scanning, and the radiation is guided to the target at the trigeminal nerve root in such a way as to avoid injury to adjacent structures. The procedure provides pain relief in about 60% of patients with TN without the need for medication; another 15% to 20% of patients experience pain relief with small tolerable doses of medication. Radiosurgery is attractive to patients and referring physicians because of the ease of performing the procedure and the minimum risk of side effects. Radiosurgery is a destructive form of treatment of TN, but the degree of damage to the nerve root is usually minimal enough that normal facial sensation is maintained. Permanent losses of facial sensation may occur in as few as 5% of patients treated with radiosurgery, depending on the dose of radiation used for the treatment. Drawbacks of radiosurgery include delayed onset of pain relief after treatment (usually a few months) and recurrences. Radiosurgery can be repeated in the event of initial failure of the treatment or in case of recurrence after an initially successful treatment. The reasonable success rate, the ease of performance of the procedure, and the minimal risk of side effects make radiosurgery a treatment that can be recommended early in the treatment of TN, once the diagnosis has been well established, because it may provide permanent cure of the disease with minimal risk.

REFERENCES

Bagheri SC, Fairhdvash F, Perciaccante VJ. Diagnosis and treatment of patients with trigeminal neuralgia. Am-Dent Assoc 2004;135:1713–7.

Kres B, Schindler M, Rasche D, et al. MRI volumetry for the preoperative diagnosis of trigeminal neuralgia. Eur Radiol 2005;15:1344–8.

Liu JK, Apfelbaum RI. Treatment of trigeminal neuralgia. Neurosurg Clin North Am 2004;15:319–34.

Shetter AG, Aabramisk JM, Speiser BL. Microvascular decompression after gamma knife surgery for trigeminal neuralgia: Intraoperative findings and treatment outcomes. J Neurosurg 2000;102(Suppl.):259–61.

Young RF. Stereotactic procedures for facial pain. In: Apuzzo M, editor. Brain Surgery: Complication Avoidance and Management. New York: Churchill Livingstone; 1993. pp. 2097–114.

Young RF. Radiosurgery versus microsurgery for trigeminal neurlagia: Current techniques in neurosurgery. In: Salcman M, editor. Current medicine. New York: Springer; 1998. pp. 35–43.

Young RF, Vermeulen SS, Grimm P, et al. Gamma knife radiosurgery for treatment of trigeminal neuralgia: Idiopathic and tumor related. Neurology 1997;48:608–14.

Young RF, Vermeulen SS, Posewitz A. Gamma knife radiosurgery for treatment of trigeminal neuralgia. Stereotact Funct Neurosurg 1998;70:192–9.

Acute Peripheral Facial Paralysis (Bell's Palsy)

Method of
Bryan K. Ward, MD, and Barry M. Schaitkin, MD

Acute facial nerve paralysis (i.e., Bell's palsy) manifests as an acute onset of facial muscle weakness. The condition is named for the Scottish surgeon Sir Charles Bell. In 1821, he described paralysis of the muscles of facial expression after facial trauma. The name *Bell's palsy* was later given to this common atraumatic cause of facial paralysis. Although there are numerous causes of facial paralysis, approximately two thirds of cases are idiopathic acute facial nerve paralysis, or Bell's palsy (Fig. 1).

DIFFERENTIAL DIAGNOSIS OF ACUTE FACIAL NERVE PARALYSIS

Idiopathic (65%)

- Bell's palsy

Infection (associated with Bell's palsy)

- Herpes zoster, herpes simplex, borreliosis (commonly associated)
- Epstein-Barr, HIV, cytomegalovirus virus, mycoplasma pneumonia, tuberculosis, Kawasaki syndrome (uncommonly associated)
- Acute and chronic suppurative otitis media (rare since introduction of antibiotics)

Trauma (25%)

- Temporal bone fracture, penetrating wound

Neoplasms (5%)

- Parotid gland, metastases (skin, breast, lung, kidney, colon), cholesteatoma, schwannoma

Metabolic and toxic

- Diabetes, thyroid disease, alcoholism, carbon monoxide

Other rare causes

- Sarcoidosis, multiple sclerosis, amyloidosis, Wegener's granulomatosis, Sjögren's disease, Guillain-Barré syndrome, Melkersson-Rosenthal syndrome

---

FIGURE 1. Causes of facial nerve palsy. *Abbreviation:* HIV = human immunodeficiency virus.

The incidence of Bell's palsy is 1 case per 3000 people per year. It occurs most commonly in persons between the ages of 15 and 40 years and less commonly in children younger than 15 years. Diabetics and pregnant women are at increased risk, with pregnant women three times as likely to develop Bell's palsy compared with nonpregnant women, particularly in the third-trimester and postpartum periods.

The mechanism of Bell's palsy is still unconfirmed, but there are hypotheses. One theory is that inflammation of the facial nerve causes entrapment along its course through the fallopian canal, leading to secondary ischemia and nerve damage. Another theory involves viral infection causing direct interference with neural function without nerve compression.

Numerous viruses have been associated with acute facial nerve paralysis. Evidence points to an association with herpesvirus, but no direct causality in humans has been shown. Using a mouse model, Sugita and colleagues were able to demonstrate transient facial weakness in mice inoculated with a strain of herpes simplex virus type 1 (HSV-1). The greatest evidence for a viral association with Bell's palsy in humans is the work by Murakami and associates, in which endoneural fluid from 10 of 13 patients tested positive by polymerase chain reaction (PCR) assay for HSV-1 DNA after surgical decompression of the facial nerve. PCR testing of endoneural fluid from 7 patients with Ramsay-Hunt syndrome showed the samples to be positive varicella-zoster virus (i.e., human herpesvirus 3).

A temporal relationship between viral reactivation and the onset of Bell's palsy has not been confirmed. PCR studies have demonstrated a link but cannot differentiate latent from active infections. Perhaps the strongest evidence for a viral cause of Bell's palsy comes from a clustering of cases in Switzerland after the administration of an inactivated nasal influenza vaccination. A matched case-control study showed that 27.7% of 68 patients with Bell's palsy during the study had received the vaccine, compared with 1.1% of controls. The risk for those who received the vaccination was highest at 30 to 60 days, and this increased risk did not exist for those who received the parenteral form.

Clinical Presentation

Bell's palsy has been described as "peas in a pod" because of its typical clinical presentation. Patients may initially experience pain behind the ear or in the ear canal that precedes facial muscle weakness. The patient may have a history of recent upper respiratory infection. Weakness progresses within 48 hours to complete or near-complete paralysis of all the muscles of facial expression, almost always unilaterally. Other possible symptoms include hyperacusis on the affected side due to paresis of the stapedius muscle, ipsilateral impaired taste in the anterior tongue due to dysfunction of the chorda tympani nerve, and decreased tearing from interrupted parasympathetic input to the lacrimal gland. Palsies of other cranial nerves have been associated with Bell's palsy, although this relationship is controversial.

Not all facial paralysis is Bell's palsy. Because the cause of Bell's palsy is probably viral, which has no available diagnostic test, other forms of acute facial paralysis must first be considered. Any patient with acute facial paralysis but without the typical clinical presentation of Bell's palsy should be further evaluated. Atypical presentations have been described by Mark May as lima beans in a pea pod, and they require further investigation. The time of onset of the facial weakness is important. Slowly progressive weakness and recurrent or persistent paralysis should raise suspicion of a neoplasm involving the facial nerve. Other findings suggesting a tumor include a parotid mass on physical examination, the isolated weakness of a single peripheral branch of the nerve, muscle twitching preceding paralysis, and a history of any previous malignancy. The patient should be asked about past trauma, a draining ear, vertigo, hearing loss, tinnitus, tick exposure, and other neurologic complaints.

Patients with more severe pain likely have herpes zoster oticus (i.e., Ramsay Hunt syndrome), which is diagnosed by the presence of vesicles that usually occur in the external auditory canal or on the auricle. Ramsay Hunt patients may also have vestibulocochlear nerve symptoms, such as hearing loss, vertigo, or tinnitus. These symptoms are not found in patients with Bell's palsy.

Lyme disease and sarcoidosis are two commonly discussed but uncommon causes of facial paralysis. Borreliosis can cause facial paralysis in up to 11% of all cases of Lyme disease, a third of which manifest bilaterally. If the patient does not demonstrate other symptoms of Lyme disease, it is unlikely to be the cause of facial paralysis. Lyme titers are not recommended unless a patient also has other symptoms, such as rash, arthritis, or heart block.

Sarcoidosis is another rare cause of bilateral facial paralysis; facial paralysis occurs in less than 5% of patients with sarcoidosis. Patients can present with a rare syndrome of sarcoidosis called Heerfordt's syndrome or uveoparotid fever, which includes uveitis, parotitis, and facial nerve paralysis.

Evaluation

When evaluating a patient for Bell's palsy, it is helpful to think about the course of the facial nerve. The commands for facial expression are initiated in the cerebral cortex at the lateral precentral gyrus and cross as corticobulbar fibers. The fibers supplying the lower face cross only once, whereas the fibers ultimately supplying the forehead cross twice and provide bilateral cortical innervation. A central cause of acute facial paralysis usually affects only the lower face on the contralateral side. Patients with cortical lesions may have some emotional or involuntary response in the affected side because these fibers are thought to arise more caudally in the thalamus.

From descending corticobulbar fibers, the facial nerve arises in the pons near the abducens nerve. Simultaneous facial muscle and lateral rectus muscle weakness suggests a pontine lesion. At the cerebellopontine angle, the facial nerve joins the vestibulocochlear nerve before entering the temporal bone. As a result of this proximity to other cranial nerves, performing a detailed cranial nerve examination is important for localizing mass lesions that may cause facial paresis.

The facial nerve then enters the temporal bone and travels 3 to 4 mm through the narrowest portion of the temporal bone, called the fallopian canal. The meatal segment is the narrowest portion of the canal and is a common site of injury during temporal bone fractures. This segment is thought to be the site of nerve compression by edema in Bell's palsy. Otoscopic examination of the auditory canal and tympanic membrane can help diagnose other causes of facial nerve damage in this area, such as acute or chronic otitis media, trauma, or masses such as cholesteatomas or glomus jugulare tumors.

The nerve exits the temporal bone through the stylomastoid foramen and enters the parotid gland, where it branches into terminal segments. Palpation of the parotid gland is important to evaluate for signs of neoplasms that can invade the facial nerve and cause paresis. Evaluation of the integrity of each of the five terminal branches is accomplished by asking the patient to elevate the brow, tightly close the eyes, show the teeth, pucker the lips, and tense the neck. Before emerging from the temporal bone, the facial nerve is not organized into distinct branches; therefore, any lesion with a distinct branch weakness can be caused only by parotid pathology.

Most patients with typical Bell's palsy do not require any additional work-up. In atypical cases, computed tomography (CT) or magnetic resonance imaging (MRI) may be beneficial for evaluating masses or other potential surgical causes of facial nerve paralysis. Electrodiagnostic testing can be performed on patients with acute facial nerve paralysis for diagnostic and prognostic purposes, but it is typically reserved for patients with complete paralysis. Electroneurography involves stimulating the facial nerve at the stylomastoid foramen and recording combined action potentials from electrodes placed over the affected muscles. This test is usually performed in the first 10 days after the onset of symptoms to evaluate nerve degeneration. More than 90% nerve degeneration combined with the absence of voluntary motor unit action potentials indicates a poor prognosis and a point at which surgical decompression may be beneficial, but surgery remains controversial.

CURRENT DIAGNOSIS

- Acute facial paralysis (Bell's palsy) is a symptomatically defined diagnosis of exclusion.
- Full head and neck examination, including cranial nerves and House-Brackmann assessment, should be performed on all patients with acute facial paralysis.
- Patients with atypical features, such as prolonged paralysis, recurrent paralysis, or isolated branch weakness, should be evaluated with CT or MRI and evaluated by a specialist.

Clinical Course

Bell's palsy typically progresses to maximal weakness within 48 hours, but this progression may take up to 2 weeks. Approximately 85% of patients begin recovery within 3 weeks. No recovery within 3 weeks portends a poorer prognosis. Without treatment, 71% of patients with Bell's palsy will recover fully. An often-cited 1982 study by Pieterson and colleagues followed 1011 patients with Bell's palsy and revealed that the prognosis for full recovery depends on the severity of the initial paralysis. Clinically, the House-Brackmann (HB) scale is an accepted objective measure of this subjective clinical assessment of severity (Fig. 2).

In addition to severity of paralysis, other factors may affect the prognosis for recovery from facial paralysis. Ramsay Hunt syndrome causes more severe paralysis and has a poorer outcome. Gillman and coworkers showed that pregnant women who develop Bell's palsy might also have a poorer prognosis if complete paralysis develops (52% recovering to HB I or II, compared with 80% in a nonpregnant population). Diabetics may also have a poorer prognosis. Although the reason for this poorer prognosis is unknown, a possible explanation may involve patient compliance during steroid administration and resultant uncontrolled hyperglycemia.

Treatment

PHARMACOLOGIC THERAPY

The rationale for treatment with steroids originates with observations during surgery of facial nerve swelling in patients with Bell's palsy and the presumption that this edema contributes to facial paralysis.

HOUSE-BRACKMANN FACIAL NERVE GRADING SYSTEM

Grade I: Normal function
- Normal facial function in all areas

Grade II: Mild dysfunction
- Slight weakness noticeable on close inspection; may have very slight synkinesis

Grade III: Moderate dysfunction
- Obvious weakness or disfiguring asymmetry; normal symmetry and tone at rest; incomplete eye closure

Grade IV: Moderately severe dysfunction
- Obvious weakness or disfiguring asymmetry; normal symmetry and tone at rest; incomplete eye closure

Grade V: Severe dysfunction
- Only barely perceptible motion; asymmetry at rest

Grade VI: Total paralysis
- No movement

FIGURE 2. House-Brackmann facial nerve grading system.

Many studies have indicated a benefit for glucocorticoids over placebo in patients with Bell's palsy, although the data initially were conflicting. Because most patients with Bell's palsy do well without any intervention, demonstrating improvement requires much larger studies than were originally performed.

A double-blind, randomized, controlled trial by Sullivan and colleagues assessed the benefit of prednisolone (Millipred)[1] and acyclovir (Zovirax)[1] in the early treatment of Bell's palsy in a large population. The study had four arms consisting of acyclovir alone, prednisolone alone, acyclovir plus prednisolone, and placebo, with all treatments given within 72 hours of the development of symptoms. At 3 months and 9 months of follow-up, patients who received prednisolone were more likely to have a complete recovery than those who received placebo. The number of patients with facial paralysis needed to treat to obtain one additional full recovery was six at 3 months and eight at 9 months. As a result, early treatment with glucocorticoids for patients with Bell's palsy is recommended.

Results of trials of antiviral therapies have had conflicting results. Because Bell's palsy was strongly associated with viral infections, antiviral medications became a preferred treatment, regardless of the lack of evidence demonstrating their effectiveness. Numerous studies have indicated a role for early steroid treatment in improving long-term recovery of patients with Bell's palsy, but the role of antivirals remains controversial. The Sullivan study indicated no advantage for acyclovir over placebo, alone or combined with glucocorticoids. The results of this study, however, conflict with another large, randomized, controlled trial by Hato and associates, in which patients were given valacyclovir (Valtrex[1] 500 mg twice daily for 5 days) or placebo and prednisolone. In this study, an overall benefit was seen for valacyclovir with prednisolone over prednisolone alone, including a marked improvement in percent of patients with complete facial paralysis who had full recovery among those (90.1% versus 75.0%). Although these outcomes are compelling, no study findings have been adopted as the gold standard. The use of valacyclovir should receive further investigation. Prednisone is used universally, and antivirals continue to be commonly employed.

Although the Sullivan study indicated no role for acyclovir in the treatment of Bell's palsy, valacyclovir may provide benefit because of its lack of first-pass metabolism and its better pharmacokinetic profile. Cost remains a factor because antivirals are considerably more expensive than corticosteroids. Valacyclovir may provide benefit, but it should be reserved for those with complete facial paralysis in the first 72 hours.

SURGICAL THERAPY

The surgical treatment of Bell's palsy is usually performed by a neuro-otologist who decompresses the facial nerve at its narrowest point in the fallopian canal using a middle fossa approach. Beginning with surgeons Balance and Duel in the 1930s, some of the earliest treatments for Bell's palsy were surgical decompression. These approaches began to wane as steroids became popular. Surgical decompression of the facial nerve is still performed, but it remains controversial. Electrical testing is used to determine potential surgical benefit, which is performed only in cases of complete facial paralysis. A retrospective study by Gantz and colleagues of 54 patients who elected to undergo decompression surgery demonstrated surgical benefit for those with complete facial paralysis and more than 90% degeneration as determined by electroneurography at 10 days and with no voluntary motor unit action potentials on electromyography. Of those who chose surgical decompression by a middle fossa approach, 91% achieved HB grade I or II results, compared with 42% who chose medical therapy with corticosteroids. The risks associated with this procedure include hearing loss, further facial nerve injury, cerebrospinal fluid leak, and seizures.

OTHER THERAPY

Eye care is needed. Patients for whom the eyelids cannot appose are at increased risk for drying and corneal ulceration. These patients need to be monitored for exposure keratitis, which may require referral to an ophthalmologist. Symptoms include blurred vision,

CURRENT THERAPY

- Corticosteroid therapy initiated within 72 hours of the onset of paralysis increases the likelihood of recovery of patients with Bell's palsy (prednisolone[1] 20 mg twice daily for 7 days or prednisone 60–80 mg daily for 7 days).
- Although the use of acyclovir (Zovirax)[1] remains controversial, valacyclovir (Valtrex)[1] may provide benefit for patients with more severe facial paralysis (500 mg twice daily for 7 days).
- Eye care with artificial tears, barrier protection, and ophthalmic ointments at night can prevent exposure keratitis.

[1]Not FDA approved for this indication.

photophobia, irritation, and epiphora (i.e., tearing). Use of artificial tears while awake and ophthalmic ointments at night can prevent drying. Protective glasses should be worn during the day. If necessary, a gold weight may aid in closing the affected eye.

Nerve stimulation has been used to aid recovery of facial nerve function; however, there have been no studies to show its effectiveness. Because cases of hemifacial spasm have been reported after electrical stimulation, it is not recommended for treatment of Bell's palsy. Management of Bell's palsy can usually be handled by the primary care physician in an outpatient setting. These patients should be followed for at least 6 months to monitor for improvement or progression of paralysis. Patients who fail to improve or who have atypical symptoms should be referred to an otolaryngologist with expertise in facial paralysis.

Although most patients with Bell's palsy recover without impairment, 30% suffer some permanent change, and 15% are left with substantial deficits. Facial paralysis greatly affects the individual's ability to interact socially. In addition to psychiatric concerns such as depressed mood and anxiety, patients may experience difficulty with maintaining employment and relationships. Regional centers offer facial physical therapy by therapists specializing in these problems. Facial reanimation procedures may aid cosmetically, but they are performed only in a small percentage of patients. Botulinum toxin (Botox)[1] injections and physical therapy are the primary therapies offered for late sequelae; nevertheless, patients with persistent paresis after Bell's palsy may require long-term psychosocial care.

REFERENCES

Gantz BJ, Rubinstein JT, Gidley P, Woodworth G. Surgical management of Bell's palsy. Laryngoscope 1999;109:1177–88.

Gillman GS, Schaitkin BM, May M, Klein SR. Bell's palsy in pregnancy: A study of recovery outcomes. Otolaryngol Head Neck Surg 2002;126:26–30.

Hato N, Yamada H, Kohno H, et al. Valacyclovir and prednisolone treatment for Bell's palsy: A multicenter, randomized, placebo-controlled study. Otol Neurotol 2007;28:408–13.

House JW, Brackmann DE. Facial nerve grading system. Otolaryngol Head Neck Surg 1985;93:146–7.

May M, Schaitkin BM. The Facial Nerve. 2nd ed. New York: Thieme Medical Publishers; 2000.

Murakami S, Mizobuchi M, Narashiro Y, et al. Bell's palsy and herpes simplex virus: Identification of viral DNA in endoneurial fluid and muscle. Ann Intern Med 1996;124:27–30.

Mutsch M, Zhou W, Rhodes P, et al. Use of the inactivated intranasal influenza vaccine and the risk of Bell's palsy in Switzerland. N Engl J Med 2004;350:896–903.

Peitersen E. The natural history of Bell's palsy. Am J Otol 1982;4:107–11.

Sugita T, Murakami S, Yanagihara N, et al. Facial nerve paralysis induced by herpes simplex virus in mice; an animal model of acute and transient facial paralysis. Ann Otol Rhinol Laryngol 1995;104:574–81.

Sullivan FM, Swan IRC, Donnan PT, et al. Early treatment with prednisolone or acyclovir in Bell's palsy. N Engl J Med 2007;357:1598–607.

[1]Not FDA approved for this indication.

[1]Not FDA approved for this indication.

Parkinsonism

Method of
Rajesh Pahwa, MD, and Kelly E. Lyons, PhD

Clinical Features

Parkinsonism is a clinical syndrome with the cardinal motor signs of bradykinesia, rigidity, tremor, and postural instability. A diagnosis of parkinsonism requires the presence of at least two of the four cardinal features. Other motor features can include hypomimia, decreased blink rate, speech difficulties including hypophonia and dysarthria, micrographia, no or reduced arm swing, shuffling and short steps, freezing, festination, difficulty turning in bed, and stooped posture or kyphosis. Common autonomic features include orthostatic hypotension, dysphagia, constipation, urinary frequency and urgency, incontinence, nocturia, sexual dysfunction, and thermoregulatory dysfunction. Sensory symptoms such as anosmia, visual difficulties, pain, and paresthesias can also occur with parkinsonism. Sleep disturbances including insomnia, fragmented sleep, excessive daytime sleepiness, vivid dreaming, and an increased incidence of sleep disorders are common. Finally, neuropsychiatric disturbances such as anxiety, depression, dementia, and psychosis are often seen with parkinsonism.

Differential Diagnosis

There are many possible causes of parkinsonism (Box 1). Diagnosis is based primarily on clinical examination, medical history, family history and past and current medication use. The most common cause of parkinsonism is Parkinson's disease (PD). PD is a slowly progressive neurodegenerative disease generally with unilateral onset. It is estimated that 0.03% of the general population, 3% older than 65 years and 10% older than 80 years develop PD, with an estimated 50,000 new cases diagnosed each year.

BOX 1   Causes of Parkinsonism

Degenerative Disorders
Parkinson's disease (sporadic and familial)
Parkinson-plus syndromes
- Progressive supranuclear palsy (PSP)
- Multiple system atrophy (MSA)
- Corticobasal degeneration (CBD)
- Dementia with Lewy bodies (DLB)

Other Degenerative Disorders
Hallervorden–Spatz disease
Huntington's disease
Lubag (X-linked dystonia–parkinsonism)
Neuroacanthocytosis
Parkinsonism–ALS–dementia complex of Guam
Spinocerebellar ataxias
Wilson's disease

Secondary Parkinsonism
Drug-induced
Infectious (e.g., Creutzfeld–Jakob disease)
Metabolic (e.g., parathyroidism)
Structural (e.g., hydrocephalus, trauma, tumor)
Toxin-induced
Vascular

ALS = amyotrophic lateral sclerosis.

 CURRENT DIAGNOSIS

Cardinal Motor Signs
- Bradykinesia
- Postural instability
- Rigidity
- Tremor

Autonomic Dysfunction
- Cardiovascular (e.g., orthostatic hypotension)
- Gastrointestinal (e.g., dysphagia, drooling, constipation, delayed gastric emptying)
- Sexual (e.g., erectile dysfunction, decreased desire and arousal)
- Thermoregulatory (e.g., hyperhydrosis)
- Urologic (e.g., increased urinary frequency and urgency, incontinence, nocturia)

Neuropsychiatric Dysfunction
- Anxiety
- Depression
- Dementia
- Psychosis

Sensory Dysfunction
- Olfactory disturbance (e.g., anosmia)
- Pain
- Paresthesia
- Visual disturbances (e.g., abnormal eye movements, blurred or double vision)

Sleep Dysfunction
- Excessive daytime sleepiness
- Insomnia or fractionated sleep
- Sleep disorders (e.g., REM behavior disorder, sleep apnea, restless legs syndrome)

REM = rapid eye movement.

PD is a clinical diagnosis based on the presence of two of three cardinal symptoms of bradykinesia, rigidity, and tremor with a positive response to carbidopa/levodopa (Sinemet). Several features suggest a diagnosis of a form of parkinsonism other than PD (Table 1). The most common features include a poor response to levodopa, falling as an early symptom, symmetrical onset of symptoms, rapid progression, lack of tremor, and early autonomic symptoms such as urinary incontinence and symptomatic orthostatic hypotension.

PARKINSON-PLUS SYNDROMES

The Parkinson-plus syndromes, progressive supranuclear palsy (PSP), multiple system atrophy (MSA), corticobasal degeneration (CBD), and dementia with Lewy bodies (DLB), can be difficult to differentiate from PD and are often, especially early in the disease course, misdiagnosed as PD.

PSP is a slowly progressive neurodegenerative disease occurring after the age of 40 years; however, the disease course is generally more rapid than that of PD. It can manifest with bradykinesia, rigidity, hypomimia, hypophonia and postural instability with falling, often in the first year. The onset of PSP is often symmetrical, minimal to no rest tremor is observed, and the response to levodopa is poor. As the disease progresses, vertical gaze limitations and other eye movement abnormalities along with dysarthria and dysphagia generally occur. Neck rigidity is usually greater than limb rigidity, and the neck can be held in an extended posture. Frontal dementia and apathy are also commonly seen with PSP.

MSA is a neurodegenerative disorder with various combinations of parkinsonian, autonomic, cerebellar, and pyramidal signs. The

TABLE 1 Features Indicating a Form of Parkinsonism Other Than Parkinson's Disease

Feature	Possible Diagnosis
Acute onset	Vascular, drug or toxin-induced, psychogenic
Alien limb	Corticobasal degeneration
Apraxia	Corticobasal degeneration
Ataxia	Multiple system atrophy
Autonomic disturbances (early in disease course)	Multiple system atrophy
Dementia (within 1 y of parkinsonian signs)	Dementia with Lewy bodies
Gaze palsies	Progressive supranuclear palsy, corticobasal degeneration, multiple system atrophy, dementia with Lewy bodies
Hallucinations (unrelated to drug use)	Dementia with Lewy bodies
Pyramidal signs	Multiple system atrophy, vascular
Postural instability (early in disease course)	Progressive supranuclear palsy, multiple system atrophy
Symmetrical onset	Progressive supranuclear palsy, multiple system atrophy
Stepwise worsening	Vascular
Tremor minimal or absent	Progressive supranuclear palsy, vascular
Young onset (<40 y of age)	Drug induced, Wilson's disease

BOX 2 Medications That Can Cause Parkinsonism

Antipsychotics
Acetophenazine (Tindal)[2]
Aripiprazol (Abilify)
Chlorpromazine (Thorazine)
Chlorprothixene (Taractan)
Fluphenazine (Permitil, Prolixin)
Haloperidol (Haldol)
Loxapine (Loxitane)
Mesoridazine (Serentil)
Molindone (Moban)

Antiemetics
Metoclopramide (Reglan)
Prochlorperazine (Compazine)

Miscellaneous
Amiodarone (Cordarone)
Amoxapine (Asendin)
Divalproex (Depakote)
Lithium (Eskalith)
Olanzapine (Zyprexa)
Perphenazine (Trilafon)
Perphenazine + amitriptyline (Etafron, Triavil)
Procaine (Novocain)
Promethazine (Phenergan)
Risperidone (Risperdal)
Thioridazine (Mellaril)
Thiothixene (Navane)
Trifluoperazine (Stelazine)
Trifluopromazine (Vesprin)
Ziprasidone (Geodon)

[2]Not available in the United States.

disease course is generally more rapid than that of PD, and it generally affects people in their 50s and 60s. It is estimated that 80% of MSA patients have predominantly parkinsonian (MSA-P) features and 20% have predominantly cerebellar features (MSA-C). Autonomic symptoms most commonly include orthostatic hypotension, urinary incontinence or partial bladder emptying, and erectile dysfunction. Parkinsonian features can include bradykinesia, rigidity, postural instability, and tremor. In addition, orofacial dystonia, antecollis, and a jerky postural tremor can occur. MSA generally responds poorly to levodopa; an initial response may be observed, but it is rarely sustained. Cerebellar features include gait and limb ataxia, ataxic dysarthria, and sustained gaze-evoked nystagmus.

CBD is a progressive, asymmetric disorder affecting persons in their 60s and 70s. The cortical signs include cortical sensory loss, alien limb phenomenon, apraxia, frontal release reflexes, visual or sensory hemineglect, cognitive dysfunction, and dysphasia. The basal ganglia signs include akinesia, rigidity, action or postural tremor, limb dystonia, athetosis, postural instability, falling, and orolingual dyskinesia. Additional signs include hyperreflexia, impaired ocular motility, dysarthria, focal reflex myoclonus, blepharospasm, and dysphagia. CBD does not respond to levodopa.

DLB can be difficult to differentiate from PD dementia (PDD). In general, if the dementia and motor features occur within a year of each other, a diagnosis of DLB rather than PDD is made. DLB results in a progressive decline in cognition that is severe enough to interfere with activities of daily living. It is not uncommon to see fluctuations in cognition with significant variability in attention and alertness and recurrent visual hallucinations. Motor symptoms consistent with parkinsonism are also present. Additional supportive features include frequent falling, syncope, transient loss of consciousness, delusions, REM sleep behavior disorder, and depression. In DLB, the response to levodopa is variable, but few patients have the strong positive response seen in PD.

DRUG-INDUCED PARKINSONISM

Drug-induced parkinsonism occurs in 20% to 40% of patients taking dopamine-blocking agents. The most common offenders are antipsychotics and antiemetics, although other miscellaneous drugs have been reported to cause drug-induced parkinsonism (Box 2). Drug-induced parkinsonism generally has a subacute, asymmetrical onset and can resolve without discontinuation of the offending agent; however, it is best if the offending agent can be stopped. It also tends to be more common and more severe in older persons. Anticholinergics can be helpful with drug-induced symptoms in some patients, as can dopaminergic drugs; however, these drugs can worsen nausea and hallucinations.

Treatment

Although there are multiple treatment options that can improve PD symptoms, there is no known treatment for the other forms of parkinsonism. Often the same medications that are used for PD are tried for other forms of parkinsonism without significant improvement in symptoms. Occasionally, MSA initially responds to PD medications; however, the response is not sustained. In fact, a dramatic and sustained response to antiparkinsonian therapy usually confirms the diagnosis of PD. Symptomatic medical or surgical therapy is the basis of the management of PD. There is increasing attention being focused on the management of nonmotor symptoms of PD such as dementia, depression, psychosis, dysautonomia, and sleep disturbances.

MEDICATIONS

Currently available PD medications include carbidopa/levodopa, monoamine oxidase type B (MAO-B) inhibitors, dopamine agonists, catechol-O-methyl transferase (COMT) inhibitors, anticholinergics, and the antiviral drug amantadine (Symmetrel).

Levodopa

Dopamine is one of the main neurotransmitters that is reduced in PD, and treatment to date has focused on restoring or manipulating this neurotransmitter. Oral dopamine is metabolized and cannot be used as

CURRENT THERAPY

- Dopamine precursor (levodopa)
- MAO-B inhibitors
- Dopamine agonists
- COMT inhibitors
- Amantadine
- Anticholinergics

COMT = catechol-*O*-methyl transferase; MAO = monoamine oxidase.

treatment in PD. Levodopa, which is the precursor of dopamine, is considered the gold standard for the symptomatic treatment of PD. Orally administered levodopa is mainly absorbed in the upper gastrointestinal tract. Levodopa is metabolized in the periphery mainly to dopamine by aromatic amino acid decarboxylase (AAAD) and to 3-*O*-methyldopa (3-OMD) by the COMT enzyme. Once levodopa crosses the blood-brain barrier, it is converted to dopamine intraneuronally.

Orally administered levodopa is almost completely absorbed from the gut. Due to metabolism by AAAD and COMT, less than 5% of an oral dose of levodopa crosses the blood–brain barrier. Hence, levodopa is combined with carbidopa, an AAAD inhibitor. Because carbidopa does not cross the blood–brain barrier, it does not inhibit the conversion of levodopa to dopamine in the brain. The half-life of levodopa is approximately 50 minutes, but when administered with carbidopa it increases to 90 minutes. Approximately 70 to 100 mg of carbidopa is required to saturate peripheral decarboxylase to reduce the peripheral side effects of dopamine, such as nausea and vomiting.

Levodopa improves all the cardinal motor features of PD including tremor, bradykinesia, and rigidity. It is the most efficacious medication for PD. Levodopa does not generally improve nonmotor symptoms such as depression or dementia, nor does it improve axial motor symptoms such as speech or swallowing difficulties, freezing of gait and postural instability.

Carbidopa/levodopa is available in dosages of 10/100 mg, 25/100 mg, and 25/250 mg tablets. The initial dose of carbidopa/levodopa is generally one 25/100 mg tablet three times per day. It is advisable to initiate carbidopa/levodopa slowly, starting with one half of a 25/100 mg tablet twice a day for 1 week and then increasing by one-half tablet daily until symptoms are well controlled. Carbidopa/levodopa is also available in an orally dissolvable formulation (Parcopa). This formulation is available in the same strengths as immediate-release carbidopa/levodopa and has similar safety and efficacy. It is particularly useful in patients with swallowing difficulties.

There is also a controlled-release formulation of carbidopa/levodopa (Sinemet-CR) in doses of 25/100 mg and 50/200 mg. This formulation is generally started with 25/100 mg/day and increased to a typical dose of 25/100 mg three times per day or 50/200 mg twice a day. Controlled-release preparations are not as well absorbed, and the bioavailability is 20% to 30% lower than standard preparations. These formulations do not provide any major advantage over the standard formulations.

One of the biggest limitations to the long-term use of levodopa is the development of motor fluctuations and dyskinesia. Approximately 50% of PD patients develop these motor complications after 5 years of levodopa use. Motor fluctuations include end-of-dose wearing-off and random on/off phenomena. When levodopa is initiated, patients generally have a stable control of PD symptoms during the day. However, over a period of months to years, they experience improvement in the PD symptoms for only a few hours after levodopa ingestion and the effects of the drug wear off before the next dose, which is required before the symptoms improve again. This is known as *end-of-dose wearing off*. As the disease progresses, the number of hours of benefit with each dose of levodopa decreases and the patient often requires multiple doses throughout the day. Random on/off fluctuations are rapid transitions (over seconds) between the on state (when the PD symptoms are under good

control) and off state (when PD symptoms are present), and these are usually unpredictable and unrelated to the timing of levodopa.

Dyskinesia is another long-term motor complication of levodopa therapy. Dyskinesia involves involuntary movements such as chorea, dystonia, and ballismus. The most common types of dyskinesia are peak-dose dyskinesia, wearing-off dystonia, and diphasic dystonia/dyskinesia. Peak-dose dyskinesia is the most common form of dyskinesia and occurs when dopamine levels are at their peak. These movements consist of involuntary choreiform movements of the arms, legs, trunk, and head. Wearing-off dystonia is the painful dystonic movements that occur when dopamine levels are low, usually between levodopa dosing, in the middle of the night, or early in the morning before levodopa is taken. Diphasic dystonia/dyskinesia is uncommon and occurs when dopamine levels are rising or falling.

Common acute adverse effects with carbidopa/levodopa include nausea, vomiting, somnolence, and orthostatic hypotension. Other side effects include skin rash, diaphoresis, cardiac arrhythmias, and pedal edema. Psychiatric side effects include confusion, vivid dreams, nightmares, hallucinations, and delusions.

Dopamine Agonists

Dopamine agonists are drugs that directly stimulate the postsynaptic dopamine receptors. After levodopa, dopamine agonists are the most efficacious symptomatic therapy for PD. Dopamine agonists were initially used as an adjunctive therapy to levodopa; however, currently they are increasingly used as both initial monotherapy and as adjunctive therapy. Studies have demonstrated that initial use of dopamine agonists as monotherapy for PD delays the onset of motor fluctuations and dyskinesia. Dopamine agonists also reduce off time in PD patients on levodopa therapy with motor fluctuations.

Commonly used dopamine agonists include pramipexole (Mirapex) and ropinirole (Requip and Requip XL). Other dopamine agonists include bromocriptine (Parlodel), pergolide (Permax),[2] apomorphine (Apokyn), and the rotigotine transdermal system (Neupro).[2]

Bromocriptine

Bromocriptine is an ergoline dopamine agonist and was the first dopamine agonist approved for use in the United States in 1978. Bromocriptine is mainly a D_2 agonist with weak D_1 antagonist properties. It is rapidly absorbed, with a half-life is between 3 and 8 hours. Peak drug plasma levels are reached in 1 to 2 hours. Due to the risk of ergot-related side effects, bromocriptine is rarely used in clinical practice. It is generally started at 1.25 mg once per day and titrated over several weeks to a maximum dose of 10 to 40 mg/day divided into three or four doses.

Pergolide

Pergolide is an ergot-derived dopamine agonist that was withdrawn from the United States market due to concerns of cardiac valvular fibrosis. Patients previously exposed to pergolide might be at risk and should undergo echocardiogram screening.

Pramipexole

Pramipexole is a nonergot dopamine agonist approved for use as monotherapy and adjunctive therapy in PD. Pramipexole mainly acts on the D_2, D_3, and D_4 dopamine receptors. It has a half-life of 8 to 12 hours and reaches peak drug plasma concentration in approximately 2 hours. Pramipexole is excreted in the urine mostly unchanged. It is initiated at 0.125 mg three times per day and slowly increased over several weeks to a maximum dose of 1.5 mg three times per day (Table 2). An extended-release formulation, pramipexole extended release (Mirapex ER) is also available, allowing once-daily dosing.

Ropinirole

Ropinirole is also a nonergot dopamine agonist approved for both monotherapy and adjunctive therapy in PD. It has affinity for the D_2 family of dopamine receptors and no effect on the D_1 or D_5 dopaminergic

[2]Not available in the United States.

TABLE 2 Dopamine Agonist Titration Schedules

Week	Pramipexole (Mirapex)*	Ropinirole (Requip)	Ropinirole Extended Release (Requip XL)
1	0.125 mg tid	0.25 mg tid	2 mg qd
2	0.25 mg tid	0.5 mg tid	4 mg qd
3	0.5 mg tid	0.75 mg tid	6 mg qd
4	0.75 mg tid	1.0 mg tid	8 mg qd
5	1.0 mg tid	1.5 mg tid	12 mg qd
6	1.25 mg tid	2.0 mg tid	16 mg qd
7	1.5 mg tid	2.5 mg tid	20 mg qd
8		3.0 mg tid	24 mg qd
Maximum	1.5 mg tid	8.0 mg tid	24 mg qd

*Pramipexole extended release has the same titration schedule as the immediate-release formulation but is taken once daily rather than 3 times daily.

receptors. The plasma half-life of ropinirole is approximately 6 hours, and peak drug plasma concentrations occur in 1 to 2 hours. Ropinirole is initiated at 0.25 mg three times per day and gradually increased over several weeks to a maximum dose of 8 mg three times per day. An extended release formulation, ropinirole prolonged release (Requip XL) is also available, allowing once daily dosing (see Table 2).

Rotigotine

Rotigotine was the first transdermal PD medication approved for use in the United States; however, it was withdrawn from the market in 2008 due to manufacturing issues. It is currently available in the European Union but requires cold chain storage and distribution. It is a nonergot dopamine agonist currently approved for early PD. It mainly acts on the D_3, D_2, and D_1 receptors but also has action on the D_4 and D_5 receptors. It is continuously absorbed over 24 hours with stable plasma levels and a half-life of 5 to 7 hours. Rotigotine is initiated at 2 mg per 24 hours and over a period of 3 weeks can be increased to a maximum of 6 mg per 24 hours. The patch is changed daily. The transdermal patch is applied to different body locations, which should change daily, avoiding application to a previous location for at least 14 days to reduce the incidence of skin reactions.

Apomorphine

Apomorphine is approved for advanced PD as a rescue therapy for severe off periods. It is the only subcutaneous injection for PD available in the United States. It is a nonergot, fast-acting dopamine agonist with a high affinity for D_4 receptors, moderate affinity for D_2, D_3, D_5 receptors, and low affinity for D_1 receptors. Apomorphine is rapidly absorbed in 10 to 60 minutes, has a half-life of approximately 40 minutes, and provides an effect for up to 90 minutes. It can be given every 2 hours; however, there are limited data for use exceeding five times per day. A test dose of 2 mg (0.2 mL) is given under medical supervision during an off state, and the dose is titrated by 0.1 mL increments up to a maximum single dose of 0.6 mL.

Apomorphine is an emetic and can cause severe nausea and vomiting; therefore, an antiemetic such as trimethobenzamide (Tigan)[1] should be used for 3 days before administration and for at least 6 weeks after administration of apomorphine. Due to severe hypotension and possible loss of consciousness, apomorphine should not be used with 5-HT_3 antagonists like ondansetron (Zofran), granisetron (Kytril), dolasetron (Anzemet), palonosetron (Aloxi), and alosetron (Lotronex).[11]

Adverse Effects

All dopamine agonists have similar side effects except for the long-term risks of pulmonary fibrosis, retroperitoneal fibrosis, and cardiac valvular fibrosis associated only with the ergot dopamine agonists.

[1]Not FDA approved for this indication.
[11]Required to enroll in the manufacturer's prescribing program.

Adverse effects may be dose and time dependent, and they often occur when therapy is initiated. Common adverse effects include nausea, vomiting, dizziness, somnolence, insomnia, peripheral edema, and orthostatic hypotension. Central adverse effects are mainly psychiatric such as hallucinations, confusion, mood changes, depression, irritability, euphoria, vivid dreams, sleep disturbances, inappropriate sexual behavior, delusions, agitation, and paranoid psychosis. There have been reports of patients falling asleep during activities of daily living, including while operating motor vehicles, and of impulsive disorders like gambling, eating, shopping, and sexual behavior with dopamine agonists.

Catechol-O-Methyl Transferase Inhibitors

COMT inhibitors are drugs that increase the half-life of levodopa by reducing its metabolism. Using COMT inhibitors with levodopa prolongs the action of individual doses of levodopa. Tolcapone (Tasmar) and entacapone (Comtan) are both specific and reversible inhibitors of COMT, and they increase the area under the levodopa plasma concentration/time curve. At therapeutic doses, entacapone only acts peripherally and does not affect central COMT activity. Tolcapone can pass the blood-brain barrier and block central COMT in addition to its peripheral actions.

Tolcapone

Tolcapone (Tasmar) has a half-life of approximately 2 to 3 hours, and the time to maximum plasma concentration is approximately 2 hours. It is initiated at 100 mg three times a day and increased to 200 mg three times a day if needed. Tolcapone should always be used with levodopa.

The majority of the adverse effects related to tolcapone are dopaminergic in nature. Dyskinesia, nausea, hallucinations, insomnia, anorexia, and orthostatic hypotension are common. These adverse effects are usually improved by reduction in the levodopa dose. Diarrhea as an adverse effect usually begins at 6 to 12 weeks but can appear as early as 2 weeks after tolcapone is started. If the diarrhea is bothersome, therapy must be discontinued. Urine discoloration is a harmless side effect that occurs in less than 10% of patients.

Significant increases in liver enzymes have been reported, and after FDA approval, there were three cases of fatal liver injury reported with the use of tolcapone. This led to strict guidelines regarding the use of tolcapone: it may only be used in PD patients who have tried all other antiparkinsonian medications, and serum ALT and AST should be tested at baseline, every 2 to 4 weeks for the first 6 months, and then as clinically indicated. Tolcapone should be discontinued if the patient does not have a response or if there is a two times increase in the upper limit of ALT and AST.

Entacapone

Entacapone (Comtan) is approved for the management of motor fluctuations in PD. Its half-life is approximately one half hour (0.4–0.7 hours). It reduces the peripheral metabolism of levodopa and prolongs the levodopa half-life from 1.3 to 2.4 hours. It is initiated at 200 mg with each dose of levodopa for a maximum of eight doses per day.

The side effects of entacapone are similar to those of tolcapone and mostly related to increased dopaminergic stimulation. Dyskinesia, nausea, vomiting, and hallucinations are the most commonly seen dopaminergic adverse effects. These side effects can usually be reduced or eliminated by decreasing the levodopa dose. There is no known hepatotoxicity associated with entacapone and no requirement for liver enzyme monitoring.

Carbidopa/Levodopa/Entacapone

The triple combination carbidopa/levodopa/entacaopone (Stalevo) is available in six different combinations: Stalevo 50 (carbidopa 12.5 mg/levodopa 50 mg/entacapone 200 mg), Stalevo 75 (carbidopa 18.75 mg/levodopa 75 mg/entacapone 200 mg), Stalevo 100 (carbidopa 25 mg/levodopa 100 mg/entacapone 200 mg), Stalevo 125 (carbidopa 31.25 mg/levodopa 125 mg/entacapone 200 mg), Stalevo 150 (carbidopa 37.5 mg/levodopa 150 mg/entacapone 200 mg), and Stalevo 200 (carbidopa 50 mg/levodopa 200 mg/entacapone 200 mg). This triple combination is indicated in PD patients as a substitute for immediate-release carbidopa/levodopa and entacapone previously administered separately. It can also replace immediate-release carbidopa/levodopa (without entacapone) in patients experiencing end-of-dose wearing-off who are taking 600 mg or less of levodopa and are not having dyskinesia. The adverse effects are similar to those seen with carbidopa/levodopa and entacapone used separately.

Monoamine Oxidase B (MAO-B) Inhibitors

Selegiline (Eldepryl), orally disintegrating selegiline (Zelapar), and rasagiline (Azilect) are the MAO-B inhibitors available in United States. They are selective irreversible MAO-B inhibitors. MAO-B inhibitors increase the half-life of levodopa by blocking the metabolism of dopamine by MAO-B.

Selegiline

Selegiline is an irreversible MAO-B inhibitor and has an elimination half-life of approximately 2 hours. However, because the drug irreversibly inhibits MAO-B, the therapeutic benefits are lost after the enzyme is regenerated. The major plasma metabolites of selegiline are N-desmethylselegiline (the only metabolite with MAO-B inhibiting properties), L-amphetamine, and L-methamphetamine. Selegiline is approved as an adjunct treatment to levodopa; however, it is also used as monotherapy in early disease. The typical dose is 5 mg with breakfast and lunch.

Selegiline is generally well tolerated. The most common adverse effects include nausea, dizziness, insomnia, constipation, excessive sweating, confusion, hallucinations, dry mouth, and orthostatic hypotension. When used as an adjunct to levodopa therapy, an increase in dyskinesia can occur, as well as increases in other levodopa-related side effects.

Orally Disintegrating Selegiline

The orally disintegrating selegiline tablet is available for oral administration (not to be swallowed) in the strength of 1.25 mg. It is approved for use in advanced PD with motor fluctuations. The initial dose is 1.25 mg a day, which can be increased to 2.5 mg per day if clinically indicated. Selegiline disintegrates within seconds after placement on the tongue and is rapidly absorbed. The pregastric absorption of orally disintegrating selegiline and the avoidance of first-pass metabolism results in higher concentrations of selegiline and lower concentrations of its metabolites compared with the 5-mg swallowed selegiline tablet. Side effects are similar to those reported with selegiline tablets. There are no data on the use of orally disintegrating selegiline as monotherapy in PD.

Rasagiline

Rasagiline is an irreversible MAO-B inhibitor. It is rapidly absorbed and reaches peak plasma concentrations in approximately 1 hour. Its half-life is approximately 3 hours, but because it irreversibly inhibits MAO-B, the therapeutic benefit is not dependent on its half-life. It is approved as monotherapy in early disease (1 mg/day) and in PD patients with advanced disease experiencing motor fluctuations (0.5 mg/day, which can be increased to 1 mg/day as needed).

The most commonly observed adverse events with rasagiline monotherapy were flu syndrome, arthralgia, depression, dyspepsia, and falls. As an adjunct to levodopa, the common adverse effects included dyskinesia, accidental injury, weight loss, postural hypotension, vomiting, anorexia, arthralgia, abdominal pain, nausea, constipation, dry mouth, rash, ecchymosis, somnolence, and paresthesia.

Contraindications

Although MAO inhibitors used in the treatment of PD are specific MAO-B inhibitors, at higher than recommended doses or as an idiosyncratic reaction, MAO-A can also be inhibited. Hence, certain medications should not be used with these medications: analgesics such as meperidine (Demerol), tramadol (Ultram), methadone (Dolophine, Methadose), and propoxyphene (Darvon); the antitussive agent dextromethorphan (found in many over-the-counter cough medicines); St. John's wort, mirtazapine (Remeron), and cyclobenzaprine (Flexeril); and other MAO inhibitors.

Anticholinergics

Anticholinergics were the first class of drugs used for the treatment of PD. They work mainly on the muscarinic acetylcholine receptors. The exact mechanism of action of anticholinergics is unclear. It is believed that there is antagonism between the effects of dopamine and acetylcholine in the basal ganglia and that anticholinergics work by correcting the disequilibrium between striatal dopamine and acetylcholine activity.

A number of anticholinergics are available. They are generally well absorbed after oral administration and usually require dosing two or three times a day. The commonly used anticholinergics for PD include biperiden (Akineton), trihexyphenidyl (Artane), benztropine (Cogentin), and procyclidine (Kemadrin). Anticholinergics should be started at low doses and increased very slowly. Anticholinergics are mildly beneficial in the management of PD and mainly help tremor without significantly affecting bradykinesia or rigidity. Anticholinergics are mainly used in young patients due to safety concerns.

Anticholinergics are contraindicated in patients with narrow-angle glaucoma, tachycardia, prostate hypertrophy, gastrointestinal obstruction, and megacolon. Common side effects include blurring of vision, nausea, constipation, urinary retention, and dry mucous membranes in the mouth and eyes. Acute confusion, hallucinations, psychosis, and sedation can occur. All central adverse effects are more likely to occur in patients with advanced age and in patients with impaired cognitive function.

Amantadine

Amantadine (Symmetrel) was initially marketed as an antiviral agent but was reported to be helpful for tremor, rigidity, and bradykinesia in PD. Since then, the efficacy of amantadine both as monotherapy and in combination with levodopa in the treatment of PD has been demonstrated. There are several modes of action of amantadine, but the exact mechanism in PD is unknown. Presynaptically, amantadine enhances the release of stored catecholamines from dopaminergic terminals and inhibits the reuptake process. Postsynaptically, amantadine exerts a direct effect on dopamine receptors. In addition, it is believed that amantadine has anticholinergic effects and N-methyl-D-aspartate (NMDA) glutamate receptor blockade.

Amantadine is quickly absorbed, with peak blood levels 2 to 4 hours after an oral dose. It should be used with caution in patients with impaired renal function and should not be used in patients with renal failure. The usual dose is 200 to 300 mg/day in divided doses. In early PD, amantadine has mild antiparkinsonian benefits on tremor, bradykinesia, and rigidity. In advanced PD, amantadine has been reported to be efficacious in improving dyskinesia. Common side effects include dizziness, anxiety, impaired coordination, insomnia, and nervousness. Nausea and vomiting occur in 5% to 10% of patients. In some patients, pedal edema and livedo reticularis can be bothersome and can lead to discontinuation of therapy.

DEEP BRAIN STIMULATION

When motor fluctuations and dyskinesia cannot be adequately controlled with medications, surgery may be an option for appropriate patients. Deep brain stimulation (DBS) involves implanting a stimulating electrode into the brain. There are three possible DBS targets for treating PD. DBS of the thalamus results in marked improvement in tremor but does not improve bradykinesia, rigidity, or drug-induced dyskinesia and only minimally improves activities of daily living. DBS of the globus pallidus interna improves all of the cardinal symptoms of PD (tremor, rigidity, bradykinesia) and markedly reduces dyskinesia. DBS of the subthalamic nucleus is the most commonly performed DBS procedure for PD and results in improvements in all the cardinal motor symptoms of PD, motor fluctuations, and dyskinesia, while allowing a substantial decrease in antiparkinsonian medications.

Candidates for Deep Brain Stimulation

Thalamic stimulation is rarely used for PD and may be recommended for patients who have disabling, medication-resistant tremor with minimal signs of bradykinesia and rigidity. Patients who have levodopa-responsive PD and medication-resistant motor fluctuations and dyskinesia are appropriate candidates for pallidal or subthalamic stimulation. For DBS procedures, patients should not have significant cognitive, psychiatric, or behavioral problems, such as dementia or severe depression.

Adverse Events

In general, all DBS procedures have similar adverse effects. These adverse effects can be categorized as surgical, device-related, and stimulation-related complications. The experience of the neurosurgeon and proper patient selection generally reduce the occurrence of adverse events. Serious surgical complications can occur in 1% to 2% of patients and include intracranial bleeds, strokes, and seizures. Infections have been reported in 5% to 8% of patients. Device-related events can occur in up to 25% of patients. These include lead reposition due to incorrect placement, lead displacement, erosion of the skin over the lead or the extension, breakage of the lead or the extension, or malfunction of the implanted pulse generator. Adverse effects related to stimulation depend on the location of the electrode and the stimulus intensity, and they usually improve with stimulation adjustments.

MANAGEMENT

Early Disease

Multiple options are available in initiating therapy in a patient with newly diagnosed PD. Anticholinergics are rarely used due to concerns of adverse effects. Patients with mild symptoms are generally initiated with an MAO-B inhibitor and occasionally may be initiated on amantadine. However, if a patient has functional impairment, an MAO-B inhibitor, dopamine agonist, or levodopa is initiated. If the symptoms are causing significant functional disability, in young patients, a dopamine agonist such as ropinirole, ropinirole extended release, pramipexole, or pramipexole extended release is initiated. In older patients, especially those with cognitive impairment, levodopa is initiated. As the disease progresses, patients often end up on combination therapy.

Advanced Disease

There are multiple treatment options for patients on levodopa who develop motor fluctuations. These include increasing the dose or dosing frequency of levodopa and providing adjunctive therapy with dopamine agonists, COMT inhibitors, or MAO-B inhibitors. Often, patients end up taking medications from each of these classes. Amantadine is the only drug reported to improve dyskinesia. If motor fluctuations and dyskinesia cannot be managed with medications, DBS may be considered in some patients.

REFERENCES

Litvan I. Atypical Parkinsonian Disorders: Clinical and Research Aspects. Totowa, NJ: Humana Press; 2005.

Miyasaki JM, Martin W, Suchowersky O, et al. Practice parameter: Initiation of treatment for Parkinson's disease: An evidence-based review. Neurology 2002;58:11–7.

Olanow CW, Watts RL, Koller WC. An algorithm (decision tree) for the management of Parkinson's disease (2001): Treatment guidelines. Neurology 2001;56(Suppl. 5):S1–8.

Pahwa R, Factor SA, Lyons KE, et al. Practice parameter: Treatment of Parkinson disease with motor fluctuations and dyskinesia (an evidence-based review). Neurology 2006;66:983–95.

Pahwa R, Lyons KE. Handbook of Parkinson's Disease. 4th ed. New York: Informa Healthcare; 2007.

Suchowersky O, Reich S, Perlmutter J, et al. Practice parameter: Diagnosis and prognosis of new onset Parkinson disease (an evidence-based review). Neurology 2006;66:968–75.

Peripheral Neuropathies

Method of
Kerrie Schoffer, MD, FRCPC

Disorders of the peripheral nerve system (PNS) include pathology affecting the spinal cord roots (radiculopathies), the dorsal root ganglia (neuronopathies), the brachial, lumbar, and sacral plexuses (plexopathies), and the terminal nerve (mononeuropathies) or nerves (polyneuropathies). They are among the most common and challenging problems in medical practice, with literally hundreds of conceivable causes. An organized diagnostic approach consists of first categorizing the neuropathy based on clinical and electrophysiologic assessments and then performing a tailored diagnostic evaluation. However astute the diagnostician, the cause of a neuropathy might not found in up to 20% of patients.

Anatomy

Four types of fibers are found in the PNS: motor, large fiber sensory, small fiber sensory, and autonomic. Motor fibers extend peripherally to the neuromuscular junction of their respective muscles and have their cell bodies in motor neurons located in the spinal cord. Conversely, sensory fibers receive information from peripheral sensory receptors and transfer this to cell bodies in the dorsal root ganglia, located near, but outside, the spinal cord. Large, myelinated sensory fibers supply information regarding position and vibration. Small myelinated axons, composed of autonomic and sensory fibers, are responsible for light touch, pain, temperature, and parasympathetic and sympathetic information.

Damage can occur to the cell bodies (neuronopathy), nerve fibers (axonopathy), or to the surrounding myelin sheath (myelinopathy). Myelinopathies principally affect only the coating around the nerve, and an axonopathy results in degeneration of both the axon and myelin. The most distal segments usually degenerate first, in a process termed *Wallerian degeneration*, resulting in a dying-back neuropathy and a stocking and glove clinical pattern. Neuronopathies affect either the motor neuron or dorsal root ganglion and result in degeneration of both peripheral and central processes.

Five-Step Approach to Neuropathies

When evaluating neuropathy, the differential diagnosis can be limited by asking five key questions:

- What is the *fiber type* involved (motor, large sensory, small sensory, autonomic, combination)?
- What is the *pattern of distribution* (distal or proximal, symmetric or asymmetric)?
- What is the *temporal course* (acute, chronic, progressive, stepwise, relapsing remitting)?
- Are there any *key features* pointing to a specific etiology?
- What is the *pathology* (axonal, demyelinating)?

FIBER TYPE

The PNS produces symptomatology in only two ways: negative symptoms (weakness, numbness), which reflects loss of nerve signaling; or positive symptoms (tingling, burning) due to inappropriate spontaneous nerve activity. Box 1 lists symptoms and signs that suggest localization to the peripheral nerves and point specifically to motor, sensory, or autonomic involvement. When inquiring about symptoms, it is important to ask the patient to be as specific as possible. Many patients simply describe an area as numb when, in fact, they are experiencing tingling or even weakness.

A detailed motor examination should include inspection for atrophy, particularly in the distal extensor digitorum brevis and first dorsal interosseous muscles, and for fasciculations (visible twitches of muscle), which are best seen using tangential light. Strength should be tested against resistance, as well as with active maneuvers such as walking on the heels and toes to assess distal strength, and rising from a squatting position to examine proximal muscles. Facial muscles should also be tested. When assessing deep tendon reflexes, ensure the reflex is truly absent by asking the patient to concurrently perform a Jendrassic maneuver (pulling against interlocking fingers) or clench the jaw. Note that the reflex arc consists of large-diameter afferent sensory input as well as motor nerve output, so that dysfunction of either can impair reflexes. Tone is sometimes reduced in peripheral nerve diseases.

On sensory examination, sensation should be tested with a pin and a 128-Hz vibratory tuning fork, beginning at the big toe level and moving progressively more proximal. Likewise, position testing should begin distally, with fingers placed on the lateral sides of the big toe and progressively smaller movements tested. Severe loss of position sense can result in athetoid movements of the fingers when the eyes are closed (pseudoathetosis) or a positive Romberg's sign. Temperature can be tested informally by placing

a cold tuning fork on the skin. Foot injuries may be apparent with severe sensory loss.

Other important signs include high arches and hammertoe deformities, which suggest a long-standing neuropathy causing differences in muscular force. Demyelinating neuropathies, amyloidosis, and leprosy can cause nerve thickening, which is felt best in the dorsal cutaneous nerve of the foot or the great auricular nerve. Superficial nerves, such as the ulnar nerve at the elbow, can be palpated when appropriate. Postural blood pressure should be assessed for a blood pressure drop more than 20 mm Hg systolic or more than 10 mm Hg diastolic, following 5 minutes of supine rest at a minimum, to test autonomic functioning.

Several other levels of the nervous system can mimic symptoms of PNS disease. Myelopathy and motor neuron disease can manifest with weakness similar to motor neuropathies, although upper motor neuron features such as spasticity and increased reflexes are clues. Myopathies can also cause weakness, but usually more proximal than distal and without any sensory impairment. Isolated sensory involvement should be a red flag that the dorsal root ganglia may be the site of involvement rather than the peripheral nerve, particularly important because neuronopathies have a limited differential.

PATTERN OF DISTRIBUTION

The pattern of distribution should be classified in two ways: symmetric or asymmetric and distal or proximal. Putting this together with the fiber type, six patterns of PNS disorders can be appreciated, with specific differentials (Table 1).

The symmetric distal sensorimotor neuropathy (pattern 1) manifests in a stocking-and-glove distribution and is the most common type of polyneuropathy. Once the level of the upper calves is reached, fibers of the same length in the fingertips begin to be affected. Sensorimotor polyneuropathies that affect both the distal and proximal nerves (pattern 2) should alert the physician to think of inflammatory neuropathies, such as Guillain-Barré syndrome (GBS) and chronic inflammatory demyelinating polyneuropathy (CIDP).

Asymmetric patterns (pattern 3) are often a result of trauma or compression, such as that seen in mononeuropathies, radiculopathies, and plexopathies. A pattern that affects multiple anatomically separated nerves is termed *mononeuritis multiplex* and is usually the result of a more diffuse process, such as diabetes or vasculitis.

Predominant motor neuropathies (pattern 4) are often proximal, such as diabetic amyotrophy. An exception is lead neuropathy, which affects motor fibers in a distal radial and peroneal distribution. Pure sensory neuropathies (pattern 5) are more likely to be distal, with the exception of a rare few such as Tangier disease, which manifests with a bathing-suit pattern. Neuropathies with autonomic impairment have a limited differential (pattern 6).

Additionally, involvement of the cranial nerves is only seen in a few causes of neuropathy. GBS, CIDP, Lyme disease, sarcoidosis, HIV-associated neuropathy, and Tangier disease are examples.

TEMPORAL COURSE

Acute neuropathies are relatively rare and suggest an etiology such as GBS, acute intermittent porphyria, ischemia, toxins (thallium toxicity), drugs, or infections (diphtheric neuropathy). Subacute onset (>8 weeks) is seen in nutritional deficiencies, metabolic neuropathies, paraneoplastic syndromes, and CIDP. A chronic course is typical of hereditary neuropathies, a stepwise pattern can be seen in mononeuropathy multiplex, and a relapsing-remitting course occurs with intermittent exposure to a toxin or drug and in CIDP.

KEY SIGNS

Sometimes, there is a key classic feature on history or examination that significantly narrows the differential immediately. Box 2 includes a checklist of items for inquiry and observation during assessment of neuropathy.

BOX 1 — Signs and Symptoms of Peripheral Nervous System Disease by Fiber Type

Motor
- Cramps
- Fasciculations
- Hyporeflexia
- Hypotonia
- Muscle atrophy
- Myokymia
- Pes cavus
- Weakness

Large Fiber Sensory
- Decreased vibration and position
- Hyporeflexia
- Pins and needles
- Tingling
- Unsteady gait, especially at night or with eyes closed

Small Fiber Sensory
- Burning
- Decreased pain sensation
- Decreased temperature sensation
- Jabbing

Autonomic
- Decreased or increased sweating
- Heat intolerance
- Impotence
- Postural hypotension
- Urinary retention

TABLE 1   Causes of Neuropathy by Pattern Type

Causes	Potentially Useful Tests
Sensorimotor	
Symmetric and Distal	
Metabolic disorders	OGTT, LFT, creatinine, TSH, vitamin B$_{12}$
Hereditary disorders (CMT)	EMG/NCS
Infections (HIV, leprosy)	HIV test, review of medical and social history
Toxins (drugs, alcohol, arsenic, thallium)	
Symmetric and Proximal and Distal	
Inflammatory neuropathies (GBS, CIDP)	EMG/NCS, CSF
Asymmetric	
Mononeuropathy, radiculopathy, plexopathy	EMG/NCS
Mononeuritis multiplex	ANA, RF, ESR, ANCA, nerve bx
Vasculitis	
Diabetes	OGTT
HIV	HIV test
Multifocal CIDP	CSF
Rare: porphyria, leprosy, HNPP	
Pure Motor	
Proximal	
Diabetic amyotrophy	OGTT
MMNCB	EMG/NCS
Motor variants of GBS, CIDP, MGUS	CSF, SPE, IF
Lymphoma	CBC
Distal	
Rare: Lead toxicity, porphyria	
Pure Sensory	
Neuropathies	
Nonsystemic vasculitis neuropathy	Nerve bx
Chronic gluten enteropathy	Antigliadin antibodies
Vitamin E deficiency	Vitamin E level
Distal, demyelinating, symmetric neuropathy	SPE, IF
Rare: primary biliary cirrhosis, Crohn's disease	
Neuronopathies	
Paraneoplastic neuronopathy	Anti-Hu/CV2, Imaging
Sjögren's syndrome	Lip biopsy
HIV-related sensory neuronopathy	HIV test
Miller Fisher variant	EMG/NCS
Drugs (see Box 4)	Medication review
Autonomic	
Diabetes	OGTT
GBS	EMG/NCS
Paraneoplastic sensory neuropathy	Anti-Hu, CV2, imaging
HIV-related neuropathy	HIV test
Vincristine (Oncovin)	Medication review
Thiamine deficiency	Alcohol history
Rare: porphyria, hereditary autonomic neuropathy, amyloidosis	

Abbreviations: ANA = antinuclear antibodies; ANCA = antineutrophilic cytoplasmic antibodies; bx = biopsy; CBC = complete blood count; CIDP = chronic inflammatory demyelinating polyneuropathy; CMT = Charcot-Marie-Tooth disease; CSF = cerebrospinal fluid; EMG/NCS = electromyography/nerve conduction studies; ESR = erythrocyte sedimentation rate; GBS = Guillain-Barré syndrome; HIV = human immunodeficiency virus; HNPP = hereditary neuropathy with liability to pressure palsies; IF = immunofixation; LFT = liver function tests; MGUS = monoclonal gammopathy of unknown significance; MMNCB = multifocal motor neuropathy with conduction blocks; OGTT = oral glucose tolerance test; RF = rheumatoid factor; SPE = serum protein electrophoresis; TSH = thyroid-stimulating hormone.

BOX 2   Key Diagnostic Features

Medical History
- Connective tissue disease
- Diabetes
- Renal disease
- Thyroid disease

Surgical History, Trauma
- Compression neuropathies

Medication History
- Drug-induced neuropathy

Family History, High Arches
- Inherited neuropathy

Nutrition, Alcohol Use
- Alcoholic neuropathy
- Vitamin deficiency

Occupational Exposures
- Toxic neuropathy

History of Weight Loss
- Amyloidosis
- HIV
- Malignancy

Recent Infection, Travel
- Diphtheria
- Guillain-Barré syndrome
- HIV
- Leprosy
- Lyme disease

Dry Eyes and Mouth
- Sarcoidosis

Severe Pain
- Amyloidosis
- Diabetes
- Guillain-Barré syndrome
- HIV
- Vasculitis

Skin Lesions
- Anesthetic patches (leprosy)
- Bullous lesions (porphyria)
- Hyperpigmentation (osteosclerotic myeloma)
- Mee's lines (arsenic or thallium poisoning)
- Orange tonsils (Tangier disease)
- Angiokeratomas (Fabry's disease)

PATHOLOGY AND THE ROLE OF NEUROPHYSIOLOGY

Nerve conduction studies (NCSs) and electromyography (EMG) are highly specialized tests that are performed principally by neurologists. NCSs electrically activate peripheral nerves at particular sites and then assess for abnormal transmission from the stimulation point to the final muscle response. EMG involves placing a small needle into the muscle to observe both the sound and appearance of the muscle at rest and with motor units firing. Because NCSs can only be performed at points where the nerve is superficial (most often distal), EMG is needed to assess for more proximal damage such as radiculopathy. EMG can also rule out other mimics of PNS disease, such as myopathy.

- Charcot-Marie-Tooth disease
- Hereditary neuropathy with liability to pressure palsies
- Inflammatory neuropathies
- Monoclonal gammopathies and paraproteinemias
- Multifocal motor neuropathy with conduction block
- Neuropathies caused by drugs such as amiodarone (Cordarone) and suramin[2]
- Neuropathies caused by infections (diphtheria) or toxins (arsenic)

[2]Not available in the United States.

For the general physician, the most important thing is being able to interpret the results of these tests. Often, a report will be received back such as: "There is evidence of a symmetric distal axonal sensorimotor neuropathy." An NCS/EMG study should be able to specify the distribution and if motor or sensory fibers are involved. Autonomic and small sensory fibers are not tested well by EMG, so the diagnosis of these types of neuropathies is often clinical or requires more specialized testing. Thus, a normal NCS/EMG does not rule out neuropathy.

A further feature that electrophysiology can add is whether the pathology is demyelinating or axonal. Demyelination is characterized by slowed conduction velocity, temporal dispersion of the muscle action potential, and conduction block. Hereditary demyelinating neuropathies, such as Charcot-Marie-Tooth disease, do not show the latter two features, which are only seen in acquired neuropathies. Axonal disease is characterized by modest slowing of velocities, and more marked reduction in the amplitudes of the muscle and sensory action potentials. On EMG, there are fibrillations within 3 weeks of the neuropathic injury, indicating spontaneous firing of denervated muscle. Enlarged and prolonged motor unit potentials indicate subsequent regeneration, which occurs after several weeks to months.

Demyelination has a limited differential (Box 3), and often a better prognosis, because myelin can start to regenerate within a few days. Axonal regeneration proceeds at a far slower rate of 1 to 3 μm/day, and nerves with proximal lesions must go a long distance to reinnervate their muscle and might never reach their goal.

Investigations

Once the neuropathy has been subclassified, investigations for the specific causes in that pattern class should be undertaken (see Table 1). Several recent papers suggest that 2-hour oral glucose tolerance testing (OGTT) is the best test for glucose intolerance due to the relatively low sensitivity of serum glucose levels and glycosylated hemoglobin (HbA1c). Likewise, vitamin B_{12} levels have a low sensitivity, and serum metabolites methylmalonic acid (MMA) and homocysteine (Hcy) should be measured in patients with a result less than 300 pg/mL to improve diagnostic accuracy. These metabolites can be falsely increased with hypovolemia, renal insufficiency, hypothyroidism, and increased age, but a return to normal levels 1 to 2 weeks after beginning replacement therapy indicates this is the cause. The combination of elevated gastrin and anti–parietal cell antibodies may be used to diagnose pernicious anemia. The yield of general testing for other vitamin deficiencies in polyneuropathy is relatively low.

Antinuclear antibodies (ANA) probably are usually only significant in the context of suggestive features (abrupt onset, mononeuropathy multiplex pattern, arthralgia or arthritis, fevers, rash, or renal abnormalities) because they are positive in about 3% of normal patients. However, referral to a rheumatologist should be considered with a very high titer (>1:1280).

The erythyrocyte sedimentation rate (ESR) is often elevated, especially in older patients. Rates greater than 70 mm/hour tend to be more meaningful, particularly with a mononeuritis multiplex pattern.

Serum protein electrophoresis lacks sensitivity, and immunofixation should be ordered if there is high suspicion of a paraproteinemia. If an elevated monoclonal antibody is found, a 24-hour urine test for Bence Jones proteinuria, skeletal survey, CBC, renal function tests, and serum calcium should be ordered. If the M protein is greater than 2.5 g/dL or if abnormalities are detected on these tests, referral to a hematologist for bone marrow aspiration is required. Polyclonal antibodies are not associated with neuropathy.

If there is suspicion of amyloidosis, a rectal, abdominal fat, or sensory nerve biopsy can be undertaken. Sural nerve biopsy is reserved for difficult diagnostic situations because it causes a permanent area of numbness with possible dysesthesias over the biopsied area. Suspicion of vasculitis is the most common indication, but pathology can also be seen in leprosy and with tumor infiltrate.

In approximately 20% of patients, an underlying cause of neuropathy is not found. These patients are said to have a cryptogenic sensory or sensorimotor neuropathy. A distinct clinical picture has emerged, most commonly of a patient in the sixth or seventh decade, manifesting with distal dysesthesias and possibly with mild weakness and sensory ataxia. These patients tend not to develop significant disability, and treatment is mainly for neuropathic pain.

Treatment

MONONEUROPATHIES

The most common cause of mononeuropathy is nerve compression, and surgical treatment is often a consideration for these patients. The four most common locations are median neuropathy at the wrist (carpal tunnel syndrome), ulnar neuropathy at the elbow, peroneal neuropathy at the fibular head, and facial nerve palsy (Bell's palsy).

Carpal tunnel syndrome manifests with pain and numbness principally in the first three digits, although it is often poorly localized. Classic features include pain at night and shaking out the hand to relieve pain. For milder symptoms, a nighttime splint, which prevents wrist flexion and high pressure in the carpal tunnel, is often helpful. Local corticosteroid injections can provide relief, and surgical decompression has a very high success rate.

Ulnar neuropathy manifests with numbness of the fourth and fifth digits and wasting of the interosseous muscles, often with pain localized to the elbow. Peroneal neuropathies manifest with foot drop and numbness on the dorsum of the foot. In both cases, avoidance of pressure over the nerve often leads to improvement. Surgery might improve symptoms, but less reliably so than carpal tunnel surgery.

Bell's palsy is an inflammatory rather than compressive process, presumably due to a viral etiology. Treatment is controversial, but early (within 14 days) use of prednisone[1] 60 mg daily, decreasing by 10 mg steps every 2 days, along with acyclovir (Zovirax)[1] 800 mg five times daily for 7 days has been advocated. About 15% of patients have residual facial weakness.

[1]Not FDA approved for this indication.

GUILLAIN-BARRÉ SYNDROME

GBS often begins following gastroenteritis with *Campylobacter jejuni*, or an upper respiratory tract infection, due to a presumed autoimmune response directed against myelin. The incidence is 1 or 2 per 100,000 persons per year. Characteristic features are ascending weakness, areflexia, and sensory and autonomic symptoms progressing over a few days up to 4 weeks. Facial diplegia and pain can occur. Electrophysiology shows acute demyelination with conduction blocks, and cerebrospinal fluid (CSF) reveals an increase in protein with a cell count of less than 5 white blood cells (cytoalbuminologic dissociation) in more than 80% of patients after 2 weeks. A CSF pleocytosis of more than 10 lymphocytes/mm^3 should alert the physician to another cause such as sarcoidosis, Lyme disease, or early HIV.

The Miller-Fisher variant is characterized by specific clinical features of sensory ataxia, areflexia, and ophthalmolplegia. *C. jejuni* infection has been correlated with more severe variants, such as acute motor axonal neuropathy (AMAN) and acute motor and sensory axonal neuropathy (AMSAM), which damage axons in addition to myelin. *C. jejuni*–related GBS correlates with anti-GM1 antibodies, although they are not prognostic or specific. Recovery can take months to years. Only 20% of patients are left without residual deficit. About 5% to 10% have significant persistent disability, and the mortality rate is 5%.

During early treatment, patients might require admission to intensive care, with close monitoring of pulmonary function tests for respiratory compromise. Diaphragmatic weakness correlates with neck flexion and extension and shoulder abduction. The patient should be intubated when the forced vital capacity (FVC) declines to less than 15 mL/kg or when negative inspiratory flow (NIF) is less than −20 to −30. Monitoring of the cardiac rhythm is important due to dysautonomia.

The preferred treatment is intravenous immunoglobulin (IVIg)[1] at a dose of 0.4 g/kg/day for 5 days. This is generally well tolerated, and adverse side effects such as myalgia, headache, or flu-like symptoms often resolve with a reduced infusion rate. If IVIg is contraindicated (renal failure, IgA deficiency), plasmapheresis can be initiated with four alternate-day exchanges over 7 to 10 days for a total of 200 to 250 mL/kg. Both plasmapheresis and IVIg continue to work for several weeks after the treatment period, but if patients experience a secondary worsening after successful treatment, a second dose may be initiated. Steroids were reviewed recently by a Cochrane systematic review and were not found to be of benefit in GBS.

CHRONIC INFLAMMATORY DEMYELINATING POLYNEUROPATHY

This neuropathy is pathologically similar to GBS, but progression is longer than 8 weeks, often with a relapsing-remitting course. Symmetric distal and proximal weakness and sensory impairment, hyporeflexia, and cytoalbuminergic dissociation in the CSF is the classic presentation, although there are variants.

Treatment is either IVIg[1] or prednisone. IVIg is given initially at 0.4 g/kg/day for 5 days, then the dose and frequency are reduced over time. Prednisone is given 1 mg/kg/day until improvement, followed by a slow tapering of 5 mg every 2 to 3 weeks over a period of months. Response is usually seen within 4 weeks. Refractory patients have been treated with repeated plasmapheresis treatments or immunosuppressive therapy with cyclosporine (Sandimmune).[1]

MULTIFOCAL MOTOR NEUROPATHY

Multifocal motor neuropathy (MMN) is not a common disorder but is important not to mistake for motor neuron disease because it has a very different prognosis and treatment. Patients present with progressive asymmetric distal weakness, often of the arm, without sensory loss and with less atrophy than would be expected for the degree of weakness. Unlike motor neuron disease, there are no upper motor neuron signs. It is different from multifocal acquired demyelinating sensory and motor neuropathy (MADSAM), an asymmetric variant of CIDP, in that loss of reflexes and weakness involves only the affected limb, there is a relatively normal CSF protein concentration, and sensory nerve conduction studies are normal. Diagnosis is supported by finding conduction blocks in sites not usually associated with compression. The GM1 antibody is elevated in 60% of cases. Repeated treatments with IVIg[1] or cyclophosphamide (Cytoxan)[1] are common choices. Rituximab (Rituxan),[1] a monoclonal antibody, has also been used. Prednisone classically worsens the condition.

DIABETIC NEUROPATHY

Diabetes is one of the most common causes of neuropathy. Patients can present with a symmetric distal neuropathy, autonomic proximal diabetic neuropathy, mononeuritis multiplex, compressive and cranial neuropathies, and trunk polyradiculopathies.

The distal symmetric sensory polyneuropathy (DSPN) correlates with the duration of the diabetes, control of hyperglycemia, and presence of retinopathy and nephropathy. The exact etiology is unknown, but theories include a metabolic process involving aldose reductase, ischemic damage, or an immunologic disorder. Typical symptoms include lancinating pains or burning, worse at night, and possible dysautonomia. Atrophy may be noted in the foot muscles, but severe weakness is atypical. NCS may be normal because small fibers are primarily affected. Treatment includes blood sugar control to limit progression and symptom control for neuropathic pain. Gabapentin (Neurontin)[1] and tricyclic antidepressants are common choices (see later). Drugs such as QR-333, a topical compound that contains quercetin, a flavonoid with aldose reductase–inhibitor effects, are being investigated specifically for diabetic neuropathy.

Autonomic neuropathy is treated symptomatically, with fludrocortisone (Florinef)[1] 0.1 mg/day for orthostatic hypotension metoclopramide (Reglan) 10 mg before meals for gastroparesis, and sildenafil (Viagra) 25 mg 1 hour before sexual intercourse for impotence.

Proximal diabetic neuropathy (diabetic amyotrophy) manifests typically with unilateral pain in the anterior thigh followed by stepwise progression over weeks to months of quadriceps weakness, atrophy of the proximal leg muscles, and a reduced knee reflex, with occasional contralateral leg involvement. The erythrocyte sedimentation rate (ESR) may be elevated and CSF protein mildly increased (120 mg/dL on average). NCS and EMG reflect multifocal active axonal damage (fibrillations) to the lumbar plexus and roots. Small retrospective studies have reported that IVIg[1] and other forms of immunosuppressive therapy are effective in treating patients with proximal diabetic neuropathy. A short course of corticosteroids (prednisone[1] 50 mg/day for 1 week, then tapering by 10 mg/week) can be used to ease pain in severe cases, with close monitoring of the glucose level, but overall prognosis is quite good, ranging from 1 to 18 months of recovery phase (mean of 6 months) and partial or complete restoration of strength in approximately 70% of patients.

PARAPROTEINEMIC NEUROPATHIES

Multiple myeloma, Waldenström's macroglobulinemia, cryoglobulinemia, osteosclerotic myeloma (POEMS syndrome), and monoclonal gammopathy of unknown significance (MGUS) are associated with monoclonal antibodies directed at PNS components, such as myelin-associated glycoprotein (MAG). Neuropathies associated with an immunoglobulin (Ig)M monoclonal protein (approximately 60%) are typically distal, demyelinating, and symmetric, whereas IgG (30%) and IgA (10%) gammopathies can be axonal or demyelinating. In terms of treatment, the distal demyelinating neuropathy of IgM paraproteinemias tends to be treatment refractory. IgG and IgA gammopathies can mimic the demyelination pattern seen in CIDP, and patients with any antibody and this pattern should receive immunotherapy as recommended for CIDP (see earlier). Axonal neuropathies and IgM, IgG, or IgA gammopathies have a less clear relationship and are typically not responsive to treatment.

---

[1]Not FDA approved for this indication.

HEREDITARY NEUROPATHIES

Charcot-Marie-Tooth (CMT) disease is among the most common of genetic neuromuscular disorders, and more than 30 genes have been identified. Clues are a history of difficulty running in childhood, high arches, hammertoes, ankle weakness, and nerve hypertrophy developing in teenage years. Depending on the subtype, the neuropathy may be axonal or demyelinating, but the most common type (CMT-1) is caused by an autosomal dominant gene encoding peripheral myelin protein 22 and is easily diagnosed by the relatively uniform slowing on nerve conduction velocities (<25% of lower limits of normal). Patients have a mild course and remain ambulatory throughout life in most cases.

Hereditary neuropathy with liability to pressure palsies (HNPP) is another dominantly inherited neuropathy in which patients have recurrent episodes of isolated mononeuropathies, typically affecting, in order of decreasing frequency, the common peroneal, ulnar, radial, and median nerves. Most attacks are sudden onset, painless, and followed by complete recovery. There is no treatment other than preventive measures.

TOXIC AND NUTRITIONAL NEUROPATHIES

Treatment of toxic and nutritional neuropathies involves detection and removal of the underlying cause. A thorough review of medications, occupational exposures, and nutritional risk factors is essential (Box 4). Drug toxicity is much more common than environmental toxicity. Incidence of neuropathy does not always correlate with the dosage and duration of exposure. For instance, amiodarone neuropathy has been reported with dosages as low as 200 mg/day and durations as short as 1 month. Symptoms might not improve, or might even worsen, for several weeks after the drug is stopped before improvement starts, a phenomenon known as *coasting*.

Cisplatin can cause a neuropathy that overlaps in symptomatology with paraneoplastic sensory neuronopathy, and dapsone is associated with a motor axonopathy. Gold neuropathy can have prominent myokymia and can mimic GBS.

Specific treatments for drug-induced neuropathies include cyanocobalamin (vitamin B_{12})[1] for nitrous oxide neuropathy and pyridoxine (vitamin B_6)[1] for hydralazine and isoniazid neuropathies. Excessive vitamin B_6 can also *cause* a neuropathy. Glutamine[7] and vitamin E[1] 300 mg twice a day has shown promise for paclitaxel neuropathy, and neuroprotective agents such as nerve growth factor are being investigated for cisplatin-induced neuropathy. Tacrolimus can cause a CIDP-like neuropathy that responds to IVIg[1] or plasmapheresis.

One of the most common nutritional neuropathies is caused by thiamine deficiency and is associated with alcohol consumption of at least 100 g per day. Patients present with burning feet, and early alcohol abstinence and treatment with thiamine denotes better chance of recovery. Vitamin B_{12} deficiency is vital not to miss and can manifest with a subacute combined degeneration, whereby patients have a superimposed myelopathy and neuropathy (spasticity but reduced reflexes). Sudden-onset symptoms, particularly in the feet and hands simultaneously, are also suggestive.

METABOLIC AND INFECTIOUS NEUROPATHIES

Peripheral neuropathy can complicate renal failure, hypothyroidism, biliary cirrhosis, porphyria, Tangier disease, Fabry's disease, and mitochondrial diseases.

Early in the course, HIV can manifest as a GBS-like syndrome, although with CSF pleocytosis. This typically responds to IVIg[1] and plasmapheresis. In later stages, patients might develop a distal symmetric polyneuropathy, although it is important to determine if this might be due to nucleoside reverse transcriptase inhibitors, nutritional deficiency, or infection. Cranial neuropathies, sensory neuronopathy, lumbosacral polyradiculopathies, and mononeuritis multiplex also occur.

Leprosy is the most common treatable neuropathy worldwide. Tuberculoid leprosy leads to hypopigmented patches with loss of

---

BOX 4 Causes of Toxic and Nutritional Neuropathies

Drug Toxins
Axonal
- Colchicine
- Dapsone
- Disulfiram
- Ethambutol
- Hyralazine
- Isoniazid
- Metronidazole
- Nitrofurantoin
- Nitrous oxide
- Nucleosides
- Paclitaxel
- Phenytoin
- Tacrolimus
- Vincristine

Demyelinating
- Amiodarone (Cordarone)
- Chloroquine (Aralen)
- Gold
- Suramin[2]

Neuronopathy
- Cisplatin (Platinol-AQ)
- Pyridoxine (vitamin B_6)
- Thalidomide (Thalomid)

Environmental Toxins
- Acrylamide (plastics)
- Allyl chloride (insecticides)
- Arsenic
- Carbon disulfide (cellophanes)
- Ethylene glycol (antifreeze)
- Ethylene oxide (sterilizer)
- Hexacarbons (glue)
- Lead
- Mercury
- Methyl bromide (fumigant)
- Organophosphates (insecticides)
- Thallium (pesticides)
- Trichloroethylene (drycleaning)
- Vacor (rodenticide)

Vitamin Deficiencies
- B_1 (alcoholism)
- B_3 (alcoholism)
- B_6 (isoniazid use)
- B_{12} (vegans, pernicious anemia)
- E (cholestasis and abetalipoproteinemia)

[2]Not available in the United States.

---

pain and temperature sensation. Lepromatous leprosy, a more severe form seen in immunosuppressed persons, can cause ulnar, common peroneal, and facial neuropathies. Treatment involves a long-term multidrug regimen of dapsone and rifampin (Rifadin).[1]

Herpes zoster can cause a postherpetic neuralgia, defined as pain persisting for more than 6 weeks after the rash appears. Early treatment with acyclovir (Zovirax) (800 mg five times daily for 7 days) can reduce the duration of the acute phase. Chronic discomfort is treated with medications for neuropathic pain (see later).

Lyme disease, caused by *Borrelia burgdorferi*, begins with erythema migrans, followed by multifocal peripheral and cranial neuropathies, particularly facial diplegia. CSF lymphocytic pleocytosis plus serologic demonstration of *B. burgdorferi* infection on serum or CSF are the diagnostic features. Early stages are treated with a 3-week course of doxycycline[1] 100 mg twice daily, and intravenous penicillin G[1] should be given in the late stages.

CARCINOMATOUS NEUROPATHY

Tumors can cause neuropathy by compression, metastatic spread, paraneoplastic antibodies, hemorrhage, and treatment with chemotherapy or radiation therapy. A distal sensorimotor neuropathy is associated with many different tumors and seldom precedes tumor diagnosis. Pathogenesis can include toxic, nutritional, and immunologic causes. A sensory neuronopathy is less common, but often precedes tumor diagnosis, thus warranting a careful work-up. Lung, breast, ovary, and gastrointestinal tract cancers are the most likely associated types. Imaging and paraneoplastic antibodies (particularly anti-Hu and anti-CV2, most commonly associated with lung cancer) may help in making the diagnosis. Treatment focuses on the underlying neoplasm.

VASCULITIC NEUROPATHY

Vasculitis can be primary (polyarteritis nodosa, Wegener's granulomatosis, Churg-Strauss syndrome, microscopic polyangitis) or secondary (connective tissue diseases, systemic infections, drug reactions). It classically manifests with a painful mononeuritis multiplex with asymmetric patchy features, reflecting multifocal ischemic damage. If the patient's vasculitis is restricted to the PNS, serologic testing for these disorders is often negative. In this case, a sural nerve biopsy might reveal fibrinoid necrosis and perivascular inflammation.

Treatment needs to be carefully undertaken with intravenous methylprednisolone (Solu-Medrol)[1] for 3 days followed by oral prednisone. In many cases, other immunosuppressive drugs are eventually used.

Neuropathic Pain

Often pain is the most predominant and distressing feature of neuropathy. Several classes of medications can be tried (Table 2), although it is important to counsel the patient that complete abolition of pain is unlikely. A trial period should be for at least 6 to 8 weeks before concluding that the patient does not respond. A combination of agents with different mechanisms can have an advantage over monotherapy for the nonresponsive patient.

First-line treatment is generally with tricyclic antidepressants. Serotonin and noradrenaline reuptake inhibitors such as amitriptyline[1] (Elavil), imipramine[1] (Tofranil), and clomipramine[1] (Anafranil) may be marginally more effective than those with relatively selective noradrenergic effects such as desipramine and nortriptyline. However, nortriptyline and desipramine are less sedating. Selective serotonin reuptake inhibitors appear to be less effective. Second-line antidepressants include venlafaxine[1] (Effexor), bupropion[1] (Wellbutrin), and the recently approved duloxetine (Cymbalta), which have the advantage of better tolerability due to less muscarinic, histaminergic, and α-adrenergic affinity.

The typical next class of medications to try is the antiepileptics. Gabapentin[1] is a common choice and is generally well tolerated. Pregabalin (Lyrica) is a newer related agent that, unlike gabapentin, exhibits linear pharmacokinetics and can be initiated at a therapeutic dose without a long titration. Second-line choices include lamotrigine[1] (Lamictal), carbamazepine[1] (Tegretol), and topiramate[1] (Topamax). Valproate[1] (Depacon) and zonisamide[1] (Zonegran) have limited evidence, and phenytoin[1] (Dilantin) can cause neuropathy. Oxcarbazepine[1] (Trileptal), like carbamazepine, slows the recovery rate of voltage-activated sodium channels, but it also inhibits high-threshold N-type and P/Q-type calcium channels and reduces glutamatergic transmission. As a result, it can modulate both peripheral and central neuropathic pain pathways, and several studies into its efficacy are under way.

Topical creams, such as capsaicin (Zostrix), an extract of chili, can be tried. Capsaicin works by depleting substance P and can temporarily worsen pain by causing a burning sensation. Lidocaine[1] (Xylocaine) can be also used topically.

Other agents for severe neuropathies include opioid agents, such as tramadol (Ultram), which has low-affinity binding for μ-opioid receptors coupled with mild inhibition of norepinephrine and serotonin reuptake. Slow-release opioids, such as oxycodone (OxyContin) 30 to 60 mg/day, can help, and risk of addiction is low in this population. Glutamate antagonists, such as dextromethorphan[1] (Delsym), have shown benefit in some studies, as has mexiletine[1] (Mexitil), a class IB antiarrhythmic agent and oral analogue of lidocaine. Nonpharmacologic therapies, such as transcutaneous electrical nerve stimulation (TENS) and acupuncture, might also provide adjunctive relief.

---

[1]Not FDA approved for this indication.

[1]Not FDA approved for this indication.

TABLE 2 Select Neuropathic Pain Medications

Drug	Dosage	Side Effects
Amitriptyline (Elavil)[1]	10 mg/d, increasing weekly by 10 mg, up to 150 mg/d	Dry mouth, sedation, urinary retention, cardiac arrhythmias, orthostatic hypotension, constipation, weight gain Contraindications: cardiac arrhythmias, CHF, recent MI, narrow angle glaucoma, urinary retention
Capsaicin (Zostrix)	0.075% cream applied tid to qid	Sneezing, coughing, rash, skin irritation
Carbamazepine (Tegretol)[1]	100 mg bid, increasing by 100 mg weekly Max: 1200 mg/d	Somnolence, dizziness, nausea, gait changes, urticaria, hyponatremia, pancytopenia, hepatic dysfunction Obtain baseline and 6-wk CBC and LFT
Gabapentin (Neurontin)[1]	300 mg on day 1, 600 mg on day 2, 900 mg on day 3 Max: 3600 mg/d	Sedation, fatigue, dizziness, confusion, tremor, weight gain, peripheral edema, headache Reduce dose in renal insufficiency
Lamotrigine (Lamictal)[1]	25 mg at night for 2 wk, increasing weekly by 25–50 mg Max: 400 mg/d	Severe rash (especially if increased too quickly), dizziness, unsteadiness, drowsiness, diplopia
Tramadol (Ultram)	50 mg bid Titrate 50 mg every 3–7 d, using a tid or qid schedule Max: 100 mg qid	Constipation, headache, nausea Risk of seizures with neuroleptics and antidepressants Reduce dose with hepatic or renal dysfunction

[1]Not FDA approved for this indication.
Abbreviations: CBC = complete blood count; CHF = congestive heart failure; LFT = liver function test; max = maximum; MI = myocardial infarction.

REFERENCES

Donofrio PD, Albers JW. AAEM minimonograph 34. Polyneuropathy: Classification by nerve conduction studies and electromyography. Muscle Nerve 1990;13:889–903.

Dworkin RH, Backonja M, Rowbotham MC, et al. Advances in neuropathic pain: Diagnosis, mechanisms, and treatment recommendations. Arch Neurol 2003;60:1524–34.

Grant I, Benstead TJ. Differential diagnosis of peripheral neuropathy. In: Dyck PJ, Thomas PK, editors. Peripheral Neuropathy. Philadelphia: Saunders; 2005.

Poncelet AN. An algorithm for the evaluation of peripheral neuropathy. Am Fam Physician 1997;57(4):755–64.

Stewart JD. Focal peripheral neuropathies. New York: Raven; 1993.

Management of Head Injuries

Method of
Todd W. Vitaz, MD

Traumatic brain injury (TBI) most commonly results from motor vehicle crashes (MVC) and typically affects males in the 2nd through 4th decades of life. These sudden random acts can have long-lasting effects on the patient and family, but these events also impact society as a whole when a young, viable working-age individual becomes suddenly disabled and dependent on the care of others. TBI has no regard for age or gender, however, and can be seen in infants as a result of nonaccidental trauma as well as in geriatric patients following falls. The management of these patients can become extremely complicated and often requires the close interaction of numerous different health care providers ranging from trauma, orthopedic, and neurologic surgeons to nurses, social workers, speech, occupational, and physical therapists. Unfortunately, current interventions are still limited to the avoidance or minimization of secondary injury and rehabilitative intervention. However, when these patients are managed with aggressive, comprehensive, multidisciplinary approaches, the outcomes at times can be rewarding.

TBI can be categorized based on numerous factors. Most commonly it is differentiated based on mechanism and injury type (closed versus penetrating), whether it has occurred with or without systemic injuries (isolated versus multisystem), and the severity (mild, moderate, severe). The Glasgow Coma Scale (GCS) (Table 1), which was initially developed as a prognostic indicator following closed head injury, has become the principal triage tool for evaluating these patients. Patients are scored based on their best response in each of the three categories (eye opening, verbal responses, and

TABLE 1 Glasgow Coma Scale

Best Motor Score	Best Verbal Response	Best Eye Opening
6 Obeys commands	5 Normal speech	4 Spontaneous
5 Localizes to pain	4 Confused	3 To voice
4 Withdraws to pain	3 Inappropriate words	2 To pain
3 Flexor posturing	2 Incomprehensible sounds	1 No eye opening
2 Extensor posturing	1 No verbal response	
1 No motor response	Intubated patients receive a 1 with the suffix T added to score	

motor score) and then subdivided into mild (13 to 15), moderate (9 to 12), and severe (3 to 8). One caveat to this assessment tool is that it can be affected by numerous alterations: hypoxia, hypotension, hypothermia, intoxication, infection, and other metabolic derangements, which are commonly seen in the trauma population.

Pathology

Another common classification system following TBI is based on pathophysiologic findings. Concussion commonly occurs following mild or moderate TBI as the result of transient (typically seconds to minutes) neurologic dysfunction in the setting of a normal computed tomography (CT) scan. Brief loss of consciousness, commonly with amnesia regarding the event, is not uncommon and is often associated with nausea, vomiting, headache, dizziness, and transient visual obscuration. These symptoms may persist for several hours to weeks as part of the *postconcussive syndrome* and, in rare instances, especially following repetitive injury, these alterations may become long-lasting. As a result of these persistent problems, in addition to a better understanding of the neurocognitive effects following this type of injury, there has been an enormous emphasis placed on their prevention (see text following).

Skull fractures may occur in isolation or be associated with other types of brain injuries. They are commonly classified based on whether they are open (overlying laceration) or closed, linear or comminuted, nondepressed or depressed. Skull fractures occur either as the result of a large force directed to a small area (i.e., depressed skull fracture following a blow to the head with a golf club) or when larger forces are dissipated throughout the skull resulting in fracture through the weakest area (linear fractures through frontal skull base, petrous, or squamous temporal bone). Linear fractures are commonly associated with raccoon eyes (frontal skull base fractures), Battle's sign (posterior skull base fracture), cerebrospinal fluid leak (otorrhea or rhinorrhea) or olfactory, facial or acoustic nerve injury (amnesia, facial palsy, sensorineuronal deafness).

In addition, temporal bone fractures may also be associated with epidural hematomas (EDHs). These extra-axial blood clots are most commonly caused by laceration of the middle meningeal artery and result in accumulation of *high-pressure arterial bleeding* in the potential space between the dura and skull. EDHs are more commonly seen in younger individuals probably because of the decreased skull thickness and lack of adhesions between the skull and dura mater in this population. Commonly, these lesions appear on CT scan as lens-shaped, extra-axial hematomas most often in the temporal region and can be rapidly expansive secondary to the high-pressure arterial bleeding. The clinical course in these patients is classically described by a brief loss of consciousness from the initial concussion, followed by a "lucid interval" in which the patient may be awake and alert, which then gives way to another episode of decreased mental status that may be rapidly progressive and associated with signs of brain stem compression (flexor or extensor posturing, dilated nonreactive pupil). EDHs are usually treated surgically unless they are extremely small and constitute one of the few true neurosurgical emergencies where mere minutes may make an enormous difference in the patient's outcome.

Unlike EDHs, subdural hematomas (SDHs) are often associated with other types of brain injury and thus typically involve an altered level of consciousness (LOC) from the onset. SDHs are typically caused by bleeding from bridging veins that get torn when the brain moves within its cerebrospinal fluid (CSF) buffer while the veins remain tethered at their dural insertions; however, other causes such as venous or arterial hemorrhage from a brain laceration also exist. CT scanning reveals that these lesions commonly appear more crescent-shaped but never cross the dural boundaries (falx or tentorium). Unlike the high-pressure EDHs, SDHs typically expand at a slower rate but still cause devastating neurologic dysfunction from compression of the underlying brain. In addition mortality rates tend to be higher with worse outcome for SDH as a result of the common underlying brain injury. Once again these extra-axial clots frequently require surgical evacuation unless they are small and fail to have substantial compression on the underlying brain, where they are managed with serial imaging and close neurologic observation. In patients for whom a small SDH is not treated surgically, the physician must remain cognizant of the fact that a small proportion of these will increase in size between 1 and 4 weeks following the trauma and can be a cause of delayed deterioration or increased headache and new neurologic findings.

Intraparenchymal hematomas occur quite commonly following TBI and can be either hemorrhagic or nonhemorrhagic. These lesions range in size from 1 to 2 mm, up to several centimeters, and can cause a full range of symptoms and neurologic findings based on their location, size, and degree of compression on surrounding structures. Just like extra-axial hematomas, these lesions may increase in size and commonly coalesce or mature and *blossom* during the first 12 to 24 hours following the trauma. In addition, larger hematomas incite an inflammatory reaction in the surrounding brain resulting in increased edema around the lesion, which may result in increases in the intracranial pressure (ICP) (commonly seen on postinjury days [PIDs] 3 to 7). Management of these lesions depends on their size, location, and associated findings and ranges from serial observation and repeat imaging, surgical evacuation of the hematoma, or decompressive craniectomy with or without lobectomy.

The final category of pathologic abnormalities following TBI occurs as the result of shear injury to the axons themselves, called diffuse axonal injury (DAI). This is caused by either acceleration and deceleration or rotational forces to the axons resulting in micro- or macroscopic areas of injury and axonal transection. Most commonly this is encountered in the setting where a patient clinically has signs of a severe TBI, often with a GCS score less than 6; however, the CT scan is either unimpressive or shows only small areas of petechial hemorrhage. In addition ICP recording typically shows normal or only slightly elevated values. Magnetic resonance imaging (MRI) is commonly used in this subset of patients and can be used as a predictive indicator for determining the severity of injury, especially if CT is negative. MRI commonly shows areas of increased intensity on fluid attenuation inversion recovery (FLAIR) and T2-weighted sequences in the brainstem, diencephalon, deep white matter tracts, or corpus callosum. Recovery following this type of injury is variable and depends more on the injury location (reticular activating system of brainstem versus supratentorial white matter tracts) rather than the injury volume.

In addition to these abnormalities, patients with TBI are also at risk for damage to the spinal cord and vertebral and carotid arteries. Thus, patients with altered LOC should be assumed to have spinal instability and possible spinal cord injury (SCI); they should remain immobilized until the absence of these can be confirmed. The incidence of carotid and vertebral artery injury associated with severe TBI is unknown, but patients with facial or cervical fractures and those with soft tissue neck or chest injury (seat belt sign) have been found to be at higher risk. The appropriate screening for and treatment of these injuries have become a topic of intense debate in recent years but should be suspected in a patient with focal neurologic findings without identifiable cause on other imaging.

INTRACRANIAL PRESSURE AND THE MONROE-KELLIE DOCTRINE

Regardless of the pathophysiologic type of injury, the end result commonly is the generation of increases in the ICP, which can then lead to secondary brain injury. ICP dynamics are easily understood if one considers the principles of the volume pressure relationships outlined by the Monroe-Kellie doctrine. The basis of this principle resides on the fact that the skull is a fixed and rigid volume; because of this any changes to the volume of its contents will directly affect the pressure within this rigid space. In simplest terms the intracranial cavity contains blood, water, and tissue. Blood may be intravascular (IV) or extravascular (EV) in the case of extra-axial blood clots; water includes not only cerebrospinal fluid, which may build up in cases of hydrocephalus, but also edema following traumatic injuries; brain parenchyma typically compromises the tissue component but in select instances tumors or cysts may also fall into this category.

 CURRENT DIAGNOSIS

Classification of Head Injuries

- Closed versus penetrating
- Isolated versus multisystem injuries
- Severity
  - Mild (GCS 13–15)
  - Moderate (GCS 9–12)
  - Severe (GCS 3–8)

Pathologic Findings with Closed Head Injuries

- Skull fractures
- Epidural hematomas
- Subdural hematomas
- Parenchymal contusions
- Intraparenchymal hematomas
- Diffuse axonal injury

As increases in any or all three of these categories occur, the pressure inside the cranial cavity increases proportionally. At first compensatory changes occur, which accommodate for these increases, resulting in only mild pressure changes; however, eventually a critical volume is reached where the compensatory mechanisms are saturated, resulting in rapid and dramatic pressure changes. The following scenario illustrates these principles. A patient is involved in a motor vehicle crash and suffers a head injury with a small epidural hematoma. Initially he is awake and alert without any focal neurologic findings. The epidural hematoma creates an increase in the EV blood component of the Monroe-Kellie doctrine; however, compensatory changes in intracranial CSF volume result in decreases in the water component, thus preventing significant changes in ICP. However, the hematoma continues to enlarge, causing increases in ICP exhibited clinically by slow deterioration in the patient's level of consciousness. The patient is now intubated and mildly hyperventilated causing vasoconstriction, thereby decreasing the intravascular blood component and reducing ICP with an improvement in the patient's neurologic condition. Unfortunately, as the operating room (OR) is being prepared, the patient suffers a rapid decrease in his level of conscious, becoming unresponsive with flexor posturing and a nonreactive pupil. Although the hematoma has expanded at a constant rate over time, the rapid change in the patient's condition is the result of him reaching the critical point where all compensatory mechanisms have been exhausted, thus causing profound rapid changes in the patient's ICP.

Treatment of Elevated Intracranial Pressure

Acute changes in ICP result in altered LOC, and at times other localizing neurologic findings such as *blown* (dilated, nonreactive) pupils and flexor or extensor posturing, and such findings may be the sign of impending herniation and death without immediate intervention. In a patient without a ventricular drain already in place, hyperventilation is the most rapid mechanism for acutely lowering elevated ICP. Currently, aggressive hyperventilation ($Pco_2 < 30$) is recommended only for short durations in cases of impending cerebral herniation while patients are being stabilized. As stated previously, hyperventilation causes vasoconstriction, which reduces intravascular blood within the cranial vault and almost instantaneously lowering ICP. However, several studies have now shown that the routine use of aggressive hyperventilation in the management of patients with severe closed head injury (CHI) results in decreased outcomes because of hypoxic injury and possible stroke caused by the sustained hyperventilation. Our current practice is to maintain Pco_2 values between 35 and 38 with controlled ventilation in all patients with severe CHI; because of this we leave all these patients intubated and mechanically ventilated until their ICPs normalize and all other therapies are withdrawn.

Adequate sedation and pain control are also important elements of ICP control. Patients who are restless and agitated will have higher ICPs than similar patients who are resting quietly in bed. Another important point is the prevention of venous congestion. This occasionally is evident in cervical collars, which are fastened too tight or with the use of trach ties that are wrapped too tightly around the neck to hold the endotracheal tube in place.

Several medications are available for the treatment of elevated ICP with the most common one being mannitol. Although this agent acts as an osmotic diuretic and helps pull excess interstitial fluid into the vascular space and thus lower ICP, there are several other hypothetical mechanisms that probably also increase its efficacy such as increasing RBC flexibility, decreasing RBC and platelet clumping in small arterioles and capillaries, and increasing intravascular volume, thus improving cardiac function. Other diuretics such as furosemide (Lasix)[1] or urea (Ureaphil) may also be used but have less dramatic effects on ICP. Hypertonic saline (NaCl 3% to 5%)[1] has also been used more recently by some physicians and has been shown to have many of the same effects as mannitol.

CSF diversion is one of the simplest, quickest acting methods for decreasing ICP especially if a ventricular drain is already in place. The emergent surgical evacuation of mass lesions such as large epidural, subdural, or intraparenchymal hematomas is also extremely effective for controlling ICP, and in many instances it is also life-saving. However, in some instances, underlying brain injury or stroke from prolonged brain compression may be exhibited as massive intraoperative brain swelling and in these instances may necessitate that the bone flap be left off (craniectomy).

Management of Severe Closed Head Injury

The current recommendations of the Brain Trauma Foundation Guidelines for the management of closed head injuries call for the placement of ICP monitors in all patients who fall into the severe category (GCS score <9). At our institution we routinely place combination intraventricular monitors and drains in all patients with a postresuscitation GCS score of less than 7. Monitors are inserted into patients with a GCS score of 7 to 9 on an individual basis depending on whether there are distracting reasons, such as intoxication, to cause the altered LOC. If patients are intubated and not following commands but are purposeful in their movements, we will sometimes elect not to place a ventriculostomy and follow the patient's clinical course over several hours. Other factors include CT findings and the need to go to the operating room during the acute period for the treatment of other life-threatening injuries, age, or for heavy sedation secondary to other injuries or pulmonary problems. At times patients in this GCS range will be given 6 to 12 hours and treated medically to see whether or not they improve prior to placement of an ICP monitor.

---

[1]Not FDA approved for this indication.

CURRENT THERAPY

Management of Elevated Intracranial Pressure

- Prevention of venous engorgement
- CO_2 control (mild hyperventilation)
- Sedation and pain control
- Cerebrospinal fluid drainage
- Mannitol
- Lasix
- Hypertonic saline
- Decompressive craniectomy
- Pentobarbital coma

Once an ICP monitor and drain have been placed elevations in ICP are treated in a systematic order. Target values include attempts to keep ICP less than 15 to 20 and cerebral perfusion pressure (CPP) greater than 60. Low CPP (CPP = mean arterial blood pressure [MAP] − ICP) is caused by either elevated ICP or low MAP. For patients with low MAP or uncontrolled ICP, vasopressors may be used to increase blood pressure (BP) and central venous pressure. At the University of Louisville, dopamine (Intropin) is used as a first line agent, followed by phenylephrine (Neo-Synephrine) and norepinephrine (Levophed) in refractory cases. ICP elevations are initially treated with adequate sedation and pain control, such as midazolam (Versed),[1] propofol (Diprivan), and/or morphine (Lioresal),[1] to prevent agitation and elevated airway pressures, which can further increase ICP and intermittent CSF diversion. In cases where this fails to control ICP, mannitol is then added to the treatment protocol along with more continuous CSF diversion and finally chemical paralysis. Mannitol is administered as a bolus infusion in doses ranging from 0.25 to 1.0 mg/kg body weight every 4 to 8 hours with the endpoints being either ICP control or measured serum osmolarity greater than 315 mOsmL.

Patients who continue to have sustained increases in their ICP despite these interventions are considered to have refractory ICP and at our facility are considered for one of two potential salvage treatments. Pentobarbital (Nembutal)[1] coma has been used successfully on occasion in young patients without mass lesions to decrease the metabolic demands of the brain during these periods of sustained ICP. Patients need to be chosen wisely for this therapy because it carries enormous risks in addition to the possibility of preserving the patient in a long-term, nonfunctional, persistent vegetative state. Initiation of pentobarbital (Nembutal)[1] coma causes severe hypotension, and patients almost always require the use of pressors in addition to volume expansion. At our facility we also place all of these patients on a Rotorest bed in an attempt to minimize the pulmonary complications that frequently occur with the use of this technique.

The second salvage therapy is decompressive craniectomy. This procedure involves the removal of a significant area of skull, typically almost an entire hemisphere or both frontal regions with opening of the dura. This permits the injured swollen brain to herniate through the opening and is the only intervention that increases the volume of the intracranial compartment, thereby reducing pressure. In addition this technique allows for the evacuation of large hemorrhagic contusions, or in cases of extreme ICP elevations it can be coupled with either frontal or temporal lobectomy. Once again, patients must be selected carefully for this intervention. Decompressive craniectomy is used much more frequently than pentobarbital (Nembutal)[1] coma at our institution. We use this strategy for patients with elevated ICP—more than 30 to 40 for more than 30 minutes—or a significant change in neurologic condition that is nonresponsive to all other interventions. In order for either of these two salvage approaches to be effective, they must be used at the first signs of refractory ICP prior to the occurrence of complications such as ischemic infarcts or brainstem compression or hemorrhage.

Patients treated with decompressive craniectomies are at risk for significant alterations in CSF dynamics that may result in delayed deterioration. Signs of hydrocephalus either in the form of ventriculomegaly or extra-axial or interhemispheric CSF fluid collections will be evident in 50% to 80% of these patients. When necessary these patients will be treated with external ventricular or subdural drains followed by early cranioplasty (replacement of the bone plate). In many instances these changes will resolve following cranioplasty and therefore avoid the need for ventriculoperitoneal shunting, with its associated risks and complications.

All patients with abnormal head CT scans (regardless of GCS score) are treated with close neurologic observation most commonly in an intensive care unit (ICU) setting, serial CT scans (4 to 6 hours later and on PID 1), and placed on 7 days of phenytoin (Dilantin). Temkin and colleagues showed that patients with post-traumatic

---

[1]Not FDA approved for this indication.

intracranial hemorrhage were at increased risk of suffering seizures in the acute period; treatment with antiepileptics beyond 7 days did not decrease the risk of these patients from developing epilepsy or delayed seizures but there were increased risks associated with side effects from medication administration. Patients who experience a seizure following CHI (with the exception of acute post-traumatic seizures) should be maintained on antiepileptics for at least 3 to 6 months and possible indefinitely depending on their clinical condition and EEG results. Patients with acute post-traumatic seizures (within the first several minutes following the event) are not felt to be at increased risk for developing further seizures and receive the routine 7-day treatment. At the University of Louisville we have found that changing phenytoin dosing to a weight-based schedule (15 mg/kg load, 2 mg/kg every 8 hours unless elderly [$\geq$70 years old], then 2 mg/kg every 12 hours) increases the chance of achieving a therapeutic dose earlier in the treatment course and lowers the costs of monitoring these agents.

Finally, the treatment of these patients requires a tight-knit group of specialists and ancillary service providers with open communication channels. We have found that the use of a time-independent phased outcome clinical pathway helps maximize the level of patient care and maintain cost-effectiveness. By using such an approach all routine interactions are initiated at the time of admission and each care provider has a clear role and responsibility; one of the most important aspects of this system is the creation of a clinical coordinator whose responsibility includes ensuring that all aspects of patient care and family education are completed at the appropriate intervals. We believe another key component of this is our philosophy toward early feeding (prior to PID 3) and early tracheotomy and percutaneous endoscopic gastrostomy (PEG) feeding tube placement in a majority of these individuals (PID 4). We have shown that such an aggressive approach to these issues helps reduce infectious complications and minimizes length of ICU stay.

Treatment of Mild and Moderate Traumatic Brain Injury

In many circumstances patients with moderate TBI are treated almost as though they had severe TBI, with the exception of invasive ICP monitoring. Many patients will be intubated at the time of admission and require sedation and adequate pain management. This can be difficult because it is of utmost importance to maintain the ability to perform serial neurologic examinations. Therefore, we commonly use a combination of propofol (Diprivan) infusions and intermittent morphine (Lioresal)[1] injections in these patients, thereby allowing hourly assessment of neurologic function. We have found that a subset of patients (older than age 45 years, multisystem trauma, presence of early pneumonia) with moderate TBI requires more aggressive treatment with early tracheostomy and PEG tube placement and at times ICP monitors.

The subset of patients with moderate TBI who are not intubated at the time of admission are also watched closely in the ICU. Once again, close monitoring of neurologic function and vigorous pulmonary toilet is of key importance because some patients may be lethargic and are at risk of pulmonary decompensation. We have found ipratropium (Atrovent)[1] and albuterol (Proventil)[1] nebulizers and early mobilization minimize pulmonary problems. Patients with progressive lethargy, worsening neurologic function, hypoxia, hypercapnia, or the inability to protect their airways are intubated and placed on mechanical ventilation. Once again, patients unable to tolerate a diet by PID 3 have a nasogastric feeding tube placed to allow for early enteral nutritional support; however, PEG tubes are not placed until later in the hospital course in the predischarge phase because many patients in this category will improve throughout their hospitalization and be able to tolerate an oral diet by the time of discharge.

Patients with mild TBI are treated over a much wider continuum, ranging from discharge from the emergency room (ER) with

appropriate adult supervision to observation in the ICU to immediate surgical treatment of surgical mass lesions. The two most important factors in determining treatment algorithms for these patients are presence or absence of abnormal CT findings and neurologic function, with associated symptoms such as nausea, vomiting, dizziness, or visual problems. Headache is a common complaint in all of these patients and must be taken in context with other complaints and imaging results. Patients with severe headaches, dizziness, and vomiting (postconcussive syndrome) may commonly require a brief hospital stay to allow for delayed imaging and at least partial resolution of some of the complaints.

Early and Delayed Neurologic Changes

Any patient suffering a significant neurologic injury requires close neurologic monitoring. Although most patients remain unchanged or show gradual improvement in the early phases, a small percentage will show signs of neurologic deterioration. At first these signs may be subtle (agitation, mild increase in lethargy, protracted vomiting); but eventually they may become more profound and can be precursors to impending neurologic demise and death. When these changes are the result of either expanding mass lesions or increases in ICP, treatment instituted in the early phases is more likely to be more successful compared to instances when interventions are performed under conditions associated with cerebral herniation syndromes. Thus any patient showing persistent signs of neurologic decline should be promptly evaluated by a physician and many may also require repeat CT scanning.

However, not all neurologic changes are the result of changes in ICP or expansion of mass lesions, and such irregularities may be caused by a long list of other metabolic or neurologic conditions. Some of the more common causes are seizures, strokes (especially from carotid or vertebral dissections), electrolyte imbalances, hypoxia, hypercarbia, fever, excess sedation, or drug and/or alcohol withdrawal.

Concussions and Sports-Related Injuries: Return to Play Guidelines

Over the past 2 decades, the knowledge regarding the detrimental effects of repetitive mild head injuries has led to intense public debate concerning whether athletes should be allowed to return to play following such injuries. Concussions are not uncommon among participants of competitive sports including football, hockey, baseball, and soccer. Concerns regarding the full negative impact of repetitive, almost innocuous injury have led many youth soccer leagues to ban or modify rules regarding *heading* of the ball. In addition, other concerns exist following more severe concussions such as development of other life-threatening neurologic injuries such as subdural or epidural hematomas, development of the double-impact syndrome (rapid uncontrolled increases in ICP following sequential minor traumas), and the long-term neuropsychological impact of these injuries. As a result of these concerns, the guidelines concerning when and if an athlete should be allowed to return to play have undergone modification since development of the earlier criteria. Because of these frequent changes, readers are encouraged to check with their local medical agencies or recent publications and Internet sources if faced with these issues. In short, if a player loses consciousness or has persistent symptoms (>15 to 20 minutes), he or she should not be allowed to return to play on that day or even not for 1 to 2 weeks following the complete resolution of all symptoms. It should also be stressed that an individual may have a concussion without loss of consciousness and that concussion is defined as any transient change in mental status. To this end many organizations including the National Football League have developed a sideline neuropsychological screening test that can often help illustrate these deficits even when the athlete appears normal.

---

[1]Not FDA approved for this indication.

Restorative Therapies

Patients suffering any type of TBI can have long-lasting cognitive, psychological, and emotional dysfunction in addition to their functional and neurologic deficits. Although most people assume that the resolution of decreased alertness and consciousness symbolizes resolution of the overall neurologic injury, this is not the case in most patients. In our series of patients with moderate TBI, we found that almost 50% of patients at median follow-up of 27 months complained of persistent emotional or cognitive problems that interfered with their lifestyle despite the fact that they all were discharged from the hospital with a GCS score of 14 to 15. Long-term speech and cognitive therapies as well as individual, group, and family counseling will be helpful for many of these patients.

In the late hospital and early rehabilitative stages, numerous pharmacologic agents may be helpful to overcome some of the neurologic side effects following TBI. Patients with autonomic storms (intermittent episodes of diaphoresis, tachycardia, fever, agitation) may respond to adrenergic antagonists such as clonidine (Catapres)[1] or propanolol (Inderal),[1] in addition to volume resuscitation, morphine (Lioresal),[1] baclofen,[1] and bromocriptine (Parlodel).[1] Patients with hypoarousal are treated with amantadine[1] (Symmetrel), 100 mg at 8 am and 12 pm, and bromocriptine,[1] 5 to 15 mg every day. Trazodone (Desyrel), 50 to 100 mg at bedtime, may be helpful in restoring sleep-wake cycles, whereas risperidone (Risperdal),[1] olanzapine (Zyprexa),[1] and quetiapine (Seroquel)[1] may be helpful to control agitation and combativeness during the subacute recovery phases.

Future Considerations

The previously mentioned treatment strategies include what is considered common practice at the University of Louisville; however, newer, more aggressive treatments and monitoring capabilities are always being developed. Some of the newer monitoring systems under development include cerebral oximetry measurements (frequently through invasive indwelling catheters) or cerebral microdialysis systems, in which continuous assessments are performed to determine the concentrations of critical markers such as lactate in the brain or CSF. Both of these methods provide physiologic feedback for the metabolic environment of the brain, are sensitive enough to predict changes in regional oxygenation, and have been found to be correlated with outcomes in small nonrandomized studies.

---

[1]Not FDA approved for this indication.

REFERENCES

Brain Trauma Foundation. Management and Prognosis of Severe Traumatic Brain Injury. New York: Brain Trauma Foundation; 2000.

Mcilvoy L, Spain DA, Raque G, et al. Successful incorporation of the Severe Head Injury Guidelines into a phased-outcome clinical pathway. J Neurosci Nurs 2001;33(2):72–8 82.

Miller PR, Fabian TC, Bee TK, et al. Blunt cerebrovascular injuries: Diagnosis and treatment. J Trauma 2001;51(2):279–86.

Temkin NR, Dikmen SS, Wilensky AJ, et al. A randomized, double-blind study of phenytoin for the prevention of post-traumatic seizures. N Engl J Med 1990;323:497–502.

Vitaz TW, McIlvoy L, Raque GH, et al. Development and implementation of a clinical pathway for severe traumatic brain injury. J Trauma 2001;51(2):369–75.

Vitaz TW, McIlvoy L, Raque GH, et al. Development and implementation of a clinical pathway for spinal cord injuries. J Spinal Disord 2001;14(3):271–6.

Vitaz TW, Jenks J, Raque GH, Shields CB. Outcome following moderate traumatic brain injury. Surg Neurol 2003;60(4):285–91.

Traumatic Brain Injury in Children

Method of
Stephen R. Deputy, MD

Traumatic brain injury (TBI) is one of the leading causes of death and disability among children, adolescents, and young adults. An estimated 185 per 100,000 children (ages 0 to 14 years) and 550 per 100,000 adolescents (ages 15 to 19 years) are hospitalized each year for TBI. The etiology of TBI varies depending on the age of the patient, with younger children more likely to be injured from falls and pedestrian injuries, and adolescents more often injured in motor vehicle accidents and assaults. Inflicted TBI (shaking-impact syndrome of infancy) is the leading cause of injury-related deaths in children younger than 4 years of age and accounts for 80% of deaths from head trauma in children younger than 2 years of age.

Types and Severity of Head Injury

Closed head injury is the most common type of TBI seen in children. Forces from rapid deceleration are applied diffusely throughout the brain and consciousness is frequently impaired. *Open head injuries*, in which the dura is breached, are caused by focal penetrating forces, and the risk of post-traumatic epilepsy is relatively high.

Primary brain injury is caused by the mechanical forces of the trauma itself. Diffuse axonal injury is an example of primary brain injury. During rapid deceleration, angular forces applied to the head cause the brain to rotate about its center of gravity. Shifting regions of differing densities within the brain itself result in shearing along planes such as the gray-white junction, corpus callosum, and brainstem. The shearing of axons effectively serves to "disconnect" the cortex from the brainstem and consciousness becomes impaired. Translational (straight-line) forces applied to the head produce impact-loading contact phenomena, resulting in focal injuries to the scalp, skull, and brain, such as lacerations, skull fractures, cerebral contusions, and epidural hematomas. *Subdural hematomas* may occur because of tearing of fragile dural bridging veins during rapid decelerations.

Secondary brain injury follows and is the consequence of primary injury. Examples include hypoxic-ischemic injury (secondary to low cerebral perfusion pressure or anoxia), disrupted cerebral autoregulation, seizures or status epilepticus, diffuse cerebral edema, hydrocephalus, and raised intracranial pressure. The goal of treatment for TBI is to reduce or prevent secondary brain injury from occurring because the primary brain injury has already happened at the time of trauma and cannot be altered.

The severity of TBI can be broken down into mild, moderate, and severe. *Mild* TBI is defined as head trauma with an initial Glasgow Coma Scale (GCS) score of 13 to 15. *Moderate* TBI occurs with an initial GCS score of 9 to 12. *Severe* TBI occurs with an initial GCS score of 8 or less. The GCS is modified for use in infants under the age of 36 months (Table 1).

Special attention should be given to those infants with TBI who do not show evidence of external facial or head trauma and who may not be presented by their caregivers as having a history of head injury. The *shaking-impact syndrome* is usually found in infants younger than 3 years of age with a peak incidence in infants younger than 1 year of age. Presenting symptoms include irritability, lethargy, or coma, apnea or breathing irregularities, and seizures. Retinal hemorrhages may be found in from 65% to 95% of these patients and should be actively looked for with a dilated funduscopic examination in any case where head trauma is suspected. Computed tomography (CT) imaging most commonly shows evidence of acute or remote subdural hematomas with or without evidence of cerebral infarction. Workup should include a skeletal survey to look for evidence of skull, posterior rib,

TABLE 1 Glasgow Coma Scale for Children

Score	Eyes Open	Best Verbal Response	Best Verbal Response	Best Motor Response (<36 mo)	Best Motor Response (<36 mo)
6	—	—	—	Follows commands	Normal spontaneous movements
5	—	Oriented and converses	Coos and babbles	Localizes pain	Withdraws to touch
4	Spontaneously	Confused	Irritable to pain	Withdraws to pain	Withdraws to pain
3	To verbal commands	Inappropriate words	Cries to pain	Flexor posturing	Flexor posturing
2	To painful stimuli	Nonspecific sounds	Moans to pain	Extensor posturing	Extensor posturing
1	None	None	None	No response	No response

or long bone fractures of different healing stages. Infants may be more susceptible to shaking-impact syndrome given their relatively large head size compared to their underdeveloped neck musculature. Infants also have thinner skulls, and translational forces may cause more severe contusions. Relatively longer subdural veins that bridge the infant's enlarged subarachnoid spaces can be easily lacerated from angular forces, resulting in subdural hematomas.

Management of Traumatic Brain Injury in Children

MILD TRAUMATIC BRAIN INJURY

Mild TBI accounts for more than 90% of all pediatric admissions for TBI. Children in this category should have a GCS score of 15 upon arrival to the emergency room, no focal neurologic deficits, and no signs of increased intracranial pressure (ICP). These children may have had a brief loss of consciousness (less than 1 minute), amnesia for the event, an immediate impact seizure, vomiting, or lethargy (as long as the GCS score is 15 during the evaluation). Children without loss of consciousness or amnesia may be observed or sent home with competent caregivers without performing neuroimaging studies. Vigilance for any change in the child's neurologic status should be maintained for up to 72 hours after the injury. If there has been a brief loss of consciousness or amnesia for the event, the risk of intracranial hemorrhage is still relatively low, and it is up to the discretion of the treating physician whether CT imaging is warranted.

Clinical predictors of intracranial hemorrhage are less reliable for children under the age of 2 years, and nonaccidental trauma also comes into consideration in this age group. Therefore, most children under the age of 2 years with TBI should undergo CT imaging followed by careful observation.

MODERATE TRAUMATIC BRAIN INJURY

Patients who fall within the moderate category generally need more intensive monitoring and medical management to avoid secondary brain injuries. As with all critical illness, attention should first be paid to following the ABCs (airway, breathing, circulation).

Airway

Patients with a GCS score of 9 or greater usually do not require endotracheal intubation for airway protection, although they should be kept NPO (nothing by mouth) in case of clinical deterioration.

Breathing

Hypoxemia and hypoventilation may increase ICP, so supplemental oxygen by nasal cannula may be helpful.

Circulation

It is important to avoid hypotension to maintain adequate cerebral perfusion pressure (CPP). Isotonic intravenous fluids should be provided with care to avoid fluid overload, hypoglycemia, or hyperglycemia. Careful attention should be paid to fluid and sodium balance because these patients may be at risk for developing diabetes insipidus. Likewise, the head of the bed should be raised to 30 degrees and the patient's head kept midline to optimize venous return from the cranium to the right side of the heart. Sedation with short-acting sedatives (propofol [Diprivan] or midazolam [Versed]) or opioids may be necessary to avoid agitation, which can also reduce venous return to the heart.

Early post-traumatic seizures are fairly rare in children with moderate TBI. The need for empirical anticonvulsant therapy in this group remains controversial and should be reserved for those patients in whom raised intracranial pressure is of concern. Likewise, empirical use of mannitol has little clinical support for this group.

SEVERE TRAUMATIC BRAIN INJURY

Patients in the severe group are at the highest risk for secondary brain injuries. The following additional interventions are recommended.

Airway

By definition, these patients have a GCS score of 8 or lower and require endotracheal intubation for airway protection.

Breathing

Hyperventilation with a goal Pco_2 of 26 to 30 mm Hg should be performed only if there is impending brainstem herniation or to bridge the gap until more definitive neurosurgical intervention can be performed to lower intracranial pressure. The benefit of hyperventilation is generally short lived (1 to 24 hours) and may worsen local ischemia following trauma or acute stroke.

Circulation

In the setting of suspected raised intracranial pressure, the goal of fluid and blood pressure management should be to maintain the cerebral perfusion pressure greater than 50 to 70 mm Hg. Recall that CPP equals MAP (mean arterial blood pressure) minus ICP. Because children generally have a lower MAP than adults, it is not always necessary to provide vasopressor therapy to keep the CPP above 70 mm Hg unless there is evidence of raised ICP. Invasive intracranial pressure monitoring should be considered if the GCS score is lower than 8 or in the setting of elevated ICP to optimize CPP.

Other Techniques to Lower Intracranial Pressure

NEUROSURGICAL

Obvious mass lesions, such as hydrocephalus, subdural and epidural hematomas, and contused cortical tissue should be surgically evacuated whenever feasible. CT scanning is able to identify most of these surgical lesions. Decompressive craniectomy is now used more frequently to relieve pressure when multifocal contusions or diffuse cerebral edema is present. As mentioned earlier, ICP monitoring is usually warranted for all severe TBI patients.

CURRENT DIAGNOSIS

- Children under the age of 2 years with traumatic brain injury (TBI) may require neuroimaging because clinical predictors of intracranial hemorrhage are less reliable in this age group.
- Children under the age of 1 year presenting with lethargy, irritability, apnea, or seizures should be evaluated with computed tomography (CT) imaging and a dilated funduscopic examination to rule out shaking-impact syndrome.

OSMOTHERAPY

Mannitol (20% solution) may be given as an initial bolus of 0.5 to 1 g/kg. Repeat doses of 0.25 to 0.5 g/kg are given every 6 to 8 hours as needed to maintain the serum osmolality and sodium levels to less than or equal to 320 mOsmL and 150 mEq, respectively. Osmotic diuretics should be used with caution in patients with renal insufficiency. The beneficial effects occur within minutes, peak at 1 hour, and last 4 to 24 hours. Potential disadvantages include worsening of focal cerebral edema in areas where the blood-brain barrier is disrupted.

BARBITURATES

Sedating agents may lower ICP by reducing pain as well as by making the brain metabolically less active. Pentobarbital is given as a loading dose of 5 to 20 mg/kg, followed by a continuous infusion of 1 to 4 mg/kg per hour. Continuous EEG monitoring to maintain a burst suppression pattern is warranted with this therapy. Potential disadvantages include systemic hypotension and a long half-life that may interfere with the declaration of brain death.

ANTICONVULSANT THERAPY

Children with severe TBI are at a high risk for early post-traumatic seizures, which can further elevate the ICP. It is generally recommended empirically to load these children with 20 mg/kg of intravenous phenytoin (Cerebyx). Maintenance therapy can be achieved with 5 mg/kg per day divided every 8 hours with target blood levels of 10 to 20 mg/dL.

HYPOTHERMIA

More centers are including hypothermia as an option for patients with elevated ICP not responsive to medical or surgical management. The best method of cooling (i.e., whole body versus head only) and the optimal core temperature are not established for children.

CURRENT THERAPY

- Children with mild TBI and a GCS score of 15 at presentation can usually be observed clinically without the need for neuroimaging.
- The goal of treatment for TBI is to minimize *secondary* brain injury.
- In the setting of raised ICP, it is important to maintain CPP above 50 to 70 mm Hg.
- Early post-traumatic seizures are relatively frequent in open head injury and in severe TBI. They should be empirically treated in any patient in whom raised ICP is a concern.
- Direct intracranial pressure monitoring should be considered in any TBI patient with a GCS score of 8 or less.

Abbreviations: CPP = cerebral perfusion pressure; ICP = intracranial pressure; GCS = Glasgow Coma Scale; TBI = traumatic brain injury.

Of note, apart from neurosurgical interventions, none of the techniques just described are shown definitively to reduce morbidity or mortality in children with severe TBI.

REFERENCES

Annegers JF, Grabow JD, Grover RV, et al. Seizures after head trauma: A population study. Neurology 1980;30:683–9.

Bruce DA, Zimmerman RA. Shaken impact syndrome. Pediatr Ann 1989;18:482–94.

Committee on Quality Improvement. American Academy of Pediatrics: The management of minor closed head injury in children. Pediatrics 1999;104 (6):1407–15.

Deputy SR. Shaking-impact syndrome of infancy. Semin Pediatr Neurol 2003;10(2):112–9.

Kraus JF, Nourjah P. The epidemiology of uncomplicated brain injury. J Trauma 1988;28:1637–43.

Schutzman SA, Barnes P, et al. Evaluation and management of children younger than two years old with apparently minor head trauma: Proposed guidelines. Pediatrics 2001;107:983–93.

Brain Tumors

Method of
Douglas E. Ney, MD, and Andrew B. Lassman, MD

More than 64,000 primary brain tumors were diagnosed between 1998 and 2002, yielding an incidence of 14.8 brain tumors per 100,000 people. For children and men between 20 and 39 years old, these tumors represent the second leading cause of death. Metastatic disease is much more common, with more than 100,000 symptomatic intracranial metastases diagnosed every year. Data suggest that the incidence of primary and metastatic tumors is increasing, although this may partially reflect advances in diagnosis.

Patients with brain tumors typically develop signs over a period of weeks to months, although occasionally onset is abrupt (e.g., seizure). Initial symptoms typically are nonspecific and are related to the anatomic location of the tumor. Frontal tumors may be particularly difficult to diagnosis because they may involve symptoms of personality or mood changes, which may be misdiagnosed as depression. Other common signs include headache, nausea, vomiting, seizures, weakness, double vision, tinnitus, personality change, confusion, and difficulty walking.

Magnetic resonance imaging (MRI) remains the gold standard for imaging brain tumors. It gives the best anatomic detail of the brain and enables superior localization. Ultimately, definitive diagnosis is based on histopathologic characteristics (Table 1). Noninvasive techniques being developed to assist in treatment planning include magnetic resonance spectroscopy, which allows biochemical measurement of a region of interest, and the findings may correlate with tumor histology. Perfusion MRI helps to determine tumor vascularity, which may be a marker for tumor grade. However, it is unclear how best to incorporate magnetic resonance spectroscopy or perfusion into routine clinical care. Computed tomography (CT) is helpful in characterizing calcification, which is more common in oligodendrogliomas than in astrocytomas, and identifying hemorrhage. It is also superior for determining bony involvement of the skull. Positron emission tomography (PET) provides metabolic imaging of tumors, and uptake of radiolabeled isotopes may increase in proportion to tumor grade.

Gliomas

Gliomas are tumors that resemble glia such as astrocytes, ependymal cells, and oligodendrocytes. Together, gliomas account for 40% of all primary brain tumors and 78% of all malignant brain tumors.

TABLE 1 WHO Classification of Common Primary Brain Tumors

Histologic Class	Subtype	WHO Grade
Astrocytic tumors	Subependymal giant cell astrocytoma	I
	Pilocytic astrocytoma	I
	Pleomorphic xanthoastrocytoma	I
	Astrocytoma	II
	Anaplastic astrocytoma	III
	Glioblastoma	IV
Oligodendroglial tumors	Oligodendroglioma	II
	Anaplastic oligodendroglioma	III
	Oligoastrocytoma	II
	Anaplastic oligoastrocytoma	III
Ependymal tumors	Subependymoma	I
	Myxopapillary ependymoma	I
	Ependymoma	II
	Anaplastic ependymoma	III
Meningeal tumors	Meningioma	I
	Atypical meningioma	II
	Anaplastic or malignant meningioma	III
	Hemangiopericytoma	II
	Anaplastic hemangiopericytoma	III
	Hemangioblastoma	I

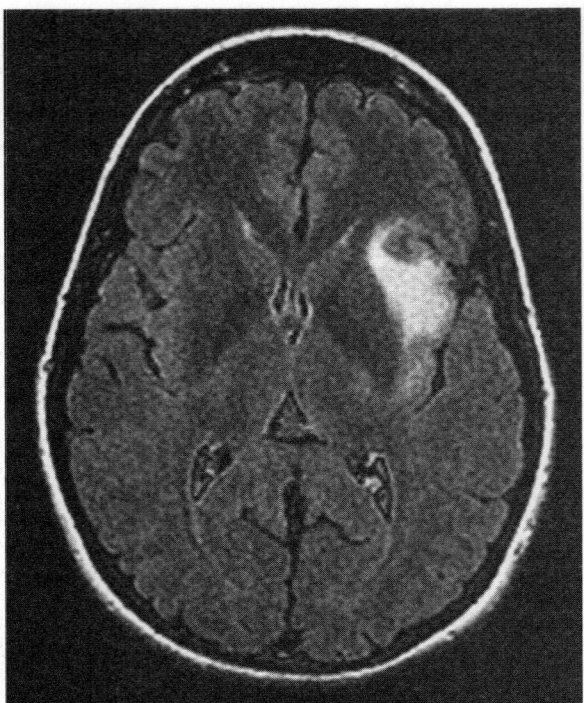

FIGURE 1. FLAIR MRI sequence of a brain shows a low-grade (WHO grade II) astrocytoma.

Gliomas are classified by histologic type and by levels of aggressiveness. Histologically, astrocytomas comprise most gliomas, and oligodendrogliomas represent only 10%.

LOW-GRADE GLIOMAS

World Health Organization (WHO) grade I astrocytomas, most commonly juvenile pilocytic astrocytomas, typically arise in the cerebellum of children and may be amenable to surgical cure. Their biology is different from the other gliomas (WHO grades II through IV), which are all diffusely infiltrating tumors without clean margins between tumor tissue and normal brain, making surgical cure impossible.

In adults, most low-grade gliomas are supratentorial, and they appear as nonenhancing masses on brain MRI (Fig. 1). After maximal surgical resection, low-grade (WHO grade II) astrocytomas and oligodendrogliomas usually are treated with radiation therapy (RT). A dose of approximately 50 Gy is standard because higher doses increase toxicity without improving survival. The timing of RT remains controversial because it may prolong progression-free survival but not overall survival. Observation may be a reasonable approach in young and otherwise healthy patients with small tumors that have predominantly oligodendroglial histology, who have undergone gross total resection, and who are asymptomatic. Older patients with poor performance status, neurologic symptoms, and large, bi-hemispheric tumors not amenable to extensive resection should undergo RT. Chemotherapy is not routinely used at diagnosis except in a research setting, although the use of temozolomide (Temodar), an oral alkylating agent that is generally well tolerated, is an emerging treatment (Table 2).

In almost all cases, WHO grade II gliomas are incurable diseases. With time, tumors accumulate molecular oncogenic abnormalities, leading to more aggressive behavior. In this manner, they transform into high-grade gliomas.

HIGH-GRADE GLIOMAS

Anaplastic (WHO grade III) astrocytomas are treated with RT, although some clinicians treat them analogously to glioblastoma (GBM) with irradiation and temozolomide. Treatment of anaplastic oligodendrogliomas or oligoastrocytomas is controversial, but commonly used approaches include RT, chemotherapy, and chemoradiation therapy. Two trials demonstrated that the addition of

chemotherapy with the combination of procarbazine (Matulane),[1] lomustine (CCNU, CeeNU), and vincristine (Oncovin)[1] (PCV regimen) to RT likely prolongs progression-free but not overall survival (see Table 2). It remains controversial whether the improvement in progression-free survival outweighs the potential toxicity of the PCV regimen. Temozolomide has become the most commonly used form of chemotherapy for oligodendrogliomas, but a direct comparison with PCV has not been conducted.

GBM (WHO grade IV) is the most common glioma subtype (>50% of all gliomas), and it is also the most aggressive, with an average survival of about 1 year. GBMs can arise from lower-grade gliomas (i.e., secondary GBMs). Alternatively, tumors can manifest as GBM first without a history of a lower-grade glioma (i.e., de novo or primary GBMs). Primary and secondary GBMs are histologically identical and are treated in the same manner.

The current standard of care for patients with GBM who are younger than 70 years and have good baseline performance status is maximal surgical resection followed by RT to a dose of approximately 60 Gy, with concurrent and adjuvant temozolomide (see Table 2). The typical MRI appearance involves a contrast-enhancing abnormality with a necrotic center (Fig. 2). Fluid attenuation inversion recovery (FLAIR) imaging shows an abnormality encompassing a nonenhancing tumor and surrounding edema (Fig. 3). Compared with treatment with surgery and RT, the addition of temozolomide administered concurrently with RT and for 6 months after RT improves median survival from 12.1 to 14.6 months. Although modest, this benefit is sustained, with 2-year survival rates of 10% and 27% for those treated with RT alone and RT with temozolomide, respectively. Some advocate placement of carmustine (BCNU)-containing wafers (Gliadel) into the operative bed, and this approach is associated with a prolongation of survival, although it can also contribute to wound-healing difficulties.

Older patients or those with poor performance status may benefit from postoperative RT and temozolomide. However, they are sometimes treated with an abbreviated course of RT (fewer fractions and higher dose per fraction) or occasionally with temozolomide alone.

---

[1]Not FDA approved for this indication.

TABLE 2 Common Chemotherapy Regimens for Brain Tumors

Regimen	Generic Name	Trade Name	Dose
Temozolomide	Temozolomide	Temodar	75 mg/m² daily during radiotherapy for approximately 6 weeks 150–200 mg/m², days 1–5 of 28 not during radiotherapy
PCV	Procarbazine	Matulane¹	60 mg/m²/day (oral), days 8–21 of 56
	Lomustine	CCNU, CeeNU	110 mg/m² (oral), day 1 of 56
	Vincristine	Oncovin¹	1.4 mg/m² (2-mg cap) IV, days 8 and 29 of 56
Bevacizumab +/–	Bevacizumab	Avastin	10 mg/kg, days 1 and 8 of 14
Irinotecan	Irinotecan	CPT-11, Camptosar¹	125 mg/m²* or 340 mg/m²,† days 1 and 8 of 14

¹Not FDA approved for this indication.
Patients not taking* or taking† concurrent hepatic P-450 enzyme-inducing antiseizure drugs such as phenytoin (Dilantin), fosphenytoin (Cerebyx), phenobarbital, primidone (Mysoline), carbamazepine (Tegretol, Carbatrol), or oxcarbazepine (Trileptal).

For recurrent or progressive disease, repeat resection with or without intracavitary carmustine wafer placement, intravenous carmustine (BiCNU), and temozolomide for naive patients are accepted standard options. However, their relatively poor efficacy rates lead many patients to participate in clinical trials. Results with antiangiogenic therapy, such as bevacizumab (Avastin) have generated enthusiasm, but serious toxicity (especially thromboembolic events) occurs in a substantial minority of patients. Bevacizumab recently received accelerated FDA approval for progressive GBM.

Brainstem gliomas are a heterogeneous group of tumors that account for less than 5% of all gliomas. Most occur in childhood, although the prognosis is usually better in adults. Imaging is usually sufficient for diagnosis. Surgery is restricted to biopsy alone, usually only when diagnosis is in question. Treatment for large or symptomatic lesions consists of RT. No chemotherapeutic regimens have been beneficial in treating brainstem gliomas.

Several factors are important in determining prognosis for patients with gliomas, including age, performance status, tumor histology and grade, extent of surgery, and presence of neurologic deficits. In adults, median survival for low-grade (WHO grade II) and anaplastic (WHO grade III) astrocytomas is about 5 and 2 years, respectively. Oligodendrogliomas are associated with longer survival times than astrocytomas of the same grade. For example, low-grade and anaplastic oligodendrogliomas have median survival times of about 10 and 4 years, respectively. However, there is a wide range of survival times for oligodendrogliomas, and the prognosis in part depends on molecular analysis of tumor tissue. Loss of heterozygosity of chromosomes 1p and 19q in oligodendrogliomas has been associated with better overall survival and better response to treatment. O6-Methylguanine DNA methyltransferase (MGMT) promoter methylation appears to correlate with increased sensitivity to temozolomide and improved prognosis, especially for GBM.

Meningiomas

Meningiomas account for approximately 30% of all brain tumors, with an incidence of 4.5 tumors per 100,000 people, and they represent the most common primary brain tumor. They occur most often in the elderly population and affect women two to three times more often than men. One identifiable risk factor is previous cranial irradiation.

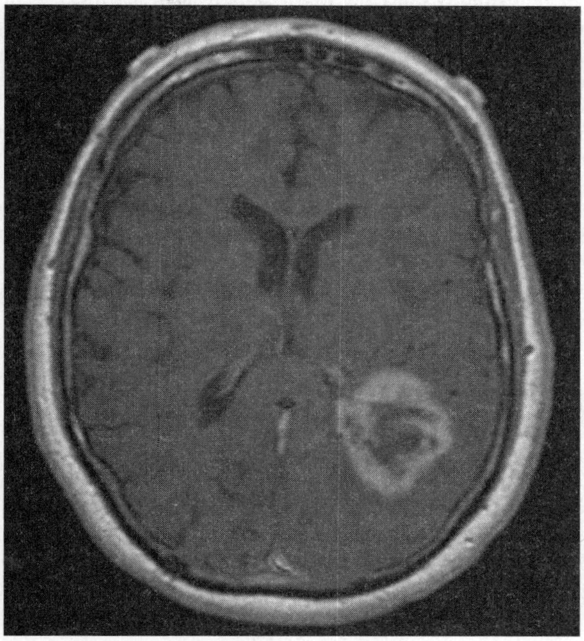

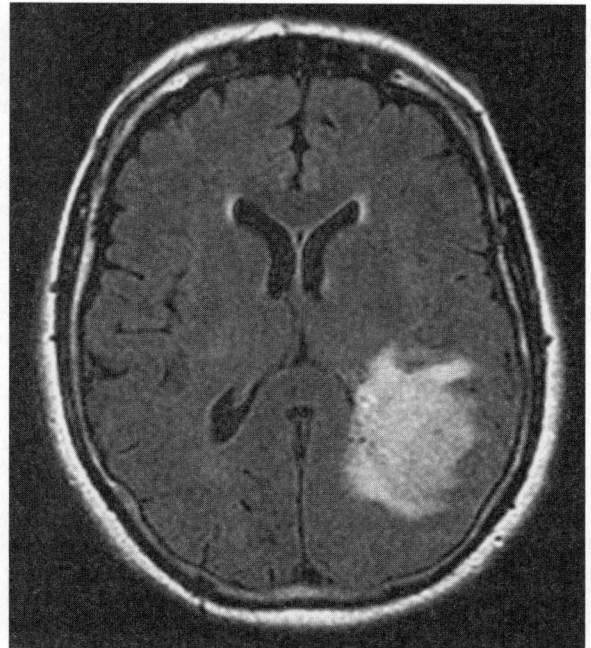

FIGURE 2. Contrast-enhanced MRI shows the typical appearance of a glioblastoma.

FIGURE 3. FLAIR MRI sequence (same patient as in Figure 2) shows a nonenhancing tumor and surrounding edema.

Meningiomas arise from arachnoid cap cells of the meninges. Loss of genetic material from chromosome 22 has been reported in the development of meningiomas. Accumulation of other chromosomal mutations may lead to the development of atypical or anaplastic meningiomas. Radiation-induced meningiomas usually are atypical or anaplastic.

Many histologic subtypes of meningioma exist, but grading has been the source of much debate. The WHO classifies meningiomas as benign (grade I), atypical (grade II), or anaplastic (grade III). Grading largely depends on the amount of mitotic activity in the tumor. Together, atypical and anaplastic meningiomas account for less than 10% of meningiomas.

Meningiomas are slow-growing tumors, and many are asymptomatic and discovered incidentally. In these cases, the decision to treat may be controversial, and observation is frequently recommended. However, treatment is usually indicated for patients presenting with neurologic symptoms or unusual radiographic features. Surgery remains the primary treatment modality. Surgery with curative intent requires complete excision. Because meningiomas are highly vascular tumors, they are sometimes embolized preoperatively.

After surgery, benign meningiomas undergoing complete excision usually do not warrant RT. However, RT may be useful for subtotal resections. If the tumor recurs, RT may be undertaken after a second resection. Atypical or malignant meningiomas always require RT. Chemotherapy has little established role in treatment of meningiomas. Hydroxyurea (Hydrea)[1] offers modest benefit for otherwise refractory disease. Other agents are under investigation.

Primary Central Nervous System Lymphoma

Primary central nervous system lymphoma (PCNSL) is a non-Hodgkin's lymphoma involving any part of the craniospinal axis and the eyes, usually without evidence of systemic disease. It accounts for 3% of all intracranial tumors and has an incidence of approximately 0.5 per 100,000 people. Two populations are affected by PCNSL: the immunocompetent and the immunocompromised. Whether congenital or acquired, immune suppression is the major established risk factor for this disease. Most PCNSLs in the immunosuppressed population are related to latent Epstein-Barr virus infection.

The treatment of PCNSL involves multiple modalities. Surgery is used only to make the diagnosis, usually by stereotactic biopsy. Debulking of tumor is not undertaken except when there is diagnostic confusion or impending herniation from large tumors causing increased intracranial pressure. In contrast to treatment of other brain tumors, corticosteroids can have a direct effect on lymphoma cells, leading to significant improvement and sometimes to resolution of the tumor burden. Corticosteroids should be withheld until after biopsy, if medically safe. The use of corticosteroids alone, however, rarely produces sustainable remission. Although it is a radiosensitive tumor, it is unclear whether whole-brain radiotherapy (WBRT) along with chemotherapy is superior to chemotherapy alone. Given the risk of delayed neurotoxicity, particularly in those older than 60 years, WBRT is often deferred and later used for relapsing disease. For ocular lymphoma, however, irradiation of the globes usually is typically considered mandatory.

The mainstay of chemotherapy is high-dose methotrexate, although ideal regimens continue to be under investigation. Doses from 3 to 8 g/m^2 are routinely used[3] to attain high tissue concentrations across the blood-brain barrier. Most regimens still use this as the basis of therapy, adding additional agents such as vincristine (Oncovin),[1] procarbazine (Matulane),[1] and cytarabine (Tarabine).[1] Other agents that cross the blood-brain barrier, such as temozolomide (Temodax),[1] are being investigated, as is the B-cell antibody rituximab (Rituxan).[1]

Outcome is worse for patients older than 60 years, those who are immunocompromised, and those with poor pretreatment performance status. WBRT produces a median survival of 12 to 18 months, whereas methotrexate-based regimens produce a median survival of 40 to 60 months. The risk of relapse approaches 50%, usually occurring within the first 2 years of diagnosis. There is no consensus strategy to manage relapsed PCNSL, but treatment may consist of any of the modalities used to treat a first occurrence, including prior chemotherapy.

Metastatic Disease

Metastatic disease remains the most common intracranial neoplasm, with approximately 200,000 people diagnosed every year. Approximately one half of patients have one metastasis, and the remaining patients have multiple lesions. Cancers of the lung, breast, and skin (melanoma) most commonly metastasize to the brain. Renal cell carcinoma and colon cancers also are common primary tumors. Diagnosis of a brain metastasis in a patient without a known primary cancer should always prompt a systemic evaluation.

Supportive treatment is based on the type and severity of symptoms. Symptomatic brain edema is frequently encountered in this population and usually is managed with corticosteroids such as dexamethasone (Decadron) in dosages between 16 and 100 mg/day.[3] Patients who are on corticosteroids for an extensive period (>6 weeks) should receive prophylaxis against *Pneumocystis jiroveci* pneumonia. Prophylactic anticonvulsants are not given unless the patient develops seizures.

Anti-convulsant use of surgery for patients with one brain metastasis is well established. Patients who undergo resection followed by WBRT (typically 30 to 35 Gy in 10 to 15 fractions) have improved survival, reduced local recurrence rates, and longer functional independence than patients undergoing WBRT alone. Whether patients who undergo complete resection should receive postoperative WBRT remains controversial because of concerns about long-term neurotoxicity from RT. However, postoperative WBRT clearly reduces local and whole-brain recurrence rates.

For patients with multiple metastases, WBRT is a standard approach, although surgical resection of up to three discrete lesions has been advocated by some, especially if there is a dominant lesion amenable to resection. Stereotactic radiosurgery (SRS) is increasingly used in the treatment of brain metastases. It involves high-dose radiation delivered to small areas of disease, and it may be most effective against tumors that are relatively resistant to standard RT. SRS is limited in that only lesions that are less than 3 cm (at most 4 cm) are amenable to treatment without substantially increasing the risk of toxicity. Chemotherapy may be beneficial, particularly among chemotherapy-naive patients and those with chemosensitive primary tumors (e.g., breast, lung). Standard regimens are those that are useful in the treatment of the underlying disease as long as they penetrate the blood-brain barrier. Agents such as temozolomide[1] and tyrosine kinase inhibitors are under investigation.

For untreated patients, median survival is 1 to 2 months. RT alone yields a meager median survival of 4 to 6 months, although most will experience neurologic improvement. Patients with a single brain metastasis that is excised, and who have systemic disease under good control, have a 10% to 15% 5-year survival rate.

Leptomeningeal Disease

Leptomeningeal disease results from infiltration of the covering of the brain with malignant cells, which usually are metastatic from an extrameningeal primary tumor. It can involve any area of the brain or spinal cord. Like solid brain metastases, the incidence of leptomeningeal metastases is increasing despite increased survival from systemic cancers. The increase is likely related to the poor penetrance

---

[1]Not FDA approved for this indication.
[3]Exceeds dosage recommended by the manufacturer.

---

[1]Not FDA approved for this indication.
[3]Exceeds dosage recommended by the manufacturer.

of systemic chemotherapies through the blood-brain barrier, allowing malignant cells to grow within the CNS as a sanctuary site.

Treatment of leptomeningeal disease is largely palliative. Corticosteroids and RT may alleviate neurologic symptoms. Despite the diffuse nature of the disease, focal RT to affected areas, such as WBRT for patients with headache or cranial neuropathies, may be helpful. In cases of cerebrospinal fluid blockade, hydrocephalus may develop, which sometimes requires ventriculoperitoneal shunting, although WBRT or focal RT to painful or bulky areas of spinal leptomeningeal disease may be helpful. Intrathecal treatment with methotrexate (Methotrexate LPF),[1] cytarabine (in free and depot formulations [Tarabine PFS, DepoCyt]),[1] and systemic chemotherapy have been used in patients able to tolerate such therapy. Ideally, intrathecal chemotherapy should be administered through an Ommaya reservoir. Systemic therapy with high-dose (3.5 g/m^2 body surface area)[3] intravenous methotrexate[1] may be helpful, especially for patients with breast cancer.

Prognosis depends performance status, bulk of CNS disease, extent of systemic cancer, and tumor type. Patients with breast cancer and lymphoma may survive longer than most, for whom the average is at best a few months.

---

[1]Not FDA approved for this indication.
[11]Required to enroll in the manufacturer's prescribing program.

REFERENCES

Abrey LE, Ben-Porat LL, Panageas KS, et al. Primary central nervous system lymphoma: The Memorial Sloan-Kettering Cancer Center prognostic model. J Clin Oncol 2006;24:5711–5.

Central Brain Tumor Registry of the United States. Statistical report: Primary brain tumors in the United States, 1998–2002, Available at http://www.cbtrus.org [accessed July 2009].

Gavrilovic IT, Posner J. Brain metastases: Epidemiology and pathophysiology. J Neurooncol 2005;75:5–14.

Gilbert MR, Lang FF. Anaplastic oligodendroglial tumors: A tale of two trials. J Clin Oncol 2006;24:2689–90.

Karim AB, Maat B, Hatlevoll R, et al. A randomized trial on dose-response in radiation therapy of low-grade cerebral glioma: European Organization for Research and Treatment of Cancer (EORTC) study 22844. Int J Radiat Oncol Biol Phys 1996;36:549–56.

Louis DN, Ohgaki H, Wiestler OD, et al. WHO Classification of Tumours of the Central Nervous System. 4th ed. Lyon: International Agency for Research on Cancer; 2007.

Patchell RA, Tibbs PA, Regine WF, et al. Postoperative radiotherapy in the treatment of single metastases to the brain: A randomized trial. JAMA 1998;280:1485–9.

Patchell RA, Tibbs PA, Walsh JW, et al. A randomized trial of surgery in the treatment of single metastases to the brain. N Engl J Med 1990; 322:494–500.

Stupp R, Mason WP, van den Bent MJ, et al. Radiotherapy plus concomitant and adjuvant temozolomide for glioblastoma. N Engl J Med 2005; 352:987–96.

van den Bent MJ, Afra D, de Witte O, et al. Long-term efficacy of early versus delayed radiotherapy for low-grade astrocytoma and oligodendroglioma in adults: The EORTC 22845 randomised trial. Lancet 2005; 366:985–90.

Vredenburgh JJ, Desjardins A, Herndon JE, et al. Bevacizumab plus irinotecan in recurrent glioblastoma multiforme. J Clin Oncol 2007;25:4722–9.

Westphal M, Ram Z, Riddle V, et al. Gliadel wafer in initial surgery for malignant glioma: Long-term follow-up of a multicenter controlled trial. Acta Neurochir (Wien) 2006;148:269–75.

The Locomotor System

Rheumatoid Arthritis

Method of
Arthur Kavanaugh, MD, and
Venkata Sri Cherukumilli, BS

Rheumatoid arthritis (RA) is a progressive, systemic inflammatory disease that affects about 0.5% to 1% of the population worldwide. RA is associated with substantial morbidity and accelerated mortality, and it exerts a tremendous economic toll on affected patients, their families, and society. Women are three to four times more likely to be affected than men. The peak age of onset is between 40 and 60 years, but it is possible to get RA at any age, and it affects the elderly and young children.

Even though there has been progress in deciphering the cellular and molecular mechanism of RA, the cause is still not fully defined. RA is characterized by synovial and vascular proliferation with the formation of pannus tissue, which results in damage to articular cartilage and adjacent subchondral bone. Activation of specific $CD4^+$ T cells, potentially in response to unidentified antigens, in an immunogenetically susceptible individual is hypothesized to be an early event in this process. Activated T cells orchestrate a cell-mediated immune response, stimulating and interacting with monocytes or macrophages, synovial fibroblasts, osteoclasts, B cells, and many other cell types. The cascade of inflammatory mediators that is released contributes to the sustenance of the ongoing immune activation and directly causes signs, symptoms, and sequelae of the disease, such as destruction of joints. Joint destruction, which may be considered the sequela of untreated inflammation over time, correlates directly with functional disability. Impaired function correlates with many key outcomes, such as increased mortality and greater costs.

Diagnosis

RA diagnosis is mainly clinical based on physical findings, patient history, and ongoing observation of symptoms, signs, and response to therapy. The American College of Rheumatology (ACR) classification for the diagnosis of RA requires at least four of seven features to be present, and the first four criteria must be present for at least 6 weeks (see Current Diagnosis box).

Treatment

The main goals of treatment for RA are to alleviate pain, prevent or limit joint damage, optimize quality of life, avoid complications of therapy, and improve or preserve function. Novel therapies with specific targets are being designed based on the improved understanding of the pathophysiology of RA. Adoption of an aggressive approach early in the course of the disease is thought to be the best way to prevent irreversible joint damage and to spare patients years of pain and discomfort. Remission, once a purely hypothetical consideration, is now considered to be an appropriate and attainable goal, largely due to the introduction of new therapies, particularly biologic agents, and new treatment paradigms, particularly the frequent assessment of disease activity with resultant changes in treatment to achieve low disease activity.

Treatment response in clinical trials is typically measured using the ACR criteria for measuring improvement of arthritis. The ACR20 refers to 20% improvement in tender and swollen joint counts and 20% improvement in three of the five additional measures: patient and physician global assessments of arthritis, pain, disability, and an acute-phase reactant, such as the erythrocyte sedimentation rate (ESR) or C-reactive protein (CRP). Variations that define higher levels of response—the ACR50 and ACR70, which require improvements in individual measures exceeding 50% and 70%, respectively—are more stringent outcomes. The Health Assessment Questionnaire (HAQ) and Short Form 36 (SF-36) are used to calculate functional disability and health-related quality of life, respectively. Joint damage in patients with RA is assessed by quantifying radiographic changes characteristic of RA, including joint space narrowing and periarticular bony erosions.

Treatment of RA begins after the diagnosis is established, baseline activity is assessed, and prognosis is estimated. Therapy is initiated with patient education about the disease and the treatments available. Symptoms can be controlled to some extent with nonsteroidal anti-inflammatory drugs (NSAIDs) and low-dose oral glucocorticoids or

CURRENT DIAGNOSIS

- Morning stiffness in and around the joint that lasts for 1 hour before maximal improvement
- Arthritis (i.e., soft tissue swelling or fluid) in three or more joint areas simultaneously observed by a physician
- Arthritis involving the wrist, metacarpophalangeal, or proximal interphalangeal joints
- Symmetrical arthritis that involves same joint areas on both sides of the body
- Rheumatoid nodules (i.e., subcutaneous nodules over bony prominences, extensor surfaces, or in juxtaarticular regions) observed by a physician
- Positive serum rheumatoid factor test result
- Radiographic changes typical of RA on the posteroanterior hand and wrist

glucocorticoid joint injections. Ideally, disease-modifying antirheumatic drugs (DMARDs) should be started soon after diagnosis is established (e.g., within 3 months). Further care is determined by assessing disease activity and response to treatment. The Current Therapy box lists commonly used treatments for RA and includes trade names and usual maintenance doses for these drugs.

ANALGESICS AND NONSTEROIDAL ANTIINFLAMMATORY DRUGS

Analgesics (e.g., acetaminophen, tramadol [Ultram], opioids) are used to relieve pain, but they do not reduce inflammation or prevent joint destruction. NSAIDs (e.g., aspirin, ibuprofen [Motrin], naproxen [Naprosyn], ketoprofen [Orudis], piroxicam [Feldene], diclofenac [Voltaren], celecoxib [Celebrex]) reduce pain and inflammation (at higher doses) but do not slow joint damage. These drugs are used as adjuncts but are not usually the sole treatment for RA because they do not prevent disease progression.

Although many analgesics and NSAIDs are available over the counter and are perceived by patients to be benign, they are not risk free. Narcotic analgesics should be used with caution because of their potential for habituation and toxicity with chronic use. NSAIDs work by inhibiting cyclooxygenase enzyme isoforms COX-1 and COX-2. COX-1 is constitutively expressed by many cells, whereas COX-2 production is usually increased at sites of inflammation. Side effects with chronic use of NSAIDs include gastrointestinal irritation, rash, fluid retention, and the potential for renal toxicity. Acetaminophen (Tylenol), a non-NSAID COX inhibitor, does not cause gastrointestinal irritation, but it may cause severe hepatotoxicity, and it potentially interacts with warfarin (Coumadin). The frequency of NSAID-induced ulcers can be reduced with concomitant use of proton pump inhibitors or misoprostol (Cytotec). COX-2 inhibitors were developed because their more specific activity was expected to control signs and symptoms of arthritis with less risk of gastrointestinal complications. However, two of the three COX-2 inhibitors approved in the United States were withdrawn due to concerns about thrombotic and atherosclerotic toxicities; the remaining available COX-2 inhibitor, celecoxib, seems to have a safety profile comparable to other NSAIDs in that regard.

GLUCOCORTICOIDS

Oral glucocorticoids at lower doses (e.g., <10 mg prednisone equivalent per day) are often used to control pain, inflammation, and stiffness, and they potentially can slow progression of joint damage. However, because of the possibility of significant side effects, especially with long-term use at a high dose, glucocorticoids are most commonly used for short-term treatment of very active or aggressive RA, usually in combination with NSAIDs and DMARDs. They are often tapered when the disease is under control.

Side effects of glucocorticoids include changes to appetite and weight, glucose intolerance or hyperglycemia, infection, osteoporosis, mood and sleep disturbances, hypertension, suppression of the hypothalamic-pituitary axis, and interference with wound healing, among others. Administering calcium and vitamin D supplementation, bisphosphonates, calcitonin (Miacalcin),[1] parathyroid hormone (teriparatide [Forteo]),[1] and estrogen[1] or testosterone[1] replacement can reduce the risk of bone loss in patients taking corticosteroids.

Intraarticular glucocorticoid injections can provide dramatic but usually temporary clinical improvement in patients who have a disease flare in a single or a few joints. Most clinicians think that no more than one injection in any 3-month period should be made in a given joint. The need for more repeated injections suggests that the overall treatment plan requires reevaluation.

DISEASE-MODIFYING ANTIRHEUMATIC DRUGS

DMARDs are the mainstay of treatment for RA because they can modify various aspects of the immune and inflammatory responses, potentially controlling signs and symptoms of disease and slowing its progression. Extensive clinical studies of DMARDs have

[1]Not FDA approved for this indication.

demonstrated reductions in joint damage, preservation of joint function, and higher rates of productivity. DMARDs are considered first-line therapy for all patients with newly diagnosed RA. The standard of care is to initiate DMARD therapy early, such as within the first 3 months of disease for patients with established RA who, despite adequate treatment with NSAIDs, have ongoing joint pain, significant morning stiffness or fatigue, active synovitis, evidence of active inflammation (e.g., persistent elevation of the ESR or CRP level, actively inflamed joints) or radiographic joint damage. Because DMARDs may take 2 to 6 months to reach full effect, NSAIDs and sometimes glucocorticoids can be used in the interim to reduce pain and swelling. The duration of DMARD use may be limited by loss of efficacy or development of toxicity.

Methotrexate (Rheumatrex) is the most commonly used DMARD because of its oral, once-weekly administration; well-defined safety profile; demonstrated efficacy; and low cost. Sulfasalazine (Azulfidine EN-tabs) or hydroxychloroquine (Plaquenil) tends to be used in persons whose disease is considered milder or more slowly progressive. They are also used in combination with methotrexate for aggressive disease. Leflunomide (Arava) was shown in several phase III trials to offer comparable efficacy to methotrexate and sulfasalazine against active RA. Older drugs in this class (e.g., parenteral or oral gold [aurothiomalate or auranofin], azathioprine [Imuran], D-penicillamine [Cuprimine]) were shown to be effective in older clinical trials, but they are less commonly used now largely due to tolerability issues.

In RA, methotrexate's mechanism of action may be related to its inhibition of inflammation, presumably by increasing the local release of adenosine. Clinical response may take 6 to 8 weeks to be seen. The mean dose used among RA patients worldwide is approximately 17.5 mg/week, although many clinicians initiate therapy at lower doses to help ensure tolerability. Most clinicians consider 25 mg/week to be a maximum dose. Higher doses are not clearly associated with better disease control but may be associated with more toxicity. Parenteral administration may be used at doses higher than 15 mg/week because of more predictable absorption. Many RA patients have taken methotrexate successfully for years, attesting to its efficacy and safety.

Leflunomide is a prodrug that is actively metabolized after oral administration. This active metabolite inhibits dihydroorotate dehydrogenase, which interferes with pyrimidine synthesis and ultimately leads to inhibition of activated T cells and other cells. To minimize toxicity, the maintenance dose of 20 mg/day can be reduced to 10 mg/day.

Although DMARDs represent a major advance in the management of RA, they are not without risks or limitations. Methotrexate is associated with rare but serious side effects, including bone marrow suppression, hypersensitivity pneumonitis, and hepatotoxicity. It may also slightly increase the risk of infection. It must be used with caution in patients with preexisting liver disease, renal impairment, significant pulmonary disease, or alcohol abuse. Less serious but common side effects of methotrexate include stomatitis, gastrointestinal effects, headache, fatigue, and liver transaminase elevations. Folic acid supplementation can prevent many of the minor side effects. Leflunomide can lead to elevated liver enzyme levels, weight loss, hypertension, diarrhea, reversible alopecia, and myelosuppression. Leflunomide inhibits cytochrome P-450 (CYP) 2C9, so there is a theoretical potential for interactions with other drugs that are also CYP2C9 substrates. Methotrexate and leflunomide necessitate regular monitoring of liver enzymes and complete blood cell counts at regular intervals. Treatment should be stopped for any persistent or severe abnormalities.

Other side effects seen with various DMARDs include gastrointestinal intolerance and rash. Although antimalarial drugs (e.g., hydroxychloroquine) have been reported to cause ocular toxicity, with current dosages and preparations, this reaction is rare. Sulfasalazine may cause cutaneous adverse events (e.g., urticaria, maculopapular rash, photosensitivity) and hematologic side effects. Cyclosporine's use has been limited by its toxicity, which includes headache, tremors, hypertension, and renal insufficiency. Patients taking cyclosporine (Neoral) require regular monitoring of blood pressure and serum creatinine levels. Some DMARDs (e.g., cyclophosphamide [Cytoxan],[1] chlorambucil [Leukeran],[1] azathioprine) may promote the development of secondary malignancies. Some DMARDs are teratogenic and abortifacient and therefore should not be used during pregnancy or breast-feeding and must be discontinued for an appropriate amount of time, typically 3 months or more, before any attempts to conceive.

BIOLOGIC RESPONSE MODIFIERS

The introduction of biologic agents was driven largely by three factors: recognition of the unmet clinical need for more effective treatments based on an appreciation of the significantly poor outcomes of uncontrolled RA; improved understanding of the immunopathogenesis of RA; and advances in biopharmaceutical science allowing the development of specific inhibitors of relevant targets within the dysregulated immune system.

Traditional therapies such as NSAIDs, corticosteroids, and DMARDs may help ameliorate the symptoms of RA, but they rarely induce sustained remission, and they can have toxicities that prevent their long-term use. Newer therapies, many of which are large protein molecules such as monoclonal antibodies or soluble receptor constructs, are referred to as biologic agents. Biologic agents, particularly inhibitors of tumor necrosis factor (TNF), have changed the treatment paradigm for RA. They can inhibit various components of the immune system and inflammatory response that are central to the pathogenesis of RA. The goal is to adopt an early, proactive approach to treatment to prevent the damage from chronic synovial inflammation. Studies have shown that biologic agents can slow disease progression, control signs and symptoms of disease, improve function, and improve quality of life. They are typically used in combination with DMARDs, most commonly methotrexate, to potentiate treatment responses. This newer class of antirheumatic drugs can be further subclassified according to their specific target or mechanism.

Tumor Necrosis Factor-α Inhibitors

Use of TNF-α inhibitors in combination with methotrexate is considered by many to be the gold standard for treatment of RA. TNF-α is a soluble 17-kDa protein homotrimer that binds to two receptors: type 1 TNF receptor and type 2 TNF receptor. A versatile, multipotent cytokine, it induces production of other inflammatory cytokines such as interleukin-1 (IL-1), IL-6, and granulocyte-monocyte colony-stimulating factor (GM-CSF) and chemokines such as IL-8. TNF-α causes tissue destruction by promoting release of matrix metalloproteinases, upregulates cell trafficking through adhesion molecules and chemokines, increases the breakdown of proteoglycans in the cartilage, and potentiates osteoclast differentiation and activation. There is abundant evidence that TNF inhibition dramatically improves patient outcomes for RA and other autoimmune systemic inflammatory conditions, including psoriasis, psoriatic arthritis, ankylosing spondylitis, and inflammatory bowel disease.

Most RA patients respond to TNF-α inhibitors with a reduction in signs and symptoms, improved quality of life, and preservation of functional status; some even achieve clinical remission of disease. Radiographic evidence shows that TNF-α inhibitors inhibit radiographic disease progression to an extent not seen with any previous agents. From an immunologic standpoint, TNF-α inhibitors do not represent a cure, and maintenance of clinical efficacy almost always requires continued therapy, certainly for patients with long-standing RA. Five of the available biologic agents are inhibitors of TNF-α: infliximab (Remicade), etanercept (Enbrel), adalimumab (Humira), golimumab (Simponi), and certolizumab pegol (Cimzia).

Infliximab, a chimeric human/mouse monoclonal anti-TNF-α monoclonal antibody, was shown to be effective initially in open trials, followed soon by double-blind, placebo-controlled, randomized clinical trials. Inhibition in the progression of joint damage and improvement in health-related quality of life and functional status were observed in patients treated with infliximab. It is used mostly in combination with methotrexate, which decreases immunogenicity and produces synergy in clinical outcomes.

Etanercept is a recombinant form of the human receptor that is fused to the Fc fragment of the human immunoglobulin G1. Clinical trials have shown etanercept to be effective in improving the signs and symptoms of RA when used as monotherapy and in combination with methotrexate; it also inhibits disease progression and optimizes functional status and quality of life.

Adalimumab is a human anti-TNF-α monoclonal antibody. The efficacy of adalimumab on the signs and symptoms of RA has been proved in various studies, and it has demonstrated benefit in terms of improving quality of life and functional status and in attenuating the progression of joint damage.

Certolizumab pegol is a PEGylated Fab' fragment of a humanized monoclonal anti-TNF antibody. Golimumab is a human anti-TNFα monoclonal antibody. Both of these recently approved agents have been shown to improve signs and symptoms of disease and physical function, and to prevent disease progression in patients with active RA.

TNF antagonists exhibit a rapid onset of action, provide significant clinical response, improve quality of life, and most importantly, substantially inhibit radiographic progression of disease. Most patients on TNF antagonists are still treated with methotrexate because studies have shown that TNF antagonists work better in this combination. There are some safety concerns because reports of opportunistic infections, tuberculosis, lymphoma, administration reactions, immune or autoimmune responses, and demyelinating syndromes have emerged with TNF antagonist treatment. Some patients do fail to respond or eventually lose the ability to respond. Other biologic agents can be effective for patients who fail anti-TNF therapy.

Interleukin-1 Receptor Antagonist

IL-1 appears to have a prominent role in synovial inflammation and displays many overlapping effects with TNF-α. RA patients have increased levels of IL-1 in the plasma and synovial fluid, and its concentration has been correlated with disease activity. Similar to TNF-α, IL-1 can activate a variety of inflammatory cells and mediators using some overlapping signal transduction pathways.

Anakinra is a subcutaneously administered IL-1 receptor antagonist. Anakinra has been shown in several studies to reduce the signs and symptoms of RA; however, the extent of improvement is less than that seen with TNF antagonists. Combination therapy with anti-IL-1 and anti-TNF is contraindicated because of an observed increase in the risk of adverse events in a study in which patients were treated with anakinra and etanercept. Anakinra usually is well tolerated, and the most common side effect is injection site reactions. The need for daily injectable administration and the modest efficacy compared with TNF inhibitors have limited the use of anakinra. Tocilizumab is a recently approved humanized anti-IL-6 receptor monoclonal antibody. It has been shown to reduce signs and symptoms and improve functional status and to inhibit radiographic progression in patients with active RA.

B-Cell Directed Therapy

Mounting evidence suggests that B cells play an active role in RA. B cells can accumulate in the synovium, form aggregates, produce autoantibodies such as rheumatoid factor (RF), and function as antigen-presenting cells that aid in the activation of CD4+ T cells. These findings provide the rationale for targeting B cells in RA patients. Rituximab (Rituxan) is a monoclonal antibody directed against the CD20 antigen found on the surface of B cells. When bound to CD20, rituximab depletes B cells through various mechanisms, including complement-mediated lysis, antibody-dependent cytotoxicity, and apoptosis.

Rituximab treatment induced depletion of peripheral-blood B cells for 6 months or longer, but the levels of immunoglobulins in the serum (IgG, IgA, IgM) did not change substantially. RF levels decreased substantially. Despite the prolonged depletion of peripheral-blood B cells, the overall incidence of infection was similar in the control group and the rituximab groups. However, an increased rate of infusion-related reactions was identified for the rituximab group compared with the placebo group. In patients with active RA who failed one or more anti-TNF-α therapies, rituximab significantly reduced signs, symptoms, fatigue, and disability and improved health-related quality of life.

---

[1]Not FDA approved for this indication.

CURRENT THERAPY

Nonpharmacologic Treatment

- Patient and family education and longitudinal supportive care by physicians and their staff
- Physical therapy and occupational therapy for patients with compromised activities of daily living
- Dynamic and aerobic conditioning exercises to improve mobility, strength, and psychological well-being

Pharmacologic Treatment

NSAIDs and Selective Cyclooxygenase 2 (COX-2) Inhibitors

- Improve joint function by reducing joint pain and swelling

Glucocorticoids

- Can relieve signs and symptoms of disease, and may slow progression
- Use low-dose glucocorticoids, such as <10 mg of prednisone daily or the equivalent
- Local injections of depot formulations of corticosteroids
- Bridge therapies for flares or when starting treatment

Disease-Modifying Antirheumatic Drugs (DMARDs)

- Can preserve joint integrity and function by reducing joint damage
- Commonly used DMARDs:
  - Methotrexate (Rheumatrex) PO 7.5 to 25 mg/week; injectable 7.5 to 25 mg/week
  - Hydroxychloroquine (Plaquenil) 200 mg twice daily
  - Sulfasalazine (Azulfidine-EN Tabs)[3] 1000 mg twice or three times daily
  - Leflunomide (Arava) 20 mg/day in a single dose, if tolerated; otherwise, 10 mg/day
  - Cyclosporine A (Neoral)[3] ≈2.5 to 4.5 mg/kg/day in divided doses (twice daily)
  - Combinations of DMARDs that have been effective in RA include methotrexate plus cyclosporine, methotrexate plus leflunomide, and methotrexate plus sulfasalazine plus hydroxychloroquine.

[3]Exceeds dosage recommended by the manufacturer.

Biologic Response Modifiers (Biologics)

- Commonly used in combination with methotrexate or less commonly with other DMARDs
- Slow or prevent disease progression (particularly TNF inhibitors) and can induce remission
- TNF-α inhibitors:
  - Infliximab (Remicade) intravenous infusion of doses between 3 and 10 mg/kg (mean dose, ≈5 mg/kg) with additional similar doses at 2 and 6 weeks after the first infusion and then every 8 weeks thereafter
  - Etanercept (Enbrel) = SQ injection 50 mg/week (given as a single dose of 50 mg once per week or 25 mg biweekly)
  - Adalimumab (Humira) SQ injection 40 mg every other week (also approved for use weekly)
- Interleukin-1 receptor antagonist: anakinra (Kineret) SQ injection 100 mg/day
- Anti-CD20 antibody: rituximab (Rituxan) two 1000-mg IV infusions separated by 2 weeks; further treatments are typically given after 6 months when disease activity recurs
- CTLA-4-immunoglobulin: abatacept (Orencia) IV infusion for initial dose, followed by doses 2 and 4 weeks later, with further doses every 4 weeks thereafter; dosage between 500 and 1000 mg based on weight (dose approximates 10 mg/kg)

Surgical Treatment

- Surgery is used for patients with intolerable pain, loss of range of motion, or structural joint damage that leads to limitation of function.
- Procedures include joint fusion, synovectomy, total joint arthroplasty, and partial joint replacement or remodeling.

T-Cell Directed Therapy

T-cell activation plays a central role in the pathogenesis of RA. For example, the rheumatoid synovium contains a preponderance of CD4[+] T cells. It is thought that these cells are stimulated by arthritogenic antigens to initiate synovial inflammation. Cytotoxic T lymphocyte–associated antigen 4 (CTLA4) is expressed on the surface of T cells within days after they have become activated. CTLA4 binds to and prevents CD80 and CD86 from binding to CD28, thereby effectively blocking the costimulatory signal required for activation of T cells. Blocking CD28 costimulation has been shown to induce T-cell anergy.

Abatacept (Orencia), an inhibitor of T-cell costimulation, is a fusion protein construct consisting of the extracellular component of CTLA4 fused to the Fc region of human IgG, which increases its half-life. The high affinity of CTLA4-Ig for CD28 prevents B7-mediated costimulation. Abatacept has improved signs and symptoms of disease, helped to maintain physical function, and reduced progression of joint damage in patients with active disease despite concomitant methotrexate. Similarly, it improved signs and symptoms, physical function, and health-related quality of life in RA patients refractory to TNF-α inhibition.

Biologic agents have different mechanisms, methods of delivery, and side effects. A patient who does not respond to or cannot tolerate one may still have a good outcome with another. Although they are commonly used in combination with methotrexate, biologic agents usually are not given in combination with each other, because this approach may increase risk without much increase in benefit. Because biologic agents modulate part of the immune response, there is concern about potential side effects related to impaired immune function, such as increased risk of minor and serious infections and secondary malignancies.

Biologic agents require parenteral administration: subcutaneous injections (e.g., etanercept, adalimumab, anakinra certolizumab, golimumab) or intravenous infusions (e.g., infliximab, abatacept, rituximab, tocilizumab). These routes are less convenient than orally administered drugs and can be associated with administration reactions, such as injection-site or infusion reactions. Biologic agents are also more expensive than traditional DMARDs, which has affected their use. However, the increased clinical benefit seen with these agents needs to be considered in any comprehensive cost-efficacy analysis.

Conclusions

RA is a prevalent disease and a leading cause of physical disability. There is no cure for RA. However, with available agents applied appropriately, clinical remission is the goal of therapy and is a realistic expectation for some patients. When remission is not achieved, the rheumatologist must look for the most effective combination of therapies to alleviate pain, maintain function, and maximize quality of life. Methotrexate is still the mainstay of long-term care, but newer biologic DMARDs provide additional benefits. The role of biologic agents is still evolving. Their use is often reserved for patients who fail to respond to methotrexate, but the trend is toward earlier use of these agents. NSAIDs and glucocorticoids are useful for bridge therapy in patients with acute symptoms, especially while waiting for DMARDs to reach their maximal effect. Patients should be evaluated periodically for evidence of disease activity and progression and for drug toxicity. The management strategy should be changed if there is progressive joint damage, evidence of ongoing activity after 3 months of maximal treatment, or if treatment is poorly tolerated.

REFERENCES

American College of Rheumatology Subcommittee on Rheumatoid Arthritis Guidelines. Guidelines for the management of rheumatoid arthritis: 2002 update. Arthritis Rheum 2002;46:328–46.

Arnett FC, Edworthy SM, Bloch DA, et al. The American Rheumatism Association 1987 revised criteria for the classification of rheumatoid arthritis. Arthritis Rheum 1988;31:315–24.

Chang J, Kavanaugh A. Novel therapies for rheumatoid arthritis. Pathophysiology 2005;12:217–25.

Doan QV, Chiou CF, Dubois RW. Review of eight pharmacoeconomic studies of the value of biologic DMARDs (adalimumab, etanercept, and infliximab) in the management of rheumatoid arthritis. J Manag Care Pharm 2006;12: 555–69.

Felson DT, Anderson JJ, Boers M, et al. for the American College of Rheumatology: Preliminary definition of improvement in rheumatoid arthritis. Arthritis Rheum 1995;38:727–35.

Olsen NJ, Stein M. New drugs for rheumatoid arthritis. N Engl J Med. 2004;350:2167–79.

Scott D, Kingsley G. Biologics in Rheumatoid Arthritis. Inflammatory Arthritis in Clinical Practice. London: Springer; 2007.

Juvenile Idiopathic Arthritis

Method of
James N. Jarvis, MD

The term *juvenile idiopathic arthritis* (JIA) is now the internationally accepted term to describe a family of illness characterized by chronic inflammation of synovial membranes. It replaces, but does not completely overlap, the diagnostic classification system that used the term *juvenile rheumatoid arthritis*. Three major phenotypes of JIA are recognized: oligoarticular, polyarticular, and systemic. In addition, the accepted international classification scheme recognizes other subtypes (e.g., enthesitis-associated arthritis, which overlaps the family of conditions previously designated *spondyloarthropathies*) that have distinct clinical phenotypes and that the clinician must recognize against the general background of children presenting with musculoskeletal complaints. Because each of these subtypes represents a distinct phenotype based on presentation, age of onset, differential diagnosis, and therapy, each of these illnesses is described as a distinct entity.

Oligoarticular Juvenile Idiopathic (Pauciarticular) Arthritis (Pauciarticular Juvenile Rheumatoid Arthritis)

EPIDEMIOLOGY

Oligoarticular JIA (*pauciarticular JRA* under the old American College of Rheumatology criteria) is typically a disease of preschoolers of European descent. This subtype of JIA is quite rare in African American children, children from the Indian subcontinent, and Native American children.

RISK FACTORS

Specific human leukocyte antigen (HLA) alleles, particularly in the class II locus, are known to confer risk for this JIA subtype. However, different alleles are seen in different ethnic subgroups, even in European populations. Thus, the presence of specific HLA alleles is not clinically useful for the diagnosis of most forms of monoarticular JIA. Older boys presenting with monoarthritis might, in fact, have what is now termed enthesitis-associated arthritis (EAA), for which the presence of class I HLA allele B27 can often be a diagnostic clue, because this allele is a major risk factor for developing EAA.

Young age (onset before the age of 3 years) and the presence of antinuclear antibodies (ANA) are specific risk factors for the development of uveitis in children with established disease. Slit-lamp examination (see "Complications," later) are recommended every 4 months for children in this high-risk group.

PATHOPHYSIOLOGY

The pathophysiology of this form of JIA is not well understood. Once generally accepted as an autoimmune disease, the high percentage of autoantibodies (especially ANA) in perfectly healthy children makes it more difficult to assess their pathologic significance in children with arthritis. Under any circumstances, what is generally accepted is that leukocyte invasion of the synovium transforms it into a growing, locally invasive tissue that secretes cytokines (thus sustaining the inflammatory process) and proteolytic enzymes that can injure surrounding joint structures.

PREVENTION

This illness is not known to be preventable.

CLINICAL MANIFESTATIONS

Children with pauciarticular JIA typically present with a combination of relatively painless joint swelling, often in combination with gait disturbance. The gait disturbance, when present, is typically more prominent after periods of inactivity (e.g., first thing in the morning or after a nap). Verbalized musculoskeletal pain is almost never a prominent presenting complaint. Although children seldom verbalize pain, they might express some distress when the affected joint is moved.

DIAGNOSIS

This illness typically occurs in preschool children, with a female-to-male ratio of about 3:1. In older children and teenagers with monoarticular disease, diagnoses other than JIA should be considered. Children typically present with relatively painless swelling of a lower extremity joint.

Gait disturbance, most prominent after periods of inactivity (e.g., first thing in the morning or after an afternoon nap) is often a prominent symptom. Careful palpation of lower extremity joints typically reveals warm, thickened synovial tissue. An effusion might or might not be present if the affected joint is a knee. Laboratory tests are not particularly helpful, except in excluding other diagnoses (e.g., Lyme disease, leukemia).

The diagnosis is typically established on the basis of the history and physical examination. Laboratory studies may be necessary to exclude other causes of monoarticular or oligoarticular joint swelling, particularly in children not in the typical demographic (e.g., older children or children of non-European ancestry). No single laboratory test or set of laboratory tests establishes the diagnosis. ANA and rheumatoid factor (RF) tests are particularly unhelpful, because of the low positive predictive value of the former and the low positive and negative predictive values of the latter.

DIFFERENTIAL DIAGNOSIS

In a typical clinical setting, the diagnosis is usually straightforward. In areas of North America and Europe where Lyme disease is endemic, Lyme disease is a more-common cause of monoarticular

CURRENT DIAGNOSIS

- Isolated musculoskeletal pain is almost never the presenting complaint of children with chronic forms of arthritis. Relatively *painless* joint swelling, often associated with gait disturbance, is more common.
- The laboratory has very limited use in making the diagnosis of juvenile idiopathic arthritis (JIA). Anti-nuclear antibody (ANA) tests have limited utility because they are so commonly positive in perfectly healthy children (as many as 30%), and the titers that healthy children have directly overlap those seen in children with JIA. Thus, the test cannot discriminate a healthy child from one with JIA and should not be used for that purpose. Rheumatoid factor (RF) tests have the opposite problem: They are seldom positive in children with JIA, and only the minority of children with positive RF tests have JIA or any other rheumatic disease. The low positive and negative predictive values of the test make it virtually useless for diagnostic purposes. This test should never be ordered as a means of evaluating musculoskeletal pain in children.
- The hallmark for making the diagnosis of JIA is the presence of warm, thickened synovial membranes that can be palpated around the joints of affected children. The presence of hypertrophic synovial tissue around the joint(s) of a child with a typical history and clinical setting is virtually diagnostic of JIA.

joint swelling than oligoarticular JIA. Lyme arthritis can usually be established or excluded on the basis of a screening enzyme-linked immunosorbent assay (ELISA) and Western blot analysis. In preschoolers presenting with severe musculoskeletal pain in a lower extremity joint, acute lymphocytic leukemia should be considered and investigated with one or more complete blood counts (CBC, performed serially), a serum lactate dehydrogenase (LDH), and possibly plain films to examine for periosteal elevation around the affected joint. In children from ethnic groups not typically within the oligoarticular JIA risk group (e.g., Native American children), a more determined search for nonrheumatic causes of monoarticular arthritis (e.g., tuberculosis) may be advisable.

TREATMENT

The goals of treatment are to rapidly re-establish normal function, prevent further intrusiveness of the disease process into normal activities, and prevent damage to the affected joint(s) and atrophy of the surrounding muscles. Rapid restoration of normal function is increasingly being addressed by the use of intraarticular steroid injections. Daily administration of nonsteroidal antiinflammatory drugs (NSAIDs; e.g., naproxen [Naprosyn], 10-20[3] mg/kg/day) can often

---

[3]Exceeds dosage recommended by the manufacturer.

CURRENT THERAPY

- Nonsteroidal antiinflammatory drugs
- Systemic glucocorticoids in select instances
- Oral or subcutaneous methotrexate (particularly for polyarticular disease)
- Anti-TNF (tumor necrosis factor) therapies, particularly for polyarticular disease
- Anti-IL-1 (interleukin-1) therapies, particularly in systemic disease

accomplish this same aim but take considerably longer to demonstrate efficacy. In a few cases, synovitis is intractable even with the combination of NSAIDs and joint injection, and in these cases, methotrexate, given either orally or subcutaneously at 10 to 20 mg/m[2]/week, typically provides good disease control. Treatment of uveitis is discussed later.

MONITORING

The disease process itself is monitored by interim histories and physical examinations. Slit-lamp examinations are a critical component of the monitoring of all children with JIA, because uveitis is typically indolent and asymptomatic. Children on daily NSAIDs should have a CBC (to monitor for occult blood loss) as well as comprehensive metabolic panel and urinalysis (to monitor for renal toxicity) at least twice a year. The same laboratory studies should be performed in children on methotrexate, although pediatric rheumatologists typically monitor more frequently (every 3-4 months) in children on that drug.

COMPLICATIONS

Before effective therapies were available, muscle atrophy and joint contracture were common complications of this form of JIA. Such sequelae are rare with current approaches to treatment. Uveitis remains the single most common and serious complication of this form of JIA and, even with new and more-aggressive therapies, uveitis often results in loss of some visual acuity in the affected eye(s). Diagnosis of this complication can only be made under slit-lamp examination, because signs and symptoms develop only later, when visual acuity is already severely compromised. Children in the highest risk group should have slit lamp examinations at least three times per year. The high-risk group includes children with a new diagnosis, who are 3 years of age or younger, and who are ANA positive; note that the ANA in this setting is used for prognostic, not diagnostic, purposes. The risk of uveitis is lifelong, and slit-lamp examinations should continue on a yearly basis throughout adulthood.

First-line therapy for uveitis typically includes topical corticosteroids. However, methotrexate and anti–tumor necrosis factor (TNF) monoclonal antibodies (infliximab [Remicade],[1] adalimumab [Humira]) have been shown to be effective in children with disease that is refractory, persistent, or recurrent.

Polyarticular Juvenile Idiopathic Arthritis

EPIDEMIOLOGY

Polyarticular JIA occurs in all age groups (although cases diagnosed in children younger than 1 year of age are rare) and in all ethnic groups. Polyarticular disease is further subcategorized based on the presence or absence of immunoglobulin M (IgM) RFs detected by standard laboratory tests. RF-positive children tend to be older (school-aged children and adolescents) and have severe synovitis, morning stiffness, and other constitutional symptoms. This subtype is more strongly represented among African American and Native American patients, where it represents as many as 50% of all cases of polyarticular JIA. It is rare in European and European-descended children, representing only 10% of all cases of JIA in that population.

RF-negative JIA occurs at all ages in European and European-descended children, from preschool ages to adolescence. African American and Native American children tend to be school-aged or adolescents.

RISK FACTORS

Specific HLA class II alleles are known to confer risk for RF-negative polyarticular JIA, but, as with pauciarticular disease, these associations vary among different ethnic groups and are not sufficiently

---

[1]Not FDA approved for this indication.

strong to be useful diagnostically. Alleles subsumed under the HLA-DR4 group are associated with RF-positive disease, particularly in Native Americans.

PATHOPHYSIOLOGY

The pathophysiology of polyarticular JIA is poorly understood. Once thought to be a typical autoimmune disease in which autoreactive T cells initiate an immune reaction against (unknown) joint or synovial antigens, that concept has come under challenge. Disease biomarker studies have suggested an important role for innate immunity in this JIA subtype, particularly monocytes and neutrophils. Under any circumstances, leukocyte infiltration of the synovium transforms it into a proliferating, invasive, and immunologically active tissue. Secretion of both cytokines and proteolytic enzymes plays an important role in causing local tissue damage. Gene expression profiling studies of peripheral blood suggest important roles for interferon (IFN)-γ and TNF-α in either initiating or sustaining the chronic inflammatory response.

PREVENTION

This illness is not known to be preventable. Given the strong association between tobacco smoking and HLA-DR4–positive RA in adults, it is possible that measures used to prevent tobacco abuse could reduce the incidence of disease in high-risk populations, such as members of specific Native American tribes.

CLINICAL MANIFESTATIONS

Because of the wide age range affected, clinical manifestations vary significantly for this JIA subtype. Preschoolers typically present with joint swelling and gait disturbance. Failure to gain or loss of major motor milestones is a fairly rare but well-described presentation in this age group. Joint swelling is the most common presenting complaint in older children and adolescents. Less than 20% of children with JIA verbalize pain at all on initial presentation. Morning stiffness lasting for an hour or more is typically seen in all age groups. Older children with wrist or finger involvement (or both) commonly complain of difficulty with fine motor tasks, such as playing a musical instrument.

DIAGNOSIS

As with oligoarticular JIA, musculoskeletal pain is not a common complaint at presentation in children with polyarticular JIA. Joint swelling, gait disturbance, or, in younger children, loss of (or failure to achieve) major motor milestones are more common presentations.

As with oligoarticular JIA, the laboratory is of limited utility. The diagnosis is made on the basis of the history and physical examination. The critical physical finding in polyarticular JIA is the presence of warm, thickened synovial membranes, typically including both large (knees, ankles) and small (fingers, toes) joints.

The diagnosis is established on the basis of a typical history (swelling in multiple joints, morning stiffness) and a physical examination demonstrating warm, thickened synovial membranes around multiple joints. Involvement of at least one wrist and small joints of the hands is typical. As with all other forms of childhood-onset arthritis, the laboratory is only of marginal use in making the diagnosis and is more useful in excluding other diagnoses. RF tests are singularly unhelpful and should not be ordered for diagnostic purposes. ANA tests are helpful only in excluding the diagnosis of systemic lupus erythematosus (SLE; see later under "Differential Diagnosis"). Thrombocytosis and mild anemia may be seen in severely affected children, but in such cases the history and physical examination have usually established the diagnosis without need of the laboratory.

DIFFERENTIAL DIAGNOSIS

Acute postinfectious arthritis can mimic polyarticular JIA. A distinguishing feature of postinfectious arthritis is the prominence of joint pain as a presenting complaint. Acute rheumatic fever (RF)

occasionally mimics polyarticular JIA, but the joint swelling of acute RF is typically exceptionally painfully and migratory (i.e., swelling moves from joint to joint and seldom lasts more than 24 hours in any given joint).

Acute leukemia occasionally manifests with painful swelling in multiple joints and should be considered in a child with swelling and severe musculoskeletal pain.

SLE is another entity that can present with swelling in multiple joints and constitutional symptoms. ANA tests may be helpful in establishing this diagnosis if the titer is 1:1080 or more. Titers between 1:320 and 1:640 are ambiguous, because these results can be seen in healthy children and in children with JIA. Serum C3 and C4 levels and a urinalysis should always be drawn when an ANA test is being requested for diagnostic purposes, because most children with SLE have low serum complement levels and an abnormal urinalysis. Thus, abnormal results from these tests can often clarify the ambiguity that emerges with ANA titers between 1:320-1:640.

TREATMENT

The goals of therapy for polyarticular JIA are identical to those for pauciarticular JIA: to rapidly reestablish normal function, prevent further intrusion of the disease process into normal activities, and prevent damage to the affected joint(s) and atrophy of the surrounding muscles. Very few children with polyarticular JIA have adequate clinical responses on NSAIDs alone, although these drugs (most commonly naproxen, 10 to 20[3] mg/kg/day in two divided doses) are often used.

More-aggressive treatment approaches are now typical in pediatric rheumatology, supported by recently published data that demonstrate that only 5% of children with this disease achieve remission within 5 years. Combinations of methotrexate (10-20 mg/m² given orally or subcutaneously), NSAIDs, and oral steroids are often used in children as first-line treatment. Joint injections with triamcinolone (Aristopan) are used to quickly restore function when activities of daily living or comfort are compromised by synovitis in one or a few joints. TNF inhibitors (etanercept [Enbrel], infliximab,[1] adalimumab) have all shown efficacy in children who have failed methotrexate, and there is a growing trend to use these drugs earlier in the disease course or even at presentation in severely affected children.

There is limited experience in pediatric rheumatology with the IL-1 inhibitor anakinra (Kineret),[1] in polyarticular in JIA, and many children find the required daily injections burdensome. Inhibitors of T cell costimulation signals (e.g., abatacept [Orencia]) have shown some efficacy in children but are generally reserved for children who have failed other therapies. Autologous stem cell transplantation has been shown to be efficacious in children who have failed multiple therapies and have a poor quality of life because of severe, persistent synovitis.

MONITORING

Monitoring for NSAIDs and methotrexate is described under the section on oligoarticular arthritis. Potential hepatic, renal, and bone marrow toxicities of TNF inhibitors are monitored exactly as is done for methotrexate. Because the TNF inhibitors can unmask latent tuberculosis, a PPD is required before starting anti-TNF therapy. All children with polyarticular JIA should be monitored for uveitis through routine slit-lamp examinations (see below).

Children on methotrexate and etanercept (with or without concomitant corticosteroid therapy) should be considered immunosuppressed. Thus, fever, unexplained pulmonary infiltrates, or other signs of infection might need to be investigated more vigorously than in an otherwise healthy child. Fever is almost never a sign of the underlying arthritis.

COMPLICATIONS

Uveitis is a complication of all forms of JIA, including polyarticular JIA. As with oligoarticular JIA, younger children who are ANA positive are at highest risk for this complication, and routine slit-lamp

---

[1]Not FDA approved for this indication.
[3]Exceeds dosage recommended by the manufacturer.

examinations are recommended. Treatment of uveitis is described in the section on oligoarticular arthritis. Anemia of chronic inflammation is often seen in children with severe polyarticular JIA. The most efficient way of treating this complication is to resolve the inflammatory process as rapidly as possible, and providing oral iron can attenuate or resolve this problem.

A severe, albeit rare, complication of polyarticular JIA is an entity called *macrophage activation syndrome*. This severe, sometimes fatal, complication is described in detail in the section on systemic disease.

Severe joint destruction is becoming rare in children with polyarticular JIA, but it still occurs, particularly in children who are RF positive. Joint replacement surgery has sometimes been useful in this setting.

Systemic-Onset Juvenile Idiopathic Arthritis

EPIDEMIOLOGY

All age groups are affected by systemic-onset JIA. This is one of the few forms of JIA that affects boys and girls equally. After RF-positive polyarticular JIA, this is the rarest form of JIA. However, this form of JIA may be proportionally more common in some Asian countries, including Japan.

RISK FACTORS

There are no known risk factors for this illness. Unlike other types of JIA, there are no convincing HLA associations with this subtype.

PATHOPHYSIOLOGY

As with all the other forms of JIA, the pathophysiology of this illness is poorly understood. Mouse models that overexpress human IL-6 mimic many of the features of the human illness, including growth failure. The importance of IL-6 has been corroborated in gene-expression studies from Japan. Gene-expression profiling in affected children also demonstrates a prominent role for IL-1 and IL-1–regulated genes. These findings together suggest an important role for innate immunity in disease pathogenesis. How these findings fit together, or how they explain the chronic synovitis that eventually evolves during or after the febrile phase of the disease, remains to be elucidated.

PREVENTION

There are no known preventive measures for systemic-onset JIA.

CLINICAL MANIFESTATIONS

Children typically present with fever and rash. The fever commonly occurs at regular intervals, once, twice, or three times a day. When the fever is present, the child can appear to be quite ill. In contrast, between febrile episodes, the child can appear active, playful, and near normal. The patterned occurrence of the fever and the child's often-robust appearance between febrile episodes are important clues to the diagnosis. Once the febrile episodes begin, they invariably occur daily. Other diagnoses should be pursued in a child with intermittent fever who goes entire days without a febrile episode. The characteristic salmon-colored rash may be present all the time or appear only with the fever. In cases where the rash is continuously present, it can become more prominent during febrile periods. The rash is macular, often confluent in areas, and present on the trunk and extremities but not usually the palms and soles.

The synovitis might appear at the time of the fever and rash or only appear days, weeks, or months later. The presence of joint pain is not diagnostically useful, because many febrile children have this complaint. The presence of morning stiffness or gait disturbance should prompt a very careful examination of the lower extremities for proliferative synovium around the knees, ankles, or small joints of the feet.

An acute phase response is quite typical, and its absence should lead to the pursuit of other diagnoses. White blood cell counts of more than 20,000/mm^3 are common, and counts below 15,000 mm^3 relatively uncommon. Platelet counts are typically greater than 500,000/mm^3, and it is not unusual to see erythrocyte sedimentation rates of more than 80 mm/hour.

DIAGNOSIS

Fever and rash are the typical presenting complaints in children with systemic-onset JIA. The fever typically occurs daily, not intermittently. Other diagnostic entities (e.g., Epstein-Barr virus [EBV] infection) should be considered in children with intermittent fever. The fever typically occurs regularly, in a once, twice, or (more rarely), thrice daily pattern. When the fever is present, the child usually appears quite ill; affected children appear surprisingly well in periods between febrile episodes. Querying parents and caretakers for this very typical feature of the disease can be useful diagnostically. The rash, when present, typically intensifies when the fever is present. A brisk acute phase response is typically seen. White blood cell counts of more than 20,000/mm^3 and platelet counts of more than 500,000/mm^3 are common.

The diagnosis is made based on the history and physical examination and the exclusion of other explanations for fever. The diagnosis can be challenging to make in children who have not yet developed synovitis. This is one form of JIA where the laboratory can be somewhat helpful, because the absence of leukocytosis and thrombocytosis make systemic onset JIA less likely. Determined efforts to exclude infection, malignancy, and other inflammatory disorders (e.g., Kawasaki's disease) are often required before the diagnosis of systemic-onset JIA can be established.

DIFFERENTIAL DIAGNOSIS

The differential diagnosis for systemic JIA is broad and includes infectious (e.g., EBV and cytomegalovirus [CMV] infection), malignant (e.g., lymphoma, neuroblastoma, and leukemia), and other inflammatory (e.g. Kawasaki's disease) etiologies. The latter can be difficult to exclude in a toddler and, thus, the importance of the details of the history and physical; for example, toddlers with Kawasaki's disease are typically irritable even when they are afebrile, but children with systemic-onset JIA often appear quite comfortable between febrile episodes. Younger children (younger than 10 years) might not make the heterophile antibody that is detected in the monospot test for EBV, and antibody titers to specific EBV antigens (usually available in standard EBV antibody panels) should be requested to exclude this diagnosis. Bone marrow examination may be required to exclude malignancy, especially if corticosteroid therapy is anticipated.

TREATMENT

Corticosteroids, given either as daily oral prednisone (1-2 mg/kg/day) or as methylpredisolone (Medrol) pulses (500 mg/m^2/dose) are usually effective in controlling the systemic symptoms. In Japan, where systemic disease is quite common, anti–IL-6 monoclonal antibody therapy with tocilizumab (Actemra)[1] has been shown to be effective in controlling both systemic and articular disease. Clinical trials of tocilizumab are under way in North America. Recent work has also shown promising results for the IL-1 receptor antagonist anakinra,[1] based on measured clinical efficacy and responses measured by gene expression profiling. Methotrexate (10-20 mg/m^2/week) remains a standard treatment for persistent articular disease, which is typically treated using approaches much like those used for polyarticular disease. Cyclosporine (Neoral)[1] has demonstrated some efficacy for both systemic and articular disease in children who have failed other agents.

MONITORING

Monitoring is the same as for polyarticular JIA. Uveitis is not as common in systemic-onset JIA as in other forms of JIA.

---

[1]Not FDA approved for this indication.

COMPLICATIONS

The hematologic and articular complications of systemic-onset JIA are essentially the same as those seen in polyarticular disease. A serious, sometimes lethal, complication of systemic JIA is macrophage activation syndrome. Macrophage activation syndrome comprises endothelial cell activation and hepatic and cerebral dysfunction typically heralded by otherwise unexplained decreases in serum hemoglobin, white blood cell, and platelet counts. Elevations in serum ASL/ALT and serum ferritin are other diagnostic clues. Bone marrow aspiration might reveal erythrophagocytic macrophages; their presence is diagnostic, but their absence does not exclude macrophage activation syndrome and should not delay therapy. The development of macrophage activation syndrome should be considered a medical emergency, and affected children should be referred immediately to facilities with experience in caring for this complication.

Enthesitis-Associated Arthritis

EPIDEMIOLOGY

Enthesitis-associated arthritis describes a group of arthritides characterized by male predilection, involvement of the axial skeleton (e.g., hips, sacroiliac joints, cervical spine), extraarticular inflammation (bursae, tendon insertions or enthuses, plantar fascia), and acute uveitis. This is the most common form of childhood-onset arthritis on the Indian subcontinent and in some Native American tribes. It might also be more common among children from Mexico and Central America than it is among European and European-descended children.

RISK FACTORS

HLA-B27 represents an important risk factor in all populations. Between 80% and 90% of European Americans with enthesitis-associated arthritis are HLA-B27 positive. African American patients are less commonly HLA-B27 positive (60% to 70%), so the absence of HLA-B27 should not exclude the diagnosis in this population.

PATHOPHYSIOLOGY

Current evidence suggests a causative role for HLA-B27. Rats expressing the human HLA-B27 gene develop a clinical picture nearly identical to the human disease. HLA-B27 transgenic rats raised in germ-free environments do not develop the disease, suggesting that normal commensural flora, particularly intestinal flora, play an important role. The connection between gastrointestinal flora and human disease is corroborated by the development of postinfectious arthritic syndromes (e.g., Reiter's syndrome) in HLA-B27-positive adolescents and adults after salmonella, shigella, or chlamydia infection. Finally, the high prevalence of arthritis strongly resembling enthesitis-associated arthritis in patients with inflammatory bowel disease suggests a link between the arthritis and loss of integrity of the gastrointestinal mucosal barrier. Recent research interest has therefore focused on antigen processing by gut-associated lymphoid tissue, although no single pathogenic model has emerged.

PREVENTION

There are no known preventive measures.

CLINICAL MANIFESTATIONS

Enthesitis-associated arthritis demonstrates a wide variety of clinical presentations. The practitioner may be confronted with a preschool or school-aged boy with monoarticular joint swelling virtually indistinguishable from oligoarticular JIA (male sex and the older age of the child may be important diagnostic clues). School-aged and adolescent patients often present with unilateral or bilateral hip pain. The pain is characteristically worse in the morning and better with activity, which helps distinguish it from other causes of hip pain in teens (e.g., slipped capital femoral epiphysis), which typically cause pain that is worse with activity and better with rest. Finally, some patients present with an acute polyarthritis very similar to polyarticular JIA. Selective involvement of the distal interphalangeal joints of the fingers with sparing of the proximal interphalangeal joints is a typical pattern. Low back pain is very seldom a presenting complaint, unlike in adults with HLA-B27–mediated forms of arthritis.

DIAGNOSIS

The disease typically occurs as a monoarthritis, often involving the hip. This is the only form of JIA where pain is typically a prominent presenting complaint. Hip pain, made worse with rest and better with activity, is a common presenting complaint. Unlike in adults, back pain is only an infrequent presenting complaint in children. The diagnosis is supported (but not established) by the presence of HLA-B27 on peripheral blood leukocytes.

As with all the other forms of JIA, the diagnosis is established on the basis of the history and physical examination. Hip disease typically is associated with pain on internal and external rotation of the affected hip(s), with some loss of range of motion. The presence of extraarticular inflammation (e.g., pain or swelling around the Achilles tendons, plantar fasciitis, bursitis of the hips or shoulders) can be helpful diagnostic clues. Nail pitting, sometimes with frank onycholysis, is sometimes seen. Diffuse swelling of a single toe (sausage toe) is a characteristic finding, as is painful arthritis of the first metatarsophalangeal joint.

The laboratory can be helpful in making the diagnosis. HLA-B27 is present in 80% to 90% of patients of European descent. Elevations in erythrocyte sedimentation rate or anemia associated with chronic inflammation are sometimes seen. Imaging studies of the hips can show cartilage loss with or without periarticular demineralization. Changes in the sacroiliac joints are seldom seen at presentation but they can evolve over the course of the disease; their appearance strongly supports the diagnosis.

DIFFERENTIAL DIAGNOSIS

Because of the broad spectrum of clinical presentations, the differential diagnosis is likewise broad. Transient synovitis of the hip must be considered in younger children complaining of hip pain. In older children, this same complaint can raise the possibility of Legg-Calvé-Perthes disease, slipped capital femoral epiphysis, idiopathic avascular necrosis, or axial skeletal tumors (e.g., Ewing's sarcoma). Hip pain in children is almost always an indication for obtaining plain films.

Oligoarticular JIA and polyarticular JIA are almost always considered in patients presenting with peripheral arthritis. Acute, self-limited, postinfectious arthritis is sometimes in the differential diagnosis.

TREATMENT

Therapeutic goals and approaches are virtually identical to those for polyarticular JIA.

MONITORING

See the section on polyarticular JIA.

COMPLICATIONS

Acute, painful uveitis is a common complication of this form of arthritis and can even be the presenting complaint. Pain; red, inflamed sclerae; and photophobia almost invariably lead patients to seek medical attention quickly. Most patients with acute uveitis respond well to topical corticosteroids. Inflammation of the genital tract (sterile urethritis, balanitis) are less-common complications.

Progressive joint destruction, particularly in affected hips, can occur even with aggressive management. Sacroiliitis can be seen in older patients or patients with long-standing disease. Frank ankylosis of the spine is rare before adulthood.

Acknowledgment

Special thanks to Ms. Lucy Chen for proofreading and editing and for helpful comments on this chapter.

REFERENCES

Allantaz F, Chaussabel D, Stichweh D, et al. Blood leukocyte microarrays to diagnose systemic onset juvenile idiopathic arthritis and follow the response to IL-1 blockade. J Exp Med 2007;204:2131–44.

Foster CS. Diagnosis and treatment of juvenile idiopathic arthritis-associated uveitis. Curr Opin Ophthalmol 2003;14:395–8.

Hashkes PJ, Laxer RM. Update on the medical treatment of juvenile idiopathic arthritis. Curr Rheum Rep 2006;8:450–8.

Hayward K, Wallace CA. Recent developments in anti-rheumatic drugs in pediatrics: treatment of juvenile idiopathic arthritis. Arthritis Res Ther 2009;11:216.

Ilowite NT. Update on biologics in juvenile idiopathic arthritis. Curr Opin Rheumatol 2008;20:613–8.

Jarvis JN. Commentary: Ordering laboratory tests for suspected rheumatic disease. Pediatr Rheumatol 2008;6:19.

McGhee JL, Kickingbird L, Jarvis JN. Clinical utility of ANA tests in children. BMC Pediatr 2004;4:13.

McGhee JL, Burks F, Sheckels J, Jarvis JN. Identifying children with chronic arthritis based on chief complains: Absence of predictive value for musculoskeletal pain as an indicator of rheumatic disease in children. Pediatrics 2002;110:354–9.

Tse SM, Laxer RM. Juvenile spondyloarthropathy. Curr Opin Rheumatol 2003;15:374–9.

Ankylosing Spondylitis

Method of
John D. Reveille, MD

The term *ankylosing spondylitis* (AS) comprises a group of chronic inflammatory diseases characterized by spinal and peripheral joint oligoarthritis, inflammation of the attachments of ligaments and tendons to bones (enthesitis), and, at times ocular or cardiac manifestations.

Epidemiology

The prevalence of AS parallels the frequency of HLA-B27. AS occurs in 0.2% to 0.5% of persons of European descent and eastern Asian descent, with B27 seen in 8% and 6%, respectively. Higher incidences of AS are reported in eastern Europe and Scandinavia, where HLA-B27 is more common, and in certain Native American groups. AS is rare in Africans and Japanese, where HLA-B27 is rare. Men are affected three times more commonly than women.

Pathophysiology

AS is caused primarily by genetic factors, with a sibling recurrence risk ratio as high as 82 and twin-based studies estimating disease heritability to exceed 90%. The major histocompatibility complex (MHC) gene HLA-B27 confers the greatest known risk for AS and is found in up to 90% of patients of European and East Asian ancestry (although AS patients from the Middle East and Africa have lower B27 frequencies).

How HLA-B27 contributes to the pathogenesis of AS is not known. One theory is the arthritogenic peptide hypothesis: that AS results from HLA-B27 binding a unique peptide or a set of antigenic peptides derived from either triggering microorganisms or from self proteins. Another possibility is that HLA-B27 heavy chains self associate to form homodimers, which can result in a proinflammatory unfolded protein response. A third hypothesis is that AS results from a gut infection, given that HLA-B27–positive persons are more efficient at dealing with certain infections (hepatitis C and HIV) and less efficient at dealing with others (*Salmonella, Shigella, Chlamydia* species, and others). Older studies have implicated *Klebsiella pneumoniae*, although recent data have not borne this out. How these factors initiate disease onset is not known.

Less than 5% of HLA-B27–positive people in the general population develop AS or other spondyloarthritis, as opposed to 20% of HLA-B27–positive relatives of AS patients. Family studies have suggested that HLA-B27 forms only about 40% of the overall risk for AS. Other MHC genes, such as HLA-B60 *(B*4001)*, have also been seen in both white and Asian AS patients.

Non-MHC genes have been implicated in AS susceptibility, such as endoplasmic reticulum aminopeptidase (ERAP1-involved in trimming peptides to the optimal length for loading onto the peptide binding groove for MHC class I presentation), interleukin 23 receptor (a key cytokine involved in the differentiation of naïve CD4$^+$ T cells into T_H17 helper T cells) and interleukin-1α (IL-1α), a proinflammatory cytokine in the T_H1 response. In addition, a genome-wide association study has identified AS susceptibility loci in two gene deserts at chromosome 2p15 and 21q22 as well as the genes *ANTXR2* (encoding capillary morphogenesis protein-2) and *IL1R2* (which acts as a decoy receptor, interfering with the binding of IL-1 to IL-1R1), in addition to strong association with the MHC and with *IL23R* and *ERAP1*. This suggests a major role for the IL-23 and IL-1 cytokine pathways in AS susceptibility.

Clinical Manifestations

The hallmark of AS is inflammatory back pain. This pain is classically characterized as a dull pain in the low back or in the buttocks and hips that begins before the age of 40 years, has an insidious onset, and lasts longer than 3 months. Inflammatory back pain is associated with morning stiffness lasting 30 minutes or longer, which responds readily to nonsteroidal antiinflammatory drugs (NSAIDs), is relieved with activity and worsened with rest, and often awakens the patient during the second half of the night. As the disease progresses, patients can develop limitation of spinal mobility, loss of lumbar and cervical lordosis, and kyphotic deformities of the spine. This limitation of motion is initially the result of axial inflammation and muscle spasm but is contributed to over time by ossification of the ligamentous structures and ultimately bony fusion of the sacroiliac joints, apophyseal joints, and the outer fibers of the annulus fibrosis of the intervertebral disks.

Arthritis of the hips occurs in approximately 50% of patients with AS. About 10% of AS patients have arthritis of the joints of the hands, feet, wrists, and ankles. Enthesitis, inflammation of tendinous or ligamentous insertions onto bone, is one of the most characteristic findings of the AS and other spondyloarthritides, especially in the Achilles tendon and the plantar fascial insertions, although involvement of the ligamentous and tendinous insertions onto the pelvic bones is also encountered. Dactylitis or sausage digits—fusiform swelling of the entire digit due to inflammation and swelling of the flexor tenosynovium—also occasionally occurs.

AS also affects the gastrointestinal tract and eyes. About 6% of AS patients have inflammatory bowel disease (Crohn's disease or ulcerative colitis), and asymptomatic bowel inflammation is seen on ileocolonoscopy in up to 50% of patients with AS. Anterior uveitis occurs in about 40% of AS patients. It is usually unilateral with sudden onset, manifesting as a painful red eye with photophobia and blurred vision. It can recur periodically, although is rarely associated with permanent loss of vision. Similarly, about 10% of AS patients have psoriasis.

Diagnosis

The diagnosis of AS rests on the presence of inflammatory spinal pain or restriction of spinal and chest wall motion occurring in the setting of radiographic sacroiliitis (sclerosis, erosion, and even ankylosis of the sacroiliac joints). Plain radiographs of the spine show

Romanus lesions (shiny corners) and squaring of the vertebral body owing to erosions at the attachments of the spinal ligaments early in disease, followed by formation of syndesmophytes owing to ossification of the outer layer of the annulus fibrosis and eventual ankylosis of the spine, producing a bamboo spine appearance.

Abnormalities on standard radiographs typically are not seen until up to 8 to 11 years after disease onset, leading to a significant delay in diagnosis and initiation of therapy. Radiographic changes can be detected with magnetic resonance imaging (MRI) years before the appearance of radiographic disease, with bone marrow edema adjacent to the inflamed sacroiliac joint and spinal joints. This preradiographic disease has resulted in the concept of axial spondyloarthritis, for which new criteria have been developed based on the presence of inflammatory back pain accompanied by the presence of a positive MRI or HLA-B27 typing and other spondyloarthritis features (e.g., uveitis, enthesitis).

Differential Diagnosis

Diffuse idiopathic skeletal hyperostosis (DISH) is a disease of older persons, predominantly men, characterized by low back pain and stiffness. Characteristic findings are flowing calcification and ossification along the anterolateral segment of at least four contiguous vertebral bodies with the relative preservation of intervertebral disk height and the absence of apophyseal joint ankylosis. The sacroiliac joints are characteristically spared or show degenerative changes but not erosion or fusion, and the back pain is usually mechanical in nature.

Osteitis condensans ilii is a condition primarily noted in young multiparous women. It consists of increased bone density generally confined to a triangular area along the inferior aspect of the ilium adjacent to the sacroiliac joint. It is usually asymptomatic, and erosions and intra-articular ankylosis are rare.

Ochronosis is a rare hereditary metabolic disease in which the enzyme homogentisic acid oxidase is absent. It is characterized by abnormal pigmentation of the sclerae and ears. Ochronotic arthropathy manifests in the fourth decade, especially in the hips, knees, and shoulders. Although the spine can appear fused as in AS, characteristic findings include loss of disk height and calcification of the disks, which are not seen in AS.

Treatment

A great deal of educational information is available for patients (www.spondylitis.org). Unsupervised recreational exercise improves pain and stiffness, and back exercise improves pain and function in patients with AS, but these effects differ with disease duration. Health status is improved when patients perform recreational exercise at least 30 minutes per day and back exercises at least 5 days per week.

NSAIDs, used in high (antiinflammatory) doses on a daily basis, remain the starting point of treatment of spondylitis, and up to half of AS patients attain satisfactory symptom control with these agents alone. There are no strong data to suggest the superiority of any specific NSAID in patients with AS.

Disease-modifying antiinflammatory drugs (DMARDs), especially sulfasalazine (Azulfidine)[1] in doses of 2 to 3 g/day, but also methotrexate (Trexall)[1] (up to 25 mg once a week) and leflunomide ([Arava])[1] 20 mg per day) are effective in the treatment of peripheral joint involvement in AS, although not in axial disease.

Glucocorticoids such as prednisone (5-15 mg/day) are occasionally used by clinicians to augment the effect of NSAIDs, although owing to unproven efficacy and side effects, including osteoporosis, they are not recommended unless other treatments are not available. Intraarticular and peritendinous injections of depot steroids can provide relief of local flares, although injecting around the Achilles tendon is not recommended because of the risk of tendon rupture.

TNF-α blockers have become a mainstay in AS treatment for those not responding to NSAIDs and DMARDs. Currently four are approved by the FDA for use in AS. Three are injected subcutaneously, including the soluble TNF-α receptor etanercept (Enbrel), given at 50 mg weekly, and the TNF-α monoclonal antibodies adalimumab (Humira) 40 mg every 2 weeks and golimumab (Simponi) 50 mg once a month. In addition, the TNF-α monoclonal antibody infliximab (Remicade) is infused at 5 mg/kg every 6 to 8 weeks intravenously. These medications have been shown to be beneficial in both the axial and peripheral manifestations of AS. Onset of action is rapid, and improvement is seen not only clinically but also on MRI, with clearing of bone marrow edema. Anti-TNF treatment is expensive, and complications can include infusion or injection site reactions, infections (especially from *Mycoplasma tuberculosis*), lymphoma (though not other malignancies), and the development of antinuclear antibodies following anti-TNF treatment, although reports of patients developing systemic lupus erythematosus or other connective tissue disease are extremely rare.

Patients with AS also require surgical treatment on occasion. Total hip arthroplasty is the most common surgical procedure in patients with AS, and heterotopic new bone formation can be a potential problem. Patients with AS are at increased risk for vertebral fracture, often resulting in neurologic compromise due to osteoporosis. In general, halo vest immobilization is recommended. Surgical intervention may be necessary when neurologic impairment is seen. Also, osteotomies (open, polysegmental, and closing wedge) are occasionally employed to correct the fixed kyphotic deformities seen in patients with advanced AS.

Monitoring

The most widely used clinical measure of disease activity is the Bath Ankylosing Spondylitis Disease Activity (BASDI) measure, a self-reported questionnaire consisting of six 10-cm horizontal visual

[1]Not FDA approved for this indication.

analogue scales. It measures severity of fatigue, spinal and peripheral joint pain, localized tenderness, and morning stiffness. Functional impairment is measured by the Bath Ankylosing Spondylitis Functional Index (BASFI), another self-reported questionnaire with ten 10-cm visual analogue scales, including eight AS-specific questions and two on coping and daily life. Spinal mobility can be assessed by specific physical examination maneuvers, such as the Schober test, which measures lumbar flexion; chest wall expansion, which assess costovertebral joint involvement; the occiput-to-wall measurement, which assesses cervical extension; and the lateral bending maneuver.

Laboratory markers of disease include C-reactive protein (CRP) and erythrocyte sedimentation rate (ESR). Radiographic severity is measured by the Modified Stoke Ankylosing Spondylitis Spinal Score (mSASSS), a detailed scoring system comparable to the Sharp Score in rheumatoid arthritis. However, standard radiographs are complicated by low sensitivity to change and are not useful in gauging disease activity. MRI scanning is more helpful, particularly in measuring disease activity.

Complications

Cardiac manifestations, including conduction abnormalities and aortic valvular insufficiency, occasionally are seen in AS patients. The spectrum of pulmonary involvement in AS ranges from restricted chest wall movement from costovertebral joint fusion to a rare upper lobe–predominant interstitial lung disease. Other complications of AS include osteoporosis; spinal fracture, often accompanied by neurologic compromise; atlantoaxial subluxation; cauda equina syndrome; secondary amyloidosis; sleep disturbance; and depression.

REFERENCES

Braun J, Kalden JR. Biologics in the treatment of rheumatoid arthritis and ankylosing spondylitis. Clin Exp Rheumatol 2009;27(4 Suppl. 55):S164–7.
Harper BE, Reveille JD. Spondyloarthritis: Clinical suspicion, diagnosis, and sports. Curr Sports Med Rep 2009;8(1):29–34.
Reveille JD. Recent studies on the genetic basis of ankylosing spondylitis. Curr Rheumatol Rep 2009;11(5):340–8.
Reveille JD, Arnett FC. Spondyloarthritis: Update on pathogenesis and treatment. Am J Med 2005;118(6):592–603.
Reveille JD, Sims AM, Danoy P, et al. Genomewide association study of ankylosing spondylitis identifies multiple non-MHC susceptibility loci. Nat Genet 2010;42(2):123–7.
Rudwaleit M, van der Heijde D, et al. The development of Assessment of SpondyloArthritis international Society classification criteria for axial spondyloarthritis (part II): Validation and final selection. Ann Rheum Dis 2009;68(6):770–6.

Temporomandibular Disorders

Method of
Jeffrey P. Okeson, DMD

Temporomandibular disorder (TMD) is a collective term that includes a number of clinical complaints involving the muscles of mastication, the temporomandibular joints (TMJs) and associated orofacial structures. Other commonly used terms are Costen's syndrome, TMJ dysfunction, and craniomandibular disorders. Temporomandibular disorders are a major cause of nondental pain in the orofacial region and are considered a subclassification of musculoskeletal disorders. In many TMD patients the most common complaint is not with the TMJs but rather the muscles of mastication. Therefore, the terms TMJ dysfunction or TMJ disorder are actually inappropriate for many of these complaints. It is for this reason that the American Dental Association adopted the term *temporomandibular disorder.*

Signs and symptoms associated with TMDs are a common source of pain complaints in the head and orofacial structures. These complaints can be associated with general joint problems and somatization. Approximately 50% of patients suffering with TMDs do not first consult with a dentist but seek advice for the problem from a physician. The family physician should be able to appropriately diagnose many TMDs. In many instances the physician can provide valuable information and simple therapies that will reduce the patient's TMD symptoms. In other instances, it is appropriate to refer the patient to a dentist for additional evaluation and treatment.

Epidemiology

Cross-sectional population-based studies reveal that 40% to 75% of adult populations having at least one sign of TMJ dysfunction (e.g., jaw movement abnormalities, joint noise, tenderness on palpation), and approximately 33% have at least one symptom (e.g., face pain, joint pain). Many of these signs and symptoms are not troublesome for the patient, and only 3% to 7% of the population seeks any advice or care. Although in the general population women seem to have only a slightly greater incidence of TMD symptoms, women seek care for TMD more often than men at a ratio ranging from 3:1 to 9:1. For many patients TMDs are self-limiting, or are associated with symptoms that fluctuate over time without evidence of progression. Even though many of these disorders are self-limiting, the health care provider can provide conservative therapies that will minimize the patient's painful experience.

Signs and Symptoms

The primary signs and symptoms associated with TMD originate from the masticatory structures and are associated with jaw function (Box 1). Pain during opening of the mouth or during chewing is common. Some persons even report difficulty speaking or singing. Patients often report pain in the preauricular areas, face, or temples. TMJ sounds are often described as clicking, popping, grating, or crepitus and can produce locking of the jaw during opening or closing. Patients commonly report painful jaw muscles and, on occasion they even report a sudden change in their bite coincident with the onset of the painful condition.

It is important to appreciate that pain associated with most TMDs is increased with jaw function. Because this is a condition of the musculoskeletal structures, function of these structures generally increases the pain. When a patient's pain complaint is not influenced by jaw function, other sources of orofacial pain should be suspected.

BOX 1   Common Primary and Secondary Symptoms Associated with Temporomandibular Disorders

Primary Symptoms

Facial muscle pain
Preauricular (TMJ) pain
TMJ sounds: jaw clicking, popping, catching, locking
Limited mouth opening
Increased pain associated with chewing

Secondary Symptoms

Earache
Headache
Neckache

Abbreviation: TMJ = temporomandibular joint.

The spectrum of TMD often includes commonly associated complaints such as headache, neckache, or earache. These associated complaints are often referred pains and must be differentiated from primary pains. As a general rule, referred pains associated with TMDs are increased with any activity that provokes the TMD pain. Therefore, if the patient reports that the headache is aggravated by jaw function, it could very well represent a secondary pain related to the TMD. Likewise, if the secondary symptom is unaffected by jaw use, one should question its relationship to the TMD and suspect two separate pain conditions. Pain or dysfunction due to non-musculoskeletal causes such as otolaryngologic, neurologic, vascular, neoplastic, or infectious disease in the orofacial region is not considered a primary TMD even though musculoskeletal pain may be present. However, TMDs often coexist with other craniofacial and orofacial pain disorders.

Anatomy and Pathophysiology

The TMJ is formed by the mandibular condyle fitting into the mandibular fossa of the temporal bone. The movement of this joint is quite complex as it allows hinging movement in one plane and at the same time allows gliding movements in another plane.

Separating these two bones from direct articulation is the articular disk. The articular disk is composed of dense fibrous connective tissue devoid of any blood vessels or nerve fibers. The articular disk is attached posteriorly to a region of loose connective tissue that is highly vascularized and well innervated, known as the retrodiskal tissue. The anterior region of the disk is attached to the superior lateral pterygoid muscle.

The movement of the mandible is accomplished by four pairs of muscles called the muscles of mastication: the masseter, temporalis, medial pterygoid, and lateral pterygoid. Although not considered to be muscles of mastication, the digastric muscles also play an important role in mandibular function. The masseter, temporalis, and medial pterygoid muscles elevate the mandible and therefore provide the major forces used for chewing and other jaw functions. The inferior lateral pterygoid muscles provide protrusive movement of the mandible, and the digastric muscles serve to depress the mandible (open the mouth).

When discussing the pathophysiology of TMD one needs to consider two main categories: joint pathophysiology and muscle pathophysiology. Because etiologic considerations and treatment strategies are different for these conditions, they are presented separately.

PATHOPHYSIOLOGY OF INTRACAPSULAR TMJ PAIN DISORDERS

Several common arthritic conditions such as rheumatoid arthritis, traumatic arthritis, hyperuricemia, and psoriatic arthritis can affect the TMJ. These conditions, however, are not nearly as common as local osteoarthritis. As with most other joints, osteoarthritis results from overloading the articular surface of the joint, thus breaking down the dense fibrous articular surface and ultimately affecting the subarticular bone. In the TMJ, this overloading common occurs as a result of an alteration in the morphology and position of the articular disk. In the healthy TMJ the disk maintains its position on the condyle during movement because of its morphology (i.e., the thicker anterior and posterior borders) and interarticular pressure maintained by the elevator muscles. If, however, the morphology of the disk is altered and the diskal ligaments become elongated, the disk can be displaced from its normal position between the condyle and fossa. If the disk is displaced, normal opening and closing of the mouth can result in an unusual translatory movement between the condyle and the disk, which is felt as click or pop. Disk displacements that result in joint sounds might or might not be painful. When pain is present it is thought to be related to either loading forces applied to the highly vascularized retrodiskal tissues or a general inflammatory response of the surrounding soft tissues (capsulitis or synovitis).

PATHOPHYSIOLOGY OF MASTICATORY MUSCLE PAIN DISORDERS

The muscles of mastication are a very common source of TMD pain. Understanding the pathophysiology of muscle pain, however, is very complex and still not well understood. The simple explanation of muscle spasm does not account for most TMD muscle pain complaints. It appears that a better explanation would involve a central nervous system affect on the muscle that results in an increase in peripheral nociceptive activity originating from the muscle tissue itself. This explanation more accurately accounts for the high levels of emotional stress that are commonly associated with TMD muscle pain complaints. In other words, an increase in emotional stress activates the autonomic nervous system, which in turn seems to be associated with changes in muscle nociception.

These masticatory muscle pain conditions are further complicated when one considers the unique masticatory muscle activity known as bruxism. Bruxism is the subconscious, often rhythmic, grinding or gnashing of the teeth. This type of muscle activity is considered to be parafunctional and can also occur as a simple static loading of the teeth known as clenching. This activity commonly occurs while sleeping but can also be present during the day. These parafunctional activities alone can represent a significant source of masticatory muscle pain, and certainly bruxism in the presence of central nervous system–induced muscle pain can further accentuate the patient's muscle pain complaints.

Etiology

Because TMD represents a group of disorders, any of several etiologies may be associated. Problems arising from intracapsular conditions (clicking, popping, catching, locking) may be associated with various types of trauma. Gross trauma, such as a blow to the chin, can immediately alter ligamentous structures of the joint, leading to joint sounds. Trauma can also be associated with a subtler injury such as stretching, twisting or compressing forces during eating, yawning, yelling, or prolonged mouth opening.

When the patient's chief complaint is muscle pain, etiologic factors other than trauma should be considered. Masticatory muscle pain disorders have etiologic considerations similar to other muscle pain disorders of the neck and back. Emotional stress seems to play a significant role for many patients. This can explain why patients often report that their painful symptoms fluctuate greatly over time.

Although most TMD patients do not have a major psychiatric disorder, psychological factors can certainly enhance the pain condition. The clinician needs to consider such factors as anxiety, depression, secondary gain, somatization, and hypochondriasis. Psychosocial factors can predispose certain person to TMD and can also perpetuate TMD once symptoms have become established. A careful consideration of psychosocial factors is therefore important in the evaluation and treatment of every TMD patient.

TMDs have a few unique etiologic factors that differentiate them from other musculoskeletal disorders. One such factor is the occlusal relationship of the teeth. Traditionally it was thought that malocclusion was the primary etiologic factor responsible for TMD. Recent investigations, however, do not support this concept. Still, in certain instances occlusal instability of the teeth can contribute to a TMD. This may be true in patients with or without teeth. Poorly fitting dental prostheses can also contribute to occlusal instability. The occlusal condition should especially be suspected if the pain problem began with a change in the patient's occlusion (e.g., following a dental appointment).

History and Examination

All patients reporting pain in the orofacial structures should be screened for TMD. This can be accomplished with a brief history and physical examination. The screening questions and examination

BOX 2   Recommended Screening Questionnaire for Temporomandibular Disorder

All patients reporting pain in the orofacial region should be screened for TMD with a questionnaire that includes these questions. The decision to complete a comprehensive history and clinical examination depends on the number of positive responses and the apparent seriousness of the problem for the patient. A positive response to any question may be sufficient to warrant a comprehensive examination if it is of concern to the patient or viewed as clinically significant by the physician.

1. Do you have difficulty, pain, or both when opening your mouth, for instance when yawning?
2. Does your jaw get stuck or locked or go out?
3. Do you have difficulty, pain, or both when chewing, talking, or using your jaws?
4. Are you aware of noises in the jaw joints?
5. Do your jaws regularly feel stiff, tight, or tired?
6. Do you have pain in or about the ears, temples, or cheeks?
7. Do you have frequent headaches, neckaches, or toothaches?
8. Have you had a recent injury to your head, neck, or jaw?
9. Have you been aware of any recent changes in your bite?
10. Have you been previously treated for unexplained facial pain or a jaw joint problem?

Abbreviation: TMD = temporomandibular disorder.

BOX 3   Recommended Screening Examination Procedures for Temporomandibular Disorder

All patients with face pain should be briefly screened for TMD using this or a similar cursory clinical examination. The need for a comprehensive history and clinical examination depends on the number of positive findings and the clinical significance of each finding.

1. Palpate for pain or tenderness in the masseter and temporalis muscles.
2. Palpate for pain or tenderness in the preauricular (TMJ) areas.
3. Measure the range of mouth opening. Note any incoordination in the movements.
4. Auscultate and palpate for TMJ sounds (i.e., clicking or crepitus).
5. Note excessive occlusal wear, excessive tooth mobility, buccal mucosal ridging, or lateral tongue scalloping.
6. Inspect symmetry and alignment of the face, jaws, and dental arches.

Abbreviation: TMJ = temporomandibular joint.

are performed to rule in or out the possibility of a TMD. If a positive response is found, a more extensive history and examination is indicated. Box 2 lists questions that should be asked during a screening assessment for TMD. Any positive response should be followed by additional clarifying questions.

Patients experiencing orofacial pain should also be briefly examined for any clinical signs associated with TMD. The clinician can easily palpate a few sites to assess tenderness or pain as well as assess for jaw mobility. The masseter muscles can be palpated bilaterally while asking the patient to report any pain or tenderness. The same assessment should be made for the temporal regions as well as the preauricular (TMJ) areas. While the examiner's hands are over the preauricular areas the patient should repeatedly open and close the mouth. The presence of joint sounds should be noted and whether these sounds are associated with joint pain.

A simple measurement of mouth opening should be made. This can be accomplished by placing a millimeter ruler on the lower anterior teeth and asking the patient to open as wide as possible. The distance should be measured between the maxillary and mandibular anterior teeth. It is generally accepted that less than 40 mm is a restricted mouth opening.

It is also helpful to inspect the teeth for significant wear, mobility, or decay that may be related to the pain condition. The clinician should examine the buccal mucosa for ridging and the lateral aspect of the tongue for scalloping. These are often signs of clenching and bruxism. A general inspection for symmetry and alignment of the face, jaws, and dental arches may also be helpful. A summary of this screening examination is shown in Box 3.

Treatment

Most recent studies suggest that TMDs are generally self-limiting and symptoms often fluctuate over time. Understanding this natural course does not mean these conditions should be ignored. TMD

can be a very painful condition leading to a significant decrease in the patient's quality of life. Understanding the natural course of TMD does suggest, however, that therapy might not need to be very aggressive. In general, initial therapy should begin very conservatively and only escalate when therapy fails to relieve the symptoms.

When the physician identifies a patient with a TMD, he or she has two options. The physician can elect to treat the patient or refer the patient to a dentist who specializes in TMD for further evaluation and treatment. The decision to refer the patient should be based on whether the patient needs any unique care provided only in a dental office. The following are some indications for referral to a dentist:

- History of trauma to the face related to the onset of the pain condition
- The presence of significant TMJ sounds during function
- A feeling of jaw catching or locking during mouth opening
- The report of a sudden change in the occlusal contacts of the teeth
- The presence of significant occlusal instability
- Significant findings related to the teeth (e.g., tooth mobility, tooth sensitivity, tooth decay, tooth wear)
- Significant pain in the jaws or masticatory muscles upon awaking.
- The presence of an orofacial pain condition that is aggravated by jaw function and has been present for more than several months.

The specific therapy for a TMD varies according to the precise type of disorder identified. In other words, masticatory muscle pain is managed somewhat differently than intracapsular pain. Generally, however, the initial therapy for any type of TMD should be directed toward the relief of pain and the improvement of function. This initial conservative therapy can be divided into three general types: patient education, pharmacologic therapy, and physical therapy.

PATIENT EDUCATION

It is very important that patients have an appreciation for the factors that may be associated with their disorder, as well as the natural course of the disorder. Patients should be reassured, and if necessary, convinced by appropriate tests, that they are not suffering from a malignancy. Properly educated patients can contribute greatly to their own treatment. For example, knowing that emotional stress is an influencing factor in many TMDs can help the patient understand the reason for daily fluctuations of pain intensity. Attention should be directed toward changing their response to stress or, when possible, reducing their exposure to stressful conditions. Patients with pain during chewing should be told to begin a softer diet, chew slower, and eat smaller bites. As a general rule the patient should be told "if it hurts, don't do it." Continued pain can contribute to the cycling of pain and should always be avoided. The patient should be instructed to let the jaw muscles relax, maintaining the teeth apart. This will discourage clenching activities and minimize loading of the teeth and joints.

When pain is associated with a clicking TM joint, the patient should be informed of the biomechanics of the joint. This information often allows the patient to select functional activities that are less traumatic to the joint structures. For example, some patients may report that the pain and clicking are less when they chew on a particular side of the mouth. When this occurs, they should be encouraged to continue this type of chewing.

PHARMACOLOGIC THERAPY

Pharmacologic therapy can be an effective adjunct in managing symptoms associated with TMDs. Patients should be aware that medication alone will not likely solve or cure the problem. Medication, however, in conjunction with appropriate physical therapy and definitive treatment, does offer the most complete approach to many TMD problems. Mild analgesics are often helpful for many TMDs. Control of pain is not only appreciated by the patient but also reduces the likelihood of other complicating pain disorders such as muscle co-contraction, referred pain, and central sensitization.

Nonsteroidal antiinflammatory drugs (NSAIDs) are very helpful with many TMDs. Included in this category are aspirin, acetaminophen (Tylenol), and ibuprofen. Ibuprofen (Motrin, Advil, Nuprin) is often very effective in reducing musculoskeletal pains. A dosage of 600 to 800 mg three times a day for 3 to 5 days commonly reduces pain and stops the cyclic effects of the deep pain input. For patients with gastrointestinal issues, short-term use of a cyclooxygenase-2 (COX-2) inhibitor such as celecoxib (Celebrex) can also be useful.

PHYSICAL THERAPY

In many patients with TMD, symptoms are relieved with very simple physical therapy methods. Simple instructions for the use of moist heat or cold can be very helpful. Surface heat can be applied by laying a hot moist towel over the symptomatic area. A hot water bottle wrapped inside the towel will help maintain the heat. This combination should remain in place for 10 to 15 minutes, not to exceed 30 minutes. An electric heating pad may be used, but care should be taken not to leave it on the face too long. Patients should be discouraged from using the heating pad while sleeping because prolonged use is likely.

Like thermotherapy, coolant therapy can provide a simple and often effective method of reducing pain. Ice should be applied directly to the symptomatic joint or muscles and moved in a circular motion without pressure to the tissues. The patient will initially experience an uncomfortable feeling that will quickly turn into a burning sensation. Continued icing will result in a mild aching and then numbness. When numbness begins the ice should be removed. The ice should not be left on the tissues for longer than 5 minutes. After a period of warming a second cold application may be desirable.

The physician should be aware that many TMDs respond to the use of orthopedic appliances such as occlusal appliances, bite guards, and splints. These appliances are made by the dentist and are custom fabricated for each patient. Several types of appliances are available. Each is specific for the type of TMD present. The dentist should be consulted for this type of therapy.

OTHER THERAPEUTIC CONSIDERATIONS

Sometimes TMDs become chronic and, as with other chronic pain conditions, might then be best managed by a multidisciplinary approach. If the patient reports a long history of TMD complaints, the physician should consider referring the patient to a dentist associated with a team of therapists, such as a psychologist, physical therapist, and even a chronic pain physician. Generally, patients with chronic TMD are not managed well by the simple initial therapies discussed in this chapter. Often other factors, such as mechanical

conditions within the TM Js or psychological factors need to be addressed. The physician who attempts to manage these conditions in the private practice setting can become very frustrated with the results. It is therefore recommended that if the patient's history suggests chronicity or if initial therapy fails to reduce the patient's symptoms, referral is indicated.

REFERENCES

de Leeuw RE. Orofacial Pain: Guidelines for Assessment, Diagnosis and Management. 4th ed. Chicago: Quintessence; 2008.

Okeson JP. Management of Temporomandibular Disorders and Occlusion. 6th ed. St. Louis: Mosby; 2008.

Okeson JP. Bell's Orofacial Pains. 6th ed. Chicago: Quintessence; 2005.

Scrivani SJ, Keith DA, Kaban LB. Temporomandibular disorders. N Engl J Med 2008;359(25):2693–705.

Bursitis, Tendinitis, Myofascial Pain, and Fibromyalgia

Method of
Keith K. Colburn, MD

Soft tissue rheumatism is a term that describes musculoskeletal pain and other symptoms not caused by arthritis. Bursitis, tendinitis, myofascial pain syndrome, and fibromyalgia belong to this group of disorders. These maladies can occur in the absence of systemic disease. They are associated with persistent mild trauma and overuse of muscles, bursae, tendons, entheses, ligaments, and fascia. Localized tendinitis or bursitis are very specific and may be self-limiting, relieved by topical or oral antiinflammatory medications, or treated with a well-placed injection. Fibromyalgia is more diffuse and may be very difficult to treat. There are no abnormal laboratory tests consistently associated with soft tissue rheumatism. Radiologic tests and scans can show abnormalities of soft tissue; however, it is only occasionally necessary to do expensive tests to get an accurate diagnosis of these conditions. Diagnosis requires a good history and a careful physical examination of the musculoskeletal system.

Bursitis and Tendinitis

Bursitis and tendinitis can occur in any one of hundreds of locations throughout the body. A bursa is a synovial membrane–lined sac containing synovial fluid found in areas of potential friction, such as where tendons, ligaments, and bone rub against each other. Bursitis and tendinitis are considered together by regions of the body because diagnosis and treatment share some common principles.

GENERAL PRINCIPLES

Diagnosis

Localized tenderness is usually palpated directly over an affected bursa or tendon. Most often, active range of motion in the affected tendon or bursa is painful, but unlike with arthritis, passive range of motion is often painless. Blood tests and x-rays are usually normal.

Treatment

Use conservative measures first in treating bursitis and tendinitis. These include rest, modifying wear-and-tear activities, heat or ice (or both), physical therapy, weight loss, splinting, topical analgesics,

CURRENT DIAGNOSIS

Bursitis and Tendinitis

- Localized tenderness is usually palpated directly over an affected bursa or tendon.
- Most often, active range of motion in the affected tendon or bursa is painful, but unlike with arthritis, passive range of motion is often painless.
- With a few exceptions, blood tests and x-rays are usually normal.

Fibromyalgia

- Typical presentation includes a greater than 3 month history of chronic, widespread pain both above and below the waist and on both sides of the body in the absence of another condition to explain the pain.
- Diagnosis requires the presence of at least 11 of 18 tender points by digital palpation at previously published locations.
- Signs and symptoms include sleep disturbance, fatigue, paresthesias, stiffness, depression, dry eyes and mouth, Raynaud's syndrome, and headaches.

CURRENT THERAPY

Bursitis and Tendinitis

- Use conservative measures first: rest, modifying wear and tear activities, applying heat or ice or both, physical therapy, weight loss, splinting, topical analgesics, nonsteroidal antiinflammatory drugs (NSAIDs) and well-placed lidocaine injections with or without corticosteroids.
- Corticosteroid injections are best administered after 1-10 mL of lidocaine has been injected with a separate syringe, leaving the needle in place while changing the syringe. This prevents subcutaneous fat atrophy at the injection site from the corticosteroid. Inject around, not into a tendon to avoid tendon rupture.
- For the patient's comfort use a 25- or 27-gauge needle of appropriate length. Ethyl chloride spray on the skin obscures the pain of the needle stick. Adding sodium bicarbonate[1] to the syringe neutralizes the stinging sensation of lidocaine.
- Surgery for bursitis and tendinitis are reserved for cases unresponsiveness to conservative measures.

Fibromyalgia

- Daily aerobic exercise, starting with as little as 5 minutes at first, progressing to between 30 to 60 minutes, but even some exercise is beneficial
- Medication includes tramadol (Ultram) 50 mg, progressively up to 8 tablets daily in divided doses, for pain and zolpidem (Ambien) 10 mg at bedtime
- Psychological therapy to help with coping mechanisms and to aid in family support systems
- Medications that may be added onto, or substituted for, one of the first-line medications include pregabalin (Lyrica) 150 mg three times daily or gabapentin (Neurontin)[1] 1800 to 3600 mg daily in progressive, divided doses, primarily for pain; amitriptyline (Elavil) 10 to 200[3] mg or trazodone (Desyrel) 25 to 250 mg at bedtime; a selective serotonin reuptake inhibitor, such as sertraline (Zoloft) 50 mg daily.[1]
- Other tested and possibly helpful therapies include muscle relaxants including tizanidine (Zanaflex)[1] 4-8 mg three times daily, baclofen (Lioresal)[1] 10 to 20 mg three times daily, or cyclobenzaprine (Flexeril)[1] 10 mg at bedtime; Newer antidepressants such as duloxetine (Cymbalta) 60 mg twice daily[3] and milnacipran (Savella) 50 mg twice daily; and magnesium 500 mg combined with malic acid[7] 1200 to 2400 mg daily for fatigue.
- Avoid narcotics, NSAIDs (rarely helpful), prolonged bed rest and inactivity, and expensive or dangerous alternative therapies.

---

[1]Not FDA approved for this indication.
[3]Exceeds dosage recommended by the manufacturer.
[7]Available as a dietary supplement.

---

nonsteroidal antiinflammatory drugs (NSAIDs), and well placed lidocaine (Xylocaine) injections with or without corticosteroids. There are numerous NSAID preparations including naproxen (Naprosyn) 500 mg twice daily, ibuprofen (Motrin)[1] 400 to 800 mg every 6 to 8 hours, and the cyclooxygenase (COX)-2 selective agents including celecoxib (Celebrex)[1] 100 to 200 mg once or twice daily. If the patient is taking aspirin, even a baby aspirin, the COX-2 effect is eliminated. A proton pump inhibitor such as lansoprazole (Prevacid) 15 to 30 mg daily with a traditional NSAID gives the equivalent gastrointestinal protection of the COX-2 agents.

Corticosteroid injections using 0.5-1.0 mL of methylprednisolone acetate (Depo-Medrol) or triamcinolone acetonide (Kenalog-40) are best administered after 1 to 10 mL of lidocaine (Xylocaine) has been injected with a separate syringe, leaving the needle in place while changing the syringe. This prevents subcutaneous fat atrophy at the injection site from the corticosteroid. Inject around, not into, a tendon to avoid tendon rupture.

For the patient's comfort, a 25- or 27-gauge needle of appropriate length should be used. Ethyl chloride spray on the skin obscures the pain of the needle stick. Adding sodium bicarbonate[1] to the syringe neutralizes the stinging sensation of lidocaine.

Surgery for bursitis and tendinitis are reserved for cases unresponsive to conservative measures.

SPECIFIC AREAS

Shoulder Region

Shoulder pain is a common problem that increases with age. Because the shoulder has an extensive range of motion, it is one of the most unstable joints in the body.

Rotator cuff tendinitis or the impingement syndrome is reported to be the most common cause of shoulder pain, but in our rheumatology clinics, bicipital tendinitis seems to be a more common cause of shoulder pain. Subacromial bursitis may be secondarily present with the impingement syndrome. Pain on active abduction and internal rotation of the glenohumeral joint and aching over the deltoid area are the main symptoms of this condition. The impingement syndrome may be acute from a recent injury or chronic with calcific tendinitis sometimes seen on x-rays.

Rotator cuff tears may be partial or complete, acute or chronic, extremely painful or hardly felt. Weakness and pain on abduction, night pain, and tenderness on palpation can indicate the presence of a torn rotator cuff. The diagnosis may be established by a shoulder arthrogram, ultrasonography, or magnetic resonance imaging (MRI). Incomplete tears often are best treated by conservative means; over time they often become complete tears. Complete tears can often be surgically repaired, especially if they are acute and occur in younger patients.

---

[1]Not FDA approved for this indication.

Bicipital tendinitis often manifests as anterior shoulder pain. Often the pain is diffuse or felt as referred pain to the posterior shoulder or subacromial area. Rolling the long head of the inflamed biceps tendon under the examiner's thumb elicits localized tenderness. Rupture of the long head of the biceps tendon manifests as an enlargement of the distal end of the biceps muscle. This complication is usually not repaired except in a young person because it results in only a minor loss of strength in the biceps muscle.

Adhesive capsulitis or frozen shoulder manifests as generalized pain and tenderness of the shoulder area with a marked loss of active and passive range of motion and muscle atrophy. Inflammatory arthritis, diabetes, immobility, low pain threshold, depression, or improper treatment of a painful shoulder can result in a frozen shoulder. Arthrography demonstrates a contracted joint capsule space. Less-common painful conditions associated with the shoulder region include the thoracic outlet syndrome, brachial plexopathy, and neuropathies.

Anterior Chest Wall

Pain in the anterior chest wall is common and often needs to be differentiated from cardiac, pulmonary, or gastrointestinal pain. Point tenderness helps delineate actual chest wall pain from internal organ generated pain. Costochondritis (Tietze's syndrome) is manifested by tenderness at the costochondral junction of the anterior ribs. Xiphodynia is characterized by tenderness and pain over the xiphoid area.

Elbow Region

Olecranon bursitis occurs with repetitive mild trauma and abrasion over the elbow or with an inflammatory condition including gout, pseudogout, rheumatoid arthritis, or an infection. Aspiration of an uninfected bursa alone or combined with an injection of a corticosteroid is the usual treatment. Crystal identification with a polarized microscope is helpful to differentiate gout or pseudogout from infection. Antibiotic treatment, after a Gram stain and culture of purulent fluid, is indicated in a suspected infected bursa.

Lateral epicondylitis or tennis elbow and medial epicondylitis or golfer's elbow are common findings in the repetitive use of one's arms. Tenderness is elicited by pressing the extensor or flexor tendons 1 to 2 cm distal to the epicondyle. Shaking hands or lifting a bag causes pain in the same location. A soft forearm brace may be helpful if patients would prefer not to have an injection of the tender spot.

Ulnar nerve entrapment and tendinitis of the musculotendinous insertion of the biceps are conditions also found in the elbow region.

Hand and Wrist Region

A ganglion is a cyst arising from a tendon sheath or a joint, commonly located on the dorsum of the wrist. It is lined with synovium and contains a thick, jelly-like liquid. de Quervain's tenosynovitis is inflammation and tenderness of the sheath of the abductor pollicis longus and extensor pollicis brevis tendons located over the radial styloid. Repetitive trauma, pregnancy, and systemic rheumatoid diseases are causes for this disorder.

Carpal tunnel syndrome caused by the compression of the median nerve by the surrounding structures in the wrist is the most common cause of numbness and tingling in the hands. A positive Tinel's or Phalen's sign with a confirming nerve conduction test makes the diagnosis fairly simple. Trauma, pregnancy, and a host of metabolic or inflammatory diseases are often responsible for this condition. Treatment starts with wrist splinting at night. The use of 200 mg of vitamin B_6 (pyridoxine)[1] daily until the symptoms subside may be controversial, but in my opinion it often seems to be very helpful. If these measures are unsuccessful, a corticosteroid injection on the ulnar side of the carpal tunnel, a few millimeters away from the median nerve, usually relieves the numbness and tingling, often for months. In many patients, surgery is eventually required to release the median nerve.

---

[1]Not FDA approved for this indication.

Other, less-common hand and wrist soft tissue problems include pronator teres syndrome, anterior interosseous nerve syndrome, radial nerve palsy, ulnar nerve entrapment at the wrist, volar flexor tenosynovitis, and Dupuytren's contractures.

Hip Region

The trochanteric bursa lies on the posterior portion of the greater trochanter. Pain from trochanteric bursitis is felt in the trochanteric area and lateral thigh, and it is often inaccurately thought to be hip joint pain. Hip joint pain is usually felt in the groin and high in the buttock. Excessive trauma to the bursal area, such as an unusual amount of exercise like an excessively long hike, can precipitate trochanteric bursitis. Osteoarthritis of the lumbar spine or hip, scoliosis or leg length discrepancies, and age can contribute to trochanteric bursitis.

Ilopsoas (iliopectineal) bursitis causes groin and anterior thigh pain and is made worse on passive hyperextension, and sometimes flexion, of the hip with resistance.

Ischial (ischiogluteal) bursitis or weaver's bottom is caused by trauma or sitting a long time on hard surfaces. Pain from ischial bursitis is felt down the back of the thigh, with point tenderness over the ischial tuberosity. Soft seating cushions and a corticosteroid injection of the bursa usually helps the pain.

Piriformis syndrome manifests as pain over the buttocks, sometimes radiating down the back of the thigh and leg. Trauma is usually involved in the etiology. The diagnosis is often made on rectal or vaginal examination.

Meralgia paresthetica is caused by the compression of the lateral femoral cutaneous nerve (L2-L3). It causes intermittent burning pain, hyperesthesia, and numbness of the anterolateral thigh. This syndrome is seen most often in patients with obesity, diabetes, or pregnancy.

Knee Region

Popliteal cysts or Baker's cysts are associated with knee joint effusions, causing a synovial herniation into the popliteal fossa. The cyst can rupture and dissect down the calf, often to the ankle, where it can leave a purpuric crescent sign beneath the malleolus. A ruptured Baker's cyst is acutely painful and must be differentiated from thrombophlebitis. An arthrogram or ultrasound examination of the knee may be used to diagnose a Baker's cyst with or without a rupture. An ultrasound for a DVT or venogram can exclude concomitant thrombophlebitis if necessary. Surgical removal of the cyst may be necessary if an injection of a corticosteroid is ineffective.

Anserine bursitis is diagnosed by tenderness over the medial aspect of the knee an inch or two below the joint line and predominantly occurs in obese, middle-aged to elderly women with osteoarthritis of the knee and in patients with fibromyalgia.

Prepatellar bursitis or housemaid's knee presents as a mildly tender swelling over the patella. It is usually caused by trauma from frequent kneeling. Aspiration of the bursa is important because septic prepatellar bursitis is occasionally present. Because this bursa does not communicate with the knee joint, treatment with oral antibiotics appropriate for the organism cultured is adequate. For sterile bursitis, an injection of a corticosteroid is helpful as protection of the knee from trauma.

Less-common painful soft tissue conditions of the knee include patellar tendinitis, popliteal tendinitis, medial plica syndrome, rupture of the quadriceps tendon and infrapatellar tendon, and patellofemoral pain syndrome (chondromalacia patellae).

Ankle and Foot Region

Achilles tendinitis has two predominant causes. One is trauma; the other is a group of inflammatory conditions including rheumatoid arthritis, ankylosing spondylitis, reactive arthritis, and pseudogout. Tenderness, pain, and swelling occur proximal to or at the Achilles tendon attachment to the calcaneus. Shoe corrections, heel lifts, a splint with plantar flexion, and careful stretching of the tendon constitute the safest treatments. The inflamed Achilles tendon is vulnerable to rupture, especially if a corticosteroid is injected around it (which is not recommended). The differential diagnosis of Achilles tendinitis includes retrocalcaneal bursitis and subcutaneous Achilles bursitis.

Plantar fasciitis is characterized by burning, lancing, or aching pain and tenderness over the plantar surface of the heel from a variety of kinds of trauma or overuse.

Tarsal tunnel syndrome is caused by compression of the posterior tibial nerve, posterior and inferior to the medial malleolus. A positive Tinel's sign may be elicited by percussion over the entrapment site. Numbness, paresthesias and burning pain are felt from the toes to the medial malleolus. Changing shoes and using conservative therapy, such as NSAIDSs, topical analgesics or local steroid injections might help in the treatment of this condition, but surgery is often needed to decompress the nerve and provide relief.

Morton's neuroma is an entrapment neuropathy of the interdigital nerve most commonly found between the third and fourth toes. This condition is often detected in middle-aged women wearing high heels or tight shoes. Pain is often felt in the fourth toe as a burning, aching pain with paresthesias. Treatment consists of a metatarsal bar or a corticosteroid injection in the web space of the toe where the tenderness is palpated. If these are unsuccessful, surgery to remove the neuroma may be necessary.

Other causes of nonarthritic foot pain include posterior tibial tendinitis, hallux valgus, bunionette (tailor's bunion) of the fifth toe, hammer toes, metatarsalgia, pes planus (flat foot), pes cavus (claw foot), and a variety of tendon ruptures or displacements including the Achilles, posterior tibialis and the peroneal tendons.

Myofascial Pain Syndrome

Myofascial pain syndromes are often referred to as localized or regional fibromyalgia. They include regional pain disorders including chronic whiplash, repetitive strain syndrome, and temporomandibular joint syndrome. Myofascial pain is characterized by the presence of trigger points, defined as localized areas of deep muscle tenderness located in a taut band in the muscle. Unlike in the tender points of fibromyalgia, when these are palpated the pain is referred to distant zones of perceived pain. Treatment includes injecting the trigger points (see the treatments for bursitis and tendinitis) and often adding the treatment modalities outlined in the fibromyalgia section.

Complex Regional Pain Syndromes

Formerly referred to as reflex sympathetic dystrophy, Sudek's atrophy, causalgia, or shoulder–hand syndrome, among other terms, this condition was named complex regional pain syndrome in 1995. It is described as regional pain usually related to nerve injury, trauma, surgery, myocardial infarction, or stroke. The pain is usually worse than should be expected from the inciting injury. It is associated with pain, edema, and skin temperature and color changes. Treatment is complex and requires the help of physiatrists, physical therapists, and pain clinics.

Fibromyalgia Syndrome

Fibromyalgia is a chronic, diffuse pain syndrome of unknown etiology. It is characterized by widespread musculoskeletal pain of variable intensity and specific tender points to palpation (see later). Fibromyalgia is associated with a lack of deep sleep and a relative intolerance of physical activities due to pain.

CLINICAL MANIFESTATIONS AND DIAGNOSIS

Signs and symptoms include sleep disturbance, fatigue, paresthesias, stiffness, depression, dry eyes and mouth, Raynaud's syndrome, and headaches. Primary fibromyalgia is remarkable for the lack of

---

> **BOX 1   Conditions Associated or Concurrent with Fibromyalgia**
>
> **Conditions Associated with Fibromyalgia**
> Hypothyroidism
> Polymyalgia rheumatica
> Tapering off corticosteroids
> Drugs: lipid-lowering and antiviral agents
> Cervical stenosis (?)
> Malignancy
> Viral infections: parvovirus, Lyme disease, hepatitis C, others
>
> **Conditions Concurrent with Fibromyalgia**
> Chronic fatigue syndrome
> Autoimmune diseases such as systemic lupus erythematosus or rheumatoid arthritis
> Myofascial pain syndrome
> Irritable bowel syndrome
> Gulf War syndrome
> Migraine headaches
> Interstitial cystitis

abnormal laboratory and radiologic tests routinely done for rheumatologic diseases. Secondary fibromyalgia, fibromyalgia linked to another disease, can improve when the primary disease is treated. Concurrent fibromyalgia or fibromyalgia coexisting together with other conditions (Box 1) including approximately 30% of patients with rheumatoid arthritis and systemic lupus erythematosus might not respond to treatment of the other disease.

Presentation includes a history of chronic, widespread pain both above and below the waist and on both sides of the body in the absence of another condition to explain the pain and that has lasted longer than 3 months. The diagnosis is based on the presence of at least 11 out of 18 tender points by digital palpation at previously published locations. Tender point sites include bilateral locations on the occiput, anterior lower neck (C-5-C7), trapezius, supraspinatus, second anterior costochondral junction, lateral epicondyle, buttocks in the upper outer quadrant, greater trochanters and medial fat pad of the knees. Digital palpation of the tender points is done at about 4 kg of force, which is roughly enough pressure to blanch the thumbnail.

TREATMENT

It is extremely important that patients are made aware by the treating physician that they own this diagnosis and it requires effort on their part to get better. Treatment with narcotics should be avoided if at all possible because they seldom relieve pain caused by fibromyalgia for an adequate length of time. Self-motivated patients might find relief for a significant portion of their discomfort in combining aerobic exercise with a well-thought-out drug and psychological treatment program. Refer patients to support groups backed by organizations like the Arthritis Foundation.

Initial Treatment

Daily aerobic exercise, starting with as little as 5 minutes at first, progressing to between 30-60 minutes, is ideal. Emphasize to patients that without the progressive aerobic exercise part of treatment—walking, swimming in warm water, bicycling, jogging, or other exercise—they are unlikely to improve very much no matter what medications they take. It usually takes 6 to 12 months of exercise by unusually motivated patients to attain the level of fitness that is likely to diminish most or all the pain. Even some exercise is still beneficial.

Tramadol (Ultram) 50 mg, progressively titrated up to 8 tablets daily in divided doses, may be given for pain. Zolpidem (Ambien) 10 mg at bedtime can help with sleep disturbances. This drug is less habit forming and gives the deepest (i.e. state 3 or 4) sleep of any sleeping medications.

Psychological therapy should be considered to help with coping mechanisms and to aid in family support systems.

Second-line Treatment

Other medications may be added onto, or substituted for, one of the first-line medications depending on drug interactions and efficacy. Pregabalin (Lyrica) 150 mg three times a day (this is the first medication approved by the FDA primarily for the treatment of fibromyalgia) or gabapentin (Neurontin)[1] 1800 to 3600 mg daily in progressive, divided doses, may be used primarily for pain. Amitriptyline (Elavil) 10 to 200[3] mg or trazodone (Desyrel) 25 to 250 mg at bedtime may help with sleep disturbance,[1] depression, and mild pain relief.[1] A selective serotonin reuptake inhibitor (SSRI), such as sertraline (Zoloft) 50 mg daily, may be useful for depression and mild pain relief.[1]

Other Tested and Possibly Helpful Treatments

Muscle relaxants including tizanidine (Zanaflex)[1] 4 to 8 mg three times a day, baclofen (Lioresal)[1] 10 to 20 mg three times a day, or cyclobenzaprine (Flexeril)[1] 10 mg at bedtime may be helpful for pain and rest. Newer antidepressants such as duloxetine (Cymbalta) (now approved by the FDA for fibromyalgia) 60 mg twice daily[3] for pain and secondarily for depression, and the newest FDA-approved drug for fibromyalgia, milnacipran (Savella) 50 mg twice daily (starting at 10 mg/day and titrated to arrive at the recommended dose in 1 week) may be helpful. Magnesium 500 mg combined with malic acid[7] 1200 to 2400 mg daily might be helpful for fatigue.

Treatments to Avoid

Narcotics should be avoided. NSAIDs are rarely helpful. Prolonged bed rest and inactivity are counterproductive. Expensive or dangerous alternative therapies should be avoided.

---

[1]Not FDA approved for this indication.
[3]Exceeds dosage recommended by the manufacturer.
[7]Available as a dietary supplement.

REFERENCES

Biundo Jr JJ. Regional rheumatic pain syndromes. In: Klippel JH, Stone JH, Crofford LJ, White PH, editors. Primer on the Rheumatic Diseases. 13th ed. Atlanta: Arthritis Foundation; 2008. p. 68–86.
Dadabhoy D, Clauw DJ. The fibromyalgia syndrome. In: Klippel JH, Stone JH, Crofford LJ, White PH, editors. Primer on the Rheumatic Diseases. 13th ed. Atlanta: Arthritis Foundation; 2008. p. 87–93.
Fransen J, Russell IJ. Medical management of fibromyalgia. In: Fransen J, Russell IJ, editors. The Fibromyalgia Help Book. St. Paul: Smith House Press; 1996. p. 35–58.
Goldenberg DL. Fibromyalgia and related syndromes. In: Hochberg MC, Silman AL, Smolen JS, et al, editors. Rheumatology. 3rd ed. St Louis: Mosby; 2003. p. 701–12.
Sheon RP. Overview of soft tissue rheumatic disorders. 2009. UpToDate, online 17.3, www.uptodate.com.

Osteoarthritis

Method of
David H. Neustadt, MD

Osteoarthritis (OA) (degenerative joint disease) is the most commonly encountered rheumatic disorder and the major cause of disability and reduced activity after 50 years of age. Radiographic evidence of OA is found in up to 85% of people older than 65 years. Autopsies indicate evidence of OA in weight-bearing joints of almost all persons by the age of 45 years.

CURRENT DIAGNOSIS

- Enhanced understanding and knowledge of the pathogenesis of osteoarthritis have led to increasing optimism for the 20 to 30 million osteoarthritis sufferers in the United States.
- Osteoarthritis is now known to involve inflammatory mechanisms, not mechanical wear and tear, as believed in the past.

In spite of the evidence of pathologic changes of OA found in Java and Neanderthal human skeletons and dinosaur skeletons, OA was confused with rheumatoid arthritis (RA) until the turn of the 20th century. It is characterized pathologically by involvement of cartilage, varying from fissures and microfibrillations in early disease to erosive destruction in advanced disease. Weight-bearing or shearing forces are transmitted to the subchondral bone, leading to sclerosis, cyst formation, and bone remodeling. Osteophytes (spurs) develop at the margins of joints, and new cartilage proliferates over these bony spurs.

An inflammatory component is present in most patients with symptomatic OA. The traditional belief that OA is simply a wear-and-tear condition associated with the stress of advancing years is not tenable. This mistaken belief is considered the major reason for the relatively slow progress of cartilage and bone research and investigation into the etiology and pathogenesis of OA. During the past decade, much new knowledge on cartilage, including metabolic changes, genetic mutations, metalloproteinases, and possible diagnostic biomarkers and inflammatory mediators, has fostered considerable excitement and interest in new approaches for the prevention, monitoring, and treatment of OA.

Although the cause of OA is unknown, contributing factors include heredity, trauma, overweight, overuse of joints, and aging. OA may be classified into primary (idiopathic) and secondary forms. Secondary OA results from trauma or repetitive overuse of a specific joint; in an inflammatory form of arthritis such as RA, repeated attacks of gout, or septic arthritis; developmental problems such as congenital dysplasia of a hip or slipped capital femoral epiphysis; or metabolic and miscellaneous causes including hemophiliac arthropathy, ochronosis (alkaptonuria), and osteonecrosis. Thus, OA may be considered a (final) common pathway resulting from a host of many different problems.

Joints commonly affected in OA include the large weight-bearing and frequently used joints, such as the hips and knees, spine, distal interphalangeal (DIP) joints (Heberden's nodes), and trapeziometacarpal (carpometacarpal thumb base) and first metatarsophalangeal joint (bunion). Joints often spared in OA include the metacarpals, the wrists, the shoulders, and the ankles (except in ballet dancers).

Clinical Features

The onset of OA is insidious, and the course is slowly progressive. Clinical features include variable pain and mild stiffness, with associated limited motion; bony enlargement with or without tenderness; synovitis of the knees; and functional impairment with malalignment (varus or valgus deformities) when advanced involvement of the knees or hips develops. There are no specific laboratory abnormalities or specific (disease) markers of the disease, except in ochronosis.

Radiographs and other imaging procedures demonstrate evidence of OA, manifested chiefly by a narrowed joint space (loss of cartilage), osteophyte formation, and secondary subchondral sclerosis. There may be a poor correlation between symptoms and underlying abnormal structural findings on x-ray images. Special subsets of OA and significant associated conditions include inflammatory (cystic erosive) OA, calcium pyrophosphate dihydrate disease (chondrocalcinosis), and diffuse idiopathic skeletal hyperostosis (DISH).

Treatment

The optimal management program for OA should be individualized to the specific problems and clinical syndromes presented by each patient (Box 1).

GENERAL CONSIDERATIONS

Realistic reassurance that the patient does not have a serious, potentially crippling disease such as RA and adequate understanding of what to expect are of paramount importance for successful management. Education of the patient is the basic foundation of the treatment program. The updated OA booklet provided by the National Arthritis Foundation is an available useful supplement to education. Involving spouses and other family members in coping skills training may be helpful. Understanding the patient's problem permits reasonable delegation of responsibilities for chores and engaging in activities. Patients and spouses who are better informed about the disease and its outlook are generally better able to cope with the condition. Cognitive behavior techniques can help patients confront the variability of symptoms, the effects of rest and exercise, and emotional aspects.

PROPHYLACTIC MEASURES

Reducing the impact of the load and shearing force on an osteoarthritis joint not only can diminish symptoms but also can retard progression of the disease. Explaining the biomechanical factors enables the patient to understand the need for rest and protection of the affected joints. Weight reduction by dietetic means is strongly encouraged for the obese patient. Protective and preventive measures for the knee include avoiding weight-bearing knee bending, stair climbing, jogging, and prolonged walking. Knee loading during weight bearing can be avoided by using a high chair or stool, elevated toilet seat, knee supports or braces, and walking devices (Box 2).

NONPHARMACOLOGIC THERAPY

The most important aspect is specific instructions for balanced rest and exercise (preferably at home). Exercises should be mainly isometric (nonmovement), such as quadriceps muscle strengthening, stretching, and range-of-motion exercises.

Instructions should be given for joint protection with measures to conserve energy and on the use of any needed assistive aids, such as canes, crutches, walkers, splints, back supports and braces, cervical supporting collars, and proper shoes with any needed modifications and orthotics.

BOX 1   Comprehensive Management Program for Osteoarthritis

Education of the patient and family
Coping measures: Rest and modification of activities of daily living
Measures to reduce joint loading
Physical therapy, occupational therapy, assistive devices
Pharmacotherapy
Intraarticular therapy (steroids, hyaluronan)
Surgery

BOX 2   Measures to Protect Knees

Avoid knee bending when weight bearing
Avoid steps when possible
Use high chair or high stool
Use elevated toilet seat
Use cane, crutches, or walker for prolonged walking
Do isometric quadriceps muscle-strengthening exercises

CURRENT THERAPY

- Although there is no cure for osteoarthritis, coping strategies including simple measures such as weight reduction and modification of activities to reduce stress and load on the joints should be emphasized.
- Pharmacotherapy includes acetaminophen (Tylenol), other simple analgesics, and judicious use of nonsteroidal antiinflammatory drugs. Opioids should be avoided.
- When usual medical measures fail to control the pain of osteoarthritis, intraarticular injections of a corticosteroid is the next step.
- A painful effusion is the major indication for arthrocentesis, aspiration, and if fluid is not infectious, instillation of a corticosteroid preparation.
- After a corticosteroid injection for knee osteoarthritis, increased therapeutic response results if a postinjection rest regimen is imposed. The patient remains in bed or at rest for 3 days and then uses walking devices (cane or crutches) for 2 to 3 weeks.
- The main factors that influence the therapeutic response from a series of hyaluronan injections are the extent of loss of cartilage and severity of the osteoarthritis disease in the affected knee.
- Total knee and hip replacement procedures are considered when nonoperative management fails to adequately control symptoms and pain.

Heat modalities should be prescribed in the form of hot showers or tub soaks, hot packs such as a Bed Buddy (microwavable cervical collar or back wrap), and a warm pool for water aerobic exercises. These measures ameliorate discomfort and facilitate the exercise program. Diathermy, short wave, and ultrasound methods are relatively expensive and of questionable benefit. The use of a hot tub or whirlpool bath, especially after exercise or work, may be of palliative benefit.

Job and recreational activities must be assessed and modified if necessary to avoid overuse of affected joints. Sexual counseling may be needed, especially in some patients with severe knee, hip, or back involvement.

PHARMACOTHERAPY

The basic program of education and reassurance of the patient, joint rest and protection, and physical measures can control symptoms in some patients with early mild OA. Many patients, however, require drug therapy. Although no available drugs predictably reverse or halt the inexorable progression of the disease, the drugs do reduce pain and inflammation, enhancing the patient's quality of life.

Analgesics

Some patients with OA have minimal inflammation and can be managed with analgesics alone. Analgesic agents (non-narcotic) currently available include acetaminophen (Tylenol), propoxyphene (Darvon), and tramadol (Ultram). Effective dosages of acetaminophen are 1.0 to 1.3 g administered every 8 hours or three or four times daily (do not exceed 4 g/day). Adverse effects are rare, but caution must be exercised in patients who have preexisting renal or liver conditions. Propoxyphene is effective, especially in combination with acetaminophen (Darvocet-N 100), and may be given in a dosage of 1 tablet every 4 to 6 hours for supplementary analgesia. Side effects are usually minimal, with the patient occasionally intolerant because of nausea or lightheadedness. Tramadol can be given in 50-, 100-, 200-, or 300-mg tablets up to two to three times daily for pain relief (do not exceed 400 mg of immediate-release tablets per day or 300 mg of extended-release tablets per day). These drugs are generally well tolerated, and nausea, vomiting, and dizziness are the most common adverse effects. A combination preparation, Ultram 37.5 plus acetaminophen (Ultracet), is available. I advise avoiding regular use of opioids. Opioids may be needed occasionally for intense pain, but the benefits are limited owing to the common gastrointestinal adverse events and the potential for addiction.

Antiinflammatory Agents

A much-discussed report compared acetaminophen 4 g/day with ibuprofen (Advil, Motrin) 1200 to 2400 mg/day, in OA of the knee. The clinical results demonstrated no significant difference in efficacy among the three treatment groups. Critical analysis of this comparative study, however, discloses a short duration of the treatment trial (4 weeks) and a relatively low antiinflammatory dosage (up to 2400 mg) of ibuprofen. In my experience and that of many others, pain in OA patients is often not adequately controlled with pure analgesics, whereas nonsteroidal antiinflammatory drugs (NSAIDs) in adequate dosage can provide significant clinical improvement.

Nonacetylated salicylates are widely used in OA. Compounds currently available include salsalate, choline magnesium trisalicylate, and magnesium salicylate. These agents are weak prostaglandin (cyclooxygenase) inhibitors, thus avoiding the anticlotting effect and potential adverse effect on the gastrointestinal tract and kidneys. Side effects are relatively uncommon and minor with nonacetylated salicylates when administered in a dosage of 1 to 1.5 g twice daily. Gastrointestinal and cardiovascular problems have not been reported. Salicylism with ototoxicity is a rare side effect.

If simple analgesics and salsalate fail to provide adequate relief, one of the many currently available NSAIDs may be selected for a therapeutic trial. Clinical trials with naproxen, diclofenac, and sulindac showed significantly greater improvement of the NSAID when compared with high-dose acetaminophen. The chief limiting factor in the use of NSAIDs is the possible induced gastric pathologic changes, disturbed renal function, and potential increased cardiac events.

Cost and compliance also must be given consideration. Many of the NSAIDs are now available in dosage forms that can be given once or twice daily, which helps overcome the compliance problem.

Currently available NSAIDs are all similar in their proposed mechanism of action but vary considerably in their pharmocokinetics, dosage, clinical response, and side effects. The variability of the effects of different NSAIDs in patients is significant and unpredictable. All NSAIDs are metabolized in the liver, except two available compounds, sulindac (Clinoril) and nabumetone (Relafen), which are prodrugs that are not converted to active drugs until after absorption and hepatic biotransformation. The prodrug effect might partially spare the gastrointestinal tract and also produces less suppression of renal prostaglandins. Etodolac (Lodine) reportedly has fewer gastric complications, and endoscopy does not demonstrate the typical gastric erosions found in the gastric mucosa of the majority of patients taking older NSAIDs.

Concomitant prophylactic use of misoprostol (Cytotec) has been recommended to protect gastric mucosa in patients with a previous history of peptic ulcer or gastrointestinal bleeding. Unfortunately, misoprostol causes cramps and diarrhea in a relatively high percentage of patients. A gastroprotective agent, such as a proton pump inhibitor, will reduce the risk of gastrointestinal adverse effects.

The question of potential deleterious effect on cartilage versus chondroprotective properties by various NSAIDs remains controversial.

Cyclooxygenase 2 Inhibitors

Prostaglandin synthesis in humans is catalyzed by two enzyme forms of cyclooxygenase: cyclooxygenase 1 (COX-1) and cyclooxygenase 2 (COX-2).

COX-1 is constitutively expressed and is considered responsible for suppression of physiologic functions including gastric mucosal protection. In contrast, COX-2 is induced by inflammatory mediators and is responsible for inflammation without any significant effect on the gastric mucosa. The development of agents that selectively inhibit the COX-2 pathway without significant gastrointestinal adverse effects was considered an extremely important advance.

Currently only one COX-2–specific inhibiting NSAID is FDA approved and available. Celecoxib (Celebrex) is equivalent to the older nonselective NSAIDs with regard to therapeutic effectiveness, but the risk of gastrointestinal toxicity and adverse effects on platelet aggregation is lessened. The risk of renal side effects is probably comparable with that of the conventional NSAIDs. A trial assessing the effect of celecoxib on cardiovascular events found a slightly higher risk of cardiovascular events but chiefly only at higher doses (400 mg/day or greater). Celecoxib can be used with low-dose aspirin (81 mg) daily and anticoagulants including warfarin (Coumadin).

INTRAARTICULAR INJECTIONS

Corticosteroids

After many years of controversy concerning intraarticular corticosteroid therapy in OA, there is now consensus that this form of therapy is of considerable value when it is indicated and skillfully administered. Although early on it is still preferable to attempt to control symptoms by simple measures with oral therapy, rather than by local injection, when faced with relatively acute painful conditions such as synovitis of the knee or inflamed Heberden's nodes, quick and sometimes lasting relief can be obtained with intrasynovial steroid injection. This form of treatment is considered an adjunct to a conventional management program.

A painful knee effusion is the most common indication for arthrocentesis followed by a local corticosteroid injection. The remote potential deleterious effect of instability developing in the knee can be avoided by giving injections at infrequent intervals and prescribing a strict postinjection rest regimen. Specific instructions are given to the patient to refrain from weight-bearing activity for 3 days, except getting up for meals and going to the bathroom. The patient is advised to reduce loading of the injected knee by using a cane or crutches with a three-point gait during weight bearing for 2 to 3 weeks after the procedure. This rest regimen delays escape of the steroid suspension from the joint cavity and promotes a longer duration of response to the injection. I have observed numerous patients with OA of the knee associated with large recurrent synovitis who had been given three to five or more local injections with only transient benefit. When a strict postinjection rest program was imposed, these patients obtained substantial improvement in the duration of the effect, and some achieved indefinite "cures." The remote risk of introducing infection from the procedure is minimized by adhering to a meticulous aseptic technique.

Another important indication for arthrocentesis and intraarticular steroid therapy is OA associated with crystal synovitis due to calcium pyrophosphate dihydrate disease (CPPD) or pseudogout. Diagnosis is confirmed by radiographic findings of chondrocalcinosis and polarized microscopic identification of the specific crystals in the fluid. Treatment, including aspiration and administration of intraarticular steroids, is usually successful in controlling the acute synovitis.

Hyaluronans (Hyaluronic Acid, Hyaluronate)

Intraarticular hyaluronan, approved by the FDA in 1997 as a new procedure for clinical use in OA of the knee, represents a valuable addition to the therapeutic armamentarium for the treatment of OA. The clinical use of intraarticular hyaluronan in painful OA of the knee was introduced in Europe in the 1990s. The mechanism of action of hyaluronate is termed *viscosupplementation* in an effort to restore normal viscoelastic properties to the pathologically altered synovial fluid. Other possible beneficial effects include protection of the chondrocytes, antiinflammatory effects, and improvement of the mechanics of joint motion.

Numerous preparations of FDA approved hyaluronan preparations are in wide use in the United States. Initially, all hyaluronans were extracted from rooster combs. Table 1 lists the more common hyaluronans that are available for injecting knee osteoarthritis. The hyaluronan products are injected in a series of three, four, or five at weekly intervals in accordance with the patient's response. All the hyaluronans are highly purified natural preparations except Hylan

TABLE 1 Some Common FDA-Approved Hyaluronans and Their Molecular Weights

Product	MW (kDa)	Dose (Weekly)
Hylan G-F20 (Synvisc)	5000–6000	3 × 16 mg
High-molecular-weight hyaluronan (Orthovisc)	1000–2900	3–4 × 30 mg
Sodium hyaluronate (Hyalgan)	500–720	3–5 × 20 mg
Sodium hyaluronate (Supartz)	620–1200	5 × 25 mg
1% Sodium hyaluronate (Euflexxa)*	2400–3600	3 × 20 mg

*Derived from biological fermentations.

G-F20, which is cross-linked with added formaldehyde and vinyl sulfone in an effort to increase retention in the joint cavity. Effectiveness and duration of improvement are similar with all the products. Undesirable complications and adverse effects are limited to rare local mild pain, with the exception of the cross-linked Hylan G-F20, which can cause a severe acute inflammatory reaction (SAIR, or pseudoseptic reaction) in approximately 2% to 8% of patients injected with the product.

Newer hyaluronan products are non–animal-derived preparations that are developed from biological fermentation of streptococcal origin. Until recently, these hyaluronans have been available only in Europe. One of these products (Euflexxa) has been approved by the FDA for use in the United States. This preparation would be especially useful in the rare patient who is allergic to avian products. Hyaluronan therapy has been studied in other specific joints including the hip, shoulder, ankle, and first carpometacarpal joints. Approval from the FDA is expected. Drawbacks of intraarticular hyaluronan include difficulty injecting and limited response in patients with extreme obesity and severe advanced osteoarthritis of the knee (grade 4 Kellgren classification). Re-treatment with intraarticular hyaluronic acid 1 year after the first series is safe and effective in patients whose initial course of therapy was successful. A new hyaluronan preparation (Monovisc) has been developed, containing 4 or 5 times the amount of hyaluronan used in the usual knee injection, which is given in a series of 3 or 4 weekly injections. The approach, if effective, would simplify the procedure, especially for "needle shy" patients. The treatment is available in Europe but is not FDA approved as yet for use in the United States.

JOINT LAVAGE AND ARTHROSCOPY

Lavage of the arthritic knee may be performed with arthroscopic visualization. The authors of a recent double-blind, sham-controlled evaluation concluded that "most, if not all" of the effects of tidal irrigation seem to be attributable to a placebo effect. Arthroscopy permits inspection of the joint cavity. Associated abnormalities such as ligamentous and meniscal tears can be observed in conjunction with osteoarthritis. Calcified loose bodies can be removed, and débridement can be carried out.

TREATMENT OF CYSTIC EROSIVE (INFLAMMATORY) OSTEOARTHRITIS

Cystic erosive OA is the genetically determined clinical syndrome manifested by the lumpy-bumpy fingers with involvement of the DIP joints (Heberden's nodes) and proximal interphalangeal joints (Bouchard's nodules). It rarely causes significant pain except during the early developing stage. It is important to strongly reassure the patient that this is not a serious crippling disease, emphasizing the distinction of the knobby nodes from the swelling of the synovitis of RA. However, if the thumb base joint (trapeziometacarpal, first carpometacarpal) is involved, abduction splinting or local injection may be necessary for relief of pain.

Occasionally, when OA of the fingers is symptomatic, warm soaks; application of an analgesic balm, such as triethanolamine, after the warm soaks; and the wearing of spandex gloves during sleep at night are sometimes useful. When a digital node is inflamed, local instillation of a few drops of a corticosteroid suspension often provides prompt relief.

If symptoms persist, a cautious trial with one of the topical analgesic pepper plant creams (capsaicin) such as Zostrix may be worthwhile. Capsaicin is an inhibitor of substance P, the neuropeptide pain mediator. The topical cream is safe, and a local burning or transient stinging sensation during application is the only troublesome adverse effect. The stinging diminishes with use after a few days.

NEW APPROACHES

Disease-Modifying Drugs

The purpose of the investigational disease-modifying drugs is to play a role in either enhancing the biosynthesis of cartilage matrix or preventing enzymatic degradation and inhibiting catabolic cytokine activity in an attempt to induce cartilage repair and restore joint homeostasis.

Tetracycline (Sumycin)[1] and its congeners (doxycycline (Vibramycin),[1] minocycline (Dynacin)[1]) have shown evidence of inhibiting enzymatic degradation of cartilage, including that by stromelysin, collagenase, and gelatinase, in dog, guinea pig, and rabbit models of OA. A proposed long-term clinical trial in human subjects is in progress.

Hydroxychloroquine (Plaquenil)[1] and chloroquine (Aralen)[1] have been administered successfully for many years in RA and systemic lupus erythematosus. Recently, anecdotal and retrospective uncontrolled studies have reported the efficacy of hydroxychloroquine in retarding the progression of inflammatory (cystic) erosive OA. It has been suggested that the beneficial action of hydroxychloroquine is due to its inhibitory effects on lysosomal enzymes and the secretion of interleukin-1. Experience thus far suggests that this agent may be promising in inflammatory OA.

Other novel therapeutic approaches that are under study but lack conclusive significant data at this time include insulin-like growth factors, transforming growth factor-β, and glucosamine, a proteoglycan component and a growth factor for cartilage. In ongoing studies, an antinerve growth factor antibody, fully humanized, effectively reduces pain and improves function in subjects with knee osteoarthritis. Undesirable effects so far are minor, including a rare transient mild peripheral neuritis.

Chondrocyte Transplantation

Chondrocyte transplantation was initially developed and carried out in Sweden for localized cartilage damage resulting from trauma in young subjects. A subsequent report described relatively successful treatment of 23 patients who had chondral defects of the knee and were given autologous chondrocyte transplantation combined with periosteal grafting. The expectation that the procedure will "cure" OA lesions remains an unmet possibility for the future. Regeneration of articular cartilage is a complex process and will require long-term evaluation of the function of the new cartilage and prospective controlled clinical studies to confirm the value of the procedure.

Gene Therapy

Gene therapy is an exciting new technology that holds promise for the future but requires considerable further investigation and refinement. Techniques to introduce gene transfer in conjunction with autologous cultured chondrocytes are being explored.

Glucosamine and Chondroitin Sulfate

Glucosamine[7] and chondroitin[7] sulfate are over-the-counter nutraceuticals (dietary supplements) that have considerable anecdotal data touting their symptom-modifying effects. Some reports have suggested

---

[1]Not FDA approved for this indication.
[7]Available as a dietary supplement.

that glucosamine can retard or modify structural changes of OA, but convincing evidence for this effect is lacking. The drugs are well tolerated and have no significant adverse effects. Recently published studies have no evidence or significant data demonstrating that either of these preparations used alone or in combination prevents or reduces pain in osteoarthritis of the knee. Further observations with long-term randomized, double-blind studies are needed to confirm any value of these popular but unproved medications.

SURGERY

When appropriate medical (nonoperative) management fails to adequately control pain, and functional disability significantly interferes with lifestyle, surgical options should be considered.

Available procedures include osteotomy for joint malalignment (varus knee deformities); arthroscopy, especially for specific lesions such as calcified loose bodies or meniscal tears; and arthrodesis (fusion) for unstable joints, when joint replacement is not indicated or declined. Arthrodesis may be the optimal procedure in young, overweight, active patients with severe OA involving a single knee.

Partial or total arthroplasty, especially total knee and hip replacement, may be carried out in patients in whom medical management fails to adequately control symptoms. An estimated 125,000 total hip replacements, most of which are for OA, are performed each year in the United States. Total knee replacement (total knee arthroplasty) is an increasingly gratifying operation for advanced knee OA. Innovative approaches and new techniques, including the development of minimal invasive procedures (MIS), bodes well for the future.

REFERENCES

Mandell BF, Lipani J. Refractory osteoarthritis. Differential diagnosis and therapy. Rheum Dis Clin North Am 1995;21:163–78.

Neustadt DH. Intra-articular injections for osteoarthritis of the knee. Cleve Clin J Med 2006;73:897–910.

Neustadt DH. Current approach to therapy for osteoarthritis of the knee. Louisville Med 2004;51:341–3.

Neustadt DH, Altman RD. Intra-articular therapy. In: Moskowitz RW, Howell DS, Goldberg VM, et al, editors. Osteoarthritis, Diagnosis and Medical/Surgical Management. 4th ed. Philadelphia: Lippincott Williams & Wilkins; 2007. pp. 287–301.

Poole AR, Howell DS. Etiopathogenesis of osteoarthritis. In: Moskowitz RW, Howell DS, Goldberg VM, et al, editors. Osteoarthritis, Diagnosis and Medical/Surgical Management. 4th ed. Philadelphia: Lippincott Williams & Wilkins; 2007. pp. 27–49.

Sharma L, Kapoor D, Issa S. Epidemiology of osteoarthritis. In: Moskowitz RW, Howell DS, Goldberg VM, et al, editors. Osteoarthritis, Diagnosis and Medical/Surgical Management. 4th ed. Philadelphia: Lippincott Williams & Wilkins; 2007. pp. 1–26.

Steinbrocker O, Neustadt DH. Aspiration and Injection Therapy. Arthritis and Musculoskeletal Disorders: A Handbook on Technique and Management. Hagerstown MD: Harper & Row; 1972.

Polymyalgia Rheumatica and Giant Cell Arteritis

Method of
Barri J. Fessler, MD, MSPH

Polymyalgia rheumatica (PMR) and giant cell arteritis (GCA) are systemic inflammatory disorders of unknown etiology. Each condition can occur in isolation or in conjunction with the other; 15% to 20% of patients with PMR have GCA, and 40% to 60% of patients with GCA have PMR. For both conditions, onset is in people older than 50 years, women are more commonly affected than men, and significant elevations in acute phase reactants are typically seen in the majority of patients. The prevalence of GCA is highest in Scandinavian countries and regions with people of Northern European descent. It is rare in blacks and Hispanics.

Polymyalgia Rheumatica

CLINICAL PRESENTATION

PMR is characterized by aching, pain, and stiffness in the muscles of the neck, shoulder, and hip girdle. Symptoms initially may be unilateral but they eventually become bilateral. The pain typically radiates toward the elbows and knees. Weakness is not a feature of PMR. Fatigue, anorexia, weight loss, and low-grade fevers may be seen. Half of patients develop an asymmetric arthritis affecting the knees and wrists or diffuse pitting edema of the hands and feet. The erythrocyte sedimentation rate (ESR) is usually more than 40 mm/h; up to 20% of patients have a normal ESR.

DIAGNOSIS

The diagnosis of PMR depends upon a combination of symptoms, elevated ESR, exclusion of other diseases, and response to corticosteroids. Diseases to be excluded include elderly-onset rheumatoid arthritis, spondyloarthropathy, crystal-induced arthritis, polymyositis, malignancy, and infection.

TREATMENT

Treatment of PMR is with moderate doses of corticosteroids (e.g., prednisone[1] 15-20 mg daily). The majority of patients experience rapid and dramatic relief of symptoms within 24 to 48 hours. If there

---

[1]Not FDA approved for this indication.

CURRENT DIAGNOSIS

Polymyalgia Rheumatica

- Age at onset is 50 years or older.
- Symptoms include pain and stiffness in neck, bilateral shoulders and upper arms, hips and proximal thighs. Weakness is *not* a feature of Polymyalgia rheumatica and should prompt a search for other diagnoses.
- Erythrocyte sedimentation rate is ≥40 mm/h.*
- Exclude other diagnoses that can cause similar symptoms.
- Up to 20% of patients with Polymyalgia rheumatica also have giant cell arteritis.

Giant Cell Arteritis

- Age at onset is 50 years or older.
- Symptoms can include new-onset headache, jaw claudication, scalp tenderness, and vision loss or diplopia.
- Fevers, anorexia, weight loss, or hoarseness may also be present.
- Polymyalgia rheumatica is seen in 40% to 60% of patients with giant cell arteritis.
- The temporal artery may be tender to palpation or have decreased pulsations.
- Erythrocyte sedimentation rate is at least 40 mm/hour. *
- Temporal artery biopsy is the gold standard for diagnosis; however, the biopsy may be negative owing to patchy involvement of the arteries.
- Giant cell arteritis can present as a fever of unknown origin.

---

*A normal sedimentation rate may be seen in up to 20% of patients and should not exclude a diagnosis.

CURRENT THERAPY

Polymyalgia Rheumatica

- Corticosteroids (e.g., prednisone[1] 15-20 mg daily) are used with a gradual taper. If prednisone is tapered too rapidly, the symptoms will return. Patients are generally treated for at least 1 year.
- Rarely are higher doses of prednisone required. If symptoms do not respond to prednisone 30 mg daily, the diagnosis should be reevaluated.

Giant Cell Arteritis

- Corticosteroids (e.g., prednisone[1] at 1 mg/kg/day or 60 mg daily) are followed by a gradual taper.
- Patients are generally on treatment for at least 1 to 2 years. Some patients require low doses of prednisone indefinitely.
- One aspirin[1] daily, unless contraindicated (possibly with a proton pump inhibitor in high-risk patients), is used to decrease the risk of ischemic events.
- Prophylaxis for steroid-induced osteoporosis includes calcium, vitamin D, and a bisphosphonate unless contraindicated.

---

[1]Not FDA approved for this indication.

is no clinical improvement, the prednisone dose can be increased to 30 mg daily. If there is still no response, the diagnosis of PMR needs to be questioned. Following relief of symptoms the prednisone is gradually tapered in small increments every 2 to 4 weeks; relapse is common if taper is too rapid. Successful tapering is based on suppression of symptomatology, not the level of the ESR. Treatment duration is typically 1 to 2 years.

Giant Cell Arteritis

CLINICAL PRESENTATION

GCA, also known as temporal arteritis, is a vasculitis characterized by granulomatous inflammation in the wall of medium and large arteries especially the proximal aorta and its branches. It typically manifests with new-onset severe headache, usually located over the temporal area, which is constant and interferes with sleep. The temporal artery may be thickened, nodular, and tender, with diminished or absent pulsation. The vertebral, ophthalmic, posterior ciliary, and central retinal arteries and the internal and external carotid arteries may be affected in addition to the temporal artery. Half of patients have jaw claudication or scalp tenderness (or both). Symptoms of PMR are common, occurring in 40% to 60% of patients with GCA.

Vision disturbances (e.g., diplopia, amaurosis fugax) due to optic nerve ischemia can occur as an early manifestation or during the tapering of corticosteroids. Vision loss may be irreversible if not treated expeditiously.

Fever, malaise, and weight loss may be present. Rarely GCA manifests as a fever of unknown origin (FUO), without the other more typical symptoms.

Aortic arch involvement occurs in 10% to 15% and can manifest with claudication of the arms or legs, with bruits present over affected arteries. Strokes are seen in 3% to 7% of patients owing to ischemia in the vertebrobasilar or carotid arteries. Thoracic aortic aneurysms can develop years after initial diagnosis of GCA and are an important late complication.

DIAGNOSIS

Laboratory testing demonstrates an elevated ESR ($\geq$50 mm/hour) in 80% of patients. A normal ESR does not rule out the diagnosis. Anemia of chronic disease is often present.

A temporal artery biopsy should be obtained, if possible, but should not delay onset of treatment. Because the arterial inflammation occurs in a patchy distribution, a temporal artery biopsy of 3 to 4 cm in length should be obtained to minimize the false-negative rate. Histopathologic evidence is the gold standard for diagnosis; however, the diagnosis of GCA may be established clinically based on characteristic signs and symptoms without a biopsy.

TREATMENT

Treatment with high-dose corticosteroids (e.g., prednisone[1] 60 mg daily or 1 mg/kg/day equivalent) is initiated once the diagnosis of GCA is entertained; treatment should not be postponed while awaiting temporal artery biopsy. If vision loss has occurred, some advocate treatment with intravenous methylprednisolone (Solu-Medrol)[1] (1000 mg daily for 3 days) followed by high-dose daily oral prednisone. Alternate-day treatment is not recommended owing to the higher rate of disease flare. Following clinical response, corticosteroids are tapered gradually every 2 to 4 weeks. Relapse of symptoms can occur at any time in up to 60% of patients. The decision to increase the dose of steroids is based on recurrence of clinical symptoms; an elevated ESR in the absence of symptoms is not a reason to increase the prednisone dose. Treatment duration is usually 1 to 2 years; however, a subset of patients require chronic steroid treatment. Aspirin,[1] unless contraindicated, is an important adjunctive treatment because studies suggest a decreased risk of vision loss and central nervous systemic events.

---

[1]Not FDA approved for this indication.

REFERENCES

Dasgupta B, Matteson EL. Maradit-Kremers: Management guidelines and outcome measures in polymyalgia rheumatica. Clin Exp Rheumatol 2007;25:S130–6.

Gonzalez-Gay MA, Vazquez-Rodriguez TR, Gomez-Acebo I, et al. Strokes at time of disease diagnosis in a series of 287 patients with biopsy-proven giant cell arteritis. Medicine (Baltimore) 2009;88:227–35.

Hernandez-Rodriguez J, Cid MC, Lopez-Soto A, et al. Treatment of polymyalgia rheumatica: A systematic review. Arch Intern Med 2009;169:1839–50.

Marie I, Proux A, Duhaut P, et al. Long-term follow-up of aortic involvement in giant cell arteritis. Medicine (Baltimore) 2009;88:182–92.

Michet CJ, Matteson EL. Polymyalgia rheumatica. BMJ 2008;336:765–9.

Salvarani C, Cantini F, Hunder G. Polymyalgia rheumatica and giant cell arteritis. Lancet 2008;372:234–45.

Warrington KJ, Matteson EL. Management guidelines and outcome measures in giant cell arteritis. Clin Exp Rheumatol 2007;25:S137–41.

Osteomyelitis

Method of
Brian K. Albertson, MD, and
George D. Harris, MD, MS

Osteomyelitis is a disease of the bone that has changed over the years from a primarily hematogenous disease with high mortality to one of high morbidity. Since the introduction of antibiotics, the incidence of hematogenous osteomyelitis has declined, whereas infection from direct inoculation has increased, especially in those with diabetes. Several methods are used to classify osteomyelitis; most separate the illness into acute or chronic types and hematogenous or contiguous types. Local extension may occur from spread from adjacent structures, or direct implantation of organisms may occur, as seen in cases of trauma or surgical procedures.

The Cierny-Mader system assigns the patient to one of several groups based on the anatomy of the infection and health of the host, including the increased risk for patients who have peripheral arterial obstructive disease or diabetes mellitus. Patients are further separated according to systemic and local factors that may influence disease progression or healing, such as diabetes, extremes of age, and tobacco use. In diabetic patients, osteomyelitis is most commonly caused by overlying lower limb cellulitis. In the nondiabetic adult patient, vertebral osteomyelitis is most common.

The Cierny-Mader classification allows the clinician to use tested treatment protocols, including chemotherapy, surgery, and adjunctive therapies, that are most effective for a specific class of disease and for the host status. The Cierny-Mader system divides the patients into four anatomic groups. Stage 1, or medullary osteomyelitis, is confined to the endosteum of the bone and is often hematogenous. State 2, or superficial osteomyelitis, is localized to the surface of the bone. This is a true contiguous lesion. Stage 3, or localized osteomyelitis, involves cortical sequestration or cavitation, or both, and is a full-thickness lesion that extends into the medullary region. Stage 4, or diffuse osteomyelitis, involves the hard and soft tissues ("through and through"), and it requires surgical débridement of the affected bone to remove all the infected tissue.

For treatment to be successful, the patient must be physiologically able to heal any wounds, defend against contamination or infection, and tolerate the stress of treatment. The hosts are classified as A, B, or C, depending on the ability to resist infections. Those with good immunity are classified as an A host, whereas a B host is compromised locally (B_L) or systemically (B_S); Table 1 shows the physiologic classifications. The final class assigns a C rating to patients whose treatment is more detrimental than the disability from the disease. These patients may require suppressive or no treatment. The clinical stages are adjusted during the course of therapy as conditions change, allowing adjustment of the treatment protocol to optimize therapy.

A much simpler system described by Waldvogel classifies the patient by duration (i.e., acute or chronic) and the mechanism of inoculation (i.e., hematogenous or contiguous). Contiguous infections are further classified as those with or without vascular insufficiency. However, this classification does not provide guidance for specific surgical or antibiotic therapy.

TABLE 1 Cierny-Mader Classification System

Feature	Examples
Anatomic type	Stage 1: medullary osteomyelitis
	Stage 2: superficial osteomyelitis
	Stage 3: localized osteomyelitis
	Stage 4: diffuse osteomyelitis
Physiologic class	A: normal (healthy) host
	B: compromised host
	B_S: systemically compromised
	B_L: locally compromised
	C: treatment worse than disease
Factors affecting host status	
Systemic	Malnutrition
	Renal and hepatic failure
	Diabetes mellitus
	Chronic hypoxia
	Immune disease
	Malignancy
	Extremes of age
	Immunosuppression
Local	Chronic lymphedema
	Venous stasis
	Major vessel compromise
	Arteritis
	Extensive scarring
	Radiation fibrosis
	Small-vessel disease
	Neuropathy
	Tobacco use

Epidemiology

Acute hematogenous osteomyelitis is usually seen in male children of lower socioeconomic class before the age of 2 years or between 8 and 12 years. There may be some genetic influences. Aboriginal children in Western Australia are known to suffer from acute hematogenous osteomyelitis at a rate nearly four times that of Western European children living in the same neighborhood. An acute infection will progress to chronic osteomyelitis if it is not treated.

Chronic osteomyelitis is usually the result of direct inoculation (e.g., trauma, surgery). Its epidemiology is less clearly described, except in diabetic foot infections. It is estimated that 11 million people in the United States suffer from diabetes. Annually, more than 300,000 of them develop a foot ulcer, and nearly one third of those require amputations. In 2002, osteomyelitis was estimated to cost the citizens of the United States more than $2.3 billion dollars. This major public health problem is expected to increase as the incidence of adults with diabetes increases. Because chronic infection can persist for life, it is important to have early identification and treatment to ensure the best possible outcome.

Pathogenesis

The presence of bacteria in an open wound is not sufficient to cause infection. It is the compromised blood supply of traumatized tissue leading to necrosis and subsequent bacterial adherence that promotes the infection. Trauma can delay the inflammatory response to bacteria, depress cell-mediated immunity, and impair chemotaxis, superoxide production, and the microbial killing capacity of polymorphonuclear neutrophils (PMNs). Osteomyelitis usually involves the metaphysic, which is well vascularized and has significant bone growth.

In acute osteomyelitis, signs or symptoms are usually abrupt. Local infection is characterized by edema, vascular congestion, and small-vessel thrombosis. This leads to increased pressure within the intramedullary canal, allowing extravasation through the Havers and Volkmann canals to the periosteum. In children, the periosteum is usually more flexible and easier to detect radiographically; in adults, the bone matrix is more firmly attached to the periosteum. Untreated, the suppurative infection can reach adjacent soft tissue, leading to a cellulitis. The presence of a Brodie or intraosseous abscess without extravasation into surrounding tissue is classified as subacute pyogenic osteomyelitis. The resulting infection can lead to sequestration involving large areas of bone destruction and dead bone, with reactive bone formation leading ultimately to chronic osteomyelitis.

Chronic osteomyelitis is usually polymicrobial and is characterized by the presence of necrotic bone, new bone growth, and exudation of polymorphonuclear leukocytes, plasma cells, and other infection-fighting cells. The involucrum (i.e., layer of reactive competent bone that covers dead bone) is often dotted with tracts that allow pus to pass into surrounding tissue or to form a sinus tract to the skin surface. These sinus tracts are often contaminated with numerous organisms that do not reflect those found with direct sampling. This repetitive process of bone loss and growth and the involucrum explains why chronic osteomyelitis is difficult to eradicate with antibiotics alone. The antibiotics cannot penetrate avascular areas.

Etiology

CHILDREN

In children of all ages, the most common bacterial pathogen is *Staphylococcus aureus*, followed by *Streptococcus pneumoniae* and *Kingella kingae*. However, age and chronic illness allow other organisms to flourish; *Salmonella* and pneumococcal disease (*S. pneumoniae*) are common in patients with sickle cell disease. *Pasteurella multocida, Streptococcus* species, and anaerobes often are identified after animal or human bites. In children, most cases arise hematogenously and are characteristically seen in the metaphysis of long bones (i.e., femur, tibia, and humerus), accounting for 68% of childhood infections.

The exact mechanism is unclear, but it is thought that the extensive branching of the nutrient-rich arteries at the metaphyses of the long bones leads to sluggish blood flow and ultimate bacterial seeding. Possible routes include the formation of small hematomas in the metaphysis, allowing microbial seeding after transient bacteremia; penetrating injuries or surgical manipulation, causing direct inoculation of bacteria into bone; and local invasion from a contiguous focus of infection.

ADULTS

Most infections in adults arise by direct inoculation from sources such as trauma, prosthetic joints, open fractures, and diabetic foot infections. The most common organism remains *S. aureus*. Other organisms to consider include *Staphylococcus epidermis*, *Pseudomonas aeruginosa*, *Escherichia coli*, and *Serratia marcescens*. Most contiguous, related infections are polymicrobial.

Clinical Manifestations

The severity of the signs and symptoms depends on the location of the infection, the patient's age, and any comorbidities. Patients may experience many, few, or no symptoms. Classically, there are marked pain, tenderness, and swelling. Fever and leukocytosis are also common.

Vertebral osteomyelitis often causes severe pain, fever, and disability, whereas osteomyelitis of the foot rarely causes pain. An epidural abscess causes pain and neurologic deficits, whereas vertebral osteomyelitis without abscess formation has no neurologic deficits.

Children often present with systemic symptoms (e.g., fever, weight loss, pain). Pseudoparalysis may be the only sign in a newborn, but toddlers often exhibit pain, fever, erythema, edema, or warmth, or they may suddenly stop walking. In contrast, patients with chronic osteomyelitis may exhibit localized signs and symptoms, including nonhealing ulcers, purulence from sinus tracts, soft tissue edema and pain, abscesses, erythema, pain, and fatigue. Generalized signs and symptoms may be seen early in the disease, but they are unlikely in the later or chronic stages.

Diagnosis

LABORATORY TESTS

A bone biopsy remains the gold standard when diagnosing osteomyelitis. However, there is a high false-negative rate, and the negative predictive value is close to 65%, mainly due to the organism's patchy distribution. No specific laboratory test can be recommended. However, testing acute-phase reactants (e.g., erythrocyte sedimentation rate [ESR], C-reactive protein [CRP], leukocyte count with a differential count) can strongly suggest (positive predictive value of 100%) osteomyelitis if the ESR value is greater than 70 mm/hour in the absence of an inflamed ulcer. However, these tests lack specificity, and it may take several days to demonstrate significantly elevated levels. All patients should have blood cultures performed. A positive blood culture with a suspicious physical finding can suggest a bone infection, but only one half of the cases have a positive test result. Blood cultures, like bone biopsies, can be affected by recent antibiotic exposure.

RADIOLOGY

There is no one imaging modality routinely recommended to diagnose osteomyelitis, often requiring more than one technique. Plain film radiography should always be the initial study, and the result can be diagnostic if positive. However, changes (usually along the metaphysic) typically require at least 1 to 2 weeks to be seen radiographically.

Positron emission tomography (PET) is the most specific and sensitive of imaging techniques, but its high cost and lack of availability

makes it impractical for most clinicians. The best choice for imaging depends on the age of the patient, duration of symptoms, suspected location of infection (if known), and concurrent or previous medical conditions.

Plain radiographs are the most available, least expensive, and easiest to obtain, but they lack sensitivity (43%–75%), and a negative result does not exclude the diagnosis. However, they have reasonable specificity (75%–83%), and a positive finding can confirm the diagnosis or provide clues to alternative pathology, such as a tumor. Bony changes can take between 10 and 21 days to become visible on plain films; however, soft tissue changes can be seen in as little as 3 days. The soft tissue changes are especially important in neonates and children because focal soft tissue swelling around the bony metaphysis may be the first sign of bone involvement.

Radionuclide imaging (i.e., triple-phase bone scan, leukocyte scintigraphy, and PET) is a preferred method of advanced imaging, and it has several advantages compared with other techniques. Young children often complete the examination without sedation, and prosthetic joints do not produce the artifact commonly seen on magnetic resonance imaging (MRI) and computed tomography (CT) scans. Positive results can be seen 24 to 48 hours after onset of symptoms, and a negative examination result effectively rules out osteomyelitis.

The triple-phase bone scan (technetium 99m diphosphonate) is often the examination of choice (sensitivity of 73%–100%), and it can distinguish between cellulitis and osteomyelitis when complications are absent. However, the sensitivity decreases dramatically when other conditions are present (i.e., trauma, diabetes, or recent surgery), and it has been reported to be as low as 38%. Bone scans usually lack the specificity (25%–90%) of other modalities, fail to provide detailed pictures of complex anatomy, and can be influenced by poor circulation. The examination takes up to 48 hours to complete and often requires the patient to make many trips to the facility. In the early phase, uptake is greatest in areas of acute inflammation. In the next phase, uptake occurs in areas of soft tissue inflammation, and in the late (delayed) phase, uptake remains in the presence of osteomyelitis.

Leukocyte scintigraphy using gallium 67 has a higher specificity (80%–90%) than triple-phase scanning (67%) in the peripheral skeleton, but it decreases to 25% when looking at the axial skeleton. Leukocyte scintigraphy is the preferred method when evaluating patients with previous joint replacements, diabetes, or trauma.

CURRENT DIAGNOSIS

- A bone biopsy remains the gold standard when diagnosing osteomyelitis.
- All patients should have blood cultures performed.
- No one imaging modality is routinely recommended to diagnose osteomyelitis.
- Plain film radiography should always be the initial study and can be diagnostic if positive.
- Magnetic resonance imaging (MRI) can detect acute osteomyelitis as early as 3 days.

CURRENT THERAPY

- The Cierny-Mader classification system provides an easy-to-use algorithm for treatment (Box 1).
- The most important factor in any treatment is identification of the organism.
- The optimal duration of antibiotic therapy remains undefined, with most authorities recommending treatment for about 6 weeks.
- Hematogenous osteomyelitis is usually monomicrobial, whereas contiguous infections are usually polymicrobial.

BOX 1 Management of Suspected Osteomyelitis

History and physical findings suggesting osteomyelitis
Nonhealing ulcer present
Yes
Is bone visible or accessible by sterile probe?
Yes
Osteomyelitis
No
No
Plain radiography
Positive
Osteomyelitis
Treat empirically
Bone biopsy
Adjust treatment if appropriate
No
Highly suspicious
Further evaluation
Less suspicious
Repeat radiologic examination in 2 weeks
Further evaluation
ESR >70 mm/h
Yes
Osteomyelitis
No
Blood cultures
Positive
Treat accordingly
Source suspected
MRI of suspected part
Source site unknown
Bone scan
Negative
Bone scan
Bone scan
Source located
Yes
Bone biopsy
Treat accordingly
Treat empirically until biopsy or culture provides sensitivities
Consider MRI or CT scan if surgery considered
No source
Consider alternative pathology

MRI can detect acute osteomyelitis as early as 3 days. It is nearly as sensitive (82%–100%) and specific (75%–96%) as radionuclide studies. MRI allows tracking of disease progress and response to treatment. MRI can be used to date osteomyelitis. Some patients with osteomyelitis are treated and later develop another episode. The MRI can distinguish whether the second episode is a new infection or a recurrence of the previous infection. It also provides detailed visualization of complex anatomy and critical structures, allowing surgeons to map any planned surgical intervention.

CT is rarely used for osteomyelitis, except when sequestered bone is suspected or for interventional procedures. Sinography can be used to map sinus tracts with fluoroscopy or combined with CT. Ultrasound is sometimes used in children and can be helpful in differentiating acute from chronic infections. It provides guidance during drainage, aspirations, or biopsies of the affected bone, and it is a noninvasive method to monitor soft tissue involvement in chronic illness.

Treatment

Older methods, such as closed suction drains, are no longer commonly used because of long hospital stays and the risk of contamination, and newer modalities, such as hyperbaric oxygen therapy, have failed to live up to expectations. The Cierny-Mader classification system provides a straightforward algorithm for treatment. However, the most important factor in any treatment is the identification of the causative organism.

ANTIBIOTIC THERAPY

Unlike chronic infections, acute infections require hospitalization for initiation of therapy and supportive care. Serial examinations should be undertaken to assess the success of treatment and monitor for systemic signs or symptoms. Cultures of blood and bone should be obtained to guide therapy. Laboratory studies can be followed, but other than CRP levels, they fail to provide significant data. The CRP value can be expected to decrease 24 to 48 hours after initiation of appropriate antibiotic therapy. A lack of response may indicate inappropriate therapy or an occult abscess, and the physician should reconsider surgery if previously delayed.

The medical literature remains inconclusive about the antibiotic treatment of osteomyelitis, especially when trying to determine the best agents, route, or duration of antibiotic therapy. Although the optimal duration of antibiotic therapy remains undefined, most authorities recommend treatment for about 6 weeks (Table 2).

TABLE 2 Antibiotics for Osteomyelitis

Organism	Preferred Drug	Alternative Drugs
Staphylococcus aureus	Nafcillin (Unipen) 1–2 g IV or IM q4h	Cefazolin, vancomycin, clindamycin
Methicillin-resistant S. aureus	Vancomycin (Vancocin) 1 g q8h	Trimethoprim-sulfamethoxazole (Bactrim)[1] plus rifampin (Rifadin)[1]
Streptococcus pneumoniae, group A β-hemolytic streptococci	Penicillin G (Pfizerpen)[1] 2 million units IV q4h	Cefazolin, vancomycin, clindamycin
Enterococci, Haemophilus influenzae β-lactamase negative	Cefotaxime (Claforan) 2 g q6h	Trimethoprim-sulfamethoxazole, ceftriaxone
H. influenzae β-lactamase positive, Klebsiella pneumoniae	Ceftriaxone (Rocephin) 2 g q24h	Trimethoprim-sulfamethoxazole, ciprofloxacin, piperacillin (Pipracil), imipenem (Primaxin)
Escherichia coli	Cefazolin (Ancef) 2 g q8h	Ciprofloxacin, ceftriaxone, imipenem
Pseudomonas aeruginosa	Ciprofloxacin (Cipro) 400 mg q12h	Piperacillin plus aminoglycoside, aztreonam (Azactam)[1]
Salmonella	Choose ampicillin, ceftriaxone, imipenem (Primaxin), or ciprofloxacin, depending on sensitivities	
Bacteroides spp.	Clindamycin (Cleocin) 600 mg q6h	Imipenem, metronidazole (Flagyl)
Serratia marcescens	Ceftriaxone (Rocephin) 2 g q24h	Imipenem, trimethoprim-sulfamethoxazole, ciprofloxacin

Modified from Cohen J, Powderly WG (eds): Infectious Diseases, 2nd ed. St Louis, Mosby, 2003.
[1]Not FDA approved for this indication.

After the infection is under control, the physician may switch the patient to an oral antibiotic for 3 to 12 months (i.e., a fluoroquinolone with or without rifampin [Rifadin][1]). However, treatment can be as short as 3 weeks for uncomplicated acute, hematogenous osteomyelitis. Management can include oral preparations after a short parenteral course, provided the drug has high bioavailability and the organism is susceptible. A microbiologic diagnosis (preferably by bone biopsy) is essential so the choice of antibiotic accounts for the specific organism, the host status, and least toxic medication for the individual. Hematogenous osteomyelitis is usually monomicrobial, whereas contiguous infections are usually polymicrobial and may include *Pseudomonas* in certain populations.

For methicillin-sensitive *S. aureus*, nafcillin (Unipen) or a first- or second-generation cephalosporin can be implemented. For methicillin-resistant *S. aureus*, vancomycin (Vancocin) is recommended. For an anaerobic infection, clindamycin (Cleocin) is a good choice.

SURGERY

Bones can heal in the presence of active infection. However, in the presence of obvious signs of infection, such as an abscess or Cierny-Mader stage 3 or 4 disease, acute surgical débridement and irrigation are warranted. The goals of surgery include drainage, débridement, and stabilization. After successful débridement and stabilization, antibiotic therapy is initiated and continued until adequate healing has occurred, usually 6 weeks. If débridement is unsuccessful, inert substances must be completely removed and tissue débrided. Antibiotics should be placed in contact with the bone using a polymethylmethacrylate antibiotic (PMMA) bead chain or other biodegradable delivery systems to achieve higher local antibiotic concentrations. The site needs to be stabilized with an external fixator, and staged reconstruction should be initiated.

[1]Not FDA approved for this indication.

REFERENCES

Berendt A, Norden C. Acute and chronic osteomyelitis. In: Cohen J, Powderly WG, editors. Infectious Diseases, 2nd ed. St Louis: Mosby; 2003.

Cierny GII, Mader JT, Pennick JJ. A clinical staging system for adult osteomyelitis. Contemp Orthop 1985;10:17–37.

Kaplan SL. Osteomyelitis in children. Infect Dis Clin North Am 2005;19: 787–97.

Krogstad P. Osteomyelitis and septic arthritis. In: Feigin RD, Cherry JD, Demmler GJ, et al., editors. Textbook of Pediatric Infectious Diseases, 5th ed. Philadelphia: WB Saunders; 2004. p. 713–36.

Lampe RM. Osteomyelitis. In: Behrman RE, Kliegman RM, Jenson HB, Stanton BF, editors. Nelson Textbook of Pediatrics, 18th ed. Philadelphia: WB Saunders; 2007.

Lazzarini L, Lipsky BA, Mader JT. Antibiotic treatment of osteomyelitis: What have we learned from 30 years of clinical trials? Int J Infect Dis 2005;9: 127–38.

Lipsky B, Weigelt J, Gupta V, et al. Skin, soft tissue, bone, and joint infections in hospitalized patients: Epidemiology and microbiological, clinical, and economic outcomes. Infect Control Hosp Epidemiol 2007;28:1290–8.

Pineda C, Vargas A, Rodriguez A. Imaging of osteomyelitis: Current concepts. Infect Dis Clin North Am 2006;20:789–825.

Waldvogel FA, Medoff G, Swartz MN. Osteomyelitis: A review of clinical features, therapeutic considerations and unusual aspects. N Engl J Med 1970;282:198–206.

White LM, Schweitzer ME, Deely DM, Gannon F. Study of osteomyelitis: Utility of combined histologic and microbiologic evaluation of percutaneous biopsy samples. Radiology 1995;197:840–2.

Ziran BH. Osteomyelitis. J Trauma 2007;62(Suppl.):S59–60.

Common Sports Injuries

Method of
Douglas DiOrio, MD, and Julie Shott, MD

Ankle Injuries

The ankle is the most frequently injured joint among athletes. In the primary care setting, the ankle sprain is the most commonly presenting musculoskeletal injury and accounts for 30% of all musculoskeletal visits.

Understanding the anatomy of the ankle is important for evaluating ankle injuries. The ankle is a hinge joint where three bones come together: the fibula, the tibia, and the talus. The lateral stability of the ankle is provided by the anterior talofibular ligament (ATFL), the calcaneofibular ligament (CFL), and the posterior talofibular ligament (PTFL). The ATFL is the most commonly injured ligament in the ankle. The medial stability of the ankle comes from the deltoid ligament.

When a patient presents with ankle pain, a complete history is necessary. This includes determining the mechanism of injury, such as whether the injury resulted from an inversion, eversion, plantar, or dorsiflexion mechanism. It is also important to know if the patient could bear weight on the affected ankle immediately after the injury, where the patient felt the pain, when the swelling began, and a description of the type of pain.

A thorough examination of the injured ankle should be undertaken. The normal ankle also should always be examined and compared with the injured one. The ankle examination begins with a visual inspection for swelling, deformity, or ecchymosis. Passive and active range of motion and strength should be ascertained, although it is likely to be abnormal in most acute ankle sprains. Palpation of the ankle ligaments usually can pinpoint the source of injury in ankle sprains. Palpation of the medial and lateral malleoli and their physes and palpation of the proximal fifth metatarsal and the navicular should be done to rule out injury to the bones. Not all ankle injuries necessitate a radiograph. The Ottawa Ankle Rules can aid decision making about whether a foot or ankle radiograph is needed. These rules state that films are recommended if any of the following are positive: inability to walk four steps immediately after injury or in the office, tenderness of the distal 6 cm of the tibia or fibula, midfoot or navicular tenderness, tenderness over the proximal fifth metatarsal, age older than 55 years, or skeletal immaturity. A positive history of weight bearing immediately after the injury followed by a later increase in pain and swelling suggests an ankle sprain over a fracture.

LATERAL INVERSION SPRAIN

The lateral inversion sprain accounts for 80% to 85% of all ankle sprains. The mechanism of injury with a lateral inversion sprain is plantar flexion, inversion, and internal rotation of the ankle, which results in stretching and tearing of the three lateral ligaments. In a lateral inversion sprain, the ligaments are usually torn in the same order: ATFL, CFL, and PTFL. The patient often has acute pain after "twisting" the ankle. The area is tender over the ATFL and possibly over the CFL and the PTFL if those ligaments are involved.

MEDIAL EVERSION SPRAIN

Although the medial eversion sprain accounts for less than 10% of all ankle sprains, it accounts for more than 75% of all ankle fractures. The mechanism of injury with the medial eversion sprain is external rotation of the leg and dorsiflexion of the ankle and pronation, leading to injury of the deltoid ligament. The patient has pain over the deltoid ligament. It is important to rule out a fracture with any medial compartment injury, including a medial eversion sprain.

Treatment of medial and lateral ankle sprains includes protecting the joint and controlling the pain and swelling with RICE maneuvers:

rest, ice, compression, and elevation. Patients may need crutches, an air cast, or a lace-up ankle brace to assist with ambulation.

For an adult, pain control can be initiated with acetaminophen (Tylenol) 1000 mg PO every 6 to 8 hours or ibuprofen (Motrin) 600 mg PO every 8 hours. For stable ankle sprains, adequate pain control is important to ensure that the patient begins early mobilization and rehabilitation. Rehabilitation of the ankle injury progresses to include regaining full motion, strength, and proprioception. This can be achieved through formal physical therapy or a home exercise program. The exercises focus on range of motion, resisted strength, and proprioception. They include a specific progression of exercises from standing on one foot with eyes open and then with eyes closed, to standing on uneven surfaces, and to standing on one foot and squatting. After the injured ankle has regained full range of motion and strength, the patient can gradually return to sport-specific activities. Appropriate and complete rehabilitation limits the chances the patient will repeatedly sprain his or her ankles.

Knee Injuries

ANTERIOR CRUCIATE LIGAMENT TEAR

The anterior cruciate ligament (ACL) is the key stabilizing ligament in the knee. Tears of the ACL are common among patients engaging in sports. Although ACL tears are seen in all agility sports, they occur most commonly in football, basketball, soccer, and gymnastics. Female athletes have a higher incidence of ACL tears (2.4–9.7 times) than their male counterparts. The ACL tear can be an isolated injury to the knee, or it can also involve meniscal or medial collateral ligament (MCL) injury. Fifty percent of ACL tears are associated with a meniscal tear, with the lateral meniscus tearing four times more commonly than the medial meniscus. Most commonly, the mechanism of an ACL tear involves a noncontact situation in which the athlete pivots on a planted foot, lands from a jump, or decelerates suddenly. It also can occur after a sudden valgus impact to the knee.

The classic history for a patient with an ACL tear is that the patient hears an audible "pop" or feels the knee "give out," and the patient has immediate pain and is unable to continue the activity. A thorough examination of the injured knee is important. The normal knee should always be examined and compared with the injured one. With an ACL tear, the patient often develops a hemarthrosis that is seen as a large, tense effusion. Athletes with an ACL tear have a positive Lachman's test result, although the effusion and muscle spasm may limit the examination. The Lachman's test is performed by flexing the knee to 15 degrees, holding the femur stable, and then drawing the tibia forward, assessing for laxity and the quality of the end point of the ACL. A positive test result has laxity and no discrete end point compared with the uninjured side. The athlete also has restricted movement, especially a loss of extension of the knee. There may be diffuse, mild tenderness of the knee. Medial or lateral joint line tenderness may be seen if there is an associated medial or lateral meniscal tear. Lateral joint line tenderness may also be seen because the subluxing knee stretches the lateral joint capsule.

If an ACL rupture is suspected, anteroposterior and lateral radiographs of the knee should be obtained to rule out the possibility of a tibial spine avulsion. Magnetic resonance imaging (MRI) may be needed if the diagnosis of ACL rupture is not clear or if associated injury to the cartilage is suspected. Eighty percent of ACL tears have a bone bruise visible on MRI, and most of these involve the lateral femoral condyle.

Treatment of patients with ACL tears includes referral to an orthopedic surgeon to discuss the possibility for reconstructive surgery. Athletes who wish to return to competitive sports participation are candidates for surgery. Not all patients with ACL tears need surgery. Depending on the patient's age and activity level, the patient may be treated conservatively without surgery. Until the patient is seen by the orthopedic surgeon, he or she can be placed on crutches and in a knee brace, as needed for comfort. The patient should be instructed to ice the injured knee several times each day for 20 minutes per session. Range-of-motion exercises are essential in the first week after the injury to ensure that the patient regains full extension of the knee. The patient can also do exercises to contract the hamstring and quadriceps muscles to help preserve muscle mass.

MEDIAL COLLATERAL LIGAMENT SPRAIN

An MCL sprain is another common injury to the knee. It results from a valgus stress to a partially flexed knee. It is common in football, wrestling, and basketball. If the force to the knee is severe, the ACL also may be injured. Patients with an MCL sprain present with pain over the medial aspect of the knee. MCL tears are graded I through III, depending on their severity. Stretching of the MCL fibers without an increase in joint laxity is classified as a grade I sprain. A grade II MCL sprain has partial tearing of the MCL fibers with increased laxity on valgus stress testing. A grade III sprain is a complete rupture of the MCL ligament fibers.

On examination, a patient with a grade I sprain has point tenderness along any point on the MCL but does not have swelling or increased laxity of the joint with valgus testing. A patient with a grade II MCL sprain presents with pain and swelling over the medial aspect of the knee, with point tenderness over the MCL and with pain and increased laxity with valgus stress testing at 30 degrees of knee flexion. On examination, an end point of the MCL is felt. A grade III MCL sprain is complete rupture of the MCL ligament fibers, and no end point of the MCL is felt with valgus stress testing. Any increased laxity at 0 degrees of flexion with valgus stress testing points to a coexisting ACL injury. Radiographs are indicated if the patient has significant swelling to rule out an avulsion fracture.

Treatment of isolated MCL tears is conservative. The more severe the MCL injury, the longer the period of rehabilitation will be. The patient should be instructed to ice his or her knee three times each day for 20 minutes per session during the initial injury period. The patient should use crutches until he or she is able to walk with a normal gait. A hinged knee brace can provide support and protection to the knee during the healing process. During the first week after the injury, it is important to control swelling, work on range-of-motion exercises, and develop quadriceps strength. By 2 weeks after the injury, all swelling should be gone, and the patient should have full flexion range of motion. The patient should work on quadriceps strength after the injury, and a stationary bike is an excellent rehabilitation tool. The patient can return to sports when he or she has full range of motion, has full strength (compared with the uninjured side), and is able to do sport-specific drills with proper form. Rehabilitation times vary and may take 6 to 8 weeks for grade II sprains and up to 12 weeks for grade III sprains.

Hand Injuries

SCAPHOID FRACTURES

The most common carpal bone fractured is the scaphoid, accounting for 70% of all carpal fractures. Patients present with wrist pain after a fall on an outstretched hand. Many patients have a delay in presentation because they think they "sprained" their wrist and it will get better. It is important to diagnose this problem because a fractured scaphoid is vulnerable to nonunion and avascular necrosis. The blood supply to the scaphoid is from a recurrent interosseous blood supply that enters the bone distally and runs proximally. A more proximal fracture has a higher chance of delayed healing and a higher risk of avascular necrosis.

On physical examination, the hallmark sign of a scaphoid fracture is tenderness in the anatomic snuffbox, an area on the hand bordered ulnarly by the tendons of the extensor pollicis longus and the abductor pollicis longus and radially by the tendons of the extensor pollicis brevis. Other physical signs include possible pain with palpation of the scaphoid tubercle, swelling, and a loss of grip strength. If the patient has tenderness in the snuffbox, radiographs are mandated. Posteroanterior, lateral, and scaphoid views are recommended. A negative radiographic result *cannot* rule out a clinically suspected scaphoid fracture. If this occurs, initial treatment for a possible scaphoid fracture is indicated with a thumb spica splint or thumb spica cast. The patient is reassessed at 2 weeks, and radiographs are again obtained.

Treatment of a scaphoid fracture is based on the fracture location and whether there is any degree of displacement. If a suspected fracture does not have a radiographic abnormality, initial treatment for a scaphoid facture is begun; early immobilization with a short-arm thumb spica cast is maintained for 2 weeks. After 2 weeks, repeat radiographs are obtained. If a fracture is seen, definitive treatment for the scaphoid fracture is followed. If the radiographs are still negative but the physical examination still shows signs of a possible scaphoid fracture (i.e., snuffbox tenderness), a computed tomography (CT) scan or MRI should be obtained. If radiographs are negative and the physical examination is improved (i.e., no pain in the anatomic snuffbox), concern about a possible scaphoid fracture drops.

A patient with a stable, nondisplaced fracture (<1 mm of displacement) of the distal third of the scaphoid should be placed in a short-arm thumb spica cast for 6 weeks. A patient with a nondisplaced fracture of the middle or proximal third of the scaphoid should be placed in a long-arm thumb spica cast for 6 weeks, followed by a short-arm thumb spica cast until healing is visible on radiographs. Typically, these patients have a total of approximately 10 to 12 weeks of immobilization.

An unstable, displaced scaphoid fracture is a fracture that has a step-off or angulation of 1 mm or more. Patients with these fractures should be referred for an orthopedic consultation, as should patients with nonunion fractures and patients showing signs of early avascular necrosis.

After successful treatment of a scaphoid fracture, mobilization and strengthening of the wrist are necessary. Rehabilitation should begin immediately after cast removal.

Finger Injuries

MALLET FINGER

A mallet finger has an extension lag at the distal interphalangeal (DIP) joint caused by a loss of continuity of the terminal extensor digitorum tendon (EDT) at its insertion. This can be the result of stretching, rupture, or avulsion of the EDT, or it can be caused by a fracture of the distal phalange where the EDT inserts. The most common mechanism of injury is a blunt force to a slightly flexed fingertip, such as when a ball hits a distal finger. Often, the patient thinks he or she "jammed" the finger. The most common finger to be involved is the middle finger, although any finger can be affected. Although this is not a common sports injury, it is important because prompt diagnosis of the condition is necessary to ensure a full recovery for the patient.

When the patient presents for evaluation of this injury, each joint of the finger should be isolated and examined separately. The physical examination of a mallet finger shows that the affected joint sits in an abnormally flexed position, and the patient is unable to actively extend the DIP joint from this flexed position. Passive extension of the joint should be normal. Radiographs (i.e., anteroposterior, lateral, and oblique) are necessary to check for a possible avulsion fracture.

Treatment of a mallet finger is done by splinting the digit in hyperextension at the DIP joint. This can be accomplished by using a stack splint. If there is a bony avulsion, the patient should wear the stack splint continuously for 6 weeks. If there is no bony avulsion, the splint should be worn continuously for 8 weeks, followed by an additional 6 to 8 weeks with splinting at night and during athletic activities. Surgery is indicated if there is volar subluxation of the distal phalanx and a bony avulsion. The joint must be maintained in hyperextension at all times, even when taking the splint off to clean the finger. Any bending of the affected joint will restart the time of treatment to time zero and affect the chances for full healing.

JERSEY FINGER

Jersey finger is the term used to describe the disruption of the flexor digitorum profundus (FDP) tendon from the distal phalangeal base on the volar aspect of the hand. Typically, the mechanism of injury is an actively flexed DIP joint that is forcibly extended, as can occur when an athlete grabs onto another player's jersey. The usual history is that the patient hears a snap at the time of the injury. Although this type of injury can occur on any finger, in 75% of cases, the injury involves the fourth finger.

The patient presents with pain and swelling and an inability to actively flex the DIP joint of the affected finger. There may be fullness or pain proximal to the insertion of the DIP if the tendon retracted proximally. There may also be a palpable nodule, which represents the tendon at any point from the palm up to the DIP joint. Radiographs should be obtained to rule out the possibility of an avulsion fracture of the proximal DIP where the FDP inserts.

Treatment of a Jersey finger injury is surgery. The patient should be referred to an orthopedic surgeon so that repair of the finger can occur within 7 to 10 days of the injury. Operative intervention is less successful when the injury was initially missed and it became chronic in nature.

Overuse Syndromes

PATELLOFEMORAL PAIN SYNDROME

Patellofemoral pain syndrome (PFPS) is the most common diagnosis for patients with anterior knee pain who present to a primary care office. PFPS accounts for 25% to 40% of all knee problems of persons presenting to sports medicine centers. The terms *chondromalacia patella* and *runner's knee* are common synonyms for PFPS.

The patella is controlled by the quadriceps muscles as it moves through the femoral groove during flexion and extension of the knee. There can be a lack of control with quadriceps weakness or inhibition due to pain around the knee. This can cause PFPS and propagate it. Further pain leads to further inhibition of the quadriceps, which leads to further abnormal patellar tracking. Risk factors for PFPS include muscle dysfunction; patellar hypermobility; poor quadriceps, hamstring, or iliotibial band flexibility; training errors or overuse; trauma; malalignment; and altered biomechanics of the lower extremity.

The patient with PFPS presents to the physician complaining of unilateral or bilateral anterior knee pain. The pain is described as "all around," "behind," or "underneath" the patella. Rarely, an intraarticular effusion may be present. The pain is typically worse with walking, running, ascending or descending stairs, squatting, and sitting for prolonged periods (i.e., theatre sign). Patients may also complain of stiffness. Knee locking is not characteristic of PFPS and points to another diagnosis. The physical examination may reveal tenderness at the medial or lateral patellar facets. If the patient has pain only after activity, the examination findings may be benign, and the diagnosis needs to be based on the patient's history alone. Radiographs are not routinely indicated for PFPS but may be used for patients with a history of trauma or surgery, those with an effusion, or those who are not getting better after initial treatment.

Treatment of patellofemoral pain syndrome is done primarily through strengthening the quadriceps muscles and hip rotators. This can be accomplished through physical therapy. While the exercises are being done to strengthen the muscles, other activities are undertaken to reduce the pain of PFPS: resting from aggravating activities, using ice and nonsteroidal antiinflammatory medications as needed, and participating in other modalities such as ultrasound for pain relief. Runners may benefit from being properly fitted for running shoes.

ILIOTIBIAL BAND SYNDROME

The most common cause of lateral knee pain in an athlete is iliotibial band syndrome. Although any athlete who that participates in repetitive knee flexion activities can develop iliotibial band syndrome, it is most commonly seen in long distance runners and cyclists. The iliotibial band is made up of fascia from the hip abductors, extensors, and flexors. It originates at the anterior iliac crest outer lip and runs distally to insert at Gerdy's tubercle over the lateral aspect of the proximal tibia. The functions of the iliotibial band include helping with hip abduction, hip internal rotation, and knee flexion and extension, depending on the angle of the knee.

The patient with iliotibial band syndrome presents with pain or an ache over the lateral aspect of the knee that is worse with running, especially during long runs or downhill running. Risk factors for the development of iliotibial band syndrome include having iliotibial band tightness, putting in high weekly mileage (with running or biking), and having muscle weakness of the knee flexors, knee extensors, and hip abductors.

On physical examination, the patient may have tenderness over the lateral epicondyle of the femur about 1 inch above the joint line and at Gerdy's tubercle on the proximal tibia. Repeatedly flexing and extending the knee may reproduce the patient's symptoms. Ober's test may demonstrate iliotibial band tightness. The strength of the major muscle groups in the lower extremity must be tested, because hip abduction weakness may be identified. Radiographic imaging is usually not necessary for iliotibial band syndrome.

Iliotibial band syndrome is treated by physical therapy to strengthen the hip abductors, internal rotators, and knee flexors and extensors. Symptomatic relief of pain can be obtained through routine icing, antiinflammatory medications (e.g., ibuprofen [Motrin] 600 mg PO every 8 hours as needed), and physical therapy modalities such as ultrasound or electrical stimulation. The patient with iliotibial band syndrome may also use a foam roller on the lateral thigh along the length of the iliotibial band to stretch it. Runners should wear properly fitting running shoes.

LATERAL EPICONDYLITIS: TENNIS ELBOW

The patient who presents with lateral elbow pain may have lateral epicondylitis, also called *tennis elbow*. Tennis elbow is a tendinopathy of the extensor tendons that occurs from repeated wrist extension against resistance. This is a common injury for racket sport participants and for individuals who participate in occupational activities such as computer use and recreational activities such as sewing and knitting. Many processes can lead to the development of this tendinopathy, including overuse, poor technique, heavy racquets, grips that are too small, and a poor blood supply to the extensor tendons. When the tendinopathy becomes a chronic problem, it becomes a tendinosis. Although tendinosis may affect patients of any age, its peak incidence occurs between the ages of 40 and 50 years.

The patient with lateral epicondylitis usually describes a gradual onset of pain after the start of a new activity that involved repeated wrist extension or the sudden onset of pain after the patient overexerted his or her wrist extensors by lifting a heavy object. On physical examination, the patient has maximal point tenderness approximately 1 to 2 cm distal to the lateral epicondyle. The extensor muscles may also be tight and hypersensitive. The patient may have pain with resisted wrist extension, especially with the wrist pronated and radially deviated (i.e., Mill's test), and with resisted third digit extension. Occasionally, grip strength testing can cause pain.

No single treatment has been found to be 100% effective in treating lateral epicondylitis. A combination of several treatments results in resolution of symptoms in most cases. As with most soft tissue injuries, the treatment goals are pain control, restoration of range of motion and strength, correction of the predisposing factors (e.g., poor racquet technique), and a gradual return to full activity. Regular icing decreases inflammation. Physical therapy can help a patient with stretching and strengthening, and pain management can be achieved through physical therapy modalities such as ultrasound and electrical stimulation. Strengthening treatment initially focuses on isometric contraction of the wrist extensors and progresses to concentric and then to eccentric exercises. Soft tissue therapy such as myofascial release has been helpful. Acupuncture has provided short-term relief of lateral elbow pain. Corticosteroid injections are controversial and should be reserved for the patient who does not improve after 3 months of rehabilitation. Surgery should be reserved for patients with pain that lasts through at least 12 months of conservative treatment. Surgery involves the release of the tendon from the lateral epicondyle.

MEDIAL EPICONDYLITIS: GOLFER'S ELBOW

Although medial epicondylitis is not as common as lateral epicondylitis, it is still a fairly common injury seen in participants of certain sports such as golf, tennis, and racquetball. It is an injury that occurs in individuals who have had excessive activity of the wrist flexors and pronator teres.

The patient presents with a history of medial elbow pain. On physical examination, the patient has localized tenderness at or below the medial epicondyle. The patient has pain with resisted wrist flexion and pain with resisted forearm pronation. The flexor muscle group may have tight banding.

Treatment is the same as that for lateral epicondylitis. Athletes in golf and tennis also need to ensure that they are using appropriate technique (e.g., golf swing technique, the tennis forehand shot). Entrapment of the ulnar nerve in the scar tissue of an individual with medial epicondylitis is a concern, and it can be treated with neural stretching exercises.

REFERENCES

Brucker P, Khan K. Clinical Sports Medicine. 3rd ed. Sydney, Australia: McGraw-Hill; 2006.

Dixit S, DiFiori JP, Burton M, Mines B. Management of patellofemoral pain syndrome. Am Fam Physician 2007;75:194–202.

Eiff MP, Hatch RL, Calmbach WL. Fracture Management for Primary Care. 2nd ed. Philadelphia: WB Saunders; 2003.

McKeag DB, Moeller JL. ACSM's Primary Care Sports Medicine. New York: Lippincott Williams & Wilkins; 2007.

Peterson JJ. Injuries of the fingers and thumb in the athlete. Clin Sports Med 2006;25:527–42.

Pommering TL, Kluchurosky L, Hall SL. Ankle and foot injuries in the pediatric and adult athlete. Prim Care 2005;32:133–61.

Obstetrics and Gynecology

Antepartum Care

Method of
Kirk D. Ramin, MD, and Jessica P. Swartout, MD

Antepartum Care

Ideally, antepartum care commences 3 months before actual conception with the recommendation that women who are sexually active and not using contraception should begin taking daily multivitamin or folic acid supplements. The most convincing trials of this were performed in Europe and China when it was concluded that women of reproductive age should take multivitamin supplements containing 0.4 mg of folate daily. Women with histories of children with neural tube defects or other anomalies should increase this dose to 4 mg of folate in the periconceptional period to reduce risks of recurrence.

Preconception counseling should also include an accurate assessment of preexisting maternal medical conditions. This is the ideal time to stress changes in factors that respond to early intervention: quitting smoking, refraining from alcohol or drug abuse, treating gum disease, and avoiding teratogens. Alcohol is a known teratogen. Immunization status should be reviewed and vaccines should be administered as appropriate. Special consideration is given to patients with thyroid disease. Concern focuses on associations with low intelligence quotients (IQs) in children conceived by hypothyroid mothers. Patients with diabetes should be counseled that the increased risk of birth defects is directly related to the level of glucose control at conception.

High-risk obstetric referrals may be offered to women with potential for obstetric complications suggested by conditions listed in Box 1. Identification of the high-risk patient is critical to avoiding adverse outcomes.

In most cases, a woman's pregnancy is a normal event that is complicated by potentially dangerous disease in a minority of cases. The physician who manages pregnant patients must follow the normal changes that occur during antepartum care, so that abnormalities can be recognized and treated appropriately. Additionally, routine prenatal care offers multiple opportunities for patient education, primary intervention, and appropriate monitoring of the low-risk pregnancy in the setting of the family and community. For some women, antepartum care is part of their own continuum in a long-term primary care relationship with caregivers.

Timeline of Routine Antepartum Care

FIRST VISIT AND EARLY CARE

History

After pregnancy is confirmed, it is extraordinarily important to determine the duration of pregnancy and the estimated date of confinement (EDC). Further care is heavily predicated on this estimate. The history begins with ascertaining the first day of the last menstrual period and calculating the EDC by assuming duration of pregnancy averages 280 days (40 weeks).

The documentation of prior obstetric history includes prior complications, route of delivery, and estimated birth weights. Maternal medical disorders are often exacerbated by pregnancy; cardiovascular, renal, and endocrine disorders require evaluation and counseling concerning possible treatments required. A history of previous gynecologic surgery, including cesarean delivery, is important to consider. A family history of twinning, diabetes mellitus, familial disorders, or hereditary disease is relevant.

Current medications (prescription and nonprescription) are reviewed. Certain prescription medications are known teratogens and should be discontinued. Examples include isotretinoin (Accutane), tetracycline (Sumycin), quinolone antibiotics (ciprofloxacin [Cipro], levofloxacin [Levaquin]), and warfarin (Coumadin). Angiotensin-converting enzyme (ACE) inhibitors should not be used during the second and third trimesters, and the FDA has recently raised doubt

---

BOX 1 Potential Indications for High-Risk Referral

- Current disease involving renal, cardiac, or endocrine systems
- Fetal anomalies
- History of preterm delivery
- Incompetent cervix
- Isoimmunization
- Known carrier of genetic disorder
- Multiple gestation
- Placenta previa after 28 weeks
- Prior intrauterine fetal demise or stillbirth
- Systemic diseases such as hypertension, diabetes, or asthma
- Third-trimester bleeding

about their use in the first trimester. According to the approved label, ACE inhibitors are labeled pregnancy category C for the first trimester and pregnancy category D during the second and third trimesters. On June 8, 2006, the FDA issued an alert that infants whose mothers had taken an ACE inhibitor during the first trimester had an increased risk of major congenital malformations.

Honest discussion of substance abuse (alcohol, tobacco, and illicit drugs) is an integral part of the patient interview. Counseling patients about smoking cessation is vital in early pregnancy. Smoking increases the risk of fetal death or damage in utero. It is also associated with increased risk of placental abruption and placenta previa, each of which put both mother and child at risk.

Examination

Physical examination begins with a thorough general examination to assess maternal well-being including body mass index (BMI) and blood pressure (BP). The BMI is calculated by dividing weight in kilograms by height in meters squared. The BMI of a patient is categorized as underweight (under 19.8), normal weight (19.8 to 25), overweight (25 to 30), or obese (over 30). A brief fundoscopic examination might reveal signs of hypertension-induced changes.

Breast examination may be significant for changes in pregnancy that result from hormonal responses by the mammary ducts. These changes include engorgement and vascular prominence, occasionally resulting in mastodynia. Enlargement of areolar sebaceous glands (Montgomery's tubercles) occurs between 6 and 8 weeks' gestation.

A pelvic examination is performed with attention to the adequacy of pelvis and evaluation for adnexal masses. Numerous changes in the pelvic organs occur in pregnancy. For example, congestion of the pelvic vasculature (Chadwick's sign) causes bluish discoloration of the vagina and cervix. Softening of the cervix due to increased vascularity of the cervical tissue (Goodell's sign) can occur as early as 4 weeks. The uterus is palpable at the pubic symphysis at 8 weeks.

Portable devices using Doppler effect will reliably detect fetal heart tones at a rate of 120 to 160 beats per minute as early as 8 weeks.

Laboratory Studies

Routine laboratory studies ordered at the first visit include complete blood count (CBC) with differential, ABO and Rh typing, red cell antibody screen, rubella immunoglobulin (Ig)G, hepatitis B surface antigen (HBsAg), syphilis serology, and HIV 1 and HIV 2 antibody screens. Patients may refuse HIV testing, but all patients are counseled and offered the option for screening. A Papanicolaou (Pap) smear is performed in conjunction with cultures for chlamydia and gonorrhea.

A midstream urinalysis checks for the presence of protein or glucose. A microscopic examination of the urine is performed to rule out infection or asymptomatic bacteriuria. A baseline 24-hour urine protein collection and serum creatinine should be collected from all patients with hypertension, diabetes, or other preexisting renal disease.

Other Studies

Special-purpose studies are also considered in early gestation. First-trimester screening with nuchal translucency should be offered to all women older than 35 years between 11 and 14 weeks' gestation. The first-trimester screen uses the nuchal translucency and maternal serum-free β–human chorionic gonadotropin (hCG) and pregnancy-associated plasma protein A (PAPP-A) and detects up to 85% of Down syndrome and trisomy 18 cases.

Chorionic villus sampling (CVS) may be offered at 10 to 13 weeks to women older than 35 years, to those with abnormal first-trimester screens, and to those with abnormal pedigrees. From this, placental tissue may be subjected to chromosomal, metabolic, or DNA study. CVS cannot be used for diagnosis of neural tube defects, because this requires measuring alpha fetoprotein (AFP) levels in maternal serum at a later date.

Patients with tuberculosis exposure may be assessed for active tuberculosis with skin testing (if not vaccinated with bacille Calmette-Guérin [BCG]) and chest x-ray. Serologic assessment for toxoplasmosis, cytomegalovirus, and varicella immunity is not routinely indicated.

Screening for genetic disorders may be undertaken if concern exists based on racial or ethnic background (hemoglobinopathies, β-thalassemia, α-thalassemia, Tay-Sachs disease) or familial background (cystic fibrosis, fragile X, Duchenne's muscular dystrophy).

Follow-up

Follow-up visits are scheduled once monthly until 28 weeks' gestation, and then patients are followed twice monthly until 36 weeks. Visits are then scheduled at weekly intervals until delivery. At each visit, weight gain, edema, BP, fundal height, Leopold's maneuvers, and fetal heart tones are recorded. Because BP tends to decrease during the second trimester, increases of 30 mm Hg systolic or 15 mm Hg diastolic over first trimester pressures are abnormal. Interval history includes questions about diet, sleeping patterns, and fetal movement. Warning signs such as bleeding, contractions, leaking of fluid, headache, or visual disturbances are reviewed.

15 TO 18 WEEKS' GESTATION

Alpha Fetoprotein Testing

Maternal serum AFP testing is offered for all pregnancies at 16 to 18 weeks as a means of screening for open neural tube defects or chromosomal trisomy. In pregnancy, AFP is produced in sequence by the fetal yolk sac, the fetal gastrointestinal tract, and the fetal liver. AFP in the maternal serum occurs via placental exchange and transamniotic diffusion.

High levels of AFP are associated with various fetal anomalies including neural tube defects, multiple gestations, and ventral wall defects. Unexplained elevation of AFP has been associated with poor fetal growth, fetal loss, and preeclampsia. In cases with unexplained elevation of AFP, maternal and fetal surveillance should be increased. Low levels of AFP are associated with increased risk of Down syndrome.

The interpretation of this test depends on the gestational age; even if timed correctly, it is known to have a moderate level of false-positive results. Expanded serum markers of AFP, unconjugated estriol, inhibin A, and β-hCG are available to more accurately screen for Down syndrome, but detection is only about 60%, and false-negative results remain at 5%.

Amniocentesis

A more certain diagnosis is available via ultrasound-guided transabdominal amniocentesis at 16 to 18 weeks. Chromosomes from fetal cells are subjected to culture for karyotype and fluorescent in-situ hybridization (FISH) analysis, which detects trisomies 13, 18, 21, and abnormal numbers of sex chromosomes.

Physical Findings

Interval changes in the physical examination now include the start of colostrum secretion, which can begin as early as 16 weeks' gestation.

Chloasma is darkening of the skin over the forehead, bridge of the nose, or cheekbones and is more obvious in those with dark complexions. It can begin to manifest at this time, and is intensified by exposure to sunlight. Darkening of the skin in the areolae and nipples becomes more accentuated. A darkened line appears in the lower midline of the abdomen from the umbilicus to the pubis (linea nigra). The basis of these changes is stimulation of melanophores by increased melanocyte-stimulating hormone.

At 15 to 20 weeks, abdominal enlargement can appear more rapid as the uterus rises out of the pelvis and into the abdomen.

18 TO 20 WEEKS' GESTATION

Physical Findings

The mother might detect fetal movements (quickening) at around 20 weeks. The uterus is palpable at 20 weeks at the umbilicus, and ballottement reveals a fetus floating in amniotic fluid. Measurements that are 2 cm smaller than expected for week of gestation are suspicious for oligohydramnios, intrauterine growth restriction, fetal anomaly, or abnormal fetal lie. Conversely, measurements 2 cm larger than expected can indicate multiple gestation, polyhydramnios, or fetal macrosomia. These rules apply for the gestational ages of 18 to 32 weeks. Either condition can be fully evaluated with ultrasound examination and consultation with an obstetrician or maternal-fetal medicine specialist.

Laboratory Studies

Increased surveillance for preeclampsia includes testing for urine protein in patients with BP greater than 140/90 mm Hg or in those with weight gains greater than 3 pounds/week. Evaluation is also necessary for clinical signs of upper extremity edema, right upper quadrant tenderness, headaches, or vision changes. Proteinuria of more than 300 mg in 24 hours can indicate renal dysfunction or the onset of preeclampsia.

Ultrasonography

Sonography has long established itself as the single most useful technology in monitoring pregnancy and diagnosing complications. It is for this reason that basic level ultrasound is offered at 18 to 20 weeks to evaluate growth, placentation, amniotic fluid volume, and fetal anatomy. If earlier dating of the pregnancy is uncertain, this is an opportunity to confirm or refute prior estimates. If anomalous conditions are discovered or the patient has a history of diabetes, advanced maternal age, or has prior children with anomalies, more comprehensive ultrasonography becomes necessary.

28 WEEKS' GESTATION

Physical Findings

New physical examination findings at this time include the onset of stretch marks (striae) of the breasts and abdomen. These are caused by separation of underlying collagen tissue, a response to increased adrenocorticosteroid. The ligamentous structures of the pelvis also undergo slight but definite relaxation of the joints, a progesterone effect. As the uterus enlarges, it often rotates to the right. Fundal size roughly correlates with the estimated gestational age at 26 to 34 weeks. Braxton Hicks contractions, characterized as painless uterine tightening, increase in regularity. The fetal outline can be easily palpated through the maternal abdominal wall.

Laboratory Studies

A CBC for anemia and a 1-hour glucose tolerance test (after ingestion of 50 g of glucose) is scheduled to detect patients at risk for developing gestational diabetes. If the screening test is abnormal, a 3-hour test is performed to confirm the diagnosis. Two or more abnormal values on this test are considered diagnostic of gestational diabetes mellitus.

A repeat Rh antibody is checked at this time in Rh-negative mothers. Those who remain unsensitized in the third trimester receive a first dose of Rho(D) immune globulin (RhoGAM) to prevent maternal isoimmunization to fetal red blood cells. A 300 μg dose is sufficient for 15 mL of red cells (equivalent to 30 mL of whole blood).

Follow-up

Return visits at 2-week intervals are now initiated, and the patient is oriented to the labor and delivery ward. Precautions are given regarding the onset of conditions listed in Box 2. The onset of any of these should prompt immediate medical attention.

36 WEEKS' GESTATION

Physical Findings

Patients might complain of increased vaginal discharge at this time in their pregnancy, a physiologic consequence of hormone stimulation. The discharge consists mainly of epithelial cells and cervical mucus and is treated with reassurance. Discharge accompanied by itching, burning, or malodor should be evaluated and treated accordingly, however.

BOX 2 Warning Signs and Symptoms Prompting Medical Attention

- Burning with urination
- Chills or fever
- Prolonged vomiting or inability to keep liquids down
- Pronounced decrease in fetal movements
- Rhythmic cramping pains (>6/h)
- Rupture of membranes
- Severe abdominal, pelvic, or back pain
- Signs of preeclampsia (headache, edema, right upper quadrant pain)
- Vaginal bleeding

Laboratory Studies

Vaginal and rectal cultures are collected to evaluate for the presence of group B Streptococcus (GBS) at 35 to 37 weeks. GBS organisms are implicated in preterm labor, amnionitis, endometritis, and wound infection. If cultures are positive, the patient will be given antibiotic prophylaxis during active labor in efforts to protect the newborn against vertical transmission, resulting in newborn sepsis.

Follow-up

Follow-up visits are planned on a weekly basis with emphasis on weight gain, BP, and signs of preeclampsia. Review of precautions regarding infection, pregnancy loss, and symptoms of preeclampsia completes the visit.

POST-TERM GESTATION

About 3% to 12% of pregnancies continue beyond 43 weeks of gestation and are considered post-term. Although some of these may be due to inaccurate dating, some patients clearly progress to excessively long gestations that are a significant risk to the fetus. Increased antepartum surveillance by cervical examination, fetal heart rate testing (see the discussion of contraction stress testing), and biophysical profile should be initiated between 41 and 42 weeks. Even if fetal testing is reassuring, patients with reliable dating greater than 41 weeks are candidates for induction of labor.

Common Concerns of the Antenatal Period

BLEEDING

About one half of pregnant women experience some form of bleeding during the pregnancy; often this is benign. Patients also have a heightened awareness of symptoms that previously may have gone unnoticed in the nonpregnant state. Efficient and competent evaluation, followed by compassion and reassurance when prudent, allays many fears and provides clear direction. Spotting due to bleeding at the implantation site occurs from the time of implantation (about 6 days after fertilization) until 29 to 35 days after the last menstrual period in many women. Some women have unexplained cyclic bleeding throughout pregnancy. Usually, cardiac activity on ultrasound and appropriate β-hCG levels confirm a viable early pregnancy. First-trimester bleeding in lieu of these findings may be a sign of spontaneous miscarriage or ectopic pregnancy. Vaginal bleeding in late pregnancy is covered in other articles.

NAUSEA

Nausea is a common symptom that occurs in most pregnancies. It is heightened before 14 weeks' gestation and is largely benign. The etiology is not well understood but likely is related to elevating levels of β-hCG. Its moniker "morning sickness" is misleading, because nausea of pregnancy can occur at any time during the day. Aggravating factors vary with the individual patient; success varies with interventions designed to reduce symptoms.

Uncomplicated nausea may be responsive to small nonfatty portions at mealtime. Pyridoxine (vitamin B$_6$)[1] tablets 12.5 mg twice a day or doxylamine (Unisom)[1] 12.5 mg twice a day are safe in pregnancy and may be helpful. Antiemetic drugs in the outpatient setting are a measure of last resort.

Inability to control protracted vomiting in conjunction with clinical dehydration can require hospitalization for intravenous fluids and treatment of hyperemesis gravidarium. Extreme nausea and vomiting or nausea and vomiting that persists beyond 18 to 20 weeks' gestation may be signs of multiple gestation, thyroid disease, or molar pregnancy.

NUTRITION AND WEIGHT GAIN

The mother's nutrition is a vital factor in the development of the fetus from preconception through the postpartum period. Therefore, the pregnant woman should be advised to eat a balanced diet and should be informed of the additional 300 kcal/day needed during pregnancy. The American College of Obstetricians and Gynecologists (ACOG) recommends a target weight gain of 10 to 12 kg (22–27 lb) during pregnancy. They also advise that underweight women might need to gain more and obese women should gain less. Nutritional requirements for protein are 80 g/day, for calcium are 1500 mg/day, for iron are 30 mg/day, and for folate are 0.4 mg/day (4 mg/day in some cases). Patients with seizure disorders managed with valproic acid (Depakene) or carbamazepine (Tegretol) are also at risk and might benefit from the higher dose of folate.

HEARTBURN

Heartburn in the form of reflux esophagitis is caused by the enlarging uterus displacing the stomach and by progesterone's relaxation of the lower esophageal sphincter. Treatment consists of taking antacids, decreasing exacerbating factors such as spicy foods, eating more frequently but in smaller quantities, limiting eating before bedtime, and taking H$_2$-receptor inhibitors.

URINARY SYMPTOMS

Urinary frequency, nocturia, and bladder irritability are common complaints due to progesterone-mediated relaxation of smooth muscle and subsequent altered bladder function. Later in pregnancy, urinary frequency becomes even more prominent from pressure on the bladder by the enlarging uterus and the fetal presenting parts, such as when the fetal head descends into the pelvis.

Dysuria, however, is often a sign of infection that requires antibiotic treatment. Bacteriuria combined with urinary stasis from altered bladder function predisposes the patient to pyelonephritis. Although simple urinary tract infections are treated on an outpatient basis, pyelonephritis remains the most common nonobstetric cause for hospitalization during antenatal care.

Patients with a diagnosis of pyelonephritis require hospitalization, aggressive fluid replacement, and IV antibiotics until they remain afebrile for longer than 24 hours. Close monitoring of maternal respiratory status is important because these women are at risk for acute respiratory distress syndrome (ARDS). All patients should complete a 10-day course of antibiotic treatment. After treatment has been completed, suppressive therapy should be continued until delivery.

INFECTION

Two infections of special note are HIV and bacterial vaginosis (BV). HIV transmission to the newborn can be reduced significantly with appropriate infectious disease and maternal-fetal medicine specialty management. Appropriate treatment of BV in women at high risk for preterm delivery or recurrent loss can significantly reduce either of these untoward outcomes. Debate exists as to whether or not low-risk women should be screened.

Chlamydia trachomatis is an obligate intracellular bacterium and is the most common sexually transmitted bacterial infection in women of reproductive age. It may be associated with urethritis, mucopurulent cervicitis, and acute salpingitis, or it may be clinically silent. Perinatal transmission is clearly associated with neonatal conjunctivitis (leading to blindness) and pneumonia and is likely associated with preterm delivery, premature rupture of membranes, and perinatal mortality. Diagnosis is confirmed by polymerase chain reaction (PCR) during routine screening. Doxycycline should be avoided in pregnancy, and erythromycin is associated with gastrointestinal upset, so treatment with azithromycin is often appropriate.

Gonococcal infection is associated with concomitant chlamydia infection in about 40% of infected pregnant women. It is usually limited to the lower genital tract, including the cervix, urethra, and periurethral or vestibular glands. Because of an association between gonococcal cervicitis and septic spontaneous abortion, and because preterm delivery, premature rupture of membranes, and postpartum infection are more common with gonococcal infection, routine cultures are appropriate at the first antenatal visit. Because some strains have rendered some β-lactam drugs ineffective for therapy, the recommendation for uncomplicated gonococcal infection is intramuscular ceftriaxone 125 mg.

Vaginosis due to *Candida albicans* can become symptomatic with caseous white discharge and vaginal itching or burning, and it may be associated with red satellite lesions on the vulva. Marked inflammation of the vagina and introitus may be noted. Topical application of over-the-counter antifungal creams such as miconazole nitrate (Monistat) or nystatin (Mycostatin) is generally helpful in controlling the imbalance of vaginal flora.

Cytomegalovirus is a ubiquitous DNA herpes virus that is transmitted horizontally between humans by droplet infection. It is transmitted vertically from mother to fetus and is the most common cause of perinatal infection. The virus becomes latent after primary infection, with periodic reactivation and viral shedding. Infection is usually clinically silent. Many of the affected infants have died from infection, and most of the survivors have severe handicaps, including mental retardation, blindness, and deafness. Serious sequelae are more common among primary infections. The syndrome of congenital cytomegalovirus infection includes low birth weight, microcephaly, intracranial calcifications, chorioretinitis, mental and motor retardation, sensorineural deficits, hepatosplenomegaly, jaundice, hemolytic anemia, and thrombocytopenic purpura. Confirmation of primary infection is suggested by a fourfold increase of IgG titers in paired acute and convalescent sera or by detecting IgM cytomegalovirus antibodies. There is no effective therapy for maternal infection.

Human parvovirus B19 causes erythema infectiosum, or fifth disease. This is a single-stranded DNA virus that is heralded by the appearance of clinical findings of bright red macular rash and accompanying arthralgias. Acute infection is confirmed by IgM-specific antibody and can prompt adverse pregnancy outcomes, including spontaneous miscarriage and fetal death.

Rubella, also known as German measles, is directly responsible for spontaneous miscarriage and severe congenital malformations. Although large epidemics of rubella are nonexistent in the United States because of immunization, the disease can still affect the up to 25% of susceptible women. Absence of rubella antibody indicates susceptibility. Vaccination involves an attenuated live virus (MMR) and therefore is avoided in pregnancy. Vaccination of nonpregnant susceptible women (including those during the postpartum period) and hospital personnel continues to be the mainstay of therapy. Detection by IgM-specific antibody confirms recent infection. Congenital rubella syndrome (CRS) is a severe example of antenatal infection and includes one or more of the conditions listed in Box 3.

Varicella-zoster virus, the etiologic agent of childhood chickenpox, is a DNA herpes virus that remains latent in the dorsal root ganglia and may be reactivated years later to cause herpes zoster or shingles. Infection early in pregnancy can lead to severe congenital malformations including chorioretinitis, cerebral cortical atrophy, hydronephrosis, and cutaneous and bony leg defects. Varicella-zoster immunoglobulin (VZIg) 125 U/10 kg can attenuate varicella infection if given within 96 hours.

---

[1]Not FDA approved for this indication.

BOX 3　Conditions Associated with Congenital Rubella Syndrome

- Central nervous system defects (meningoencephalitis)
- Chromosomal abnormalities
- Chronic diffuse interstitial pneumonitis
- Eye lesions
  - Cataracts
  - Glaucoma
  - Microphthalmia
- Heart disease
  - Patent ductus arteriosus
  - Septal defects
  - Pulmonary artery stenosis
- Hepatic dysfunction
  - Hepatitis
  - Hepatosplenomegaly
  - Jaundice
- Osseous changes
- Retarded growth
- Sensorineural deafness
- Thrombocytopenia and anemia

Genital herpes simplex virus (HSV) may be confirmed by tissue culture if active lesions are present; in this event, cesarean delivery is indicated because the fetus is at risk for acquiring the virus during passage through the birth canal. Oral or topical acyclovir can improve symptoms. If no lesions and no prodromal symptoms are present, vaginal delivery is recommended.

Trichomonas vaginalis can be found in 20% to 30% of pregnant patients, but only a small number complain of discharge or irritation. This flagellated, oval, motile organism can be seen on normal saline wet prep and is evident clinically by presence of a foamy or greenish discharge accompanied by multiple cervical petechiae. Treatment is oral metronidazole.

Prenatally acquired infection caused by the protozoan parasite *Toxoplasma gondii* can result in the presence of abnormalities such as microcephalus or hydrocephalus at birth, development of jaundice with hepatosplenomegaly or meningoencephalitis in early childhood, or delayed appearance of ocular lesions such as chorioretinitis in later childhood. Exposure to the parasite is through eating undercooked meat, gardening in soil that is potentially contaminated by mammalian feces, or cleaning a cat's litter box.

VARICOSE VEINS

Pressure by the enlarged uterus on venous return from the legs and progesterone-mediated vasodilation can lead to prominent varicosities and edema of the legs or vulva. Any concern for deep vein thrombosis should be ruled out by examination for erythema, edema, cords, or tenderness. Doppler ultrasound may be indicated in equivocal findings of the lower extremities. Benign varicosities almost invariably return to normal after delivery, thus limiting the need for intervention in the antepartum period. Edema of the lower extremities is common, responds to elevation, and must be differentiated from facial or hand edema accompanying preeclampsia. Hemorrhoids are manifestations of the varicosities of the rectal veins. Treatment focuses on stool softeners, sitz baths, and over-the-counter topical preparations.

CONSTIPATION

Bowel transit time and relaxation of intestinal smooth muscle are both increased due to progesterone effects, resulting in overall slowing of bowel function. If pronounced, this can lead to constipation. Dietary management of this condition is centered around recommendations for increased fluids and high-fiber foods. Enemas and laxatives are avoided.

UPPER EXTREMITY DISCOMFORT

Periodic numbness and tingling of the fingers is due to exacerbations of carpal tunnel compression exacerbated by tissue edema. Splinting of the affected hand at night is indicated, with anticipation of resolution during postpartum diuresis.

CURRENT DIAGNOSIS

- Pregnancy evaluation should begin 3 months before conception with optimization of underlying medical conditions and commencement of prenatal vitamins with 400 µg of folic acid.
- Preconception counseling with a specialist in high-risk pregnancies should be considered in all patients with underlying medical conditions, if possible.
- The first prenatal visit should include a review of the medical and obstetric histories, current medications, herbal remedies, and tobacco, alcohol, and drug use.
- Prenatal laboratory studies should be done at the first visit after a pregnancy is confirmed with a urine pregnancy test. These studies include hemoglobin, platelet count, type and screen, rubella status, and hepatitis B testing. All women should be offered screening for HIV. High-risk patients should be screened for hepatitis C, gonorrhea, and chlamydia.
- Genetic screening should be offered based on ethnic background and family history.
- Both first-trimester screening (nuchal translucency combined with maternal serum PAPP-A/free β-hCG) and second-trimester quadruple screen should be offered to all patients. These tests aid in diagnosis of chromosome abnormalities. If a patient opts for a first-trimester screen, it is important to perform an AFP screen in the second trimester to screen for neural tube defects.
- Appropriate weight gain in pregnancy depends on maternal BMI before pregnancy. In patients with a normal BMI, a 25- to 35-pound weight gain is recommended. Underweight patients are encouraged to gain 30 to 40 pounds, and overweight patients are encouraged to gain no more than 25 pounds.
- Prenatal visits should begin at 8 to 12 weeks' gestation and continue monthly until 24 weeks. Visits should then be every 2 weeks until 36 weeks and then weekly. Each visit should include assessment of maternal weight, BP, urinalysis for protein and glucose, fundal height measurement, documentation of fetal heart tones, and review of symptoms of preterm labor and preeclampsia.
- All patients should undergo a glucose challenge test at 24 to 28 weeks. This is done by administering a 50-g load of glucose and obtaining a serum sample 1 hour after administration. A level greater than 140 mg/dL is considered abnormal, and a 3-hour glucose tolerance test is indicated. If a woman demonstrates abnormalities in two of the four values, gestational diabetes is diagnosed.

Abbreviations: AFP = alpha fetoprotein; BMI = body mass index; BP = blood pressure; hCG = human chorionic gonadotropin; PAPP-A = pregnancy-associated plasma protein A.

CURRENT THERAPY

- Administration of the inactivated influenza vaccine (Fluzone, Fluvirin, Fluvarix) is recommended in all pregnant patients, regardless of trimester, who will be pregnant during the flu season.
- Folic acid supplementation should begin before conception. The recommended dose is 400 µg daily. In patients with a previous pregnancy complicated by a neural tube defect, 4 mg daily is recommended to prevent recurrence of a neural tube defect.
- Pyelonephritis requires hospitalization and IV antibiotics in all pregnant patients. IV antibiotics should be continued until the patient is afebrile for longer than 24 hours. Oral antibiotics should then be commenced to complete a 10-day course. All patients should continue on suppressive antibiotic therapy until delivery.
- All patients with HIV should be treated with antiretroviral therapy regardless of gestation. Intrapartum zidovudine is recommended for all patients with HIV.

BACKACHE AND PELVIC DISCOMFORT

Endocrine relaxation of ligamentous structures coupled with an offset center of gravity create exaggerated spinal curve, joint instability, and compensatory back pain. Most women experience some form of this discomfort as pregnancy progresses. Advice given for improvements in posture, local heat, acetaminophen, and massage may be helpful. Minimizing the time spent standing can have a positive effect. Round ligament pain usually occurs during the second trimester and is described as sharp bilateral or unilateral groin pain. It may be exacerbated by change in position or rapid movement and might respond to similar measures. These routine aches and pains of pregnancy must be differentiated from rhythmic cramping pains originating in the back. The latter may be a sign of preterm labor requiring appropriate evaluation.

LEG CRAMPS

Leg cramps in the form of recurrent muscle spasms in pregnancy are believed to be due to lower levels of serum calcium or higher levels of serum phosphorus. The calves are most commonly involved and attacks are more frequent at night and in the third trimester. There are no data from controlled trials to show benefit over placebo for treatment targeted toward reduced phosphate and increased calcium or magnesium intake. Local heat, putting the affected muscle on stretch, acetaminophen, and massage can be helpful in acute events.

INTERCOURSE

In general, intercourse is considered safe in pregnancy. The exception to this rule is found in patients who are experiencing uterine bleeding, or postcoital cramps, and spotting. It may be wise to avoid intercourse in couples who are at risk for special circumstances. Firmer recommendations can be made in instances of placenta previa or known rupture of membranes; in these instances intercourse should not occur.

DENTAL CARE

Ideally, women should have dental care completed before conception. However, dental procedures under local anesthesia may be carried out at any time during the pregnancy. Use of nitrous oxide inhalants is to be avoided, however. Long procedures should be postponed until the second trimester. Antibiotics are given for dental abscesses and in cases of rheumatic heart disease or mitral valve prolapse.

X-RAYS, IONIZING RADIATION, AND IMAGING

The adverse effects of ionizing radiation are dose dependent, but there is no single diagnostic procedure that results in a dose of radiation high enough to threaten the fetus or embryo. Diagnostic radiation of less than 5000 mrad is considered by ACOG to have minimal teratogenic risk, and if medically indicated, x-ray imaging may be performed safely. For example, patients may undergo chest x-rays as indicated; a dose of 0.05 mrad is typical exposure. Patients receiving dental x-rays are additionally protected by a lead apron. Still, the need for x-ray films should be evaluated for risks and potential benefits in the individual pregnant patient to conservatively protect the mother and fetus from theoretical genetic or oncogenic risk. MRI is considered safe due to its mechanism of action, which is a nonionizing form of radiation. Radioactive iodine (^{131}I) is contraindicated in pregnancy.

IMMUNIZATION

Live virus vaccines must be avoided during pregnancy because of possible effects on the fetus. These include measles, mumps, rubella (MMR) and yellow fever (VF-Vax). The risks to the fetus from the administration of rabies vaccine (RabAvert, IMOVAX) are unknown. The varicella vaccine (Varivax) is not recommended in pregnancy.

Diphtheria and tetanus toxoid (Td) may be administered in pregnancy if exposure to pathogens is likely. The hepatitis B vaccine (Engerix B, Recombivax HB) series is safe and may be given in pregnancy to women at risk. The inactivated influenza vaccine (Fluzone, Fluvirin, Fluvarix) is also recommended in all women during any trimester they will be pregnant during the flu season.

Tests of Fetal Well-Being

A primary goal in antepartum care is the competent management of patient care extended to both mother and baby in order to reduce the risk of fetal demise after 24 weeks, ensure optimal conditions for term delivery after 37 weeks, and intervene for evolving conditions threatening the well-being of either patient. Any pregnancy that may be at increased risk for antepartum fetal compromise is a candidate for tests of fetal well-being performed weekly, beginning at 28 to 32 weeks. Some conditions requiring antepartum testing are listed in Box 4.

NONSTRESS TEST

The nonstress test consists of fetal heart rate monitoring in the absence of uterine contractions. A reactive tracing is one in which heart rate accelerations of 15 bpm above the baseline of 120 to 160 bpm are of at least 15 seconds' duration. Two of these accelerations must be observed in a 20-minute period. False-positive nonreactive tracings are more common before 28 weeks' gestation.

CONTRACTION STRESS TEST

The requirements for a reactive tracing are combined with tocodynamometer recordings of three contractions of 40 seconds or more duration in a 10-minute period. If no contractions are present, they may be induced via nipple stimulation or intravenously administered oxytocin. Relative contraindications to this test are preterm premature rupture of membranes, classic uterine incision scar, placenta

---

BOX 4   Conditions That Prompt Further Testing

- Decreased fetal movements
- Fetal growth restriction
- Hypertensive disorders
- Insulin-dependent diabetes mellitus
- Multiple gestation with discordant fetal growth
- Oligohydramnios or polyhydramnios
- Post-term pregnancy
- Prior loss or stillbirth

TABLE 1 Possible Results of the Contraction Stress Test

Result	Description
Negative	No late decelerations
Positive	Late decelerations follow 50% of contractions
Equivocal	Intermittent or variable decelerations
Unsatisfactory	<3 contractions in 10 minutes

previa, and unexplained vaginal bleeding. The results of the contraction stress test are categorized in Table 1.

BIOPHYSICAL PROFILE

The biophysical profile consists of a nonstress test with ultrasound observations. A total of ten points is given for the following elements (two points each):

- Reactive nonstress test
- Presence of fetal breathing movements of 30 seconds or more in 30 minutes
- Fetal movement defined as three or more discrete body or limb movements within 30 minutes
- Fetal tone defined as one or more episodes of fetal extremity extension and return to flexion
- Quantification of amniotic fluid volume, defined as a pocket of fluid that measures at least 2 cm by 2 cm

Antepartum Hospitalization

Pregnant patients with complications requiring hospitalization are admitted to a high-risk antepartum floor in close proximity to the labor and delivery area. Specialists in maternal-fetal medicine are intimately involved in the care plans of these patients.

REFERENCES

American College of Obstetricians and Gynecologists. Compendium of Selected Publications. Atlanta: American College of Obstetricians and Gynecologists; 2007.

Carpenter MW, Coustan DR. Criteria for screening tests for gestational diabetes. Am J Obstet Gynecol 1982;144(7):763–73.

Centers for Disease Control and Prevention. Influenza: Information for Health Professionals, Available at http://www.cdc.gov/flu/ [accessed July 13, 2007].

Cunningham FG, Leveno KL, Bloom SL, et al. Williams Obstetrics. 22nd ed. New York: McGraw-Hill; 2005.

Lopez A, Dietz VJ, Wilson M, et al. Preventing congenital toxoplasmosis. MMWR Recomm Rep 2000;49(RR-2):59–68.

Wald NJ, Rodeck C, et al. First and second trimester antenatal screening for Down's syndrome. The results of the Serum, Urine and Ultrasound Screening Study. J Med Screen 2003;10(2):56–104.

Ectopic Pregnancy

Method of
Gary H. Lipscomb, MD

In the United States, the incidence of ectopic pregnancies has increased dramatically during the last several decades. Commonly cited risks include prior pelvic inflammatory disease (PID), previous tubal surgery, intrauterine device (IUD) use, previous ectopic pregnancy, ovulation induction and in vitro fertilization, progestin-containing contraceptives, smoking, previous abdominal surgery, in utero diethylstilbestrol (DES) exposure, and previous induced abortion.

A high degree of suspicion is necessary for the early diagnosis of an ectopic pregnancy. Almost all ectopic pregnancies have episodes of vaginal bleeding or lower abdominal pain prior to rupture. Such patients are appropriate candidates to evaluate for ectopic pregnancy. Figure 1 illustrates a diagnostic algorithm that is useful in efficiently coordinating and interpreting the tests used in the diagnosis of ectopic pregnancy.

Diagnosis

Serum progesterone levels are helpful as an initial screening test for ectopic pregnancy. Levels higher than 25 ng/mL are associated with ectopic pregnancy in only 1% to 2% of cases; levels less than 5 ng/mL are associated with a nonviable pregnancy (either intrauterine or ectopic) more than 99% of the time. If progesterone levels are not readily available in a timely manner, however, human chorionic gonadotropin (hCG) levels alone may be used.

Levels of hCG rise in an essentially linear fashion until after 41 days of gestation. By this gestational age, an intrauterine pregnancy (IUP) should be seen on ultrasound. In 85% of normal pregnancies, hCG doubles approximately every 2 days, rising at least 66% in 48 hours. However, 15% of normal IUPs rise less than this in 48 hours. Conversely, 15% of ectopic pregnancies rise more than 66%. But a rise of less than 50% is associated with an abnormal pregnancy 99.9% of the time.

Because the interassay variability of hCG is 15%, a change of less than this amount is considered a plateau. Plateaued levels are the most predictive of ectopic pregnancy. The use of a urine pregnancy test to rule out the possibility of phantom hCG is strongly recommended prior to surgical or medical treatment. This phenomenon, caused by heterophilic serum antibodies, produces false-positive hCG levels usually less than 1000 IU/L.

The sonographic identification of an intrauterine gestational sac essentially excludes an ectopic pregnancy. A viable IUP should always be visualized at an hCG titer of 2000 IU/L by transvaginal scan and by 6500 IU/L with transabdominal ultrasound. An adnexal mass, in a patient with a presumed ectopic pregnancy and hCG levels less than 2000 IU/L, should not automatically be assumed to be an ectopic without the presence of a yolk sac, fetal pole, or cardiac activity. Such masses are frequently corpus luteum cysts associated with an early IUP.

Except in the rare case of heterotopic pregnancy, the identification of chorionic villi in uterine contents essentially eliminates the diagnosis of ectopic pregnancy. The use of dilation and curettage (D&C) also eliminates giving methotrexate unnecessarily to a patient with a failed IUP.

A D&C is particularly important in patients with hCG titers below the discriminatory zone of ultrasound. In these patients, the appropriate use of hCG doubling times and serum progesterone levels is necessary to avoid interrupting a viable IUP. Patients with

CURRENT DIAGNOSIS

- Screening for symptomatic patients or those with risk factors
- Diagnostic algorithm to coordinate testing
- hCG titers every 48 hours
- Ultrasound at hCG level of 2000 mIU/mL
- D&C for inappropriate hCG rise (<50% in 48 hours) below 2000 mIU/mL

Abbreviations: D&C = dilation and curettage; hCG = human chorionic gonadotropin.

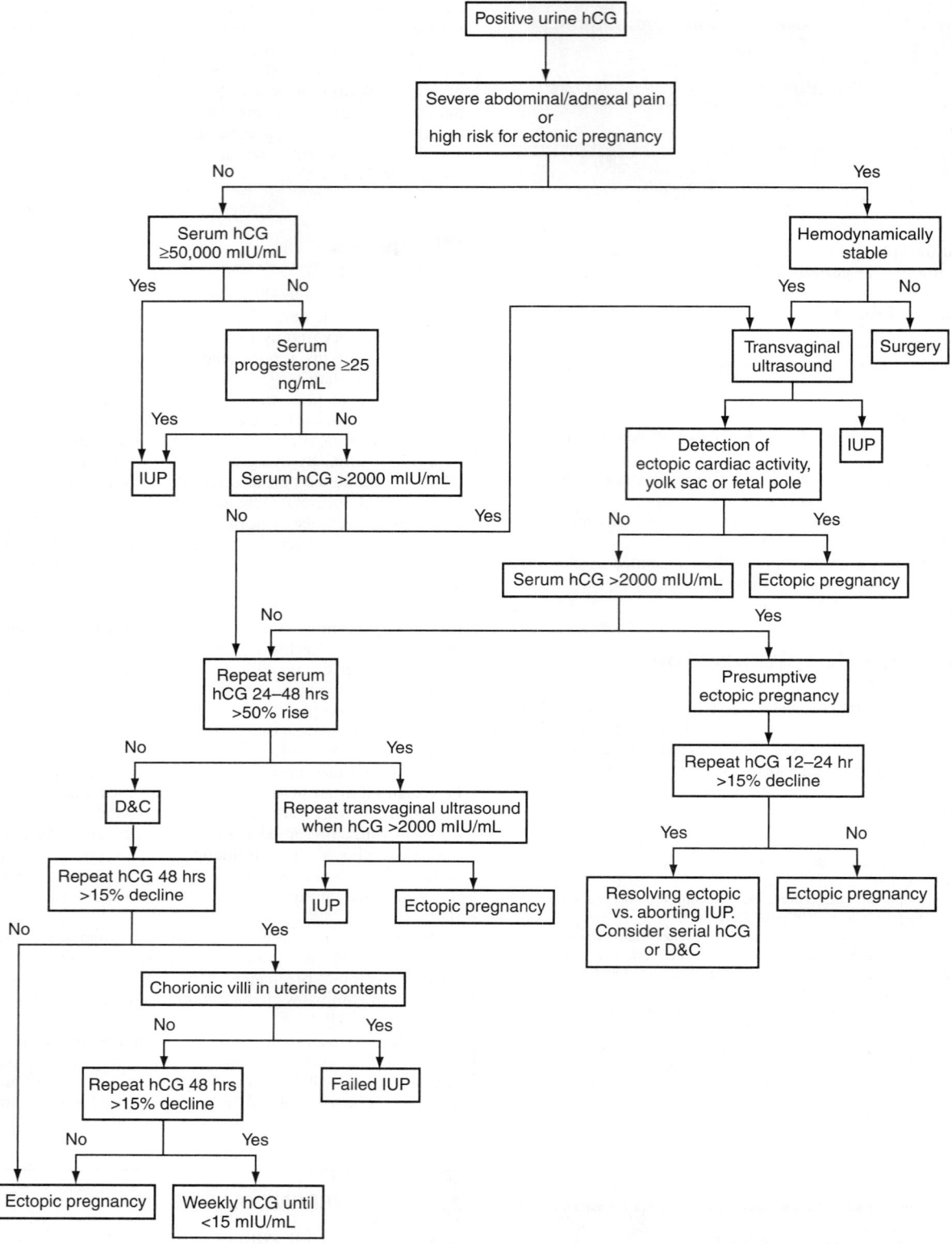

FIGURE 1. University of Tennessee Diagnostic Algorithm. D&C = dilation and curettage; hCG = human chorionic gonadotropin.

hCG titers that plateau (less than 15% change) or an hCG rise of less than 50% in 48 hours should undergo D&C to differentiate between a failed IUP and an ectopic pregnancy. Villi is absent on final histology in up to 50% of these cases. Because only the presence of villi is diagnostic, those without villi require serial hCG titers. While awaiting final histologic pathology, hCG titers are also followed. As noted in the ectopic algorithm, a serum hCG drawn after D&C is followed by a repeat level in 12 to 24 hours. Rising or inappropriately falling levels after D&C are considered diagnostic of an ectopic pregnancy.

Laparoscopy remains the gold standard for the diagnosis of ectopic pregnancy. It should be employed in any patient with suspected ectopic rupture, unreliable patients, or any others suspected of ectopic pregnancy for which the diagnostic algorithms are inappropriate.

CURRENT THERAPY

- Surgery: treatment of choice for unstable patients
- Methotrexate success: correlation with hCG levels
- Multidose methotrexate: 1 mg/kg body weight IM alternate days with leucovorin 0.1 mg/kg IM until hCG declines 15%
- Multidose treatment follow-up: daily hCG until decline, then weekly
- Single-dose methotrexate: 50 mg/m² based on actual body weight
- Single-dose treatment follow-up: hCG on days 1, 4, 7, then weekly if 15% decline between days 4 and 7

Abbreviations: hCG = human chorionic gonadotropin; IM = intramuscularly.

Treatment

Surgery is the classic treatment for ectopic pregnancy and remains the treatment of choice in hemodynamic unstable patients, those desiring no further pregnancies, or those who are unsuitable or unwilling to risk medical therapy.

Medical therapy with methotrexate[1] is an acceptable option to surgical therapy. Reported success rates range from 75% to 96%, with an average of approximately 90%. Whether a multidose or single-dose methotrexate protocol is most effective remains debatable, but single-dose methotrexate is the most popular because of its ease of use and low incidence of side effects.

Contraindications to medical therapy remain ill defined, but Boxes 1 and 2 note frequently used contraindications. The hCG level is the single factor most predictive of failure. With hCG levels of 5000 to 9999, success rates fall to approximately 87%, further dropping to 82% for levels 10,000 to 14,999 and 68% if more than 15,000. These levels can be used to counsel patients about the risk of failure.

MULTIDOSE METHOTREXATE

Intramuscular methotrexate, 1 mg/kg of actual body weight, alternating with citrovorum rescue factor (Leucovorin), 0.1 mg/kg, is given daily and continued until a 15% decline in two consecutive daily hCG titers. Human chorionic gonadotropin levels are then followed weekly. A repeat course of methotrexate/citrovorum is given if levels fall to less than 15% or rise between two consecutive hCG titers.

SINGLE-DOSE METHOTREXATE PROTOCOL

Methotrexate, 50 mg/m² based on actual body weight, is given intramuscularly. The day methotrexate is given is considered day 1. A repeat hCG is performed on days 4 and 7. If there is an appropriate decline, hCG levels are followed weekly. If the hCG level declines less

[1] Not FDA approved for this indication.

than 15% between days 4 and 7, a second dose of methotrexate is given and the protocol restarted at a new day 1. Although this protocol is referred to as "single-dose methotrexate," approximately 20% of patients require more than one treatment cycle.

In conclusion, the incidence of ectopic pregnancy has reached epidemic proportions in the United States. Nevertheless, the mortality associated with this disease is steadily declining. This decline is primarily because of earlier diagnosis that allows treatment prior to rupture. This earlier diagnosis is the result of improved assays for progesterone, hCG, transvaginal ultrasound, and the use of diagnostic algorithms that do not require the use of laparoscopy. Once diagnosed, numerous treatment options are now available, including the option of medical therapy. Future developments ideally will provide for an even earlier diagnosis as well as data on the optimum candidates for each form of treatment.

REFERENCES

Brenaschek G, Rudelstorfer R, Csaicsich P. Vaginal sonography versus serum human chorionic gonadotropin in early detection of pregnancy. Am J Obstet Gynecol 1988;158:608–12.
Kadar N, Freedman M, Zacher M. Further observation on the doubling time of human chorionic gonadotropin in early asymptomatic pregnancy. Fertil Steril 1980;54:783–7.
Lipscomb GH, McCord ML, Huff G, et al. Predictors of success of methotrexate treatment in women with tubal ectopic pregnancies. N Engl J Med 1999;341:1874–8.
Lipscomb GH, Stovall TS, Ling FW. Nonsurgical treatment of ectopic pregnancy. N Engl J Med 2000;343:1325–9.
Stovall TS, Ling FW, Buster JE. Nonsurgical diagnosis and treatment of tubal pregnancy. Fertil Steril 1990;54:537–8.
Stovall TG, Ling FW, Gray LA, et al. Methotrexate treatment of unruptured ectopic pregnancy: A report of 100 cases. Obstet Gynecol 1991;77:749–53.

Vaginal Bleeding in Late Pregnancy

Method of
Jami Star Zeltzer, MD

Vaginal bleeding in late pregnancy complicates approximately 6% of pregnancies and is associated with increased maternal and fetal morbidity and mortality. Excluding labor, the most likely causes are placenta previa and placental abruption, followed by uterine rupture and vasa previa; less common etiologies include trauma, cervical lesions, and coagulopathy. The primary focus in obstetric hemorrhage, regardless of cause, is maternal hemodynamic assessment and stabilization. Given the extraordinary blood flow to the uterus at term (600 to 800 mL/min), exsanguination can occur rapidly. Additionally, redistribution of maternal blood flow may lead to fetal hypoxia.

Early maternal signs of hemodynamic compromise include tachycardia and tachypnea; later, hypotension, weakened pulses, and oliguria ensue, along with evidence of fetal compromise. Further decompensation can ultimately result in the death of both mother and fetus. Guidelines for restoration of maternal circulating volume are approximately 3 mL of intravenous crystalloid, (i.e., normal saline or Ringer's solution) per 1 mL of blood lost (often underestimated). Laboratory evaluation includes a complete blood count, blood type, and crossmatch; in the setting of thrombocytopenia (less than 100,000 platelets), coagulation studies (prothrombin time [PT], partial thromboplastin time [PTT], fibrinogen, fibrin degradation products [FDPs]) are recommended. Packed red blood cells, fresh-frozen plasma, platelets, and/or cryoprecipitate are given to maintain maternal hemoglobin near 10 g/dL and correct coagulopathy (unlikely if whole blood is observed to clot in less than 8 minutes). Additional measures include administration of oxygen, lateral displacement of the uterus and, rarely, vasopressors. Fetal evaluation and treatment, including consideration of delivery, follow stabilization of the mother.

Placenta Previa

Placenta previa, or the implantation of the placenta adjacent to or covering the internal os, complicates approximately 0.5% of all deliveries. The degree of placenta previa may be:

- Complete (internal os covered entirely)
- Partial (portion of internal os covered)
- Marginal (placental edge at cervix or less than 2 cm away)
- Low lying (not a true previa, where the placental edge implants in the lower uterine segment but doesn't reach the cervix)

Box 1 lists the risk factors. The pathophysiology appears to involve endometrial damage, with resulting limitation of healthy uterine tissue for implantation.

The hallmark symptom is painless vaginal bleeding, presumably initiated by development of the lower uterine segment. Usually, this occurs by 29 to 30 weeks' gestation, although in approximately 33% of cases, there is no bleeding until labor. The first bleed may be self-limited, but rebleeding complicates approximately 60% of cases. The diagnosis is often made in the absence of symptoms on routine ultrasound. The incidence of placenta previa is 5% to 10% in mid-gestation; this resolves in most cases with development of the lower uterine segment (*placental migration*). When asymptomatic, expectant management is appropriate, although vaginal precautions after 28 weeks' gestation may be advised.

When a patient presents with third-trimester bleeding, speculum exams are contraindicated until placenta previa is ruled out. The most accurate method of diagnosis is transvaginal ultrasound, which is safe in experienced hands; transperineal or transabdominal ultrasound carry greater risks of false-positive and false-negative results.

Observation in the hospital is recommended following a bleed, during which time approximately 50% of patients will deliver. Steroids are indicated for enhancement of fetal lung maturation. Tocolysis can

be administered if the mother and fetus are stable, but betasympathomimetics should be avoided in order to minimize cardiovascular effects. Outpatient management is acceptable if bleeding ceases, as long as the patient is compliant and has ready access to a hospital. Serial ultrasound assessment is recommended because there is an increased risk of intrauterine growth restriction. Transfusion should be offered to maintain hemoglobin greater than 10 mg/dL.

Urgent delivery by cesarean section is indicated when there is ongoing maternal hemorrhage or evidence of fetal compromise. In the stable patient, a planned cesarean section can be performed at 35 to 36 weeks, generally after an amniocentesis is performed to confirm fetal lung maturity. Vaginal delivery may be attempted if delivery is imminent, or with marginal previa, although a double setup for emergent cesarean section is advised. In the setting of fetal demise, vaginal delivery is preferable.

Placenta previa predisposes to postpartum hemorrhage, either from atony of the lower uterine segment or inability to remove the placenta because of absence of the decidua basalis. The most common form of this latter condition is placenta accreta, where the trophoblast adheres to the myometrium. Less common forms include placenta increta (the trophoblast invades the myometrium) and placenta percreta (trophoblast invades uterine serosa and/or adjacent organs). The primary risk factor for placenta accreta is the number of previous cesarean sections, with an incidence approaching 40% in patients with two prior cesarean sections and a placenta previa. Other risk factors include age, parity, and history of curettage. Color Doppler ultrasound and magnetic resonance imaging (MRI) are helpful but not always definitive for diagnosis. If placenta accreta is suspected, preparations can be made for scheduled delivery with trained personnel and blood products available. At delivery, the placenta should be left in place if a cleavage plane cannot be developed easily. Cesarean–hysterectomy is often required for hemostasis, although conservative management, including preoperative and intraoperative selective embolization and/or use of methotrexate, has been reported. With placenta percreta, bladder invasion may require cystoscopy and urologic repair.

Placental Abruption

Abruption of the placenta, or separation of the normally implanted placenta before birth, complicates 1% to 2% of pregnancies. Bleeding into the decidua basalis, with subsequent separation of varying amounts of placental tissue from the endometrium, may result in fetal compromise and/or demise. The exact pathophysiology is unclear. Box 2 lists the risk factors.

Vaginal bleeding in the second half of pregnancy is assumed to be caused by placental abruption, once placenta previa and other rare

---

BOX 1 Risk Factors for Placenta Previa

- Advancing maternal age
- Ethnic background (increased in Asians)
- Multiparity
- Multiple gestation
- Previous curettage
- Prior cesarean section (increases with number of sections)
- Prior placenta previa
- Smoking

BOX 2 Risk Factors for Placental Abruption

- Chorioamnionitis
- Cocaine use
- Ethnic background (highest in blacks)
- Hypertension
- Male fetal gender
- Multiple gestation
- Parity
- Polyhydramnios (rapid decompression at membrane rupture and/or therapeutic amniocentesis)
- Preterm premature rupture of membranes
- Previous cesarean section
- Smoking
- Trauma, including domestic violence
- Unexplained elevated second trimester alpha-fetoprotein
- Uterine anomalies/short umbilical cord

causes are ruled out. Concealed hemorrhage, present in 10% to 20% of cases, can complicate the diagnosis. Abdominal pain, back pain, uterine contractions (often described as low amplitude, high frequency), hypertonus, uterine tenderness, and/or idiopathic premature labor may be present. While ultrasound can identify placenta previa, it cannot be relied upon to definitively diagnose abruption, as clot is sonographically visible in less than 50% of cases. The differential diagnoses include uterine rupture, appendicitis, and chorioamnionitis, as well as other causes of abdominal pain.

Most commonly, bleeding is not profuse and, if the episode is self-limited, expectant management of a preterm gestation includes observation, serial fetal growth assessment, fetal well-being testing, and steroid therapy to accelerate fetal lung maturation. With ongoing significant blood loss, stabilization of the mother, fetal assessment, and laboratory evaluation are indicated. Coagulopathy is rare in the absence of fetal demise. If tocolysis is required, betasympathomimetics should be avoided, as they may mask maternal cardiovascular decompensation.

Vaginal delivery is appropriate if mother and fetus are stable. Amniotomy may decrease extravasation of blood into the myometrium by head compression. Not uncommonly, effacement will precede dilatation; oxytocin (Pitocin) is acceptable for labor dysfunction. In the event of an intrauterine demise, vaginal delivery is preferred. Acute hemorrhage requires immediate cesarean delivery, with blood and coagulation factor replacement as needed.

Potential complications of abruption include hemorrhagic shock, disseminated intravascular coagulation (unlikely unless there is greater than 2000 mL blood loss and/or fetal demise), ischemic necrosis of maternal organs (especially kidney), and Couvelaire uterus (extravasation of blood into uterine muscle). Recurrence is approximately 5% to 15%, increasing with each subsequent event. There are no known preventive measures other than correcting modifiable risk factors. Research into the association between thrombophilia and abruption is ongoing, but in absence of other risk factors, a work-up for hypercoagulability may be considered.

Vasa Previa

Vasa previa is a rare condition (estimated 1 in 2500 deliveries) in which fetal blood vessels cross over the membranes in advance of the presenting part. This is most often associated with velamentous insertion of the umbilical cord (vessels reach the placenta after coursing through the membranes rather than by direct insertion); Box 3 lists the risk factors. Vasa previa carries a profound risk of fetal mortality from exsanguination, particularly at the time of membrane rupture (fetal blood volume at term is approximately 250 mL). Even in the absence of bleeding, vessel compression may result in compromise of the fetal circulation.

Signs include hemorrhage, as well as fetal heart rate abnormalities. A high index of suspicion is required, and advances in imaging techniques (color Doppler, transvaginal ultrasound) make prenatal diagnosis possible. If there is unexplained bleeding, an Apt test or Kleihauer-Betke test can identify fetal red blood cells. If the diagnosis of vasa previa is strongly suspected at term, or if hemorrhage is significant, prompt cesarean delivery is recommended, followed by neonatal resuscitation.

BOX 4 Uterine Rupture

Risk Factors
Previous cesarean section (especially classical)
Use of oxytocin, prostaglandins, or misoprostol
Multiparity
Midforceps application
Breech version/extraction
Placental abruption
Shoulder dystocia
Placenta percreta
Müllerian duct anomalies
History of pelvic radiation

Differential Diagnoses
Appendicitis
Biliary colic
Pancreatitis
Peptic ulcer disease
Intestinal obstruction
Ovarian torsion
Placental abruption
Urinary tract disorders

Uterine Rupture

Most often reported following prior cesarean section, uterine rupture can also occur in an unscarred uterus (1 in 8000 to 1 in 15,000 deliveries). This phenomenon implies complete separation of the uterine wall (as compared to uterine dehiscence), with or without expulsion of the fetus. Box 4 lists risk factors and differential diagnoses.

Common signs and symptoms include abdominal pain/tenderness and vaginal bleeding; additional complaints include epigastric or shoulder pain, abdominal distention, and constipation. The fetal tracing may show sudden variable decelerations or abrupt and prolonged bradycardia, often accompanied by recession of the presenting part. Maternal and fetal morbidity and mortality are high, particularly with delayed diagnosis. Treatment is urgent cesarean delivery, with repair of the uterus and/or hysterectomy as needed. Repeat cesarean section is advised in the future because of the risk for recurrence.

Hypertensive Disorders of Pregnancy

Method of
Brenda Stokes, MD

Hypertensive disorders of pregnancy are the most common medical disorder in pregnancy. Hypertension is estimated to occur in 5% to 12% percent of all pregnancies. It is a major cause of maternal and fetal morbidity and mortality. The hypertensive disorders of pregnancy are classified as shown in Box 1.

Pregnancy-induced or gestational hypertension is the most common cause of hypertension in pregnancy. It is defined as a systolic blood pressure of more than 140 mm Hg and diastolic blood pressure

---

BOX 3 Risk Factors for Vasa Previa

- Bilobed placenta
- In vitro fertilization
- Low-lying placenta
- Multiple pregnancy
- Succenturiate lobe
- Velamentous insertion of umbilical cord

BOX 1 Hypertensive Disorders of Pregnancy

- Gestational (pregnancy-induced) hypertension
- Preeclampsia and eclampsia
- Chronic hypertension
- Preeclampsia superimposed on chronic hypertension

of more than 90 mm Hg on two different measurements at least 6 hours apart. The measurements should be done no more than 1 week apart. This is further classified as mild or severe disease. Mild disease usually develops later in pregnancy. The pregnancy outcomes with mild disease usually are good. Severe disease is associated with a higher morbidity in pregnancy than women with mild preeclampsia. Women with severe disease have rates of preterm delivery, small for gestational age infants, and abruption similar to those for women with severe preeclampsia.

Clinical Characteristics and Diagnosis

Preeclampsia is defined as hypertension developing after 20 weeks' gestation and with proteinuria. Hypertension is defined the same for preeclampsia as for gestational hypertension. Proteinuria is defined as excretion of 300 mg or more of protein in a 24-hour urine collection. Preeclampsia is further divided into mild or severe disease. Multiple risk factors have been associated with the development of preeclampsia. Box 2 lists some of the common risk factors.

There are many theories about the cause of preeclampsia. For example, ongoing investigations suggest that preeclampsia may be an autoimmune disorder caused by pregnancy-induced autoantibodies that activate the angiotensin II receptor type 1a (AT1 receptor). Women with preeclampsia have been found to have autoantibodies that bind and stimulate AT1 receptors. In one study, injection of these AT1 autoantibodies into pregnant mice caused all of the main features of preeclampsia, including hypertension, glomerular endotheliosis, proteinuria, placental abnormalities, and reduced fetal size. There is definitely a relationship between abnormal placentation and preeclampsia, but it is unclear if this is a cause or an effect. For example, a genetic deficiency of an estradiol metabolite, 2-methoxyestradiol (2-ME), may underlie the placental effects in preeclampsia, suggesting that therapeutic supplementation may prevent or treat the disorder. Serum levels of 2-ME were greatly reduced in a model of preeclampsia, resulting from a lack of placental catechol-O-methyltransferase (COMT) expression. In normal pregnant women, levels of 2-ME are elevated during the third trimester, but in women with preeclampsia, 2-ME levels are lower, and placental expression of COMT protein expression is reduced. This suggests that the actions of COMT and 2-ME are central to proper vascular function in the placenta.

Preeclampsia affects multiple maternal organ systems. It causes proteinuria and can rarely lead to renal failure. Hyperreflexia, grand mal seizures, hemorrhagic stroke (rare), and visual disturbances, including transient blindness, can occur. The vascular system becomes contracted, which increases the hematocrit. Thrombocytopenia, coagulation abnormalities, and hemolysis can occur. Heart failure and pulmonary edema are late complications. Abnormal liver transaminase levels with hepatic congestion and hepatic rupture can also occur.

BOX 2   Risk Factors for the Development of Preeclampsia

- Nulliparity
- New partner
- Obesity
- Multiple gestation
- Family history of preeclampsia
- Chronic hypertension
- Renal disease
- Diabetes mellitus
- Presence of thrombophilias
- Previous history of preeclampsia
- Abnormal uterine Doppler studies at 18 and 24 weeks' gestation
- Maternal age ≥40 years

CURRENT DIAGNOSIS

- Hypertensive disorders of pregnancy are the most common medical disorder in pregnancy.
- Hypertensive disorders of pregnancy are a major cause of maternal and fetal morbidity and mortality.
- Clinicians providing care for pregnant patients should be aware of the signs and symptoms of preeclampsia and screen for them at every visit.

Preeclampsia also affects the developing fetus. Decreased placental perfusion leads to an increased incidence of intrauterine growth restriction and placental abruption. Oligohydramnios can develop as a result of the poor placental perfusion.

The initial signs and symptoms of preeclampsia vary. Patients typically present with increased blood pressure and proteinuria. Peripheral nondependent edema is common, as is weight gain. Symptoms may include epigastric or right upper quadrant abdominal pain, headaches, and visual disturbances. Most patients present with mild preeclampsia. However, some present with severe disease, which requires prompt diagnosis and treatment. Preeclampsia can manifest antepartum, intrapartum, or postpartum.

An increased rate of maternal and fetal morbidity and mortality is associated with preeclampsia. The rate depends on the severity of maternal disease and the gestational age of the fetus at diagnosis. Mild preeclampsia has been associated with fetal outcomes similar to those for normotensive patients. Patients with mild preeclampsia have a higher rate of cesarean delivery. Severe disease is associated with an increased risk of maternal morbidity and mortality and a higher rate of premature delivery, abruption, and small for gestational age infants. Because of the potential morbidity and mortality associated with preeclampsia, there is interest in early diagnosis and primary prevention in patients at high risk for the disease.

Prevention and Treatment

Many different therapies have been studied for primary prevention of preeclampsia in patients who are at high risk for the disease. Calcium[1] supplementation of 2 g/day or less has been studied, and the incidence of preeclampsia and gestational hypertension has been reduced. The benefit is seen more in patients at high risk for gestational hypertension and in women with a low dietary intake of calcium. Antioxidant supplementation, mostly with vitamins C[1] and E,[1] during pregnancy has been evaluated for preventing preeclampsia. A Cochrane systematic review of many studies failed to show any benefits for using antioxidants in pregnancy to prevent preeclampsia or its complications. A prospective cohort study showed a reduction in preeclampsia with supplementation of a multivitamin with folic acid[1] in the second trimester. Antiplatelet therapy, mainly low-dose aspirin,[1] has been moderately effective in reducing the incidence of preeclampsia and its complications in women at high risk for the disease. Physical activity has been studied for the prevention of preeclampsia, but the results have been inconclusive.

Preeclampsia can occur as mild or severe disease. Table 1 shows the clinical manifestations for each type. Disease is considered mild unless any of the criteria is met for severe disease.

The management of preeclampsia, especially severe disease, is controversial. Suggested management plans for mild and severe disease are presented in Figure 1. The recommendations are based on the best available data of maternal and fetal outcomes. The management of preeclampsia depends on the gestational age of the fetus at diagnosis and the severity of illness in the mother. Although some cases can occur in the postpartum period, delivery of the fetus is the definitive treatment for preeclampsia in other situations. Conservative management is

---

[1]Not FDA approved for this indication.

TABLE 1 Classification of Preeclampsia

Feature	Mild Disease	Severe Disease
CNS symptoms	Headache, hyperreflexia	Seizures, blurred vision, scotomas, headache, clonus, irritability
Proteinuria	≥300 mg/24 hours	>5 g/24 hours
Liver function	Normal transaminase levels	Elevated transaminase levels, epigastric pain, liver rupture
Platelet level	>100,000/hpf	<100,000/hpf
Hemoglobin level	Normal	Elevated level, hemolysis, DIC
Blood pressure	<160/110 mm Hg	>160/110 mm Hg
Fetal status	Normal AFI, fetal testing, and growth	IUGR, oligohydramnios, signs of fetal distress, abruption, fetal demise

Abbreviations: AFI = amniotic fluid index; CNS = central nervous system; DIC = disseminated intravascular coagulation; hpf = high-power field; IUGR = intrauterine growth restriction.

recommended in pregnancies less than 38 weeks' gestation and mothers with mild disease. Although bed rest is recommended, there is no evidence to support this. Care includes daily blood pressure checks and urine dipstick determinations for protein. Patients with mild disease can be managed on an inpatient or outpatient basis. Laboratory evaluation, which includes a 24-hour urine collection for total protein and blood testing, should be obtained for all patients at least twice weekly. Daily fetal kick counts are advised with antenatal fetal testing twice weekly. Serial obstetric ultrasound evaluations are recommended to monitor fetal growth at baseline and then every 3 weeks.

Severe preeclampsia is managed aggressively because of the increased risk of maternal and fetal morbidity. The primary goal in management is the health and well-being of the mother and then the delivery of a mature fetus. All patients with severe preeclampsia require immediate hospitalization. Intravenous magnesium sulfate infusion is recommended for seizure prophylaxis. Antihypertensive medications are recommended to treat systolic blood pressure higher than 160 mm Hg and diastolic blood pressure higher than 110 mm Hg. Corticosteroids are recommended for patients at gestational ages between 22 and 34 weeks. Daily maternal and fetal evaluations with laboratory testing and antepartum fetal testing are recommended. Obstetric ultrasound scans are used to evaluate intrauterine fetal growth restriction (IUGR), oligohydramnios, and abruption.

Choice of the mode of delivery of the fetus is based on the gestational age and the maternal and fetal status. Vaginal delivery is the preferred route of delivery in a patient with preeclampsia. Cesarean delivery should be considered for premature infants, for severe IUGR,

and for severe disease with an unfavorable cervix. Continuous fetal monitoring should be instituted intrapartum. Epidural or spinal anesthesia is preferred for cesarean delivery. If necessary, maternal transfer should be considered to an institution that has the ability to care for the newborn infant, who may be premature, and the mother, who may need intensive care monitoring after delivery.

Intravenous magnesium sulfate infusion is typically initiated for seizure prophylaxis intrapartum and continued postpartum. Its use in mild preeclampsia is controversial because the data are not clear about whether the benefits outweigh the risks. The total intravenous fluid rate needs to be monitored closely and usually does not exceed 150 mL/hour. Magnesium sulfate is started as a bolus infusion of 4 to 6 g over 15–20 minutes and then continued at a rate of 1–2 g/hour. Magnesium toxicity needs to be monitored. Box 3 lists clinical signs of magnesium toxicity. Therapeutic levels are 4 to 8 mg/dL. Urine output should be monitored closely. Calcium gluconate should be available to reverse toxicity if needed. It is administered intravenously as 1 g over 2 minutes. The magnesium sulfate infusion is usually continued for 24 hours postpartum but should be continued longer if clinically indicated.

Blood pressure is monitored closely in the patient with preeclampsia. Treatment is indicated for systolic blood pressure higher than 160 mm Hg and diastolic blood pressure higher than 110 mm Hg. Traditionally, intravenous hydralazine (Apresoline) or labetalol (Trandate) have been used. Oral nifedipine (Procardia) also has been effective.

Eclampsia occurs in the setting of preeclampsia when seizures or coma develop without other identified causes. It can be associated with mild or severe disease, and it can occur antepartum, intrapartum,

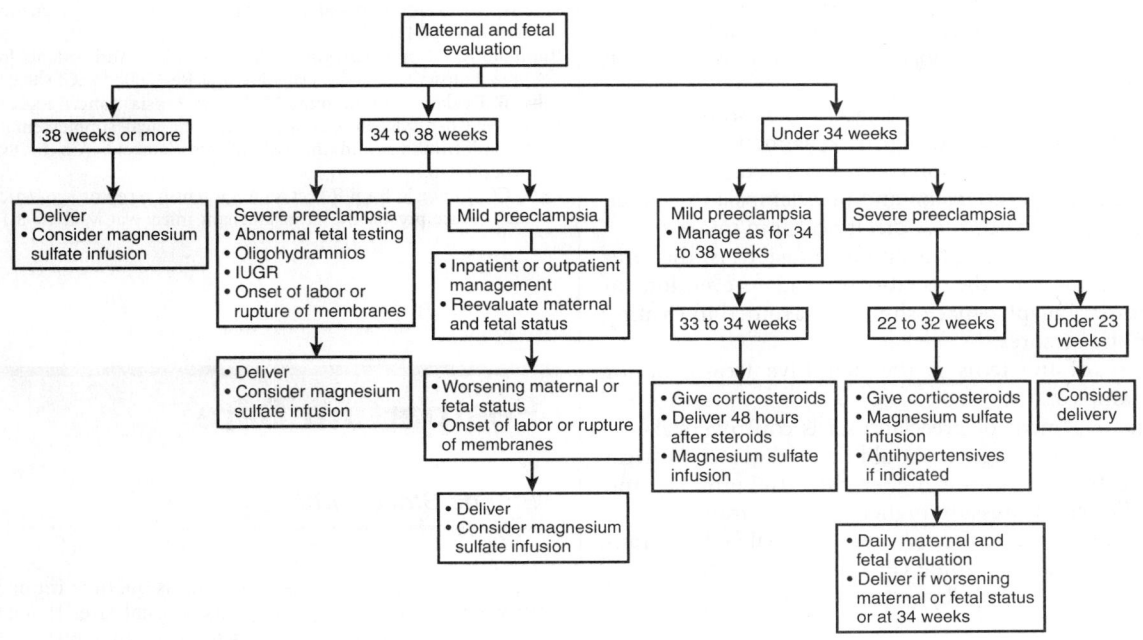

FIGURE 1. Management of preeclampsia. *Abbreviation:* IUGR = intrauterine growth restriction.

BOX 3 Signs of Magnesium Toxicity, Listed Progressively with Increasing Magnesium Levels

- Loss of deep tendon reflexes
- Somnolence and slurred speech
- Decreased respiratory rate <12 breaths/min
- Decreased urine output
- Pulmonary edema

---

or postpartum. The pathophysiology is unknown but is thought to include cerebral edema, ischemia, hemorrhage, or transient cerebral arterial vasospasm.

Eclampsia is managed by controlling blood pressure and preventing recurrent seizures. Intravenous magnesium sulfate infusion is the agent of choice for treatment of eclampsia and prevention of recurrent seizures. The maternal airway should be protected and supplemental oxygen given. Fetal heart rate abnormalities, usually fetal bradycardia, may occur but heart rate typically returns to baseline after the seizure. Immediate delivery is not always necessary if the infant and mother are stabilized. Polypharmacy to treat the seizures should be avoided because it only increases maternal side effects.

HELLP syndrome, a form of severe preeclampsia, is defined as hemolysis, elevated liver enzymes, and low platelets. It can sometimes be misdiagnosed when it occurs early in pregnancy and the blood pressure is not elevated. It should be managed the same as severe preeclampsia.

Chronic hypertension occurs in approximately 1% to 5% of pregnancies. Patients with chronic hypertension are at increased risk for complications in pregnancy, including preeclampsia. It is defined as hypertension diagnosed before pregnancy or before 20 weeks' gestation. It can also be diagnosed retrospectively postpartum when elevated blood pressure persists. It is associated with an increased risk of abruption, poor perinatal outcomes, and superimposed preeclampsia. Early prenatal care and close maternal and fetal monitoring are required.

CURRENT THERAPY

- Mild to moderate hypertension in pregnancy does not require treatment.
- Antihypertensive drug selection should be based on the clinician's familiarity with the medication.
- Angiotensin-converting enzyme (ACE) inhibitors and angiotensin receptor blockers are contraindicated in pregnancy.
- Low-dose aspirin[1] is beneficial in the prevention of preeclampsia in selected high-risk women.
- Calcium[1] supplementation is beneficial in the prevention of gestational hypertension and preeclampsia in women at high risk and with a low dietary calcium intake.
- Magnesium sulfate intravenous infusion is the preferred agent for the treatment and prevention of eclampsia. Polypharmacy should be avoided in treating eclamptic seizures.
- Delivery of the fetus is the definitive treatment for preeclampsia.
- The management of preeclampsia is controversial.
- Antihypertensive agents should be used acutely to treat systolic blood pressure higher than 160 mm Hg and diastolic blood pressure higher than 110 mm Hg.
- Intravenous hydralazine (Apresoline), labetalol (Trandate), and oral nifedipine (Procardia) have been effective in treating severe hypertension in pregnancy.

---

[1]Not FDA approved for this indication.

It is unclear whether treatment of chronic hypertension affects pregnancy outcomes, especially for women with mild hypertension. Maternal and fetal outcomes are generally good despite mild hypertension. Antihypertensive medications can reduce the risk of severe hypertension but do not reduce other complications. Medications usually can be discontinued in early pregnancy. Antihypertensive medication is chosen based on the clinician's preference and experience if indicated. Angiotensin-converting enzyme (ACE) inhibitors and angiotensin receptor blockers are contraindicated in pregnancy.

Summary

Hypertensive disorders of pregnancy are the most common medical problems encountered during pregnancy. Hypertension is associated with increased maternal and fetal morbidity and mortality. Close monitoring and appropriate timing of delivery are required to ensure the best possible maternal and fetal outcomes.

REFERENCES

Abalos E, Duley L, Steyn DW, Henderson-Smart DJ. Antihypertensive drug therapy for mild to moderate hypertension during pregnancy. Cochrane Database Syst Rev 2007;(1):CD002252.

Askie LM, Duley L, Henderson-Smart DJ, Stewart L. for the PARIS Collaborative Group. Antiplatelet agents for prevention of preeclampsia: A meta-analysis of individual patient data. Lancet 2007;369:1791–8.

Duley L, Henderson-Smart DJ, Meher S. Drugs for treatment of very high blood pressure during pregnancy. Cochrane Database Syst Rev 2006;(3):CD001449.

Duley L, Meher S, Abalos E. Management of preeclampsia. BMJ 2006;332:463–538.

Hofmeyr GJ, Atallah AN, Duley L. Calcium supplementation during pregnancy for preventing hypertensive disorders and related problems. Cochrane Database Syst Rev 2006;(3):CD001059.

Leeman L, Fontaine P. Hypertensive disorders of pregnancy. Am Fam Physician 2008;78:93–100.

Kanasaki K, Palmsten K, Sugimoto H. Deficiency in catechol-O-methyltransferase and 2-methoxyoestradiol is associated with pre-eclampsia. Nature 2008;453:1117–21.

Meher S, Duley L. Exercise or other physical activity for preventing preeclampsia and its complications. Cochrane Database Syst Rev 2006;(2):CD005942.

Roberts JM, Pearson G, Cutler J, Lindheimer M. Summary of the NHLBI working group on research on hypertension during pregnancy. Hypertension 2003;41:437–45.

Rumbold A, Duley L, Crowther CA, Haslam RR. Antioxidants for preventing preeclampsia. Cochrane Database Syst Rev 2008;(1):CD004227.

Sabai B, Dekker G, Kupferminc M. Pre-eclampsia. Lancet 2005;365:785–99.

Wen SW, Chen XK, Rodger M, et al. Folic acid supplementation in early second trimester and the risk of preeclampsia. Am J Obstet Gynecol 2008;198:45.

Zhou CC, Zhang Y, Irani RA, et al. Angiotensin receptor agonistic autoantibodies induce pre-eclampsia in pregnant mice. Nat Med 2008;14:810–2.

Postpartum Care

Method of
Brenda Stokes, MD

The postpartum period, or puerperium, is the time immediately after birth when the uterus returns to its normal size. It starts with the delivery of the placenta and ends 6 weeks after birth. This chapter reviews specific concerns and problems that arise in the postpartum period.

BOX 1 Etiology of Postpartum Hemorrhage

Uterine atony
Lacerations
Retained products of conception
Coagulation disorders

Postpartum Hemorrhage

The World Health Organization defines postpartum hemorrhage as 500 mL or more of blood loss in the first 24 hours after delivery. Postpartum hemorrhage occurs in approximately 30% to 40% of all deliveries. It continues to be a major cause of maternal morbidity and mortality in both developed and developing countries.

Early recognition and treatment are essential in preventing complications from postpartum hemorrhage. The amount of blood loss following a delivery is difficult to measure accurately. It is typically estimated by visual inspection. Brisk vaginal bleeding following birth should trigger an investigation for its etiology.

The etiology of postpartum hemorrhage is shown in Box 1. Uterine atony is the most common cause of immediate postpartum hemorrhage. Once brisk bleeding is identified, a careful examination for the cause is performed. Palpation of the uterine fundus is done to assess the tone of the uterus. Bimanual uterine massage both confirms and treats uterine atony. The medications listed in Table 1 are oxytocics used to control vaginal bleeding due to uterine atony. Emptying the bladder with catheterization is useful to keep the uterus contracted. Surgical methods are considered if medications and uterine massage fail to control the bleeding. A careful inspection of the vagina and cervix for lacerations needs to be done. Manual curettage of the uterus can be performed immediately postpartum under appropriate anesthesia.

Breast-Feeding

Breast-feeding has many benefits for both the infant and mother. Breast milk provides the proper nutrition for the infant and protection against certain infectious diseases. Breast-feeding enhances maternal infant bonding and can delay ovulation.

Mothers need support for initiation and continuation of breast-feeding. Both social and professional support systems are invaluable resources for lactating mothers.

Common breast-feeding problems include sore nipples, breast engorgement, blocked milk ducts, and infections. Sore nipples are usually due to improper latch-on of the infant during feeding. This will improve after correction of the latch-on. Breast engorgement usually responds to emptying the breasts by feeding or pumping.

Blocked milk ducts can be confused with infections. A blocked milk duct appears as a localized area of tenderness and erythema in one breast. It responds to warm compresses and gentle massage to express the breast milk and unclog the duct. Mastitis manifests as an erythematous, tender, hard area on one breast. Most women have systemic symptoms, such as fever and chills. Narrow-spectrum

CURRENT DIAGNOSIS

- Recognize and treat postpartum hemorrhage early.
- Uterine atony is the most common cause of immediate postpartum hemorrhage.
- Return to normal diet and physical activity can occur just after birth.
- Endometritis is the most common cause of puerperal fever.
- Screen for postpartum depression several times throughout the postpartum period.
- Address postpartum contraception early after delivery.

antibiotics can be used in most cases. Breast-feeding should be continued on both breasts. If the mother is unable to breast-feed, both breasts should be emptied by a breast pump. A breast abscess can develop as a complication of mastitis and must be surgically drained.

Nutrition and Activity

There are no dietary restrictions in healthy women in the postpartum period. Lactating women need to increase the protein, calories, and calcium in their diet. Physical activity is recommended in pregnancy and should be continued in the postpartum period. Less active women tend to retain more weight at 1 year postpartum than active women.

Puerperal Infections

Uterine infection, which is referred to as *endometritis*, is a common cause of puerperal fever. It is more common following a cesarean delivery. Diagnosis is made from history and physical examination. Fever is the typical manifesting symptom. Uterine tenderness is usually present. Endometritis is a polymicrobial infection. Broad-spectrum intravenous antibiotics are required for treatment. Intravenous antibiotics should be continued for 24 hours after defervescence. Oral antibiotics are not needed following the initial intravenous antibiotics. Complications of endometritis include pelvic infections, pelvic abscess, and septic pelvic thrombophlebitis.

Contraception

Postpartum contraception needs to be addressed with every patient because most will become sexually active before the traditional 6-week postpartum visit. The choice of contraception depends on patient preference, desire for future fertility, and clinical considerations. Table 2 lists methods of postpartum contraception and precautions specific to the postpartum period.

TABLE 1 Medications Used in the Treatment of Postpartum Hemorrhage

Medication	Dosage	Route	Dosing Interval	Cautions and Contraindications
Oxytocin (Pitocin)	10 units IM, 10–40 units/ 1000 mL IV fluids	IV, IM	One dose IM, IV rate as needed to control bleeding	Hypersensitivity to drug or class
Carboprost tromethamine (Hemabate)	250 µg	IM	Every 15–90 min up to 2 mg total	Active cardiac, pulmonary, liver, or renal disease
Methylergonovine (methergine)	0.2 mg	IM, oral	Every 2–4 h up to 5 doses IM, oral tid-qid for 3–7 d	Hypertension

TABLE 2 Methods of Postpartum Contraception

Method of Contraception	When to Start	Precautions in Postpartum Period
Barrier methods: Condoms, diaphragm, cervical cap	At the resumption of sexual activity	Diaphragm or cervical cap will need to be refitted about 6 wk postpartum
Progesterone-only pills (Micronor), injectable (Depo-Provera), or implant (Implanon)	Any time after 24 h postpartum	Pills need to be taken the same time every d Can cause irregular prolonged bleeding postpartum Does not interfere with lactation
Combined oral contraceptive pills, patch (Ortho-Evra), or vaginal ring (NuvaRing)	4 wk postpartum	Decreases breast milk production Not advised if high risk of thromboembolic disease
Intrauterine device or system, progesterone containing (Mirena) or copper T (ParaGard)	Immediately postpartum or 6 wk postpartum	Increased risk of expulsion if inserted immediately postpartum Not advised if high risk of infection or previous ectopic pregnancy
Sterilization: Male or female (transabdominal or transcervical [Essure])	Male anytime, but ideally during the antepartum period. Female after delivery but before hospital discharge or 6 wk postpartum	Future fertility not desired Requires surgery Transcervical sterilization is an outpatient procedure but requires follow-up testing
Lactational amenorrhea method	Can be effective if exclusively breastfeeding up to 6 mo	Not reliable Ovulation can resume at any time
Natural family planning	After onset of first menses	None

Medical Complications

Hypertension and preeclampsia can occur in the postpartum period with persistently elevated blood pressures. Blood pressure is highest 3 to 6 days postpartum. According to a 2005 Cochrane review of trials for treatment and prevention of postpartum hypertension, there are no reliable data to guide its treatment. Significantly elevated blood pressures should be treated as indicated. Evaluation for preeclampsia should be performed postpartum when suspected based on typical symptoms.

Peripartum cardiomyopathy can occur any time from the last month of pregnancy to 5 months postpartum. Diagnosis is made when heart failure develops during this time with no other identifiable cause or preexisting heart failure. Echocardiography is used to document left ventricular systolic dysfunction.

Gestational diabetes complicates approximately 2% to 14% of all pregnancies. Postpartum glucose tolerance testing in gestational diabetics is recommended by the American College of Obstetricians and Gynecologists and the American Diabetes Association. This can be completed at the 6-week postpartum visit.

Other medical problems that can occur in the postpartum period include venous thromboembolic disease, urinary retention, and other infections. These should be identified and treated as appropriate based on the patient's symptoms.

CURRENT THERAPY

- Postpartum hemorrhage usually responds to uterine massage and oxytocics.
- Social and professional support systems are key factors in successful continuation of breast-feeding.
- Oral antibiotics are not necessary after intravenous treatment of endometritis.
- All methods of contraception are acceptable choices postpartum with a few special considerations.

Mood Disorders

Postpartum depression is a common problem that can negatively affect both the mother and infant. Early diagnosis and treatment are important to prevent any negative effects on the child or mother. It is important to screen for depression several times during the postpartum period. The baby blues is very common in the first week after birth and resolves without treatment. Symptoms in patients at high risk for postpartum depression or those that persist after the first week should be treated.

Treatment of postpartum depression should be individualized. Treatment consists of social support and counseling with or without medications. Psychosocial and psychological interventions are associated with a decreased likelihood of depressive symptoms at 1 year postpartum. Antidepressants may be used in the postpartum period but might need to be adjusted during lactation.

Postpartum psychosis is uncommon but potentially dangerous for the mother and infant. The risk of suicide and homicide is high. Inpatient treatment is recommended for postpartum psychosis.

REFERENCES

Britton C, McCormick FM, Renfrew MJ, et al. Support for breastfeeding mothers. Cochrane Database Syst Rev 2007;(1):CD001141.

Committee on Health Care for Underserved Women; Committee on Obstetric Practice. Breastfeeding: Maternal and infant aspects. Int J Gynaecol Obstet 2001;74:217–32.

Dennis CL, Hodnett E. Psychosocial and psychological interventions for treating postpartum depression. Cochrane Database Syst Rev 2007;(4):CD006116.

French LM, Smaill FM. Antibiotic regimens for endometritis after delivery. Cochrane Database Syst Rev 2004;(4):CD001067.

Grimes DA, Schulz KF, Van Vliet H, et al. Immediate post-partum insertion of intrauterine devices. Cochrane Database Syst Rev 2001;(2):CD003036.

Magee L, Sadeghi S. Prevention and treatment of postpartum hypertension. Cochrane Database Syst Rev 2005;(1):CD004351.

Olson CM, Strawderman MS, Hinton PS, Pearson TA. Gestational weight gain and postpartum behaviors associated with weight change from early pregnancy to 1 year postpartum. Int J Obes Relat Metab Disord 2003;27:117–27.

Oyelese Y, Scorza WE, Mastrolia R, Smulian JC. Postpartum hemorrhage. Obstet Gynecol Clin North Am 2007;34:421–41.

Ro A, Frishman WH. Peripartum cardiomyopathy. Cardiol Rev 2006;14:35–42.

Russell MA, Phipps MG, Olson CL, et al. Rates of postpartum glucose testing after gestational diabetes mellitus. Obstet Gynecol 2006;108:1456–62.

Resuscitation of the Newborn

Method of
Stacey Hinderliter, MD, and David Gregory, MD

The changes that occur in the transition from fetus to newborn are unmatched in any other time of life. Most newborns manage to make this transition on their own, but about 10% require some assistance. Approximately 1% of newborns require extensive resuscitative measures to survive. The approach to resuscitation in infants is similar to that in adults, consisting of evaluation and intervention when needed for the infant's airway, breathing, and circulation. Every birth should be attended by personnel trained in neonatal resuscitation. Specific training and certification are offered by the American Heart Association's Neonatal Resuscitation Provider (NRP) course.

Transition from Fetal to Extrauterine Life

The environment of the fetus differs greatly from that of the infant after birth. The fetus depends on receiving oxygen and nutrients from the mother through the placental circulation. The fetus experiences relative hypoxia and almost constant body temperature in the amniotic fluid. The fetal lungs are filled with fluid and do not participate in the exchange of oxygen and carbon dioxide. Several adaptations in the fetus permit survival in this environment.

Oxygenated blood from the mother enters the fetus by means of the placenta through the umbilical vein. Most of this oxygenated blood bypasses the liver through the ductus venosus and enters the inferior vena cava. On entering the right atrium, this oxygenated blood is directed toward the patent foramen ovale into the left atrium, bypassing the fetal lungs. Fetal blood also passes through the right atrium into the right ventricle and then into the pulmonary artery. The vascular resistance and blood pressure of the pulmonary vessels in the fetal lung are higher than in the aorta and systemic circulation; most of the blood is therefore shunted away from the lungs through the ductus arteriosus into the ascending aorta. Only a small amount of fetal blood passes through the lungs to the left atrium and then to the left ventricle. The umbilical arteries branch off from the internal iliac arteries and return fetal blood to the placenta. The functional organ for gas exchange of oxygen and carbon dioxide in the fetus is the placenta.

At birth, the newborn is no longer connected to the placenta, and the lungs become the only source of oxygen. The first breaths of the infant cause the fluid in the lung alveoli to be replaced with air. The umbilical arteries and veins constrict at birth and are eventually clamped. This increases the vascular resistance and blood pressure of the systemic circulation. As the oxygen level in the alveoli increases, the blood vessels in the lung start to relax, decreasing pulmonary vascular resistance. Blood in the pulmonary artery travels toward the lung and away from the ductus arteriosus because the blood pressure in the systemic circulation is higher than that in the pulmonary circulation. Increased blood flow to the lungs allows the oxygen from the alveoli to enter the infant's blood, increasing the Po_2. Oxygenated blood enters the left heart through the pulmonary vein and is delivered to the rest of the infant's tissues through the aorta.

Although the initial steps in this transition occur within a few minutes of birth, the entire process may not be completed for several hours to days. The ductus venosus, foramen ovale, and ductus arteriosus remain potentially patent and do not completely involute for days or weeks. Changes in the infant's systemic and pulmonary pressures can result in blood flow through these channels in the infant.

Transition can be prevented or delayed in several circumstances. The infant may not breathe adequately, in which case the lung fluid is not forced out of the alveoli. Material such as meconium may block air from entering the alveoli. If the lungs do not fill with air, hypoxia will quickly develop. Systemic hypotension due to excessive blood loss, poor cardiac function, or bradycardia prevents the change in the direction of blood flow that is necessary to promote blood flow into the lungs. Failure of the lungs to expand or hypoxia can prevent relaxation of the pulmonary blood vessels, resulting in a high pulmonary vascular resistance. This leads to decreased blood flow to the lungs and worsening of hypoxia.

Risk Factors for Newborn Resuscitation

A number of prenatal and intrapartum factors are associated with a higher chance that the infant will have a delay in transition and require resuscitation. These characteristics are summarized in Table 1. Some, such as severe maternal hypertension or toxemia, can directly affect the placenta blood vessels, resulting in decreased oxygen delivery to the fetus. Complications during labor, including placental abruption, chorioamnionitis, and premature labor, can affect the condition of the infant at the time of birth. Symptoms of fetal compromise, such as fetal bradycardia and meconium staining of the amniotic fluid, are warning signs for a possible need for resuscitation. Maternal age, lack of prenatal care, substance use, and other maternal issues can also affect the newborn infant in a multifactorial fashion. However, some infants *with no risk factors* need resuscitation; therefore, preparations for neonatal resuscitation should be made during all deliveries.

TABLE 1 Risk Factors for Newborn Resuscitation

Prenatal Factors	Intrapartum Factors
Maternal	Placental
Diabetes, preexisting	Placenta previa
Chronic hypertension	Abruption of the placenta
Infection	Premature or prolonged
Cardiac, renal, pulmonary, thyroid, or neurologic disease	rupture of membranes
	Chorioamnionitis
Drug therapy	Fetal
Substance use	Macrosomia
Lack of prenatal care	Low birth weight
Age <16 or >35 years	Breech or other abnormal
Previous fetal or neonatal death	presentation
	Persistent fetal bradycardia
Pregnancy	Non-reassuring fetal heart rate
Bleeding in second or third trimester	patterns
Pregnancy-induced hypertension	Labor
	Premature labor
Toxemia	Precipitous labor
Gestational diabetes	Prolonged labor (>24 h)
Fetal anemia or isoimmunization	Prolonged second stage of labor (>2 h)
	Prolapsed cord
Polyhydramnios	Emergency cesarean section
Oligohydramnios	Forceps or vacuum-assisted
Fetal hydrops	delivery
Postterm gestation	Other
Multiple gestation	Meconium-stained amniotic
Size-date discrepancy	fluid
Diminished fetal activity	General anesthesia
Fetal malformation or abnormality	Narcotics given within 4 h of delivery
	Uterine hyperstimulation
	Severe intrapartum bleeding

Reaction to Hypoxia and Asphyxia

Normally at birth, the newborn makes vigorous efforts to breathe. The process of leaving the warm, dark, and liquid environment in utero is replaced by cold air, dryness, and bright lights. Drying the infant with towels and suctioning the mouth and nose are all the assistance that most newborns require. The end result of any mechanism that delays transition is a period of hypoxia for the fetus or newborn infant. Laboratory studies have shown that the first sign of oxygen deprivation in the newborn is a change in the breathing pattern. After an initial period of rapid breathing attempts, cessation of breathing occurs. This is called *primary apnea*. Stimulation by drying the infant or slapping the feet can cause breathing to resume. If hypoxia continues after primary apnea has occurred, the infant will make attempts at gasping and then stop breathing. This is called *secondary apnea*. Stimulation does not affect secondary apnea. Assisted ventilation is necessary to provide breaths to the newborn to reverse the hypoxia. The infant's heart rate starts to decrease when primary apnea occurs. The heart rate increases with stimulation if the infant has primary apnea, and blood pressure is maintained. With continued hypoxia, the heart rate continues to drop, and hypotension develops. If assisted ventilation is not adequate to increase the infant's heart rate, chest compressions will be required.

When a newborn becomes apneic, it is not readily apparent whether the infant has primary or secondary apnea. The approach to resuscitation therefore requires that any apneic event in a newborn be treated using the same sequence of interventions. If the apneic infant responds to simple stimulation, the diagnosis is primary apnea, and no further intervention is required. If the infant does not improve with stimulation, secondary apnea has occurred, and more intensive intervention is needed.

CURRENT DIAGNOSIS

- The transition from intrauterine to extrauterine life at birth requires effective breathing by the infant to expand the lungs and oxygenate the blood. All newborn infants are at risk for delays in this process, prompting a need for resuscitation.
- The fetal and newborn response to hypoxia is to develop apnea. If primary apnea is diagnosed, it can be corrected by gentle stimulation and oxygen delivery. If hypoxia persists, secondary apnea will occur. It is not readily apparent whether a newborn has primary or secondary apnea, and the approach to resuscitation therefore requires that any apneic event be treated using the same sequence of interventions.
- Basic newborn resuscitation includes drying the infant, providing warmth, suctioning the airway, and providing gentle stimulation. Infants who do not respond to these interventions need more assistance. Establishment of effective ventilation spontaneously by the newborn or with assistance by positive-pressure ventilation is the most important step in newborn resuscitation.
- Reassessment of the infant's heart rate, respiratory effort, color, and tone every 30 seconds during resuscitation is crucial to determine the next appropriate intervention. Apgar scoring should *not* be used to guide newborn resuscitation.
- If application of positive-pressure ventilation does not improve the infant's heart rate, chest compressions or drug therapy, or both, may be required. A team approach is needed to coordinate these interventions, and ongoing reassessment is necessary to determine cardiorespiratory and hemodynamic status. Subsequent assessment and treatment should be performed in an intensive care setting.

Sequence of Newborn Resuscitation

INITIAL STEPS AND BASIC RESUSCITATION

Resuscitation of the newborn starts with knowledge of two essential risk factors: Is the infant at *term gestation*, and is the amniotic fluid stained with *meconium*? The answers to these questions will affect the approach to care. Resuscitation when fluid is meconium stained is discussed later in this chapter. The information presented here refers to term infants with clear amniotic fluid. More information regarding the care of premature infants is discussed in a later section.

The next step is to determine whether the infant is crying vigorously and whether there is good muscle tone. This quick assessment should be performed simultaneously with the initial steps of resuscitation: providing warmth, positioning and clearing (if needed) the airway, drying and stimulating the infant.

The newborn should be placed under a radiant warmer to prevent heat loss and to allow easy observation. Although warm blankets or towels can be used to dry the infant, they should not be left in place to cover the infant. The newborn should be placed on the back with the neck slightly extended in the "sniffing" position (Fig. 1). This facilitates air entry into the lungs by lining up the posterior pharynx, larynx, and trachea. Hyperextension or hyperflexion of the neck can obstruct air entry into the lungs.

If the newborn is crying vigorously, secretions can be removed by wiping the nose and the mouth with a towel or gentle suctioning of the mouth and nose with a bulb syringe or suction catheter. Deep or vigorous suctioning can be detrimental to the infant because of stimulation of the vagus nerve, causing bradycardia or apnea.

Drying the infant, slapping the feet, and rubbing the back are appropriate forms of stimulation. More forceful methods of stimulation can harm the infant. Primary apnea, if present, will respond to stimulation in less than 30 seconds. Prolonged apnea will require positive-pressure ventilation (PPV).

Evaluating the infant's response to resuscitation is essential. The Apgar score is a traditional method for evaluating newborn status at 1 and 5 minutes after delivery. However, effective resuscitation demands that evaluation of the newborn's status not be delayed until 1 minute of age, and Apgar scores therefore should *not* be used to guide resuscitative efforts. Within 30 seconds of delivery, the infant's need for PPV must be assessed. Establishment of effective ventilation spontaneously by the newborn or with assistance by PPV is the most important step in newborn resuscitation. The respiratory status, heart rate, and color should be determined. The chest wall should move with each breath, and the newborn should be breathing spontaneously. Heart rate can be assessed by feeling for a pulse at the base

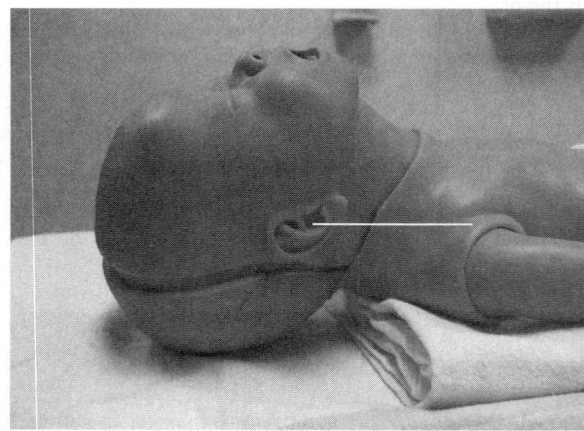

FIGURE 1. The sniffing position. Positioning the infant on the back with the neck slightly extended brings the posterior pharynx, larynx, and trachea in line (*white line*) to facilitate air entry into the lungs.

of the umbilical cord. If this pulse cannot be felt, a stethoscope can be used to listen for the heartbeat. The heart rate should be greater than 100 beats/min. Peripheral cyanosis (i.e., blueness of the hands and feet) is acceptable in the initial period after delivery. Central cyanosis in which the lips and trunk are blue indicates hypoxemia and the need for more resuscitation efforts.

RESPIRATORY SUPPORT AND POSITIVE-PRESSURE VENTILATION

If the infant is breathing with a heart rate higher than 100 beats/min but has central cyanosis, free-flowing oxygen delivery is indicated. This can be administered with a facemask or by holding oxygen tubing or a flow-inflating bag and mask close to the infant's face. *A self-inflating bag and mask cannot be used to give free-flowing oxygen.* If the newborn is apneic, not breathing effectively, or has a heart rate less than 100 beats/min, PPV using a self-inflating bag, flow-inflating (or anesthesia) bag, or a T-piece resuscitator is required. Use of a flow-inflating bag requires a compressed gas source and considerable practice to be used effectively. A T-piece resuscitator needs special equipment and a compressed gas source. Most delivery rooms are equipped with self-inflating bags (Fig. 2) because they are easy to use and can be fitted with a pressure-release valve to decrease overinflation. A reservoir must be used with a self-inflating bag to provide 100% oxygen.

The facemask should cover the infant's nose, mouth, and tip of chin, but not the eyes (Fig. 3). Multiple sizes should be available. A tight seal between the infant's skin and the facemask is needed, but excessive pressure can bruise the face. The mask can be held in place using the thumb and index finger in a C-shaped position on top of the mask, with the remaining fingers in an E-shaped position below the infant's chin (Fig. 4). Inspiratory pressures of 20 to 30 cm H_2O are usually needed when squeezing the bag to make the infant's chest rise. A pressure gauge can be connected to the self-inflating bag for monitoring inspiratory pressure. The heart rate and color of the infant should rapidly improve if enough pressure is being given. An assistant can also use a stethoscope to listen to breath sounds for air movement. Breaths should be given at a rate of 40 to 60 breaths/min.

Traditionally, 100% oxygen has been used in newborn resuscitation. However, several randomized, controlled studies enrolling term and near-term infants have shown that room air can be used initially with oxygen as a backup if room air fails. A meta-analysis of these trials showed a benefit for the use of room air. Providing oxygen at concentrations between room air and 100% requires the use of compressed air, oxygen, and blenders by experienced personnel. Not all facilities have these items available. The current recommendation is that initially using room air or 100% oxygen is acceptable and that ensuring adequate ventilation is the priority.

After 30 seconds of PPV, the infant should be reevaluated. Ventilation with a bag and mask can be stopped when the newborn has a heart

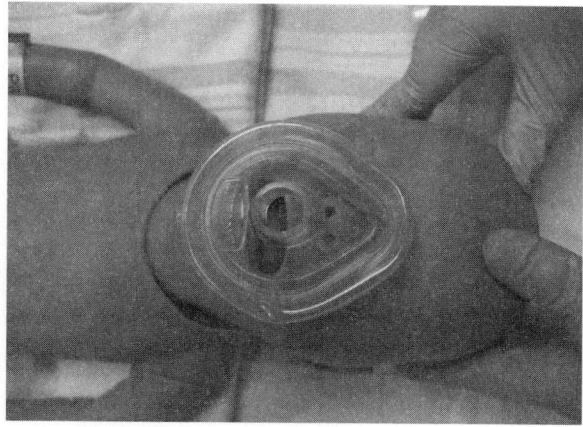

FIGURE 3. Facemask. Choose a size that covers the infant's mouth and nose.

rate higher than 100 beats/min, spontaneous breathing, improved color, and good muscle tone. Supplemental oxygen should still be given to the infant. If the newborn is not improving, reassess the seal between the face mask and the infant's skin, look for airway blockage by repositioning and suctioning, or increase the pressure being used to inflate the bag. If these steps do not improve the infant's heart rate and color, endotracheal (ET) intubation may be required.

ET intubation is a technical skill that must be learned and practiced to maintain competency. Effective ventilation can be given with a bag and mask approach to most newborns. This skill is easily mastered and maintained. If an infant is responding well to bag and mask ventilation, it can be continued for longer periods; however, some air may escape into the esophagus and into the stomach. This may cause gastric distention, which can prevent full expansion of the lungs and cause vomiting and aspiration. An orogastric tube can be placed in the stomach and left open to air to vent any air introduced into the infant's stomach during bag and mask ventilation.

CHEST COMPRESSIONS

After 30 seconds of effective PPV, the heart rate should be assessed. If the heart rate dips below 60 beats/min, chest compressions are needed to support the circulation. The thumb technique (Fig. 5) is preferred, but the two-finger technique (Fig. 6) can be used, especially when placement of an umbilical venous catheter is required. Two people are required to give PPV and chest compressions effectively. To coordinate the breaths and chest compressions, three compressions are given followed by one breath, and this sequence is repeated to give the infant

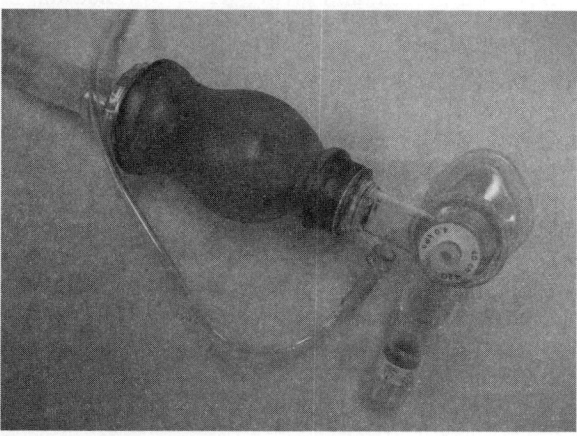

FIGURE 2. Self-inflating bag with infant mask and reservoir. This type of device is available in most delivery rooms.

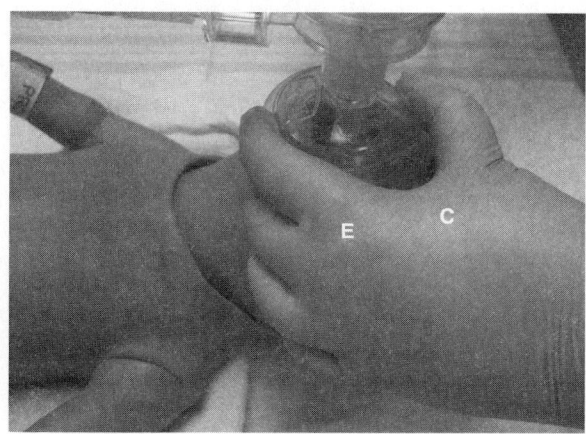

FIGURE 4. Facemask placement. The thumb and index finger are held in a C-shaped position on top of the mask, and the remaining fingers are held in an E-type position under the chin.

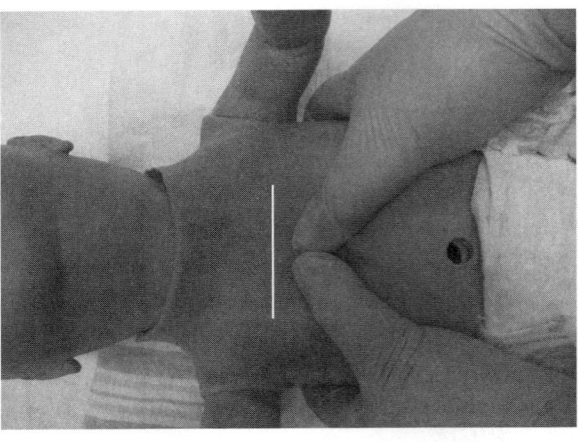

FIGURE 5. Thumb technique. The hands encircle the torso, and the thumbs are placed on top of the lower sternum above the xyphoid process and below a line drawn between the nipples *(white line)*.

90 compressions and 30 breaths/min. The thumb or fingers are placed on the lower third of the infant's sternum but above the xyphoid process. The sternum is depressed to a depth of one third of the infant's anteroposterior chest diameter. The purpose of chest compressions is to squeeze the heart between the sternum and the spine, forcing blood in and out of the heart and to the body. The direction of the compressions should be perpendicular to the chest surface, and the fingers should not be lifted off of the chest after the correct placement is obtained. Incorrect methods during chest compressions can cause rib fracture and liver laceration.

After 30 seconds of chest compressions, the infant's heart rate, color, breathing, and tone are reassessed. If the heart rate is higher than 60 beats/min, chest compressions can be stopped, although PPV may still be needed. If the heart rate is not improving, the following problems must considered: ventilation is not adequate, 100% oxygen concentration is not being given, or the compressions may not be deep enough or well coordinated with the breaths.

MEDICATIONS FOR NEWBORN RESUSCITATION

If the newborn heart rate remains below 60 beats/min despite PPV and chest compressions, epinephrine (Adrenalin) can be used to stimulate the newborn heart. Fewer than 2 of 1000 infants will require this step in resuscitation. Epinephrine can be administered by ET tube, but *intravenous administration is preferred.*

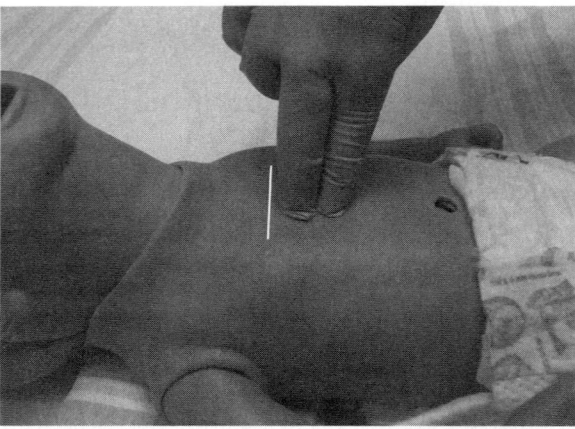

FIGURE 6. Two-finger technique. The index and middle finger are used to apply pressure on the lower third of the sternum above the xyphoid process and below a line drawn between the nipples *(white line)*.

A catheter can be quickly inserted into the umbilical vein for intravenous access. A 3.5 or 5 F catheter prefilled with saline and connected to a 3-way stopcock is inserted about 2 to 4 cm into the umbilical vein using sterile technique. After blood is aspirated, insertion of the catheter is stopped, and the epinephrine is given, followed by a saline flush. The concentration of epinephrine used in neonatal resuscitation is 1:10,000. The intravenous dose is 0.01 to 0.03 mg/kg (0.1 to 0.3 mL/kg) (Table 2). A dose of epinephrine can be given through the ET tube during the umbilical vein catheterization. The ET dose of epinephrine is 0.03 to 0.1 mg/kg (0.3 to 1 mL/kg). *These higher doses are for ET use only.* Because lung absorption of epinephrine varies, the intravenous route using the umbilical vein is preferred.

During umbilical vein cannulation, PPV and chest compressions are continued. More personnel will be needed to place the catheter and draw up the medications and saline flushes. After an intravenous dose of epinephrine, the infant's heart rate, respirations, color, and tone are reevaluated. The heart rate should increase to more than 60 beats/min. If the heart rate does not respond, the dose of epinephrine can be repeated every 3 to 5 minutes. The effectiveness of ventilation and compressions should be reassessed. If the infant appears pale, has delayed capillary refill, or decreased pulses, shock may be present. Infant blood loss might have occurred during delivery from placental problems or other sources. Administration of a volume expander such as normal saline or Ringer's lactate at 10 mL/kg over 5 to 10 minutes can improve circulation. If anemia is suspected, O negative blood can be given. Volume expansion should be used cautiously because there is evidence from animal studies for poorer outcomes when volume expansion is used in the absence of hypovolemia.

Newborns, especially premature infants, are at risk for hypoglycemia. Blood from the infant's heel or the umbilical vein can be tested at the bedside and intravenous 10% dextrose (2 to 5 mL/kg) given for glucose levels below 40 g/dL. In cases of severe metabolic acidosis, administration of sodium bicarbonate may be considered, but only if ventilation is adequate because sodium bicarbonate produces carbon dioxide. It is also caustic and should *never* be given in the ET tube. There is no evidence that use of sodium bicarbonate benefits the neonate, and its use during resuscitation in the delivery room is not recommended.

After resuscitation, newborns should be monitored in an intensive care setting. These infants are at risk for several complications, such as infection, metabolic abnormalities, and seizures.

CURRENT THERAPY

- Initial resuscitation therapy for all newborns includes drying the infant, providing warmth, suctioning the nose and mouth, and giving gentle stimulation.
- If the infant is breathing vigorously but has central cyanosis, oxygen should be administered.
- If the infant is apneic, breathing slowly, or gasping, positive-pressure ventilation (PPV) with a mask and bag should be administered. Infants with meconium-stained amniotic fluid who are apneic should receive suctioning of the trachea by endotracheal intubation before PPV.
- If the infant's heart rate drops below 60 beats/min, chest compressions should be initiated using the thumb or two-finger technique.
- If the heart rate remains less than 60 beats/min despite PPV and chest compressions, IV epinephrine (Adrenalin) and other medications should be given using an umbilical venous catheter.
- Reassessment of the newborn every 30 seconds during resuscitation is required to adjust therapy as indicated.

TABLE 2 Drugs for Newborn Resuscitation

Drug	Concentration	Dose	Indications	Comments
Epinephrine	1:10,000	0.01–0.03 mg/kg IV = 0.1–0.3 mL/kg IV route preferred 0.03–0.1 mg/kg ETT	Asystole Bradycardia that does not improve with PPV and chest compressions Shock	May repeat every 3–5 min
Volume expanders	Normal saline Ringer's lactate O negative blood	10 mL/kg IV	Hypovolemia	Crossmatch blood to mother if possible Repeat if needed
Glucose	10% Dextrose	2–5 mL/kg IV	Hypoglycemia	Monitor glucometer or venous glucose levels
Naloxone (Narcan)		0.1 mg/kg IV	Maternal administration of narcotics <4 h before delivery and newborn respiratory depression	Use PPV first, then give naloxone; repeated doses may be needed May cause opioid withdrawal in newborns born to addicted mothers
Sodium bicarbonate	0.5 mEq/mL	1–2 mEq/kg IV	Severe metabolic acidosis with adequate ventilation	Infuse slowly No evidence of benefit

Abbreviations: ETT = endotracheal tube; IV = intravenous; PPV = positive-pressure ventilation.

Special Considerations

Some newborns do not respond to resuscitation because of specific problems. Infants with upper airway obstruction from micrognathia can be helped by a nasopharyngeal airway and placement of the infant in the prone position. Choanal atresia can be treated by placing an oral airway. Absence of breath sounds on one side of the chest can indicate a pneumothorax, requiring needle aspiration of the chest. An infant with a scaphoid abdomen and decreased breath sounds may have a diaphragmatic hernia. These infants should be intubated, and PPV by mask and bag should not be used. If the mother has received narcotics shortly before the delivery, the narcotic may be the cause of respiratory depression in the infant. These infants need *PPV and respiratory support first.* After resuscitation, intravenous naloxone (Narcan) at 0.1 mg/kg can be given. Prolonged ventilation and multiple doses of naloxone may be needed.

ENDOTRACHEAL INTUBATION

Intubation of the newborn requires preparation that can be performed while the infant is being ventilated by bag and mask. The ET tube should not be placed unless the glottis is visualized by direct laryngoscopy. To ensure that the tube is in the trachea, a carbon dioxide (CO_2) detector should be used. Listening for equal breath sounds and looking for vapor condensation in the ET tube during exhalation can help, but an increase in the infant's heart rate or a positive detection of CO_2 is most reliable.

Intubation should be performed as quickly as possible, with a goal of 20 seconds from insertion of the laryngoscope to the connection of the ET tube to the resuscitation bag. Complications of intubation include worsening of hypoxia and bradycardia, pneumothorax, contusions, perforation of the trachea or esophagus, and infection. After the infant has been intubated, deterioration in the infant's status should prompt an organized sequence to assess the adequacy of ventilation using the mnemonic DOPE:

Dislodged (D): Is the tube in the right bronchus or out of the trachea?
Obstructed (O): Is the tube obstructed by secretions or blood?
Pneumothorax (P) and *esophagus* (E): Is the tube in the esophagus?

An alternative to intubation is placement of a laryngeal mask airway. This type of airway does not require laryngoscopy. A soft inflatable mask that is attached to a flexible airway tube is placed in the hypopharynx such that the air in the tube is directed into the larynx and away from the esophagus. However, this type of airway cannot be used to suction meconium from the trachea.

PREMATURE INFANTS

Infants born before 37 weeks' gestation are at increased risk for complications and the need for resuscitation. Premature lungs may lack surfactant, making ventilation difficult. Immature brain development may decrease the drive to breathe. Weak muscles make respiratory efforts less effective. Thin skin and decreased subcutaneous fat make temperature regulation a challenge. Premature infants often have infections such as pneumonia or sepsis. The blood vessels in their brains are fragile and can easily bleed during periods of blood pressure variation. The lower birth weights of premature newborns also require smaller sizes of equipment for resuscitation such as facemasks, suction catheters, endotracheal tubes, and umbilical catheters. Oxygen concentrations less than 100% are often used to protect the premature infant from oxygen toxicity. Many personnel trained in newborn resuscitation should be present at the delivery of a high-risk premature infant.

MECONIUM STAINING OF THE AMNIOTIC FLUID

Meconium is formed in the newborn gastrointestinal system during gestation. Intrauterine stress can cause release of meconium into the amniotic fluid. Aspiration of meconium-stained amniotic fluid into the lungs can result in severe pneumonitis and lung injury. The approach to resuscitation for an infant with meconium-stained fluid depends on the *condition of the infant immediately after birth.* There is no evidence that the consistency of meconium-stained fluid (i.e., thick or thin) should change these approaches.

Crying and Vigorous Infant

If the newborn with meconium-stained amniotic fluid has normal respiratory effort and muscle tone with a heart rate higher than 100 beats/min, *gentle* mouth and nose suctioning can be performed using a bulb syringe or suction catheter, similar to the initial resuscitation steps for all infants. Deep and prolonged suctioning should be avoided. ET intubation is not required for vigorous infants with meconium-stained amniotic fluid.

Depressed Infant

Newborns who are gasping or apneic, have poor muscle tone, and have a heart rate less than 100 beats/min require direct suctioning of the trachea to prevent aspiration of the meconium-stained fluid. A laryngoscope is inserted, and a 12- or 14-F catheter is used to suction the mouth and posterior pharynx. After visualizing the glottis, an ET tube is inserted and attached to a suction source. Suction is applied as the ET tube is withdrawn (Fig. 7). This maneuver may

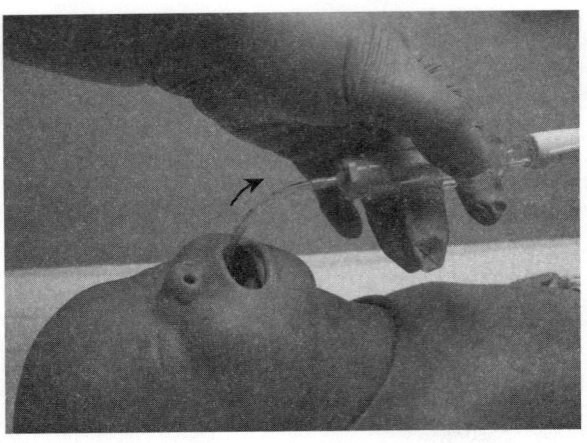

FIGURE 7. The meconium aspirator is attached to a suction source and connected to the endotracheal (ET) tube inserted into the infant's trachea. The thumb is used to occlude the suction-control port to apply suction to the ET tube while gradually withdrawing the ET tube from the trachea (arrow).

be repeated until the suctioned fluid is clear unless the infant requires resuscitation (e.g., apneic, heart rate <100 beats/min, decreased muscle tone, cyanotic). After ET suctioning, a bag and mask can be used to provide PPV for the infant if needed. The usual sequence of newborn resuscitation is then followed.

NEWBORN RESUSCITATION OUTSIDE OF THE DELIVERY ROOM

Resuscitation of infants born at home, in an emergency room, in an ambulance, or otherwise outside of a delivery room setting should proceed according to the same principles as in the delivery room. Providing warmth, suctioning the airway, and providing stimulation

TABLE 3 Equipment for Newborn Resuscitation

Type of Use	Equipment
General	Sterile towels
	Radiant warmer or heat lamps
	Pulse oximeter
	Cardiorespiratory monitor
	Sterile gowns, gloves
Airway	Bulb syringe
	Suction catheters (5, 8, 10, 12, 14 F)
	Suction source with manometer
	Oral and nasopharyngeal airways (newborn sizes)
	Laryngoscope and straight blades sizes 0 and 1
	Endotracheal tubes (sizes 2.5, 3.0, 3.5, 4.0)
	Meconium suction device
Ventilation	Face masks (premature, newborn, and infant sizes)
	Self-inflating bag (450–750 mL) with oxygen reservoir and manometer
	Oxygen source
	Orogastric tubes (8, 10 F)
	Carbon dioxide (CO_2) indicator
	Chest tubes (8 and 10 F)
Circulation	Umbilical catheters (3.5 and 5 F)
	Umbilical catheter tray (sterile scissors, scalpel, forceps, umbilical tape)
	Three-way stopcock
	Syringes (1, 3, 5, 10 mL)
	Normal saline
	Epinephrine 1:10,000
	10% Dextrose
	Naloxone (Narcan)
	Sodium bicarbonate (0.5 mEq/mL)
	Ringer's lactate

are usually adequate measures. Establishing effective ventilation using a bag and mask is the most important step if the infant fails to breathe on its own. Emergency providers should be familiar with resuscitation of the newborn, and basic equipment (Table 3) should be available.

WITHHOLDING AND WITHDRAWING NEWBORN RESUSCITATION

Newborns should be offered resuscitation at delivery except in extreme circumstances. Newborn resuscitation should not be used if the infant has a condition that is incompatible with survival, such as a confirmed gestational age of less than 23 completed weeks, birth weight less than 400 g, or congenital anomalies associated with certain death or extreme morbidity.

In most situations, initial resuscitation can provide time to observe the infant's response to interventions and to discuss the infant's condition with the parents. Techniques for obstetric dating of pregnancies are accurate only to ±1 to 2 weeks, and estimates of fetal weight are accurate only to ±100 to 200 g. Care must be taken before deciding to withhold resuscitation from a newborn. Ongoing conversation between parents and medical caregivers allows mutual decision making. Withdrawal of care is indicated if continued support is futile. After 10 minutes of asystole (heart rate of 0), newborns are very unlikely to survive.

REFERENCES

American Academy of Pediatrics Committee on Fetus and Newborn. EF Bel. Noninitiation or withdrawal of intensive care for high-risk newborns. Pediatrics 2007;119:401.

American Heart Association. 2005 American Heart Association (AHA) guidelines for cardiopulmonary resuscitation (CPR) and emergency cardiovascular care (ECC) of pediatric and neonatal patients: Neonatal resuscitation guidelines. Pediatrics 2006;117:e1029.

Aschner JL, Poland RL. Sodium bicarbonate: Basically useless therapy. Pediatrics 2008;122:831.

Bassam H, Mercer BM, Livingston JC, et al. Outcome after successful resuscitation of babies born with Apgar scores of 0 at both 1 and 5 minutes. Am J Obstet Gynecol 2000;182:1210.

Escobedo M. Moving from experience to evidence: Changes in US Neonatal Resuscitation Program based on International Liaison Committee on Resuscitation Review. J Perinatol 2008;28:835.

Field DJ, Dorling JS, Manktelow BN, et al. Survival of extremely premature babies in a geographically defined population: Prospective cohort study of 1994–99 compared with 2000–05. BMJ 2008;336:1221.

Halliday HL. Endotracheal intubation at birth for preventing morbidity and mortality in vigorous, meconium-stained infants born at term. Cochrane Database Syst Rev 2001;(1):CD000500.

Jain L, Ferre C, Vidyasagar D, et al. Cardiopulmonary resuscitation of apparently stillborn infants: Survival and long-term outcome. J Pediatr 1991;118:778.

Wiswell TE, Gannon CM, Jacob J, et al. Delivery room management of the apparently vigorous meconium-stained neonate: Results of the multicenter, international collaborative trial. Pediatrics 2000;105:1.

Care of the High-Risk Neonate

Method of
Paul S. Kingma, MD, PhD

The maturation of the fetus and transition to neonatal life requires the precise coordination of an immensely complex cascade of biochemical and physiologic events. As a result, the late fetal and early neonatal period is also the time of life exhibiting the highest mortality rate of any pediatric age interval. The infant mortality rate includes both the neonatal (days 1-28) and the postneonatal (days 28-365) periods and is expressed as the number of deaths per 1000 live births. Despite considerable advances in neonatal and obstetrics care over the past few decades, the infant mortality rate in the United States in 2006 was 6.7 per 1000 live births, with congenital malformations and prematurity or low birth weight as the top two causes of infant death. Early identification and initiation of appropriate care of these high-risk neonates is essential to improving their outcome.

Care of the high-risk neonate begins with appropriate delivery, management, and resuscitation of the infant. The goals of resuscitation are to maintain or establish effective ventilation and oxygenation, maintain or restore adequate cardiac output and tissue perfusion, and maintain or restore normal body temperature. The steps needed to achieve these goals are based on the common ABC (airway, breathing, circulation) principles that are relevant to all infants. However, after adequate resuscitation, the care of the high-risk neonate is dictated by the diagnosis of the infant's problem. Most of these diagnoses and the treatment approach for each can be categorized into prematurity, abnormal transition, infection, intestinal malformations, and pulmonary hypoplasia.

Prematurity

EPIDEMIOLOGY

The mean duration of a spontaneous singleton pregnancy is 40 postmenstrual weeks. An infant delivered before the completion of the 37th week is considered preterm. Preterm infants can be further classified according to birth weight: low birth weight (LBW) if less than 2500 g, very low birth weight (VLBW) if less than 1500 g, and extremely low birth weight (ELBW) if less than 1000 g. The rate of preterm births increased to 12.8 percent in 2006, up 20% since 1990. This is a result mostly of increases in late preterm births which, in turn, can be attributed to a significant rise in both indicated preterm births and multifetal gestations associated with assisted reproductive technology.

CLINICAL MANIFESTATIONS AND TREATMENT

Besides the risk for death, prematurity is also associated with an increased risk of morbidity in nearly every organ system, and this risk increases dramatically as both the gestational age and birth weight decrease. The approach to the common problems associated with the premature neonate is presented in Box 1.

COMPLICATIONS

One of the most difficult decisions faced by families and health care professionals regards the treatment of infants at the threshold of viability. Although this threshold has decreased since the 1970s, most neonatologists recognize 22 to 24 weeks' gestation as the limit of viability. Survival rates for infants born at 23 weeks' gestation (23 0/7 to 23 6/7 days) range from 15% to 30%, whereas survival increases to between 30% and 55% for infants born at 24 weeks' gestation. Within this group of survivors, 30% to 50% will have moderate to severe disability, including blindness, deafness, developmental delays, and cerebral palsy. The American Academy of Pediatrics recommends that decisions regarding life-sustaining treatment of these infants should be based on the best interests of the newborn, and the Academy also recognizes that parents should have the primary role in choosing aggressive versus palliative care of their infant. Making decisions within this gestational range requires accurate information regarding the mortality and morbidity risks for this population and thorough communication with the family.

Abnormal Transition

The transition from fetal to neonatal life involves a dramatic process of pulmonary adaptation that includes evacuation of fluid from the lungs, expansion of the lungs with air, decreasing pulmonary vascular resistance, and initiating respiratory effort. Often, this transition is delayed or disrupted and the respiratory status of the newborn is compromised. A few conditions associated with an abnormal transition are reviewed.

TRANSIENT TACHYPNEA OF THE NEWBORN
Epidemiology

Transient tachypnea of the newborn (TTN) is a mild condition affecting term and late preterm infants and is the most common respiratory cause of admission to the special care nursery. By definition, TTN is self-limiting, rarely causes hypoxic respiratory failure (hypoxia requiring ventilator support), and has no increased risk of pulmonary dysfunction later in life.

Risk Factors

TTN is classically seen in term or late preterm infants, especially after cesarean birth before the onset of spontaneous labor.

Pathophysiology

Traditional explanations for the pathophysiology of TTN involve impaired fluid clearance from the lungs because of decreased Starling forces and pulmonary squeeze normally encountered during movement through the birth canal. However, the bulk of pulmonary fluid clearance during labor is mediated by activation of sodium channels in the respiratory epithelial cells. In addition, some studies suggest TTN might also involve a mild surfactant deficiency.

Clinical Manifestation

TTN usually manifests with significant grunting along with tachypnea, nasal flaring, mild retractions, and mild hypoxia.

Diagnosis

TTN is primarily a clinical diagnosis. Chest x-rays often demonstrate mild pulmonary congestion, with small accumulations of extrapleural fluid, especially in the minor fissure on the right side. Symptoms usually improve rapidly and resolve within the first 24 to 36 hours.

Differential Diagnosis

TTN is a diagnosis of exclusion and it is important that other potential causes of respiratory distress in the newborn such as infection, pneumothorax, meconium aspiration, polycythemia, and congenital heart disease are excluded.

Treatment

Management is mainly supportive. Supplemental oxygen is provided to keep the O_2 saturations greater than 88%. Continuous positive airway pressure is rarely needed and may increase the risk of pneumothorax in this population. If symptoms last longer than 2 to 3 hours, infants are usually given intravenous fluids and not fed orally until their tachypnea resolves.

MECONIUM ASPIRATION
Epidemiology

Meconium stained amniotic fluid occurs in 12% to 15% of all deliveries, and this rate increases in postterm gestation and in African American infants. In contrast to meconium-stained amniotic fluid, meconium aspiration syndrome is rare, occurring in 2% of deliveries with meconium-stained amniotic fluid, although the reported incidence varies and trends suggest this incidence is decreasing.

Risk Factors

Risk factors for meconium aspiration include meconium stained fluid, in utero stress, and postterm gestation.

BOX 1   Common Problems and Treatment in Premature Infants

Delivery Room

Anticipation and preparation is key. The delivery team should include a neonatologist, neonatal nurse, and respiratory therapists. Dry and warm the infant immediately. Ventilate with a bag mask if the heart rate is low or there is no respiratory effort. Use mask continuous positive airway pressure (CPAP) if the heart rate is good and the infant has good respiratory effort. Intubate if there is no response from bag mask ventilation. Avoid high pressures.

Pulmonary

Respiratory distress syndrome owing to surfactant deficiency is common in preterm infants. Care is supportive with supplemental oxygen, CPAP, or gentle ventilation as needed. To reduce risk of chronic lung disease, use the lowest support needed to achieve oxygen saturations of 88% to 92% and $Paco_2$ of 50 to 65 mm Hg. Use exogenous surfactant when indicated. Apnea is common and is treated with caffeine citrate (Cafcit) 20 mg/kg bolus, 5 mg/kg every 24 hours maintenance.

Cardiovascular

Hypotension can require inotropic (epinephrine or dopamine) support. Avoid large fluid boluses in extremely-low-birth-weight (ELBW) infants. Some hypotensive preterm infants are adrenal deficient and might respond to hydrocortisone (Solu-Cortef). Patent ductus arteriosus (PDA) occurs in 50% of ELBW infants. Medical treatment consists of fluid restriction and indomethacin (Indocin IV, 0.2 mg/kg/dose for four doses[3]). Surgical ligation of the PDA may be needed.

Nutrition

Parenteral nutrition is required in most infants younger than 32 weeks' gestation while enteral feedings are increased and will require placement of a percutaneous central venous catheter. Premature infants require higher-calorie (24 to 30 calories/ounce) preterm formula or human milk supplemented with preterm fortifiers.

Fluids and Electrolytes

Total fluid requirements for premature infants start at 80 mL/kg/day of $D_{7.5}W$ or $D_{10}W$ on day 1 of life and increase by 20 mL/kg/day each day to a maximum of 140 to 160 mL/kg/day. Fluid intake needs can vary depending on the clinical status of the infant. Sodium and potassium supplements are added on day 2. Hypernatremia is caused by increased free water loss.

Gastrointestinal

Necrotizing enterocolitis is a devastating complication of prematurity and is characterized by abdominal distention, feeding intolerance, bloody stools, and evidence of pneumatosis intestinalis, portal venous gas, and/or free air on abdominal radiographs. Early medical management includes decompressing the bowel, stopping enteral feedings, and giving intravenous antibiotics. Surgery is indicated in patients with intestinal perforation or failed medical treatment.

Anemia

Because of frequent blood draws and delayed activation of erythropoiesis, most ELBW infants require a transfusion of packed red blood cells (10 to 20 mL/kg) during their hospital stay.

Hyperbilirubinemia

Bilirubin central nervous system toxicity occurs at a lower level in preterm infants, and as a result phototherapy needs to be initiated sooner in this population.

Central Nervous System

Intraventricular hemorrhage remains a significant problem in premature infants. The risk increases with decreasing gestational age, stress, sepsis, birth asphyxia, rapid shifts in volume status, and hypotension. A head ultrasound should be obtained at 7 to 10 days of age to evaluate for intraventricular hemorrhage and afterward as needed depending on the severity of the findings.

Pathophysiology

Traditional explanations for the pathophysiology of meconium aspiration syndrome suggest that fetal stress leads to passage of meconium in utero. Once this meconium is aspirated, it can cause airway obstruction, pneumothorax, chemical pneumonitis, and pulmonary hypertension. However, recent reports that describe infants born through clear amniotic fluid with respiratory distress and other clinical findings similar to meconium aspiration syndrome suggest this traditional explanation may be incorrect.

Clinical Manifestation

Meconium aspiration syndrome manifests as severe respiratory failure and pulmonary hypertension.

Diagnosis

By definition, the diagnosis of meconium aspiration syndrome includes delivery through meconium-stained amniotic fluid along with respiratory distress and a characteristic chest x-ray appearance of patchy infiltrates with areas of hyperlucency throughout the lung fields.

Differential Diagnosis

Other potential causes of respiratory distress in the newborn such as infection, surfactant deficiency, pneumothorax, and congenital heart disease must be considered.

Treatment

Until recently, aggressive suctioning of the airway in infants delivered through meconium stained fluid was considered the key to preventing meconium aspiration syndrome. Now the Neonatal Resuscitation

Program protocol for delivery room management no longer recommends tracheal suctioning for vigorous infants (depressed infants should have their airways cleared as needed), implying that establishment of ventilation should take precedence over attempting to suction an unobstructed airway.

The treatment of meconium aspiration syndrome has dramatically improved in recent years, leading to decreases in morbidity, mortality, and the use of extracorporeal membrane oxygenation (ECMO). Most of these advances have come from treatment of pulmonary hypertension with selective pulmonary vasodilators such as inhaled nitric oxide (iNO). These agents improve oxygenation, which in turn decreases the need for ventilator support and the risk of air leak and chronic lung disease. Administration of exogenous surfactant (Survanta) may be another useful treatment modality.

PERSISTENT PULMONARY HYPERTENSION OF THE NEWBORN

Epidemiology

Persistent pulmonary hypertension of the newborn (PPHN) occurs when the normal cardiopulmonary transition of the delivered infant fails. Estimates indicate that severe PPHN occurs in 2 per 1000 liveborn term infants, but PPHN complicates the clinical course of up to 10% of all neonates with respiratory failure.

Risk Factors

Risk factors for developing PPHN include sepsis, pneumonia, congenital malformations, and all conditions associated with pulmonary hypoplasia.

Pathophysiology

At delivery, the normal decrease in pulmonary vascular resistance requires relaxation of pulmonary arteriolar smooth muscle, distention of alveoli, and a change in endothelial cell shape. When pulmonary development is hypoplastic or the fetus experiences significant intrauterine stress or hypoxemia, there is an increase in both pulmonary arteriole reactivity and proliferation of medial smooth muscle of the pulmonary vessels. When these vessels are subjected to hypoxemia or acidosis, they are more prone to constriction, which subsequently induces right-to-left shunting of deoxygenated blood.

Clinical Manifestation

PPHN typically manifests with severe hypoxemia in the setting of respiratory failure with a more than 5% differential in preductal and postductal oxygen saturations. Often, hypotension secondary to right heart failure and decreased left ventricular filling is also present. PPHN symptoms may be isolated or occur in combination with the primary cause of stress or respiratory failure.

Diagnosis

PPHN is diagnosed with an echocardiogram, which reveals elevated right ventricular pressures and right-to-left shunting across the foramen ovale and ductus arteriosus. In severe PPHN, right ventricular pressures are equal to or greater than systemic pressures.

Differential Diagnosis

The primary cause of stress or respiratory failure in PPHN such as sepsis, pneumonia, and pulmonary hypoplasia must always be considered. In addition, congenital heart disease must be excluded.

Treatment

The first goal of PPHN therapy is optimal oxygenation and ventilation. However, care must be taken not to induce significant overdistention of alveoli and pulmonary injury. Often the short-term benefit of improving carbon dioxide levels or oxygen saturations by a few points is not worth the risk of lung injury and bronchopulmonary dysplasia. As a result, targeting an oxygen saturation of 88% to 92%, arterial pH levels of 7.25 to 7.35, and carbon dioxide levels of

50 to 65 mm Hg usually achieves a good balance between short-term and long-term goals.

The treatment of PPHN has significantly improved since the turn of the 21st century owing to pharmacologic interventions that specifically reduce pulmonary vascular resistance. Of these, iNO (dose 5-20 ppm) is the best studied and has demonstrated a clear benefit in the setting of PPHN caused by meconium aspiration syndrome or sepsis. Other pulmonary vasodilators, including sildenafil (Revatio),[1] bosentan (Tracleer),[1] and prostacyclin (epoprostenol, Flolan)[1] are increasing in use. When adequate ventilation and pulmonary vasodilators fail in patients with PPHN, ECMO may be considered.

HYPOXIC-ISCHEMIC ENCEPHALOPATHY

Epidemiology

Despite significant advances in obstetric and neonatal care, the incidence of hypoxic-ischemic encephalopathy (HIE) remains at 1 to 2 infants per 1000 term births. Although HIE was once thought to result from brain injury sustained only during the perinatal period, recent data show that most brain injury occurs well before labor and only 10% of neonatal brain injury is related to perinatal or intrapartum events.

Risk Factors

Several clinical measures such as fetal heart rate abnormalities, meconium-stained amniotic fluid, low Apgar scores, large size for gestational age, and the need for resuscitation in the delivery room suggest an increased risk for developing HIE. However, all of these indicators have a very high false-positive rate and therefore do not reliably identify infants who will develop HIE.

Pathophysiology

The brain injury referred to as HIE occurs when oxygen delivery to the brain is insufficient to meet the metabolic demands, resulting in hypoxia, hypercarbia, and metabolic acidosis. This asphyxia is due most often to an interruption of placental blood flow or gas exchange. Although HIE is initiated by a hypoxic event, a growing body of evidence now suggests that there is also a reperfusion phase of brain injury, and several emerging neuroprotective therapies are targeting this phase of injury.

Clinical Manifestation

HIE is clinically characterized by a depressed level of consciousness, seizures and abnormalities in muscle tone (hypotonia initially followed by hypertonia), reflexes (usually decreased initially), and respiratory effort. If other organ systems are involved, infants can also present with signs of heart, kidney, and liver failure.

Diagnosis

HIE is a clinical diagnosis. The Sarnat staging system is often used to classify the severity of the brain injury. Sarnat stage 1 infants have a good prognosis. Sarnat stage 2 infants have long-term neurologic impairment in 20% to 25% of cases, and more than 80% of Sarnat stage 3 infants develop long-term neurologic sequelae. Although brain imaging studies such as magnetic resonance imaging (MRI) are often used to assess the location and severity of brain injury, correlating MRI findings with long-term neurologic outcome is difficult.

Differential Diagnosis

The findings of HIE usually result from hypoxic injury, but they can also result from exposure to toxins or from metabolic, neuromuscular, and chromosomal abnormalities.

Treatment

First-line therapy in infants with HIE is supportive. Adequate ventilation and systemic perfusion should be established using ventilator

---

[1]Not FDA approved for this indication.

and inotropic support as needed. If seizures occur, phenobarbital is a good first-line antiepileptic agent in these infants.

Cooling therapy is being studied as a potential therapy for HIE infants. In infants with moderate to severe HIE, whole-body cooling decreased the risk of death or moderate to severe disability by 18%. Current recommendations suggest the following clinical parameters in order to qualify for cooling: gestational age 36 weeks or older, umbilical artery pH less than 7.00 or a base deficit at least 16 mEq/L, and evidence of an abnormal neurologic examination, seizures, or abnormal electroencephalogram (EEG).

Infection

Epidemiology

Neonatal sepsis is a significant cause of morbidity and mortality in term and preterm infants, and the risk of infection increases as the gestational age decreases. Neonatal sepsis is generally divided into two categories: early and late onset. Early-onset sepsis occurs in the first 3 days of life at a rate of approximately 1.9% of VLBW infants. Early-onset sepsis is caused by bacteria residing in the mother's genitourinary tract such as *Escherichia coli*, group B *Streptococcus* (GBS), and *Listeria monocytogenes*. The incidence of GBS disease has significantly decreased since the institution of screening and treatment for GBS colonization in mothers during the third trimester. Late-onset sepsis occurs between days 3 and 28 and is more common, with an incidence of 21% of VLBW infants. Late-onset sepsis is caused by a variety of bacteria including *Staphylococcus epidermidis*, *Staphylococcus aureus*, *Escherichia coli*, *Klebsiella*, *Enterococcus*, *Pseudomonas*, and *Streptococcus pneumoniae*. Ultimately 18% to 36% of infected VLBW infants die; those who survive have a significantly prolonged hospital stay and increased morbidity when compared to uninfected infants.

Risk Factors

The risk for neonatal infection is inversely proportional to gestational age. African American race and male sex are additional risk factors for neonatal infection. Specific risk factors for early-onset sepsis include prolonged rupture of membranes (>24 hours), chorioamnionitis, maternal infection, and prematurity. The risk for late-onset sepsis is increased by the presence of central venous catheters, peripheral intravenous catheters, endotracheal tubes, umbilical vessel catheters, and electronic monitoring devices.

Pathophysiology

Although infants are protected by maternal antibodies transferred across the placenta during the third trimester, compared with older children or adults, the neonatal immune system is still deficient. Innate immunity is defective at several levels. Skin and mucosal barriers are poorly developed, and bacterial translocation across these barriers is common. Antibacterial proteins such as lysozyme, lactoferrin, and lectins are decreased. Neutrophil chemotaxis, phagocytosis, and intracellular killing are limited. In addition to these defects in innate immunity, humoral and cell-mediated immune functions are also poorly developed.

Clinical Manifestation

Neonatal sepsis can manifest with a variety of nonspecific signs including lethargy, poor feeding, temperature instability, decreased tone, increased work of breathing, apnea, cyanosis, bradycardia, tachycardia, abdominal distention, and altered perfusion. Petechiae and purpura may be present during disseminated intravascular coagulation. Although fever and localizing symptoms are common in older children and adults with infection, neonatal sepsis rarely manifests with these symptoms.

Diagnosis

The gold standard for diagnosing sepsis is a positive blood culture. However, the sensitivity of a blood culture in an infected neonate is between 30% and 60% depending on the volume of blood used for the culture. Therefore, the diagnosis of sepsis in the neonate is more often based on clinical suspicion than laboratory evaluation.

All infants in whom sepsis is suspected should have a thorough clinical examination to evaluate the infant for signs of infection and assess his or her clinical stability. A complete blood count (CBC), cerebrospinal fluid (CSF) culture, and urine culture can also be sent as part of the work-up for neonatal infection, but the value of each of these tests is uncertain. A white blood cell count less than 5000 or greater than 40,000, a total neutrophil count less than 1000, and a band neutrophil count of greater than 20% all correlate with an increased risk of infection, but these tests have a sensitivity for detecting infection that is less than 50%. In addition, because CBC values are often abnormal in healthy neonates, the positive predictive value of an abnormal CBC is less than 18%. Therefore, a normal CBC only weakly supports that the infant is uninfected, and likewise an abnormal CBC only weakly supports the diagnosis of infection.

Many institutions send a CSF for culture, Gram stain, cell count, and protein and glucose levels as part of the evaluation of every infant with suspected sepsis. In contrast, some institutions only send CSF for analysis if the blood culture is positive. The latter method is based on the assumption that because of the inability to isolate infections and the poorly developed blood–brain barrier in the neonate, all neonates with meningitis also have positive blood cultures. This approach is refuted by studies that demonstrate negative blood cultures in up to 50% of infants with meningitis. However, these same studies demonstrate that the incidence of meningitis is the same with either approach; therefore there may be little benefit to subjecting every neonate with suspected sepsis to a lumbar puncture.

Differential Diagnosis

The differential diagnosis of neonatal sepsis includes respiratory distress syndrome, TTN, PPHN, metabolic disorders, and congenital heart disease.

Treatment

Ampicillin and gentamicin for 10 to 14 days remains the most effective first-line therapy against most organisms responsible for early-onset sepsis. The antibiotic choice can be tailored once the identity of the organism and antibiotic sensitivities are determined. If meningitis is present, improved penetration of the blood–brain barrier with a third-generation cephalosporin is recommended. Late-onset sepsis is treated with a similar approach but the antibiotic choice may be modified depending on the exposure history of the infant and the indigenous microbiologic flora of the hospital. If methicillin-resistant *Staphylococcus* species are common, vancomycin (Vancocin) may be warranted as a first-line agent in late-onset sepsis. If signs of infection persist despite aggressive antibacterial treatment, a fungal infection may be present, which is treated with amphotericin B (Fungizone).

After initiating appropriate antibiotic coverage, the remaining therapy for neonatal sepsis is supportive. Adequate oxygenation and ventilation can require ventilator support. Blood pressure and urine output are monitored to determine the need to treat septic shock with fluids or inotropic agents. Pulmonary vasodilators may be needed to treat exacerbations of pulmonary hypertension associated with sepsis.

Intestinal Malformations

INTESTINAL OBSTRUCTION

Epidemiology

Obstruction of the gastrointestinal tract can be complete (atresia) or partial (stenosis) and occur at any point from the esophagus to the anus. Obstruction of the intestinal tract occurs in 1 out of 1500 live births.

Esophageal atresia occurs in 1 out of 4000 live births. Of infants with esophageal atresia, 85% have a tracheoesophageal fistula and approximately 40% of infants with tracheoesophageal fistula have other associated anomalies as part of the VACTERL syndrome, which includes vertebral, anal, cardiac, tracheal, esophageal, renal, and limb anomalies.

Duodenal atresia occurs in 1 out of 5000 live births and is often associated with trisomy 21. Seventy percent of duodenal atresia cases are associated with other malformations such as cardiac anomalies, intestinal malrotation, annular pancreas and imperforate anus. In the jejunum and ileum, atresia is more common than stenosis, and ileal lesions are more common than jejunal lesions. Malrotation is associated with other gastrointestinal lesions including duodenal atresia, gastroschisis, omphalocele, and congenital diaphragmatic hernia.

Hirschsprung's disease occurs in 1 out of 5000 live births and is the most common cause of large bowel obstruction in neonates. It is more common in boys, siblings of infants with Hirschsprung's disease, and infants with trisomy 21.

Imperforate anus occurs in 1 out of 5000 live births.

Pathophysiology

All intestinal atresia or stenosis occurs as a result of either an incomplete formation during development or a vascular accident in utero. Regardless of the location or cause, the obstruction will lead to dilation of the bowel proximal to the narrowing and atrophy of the bowel distally. If the proximal bowel is not decompressed, distention can lead to injury and necrosis.

Malrotation is caused by the incomplete rotation and fixation of the bowel as it returns to the abdominal cavity during development, with abnormally fixed bands crossing the duodenum. Malrotated intestine is at increased risk for volvulus, which causes strangulation of the superior mesenteric artery and occlusion of blood flow to the intestine.

Hirschsprung's disease is caused by defective migration of neural crest cells to the distal colon, resulting in a distal segment of colon that is aganglionic and dysfunctional.

Clinical Manifestation

Infants with atresia or stenosis of the intestinal tract present with signs of obstruction. Infants with esophageal atresia present with excessive oral secretions, inability to feed, gagging, and respiratory distress when feeding is attempted. Infants with duodenal atresia present with abdominal distention and vomiting shortly after the first feeding. Patients with jejunal and ileal atresia also present with abdominal distention and vomiting, but the emesis may be delayed until the second or third feeding.

Malrotation and volvulus manifest as abdominal distention and bilious emesis. As this condition rapidly progresses, hematochezia, hypotension, and disseminated intravascular coagulation can develop.

Hirschsprung's disease can manifest with failure to pass meconium in the first 24 hours of life, constipation, abdominal distention, explosive stool output with rectal examination, vomiting, and poor feeding.

Imperforate anus manifests with abdominal distention, lack of stool output, and the finding of imperforate anus on clinical examination.

Diagnosis

The diagnosis of esophageal fistula is often suggested by clinical symptoms and the inability to pass a feeding catheter into an infant with poor feeding skills. The diagnosis is then confirmed by chest radiographs with a feeding catheter looped in the obstructed proximal esophagus.

Duodenal atresia is diagnosed by the characteristic duodenal gaseous distention on radiograph (the double bubble sign) and contrast radiographic study of the upper gastrointestinal tract. Malrotation, jejunal atresia, and ileal atresia are all suggested by plain radiographs showing distention of the proximal small bowel and confirmed by contrast radiographic study of the upper gastrointestinal tract. If true bilious emesis occurs and malrotation is suspected, these patients are considered a medical emergency because the integrity of the bowel

will be quickly compromised by vascular occlusion and these patients will rapidly progress to a fulminant and even fatal condition without surgical intervention.

Hirschsprung's disease is suggested by clinical history and examination, plain radiograph revealing intestinal distention, and contrast radiograph of the distal bowel revealing proximal dilation and distal narrowing of the aganglionic segment. The diagnosis is confirmed by rectal biopsy revealing the absence of ganglia.

Imperforate anus is diagnosed by clinical examination.

Treatment

The first stage of therapy in all intestinal obstructions is to decompress the tract proximal to the obstruction with a repogle and stabilize the infant with intravenous fluids. The infant should be evaluated for associated anomalies, when indicated, by echocardiogram and renal ultrasound. Once the infant is stable, the obstruction is repaired by surgical removal of the lesion or dysfunctional bowel and reanastomosis. Often the defect can be repaired primarily, but in certain severe cases a diverting ostomy is required until the final repair can be completed.

Complications

In severe cases, intestinal obstruction is complicated by compromise of significant segments of bowel, requiring removal of large portions of the intestinal tract. When large sections are removed, absorption of nutrients is deficient and long-term parental nutrition may be needed.

GASTROSCHISIS AND OMPHALOCELE

Epidemiology

The combined incidence of omphalocele and gastroschisis is 1 in 4000 live births. Of these two defects, gastroschisis is more common. In infants with omphalocele, 35% have other gastrointestinal defects and 20% have congenital heart defects. Other anomalies including trisomies 13 and 18, urinary tract anomalies, and Beckwith-Wiedemann syndrome are associated with omphalocele. In contrast, associated congenital or chromosomal anomalies are rare in gastroschisis patients, but these patients do have higher rates of malrotation, intestinal atresia, and necrotizing enterocolitis.

Risk Factors

Pregnancies complicated by infection, young maternal age, smoking, or drug abuse can increase the rate of gastroschisis. Interestingly, owing to unknown causes, the incidence of gastroschisis has increased in recent years.

Pathophysiology

Gastroschisis is caused by a cleft in the abdominal wall to the right of the umbilical cord that allows abdominal contents to herniate into the amniotic fluid. By definition, gastroschisis is not covered by a sac. In addition to being at risk for torsion and necrosis during this herniated state, the prolonged exposure of the bowel to the amniotic fluid causes a severe inflammatory response that results in intestinal injury and ileus.

Omphalocele results when the abdominal contents herniate through the base of the umbilical cord into a sac covered by peritoneum and amniotic membrane. The sac covering the defect is thin and can rupture in utero or during delivery. The size of the defect can range from small (containing only a small amount of intestine), to large (containing most of the abdominal organs), to giant (containing the majority of the liver). Giant omphaloceles are rare (1 in 10,000 births) and are often associated with pulmonary hypoplasia.

Clinical Manifestation and Diagnosis

Polyhydramnios is noted in utero in both conditions. Ten percent of infants with omphalocele and 60% of those with gastroschisis are born prematurely. Diagnosis of gastroschisis and omphalocele is initially made by prenatal ultrasound and confirmed by physical examination after delivery. Early prenatal diagnosis allows proper counseling of the family and referral to a tertiary care center for further management. Infants with omphalocele are also at risk for congenital heart defects and should be evaluated by echocardiogram. Infants with gastroschisis should be evaluated for areas of intestinal torsion, necrosis, or atresia at the time of their initial physical examination.

Treatment

Cesarean section is recommended in giant omphalocele to decrease the risk of rupture of the omphalocele sac, but cesarean section does not improve the outcome in smaller omphaloceles or gastroschisis. If the infant is stable, small omphalocele defects can be closed primarily, but larger defects require a staged repair and can be postponed as long as the sac is intact. Treatment of the intact omphalocele before closure includes intestinal decompression with a repogle to minimize gastrointestinal distention. Although protocols for topical care of the omphalocele sac vary, many cover the sac with petroleum-impregnated gauze and then wrap the sac with gauze to support the viscera on the abdominal wall. Prognosis worsens if the sac is ruptured; therefore there should be no attempt to reduce the omphalocele.

Initial treatment of gastroschisis involves placement of a nasogastric tube to suction, covering the exposed intestine with saline-soaked gauze, and wrapping the exposed intestine and lower half of the infant with a sterile bag to minimize fluid loss and injury to the bowel. Aggressive fluid management is required to compensate for extra fluid loss from the exposed bowel. Many institutions place the infant on antibiotics to cover for infection caused by bowel flora.

In 10% of infants with gastroschisis, single-stage primary closure is possible. In most infants with gastroschisis, a silicone elastic silo is placed over the exposed bowel, allowing gradual reduction of the intestine into the abdomen over a period of several days. Once the bowel is completely reduced, the defect is surgically closed. Postsurgical care of infants with gastroschisis involves a prolonged recovery phase of the bowel during which the infants will require parenteral nutrition and a gradual advancing of enteral feeds.

Pulmonary Hypoplasia

EPIDEMIOLOGY

Lung development begins during the first trimester, progresses through several rounds of branching morphogenesis during the remaining months of gestation, and is not completed until the second or third year of life. Perturbation of lung development during any phase of gestation can result in pulmonary hypoplasia. Because of the variety of conditions associated with pulmonary hypoplasia, the true incidence is unknown.

RISK FACTORS

The most common risk factors for pulmonary hypoplasia include prolonged rupture of membranes, fetal renal dysplasias and obstructive uropathies, congenital diaphragmatic hernia, and congenital cystic lung lesions.

PATHOPHYSIOLOGY

For lung development to proceed normally, the volume of the thorax must be adequate for lung expansion, and amniotic fluid must enter the lung through fetal breathing. Conditions that externally compress the lung (congenital diaphragmatic hernia, cystic lung lesions, pleural effusions with fetal hydrops, malformations of the thorax, abdominal mass lesions) or conditions that decrease amniotic fluid levels (prolonged rupture of membranes, renal agenesis, cystic kidney disease, and urinary tract obstruction) inhibit the branching morphogensis of the lung and development of the gas exchange interface. As a result, hypoplastic lungs have reduced lung weight and alveolar number, fewer branchings of airways, fewer pulmonary arteries, and an increase in both pulmonary arteriole reactivity and proliferation of medial smooth muscle in pulmonary vessels.

CLINICAL MANIFESTATION

In addition to the manifestations associated with the primary disease, infants with pulmonary hypoplasia also present with significant respiratory and cardiac signs. The presentation is highly dependent on the severity of the pulmonary hypoplasia. Most infants with pulmonary hypoplasia present with increased work of breathing and significant hypoxia and acidosis. Shunting across the ductus arteriosus is evident on pre- and postductal oxygen saturations. Hypotension secondary to right heart failure and decreased left ventricular filling is often present.

DIAGNOSIS

The diagnosis is based on a clinical history of an anomaly associated with pulmonary hypoplasia. Chest radiographs reveal small bell-shaped lungs or space-occupying chest mass depending on the cause of the hypoplasia. Pulmonary hypertension is often evident on echocardiogram.

DIFFERENTIAL DIAGNOSIS

The differential diagnosis of pulmonary hypoplasia includes pneumonia, cyanotic congenital heart disease, primary PPHN, and sepsis.

TREATMENT

In the fetus with pulmonary hypoplasia, a few interventions can improve prognosis. These include serial amnioinfusions in the setting of prolonged rupture of membranes and nephrostomy tubes in obstructive uropathy.

A portion of these infants have relatively mild disease and require only minimal support; however, many have profound hypoxia as a result of severe pulmonary hypertension. In these infants, the first goal is to establish adequate oxygenation and ventilation. However, care must be taken not to induce significant overdistention of alveoli and pulmonary injury. Targeting an oxygen saturation of 88% to 92%,

CURRENT DIAGNOSIS

- Evaluation of the high-risk infant begins with the prenatal and perinatal history.
- Initial assessment in the delivery room should focus on the status of airway, breathing, and circulation.
- Neonatal signs are often systemic, nonspecific, and overlapping.
- Common neonatal problems involve prematurity, abnormal transition, infection, intestinal malformations, or pulmonary hypoplasia.

CURRENT THERAPY

- Most neonatal respiratory problems are treated with gentle supportive therapy.
- Ampicillin and gentamicin remain the most effective first-line therapy against most organisms responsible for sepsis in neonates.
- Selective pulmonary vasodilators have significantly improved the outcome in infants with pulmonary hypertension.
- Cooling therapy should be considered in infants with hypoxic brain injury.
- Initial therapy of intestinal obstruction requires decompression of proximal bowel and stabilization with intravenous fluids.

arterial pH levels of 7.25 to 7.35, and carbon dioxide levels of 50 to 65 mm Hg usually achieves a good balance between short-term benefit and long-term pulmonary injury. Pulmonary vasodilators have significantly improved the care of infants, with pulmonary hypertension associated with pulmonary hypoplasia. Of these, inhaled nitric oxide, 5 to 20 ppm, is the best studied. Other pulmonary vasodilators, including sildenafil,[1] bosentan,[1] and prostacyclin,[1] are increasing in use. Often long-term pulmonary vasodilators are needed to promote lung remodeling and growth.

In patients with congenital diaphragmatic hernia, distention of the bowel that is herniated into the thorax can significantly compromise the respiratory status of the infant. Therefore, at delivery, the infant should be intubated immediately and have a repogle placed to facilitate decompression of the bowel. In addition, bag-mask ventilation in infants with unrepaired congenital diaphragmatic hernia should be avoided.

---

[1]Not FDA approved for this indication.

REFERENCES

Greenberg JM, Donovan EF, Warner BB, et al. Neonatal morbidities of prenatal and perinatal origin. In: Creasy R, Resnik R, Iams J, editors. Creasy and Resnik's maternal-Fetal Medicine: Principles and Practice. 6th ed. Philadelphia: Saunders; 2009. pp. 1197–228.

Klaus MH, Fanaroff AA. Care of the high-risk neonate. 5th ed. Philadelphia: WB Saunders; 2001.

Ledbetter DJ. Gastroschisis and omphalocele. Surg Clin North Am 2006;86 (2):249–60, vii.

Orford J, Cass DT, Glasson MJ. Advances in the treatment of esophageal atresia over three decades: the 1970s and the 1990s. Pediatr Surg Int 2004;20 (6):402–7.

Shankaran S, Johnson Y, Langer JC, et al. Outcome of extremely-low-birth-weight infants at highest risk: Gestational age ≤24 weeks, birth weight ≤750 g, and 1-minute Apgar ≤3. Am J Obstet Gynecol 2004;191(4):1084–91.

Steinhorn RH. Neonatal pulmonary hypertension. Pediatr Crit Care Med 2010;11(Suppl. 2):S79–84.

Stoll BJ, Hansen N, Fanaroff AA, et al. Late-onset sepsis in very low birth weight neonates: the experience of the NICHD neonatal research network. Pediatrics 2002;110(2 Pt 1):285–91.

Normal Infant Feeding

Method of
Meg Begany, RD, CSP, LDN, and
Maria Mascarenhas, MBBS

Adequate and appropriate nutrition is especially critical during infancy. Infancy, defined as birth to 1 year of age, is characterized by the period of most rapid growth and development during the life cycle. In addition, recent research shows that nutrition during infancy can influence risk factors for disease at other stages of the life cycle.

Infant Feeding

For the healthy term infant, the suck-swallow and rooting reflexes are present at birth, and thus liquid feedings can be initiated almost immediately following delivery.

BREAST-FEEDING

The American Academy of Pediatrics (AAP) recommends human milk as the feeding of choice for nearly all infants whenever possible and mutually desirable for the mother and infant. Successful lactation and breast-feeding requires a supportive environment for the mother provided by the medical practitioner, including instruction and counseling. The World Health Organization (WHO) Expert Consultation on the Optimal Duration of Exclusive Breastfeeding, which considered the results of a systematic review of the evidence, concluded that human milk is recommended as the exclusive source of nutrition for the first 6 months and continuing human milk in combination with complementary foods until at least 12 months of age. The nutrient needs of the full-term normal birth weight infant can be met by human milk alone, with few exceptions, for the first 6 months if the mother is well nourished. The benefits of breast-feeding over formula feeding are well established and include enhanced maturity and motility of the gastrointestinal tract; maternal–infant bonding; monetary savings; facilitated fat, protein, and carbohydrate digestion and absorption; passive immunity; improved cognitive development; and decreased incidence of otitis media and respiratory and gastrointestinal disease. Further potential benefits, such as lower risk of overweight in children and adults, as well as decreased risk of cardiovascular disease in adulthood, were demonstrated in recent research.

Breast-feeding should be offered as early as possible after birth and then every 2 to 3 hours until satiety for approximately 10 to 15 minutes per breast during the first few weeks. Less frequent feedings may occur once breast-feeding is established. Intervals of more than 5 hours in between breast-feeding should be avoided during the first few weeks, including at night. Adequacy of breast-feeding is demonstrated when the infant has feedings 8 to 12 times per day, at least 6 to 8 wet diapers per day, regular stooling pattern, and is growing along established growth curves.

The composition of breast milk varies from individual to individual, as well as within the same individual, with composition changes occurring with stage of lactation, time of day, maternal diet, and time elapsed since feeding began. Milk production tends to be higher during the daytime, and fat content is increased toward the end of a feeding. On average, breast milk provides approximately 20 calories per ounce.

Contraindications to breast-feeding include maternal infections by organisms known to be transmitted to the infant via breast milk (e.g., HIV); maternal exposure to drugs, foods, or environmental agents that are excreted in human milk and harmful to the infant; and inborn errors of metabolism that are exacerbated by components present in human milk (e.g., galactosemia).

INFANT FORMULA

When a mother chooses not to breast-feed or human milk is not an option, infant formula is an appropriate substitute. Although the composition of infant formula does not exactly duplicate that of breast milk, the composition of infant formulas continues to evolve in an effort to do so. The addition of docosahexaenoic acid (DHA) and arachidonic acid (ARA) is a recent modification to infant formula. Unlike breast milk, infant formulas prior to 2002 contained only the precursor essential fatty acids, linoleic and α-linolenic acids, from which DHA and ARA had to be synthesized. Multiple studies in both preterm and term infants have demonstrated significantly lower levels of DHA and ARA in the erythrocytes of formula-fed infants compared to their breast-fed counterparts. This suggested that infant formula containing only the precursors, α-linolenic acid and linoleic acid, could be ineffective in allowing adequate synthesis of DHA and ARA. Thus multiple studies have been published comparing visual acuity, developmental outcomes, and growth of infants fed DHA and ARA supplemented and unsupplemented formula or breast milk. Some of these studies, but not all, found short-term improvements in visual and cognitive functions in both preterm and term infants. However, no long-term benefits were demonstrated. Although the single supplementation of DHA alone resulted in ARA deficiency status and poor growth in premature infants, the balanced supplementation of both DHA and ARA consistently do not show any adverse effect on growth.

Both iron-fortified and low-iron formulas are commercially available. The AAP has stated that there is no role for the use of low-iron formulas in infant feeding and recommends that all formulas fed to infants be fortified with iron. Well-controlled studies failed to show a benefit, in terms of feeding tolerance, related to the use of low-iron formula. The amount of iron present in iron-fortified formulas meets the iron requirements through the entire first year.

Infant formula should be prepared and stored with careful attention to the manufacturer's guidelines to prevent the risk of bacterial growth.

VITAMIN AND MINERAL SUPPLEMENTATION

The majority of vitamin and mineral requirements for infants are met in full by breast milk or infant formula. Guidelines for supplementation of vitamin K, vitamin D, iron, and fluoride are established. A single dose of vitamin K is typically given to all infants intramuscularly at birth to prevent hemorrhagic disease of the newborn.

In a 2008 report, the AAP advised that all infants and children have a minimum daily intake of 400 IU of vitamin D beginning in the first few days of life. This new recommendation replaces the prior report that recommended 200 IU of vitamin D per day. Adequate vitamin D is essential for the prevention and treatment of rickets, and evidence has shown that supplementation may have lifelong health benefits. A multivitamin or tri-vitamin preparation can be used. Alternatively, solitary vitamin D drops are now available in a cost-effective, easy-to-dose form (Carson Laboratories).

The iron requirements for formula-fed infants are met through iron-fortified formula. Although the iron content of human milk is minimal, its bioavailability is high. However, the iron body stores of the breast-fed infant diminish by 4 to 6 months of age, and thus an additional iron source is recommended at this age. Iron needs of the breast-fed infant can be met with the introduction of complementary foods when foods with good sources of iron are included (e.g., meat, fish, iron-fortified cereal, whole grains, and dark leafy green vegetables).

Fluoride supplementation is recommended at 6 months of age for both breast-fed infants and formula-fed infants who receive exclusively ready-to-feed formulas or whose water supply contains less than 0.3 ppm of fluoride.

INTRODUCTION OF COMPLEMENTARY FOODS

At approximately 6 months of age, human milk or infant formula can no longer supply all of an infant's nutrition requirements, and complementary foods are needed to ensure adequate nutrition and growth. It is the micronutrients, rather than energy and protein, which are likely to become lacking. The ability to digest and absorb carbohydrates, proteins, and fats is mature by 6 months of age.

Trypsin and chymotrypsin activities increase during the first 4 months of life. Age should not be the only factor in determining the timing of introduction of complementary feeding, but rather the timing should be determined by individual physical and psychological readiness of the infant, as well as rate of maturation of the nervous system, intestinal tract, and kidneys. Before spoon feedings are introduced, the infant should exhibit trunk stability, head control, and disappearance of the extrusion reflex. At approximately 5 to 6 months, an infant is able to indicate a desire for food by leaning forward and opening his or her mouth to indicate hunger and leaning back and turning away to show disinterest or satiety. Muraro et al. state that introduction of complementary feedings prior to 4 months of age is associated with an increased risk of atopic eczema and cow's milk protein allergy. There are presently no controlled studies showing an allergy preventative effect of restrictive diets after 6 months of age. Studies suggest that introducing complementary foods prior to 6 months does not result in increased caloric intake and has no growth advantage because the infant will displace breast milk to maintain the same level of caloric intake. Although it is possible to meet the nutrition needs of the infant solely from infant formula through the entire first year, delay of introduction of solids can lead to feeding aversions and food refusal. All infants need exposure to a variety of tastes, textures, and foods to develop appropriate feeding practices and a wider acceptance of new foods. In addition to adequate nutrition, the feeding relationship between the infant and caregiver is vital for normal growth and development.

To observe for symptoms of intolerance, only one new food should be introduced every 3 days. Because of its hypoallergenicity, infant rice cereal is often introduced as the first feeding. However, if spoon feeding is initiated at 6 months of age, gastrointestinal and renal development is mature enough to allow feedings from multiple food groups. Despite enhanced bioavailability, breast milk is relatively low in iron and zinc. Because low liver reserves of zinc at birth may predispose some infants to zinc deficiency, similar to the situation for iron, meat may be the ideal first food to provide these nutrients at the levels needed. Dr. Samuel Fomon states that unless there is a strong family history of allergy, introduction of soft-cooked red meats is desirable by 5 to 6 months of age. Furthermore, the proportion of Dietary Reference Intakes that needs to be supplied by complementary foods is highest for iron, zinc, phosphorus, and magnesium. Regardless of the food choice for the first feeding, the consistency should be thin and liquid/pureed. Thinning foods with breast milk or infant formula can enhance acceptability of the food by the infant. Repeated exposure to a new food may be necessary before it is accepted.

By 9 months of age, finely chopped foods and finger foods can be added to the infant's diet. At 12 months of age, rotary chewing is well

---

ⓒ CURRENT THERAPY

Infant Formula Composition and Indications

FORMULA	EXAMPLES	INDICATIONS	CHARACTERISTICS
Milk based	Enfamil LIPIL, Enfamil PREMIUM Newborn, Enfamil PREMIUM Infant, Enfamil PREMIUM with Triple Health Guard, Similac Advance, Good Start Gentle PLUS, Good Start Protect PLUS, Enfamil Gentlease, Similac Organic, Similac Sensitive, Enfamil A.R., Enfamil RestFull, Similac Sensitive RS, Similac Sensitive for Spit-Up (thickness with gastric pH)	Breast milk substitute for term infants	Ready to feed, powder, or liquid concentrate Variable whey-to-casein ratio 20 kcal/oz May contain DHA/ARA
Soy based	Enfamil ProSobee, Similac Sensitive Isomil Soy, Good Start Soy PLUS, Similac Expert Care-for Diarrhea	Breast milk substitute for infants with lactose intolerance or milk protein allergy*	Lactose free; some sucrose free Ready to feed, powder, or liquid concentrate 20 kcal/oz May contain DHA/ARA May contain fiber

Formula	Examples	Indications	Characteristics
Premature (hospital grade)	Enfamil Premature, Similac Special Care, Good Start Premature 24	Breast milk substitute for low-birth-weight hospitalized preterm infants	Low lactose High calcium and phosphorus Contain MCT 20, 24, or 30 kcal/oz Contain DHA/ARA
Human milk fortifiers	Similac Human Milk Fortifier, Enfamil Human Milk Fortifier, Similac Special Care 30	Fortification of human milk for low-birth-weight preterm infants	Increase calorie, protein, and vitamin/mineral content of breast milk Contain MCT
Premature transitional	Similac Expert Care NeoSure, Enfamil EnfaCare	Breast milk substitute for preterm infants >2.5 kg or discharge formula for preterm infants (used until 6–12 mo corrected age or until catch-up growth is completed)	22 kcal/oz Ready to feed or powder Contain DHA/ARA Vitamin and mineral content between that of term and premature formulas
Hypoallergenic	Nutramigen, Nutramigen AA, Nutramigen with Enflora LGG	Milk or soy protein allergy	Hydrolyzed protein or free amino acids Ready to feed, powder, or liquid concentrate Sucrose free, lactose free No MCT May contain DHA/ARA
Protein hydrolysate with MCT	Similac Expert Care Alimentum, Pregestimil	Malabsorption Short bowel syndrome Allergy	Lactose free Hydrolyzed protein Contain MCT May contain DHA/ARA Ready to feed or powder
Amino-acid based	Neocate Infant with DHA and ARA, EleCare	Malabsorption Short bowel syndrome Allergy	Lactose free Free amino acids May contain MCT May contain DHA/ARA Powder only
Fat modified	Monogen, Enfaport, Similac Expert Care Alimentum, Pregestimil	Defects in digestion, absorption, or transport of fat	Contain increased % of kcals as MCT
Carbohydrate modified	RCF, Product 3232 A, KetoCal	Simple sugar intolerance Ketogenic diet	Requires addition of complex carbohydrate to be complete
Amino acid modified	Multiple products (e.g., Cyclinex-1, MSUD Analog, Phenyl-Free)	Inborn errors of metabolism	Low or devoid of specific amino acids that cannot be metabolized
Electrolyte modified	Similac PM 60/40	Renal or other disease, state requiring low renal solute load	Decreased potassium content Decreased calcium and phosphorus content May be low iron content

*Children allergic to milk protein may also be allergic to soy protein.
Abbreviations: ARA = arachidonic acid; DHA = docosahexaenoic acid; MCT = medium chain triglycerides; MSUD = maple syrup urine disease.

controlled, and many infants can progress to table foods. Choking hazards that are round and hard, such as grapes, nuts, popcorn, hot dogs, and hard candy, should be avoided.

For the average healthy infant, meals of complementary foods should be provided two to three times per day from 6 to 8 months of age and three to four times per day from 9 to 12 months of age, with addition of nutritious snacks once or twice per day as desired. Vegetarian diets cannot meet nutrient needs at this age unless fortified products or nutrient supplements are provided. Estimates of the energy gap that must be filled by complementary food in industrialized countries is approximately 130 kcal/day at 6 to 8 months, 310 kcal/day at 9 to 11 months and 580 kcal/day at 12 to 23 months of age.

Juice is not a necessary component of the diet and may displace the intake of nutrient-dense breast milk or formula. In addition, offering juice by bottle can contribute to dental caries. If juice is provided, it should be limited to 4 to 8 ounces per day and should not be given prior to 6 months of age.

Whole cow's milk should not be introduced before 12 months of age because of its low iron content, high renal solute load, potential for causing gastrointestinal bleeding, and increased risk of cow's milk protein allergy. Furthermore, cow's milk is a poor source of vitamin C, vitamin E, and essential fatty acids. Breast-fed infants weaned before 12 months of age should receive an iron-fortified infant formula rather than cow's milk.

Nutritional Requirements

Because of the rapid rate of growth and development during infancy, nutrient needs per unit of body weight are very high in comparison to that of the older child or adult. An infant's energy or caloric requirement depends on many factors, including resting energy expenditure, body size and composition, physical activity, age, sex, and genetics. In general, an infant's hunger and satiety cues should guide decisions on when and how much to feed because infants are capable of regulating their intake to meet their caloric needs. The dietary reference intakes (DRIs) for healthy term infants provide the following equations to calculate estimated energy requirements (EERs):

$$0-3 \text{ months } (89 \times \text{weight [kg]} - 100) + 175 \text{ kcal}$$
$$4-6 \text{ months } (89 \times \text{weight [kg]} - 100) + 56 \text{ kcal}$$
$$7-12 \text{ months } (89 \times \text{weight [kg]} - 100) + 22 \text{ kcal}$$

Based on the above equations and reference weights ranging from 4.2 to 10.3 kg, estimated energy requirements for the healthy term infant range from 438 to 572 kcal/day (95 to 107 kcal/kg) at birth to 3 months, from 508 to 645 kcal/day (~82 kcal/kg) at 4 to 6 months, and from 608 to 844 kcal/day (~80–82 kcal/kg) at 7 to 12 months of age. Individual needs and growth patterns may necessitate modification of these requirements. The DRIs for protein were based on protein intake of the exclusively breast-fed infant from 0 to 6 months of age. Infant formula provides higher levels of protein than breast milk, which accounts for the decreased efficiency of absorption compared with that of breast milk. The contribution of complementary foods to total protein intake in the latter 6 months of infancy was considered in establishing the DRIs for this age. The DRI for protein is 9.1 g/day (~1.52 g/kg) from birth to 6 months and 11 g/day (~1.22 g/kg) from 7 to 12 months. Caloric distribution during infancy is recommended to be 40% to 50% fat, 7% to 11% protein, and 40% to 55% carbohydrate. The water-to-energy ratio should be 1.5 mL/kcal. Both human milk and infant formulas are models of this distribution. Hydration requirements are met by breast milk or infant formula without further addition of water to the diet, except potentially during periods of illness with fever, diarrhea, or emesis.

Growth

Growth velocity of weight, length, and head circumference is a general indicator of adequacy of kilocalorie, protein, and micronutrient intakes during infancy. Weight, length, and head circumference should be monitored serially during infancy and plotted on the gender-specific 2006 World Health Organization (WHO) Growth Charts. Breast-fed infants tend to gain less weight and usually are leaner than formula-fed infants in the second half of infancy. This difference does not seem to be the result of nutritional deficits but rather infant self-regulation of energy intake.

Obesity is increasing among children in the United States. High rates of weight gain during the first few months of life are associated with obesity in childhood and early adulthood. Optimal nutrition and growth during infancy should be promoted by encouraging healthy eating patterns in the infant to prepare for a healthy lifestyle later in life. Early identification and intervention may be a key component for establishing appropriate weight gain patterns.

Although no consensus exists on universal criteria to define failure to thrive, careful evaluation should occur when weight is less

CURRENT DIAGNOSIS

Expected Growth Velocity during Infancy

Age	Weight Gain (g/d)	Length (cm/mo)	Head Circumference (cm/wk)
0–3 mo	25–35	2.5–3.5	0.3–0.6
3–6 mo	15–21	1.6–2.5	0.2–0.5
6–12 mo	10–13	1.2–1.7	0.1–0.4

than the 5th percentile or falls more than two major percentiles from a previously established growth channel. In addition, relationship of weight to height must be considered. Prompt intervention with nutritional rehabilitation is essential to prevent illness, growth stunting, cognitive delay, and social and behavioral problems.

For the treatment of either over- or undernutrition, a multidisciplinary team approach involving the physician, dietitian, psychologist, and social worker, along with community services, can often be beneficial and necessary.

In conclusion, infant feeding during the first year of life is a complex process, and guidelines are based on developmental, nutritional, and social factors. Human milk is superior to infant formula and should be the feeding of choice for all infants. Although infant formulas do not exactly duplicate breast milk, the composition of infant formulas continues to evolve in an effort to do so. Complementary foods should be introduced at 6 months of age. Cow's milk should not be introduced until 1 year of age. Careful attention should be paid to growth and nutritional status throughout infancy, with prompt attention to any deviation from expected growth patterns.

REFERENCES

American Academy of Pediatrics, Committee on Nutrition. Iron fortification of infant formulas. Pediatrics 1999;104:119–23.

American Academy of Pediatrics, Section on Breastfeeding. Breastfeeding and the use of human milk. Pediatrics 2005;115:496–506.

Dewey KG. Nutrition, growth and complementary feeding of the breastfed infant. Pediatr Clin North Am 2001;48:87–104.

Foman SJ. Feeding normal infants: Rationale for recommendations. J Am Diet Assoc 2001;101:1002–5.

Institute of Medicine, Food and Nutrition Board. Dietary Reference Intakes for Energy, Carbohydrate, Fiber, Fat, Fatty Acids, Cholesterol, Protein, and Amino Acids. Washington, DC: National Academies Press; 2005.

Kleinman RE, editor. Pediatric Nutrition Handbook. 5th ed. Elk Grove Village, Ill: American Academy of Pediatrics, Committee on Nutrition; 2003.

Michaelsen KF. Cows' milk in complementary feeding. Pediatrics 2000;106: 1302–3.

Muraro A, Dreborg S, Halken S, et al. Dietary prevention of allergic diseases in infants and small children. Part III: Critical review of published peer-reviewed observational and interventional studies and final recommendations. Pediatr Allergy Immunol 2004;15:291–307.

PAHO and WHO. Guiding Principles for Complementary Feeding of the Breastfed Child. Washington, DC: Pan American Health Organization and World Health Organization; 2003.

Samour PQ, King K, editors. Handbook of Pediatric Nutrition. 3rd ed. Sudbury, Mass: Jones and Bartlett; 2005.

Slaughter CW, Bryant AH. Hungry for love: The feeding relationship in the psychological development of young children. Permanente J 2004;8:23–9.

Wagner CL, Greer FR, et al. Prevention of rickets and vitamin D deficiency in infants, children, and adolescents. Pediatrics 2008;122:1142–52.

WHO Child Growth Standards (http://www.who.int/childgrowth/en). Published by the Centers for Disease Control and Prevention, November 1, 2009. Retrieved from http://www.cdc.gov/growthcharts/who_charts.htm.

WHO Working Group on the Growth Reference Protocol and the WHO Task Force on Methods for the Natural Regulation of Fertility. Growth of healthy infants and the timing, type, and frequency of complementary foods. Am J Clin Nutr 2002;76:620–7.

Diseases of the Breast

Method of
*Paniti Sukumvanich, MD, and
Patrick Borgen, MD*

Benign Diseases of the Breast

Benign diseases of the breast historically are subdivided into proliferative and nonproliferative lesions (Table 1). In a study by Dupont and Page, patients with breast biopsies yielding nonproliferative lesions had no increased risk of subsequent breast cancer. In contrast, proliferative lesions were associated with a minimal to a fivefold increased risk of breast cancer. In clinical practice, of the proliferative lesions, only atypical epithelial lesions increase breast cancer risk significantly. Appropriate treatment and counseling of patients depend on the risk of breast cancer associated with these benign breast diseases.

Nonproliferative Lesions

Nonproliferative lesions comprise mild hyperplasia without atypia, squamous or apocrine metaplasia, duct ectasia, mastitis, and cysts. In the study of 3303 patients by Dupont and Page, only 2.2% of patients with nonproliferative lesions had breast cancer following a benign breast biopsy with a mean follow-up time of 17 years (Figure 1).

BREAST CYSTS AND FIBROCYSTIC BREAST DISEASE

Fibrocystic breast disease is a benign process in which generalized microcystic formation with stromal proliferation leads to increased breast nodularity. Cysts within the breast are most common in perimenopausal women 50 to 59 years of age as well as premenopausal women. Postmenopausal women not on hormone replacement therapy are unlikely to develop cysts in their breasts. Benign cysts are often tender and fluctuate in size with the menstrual cycle. Cysts may be detected either on physical examination as a palpable, smooth, mobile nodule or by breast ultrasound. They may appear as a solitary nodule or in a cluster. Ultrasonographic appearance of simple benign cysts is that of an anechoic, round or oval, well-circumscribed mass with posterior enhancement. If the mass has all

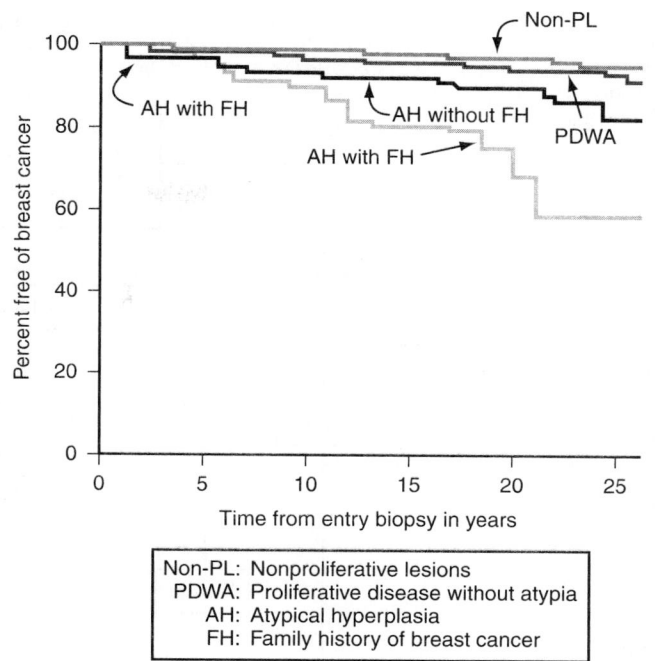

FIGURE 1. Nonproliferative lesions in breast cancer.

four criteria, the accuracy of ultrasound is close to 100% for the diagnosis of a simple benign cyst. Cysts that appear complex, with internal echoes, thick septations, and irregular walls, are suspicious for breast carcinoma and should be examined surgically or with an ultrasound-guided biopsy. Confirmation of the diagnosis can be made by fine-needle aspiration (FNA) of the cystic fluid. Bloody fluid may be an indication for a biopsy. In a study of 6782 cyst aspirates, Ciatto and colleagues found that cytologic examination identified atypical cells in 1677 specimens. Of these specimens, only 0.3% of these cases had clinically and radiologically negative intracystic papillomas. Cytologic examination was positive in only 0.1% of these cases. Thus fluid from cyst aspirations are not sent routinely for cytologic examination. Figure 2 describes the management of suspected cysts.

MASTITIS AND DUCT ECTASIA

Mastitis is divided into lactational or nonlactational. Lactational mastitis can occur from the reflux of bacteria into the breast during breast-feeding. The causative bacteria are usually gram-positive cocci. Patients should be treated with antibiotics with the appropriate coverage and can continue to nurse or pump the breast to prevent engorgement. Nursing mothers can continue to breast-feed because the infant is not at risk for infection. Nonlactational (periductal) mastitis can be caused by duct ectasia, which occurs when the milk ducts become congested with secretions and debris, resulting in a periductal inflammation. These patients may present with greenish nipple discharge, nipple retraction, and subareolar noncyclical pain. The treatment of nonlactational mastitis includes broad-spectrum antibiotics to cover for gram-positive cocci and skin anaerobes. Total duct excision and eversion of the nipple may be necessary to treat recurrent periductal mastitis.

Proliferative Benign Breast Diseases

Proliferative breast diseases include moderate or florid hyperplasia, microglandular and sclerosing adenosis, papilloma, fibroadenoma, and atypical ductal and lobular hyperplasia. All proliferative lesions have an increased risk of subsequent breast cancer after biopsy except for fibroadenoma. Overall, with a median follow-up of 17 years, 5.3%

TABLE 1 Benign Diseases of the Breast

	Increase in Breast Cancer Risk
Nonproliferative Lesions	
Mild hyperplasia without atypia	None
Squamous or apocrine metaplasia	None
Duct ectasia	None
Mastitis	None
Cysts	None
Proliferative Lesions	
Fibroadenoma	None
Moderate or florid hyperplasia	Minimal
Microglandular adenosis	Minimal
Sclerosing adenosis	Minimal
Papilloma	Minimal
Atypical ductal hyperplasia	4- to 5-fold
Atypical lobular hyperplasia	5.8-fold

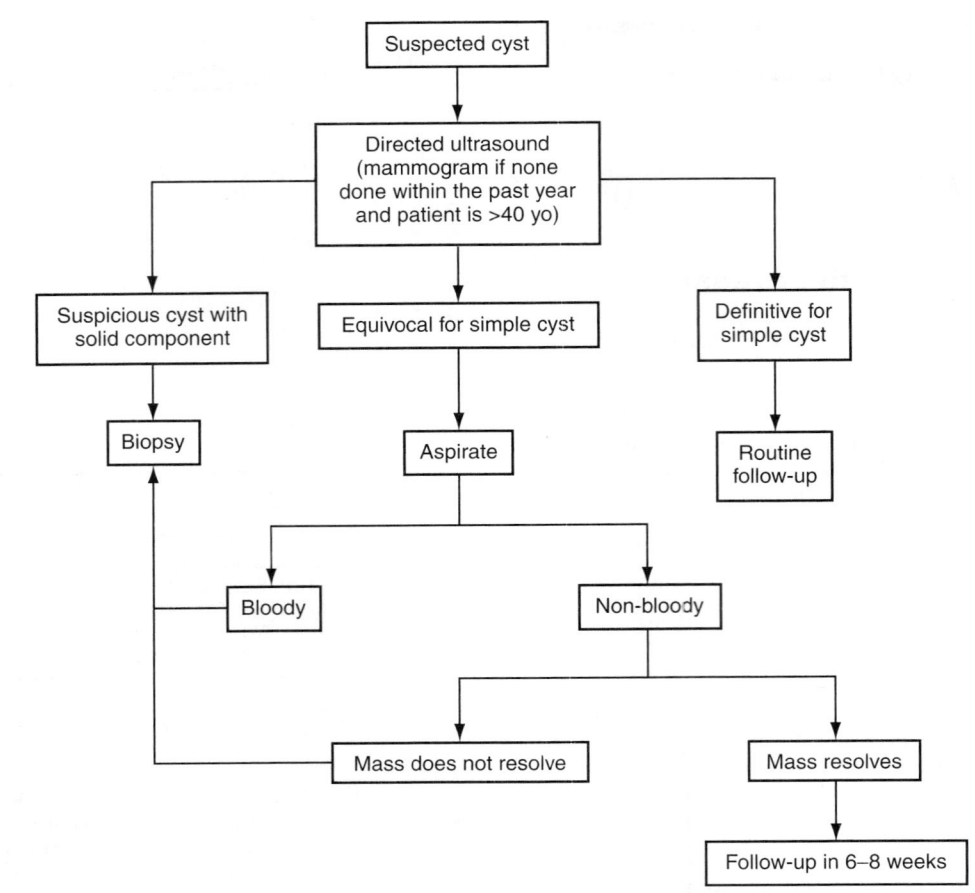

FIGURE 2. Algorithm for the management of suspected cysts.

of patients with proliferative lesions develop breast cancer. This percentage increases to 12.9% in the presence of atypia (see Figure 1). Patients with moderate or florid hyperplasia, sclerosing adenosis, and solitary papilloma without atypia carry a minimal increase in risk of developing breast cancer over the general population. These patients are not classified as high risk. But the risk of subsequent breast cancer is increased by four- to fivefold in the presence of atypia. Atypical lobular hyperplasia carries a higher risk than atypical ductal hyperplasia, with a relative risk as high as 5.8. This increased risk applies to the contralateral breast because subsequent breast carcinomas are evenly divided between both breasts.

PROLIFERATIVE LESIONS WITH NO INCREASED RISK OF SUBSEQUENT CANCER: FIBROADENOMA

Fibroadenomas are benign tumors commonly found in young women (less than 30 years of age with a peak incidence at 21 to 25 years of age). They are characteristically detected on physical examination as well-circumscribed, rubbery, highly mobile, palpable masses. On mammograms, these lesions may appear as a well-circumscribed mass. Involution of fibroadenomas in the elderly can lead to hyalinization and dense popcorn-like calcification on mammograms. Fibroadenomas pose no increased risk of breast cancer and do not mandate surgical removal unless desired by the patient. Pregnancy can increase the size of these lesions; thus it may be reasonable to remove them prior to a planned pregnancy. Removal may facilitate follow-up, given the inability to follow breast masses adequately during pregnancy. Other types of fibroadenomas include juvenile and giant fibroadenomas. Juvenile fibroadenomas occur in adolescent women and can grow larger than 5 cm in diameter. These lesions are not malignant; given their large size, however, surgical excision may be needed to prevent

asymmetry of the breasts. Giant fibroadenomas are large fibroadenomas found in the lactating breast or in the breasts of pregnant patients. These lesions may regress in size once hormonal stimulation subsides. Lesions that remain large can be excised surgically. Fibroadenomas and phyllodes tumors may be linked. Any rapidly enlarging fibroadenoma should be considered for surgical excision to rule out phyllodes tumor because it is difficult clinically to differentiate fibroadenoma from phyllodes tumor.

PROLIFERATIVE LESIONS WITH MINIMAL INCREASED RISK OF SUBSEQUENT BREAST CANCER

Multiple Peripheral Papillomas

Multiple peripheral papillomas are lesions that occur in the peripheral ducts. They most commonly present as a mass but may also present with nipple discharge. Complete excisional removal should be considered to rule out a papillary carcinoma of the breast. Approximately 10% to 33% of patients have subsequent breast cancer; thus close follow-up of these patients is warranted.

Sclerosing and Microglandular Adenosis

Sclerosing adenosis occurs as result of the proliferation of stromal tissue along with small terminal ductules. Often these lesions are picked up incidentally, but they may also present as microcalcifications on mammogram or as a mass (termed *adenosis tumor*). Sclerosing adenosis may be confused with a tubular carcinoma. Staining with immunohistochemical (IHC) markers such as actin, smooth muscle myosin heavy chain p63, or calponin may be helpful in distinguishing between the two lesions because only sclerosing adenosis contains myoepithelial cells. Microglandular adenosis is an uncommon lesion that may be mistaken for tubular carcinoma on histologic examination, and it can increase the patient's subsequent breast cancer risk. Concomitant breast cancer has been reported, so complete surgical excision should be considered for these lesions.

PROLIFERATIVE LESIONS WITH A FOUR- TO FIVEFOLD RISK OF SUBSEQUENT BREAST CANCER: ATYPICAL DUCTAL AND LOBULAR HYPERPLASIA

Atypical ductal and lobular hyperplasia are very similar to their in situ counterparts. These lesions are termed *atypical hyperplasia* because they lack some of the microscopic features of in situ disease. The distinction between atypical hyperplasia and carcinoma in situ is sometimes hard to make. In a study by Rosai, five expert breast cancer pathologists reviewed 17 cases of ductal or lobular lesions. In no case did all five agree on a diagnosis. Four out of the five were able to agree on a diagnosis in three cases (18%). In one third of the patients, the diagnosis ran the gamut from hyperplasia without atypia to carcinoma in situ. Despite such difficulty, the diagnosis of atypical hyperplasia is on the rise as mammographic screening becomes more popular. Atypical hyperplasia, which is detected secondary to microcalcifications or by serendipity, carries the highest risk of subsequent breast carcinoma among all proliferative lesions of the breast, with a four- to fivefold increased risk over the general population. Atypical lobular hyperplasia carries a higher risk than atypical ductal hyperplasia, with a relative risk as high as 5.8. This risk applies to the contralateral breast as well as the ipsilateral breast. Surgical excision of atypical hyperplasia on a core biopsy is recommended because 20% of patients are found to have breast cancer at time of surgical excision for atypical hyperplasia. It is not necessary to achieve negative margins for these lesions.

OTHER BENIGN BREAST LESIONS: FAT NECROSIS, HAMARTOMA, MONDOR'S DISEASE, RADIAL SCARS, AND PSEUDOANGIOMATOUS STROMAL HYPERPLASIA

Other benign lesions of the breast include fat necrosis, hamartoma, Mondor's disease, radial scars, and pseudoangiomatous stromal hyperplasia (PASH). Trauma to the breast may lead to fat necrosis and can be mistaken for carcinomas on clinical examination. Fat necrosis lesions present clinically as painless, irregular masses with or without associated skin changes such as skin thickening. These lesions can be normal or may have rim calcifications on mammograms. No further treatment is needed when a core biopsy definitively makes the diagnosis of fat necrosis.

Hamartomas are benign lesions that are often picked up on a mammogram. The fatty composition of the mass makes these lesions clinically occult. They can be mistaken for fibroadenomas on mammograms. Hamartomas can be left alone without histologic confirmation if diagnosed definitively on a mammogram.

Mondor's disease is a thrombophlebitis of the superficial breast veins that presents as a palpable tender cord leading to the axilla. In a study of 63 cases, 8 patients (25%) had an underlying malignancy; thus a mammogram should be done to rule out the presence of breast carcinoma.

Radial scars are benign lesions whose etiology is unknown. They are often mistaken for breast carcinoma on mammograms because of their stellate appearance. Radial scars may also mimic breast carcinoma histologically. Staining for myoepithelial cells can help distinguish between invasive carcinoma and a radial scar. Radial scars carry a 1.5-fold increase in risk of subsequent breast carcinoma, so these lesions should be considered markers of future disease.

First described in 1986, PASH is a benign proliferative lesion that may present as an incidental finding or a mobile breast mass. It can occur in all ages and also in men. On a mammogram, PASH appears as a round noncalcified mass. Histologically, PASH may be mistaken for low-grade angiosarcoma. Unlike angiosarcoma, however, there should be no evidence of mitosis or cytologic atypia in PASH specimens. The role of hormones in the pathogenesis of PASH is controversial. Although these lesions tend to occur in young patients or in

elderly patients on hormone therapy, most cases tend to be negative for estrogen receptors. The treatment for PASH is complete surgical excision. Approximately 7% of cases recur despite adequate treatment.

Risk Factors for Breast Cancer

An estimated 80% of women in whom breast cancer develops have no documented risk factors or determinants. Risk factors cannot be changed, whereas risk determinants can be altered to decrease a person's risk of subsequent breast cancer. Common risk factors include a familial history of breast cancer, personal breast biopsy history, menarche before 12 years of age, menopause after 55 years of age, increasing age, geographical location, and mutations of the BRCA1 or BRCA2 genes. Women known to have the BRCA1 or BRCA2 genetic mutation have an 85% lifetime risk of breast cancer as well as an increased risk of ovarian cancer. BRCA1 carriers are at a higher risk for developing ovarian cancer than BRCA2 (60% versus 20%, respectively). The risk determinants for breast cancer include reproductive factors such as nulliparity and first pregnancy after the age of 30 years and previous radiation exposure. Previous therapy for lymphoma, especially during adolescence, elevates a woman's risk of subsequent breast cancer.

Screening Techniques

Screening for breast cancer includes mammography, ultrasound, breast self-examination (BSE), and physical examination by a physician. Multiple studies such as the Göthenborg and Malmö trials show a reduction in breast cancer mortality from 30% to 40% in patients 40 to 49 years of age who undergo screening mammograms. A meta-analysis of six randomized trials indicates a 30% reduction in breast cancer mortality in patients 50 to 69 years of age. The sensitivity of mammograms depends on the patient's age and ranges from 53% to 81% in women 40 to 49 years of age to 73% to 81% in patients 50 years of age or older. An estimated 10% to 15% of breast cancer cases are not detectable on screening mammography, thus emphasizing the importance of physical breast examination by a physician and BSE that include both visual inspection and manual examination of the breast. On inspection, signs of breast malignancy include skin or nipple retraction or discoloration, nipple discharge/crusting, or peau d'orange edema of the breast. On palpation, any asymmetric mass of the breast or axilla may be regarded as a potential malignancy that deserves further evaluation.

Current recommendations are for a woman to start performing BSE at 18 years of age, have a yearly physical exam, and initiate annual mammography at 40 years of age. Little data exist on what should be the upper age limit of mammogram screening. Given that breast density decreases with age and breast cancer increases with age, mammograms should be even more sensitive and specific in the older age group. For these reasons, mammograms may be continued in very elderly patients as long as the patient is not suffering from any major co-morbidities. In patients who have a very high risk of breast cancer, such as BRCA carriers, screening should start 10 years earlier than the age of onset of an affected relative or at the age of 35. Kriege screened 1909 patients (including 358 BRCA mutation carriers) who had more than a 15% lifetime risk of developing breast cancer. These patients had a biannual breast exam as well as annual mammogram and breast magnetic resonance imaging (MRI). In this population, mammograms had a sensitivity of 33% with a specificity of 95%. Breast MRI had significantly higher rates of sensitivity and specificity at 80% and 90%, respectively. Given these findings, breast MRI should be a part of the screening exam for these high-risk patients. MRI is recommended as a standard screening test in BRCA heterozygotes. Routine surveillance in high-risk patients includes a 6-month interval alternating between breast MRI and mammograms. Patients with a history of mantle radiation for lymphoma should start annual screening at 25 years of age and biannual screening 10 years after receiving radiation therapy.

Workup of a Breast Mass

DOMINANT PALPABLE MASS

The workup of a dominant palpable breast mass depends on the patient's menopausal status and the degree of suspicion. It is not unreasonable to follow a premenopausal patient with a nonsuspicious mass over one menstrual cycle and then reexamine her. Suspicious lesions present as a hard, nontender, irregular mass or as a mass in a high-risk patient. Palpable masses in postmenopausal patients may also warrant a workup. FNA should not be performed prior to diagnostic imaging because it may result in a hematoma that could obscure the image of the mass. Certain benign lesions on core biopsy should be excised, including lobular carcinoma in situ (LCIS), atypical ductal hyperplasia (ADH), radial scars, sclerosing papillary lesions, columnar cell hyperplasia with atypia, and PASH (Figure 3). Twenty percent of surgeries performed for atypical ductal hyperplasia have concurrent carcinoma in the specimen. Patients with a high-risk proliferative lesion should have close follow-up after surgery including physical examinations. Negative findings on a mammogram do not preclude the diagnosis of cancer because 10% of cancers are occult mammographically. This number drops to 3% when a lesion is occult both mammographically and ultrasonographically. An alternative to core biopsies in younger women is the use of the triple test: a physical exam in conjunction with breast imaging (mammogram or ultrasound) and FNA. When all three components indicate the mass is benign, the negative predictive value is 100%. In a study by Morris, a triple test score assigns points to each component of the test. One point is given for benign findings, 2 points for suspicious findings, and 3 points for malignant findings. When added together, masses with scores of 4 or less are found to be benign. The triple test should only be used in women 40 years of age or younger because the incidence of breast cancer increases dramatically after that cutoff.

MASSES REVEALED ON SCREENING MAMMOGRAMS

The American College of Radiology's classification lexicon, the Breast Imaging Reporting and Data System (BI-RADS), is used in breast imaging (Table 2). BI-RADS 0 means the assessment is incomplete and more workup is needed. BI-RADS 1 indicates a normal mammogram. Mammograms with BI-RADS 2 signify benign findings. Patients with BI-RADS 3 have a 1% to 2% risk of malignancy and should have short-term follow-up with another mammogram in 6 months. BI-RADS 4 indicates the presence of suspicious lesions with a 20% to 40% probability of a malignant lesion. BI-RADS 5 is highly suggestive of cancer with a greater than 95% chance of harboring an underlying malignant lesion. BI-RADS 6, recently added as a category, indicates known malignant disease. BI-RADS 4 and 5 both indicate a biopsy.

A core biopsy via ultrasound guidance may be attempted first. A stereotactic core biopsy should be considered if this is not possible. Stereotactic biopsies may be impossible in patients with lesions that are very superficial or close to the chest wall or in patients with very small breasts that compress to less than 3 cm or who are unable to lie still for the procedure. In such situations, surgical excision with needle localization is warranted. In studies comparing surgical excision to core biopsies, the concordance rate is close to 100%. The surgeon

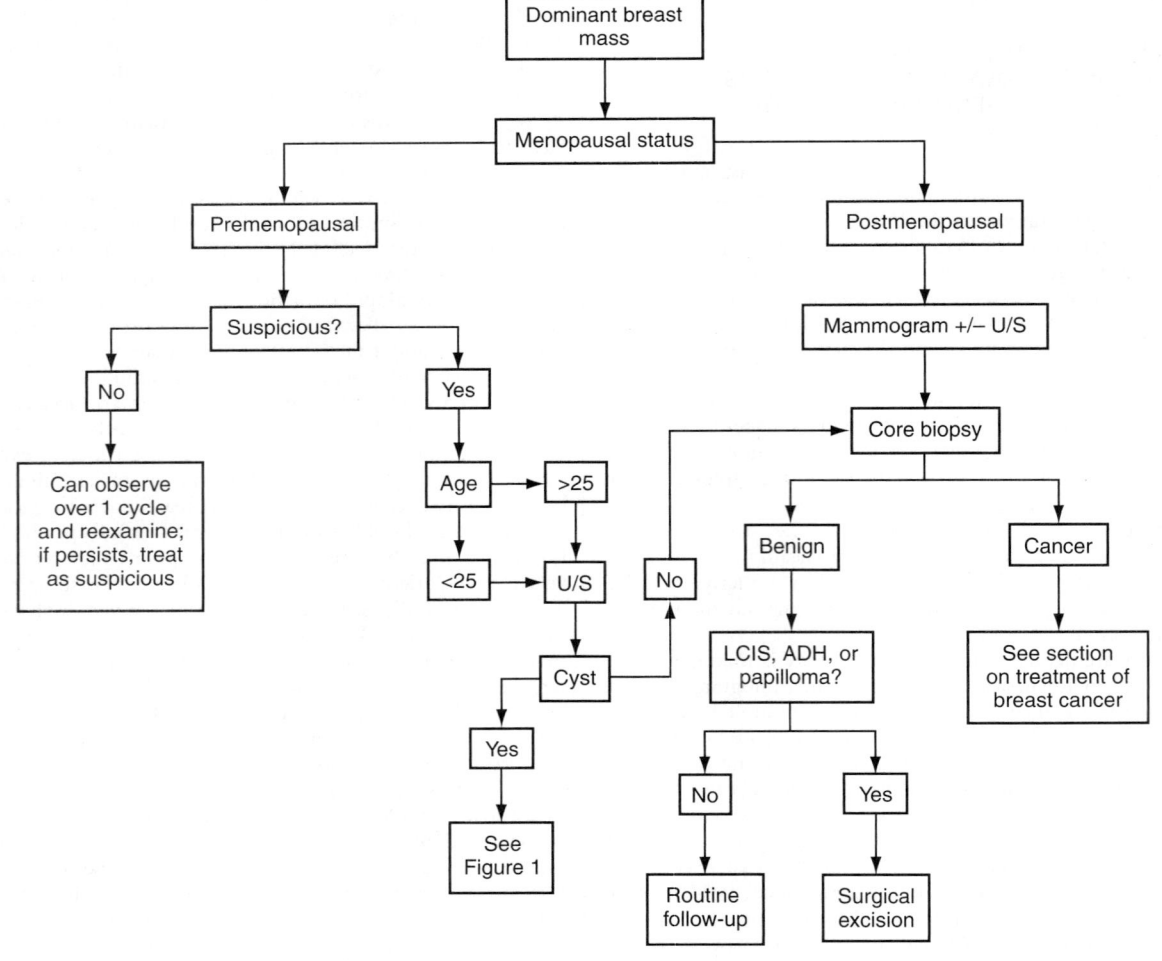

FIGURE 3. Algorithm for workup of a breast mass. ADH = atypical ductal hyperplasia; LCIS = lobular cancer in situ; U/S = ultrasound.

TABLE 2 BI-RADS Mammography Classification

BI-RADS Category	Definition	Risk of Malignancy	Recommended Follow-Up
0	Incomplete assessment	N/A	Further workup
1	Negative study	N/A	Repeat mammogram in 1 y
2	Benign	N/A	Repeat mammogram in 1 y
3	Probably benign	<2%	Repeat mammogram in 6 mo
4	Suspicious	20%	Biopsy should be considered
5	Highly suggestive of malignancy	90%	Appropriate action should be taken
6	Known biopsy-proven malignancy	N/A	Appropriate action should be taken

Abbreviation: BI-RADS = Breast Imaging Reporting and Data System.

can obviate the need for multiple surgeries in the same patient by performing a core biopsy for diagnosis. High-risk proliferative lesions, such as LCIS, atypical ductal hyperplasia, radial scars, sclerosing papillary lesions, columnar cell hyperplasia with atypia, and PASH, should be considered for an excisional biopsy if the diagnosis is made by a core biopsy.

In Situ Diseases

LOBULAR CARCINOMA IN SITU

Lobular carcinoma in situ (LCIS) should be considered a marker for future breast cancer risk and not an early noninvasive lobular cancer. This disease is most commonly seen in premenopausal women, with a peak incidence in women 40 to 50 years of age. Only 10% of LCIS occurs in postmenopausal women. Unlike ductal carcinoma in situ, LCIS is often found incidentally because typically no clinical or radiologic abnormalities are seen at time of diagnosis. In 50% of patients, LCIS is a multifocal finding. In 30% of patients, it can be found in the contralateral breast. Patients with LCIS are at 8 to 10 times the risk of the general population for subsequent breast cancer. Their overall lifetime risk is as high as 30% to 40% for the development of invasive breast cancer. In a meta-analysis, 15% of patients developed breast cancer in the ipsilateral breast, and 9.3% of patients developed cancer in the contralateral breast. The type of breast cancer can be either ductal or lobular, although the majority is ductal.

DUCTAL CARCINOMA IN SITU

Ductal carcinoma in situ (DCIS), or intraductal carcinoma, is a noninvasive breast cancer and designated stage 0. Historically, DCIS represented only approximately 5% of breast cancer cases, whereas today it constitutes 20% to 30% of all cases. This rise is predominantly attributed to the increasing use of screening mammography because DCIS is most often detected as mammographic microcalcifications. It tends to occur at a later age than LCIS and is not considered a multifocal or bilateral disease. Unlike LCIS, DCIS should be considered a true precursor lesion because if left untreated, approximately 60% to 100% of DCIS cases progress to invasive carcinoma.

TREATMENT FOR IN SITU DISEASE

Lobular Carcinoma in Situ

LCIS should be treated as a marker for increased breast cancer risk. Surgery in an attempt to achieve negative margins is not warranted for LCIS. The NSABP P-1 (the National Surgical Adjuvant Breast and Bowel Project) randomized trial examined the role of tamoxifen (Nolvadex) as a chemopreventive agent in high-risk patients, including those with LCIS. Women taking tamoxifen had a 50% reduction in the subsequent risk of breast cancer without any improvement in overall survival. The main risks of tamoxifen include increased risk of thromboembolic disease and endometrial cancer. The rate of pulmonary embolism was 3 in 1000 patients in the tamoxifen group versus 1 in 1000 in the placebo group. The rate of deep-vein thromboembolism was 5 in 1000 patients in the tamoxifen group

versus 3 in 1000 in the placebo group. Endometrial cancer was seen in 9 in 1000 patients in the tamoxifen group versus 3.5 in 1000 in the placebo group. The decision to use tamoxifen as a chemopreventive agent should be made on an individual basis given these side effects. The highest reduction in breast cancer occurred in the LCIS group with a 70% reduction in risk. Despite this, no difference in survival was seen between the tamoxifen and placebo group.

Ductal Carcinoma in Situ

Treatment of DCIS has evolved from simple mastectomy to lumpectomy with radiation therapy. A simple mastectomy is associated with a 1% local recurrence rate. Thus it is still considered a viable option in patients who do not desire or are ineligible for breast conservation therapy (BCT). No difference in survival is seen in patients treated with mastectomy versus BCT. The NSABP B-17 randomized trial examined the role of lumpectomy with and without radiotherapy for the treatment of DCIS. The addition of radiotherapy decreased the recurrence rate from 16.4% to 7% with 8 years of follow-up. More importantly, it decreased the rate of invasive carcinoma from 8% to 2%. The 5-year event-free survival with lumpectomy and radiation is 84%. Limited data support excision alone in small well-differentiated DCIS with surgical margins of at least 1 cm. Silverstein showed in retrospective studies that the recurrence rate in such patients is approximately 4%. Routine axillary lymph node dissection (ALND) is not recommended for DCIS because only 1% of patients have positive axillary nodes. Recent studies, however, show that sentinel lymph node biopsy may have a role in the management of selected patients with DCIS. This is especially true in patients receiving a mastectomy as definitive treatment or if there is a question of microinvasion on the core biopsy. Patients with DCIS and microinvasion can have anywhere from a 3% to 20% incidence of nodal involvement. Indications for a sentinel node biopsy include extensive calcifications, a palpable lesion, patients undergoing mastectomy as treatment for DCIS, and lesions for which the pathology reads "can not rule out microinvasion." Tamoxifen (Nolvadex) can also be considered in cases of DCIS that are estrogen receptor positive. The NSABP B-24 randomized trial examined the utility of tamoxifen in patients treated with lumpectomy and radiotherapy. Ipsilateral tumor recurrences decreased from 13.4% without tamoxifen to 8.2% with tamoxifen. The incidence of invasive cancer was reduced by 47%. No difference in survival was observed between the placebo and the tamoxifen group. Side effects are similar to that of the NSABP P-1 trial.

Invasive Breast Cancer

INCIDENCE

An estimated 1 in 9 women living in the United States who survive to 90 years of age will develop breast cancer. The average age at diagnosis is 64 years of age and increases along with age.

The American Joint Committee on Cancer TMN (tumor, metastasis, node) system designates breast cancer as stage 0, I, II, III, or IV. This system categorizes breast cancer by its invasive or noninvasive

TABLE 3 Overall Survival in Breast Cancer Patients

Stage	10-Year Overall Survival	15-Year Overall Survival
I	74%–95%	64%
II	76%	62%
IIA	81%	72%
IIB	70%	52%
III	50%	40%
IIIA	59%	49%
IIIB	36%	18%
IIIC	36%	18%
IV	18%	18%

Adapted from Rosen PP, et al. J Clin Oncol 1989;355–366; Woodward WA, Strom EA, Tucker SL, et al. Changes in the 2003 American Joint Committee on Cancer staging for breast cancer, dramatically affect stage-specific survival. J Clin Oncol 2003;21:3244–3248.

character, tumor size, axillary lymph node status, and the presence of metastatic disease (see Table 2). Overall survival with breast cancer is related to stage (Table 3).

HISTOLOGY

The most common type of infiltrating carcinoma is ductal carcinoma-not otherwise specified (IFDC-NOS), which represents 85% of all invasive breast cancer. Infiltrating lobular carcinoma originates from the lobular structures of the breast and accounts for 15% of all invasive breast cancer. Other less common subtypes represent less than 10% and include tubular, medullary, mucinous, and papillary carcinoma. Additional rare subtypes of breast cancer include inflammatory carcinoma, malignant phyllodes tumor, sarcoma, lymphoma, and Paget disease.

BREAST CANCER STAGING

In 2003 the American Joint Committee on Cancer (AJCC) revised their staging system on breast cancer. This latest revision stresses the importance of nodal status as a prognostic factor by making several changes in how it is classified within the staging system. Major changes to the staging system include the following:

- Designation is made for isolated tumor cells (ITCs), which are differentiated from micrometastasis and defined as "single tumor cells or small cell clusters not greater than 0.2 mm, usually detected only by IHC (immunohistochemistry) or molecular methods, but which may be verified on H&E (hematoxylin-eosin) stains. ITCs do not usually show evidence of malignant activity, e.g., proliferation or stromal reaction." ITCs are designated as pN0 with modifiers for positive or negative IHC (i−, i+) and molecular findings (mol−, mol+).
- Internal mammary nodes (IMNs) are reclassified based on how they are detected and whether or not there is concomitant axillary lymph node metastasis. Detection of IMNs by sentinel node biopsy alone is classified as pN1b in the absence of positive axillary nodes or pN1c in the presence of positive axillary nodes. Internal mammary nodes detected by imaging studies (excluding lymphoscintigraphy) or by clinical exam are classified as pN2b in the absence of positive axillary nodes or pN3b in the presence of positive axillary nodes.
- Supraclavicular nodal involvement is now reclassified as N3 disease; thus a patient with supraclavicular nodal involvement does not automatically have stage IV disease.
- Infraclavicular nodal involvement is added as N3 disease.
- Axillary lymph node involvement is now classified by the number of nodes involved. Involvement of 1 to 3 axillary nodes is considered pN1 disease. Involvement of 4 to 9 axillary nodes is considered pN2 disease. Involvement of greater than 10 axillary nodes is considered pN3 disease.

Staging of breast cancer can be divided into clinical staging versus pathologic staging. Factors used for clinical staging include the size of the tumor within the breast, presence or absence of pathologically confirmed lymph nodes, and presence or absence of distant metastasis. There are five stages for breast cancer. Stage 0 is defined as the presence of in situ disease only, without evidence of nodal or distant metastasis. Stage I is considered breast cancer confined to the breast, regardless of tumor size. Exception to this general characterization includes tumors with extension to the chest wall or skin or inflammatory breast cancers. These tumors are at least stage IIIB. Stage II is considered a breast cancer of any size with pathologically positive ipsilateral mobile axillary nodes. Stage IIIA is considered a breast cancer of any size with pathologically positive ipsilateral fixed axillary nodes or clinically apparent internal mammary nodes in the absence of positive axillary nodes. Also any large tumors (bigger than 5 cm) with any type of positive axillary or internal mammary nodes are considered stage IIIA. Stage IIIB tumors are breast tumors with extension to the skin or chest wall or inflammatory breast cancer. Involvement of the pectoralis major or minor muscle does not constitute chest wall involvement. Stage IIIC tumors are breast cancers of any size with either positive infraclavicular or supraclavicular nodes or positive internal mammary nodes in the presence of positive axillary nodes. Stage IV connotes any breast cancers with distant metastasis (see Figure 3).

Pathologic staging of breast cancer is more complicated and differs from clinical staging in that the number of nodes involved as well as how nodal metastasis is detected are used in stage designation of nodal status (Figures 4 and 5).

SURGICAL TREATMENT OF THE BREAST

A significant paradigm shift in the treatment of breast cancer has occurred over the past several decades. The Halsted paradigm, popularized at the beginning of the 20th century, hypothesized that breast cancer spreads in a contiguous fashion from the breast to the axillary lymph nodes and then to distant sites elsewhere in the body. The Fisher paradigm, which views breast cancer as systemic from very early in the course of the disease, modified this theory; the axillary lymph nodes act not as a barrier but as indicators of disease aggressiveness. Both paradigms are correct and incorrect. At a certain point in the evolution of a breast cancer, the disease changes from a local disease to a systemic disease. The Halsted paradigm promotes more intensive local treatment to eradicate the cancer, whereas the Fisher paradigm promotes less aggressive local treatment with the addition of systemic treatment in most women, even with relatively early disease. Because of this philosophy change and the detection of earlier disease through diligent screening techniques, surgical treatment of breast cancer is progressing toward less radical surgery and more adjuvant therapy, with equal or better outcomes. Recent mammograms of both breasts should be reviewed for any other suspicious lesions. There may be a slight increase in synchronous breast cancer in patients with invasive lobular cancer, although the rate of

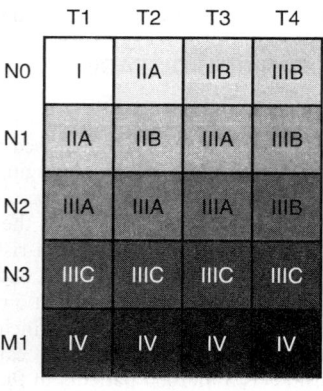

FIGURE 4. Pathologic staging of breast cancer.

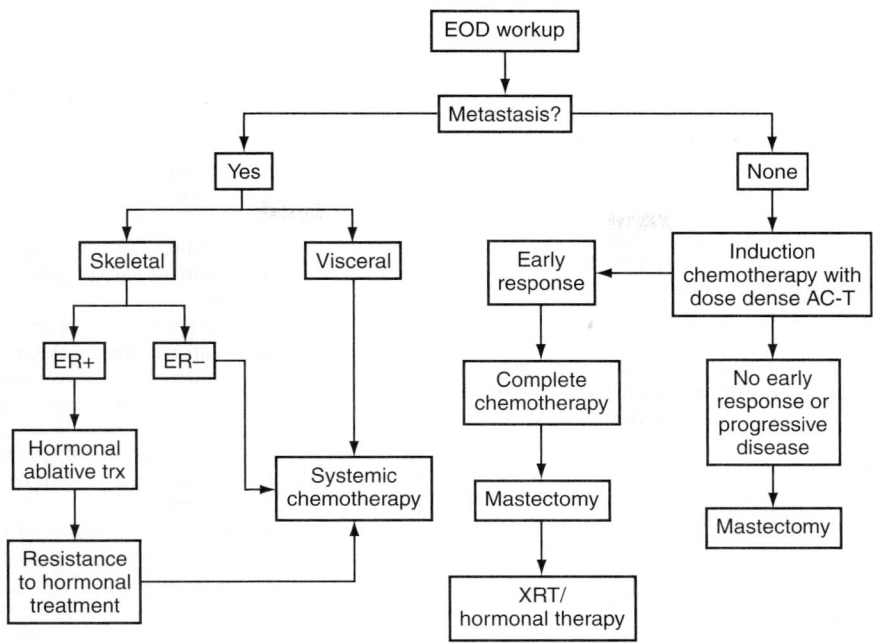

FIGURE 5. Algorithm for treatment of locally advanced breast cancer (LABC). AC-T = Adriamycyin and cyclophosphamide plus Taxol; EOD = extent-of-disease; trx = treatment; XRT = x-radiation therapy.

contralateral breast cancer is equal to that of invasive ductal carcinoma over the lifetime of the patient. The risk of distant metastasis is 25% to 50% in patients with inflammatory breast cancer.

Breast Conservation Therapy

Most small noninvasive and invasive breast cancers are treated by BCT, which consists of wide local excision with negative surgical margins and irradiation of the breast. The NSABP B-06, Milan I and Milan II, as well as other clinical trials, show no statistically significant difference in patient survival with mastectomy or BCT.

The addition of radiation treatment to wide local excision in patients with noninvasive and invasive carcinoma is currently the standard of treatment. The NSABP B-06 randomized trial evaluated local recurrence of small invasive tumors with and without irradiation after lumpectomy. It found that patients who did not undergo radiation therapy had significantly higher rates of local recurrence. With BCT, incidence of recurrence in the treated breast is 7% at 5 years, 14% at 10 years, and 20% at 20 years. Local recurrence rate is much lower in patients treated with mastectomy, with an overall incidence of 5% to 10%. The majority of recurrences occur in the first 3 years after surgery. Contraindications to BCT include tumor of any size that cannot be adequately excised with significant deformity to the breast, multicentric disease, noncompliant patient, first- or second-trimester pregnant patient, history of significant collagen vascular disease, and history of previous radiation therapy to the chest wall. If both BCT and mastectomy are viable options, the patient's preference should also play a role in the decision to proceed with BCT versus a mastectomy.

MASTECTOMY

A patient with contraindications to breast conservation should have a mastectomy with or without immediate reconstruction. Total mastectomy surgically removes the breast parenchyma, pectoral fascia, nipple, and the areola complex. A modified radical mastectomy includes axillary dissection. A radical mastectomy, rarely done today, includes removal of the pectoralis major and minor muscles and axillary dissection.

BREAST RECONSTRUCTION

Any patient recommended to have a mastectomy should be offered the option of immediate or delayed reconstruction and referred to a plastic and reconstructive surgeon to discuss which techniques are appropriate. One commonly used method of breast reconstruction is a tissue expander breast implant. A tissue expander is placed beneath the pectoralis muscles, and expansions are performed over a period of several weeks to months to stretch the subpectoral pocket to accommodate the permanent implant. The permanent saline or silicone implant is then inserted as a secondary procedure.

Another method of breast reconstruction is the transverse rectus abdominis myocutaneous (TRAM) flap, which involves the transfer of skin, fat, and muscle from the lower part of the abdomen to create a reconstructed breast. This procedure can be performed as a free flap with the arterial and venous supply anastomosed to vessels in the axilla or as a pedicle flap with the arterial and venous supply from the superior epigastric vessels. Other types of flap reconstructions include latissimus dorsi or gluteal flaps. Reconstruction of the nipple and areola is often performed as a later procedure.

SURGICAL TREATMENT OF THE AXILLA

The status of the axilla should be assessed for metastases in any patient with invasive breast cancer for several reasons. The status of the axillary lymph nodes is important in determining the patient's stage of disease. The presence or absence of axillary lymph node metastases is predictive of the prognosis and facilitates decisions by the medical oncology team regarding adjuvant therapy. Relapse-free survival is closely related to the number of lymph nodes that are positive. In a study of 2873 patients, Hilsenbeck found that the relapse-free survival at 5 years was 80% in patients with node-negative disease. This number decreased to 70%, 60%, and 40% with 1 to 3 positive nodes, 4 to 9 positive nodes, and more than 10 positive nodes, respectively. Nodal status is now incorporated into the sixth revision of the AJCC staging system. Surgical removal of metastatic nodes in the axilla significantly decreases the possibility of axillary recurrence. ALND may improve overall survival, but this issue is debated in the medical literature.

Sentinel Lymph Node Biopsy

Axillary dissection traditionally was performed on all patients with invasive breast cancer. Today, sentinel lymphadenectomy, or sentinel lymph node (SLN) biopsy, identifies the first, or sentinel, lymph node or nodes in the axillary chain to receive drainage from the breast cancer and thus the most likely to contain metastases. The SLN biopsy is performed by injecting isosulfan blue dye and/or radioactive isotope to localize the sentinel lymph node.

The sentinel node can be identified in 95% of all cases. Multiple studies show that SLN biopsy can predict accurately the presence of axillary metastases in T1-2 breast cancer with a false-negative rate of 5% and an accuracy rate of 95%. The false-negative rate of SLN biopsy can be decreased to 1% to 3% if any palpable node is removed along with any hot or blue nodes. The SLN biopsy, a less invasive way to assess the status of the axilla, is associated with fewer complications than an axillary node dissection. Areas of controversy in SLN biopsy include T3, palpable suspicious axillary lymph nodes, and previous neoadjuvant therapy. In a study by Specht, 25% of palpable suspicious axillary lymph nodes proved benign on final pathology. Previous axillary dissection is not a strict contraindication per se because 75% of these patients can still have an identifiable sentinel node. The success rate depends on the number of nodes previously removed, with a success rate of 87% when fewer than 10 nodes are removed versus a success rate of 47% when more than 10 nodes are removed. Contraindications to SLN biopsy include T4 breast cancer and pregnancy. SLN biopsy is contraindicated in pregnancy because of the lack of data regarding fetal safety, although computer models suggest the amount of radiation exposure to the fetus is negligible.

Axillary Dissection

Patients who have metastatic cells on SLN biopsy typically undergo complete ALND. Alternatively, if a patient is not a candidate for SLN biopsy, ALND should be considered. Axillary dissection involves the removal of 10 to 30 lymph nodes from the axilla. The potential risk of axillary dissection includes the accumulation of a seroma, ipsilateral arm lymphedema, and numbness around the area of the intercostal brachial innervation if the nerve is sacrificed at the time of surgery. Because of the lifetime increased chance of arm lymphedema and possible infection, patients should avoid any trauma or procedures such as venipuncture or blood pressure measurements on the ipsilateral arm.

Adjuvant Therapy

Adjuvant therapy is used to treat patients with a demonstrable likelihood for the development of metastatic disease. Most medical oncologists consider this risk sufficient in node-negative patients with a tumor diameter of 1 cm or larger and in those with nodal metastases to justify adjuvant chemotherapy or hormonal therapy. Most commonly used cytotoxic regimens include CMF (cyclophosphamide [Cytoxan], methotrexate, and 5-FU [fluorouracil]) for 6 cycles or AC-T for 8 cycles (4 cycles of doxorubicin [Adriamycin] and cyclophosphamide followed by 4 cycles of paclitaxel [Taxol]). There appears to be a slight improvement of 3% in overall survival favoring the anthracycline-containing regimen over the CMF regimens. In the elderly population, the CMF regimen may be easier to tolerate than the AC-T regimens. In a recent study, a dose dense regimen of AC-T results in a slight improvement of disease-free and overall survival. Dose-dense regimen involves giving the chemotherapy in cycles every 2 weeks, with bone marrow support such as G-CSF (Neupogen), as opposed to the traditional cycles every 3 weeks. The improvement in survival is approximately 3%. In the Early Breast Cancer Trialists' Collaborative Group (EBCTCG) meta-analysis, adjuvant chemotherapy appears the most beneficial for women younger than 50 years of age. Combination chemotherapy resulted in the improvement of 10-year-overall survival from 71% in node-negative patients not receiving chemotherapy to 78% in those that did receive chemotherapy. This increase was even more dramatic in node-positive patients, with an improvement of overall survival from 42% to 53%. A much smaller effect was seen in patients older than 50 years of age. In this group of patients, survival was increased from 67% to 69% when node-negative patients not receiving chemotherapy were compared to those receiving chemotherapy. In node-positive elderly patients, improvement in overall survival was also minimal, with an increase of survival from 47% to 49% with chemotherapy.

Hormonal therapy, such as tamoxifen, is a commonly used adjuvant treatment in early breast cancer patients with estrogen receptor–positive tumors. The EBCTCG meta-analysis looking at the role of tamoxifen in the premenopausal patients found that tamoxifen results in an absolute improvement of 10-year overall survival of 5.6% in node-negative patients and 10.9% in node-positive patients. This effect is even greater in the postmenopausal population, with a 26% proportional reduction in 10-year mortality rates. The recommended length of treatment for node-negative patients is 5 years. Additionally, tamoxifen can be used as a chemopreventive agent to decrease the chance of an additional ipsilateral tumor developing in patients undergoing breast conservation or to decrease the possibility of contralateral breast cancer.

More recently, three large randomized trials of aromatase inhibitors, such as anastrozole (Arimidex), exemestane (Aromasin), and letrozole (Femara), was published. In the ATAC (Arimidex, Tamoxifen, Alone or in Combination) trial, patients on anastrozole had a statistically significant longer disease-free interval when compared with patients on tamoxifen alone (hazard ratio of 0.83). No difference in survival was seen between the two groups. In another large study, patients on tamoxifen for 2 to 3 years were randomized to continuing tamoxifen versus switching to exemestane for a total of 5 years of therapy. There appeared to be an improvement in disease-free survival in the aromatase inhibitor arm (hazard ratio of 0.68). No difference in survival was seen, and given the early stoppage and cross-over of patients, no survival data will be obtainable from this study. Yet another large double-blinded randomized trial involved patients who had finished a 5-year course of tamoxifen and were then randomized to receiving letrozole versus placebo. The trial was stopped at a mean follow-up of 2.4 years secondary to a significant improvement in disease-free survival in the letrozole arm (hazard ratio of 0.57). Again, no difference in survival was seen. Aromatase inhibitors are useful only in postmenopausal patients. Premenopausal patients may benefit from an aromatase inhibitor only after ovarian ablation.

Recommendations regarding tamoxifen, aromatase inhibitors, and chemotherapy depend on the clinical judgment of the treating medical oncologist. In general, if adjuvant chemotherapy is given, it should take place prior to the initiation of radiotherapy. Consideration should be given to the likelihood of systemic recurrence based on nodal status, tumor size, and tumor grade. Estrogen receptor positivity of the tumor is predictive of a response to hormonal therapy, and HER2-neu may determine the type of appropriate chemotherapy. Another factor is the patient's age and any co-morbid diseases that would decrease the patient's tolerance to a course of chemotherapy.

Surveillance After a Diagnosis of Breast Cancer

Surveillance should continue alter diagnosis and treatment of breast cancer to detect local recurrence or a new primary breast cancer in either the ipsilateral or contralateral breast. The National Comprehensive Cancer Network guidelines recommend that patients continue diligent monthly self-examinations and that a physician perform a physical examination at 6-month intervals to assess for evidence of local recurrence and symptoms of metastatic disease. The ipsilateral arm should be evaluated to detect early signs of lymphedema and initiate appropriate management. Bilateral mammograms should be obtained every year. Bone and computed tomographic scans and other tumor markers should be performed only on patients with symptomatic systemic disease because of the lack of evidence of improved survival with early detection of distant metastases.

Special Topics in Breast Disease

PHYLLODES TUMOR

Phyllodes tumor (cystosarcoma phyllodes) is a fibroepithelial lesion that can be either benign or malignant. It is a rare tumor of the breast accounting for 1% of all cases. The mean age of patients is 54 years of age. These tumors often present as a breast mass on clinical and mammographic examination, and they are considered benign or malignant depending on stromal cellularity, mitotic activity, presence of necrosis, and type of borders. Treatment is complete excision without axillary node dissection. Metastases secondary to malignant phyllodes are hematogenous and primarily travel to the lungs. It is important to obtain negative margins. A mastectomy occasionally may be warranted for large lesions. Patients with malignant phyllodes have an 80% chance of 5-year survival as opposed to more than 95% for benign phyllodes.

NIPPLE DISCHARGE

Nipple discharge can occur at any age and presents as a bloody, serous, or milky discharge. Only 6% to 12% of patients with a nipple discharge are found to have an underlying malignancy. This risk is slightly elevated if the discharge is bloody. The most common cause of serous or serosanguineous nipple discharge is a benign intraductal papilloma. Numerous drugs can also cause nipple discharge, such as phenothiazine, tricyclic antidepressants, reserpine, butyrophenones, cimetidine (Tagamet), verapamil (Calan), metoclopramide (Reglan), thiazides, and hormone replacement therapy. The most common underlying malignancy is DCIS. Ductograms may be useful in locating the papilloma. When the nipple discharge is unilaterally persistent, spontaneous, or postmenopausal, further workup may be considered. Other suspicious nipple discharges are those confined to one duct or that are bloody or serous. In general, the evaluation of nipple discharge should begin with a clinical examination and a mammogram. Cytologic examination of the discharge has a low sensitivity for detection of underlying malignancy and should be not be used in the workup. Treatment consists of a major duct excision.

GYNECOMASTIA

Gynecomastia is the unilateral or bilateral benign enlargement of male breast tissue. The etiology is often related to various substances, including exogenous hormones, cimetidine (Tagamet), thiazides, digoxin, theophylline, phenothiazines, alcohol, and marijuana use; it may also be idiopathic. The main concern is to rule out the diagnosis of male breast cancer. Once breast cancer is excluded, no treatment is indicated. If medication and lifestyle etiologies are eliminated without remission of the gynecomastia, the excess breast tissue may be surgically removed for cosmetic considerations or for breast pain.

MALE BREAST CANCER

Carcinoma of the male breast represents 1% of all breast cancers. Because men are not routinely screened for breast cancer, the diagnosis is often delayed. The most common manifestation of male breast cancer is a painless, firm, subareolar breast mass. The differential diagnosis includes gynecomastia. Breast imaging with mammography and/or ultrasound may be helpful in rendering a diagnosis inasmuch as the appearance of male breast cancer is a stellate, irregular solid mass. Any suspicious breast mass in a male patient should undergo diagnostic biopsy. If a malignancy is diagnosed, standard treatment is mastectomy with assessment of the axillary nodes by SLN biopsy or ALND. Most cases of male breast cancer are estrogen receptor positive, and recommendations for adjuvant chemotherapy or hormonal therapy should be based on criteria similar to those for breast cancer in female patients.

BREAST CANCER IN PREGNANCY

Pregnancy-associated breast cancer represents less than 2% of all breast cancer diagnoses. The breast cancer frequently is diagnosed at a late stage because of the difficulty of examining the breast in pregnant women and the avoidance of mammography during pregnancy. Any suspicious lesion noted during pregnancy should be subjected to biopsy in the same fashion as in a nongravid woman. Radiation therapy should not be administered during pregnancy, so breast conservation is generally contraindicated unless the diagnosis is made within a few weeks of delivery. Surgical treatment with mastectomy and ALND is the standard treatment of breast cancer during pregnancy. Adjuvant chemotherapy can be delivered with selective agents during the second and third trimesters. The prognosis is similar to that of nongravid women in whom breast cancer is diagnosed at a comparable stage.

INFLAMMATORY BREAST CANCER

The classic manifestation of inflammatory breast cancer is erythema, edema, peau d'orange, and color of the breast resembling an infectious process. Malignant cells within the dermal lymphatic vessels of the breast confirm the diagnosis. The usual pathology of the associated carcinoma is IFDC-NOS. Inflammatory carcinoma is a very aggressive type of breast cancer, with over 90% of patients having positive axillary lymph nodes at diagnosis. The recommended treatment is multimodality therapy, with chemotherapy preceding surgery. Surgical treatment is mastectomy followed by radiation therapy and often additional chemotherapy.

LOCALLY ADVANCED BREAST CANCER

Patients with N2 or N3 nodal status or those with four or more positive axillary nodes, T3 or T4 tumors, or involvement of the pectoralis fascia have locally advanced breast cancer (LABC). The recommended treatment for patients is neoadjuvant chemotherapy, which is administered before surgical treatment, although it has no impact on overall survival. An extent-of-disease (EOD) workup should be done in patients with LABC and includes a computed tomography (CT) of the chest, abdomen, and pelvis along with a bone scan. Figure 5 provides an algorithm for the treatment of LABC.

Endometriosis

Method of
David L. Olive, MD

Endometriosis is one of the most common diseases encountered by the practicing gynecologist, yet it is also one of the most vexing. Researchers have been searching for answers to even the most fundamental questions regarding this disease for well over a century; even today huge gaps remain in the understanding of this disorder.

Definition

Endometriosis is defined as the presence of endometrial glands and stroma outside the endometrial cavity and uterine musculature. The requirement for both glands and stroma is an arbitrary standard, and it is unclear whether either component of endometrium alone, if placed ectopically, can result in the symptoms and signs of endometriosis.

Two related diseases are also frequently observed. Adenomyosis is the presence of endometrial glands and stroma within the myometrium. This disorder is epidemiologically and pathogenically distinct from endometriosis, but the resulting symptoms (and medical treatments) are similar. Endosalpingiosis is identical to endometriosis in location and appearance but histologically resembles tubal glands and stroma. This latter abnormality has been poorly studied, and to date, little is known regarding the distinction between endometriosis and endosalpingiosis.

Genetics

Evidence continues to accumulate that endometriosis has a genetic basis. Evidence for this includes familial clustering, concordance in monozygotic twins, and increased prevalence among first-degree relatives. A search was recently undertaken to identify the gene or genes responsible for susceptibility to endometriosis. Although suggestive linkages were discovered, no genes have been firmly identified as instrumental in this disorder. It is hoped, however, that genetic research will eventually uncover information critical to understanding the molecular and cellular basis of this disease.

Pathogenesis

The pathogenesis of endometriosis is a controversial subject inspiring many researchers to investigate it. Over the last 25 years considerable advancement has been made, providing solid clues to the understanding of the disease process. Today, a clear picture is beginning to emerge regarding how women develop endometriosis.

HISTOGENESIS

Leading researchers in the field have proposed numerous theories of histogenesis. The primary theory of histogenesis is transplantation of shed uterine endometrium to ectopic locations. A number of routes of dissemination of the tissue are proposed, including lymphatic dissemination, vascular spread, iatrogenic transplantation, and retrograde menstruation.

A critical aspect of this theory is that cast-off endometrium cells remain viable and capable of implanting. Furthermore, it proposes that the tissue distribution has the capacity to sustain implantation. Considerable research has established that shed endometrial cells are viable in vitro. In vitro studies of endometrial attachment to peritoneum also support the concept of transplantation, attachment, and invasion.

Additional theories of histogenesis include coelomic metaplasia and induction of endometriosis. However, little scientific evidence indicates that either route is a viable etiology of the disease, much less a common method for development.

ETIOLOGY AND MAINTENANCE

Retrograde menstruation is a well-established phenomenon. Data available from women undergoing peritoneal dialysis and laparoscopy at the time of menses suggest that 76% to 90% of women have retrograde flow. This mechanism is considered a critical first step in the initiation of much if not most endometriosis by a wide variety of epidemiologic and anatomic data. However, the majority of women do not have endometriosis. The question that arises is "Why not?"

Because the placement of menstrual debris into the peritoneal cavity happens with each menses, a mechanism must exist to eliminate this tissue. The prime candidate for removal of endometrial cells is cell-mediated cytotoxicity. Deficient cytotoxic response to ectopic endometrium is suggested as a mechanism for allowing implantation and growth. It is also postulated that factors positively affecting growth and maintenance may be altered to enhance the risk of endometriosis. Current evidence suggests that a variety of cytokines, including monocyte chemotactic protein-1, interleukin-8, and regulated on activation, T-cell expressed and secreted (RANTES) are overexpressed in women with endometriosis, resulting in the attraction and activation of macrophages. The source of this cytokine increase could be one or more of several tissues: Endometrium, peritoneal mesothelium, and macrophages themselves could be the primary aberrancy by which this cascade is begun.

Other abnormalities are speculated to promote endometriosis. These include abnormal expression of matrix metalloproteinases and the enzyme aromatase, which could locally produce a hyperestrogenic proimplantation environment. The mechanisms by which these abnormalities may cause disease as well as the source of such alterations are under investigation.

Prevalence and Epidemiology

Endometriosis is a disease found almost exclusively in reproductive-age women. The mean age at diagnosis is reported to be from 25 to 29 years, although this figure depends on the diagnostic method. Because traditional diagnosis requires laparoscopy, it is likely that the disease is frequently present in even younger patients for whom many gynecologists do not readily schedule surgery.

Although rare in the premenarcheal female, adolescent endometriosis is a relatively common entity. Endometriosis is found in 47% to 65% of women younger than 20 years with chronic pelvic pain or dyspareunia.

Endometriosis is associated with increased exposure to menstruation typified by earlier menarche, more frequent menses, longer menses, fewer pregnancies, later initial pregnancy, and less breast-feeding. In addition, factors known to decrease the amount of menses or lower estrogen levels also reduce the risk: oral contraceptive use, irregular menses/oligomenorrhea, stress, exercise, and cigarette smoking (Box 1).

Postmenopausal endometriosis seldom occurs; this age group represents only 2% to 4% of all women requiring laparoscopy for endometriosis. The majority of such cases are a sequela to reactivation of disease by hormone replacement therapy; this is not true in all cases.

Clinical Presentation

Endometriosis is associated with a wide array of presenting signs and symptoms, although many women with physical manifestations of the disease remain completely asymptomatic. Commonly, the severity of symptoms does not correlate with the stage of endometriosis; extensive disease sometimes causes only minimal symptoms, and in others, minimal disease can be associated with severe symptoms. Some symptoms may strongly suggest the presence of endometriosis, but none are pathognomonic of this disorder. Because endometriosis most commonly involves the pelvis, infertility, dysmenorrhea, pelvic pain, dyspareunia, and menstrual dysfunction are common clinical presentations. When the ovary is severely involved, an ovarian cyst or pelvic mass may be the initial sign of endometriosis.

Pelvic pain is the most frequent complaint for endometriosis patients. This generally presents as secondary dysmenorrhea, worsening primary dysmenorrhea, dyspareunia, or even noncyclic lower abdominal pain, chronic pelvic pain, and backaches. In addition, pain may be site specific when endometriosis is found in unusual locations outside of the pelvis.

Only rarely are physical findings specific for endometriosis. Localized cul-de-sac and uterosacral ligament tenderness may frequently be detected. Thickened, nodular uterosacral ligaments or rectovaginal masses may be palpable. Adnexal enlargement or tenderness may reflect ovarian involvement. Retroverted fixation of the uterus may be noted with posterior cul-de-sac obliteration by the disease.

BOX 1 Epidemiology of Endometriosis

Increased risk with:
- Menses >6 d
- More menses

Decreased risk with:
- Increased parity
- Irregular menses
- Oral contraceptives
- Late menarche
- Exercise
- Smoking

Cutaneous manifestations may be present, with apparent lesions on the perineum or vagina, or, less commonly, in the inguinal region, the umbilical area, or at the site of surgical scars. They should be suspected whenever a scar or lesion is associated with cyclical pain, tenderness, swelling, or bleeding.

Diagnosis

The current gold standard for the definitive diagnosis of endometriosis is laparoscopy. However, because of the heterogeneity in appearance of endometriosis lesions, the accuracy of laparoscopic diagnosis is variable and depends on the ability of the surgeon to recognize the disease. Although histologic confirmation would be ideal to ensure the presence of disease, this is infrequently accomplished because of the reticence of surgeons to excise endometriosis lesions.

Ultrasound is most useful for the detection of ovarian endometriomas, although the appearance of a cystic structure with heightened echogenicity is certainly not limited to this form of endometriosis. Structures often confused with endometriomas include corpora lutea, hemorrhagic cysts, unilocular dermoid cysts, and other benign cystic neoplasias. Ultrasound is not currently useful for identifying focal implants.

Magnetic resonance imaging (MRI) demonstrates significant potential in the diagnosis of endometriosis. MRI is clearly of value in diagnosing the ovarian endometrioma, and as technology improves, the potential for detecting peritoneal lesions will increase.

Treatment

MEDICAL THERAPY

The first drug to be approved for the treatment of endometriosis in the United States was danazol (Danocrine), a derivative of testosterone. It was originally thought to produce a pseudomenopause, but subsequent studies have revealed that the drug acts primarily by diminishing the midcycle luteinizing hormone (LH) surge, creating a chronic anovulatory state. The recommended dosage of danazol for the treatment of endometriosis is 600 to 800 mg/day; however, these doses have substantial androgenic side effects such as increased hair growth, mood changes, adverse serum lipid profiles, deepening of the voice (possibly irreversible), and, rarely, liver damage (possibly irreversible and life threatening) and arterial thrombosis. Studies of lower doses as primary treatment for endometriosis-associated pain have been uncontrolled or with small numbers and thus contain information of limited value.

Progestogens are a class of compounds that produce progesterone-like effects on endometrial tissue. A large number of progestogens exist, ranging from those chemically derived from progesterone (progestins), such as medroxyprogesterone acetate (MPA), to 19-nortestosterone derivatives such as norethindrone and norgestrel. The proposed mechanism of action of these compounds causes initial

CURRENT DIAGNOSIS

- Symptoms associated with endometriosis are primarily those of pain and infertility, although site-specific symptoms and signs may exist when the disease is in unusual locations.
- The standard for diagnosis is laparoscopic visualization; however, this method has a high false-positive and false-negative rate. The only method to confirm the disease absolutely is excisional biopsy.

CURRENT THERAPY

- Both medical and surgical therapies are efficacious in the treatment of endometriosis-associated pain. It is unclear which offers the better approach.
- Combined medical/surgical therapy may offer an advantage over surgery alone, if the medication is used at least 6 months postoperatively.
- Medical therapy has no role in the treatment of endometriosis-associated infertility.
- Surgical therapy for endometriosis-associated infertility appears to be of value for all stages of disease, but its relative value compared to assisted reproduction is not yet determined.

shedding of endometrial tissue followed by eventual atrophy. The most extensively studied progestational agent for the treatment of endometriosis is medroxyprogesterone (dep-subQ Provera 104), which is currently approved by the Food and Drug Administration (FDA) for use in treating endometriosis in a depot subcutaneous form. A common side effect is transient breakthrough bleeding, which occurs in 38% to 47% of patients. This is generally well tolerated and, when necessary, can be adequately treated with supplemental estrogen or an increase in the progestogen dose. Other side effects include nausea (0% to 80%), breast tenderness (5%), fluid retention (50%), and depression (6%). A recent approach to treating endometriosis with progestogen is the use of a progestogen-containing intrauterine contraceptive device[1] (Mirena).

The combination of estrogen and progestogen for therapy of endometriosis, the so-called pseudopregnancy regimen, has been used for 40 years. The most commonly used pseudopregnancy regimen today is the oral contraceptive pill[1] (OCP); in fact, it is the most commonly prescribed treatment for endometriosis symptoms. Like progestational therapy, pseudopregnancy is believed to produce initial decidualization and growth of endometrial tissue, followed in several months by atrophy.

Gonadotropin-releasing hormone (GnRH) agonists are analogues of the hormone GnRH. This hypothalamic hormone is responsible for stimulating the pituitary gland to secrete follicle-stimulating hormone (FSH) and LH, two hormones necessary for normal ovarian function. GnRH is secreted in a pulsatile manner; the correct pulse results in stimulation of FSH and LH release, whereas too high or too low a pulse rate results in a decrease in pituitary hormone secretion. GnRH agonists are modified forms of GnRH that bind to the pituitary receptors and remain for a lengthy period. Thus, they are identified by the pituitary as rapidly pulsatile GnRH, and after initial stimulation of FSH and LH secretion, result in a shutdown (downregulation) of the pituitary and no stimulation of the ovary. The result is a hypoestrogenic state similar to that of menopause, producing endometrial atrophy and amenorrhea. The agonist can be given intranasally (naferelin [Synarel]), subcutaneously (goserelin [Zoladex]), or intramuscularly (IM) (leuprolide acetate [Lupro Depot]), depending on the specific product, with frequency of administration ranging from twice daily to every 3 months. The side effects are those of hypoestrogenism such as transient vaginal bleeding, hot flashes, vaginal dryness, decreased libido, breast tenderness, insomnia, depression, irritability and fatigue, headache, osteoporosis, and decreased skin elasticity; these are dose dependent.

A recent modification of GnRH agonist treatment is to add back small amounts of steroid hormone in a manner similar to that used in the treatment of postmenopausal women. The theory is that the requirement for estrogen is greater for endometriosis than is needed by the brain (to prevent hot flashes), the bone (to prevent osteoporosis), and other tissues deprived of this hormone. With this approach

[1]Not FDA approved for this indication.

there is an equivalent rate of pain relief with far fewer side effects than GnRH agonist alone. Estrogen as a solitary add-back, however, is less effective and thus not indicated.

SURGICAL THERAPY

Most surgeons performing surgery for endometriosis must choose one of two possibilities: conservative surgery, where the patient's future fertility remains an option, or definitive surgery. The latter procedure generally involves removal of the female gonads, a hysterectomy, or a combination of the two. The general perception is that definitive surgery is more effective over time than conservative treatment, but it must be reserved for patients in whom fertility or continued endocrine function is deemed less important than relief of pain symptoms.

When conservative surgery is desired, the first technical issue confronted is method of access. Traditionally, laparotomy was used for endometriosis surgery. However, recently, most surgeons performing extensive surgery for endometriosis have favored a laparoscopic approach because of improved magnification of disease with a resulting increase in surgical precision.

Surgical destruction of endometriosis lesions can be accomplished in a variety of ways: Excision, vaporization, and fulguration/desiccation have all been used. Excision is generally thought to be the most complete of these techniques, but no comparative trials have assessed the relative efficacy of each approach.

Endometriomas, or ovarian cysts formed from endometriosis, are commonly present in the patient with endometriosis. The ovaries should first be freed of all adhesions when operating on endometriomas. The endometrioma may open spontaneously during this process; if not, incision and drainage is indicated. At this point, the cyst wall may be stripped, excised, or drained.

TREATMENT RESULTS

Medical therapy is effective against endometriosis-associated pain. Placebo-controlled randomized clinical trials (RCTs) have proven that danazol and medroxyprogesterone reduce pain significantly better than no treatment for up to 6 months following discontinuation of the drug. No good data exist for longer follow-up periods. Numerous randomized trials have compared medical therapies to one another. In 15 RCTs comparing danazol to GnRH agonists, no difference was demonstrated between the two as first-line drugs. Similarly, little difference was seen when GnRH agonists were compared to oral contraceptives, progestogens, or gestrinone.

Several trials have addressed the efficacy of combined add-back therapy and GnRH agonist treatment during 6-month treatment periods. In general, pain was relieved as effectively with the combination as with GnRH agonist alone, and it significantly reduced the side effects of the GnRH agonist. The results were similar in three longer trials of approximately 1-year duration (Figure 1). The amelioration of side effects with maintenance of efficacy seems to be even when the add-back therapy is begun during the first month of treatment, suggesting that an add-back-free interval at the beginning of a treatment cycle is unnecessary.

Although the studies just described randomize patients for initial therapy of endometriosis-associated pain, one study examined the value of GnRH agonist in patients failing primary therapy. Ling and colleagues treated women having failed to obtain relief with OCPs with either GnRH agonist or placebo. Those treated with active drug responded significantly better than those given placebo, with more than 80% experiencing pain relief in 3 months (Figure 2). Of interest is the fact that the therapy seemed to be beneficial whether or not endometriosis was seen at laparoscopy.

Most of the established medical therapies used to treat endometriosis have been applied to the problem of subfertility in women with this disease. These medications inhibit ovulation, and thus they are used to treat the disease for a period of time prior to allowing an attempt at conception. Five randomized trials with six treatment arms have compared one of these medical treatments for endometriosis to placebo or no treatment with fertility as the outcome measure. Another eight RCTs compared danazol to a second medication. These

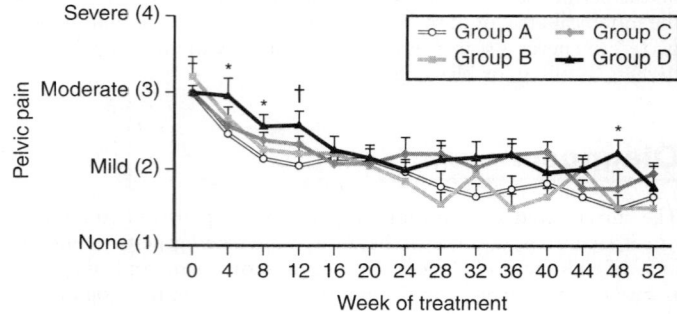

MEAN PELVIC PAIN SCORE AT EACH VISIT

* $P \le 05$ ⎱ Change from baseline
† $P \le 01$ ⎰ compared with Group A

FIGURE 1. Pain relief from gonadotropin-releasing hormone (GnRH) agonist (Group A) and three different add-back therapies. (High dose progestin, low dose estrogen/progestin, higher dose estrogen/progestin). No difference is seen among the groups in the amount of pain relief. (From Hornstein MD, Surrey ES, Weisberg GW, Casino LA: et al: Leuprolide acetate depot and hormonal add-back in endometriosis: A 12-month study. Lupron Add-Back Study Group. Obstet Gynecol 1998;91[1]:16–24.)

latter trials were summarized by a meta-analysis by Hughes et al. and modified by Olive and Pritts to include loss of fertility while on the medications (Figure 3). The data clearly show that medical therapy for endometriosis has not proven to be of value, and in fact may be counterproductive, to the subfertile patient.

Only two studies have investigated surgery for endometriosis-associated pain versus sham surgery. Sutton and colleagues assessed the efficacy of laser laparoscopic surgery in the treatment of pain associated with minimal, mild, or moderate endometriosis. They found that there was no difference in pain at 3 months follow-up, but by 6 months a clear-cut advantage was seen for surgery. Abbott and colleagues evaluated excision of endometriosis versus diagnostic laparoscopy and had nearly identical results at 6 months. Thus, both techniques were proven better than no therapy.

Conservative surgery was used extensively in an attempt to enhance fertility. Most studies, however, are uncontrolled and of poor quality. Two randomized trials were performed to examine the value

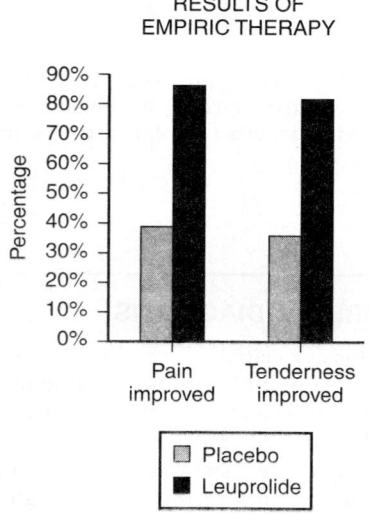

RESULTS OF EMPIRIC THERAPY

FIGURE 2. Patients with pain relief from empirical gonadotropin-releasing hormone (GnRH) agonist or placebo.

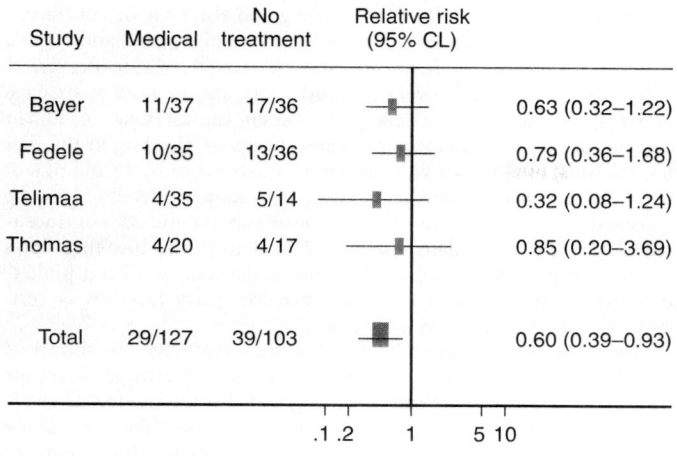

Study	Medical	No treatment	Relative risk (95% CL)
Bayer	11/37	17/36	0.63 (0.32–1.22)
Fedele	10/35	13/36	0.79 (0.36–1.68)
Telimaa	4/35	5/14	0.32 (0.08–1.24)
Thomas	4/20	4/17	0.85 (0.20–3.69)
Total	29/127	39/103	0.60 (0.39–0.93)

FIGURE 3. Meta-analysis of all randomized trials comparing medical therapy versus no treatment or placebo for endometriosis-associated infertility. Note that the untreated group has a significantly better pregnancy rate.

of ablation of early-stage endometriosis versus sham surgery, with contradictory results. When combined into a meta-analysis, surgical treatment of early-stage endometriosis still appears to provide a significant improvement in pregnancy rates. No such trials exist for more extensive disease; expert opinion would suggest that surgery will enhance fertility but may be inferior to advanced reproductive technologies.

The use of medical therapies for endometriosis is not restricted to their use as stand-alone agents. Clinicians frequently have used drugs in combination with surgical treatment of the disease. Numerous trials have examined the issue of postoperative medical therapy as an effective adjunct for pain. Those that have treated patients for at least 6 months after surgery showed efficacy, but in those studies where only 3 months of postoperative treatment was performed, no benefit was seen. Results are similar for all medications (Table 1).

In summary, endometriosis is an enigmatic disease that has long frustrated clinicians and patients. However, great strides in the understanding of this disorder are being made. The coming years are likely to produce a plethora of new treatment approaches targeting the biologic basis of this disease. In this regard, better understanding will undoubtedly result in renewed hope for the patient suffering from the ravages of endometriosis.

TABLE 1 Postoperative Medical Therapy

Drug	Duration of Treatment	Studies	Findings
OCPs	6 mo	1	NS at 24, 36 mo
Medroxy-progesterone, 100 mg/d	6 mo	1	$p < 0.05$ at 6 mo
Danazol, 600 mg/d	3 mo	1	NS at 6 mo
Danazol, 600 mg/d	6 mo	1	$p < 0.05$ at 6 mo
Danazol, 100 mg/d	6 mo	1	$p < 0.05$ at 24 mo
GnRH-a	3 mo	1	NS at 6 mo
GnRH-a	6 mo	2	$p = 0.008$ at 12 mo

Abbreviations: GnRH = gonadotropin-releasing hormone; NS = not significant; OCPs = oral contraceptive pills.

REFERENCES

Abbott JA, Hawe J, Hunter D, et al. Laparoscopic excision of endometriosis: A randomized, placebo controlled trial. Fertil Steril 2004;82:878–84.

Hornstein MD, Surrey ES, Weisberg GW, Casino LA. Lupron Add-Back Study Group. Leuprolide acetate depot and hormonal add-back in endometriosis: a 12-month study. Obstet Gynecol 1998;91:16–24.

Hughes E, Ferorkow D, Collins J, Vandekerckhone P. Ovulation suppression for endometriosis (Cochrane review). In: The Cochrane Library (issue 1). Oxford, England: Update Software; 2000.

Jacobson TZ, Barlow DH, Koninclex PR, et al. Laparoscopic surgery for subfertility associated with endometriosis. Cochrane Database Syst Rev 2002; (4):CD001398.

Jansen RPS, Russel P. Nonpigmented endometriosis: Clinical, laparoscopic and pathologic definition. Am J Obstet Gynecol 1986;155:1154.

Ling FW. Randomized controlled trial of depot leuprolide in patients with chronic pelvic pain and clinically suspected endometriosis. Obstet Gynecol 1999;93:51–8.

Moghissi KS, Schlaff WD, Olive DL, et al. Goserelin acetate (Zoladex) with or without hormone replacement therapy for the treatment of endometriosis. Fertil Steril 1998;69:1056–62.

Olive DL, Pritts EA. The treatment of endometriosis: a review of the evidence. Ann NY Acad Sci 2002;955:360–72.

Olive DL, Pritts EA. Treatment of endometriosis. N Engl J Med 2001;345: 266–75.

Sampson JA. Perforating hemorrhagic (chocolate) cysts of the ovary. Arch Surg 1921;3:245.

Sutton CJG, Ewen SP, Whitelaw N, Haines P. Prospective, randomized, double-blind, controlled trial of laser laparoscopy in the treatment of pelvic pain associated with minimal, mild, or moderate endometriosis. Fertil Steril 1994;62:696.

Abnormal Uterine Bleeding

Method of
Beth W. Rackow, MD, and Aydin Arici, MD

Abnormal uterine bleeding is a common disorder among reproductive-age women. Although abnormal bleeding involves a broad differential diagnosis, approximately 33–50% of women with abnormal bleeding are found to have a systemic disorder that affects the hypothalamic-pituitary-ovarian axis and hence makes them anovulatory. Normal menstrual bleeding predictably occurs at the end of an ovulatory cycle because of estrogen and progesterone withdrawal; the bleeding lasts up to 7 days, with a cycle interval of 24 to 35 days. Abnormal bleeding may present with altered intervals between menstrual cycles or changes in volume or duration of menstrual blood flow.

Evaluation of the woman with abnormal uterine bleeding must consider a broad differential diagnosis that includes a complication of pregnancy, cervical and uterine pathology (polyps, leiomyomas, adenomyosis, malignancies, chronic endometritis, congenital anomalies), infectious etiologies (sexually transmitted infections, vaginitis), endocrinopathies (thyroid or androgen disorders, hyperprolactinemia), medications (exogenous hormonal therapy, anticoagulants, antibiotics, glucocorticoids, tamoxifen [Nolvadex], herbal supplements), bleeding diathesis, systemic illness (liver or renal disease), and genital trauma or foreign bodies. A thorough menstrual history is essential and should include details about past and present length of intermenstrual intervals, regularity of menses, volume and duration of bleeding, onset of abnormal bleeding, factors associated with change in bleeding (postcoital, contraceptive method, postpartum, new medical diagnosis, change in weight), and associated symptoms such as premenstrual symptoms, dysmenorrhea, dyspareunia, pelvic pain, hirsutism, or galactorrhea. A complete medical history, list of medications, and review of systems help identify any systemic illness or medication effect contributing to the abnormal bleeding. The physical exam should include careful inspection of the external genitalia, vagina, and cervix and a bimanual exam to palpate the uterus and adnexa to assess size, contour, and tenderness.

Laboratory evaluation provides further information. A negative pregnancy test (preferably quantitative) rules out bleeding because of a pregnancy complication. A complete blood count evaluates for anemia and thrombocytopenia, and is important with prolonged or heavy bleeding. Endocrine testing may include serum thyroid stimulating hormone, prolactin, testosterone levels, and further evaluation as indicated. Coagulation studies (prothrombin, partial thromboplastin, bleeding time, and von Willebrand disease testing) should be performed in adolescents, women with unexplained menorrhagia, and those with a personal or family history concerning for a bleeding disorder. In the setting of a systemic disorder such as chronic liver or renal disease, appropriate testing should be performed.

An endometrial biopsy should be performed in women at high risk for hyperplasia and cancer based on age (35 years and older) and duration of unopposed estrogen exposure. Young women (less than 35 years old) with chronic anovulation, thus prolonged estrogen exposure, should also undergo endometrial biopsy because they can develop endometrial hyperplasia and cancer. If the biopsy reveals secretory endometrium, and not proliferative endometrium, this suggests that ovulation has occurred. A Pap smear, cervical cultures, and wet mount should also be performed as indicated.

A history of regular menstrual cycles with an increasing volume or duration of bleeding, or intermenstrual bleeding, is suggestive of an anatomic cause of abnormal bleeding. Transvaginal ultrasonography provides detailed assessment of the uterus and endometrium. Pathology such as leiomyomas and polyps can be identified, and size and location determined. Although an endometrial biopsy may not be necessary if the endometrium is thin (less than 5 mm), clinical suspicion of endometrial pathology takes precedence. Sonohysterography (or saline-infusion sonography) involves ultrasonographic assessment of the uterus and endometrium while sterile saline distends the uterine cavity. This procedure has high sensitivity and specificity for detecting uterine and endometrial pathology and is comparable to hysteroscopy. Hysteroscopy can simultaneously diagnose and treat intrauterine pathology, but involves an invasive procedure. During assessment of uterine anatomy, it is important to recognize when anatomic abnormalities, such as leiomyomas, are present but not contributing to the bleeding.

Anovulatory Uterine Bleeding

A menstrual history that reveals irregular, infrequent, unpredictable bleeding, a varying amount and duration of bleeding, and no reliable premenstrual symptoms is often sufficient to diagnose anovulatory bleeding. Considered a systemic disorder, anovulatory bleeding occurs because of a variety of endocrinologic, neurochemical or pharmacologic processes. Estrogen breakthrough is the most common scenario: persistently high estrogen levels stimulate overgrowth of an endometrium that is fragile without the stabilizing, growth-limiting effects of progesterone, and focal areas of the endometrium breakdown, bleed, and subsequently heal because of estrogen effect. Therefore, synchronous and complete endometrial shedding does not occur. This pattern of bleeding is common in women with polycystic ovary syndrome, in postmenarchal adolescents, and in perimenopausal women. Other conditions associated with anovulation include thyroid disorders, hyperprolactinemia, androgen disorders, psychological or physical stress, eating disorders, dramatic weight changes, and insulin resistance.

Management of anovulatory bleeding involves treating both the cause of anovulation and the abnormal bleeding. Progestins are the foundation of this medical therapy. Cyclic courses of progestin stabilize the estrogen-stimulated endometrium and result in withdrawal bleeding after the progestin course. Medications used for a 10–14 day course each month include medroxyprogesterone acetate (Provera), 10 mg, and norethindrone acetate (Aygestin), 5 mg. If bleeding does not occur after progestin withdrawal, the woman may also be hypoestrogenic, and further evaluation is indicated. Estrogen-progestin contraceptives effectively cause regular withdrawal bleeding and may decrease the volume of bleeding and also provide contraception. Combined contraceptives are available in pill, patch, and vaginal ring preparations. Medroxyprogesterone acetate (Depo-Provera),[1] 150 mg intramuscularly every 3 months, can also be used to manage anovulatory bleeding, especially if women cannot take combined contraceptives. This therapy may cause irregular bleeding in the first few months, but 50% of women report amenorrhea by 12 months of use. Treatment of prolonged heavy anovulatory bleeding can be achieved with either low-dose monophasic combined contraceptives,[1] one pill twice daily for 5 to 7 days until the bleeding slows or stops, followed by routine daily use if desired, or with a higher-dose course of progestin therapy. Once the heavy bleeding is controlled, further evaluation is warranted.

Estrogen therapy is indicated for the treatment of abnormal bleeding with a thinned endometrium due to low estrogen levels or prolonged bleeding. This can be accomplished with conjugated estrogens (Premarin),[1] 1.25 mg, or micronized estradiol (Estrace),[1] 2 mg daily for 7 to 10 days. Similarly, estrogen (a 7- to 10-day course) can be used to treat progestin breakthrough bleeding in the setting of long-acting progestin therapy (medroxyprogesterone acetate [Depo-Provera]).

Ovulatory Uterine Bleeding

Heavy or prolonged bleeding may occur during ovulatory cycles, and often no specific etiology is identified; local defects in endometrial hemostasis are implicated. A number of medical and surgical therapies are effective in this situation. Nonsteroidal anti-inflammatory drugs (NSAIDs), such as ibuprofen (Motrin),[1] naproxen (Aleve),[1] or mefenamic acid (Ponstel),[1] decrease menstrual blood loss by inhibiting prostaglandin synthesis, and thus altering the balance of factors required for endometrial hemostasis. NSAIDs may decrease blood loss by 20% to 40%, and should be initiated just prior to the onset of menses and continued for 3 to 5 days. Similarly, combined contraceptives can reduce menstrual flow by 40% to 60%. Another option is the levonorgestrel-releasing intrauterine system (Mirena)[1]; the local progestin effect on the endometrium is profound and can reduce menstrual blood loss by 75% to 90% in women with heavy bleeding. Gonadotropin-releasing hormone agonists produce a hypoestrogenic state and thus cause amenorrhea as well as shrinkage of myomas, if present. This therapy is best reserved for short-term management of heavy bleeding and severe anemia prior to a surgical procedure because of its cost and significant side effects such as menopausal symptoms and bone demineralization. The only FDA-approved nonhormonal treatment for heavy menstrual bleeding (menorrhagia) is tranexamic acid (Lysteda), an antifibrinolytic agent; two 650-mg tablets are taken for up to 5 days per month during menses.

Intermenstrual bleeding can also occur during ovulatory cycles. This abnormal bleeding can be caused by anatomic abnormalities, infection, or the preovulatory decline in estrogen. Conjugated estrogens (Premarin),[1] 1.25 mg, or micronized estradiol (Estrace), 2 mg for 2 to 3 days midcycle or 7 to 10 days for persistent break-through bleeding, may be effective.

For women who fail medical therapy or for those who do not desire future fertility, surgical management is appropriate. The definitive procedure is hysterectomy, but this surgery carries a significant risk of complications and involves longer recovery time. Endometrial ablation by hysteroscopic, thermal, or cryosurgical techniques is a less invasive procedure for the management of abnormal bleeding, and should be reserved for women who do not desire future fertility. These techniques can result in significantly reduced bleeding and dysmenorrhea, and even amenorrhea, but approximately 20% of women require additional procedures. Women with menorrhagia attributed to uterine myomas can be managed with myomectomy (hysteroscopic, laparoscopic, or abdominal procedures as indicated) or

---

[1]Not FDA approved for this indication.

CURRENT DIAGNOSIS

- Detailed medical and menstrual history
- Thorough physical and gynecologic examination
- Pregnancy test for all reproductive-age women
- Determination of ovulatory status based on menstrual history
- Laboratory evaluation: complete blood count, endocrine studies, coagulation profile
- Endometrial sampling if high risk for hyperplasia or cancer
- Imaging studies to evaluate anatomy

uterine artery embolization. Currently, pregnancy is not recommended after the latter option because few data are available on postprocedure pregnancy outcomes.

Uterine Hemorrhage

Acute heavy bleeding requires high-dose estrogen therapy. Women who need inpatient management should receive conjugated estrogens (Premarin), 25 mg intravenously every 4 hours for 24 hours or until the bleeding decreases. A Foley catheter balloon (30 cc) can be placed in the uterine cavity to tamponade the bleeding. Additionally, dilation and curettage can be performed to help stop acute uterine hemorrhage. If stable for outpatient management, women can receive conjugated estrogens (Premarin),[1] 1.25 mg, or micronized estradiol (Estrace),[1] 2 mg every 4 to 6 hours for 24 hours, and when the bleeding is controlled, the dose is tapered to once daily for 7 to 10 days. Another effective regimen uses high-dose combination contraceptives[1] (3 to 4 pills daily) until the bleeding is decreased, followed by a taper to 1 pill daily for several weeks. Estrogen therapy should be followed by progestins or combined contraceptives to stabilize the estrogen-stimulated endometrium.

When evaluating a woman with abnormal uterine bleeding, a thorough history and evaluation are essential to help narrow the differential diagnosis. A number of medical and surgical treatments are available for the management of abnormal uterine bleeding, but the range of options may be limited by a woman's fertility plans.

[1]Not FDA approved for this indication.

CURRENT THERAPY

- Progestins
  Cyclic or intermittent use
  Prolonged therapy
  Progestin-releasing intrauterine device (IUD) (Mirena)[1]
- Estrogens[1]
  Intermittent use
  High-dose course for acute heavy bleeding
- Estrogen-progestin contraceptives[1]
  Cyclic use
  High-dose course with taper for heavy bleeding
- Other therapies
  Nonsteroidal anti-inflammatory drugs[1]
  Tranexamic acid (Lysteda)
  Gonadotropin-releasing hormone agonists
- Surgical options
  Endometrial ablation
  Myomectomy
  Uterine artery embolization
  Hysterectomy

[1]Not FDA approved for this indication.

REFERENCES

American College of Obstetricians and Gynecologists. Management of anovulatory bleeding. ACOG Practice Bulletin, no. 14, March 2000.

Bayer SR, DeCherney AH. Clinical manifestations and treatment of dysfunctional uterine bleeding. JAMA 1993;269:1823–8.

Berek JS, editor. Benign diseases of the female reproductive tract. In: Berek JS, editor. Novak's Gynecology. Philadelphia: Lippincott Williams & Wilkins; 2002. pp. 351–73.

Bonnar J, Sheppard BL. Treatment of menorrhagia during menstruation: Randomised controlled trial of ethamsylate, mefenamic acid, and tranexamic acid. BMJ 1996;313:579–82.

Dickersin K, Munro MG, Clark M, et al. Hysterectomy compared with endometrial ablation for dysfunctional uterine bleeding: A randomized controlled trial. Obstet Gynecol 2007;110:1279–89.

Farquhar CM, Lethaby A, Sowter M, et al. An evaluation of risk factors for endometrial hyperplasia in premenopausal women with abnormal menstrual bleeding. Am J Obstet Gynecol 1999;181:525–9.

Kouides PA, Conard J, Peyvandi F, et al. Hemostasis and menstruation: Appropriate investigation for underlying disorders of hemostasis in women with excessive menstrual bleeding. Fertil Steril 2005;84:1345–51.

Munro MG. Dysfunctional uterine bleeding: Advances in diagnosis and treatment. Curr Opin Obstet Gynecol 2001;13:475–89.

Munro MG. Medical management of abnormal uterine bleeding. Obstet Gynecol Clin North Am 2000;27:287–304.

Shwayder JM. Pathophysiology of abnormal uterine bleeding. Obstet Gynecol Clin North Am 2000;27:219–34.

Speroff L, Fritz M. Dysfunctional uterine bleeding. In: Clinical Gynecologic Endocrinology and Infertility. Philadelphia: Lippincott Williams & Wilkins; 2005. pp. 548–71.

Wallach EE, Vlahos NF. Uterine myomas: An overview of development, clinical features and management. Obstet Gynecol 2004;104:393–406.

Infertility

Method of
Steven R. Williams, MD

Absence of desired conception despite 12 months of unprotected intercourse generally defines infertility. Historical and physical factors allow the physician to adjust this definition to the individual patient. For example, women with longstanding amenorrhea or known distal hydrosalpinges should consider intervention before 12 months has elapsed. However, a young couple (22 years of age) with a negative history can be encouraged to try a bit longer than 12 months before evaluation begins. After 6 months of trying, approximately 45% of couples achieve pregnancy, and after 12 months of trying, approximately 85% will conceive. Pregnancy can occur with sex 6 days before ovulation, although one study found no pregnancies were conceived from sex the day after ovulation. Thus we recommend couples trying for a baby should plan to be active together every other day starting about 6 days before ovulation is expected (cycle day 8) until 2 to 3 days after ovulation has happened (cycle day 18). If the mood were to strike more often, that's fine with us; if the mood strikes less often, we can still be comfortable given the 6-day interval previously described. As in all of medicine, important historical points can guide the direction of the evaluation and treatment of the infertile couple.

Male-factor historical points include fathering past pregnancies or miscarriages, sexual function, urologic or hernia surgery, infections, medications, and tobacco use. Semen analysis remains the most important test for male factor evaluation. The World Health Organization (WHO) reports normal males to have more than 20 million sperm per cc with greater than 50% motility. It is probably best to advise 48 hours of abstinence before collection of the sample. A urologic exam and evaluation is indicated with abnormal counts. Modern in vitro fertilization (IVF) treatments can achieve pregnancies as long as any sperm at all can be isolated, even if that means

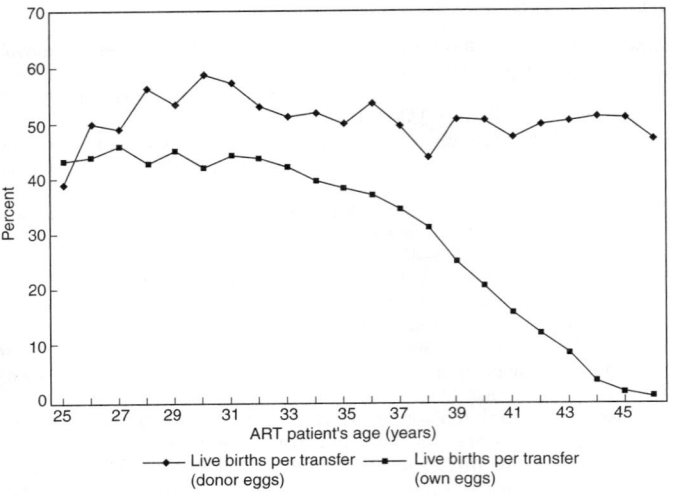

FIGURE 1. Live births per transfer for ART cycles using fresh embryos from own and donor eggs, by ART patient's age, 2002. ART = assisted reproductive technology.

surgical aspiration. Before pursuing assisted reproduction for severely low counts, genetic testing will be recommended because severely low counts can predict higher rates of cystic fibrosis carrier status, balanced translocation, and perhaps microdeletions of the Y chromosome.

A women's age has a strong correlation with fertility success. Figure 1 compares the live birth rate when IVF patients used their own eggs fertilized with their partner's sperm compared to the rate when young oocyte donor's eggs are fertilized with the IVF patient's partner's sperm and the resultant embryos transferred into the IVF patient's uterus. One must conclude from these data that the majority of the decline in success is related to oocyte quality, as anyone can expect the success of a woman 25 years of age who uses the oocytes from a woman 25 years of age! Follicle-stimulating hormone (FSH) measured on day 3 of the menstrual cycle correlates well with ovarian reserve and is commonly ordered for women more than 30 years of age with infertility. In our office, day-3 FSH values lower than 9 mU/mL are reassuring with respect to ovarian reserve, whereas values greater than 20 mU/mL are rarely associated with future fertility success using that patient's eggs.

Previous full-term deliveries are reassuring, whereas recurrent abortions or preterm deliveries can predict a uterine issue. Pelvic infections, intrauterine device (IUD) use, previous abdominal surgery, dysmenorrhea, or dyspareunia can predict tubal obstruction. This is explored with hysterosalpingography (HSG). After sterile preparation of the cervix, a sterile cannula is inserted, and under fluoroscopic guidance radiograph contrast is injected. The dye reveals the contour of the uterine cavity and displays uterine septa and intracavitary lesions such as fibroids or polyps. It then fills into the fallopian tubes and spills into the abdominal cavity. Most women describe the discomfort of the test as a severe menstrual cramp that lasts for several minutes. Pain is reduced by slow injection of the dye, gentle tissue handling, and pretreatment with nonsteroidal antiinflammatory drugs (NSAIDs). Many authors suggest that the procedure itself has a fertility-enhancing effect. The American College of Obstetricians and Gynecologists (ACOG) suggests prophylaxis with doxycycline (Vibramycin)[1] 100 mg twice daily orally for 5 days after HSG if dilated tubes are demonstrated; no prophylaxis is indicated in a normal study. Abnormal uterine cavities can be further evaluated with saline infusion hysterograms or magnetic resonance imaging (MRI). Many uterine abnormalities can be treated completely with hysteroscopic surgery. Unilateral tubal disease noted on the HSG predicts subtle decreases in future fertility in these

---

[1]Not FDA approved for this indication.

CURRENT DIAGNOSIS

- Medical history can guide fertility testing.
- Simple laboratory and radiograph tests can determine infertility causes.

women compared with women with normal tubes. Bilateral tubal disease discovered on HSG predicts dramatic declines in fertility. Tubal patency established by HSG does not rule out peritubal adhesions that can affect fertility. Laparoscopy is an outpatient surgical procedure that can be used to further evaluate tubal abnormalities seen on HSG or to look for undetected peritubal adhesions. Laparoscopy also will detect endometriosis.

Endometriosis is noted in approximately 1 in 30 laparoscopies performed for tubal ligation (presumably for fertile women), although one third of women undergoing infertility evaluations will have endometriosis. Surgical treatment of minimal or mild endometriosis does appear to help with subsequent fertility somewhat. A prospective study of infertile women found to have mild or minimal endometriosis noted at laparoscopy showed a 31% pregnancy rate in the next 9 months for patients randomized to treatment versus a 17% pregnancy rate in the next 9 months for women randomized to no treatment.

Irregular menstruation generally indicates irregular ovulation and diminished fertility. Even with regular menstruations, serum progesterone measurements in the luteal phase (6 to 8 days after ovulation) should be greater than 10 ng/mL for the "most fertile" of ovulations. If it is not, thyroid and prolactin studies should be ordered and induction of ovulation with clomiphene citrate (Clomid) considered. Clomiphene citrate in a 50-mg dose is taken orally for 5 days starting on menstrual day 3. Serum luteal phase progesterone is drawn 7 days after ovulation and is expected to be greater than 10 ng/dL. If it is, refills for 2 more months of treatment are written. If it is not, we recommend increasing the dose of clomiphene citrate to 100 mg daily for 5 days and repeating the luteal phase progesterone assay. If still not greater than 10 ng/dL, clomiphene citrate at 150 mg daily can be tried. If the patient is still anovulatory, referral to a gynecologist or reproductive endocrinologist is considered. For resistant patients, adjunctive treatments with the clomiphene citrate can include ultrasound monitoring with HCG injections when mature follicles are noted or adding insulin-sensitizing agents or glucocorticoids. Clomiphene ovulation induction yields approximately a 70% ovulation rate and, in young couples, approximately an 8% pregnancy rate per month. One in ten clomiphene citrate pregnancies are twins, although triplets and quadruplets are very rare on this therapy. Side effects of clomiphene citrate include hot flushes, emotional lability, mittelschmerz, headache, and sleep disturbance. Discontinue the drug if the patient experiences severe visual disturbance. Because the majority of clomiphene citrate pregnancies happen early in treatment, referral to reproductive specialists should be considered if the patient is not pregnant after 3 months of treatment.

Gonadotropin ovulation induction is available for women who failed to ovulate using clomiphene citrate or did not conceive on that therapy. This medication is the natural hormone used to initiate ovulation; therefore, response and pregnancy rates are better than with clomiphene citrate. Unfortunately, dramatic increases in multiple pregnancy are associated with these medications, and often they are quite expensive. One large study reviewed success and multiple pregnancy rates in patients treated with gonadotropin ovulation induction.

CURRENT THERAPY

- Clomiphene citrate is a low risk treatment option when indicated.
- Assisted reproduction is delivering more and more babies with fewer multiples.

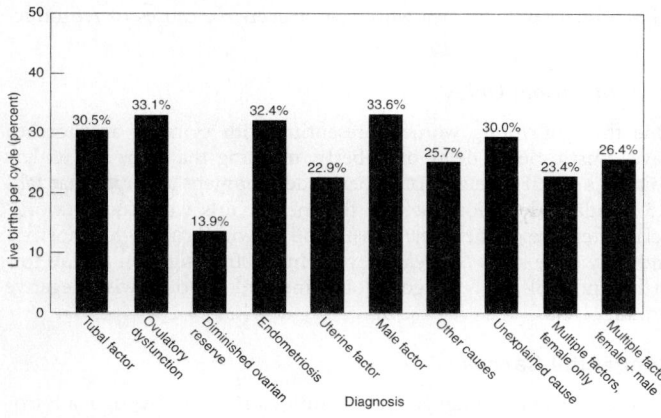

FIGURE 2. Live birth rates among women who had ART cycles using fresh nondonor eggs or embryos, by diagnosis, 2002. ART = assisted reproductive technology.

The authors concluded the protocols employed with gonadotropin ovulation induction lead to an unacceptably high incidence of higher-order multiple pregnancies and raised the question whether that treatment could be replaced by IVF.

IVF involves induction of ovulation with gonadotropin in hopes of retrieving multiple oocytes. Ovarian response is monitored with pelvic ultrasounds and serum estradiol measurements. When the oocytes are mature, HCG is given to trigger the completion of oocyte development. Then transvaginal ultrasound is used to guide an aspirating needle through the posterior cul-de-sac and into the ovaries for aspiration of the oocytes. The procedure takes approximately 15 minutes under local anesthesia and is often performed in an office setting. Oocytes are then inseminated in the lab with the husband's sperm and cultured. In certain circumstances (very low sperm count, surgically aspirated sperm, previous failed fertilization) the oocytes can be directly injected with the sperm via intracytoplasmic sperm injection (ICSI). The resultant embryos are then cultured for 2 to 5 days and then transferred into the uterus via a simple transcervical approach. IVF thus allows embryo development without tubal ovarial interaction, making it a great choice for patients with tubal disease or endometriosis. In fact, nothing we can find at laparoscopy that was not discovered by pelvic ultrasound and HSG will affect IVF success (Figure 2). We are developing protocols that reduce the numbers of embryos transferred for couples at high risk for multiple pregnancy to one. I believe that in the future IVF will replace both gonadotropin ovulation induction and the need for laparoscopy for treatment of infertility. The 2001 Centers for Disease Control (CDC) report on assisted reproductive technology (ART) success reported national average live birth rates in the high 30% per cycle start for women younger than 35 years of age. Some individual centers are reporting live birth rates in the 50% range. IVF is a very effective and increasingly safer alternative to older treatments for refractory infertility.

REFERENCES

American College of Obstetrics and Gynecology. Antibiotic prophylaxis for gynecologic procedures. ACOG Practice Bulletin 2003;23.

Centers of Disease Control. 2002 Assisted reproductive technology success rates, National summary and fertility clinic reports. Atlanta: Center for Disease Control; 2002.

Gleicher N, Oleske DM, Tur-Kaspa I, et al. Reducing the risk of higher order multiple pregnancy after ovarian stimulation with gonadotropins. N Engl J Med 2000;343:2–7.

Jain T, Soules MR, Collins JA. Comparison of basal follicle-stimulating hormone versus the clomiphene citrate challenge test for ovarian reserve testing. Fertil Steril 2004;82:180–225.

Jordan J, Craig K, Clifton DK, et al. Luteal phase defect: The sensitivity and specificity of diagnostic methods in common clinical use. Fertil Steril 1995;63:427–8.

Marcoux S, Maheux R, Berube S. Laparoscopic surgery in infertile women with minimal or mild endometriosis. Canadian collaborative group on endometriosis. N Engl J Med 1997;337:217–22.

Mol BW, Swart P, Bossuyt BM, et al. Is hysterosalpingography an important tool in predicting fertility outcome? Fertil Steril 1997;67:663–9.

Schwabe MG, Shapiro SS, Haning RV Jr. Hysterosalpingography with oil contrast medium enhances fertility in patients with infertility of unknown etiology. Fertil Steril 1983;40:604–6.

Trimbos JB, Trimbos-Kemper GC, Peters AA, et al. Findings in 200 consecutive asymptomatic women, having a laparoscopic sterilization. Arch Gynecol Obstet 1990;247:121–4.

Wilcox AJ, Weinberg CR, Baird DD. Timing of sexual intercourse in relation to ovulation. Effects on the probability of conception, survival of the pregnancy, and sex of the baby. N Engl J Med 1995;333:1517–21.

Amenorrhea

Method of
Vickie Martin, MD, and Robert L. Reid, MD

Amenorrhea, simply put, is the absence of menses. It can be classified as either primary (when a woman of reproductive age has never had menstruation) or secondary (when amenorrhea occurs after menstruation has been established). There are normal situations in which amenorrhea is expected (physiologic amenorrhea): during pregnancy, during lactation, and at the onset of menopause. Approximately 5% of reproductive-age women experience amenorrhea at times other than these, which warrants investigation. Women with amenorrhea often present with significant apprehension and anxiety. Thus, an appropriate but timely workup and diagnosis are required. The clinician must have a systematic approach for evaluating such women to ensure that important causes of amenorrhea are identified. As always, a detailed history, a targeted physical examination, and selective use of simple diagnostic tests are required.

Definition

Amenorrhea may be defined as the absence of menstruation for 3 or more months in women with past menses (secondary amenorrhea) or the absence of menarche by the age of 16 years in girls who have never menstruated (primary amenorrhea). Infrequent menstruation, termed *oligomenorrhea*, may have similar causes and also warrants investigation.

Menstrual Cycle

A clear working knowledge of the menstrual cycle and its physiology is mandatory for the clinician in these circumstances. Menstruation normally results when a cascade of hormonal signals from the hypothalamus (gonadotropin-releasing hormone [GnRH]) to cause pituitary release of luteinizing hormone (LH) and follicle-stimulating hormone (FSH). These in turn stimulate the development of an egg-containing ovarian follicle. Estrogen from this follicle results in steady growth of the endometrial lining over a 2-week period (follicular phase). When ovulation occurs, the follicle (now called the corpus luteum) develops the ability to produce a second hormone, progesterone.

The secretion of estrogen and progesterone for the next 2-week period causes the endometrial lining to become lush (decidualized) in preparation for implantation of a pregnancy. If pregnancy fails to occur, the corpus luteum undergoes a spontaneous demise, the endometrium no longer has adequate hormonal support to survive, and the tissue is sloughed synchronously over the next 5 to 7 days as menstrual flow. The final steps of this process require a means of egress for blood, implying a normal uterus with a patent cervix and vagina (the outflow tract).

Etiology

Different classification systems have been employed. One system defines the type of amenorrhea based on the level of FSH in circulation. For example, high FSH levels indicate that the hypothalamus and pituitary are fully functioning but that the ovary is not responding (similar to menopause). The gonadotropin (FSH) levels are high and the ovary (gonad) is not functioning, which is termed *hypergonadotropic hypogonadism. Hypogonadotropic hypogonadism* refers to the situation where FSH levels are very low due to some central disturbance of hypothalamic or pituitary function. The problem with this classification is that normal FSH levels are often low and the distinction between hypogonadotropic and eugonadotropic causes of amenorrhea can be difficult.

A simple way to consider causes of amenorrhea is to divide the processes that regulate menstruation (the hypothalamic-pituitary-ovarian axis [HPO axis]) into compartments (Figure 1) and then consider possible contributory factors for disruption of normal processes at each of these levels. Always consider the possibility that amenorrhea may be due to unexpected pregnancy before moving on to a full investigation.

HYPOTHALAMIC COMPARTMENT

The hypothalamus integrates a wide variety of signals from the brain and is ultimately responsible for turning on or off the hormonal cascade necessary for triggering ovulatory and menstrual function. In adolescents, the development of breasts (thelarche) between ages 8 and 10 years is usually the first sign that the HPO axis has turned on and first menstruation (menarche) typically follows within 3 to 5 years. All girls with primary amenorrhea by age 14 years, particularly if 5 or more years have passed since the first evidence of pubertal development, warrant careful investigation, because girls with primary amenorrhea on the basis of constitutional delay cannot readily be differentiated on clinical history from the two thirds of patients

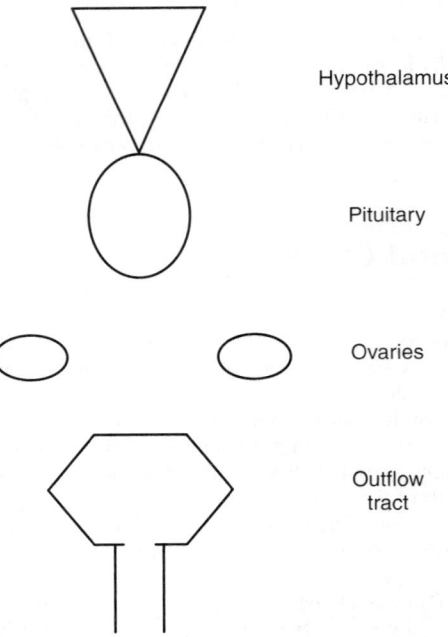

Hypothalamus

Pituitary

Ovaries

Outflow tract

FIGURE 1. The four compartments to consider when evaluating amenorrhea.

with primary amenorrhea who have irreversible causes of reproductive failure.

Constitutional Delay

One third of young women presenting with primary amenorrhea have constitutional delay of puberty, meaning that they are undergoing a normal sequence of pubertal development at a rate that falls 2.5 standard deviations behind the mean. Girls with constitutional delay often present between ages 13 and 16 with primary amenorrhea and only early signs of breast development. Investigation reveals low to low-normal levels of gonadotropins and an otherwise negative workup.

Congenital Causes

A variety of unusual congenital conditions result in hypogonadotropic hypogonadism and primary amenorrhea. These conditions may be caused by deficiency of GnRH production or by abnormalities of the GnRH receptor. A Kallman's-like syndrome has been identified in some affected women who present with anosmia and a complete lack of pubertal development.

Acquired Causes

Acquired diseases can lead the hypothalamus to shut down the reproductive hormonal cascade, resulting in amenorrhea, which may be primary or secondary, depending on when they develop. Nutritional deprivation (including eating disorders), excessive caloric demand due to participation in demanding sports, and extreme psychological stress are common reasons for delayed activation of reproductive processes by the hypothalamus. Less commonly, systemic illnesses, including malabsorption states, active autoimmune diseases, and rare hypoxemic states related to congenital heart malformations or severe anemias (sickle cell disease), can lead to amenorrhea.

PITUITARY COMPARTMENT

Lesions of the pituitary stalk that interrupt normal delivery of GnRH to the pituitary include those resulting from head trauma, rare stalk tumors such as craniopharyngiomas, or from the surgery to remove these.

Pituitary causes of amenorrhea are almost always due to oversecretion of prolactin. Hyperprolactinemia resulting in amenorrhea, if associated with central retro-orbital headache and bitemporal hemianopia, can result from a prolactin-producing tumor.

Other causes of hyperprolactinemia originate outside the pituitary. For example, primary hypothyroidism, breast or chest wall lesions (or piercings) in the T4-6 dermatome, renal failure, and a variety of medications have all been linked to hyperprolactinemia. Medications that can cause hyperprolactinemia include dopamine receptor antagonists (phenothiazines, butyrophenones, thioxanthenes, risperidone, metoclopramide, sulpiride,[2] pimozide), dopamine-depleting agents (e.g., methyldopa, reserpine), H₂-blockers (cimetidine), opiates, and cocaine.

Rarely, other pituitary conditions result in amenorrhea. In empty sella syndrome, radiologic examination reveals an apparently empty sella due to pituitary regression from some vascular or other insult. Other conditions include Sheehan syndrome (postpartum pituitary necrosis), pituitary apoplexy (massive pituitary infarction), and radiation-induced hypopituitarism. In each of these situations, amenorrhea is usually part of a larger picture of endocrine disruption.

OVARIAN COMPARTMENT

Depletion of eggs from the ovary before or after puberty results in primary or secondary amenorrhea, respectively. FSH levels are markedly elevated in these cases, as the hypothalamus and pituitary try to elicit follicular development from the unresponsive ovary. Destruction of oocytes by any of several environmental insults, including

[2]Not available in the United States.

ionizing radiation, various chemotherapeutic (especially alkylating) agents, and certain viral infections can accelerate follicular atresia.

Primary amenorrhea in a woman with evidence of gonadal failure should elicit a search for a chromosomal abnormality. It is known that two intact X chromosomes are needed for maintenance of ovarian function. A variety of X chromosome structural abnormalities have been identified in women with premature ovarian failure, including complete absence of one X chromosome (Turner's syndrome).

Elevated FSH occurs in association with a normal karyotype. These women have normal 46,XY or 46,XX karyotypes without the phenotypic abnormalities of Turner's syndrome. Those with a Y chromosome should have their gonads removed because of the potential for malignant transformation.

Several rare inherited enzymatic defects also may be associated with premature ovarian failure. These include partial deficiencies in four enzymes in the steroidogenic pathway—17α-hydroxylase, 17,20-desmolase, 20,22-desmolase, and aromatase—and galactosemia.

Premature ovarian failure may be associated with a number of autoimmune disorders. Most commonly associated with thyroiditis, ovarian failure also occurs in women with polyglandular failure, including hypoparathyroidism, hypoadrenalism, and mucocutaneous candidiasis.

Though it is not exclusively an ovarian disorder, it is useful to consider polycystic ovary syndrome (PCOS) in the ovarian compartment for the purpose of completeness in considering possible diagnoses. PCOS is one of the most common causes of secondary amenorrhea. Typically, women suffering from this condition are overweight (although one third have normal body weight) and have clinical features of hyperandrogenism (acne and hirsutism), hyperinsulinism (acanthosis nigricans), and hyperestrogenism (watery cervical mucus). Months of amenorrhea may be punctuated by episodes of heavy and prolonged menstrual bleeding as an estrogen-thickened endometrium sheds irregularly over several weeks.

OUTFLOW TRACT COMPARTMENT

Congenital abnormalities of development of the reproductive outflow tract can cause amenorrhea. Complete absence of a uterus can be due to isolated müllerian agenesis or it can manifest in phenotypic females with a 46,XY karyotype who have complete androgen insensitivity. Developmental abnormalities can include cervical atresia, tranverse vaginal septum, and imperforate hymen. These latter abnormalities may be associated with cyclic menstrual pain in the absence of bleeding (cryptomenorrhea). Similarly, monthly cramps can occur with cervical stenosis following trachelectomy or conization. Uterine synechiae due to a vigorous curettage in the face of a postpartum or postabortion endometritis can result in obliteration of the uterine cavity and secondary amenorrhea with or without monthly menstrual-like cramps.

OTHER CAUSES

Pregnancy must always be considered in a sexually active female patient presenting with secondary amenorrhea. Hormonal suppression of the endometrium can be accomplished with a variety of medications. The progestin component of the cyclic oral contraceptive gradually results in a thinner and thinner endometrium, which can ultimately result in pill-withdrawal amenorrhea. Other medications, including danazol, medroxyprogesterone, and long-acting GnRH agonists can result in amenorrhea.

Diagnosis

HISTORY

A search for clues as to the etiology should start with a personal developmental history in the amenorrheic teen and with a menstrual and reproductive history in the older amenorrheic woman. Events in the 3 to 6 months preceding the onset of amenorrhea are often critical. Rapid weight gain or loss or a marked change in energy

---

BOX 1 A Compartmental Approach to Systems Review

Hypothalamic Compartment
- Changes in temperature regulation, sleep, appetite, thirst
- Headache or visual field defects

Pituitary Compartment
- Central retro-orbital headache, bitemporal hemianopa a
- Galactorrhea
- Features of hypothyroidism
- Medications affecting prolactin

Ovary Compartment
- Hot flushes
- Insomnia
- Night sweats
- Vaginal dryness

Outflow Compartment
- Cyclic cramps
- Possibility of pregnancy
- Recent gynecologic procedures (dilation and curettage, cervical laser or conization)

---

expenditure through exercise may be important. Systems review should examine possible disruption to any of the compartments (Box 1). Inquiry about general health, risk of pregnancy, and use of medication (including illicit drugs) is important.

PHYSICAL EXAMINATION

Height, weight, and body mass index (BMI) should be determined. Body habitus often provides an important clue to which patients are amenorrheic due to excessive physical or nutritional stress (eating disorder or malnutrition). In primary amenorrhea, examination for the stage of breast and pubic hair development (Tanner staging) can indicate whether there has been delay or disruption to the entire process of pubertal development. Restriction of later visual fields to examination by confrontation, the presence of galactorrhea, or evidence of recent scars or lesions in the region of the breast (such as zoster) can implicate hyperprolactinemia. The thyroid gland should be palpated and features of hypothyroidism sought. A lower abdominal mass may be due to pregnancy, hematocolpos or hematometra.

The gynecologic examination should be tailored to the patient. The external genitalia should be evaluated for pubic hair, acanthosis nigricans, and clitoral size. The hymen should be visualized; an imperforate hymen usually shows a bluish central bulge. Estrogenization of the tissues (presence of leukorrhea, thickened mucosa, or watery cervical mucus) can be assessed with speculum examination (choosing a speculum size appropriate to the sexual maturity of the patient). Visualization of the cervix in most circumstances is sufficient to rule out an outflow compartment problem.

INVESTIGATIONS

Initial Investigations

Initial investigation for any patient with amenorrhea or oligomenorrhea includes follicle-stimulating hormone (FSH), prolactin (PRL), thyroid stimulating hormone (TSH), and a sensitive pregnancy test if pregnancy is a possibility.

Ultrasonography can be helpful when an internal examination cannot be performed. When a congenital anomaly is considered, magnetic resonance imaging (MRI) can provide more definitive information.

CURRENT DIAGNOSIS

- Always consider the possibility of pregnancy in any woman presenting with secondary amenorrhea.
- Secondary amenorrhea is most commonly the result of some significant lifestyle change (weight gain or loss, stress, excessive exercise) or illness (with marked weight loss) in the preceding 6 months.
- Obesity and features of androgen excess are most often related to polycystic ovary syndrome (PCOS).
- Because constitutional delay of puberty is found in only one third of girls presenting with delayed menarche, an investigation should be initiated at the time of presentation rather than waiting until the girl is 16 years old (meeting the definitional criteria).
- Primary amenorrhea, particularly with the absence of other features of pubertal development (breasts and pubic and axillary hair) suggests ovarian failure.
- When amenorrhea due to ovarian failure (high FSH) occurs before age 35 years, a karyotype is indicated. If Y chromosome material is identified on karyotype, gonadectomy is required to reduce the risk of malignancy in the gonadal tissues.

Follow-up Investigations

A low normal FSH in the presence of a normal outflow tract should elicit a more detailed search for hypothalamic disruptors (such as nutritional, physical, or psychological stress). In a patient who has low FSH in conjunction with an elevated PRL and who is not taking medications known to increase PRL and whose TSH is normal, lesions of the hypothalamus or pituitary should be excluded with CT or MRI.

An elevated FSH indicates ovarian failure and should elicit a search for possible explanations such as past surgery, exposure to radiation or chemotherapy, or genetic causes. With an elevated FSH, a karyotype is usually indicated unless there is some obvious cause for loss of ovarian function. If the karyotype reveals any Y chromosome material, then, at the appropriate age, referral to a gynecologist is necessary for counseling and gonadectomy to reduce the risk of gonadoblastoma and dysgerminoma.

Evidence of outflow tract obstruction on pelvic examination or the possibility of cervical stenosis (cyclic dysmenorrhea without bleeding after a cervical surgical procedure such as a loop excision, cone biopsy, or trachelectomy) or Asherman's syndrome (obliteration of the endometrial cavity following a postpregnancy or postabortion dilation and curettage) merits referral to a gynecologist for further assessment and management.

Secondary amenorrhea related to weight gain or obesity, particularly when associated with features of acne and hirsutism, suggests the polycystic ovary syndrome. Management depends on whether the patient is seeking menstrual cycle regulation and relief from hirsutism (cyclic progestational therapy or an oral contraceptive plus an anti-androgen) or pregnancy (weight loss and fertility medication such as clomiphene citrate [Clomid]).

REFERENCES

Rebar RW. Evaluation of amenorrhea, anovulation and abnormal bleeding. March 26, 2006. Available at http://endotext.org/female/female4/femaleframe4.htm [accessed June 15, 2007].
Reid RL. Amenorrhea. In: Copeland L, Jarrell J, McGregor J, editors. Textbook of Gynecology. 2nd ed. Philadelphia: WB Saunders; 1997. pp. 365–90.
Reindollar R, Lalwani S. Abnormalities of female pubertal development. November 21, 2002. Available at http://endotext.org/female/female2/femaleframe2.htm [accessed June 15, 2007].

Dysmenorrhea

Method of
David R. Harnisch, Sr., MD

Dysmenorrhea, which is difficult and painful menstruation, is the most common gynecologic problem in menstruating women. It is divided into primary and secondary forms. *Primary dysmenorrhea* is dysmenorrhea due to a functional disturbance and not to inflammation, new growths, or anatomic factors. It may be referred to as intrinsic, functional, or essential. *Secondary dysmenorrhea* results from inflammation, infection, tumor, or anatomic factors. Primary dysmenorrhea is so common as to be normative, and in some published studies, it has been prevalent in 90% of the studied population. It becomes significant when it leads to loss of pleasure or diminishment in functional capacity. At worst, it can lead to significant absenteeism from school, work, or other social obligations or activities.

Primary Dysmenorrhea

Primary dysmenorrhea, or a painful cramping sensation in the lower abdomen, may be accompanied by a variety of other symptoms, including nausea, vomiting, headaches, malaise, dizziness, sweating, fatigue, bowel changes, and anxiety associated with the anticipation and experience of the pain. These symptoms occur just before the onset of menses and usually resolve within 48 to 72 hours.

Primary dysmenorrhea usually begins within 6 to 12 months of menarche and is associated with the establishment of ovulatory cycles. It has a greater prevalence in adolescence, with some easing of symptoms in adulthood and often a significant decrease in prevalence after childbirth.

The primary mechanism of the pain of primary dysmenorrhea is thought to be a prostaglandin-mediated event. Prostaglandins are produced during the secretory phase of the cycle, leading to uterine contractions and vasoconstriction with an associated degree of uterine ischemia. Vasopressin and leukotrienes may also play a role in generating the symptoms of primary dysmenorrhea and may ultimately lead to some novel therapies.

Significant risk factors for developing dysmenorrhea include tobacco use, heavy menses, depression or anxiety, attempts at weight loss, age younger than 20 years, and disruption of a patient's social supports. If the standard treatment measures instituted for the management of primary dysmenorrhea are successful in relieving the symptoms, the diagnostic evaluation may end there. If the symptoms do not resolve simply, secondary causes should be investigated.

DIAGNOSIS

The initial approach to the diagnosis and ultimately to treatment is a thorough history. Patients with a classic history of onset of pain with regard to menarche and timing of pain with regard to the menstrual flow and an otherwise noncontributory review or systems and past medical history may not need an extensive physical examination or laboratory testing. This is especially significant for the young, virginal patient because a complete gynecologic examination may be extremely disconcerting to her. Because pain is often a symptom

CURRENT DIAGNOSIS

- Painful cramping sensation in the lower abdomen
- Occurs just before or during the menses and lasts 1 to 3 days
- Usually unaccompanied by other pathologic pelvic conditions

found in young girls, parental assistance in obtaining the history may be necessary. One of the risk factors is a positive family history of primary dysmenorrhea. If the history deviates from the classic script of primary dysmenorrhea, a more detailed evaluation of the patient may be necessary before starting a trial of therapy.

TREATMENT

Treatment for primary dysmenorrhea involves patient education and reassurance and the use of antiprostaglandins in the form of nonsteroidal antiinflammatory drugs (NSAIDs). Many young women have already begun self-treatment with NSAIDs before visiting the physician, but it is the provider's responsibility to ensure that adequate appropriate treatment regimens are instituted and followed.

Although research has been done implicating many different NSAIDs as possible treatment agents, starting with mefenamic acid (Ponstel), experience shows that any of the NSAIDs may be effective in the treatment of primary dysmenorrhea. However, some patients may find that they respond better to a nonsteroidal drug of a different class. The key to successful institution of therapy is to get therapy started before the typical symptoms of dysmenorrhea begin. Therapy is less successful after dysmenorrhea has begun. Table 1 lists some of the NSAIDs for the treatment of dysmenorrhea and their effective dosage ranges. This is not an inclusive listing, but representatives of each of the six classes of NSAIDs are listed. Notice that aspirin typically is not used because it is not potent enough in the standard dosage.

Effectiveness varies for drugs within each class. Therapy should be tailored to the individual. If a patient does not respond to one of the classes of NSAIDs, an agent from another class should be substituted and trialed. As a group, NSAIDs are 65% to 100% effective in treating the symptoms of dysmenorrhea.

Although NSAIDs are the mainstay of treatment, have a relatively low cost, and can be used on an intermittent basis with ease, some patients may be candidates for or desire to use other therapies, especially if the NSAID trials are ineffective. Alternate therapies may include oral contraceptive pills or injectable contraceptives if the patient has no contraindication to them. Decreased ovulation and thinning of the endometrial lining of the uterus may result in a

CURRENT THERAPY

- Nonsteroidal antiinflammatory drugs
- Hormonal modalities
- Complementary and alternative medicines

decrease in endometrial volume, along with a decrease in prostaglandin levels. These hormonal options may be more effective when used in combination with NSAIDs. Alternate therapies are listed in Table 2.

Secondary Dysmenorrhea

Dysmenorrhea that does not resolve with NSAIDs or hormonal agents or that a comprehensive evaluation links to inflammation, infection, tumor, or anatomic factors is referred to as secondary dysmenorrhea. Causes include endometriosis, cervical stenosis, pelvic inflammatory disease, ovarian cysts, imperforate hymen, congenital obstruction of the vaginal outflow tract, adenomyosis, endometrial polyps, pelvic congestion, intrauterine devices, fibroids, and pelvic adhesions.

Characteristics that may point to a diagnosis of secondary dysmenorrhea include dysmenorrhea beginning during the first one or two cycles after menarche, pain that begins after age 25, later onset after a history of painless menstruation, any pelvic abnormality identified on the physical examination, infertility, heavy menstrual flow or irregular cycles, nulliparity, depression, and dyspareunia.

Some nongynecologic entities can manifest with or mimic dysmenorrhea. A partial list includes irritable bowel syndrome, psychogenic disorders, interstitial cystitis, inflammatory bowel syndrome, conditioned behavior, stress, and tension.

If primary treatments fail to relieve symptoms, a more extensive workup is indicated. It can encompass a complete physical examination, including a complete gynecologic rectovaginal examination and cytologic and microbiologic testing. Pelvic ultrasound or computed

TABLE 1 Nonsteroidal Antiinflammatory Drugs for the Treatment of Dysmenorrhea

Drug Class	Medication Name	Typical Dosages	Maximum Dosages
Propionate	Ibuprofen (Motrin, Advil)	400–800 q4–6h	2400 mg/d
Propionate	Naproxen (Naprosyn)	500 mg first dose, then 250 mg q6–8h prn	1250 mg/d
Acetic acid	Indomethacin (Indocin)[1]	25–50 mg PO tid	150 mg
Fenamate	Mefenamic acid (Ponstel)	500 mg first dose, then 250 mg q6h	For 3 days
Oxicam	Piroxicam (Feldene)[1]	20 mg qd	20 mg/d
Cyclooxygenase type 2 (COX-2) inhibitor	Celecoxib (Celebrex)	400 mg load, then 200 mg bid; may take additional 200 mg on day 1	Varies
Salicylate	Aspirin[1]	325–650 mg q4–6h	4 g/d

TABLE 2 Potential Therapeutic Options for Dysmenorrhea

Type of Interaction	Therapy
Surgical	Presacral neurectomy, laparoscopic uterosacral nerve ablation, oophorectomy, hysterectomy
Electrical	Transcutaneous electrical nerve stimulation (TENS)
Manual	Acupuncture, acupressure, heat-producing patches
Complementary and alternative	Omega-3 fatty acids,[1,7] exercise, Toki-shakuyaku-san[1,7]
Traditional medications	Transdermal nitroglycerin (NitroDur),[1] thiamine,[1] magnesium supplements,[1] vitamin E,[1] terbutaline (Brethine),[1] nifedipine (Procardia),[1] danazol (Danocrine),[1] leuprolide (Lupron),[1] levonorgestrel-releasing intrauterine device (Mirena),[1] glyceryl trinitrate (nitroglycerin),[1] selective serotonin reuptake inhibitors[1]

[1]Not FDA approved for this indication.
[7]Available as a dietary supplement.

tomography may be used for the evaluation, and the patient may be referred for laparoscopy or sonohysterography. Magnetic resonance imaging can be done, but it is less sensitive than other modalities, especially in the diagnosis of endometriosis. In the evaluation for secondary dysmenorrhea, it is important to rule out causes such as tumors or cysts. If the history or physical examination findings suggest further evaluation, cystoscopy or colonoscopy may be in order.

REFERENCES

American College of Obstetricians and Gynecologists (ACOG). Practice Bulletin Number 51: Chronic Pelvic Pain. Washington, DC: ACOG; 2004.
Coco AS. Primary dysmenorrhea. Am Fam Physician 1999;60:489–96.
Edmundson LD. Dysmenorrhea, Available at http://www.emedicine.com/emerg/topic156.htm [accessed July 2009].
French L. Dysmenorrhea. Am Fam Physician 2005;71:285–91, 292.
Smith RP, Kaunitz AM. Pathogenesis, clinical manifestations, and diagnosis of primary dysmenorrhea in adult women, Available at http://www.uptodate.com/online/index.do [accessed September 2008].
Smith RP, Kaunitz AM, et al. Treatment of primary dysmenorrhea in adult women, Available at http://www.uptodate.com/online/index.do [accessed September 2008].
Stenchever A. Primary and secondary dysmenorrhea and premenstrual syndrome. In: Stenchever A, Droegemueller W, Herbst AL, Mishell DR, editors. Comprehensive Gynecology. 4th ed. St Louis: Mosby; 2001. pp. 1065–70.
Wellberry C. Diagnosis and treatment of endometriosis. Am Fam Physician 1999;60:1753–68.

Premenstrual Syndrome

Method of
Ellen W. Freeman, PhD

The premenstrual syndromes (PMS) are characterized by mood, behavioral, and physical symptoms that occur from several days to 2 weeks before menses and remit with the menstrual flow. The term *PMS* as used by clinicians and the general public is generic, imprecise, and commonly applied to numerous symptoms. Included symptoms range from the mild and normal physiologic changes of the menstrual cycle to clinically significant symptoms that limit or impair normal functioning. In recent years, randomized controlled trials and other well-designed studies have defined diagnostic criteria for PMS and identified effective treatments for this disorder.

Based on scientific evidence at this time, serotonergic antidepressants are considered the primary treatment for clinically significant PMS, and particularly its severe form termed *premenstrual dysphoric disorder* (PMDD). This review focuses on PMS and its treatment with serotonergic antidepressants. It is not a comprehensive review of all treatments or associated literature. Other recent reviews may guide the reader to further information and other treatments for PMS and PMDD.

Symptoms

Numerous symptoms were traditionally attributed to PMS. This plethora is related in part to the absence of a clear diagnosis that distinguishes PMS from other co-morbid conditions. Many disorders, both physical and psychiatric, are exacerbated premenstrually or occur as a co-morbid disorder with PMS. When a careful diagnosis is made to distinguish PMS from other conditions, a much smaller group of symptoms appear to be typical of the disorder (Box 1).

Mood symptoms are usually the main complaint (irritability, anxiety, tension, mood swings, feeling out of control, depression), but behavioral symptoms (e.g., decreased interest, fatigue, poor

---

> **BOX 1   Symptoms of Premenstrual Syndrome**
>
> Affective
> - Irritability
> - Anxiety
> - Angry outbursts
> - Confusion
> - Social withdrawal
> - Depression
>
> Somatic
> - Bloating
> - Swelling
> - Breast tenderness
> - Headache
>
> From American College of Obstetricians and Gynecologists (ACOG) Practice Bulletin 15, 2001.

concentration, poor sleep) and physical symptoms, most commonly breast tenderness and abdominal swelling, are also present. Several recent studies suggest that irritability is the cardinal symptom of PMS. Although depressive symptoms such as low mood, fatigue, sleep difficulties, and poor concentration are frequent complaints of women with PMS, the growing evidence indicates that PMS is not a simple variant of depression but has distinct mechanisms that differ from those of depressive disorders.

Prevalence

Surveys indicate that PMS is among the most common health problems reported by reproductive-age women. Current estimates from epidemiologic data indicate that approximately 25% of women experience severe and clinically significant premenstrual symptoms, although only 6% to 8% of menstruating women meet the stringent and predominantly dysphoric criteria for PMDD.

Morbidity

The morbidity of PMS is related to its severity, chronicity, and resulting distress that affect work, personal relationships, or daily activities. The level of impairment is significantly above community norms and similar to that of other health problems such as major depressive disorder. Studies consistently demonstrate that the greatest impairment or distress resulting from PMS is in relationships with the partner or children and in the effectiveness of work.

Etiology

The etiology of PMS remains undefined, although the monthly cycling of the reproductive hormones appears to have an essential role in the disorder. While circulating levels of the hormones are in normal range, the dominant theory is that some women have an underlying vulnerability to the normal fluctuations of one or more of these hormones. It is further believed that PMS involves central nervous system–mediated interactions of the reproductive steroids with neurotransmitters. The principal research evidence at this time supports the involvement of reproductive hormones, serotonergic dysregulation, and possibly dysregulation of GABAergic receptor functioning.

Diagnosis

A diagnosis of PMS is determined primarily by the *timing* and the *severity* of the symptoms. These factors, together with an assessment of whether other physical or psychiatric disorders may account for

Presenting symptoms:

- Consistent with premenstrual syndrome
- Restricted to the luteal phase
- Cause impairment or distress
- Not an exacerbation of another disorder
- Confirmed by 2 cycles of daily symptom rating

From American College of Obstetricians and Gynecologists (ACOG) Practice Bulletin 15, 2001.

the symptoms, are more important for the diagnosis than the particular symptoms, which are typically nonspecific and must be assessed for their relationship to the menstrual cycle.

Box 2 lists the diagnostic criteria for PMS presented by the American College of Obstetricians and Gynecologists in 2000. These criteria indicate that PMS symptoms must be experienced during the 5 days before menses and abate during the menstrual flow. The symptoms should cause identifiable impairment or distress, be confirmed by prospective reports recorded daily by the woman for at least two menstrual cycles, and not be accounted for by other disorders.

The diagnostic criteria for premenstrual dysphoric disorder (PMDD) are listed in the *Diagnostic and Statistical Manual of Mental Disorders*, Fourth Edition *(DSM-IV)*. Importantly, the Food and Drug Administration (FDA) has approved medications only for the indication of PMDD and not for the indication of PMS at the present time. The PMDD criteria are intended to diagnose a severe, dysphoric form of PMS and require 5 of 11 listed symptoms including at least one of the mood symptoms. Physical symptoms, regardless of the number, are considered a single symptom in meeting the diagnostic criteria. The 11 PMDD symptoms are depressed mood, anxiety or tension, mood swings, anger or irritability, decreased interest, concentration difficulties, fatigue, appetite change or food cravings, sleep disturbance, feeling overwhelmed, and physical symptoms. At least five of these symptoms must each be severe premenstrually and abate with the menstrual flow. The symptoms must markedly interfere with functioning, be confirmed by daily symptom reports for at least two menstrual cycles, and not be an exacerbation of another physical or mental disorder.

CURRENT DIAGNOSIS

- Confirm that symptoms occur premenstrually and abate following menses.
- Confirm that symptoms are clinically significant and impair daily activities and/or cause problems for the woman.
- Obtain a medical history and conduct a physical examination to determine that other disorders are not causing the symptoms.
- Assess depression, stress, substance abuse, and other diagnoses that could cause the symptoms.
- Ask the woman to maintain a daily symptom report for two or more menstrual cycles to confirm the reported symptoms and their relation to the menstrual cycle.
- Perform laboratory tests only as needed to confirm general good health or rule out other suspected conditions.

To diagnose PMS, a medical history should be obtained and a complete physical with gynecologic examination performed. PMS is understood to occur in ovulatory menstrual cycles; cycles that are irregular or outside the normal range are an indication for further gynecologic investigation. Co-morbid conditions such as dysmenorrhea, endometriosis, uterine fibroids, pelvic inflammatory disease, thyroid disorders, migraine, diabetes, mood disorders, substance abuse, and numerous other possibilities should be identified. It may be difficult to determine whether the symptoms under investigation are an exacerbation of a co-morbid condition or superimposed on another condition. In either case, the usual recommendation is to treat the ongoing condition first, then reassess and possibly add treatment for the symptoms that arise premenstrually.

No laboratory test identifies PMS and none should be routinely performed for diagnosis. Laboratory tests that indicate or confirm other possible disorders are useful if suggested by the individual woman's symptom presentation or medical findings.

The key diagnostic tool for evaluating premenstrual symptoms is the daily symptom report. The diagnostic criteria for both PMS and PMDD include a daily symptom report that is kept by the woman for at least two menstrual cycles to confirm that the woman's reported symptoms are linked to the menstrual cycle in the requisite pattern. Numerous symptom reports appropriate for this diagnosis are identified in the medical literature on PMS and PMDD. It is important that the ratings indicate the severity of each symptom (and not simply check the presence or absence of symptoms).

It is informative to use two visits for the diagnostic evaluation. Although counterintuitive, seeing the patient following menses when PMS symptoms have abated is instructive. If symptoms are absent, it provides strong evidence for the diagnosis. If symptoms are present in the follicular phase, the type and severity of the symptoms are important diagnostic information for identifying other physical or mental disorders that may be the primary focus of treatment.

Treatment

SELECTIVE SEROTONIN REUPTAKE INHIBITORS

Serotonergic antidepressants are the primary treatment for severe PMS and PMDD at this time. Modulating serotonergic function is consistent with a leading theoretical view that the normal gonadal steroid fluctuations of the menstrual cycle are associated with an abnormal serotonergic response in vulnerable women. A meta-analysis of randomized controlled trials of selective serotonin reuptake inhibitors (SSRIs) in treatment of PMS and PMDD determined that these drugs were an effective first-line therapy, with both a statistically significant and clinically meaningful difference from placebo. The FDA has approved fluoxetine (Sarafem), sertraline (Zoloft), and paroxetine (Paxil) for the indication of PMDD. Other randomized, placebo-controlled, double-blind trials showed efficacy for citalopram (Celexa[1]), venlafaxine (Effexor[1]) (a selective serotonin-norepinephrine reuptake inhibitor [SNRI]), and clomipramine (Anafranil[1]) (a tricyclic antidepressant) for treatment of PMS and PMDD.

Effective doses of SSRIs are consistently at the low end of the dose range for depressive disorders in all reports of PMS and PMDD treatments. Significant response is often seen in the first menstrual cycle of treatment, with smaller increments with or without dose adjustments in the second and third treatment cycles. If there is not sufficient response in the first treated menstrual cycle, the dose should be increased in the next cycle unless precluded by side effects.

Side effects are common with the initiation of an SSRI but are usually transient and abate within 1 to 2 weeks of continued treatment. The most common side effects include headache, nausea, insomnia, fatigue or lethargy, diarrhea, decreased concentration, dizziness, and decreased libido or delayed orgasm. The sexual side effects of SSRIs have received considerable attention, although it is often difficult to determine the extent to which sexual effects are

---

[1]Not FDA approved for this indication.

CURRENT THERAPY

SSRI	Range Studied (mg)	Mean Dose (mg/d)
Citalopram (Celexa[1])	10–30	20
Escitalopram (Lexapro[1])	10–20	15
Fluoxetine (Prozac,[1] Sarafem*)	10–60	20
Paroxetine (Paxil[1])	10–30	20
Paroxetine-CR* (Paxil-CR)	12.5, 25	NA[†]
Sertraline (Zoloft*)	50–150	75
SNRI		
Venlafaxine (Effexor[1])	37.5–200	112.5

[1]Not FDA approved for this indication.
*FDA approved for the indication of premenstrual dysphoric disorder (PMDD).
[†]Not applicable because of fixed-dose study.

related to the medication or to preexisting conditions. The incidence of decreased sexual interest or delayed orgasm in the few published reports of PMS patients is approximately 9% to 16%, which is notably lower than the rates reported with the use of SSRIs by depressed patients. Another important issue is the lack of any well-controlled clinical trials of SSRI treatment for PMS and PMDD in adolescents. Whether SSRIs are safe and effective for this indication in women younger than 18 years is not demonstrated.

Luteal Phase Dosing

The use of medication only in the symptomatic luteal phase of the menstrual cycle is particularly important in PMS because of the cyclic pattern of the symptoms, which occur only in the premenstrual phase and abate following menses. Efficacy of luteal phase administration of the SSRIs is demonstrated in multiple trials: three large multicenter, randomized, placebo-controlled trials that examined fluoxetine (Sarafem), paroxetine (Paxil), and sertraline (Zoloft); a trial that directly compared continuous and luteal phase administration of sertraline; and multiple preliminary studies.

Luteal phase administration of an SSRI is typically initiated 14 days prior to the expected onset of menstrual bleeding and concluded within several days of bleeding, using a taper for increased doses. As with continuous dosing, the SSRI doses are usually at the low end of the dose range.

One preliminary study compared symptom-onset dosing (mean of 6 days before menses) to luteal phase dosing and found no difference between the two dosing regimens in improvement overall, although there was suggestion that women with more severe symptoms may respond better to full luteal phase dosing.

Side effects may be less frequent with an intermittent dosing regimen because they may not occur when not taking the medication. However, some women experience recurring side effects when dosing is resumed, and discontinuation symptoms might also occur with the stop-start dosing pattern. At this time, no systematic data confirm discontinuation symptoms with the intermittent dosing regimen.

Insufficient Response to Selective Serotonin Reuptake Inhibitors

Approximately 60% of PMS and PMDD patients in controlled studies respond well to an SSRI. There are no clear predictors of response. An adequate trial of an SSRI for PMS and PMDD is at least two menstrual cycles at a dose level of demonstrated efficacy, with a third cycle when there is partial response. If a woman has an insufficient response or unacceptable side effects, it is reasonable to try another SSRI. Although the SSRIs are similar in their structure and have

similar response rates and side-effect profiles, an individual patient may respond better to one SSRI versus another.

Other approaches to a poor treatment response include augmenting the SSRI with another medication to address the nonresponding symptoms, but there is no systematic information on this in PMS or PMDD treatment. Switching to another class of medication, such as anxiolytics, is suggested, but no data indicate whether nonresponders to SSRIs will respond to another class of medication. Nonresponse may also be related to other co-morbid disorders. A thorough review of the diagnosis and adjustments of the premenstrual doses of medication for both the primary disorder and PMS should be considered before pursuing other treatments.

OTHER TREATMENTS

Hormonal

In spite of the evidence for hormonal involvement in PMS and PMDD, traditional oral contraceptives (OCs) do not show efficacy for the disorder. However, recent data indicate that shortening or omitting the placebo week in the traditional OC pill pack may effectively treat PMS and PMDD. The FDA has approved the oral contraceptive YAZ, a 24/4-day combination pill, to treat PMDD.

Gonadotropin-releasing hormone (GnRH) agonists such as depot leuprolide[1] (Lupron) and buserelin[2] (Suprefact) are effective for PMS and PMDD but are of limited usefulness because of the risks associated with low estrogen levels that result from these treatments. Although add-back therapy using low-lose estrogen and progesterone together with the GnRH agonist did not appear to reduce efficacy in a meta-analysis, there are no definitive data on the safety and efficacy of this approach in long-term treatment. The historic use of progesterone has failed to show efficacy for the mood and behavioral symptoms of PMS in numerous controlled trials.

Anxiolytics

Alprazolam[1] (Xanax) and buspirone[1] (Buspar) showed modest efficacy for PMS in some studies but not others. Although these medications offer an alternative to antidepressants, the response rates appear much lower, and it is not known whether a PMS patient who does not respond to antidepressants will respond to an anxiolytic. The risk of dependency with alprazolam should be considered. Dosing should be strictly limited to the luteal phase, and the patient should have no history of substance abuse.

Nonpharmacologic

Calcium supplementation[1] (600 mg twice daily) reduced PMS symptoms significantly more than placebo. Calcium offers a dietary supplement approach that may be beneficial for some women with PMS, although there are no predictors of which women will respond well to this therapy. Other complementary and alternative therapies may be helpful for some women, but there is no convincing evidence of their efficacy for PMS.

Behavioral treatments that facilitate coping or reduce stress may reduce PMS symptoms. Cognitive-behavioral therapy is effective for PMS, and in one study it was as effective as the SSRI fluoxetine after 6 months of treatment.

TREATMENT DURATION

All published studies of treatment efficacy for PMS and PMDD are based on acute treatment of 2 to 3 months' duration. Several small pilot investigations suggest that PMS symptoms are likely to return within several months after medication is stopped. It also appears that PMS symptoms do not resolve spontaneously but continue for many years. These observations of PMS as a chronic condition and the swift return of symptoms following the cessation of medication suggest that treatment can be expected to be long term. In a controlled study that compared 4 months to 1 year of SSRI treatment, approximately half of the patients who improved with SSRI treatment relapsed within 6 to 8 months after

[1]Not FDA approved for this indication.
[2]Not available in the United States.

discontinuing medication. Longer treatment was marginally better at preventing relapse. Patients with more severe symptoms before treatment were the most likely to relapse, while patients who experienced symptom remission with treatment were least likely to relapse.

The SSRIs are currently the first-line treatment for severe PMS and PMDD. Continuous dosing and luteal phase dosing regimens are similarly effective for these disorders when the symptoms are clearly limited to the luteal phase of the menstrual cycle. Hormonal treatments have lacked consistent scientific evidence of their efficacy or safety or both for PMS treatment. Several new oral contraceptives that decrease or omit the placebo interval may provide an effective alternative to antidepressant medications. Evidence indicates that long-term maintenance of the medication may be required for PMS and PMDD.

REFERENCES

ACOG Practice Bulletin. Premenstrual syndrome. Int J Gynecol Obstet 2001; 73(2):183–90.

Brown J, O'Brien PM, Marjoribanks J, Wyatt K. Selective serotonin reuptake inhibitors for premenstrual syndrome. Cochrane Database Syst Rev 2009;2:CD001396.

Dell DL. Premenstrual syndrome, premenstrual dysphoric disorder, and premenstrual exacerbation of another disorder. Clin Obstet Gynecol 2004;47 (3):568–75.

Freeman EW. Luteal phase administration of agents for the treatment of premenstrual dysphoric disorder. CNS Drugs 2004;18(7):453–68.

Freeman EW, Rickels K, Sammel MD, Lin H, Sondheimer SJ. Time to relapse after short-term or long-term treatment of severe premenstrual syndrome with sertraline. Arch Gen Psychiatry 2009;66(5):537–44.

Girman A, Lee R, Kligler B. An integrative medicine approach to premenstrual syndrome. Am J Obstet Gynecol 2003;188(5 Suppl.):S56–65.

Grady-Weliky TA. Premenstrual dysphoric disorder. N Engl J Med 2003;348 (5):433–8.

Halbreich U. The etiology, biology, and evolving pathology of premenstrual syndromes. Psychoneuroendocrinology 2003;28(Suppl. 3):55–99.

Johnson SR. Premenstrual syndrome, premenstrual dysphoric disorder, and beyond: A clinical primer for practitioners. Obstet Gynecol 2004;104(4):845–59.

Whelan AM, Jurgens TM, Naylor H. Herbs, vitamins and minerals in the treatment of premenstrual syndrome: A systematic review. Can J Clin Pharmacol 2009;16:c407–29.

Menopause

Method of
Irina Burd, MD, PhD; Stacey A. Scheib, MD; and Krystene I. Boyle, MD

Menopause is the physiologic process characterized by a marked decrease in the number of oocytes, subsequent follicular depletion, decreased ovarian estrogen secretion, and finally cessation of menses. For 95% of women, menopause occurs between the ages of 45 and 55, with a mean age of 51. Time of menopause is influenced by genetic as well as environmental factors (Box 1). Menopause before age 40 years is considered premature ovarian failure.

Diagnosis

Menopause is defined clinically as 12 months of amenorrhea following the last menstrual period in the absence of other causes. The Staging of Reproductive Aging Workshop (STRAW) has provided a beneficial staging system to help categorize patients (Box 2).

The differential diagnosis for menopause includes thyroid disease, pregnancy, hyperprolactinemia, medications, carcinoid, pheochromocytoma, or underlying malignancy, which are important in considering the diagnosis algorithm (Box 3). Follicle-stimulating hormone (FSH) and estradiol are commonly measured to diagnose menopause and are often misleading because they can fluctuate vastly in the perimenopausal period.

BOX 1 Factors That Influence the Timing of Menopause

- Alcohol abuse
- Chemotherapy
- Cigarette smoking
- Contraception
- Family history of early menopause
- Galactose consumption
- Obesity
- Parity
- History of pelvic irradiation
- Physiologic and psychological stresses (e.g., living at high altitudes, depression)
- Race
- Shorter cycle length during adolescence
- Type 1 diabetes mellitus

BOX 2 STRAW Staging System

- Perimenopause
  - Stage −2 (early): Variable cycle length (>7 days from normal cycle)
  - Stage −1 (late): ≥2 skipped cycles and amenorrhea interval ≥60 days
- Menopause
  - Stage +1 (early): First 5 years after final menstrual period
  - Stage +2 (late): 5 years after final menstrual period until death

Abbreviation: STRAW = Stages of Reproductive Aging Workshop.

BOX 3 Algorithm for the Diagnosis of Menopause

Older than 45 years
- No symptoms suggestive of hyperthyroidism: No further diagnostic evaluation
- With symptoms suggestive of hyperthyroidism: Check serum TSH, T3, free T4

Younger than 45 years
- Oligomenorrhea or amenorrhea workup: Check serum hCG, prolactin, TSH, FSH

Younger than 40 years
- Complete evaluation for premature ovarian failure

Abbreviations: FSH = follicle-stimulating hormone; hCG = human chorionic gonadotropin; T3 = triiodothyronine; T4 = thyroxine; TSH = thyroid-stimulating hormone.

Systemic Manifestations of Menopause

VASOMOTOR SYMPTOMS

Hot flushes are the most common symptom associated with menopause. They are self-limited sensations of generalized heat that last 2 to 4 minutes and vary widely among people and across cultures. Without treatment, they resolve within 1 to 5 years.

CURRENT DIAGNOSIS

- For women older than 45 years who have menopausal symptoms, no further workup is necessary unless there are symptoms of hyperthyroidism.
- For women younger than 45 years, proceed with an oligomenorrhea or amenorrhea workup: Check serum hCG, prolactin, TSH, and FSH.
- Women younger than 40 years should have a complete evaluation for premature ovarian failure.
- Common symptoms of menopause include abnormal bleeding, hot flushes, genitourinary complaints, sleep disturbances, mood disturbances, joint pain, and difficulty concentrating.
- FSH and estradiol levels can be misleading and so should not be used to make the diagnosis.

Abbreviations: FSH = follicle-stimulating hormone; hCG = human chorionic gonadotropin; TSH = thyroid-stimulating hormone.

BOX 4 Risk Factors for Osteoporosis

Modifiable Risk Factors
- Chronic corticosteroid use
- Cigarette smoking
- Early menopause (before age 45 years)
- High alcohol intake
- High caffeine intake
- Low body weight (<127 pounds)
- Low dietary calcium intake
- Low vitamin D intake
- Premenopausal amenorrhea (>1 y)
- Sedentary lifestyle

Nonmodifiable Risk Factors
- Dementia
- Family history of osteoporosis
- Poor general health
- White or Asian ethnicity

SLEEP DISTURBANCES

Sleep disturbances often occur in menopause as a result of hot flushes arousing the woman from sleep. When the hot flushes are treated, sleep usually improves. Persistent sleep disturbances can lead to more serious symptoms such as difficulty concentrating, fatigue, mood disturbances, depression, and other psychological symptoms.

GENITOURINARY SYMPTOMS

Estrogen deficiency leads to atrophy of the urethral and vaginal epithelium. Vaginal atrophy can result in vaginal dryness, itching, irritation, and dyspareunia. The pH in the vagina also increases and, with vaginal atrophy, can lead to recurrent vaginal infections. Decreasing elasticity of the vaginal wall elasticity can result in a shorter and narrower vagina, especially without continued sexual activity. The lack of estrogen affects blood flow to the vagina and vulva, which in turn causes decreased lubrication and neuropathy. These are both reversible with estrogen replacement therapy, especially vaginal therapy.

Incontinence incidence increases with age but has not been clearly associated with menopause. The theory is that atrophy of the urethral epithelium results in diminished urethral mucosal seal, loss of compliance, and irritation. These are believed to contribute to stress and urge incontinence. These patients also report recurrent urinary tract infections; this is probably related to the increase in vaginal pH.

ABNORMAL BLEEDING

Even though most postmenopausal bleeding is due to atrophy, during the perimenopausal period the endometrium may be exposed to unopposed estrogen that can result in anovulatory bleeding or endometrial hyperplasia. If this occurs, endometrial biopsy is needed to rule out endometrial hyperplasia or cancer. A transvaginal ultrasound can also be used as a screening tool first and then be followed by an endometrial biopsy if the endometrial thickness is greater than 4 mm.

MOOD DISTURBANCES

In the Study of Women's Health Across the Nation (SWAN), higher risks of mood symptoms were found in perimenopausal women. The strongest risks of depression associated with menopause are a prior history of depression and premenstrual syndrome. Depression might not be entirely related to the physiology of menopause but may be a result of stressors concomitantly occurring around the time of menopause, such as children leaving home, dealing with aged parents, and midlife adjustment.

MENSTRUAL MIGRAINES

Menstrual migraines are believed to be related to decreased estrogen levels around the time of menses. Because menopause is related to a decrease in estrogen, menstrual migraines can increase in intensity and frequency.

BALANCE AND OSTEOPOROSIS

Estrogen deficiency can have an effect on the central nervous system by impairing balance. Along with osteoporosis, loss of balance remains one of the big causes of fractures in menopausal women. There are multiple risk factors for osteoporosis, modifiable and nonmodifiable (Box 4).

OTHER EFFECTS

Other long-term issues that are believed to be related to menopause include cardiovascular disease and dementia.

Treatment

HORMONE REPLACEMENT THERAPY

Until relatively recently, long-term estrogen and combined estrogen and progestin therapy was routinely given to postmenopausal women. Hormone replacement therapy (HRT) was believed to prevent cardiovascular disease and osteoporosis. The Women's Health Initiative (WHI) was a set of clinical trials, whose results were first published in 2002, that resulted in a dramatic change in clinical practice. The study was designed to see if there was a decrease in cardiovascular risk with conjugated equine estrogen (CEE [Premarin]) in patients without a uterus or in combination with medroxyprogesterone acetate (MPA [Provera]). The CEE-MPA (Prempro) arm of the trial was stopped early after 5 years because of the increased risks for breast cancer, coronary heart disease (CHD) (29%), stroke (41%) and venous thromboembolism (VTE) (33%), even though there was a reduction in risk of hip and vertebral fractures and colon cancer. There was also an increased risk of stroke (39%) and VTE (33%) in the CEE-alone arm after 7-year follow-up, but there was no difference in heart disease.

The Heart and Estrogen/progestin Replacement Studies (HERS I and II trials) looked at secondary prevention in postmenopausal women with known CHD, which showed that there was not a reduction of CHD events with CEE-MPA. Both the WHI and HERS studies revealed an increase in the number of VTEs.

CURRENT THERAPY

- CEE or 17-β estradiol plus MPA, as either continuous or cyclic short-term therapy lasting no more than 5 years is a first-line treatment for vasomotor symptoms in a patient with no contraindications.
- Locally active estrogen-containing compounds are available for treating urogenital symptoms.
- SERMs provide an alternative for treating menopausal symptoms, specifically osteoporosis. Raloxifene has less antiresorptive action than the bisphosphonates (e.g., alendronate) and should be given to patients who do not tolerate bisphosphonates.
- Alendronate increases BMD in the vertebral spine and femoral neck more than raloxifene, but patients taking both alendronate and raloxifene increased their BMD the most.
- More research is needed in the use of androgen replacement in menopause, although some evidence suggests that it might improve libido.

Abbreviations: BMD = bone mineral density; CEE = conjugated equine estrogen; MPA = medroxyprogesterone acetate; SERM = selective estrogen-receptor modulator.

In the WHI Memory Study (WHIMS), with CEE and CEE-MPA there was an increased risk of dementia compared with placebo, but this was in an older postmenopausal population. Epidemiologic studies indicate that estrogen may be neuroprotective if initiated earlier. Therefore, therapy should not initiated after age 65 years.

As a result of these studies and the recommendations of the North American Menopause Society, the only use for estrogen therapy, either alone or combined with progestin, is for control of menopausal symptoms, particularly hot flushes, vaginal dryness, urinary symptoms, joint pain, skin changes, and emotional lability. Studies are inconclusive whether CEE alone or CEE-MPA is beneficial for incontinence. Contraindications to estrogen therapy are a history of endometrial cancer, liver disease, breast cancer, CHD, history of VTE or stroke, or high risk of any of the above. In the Nurses' Health Study, an increased incidence of new onset of asthma that may be dose related and development of systemic lupus erythematosus might result from estrogen therapy.

The absolute risk of an adverse event is extremely low. For a 50-year-old woman on combined estrogen-progestin, estimated risk is 1:1000 at 1 year and 1:200 at 5 years. This absolute risk doubles for a 60 year-old woman. The goal of treatment is a short-term therapy, lasting no more than 5 years. Therapy should be tapered, decreasing by one pill every 1 or 2 weeks, so that there is no rebound in menopausal symptoms.

Progestin should be added to HRT for any woman with a uterus in order to prevent endometrial hyperplasia and cancer. The Postmenopausal Estrogen/Progestin Interventions (PEPI) trial showed a statistically significant reduction in the incidence of simple, complex, and atypical endometrial hyperplasia with CEE-MPA therapy compared with CEE alone. The only recommended progestin at this time is MPA 2.5 mg/day. Alternative progestin doses, less frequent administration, and alternative routes of administration have not been studied and thus might not be able to prevent endometrial hyperplasia or cancer; if these are used, closer endometrial surveillance is necessary.

Women with premature ovarian failure should be given hormonal therapy, and risks and benefits should be reassessed at age 50 years.

More research is needed the in use of androgen replacement in menopause, although some evidence suggests that it might improve libido.

Alternative therapy has been proposed for menopausal symptoms (Table 1 and Box 5).

TABLE 1 Treatment of Vasomotor Symptoms

Treatment	Suggested Dose	Possible Side Effects
Hormones		
CEE (Premarin) or 17-β estradiol, plus MPA (Provera), either continuous or cyclic	CEE 0.3 mg/d *or* Estradiol 0.5 mg PO qd *or* Estradiol 0.05 mg patch qd *plus* MPA 2.5 mg/d or for 12–14 d/mo	See text
MPA	20 mg/d[3] oral or 150 mg IM (Depo-Provera)[1] q3 mo	Mood disturbances, breast tenderness, alopecia
Megestrol acetate (Megace)[1]	20 mg bid	Vomiting, diarrhea, flatulence
Selective Serotonin Reuptake Inhibitors		
Paroxetine (Paxil, Paxil CR)[1]	10–20 mg/d or 12.5–25 mg CR/d	Fatigue, dry mouth, nausea, decreased libido
Fluoxetine (Prozac)[1]	20 mg/d	
Venlafaxine (Effexor, Effexor XR)[1]	37.5–75 mg XR/d	
Other Medications		
Gabapentin (Neurontin)[1]	300–900 mg/d	Dizziness, somnolence, peripheral edema
Clonidine (Catapres TTS)[1]	0.1 mg/24 h wk patch	Orthostatic hypotension, drowsiness
Dietary Supplements		
Vitamin E[1]	800 IU/d	Fatigue, weakness, diarrhea
Black cohosh[7]		Gastrointestinal complaints, dizziness
Evening primrose oil[7]		
Other Interventions		
Acupuncture or acupressure		
Exercise		
Lifestyle interventions (e.g., layered clothing, fans, air conditioners)		

[1]Not FDA approved for this indication.
[3]Exceeds dosage recommended by the manufacturer.
[7]Available as a dietary supplement.
Abbreviations: CEE = conjugated equine estrogen; MPA = medroxyprogesterone acetate.

BISPHOSPHONATES

Bisphosphonates impair osteoclastic bone resorption and are used to treat osteoporosis (Box 6). The most common side effects are bone pain and upper gastrointestinal disorders such as dysphagia, esophagitis, and esophageal or gastric ulcer. They are contraindicated in patients with renal impairment, uncorrected hypocalcemia, or sensitivity to the drug components. There have been no randomized, controlled studies comparing one type of bisphosphonate with another.

SELECTIVE ESTROGEN RECEPTOR MODULATORS

Selective estrogen receptor modulators (SERMs) provide an alternative for treating menopausal symptoms, specifically osteoporosis (Box 6). SERMs bind to the estrogen receptor, but they have tissue-specific properties. The two SERMs that have been studied the most are raloxifene (Evista) and tamoxifen (Nolvadex). Raloxifene's mechanism for tissue-specific activity is not fully clear. Tamoxifen probably works by variable gene expression in different cell types.

Raloxifene

Two major double-blinded, placebo-controlled trials, one in the United States and one in Europe, have looked at raloxifene versus placebo, measuring bone mineral density (BMD), markers of bone turnover, and serum lipid levels. In all treatment arms in both studies, BMD was significantly increased and serum concentrations of both total and low-density lipoprotein (LDL) cholesterol were significantly decreased compared with placebo. In both trials there was no difference in complaints of breast pain or vaginal bleeding and no difference in endometrial thickness.

In the longer-term Multiple Outcomes of Raloxifene Evaluation (MORE) study, there was a relative risk reduction in vertebral fractures but not for nonvertebral fractures. The risk of invasive, but not noninvasive, breast cancer appeared to decrease, most likely due to the antagonistic effect of raloxifene. There was no increase in endometrial cancer. The relative risk of thromboembolic disease was 3.1 compared with placebo, but it appears that the risk is less than that with tamoxifen. There was no difference in cardiovascular events, except there was a decrease in the subset of women at greatest risk.

In a study looking at osteoporosis in postmenopausal women, patients on alendronate (Fosamax) increased their BMD in the

vertebral spine and femoral neck more than patients on raloxifene, but patients taking both medications increased their BMD the most. CEE had a better effect on BMD compared with raloxifene in hysterectomized postmenopausal women. Raloxifene has less antiresorptive action than the bisphosphonates (e.g., alendronate) and should be given to patients who do not tolerate bisphosphonates.

Raloxifene significantly increased the occurrence of hot flushes compared with placebo in all the studies. Other side effects of raloxifene noted were influenza-like symptoms, peripheral edema, and leg cramps. It does not appear to affect vaginal symptoms, urinary symptoms, gallbladder disease, cognitive decline, or cataracts.

The recommended starting dose is 60 mg/day.

Tamoxifen

Tamoxifen[1] has demonstrated some benefit for osteoporosis, but estrogen and bisphosphonates have shown a greater increase in lumbar spine BMD. In the National Surgical Adjuvant Breast and Bowel Project (NSABP) P-1 Trial, women on tamoxifen had fewer hip, wrist, and vertebral fractures at 7-year follow-up. In this study there was not a significant difference in the occurrence of cardiovascular events. Total and LDL cholesterol were significantly decreased on tamoxifen.

In combination with adjuvant therapy for estrogen receptor–positive breast cancer, tamoxifen can decrease the risk of recurrence and death and aid those with metastatic disease.

As with raloxifene, patients taking tamoxifen have a greater risk for VTE. This association is found particularly in patients who are concomitantly receiving chemotherapy.

The main difference between raloxifene and tamoxifen is that tamoxifen use is associated with a greater risk of endometrial cancers, especially uterine sarcoma. This risk depended on length of treatment. As a result, the American College of Obstetrics and Gynecologists (ACOG) has recommendations regarding monitoring women taking tamoxifen (Box 7), but these are not evidence based. For prevention, an intrauterine levonorgestrel could be placed. Even though there is evidence to suggest that tamoxifen is effective in preventing and treating osteoporosis, it is not approved by the FDA except for the prevention and treatment of breast cancer.

---

[1]Not FDA approved for this indication.

REFERENCES

American College of Obstetricians and Gynecologists. Tamoxifen and endometrial cancer. ACOG Committee Opinion 232. Washington, DC: American College of Obstetricians and Gynecologists; 2000.

American College of Obstetricians and Gynecologists Task Force. Hormone Therapy. Obstet Gynecol 2004;104(Suppl. 4):S1–129.

Barnabei VM, Cochrane BB, Aragaki AK, et al. Menopausal symptoms and treatment-related effects of estrogen and progestin in the Women's Health Initiative. Obstet Gynecol 2005;105:1063–73.

Barrett-Connor E, Cauley JA, Kulkarni PM, et al. Risk-benefit profile for raloxifene: 4-Year data from the Multiple Outcomes of Raloxifene Evaluation (MORE) randomized trial. J Bone Miner Res 2004;19:1270–5.

Grady D, Herrington D, Bittner V, et al. Cardiovascular disease outcomes during 6.8 years of hormone therapy: Heart and Estrogen/Progestin Replacement Study follow-up (HERS-II). JAMA 2002;288:49–57.

Hulley S, Grady D, Bush T, et al. for the Heart and Estrogen/Progestin Replacement Study (HERS) Research Group. Randomized trial of estrogen plus progestin for secondary prevention of coronary heart disease in postmenopausal women. JAMA 1998;280:605–13.

North American Menopause Society. Treatment of menopause-associated vasomotor symptoms: Position statement of The North American Menopause Society. Menopause 2004;11:11–33.

Soules MR, Sherman S, Parrott E, Rebar R. Executive summary: Stages of Reproductive Aging Workshop (STRAW). Fertil Steril 2001;76:874–8.

Women's Health Initiative Steering Committee. Effects of conjugated equine estrogen in postmenopausal women with hysterectomy. JAMA 2004;291:1707–12.

Writing Group for the PEPI Trial. Effects of estrogen or estrogen/progestin regimens on heart disease risk factors in postmenopausal women. The Postmenopausal Estrogen/Progestin Interventions (PEPI) Trial. JAMA 1995;273:199–208.

Writing Group for the Women's Health Initiative Investigators. Risks and benefits of estrogen plus progestin in healthy postmenopausal women: Principal results from the Women's Health Initiative randomized controlled trial. JAMA 2002;288:321–33.

Vulvovaginitis

Method of
Christine Hudak, MD

From a medical perspective, it is tempting to consider vulvovaginitis a minor problem. However, to the woman affected, getting relief is quite important. In addition to the immediate physical discomfort and potential risks in pregnancy, those with untreated vaginitis can experience body image issues and sexual problems. Evaluation of vaginitis accounts for more than 10 million office visits a year in the United States, so proper diagnosis and management are essential. This article addresses the most common causes of vaginitis: bacterial vaginosis (40%–50% of cases), candidiasis (20%–25%), and trichomoniasis (15%–20%.) Of these three, only trichomoniasis is sexually transmitted, although all have been associated with other sexually transmitted infections.

Symptoms of vaginitis most commonly include vaginal redness, itching, and discharge that may be malodorous. Trichomoniasis can also cause dysuria, dyspareunia, and postcoital bleeding. Candidal infections can also produce vulvar redness, itching, dysuria, and dyspareunia.

Identifying the etiology of vaginitis is primarily based on patient history, pelvic examination, vaginal pH measurement, and microscopic evaluation of the discharge. Even in expert hands, the sensitivity of a 0.9% normal saline and 10% KOH slide preparations is 50% to 60%. Culture and newer office-based testing options are also available.

Bacterial Vaginosis

Bacterial vaginosis is not an infection but rather a shift in the normal bacterial vaginal flora. There is a decrease of lactobacilli and an overgrowth of *Gardnerella vaginalis*, *Mycoplasma hominus*, and anaerobes. Factors that are associated with bacterial vaginosis include multiple sex partners, a new sex partner, and douching.

Clinical indicators of bacterial vaginosis include Amsel's criteria: abnormal gray discharge, vaginal pH greater than 4.5, a positive amine test, and more than 20% clue cells on normal saline microscopy. If two or three of the criteria are present, the clinical diagnosis of bacterial vaginosis can be made with a 90% sensitivity and 77% specificity. (The amine test is commonly referred to as the *whiff test*

and is positive if the addition of KOH to a sample of the discharge produces a strong fishy odor.) Additional microscopic findings can include a large amount of coccobacillary bacteria and a lack of lactobacilli.

A recent meta-analysis evaluating the accuracy of signs and symptoms of vaginitis to determine etiology found that in patients with the symptom of vaginal odor, the likelihood ratio for having bacterial vaginosis was 1.6 with a sensitivity of 97% and a specificity of 40%. The use of culture for the diagnosis of bacterial vaginosis is not recommended because the organisms in question are all normal vaginal flora. There is also a rapid office test available (QuickVue Advance *G. vaginalis* test) for CLIA (Clinical Laboratory Improvement Admendment) moderately complex labs. Changes suggesting bacterial vaginosis reported on a Papanicolaou (Pap) smear do not require treatment unless the patient is symptomatic.

In addition to causing vaginitis, bacterial vaginosis has also been associated with pelvic inflammatory disease, infections after gynecologic surgery, and acquisition of sexually transmitted infections such as herpes and HIV. Treatment for bacterial vaginosis prior to hysterectomy and abortion decreases the postoperative infection rate.

In pregnant patients, bacterial vaginosis has been associated with premature rupture of membranes (PROM), prematurity, chorioamnionitis, and low birth weight. In symptomatic patients, the treatment of bacterial vaginosis decreases those risks, though the current data do not support screening asymptomatic patients during pregnancy. The exception may be for women at high risk for preterm delivery. Several studies demonstrated that screening and treating asymptomatic pregnant women for bacterial vaginosis decreased the risk of prematurity and PROM, although one study did not show a benefit.

Box 1 summarizes the 2006 Centers for Disease Control and Prevention (CDC) recommendations for treating bacterial vaginosis. Because this is not a sexually transmitted infection, treatment of the partner is not recommended.

Vulvovaginal Candidiasis

Vulvovaginal candidiasis is the second most common etiology of clinical vaginitis. Symptoms of candidiasis are vaginal itching, irritation, a thick white discharge, dysuria, and dyspareunia. With the availability of over-the-counter antifungal treatments, many women self-diagnose and treat their symptoms. Unfortunately, the accuracy of self-diagnosis is not very good. If women have had a prior episode of candidiasis, they correctly identify recurrence 36% of the time. With no prior episode, self-diagnosis accuracy drops to 9%. Women

---

BOX 1   Treatment of Bacterial Vaginosis

Nonpregnant Patients
Recommended Regimens
Metronidazole (Flagyl): 500 mg PO bid × 7 days
Metronidazole gel 0.75% (MetroGel-Vaginal): 1 applicator (5 g) intravaginally qhs × 5 days
Clindamycin cream 2% (Cleocin): 1 applicator (5 g) intravaginally qhs × 7 days

Alternative Regimens
Clindamycin (Cleocin): 300 mg PO bid × 7 days
Clindamycin ovules (Cleocin): 100 g intravaginally qhs × 3 days

Pregnant Patients
Metronidazole (Flagyl): 500 mg PO bid × 7 days
Metronidazole: 250 mg PO tid × 7 days
Clindamycin (Cleocin): 300 mg PO bid × 7 days

treating themselves empirically for candidiasis can delay treatment of other more serious disorders. Although self-treatment may be a good option for some, it is important for patients to be evaluated by a physician if the initial treatment fails.

Similarly, physicians are not very accurate at making the diagnosis from symptoms and physical examination findings alone. The most predictive signs and symptoms are thick white curdlike discharge and vulvar inflammation. Microscopy with 10% KOH demonstrates blastospores or pseudohyphae and few (if any) leukocytes. Vaginal pH is typically normal in the presence of candidiasis, 4 to 4.5. The sensitivity of microscopy has been estimated at 65% and varies with the experience of the physician.

Most candidiasis is caused by *Candida albicans*, although non-albicans types can also cause symptoms. *Candida* is normal flora in the vagina and so is not a sexually transmitted infection but rather an overgrowth phenomenon like bacterial vaginosis. Culture is typically reserved for women who do not respond to treatment and is especially helpful when identifying non-albicans infections. *Candida glabrata* does not form the typical pseudohyphae seen on microscopy of *C. albicans*.

The CDC divides candidiasis into two categories: complicated and uncomplicated. Patient risk factors for complicated candidiasis include pregnancy, diabetes (or other serious medical conditions) and immunocompromised status. Other characteristics of complicated candidiasis are the suspicion of a non-albicans infection, a severe infection, or infection that recurs four or more times a year. Treatment recommendations are different for complicated and uncomplicated candidiasis. Partners of women with candidiasis do not need to be treated because this is not a sexually transmitted infection. Candidiasis has not been associated with any pregnancy risks.

Boxes 2 and 3 summarize the 2006 CDC recommendations for treatment of candidiasis.

BOX 2 Treatment of Uncomplicated Vulvovaginal Candidiasis

1-Day Therapy

Fluconazole (Diflucan): 1 150-mg tablet PO
Butoconazole 2% SR cream (Gynazole-1): 1 applicator (5 g) intravaginally × 1
Tioconazole 6.5% cream (Monistat-1, Vagistat-1): 1 applicator (4.6 g) intravaginally × 1
Miconazole 1200 mg suppository (Monistat-1 Combination Pack): 1 suppository intravaginally × 1

3-Day Therapy

Butoconazole 2% cream (Femstat-3, Mycelex 3) 1 applicator (5 g) intravaginally qhs × 3 days
Terconazole 0.8% cream (Terazol-3), 1 applicator (5 g) intravaginally qhs × 3 days
Clotrimazole 200 mg vaginal tablet (Gyne-Lotrimin-3) 1 tablet intravaginally qhs × 3 days
Miconazole 200 mg suppository (M-zole 3 combo pack) 1 suppository intravaginally qhs × 3 days
Terconazole 80 mg suppository (Terazol-3) 1 suppository intravaginally qhs × 3 days

7-Day+ Therapy

Clotrimazole 1% cream (Gyne-Lotrimin 7, Mycelex-7): 1 applicator (5 g) intravaginally qhs × 7–14 days
Miconazole 2% cream Femizol-M, Monistat-7): 1 applicator (5 g) intravaginally qhs × 7 days
Terconazole 0.4% cream (Terazol-7) 1 applicator (5 g): intravaginally × 7 days
Clotrimazole 100 mg tab (Mycelex-7 Combo pack): 1 tab intravaginally qhs × 7 days
Miconazole 100 mg suppository (Monistat 7): 1 suppository intravaginally qhs × 7 days
Nystatin 100,000 U tab: 1 tab intravaginally qhs × 14 days

BOX 3 Treatment of Complicated Vulvovaginal Candidiasis

Treatment Regimens

Fluconazole (Diflucan) 100-, 150-, or 200-mg tablet: 1 tablet PO q 3 days × 3 doses
Topical azole cream, tablet or suppository: 1 dose intravaginally qhs × 7–14 days

Maintenance Regimens

Fluconazole 100-, 150-, or 200-mg tablet: 1 tablet PO every week × 6 months
Clotrimazole 200-mg suppository (Gyne-Lotrimin 3): 1 suppository intravaginally qhs 2×/week
Butoconazole 2% cream (Femstat-3, Mycelex-3): 1 applicator (5 g) intravaginally qhs × 3 days

---

Non-albicans infections such as those caused by *C. glabrata* are only about 50% responsive to the azoles. For azole treatment failure, 600 mg vaginal boric acid capsules[6] can be used daily for 14 days. Topical flucytosine cream[1,6] has also been used successfully in resistant infections. For recurrent candidiasis, maintenance regimens are suggested by the CDC, although there is a high rate of relapse once the medications are discontinued.

Trichomonas Vaginitis

Trichomoniasis is sexually transmitted and caused by the flagellated protozoan, *Trichomonas vaginalis*. Women may be asymptomatic (as their partners often are) or report symptoms of malodorous yellow-green discharge, itching, dysuria, dyspareunia, and postcoital bleeding.

Diagnosis in women is most commonly made by viewing motile trichomonads microscopically, which has a sensitivity of 60% to 70%. A large number of white blood cells can also be seen on the wet preparation. Vaginal pH is typically higher than normal. Office point-of-care testing kits are available, including the OSOM Trichomonas Rapid Test and the Affirm VP III (the last tests for *T. vaginalis*, *G. vaginalis*, and *C. albicans*). Samples may also be sent for culture of trichomonas, although they are not commonly used clinically.

In men, urethral swab, urine, or semen can be cultured if necessary because the wet preparation and microscopy are not sensitive. Physicians might consider empirically treating the partner to decrease the rate of reinfection.

In pregnant patients, *Trichomonas* infection is associated with harmful outcomes such as PROM, preterm delivery, and low-birth-weight babies. Curiously, studies that have been done to date do not show a decrease in these outcomes when women have been treated. Those studies had some limitations, and there is no current

---

[1]Not FDA approved for this indication.
[6]May be compounded by pharmacists.

CURRENT DIAGNOSIS

- Bacterial vaginosis: pH, >4.5; 20% clue cells, malodorous discharge
- Vulvovaginal candidiasis: pH, 4–4.5; pseudohyphae, blastospores, thick curdlike discharge, vulvar inflammation
- *Trichomonas* vaginitis: pH, >4.5; motile, flagellated trichomonads, many WBCs, yellow discharge, vulvovaginal inflammation

---

BOX 4 Treatment of Trichomoniasis

Recommended Regimens

Metronidazole (Flagyl) 2 g PO × 1 dose *or*
Tinidazole (Tindamax) 2 g PO × 1 dose

Alternative Regimen

Metronidazole 500 mg PO bid × 7 days

---

recommendation about the necessity of treatment in pregnancy. However, the most common medication for treatment, metronidazole (Flagyl), is Category B and considered safe for use in all trimesters.

Box 4 summarizes the 2006 CDC recommendations for treatment of *Trichomonas* vaginitis.

Tinidazole (Tindamax) is newly approved in the United States for the treatment of trichomoniasis and is as efficacious as metronidazole. Resistance to metronidazole is estimated to be less than 5%, and this can often be overcome with a higher dose of metronidazole or by treating with tinidazole due to its longer half-life. Topical preparations of metronidazole (MetroGel-Vaginal, Vandazole) are not very successful in treating *Trichomonas* and are not recommended. Follow-up testing is not required for patients who are asymptomatic after treatment.

REFERENCES

ACOG Committee on Practice Bulletins—Gynecology. ACOG Practice Bulletin. Clinical management guidelines for obstetrician-gynecologists, Number 72, May 2006: Vaginitis. Obstet Gynecol 2006;107:1195–206.

Anderson MR, Klink K, Cohrssen A. Evaluation of vaginal complaints. JAMA 2004;291(11):1368–79.

Centers for Disease Control and Prevention. Workowski KA, Berman SM. Sexually transmitted diseases treatment guidelines, 2006. MMWR Recomm Rep 2006;55(RR-11):1–94.

Owen MK, Clenney TL. Management of vaginitis. Am Fam Physician 2004; 70:2125–32, 2139–40.

Chlamydia trachomatis

Method of
Catherine Stevens-Simon, MD*

The Scope of the Problem

Responsible for more than 3 million infections each year in the United States, *Chlamydia trachomatis* poses a public health problem of epidemic proportions. Because of the large reservoir of undiagnosed, asymptomatic infections, the number of reported cases significantly underestimates the true prevalence of this infection. Nonetheless, *C. trachomatis* is not only the most commonly reported bacterial sexually transmitted disease (STD) in the United States but also the nation's most commonly reported bacterial infection. It is difficult to give meaningful prevalence figures because the proportion of infected individuals depends on the characteristics of the population studied and how they are studied. In addition, whereas passive surveillance systems indicate that the prevalence of this infection has risen precipitously over the last decade, studies conducted at

---

*Deceased.

---

sentinel surveillance sites demonstrate a decline, which suggests that expanded screening, increased reporting, and improved test sensitivity mask a true decrease in prevalence in some sectors of American society. The epidemiologic characteristics and clinical manifestations of chlamydial infections in the United States reflect the fact that most infections are sexually transmitted and that prevalent stereotypes have an affinity for columnar epithelium. Teenage girls are most susceptible to these infections because of the following factors:

- At their age, the columnar epithelium is prominent on the ectocervix.
- Some experience a high level of unprotected, serially monogamous sexual activity with older men whose sexual risk profiles they rarely investigate.

With these two factors combined, teenage girls are at maximal biologic and social risk. Although the national prevalence of chlamydial infections in this population is unknown, school- and clinic-based studies suggest a range of 8% to 26% (compared to 3% to 5% in sociodemographically similar young adult women), with the highest age-specific prevalence reported among adolescents ages 14 to 15 years. Although readily eradicable, the economic and human costs of these infections are staggering. Annual expenditures are estimated to exceed $1.5 billion, with 75% of the cost devoted to treating sequelae of cervical infections that were initially uncomplicated. Because the majority of severe consequences of untreated infections occur in women, and as much as 66.6% of tubal factor infertility and 33.3% of ectopic pregnancies in the United States are attributed to chlamydial infections, it is estimated that every dollar spent on screening and treating asymptomatic young women and their sex partners saves approximately $12. Although this uniquely positions primary health care providers to prevent the costly sequelae of chlamydial infections, given their prevalence among teenagers, expansion of screening and treatment programs to nontraditional settings such as schools, juvenile detention centers, and drug treatment facilities is likely to be a critical component of any national strategy to ontrol this infection.

Clinical Presentation

Chlamydial infections are an excellent example of the dependence of the clinical manifestations of disease on the intrinsic properties of the pathogen and host. In Western industrialized countries, virtually all chlamydial infections are either sexually transmitted or vertically transmitted at birth. They are caused by nonlymphogranuloma venereum stereotypes that have an affinity for columnar epithelium and can only survive by a cytotoxic, replicative cycle that evokes a variable immune response in the host. Hence, in the United States, the endocervix, urethra, rectum, and conjunctiva are preferentially affected, and clinical manifestations range from asymptomatic to florid inflammatory conditions with severe reproductive consequences. *Chlamydia* should be suspected in these populations:

- Women and men with dysuria and pyuria
- Women with dyspareunia; abnormal vaginal discharge; postcoital, irregular menstrual, or breakthrough contraceptive bleeding; and lower abdominal or pelvic pain
- Infants with conjunctivitis or a staccato cough

These signs and symptoms are neither a sensitive nor a specific indication of infection, however. Indeed, because nearly 90% of chlamydial infections are asymptomatic and *C. trachomatis* is isolated from less than 33.3% of women with mucopurulent cervicitis and less than 50% of men with nongonococcal urethritis, such complaints are unreliable predictors of infection. In women, the most common sign is mucopurulent cervicitis, a nonspecific clinical syndrome characterized by erythema, edema, and friability of the ectocervix and purulent endocervical exudate. Mucopurulent cervicitis, however, is also caused by other STDs and noninfectious factors (i.e., cyclical fluctuations in gonadal hormones), which increase the size of the cervical ectropion or the resident population of cervical leukocytes.

Other clinical manifestations of lower genital tract chlamydial infections in women include urethritis and bartholinitis. Although pelvic inflammatory disease (PID) is a polymicrobial infection, *C. trachomatis* is also often involved, and, conversely, PID is the most common complication of chlamydial cervicitis. The estimated incidence ranges from 10% to 40% in untreated women. Young age and prolonged or recurrent infection significantly increase, whereas treatment of asymptomatic infections significantly decreases both disease severity and sequelae, such as salpingo-oophoritis, perihepatitis (Fitz-Hugh-Curtis syndrome), infertility, ectopic pregnancy, and chronic pelvic pain. Adverse outcomes associated with chlamydial infections during pregnancy include preterm labor, premature rupture of the placental membranes, low-birth-weight delivery, neonatal death, postpartum or postabortal endometritis, and vertical transmission to infants. In the infected infants, 30% to 50% develop conjunctivitis, 15% to 20% develop nasopharyngitis, and 5% to 10% develop pneumonia.

In men, the most common clinical manifestation is urethritis, the symptoms of which typically commence 1 to 3 weeks after exposure and range from mild dysuria to frank penile discharge. Other clinical syndromes in men include epididymitis, prostatitis, acute proctocolitis, and Reiter syndrome (urethritis, conjunctivitis, arthritis, and mucocutaneous lesions). These suppurative complications rarely require inpatient therapy and are far less common than those encountered in women. Nonetheless, sequelae ranging from urethral strictures to infertility do occur. Nongenital clinical manifestations, such as conjunctivitis, tenosynovitis, and arthritis, are uncommon among adults in the United States.

Diagnosis and Screening

In the United States, testing for both symptomatic and asymptomatic chlamydial infections is done with ligase chain reaction (LCR), polymerase chain reaction (PCR), and other nucleic acid amplification techniques (NAATs) because they do not require the presence of intact organisms. Urine, cervical, vaginal, or urethral fluids can be used as the analyte for these tests; specimens are stable and easy to transport; and results can be obtained within a day. This is a major advantage over the stringent collection, transport, and 3-day growth period culturing requirements associated with this fastidious organism. Although nonculture assays, non-NAATs, and rapid diagnostic tests capable of making a diagnosis within 30 minutes are available, these assays are too insensitive to be recommended for routine testing.

The signs and symptoms of chlamydial infection are nonspecific and often persist for weeks after documented eradication of the pathogen. Because of this, leukocyte, esterase-positive urine dipsticks, leukocyte-laden vaginal wet mounts, and endocervical Gram stains should be regarded as no more than a trigger for testing. Although concerns about the consequences of underdiagnosis and undertreatment typically overshadow concerns about the consequences of overdiagnosis and overtreatment, therapeutic decisions should not be based on these poorly standardized tests. Indeed, given their low positive predictive value for chlamydial infections, the adverse psychological effects of being diagnosed with an STD, and the serious public health problems that the indiscriminate use of antibiotics creates—even in settings where the prevalence of chlamydial infections is high and patient follow-up is uncertain and in resource-poor clinics where NAATs are unavailable—enthusiasm for the practice of diagnosing chlamydial infections empirically. This must be tempered by the knowledge that to prevent one individual from suffering the sequelae of an untreated infection, hundreds will needlessly suffer the adverse psychosocial consequences of an STD diagnosis. This is true even when the diagnosis is made based on characteristic symptom complexes, suggestive leukocyte esterase urine dipsticks, and/or vaginal wet mounts. Thus, with sensitivities and specificities fluctuating approximately 98% on male urethral and urine specimens as well as on female cervical specimens, NAATs are currently the best chlamydial tests available. However, because the sensitivity of these assays for detecting infections in women is significantly lower when urine

CURRENT DIAGNOSIS

- Signs and symptoms are neither a sensitive nor a specific indication of chlamydial infection and often persist for weeks after documented eradication of the pathogen.

  Most chlamydial infections are asymptomatic.
  Chlamydia trachomatis is isolated from less than half of women and men with the most common signs and symptoms (mucopurulent cervicitis and urethritis).
- *Chlamydia* should be suspected in:
  Women and men with dysuria and pyuria.
  Women with dyspareunia, abnormal vaginal discharge, abnormal bleeding, and lower abdominal or pelvic pain; infants with conjunctivitis or a staccato cough
- Routine periodic screening with nucleic acid amplification techniques (NAATs) is the only reliable way to diagnose this infection.

(80% to 95%) or patient- or provider-collected vaginal fluid (70% to 85%) is the analyte, endocervical specimens should be used, except in screening situations where it is impractical to perform pelvic examinations. Thus every case diagnosed on a urine or vaginal specimen is a bonus.

Despite consensus about how to screen, uncertainty continues about whom to screen and how frequently to screen them. Pregnant women and sexually active women younger than 25 years of age are the only groups for whom there is good evidence that the benefits of screening outweigh the harms. Specifically, when prevalence rates exceed 2%, testing and treating these individuals for asymptomatic chlamydial infections is a cost-effective preventive measure that:

- Averts PID and associated medical complications.
- Reduces transmission to sex partners.
- Reduces the risk of acquiring HIV.
- Lowers the prevalence of *Chlamydia* in the community.

It is unlikely that these benefits reflect factors other than screening (i.e., increased condom use) because knowledge of sexual risk behavior adds nothing to predictive algorithms that include age and prior STD history. However, because of the highly infectious nature of this bacterium, the lack of a vaccine, and the failure of the human immune system to build up resistance to the bacteria, reinfection of effectively treated individuals tends to diminish short-term efficacy, making long-term periodic screening a prerequisite of cost efficacy.

The only other caveat is that most cost-effectiveness analyses are based on culture-proven disease and therefore may reflect a larger inoculum than infections diagnosed by NAAT assays, which can detect extremely low levels of viable and nonviable organisms. Thus further research is needed to determine if and how inoculum size affects disease presentation and to define the clinical and public health significance of NAAT-detectable infections. Specifically, studies comparing transmission rates and the clinical consequences of infections that are detected only by NAAT assay versus those that are detected by traditional assays are still needed to prove that routine, periodic, urine-based screening of asymptomatic individuals is a cost-effective way to control chlamydial infections at the population level. Moreover, because identifying infected individuals is only the first step in effective disease control, it is also important to demonstrate that once identified, the majority of these asymptomatically infected individuals and their sex partners can be contacted and treated. The randomized trial data that determine how frequently community members should be screened to lower chlamydial infections at the population level are lacking; however, observational studies consistently indicate that among sexually active teens the median time between first and repeat infections is approximately 6 months. Based on these data, biannual screening seems reasonable for women at this age (older than 25 years). Because the risk of reinfection is inversely related to age, it is unclear whether this recommendation should be extended to young adults. Nevertheless, a history of prior infection predicts reinfection regardless of sexual risk behavior, and in women repeat infections are implicated in the pathogenesis of upper genital tract damage. It may be wise, therefore, to rescreen all women who were treated for chlamydial infections at 6-month intervals.

Developing selective screening criteria is a vigorously pursued public health goal. With the exception of age, however, no single demographic or behavioral risk factor or combination of risk factors consistently identifies a group of young, sexually active women who should not be screened. The utility of more selective screening is limited by the high proportion of missed infections.

Parallel evidence to support screening asymptomatic men may be lacking because before the introduction of urine screening men were not routinely tested for chlamydial infection. But because the cost of treating men is lower than the cost of treating women, a greater proportion of infected men are symptomatic than women, and the harm associated with misdiagnoses is not inconsequent, it will undoubtedly be more difficult to justify routine periodic male screening. However, false-negative test results create a reservoir of untreated disease that is likely to contribute disproportionately to the spread of *C. trachomatis*; but the psychosocial consequences of false-positive test results can range from dysphoric feelings and decreased self-esteem to the disruption of romantic relationships and domestic violence. Moreover, if treatment is initiated inappropriately, the adverse effects of drug reactions and bacterial resistance caused by antibiotic overuse must be taken into account. Thus, until more data become available, the United States Preventive Services Task Force recommends symptom-based screening for all men and for women older than 25 years of age who do not exhibit other characteristics associated with a high prevalence of chlamydial infections (i.e., unmarried status, African American race, a history of STDs, a history of new or multiple sex partners, cervical ectopy, and inconsistent condom use).

Treatment

Recommendations for antibiotic treatment of chlamydial infections depend on the clinical syndrome. Box 1 summarizes the options for outpatient therapy of uncomplicated genital tract infections in men and women. However, because humans do not develop a natural immunity to chlamydia, treated patients remain at risk for reinfection. For this reason therapy should not be considered complete until all recent sexual contacts are treated and the patient is counseled about future disease prevention. An estimated 70% of the male partners of women with chlamydial cervicitis are infected, and, conversely, approximately 30% of the female partners of *Chlamydia*-infected men are infected. Treatment is recommended for the most recent sex partner and all other individuals who had sexual contact

---

BOX 1   *Chlamydia trachomatis*: Recommended Treatment Regimens by Clinical Syndrome

Asymptomatic, Cervicitis, Urethritis*
- First-choice regimen
- Azithromycin (Zithromax), 1 g orally in a single dose
  or
- Doxycycline (Vibramycin), 100 mg orally twice a day for 7 days

Alternative Regimens (One of the Following)
- Erythromycin base (E-Mycin), 500 mg orally four times a day for 7 days
- Erythromycin ethylsuccinate (EES), 800 mg orally four times a day for 7 days
- Ofloxacin (Floxin), 300 mg orally twice a day for 7 days
- Levofloxacin (Levaquin),[1] 500 mg orally for 7 days

Epididymitis
- Ceftriaxone (Rocephin),[1] 250 mg intramuscularly (single dose)
  or
- Doxycycline,[1] 100 mg orally twice a day for 7 days

Outpatient Pelvic Inflammatory Disease
- Ceftriaxone, 250 mg intramuscularly (single dose)
  plus
- Doxycycline, 100 mg orally twice a day for 14 days *with or without*
- Metronidazole (Flagyl), 500 mg orally twice a day for 14 days

Alternative Regimens
- Ceftriaxone, 250 mg intramuscularly (single dose)
  or
- Cefoxitin (Mefoxin), 2 g intramuscularly (single dose)
  plus
- Probenecid, 1 g orally
  plus
- Doxycycline, 100 mg orally twice a day for 14 days *with or without*
- Metronidazole, 500 mg orally twice a day for 14 days

Inpatient Pelvic Inflammatory Disease[†]
- Cefotetan (Cefotan), 2 g intravenously every 12 hours
  or
- Cefoxitin, 2 g intravenously every 6 hours
  plus
- Doxycycline,[1] 100 mg orally or intravenously every 12 hours

Alternative Regimens
- Clindamycin, 900 mg intravenously every 8 hours
  plus
- Gentamicin,[1] 2 g/kg of body weight loading dose, then 1.5 mg/kg of body weight every 8 hours. Treatment should be continued for 24 to 48 hours after significant clinical improvement occurs and then should consist of oral therapy with doxycycline, 100 mg orally twice a day for 14 days, or clindamycin, 450 mg orally four times a day, for a total of 14 days.

Providers should consult the Centers for Disease Control and Prevention's website at: http://www.cdc.gov/std/treatment for up-to-treatment recommendations.
[1]Not FDA approved for this indication.
*Pregnancy: Doxycycline, erythromycin estolate (Ilosone), and ofloxacin are contraindicated, and repeat testing 3 weeks after completion of therapy is recommended because antibiotics may be less efficacious. HIV infection: Patients who have chlamydial infection and who also are infected with HIV should receive the same treatment regimen as those who are HIV-negative.
[†]Studies indicate that the efficacy of inpatient and outpatient treatment is comparable in terms of fertility and other long-term health outcomes. Criteria for inpatient treatment include surgical emergencies, pregnancy, unresponsive to oral antimicrobial therapy, unable to follow or tolerate an outpatient oral regimen, severe illness, nausea and vomiting, or high fever, or tubo-ovarian abscess.

CURRENT THERAPY

- Antibiotic treatment is easy to summarize in tabular form but is ineffective if given in isolation of sexual network.
  - Large reservoir of asymptomatically infected partners and potential partners undermines the effectiveness of individual treatments.
  - Half of all chlamydial infections occur in previously treated persons.
- Therapy is not complete until all recent sexual contacts are treated and the patient is counseled about disease prevention.
- Prevalence of *Chlamydia trachomatis* in the sexual network is the best predictor of infection.
- Whom an individual has sexual intercourse with puts him or her at higher risk for acquisition of this infection than how they do so.
- For disease prevention, condoms are plan B. Plan A is choosing low-risk sexual partners.

with the infected person during the 60 days preceding the onset of symptoms or diagnosis. Also, partners should abstain from sexual intercourse for a week after they complete treatment.

Although patient-delivered partner treatment is as effective as partner notification, partners are more likely to be treated if informed by physicians rather than by the patients. This is because only 65% (approximately) of women with known chlamydial infections refer their sex partners for therapy, and even fewer (approximately 45%) infected men do so. Because the cure rate for single-dose azithromycin (Zithromax) therapy is close to 100% and the medication can easily be administered under medical supervision, a test of cure 3 weeks after treatment—NAATs remain positive for this long despite successful eradication of infection—is only recommended for pregnant women (among whom antibiotic efficacy may be reduced) and when compliance is in doubt.

Approximately 50% of all chlamydial infections occur in previously treated persons. Demographic characteristics, such as age and a past history of chlamydial infection, are better predictors of infection than behavioral risk factors, such as multiple sexual partners and the failure to use condoms consistently. Being involved with a sexual network in which *Chlamydia* is hyperendemic appears to put individuals at greater risk for infection than unsafe sexual behavior in the general population. Hence, to control the spread of *C. trachomatis*, it may be necessary to:

- Extend screening and treatment beyond recent partners to include the group of core transmitters in the infected individual's sexual network.
- Help STD patients learn to choose less risky sex partners by promoting sexual health communication within partnerships.

Although the debate about the content and duration of counseling necessary to achieve this goal is ongoing, there is a growing consensus that brief (5 minutes), personalized (provider-delivered and client-centered) counseling sessions—aimed at personal risk reduction and increasing awareness of partner risk behavior—are more effective than the conventional didactic approach to STD prevention education. They are certainly as effective as more prolonged sessions, which are difficult to conduct in busy public health clinics.

REFERENCES

Aral SO, Hughes JP, Stoner B, et al. Sexual mixing patterns in spread of gonococcal and chlamydial infections. Am J Pub Health 1999;89:825–33.
Biro F, Workowski K, Blythe MJ, Lara-Torre E. NASPAG/JPAG roundtable discussion annual clinical meeting 2003. Philadelphia, PA: Sexually transmitted diseases (STD) treatment guidelines 2002. J Pediatr Adolesc Gynecol 2004;17:143–6.
Cates Jr W. Contraception, unintended pregnancies, and sexually transmitted diseases: Why isn't a simple solution possible? Am J Epidemiol 1996;143:311–8.
Critchlow CW, Wolner-Hanssen P, Eschenbach DA, et al. Determinants of cervical ectopia and cervicitis: Age, oral contraception, specific cervical infection, smoking, and douching. Am J Obstet Gynecol 1995;173:534–43.
Duncan B, Hart G, Scoular A, Bigrigg A. Qualitative analysis of psychosocial impact of diagnosis of Chlamydia trachomatis. Implications for screening. BMJ 2001;322:195–229.
Ford CA, Viadro CI, Miller WC. Testing for chlamydial and gonorrheal infections outside of clinic settings. A summary of the literature. Sex Transm Dis 2004;31:38–51.
Kamb ML, Fishbein M, Douglas Jr JM, et al. Efficacy of risk-reduction counseling to prevent human immunodeficiency virus and sexually transmitted diseases: A randomized controlled trial for the Project RESPECT Study Group. JAMA 1998;280:1161–7.
Peipert JF. Clinical practice. Genital chlamydial infections. N Engl J Med 2003;349:2424–30.
Rietmeijer CA, Van Bemmelen R, Judson FN, Douglas JM. Incidence and repeat infection rates of Chlamydia trachomatis among male and female patients in an STD clinic. Sex Transm Dis 2002;29:65–72.
U.S. Preventive Services Task Force. Screening for chlamydial infection: Recommendations and rationale. Am J Prev Med 2001;20(3S):90–4.

Pelvic Inflammatory Disease

Method of
Adrianne Williams Bagley, MD, and Maria Trent, MD, MPH

Pelvic inflammatory disease (PID) is a spectrum of disorders characterized by an infection of the female upper genital tract. Organs that may be affected include the uterus (endometritis, parametritis), fallopian tubes (salpingitis), and ovaries (oophoritis, tubo-ovarian abscesses [TOAs]), or the infection may involve the pelvic peritoneum.

Epidemiology

Approximately 800,000 women per year are diagnosed with PID. Up to 20% of cases occur in teenagers. Risk factors associated with development of PID mirror the risk factors that increase the likelihood of acquiring a sexually transmitted infection. These risk factors include having multiple sex partners and inconsistent or incorrect use of condoms. Douching and use of intrauterine devices are also associated with PID. Women with a prior diagnosis of PID are at higher risk of developing future episodes.

Pathophysiology

The infection of the female upper genital tract that characterizes PID is caused by the ascent of infectious organisms from the vagina and cervix. It is postulated that the ascent of organisms may occur more readily during menses because of reflux of blood in the fallopian tubes, and studies show a temporal relationship between menses and the subsequent diagnosis of PID.

The infectious agents most often implicated in PID are the sexually transmitted organisms *Neisseria gonorrhoeae* and *Chlamydia trachomatis*. However, PID may be a polymicrobial infection. Other contributing infectious etiologies include anaerobic bacteria such as *Bacteroides* and *Peptostreptococcus* species, *Gardnerella vaginalis*, *Haemophilus influenzae*, *Streptococcus* species, *Mycoplasma hominis*, *Ureaplasma urealyticum*, enteric gram-negative bacilli, and cytomegalovirus.

Diagnosis

The diagnosis of PID is made based on clinical assessment; therefore, a detailed history, careful examination, and the use of additional supportive diagnostic tests are warranted. Patients may present with varied nonspecific complaints including lower abdominal pain, vaginal discharge, and irregular menses or bleeding with sexual intercourse. Patients may or may not be febrile, experience vomiting or diarrhea, or have urinary symptoms. The differential diagnosis includes processes that affect not only the reproductive tract but also the gastrointestinal and urinary tracts. The differential diagnosis includes but is not limited to ovarian cyst, endometriosis, dysmenorrhea, ectopic pregnancy, septic or threatened abortion, gastroenteritis, appendicitis, diverticulitis, constipation, inflammatory bowel disease, irritable bowel syndrome, urethritis, cystitis, pyelonephritis, and nephrolithiasis.

The 2006 Centers for Disease Control and Prevention (CDC) guidelines recommend empirical treatment for PID in sexually active women with minimum diagnostic criteria of uterine tenderness, adnexal tenderness, or cervical motion tenderness, in whom no other cause can be identified. Additional supportive criteria may be used to increase the specificity of diagnosis; these criteria include oral temperature greater than 38°C (101°F), abnormal cervical or vaginal mucopurulent discharge, presence of white blood cells on saline wet mount of vaginal secretions, elevated erythrocyte sedimentation rate (ESR) or Creactive protein (CRP), and documented cervical infection with *N. gonorrhoeae* or *C. trachomatis*. However, if cervical infection with *N. gonorrhoeae* or *C. trachomatis* is not found, these organisms can still be responsible for upper genital tract infection. Additional diagnostic tests may include complete blood cell count (CBC) with differential, urine dipstick or urinalysis, urine culture, and urine pregnancy test. Pelvic ultrasonography should be obtained if there is evidence of a pelvic mass on examination or if there is adnexal tenderness in the setting of high fever, elevated white blood cell count, or elevated CRP or ESR; this constellation of findings may suggest a TOA.

Treatment

Treatment should be initiated promptly for the patient with suspected PID to prevent complications, which include chronic pelvic pain, ectopic pregnancy, and infertility. Antibiotic treatment is broad spectrum to ensure coverage of typical pathogens, namely *N. gonorrhoeae*, *C. trachomatis*, and anaerobes. With prompt appropriate medical treatment, the future reproductive ability of the patient may be protected.

The Current Therapy box outlines the 2006 CDC treatment guidelines for inpatient treatment. Hospitalization for parenteral treatment is reserved for patients for whom surgical causes of abdominal pain cannot be excluded, patients who are pregnant, patients who fail outpatient regimens (unable to follow or tolerate an outpatient regimen, no clinical response to oral antibiotics after 72 hours), patients with severe illness, nausea, vomiting, or high fever, and patients with a TOA. Patients younger than 16 years and those with extenuating social circumstances may also be candidates for inpatient treatment.

CURRENT DIAGNOSIS

- Pelvic inflammatory disease is a clinical diagnosis.
- The minimum diagnostic criterion is one or more of the following clinical findings: uterine tenderness, adnexal tenderness, *or* cervical motion tenderness in the patient in whom no other cause can be identified.
- The use of additional supportive criteria can increase the accuracy of the diagnosis.

CURRENT THERAPY

Inpatient Treatment for Pelvic Inflammatory Disease

Regimen A:
- Cefotetan (Cefotan), 2 g IV q12h, *or* cefoxitin (Mefoxin), 2 g IV q6h, *plus* doxycycline (Vibramycin), 100 mg PO or IV q12h

Regimen B:
- Clindamycin (Cleocin), 900 mg IV q8h, *plus* gentamicin (Garamycin) loading dose: 2 mg/kg IV/IM, followed by maintenance dose: 1.5 mg/kg IV q8h. Single daily dosing may be substituted.

Alternative Regimen:
- Ampicillin/Sulbactam (Unasyn) 3 g IV q6h *plus* doxycycline (Vibramycin) 100 mg PO or IV q12h.

Note: Parenteral therapy for PID should be considered for 24 hours following clinical improvement, and patients should be discharged home on an oral course of doxycycline (Vibramycin) 100 mg PO bid, or clindamycin (Cleocin) 450 PO qid to complete 14 days.

Outpatient Treatment for Pelvic Inflammatory Disease

Recommended Oral Regimens:
- Ceftriaxone (Rocephin), 250 mg IM in a single dose, *or*
- Cefoxitin (Mefoxin), 2 g IM in a single dose, with probenecid, 1 g PO in a single dose, *or*
- Other parenteral third-generation cephalosporins (ceftizoxime [Cefizox] or cefotaxime [Claforan]) *plus* doxycycline (Vibramycin), 100 mg PO bid for 14 days, *with or without* metronidazole (Flagyl), 500 mg PO bid for 14 days.

Alternative Oral Regimens:
- Levofloxacin (Levaquin) 500 mg PO once daily for 14 days or ofloxacin (Floxin) 400 mg PO bid for 14 days with or without metronidazole (Flagyl) 500 mg PO bid for 14 days, if the community prevalence and individual risk of gonorrhea are low (see CDC Sexually Transmitted Disease Treatment Guidelines, 2006). Testing for *N. gonorrhoeae* must be performed prior to treatment. If NAAT test is positive, parental cephalosporin is recommended. If culture is positive for *N. gonorrhoeae*, treatment should be based on antimicrobial susceptibility. If antimicrobial susceptibility cannot be obtained or culture is quinolone resistant *N. gonorrhoeae* (QRNG), parenteral cephalosporin is recommended.

Note: Recommendations from the Centers for Disease Control and Prevention 2006 Sexually Transmitted Diseases Treatment Guidelines are available at http://www.cdc.giv/std/treatment.
Abbreviations: IM = intramuscular; IV = intravenous; PO = orally.

Outpatient treatment for PID is appropriate in most cases for patients who do not meet the criteria for hospitalization. Metronidazole (Flagyl) is often included as part of the treatment regimen to provide anaerobic coverage, and it is an appropriate adjunct medication in patients who also have evidence of bacterial vaginosis on saline wet mount.

FOLLOW-UP

Patients treated with outpatient therapy should be reevaluated in 48 to 72 hours to assess response to treatment. At this visit, the medical provider can review medication adherence, readdress partner notification, review the importance of safe sexual practices, discuss related family planning issues, answer questions that the patient may have about the diagnosis, and reexamine the patient to ensure that she is improving on the current therapeutic regimen. Patients who are not improving on oral antibiotics or who have been unable to adhere with the outpatient regimen may need additional diagnostic testing for complications and hospitalization for parental treatment.

Patients being treated for PID should be advised to abstain from sexual intercourse throughout the course of treatment. All sexual partners within the past 60 days should be tested and empirically treated for both *N. gonorrhoeae* and *C. trachomatis*.

Potential Complications

Short-term complications of PID include TOA and Fitz-Hugh–Curtis syndrome. Patients with TOA require hospitalization for parenteral treatment. Fitz-Hugh–Curtis syndrome is a perihepatitis that may result from spread of *N. gonorrhoeae* or *C. trachomatis* and is characterized by right upper quadrant pain.

Long-term complications of PID include chronic pelvic pain, tubal infertility secondary to scarring, and ectopic pregnancy. Patients with a history of PID have a 6- to 10-fold increased risk of ectopic pregnancy.

Prevention

Primary prevention of PID can be best accomplished by prevention of sexually transmitted infections. Sexually active women should undergo routine screening for gonorrhea and *Chlamydia* and be instructed about the importance of proper condom usage. Secondary prevention can be accomplished with partner notification and empirical treatment using antibiotics with adequate coverage for infections caused by *N. gonorrhoeae* and *C. trachomatis*.

REFERENCES

American Academy of Pediatrics. Pelvic inflammatory disease. In: Pickering LK, editor. Red Book: 2003 Report of the Committee on Infectious Diseases. 26th ed. Elk Grove Village, Ill: American Academy of Pediatrics; 2003. pp. 468–72.

Centers for Disease Control and Prevention. Sexually transmitted disease treatment guidelines 2006. MMWR 2006;55(No. RR-11):56–61.

Ness RB, Soper DE, Holley RL, et al. Effectiveness of inpatient and outpatient treatment strategies for women with pelvic inflammatory disease: Results from the pelvic inflammatory disease evaluation and clinical health (PEACH) randomized trial. Am J Obstet Gynecol 2002;186(5):929–37.

Rein DB, Kassler WJ, Irwin KL, et al. Direct medical costs of pelvic inflammatory disease and its sequelae: Decreasing, but still substantial. Obstet Gynecol 2000;95(3):397–402.

Shrier LA. Bacterial sexually transmitted infections: Gonorrhea, chlamydia, pelvic inflammatory disease, and syphilis. In: Emans SJ, Laufer MR, Goldstein DP, editors. Pediatric and Adolescent Gynecology. 5th ed. Lippincott-Raven; 2004. pp. 583–98.

Trent M, Chung S, Forrest L, Ellen JE. Subsequent pelvic inflammatory disease (PID) and sexually transmitted infections after outpatient treatment for PID in pediatric ambulatory settings. Arch Pediatr Adolesc Med 2008; 162(11):1022–5.

Trent MA, Ellen JM, Walker A. Pelvic Inflammatory disease in adolescents—care delivery in pediatric ambulatory settings. Pediatr Emerg Care 2005; 21(7):431–6.

Trent M, Judy SL, Ellen JM, Walker A. Use of an institutional intervention to improve quality of care for adolescents treated in pediatric ambulatory settings for pelvic inflammatory disease. J Adolesc Health 2006;39(1):50–6.

Update to CDC's sexually transmitted diseases treatment guidelines, 2006. Fluoroquinolones no longer recommended for treatment of gonococcal infections. MMWR Weekly April 13, 2007;56(14):332–6.

Uterine Leiomyomas

Method of
Tod C. Aeby, MD, and Stella Dantas, MD

Epidemiology

Uterine leiomyomas are the most common pelvic tumor in women. They affect approximately 20% of women older than 35 years of age and 40% of women older than 50 years of age, although they are found any time from puberty through menopause. Survey studies involving histologic examination of the uterus suggest they are present in more than 80% of women. Nulliparity, early menarche, and African American ethnicity increase the risk of developing leiomyomas. The incidence among women of African descent is not as high in countries other than the United States, which suggests possible dietary, environmental, and genetic influences on development. Risk is also increased in women with a higher body mass index, presumably because of the increased estrogen production in adipocytes. Pregnancy reduces the risk of developing leiomyomas.

Pathophysiology

The etiology of uterine leiomyomas is not completely understood, but development is thought to be a multistep process. They are benign monoclonal tumors of the smooth muscle of the myometrium that presumably derive from a normal myocyte. Estrogen and progesterone, in concert with local growth factors, lead to a somatic mutation of normal myometrium to a leiomyoma. Some growth factors that cause leiomyoma proliferation are epidermal growth factors, insulin-like growth factors, heparin-binding growth factors, and transforming growth factor-β. Leiomyomas develop during the reproductive years and increase in size during pregnancy. Growth usually ceases in menopause, and leiomyomas then decrease in volume. This supports the theory that estrogen and progesterone promote growth.

Symptoms and Signs

Most uterine leiomyomas are asymptomatic. They are categorized into subgroups based on their anatomic relationship and position in the uterus, and symptoms usually depend on those relationships. They can be subserosal, intramural, submucosal, or pedunculated. The most common symptom is abnormal uterine bleeding, usually menorrhagia, occurring in 30% of women with leiomyomas. The cause of the abnormal bleeding is not totally clear but may be the result of abnormal growth and function of the endometrium near the leiomyoma and local interference with normal physiologic mechanisms for hemostasis.

Pelvic pain and increasing pelvic pressure occur in 30% of women with leiomyomas. Other symptoms include dysmenorrhea, postcoital bleeding, and dyspareunia. Pain can be caused by leiomyomas outgrowing their blood supply and becoming necrotic. This red degeneration is common in pregnancy. Patients may have an increasing abdominal girth and pressure symptoms as a result of large fibroids. Pressure on adjacent organs such as the bladder or bowel can cause urinary frequency and urgency or constipation. Rarely, an enlarged uterus causes a palpable kidney secondary to hydronephrosis from ureteral obstruction. Patients also may be lethargic from anemia secondary to menorrhagia. Leiomyomas may also be associated with infertility, although the relationship is controversial.

CURRENT DIAGNOSIS

- Abnormal uterine bleeding, postcoital spotting
- Pelvic pain, pressure, dysmenorrhea and dyspareunia
- Urinary frequency and urgency, constipation
- Lethargy
- Infertility
- Physical findings: Enlarged, irregular, and firm uterus
- Ultrasound: Diagnostic imaging modality of choice
- Saline infusion sonohysterography and/or hysteroscopy: Used to evaluate the uterine cavity

A rapidly enlarging uterus should raise concern for malignant transformation. But leiomyosarcomas are extremely rare, occurring in less than 0.1% of women operated on for presumed leiomyomas.

Diagnosis

Uterine leiomyomas are typically diagnosed at pelvic exam when an enlarged and irregularly shaped uterus is noted. Abdominal and transvaginal ultrasound is often helpful in making the diagnosis and in differentiating leiomyomas from adnexal masses or other pelvic pathology. Serial ultrasounds also can be used to monitor their growth. During a pelvic exam, it may not be possible to palpate ovaries next to an enlarged uterus, but an adnexal tumor can be suspected if the mass moves independently of the uterus. Submucosal leiomyomas are diagnosed using saline infusion sonohysterography and hysteroscopy. Definitive diagnosis requires histologic examination.

Management

For the most part, asymptomatic leiomyoma should be managed expectantly. The approaches to the patient experiencing problems fall into the three general categories of medical management, conservative procedures, and hysterectomy. The choice should be individualized to the patient, based on the severity of her symptoms, her plans for future childbearing, and her personal interest in retaining her uterus. Other causes of abnormal bleeding should be considered.

Current medical therapy is limited to the use of gonadotropin-releasing hormone (GnRH) analogues and antagonists (i.e., leuprolide

acetate [Lupron Depot], 3.75 mg monthly; nafarelin acetate [Synarel],[1] 200 µg intranasally twice a day; and goserelin acetate implant [Zoladex],[1] 3.6-mg implant monthly, cetrorelix [Cetrotide]).[1] These expensive medications are shown to decrease the uterine size by up to 65%, allowing for easier or more conservative surgical treatments. The progesterone antagonist mifepristone (Mifeprex)[1] is also effective but not currently available for this purpose in the United States. GnRH therapy has significant side effects, mostly related to the induced hypoestrogenic state. To preserve bone density the duration of therapy must be limited. Additionally, the uterus rapidly returns to its enlarged size when the therapy is discontinued. These medications are a very effective means of inducing amenorrhea to allow for correction of an anemia prior to surgery.

Conservative procedures include myomectomy or myolysis (surgical removal or destruction of the individual fibroids while preserving the uterus), uterine artery embolization, and endometrial ablation. Each of these approaches has different risks, benefits, and complications (Table 1).

Hysterectomy remains the most common treatment for women with symptomatic leiomyoma and offers the advantage of a complete and definitive cure. The uterus can be removed through the vagina (with or without the aid of laparoscopic techniques) or through an abdominal incision. The route of removal largely depends on the size of the uterus, the patient's medical and surgical history, and the experience and preference of her surgeon.

---

[1]Not FDA approved for this indication.

CURRENT THERAPY

- Only symptomatic leiomyomas require treatment.
- Medical therapy is for temporizing and making invasive procedures easier or more effective.
- Conservative procedures include myomectomy, myolysis, hydrothermal endometrial ablation, and uterine artery embolization.
- Hysterectomy is the only definitive therapy for leiomyomata.
- Choice of treatment should be made considering the severity of symptoms and respecting the patient's preferences.

TABLE 1 Comparison of Various Procedures for the Treatment of Symptomatic Uterine Leiomyoma

Therapy	Success Rate	Complication Rate	Possibility of Future Childbearing	Comments
Hysterectomy	100%	40%	No	Recovery time varies depending on the route of removal.
Myomectomy and myolysis	75%	39%	Yes	Can be associated with significant blood loss and can result in an unplanned hysterectomy. Recurrent leiomyomas are common.
Myolysis	62%–97%*	3%*	Not currently recommended	Several methods for myolysis are available, including bipolar electrocautery, laser energy, and cryotherapy.
Uterine artery embolization	77%–91%	5%	Not currently recommended	Complication rates are low but can be severe, including infection, sepsis, and nontarget tissue necrosis. A few deaths have been reported.
Hydrothermal endometrial ablation	80%–91%*	1%–2%	No	Hysteroscopic resection of submucosal leiomyomas, prior to endometrial ablation, improves success rates. Several methods are available, including hydrothermal, balloon, bipolar electrocautery, cryotherapy, and microwave endometrial ablation. Pregnancies have occurred after these procedures, so contraception is still required.

*Best estimate based on limited studies.

REFERENCES

Buttram Jr VC, Reiter RC. Uterine leiomyomata: Etiology, symptomatology, and management. Fertil Steril 1981;36:433–45.

Felberbaum RE, Germer U, Ludwig M, et al. Treatment of uterine fibroids with a slow-release formulation of the gonadotrophin-releasing hormone antagonist Cetrorelix. Hum Reprod 1998;13(6):1660–8.

Goldfarb HA. Bipolar laparoscopic needles for myoma coagulation. J Am Assoc Gynecol Laparosc 1995;2(2):175–9.

Lethaby A, Vollenhoven B, Sowter M. Pre-operative GnRH analogue therapy before hysterectomy or myomectomy for uterine fibroids. The Cochrane Database Syst Rev 2001;(2):CD000547. DOI: 10.1002/14651858.CD000547.

Parker WH, Fu YS, Berek JS. Uterine sarcoma in patients operated on for presumed leiomyoma and rapidly growing leiomyoma. Obstet Gynecol 1994;83:414.

Pron G, Bennett J, Common A, et al. Ontario Uterine Fibroid Embolization Collaboration Group. The Ontario Uterine Fibroid Embolization Trial: II. Uterine fibroid reduction and symptom relief after uterine artery embolization for fibroids. Fertil Steril 2003;79(1):120–7.

The Hydro Therm Ablator system for management of menorrhagia in women with submucous myomas: 12- to 20-month follow-up. J Am Assoc Gynecol Laparosc 2003;10(4):521–7.

Cancer of the Endometrium

Method of
Dan-Arin Silasi, MD, and Masoud Azodi, MD

Epidemiology

In the United States, endometrial cancer is the most common malignancy of the female reproductive tract. In 2008, the American Cancer Society estimated that endometrial cancer was diagnosed in 40,100 women, and 7470 deaths were caused by this disease. Endometrial cancer ranks eighth in cause of cancer deaths for women.

Although it has been described to occur as early as age 16 years, it is primarily a disease of the postmenopausal woman. Only 25% of the cases occur in premenopausal patients.

Classification

Two types of endometrial cancer have been described.

TYPE I CANCER

Type I has endometrioid histology and is the more common form. These tumors often arise in the background of chronically estrogen-stimulated endometrium; progesterone has a protective effect. Most commonly, an excess estrogenic environment occurs when steroid hormone precursors are converted by aromatase in adipose cells into estrone, a weak estrogen. This explains why type I uterine cancer is strongly linked to obesity. Other conditions related to a hyperestrogenic status are chronic anovulation, nulliparity, late menopause, iatrogenic estrogen administration, and estrogen-secreting tumors such as granulosa-cell tumors. Tamoxifen (Nolvadex) is a selective-estrogen receptor (ER) modulator that exhibits antiestrogenic properties on the breast tissue and estrogenic effects on the endometrium. Its use in the treatment of ER–positive breast cancers is an established risk factor for uterine cancer.

Type I cancers have a more indolent course when compared to type II, are better differentiated, and have a better prognosis. Seventy-five percent of patients with type I cancers present with stage I disease.

Type I endometrioid carcinomas are diploid in 80% of cases, and they often exhibit a mutation of the PTEN tumor suppressor gene, microsatellite instability, and ER and progesterone-receptor (PR) positivity.

A genetic predisposition for uterine cancer accounts for less than 5% of all cases. The most common is the hereditary nonpolyposis colorectal syndrome, which is caused by a germline mutation of the DNA repair genes. Members of families with these mutations are affected mostly by colorectal adenocarcinomas, but endometrial cancer is second in incidence.

TYPE II CANCER

Type II cancers encompass clear cell carcinoma and papillary serous carcinoma. Endometrioid carcinomas with architectural grade 3 are also classified as type II. Obesity and exposure to excess estrogen are not established risk factors. These cancers occur at ages older than type I, are characterized by aggressive behavior, and occur commonly in a background of atrophic endometrium.

Less than 10% of all endometrial cancers are of the papillary serous variety, but they cause 40% of deaths from endometrial cancer. Metastatic disease can occur even when the primary tumor is confined to an endometrial polyp. Only 55% of patients present with stage I disease, and 40% present with metastatic disease.

Uterine papillary serous carcinoma has a histologic appearance similar to ovarian serous papillary cancer and has the same pattern of spread. However, ovarian cancer has a much better response to chemotherapy.

At the molecular level, *p53* overexpression is encountered in 90% of tumors, *PTEN* mutations are rare, and half exhibit *HER-2/neu* overexpression. They are ER and PR negative. Type II tumors are often aneuploid.

Clear cell carcinomas are characterized by aggressive behavior and account for 4% of all uterine cancers and 8% of deaths. *PTEN* or *p53* mutations are present in less than 20%.

Clinical Presentation

The majority of patients with endometrioid cancer present with abnormal vaginal bleeding. This is often the only symptom, but fortunately it appears early in the course of the disease, especially for the type I carcinomas. For most women, postmenopausal bleeding prompts them to seek medical attention, and this accounts for the diagnosis at stage I in 75% of the patients.

For menstruating women, a change in the bleeding pattern, spotting, or frank intermenstrual bleeding requires investigation. In anovulatory patients, of whom a significant proportion are obese or morbidly obese, the absence of menses for long periods of time, interspersed with spotting or episodes of heavy vaginal bleeding, can be an indicator of endometrial pathology, including malignancy.

Advanced disease, with spread to and beyond the pelvic organs, can manifest with pelvic pressure, pain, or urinary and bowel symptoms.

Diagnosis

No screening methods for endometrial cancer exist.

Abnormal vaginal bleeding, whether it is postmenopausal, irregular, or the absence of menses in a nonpregnant premenopausal woman, is routinely assessed by endometrial biopsy. This can be performed in the office using a small-bore rigid or flexible catheter and is 95% as accurate as dilation and curettage (D&C). Fractional D&C with or without hysteroscopic guidance is another approach used to obtain an endometrial and endocervical specimen.

The finding of endometrial cells on cytologic examination of the cervix (Papanicolaou [Pap] smear) in a postmenopausal woman can be an indicator of uterine carcinoma and requires endometrial sampling. For premenopausal women, an endometrial biopsy is indicated only when the endometrial cells on the Pap smear are abnormal.

CURRENT DIAGNOSIS

- Most patients with uterine cancer are postmenopausal, and bleeding occurs early in the course of the disease.
- Postmenopausal vaginal bleeding is evaluated by endometrial biopsy.
- In premenopausal patients, especially obese women, irregular bleeding, including absence of menses, requires diagnostic evaluation.
- The presence of endometrial cells on a Papanicolaou (Pap) smear in premenopausal women is an indication for biopsy only when they are abnormal.
- The biopsy can be performed in the office and requires no sedation or analgesia.
- When it is not possible to obtain an adequate sample because of severe genital atrophy, obesity, or pain, operative dilation and curettage should be performed.

When the endometrial biopsy detects changes of endometrial hyperplasia with nuclear atypia, up to 25% of patients harbor an undetected uterine carcinoma. This is invariably well differentiated and early stage.

Rarely, carcinoma is discovered in the surgical specimen after hysterectomy was performed for other indications.

Imaging techniques are of limited value for the diagnosing endometrial cancer. Carcinoma is unlikely to be present when the endometrial thickness in a postmenopausal woman measures less than 5 mm by transvaginal ultrasound

Staging

Uterine cancer is staged surgically. In 2009, the Committee on Gynecologic Oncology of the International Federation of Gynecology and Obstetrics revised the 1988 staging system for endometrial cancer (Table 1).

TABLE 1 Staging System for Endometrial Cancer

Stage	Description
Stage I	
I*	Tumor confined to the corpus uteri
IA*	No or less than half myometrial invasion
IB*	Invasion equal to or more than half of the myometrium
Stage II	
II*	Tumor invades cervical stroma but does not extend beyond the uterus[†]
Stage III	
III*	Local and/or regional spread of the tumor
IIIA*	Tumor invades the serosa of the corpus uteri and/or adnexae[‡]
IIIA*	Tumor invades the serosa of the corpus uteri and/or adnexae[‡]
IIIB*	Vaginal and/or parametrial involvement[‡]
IIIC*	Metastases to pelvic and/or para-aortic lymph nodes[‡]
IIIC1*	Positive pelvic nodes
IIIC2*	Positive para-aortic lymph nodes with or without positive pelvic lymph nodes
Stage IV	
IV*	Tumor invades bladder and/or bowel mucosa, and/or distant metastases
IVA*	Tumor invasion of bladder and/or bowel mucosa
IVB*	Distant metastases, including intra-abdominal metastases and/or inguinal lymph nodes

*G1, G2, or G3.
[†]Endocervical glandular involvement only should be considered as stage I and no longer as stage II.
[‡]Positive cytology must be reported separately without changing the stage.

Treatment

SURGICAL TREATMENT

Comprehensive surgical staging for carcinoma of the corpus uteri includes exploration of the peritoneal cavity, hysterectomy, resection of the ovaries and fallopian tubes, and pelvic and periaortic lymph node dissection. At the beginning of each operation, a cytologic evaluation of the abdominal cavity is performed. In addition to these procedures, omentectomy and peritoneal biopsies are often performed for type II uterine cancers. When intraabdominal metastatic disease is encountered, resection of all masses is indicated.

Controversy exists regarding the necessity and extent of lymph node dissection, especially for early type I cancers. There is consensus, however, that the most accurate evaluation of lymph node involvement is by lymphadenectomy and pathologic review. Two large prospective trials conducted in Europe randomized patients to hysterectomy and lymphadenectomy or hysterectomy only and found no difference in survival and recurrence rate. However, all patients were treated with radiation postoperatively. In the United States, a retrospective study of 12,000 patients found a survival benefit for patients who underwent lymph node dissection.

The surgical staging can be performed by laparotomy or laparoscopy. A body of literature exists that recognizes minimally invasive surgery as a better treatment option where applicable. A Gynecologic Oncology Group (GOG) study has shown that the number of lymph nodes and the incidence of lymph node metastases were similar for both operative approaches. Laparoscopy has the advantage of a shorter hospital stay, less postoperative pain, lesser incidence of incisional hernias, faster recovery, and faster return to regular activities.

Main deterrents to a laparoscopic approach are obesity, prior abdominal surgeries, and long learning curve for the operator. In our experience, since the introduction of the robotic surgical system in clinical practice, these factors have had no impact on the patients' care. At Yale New Haven Hospital, the hospital course and postoperative outcomes of obese and morbidly obese patients who underwent robotic surgery was no different than that of patients with a body mass index in the normal range. The median postoperative hospital stay for patients with malignant obesity was 1.2 days.

ADJUVANT THERAPY

Early-Stage Disease

Adjuvant radiation therapy is recommended for type I cancers when the tumors are high-grade, penetrate deep into the myometrium, involve the cervix, or show evidence of lymphovascular space invasion. The treatment can be in the form of external beam pelvic radiation or brachytherapy to the vaginal apex and superior vagina.

CURRENT THERAPY

- Most patients with endometrial cancer present with stage I disease and surgery is the mainstay of therapy
- Conventional or robotic laparoscopic approaches have faster postoperative recovery.
- The current standard is pelvic and periaortic lymphadenectomy in addition to hysterectomy and adnexectomy.
- Controversy exists regarding the need and extent of lymph node dissection, especially for patients with low-grade endometrioid cancers.
- Adjuvant radiation therapy is recommended for type I cancers when the tumors are high-grade, penetrate deep into the myometrium, involve the cervix, or show evidence of lymphovascular space invasion.
- Platinum-based chemotherapy is indicated for uterine papillary serous and clear cell cancers, even for stage IA.

Platinum-based chemotherapy is indicated for uterine papillary serous and clear cell cancers, even for stage IA.

Metastatic Disease

Cytotoxic chemotherapy is the mainstay of therapy for metastatic carcinoma of the endometrium. Systemic therapy was found to be superior to whole abdominal radiation. Regardless of the regimen chosen, response rates are modest. Median values of progression-free intervals do not exceed 6 months, and overall survival does not exceed 12 months.

Single-Agent Therapies

Single-agent therapies with doxorubicin (Adriamycin),[1] cisplatin (Platinol),[1] carboplatin (Paraplatin),[1] and paclitaxel (Taxol)[1] have response rates of 20% and higher. Pegylated liposomal doxorubicin (Doxil)[1] has poor activity against metastatic endometrial cancer.

Combination Chemotherapy

Both the GOG and EORTC (European Organisation for Research and Treatment of Cancer) have completed phase III trials that investigated differences in responses to doxorubicin versus doxorubicin and cisplatin. The response rates were 25% versus 42% for GOG and 17% versus 43% for EORTC. Although these differences were statistically significant, no benefit in overall survival was noted.

In another GOG trial, the response rate of patients treated with a three-drug regimen, doxorubicin, cisplatin, and paclitaxel, was 57%, whereass the doxorubicin and cisplatin arm showed a response rate of 34%. Toxicity was higher in the three-drug arm, and the GOG final statistical report in January 2007 showed that the addition of paclitaxel to doxorubicin and cisplatin following surgery and volume-directed radiation did not increase survival.

The combination of carboplatin and paclitaxel is often prescribed for metastatic and recurrent endometrial cancer. Response rates range from 46% to 78%. In the current phase III GOG protocol for recurrent endometrial cancers, the combination of doxorubicin, cisplatin, and paclitaxel (control arm) is being compared to carboplatin and paclitaxel.

Progestin Treatment

Endometrial cancers with low histologic grade, the presence of PR, and a longer interval to develop metastases after treatment of the primary tumor are more likely to respond to progesterone treatment, usually administered as oral megestrol acetate (Megace).

OTHER TREATMENTS

From the selective estrogen-receptor modulators, tamoxifen[1] alone has modest efficacy in the treatment of metastatic endometrial cancer. Tamoxifen was also added to progestins to prevent downregulation of PR that occurs with progesterone treatment. Response rates were higher than for progesterone alone, but progression-free intervals and overall survival were similar.

Two aromatase inhibitors, anastrozole (Arimidex)[1] and letrozole (Femara),[1] were investigated in phase II trials and demonstrated minimal activity.

A gonadotropin-releasing hormone agonist, goserelin acetate (Zoladex),[1] has shown insufficient activity.

MOLECULAR THERAPY

Trastuzumab (Herceptin)[1] has not shown activity in a GOG study investigating its efficacy in the treatment of *HER-2/neu*-positive endometrial cancer.

Erlotinib (Tarceva),[1] an epidermal growth factor receptor (EGFR) inhibitor, demonstrated some activity, and cetuximab (Erbitux)[1] is currently being investigated.

---

[1]Not FDA approved for this indication.

A GOG phase II trial of the antiangiogenic agent bevacizumab (Avastin)[1] has been completed; results are pending. Sorafenib (Nexavar)[1] has shown modest activity.

Other agents investigated that have shown clinical responses were the fusion protein VEGF-Trap, and mTOR (mammalian target of rapamycin) inhibitors such as everolimus (RAD-001 [Afinitor])[1] and AP23573.

RECURRENT DISEASE

The most common site for recurrence, especially for type I cancers, is at the vaginal apex. When the recurrent cancer occurs in the form of surgically resectable masses, surgery is followed by systemic chemotherapy. Unresectable metastatic disease is treated with systemic therapy.

---

[1]Not FDA approved for this indication.

REFERENCES

FIGO Committee on Gynecologic Oncology. Revised FIGO staging for carcinoma of the vulva, cervix, and endometrium. Int J Gynecol Obstet 2009;105:103–4.

Fowler W, Mutch D. Management of endometrial cancer. Women's Health 2008;4(5):479–89.

Lowe MP, Johnson PR, Kamelle SA, et al. A multiinstitutional experience with robotic-assisted hysterectomy with staging for endometrial cancer. Obstet Gynecol 2009;114:236–43.

Mendivil A, Schuler KM, Gehrig PA. Non-endometrioid adenocarcinoma of the uterine corpus: A review of selected histological subtypes. Cancer Control 2009;16(1):46–52.

Writing Committee on behalf of the ASTEC Study Group. Efficacy of systematic pelvic lymphadenectomy in endometrial cancer (MRC ASTEC trial): A randomised study. Lancet 2009;373:125–36.

Cervical Cancer

Method of
*Lucybeth Nieves-Arriba, MD, and
Peter G. Rose, MD*

Epidemiology

Worldwide, cervical cancer is the second most common cancer in women. It is the greatest cancer killer of young women and the most common cause of death from cancer in women in the developing world. Worldwide in 2007, among the 555,100 new cases of cervical cancer, the highest incidence rates were in Africa, Central and South America, and Asia. In the United States, it is estimated that approximately 12,200 new cases were diagnosed and 4,210 patients died from cervical cancer in 2010. Significant disparities in incidence and stage at time of diagnosis have been identified among different ethnic groups—African Americans, Asian Americans, European Americans, and Latin Americans—in the United States. Factors that increase the risk of cervical cancer include early age at first coitus, multiple sexual partners, history of sexually transmitted diseases, low socioeconomic status, cigarette smoking, immunosuppression, and Fanconi's syndrome.

Pathophysiology

Cervical cancer occurs secondary to viral transformation of the surface (epithelial) cells by high-risk types of the human papillomavirus (HPV), and it is the only gynecologic cancer that can be prevented by regular screening. Persistent infection with high-risk HPV has been identified as the essential factor in the pathogenesis of the majority of cervical cancers. The virus's ability to transform human epithelium is been associated with the expression of two viral gene products, E6 and E7, which interact with p53 (a tumor-suppressor protein) and retinoblastoma protein (pRB), respectively, and affect control mechanisms of the cell cycle.

The prevalence of genital HPV infection in the world is estimated to be 400 million. Data from the National Health and Nutrition Examination Survey (NHANES) estimate the prevalence of HPV infection among girls and women in the United States aged 14 to 59 years is 26.8%. In about 90% of cases, the high-risk HPV infection is cleared by the immune system within 16 months. HPV infections in girls and younger women are more likely transient and therefore less likely to be associated with significant cervical lesions.

Prevention and Screening

Recent advances in molecular biology have allowed the development of viral-like particles using the L1 protein (major immunogenic capsid protein) of the HPV virus. Current vaccines, Gardasil (approved 2006) and Cervarix (approved 2009) contain two high-risk genotypes, HPV-16 and HPV-18, and could theoretically prevent 70% of cervical cancer cases. The Gardasil vaccine also contains two low-risk genotypes, HPV-6 and HPV-11, to prevent viral genital warts. The vaccines were FDA approved to use in girls and women between the ages of 9 and 26 years. If all children younger than 12 years were vaccinated, the most optimistic predictions expect a major effect on the cancer incidence will not be seen for 30 years. In 2009 HPV vaccination of males in the same age group was approved.

The current standard screening algorithm in the United States for preventing cervical cancer is presented in Table 1. Women with abnormal cytology are referred for a colposcopic examination. The colposcopic examination is used to guide biopsies of the exocervix, and in most cases an endocervical biopsy is also performed. The biopsy results then determine the type of follow-up and or therapy required.

Staging

The International Federation of Gynecology and Obstetrics (FIGO) defined the most commonly accepted staging of cervical cancer. This staging is based on a careful clinical examination and the results of specific radiologic studies and procedures. FIGO's latest update (2009) is summarized in Table 2.

In cervical cancer, primary lesions initially progress to lymphatics in the parametrium and pelvic nodes and then extend laterally to the pelvic side wall, bladder, and rectum. The two major spread patterns identified in cervical cancer include direct extension and lymphatic spread.

Diagnosis

The initial work-up for cervical cancer depends on whether a cervical lesion is visible. Patients without a visible cervical lesion require a cone biopsy to diagnose stage IA1 or IA2 tumor. Patients with a cervical lesion are assessed by history and physical examination and possibly by examination under anesthesia for biopsy, cystoscopy, sigmoidoscopy, and conventional imaging (chest x-ray, intravenous pyelogram). Other imaging modalities including computed tomography (CT), magnetic resonance imaging (MRI), and fluorodeoxyglucose positron emission tomography (FDG-PET) are useful in evaluating nodal or other metastatic sites but are not incorporated in the FIGO staging system owing to their limited availability worldwide. MRI performed significantly better than CT in detecting parametrial invasion, presence of bladder or rectal invasion, and identification of women suitable for fertility-preserving surgery. PET-CT is the most sensitive modality in identifying nodal metastasis or metastatic disease assisting with radiotherapy planning and evaluation of metabolic response to therapy. A 3-month post-therapy PET scan is highly predictive of long-term survival outcome.

Treatment

Multiple factors including tumor stage, size, histologic features (lymphovascular space invasion [LVSI], nonsquamous components, and depth of cervical stromal invasion), and evidence of lymph node metastasis influence the choice of treatment for cervical cancer. Patients with stage IA1 cervical cancer have undergone a cone biopsy and pathology demonstrates 3 mm of invasion or less, less than 7 mm width, no LVSI, and negative margins. Patients with this extent of disease can safely be treated with a less-radical hysterectomy, an extrafascial hysterectomy. Pelvic lymphadenectomy is not recommended owing to the low risk of pelvic node metastasis (less than 1%). In patients who desire to retain fertility, a cone biopsy may be considered. Wright and colleagues reported on 1409 women from the SEER database who were younger than 40 years and had stage IA1 cancer. The 5-year survival was 98% among 568 who underwent cone biopsy alone versus 99% among 841 who underwent hysterectomy.

CURRENT DIAGNOSIS

- New recommendations for cytology screening recommend starting screening at 21 years of age.
- Initial work up must include a biopsy.
- Imaging techniques including magnetic resonance imaging and positron emission tomography–computed tomography can assist in treatment planning.

TABLE 1 Cervical Cytologic Screening Guidelines from the American College of Obstetricians and Gynecologists

Age (y)	Recommendation for Cytologic Screening	Comments
Younger than 21	Avoid screening	
21 to 29	Screen every 2 y	
30 to 65 or 70	May screen every 3 y*	This recommendation applies only to women with 3 consecutive cytologic tests; exceptions include women with HIV infection, compromised immunity, a history of cervical intraepithelial neoplasia grade 2 or 3, or exposure to DES in utero.
Between 65 and 70	May discontinue screening	This recommendation applies only to women with ≥3 consecutive negative cytologic tests and no abnormal tests in the preceding 10 y; exceptions include women with multiple sexual partners

Abbreviation: DES = diethylstilbestrol.
Adapted from American College of Obstetricians and Gynecologists (ACOG). Cervical cytology screening. Washington (DC): American College of Obstetricians and Gynecologists (ACOG); 2009 Dec. 12 (ACOG practice bulletin; no. 109).

TABLE 2   Revised FIGO Staging for Carcinoma of the Cervix

Stage	Criteria
Stage I	
I	The carcinoma is strictly confined to the cervix
IA	Invasive carcinoma, which can be diagnosed only by microscopy, with deepest invasion ≤5 mm and largest extension ≥7 mm
IA1	Measured stromal invasion of ≤3 mm in depth and extension of ≤7 mm
IA2	Measured stromal invasion of >3 mm in depth and extension of >7 mm
IB	Clinically visible lesions limited to the cervix or preclinical cancers greater than stage IA
IB1	Clinically visible lesion ≤4 cm in greatest dimension
IB2	Clinically visible lesion >4 cm in greatest dimension
Stage II	
II	Cervical carcinoma invades beyond the uterus, but not to the pelvic wall or to the lower third of the vagina
IIA	Without parametrial invasion
IIA1	Clinically visible lesion ≤4 cm in greatest dimension
IIA2	Clinically visible lesion >4 cm in greatest dimension
IIB	With obvious parametrial invasion
Stage III	
III	The tumor extends to the pelvic wall and/ or involves lower third of the vagina and/ or causes hydronephrosis or nonfunctioning kidney
IIIA	Tumor involves lower third of the vagina, with no extension to the pelvic wall
IIIB	Extension to the pelvic wall and/ or hydronephrosis or nonfunctioning kidney
Stage IV	
IV	The carcinoma has extended beyond the true pelvis or has involved (biopsy proven) the mucosa of the bladder or rectum; a bullous edema, as such, does not permit a case to be allotted as stage IV
IVA	Spread of the growth to adjacent organs
IVB	Spread to distant organs

Adapted from Pecorelli S: Revised FIGO staging for carcinoma of the vulva, cervix, and endometrium. Int J Gynaecol Obstet 2009;105(2):103-104. Erratum in Int J Gynaecol Obstet 2010;108(2):176.

CURRENT THERAPY

- Despite recent availability of human papilloma virus (HPV) vaccination (Gardasil, Cervarix) and advances in screening, cervical cancer remains a significant global health problem, especially in underserved populations.
- Improved understanding of the disease has allowed more conservative treatment of selected patients with early-stage disease.
- For advanced and high-risk cervical cancer, chemoradiation has had a significant impact on survival.

Patients with stage IA2 to IB1 are generally treated with radical hysterectomy; in patients who are not candidates for surgery owing to comorbidities, radiation therapy is used. In patients with high-risk criteria after surgery—positive surgical margin, parametrial involvement, and positive pelvic nodes—cisplatin-based[1] chemoradiation, based on a positive randomized trial, is recommended. Those with intermediate risk factors including tumor size, cervical stromal invasion, and lymphovascular invasion had an improved progression-free survival with adjuvant radiation.

Radical trachelectomy—laparoscopic, vaginal or open—in conjunction with lymphadenectomy is a reasonable alternative treatment for select young patients with stage IA2 and IB1 who desire to maintain their childbearing capacity. The criteria used for patient selection include early-stage cervical cancer with a lesion less than 2 cm, no lymphovascular invasion, and no lymph node metastasis. Reports comparing radical trachelectomies with matched controls identified increased complications (25% versus 3%) and overall less-radical dissection.

Treatment of stage IB2 cancer of the cervix varies depending on the bulkiness and shape of the lesion. Surgery and chemoradiation therapy have advantages and disadvantages. Finan and colleagues reported that up 72% of patients with stage IB2 disease who were treated with surgery received adjuvant radiation owing to high-risk factors identified in pathologic evaluation of specimens. In a randomized Gynecologic Oncology Group trial, 94% of patients with IB2 cervical cancer who underwent radical hysterectomy had high or intermediate risk factors warranting adjuvant radiation.

In 1999 the National Cancer Institute (NCI) initiated a clinical alert recommending that concurrent cisplatin-based[1] chemotherapy be given with radiotherapy to women with cervical cancer based on five randomized studies, and this established a new standard of care (Table 3).

It is estimated that approximately 35% of patients with invasive cervical cancer will have recurrent or persistent disease, with most recurrences occurring in the first 2 years following primary therapy. Recurrence can be expected in 10% to 20% of patients treated with radical hysterectomy in contrast to 30% to 50% treated for more-advanced disease primarily with radiation plus concurrent chemotherapy. The site of the recurrence can direct further treatment. Patients with central pelvic recurrences after surgery are candidates for curative radiation; after primary treatment with radiation therapy patients may be candidates for curative radical surgery (exenteration). Prognosis is more favorable for patients undergoing exenteration when there is a small (less than 3 cm) central recurrence, no sidewall involvement, and longer than 2 years of disease-free interval. Those with small recurrences limited to the cervix or upper vagina can occasionally be treated with radical hysterectomy and upper vaginectomy.

However, most recurrences are distant, involving the lung, bone, abdominal cavity, and supraclavicular lymph nodes. Recurrences within irradiated areas have a poor response to therapy (0% to 5%). Recurrences in the nonirradiated areas respond better to chemotherapy, with response rates of 25% to 70%. The use of chemotherapy in the treatment of recurrent cervical cancer is challenging because agents are only moderately active and patients can present with renal impairment secondary to obstructive uropathy, resulting in altered excretion with increased toxicity from chemotherapeutic agents. Table 4 compars results of randomized chemotherapy trials for the treatment of recurrent cervical cancer.

[1]Not FDA approved for this indication.

[1]Not FDA approved for this indication.

TABLE 3 Randomized Trials of Cisplatin-based Chemoradiation

Treatment	Stage	Survival Type	Survival Percentage	Significance
Gynecology Oncology Group 85				
RT/5FU[1] infusion/bolus cisplatin[1]	IIB-IVA	3 y PFS	67%	$P = 0.033$
RT/oral HU[1]			57%	
Gynecology Oncology Group 109				
Rad hyst/RT	IA2-IIA	Est. 4-y	63%	$P = 0.003$
Rad hyst/RT/cisplatin[1]/5-FU[1]			80%	
Radiation Therapy Oncology Group 9001				
RT	IIB-IVA	DFS	40%	$P < 0.001$
RT/5-FU[1]/cisplatin[1]			67%	
Gynecology Oncology Group 120				
RT + cisplatin[1]	IIB-IVA	3-y PFS	67%	$P < 0.001$
RT + cisplatin[1]/5FU[1]/HU[1]			64%	
RT + HU[1]			47%	
Gynecology Oncology Group 123				
RT+ TAH	IB$_2$	3 yr PFS	74%	$P < 0.001$
RT+ cisplatin[1]+ TAH			83%	
Pearcey et al				
RT + cisplatin[1]	IB-IVA >5 cm	5-y DFS	62%	$P = 0.42$
RT			58%	

[1]Not FDA approved for this indication.
DFS = disease-free survival; 5-FU = fluorouracil (Adrucil); HU = hydroxyurea; PFS = progression free survival; rad hyst = radical hysterectomy; RT = radiotherapy; TAH = total abdominal hysterectomy.

TABLE 4 Phase III Trials Comparing Cisplatin Doublets and Cisplatin Alone to Treat Metastatic or Recurrent Cervical Carcinoma

Study	Stage	Response Rate (%)	Progression-Free Survival (mo)	Overall Survival (mo)
Gynecology Oncology Group 110				
Cisplatin[1]	IVB or recurrent	18	3.2	8
Cisplatin/mitolactol[8]		21	3.3	7.3
Cisplatin/ifosfamide (Ifex)[1]		31	8.3	4.6
Significance		$P = 0.004$	$P = 0.003$	$P = 0.835$
Gynecology Oncology Group 149				
Cisplatin/bleomycin[1]/ifosfamide	IVB or recurrent	31	5.1	8.4
Cisplatin/ifosfamide		32	4.6	8.5
Significance		$P = 0.42$	$P = 0.495$	$P = 0.79$
Gynecology Oncology Group 169				
Cisplatin	IVB or recurrent	19	2.8	8.8
Cisplatin/paclitaxel (Taxol)[1]		36	4.8	9.7
Significance		$P = $ NS	$P = $ NS	$P = $ NS
Gynecology Oncology Group 179				
Cisplatin	IVB or recurrent	13	2.9	6.5
Cisplatin/topotecan (Hycamtin)[1]		27	4.6	9.4
Cisplatin/methotrexate[1]/vinblastine (Velban)[1]/ doxorubicin (Adriamycin)[1]				
Significance		$P = 0.004$	$P = 0.014$	$P = 0.017$
Gynecology Oncology Group 204				
Cisplatin/paclitaxel versus				
Cisplatin/vinorelbine (Navelbine)[1]			HR[†] = 1.35	NR
Cisplatin/gemcitabine (Gemzar)[1]			HR[†] = 1.43	NR
Cisplatin/topotecan	IVB or recurrent		HR[†] = 1.28	NR

[1]Not FDA approved for this indication.
[8]Orphan drug in the United States.
[†]Hazard ratio for PFS for experimental arms to cisplatin/paclitaxel.
NR = not reported; NS = not significant.

Conclusion

Adherence to current screening guidelines should allow early cervical cancer or precancerous detection. However, most patients with cervical cancer have not participated in regular screening and present with a variety of disease extents.

REFERENCES

American Cancer Society. Cancer Facts and figures, Available at http://www.cancer.org/Research/CancerFactsFigures/CancerFactsFigures/index [accessed August 12, 2010].

American College of Obstetricians and Gynecologists (ACOG). Cervical cytology screening, Washington (DC): American College of Obstetricians and Gynecologists (ACOG); Dec. 2009. 12 p. (ACOG practice bulletin; no. 109). Available at http://guideline.gov/content.aspx?id=15274 [accessed August 12, 2010].

Bloss JD, Blessing JA, Behrens BC, et al. Randomized trial of cisplatin and ifosfamide with or without bleomycin in squamous carcinoma of the cervix: A Gynecologic Oncology Group study. J Clin Oncol 2002;20:1832–7.

Covens A, Shaw P, Murphy J, et al. Is radical trachelectomy a safe alternative to radical hysterectomy for patients with stage IA-B carcinoma of the cervix? Cancer 1999;86:2273–9.

Dunne EF, Unger ER, Sternberg M, et al. Prevalence of HPV infection among females in the United States. JAMA 2007;297(8):813–9.

Finan MA, Decesare S, Fiorica JV, et al. Radical hysterectomy for stage IB1 vs IB2 carcinoma of the cervix: does the new staging system predict morbidity and survival? Gynecol Oncol 1996;62(2):139–47.

Keys HM, Bundy BN, Stehman FB, et al. Cisplatin, radiation, and adjuvant hysterectomy compared with radiation and adjuvant hysterectomy for bulky stage IB cervical carcinoma. N Engl J Med 1999;340(15):1154–61. Erratum in N Engl J Med 1999;341(9):708.

Long HJ 3rd, Bundy BN, Grendys EC, et al. Randomized phase III trial of cisplatin with or without topotecan in carcinoma of the uterine cervix: A Gynecologic Oncology Group study. J Clin Oncol 2005;23(21):4626–33.

Monk BJ, Sill MW, McMeekin DS, et al. Phase III trial of four cisplatin-containing doublet combinations in stage IVB, recurrent, or persistent cervical carcinoma: A Gynecologic Oncology Group study. J Clin Oncol 2009;27(28):4649–55.

Moore DH, Blessing JA, McQuellon RP, et al. Phase III study of cisplatin with or without paclitaxel in stage IVB, recurrent, or persistent squamous cell carcinoma of the cervix: A Gynecologic Oncology Group study. J Clin Oncol 2004;22(15):3113–9.

Morris M, Eifel PJ, Lu J, et al. Pelvic radiation with concurrent chemotherapy compared with pelvic and para-aortic radiation for high-risk cervical cancer. N Engl J Med 1999;340(15):1137–43.

National Cancer Institute. Cervical cancer. Available at: http://www.cancer.gov/cancertopics/types/cervical [accessed August 12, 2010].

Omura GA, Blessing JA, Vaccarello L, et al. Randomized trial of cisplatin versus cisplatin plus mitolactol versus cisplatin plus ifosfamide in advanced squamous carcinoma of the cervix: A Gynecologic Oncology Group study. J Clin Oncol 1997;15(1):165–71.

Pearcey R, Brundage M, Drouin P, et al. Phase III trial comparing radical radiotherapy with and without cisplatin chemotherapy in patients with advanced squamous cell cancer of the cervix. J Clin Oncol 2002;20(4):966–72.

Pecorelli S. Revised FIGO staging for carcinoma of the vulva, cervix, and endometrium. Int J Gynaecol Obstet 2009;105(2):103–4. Erratum in Int J Gynaecol Obstet 2010;108(2):176.

Peters 3rd WA, Liu PY, Barrett 2nd RJ, et al. Concurrent chemotherapy and pelvic radiation therapy compared with pelvic radiation therapy alone as adjuvant therapy after radical surgery in high-risk early-stage cancer of the cervix. J Clin Oncol 2000;18(8):1606–13.

Rose PG, Bundy BN, Watkins EB, et al. Concurrent cisplatin-based radiotherapy and chemotherapy for locally advanced cervical cancer. N Engl J Med 1999;340(15):1144–53.

Whitney CW, Sause W, Bundy BN, et al. Randomized comparison of fluorouracil plus cisplatin versus hydroxyurea as an adjunct to radiation therapy in stage IIB-IVA carcinoma of the cervix with negative para-aortic lymph nodes: A Gynecologic Oncology Group and Southwest Oncology Group study. J Clin Oncol 1999;17(5):1339–48.

Wright JD, Nathavithrana R, Lewin SN, et al. Fertility-conserving surgery for young women with stage IA1 cervical cancer: Safety and access. Obstet Gynecol 2010;115(3):585–90.

Neoplasms of the Vulva

Method of
Susan A. Davidson, MD

The female external genitalia includes the mons pubis, labia majora, labia minora, clitoris, perineal body, and the structures of the vaginal introitus or vestibule. Whether benign or malignant, vulvar neoplasms are uncommon, occur at all ages, and have varying characteristics. Therefore liberal use of biopsies is usually required for diagnosis and to guide treatment.

Benign Cystic Neoplasms

Benign cystic lesions of the vulva include Bartholin's duct cyst, sebaceous and epidermal inclusion cysts, mucinous cysts, Skene duct cysts, and cysts of the canal of Nuck. Bartholin's duct cyst, located in the posterior labia near the vaginal introitus, is most common. Treatment is usually not required in asymptomatic young women (<40 years). If the cyst is symptomatic or infected, however, drainage by marsupialization or use of a Word catheter, is indicated. Bartholin's gland carcinomas are rare, especially in women younger than 40 years of age. But if the mass feels firm or nodular, it should be biopsied.

Sebaceous and epidermal inclusion cysts are also common. They are prone to infection but rarely malignant. If an infection develops, they should be incised and drained. Mucinous cysts are rare and possibly arise from the minor vestibular glands. They are located anteriorly on the vulva, typically on the inner labia minora. Skene duct cysts are located next to the urethra. Excision of these cysts is necessary only if symptomatic.

Cysts of the canal of Nuck are located in the anterior portion of the labia majora at the termination of the insertion of the round ligament. These cysts represent herniation of the peritoneum through the inguinal canal and contain peritoneal fluid. If symptomatic, excision must be accompanied by closure of the fascial defect to prevent recurrence.

Benign Solid Neoplasms

The benign solid tumors of the vulva include fibromas, myomas, lipomas, hidradenomas, syringomas, myoblastomas, vestibular adenomas, and angiomas, among others. Benign pigmented lesions, such as nevi and seborrheic keratoses, may occasionally be found. Malignancy is rare, but most should be excised for diagnostic and therapeutic purposes.

CONDYLOMA ACUMINATUM

Vulvar condyloma acuminatum is a sexually transmitted verrucous lesion of the vulva caused by human papilloma virus (HPV), most frequently types 6 and 11. These lesions are warty growths that frequently cover large areas of the vulva. Smoking and immunosuppression are risk factors. Representative biopsies should be obtained to document disease and rule out malignancy. Wide local excision can be used for small lesions, although these growths are usually best treated by ablation.

Chemical ablative techniques include topical application of trichloroacetic acid (Tri-Chlor), podofilox (0.5%, Condylox), 5-fluorouracil[1] (1%, Fluoroplex or 5%, Efudex),[1] or imiquimod (5%, Aldara). Podophyllin can be applied twice daily for 3 days, repeated weekly for 4 weeks. Imiquimod can be applied three times per week for up to

---

[1]Not FDA approved for this indication.

16 weeks. Podophyllin and 5-fluorouracil should not be used in women who could become pregnant. Surgical ablative therapies include CO_2 laser vaporization and use of the Cavitron ultrasonic aspirator (CUSA), especially for extensive disease.

Intraepithelial Neoplasms of the Vulva

VULVAR INTRAEPITHELIAL NEOPLASIA

Vulvar intraepithelial neoplasia (VIN) is a dysplastic condition of the squamous epithelium whose incidence is increasing, especially in younger women. Risk factors are HPV types 16 and 18, smoking, and immunosuppression. Symptoms include pruritus (most common), pain, a noticeable lesion, and discoloration. Most patients with HPV-related disease have multifocal lesions including vaginal and cervical dysplasia. The most common location is in the area of the posterior fourchette and perineal body. Typical findings are raised white, gray, red, or mottled lesions; application of 4% acetic acid for several minutes can help identify faint lesions and outline abnormal vascular patterns. Diagnosis of VIN is made by punch biopsies through full thickness of the epithelium to rule out invasion, present in 20% of patients with VIN III (full-thickness dysplasia or carcinoma in situ). Of those patients with invasion, half (10% of VIN III) have invasion more than 1 mm.

Treatment of VIN can be categorized into excisional and ablative therapies. Patients at risk for microinvasion (unifocal disease, raised lesions, older age, and prior radiation) should have the lesion excised completely if possible. Skinning vulvectomy is rarely used because of psychological and sexual consequences related to scarring and disfigurement.

The ablative therapies can be divided into mechanical and chemical. The mechanical method most commonly used is the CO_2 laser, although use of the CUSA is also described. Both can ablate large or multifocal lesions successfully with an excellent cosmetic and functional outcome. The chemical method most commonly used is topical 5-fluorouracil (5%, Efudex).[1] Because of its teratogenic potential, it should not be used in women who could become pregnant. It can be applied on two consecutive nights weekly for 10 weeks. An alternative ablative therapy is use of imiquimod[1] (Aldara), as described earlier. Because of the irritation caused by these topical therapies, many patients have problems with treatment compliance. Residual disease should be excised to rule out invasion.

Patients with VIN frequently have recurrent disease, regardless of the treatment method used (Table 1). Continued smoking increases this risk, so patients should be counseled in smoking cessation. In those patients whose cancers recur and are retreated, subsequent 5-fluorouracil prophylaxis, with a single application biweekly, is used successfully to minimize further recurrences.

PAGET'S DISEASE

Paget's disease of the vulva is an uncommon condition characterized by a patchy, eczematoid lesion that frequently covers much of the vulva. Most patients are postmenopausal and present with

[1]Not FDA approved for this indication.

TABLE 1 Recurrence of Vulvar Intraepithelial Neoplasia III

Treatment Method	% Recurrence
Chemical ablation	20–40
Mechanical ablation	20–40
Wide local excision	
Negative margin	15–25
Positive margin	30–45

TABLE 2 Incidence of Regional Node Metastases by Tumor Diameter

Tumor Diameter (cm)	% Positive Inguinal Nodes
<1	0–15
5–20	
25–35	
35–50	
≥50	≥50

complaints of pruritus. Although Paget's disease is an in situ disease process, 15% to 25% of patients have an underlying malignancy, usually an adenocarcinoma of the apocrine glands but occasionally an invasive Paget's. In addition, up to 30% of patients have a synchronous adenocarcinoma of the breast, colon, rectum, or upper genital tract. Screening for these cancers is therefore recommended. To assess for invasion, the lesion should be excised via wide local excision or simple vulvectomy with at least 5 mm of the adjacent subcutaneous tissue. Achieving negative margin status is frequently difficult. However, the risk of recurrence is approximately 30% whether margins are negative or positive. Thus expectant management, reserving treatment for symptomatic recurrences, is usually recommended.

Invasive Vulvar Lesions

Less than 5% of gynecologic cancers arise on the vulva. Approximately 85% are squamous cell carcinomas. The etiology of this type appears mixed. Up to 50% evolve from VIN III and are usually associated with HPV-16. These women are slightly younger (age 45–52 years). Most arise in older women (age 60–69 years), and suggested risk factors include immunosuppression, hypertension, diabetes mellitus, obesity, and chronic vulvar inflammation. Other histologic types are melanomas (5% to 10%), basal cell carcinomas (2% to 3%), adenocarcinomas (1%), and sarcomas (1% to 2%). Most patients present with a combination of symptoms, including pruritus, discomfort, and complaints of a mass. Examination frequently reveals a suspicious lesion, which should be biopsied for diagnosis. Vulvar cancers typically spread by local extension and lymphatic dissemination. Factors that influence dissemination include tumor size (Table 2), depth of invasion (Table 3), lymphovascular space invasion, and tumor grade. Staging is surgical and classified using the tumor, nodes, and metastasis (TNM) system (Box 1) as well as the International Federation of Gynecology and Obstetrics (FIGO) system (Box 2).

SQUAMOUS CELL CARCINOMAS AND ADENOCARCINOMAS

Surgical management of squamous cell carcinomas and adenocarcinomas depends on the size, depth of invasion, and location of the lesion. The vulvar lesion is managed with a radical excision. Management of the groins is based on depth of invasion. Lesions with invasion of <1 mm have minimal risk of lymphatic spread and do not require lymphadenectomy. All others require surgical assessment of the lymph nodes. Lesions located in the midline structures require bilateral groin dissection, whereas lateral lesions are managed with

TABLE 3 Incidence of Regional Node Metastases by Depth of Tumor Invasion

Depth of Invasion (mm)	% Positive Inguinal Nodes
<1	1–5
1–3	10–15
3–5	15–30
5–10	30–45
>10	>40

BOX 1 TNM Classification of Vulvar Carcinoma

T	Primary tumor
Tis	Carcinoma in situ
T1	Confined to vulva, diameter ≤2 cm
T2	Confined to vulva, diameter >2 cm
T3	Adjacent spread to urethra, vagina, perineum, or anus (any size)
T4	Infiltration of upper urethral mucosa, bladder, rectum, or bone
N	Regional lymph nodes
N0	No lymph node metastases
N1	Unilateral regional lymph node metastasis
N2	Bilateral regional lymph node metastasis
M	Distant metastases
M0	No clinical metastases
M1	Distant metastasis (including pelvic lymph node metastasis)

Abbreviation: TNM = tumor, node, metastasis.

ipsilateral groin dissection. This surgical approach is associated with significant morbidity including disfigurement, wound breakdown, and problems with lymphocysts and chronic lymphedema. For patients with very large lesions or lesions in sensitive areas such as the clitoris, preoperative radiation, followed by less radical excision of residual disease, may minimize problems with the vulvar wound. Current investigations are ongoing in the use of sentinel lymph node dissections as a method of minimizing the groin morbidity without sacrificing survival. Positive vulvar margins or metastases to lymph nodes are managed with postoperative radiation. Survival depends on stage at diagnosis (Table 4).

BOX 2 FIGO Classification (With Corresponding TNM Classification) for Vulvar Carcinoma

Stage I (T1N0M0)	Tumor confined to vulva and/or perineum, 2 cm in greatest dimension; nodes are negative
Stage IA	Stromal invasion no greater than 1 mm
Stage IB	Stromal invasion >1 mm
Stage II (T2N0M0)	Tumor confined to the vulva and/or perineum, >2 cm in greatest dimension; nodes are negative
Stage III	
T3N0M0	Tumor of any size with adjacent spread to the lower urethra and/or the vagina or the anus
T3N1M0	Unilateral regional lymph node metastasis
T2N1M0	
Stage IVA	
T1N2M0	Tumor invades any of the following: upper urethra, bladder mucosa, rectal mucosa, pelvic bone, and/or bilateral regional node metastasis
T2N2M0	
T3N2M0	
T4 any N M0	
Stage IVB	
Any T any N M1	Any distant metastasis including pelvic lymph nodes

Abbreviations: FIGO = International Federation of Gynecology and Obstetrics; TNM = tumor, node, metastasis.

TABLE 4 Survival Rate by FIGO Stage for Patients With Invasive Squamous Cell Vulvar Cancer

FIGO Stage	% Surviving 5 Years
I	70–90
II	50–80
III	30–50
IV	10–15

Abbreviation: FIGO = International Federation of Gynecology and Obstetrics.

MALIGNANT MELANOMA

Malignant melanoma is the second most common vulvar malignancy. Most patients have disease on the mucosal surfaces of the vulvar introitus, clitoris, and labia minora. The vulvar lesion is treated by radical excision, but management of the groins is controversial. The risk of spread is significant with a tumor thickness greater than 0.75 mm, but survival at 5 years is only approximately 10% with groin node metastases. Some argue against node dissection for this reason. However, given some long-term survivors with modern melanoma therapy, either lymphadenectomy or sentinel lymph node dissection, as is done for other cutaneous melanomas, appears indicated.

VERRUCOUS CARCINOMA

Verrucous carcinoma is a large exophytic tumor that resembles giant condyloma acuminatum. It is a variant of squamous carcinomas but has an excellent prognosis because of the lack of metastases. Verrucous carcinomas have a high tendency to recur and should be managed with radical local excision.

CURRENT DIAGNOSIS

- Most cystic lesions are benign. Excision is reserved for symptomatic cysts and suspicious Bartholin's gland cysts, especially in women older than 40 years of age.
- All solid lesions should be biopsied for diagnostic purposes.
- Multifocal disease requires multiple biopsies to rule out invasive disease.
- Most premalignant and malignant lesions cause pruritus, discomfort, or a noticeable lesion.
- The vagina and cervix in women with dysplastic or malignant vulvar lesions should be evaluated.

CURRENT THERAPY

- Benign solid lesions should be excised.
- After ablative treatment of vulvar intraepithelial neoplasia (VIN), excise any residual lesions to rule out occult invasive disease.
- Avoid podophyllin and 5-fluorouracil in women of reproductive potential.
- Rule out synchronous neoplasms in women with Paget's disease.
- Invasion more than 1 mm requires radical excision and lymph node evaluation.

BASAL CELL CARCINOMA

Basal cell carcinomas typically occur in elderly white women, are commonly located on the labia majora, and have characteristics similar to basal cell carcinomas at other sites. Treatment is wide local excision only because metastases are rare. Basal cell carcinomas are prone to local recurrence, however. A malignant squamous component must be ruled out because it should be managed as a squamous cell carcinoma.

SARCOMAS

Leiomyosarcoma is the most common vulvar sarcoma and usually arises in the labia majora. Malignant fibrous histiocytoma is the second most common. Management of these lesions is radical vulvar excision.

REFERENCES

Garland SM. Imiquimod. Curr Opin Infect Dis 2003;16:85–9.

Homesley HD, Bundy BN, Sedlis A, et al. Prognostic factors for groin node metastasis in squamous cell carcinoma of the vulva (a Gynecologic Oncology Group study). Gynecol Oncol 1993;49:279–83.

Krebs HB. The use of topical 5-fluorouracil in the treatment of genital condylomas. Obstet Gynecol Clin North Am 1987;14(2):559–68.

Modesitt SC, Waters AB, Walton L, et al. Vulvar intraepithelial neoplasia III: Occult cancer and the impact of margin status on recurrence. Obstet Gynecol 1998;92(6):962–6.

Phillips GL, Bundy BN, Okagaki T, et al. Malignant melanoma of the vulva treated by radical hemivulvectomy, a prospective study of the Gynecologic Oncology Group. Cancer 1994;73:2626–32.

Tebes S, Cardosi R, Hoffman M. Paget's disease of the vulva. Am J Obstet Gynecol 2002;187:281–4.

Trimble CL, Trimble EL, Woodruff JD. Diseases of the vulva. In: Hernandez E, Atkinson BE, editors. Clinical Gynecologic Pathology. Philadelphia: WB Saunders; 1995. p. 1–90.

Wright VC, Chapman WB. Colposcopy of intraepithelial neoplasia of the vulva and adjacent sites. Obstet Gynecol Clin North Am 1993;20(1):231–55.

Ovarian Cancer

Method of
Peter G. Rose, MD

Ovarian cancer is the seventh most common cancer and the fourth most common cause of cancer death for women. It is the second most common gynecologic cancer and the deadliest. In the United States, it is estimated that approximately 21,880 patients will be diagnosed and 13,850 patients will die from ovarian cancer in 2010.

Epidemiology

Ovarian cancers are heterogeneous tumors. Germ cell tumors occur most frequently in the second and third decades of life, stromal tumors occur in a bimodal distribution, and epithelial tumors increase in frequency with increasing age, with the median occurrence in the sixth and seventh decades of life. Approximately 10% of epithelial ovarian cancers are related to the *BRCA* gene mutation, and a small percentage of the tumors are associated with the hereditary nonpolyposis colon cancer (HNPCC) syndrome.

Screening

No effective screening programs have been established for ovarian cancer because of its rarity and nonspecific symptoms. Most ovarian cancer patients present with symptoms of dyspepsia, vague abdominal discomfort, gas, distention, early satiety, anorexia, increasing abdominal girth, change in bowel pattern, urinary frequency, and pain. However, in a primary care setting, 72% of women had recurring symptoms, with a median number of two symptoms. Goff and colleagues found that the most common were back pain (45%), fatigue (34%), bloating (27%), constipation (24%), abdominal pain (22%), and urinary symptoms (16%). A prospective study of screening by symptoms is planned.

Because patients with early-stage disease have a significantly better prognosis, identifying the disease as early as possible would be ideal. Most of the cancers diagnosed in screening studies were advanced-stage disease. Screening based on high-risk family history or *BRCA* gene mutation status also resulted in most detected cancers being advanced stage. Because of this pattern of late detection, prophylactic surgery to remove the fallopian tubes and ovaries remains the most effective way to reduce the risk of gynecologic cancer among high-risk patients. Patients with the HNPCC syndrome are at increased risk for uterine and ovarian cancer, and therefore removal of the uterus, fallopian tubes, and ovaries is advised.

Germ Cell Tumors

Germ cell tumors comprise 2% of ovarian cancers and are usually seen in adolescents and young adults. Treatment involves oophorectomy and staging surgery (Table 1), including omentectomy, peritoneal biopsies, and pelvic and paraaortic lymphadenectomy. These tumors are usually unilateral, and conservation of the uterus and contralateral ovary is the standard of care. Because these tumors are most often found unexpectedly, staging surgery is rarely performed.

Tumor histologies include dysgerminoma (40%), endodermal sinus tumor (22%), immature teratoma (20%), mixed tumors (14%), polyembryoma (<1%), and choriocarcinoma (<1%). Dysgerminomas have the best prognosis. They can be observed during the early stage and can be effectively treated with chemotherapy without bleomycin in the advanced stage. For patients with nondysgerminomatous tumors without gross residual disease, prospective trials have demonstrated that bleomycin (Blenoxane),[1] etoposide

---

[1]Not FDA approved for this indication.

TABLE 1 FIGO Staging for Carcinoma of the Ovary

Stage	Description
I	Growth limited to the ovaries
Ia	Growth limited to one ovary
Ib	Growth limited to both ovaries
Ic	Stage Ia or Ib with tumor on surface of ovaries, or with capsule ruptured, or with ascites present containing malignant cells
II	With pelvic extension
IIa	Extension to reproductive organs
IIb	Extension to other pelvic tissues
IIc	Stage IIa or IIb with tumor on surface of ovaries, or with capsule(s) ruptured, or with ascites present containing malignant cells
III	Tumor outside the pelvis or positive retroperitoneal or inguinal nodes
IIIa	Microscopic seeding of abdominal peritoneal surfaces
IIIb	Macroscopic disease measuring less than 2 cm in diameter
IIIc	Macroscopic disease measuring greater than 2 cm in diameter or positive retroperitoneal or inguinal nodes
IV*	Extraabdominal extension

*If a pleural effusion is present, there must be positive cytology or parenchymal liver metastasis.
Abbreviation: FIGO = International Federation of Gynecology and Obstetrics.

(Toposar),[1] and cisplatin (Platinol AQ) chemotherapy is associated with a survival rate of 98%. Low-grade and low-stage immature teratomas can be observed.

Stromal Tumors

Stromal tumors comprise 2% of ovarian cancers and are seen in young and older patients. Their treatment depends on the extent of disease and the reproductive potential of the patient. Conservation of the uterus and contralateral ovary is usually appropriate for young patients. Staging surgery, including omentectomy, peritoneal biopsies, and pelvic and paraaortic lymphadenectomy, is usually recommended. However, based on the patterns of recurrence, the role of lymphadenectomy has been questioned. Advanced-stage and recurrent stromal tumors are often treated like germ cell tumors, using a chemotherapy regimen of bleomycin,[1] etoposide,[1] and cisplatin. Paclitaxel (Taxol) is also active against stromal tumors, and some investigators have used carboplatin (Paraplatin) and paclitaxel for therapy.

Epithelial Ovarian Cancer

Epithelial ovarian cancer, also known as ovarian carcinoma, arises from the surface epithelium of the ovary. This epithelium is derived from pelvic peritoneum that envelops the ovarian tissue as it migrates during embryologic development from the supragonadal ridge to the pelvis. The ovarian epithelium is identical to other peritoneum, and peritoneal carcinomas are biologically equivalent to ovarian carcinoma. Approximately 15% of all ovarian carcinomas are borderline tumors, which are noninvasive and indolent in their behavior.

Borderline and invasive epithelial tumors of the ovary can be classified by their stage, histologic type, and histologic grade. Molecular studies have demonstrated that borderline and low-grade tumors are similar and distinct from high-grade carcinomas. Low-grade tumors are characterized by *KRAS* and *BRAF* mutations, whereas high-grade tumors have *TP53* mutations. Ovaries and tubes removed prophylactically in genetically predisposed individuals demonstrate frequent *TP53* mutations in the fallopian epithelium but not the ovarian surface epithelium, and the tubal epithelium has been proposed as the source of high-grade serous carcinomas.

The distinction of ovarian, peritoneal, and tubal carcinomas is more anatomic than functional, because these tumors are treated and behave similarly. Tumor histologies include serous (60%), endometrioid (20%), mucinous (3%), clear cell (2%), transitional (1%), and Brenner (1%). Advanced-stage or recurrent mucinous and clear cell tumors respond poorly to chemotherapy and have a poorer prognosis compared with other histologies.

CURRENT DIAGNOSIS

- Evaluate patients by family history of breast and ovarian cancer; seek genetic consultation.
- Evaluate for symptoms of ovarian cancer, including back pain, fatigue, bloating, constipation, abdominal pain, and urinary symptoms.
- Perform a follow-up assessment for any abnormal imaging results.
- Routine screening is not recommended.

---

[1]Not FDA approved for this indication.

Treatment

SURGERY

Ovarian cancer is typically treated with primary surgery to establish the diagnosis, determine the extent of disease, and remove as much cancer as possible before initiation of chemotherapy for advanced-stage disease. The surgical procedure indicated depends on the disease extent at presentation. For patients with apparent early-stage disease, staging surgery, including omentectomy, peritoneal biopsies, and pelvic and paraaortic lymphadenectomy, should be performed. For patients with limited metastatic disease, omentectomy and pelvic and paraaortic lymphadenectomy may affect staging and prognosis. For patients with advanced-stage disease, the goal of surgery is maximal tumor resection (i.e., cytoreduction or debulking). Retrospective data demonstrate improved survival for patients with no or minimal residual disease. The extent of surgery necessary to accomplish maximal tumor reduction varies from patient to patient. Intestinal surgery is often required, and sigmoid resection is the most common intestinal procedure.

After surgery, patients are evaluated for adjuvant chemotherapy based on disease stage and histologic findings. Borderline tumors are observed unless they have invasive metastatic implants. Patients with invasive tumors at low risk for recurrence (i.e., stage IA or IB with low-grade histology) are also observed. In view of the similar molecular profile of grade 2 and 3 histologies, treatment of grade 2 tumors should be considered.

CHEMOTHERAPY

Based on the results of randomized trials, primary chemotherapy consists of a platinum compound (i.e., carboplatin or cisplatin) and a taxane (i.e., paclitaxel or docetaxel [Taxotere][1]). In cases of advanced-stage disease, a minimum of six courses of a platinum/taxane doublet is given. For patients with suboptimal stage III and IV disease (i.e., residual tumor or tumors >1 cm in the greatest dimension), the median progression-free and overall survival times are 18 and 38 months, respectively. For patients with optimal residual disease (i.e., residual tumor or tumors <1 cm in greatest diameter), the median progression-free and overall survival times are 20.7 and 57.4 months, respectively.

In the late 1990s, several active second-line chemotherapy agents were approved for ovarian cancer. A very large, five-arm, randomized trial evaluating these agents in triplet or doublet combinations with carboplatin and paclitaxel failed to demonstrate an improvement. The number of courses of treatment is individualized based on radiologic and tumor marker response. After a complete clinical response, patients are observed. Clinical factors favorably affecting survival after treatment for advanced-stage disease included no or minimal residual disease, germline *BRCA* mutation, nonmucinous or non–clear cell tumor histology, better performance status, and younger age.

Neoadjuvant chemotherapy with a platinum/taxane doublet for patients with apparent advanced-stage disease is used for those who are elderly and compromised or those with serious medical comorbidities. Neoadjuvant chemotherapy is also used by some investigators for patients with extensive disease. Patients who respond favorably can then be considered for interval debulking surgery. A randomized trial comparing primary surgery with neoadjuvant chemotherapy demonstrated similar progression-free and overall survival times of 12 and 30 months, respectively.

Intraperitoneal chemotherapy has demonstrated efficacy in three large randomized trials and has been advocated by a National Cancer Institute Clinical Alert. The latest study, which used intraperitoneal cisplatin[1] and intravenous paclitaxel on day 1 and intraperitoneal paclitaxel[1] on day 6, reported progression-free and overall survival times of 23.8 and 65.6 months, respectively, compared with 18.3 and 49.7 months for the control group. However, trial design

---

[1]Not FDA approved for this indication.

and increased toxicity with the most recent intraperitoneal regimen has limited its acceptance in clinical practice.

Second-look laparotomy or laparoscopy used in the past to determine pathologic response has not been shown to affect disease outcome.

CONSOLIDATION OR MAINTENANCE THERAPY

Despite the high response rate to primary chemotherapy, advanced-stage ovarian cancer patients are at significant risk for recurrent disease. Maintenance therapy with paclitaxel for 12 months produced a superior progression-free survival compared with treatment for 3 months. However, seven other maintenance trials with paclitaxel, topotecan (Hycamtin),[1] or biologic agents have had negative results. An ongoing trial powered to evaluate progression-free and overall survival is evaluating maintenance therapy with one of two taxane compounds compared with observation.

BIOLOGIC THERAPY

Among the numerous biologic agents that have been studied in ovarian cancer, bevacizumab (Avastin),[1] an antibody against the vascular endothelial growth factor (VEGF), has demonstrated the most activity. After demonstration of activity against recurrent disease, ongoing trials in the United States and Europe are evaluating its role in combination with carboplatin and paclitaxel and as single-agent maintenance.

TREATMENT OF RECURRENT DISEASE

Although recurrent disease is incurable, patients may benefit from interventions. The potential for successful treatment of recurrent ovarian carcinoma is determined by response to prior therapy and the duration of the treatment-free interval. Secondary cytoreductive surgery has been used and is most effective for patients with a long treatment-free interval (>12 months), isolated site of recurrence, prior complete response to chemotherapy, and good performance status. Very late recurrences may represent second primaries.

CURRENT THERAPY

Primary Disease

- Primary surgery with comprehensive staging or maximal cytoreduction
- Intravenous platinum or taxane, or both (patients with optimal and suboptimal residual disease)
- Intraperitoneal platinum with intravenous or intraperitoneal taxane (patients with optimal residual stage III disease)
- Neoadjuvant chemotherapy with interval debulking

Recurrent Disease

- Platinum combination for recurrence after more than 6 months off therapy
- Nonplatinum single-agent therapy for recurrence after less than 6 months off therapy
- Radiation therapy as needed for disease palliation

---

[1]Not FDA approved for this indication.

Second-line chemotherapy that includes retreatment with a platinum compound is most effective in patients with a treatment-free interval of 6 months or more, and better response rates have been seen with longer treatment-free intervals. In this patient population, platinum in combination with paclitaxel or gemcitabine (Gemzar) is appropriate based on randomized trial data.

Patients can be repeatedly treated with a platinum compound until they develop resistant disease or intolerance to the adverse effects. Numerous other agents may be effective in controlling disease progression. Radiation therapy is used as needed for disease palliation.

End-of-Life Care

Progressive disease can manifest as intestinal obstruction, unrelenting ascites, or pleural effusions. Percutaneous gastrostomy for drainage of effusions or ascites may provide symptomatic relief. Shifting from active treatment to a goal of palliation with attention to quality of life is appropriate at this point.

REFERENCES

Armstrong DK, Bundy B, Wenzel L, et al. for the Gynecologic Oncology Group. Intraperitoneal cisplatin and paclitaxel in ovarian cancer. N Engl J Med 2006;354:34–43.

Bookman MA, Brady MF, McGuire WP, et al. Evaluation of new platinum-based treatment regimens in advanced-stage ovarian cancer: A phase III trial of the Gynecologic Cancer Intergroup. J Clin Oncol 2009;27:1419–25.

Brown J, Sood AK, Deavers MT, et al. Patterns of metastasis in sex cord-stromal tumors of the ovary: Can routine staging lymphadenectomy be omitted? Gynecol Oncol 2009;113:86–90.

Fishman DA, Cohen L, Blank SV, et al. The role of ultrasound evaluation in the detection of early-stage epithelial ovarian cancer. Am J Obstet Gynecol 2005;192:1214–22.

Goff BA, Mandel LS, Melancon CH, Muntz HG. Frequency of symptoms of ovarian cancer in women presenting to primary care clinics. JAMA 2004;291:2705–12.

Markman M, Liu PY, Wilczynski S, et al. Phase III randomized trial of 12 versus 3 months of maintenance paclitaxel in patients with advanced ovarian cancer after complete response to platinum and paclitaxel-based chemotherapy: A Southwest Oncology Group and Gynecologic Oncology Group trial. J Clin Oncol 2003;21:2460–5.

McGuire WP, Hoskins WJ, Brady MF, et al. Cyclophosphamide and cisplatin versus paclitaxel and cisplatin: A phase III randomized trial in patients with suboptimal stage III/IV ovarian cancer. N Engl J Med 1996;334:1–6.

Ozols RF, Bundy BN, Greer BE, et al. Phase III trial of carboplatin and paclitaxel compared with cisplatin and paclitaxel in patients with optimally resected stage III ovarian cancer: A Gynecologic Oncology Group study. J Clin Oncol 2003;21:3194–200.

Parmar MK, Ledermann JA, Colombo N, et al. ICON and AGO Collaborators. Paclitaxel plus platinum-based chemotherapy versus conventional platinum-based chemotherapy in women with relapsed ovarian cancer: The ICON4/AGO-OVAR-2.2 trial. Lancet 2003;361:2099–106.

Partridge E, Kreimer AR, Greenlee RT, et al. Results from four rounds of ovarian cancer screening in a randomized trial. Obstet Gynecol 2009;113:775–82.

Pfisterer J, Plante M, Vergote I, et al., for AGO-OVAR; NIC CTG; EORTC GCG. Gemcitabine plus carboplatin compared with carboplatin in patients with platinum-sensitive recurrent ovarian cancer: An intergroup trial of the AGO-OVAR, the NCIC CTG, and the EORTC GCG. J Clin Oncol 2006;24:4699–707.

Vergote I, Trope CG, Amant F, et al. Neoadjuvant chemotherapy or primary surgery in stage IIIC or IV ovarian cancer. N Engl J Med 2010;363:943–53.

Winter WE, Maxwell GL, Tian C, et al. Prognostic factors for stage III epithelial ovarian cancer: Gynecologic Oncology Group Study. J Clin Oncol 2007;25:3621–7.

Psychiatric Disorders

Alcoholism

Method of
Richard N. Rosenthal, MD

Epidemiology

Alcohol-use disorders are among the most prevalent mental disorders in the population, occurring at frequencies that rival those of mood and anxiety disorders. In any year, almost 8½% of the U.S. population older than 18 years meets criteria for a formal alcohol use disorder (alcohol abuse or dependence), and almost 4% meets criteria for alcohol dependence.

Economic and Medical Sequelae

Alcohol use disorders are important to identify and treat for several reasons. The first is the direct negative impact of chronic heavy alcohol exposure on cognitive, physical, social, and vocational functioning. The second is the well-described long-term medical sequelae of alcohol dependence such as hepatic cirrhosis, pancreatitis, and dementia. Chronic heavy drinking, even in the absence of a formal diagnosis of alcohol dependence, is associated with an increased risk of diabetes mellitus, hypertension, gastrointestinal bleeding, hemorrhagic stroke, and several forms of carcinoma. The third reason for identification and treatment is the public impact of alcohol use disorders, which covers associated traumatic injuries from motor vehicle and job-related accidents, alcohol-related crime, and their associated economic costs. More than $180 billion is lost to the U.S. economy each year due to alcohol-related crime, injury, health care costs, and lost productivity in the workplace.

Screening

SCREENING RATIONALE

Screening for alcohol problems arrays patients on a continuum from abstinence to dependence and is a highly efficient way to identify patients who are at acute risk for the effects of alcohol abuse and dependence as well as those who do not currently meet formal alcohol-related diagnoses but who are at risk for long-term medical and social consequences of heavy alcohol exposure (Box 1). The U.S. Preventative Services Task Force (USPSTF) found that screening could accurately identify patients whose levels or patterns of alcohol consumption do not meet criteria for alcohol dependence but that place them at risk for increased morbidity and mortality. The USPSTF also found good evidence that brief interventions that consist of behavioral counseling and follow-up can reduce alcohol consumption for 6 to 12 months or longer and that the benefits outweigh any potential harms. Thus, it is recommended that alcohol screening and brief interventions be performed in primary care settings to reduce alcohol problems for adults, including pregnant women.

BRIEF SCREENING

Every patient should be asked about alcohol use. Because drinking is normative in the United States, if drinking is denied, it is useful to determine if the patient used to drink but has stopped because of a past problem. After determining if a patient currently uses any alcohol, the simplest strategy is to ask about the number of heavy drinking days in the past year, where heavy drinking is defined as more than four drinks for men and more than three drinks for women in one day. If that threshold is reached, which corresponds to at-risk or hazardous drinking, then further evaluation of alcohol-related problems is indicated through the use of screening instruments. A standard drink is the same amount of alcohol contained in different volumes of alcoholic beverages (Box 2).

BOX 1   Current Risk Terms

Abstinence
- No alcohol use

Moderate Drinking
- Men: No more than 2 standard drinks per drinking d
- Women: No more than 1 standard drink per drinking d
- Elderly persons (>65 y): No more than 1 standard drink per drinking d

Risky or Hazardous Drinking
- Men
  - More than 4 standard drinks per drinking d
  - More than 14 standard drinks per wk
- Women
  - More than 3 standard drinks per drinking d
  - More than 7 standard drinks per wk
- Elderly persons (>65 y):
  - More than 3 standard drinks per drinking d
  - More than 7 standard drinks per wk

BOX 2 Standard Drinks

Each equivalent drink contains about 14 g of pure alcohol:
- 12 oz of beer or wine cooler
- 8–9 oz of malt liquor
- 5 oz of wine
- 3 to 4 oz of fortified wine (e.g., port)
- 1½ oz of 80-proof distilled spirits (or 1 jigger of liquor before mixing)

The Alcohol Use Disorders Identification test (AUDIT) (Table 1) is a 10-item screen developed by the World Health Organization. Given its length, the AUDIT can be used as a self-report screener that patients can fill out in the waiting area before seeing the clinician. The minimum score is 0 and the maximum score is 40. A score of 8 or more for men or 4 or more for women, adolescents, and persons older than 65 years, like a positive endorsement of any heavy drinking days, indicates the need for further evaluation of alcohol use and an increased risk of an alcohol use disorder. For brevity, the AUDIT-C, a truncated version of the AUDIT consisting of the first three AUDIT questions focused on alcohol consumption, can be used as a part of a waiting-room health history form. A score of 6 or more for men or 4 or more for women on the AUDIT-C indicates a need for further evaluation.

Asking about alcohol consumption during a routine clinical interview is best bundled with other questions about lifestyle and health, such as diet, smoking, and exercise. In addition to giving the patient a pre-examination questionnaire to fill out such as the AUDIT, another screening strategy is to ask the CAGE questions (Box 3) during the clinical examination. A positive answer to any of these questions also indicates the need for further evaluation of alcohol use. Two or more CAGE questions answered affirmatively identifies a patient at high risk for alcohol dependence. Because the CAGE screens for consequences, it is not as sensitive for risky drinking.

There are other question sets that are more sensitive than the CAGE in specific demographic subsets, and these can also be easily asked during a routine history. The five-item TWEAK questionnaire (Table 2) may be a more optimal screening questionnaire for identifying women (including pregnant women) with risky drinking or alcohol-use disorders in racially mixed populations. The CRAFFT (Box 4) is a 6-item question set that has high sensitivity in screening adolescents for alcohol and other substance-abuse problems. For patients older than 65 years, the Short Michigan Alcoholism Screening Test—Geriatric (S-MAST-G) (Box 5) is useful in identifying those at risk for alcohol problems, because these patients might not need the same volumes of alcohol intake as others to develop alcohol-related problems. To complete the initial screening, one should compute the average number of drinks per week by multiplying the days per week on average that the patient drinks by the number of drinks consumed on a typical drinking day.

Laboratory testing for elevations of alanine aminotransferase (ALT), aspartate aminotransferase (AST), γ-glutamyltransferase (GGT), or carbohydrate-deficient transferrin (CDT) have no incremental sensitivity over those of validated screening instruments, and they may be better suited to monitoring patients already in treatment for alcohol-use disorders. The patient must still be asked about quantity and frequency of alcohol use. However, laboratory testing can provide indicators of covert heavy drinking (e.g., elevated GGT

TABLE 1 Alcohol Use Disorders Identification Test (AUDIT)

Questions	Scoring				
	0	1	2	3	4
Consumption (AUDIT-C)					
How often do you have a drink containing alcohol?	Never	Monthly or less	2 to 4 times a month	2 to 3 times a week	4 or more times a week
How many drinks containing alcohol do you have on a typical day when you are drinking?	1 or 2	3 or 4	5 or 6	7 to 9	10 or more
How often do you have five or more drinks on one occasion?	Never	Less than monthly	Monthly	Weekly	Daily or almost daily
Personal Consequences					
How often during the last year have you found that you were not able to stop drinking once you had started?	Never	Less than monthly	Monthly	Weekly	Daily or almost daily
How often during the last year have you failed to do what was normally expected of you because of drinking?	Never	Less than monthly	Monthly	Weekly	Daily or almost daily
How often during the last year have you needed a first drink in the morning to get yourself going after a heavy drinking session?	Never	Less than monthly	Monthly	Weekly	Daily or almost daily
How often during the last year have you had a feeling of guilt or remorse after drinking?	Never	Less than monthly	Monthly	Weekly	Daily or almost daily
How often during the last year have you been unable to remember what happened the night before because of your drinking?	Never	Less than monthly	Monthly	Weekly	Daily or almost daily
Social Consequences					
Have you or someone else been injured because of your drinking?	No		Yes, but not in the last year		Yes, during the last year
Has a relative, friend, doctor, or other health care worker been concerned about your drinking or suggested you cut down?	No		Yes, but not in the last year		Yes, during the last year

Scoring and Interpretation
Add all scores to obtain a total: >8 points for men or >4 points for women indicates a high risk of alcohol use disorder.
AUDIT-C (first three AUDIT questions): >6 points for men or >4 points for women indicates a need for further evaluation.

- Have you ever felt that you should *Cut down* on your drinking?
- Have people *Annoyed* you by criticizing your drinking?
- Have you ever felt bad or *Guilty* about your drinking?
- Have you ever taken a drink *(Eye opener)* first thing in the morning to steady your nerves or to get rid of a hangover?

One yes response indicates need for further assessment. Two yes responses indicate risk of an alcohol use disorder.

CURRENT DIAGNOSIS

Risky or Hazardous Drinking (Need Further Evaluation)

- Men who drink more than four standard drinks per day or 14 standard drinks per week
- Women and those older than 65 years who drink more than three standard drinks per day or more than seven standard drinks per week
- Drinking concurrent with any medical condition where alcohol is contraindicated

Alcohol Abuse

- Repeated failure to fulfill obligations at home, school, or work
- Increased risk of physical harm
- Legal problems or interpersonal problems in any year

Alcohol Dependence (Three or More in Any Year)

- Cannot cut down or stop
- Decreased time spent in other usual activities
- Drinking despite physical or psychological consequences
- Drinking more than intended
- Physical tolerance
- Preoccupied with drinking
- Withdrawal episodes

and CDT) when the patient does not reveal the extent of alcohol intake. CDT, which is perturbed less than other indices by nonalcoholic liver disease, may be a more specific and sensitive indicator of heavy drinking.

Diagnosis

Screening can identify those who are at risk for the sequelae of risky or hazardous drinking and who might benefit from a brief intervention conducted in the primary care office, but only a diagnostic evaluation can confirm the clinician's suspicion that the patient's use of alcohol meets syndromal criteria and warrants specific medical and psychosocial treatment beyond the brief intervention. If, during the last 12 months, alcohol has contributed to repeated episodes of failure to fulfill obligations at home, school or work, episodes of increased risk of physical harm, arrests or other legal problems, or recurrent problems with significant others, then the patient has a diagnosis of alcohol abuse, according to *Diagnostic and Statistical Manual of Mental Disorders*, Fourth Edition (Text Revision) (DSM-IV-TR) criteria (Table 3). The patient has a diagnosis of alcohol dependence if he or she has three or more of the following criteria over a 12-month period: physical tolerance, symptoms of withdrawal, repeatedly drinking more than intended, unsuccessful reduction or quit attempts, increased time drinking or recovering from drinking, reduced time in other pleasurable or important activities, and continued drinking despite physical or psychological problems.

Rates of co-occurring mood and anxiety disorders are especially high among those with alcohol-use disorders. Untreated mood and anxiety disorders tend to have a negative impact on alcoholism recovery. Among treatment-seeking patients in the National Epidemiologic Survey on Alcohol and Related Conditions (NESARC) sample with a current alcohol use disorder, 40% had at least one current independent mood disorder, and more than one third had at least one current independent anxiety disorder. Heavy alcohol intake can also induce symptoms of mood and other mental disorders. To differentiate alcohol-induced symptoms from independent disorders, it is optimal to reassess symptoms of a mental disorder several weeks after cessation or significant reduction of alcohol intake.

Brief Intervention

INTENTION

Although risky or hazardous drinking is not a formal diagnosis, it describes a group with a higher likelihood to develop alcohol problems with risk for accidents, injuries, and social and health problems compared with the general population (see Box 1). Thus, even without a formal diagnosis, it is beneficial to help the patient with risky drinking to change his or her drinking behavior. Several well-described short interchanges between the clinician and the patient, organized under the rubric of *brief interventions*, have been validated in randomized trials as decreasing alcohol intake in those who drink too much but do not have a diagnosis of alcohol dependence. Brief intervention has been demonstrated to reduce weekly alcohol use, frequency of binging, liver enzymes associated with heavy drinking, blood pressure, emergency department visits, hospital days, and psychosocial problems, typically for 6 to 12 months, and to reduce drinking and hospital days at up to 4 years in one study. Because most at-risk patients seen in primary care settings are subsyndromal for alcohol-use disorders, the typical clinical interaction related to alcohol will be that of screening and then a brief intervention for positive cases. The two are typically referred to together under the acronym SBI (screening and brief intervention).

The basic intention of a brief intervention is to educate the patient about the risks of heavy alcohol use in such a way as to motivate him or her to reduce weekly alcohol consumption. The standard

TABLE 2 TWEAK Questionnaire

Feature	Question	Answer	Score
Tolerance	How many drinks does it take before you begin to feel the first effects of alcohol?	≥3	2
Worry	Have your friends or relatives worried or complained about your drinking in the past year?	Yes	2
Eye-opener	Do you sometimes take a drink in the morning when you first get up?	Yes	1
Amnesia	Are there times when you drink and afterward you can't remember what you said or did?	Yes	1
Kut	Do you sometimes feel the need to cut down on your drinking?	Yes	1

Scoring and interpretation: Two or more points indicate a possible alcohol problem.

BOX 4   CRAFFT Questionnaire

- Have you ever ridden in a **C**ar driven by someone (including yourself) who was high or had been using alcohol or drugs?
- Do you ever use alcohol or drugs to **R**elax, feel better about yourself, or fit in?
- Do you ever use alcohol or drugs while you are **A**lone?
- Do you ever **F**orget things you did while using alcohol or drugs?
- Do your **F**amily or **F**riends ever tell you that you should cut down on your drinking or drug use?
- Have you ever gotten into **T**rouble while you were using alcohol or drugs?
  One yes response indicates need for further assessment. Two yes responses indicate risk of alcohol-use disorder.

initial brief intervention takes about 15 minutes and consists of feedback, advice, and goal setting. It can be performed wholly in the primary care setting by the physician or other members of the health delivery team. Including alcohol screening, the USPSTF suggests five as to conducting SBI: *assess* the patient's alcohol consumption with a screening tool and clinical evaluation as indicated; *advise* reduction of alcohol consumption to appropriate levels, including abstinence if indicated; *agree* on individual goals for reducing alcohol use, including abstinence if indicated; *assist* patients in obtaining the motivation, skills, or supports needed to institute changes in drinking; and *arrange* for follow-up support, including specialty treatment referral for dependent patients. The most effective interventions are multicontact ones that provide ongoing assistance and follow-up.

PROCEDURE

Assess

Screen patients with the AUDIT or with the CAGE, TWEAK, CRAFFT, or S-MAST-G questionnaires as appropriate, and compute average drinks per week.

BOX 5   S-MAST-G Questionnaire

- When talking with others, do you ever underestimate how much you actually drink?
- After a few drinks, have you sometimes not eaten or been able to skip meals because you didn't feel hungry?
- Does having a few drinks help decrease your shakiness or tremors?
- Does alcohol sometimes make it hard for you to remember parts of the day or night?
- Do you usually take a drink to relax or calm your nerves?
- Do you drink to take your mind off your problems?
- Have you ever increased your drinking after experiencing a loss in your life?
- Has a doctor or nurse ever said that he or she was worried or concerned about your drinking?
- Have you ever made rules to manage your drinking?
- When you feel lonely, does having a drink help?
  Two or more yes responses indicate a probable alcohol problem.

Abbreviation: S-MAST-G = Short Michigan Alcoholism Screening Test—Geriatric.

Advise

Give feedback in the form of expression of concern, direct conclusions, and recommendations. Present medical findings, such as elevated liver enzymes, to back up conclusive statements such as "I'm concerned that your alcohol intake exceeds safe limits." Show the patient information comparing use with population norms and the associated health risks. Educate the patient about how alcohol can lead to medical, psychosocial, and legal consequences. Where possible, link the patient's current symptoms to alcohol use. Recommend appropriate and specific changes in behavior, such as "I strongly recommend you cut down your drinking," or in the case in which any drinking places the patient at high risk, "I strongly suggest you quit drinking."

Agree

Determine the patient's readiness to change drinking behavior, such as asking, "Do you think that cutting down on your drinking is something you are willing to talk about?" If the patient is ambivalent, avoid labeling the patient's behavior with a diagnosis at this stage, which can increase resistance to change, but encourage the patient to reflect on the positive reasons for drinking and the negative consequences of drinking. Offer concerns that continued drinking at the same level will impede the patient's achievement of goals such as decreased gastric distress or improved sleep patterns.

Empathic listening is generally more effective than a confrontational approach, and it is useful to express optimism about the patient's capacity to change. Elicit what the patient's concerns are about cutting down or quitting. Avoid arguing or challenging when the patient is unready to change, but schedule a follow-up visit to continue the dialogue and reassess drinking behavior. Restate your commitment to help when the patient is ready and that you remain open to questions.

When the patient concurs that a change in drinking would be beneficial, agree on a specific goal to cut down to particular daily and weekly limits for low-risk drinking or to stop drinking, if indicated, for a specific period of time. The agreement should be recorded and a copy given to the patient both as a reminder and motivator for behavioral change.

Assist

Work with the patient to formulate concrete steps to implement the drinking reduction plan. These steps include how to avoid high-risk drinking situations, how to keep a record of alcohol intake, and who can support the patient in meeting his or her goals. Provide resources in the form of patient educational materials, examples of which can be downloaded from the National Institute of Alcohol Abuse and Alcoholism (NIAAA) website (www.niaaa.nih.gov).

Arrange

Set up follow-up support and counseling visits or refer patients meeting dependence criteria for specialty treatment. Advise the patient to seek immediate medical treatment if withdrawal symptoms occur.

Treatment

DETOXIFICATION

Put simply, detoxification is medical stabilization that offers an opportunity to engage patients in alcoholism treatment, but it is not in itself treatment for alcohol dependence. Patients who drink more than 250 grams of alcohol daily are likely to experience physiologic withdrawal symptoms on cessation of drinking, but volume is not the only predictor of withdrawal severity. Although often mild, untreated alcohol withdrawal can result in seizures or delirium tremens (DTs), with increased risk of mortality.

TABLE 3 Diagnosis of Alcohol-Use Problems

Criteria	Typical Symptoms and History
Alcohol Abuse (≥1 in the last 12 months)	
Alcohol has caused or contributed to repeated:	
Failure to fulfill obligations at home, school, or work	Hangovers at work, truancy at school, missing appointments
Episodes of increased risk of physical harm	Driving, swimming, or operating machinery under the influence D of alcohol
Arrests or other legal problems	Public intoxication, DUI or DWI
Problems with significant others	Spousal strife, physical fights
Alcohol Dependence (≥3 in the last 12 mo)	
Development of physical tolerance	Drinks more for the same effect
Episodes of withdrawal syndrome (see below)	Morning shakes, nausea, anxiety
Drinking more than intended repeatedly	Binging episodes
Unsuccessful efforts to cut down or stop drinking	Failed New Year's resolution
Increased time planning for drinking, drinking, or recovering from drinking	Instead of being with kids, spends weekend mornings sleeping in
Reduced time in other pleasurable or important activities	Stopped socializing with friends, withdrew from hobby group
Drinking persists despite physical or psychological problems	Developed depressed mood, but kept on drinking
Alcohol Withdrawal (≥2 within hours to days after lowered blood alcohol levels)	
Autonomic hyperactivity	Heart rate ≥100 bpm, diaphoresis
Hand tremor	Hands shake when extended
Insomnia	Difficulty falling asleep
Nausea or vomiting	Feels queasy
Anxiety	Spontaneous report of fear
Psychomotor agitation	Inability to keep still, pacing
Hallucinations or illusions	Reports visual disturbances
Seizures	Tonic-clonic movements

Assessment

The Clinical Institute Withdrawal Assessment for Alcohol scale, Revised (CIWA-Ar) is a public domain scale that scores 10 signs and symptoms of withdrawal by severity ranging from not present to severe (Box 6). A score of less than 8 indicates mild withdrawal, characterized by increased autonomic activity with low-grade anxiety, diaphoresis, agitation, nausea, and elevated blood pressure, temperature, and heart rate. Scores of 8 to 15 indicate moderate withdrawal, and scores of 15 or more indicate more severe withdrawal states. In severe withdrawal, in the context of autonomic hyperarousal, the patient can become disoriented and have a clouded sensorium, the hallmarks of delirium.

Prior history of severe withdrawal, such as DTs, is a reasonable predictor of similar future responses to alcohol withdrawal. Risk for withdrawal delirium is increased if the patient has a heart rate of greater than 120 bpm before treatment, a current infectious disease, withdrawal symptoms in the context of a blood alcohol concentration greater than 100 mg/dL, a prior history of either delirium or seizures, or a high CIWA-Ar score, indicating severe autonomic hyperactivity. Patients who have severe withdrawal symptoms, who are at high risk for seizures, or who have a medical condition likely to be exacerbated by withdrawal, such as type 1 diabetes or coronary artery disease, should have medically supervised inpatient detoxification.

CURRENT THERAPY

All At-Risk Patients

- Assess: Screen patients with standard instruments and compute average standard drinks per week.
- Advise: Give feedback, express concern, present findings and conclusions, and recommend specific behavioral changes.
- Agree: Determine the patient's readiness to change, encourage reflection, listen empathically, elicit patient concerns, avoid arguing, express optimism, set a specific reduction or abstinence goal.
- Assist: Formulate concrete implementation plan, including avoiding high-risk situations, recording alcohol intake, and eliciting family and community support for patient goals.
- Arrange: Set up follow-up visits and refer patients meeting dependence criteria for specialty treatment.

Additionally for Alcohol-Dependent Patients

- Offer or arrange for detoxification if indicated.
- Offer or arrange for specialty alcoholism treatment and/or mutual help groups.
- Offer pharmacotherapy to support maintenance of abstinence: naltrexone, acamprosate, or disulfiram.
- Offer medication management support during follow-up visits.

Pharmacologic Therapy

Alcohol withdrawal is best treated with sedative hypnotic medications that are cross-tolerant with alcohol, such as benzodiazepines. Longer-acting benzodiazepines such as diazepam (Valium) and chlordiazepoxide (Librium) are easier to titrate against withdrawal symptoms and give a gradual offset in plasma concentration, but shorter-acting benzodiazepines such as lorazepam (Ativan)[1] are less likely to oversedate the patient. Rapid-onset benzodiazepines have a higher abuse liability and are generally best avoided. However, patients with severe hepatic impairment (elevated total bilirubin) are best treated with benzodiazepines that are not oxidized by the liver, such as oxazepam (Serax) or lorazepam.

Typical dosing is chlordiazepoxide 50 to 100 mg, diazepam 10 to 20 mg, oxazepam 20 to 40[3] mg, or lorazepam[1] 2 to 4 mg. The typical front-loading style of dosing is to administer medication at the higher end of the dose range every 1 to 2 hours so that the CIWA-Ar score is less than 8 for 24 hours.

With long-acting medications, once symptoms subside, there is often no need to taper doses. The short-acting benzodiazepines and long-acting benzodiazepines given to patients at high-risk for seizures

---

[1]Not FDA approved for this indication.
[3]Exceeds dosage recommended by the manufacturer.

BOX 6   Clinical Institute Withdrawal Assessment for Alcohol Scale, Revised (CIWA-Ar)

Patient:_____ Date:_____ Time:_____ (24-hour clock, midnight = 00:00)

Pulse or heart rate, taken for one minute:_____ Blood pressure:_____ mm Hg

Nausea and Vomiting – Ask, "Do you feel sick to your stomach? Have you vomited?" Observation:
0 no nausea and no vomiting
1 mild nausea with no vomiting
2
3
4 intermittent nausea with dry heaves
5
6
7 constant nausea, frequent dry heaves, and vomiting

Tremor – Arms extended and fingers spread apart. Observation:
0 no tremor
1 not visible, but can be felt fingertip to fingertip
2
3
4 moderate, with patient's arms extended
5
6
7 severe, even with arms not extended

Paroxysmal Sweats – Observation:
0 no sweat visible
1 barely perceptible sweating, palms moist
2
3
4 beads of sweat obvious on forehead
5
6
7 drenching sweats

Anxiety – Ask, "Do you feel nervous?" Observation:
0 no anxiety, at ease
1 mild anxious
2
3
4 moderately anxious, or guarded, so anxiety is inferred
5
6
7 equivalent to acute panic states as seen in severe delirium or acute schizophrenic reactions

Agitation – Observation:
0 normal activity
1 somewhat more than normal activity
2
3
4 moderately fidgety and restless
5
6
7 paces back and forth during most of the interview or constantly thrashes about

Tactile Disturbances – Ask, "Have you any itching, pins and needles sensations, any burning, any numbness, or do you feel bugs crawling on or under your skin?" Observation:
0 none
1 very mild itching, pins and needles, burning, or numbness
2 mild itching, pins and needles, burning, or numbness
3 moderate itching, pins and needles, burning, or numbness
4 moderately severe hallucinations
5 severe hallucinations
6 extremely severe hallucinations
7 continuous hallucinations

Auditory Disturbances – Ask, "Are you more aware of sounds around you? Are they harsh? Do they frighten you? Are you hearing anything that is disturbing to you? Are you hearing things you know are not there?" Observation:
0 not present
1 very mild harshness or ability to frighten
2 mild harshness or ability to frighten
3 moderate harshness or ability to frighten
4 moderately severe hallucinations
5 severe hallucinations
6 extremely severe hallucinations
7 continuous hallucinations

Visual Disturbances – Ask, "Does the light appear to be too bright? Is its color different? Does it hurt your eyes? Are you seeing anything that is disturbing to you? Are you seeing things you know are not there?" Observation:
0 not present
1 very mild sensitivity
2 mild sensitivity
3 moderate sensitivity
4 moderately severe hallucinations
5 severe hallucinations
6 extremely severe hallucinations
7 continuous hallucinations

Headache, Fullness in Head – Ask, "Does your head feel different? Does it feel like there is a band around your head?" Do not rate for dizziness or lightheadedness. Otherwise, rate severity:
0 not present
1 very mild
2 mild
3 moderate
4 moderately severe
5 severe
6 very severe
7 extremely severe

Orientation and Clouding of Sensorium – Ask, "What day is this? Where are you? Who am I?"
0 oriented and can do serial additions
1 cannot do serial additions or is uncertain about date
2 disoriented for date by no more than 2 calendar days
3 disoriented for date by more than 2 calendar days
4 disoriented for place or person

Total CIWA-Ar Score_____
Rater's Initials_____
Maximum Possible Score: 67

The CIWA-Ar *is not* copyright and may be reproduced freely. This assessment for monitoring withdrawal symptoms requires approximately 5 minutes to administer.

From Sullivan JT, Sykora K, Schneiderman J, Naranjo CA, Sellers EM: Assessment of alcohol withdrawal: The revised Clinical Institute Withdrawal Assessment for Alcohol scale (CIWA-Ar). Br J Addiction 1989;84:1353–1357.

or DTs are best given on a fixed-dose regimen of four times daily for the first 24 hours, with the patient reassessed 1 to 2 hours after each dose, and additional medication given as needed. On days 2 and 3, 50% of the dose can be given four times daily.

Long-acting barbiturates, such as phenobarbital,[1] can be also used on a fixed-dose regimen of 60 mg every 4 to 6 hours, with a loading dose of 120 mg orally or intramuscularly every hour for acute withdrawal symptoms (e.g., pulse >110 bpm) or a CIWA-Ar score of 10 or more.

Anticonvulsants such as carbamazepine (Tegretol),[1] valproate (Depakote),[1] or gabapentin (Neurontin)[1] have also been used effectively in uncomplicated withdrawal, but they are unproved in preventing withdrawal-related seizures and in treating DTs.

Although phenothiazines and haloperidol are somewhat effective compared with benzodiazepines in reducing withdrawal symptoms such as agitation, they are not as protective against seizures or delirium and thus are not recommended.

Thiamine (vitamin B$_1$) supplementation of 100 mg/day for 3 days can counteract the thiamine deficiencies that are common in alcoholic patients.

PSYCHOSOCIAL INTERVENTIONS FOR ALCOHOL DEPENDENCE

In addition to brief interventions for risky alcohol use, the most opportune and practical psychosocial intervention that the primary care office can provide is clinical behavioral support for pharmacotherapy for alcohol dependence. Simply put, medication management support consists initially of feedback to the patient of screening and medical evaluation results and the negative health effects of continued heavy drinking, as in a brief intervention. The patient is then given the basis for the diagnosis of alcohol dependence, the rationale for abstinence, and recommendation for pharmacotherapy. The patient is given information about medication and the appropriate prescriptions and is encouraged to seek community support for sobriety in mutual help groups such as Alcoholics Anonymous or to follow a plan such as Rational Recovery. Follow-up visits consist of assessment of medication side effects, patient adherence to the medication regimen, assessment of abstinence or quantity and pattern of alcohol intake, and assessment of overall functioning. Problems with medication adherence are identified and addressed.

There are evidence-based psychosocial interventions that are typically performed in the context of specialty programs for alcohol dependence, but they can be offered by clinical personnel in the context of the physician's office. Cognitive behavior therapy, network therapy, behavioral family therapy, and motivational interviewing are effective approaches for the treatment of alcohol dependence. Motivational interviewing is especially adaptable for use in primary care settings in that it is an approach to interacting with the alcohol-dependent patient that can be learned quickly and executed by any staff with clinical contact. A motivational enhancement manual can be accessed at the NIAAA website (http://www.niaaa.nih.gov/).

MEDICATION MANAGEMENT OF ALCOHOL DEPENDENCE

There are currently four FDA-approved medications for the treatment of alcohol dependence. Any of these medications can and should be given concurrently with other interventions such as psychosocial treatment or mutual help groups.

Disulfiram (Antabuse) works by inhibiting the metabolism of ethyl alcohol, causing a buildup of acetaldehyde, a noxious substance, which causes a strong stereotypic aversive response (flushing, diaphoresis, nausea, tachycardia) in the patient. Standard dosing is 250 mg/day (range, 125–500 mg). The major clinical concern with disulfiram is patient noncompliance with the medication regimen. Thus, it is most likely to be effective when there is a concrete method

for supporting compliance in place, such as directly observed therapy by a spouse or in a clinic.

More recently, the opioid antagonist naltrexone (ReVia, Depade) was approved for the treatment of alcohol dependence. It is dosed at 50 mg once daily. Naltrexone reduces days of heavy drinking and can reduce alcohol craving. Naltrexone in a long-acting intramuscular formulation (Vivitrol) allows once-monthly dosing (380 mg) and reduces the risk of noncompliance. It reduces heavy drinking overall and helps maintain abstinence in those who are abstinent at initial drug administration. Both oral and IM naltrexone formulations carry FDA black-box warnings related to findings of reversible elevations of liver enzymes at three to six times the standard dosage; however, naltrexone is safe at the recommended dose.

Acamprosate (Campral) is a taurine analogue that has been demonstrated to reduce relapse to any drinking as well as reducing heavy drinking in nonabstinent patients. It is dosed as two 333-mg tablets three times a day to patients who have ceased alcohol intake. It is excreted unchanged through the kidneys and has no interactions with other medications. Side effects are benign, and the most frequent is loose stools, which are mild to moderate and self-limited.

Topiramate[1] (Topamax) titrated over 5 weeks between 50 mg and 300 mg daily appears to reduce heavy drinking and days of any drinking over the short term (12 weeks) in alcohol-dependent patients who have not established abstinence prior to treatment. Common side effects include paresthesias, taste perversion, decreased appetite, and difficulty concentrating.

---

[1]Not FDA approved for this indication.

REFERENCES

American Psychiatric Association. Diagnostic and statistical manual of mental disorders. 4th ed. text revision. Washington, DC: American Psychiatric Association; 2000.

Bertholet N, Daeppen J-B, Wietlisbach V, et al. Reduction of alcohol consumption by brief alcohol intervention in primary care systematic review and meta-analysis. Arch Intern Med 2005;165:986–95.

Bradley KA, Boyd-Wickizer J, Powell SH, Burman ML. Alcohol screening questionnaires in women: A critical review. JAMA 1998;280:166–71.

Chang G, Kosten TR. Detoxification. In: Lowinson JH, Ruiz P, Millman RB, Langrod JG, editors. Substance Abuse: A Comprehensive Textbook. Philadelphia: Lippincott Williams & Wilkins; 2004. p. 579–87.

Fleming MF, Mundt MP, French MT, et al. Brief physician advice for problem drinkers: Long-term efficacy and cost-benefit analysis. Alcohol Clin Exp Res 2002;26:36–43.

Grant BF, Stinson FS, Dawson DA, et al. Prevalence and co-occurrence of substance use disorders and independent mood and anxiety disorders: Results from the National Epidemiologic Survey on Alcohol and Related Conditions. Arch Gen Psychiatry 2004;61:807–16.

Johnson BA, Rosenthal N, Capece JA, et al. Topiramate for treating alcohol dependence: A randomized controlled trial. JAMA 2007;298:1641–51.

Knight JR, Sherritt L, Shrier LA, et al. Validity of the CRAFFT substance abuse screening test among adolescent clinic patients. Arch Pediatr Adolesc Med 2002;156(6):607–14.

Maisto SA, Saitz R. Alcohol use disorders: Screening and diagnosis. Am J Addict 2003;12(Suppl. 1):S12–25.

McCaul ME, Petry NM. The role of psychosocial treatments in pharmacotherapy for alcoholism. Am J Addict 2003;12(Suppl. 1):S41–52.

National Institute on Alcohol Abuse and Alcoholism. Helping patients who drink too much: a clinician's guide, Rockville, MD: National Institute on Alcohol Abuse and Alcoholism; 2005. Available at http://pubs.niaaa.nih.gov/publications/Practitioner/CliniciansGuide2005/guide.pdf (accessed June 15, 2007).

Saitz R. Unhealthy alcohol use. N Engl J Med 2005;352:596–607.

Saunders JB, Aasland OG, Babor TF, et al. Development of the Alcohol Use Disorders Screening Test (AUDIT) WHO collaborative project on early detection of persons with harmful alcohol consumption. Addiction 1993;88:791–804.

Sullivan JT, Sykora K, Schneiderman J, et al. Assessment of alcohol withdrawal: The revised Clinical Institute Withdrawal Assessment for Alcohol scale (CIWA-Ar). Br J Addict 1989;84:1353–7.

U.S. Preventive Services Task Force. Screening and behavioral counseling interventions in primary care to reduce alcohol misuse: Recommendation statement. Ann Intern Med 2004;140:554–6.

---

[1]Not FDA approved for this indication.

Drug Abuse

Method of
William Greene, MD, and Mark S. Gold, MD

Epidemiology

Widespread pathologic use of intoxicating substances, both legal and illegal, remains one of the greatest public health concerns facing our nation. According to the 2008 National Survey on Drug Use and Health, 20.1 million Americans (8.0% of the population) aged 12 years and older used an illicit drug within the past month. By order of frequency, these include marijuana, nonmedical use of prescription drugs, cocaine, hallucinogens, inhalants, and heroin. In addition, 70.9 million Americans (28.4%) aged 12 years and older used tobacco within the past month, mostly in the form of cigarettes. Each year in the United States, approximately 440,000 people die of an illness attributable to cigarette smoking, making this the foremost cause of preventable death. The estimated annual economic cost of drug abuse (excluding alcohol) is $349 billion in the United States alone: $181 billion for illicit drugs and $168 billion for tobacco. These costs include only direct health-related, crime-related, and lost-productivity costs, thus underestimating the full impact of drug abuse on society.

From 2002 to 2008, the rate of past-month cigarette use among 12- to 17-year-olds has steadily dropped from 13.0% to 9.1%. The 2008 Monitoring the Future survey data confirm that cigarette smoking has continued to fall to the lowest rate in the survey's history (i.e., past month use among 12th graders is now at 20%). Since 2000, overall rates of illicit drug use have slowly dropped, but use of marijuana has recently slowed its rate of decline and initiation of illicit prescription drugs is now on the rise. In 2006, new users of illicit prescription drugs caught up with new users of marijuana for the first time; currently, more adolescents begin illicit drug use with prescription drugs than any other class, including marijuana. Although overall drug-use rates are generally improving, as of 2008, 47% of 12th graders still report having used an illicit drug at some point in their life. Despite recent advances in our understanding and treatment of substance use disorders, drug abuse remains an epidemic.

Diagnosis

For practical treatment planning, it is useful for clinicians to distinguish between two substance-use disorders defined in the DSM-IV-TR: substance abuse and substance dependence (Box 1). Substance abuse is considered to be under voluntary control, and essentially involves recurrent problematic use. On a societal level, substance abuse is arguably the larger concern, because it is more prevalent and contributes to more overall morbidity and mortality. However, on an individual patient level, substance dependence ("addiction") is clearly the more-severe diagnosis. Physiologic dependence (presence of tolerance or withdrawal) is neither sufficient nor necessary to diagnose substance dependence. The hallmark feature of substance dependence is loss of control, and this disorder is now widely recognized as a chronic *brain disease*. Substance dependence is characterized by a dysfunctional reward pathway and is considered a medical problem beyond the realm of voluntary control. It is a disease with no known cure but for which sustained remission is possible with appropriate treatment.

Tobacco and Nicotine

Nicotine is the main addictive component in tobacco, which is administered via smoking (e.g., cigarettes, cigars, pipes, bidis, hookah) or in smokeless formulations (e.g., dip, snuff, snus, chew). However,

---

BOX 1   DSM-IV-TR Criteria for Substance Dependence, Substance Abuse

Substance Dependence ("Addiction")
Three or more in a 12-month period
- Tolerance (needing more for same effect, or diminished effect with same amount)
- Characteristic withdrawal symptoms
- Substance taken in larger amount or for longer period than intended
- Persistent desire or unsuccessful efforts to cut down or control use
- Great deal of time spent in activities to obtain, use, or recover
- Important social, occupational, or recreational activities given up or reduced
- Use continues despite knowledge of having a physical or psychological problem worsened by the substance

Substance Abuse
One or more in a 12-month period; symptoms must never have met dependence criteria for the same class
- Recurrent use resulting in failure to fulfill major role obligation at work, home, or school
- Recurrent use in physically hazardous situations
- Recurrent substance related legal problems
- Continued use despite persistent or recurrent social or interpersonal problems caused or exacerbated by substance

---

smoking tobacco is clearly not equivalent to taking nicotine. Cigarette smoking causes nicotine, brain monoamine oxidase (MAO), and other effects in the smoker, some due to the smoke and others due to nicotine.

Following administration, nicotine rapidly binds to nicotinic acetylcholine receptors in the central nervous system (CNS), where it acts as a mild psychostimulant and mood modulator in a nonimpairing, yet profoundly addictive manner. When the user is tired, smoking has a stimulating effect. When the user is anxious or stressed, smoking exerts a calming effect. Smoking is injection without a needle, and owing to its short half-life, repeated self administration serves to effectively relieve unpleasant withdrawal symptoms from the nicotine itself. Repeated use quickly leads to both physiologic and psychological dependence.

As with other drugs of abuse, cue-induced cravings play an important role in maintaining the addiction. For example, the smell of the smoke, the sound of a lighter, and the feel of a cigarette on the lips all contribute to an overall process addiction beyond just addiction to the nicotine itself. Tobacco use is also strongly associated with alcohol use, with which it has synergistic toxic effects.

Toxicities from tobacco use are well described and include severe pulmonary disease, cardiovascular disease, and carcinomas of the upper aerodigestive tract and bladder. Even secondhand smoke, previously considered harmless, is now correctly regarded as a serious health risk to the nonsmoker and a "drug" itself.

Although quitting remains difficult for even the most motivated tobacco users, effective treatments for nicotine dependence now exist. Clinical trials indicate a combination of counseling and medications offers the best chance for success and should be offered to patients who are willing to make a quit attempt. A wide range of FDA-approved nicotine replacement therapies are readily available and have similar rates of efficacy (Table 1). Patches (Nicoderm CQ), gums (Nicorette), and lozenges (Commit) are available over the counter, but the nasal spray (Nicotrol NS) and inhaler (Nicotrol Inhaler) are available by prescription only.

Nonnicotine prescription medications with proven efficacy are available. Bupropion HCl (Wellbutrin) is an antidepressant that was serendipitously noted to dramatically reduce nicotine cravings

TABLE 1 Pharmacotherapy for Nicotine Dependence

Drug	Mechanism of Action	Dosage	Instructions	Comments
Nicotine patch (Nicoderm CQ)	NRT	7 mg, 14 mg, 21 mg	1 patch daily	Tapering doses recommended to discontinue
Nicotine gum (Nicorette)	NRT	2 mg, 4 mg	Chew slightly then "park" on oral mucosa	Tapering doses recommended to discontinue
Nicotine lozenge (Commit)	NRT	2 mg, 4 mg	Absorbed through oral mucosa; minimize swallowing	Tapering doses recommended to discontinue
Nicotine inhaler (Nicotrol Inhaler)	NRT	4 mg/cartridge	6-16 cartridges/day	By prescription only; tedious administration
Nicotine nasal spray (Nicotrol NS)	NRT	0.5 mg/spray	1-2 sprays each nostril q1h; max 80 sprays/day	By prescription only
Bupropion HCl (Wellbutrin,[1] Zyban)	Inhibits reuptake of NE and DA	150 mg SR tab, 300 mg XL tab	300 mg PO (divided qd-bid) daily × 7-12 wk	Helps with comorbid depression; can help prevent weight gain
Varenicline (Chantix)	Partial agonist at $\alpha_4\beta_2$ nicotinic acetylcholine receptor	0.5 mg, 1 mg	0.5 mg PO qd × 3 d, then 0.5 mg PO bid × 4 d, then 1 mg PO bid × 11 wk	May smoke during 1st wk; may continue additional 12 wk
Nicotine vaccine (NicVAX)	Antibody sequestration of nicotine	n/a	n/a	In clinical trials

[1]Not FDA approved for this indication.
Abbreviations: DA = dopamine; max = maximum; n/a = not applicable; NE = norepinephrine; NRT = nicotine replacement therapy; SR = sustained release; XL = extended release.

in some patients, and it is now widely used for this purpose (as Zyban). Varenicline (Chantix) was specifically developed to treat nicotine dependence and represents a considerable advancement, with improved smoking cessation rates. It acts as a partial agonist at the nicotine receptor and effectively serves to satisfy cravings while simultaneously blocking the effects of exogenously administered nicotine. Although probably the most effective agent, varenicline carries significant risk of psychiatric side effects. The "nicotine vaccine" (NicVAX),[5] a novel approach, is currently in phase III clinical trials, and appears promising.

Nicotine replacement, bupropion, and varenicline are all considered first-line pharmacotherapy. Bupropion, but not varenicline, may also be used in combination with nicotine-replacement therapies. All pharmacotherapy options are enhanced with coadministration of counseling or behavioral therapies. Helpful resources for patients interested in quitting include www.smokefree.gov (a government website dedicated to helping people quit smoking), 1-800-QUIT-NOW (a free phone-based services with coaches and educational materials), and a variety of resources available through the American Cancer Society and American Heart Association.

Cannabis

Cannabis (marijuana, pot, weed, grass, ganja, hash) remains the most-used illicit drug in the world. In Americans older than 12 years, 41% have used cannabis at least once, and 6.1% have used it in the past month. Cannabis is readily harvested from *Cannabis sativa*, and typically it is smoked, although it may also be ingested or vaporized. Despite a recent trend advocating legitimate medicinal use, it is still listed in Schedule I by the Drug Enforcement Agency (DEA), with high potential for abuse and no currently accepted medical use. $\triangle$-9-Tetrahydrocannabinol (THC) is the active ingredient, which exerts its desired psychoactive effects at CB_1 receptors diffusely throughout the CNS. Marijuana's THC concentration has been steadily increasing owing to selective plant breeding. Annual analysis of DEA seizures indicates average THC concentrations increased from approximately 1% in 1975 to approximately 10% in 2008. To what extent this makes the drug more dangerous or more addictive remains unclear.

Acute psychoactive effects of cannabis include euphoria, relaxation, heightened sensations, increased appetite, distorted sense of time, slowed reaction time, illusions and hallucinations, paranoia, and anxiety. Acute somatic effects include conjunctival injection, xerostomia, increased heart rate and blood pressure, muscle relaxation, and reduced intraocular pressure. There is no known risk of dangerous overdose, and withdrawal symptoms are generally mild but include irritability, cravings, diminished appetite, and insomnia. Cannabis is now recognized as unequivocally addictive. Abusers of this drug rapidly develop tolerance, and commonly demonstrate loss of control and continued use despite negative consequences—the hallmarks of addiction. It is estimated that 290,000 Americans sought treatment for cannabis as their primary drug of choice in 2006.

Not surprisingly, with more than 400 chemicals identified in its smoke, cannabis is dangerous with respect to long-term health. Chronic cannabis use is associated with lung cancer, chronic obstructive pulmonary disease, cardiovascular disease, impaired immunity, persistent disruption of memory and attention, and various psychiatric disorders, most commonly anxiety disorders and depressive disorders. There is a growing body of evidence that cannabis abuse can lead to lasting psychosis (i.e. schizophrenia) in predisposed persons.

Currently, treatment of cannabis dependence remains entirely psychosocial. Various existing drugs (including fluoxetine [Prozac],[1] lithium,[1] buspirone [Buspar][1]) have been investigated. However, well-controlled clinical trials to support their use are lacking. Preliminary data suggest that dronabinol (Marinol)[1] may be of some utility in relieving cravings and withdrawal symptoms without causing intoxication. Rimonabant (Acomplia),[2] a CB_1 antagonist used for weight loss in Europe, showed promise but has failed to achieve FDA approval due to psychiatric side effects.

Cocaine and Other Stimulants

As a class, cocaine and other stimulants work primarily by enhancing dopamine transmission in a dose-dependent fashion, either directly (amphetamines) or by blocking reuptake (cocaine). Cocaine and a

---

[5]Investigational drug in the United States.

[1]Not FDA approved for this indication.
[2]Not available in the United States.

variety of amphetamines (e.g., amphetamine [Adderall], methamphetamine [Desoxyn], methylphenidate [Methylin, Ritalin]) are available for legitimate medical use as Schedule II drugs. Cocaine (in solution) is still used as a topical anesthetic, and amphetamine derivatives are used to treat attention-deficit/hyperactivity disorder (ADHD), narcolepsy (amphetamine and methylphenidate), and obesity (methamphetamine only). Any of these agents may be abused and carry significant potential for addiction. Even newer "safer" agents such as modafinil (Provigil) and armodafinil (Nuvigil) are associated with abuse and dependency, albeit less commonly than with traditional stimulants.

Prescription stimulant abuse can involve using excessive doses to achieve a euphoric high, or via nonmedical use or diversion of prescriptions (e.g., students sharing medication to facilitate studying). When taken at prescribed doses for an appropriate condition, even methamphetamine is generally safe and effective. In contrast, when it is synthesized in clandestine laboratories and smoked or injected in extreme quantities, methamphetamine (crystal meth, ice, crank, speed) is alarmingly dangerous. No other commonly abused drug is so strongly associated with permanent brain damage, resembling that seen in traumatic brain injury victims. As ADHD becomes more recognized and treated, physicians must be aware of the potential for abuse of their well-intentioned prescriptions. To this end, several recent pharmacologic developments have introduced improved options for treatment. Time-released formulations of methylphenidate (Concerta) and amphetamine/dextroamphetamine (Adderall XR) are considered to have less abuse potential than the short-acting formulations. Better still, the formulation of lisdexamfetamine (Vyvanse) includes the amino acid lysine coupled with the amphetamine molecule, consequently acting as a prodrug with the least abuse potential of all ADHD stimulants.

Cocaine and other stimulants induce sympathomimetic effects including tachycardia, hypertension, mydriasis, and diaphoresis. These drugs are commonly associated with seizures, myocardial infarction, hemorrhagic strokes, dyskinesias and dystonias, and psychosis when taken at the doses typically used to achieve euphoria. Withdrawal is generally experienced as a crash and includes fatigue, depressed mood, increased appetite, and cravings. Considered nonaddictive until about 1980, cocaine is now widely recognized as one of the most addictive drugs, particularly in the base form (crack or freebase). MDMA, or ecstasy, shares the pharmacodynamic properties of the stimulants, combined with serotoninergic effects of the hallucinogens.

Currently, no medication has demonstrated efficacy in treating cocaine or stimulant dependence. Pharmacologic treatment remains symptomatic during the acute withdrawal phase. Stimulant-induced psychosis and mania respond well to traditional psychotropics when warranted; however, to date, no medications have reliably demonstrated efficacy in preventing relapse. A "cocaine vaccine,"[5] which enlists the immune system to develop antibodies rendering cocaine useless, is currently in phase II clinical trials and holds promise for the future. In the meantime, traditional psychosocial treatments remain the mainstay of clinical care.

Opioids

Opioids are categorized as endogenous (endorphins, enkephalins, dynorphins), opium alkaloids (morphine, codeine), semisynthetic (heroin, oxycodone [Roxicodone, OxyContin]), or synthetic (methadone [Dolophine], fentanyl [Sublimaze, Duragesic]). The last three categories have a wide range of clinical uses including analgesia, anesthesia, antidiarrhea, cough suppression, and detoxification and maintenance therapy.

Opioids exert their clinical effect at mu, delta, and kappa opioid receptors. The effect on mu receptors is considered the most important, with its activation directly linked to both analgesic and euphoric effects. Most humans subjectively experience opioids with a neutral to aversive response. However, when used in sufficient quantities by genetically vulnerable persons, some users experience energy, relief of emotional pain, and a euphoria many describe as a "total body orgasm." Intoxication manifests with miosis, impaired consciousness, slurred speech, bradycardia, and depressed respiration. Overdose is potentially fatal via respiratory depression, but it is quite amenable to treatment with repeated doses of intravenous naloxone (Narcan). The withdrawal syndrome is characterized by a constellation of miserable, but not life-threatening, symptoms including mydriasis, piloerection, muscle cramps, diaphoresis, vomiting, lacrimation, rhinorrhea, chills, insomnia, cravings, and autonomic hyperactivity.

Since pain was recognized as "the fifth vital sign" in the 1990s, concurrent with heavy marketing campaigns from pharmaceutical companies, the United States has experienced a veritable explosion of widespread opioid prescribing for nonmalignant pain. An entire industry of pain management has developed, with the unfortunate side effect of having a sizable proportion of its output being used nonmedically. It is important for prescribers to recognize that the abuse potential of prescription opioids matches, or even exceeds, that of heroin. Today, a 1-month prescription of time-released oxycodone prescribed at 80 mg three times daily has a street value of approximately $3600.

The most common method of abuse involves simply taking more than prescribed, usually by the appropriate route of administration. Alternatively, opioid abusers commonly take their medications via nasal insufflation or inject them intravenously. The time-release property of certain medications, such as oxycodone, is easily circumvented by crushing the pills, which greatly enhances the euphoric effect. Even transdermal fentanyl patches (Duragesic) are abused via any number of methods such as applying heat to a worn patch, employing complex extraction techniques described on the Internet, or simply sucking on the patch itself (a common finding by the coroner). Once the prescription is finished early, the user must either supplement the supply or face the unpleasant effects of withdrawal.

There is no shortage of easy methods to obtain opiates illegally. These include seeing multiple prescribers (doctor shopping), purchasing online at foreign "pharmacies," and general trade or purchase on the black market. Also alarming is the growing problem of diversion from hospitals and pharmacies by health care professionals, who are not immune to the disease of addiction. Many states are implementing controlled substance databases aimed to curb the problem of abuse of opioids and other prescription drugs.

Acute detoxification from opioids is achieved via one of two basic strategies: symptomatic treatment with unrelated medications, or substitution with a cross tolerant (opioid) drug with less abuse potential (Table 2). The first strategy may employ the use of clonidine (Catapres),[1] an α_2-adrenergic agonist, to help with the autonomic component of withdrawal. This is commonly done in combination with other symptomatic treatments on an as-needed basis, such as diazepam (Valium) for anxiety, loperamide (Imodium) for diarrhea, and promethazine (Phenergan)[1] or ondansetron (Zofran)[1] for nausea.

The second strategy typically involves either methadone or buprenorphine (Subutex). Methadone, a pure mu agonist with a half-life of about 36 hours, is usually started in the 20- to 30-mg range and titrated cautiously by 10 mg every 4 to 7 days. Maintenance therapy with methadone occurs only in highly regulated methadone clinic settings. Buprenorphine, a partial agonist at the mu receptor (and kappa antagonist) is administered sublingually and has a half-life similar to methadone's. It was approved in 2002 for office-based treatment of opioid addiction, making pharmacotherapy much more widely available. Caution should be used to not administer buprenorphine too soon (before onset of withdrawal syndrome), or acute withdrawal can actually be precipitated. Buprenorphine is available either alone or in combination with naloxone. Here, the role of naloxone is solely to deter intravenous abuse, because naloxone is inactive when taken as sublingually as prescribed.

Buprenorphine and methadone are useful in managing acute withdrawal, as well as long-term (months to years) maintenance

---

[5]Investigational drug in the United States.

[1]Not FDA approved for this indication.

TABLE 2 Useful Medications in Treating Opioid Use Disorders

Drug	Utility	Forms	Administration	Notes
Naloxone (Narcan)	Overdose; additive to prevent abuse[1]	SC, IM, IV	0.4-2 mg q2-3min prn	$T_{1/2}$ = 1 h, wears off quickly
Naltrexone (ReVia, Vivitrol[1])	Prevention of relapse	PO, IM	ReVia: 50-100 mg PO daily; Vivitrol: 380 mg IM q4wk	Potential for hepatotoxicity; precipitates withdrawal; useful for ETOH as well
Clonidine (Catapres, Catapres-TTS patch)	Withdrawal	PO, transdermal	0.1-0.2 mg PO tid prn 0.1-0.3 mg/24 h transdermal via weekly patch	Monitor for hypotension
Methadone (Dolophine)	Withdrawal; maintenance	PO	Start 20-30 mg PO qd Target 80-120+ mg PO qd	Restricted to methadone clinics
Buprenorphine (Subutex, Suboxone [with naloxone], Buprenex Injection[1])	Withdrawal; maintenance	SL, IM, IV	Start 2-4 mg SL qd-bid Target 4-32 mg SL daily divided qd-tid	Requires special DEA certification

[1]Not FDA approved for this indication.
Abbreviations: DEA = Drug Enforcement Administration; ETOH = ethanol.

therapy for preventing relapse to heroin or the opioid of choice. As maintenance therapy, these agents serve to block euphoria, satisfy cravings, and reduce illicit use, with consequent verifiable harm reduction. Buprenorphine, with a built-in ceiling effect owing to its unique pharmacology, is much safer than methadone, which is often fatal in overdose. Increasingly, buprenorphine is being used as an analgesic as well[1], and it may be an ideal choice in patients with comorbid pain and addiction who have demonstrated an inability to safely use other opioids.

Also approved for prevention of opioid relapse is naltrexone, an opioid antagonist, which is available in oral (ReVia) and intramuscular depot formulations (Vivitrol).[1]

Sedative-Hypnotics

This class of drugs includes a wide array of compounds (benzodiazepines, barbiturates, and various related compounds) (Table 3), most of which have at least some potential for abuse. Overall, these medications do much more good than harm, and are useful in treating anxiety disorders, insomnia, seizures, and muscle spasms. They are also important in managing withdrawal states and as a component of surgical anesthesia. These drugs act as CNS depressants, and their primary mechanism of action is to enhance inhibitory GABA neurotransmission. The risk of toxicity is by respiratory depression, which is magnified by concomitant use of opioids or other CNS depressants, such as alcohol.

Sedative-hypnotic intoxication and withdrawal states closely resemble those of alcohol, except for a more protracted time course of withdrawal. Anxiety, restlessness, insomnia, tremor, nystagmus, tachycardia, and hypertension usually appear 2 to 12 hours after the last dose, and symptoms gradually resolve over 1 to 2 weeks. Withdrawal seizures, psychosis, and delirium are fairly common. Detoxification is best accomplished on an inpatient basis and typically involves tapering doses of a long-acting benzodiazepine (e.g., clonazepam [Klonopin], diazepam, chlorazepate [Tranxene]) at a rate of about 10% of initial daily requirement per day. Acute sedative overdose is managed primarily with supportive care and airway management. Flumazenil (Romazicon) 0.2 to 0.5 mg/min IV may be used with caution for acute overdose of benzodiazepines, because it can precipitate severe acute withdrawal symptoms.

TABLE 3 Common Sedative-Hypnotics, Equivalent Dose Conversions

Generic Name	Trade Name	Dose (mg)
Benzodiazepines		
Diazepam	Valium	10
Alprazolam	Xanax, Niravam	0.5-1
Lorazepam	Ativan	2
Clonazepam	Klonopin	1-2
Chlordiazepoxide	Librium	25
Clorazepate	Tranxene	7.5
Oxazepam	Serax	10-15
Temazepam	Restoril	15
Triazolam	Halcion	0.25
Flurazepam	Dalmane	15
Barbiturates		
Phenobarbital	n/a	30
Pentobarbital	Nembutal	100
Secobarbital	Seconal	100
Butalbital (with caffeine and aspirin or acetaminophen)	Fiorinal, Fioricet	100
Amobarbital	Amytal	100
Related Compounds		
Carisoprodol	Soma	700
Meprobamate	Miltown, Equanil	1,200
Chloral hydrate	Noctec	500
Methaqualone[2]	Quaalude	300
Ethchlorvynol[2]	Placidyl	500
Zolpidem	Ambien	20
Zaleplon	Sonata	20
Eszopiclone	Lunesta	3

[2]Not available in the United States.

Since their introduction in the 1960s, benzodiazepines have largely replaced barbiturates owing to their enhanced safety profile. However, barbiturates still in common use include phenobarbital and butalbital. Phenobarbital, used mainly for treating seizures, is considered to have low potential for abuse. Butalbital, compounded with caffeine plus acetaminophen or aspirin (Fioricet, Fiorinal), has moderate abuse potential, typically in combination with other drugs. Carisoprodol (Soma), although not a barbiturate, is metabolized into meprobamate, a barbiturate-like drug. Commonly taken in combination with opioids and other sedatives, carisoprodol is highly abused.

---

[1]Not FDA approved for this indication.

Alprazolam (Xanax) stands out among its peers as the single most abused, most addictive, and yet currently most prescribed sedative-hypnotic. Its rapid onset (T_{max} 1-2 hours) and relatively short half life (6-14 hours) contribute to its abuse liability and propensity for withdrawal seizures. Diazepam, historically the most prescribed sedative, also has relatively rapid onset and significant abuse potential, but its long half life makes it an ideal agent for use in treating withdrawal from other sedatives. Flunitrazepam (Rohypnol, "roofies") is a benzodiazepine that causes anterograde amnesia and is now illegal in the United States owing to its use in drug-facilitated sexual assaults.

γ-Hydroxybutyric acid (GHB) and baclofen (Lioresal) also act as GABAergic CNS depressants, with intoxication and withdrawal states consistent with the class. Oddly, GHB is considered a Schedule I drug with high abuse potential and no accepted medical use, but GHB marketed as sodium oxybate (Xyrem) is available as a Schedule III drug (with special restrictions) when used to treat narcolepsy. Baclofen, on the other hand, appears to have rather low abuse potential and may actually play a role in the treatment of alcoholism.[1]

Relatively new drugs such as zolpidem (Ambien), zaleplon (Sonata), and eszopiclone (Lunesta) are benzodiazepine-like drugs with CNS depressant activity, approved for short-term treatment of insomnia, and have at least some potential for abuse and dependence. Clonazepam is generally considered to have the lowest potential for euphoria and abuse and is the agent of choice if a benzodiazepine must be given to patients with a relative contraindication, such as a history of any drug abuse or dependence.

Conclusion

Despite intensive supply-reduction strategies, improved primary prevention efforts, and the many recent pharmacotherapy advances, drug abuse remains largely unchanged in its overall scale. The one notable exception is the significant reduction in tobacco use seen since the turn of the century. It is estimated that 25% of patients seen in office settings and 50% of those seen in emergency department settings have active problems related to substance abuse. All patients in primary care settings must be screened for tobacco, alcohol, and illicit drug abuse. Patients should be asked directly about substance use at the initial point of contact (e.g., emergency departments, primary care offices.), and clinicians should maintain a healthy degree of skepticism toward patients' responses, remembering that most patients minimize substance use. Urine drug screening should be considered part of any comprehensive medical workup. A variety of affordable quick-screen kits are available, which can be sent out for laboratory confirmation of positive results.

Physicians and other health care professionals are in a unique position to intervene on drug abuse at the individual level, because it is encountered commonly in clinical practice. The problem must first be identified, and depending on the skill set of the primary provider, patients should be treated or referred to an appropriate treatment provider. There is an initiative to incorporate formal SBIRT (screening, brief intervention, and referral to treatment) into routine clinical practice (current procedural terminology [CPT] codes and reimbursement schedule for screening and brief intervention may be located online at http://sbirt.samhsa.gov/coding.htm). Screening may involve written or verbal assessment of substance use to determine whether the patient exhibits problematic levels of use. The brief intervention aspect of SBIRT targets those with nondependent substance use and provides effective strategies for intervention before the need for more extensive or specialized treatment. Referral to specialized treatment is recommended for patients with severe substance use or dependence. Data suggest this approach is successful in modifying problematic substance-use behavior. In addition to formal treatment, physician referral to local 12-step recovery meetings (Alcoholics Anonymous, Narcotics Anonymous) has proved beneficial. Local chapters provide physicians with names and telephone numbers of members willing to welcome newcomers (www.aa.org).

---

[1]Not FDA approved for this indication.

Physicians are usually well equipped to treat the sequelae of drug abuse, but they often forget that addiction is a treatable disease entity itself. Treatment ranges in intensity along a continuum from medically managed inpatient detoxification to partial hospitalization to intensive outpatient to outpatient care. The American Society of Addiction Medicine provides patient placement criteria that dictate the appropriate level of treatment based on a multidimensional assessment. Health care professionals should be familiar with the treatment centers in their area, which can place the patient in the appropriate level of care.

It is important to remember that relapse is a characteristic of addiction and does not equate to treatment failure, but rather indicates a need for adjustment in treatment level or monitoring. Other chronic diseases, such as diabetes or hypertension, necessitate ongoing monitoring and adjustment of treatment interventions as needed, and so is the case with addiction. Recently published data on the treatment and monitoring of recovering physicians (a subgroup of addicts that boasts a 5-year success rate greater than 78%) teaches us the lesson that adequate initial treatment coupled with ongoing monitoring is critical. Sustained recovery from substance dependence is attainable and is characterized by voluntary sobriety, improved personal health, and improved citizenship.

REFERENCES

American Psychiatric Association. Diagnostic and statistical manual of mental disorders. 4th ed. text revision. Washington, DC: American Psychiatric Association; 2000.

Centers for Disease Control and Prevention. Annual smoking-attributable mortality, years of potential life lost, and productivity losses—United States, 1997–2001. MMWR 2005;54(25):625–8.

DuPont RL, McLellan AT, White WL, et al. Setting the standard for recovery: Physicians health programs. J Subst Abuse Treat 2009;36(2):159–71.

Fowler JS, Volkow ND, Wang GJ, et al. Neuropharmacological actions of cigarette smoke: Brain monoamine oxidase B (MAO B) inhibition. J Addict Dis 1998;17(1):23–4.

Gold MS, Kobeissy FH, Wang KK, et al. Methamphetamine- and trauma-induced brain injuries: Comparative cellular and molecular neurobiological substrates. Biol Psychiatry 2009;66(2):118–27.

Haney M, Hart CL, Foltin RW. Effects of baclofen on cocaine self-administration: Opioid- and nonopioid-dependent volunteers. Neuropharmacology 2006;31:1814–21.

Johnston LD, O'Malley PM, Bachman JG, Schulenberg JE. Monitoring the Future: National results on adolescent drug use: Overview of key findings, 2008. Bethesda, MD: National Institute on Drug Abuse (NIH Publication No. 09-7401); 2009.

Office of National Drug Control Policy. The Economic Costs of Drug Abuse in the United States: 1992-2002. Washington, DC: Executive Office of the President (Publication No. 207303); 2004.

Small E, Shah HP, Davenport JJ, et al. Tobacco smoke exposure induces nicotine dependence in rats. Psychopharmacology (Berl) 2010;208(1):143–58.

Substance Abuse Health and Services Administration. Results from the 2008 National Survey on Drug Use and Health: National Findings. Rockville, MD: Office of Applied Studies (NSDUH Series H-36; DHHS Publication No. SMA09-4434); 2008.

Anxiety Disorders

Method of
Natalie C. Blevins, PhD, and
Andrew W. Goddard, MD

Epidemiology

Anxiety disorders are among the most prevalent psychiatric disorders in the world. In the United States, it is estimated that an anxiety disorder is diagnosed in approximately 16 million adults each year and approximately 30 million meet criteria for an anxiety disorder over the course of their lifetimes. Second to depression, anxiety disorders are the most common mental health problems seen by physicians in the general medical setting. In fact, patients with anxiety are more likely to present initially to a general practitioner's office than to a mental health care provider.

Anxiety disorders tend to be chronic and disabling, and they impose a high individual and social burden. It has been estimated that the United States spends approximately $40 billion to $60 billion per year for costs associated with anxiety disorders. These include not only direct costs associated with treatment but also indirect costs associated with lost productivity. Thus, the importance of early detection and treatment is critically important.

Risk Factors

Risk factors found to be associated with anxiety disorders include past personal or family history of anxiety; recent increase in stressful life events; lack or perceived lack of social support; ineffective emotional coping strategies; being female; experiencing childhood adversity, including trauma or witnessing a traumatic event; having a chronic health condition or serious illness; having an acute or chronic pain condition; and substance abuse. Although a genetic predisposition to developing an anxiety disorder is likely, environmental stressors clearly play a role. Research has also shown that patients suffering from anxiety are generally more sensitive to physiologic changes than nonanxious patients. This heightened sensitivity leads to diminished autonomic flexibility, which may be the result of faulty central information processing in anxiety-prone persons.

Pathophysiology

Anxiety symptoms and the resulting disorders are believed to be due to dysregulation of neuronal activity with the CNS fear circuit. Physical and emotional manifestations of this dysregulation are the result of a state of hyperarousal. Several neurotransmitter systems have been implicated in the genesis of this state.

The most commonly considered are the serotoninergic and noradrenergic neurotransmitter systems. Very simply, it is believed that an underactivation of the serotoninergic system and an overactivation of the noradrenergic system are involved. These systems regulate and are regulated by other pathways and neuronal circuits in various regions of the brain, including the locus caeruleus and limbic structures, resulting in dysregulation of physiologic arousal and the emotional experience of this arousal. Disruption of the γ-aminobutyric acid (GABA) system has also been implicated because of the response of many of the anxiety-spectrum disorders to treatment with benzodiazepines.

There has also been some interest in the role of corticosteroid regulation and its relation to symptoms of fear and anxiety. Corticosteroids might increase or decrease the activity of certain neural pathways, affecting not only behavior under stress but also the brain's processing of fear-inducing stimuli. The stress response is hardwired into the brain and is most often triggered when survival of the organism is threatened. The stress response, however, can be triggered not only by a physical challenge or threat but also by the mere anticipation (or fear) of threat. As a result, when humans chronically and erroneously believe that a threatening event is about to occur, they begin to experience the physical and psychological symptoms of anxiety and panic.

Finally, a subcortical neural structure, the amygdala, serves an important role in coordinating the cognitive, affective, neuroendocrine, cardiovascular, respiratory, and musculoskeletal components of fear and anxiety responses (fear expression). It is central to registering the emotional significance of stressful stimuli and creating emotional memories. The amygdala receives input from neurons in the sensory cortex. When activated, the amygdala stimulates regions of the midbrain and brain stem, causing autonomic hyperactivity, which can be correlated with the physical symptoms of anxiety.

Prevention

No biological markers are specific enough yet to detect anxiety early, and there is no available evidence to suggest that current medications prove efficacious in preventing these disorders. Therefore, it is important to screen for specific risk factors, such as family history and substance abuse. If an person is anxiety-prone, he or she should first be encouraged to adopt healthy lifestyle habits. Physical activity has been shown to relieve tension and anxiety. These patients should also be encouraged to avoid stimulants such as caffeine and nicotine, which can exacerbate symptoms. It is also recommended that anxiety-prone persons reduce subjective levels of stress by learning effective methods of relaxation and other stress-management skills.

Clinical Manifestations

Anxiety is characterized by subjective feelings of worry, dread, or anticipation and can include hypervigilance and avoidance of anxiety-producing situations. The physical symptoms can include jitteriness or shakiness, trembling, muscle aches and tension, sweating, cold or clammy hands, dizziness, or vertigo; fatigue; racing or pounding heart, hyperventilation; sensation of a lump in the throat, choking sensation, dry mouth; numbness and tingling in hands, feet, or other body part; upset stomach, nausea, vomiting, or diarrhea; decreased sexual desire; and sleep and appetite disturbances.

Psychological symptoms include unrealistic or excessive worry, apprehension, exaggerated startle response, hypervigilance, and distractibility. Patients often express feelings of impatience, irritability, and fear. Some patients exhibit phobias such as fear of being far from home or fear of social contact. Others express fear of falling asleep owing to recurrent nightmares. These symptoms cause significant distress and impairment of function.

Diagnosis

An anxiety disorder diagnosis is arrived at when a patient meets the specific diagnostic criteria outlined in the *Diagnostic and Statistical Manual of Mental Disorders,* Fourth Edition, Text Revision (DSM-IV-TR). The four most common anxiety disorders seen in primary care are generalized anxiety disorder, panic disorder, social anxiety disorder, and posttraumatic stress disorder.

GENERALIZED ANXIETY DISORDER

Persons with generalized anxiety disorder (GAD) experience uncontrollable, excessive anxiety and worry involving several areas of functioning on most days for at least 6 months. The anxiety must be

CURRENT DIAGNOSIS

- A thorough history is required to ensure the patient meets DSM-IV-TR criteria for an anxiety disorder. Symptoms that persist and are associated with significant distress and impairment of functioning are likely caused by an anxiety disorder that warrants treatment.
- Anxiety is characterized by subjective feelings of worry, dread, or anticipation and can include hypervigilance and avoidance of anxiety-producing situations. Physical symptoms often include jitteriness, restlessness, muscle aches and tension, sweating, dizziness, fatigue, racing heart, hyperventilation, dry mouth, nausea, decreased sexual desire, and sleep and appetite disturbances.
- Relevant medical examination and laboratory work may be indicated to rule out organic causes, substance abuse, or withdrawal.

associated with at least three of the following symptoms: restlessness, fatigue, impaired concentration, irritability, muscle tension, or sleep problems. Patients tend to express chronic excessive nervousness, exaggerated worry, tension, and irritability that appear to have no cause or are more intense than the situation warrants. Physical signs such as headaches, trembling, twitching, or sweating often develop, which lead to further worries. GAD symptoms tend to wax and wane over time, with short-term exacerbations of acute anxiety in response to stress. Symptoms show substantial overlap with those of other medical and psychological disorders, particularly major depressive disorder, substance abuse disorders, and other anxiety disorders, which tends to complicate diagnosis.

PANIC DISORDER

Panic disorder is marked by recurrent, unexpected panic attacks with persistent concern about future attacks or worries about their implications or consequences. A panic attack is a period of intense fear, developing abruptly and peaking within 10 minutes. Diagnosis requires at least four of the following: chest pain or discomfort; chills or hot flushes; derealization (feeling of unreality) or depersonalization (being detached from oneself); fear of losing control; feeling dizzy, unsteady, lightheaded, or faint; feeling of choking; nausea; palpitations; paresthesias; sensations of shortness of breath or smothering; sense of impending doom; sweating; or trembling or shaking.

Patients with panic disorder often seek medical treatment because they fear that their physical symptoms are caused by a heart attack. The anticipatory anxiety and intense fear of future attacks can lead to phobic avoidance. The combination of panic symptoms and the phobic avoidance can impair the patient's occupational, social, and family functioning. Sometimes, panic disorder leads to agoraphobia, which can be disabling. Patients with agoraphobia often refuse to leave their home for fear of being in a situation in which they might experience anxiety or panic and from which escape might be difficult or embarrassing.

SOCIAL ANXIETY DISORDER

Social phobia or social anxiety disorder is manifested by excessive, persistent fear of social and performance situations that is so severe that it disrupts daily life and relationships. Persons with social anxiety have a persistent, intense, and ongoing fear of being extremely embarrassed or being watched, judged by others, or humiliated by their own actions. Exposure to the feared social situation provokes anxiety, which can take the form of a panic attack. The person recognizes that the fear is excessive or unreasonable.

POSTTRAUMATIC STRESS DISORDER

Posttraumatic stress disorder (PTSD) develops after a person experiences, witnesses, or confronts a physically or psychologically distressing event. The event might involve actual or threatened death or serious injury or a threat to the physical integrity of self or others. The person's response to the threat involved intense fear, helplessness, or horror. PTSD is diagnosed in a person who displays symptoms associated with re-experiencing the traumatic event, including recurrent and intrusive distressing recollections, nightmares, or a sense of reliving the experience through flashbacks. The person must also display a consistent pattern of avoidance of themes associated with the traumatic event (thoughts, feelings, conversations, activities, places, or people), hyperarousal and autonomic hyperactivity that can manifest in difficulties with sleep or concentration, irritability, hypervigilance and an exaggerated startle response. The diagnosis is made if the symptoms have been present for at least 1 month and cause clinically significant distress or impairment in functioning.

Differential Diagnosis

It is important to perform a thorough medical workup when initially assessing the patient with anxiety symptoms. The differential diagnosis can include several organic causes, such as endocrine

---

> ### BOX 1   Medical Conditions Often Associated with Anxiety Symptoms
>
> **Cardiopulmonary**
> Angina
> Mitral valve prolapse
> Pulmonary embolism
> Chronic obstructive pulmonary disease (COPD)
> Asthma
>
> **Endocrine**
> Hyperthyroidism
> Pheochromocytoma
> Cushing's syndrome
> Menopause
>
> **Gastrointestinal**
> Gastroesophageal reflux
> Irritable bowel syndrome (IBS)
> Gastritis
>
> **Neurologic**
> Dementia
> Substance intoxication or withdrawal
> Seizure disorder
> Migraine

dysfunction, intoxication or withdrawal, hypoxia, metabolic abnormalities, and neurologic disorders. It is also important to rule out other comorbid psychiatric disorders. Severe depression, bipolar disorder, prodromal schizophrenia, delusional disorder, and adjustment disorder can often accompanied by severe anxiety. Many organic causes can be ruled out by a thorough history and basic laboratory work, including thyroid-stimulating hormone, urine toxicology, electrocardiogram, complete blood count, and metabolic panel. The most common medical conditions associated with anxiety are presented in Box 1.

The list of drugs suspected of causing anxiety is extensive. Drugs commonly associated with anxiety include stimulants such as amphetamine, cocaine, methamphetamine, and caffeine. Drugs such as lysergic acid diethylamide (LSD) and 3,4-methylenedioxymethamphetamine (MDMA, or "ecstasy") can also cause acute and chronic anxiety. Prescription medications to consider include sympathomimetics, antihypertensives, and nonsteroidal antiinflammatory drugs (NSAIDs).

Treatment and Monitoring

Treatment for a patient with an anxiety disorder begins with education. The practice guidelines for panic disorder recommend education of the family as well. Many people are confused by the symptoms and behavior and are reassured to know they are not alone and that there are effective interventions. The patient should receive an appropriate medical work-up, such as a physical examination, and studies (e.g., electrocardiogram, thyroid-stimulating hormone) when indicated. After ruling out a medical condition, developing a working alliance with the patient provides a basis for ongoing management and prevents further inappropriate use of the medical system.

A combination of psychotherapy and medication management is recommended in all of the anxiety disorders. Cognitive-behavioral therapy (CBT) has the strongest empiric support of all the psychotherapies, but it requires commitment to treatment on the part of the patient. Its efficacy is also contingent on the ability of the therapist and the length of therapy, with a 78% response rate in panic-disorder patients who have committed to 12 to 15 weeks of therapy. Studies show that when compared with patients undergoing

CURRENT THERAPY

- Educate the patient and family members about treatment options as well as realistic treatment expectations and reassure them of the absence of medical causes.
- First-line treatment is a selective serotonin reuptake inhibitor (SSRI), starting at low doses with careful titration so as not to exacerbate anxiety symptoms.
- Initiate cognitive-behavioral therapy (CBT) along with medication to significantly increase response rates.
- Consider short-term, high-potency benzodiazepine use in more severe cases. Use medications with longer half-lives to minimize withdrawal effects.
- Refer to a psychiatrist in difficult cases or for patients with a less-than-expected response to treatment.

monotherapy, patients treated with a combination of CBT and medication experience nearly twice the remission rate.

The selective serotonin reuptake inhibitors (SSRIs) have been shown to be the best-tolerated medications, and response rates are significantly higher than placebo for panic disorder, PTSD, social anxiety disorder, and GAD. This class of medication includes fluoxetine (Prozac), fluvoxamine (Luvox), citalopram (Celexa), escitalopram (Lexapro), paroxetine (Paxil), and sertraline (Zoloft). Some improvement should be noted within 3 or 4 weeks, and the dose should be increased if no improvement is seen. In all of the anxiety disorders, SSRIs should be started at low doses and gradually titrated up to therapeutic levels to avoid an initial exacerbation of anxiety. Pharmacotherapy options for the treatment of GAD are presented in Table 1.

Benzodiazepines, which have been used commonly in the past to treat anxiety disorders, continue to be useful in the short-term management of symptoms until acceptable reduction of symptoms is achieved with an SSRI or CBT. The tolerability and lack of addiction potential make the SSRIs more desirable for long-term management, but the delay in response makes short-term symptom relief with a benzodiazepine desirable for those with the greatest impairment. Because of the risk for rebound anxiety when withdrawing from benzodiazepines with short half-lives, such as alprazolam (Xanax), many prefer the longer-acting benzodiazepines, such as clonazepam (Klonopin).

If the patient does not respond to the combination of CBT and medication, a reevaluation of symptoms might reveal a comorbid disorder missed on the first examination. Comorbid psychiatric disorders significantly lower the likelihood of recovery from anxiety and increase recurrence rates. Many clinicians try switching between SSRIs before considering the next step in treatment. A referral to a psychiatrist for further evaluation and management may be necessary if none of these strategies works. Treatment-refractory anxiety can be extremely frustrating for both the patient and clinician. This can lead to increased dependence on benzodiazepines and an escalation of doses required for the same effect.

When approaching the start of therapy, the clinician should reassure the patient that effective treatment is available, but that patience may be necessary until the right combination of modalities is found. Although all of the anxiety disorders display a significant amount of chronicity, most patients have an improved outcome with appropriate treatment. Response rates improve when comorbidity is low. Patients with an earlier onset of symptoms (childhood or adolescence) can generally expect a more chronic course and may be more difficult to treat. In some of the disorders (e.g., PTSD, panic disorder), patients can have a spontaneous remission of symptoms or can continue to function despite the symptoms. However, time to resolution of symptoms is shortened and overall functioning can improve with treatment.

Pharmacotherapy often helps to prevent relapse, and rates are improved when effective treatment is continued for 12 months. When considering termination of pharmacologic treatment, the risk for relapse in all of the disorders should be discussed with the patient. When discontinuing the SSRIs, a slow taper is recommended, with close monitoring for withdrawal symptoms (e.g., headache, gastrointestinal upset, restlessness, and other flulike symptoms). Also monitor for rebound anxiety symptoms. If relapse occurs, reinstituting treatment is indicated, and many patients opt for indefinite treatment to maintain remission of symptoms. Lifelong management with pharmacotherapy or psychotherapy, or both, is not unusual for many patients. For many, a maximum reduction of symptoms, rather than a full remission, is an acceptable outcome.

Complications

Untreated anxiety disorders can lead to, or worsen, other mental and physical health conditions, including bruxism (teeth grinding), cognitive impairment, depression, gastrointestinal disorders, headache, insomnia, heart disease, substance abuse, and significantly impaired quality of life.

Conclusion

Anxiety disorders are highly prevalent. These conditions can be disabling and costly to the patient and to the health care system. Despite the prevalence of anxiety disorders, patients often remain undiagnosed and untreated, and patients with unrecognized anxiety disorders tend to be high users of general medical care. Patients with anxiety disorders can present with multiple somatic complaints and comorbid disorders, causing great effort and expense in identifying the cause of unexplained symptoms. Once anxiety disorders are identified, patients may be treated using well-tested and efficacious pharmacologic and psychotherapeutic treatments. Helpful resources for patients and families are listed in Table 2.

TABLE 1 Pharmacotherapy for the Treatment of Generalized Anxiety Disorder

Drug	Starting Dose	Target Dose
Selective Serotonin Reuptake Inhibitors		
Paroxetine (Paxil)*	10 mg qd	10-60 mg qd
Escitalopram (Lexapro)*	5-10 mg qd	10-20 mg qd
Sertraline (Zoloft)	12.5-25 mg qd	50-200 mg qd
Fluoxetine (Prozac)	10 mg qd	20-40 mg qd
Serotonin-Norepinephrine Reuptake Inhibitors		
Venlafaxine (Effexor XR)*	37.5 mg qAM	150-300[3] mg qAM
Duloxetine (Cymbalta)*	30 mg qd	60-90 mg qd
Other		
Buspirone (BuSpar)	5 mg bid-tid	10 mg tid

[3]Exceeds dosage recommended by the manufacturer.
*FDA indication for GAD.

TABLE 2 Helpful Resources for Patients with Anxiety Disorders

Organization	Website
Anxiety Disorders Association of America	www.adaa.org
Association for Behavioral and Cognitive Therapies	www.abct.org
National Institute of Mental Health	www.nimh.nih.gov/index.shtml

REFERENCES

American Psychiatric Association. Diagnostic and statistical manual of mental disorders. 4th ed. text revision. Washington, DC: American Psychiatric Association; 2000.

American Psychiatric Association. Practice guideline for the treatment of patients with panic disorder. 2nd ed. Washington, DC: American Psychiatric Association; 2009.

Campbell-Sills L, Stein MB. Guideline watch: Practice guidelines for the treatment of patients with panic disorder. Arlington, VA: American Psychiatric Association; 2006.

Gabbard GO. Treatment of psychiatric disorders. 3rd ed. vols. 1–2. Washington, DC: American Psychiatric Publishing; 2001.

Goddard AW, Coplan JD, Shekhar A, et al. Principles of the pharmacotherapy of anxiety disorders. In: Charney DS, Nestler EJ, editors. The Neurobiology of Mental Illness. 2nd ed. New York: Oxford University Press; 2004. p. 661–82.

Kessler RC, Berglund P, Demler O, et al. Lifetime prevalence and age-of-onset distributions of DSM-IV disorders in the National Comorbidity Survey Replication. Arch Gen Psychiatry 2005;62:593–602.

Kroenke K, Spitzer RL, Williams JBW, et al. Anxiety disorders in primary care: Prevalence, impairment, comorbidity, and detection. Ann Intern Med 2007;146:317–25.

Lépine JP. The epidemiology of anxiety disorders: Prevalence and societal costs. J Clin Psychiatry 2002;63(Suppl. 14):4–8.

Sadock BJ, Sadock VA. Kaplan and Sadock's synopsis of psychiatry: Behavioral sciences/clinical psychiatry. 10th ed. Philadelphia: Lippincott Williams & Wilkins; 2007.

Stein MB. Attending to anxiety disorders in primary care. J Clin Psychiatry 2003;64(Suppl. 15):35–9.

Bulimia Nervosa

Method of
James Lock, MD

Bulimia nervosa is characterized by binge eating episodes, followed by inappropriate compensatory behaviors, such as self-induced vomiting, laxative or diuretic misuse, fasting, and excessive exercise. A sense of loss of control about overeating accompanies these episodes of binge eating. These behaviors are associated with overvaluation of shape and weight. The episodes must occur at a frequency of two times per week for 3 months to meet diagnostic thresholds.

Bulimic behaviors usually have their onset during middle adolescence (14–16 years old). Full-syndrome bulimia nervosa is most common during late adolescence and young adulthood (17–24 years old). Onset of bulimia nervosa is rare in younger children, although not unknown. The point prevalence of bulimia nervosa is 1% to 2% among females. Male patients account for about 10% of bulimia nervosa cases.

It is common for other psychiatric disorders to coexist with bulimia nervosa, particularly depression, anxiety disorders, and substance use. Common physical health problems associated with bulimia nervosa include electrolyte disturbances, loss of dental enamel, and esophageal tears. The use of ipecac to induce vomiting can lead to serious cardiac and skeletal myopathies. Frequent laxative use can cause metabolic acidosis and elevated serum amylase levels, and it can lead to dependence on laxatives for bowel emptying. Amenorrhea, infertility, osteoporosis, and dehydration are other possible outcomes.

Common characteristics associated with bulimia nervosa include impulsivity, interpersonal problems, substance use, and personality disorders. These related problems usually occur about the same time or after the onset of bulimia nervosa and many remit after treatment. In patients who abuse substances, most begin substance use as a means to control appetite and weight.

Etiology

Bulimia nervosa is best understood as a multiply determined phenomenon that includes biologic, psychological, familial, and sociocultural factors. Evidence for a biologic basis can be found in genetic,

neurotransmitter, and neuroimaging studies. Bulimia nervosa clusters in families, supporting a genetic basis for the disorder. Twin studies document that one half of the variance in heritability is accounted for by genetic factors. There is also evidence of reduced serotonin levels in individuals with bulimia nervosa. Imaging studies have found disturbances in the orbital-frontal serotonergic circuits in these patients. These areas of the brain are associated with behavioral dyscontrol.

Psychological factors likely contribute to the cause of bulimia nervosa. Low self-esteem and increased sensitivity to peer rejection are highly associated with the disorder, as are personality characteristics of impulsivity, perfectionism, and interpersonal relationship instability. Family dynamics are also implicated. Parental obesity and familial criticism about weight, shape, and eating, as well as familial emphasis on appearance and achievement, appear to increase risk for the disorder. Families of patients are often characterized as unorganized, conflict ridden, and lacking in warmth.

Sociocultural factors appear to contribute to the increased risk for bulimia nervosa. Intensified pressures for women to be thin, as portrayed in magazine and television advertisements, contribute to increased rates of the disorder. These pressures may be increasing for men as the print and video media present male models with increased muscularity and less body fat.

Diagnosis

Clinicians must review the history and current status of the patient's eating disorder pathology, such as restriction, binge eating, purging, and other compensatory behaviors; height and weight trends; weight and shape concerns; history of weight control measures; and motivation for seeking current treatment. Examination of possible triggers for dieting and weight concerns should be explored, including past experiences with teasing about weight; family culture around food, weight, and eating; interpersonal relationship stressors; and occupational risks (e.g., food service worker, model, athlete). It is important to review any contributing medical symptoms, such as fatigue, headaches, bloating, constipation, and irregular menstrual status. Common comorbid mental health problems, particularly depression, anxiety, substance abuse, and personality disorders, must also be assessed.

Several self-report standardized interviews may be useful in making the diagnosis. Two of the most widely used measures are the Eating Attitudes Test and the Eating Disorders Inventory-2. A third commonly used self-report measure is the Bulimia Test–Revised. These self-report measures are best used to augment the clinical interview to refine information specific to eating-related symptoms and psychopathology.

Treatment

THERAPY FOR ADOLESCENT BULIMIA NERVOSA

Because bulimia nervosa has the potential for serious physical, emotional, and social consequences, treatment entails attention to this range of possible difficulties. Research has focused almost exclusively

CURRENT DIAGNOSIS

- Binge eating episodes (i.e., eating more than an average person would in the same setting) accompanied by a sense of being unable to cease eating occur at least twice each week for 3 months.
- Purging episodes (i.e., vomiting, laxative use, diuretics, enemas, overexercise) occur at least twice each week for 3 months.
- Overvaluation of shape and weight is a source of self-worth and self-esteem.
- Weight is in the normal range (i.e., patient is not experiencing an episode of anorexia nervosa).

on adults with the disorder. More than 70 controlled treatment trials have enrolled adults with bulimia nervosa, whereas only two randomized trials have enrolled adolescents. Treatment studies have focused on psychotherapy, mostly cognitive-behavioral therapy (CBT), and medications. Both approaches appear to be efficacious.

The main premise of CBT is that dysfunctional attitudes toward body shape and weight are the maintaining factors for the bulimia nervosa. As a result of these distorted ideas, there is an overvaluing of appearance, particularly thinness. This overvaluation leads to dissatisfaction with current body weight and shape, which is followed by attempts to control shape and weight by excessive dieting. Excessive dieting triggers a sense of psychological deprivation and real physiologic deprivation. Excessive dieting also increases feelings of hunger. Feelings of hunger increase the need to eat, which increases the probability of binge eating. After a binge has been completed, fears of weight gain are followed by purging (e.g., vomiting, laxatives, diuretic, enemas, extreme exercise) as an attempt to allay these anxieties. The combination of psychological and physical stresses often increases moodiness and depression.

CBT has been subjected to a large number of randomized, controlled trials and is considered the most effective psychotherapeutic approach for bulimia nervosa. Studies have found that CBT is more effective than no therapy, nondirective therapy, pill placebo, manualized psychodynamic therapy (i.e., supportive-expressive), stress management, and antidepressant treatment. Treatment response to CBT is generally good, with 50% of patients recovered and an additional 20% much improved by the end of treatment. Longer-term follow-up studies suggest that these improvements are sustained over time. At 5 years after treatment, about 60% of patients no longer had bulimia nervosa. In a meta-analysis of nine double-blind, placebo-controlled medication trials (870 subjects) and 26 randomized psychosocial studies (460 subjects), CBT was found to produce significantly greater improvements in binge eating, purging frequency, depression, and eating attitudes than comparison treatments.

The use of CBT for adolescents with bulimia nervosa treated with CBT has limited systematic support. Only two studies are available, but both provide preliminary evidence that CBT is acceptable and feasible as a treatment for these patients. Case series data on 40 adolescents treated with CBT found that 56% were recovered (i.e., absence of binge eating or purging) at the end of treatment. One randomized, controlled trial compared a self-help version of CBT (CBT-GSC) with family therapy. This study concluded that CBT-GSC was as effective (with rates of recovery of 36%) as family therapy for adolescent bulimia nervosa and was a more cost-effective treatment.

Interpersonal psychotherapy (IPT) modified for bulimia nervosa has been shown to be an effective therapy for the disorder. IPT focuses on the interpersonal context within which the eating disorder developed and is maintained with the aim of helping the patient make specific changes in identified interpersonal problem areas. Little attention is paid to eating habits or attitudes toward weight and shape, nor does the treatment contain any of the specific behavioral or cognitive procedures that characterize CBT. Because interpersonal success is closely linked to societal mandates about physical attractiveness, body shape and weight become critical determinants of self-esteem for adolescents, especially for girls. The relevance of IPT is supported by the findings of laboratory research showing that individuals with eating disorder symptoms seem particularly vulnerable to interpersonal stressors.

CBT was compared with IPT in a large, multisite trial enrolling 220 patients with bulimia nervosa. In this trial, CBT was superior to IPT at the end of treatment, but on follow-up, no differences were found between the two treatments. These studies suggested that bulimia nervosa was responsive to IPT and CBT, but that the improvements associated with IPT were slower to develop. IPT for adolescents with the disorder remains unexamined.

An approach specifically designed for adolescents is family-based treatment for bulimia nervosa (FBT-BN). The use of families to directly change dysfunctional eating behaviors in adolescents was used first with adolescents with anorexia nervosa. FBT-BN used parents to help their adolescent children stop binge eating and purging by directly monitoring these behaviors to prevent and disrupt them.

CURRENT THERAPY

- Cognitive-behavioral therapy (CBT) is the best-evidenced approach for bulimia nervosa.
- Interpersonal psychotherapy may be an alternative treatment if CBT is not effective or acceptable.
- Family-based treatment for bulimia nervosa is useful for adolescents.
- Antidepressants are useful but are not as effective as CBT and are a second-line treatment. However these medications may be used to augment psychological treatments or as an alternative when psychological treatments are not effective, are refused, or are not available.
- Serotonin reuptake inhibitors (SSRIs) are the recommended antidepressants. Relatively high doses are used, similar to the dosages used in the treatment of obsessive-compulsive disorder.

This form of family therapy does not focus on the cause of bulimia nervosa, but it assumes that most of the challenges of adolescence (e.g., peer relationships, increased autonomy, increased risk taking) are adversely affected by the disorder. Limited data are available to support the use of this approach with adolescents with bulimia nervosa in the form of pilot studies and two randomized clinical trials of moderate size. One study found that FBT-BN was superior to individual therapy for patients achieving abstinence at the end of treatment (40% versus 18%) and at follow-up (30% versus 10%).

PHARMACOTHERAPY

The use of antidepressant medications has also been examined. Studies include double-blind, placebo-controlled trials of antidepressants for adults. Most types of antidepressants are superior to placebo in reducing binge frequency. Mood disturbance, which is commonly associated with bulimia nervosa, improved with medication. However, controlled studies that examined the relative contributions to symptomatic change in combined treatment with CBT and antidepressants suggest that the additional benefit of medications over CBT alone is quite small. Unfortunately, only one small case series examined the use of antidepressants in adolescents. This pilot study found that fluoxetine (Prozac) was well tolerated, appeared to decrease binge eating and purging, and was acceptable to the patients and their parents.

REFERENCES

Agras WS, Walsh BT, Fairburn CG, et al. A multicenter comparison of cognitive-behavioral therapy and interpersonal psychotherapy for bulimia nervosa. Arch Gen Psychiatry 2000;57:459–66.

Bulik CM. Genetic and biological risk factors. In: Thompson J, editor. Handbook of Eating Disorders and Obesity. Hoboken, NJ: John Wiley & Sons; 2004. pp. 3–16.

Fairburn CG, Brownell K. Eating Disorders and Obesity: A Comprehensive Handbook. New York: Guilford Press; 2002.

Fairburn CG, Marcus MD, Wilson GT. Cognitive-behavioral therapy for binge eating and bulimia nervosa: A comprehensive treatment manual. In: Fairburn CG, Wilson GT, editors. Binge Eating: Nature, Assessment, & Treatment. New York: Guildford Press; 1993. pp. 361–404.

Hoek H, Hoeken DV. Review of prevalence and incidence of eating disorders. Int J Eat Disord 2003;34:383–96.

Le Grange D, Crosby R, Rathouz P, Leventhal B. A randomized controlled comparison of family-based treatment and supportive psychotherapy for adolescent bulimia nervosa. Arch Gen Psychiatry 2007;64:1049–56.

Le Grange D, Lock J. Treating Bulimia in Adolescence. New York: Guilford Press; 2007.

Lilenfeld L, Kaye WH, Greeno C, et al. A controlled family study of anorexia nervosa and bulimia nervosa: Psychiatric disorders in first-degree relatives and effects of proband comorbidity. Arch Gen Psychiatry 1998;55:603–10.

Lock J. Adjusting cognitive behavioral therapy for adolescent bulimia nervosa: Results of a case series. Am J Psychother 2005;59:267–81.

Stein D, Kaye WH, Matsunaga H, et al. Eating-related concerns, moods, personality traits in recovered bulimia nervosa subjects: A replication study. Int J Eat Disord 2002;32:225–9.

Delirium

Method of
Arna Banerjee, MD, and
Pratik Pandharipande, MD, MSCI

Delirium is defined by the *Diagnostic and Statistical Manual of Mental Disorders*, Fourth Edition (DSM-IV) as a disturbance of consciousness with inattention, accompanied by a change in cognition or perceptual disturbances that develop over a short period (hours to days) and that fluctuate over time (Box 1). Although dysfunction of other organ systems continues to receive more clinical attention, delirium is recognized to be a significant contributor to morbidity, including longer hospitalizations, higher costs, and prolonged cognitive impairment. More alarmingly, delirium is an independent predictor of higher mortality for hospitalized and critically ill patients. Data show that patients who manifest some but not all the diagnostic features of delirium (i.e., subsyndromal delirium) have higher morbidity and mortality rates than those who are normal, although they fare better than those meeting the full criteria for delirium.

Prevalence and Subtypes

The prevalence of delirium at hospital admission ranges from 14% to 24%, with incident rates up to 60% among general hospital populations, especially in older patients and those in nursing homes or post-acute care settings. Although the overall prevalence of delirium in the community is only 1% to 2%, the prevalence increases with age, rising to 14% among those older than 85 years. The prevalence of delirium in medical and surgical intensive care unit (ICU) cohort studies is 20% to 80%, depending on the severity of illness and the need for mechanical ventilation. Despite high prevalence rates in the ICU, delirium often goes unrecognized by clinicians, or its symptoms are incorrectly attributed to dementia or depression, or they are considered an expected, inconsequential complication of critical illness.

Delirium can be categorized according to psychomotor behavior (Table 1). In non-ICU settings, the prevalences are 30% for the hyperactive subtype, 24% for the hypoactive subtype, and 46% for the mixed subtype. In the ICU, the rates are 1.6% for the hyperactive subtype, 43.5% for the hypoactive subtype, and 54.1% for the mixed subtype.

Pathogenesis and Risk Factors

The pathophysiology of delirium is poorly understood, although there are several hypotheses. Imbalance or derangement of multiple neurotransmitter systems has been implicated in the pathophysiology

---

BOX 1   DSM-IV Criteria for Delirium

- Disturbance of consciousness (i.e., reduced clarity of awareness of the environment) with reduced ability to focus, sustain, or shift attention)
- A change in cognition (e.g., memory deficit, disorientation, language disturbance) or development of a perceptual disturbance that is not better accounted for by a preexisting, established, or evolving dementia
- The disturbance develops over a short period (usually hours to days) and tends to fluctuate during the course of the day.

Abbreviation: DSM-IV = *Diagnostic and Statistical Manual of Mental Disorders*, Fourth Edition.

TABLE 1 Subtypes of Delirium

Subtype	Characteristics
Hyperactive	Agitation
	Restlessness
	Attempts to remove catheters and tubes
	Hitting
	Biting
	Emotional lability
Hypoactive	Withdrawal
	Flat affect
	Apathy
	Lethargy
	Decreased responsiveness
Mixed	Concurrent or sequential appearance of hyperactive and hypoactive delirium

of delirium, with the greatest focus on dopamine, γ-aminobutyric acid (GABA), and acetylcholine. Dopamine is thought to increase the excitability of neurons, and acetylcholine and GABA decrease neuronal excitability. An excess of dopamine or depletion of acetylcholine has been associated with delirium. Other postulated mechanisms of delirium include serotonin imbalance, endorphin hyperfunction, and increased central noradrenergic activity.

Another hypothesis enlists inflammatory mediators. The inflammatory mediators produced during critical illness (e.g., tumor necrosis factor-α, interleukin-1, other cytokines and chemokines) potentially initiate a cascade of endothelial damage, thrombin formation, and microvascular compromise that may play a role in delirium.

Impaired oxidative metabolism may play a role in the pathophysiology of delirium. Early hypotheses attempted to explain delirium as a behavioral manifestation of a "widespread reduction of cerebral oxidative metabolism resulting in an imbalance of neurotransmission." Investigators hypothesized that delirium was the result of "cerebral insufficiency" (i.e., global failure of cerebral oxidative metabolism), a factor that is known to be important in the pathogenesis of multiple organ dysfunction in critical illness.

Other investigators looked at cholinergic deficiency. Impaired oxidative metabolism in the brain results in a cholinergic deficiency. The finding that hypoxia impairs acetylcholine synthesis supports this hypothesis. The reduction in cholinergic function results in an increase in the levels of glutamate, dopamine, and norepinephrine in the brain. Serotonin and GABA are reduced, contributing to delirium.

Neurotransmitter levels and function can be affected by changes in the plasma concentrations of various amino acid precursors. Amino acid entry into the brain is regulated by a sodium-independent large neutral amino acid transporter type 1 (LAT1). Increased cerebral uptake of tryptophan and phenylalanine, compared with that of other large neutral amino acids, can lead to elevated levels of dopamine and norepinephrine, two neurotransmitters that have been implicated in the pathogenesis of delirium.

The causes of delirium are multifactorial. The risk factors can be divided into predisposing factors (i.e., host factors) and precipitating factors (Table 2).

Diagnosis

Delirium affects more than one third of hospitalized patients, but it remains underdiagnosed and is often inappropriately evaluated and managed. The diagnosis of delirium is primarily clinical and is based on careful bedside observation of key features (Table 3).

Diagnosis of delirium is a two-step process. Level of arousal is first measured, and if the patient is arousable, delirium evaluation can be performed by instruments such as the Confusion Assessment

CURRENT DIAGNOSIS

- Delirium is a disturbance of consciousness with inattention, accompanied by a change in cognition or perceptual disturbances that develop over a short period and fluctuate over days.
- Three delirium subtypes depend on the psychomotor behavior: hyperactive, hypoactive, and mixed.
- The pathophysiology of delirium is poorly understood, although inflammation, cholinergic imbalances, and neurotransmitter disturbances are leading hypotheses.
- Delirium affects more than one third of hospitalized patients, but it remains underdiagnosed and often is inappropriately evaluated and managed.
- Diagnosis of delirium is a two-step process. Level of arousal is measured, and if the patient is arousable, delirium evaluation is performed using instruments such as the Confusion Assessment Method or the Delirium Rating Scale–Revised 98 (DRS-R 98).

Method (Table 4) or the Delirium Rating Scale–Revised 98 (DRS-R 98). The DRS-R 98 provides a measure of severity of delirium in addition to being used to diagnose delirium. It is a 16-item, clinician-rated scale with 13 severity items and 3 diagnostic items. In the ICU, delirium can be diagnosed by using a sedation scale to assess arousal, followed by the Confusion Assessment Method for the ICU (CAM-ICU) or the Intensive Care Delirium Screening Checklist (ICDSC); both instruments are reliable and have been validated in critically ill patients.

Prevention

Nonpharmacologic and pharmacologic approaches have been studied to prevent delirium in hospitalized patients (Table 5). A study in 1999 demonstrated that a unit-based proactive multicomponent intervention, the Hospital Elder Life Program (HELP), reduced the incidence of delirium by 40% among hospitalized patients 70 years old or older. The protocol focused on optimization of risk factors with the following methods: repeated reorientation of the patient by trained volunteers and nurses, provision of cognitively stimulating activities for the patient three times per day, a nonpharmacologic sleep protocol to enhance normalization of sleep-wake cycles, early mobilization activities and range-of-motion exercises, timely removal of catheters and physical restraints, early correction of dehydration, earwax disimpaction, and institution of the use of eyeglasses, magnifying lenses, and hearing aids. Other studies have had similar or limited benefits in reducing the incidence of delirium or the severity and duration (see Table 5).

Treatment

A multidisciplinary, multifactorial approach to treatment is the most successful, because many factors contribute to delirium. Several interventions, even if individually small, may yield marked clinical

TABLE 2 Risk Factors for Delirium

Host Factors	Factors of Critical Illness	Iatrogenic Factors
Age 65 years or older	Acidosis	Immobilization
Male sex	Anemia	Medications (e.g., opioids, benzodiazepines)
Alcoholism	Fever, infection, sepsis	
ApoE4 polymorphism	Hypotension	Anticholinergic drugs
Cognitive impairment	Metabolic disturbances (e.g., sodium, calcium, blood urea nitrogen, bilirubin)	Alcohol or drug withdrawal
Dementia	Respiratory disease	Sleep disturbances
History of delirium	Great severity of illness	
Depression		
Hypertension		
Smoking		
Vision or hearing impairment		

TABLE 3 Clinical Features of Delirium

Feature	Description
Acute onset	Occurs abruptly, usually over a period of hours to days
Fluctuating course	Symptoms seem to come and go or increase and decrease in severity over a 24-hour period
	Characteristic lucid intervals
Inattention	Difficulty focusing, sustaining, and shifting attention
	Difficulty maintaining conversation or following commands
Disorganized thinking	Disorganized or incoherent speech
	Rambling, irrelevant conversation
	Unclear or illogical flow of ideas
Altered level of consciousness	Reduced clarity of awareness of the environment
Cognitive deficits	Disorientation, memory deficits, and language impairment
Perceptual disturbances	Illusions and hallucinations in 30% of patients
Psychomotor disturbances	Hypoactive, hyperactive, and mixed
Altered sleep-wake cycle	Daytime drowsiness, nighttime insomnia, fragmented sleep
Emotional disturbances	Symptoms of fear, paranoia, anxiety, depression, irritability, apathy, anger, or euphoria

TABLE 4 Confusion Assessment Method Diagnostic Algorithm

Feature*	Description	Diagnostic Relevance
1	Acute onset or fluctuating course	This feature is usually obtained from a family member or nurse and is shown by positive responses to the following questions: Is there evidence of an acute change in mental status from the patient's baseline? Did the (abnormal) behavior fluctuate during the day; that is, did it tend to come and go or increase and decrease in severity?
2	Inattention	This feature is demonstrated by a positive response to the following question: Did the patient have difficulty focusing attention, such as being easily distractible or having difficulty keeping track of what was being said?
3	Disorganized thinking	This feature is shown by a positive response to the following question: Was the patient's thinking disorganized or incoherent, such as rambling or irrelevant conversation, unclear or illogical flow of ideas or unpredictable switching from subject to subject?
4	Altered level of consciousness	This feature is demonstrated by any answer other than "alert" to the following question: Overall, how would you rate this patient's level of consciousness? Possible answers: alert (normal), vigilant (hyperalert), lethargic (drowsy, easily aroused), stupor (difficult to arouse), or coma (unarousable)

*Diagnosis of delirium by the Confusion Assessment Method requires the presence of features 1 and 2 plus feature 3 or 4.

TABLE 5 Models of Care for Delirium: Summary of Evidence

Model	Approach	Outcome	Comments
Hospital Elder Life Program (HELP)	Proactive	40% Reduction in incident delirium	No benefit in shortening the duration or severity of delirium
Geriatric consultation for hip fracture patients	Proactive	36% Reduction in incident delirium	No benefit in shortening the duration or severity of delirium
Reorganization of care: nurse-led programs, patient-centered care	Proactive	No reduction in incidence Reduced severity and duration of delirium	Overall hospital length of stay shortened; some mortality benefit
Low-dose prophylactic haloperidol (Haldol)[1] in high-risk hip surgery patients	Proactive	No reduction in delirium incidence Reduced severity and duration of delirium	Haloperidol (1.5 mg/d) well tolerated, with minimal side effects
Specialized delirium management team	Treatment	No significant benefit in any outcomes measured	Intervention may have been of insufficient duration or intensity; no difference observed

[1]Not FDA approved for this indication.

TABLE 6 Pharmacologic Treatment of Delirium in Hospitalized patients

Class and Drug	Dose
Antipsychotics	
Haloperidol (Haldol)[1]	0.5–1.0 mg PO twice daily, with additional doses every 4 hours as needed up to a maximum to 20 mg 0.5–1.0 mg IM; observe after 30–60 min and repeat if needed.
Atypical Antipsychotics	
Risperidone (Risperdal)[1]	0.25–1 mg PO daily or twice daily
Olanzapine (Zyprexa)[1]	2.5–10 mg PO daily or twice daily
Quetiapine (Seroquel)[1]	25–50 mg PO daily or twice daily
Ziprasidone (Geodon)[1]	20–40 mg PO once daily to twice daily
Benzodiazepines	
Lorazepam (Ativan)[1]	0.5–1 mg PO, with additional doses every 4 hours as needed. Reserve for use in alcohol withdrawal, Parkinson's disease, and neuroleptic malignant syndrome.
Antidepressants	
Trazodone (Desyrel)[1]	25–150 mg PO at bedtime

[1]Not FDA approved for this indication.

improvement. Medications should be used only after giving adequate attention to correction of modifiable contributing factors (e.g., sleep disturbance, deliriogenic medications, restraints).

Delirium may be a manifestation of an acute, life-threatening problem that requires immediate attention (e.g., hypoxia, hypercarbia, hypoglycemia, metabolic derangements, shock). After addressing these concerns, delirious patients should be considered for nonpharmacologic interventions and their acute symptoms managed by pharmacologic protocols if necessary (Table 6 and Fig. 1). Although the agents used to treat delirium are intended to improve cognition, they have psychoactive effects that may further cloud the sensorium and promote a longer overall duration of cognitive impairment. All typical and atypical antipsychotics can cause extrapyramidal symptoms and prolonged QT on electrocardiogram.

Conclusions

Delirium is a common brain dysfunction in hospitalized and critically ill patients contributing to increased morbidity and mortality. The pathophysiology of delirium remains unclear and is the focus of ongoing research. Protocols and evidence-based strategies for prevention and treatment of delirium will emerge from ongoing randomized clinical trials of nonpharmacologic and pharmacologic strategies.

```
┌─────────────────────────────────┐
│ Diagnosis of delirium using     │
│ instruments such as             │
│ CAM or DRS-R 98                 │
└─────────────────────────────────┘
              │
              ▼
┌─────────────────────────────────┐
│ Evaluate for potential          │
│ causes of delirium              │
└─────────────────────────────────┘
              │
              ▼
┌─────────────────────────────────┐
│ Discontinuation of triggers     │
│ of delirium                     │
└─────────────────────────────────┘
```

Nonpharmacological management
- Treatment of precipitating factors—hypoxia, hypercarbia, hypoglycemia, metabolic derangements, shock
- Provision of a supportive environment—correct sleep disturbances, vision and hearing modification
- Reevaluate requirement of bladder catheter and restraints
- Maintenance of nutrition
- Prevention of dehydration

Pharmacological management
- 0.5–1.0 mg twice daily orally, with additional doses every 4 hours
- Risperidone 0.25–1.0 mg twice daily
- Olanzapine 2.5 to 10.0 mg once daily or twice daily
- Quetiapine 25–50 mg once daily or twice daily
- Ziprasidone 20–40 mg once daily to twice daily
- Benzodiazepines should be reserved for patients with alcohol withdrawal
- Monitor for side effects

Drugs: evaluate the use of sedatives (e.g., benzodiazepines or opiates) and medications with anticholinergic activity, abrupt cessation of smoking or alcohol, withdrawal from chronically used sedatives

Elderly: age >65, preexisting dementia, or mild cognitive impairment or depression

Laboratory abnormalities: hyponatremia, azotemia, hyperbilirubinemia, hypocalcemia, and metabolic acidosis

Infection: Sepsis, especially urinary, respiratory tract infections, reevaluate the use of bladder catheters

Respiratory: consider respiratory failure (P_{CO_2} greater than 45 mm Hg or P_{O_2} less than 55 mm Hg or oxygen saturation less than 88%), chronic obstructive pulmonary disease, ARDS, pulmonary embolism

Intracranial perfusion: consider presence of hypertension or hypotension, hemorrhage, stroke, tumor

Urinary/fecal retention: consider urinary retention or fecal impaction, especially in elderly and in postoperative patients

Myocardial: myocardial infarction, acute heart failure, arrhythmia

Sleep and sensory deprivation: consider the alterations of the sleep cycle and sleep deprivation, consider the nonavailability of glasses (poor vision), consider the nonavailability of hearing devices (poor hearing), reevaluate the use of restraints

*Adapted from www.icudelirium.org with permission.

FIGURE 1. Treatment algorithm for hospitalized patients with delirium. *Abbreviations:* ARDS = acute respiratory distress syndrome; CAM = Confusion Assessment Method; DRS-R 98 = Delirium Rating Scale–Revised 98,

CURRENT THERAPY

- A multidisciplinary, multifactorial approach is the most successful, because many factors contribute to delirium.
- Medications should be used only after giving adequate attention to correction of modifiable contributing factors.
- The nonpharmacologic components of treatment include
    - Treatment of precipitating factors such as hypoxia, hypercarbia, hypoglycemia, metabolic derangements, and shock
    - Provision of a supportive environment (correction of sleep disturbance, restraints, maintaining familiar surroundings)
    - Maintenance of nutrition
    - Prevention of dehydration
    - Discontinuation of pharmacologic agents known to cause delirium
- Pharmacologic treatments include the following:
    - Haloperidol (Haldol)[1] is considered to be the first-line drug and should be started at a low dose.
    - Atypical antipsychotics have been used when the risk for adverse events such as QTc prolongation or extrapyramidal side effects are estimated to be high. These drugs include olanzapine (Zyprexa),[1] risperidone (Risperdal),[1] quetiapine (Seroquel),[1] and ziprasidone (Geodon).[1]
    - Benzodiazepines should be used only in cases of delirium associated with alcohol withdrawal.

[1]Not FDA approved for this indication.

REFERENCES

American Psychiatric Association. Diagnostic and statistical manual of mental disorders. 4th ed. text revision (DSM-IV-TR). Washington, DC: American Psychiatric Association; 2000.

Ely EW, Shintani A, Truman B, et al. Delirium as a predictor of mortality in mechanically ventilated patients in the intensive care unit. JAMA 2004;291(14):1753–62.

Engel GL, Romano J. Delirium, a syndrome of cerebral insufficiency. J Chronic Dis 1959;9(3):260–77.

Girard T, Pandharipande P, Ely EW. Delirium in the intensive care unit. Crit Care 2008;12(Suppl. 3):S3.

Inouye SK. Delirium in older persons. N Engl J Med 2006;354(11):1157–65.

Maldonado JR. Delirium in the acute care setting: Characteristics, diagnosis and treatment. Crit Care Clin 2008;24(4):657–722.

Marcantonio ER. Clinical management and prevention of delirium. Psychiatry 2005;4(1):68–72.

Meagher DJ, Hanlon DO, Mahony EO, et al. Relationship between symptoms and motoric subtype of delirium. J Neuropsychiatry Clin Neurosci 2000;12:51–6.

Morandi A, Gunther ML, Ely EW, Pandharipande P. The pharmacological management of delirium in critical illness. Current Drug Ther 2008;3: 148–57.

Nayeem K, O'Keeffe ST. Delirium. Clin Med 2003;3(5):412–5.

Peterson JF, Pun BT, Dittus RS, et al. Delirium and its motoric subtypes: A study of 614 critically ill patients. J Am Geriatr Soc 2006;54(3):479–84.

Tropea J, Slee J-A, Brand CA, et al. Clinical practice guidelines for the management of delirium in older people in Australia. Australas J Ageing 2008;27:150–6.

Truman B, Ely EW. Monitoring delirium in critically ill patients: Using the Confusion Assessment Method for the ICU. Crit Care Nurse 2003;23:25–36.

Trzepacz PT. General instructions for use of the DRS-R-981998.

Trzepacz PT. Update on the neuropathogenesis of delirium. Dement Geriatr Cogn Disord 1999;10:330–4.

Mood Disorders

Method of
Paul R. Kelley, MD, and Jill D. McCarley, MD

Disorders of mood are ubiquitous, spreading misery, impairment, and death through every culture on Earth. Approximately 21 million American adults suffer from a mood disorder in a given year, according to the National Institute of Mental Health. Major depression has a median age of onset of 32 years, affecting 6.7% of adults, and bipolar disorder's median age of onset is approximately 25 years and affects 2.6% of adults in the United States. Due to the prevalence of mood disorders, only a minority of sufferers receive ongoing psychiatric treatment. They instead seek help from their primary care providers, who provide most of the psychotropic medications prescribed. Approximately one in 10 patients seen in a primary care setting has a major depressive disorder. Most patients with mood disorders are treated by primary care providers, so it is essential that mood disorders are recognized and properly treated. The World Health Organisation reports, "Major Depressive Disorder is the leading cause of disability and the 4th leading contributor to the global burden of disease."

Suicide

In 2006, 33,300 people killed themselves in this country. Women attempt suicide twice as often as men, but men actually die from suicide at four times the rate of women. Older white men are at the highest risk for death by suicide. Most people who commit suicide suffer from depression. Other risk factors include substance abuse, the presence of severe anxiety or panic, a major loss or disease, and a history of suicide attempts. Alarmingly, more than half of these people have seen their physicians within a month of their death.

Diagnosis

The *Diagnostic and Statistical Manual of Mental Disorders*, Fourth Edition, Text Revision (DSM-IV-TR) lists the mood disorders and their diagnostic criteria (Box 1). They fall into three areas: major depression, mood instability disorders (including bipolar disorder), and mood disorders associated with a medical condition or induced by a substance. Adjustment disorders can also feature a depressed mood.

CURRENT DIAGNOSIS

- Screen for mood disorders if your patient seems anergic, withdrawn, irritable or sad, agitated, pressured or if significantly different.
- Directly ask: "You seem sad, let's talk."
- Laboratory studies: Get TSH, T4, CBC, B-12 level
- Empathic responses are essential. First, connect with your patient: "You seem overwhelmed [distraught, really down]." Then, reassure and support.
- Explore suicide risk. Ask directly. If suicide risk is found, strongly consider referral to a psychiatrist and/or immediate hospitalization.
- Rule out bipolar mania or hypomania before initiating antidepressant therapy. If bipolar disorder is found, see treatment options.
- Explore for psychosis. If psychosis is found, strongly consider referral to a psychiatrist or immediate hospitalization.
- Involve supportive family as treatment team members.

BOX 1   DSM-IV-TR Criteria for Major Depressive Episode

A. Five (or more) of the following symptoms have been present during the same 2-week period and represent a change from previous functioning; at least one of the symptoms is either depressed mood or loss of interest or pleasure. *Note:* Do not include symptoms that are clearly caused by a general medical condition, mood-incongruent delusions, or hallucinations.
  1. Depressed mood most of the day, nearly every day, as indicated by either subjective report (e.g., feels sad or empty) or observation made by others (e.g., appears tearful). *Note:* In children and adolescents, can be irritable mood.
  2. Markedly diminished interest or pleasure in all, or almost all, activities most of the day, nearly every day (as indicated by either subjective account or observation made by others)
  3. Significant weight loss when not dieting or weight gain (e.g., a change of more than 5% of body weight in a month), or decrease or increase in appetite nearly every day. *Note:* In children, consider failure to make expected weight gains.
  4. Insomnia or hypersomnia nearly every day
  5. Psychomotor agitation or retardation nearly every day (observable by others, not merely subjective feelings of restlessness or being slowed down)
  6. Fatigue or loss of energy nearly every day
  7. Feelings of worthlessness or excessive or inappropriate guilt (which may be delusional) nearly every day (not merely self-reproach or guilt about being sick)
  8. Diminished ability to think or concentrate, or indecisiveness, nearly every day (either by subjective account or as observed by others)
  9. Recurrent thoughts of death (not just fear of dying), recurrent suicidal ideation without a specific plan, or a suicide attempt or a specific plan for committing suicide
B. The symptoms do not meet criteria for a mixed episode.
C. The symptoms cause clinically significant distress or impairment in social, occupational, or other important areas of functioning.
D. The symptoms are not due to the direct physiologic effects of a substance (e.g., a drug of abuse, a medication) or a general medical condition (e.g., hypothyroidism).
E. The symptoms are not better accounted for by bereavement (i.e., after the loss of a loved one); the symptoms persist for longer than 2 months or are characterized by marked functional impairment, morbid preoccupation with worthlessness, suicidal ideation, psychotic symptoms, or psychomotor retardation.

Major Depression

RISK FACTORS

Children of one parent with depression have an approximately 30% chance of developing major depression, a rate approximately five times that of the adult population. This risk more than doubles when both parents have a mood disorder. Lower socioeconomic status and being female are risk factors for unipolar depression. Psychological and physical stressors, such as divorce, significant loss, medical disease, and drug abuse are also associated with the development of depression.

PATHOPHYSIOLOGY

The neuroscience involved in the pathophysiology of the mood disorders is complex and the subject of enormous research effort. For years it has been known that the paucity of certain neurotransmitters in specific areas of the brain is associated with depression. The study of three primary neurotransmitters—norepinephrine, serotonin, and dopamine—has resulted in numerous antidepressant medications that increase the bioavailability of the targeted neurotransmitters.

TREATMENT

General Considerations

Treatment of major depression starts when the physician educates the patient about depression and treatment options. Patients may be offered antidepressants, psychotherapy of certain types, electroconvulsive therapy (ECT), or experimental approaches such as vagus

---

 CURRENT THERAPY

Major Depression

- Always treat clinical depression in a consenting patient.
- Mild depression (dysthymia) should be treated as aggressively as more serious depression.
- Treat aggressively and with adequate trials.
- A response usually takes 2 to 3 weeks.
- If an antidepressant has failed an adequate trial, adjunctive therapy might be in order.
- Only abruptly stop an antidepressant in an emergency.
- Early energy improvement can raise suicide risk.
- Never give another antidepressant within 2 weeks of a monoamine oxidase inhibitor.

Bipolar Disorder

- Treatment is usually management rather than cure.
- Treatment is built around mood stabilizers.
- Consider referral to a psychiatrist.
- Aggressively treat substance abuse in a patient with bipolar disorder.
- Counsel stability in life style, especially in sleep hygiene and drug and alcohol use.

Substance-Induced Mood Disorders

- Treating substance-induced mood disorders is most effective when the offending substance is either reduced or stopped.

Mood Disorder Due to a General Medical Condition

- Useful screening laboratory tests include thyroid-stimulating hormone, complete blood count, liver function tests, fasting glucose and serum albumin, serum calcium, vitamin B_{12}, and urinalysis.
- Treatment of the causative disorder is essential.

---

nerve stimulation and transcranial magnetic stimulation. Always treat clinical depression in a consenting patient. Never surrender to the destructive notion of "Who wouldn't be depressed if they were paralyzed or dying." Depression is a miserable, impairing condition that worsens all other comorbid disorders and, whether mild or severe, a patient with depression always deserves treatment.

At this time there is considerable support for the use of antidepressant medication in combination with either cognitive-behavioral therapy (CBT) or interpersonal therapy as being the most effective approach to the treatment of serious depression. Mild to moderate depression responds to CBT and interpersonal therapy but usually more slowly than with medications alone. If medications are used without psychotherapy, the medication response is added to the 30% to 50% placebo response, resulting in almost 70% of patients showing significant improvement or achieving remission.

Always ask about psychotic symptoms in depressed patients. If psychotic symptoms are present (usually auditory hallucinations, paranoia, delusions or cognitive impairment), add a new-generation antipsychotic to the existing antidepressant. Consider hospitalization for patients with a psychotic depression.

Rule out bipolar depression before starting antidepressant medications. Antidepressants can destabilize a person with a bipolar disorder, and they often produce limited benefits. Explore for history of mania. Weigh risks and benefits. Consult a psychiatrist if doubts persist.

Rule out comorbid substance abuse. Patients do not recover if addiction is not under control. Furthermore, the risk of suicide is much higher with comorbid substance abuse, and hospitalization should be strongly considered.

Treatment Planning and Progress

Treat aggressively and with adequate trials. If you decide to treat depression do it aggressively (and safely) regardless of the severity of the symptoms. Selection of an antidepressant should usually be based on the patient's needs and expected side effects (Table 1). For instance, avoid tricyclic antidepressants (TCAs) with suicidal patients because they are commonly lethal in overdose. Typically, selective serotonin reuptake inhibitors (SSRIs) are very effective if a patient's depression is accompanied by anxiety or panic. Other factors to consider might be a blood relative's response to an antidepressant and the patient's own medication history and health.

Talk to your patient. When starting or changing antidepressant therapy, tell your patient a response usually takes 2 to 3 weeks. Discuss side effects and risks and benefits. Then see the patient again in 3 weeks to judge progress. Increase the dose of the tolerated antidepressant every 2 or 3 weeks until the maximum level is reached or the patient notices significant improvement. This is an adequate trial.

If an antidepressant has failed an adequate trial, adjunctive therapy might be in order. You may add an antidepressant to the existing medication, keeping the first antidepressant at the same or slightly reduced dose. Slowly cross taper the two medications, reducing the first medication slowly while increasing the second antidepressant. Add an adjunctive agent such as lithium[1] (300 to 900 mg at bedtime), a new-generation antipsychotic in low dose at bedtime, a benzodiazepine (considering the obvious drawbacks), or liothyronine (Cytomel)[1] at 5 µg every morning. Again, give 2 or 3 weeks for an adequate trial.

Duration of treatment for treatment of a first clinical depression should be from 8 to 12 months, starting from the point of full remission of depressive symptoms. It has been well established that if maintenance therapy continues for a minimum of 6 months after the achievement of full remission of symptoms, there is a significantly less chance of a future episode of depression. If the patient has had an extremely severe depression or recurrent episodes, lifelong treatment (at adequate-trial dose levels) should be considered.

Do not trigger rebound symptoms. Only abruptly stop an antidepressant in an emergency (if it has been taken for longer than a month). Always taper the medication over 2 to 6 weeks if it must be discontinued.

---

[1]Not FDA approved for this indication.

TABLE 1 Selective Serotonin Reuptake Inhibitors

Medication	Daily Dosage Range	Significant Attribute	Typical Side Effects*	Comorbid Conditions
Citalopram[†] (Celexa)	20-40 mg	Simple dosing	Akathisia, weight gain or loss, nausea, diarrhea, activation and insomnia or sedation	Generalized anxiety,[1] panic disorder,[1] OCD[1]
Escitalopram (Lexapro)	10-20 mg	Simple dosing	Akathisia, weight gain or loss, nausea, diarrhea, activation and insomnia or sedation	Generalized anxiety,[1] panic disorder,[1] OCD[1]
Fluoxetine (Prozac)	10-80 mg	Extreme duration of action	Akathisia, weight gain or loss, nausea, diarrhea, activation and insomnia or sedation	Panic disorder, anorexia,[1] bulimia, OCD, PMDD, generalized anxiety,[1] social anxiety[1]
Paroxetine (Paxil)	10-40 mg IR, CR	Paninhibitor of hepatic CYP enzymes	Akathisia, weight gain or loss, nausea, diarrhea, activation and insomnia or sedation	Panic disorder, social anxiety, generalized anxiety (IR), OCD (IR), PTSD (IR), PMDD (CR)
Fluvoxamine (Luvox)	50-300 mg	Usually used to treat OCD	Akathisia, weight gain or loss, nausea, diarrhea, activation and insomnia or sedation	Generalized anxiety,[1] panic disorder,[1] OCD[1]
Sertraline (Zoloft)	25-200 mg	Large effective dose range	Akathisia, weight gain or loss, nausea, diarrhea, activation and insomnia or sedation	Social phobia, panic disorder, PTSD, OCD, PMDD, generalized anxiety[1]
Trazodone (Desyrel)	25-400 mg Up to 600 mg in hospital settings	Used only as a sleep aid due to sedation and short duration	No anticholinergic effects, significant postural hypotension, priapism (rare)	

[1]Not FDA approved for this indication.
*Side effects are common but mild and often disappear in less than 10 days. Sexual side effects occur in about 40%.
[†]Citalopram is indicated for major depressive disorder only.
Abbreviations: CR = controlled release; CYP = cytochrome P-450; IR = immediate release; OCD = obsessive–compulsive disorder; PMDD = premenstrual dysphoric disorder; PTSD = posttraumatic stress disorder.

Mild depression (dysthymia) should be treated as aggressively as more serious depression. Patients with dysthymia often fail to recognize that their chronic misery is a treatable disorder or that their misery can worsen into severe major depression.

Selective Serotonin Reuptake Inhibitors

The selective serotonin reuptake inhibitors (SSRIs) act to increase the availability of serotonin (5-HT) at the synapse. These medications are often inhibitors of cytochrome P-450 enzymes, especially paroxetine (Paxil) and fluoxetine (Prozac) (see Table 1). Take note of drug-drug interactions when prescribing them concurrently with other medications.

The side-effect profile of SSRIs is quite benign for most patients. The most common are mild: jitteriness, gastrointestinal disturbances, lightheadedness, weight change, (gain more than loss), and sedation or activation, (activation more than sedation). In addition, approximately 40% of both sexes experience sexual side effects. Often, taking the medication at the right time of day or night and taking it with food minimizes the untoward effects.

If the depressed patient has significant anxiety, panic or obsessive–compulsive disorder, the SSRI medications are particularly helpful and should be strongly considered. Doses higher than necessary for remission of depressed mood are usually necessary for comorbid anxiety, panic or obsessive–compulsive disorder.

Serotonin and Norepinephrine Reuptake Inhibitors

Serotonin and norepinephrine reuptake inhibitors (SNRIs) combine selective inhibition of 5-HT reuptake and inhibition of norepinephrine reuptake (Table 2). These medications share the side effects of the SSRIs, and at higher doses they can increase blood presure. Caution should be used for this reason in at-risk populations, and vital signs should be monitored.

Side Effects, Suicide, and Follow-up

Initially, patients expect improvement and instead might experience uncomfortable side effects. Your patients should know to expect this and that the side effects will usually dissipate.

Early energy improvement can raise suicide risk. Not all symptoms of depression respond equally or at the same rate. For instance, anergia might improve faster than mood, giving patients energy to act on suicidal ideation.

Schedule a follow-up appointment every 2 or 3 weeks until the patient is significantly improved to help with compliance and prevent a poor outcome.

Bipolar Disorder

RISK FACTORS

First-degree relatives of a person with bipolar disorder are seven times more likely to have the disorder than the general population. Interestingly, bipolar disorder is much more commonly seen in higher socioeconomic groups than in the general population. Major stressing events such as interpersonal loss can precipitate either a bipolar depression or a manic state. Men and women get bipolar disorder in equal numbers, but women have more depressive cycles and rapid cycling, whereas men experience a higher percentage of mania.

GENERAL CONSIDERATIONS

Untreated, bipolar disorder worsens over time. Patients with a relatively mild bipolar II condition might at any time switch to full blown bipolar disorder. Bipolar disorder is often as impairing as schizophrenia. It is common for patients in either or both the manic and the depressive states to experience psychosis, complete with hallucinations, delusions, paranoia, and disorders of cognition. A characteristic of bipolar that usually separates it from schizophrenia

TABLE 2 Serotonin and Norepinephrine Reuptake Inhibitors and Bupropion

Medication	Daily Dosage Range	Significant Attributes	Typical Side Effects*	Comorbid Conditions
Desvenlafaxine (Pristiq)	50 mg, ER	Possibly a bit faster onset	Headache, dizziness, GI problems (e.g., nausea, diarrhea, constipation)	
Duloxetine (Cymbalta)	20-120 mg	Effective also at higher doses for neurogenic pain Do not take with thioridazine (Mellaril) Contraindicated in patients with narrow-angle glaucoma	Headache, dizziness, GI problems (e.g., nausea, diarrhea, constipation)	Neurogenic pain, fibromyalgia
Mirtazepine (Remeron)	15-45 mg	Excellent sleep aid at lower doses	No sexual side effects Weight gain, sedation, flulike symptoms, decreased ability to fight infection (fever, chill, sore throat), mouth sores	
Venlafaxine (Effexor)	37.5-300 mg, ER	Possibly a bit faster onset	Headache, dizziness, GI problems (e.g., nausea, diarrhea, constipation); weight loss > gain; restlessness, blurred vision	Generalized anxiety (ER), panic disorder (ER), social anxiety, OCD[1]
Bupropion (Wellbutrin)	100-450 mg, ER	Lower seizure threshold at highest doses Do not exceed 450 mg/d	No sedation, some activation, no weight gain, no sexual side effects, restlessness, insomnia, dry mouth	Smoking cessation[†] (Zyban)

[1]Not FDA approved for this indication.
*Side effects are common but mild and often disappear in less than 10 days. Weight gain, sexual dysfunction, and hypertension can occur and persist.
[†]Specific FDA approval for this indication.
Abbreviations: ER = extended release available; OCD = obsessive–compulsive disorder.

is that between episodes, many patients are totally symptom free. Most patients, especially women, experience more depressive episodes than manic, particularly later in life. Episodes of both depression and mania can last from days to months. Using current therapeutic treatments, 60% to 75% of patients with bipolar disorder can live useful and productive lives.

DIAGNOSIS

To meet the criteria of the DSM IV-TR for bipolar disorder, your patients must experience at least one major depressive episode and at least one full manic episode (bipolar I) or a hypomanic episode (bipolar II) in their lifetime (Box 2). The depressive episode is identical to an episode of unipolar depression. For this reason, a good history, exploring for past mania or hypomania, often with collateral information, should be undertaken with every depressed patient. Most patients have had several episodes of depression before their first manic experience. Always suspect bipolar disorder in patients with recurrent depressive episodes. Bipolar disorder is underdiagnosed. Investigation of family history often offers the first indication of a bipolar disorder.

A manic episode is a distinct period of abnormally and persistently elevated, expansive, or irritable mood, lasting at least 1 week (or any duration if hospitalization is necessary). The mood change is usually accompanied by a significantly elevated level of energy and activity. A common early red flag for a developing mania is a drop in need for sleep. A mixed episode is characterized by the criteria for a manic episode in conjunction with those for a major depressive episode (depressed mood, loss of interest or pleasure in

---

BOX 2   DMS-IV-TR Criteria for a Manic Episode

A. A distinct period of abnormally and persistently elevated, expansive, or irritable mood, lasting at least 1 week (or any duration if hospitalization is necessary).
B. During the period of mood disturbance, three (or more) of the following symptoms have persisted (four if the mood is only irritable) and have been present to a significant degree:
   1. Inflated self-esteem or grandiosity
   2. Decreased need for sleep (e.g., feels rested after only 3 hours of sleep)
   3. More talkative than usual or pressure to keep talking
   4. Flight of ideas or subjective experience that thoughts are racing
   5. Distractibility (i.e., attention too easily drawn to unimportant or irrelevant external stimuli)
   6. Increase in goal-directed activity (either socially, at work or school, or sexually) or psychomotor agitation
   7. Excessive involvement in pleasurable activities that have a high potential for painful consequences (e.g., engaging in unrestrained buying sprees, sexual indiscretions, or foolish business investments)
C. The symptoms do not meet criteria for a mixed episode.
D. The mood disturbance is sufficiently severe to cause marked impairment in occupational functioning or in usual social activities or relationships with others, or to necessitate hospitalization to prevent harm to self or others, or there are psychotic features.
E. The symptoms are not due to the direct physiological effects of a substance (e.g., a drug of abuse, a medication, or other treatment) or a general medical condition (e.g., hyperthyroidism).

nearly all activities) and is sufficiently severe to cause marked impairment or psychosis. The symptoms are not due to the direct physiologic effects of a substance or a general medical condition.

TREATMENT

Treatment is usually management rather than cure. Significantly reducing severity and frequency of episodes is the goal, and occasionally the more fortunate patients live symptom free for many years. Treatment is built around mood stabilizers, and all mood stabilizers act to treat current and prevent future mania and depression. Lithium carbonate is the gold standard for bipolar treatment, and no medication has shown itself to be superior to lithium, although the side-effect profile of lithium often supports the use of other mood stabilizers.

Two additional classes of medications are extensively used (often off-label) by psychiatrists to successfully treat this condition. The antiseizure medications—valproate, (divalproex sodium, Depakote),[1] carbamazepine (Tegretol),[1] and lamotrigine (Lamictal)—have shown efficacy equal to lithium in many studies. The new-generation antipsychotics are also used. These include aripiprazole (Abilify), olanzapine (Zyprexa), risperidone (Risperdal), quetiapine (Seroquel), and ziprasidone (Geodon). Oxcarbazepine (Trileptal)[1], topiramate (Topamax)[1] and gabapentin (Neurontin)[1] are also used as mood stabilizers, but there is little evidence that they are effective.

Bipolar episodes that combine elements of both mania and depression, mixed episodes, or rapid-cycling patterns (more than four episodes a month) are particularly difficult to treat. Often these patients require a combination of mood stabilizers. There is a mild variant of bipolar disorder called cyclothymia, which is often thought of as less-impairing form of mood disorder. Even so, consider a mood stabilizer if the patient feels that his or her life is being affected in a detrimental way.

Consider referral to a psychiatrist if your patient has a bipolar disorder. The disorder and treatment are complicated, and there are enormous risks to both patient and doctor. Hospital treatment is indicated if your bipolar patient is suicidal or psychotic or has a comorbid addiction.

Always aggressively treat substance abuse in your patient with a bipolar disorder. Patients always do poorly with bipolar disorder if they are abusing drugs.

Medication

Avoid using antidepressants unless the patient is first established on a mood stabilizer. The risk of downstream mood destabilization with antidepressants should be carefully considered.

Avoid rapid mood stabilizer decreases once treatment is established. Avoid stopping a mood stabilizer once it is established unless you first obtain several months of coverage of the replacement mood stabilizer. When one mood stabilizer is inadequate, consider adding another instead of risking additional instability by stopping the first.

Often your choice of mood stabilizers depends on the expected side effects of the medications and your patient's needs. Always bring your patient and often their family into determining in the treatment choices.

Adjunctive Treatment

Counsel stability in life style, especially in sleep hygiene and drug and alcohol use for your bipolar patient. Individual and family counseling and education about the disorder can be very important for your patient.

Acute Episode

The primary medication for treating an acute episode of mania or bipolar depression with psychotic features should be a new-generation antipsychotic alone or in combination with lithium, valproate, or carbamazepine[1] (Table 3).

Substance-Induced Mood Disorders

A prominent and persistent mood disorder characterized by a depressed mood, significant anhedonia, or an elevated, expansive, or irritable mood associated with drug or medication use, and during or within a month of intoxication, or withdrawal, meets the criteria for a substance-induced mood disorder. Meeting the full criteria for a DSM IV-TR major depression or bipolar disorder is not necessary.

Current neurophysiologic models of affective disorders helping to explain these disorders include models of catecholamine depletion, tryptophan depletion, and changes within the hypothalamic-pituitary-adrenal axis. People with a predisposition to mood disorders are thought to more easily fall victim to these drug-induced problems.

Medications and drugs that cause depression include alcohol, corticosteroids, digoxin, benzodiazepines, opiates, interferon β1b (Beta-seron, Extavia), peginterferon alfa-2b (PEG-Intron), amantadine (Symmetrel), isocarboxazid (Marplan), β-blockers, and melatonin.[7]

Mania, either temporary or a full manic episode in patients who are predisposed, can be triggered by amphetamines (and similar drugs such as ephedrine[2] and cocaine), corticosteroids, and the antidepressants. Triggering antidepressants, in order of descending risk, TCAs, SSRIs, monoamine oxidase inhibitors (MAOIs), and SNRIs.

Treating substance-induced mood disorders is most effective when the offending substance is either reduced or stopped. In the case of withdrawal symptoms, baseline mood should return within a few days to a month of discontinuing the substance.

The brief use of ameliorating medications for psychotic symptoms (low-dose antipsychotics), severe anxiety (benzodiazepines) may be considered. Without a history of recurrent depressions, antidepressant medication is usually not started until ample time is given for the patient to recover.

Mood Disorder Due to a General Medical Condition

A mood disorder due to a general medical condition is diagnosed when the clinician believes a specific general medical condition causes symptoms suggesting a manic, hypomanic, or major depressive episode. A prominent and persistent mood disorder characterized by a depressed mood, significant anhedonia, or an elevated, expansive, or irritable mood that is the direct physiologic consequence of a general medical condition is based on evidence from the history, physical examination, or laboratory findings.

Depressive symptoms can be caused by hypothyroidism, HIV infection and AIDS, systemic lupus erythematosus, dementing illness, delirium, Parkinson's disease, epilepsy, emphysema, asthma, vitamin B_{12} deficiency, or hypercortisolism. Other conditions associated with mood disorders are: stroke, myocardial infarction, diabetes, and viral illness.

Mania-like symptoms are sometimes associated with delirium, stroke, hyperthyroidism, or vitamin B_{12} deficiency. A deterioration in mental status of an elderly woman with depression, mania-like symptoms, or psychosis is reason to screen for urinary tract infection. Sleep deprivation can hasten mania.

Useful screening laboratory tests for identifying physical disease in psychiatric patients include thyroid-stimulating hormone, complete blood count, liver function tests, fasting glucose and serum albumin, serum calcium, vitamin B_{12}, and urinalysis.

Treatment of the causative disorder is essential. Medications such as antipsychotics and benzodiazepines are sometimes required for a limited time. In the case of depression from vitamin B_{12} and thyroid deficiencies, antidepressants can prove very helpful. Their use can

---

[1]Not FDA approved for this indication.

[2]Not available in the United States.
[7]Available as dietary supplement.

TABLE 3 Medications Used in Bipolar Disorder

Medication	Dosage Range	Blood Levels	Lab Tests	Significant Attributes	Typical Side Effects	Caution	Comments
Lithium carbonate (Lithobid, Lithonate), ER	300-800 mg/d	0.4-1.2 mEq/L >1.6 mEq/L often toxic	CBC, LFTs, BUN, TSH, T₄, creatinine, EKG, blood levels q6mo	Effective antidepressant, cheap Blood levels rise as sodium drops and drop as sodium rises, a significant association	Tremors, polyuria, nausea, sedation, confusion, memory loss	Toxic symptoms = being drunk Ataxia, confusion, slurred speech, nausea, vomiting, diarrhea, weakness, fetal risk Caution w/NSAIDs, metronidazole (Flagyl), diuretics	ER form available
Valproate[1] (Depakote)	500-1000 mg/day	50-120 µg/mL >130 µg/mL often toxic	LFTs, platelets, blood levels q6mo	Phenytoin, carbamazepine, and phenobarbital induce metabolism of valproate Metabolism of numerous drugs inhibited by valproate Check drug–drug interactions	Sedation, nausea, dizziness, vomiting, asthenia, abdominal pain, rash, dyspepsia	Hepatotoxicity, teratogenicity, pancreatitis, thrombocytopenia, FR	
Carbamazepine[1] (Tegretol)	200-800 mg/day	5-10 µg/mL	CBC, liver function, BUN, urinalysis Check blood levels and lab values q6mo	CYP 3A4 inhibitors and inducers affect carbamazepine level Carbamazepine induces CYP activity Check drug–drug interactions	Sedation, dizziness, unsteadines, nausea, blood pressure changes	Aplastic anemia, agranulocytosis and porphyria, FR, BCP, TEN, SJS	Carbamazepine ER (Equetro) is the only carbamazepine product approved for acute manic and mixed episodes associated with bipolar I disorder
Lamotrigine[1] (Lamictal)[1]	200-400 mg/day	Blood levels not helpful Follow PDR dose increases closely		Numerous drugs induce metabolism, valproate inhibits it Lamotrigine induces valproate's metabolism Indicated for maintanance, not acute episodes Check drug–drug interactions	Headache, ataxia, dizziness, sedation, diplopia, nausea (especially if given with valproate) rash	SJS, rapid dose increases can increase risk Hypersensitivity reactions, acute multiorgan failure, blood dyscrasias	ER form available Lamictal XR is only indicated for seizures
Aripiprazole (Abilify)	2-30 mg/day	Blood levels not helpful		Indicated for acute and maintenance treatment of manic and mixed episodes with or without psychotic features	Nausea, vomiting, constipation, headache, dizziness, akathisia, anxiety, insomnia and restlessness. QTc interval increase	IME, NMS, TD, but much less than 1st-generation neuroleptics	liquid form and IM form available

Continued

Mood Disorders

1137

TABLE 3 Medications Used in Bipolar Disorder—Cont'd

Medication	Dosage Range	Blood Levels	Lab Tests	Significant Attributes	Typical Side Effects	Caution	Comments
Olanzapine (Zyprexa)	2.5-20 mg/day	Blood levels not helpful	Monitor blood glucose, lipids	Indicated for acute and maintenance treatment of manic and mixed episodes with or without psychotic features Carbamazepine induces metabolism, fluvoxamine inhibits	Orthostasis, asthenia, dry mouth, constipation, weight gain, dizziness, akathisia	IME, risk of metabolic syndrome and diabetes. NMS, TD, but much less than 1st-generation neuroleptics	Zydis form orally dissolves IM form available
Risperidone (Risperdal)	1-9 mg/day	Blood levels not helpful	Monitor blood glucose, lipids	Indicated for short-term treatment of acute manic or mixed episodes Phenytoin, rifampin, phenobarbital induce metabolism Paroxetine and fluoxetine inhibit metabolism Check drug-drug interactions	Orthostasis, paranoia, sedation, dizziness, EPSE, dispepsia, nausea	IME, can elevate prolactin levels Mild risk of metabolic syndrome and diabetes NMS, TD, but much less than 1st-generation neuroleptics	M-Tab is orally dissolving form Consta is depot IM form
Quetiapine (Seroquel)	25-800 mg/d	Blood levels not helpful	Monitor blood glucose, lipids	Indicated for acute and maintenance treatment of manic and mixed episodes with or without psychotic features Phenytoin, carbamazepine, and phenobarbital induce metabolism Check drug-drug interactions	Sedation, dizziness, orthostasis, dry mouth, constipation, ↑ALT, weight gain, dyspepsia	IME, mild to moderate risk of metabolic syndrome and diabetes NMS, TD, but much less than 1st-generation neuroleptics	ER available ER in 1 hs dose or IR in divided doses
Ziprasidone (Geodon)	40-80 mg bid	Blood levels not helpful		Carbamazepine induces ziprasidone metabolism, ketoconazole inhibits Ziprasidone has little effect on other medications	EPSE, orthostasis, akathisia, anxiety, depression, weight gain, dizziness, dystonia, rash, vomiting, ↑QTc interval	IME, NMS, TD, but much less than 1st-generation neuroleptics	IM[1] available, but indicated only for acute agitation

[1]Not FDA approved for this indication.
Abbreviations: ↑ = increase(s); ALT = alanine aminotransferase; BCP = (reduces effectiveness of) birth control pills, BUN = blood urea nitrogen; CBC = complete blood count; CYP = cytochrome P-450 (system); EPSE = extrapyramidal side effects; ER = extended release form; FR = fetal risk, IME = increased mortality with elderly dementia with psychosis; IR = immediate release form; lab = laboratory; LFT = liver function test; NMS = neuroleptic malignant syndrome; PDR = *Physicians' Desk Reference*; SJS = Stevens-Johnson syndrome; TD = tardive dyskinesia; TEN = toxic epidermal necrolysis.

usually be limited to 6 to 12 months beyond the cessation of symptoms, but as with all depressions, treatment should be aggressive, using the adequate clinical trial model.

Summary

Mood disorders are ubiquitous, impairing, and often deadly. Their presence requires immediate exploration and almost always treatment. Never undertreat depression and never stop mood stabilizers in bipolar patients without considering the potential consequences of instability. Always screen for suicide and psychosis, and always approach your patients with empathy.

REFERENCES

American Psychiatric Association. Diagnostic and statistical manual of mental disorders. 4th ed. text revision. Washington, DC: American Psychiatric Association; 2000.

American Psychiatric Association. Practice guideline for the treatment of patients with bipolar disorder (revision). Am J Psychiatry 2002;159(Suppl. 4):1–50.

Busch AB, Frank RG, Sachs G, Normand SLT. Bipolar-I patient characteristics associated with differences in antimanic medication prescribing. Available at http://cme.medscape.com/viewarticle/588069 [accessed August 25, 2010].

Cole SA, Christensen JF, Cole MR, et al. Depression. In: Feldman MD, Christensen JF, editors. Behavioral Medicine. 3rd ed. New York: McGraw-Hill; 2007. pp. 199–226.

Conway MW, Miller MN. Mood Disorders. In: Rakel RE, Bope ET, editors. Conn's Current Therapy 2006. Philadelphia: Saunders; 2006. pp. 1300–8.

Gruenberg AM, Goldstein RD. Mood disorders: Depression. In: Tasman A, Kay J, Lieberman JA, editors. Psychiatry. 2nd Edition. Vol. 2. Chichester, UK: John Wiley & Sons, 2003. pp. 1207–36.

Joska JA, et al. Phenomenology of mood disorders. In: Hales RE, et al., eds. The American Psychiatric Publishing Textbook of Psychiatry. 5th ed. Arlington, VA: American Psychiatric Association, 2008. pp. 457–503.

Thase ME, MacFadden W, Weisler RH, et al. Efficacy of quetiapine monotherapy in bipolar I and II depression: A double-blind, placebo-controlled study. J Clin Psychopharmacol 2006;26:600–9.

Schizophrenia

Method of
Brian Miller, MD, MPH, and Peter Buckley, MD

Schizophrenia is a complex, chronic, and often severe psychiatric disorder that is a leading cause of disability worldwide. Although the literal translation of the word *schizophrenia* is "split mind," patients with this disorder do not have a "split personality" or a multiple personality disorder. Schizophrenia is a psychotic disorder that interferes with a person's thinking, mood, behavior, and interpersonal relations. Schizophrenia often has devastating, lifelong consequences for affected individuals and their families, and it is associated with an increased risk of premature mortality, including deaths from suicide and cardiovascular disease. In this chapter, the epidemiology and diagnosis of schizophrenia are reviewed. We then discuss pharmacologic and psychosocial treatments for schizophrenia in the context of a chronic disease model. The risks of medical and substance-use comorbidity and suicidality are also highlighted.

Epidemiology and Risk Factors

The cause of schizophrenia is not known, but it is thought to involve interactions between genetic (or epigenetic) and environmental factors, including developmental problems that occur during gestation. The lifetime prevalence of schizophrenia is approximately 1% and

is equal for men and women. The usual age of onset is in the late teens or early 20s to late 30s, although schizophrenia can have onset before age 10 (early onset) or after age 45 (late onset). The age of onset is usually younger for men than women.

Several lines of evidence support a genetic contribution to the risk of schizophrenia. There is a 40% lifetime risk of schizophrenia in a child of two parents with schizophrenia. Twin-twin concordance is 50% for monozygotic twins and 12% for dizygotic twins. A meta-analysis found "strong epidemiologic credibility" for four candidate genes: *DRD1, DTNBP1, MTHFR,* and *TPH1,* although numerous other genes have been implicated. There are likely multiple candidate genes that increase the risk of schizophrenia, each with a small effect size.

Replicated environmental risk factors for schizophrenia include season of birth (i.e., winter), advanced paternal age, prenatal stress throughout gestation (e.g., famine and acute maternal stress in the first trimester, second-trimester influenza exposure, loss of the father in the second or third trimester), obstetric complications (e.g., gestational diabetes, low birth weight, asphyxia), severe childhood abuse, and cannabis use. It remains unclear whether some of these risk factors are causal or represent early manifestations of schizophrenia.

Diagnosis

There are three primary symptom domains in schizophrenia: positive, negative, and cognitive. Positive symptoms are abnormalities of thought content, including hallucinations (i.e., abnormal sensory perceptions in the absence of external stimuli) and delusions (i.e., fixed, false beliefs) and disorganized thinking and behavior. Hallucinations are most commonly auditory, but they can occur in any sensory modality. Negative symptoms include impairments in motivation (i.e., avolition), emotional expression (i.e., blunted affect), speech (i.e., alogia), and the ability to experience pleasure (i.e., anhedonia). Cognitive symptoms include impairments in attention, language, memory, processing speed, and executive function.

The most commonly used diagnostic criteria for schizophrenia are derived from the *Diagnostic and Statistical Manual of Mental Disorders,* Fourth Edition, Text Revision (DSM-IV-TR). These criteria include the presence of two or more characteristic symptoms (i.e., delusions, hallucinations, disorganized speech, disorganized behavior, or negative symptoms) for a significant portion of time during a 1-month period, with continuous signs of the disturbance persisting for at least 6 months. During this period, there is significant impairment in one or more major areas of functioning, including work, interpersonal relations, and self-care. It must also be established that the disorder is not better accounted for by a primary mood disorder, schizoaffective disorder, substance intoxication or withdrawal, or another general medical condition. Delusions and

CURRENT DIAGNOSIS

- Three primary symptom domains:
  - Positive (i.e., hallucinations, delusions, and disorganized thought and behavior)
  - Negative (i.e., blunted affect, anhedonia, alogia, and avolition)
  - Cognitive (i.e., attention, language, memory, and processing speed)
- Symptoms lasting for 1 month and continuous signs of illness for 6 months
- Significant impairment of one or more major areas of functioning (work, interpersonal relations, or self-care)
- Ensure that psychosis is not caused by a primary mood disorder, schizoaffective disorder, substance intoxication or withdrawal, or a general medical condition

hallucinations, although common, are not required for the diagnosis. Although cognitive symptoms are not required for the diagnosis, they are a significant cause of illness-related disability. A diagnosis of schizophrenia is most definitively made by interviewing the patient, obtaining collateral history from family and friends, and completing a medical work-up (i.e., physical examination with routine blood and urine tests).

Treatment

There is no cure for schizophrenia. Although there is significant clinical heterogeneity within the disorder, schizophrenia is usually a chronic condition that requires long-term treatment. Comprehensive treatment involves outpatient medication management and therapy, psychosocial interventions, involvement of the family and other support system, inpatient care for acute crisis intervention or illness exacerbation, and collaboration with primary care physicians.

Antipsychotic medications play an important role in the pharmacologic management of schizophrenia. First-generation antipsychotics have been in clinical use since the introduction of chlorpromazine (Thorazine) in the 1950s. These agents block the dopamine D_2 receptor, and common side effects include extrapyramidal side effects (e.g., parkinsonism, dystonia). The second-generation antipsychotics (SGAs), in addition to D_2 receptor blockade, are also serotonin 5-HT_2 receptor antagonists. Although the risk of extrapyramidal side effects is lower with the use of SGAs than with first-generation antipsychotics, the SGAs are associated with a heightened risk of weight gain and the metabolic syndrome. Table 1

TABLE 1 Antipsychotic Medications

Agent	Mechanism of Action*	Typical Dosing	Side Effects[†]	Side Effects[†]	Comments
First Generation					
Haloperidol (Haldol)	D_2-antagonist	1.5–15 mg/d	EPS/TD Akathisia	NMS Hyperprolactinemia	PO, IM, IV, and long-acting injection formulations
Second Generation					
Aripiprazole (Abilify)	Partial D_2-agonist and antagonist	10–30 mg/d	Weight gain (+) Dyslipidemia (+) Glucose dysregulation (+)	Sedation EPS/TD Akathisia	PO, rapid-dissolving PO, and IM formulations
Asenapine (Saphris)	D_2-antagonist/ 5-HT_2 antagonist	10–20 mg/ day	Weight gain (+) Dyslipidemia (+) Glucose dysregulation (+)	Sedation EPS/TD Akathesia	Rapid-dissolving PO, and IM formulations
Clozapine (Clozaril)	D_2-antagonist/ 5-HT_2 antagonist	300–900 mg/d	Weight gain (+++) Dyslipidemia (+++) Glucose dysregulation (++) Agranulocytosis Sedation	Orthostatic hypotension Seizures Myocarditis EPS/TD	PO and rapid-dissolving PO formulations
Olanzapine (Zyprexa)	D_2-antagonist/5-HT_2 antagonist	5–20 mg/d	Weight gain (+++) Dyslipidemia (+++) Glucose dysregulation (++)	Sedation EPS/TD	PO, rapid-dissolving PO, and IM formulations
Paliperidone (Invega)	D_2-antagonist/5-HT_2 antagonist	6–12 mg/d	Weight gain (+) Dyslipidemia (+) Glucose dysregulation (+)	EPS/TD	PO formulation Active metabolite of risperidone (Risperdal)
Quetiapine (Seroquel)	D_2-antagonist/5-HT_2 antagonist	400–800 mg/d	Weight gain (++) Dyslipidemia (+) Glucose dysregulation (+)	Sedation EPS/TD Orthostatic hypotension	PO and ER formulations
Risperidone (Risperdal)	D_2-antagonist/5-HT_2 antagonist	2–6 mg/d	Weight gain (++) Dyslipidemia (+) Glucose dysregulation (+)	EPS/TD Hyperprolactinemia	PO, PO liquid, rapid-dissolving PO, and long-acting injection formulations
Ziprasidone (Geodon)	D_2-antagonist/5-HT_2 antagonist	80–160 mg/ d with food	Weight gain (+) Dyslipidemia (+) Glucose dysregulation (+)	QTc prolongation EPS/TD	PO and IM formulations

*All first-generation and second-generation antipsychotics have an FDA black box warning for an "association with an increased risk of mortality in elderly patients treated for dementia-related psychosis."

[†]EPS and TD are possible side effects with all antipsychotics, but they occur less frequently with second-generation than first-generation drugs.

Abbreviations: D_2 = dopamine D_2 receptor; EPS = extrapyramidal side effects; ER, extended release; 5-HT_2 = serotonin 5-HT_2 receptor; NMS = neuroleptic malignant syndrome; TD = tardive dyskinesia; + = mild or low risk; ++ = moderate risk; +++ = severe risk.

provides a more detailed description of antipsychotic medications. The Texas Medication Algorithm Project (TMAP) recommends a trial of a single (non-clozapine) SGA for newly diagnosed patients with schizophrenia or for patients never before treated with an SGA. However, neither the TMAP nor the American Psychiatric Association (APA) guidelines for the treatment of schizophrenia preferentially endorse a particular antipsychotic. Clozapine (Clozaril) is primarily used for treatment-refractory schizophrenia, usually defined as a lack of or partial response to an adequate trial of two or three antipsychotics.

Adjunctive medications may play an important role in the pharmacologic treatment of some patients with schizophrenia. The drugs include antidepressants for depression and anxiety, mood stabilizers for depression or mood elevation, benzodiazepines for anxiety or agitation, β-blockers for akathisia, and anticholinergics for extrapyramidal side effects.

Medication nonadherence is a major treatment issue for patients with schizophrenia at all phases of the illness. Reasons for nonadherence are complex and multifaceted but may include medication side effects, impaired insight into illness, psychopathology in all three symptom domains, lack of efficacy, and comorbid substance use. More than 70% of patients in the Clinical Antipsychotic Trials of Intervention Effectiveness (CATIE) schizophrenia trial discontinued medication within the first 18 months of treatment. Medication nonadherence leads to dramatically increased risk of illness relapse, hospitalization, and suicidal behavior, and it should be routinely assessed in clinical visits. The use of rapid-dissolving oral or long-acting injectable medications may improve adherence for some patients.

Psychosocial interventions are a cornerstone of the comprehensive treatment of patients with schizophrenia, and when used in combination with medication, they are more effective than antipsychotics alone. Psychotherapy, including cognitive-behavioral therapy, supportive therapy, and group therapy, promotes improved illness management and medication adherence. Involvement of the patient's family or support system in care, including family-based therapies and psychoeducation, has increased medication adherence and decreased illness relapse rates. Psychosocial rehabilitation, which may include assertive community treatment, social skills training, vocational rehabilitation, and cognitive remediation, can help maximize patients' psychosocial function.

Although there is no typical patient with schizophrenia, the clinical course is often characterized by acute relapses of illness with interepisode absence or attenuation of symptoms. Many factors increase a patient's risk of illness relapse, including medication nonadherence, psychosocial stressors, substance use, medical illnesses such as infections, and the natural history of the disorder itself. Hospitalization may be required for acute exacerbations of psychotic symptoms, including hallucinations, delusions, and impaired self-care. Hospitalization may also be required if patients represent an acute danger to themselves or others.

The concept of the recovery model and recovery-oriented care is a movement that is transforming the delivery of mental health services. Integral to the recovery model are certified peer specialists (CPSs). CPSs are licensed professionals who have progressed in their own recovery from mental illness and work to assist patients with schizophrenia and other mental illness in regaining control over their own lives and over their own recovery process. CPSs provide peer support services, serve as consumer advocates, are a resource for psychoeducation, and offer the unique perspective of their individual experiences.

Comorbidity

Schizophrenia is associated with an increased risk of premature mortality, and cardiovascular disease is a leading cause of death in this patient population. Many factors contribute to this risk, including

CURRENT THERAPY

- Antipsychotic medication, with monitoring for medication adherence and side effects
- Adjunctive medications as needed, including antidepressants, mood stabilizers, benzodiazepines, β-blockers, and anticholinergics
- Aggressive monitoring for and management of medical comorbidities, substance use disorders, and suicidality, including collaboration with a primary care physician
- Psychosocial interventions
- Involvement of family and support system in care
- Long-term treatment, including outpatient medication management and therapy, with inpatient care for acute crisis intervention or illness exacerbation

a high prevalence of smoking, poor health habits, poor health care, medication side effects, and perhaps the pathophysiology of the disorder itself. SGAs as a class are associated with weight gain and an increased risk of the metabolic syndrome. More than 40% of the 1460 patients in the CATIE schizophrenia trial met the criteria for the metabolic syndrome at baseline. Recommendations for monitoring of patients on SGAs, based on a consensus statement from the American Diabetes Association and the American Psychiatric Association, are described in Table 2. Primary care physicians play an important collaborative role with psychiatrists in the detection and management of metabolic disturbances in patients with schizophrenia to minimize the cardiovascular risks associated with these comorbidities.

Patients with schizophrenia are at an increased risk for suicide, which is a leading cause of premature mortality. The prevalence of completed suicide attempts among patients with schizophrenia is about 10%, and suicide attempts occur with even greater frequency. Clinicians should routinely assess patients for suicidal ideation, and if present, explore risk factors for completed suicide, which include a suicidal plan and intent, previous suicide attempts, a family history of suicide, access to lethal means, social isolation, and comorbid substance use. Medications, psychotherapy, and hospitalization may be required.

Comorbid substance-use disorders predominate among patients with schizophrenia; the estimated prevalence is 40% to 50%. Common substances of abuse include alcohol, marijuana, and cocaine. Patients with schizophrenia and comorbid substance use are at increased risk for medication nonadherence, illness relapse, hospitalization, suicidal and violent behavior, and an overall poor response to treatment. Up to 90% of patients with schizophrenia are tobacco users, which contributes to the increased risk of medical comorbidity. Clinicians are encouraged to routinely screen for and address substance use in their treatment plans.

Conclusions

Schizophrenia is a complex, heterogeneous, and chronic psychiatric disorder. Comprehensive treatment usually involves long-term medication management and therapy, education for patients and their families, and psychosocial interventions. Primary care physicians play an important collaborative role in the detection and management of medical comorbidities, substance-use disorders, and suicidality. Physicians, patients, and families are encouraged to become involved in the National Alliance on Mental Illness (NAMI; www.nami.org), which is a tremendous resource for help, support, education, and advocacy for patients with schizophrenia and other mental illness.

TABLE 2 Monitoring Second-Generation Antipsychotics (Excluding Clozapine)

Feature	Baseline	4 Weeks	8 Weeks	12 Weeks	Quarterly	Annually	If Symptoms Arise	Every 5 Years	Other
Personal and family history*	X					X			
Pregnancy test†	X						X		
Weight and body mass index	X	X	X	X	X				
Waist circumference	X					X			
Blood pressure	X			X		X			
Fasting glucose and HgbA$_{1C}$	X			X		X			
Fasting lipid panel	X			X				X	
Electrocardiogram‡	X						X		
Prolactin	X						X		
Complete blood cell count with differential§									X

*Including obesity, diabetes, hypertension, and dyslipidemia.
†In all women of childbearing age.
‡For patients taking ziprasidone (Geodon), which may prolong the QTc interval, and clozapine (Clozaril).
§For patients taking clozapine (Clozaril). Complete blood cell count with a differential cell count is required at baseline, then weekly for 6 months, then every other week for 6 months, and then monthly thereafter. White blood cell count must be $\geq 3500/mm^3$, and absolute neutrophil count must be $\geq 2000/mm^3$ due to risk of agranulocytosis. More frequent assessments may be warranted based on clinical status.

REFERENCES

Allen NC, Bagade S, McQueen MB, et al. Systematic meta-analyses and field synopsis of genetic association studies in schizophrenia: The SzGene database. Nat Genet 2008;40:827.

American Diabetes Association, American Psychiatric Association, American Association of Clinical Endocrinologists, North American Association for Studies on Obesity. Consensus development conference on antipsychotic drugs and obesity and diabetes. J Clin Psychiatry 2004;65:267.

American Psychiatric Association. Practice guideline for the treatment of patients with schizophrenia, 2nd edition. Am J Psychiatry 2004;161 (Suppl):1717.

Brown S. Excess mortality of schizophrenia. A meta-analysis. Br J Psychiatry 1997;171:502.

Buchanan RW, Carpenter WT. Schizophrenia and other psychotic disorders. In: Sadock BJ, Sadock VA, editors. Kaplan and Sadock's Comprehensive Textbook of Psychiatry. 8th ed. Philadelphia: Lippincott Williams & Wilkins; 2005. pp. 1329–45.

Green A. Schizophrenia and comorbid substance use disorder: Effects of antipsychotics. J Clin Psychiatry 2005;66:21.

Leucht S, Corves C, Arbter D, et al. Second-generation versus first-generation antipsychotic drugs for schizophrenia: A meta-analysis. Lancet 2009;373:31.

Lieberman JA, Stroup TS, McEvoy JP, et al. Effectiveness of antipsychotic drugs in patients with chronic schizophrenia. N Engl J Med 2005;353:1209.

McEvoy JP, Meyer JM, Goff DC, et al. Prevalence of the metabolic syndrome in patients with schizophrenia: Baseline results from the clinical antipsychotic trials of intervention effectiveness (CATIE). Schizophr Res 2005;80:19.

Messias EL, Chen CY, Eaton WW. Epidemiology of schizophrenia: Review of findings and myths. Psychiatr Clin North Am 2007;30:323.

Panic Disorder

Method of
Lakshmi Ravindran, MD, and
Murray B. Stein, MD

Lifetime prevalence estimates of panic disorder (PD), with or without agoraphobia, vary worldwide from 1.6% to 2.2%, but epidemiologic studies suggest that approximately 5% of U.S. adults will meet the criteria for panic disorder in their lifetimes. Although reasons for this discrepancy are not clear, differences in study methodology, diagnostic criteria, and cultural manifestations of panic may play a role.

Diagnosis

Panic attacks, the core feature of PD, are abrupt surges in anxiety characterized by physical and cognitive symptoms (Box 1). These symptoms build to a climax, usually within 10 to 15 minutes, before eventually dissipating over the next several minutes or hours. Although isolated panic attacks are not uncommon, with a lifetime prevalence of up to 23% reported for the general population, the attacks seen in PD are recurrent, may not have a precipitant, and are accompanied by persistent concerns and changes in behavior. Characteristic concerns seen in PD include fear of having more attacks or fears about what the attacks mean for the person's medical or mental health, whereas behavioral changes usually involve avoidance of activities or places that become associated with the attack itself or with its perceived triggers.

When avoidance becomes excessive, agoraphobia ("fear of the marketplace") may be diagnosed; it can be found in up to 50% of people with PD. Individuals with agoraphobia often restrict their excursions into novel or public places for fear of experiencing and displaying panic symptoms in front of strangers without possibility

BOX 1 Typical Symptoms of a Panic Attack

Physical Symptoms
- Palpitations, pounding heart, or rapid heartbeat
- Difficulty breathing (e.g., feeling smothered)
- Choking
- Chest pain
- Sweating
- Chills or hot flushes
- Nausea or abdominal discomfort
- Difficulty swallowing
- Dizziness, lightheadedness, or feeling faint
- Paresthesias (i.e., numbness, prickling, or tingling) in the extremities or the face
- Trembling or shaking

Cognitive Symptoms
- Fear of going crazy
- Fear of dying
- Fear of losing control
- Perceptual abnormalities
- Feeling detached from one's body (i.e., depersonalization)
- Feelings of unreality regarding objects outside one's body (i.e., derealization)
- Sense of impending doom
- Feelings of paralyzing terror

of escape. In extreme cases, individuals may become housebound. If left untreated, PD may cause considerable losses in quality of life and overall function, not to mention the societal costs that result.

Lifetime prevalence rates of PD are consistently greater in females, with reports of a twofold greater risk compared with males. Although the onset of PD may occur across a wide age span, the age of onset commonly reported is late adolescence and the early 20s. The National Comorbidity Survey-Replication (NCS-R) reports a median age of onset for PD of 24 years. Rarely, PD may begin in childhood and early adolescence, although this has been associated with the subsequent development of comorbid psychiatric illness. The new onset of panic attacks in older adults (>60 years) is also atypical and more likely to be related to another psychiatric or medical illness rather than primary PD.

The risk for development of PD has a genetic component. Evidence from twin and family studies suggests the heritability of PD is approximately 40%, with first-degree relatives of probands with PD at a sevenfold greater risk of also developing PD compared with the general population. This risk is substantially higher in families in which the proband had early-onset PD.

Because genetic patterns do not fully explain the incidence of PD, a stress-diathesis model has been proposed in which environmental stressors are presumed to play a role in precipitating and maintaining the illness in at-risk individuals. Some studies have reported that up to 80% of individuals described the occurrence of a stressful life event in the year preceding the onset of PD, with most subjects believing a direct connection existed between the two events.

Several other risk factors for PD have been identified. Anxiety sensitivity is a traitlike construct referencing an individual's tendency to specifically fear the physiologic symptoms of anxiety (e.g., palpitations, shortness of breath, sweating) because of the concern that they represent indications of a harmful or negative consequence (e.g., "I am having a heart attack"). Elevated anxiety sensitivity is a risk factor for different anxiety disorders, including PD, as is the personality trait of neuroticism (i.e., tendency to readily experience negative emotions such as anger or anxiety). Other risk factors for PD include a history of heavy smoking in adolescence or a history of childhood abuse.

Psychiatric comorbidity with PD is extremely common, with more than 83% reporting one or more lifetime comorbid conditions (NCS-R), although rates are even higher with a diagnosis of PD with agoraphobia. Other anxiety disorders were identified as the most frequent lifetime comorbidity, followed by mood disorders. Much attention has been focused on comorbidity with major depressive disorder (MDD) because 34.1% of individuals with PD report a lifetime history of MDD, and there is a higher risk for PD with agoraphobia (38.5%). In one third of cases, PD precedes MDD; the reverse occurs in another third; and in the final third, the two conditions may occur together. Comorbid depression is also associated with poorer outcomes in both conditions, including worse levels of disability, greater time to response, lower rates of remission, increased risk of substance abuse or additional comorbidity, and greater suicide risk. PD itself is associated with elevated risk of suicide attempts within the past year, independent of the presence of depression. A suspected diagnosis of PD should include a thorough suicide risk assessment.

Differential Diagnosis

A variety of medical and psychiatric illnesses may manifest with panic attacks or panic-like symptoms. Differentiating between these isolated panic attacks and PD poses a diagnostic challenge. Isolated panic attacks are discrete attacks that are not followed by persistent concerns about more attacks or avoidant behavior, nor are there any resultant changes in the patient's overall level of functioning. Distinguishing PD from other disorders may be more difficult (Table 1). The frightening presence of chest pain, palpitations, or respiratory difficulties during a panic attack may be why individuals with PD present with somatic symptoms as their primary complaint.

A complete history and thorough physical examination are key in ruling out the possibility of underlying medical illness, substance intoxication, or drug withdrawal. Simple laboratory investigations may be helpful in initially ruling out serious illness. For instance, a preliminary work-up that includes a complete blood cell count, basic chemistry panel, thyroid-stimulating hormone (TSH) determination, chest radiograph, electrocardiogram or Holter monitor, and urine toxicology screen can rule out a large number of the differential diagnoses. More complex investigations, such as electroencephalography, computed tomography, or assay of urinary catecholamines, may be performed based on specific indications from the clinical examination. Atypical symptoms, new-onset symptoms in older individuals, and accompanying physical signs may suggest an underlying medical cause.

Although medical illness can mimic, precipitate, or exacerbate preexisting panic symptoms, PD may also aggravate perception of and vigilance about medical symptoms and may influence the

CURRENT DIAGNOSIS

- Presence of recurrent unexpected panic attacks
- Anticipatory anxiety about future attacks
- Fears about medical or psychological implications of an attack
- May engage in avoidance behavior
- Frequently presents with concern about somatic symptoms rather than panic
- New-onset panic attacks common in people in their late teens or early 20s but rare in older adults
- Commonly comorbid with other psychiatric disorders
- Always should assess suicide risk
- Panic attacks occurring in psychiatric disorders other than panic disorder

TABLE 1 Differential Diagnosis of Panic Attacks

Diagnostic Feature	Possible Diagnoses
Psychiatric	Mood disorder (e.g., major depression, bipolar disorder)
	Other anxiety disorder (e.g., social anxiety disorder, specific phobia, posttraumatic stress disorder, generalized anxiety disorder, obsessive compulsive disorder)
	Agoraphobia without panic disorder
	Psychotic disorder
	Somatoform disorder
	Factitious disorder
Cardiac	Angina or myocardial infarction
	Arrhythmia
	Mitral valve prolapse
	Labile hypertension
	Congestive heart failure
Endocrine	Adrenal dysfunction
	Thyroid disorder (i.e., hypothyroid or hyperthyroid)
	Hypoglycemia
	Hyperparathyroidism
Respiratory	Chronic obstructive pulmonary disease
	Asthma
	Pulmonary embolus
Neurologic	Seizure disorder (e.g., temporal lobe epilepsy)
	Pheochromocytoma
	Vestibular dysfunction
Substance intoxication	Excess caffeine use
	Psychostimulants (e.g., L-dopa, cocaine, amphetamines)
	Cannabis use
Substance withdrawal	Caffeine withdrawal
	Nicotine withdrawal
	Alcohol or sedative withdrawal
	Opioid withdrawal

outcome of physical illness. For instance, PD in patients with comorbid asthma has been associated with worse quality of life, increased use of respiratory medication, and increased hospitalization rates. The presence of comorbid PD is more frequently found in certain medical illnesses, such as respiratory disease, vestibular dysfunction, thyroid disorders (i.e., hypothyroidism and hyperthyroidism), cardiac disease, chronic pain, migraines, and irritable bowel syndrome.

Panic attacks often form part of the presentation of psychiatric illnesses, particularly of other anxiety disorders and major depression. A careful history documenting the onset, course, possible triggers, and accompanying symptoms is vital in establishing the diagnosis. For instance, the presence of situationally specific panic attacks can suggest a specific phobia or may occur as part of posttraumatic stress disorder when individuals are exposed to reminders of traumatic events, whereas new-onset panic attacks and excessive worry in a 50-year-old patient with accompanying symptoms of disturbances in sleep and appetite and with psychomotor changes may suggest MDD. Although uncommon (U.S. lifetime prevalence estimated at 0.17%–0.8%), some individuals may be diagnosed with agoraphobia without ever meeting the criteria for PD; this diagnosis remains controversial in the psychiatric community.

Treatment

Effective pharmacologic and psychotherapeutic strategies exist for the treatment of PD. Regardless of the modality chosen, aims of treatment include decreased frequency and eventual elimination of panic attacks, eradication of anticipatory anxiety and associated phobic avoidance, correction of faulty cognitions about panic, and return to optimal psychosocial function. Initial choice of treatment modality may depend on a number of factors, including patient and physician preference, severity of symptoms, presence of comorbidity, availability of a therapist, and cost. There is insufficient evidence to recommend one modality (psychotherapy versus medication) over another as a first-line intervention during the acute phase. Figure 1 provides a suggested algorithm for the acute treatment of PD.

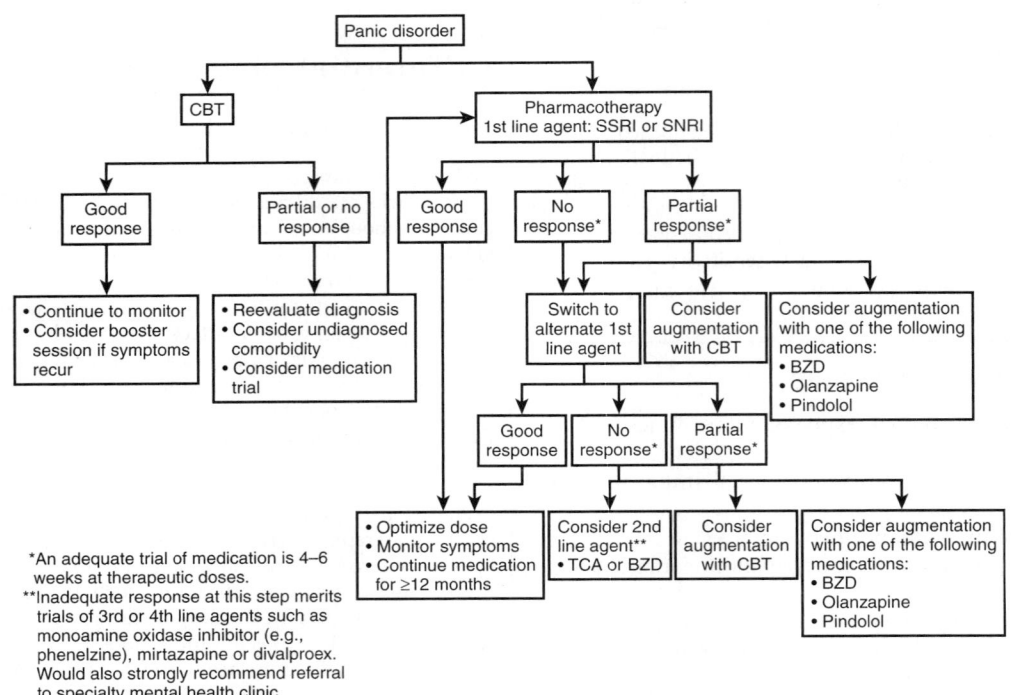

*An adequate trial of medication is 4–6 weeks at therapeutic doses.
**Inadequate response at this step merits trials of 3rd or 4th line agents such as monoamine oxidase inhibitor (e.g., phenelzine), mirtazapine or divalproex. Would also strongly recommend referral to specialty mental health clinic.

FIGURE 1. Suggested algorithm for the acute treatment of panic disorder. *Abbreviations:* BZD = benzodiazepine; CBT = cognitive-behavioral therapy; SNRI = serotonin-norepinephrine reuptake inhibitor; SSRI = selective serotonin reuptake inhibitor; TCA = tricyclic antidepressant.

PHARMACOTHERAPY

Table 2 summarizes common medications used in the treatment of PD. A meta-analysis showed that selective serotonin reuptake inhibitors (SSRIs), tricyclic antidepressants (TCAs), and benzodiazepines had similar tolerability and efficacy in the treatment of PD. However, there may be clinical rationale for the choice of one medication class over another. Because benzodiazepines have limited benefit for mood symptoms, have the potential to be abused, and may cause psychomotor side effects, antidepressants may be the preferred treatment for patients with psychiatric comorbidity (particularly depressive or anxious disorders), a history of past or present substance abuse, older patients, or those with a history for a specific antidepressant agent. In contrast, benzodiazepines may be preferred in patients with severe physical symptoms of anxiety or with comorbid bipolar disorder or where there is an urgent need for onset of action. A temporary course of benzodiazepines may be prescribed at the time of SSRI initiation to provide some symptomatic relief while the SSRI takes effect and to alleviate potential SSRI side effects that mimic anxiety (e.g., nausea, dizziness, agitation). In some cases as-needed use of benzodiazepines may be helpful, such as in patients with rare panic symptoms that are otherwise not troublesome or for periodic breakthrough symptoms. However, using benzodiazepines on a regular schedule usually is preferred. Monotherapy with β-blockers or the partial 5-HT$_{1A}$ agonist, buspirone (BuSpar),[1] has not shown efficacy for PD.

If symptom remission and return to optimal psychosocial function are achieved, clinicians should maintain patients on the optimized dose of medication for a minimum of 12 months. At that time, the clinician may attempt a very slow taper off medication (to minimize discontinuation or withdrawal symptoms) with close monitoring for symptom recurrence. A reasonable taper schedule may be 25% decreases in dose every 4 to 8 weeks, with a more gradual taper for benzodiazepines (e.g., 10% decreases every 1 to 2 weeks).

---

[1]Not FDA approved for this indication.

TABLE 2 Common Medications Used to Treat Panic Disorder

Medication (Trade Name)	Recommended Initial Dose (mg/day)	Recommended Dose Range (mg/day)
Citalopram (Celexa)[1]	5–10	20–60
Escitalopram (Lexapro)[1]	5	10–20
Fluoxetine (Prozac)	5–10	20–60
Fluvoxamine (Luvox)[1]	50	100–300
Paroxetine (Paxil)	5–10	20–60
Paroxetine (Paxil CR)	6.25	25–75
Sertraline (Zoloft)	25	50–200
Venlafaxine XR (Effexor XR)	37.5	75–225
Tricyclic Antidepressants		
Clomipramine (Anafranil)[1]	25	75–250
Imipramine (Tofranil)[1]	25	75–250
Monoamine Oxidase Inhibitors		
Phenelzine* (Nardil)[1]	15	45–90†
Benzodiazepines		
Alprazolam (Xanax)	0.25 tid	2–4‡
Lorazepam (Ativan)[1]	0.25 tid	2–8‡
Clonazepam (Klonopin)	0.25 bid	1–2‡

[1]Not FDA approved for this indication.
*Dietary restrictions required (low-tyramine diet); 2-week washout required before initiation and after termination of monoamine oxidase inhibitor trial.
†Usually administered three times daily.
‡Total daily dosage is divided across 2 to 4 doses/day.

PSYCHOTHERAPY

Among the psychotherapies available, cognitive-behavioral therapy (CBT) has the greatest evidence to support its use. Two schools of CBT for PD predominate (i.e., panic control treatment [PCT] and cognitive therapy for panic [CTP]), although many therapists use elements of both. PCT, developed by Barlow and Craske, consists of three key components. First, psychoeducation provides patients with an understanding of the pathophysiology underlying panic attacks. This allows patients to link physiologic system changes with the production of somatic symptoms (e.g., palpitations, dizziness) and accompanying anxious thoughts (e.g., "I am going to lose consciousness.") and to understand how these factors may interact to reinforce each other. Second, cognitive restructuring teaches patients to identify erroneous beliefs about panic and to use logic and reasoning to correct distorted cognitions that overestimate the threat and consequences of panic attacks. Third, patients undergo interoceptive exposure—systematic, repeated exposure to feared internal cues (i.e., physical symptoms of panic)—which facilitates progressive desensitization and normalization of these sensations. Additional relaxation strategies, such as progressive muscle relaxation or deep breathing, which are useful for lowering general anxiety, may be used. When agoraphobia is also present, graded in vivo exposure of avoided situations may be incorporated into the treatment.

CTP, developed by Clark, is based on the premise that recurrent panic attacks are common in individuals with a habitual tendency to misinterpret normal bodily sensations (e.g., dizziness) as signs of imminent, potentially harmful events (e.g., a stroke). A positive-feedback loop is created when these misperceptions result in intense anxiety, which reinforces the intensity of the physical symptoms and arousal until a panic attack results. Although more reliant on cognitive techniques to correct misappraisals of physical symptoms, CTP also emphasizes psychoeducation to explain the creation of the vicious cycle. Patients become more aware of the sequence of events leading to the panic attack through the explanation of the vicious cycle. As with PCT, patients are encouraged to logically examine the basis of their fears and realistically evaluate their likelihood. Patients are taught to develop alternative rational explanations for the symptoms. Over time, the strength of beliefs that perpetuate the cycle is weakened and may be eliminated. CTP may also involve the use of exposure-based behavioral experiments to reinforce corrective learning.

PCT and CTP are time-limited interventions accomplished over 12 to 16 1-hour sessions. Periodic "booster" sessions, usually yearly, may be of benefit in cases of symptom recurrence.

 CURRENT THERAPY

- Pharmacotherapy and cognitive-behavioral therapy (CBT) are effective for panic disorder.
- Recommended first-line antidepressant agents include selective serotonin reuptake inhibitors or venlafaxine XR (Effexor XR).
- To maximize tolerability, initiate antidepressants at 25% to 50% of the usual starting dose, but aim to reach antidepressant dose ranges similar to those used in major depression.
- To minimize side effects of agitation when antidepressants are initiated, consider temporary use of a benzodiazepine.
- Goal is symptom remission to minimize risk of relapse.
- If patients improve, treat for a minimum of 12 months.
- If discontinuing medications, use a very slow taper while monitoring closely for recurrence.
- In cases of treatment resistance, consider treatment noncompliance and undiagnosed comorbid disorders (e.g., substance use, medical illness), and consider reevaluation of the diagnosis.

Course and Prognosis

PD tends to follow a chronic course with a waxing and waning pattern. During periods of stress, the chance of recurrence or exacerbation is high. Follow-up studies of patients treated for PD suggest that at 4-year follow-up, about 30% of patients maintain remission, 40% to 50% continue to experience mild to moderate symptoms, and approximately 20% report persistent and more severe symptoms. Although CBT and pharmacotherapy appear to be relatively equivalent during the acute phase of treatment, some evidence suggests that CBT may prolong periods of remission in patients with PD but may not necessarily prevent recurrence. Among patients who were treated with CBT, 39% experienced a recurrence at 10 years, whereas among those treated with medications, the same proportion relapsed within 6 months. A meta-analysis did find an advantage for combined treatment (i.e., psychotherapy and pharmacotherapy) delivered in the acute phase over either psychotherapy or pharmacotherapy alone; however, after treatments were discontinued, no differences were observed between those who received combined treatment and those who received psychotherapy alone, although both groups did better than those on pharmacotherapy alone.

It has been suggested that rather than the duration of treatment, the level of symptom severity at the time of treatment discontinuation is the key factor in reducing recurrence, highlighting the importance of aiming for symptomatic remission. A course of CBT provided before medication discontinuation may enhance the odds of longer-term remission.

Among adults with PD, several negative prognostic factors have been identified: presence of comorbid depression, generalized anxiety, or personality disorder; longer duration of illness; greater levels of avoidance; low levels of social support; and more intense fears about social catastrophes after a panic attack (e.g., "People will laugh at me"). The presence of agoraphobia with PD has been associated with more severe symptoms, chronicity, and limited response to treatment.

REFERENCES

Barlow DH, Craske MG. Mastery of Your Anxiety and Panic. Albany, NY: Graywind Publications; 1989.

Clark DM. A cognitive approach to panic. Behav Res Ther 1986;24:461–70.

Furukawa TA, Watanabe N, Churchill R. Psychotherapy plus antidepressant for panic disorder with or without agoraphobia: Systematic review. Br J Psychiatry 2006;188:305–12.

Grant BF, Hasin DS, Stinson FS, et al. The epidemiology of DSM-IV panic disorder and agoraphobia in the United States: Results from the National Epidemiologic Survey on Alcohol and Related Conditions. J Clin Psychiatry 2006;67:363–74.

Kessler RC, Berglund P, Demler O, et al. Lifetime prevalence and age-of-onset distributions of DSM-IV disorders in the National Comorbidity Survey Replication. Arch Gen Psychiatry 2005;62:593–602.

Kessler RC, Chiu WT, Jin R, et al. The epidemiology of panic attacks, panic disorder, and agoraphobia in the National Comorbidity Survey Replication. Arch Gen Psychiatry 2006;63:415–24.

Manfro GG, Otto MW, McArdle ET, et al. Relationship of antecedent stressful life events to childhood and family history of anxiety and the course of panic disorder. J Affect Disord 1996;41:135–9.

Mitte K. A meta-analysis of the efficacy of psycho- and pharmacotherapy in panic disorder with and without agoraphobia. J Affect Disord 2005;88:27–45.

Smoller JW, Gardner-Schuster E, Covino J. The genetic basis of panic and phobic anxiety disorders. Am J Med Genet C Semin Med Genet 2008;148:118–26.

Stein MB, Goin MK, Pollack MH, et al. Practice guidelines for the treatment of patients with panic disorder, Washington, DC: American Psychiatric Publishing; 2009. Available at http://www.psychiatryonline.com/pracGuide/pracGuideTopic_9.aspx (accessed July 2009).

Physical and Chemical Injuries

Burn Treatment Guidelines

Method of
Barbara A. Latenser, MD

The initial management of the severely burned patient follows guidelines established by the American College of Surgeons (ACS). It is crucial that the patient be managed properly in the early hours after injury because the initial management of a seriously burned patient can significantly affect the long-term outcome. Optimal burn-care criteria have been established and refined by the American Burn Association (ABA) over the past 20 years.

Because of regionalization, it is common for the initial care of the seriously burned patient to occur outside the burn center. Burns are a specialized form of trauma. Therefore, the ABCs (airway, breathing, circulation) are the same as for the trauma patient: airway with cervical spine immobilization if appropriate, breathing, circulation, disability, and exposure. Also, the burn patient could be a victim of associated trauma. It is easy to be sidetracked by the obvious thermal injury. Only after the primary and secondary surveys have been performed should you evaluate the severity of the burn injury. Obtain as much information as possible regarding the incident and about the patient. An easy way to remember the information is the mnemonic AMPLE:

- Allergies
- Medications
- Past medical history
- Last meal
- Events

Universal precautions appropriate for each burn patient must be implemented by every member of the health care team.

The most commonly used guide for making an initial estimate of the second- and third-degree burns is the Rule of Nines (Figure 1). Various anatomic regions are roughly 9% of the total body surface area (TBSA) or multiples thereof. To calculate scattered burn areas, the patient's palm, including fingers, represents approximately 1% of the TBSA. A much more precise estimate of TBSA burn is provided by the Lund-Browder Classification (Figure 2). By drawing in the areas that are burned, the TBSA burn necessary for calculating resuscitation requirements can be determined. The consensus formula for the first 24 hours postburn is:

4 mL lactated Ringer's × body weight in kg × percent TBSA burn

Half the calculated amount is given in the first 8 hours and the rest over the remaining 16 hours. Patients with burns on more than 20% TBSA are prone to gastric dilatation and should have a nasogastric (NG) tube. To determine hourly urine output, a urinary catheter is necessary. Intravenous (IV) morphine sulfate is indicated for control of pain associated with burns. Intramuscular (IM) or subcutaneous (SC) routes of drug administration should not be used as absorption is erratic. To calculate fluid needs, weigh the patient or estimate the preinjury weight. Reliable peripheral veins should be used to establish an IV line. Use vessels underlying burned skin if necessary. If it is impossible to establish peripheral IV access, an intraosseous line may be necessary, and may be used in any age patient. If unable to insert an intraosseous line, central venous access may be necessary using a short, fluid infusion line made specifically for large volume resuscitations.

The burn wound should be covered with a clean, dry sheet to prevent air currents from causing pain in partial-thickness burns and to decrease fluid losses and hypothermia. Although there are many common topical antimicrobials in use, the optimal dressing prior to burn center transfer is plastic wrap such as Saran Wrap. Topical antimicrobials will just have to be washed off on arrival to the burn center, causing patient discomfort and mechanical trauma to the wound. Cold applications are appropriate only in small burns because they rapidly lead to hypothermia. Ice should never be applied because it will deepen the zone of ischemia in a thermal injury.

Escharotomies and/or fasciotomies are rarely required prior to burn center transfer, unless transfer is delayed beyond 24 hours. Patients most at risk are those with large TBSA burns, circumferential full-thickness burns, and those with electrical injury. Circumferential chest/abdominal burns may restrict ventilatory excursion. A child has a more pliable rib cage and may need an escharotomy earlier than an adult burn. If you are considering performing an escharotomy, confer with the accepting burn physician before proceeding.

So how do you know which patients should be referred to a burn center? To guide your decision making there are currently 10 burn unit referral criteria. You should have a written transfer agreement in place with a referral burn unit. The agreement should specify which patients will be referred, what stabilization is expected, who arranges transportation, and what the patient will need during transport.

Partial-Thickness Burns on More Than 10% Total Body Surface Area

Second-degree or partial-thickness burns involve a variable portion of dermis. The skin may be red, blistered, and edematous. Because sensory nerves are damaged and/or exposed, these wounds are typically extremely painful. Healing time is proportional to the depth of dermal injury. Scarring is minimal if healing occurs in 14 days or less. With closure time beyond 3 weeks, scarring will occur, the degree being greater in darker skinned individuals.

Proper fluid management is critical to the survival of patients with extensive burns. Fluid resuscitation is aimed at maintaining tissue perfusion and organ function while avoiding the complications of inadequate or excessive fluid therapy. Shock and organ failure, most commonly acute renal failure, may occur as a consequence of hypovolemia in a patient with an extensive burn who is inadequately

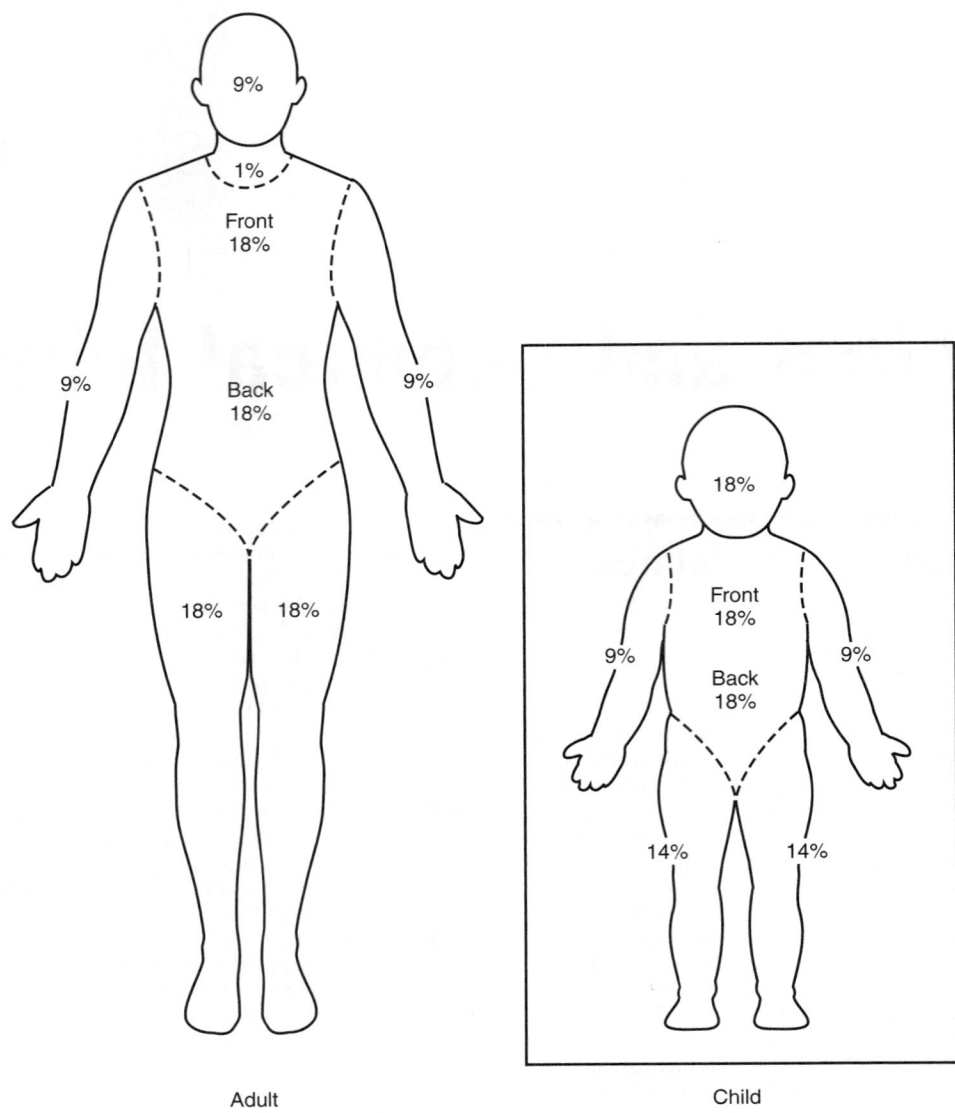

Adult

Child

FIGURE 1. Rule of Nines.

resuscitated. The increase in capillary permeability caused by the burn is greatest in the immediate postburn period and diminution in effective blood volume is most rapid at that time. A marked increase in peripheral vascular resistance accompanied by a decrease in cardiac output occurs in the first 18 to 24 hours postinjury.

In the presence of increased capillary permeability, colloid content of the resuscitation fluid exerts little influence on intravascular retention during the initial hours postburn. Crystalloid fluid is the initial resuscitation of burn patients. *Always* remember, estimates are inexact. Each patient reacts differently to burn injury and resuscitation. The actual volume of fluid infused should be varied from the calculated volume as indicated by physiologic monitoring. The patient's general condition reflects the adequacy of fluid resuscitation and should be assessed and reassessed. Mental status, anxiety, and restlessness may be signs of hypoxemia, hypovolemia, or pain.

Although urine output does not guarantee tissue perfusion, it remains the most readily available and generally reliable guide to resuscitation. Adults should produce 0.5 mL/kg per hour of urine. Children should produce 1.0 mL/kg per hour of urine, and infants 12 months or younger should produce 2.0 mL/kg per hour of urine. Oliguria is most frequently the result of inadequate fluid administration. Diuretics are contraindicated; the rate of resuscitation should be increased. During the first 24 hours, neither the hemoglobin nor the hematocrit is a reliable guide to resuscitation, and using either leads to over-resuscitation. For resuscitation failures or patients with large burns (>30% TBSA), colloid should be added. One method is hetastarch at 20 mL/kg/day for adults and 15 mL/kg/day for children. Hetastarch should be given only for 24 hours due to the increased bleeding risks.

Measuring blood pressure (BP) by a sphygmomanometer may be misleading in a burned limb with progressive edema formation. As the swelling increases, the signal becomes diminished. If fluid infusion is increased based on this finding, edema formation may be exaggerated. Even intra-arterial monitoring may be unreliable in patients with massive burns because of peripheral vasoconstriction secondary to marked elevation of catecholamines. Heart rate is also of limited usefulness in monitoring fluid therapy. The level of tachycardia depends on the normal heart rate in each child.

Burns That Involve the Face, Hands, Feet, Genitalia, Perineum, or Major Joints

Facial burns are considered a serious injury. The possibility of respiratory tract damage must be considered. Because of the rich blood supply and loose areolar tissue of the face, facial burns are associated

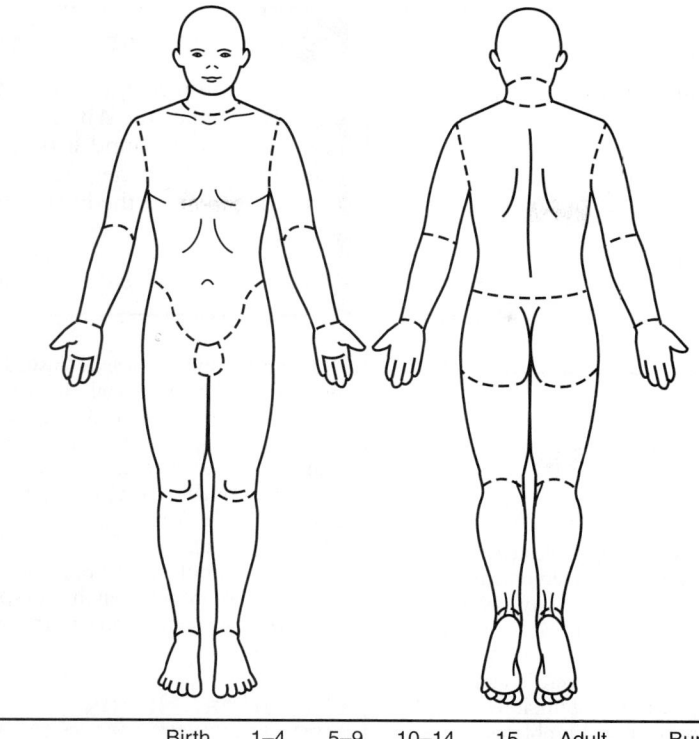

	Birth 1 yr.	1–4 yrs.	5–9 yrs.	10–14 yrs.	15 yrs.	Adult	Burn size estimate
Head	19	17	13	11	9	7	
Neck	2	2	2	2	2	2	
Anterior trunk	13	13	13	13	13	13	
Posterior trunk	13	13	13	13	13	13	
Right buttock	2.5	2.5	2.5	2.5	2.5	2.5	
Left buttock	2.5	2.5	2.5	2.5	2.5	2.5	
Genitalia	1	1	1	1	1	1	
Right upper arm	4	4	4	4	4	4	
Left upper arm	4	4	4	4	4	4	
Right lower arm	3	3	3	3	3	3	
Left lower arm	3	3	3	3	3	3	
Right hand	2.5	2.5	2.5	2.5	2.5	2.5	
Left hand	2.5	2.5	2.5	2.5	2.5	2.5	
Right thigh	5.5	6.5	8	8.5	9	9.5	
Left thigh	5.5	6.5	8	8.5	9	9.5	
Right leg	5	5	5.5	6	6.5	7	
Left leg	5	5	5.5	6	6.5	7	
Right foot	3.5	3.5	3.5	3.5	3.5	3.5	
Left foot	3.5	3.5	3.5	3.5	3.5	3.5	

Total BSAB _____

FIGURE 2. Lund-Browder Classification of Burn Size.

with extensive edema formation. To minimize this edema, keep the head of the bed elevated at 30°. Cool saline compresses on the face may also help. Careful examination of the eyes should be completed as soon as possible because the rapid onset of eyelid swelling will make this difficult. Fluorescein should be used to identify corneal injury. Chemical burns to the eyes should be rinsed with copious amounts of saline. Burns of the ears require examination of the external auditory canal and ear drum before swelling occurs.

Minor burns of the hands may result in only temporary disability and inconvenience. More extensive thermal injury may cause permanent loss of function. Monitoring the digital and palmar pulses with an ultrasonic flowmeter is the most accurate means of assessing perfusion of the tissues in the hand. The burned extremity should be elevated above the heart to minimize edema formation. Digital escharotomies are not indicated prior to transfer to a burn center. Contact the accepting burn center physician if you are concerned about the extent of the digital injury. As with burns of the upper extremity, it is important to assess the circulation and neurologic function of the feet on an hourly basis.

CURRENT DIAGNOSIS

- Maintain a high index of suspicion
- Remember the ABCs
- Rule out concomitant trauma
- Establish size and depth of burn
- Be wary of chemical and electrical burns, which may be misleading
- Establish resuscitation requirements

Abbreviations: ABC = airway with cervical spine immobilization if appropriate, breathing, circulation, disability, and exposure.

CURRENT THERAPY

- Communicate with your burn center early and often
- Remember the ABCs
- Cover the wound with Saran Wrap
- Prevent hypothermia
- Transport to the burn center

Abbreviations: ABC = airway with cervical spine immobilization if appropriate, breathing, circulation, disability, and exposure.

Third-Degree Burns in Any Age Group

A full-thickness or third-degree burn occurs with destruction of the entire epidermis and dermis, leaving no dermal elements to repopulate. A characteristic initial appearance is a waxy white color. Full-thickness injuries require emergent management. In most cases, treatment of the wound requires surgical skin grafting. Deep partial-thickness and full-thickness burns heal with severe scarring if not treated by surgical excision and skin grafting for optimal recovery. Disfigurement is common, and long-term functional problems can persist for years. There is also a high risk of infection, because an unexcised full-thickness burn behaves like an undrained abscess.

Electric Burns, Including Lightning Injury

Electrical burns can be divided into flash (typical thermal injury) and high-tension injury. The latter, caused by more than 1000 volts, produces clinically characteristic entry and exit wounds. They are usually ischemic, painless, and dry; wounds of entry may appear charred and the exit explosive. Deep-muscle injury may be present even when skin appears normal. Findings that suggest electrical injury include loss of consciousness, paralysis or mummification of an extremity, loss of peripheral pulses, flexor surface burns, myoglobinuria, serum creatine kinase (CK) more than 1000, and cardiopulmonary arrest at the scene. Electrical injuries can produce vascular thrombosis, muscle tetany causing fractures, and internal organ damage. In addition to other interventions, obtain a 12-lead electrocardiogram (ECG), cardiac enzymes, and evaluate the urine for myoglobin. If there is evidence of myoglobin from muscle damage, the urine output should be maintained at 2 mL/kg per hour until the urine grossly clears to prevent acid hematin deposition in the kidney and irreversible renal damage. Compartment pressures must be monitored. If a compartment syndrome develops, contact your burn center physician because fasciotomy may be required. The most serious immediate problem associated with electrical injuries is ventricular fibrillation, asystole, or other dysrhythmias. Life-threatening arrhythmias are treated according to advanced cardiac life support (ACLS) protocols. Survival of contact with voltage greater than 70,000 volts is uncommon.

The approximate electrical potential of a lightning bolt is 20 million volts. Lightning injury can produce an enormous spectrum of clinical symptoms and signs ranging from common (cardiac asystole, respiratory arrest, arborescent markings) to the rare (disseminated intravascular coagulation [DIC], intracerebral hemorrhage). Immediate neurologic manifestations include agitation, amnesia, loss of consciousness, or motor disturbances. The eyes are particularly vulnerable to injury from electrical current, and symptoms closely correlate with the extent of the central nervous system (CNS) injury. Vitreous hemorrhage, iridocyclitis, retinal tear, macular puncture, and retinal detachment have been reported.

Lightning injuries are not usually associated with deep burns but most often with superficial injury to the skin and underlying soft tissue called *ferning*. The feathering type of burn appears as an arborescent, branching skin marking that disappears within a few hours. Pathognomonic of lightning injury, they may be of great diagnostic value in a comatose patient. Often the respiratory arrest lasts longer than the cardiac arrest. Severely injured victims often present in asystole or ventricular fibrillation. Cardiac resuscitation may occasionally be successful; but direct brain trauma as well as blunt trauma, skull fracture, and intracranial injuries, are common in these patients. The prognosis for recovery in this group is usually poor.

Chemical Burns

Health care providers must wear protective clothing when caring for patients with potential chemical injury. The initial appearance of a chemical burn is usually deceptively benign. The severity of a chemical injury is related to the agent, concentration, volume, duration of contact, and mechanisms of action of the agent. Immediate irrigation decreases the concentration and duration of contact, reducing the severity of injury. If the agent is a powder, brush it off and irrigate with water. Irrigation should continue through emergency evaluation in the hospital and in general until evaluation in a burn center, especially for an alkali or if an unknown agent. Neutralizing agents are contraindicated because of the potential for heat generation, thereby giving the patient both a chemical and a thermal injury!

Acid burns are less severe than alkali burns. They are found in many household products including bathroom cleansers, drain cleaners, and swimming pool acidifiers. Tissue is damaged by coagulation necrosis and protein precipitation. Once a layer of eschar is formed, the burning process is self-limiting. The exception to this rule is hydrofluoric acid (HA), which is used to etch glass, make Teflon, and to remove rust. The pathogenesis of tissue damage in HA burns is distinct from other acids. HA readily crosses lipid membranes and has a potent diffusing capacity into the tissues. The molecule releases the freely dissociable fluoride ion, which produces extensive liquefactive necrosis of the soft tissues. Fluoride rapidly binds free calcium in the blood, and death from hypocalcemia may occur. Treatment is intra-arterial calcium gluconate[1] (or calcium chloride)[1] administered until the characteristic *pain out of proportion to the burn* has resolved. Even small areas of contact may result in profound hypocalcemia and death. Cardiac monitoring and frequent serum calcium determinations are indicated.

Alkalis damage tissue by liquefaction necrosis and protein denaturation. Tissue pH abnormalities may persist for 12 hours postburn, allowing deeper spread of the chemical and more severe burns. Examples would include the hydroxides, caustic sodas, and ammonium compounds found in oven cleaners, fertilizer, and cement. Wet cement damages skin in three ways: allergic dermatitis as a reaction to chromate ions, abrasions caused by the gritty nature of the cement, and as an alkali with a pH of 12.5. The ability of cement to cause such injury is not well recognized, even by professional users. With the

---

[1]Not FDA approved for this indication.

increased media interest in do-it-yourself projects, it is likely this problem will increase.

Organic compounds such as creosote and petroleum products produce contact chemical burns as well as systemic toxicity. Gasoline and diesel fuel are petroleum products that may produce a full-thickness burn that initially appears as only partial thickness. Organic compounds cause cutaneous damage by delipidation because of their fat solvent action on cell membranes. After a motor vehicle crash involving petroleum products, always look for petroleum exposure in the lower extremities, back, and buttocks. Systemic effects include elevated liver enzymes and decreased urinary output.

Inhalation Injury

Smoke inhalation injuries are the leading cause of fatalities from burn injuries, accounting for some 80% of all fire-related deaths. The major forms of inhalation injuries are carbon monoxide (CO) toxicity, injury to the upper airway, and pulmonary parenchymal damage. Each has different symptoms and signs, treatment, and prognosis. The compromised airway is protected by tracheal intubation, and respiratory failure is treated with assisted ventilation. Inhalation injury is manifested by the pathology and dysfunction that rapidly become evident in the airways, lungs, and respiratory system after inhaling the products of incomplete combustion. Patients receiving massive fluid resuscitation can develop upper airway edema with subsequent asphyxiation.

Immediate medical attention and diagnosis depend on a high index of suspicion, an appropriate history, careful examination of the upper airway, the presence of clinical symptoms, and suggestive arterial blood gases. An inhalation injury is suspected in any patient with full-thickness facial burns or with any burns combined with a history of being confined within an enclosed space. Other classic signs are soot or carbonaceous sputum, stridor or hoarseness, or blistering of the pharynx or vocal cords. Late signs include grunting, nasal flaring, retractions, wheezes, and rales. Use of prophylactic antibiotics and steroids is discouraged.

The effect of CO poisoning may be exhibited by respiratory symptoms and CNS findings such as altered level of consciousness, seizures, or coma. Cardiovascular effects include diminished cardiac output evidenced by decreased perfusion and hypotension. There is much controversy regarding hyperbaric oxygen therapy, but there are no objective data proving the efficacy of hyperbaric oxygen in CO poisoning. At this time, hyperbaric oxygen treatment for acute CO toxicity should be restricted to randomized prospective studies. The correct treatment is administering 100% oxygen, thereby decreasing the CO half-life from 4 hours to 45 minutes.

Burn Injury in Patients with Preexisting Medical Disorders That Could Complicate Management, Prolong Recovery, or Affect Mortality

Peripheral vascular disease can lead to a decrease in wound blood flow. Diabetes, through high glucose, will impede capillary flow. Optimum control of the blood glucose is needed to optimize blood flow. A local decrease in wound-tissue oxygen tension is recognized to be a major wound-healing impediment because all phases of healing are oxygen dependent, including local infection control. Most common causes are a decrease in systemic blood volume and oxygen delivery, decrease in hemoglobin saturation, eschar on the wound surface, or infection. Treatment modalities need to focus first on correction of systemic abnormalities: correct cardiovascular and lung function, correct large vessel obstructive disease impeding wound flow, aggressive wound débridement, and eliminate tissue exudates. Patients with preexisting cardiac disease are particularly sensitive to fluids and may tolerate the necessary fluid resuscitation poorly.

Any Patient With Burns and Concomitant Trauma (Such as Fractures) in Which the Burn Injury Poses the Greatest Risk of Morbidity and Mortality

In such cases, if the trauma poses the greater immediate risk, the patient may be initially stabilized in a trauma center before being transferred to a burn unit. Physician judgment will be necessary in such situations and should be in concert with the regional medical control plan and triage protocols.

Most burn-trauma publications cite a 5% frequency of burn-trauma patient. Because burn trauma is rare outside of a major conflict or disaster, most centers see only a few patients annually. By definition, child abuse falls into the burn-trauma category. It may be the burn injury that prompts relatives or neighbors to bring the child to the hospital or report the family to authority. The visibility of the injury may instigate corrective action. In a 44-month review we saw 120 cases of burns and trauma. Although motor vehicle crashes (MVCs) can result in fracture, soft tissue, and thermal injury, unique to this burn-trauma population was that the MVC injury was frequently a result of assault. With the graying of America, elder abuse may become a larger societal problem.

Burned Children in Hospitals Without Qualified Personnel or Equipment for the Care of Children

Each year more than 2500 children die and 10,000 more sustain permanent disability from thermal injury. Children are not just little adults! They respond differently than adults to severe trauma, maintaining normal vital signs longer but decompensating rapidly. Because of the smaller cross-sectional diameter of the pediatric airway, it takes much less edema to compromise a pediatric airway. If intubation is required, the most experienced pediatric airway manager should intubate the child because repeated attempts may create sufficient airway edema as to cause obstruction. Anatomical airway differences make intubation by the inexperienced even more difficult.

The greater surface area per unit of body mass of children necessitates the administration of relatively greater amounts of resuscitation fluid. The surface area/body mass relationship of the child also defines a lesser intravascular volume per unit surface area burned. This makes the burned child more susceptible to fluid overload and hemodilution. Hypoglycemia may occur if the limited glycogen stores of the child are rapidly exhausted by the early postburn elevation of circulating levels of steroids and catecholamines. Infants should receive maintenance fluids with 5% dextrose in addition to the resuscitation fluids outlined in the consensus formula. Children younger than 2 years of age have disproportionally thin skin so that exposures that would produce only partial-thickness burns in older patients produce full-thickness injuries. Children have a relatively small muscle mass, hampering intrinsic heat generation. Children younger than 6 months of age are unable to shiver and thus are even more prone to develop hypothermia.

Stress for the burned child not only includes the body surface area (BSA) burn and the pain that is involved but also the separation from parents and loved ones. This escalates especially if the parents were also burned in the fire. Emergency management of each pediatric burn patient requires an individual care plan. Early consultation with the burn center physician is advised.

Burn Injury in Patients Who Will Require Special Social, Emotional, and/or Long-Term Rehabilitative Intervention

Failure to recognize the thermal manifestations of child abuse not only negates protection of the child but predicates potential lethal injury. Awareness of the patterns of abuse, the behavior patterns of the parents, and the physical manifestations will protect the child by early recognition and reporting. Physical child abuse victims frequently present with thermal injuries of varying degrees. The history of injury should correlate with the physical findings. The history also becomes important in identifying repetitious hospital visits for accidental injury. Not infrequently, the hospital visits will be made at different hospitals to avoid disclosure and identification.

The events leading to an injury are extremely important in the initial evaluation of an infant or child. *Always* consider the potential for child abuse. The incidence of child abuse is approximately 10% of all children presenting to an emergency department (ED), with a mortality rate less than 1%. Abused children present with a higher median Injury Severity Score, more severe injuries of the head and integument, longer hospital lengths of stay, and a high mortality rate.

A burn of any magnitude can be a serious injury. Health care providers must be able to assess the injuries rapidly and develop a priority-based plan of care. The plan of care is determined by the type, extent, and degree of burn as well as by available resources.

Burn care is complex. It involves a multisystem assessment and appropriate intervention. The first 24 hours of management are perhaps the most critical for patient survival. Burn centers provide optimal care in a cost-effective, multidisciplinary manner. Every health care provider must know how and when to contact the closest burn center. If the attending physician determines that the patient should be treated at the burn center, the extent of treatment provided at the referring hospital—and the method of transport to the burn center—should be decided in consultation with the burn center physician. A complete list of verified burn centers is available at http://ameriburn.org.

REFERENCES

Advanced Burn Life Support Course. American Burn Association, 625 N. Michigan Ave., Suite 1530, Chicago, IL. 60611. 2001.

American College of Surgeons Committee on Trauma. Resources for optimal care of the injured patient: 1999. Chicago: American College of Surgeons; 1999.

Andrews CJ, Cooper MA, Darveniza M, Mackerras D, editors. Lightning injuries: Electrical, medical, and legal aspects. Boca Raton, Fla: CRC Press; 1992.

Burd A. Hydrofluoric acid—revisited. Burns 2004;30(7):720–2.

Chang DC, Knight V, Ziegfeld S, et al. The tip of the iceberg for child abuse: The critical roles of the pediatric trauma service and its registry. J Trauma 2004;57(6):1189–98.

Heimbach DM. Regionalization of burn care: A concept whose time has come. J Burn Care Rehabil 2003;24(3):173–4.

Latenser BA, Iteld L. Smoke inhalation injury. Seminars in Respiratory and Critical Care Medicine 2001;22(1):13–22.

Luce EA, editor. Clinics in plastic surgery. An international quarterly. Burn care and management. Philadelphia: WB Saunders; 2000.

Varghese TK, Kim AW, Kowal-Vern A, Latenser BA. Frequency of burn-trauma patients in an urban setting. Arch Surg 2003;138:1292–6.

High-Altitude Illness

Method of
James A. Litch, MD, DTMH

Decreased partial pressure of oxygen at high altitude results in pronounced physiologic responses that range from beneficial to pathologic. Slow ascent normally leads to acclimatization. High-altitude illness is a collective term for a cluster of acute clinical syndromes that are a direct consequence of rapid ascent to high altitude above 2500 m. The acute syndromes affecting the brain include acute mountain sickness (AMS) and high-altitude cerebral edema (HACE). The acute syndrome affecting the lung is high-altitude pulmonary edema (HAPE). All unacclimatized sojourners to high altitude are potentially at risk. The characteristic cerebral and pulmonary abnormalities are not subtle, but when unrecognized or ignored, they may progress to death. Each year millions travel to high-altitude locations on every continent, resulting in morbidity and mortality with associated economic consequences.

Normal Acclimatization

It is not uncommon for normal acclimatization of novice healthy visitors to high altitude to cause concern that they are experiencing a health problem. Normal acclimatization includes immediate hyperventilation, shortness of breath with moderate excursion, and a decreased work capacity. These are followed by diuresis, disturbed sleep (including periodic breathing), and peripheral/facial edema. It is important to recognize the signs of normal acclimatization so reassurance and education may be appropriately provided.

Incidence and Risk Factors

Determinants of whether high-altitude illness will occur are individual susceptibility, rate of ascent, altitude reached, and sleep altitude. Incidence rates of AMS reported in literature are difficult to compare because of variability in methodology and rates of ascent. Reported incident figures for AMS following ascent by hiking, vehicle, or flying range from 10% to 40% at 2700 to 3000 m, and from 40% to 95% at 3800 to 4000 m. HACE and HAPE are both far less common than mild AMS, but actual incident rates are unavailable. HAPE can occur as low as 2500 m. HACE is rare below 3600 m. Most cases of HACE and HAPE are preceded by AMS.

Risk factors for altitude illness include a history of previous high-altitude illness, residence at altitude below 1000 m, physical exertion, and preexisting cardiopulmonary conditions. Traveling in a large group presents a risk because a tight itinerary often does not allow time for acclimatization, and members are reluctant to declare symptoms for fear of being left behind. Children appear to carry the same risk for altitude illness as adults, but persons over 50 years of age seem less susceptible, possibly because of a more cautious ascent profile. There appears to be little or no gender difference for AMS, but women may be less susceptible to HAPE. Heavy physical exertion at exceedingly high altitude appears to be an important risk factor for HAPE. Rapid ascent, especially by flying or driving to altitude, places sojourners at risk for altitude illnesses.

Prevention of Altitude Illnesses

Gradual ascent to altitude over several days to allow for acclimatization reduces the likelihood of acute mountain sickness. Ascent rates of less than 300 m per day at altitudes of more than 2500 m is a common recommendation; but individuals will still experience altitude illness when abiding to this recommendation. However, the critical understanding to prevent serious life-threatening altitude illness (HAPE and HACE) is to halt further ascent until symptoms resolve.

Medications are available to help prevent the symptoms of AMS when rapid ascent (<24 hours) to altitudes more than 3000 m is anticipated, or for those with a past history of AMS with a similar ascent profile. These agents are started the evening before ascent and continued for 2 to 3 days. The most commonly used medications are acetazolamide (Diamox) (125 to 250 mg twice a day), acetaminophen[1] (325 mg four times a day), or aspirin[1] (325 mg three

---

[1]Not FDA approved for this indication.

times a day). Acetazolamide (Diamox) is particularly useful because it actually improves oxygenation, has a positive impact on the quality of sleep at high altitude, and is effective for periodic breathing that occurs during sleep. However, these medications do not protect against the development of life threatening altitude illness: HAPE and HACE. Other medications have been suggested for use in preventing altitude illness. Randomized double blinded placebo-controlled trails of ginkgo biloba[1] and acetazolamide (Diamox) have shown no benefit from ginkgo biloba over placebo, and reduced incidence and severity of AMS symptoms from acetazolamide (Diamox). Dexamethasone (Decadron),[1] a potent steroid, is generally best avoided as a prevention measure against AMS during ascent so it may be used, if needed, for treatment of HACE along with descent.

Nifedipine (Adalat, Procardia)[1] has been studied for use in prevention of HAPE and found to be of benefit for persons with a history of recurrent HAPE. Studies are under way to evaluate sildenafil citrate (Viagra),[1] an agent that selectively lowers pulmonary artery pressure, in the prevention of HAPE. In addition, inhaled salmeterol (Serevent)[1] has been found effective for the prevention of HAPE in a small group of climbers who had previously shown susceptibility to HAPE. However, these high-risk individuals would do far better with cautious gradual ascent, rather than relying on a medication with limited effect for a life-threatening condition.

Several nonmedication measures that can prevent or ameliorate symptoms of high-altitude illness include the following:

- Begin a high-carbohydrate diet one or two days before the climb and maintain during the ascent
- Adapt plans to realistically reflect the decreased work capacity at high altitude
- Reschedule or slow the ascent should an upper respiratory or other active infection present
- Avoid overexertion during ascent by maintaining a reasonable pace and not overloading with nonessential gear
- Maintain adequate hydration on the climb to offset increased fluid loss at altitude
- Avoid nonessential medications and remedies
- Provide good ventilation for camp stoves used in confined places
- Allow for several days of altitude exposure the week prior to ascent to high altitude

Acute Mountain Sickness and High-Altitude Cerebral Edema

AMS is defined as a headache in the setting of recent altitude gain and typical symptoms which include anorexia, nausea, vomiting, insomnia, dizziness, or fatigue (Current Diagnosis box). Symptoms are nonspecific, and there is an absence of physical findings. The differential diagnosis is extensive and other conditions should be considered (Box 1). Pulse oximetry values may be high, normal, or low for the altitude and do not correlate to severity of symptoms. A careful and detailed history is essential to steer diagnostic decision making. Often in outdoor settings multiple conditions can be present such as AMS and dehydration. Rapid resolution of symptoms during treatment with oxygen is very specific to AMS. Early recognition of AMS is a key principle in remote areas with limited support.

AMS is not life threatening, but ignoring it can be. Progressive neurologic deterioration may occur over hours or days as dangerous collections of fluid develop in the brain leading to HACE. HACE presents with truncal ataxia, confusion, and hallucination in the setting of recent altitude gain. The period of time from initial ataxia and confusion to onset of coma may be as little as 8 to 12 hours. If descent or oxygen supplementation is not accomplished within hours, coma and death can ensue from brain herniation. A presumptive and/or rigid diagnosis of HACE in the setting of progressive neurologic

| BOX 1 | Differential Diagnosis of High-Altitude Illnesses |

Acute Mountain Sickness and High-Altitude Cerebral Edema
- Alcohol intoxication
- Brain tumor
- CO inhalation
- CNS infection
- Cerebral vascular accident
- Dehydration
- Diabetic ketoacidosis
- Exhaustion
- Hypoglycemia and insulin shock
- Hyponatremia
- Hypothermia
- Migraine
- Narcotics
- Poisoning
- Psychosis
- Sedatives overdose
- Seizures
- Subarachnoid hemorrhage
- Transient ischemic attack

High-Altitude Pulmonary Edema
- Adult respiratory distress syndrome
- Asthma
- Bronchitis
- Congestive heart failure
- Myocardial infarction
- Pneumonia (infection or aspiration)
- Poisoning
- Pulmonary embolus
- Respiratory failure

Abbreviations: CNS = central nervous system; CO = carbon monoxide.

deterioration has led to tragic situations when other life-threatening conditions were actually present (see Box 1). Details of the initial presentation, response to immediate descent/supplemental oxygen, and recognition of additional signs can guide clinical decision making while maintaining a high index of suspicion for other neurologic conditions. Patients with persistent symptoms after descent require prompt evacuation and thorough evaluation. In addition, HAPE may develop concurrently with HACE resulting in shortness of breath while at rest and a further reduction of oxygen delivery to the body.

Definitive diagnosis is available using imaging studies such as CT and MRI. However, these have limited application, because the condition should have greatly improved from oxygen/descent before the opportunity presents to obtain the study. Neuroimaging demonstrates vasogenic edema in individuals with moderate to severe AMS or HACE.

Management of AMS is directed at limiting further hypoxia by halting ascent, and providing additional oxygen should symptoms persist or progress to HACE. Acetazolamide (Diamox) is helpful for the treatment of AMS. For the management of HACE improved oxygenation is the definitive treatment. There are several methods of oxygen delivery: (1) descent, (2) supplemental oxygen via cylinder or concentrator, and/or (3) portable hyperbaric bag. These may be combined or applied in series depending on resources, location, and logistic support. Concomitant pharmacologic treatment with dexamethasone (Decadron)[1] and acetazolamide (Diamox) aid recovery. Persons with suspected HACE who do not rapidly recover during

---

[1] Not FDA approved for this indication.

[1] Not FDA approved for this indication.

CURRENT DIAGNOSIS

- Acute mountain sickness—In the setting of a recent gain in altitude, the presence of headache and at least one of the following: GI symptoms (anorexia, nausea, or vomiting), fatigue or weakness, dizziness or light-headedness, or difficulty sleeping
- High-altitude cerebral edema—In the setting of a recent gain in altitude, the presence of a change in mental status and/or ataxia in a person with AMS, or the presence of both mental status change and ataxia in a person without AMS
- High-altitude pulmonary edema—In the setting of a recent gain in altitude, the presence of at least two of the following symptoms: dyspnea at rest, cough, weakness or decreased exercise performance, chest tightness, or congestion; and two of the following signs: rales or wheezing in at least one lung field, central cyanosis, tachypnea, or tachycardia

*The Lake Louise Consensus on the Definition and Quantification of Altitude Illness.
Abbreviations: AMS = acute mountain sickness; GI = gastrointestinal.

treatment or those with focal neurologic deficits should be hospitalized and undergo comprehensive neurologic evaluation including magnetic resonance imaging (MRI). The Current Therapy box summarizes management of HACE.

High-Altitude Pulmonary Edema

HAPE is defined as noncardiogenic edema resulting from hypoxia-induced changes in the pulmonary circulation. HAPE is commonly preceded by AMS, and 20% of individuals with HAPE develop HACE. Early symptoms of HAPE include decreased exercise performance beyond that expected for the altitude, often accompanied with a dry cough (see Current Diagnosis Box). Progression is rapid with even minimal continued physical activity without descent. The hallmark of progression requiring prompt action is dyspnea at rest. Rales are present at this stage. Resting pulse oximetry reveals below-normal oxygen saturation for the altitude. Tachypnea and tachycardia beyond that expected for the altitude also are present. Pink, frothy sputum develops late in the illness. Early diagnosis is important because progression of the illness further limits oxygenation and worsens the degree of hypoxemia causing the condition.

HAPE is a life-threatening emergency; immediate improvement in oxygenation is critical to arrest the progression and is the definitive treatment. In medical facilities high-flow supplemental oxygen while at rest and sitting in an upright position should be initiated immediately during the initial assessment of the patient. Response may be assessed by pulse oximetry and resting respiratory rate. Despite prompt improvement during the first few hours of treatment, maintenance of oxygenation (oxygen saturation greater than 90%) with low-flow supplemental oxygen and rest is often required for 2 to 3 days unless descent is achieved. For vacationers to high-altitude resort areas, this oxygen requirement can be maintained outside the hospital using a cylinder or concentrator as an alternative to descent for informed individuals that wish to remain in the locale of family and friends. A continued requirement of high-flow oxygen of 4 to 5 L per minute or more to maintain oxygen saturation greater than 90%, or concurrent HACE, requires hospitalization. Antibiotics are indicated if infection is suspected. Endotracheal intubation and mechanical ventilation are rarely indicated. The differential diagnosis is extensive, and a high index of suspicion for other conditions should be maintained throughout the treatment course (see Box 1).

CURRENT THERAPY

Acute Mountain Sickness

- Halt ascent, do not exceed light activity level, oral hydration.
- Administer acetazolamide (Diamox) 250 mg PO bid.
- Administer analgesics and antiemetics.
- If readily available, administer oxygen 1 to 2 L per minute as needed to resolve symptoms.
- If no improvement after 24 hours, descend to altitude where person last slept without symptoms until fully recovered.

High-Altitude Cerebral Edema

- Administer oxygen 2 to 4 L per minute.
- In remote mountain areas, prepare for immediate descent of at least 600 m by ground or aircraft, and if oxygen unavailable, use portable hyperbaric chamber.
- Monitor at all times, and replenish/maintain hydration as needed.
- Administer dexamethasone (Decadron) 8 mg IM, IV, or PO × 1 dose, then 4 mg q6h.
- Administer acetazolamide (Diamox) 250 mg PO bid.

High-Altitude Pulmonary Edema

- Administer oxygen initially 4 to 6 L per minute, then titrate to keep arterial oxygen saturation more than 90%.
- In remote mountain areas, prepare for immediate descent of at least 600 m by ground or aircraft; and if oxygen unavailable, use portable hyperbaric chamber on incline with head end elevated.
- Sit upright at 45 degree angle, strict rest, and monitor at all times.
- Administer nifedipine (Adalat, Procardia) 10 mg PO initially, then 30 mg extended release q12h *IF* oxygen unavailable *AND* IV fluid resuscitation immediately available.
- Administer salmeterol (Serevent) inhaler, 1 puff bid *OR* albuterol (Proventil) inhaler, 4 to 6 puffs q4h.
- Administer dexamethasone (Decadron) 8 mg IM, IV or PO × 1 dose, then 4 mg q6h *IF* suspect or unsure if HACE is also present.

Abbreviations: bid = twice daily; IM = intramuscular; IV = intravenous; PO = orally; q = every.

In remote areas oxygen may be administered by:

- Descent with minimal exertion
- Supplemental oxygen via cylinder or concentrator
- Portable hyperbaric bag placed on an incline to keep the head elevated

Because of a lack of equipment, immediate descent may be the only option available. In late stages more than one oxygen modality may need to be employed concurrently. These efforts place great strain on the limited resources of groups traveling in remote areas. It is common for the shared concern and cooperation among group members (tourists/staff/porters) to disintegrate or for groups to discover that they are woefully unequipped to handle HAPE. As a result fatal outcomes are common when HAPE presents in remote settings.

Pharmacologic treatment is directed at agents that reduce pulmonary artery pressure and thereby may improve oxygenation in HAPE. Medications including nifedipine (Adalat, Procardia),[1] nitric oxide

[1]Not FDA approved for this indication.

(INO$_{max}$),[1] epoprostenol (Flolan),[1] and sildenafil (Viagra)[1] have been studied for use in treatment of HAPE. Current clinical experience warrants consideration of nifedipine (Adalat, Procardia) as an adjunct treatment for HAPE when immediate supplemental oxygen is unavailable or descent is delayed. Vascular access and intravenous (IV) fluid should be immediately available if nifedipine (Adalat, Procardia) is administered because patients are often intravascularly depleted and risk a severe hypotensive event that could be devastating in the setting of concomitant HACE. Sildenafil citrate (Viagra)[1] can also selectively lower pulmonary artery pressure with less effect on systemic blood pressure, and is under study for the treatment of HAPE. Inhaled β-agonists, salmeterol (Serevent),[1] and albuterol (Proventil)[1] are currently under study for treatment of HAPE because β-agonists increase the clearance of fluid from the alveolar space and might lower pulmonary artery pressure. The Current Therapy box summarizes the management of HAPE.

Reascent After Altitude Illness

Mild AMS is common and indicative of an ascent rate that is too rapid for a given person. Further ascent should not resume until full resolution of all symptoms. Future trips with similar ascent profiles warrant consideration of prophylaxis with acetazolamide (Diamox).

After episodes of HACE and HAPE resolve fully, reascent has been successful for many patients, some reaching exceptionally high summits. Caution is warranted, however. Persons should be advised to ascend more slowly and to recognize and act appropriately for early signs of altitude illness. Persons with multiple episodes of HAPE may benefit during subsequent ascent from prophylaxis with nifedipine (Adalat, Procardia)[1] and potentially with salmeterol (Serevent)[1] while stressing the value of cautious gradual ascent over medication. Recurrent HAPE or HAPE occurring at altitudes below 3000 m should prompt evaluation to rule out cardiac or pulmonary shunts, valvular disease, or pulmonary hypertension.

---

[1]Not FDA approved for this indication.

REFERENCES

Bartsch P, Merki B, Hofstetter D, et al. Treatment of acute mountain sickness by simulated descent: A randomized controlled trial. BMJ 1993;306:1098–101.

Chow T, Browne V, Heileson HL, et al. Ginkgo biloba and acetazolamide prophylaxis for acute mountain sickness: A randomized placebo-controlled trial. Arch Intern Med 2005;165:296–301.

Consensus Group. The Lake Louise consensus on the definition and quantification of altitude illness. In: Sutton JR, Coates G, Houston CS, editors. Hypoxia and mountain medicine. Burlington, VT: Queen City Printers; 1992. p. 327–30.

Larson EB, Roach RC, Schoene RB, Hornbein TF. Acute mountain sickness and acetazolamide—Clinical efficacy and effect on ventilation. JAMA 1982;248:328–32.

Litch JA. Endotracheal intubation and mechanical ventilation following respiratory arrest from high altitude pulmonary edema. West J Med 1999;170 (3):174–6.

Litch JA, Basnyat B, Zimmerman M. Subarachnoid hemorrhage at high altitude. West J Med 1997;167(3):180–1.

Litch JA, Bishop RA. Re-ascent following resolution of high altitude pulmonary edema (HAPE). High Alt Med Biol 2001;2(1):53–5.

Litch JA, Bishop RA. Oxygen concentrators for the delivery of supplemental oxygen in remote high altitude areas. Wilderness Environ Med 2000;11 (3):189–91.

Oelz O, Maggiorini M, Ritter M, et al. Prevention and treatment of high altitude pulmonary edema by a calcium channel blocker. Int J Sports Med 1992;13(Suppl. 1):S65–8.

Pollard AJ, Niermeyer S, Barry P, et al. Children at high altitude: An international consensus statement by an ad hoc committee of the International Society of Mountain Medicine. High Alt Med Biol 2001;2(3):389–403.

Rabold MB. Dexamethasone for prophylaxis and treatment of acute mountain sickness. West J Med 1992;3:54–60.

Sartori C, Allemann Y, Duplain H, et al. Salmeterol for the prevention of high-altitude pulmonary edema. N Engl J Med 2002;346(21):1631–6.

Disturbances Caused by Cold

Method of
Frederick K. Korley, MD, and
Jerrold B. Leikin, MD

Accidental Hypothermia

Hypothermia is classically defined as a reduction in the body's core temperature below 95.0°F (35.0°C). Most reported cases of hypothermia are due to exposure to low ambient temperatures (accidental hypothermia). Other causes of hypothermia include sepsis, severe hypothyroidism, diabetic ketoacidosis, multisystem trauma, and prolonged cardiac arrest.

EPIDEMIOLOGY

Risk factors for developing hypothermia include extremes of age (the elderly might not be able to remove themselves from cold environments, and young children lose heat more rapidly due to their increased total body surface area), major trauma, homelessness, psychiatric illness, and drug and alcohol abuse (Box 1). Cold-related deaths also are reported in military combatants and outdoor winter sports participants. Several drugs and chemicals can predispose to hypothermia (Box 2). Alcohol is the most common intoxicant associated with hypothermia due to its ability to cause cutaneous vasodilation, impairment of shivering, and impairment of adaptive behavior.

Between 1979 and 2002, a total of 16,555 deaths in the United States, an average of 689 per year, were attributed to exposure to low environmental temperatures. In 2002, of the 646 hypothermia-related deaths reported, 66% occurred in male patients, 52% of all decedents were aged 65 years or younger, 45% of the deaths occurred among white male patients, and 14% occurred among black male patients. The states of Alaska, New Mexico, North Dakota, and Montana had the largest overall death rates due to hypothermia in 2002. The lowest recorded core temperature in a pediatric survivor of accidental hypothermia is 57.9°F (14.4°C) and the lowest is 56.7°F (13.7°C) in an adult survivor.

PATHOPHYSIOLOGY

The normal range of human core temperature is 97.5°F (36.4°C) to 99.5°F (37.5°C). Humans are thus warm-blooded and are normally able to maintain their body temperature by heat-generating mechanisms and heat-conserving behavior. These compensatory responses, however, can be overwhelmed under extreme environmental conditions, leading to hypothermia.

The anterior hypothalamus coordinates the nonshivering heat conservation and dissipation mechanisms, and the posterior hypothalamus coordinates shivering thermogenesis. Heat loss usually occurs by four mechanisms: About 55% to 65% of heat is lost by radiation, 25% to 30% by evaporation from the skin and respiratory tract, and 10% to 15% by conduction and convection. The amount of heat lost via conduction is markedly increased in cold-water immersion (by about 32 times). Each organ system is affected uniquely by hypothermia.

The Cardiovascular System

One of the initial heat-conserving mechanisms is peripheral vasoconstriction to decrease blood flow to the skin. There are also initial increases, in heart rate and blood pressure due to a catecholamine surge. At core temperatures below 82.4°F (28.0°C), bradycardia can occur. The myocardium also becomes irritable, predisposing it to arrhythmias. Atrial arrhythmias can occur with a slow ventricular response and they can precede ventricular arrhythmias and asystole at core temperatures below 77.0°F (25.0°C). The characteristic Osborn

BOX 1 Factors Predisposing to Hypothermia or Frostbite

Physiologic

Decreased Heat Production
- Age extremes (infants, elderly)
- Dehydration or nalnutrition
- Diaphoresis or hyperhidrosis
- Endocrinologic insufficiency
- Hypoxia
- Insufficient fuel
- Overexertion
- Physical conditioning
- Prior cold injury
- Trauma (multisystem or extremity)

Increased Heat Loss

Burns
- Dermatologic malfunction
- Cold infusions
- Emergency resuscitation
- Poor acclimatization or conditioning
- Shock
- Vascular diseases

Impaired Thermoregulation
- Central nervous system trauma or disease
- Metabolic disorders
- Pharmacologic or toxicologic agents
- Sepsis
- Spinal cord injury

Psychological
- Fatigue
- Fear or panic
- Hunger
- Intense concentration on tasks
- Intoxicants
- Mental status or attitude
- Peer pressure

Environmental
- Altitude with or without associated conditions
- Ambient temperature or humidity
- Duration of exposure
- Heat loss (conductive, evaporative, radiative, convective)
- Quantity of exposed surface area
- Wind chill factor

Mechanical
- Constricting or wet clothing or boots
- Inadequate insulation
- Immobility or cramped positioning

or J waves (a hump seen at the QRS-ST junction) may be seen on the electrocardiogram (ECG) at core temperatures below 89.6°F (32.0°C).

The Renal System

Renal blood flow is increased by peripheral vasoconstriction, leading to cold-induced diuresis. Antidiuretic hormone activity is usually inhibited. This results in intravascular volume depletion, subsequent vasodilation, to increase renal blood flow, and ultimately acute renal failure.

The Respiratory System

At core temperatures below 82.4°F (28°C), minute ventilation is reduced; bronchorrhea can occur, with a loss of cough and gag reflexes leading to an increased risk for aspiration. Apnea can then result.

The Central Nervous System

Cerebral metabolism is depressed 6% to 7% per 1°C decrease in core temperature. Cerebrovascular autoregulation remains intact until below 77.0°F (25.0°C), which helps maintain cortical blood flow. Electroencephalographic activity is clearly not prognostic, and it silences around 66.2°F to 68.0°F (19.0°C–20.0°C).

CLINICAL PRESENTATION

Accidental hypothermia is classified as mild at body temperatures of 90°F (32.2°C) to 95°F (35°C), moderate at body temperatures of 82.4°F (28.0°C) to 90°F (<32.2°C), or severe at body temperatures less than 28°C (82.4°F).

In general, a patient's symptoms depend on the severity of the temperature drop. Patients with mild hypothermia can develop vigorous shivering and cold diuresis. Those with moderate hypothermia can have a paradoxical decrease in shivering, slurred speech, hyporeflexia, and confusion. They may have Osborn J waves on the ECG. They are also at risk for intravascular thrombosis. Splanchnic vasoconstriction, gastric erosions, hepatic necrosis, and pancreatitis can occur.

During severe hypothermia, shivering gives way to rigor, minute ventilation decreases, and heart rate and cardiac output decrease. Cardiac instability can be seen at this stage and can manifest in the form of arrhythmias, heart blocks, and eventually asystole. Neurologically, the patient's mental status declines. He or she might attempt to undress (paradoxical undressing) and might respond only to painful stimuli, have decreased gag reflexes, and eventually become apenic. Generally, at about 68.0°F (20.0°C), patients become totally neurologically unresponsive, lose corneal and ocular reflexes, and can have a flat electroencephalograph (EEG).

EMERGENCY DEPARTMENT EVALUATION

Typically, the source of hypothermia is revealed from the patient's history; however, it is very important to rule out secondary causes of hypothermia such as sepsis, hypothyroidism, central nervous system (CNS) lesions, and hypoglycemia among others. All patients arriving in the emergency department with hypothermia need a complete evaluation to rule out traumatic injuries and drug or toxin ingestion or overdose.

As in all resuscitation, attention should be paid to the ABCs (airway, breathing and circulation). Respiratory failure should be treated with endotracheal intubation and mechanical ventilation. Hypotension can be treated initially with warmed fluids. Placing the patient in a warm environment, removing all cold and wet clothes, and remembering to cover up the patient after he or she has been exposed should help avoid further heat loss.

The temperature should be confirmed by checking a core temperature (e.g., rectal, bladder, or esophageal), using a thermometer capable of recording very low temperatures. Patients should be placed on a cardiac monitor and an ECG should be obtained. Laboratory testing is especially useful in the postresuscitative period when complications begin. Laboratory tests should include a complete blood count (CBC), a chemistry panel, creatine phosphokinase (CPK) to evaluate for rhabdomyolysis, a coagulation profile, blood type and screen, an arterial blood gas (ABG), and a drug screen. A Foley catheter should be placed to access urinary output.

REWARMING STRATEGIES

There are several methods of rewarming. The method of choice usually depends on the severity of hypothermia. During rewarming, the patient should be placed on a cardiac monitor with frequent measurements of blood pressure and temperature (via a rectal probe) for easy detection of complications of rewarming such as rewarming-related hypotension, arrhythmias, and core temperature after-drop.

BOX 2   Drugs and Chemicals That Can Cause Hypothermia

Medicinals

Acetaminophen (Tylenol)
Amphotericin B (Fungizone)
Azithromycin (Zithromax)
Baclofen (Lioresal)
Barbiturates
Benzodiazepines
β-Adrenergic blocking agents
Bethanechol (Urecholine)
Biperiden (Akineton)
Bromocriptine (Parlodel)
Carbamazepine (Tegretol)
Chloral hydrate (Noctec)
Chlorpromazine (Thorazine)
Clonidine (Catapres)
Colchicine
Diltiazem (Cardizem)
Ethchlorvynol (Placidyl)
Ethyl alcohol
Fenoprofen (Nalfon)
Fluphenazine (Prolixin)
Fosphenytoin (Cerebyx)
Gallium nitrate (Ganite)
Glutethimide (Doriden)[2]
Guanabenz (Wytensin)
Guanfacine (Tenex)
Haloperidol (Haldol)
Heroin
Ibuprofen (Advil, Motrin)
Insulin preparations
Interferon-β-1 b (Betaseron)
Lithium (Eskalith, Lithobid)
Loxapine (Loxapac, Loxitane)
Magnesium sulfate
Maprotiline (Ludiomil)
Mefenamic acid (Ponstel)
Methyldopa (Aldomet)
Methyprylon (Noludar)[2]
Moricizine (Ethmozine)

Morphine sulfate
Naphazoline (Naphcon)
Omeprazole (Prilosec)
Oxymetazoline (Afrin)
Phencyclidine
Phenol
Phenytoin (Dilantin)
Pilocarpine (Salagen)
Prazosin (Minipress)
Propoxyphene (Darvon)
Rauwolfia serpentine
Reserpine
Salicylate
Terazosin (Hytrin)
Tetracycline (Sumycin)
Tetrahydrozoline (Visine, Opti-Clear)
Thioridazine (Mellaril)
Tretinoin (Topical) (Retin A)
Tricyclic antidepressants
Valproic acid and derivatives
   (Depakene)
Zinc sulfate

Nonmedicinals

Acrylamide
Aldicarb
Amitraz
Barium
Bromophos
Carbon disulfide
Carbon monoxide
Chloralose
Chlorfenvinphos
Chloryrifos
Coumaphos
Cyanide
Diazinon
Dichlorvos

Dicrotophos
Dioxathion
Disulfoton
Ether
Ethion
Fensulfothion
Fenthion
Hexachlorobenzene
Hydrogen sulfide
Isopropyl alcohol
Lewisite
Malathion
Methidathion
Methiocarb
Methomyl
Methylparathion
Nickel
Parathion
Profenofos
Pyrimidifen
Sodium azide
Terbufos
Tetraethyl-pyrophosphate

Biologicals

Ackee fruit poisoning
Ciguatera food poisoning
Delphinium
Lobelia
Marijuana (Cannabis)
Monkshood
Nutmeg
Star of Bethlehem (Hippobroman
   longiflora)
Tetrodotoxin food poisoning
White chameleon

[2]Not available in the United States.

Passive External Warming

Passive external warming is ideal for patients with mild hypothermia who are otherwise healthy. It uses the patient's endogenous heat production for rewarming and it involves simple, logical passive maneuvers that minimize heat dissipation. When using this method, all wet clothing should be removed, the ambient core temperature should exceed 70.0°F (21.0°C), and the patient should be covered with insulating materials. Patients warmed easily using this method can be safely discharged.

Active External Rewarming

Active external rewarming is controversial. It involves exposing the skin of the patient to exogenous heat sources. Radiant heat, thermal mattresses, electric heating blankets, and forced-air heating blankets are some of the available techniques.

This method has a number of disadvantages. First, burn injuries can occur to the vasoconstricted skin. Second, any sort of immersion can hinder monitoring and other resuscitative activities. Finally and most important, active external rewarming produces a phenomenon called *core temperature after-drop*. This refers to a drop in core temperature as a result of sudden peripheral vasodilation. This causes cold, acidic blood to return to the core. Hypotension and potentially fatal dysrhythmias can result. Focusing on rewarming the trunk only (rather than the trunk and extremities) can prevent these

CURRENT DIAGNOSIS

- Accidental hypothermia may be classified as mild, moderate, or severe.
- The measured temperature should be the core body temperature.
- The method of rewarming depends on the severity of the temperature drop.
- The complications of rewarming include arrhythmias, rewarming-related hypotension, core temperature after drop, and rhabdomyolysis.
- Patients can only be declared dead after they are warm and dead.

temperature gradients. In general, active external rewarming is used in conjunction with active core rewarming.

Active Core Rewarming

Active core rewarming involves techniques to deliver direct heat internally. It should be used in patients with moderate to severe hypothermia. The simplest method entails the administration of heated, humidified oxygen at 107.6°F to 114.8°F (42.0°C–46.0°C) and intravenous saline solution warmed to 109.4°F (43.0°C). Saline should be administered via a central line at 150 to 200 mL/hour. Gastric, bladder, and colonic irrigations have been used but their relatively small surface areas usually limit their effect.

Another method of active core rewarming is pleural irrigation using two large-bore (36°F or greater) thoracostomy tubes. One tube is placed at the midclavicular line and is connected to saline to 107.6°F (42.0°C). The other tube is placed at the posterior axillary line and connected to a chest tube drainage kit.

A more aggressive method of active core rewarming is via peritoneal lavage and dialysis. This can be accomplished using a standard diagnostic peritoneal lavage (DPL) kit and introducing an 8-F catheter into the peritoneum using Seldinger's technique. The crystalloid dialysate should be warmed to 104.0°F to 113.0°F (40.0°C–45.0°C). This method affords the added advantage of allowing the serum potassium level to be adjusted.

The most efficient and physiologic active core rewarming method is via extracorporeal warming or heated cardiopulmonary bypass. This is the method of choice for the most severe cases, patients with severe rhabdomyolysis, and for patients who require cardiopulmonary resuscitation.

Most arrhythmias are corrected by rewarming. Atropine is typically ineffective for associated bradydysrhythmias. Ventricular tachycardia and fibrillation require electrocardioversion and the use of bretylium,[2] if it is available. The safety of amiodarone (Cordarone) in these situations is questionable. Dopamine (Intropin) may be an effective vasopressor. Empiric antibiotics may be given. However, the empiric use of levothyroxine (Synthroid)[1] and corticosteroids may be hazardous. Phenytoin (Dilantin)[1] might have cardiac-depressant qualities in the moderately hypothermic patient. Box 3 demonstrates drugs with possible decreased metabolism or clearance with increase in toxicity in hypothermia.

Indicators of grave prognosis include development of profound hyperkalemia (serum potassium >10 mEq/L), underlying medical conditions, intravascular thrombosis (fibrinogen <59 mg/dL), pH less than 6.5, and a core temperature less than 50.0°F to 53.6°F (10.0°C–12.0°C).

Peripheral Cold Injuries

Peripheral cold injuries span a spectrum ranging from minimal to severe tissue damage. Freezing and nonfreezing syndromes can cause these injuries. Frostnip and frostbite are caused by exposure to freezing temperatures. *Frostnip* refers to the numbness and blue-white discoloration of the face and extremities that occur during exposure to freezing temperatures. It is a precursor to frostbite. It is characterized by reversible skin changes including blanching and numbness with no permanent tissue damage, unlike frostbite. Nonfreezing injuries depend on whether the ambient environment during exposure was wet (trench or immersion foot) or dry (pernio or chilblain).

---

[1]Not FDA approved for this indication.
[2]Not available in the United States.

BOX 3   **Drugs Displaying Reduced Metabolism or Clearance in Hypothermia**
• Atropine • Digoxin • D-Tubocurarine • Fentanyl (Sublimaze, Duragesic) • Gentamicin (Garamycin) • Lidocaine (Xylocaine) • Phenobarbital • Procaine • Propranolol (Inderal) • Sulfanilamide (AVC Cream) • Suxamethonium (Succinylcholine, Anectine)

PATHOPHYSIOLOGY

During exposure to cold temperatures, the core body temperature is preserved to the detriment of the extremities. Frostbite occurs in four stages: prefreeze, freeze-thaw, vascular stasis, and late ischemic stages. The prefreeze phase occurs when the temperature of the extremities falls below 50.0°F (10.0°C) and cutaneous sensation is lost. Vasoconstriction also occurs along with leakage of intracellular fluid into the interstitium. The freeze-thaw phase begins at the freezing point of water (32.0°F or 0°C) with the formation of ice crystals extracellularly. This further enhances the exit of water from the intracellular space under osmotic forces, resulting in cell shrinkage and ultimately damage. During the vascular stasis phase, plasma leakage and formation of ice crystals continue. Arachidonic acid break down products are then released from underlying damaged tissue. Both prostaglandin $F_{2\alpha}$ and thromboxane A_2 produce platelet aggregation, leukocyte immobilization, and vasoconstriction. Endothelial cells are sensitive to cold injury, and the microvasculature becomes distorted and clogged, leading to tissue ischemia. The late ischemic phase is characterized by ischemia, thrombosis, continued shunting, gangrene, autonomic dysfunction, and denaturation of tissue proteins. The tissue can eventually mummify and demarcate more than 60 to 90 days later.

CLINICAL PRESENTATION

The face and ears are the most common sites prone to cold injury, followed by the hands and feet.

Frostnip and Frostbite

Patients with frostnip usually have blanching and numbness of their fingertips. Frostbite has been classified as superficial, affecting the skin and subcutaneous tissue, or deep, affecting the bones, joints, and tendons. When a superficial frostbite is rewarmed, the skin can form a clear blister; however, when a deep frostbite is rewarmed, it can form a hemorrhagic blister. This classification, however, has no therapeutic or prognostic value given that frostbites can initially appear benign. Many weeks can pass before the demarcation between viable and nonviable tissues becomes apparent.

Although no prognostic factors can be entirely predictive, favorable factors include retained sensation, normal skin color, and clear rather than cloudy fluid in the blisters, if present. Poor prognostic features include nonblanching cyanosis, firm skin, and dark, fluid-filled blisters. Patients can present with pain, numbness, and a clumsy "chunk of wood" sensation in the affected extremity. The pain is initially described as a dull ache and evolves to become a throbbing sensation in about 48 to 72 hours.

Chilblain

Chilblain results from repetitive exposure to cold dry air. It manifests as erythematous or cyanotic lesions often referred to as *cold sores*. These lesions usually develop on exposed surfaces after a delay of 12 to 14 hours and are characterized by pruritus and burning paresthesias. Young women, especially those with Raynaud's phenomenon, are at risk.

Trench Foot and Immersion Foot

Trench foot occurs as a result of prolonged exposure to a damp, cold, nonfreezing environment. It has been classically described among soldiers in World War I, many of whom were confined to cold and damp trenches for prolonged periods. Symptoms include numbness and painful paresthesias that can progress to a throbbing and burning sensation. Initial evaluation reveals a cold, pale extremity, with or without vesicles or bullae.

Immersion foot may be considered the sailor's counterpart to trench foot. It occurs after prolonged immersion in cold water at temperatures above freezing.

TREATMENT

Treatment of frostbite should begin with removing all wet or frozen clothing. For patients with moderate and severe hypothermia as described above, initial resuscitative efforts should be geared toward

CURRENT THERAPY

Mild Hypothermia: 32.2°C (90°F) to 35°C (95°F)

- Passive external rewarming
  - Remove wet clothing.
  - Ambient temperature should exceed 21.0°C (70.0°F).
  - Cover patient with insulating material.

Moderate Hypothermia: 28°C (82.4°F) to 32.2°C (90°F)

- Active external rewarming
  - Radiant heat
  - Thermal mattresses
  - Electric heating blankets
  - Forced-air heating blankets
- Active core rewarming
  - Warmed humidified oxygen
  - Warmed intravenous saline
  - Bladder, colonic, and gastric irrigation
  - Pleural cavity lavage

Severe Hypothermia: Less than 28°C (82.4°F)

- Aggressive active core rewarming
  - Warmed, humidified oxygen
  - Warmed intravenous saline
  - Bladder, colonic, and gastric irrigation
  - Pleural cavity lavage
  - Peritoneal lavage or dialysis
  - Extracorporeal warming or heated cardiopulmonary bypass

Frostnip

- Gentle rewarming
- Usually self-resolving

Frostbite

- Warm-water immersion
- Débride broken vesicles
- Apply topical aloe vera or antibiotic ointment
- Use NSAIDs for pain
- Update tetanus status

Chilblain

- Gentle rewarming
- Nifidipine (procardia)

Trench Foot

- Dry the foot
- Gentle rewarming

Abbreviation: NSAID = nonsteroidal antiinflammatory drug.

---

raising their core temperature. The patient should be moved to a warm environment and all wet clothing should be removed. The frozen extremity should be rewarmed by immersion in circulation water at 104.0°F to 108.0°F (40.0°C–42.0°C) for about 15 to 30 minutes. Given the risks of thermal injury, the frozen parts should not be exposed to direct or dry heat (such as hair dryers, heating pads, or heat lamps). Do not rub or massage the affected area. The process should be continued until the extremity appears warm and well perfused. Due to the pain associated with reperfusion, there may be the temptation to abruptly abort the rewarming process. This can, however, promote further tissue damage. Parenteral analgesic medications (nonsteroidal antiinflammatory drugs [NSAIDs] and opioids) may be administered as needed to make this process more tolerable.

Almost all authors agree that hemorrhagic blisters should not be débrided because of the risk of secondary desiccation of deep dermal layers, extending the injury. Débriding broken vesicles or bullae is also widely accepted; however, clear, intact vesicles may be broken and débrided or left intact. Topical aloe vera ointment (Dermaide Aloe) (a thromboxane inhibitor) or topical antibiotic ointments may be applied. The injured tissue should be loosely covered with sterile, dry, nonadherent dressing. Hands and feet may be splinted and elevated to reduce edema. Because the damaged tissue is tetanus prone, patients whose tetanus status has not been updated need a tetanus shot (Td).

Adjunctive agents that have been used for their antithrombotic and vasodilative properties with varying success include heparin,[1] steroids,[1] NSAIDs,[1] dimethylsulfoxide (DMSO),[1] nonionic detergents,[1] dipyridamole (Persantine),[1] calcium channel blockers,[1] pentoxifylline (Trental),[1] and phenoxybenzamine (Dibenzyline).

Surgical consultation is appropriate for guiding long-term management, because some patients might need débridement of infections or skin grafts for nonhealing wounds. A sympathetic nerve block can relieve painful and refractory vasospasms.

Chilblain (pernio) may be treated with nifidipine (Procardia)[1] at an oral dose of 20 to 60 mg daily.

SEQUELAE

Late sequelae of frostbite include cold hypersensitivity, numbness, pain, and decreased sensation. This is a result of early neuronal damage and abnormal sympathetic tone. Patients with chronic symptoms should be advised to avoid nicotine and cold exposure while using NSAIDs. Tissue demarcation can occur 60 to 90 days after initial injury. Amputation decisions should be deferred unless there is supervening sepsis or gangrene. The ultimate tissue salvage after a spontaneous slough usually far exceeds the most optimistic initial estimates.

Therapeutic Hypothermia

Therapeutic hypothermia for reducing anoxic brain injury has been increasingly used in clinical practice in post–cardiac arrest states. The usual scenarios for such a practice are in patients with suspected postanoxic injuries following cardiopulmonary resuscitation, traumatic brain injuries associated with elevation of intracranial pressure, stroke, and various perioperative situations (such as vascular surgery). Hypothermia can reduce the metabolic oxygen utilization rate in the brain by 6% for every 1°C reduction in brain temperature (over 82.4°F or 28°C) due to reduced normal cerebral electrical activity and suppression of chemical reactions (such as free radical and glutamate production along with calcium shifts) associated with reperfusion injury. Cooling is usually initiated within 6 hours following return of spontaneous circulation, with moderate hypothermia (82.4°F to 90°F or 28°C to 32.2°C) for induction. Intravenous cooling techniques (infusion of 30 mL/kg of crystalloid solution at 4°C over 30 minutes) or extracorporeal cooling methods have been used. An intravascular heat-exchange device has also been developed. Shivering is prevented via neuromuscular blockade and sedation. Temperature can be monitored by a bladder temperature probe or through a central pulmonary catheter.

---

[1]Not FDA approved for this indication.

REFERENCES

Aslam AF, Aslam AK, Vasavada BC, Khan IA. Hypothermia: Evaluation, electrocardiographic manifestations, and management. Am J Med 2006;119 (4):297–301.

Bhagat H, Bithal PK, Chouhan RS, Arora R. Is phenytoin administration safe in a hypothermic child? J Clin Neurosci 2006;13(9):953–5.

Centers for Disease Control and Prevention (CDC). Hypothermia-related deaths—United States, 2003–2004. MMWR Morb Mortal Wkly Rep 2005;54(7):173–5.

Danzl DF. Hypothermia. Semin Respir Crit Care Med 2002;23(1):57–68.

Danzl DF, Pozos RS. Accidental hypothermia. N Engl J Med 1994;331(26): 1756–60.

Ervasti O, Juopperi K, Ketlumen P, et al. The occurance of frostbite and its risk factors in young men. Int J Circumpolar Health 2004;63(1):71–80.

Gilbert M, Busund R, Skagseth A, et al. Resuscitation from accidental hypothermia of 13.7 degrees C with circulatory arrest. Lancet 2000;355 (9201):375–6.

Lloyd EL. Accidental hypothermia. Resuscitation 1996;32:111–24.

McCauley RD, Smith DJ, Robson MC, et al. Frostbite and other cold-induced injuries. In: Auerbach PS, editor. Wilderness medicine: Management of wilderness and environmental emergencies. 3rd ed. St Louis: Mosby; 1995. p. 129–45.

McDonagh DL, Allen IN, Keifer JC, Warner DS. Induction of hypothermia after intraoperative hypoxic brain insult. Anesth Analg 2006;103(1):180–1.

Nolan JP, Morley PT, Vanden Hoek TL, Hickey RW, et al. International Liaison Committee on Resuscitation: Therapeutic hypothermia after cardiac arrest: An advisory statement by the advanced life support task force of the International Liaison Committee on Resuscitation. Circulation 2003;108:118–21.

Ulrich AS, Rathlev NK. Hypothermia and localized cold injuries. Emerg Med Clin North Am 2004;22(2):281–98.

Disturbances Caused by Heat

Method of
John F. Coyle II, MD

Exertional Heat Stroke

Heat stroke is an illness caused by failure of thermoregulation with elevation of core temperature to 40.6°C (105°F) or more, associated with central nervous system dysfunction. Heat stroke is traditionally subdivided into *exertional* and *classic* (or *nonexertional*) forms.

Exertional heat stroke is a sporadic illness triggered by exercise in warm environmental conditions that add to the thermal load produced by muscular contraction. It mainly strikes manual laborers, soldiers in training, and athletic competitors; indeed, it is the third leading cause of death among high school and college athletes in the United States. Exertional heat stroke may occur at moderate temperatures, especially if humidity is high, but both exertional and classic heat strokes most likely develop in conditions of high heat. The incidence of heat stroke increases exponentially when heat stress exceeds a boundary value. Appearance of the first case should sound an alarm that conditions have become dangerous, and more cases should be anticipated. The typical heat stroke victim is highly motivated, poorly conditioned, obese, and not acclimatized. Fatigue and sleep deprivation are commonly encountered, and recent or ongoing febrile or dehydrating illness increases risk. Dehydration may play a role, especially if severe. The use of certain medicines also increases risk, most notably those that decrease cardiac output (β-blockers), promote dehydration (diuretics), affect hypothalamic control (major tranquilizers, neuroleptics, alcohol), inhibit sweating (anticholinergics, tricyclic antidepressants, antihistamines), or increase thermogenicity (amphetamines, cocaine).

Prevention is the ideal treatment. Because behavior is the most powerful thermoregulatory mechanism, education and empowerment have the greatest preventive potential. To avoid exertional heat stroke, organizers should schedule vigorous exercise in the coolest hours of the day (shortly after dawn or after nightfall, in difficult seasons). Exercise level should be governed by athlete fitness, acclimatization, hydration status, and freedom from intercurrent illness. Clothing should be appropriate for exercise conditions. Medication use that might interfere with effective thermoregulation should be recognized, and medical personnel must be charged with the responsibility for stopping any participant who appears to be decompensating.

Triage of those with exertional heat stroke is highly variable. Runners who are plunged unconscious into an ice water bath at the end of a race often respond promptly to treatment, reawaken, and are sometimes sent home without hospitalization. A less-favorable response necessitates hospital admission.

Classic (Nonexertional) Heat Stroke

Classic (nonexertional) heat stroke usually occurs during heat waves that cause passive warming by exposure to unrelenting hot and humid conditions, afflicting urban dwellers who are elderly, infirm, solitary, and poor. Heat waves tend to be "silent and invisible killers of silent and invisible people." Their housing lacks air-conditioning or they do not use it because of expense or confusion. Alcoholism and chronic illness, especially mental illness, predispose people to heat stroke. Young children are susceptible, reflecting their high surface-to-volume ratio, relatively inefficient sweat glands, and dependent status. Classic heat stroke requires preventive measures at the community level. Those with chronic illness and substance abuse history are at highest risk, and they may be the most difficult to contact. Although ventilation fans are of little help in hot and humid conditions, a few hours spent in air-conditioned rooms each day can significantly reduce the likelihood of heat stroke. Whether this is primarily a physiologic or a sociologic effect is unclear. Patients with classic heat stroke usually respond slowly to treatment and require hospital admission.

Pathophysiology

The pathophysiology of heat stroke is incompletely understood. Although a vast number of runners in a marathon may develop dehydration and a high core temperature, very few proceed to heat stroke. Excessive heat is a noxious agent that causes direct cell injury. The severity of heat stroke is related to the degree and duration of temperature elevation above 41.6°C (106.9°F). Exercise lowers the thermal threshold for heat stroke because of hormonal effects and

---

  CURRENT DIAGNOSIS

- Heat stroke often occurs in the first 2 hours of exercise and may occur in so-called moderate heat stress conditions.
- Heat stroke may occur in sedentary urban dwellers during heat waves, especially in the presence of drug or alcohol use, senility, or in young children.
- Abnormal mental status (coma, delirium, agitation, confusion, combativeness) is a constant feature of heat stroke.
- Rectal temperature should be checked immediately. Axillary and aural temperatures may be misleadingly low. A rectal temperature of 40.6°C (105°F) or more is required for diagnosis of heat stroke, but delayed measurement may produce a misleadingly low temperature.
- The trap of proceeding with complex diagnostic procedures (such as computed tomographic scans) before core temperature is assessed and lowered to less than 39°C (102.2°F) should be avoided.
- After cooling measures are instituted, blood samples should be obtained to assess coagulation status, hepatic function, renal function, likelihood of infection, acid-base status, and muscle injury.

competing demands of organ systems as blood flow is directed away from the viscera to the active muscles and the skin. Gut ischemia may result in release of bacterial polysaccharides into the blood. What happens next is a complex interplay of factors including cytokines, bacterial polysaccharides, and heat shock proteins. As endothelial abnormalities accumulate, there is precipitation of a cascade of events including activation of the coagulation system and vascular dilation, resulting in hypotension and coagulation disorders. These events in many respects mimic sepsis.

Because the brain is extremely sensitive to heat stress, the first signs of heat stroke are neurologic. Judgment is impaired, and the chance for self-diagnosis is greatly reduced. After loss of consciousness, muscular activity is markedly diminished, but temperature may remain elevated for hours. Multisystem injury may follow, with the possibility of neurologic, pulmonary, cardiac, hepatic, renal, vascular, hematologic, and immunologic damage. A high percentage of classic heat stroke patients suffer infection within 36 hours of hospital admission.

Treatment

Treatment of heat stroke can be summarized easily:

- Lower rectal temperature immediately to 39°C (102.2°F).
- Support organ systems injured by heat, hypotension, inflammation, and coagulopathy.

There is a *golden hour* after the onset of heat stroke in which therapy can be extremely effective. When treating a patient outside of the hospital, the patient should be moved to a shaded area, clothes removed, and the person covered with water and fanned. When resources become available, the simplest treatment appears to be cold-water immersion in a shallow tub, with patient head, arms, and lower legs outside the tub. The high efficiency of this method comes from two properties of water: It has 25 times the thermal conductivity of air, and it makes perfect contact with all skin surfaces. In addition, the hydrostatic properties of water tend to reduce the risk of hypotension. Other methods of cooling include skin wetting with fanning, application of total-body ice packs (24 ice packs, with special emphasis on the neck, armpits, and groin), or use of a body-cooling unit (evaporation and convection).

Assessment of the patient with presumed heat stroke should be delayed pending initiation of cooling. Determination of rectal temperature, heart rate, and blood pressure can be carried out while the patient is being cooled. Oral and tympanic membrane temperatures cannot be used because they may be misleadingly low. Rectal temperature should be measured every 5 to 10 minutes, and the patient should be removed from cooling when 39°C (102.2°F) is reached, to avoid overshoot hypothermia. Hydration with normal saline or lactated Ringer's solution should be started after initiation of cooling, and most patients require 1 L in the first hour of treatment. Further rehydration needs to be guided by estimated water losses, and in difficult cases placement of a central venous monitoring catheter may be needed. Overhydration may promote cerebral edema, pulmonary edema, and hyponatremia.

Seizures, which occur commonly, should be managed with diazepam (Valium), 5 mg intravenously (IV). Shivering may also be treated with diazepam. The patient must be monitored closely with use of this medication, which occasionally promotes hypotension. Hypotension should be treated with cooling and volume expansion. If blood pressure remains depressed, pressors may be needed. For patients with prolonged exertional heat stroke, mannitol, 0.25 g/kg, or furosemide (Lasix), 0.5 to 1 mg/kg, should be given after volume expansion is carried out to minimize the adverse effects of rhabdomyolysis on renal function.

In patients with severe multiorgan damage, disseminated intravascular coagulation (DIC) is a common finding. Bleeding in DIC should be treated with transfusion of fresh-frozen plasma, cryoprecipitate, and platelet concentrates as needed. There is no role for heparin or thrombolytics in DIC in this setting. Adult respiratory distress

CURRENT THERAPY

- Injury because of heat stroke is related to both the magnitude and duration of core temperature elevation.
- After elevated rectal temperature is documented, treatment should not be delayed. In particular, it should not be delayed to start an intravenous line or to carry out advanced testing such as computed tomography or other radiograph study.
- Ideal treatment for heat stroke is cold-water immersion in a low tub, such as a child's wading pool, with the patient's arms, legs, and head hanging out of the tub.
- If low tub immersion is not available, constant flowing of cold water from a tap over the patient with drainage through a slotted Gurney cart in the presence of constant high-velocity electric fanning can be effective.
- Applying ice packs to the axillae, groins, trunk, and as many other skin surfaces as possible can be useful, but this method of cooling is not as efficient as cold-water immersion or constant cold-water flow because of reduced contact surface and limited thermal gradient.
- Rectal temperature should be checked every 5 minutes during cooling. Cooling measures are discontinued when rectal temperature reaches 39°C (102.2°F) to avoid excessive cooling. Clinicians should watch for rebound temperature elevation after cooling is discontinued.
- Clinicians should be prepared to support the patient through multisystem organ failure. Hemorrhage should be treated with transfusion of red blood cells, platelets, fresh-frozen plasma, and clotting factors. Heparin has no role in treatment of this consumptive coagulopathy. Volume expansion may be needed. Prolonged ventilator support and hemodialysis may be required.
- Medications that may be needed are diazepam (Valium), 5 mg intravenously (IV), for seizures; pressors; and mannitol, 0.25 g/kg IV, and furosemide (Lasix), 0.5 to 1.0 mg/kg IV, for renal protection from rhabdomyolysis, but only after adequate volume expansion is achieved.

syndrome tends to occur in conjunction with DIC, and prolonged ventilator support may be required. Hepatic failure in heat stroke is usually transient. Renal failure may necessitate emergency hemodialysis. No evidence supports use of anti-inflammatory agents or antipyretic agents in heat stroke. Use of strategies that are helpful in sepsis may ultimately find a role in treatment of heat stroke, but such treatments should be considered experimental at this time.

Prognosis can be estimated by time to recovery of consciousness (shorter is better) and elevation of liver enzymes (lactate dehydrogenase [LDH] at 24 hours less than three times normal is a good prognostic sign).

Heat stroke should usually be regarded as an accident, like drowning. The population at highest risk is readily defined, but because of the rarity of this ailment it is difficult to maintain a high level of preparedness for its prevention and treatment. Once encountered, heat stroke must be treated with much the same urgency as cardiac arrest because prompt cooling can sometimes make the crisis little more than an inconvenience. After the process of systemic injury becomes established, heat stroke's cascade of microvascular dysfunction can take on a life of its own, eventuating in a desperate struggle against multisystem failure and a high mortality rate.

REFERENCES

Bouchama A, Knochel JP. Heat stroke. N Engl J Med 2002;346(25):1978–88.

Crandall CG, Vongpatanasin W, Victor RG. Mechanism of cocaine-induced hyperthermia in humans. Ann Intern Med 2002;136(11):785–91.

Dematte JE, O'Mara K, Buescher J, et al. Near-fatal heat stroke during the 1995 heat wave in Chicago. Ann Intern Med 1998;129(3):173–81.

Eichner ER. Treatment of suspected heat illness. Int J Sports Med 1998;19 (Suppl. 2):S150–3.

Epstein Y, Moran DS, Shapiro Y. Exertional heatstroke in the Israeli Defence Forces. In: Pandolf KB, Burr RE, editors. Medical aspects of harsh environments. U.S. Defense Dept., Army, Office of the Surgeon General; 2001. pp. 281–92. Available free online: http://www.bordeninstitute.army.mil/medaspofharshenvrnmnts/

Gaffin SL, Hubbard RW. Pathophysiology of heatstroke, In: Pandolf KB, Burr RE, editors. Medical aspects of harsh environments. U.S. Defense Dept., Army, Office of the Surgeon General; 2001. pp. 161–208. Available free online: http://www.bordeninstitute.army.mil/medaspofharshenvrnmnts/

Gardner JW, Kark JA. Clinical diagnosis, management and surveillance of exertional heat illness, In: Pandolf KB, Burr RE, editors. Medical aspects of harsh environments. U.S. Defense Dept., Army, Office of the Surgeon General; 2001. pp. 221–79. Available free online: http://www.bordeninstitute.army.mil/medaspofharshenvrnmnts/

Klinenberg E. Review of heat wave: Social autopsy of disaster in Chicago. N Engl J Med 2003;348(7):666–7.

Shephard RJ, Shek PN. Immune dysfunction as a factor in heat illness. Crit Rev Immunol 1999;19(4):285–302.

Spider Bites and Scorpion Stings

Method of
Anne-Michelle Ruha, MD

Spider Bites

The majority of spiders native to the United States are incapable of envenomating humans. Important exceptions are *Latrodectus* and *Loxosceles* spiders, which produce clinical envenomations that, on rare occasion, are life-threatening.

BROWN RECLUSE SPIDER

The most famous and abundant *Loxosceles* spider in the United States is *Loxosceles reclusa*, known as the brown recluse or fiddleback spider, due to the violin-shaped marking on its cephalothorax. The brown recluse inhabits the midwestern United States, with a range extending from east Texas to west Georgia and reaching north to southern Iowa. Bites from this nonaggressive spider are defensive, and they generally occur when spiders become trapped in clothes or bedsheets. The risk of a bite, even in heavily infested homes, appears to be very small. Most diagnoses of brown recluse bites, including many published in the medical literature, are likely erroneous, occurring in nonendemic areas without identification of the spider. Other *Loxosceles* species found in the United States are even less likely to bite because they avoid human dwellings. Evidence supporting an association between other native spider species and necrotic wounds is weak.

Although the majority of brown recluse bites do not produce significant injury, some result in loxoscelism, which ranges from minor dermonecrosis to, very rarely, life-threatening illness. The venom component thought responsible for loxoscelism is sphingomyelinase D, which affects platelets and cell membranes and activates inflammatory mediators. The first signs of dermonecrosis are often erythema, pruritus, and pain at the bite site. Over hours the site becomes pale and edematous. Erythema can progress and spread gravitationally. A vesicle can develop, form an eschar, and slough over

CURRENT DIAGNOSIS

Black Widow Bite

- Target lesion, not always present
- Generalized pain and muscle cramps
- Hypertension, regional diaphoresis

Brown Recluse Bite

- Unlikely to occur outside of endemic areas
- Cyanotic or blistering wound within area of pallor surrounded by erythema
- Systemic loxoscelism associated with rash, fever, hemolysis, renal failure

Bark Scorpion Sting

- Absence of lesion or local inflammatory reaction
- Painful paresthesias
- Disconjugate, roving eye movements are characteristic
- Restlessness, agitation, and involuntary jerking of muscles

days to weeks. In the first days after the bite, a sunken bluish wound surrounded by a ring of pallor and then erythema is characteristic. Some patients develop a generalized maculopapular rash. Although most necrotic lesions are not serious, some can enlarge to 40 cm and leave a significant scar. Obese persons are at risk for more-severe lesions.

Very rarely, systemic loxoscelism develops within 48 hours of the bite, characterized by fever, myalgias, and hemolysis. Vomiting and diarrhea can occur, and some patients develop a diffuse erythroderma. Renal failure, disseminated intravascular coagulation, and death can result. Death from massive hemolysis is rare and is more likely to occur in children.

Diagnosis of loxoscelism depends on recognition of signs and symptoms in combination with positive identification of the spider when possible. Alternative etiologies for necrotic wounds are much more common than necrotic arachnidism, especially in nonendemic areas. The differential diagnosis of brown recluse bite is large and includes infectious causes, neoplastic disease, and vascular disease.

Treatment is supportive. Most wounds heal without intervention, although a scar might remain. Early surgical excision, dapsone,[1]

---

[1]Not FDA approved for this indication.

CURRENT THERAPY

Black Widow Bite

- Opioid analgesics to control pain
- Benzodiazepines to control muscle cramping and anxiety
- Anti-*Latrodectus* antivenom (Antivenin) for persistent severe symptoms

Brown Recluse Bite

- General wound care
- If surgical excision is required, perform after 6 to 8 weeks
- Antibiotics only if infected

Bark Scorpion Sting

- Close attention to airway
- Opioid analgesics to control pain
- Benzodiazepines to control agitation
- Anti-*Centruroides* antivenom,[5] if available

---

[5]Investigational drug in the United States.

hyperbaric oxygen, or prophylactic antibiotics cannot be recommended owing to lack of convincing evidence. Patients should receive tetanus prophylaxis (Td) and general wound care. In severe cases, healing can take months and require surgical intervention, which should occur 6 to 8 weeks following the bite after the wound is fully demarcated.

BLACK WIDOW SPIDERS

Latrodectus, or widow, spiders are, medically, the most important group of spiders in the world. Native black widow spiders are shiny black with a red hourglass pattern on their ventral surface. They can reside in or near human structures, leading to contact with humans and subsequent bites.

α-Latrotoxin in venom causes neurotransmitters to be released from synaptic vesicles. This results in a combination of neuromuscular and autonomic effects unique to *Latrodectus* bites, termed *latrodectism.* Bites are inconsistently felt, and they might or might not leave visible puncture marks and a target-like lesion. Pain can progress locally or become generalized within several hours. Severe muscle pain, particularly involving the abdomen and back, is common. Other findings include hypertension, tachycardia, tremor, localized or diffuse diaphoresis, periorbital edema, and urinary retention. Less commonly, vomiting, fever, priapism, paresthesias, and fasciculations occur. Rhabdomyolysis can result from increased muscle activity. Rarely, acute cardiomyopathy, cardiac ischemia, and pulmonary edema occur. Deaths are uncommon but reported.

Diagnosis of latrodectism is based on history of a spider bite and consistent clinical findings. In the absence of a witnessed bite, diagnosis can be difficult. Sudden onset and rapid progression of symptoms should raise suspicion. Infectious and surgical etiologies must be considered in a febrile or vomiting patient. Similar neuromuscular and autonomic findings might also be seen with intoxication by stimulant drugs and scorpion envenomations, and these should be considered in the differential.

Latrodectism typically resolves within 2 to 7 days. Opioid analgesics are often required to treat pain. Severe symptoms require intravenous opioids for adequate pain control and benzodiazepines for muscle spasms and anxiety. If symptoms are life-threatening or not controlled with these therapies, antivenom (Antivenin [*Latrodectus mactans*, equine origin], Merck, Boston, Mass.) should be considered. One vial reverses symptoms of envenomation. This whole-immunoglobulin product can produce acute hypersensitivity and should be administered in a monitored setting. Risks and benefits must be weighed before using this product. If antivenom is not an option or the patient is critically ill, care is supportive, including oxygen and airway support as needed, antihypertensives, antiemetics, and other symptomatic treatment.

TARANTULAS

Tarantulas are common pets and are generally harmless. Bites may be painful, but envenomation by native species has not been reported. Most injury to humans resulting from interaction with tarantulas is secondary to trauma and inflammation caused by barbed abdominal hairs that the spiders eject defensively when threatened. If the hairs embed in the skin, a rash and pruritus can result. They can also embed in the cornea or be transferred there by rubbing the eyes after handling a tarantula. Ophthalmia nodosa, iritis, and keratouveitis have all been reported following exposure to tarantula hairs.

Treatment of embedded corneal hairs entails referral to an ophthalmologist and removal of the hairs if possible. Topical steroids are generally recommended, and some authors also recommend topical antibiotics.

Scorpion Stings

The bark scorpion, *Centruroides sculpturatus,* is the only native scorpion capable of producing a life-threatening envenomation. This small (<3 inch), yellowish-brown scorpion is found throughout Arizona and in bordering areas of surrounding states.

The scorpion seeks cool, dark environments and commonly enters homes. It injects venom by thrusting its stinger, located at the tip of its tail, toward the victim. The neurotoxic venom increases release of neurotransmitters that act at the neuromuscular junction and autonomic nerve endings.

Most stings are minor, producing local pain and paresthesias. Less than 5% of stings result in neurotoxicity, and the majority of these occur in children. Stings typically do not produce a visible skin lesion, although on rare occasion a small red mark is noted. Pain is immediate, and in a grade 1 envenomation remains local and resolves quickly. Grade 2 envenomations involve pain and paresthesias distal from the sting site, which can persist for days to weeks.

Most severe envenomations affect children younger than 5 years. Symptoms develop within 5 to 45 minutes and can progress for 4 hours. Infants and toddlers can exhibit sudden agitation and crying and transient vomiting, and they might rub their face and ears in response to paresthesias. If the child is verbal, complaints of burning pain and sensation of tongue swelling are common. Sinus tachycardia, hypertension, low-grade fever, and hypersalivation are common, and some children develop stridor. Restlessness, agitation, and twisting of the trunk with thrashing of the extremities is typical, as are tongue fasciculations and dysconjugate eye movements, or opsoclonus. Patients are conscious but often keep their eyes closed owing to diplopia. Presence of cranial nerve findings or neuromuscular agitation constitute a grade 3 envenomation; both are present in grade 4 envenomation. Severe envenomation may be associated with pulmonary edema, rhabdomyolysis, and aspiration pneumonia. Respiratory failure can occur due to several factors, including loss of tongue and respiratory muscle control, hypersalivation, and use of respiratory depressant medications.

Diagnosis often relies on recognition of symptoms, because children might not report a sting. Characteristic findings in regions inhabited by this scorpion usually make diagnosis straightforward. Differential diagnosis includes seizures or amphetamine toxicity. If a suspected envenomation does not follow the expected clinical course, a urine drug screen should be obtained.

Patients with grade 4 envenomation must be monitored for respiratory compromise in an emergency department or intensive care unit. If available, anti-*Centruroides* antivenom[5] should be administered, because it reverses neurotoxicity within 1 to 2 hours. Short-acting opioids and benzodiazepines (fentanyl [Sublimaze][1] and midazolam [Versed][1]) may be used as needed to control pain and agitation until antivenom takes effect. Anti-*Centruroides* antivenom, currently undergoing clinical trials in the United States, may be available in the future. As with all antivenoms, acute hypersensitivity reactions are possible, so antihistamines and epinephrine (Adrenalin) must be accessible. Serum sickness can also develop up to 3 weeks after receiving antivenom.

If antivenom is not an option, longer-acting medications (morphine and lorazepam [Ativan][1]) may be used to control pain and agitation. Intubation and mechanical ventilation is sometimes necessary owing to venom effects and respiratory depression from the medications used to control symptoms. While the patient is intubated, continuous infusion of sedative, analgesic, and muscle relaxing agents may be necessary until signs and symptoms of envenomation resolve. This typically occurs within 24 hours, although residual medication effects can require prolonged observation.

---

[1]Not FDA approved for this indication.
[5]Investigational drug in the United States.

REFERENCES

Bernardino CR, Rapuano C. Ophthalmia nodosa caused by casual handling of a tarantula. CLAO 2000;26(2):111–2.

Boyer LV, Theodorou AA, Berg RA, et al. Antivenom for critically ill children with neurotoxicity from scorpion stings. N Engl J Med 2009;360(20):2090–8.

Clark RF, Wethern-Kestner S, Vance MV, Gerkin R. Clinical presentation and treatment of black widow spider envenomation: A review of 163 cases. Ann Emerg Med 1992;21(7):782–7.

Curry SC, Vance MV, Ryan PJ, et al. Envenomation by the scorpion *Centruroides sculpturatus*. J Toxicol Clin Toxicol 1983-1984;21(4–5):417–49.

Furbee RB, Kao LW, Ibrahim D. Brown recluse spider envenomation. Clin Lab Med 2006;26:211–26.

Vetter RS. Spiders of the genus *Loxosceles (Araneae, Sicariidae):* A review of biological, medical and psychological aspects regarding envenomations. J Arachnol 2008;36:150–63.

Vetter RS, Isbister GK. Medical aspects of spider bites. Annu Rev Entomol 2008;53:409–29.

Vetter RS, Isbister GK. Do hobo spider bites cause dermonecrotic injuries? Ann Emerg Med 2004;44(6):605–7.

Watts P, Mcpherson R, Hawksworth NR. Tarantula keratouveitis. Cornea 2000;19(3):393–4.

Venomous Snakebite

Method of
Steven A. Seifert, MD, FAACT, FACMT

Two families of venomous snakes are native to the United States. The Viperidae family (viperids) is composed of three genera and more than 30 species of rattlesnakes, copperheads, and cottonmouths. The Elapidae family (elapids) is composed of two genera and several species of coral snakes.

Each year, there are approximately 4750 venomous bites by native species reported to U.S. poison centers, with fewer than 10 deaths. Ninety-eight percent of these bites are from viperids, and a single Crotalidae polyvalent immune FAB (ovine) antivenom (CroFab, Protherics, Brentwood, Tenn.) is effective against all native species in this family. There is also a single antivenom (Antivenin [*Micrurus fulvius*], equine origin, Wyeth Laboratories, Marietta, Pa.) against coral snakes, which are usually easily recognized by their distinctive markings. After a bite, it is not necessary to capture or further identify the snake, because this will only increase the likelihood of additional envenomations and victims.

There are approximately 50 additional bites per year by a wide variety of nonnative venomous species of snakes housed in zoos, academic institutions, and private collections. Identification of the biting species in these cases is usually not an issue.

Diagnostic and Management Overview

TAKING ACTION

Only a few actions can be undertaken in the field to reduce morbidity or mortality from a venomous snakebite. Most "treatments" that have been advocated—cutting, sucking, or applying tourniquets, heat, cold, or electricity—have no proven efficacy and are much more likely to result in additional tissue injury and delay of definitive therapy. Appropriate local injury management—primarily removal of jewelry, splinting of the extremity, and measures to retard venom entry into central circulation until definitive therapy can be undertaken *in carefully selected cases*—and expeditious transport to a health care facility can produce optimal outcomes.

Definitive management for native venomous snakes in the United States is achieved with appropriate local wound care and antivenom, which is composed of antibodies raised in a host animal (i.e., horses or sheep) against snake venom components. Because native viperids inhabit every state except Maine, every hospital should stock or have ready access to this antivenom.

No FDA-approved elapid antivenom is currently being manufactured in the United States. Older stocks of a previously produced antivenom (Antivenin) are still available at many hospitals in endemic areas (e.g., Florida, Georgia, Alabama, Louisiana, Texas), but they are rapidly being depleted, and existing stocks eventually will be consumed or pass their expiration dates. Foreign-produced antivenoms against related coral snake species may have efficacy against U.S. snakes.

An even more difficult situation results from exotic envenomations, for which the appropriate antivenom (if one exists) is certain to be a non–FDA-approved product and may be located at a zoo or other non–health care source quite distant from the location of the envenomation.

Antivenom, local wound care, and symptomatic and supportive care are the mainstays of envenomation management. A regional poison center should be contacted for information and assistance in managing any venomous snake exposure, including locating an appropriate antivenom. Poison centers have personnel who are experienced at assessing and managing envenomations and have access to a database, the Antivenom Index, which lists sources of non–FDA-approved antivenoms. Poison centers can be contacted from anywhere in the United States by calling 800-222-1222.

SNAKE IDENTIFICATION

Beyond determining whether the victim has been bitten by a coral snake or a viperid, it is relatively immaterial to know the species of the offending snake. A photo taken with a cell phone may be of some value to the treating physician, but it should be obtained only if it can be done safely and without causing a delay in transporting the patient. Viperid snakes are easily differentiated from coral snakes by virtue of the latter's distinctive color pattern of red, yellow, and black bands. It can be difficult to differentiate a coral snake from nonvenomous snakes that have similar markings. The ditty "red on yellow, kill a fellow; red on black, venom lack," which describes the red band being surrounded on either side by yellow or black, is accurate only for North American coral snakes. South American coral snakes have the opposite pattern.

Because all viperid envenomations are treated with a single product and the physical findings or laboratory evaluation is all that is required to determine that the snake is venomous, attempting to kill or capture the snake is unlikely to add additional information to treatment decisions but is likely to result in the individual being bitten a second time or other individuals becoming bite victims. Differences in the appearance of the bite wound (e.g., fang punctures, swelling, ecchymosis) and the observation of signs and symptoms are usually sufficient to determine whether the biting snake was venomous and to guide therapy.

For future reference, remember this advice: "Red on yellow, leave it alone. Red on black, leave it alone. Slithers on the ground, LEAVE IT ALONE."

FACTORS AFFECTING TOXICITY AND THE SEVERITY OF ENVENOMATION

Many factors govern whether an envenomation occurs after a bite, the signs and symptoms that develop, and the overall severity of effects. Up to 25% of viperid bites and up to 50% of elapid bites do not result in an envenomation. Barriers to fang penetration and other factors may result in no venom being injected. Patients must be watched for a sufficient length of time (i.e., 8 hours in a viperid bite and 24 hours in a coral snakebite) to ensure that this has been the case.

If an envenomation has occurred, the family and species of snake generally determines the spectrum of symptoms and signs. The amount of venom, specific venom components, and the underlying health status of the victim determine severity.

Viperid Envenomations

EPIDEMIOLOGY AND RECOGNITION

Viperid snakes are distributed throughout North America, with the apparent exception of Maine. Bites are more common in southern states and during summer months, but they occur year-round and may occur at any time and in any location with captive collections. The various genera and species of viperids in the United States have relatively stable geographic ranges, with much overlap. Many different species of venomous snakes may inhabit any given area. Nonvenomous or mildly venomous colubrid snakes are also native to the United States. Viperids, also called pit vipers (i.e., rattlesnakes, copperheads, and cottonmouths), may be recognized by a generally triangular-shaped head, the so-called pit (an infrared heat-detection organ) located approximately midway between the nostril and the eye, and pupils shaped like those of a cat (not round).

Pit vipers have large, movable fangs through which venom is injected into the victim. Because fangs are curved, venom is usually injected subcutaneously, rather than into deeper muscle compartments. Because of anatomic and other physical factors, bite wounds may appear as scratches or as one or more punctures. Envenomation may occur with a break in the skin.

Viperid venom is complex, consisting of dozens of proteolytic enzymes, small peptides, phospholipases, and other elements responsible for the spectrum of clinical effects seen. There is a great variability in this complex poison between species, within species, and even within a single specimen over the course of a season and lifespan.

CLINICAL EFFECTS

The spectrum of clinical effects is based on the specific genus or species of viperid and is unpredictable, ranging in any given event from a nonenvenomation (up to 25% of bites) to life-threatening reactions. Viperid snake envenomation invariably results in tissue injury, manifested by pain and progressive swelling, and it may include ecchymosis, elevated tissue and compartment pressures, tissue necrosis, and tissue loss. The complete absence of local effects can be used as a reliable marker of nonenvenomation in a viperid bite as long as a sufficient period (8–10 hours) of observation has occurred.

Systemic effects may occur, including hematologic, neurologic, cardiovascular, and nonspecific findings. Rattlesnake envenomations are more likely to result in hematologic effects, such as thrombocytopenia, hypofibrinogenemia, or prolongation of the prothrombin time (PT) or activated partial thromboplastin time (aPTT), and are more likely to produce neurologic effects, such as muscle fasciculation or weakness, compared with copperhead or cottonmouth envenomations, but these effects can be seen with any viperid snake. Hypotension from direct myocardial depression or from type 1 hypersensitivity (i.e., anaphylactic or anaphylactoid) reactions may occur with any viperid exposure. Nausea, vomiting, diaphoresis, anxiety, and other nonspecific effects may be seen.

DURATION OF CLINICAL EFFECTS

Local effects may develop rapidly or may not be apparent for many hours. Progression may occur for 24 to 36 hours, with resolution of tissue injury occurring over 3 to 6 weeks. Complications of tissue necrosis or infection have their own time frame of resolution. Hematologic effects usually begin within 1 to 2 hours of envenomation. If antivenom is given within this time frame, the detection of those effects may be masked and become apparent only after unbound antivenom has been eliminated from the body, usually 2 to 4 days after treatment. Hematologic effects may persist for 1 to 3 weeks after an envenomation. Neurologic and other systemic effects tend to occur within a few hours of envenomation and resolve over 24 to 36 hours.

SEVERITY OF ENVENOMATION

Untreated, local injury worsens over time, with proximal progression of tissue injury. Hematologic effects can be profound, resulting in spontaneous hemorrhage. Hypotension may be profound and can result in death. Neurologic and other systemic effects are rarely life-threatening events. Because of changes in basic medical care and health care systems, it is not directly applicable to compare case-fatality rates before the introduction of antivenom (1950) with what can be expected today. However, at that time, there were several hundred deaths per year in the United States from viperid envenomations.

MANAGEMENT

Determining Whether Envenomation Has Occurred and Its Severity

Because of the unpredictability of envenomation and the variability of possible clinical effects, each viperid bite must be assessed and responded to individually (Box 1). It is important to determine whether an envenomation has occurred. If there are no signs or symptoms of envenomation, there is no indication for antivenom or other specific treatment. The severity of the envenomation helps to determine the amount of antivenom required to counter and neutralize venom effects, but this may not be immediately apparent, because envenomations tend to progress over time, and what may at first appear to be mild venom effects may progress to a severe envenomation.

Initial Hospital Management

On arrival at the hospital, jewelry should be removed and the bitten extremity loosely splinted. The wound should be cleaned, and a radiograph should be obtained to rule out a foreign body (Box 2). Tetanus status should be updated if needed. In the absence of other factors, the extremity should be maintained slightly below heart level until antivenom is started and then should be elevated. If there are immediate life-threatening effects (e.g., anaphylaxis, hypotension), the extremity should be placed in an inferior position and consideration given to impeding venom entry into central circulation by means of a lymphatic constriction band or pressure immobilization bandage, weighing the potential benefit against the possible risk of increased local tissue injury from increasing venom concentration and duration in the tissues. Patients often require opioid-level pain relief.

At least one large intravenous line should be initiated and crystalloid infused as needed. Initial hospital therapy, including a first dose of antivenom, should be provided in an area capable of close monitoring of vital signs and capable of managing life-threatening reactions; this usually is an emergency department. Whether an intensive care unit (ICU) or similar patient care area is used for subsequent management depends on the clinical situation.

Indications for Antivenom

Because of the safety of the current FDA-approved antivenom and its ability to stop proximal progression of local tissue injury, all patients with signs of progressive local envenomation effects and those with significant systemic effects are candidates for treatment with antivenom.

Depending on the original indication for treatment, initial control of envenomation effects is the goal of the loading dose of antivenom. The only FDA-approved viperid antivenom for North American pit viper envenomation is Crotalidae Polyvalent Immune Fab (Ovine) Antivenin (CroFab), which is an ovine-based Fab antivenom. The incidence of type 1 hypersensitivity reactions is approximately 6%. There are rare reports of IgE-mediated type 1 hypersensitivity reactions on repeat exposure in individuals who were previously treated with CroFab, but most people who have been previously treated do

---

BOX 1   Prehospital Management of Viperid Envenomation

- Remove jewelry.
- Splint the extremity and maintain just below heart level.
- Expeditiously transport to a health care facility.
- Consider use of lymphatic constriction band (blood pressure cuff at 15–25 mm Hg) *for life-threatening effects only.*
- Obtain intravenous access if possible.
- Do not use cutting, sucking, heat, cold, or other local "therapies."

BOX 2   Hospital Diagnosis and Initial Management for Viperid Envenomation

- Remove jewelry.
- If an arterial or venous tourniquet has been placed, convert to a lymphatic constriction band.
- Obtain intravenous access, and use crystalloid as indicated.
- Obtain CBC with platelet count, PT or INR, aPTT, and fibrinogen level q6–12h for 1 day and then daily if values are abnormal. An initial D-dimer value (or fibrin degradation products) should be obtained to detect fibrinogenolytic activity that may not yet have produced hypofibrinogenemia.
- Determine whether an envenomation has occurred.
- Determine severity based on the family or species of snake, age and health status of the victim, and development and rate of progression of signs and symptoms (e.g., local injury, hematologic abnormalities, hypotension and other systemic effects).
- Determine the tetanus vaccination status and update if necessary.
- Seek consultation from a poison center: 800-222-1222.
- If a pressure immobilization or lymphatic constriction band was placed before arriving at the hospital, determine whether antivenom is indicated, and remove the band after the antivenom infusion is started.
- If there are minimal or no signs of envenomation or if the bands are placed inappropriately, remove them under close observation.
- Determine whether antivenom is indicated, and administer per protocol.
- Provide basic wound care (i.e., cleaning and radiograph), and determine whether local injury requires specific management.
- Determine whether hematologic or other systemic effects require specific management.

Abbreviations: aPTT = activated partial thromboplastin time; CBC = complete blood cell count; INR = international normalized ratio; PT = prothrombin time.

not develop an adverse reaction to subsequent administrations. The incidence of type 3 hypersensitivity reactions ("serum sickness") is also approximately 6%. Pretreatment sensitivity testing is not required or recommended. The half-life of this antivenom is approximately 18 to 24 hours, which is considerably shorter than IgG or F(ab')2 antivenoms, and it is responsible for the recurrence of hematologic effects in approximately 70% of patients with an initial coagulopathy.

For moderate to severe envenomations, antivenom is administered as an intravenous solution, with 4 to 6 vials diluted into 250 to 500 mL of D_5W or normal saline. Treatment of life-threatening envenomations may be started with 10 to 12 vials. The infusion should be run slowly for the first 5 to 10 minutes, and the patient should be observed closely for a type 1 hypersensitivity reaction. If such a reaction occurs, the infusion should be slowed or stopped, depending on the severity, and appropriate symptomatic treatment should be started with H_1- and H_2-blockers, epinephrine, corticosteroids, and other supportive measures, as needed. It should be determined whether antivenom is still required, and if so, it should be restarted at a slower rate or higher dilution, or both. If a reaction does not occur, the infusion is concluded over 1 hour.

Treatment of Local Tissue Injury

If the antivenom is given exclusively for local findings, the syndromic response to envenomation is deemed to be controlled if there is cessation of proximal progression of edema at the end of the infusion. There is often some redistribution of existing tissue edema, and continued proximal progression is usually distinguishable by a raised, tender, and perhaps erythematous leading edge of edema. If antivenom is being given for hematologic effects, cessation of worsening or reversal should be seen. Often, thrombocytopenia rebounds dramatically. Hypofibrinogenemia may not rebound as quickly or merely stabilize, because the liver must manufacture new fibrinogen. Although an elevated D-dimer value indicates fibrinogenolytic activity, it is not an independent indicator for antivenom treatment.

Other systemic effects may serve as indicators for antivenom use, and they should show control by the end of the initial infusion. If initial control is not deemed to have occurred, additional doses of antivenom should be administered until initial control is determined to have occurred. Most patients achieve initial control with 4 to 12 vials of antivenom, although more may be required.

Maintenance Doses

Because of the rapid decline of antivenom levels resulting from the larger volume of distribution of Fab antivenoms, after initial control is achieved, maintenance dosing of 2 vials every 6 hours for three doses is commenced. This usually maintains adequate antivenom serum levels to prevent recurrence of local tissue injury progression. If progression does recur, an additional 2 vials of antivenom usually are sufficient to control local worsening. Tissue pressures may be increased, and elevated muscle compartment pressures may be identified when measured directly. My colleagues and I do not routinely measure tissue or compartment pressures. When pressures are measured and demonstrated to be elevated, it should be remembered that the mechanisms of these phenomena are different from other muscle compartment syndromes. For example, extensive edema in the subcutaneous space circumferentially in an extremity may elevate compartment pressures by extrinsic compression. Case reports and series suggest that additional antivenom and extremity elevation result in reduced tissue and compartment pressures. Intracompartmental injection of venom can result in a true compartment syndrome. However, there is no evidence that fasciotomy is beneficial in this setting, and there are animal data to suggest that it may result in worse clinical outcomes.

Bleb formation at the site of a bite is not an important sign in and of itself, although it may suggest significantly elevated tissue pressures resulting in dermal-epidermal separation or the presence of tissue necrosis. Bleb fluid may contain unneutralized venom. It is reasonable to unroof blebs at or near the bite site and to débride obviously necrotic tissue that usually becomes apparent several days after the bite.

Antibiotics

The incidence of culture-proven infection in U.S. viperid bites is low, probably less than 5%. There are no data to support the use of prophylactic antibiotics, and it is best to limit the opportunities for adverse drug effects. It is often difficult to distinguish inflammatory venom effects from infection starting on the second day after an envenomation. If antibiotics are prescribed, a first-generation, broad-spectrum agent should be used.

Long-Term Local Tissue Effects

The edema and tissue injury produced by most North American viperid envenomations usually resolves within 1 to 2 months, and a return to normal function can be anticipated. However, tissue necrosis or deep tissue injury may result in longer-term or even permanent structural and functional disability. Loss of tissue may occur, including digits and other parts of extremities, although this is rare and may be associated with prehospital application of tourniquets or other imprudent surgical interventions, delayed care, or complications such as infections. Some victims engage in behaviors that result in multiple envenomations, and this may increase the risks of long-term tissue injury.

Hematologic Abnormalities and Bleeding

One or more hematologic abnormalities may occur with native viperid envenomation (Box 3). Significant decreases in platelet count or fibrinogen concentrations are independent indications for antivenom treatment. Isolated, mild prolongations of PT or aPTT may not require antivenom treatment. However, these effects may be progressive or indicate an impending hypofibrinogenemia, and early antivenom treatment may prevent severe abnormalities. Even if platelets, fibrinogen, and intrinsic and extrinsic clotting systems are involved, the end result is not a true disseminated intravascular coagulopathy, because there is no true intravascular coagulation. Sufficient platelets, fibrinogen, and thrombin are usually available for hemostasis, and clinically significant bleeding is rarely seen. However, severe depletion of individual clotting elements or a combination of hematologic abnormalities can result in bleeding.

The management of initial or persistent laboratory abnormalities is achieved with additional antivenom. Administration of blood products (e.g., fresh-frozen plasma [FFP], platelet concentrates, other blood products) should be reserved for clinically significant bleeding and be given in conjunction with additional antivenom, because transfused elements are similarly likely to be consumed by venom activity. Ecchymoses in damaged tissues, expansion of the vascular volume from crystalloid administration, and red blood cell hemolysis from hemolytic venom factors may produce an anemia that may rarely require a red blood cell transfusion.

Recurrence of Hematologic Effects

Approximately 70% of patients who develop an initial hematologic effect will have a recurrence of those effects 2 to 4 days after initial treatment. The severity of the recurrence is usually similar to the initial effects. A person who presented with a severe thrombocytopenia is likely to return with recurrent severe thrombocytopenia. The mechanism is recurrent unneutralized venomemia after elimination of unbound Fab antivenom. The recurrent effects may be milder, because there is less venom in the body and severity is a function of venom effect and the body's ability to produce factors such as platelets or fibrinogen in excess of their rate of consumption. Recurrent effects may be more severe, however, or even appear to be occurring de novo if the patient was treated soon after envenomation, blunting the acute effects of the venom and masking the true severity of the envenomation.

Patients who present with severe early hematologic effects or who are treated with antivenom within 1 to 2 hours of envenomation are at risk for severe recurrent effects and should be followed closely after discharge. Although the incidence of significant bleeding is low, even with profound laboratory abnormalities, it seems prudent to administer additional antivenom if the platelet count is less than 25,000, the fibrinogen level is less than 50 mg/dL, the PT or PTT values indicate nonclotting, or there is a combination of significant defects in coagulation, or there are underlying medical conditions that make hemorrhage more likely, such as advanced age, hypertension, or a bleeding diathesis. Additional antivenom can be given on an outpatient basis, although patients with any significant bleeding or at high risk for bleeding should be readmitted. Two vials of antivenom should be given, with daily follow-up until hematologic laboratory values are improving, which may take 2 to 3 weeks in some cases.

DISPOSITION

Patients whose local effects are regressing and do not have complications, such as infection or necrosis, and whose hematologic and other systemic effects are controlled may be discharged. Typically, this occurs between 36 and 48 hours after envenomation. Ongoing pain relief may be required, with an effort to transition to nonopioid agents during the first week, and the patient should be warned to watch for signs of serum sickness. Occupational or physical therapy should be arranged to maximize return of function, and follow-up for local and systemic effects should be arranged.

Elapid Envenomations

EPIDEMIOLOGY AND RECOGNITION

U.S. coral snakes can be recognized by their distinctive band pattern, with a red band seeming to be placed on top of a larger yellow band. This color pattern applies only to North American coral snakes. Each year, there are approximately 75 to 100 bites by coral snakes in the United States. Two genera and several species inhabit the United States, with the *Micrurus* genus responsible for most bites in Florida, Texas, Georgia, Louisiana, Alabama, and some neighboring states. A smaller genus, *Micruroides*, is found in Arizona and New Mexico, but it is responsible for very few bites, and there have been no reports of serious envenomations in recent years. Bites are more common during the warmer months.

Elapids have relatively short, fixed fangs, which may decrease the rate of envenomation. More than one puncture, deep punctures, and a history of the snake hanging on increases the risk of envenomation.

CLINICAL EFFECTS

Envenomation by the coral snake produces primarily neurologic toxicity from presynaptic toxins initially producing bulbar muscle weakness, ptosis, diplopia, and dysphagia. These effects can begin within 15 to 30 minutes or may be delayed up to 24 hours after an envenomation. Muscle weakness and paralysis progress to include respiratory muscles, and they can result in respiratory arrest and death. Typical of presynaptic toxins, effect progression can be arrested with the use of antivenom, but the effects are not rapidly reversed. Typically, there is no or little local tissue injury, and the absence of local injury cannot be used to exclude envenomation. Likewise, there is

---

> ### BOX 3   Management of Hematologic Effects and Recurrence in Viperid Envenomation
>
> - Administer 4 to 6 vials of antivenom (Crotalidae Polyvalent Immune Fab [Ovine]) for significant abnormalities of platelet count, PT or INR, aPTT, or fibrinogen. An elevated D-dimer value indicates accelerated fibrinogen breakdown and should prompt close monitoring of the fibrinogen concentrations, but it is not an independent indication to treat with antivenom.
> - Administer additional antivenom in 4- to 6-vial increments until there is reversal of hematologic abnormalities. Replacement of platelets, clotting factors, or fibrinogen may be gradual, and a positive trend indicates neutralization of venom or replacement in excess of venom effect.
> - Patients with initial hematologic effects or who were treated within 1 to 2 hours of envenomation are at risk for recurrent effects 2 to 4 days after treatment and should be followed closely: every other day until no recurrence at 4 days or daily for declining parameters.
> - Consider treating recurrent hematologic abnormalities with additional antivenom. Indications include platelets <25,000/mm³; fibrinogen <50 mg/dL; INR >5; aPTT >150 seconds; and lesser abnormalities involving more than one parameter.
> - Consider readmission for severe abnormalities, other risk factors (e.g., uncontrolled hypertension, advanced age, other bleeding diatheses), or clinically significant bleeding.
> - Administer blood products *plus* additional antivenom for significant bleeding.
>
> *Abbreviations:* aPTT = activated partial thromboplastin time; INR = International Normalized Ratio; PT = prothrombin time.

usually no effect on hematologic function, and other systemic effects are rare. Patients cannot be assumed to have eluded envenomation by a coral snake because they lack these symptoms, and patients should be observed for at least 24 hours before concluding that an envenomation has not occurred.

Because of changes in basic medical care and health care systems, it is not directly applicable to compare case-fatality rates before the introduction of antivenom (1967) with what can be expected today. However, at that time, the case-fatality rate was approximately 10%.

MANAGEMENT

Because of the potential for rapid progression of motor paralysis and respiratory compromise, the difficulty of reversing paralysis after it is established, and the lack of local effects, it is reasonable to attempt to retard venom progression into the circulation until a decision regarding antivenom can be made. A pressure immobilization band (i.e., elastic bandage wrapped from an extremity's tip to trunk with the degree of tension used for sprains) is used for this purpose for elapid envenomations elsewhere in the world (Boxes 4 and 5). However, the proper technique requires training, and the infrequency of these bites makes teaching and retention of such skills problematic. A blood pressure cuff inflated to 15 to 25 mm Hg may also retard venom

---

BOX 4   Prehospital Management of Elapid Envenomation

- Remove jewelry.
- Splint the extremity and maintain just below heart level.
- Expeditiously transport to a health care facility.
- Apply a pressure immobilization bandage (i.e., 3- to 4-inch crepe bandage at lymphatic pressure from the tip of the extremity to the trunk) or a lymphatic constriction band (i.e., wide rubber band or blood pressure cuff at 15–25 mm Hg) proximal to the bite site.
- Obtain intravenous access if possible.
- Do not use cutting, sucking, heat, cold, or other local "therapies."

BOX 5   Hospital Diagnosis and Initial Management of Elapid Envenomation

- Remove jewelry.
- If an arterial or venous tourniquet has been placed, convert to a lymphatic constriction band.
- Obtain intravenous access, and use crystalloid as indicated.
- Determine whether an envenomation has occurred.
- Determine severity based on the family or species of snake, the age and health status of the victim, and the rate of progression of signs or symptoms (i.e., paralysis and other neurologic effects).
- Determine the tetanus vaccination status and update if necessary.
- Seek consultation from a poison center: 800-222-1222.
- If a pressure immobilization band or lymphatic constriction band has been placed before arrival at the hospital, determine whether antivenom is needed, and begin antivenom infusion before removing the band.
- Determine whether antivenom is indicated, and administer per protocol.
- Provide basic wound care (i.e., cleaning and radiograph), and determine whether local injury requires specific management.
- Determine whether other systemic effects require specific management.

---

entry into circulation, and it can be a more reliable and easily taught technique, although it has not been validated in clinical studies.

Standard wound care should be performed, including cleansing the wound, obtaining a radiograph, and updating the tetanus status, if needed. Wound infection is uncommon, and prophylactic antibiotics are not recommended.

Because the first signs of envenomation can be rapidly progressive neurotoxicity and because of the difficulty of reversing paralysis, some authorities have proposed administering antivenom in cases in which an envenomation is possible, before the appearance of any clinical symptoms. Others have pointed to the infrequency of respiratory muscle paralysis resulting in the need for intubation and respiratory support and to possible geographic differences in snake toxicity, and they have counseled observation and antivenom treatment only after envenomation has been confirmed by progressive symptoms. Recent analysis of the national database has not demonstrated a significant difference in clinical severity between Florida and Texas coral snake envenomations, which supports early treatment. However, the impending loss of an FDA-approved coral snake antivenom (Antivenin)[2] is likely to result in delays of many hours before antivenom can be administered, if it is available at all. Aggressive and meticulous respiratory support, including intubation and ventilation that may be needed for days to weeks, should ultimately result in survival of even severe neurotoxic envenomations. If an FDA-approved coral snake antivenom is not available, there may be a clinical trial of an investigational coral snake antivenom in progress. Clinical trials can be located at: www.clinicaltrials.gov.

Exotic Snakebite

EPIDEMIOLOGY AND CLINICAL EFFECTS

In the United States, most exotic snake envenomations occur in private collections. These are not usually known to authorities or health care providers until an envenomation occurs, and they may involve the collection owner or family members, including children. They may occur in any locale, and victims may present to any health care facility.

Viperid and elapid snakes, which account for the bulk of venomous bites worldwide, have patterns of venom activity similar to those of their North American counterparts, with some variation and with generally greater toxicity for some non-U.S. species. Some nonnative elapids, such as cobras, mambas, black snakes, or taipans, produce much higher rates of respiratory paralysis and may produce much greater local tissue injury than U.S. coral snakes. Similarly, envenomation from some nonnative viperids, such as *Bothrops*, *Echis*, or *Bitis* species, or from an African colubrid, such as the boomslang, results in a greater risk of bleeding. Some of these species may directly activate prothrombin (e.g., *Echis* species, *Bothrops* species) and factor X (e.g., *Vipera* species, *Dispholidus* species), leading to a true disseminated intravascular coagulopathy with intravascular thrombosis, marked organ dysfunction, and potentially, death.

MANAGEMENT

The specific management of exotic envenomations is beyond the scope of this chapter. Not all venomous exotic snakes have antivenoms, and even for snakes with antivenoms, none may be available in the United States, but zoos stock antivenoms for snakes in their collections. An updateable online database, the Antivenom Index, lists these antivenoms and is accessible by regional poison centers. For information on exotic antivenoms and assistance in managing an exotic snake envenomation, the regional poison center should be contacted (1-800-222-1222).

---

[2]Not available in the United States.

REFERENCES

Boyer LV, Seifert SA, Cain JS. Recurrence phenomena after immunoglobulin therapy for snake envenomations. Part 2. Guidelines for clinical management with Crotaline Fab antivenom. Ann Emerg Med 2001;37:196–201.

Boyer LV, Seifert SA, Clark RF, et al. Recurrent and persistent coagulopathy following pit viper envenomation. Arch Intern Med 1999;159(7):706–10.

Gold BS, Barish RA, Dart RC. North American snake envenomation: Diagnosis, treatment, and management. Emerg Med Clin North Am 2004;22 (2):423–43 ix.

Kitchens CS, Van Mierop LH. Envenomation by the Eastern coral snake (*Micrurus fulvius fulvius*). A study of 39 victims. JAMA 1987;258(12):1615–8.

Seifert SA, Boyer LV. Recurrence phenomena after immunoglobulin therapy for snake envenomations. Part 1. Pharmacokinetics and pharmacodynamics of immunoglobulin antivenoms and related antibodies. Ann Emerg Med 2001;37(2):189–95.

Seifert SA, Boyer LV, Dart RC, et al. Relationship of venom effects to venom antigen and antivenom serum concentrations in a patient with *Crotalus atrox* envenomation treated with a Fab antivenom. Ann Emerg Med 1997;30(1):49–53.

Seifert SA, Oakes JA, Boyer LV. Toxic Exposure Surveillance System (TESS)-based characterization of U.S. non-native venomous snake exposures, 1995–2004. Clin Toxicol (Phila) 2007;45(5):571–8.

Marine Poisonings, Envenomations, and Trauma

Method of
Allen Perkins, MD, MPH

The United States has more than 80,000 miles of coastline, and more people are enjoying water-dependent recreation activities such as scuba diving, snorkeling, and surfing. As a consequence, people are more likely to suffer trauma, envenomation, or poisoning related to an encounter with a marine creature, which will come to the attention of a physician. The science of marine medicine is limited; hence, treatment of these conditions is largely based on case reports and expert opinion; very few randomized, controlled studies are available. Misdiagnosis is common, especially when the patient has returned from vacationing or when the patient has been poisoned by improperly handled seafood. This article describes common ailments and injuries occurring as a consequence of direct contact with sea creatures and discusses management and prevention.

Ingestions

CIGUATERA

Epidemiology

Ciguatera poisoning is the most commonly reported marine toxin disease in the world. It is caused by human ingestion of reef fish that have bioaccumulated sufficient amounts of the dinoflagellate *Gambierdiscus toxicus*, either through direct ingestion or through ingestion of smaller reef fish. Although limited to tropical regions, it is heat and cold tolerant, is lipid soluble, and can survive transport to other areas. The toxin becomes more concentrated as it passes up the food chain; fish such as amberjack, grouper, and snapper pose less of a risk than predatory fish such as barracuda and moray eel. Ciguatera poisoning affects at least 50,000 people worldwide annually, and there are several thousand cases of poisoning in Puerto Rico, the U.S. Virgin Islands, Hawaii, and Florida each year.

Clinical Features

Patients can exhibit a primarily gastrointestinal (diarrhea, abdominal cramps, and vomiting), neurologic (parasthesias, diffuse pain, blurred vision), cardiac (bradycardia), or mixed pattern of symptoms. Additionally, a cold sensation reversal, in which a patient perceives the cold temperatures as a hot sensation and vice versa, occurs in 80% of patients and is considered pathognomonic for ciguatera poison (Box 1).

BOX 1 Symptom Patterns Associated With Ciguatera Poisoning

Gastrointestinal Pattern

Onset 15 minutes to 24 hours, typically worsens, lasts 1–2 days and resolves
- Nausea and/or vomiting
- Profuse, watery diarrhea
- Abdominal pain

Neurologic Pattern

Onset up to 24 hours after ingestion, commonly nonphysiologic pattern, can last several months
- Numbness and paresthesias
- Vertigo
- Ataxia
- Severe weakness or lethargy
- Severe myalgia
- Decreased vibration and pain sensations
- Diffuse pain pattern
- Cold sensation reversal
- Coma

Cardiovascular Pattern

Onset up to 24 hours after ingestion is uncommon but occurs rapidly
- Bradycardia
- Hypotension
- Cardiovascular collapse

The attack rate is high. As many as 80% to 100% of people who ingest affected fish develop symptoms depending on the size of the fish and the toxin load. Ingestion of internal organs where the toxin accumulates (e.g., liver, roe) is associated with more severe symptoms, but avoiding these organs is not protective. The symptoms are also related to the number of exposures over time, and patients typically have more severe symptoms with subsequent exposures. There is no age-related susceptibility, and no immunity is acquired through exposure.

Symptoms typically begin 1 to 6 hours after ingestion, although a delay of 12 to 24 hours can occur. Duration is 7 to 14 days, and neurologic symptoms occasionally persist for months to years. Chronic ciguatera syndrome can also occur as a constellation of symptoms such as general malaise, depression, headaches, muscle aches, and dysesthesias in the extremities. Patients with chronic disease report recurrences with ingestion of fish, ethanol, caffeine, and nuts up to 6 months after the acute illness resolves.

Diagnosis

The diagnosis should be entertained in any patient who has neurologic, gastrointestinal, or cardiac symptoms and a history of ingesting predatory fish within the past 24 hours. The symptom constellation can be similar to other ingestions, such as certain shellfish toxins,

---

CURRENT DIAGNOSIS

- History of exposure is necessary for diagnosis.
- Ingested toxins can cause unusual symptoms, predominately gastrointestinal.
- Jellyfish envenomation is very painful but almost always self-limited.
- Trauma management follows principles of dirty wounds.
- Specific marine pathogens should be covered if contamination is suspected.

and differentiation requires knowledge of the patient's diet for the previous day. Additionally, scombroid and type E botulinum poisoning should be considered, but these are unlikely if the patient did not ingest ill-appearing game. Other poisonings, such as organophosphates, can produce a similar symptom complex. There are no currently available clinical assays to assist in making the diagnosis, which is based on clinical suspicion and knowledge of the patient's diet history.

Treatment

If ciguatera poisoning is suspected soon after ingestion, I would consider gut decontamination with activated charcoal (Actidose-Aqua) because it can reduce the toxin load and subsequent symptoms. Initial symptomatic treatment typically consists of fluid replacement to replace gastrointestinal losses.

Atropine (AtroPen) is used in patients who have bradycardia. Temporary electrical pacing may be used for refractory symptoms, and pressors may be needed in cases of severe hypotension. Neurologic symptoms are problematic because of their extended course as well as their severity. Mannitol (Osmitrol)[1] is often cited as effective in reducing the duration of neurologic symptoms, but I would use it with caution because the only double-blind trial failed to show any benefit. Nifedipine (Procardia)[1] (adult dose 10–20 mg three times daily) shows some theoretical promise in this regard, but there have been no studies in humans at this time. There are many local remedies used throughout the world that are said to be successful, which likely attests to the self-limited course of the ingestion in most cases. Table 1 offers more details regarding treatments currently used for ciguatera poisoning.

Prevention

Prevention is difficult except by avoiding ingestion of affected reef fish. The toxin is not deactivated by cooking, freezing, smoking, or salting. There are no outward signs of ciguatera: The fish look, taste, and smell normal. Although several commercial assays are available, they are neither sensitive nor specific enough to be relied on to prevent ciguatera poisoning.

To decrease the risk of ciguatera poisoning, I recommend the following steps: Avoid warm-water reef fish, especially those caught where ciguatera poisoning is known to occur; avoid moray eel injection; avoid ingesting large game fish; avoid consuming the internal organs; and limit the amount of initial ingestion if you are in an area

where ciguatera is known to occur. Additionally, patients travelling to distant locales should be made aware that, although the vast majority of cases result from direct ingestion, there have been cases of ciguatera passed through sexual contact and through breast milk, so they should be wary of body fluid contact if ciguatoxin is endemic to the area, if for no other reasons.

SCOMBROID

Epidemiology

Scombroid poisoning (also known as histamine fish poisoning) results from improper handling of certain fish between the time the fish is caught and the time it is cooked. In the United States it is most common in Hawaii and California. Improper preservation and refrigeration lead to histamine and histamine-like substances being produced in the dark meat of certain fish through a conversion of histidine to histamine by bacterial decarboxylases. Members of the family Scombridae, such as tuna and mackerel, contain the highest amounts of this substance, but both scombroid and nonscombroid fish have been associated with the disease. The production of toxins requires the introduction of bacteria during the handling process, primarily during storage at high temperatures. It is the total amount of histamine, the presence of other biogenic amines, and individual susceptibility that determine the severity of the symptoms.

Clinical Features

The patient develops a histamine reaction 20 to 30 minutes after ingestion. Symptoms can be cutaneous, gastrointestinal, neurologic, or hemodynamic or any combination of these. Cutaneous (flushing, urticaria and conjunctival injection, and localized edema; gastrointestinal symptoms include dry mouth, nausea, vomiting, diarrhea, and abdominal cramping; neurologic symptoms include severe headache and dizziness; and hemodynamic symptoms include palpitations and hypotension. In severe cases there can be bronchospasm and respiratory distress. These symptoms typically come on rapidly (within several minutes) and last less than 6 to 8 hours. Flushing is the most consistent clinical sign, occurring on exposed areas so it typically resembles sunburn. Diarrhea is also very common, occurring in 75% of symptomatic patients.

Diagnosis

As with ciguatera, the diagnosis is one of history. If the time between ingestion and illness is short and the patient has ingested a type of fish previously implicated in scombroid, then a tentative diagnosis can be made. The diagnosis is often confused with an allergic reaction. It can be distinguished from allergy by the lack of a previous

---

[1]Not FDA approved for this indication.

TABLE 1 Treatment for Ciguatera Poisoning

Drug	Dose	Indication
Activated charcoal (Actidose-Aqua)	Children <1 y: 1 g/kg Children 1–12 y: 25–50 g Adults: 25–100 g	Gut emptying and decontamination More effective in first hour
Antiemetics (no preference)	Administer per dosing recommendations	Intractable nausea and/or vomiting
Intravenous fluid bolus and infusion (normal saline or lactated Ringer's as initial)	Per volume replacement protocols	Hypovolemia
Atropine (AtroPen)	0.5–1.0 mg IV every 3–5 min to a maximum dose of 0.04 mg/kg per episode Maximum total dose: 3 mg for adults, 2 mg for adolescents, 1 mg for young children	Bradycardia
Pressors: Dopamine (Intropin), dobutamine (Dobutrex), epinephrine	Varies with clinical response	Hypotension, shock
Antihistamines (no preference)	Administer per dosing recommendations	Pruritus
Mannitol (Osmitrol)[1]	1 g/kg of a 20% solution given IV over several h Adult dose: 25–100 g, titrate to urinary output of 100 mL/h	Neurologic symptoms, double-blind study did not show benefit
Amitriptyline (Elavil)[1]	25–75 mg PO bid for patients >25 kg	Pruritus, dysesthesias

[1]Not FDA approved for this indication.

allergic reaction as well as by testing the remaining fish for histamine, although testing is rarely warranted.

Treatment

Treatment is the same as for any histamine reaction, the cornerstone of which is antihistamine. Diphenhydramine (Benadryl) 50 mg for adults and 0.5–1 mg/kg/dose for children, repeated every 4 hours until symptoms abate, is delivered either intravenously or intramuscularly in severe cases and orally for milder cases. For severe cases, cimetidine (Tagamet)[1] 300 mg for adults, 20 mg/kg for children, either orally or intravenously, might be added for more complete histamine-receptor blockade. In cases where ingestion was recent, consider induced emesis using syrup of ipecac: 15 mL for children younger than 12 years or 30 mL otherwise. Most patients require only reassurance, and pharmacologic treatment will be unnecessary. It should be stressed to the patient that this is not an *allergic* reaction to fish, because the histamine is exogenous. Prevention is possible in regions where food storage and preparation are monitored through identification and removal of suspect fish.

OTHER INGESTED TOXINS

In addition to the toxins just discussed, ingestion of certain other marine creatures can lead to problems.

Ingestion of bivalves harvested from contaminated waters has been associated with hepatitis A, Norwalk virus, *Vibrio parahaemolyticus* and *Vibrio vulnificus* infections, the latter two particularly problematic and occasionally fatal in immunocompromised patients. I counsel patients likely to be immunocompromised, including diabetics and those with known liver disease, to avoid uncooked bivalves.

Shellfish are occasionally known to contain one or more of several toxins acquired through bioaccumulation of certain algae. These dinoflagellates tend to bloom in summer months. The symptoms occur immediately after ingestion and last several hours and are typically neurologic or gastrointestinal, or both. The shellfish poisoning syndromes are known as paralytic, neurologic, diarrheal, or amnestic depending on the predominant symptom. The care is typically supportive. Public health officials typically monitor local mollusk populations fairly carefully and alert the public to possible hazards.

Ingestion of the flesh of certain puffer fish has been associated with tetrodotoxin poisoning. The flesh of the fish (fugu) is considered a delicacy. The toxin builds up in internal organs such as the liver and the roe. If the toxin is ingested, it is likely to be fatal but there are certified chefs who are trained in avoiding the toxin when preparing the dish. Despite this precaution, as many as 50 deaths occur in Japan annually from exposure to this toxin. Avoiding this puffer fish and avoiding the ingestion of certain other exotic animals (such as the blue-ringed octopus) eliminate the risk of acquiring this toxin.

Envenomations

Many marine creatures are venomous, and beachgoers experience clinically significant envenomations with some regularity. Jellyfish and related creatures (Cnidarians), sea urchins (Echinodermata), and stingrays (Chondrichthyes) are some of the more commonly identified marine animals involved with envenomations.

JELLYFISH

These invertebrates have stinging cells called *nematocytes*, which carry nematocysts that continue to function when separated from the larger organism. For example, jellyfish nematocysts can sting if the tentacle is separated and after the jellyfish is dead. The venom is antigenic and causes a reaction of a dermatonecrotic, hemolytic, cardiopathic, or neurotoxic nature. The severity of the reaction depends on several variables, including the number of nematocysts that discharge, the toxicity of the coelenterate involved, and each patient's unique antigenic response.

---

[1]Not FDA approved for this indication.

Clinical Features

Although occasionally fatal as a consequence of an anaphylactic response in the United States and Caribbean, the primary concern in these areas with contact is pain, which is almost always self-limiting. Other less common symptoms include parasthesias, nausea, headaches, and chills. The symptoms may last up to 2 to 3 days. Certain Pacific jellyfish primarily found in the waters around Australia have a more potent toxin and are much more likely to cause death (which is still very uncommon). Additionally, the Irukandji syndrome, which occurs in the Pacific, is a suite of symptoms including muscle spasms, vomiting, hypertension, incessant coughing, and occasionally heart failure and brain hemorrhage. Almost all exposed people, regardless of the geographic location, do not have a severe reaction, and the principles of first aid are primarily the same throughout the world.

Treatment

In my experience, treatment is mostly concerned with limiting pain and neurologic symptoms, because anaphylaxis and other severe reactions are rare, and the following general guidelines can be applied. In the field, either the victim or a companion should remove any visible tentacles. To do so requires using care, with gloves or forceps being optimal to prevent further stings. If a towel is used, any nematocysts remaining on the towel can still discharge. Salt water can be used to wash off the nematocysts. Urine, household vinegar, fresh water, and rubbing with sand should be avoided.

Should the victim present to the physician's office or emergency department, topical lidocaine (4%)[1] should be liberally applied for 30 minutes or until the pain subsides followed by removal of the nematocysts, usually through use of the gloved hand or with forceps. Another method for removing the nematocysts is to apply shaving cream or baking soda slurry to the area and scrape off the nematocysts with a razor. Applications of cold, in the form of an ice pack, and immesion in hot water have variously been shown to improve pain, but because of the self-limited nature of the discomfort it is hard to gauge an optimum therapy. Either is probably

---

[1]Not FDA approved for this indication.

 CURRENT THERAPY

Ingestions

- Avoidance is the best strategy.
- Early decontamination with activated charcoal (Actidose-Aqua) can reduce duration of symptoms.
- Symptomatic care is generally sufficient.

Jellyfish

- Remove visible stingers.
- Control pain with topical analgesia.

Trauma

- Avoiding water at feeding time can help to avoid injury.
- If envenomation is suspected, consider hot water immersion.
- Tetanus status should be checked.
- Antibiotic coverage should take marine pathogens into account.

acceptable until the patient is comfortable. Meat tenderizer has been found to be ineffective. Local anesthetics, antihistamines, and steroids are all used to control prolonged symptoms based on anecdotal experience. Antibiotics are not generally necessary. In the rare cases of cardiovascular collapse, supportive care and principles of treatment of anaphylaxis should be followed. A delayed hypersensitivity reaction can occur 1 to 3 days out, which will almost certainly be self-limited and can be treated with oral antihistamines and topical steroids if symptoms are severe.

Sea bather's itch is a form of jellyfish sting caused by the larvae of the thimble jellyfish. It is characterized by a painful, itchy rash under the edges of the bathing suit or wet suit. It can occasionally progress to a popular rash. Topical steroids can be used to relieve symptoms.

Prevention

Prevention is mostly a matter of common sense. Staying away from the organism (the tentacles can extend several meters from the body of the organism) and staying out of the water when jellyfish are known to be present are the most effective. There is a commercially available product, Safe Sea, which has been shown to reduce the number of nematocyst discharges and thus the severity of the sting should a swimmer need to be in the water when jellyfish are present. Wetsuits and other protective gear are ineffective.

ECHINODERMS

The Echinoderm family includes sea urchins. Urchins have toxin-coated spines that break off, leaving calcareous material in the wound, which can potentially cause infection. Symptoms include local pain, burning, and local discoloration. The discoloration is thought to be a temporary tattooing of the skin resulting from dye in the spines; absence of a spine is indicated if the discoloration spontaneously resolves within 48 hours. Theoretically, hot water disables the toxin, although there is no evidence in humans that it is effective. If a spine is present and easily accessible, it should be removed with fingers or forceps. If it is close to a joint or neurovascular structure it should be surgically removed. If the spines do not cause symptoms, retained pieces will likely reabsorb into the skin.

STINGRAYS

Although many fish are venomous, stingrays are the most clinically important, accounting for an estimated 1500 mostly minor injuries in the United States annually. These creatures partially bury themselves in the shallow, sandy bottom of the ocean, leading water enthusiasts to accidentally step on them or grab at what they think is a seashell.

Clinical Features

Stingrays have a spine at the base of their tail, which contains a venom gland. The spine, including the venom gland, is broken off and may be left in the resulting wound. The venom has vasoconstrictive properties that can lead to cyanosis and necrosis with poor wound healing and infection. Symptoms can include immediate and intense pain, salivation, nausea, vomiting, diarrhea, muscle cramps, dyspnea, seizures, headaches, and cardiac arrhythmias. Fatalities are rare and mostly a consequence of exsanguination at the scene or penetration of a vital organ.

Treatment

Home care should include rinsing the area thoroughly with fresh water if available (salt water if not) and removing any foreign body. If the damage is minimal the victim may soak the wound in warm water at home. The victim should watch for signs of infection and seek care for excessive bleeding, retained foreign body, or infection.

For severe wounds that lead the victim to seek medical attention, treatment should include achieving hemostasis followed by submersion of the affected region in hot but not scalding water (42–45°C, 108–113°F) for 30 to 90 minutes or until the pain resolves. Spines and stingers are typically radiopaque, so radiographs or an ultrasound should be obtained if a retained spine is suspected. The wound should be thoroughly cleansed, and delayed closure should be allowed. Tetanus immunization status should be reviewed and updated as appropriate. Surgical exploration may be necessary to remove residual foreign bodies. Prophylactic antibiotics are typically not necessary unless there is a residual foreign body or if the patient is immunosuppressed. If the wound becomes infected, *Staphylococcus* and *Streptococcus* species are the most common pathologic organisms. Unique to the marine environment are *Vibrio vulnificus* and *Mycobacterium marinum*, and antibiotic coverage should include coverage for all of these (Table 2).

OTHER VENOMOUS SEA CREATURES

Seasnakes are venomous creatures found most commonly in the Indo-Pacific area. Bites are uncommon (and envenomation is even less common), but should they occur, the toxin is very potent. The care is supportive. There is antivenom, which may be available in areas where the snakes are endemic.

Certain other fish and octopi have been associated with envenomation and occasional death. Most are tropical such as the stonefish, scorpionfish, and rabbitfish and the blue-ringed octopus. Certain varieties of catfish have venom as well. Envenomations, are rare

TABLE 2 Antibiotic Choices in Marine Injuries

	Dosage	
Drug	**Pediatric**	**Adult**
Outpatient Management		
Ciprofloxacin (Cipro)	20–30 mg/kg/day PO × 14 d[1]	500 mg PO bid × 14 d
Levofloxin (Levaquin)		750 mg PO qd × 14 d
Doxycycline (Vibramycin, Doryx)	>8 y: 2.2 mg/kg PO qd × 14 d	100 mg bid × 14 d
Inpatient Management		
Preferred		
Ceftazidime (Fortaz, Tazicef)	150 mg/kg/d q8h	1 g IV q8h
plus		
PO or IV quinolone or doxycycline	150 mg/kg/d q8h	1 g IV q8h
Alternative		
Gentamicin	Typically based on institutional protocol and adjusted based on serum levels	Typically based on institutional protocol and adjusted based on serum levels
plus		
TMP-SMX (Bactrim, Cotrim, Septra)	8–10 mg/kg/d TMP	8–10 mg/kg (lean body mass)/d TMP

[1]Not FDA approved for this indication.
TMP-SMX = trimethoprim-sulfamethoxazole.

and if they occur, treatment is based on good first-aid principles and antivenom where available (mostly in tropical areas).

Certain cone shells contain a toxin that can be fatal. This toxin is injected by the mollusk into the victim from a proboscis, which it extends from the small end of the cone. Treatment is primarily supportive.

Trauma

Abrasions, bites, and lacerations are usually the result of a marine animal's instinct to protect itself against a perceived danger. The most commonly involved marine animals are octopi, sharks, moray eels, and barracuda. The trauma alone creates problems for patients but the trauma can be further complicated by envenomation. It is often difficult to identify the marine animal involved in the attack. Treatment is for the most part symptomatic, with local cleansing and topical dressing usually sufficing. If the wound becomes infected, antibiotics should cover common organisms (see Table 2).

ENVIRONMENTAL HAZARDS

Abrasions from the ambient environment are also common. These wounds should be thoroughly cleansed with soap and water and a topical antibiotic applied, because the wounds can contain toxins and are commonly contaminated with bacteria. Coral contains nematocysts and also has very sharp edges. Scuba divers in particular suffer from coral cuts in the course of their recreational diving. If these wounds become infected, coverage for *Vibrio* species should be included as well.

SHARKS

Although shark attacks receive a lot of publicity, there are only around 50 such attacks worldwide annually and they result in fewer than 10 deaths. The majority of the deaths are in South Africa. Typically these attacks involve the tiger, great white, gray reef, and bull sharks. Attacks occur in shallow water within 100 feet of shore during the evening hours when sharks tend to feed. Common sense dictates avoiding areas where aggressive shark feeding has been noted.

Sequelae of a shark attack range from abrasions to death from hemorrhage. Abrasions and lacerations can occur when sharks brush or aggressively investigate humans. Soft tissue damage, fractures, and neurovascular damage result from such attacks. The majority of attacks result in minor injuries that require simple suturing. Morbidity increases in wounds that are greater than 20 cm or where more than one myofascial compartment is lost. General principles of first aid in marine animal injuries are found in Box 2. Although it would seem self-evident, practices such as urinating on the injury, applying oil or gasoline to injuries, and application of any strong oxidizing agents, such as strong bases or acids should be counseled against when doing patient education regarding self-care.

REFERENCES

Birsa L, Verity P, Lee R. Evaluation of the effects of various chemicals on discharge of and pain caused by jellyfish nematocysts. Comp Biochem and Physiol Part C: Toxicology & Pharmacology 2010;151:426–30.

Centers for Disease Control and Prevention. Management of *Vibrio vulnificus* wound infection. Available at http://www.bt.cdc.gov/disasters/hurricanes/katrina/vibriofaq.asp (accessed June 13, 2008).

Edmonds C. Marine animal injuries. In: Bove AA, editor. Bove and Davis' Diving Medicine. 4th ed. Philadelphia: Saunders; 2004. pp. 287–318.

Fleming LE. Ciguatera fish poisoning, In: Miami FL, editor. National Institute of Environmental Health Sciences, Marine and Freshwater Biomedical Sciences Center; 2006 available at http://www.rsmas.miami.edu/groups/niehs/science/ciguatera.htm (accessed June 14, 2008).

Isbister GK. Venomous fish stings in tropical northern Australia. Am J Emerg Med 2001;19:561–5.

Lahey T. Invasive *Mycobacterium marinum* infections, Emerg Infect Dis [serial online] 2003. November; Available at http://www.cdc.gov/ncidod/EID/vol9no11/03-0192.htm (accessed June 14, 2008).

Lehane L, Olley J. Histamine (scombroid) fish poisoning: A review in a risk-assessment framework. Canberra, Australia: National Office of Animal and Plant Health; 1999.

Lynch PR, Bove AA. Marine poisonings and intoxications. In: Bove AA, editor. Bove and Davis' Diving Medicine. 4th ed. Philadelphia: Saunders; 2004. pp. 287–318.

Perkins A, Morgan S. Poisonings, envenomations, and trauma from marine creatures. Am Fam Physician 2004;69:885–90.

Thomas C, Scott SA. All Stings Considered: First Aid and Medical Treatment of Hawaii's Marine Injuries. Honolulu: University of Hawaii Press; 1997.

Thomas CS, Scott SA, Galanis DJ, Goto RS. Box jellyfish *Carybdea alata* in Waikiki. The analgesic effect of Sting-Aid, Adolph's meat tenderizer and fresh water on their stings: A double-blinded, randomized, placebo-controlled clinical trial. Hawaii Med J 2001;60:205–10.

Thomas CS, Scott SA, Galanis DJ, Goto RS. Box jellyfish *Carybdea alata* in Waikiki. Their influx cycle plus the analgesic effect of hot and cold packs on their stings to swimmers at the beach: A randomized, placebo-controlled, clinical trial. Hawaii Med J 2001;60:100–7.

Medical Toxicology: Ingestions, Inhalations, and Dermal and Ocular Absorptions

Method of
Howard C. Mofenson, MD; Thomas R. Caraccio, PharmD; Michael McGuigan, MD; and Joseph Greensher, MD

Introduction and Epidemiology

According to the national Toxic Exposure Surveillance System (TESS), over 2.4 million potentially toxic exposures were reported last year to Poison Control Centers throughout the United States. Poisonings were responsible for 1183 deaths and more than 500,000 hospitalizations. Poisoning accounts for 2% to 5% of pediatric hospital admissions, 10% of adult admissions, 5% of hospital admissions in the elderly (>65 years of age), and 5% of ambulance calls. In one urban hospital, drug-related emergencies accounted for 38% of the emergency department visits. An evaluation of a medical intensive care unit and step-down unit over a 3-month period indicated that poisonings accounted for 19.7% of admissions.

BOX 2 Management of Marine Trauma

Remove the victim from the water.
Ensure airway control.
Control bleeding.
Do not remove the wet suit if the victim is wearing one.
Attempt to identify the animal involved in the injury.
If the injury is severe, transport the victim to a hospital.
If envenomation is suspected, consider hot water immersion.
Irrigate the wound with normal saline.
Perform surgical débridement of the wound as appropriate.
If sutures must be placed, place them loosely and allow drainage. Primary suturing should be avoided in puncture wounds, crush injuries, and wounds in the distal extremities.
Start appropriate antibiotics if indicated.

The largest number of fatalities resulting from poisoning reported to the TESS are caused by analgesics. The other principal toxicologic causes of fatalities are antidepressants, sedative hypnotics/antipsychotics, stimulants/street drugs, cardiovascular agents, and alcohols. Less than 1% of overdose cases reaching the hospitals result in fatality. However, patients presenting in deep coma to medical care facilities have a fatality rate of 13% to 35%. The largest single cause of coma of inapparent etiology is drug poisoning.

Pharmaceutical preparations are involved in 50% of poisonings. The number one pharmaceutical agent involved in exposures is acetaminophen. The severity of the manifestations of acute poisoning exposures varies greatly depending on whether the poisoning was intentional or unintentional. Unintentional exposures make up 85% to 90% of all poisoning exposures. The majority of cases are acute, occurring in children younger than 5 years of age, in the home, and resulting in no or minor toxicity. Many are actually ingestions of relatively nontoxic substances that require minimal medical care. Intentional poisonings, such as suicides, constitute 10% to 15% of exposures and may require the highest standards of medical and nursing care and the use of sophisticated equipment for recovery. Intentional ingestions are often of multiple substances and frequently include ethanol, acetaminophen, and aspirin. Suicides make up 54% of the reported fatalities. About 25% of suicides are attempted with drugs. Sixty percent of patients who take a drug overdose use their own medication and 15% use drugs prescribed for close relatives. The majority of the drug-related suicide attempts involve a central nervous system (CNS) depressant, and coma management is vital to the treatment.

Assessment and Maintenance of the Vital Functions

The initial assessment of all patients in medical emergencies follows the principles of basic and advanced cardiac life support. The adequacy of the patient's airway, degree of ventilation, and circulatory status should be determined. The vital functions should be established and maintained. Vital signs should be measured frequently and should include body core temperature. The assessment of vital functions should include the rate numbers (e.g., respiratory rate) and indications of effectiveness (e.g., depth of respirations and degree of gas exchange). Table 1 gives important measurements and vital signs.

Level of consciousness should be assessed by immediate AVPU (Alert, responds to Verbal stimuli, responds to Painful stimuli, and Unconscious). If the patient is unconscious, one must assess the severity of the unconsciousness by the Glasgow Coma Scale (Table 2).

If the patient is comatose, management requires administering 100% oxygen, establishing vascular access, and obtaining blood for pertinent laboratory studies. The administration of glucose, thiamine, and naloxone, as well as intubation to protect the airway, should be considered. Pertinent laboratory studies include arterial blood gases (ABG), electrocardiography (ECG), determination of blood glucose level, electrolytes, renal and liver tests, and acetaminophen plasma concentration in all cases of intentional ingestions. Radiography of the chest and abdomen may be useful. The severity of a stimulant's effects can also be assessed and should be documented to follow the trend.

The examiner should completely expose the patient by removing clothes and other items that interfere with a full evaluation. One should look for clues to etiology in the clothes and include the hat and shoes.

Prevention of Absorption and Reduction of Local Damage

EXPOSURE

Poisoning exposure routes include ingestion (76.8%), dermal (8%), ophthalmologic (5%), inhalation (6%), insect bites and stings (4%), and parenteral injections (0.5%). The effect of the toxin may be local, systemic, or both.

Local effects (skin, eyes, mucosa of respiratory or gastrointestinal tract) occur where contact is made with the poisonous substance. Local effects are nonspecific chemical reactions that depend on the chemical properties (e.g., pH), concentration, contact time, and type of exposed surface.

Systemic effects occur when the poison is absorbed into the body and depend on the dose, the distribution, and the functional reserve of the organ systems. Shock and hypoxia are part of systemic toxicity.

TABLE 1 Important Measurements and Vital Signs

Age	Body Surface Area (m²)	Weight (kg)	Height (cm)	Pulse (bpm) Resting	Hypotension	Blood Pressure Hypertension Significant	Severe	Respiratory Rate (rpm)
Newborn	0.19	3.5	50	70–190	<60/40	>96	>106	30–60
1 mo–6 mo	0.30	4–7	50–65	80–160	<70/45	>104	>110	30–50
6 mo–1 y	0.38	7–10	65–75	80–160	<70/45	>104	>110	20–40
1–2 y	0.50–0.55	10–12	75–85	80–140	<74/47	>112/74	>118/82	20–40
3–5 y	0.54–0.68	15–20	90–108	80–120	<80/52	>116/76	>124/84	20–40
6–9 y	0.68–0.85	20–28	122–133	75–115	<90/60	>122/82	>130/86	16–25
10–12 y	1.00–1.07	30–40	138–147	70–110	<90/60	>126/82	>134/90	16–25
13–15 y	1.07–1.22	42–50	152–160	60–100	<90/60	>136/86	>144/92	16–20
16–18 y	1.30–1.60	53–60	160–170	60–100	<90/60	>142/92	>150/98	12–16
Adult	1.40–1.70	60–70	160–170	60–100	<90/60	>140/90	>210/120	10–16

Data from Nadas A: Pediatric Cardiology, 3rd ed. Philadelphia, WB Saunders, 1976; Blumer JL (ed): A Practice Guide to Pediatric Intensive Care. St Louis, Mosby, 1990; AAP and ACEP: Respiratory Distress in APLS Pediatric Emergency Medicine Course, 1993; Second Task Force: Blood pressure control in children–1987, Pediatr 79:1, 1987; Linakis JG: Hypertension. In Fliesher GR, Ludwig S (eds); Textbook of Pediatric Emergency Medicine, 3rd ed. Baltimore, Williams & Wilkins, 1993.

TABLE 2 Glasgow Coma Scale

Scale	Adult Response	Score	Pediatric, 0–1 Years
Eye opening	Spontaneous	4	Spontaneous
	To verbal command	3	To shout
	To pain	2	To pain
	None	1	No response
Motor response			
To verbal command	Obeys	6	
To painful stimuli	Localized pain	5	Localized pain
	Flexion withdrawal	4	Flexion withdrawal
	Decorticate flexion	3	Decorticate flexion
	Decerebrate extension	2	Decerebrate flexion
	None	1	None
Verbal response: adult	Oriented and converses	5	Cries, smiles, coos
	Disoriented but converses	4	Cries or screams
	Inappropriate words	3	Inappropriate sounds
	Incomprehensible sounds	2	Grunts
	None	1	Gives no response
Verbal response: child	Oriented	5	
	Words or babbles	4	
	Vocal sounds	3	
	Cries or moans to stimuli	2	
	None	1	

Data from Teasdale G, Jennett B: Assessment of coma impaired consciousness. Lancet 2:83, 1974; Simpson D, Reilly P: Pediatric coma scale. Lancet 2:450, 1982; Seidel J: Preparing for pediatric emergencies. Pediatr Rev 16:470, 1995.

DELAYED TOXIC ACTION

Therapeutic doses of most pharmaceuticals are absorbed within 90 minutes. However, the patient with exposure to a potential toxin may be asymptomatic at this time because a sufficient amount has not yet been absorbed or metabolized to produce toxicity at the time the patient presents for care.

Absorption can be significantly delayed under the following circumstances:

1. Drugs with anticholinergic properties (e.g., antihistamines, belladonna alkaloids, diphenoxylate with atropine [Lomotil], phenothiazines, and tricyclic antidepressants).
2. Modified release preparations such as sustained-release, enteric-coated, and controlled-release formulations have delayed and prolonged absorption.
3. Concretions may form (e.g., salicylates, iron, glutethimide, and meprobamate [Equanil]) that can delay absorption and prolong the toxic effects. Large quantities of drugs tend to be absorbed more slowly than small quantities.

Some substances must be metabolized into a toxic metabolite (acetaminophen, acetonitrile, ethylene glycol, methanol, methylene chloride, parathion, and paraquat). In some cases, time is required to produce a toxic effect on organ systems (*Amanita phalloides* mushrooms, carbon tetrachloride, colchicine, digoxin [Lanoxin], heavy metals, monoamine oxidase inhibitors, and oral hypoglycemic agents).

Initial Management

1. Stabilization of airway, breathing, and circulation and protection of same.
2. Identification of specific toxin or toxic syndrome.
3. Initial treatment: D50W; consider thiamine, naloxone (Narcan), oxygen, and antidotes if needed.
4. Physical assessment.
5. Decontamination: Gastrointestinal tract, skin, eyes.

DECONTAMINATION

In the asymptomatic patient who has been exposed to a toxic substance, decontamination procedures should be considered if the patient has been exposed to potentially toxic substances in toxic amounts.

Ocular exposure should be immediately treated with water irrigation for 15 to 20 minutes with the eyelids fully retracted. One should not use neutralizing chemicals. All caustic and corrosive injuries should be evaluated with fluorescein dye and by an ophthalmologist.

Dermal exposure is treated immediately with copious water irrigation for 30 minutes, not a forceful flushing. Shampooing the hair, cleansing the fingernails, navel, and perineum, and irrigating the eyes are necessary in the case of an extensive exposure. The clothes should be specially bagged and may have to be discarded. Leather goods can become irreversibly contaminated and must be abandoned. Caustic (alkali) exposures can require hours of irrigation. Dermal absorption can occur with pesticides, hydrocarbons, and cyanide.

Injection exposures (e.g., snake envenomation) can be treated with venom extracts. Venom extractors can be used within minutes of envenomation, and proximal lymphatic constricting bands or elastic wraps can be used to delay lymphatic flow and immobilize the extremity. Cold packs and tourniquets should not be used and incision is generally not recommended. Substances of abuse may be injected intravenously or subcutaneously. In these cases, little decontamination can be done.

Inhalation exposure to toxic substances is managed by immediate removal of the victim from the contaminated environment by protected rescuers.

Gastrointestinal exposure is the most common route of poisoning. Gastrointestinal decontamination historically has been done by gastric emptying: induction of emesis, gastric lavage, administration of activated charcoal, and the use of cathartics or whole bowel irrigation. No procedure is routine; it should be individualized for each case. If no attempt is made to decontaminate the patient, the reason should be clearly documented on the medical record (e.g., time elapsed, past peak of action, ineffectiveness, or risk of procedure).

Gastric Emptying Procedures

The gastric emptying procedure used is influenced by the age of the patient, the effectiveness of the procedure, the time of ingestion (gastric emptying is usually ineffective after 1 hour postingestion), the patient's clinical status (time of peak effect has passed or the patient's condition is too unstable), formulation of the substance ingested (regular release versus modified release), the amount ingested, and the rapidity of onset of CNS depression or stimulation (convulsions). Most studies show that only 30% (range, 19% to 62%) of the ingested toxin is removed by gastric emptying under optimal conditions. It has not been demonstrated that the choice of procedure improved the outcome.

A mnemonic for gathering information is STATS:

S—substance
T—type of formulation
A—amount and age
T—time of ingestion
S—signs and symptoms

The examiner should attempt to obtain AMPLE information about the patient:

A—age and allergies
M—available medications
P—past medical history including pregnancy, psychiatric illnesses, substance abuse, or intentional ingestions
L—time of last meal, which may influence absorption and the onset and peak action
E—events leading to present condition

The intent of the patient should also be determined.

The Regional Poison Center should be consulted for the exact ingredients of the ingested substance and the latest management. The treatment information on the labels of products and in the *Physicians' Desk Reference* are notoriously inaccurate.

Ipecac Syrup

Syrup of ipecac–induced emesis has virtually no use in the emergency department. Although at one time it was considered most useful in young children with a recent witnessed ingestion, it is no longer advised in most cases. Current guidelines from the American Association of Poison Control Centers have significantly limited the indications for inducing emesis because the risk most often exceeds the benefit derived from this procedure. The Poison Control Center should be called if inducting emesis is being considered.

Contraindications or situations in which induction of emesis is inappropriate include the following:

- Ingestion of caustic substance
- Loss of airway protective reflexes because of ingestion of substances that can produce rapid onset of CNS depression (e.g., short-acting benzodiazepines, barbiturates, nonbarbiturate sedative-hypnotics, opioids, tricyclic antidepressants) or convulsions (e.g., camphor [Ponstel], chloroquine [Aralen], codeine, isoniazid [Nydrazid], mefenamic acid, nicotine, propoxyphene [Darvon], organophosphate insecticides, strychnine, and tricyclic antidepressants)
- Ingestion of low-viscosity petroleum distillates (e.g., gasoline, lighter fluid, kerosene)
- Significant vomiting prior to presentation or hematemesis
- Age under 6 months (no established dose, safety, or efficacy data)
- Ingestion of foreign bodies (emesis is ineffective and may lead to aspiration)
- Clinical conditions including neurologic impairment, hemodynamic instability, increased intracranial pressure, and hypertension
- Delay in presentation (more than 1 hour postingestion)

The dose of syrup of ipecac in the 6- to 9-month-old infant is 5 mL; in the 9- to 12-month-old, 10 mL; and in the 1- to 12-year-old, 15 mL. In children older than 12 years and in adults, the dose is 30 mL. The dose can be repeated once if the child does not vomit in 15 to 20 minutes. The vomitus should be inspected for remnants of pills or toxic substances, and the appearance and odor should be documented. When ipecac is not available, 30 mL of mild dishwashing soap (not dishwasher detergent) can be used, although it is less effective.

Complications are very rare but include aspiration, protracted vomiting, rarely cardiac toxicity with long-term abuse, pneumothorax, gastric rupture, diaphragmatic hernia, intracranial hemorrhage, and Mallory-Weiss tears.

Gastric Lavage

Gastric lavage should be considered only when life-threatening amounts of substances were involved, when the benefits outweigh the risks, when it can be performed within 1 hour of the ingestion, and when no contraindications exist.

The contraindications are similar to those for ipecac-induced emesis. However, gastric lavage can be accomplished after the insertion of an endotracheal tube in cases of CNS depression or controlled convulsions. The patient should be placed with the head lower than the hips in a left-lateral decubitus position. The location of the tube should be confirmed by radiography, if necessary, and suctioning equipment should be available.

Contraindications to gastric lavage include the following:

- Ingestion of caustic substances (risk of esophageal perforation)
- Uncontrolled convulsions, because of the danger of aspiration and injury during the procedure
- Ingestion of low-viscosity petroleum distillate products
- CNS depression or absent protective airway reflexes, without endotracheal protection
- Significant cardiac dysrhythmias
- Significant emesis or hematemesis prior to presentation
- Delay in presentation (more than 1 hour postingestion)

Size of Tube

The best results with gastric lavage are obtained with the largest possible orogastric tube that can be reasonably passed (nasogastric tubes are not large enough to remove solid material). In adults, a large-bore orogastric Lavacuator hose or a No. 42 French Ewald tube should be used; in young children, orogastric tubes are generally too small to remove solid material and gastric lavage is not recommended.

The amount of fluid used varies with the patient's age and size. In general, aliquots of 50 to 100 mL per lavage are used in adults. Larger amounts of fluid may force the toxin past the pylorus. Lavage fluid is 0.9% saline.

Complications are rare and may include respiratory depression, aspiration pneumonitis, cardiac dysrhythmias as a result of increased vagal tone, esophageal-gastric tears and perforation, laryngospasm, and mediastinitis.

Activated Charcoal

Oral activated charcoal adsorbs the toxin onto its surface before absorption. According to recent guidelines set forth by the American Academy of Clinical Toxicology, activated charcoal should not be used routinely. Its use is indicated only if a toxic amount of substance has been ingested and is optimally effective within 1 hour of the ingestion. Because of the slow absorption of large quantities of toxin, activated charcoal may be beneficial after 1 hour postingestion.

Activated charcoal does not effectively adsorb small molecules or molecules lacking carbon (Table 3). Activated charcoal adsorption may be diminished by milk, cocoa powder, and ice cream.

There are a few relative contraindications to the use of activated charcoal:

1. Ingestion of caustics and corrosives, which may produce vomiting or cling to the mucosa and falsely appear as a burn on endoscopy.
2. Comatose patient, in whom the airway must be secured prior to activated charcoal administration.
3. Patient without presence of bowel sounds.

Note: Activated charcoal was shown not to interfere with effectiveness of *N*-acetylcysteine in cases of acetaminophen overdose, so it is no longer contraindicated as was thought in the past.

TABLE 3 Substances Poorly Adsorbed by Activated Charcoal

C   Caustics and corrosives
H   Heavy metals (arsenic, iron, lead, mercury)
A   Alcohols (ethanol, methanol, isopropanol) and glycols (ethylene glycols)
R   Rapid onset of absorption (cyanide and strychnine)
C   Chlorine and iodine
O   Others insoluble in water (substances in tablet form)
A   Aliphatic hydrocarbons (petroleum distillates)
L   Laxatives (sodium, magnesium, potassium, and lithium)

The usual initial adult dose is 60 to 100 g and the dose for children is 15 to 30 g. It is administered orally as a slurry mixed with water or by nasogastric or orogastric tube. *Caution*: Be sure the tube is in the stomach. Cathartics are not necessary.

Although repeated dosing with activated charcoal may decrease the half-life and increases the clearance of phenobarbital, dapsone, quinidine, theophylline, and carbamazepine (Tegretol), recent guidelines indicate there is insufficient evidence to support the use of multiple-dose activated charcoal unless a life-threatening amount of one of the substances mentioned is involved. At present there are no controlled studies that demonstrate that multiple-dose activated charcoal or cathartics alter the clinical course of an intoxication. The dose varies from 0.25 to 0.50 g/kg every 1 to 4 hours, and continuous nasogastric tube infusion of 0.25 to 0.5 g/kg/h has been used to decrease vomiting.

Gastrointestinal dialysis is the diffusion of the toxin from the higher concentration in the serum of the mesenteric vessels to the lower levels in the gastrointestinal tract mucosal cell and subsequently into the gastrointestinal lumen, where the concentration has been lowered by intraluminal adsorption of activated charcoal.

Complications of treatment with activated charcoal include vomiting in 50% of cases, desorption (especially with weak acids in intestine), and aspiration (at least a dozen cases of aspiration have been reported). There are many cases of unreported pulmonary aspirations and "charcoal lungs," intestinal obstruction or pseudoobstruction (three case reports with multiple dosing, none with a single dose), empyema following esophageal perforation, and hypermagnesemia and hypernatremia, which have been associated with repeated concurrent doses of activated charcoal and saline cathartics. Catharsis was used to hasten the elimination of any remaining toxin in the gastrointestinal tract. There are no studies to demonstrate the effectiveness of cathartics, and they are no longer recommended as a form of gastrointestinal decontamination.

Whole-Bowel Irrigation

With whole bowel irrigation, solutions of polyethylene glycol (PEG) with balanced electrolytes are used to cleanse the bowel without causing shifts in fluids and electrolytes. The procedure is not approved by the U.S. Food and Drug Administration for this purpose.

Indications

The procedure has been studied and used successfully in cases of iron overdose when abdominal radiographs reveal incomplete emptying of excess iron. There are additional indications for other types of ingestions, such as with body-packing of illicit drugs (e.g., cocaine, heroin).

The procedure is to administer the solution (GoLYTELY or Colyte), orally or by nasogastric tube, in a dose of 0.5 L per hour in children younger than 5 years of age and 2 L per hour in adolescents and adults for 5 hours. The end point is reached when the rectal effluent is clear or radiopaque materials can no longer be seen in the gastrointestinal tract on abdominal radiographs.

Contraindications

These measures should not be used if there is extensive hematemesis, ileus, or signs of bowel obstruction, perforation, or peritonitis. Animal experiments in which PEG was added to activated charcoal indicated that activated charcoal-salicylates and activated charcoal-theophylline combinations resulted in decreased adsorption and desorption of salicylate and theophylline and no therapeutic benefit over activated charcoal alone. Polyethylene solutions are bound by activated charcoal in vitro, decreasing the efficacy of activated charcoal.

Dilutional treatment is indicated for the immediate management of caustic and corrosive poisonings but is otherwise not useful. The administration of diluting fluid above 30 mL in children and 250 mL in adults may produce vomiting, reexposing the vital tissues to the effects of local damage and possible aspiration.

Neutralization is not proven to be either safe or effective.

Endoscopy and surgery have been required in the case of body-packer obstruction, intestinal ischemia produced by cocaine ingestion, and iron local caustic action.

Differential Diagnosis of Poisons on the Basis of Central Nervous System Manifestations

Neurologic parameters help to classify and assess the need for supportive treatment as well as provide diagnostic clues to the etiology. Table 4 lists the effects of CNS depressants, CNS stimulants, hallucinogens, and autonomic nervous system anticholinergics and cholinergics.

Central nervous system depressants are cholinergics, opioids, sedative-hypnotics, and sympatholytic agents. The hallmarks are lethargy, sedation, stupor, and coma. In exception to the manifestations listed in Table 4, (a) barbiturates may produce an initial tachycardia; (b) convulsions are produced by codeine, propoxyphene (Darvon), meperidine (Demerol), glutethimide, phenothiazines, methaqualone, and tricyclic and cyclic antidepressants; (c) benzodiazepines rarely produce coma that will interfere with cardiorespiratory functions; and (d) pulmonary edema is common with opioids and sedative-hypnotics.

The CNS stimulants are anticholinergic, hallucinogenic, sympathomimetic, and withdrawal agents. The hallmarks of CNS stimulants are convulsions and hyperactivity.

There is considerable overlapping of effects among the various hallucinogens, but the major hallmark manifestation is hallucinations.

Guidelines for In-Hospital Disposition

Classification of patients as high risk depends on clinical judgment. Any patient who needs cardiorespiratory support or has a persistently altered mental status for 3 hours or more should be considered for intensive care.

Guidelines for admitting patients older than 14 years of age to an intensive care unit, after 2 to 3 hours in the emergency department, include the following:

1. Need for intubation
2. Seizures
3. Unresponsiveness to verbal stimuli
4. Arterial carbon dioxide pressure greater than 45 mm Hg
5. Cardiac conduction or rhythm disturbances (any rhythm except sinus arrhythmia)
6. Close monitoring of vital signs during antidotal therapy or elimination procedures
7. The need for continuous monitoring

TABLE 4 Agents with Central Nervous System (CNS) Effects

Agents	General Manifestations	Agents	General Manifestations
CNS Depressants	Bradycardia	**Hallucinogens**	Tachycardia and dysrhythmias
Alcohols and glycols (S-H)	Bradypnea	Amphetamines[‡]	Tachypnea
Anticonvulsants (S-H)	Shallow respirations	Anticholinergics	Hypertension
Antidysrhythmics (S-H)	Hypotension	Cardiac glycosides	Hallucinations, usually visual
Antihypertensives (S-H)	Hypothermia	Cocaine	Disorientation
Barbiturates (S-H)	Flaccid coma	Ethanol withdrawal	Panic reaction
Benzodiazepines (S-H)	Miosis	Hydrocarbon inhalation (abuse)	Toxic psychosis
Butyrophenones (Syly)	Hypoactive bowel sounds	Mescaline (peyote)	Moist skin
β-Adrenergic blockers (Syly)		Mushrooms (psilocybin)	Mydriasis (reactive)
Calcium channel blockers (Syly)		Phencyclidine	Hyperthermia
Digitalis (Syly)			Flashbacks
Opioids			
Lithium (mixed)			
Muscle relaxants			
Phenothiazines (Syly)		**Anticholinergics**	Tachycardia, dysrhythmias (rare)
Nonbarbiturate/benzodiazepine		Antihistamines	Tachypnea
glutethimide, methaqualone,		Antispasmodic gastrointestinal preparations	Hypertension (mild)
methyprylon, sedative-hypnotics		Antiparkinsonian preparations	Hyperthermia
(chloral hydrate, ethchlorvynol, bromide)		Atropine	Hallucinations ("mad as a hatter")
Tricyclic antidepressants (late Syly)		Cyclobenzaprine (Flexeril)	Mydriasis (unreactive)
		Mydriatic ophthalmologic agents	("blind as a bat")
		Over-the-counter sleep agents	Flushed skin ("red as a beet")
CNS Stimulants	Tachycardia	Plants (Datura spp)/mushrooms	Dry skin and mouth ("dry as a bone")
Amphetamines (Sy)	Tachypnea and dysrhythmias	Phenothiazines (early)	Hypoactive bowel sounds
Anticholinergics*	Hypertension	Scopolamine	Urinary retention
Cocaine (Sy)	Convulsions	Tricyclic/cyclic antidepressants (early)	Liliputian hallucinations ("little people")
Camphor (mixed)	Toxic psychosis		
Ergot alkaloids (Sy)	Mydriasis (reactive)		
Isoniazid (mixed)	Agitation and restlessness	**Cholinergics**	Bradycardia (muscarinic)
Lithium (mixed)	Moist skin	Bethanechol (Urecholine)	Tachycardia (nicotinic effect)
Lysergic acid diethylamide (H)	Tremors	Carbamate insecticides (Carbaryl)	Miosis (muscarinic)
Hallucinogens (H)		Edrophonium	Diarrhea (muscarinic)
Mescaline and synthetic analogs		Organophosphate insecticides (Malathion, parathion)	Hypertension (variable)
Metals (arsenic, lead, mercury)		Parasympathetic agents (physostigmine, pyridostigmine)	Hyperactive bowel sounds
Methylphenidate (Ritalin) (Sy)		Toxic mushrooms (Clitocybe spp.)	Excess urination (muscarinic)
Monoamine oxidase inhibitors (Sy)			Excess salivation (muscarinic)
Pemoline (Cylert) (Sy)			Lacrimation (muscarinic)
Phencyclidine (H)†			Bronchospasm (muscarinic)
Salicylates (mixed)			Muscle fasciculations (nicotinic)
Strychnine (mixed)			Paralysis (nicotinic)
Sympathomimetics (Sy) (phenylpropanolamine,			
theophylline, caffeine, thyroid)			
Withdrawal from ethanol, β-adrenergic blockers,			
clonidine, opioids, sedative-hypnotics (W)			

*Anticholinergics produce dry skin and mucosa and decreased bowel sounds.
†Phencyclidine may produce miosis.
‡The amphetamine hybrids are methylene dioxymethamphetamine (MDMA, ecstasy, "Adam") and methylene dioxyamphetamine (MDA, "Eve"), which are associated with deaths.
Abbreviations: H = hallucinogen; S-H = sedative-hypnotic; Sy = sympathomimetic; Syly = sympatholytic; W = withdrawal.

8. QRS interval greater than 0.10 second, in cases of tricyclic antidepressant poisoning
9. Systolic blood pressure less than 80 mm Hg
10. Hypoxia, hypercarbia, acid-base imbalance, or metabolic abnormalities
11. Extremes of temperature
12. Progressive deterioration or significant underlying medical disorders

Use of Antidotes

Antidotes are available for only a relatively small number of poisons. An antidote is not a substitute for good supportive care. Table 5 summarizes the commonly used antidotes, their indications, and their methods of administration. The Regional Poison Control Center can give further information on these antidotes.

Enhancement of Elimination

The acceptable methods for elimination of absorbed toxic substances are dialysis, hemoperfusion, exchange transfusion, plasmapheresis, enzyme induction, and inhibition. Methods of increasing urinary excretion of toxic chemicals and drugs have been studied extensively, but the other modalities have not been well evaluated.

In general, these methods are needed in only a minority of cases and should be reserved for life-threatening circumstances when a definite benefit is anticipated.

DIALYSIS

Dialysis is the extrarenal means of removing certain substances from the body, and it can substitute for the kidney when renal failure occurs. Dialysis is not the first measure instituted; however, it may be lifesaving later in the course of a severe intoxication. It is needed in only a minority of intoxicated patients.

Peritoneal dialysis uses the peritoneum as the membrane for dialysis. It is only 1/20 as effective as hemodialysis. It is easier to use and less hazardous to the patient but also less effective in removing the toxin; thus it is rarely used except in small infants.

Hemodialysis is the most effective dialysis method but requires experience with sophisticated equipment. Blood is circulated past a semipermeable extracorporeal membrane. Substances are removed by diffusion down a concentration gradient. Anticoagulation with heparin is necessary. Flow rates of 300 to 500 mL/min can be achieved, and clearance rates may reach 200 or 300 mL/min.

Dialyzable substances easily diffuse across the dialysis membrane and have the following characteristics: (a) a molecular weight less than 500 daltons and preferably less than 350; (b) a volume of distribution less than 1 L/kg; (c) protein binding less than 50%; (d) high water solubility (low lipid solubility); and (e) high plasma concentration and a toxicity that correlates reasonably with the plasma concentration. Considerations for hemodialysis and hemoperfusion are cases of serious ingestions (the nephrologist should be notified immediately), and cases involving a compound that is ingested in a potentially lethal dose and the rapid removal of which may improve the prognosis. Examples of the latter are ethylene glycol 1.4 mL/kg 100% solution or equivalent and methanol 6 mL/kg 100% solution or equivalent. Common dialyzable substances include alcohol, bromides, lithium, and salicylates.

The patient-related criteria for dialysis are (a) anticipated prolonged coma and the likelihood of complications; (b) renal compromise (toxin excreted or metabolized by kidneys and dialyzable chelating agents in heavy metal poisoning); (c) laboratory confirmation of lethal blood concentration; (d) lethal dose poisoning with an agent with delayed toxicity or known to be metabolized into a more toxic metabolite (e.g., ethylene glycol, methanol); and (e) hepatic impairment when the agent is metabolized by the liver, and clinical deterioration despite optimal supportive medical management.

Table 6 gives plasma concentrations above which removal by extracorporeal measures should be considered.

The contraindications to hemodialysis include the following: (a) substances are not dialyzable; (b) effective antidotes are available; (c) patient is hemodynamically unstable (e.g., shock); and (d) presence of coagulopathy because heparinization is required.

Hemodialysis also has a role in correcting disturbances that are not amenable to appropriate medical management. These are easily remembered by the "vowel" mnemonic:

A—refractory acid-base disturbances
E—refractory electrolyte disturbances
I—intoxication with dialyzable substances (e.g., ethanol, ethylene glycol, isopropyl alcohol, methanol, lithium, and salicylates)
O—overhydration
U—uremia

Complications of dialysis include hemorrhage, thrombosis, air embolism, hypotension, infections, electrolyte imbalance, thrombocytopenia, and removal of therapeutic medications.

HEMOPERFUSION

Hemoperfusion is the parenteral form of oral activated charcoal. Heparinization is necessary. The patient's blood is routed extracorporeally through an outflow arterial catheter through a filter-adsorbing cartridge (charcoal or resin) and returned through a venous catheter. Cartridges must be changed every 4 hours. The blood glucose, electrolytes, calcium, and albumin levels; complete blood cell count; platelets; and serum and urine osmolarity must be carefully monitored. This procedure has extended extracorporeal removal to a large range of substances that were formerly either poorly dialyzable or nondialyzable. It is not limited by molecular weight, water solubility, or protein binding, but it is limited by a volume distribution greater than 400 L, plasma concentration, and rate of flow through the filter. Activated charcoal cartridges are the primary type of hemoperfusion that is currently available in the United States.

The patient-related criteria for hemoperfusion are (a) anticipated prolonged coma and the likelihood of complications; (b) laboratory confirmation of lethal blood concentrations; (c) hepatic impairment when an agent is metabolized by the liver; and (d) clinical deterioration despite optimally supportive medical management.

The contraindications are similar to those for hemodialysis.

Limited data are available as to which toxins are best treated with hemoperfusion. Hemoperfusion has proved useful in treating glutethimide intoxication, phenobarbital overdose, and carbamazepine, phenytoin, and theophylline intoxication.

Complications include hemorrhage, thrombocytopenia, hypotension, infection, leukopenia, depressed phagocytic activity of granulocytes, decreased immunoglobulin levels, hypoglycemia, hypothermia, hypocalcemia, pulmonary edema, and air and charcoal embolism.

HEMOFILTRATION

Continuous arteriovenous or venovenous hemodiafiltration (CAVHD or CVVHD, respectively) has been suggested as an alternative to conventional hemodialysis when the need for rapid removal of the drug is less urgent. These procedures, like peritoneal dialysis, are minimally invasive, have no significant impact on hemodynamics, and can be carried out continuously for many hours. Their role in the management of acute poisoning remains uncertain, however.

PLASMAPHERESIS

Plasmapheresis consists of removal of a volume of blood. All the extracted components are returned to the blood except the plasma, which is replaced with a colloid protein solution. There are limited clinical data on guidelines and efficacy in toxicology. Centrifugal and membrane separators of cellular elements are used. It can be as effective as hemodialysis or hemoperfusion for removing toxins that have high protein binding, and it may be useful for toxins not filtered by hemodialysis and hemoperfusion.

TABLE 5 Initial Doses of Antidotes for Common Poisonings

Antidote	Use	Dose	Route	Adverse Reactions/Comments
N-Acetyl Cysteine (NAC, Mucomyst): Stock level to treat 70 kg adult for 24 h: 25 vials, 20%, 30 mL	Acetaminophen, carbon tetrachloride (experimental)	140 mg/kg loading, followed by 70 mg/kg every 4 h for 17 doses 150 mg/kg in 200 mL of D_5W over 1 hr, then 50 mg/kg in 1 liter D_5W over 16 hr	PO IV	Nausea, vomiting. Dilute to 5% with sweet juice or flat cola. Useful for those who cannot tolerate oral route.
Atropine: Stock level to treat 70 kg adult for 24 h: 1 g (1 mg/mL in 1, 10 mL)	Organophosphate and carbamate pesticides: bradydysrhythmics, β-adrenergics, calcium channel blockers/nerve agents	*Child:* 0.02–0.05 mg/kg repeated q5–10 min to max of 2 mg as necessary until cessation of secretions *Adult:* 1–2 mg q5–10 min as necessary. Dilute in 1–2 mL of 0.9% saline for ET instillation. *IV infusion dose:* Place 8 mg of atropine in 100 mL D_5W or saline. Conc. = 0.08 mg/mL; dose range = 0.02–0.08 mg/kg/h or 0.25–1 mL/kg/h. Severe poisoning may require supplemental doses of IV atropine intermittently in doses of 1–5 mg until drying of secretions occurs.	IV/ET	Tachycardia, dry mouth, blurred vision, and urinary retention. Ensure adequate ventilation before administration.
Calcium Chloride (10%): Stock level to treat 70 kg adult for 24 h: 10 vials 1 g (1.35 mEq/mL)	Hypocalcemia, fluoride, calcium channel blockers, β-blockers, oxalates, ethylene glycol, hypermagnesemia	0.1–0.2 mL/kg (10–20 mg/kg) slow push every 10 min up to max 10 mL (1 g). Since calcium response lasts 15 min, some may require continuous infusion 0.2 mL/kg/h up to maximum of 10 mL/h while monitoring for dysrhythmias and hypotension.	IV	Administer slowly with BP and ECG monitoring and have magnesium available to reverse calcium effects. Tissue irritation, hypotension, dysrhythmias from rapid injection. Contraindications: digitalis glycoside intoxication.
Calcium Gluconate (10%): Stock level to treat 70 kg adult for 24 h: 20 vials 1 g (0.45 mEq/mL)	Hypocalcemia, fluoride, calcium channel blockers, hydrofluoric acid; black widow envenomation	0.3–0.4 mL/kg (30–40 mg/kg) slow push; repeat as needed to max dose 10–20 mL (1–2 g).	IV	Same comments as calcium chloride.
Infiltration of Calcium Gluconate	Hydrofluoric acid skin exposure	Dose: Infiltrate each square cm of affected dermis/subcutaneous tissue with about 0.5 mL of 10% calcium gluconate using a 30-gauge needle. Repeat as needed to control pain.	Infiltrate	
Intra-arterial Calcium Gluconate	Hydrofluoric acid skin exposure	Infuse 20 mL of 10% calcium gluconate (not chloride) diluted in 250 mL D_5W via the radial or brachial artery proximal to the injury over 3–4 h.		Alternatively, dilute 10 mL of 10% calcium gluconate with 40–50 mL of D_5W.
Calcium Gluconate Gel: Stock level: 3.5 g	Hydrofluoric acid skin exposure	2.5 g USP powder added to 100 mL water-soluble lubricating jelly, e.g., K-Y Jelly or Lubifax (or 3.5 mg into 150 mL). Some use 6 g of calcium carbonate in 100 g of lubricant. Place injured hand in surgical glove filled with gel. Apply q4h. If pain persists, calcium gluconate injection may be needed (above).	Dermal	Powder is available from Spectrum Pharmaceutical Co. in California: 800-772-8786. Commercial preparation of Ca gluconate gel is available from Pharmascience in Montreal, Quebec: 514-340-1114.

	Indication	Route	Dose	Comments
Cyanide Antidote Kit: Stock level to treat 70 kg adult for 24 h: 2 Lilly Cyanide Antidote kits	Cyanide Hydrogen sulfide (nitrites are given only) Do not use sodium thiosulfate for hydrogen sulfide Individual portions of the kit can be used in certain circumstances (consult PCC)	Inhalation	Amyl nitrite: 1 crushable ampule for 30 sec of every min. Use new amp q3 min. May omit step if venous access is established.	If methemoglobinemia occurs, do not use methylene blue to correct this because it releases cyanide.
	Cyanide Hydrogen sulfide (nitrites are given only) Do not use sodium thiosulfate for hydrogen sulfide Individual portions of the kit can be used in certain circumstances (consult PCC)	IV	Sodium nitrite: *Child:* 0.33 mL/kg of 3% solution if hemoglobin level is not known, otherwise based on tables with product. *Adult:* up to 300 mg (10 mL). Dilute nitrite in 100 mL 0.9% saline, administer slowly at 5 mL/min. Slow infusion if fall in BP.	If methemoglobinemia occurs, do not use methylene blue to correct this because it releases cyanide.
	Cyanide Hydrogen sulfide Do not use sodium thiosulfate for hydrogen sulfide Individual portions of the kit can be used in certain circumstances (consult PCC)	IV	Sodium thiosulfate: *Child:* 1.6 mL/kg of 25% solution, may be repeated every 30–60 min to a maximum of 12.5 g or 50 mL in adult. Administer over 20 min.	Nausea, dizziness, headache. Tachycardia, muscle rigidity, and bronchospasm (rapid administration).
Dantrolene Sodium (Dantrium): Stock level to treat 70 kg adult for 24 h: 700 mg, 35 vials (20 mg/vial)	Malignant hyperthermia	IV/PO	2–3 mg/kg IV rapidly. Repeat loading dose every 10 min. If necessary up to a maximum total dose of 10 mg/kg. When temperature and heart rate decrease, slow the infusion 1–2 mg/kg every 6 h for 24–28 h until all evidence of malignant hyperthermia syndrome has subsided. Follow with oral doses 1–2 mg/kg four times a day for 24 h as necessary.	Hepatotoxicity occurs with cumulative dose of 10 mg/kg. Thrombophlebitis (best given in central line). Available as 20 mg lyophilized dantrolene powder for reconstruction, which contains 3 g mannitol and sodium hydroxide in 70-mL vial. Mix with 60 mL sterile distilled water without a bacteriostatic agent and protect from light. Use within 6 hours after reconstituting.
Deferoxamine (Desferal): Stock level to treat 70 kg adult for 24 h: 17 vials (500 mg/amp)	Iron	Preferred IV: avoid therapy >24 h	IV infusion of 15 mg/kg/h (3 mL/kg/h: 500 mg in 100 mL D₅W) max 6 g/d Rates of >45 μg/kg/h if conc >1000 μg/dL.	Hypotension (minimized by avoiding rapid infusion rates) DFO challenge test 50 mg/kg is unreliable if negative.
Diazepam (Valium): Stock level to treat 70 kg adult for 24 h: 200 mg, 5 mg/mL; 2, 10 mL	Any intoxication that provokes seizures when specific therapy is not available, (e.g., amphetamines, PCP, barbiturate and alcohol withdrawal). Chloroquine poisoning	IV	Adult, 5–10 mg IV (max 20 mg) at a rate of 5 mg/min until seizure is controlled. May be repeated 2 or 3 times. Child, 0.1–0.3 mg/kg up to 10 mg IV slowly over 2 min.	Confusion, somnolence, coma, hypotension. Intramuscular absorption is erratic. Establish airway and administer 100% oxygen and glucose.
Digoxin-Specific Fab Antibodies (Digibind): Stock level to treat 70 kg adult for 24 h: 20 vials	Digoxin, digitoxin, oleander tea with the following: (1) Imminent cardiac arrest or shock (2) Hyperkalemia >5.0 mEq/L (3) Serum digoxin >5 ng/mL (child) at 8–12 h post ingestion in adults (4) Digitalis delirium (5) Ingestion over 10 mg in adults or 4 mg in child (6) Bradycardia or second- or third-degree heart block unresponsive to atropine (7) Life-threatening digitoxin or oleander poisoning	IV	(1) If amount ingested is known total dose × bioavailability (0.8) = body burden. The body burden + 0.6 (0.5 mg of digoxin is bound by 1 vial of 38 mg of Fab) = # vials needed. (2) If amount is unknown but the steady state serum concentration is known in ng/mL: Digoxin: ng/mL (5.6 L/kg Vd) × (wt kg) = μg body burden. Body burden + 100 = mg body burden/0.5 = # vials needed. Digitoxin body burden = ng/mL × (0.56 L/kg Vd) × (wt kg) Body burden + 1000 = mg body burden/0.5 = # vials needed. (3) If the amount is not known, it is administered in life-threatening situations as 10 vials (400 mg) IV in saline over 30 min in adults. If cardiac arrest is imminent, administer 20 vials (adult) as a bolus.	Allergic reactions (rare), return of condition being treated with digitalis glycoside. Administer by infusion over 30 min through a 0.22-μ filter. If cardiac arrest imminent, may administer by bolus. Consult PCC for more details.

Continued

TABLE 5 Initial Doses of Antidotes for Common Poisonings—Cont'd

Antidote	Use	Dose	Route	Adverse Reactions/Comments
Dimercaprol (BAL in Peanut Oil): Stock level to treat 70 kg adult for 24 h: 1200 mg (4 amps—100 mg/mL 10% in oil in 3 mL amp)	Chelating agent for arsenic, mercury, and lead	3–5 mg/kg q4h usually for 5–10 d	Deep IM	Local infection site pain and sterile abscess, nausea, vomiting, fever, salivation, hypertension, and nephrotoxicity (alkalinize urine).
2,3 Dimercaptosuccinic Acid (DMSA Succimer): 100 mg/capsule: 20 capsules	Used as a chelating agent for lead, especially blood lead levels >45 μg/dL. May also be used for symptomatic mercury exposure	10 mg/kg 3 × daily for 5 days followed by 10 mg/kg 2 × daily for 14 days.	PO	Precautions: monitor AST/ALT; use with caution in G6PD-deficient patients. Avoid concurrent iron therapy. Relatively safe antidote, rarely severe, uncommon minor skin rashes may occur.
Diphenhydramine (Benadryl): Antiparkinsonian action. Stock level to treat a 70 kg adult for 24 h: 5 vials (10 mg/mL, 10 mL each)	Used to treat extrapyramidal symptoms and dystonia induced by phenothiazines, phencyclidine, and related drugs	*Children:* 1–2 mg/kg IV slowly over 5 min up to maximum 50 mg followed by 5 mg/kg/24 h orally divided every 6 h up to 300 mg/24 h. *Adults:* 50 mg IV followed by 50 mg orally four times daily for 5–7 d. *Note:* Symptoms abate within 2–5 min after IV.	IV	Fatal dose: 20–40 mg/kg. Dry mouth, drowsiness.
Ethanol (Ethyl Alcohol): Stock level to treat 70 kg adult for 24 h: 3 bottles 10% (1 L each)	Methanol, ethylene glycol	10 mL/kg loading dose concurrently with 1.4 mL/kg (average) infusion of 10% ethanol (consult PCC for more details)	IV	Nausea, vomiting, sedation. Use 0.22-μ filter if preparing from bulk 100% ethanol.
Flumazenil (Romazicon): Stock level to treat 70 kg adult for 24 h: 4 vials (0.1 mg/mL, 10 mL)	Benzodiazepines (may also be beneficial in the treatment of hepatic encephalopathy)	Administer 0.2 mg (2 mL) IV over 30 sec (pediatric dose not established, 0.01 mg/kg), then wait 3 min for a response, then if desired consciousness is not achieved, administer 0.3 mg (3 mL) over 30 sec, then wait 3 min for response, then if desired consciousness is not achieved, administer 0.5 mg (5 mL) over 30 sec at 60-sec intervals up to a maximum cumulative dose of 3 mg (30 mL) (1 mg in children). Because effects last only 1–5 h, if patient responds, monitor carefully over next 6 h for resedation. If multiple repeated doses, consider a continuous infusion of 0.2–1 mg/h.	IV	Nausea, vomiting, facial flushing, agitation, headache, dizziness, seizures, and death. It is not recommended to improve ventilation. Its role in CNS depression needs to be clarified. It should not be used routinely in comatose patients. It is **contraindicated** in cyclic antidepressant intoxications, stimulant overdose, long-term benzodiazepine use (may precipitate life-threatening withdrawal), if benzodiazepines are used to control seizures, in head trauma.
Folic Acid (Folvite): Stock level to treat 70 kg adult for 24 h: 4 100-mg vials	Methanol/ethylene glycol (investigational)	1 mg/kg up to 50 mg q4h for 6 doses.	IV	Uncommon
Fomepizole (4-MP, Antizol): Stock level to treat 70 kg adult: 4 1.5-mL vials (1 g/mL)	Ethylene glycol Methanol	Loading dose: 15 mg/kg (0.015 mL/kg) IV followed by maintenance dose of 10 mg/kg (0.01 mL/kg) every 12 h for 4 doses, then 15 mg/kg every 12 h until ethylene glycol levels are <20 mg/dL. Fomepizole can be given to patients undergoing hemodialysis (dose q4h).	IV	Suggested: co-administer folate 50 mg IV (child 1 mg/kg), thiamine 100 mg/d (child 50 mg), and pyridoxine 50 mg IV/IM q6h until intoxication is resolved. Monitor for urinary oxalate crystals. Adverse reactions include headache, nausea, and dizziness. Antizole should be diluted in 100 mL 0.9% saline or D₅W and mixed well. Antizole should not be given undiluted.
Glucagon: Stock level to treat 70 kg adult for 24 h: 10 vials, 10 units	β-Blocker, calcium channel blocker	3–10 mg in adult, then infuse 2–5 mg/h (0.05–0.1 mg/kg in child, then infuse 0.07 mg/kg/h) Large doses up to 100 mg/24 h used	IV	Use D₅W, not 0.9% saline, to reconstitute the glucagon (rather than diluent of Eli Lilly, which contains phenol). Vomiting precautions.

Antidote	Indication	Route	Dose	Comments
Magnesium Sulfate: Stock level to treat 70 kg adult for 24 h: approx 25 g (50 mL of 50% or 200 mL of 12.5%)	Torsades de pointes	IV	*Adult:* 2 g (20 mL or 20%) over 20 min. If no response in 10 min, repeat and follow by continuous infusion 1 g/h. *Children:* 25–50 mg/kg/24 h initially and maintenance is (30–60 mg/kg/24 h) (0.25–0.5 mEq/kg/24 h) up to 1000 mg/24 h. (Dose not studied in controlled fashion.)	Use with caution if renal impairment is present.
Methylene Blue: Stock level to treat 70 kg adult for 24 h: 5 amps (10 mg/10 mL)	Methemoglobinemia	IV	0.1–0.2 mL/kg of 1% solution, slow infusion, may be repeated every 30–60 min	Nausea, vomiting, headache, dizziness.
Naloxone (Narcan): Stock level to treat 70 kg adult for 24 h: 3 vials (1 mg/mL, 10 mL)	Comatose patient; decreased respirations <12; opioids	IV, ET	In postoperative opioid depression reversal, IV 0.1–0.5 μg/kg every 2 min as needed and may repeat up to a total dose of 1 μg/kg. In **suspected overdose,** administer IV 0.1 mg/kg in a child younger than 5 years of age up to 2 mg, in older children and adults administer 2 mg every 2 min up to a total of 10–20 mg. Can also be administered into the endotracheal tube. If no response by 10 mg, a pure opioid intoxication is unlikely. If **opioid abuse** is suspected, **restraints** should be in place before administration; **initial dose** 0.1 mg to avoid withdrawal and violent behavior. The initial dose is then doubled every minute progressively to a total of 10 mg. A **continuous infusion** has been advocated because many opioids outlast the short half-life of naloxone (30–60 min). The **naloxone infusion hourly rate** to produce a response is equal to the effective dose required (improvement in ventilation and arousal). An additional dose may be required in 15–30 min as a bolus.	**Larger doses** of naloxone may be required for more poorly antagonized synthetic opioid drugs: buprenorphine (Buprenex), codeine, dextromethorphan, fentanyl, pentazocine (Talwin), propoxyphene (Darvon), diphenoxylate, nalbuphine (Nubain), new potent "designer" drugs, or long-acting opioids such as methadone (Dolophine). **Complications.** Although naloxone is safe and effective, there are rare reports of complications (<1%) of pulmonary edema, seizures, hypertension, cardiac arrest, and sudden death. The infusions are titrated to avoid respiratory depression and opioid withdrawal manifestations. Tapering of infusions can be attempted after 12 h and when the patient is stable.
Physostigmine (Antilirium): Stock level to treat 70 kg adult for 24 h: 2–4 mg (2 mL each)	Anticholinergic agents (not routinely used, only indicated if life-threatening complications)	IV	*Child:* 0.02 mg/kg slow push to max 2 mg q30–60 min. *Adult:* 1–2 mg q5 min to max 6 mg.	Bradycardia, asystole, seizures, bronchospasm, vomiting, headaches. Do not use for cyclic antidepressants.
Pralidoxime (2PAM, Protopan): Stock level to treat 70 kg adult for 24 h: 12 vials (1 g per 20 mL)	Organophosphates/nerve agents	IV	Child ≤12 y, 25–50 mg/kg max (4 mg/min); >12 y, 1–2 g/dose in 250 mL of 0.9% saline over 5–10 min. Max 200 mg/min. Repeat q6–12h for 24–48h. Max adult 6 g/d. Alternative: Maintenance infusion 1 g in 100 mL, of 0.9% saline at 5–20 mg/kg/h (0.5–12 mL/kg/h) up to max 500 mg/h or 50 mL/h. Titrate to desired response. End point is absence of fasciculations and return of muscle strength.	Nausea, dizziness, headache; tachycardia, muscle rigidity, bronchospasm (rapid administration).
Pyridoxine (Vitamin B₆): Stock level to treat 70 kg adult for 24 h: 100 mg/mL 10% solution. For a 70 kg patient, 10 g = 10 vials	Seizures from isoniazid or *Gyromitra* mushrooms, ethylene glycol	IV	*Isoniazid: Unknown amt ingested:* 5 g (70 mg/kg) in 50 mL D₅W over 5 min + diazepam 0.3 mg/kg IV at rate of 1 mg/min in child or 10 mg dose at rate up to 5 mg/min in adults. Use different site (synergism). May repeat q5–20 min until seizure controlled. Up to 375 mg/kg have been given (52 g). *Known amount:* 1 g for each gram isoniazid ingested over 5 min with diazepam (dose above). *Gyromitra mushroom:* Child 25 mg/kg or 2–5 g, adults IV over 15–30 min to max 20 g.	After seizure is controlled, administer remainder of pyridoxine 1 g/1 g isoniazid total 5 g as infusion over 60 min. Adverse reactions uncommon; do not administer in same bottle as sodium bicarbonate. For *Gyromitra* mushrooms, some use PO 25 mg/kg/d early when mushroom ingestion is suspected.

TABLE 5 Initial Doses of Antidotes for Common Poisonings—Cont'd

Antidote	Use	Dose	Route	Adverse Reactions/Comments
Sodium Bicarbonate (NaHCO₃): Stock level to treat 70 kg adult for 24 h: 10 ampules or syringes (500 mEq)	Tricyclic antidepressant cardiotoxicity (QRS >0.12 sec; ventricular tachycardia, severe conduction disturbances); metabolic acidosis; phenothiazine toxicity *Salicylate:* to keep blood pH 7.5–7.55 (not >7.55) and urine pH 7.5–8.0. Alkalinization recommended if salicylate conc. >40 mg/dL in acute poisoning and at lower levels if symptomatic in chronic intoxication, 2 mEq/kg will raise blood pH 0.1 unit	*Ethylene glycol:* 100 mg IV daily. 1–2 mEq/kg undiluted as a bolus. If no effect on cardiotoxicity, repeat twice a few minutes apart *Adult* with clear physical signs and laboratory findings of acute moderate or severe salicylism: Bolus 1–2 mEq/kg followed by infusion of 100–150 mEq NaHCO₃ added to 1 L of 5% dextrose at rate of 200–300 mL/h *Child:* Bolus same as adult followed by 1–2 mEq/kg in infusion of 20 mL/kg/h 5% dextrose in 0.45% saline. Add potassium when patient voids. Rate and amount of the initial infusion, if patient is volume depleted: 1 h to achieve urine output of 2 mL/kg/h and urine pH 7–8. In mild cases without acidosis and urine pH >6, administer 5% dextrose in 0.9% saline with 50 mEq/L or 1 mEq/kg NaHCO₃ as maintenance to replace ongoing renal losses. If acidemia is present and pH <7.2, add 2 mEq/kg as loading dose followed by 2 mEq/kg q3–4h to keep pH at 7.5–7.55. If acidemia is present, recommend isotonic NaHCO₃, 3 ampules to 1 L of D₅W @ 10–15 mL/kg/h or sufficient to produce normal urine flow and a urine pH of 7.5 or higher.	IV	Monitor sodium, potassium, and blood pH because fatal alkalemia and hyponatremia have been reported. Monitor both urine and blood pH. Do not use the urine pH alone to assess the need for alkalinization because of the paradoxical aciduria that may occur. Adjust the urine pH to 7.5–8 by NaHCO₃ infusion. After urine output established, add potassium 40 mEq/L.
	Long-acting barbiturates: Phenobarbital and primidone (Mysoline). *Note:* Alkalinization is ineffective for the short- or intermediate-acting barbiturates	NaHCO₃: 2 mEq/kg during the first hour or 100 mEq in 1 L of D₅W with 40 mEq/L potassium at a rate of 100 mL/h in adults. Adequate potassium is necessary to accomplish alkalinization	IV	Additional sodium bicarbonate and potassium chloride may be needed. Adjust the urine pH to 7.5–8 by NaHCO₃ infusion.
Thiamine: 100 mg/mL, 2 vials	Thiamine deficiency, ethylene glycol poisoning, alcoholism	100 mg IV followed with 100 mg V/IM for 5–7 days in an alcoholic and followed by 100 mg/d orally.	IV/IM	
Vitamin K₁ (Aqua Mephyton): 10 mg/1–5 mL; 5-mg tablets	Warfarin anticoagulant or rodenticide toxicity	Oral 0.4 mg/kg/dose child, 10–25 mg adults. If evidence of bleeding, administer vitamin K₁ SC, IV 0.6 mg/kg/dose child and up to 25–50 mg adults for 6 hours depending on severity.	PO/SC, IV	Give vitamin K daily until PT/INR are normal. Examine stools and urine for evidence of bleeding.

Abbreviations: ALT = alanine aminotransferase; amp = ampule; AST = aspartate aminotransferase; BAL = British anti-Lewisite; BP = blood pressure; conc. = concentration; ECG = electrocardiogram; ET = endotracheal; G6PD = glucose-6-phosphate dehydrogenase; IM = intramuscular; IV = intravenous; PCC = poison control center; PO = oral; PT = prothrombin time; SC = subcutaneous.

TABLE 6 Plasma Concentrations Above Which Removal by Extracorporeal Measures Should Be Considered

Drug	Plasma Concentration	Protein Binding (%)	Volume Distribution (L/kg)	Method of Choice
Amanitin	NA	25	1.0	HP
Ethanol	500–700 mg/dL	0	0.3	HD
Etchlorvynol	150 μg/mL	35–50	3–4	HP
Ethylene glycol	25–50 μg/mL	0	0.6	HD
Glutethimide	100 μg/mL	50	2.7	HP
Isopropyl alcohol	400 mg/dL	0	0.7	HD
Lithium	4 mEq/L	0	0.7	HD
Meprobamate (Equanil)	100 μg/mL	0	NA	HP
Methanol	50 mg/dL	0	0.7	HD
Methaqualone	40 μg/dL	20–60	6.0	HP
Other barbiturates	50 μg/dL	50	0–1	HP
Paraquat	0.1 mg/dL	poor	2.8	HP > HD
Phenobarbital	100 μg/dL	50	0.9	HP > HD
Salicylates	80–100 mg/dL	90	0.2	HD > HP
Theophylline		0	0.5	
Chronic	40–60 μg/mL			HP
Acute	80–100 μg/mL			HP
Trichlorethanol	250 μg/mL	70	0.6	HP

Data from Winchester JF: Active methods for detoxification. In Haddad LM, Winchester JF (eds). Clinical Management of Poisoning and Drug Overdose, 2nd ed. Philadelphia, WB Saunders, 1990; Balsam L, Cortitsidis GN, Fienfeld DA: Role of hemodialysis and hemoperfusion in the treatment of intoxications. Contemp Manage Crit Care 1:61, 1991.

Note: Cartridges for charcoal hemoperfusion are not readily available anymore in most locations. So hemodialysis may be substituted in these situations. In mixed or chronic drug overdoses, extracorporeal measures may be considered at lower drug concentrations.

Abbreviations: HD = hemodialysis; HP = hemoperfusion; HP > HD = hemoperfusion preferred over hemodialysis.

Plasmapheresis has been anecdotally used in treating intoxications with the following agents: paraquat (removed 10%), propranolol (removed 30%), quinine (removed 10%), L-thyroxine (removed 30%), and salicylate (removed 10%). It has been shown to remove less than 10% of digoxin, phenobarbital, prednisolone, and tobramycin. Complications include infection; allergic reactions including anaphylaxis; hemorrhagic disorders; thrombocytopenia; embolus and thrombus; hypervolemia and hypovolemia; dysrhythmias; syncope; tetany; paresthesia; pneumothorax; acute respiratory distress syndrome; and seizures.

Supportive Care, Observation, and Therapy for Complications

ALTERED MENTAL STATUS

If airway protective reflexes are absent, endotracheal intubation is indicated for a comatose patient or a patient with altered mental status. If respirations are ineffective, ventilation should be instituted, and if hypoxemia persists, supplemental oxygen is indicated. If a cyanotic patient fails to respond to oxygen, the practitioner should consider methemoglobinemia.

HYPOGLYCEMIA

Hypoglycemia accompanies many poisonings, including with ethanol (especially in children), clonidine (Catapres), insulin, organophosphates, salicylates, sulfonylureas, and the unripe fruit or seed of a Jamaican plant called ackee. If hypoglycemia is present or suspected, glucose should be administered immediately as an intravenous bolus. Doses are as follows: in a neonate, 10% glucose (5 mL/kg); in a child, 25% glucose 0.25 g/kg (2 mL/kg); and in an adult, 50% glucose 0.5 g/kg (1 mL/kg).

A bedside capillary test for blood glucose is performed to detect hypoglycemia, and the sample is sent to the laboratory for confirmation. If the glucose reagent strip visually reads less than 150 mg/dL, one administers glucose. Venous blood should be used rather than capillary blood for the bedside test if the patient is in shock or is hypotensive. Large amounts of glucose given rapidly to nondiabetic patients may cause a transient reactive hypoglycemia and hyperkalemia and may accentuate damage in ischemic cerebrovascular and cardiac tissue. If focal neurologic signs are present, it may be prudent to withhold glucose, because hypoglycemia causes focal signs in less than 10% of cases.

THIAMINE DEFICIENCY ENCEPHALOPATHY

Thiamine is administered to avoid precipitating thiamine deficiency encephalopathy (Wernicke-Korsakoff syndrome) in alcohol abusers and in malnourished patients. The overall incidence of thiamine deficiency in ethanol abusers is 12%. Thiamine 100 mg intravenously should be administered around the time of the glucose administration but not necessarily before the glucose. The clinician should be prepared to manage the anaphylaxis that sometimes is caused by thiamine, although it is extremely rare.

OPIOID REACTIONS

Naloxone (Narcan) reverses CNS and respiratory depression, miosis, bradycardia, and decreased gastrointestinal peristalsis caused by opioids acting through μ, κ, and δ receptors. It also affects endogenous opioid peptides (endorphins and enkephalins), which accounts for the variable responses reported in patients with intoxications from ethanol, benzodiazepines, clonidine (Catapres), captopril (Capoten), and valproic acid (Depakote) and in patients with spinal cord injuries. There is a high sensitivity for predicting a response if pinpoint pupils and circumstantial evidence of opioid abuse (e.g., track marks) are present.

In cases of suspected overdose, naloxone 0.1 mg/kg is administered intravenously initially in a child younger than 5 years of age. The dose can be repeated in 2 minutes, if necessary up to a total dose of 2 mg. In older children and adults, the dose is 2 mg every

2 minutes for five doses up to a total of 10 mg. Naloxone can also be administered into an endotracheal tube if intravenous access is unavailable. If there is no response after 10 mg, a pure opioid intoxication is unlikely. If opioid abuse is suspected, restraints should be in place before the administration of naloxone, and it is recommended that the initial dose be 0.1 to 0.2 mg to avoid withdrawal and violent behavior. The initial dose is then doubled every minute progressively to a total of 10 mg. Naloxone may unmask concomitant sympathomimetic intoxication as well as withdrawal.

Larger doses of naloxone may be required for more poorly antagonized synthetic opioid drugs: buprenorphine (Buprenex), codeine, dextromethorphan, fentanyl and its derivatives, pentazocine (Talwin), propoxyphene (Darvon), diphenoxylate, nalbuphine (Nubain), and long-acting opioids such as methadone (Dolophine).

Indications for a continuous infusion include a second dose for recurrent respiratory depression, exposure to poorly antagonized opioids, a large overdose, and decreased opioid metabolism, as with impaired liver function. A continuous infusion has been advocated because many opioids outlast the short half-life of naloxone (30 to 60 minutes). The hourly rate of naloxone infusion is equal to the effective dose required to produce a response (improvement in ventilation and arousal). An additional dose may be required in 15 to 30 minutes as a bolus. The infusions are titrated to avoid respiratory depression and opioid withdrawal manifestations. Tapering of infusions can be attempted after 12 hours and when the patient's condition has been stabilized.

Although naloxone is safe and effective, there are rare reports of complications (less than 1%) of pulmonary edema, seizures, hypertension, cardiac arrest, and sudden death.

AGENTS WHOSE ROLES ARE NOT CLARIFIED

Nalmefene (Revex), a long-acting parenteral opioid antagonist that the Food and Drug Administration has approved, is undergoing investigation, but its role in the treatment of comatose patients and patients with opioid overdose is not clear. It is 16 times more potent than naloxone, and its duration of action is up to 8 hours (half-life 10.8 hours, versus naloxone 1 hour).

Flumazenil (Romazicon) is a pure competitive benzodiazepine antagonist. It has been demonstrated to be safe and effective for reversing benzodiazepine-induced sedation. It is not recommended to improve ventilation. Its role in cases of CNS depression needs to be clarified. It should not be used routinely in comatose patients and is not an essential ingredient of the coma therapeutic regimen. It is contraindicated in cases of co-ingestion of cyclic antidepressant intoxication, stimulant overdose, and long-term benzodiazepine use (may precipitate life-threatening withdrawal) if benzodiazepines are used to control seizures. There is a concern about the potential for seizures and cardiac dysrhythmias that may occur in these settings.

Laboratory and Radiographic Studies

An electrocardiogram (ECG) should be obtained to identify dysrhythmias or conduction delays from cardiotoxic medications. If aspiration pneumonia (history of loss of consciousness, unarousable state, vomiting) or noncardiac pulmonary edema is suspected, a chest radiograph is needed. Electrolyte and glucose concentrations in the blood, the anion gap, acid-base balance, the arterial blood gas (ABG) profile (if patient has respiratory distress or altered mental status), and serum osmolality should be measured if a toxic alcohol ingestion is suspected. Table 7 lists appropriate testing on the basis of clinical toxicologic presentation. All laboratory specimens should be carefully labeled, including time and date. For potential legal cases, a "chain of custody" must be established. Assessment of the laboratory studies may provide a due to the etiologic agent.

TABLE 7 Patient Condition/Systemic Toxin and Appropriate Tests

Condition	Tests
Comatose	Toxicologic tests (acetaminophen, sedative-hypnotic, ethanol, opioids, benzodiazepine), glucose.
Respiratory toxicity	Spirometry, FEV_1, arterial blood gases, chest radiograph, monitor O_2 saturation
Cardiac toxicity	ECG 12-lead and monitoring, echocardiogram, serial cardiac enzymes (if evidence or suspicion of a myocardial infarction), hemodynamic monitoring
Hepatic toxicity	Enzymes (AST, ALT, GGT), ammonia, albumin, bilirubin, glucose, PT, PTT, amylase
Nephrotoxicity	BUN, creatinine, electrolytes (Na, F, Mg, Ca, PO_4), serum and urine osmolarity, 24-hour urine for heavy metals if suspected, creatine kinase, serum and urine myoglobin, urinalysis and urinary sodium
Bleeding	Platelets, PT, PTT, bleeding time, fibrin split products, fibrinogen, type and match

Abbreviations: ALT = alanine transaminase; AST = aspartate transaminase; BUN = blood urea nitrogen; ECG = electrocardiogram; FEV_1 = forced expiratory volume at 1 second; GGT = γ-glutamyltransferase; PT = prothrombin time; PTT = partial thromboplastin time.

ELECTROLYTE, ACID-BASE, AND OSMOLALITY DISTURBANCES

Electrolyte and acid-base disturbances should be evaluated and corrected. Metabolic acidosis (usually low or normal pH with a low or normal/high $PaCO_2$ and low HCO_3) with an increased anion gap is seen with many agents in cases of overdose.

The anion gap is an estimate of those anions other than chloride and HCO_3 necessary to counterbalance the positive charge of sodium. It serves as a clue to causes, compensations, and complications. The anion gap (AG) is calculated from the standard serum electrolytes by subtracting the total CO_2 (which reflects the actual measured bicarbonate) and chloride from the sodium: $(Na - [Cl + HCO_3]) = AG$. The potassium is usually not used in the calculation because it may be hemolyzed and is an intracellular cation. The lack of anion gap does not exclude a toxic etiology.

The normal gap is usually 7 to 11 mEq/L by flame photometer. However, there has been a "lowering" of the normal anion gap to 7 ± 4 mEq/L by the newer techniques (e.g., ion selective electrodes or colorimetric titration). Some studies have found anion gaps to be relatively insensitive for determining the presence of toxins.

It is important to recognize anion gap toxins, such as salicylates, methanol, and ethylene glycol, because they have specific antidotes, and hemodialysis is effective in management of cases of overdose with these agents.

Table 8 lists the reasons for increased anion gap, decreased anion gap, or no gap. The most common cause of a decreased anion gap is laboratory error. Lactic acidosis produces the largest anion gap and can result from any poisoning that results in hypoxia, hypoglycemia, or convulsions.

Table 9 lists other blood chemistry derangements that suggest certain intoxications.

Serum osmolality is a measure of the number of molecules of solute per kilogram of solvent, or mOsm/kg water. The osmolarity is molecules of solute per liter of solution, or mOsm/L water at a specified temperature. Osmolarity is usually the calculated value and osmolality is usually a measured value. They are considered interchangeable where 1 L equals 1 kg. The normal serum osmolality is 280 to 290 mOsm/kg. The freezing point serum osmolarity measurement specimen and the serum electrolyte specimens for calculation should be drawn simultaneously.

TABLE 8 Etiologies of Metabolic Acidosis

Normal Anion Gap Hyperchloremic	Increased Anion Gap Normochloremic	Decreased Anion Gap
Acidifying agents	Methanol	Laboratory error[†]
Adrenal insufficiency	Uremia*	Intoxication—bromine, lithium
Anhydrase inhibitors	Diabetic ketoacidosis*	Protein abnormal
Fistula	Paraldehyde,* phenformin	Sodium low
Osteotomies	Isoniazid	
Obstructive uropathies	Iron	
Renal tubular acidosis	Lactic acidosis[†]	
Diarrhea, uncomplicated*	Ethanol,* ethylene glycol*	
Dilutional	Salicylates, starvation solvents	
Sulfamylon		

*Indicates hyperosmolar situation. Studies have found that the anion gap may be relatively insensitive for determining the presence of toxins.
[†]Lactic acidosis can be produced by intoxications of the following: carbon monoxide, cyanide, hydrogen sulfide, hypoxia, ibuprofen, iron, isoniazid, phenformin, salicylates, seizures, theophylline.

TABLE 9 Blood Chemistry Derangements in Toxicology

Derangement	Toxin
Acetonemia without acidosis	Acetone or isopropyl alcohol
Hypomagnesemia	Ethanol, digitalis
Hypocalcemia	Ethylene glycol, oxalate, fluoride
Hyperkalemia	β-Blockers, acute digitalis, renal failure
Hypokalemia	Diuretics, salicylism, sympathomimetics, theophylline, corticosteroids, chronic digitalis
Hyperglycemia	Diazoxide, glucagon, iron, isoniazid, organophosphate insecticides, phenylurea insecticides, phenytoin (Dilantin), salicylates, sympathomimetic agents, thyroid vasopressors
Hypoglycemia	β-Blockers, ethanol, insulin, isoniazid, oral hypoglycemic agents, salicylates
Rhabdomyolysis	Amphetamines, ethanol, cocaine, or phencyclidine, elevated creatine phosphokinase

The serum osmolal gap is defined as the difference between the measured osmolality determined by the freezing point method and the calculated osmolarity. It is determined by the following formula:

$$(Sodium \times 2) + (BUN/3) + (Glucose/20)$$

where BUN is blood urea nitrogen.

This gap estimate is normally within 10 mOsm of the simultaneously measured serum osmolality. Ethanol, if present, may be included in the equation to eliminate its influence on the osmolal gap (the ethanol concentration divided by 4.6; Table 10).

The osmolal gap is not valid in cases of shock and postmortem state. Metabolic disorders such as hyperglycemia, uremia, and dehydration increase the osmolarity but usually do not cause gaps greater than 10 mOsm/kg. A gap greater than 10 mOsm/mL suggests that unidentified osmolal-acting substances are present: acetone, ethanol, ethylene glycol, glycerin, isopropyl alcohol, isoniazid, ethanol, mannitol, methanol, and trichloroethane. Alcohols and glycols should be sought when the degree of obtundation exceeds that expected from the blood ethanol concentration or when other clinical conditions exist: visual loss (methanol), metabolic acidosis (methanol and ethylene glycol), or renal failure (ethylene glycol).

A falsely elevated osmolar gap can be produced by other low molecular weight un-ionized substances (dextran, diuretics, sorbitol, ketones), hyperlipidemia, and unmeasured electrolytes (e.g., magnesium).

Note: A normal osmolal gap may be reported in the presence of toxic alcohol or glycol poisoning, if the parent compound is already metabolized. This situation can occur when the osmolar gap is measured after a significant time has elapsed since the ingestion. In cases of alcohol and glycol intoxication, an early osmolar gap is a result of the relatively nontoxic parent drug and delayed metabolic acidosis, and an anion gap is a result of the more toxic metabolites. The serum concentration is calculated as

$$mg/dL = mOsm\ gap \times MW\ of\ substance\ divided\ by\ 10.$$

RADIOGRAPHIC STUDIES

Chest and neck radiographs are useful for suspected pathologic conditions such as aspiration pneumonia, pulmonary edema, and foreign bodies and to determine the location of the endotracheal tube. Abdominal radiographs can be used to detect radiopaque substances.

The mnemonic for radiopaque substances seen on abdominal radiographs is CHIPES:

C—chlorides and chloral hydrate
H—heavy metals (arsenic, barium, iron, lead, mercury, zinc)

TABLE 10 Conversion Factors for Alcohols and Glycols

Alcohols/ Glycols	1 mg/dL in Blood Raises Osmolality mOsm/L	Molecular Weight	Conversion Factor
Ethanol	0.228	40	4.6
Methanol	0.327	32	3.2
Ethylene glycol	0.190	62	6.2
Isopropanol	0.176	60	6.0
Acetone	0.182	58	5.8
Propylene glycol	not available	72	7.2

Example: Methanol osmolality. Subtract the calculated osmolality from the measured serum osmolarity (freezing point method) = osmolar gap × 3.2 (one-tenth molecular weight) = estimated serum methanol concentration.
Note: This equation is often not considered very reliable in predicting the actual measured blood concentration of these alcohols or glycols.

I—iodides
P—PlayDoh, Pepto-Bismol, phenothiazine (inconsistent)
E—enteric-coated tablets
S—sodium, potassium, and other elements in tablet form (bismuth, calcium, potassium) and solvents containing chlorides (e.g., carbon tetrachloride)

TOXICOLOGIC STUDIES

Routine blood and urine screening is of little practical value in the initial care of the poisoned patient. Specific toxicologic analyses and quantitative levels of certain drugs may be extremely helpful. One should always ask oneself the following questions: (a) How will the result of the test alter the management? and (b) Can the result of the test be returned in time to have a positive effect on therapy?

Owing to long turnaround time, lack of availability, factors contributing to unreliability, and the risk of serious morbidity without supportive clinical management, toxicology screening is estimated to affect management in less than 15% of cases of drug overdoses or poisonings. Toxicology screening may look specifically for only 40 to 50 drugs out of more than 10,000 possible drugs or toxins and more than several million chemicals. To detect many different drugs, toxic screens usually include methods with broad specificity, and sensitivity may be poor for some drugs, resulting in false-negative or false-positive findings. On the other hand, some drugs present in therapeutic amounts may be detected on the screen, even though they are causing no clinical symptoms. Because many agents are not sought or detected during a toxicologic screening, a negative result does not always rule out poisonings. The specificity of toxicologic tests is dependent on the method and the laboratory. The presence of other drugs, drug metabolites, disease states, or incorrect sampling may cause erroneous results.

For the average toxicologic laboratory, false-negative results occur at a rate of 10% to 30% and false-positives at a rate of 0% to 10%. The positive screen predictive value is approximately 90%. A negative toxicology screen does not exclude a poisoning. The negative predictive value of toxicologic screening is approximately 70%. For example, the following benzodiazepines may not be detected by some routine immunoassay benzodiazepine screening tests: alprazolam (Xanax), clonazepam (Klonopin), temazepam (Restoril), and triazolam (Halcion).

The "toxic urine screen" is generally a qualitative urine test for several common drugs, usually substances of abuse (cocaine and metabolites, opioids, amphetamines, benzodiazepines, barbiturates, and phencyclidine). Results of these tests are usually available within 2 to 6 hours. Because these tests may vary with each hospital and community, the physician should determine exactly which substances are included in the toxic urine screen of his or her laboratory. Tests for ethylene glycol, red blood cell cholinesterase, and serum cyanide are not readily available.

For cases of ingestion of certain substances, quantitative blood levels should be obtained at specific times after the ingestion to avoid spurious low values in the distribution phase, which result from incomplete absorption. The detection time for drugs is influenced by many variables, such as type of substance, formulation, amount, time since ingestion, duration of exposure, and half-life. For many drugs, the detection time is measured in days after the exposure.

Common Poisons

ACETAMINOPHEN (PARACETAMOL, *N*-ACETYL-PARAAMINOPHENOL)

Toxic Mechanism

At therapeutic doses of acetaminophen, less than 5% is metabolized by P450-2E1 to a toxic reactive oxidizing metabolite, *N*-acetyl-p-benzoquinoneimine (NAPQI). In a case of overdose, there is insufficient glutathione available to reduce the excess NAPQI into nontoxic conjugate, so it forms covalent bonds with hepatic intracellular proteins to produce centrilobular necrosis. Renal damage is caused by a similar mechanism.

Toxic Dose

The therapeutic dose of acetaminophen is 10 to 15 mg/kg, with a maximum of five doses in 24 hours for a maximum total daily dose of 4 g. An acute single toxic dose is greater than 140 mg/kg, possibly greater than 200 mg/kg in a child younger than age 5 years. Factors affecting the P450 enzymes include enzyme inducers such as barbiturates and phenytoin (Dilantin), ingestion of isoniazid, and alcoholism. Factors that decrease glutathione stores (alcoholism, malnutrition, and HIV infection) contribute to the toxicity of acetaminophen. Alcoholics ingesting 3 to 4 g/d of acetaminophen for a few days can have depleted glutathione stores and require *N*-acetylcysteine therapy at 50% below hepatotoxic blood acetaminophen levels on the nomogram.

Kinetics

Peak plasma concentration is usually reached 2 to 4 hours after an overdose. Volume distribution is 0.9 L/kg, and protein binding is less than 50% (albumin).

Route of elimination is by hepatic metabolism to an inactive nontoxic glucuronide conjugate and inactive nontoxic sulfate metabolite by two saturable pathways; less than 5% is metabolized into reactive metabolite NAPQI. In patients younger than 6 years of age, metabolic elimination occurs to a greater degree by conjugation via the sulfate pathway.

The half-life of acetaminophen is 1 to 3 hours.

Manifestations

The four phases of the intoxication's clinical course may overlap, and the absence of a phase does not exclude toxicity.

- Phase I occurs within 0.5 to 24 hours after ingestion and may consist of a few hours of malaise, diaphoresis, nausea, and vomiting or produce no symptoms. CNS depression or coma is not a feature.
- Phase II occurs 24 to 48 hours after ingestion and is a period of diminished symptoms. The liver enzymes, serum aspartate aminotransferase (AST) (earliest), and serum alanine aminotransferase (ALT) may increase as early as 4 hours or as late as 36 hours after ingestion.
- Phase III occurs at 48 to 96 hours, with peak liver function abnormalities at 72 to 96 hours. The degree of elevation of the hepatic enzymes generally correlates with outcome, but not always. Recovery starts at about 4 days unless hepatic failure develops. Less than 1% of patients with a history of overdose develop fulminant hepatotoxicity.
- Phase IV occurs at 4 to 14 days, with hepatic enzyme abnormalities resolving. If extensive liver damage has occurred, sepsis and disseminated intravascular coagulation may ensue.

Transient renal failure may develop at 5 to 7 days with or without evidence of hepatic damage. Rare cases of myocarditis and pancreatitis have been reported. Death can occur at 7 to 14 days.

Laboratory Investigations

The therapeutic reference range is 10 to 20 μg/mL. For toxic levels, see the nomogram presented in Figure 1.

Appropriate and reliable methods for analysis are radioimmunoassay, high-pressure liquid chromatography, and gas chromatography. Spectroscopic assays often give falsely elevated values: bilirubin, salicylate, salicylamide, diflunisal (Dolobid), phenols, and methyldopa (Aldomet) increase the acetaminophen level. Each 1 mg/dL increase in creatinine increases the acetaminophen plasma level 30 μg/mL.

If a toxic acetaminophen level is reached, liver profile (including AST, ALT, bilirubin, and prothrombin time), serum amylase, and blood glucose must be monitored. A complete blood cell count (CBC); platelet count; phosphate, electrolytes, and bicarbonate level measurements; ECG; and urinalysis are indicated.

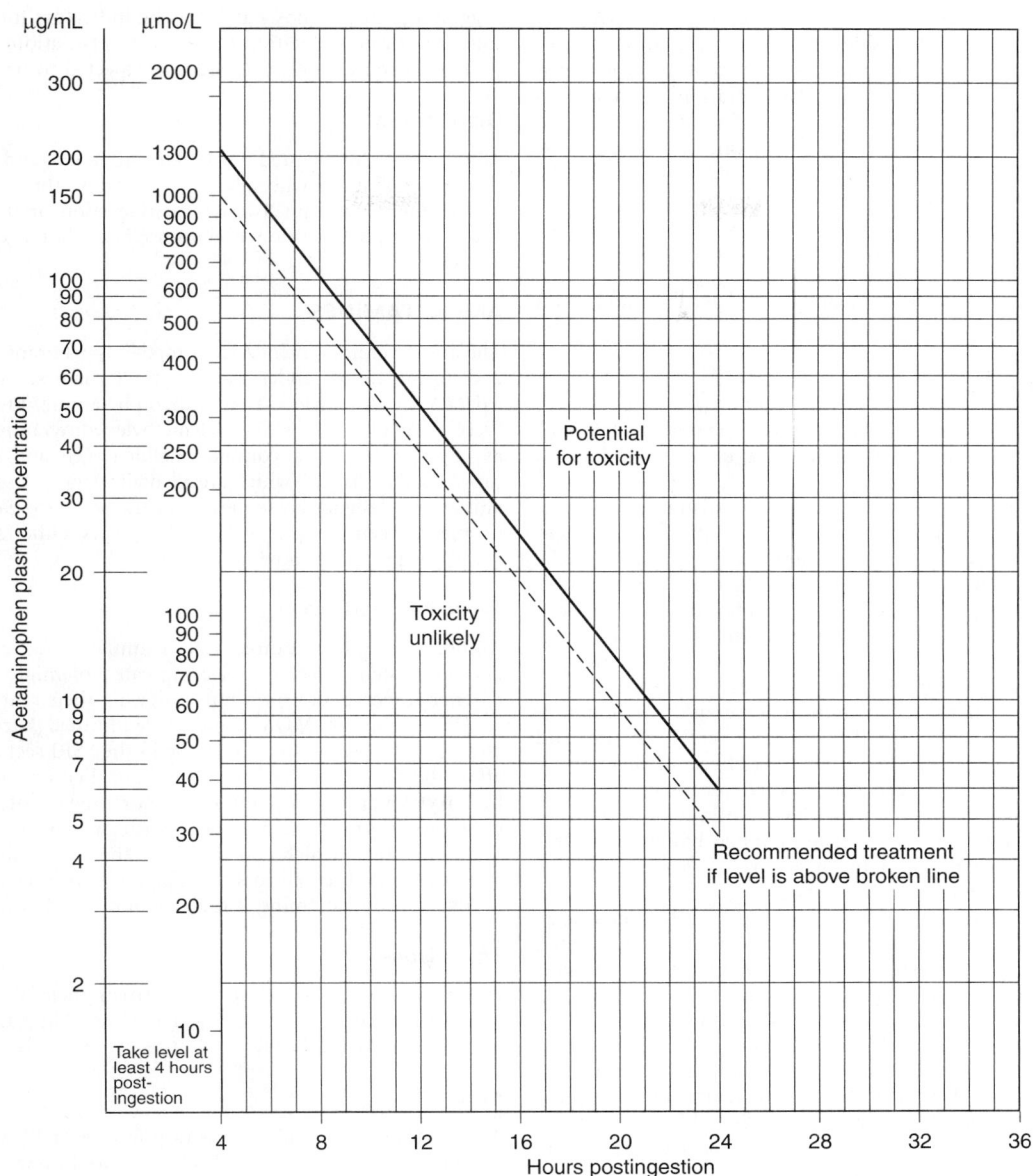

FIGURE 1. Nomogram for acetaminophen intoxication. *N*-acetylcysteine therapy is started if levels and time coordinates are above the lower line on the nomogram. Continue and complete therapy even if subsequent values fall below the toxic zone. The nomogram is useful only in cases of acute single ingestion. Levels in serum drawn before 4 hours may not represent peak levels. (From Rumack BH, Matthew H: Acetaminophen poisoning and toxicity. Pediatrics 55:871, 1975.)

Management

Gastrointestinal Decontamination

Although ipecac-induced emesis may be useful within 30 minutes of ingestion of the toxic substance, we do not advise it because it could result in vomiting of the activated charcoal. Gastric lavage is not necessary. Studies have indicated that activated charcoal is useful within 1 hour after ingestion. Activated charcoal does adsorb *N*-acetylcysteine (NAC) if given together, but this is not clinically important.

However, if activated charcoal needs to be given along with NAC, separate the administration of activated charcoal from the administration of NAC by 1 to 2 hours to avoid vomiting.

N-*Acetylcysteine (Mucomyst)*

NAC (Table 11), a derivative of the amino acid cysteine, acts as a sulfhydryl donor for glutathione synthesis, as surrogate glutathione, and may increase the nontoxic sulfation pathway resulting in conjugation of NAPQI. Oral NAC should be administered within the first 8 hours

TABLE 11 Protocol for *N*-Acetylcysteine Administration

Route	Loading Dose	Maintenance Dose	Course	FDA Approval
Oral	140 mg/kg	70 mg/kg every 4 h	72 h	Yes
Intravenous	150 mg/kg over 15 min	50 mg/kg over 4 h followed by 100 mg/kg over 16 h	20 h	Yes

after a toxic amount of acetaminophen has been ingested. NAC can be started while one awaits the results of the blood test for acetaminophen plasma concentration, but there is no advantage to giving it before 8 hours. If the acetaminophen concentration result after 4 hours following ingestion is above the upper line on the modified Rumack-Matthew nomogram (see Figure 1), one should continue with a maintenance course. Repeat blood specimens should be obtained 4 hours after the initial level is measured if it is greater than 20 mg/mL, which is below the therapy line, because of unexpected delays in the peak by food and co-ingestants. Intravenous NAC (see Table 11) is approved in the United States.

There have been a few cases of anaphylactoid reaction and death by the intravenous route.

Variations in Therapy

In patients with chronic alcoholism, it is recommended that NAC treatment be administered at 50% below the upper toxic line on the nomogram.

If emesis occurs within 1 hour after NAC administration, the dose should be repeated. To avoid emesis, the proper dilution from 20% to 5% NAC must be used, and it should be served in a palatable vehicle, in a covered container through a straw. If this administration is unsuccessful, a slow drip over 30 to 60 minutes through a nasogastric tube or a fluoroscopically placed nasoduodenal tube can be used. Antiemetics can be used if necessary: metoclopramide (Reglan) 10 mg per dose intravenously 30 minutes before administration of NAC (in children, 0.1 mg/kg; maximum, 0.5 mg/kg/d) or ondansetron (Zofran) 32 mg (0.15 mg/kg) by infusion over 15 minutes and repeated for three doses if necessary. The side effects of these antiemetics include anaphylaxis and increases in liver enzymes.

Some investigators recommend variable durations of NAC therapy, stopping the therapy if serial acetaminophen blood concentrations become nondetectable and the liver enzyme levels (ALT and AST) remain normal after 24 to 36 hours.

There is a loss of efficacy if NAC is initiated 8 or 10 hours postingestion, but the loss is not complete, and NAC may be initiated 36 hours or more after ingestion. Late treatment (after 24 hours) decreases the rates of morbidity and mortality in patients with fulminant liver failure caused by acetaminophen and other agents.

Extended relief formulations (ER embossed on caplet) contain 325 mg of acetaminophen for immediate release and 325 mg for delayed release. A single 4-hour postingestion serum acetaminophen concentration can underestimate the level because ER formulations can have secondary delayed peaks. In cases of overdose of the ER formulation, it is recommended that additional acetaminophen levels be obtained at 4-hour intervals after the initial level is measured. If any level is in the toxic zone, therapy should be initiated.

It is recommended that pregnant patients with toxic plasma concentrations of acetaminophen be treated with NAC to prevent hepatotoxicity in both fetus and mother. The available data suggest no teratogenicity to NAC or acetaminophen.

Indications for NAC therapy in cases of chronic intoxication are a history of ingestion of 3 to 4 g for several days with elevated liver enzyme levels (AST and ALT). The acetaminophen blood concentration is often low in these cases because of the extended time lapse since ingestion and should not be plotted on the Rumack-Matthew nomogram. Patients with a history of chronic alcoholism or those on chronic enzyme inducers may also present with elevated liver enzyme levels and should be considered for NAC therapy if they have a history of taking acetaminophen on a chronic basis, because they are considered to be at a greater risk for hepatotoxicity despite a low acetaminophen blood concentration.

Specific support care may be needed to treat liver failure, pancreatitis, transient renal failure, and myocarditis.

Liver transplantation has a definite but limited role in patients with acute acetaminophen overdose. A retrospective analysis determined that a continuing rise in the prothrombin time (4-day peak, 180 seconds), a pH of less than 7.3 2 days after the overdose, a serum creatinine level of greater than 3.3 mg/dL, severe hepatic encephalopathy, and disturbed coagulation factor VII/V ratio greater than 30 suggest a poor prognosis and may be indicators for hepatology consultation for consideration of liver transplantation.

Extracorporeal measures are not expected to be of benefit.

Disposition

Adults who have ingested more than 140 mg/kg and children younger than 6 years of age who have ingested more than 200 mg/kg should receive therapy within 8 hours postingestion or until the results of the 4-hour postingestion acetaminophen plasma concentration are known.

AMPHETAMINES

The amphetamines include illicit methamphetamine ("Ice"), diet pills, and formulations under various trade names. Analogues include MDMA (3,4 methylenedioxymethamphetamine, known as "ecstasy," "XTC," "Adam") and MDA (3,4-methylenedioxyamphetamine, known as "Eve"). MDA is a common hallucinogen and euphoriant "club drug" used at "raves," which are all-night dances. Use of methamphetamine and designer analogues is on the rise, especially among young people between the ages of 12 and 25 years. Other similar stimulants are phenylpropanolamine and cocaine.

Toxic Mechanism

Amphetamines have a direct CNS stimulant effect and a sympathetic nervous system effect by releasing catecholamines from α- and β-adrenergic nerve terminals but inhibiting their reuptake.

Hallucinogenic MDMA has an additional hazard of serotonin effect (refer to serotonin syndrome in the SSRI section). MDMA also affect the dopamine system in the brain. Because of its effects on 5-hydroxytryptamine, dopamine, and norepinephrine, MDMA can lead to serotonin syndrome associated with malignant hyperthermia and rhabdomyolysis, which contributes to the potentially life-threatening hyperthermia observed in several patients who have used MDMA.

Phenylpropanolamine stimulates only the β-adrenergic receptors.

Toxic Dose

In children, the toxic dose of dextroamphetamine is 1 mg/kg; in adults, the toxic dose is 5 mg/kg. The potentially fatal dose of dextroamphetamine is 12 mg/kg.

Kinetics

Amphetamine is a weak base with pKa of 8 to 10. Onset of action is 30 to 60 minutes, and peak effects are 2 to 4 hours. The volume distribution is 2 to 3 L/kg.

Through hepatic metabolism, 60% of the substance is metabolized into a hydroxylated metabolite that may be responsible for psychotic effects.

The half-life of amphetamines is pH dependent—8 to 10 hours in acid urine (pH <6.0) and 16 to 31 hours in alkaline urine (pH >7.5). Excretion is by the kidney—30% to 40% at alkaline urine pH and 50% to 70% at acid urine pH.

Manifestations

Effects are seen within 30 to 60 minutes following ingestion.

Neurologic manifestations include restlessness, irritation and agitation, tremors and hyperreflexia, and auditory and visual hallucinations. Hyperpyrexia may precede seizures, convulsions, paranoia, violence, intracranial hemorrhage, psychosis, and self-destructive behavior. Paranoid psychosis and cerebral vasculitis occur with chronic abuse.

MDMA is often adulterated with cocaine, heroin, or ketamine, or a combination of these, to create a variety of mood alterations. This possibility must be taken into consideration when one manages patients with MDMA ingestions, as the symptom complex may reflect both CNS stimulation and CNS depression.

Other manifestations include dilated but reactive pupils, cardiac dysrhythmias (supraventricular and ventricular), tachycardia, hypertension, rhabdomyolysis, and myoglobinuria.

Laboratory Investigations

The clinician should monitor ECG and cardiac readings, ABG and oxygen saturation, electrolytes, blood glucose, BUN, creatinine, creatine kinase, cardiac fraction if there is chest pain, and liver profile. Also, one should evaluate for rhabdomyolysis and check urine for myoglobin, cocaine and metabolites, and other substances of abuse. The peak plasma concentration of amphetamines is 10 to 50 ng/mL 1 to 2 hours after ingestion of 10 to 25 mg. The toxic plasma concentration is 200 ng/mL. When the rapid immunoassays are used, cross-reactions can occur with amphetamine derivatives (e.g., MDA, "ecstasy"), brompheniramine (Dimetane), chlorpromazine (Thorazine), ephedrine, phenylpropanolamine, phentermine (Adipex-P), phenmetrazine, ranitidine (Zantac), and Vicks Inhaler (L-desoxyephedrine). False-positive results may occur.

Management

Management is similar to management for cocaine intoxication. Supportive care includes blood pressure and temperature control, cardiac monitoring, and seizure precautions. Diazepam (Valium) can be administered. Gastrointestinal decontamination can be undertaken with activated charcoal administered up to 1 hour after ingestion.

Anxiety, agitation, and convulsions are treated with diazepam. If diazepam fails to control seizures, neuromuscular blockers can be used and the electroencephalogram (EEG) monitored for nonmotor seizures. One should avoid neuroleptic phenothiazines and butyrophenone, which can lower the seizure threshold.

Hypertension and tachycardia are usually transient and can be managed by titration of diazepam. Nitroprusside can be used for hypertensive crisis at a maximum infusion rate of 10 μg/kg/minute for 10 minutes followed with a lower infusion rate of 0.3 to 2 mg/kg/minute. Myocardial ischemia is managed by oxygen, vascular access, benzodiazepines, and nitroglycerin. Aspirin and thrombolytics are not routinely recommended because of the danger of intracranial hemorrhage. It is important to distinguish between angina and true ischemia. Delayed hypotension can be treated with fluids and vasopressors if needed. Life-threatening tachydysrhythmias may respond to an α-blocker such as phentolamine (Regitine) 5 mg IV for adults or 0.1 mg/kg IV for children and a short-acting β-blocker such as esmolol (Brevibloc) 500 μg/kg IV over 1 minute for adults, or 300 to 500 μg/kg over 1 minute for children. Ventricular dysrhythmias may respond to lidocaine or, in a severely hemodynamically compromised patient, immediate synchronized electrical cardioversion.

Rhabdomyolysis and myoglobinuria are treated with fluids, alkaline diuresis, and diuretics. Hyperthermia is treated with external cooling and cool 100% humidified oxygen. More extensive therapy may be needed in severe cases. If focal neurologic symptoms are present, the possibility of a cerebrovascular accident should be considered and a CT scan of the head should be obtained.

Paranoid ideation and threatening behavior should be treated with rapid tranquilization using a benzodiazepine. One should observe for suicidal depression that may follow intoxication and may require suicide precautions.

Extracorporeal measures are of no benefit.

Disposition

Symptomatic patients should be observed on a monitored unit until the symptoms resolve and then observed for a short time after resolution for relapse.

ANTICHOLINERGIC AGENTS

Drugs with anticholinergic properties include antihistamines (H_1 blockers), neuroleptics (phenothiazines), tricyclic antidepressants, antiparkinsonism drugs (trihexyphenidyl [Artane], benztropine [Cogentin]), ophthalmic products (atropine), and a number of common plants.

The antihistamines are divided into the sedating anticholinergic types, and the nonsedating single daily dose types. The sedating types include ethanolamines (e.g., diphenhydramine [Benadryl], dimenhydrinate [Dramamine], and clemastine [Tavist]), ethylenediamines (e.g., tripelennamine [Pyribenzamine]), alkyl amines (e.g., chlorpheniramine [Chlor-Trimeton], brompheniramine [Dimetane]), piperazines (e.g., cyclizine [Marezine], hydroxyzine [Atarax], and meclizine [Antivert]), and phenothiazine (e.g., Phenergan). The nonsedating types include astemizole (Hismanal), terfenadine (Seldane), loratadine (Claritin), fexofenadine (Allegra), and cetirizine (Zyrtec).

The anticholinergic plants include jimsonweed (*Datura stramonium*), deadly nightshade (*Atropa belladonna*), henbane (*Hyoscyamus niger*), and antispasmodic agents for the bowel (atropine derivatives).

Toxic Mechanism

By competitive inhibition, anticholinergics block the action of acetylcholine on postsynaptic cholinergic receptor sites. The toxic mechanism primarily involves the peripheral and CNS muscarinic receptors. H_1 sedating-type agents also depress or stimulate the CNS, and in large overdoses some have cardiac membrane–depressant effects (e.g., diphenhydramine [Benadryl]) and α-adrenergic receptor blockade effects (e.g., promethazine [Phenergan]). Nonsedating agents produce peripheral H_1 blockade but do not possess anticholinergic or sedating actions. The original agents terfenadine (Seldane) and astemizole (Hismanal) were recently removed from the market because of the severe cardiac dysrhythmias associated with their use, especially when used in combination with macrolide antibiotics and certain antifungal agents such as ketoconazole (Nizoral), which inhibit hepatic metabolism or excretion. The newer nonsedating agents, including loratadine (Claritin), fexofenadine (Allegra), and cetirizine (Zyrtec), have not been reported to cause the severe drug interactions associated with terfenadine and astemizole.

Toxic Dose

The estimated toxic oral dose of atropine is 0.05 mg/kg in children and more than 2 mg in adults. The minimal estimated lethal dose of atropine is more than 10 mg in adults and more than 2 mg in children. Other synthetic anticholinergic agents are less toxic, and the fatal dose varies from 10 to 100 mg.

The estimated toxic oral dose of diphenhydramine (Benadryl) in a child is 15 mg/kg, and the potential lethal amount is 25 mg/kg. In an adult, the potential lethal amount is 2.8 g. Ingestion of five times the single dose of an antihistamine is toxic.

For the nonsedating agents, an overdose of 3360 mg of terfenadine was reported in an adult who developed ventricular tachycardia and fibrillation that responded to lidocaine and defibrillation. A 1500-mg overdose produced hypotension. Cases of delayed serious dysrhythmias (torsades de pointes) have been reported with doses of more than 200 mg of astemizole. The toxic doses of fexofenadine (Allegra), cetirizine, and loratadine (Claritin) need to be established.

Kinetics

The onset of absorption of intravenous atropine is in 2 to 4 minutes. Peak effects on salivation after intravenous or intramuscular administration are at 30 to 60 minutes.

Onset of absorption after oral ingestion is 30 to 60 minutes, peak action is 1 to 3 hours, and duration of action is 4 to 6 hours, but symptoms are prolonged in cases of overdose or with sustained-release preparations.

The onset of absorption of diphenhydramine is in 15 minutes to 1 hour, with a peak of action in 1 to 4 hours. Volume distribution is 3.3 to 6.8 L/kg, and protein binding is 75% to 80%. Ninety-eight percent of diphenhydramine is metabolized via the liver by *N*-demethylation. Interactions with erythromycin, ketoconazole (Nizoral), and derivatives produce excessive blood levels of the antihistamine and ventricular dysrhythmias.

The half-life of diphenhydramine is 3 to 10 hours.

The chemical structure of nonsedating agents prevents their entry into the CNS. Absorption begins in 1 hour, with peak effects in 4 to 6 hours. The duration of action is greater than 24 hours.

These agents are metabolized in the gastrointestinal tract and liver. Protein binding is greater than 90%. The plasma half-life is

3.5 hours. Only 1% is excreted unchanged; 60% of that is excreted in the feces and 40% in the urine.

Manifestations

Anticholinergic signs are hyperpyrexia ("hot as a hare"), mydriasis ("blind as a bat"), flushing of skin ("red as a beet"), dry mucosa and skin ("dry as a bone"), "Lilliputian type" hallucinations and delirium ("mad as a hatter"), coma, dysphagia, tachycardia, moderate hypertension, and rarely convulsions and urinary retention. Other effects include jaundice (cyproheptadine [Periactin]), dystonia (diphenhydramine [Benadryl]), rhabdomyolysis (doxylamine) and, in large doses, cardiotoxic effects (diphenhydramine).

Overdose with nonsedating agents produces headache and confusion, nausea, and dysrhythmias (e.g., torsades de pointes).

Laboratory Investigations

Monitoring of ABG (in cases of respiratory depression), electrolytes, glucose, and the ECG should be undertaken. Anticholinergic drugs and plants are not routinely included on screens for substances of abuse.

Management

For patients in respiratory failure, intubation and assisted ventilation should be instituted. Gastrointestinal decontamination can be instituted. Caution must be taken with emesis in cases of diphenhydramine (Benadryl) overdose because of the drug's rapid onset of action and risk of seizures. If bowel sounds are present for up to 1 hour after ingestion, activated charcoal can be given. Seizures can be controlled with benzodiazepines (diazepam [Valium] or lorazepam [Ativan]).

The administration of physostigmine (Antilirium) is not routine and is reserved for life-threatening anticholinergic effects that are refractory to conventional treatments. It should be administered with adequate monitoring and resuscitative equipment available. The use of physostigmine should be avoided if a tricyclic antidepressant is present because of increased toxicity. Urinary retention should be relieved by catheterization to avoid reabsorption of the drug and additional toxicity.

Supraventricular tachycardia should be treated only if the patient is hemodynamically unstable. Ventricular dysrhythmias can be controlled with lidocaine or cardioversion. Sodium bicarbonate 1 to 2 mEq/kg IV may be useful for myocardial depression and QRS prolongation. Torsades de pointes, especially when associated with terfenadine and astemizole ingestion, has been treated with magnesium sulfate 4 g or 40 mL 10% solution intravenously over 10 to 20 minutes and countershock if the patient fails to respond.

Hyperpyrexia is controlled by external cooling. Hemodialysis and hemoperfusion are not effective.

Disposition

Antihistamine H₁ Antagonists

Symptomatic patients should be observed on a monitored unit until the symptoms resolve, then observed for a short time (3 to 4 hours) after resolution for relapse.

Nonsedating Agents

All asymptomatic children who acutely ingest more than the maximum adult dose and all symptomatic children should be referred to a health care facility for a minimum of 6 hours' observation as well as cardiac monitoring. Asymptomatic adults who acutely ingest more than twice the maximum adult daily dose should be monitored for a minimum of 6 hours. All symptomatic patients should be monitored for as long as there are symptoms present.

BARBITURATES

Barbiturates have been used as sedatives, anesthetic agents, and anticonvulsants, but their use is declining as safer, more effective drugs become available.

Toxic Mechanism

Barbiturates are γ-aminobutyric acid (GABA) agonists (increasing the chloride flow and inhibiting depolarization). They enhance the CNS depressant effect of GABA and depress the cardiovascular system.

Toxic Dose

The shorter-acting barbiturates (including the intermediate-acting agents) and their hypnotic doses are as follows: amobarbital (Amytal), 100 to 200 mg; aprobarbital (Alurate), 50 to 100 mg; butabarbital (Butisol), 50 to 100 mg; butalbital, 100 to 200 mg; pentobarbital (Nembutal), 100 to 200 mg; secobarbital (Seconal), 100 to 200 mg. They cause toxicity at lower doses than long-acting barbiturates and have a minimum toxic dose of 6 mg/kg; the fatal adult dose is 3 to 6 g.

The long-acting barbiturates and their doses include mephobarbital (Mebaral), 50 to 100 mg, and phenobarbital, 100 to 200 mg. Their minimum toxic dose is greater than 10 mg/kg, and the fatal adult dose is 6 to 10 g. A general rule is that an amount five times the hypnotic dose is toxic and an amount 10 times the hypnotic dose is potentially fatal. Methohexital and thiopental are ultrashort-acting parenteral preparations and are not discussed.

Kinetics

The barbiturates are enzyme inducers. Short-acting barbiturates are highly lipid-soluble, penetrate the brain readily, and have shorter elimination times. Onset of action is in 10 to 30 minutes, with a peak at 1 to 2 hours. Duration of action is 3 to 8 hours. The volume distribution of short-acting barbiturate is 0.8 to 1.5 L/kg; pKa is about 8. Mean half-life varies from 8 to 48 hours.

Long-acting agents have longer elimination times and can be used as anticonvulsants. Onset of action is in 20 to 60 minutes, with a peak at 1 to 6 hours. In cases of overdose, the peak can be at 10 hours. Usual duration of action is 8 to 12 hours. Volume distribution is 0.8 L/kg, and half-life is 11 to 120 hours. The pKa of phenobarbital is 7.2. Alkalinization of urine promotes its excretion.

Manifestations

Mild intoxication resembles alcohol intoxication and includes ataxia, slurred speech, and depressed cognition. Severe intoxication causes slow respirations, coma, and loss of reflexes (except pupillary light reflex).

Other manifestations include hypotension (vasodilation), hypothermia, hypoglycemia, and death by respiratory arrest.

Laboratory Investigations

Most barbiturates are detected on routine drug screens and can be measured in most hospital laboratories. Investigation should include barbiturate level; ABG; toxicology screen, including acetaminophen; glucose, electrolyte, BUN, creatinine, and creatine kinase levels; and urine pH. The minimum toxic plasma levels are greater than 10 µg/mL for short-acting barbiturates and greater than 40 µg/dL for long-acting agents. Fatal levels are 30 µg/mL for short-acting barbiturates and 80 to 150 µg/mL for long-acting agents. Both short-acting and long-acting agents can be detected in urine 24 to 72 hours after ingestion, and long-acting agents can be detected up to 7 days.

Management

Vital functions must be established and maintained. Intensive supportive care including intubation and assisted ventilation should dominate the management. All stuporous and comatose patients should have glucose (for hypoglycemia), thiamine (if chronically alcoholic), and naloxone (Narcan) (in case of an opioid ingestion) intravenously and should be admitted to the intensive care unit. Emesis should be avoided especially in cases of ingestion of the shorter-acting barbiturates. Activated charcoal followed by MDAC (0.5 g/kg) every 2 to 4 hours has been shown to reduce the serum half-life of phenobarbital by 50%, but its effect on clinical course is undetermined.

Fluids should be administered to correct dehydration and hypotension. Vasopressors may be necessary to correct severe hypotension, and hemodynamic monitoring may be needed. The patient must be observed carefully for fluid overload. Alkalinization (ion trapping) is used only for phenobarbital (pKa 7.2) but not for short-acting barbiturates. Sodium bicarbonate, 1 to 2 mEq/kg IV in 500 mL of 5% dextrose in adults or 10 to 15 mL/kg in children during the first hour, followed by sufficient bicarbonate to keep the urinary pH at 7.5 to 8.0, enhances excretion of phenobarbital and shortens the half-life by 50%. Diuresis is not advocated because of the danger of cerebral or pulmonary edema.

Hemodialysis shortens the half-life to 8 to 14 hours, and charcoal hemoperfusion shortens the half-life to 6 to 8 hours for long-acting barbiturates such as phenobarbital. Both procedures may be effective in patients with both long-acting and short-acting barbiturate ingestion. If the patient does not respond to supportive measures or if the phenobarbital plasma concentration is greater than 150 µg/mL, both procedures may be tried to shorten the half-life.

Bullae are treated as a local second-degree skin burn. Hypothermia should be treated.

Disposition

All comatose patients should be admitted to the intensive care unit. Awake and oriented patients with an overdose of short-acting agents should be observed for at least 6 asymptomatic hours; overdose of long-acting agents warrants observation for at least 12 asymptomatic hours because of the potential for delayed absorption. In the case of an intentional overdose, psychiatric clearance is needed before the patient can be discharged. Chronic use can lead to tolerance, physical dependency, and withdrawal and necessitates follow-up.

BENZODIAZEPINES

Benzodiazepines are used as anxiolytics, sedatives, and relaxants.

Toxic Mechanism

The GABA agonists produce CNS depression and increase chloride flow, inhibiting depolarization.

Flunitrazepam (Rohypnol; street name "roofies") is a long-acting benzodiazepine agonist sold by prescription in more than 60 countries worldwide, but it is not legally available in the United States.

Toxic Dose

The long-acting benzodiazepines (half-life >24 hours) and their maximum therapeutic doses are as follows: chlordiazepoxide (Librium), 50 mg; clorazepate (Tranxene), 30 mg; clonazepam (Klonopin), 20 mg; diazepam (Valium), 10 mg in adults or 0.2 mg/kg in children; flurazepam (Dalmane), 30 mg; and prazepam, 20 mg.

The short-acting benzodiazepines (half-life 10 to 24 hours) and their doses include the following: alprazolam (Xanax), 0.5 mg, and lorazepam (Ativan), 4 mg in adults or 0.05 mg/kg in children, which act similar to the long-acting benzodiazepines.

The ultrashort-acting benzodiazepines (half-life <10 hours) are more toxic and include temazepam (Restoril), 30 mg; triazolam (Halcion), 0.5 mg; midazolam (Versed), 0.2 mg/kg; and oxazepam (Serax), 30 mg.

In cases of overdose of short- and long-acting agents, 10 to 20 times the therapeutic dose (>1500 mg diazepam or 2000 mg chlordiazepoxide) have been ingested with resulting mild coma but without respiratory depression. Fatalities are rare, and most patients recover within 24 to 36 hours after overdose. Asymptomatic unintentional overdoses of less than five times the therapeutic dose can be seen. Ultrashort-acting agents have produced respiratory arrest and coma within 1 hour after ingestion of 5 mg of triazolam (Halcion) and death with ingestion of as little as 10 mg. Midazolam (Versed) and diazepam (Valium) by rapid intravenous injection have produced respiratory arrest.

Kinetics

Onset of CNS depression is usually in 30 to 120 minutes; peak action usually occurs within 1 to 3 hours when ingestion is by the oral route. The volume distribution varies from 0.26 to 6 L/kg (LA, 1.1 L/kg); protein binding is 70% to 99%. For flunitrazepam, the onset of action is in 0.5 to 2 hours, oral peak is in 2 hours, and duration 8 hours or more. The half-life of flunitrazepam is 20 to 30 hours, volume distribution is 3.3 to 5.5 L/kg, and 80% is protein bound. Flunitrazepam can be identified in urine 4 to 30 days after ingestion.

Manifestations

Neurologic manifestations include ataxia, slurred speech, and CNS depression. Deep coma leading to respiratory depression suggests the presence of short-acting benzodiazepines or other CNS depressants. In elderly persons, the therapeutic doses can produce toxicity and can have an additive effect with other CNS depressants. Chronic use can lead to tolerance, physical dependency, and withdrawal.

Laboratory Investigations

Most benzodiazepines can be detected in urine drug screens. Quantitative blood levels are not useful. Some of the immunoassay urinary screens cannot detect all of the new benzodiazepines currently available. A consultation with the laboratory analyst is warranted if a specific case occurs in which the test result is negative but benzodiazepine use is suspected by the patient's history. Situations in which benzodiazepines may not be detected include ingestion of a low dose (e.g., <10 mg), rapid elimination, and a different or no metabolite. Some immunoassay methods can produce a false-positive finding for the benzodiazepines when nonsteroidal antiinflammatory drugs (tolmetin [Tolectin], naproxen [Aleve], etodolac [Lodine], and fenoprofen [Nalfon]) are used. If this is a concern, the laboratory analyst should be consulted.

In cases in which "date rape" drugs such as flunitrazepam are suspected, a police crime or reference laboratory should be consulted for testing.

Management

Emesis and gastric lavage should be avoided. Activated charcoal can be useful only if given early before the peak time of absorption occurs. Supportive treatment should be instituted but rarely requires intubation or assisted ventilation.

Flumazenil (Romazicon) is a specific benzodiazepine receptor antagonist that blocks the chloride flow and inhibitor of GABA neurotransmitters. It reverses the sedative effects of benzodiazepines, zolpidem (Ambien), and endogenous benzodiazepines associated with hepatic encephalopathy. It is not recommended to reverse benzodiazepine-induced hypoventilation. The manufacturer advises that flumazenil be used with caution in cases of overdose with possible benzodiazepine dependency (because it can precipitate life-threatening withdrawal), if cyclic antidepressant use is suspected, or if a patient has a known seizure disorder.

Disposition

If the patient is comatose, he or she must be admitted to the intensive care unit. If the overdose was intentional, psychiatric clearance is needed before the patient can be discharged.

β-ADRENERGIC BLOCKERS (β-BLOCKERS)

β-Blockers are used in the treatment of hypertension and of a number of systemic and ophthalmologic disorders. Properties of β-blockers include the factors listed in Table 12.

Lipid-soluble drugs have CNS effects, active metabolites, longer duration of action, and interactions (e.g., propranolol). Cardioselectivity is lost in overdose. Intrinsic partial agonist agents (e.g., pindolol) may initially produce tachycardia and hypertension. Cardiac membrane depressive effect (quinidine-like) occurs in cases of overdose but not at therapeutic doses (e.g., with metoprolol or sotalol). α-Blocking effect is weak (e.g., with labetalol or acebutolol).

TABLE 12 Pharmacologic and Toxic Properties of β-Blockers

β-Blocker	Maximum Solubility	Therapeutic Plasma Level	Lipid Solubility	Intrinsic Sympathomimetic Activity (Partial Agonist)	Membrane Stabilizing Effect β-Selective β₁	β₂	Cardiac Selectivity α-Selective
Acebutolol (Sectral)	800 mg	200–2000 ng/mL	Moderate	+	+	+	+
Alprenolol[2]	800 mg	50–200 ng/mL	Moderate	2+	+	–	–
Atenolol (Tenormin)	100 mg	200–500 ng/mL	Low	–	–	2+	–
Betaxolol (Kerlone)	20 mg	NA	Low	+	–	+	–
Carteolol (Cartrol)	10 mg	NA	No	+	–	–	–
Esmolol (Brevibloc) (Class II antidysrhythmic, IV only)			Low	–	–	+	–
Labetalol (Trandate)	800 mg	50–500 ng/mL	Low	+	+/–	–	+
Levobunolol (AKBeta eyedrop) (Eye drops 0.25% and 0.5%)	20 mg	NA	No	–	–	–	–
Metoprolol (Lopressor)			Moderate	–	–	2+	–
Nadolol (Corgard)	320 mg	20–40 ng/mL	Low	–	–	–	–
Oxyprenolol[2]	480 mg	80–100 ng/mL	Moderate	2+	+	–	–
Pindolol (Visken)	60 mg	50–150 ng/mL	Moderate	3+	+/–	–	–
Propranolol (Inderal) (Class II antidysrhythmic)	360 mg	50–100 ng/mL	High	–	2+	–	–
Sotalol (Betapace) (Class II antidysrhythmic)	480 mg	500–4000 ng/mL	Low	–	–	–	–
Timolol (Blocadren)	60 mg	5–10 ng/mL	Low	–	+/–	–	–

[2]Not available in the United States.

Toxic Mechanism

β-Blockers compete with the catecholamines for receptor sites and block receptor action in the bronchi, the vascular smooth muscle, and the myocardium.

Toxic Dose

Ingestions of greater than twice the maximum recommended daily therapeutic dose are considered toxic (see Table 12). Ingestion of 1 mg/kg propranolol in a child may produce hypoglycemia. Fatalities have been reported in adults with 7.5 g of metoprolol. The most toxic agent is sotalol, and the least toxic is atenolol.

Kinetics

Regular-release formulations usually cause symptoms within 2 hours. Propranolol's onset of action is 20 to 30 minutes and peak is at 1 to 4 hours, but it may be delayed by co-ingestants. The onset of action with sustained-release preparations may be delayed to 6 hours and the peak to 12 to 16 hours. Volume distribution is 1 to 5.6 L/kg. Protein binding is variable, from 5% to 93%.

Metabolism

Atenolol (Tenormin), nadolol (Corgard), and santalol (Betapace) have enterohepatic recirculation. The duration of action for regular-acting agents is 4 to 6 hours, but in cases of overdose it may be 24 to 48 hours. The duration of action for sustained-release agents is 24 to 48 hours.

The regular preparation with the longest half-life is nadolol, at 12 to 24 hours, and the one with the shortest half-life is esmolol, at 5 to 10 minutes.

Manifestations

See "Toxic Properties" and Table 12.

Highly lipid soluble agents produce coma and seizures. Bradycardia and hypotension are the major cardiac symptoms and may lead to cardiogenic shock. Intrinsic partial agonists initially may cause tachycardia and hypertension. ECG changes include atrioventricular conduction delay or asystole. Membrane-depressant effects produce prolonged QRS and QT interval, which may result in torsades de pointes. Sotalol produces a very prolonged QT interval. Bronchospasm may occur in patients with reactive airway disease with any β-blocker because the selectivity is lost in overdose. Other manifestations include hypoglycemia (because β-blockers block catecholamine counter-regulatory mechanisms) and hyperkalemia.

Laboratory Investigations

Measurements of blood levels are not readily available or useful. ECG and cardiac monitoring should be maintained, and blood glucose and electrolytes, BUN, and creatinine levels should be monitored, as well as ABG if there are respiratory symptoms.

Management

Vital functions must be established and maintained. Vascular access, baseline ECG, and continuous cardiac and blood pressure monitoring should be established. A pacemaker must be available. Gastrointestinal decontamination can be undertaken initially with activated charcoal up to 1 hour after ingestion. MDAC is no longer recommended, based on the latest guidelines. Whole-bowel irrigation can be considered in cases of large overdoses with sustained-release preparations, but there are no studies evaluating the efficacy of intervention.

If there are cardiovascular disturbances, a cardiac consultation should be obtained. Class IA antidysrhythmic agents (procainamide, quinidine) and III (bretylium) are not recommended. Hypotension is treated with fluids initially, although it usually does not respond. Frequently, glucagon and cardiac pacing are needed. Bradycardia in asymptomatic, hemodynamically stable patients requires no therapy. It is not predictive of the future course of the disease. If the patient is unstable (has hypotension or a high-degree atrioventricular block), atropine 0.02 mg/kg (up to 2 mg) in adults, glucagon, and a pacemaker can be used. In case of ventricular tachycardia, overdrive pacing can be used. A wide QRS interval may respond to sodium bicarbonate. Torsades de pointes (associated with sotalol) may respond to magnesium sulfate and overdrive pacing. Prophylactic magnesium for prolonged QT interval has been suggested, but there are no data. Epinephrine must not be used because an unopposed α effect may occur.

Hypotension and myocardial depression are managed by correction of dysrhythmias, Trendelenburg position, fluids, glucagon, or amrinone (Inocor), or a combination of these. Hemodynamic monitoring with a Swan-Ganz catheter or arterial line may be necessary to manage fluid therapy.

Glucagon is the initial drug of choice. It works through adenyl cyclase and bypasses catecholamine receptors; therefore, it is not affected by β-blockers. Glucagon increases cardiac contractility and heart rate. It is given as an intravenous bolus of 5 to 10 mg[3] over 1 minute and followed by a continuous infusion of 1 to 5 mg/h (in children, 0.15 mg/kg followed by 0.05 to 0.1 mg/kg/h). In large doses and in infusion therapy D_5W, sterile water, or saline should be used as a dilutant to reconstitute glucagon in place of the 0.2% phenol diluent provided with some drugs. Effects are seen within minutes. It can be used with other agents such as amrinone.

Amrinone (Inocor) inhibits phosphodiesterase enzyme, which metabolizes cyclic AMP. It is administered as a bolus of 0.15 to 2 mg/kg (0.15 to 0.4 mL/kg) intravenously, followed by infusion of 5 to 10 µg/kg/min.

Hypoglycemia should be treated with intravenous glucose. Life-threatening hyperkalemia is treated with calcium (avoid if digoxin is present), bicarbonate, and glucose or insulin. Convulsions can be controlled with diazepam or phenobarbital. If bronchospasm is present, $β_2$ nebulized bronchodilators are given.

Extraordinary measures such as intra-aortic balloon pump support can be instituted. Extracorporeal measures can be undertaken. Hemodialysis for cases of atenolol, acebutolol, nadolol, and sotalol (low volume distribution, low protein binding) ingestion may be helpful, particularly when there is evidence of renal failure. Hemodialysis is not effective for propranolol, metoprolol, and timolol.

Prenalterol[2] has successfully reversed both bradycardia and hypotension but is not currently available in the United States.

Disposition

Asymptomatic patients with history of overdose require baseline ECG and continuous cardiac monitoring for at least 6 hours with regular-release preparations and for 24 hours with sustained-release preparations. Symptomatic patients should be observed with cardiac monitoring for 24 hours. If seizures or abnormal rhythm or vital signs are present, the patient should be admitted to the intensive care unit.

CALCIUM CHANNEL BLOCKERS

Calcium channel blockers are used in the treatment of effort angina, supraventricular tachycardia, and hypertension.

Toxic Mechanism

Calcium channel blockers reduce influx of calcium through the slow channels in membranes of the myocardium, the atrioventricular nodes, and the vascular smooth muscles and result in peripheral, systemic, and coronary vasodilation, impaired cardiac conduction, and depression of cardiac contractility. All calcium channel blockers have vasodilatory action, but only bepridil, diltiazem, and verapamil depress myocardial contractility and cause atrioventricular block.

Toxic Dose

Any ingested amount greater than the maximum daily dose has the potential of severe toxicity. The maximum oral daily doses in adults and toxic doses in children of each are as follows: amlodipine (Norvasc), 10 mg for adults and more than 0.25 mg/kg for children; bepridil (Vascor), 400 mg for adults and more than 5.7 mg/kg for children; diltiazem (Cardizem), 360 mg for adults (toxic dose >2 g) and more

than 6 mg/kg for children; felodipine (Plendil), 40 mg for adults and more than 0.56 mg/kg for children; isradipine (DynaCirc), 40 mg for adults and more than 0.4 mg/kg for children; nicardipine (Cardene), 120 mg for adults and more than 0.85 mg/kg for children; nifedipine (Procardia), 120 mg for adults and more than 2 mg/kg for children; nimodipine (Nimotop), 360 mg for adults and more than 0.85 mg/kg for children; nitrendipine (Baypress),[1] 80 mg for adults and more than 1.14 mg/kg for children; and verapamil (Calan), 480 mg for adults and 15 mg/kg for children.

Kinetics

Onset of action of regular-release preparations varies: for verapamil it is 60 to 120 minutes, for nifedipine 20 minutes, and for diltiazem 15 minutes after ingestion. Peak effect for verapamil is 2 to 4 hours, for nifedipine 60 to 90 minutes, and for diltiazem 30 to 60 minutes, but the peak action may be delayed for 6 to 8 hours. Duration of action is up to 36 hours. The onset of action for sustained-release preparations is usually 4 hours but may be delayed, and peak effect is at 12 to 24 hours. In cases of massive overdose, concretions and prolonged toxicity can develop.

Volume distribution varies from 3 to 7 L/kg. Hepatic elimination half-life varies from 3 to 7 hours. Patients receiving digitalis and calcium channel blockers run the risk of digitalis toxicity, because calcium channel blockers increase digitalis levels.

Manifestations

Cardiac manifestations include hypotension, bradycardia, and conduction disturbances occurring 30 minutes to 5 hours after ingestion. A prolonged PR interval is an early finding and may occur at therapeutic doses. Torsades de pointes has been reported. All degrees of blocks may occur and may be delayed up to 16 hours. Lactic acidosis may be present. Calcium channel blockers do not affect intraventricular conduction, so the QRS interval is usually not affected.

Hypocalcemia is rarely present. Hyperglycemia may be present because of interference in calcium-dependent insulin release. Mental status changes, headaches, seizures, hemiparesis, and CNS depression may occur.

Laboratory Investigations

Specific drug levels are not readily available and are not useful. Monitor blood sugar, electrolytes, calcium, ABG, pulse oximetry, creatinine, and BUN, and also use hemodynamic monitoring, ECG, and cardiac monitoring.

Management

Vital functions must be established and maintained. Baseline ECG readings should be obtained and continuous cardiac and blood pressure monitoring maintained. A pacemaker should be available. Cardiology consultation should be sought.

Gastrointestinal decontamination with activated charcoal is recommended. If a large dose of a sustained-release preparation was ingested, whole-bowel irrigation can be considered, but its effectiveness has not been investigated.

If the patient is symptomatic, immediate cardiology consult must be obtained, because a pacemaker and hemodynamic monitoring may be needed. In the case of heart block, atropine is rarely effective and isoproterenol (Isuprel) may produce vasodilation. The use of a pacemaker should be considered early.

Hypotension and bradycardia can be treated with positioning, fluids, and calcium gluconate or chloride, glucagon, amrinone (Inocor), and ventricular pacing. Calcium salts must be avoided if digoxin is present. Calcium usually reverses depressed myocardial contractility but may not reverse nodal depression or peripheral vasodilation. Calcium chloride can be given in a 10% solution, 0.1 to 0.2 mL/kg up to 10 mL in an adult, or calcium gluconate in a 10% solution 0.3 to 0.4 mL/kg up to 20 mL in an adult. Administration is intravenous, over 5 to 10 minutes. One should monitor for dysrhythmias, hypotension, and the serum ionized calcium. The aim is to increase

---

[2]Not available in the United States.
[3]Exceeds dosage recommended by the manufacturer.

[1]Not FDA approved for this indication.

calcium 4 mg/dL to a maximum of 13 mg/dL. The calcium response lasts 15 minutes and may require repeated doses or a continuous calcium gluconate infusion 0.2 mL/kg/h up to maximum of 10 mL/h.

If calcium fails, glucagon can be tried for its positive inotropic and chronotropic effect, or both. Amrinone (Inocor), an inotropic agent, may reverse the effects of calcium channel blockers. An effective dose is 0.15 mg to 2 mg/kg (0.15 to 0.4 mL/kg) by intravenous bolus followed by infusion of 5 to 10 µg/kg/min.

In case of hypotension, fluids, norepinephrine (Levophed), and epinephrine may be required. Amrinone and glucagon have been tried alone and in combination. Dobutamine and dopamine are often ineffective.

Extracorporeal measures (e.g., hemodialysis and charcoal hemoperfusion) are not useful, but extraordinary measures such as intra-aortic balloon pump and cardiopulmonary bypass have been used successfully.

For cases of calcium channel blocker toxicity that fail to respond to aggressive management, recent studies demonstrate that insulin and glucose have therapeutic value. The suggested dose range for insulin is to infuse regular insulin at 0.5 IU/kg/h with a simultaneous infusion of glucose 1 g/kg/h, with glucose monitoring every 30 minutes for at least the first 4 hours of administration and subsequent glucose adjustment to maintain euglycemia (70 to 100 mg/dL). Potassium levels should be monitored regularly, as they may shift in response to the insulin.

Disposition

Patients who have ingested regular-release preparations should be monitored for at least 6 hours and those who have ingested sustained-release preparations should be monitored for 24 hours after the ingestion. Intentional overdose necessitates psychiatric clearance. Symptomatic patients should be admitted to the intensive care unit.

CARBON MONOXIDE

Carbon monoxide is an odorless, colorless gas produced from incomplete combustion; it is also an in vivo metabolic breakdown product of methylene chloride used in paint removers.

Toxic Mechanism

Carbon monoxide's affinity for hemoglobin is 240 times greater than that of oxygen. It shifts the oxygen dissociation curve to the left, which impairs hemoglobin release of oxygen to tissues and inhibits the cytochrome oxidase enzymes.

Toxic Dose and Manifestations

Table 13 describes the manifestations of carbon monoxide toxicity. Exposure to 0.5% for a few minutes is lethal. Sequelae correlate with the patient's level of consciousness at presentation. ECG abnormalities may be noted. Creatine kinase is often elevated, and rhabdomyolysis and myoglobinuria may occur.

The carboxyhemoglobin (CoHB) expresses in percentage the extent to which carbon monoxide has bound with the total hemoglobin. This may be misleadingly low in the anemic patient with less hemoglobin than normal. The patient's presentation is a more reliable indicator of severity than the CoHB level. The manifestations listed in Table 13 for each level are in addition to those listed at the level above. The CoHB may not correlate reliably with the severity of the intoxication, and linking symptoms to specific levels of CoHB frequently leads to inaccurate conclusions. A level of carbon monoxide greater than 40% is usually associated with obvious intoxication.

Kinetics

The natural metabolism of the body produces small amounts of CoHB, less than 2% for nonsmokers and 5% to 9% for smokers.

Carbon monoxide is rapidly absorbed through the lungs. The rate of absorption is directly related to alveolar ventilation. Elimination also occurs through the lungs. The half-life of CoHB in room air (21% oxygen) is 5 to 6 hours; in 100% oxygen, it is 90 minutes; in hyperbaric pressure at 3 atmospheres oxygen, it is 20 to 30 minutes.

TABLE 13 Carbon Monoxide Exposure and Possible Manifestations

CoHB Saturation (%)	Manifestations
3.5	None
5	Slight headache, decreased exercise tolerance
10	Slight headache, dyspnea on vigorous exertion, may impair driving skills
10–20	Moderate dyspnea on exertion, throbbing, temporal headache
20–30	Severe headache, syncope, dizziness, visual changes, weakness, nausea, vomiting, altered judgment
30–40	Vertigo, ataxia, blurred vision, confusion, loss of consciousness
40–50	Confusion, tachycardia, tachypnea, coma, convulsions
50–60	Cheyne-Stokes, coma, convulsions, shock, apnea
60–70	Coma, convulsions, respiratory and heart failure, death

Laboratory Investigations

An ABG reading may show metabolic acidosis and normal oxygen tension. In cases of significant poisoning, the ABG, electrolytes, blood glucose, serum creatine kinase and cardiac enzymes, renal function tests, and liver function tests should be monitored. A urinalysis and test for myoglobinuria should be obtained. Chest radiograph can be useful in cases of smoke inhalation or if the patient is being considered for hyperbaric chamber. ECG monitoring should be maintained, especially if the patient is older than 40 years, has a history of cardiac disease, or has moderate to severe symptoms. Which toxicology studies are used is based on symptoms and circumstances. CoHB should be monitored during and at the end of therapy. The pulse oximeter has two wavelengths and overestimates oxyhemoglobin saturation in carbon monoxide poisoning. The true oxygen saturation is determined by blood gas analysis, which measures the oxygen bound to hemoglobin. The co-oximeter measures four wavelengths and separates out CoHB and the other hemoglobin binding agents from oxyhemoglobin. Fetal hemoglobin has a greater affinity for carbon monoxide than adult hemoglobin and may falsely elevate the CoHB as much as 4% in young infants.

Management

The first step is to adequately protect the rescuer. The patient must be removed from the contaminated area, and his or her vital functions must be established.

The mainstay of treatment is 100% oxygen via a non-rebreathing mask with an oxygen reservoir or endotracheal tube. All patients receive 100% oxygen until the CoHB level is 5% or less. Assisted ventilation may be necessary. ABG and CoHB should be monitored and the present CoHB level determined. *Note:* A near-normal CoHB level does not exclude significant carbon monoxide poisoning, especially if the measurement is taken several hours after termination of exposure or if oxygen has been administered prior to obtaining the sample.

The exposed pregnant woman should be kept on 100% oxygen for several hours after the CoHB level is almost 0, because carbon monoxide concentrates in the fetus and oxygen is needed longer to ensure elimination of the carbon monoxide from fetal circulation. The fetus must be monitored, because carbon monoxide and hypoxia are potentially teratogenic.

Metabolic acidosis should be treated with sodium bicarbonate only if the pH is below 7.2 after correction of hypoxia and adequate ventilation. Acidosis shifts the oxygen dissociation curve to the right and facilitates oxygen delivery to the tissues.

The decision to use the hyperbaric oxygen chamber must be made on the basis of the ability to handle other acute emergencies that may coexist in the patient and of the severity of the poisoning. The standard of care for persons exposed to carbon monoxide has yet to be determined, but most authorities recommend using the hyperbaric oxygen chamber under any of the following conditions:

- If the patient is in a coma or has a history of loss of consciousness or seizures
- If there is cardiovascular dysfunction (clinical ischemic chest pain or ECG evidence of ischemia)
- If the patient has metabolic acidosis
- If symptoms persist despite 100% oxygen therapy
- In a child, if the initial CoHB is greater than 15%
- In symptomatic patients with preexisting ischemia
- If there are signs of maternal or fetal distress regardless of CoHB level (infants and fetus are a special problem because fetal hemoglobin has greater affinity for carbon monoxide)

Although controversial, a neurologic-cognitive examination has been used to help determine which patients with low carbon monoxide levels should receive more aggressive therapy. Testing should include the following: general orientation memory testing involving address, phone number, date of birth, and present date; and cognitive testing, involving counting by 7s, digit span, and forward and backward spelling of three-letter and four-letter words. Patients with delayed neurologic sequelae or recurrent symptoms up to 3 weeks may benefit from hyperbaric oxygen chamber treatment.

Seizures and cerebral edema must be treated.

Disposition

Patients with no or mild symptoms who become asymptomatic after a few hours of oxygen therapy and have a carbon monoxide level less than 10%, and normal physical and neurologic-cognitive examination findings, can be discharged, but they should be instructed to return if any signs of neurologic dysfunction appear. Patients with carbon monoxide poisoning requiring treatment need follow-up neuropsychiatric examinations.

CAUSTICS AND CORROSIVES

The terms *caustic* and *corrosive* are used interchangeably and can be divided into acids and alkalis. The U.S. Consumer Product Safety Commission Labeling Recommendations on containers for acids and alkalis indicate the potential for producing serious damage, as follows:

- Caution—weak irritant
- Warning—strong irritant
- Danger—corrosive

Some common acids with corrosive potential include acetic acid, formic acid, glycolic acid, hydrochloric acid, mercuric chloride, nitric acid, oxalic acid, phosphoric acid, sulfuric acid (battery acid), zinc chloride, and zinc sulfate. Some common alkalis with corrosive potential include ammonia, calcium carbide, calcium hydroxide (dry), calcium oxide, potassium hydroxide (lye), and sodium hydroxide (lye).

Toxic Mechanism

Acids produce mucosal coagulation necrosis and may be absorbed systemically; they do not penetrate deeply. Injury to the gastric mucosa is more likely, although specific sites of injury for acids and alkalis are not clearly defined.

Alkalis produce liquefaction necrosis and saponification and penetrate deeply. The esophageal mucosa is likely to be damaged. Oropharyngeal and esophageal damage is more frequently caused by solids than by liquids. Liquids produce superficial circumferential burns and gastric damage.

Toxic Dose

The toxicity is determined by concentration, contact time, and pH. Significant injury is more likely with a substance that has a pH of less than 2 or greater than 12, with a prolonged contact time, and with large volumes.

Manifestations

The absence of oral burns does not exclude the possibility of esophageal or gastric damage. General clinical findings are stridor; dysphagia; drooling; oropharyngeal, retrosternal, and epigastric pain; and ocular and oral burns. Alkali burns are yellow, soapy, frothy lesions. Acid burns are gray-white and later form an eschar. Abdominal tenderness and guarding may be present if perforation has happened.

Laboratory Investigations

If acid ingestion has taken place, the patient's acid-base balance and electrolyte status should be determined. If pulmonary symptoms are present, a chest radiograph, ABG measurement, and pulse oximetry are called for.

Management

It is recommended that the container be brought to the examination, as the substance must be identified and the pH of the substance, vomitus, tears, or saliva tested.

If the acid or alkali has been ingested, all gastrointestinal decontamination procedures are contraindicated except for immediate rinse, removal of substance from the mouth, and dilution with small amounts (sips) of milk or water. The examiner should check for ocular and dermal involvement. Contraindications to oral dilution are dysphagias, respiratory distress, obtundation, or shock. If there is ocular involvement one should immediately irrigate the eye with tepid water for at least 30 minutes, perform fluorescein stain of eye, and consult an ophthalmologist. If there is dermal involvement, one should immediately remove contaminated clothes and irrigate the skin with tepid water for at least 15 minutes. Consultation with a burn specialist is called for.

In cases of acid ingestion, some authorities advocate a small flexible nasogastric tube and aspiration within 30 minutes after ingestion.

Patients should receive only intravenous fluids following dilution until endoscopic consultation is obtained. Endoscopy is valuable to predict damage and risk of stricture. The indications are controversial, with some authorities recommending it in all cases of caustic ingestions regardless of symptoms, and others selectively using clinical features such as vomiting, stridor, drooling, and oral or facial lesions as criteria. We recommend endoscopy for all symptomatic patients or patients with intentional ingestions. Endoscopy may be performed immediately if the patient is symptomatic, but it is usually done 12 to 48 hours postingestion.

The use of corticosteroids is considered controversial. Some feel they may be useful for patients with second-degree circumferential burns. They recommend starting with hydrocortisone sodium succinate (Solu-Cortef) intravenously 10 to 20 mg/kg/d within 48 hours and changing to oral prednisolone 2 mg/kg/d for 3 weeks before tapering the dose. We do not usually recommend using corticosteroids because they have not been shown to be effective.

Tetanus prophylaxis should be provided if the patient requires it for wound care. Antibiotics are not useful prophylactically. Contrast studies are not useful in the first few days and may interfere with endoscopic evaluation; later, they can be used to assess the severity of damage.

Emergency medical therapy includes agents to inhibit collagen formation and intraluminal stents. Esophageal and gastric outlet dilation may be needed if there is evidence of stricture. Bougienage of the esophagus, however, has been associated with brain abscess. Interposition of the colon may be necessary if dilation fails to provide an adequate-sized passage.

Management of inhalation cases requires immediate removal from the environment, administration of humid supplemental oxygen, and observation for airway obstruction and noncardiac pulmonary edema. Radiographic and ABG evaluation should be obtained when appropriate. Intubation and respiratory support may be required.

Certain caustics produce systemic disturbances. Formaldehyde causes metabolic acidosis, hydrofluoric acid causes hypocalcemia and renal damage, oxalic acid causes hypocalcemia, phenol causes hepatic and renal damage, and picric acid causes renal injury.

Disposition

Infants and small children should be medically evaluated and observed. All symptomatic patients should be admitted. If they have severe symptoms or danger of airway compromise, they should be admitted to the intensive care unit. After endoscopy, if no damage is detected, the patient may be discharged when he or she can tolerate oral feedings. Intentional exposures require psychiatric evaluation before the patient can be discharged.

COCAINE (BENZOYLMETHYLECGONINE)

Cocaine is derived from the leaves of *Erythroxylum coca* and *Truxillo coca*. "Body packing" refers to the placement of many small packages of contraband cocaine for concealment in the gastrointestinal tract or other areas for illicit transport. "Body stuffing" refers to spontaneous ingestion of substances for the purpose of hiding evidence.

Toxic Mechanism

Cocaine directly stimulates the CNS presynaptic sympathetic neurons to release catecholamines and acetylcholine, while it blocks the presynaptic reuptake of the catecholamines; it blocks the sodium channels along neuronal membranes; and it increases platelet aggregation. Long-term use depletes the CNS of dopamine.

Toxic Dose

The maximum mucosal local anesthetic therapeutic dose of cocaine is 200 mg or 2 mL of a 10% solution. Although CNS effects can occur at relatively low local anesthetic doses (50 to 95 mg), they are more common with doses greater than 1 mg/kg; cardiac effects can occur with doses greater than 1 mg/kg. The potential fatal dose is 1200 mg intranasally, but death has occurred with 20 mg parenterally.

Kinetics

Cocaine is well absorbed by all routes, including nasal insufflation, and oral, dermal, and inhalation routes (Table 14). Protein binding is 8.7%, and volume distribution is 1.5 L/kg.

Cocaine is metabolized by plasma and liver cholinesterase to the inactive metabolites ecgonine methyl ester and benzoylecgonine. Plasma pseudocholinesterase is congenitally deficient in 3% of the population and decreased in fetuses, young infants, the elderly, pregnant people, and people with liver disease. These enzyme-deficient individuals are at increased risk for life-threatening cocaine toxicity.

Ten percent of cocaine is excreted unchanged. Cocaine and ethanol undergo liver synthesis to form cocaethylene, a metabolite with a half-life three times longer than that of cocaine. It may account for some of cocaine's cardiotoxicity and appears to be more lethal than cocaine or ethanol alone.

Manifestations

The CNS manifestations of cocaine ingestion are euphoria, hyperactivity, agitation, convulsions, and intracranial hemorrhage. Mydriasis and septal perforation can occur, as well as cardiac dysrhythmias, hypertension, and hypotension (with severe overdose). Chest pain is frequent, but only 5.8% of patients have true myocardial ischemia and infarction. Other manifestations include vasoconstriction, hyperthermia (because of increased metabolic rate), ischemic bowel perforation if the substance is ingested, rhabdomyolysis, myoglobinuria, and renal failure. In pregnant users, premature labor and abruptio placentae can occur.

Body cavity packing should be suspected in cases of prolonged toxicity.

Mortality can result from cerebrovascular accidents, coronary artery spasm, myocardial injury, or lethal dysrhythmias.

Laboratory Investigations

Monitoring of the ECG and cardiac rhythms, ABG, oxygen saturation, electrolytes, blood glucose, BUN, creatinine, and creatine kinase levels should be maintained. One should monitor cardiac fraction if the patient has chest pain, as well as the liver profile, and the urine for myoglobin. Intravenous drug users should have HIV and hepatitis virus testing.

Urine should be tested for cocaine and metabolites and other substances of abuse, and abdominal radiographs or ultrasonogram should be ordered for body packers. If the urine sample was collected more than 12 hours after cocaine intake, it will contain little or no cocaine. If cocaine is present, cocaine has been used within the past 12 hours. Cocaine's metabolite benzoylecgonine may be detected within 4 hours after a single nasal insufflation and for up to 114 hours. Cross-reactions with some herbal teas, lidocaine, and droperidol (Inapsine) may give false-positive results by some immunoassay methods.

Management

Supportive care includes blood pressure, cardiac, and thermal monitoring and seizure precautions. Diazepam (Valium) is the drug of choice for treatment of cocaine toxicity agitation, seizures, and dysrhythmias; doses are 10 to 30 mg intravenously at 2.5 mg per minute for adults and 0.2 to 0.5 mg/kg at 1 mg per minute up to 10 mg for a child.

Gastrointestinal decontamination should be instituted, if the cocaine was ingested, by administration of activated charcoal. MDAC may adsorb cocaine leakage in body stuffers or body packers. Whole-bowel irrigation with polyethylene glycol solution (PEG) has been used in body packers and stuffers if the contraband is in a firm container. If the packages are not visible on plain radiographs of the abdomen, a contrast study or CT scan can help to confirm successful passage. Cocaine in the nasal passage can be removed with an applicator dipped in a non–water-soluble product (lubricating jelly) if this is done within a few minutes after application.

In body packers and stuffers, venous access must be secured, and drugs must be readily available for treating life-threatening manifestations until the contraband is passed in the stool. Surgical removal may be indicated if the packet does not pass the pylorus, in an asymptomatic body packer, or in the case of intestinal obstruction.

Hypertension and tachycardia are usually transient and can be managed by careful titration of diazepam. Nitroprusside may be used for severe hypertension. Myocardial ischemia is managed by oxygen, vascular access, benzodiazepines, and nitroglycerin. Aspirin and thrombolysis are not routinely recommended because of the danger of intracranial hemorrhage.

Dysrhythmias are usually supraventricular (SVT) and do not require specific management. Adenosine is ineffective. Life-threatening tachydysrhythmias may respond to phentolamine (Regitine) 5 mg IV

TABLE 14 The Different Routes and Kinetics of Cocaine

Type	Route	Onset	Peak (min)	Half-Life (min)	Duration (min)
Cocaine leaf	Oral, chewing	20–30 min	45–90	NA	240–360
Hydrochloride	Insufflation	1–3 min	5–10	78	60–90
	Ingestion	20–30 min	50–90	54	Sustained
	Intravenous	30–120 sec	5–11	36	60–90
Freebase/crack	Smoking	5–10 sec	5–11	–	Up to 20
Coca paste	Smoking	Unknown	–	–	–

bolus in adults or 0.1 mg/kg in children at 5- to 10-minute intervals. Phentolamine also relieves coronary artery spasm and myocardial ischemia. Electrical synchronized cardioversion should be considered for patients with hemodynamically unstable dysrhythmias. Lidocaine is not recommended initially but may be used after 3 hours for ventricular tachycardia. Wide complex QRS ventricular tachycardia may be treated with sodium bicarbonate 2 mEq/kg as a bolus. β-Adrenergic blockers are not recommended.

Anxiety, agitation, and convulsions can be treated with diazepam. If diazepam fails to control seizures, neuromuscular blockers can be used. The EEG should be monitored for nonmotor seizure activity. For hyperthermia, external cooling and cool humidified 100% oxygen should be administered. Neuromuscular paralysis to control seizures will reduce temperature. Dantrolene and antipyretics are not recommended. Rhabdomyolysis and myoglobinuria are treated with fluids, alkaline diuresis, and diuretics.

If the patient is pregnant, the fetus must be monitored and the patient observed for spontaneous abortion.

Paranoid ideation and threatening behavior should be treated with rapid tranquilization. The patient should be observed for suicidal depression that may follow intoxication and may require suicide precautions. If focal neurologic manifestations are present, one should consider the possibility of a cerebrovascular accident and obtain a CT scan.

Extracorporeal clearance techniques are of no benefit.

Disposition

Patients with mild intoxication or a brief seizure that does not require treatment who become asymptomatic may be discharged after 6 hours with appropriate psychosocial follow-up. If cardiac or cerebral ischemic manifestations are present, the patient should be monitored in the intensive care unit. Body packers and stuffers require care in the intensive care unit until passage of the contraband.

CYANIDE

Hydrogen cyanide is a byproduct of burning plastic and wools in residential fires. Hydrocyanic acid is the liquefied form of hydrogen cyanide. Cyanide salts can be found in ore extraction. Nitriles, such as acetonitrile (artificial nail removers), are metabolized in the body to produce cyanide. Cyanogenic glycosides are present in some fruit seeds (such as amygdalin in apricots, peaches, and apples). Sodium nitroprusside, the antihypertensive vasodilator, contains five cyanide groups.

Toxic Mechanism

Cyanide blocks the cellular electron transport mechanism and cellular respiration by inhibiting the mitochondrial ferricytochrome oxidase system and other enzymes. This results in cellular hypoxia and lactic acidosis. *Note:* Citrus fruit seeds form cyanide in the presence of intestinal β-glucosidase (the seeds are harmful only if the capsule is broken).

Toxic Dose

The ingestion of 1 mg/kg or 50 mg of hydrogen cyanide can produce death within 15 minutes. The lethal dose of potassium cyanide is 200 mg. Five to 10 mL of 84% acetonitrile is lethal. Infusions of sodium nitroprusside in rates above 2 μg/kg per minute may cause cyanide to accumulate to toxic concentrations in critically ill patients.

Kinetics

Cyanide is rapidly absorbed by all routes. In the stomach, it forms hydrocyanic acid. Volume distribution is 1.5 L/kg. Protein binding is 60%. Cyanide is detoxified by metabolism in the liver via the mitochondrial thiosulfate-rhodanase pathway, which catalyzes the transfer of sulfur donor to cyanide, forming the less toxic irreversible thiocyanate that is excreted in the urine. Cyanide is also detoxified by reacting with hydroxocobalamin (vitamin B_{12a}) to form cyanocobalamin (vitamin B_{12}).

The cyanide elimination half-life from the blood is 1.2 hours. The elimination route is through the lungs.

Manifestations

Hydrogen cyanide has the distinctive odor of bitter almonds or silver polish. Manifestations of cyanide intoxication include hypertension, cardiac dysrhythmias, various ECG abnormalities, headache, hyperpnea, seizures, stupor, pulmonary edema, and flushing. Cyanosis is absent or appears late.

Laboratory Investigations

The examiner should obtain and monitor ABGs, oxygen saturation, blood lactate, hemoglobin, blood glucose, and electrolytes. Lactic acidemia, a decrease in the arterial-venous oxygen difference, and bright red venous blood occurs. If smoke inhalation is the possible source of cyanide exposure, CoHB and methemoglobin (MetHb) concentrations should be measured.

Cyanide levels in whole blood, red blood cells, or serum are not useful in the acute management because the determinations are not readily available. Specific cyanide blood levels are as follows: smokers have less than 0.5 μg/mL; a patient with flushing and tachycardia has 0.5 to 1.0 μg/mL, one with obtundation has 1.0 to 2.5 μg/mL, and one in coma or who has died has more than 2.5 μg/mL.

Management

If the cyanide was inhaled, the patient must be removed from the contaminated atmosphere. Attendants should not administer mouth-to-mouth resuscitation. Rescuers and attendants must be protected. Immediate administration of 100% oxygen is called for and oxygen should be continued during and after the administration of the antidote. The clinician must decide whether to use any or all components of the cyanide antidote kit.

The mechanism of action of the antidote kit is twofold: to produce methemoglobinemia and to provide a sulfur substrate for the detoxification of cyanide. The nitrites make methemoglobin, which has a greater affinity for cyanide than does the cytochrome oxidase enzymes. The combination of methemoglobin and cyanide forms cyanomethemoglobin. Sodium thiosulfate provides a sulfur substrate for the rhodanese enzyme, which converts cyanide into the relatively nontoxic sodium thiocyanate, which is excreted by the kidney.

The procedure for using the antidote kit is as follows:

Step 1: Amyl nitrite inhalant perles is only a temporizing measure (forms only 2% to 5% methemoglobin) and it can be omitted if venous access is established. Alternate 100% oxygen and the inhalant for 30 seconds each minute. Use a new perle every 3 minutes.

Step 2: Sodium nitrite ampule is indicated for cyanide exposures, except for cases of residential fires, smoke inhalation, and nitroprusside or acetonitrile poisonings. It is administered intravenously to produce methemoglobin of 20% to 30% at 35 to 70 minutes after administration. A dose of 10 mL of 3% solution of sodium nitrite for adults and 0.33 mL/kg of 3% solution for children is diluted to 100 mL 0.9% saline and administered slowly intravenously at 5 mL/min. If hypotension develops, the infusion should be slowed.

Step 3: Sodium thiosulfate is useful alone in cases of smoke inhalation, nitroprusside toxicity, and acetonitrile toxicity and should not be used at all in cases of hydrogen sulfide poisoning. The administration dose is 12.5 g of sodium thiosulfate or 50 mL of 25% solution for adults and 1.65 mL/kg of 25% solution for children intravenously over 10 to 20 minutes.

If cyanide symptoms recur, further treatment with nitrites or the perles is controversial. Some authorities suggest repeating the antidotes in 30 minutes at half of the initial dose, but others do not advise this for lack of efficacy. The child dosage regimen on the package insert must be carefully followed.

One hour after antidotes are administered, the methemoglobin level should be obtained and should not exceed 20%. Methylene blue should not be used to reverse excessive methemoglobin.

Gastrointestinal decontamination of oral ingestion by activated charcoal is recommended but is not very effective because of the rapidity of absorption. Seizures are treated with intravenous diazepam. Acidosis should be treated with sodium bicarbonate if it does not rapidly resolve with therapy. There is no role for hyperbaric oxygen or hemodialysis or hemoperfusion.

Other antidotes include hydroxocobalamin (vitamin B_{12a}) (Cyanokit), which has proven effective when given immediately after exposure in large doses of 4 g (50 mg/kg) or 50 times the amount of cyanide exposure with 8 g of sodium thiosulfate. Hydroxocobalamin has FDA orphan drug approval.

Disposition

Asymptomatic patients should be observed for a minimum of 3 hours. Patients who ingest nitrile compounds must be observed for 24 hours. Patients requiring antidote administration should be admitted to the intensive care unit.

DIGITALIS

Cardiac glycosides are found in cardiac medications, common plants, and the skin of the Bufo toad.

Toxic Mechanism

Cardiac glycosides inhibit the enzyme sodium/potassium-adenosine triphosphatase (Na^+, K^+, ATPase), leading to intracellular potassium loss and increased intracellular sodium, and producing phase 4 depolarization, increased automaticity, and ectopy. There is increased intracellular calcium and potentiation of contractility. Pacemaker cells are inhibited, and the refractory period is prolonged, leading to atrioventricular blocks. There is increased vagal tone.

Toxic Dose

Digoxin total digitalizing dose, the dose required to achieve therapeutic blood levels of 0.6 to 2.0 ng/mL, is 0.75 to 1.25 mg or 10 to 15 µg/kg for patients older than 10 years of age; 40 to 50 µg/kg for patients younger than 2 years of age; and 30 to 40 µg/kg for patients 2 to 10 years of age.

The acute single toxic dose is greater than 0.07 mg/kg or greater than 2 or 3 mg in an adult, but 2 mg in a child or 4 mg in an adult usually produces only mild toxicity. One to 3 mg or more may be found in a few leaves of oleander or foxglove. Serious and fatal overdoses are more than 4 mg in a child and more than 10 mg in an adult.

Acute digitoxin ingestion of 10 to 35 mg has produced severe toxicity and death. Digitoxin therapeutic steady state is 15 to 25 ng/mL. In cases of chronic or acute-on-chronic ingestions in patients with cardiac disease, more than 2 mg may produce toxicity; however, toxicity can develop within therapeutic range on chronic therapy.

Patients at greatest risk of overdose include those with cardiac disease, those with electrolyte abnormalities (low potassium, low magnesium, low T_4, high calcium), those with renal impairment, and those on amiodarone (Cordarone), quinidine, erythromycin, tetracycline, calcium channel blockers, and β-blockers.

Kinetics

Digoxin is a metabolite of digitoxin. In cases of oral overdose, the typical onset is 30 minutes, with peak effects in 3 to 12 hours. Duration is 3 to 4 days. Intravenous onset is in 5 to 30 minutes; peak level is immediate, and peak effect is at 1.5 to 3 hours.

Volume distribution is 5 to 6 L/kg. The cardiac-to-plasma ratio is 30:1. After an acute ingestion overdose, the serum concentration is not reflective of tissue concentration for at least 6 hours or more, and steady state is 12 to 16 hours after last dose.

Sixty percent to 80% of the parent compound is excreted unchanged in the urine. The elimination half-life is 30 to 50 hours.

Manifestations

Onset of manifestations is usually within 2 hours but may be delayed up to 12 hours.

Gastrointestinal effects of nausea and vomiting are frequently present in cases of acute ingestion but may also occur in cases of chronic ingestion. The "digitalis effect" on ECG is scooped ST segments and PR prolongation; in cases of overdose, any dysrhythmia or block is possible but none are characteristic. Bradycardia occurs in patients with acute overdose with healthy hearts; supraventricular tachycardia occurs in patients with existing heart disease or chronic overdose. Ventricular tachycardia is seen only in cases of severe poisoning.

The CNS effects include headaches, visual disturbances, and colored halo vision. Hyperkalemia occurs following acute overdose and correlates with digoxin level and outcome. Among patients with serum potassium levels of less than 5.0 mEq/L, all survive. If the level is 5 to 5.5, 50% survive, and if the level is greater than 5.5, all die. Hypokalemia is commonly seen with chronic intoxication. Patients with normal digitalis levels may have toxicity in the presence of hypokalemia.

Chronic intoxications are more likely to produce scotoma, color perception disturbances, yellow vision, halos, delirium, hallucinations or psychosis, tachycardia, and hypokalemia.

Laboratory Investigations

Continuous monitoring of ECG, pulse, and blood pressure is called for. Blood glucose, electrolytes, calcium, magnesium, BUN, and creatinine levels should also be monitored. An initial digoxin level should be measured on patient presentation and repeated thereafter. Levels should be measured more than 6 hours postingestion because earlier values do not reflect tissue distribution. Digoxin clinical toxicity is usually associated with serum digoxin levels of greater than 3.5 ng/mL in adults.

An endogenous digoxin-like substance cross-reacts in most common immunoassays (not with high-pressure liquid chromatography) and values as high as 4.1 ng/mL have been reported in newborns, patients with chronic renal failure, patients with abnormal immunoglobulins, and women in the third trimester of pregnancy.

Management

A cardiology consult should be obtained and a pacemaker should be readily available.

In undertaking gastrointestinal decontamination, excessive vagal stimulation should be avoided (e.g., emesis and gastric lavage). Activated charcoal should be administered, and if a nasogastric tube is required for the activated charcoal, pretreatment with atropine (0.02 mg/kg in children and 0.5 mg in adults) should be considered.

Digoxin-specific antibody fragments (Fab, Digibind) 38 mg binds 0.5 mg digoxin and then is excreted through the kidneys. The onset of action is within 30 minutes. Problems associated with Fab therapy are mainly from withdrawal of digoxin and worsening heart failure, hypokalemia, decrease in glucose (if the patient has low glycogen stores), and allergic reactions (very rare). Digitalis administered after Fab therapy is bound and may be inactivated for 5 to 7 days.

Absolute indications for Fab therapy include the following:

- Life-threatening malignant (hemodynamically unstable) dysrhythmias
- Ventricular dysrhythmias, unstable severe bradycardia, or second- or third-degree blocks unresponsive to atropine or rapid deterioration in clinical status
- Life-threatening digitoxin and oleander poisonings
- Relative indications for Fab therapy include the following:
- Ingestions greater than 4 mg in a child and 10 mg in an adult
- Serum potassium level greater than 5.0 mEq/L
- Serum digoxin level greater than 10 ng/mL in adults or greater than 5 ng/mL in children 6 hours after an acute ingestion
- Digitalis delirium and thrombocytopenia response

Digoxin-specific Fab fragments therapy can be administered as a bolus through a 22-µm filter if the case is a critical emergency. If the case is less urgent, then it can be administered over 30 minutes. An empiric dose is 10 vials in adults and 5 vials in a child for an unknown amount ingested in a symptomatic patient with history of a digoxin overdose.

To calculate the dose in the case of a known ingestion, the following equation is used:

$$\text{Amount (total mg)} \times (0.8) \text{ body burden}$$

If liquid capsules were taken or the substance was given intravenously the 80% bioavailability figure is not used. Instead, the body burden divided by 0.5 (0.5 mg digoxin is bound by 1 vial of 38 mg of Fab) equals the number of vials needed.

If the amount is unknown but the steady state serum concentration is known, the following equations are used:

For digoxin:

$$\text{Digitoxin ng/mL} \times (5.6 \text{ L/kg Vd}) \times (\text{wt kg}) = \text{mg body burden}$$
$$\text{Body burden} \div 1000 = \text{mg body burden}$$
$$\text{Body burden}/0.5 = \text{number of vials needed}$$

For digitoxin:

$$\text{Digitoxin ng/mL} \times (0.56 \text{ L/kg Vd}) \times (\text{wt kg}) = \text{mg body burden}$$
$$\text{Body burden} \div 1000 = \text{mg body burden}$$
$$\text{Body burden}/0.5 = \text{number of vials needed}$$

Antidysrhythmic agents or a pacemaker should be used only if Fab therapy fails. For ventricular tachydysrhythmias, electrolyte disturbances should be corrected by the administration of lidocaine or phenytoin. For torsades de pointes, magnesium sulfate 20 mL 20% IV can be given slowly over 20 minutes (or 25 to 50 mg/kg in a child), titrated to control the dysrhythmia. Magnesium should be discontinued if hypotension, heart block, or decreased deep tendon reflexes are present. Magnesium is used with caution if the patient has renal impairment.

Unstable bradycardia and second-degree and third-degree atrioventricular block should be treated by Fab first. A pacemaker should be available if necessary. Isoproterenol should be avoided because it causes dysrhythmias. Cardioversion is used with caution, starting at a setting of 5 to 10 joules. The patient should be pretreated with lidocaine, if possible, because cardioversion may precipitate ventricular fibrillation or asystole.

Potassium disturbances are caused by a shift, not a change, in total body potassium. Hyperkalemia (>5.0 mEq/L) is treated with Fab only. Calcium must never be used, and insulin/glucose and sodium bicarbonate should not be used concomitantly with Fab because they may produce severe life-threatening hypokalemia. Sodium polystyrene sulfonate (Kayexalate) should not be used. Hypokalemia must be treated with caution because it may be cardioprotective. Treatment can be administered if the patient has ventricular dysrhythmias or a serum potassium level less than 3.0 mEq/L and atrioventricular block.

Extracorporeal procedures are ineffective. Hemodialysis is used for severe or refractory hyperkalemia.

One must never use antidysrhythmic types Ia (procainamide, quinidine, disopyramide [Norpace], amiodarone [Cordarone]), Ic (propafenone [Rythmol], flecainide [Tambocor]), II (β-blockers), or IV (calcium channel blockers). Class Ib drugs (lidocaine, phenytoin [Dilantin], mexiletine [Mexitil], and tocainide [Tonocard]) can be used.

Disposition

Consultation with a poison control center and a cardiologist experienced with digoxin-specific Fab fragments is warranted. All patients with significant dysrhythmias, symptoms, elevated serum digoxin concentration, or elevated serum potassium level should be admitted to the intensive care unit.

ETHANOL

Table 15 lists the features of alcohols and glycols.

Toxic Mechanism

Ethanol has CNS depressant and anesthetic effects. Ethanol stimulates the γ-aminobutyric acid (GABA) system. It promotes cutaneous vasodilation (contributes to hypothermia), stimulates secretion of gastric juice (gastritis), inhibits the secretion of the antidiuretic hormone, inhibits gluconeogenesis (hypoglycemia), and influences fat metabolism (lipidemia).

Toxic Dose

A dose of 1 mL/kg of absolute ethanol (100% ethanol, or 200 proof) gives a blood ethanol concentration of 100 mg/dL. A potentially fatal dose is 3 g/kg for children or 6 g/kg for adults. Children are more prone to developing hypoglycemia than adults.

Kinetics

Onset of action is 30 to 60 minutes after ingestion; peak action is 90 minutes on empty stomach. Volume distribution is 0.6 L/kg. The major route of elimination (>90%) is by hepatic oxidative metabolism. The first step is by the enzyme alcohol dehydrogenase, which converts ethanol to acetaldehyde. Alcohol dehydrogenase metabolizes ethanol at a constant rate of 12 to 20 mg/dL/h (12 to 15 mg/dL/h in nondrinkers, 15 to 30 mg/dL/h in social drinkers, 30 to 50 mg/dL/h in heavy drinkers, and 25 to 30 mg/dL/h in children). At very low blood ethanol concentration (>30 mg/dL), the metabolism is by first-order kinetics. In the second step, acetaldehyde is metabolized by acetaldehyde dehydrogenase to acetic acid, which is metabolized by the Krebs cycle to carbon dioxide and water. The enzyme steps are nicotinamide adenine dinucleotide-dependent, which interferes with gluconeogenesis. Less than 10% of ethanol is excreted unchanged by the kidneys. The relationship between blood ethanol concentration (BEC) and dose (amount ingested) can be calculated as follows:

TABLE 15 Summary of Alcohol and Glycol Features

	Methanol	Isopropanol	Ethanol	Ethylene Glycol
Principal uses	Gas line antifreeze, Sterno, windshield de-icer	Solvent jewelry cleaner, rubbing alcohol	Beverage, solvent	Radiator antifreeze, windshield de-icer
Specific gravity	0.719	0.785	0.789	1.12
Fatal dose	1 mL/kg 100%	3 mL/kg 100%	5 mL/kg 100%	1.4 mL/kg
Inebriation	±	2+	2+	1+
Metabolic change		Hyperglycemia	Hypoglycemia	Hypocalcemia
Metabolic acidosis	4+	0	1+	2+
Anion gap	4+	±	2+	4+
Ketosis	Ketobutyric	Acetone	Hydroxybutyric	None
Gastrointestinal tract	Pancreatitis	Hemorrhagic gastritis	Gastritis	
Osmolality*	0.337	0.176	0.228	0.190

*1 mL/dL of substances raises freezing point osmolarity of serum. The validity of the correlation of osmolality with blood concentrations has been questioned.

TABLE 16   Clinical Signs in the Nontolerant Ethanol Drinker

Ethanol Blood Concentration (mg/dL)*	Manifestations
>25	Euphoria
>47	**Mild incoordination,** sensory and motor impairment
>50	Increased risk of motor vehicle accidents
>100	Ataxia (legal toxic level in many localities)
>150	**Moderate incoordination,** slow reaction time
>200	Drowsiness and confusion
>300	Severe incoordination, stupor, blurred vision
>500	**Flaccid coma,** respiratory failure, hypotension; may be fatal

*Ethanol concentrations sometimes reported in %.
Note: mg% is not equivalent to mg/dL because ethanol weighs less than water (specific gravity 0.79). A 1% ethanol concentration is 790 mg/dL and 0.1% is 79 mg/dL. There is great variation in individual behavior at different blood ethanol levels. Behavior is dependent on tolerance and other factors.

$$BEC\ (mg/dL) = amount\ ingested\ (mL) \times$$
$$\%\ ethanol\ product \times SG\ (0.79)/Vd\ (0.6\ L/kg) \times body\ wt\ (kg)$$
$$Dose\ (amount\ ingested) = BEC\ (mg/dL) \times$$
$$Vd\ (0.6) \times body\ wt\ (kg)/\%\ ethanol \times$$
$$specific\ gravity\ (0.79)$$

Manifestations

Table 16 lists the clinical signs of acute ethanol intoxication.

Chronic alcoholic patients tolerate higher blood ethanol concentration, and correlation with manifestations is not valid. Rapid interview for alcoholism is the CAGE questions:

- C—Have you felt the need to Cut down?
- A—Have others Annoyed you by criticism of your drinking?
- G—Have you felt Guilty about your drinking?
- E—Have you ever had a morning Eye-opening drink to steady your nerves or get rid of a hangover?

Two affirmative answers indicate probable alcoholism.

Laboratory Investigations

The blood ethanol concentration should be specifically requested and followed. Gas chromatography or a breathalyzer test gives rapid reliable results if no belching or vomiting is present. Enzymatic methods do not differentiate between the alcohols. ABG, electrolytes, and glucose should be measured, the anion and osmolar gaps determined (measure by freezing point depression, not vapor pressure), and a check for ketosis made.

Management

The examiner should inquire about trauma and disulfiram use. The patient must be protected from aspiration and hypoxia. Vital functions must be established and maintained. The patient may require intubation and assisted ventilation.

Gastrointestinal decontamination plays no role in the management of ethanol intoxication.

If the patient is comatose, glucose should be administered intravenously, 1 mL/kg 50% glucose in adults and 2 mL/kg 25% glucose in children. Thiamine, 100 mg intravenously, is administered if the patient has a history of chronic alcoholism, malnutrition, or suspected eating disorders to prevent Wernicke-Korsakoff syndrome. Naloxone (Narcan) has produced a partial inconsistent response but is not recommended for known alcoholics.

General supportive care includes administration of fluids to correct hydration and hypotension and correction of electrolyte abnormalities and acid-base imbalance. Vasopressors and plasma expanders may be necessary to correct severe hypotension. Hypomagnesemia is frequent in chronic alcoholics. In case of hypomagnesemia, a loading dose of 2 g magnesium sulfate 10% is administered by intravenous solution over 5 minutes in the intensive care unit with blood pressure and cardiac monitoring and calcium chloride 10% on hand in case of overdose. This is followed with constant infusion of 6 g of 10% solution over 3 to 4 hours. Caution must be taken with the use of magnesium if renal failure is present.

Hypothermic patients should be warmed. See the section on disturbances caused by cold.

Hemodialysis can be used in severe cases when conventional therapy is ineffective (rarely needed).

Repeated or prolonged seizures should be treated with diazepam (Valium). The brief "rum fits" do not need long-term anticonvulsant therapy. Repeated seizures or focal neurologic findings may warrant skull radiographs, lumbar puncture, and CT scan of the head, depending on the clinical findings. Withdrawal is treated with hydration and large doses of chlordiazepoxide (Librium) 50 to 100 mg or diazepam (Valium) 2 to 10 mg intravenously; these doses may be repeated in 2 to 4 hours. Very large doses of benzodiazepines may be required for delirium tremens. Withdrawal can occur in presence of elevated blood ethanol concentration and can be fatal if left untreated.

Chest radiograph is warranted to determine whether aspiration pneumonia is present. Renal and liver function tests and bilirubin level measurement should be made.

Disposition

Clinical severity (e.g., intubation, assisted ventilation, aspiration pneumonia) should determine the level of hospital care needed. Young children with significant unintentional exposure to ethanol (calculated to reach a blood ethanol concentration of 50 mg/dL) should have blood ethanol concentration obtained and blood glucose levels monitored for hypoglycemia frequently for 4 hours after ingestion. Patients with acute ethanol intoxication seldom require admission unless a complication is present. However, intoxicated patients should not be discharged until they are fully functional (can walk, talk, and think independently), have suicide potential evaluated, have proper disposition environment, and have a sober escort.

ETHYLENE GLYCOL

Ethylene glycol is found in solvents, de-icers, radiator antifreeze (95%), and air-conditioning units. Ethylene glycol is a sweet-tasting, colorless, water-soluble liquid with a sweet aromatic fragrance.

Toxic Mechanism

Ethylene glycol is oxidized by alcohol dehydrogenase to glycolaldehyde, which is metabolized to glycolic acid and glyoxylic acid. Glyoxylic acid is metabolized to oxalic acid via a pyridoxine-dependent pathway to glycine and by thiamine and magnesium-dependent pathways to α-hydroxy-ketoadipic acid. The metabolites of ethylene glycol produce a profound metabolic acidosis, increased anion gap, hypocalcemia, and oxalate crystals, which deposit in tissues (particularly the kidney).

Toxic Dose

The ingestion of 0.1 mL/kg 100% ethylene glycol can result in a toxic serum ethylene glycol concentration of 20 mg/dL. Ingestion of 3.0 mL (less than 1 teaspoonful or swallow) of a 100% solution in a 10-kg child or 30 mL of 100% ethylene glycol in an adult produces a serum ethylene glycol concentration of 50 mg/dL, a concentration that requires hemodialysis. The fatal amount is 1.4 mL/kg of 100% solution.

Kinetics

Absorption is via dermal, inhalation, and ingestion routes. Ethylene glycol is rapidly absorbed from the gastrointestinal tract. Onset is usually in 30 minutes but may be delayed by co-ingestion of food and ethanol. The usual peak level is at 2 hours. Volume distribution is 0.65 to 0.8 L/kg.

For metabolism, see *Toxic Mechanism.*

The half-life of ethylene glycol without ethanol is 3 to 8 hours; with ethanol, it is 17 hours, and with hemodialysis it is 2.5 hours. Renal clearance is 3.2 mL/kg/minute. About 20% to 50% is excreted unchanged in the urine. The relationship between serum ethylene glycol concentration (SEGC) and dose (amount ingested) can be calculated as follows:

$$0.12 \text{ mL/kg of } 100\% = \text{SEGC } 10 \text{ mg/dL}$$

Manifestations

Phase I

The onset of manifestations is 30 minutes to several hours longer after ingestion with concomitant ethanol ingestion. The patient may be inebriated. Hypocalcemia, tetany, and calcium oxalate and hippuric acid crystals in urine can be seen within 4 to 8 hours but are not always present. Early, before metabolism of ethylene glycol, an osmolal gap may be present (see *Laboratory Investigations*). Later, the metabolites of ethylene glycol produce changes starting 4 to 12 hours following ingestion, including an anion gap, metabolic acidosis, coma, convulsions, cardiac disturbances, and pulmonary and cerebral edema. Because fluorescein is added to some antifreeze, the presence of fluorescence may be a clue to ethylene glycol exposure. However, it has been shown that fluorescent urine is not a reliable indicator of ethylene glycol ingestion and should not be used as a screen.

Phase II

After 12 to 36 hours, cardiopulmonary deterioration occurs, with pulmonary edema and congestive heart failure.

Phase III

Phase III occurs 36 to 72 hours after ingestion, with pulmonary edema and oliguric renal failure from oxalate crystal deposition and tubular necrosis predominating.

Phase IV

Neurologic sequelae may occur rarely, especially in patients who fail to receive early antidotal therapy. The onset ranges from 6 to 10 days after ingestion. Findings include facial diplegia, hearing loss, bilateral visual disturbances, elevated cerebrospinal fluid pressure with or without elevated protein levels and pleocytosis, vomiting, hyperreflexia, dysphagia, and ataxia.

Laboratory Investigations

Blood glucose and electrolytes should be monitored. Urinalysis should look for oxalate ("envelope") and monohydrate ("hemp seed") crystals. Urine fluorescence is not reliable as a screen. ABG, ethylene glycol, and ethanol levels, plasma osmolarity (using freezing point depression method), calcium, BUN, and creatinine should be measured. A serum ethylene glycol concentration of 20 mg/dL is toxic (ethylene glycol levels are very difficult to obtain). If possible, a glycolate level should be obtained. Cross-reactions with propylene glycol, a vehicle in many liquids and intravenous medications (phenytoin [Dilantin], diazepam [Valium]), other glycols, and triglycerides may produce spurious ethylene glycol levels. False-positive ethylene glycol values may occur with colorimetric or gas chromatography using an OV-17 column in the presence of propylene glycol.

The following equations can be used to calculate the osmolality, osmolal gap, and ethylene glycol level:

$$2(\text{Na} + \text{mEq/L}) + (\text{Blood glucose mg/dL})/20 + (\text{BUN mg/dL})/3 =$$
$$\text{Total calculated osmolality(mOsm/L)}$$

Osmolar Gap = measured osmolality (by freezing point depression method) − calculate osmolality

A gap greater than 10 is abnormal. *Note:* if ethanol is involved, add ethanol level/4.6 to the calculated equation.

An increased osmolal gap is produced by the following common substances: acetone, dextran, dimethyl sulfoxide, diuretics, ethanol, ethyl ether, ethylene glycol, isopropanol, paraldehyde, mannitol, methanol, sorbitol, and trichloroethane. Table 10 gives the conversion factors for these substances.

Although a specific blood level of ethylene glycol in milligrams per deciliter can be estimated using the equation below, this is not considered to be a reliable method and should not take the place of obtaining a measured ethylene glycol blood concentration.

$$\text{osmolar gap} \times \text{conversion factor} = \text{serum concentration}$$

Caution: The accuracy of the ethylene glycol estimated decreases as the ethylene glycol levels decrease. The toxic metabolites are not osmotically active, and patients presenting late may show signs of severe toxicity without an elevated osmolar gap.

The anion gap can be calculated using the following equation:

$$\text{Na} - (\text{Cl} + \text{HCO}_3) = \text{anion gap}$$

The normal gap is 8 to 12. Potassium is not used because it is a small amount and may be hemolyzed. Table 8 lists factors that may account for an increased or a decreased anion gap.

Management

Vital functions should be established and maintained. The airway must be protected, and assisted ventilation can be used, if necessary. Gastrointestinal decontamination has a limited role. Only gastric aspiration can be used within 60 minutes after ingestion. Activated charcoal is not effective.

Baseline measurements of serum electrolytes and calcium, glucose, ABGs, ethanol, serum ethylene glycol concentration (may be difficult to obtain readily in some institutions), and methanol concentrations should be obtained. In the first few hours, the measured serum osmolality should be determined and compared to calculated osmolality (see osmolality equation, earlier). If seizures occur, one should measure serum calcium (preferably ionized calcium) and treat with intravenous diazepam. If the patient has hypocalcemic seizures, he or she should also be treated with 10 to 20 mL 10% calcium gluconate (0.2 to 0.3 mL/kg in children) slowly intravenously, with the dose repeated as needed. Metabolic acidosis should be corrected with intravenous sodium bicarbonate.

Ethanol therapy should be initiated immediately if fomepizole (Antizol) is unavailable (see next paragraph). Alcohol dehydrogenase has a greater affinity for ethanol than ethylene glycol. Therefore, ethanol blocks the metabolism of ethylene glycol. Ethanol therapy is called for if there is a history of ingestion of 0.1 mL/kg of 100% ethylene glycol, serum ethylene glycol concentration is greater than 20 mg/dL, there is an osmolar gap not accounted for by other alcohols or factors (e.g., hyperlipidemia), metabolic acidosis is present with an increased anion gap, or there are oxalate crystals in the urine. Ethanol should be administered intravenously (the oral route is less reliable) to produce a blood ethanol concentration of 100 to 150 mg/dL. The loading dose is 10 mL/kg of 10% ethanol intravenously, administered concomitantly with a maintenance dose of 10% ethanol of 1.0 mL/kg/h. This dose may need to be increased to 2 mL/kg/h in patients who are heavy drinkers. The blood ethanol concentration should be measured hourly and the infusion rate should be adjusted to maintain a blood ethanol concentration of 100 to 150 mg/dL.

Fomepizole (Antizol, 4-methylpyrazole) inhibits alcohol dehydrogenase more reliability than ethanol and it does not require constant monitoring of ethanol levels and adjustment of infusion rates. Fomepizole is available in 1 g/mL vials of 1.5 mL. The loading dose is 15 mg/kg (0.015 mL/kg) IV; maintenance dose is 10 mg/kg (0.01 mL/kg) every 12 hours for four doses, then 15 mg/kg every 12 hours until the ethylene glycol levels are less than 20 mg/dL. The solution is prepared by being mixed with 100 mL of 0.9% saline or D₅W (5% dextrose in water). Fomepizole can be given to patients requiring hemodialysis but should be dosed as follows:

Dose at the beginning of hemodialysis:

- If <6 hours since last Antizol dose, do not administer dose
- If >6 hours since last dose, administer next scheduled dose

Dosing during hemodialysis:

- Dose every 4 hours

Dosing at the time hemodialysis is completed:

- If <1 hour between last dose and end of dialysis, do not administer dose at end of dialysis
- If 1 to 3 hours between last dose and end of dialysis, administer one half of next scheduled dose
- If >3 hours between last dose and end of dialysis, administer next scheduled dose

Maintenance dosing off hemodialysis:

- Give the next scheduled dose 12 hours from the last dose administered

Hemodialysis is indicated if the ingestion was potentially fatal; if the serum ethylene glycol concentration is greater than 50 mg/dL (some recommend at levels of >25 mg/dL); if severe acidosis or electrolyte abnormalities occur despite conventional therapy; or if congestive heart failure or renal failure is present. Hemodialysis reduces the ethylene glycol half-life from 17 hours on ethanol therapy to 3 hours. Therapy (fomepizole and hemodialysis) should be continued until the serum ethylene glycol concentration is less than 10 mg/dL, the glycolate level is nondetectable (not readily available), the acidosis has cleared, there are no mental disturbances, the creatinine level is normal, and the urinary output is adequate. This may require 2 to 5 days.

Adjunct therapy involving thiamine, 100 mg/d (in children, 50 mg), slowly over 5 minutes intravenously or intramuscularly and repeated every 6 hours and pyridoxine, 50 mg IV or IM every 6 hours, has been recommended until intoxication is resolved, but these agents have not been extensively studied. Folate, 50 mg IV (child 1 mg/kg), can be given every 4 hours for 6 doses.

Disposition

All patients who have ingested significant amounts of ethylene glycol (calculated level above 20 mg/dL), have a history of a toxic dose, or are symptomatic should be referred to the emergency department and admitted. If the serum ethylene glycol concentration cannot be obtained, the patient should be followed for 12 hours, with monitoring of the osmolal gap, acid-base parameters, and electrolytes to exclude development of metabolic acidosis with an anion gap. Transfer should be considered for fomepizole therapy or hemodialysis.

HYDROCARBONS

The lower the viscosity and surface tension of hydrocarbons or the greater the volatility, the greater the risk of aspiration. Volatile substance abuse has produced the "Sudden Sniffing's Death Syndrome," most likely caused by dysrhythmias.

Toxicologic Classification and Toxic Mechanism

All systemically absorbed hydrocarbons can lower the threshold of the myocardium to dysrhythmias produced by endogenous and exogenous catecholamines.

Aliphatic hydrocarbons are branched straight chain hydrocarbons. A few aspirated drops are poorly absorbed from the gastrointestinal tract and produce no systemic toxicity by this route. However, aspiration of very small amounts can produce chemical pneumonitis. Examples of aliphatic hydrocarbons are gasoline, kerosene, charcoal lighter fluid, mineral spirits (Stoddard's solvent), and petroleum naphtha. Mineral seal oil (signal oil), found in furniture polishes, is a low-viscosity and low-volatility oil with minimum absorption that never warrants gastric decontamination. It can produce severe pneumonia if aspirated.

Aromatic hydrocarbons are six carbon ring structures that are absorbed through the gastrointestinal tract. Systemic toxicity includes CNS depression and, in cases of chronic abuse, multiple organ effects such as leukemia (benzene) and renal toxicity (toluene). Examples are benzene, toluene, styrene, and xylene. The seriously toxic ingested dose is 20 to 50 mL in adults.

Halogenated hydrocarbons are aliphatic or aromatic hydrocarbons with one or more halogen substitutions (Cl, Br, Fl, or I). They are highly volatile and are abused as inhalants. They are well absorbed from the gastrointestinal tract, produce CNS depression, and have metabolites that can damage the liver and kidneys. Examples include methylene chloride (may be converted into carbon monoxide in the body), dichloroethylene (also causes a disulfiram [Antabuse] reaction known as "degreaser's flush" when associated with consumption of ethanol), and 1,1,1-trichloroethane (Glamorene Spot Remover, Scotchgard, typewriter correction fluid). An acute lethal oral dose is 0.5 to 5 mL/kg.

Dangerous additives to the hydrocarbons can be summed up with the mnemonic CHAMP: C, camphor (demothing agent); H, halogenated hydrocarbons; A, aromatic hydrocarbons; M, metals (heavy); and P, pesticides. Ingestion of these substances may warrant gastric emptying with a small-bore nasogastric tube.

Heavy hydrocarbons have high viscosity, low volatility, and minimal gastrointestinal absorption, so gastric decontamination is not necessary. Examples are asphalt (tar), machine oil, motor oil (lubricating oil, engine oil), home heating oil, and petroleum jelly (mineral oil).

Laboratory Investigations

The ECG, ABG, pulmonary function, serum electrolytes, and serial chest radiographs should be continuously monitored. Liver and renal function should be monitored in cases of inhalation of aromatic hydrocarbons.

Management

Asymptomatic patients who ingested small amounts of aliphatic petroleum distillates can be followed at home by telephone for development of signs of aspiration (cough, wheezing, tachypnea, and dyspnea) for 4 to 6 hours. Inhalation of any hydrocarbon vapors in a closed space can produce intoxication. The victim must be removed from the environment, have oxygen administered, and receive respiratory support.

Gastrointestinal decontamination is not advised in cases of hydrocarbon ingestion that usually do not cause systemic toxicity (aliphatic petroleum distillates, heavy hydrocarbons). In cases of ingestion of hydrocarbons that cause systemic toxicity in small amounts (aromatic hydrocarbons, halogenated hydrocarbons), the clinician should pass a small-bore nasogastric tube and aspirate if the ingestion was within 2 hours and if spontaneous vomiting has not occurred. Some toxicologists advocate ipecac-induced emesis under medical supervision instead of small-bore nasogastric gastric lavage; we do not.

Patients with altered mental status should have their airway protected because of concern about aspiration. The use of activated charcoal has been suggested, but there are no scientific data as to effectiveness and it may produce vomiting. Activated charcoal may, however, be useful in adsorbing toxic additives such as pesticides or co-ingestants.

The symptomatic patient who is coughing, gagging, choking, or wheezing on arrival has probably aspirated. The clinician should provide supportive respiratory care and supplemental oxygen, while monitoring pulse oximetry, ABG, chest radiograph, and ECG. The patient should be admitted to the intensive care unit. A chest radiograph for aspiration may be positive as early as 30 minutes after ingestion, and almost all are positive within 6 hours. Negative chest radiographs within 4 hours do not rule out aspiration.

Bronchospasm is treated with a nebulized β-adrenergic agonist and intravenous aminophylline if necessary. Epinephrine should be avoided because of susceptibility to dysrhythmias. Cyanosis in the presence of a normal arterial PaO_2 may be a result of methemoglobinemia that requires therapy with methylene blue. Corticosteroids and prophylactic antimicrobial agents have not been shown to be beneficial. (Fever or leukocytosis may be produced by the chemical pneumonitis itself.)

Most infiltrations resolve spontaneously in 1 week; lipoid pneumonia may last up to 6 weeks. It is not necessary to surgically treat pneumatoceles that develop because they usually resolve. Dysrhythmias may require α- and β-adrenergic antagonists or cardioversion.

There is no role for enhanced elimination procedures.

Methylene chloride is metabolized over several hours to carbon monoxide. See treatment of carbon monoxide poisoning. Halogenated hydrocarbons are hepatorenal toxins; therefore, hepatorenal function should be monitored. N-acetylcysteine therapy may be useful if there is evidence of hepatic damage.

Extracorporeal membrane oxygenation (ECMO) has been used successfully for a few patients with life-threatening respiratory failure. Surfactant used for hydrocarbon aspiration was found to be detrimental.

Disposition

Asymptomatic patients with small ingestions of petroleum distillates can be managed at home. Symptomatic patients with abnormal chest radiographic, oxygen saturation, or ABG findings should be admitted. Patients who become asymptomatic and have normal oxygenation and a normal repeat radiograph can be discharged.

IRON

There are more than 100 iron over-the-counter preparations for supplementation and treatment of iron deficiency anemia.

Toxic Mechanism

Toxicity depends on the amount of elemental iron available in various salts (gluconate 12%, sulfate 20%, fumarate 33%, lactate 19%, chloride 21% of elemental iron), not the amount of the salt. Locally, iron is corrosive and may cause fluid loss, hypovolemic shock, and perforation. Excessive free unbound iron in the blood is directly toxic to the vasculature and leads to the release of vasoactive substances, which produces vasodilation. In cases of overdose, iron deposits injure mitochondria in the liver, the kidneys, and the myocardium. The exact mechanism of cellular damage is not clear but is thought to be related to free radical formation.

Toxic Dose

The therapeutic dose is 6 mg/kg/d of elemental iron. An elemental iron dose of 20 to 40 mg/kg may produce mild self-limited gastrointestinal symptoms, 40 to 60 mg/kg produces moderate toxicity, more than 60 mg/kg produces severe toxicity and is potentially lethal, and more than 180 mg/kg is usually fatal without treatment. Children's chewable vitamins with iron have between 12 and 18 mg of elemental iron per tablet or 0.6 mL of liquid drops. These preparations rarely produce toxicity unless very large quantities are ingested and have never caused death.

Kinetics

Absorption occurs chiefly in the upper small intestine. Ferrous (+2) iron is absorbed into the mucosal cells, where it is oxidized to the ferric (+3) state and bound to ferritin. Iron is slowly released from ferritin into the plasma, where it binds to transferrin and is transported to specific tissues for production of hemoglobin (70%), myoglobin (5%), and cytochrome. About 25% of iron is stored in the liver and spleen. In cases of overdose, larger amounts of iron are absorbed because of direct mucosal corrosion. There is no mechanism for the elimination of iron (elimination is 1 to 2 mg/d) except through bile, sweat, and blood loss.

Manifestations

Serious toxicity is unlikely if the patient remains asymptomatic for 6 hours and has a negative abdominal radiograph. Iron intoxication can produce five phases of toxicity. The phases may not be distinct from one another.

Phase I

Gastrointestinal mucosal injury occurs 30 minutes to 12 hours postingestion. Vomiting starts within 30 minutes to 1 hour of ingestion and is persistent; hematemesis and bloody diarrhea may occur; abdominal cramps, fever, hyperglycemia, and leukocytosis may occur. Enteric-coated tablets may pass through the stomach without causing symptoms. Acidosis and shock can occur within 6 to 12 hours.

Phase II

A latent period of apparent improvement occurs over 8 to 12 hours postingestion.

Phase III

Systemic toxicity phase occurs 12 to 48 hours postingestion with cardiovascular collapse and severe metabolic acidosis.

Phase IV

Two to 4 days postingestion, hepatic injury associated with jaundice, elevated liver enzymes, and prolonged prothrombin time occur. Kidney injury with proteinuria and hematuria occur. Pulmonary edema, disseminated intravascular coagulation, and Yersinia enterocolitica sepsis can occur.

Phase V

Four to 8 weeks postingestion, pyloric outlet or intestinal stricture may cause obstruction or anemia secondary to blood loss.

Laboratory Investigations

Iron poisoning produces anion gap metabolic acidosis. Monitoring should include complete blood cell counts, blood glucose level, serum iron, stools and vomitus for occult blood, electrolytes, acid-base balance, urinalysis and urinary output, liver function tests, and BUN and creatinine levels. Blood type and match should be obtained.

Serum iron measurements taken at the proper time correlate with the clinical findings. The lavender top Vacutainer tube contains EDTA, which falsely lowers serum iron. One must obtain the serum iron measurement before administering deferoxamine. Serum iron levels of less than 350 µg/dL at 2 to 6 hours predict an asymptomatic course; levels of 350 to 500 µg/dL are usually associated with mild gastrointestinal symptoms; those greater than 500 µg/dL have a 20% risk of shock and serious iron toxicity. A follow-up serum iron measurement after 6 hours may not be elevated even in cases of severe poisoning, but a serum iron measurement taken at 8 to 12 hours is useful to exclude delayed absorption from a bezoar or sustained-release preparation. The total iron-binding capacity is not necessary.

Adult iron tablet preparations are radiopaque before they dissolve by 4 hours postingestion. A "negative" abdominal radiograph more than 4 hours postingestion does not exclude iron poisoning.

Patients who develop high fevers and signs of sepsis following iron overdose should have blood and stool cultures checked for Yersinia enterocolitica.

Management

Gastrointestinal decontamination should involve immediate induction of emesis in cases of ingestions of elemental iron of greater than 40 mg/kg if vomiting has not already occurred. Activated charcoal is ineffective. An abdominal radiograph should be obtained after emesis to determine the success of gastric emptying. Children's chewable vitamins and liquid iron preparations are not radiopaque. If radiopaque iron is still present, whole-bowel irrigation with polyethylene glycol solution should be considered. In extreme cases, removal by endoscopy or surgery may be necessary because coalesced iron tablets produce hemorrhagic infarction in the bowel and perforation peritonitis.

Deferoxamine (Desferal) in a dose of about 100 mg binds 8.5 to 9.35 mg of free iron in the serum. The deferoxamine infusion should not exceed 15 mg/kg/h or 6 g daily, but faster rates (up to 45 mg/kg) and larger daily amounts have been administered and tolerated in extreme cases of iron poisoning (>1000 mg/dL). The deferoxamine-iron complex is hemodialyzable if renal failure develops.

Indications for chelation therapy are any of the following:

- Very large, symptomatic ingestions
- Serious clinical intoxication (severe vomiting and diarrhea [often bloody], severe abdominal pain, metabolic acidosis, hypotension, or shock)
- Symptoms that persist or progress to more serious toxicity
- Serum iron level greater than 500 mg/dL

Chelation should be performed as early as possible within 12 to 18 hours to be effective. One should start the infusion slowly and gradually increase to avoid hypotension.

Adult respiratory distress syndrome has developed in patients with high doses of deferoxamine for several days; infusions longer than 24 hours should be avoided.

The endpoint of treatment is when the patient is asymptomatic and the urine clears if it was originally a positive "vin rosö" color.

For supportive therapy, intravenous bicarbonate may be needed to correct the metabolic acidosis. Hypotension and shock treatment may require volume expansion, vasopressors, and blood transfusions. The physician should attempt to keep the urinary output at greater than 2 mL/kg/h. Coagulation abnormalities and overt bleeding require blood products or vitamin K. Pregnant patients are treated in a fashion similar to any other patient with iron poisoning.

Hemodialysis and hemoperfusion are ineffective. Exchange transfusion has been used in single cases of massive poisonings in children.

Disposition

The asymptomatic or minimally symptomatic patient should be observed for persistence and progression of symptoms or development of toxicity signs (gastrointestinal bleeding, acidosis, shock, altered mental state). Patients with mild self-limited gastrointestinal symptoms who become asymptomatic or have no signs of toxicity for 6 hours are unlikely to have a serious intoxication and can be discharged after psychiatric clearance, if needed. Patients with moderate or severe toxicity should be admitted to the intensive care unit.

ISONIAZID

Isoniazid is a hydrazide derivative of vitamin B$_3$ (nicotinamide) and is used as an antituberculosis drug.

Toxic Mechanism

Isoniazid produces pyridoxine deficiency by increasing the excretion of pyridoxine (vitamin B$_6$) and by inhibiting pyridoxal 5-phosphate (the active form of pyridoxine) from acting with L-glutamic acid decarboxylase to form γ-aminobutyric acid (GABA), the major CNS neurotransmitter inhibitor, resulting in seizures. Isoniazid also blocks the conversion of lactate to pyruvate, resulting in profound and prolonged lactic acidosis.

Toxic Dose

The therapeutic dose is 5 to 10 mg/kg (maximum 300 mg) daily. A single acute dose of 15 mg/kg lowers the seizure threshold; 35 to 40 mg/kg produces spontaneous convulsions; more than 80 mg/kg produces severe toxicity. A fatal dose in adults is 4.5 to 15 g. The malnourished patients, those with a previous seizure disorder, alcoholic patients, and slow acetylators are more susceptible to isoniazid toxicity. In cases of chronic intoxication, 10 mg/kg/d produces hepatitis in 10% to 20% of patients but less than 2% at doses of 3 to 5 mg/kg/d.

Kinetics

Absorption from intestine occurs in 30 to 60 minutes, and onset is in 30 to 120 minutes, with peak levels of 5 to 8 µg/mL within 1 to 2 hours. Volume distribution is 0.6 L/kg, with minimal protein binding.

Elimination is by liver acetylation to a hepatotoxic metabolite, acetyl-isoniazid, which is then hydrolyzed to isonicotinic acid. In slow acetylators, isoniazid has a half-life of 140 to 460 minutes (mean 5 hours), and 10% to 15% is eliminated unchanged in the urine. Most (45% to 75%) whites and 50% of African blacks are slow acetylators, and, with chronic use (without pyridoxine supplements), they may develop peripheral neuropathy. In fast acetylators, isoniazid has a half-life of 35 to 110 minutes (mean 80 minutes), and 25% to 30% is excreted unchanged in the urine. About 90% of Asians and patients with diabetes mellitus are fast acetylators and may develop hepatitis on chronic use.

In patients with overdose and hepatic disease, the serum half-life may increase. Isoniazid inhibits the metabolism of phenytoin (Dilantin), diazepam, phenobarbital, carbamazepine (Tegretol), and prednisone. These drugs also interfere with the metabolism of isoniazid. Ethanol may decrease the half-life of isoniazid but increase its toxicity.

Manifestations

Within 30 to 60 minutes, nausea, vomiting, slurred speech, dizziness, visual disturbances, and ataxia are present. Within 30 to 120 minutes, the major clinical triad of severe overdose includes refractory convulsions (90% of overdose patients have one or more seizures), coma, and resistant severe lactic acidosis (secondary to convulsions), often with a plasma pH of 6.8.

Laboratory Investigations

Isoniazid produces anion gap metabolic acidosis. Therapeutic levels are 5 to 8 µg/mL and acute toxic levels are greater than 20 µg/mL. These levels are not readily available to assist in making decisions in acute overdose situations. One should monitor the blood glucose (often hyperglycemia), electrolytes (often hyperkalemia), bicarbonate, ABGs, liver function tests (elevations occur with chronic exposure), BUN, and creatinine.

Management

Seizures must be controlled. Pyridoxine and diazepam should be administered concomitantly through different IV sites. Pyridoxine (vitamin B$_6$) is given in a dose of 1 g for each gram of isoniazid ingested. If the dose ingested is unknown, at least 5 g of pyridoxine should be given intravenously. Pyridoxine is administered in 50 mL D$_5$W or 0.9% saline over 5 minutes intravenously. It must not be administered in the same bottle as sodium bicarbonate. Intravenous pyridoxine is repeated every 5 to 20 minutes until the seizures are controlled. Total doses of pyridoxine up to 52 g have been safely administered; however, patients given 132 and 183 g of pyridoxine have developed a persistent crippling sensory neuropathy.

Diazepam is administered concomitantly with pyridoxine but at a different site. They work synergistically. Diazepam should be administered intravenously slowly, 0.3 mg/kg at a rate of 1 mg/min in children or 10 mg at a rate of 5 mg/min in adults. After the seizures are controlled, the remainder of the pyridoxine is administered (1 g/1 g isoniazid) or a total dose of 5 g.

Phenobarbital or phenytoin is ineffective and should not be used.

In asymptomatic patients or patients without seizures, pyridoxine has been advised by some toxicologists prophylactically in gram-for-gram doses in cases of large overdoses (<80 mg/kg per dose) of isoniazid, although there are no studies to support this recommendation. In comatose patients, pyridoxine administration may result in the patient's rapid regaining of consciousness. Correction of acidosis may occur spontaneously with pyridoxine administration and correction of the seizures. Sodium bicarbonate should be administered if acidosis persists.

Hemodialysis is rarely needed because of antidotal therapy and the short half-life of isoniazid, but it may be used as an adjunct for cases of uncontrollable acidosis and seizures. Hemoperfusion has not been adequately evaluated. Diuresis is ineffective.

Disposition

Asymptomatic or mildly symptomatic patients who become asymptomatic can be observed in the emergency department for 4 to 6 hours. Larger amounts of isoniazid may warrant pyridoxine administration and longer periods of observation. Intentional ingestions necessitate psychiatric evaluation before the patient is discharged. Patients with convulsions or coma should be admitted to the intensive care unit.

ISOPROPANOL (ISOPROPYL ALCOHOL)

Isopropanol can be found in rubbing alcohol, solvents, and lacquer thinner. Coma has occurred in children sponged for fever with isopropanol. See Table 10 for ethanol features of alcohols and glycols.

Toxic Mechanism

Isopropanol is a gastric irritant. It is metabolized to acetone, a CNS and myocardial depressant. It inhibits gluconeogenesis. Normal propyl alcohol is related to isopropyl alcohol but is more toxic.

Toxic Dose

A toxic dose of 0.5 to 1 mg/kg of 70% isopropanol (1 mL/kg of 70%) produces a blood isopropanol plasma concentration of 70 mg/dL. The CNS depressant potency is twice that of ethanol.

Kinetics

Onset of action is within 30 to 60 minutes, and peak is 1 hour postingestion. Volume distribution is 0.6 kg/L. Isopropyl alcohol metabolizes to acetone. Its excretion is renal.

Note: The serum isopropyl concentration and amount ingested can be estimated using the same equation as is used in ethanol kinetics and substituting the specific gravity of 0.785 for isopropyl alcohol.

Manifestations

Ethanol-like inebriation occurs, with an acetone odor to the breath, gastritis, occasionally with hematemesis, acetonuria, and acetonemia without systemic acidosis.

Depression of the CNS occurs: lethargy at blood isopropyl alcohol levels of 50 to 100 mg/dL, coma at levels of 150 to 200 mg/dL, potentially death in adults at levels greater than 240 mg/dL.

Hypoglycemia and seizures may occur.

Laboratory Investigation

Monitoring of blood isopropyl alcohol levels (not readily available in all institutions), acetone, glucose, and ABG should be maintained. The osmolal gap increases 1 mOsm per 5.9 mg/dL of isopropyl alcohol and 1 mOsm per 5.5 mg/dL of acetone. The absence of excess acetone in the blood (normal is 0.3 to 2 mg/dL) within 30 to 60 minutes or excess acetone in the urine within 3 hours excludes the possibility of significant isopropanol exposure.

Management

The airway must be protected with intubation, and assisted ventilation administered if necessary. If the patient is hypoglycemic, glucose should be administered. Supportive treatment is similar to that for ethanol ingestions.

Gastrointestinal decontamination has no role in the treatment of isopropanol ingestion. Hemodialysis is warranted in cases of life-threatening overdose but is rarely needed. A nephrologist should be consulted if the bloodisopropanol plasma concentration is greater than 250 mg/dL.

Disposition

Symptomatic patients with concentrations greater than 100 mg/dL require at least 24 hours of close observation for resolution and should be admitted. If the patient is hypoglycemic, hypotensive, or comatose, he or she should be admitted to the intensive care unit.

LEAD

Acute lead intoxication is rare and usually occurs by inhalation of lead, resulting in severe intoxication and often death. Lead fumes can be produced by burning of lead batteries or use of a heat gun to remove lead paint. Acute lead intoxication also occurs from exposure to high concentrations of organic lead (e.g., tetraethyl lead).

Chronic lead poisoning occurs most often in children 6 months to 6 years of age who are exposed in their environment and in adults in certain occupations (Table 17). In the United States, the prevalence in children aged 1 to 5 years with a venous blood lead greater than 10 μg/dL decreased from 88.2% in a 1976–1980 survey to 8.9% in a 1988–1991 survey as a consequence of measures to reduce lead in the environment, particularly leaded gasoline. However, an estimated 1.7 million children between 1 and 5 years of age and more than 1 million workers in over 100 different occupations still have blood lead levels greater than 10 μg/dL.

Toxic Dose

In cases of chronic lead poisoning, a daily intake of more than 5 μg/kg/d in children or more than 150 μg/d in adults can give a positive lead balance. In 1991, the Centers for Disease Control and Prevention (CDC) recommended routine screening for all children younger than 6 years of age. In children a venous blood level greater than 10 μg/dL was determined to be a threshold of concern. The average venous blood level in the United States is 4 μg/dL. In cases of occupational exposure (see Table 17), a venous blood level greater than 40 μg/dL is indicative of increased lead absorption in adults.

Toxic Mechanism

Lead affects the sulfhydryl enzyme systems, the immature CNS, the enzymes of heme synthesis, vitamin D conversion, the kidneys, the bones, and growth. Lead alters the tertiary structure of cell proteins by denaturing them and causing cell death. Risk factors are mouthing behavior of infants and children and excessive oral behavior (pica), living in the inner city, a poorly maintained home, and poor nutrition (e.g., low calcium and iron). The CDC questionnaire given in Table 18 is recommended at every pediatric visit. If any answers to the CDC questionnaire are "positive," a blood screening test for lead should be administered. To be more accurate, however, identifying lead exposure studies have suggested that the questionnaire will have to be modified for each individual community because it has had poor sensitivity (40%) and specificity (60%) as it stands.

Table 19 lists sources of lead. The number one source is deteriorating lead-based paint, which forms leaded dust. Lead concentrations in indoor paint were not reduced to safer (0.06%) levels until 1978. Lead can also be produced by improper interior or exterior home renovation (scraping or demolition). It is found in pre-1960 built homes. The use of leaded gasoline (limited in 1973) resulted in residue from leaded motor vehicle emissions. Lead persists in the soil near major highways and in deteriorating homes and buildings. Vegetables grown in contaminated soil may contain lead.

TABLE 17 Occupations Associated With Lead Exposure

Lead production or smelting	Demolition of ships and
Production of illicit whiskey	bridges
Brass, copper, and lead foundries	Battery manufacturing
Radiator repair	Machining/grinding lead
Scrap handling	alloys
Sanding of old paint	Welding of old painted
Lead soldering	metals
Cable stripping	Thermal paint stripping of
Worker or janitor at a firing range	old buildings
	Ceramic glaze/pottery
	mixing

Modified from Rempel D: The lead-exposed worker. JAMA 262:533, 1989.

TABLE 18 CDC Questionnaire: Priority Groups for Lead Screening

1. Children age 6–72 months (was 12–36 months) who live in or are frequent visitors to older, deteriorated housing built before 1960.
2. Children age 6–72 months who live in housing built prior to 1960 with recent, ongoing, or planned renovation or remodeling.
3. Children age 6–72 months who are siblings, housemates, or playmates of children with known lead poisoning.
4. Children age 6–72 months whose parents or other household members participate in a lead-related industry or hobby.
5. Children age 6–72 months who live near active lead smelters, battery recycling plants, or other industries likely to result in atmospheric lead release.

BOX 1 Hobbies Associated With Lead Exposure

Casting of ammunition
Collecting antique pewter
Collecting/painting lead toys (e.g., soldiers and figures)
Ceramics or glazed pottery
Refinishing furniture
Making fishing weights
Home renovation
Jewelry making, lead solder
Glass blowing, lead glass
Bronze casting
Print making and other fine arts (when lead white, flake white, chrome yellow pigments are involved)
Liquor distillation
Hunting and target shooting
Painting
Car and boat repair
Burning/engraving lead-painted wood
Making stained leaded glass
Copper enameling

Oil refineries and lead-processing smelters produce lead residue. Food cans produced in Mexico contain lead solder (95% do not in United States). Lead water pipes (until 1950) and lead solder (until 1986) deliver lead-containing drinking water (calcium deposits, however, may offer some protection). Water at a consumer's tap should contain less than 15 parts per billion (ppb) of lead (Table 20).

For occupational exposure, see Table 17. The Occupational Safety and Health Administration (OSHA) standards require employers to provide showering and clothes changing facilities for personnel working with lead; however, businesses with fewer than 25 employees are exempt from the regulation. The OSHA lead standard of 1978 set a limit of 60 µg/dL for occupational exposure to lead. At a blood lead level of 60 µg/dL, a worker should be removed from lead exposure and not allowed back until his or her lead level is below 40 µg/dL. Many authorities believe that this level should be lower. The lead residue on the clothes of the workers may represent a hazard to the family. Other occupations that are potential sources of lead exposure include plumbers, pipe fitters, lead miners, auto repairers, shipbuilders, printers, steel welders and cutters, construction workers, and rubber product manufacturers.

Leaded pots to make molds for "kusmusha" tea represent lead exposure. Imported pottery lined with ceramic glaze can leach large amounts of lead into acids (e.g., citrus fruit juices).

Hobbies associated with lead exposure are listed in Box 1. Some "traditional" folk remedies or cosmetics that contain lead include the following:

- "Azarcon por empacho" ("Maria Louisa" 90% to 95% lead trioxide): a bright orange powder used in Hispanic culture, especially Mexican, for digestive problems and diarrhea.
- "Greta" (4% to 90% lead): a yellow powder "por empacho" ("empacho" refers to a variety of gastrointestinal symptoms), used in Hispanic cultures, especially Mexican.

TABLE 19 Sources of Lead

Product	Lead Content (%) by Dry Weight
Paint	0.06
Solder	0.6
Plastic additives	2.0
Priming inks	2.0
Plumbing fixtures	2.0
Pesticides	0.1
Stained glass panes	0.1
Wine bottle foils	0.1
Construction material	0.1
Fertilizers	0.1
Glazes, enamels	0.06
Toys/recreational games	0.1
Curtain weights	0.1
Fishing weights	0.1

TABLE 20 Agency Regulations and Recommendations Concerning Lead Content

Agency	Specimen	Level	Comments
CDC	Blood (child)	10 µg/dL	Investigate community
OSHA	Blood (adult)	60 µg/dL	Medical removal from work
OSHA	Air	50 µg/m^3	PEL*
	Air	0.75 µg/m^3	Tetraethyl or tetramethyl
ACGIH	Air	150 µg/m^3	TWA†
EPA	Air	1.5 µg/m^3	Three-month average
EPA	Water	15 µg/L (ppb)	5 ppb circulating
EPA	Food	100 µg/d	Advisory
FDA	Wine	300 ppm	Plan to reduce to 200 ppm
EPA	Soil/dust	50 ppm	
CPSC	Paint	600 ppm (0.06%) by dry weight	

*PEL = permissible exposure limit (highest level over an 8-hour workday).
†TWA = time-weighted average (air concentration for 8-hour workday and 40-hour workweek).
Abbreviations: ACGIH = American Conference of Governmental Industrial Hygienists; CDC = Centers for Disease Control and Prevention; CPSC = Consumer Product Safety Commission; EPA = Environmental Protection Agency; FDA = Food and Drug Administration; OSHA = Occupational Safety and Health Administration.

- "Pay-loo-ah": an orange-red powder used for rash and fever in Southeast Asian cultures, especially among Northern Laos Hmong immigrants.
- "Alkohl" (Al-kohl, kohl, suma 5% to 92% lead): a black powder used in Middle Eastern, African, and Asian cultures as a cosmetic and an umbilical stump astringent.
- "Farouk": an orange granular powder with lead used in Saudi Arabian culture.
- "Bint Al Zahab": used to treat colic in Saudi Arabian culture.
- "Surma" (23% to 26% lead): a black powder used in India as a cosmetic and to improve eyesight.
- "Bali goli": a round black bean that is dissolved in "grippe water," used by Asian and Indian cultures to aid digestion.

Cases of substance abuse involving lead poisoning have been reported, in which the patient sniffs leaded gasoline or uses improperly synthesized amphetamines.

Kinetics

Absorption of lead is 10% to 15% of the ingested dose in adults; in children, up to 40% is absorbed, especially in cases of iron deficiency anemia. With inhalation of fumes, absorption is rapid and complete. Volume distribution in blood (0.9% of total body burden) is 95% in red blood cells. Lead passes through the placenta to the fetus and is present in breast milk.

Organic lead is metabolized in the liver to inorganic lead. Its half-life is 35 to 40 days in blood; in soft tissue, the half-life is 45 days and in bone (99% of the lead), the half-life is 28 years. The major elimination route is the stool, 80% to 90%, and then renal 10% (80 g/d) and hair, nails, sweat, and saliva. Nine percent of organic lead is excreted in the urine per day.

Manifestations

Adverse health effects are given in Table 21 and include the following.

Hematologic

Lead inhibits γ-aminolevulinic acid dehydratase (early in the synthesis of heme) and ferrochelatase (transfers iron to ferritin for incorporation of iron into protoporphyrin to produce heme). Anemia is a late finding. Decreased heme synthesis starts at >40 µg/dL. Basophilic stippling occurs in 20% of severe lead poisoning.

Neurologic

Segmental demyelination and peripheral neuropathy, usually of the motor type (wrist and ankle drop), occurs in workers. A venous blood level of lead greater than 70 µg/dL (usually >100 µg/dL), produces encephalopathy in children (symptom mnemonic "PAINT": P, persistent forceful vomiting and papilledema; A, ataxia; I, intermittent stupor and lucidity; N, neurologic coma and refractory convulsions; T, tired and lethargic). Decreased cognitive abilities have been reported with a venous blood level of lead greater than 10 µg/dL, including behavioral problems, decreased attention span, and learning disabilities. IQ scores may begin to decrease at 15 µg/dL. Encephalopathy is rare in adults.

Renal

Nephropathy as a result of damaged capillaries and glomerulus can occur at a venous blood level of lead greater than 80 µg/dL, but recent studies show renal damage and hypertension with low venous blood levels. A direct correlation between hypertension and venous blood level over 30 µg/dL has been reported. Lead reduces excretion of uric acid, and high-level exposure may be associated with hyperuricemia and "saturnine gout," Fanconi's syndrome (aminoaciduria and renal tubular acidosis), and tubular fibrosis.

Reproductive

Spontaneous abortion, transient delay in the child's development (catch up at age 5 to 6 years), decreased sperm count, and abnormal

TABLE 21 Summary of Lead-Induced Health Effects in Adults and Children

Blood Lead Level (µg/dL)	Age Group	Health Effect
>100	Adult	Encephalopathic signs and symptoms
>80	Adult	Anemia
	Child	Encephalopathy
		Chronic nephropathy (e.g., aminoaciduria)
>70	Adult	Clinically evident peripheral neuropathy
	Child	Colic and other gastrointestinal symptoms
>60	Adult	Female reproductive effects
		CNS disturbance symptoms (i.e., sleep disturbances, mood changes, memory and concentration problems, headaches)
>50	Adult	Decreased hemoglobin production
		Decreased performance on neurobehavioral tests
	Adult	Altered testicular function
		Gastrointestinal symptoms (i.e., abdominal pain, constipation, diarrhea, nausea, anorexia)
	Child	Peripheral neuropathy*
>40	Adult	Decreased peripheral nerve conduction
		Hypertension, age 40–59 years
		Chronic neuropathy*
>25	Adult	Elevated erythrocyte protoporphyrin in males
15–25	Adult	Elevated erythrocyte protoporphyrin in females
>10	Child	Decreased intelligence and growth
		Impaired learning
		Reduced birth weight*
		Impaired mental ability
	Fetus	Preterm delivery

From Anonymous: Implementation of the Lead Contamination Control Act of 1988. MMWR Morb Mortal Wkly Rep 41:288, 1992.
*Controversial.

sperm morphology can occur with lead exposure. Lead crosses the placenta and fetal blood levels reach 75% to 100% of maternal blood levels. Lead is teratogenic.

Metabolic

Decreased cytochrome P450 activity alters the metabolism of medication and endogenously produced substances. Decreased activation of cortisol and decreased growth is caused by interference in vitamin conversion (25-hydroxyvitamin D to 1,25-hydroxyvitamin D) at venous blood levels of 20 to 30 µg/dL.

Other Manifestations

Abnormalities of thyroid, cardiac, and hepatic function occur in adults. Abdominal colic is seen in children at doses greater than 50 µg/dL. "Lead gum lines" at the dental border of the gingiva can occur in cases of chronic lead poisoning.

Laboratory Investigations

Serial venous blood lead measurements are taken on days 3 and 5 during treatment and 7 days after chelation therapy, then every 1 to 2 weeks for 8 weeks, and then every month for 6 months. Intravenous infusion should be stopped at least 1 hour before blood lead levels are measured. Table 22 gives a classification of blood lead concentrations in children.

TABLE 22 Classification of Blood Lead Concentrations in Children

Blood Lead (μg/dL)	Recommended Interventions
<9	None
10–14	Community intervention
	Repeat blood lead in 3 months
15–19	Individual case management
	Environmental counseling
	Nutritional counseling
	Repeat blood lead in 3 months
20–44	Medical referral
	Environmental inspection/abatement
	Nutritional counseling
	Repeat blood lead in 3 months
45–69	Environmental inspection/abatement
	Nutritional counseling
	Pharmacologic therapy
	DMSA succimer oral or CaNa$_2$EDTA parenteral
	Repeat every 2 weeks for 6–8 weeks, then monthly for 4–6 months
>70	Hospitalization in intensive care unit
	Environmental inspection/abatement
	Pharmacologic therapy
	Dimercaprol (BAL in oil) IM initial alone
	Dimercaprol IM and CaNa$_2$EDTA together
	Repeat every week

Abbreviations: BAL = British anti-Lewisite; CaNa$_2$EDTA = edetate calcium disodium; DMSA = dimercaptosuccinic acid; IM = intramuscular.

One should evaluate CBC, serum ferritin, erythrocyte protoporphyrin (>35 μg/dL indicates lead poisoning as well as iron deficiency and other causes), electrolytes, serum calcium and phosphorus, urinalysis, BUN, and creatinine. Abdominal and long bone radiographs may be useful in certain circumstances to identify radiopaque material in bowel and "lead lines" in proximal tibia (which occur after prolonged exposure in association with venous blood lead levels greater than 50 μg/dL).

Neuropsychological tests are difficult to perform in young children but should be considered at the end of treatment, especially to determine auditory dysfunction.

Management

The basis of treatment is removal of the source of lead. Cases of poisoning in children should be reported to local health department and cases of occupational poisoning should be reported to OSHA. The source must be identified and abated, and dust controlled by wet mopping. Cold water should be let to run for 2 minutes before being used for drinking. Planting shrubbery (not vegetables) in contaminated soil will keep children away.

Supportive care should be instituted, including measures to deal with refractory seizures (continued antidotal therapy, diazepam, and possibly neuromuscular blockers), with the hepatic and renal failure, and intravascular hemolysis in severe cases. Seizures are treated with diazepam followed by neuromuscular blockers if needed.

Lead does not bind to activated charcoal. One must not delay chelation therapy for complete gastrointestinal decontamination in severe cases. Whole-bowel irrigation has been used prior to treatment. Some authorities recommend abdominal radiographs followed by gastrointestinal decontamination if necessary before switching to oral therapy. Chelation therapy can be used for patients in whom venous blood level of lead is greater than 45 μg/dL in children and greater than 80 μg/dL in adults or in adults with lower levels who are symptomatic or who have a "positive" lead mobilization test result (not routinely performed at most centers) (Table 23).

Succimer (dimercaptosuccinic acid, DMSA, Chemet), a derivative of British anti-Lewisite (BAL), is an oral agent for chelation in children with a venous blood level of greater than 45 μg/dL. The recommended dose is 10 mg/kg every 8 hours for 5 days, then every 12 hours for 14 days. DMSA is under investigation to determine its role in children with a venous blood level less than 45 μg/dL. Although not approved for adults, it has been used in the same dosage. Monitoring should be maintained by CBC, liver transaminases, and urinalysis for adverse effects.

D-Penicillamine (Cuprimine) is another oral chelator that is given in doses of 20 to 40 mg/kg/d not to exceed 1 g/d. However, it is not FDA approved and has a 10% adverse reaction rate. Nevertheless, D-penicillamine has been used infrequently in adults and children with elevated venous blood lead levels.

Edetate calcium disodium (ethylene diaminetetra-acetic acid or CaNa$_2$EDTA Versenate) is a water-soluble chelator given intramuscularly (with 0.5% procaine) or intravenously. The calcium in the compound is displaced by divalent and trivalent heavy metals, forming a soluble complex, which is stable at physiologic pH (but not at acid pH) and enhances lead clearance in the urine. EDTA usually is administered intravenously, especially in severe cases. It must not be administered until adequate urine flow is established. It may redistribute lead to the brain; therefore, BAL may be given first at a venous blood lead level of greater than 55 μg/dL in children and greater than 100 μg/dL in adults. Phlebitis occurs at a concentration greater than 0.5 mg/mL. Alkalinization of the urine may be helpful. CaNa$_2$EDTA should not be confused with sodium EDTA (disodium edetate), which is used to treat hypercalcemia; inadvertent use may produce severe hypocalcemia.

TABLE 23 Pharmacologic Chelation Therapy of Lead Poisoning

Drug	Route	Dose	Duration	Precautions	Monitor
Dimercaprol (BAL in oil)	IM	3–5 mg/kg q4–6h	3–5 days	G6PD deficiency Concurrent iron therapy	AST/ALT enzymes
CaNa$_2$ EDTA (calcium disodium versenate)	IM/IV	50 mg/kg per day	5 days	Inadequate fluid intake Renal impairment Penicillin allergy	Urinalysis, BUN Creatinine Urinalysis, BUN
D-Penicillamine (Cuprimine)	PO	10 mg/kg per day increase 30 mg/kg over 2 weeks	6–20 weeks	Concurrent iron therapy; lead exposure Renal impairment	Creatinine, CBC
2,3-Dimercaptosuccinic acid (DMSA; succimer)	PO	10 mg/kg per dose 3 times daily 10 mg/kg per dose twice daily for 14 days	19 days	AST/ALT Concurrent iron therapy G6PD deficiency lead exposure	AST/ALT

Abbreviations: ALT = alanine aminotransferase; AST = aspartate transaminase; BAL = British anti-Lewisite; bid = twice daily; BUN = blood urea nitrogen; CBC = complete blood count; G6PD = glucose-6-phosphate dehydrogenase; IM = intramuscular; IV = intravenous; PO = oral; tid = three times daily.

Dimercaprol (BAL) is a peanut oil–based dithiol (two sulfhydryl molecules) that combines with one atom of lead to form a heterocyclic stable ring complex. It is usually reserved for patients in whom venous blood lead is greater than 70 µg/dL, and it chelates red blood cell lead, enhancing its elimination through the urine and bile. It crosses the blood-brain barrier. Approximately 50% of patients have adverse reactions, including bad metallic taste in the mouth, pain at the injection site, sterile abscesses, and fever.

A venous blood lead level greater than 70 µg/dL or the presence of clinical symptoms suggesting encephalopathy in children is a potentially life-threatening emergency. Management should be accomplished in a medical center with a pediatric intensive care unit by a multidisciplinary team including a critical care specialist, a toxicologist, a neurologist, and a neurosurgeon. Careful monitoring of neurologic status, fluid status, and intracranial pressure should be undertaken if necessary. These patients need close monitoring for hemodynamic instability. Hydration should be maintained to ensure renal excretion of lead. Fluids, renal and hepatic function, and electrolyte levels should be monitored.

While waiting for adequate urine flow, therapy should be initiated with intramuscular dimercaprol (BAL) only (25 mg/kg/d divided into 6 doses). Four hours later, the second dose of BAL should be given intramuscularly, concurrently with $CaNa_2EDTA$ 50 mg/kg/d as a single dose infused over several hours or as a continuous infusion. The double therapy is continued until the venous blood level is less than 40 µg/dL.

As long as the venous blood level is greater than 40 µg/dL, therapy is continued for 72 hours and followed by two alternatives: either parenteral therapy with two drugs ($CaNa_2EDTA$ and BAL) for 5 days or continuation of therapy with $CaNa_2EDTA$ alone if a good response is achieved and the venous blood level of lead is less than 40 µg/dL. If one cannot get the venous blood lead report back, one should continue therapy with both BAL and EDTA for 5 days. In patients with lead encephalopathy, parenteral chelation should be continued with both drugs until the patient is clinically stable before changing therapy. Mannitol and dexa-methasone can reduce the cerebral edema, but their role in lead encephalopathy is not clear. Surgical decompression is not recommended to reduce cerebral edema in these cases.

If BAL and $CaNa_2EDTA$ are used together, a minimum of 2 days with no treatment should elapse before another 5-day course of therapy is considered. The 5-day course is repeated with $CaNa_2EDTA$ alone if the blood lead level rebounds to greater than 40 µg/dL or in combination with BAL if the venous blood level is greater than 70 µg/dL. If a third course is required, unless there are compelling reasons, one should wait at least 5 to 7 days before administering the course.

Following chelation therapy, a period of equilibration of 10 to 14 days should be allowed and a repeat venous blood lead concentration should be obtained. If the patient is stable enough for oral intake, oral succimer 30 mg/kg/d in three divided doses for 5 days followed by 20 mg/kg/d in two divided doses for 14 days has been suggested, but there are limited data to support this recommendation. Therapy should be continued until venous blood lead level is less than 20 µg/dL in children or less than 40 µg/dL in adults.

Chelators combined with lead are hemodialyzable in the event of renal failure.

Disposition

All patients with a venous blood lead level of greater than 70 µg/dL or who are symptomatic should be admitted. If a child is hospitalized, all lead hazards must be removed from the home environment before allowing the child to return. The source must be eliminated by environmental and occupational investigations. The local health department should be involved in dealing with children who are lead poisoned, and OSHA should be involved with cases of occupational lead poisoning. Consultation with a poison control center or experienced toxicologist is necessary when chelating patients. Follow-up venous blood lead concentrations should be obtained within 1 to 2 weeks and followed every 2 weeks for 6 to 8 weeks, then monthly for 4 to 6 months if the patient required chelation therapy. All patients with venous blood level greater than 10 µg/dL should be followed at least every 3 months until two venous blood lead concentrations are 10 µg/dL or three are less than 15 µg/dL.

LITHIUM (ESKALITH, LITHANE)

Lithium is an alkali metal used primarily in the treatment of bipolar psychiatric disorders. Most intoxications are cases of chronic overdose. One gram of lithium carbonate contains 189 mg (5.1 mEq) of lithium; a regular tablet contains 300 mg (8.12 mEq) and a sustained-release preparation contains 450 mg or 12.18 mEq.

Toxic Mechanism

The brain is the primary target organ of toxicity, but the mechanism is unclear. Lithium may interfere with physiologic functions by acting as a substitute for cellular cations (sodium and potassium), depressing neural excitation and synaptic transmission.

Toxic Dose

A dose of 1 mEq/kg (40 mg/kg) of lithium will give a peak serum lithium concentration about 1.2 mEq/L. The therapeutic serum lithium concentration in cases of acute mania is 0.6 to 1.2 mEq/L, and for maintenance it is 0.5 to 0.8 mEq/L. Serum lithium concentration levels are usually obtained 12 hours after the last dose. The toxic dose is determined by clinical manifestations and serum levels after the distribution phase.

Acute ingestion of twenty 300-mg tablets (300 mg increases the serum lithium concentration by 0.2 to 0.4 mEq/L) in adults may produce serious intoxication. Chronic intoxication can be produced by conditions listed below that can decrease the elimination of lithium or increase lithium reabsorption in the kidney.

The risk factors that predispose to chronic lithium toxicity are febrile illness, impaired renal function, hyponatremia, advanced age, lithium-induced diabetes insipidus, dehydration, vomiting and diarrhea, and concomitant use of other drugs, such as thiazide and spironolactone diuretics, nonsteroidal antiinflammatory drugs, salicylates, angiotensin-converting enzyme inhibitors (e.g., captopril), serotonin reuptake inhibitors (e.g., fluoxetine [Prozac]), and phenothiazines.

Kinetics

Gastrointestinal absorption of regular-release preparations is rapid; serum lithium concentration peaks in 2 to 4 hours and is complete by 6 to 8 hours. The onset of toxicity may occur at 1 to 4 hours after acute overdose but usually is delayed because lithium enters the brain slowly. Absorption of sustained-release preparations and the development of toxicity may be delayed 6 to 12 hours.

Volume distribution is 0.5 to 0.9 L/kg. Lithium is not protein bound. The half-life after a single dose is 9 to 13 hours; at steady state, it may be 30 to 58 hours. The renal handling of lithium is similar to that of sodium: glomerular filtration and reabsorption (80%) by the proximal renal tubule. Adequate sodium must be present to prevent lithium reabsorption. More than 90% of lithium is excreted by the kidney, 30% to 60% within 6 to 12 hours.

Manifestations

The examiner must distinguish between side effects, acute intoxication, acute or chronic toxicity, and chronic intoxications. Chronic is the most common and dangerous type of intoxication.

Side effects include fine tremor, gastrointestinal upset, hypothyroidism, polyuria and frank diabetes insipidus, dermatologic manifestations, and cardiac conduction deficits. Lithium is teratogenic.

Patients with acute poisoning may be asymptomatic, with an early high serum lithium concentration of 9 mEq/L, and deteriorate as the serum lithium concentration falls by 50% and the lithium distributes to the brain and the other tissues. Nausea and vomiting may occur within 1 to 4 hours, but the systemic manifestations are usually delayed several more hours. It may take as long as 3 to 5 days for serious symptoms to develop. Acute toxicity and acute on chronic toxicity are manifested by neurologic findings, including weakness, fasciculations, altered mental state, myoclonus, hyperreflexia, rigidity, coma, and convulsions with limbs in hypertension. Cardiovascular effects are nonspecific and occur at therapeutic doses, flat T or inverted T waves, atrioventricular block, and prolonged QT interval. Lithium is not a primary cardiotoxin. Cardiogenic shock occurs secondary to CNS toxicity. Chronic intoxication is associated with manifestations at lower serum lithium concentrations. There is some correlation with manifestations, especially at higher serum lithium concentrations. Although the levels do not always correlate with the manifestations, they are more predictive in cases of severe intoxication. A serum lithium concentration greater than 3.0 mEq/L with chronic intoxication and altered mental state indicates severe toxicity. Permanent neurologic sequelae can result from lithium intoxication.

Laboratory Investigations

Monitoring should include CBC (lithium causes significant leukocytosis), renal function, thyroid function (chronic intoxication), ECG, and electrolytes. Serum lithium concentrations should be determined every 2 to 4 hours until levels are close to therapeutic range. Cross-reactions with green-top Vacutainer specimen tubes containing heparin will spuriously elevate serum lithium concentration 6 to 8 mEq/L.

Management

Vital function must be established and maintained. Seizure precautions should be instituted and seizures, hypotension, and dysrhythmias treated. Evaluation should include examination for rigidity and hyperreflexia signs, hydration, renal function (BUN, creatinine), and electrolytes, especially sodium. The examiner should inquire about diuretic and other drug use that increase serum lithium concentration, and the patient must discontinue the drugs. If the patient is on chronic therapy, the lithium should be discontinued. Serial serum lithium concentrations should be obtained every 4 hours until serum lithium concentration peaks and there is a downward trend toward almost therapeutic range, especially in sustained-release preparations. Vital signs should be monitored, including temperature, and ECG and serial neurologic examinations should be undertaken, including mental status and urinary output. Nephrology consultation is warranted in case of a chronic and elevated serum lithium concentration (>2.5 mEq/L), a large ingestion, or altered mental state.

An intravenous line should be established and hydration and electrolyte balance restored. Serum sodium level should be determined before 0.9% saline fluid is administered in patients with chronic overdose because hypernatremia may be present from diabetes insipidus. Although current evidence supports an initial 0.9% saline infusion (200 mL/h) to enhance excretion of lithium, once hydration, urine output, and normonatremia are established, one should administer 0.45% saline and slow the infusion (100 mL/h) for all patients.

Gastric lavage is often not recommended in cases of acute ingestion because of the large size of the tablets, and it is not necessary after chronic intoxication. Activated charcoal is ineffective. For sustained-release preparations, whole-bowel irrigation may be useful but is not proven. Sodium polystyrene sulfonate (Kayexalate), an ion exchange resin, is difficult to administer and has been used only in uncontrolled studies. Its use is not recommended.

Hemodialysis is the most efficient method for removing lithium from the vascular compartment. It is the treatment of choice for patients with severe intoxication with an altered mental state, those with seizures, and anuric patients. Long runs are used until the serum lithium concentration is less than 1 mEq/L because of extensive re-equilibration. Serum lithium concentration should be monitored every 4 hours after dialysis for rebound. Repeated and prolonged hemodialysis may be necessary. A lag in neurologic recovery can be expected.

Disposition

An acute asymptomatic lithium overdose cannot be medically cleared on the basis of single lithium level. Patients should be admitted if they have any neurologic manifestations (altered mental status, hyperreflexia, stiffness, or tremor). Patients should be admitted to the intensive care unit if they are dehydrated, have renal impairment, or have a high or rising lithium level.

METHANOL (WOOD ALCOHOL, METHYL ALCOHOL)

The concentration of methanol in Sterno fuel is 4% and it contains ethanol, in windshield washer fluid it is 30% to 60%, and in gas-line antifreeze it is 100%.

Toxic Mechanism

Methanol is metabolized by alcohol dehydrogenase to formaldehyde, which is metabolized to formate. Formate inhibits cytochrome oxidase, producing tissue hypoxia, lactic acidosis, and optic nerve edema. Formate is converted by folate-dependent enzymes to carbon dioxide.

Toxic Dose

The minimal toxic amount is approximately 100 mg/kg. Serious toxicity in a young child can be produced by the ingestion of 2.5 to 5.0 mL of 100% methanol. Ingestion of 5-mL 100% methanol by a 10-kg child produces estimated peak blood methanol of 80 mg/dL. Ingestion of 15 mL 40% methanol was lethal for a 2-year-old child in one report. A fatal adult oral dose is 30 to 240 mL 100% (20 to 150 g). Ingestion of 6 to 10 mL 100% causes blindness in adults. The toxic blood concentration is greater than 20 mg/dL; very serious toxicity and potential fatality occur at levels greater than 50 mg/dL.

Kinetics

Onset of action can start within 1 hour but may be delayed up to 12 to 18 hours by metabolism to toxic metabolites. It may be delayed longer if ethanol is ingested concomitantly or in infants. Peak blood methanol concentration is 1 hour. Volume distribution is 0.6 L/kg (total body water).

For metabolism, see *Toxic Mechanism*.

Elimination is through metabolism. The half-life of methanol is 8 hours; with ethanol blocking it is 30 to 35 hours; and with hemodialysis 2.5 hours.

Manifestations

Metabolism creates a delay in onset for 12 to 18 hours or longer if ethanol is ingested concomitantly. Initial findings are as follows:

- 0 to 6 hours: Confusion, ataxia, inebriation, formaldehyde odor on breath, and abdominal pain can be present, but the patient may be asymptomatic. Note: Methanol produces an osmolal gap (early), and its metabolite formate produces the anion gap metabolic acidosis (see later). Absence of osmolar or anion gap does not always exclude methanol intoxication.
- 6 to 12 hours: Malaise, headache, abdominal pain, vomiting, visual symptoms, including hyperemia of optic disc, "snow vision," and blindness can be seen.
- More than 12 hours: Worsening acidosis, hyperglycemia, shock, and multiorgan failure develop, with death from complications of intractable acidosis and cerebral edema.

Laboratory Investigation

Methanol can be detected on some chromatography drug screens if specified. Methanol and ethanol levels, electrolytes, glucose, BUN, creatinine, amylase, and ABG should be monitored every 4 hours. Formate levels correlate more closely than blood methanol concentration with severity of intoxication and should be obtained if possible.

Management

One should protect the airway by intubation to prevent aspiration and administer assisted ventilation as needed. If needed, 100%

oxygen can be administered. A nephrologist should be consulted early regarding the need for hemodialysis.

Gastrointestinal decontamination procedures have no role.

Metabolic acidosis should be treated vigorously with sodium bicarbonate 2 to 3 mEq/kg intravenously. Large amounts may be needed.

Antidote therapy is initiated to inhibit metabolism if the patient has a history of ingesting more than 0.4 mL/kg of 100% with the following conditions:

- Blood methanol level is greater than 20 mg/dL
- The patient has osmolar gap not accounted for by other factors
- The patient is symptomatic or acidotic with increased anion gap and/or hyperemia of the optic disc.

The ethanol or fomepizole therapy outlined below can be used.

Ethanol Therapy

Ethanol should be initiated immediately if fomepizole is unavailable (see *Fomepizole Therapy*). Alcohol dehydrogenase has a greater affinity for ethanol than ethylene glycol. Therefore, ethanol blocks the metabolism of ethylene glycol.

Ethanol should be administered intravenously (oral administration is less reliable) to produce a blood ethanol concentration of 100 to 150 mg/dL. The loading dose is 10 mL/kg of 10% ethanol administered intravenously concomitantly with a maintenance dose of 10% ethanol at 1.0 mL/kg/h. This dose may need to be increased to 2 mL/kg/h in patients who are heavy drinkers. The blood ethanol concentration should be measured hourly and the infusion rate should be adjusted to maintain a concentration of 100 to 150 mg/dL.

Fomepizole Therapy

Fomepizole (Antizol, 4-methylpyrazole) inhibits alcohol dehydrogenase more reliably than ethanol and it does not require constant monitoring of ethanol levels and adjustment of infusion rates. Fomepizole is available in 1 g/mL vials of 1.5 mL. The loading dose is 15 mg/kg (0.015 mL/kg) IV, maintenance dose is 10 mg/kg (0.01 mL/kg) every 12 hours for 4 doses, then 15 mg/kg every 12 hours until the ethylene glycol levels are less than 20 mg/dL. The solution is prepared by being mixed with 100 mL of 0.9% saline or D$_5$W. Fomepizole can be given to patients requiring hemodialysis but should be dosed as follows:

Dose at the beginning of hemodialysis:

- If less than 6 hours since last Antizol dose, do not administer dose
- If more than 6 hours since last dose, administer next scheduled dose

Dosing during hemodialysis:

- Dose every 4 hours

Dosing at the time hemodialysis is completed:

- If less than 1 hour between last dose and end dialysis, do not administer dose at end of dialysis
- If 1 to 3 hours between last dose and end dialysis, administer one half of next scheduled dose
- If more than 3 hours between last dose and end dialysis, administer next scheduled dose

Maintenance dosing off hemodialysis:

- Give the next scheduled dose 12 hours from the last dose administered

Hemodialysis increases the clearance of both methanol and formate 10-fold over renal clearance. A blood methanol concentration greater than 50 mg/dL has been used as an indication for hemodialysis, but recently some toxicologists from the New York City Poison Center recommended early hemodialysis in patients with blood methanol concentration greater than 25 mg/dL because it may be able to shorten the course of intoxication if started early. One should continue to monitor methanol levels and/or formate levels every 4 hours after the procedure for rebound. Other indications for early

hemodialysis are significant metabolic acidosis and electrolyte abnormalities despite conventional therapy and if visual or neurologic signs or symptoms are present.

A serum formate level greater than 20 mg/dL has also been used as a criterion for hemodialysis, although this is often not readily available through many laboratories. If hemodialysis is used, the infusion rate of 10% ethanol should be increased 2.0 to 3.5 mL/kg/h. The blood ethanol concentration and glucose level should be obtained every 2 hours.

Therapy is continued with both ethanol and hemodialysis until the blood methanol level is undetectable, there is no acidosis, and the patient has no neurologic or visual disturbances. This may require several days.

Hypoglycemia is treated with intravenous glucose. Doses of folinic acid (Leucovorin) and folic acid have been used successfully in animal investigations to enhance formate metabolism to carbon dioxide and water. Leucovorin 1 mg/kg up to 50 mg IV is administered every 4 hours for several days.

An initial ophthalmologic consultation and follow-up are warranted.

Disposition

All patients who have ingested significant amounts of methanol should be referred to the emergency department for evaluation and blood methanol concentration measurement. Ophthalmologic follow-up of all patients with methanol intoxications should be arranged.

MONOAMINE OXIDASE INHIBITORS

Nonselective monoamine oxidase inhibitors (MAOIs) include the hydrazines phenelzine (Nardil) and isocarboxazid (Marplan), and the nonhydrazine tranylcypromine (Parnate). Furazolidone (Furoxone) and pargyline (Eutonyl)[2] are also considered nonselective MAOIs. Moclobemide,[2] which is available in many countries but not the United States, is a selective MAO-A inhibitor. MAO-B inhibitors include selegiline (Eldepryl), an antiparkinsonism agent, which does not have similar toxicity to MAO-A and is not discussed. Selectivity is lost in an overdose. MAOIs are used to treat severe depression.

Toxic Mechanism

Monoamine oxidase enzymes are responsible for the oxidative deamination of both endogenous and exogenous catecholamines such as norepinephrine. MAO-A in the intestinal wall also metabolizes tyramine in food. MAOIs permanently inhibit MAO enzymes until a new enzyme is synthesized after 14 days or longer. The toxicity results from the accumulation, potentiation, and prolongation of the catecholamine action followed by profound hypotension and cardiovascular collapse.

Toxic Dose

Toxicity begins at 2 to 3 mg/kg and fatalities occur at 4 to 6 mg/kg. Death has occurred after a single dose of 170 mg of tranylcypromine in an adult.

Kinetics

Structurally, MAOIs are related to amphetamines and catecholamines. The hydrazine peak levels are at 1 to 2 hours; metabolism is hepatic acetylation; and inactive metabolites are excreted in the urine. For the nonhydrazines, peak levels occur at 1 to 4 hours, and metabolism is via the liver to active amphetamine-like metabolites.

The onset of symptoms in a case of overdose is delayed 6 to 24 hours after ingestion, peak activity is 8 to 12 hours, and duration is 72 hours or longer. The peak of MAO inhibition is in 5 to 10 days and lasts as long as 5 weeks.

---

[2]Not available in the United States.

Manifestations

Manifestations of an acute ingestion overdose of MAO-A inhibitors are as follows:

Phase I

An adrenergic crisis occurs, with delayed onset for 6 to 24 hours, and may not reach peak until 24 hours. The crisis starts as hyperthermia, tachycardia, tachypnea, dysarthria, transient hypertension, hyperreflexia, and CNS stimulation.

Phase II

Neuromuscular excitation and sympathetic hyperactivity occur with increased temperature greater than 40°C (104°F), agitation, hyperactivity, confusion, fasciculations, twitching, tremor, masseter spasm, muscle rigidity, acidosis, and electrolyte abnormalities. Seizures and dystonic reactions may occur. The pupils are mydriatic, sometimes nonreactive with "ping-pong gaze."

Phase III

CNS depression and cardiovascular collapse occur in cases of severe overdose as the catecholamines are depleted. Symptoms usually resolve within 5 days but may last 2 weeks.

Phase IV

Secondary complications occur, including rhabdomyolysis, cardiac dysrhythmias, multiorgan failure, and coagulopathies.

Biogenic interactions usually occur while the patient is on therapeutic doses of MAOI or shortly after they are discontinued (30 to 60 minutes), before the new MAO enzyme is synthesized. The following substances have been implicated: indirect acting sympathomimetics such as amphetamines, serotonergic drugs, opioids (e.g., meperidine, dextromethorphan), tricyclic antidepressants, specific serotonin reuptake inhibitors (SSRI; e.g., fluoxetine [Prozac], sertraline [Zoloft], paroxetine [Paxil]), tyramine-containing foods (e.g., wine, beer, avocados, cheese, caviar, chocolate, chicken liver), and L-tryptophan. SSRIs should not be started for at least 5 weeks after MAOIs have been discontinued.

In mild cases, usually caused by foods, headache and hypertension develop and last for several hours. In severe cases, malignant hypertension and severe hyperthermia syndromes consisting of hypertension or hyperthermia, altered mental state, skeletal muscle rigidity, shivering (often beginning in the masseter muscle), and seizures may occur.

The serotonin syndrome, which may be a result of inhibition of serotonin metabolism, has similar clinical findings to those of malignant hyperthermia and may occur with or without hyperthermia or hypertension.

Chronic toxicity clinical findings include tremors, hyperhidrosis, agitation, hallucinations, confusion, and seizures and may be confused with withdrawal syndromes.

Laboratory Investigations

Monitoring of the ECG, cardiac monitoring, CPK, ABG, pulse oximeter, electrolytes, blood glucose, and acid-base balance should be maintained.

Management

In the case of MAOI overdose, ipecac-induced emesis should not be used. Only activated charcoal alone should be used.

If the patient is admitted to the hospital and is well enough to eat, a nontyramine diet should be ordered.

Extreme agitation and seizures can be controlled with benzodiazepines and barbiturates. Phenytoin is ineffective. Nondepolarizing neuromuscular blockers (not depolarizing succinylcholine) may be needed in severe cases of hyperthermia and rigidity. If the patient has severe hypertension (catecholamine mediated), phentolamine (Regitine), a parenteral β-blocking agent, 3 to 5 mg intravenously, or labetalol (Normodyne), a combination of an α-blocking agent

and a β-blocker, 20-mg intravenous bolus, should be given. If malignant hypertension with rigidity is present, a short-acting nitroprusside and benzodiazepine can be used. Hypertension is often followed by severe hypotension, which should be managed by fluid and vasopressors. *Caution:* Vasopressor therapy should be administered at lower doses than usual because of exaggerated pharmacologic response. Norepinephrine is preferred to dopamine, which requires release of intracellular amines.

Cardiac dysrhythmias are treated with standard therapy but are often refractory, and cardioversion and pacemakers may be needed.

For malignant hyperthermia, dantrolene (Dantrium), a nonspecific peripheral skeletal relaxing agent, is administered, which inhibits the release of calcium from the sarcoplasm. Dantrolene is reconstituted with 60 mL sterile water without bacteriostatic agents. Glass equipment must not be used, and the drug must be protected from light and used within 6 hours. Loading dose is 2 to 3 mg/kg intravenously as a bolus, and the loading dose is repeated until the signs of malignant hyperthermia (tachycardia, rigidity, increased end-tidal CO_2, and temperature) are controlled. Maximum total dose is 10 mg/kg to avoid hepatotoxicity.

When malignant hyperthermia has subsided, 1 mg/kg IV is given every 6 hours for 24 to 48 hours, then orally 1 mg/kg every 6 hours for 24 hours to prevent recurrence. There is a danger of thrombophlebitis following peripheral dantrolene, and it should be administered through a central line if possible. In addition one should administer external cooling and correct metabolic acidosis and electrolyte disturbances. Benzodiazepine can be used for sedation. Dantrolene does not reverse central dopamine blockade; therefore, bromocriptine mesylate (Parlodel) 2.5 to 10 mg should be given orally or through a nasogastric tube three times a day.

Rhabdomyolysis and myoglobinuria are treated with fluids. Urine alkalinization should also be treated.

Hemodialysis and hemoperfusion are of no proven value.

Biogenic amine interactions are managed symptomatically, similar to cases of overdose. For the serotonin syndrome cyproheptadine (Periactin), a serotonin blocker, 4 mg orally every hour for three doses, or methysergide (Sansert), 2 mg orally every 6 hours for three doses, should be considered. The effectiveness of these drugs has not been proven.

Disposition

All patients who have ingested more than 2 mg/kg of an MAOI should be admitted to the hospital for 24 hours of observation and monitoring in the intensive care unit because the life-threatening manifestations may be delayed. Patients with drug or dietary interactions that are mild may not require admission if symptoms subside within 4 to 6 hours and the patients remain asymptomatic. Patients with symptoms that persist or require active intervention should be admitted to the intensive care unit.

OPIOIDS (NARCOTIC OPIATES)

Opioids are used for analgesia, as antitussives, and as antidiarrheal agents and are illicit agents (heroin, opium) used in substance abuse. Tolerance, physical dependency, and withdrawal may develop.

Toxic Mechanism

At least four main opioid receptors have been identified. The μ receptor is considered the most important for central analgesia and CNS depression. The κ and δ receptors predominate in spinal analgesia. The σ receptors may mediate dysphoria. Death is a consequence of dose-dependent CNS respiratory depression or secondary to pulmonary aspiration or noncardiac pulmonary edema. The mechanism of noncardiac pulmonary edema is unknown.

Dextromethorphan can interact with MAOIs, causing severe hyperthermia, and may cause the serotonin syndrome (see *Selective Serotonin Reuptake Inhibitors*). Dextromethorphan inhibits the metabolism of norepinephrine and serotonin and blocks the reuptake of serotonin. It is found as a component of a large number of nonprescription cough and cold remedies.

TABLE 24 Doses and Onset and Duration of Action of Common Opioids

Drug	Adult Oral Dose	Child Oral Dose	Onset of Action	Duration of Action	Adult Fatal Dose
Camphored tincture of opium	25 mL	0.25–0.50 mL/kg (0.4 mg/mL)	15–30 min	4–5 h	NA
Codeine	30–180 mg	0.5–1 mg/kg	15–30 min	4–6 h	800 mg
		>1 mg/kg is toxic in a child, above 200 mg in adult >5 mg/kg fatal in a child			
Dextromethorphan	15 mg	0.25 mg/kg	15–30 min	3–6 h	NA
	10 mg/kg is toxic				
Diacetylmorphine; street heroin is less than 10% pure	60 mg	NA	15–30 min	3–4 h	100 mg
Diphenoxylate atropine (Lomotil)	5–10 mg	NA	120–240 min	14 h	300 mg
	7.5 mg is toxic in a child, 300 mg is toxic in adult				
Fentanyl (Duragesic)	0.1–0.2 mg	0.001–0.002 mg/kg	7–8 min	Intramuscular: ½–2 h	1.0 mg
Hydrocodone with APAP (Lortab)	5–30 mg	0.15 mg/kg	30 min	3–4 h	100 mg
Hydromorphone (Dilaudid)	4 mg	0.1 mg/kg	15–30 min	3–4 h	100 mg
Meperidine (Demerol)	100 mg	1–1.5 mg/kg	10–45 min	3–4 h	350 mg
Methadone (Dolophine)	10 mg	0.1 mg/kg	30–60 min	4–12 h	120 mg
Morphine	10–60 mg	0.1–0.2 mg/kg	<20 min	4–6 h	200 mg
	Oral dose is 6 times parenteral dose, MS Contin sustained-release prep				
Oxycodone APAP (Percocet)	5 mg	NA	15–30 min	4–5 h	NA
Pentazocine (Talwin)	50–100 mg	NA	15–30 min	3–4 h	NA
Propoxyphene (Darvon)	65–100 mg	NA	30–60 min	2–4 h	700 mg

Toxic Dose

The toxic dose depends on the specific drug, route of administration, and degree of tolerance. For therapeutic and toxic doses, see Table 24. In children, respiratory depression has been produced by 10 mg of morphine or methadone, 75 mg of meperidine, and 12.5 mg of diphenoxylate. Infants younger than 3 months of age are more susceptible to respiratory depression. The dose should be reduced by 50%.

Kinetics

Oral onset of analgesic effect of morphine is 10 to 15 minutes; the action peaks in 1 hour and lasts 4 to 6 hours. With sustained-release preparations, the duration is 8 to 12 hours. Opioids are 90% metabolized in the liver by hepatic conjugation and 90% excreted in the urine as inactive compounds. Volume distribution is 1 to 4 L/kg. Protein binding is 35% to 75%. The typical plasma half-life of opiates is 2 to 5 hours, but that of methadone is 24 to 36 hours. Morphine metabolites include morphine-3-glucuronide (inactive) and morphine-6-glucuronide (active) and normorphine (active). Meperidine (Demerol) is rapidly hydrolyzed by tissue esterases into the active metabolite normeperidine, which has twice the convulsant activity of meperidine. Heroin (diacetylmorphine) is deacetylated within minutes to 6-monoacetylmorphine and morphine. Propoxyphene (Darvon) has a rapid onset of action, and death has occurred within 15 to 30 minutes after a massive overdose. Propoxyphene is metabolized to norpropoxyphene, an active metabolite with convulsive, cardiac dysrhythmic, and heart block properties. Symptoms of diphenoxylate overdose appear within 1 to 4 hours. It is metabolized into the active metabolite difenoxin, which is five times more active as a regular respiratory depressant agent. Death has been reported in children after ingestion of a single tablet.

Manifestations

Initially, mild intoxication produces miosis, dull face, drowsiness, partial ptosis, and "nodding" (head drops to chest then bobs up). Larger amounts produce the classic triad of miotic pupils (exceptions below), respiratory depression, and depressed level of consciousness (flaccid coma). The blood pressure, pulse, and bowel activity are decreased.

Dilated pupils do not exclude opioid intoxication. Some exceptions to the miosis effect include dextromethorphan (paralyzes iris), fentanyl, meperidine, and diphenoxylate (rarely). Physiologic disturbances including acidosis, hypoglycemia, hypoxia, and postictal state, or a co-ingestant may also produce mydriasis.

Usually, the muscles are flaccid, but increased muscle tone can be produced by meperidine and fentanyl (chest rigidity). Seizures are rare but can occur with ingestion of codeine, meperidine, propoxyphene, and dextromethorphan. Hallucinations and agitation have been reported.

Pruritus and urticaria are caused by histamine release by some opioids or by sulfite additives.

Noncardiac pulmonary edema may occur after an overdose, especially with intravenous heroin abuse. Cardiac effects include vasodilation and hypotension. A heart murmur in an intravenous addict suggests endocarditis. Propoxyphene can produce delayed cardiac dysrhythmias.

Fentanyl is 100 times more potent than morphine and can cause chest wall muscle rigidity. Some of its derivatives are 2000 times more potent than morphine.

Laboratory Investigations

For patients with overdose, one should obtain and monitor ABG, blood glucose, and electrolyte levels; chest radiographs; and ECG. For drug abusers, one should consider testing for hepatitis B, syphilis, and HIV antibody (HIV testing usually requires consent). Blood opioid concentrations are not useful. They confirm diagnosis (morphine therapeutic dose, 65 to 80 ng/mL; toxic, <200 ng/mL), but are not useful for making a therapeutic decision. Cross-reactions can occur with Vick's Formula 44, poppy seeds, and other opioids (codeine and heroin are metabolized to morphine). Naloxone 4 mg IV was not associated with a positive enzyme multiplied immunoassay technique urine screen at 60 minutes, 6 hours, or 48 hours.

Management

Supportive care should be instituted, particularly an endotracheal tube and assisted ventilation. Temporary ventilation can be provided by a bag-valve mask with 100% oxygen. The patient should be placed on a cardiac monitor, have intravenous access established, and have specimens for ABG, glucose, electrolytes, BUN, and creatinine levels, CBC, coagulation profile, liver function, toxicology screen, and urinalysis taken.

For gastrointestinal decontamination, emesis should not be induced, but activated charcoal can be administered if bowel sounds are present.

If it is suspected that the patient is an addict, he or she should be restrained first and then 0.1 mg of naloxone (Narcan) should be administered. The dose should be doubled every 2 minutes until the patient responds or 10 to 20 mg has been given. If the patient is not suspected to be an addict, then 2 mg every 2 to 3 minutes to total of 10 to 20 mg is administered.

It is essential to determine whether there is a complete response to naloxone (mydriasis, improvement in ventilation), because it is a diagnostic therapeutic test. A continuous naloxone infusion may be appropriate, using the "response dose" every hour. Repeat doses of naloxone may be necessary because the effects of many opioids can last much longer than naloxone does (30 to 60 minutes). Methadone ingestions may require a naloxone infusion for 24 to 48 hours. Half of the response dose may need to be repeated in 15 to 20 minutes, after the infusion has been started.

Acute iatrogenic withdrawal precipitated by the administration of naloxone to a dependent patient should not be treated with morphine or other opioids. Naloxone's effects are limited to 30 to 60 minutes (shorter than most opioids) and withdrawal will subside in a short time.

Nalmefene (Revex), an FDA-approved long-acting (4 to 8 hours) pure opioid antagonist, is being investigated, but its role in cases of acute intoxication is unclear and it could produce prolonged withdrawal. It may have a role in place of naloxone infusion.

Noncardiac pulmonary edema does not respond to naloxone, and the patient needs intubation, assisted ventilation, positive end-expiratory pressure, and hemodynamic monitoring. Fluids should be given cautiously in patients with opioid overdose because opioids stimulate the antidiuretic hormone.

If the patient is comatose, 50% glucose (3% to 4% of comatose opioid overdose patients have hypoglycemia) and thiamine should be given prior to naloxone. If the patient has seizures that are unresponsive to naloxone, one administers diazepam and examines for metabolic (hypoglycemia, electrolyte disturbances) causes and structural disturbances.

Hypotension is rare and should direct a search for another etiology. If the patient is agitated, hypoxia and hypoglycemia must be excluded before opioid withdrawal is considered as a cause. Complications to consider include urinary retention, constipation, rhabdomyolysis, myoglobinuria, hypoglycemia, and withdrawal.

Disposition

If a patient responds to intravenous naloxone, careful observation for relapse and the development of pulmonary edema is required, with cardiac and respiratory monitoring for 6 to 12 hours. Patients requiring repeated doses of naloxone or an infusion, or those who develop pulmonary edema, require intensive care unit admission and cannot be discharged from the intensive care unit until they are symptom free for 12 hours. Intravenous overdose complications are expected to be present within 20 minutes after injection, and discharge after 4 symptom-free hours has been recommended. Adults with oral overdose have delayed onset of toxicity and require 6 hours of observation. Children with oral opioid overdose should be admitted to the hospital for observation because of delayed toxicity. Some toxicologists advise restraining a patient who attempts to sign out against medical advice after treatment with naloxone, at least until the patient receives psychiatric evaluation.

ORGANOPHOSPHATES AND CARBAMATES

Cholinergic intoxication sources are insecticides (organophosphates or carbamates), some medications, and some mushrooms, Examples of organophosphate insecticides are malathion (low toxicity, median lethal dose [LD$_{50}$] 2800 mg/kg), chlorpyrifos, which has been removed from market (moderate toxicity), and parathion (high toxicity, LD$_{50}$ 2 mg/kg). Carbamate insecticides include carbaryl (low toxicity, LD$_{50}$ 500 mg/kg), propoxur (moderate toxicity, LD$_{50}$ 95 mg/kg), and aldicarb (high toxicity, LD$_{50}$ 0.9 mg/kg). Pharmaceuticals with carbamate properties include neostigmine (Prostigmin) and physostigmine (Antilirium). Cholinergic compounds also include the "G" nerve war weapons tabun (GA), sarin (GB), soman (GB), and venom X (VX).

Toxic Mechanism

Organophosphates phosphorylate the active site on red cell acetylcholinesterase and pseudocholinesterase in the serum, neuromuscular and parasympathetic neuroeffector junctions, and in the major synapses of the autonomic ganglia, causing irreversible inhibition. There are two types of organophosphate intoxication: (a) direct action by the parent compound (e.g., tetraethylpyrophosphate), or (b) indirect action by the toxic metabolite (e.g., parathoxon or malathoxon).

Carbamates (esters of carbonic acid) cause reversible carbamylation of the active site of the enzymes. When a critical amount, greater than 50%, of cholinesterase is inhibited, acetylcholine accumulates and causes transient stimulation at cholinergic synapses and sympathetic terminals (muscarinic effect), the somatic nerves, the autonomic ganglia (nicotinic effect), and CNS synapses. Stimulation of conduction is followed by inhibition of conduction.

The major differences between the carbamates and the organophosphates are as follows: (a) carbamate toxicity is less and the duration is shorter; (b) carbamates rarely produce overt CNS effects (poor CNS penetration); (c) carbamate inhibition of the acetylcholinesterase enzyme is reversible and activity returns to normal rapidly; (d) pralidoxime, the enzyme regenerator, may not be necessary in the management of mild carbamate intoxication (e.g., carbaryl).

Toxic Dose

Parathion's minimum lethal dose is 2 mg in children and 10 to 20 mg in adults. The lethal dose of malathion is greater than 1375 mg/kg and that of chlorpyrifos is 25 g; the latter compound is unlikely to cause death.

Kinetics

Absorption is by all routes. The onset of acute ingestion toxicity occurs as early as 3 hours, usually before 12 hours and always before 24 hours. Lipid-soluble agents absorbed by the dermal route (e.g., fenthion) may have a delayed onset of more than 24 hours. Inhalation toxicity occurs immediately after exposure. Massive ingestion can produce intoxication within minutes.

Metabolism is via the liver. With some pesticides (e.g., parathion, malathion), the effects are delayed because they undergo hepatic microsomal oxidative metabolism to their toxic metabolites, the -oxons (e.g., paroxon, malaoxon).

The half-life of malathion is 2.89 hours and that of parathion is 2.1 days. The metabolites are eliminated in the urine and the presence of p-nitrophenol in the urine is a clue up to 48 hours after exposure.

Manifestations

Many organophosphates produce a garlic odor on the breath, in the gastric contents, or in the container. Diaphoresis, excessive salivation, miosis, and muscle twitching are helpful clues to diagnosis.

Early, a cholinergic (muscarinic) crisis develops that consists of parasympathetic nervous system activity. DUMBELS is the mnemonic for defecation, cramps, and increased bowel motility; urinary incontinence; miosis (mydriasis may occur in 20%); bronchospasm and bronchorrhea; excess secretion; lacrimation; and seizures. Bradycardia, pulmonary edema, and hypotension may be present.

Later, sympathetic and nicotinic effects occur, consisting of MATCH: muscle weakness and fasciculation (eyelid twitching is often present), adrenal stimulation and hyperglycemia, tachycardia, cramps in muscles, and hypertension. Finally, paralysis of the skeletal muscles ensues.

The CNS effects are headache, blurred vision, anxiety, ataxia, delirium and toxic psychosis, convulsions, coma, and respiratory depression. Cranial nerve palsies have been noted. Delayed hallucinations may occur.

Delayed respiratory paralysis and neurologic and neurobehavioral disorders have been described following certain organophosphate ingestions or dermal exposure. The "intermediate syndrome" is paralysis of proximal and respiratory muscles developing 24 to

96 hours after the successful treatment of organophosphate poisoning. A delayed distal polyneuropathy has been described with ingestion of certain organophosphates, such as triorthocresyl phosphate, bromoleptophos, and methomidophos.

Complications include aspiration, pulmonary edema, and acute respiratory distress syndrome.

Laboratory Investigations

Monitoring should include chest radiograph, blood glucose (nonketotic hyperglycemia is frequent), ABG, pulse oximetry, ECG, blood coagulation status, liver function, hyperamylasemia (pancreatitis reported), and urinalysis for the metabolite alkyl phosphate paranitrophenol. Blood should be drawn for red blood cell cholinesterase determination before pralidoxime is given. The red blood cell cholinesterase activity roughly correlates with clinical severity. Mild poisoning is 20% to 50% of normal, moderate poisoning is 10% to 20% of normal, and severe poisoning is 10% of normal (>90% depressed). A postexposure rise of 10% to 15% in the cholinesterase level determined at least 10 to 14 days after the exposure confirms the diagnosis.

Management

Protection of health care personnel with clothing (masks, gloves, gowns, goggles) and respiratory equipment or hazardous material suits, as necessary, is called for. General decontamination consists of isolation, bagging, and disposal of contaminated clothing and other articles. Vital functions should be established and maintained. Cardiac and oxygen saturation monitoring are needed. Intubation and assisted ventilation may be needed. Secretions should be suctioned until atropinization drying is achieved.

Dermal decontamination involves prompt removal of clothing and cleansing of all affected areas of skin, hair, and eyes. Ocular decontamination involves irrigation with copious amounts of tepid water or 0.9% saline for at least 15 minutes. Gastrointestinal decontamination, if the ingestion was recent, involves the administration of activated charcoal.

Atropine sulfate can be given as an antidote. It is both a diagnostic and a therapeutic agent. Atropine counteracts the muscarinic effects but is only partially effective for the CNS effects (seizures and coma). Preservative-free atropine (no benzyl alcohol) should be used. If the patient is symptomatic (bradycardia or bronchorrhea), a test dose should be administered, 0.02 mg/kg in children or 1 mg in adults, intravenously. If no signs of atropinization are present (tachycardia, drying of secretions, and mydriasis), atropine should be administered immediately, 0.05 mg/kg in children or 2 mg in adults, every 5 to 10 minutes as needed to dry the secretions and clear the lungs. Beneficial effects are seen within 1 to 4 minutes and maximum effect in 8 minutes. The average dose in the first 24 hours is 40 mg, but 1000 mg or more has been required in severe cases. Glycopyrrolate (Robinul) can be used if atropine is not available. The maximum dose should be maintained for 12 to 24 hours, then tapered and the patient observed for relapse. Poisoning, especially with lipophilic agents (e.g., fenthion, chlorfenthion), may require weeks of atropine therapy. An alternative is a continuous infusion of atropine 8 mg in 100 mL 0.9% saline at rate of 0.02 to 0.08 mg/kg/h (0.25 to 1.0 mL/kg/h) with additional 1 to 5 mg boluses as needed to dry the secretions.

Pralidoxime chloride (Protopam) has both antinicotinic and antimuscarinic effects and possibly also CNS effects. Successful treatment with pralidoxime chloride may allow a reduction in the dose of atropine. Pralidoxime acts to reactivate the phosphorylated cholinesterases by binding the phosphate moiety on the esteritic site and displacing it. It should be given early before "aging" of phosphate bond produces tighter binding. However, recent reports indicate that pralidoxime chloride is beneficial even several days after the poisoning. Improvement is seen within 10 to 40 minutes. The initial dose of pralidoxime chloride is 1 to 2 g in 250 mL 0.89% saline over 5 to 10 minutes, maximum 200 mg/minute, in adults or 25 to 50 mg/kg, maximum 4 mg/kg/minute, in children younger than 12 years of age. The dose can be repeated every 6 to 12 hours for several days.

An alternative is a continuous infusion of 1 g in 100 mL 0.89% saline at 5 to 20 mg/kg/h (0.5 to 12 mL/g/h) up to 500 mg/h and titrated to desired response. Maximum adult daily dose is 12 g. Cardiac and blood pressure monitoring are advised during and for several hours after the infusion. The end point is absence of fasciculations and return of muscle strength.

Contraindicated drugs include morphine, aminophylline, barbiturates, opioids, phenothiazine, reserpine-like drugs, parasympathomimetics, and succinylcholine.

Noncardiac pulmonary edema may require respiratory support. Seizures may respond to atropine and pralidoxime chloride but often require anticonvulsants. Cardiac dysrhythmias may require electrical cardioversion or antidysrhythmic therapy if the patient is hemodynamically unstable. Extracorporeal procedures are of no proven value.

Disposition

Asymptomatic patients with normal examination findings after 6 to 8 hours of observation may be discharged. In cases of intentional poisoning, the patients require psychiatric clearance for discharge. Symptomatic patients should be admitted to the intensive care unit. Observation of milder cases of carbamate poisoning, even those requiring atropine, for 6 to 8 hours symptom-free may be sufficient to exclude significant toxicity. In cases of workplace exposure, OSHA should be notified.

PHENCYCLIDINE (ANGEL DUST)

Phencyclidine is an arylcyclohexylamine related to ketamine and chemically related to the phenothiazines. Originally a "dissociative" anesthetic banned in United States since 1979, it is now an illicit substance, with at least 38 analogs. It is inexpensively manufactured by "kitchen chemists" and is mislabeled as other hallucinogens. Improper phencyclidine synthesis may release cyanide when heated or smoked and can cause explosions.

Toxic Mechanism

The mechanism of phencyclidine is complex and not completely understood. It inhibits some neurotransmitters and causes a loss of pain sensation without depressing the CNS respiratory status. It stimulates α-adrenergic receptors and may act as a "false neurotransmitter." The effects are sympathomimetic, cholinergic, and cerebellar.

Toxic Dose

The usual dose of phencyclidine mixed with marijuana joints is 100 to 400 mg of phencyclidine. Joints or leaf mixtures contain 0.24% to 7.9% of PCP, 1 mg of PCP/150 leaves. Tablets contain 5 mg (the usual street dose). CNS effects at doses of 1 to 6 mg include hallucinations and euphoria, 6 to 10 mg produces toxic psychosis and sympathetic stimulation, 10 to 25 mg produces severe toxicity, and more than 100 mg has resulted in fatalities.

Kinetics

Phencyclidine is a lipophilic weak base, with a pKa of 8.5 to 9.5. It is rapidly absorbed when smoked and snorted, poorly absorbed from the acid stomach, and rapidly absorbed from the alkaline middle small intestine. It has an enterogastric secretion and is reabsorbed in the small intestine. The onset of action when smoked is 2 to 5 minutes, with a peak in 15 to 30 minutes. With oral ingestion, the onset is in 30 to 60 minutes and when taken intravenously it is immediate. Most adverse reactions in cases of overdose begin within 1 to 2 hours. Its duration of action at low doses is 4 to 6 hours and normality returns in 24 hours; in large overdoses, fluctuating coma may last 6 to 10 days.

Volume distribution is 6.2 L/kg. Phencyclidine concentrates in brain and adipose tissue. Protein binding is 70%. The route of elimination is by gastric secretion, liver metabolism, and 10% urinary excretion of conjugates and free phencyclidine. Renal excretion may be increased 50% with urinary acidification. The half-life is 1 hour (in cases of overdose, it is 11 to 89 hours).

Manifestations

The classic picture is bursts of horizontal, vertical, and rotary nystagmus, which is a clue to diagnosis (occurs in 50% of cases), miosis, hypertension, and fluctuating altered mental state. There is a wide spectrum of clinical presentations.

Mild intoxication with 1 to 6 mg produces drunken and bizarre behavior, agitation, rotary nystagmus, and blank stare. Violent behavior and sensory anesthesia make these patients insensitive to pain, self-destructive, and dangerous. Most are communicative within 1 to 2 hours, are alert and oriented in 6 to 8 hours, and recover completely in 24 to 48 hours.

Moderate intoxication with 6 to 10 mg produces excess salivation, hypertension, hyperthermia, muscle rigidity, myoclonus, and catatonia. Recovery of consciousness occurs in 24 to 48 hours and complete recovery in 1 week.

Severe intoxication with 10 to 25 mg results in opisthotonus, decerebrate rigidity, convulsions, prolonged fluctuating coma, and respiratory failure. Patients in this category have a high rate of medical complications. Recovery of consciousness occurs in 24 to 48 hours, with complete normality in a month. Medical complications include apnea, aspiration pneumonia, cardiac arrest, hypertensive encephalopathy, hyperthermia, intracerebral hemorrhage, psychosis, rhabdomyolysis and myoglobinuria, and seizures. Loss of memory and "flashbacks" last for months. Phencyclidine-induced depression and suicide have been reported.

Fatalities occur with ingestions of greater than 100 mg and with serum levels greater than 100 to 250 ng/mL.

Laboratory Investigations

Marked elevation of creatine kinase level may occur. Values greater than 20,000 units have been reported. Urinalysis should be monitored and urine tested for myoglobin. One should monitor the blood for creatine kinase, uric acid (an early clue to rhabdomyolysis), BUN, creatinine, electrolytes (hyperkalemia), blood glucose (20% of patients have hypoglycemia), urinary output, liver function tests, ECG, and ABG if the patient has any respiratory manifestations. Measurement of phencyclidine in the gastric juice is called for because concentrations are 10 to 50 times higher than in blood or urine. Phencyclidine blood concentrations are not helpful. Phencyclidine may be detected in the urine of the average user for 10 days to 3 weeks after the last dose. In chronic users, it can be detected for over 1 month. The analogs of phencyclidine may not produce positive test results for phencyclidine in the urine. Cross-reactions with bleach and dextromethorphan may cause false-positive urine test results on immunoassay, and cross-reaction with doxylamine may produce a false-positive finding on gas chromatography.

Management

The patient should be observed for violent, self-destructive, bizarre behavior and paranoid schizophrenia. Patients should be placed in a low sensory environment and dangerous objects should be removed from the area.

Gastrointestinal decontamination is not effective because phencyclidine is rapidly absorbed from intestines. Overtreating the mild intoxication should be avoided. There is insufficient evidence to support the use of MDAC. In cases of severe toxicity (stupor or coma), continuous gastric suction can be tried (with protection of the airway) because the drug is secreted into the gastric juice. The value of this procedure is controversial because of limited data.

The patient must be protected from harming himself or herself or others. Physical restraints may be necessary, but they should be used sparingly and for the shortest time possible because they increase risk of rhabdomyolysis. Metal restraints such as handcuffs should be avoided. For behavioral disorders and toxic psychosis, diazepam is the agent of choice. Pharmacologic intervention includes diazepam (Valium) 10 to 30 mg orally or 2 to 5 mg intravenously initially and titrated upward to 10 mg; however, up to 30 mg may be required. "Talk down" technique is usually ineffective and dangerous. Phenothiazines and butyrophenones should be avoided in the acute phase because they lower the convulsive threshold; however, they may be needed later for psychosis. Haloperidol (Haldol) administration has been reported to produce catatonia.

Seizures and muscle spasm are managed with diazepam, from 2.5 mg up to 10 mg. Hyperthermia (>38.5°C [101.3°F]) is treated with external cooling measures. Hypertension is usually transient and does not require treatment. In the case of emergent hypertensive crisis (blood pressure >200/115 mm Hg) nitroprusside can be used in a dose of 0.3 to 2 µg/kg/min. Maximum infusion rate is 10 µg/kg/min for only 10 minutes.

Acid ion trapping diuresis is not recommended because of the danger of myoglobin precipitation in the renal tubules. Rhabdomyolysis and myoglobinuria are treated by correcting volume depletion and insuring a urinary output of greater than 2 mL/kg/h. Alkalinization is controversial because of reabsorption of phencyclidine.

Hemodialysis is beneficial if renal failure occurs; otherwise, the extracorporeal procedures are not beneficial.

Disposition

All patients with coma, delirium, catatonia, violent behavior, aspiration pneumonia, sustained hypertension greater than 200/115, and significant rhabdomyolysis should be admitted to the intensive care unit until asymptomatic for at least 24 hours. If patients with mild intoxication are mentally and neurologically stable and become asymptomatic (except for nystagmus) for 4 hours, they may be discharged in the company of a responsible adult. All patients must be assessed for suicide risk before discharge. Drug counseling and psychiatric follow-up should be arranged. Patients should be warned that episodes of disorientation and depression may continue intermittently for 4 weeks or more.

PHENOTHIAZINES AND NONPHENOTHIAZINES (NEUROLEPTICS)

Toxic Mechanism

Neuroleptics have complex mechanisms of toxicity, including (a) block of the postsynaptic dopamine receptors; (b) block of peripheral and central α-adrenergic receptors; (c) block of cholinergic muscarinic receptors; (d) quinidine-like antidysrhythmic and myocardial depressant effect in cases of large overdose; (e) lowering of the convulsive threshold; (f) effect on hypothalamic temperature regulation (Table 25).

Toxic Dose

Extrapyramidal reactions, anticholinergic effects, and orthostatic hypotension may occur at therapeutic doses. The toxic amount is not established, but the maximum daily therapeutic dose may result in significant side effects, and twice this amount may be potentially fatal. Chlorpromazine (Thorazine), the prototype, may produce serious hypotension and CNS depression at doses greater than 200 mg (17 mg/kg) in children and 3 to 5 g in an adult. Fatalities have been reported after 2.5 g of loxapine (Loxitane) and mesoridazine (Serentil) and 1.5 g of thioridazine (Mellaril).

Kinetics

These agents are lipophilic and have unpredictable gastrointestinal absorption. Peak levels occur 2 to 6 hours postingestion and have enterohepatic recirculation.

The mean serum half-life in phase 1 is 1 to 2 hours and the biphasic half-life is 20 to 40 hours. Volume distribution is 10 to 40 L/kg; protein binding is 92% to 98%. Chlorpromazine taken orally has an onset of action in 30 to 60 minutes, peak in 2 to 4 hours, and duration of 4 to 6 hours. With sustained-release preparations, the onset is in 30 to 60 minutes and duration is 6 to 12 hours.

Elimination is by hepatic metabolism, which results in multiple metabolites (some are active). Metabolites can be detected in urine months after chronic therapy. Only 1% to 3% is excreted unchanged in the urine.

TABLE 25 Neuroleptics and Properties

Compound	Antipsychotic	Anticholinergic	Extrapyramidal	Hypotensive and Cardiotoxic	Sedative
Phenothiazine					
Aliphatic	1+	3+	2+	2+	3+
Chlorpromazine (Thorazine)					
Promethazine (Phenergan)					
Piperazine	3+	1+	3+	1+	1+
Fluphenazine (Prolixin)					
Perphenazine (Trilafon)					
Prochlorperazine (Compazine)					
Trifluoperazine (Stelazine)					
Piperidine	1+	2+	1+	3+	3+
Mesoridazine (Serentil)					
Thioridazine (Mellaril)					
Nonphenothiazine					
Butyrophenone	3+	1+	3+	1+	1+
Haloperidol (Haldol)					
Dibenzoxazepine	3+	1+	3+	1+	2+
Loxapine (Loxitane)					
Dihydroindolone	3+	1+	3+	1+	1+
Molindone (Moban)					
Thioxanthenes	3+	1+	3+	3+	1+
Thiothixene (Navane)					
Chlorprothixene (Taractan)					

1+ = very low activity; 2+ = moderate activity; 3+ = very high activity.

Manifestations

In cases of phenothiazine overdose, anticholinergic symptoms may be present early but are not life-threatening. Miosis is usually present (80%) if the phenothiazine has strong α-adrenergic blocking effect (e.g., chlorpromazine), but anticholinergic activity mydriasis may occur. Agitation and delirium rapidly progress into coma. Major problems are cardiac toxicity and hypotension. The cardiotoxic effects are seen more commonly with thioridazine and its metabolite mesoridazine. These agents have produced the largest number of fatalities in patients with phenothiazine overdose. Cardiac conduction disturbances include prolonged PR, QRS, and QTc intervals, U- and T-wave abnormalities, and ventricular dysrhythmias, including torsades de pointes. Seizures occur mainly in patients with convulsive disorders or with administration of loxapine. Sudden death in children and adults has been reported.

Idiosyncratic dystonic reactions are most common with the piperidine group. Reactions are not dose-dependent and consist of opisthotonos, torticollis, orolingual dyskinesia, or oculogyric crisis (painful upward gaze). These reactions are more frequent in children and women. Neuroleptic malignant syndrome occurs in patients on chronic therapy and is characterized by hyperthermia, muscle rigidity, autonomic dysfunction, and altered mental state. There is one case reported with acute overdose. The loxapine syndrome consists of seizures, rhabdomyolysis, and renal failure.

Laboratory Investigations

Monitoring should include arterial blood gases, renal and hepatic function, electrolytes, blood glucose, and creatine kinase and myoglobinemia in neuroleptic malignant syndrome. Most of these agents are detected on routine screening. Quantitative serum levels are not useful in management. Cross-reactions with enzyme multiplied immunoassay technique tests occur with cyclic antidepressants. Phenothiazines give false-negative results on pregnancy urine tests using human chorionic gonadotropin as an indicator, and give false-positive results for urine porphyrins, indirect Coombs test, urobilinogen, and amylase.

Management

Vital functions must be established and maintained. All overdose patients require venous access, 12-lead ECG (to measure intervals), cardiac and respiratory monitoring, and seizure precautions. One should monitor core temperature to detect poikilothermic effect. If the patient is comatose, intubation and assisted ventilation may be required, as well as 100% oxygen, intravenous glucose, naloxone (Narcan), and thiamine.

Emesis is not recommended. Activated charcoal can be administered if ingestion was within 1 hour. MDAC has not been proven beneficial. A radiograph of the abdomen may be useful, if the phenothiazine is radiopaque. Haloperidol (Haldol) and trifluoperazine (Stelazine) are most likely to be radiopaque. Whole-bowel irrigation may be useful when a large number of pills are visualized on radiograph or if sustained-release preparations were taken, but whole-bowel irrigation has not been evaluated in patients with phenothiazine overdose.

Convulsions are treated with diazepam or lorazepam (Ativan). Loxapine (Loxitane) overdose may result in status epilepticus. If nondepolarizing neuromuscular blockade is required, pancuronium (Pavulon) or vecuronium (Norcuron) should be used (not succinylcholine [Anectine], which may cause malignant hyperthermia), and EEG should be monitored during paralysis.

Patients with dysrhythmias should be monitored with serial ECGs. Unstable rhythms can be treated with electrical cardioversion. Class 1a antidysrhythmics (procainamide, quinidine, and disopyramide [Norpace]) must be avoided.

Hypokalemia predisposes to dysrhythmias and should be corrected aggressively. Supraventricular tachycardia with hemodynamic instability is treated with electrical cardioversion. The role of adenosine has not been defined. Calcium channel and β-blockers should be avoided.

Prolongation of the QRS interval is treated with sodium bicarbonate 1 to 2 mEq/kg by intravenous bolus over a few minutes. Torsades de pointes is treated with magnesium sulfate IV 20% solution 2 g over 2 to 3 minutes. If there is no response in 10 minutes, the dose is repeated and followed by a continuous infusion of 5 to 10 mg/min or given as an infusion of 50 mg/minute for 2 hours followed by 30 mg/minute for 90 minutes twice a day for several days, as needed. The dose in children is 25 to 50 mg/kg initially and maintenance dose is 30 to 60 mg/kg per 24 hours (0.25 to 0.50 mEq/kg per 24 hours) up to 1000 mg per 24 hours. Serum magnesium levels should be monitored.

To treat ventricular tachydysrhythmias in a stable patient, lidocaine is used. If the patient is unstable, electrical cardioversion is used. Patients with heart block with hemodynamic instability should be managed with temporary cardiac pacing.

Hypotension is treated with the Trendelenburg position and 0.9% saline. If the condition is refractory to treatment or there is a danger of fluid overload, vasopressors are administered. The vasopressor of choice is α-adrenergic agonist norepinephrine (Levophed), titrated to response. Epinephrine and dopamine should not be used because β-receptor stimulation in the presence of α-receptor blockade may provoke dysrhythmias and phenothiazines are antidopaminergic.

Hypothermia and hyperthermia are treated with external warming and cooling measures, respectively. Antipyretic drugs must not be used.

Management of the neuroleptic malignant syndrome includes the following actions:

- Immediately discontinuing the offending agent
- Hyperventilating the patient, using 100% humidified, cooled oxygen at high gas flows (at least 10 L/min) because of rapid breathing
- Administering a benzodiazepine to control convulsions and facilitate cooling measures
- Initiating appropriate mechanical cooling measures, which may include intravenous cold saline (not lactated Ringer's), ice baths, cold lavage of the stomach, bladder, and rectum, and a hypothermic blanket
- Correcting acid-base and electrolyte disturbances and treating significant hyperkalemia with hyperventilation, calcium, sodium bicarbonate, intravenous glucose, and insulin; hemodialysis may be necessary

In addition, dysrhythmias usually respond to correction of the underlying acid-base disturbances and hyperkalemia. If antidysrhythmic agents are required, calcium channel blockers must be avoided because they may precipitate hyperkalemia and cardiovascular collapse. Dantrolene sodium (Dantrium), which is a phenytoin derivative, inhibits calcium release from the sarcoplasmic reticulum and results in decreased muscle contraction. Dantrolene acts peripherally and does not reverse the rigidity or psychomotor disturbances resulting from the central dopamine blockade; it therefore is often used in combination with bromocriptine. Bromocriptine mesylate (Parlodel) acts centrally as a dopamine agonist, as does amantadine hydrochloride (Symmetrel). Bromocriptine and dantrolene have been reported to be successful in combination with cooling and good supportive measures in malignant hyperthermia.

Dosing for these agents is as follows: dantrolene sodium at 2 to 3 mg/kg IV as a bolus, then 1 mg/kg/minute to a maximum of 10 mg/kg or until the tachycardia, rigidity, increased end-tidal CO_2, and temperature elevation are controlled. *Note:* Hepatotoxicity occurs with doses greater than 10 mg/kg. To prevent symptom recurrence, 1 mg/kg should be administered every 6 hours for 24 to 48 hours after the episode. After that time, oral dantrolene can be used at a dose of 1 mg/kg every 6 hours for 24 hours as necessary. The patient should be observed for thrombophlebitis following intravenous dantrolene. It is best administered via a central line. Bromocriptine mesylate at 2.5 to 10 mg orally or via a nasogastric tube, three times a day, should be used in combination with dantrolene.

Idiosyncratic dystonic reaction can be treated with diphenhydramine (Benadryl) 1 to 2 mg/kg/dose intravenously over 5 minutes up to maximum of 50 mg intravenously; a response is noted within 2 to 5 minutes. This can be followed with oral doses for 4 to 6 days to prevent recurrence.

Extracorporeal measures (hemodialysis, hemoperfusion) are not effective in removing these agents.

Disposition

Asymptomatic patients should be observed for at least 6 hours after gastric decontamination. Symptomatic patients with cardiotoxicity, hypotension, and convulsions should be admitted to the intensive care unit and monitored for 48 hours.

SALICYLATES (ACETYLSALICYLIC ACID, SALICYLIC ACID)

Toxic Mechanism

The primary toxic mechanisms include (a) direct stimulation of the medullary chemoreceptor trigger zone and respiratory center; (b) uncoupling oxidative phosphorylation; (c) inhibition of the Krebs cycle enzymes; (d) inhibition of vitamin K dependent and independent clotting factors; (e) alteration of platelet function; and (f) inhibition of prostaglandin synthesis.

Toxic Dose

Acute mild intoxication occurs at a dose of 150 to 200 mg/kg, moderate intoxication at 200 to 300 mg/kg, and severe intoxication at 300 to 500 mg/kg. Acute salicylate plasma concentration greater than 30 mg/dL (usually >40 mg/dL) may be associated with clinical toxicity. Chronic intoxication occurs at ingestions greater than 100 mg/kg/d for more than 2 days because of accumulation kinetics. Methyl salicylate (oil of wintergreen) is the most toxic form of salicylate. A dose of 1 mL of 98% contains 1.4 g of salicylate. Fatalities have occurred with ingestion of 1 teaspoonful in children and 1 ounce in adults. It is found in topical ointments and liniments (18% to 30%).

Kinetics

Acetylsalicylic acid and salicylic acid are weak acids with a pKa of 3.5 and 3.0, respectively. Acetylsalicylic acid is absorbed from the stomach, from the small bowel, and dermally. Onset of action is within 30 minutes. Methyl salicylate and effervescent tablets are absorbed more rapidly. Salicylate plasma concentration is detectable within 15 minutes after ingestion and peaks in 30 to 120 minutes. The peak may be delayed 6 to 12 hours in cases of large overdose, overdose with enteric-coated or sustained-release preparations, and development of concretions. The therapeutic duration of action is 3 to 4 hours but is markedly prolonged in cases of overdose.

Volume distribution is 0.13 L/kg for salicylic acid but increases as the salicylate plasma concentration increases. Protein binding is greater than 90% for salicylic acid at pH 7.4 and a salicylate plasma concentration of 20 to 30 mg/dL, 75% at a salicylate plasma concentration greater than 40 mg/dL, 50% at a salicylate plasma concentration of 70 mg/dL, and 30% at a salicylate plasma concentration of 120 mg/dL.

The half-life for salicylic acid is 3 hours after a 300 mg dose, 6 hours after a 1 g overdose, and greater than 10 hours after a 10-g overdose. Elimination includes Michaelis-Menten hepatic metabolism by three saturable pathways: (a) glycine conjugation to salicyluric acid (75%); (b) glucuronyl transferase to salicyl phenol glucuronide (10%); and (c) salicyl aryl glucuronide (4%). Nonsaturable pathways are hydrolysis to gentisic acid (<1%). Ten percent is excreted unchanged.

Acidosis increases the severity of the intoxication by increasing the non-ionized salicylate that can cross membranes and enter the brain cells. In kidneys, the unionized salicylic acid undergoes glomerular filtration, and the ionized portion undergoes tubular secretion in proximal tubules and passive reabsorption in the distal tubules. Renal excretion of salicylate is enhanced by alkaline urine.

Manifestations

The ingestion of concentrated topical salicylic acid preparations (e.g., wart remover) can cause mucosal caustic injury to the gastrointestinal tract. Occult salicylate overdose should be considered in any patient with unexplained acid-base disturbance.

The manifestations of acute overdose of salicylates are as follows:

Minimal Symptoms

Tinnitus, dizziness, and deafness may occur at high therapeutic salicylate plasma concentrations of 20 to 30 mg/dL. Nausea and vomiting may occur immediately because of local gastric irritation.

Phase I. Mild manifestations occur at 1 to 12 hours after ingestion with a 6-hour salicylate plasma concentration of 45 to 70 mg/dL. Nausea and vomiting followed by hyperventilation are usually present within 3 to 8 hours after acute overdose. Hyperventilation, an increase in both rate (tachypnea) and depth (hyperpnea), is present but it may be subtle. It results in a mild respiratory alkalosis with a serum pH greater than 7.4 and urine pH greater than 6.0. Some patients may have lethargy, vertigo, headache, and confusion. Diaphoresis may be noted.

Phase II. Moderate manifestations occur at 12 to 24 hours after ingestion with a 6-hour salicylate plasma concentration of 70 to 90 mg/dL. Serious metabolic disturbances, including a marked respiratory alkalosis with anion gap metabolic acidosis, dehydration, and urine pH less than 6.0, may occur. Other metabolic disturbances include hypoglycemia or hyperglycemia, hypokalemia, decreased ionized calcium, and increased BUN, creatinine, and lactate. Mental disturbances (confusion, disorientation, hallucinations) may occur. Hypotension and convulsions have been reported.

Phase III. Severe intoxication occurs more than 24 hours after ingestion with a 6-hour salicylate plasma concentration of 90 to 130 mg/dL. In addition to the above clinical findings, coma and seizures develop and indicate severe intoxication. Pulmonary edema may occur. Metabolic disturbances include metabolic acidemia (pH <7.4) and aciduria (pH <6.0). In adults, alkalosis may persist until terminal respiratory failure.

In children younger than 4 years of age, a mixed metabolic acidosis and respiratory alkalosis develop earlier (within 4 to 6 hours) than in adults because children have less respiratory reserve and accumulate lactate and other organic acids. Hypoglycemia is more common in children.

Fatalities occur at 6-hour salicylate plasma concentrations greater than 130 to 150 mg/dL and result from CNS depression, cardiovascular collapse, electrolyte imbalance, and cerebral edema.

Chronic salicylism is more serious than acute intoxication and the 6-hour salicylate plasma concentration does not correlate well with the manifestations in both acute and chronic cases of intoxication. Chronic intoxication usually occurs with therapeutic errors in young children or the elderly with underlying illness, and the diagnosis is delayed because it is not recognized. Noncardiac pulmonary edema is a frequent complication in the elderly. The mortality rate is about 25%. Chronic salicylate poisoning in children may mimic Reye syndrome. It is associated with exaggerated CNS findings (hallucinations, delirium, dementia, memory loss, papilledema, bizarre behavior, agitation, encephalopathy, seizures, and coma). Hemorrhagic manifestations, renal failure, and pulmonary and cerebral edema may occur. The metabolic picture is hypoglycemia and mixed acid-base derangements. A chronic salicylate plasma concentration greater than 60 mg/dL with metabolic acidosis and an altered mental state is very serious.

Laboratory Investigations

All patients with intentional salicylate overdoses should have acetaminophen plasma level measured after 4 hours.

One should continuously monitor ECG, urine output, urine pH, and specific gravity. Every 2 to 4 hours in cases of severe intoxication, salicylate plasma concentration, glucose (in a case of salicylism, CNS hypoglycemia may be present despite normal serum glucose), electrolytes, ionized calcium, magnesium and phosphorous, anion gap, ABGs, and pulse oximeter should be monitored. Daily monitoring of BUN, creatinine, liver function tests, and prothrombin time should take place.

The therapeutic salicylate plasma concentration is less than 10 mg/dL for analgesia and 15 to 30 mg/dL for antiinflammatory effect. Cross-reaction with diflunisal (Dolobid) will give a falsely high salicylate plasma concentration. The Done nomogram is not considered accurate in evaluating acute or chronic salicylate intoxications.

Management

Treatment is based on clinical and metabolic findings, not on salicylate levels. Continuous monitoring of the urine pH is essential for successful alkalinization treatment. One should always obtain an acetaminophen plasma level.

Vital functions must be established and maintained. If the patient is in an altered mental state, glucose, naloxone, and thiamine are administered in standard doses. Depending on the severity, the initial studies include an immediate and a 6-hour postingestion salicylate plasma concentration, ECG and cardiac monitoring, pulse oximeter, urine (analysis, pH, and specific gravity), chest radiograph, ABGs, blood glucose, electrolytes and anion gap calculation, calcium (ionized), magnesium, renal and liver profiles, and prothrombin time. Gastric contents and stool should be tested for occult blood. Bismuth and magnesium salicylate preparations may be radiopaque on radiographs. Consultation with a nephrologist is warranted in cases of moderate, severe, or chronic intoxication.

For gastrointestinal decontamination, activated charcoal is useful (each gram of activated charcoal binds 550 mg of salicylic acid) if a toxic dose was ingested up to 4 hours postingestion. MDAC is not recommended for salicylate intoxication.

Concretions may occur with massive (usually >300 mg/kg) ingestions. If blood levels fail to decline, prompt contrast radiography of the stomach may reveal concretions that have to be removed by repeated lavage, whole-bowel irrigation, endoscopy, or gastrostomy.

Fluids and electrolyte treatment of salicylate poisonings is given in Table 26. For shock, perfusion and vascular volume should be established with 5% dextrose in 0.9% saline, then the treatment can proceed with correction of dehydration and alkalinization.

TABLE 26 Fluid and Electrolyte Treatment of Salicylate Poisoning

Type of Salicylism	Metabolic Disturbance	Blood pH	Urine pH	Hydrating Solution	Amount of NaHCO₃ (mEq/L)	Amount of Potassium (mEq/L)
Mild	Respiratory alkalosis	>7.4	>6.0	5% Dextrose, 0.45% saline	50 (adult) 1 mEq/kg (child)	20
Moderate Chronic Child <4 years	Respiratory alkalosis Metabolic acidosis	>7.4 or <7.4	<6.0	5% Dextrose in water	100 (adult) 1–2 mEq/kg (child)	40
Severe Chronic Child <4 years	Metabolic acidosis Respiratory alkalosis	<7.4	<6.0	5% Dextrose in water	150 (adult) 2 mEq/kg (child)	60
CNS Depressant Co-ingestant	Respiratory acidosis	<7.4	<6.0	5% Dextrose in water	100–150*	60

Modified from Linden CH, Rumack BH: The legitimate analgesics, aspirin and acetaminophen. In Hansen W Jr (ed): Toxic Emergencies. New York, Churchill Livingstone, 1984.
*Correct hypoventilation.

For cases of acute moderate or severe salicylism (see Table 26), adults should receive a bolus of 1 to 2 mEq/kg of sodium bicarbonate (NaHCO$_3$) followed by an infusion of 100 to 150 mEq NaHCO$_3$ added to 500 to 1000 mL of 5% dextrose and administered over 60 minutes. Children should receive a bolus of 1 to 2 mEq/kg of NaHCO$_3$ followed by an infusion of 1 to 2 mEq/kg added to 20 mL/kg of 5% dextrose administered over 60 minutes. Potassium is added after the patient voids. The goal is to achieve a urine output of greater than 2 mL/kg/hr and a urine pH of greater than 8. The initial infusion is followed by subsequent infusions (two to three times normal maintenance) of 200 to 300 mL/h in adults or 10 mL/kg/h in children. If the patient is acidotic and has a serum pH of less than 7.15, an additional 1 to 2 mEq/kg of NaHCO$_3$ is given over 1 to 2 hours; persistent acidosis may require 1 to 2 mEq/kg of bicarbonate every 2 hours. The infusion rate, the amount of bicarbonate, and the electrolytes should be adjusted to correct serum abnormalities and to maintain the targeted urine output and urinary pH. Diuresis is not as important as the alkalinization. Careful monitoring for fluid overload should take place for patients at risk of pulmonary and cerebral edema (e.g., the elderly) and because of inappropriate secretion of the antidiuretic hormone.

In patients with mild intoxication who are not acidotic and have a urine pH greater than 6, 5% dextrose in 0.45% saline should be administered as maintenance to replace ongoing fluid loss. Some toxicologists may consider adding sodium bicarbonate 50 mEq/L or 1 mEq/kg in some cases.

To achieve alkalinization, sodium bicarbonate is administered to produce a serum pH 7.4 to 7.5 and a urine pH greater than 8. Carbonic anhydrase inhibitors (acetazolamide [Diamox]) should not be used. If the patient is acidotic, additional bicarbonate may be required. About 2 mEq/kg raises the blood pH 0.1. In children, alkalinization may be a difficult problem because of the organic acid production and hypokalemia. Hypokalemic and fluid-depleted patients cannot be adequately alkalinized. Alkalinization is usually discontinued in asymptomatic patients with a salicylate plasma concentration less than 30 to 40 mg/dL but is continued in symptomatic patients regardless of the salicylate plasma concentration. A decreased serum bicarbonate but normal or high blood pH indicates respiratory alkalosis predominating over metabolic acidosis, and the bicarbonate should be administered cautiously. An alkalemic pH of 7.40 to 7.50 is not a contraindication to bicarbonate therapy because these patients have a significant base deficit in spite of elevated blood pH.

Potassium is added, 20 to 40 mEq/L, to the infusion after the patient voids. In cases of severe, late, and chronic salicylism, 60 mEq/L of potassium may be needed. When the serum potassium is below 4.0 mEq/L, 10 mEq/L should be added over the first hour. If the patient has hypokalemia less than 3 mEq/L and flat T waves and U waves, 0.25 to 0.5 mEq/kg up to 10 mEq/h is administered. Potassium should be administered under ECG monitoring. Serum potassium is rechecked after each rapidly administered dose. A paradoxical urine acidosis (alkaline serum pH and acid urine pH) indicates that potassium is probably needed.

Convulsions are treated with diazepam or lorazepam, but hypoglycemia, low ionized calcium, cerebral edema, and hemorrhage should first be excluded with a CT scan. If tetany develops, the NaHCO$_3$ therapy is discontinued and calcium gluconate 0.1 to 0.2 mL/kg 10% administered.

Pulmonary edema management consists of fluid restriction, high FiO$_2$, mechanical ventilation, and positive end-expiratory pressure.

Cerebral edema management consists of fluid restriction, elevation of the head, hyperventilation, osmotic diuresis, and administration of dexamethasone. Vitamin K$_1$ is administered parenterally to correct an increased prothrombin time (>20 seconds) and coagulation abnormalities. If the patient has active bleeding, fresh plasma and platelets are administered as needed. Hyperpyrexia is managed by external cooling measures, not antipyretics.

Hemodialysis is the choice for removal of salicylates because it corrects the acid-base, electrolyte, and fluid disturbances as well. The indications for hemodialysis include the following:

- Acute poisoning with salicylate plasma concentration greater than 100 mg/dL without improvement after 6 hours of appropriate therapy
- Chronic poisoning with cardiopulmonary disease and a salicylate plasma concentration as low as 40 mg/dL with refractory acidosis, severe CNS manifestations (coma and seizures), and progressive deterioration, especially in elderly patients
- Impairment of vital organs of elimination
- Clinical deterioration in spite of good supportive care and alkalinization
- Severe refractory acid-base or electrolyte disturbances despite appropriate corrective measures

Disposition

There are limitations of salicylate plasma levels and patients are treated on the basis of clinical and laboratory findings. Patients who are asymptomatic should be monitored for a minimum of 6 hours, and longer if enteric-coated tablets or massive overdose was taken or if there is suspicion of concretions. Those who remain asymptomatic with a salicylate plasma concentration less than 35 mg/dL may be discharged following psychiatric evaluation, if indicated. Chronic salicylate-intoxicated patients with acidosis and an altered mental state should be admitted to the intensive care unit. Patients with acute ingestion and a salicylate plasma concentration less than 60 mg/dL and mild symptoms may be able to be treated in the emergency department. Patients with moderate and severe intoxications should be admitted to the intensive care unit.

SELECTIVE SEROTONIN REUPTAKE INHIBITORS

Selective serotonin reuptake inhibitors (SSRIs) are primarily prescribed as antidepressants. SSRIs include fluoxetine (Prozac), paroxetine (Paxil), and sertraline (Zoloft).

Toxic Mechanism

The SSRIs interfere with the neuron reuptake of serotonin (5-hydroxytryptamine) at the presynaptic ganglia sites in the brain, increasing the activity of serotonin. SSRIs should not be used within 5 weeks of when a MAOI is given, nor should MAOI therapy be initiated or discontinued within 5 weeks of SSRI therapy.

Toxic Dose

The therapeutic oral dose of fluoxetine is 20 to 80 mg/d. No toxicity is seen in children with up to 3.5 mg/kg/dose orally. A fatal dose for adults is 6 g. The therapeutic dose for paroxetine is 20 to 50 mg/d. In 35 adult patients, none developed serious side effects after the ingestion of 10 to 1000 mg, and a study involving 35 children failed to demonstrate serious adverse effects at doses less than 180 mg. The therapeutic dose for sertraline is 50 mg to 200 mg/d. Patients have ingested up to 2.6 g without serious side effects. Overdose involving children who ingested less than 100 mg failed to cause adverse events.

Kinetics

Fluoxetine is well absorbed from the gastrointestinal tract, and has a peak plasma concentration at 6 to 8 hours. Volume distribution is 20 to 42 L/kg; 95% is protein bound. The half-life is 4 days (for the demethylated active metabolite norfluoxetine, the half-life is 7 to 15 days). Elimination is 80% renal. Fluoxetine and other serotonin inhibitors are inhibitors of the cytochrome P450, CYP 2D6 enzyme. Therefore interactions may occur with many other medications, such as antidysrhythmic class IC drugs (quinidine), phenytoin (Dilantin), haloperidol, lithium, tricyclic antidepressants (TCAs), β-blockers, codeine, and carbamazepine (Tegretol).

Paroxetine is almost completely absorbed from the gastrointestinal tract, with a peak in 2 to 8 hours. Protein binding is greater than 90%; volume distribution is 13 L/kg. Paroxetine undergoes extensive first-pass liver metabolism by oxidation and methylation to inactive metabolites. It inhibits the P450 system (see fluoxetine metabolism). The average half-life is 21 hours.

Sertraline peaks in 8 to 12 hours. Its volume distribution is 20 L/kg and protein binding is 98%. The average half-life of sertraline is 26 hours. It is metabolized to form a less-active metabolite, *N*-desmethylsertraline (half-life of 62 to 104 hours).

Manifestations

All SSRIs may cause serotonin syndrome, a potentially life-threatening reaction, if they are administered concurrently with an MAOI. Serotonin syndrome is caused by cerebral serotonergic stimulation and can cause severe hyperthermia, myoclonus, rhabdomyolysis, confusion, tremors, and a variety of psychological disturbances. In addition, cardiovascular complications and extrapyramidal side effects, including akathisia, dyskinesia, and Parkinson-like syndromes may occur. Also, increased suicidal ideation, seizures, sexual disorders, and hematologic disorders (platelet serotonin activity blockade leading to prolonged bleeding times) may develop. Inappropriate secretion of antidiuretic hormone resulting in hyponatremia may occur when SSRIs are administered to the elderly. This effect is usually seen within the first week of therapy.

Overdose effects are similar to the serotonin syndrome.

Laboratory Investigations

One should obtain a complete blood count (CBC), electrolytes, glucose levels, a coagulation profile, liver function tests, creatine kinase level, and an ECG.

Management

There is no specific antidote to SSRI intoxication.

Initial management consists of stabilizing vital functions, including thermoregulation. Supportive therapy and anticipation of potential life-threatening manifestations (hypotension, hyperthermia, seizures, coma, disseminated intravascular coagulation, ventricular tachycardia, and metabolic acidosis), are essential. Vital signs, EEG, creatine kinase, and blood chemistry should be monitored.

Benzodiazepines are administered to prevent and control muscle hyperactivity (diazepam [Valium] for seizures, clonazepam [Klonopin] for myoclonus). If benzodiazepine therapy fails to control muscle activity or seizures, anesthesia or nondepolarizing neuromuscular blockade may be necessary.

Electrolyte abnormalities and acid-base balance should be corrected. Fluids are used to maintain a urine output of greater than 2 mL/kg/h if there is a risk of myoglobinuria.

There are no data to support the use of gastrointestinal decontamination, although activated charcoal may be used if an ingestion has occurred within 1 hour. Hemodialysis and charcoal hemoperfusion are unlikely to be beneficial. Haloperidol (Haldol), phenothiazines, and other highly protein-bound drugs are to be avoided.

Benzodiazepine and cooling therapy can be used for hyperthermia. Serotonin antagonists, such as cyproheptadine (Periactin), may be useful in treating serotonin syndrome, although there are no controlled data. Dantrolene (Dantrium) and bromocriptine (Parlodel) are not recommended and may actually precipitate serotonin syndrome.

Disposition

Cases of ingestions in children up to 5 years of age of less than 180 mg of paroxetine (Paxil), less than 3.5 mg/kg of fluoxetine (Prozac), or less than 100 mg of sertraline (Zoloft) can be observed at home. Symptomatic patients should be admitted to the intensive care unit until asymptomatic for 24 hours. Asymptomatic patients should be observed for 6 hours. All patients should be assessed for risk of suicide before discharge. When taken chronically, SSRIs may increase cholesterol and triglycerides and decrease uric acid, so these test results should be followed.

THEOPHYLLINE

Theophylline (Slo-Phyllin) is a methylxanthine alkaloid similar to caffeine and theobromine. Aminophylline is 80% theophylline.

Theophylline is used in the acute treatment of asthma, pulmonary edema, chronic obstructive pulmonary disease, and neonatal apnea.

Toxic Mechanism

The proposed mechanisms of action include phosphodiesterase inhibition, adenosine receptor antagonism, inhibition of prostaglandins, and increase in serum catecholamines. Theophylline stimulates the central nervous, respiratory, and emetic centers and reduces the seizure threshold. It has positive cardiac inotropic and chronotropic effects, acts as a diuretic, relaxes smooth muscle, and causes peripheral vasodilation but cerebral vasoconstriction. Gastric secretions, gastrointestinal motility, lipolysis, glycogenolysis, and gluconeogenesis are all increased.

Toxic Dose

A single dose of 1 mg/kg produces a theophylline plasma concentration of approximately 2 μg/mL. The therapeutic range usually is 10 to 20 μg/mL. An acute, single dose greater than 10 mg/kg causes mild toxicity, a dose greater than 20 mg/kg causes moderate toxicity, and a dose greater than 50 mg/kg causes serious, possibly fatal toxicity. Fatalities occur at lower doses in patients with chronic toxicity, especially those with risk factors (see *Kinetics*).

Kinetics

The pKa is 9.5. Absorption from the stomach and upper small intestine is complete and rapid, with onset in 30 to 60 minutes. Peak theophylline plasma concentration occurs within 1 to 2 hours after ingestion of liquid preparations, 2 to 4 hours after ingestion of regular tablets, and 7 to 24 hours after ingestion of slow-release formulations. Volume distribution is 0.3 to 0.7 L/kg. Protein binding is 40% to 60% in adults, mainly to albumin (low albumin increases free active theophylline).

Elimination is 90% by hepatic metabolism to an active metabolite, 2-methyl xanthine. The half-life is 3.5 hours in a child and 4 to 6 hours in an adult. The half-life is shorter in smokers and patients taking enzyme-inducing drugs. Only 8% to 10% of the drug is excreted unchanged in the urine.

Risk factors that produce a longer half-life include age younger than 6 months or older than 60 years, use of enzyme-inhibitor drugs (calcium channel blockers, oral contraceptives, cimetidine [Tagamet], ciprofloxacin [Cipro], erythromycin, macrolide antibiotics, isoniazid), illness (persistent fever >38.9°C [>102°F]), viral illness, liver impairment, heart failure, chronic obstructive pulmonary disease, and influenza vaccination.

Manifestations

Acute toxicity generally correlates with blood levels; chronic toxicity does not (Table 27).

In the case of an acute, single, regular-release overdose, vomiting and occasionally hematemesis occur at low theophylline plasma concentrations. CNS stimulation includes restlessness, muscle tremors, and protracted tonic–clonic seizures, but coma is rare. Convulsions are a sign of severe toxicity and usually are preceded by gastrointestinal symptoms (except with sustained-release and chronic intoxications). Cardiovascular disturbances include cardiac dysrhythmias (supraventricular tachycardia) and transient hypertension with mild overdoses, but hypotension and ventricular dysrhythmias with severe intoxications. Rhabdomyolysis and renal failure are occasionally seen. Children tolerate higher serum levels, and cardiac dysrhythmias and seizures occur at theophylline plasma concentrations greater than 100 μg/mL. Possible metabolic disturbances include hyperglycemia, pronounced hypokalemia, hypocalcemia, hypomagnesemia, hypophosphatemia, increased serum amylase, and elevation of uric acid.

Chronic intoxication, defined as multiple doses of theophylline over 24 hours, or cases in which interacting drugs or illness interfere with theophylline metabolism are more serious and difficult to treat. Cardiac dysrhythmias and convulsions may occur at theophylline plasma concentrations of 40 to 60 μg/mL and there is no correlation with TPC. The seizures occur without warning and are protracted

TABLE 27 Theophylline Blood Concentrations and Acute Toxicity

Plasma Concentration (μg/mL)	Toxicity Degree	Manifestations
8–10	None	Bronchodilation
10–20	Mild	Therapeutic range: nausea, vomiting, nervousness, respiratory alkalosis, tachycardia
15–25		35% have mild manifestations of toxicity
20–40	Moderate	Gastrointestinal complaints and central nervous system stimulation
		Transient hypertension, tachypnea, tachycardia; 80% will have some manifestations of toxicity
60–100	Severe	Convulsions, dysrhythmias
		Hypokalemia, hyperglycemia
		Ventricular dysrhythmias, protracted convulsions, hypotension, acid-base abnormalities

Reprinted and modified from Linden CH, Rumack BH. In Toxic Emergencies (Honser W Jr [ed]): The legitimate analgesics, aspirin and acetaminophen, copyright 1984, with permission from Elsevier.

and repetitive and may produce status epilepticus. Vomiting and typical metabolic disturbances do not occur.

Differences with slow-release preparations are that few or no gastrointestinal symptoms occur, peak concentrations and convulsions may be delayed 12 to 24 hours postingestion, and convulsions occur without warning.

Laboratory Investigations

Monitoring includes vital signs, pulse oximeter, ABG, hemoglobin, hematocrit (for gastrointestinal hemorrhage), ECG and cardiac monitor, renal and hepatic function, electrolytes, blood glucose, acid-base balance, and serum albumin. Gastric contents and stools should be tested for occult blood. Samples for theophylline plasma concentration measurement should be drawn within 1 to 2 hours after ingestion of liquid preparations, 2 to 4 hours after ingestion of regular-release formulations, and 4 hours after ingestion of slow-release formulations. One should check the serum albumin level because a decrease in albumin levels may cause manifestations of toxicity despite normal theophylline plasma concentration. A single theophylline plasma concentration reading may be misleading; therefore, theophylline plasma concentration measurement should be repeated every 2 to 4 hours to determine the trend until a declining trend is reached and then monitored every 4 to 6 hours until it is below 20 μg/mL.

Management

Vital functions must be established and maintained. If the patient is in a coma or has convulsions or vomiting, he or she should be intubated immediately. The theophylline plasma concentration is obtained and repeated every 2 to 4 hours to determine peak absorption, and a theophylline bezoar should be considered if the theophylline plasma concentration fails to decline. Consultation with a nephrologist about charcoal hemoperfusion is recommended.

Gastrointestinal decontamination is warranted in the case of an acute overdose, but emesis must not be induced. Activated charcoal is the choice decontamination procedure in a dose of 1 g/kg to all patients, followed with MDAC 0.5 g/kg every 2 to 4 hours until the theophylline plasma concentration is less than 20 μg/mL. MDAC is

effective in treating acute, chronic, and intravenous overdoses. Activated charcoal shortens the half-life of theophylline by about 50% and may be indicated up to 24 hours following ingestion.

Whole-bowel irrigation with polyethylene-electrolyte solution has been recommended for cases of massive overdose, possible concretions, and ingestion of sustained-release preparations. If intractable vomiting occurs, the antiemetic metoclopramide (Reglan) (0.1 mg/kg adult dose), droperidol (Inapsine) (2.5 to 10 mg IV), or ondansetron (Zofran) (8 to 32 mg IV) is administered. Ondansetron, however, inhibits metabolism of theophylline after a few doses.

Convulsions are controlled with lorazepam (Ativan) or diazepam (Valium) and phenobarbital. Phenytoin (Dilantin) is ineffective. The convulsions in patients with chronic intoxication are often refractory and may require, in addition to anticonvulsants, neuromuscular paralyzing agents, sedation, assisted ventilation, and EEG monitoring.

Hypotension is treated with fluids and vasopressors, if necessary. Norepinephrine (Levophed) 0.05 μg/kg/min is preferred as the vasopressor over dopamine.

Supraventricular tachycardia with hemodynamic instability requires cardioversion. Low-dose β-blockers may be used but should not be used in patients with reactive airway disease or hypotension. Adenosine (Adenocard) is ineffective. For ventricular dysrhythmias, electrolyte disturbances should be corrected. Lidocaine is the treatment of choice but has the potential to cause seizures at toxic concentrations. Cardioversion may be needed.

Hematemesis is managed with sucralfate (Carafate) 1 g four times daily and/or Maalox TC 30 mL every 2 hours and blood replacement, if necessary. H_2 antihistamine blockers that are enzyme inhibitors are not used.

Fluid and metabolic disturbances should be corrected. Hyperglycemia does not require insulin therapy. Hypokalemia should be corrected cautiously, as it may be largely an intracellular shift and not total body loss. Usually adding 40 mEq potassium to a liter of fluid will suffice. The serum potassium level must be monitored closely.

Charcoal hemoperfusion is the management of choice for patients with serious intoxications. Hemoperfusion can increase the clearance twofold to threefold over hemodialysis, but hemodialysis can be used if hemoperfusion is not available. Criteria for charcoal hemoperfusion are as follows:

- Life-threatening events such as convulsions or dysrhythmias
- Intractable vomiting refractory to antiemetics
- Acute intoxications with a theophylline plasma concentration greater than 80 μg/mL or greater than 70 μg/mL 4 hours after overdose with a sustained-release formulation and greater than 40 μg/mL in the case of chronic intoxication
- Acute or chronic overdoses with a theophylline plasma concentration greater than 40 μg/mL, especially if the patient has risk factors that lengthen the half-life of the drug (see Kinetics).

Disposition

Patients with mild symptoms and a theophylline plasma concentration less than 20 μg/mL can be treated in emergency department and discharged when asymptomatic for a few hours. Any patient with acute ingestion and a theophylline plasma concentration greater than 35 μg/mL should be admitted to a monitored bed with seizure precautions and suicide precautions, if needed. If neurologic or cardiotoxic effects or a theophylline plasma concentration greater than 50 μg/mL is present, the patient should be admitted to the intensive care unit. A patient with an overdose of a sustained-release preparation, regardless of symptoms or initial theophylline plasma concentration, requires admission, monitoring, activated charcoal, and MDAC. In patients on chronic therapy, toxicity may occur at a lower theophylline plasma concentration, and these patients should not be discharged until they are asymptomatic for several hours.

TRICYCLIC AND CYCLIC ANTIDEPRESSANTS

Historically, tricyclic antidepressants are an important cause of pharmaceutical overdose fatalities. The mortality rate was reduced from 15% in the 1970s to less than 1% in the 1990s because of a better

Generic Name (Trade Name)	Adult Daily Dose (mg)	Therapeutic Range (ng/mL)	Half-Life (hours)	Toxicity*		
				Antichol	CNS	Cardiac
Tertiary Amines						
Amitriptyline (Elavil)	75–300	120–250	31–46	3+	3+	3+
Imipramine (Tofranil)	75–300	125–250	9–24	3+	3+	2+
Doxepin (Sinequan)	75–300	30–150	8–24	3+	3+	2+
Trimipramine (Surmantil)	75–200	10–240	16–18	3+	3+	2+
Secondary Amines						
Nortriptyline (Pamelor)	75–150	50–150	18–93	2+	3+	3+
Desipramine (Norpramin)	75–200	75–160	14–62	1+	3+	3+
Protriptyline (Vivactil)	20–60	70–250	54–198	2+	3+	3+
Newer Cyclic Antidepressants						
Teracyclic			30–60	1+	2+	3+
Maprotiline (Ludiomil)	75–300	—	30–60	1+	2+	3+
Trizolopyridine, a noncyclic, produces less serious cardiac and CNS toxicity						
Trazodone (Desyrel)	50–600	700	4–7	1+	1+	1+
Monocyclic Aminoketones						
Bupropion (Wellbutrin)	200–400	—	8–24	1+	3+	1+
Dibenzazepine						
Clomipramine (Anafranil)	100–250	200–500	21–32	2+	2+	2+
Dibenoxazepine						
Amoxapine (Ascendin)	150–300	200–500	6–10	1+	3+	2+

*Antichol = anticholinergic effect; CNS = central nervous system effect primarily seizures; Cardiac = cardiac effect.
Other drugs with similar structures are cyclobenzaprine, a muscle relaxant (similar to amitriptyline), and carbamazepine, an anticonvulsant (similar to imipramine); however, they cause less cardiac toxicity.

understanding of the pathophysiology of these agents and improvements in management (Table 28).

Toxic Mechanism

The major mechanisms of toxicity of the tricyclic antidepressants are (a) central and peripheral anticholinergic effects; (b) peripheral α-adrenergic blockade; (c) quinidine-like cardiac membrane stabilizing action blockade of the fast inward sodium channels; and (d) inhibition of synaptic neurotransmitter reuptake in the CNS presynaptic neurons. The tetracyclics, monocyclic aminoketones, and dibenzoxazepines possess convulsive activity and less cardiac toxicity in overdose than the older tricyclic antidepressants. Triazolopyridine has less serious cardiac and CNS toxicity.

Toxic Dose

The therapeutic dose of imipramine (Tofranil) is 1.5 to 5 mg/kg; a dose greater than 5 mg/kg may be mildly toxic; 10 to 20 mg/kg may be life threatening, although less than 20 mg/kg has produced few fatalities; greater than 30 mg/kg carries a 30% mortality rate; and at a dose greater than 70 mg/kg, patients rarely survive. In children 375 mg and in adults as little as 500 mg have been fatal. In adults, five times the maximum daily dose is toxic and 10 times is potentially fatal. Although major overdose symptoms are associated with plasma concentrations greater than 1 µg/mL (>1000 ng/mL), plasma tricyclic levels do not correlate well with toxicity; clinical signs and symptoms should guide therapy.

The relative dosage or potency equivalents are as follows: amitriptyline (Elavil) 100 mg = amoxapine (Asendin) 125 mg = desipramine (Norpramin) 75 mg = doxepin (Sinequan) 100 mg = imipramine (Tofranil) 75 mg = maprotiline (Ludiomil) 75 mg = nortriptyline (Pamelor) 50 mg = trazodone (Desyrel) 200 mg. This allows one to determine an equivalent dosage of an agent compared with another (see Table 28).

Kinetics

The tricyclic and cyclic antidepressants are lipophilic. They are rapidly absorbed from the alkaline small intestine, but absorption may be prolonged and delayed in cases of massive overdose owing to anticholinergic action. Onset varies from less than 1 hour (30 to 40 minutes) to, rarely, 12 hours. The peak serum levels are reached in 2 to 8 hours and the peak effect is in 6 hours but may be delayed 12 hours because of erratic absorption. The clinical effects correlate poorly with plasma levels.

Cyclic antidepressants are highly protein-bound to plasma glycoproteins, 98% at a pH 7.5 and 90% at 7.0. Volume distribution is 10 to 50 L/kg. The elimination route is by hepatic metabolism. The tertiary amines are metabolized into active demethylated secondary amine metabolites. The active secondary amine metabolites undergo a 15% enterohepatic recirculation and are metabolized over a period of days into nonactive metabolites. The intestinal bacterial flora may reconstitute the metabolites, which are active.

The half-life varies from 10 hours for imipramine to 81 hours for amitriptyline and 100 hours for nortriptyline. The active metabolites have longer half-lives.

Only 3% of the ingested dose is excreted in the urine unchanged.

Manifestations

There are reports of asymptomatic patients who, upon arrival to an emergency department, suddenly have a seizure, develop hemodynamically unstable dysrhythmias, and die shortly thereafter from ingestion of a tricyclic antidepressant. Most patients with severe toxicity develop symptoms within 1 to 2 hours, but symptoms may be delayed 6 hours after overdose.

Small overdoses produce early anticholinergic effects, agitation, and transient hypertension, which are not life-threatening. Large overdoses produce depression of the CNS and myocardium, convulsions, and hypotension. Death can occur within the first 2 to 6 hours following ingestion.

Some ECG screening tools for predicting cardiac or neurologic toxicity from ingestion of a tricyclic antidepressant have been developed: (a) A QRS greater than 0.10 second may produce seizures, and if greater than 0.16 second, 50% of patients may develop ventricular dysrhythmias (20% of these may be life-threatening) and seizures; (b) a terminal 40 msec of the QRS axis greater than 120 degrees in the right frontal plane may be associated with toxicity; or (c) a large

R wave greater than 3 mm in ECG lead aVR may predispose the patient to toxicity. The quinidine cardiac membrane stabilizing effect produces depression of myocardium, conduction, and ECG changes. The peripheral α-adrenergic blockade produces hypotension.

The secondary amines are metabolized to inactive metabolites. The tetracyclics produce a high incidence of cardiovascular disturbances and seizures. Monocyclic aminoketones produce seizures in doses greater than 600 mg. Dibenzoxazepines produce a syndrome of convulsions, rhabdomyolysis, and renal failure.

Laboratory Investigations

If the patient has altered mental status or ECG abnormalities, ABG, ECG, chest radiograph, blood glucose, serum electrolytes, calcium, magnesium, blood urea nitrogen, and creatinine levels, liver profile, creatine kinase level, urine output, and, in severe cases, hemodynamic monitoring are indicated. Levels of the tricyclic and cyclic antidepressants less than 300 ng/mL are therapeutic; levels greater than 500 ng/mL indicate toxicity, and levels greater than 1000 ng/mL indicate serious poisoning and are associated with QRS widening.

Management

Vital functions must be established and maintained. Even if the patient is asymptomatic, intravenous access should be established, vital signs and neurologic status monitored, and baseline 12-lead ECG and continuous cardiac monitoring obtained for at least 6 hours from admission or 8 to 12 hours postingestion. QRS interval should be measured on a limb lead ECG every 15 minutes for 6 hours postingestion.

For gastrointestinal decontamination, emesis should not be induced and gastric lavage should not be used. Activated charcoal is preferable. If the patient is in an altered mental state, the airway must be protected. Activated charcoal 1 g/kg is recommended up to 1 hour postingestion. Benefit from MDAC has not been demonstrated.

Alkalinization does not control seizures; diazepam or lorazepam should be used. Status epilepticus may require high-dose barbiturates or neuromuscular blockers with intravenous diazepam. If not successful, the patient can be paralyzed with short-term nondepolarizing neuromuscular blockers such as vecuronium (Norcuron), intubation, and assisted ventilation. A bolus of sodium bicarbonate is recommended as an adjunct to correct the acidosis produced by the seizures.

Sodium bicarbonate is administered in a dose of 1 to 2 mEq/kg undiluted as a bolus and repeated twice a few minutes apart, if needed, for "sodium loading" and alkalinization, which may increase protein binding from 90% to 98%. The sodium loading overcomes the sodium channel blockage and is more important than the alkalinization. Indications include (a) a QRS complex greater than 0.12 second, (b) ventricular tachycardia, (c) severe conduction disturbances, (d) metabolic acidosis, (e) coma, and (f) seizures. A continuous infusion of sodium bicarbonate is of limited usefulness for controlling dysrhythmias. Bolus therapy should be used as needed.

Hyperventilation alone has been recommended, but the pH elevation is not as instantaneous and there is compensatory renal excretion of bicarbonate; therefore, we do not recommend it. The combination of hyperventilation and sodium bicarbonate has produced fatal alkalemia and is not recommended. One should monitor serum potassium level (the sudden increase in blood pH can aggravate or precipitate hypokalemia), serum sodium, and ionized calcium levels (hypocalcemia may occur with alkalinization) and blood pH.

Specific cardiovascular complications should be treated as follows: Hypotension is treated with norepinephrine, a predominantly α-adrenergic drug, which is preferred over dopamine. Hypertension that occurs early rarely requires treatment. Sinus tachycardia usually does not require treatment. Supraventricular tachycardia in a patient who is hemodynamically unstable requires synchronized electrical cardioversion, starting at 0.25 to 1.0 watt-second per kg, after sedation. Ventricular tachycardia that persists after alkalinization requires intravenous lidocaine or countershock if the patient is hemodynamically unstable. Ventricular fibrillation should be treated with defibrillation. Torsades de pointes is treated with magnesium sulfate IV 20% solution, 2 g over 2 to 3 minutes, followed by a continuous infusion of 1.5 mL 10% solution or 5 to 10 mg per minute. For the treatment of bradydysrhythmias, atropine is contraindicated because of the anticholinergic activity. Isoproterenol 0.1 μg/kg/minute, used with caution, may produce hypotension. If the patient is hemodynamically unstable, a pacemaker is used.

Extraordinary measures, such as aortic balloon pump and cardiopulmonary bypass, have been successful.

Investigational treatments include FAB fragments specific for tricyclic antidepressant, which have been successful in animals. Prophylactic NaHCO$_3$ to prevent dysrhythmias is also being investigated.

Physostigmine has produced asystole, and flumazenil has produced seizures. Both are contraindicated.

Disposition

A patient with an antidepressant overdose who meets any of the following criteria should be admitted to the intensive care unit for 12 to 24 hours: (a) ECG abnormalities except sinus tachycardia, (b) altered mental state, (c) seizures, (d) respiratory depression, and (e) hypotension. Low-risk patients include those in whom the above symptoms are absent at 6 hours postingestion, those who present with minor transient manifestations such as sinus tachycardia who subsequently become and remain asymptomatic for a 6-hour period, and asymptomatic patients who remain asymptomatic for 6 hours. These patients may be discharged if the ECG remains normal, they have normal bowel sounds, and they undergo psychiatric disposition.

Even if the patient is asymptomatic upon presentation to the health care facility, intravenous access should be established, vital signs and neurologic status monitored, a baseline 12-lead ECG obtained, and cardiac monitoring continued for at least 6 hours. *Caution*: in 25% of fatal cases, the patients were initially alert and awake at presentation. However, in most cases of fatality initially deemed as sudden cardiac death, the patient, upon reexamination, actually had symptoms that were missed.

Children younger than 6 years of age with non-intentional (accidental) exposures to amitriptyline (Elavil), desipramine (Norpramin), doxepin (Sinequan), imipramine (Tofranil), or nortriptyline (Aventyl) in a dose less than 5 mg/kg, who are asymptomatic and have what are deemed reliable caregivers, can be observed at home, with close poison control follow-up for 6 hours. Parents or caregivers should be given instructions regarding signs and symptoms to be alert for. Children who are symptomatic, or who ingested greater than 5 mg/kg, should be referred to the emergency department for monitoring, observation, and activated charcoal treatment.

Appendixes

Reference Intervals for the Interpretation of Laboratory Tests

Method of
Laura J. McCloskey, PhD

Most of the tests performed in a clinical laboratory are quantitative; that is, the amount of a substance present in blood or serum is measured and reported in terms of concentration, activity (e.g., enzyme activity), or counts (e.g., blood cell counts). The laboratory must provide reference intervals to assist the clinician in the interpretation of laboratory results. These reference intervals represent the physiologic quantities of a substance (concentrations, activities, or counts) to be expected in healthy persons. Deviation above or below the reference range may be associated with a disease process, and the severity of the disease process may be associated with the magnitude of the deviation. Unfortunately, a sharp demarcation rarely exists to distinguish between physiologic and pathologic values, and the time of transition between the two is often gradual as the disease process progresses.

Defining Normal Values

The terms "normal" and "abnormal" have been used to describe laboratory values that fall inside and outside the reference range, respectively. Use of these terms is inappropriate because no good definition of normality exists in the clinical sense, and the term "normal" may be confused with the statistical term "gaussian." Reference ranges are established from statistical studies in groups of healthy volunteers. These study subjects must be free of disease, but they may have lifestyles or habits that result in variations in certain laboratory values. Examples of these variables include diet, body mass, exercise, and geographic location. Age and gender can also affect reference values.

When the data from a large cohort of healthy subjects fit a gaussian distribution, the usual statistical approach is to define the reference limits as 2 standard deviations (SD) above and below the mean. By definition, the reference range excludes the 2.5% of the population with the lowest values and the 2.5% with the highest values. Nongaussian distributions are handled by different statistical methods, but the result is similar, in that the reference range is defined by the central 95% of the population. In other words, the probability that a healthy person has a laboratory result falling outside the reference range is 1 in 20. If 12 laboratory tests are performed, the probability that at least one of the results is outside the reference range increases to about 50%, which means that all healthy persons are likely to have a few laboratory results that are unexpected. The clinician must then integrate these data with other clinical information, such as the history and physical examination, to arrive at an appropriate clinical decision.

The reference intervals for many tests (especially enzyme and immunochemical measurements) vary with the method used. Accordingly, each laboratory must establish its own reference intervals that are appropriate for the methods used.

International System of Units

During the 1980s, a concerted effort was made to introduce the International System of Units (Systéme International d'Unités; SI units). The rationale for conversion to SI units is sound. Laboratory data are scientifically more informative when the units are based on molar concentration rather than on mass concentration. For example, the conversion of glucose to lactate and pyruvate or the binding of a drug to albumin is more easily understood in units of molar concentration. Another example is illustrated as follows:

Conventional Units	SI Units
1.0 g of hemoglobin:	4.0 mmol of hemoglobin:
Combines with 1.37 mL of oxygen	Combines with 4.0 mmol of oxygen
Contains 3.4 mg of iron	Contains 4.0 mmol of iron
Forms 34.9 mg of bilirubin	Forms 4.0 mmol of bilirubin

The use of SI units would also enhance the standardization of nomenclature to facilitate global communication of medical and scientific information. The units, symbols, and prefixes used in the international system are shown in Tables 1, 2, and 3.

TABLE 1 Base SI Units

Property	Unit	Symbol
Length	Meter	m
Mass	Kilogram	kg
Amount of substance	Mole	mol
Time	Second	s
Thermodynamic temperature	Kelvin	K
Electrical current	Ampere	A
Luminous intensity	Candela	cd
Catalytic amount	Katal	kat

Abbreviation: SI = International System of Units.

1227

TABLE 2 Derived SI Units and Non-SI Units Retained for Use with SI Units

Property	Unit	Symbol
Area	Square meter	m^2
Volume	Cubic meter	m^3
	Liter	L
Mass	Kilograms per cubic meter	kg/m^3 concentration
	Grams per liter	g/L
Substance concentration	Moles per cubic meter	mol/m^3
		mol/L
Temperature	Degree Celsius	$C = K - 273.15$
Dynamic viscosity	Pascal-second	$Pa\text{-}s = 1\ kg \cdot m^{-1} \cdot s^{-1}$

Abbreviation: SI = International System of Units.

Unfortunately, problems have arisen with the implementation of SI units in the United States. The introduction of this system in 1987 prompted many medical journals to report laboratory values in both SI and conventional units in anticipation of complete conversion to SI units in the early 1990s. The lack of a coordinated effort toward this goal forced a retrenchment on the issue. Physicians continue to think and practice with laboratory results expressed in conventional units, and few, if any, hospitals or clinical laboratories in the United States use SI units exclusively. Complete conversion to SI units is not likely to occur in the foreseeable future, but most medical journals will probably continue to publish both sets of units.

TABLE 3 Standard Prefixes

Prefix	Multiplication Factor	Symbol
yocto	10^{-24}	y
zepto	10^{-21}	z
atto	10^{-18}	a
femto	10^{-15}	f
pico	10^{-12}	p
nano	10^{-9}	n
micro	10^{-6}	μ
milli	10^{-3}	m
centi	10^{-2}	c
deci	10^{-1}	d
deca	10^{1}	da
hecto	10^{2}	h
kilo	10^{3}	k
mega	10^{6}	M
giga	10^{9}	G
tera	10^{12}	T

For this reason, the values in the tables of reference ranges in this appendix are given in both conventional units and SI units.

Tables of Reference Intervals

Some of the values included in the tables that follow have been established by the Clinical Laboratories at the Thomas Jefferson University Hospital in Philadelphia and have not been published elsewhere. Other values have been compiled from the sources cited in the suggested readings. These tables are provided for information and educational purposes only. Laboratory values must always be interpreted in the context of clinical data derived from other sources, including the medical history and physical examination. One must exercise individual judgment when using the information provided in this appendix.

REFERENCES

American Medical Association. Drug evaluations annual. Chicago: American Medical Association; 1994.

Bick RL, editor. Hematology: Clinical and laboratory practice. St Louis: Mosby—Year Book; 1993.

Borer WZ. Selection and use of laboratory tests. In: Tietz NW, Conn RB, Pruden E, editors. Applied laboratory medicine. Philadelphia: WB Saunders; 1992. p. 1–5.

Campion EW. A retreat from SI units. N Engl J Med 1992;327:49.

Friedman RB, Young DS. Effects of disease on clinical laboratory tests. 3rd ed. Washington, DC: American Association for Clinical Chemistry Press; 1997.

Henry JB. Clinical diagnosis and management by laboratory methods. 19th ed. Philadelphia: WB Saunders; 1996.

Hicks JM, Young DS. DORA 97–99: Directory of rare analyses. Washington, DC: American Association for Clinical Chemistry Press; 1997.

Jacob DS, Demott WR, Grady HJ, et al, editors. Laboratory test handbook. 4th ed. Baltimore: Williams & Wilkins; 1996.

Kaplan LA, Pesce AJ. Clinical chemistry: Theory, analysis, and correlation. 3rd ed. St Louis: Mosby—Year Book; 1996.

Kjeldsberg CR, Knight JA. Body fluids: Laboratory examination of amniotic, cerebrospinal, seminal, serous and synovial fluids. 3rd ed. Chicago: ASCP Press; 1993.

Laposata M. SI Unit Conversion Guide. Boston: NEJM Books; 1992.

Scully RE, McNeely WF, Mark EJ, McNeely BU. Normal reference laboratory values. N Engl J Med 1992;327:718–24.

Speicher CE. The right test: A physician's guide to laboratory medicine. 3rd ed. Philadelphia: WB Saunders; 1998.

Tietz NW, editor. Clinical guide to laboratory tests. 3rd ed. Philadelphia: WB Saunders; 1995.

Wallach J. Interpretation of diagnostic tests: A synopsis of laboratory medicine. 6th ed. Boston: Little, Brown; 1996.

Young DS. Effects of Preanalytical variables on clinical laboratory tests. 2nd ed. Washington, DC: American Association for Clinical Chemistry Press; 1997.

Young DS. Effects of drugs on clinical laboratory tests. 4th ed. Washington, DC: American Association for Clinical Chemistry Press; 1995.

Young DS. Determination and validation of reference intervals. Arch Pathol Lab Med 1992;116:704–9.

Young DS. Implementation of SI units for clinical laboratory data. Ann Intern Med 1987;106:114–29.

Reference Intervals* for Hematology

Test	Conventional Units	SI Units
Acid hemolysis (Ham test)	No hemolysis	No hemolysis
Alkaline phosphatase, leukocyte	Total score, 14–100	Total score, 14–100
Cell counts		
Erythrocytes		
Males	4.6–6.2 million/mm^3	4.6–6.2 × 10^{12}/L
Females	4.2–5.4 million/mm^3	4.2–5.4 × 10^{12}/L
Children (varies with age)	4.5–5.1 million/mm^3	4.5–5.1 × 10^{12}/L
Leukocytes, total	4500–11,000/mm^3	4.5–11.0 × 10^9/L
Leukocytes, differential counts*		
Myelocytes	0%	0/L
Band neutrophils	3–5%	150–400 × 10^6/L
Segmented neutrophils	54–62%	3000–5800 × 10^6/L
Lymphocytes	25–33%	1500–3000 × 10^6/L
Monocytes	3–7%	300–500 × 10^6/L
Eosinophils	1–3%	50–250 × 10^6/L
Basophils	0–1%	15–50 × 10^6/L
Platelets	150,000–400,000/mm^3	150–400 × 10^9/L
Reticulocytes	25,000–75,000/mm^3 (0.5%–1.5% of erythrocytes)	25–75 × 10^9/L
Coagulation tests		
Bleeding time (template)	2.75–8.0 min	2.75–8.0 min
Coagulation time (glass tube)	5–15 min	5–15 min
D dimer	<0.5 µg/mL	<0.5 mg/L
Factor VIII and other coagulation factors	50–150% of normal	0.5–1.5 of normal
Fibrin split products (Thrombo-Welco test)	<10 µg/mL	<10 mg/L
Fibrinogen	200–400 mg/dL	2.0–4.0 g/L
Partial thromboplastin time, activated (aPTT)	20–25 s	20–35 s
Prothrombin time (PT)	12.0–14.0 s	12.0–14.0 s
Coombs' test		
Direct	Negative	Negative
Indirect	Negative	Negative
Corpuscular values of erythrocytes		
Mean corpuscular hemoglobin (MCH)	26–34 pg/cell	26–34 pg/cell
Mean corpuscular volume (MCV)	80–96 µm^3	80–96 fL
Mean corpuscular hemoglobin concentration (MCHC)	32–36 g/dL	320–360 g/L
Haptoglobin	20–165 mg/dL	0.20–1.65 g/L
Hematocrit		
Males	40–54 mL/dL	0.40–0.54 g/L
Females	37–47 mL/dL	0.37–0.47 g/L
Newborns	49–54 mL/dL	0.49–0.54 g/L
Children (varies with age)	35–49 mL/dL	0.35–0.49 g/L
Hemoglobin		
Males	13.0–18.0 g/dL	8.1–11.2 mmol/L
Females	12.0–16.0 g/dL	7.4–9.9 mmol/L
Newborns	16.5–19.5 g/dL	10.2–12.1 mmol/L
Children (varies with age)	11.2–16.5 g/dL	7.0–10.2 mmol/L
Hemoglobin, fetal	<1.0 of total	<0.01 of total
Hemoglobin A1c	3–5% of total	0.03–0.05 of total
Hemoglobin A2	1.5–3.0% of total	0.015–0.03 of total
Hemoglobin, plasma	0.0%–5.0 mg/dL	0.0–3.2 µmol/L
Methemoglobin	30%–130 mg/dL	19–80 µmol/L
Erythrocyte sedimentation rate (ESR)		
Westergren		
Males	0–15 mm/h	0–15 mm/h
Females	0–20 mm/h	0–20 mm/h
Wintrobe		
Males	0–5 mm/h	0–5 mm/h
Females	0–15 mm/h	0–15 mm/h

*Conventional units are percentages; SI units are absolute cell counts.
Abbreviation: SI = International System of Units.

Reference Intervals* for Clinical Chemistry (Blood, Serum, and Plasma)

Analyte	Conventional Units	SI Units
Acetoacetate plus acetone		
Qualitative	Negative	Negative
Quantitative	0.3–2.0 mg/dL	30–200 mol/L
Acid phosphatase, serum (thymolphthalein monophosphate substrate)	0.1–0.6 U/L	0.1–0.6 U/L
ACTH (see Corticotropin)		
Alanine aminotransferase (ALT), serum (SGPT)	1–45 U/L	1–45 U/L
Albumin, serum	3.3–5.2 g/dL	33–52 g/L
Aldolase, serum	0.0–7.0 U/L	0.0–7.0 U/L
Aldosterone, plasma		
Standing	5–30 ng/dL	140–830 pmol/L
Recumbent	3–10 ng/dL	80–275 pmol/L
Alkaline, phosphatase (ALP), serum		
Adult	35–150 U/L	35–150 U/L
Adolescent	100–500 U/L	100–500 U/L
Child	100–350 U/L	100–350 U/L
Ammonia nitrogen, plasma	10–50 µmol/L	10–50 µmol/L
Amylase, serum	25–125 U/L	25–125 U/L
Anion gap, serum calculated	8–16 mEq/L	8–16 mmol/L
Ascorbic acid, blood	0.4–1.5 mg/dL	23–85 µmol/L
Aspartate aminotransferase (AST), serum (SGOT)	1–36 U/L	1–36 U/L
Base excess, arterial blood, calculated	0±2 mEq/L	0±2 mmol/L
Bicarbonate		
Venous plasma	23–29 mEq/L	23–29 mmol/L
Arterial blood	21–27 mEq/L	21–27 mmol/L
Bile acids, serum	0.3–3.0 mg/dL	0.8–7.6 mmol/L
Bilirubin, serum		
Conjugated	0.1–0.4 mg/dL	1.7–6.8 µmol/L
Total	0.3–1.1 mg/dL	5.1–19.0 µmol/L
Calcium, serum	8.4–10.6 mg/dL	2.10–2.65 mmol/L
Calcium, ionized, serum	4.25–5.25 mg/dL	1.05–1.30 mmol/L
Carbon dioxide, total, serum or plasma	24–31 mEq/L	24–31 mmol/L
Carbon dioxide tension (Pco_2), blood	35–45 mm Hg	35–45 mm Hg
β-Carotene, serum	60–260 µg/dL	1.1–8.6 µmol/L
Ceruloplasmin, serum	23–44 mg/dL	230–440 mg/L
Chloride, serum or plasma	96–106 mEq/L	96–106 mmol/L
Cholesterol, serum or EDTA plasma		
Desirable range	<200 mg/dL	<5.20 mmol/L
Low-density lipoprotein (LDL) cholesterol	60–180 mg/dL	1.55–4.65 mmol/L
High-density lipoprotein (HDL) cholesterol	30–80 mg/dL	0.80–2.05 mmol/L
Copper	70–140 µg/dL	11–22 µmol/L
Corticotropin (ACTH), plasma, 8 AM	10–80 pg/mL	2–18 pmol/L
Cortisol, plasma		
8:00 AM	6–23 µg/dL	170–630 µmol/L
4:00 PM	3–15 µg/dL	80–410 µmol/L
10:00 PM	<50% of 8:00 AM value	<50% of 8:00 AM value
Creatine, serum		
Males	0.2–0.5 mg/dL	15–40 µmol/L
Females	0.3–0.9 mg/dL	25–70 µmol/L
Creatine kinase (CK), serum		
Males	55–170 U/L	55–170 U/L
Females	30–135 U/L	30–135 U/L
Creatine kinase MB isoenzyme, serum	<5% of total CK activity	<5% of total CK activity
	<5% of ng/mL by immunoassay	<5% of ng/mL by immunoassay
Creatinine, serum	0.6–1.2 mg/dL	50–110 µmol/L
Erythrocytes	145–540 ng/mL	330–120 nmol/L
Estradiol-17β, adult		
Males	10–65 pg/mL	35–240 pmol/L
Females		
Follicular	30–100 pg/mL	110–370 pmol/L
Ovulatory	200–400 pg/mL	730–1470 pmol/L
Luteal	50–140 pg/mL	180–510 pmol/L
Ferritin, serum	20–200 ng/mL	20–200 µg/L
Fibrinogen, plasma	200–400 mg/dL	2.0–4.0 g/L
Folate, serum	3–18 ng/mL	6.8–4.1 nmol/L
Follicle-stimulating hormone (FSH), plasma		
Males	4–25 mU/mL	4–25 U/L
Females, premenopausal	4–30 mU/mL	4–30 U/L
Females, postmenopausal	40–250 mU/mL	40–250 U/L
Gastrin, fasting, serum	0–100 pg/mL	0–100 mg/L
Glucose, fasting, plasma or serum	70–115 mg/dL	3.9–6.4 nmol/L
γ-Glutamyltransferase (GGT), serum	5–40 U/L	5–40 U/L
Growth hormone (hGH), plasma, adult, fasting	0–6 ng/mL	0–6 µg/L
Haptoglobin, serum	20–165 mg/dL	0.20–1.65 g/L

Reference Intervals* for Clinical Chemistry (Blood, Serum, and Plasma)—Cont'd

Analyte	Conventional Units	SI Units
Immunoglobulins, serum (see table, Reference Intervals for Tests of Immunologic Function)		
Iron, serum	75–175 μg/dL	13–31 μmol/L
Iron-binding capacity, serum		
Total	250–410 μg/dL	45–73 μmol/L
Saturation	20–55%	0.20–0.55
Lactate		
Venous whole blood	5.0–20.0 mg/dL	0.6–2.2 mmol/L
Arterial whole blood	5.0–15.0 mg/dL	0.6–1.7 mmol/L
Lactate dehydrogenase (LD), serum	110–220 U/L	110–220 U/L
Lipase, serum	10–140 U/L	10–140 U/L
Lutropin (LH), serum		
Males	1–9 U/L	1–9 U/L
Females		
Follicular phase	2–10 U/L	2–10 U/L
Midcycle peak	15–65 U/L	15–65 U/L
Luteal phase	1–12 U/L	1–12 U/L
Postmenopausal	12–65 U/L	12–65 U/L
Magnesium, serum	1.3–2.1 mg/dL	0.65–1.05 mmol/L
Osmolality	275–295 mOsm/kg water	275–295 mOsm/kg water
Oxygen, blood, arterial, room air		
Partial pressure (PaO_2)	80–100 mm Hg	80–100 mm Hg
Saturation (SaO_2)	95–98%	95–98%
pH, arterial blood	7.35–7.45	7.35–7.45
Phosphate, inorganic, serum		
Adult	3.0–4.5 mg/dL	1.0–1.5 mmol/L
Child	4.0–7.0 mg/dL	1.3–2.3 mmol/L
Potassium		
Serum	3.5–5.0 mEq/L	3.5–5.0 mmol/L
Plasma	3.5–4.5 mEq/L	3.5–4.5 mmol/L
Progesterone, serum, adult		
Males	0.0–0.4 ng/mL	0.0–1.3 mmol/L
Females		
Follicular phase	0.1–1.5 ng/mL	0.3–4.8 mmol/L
Luteal phase	2.5–28.0 ng/mL	8.0–89.0 mmol/L
Prolactin, serum		
Males	1.0–15.0 ng/mL	1.0–15.0 μg/L
Females	1.0–20.0 ng/mL	1.0–20.0 μg/L
Protein, serum, electrophoresis		
Total	6.0–8.0 g/dL	60–80 μg/L
Albumin	3.5–5.5 g/dL	35–55 μg/L
Globulins		
α_1	0.2–0.4 g/dL	2.0–4.0 g/L
α_2	0.5–0.9 g/dL	5.0–9.0 g/L
β	0.6–1.1 g/dL	6.0–11.0 g/L
γ	0.7–1.7 g/dL	7.0–17.0 g/L
Pyruvate, blood	0.3–0.9 mg/dL	0.03–0.10 mmol/L
Rheumatoid factor	0.0–30.0 IU/mL	0.0–30.0 kIU/L
Sodium, serum or plasma	135–145 mEq/L	135–145 mmol/L
Testosterone, plasma		
Men	300–1200 ng/dL	10.4–41.6 nmol/L
Women	20–75 ng/dL	0.7–2.6 nmol/L
Pregnant	40–200 ng/dL	1.4–6.9 nmol/L
Thyroglobulin	3–42 ng/mL	3–42 μg/L
Thyrotropin (hTSH), serum	0.4–4.8 μIU/mL	0.4–4.8 mIU/L
Thyrotropin-releasing hormone (TRH)	5–60 pg/mL	5–60 ng/L
Thyroxine, free (FT_4), serum	0.9–2.1 ng/dL	12–27 pmol/L
Thyroxine (T_4), serum	4.5–12.0 μg/mL	58–154 nmol/L
Thyroxine-binding globulin (TBG)	15.0–34.0 μg/mL	15.0–34.0 mg/L
Transferrin	250–430 mg/dL	2.5–4.3 g/L
Triglycerides, serum, after 12-h fast	40–150 mg/dL	0.4–1.5 g/L
Triiodothyronine (T_3), serum	70–190 ng/dL	1.1–2.9 nmol/L
Triiodothyronine uptake, resin (T_3RU)	25–38%	0.25–0.38
Troponin I	0.05–0.50 ng/mL	0.05–0.50 ng/mL
Urate		
(FT_4) Males	2.5–8.0 mg/dL	150–480 μmol/L
(FT_4) Females	2.2–7.0 mg/dL	130–420 μmol/L
Urea, serum or plasma	24–49 mg/dL	4.0–8.2 nmol/L
Urea nitrogen, serum or plasma	11–23 mg/dL	8.0–16.4 nmol/L
Viscosity, serum	1.1–1.8 cP	1.1–1.8 mPas-s
Vitamin A, serum	20–80 μg/dL	0.70–2.80 μmol/L
Vitamin B_{12}, serum	180–900 pg/mL	133–664 pmol/L

*Reference values can vary depending on the method and sample source used.
Abbreviations: EDTA = ethylenediaminetetraacetic acid; SI = International System of Units.

Reference Intervals for Therapeutic Drug Monitoring (Serum or Plasma)*

Analyte	Therapeutic Range	Toxic Concentrations	Proprietary Analyte Name(s)
Analgesics			
Acetaminophen	10–40 μg/mL	>150 μg/mL	Tylenol, Datril
Salicylate	100–250 μg/mL	>300 μg/mL	Aspirin, Bufferin
Antibiotics			
Amikacin	20–30 μg/mL	Peak >35 μg/mL Trough >10 μg/mL	Amkin
Gentamicin	5–10 μg/mL	Peak >10 μg/mL Trough >2 μg/mL	Garamycin
Tobramycin	5–10 μg/mL	Peak >10 μg/mL Trough >2 μg/mL	Nebcin
Vancomycin	5–35 μg/mL	Peak >40 μg/mL Trough >10 μg/mL	Vancocin
Anticonvulsants			
Carbamazepine	5–12 μg/mL	>15 μg/mL	Tegretol
Ethosuximide	40–100 μg/mL	>250 μg/mL	Zarontin
Phenobarbital	15–40 μg/mL	40–100 ng/mL (varies widely)	Luminal
Phenytoin	10–20 μg/mL	>20 μg/mL	Dilantin
Primidone	5–12 μg/mL	>15 μg/mL	Mysoline
Valproic acid	50–100 μg/mL	>100 μg/mL	Depakene
Antineoplastics and Immunosuppressives			
Cyclosporine A	150–350 ng/mL	>400 ng/mL	Sandimmune
Methotrexate, high-dose, 48 h	Variable	>1 μmol/L, 48 h after dose	
Sirolimus (within 1 h of 2-mg dose)	4.5–14 ng/mL	Variable	Rapamune
Sirolimus (within 1 h of 5-mg dose)	10–28 ng/mL	Variable	Rapamune
Tacrolimus (FK-506), whole blood	3–20 μg/L	>15 μg/L	Prograf
Bronchodilators and Respiratory Stimulants			
Caffeine	3–15 ng/mL	>30 ng/mL	Elixophyllin
Theophylline (aminophylline)	10–20 μg/mL	>30 μg/mL	Quibron
Cardiovascular Drugs			
Amiodarone (obtain specimen more than 8 h after last dose)	1.0–2.0 μg/mL	>2.0 μg/mL	Cordarone
Digoxin (obtain specimen more than 6 h after last dose)	0.8–2.0 ng/mL	>2.4 ng/mL	Lanoxin
Disopyramide	2–5 μg/mL	>7 μg/mL	Norpace
Flecainide	0.2–1.0 μg/mL	>1 μg/mL	Tambocor
Lidocaine	1.5–5.0 μg/mL	>6 μg/mL	Xylocaine
Mexiletine	0.7–2.0 μg/mL	>2 μg/mL	Mexitil
Procainamide	4–10 μg/mL	>12 μg/mL	Pronestyl
Procainamide plus NAPA (N-acetyl procainamide)	8–30 μg/mL	>30 μg/mL	
Propranolol	50–100 ng/mL	Variable	Inderal
Quinidine	2–5 μg/mL	>6 μg/mL	Cardioquin, Quinaglute
Tocainide	4–10 ng/mL	>10 ng/mL	Tonocard
Psychopharmacologic Drugs			
Amitriptyline	120–150 ng/mL	>500 ng/mL	Elavil, Triavil
Bupropion	25–100 ng/mL	Not applicable	Wellbutrin
Desipramine	150–300 ng/mL	>500 ng/mL	Norpramin
Imipramine	125–250 ng/mL	>400 ng/mL	Tofranil
Lithium (obtain specimen 12 h after last dose)	0.6–1.5 mEq/L	>1.5 mEq/L	Lithobid
Nortriptyline	50–150 ng/mL	>500 ng/mL	Aventyl, Pamelor

*Values can vary depending on the method and sample collection device used. Always consult the reference values provided by the laboratory performing the analysis.

Reference Intervals* for Clinical Chemistry (Urine)

Analyte	Conventional Units	SI Units
Acetone and acetoacetate, qualitative	Negative	Negative
Albumin		
Qualitative	Negative	Negative
Quantitative	10–100 mg/24 h	0.15–1.5 µmol/d
Aldosterone	3–20 µg/24 h	8.3–55 nmol/d
δ-Aminolevulinic acid (δ-ALA)	1.3–7.0 mg/24 h	10–53 µmol/d
Amylase	<17 U/h	<17 U/h
Amylase-to-creatinine clearance ratio	0.01–0.04	0.01–0.04
Bilirubin, qualitative	Negative	Negative
Calcium (regular diet)	<250 mg/24 h	<6.3 nmol/d
Catecholamines		
Epinephrine	<10 µg/24 h	<55 nmol/d
Norepinephrine	<100 µg/24 h	<590 nmol/d
Total free catecholamines	4–126 µg/24 h	24–745 nmol/d
Total metanephrines	0.1–1.6 mg/24 h	0.5–8.1 µmol/d
Chloride (varies with intake)	110–250 mEq/24 h	110–250 mmol/d
Copper	0–50 µg/24 h	0.0–0.80 µmol/d
Cortisol, free	10–100 µg/24 h	27.6–276 nmol/d
Creatine		
Males	0–40 mg/24 h	0.0–0.30 mmol/d
Females	0–80 mg/24 h	0.0–0.60 mmol/d
Creatinine	15–25 mg/kg/24 h	0.13–0.22 mmol/kg/d
Creatinine clearance (endogenous)		
Males	110–150 mL/min/1.73 m^2	110–150 mL/min/1.73 m^2
Females	105–132 mL/min/1.73 m^2	105–132 mL/min/1.73 m^2
Cystine or cysteine	Negative	Negative
Dehydroepiandrosterone		
Males	0.2–2.0 mg/24 h	0.7–6.9 µmol/d
Females	0.2–1.8 mg/24 h	0.7–6.2 µmol/d
Estrogens, total		
Males	4–25 µg/24 h	14–90 nmol/d
Females	5–100 µg/24 h	18–360 nmol/d
Glucose (as reducing substance)	<250 mg/24 h	<250 mg/d
Hemoglobin and myoglobin, qualitative	Negative	Negative
Hemogentisic acid, qualitative	Negative	Negative
17-Hydroxycorticosteroids		
Males	3–9 mg/24 h	8.3–25 µmol/d
Females	2–8 mg/24 h	5.5–22 µmol/d
5-Hydroxyindoleacetic acid		
Qualitative	Negative	Negative
Quantitative	2–6 mg/24 h	10–31 µmol/d
17-Ketogenic steroids		
Males	5–23 mg/24 h	17–80 µmol/d
Females	3–15 mg/24 h	10–52 µmol/d
17-Ketosteroids		
Males	8–22 mg/24 h	28–76 µmol/d
Females	6–15 mg/24 h	21–52 µmol/d
Magnesium	6–10 mEq/24 h	3–5 mmol/d
Metanephrines	0.05–1.2 ng/mg creatinine	0.03–0.70 mmol/mmol creatinine
Osmolality	38–1400 mOsm/kg water	38–1400 mOsm/kg water
pH	4.6–8.0	4.6–8.0
Phenylpyruvic acid, qualitative	Negative	Negative
Phosphate	0.4–1.3 g/24 h	13–42 mmol/d
Porphobilinogen		
Qualitative	Negative	Negative
Quantitative	<2 mg/24 h	<9 µmol/d
Porphyrins		
Coproporphyrin	50–250 µg/24 h	77–380 nmol/d
Uroporphyrin	10–30 µg/24 h	12–36 nmol/d
Potassium	25–125 mEq/24 h	25–125 mmol/d
Pregnanediol		
Males	0.0–1.9 mg/24 h	0.0–6.0 µmol/d
Females		
Proliferative phase	0.0–2.6 mg/24 h	0.0–8.0 µmol/d
Luteal phase	2.6–10.6 mg/24 h	8–33 µmol/d
Postmenopausal	0.2–1.0 mg/24 h	0.6–3.1 µmol/d
Pregnanetriol	0.0–2.5 mg/24 h	0.0–7.4 µmol/d
Protein, total		
Qualitative	Negative	Negative
Quantitative	10–150 mg/24 h	10–150 mg/d
Protein-to-creatinine ratio	<0.2	<0.2

Continued

Reference Intervals* for Clinical Chemistry (Urine)—Cont'd

Analyte	Conventional Units	SI Units
Sodium (regular diet)	60–260 mEq/24 h	60–260 mmol/d
Specific gravity		
Random specimen	1.003–1.030	1.003–1.030
24-h collection	1.015–1.025	1.015–1.025
Urate (regular diet)	250–750 mg/24 h	1.5–4.4 mmol/d
Urobilinogen	0.5–4.0 mg/24 h	0.6–6.8 μmol/d
Vanillylmandelic acid (VMA)	1.0–8.0 mg/24 h	5–40 μmol/d

*Values can vary depending on the method used.
Abbreviation: SI = International System of Units.

Reference Intervals for Toxic Substances

Analyte	Conventional Units	SI Units
Arsenic, urine	<130 μg/24 h	<1.7 μmol/d
Bromides, serum, inorganic	<100 mg/dL	<10 mmol/L
Toxic symptoms	140–1000 mg/dL	14–100 mmol/L
Carboxyhemoglobin, blood	Saturation, percent	
Urban environment	<5%	<0.05
Smokers	<12%	<0.12
Symptoms		
Headache	>15%	>0.15
Nausea and vomiting	>25%	>0.25
Potentially lethal	>50%	>0.50
Ethanol, blood	<0.05 mg/dL, <0.005%	<1.0 mmol/L
Intoxication	>100 mg/dL, >0.1%	>22 mmol/L
Marked intoxication	300–400 mg/dL, 0.3%–0.4%	65–87 mmol/L
Alcoholic stupor	400–500 mg/dL, 0.4%–0.5%,	87–109 mmol/L
Coma	>500 mg/dL, >0.5%	>109 mmol/L
Lead, blood		
Adults	<20 μg/dL	<1.0 μmol/L
Children	<10 μg/dL	<0.5 μmol/L
Lead, urine	<80 μg/24 h	<0.4 μmol/d
Mercury, urine	<10 μg/24 h	<150 nmol/d

Abbreviation: SI = International System of Units.

Reference Intervals for Tests Performed on Cerebrospinal Fluid

Test	Conventional Units	SI Units
Cells	<5 mm^3; all mononuclear	<5 × 10^6/L, all mononuclear
Protein electrophoresis	Albumin predominant	Albumin predominant
Glucose	50–75 mg/dL (20 mg/dL less than in serum)	2.8–4.2 mmol/L (1.1 mmol/L less than in serum)
IgG		
Children <14 y	<8% of total protein	<0.08 of total protein
Adults	<14% of total protein	<0.14 of total protein
IgG index	0.3–0.6	0.3–0.6
Oligoclonal banding on electrophoresis	Absent	Absent
Pressure, opening	70–180 mm H$_2$O	70–180 mm H$_2$O
Protein, total	15–45 mg/dL	150–450 mg/L

Abbreviations: Ig = immunoglobulin; SI = International System of Units.

Reference Intervals for Tests of Gastrointestinal Function

Test	Conventional Units
Bentiromide	6-h urinary arylamine excretion >57% excludes pancreatic insufficiency
β-Carotene, serum	60–250 ng/dL
Fecal fat estimation	
Qualitative	No fat globules seen by high-power microscope
Quantitative	<6 g/24 h (>95% coefficient of fat absorption)
Gastric acid output	
Basal	
Males	0.0–10.5 mmol/h
Females	0.0–5.6 mmol/h
Maximum (after histamine or pentagastrin)	
Males	9.0–48.0 mmol/h
Females	6.0–31.0 mmol/h
Ratio: basal/maximum	
Males	0.0–0.31
Females	0.0–0.29
Secretin test, pancreatic fluid	
Volume	>1.8 mL/kg/h
Bicarbonate	>80 mEq/L
D-Xylose absorption test, urine	>20% of ingested dose excreted in 5 h

Reference Intervals for Tests of Immunologic Function

Test	Conventional Units	SI Units
Autoantibodies, Serum, Adult		
Anti-CCP antibody	0–19 U	
Anti-dsDNA antibody	0–40 IU	0–40 IU
Antinuclear antibody	<1:40	
Rheumatoid factor (total IgG, IgA, IgM)	0–30 mg/dL	
Complement, Serum		
C3	85–175 mg/dL	0.85–1.75 g/L
C4	15–45 mg/dL	150–450 mg/L
Total hemolytic (CH50)	150–250 U/mL	150–250 U/mL
Immunoglobulins, Serum, Adult		
IgA	70–310 mg/dL	0.70–3.1 g/L
IgD	0.0–6.0 mg/dL	0.0–60 mg/L
IgE	0.0–430 ng/dL	0.0–430 mg/L
IgG	640–1350 mg/dL	6.4–13.5 g/L
IgM	90–350 mg/dL	0.90–3.5 g/L

Helper-to-suppressor ratio: 0.8–1.8.
Abbreviations: anti-CCP = anticyclic citrullinated peptide; dsDNA = double-stranded DNA; Ig = immunoglobulin; SI = International System of Units.

Reference Intervals for Lymphocyte Subsets, Whole Blood, Heparinized

Antigen(s) Expressed	Cell Type	Percentage	Absolute Cell Count
CD2	E rosette T cells	73–87%	1040–2160
CD3	Total T cells	56–77%	860–1880
CD3 and CD4	Helper-inducer cells	32–54%	550–1190
CD3 and CD8	Suppressor-cytotoxic cells	24–37%	430–1060
CD3 and DR	Activated T cells	5–14%	70–310
CD16 and CD56	Natural killer (NK) cells	8–22%	130–500
CD19	Total B cells	7–17%	140–370

Reference Values for Semen Analysis

Test	Conventional Units	SI Units
Volume	2–5 mL	2–5 mL
Liquefaction	Complete in 15 min	Complete in 15 min
pH	7.2–8.0	7.2–8.0
Leukocytes	Occasional or absent	Occasional or absent
Spermatozoa		
Count	60–150 × 10^6 mL	60–150 × 10^6 mL
Fructose	>150 mg/dL	>8.33 mmol/L
Morphology	80–90% normal forms	>0.80–0.90 normal
Motility	>80% motile	>0.80 motile

Abbreviation: SI = International System of Units.

Toxic Chemical Agents Reference Chart: Symptoms and Treatment

Method of
*James J. James, MD, DrPH, MHA, and
James M. Lyznicki, MS, MPH*

Toxic chemical agents are poisonous vapors, aerosols, gasses, liquids, or solids that have toxic effects on people, animals, or plants. Most of these agents are liquid at room temperature and are disseminated as vapors and aerosols. They may be released as bombs, sprayed from aircraft and boats, or disseminated by other means to intentionally create a hazard to people and the environment. Some of these agents are highly toxic and persistent, features that can render a site uninhabitable and require costly and potentially hazardous decontamination and remediation. Health effects range from irritation and burning of skin and mucous membranes to rapid cardiopulmonary collapse and death.

Efficient deployment of hazardous materials (HazMat) teams is critical to control a chemical agent attack. Although all major cities and emergency medical systems have plans and equipment in place to address this situation, physicians and other health professionals must be aware of principles involved in managing a patient or multiple patients exposed to these agents. Chemical weapon agents have a high potential for secondary contamination from victims to

responders. This requires that medical treatment facilities have clearly defined procedures for handling contaminated casualties, many of whom will transport themselves to the facility. Precautions must be used until thorough decontamination has been performed or the specific chemical agent is identified. Health care professionals must first protect themselves (e.g., by using protective suits, respiratory protection, and chemical-resistant gloves) because secondary contamination with even small amounts of these substances (particularly nerve agents such as VX) may be lethal.

Primary detection of exposure to chemical agents will be based on the signs and symptoms of the potential victim (Table 1). Confirmation of a chemical agent, using detection equipment or laboratory analyses, will take considerable time and will not likely contribute to the early management of mass casualty victims. Several patients presenting with the same symptoms should alert physicians and hospital staff to the possibility of a chemical attack. If a chemical attack occurs, most victims will likely arrive within a short time. This situation differentiates a chemical attack from a biological attack involving infectious microorganisms. Additional diagnostic clues include:

- Unusual temporal or geographic clustering of illness
- Any sudden increase in illness in previously healthy persons
- Sudden increase in nonspecific syndromes (e.g., sudden unexplained weakness in previously healthy persons; dimmed or blurred vision; hypersecretion, inhalation, or burn-like syndrome)

A coordinated communication network is critical for transmitting reliable information from the incident scene to treatment facilities. Any suspicious or confirmed exposure to a chemical weapons agent should be reported to the local health department, local Federal Bureau of Investigations office, and the Centers for Disease Control and Prevention (1-770-488-7100).

TABLE 1   Quick Reference Chart on Chemical Weapon Agents

Chemical Agent	Diagnostic Considerations	Treatment Considerations*
Cyanides Cyanogen chloride (CK) Hydrogen cyanide (AC)	• Symptom onset: rapid, seconds to minutes • Odor: bitter almond, musty, or chlorine-like • Nonspecific hypoxic and hypoxemic symptoms • Binds cellular cytochrome oxidase causing chemical asphyxia • Respiratory: shortness of breath, chest tightness, hyperventilation, respiratory arrest • GI: nausea, vomiting • Cardiovascular: ventricular arrhythmias, hypotension, cardiac arrest, shock • CNS: anxiety, headache, drowsiness, weakness, apnea, convulsions, seizure, coma • CNS effects may be confused with carbon monoxide and hydrogen sulfide poisoning • Metabolic acidosis and increased concentration of venous oxygen (patient also may present with cyanosis) • Laboratory testing: cyanide, thiocyanate, serum lactate levels; venous and arterial partial oxygen pressure	• Immediate treatment of symptomatic patients is critical • Antidote: sodium nitrite and sodium thiosulfate; repeat one-half initial doses of both agents in 30 minutes if there is inadequate clinical response • Amyl nitrate capsules are available for first aid until intravenous access is achieved • Cyanide antidone kits are commercially available • Investigational in the United States, available in Europe: hydroxycobalamin (vitamin B_{12a}) administered with thiosulfate • Activated charcoal[A] for oral exposure • Mechanical ventilation as needed • Circulatory support with crystalloids and vasopressors • Metabolic acidosis corrected with IV sodium bicarbonate • Seizures controlled with benzodiazepines

Incapacitating Agents
Agent 15
3-quinuclidinyl benzilate (BZ)
	• Symptom onset: hours
	  0–4 h: parasympathetic blockade and mild CNS effects
	  4–20 h: stupor with ataxia and hyperthermia
	  20–96 h: full-blown delirium
	  Resolution phase: paranoia, deep sleep, reawakening, crawling, climbing automatisms, eventual reorientation
	• Odorless
	• Competitive inhibitor of acetylcholine muscarinic receptor
	• Mydriasis, blurred vision, dry mouth, dry skin, possible atropine-like flush, initial rise in heart rate, decreased level of consciousness, confusion, disorientation, visual hallucinations, impaired memory
		• Antidote: physostigmine salicylate (Antilirium)[A]
		• Support, intravenous fluids

TABLE 1 Quick Reference Chart on Chemical Weapon Agents—Cont'd

Chemical Agent	Diagnostic Considerations	Treatment Considerations*
Nerve Agents Cyclohexyl sarin (GF) Sarin (GB) Soman (GD) Tabun (GA) VX	• Symptom onset: vapor (seconds), liquid (minutes or hours); symptom onset may be delayed up to 18 hours particularly for localized exposures • Odor: none (GB, VX), fruity (GA), camphor-like (GD) • Most toxic of known chemical agents • Irreversible acetylcholinesterase inhibitors • Eyes: excessive lacrimation, miosis may be present • Respiratory: rhinorrhea, bronchospasm, respiratory failure • GI: hypersalivation, nausea, vomiting, diarrhea • Skin: localized sweating • Cardiac: sinus bradycardia • Skeletal muscles: fasciculations followed by weakness, flaccid paralysis • CNS: loss of consciousness, convulsions, apnea, seizures • May be confused with organophosphate and carbamate pesticide poisoning • Laboratory testing: erythrocyte or serum cholinesterase activity to confirm exposure	• Rapid establishment of patent airway • Antidote: Atropine[A] and pralidoxime[A] chloride (Protopam chloride, 2-PAM); additional doses until bronchial secretions are cleared and ventilation improved • Early administration of 2-PAM is critical to minimize permanent agent inactivation of acetylcholinesterase (i.e., "aging") • Benzodiazepines to control nerve agent-induced seizures • Airway and ventilatory support as needed • Atropine,[A] pralidoxime,[A] and diazepam[A] are available in autoinjector kits through the U.S. military
Pulmonary or Choking Agents Acrolein Ammonia (NH3) Chlorine (CL) Choloropicrin (PS) Diphosgene (DP) Nitrogen oxides (NO$_x$) Perfluoroisobutylene (PFIB) Phosgene (CG) Sulfur dioxide (SO$_2$)	• Symptom onset: rapid or delayed; 1–24 h (rarely up to 72 h) • Odor (CG): freshly mown hay or grass • Easily absorbed via mucous membranes of eyes, nose, oropharynx. Degree of water solubility of the agent influences onset and severity of respiratory injury. • Eye and airway irritation, dyspnea, chest tightness, rhinorrhea, hypersalivation, cough, wheezing • High-dose inhalation may produce laryngospasm, pneumonitis, and acute lung injury with delayed onset ($\leq$48 h) of acute respiratory distress syndrome • Chest radiograph: hyperinflation, noncardiogenic pulmonary edema • May be confused with inhalation exposure to industrial chemicals (e.g., HCl, Cl$_2$, NH$_3$)	• No specific antidote • Supportive measures; specific treatment depends on the agent • IV fluids for hypotension; no diuretics • Ventilation with or without positive airway pressure • Bronchodilators for bronchospasm • Methylprednisolone[A] may be effective in preventing noncardiogenic pulmonary edema
Riot Control Agents Mace (CN) Tear gas (CS)	• Symptom onset: immediate • Odor: apple blossom (CN); pepper (CS) • Metallic taste • SN$_2$ alkylating agents • Burning and pain on mucosal membranes and skin • Eyes: irritation, pain, tearing, blepharospasm • Airways: burning in nose and mouth, respiratory discomfort, bronchospasm (may be delayed 36 h) • Skin: tingling, erythema • Nausea and vomiting common • CN can cause corneal opacification • No specific laboratory tests	• Supportive care • Irrigation as necessary • Persons with asthma, emphysema may need oxygen, inhaled bronchodilators, steroids, assisted ventilation • Lotions, such as calamine,[A] for persistent erythema
Vesicant or Blister Agents	• Symptoms onset: immediate (L, CX); delayed 2–48 h (H, HD) • Primary liquid hazard • May be confused with skin exposure to caustic irritants (e.g., sodium hydroxide, ammonia) • Intracellular enzyme and DNA alkylating agents • Clinical effects dependent on extent and route of exposure; effects may be delayed, appearing hours after exposure	• Immediate decontamination • Supportive care • Thermal burn-type treatment • Symptomatic management of lesions
Sulfur mustard (H) Distilled mustard (HD)	• Odor: garlic, horseradish, or mustard • Skin: erythema and blisters (may be delayed $\leq$8 h), pruritus • Eye: irritation, conjunctivitis, corneal damage, lacrimation, pain, blepharospasm • Respiratory: mild to marked acute airway damage, pneumonitis within 1–3 d, respiratory failure • GI effects (nausea, vomiting diarrhea) may be present	• No specific antidote • Skin: silver sulfadiazine[A] • Eye: homatropine[A] ophthalmic ointment • Pulmonary: antibiotics, bronchodilators, steroids • Colony stimulating factor may be helpful for leukopenia • Systemic analgesic and antipruritics • Early use of positive end-expiratory pressure or continuous positive airway pressure

Continued

TABLE 1 Quick Reference Chart on Chemical Weapon Agents—Cont'd

Chemical Agent	Diagnostic Considerations	Treatment Considerations*
	• Bone marrow stem cell suppression leading to pancytopenia and increased susceptibility to infection • Fever, sputum production • Combination with Lewisite (called mustard-Lewisite or HL) results in rapid effects of Lewisite and delayed effects of mustard agents	• Maintain fluid and electrolyte balance (do not excessively fluid resuscitate as in thermal burns)
Lewisite (L)	• Odor: fruity or geranium • More volatile than mustard • Damages eyes, skin, and airways by direct contact • Skin: gray area of dead skin within 5 min, erythema within 30 min, blistering 2–3 h, immediate irritation or burning pain on contact, severe tissue necrosis • Eye: pain, blepharospasm, conjunctival and lid edema • Airway: pseudomembrane formation, nasal irritation • Intravascular fluid loss, hypovolemia, shock, organ congestion, leukocytosis	• Antidote: British anti-Lewisite (BAL or Dimercaprol)
Phosgene oxime (CX)	• Odor: freshly mown hay • Urticant, nonvesicant agent • Vapor extremely irritating; vapor and liquid cause tissue damage upon contact • Immediate burning, irritation, wheal-like skin lesions, eye and airway damage, conjunctivitis, lacrimation, lid edema, blepharospasm • No distinctive laboratory findings	• No antidote • Parenteral methylprednisolone[A] may be effective in preventing noncardiogenic pulmonary edema • Experimental: aerosolized dexamethasone[A] and theophylline[A] for pulmonary involvement
Vomiting (Arsine-Based) Agents Adamsite (DM) Diphenylchlorarsine (DA) Diphenylcyanoarsine (DC)	• Symptom onset: All rapidly acting within minutes • Odor: none (DA), garlic (DC), burning fireworks (DM) • Primary route of absorption is through respiratory system • Arsine gas depletes erythrocyte glutathione and causes hemolysis • Eyes: conjunctival irritation, tearing, and blepharospasm • Airways: sneezing, mucosal lung irritation, edema, progressive cough, wheezing • Cardiac: tachypnea, tachycardia • GI: intestinal cramps, emesis, diarrhea • Skin: erythema, edema at the site of dermal contact • CNS: depression, syncope • Chest radiograph to rule out chemical pneumonitis	• Supportive care • Monitor for hemolysis • Wheezing or dyspnea; may need albuterol inhalation • Eye irrigation (water, normal saline, lactated Ringer's solution) in patients sustaining ocular exposure • Treat repetitive emesis with IV hydration and antiemetics • Blood transfusion may be required • Exchange transfusion may be required • Hemodialysis may be useful in decreasing arsenic level and treating renal failure

[A]Not FDA approved for this indication.

*Different situations may require different treatment and dosage regimens. Please consult other references as well as a regional poison control conter (1-800-222-1222), medical toxicologist, clinical pharmacologist, or other drug information specialist for definitive dosage information, especially dosages for pregnant women and children.

Abbreviations: CNS = central nervous system; GI = gastrointestinal.

Biologic Agents Reference Chart: Symptoms, Tests, and Treatment

Method of

James J. James, MD, DrPH, MHA, and
James M. Lyznicki, MS, MPH

Biologic weapons are devices used intentionally to cause disease or death through dissemination of microorganisms or toxins in food and water, by insect vectors, or by aerosols. Potential targets include human beings, food crops, livestock, and other resources essential for national security, economy, and defense. Unlike nuclear, chemical, and conventional weapons, the onset of a biological attack will probably be insidious. For some infectious agents, secondary and tertiary transmission may continue for weeks or months after the initial attack.

Initial detection of an unannounced biological attack will likely occur when an astute health professional notices an unusual case or disease cluster and reports his or her concerns to local public health authorities. Physicians and other health professionals should be alert to the following:

- Unusual temporal or geographic clustering of illnesses
- Sudden increase of illness in previously healthy persons
- Sudden increase in non-specific illnesses (e.g., pneumonia, flulike illness; bleeding disorders; unexplained rashes, particularly in adults; neuromuscular illness; diarrhea)

To enhance detection and treatment capabilities, physicians and other health professionals in acute care settings should be familiar with the clinical manifestations, diagnostic techniques, isolation precautions, treatment, and prophylaxis for likely causative agents (e.g., smallpox, pneumonic plague, anthrax, viral hemorrhagic fevers). Table 1 provides a quick summary of diagnostic and treatment considerations for various infectious and toxic biological agents. For some of these agents, delay in medical response could result in a potentially devastating number of casualties. To mitigate such consequences, early identification and intervention are imperative. Frontline physicians must have an increased level of suspicion regarding the possible intentional use of biological agents as well as an increased sensitivity to reporting those suspicious to public health authorities, who, in turn, must be willing to evaluate a predictable increase in false positive reports.

Medical response efforts require coordination and planning with emergency management agencies, law enforcement, health care facilities, and social services agencies. Health care agencies should ensure that physicians know whom to call with reports of suspicious cases and clusters of infectious diseases, and should work to build a good relationship with the local medical community. Resource integration is absolutely necessary to:

- Establish adequate capacity to initiate rapid investigation of an outbreak
- Educate the public
- Begin mass distribution of antibiotics and vaccines
- Ensure mass medical care
- Control public anger and fear

In an epidemic, overwhelming numbers of critically ill patients will require acute and follow-up medical care. Both infected persons and the *worried well* will seek medical attention, with a corresponding need for medical supplies, diagnostic tests, and hospital beds. The impact—or even the threat—of an attack can elicit widespread panic and civil disorder, overwhelm hospital resources, and disrupt social services.

Any suspicious or confirmed exposure to a biological weapons agent should be reported immediately to the local health department, local Federal Bureau of Investigation office, and the Centers of Disease Control and Prevention (1-770-488-7100).

1239

TABLE 1 Quick Reference Chart on Biological Weapon Agents

Disease/Agent	Diagnostic Considerations	Treatment Considerations[1]	Prophylaxis
Bacteria Anthrax *Bacillus anthracis*	Incubation period: 1–5 d (perhaps ≤60 d)[2] *Cutaneous* - Evolving skin lesion (face, neck, arms), progresses to vesicle, dispressed ulcer, and black necrotic lesions - Lethality: 20% if untreated, otherwise rarely fatal *Gastrointestinal* - Nausea, vomiting, abdominal pain, bloody diarrhea, sepsis - Lethality: approaches 100% if untreated but data are limited; rapid, aggressive treatment may reduce mortality *Inhalational* - Abrupt onset of flu-like symptoms, fever with or without chills, sweats, fatigue or malaise, non- or minimally productive cough, nausea, vomiting, dyspnea, headache, chest pain, followed in 2–5 d by severe respiratory distress, mediastinitis, hemorrhagic meningitis, sepsis, shock.[3] - Widened mediastinum on chest radiograph is characteristic for inhalational and occasionally GI anthrax.[4]	Combination therapy of ciprofloxacin (Cipro) or doxycycline (Vibramycin) plus one or two other antimicrobials should be considered with inhalational anthrax[6] Penicillin[A] should be considered if strain is susceptible and does not possess inducible β-lactamases If meningitis suspected, doxycycline (Vibramycin) may be less optimal because of poor CNS penetration Steroids may be considered for severe edema and for meningitis	Ciprofloxacin (Cipro) or doxycycline (Vibramycin) with or without vaccination If strain is susceptible, penicillin[A] or amoxicillin[A] (Amoxil) should be considered Inactivated vaccine (licensed but not readily available); six injections and annual booster

Continued

TABLE 1 Quick Reference Chart on Biological Weapon Agents—Cont'd

Disease/Agent	Diagnostic Considerations	Treatment Considerations[1]	Prophylaxis
	• Lethality: Once respiratory distress develops, mortality rates may approach 90%; begin treatment when inhalational anthrax is suspected; do not wait for confirmatory testing[5] Gram stain and culture of blood, pleural fluid, cerebrospinal fluid, ascitic fluid, vesicular fluid or lesion exudate; sputum rarely positive; confirmatory serological and PCR tests available through public health laboratory network		
Brucellosis B. abortus B. canis B. mellitensis B. suis	Incubation period: 5–60 d (usually 1–2 mo) • Non-specific flu-like symptoms, fever, headache, profound weakness and fatigue, GI symptoms such as anorexia, nausea, vomiting, diarrhea, or constipation • Osteoarticular complications common • Lethality: less than 5% even if untreated; tends to incapacitate rather than kill Blood and bone marrow culture (may require 6 wk to grow *Brucella*); confirmatory culture and serological testing available through public health laboratory network	Doxycycline (Vibramycin) plus streptomycin or rifampin[A] (Rifadin) *Alternative therapies:* Ofloxacin (Floxin)[A] plus rifampin[A] (Rifadin) Doxycycline (Vibramycin) plus gentamicin (Garamycin) TMP/SMX (Bactrim,[A] Septra) plus gentamicin (Garamycin)	Doxycycline (Vibramycin) plus streptomycin or rifampin (Rifadin) No approved human vaccine
Inhalational (Pneumonic) Tularemia *Francisella tularensis*	Incubation period: 3–5 d (range of 1–21 d) • Sudden onset of acute febrile illness, weakness, chills, headache, generalized body aches, elevated WBCs • Pulmonary symptoms such as dry cough, chest pain or tightness with or without objective signs of pneumonia • Progressive weakness, malaise, anorexia, and weight loss occurs, potentially leading to sepsis and organ failure • Largely clinical diagnosis • Lethality: ≈30–60% fatal if untreated Culture of blood, sputum, biopsies, pleural fluid, bronchial washings (culture is difficult and potentially dangerous); confirmatory testing available through public health laboratory network	Streptomycin or gentamicin (Garamycin) *Alternative therapies:* Ciprofloxacin (Cipro)[A] Doxycycline (Vibramycin) Chloramphenicol[A] (Chloromycetin)	Tetracycline Doxycycline (Vibramycin) Ciprofloxacin (Cipro)[A] Live attenuated vaccine (USAMRIID, IND) given by scarification; currently under FDA review, limited availability
Pneumonic Plague *Yersinia pestis*	Incubation period: 1–10 d (typically 2–3 d) • Acute onset of flu-like prodrome: fever, myalgia, weakness, headache; within 24 h of prodrome, chest discomfort, cough with bloody sputum, and dyspnea. By day 2 to 4 of illness, symptoms progressing to cyanosis, respiratory distress, and hemodynamic instability • Lethality: almost 100% if untreated; 20–60% if appropriately treated within 18–24 h of symptoms; begin treatment when diagnosis of plague is suspected; do not wait for confirmatory testing Gram stain and culture of blood, CSF, sputum, lymph node aspirates, bronchial washings; confirmatory serological and bacteriological tests available through public health laboratory network	Streptomycin; gentamicin (Garamycin) *Alternative therapies:* Doxycycline (Vibramycin) Tetracycline Ciprofloxacin[A] (Cipro) Chloramphenicol[A] (Chloromycetin) is first choice for meningitis except for pregnant women	Tetracycline Doxycycline (Vibramycin) Ciprofloxacin[A] (Cipro) Inactivated whole cell vaccine licensed but not readily available; injection with boosters Vaccine not effective against aerosol exposure

TABLE 1 Quick Reference Chart on Biological Weapon Agents—Cont'd

Disease/Agent	Diagnostic Considerations	Treatment Considerations[1]	Prophylaxis
Rickettsia Q-Fever *Coxiella burnetii*	Incubation period: 2–14 d (may be ≤40 days) • Nonspecific febrile disease, chills, cough, weakness and fatigue, pleuritic chest pain, pneumonia possible • Lethality: 1–3%, fatalities are uncommon even if untreated but relapsing symptoms may occur Isolation of organism may be difficult; confirmatory testing via serology or PCR available through public health laboratory network	Tetracycline Doxycycline (Vibramycin)	Tetracycline Doxycycline (Vibramycin) Inactivated whole cell[B] vaccine (IND) Skin test to determine prior exposure to *C. burnetii* recommended before vaccination
Viruses Smallpox Variola major virus	Incubation period: 7–17 d • Prodrome of high fever, malaise, prostration, headache, vomiting, delirium followed in 2–3 d maculopapular rash uniformly progressing to pustules and scabs, mostly on extremities and face • Requires astute clinical evaluation; may be confused with chickenpox, erythema multiforme with bullae, or allergic contact dermatitis • Lethality: 30% in unvaccinated persons Pharyngeal swab, vesicular fluid, biopsies, scab material for electron microscopy and PCR testing through public health laboratory network Notify CDC Poxvirus Section at 1-404-639-2184	Supportive care Cidofovir (Vistide) shown to be effective in vitro and in experimental animals infected with surrogate orthopox virus	Live attenuated vaccinia vaccine derived from calf lymph; given by scarification (licensed, restricted supply) New vaccine being developed from tissue culture Vaccination given within 3–4 d following exposure can prevent or decrease the severity of disease
Viral Encephalitis Eastern (EEE) Western (WEE) Venezuelan (VEE)	Incubation period: 2–6 d (VEE); 7–14 d (EEE, WEE) • Systemic febrile illness, with encephalitis developing in some populations • Generalized malaise, spiking fevers, headache, myalgia • Incidence of seizures and/or focal neurologic deficits may be higher after biological attack • White blood cell count may show striking leukopenia and lymphopenia • Clinical and epidemiologic diagnosis • Lethality: <10% (VEE); 10% (VVEE); 50–75% (EEE) Confirmatory test and viral isolation available through public health laboratory network	Supportive care Analgesics, anticonvulsants as needed	Several IND vaccines, poorly immunogenic, highly reactogenic
Viral Hemorrhagic Fevers (VHFs) Arenaviruses (Lassa, Junin, and related viruses) Bunyaviruses (Hanta, Congo-Crimean, Rift Valley) Filoviruses (Ebola, Marburg) Flaviviruses (yellow fever, dengue, various tick-borne disease viruses)	Incubation period: 4–21 d • Fever with mucous membrane bleeding, petechiae, thrombocytopenia, and hypotension in patients without underlying malignancies • Malaise, myalgias, headache, vomiting, diarrhea possible • Lethality: Variable depending on viral strain; 15–25% with Lassa fever to ≤90% with Ebola Confirmatory testing and viral isolation available through public health laboratory network Call CDC Special Pathogens Office at 1-404-639-1115	Supportive therapy Ribavirin (Virazole) A may be effective for Lassa fever, Rift Valley fever, Argentine hemorrhagic fever, and Congo-Crimean hemorrhagic fever	Ribavarin (Virazole)[A] is suggested for Congo-Crimean hemorrhagic fever and Lassa fever Yellow fever vaccine is the only licensed vaccine available Vaccines for some of the other VHFs exist but are for investigational use only

Continued

TABLE 1 Quick Reference Chart on Biological Weapon Agents—Cont'd

Disease/Agent	Diagnostic Considerations	Treatment Considerations[1]	Prophylaxis
Biological Toxins Botulism *Clostridium botulinum* toxin	Symptom onset: 1–5 d (typically 12–36 h) • Blurred vision, diploplia, dry mouth, ptosis, fatigue • As disease progresses, acute bilateral descending flaccid paralysis, respiratory paralysis resulting in death • Clinical diagnosis • Lethality: 60% without ventilatory support Serum and stool should be assayed for toxin by mouse neutralization bioassay, which may require several days	Intensive and prolonged supportive care; ventilation may be necessary Trivalent equine antitoxin (serotypes A, B, E, – licensed, available from the CDC) should be administered immediately after clinical diagnosis Anaphylaxis and serum sickness are potential complications of antitoxin Aminoglycosides and clindamycin (Cleocin) A must not be used	Pentavalent toxoid (A–E), yearly booster (IND, CDC) Not available to the public Antitoxin may be sufficient to prevent illness following exposure but is not recommended until patient is showing symptoms
Enterotoxin B *Staphylococcus aureus*	Symptom onset: 3–12 h • Acute onset of fever, chills headache, nonproductive cough • Normal chest radiograph • Clinical diagnosis • Lethality: probably low (few data available for respiratory exposure) Serology on acute and convalescent serum can confirm diagnosis	Supportive care	No vaccine available
Ricin Toxin *Ricinus communis*	Symptom onset: ≤6–24 h • Weakness, nausea, chest tightness, fever, cough, pulmonary edema, respiratory failure, circulatory collapse, hypoxemia resulting in death (usually within 36–72 h) • Clinical and epidemiological diagnosis • Lethality: mortality data not available but is likely to be high with extensive exposure Confirmatory serological testing available through public health laboratory network	Supportive care Treatment for pulmonary edema Gastric decontamination if toxin ingested	No vaccine available
T-2 Mycotoxins *Fusarium* *Myrothecium* *Trichoderma* *Stachybotrys* Other filamentous fungi	Symptom onset: minutes to hours • Abrupt onset of mucocutaneous and airway irritation and pain • May include skin, eyes, and GI tract; systemic toxicity may follow • Lethality: severe exposure can cause death in hours to days Consult with local health department regarding specimen collection and diagnostic testing procedures; confirmation requires testing blood, tissue, and environmental samples	Clinical support Soap and water washing within 4–6 h reduces dermal toxicity; washing within 1 h may eliminate toxicity entirely	No vaccine available

Adapted from *Biological Weapons: Quick Reference Guide.* American Medical Association; 2002. Available at http://www.amaassn.org/ama1/pub/upload/mm/415/quickreference0902.pdf.

[A] Not FDA approved for this indication.
[B] Not available in the United States.
[1] Different situations may require different dosage and treatment regimens. Please consult other references and an infectious disease specialist for definitive dosage information, especially dosages for pregnant women and children.
[2] Data from 22 patients infected with anthrax in October and November 2001 indicate a median incubation period of 4 d (range 4–7 d) for inhalational anthrax and a mean incubation of 5 d (range 1–10 d) for cutaneous anthrax.
[3] Limited data from the October/November 2001 anthrax infections indicate hemorrhagic pleural effusions to be strongly associated with inhalational anthrax; rhinorrhea was present in only 1/10 patients.
[4] Chest radiograph abnormalities include paratracheal and hilar fullness and may be subtle. Consider chest computed tomography if diagnosis is uncertain.
[5] Limited data from the 2001 terrorist-related anthrax infections indicate that early treatment significantly decreased the mortality rate.
[6] Other agents with in vitro activity suggested for use in conjunction with ciprofloxacin (Cipro) or doxycycline (Vibramycin) for treatment of inhalational anthrax include rifampin (Rifadin), vancomycin (Vancocin), imipenem (Primaxin), chloramphenicol (Chloromycetin), penicillin and ampicillin, clindamycin (Cleocin), and clarithromycin (Biaxin).
Abbreviations: CDC = Centers for Disease Control and Prevention; CNS = central nervous system; CSF = cerebrospinal fluid; GI = gastrointestinal; IND = investigational new drug; PCR = polymerase chain reaction; TMP-SMX = trimethoprim-sulfamethoxazole; USAMRIID, U.S. Army Medical Research Institute of Infectious Diseases; WBC = white blood cell.

Popular Herbs and Nutritional Supplements

Method of
Miriam M. Chan, BSc Pharm, PharmD

Popular Herbs and Nutritional Supplements

Herb or Nutritional Supplement	Common Uses	Reasonable Adult Oral Dosage*	Precautions and Drug Interactions
Aloe vera	Commonly found in skin products as a moisturizer Used topically to treat burns, wounds, skin infections, and inflammation Approved in Germany to use orally as a laxative Used orally for a variety of conditions, including diabetes, asthma, epilepsy, and osteoarthritis	For external use, apply aloe gel on the skin tid to qid For constipation, 40-170 mg of dried aloe juice or latex (corresponds to 10-30 mg hydroxyanthracene derivatives) taken in the evening For other conditions, no established dosage is documented	Aloe gel is generally well tolerated when used orally and topically Aloe gel taken orally can cause hypoglycemia in patients who are concomitantly taking antidiabetic drugs Aloe juice or latex contains anthraquinone, a cathartic laxative, and should not be taken by people with intestinal obstruction, acute intestinal inflammation, and ulcers Pregnant women should not take aloe latex because it can cause uterine contractions Oral use of aloe latex can cause abdominal cramps and diarrhea. Long-term use or abuse can cause electrolyte imbalances, albuminuria, hematuria, and pseudomelanosis coli. Prolonged use of high doses ($\geq$1 g/d) can cause nephritis, acute renal failure, and death In 2002, the FDA banned the sale of aloe-containing laxative products in the United States owing to the lack of safety data Aloe latex can reduce drug absorption of some drugs due to decreased GI transit time Aloe can decrease platelet aggregation and should be avoided at least 2 wk before surgery
Bilberry fruit	Often used orally to improve visual acuity and to treat degenerative retinal conditions Used orally to treat chronic venous insufficiency, varicose veins, and hemorrhoids Approved in Germany to use orally for acute diarrhea and topically for mild inflammation of the mucous membranes of mouth and throat	For eye conditions and circulation, 80-160 mg tid of the extract standardized to at least 25% anthocyanosides For diarrhea, 20-60 g/d of the dried, ripe berries or as a tea preparation (5-10 g of crushed dried berries in 150 mL water, brought to a boil for 10 min, then strained) For external use, 10% decoction	No known side effects reported with bilberry fruit and extract However, bilberry leaf taken in large quantities or used long-term has been shown to cause wasting, anemia, jaundice, acute excitation, disturbances of tonus, and death in animals The anthocyanidin extracts from bilberry can increase the risk of bleeding in those taking warfarin or other blood thinners
Black cohosh root	Commonly used to relieve hot flushes and other menopausal symptoms Used to treat premenstrual discomfort and dysmenorrhea	20 mg bid of the rhizome extract standardized to triterpene glycosides The German guidelines do not recommend its use for >6 mo	Black cohosh can have an estrogen-like effect and should be avoided in women with breast cancer Large doses can induce miscarriage and it is contraindicated during pregnancy It can cause GI disturbances, headache, and hypotension International case reports of liver dysfunction suspected to be associated with its use
Black haw	To relieve uterine cramps and painful periods To prevent miscarriage and ease pain that follows childbirth	For menstrual pain, 5 mL of tincture in water, taken 3-5 times daily For prevention of miscarriage, 1-2 cups of tea per day (1 tsp of dried herb in 1 cup of boiling water, steeped for 10 min)	Black haw should not be used in pregnancy because of its uterine relaxant effects The salicylate constituent in black haw could trigger allergic reactions in persons with aspirin allergies or asthma Black haw can aggravate tinnitus Large doses of black haw can prolong bleeding time

Continued

Herb or Nutritional Supplement	Common Uses	Reasonable Adult Oral Dosage*	Precautions and Drug Interactions
			The oxalic acid component of black haw can increase kidney stone formation in susceptible persons Black haw can interact with warfarin and increase risk of bleeding
Cat's claw	Used primarily to reduce pain in osteoarthritis and rheumatoid arthritis Used for a variety of health conditions, including viral infections (e.g., herpes, HIV), Alzheimer's disease, and cancer Used to support the immune system and promote kidney health Used to prevent and abort pregnancy	For osteoarthritis, 100 mg/d of the dry encapsulated extract For rheumatoid arthritis, 20 mg tid of the dry extract standardized to 1.3% pentacyclic oxindole alkaloids free of tetracyclic oxindole alkaloids For general uses, 1-3 cups of tea per day (1 g root bark boiled for 15 min in 250 mL of water) or 1 mL of tincture 2-3×/d	Avoid using cat's claw during pregnancy or breast-feeding People with autoimmune diseases and transplant recipients should avoid cat's claw owing to its immune-stimulating effects Side effects include headaches, dizziness, and vomiting Cat's claw can lower blood pressure and cause hypotension when used with antihypertensive drugs Cat's claw can inhibit CYP3A4 and increase levels of drugs metabolized by this enzyme
Chamomile flower	Used orally to calm nerves and treat GI spasms and inflammatory diseases of the GI tract Used topically to treat wounds, skin infections, and skin or mucous membrane inflammation	1 cup of freshly made tea 3 or 4 times daily (1 Tbsp or 3 g of dried flower in 150 mL boiling water for 5-10 min)	Chamomile can cause an allergic reaction, especially in people with severe allergies to ragweed or other members of the daisy family (e.g., echinacea, feverfew, milk thistle) It should not be taken concurrently with other sedatives, such as alcohol or benzodiazepines
Chaste tree berry (Chasteberry, Vitex)	For normalizing irregular menstrual periods and relieving premenstrual complaints For relieving menopausal symptoms For restoring fertility in women For treating acne associated with menstrual cycles For increasing breast milk production in lactating women	For menstrual irregularities and premenstrual complaints, 30-40 mg/d of the dried berries or an equivalent amount of aqueous-alcoholic extracts (50%-70% v/v) Dried fruit extract, standardized to 0.6% agnusides, is used in doses of 175-225 mg/d For other conditions, no established dosage documented	Chaste tree berry can have uterine-stimulant properties and should be avoided in pregnancy Women with hormone-dependent conditions (e.g., breast, uterine, and ovarian cancers; endometriosis; uterine fibroids) and men with prostate cancer should avoid chaste tree berry because it contains progestins Side effects include intermenstrual bleeding, dry mouth, headache, nausea, rash, alopecia, and tachycardia High doses (≥480 mg/d extract) can paradoxically decrease lactation Chaste tree berry is thought to have dopaminergic effects and can interact with dopamine antagonists, such as antipsychotics and metoclopramide Chaste tree berry can decrease the effects of oral contraceptives and hormone replacement therapy
Chondroitin	Orally, often used in combination with glucosamine for osteoarthritis Topically, in combination with sodium hyaluronate, as a viscoelastic agent in cataract surgery	Oral: 200-400 mg tid	Occasional mild side effects include nausea, indigestion, and allergic reactions Chondroitin derived from bovine cartilage carries a potential risk of contamination with diseased animals
Chromium	For diabetes For hypercholesterolemia Commonly found in weight-loss products Also promoted for body building	For diabetes, 100 µg bid for ≤4 mo or 500 µg bid for 2 mo For hypercholesterolemia, 200 µg tid or 500 µg bid for 2-4 mo For body building, 200-400 µg/d Chromium picolinate has been used in most studies, even though the chloride form is also available	Adverse effects are rare, but they include headaches, insomnia, sleep disturbances, irritability, and mood changes. Some patients also experience cognitive, perceptual, and motor dysfunction Long-term use of high doses (600-2400 µg/d) can cause anemia, thrombocytopenia, hemolysis, hepatic dysfunction, and renal failure Interstitial nephritis has been reported A few studies suggest that chromium can cause DNA damage Chromium competes with iron for binding to transferrin and can cause iron deficiency Antacids, H_2 blockers, and PPIs can decrease the absorption of chromium
Coenzyme Q10	As adjunctive treatment for congestive heart failure,	For heart failure, 100 mg/d in two or three divided doses For angina, 50 mg tid	Mild adverse events include gastric distress, nausea, vomiting, and hypotension

Herb or Nutritional Supplement	Common Uses	Reasonable Adult Oral Dosage*	Precautions and Drug Interactions
	angina, hypertension, and diabetes Used for reducing cardiotoxicity associated with doxorubicin Used to treat statin-induced myopathy	For hypertension, 60 mg bid For diabetes, 100-200 mg/d	Doses >300 mg/d can cause elevated liver enzyme levels Coenzyme Q10 can reduce the anticoagulation effects of warfarin Oral hypoglycemic agents and HMG-CoA reductase inhibitors can reduce serum coenzyme Q10 levels
Cranberry	To prevent and treat UTIs or *Helicobacter pylori* infections that can lead to stomach ulcers To prevent dental plaque As an antioxidant to prevent cardiovascular disease and cancer	For UTIs, 150-600 mL of cranberry juice daily or 300-400 mg of standardized extract bid For other conditions, no dosage determined	Drinking excessive amounts of juice could cause GI upset or diarrhea Prolonged use of cranberry juice in large doses increases the risk of kidney stone formation owing to its high oxalate content Cranberry can interact with warfarin and cause an increase in INR The effectiveness of PPIs may be reduced by cranberry owing to its acidity
Creatine	To enhance muscle performance, especially during short-duration, high-intensity exercise	Loading dose of 20 g/d for 5-7 d followed by a maintenance dose of ≥2 g/d An alternative dosing of 3 g/d for 28 d has been suggested	Creatine can cause gastroenteritis, diarrhea, heat intolerance, muscle cramps, and elevated serum creatinine levels Creatine is contraindicated in patients taking diuretics Concurrent use with cimetidine, probenecid, or nonsteroidal anti-inflammatory drugs increases the risk of adverse renal effects Caffeine can decrease creatine's ergogenic effects
Dehydroepi-androsterone (DHEA)	Replace low serum DHEA levels in adrenal insufficiency Treat SLE Reverse aging Used in many other conditions, including Alzheimer's disease, depression, diabetes, menopause, osteoporosis, impotence, and AIDS Used to promote weight loss Used by bodybuilders to increase muscle mass	For replacement therapy, 25-50 mg/d For SLE, 200 mg/d For antiaging and osteoporosis, 50 mg/d For other conditions, no established dosage documented	Most-common side effects are androgenic and include acne, hair loss, hirsutism, and deepening of the voice Cases of hepatitis have been reported When used in high doses, DHEA can cause insomnia, manic symptoms, and palpitations DHEA at physiologic doses increases circulating androgens in women but not in men; it also increases circulating estrogens in men and women Avoid use of DHEA in persons with a history of sex hormone–dependent malignancy Safety of DHEA in persons <30 y unknown DHEA inhibits CYP3A4 and could increase serum concentrations of drugs metabolized by this enzyme (e.g., lovastatin, ketoconazole, itraconzaole, and triazolam)
Dong quai root	Commonly used for the relief of premenstrual and menopausal symptoms Used as a "blood tonic" and a strengthening treatment for the heart, spleen, liver, and kidneys	For premenstrual and menopausal symptoms, 3-4 g/d in three divided doses For other conditions, no established dosage documented	Dong quai should not be used in pregnant women owing to its uterine stimulant and relaxant effects Women with hormone-sensitive conditions (e.g., breast, uterine, and ovarian cancers; endometriosis; uterine fibroids) should avoid dong quai because of its estrogenic effects Drinking the essential oil of dong quai is not recommended because it contains a small amount of carcinogenic constituents Dong quai contains psoralens that can cause photosensitivity and photodermatitis Dong quai contains natural coumarin derivatives that can increase the risk of bleeding in those who are taking anticoagulant or antiplatelet drugs
Echinacea	As an immune stimulant, particularly for the prevention and treatment of the common cold and influenza Supportive therapy for lower urinary tract infections	300 mg tid of *Echinacea pallida* root or 2-3 mL tid of expressed juice of *Echinace purpurea* herb	Echinacea should not be used in transplant patients and those with autoimmune disease or liver dysfunction Allergic reactions have been reported Adverse events are rare and include mild GI effects

Continued

Popular Herbs and Nutritional Supplements—Cont'd

Herb or Nutritional Supplement	Common Uses	Reasonable Adult Oral Dosage*	Precautions and Drug Interactions
	Used topically to treat skin disorders and promote wound healing	Do not use for >8 wk because echinacea can suppress immunity if used long term	It should be discontinued as far in advance of surgery as possible Echinacea can decrease effectiveness of immunosuppressants
Ephedra (ma huang)	For diseases of the respiratory tract with mild bronchospasm Promoted for weight loss and performance enhancement	1 tsp or 2 g of dried herb (15-30 mg of ephedrine) in 240 mL boiling water for 10 min In Canada, the maximum allowable dosage of ephedrine is 8 mg per dose or 32 mg/d	Ephedra contains ephedrine, which has sympathomimetic activities; consequently, it should not be used in patients who have cardiovascular disease, diabetes, glaucoma, hypertension, hyperthyroidism, prostate enlargement, psychiatric disorders, or seizures Serious adverse effects, including seizures, arrhythmias, heart attack, stroke, and death, have been associated with the use of ephedra; as a result, the FDA has banned the sale of ephedra products in the United States Because of the cardiovascular effects of ephedrine, patients taking ephedra should discontinue use at least 24 h before surgery Concurrent use of ephedra and digitalis, guanethidine, MAOIs, or other stimulants, including caffeine, is not recommended
Evening primrose oil	For PMS, especially if mastalgia is present For treatment of atopic eczema Used for other medical conditions, including rheumatoid arthritis, menopausal symptoms, Raynaud's phenomenon, Sjögren's syndrome, and diabetic neuropathy	For PMS, 2-4 g/d For atopic eczema, 6-8 g/d For rheumatoid arthritis, 2.8 g/d These doses are based on products standardized to 9% γ-linolenic acid Daily dose can be given in divided doses	Evening primrose oil can increase the risk of pregnancy complications Side effects include indigestion, nausea, soft stools, and headache Seizures have been reported in patients with schizophrenia who were taking phenothiazines and evening primrose oil concomitantly Evening primrose oil can interact with anesthesia and cause seizures Concomitant use of evening primrose oil with anticoagulant and antiplatelet drugs can increase the risk of bleeding
Fenugreek seed	For diabetes and hypercholesterolemia For constipation, dyspepsia, gastritis, and kidney ailments Approved in Germany for oral use for loss of appetite and topical use as a poultice for local inflammation	For loss of appetite, 1-2 g of the seed tid or 1 cup of tea (500 mg seed in 150 mL cold water for 3 h) several times a day Maximum 6 g/d For other conditions, no established dosage documented For topical use, 50 g powdered seed in 250 mL of hot water to form a paste	Fenugreek can cause uterine contractions and should be avoided in pregnancy Persons who have allergies to peanuts or soybeans might also be allergic to fenugreek Fenugreek can cause diarrhea and flatulence; it can also make the urine smell like maple syrup Hypoglycemia can occur if fenugreek is taken in large amounts Repeated external applications can result in undesirable skin reactions Fenugreek contains small amounts of coumarins and can interact with anticoagulants and antiplatelet drugs High mucilage content of fenugreek can affect the absorption of oral drugs; therefore, fenugreek should not be taken within 2 h of other drugs
Feverfew	For migraine headache prophylaxis For treatment of fever, menstrual problems, and arthritis	25-75 mg bid of the encapsulated dried leaf extract standardized to 0.2% parthenolide	Feverfew can induce menstrual bleeding and is contraindicated in pregnancy Fresh leaves can cause oral ulcers and GI irritation Sudden discontinuation of feverfew can precipitate rebound headache Feverfew can interact with anticoagulants and potentiate the antiplatelet effect of aspirin
Fish oils (omega-3 fatty acids)	Commonly used in the treatment of hypertriglyceridemia Used to prevent CHD and stroke	For hypertriglyceridemia, 3-5 g/d For cardioprotection, 1 g/d for patients with CHD; oily fish at least twice a week, or about 0.5 g/d for people with no known heart disease	Common side effects include fishy aftertaste, GI disturbances, belching, halitosis, and heartburn. High doses can cause nausea and loose stools Doses >3 g/d can inhibit platelet aggregation, suppress immune function,

Herb or Nutritional Supplement	Common Uses	Reasonable Adult Oral Dosage*	Precautions and Drug Interactions
	Used in many noncardiac conditions, including depression, diabetes, dysmenorrhea, rheumatoid arthritis, and IgA nephropathy Used to reduce the risk of developing age-related maculopathy, Alzheimer's disease, and cancer Promotes visual and mental development in children	For other conditions, no established dosage documented Fish oils are composed of EPA and DHA. Fish oil capsules vary widely in amounts and ratios of EPA and DHA. The most common fish oil capsules in the United States provide 180 mg of EPA and 120 mg DHA per capsule, and three capsules provide about 1 g/d of omega-3 fatty acids	worsen glycemic control, and raise LDL cholesterol levels Long-term use may be associated with weight gain Less well-controlled preparations can contain appreciable amounts of organochloride contaminants Fish oil can increase the risk of bleeding in patients taking warfarin, an antiplatelet agent, or herbs that have antiplatelet constituents (e.g., garlic, ginkgo, red clover) Fish oils can lower blood pressure and can have additive effects with antihypertensive agents Oral contraceptives can interfere with the triglyceride-lowering effects of fish oils
Flaxseed	Orally, approved in Germany for chronic constipation, irritable bowel, and other colon disorders Often used orally for hypercholesterolemia and atherosclerosis Topically, approved in Germany for painful skin inflammation	For constipation, 1 tbsp (5 g) of whole or "bruised" seeds (not ground) in 150 mL of liquid 2-3 times daily For bowel inflammation, soak 2-3 tbsp of milled flaxseed soaked in 200-300 mL water and strain after 30 min For hypercholesterolemia, 1-2 tbsp flaxseed oil daily Topical: 30-50 g flaxseed flour as poultice or compress for a moist-heat direct application to the skin	Flaxseed should be taken with plenty of water to prevent possible intestinal blockage Patients with ileus should not take flaxseed High mucilage content of flaxseed can delay absorption of other drugs taken at the same time
Garlic	To lower blood pressure and serum cholesterol To prevent atherosclerosis	Fresh clove: one 4-g clove per day Tablet: 300 mg bid to tid standardized to 0.6%-1.3% allicin	Intake of large quantities can lead to stomach complaints Garlic has antiplatelet effects, so patients should discontinue use of garlic at least 7 d before surgery Concomitant use of garlic and anticoagulants can increase the risk of bleeding
Ginger root	As an antiemetic For prevention of motion sickness	Fresh rhizome: 2-4 g/d Powdered ginger: 250 mg 3 to 4 times daily Tea: 1 cup of tea tid (0.5-1 g dried root in 150 mL boiling water for 5-10 min)	Ginger should not be used by patients with gallstones because of its cholagogic effect It can inhibit platelet aggregation; cases of postoperative bleeding have been reported Large doses of ginger can increase bleeding time in patients taking antiplatelet agents
Ginkgo biloba leaf	To slow cognitive deterioration in dementia To increase peripheral blood flow in claudication To treat sexual dysfunction associated with the use of SSRIs	60-120 mg bid of extract Egb761 standardized to 24% flavonoids and 6% terpenoids	Adverse effects are rare and can include mild stomach or intestinal upset, headache, or allergic skin reaction Ginkgo can inhibit platelet aggregation; reports of spontaneous bleeding have been published Patients should discontinue ginkgo at least 36 h before surgery Concurrent use of ginkgo and anticoagulants, antiplatelet agents, vitamin E, or garlic can increase the risk of bleeding
Ginseng root	As a tonic during times of stress, fatigue, disability, and convalescence To improve physical performance and stamina	Root: 1-2 g/d Tablet: 100 mg bid of extract standardized to 4%-7% ginsenosides A 2- to 3-week period of using ginseng followed by a 1- to 2-week rest period is generally recommended Ginseng is commonly adulterated, especially Siberian ginseng (eleuthero) products	Ginseng has a mild stimulant effect and should be avoided in patients with cardiovascular disease Tachycardia and hypertension can occur Overdosages can lead to ginseng abuse syndrome, characterized by insomnia, hypotonia, and edema Ginseng has estrogenic effects and can cause vaginal bleeding and breast tenderness Ginseng has been shown to inhibit platelets, so patients should discontinue ginseng use at least 7 d before surgery

Continued

Popular Herbs and Nutritional Supplements—Cont'd

Herb or Nutritional Supplement	Common Uses	Reasonable Adult Oral Dosage*	Precautions and Drug Interactions
			Ginseng should not be used with other stimulants Patients taking antidiabetic agents and ginseng should be monitored to avoid the hypoglycemic effects of ginseng Ginseng can interact with warfarin and cause a decreased INR Siberian ginseng can increase digoxin levels Ginseng can interact with phenelzine (an MAOI), resulting in insomnia, headache, tremulousness, and mania-like symptoms
Glucosamine	For osteoarthritis	500 mg tid with meals Glucosamine is available in the form of sulfate, hydrochloride, or N-acetyl salt Glucosamine sulfate is the form that has been used in most clinical studies	Side effects are generally limited to mild GI symptoms, including stomach upset, heartburn, diarrhea, nausea, and indigestion Glucosamine derived from marine exoskeletons may cause reactions in people allergic to shellfish Glucosamine may raise blood glucose level in patients with diabetes
Goldenseal	Often combined with echinacea to treat colds and other upper respiratory infections Used for diarrhea, dyspepsia, and gastritis Used topically as an eyewash, mouthwash, feminine cleansing product, and skin remedy	Oral: 0.5-1 g of the dried rhizome/root or 2-4 mL tincture (1:10, 60% ethanol) or 0.3-1 mL fluid extract (1:1, 60% ethanol) tid Eyewash: For trachoma infections, 2 drops of a 0.2% aqueous berberine solution tid × 3 wk	Avoid using goldenseal during pregnancy and breast feeding; berberine, the principal constituent in goldenseal, can cause uterine contractions and neonatal jaundice Avoid using goldenseal in kidney failure owing to inadequate urinary excretion of its alkaloids High dosages or long-term use can lead to nausea, vomiting, headache, hypotension, bradycardia, leucopenia, and mucosal irritation Berberine can increase the risk of bleeding in patients taking warfarin or an antiplatelet agent Be aware that other herbs containing berberine, including Chinese goldthread and Oregon grape, are sometimes substituted for goldenseal
Grape seed	For conditions related to the heart and blood vessels, such as atherosclerosis, high blood pressure, high cholesterol, and poor circulation For vision problems, diabetic neuropathy or retinopathy, and swelling after an injury or surgery For cancer prevention and wound healing	For general health purposes, 100-300 mg daily of a standardized extract (95% oligomeric proanthocanidin complexes)	Side effects include headache, dizziness, nausea, and dry, itchy scalp Concomitant use with warfarin or antiplatelet agents can increase risk of bleeding owing to the tocopherol content of grape seed oil
Hawthorn leaf with flower	Commonly used in Germany to increase cardiac output in patients with New York Heart Association stage I and II heart failure	160-900 mg water-ethanol extract (30-169 mg procyanidins or 3.5-19.8 mg flavonoids) divided into 2-3 doses	Side effects include GI upset, palpitations, hypotension, headache, dizziness, and insomnia Concomitant use with CNS depressants can have additive CNS effects Hawthorn can potentiate effects of digoxin and vasodilators
Hops	For mood disturbances such as restlessness and anxiety For sleep disturbances Commonly found in combination products with other herbal sedatives	0.5 g of cut or powdered strobile in a single dose; can be taken as tea (0.5 g in 150 mL water), fluidextract 1:1 (0.5 mL), tincture 1:5 (2.5 mL), or dry extract 6-8:1 (60-80 mg) The preparation contains at least 0.35% (v/w) essential oil	Side effects are rare but include drowsiness and allergic reactions Hops is not recommended for use during pregnancy and lactation It can potentiate the sedative effect of CNS depressants (e.g., benzodiazepines, alcohol) and other herbal tranquilizers
Horse chestnut seed	To relieve symptoms of chronic venous insufficiency	250 mg bid of extract standardized to 50 mg aescin in delayed-release form Unsafe to ingest the raw seed, which contains significant amounts of the most toxic constituent, esculin	Mild GI symptoms, headache, dizziness, and pruritus have been reported Ingestion of high doses can cause renal, hepatic, and hematologic toxicity Concomitant use with anticoagulants can increase the risk of bleeding Horse chestnut can potentiate the effects of hypoglycemic drugs

Herb or Nutritional Supplement	Common Uses	Reasonable Adult Oral Dosage*	Precautions and Drug Interactions
Kava kava	As an anxiolytic for nervous anxiety, stress, and restlessness As a sedative to induce sleep	Herb and preparations equivalent to 60-120 mg/d of kava pyrones Most clinical trials have used 100 mg tid of extract standardized to 70% kava pyrones for anxiety disorders	Kava should not be used by patients with depression Kava should be avoided in pregnant or nursing women Kava can affect motor reflexes and judgment, so it should not be taken while driving or operating heavy machinery Accommodative disturbances have been reported; kava can exacerbate Parkinson's disease Extended use can cause a temporary yellow discoloration of skin, hair, and nails Reports have linked kava use to at least 25 cases of severe liver toxicity; sale of products containing kava has been banned in Canada and several European countries Kava has been shown to have additive CNS depressant effects with benzodiazepines, alcohol, and herbal tranquilizers Kava can potentiate the sedative effects of anesthetics, so kava should be discontinued at least 24 h before surgery
Lutein	Commonly used to prevent AMD and cataracts Used to prevent skin cancer, breast cancer, and colon cancer Used to protect against cardiovascular disease	For AMD and cataracts, 6-20 mg/d of lutein from diet For other uses, no established dosage is documented Foods containing high concentrations of lutein include kale, spinach, broccoli, and romaine lettuce Not known if supplemental lutein is as effective as natural lutein Supplemental lutein in the form of esters might require a higher fat intake for effective absorption than purified lutein	No major adverse effects and drug interactions have been reported
Lycopene	Commonly used to prevent and treat prostate cancer Used for cancer prevention, arthrosclerosis prevention, and reduction of asthma symptoms	For decreasing the growth of prostate cancer, 15 mg supplement bid For prostate cancer prevention, at least 6 mg/d from tomato products (or ≥10 servings/wk) For other uses, no established dosage documented Heat processing converts lycopene in fresh tomatoes from the *trans* to the *cis* configuration. The *cis* isomer has better bioavailability Lycopene supplements usually do not specify the type and amount of isomers in their product labeling	Lycopene, when consumed in amounts found in foods, is generally considered to be safe Concomitant ingestion of β-carotene can increase lycopene absorption Lycopene may reduce cholesterol levels and potentiate the effects of statins
Melatonin	For jet lag, insomnia, shift-work disorder, and circadian rhythm disorders For other medical conditions, including depression, multiple sclerosis, tinnitus, headache, and cancer	For jet lag, 5 mg at bedtime for 2-5 d beginning the day of return For sleep disorders, 0.3-5 mg taken 2 h before bedtime Avoid melatonin from animal pineal gland owing to possibility of contamination	Avoid use in pregnancy because melatonin decreases serum luteinizing hormone concentrations and increases serum prolactin levels The common adverse reactions include headache, transient depressive symptoms, daytime fatigue and drowsiness, dizziness, abdominal cramps, irritability, and reduced alertness Concomitant use of melatonin with alcohol, benzodiazepines, or other CNS depressants can cause additive sedation Melatonin can affect immune function and interfere with immunosuppressive therapy Concomitant use with other herbs that have sedative properties (e.g., chamomile, goldenseal, hops, kava, valerian) can produce additive CNS-impairing effects

Continued

Herb or Nutritional Supplement	Common Uses	Reasonable Adult Oral Dosage*	Precautions and Drug Interactions
Milk thistle fruit	As a hepatoprotectant and antioxidant, particularly for treatment of hepatitis, cirrhosis, and toxic liver damage Used in Europe to treat hepatotoxic mushroom poisoning from *Amanita phalloides*	Average daily dose is 12-15 g of crude drug or formulations equivalent to 200-400 mg of silymarin	Adverse effects are rare but include diarrhea and allergic reactions Milk thistle can potentiate the hypoglycemic effect of antidiabetic agents
Probiotics	Prevent and treat antibiotic-associated diarrhea and acute infectious diarrhea Relieve symptoms of irritable bowel syndrome Treat atopic dermatitis for at-risk infants	Dosage varies based on preparations *Lactobacillus* sp., *Bifidobacterium* sp., *Saccharomyces boulardii* are the most widely used organisms For *Lactobacillus* sp., 10 billion CFU/d For *Lactobacillus* sp./ *Bifidobacterium* sp., 100 million to 35 billion CFU/d For *Saccharomyces boulardii*, 250-500 mg/d Quality of products varies among brands Refrigeration is required to maintain potency	Avoid use in short-gut syndrome and severe immunocompromised condition Common adverse effects include flatulence, mild abdominal discomfort, and rarely septicemia
Red clover flower	Commonly used for conditions associated with menopause, such as hot flushes, cardiovascular health, and osteoporosis Used for PMS, benign prostate hyperplasia, and cancer prevention Used topically to treat psoriasis, eczema, and other rashes	For hot flushes, 40 mg/d of the isoflavones extract (Promensil™) For other conditions, no established dosage documented	Red clover has estrogenic activity and should be avoided during pregnancy and lactation Women with hormone-dependent conditions (e.g., breast, uterine, and ovarian cancer, and endometriosis and uterine fibroids) and men with prostate cancer should also avoid taking red clover Side effects include headache, myalgia, nausea, and rash Red clover contains coumarin derivatives and can increase the risk of bleeding in those who are taking anticoagulants or antiplatelet drugs Preliminary report suggests that red clover might antagonize the effects of tamoxifen Some evidence suggests that red clover can increase the levels of drugs metabolized by the CYP3A4 isoenzyme (e.g., lovastatin, ketoconazole, itraconzaole, fexofenadine, and triazolam)
SAMe (*S*-adenosyl-L-methionine)	For treatment of osteoarthritis, depression, fibromyalgia, and liver disease	For osteoarthritis, 200 mg tid For depression and fibromyalgia, 800 mg bid For liver disease, 600-800 mg bid	Common side effects include flatulence, nausea, vomiting, and diarrhea SAMe can cause anxiety in people with depression and hypomania in people with bipolar disorder Concurrent use of SAMe and other antidepressants can cause serotonin syndrome
Saw palmetto berry	To treat symptomatic benign prostatic hyperplasia and irritable bladder	160 mg bid of extract standardized to 85%-95% fatty acids and sterols	Adverse effects are rare but include headache, nausea, and upset stomach High doses can cause diarrhea
Soy	Commonly used for cholesterol reduction in combination with a low-fat diet Used for menopausal symptoms and for prevention of osteoporosis and cardiovascular disease in postmenopausal women	For lowering cholesterol, 25-50 g/d of soy protein For hot flushes, 20-60 g/d of soy protein For osteoporosis, 40 g/d of soy protein containing 90 mg isoflavones	Soy, when consumed as whole foods (e.g., tofu or soy milk), has minimal adverse effects Consumption of large amounts soy can cause gastric complaints such as constipation, bloating, and nausea Long-term use of soy tablets containing isoflavones (150 mg/d for 5 y) have been shown to cause endometrial hyperplasia
St. John's wort	To treat mild to moderate depression Can have antiinflammatory and antiinfective activities	300 mg tid of hypericum extract standardized to 0.3% hypericin	St. John's wort should not be used in pregnancy Side effects include dry mouth, GI upset, dizziness, fatigue, and constipation

Herb or Nutritional Supplement	Common Uses	Reasonable Adult Oral Dosage*	Precautions and Drug Interactions
			St. John's wort can induce photosensitivity, especially in fair-skinned persons It can cause serotonin syndrome if used with other antidepressants, including SSRIs, or other serotoninergic drugs It has been shown to induce CYP3A4 and decrease blood levels of many drugs such as indinavir, nevirapine, cyclosporine, digoxin, theophylline, simvastatin, oral contraceptive pills, and warfarin St. John's wort should be discontinued at least 5 d before surgery to avoid any potential drug interactions
Stinging nettle root	Approved in Germany for difficulty in urination in BPH stage 1 and 2	4-6 g/day of cut root May be taken as tea (1.5 g in 150 mL boiling water for 10-20 min, tid), fluid extract 1:1 (1.5 mL tid), tincture 1:5 (5-7.5 mL tid), or dry extract 5.4-6.6:1 (0.22-0.33 g tid)	Occasionally, mild GI upsets occur No known interactions with drugs
Valerian root	Used as a mild sedative for insomnia and anxiety	2-3 g of dried root or 1-3 mL of tincture, once to several times per day Two clinical trials found 400-450 mg of the root extract effective for insomnia	Valerian has a bad odor and can cause morning drowsiness Long-term administration can lead to paradoxical stimulation including restlessness and palpitations Because of the risk of benzodiazepine-like withdrawal, valerian should be tapered over a period of several weeks before surgery It can potentiate the sedative effect of CNS depressants (e.g., benzodiazapines, alcohol) and other herbal tranquilizers

*Doses presented in the table are adapted from the German Commission E Monographs and/or data from clinical trials. Products from different manufacturers vary considerably. A reliable product should have a label clearly stating the botanical name of the herb and milligram amount contained in the product. Standardized extracts should be used whenever possible and are often disclosed on the label of quality products.

AMD = age-related macular degeneration; BPH = benign prostatic hyperplasia; CFU = colony-forming unit; CHD = coronary heart disease; CNS, central nervous system; CYP3A4 = cytochrome P450 3A4; DHA = docosahexaenoic acid; EPA = eicosapentaenoic acid; GI = gastrointestinal; HMG-CoA = 3-hydroxy-3-methylglutaryl coenzyme A; Ig = immunoglobulin; INR = international normalized ratio; LDL = low-density lipoprotein; MAOI = monoamine oxidase inhibitor; PMS = premenstrual syndrome; PPI = proton pump inhibitor; SLE = systemic lupus erythematosus; SSRIs = selective serotonin reuptake inhibitors; UTIs = urinary tract infections.

REFERENCES

Ang-Lee MK, Moss J, Yuan C. Herbal medicines and perioperative care. JAMA 2001;286:208–16.

Barnes J, Anderson LA, Phillipson JD. PDR for herbal medicines. 3rd ed. Montvale, NJ: Medical Economics; 2004.

Blumenthal M, editor. Herbal medicines: Expanded Commission E monographs. Austin, TX: American Botanical Council; 2000.

Blumenthal M, editor. The ABC clinical guide to herbs. Austin, TX: American Botanical Council; 2003.

Cupp MJ. Herbal remedies: adverse effects and drug interactions. Am Fam Phys 1999;59(5):1239–44.

Ernst E. The risk-benefit profile of commonly used herbal therapies: Ginkgo, St John's wort, ginseng, echinacea, saw palmetto, and kava. Ann Intern Med 2002;136:42–53.

Jellin JM, Gregory P, Batz F, Bonakdar R, editors. Pharmacist's Letter/Prescriber's Letter Natural Medicines Comprehensive Database (Internet). Available at Stockton, CA. Available at www.naturaldatabase.com (accessed August 24, 2010).

Klepser TB, Klepser ME. Unsafe and potentially safe herbal therapies. Am J Health-Syst Pharm 1999;56:125–38.

Kligler B, Cohrssen A. Probiotics. Am Fam Physician 2008;78(9):1073–8.

Kronenberg F, Fugh-Berman A. Complementary and alternative medicine for menopausal symptoms: A review of randomized controlled trials. Ann Intern Med 2002;137:805–13.

Mar C. An evidence-based review of the 10 most commonly used herbs. WJW 1999;171:169.

O'Hara MA, Kiefer D, Farrell K, Kemper K. A review of 12 commonly used medicinal herbs. Arch Fam Med 1998;7:523–36.

Rotblatt MD. Cranberry, feverfew, horse chestnut, and kava. West J Med 1999;171:195–8.

Smet P. Herbal remedies. N Engl J Med 2002;2046–56.

New Drugs in 2009 and Agents Pending FDA Approval

Method of
Miriam Chan, BSc Pharm, PharmD

New Drugs Approved in 2009

Generic Name	Trade Name (Manufacturer)	Strength	Dosage Form	Normal Dosage Range	Pregnancy Rating*	FDA Approval Date (m/d/y)	Indication	Classification
New Molecular Entities								
Artemether/ lumefantrine	Coartem (Novartis)	20 mg artemether/ 120 mg lumefantrine	Tablet	One dose initially and repeat the dose after 8 h, then bid × 2 d Adults ≥35 kg: 4 tabs/ dose Children ≥35 kg: 4 tabs/dose; 25 kg to <35 kg: 3 tabs/dose; 15 kg to <25 kg: 2 tabs/dose; 5 kg to <15 kg: 1 tab/dose	C	4/7/09	Treatment of acute, uncomplicated malaria infections due to *Plasmodium falciparum* in patients ≥5 kg bodyweight	Antiinfective, antimalarial
Asenapine	Saphris (Organon)	5, 10 mg	Sublingual tablet	Schizophrenia: 5 mg SL bid Bipolar disorder: 10 mg SL bid	C	8/13/09	For acute treatment of schizophrenia in adults For acute treatment of manic or mixed episodes associated with bipolar I disorder in adults	Atypical antipsychotic, dopamine and serotonin antagonist
Benzyl alcohol	Ulesfia (Sciele Pharma)	5% in 8 oz bottle	Lotion	Apply lotion to dry hair, using enough to completely saturate the scalp and hair Rinse off with water after 10 min Repeat treatment in 7 d	B	4/9/09	Topical treatment of head lice infestation in patients ≥6 m of age	Pediculicides, asphyxiant
Bepotastine besilate	Bepreve (Ista Pharms)	1.5% in 2.5-, 5-, 10- mL bottle	Ophthalmic solution	1 drop into the affected eye(s) bid	C	9/8/09	Treatment of itching associated with allergic conjunctivitis	Antihistamine, histamine H₁ receptor antagonist
Besifloxacin	Besivance (Bausch & Lomb)	0.6%, 5 mL in 7.5-mL bottle	Ophthalmic suspension	1 drop in the affected eye(s) 3 ×/d, 4-12 h apart × 7 d	C	5/28/09	Treatment of bacterial conjunctivitis	Ophthalmic antibiotic, fluoroquinolone
Dronedarone	Multaq (Sanofi Aventis)	400 mg	Tablet	400 mg bid with morning and evening meals	X	7/1/09	To reduce the risk of cardiovascular hospitalization in patients with paroxysmal or persistent atrial fibrillation or atrial flutter, with a recent episode of atrial fibrillation or flutter and associated cardiovascular risk factors (i.e., age >70, hypertension, diabetes, prior cerebrovascular accident, left atrial diameter ≥50 mm or left ventricular ejection fraction <40%), who are in sinus rhythm or who will be cardioverted	Antiarrhythmic, benzofuran derivative

Generic name	Brand (Manufacturer)	Strengths	Form	Dosing	Pregnancy category	Approval date	Indication	Classification
Everolimus	Afinitor (Novartis)	5, 10 mg	Tablet	10 mg once daily	D	3/30/09	Treatment of patients with advanced renal cell carcinoma after failure of treatment with sunitinib or sorafenib	Antineoplastic, kinase inhibitor, MTOR inhibitor
Febuxostat	Uloric (Takeda)	40, 80 mg	Tablet	40 mg qd, may increase dose to 80 mg qd after 2 wk if needed	C	2/13/09	Chronic management of hyperuricemia in patients with gout	Antigout drug, xanthine oxidase inhibitor
Iloperidone	Fanapt (Vanda Pharms)	1, 2, 4, 6, 8, 10, 12 mg	Tablet	Start at 1 mg bid, then increase to 2 mg, 4 mg, 6 mg, 8 mg, 10 mg, and 12 mg bid on days 2, 3, 4, 5, 6, and 7, respectively, to reach the 12-24 mg/day dose range	C	5/6/09	Acute treatment of schizophrenia in adults	Atypical antipsychotic agent, dopamine and serotonin antagonist
Milnacipran	Savella (Forest)	12.5, 25, 50, 100 mg	Tablet	Start at 12.5 mg qd on d 1; increase dose to 12.5 mg bid on d 2 and 3, followed by 25 mg bid on d 4 to 7, and then increase to 50 mg bid by d 7. May increase dose to 200 mg/day based on individual patient response	C	1/14/09	For the management of fibromyalgia	Antidepressant, serotonin-norepinephrine reuptake inhibitor
Pazopanib hydrochloride	Votrient (GSK)	200, 400 mg	Tablet	800 mg once daily, at least 1 h before or 2 h after a meal	D	10/19/2009	Treatment of advanced renal cell carcinoma	Tyrosine kinase inhibitor, VEGF inhibitor
Pitavastatin	Livalo (Kowa)	1, 2, 4 mg	Tablet	1-4 mg once daily	X	8/3/09	For patients with primary hyperlipidemia and mixed dyslipidemia as an adjunctive therapy to diet to reduce elevated total cholesterol, low-density lipoprotein cholesterol, apolipoprotein B, and triglycerides and to increase high-density lipoprotein cholesterol	Antilipemic, HMG-CoA reductase inhibitor
Pralatrexate	Folotyn (Allos)	20 mg/mL in 1-, 2-mL vial	Injection	30 mg/m^2 given as an IV push over 3-5 min once weekly × 6 wk in 7-week cycles. Supplement patients with vitamin B$_{12}$ 1 mg IM every 8-10 wk and folic acid 1.0-1.25 mg PO once daily	D	9/24/09	For the treatment of patients with relapsed or refractory peripheral T-cell lymphoma	Antineoplastic, folate analogue metabolic inhibitor

New Drugs in 2009 and Agents Pending FDA Approval

New Drugs Approved in 2009—Cont'd

Generic Name	Trade Name (Manufacturer)	Strength	Dosage Form	Normal Dosage Range	Pregnancy Rating*	FDA Approval Date (m/d/y)	Indication	Classification
Prasugrel	Effient (Eli Lilly & Co)	5, 10 mg	Tablet	Loading dose: 60 mg × 1 Maintenance dose: 10 mg qd with or without food Consider 5 mg qd for patients <60 kg Patients should also take aspirin 75-325 mg qd	B	7/10/09	To reduce thrombotic cardiovascular events (including stent thrombosis) in patients with acute coronary syndrome who are to be managed with PCI as follows: Patients with unstable angina or non-ST-elevation myocardial infarction Patients with ST-elevation myocardial infarction when managed with either primary or delayed PCI	Thienopyridine, a P2Y12 platelet inhibitor
Romidepsin	Istodax (Gloucester Pharms)	10 mg vial	Injection	14 mg/m² IV infusion over 4 h on d 1, 8 and 15 of a 28-day cycle Repeat cycles q28d provided that the patient continues to benefit from and tolerates the drug	D	11/5/2009	Treatment of cutaneous T-cell lymphoma in patients who have received at least one prior systemic therapy	Antineoplastic agent, histone deacetylase inhibitor
Saxagliptin	Onglyza (Bristol Myers Squibb)	2.5, 5 mg	Tablet	2.5 to 5 mg once daily	B	7/31/09	As an adjunct to diet and exercise to improve glycemic control in adults with type 2 diabetes mellitus	Antidiabetic drug, dipeptidyl peptidase-4 inhibitor
Tolvaptan	Samsca (Otsuka)	15, 30 mg	Tablet	Start at 15 mg qd; may increase the dose to 30 mg qd, after at least 24 h, to a max dose of 60 mg qd, as needed to raise serum sodium	C	5/19/09	Treatment of clinically significant hypervolemic and euvolemic hyponatremia (serum sodium <125 mEq/L or less-marked hyponatremia that is symptomatic and has resisted correction with fluid restriction), including patients with heart failure, cirrhosis, and syndrome of inappropriate antidiuretic hormone	Hyponatremic drug, selective vasopressin V₂-receptor antagonist
Telavancin	Vibativ (Astellas Pharma)	250, 750 mg vial	Injection	10 mg/kg once daily given as an IV infusion over 60 min × 7 to 14 d	C	9/11/09	Treatment of adult patients with complicated skin and skin structure infections caused by susceptible gram-positive bacteria	Antibacterial, lipoglycopeptide

Generic name	Brand (Manufacturer)	Strength	Form	Preg.	Dose	Date	Indication	Class/Mechanism
Vigabatrin	Sabril (Lundbeck)	500 mg	Powder for oral solution Tablet	C	For infantile spasms: start at 25 mg/kg bid; titrate by 25-50 mg/kg/d increments q3d up to a max of 150 mg/kg/d For complex partial seizures: start at 500 mg bid; titrate by 500-mg increments q wk to 1.5 g bid as needed	8/21/09	Monotherapy for infantile spasms in pediatric patients 1 mo to 2 y of age As adjunctive therapy in adult patients who have refractory complex partial seizures	Antiepileptic drug, γ-aminobutyric acid transaminase inhibitor
New Biologicals								
Abobotulinumtoxin A	Dysport (Ipsen Biopharm)	300, 500 U/vial	Injection	C	Cervical dystonia: 250-1000 U given IM ≥q12wk Glabellar lines: 50 U divided in 5 equal aliquots of 10 U each given IM to affected muscles	4/29/2009	Treatment of cervical dystonia in adults Temporary improvement in the appearance of moderate to severe glabellar lines associated with procerus and corrugator muscle activity in adults <65 y	Botulinum toxin, acetylcholine release inhibitor
Antithrombin	Atryn (Ovation Pharm)	1750 IU/vial	Injection	C	Individualize dosage to restore and maintain functional antithrombin activity levels at 80%-120% (0.8-1.2 IU/mL) of normal Give loading dose as a 15-min IV infusion, immediately followed by a continuous infusion of the maintenance dose	2/2009	Prevention of perioperative and peripartum thromboembolic events in patients with hereditary antithrombin deficiency	Anticoagulant, recombinant antithrombin
Canakinumab	Ilaris (Novartis)	180 mg in 6-mL vial	Injection	C	>40 kg: 150 mg 15-40 kg: 2 mg/kg, may increase to 3 mg/kg if needed Give the dose as a single SC injection q8wk	6/17/09	Treatment of cryopyrin-associated periodic syndromes in adults and children ≥4 y including familial cold autoinflammatory syndrome and Muckle-Wells syndrome	Immunomodulator, IL-1β blocker
C1 esterase inhibitor (human)	Berinert (CSL Behring)	500 U/vial	Injection	C	20 U/kg IV injection at 4 mL/min	10/9/2009	Treatment of facial or abdominal attacks of hereditary angioedema in adults and adolescents	Hematological agent, protein C1 inhibitor
Ecallantide	Kalbitor (Dyax)	10 mg/mL vial	Injection	C	30 mg, divided in 3 × 10 mg SC injections May give an additional dose of 30 mg within 24 h	11/27/2009	Treatment of acute attacks of hereditary angioedema in patients ≥16 y	Hematologic agent, plasma kallikrein inhibitor

Continued

New Drugs Approved in 2009—Cont'd

Generic Name	Trade Name (Manufacturer)	Strength	Dosage Form	Normal Dosage Range	Pregnancy Rating*	FDA Approval Date (m/d/y)	Indication	Classification
Fibrinogen concentrate (human)	RiaSTAP (CSL Behring)	900-1300 mg/vial	Injection	Calculate dose based on fibrinogen level When fibrinogen level is unknown, use 70 mg/kg Give the dose as a slow IV injection at rate ≤5 mL/min	C	1/16/2009	Treatment of acute bleeding episodes in patients with congenital fibrinogen deficiency, including afibrinogenemia and hypofibrinogenemia	Blood product derivative, fibrinogen product
Golimumab	Simponi (Centocor Ortho Biotech)	50 mg/0.5 mL in prefilled syringe 50 mg/0.5 mL in prefilled SmartJect autoinjector	Injection	50 mg SC injection once monthly	B	4/24/2009	For moderately to severely active rheumatoid arthritis in adults, in combination with methotrexate For active psoriatic arthritis in adults, alone or in combination with methotrexate For active ankylosing spondylitis in adults	Immunomodulator, tumor necrosis factor blocker
Haemophilus b conjugate vaccine	Hiberix (GSK)	1 dose/vial	Injection	0.5 mL IM injection × 1	C	8/18/2009	Active immunization as a booster dose to prevent invasive disease caused by *Haemophilus influenzae* type b in children 15 mo through 4 y of age (before 5th birthday)	Vaccine (inactivated), bacterial
Human papillomavirus vaccine	Cervarix (GSK)	Single-dose vial Prefilled syringe	Injection	3 doses (0.5 mL each) by IM injection at 0, 1, and 6 m	B	10/16/2009	Prevention of diseases caused by oncogenic human papillomavirus types 16 and 18: • cervical cancer • cervical intraepithelial neoplasia grade 2 or worse and adenocarcinoma in situ • cervical intraepithelial neoplasia grade 1 Approved for use in girls and women 10-25 y of age	Vaccine (inactivated), viral
Influenza A (H1N1) vaccine	Influenza A (H1N1) monovalent vaccine (multiple mfrs)	0.25, 0.5 mL in prefilled syringe 5-, 10-mL multidose vial 0.2-mL prefilled, single-dose sprayer	Injection, intranasal	0.5 mL IM × 1	C	9/15/09	Active immunization against influenza disease caused by pandemic (H1N1) 2009 virus in persons ≥6 mo of age	Vaccine (inactivated), viral

Generic Name	Trade Name (Manufacturer)	Dosage Form/Strength	Form	Preg.	Dosage	Date Approved	Indication	Class
Influenza virus type A and B vaccine, high dose	Fluzone High-Dose (Sanofi Pasteur)	0.5 mL prefilled, single-use syringe	Injection	C	1 dose (0.5 mL) IM once yearly	12/23/2009	Active immunization against influenza disease caused by the influenza virus subtypes A and B in persons ≥65 y of age	Vaccine (inactivated), viral
Japanese encephalitis vaccine, inactivated, absorbed	Ixiaro (Novartis)	0.5 mL single-dose syringe	Injection	B	2 doses of 0.5 mL given IM 28 d apart Complete immunization at least 1 wk before exposure to JEV	10/23/2009	Active immunization for the prevention of disease caused by JEV in persons ≥17 y of age	Vaccine (inactivated), viral
Ofatumumab	Arzerra (Glaxo)	100 mg/5 mL vial	Injection	C	12 doses given as an IV infusion Wk 1: 300 mg × 1 dose Wk 2-8: 2000 mg once weekly × 7 doses 4 wk later: 2000 mg q4wk × 4 doses	10/26/2009	Treatment of patients with chronic lymphocytic leukemia refractory to fludarabine and alemtuzumab	Antineoplastic agent, CD20 targeted monoclonal antibody
Ustekinumab	Stelara (Cenocor)	45, 90 mg vial	Injection	B	Give dose as SC injection Patients ≤100 kg, 45 mg initially and 4 wk later, followed by 45 mg q12wk Patients >100 kg, 90 mg initially and 4 wk later, followed by 90 mg q12wk	9/25/2009	Indicated for the treatment of adult patients with moderate to severe plaque psoriasis who are candidates for phototherapy or systemic therapy	Immunomodulator, human IL-12 and -23 antagonist

Significant New Esters, New Salts, or Other Derivatives

Generic Name	Trade Name (Manufacturer)	Dosage Form/Strength	Form	Preg.	Dosage	Date Approved	Indication	Class
Dexlansoprazole	Dexilant (Takeda)	30, 60 mg	Delayed-release capsule	B	Healing of EE: 60 mg qd for up to 8 wk Maintenance of healed EE: 30 mg qd for up to 6 mo Symptomatic nonerosive GERD: 30 mg qd × 4 wk	1/30/09	Healing of all grades of erosive esophagitis Maintaining healing of EE Treating heartburn associated with nonerosive GERD	GI agent, proton pump inhibitor
Ferumoxytol	Feraheme (Amag Pharms)	510 mg of elemental iron in 17 mL vial (30 mg/mL)	Injection	C	510 mg IV injection at a rate of up to 30 mg/mL/sec, followed by a second dose of 510 mg 3-8 d later	6/30/09	Treatment of iron deficiency anemia in adult patients with chronic kidney disease	Trace element, iron replacement product

Significant New Combinations

Generic Name	Trade Name (Manufacturer)	Dosage Form/Strength	Form	Preg.	Dosage	Date Approved	Indication	Class
Acyclovir/hydrocortisone	Lipsovir (Medivir)	5%/1% in 2-, 5-g tube	Cream	B	Apply 5 × per day for 5 d	7/31/09	Early treatment of recurrent herpes labialis (cold sores), to reduce the likelihood of ulcerative cold sores, and to shorten the healing time in adults and adolescents (≥12 y of age)	Dermatologic, synthetic nucleoside analogue/corticosteroid

New Drugs in 2009 and Agents Pending FDA Approval

New Drugs Approved in 2009—Cont'd

Generic Name	Trade Name (Manufacturer)	Strength	Dosage Form	Normal Dosage Range	Pregnancy Rating*	FDA Approval Date (m/d/y)	Indication	Classification
Aliskiren/valsartan	Valturna (Novartis)	150 mg/160 mg, 300 mg/ 320 mg	Tablet	1 tab qd Add-on therapy or initial therapy; start at 150 mg/160 mg; titrate as needed up to a max of 300 mg/ 320 mg Replacement therapy: may be substituted for titrated components	D	9/16/09	Treatment of hypertension as initial, add-on, or replacement therapy	Antihypertensive, direct renin inhibitor/ angiotensin II receptor blocker
Telmisartan/ amlodipine	Twynsta (Boehringer Ingelheim)	40 mg/5 mg, 40 mg/10 mg, 80 mg/5 mg, 80 mg/10 mg	Tablet	Initiate with 40 mg/5 mg or 80 mg/5 mg once daily May increase after at least 2 wk to a max dose of 80 mg/10 mg once daily	C (1st trimester) D (2nd and 3rd trimesters)	10/16/09	Treatment of hypertension alone or with other antihypertensive agents	Antihypertensive, angiotensin II receptor blocker/dihydropyridine calcium channel blocker
Amlodipine/ valsartan/ hydro- chlorothiazide	Exforge HCT (Novartis)	10/160/12.5, 5/160/25, 10/160/25, 10/320/25 mg	Tablet	Dose once daily	D	4/30/09	Treatment of hypertension (not indicated for initial therapy)	Antihypertensive, calcium channel blocker, angiotensin receptor blocker, diuretic
Metformin/ pioglitazone	Actoplus Met XR (Takeda)	15 mg/1000 mg, 30 mg/1000 mg	Tablet	Select the starting dose based on the patient's current regiment Give once daily with the evening meal Max 45 mg/2000 mg per day	C	5/12/09	As an adjunct to diet and exercise to improve glycemic control in adults with type 2 diabetes mellitus who are already treated with pioglitazone and metformin or who have inadequate glycemic control on pioglitazone alone or metformin alone	Antidiabetic, thiazolidinedione/ biguanide
Morphine/ naltrexone	Embeda (Alpharma King)	20 mg/0.8 mg, 30 mg/1.2 mg, 50 mg/2 mg, 60 mg/2.4 mg, 80 mg/3.2 mg, 100 mg/4 mg	Extended release capsule	Once or twice daily	C	8/13/09	Management of moderate to severe pain when a continuous, around-the-clock opioid analgesic is needed for an extended period	Analgesic, opioid agonist/ antagonist
Selected New Formulations								
Bromocriptine mesylate	Cycloset	0.8 mg	Tablet	Start at 1 tab qd; may increase dose weekly by one tab to a max daily dose of 2-6 tab	B	5/5/09	As an adjunct to diet and exercise to improve glycemic control in adults with type 2 diabetes mellitus	Ergot derivative, dopamine receptor agonist
Calcitriol topical ointment	Vectical (Galderma Labs)	3 μg/g, in 5-, 100-g tube	Ointment	Apply ointment to affected areas of the body bid Max dose: ≤200 g/wk	C	1/23/09	Topical treatment of mild to moderate plaque psoriasis in adults ≥18 y	Anti-psoriatic agent, vitamin D analogue

Drug	Brand (Manufacturer)	Strength	Dosage form	Dosing	Pregnancy category	Approval date	Indication	Classification
Capsaicin patch	Qutenza (Neurogesx)	8% (179 mg)	Transdermal patch	Administer by physicians only; Apply patch to the most painful skin areas, using up to 4 patches; Remove patch(s) after 60 min; May repeat treatment q 3 m prn	B	11/16/09	Management of neuropathic pain associated with postherpetic neuralgia (PHN)	Nonopioid analgesic, TRPVI channel agonist
Ciprofloxacin otic solution	Cetraxal (Wraser Pharms)	0.2% (0.5 mg/0.25 mL) in single use container	Otic solution	Instill contents of 1 single-use container into the affected ear bid × 7 d	C	5/1/09	Treatment of acute otitis externa due to susceptible isolates of Pseudomonas aeruginosa or Staphylococcus aureus	Otic, quinolone antimicrobial
Dexamethasone intravitreal implant	Ozurdex (Allergan)	0.7 mg/solid polymer drug delivery system	Ophthalmic intravitreal injection	Insert 1 implant into each affected eye by intravitreal injection under controlled aseptic conditions	C	6/17/09	Treatment of macular edema following branch retinal vein occlusion or central retinal vein occlusion	Ophthalmic implant, corticosteroid
Diclofenac sodium	Pennsaid (Nuvo Res)	1.5%	Topical solution	Apply 40 drops on each painful knee 4 × a day	C (prior to 30 wk gestation) D (starting at 30 wk gestation)	11/4/09	Treatment of signs and symptoms of osteoarthritis of the knee(s)	Analgesic, NSAID
Fentanyl	Onsolis (Meda Pharms)	200, 400, 600, 800, 1200 µg	Buccal soluble film	Start at 200 µg; titrate dose using 200 µg film increments (up to a max of four 200 µg films or a single 1200 µg film) to adequate analgesia without undue side effects; Max is 1 dose/episode; ≤ 4 doses/day; separate by at least 2 h	C	7/16/09	Management of breakthrough pain in patients with cancer, ≥18 y of age, who are already receiving and who are tolerant to opioid therapy for their underlying persistent cancer pain	Analgesic, opioid
Ganciclovir ophthalmic gel	Zirgan (Sirion)	0.15%, 5 g tube	Ophthalmic gel	1 drop in the affected eye 5 ×/day (q3h while awake) until the corneal ulcer heals, and then 1 drop 3 × per day × 7 d	C	9/15/09	Treatment of acute herpetic keratitis (dendritic ulcers)	Antiviral, guanosine derivative
Guanfacine	Intuniv (Shire)	1, 2, 3, 4 mg	Extended-release tablet	1 mg once daily; adjust dose in increments of ≤ 1 mg/wk up to 4 mg/d if needed	B	9/2/09	Treatment of attention deficit hyperactivity disorder	Cardiovascular, selective α2A-adrenergic receptor agonist

Continued

New Drugs in 2009 and Agents Pending FDA Approval

New Drugs Approved in 2009—Cont'd

Generic Name	Trade Name (Manufacturer)	Strength	Dosage Form	Normal Dosage Range	Pregnancy Rating*	FDA Approval Date (m/d/y)	Indication	Classification
Ibuprofen	Caldolor (Cumberland Pharm)	400 mg/4 mL-, 800 mg/8 mL- vial	Injection	Pain: 400-800 mg IV over 30 min q6h prn Fever: 400 mg IV over 30 min, followed by 400 mg q4-6h or 100-200 mg q4h prn Dilute drug before administration	C (prior to 30 wk gestation) D (starting at 30 wk gestation)	6/11/09	Indicated in adults to manage mild to moderate pain; moderate to severe pain as an adjunct to opioid analgesics; reduction of fever	Analgesic/antipyretic, NSAID
Levonorgestrel	Plan B One-Step (Duramed)	1.5 mg	Tablet	1 tab PO as soon as possible within 72 h after unprotected intercourse	X	7/10/09	Prevention of pregnancy following unprotected intercourse or a known or suspected contraceptive failure	Emergency contraceptive, progestin
Oxybutynin topical gel	Gelnique (Watson Labs)	100 mg/g, in 1-g sachet (1.14 mL)	Gel	Apply 1 sachet once daily to dry, intact skin on the abdomen, upper arms and shoulders, or thighs	B	1/27/09	Treatment of overactive bladder with symptoms of urge urinary incontinence, urgency, and frequency	Genitourinary agent, antimuscarinic
Paliperidone palmitate	Invega Sustenna (Johnson and Johnson)	39, 78, 117, 156, 234 mg in prefilled syringe	Extended-release injectable solution	Give as IM injection Start at 234 mg on d 1 and 156 mg 1 wk later Monthly maintenance dose: 117 mg; may adjust within the recommended range of 39-234 mg if needed	C	7/31/09	Acute and maintenance treatment of schizophrenia in adults	Atypical antipsychotic agent, benzisoxazole derivative
Olanzapine	Zyprexa Relprevv (Eli Lilly)	210, 300, 405 mg vial	Extended release injectable suspension	Give IM injection 150-300 mg q 2 wk or 405 mg q4wk	C	12/11/09	Treatment of schizophrenia	Atypical antipsychotic agent, dibenzapine derivative
Tobramycin/ dexamethasone ophthalmic suspension	TobraDex ST (Alcon)	0.3%/0.05% in 2.5, 5, 10 mL Drop-Tainers	Ophthalmic suspension	1 drop into the conjunctival sac(s) q 4-6 h During the initial 24-48 h, dosage may be increased to 1 drop q2h	C	2/13/09	For steroid-responsive inflammatory ocular conditions for which a corticosteroid is indicated and when superficial bacterial ocular infection or a risk of bacterial ocular infection exists	Ophthalmic, steroid antibiotic combination

Telbivudine oral solution	Tyzeka (Novartis)	100 mg/5 mL in 300 mL bottle	Solution	≥16 y of age: 600 mg once daily, taken orally, with or without food	B	4/28/09	Treatment of chronic HBV infection in adult patients	Antiretroviral, HBV nucleoside analogue reverse transcriptase inhibitor
Treprostinil	Tyvaso (United Therap)	0.6 mg/ mL in 2.9 mL ampule	Inhalation solution	Start at 3 breaths (18 µg) per treatment session, 4 × daily. May titrate to 9 breaths (54 µg) per treatment session as tolerated	B	7/3009	Treatment of pulmonary arterial hypertension (WHO Group I) in patients with NYHA class III symptoms, to increase walk distance	Peripheral vasodilator, prostacyclin

Abbreviations: EE = erosive esophagitis; GERD = gastroesophageal reflux disease; GI = gastrointestinal; HBV = hepatitis B virus; IL = interleukin; JEV = Japanese encephalitis virus; NSAID = nonsteroidal antiinflammatory drug; NYHA = New York Heart Association; PCI = percutaneous coronary intervention; WHO = World Health Organization.

*FDA Pregnancy Categories:

A Adequate studies in pregnant women have not demonstrated a risk to the fetus in the first trimester of pregnancy, and there is no evidence of risk in later trimesters.

B Animal studies have shown an adverse effect, but adequate studies in pregnant women have not demonstrated a risk to the fetus during the first trimester of pregnancy, and there is no evidence of risk in later trimesters.

C Animal studies have shown an adverse effect on the fetus, but there are no adequate studies in humans; the benefits from the use of the drug in pregnant women may be acceptable despite its potential risks.

D There is evidence of human fetal risk, but the potential benefits from the use of the drug in pregnant women may be acceptable despite its potential risks.

X Adverse reaction reports indicate evidence of fetal risk; the risk of use in a pregnant woman clearly outweighs any possible benefit.

No drug should be administered during pregnancy unless it is clearly needed and potential benefit outweighs potential hazard to the fetus, regardless of the pregnancy category.

Agents Pending FDA Approval

Generic Name	Trade Name (Manufacturer)	Indication
ABT-335/Rosuvastatin	No brand name (Abbott & AstraZeneca)	Treatment of mixed dyslipidemia
Albiglutide	Syncria (GSK)	Treatment of type 2 diabetes
Aleglitazar	No brand name (Roche)	Treatment of type 2 diabetes
Almorexant	No brand name (Actelion)	Treatment of primary insomnia
Alopliptin	No brand name (Takeda)	Treatment of type 2 diabetes
Apixaban	No brand name (Bristol-Myers Squibb/Pfizer)	Prevention of venous thromboembolism and prevention of stroke
Bazedoxifene	Viviant (Wyeth)	Prevention of postmenopausal osteoporosis
17α-hydroxy-progesterone caproate	Gestiva (Adeza)	Prevention of preterm delivery (before 35 wk) in women with a history of prior preterm delivery
Ceftobiprole	Zeftera (Johnson & Johnson)	Treatment of complicated skin and soft tissue infections, including diabetes-related foot infections
Cilomilast	Ariflo (GlaxoSmithKline)	Treatment of patients with COPD who are poorly responsive to albuterol
Clodronate	Bonefos (Berlex Laboratories)	Adjuvant oral treatment for reducing the occurrence of bone metastases in stage II/III breast cancer patients
Dapagliflozin	No brand name (Bristol-Myers Squibb)	Treatment of type 2 diabetes
Dimebolin	Dimebon (Pfizer)	Treatment of Alzheimer's disease
Efaproxiral	Efaproxyn (Allos Therapeutics, Inc.)	An adjunct agent to whole-brain radiation therapy for the treatment of brain metastases in patients with breast cancer
Flibanserin	No brand name (Boehringer Ingelheim)	Treatment of female sexual dysfunction
Garenoxacin mesylate	Geninax (Schering)	Treatment of acute bacterial exacerbation of chronic bronchitis, acute bacterial sinusitis, community acquired pneumonia, complicated and uncomplicated skin and skin structure infections, and complicated intra-abdominal infections
Icatibant	Firazyr (Jerini)	Treatment of hereditary angioedema
Idraparinux, biotinylated	No brand name (Sanofi-Aventis)	Treatment of deep vein thrombosis
Insulin monomer human (rDNA origin), inhaled	Afrezza Inhalation Powder (MannKind Corp)	Treatment of type 1 and type 2 diabetes mellitus in adult patients
Insulin oral spray	Oral-lyn (Generex)	Treatment of type 1 and type 2 diabetes mellitus
Lasofoxifene	Fablyn (Prizer)	Treatment of osteoporosis in postmenopausal women at increased risk of fracture
Lorcaserin	No brand name (Arena)	Treatment of obesity
Mepolizumab	Bosatria (GSK)	An anti-IL-5 monoclonal antibody for treatment of hypereosinophilic syndrome
Naproxcinod (nitronaproxen)	No brand name (NicOx SA)	Treatment of osteoarthritis
Nicotine conjugate vaccine	NicVAX (Nabi Biopharmaceuticals)	Aid to smoking cessation and prevent relapses of a treated smoker
Odanacatib	No brand name (Merck)	Treatment of osteoporosis in postmenopausal women
Rivaroxaban	Xarelto (J & J/Bayer)	Venous blood clot prevention after elective total knee and hip replacement surgery
Roflumilast	Daxas (Forest)	Treatment of COPD
Sitaxsentan sodium	Thelin (Encysive Pharmaceuticals)	Treatment of pulmonary arterial hypertension
Teplizumab	No brand name (Eli Lilly)	Treatment of type 1 diabetes
Ticagrelor	Brilinta (AstraZeneca)	Treatment for the reduction of major adverse cardiac events in patients with acute coronary syndrome
Trabectedin	Yondelis (Ortho Biotech)	Treatment of soft tissue sarcoma
Vapreotide	Sanvar IR (H3 Pharma)	Treatment of acute esophageal variceal bleeding secondary to portal hypertension
Vernakalant	Kynapid (Astellas Pharma)	For conversion of atrial fibrillation to normal sinus rhythm
Vildagliptin	Galvus (Novartis)	Treatment of type 2 diabetes

Abbreviations: COPD = chronic obstructive pulmonary disease; GL = glucagon-like peptide; IL = interleukin; VTE = venous thromboembolism.

Index

Note: Page numbers followed by *b*, *f*, and *t* indicate boxes, figures, and tables, respectively.

1263

Index

1280

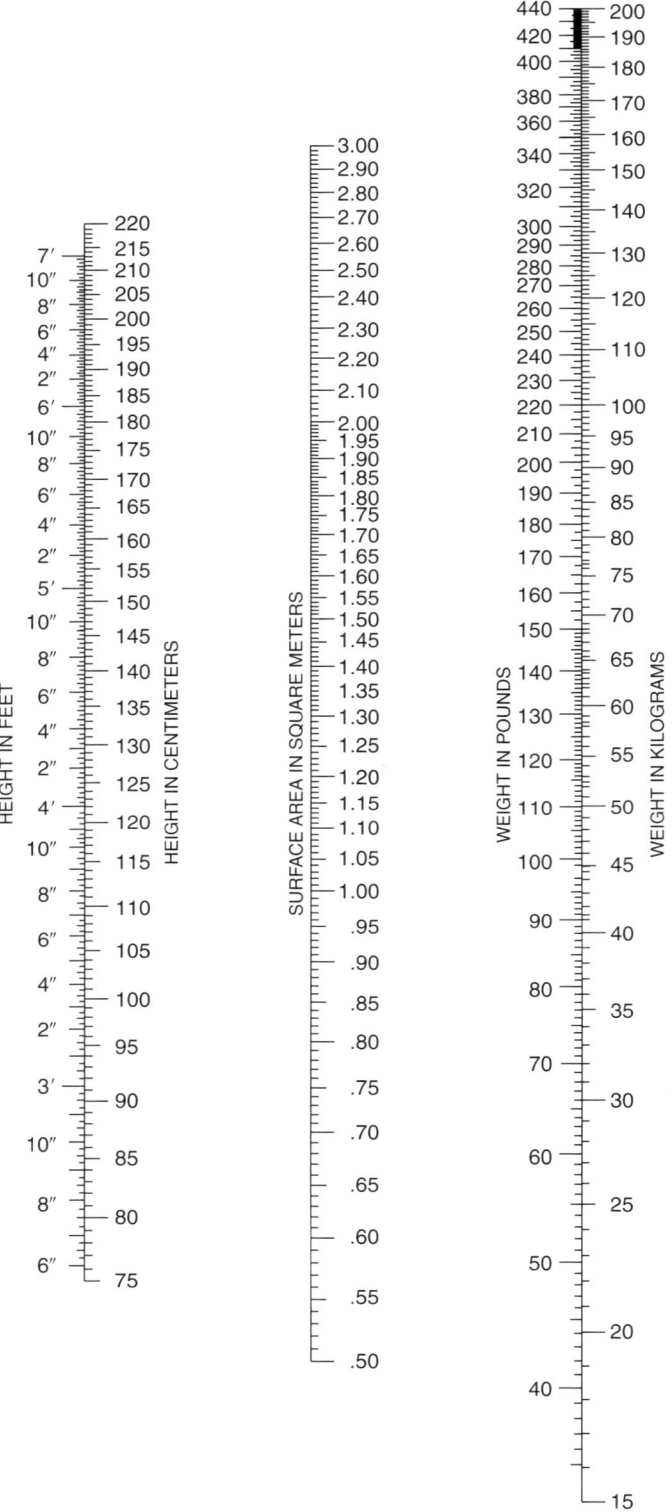

HEIGHT IN FEET   HEIGHT IN CENTIMETERS   SURFACE AREA IN SQUARE METERS   WEIGHT IN POUNDS   WEIGHT IN KILOGRAMS